Pharmacotherapy Principles & Practice

Pharmacotherapy Principles & Practice

THIRD EDITION

Editors

Marie A. Chisholm-Burns, PharmD, MPH, FCCP, FASHP

Dean and Professor
College of Pharmacy
University of Tennessee
Memphis, Tennessee

Barbara G. Wells, PharmD, FASHP, FCCP

Professor and Dean Emeritus
Executive Director Emeritus, Research Institute of
    Pharmaceutical Sciences
School of Pharmacy
The University of Mississippi
Oxford, Mississippi

Terry L. Schwinghammer, PharmD, FCCP, FASHP, FAPhA, BCPS

Professor and Chair
Department of Clinical Pharmacy
School of Pharmacy
West Virginia University
Morgantown, West Virginia

Patrick M. Malone, PharmD, FASHP

Professor and Associate Dean, Internal Affairs
College of Pharmacy
The University of Findlay
Findlay, Ohio

Jill M. Kolesar, PharmD, BCPS, FCCP

Professor
School of Pharmacy
University of Wisconsin
Director, 3P Analytical Instrumentation Laboratory
University of Wisconsin Comprehensive Cancer Center
Madison, Wisconsin

Joseph T. DiPiro, PharmD, FCCP

Professor and Executive Dean
South Carolina College of Pharmacy
University of South Carolina, Columbia
Medical University of South Carolina
Charleston and Columbia, South Carolina

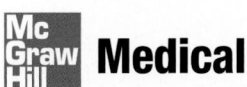 **Medical**

New York   Chicago   San Francisco   Lisbon   London   Madrid   Mexico City
Milan   New Delhi   San Juan   Seoul   Singapore   Sydney   Toronto

Pharmacotherapy Principles & Practice, Third Edition

Copyright © 2013, 2010, 2008 by The McGraw-Hill Companies, Inc. All rights reserved. Printed in China. Except as permitted under the United States Copyright Act of 1976, no part of this publication may be reproduced or distributed in any form or by any means, or stored in a data base or retrieval system, without the prior written permission of the publisher.

1 2 3 4 5 6 7 8 9 0   CTP/CTP   18 17 16 15 14 13

ISBN 978-0-07-178046-9
MHID 0-07-178046-7

This book was set in Minion by Cenveo Publisher Services.
The editors were Michael Weitz and Peter J. Boyle.
The production supervisor was Catherine H. Saggese.
Art management was by Armen Ovsepyan.
Project management was provided by Nidhi Chopra, Cenveo Publisher Services.
The designer was Alan Barnett.
China Translation & Printing Services, Ltd., was printer and binder.

Library of Congress Cataloging-in-Publication Data

Pharmacotherapy principles & practice / editors, Marie A. Chisholm-Burns ... [et al.]. — 3rd ed.
    p. ; cm.
  Pharmacotherapy principles and practice
  Includes bibliographical references and index.
    ISBN 978-0-07-178046-9 (hardback : alk. paper)   I. Chisholm-Burns, Marie A.   II. Title:
Pharmacotherapy principles and practice.
  [DNLM: 1. Drug Therapy. WB 330]
  615.5′8—dc23   2012034899

McGraw-Hill books are available at special quantity discounts to use as premiums and sales promotions, or for use in corporate training programs. To contact a representative please e-mail us at bulksales@mcgraw-hill.com.

CONTENTS

Marie A. Chisholm-Burns, BS Pharm, PharmD, MPH, FCCP, FASHP, is Dean and Professor at the University of Tennessee College of Pharmacy. She received her BS and PharmD degrees from the University of Georgia, and completed a residency at Mercer University Southern School of Pharmacy and at Piedmont Hospital in Atlanta, Georgia. She has served in elected positions in numerous professional organizations. Dr. Chisholm-Burns has greater than 250 publications and more than $8 million in external funding as principal investigator. In 2008 and 2011, textbooks co-edited by Dr. Chisholm-Burns, *Pharmacotherapy Principles and Practice* and *Pharmacy Management, Leadership, Marketing, and Finance,* respectively, received the Medical Book Award from the American Medical Writers Association. She has also received numerous awards and honors including the Robert K. Chalmers Distinguished Pharmacy Educator Award from the American Association of Colleges of Pharmacy, the Clinical Pharmacy Education Award from the American College of Clinical Pharmacy, the Daniel B. Smith Practice Excellence Award from the American Pharmacists Association, the Nicholas Andrew Cummings Award from the National Academies of Practice, the Award of Excellence from the American Society of Health-System Pharmacists, and the Rufus A. Lyman Award for most outstanding publication in the American Journal of Pharmaceutical Education (in 1996 and 2007). Dr. Chisholm-Burns lives in Memphis, is married, and has one child, John Fitzgerald Burns Jr. She enjoys writing, cycling, and playing chess.

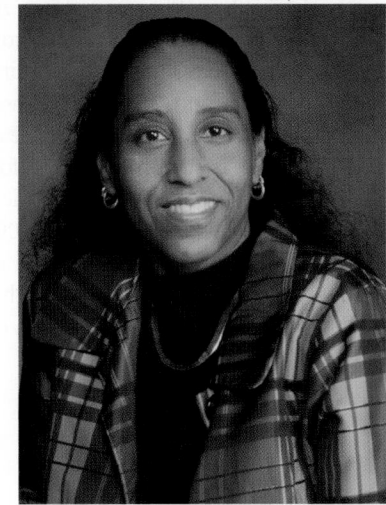

Barbara G. Wells, BS Pharm, PharmD, FCCP, FASHP, is Dean and Professor Emeritus at the University of Mississippi School of Pharmacy and Executive Director Emeritus of the Research Institute of Pharmaceutical Sciences. She completed a residency in psychiatric pharmacy practice at the University of Tennessee. She is a past president and chair of the Board of the American Association of Colleges of Pharmacy (AACP) and the American College of Clinical Pharmacy (ACCP). She is a past member of the NIH Advisory Committee on Research on Women's Health and of the FDA Psychopharmacologic Drugs Advisory Committee. Her primary instructional interests are in psychiatric therapeutics, and she has received six teaching awards, including the Robert K. Chalmers Distinguished Pharmacy Educator Award from AACP and the Paul F. Parker Award from ACCP. Other books that she coedits are *Pharmacotherapy: A Pathophysiologic Approach* and the *Pharmacotherapy Handbook*. She enjoys a leisurely or working weekend on her houseboat named Euphoria on Pickwick Lake.

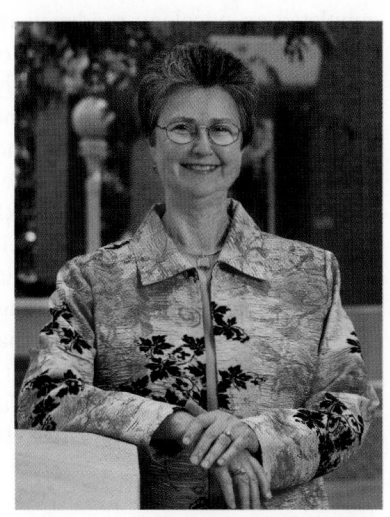

Terry L. Schwinghammer, BS Pharm, PharmD, BCPS, FCCP, FASHP, FAPhA is Professor and Chair of the Department of Clinical Pharmacy at the West Virginia University School of Pharmacy. He received his BS and PharmD degrees from Purdue University and completed a pharmacy residency at Indiana University Hospitals. He has practiced in adult inpatient and ambulatory care settings. Dr. Schwinghammer is a past recipient of the APhA-APPM Distinguished Achievement Award in Clinical/ Pharmacotherapeutic Practice and is a Distinguished Practitioner in the National Academies of Practice. His teaching focuses on pharmacotherapy of rheumatic diseases and physical assessment. In addition to authoring over 60 publications, he is coeditor of the *Pharmacotherapy Casebook* and *Pharmacotherapy Handbook* and is Editor-in-Chief of AccessPharmacy (www.AccessPharmacy.com). He has been elected to membership in the Rho Chi Pharmaceutical Honor Society and the Phi Lambda Sigma Pharmacy Leadership Society. He was named a Distinguished Alumnus of Purdue University in 2004. His hobby is collecting apothecary antiques, and he enjoys boating and water skiing with his family.

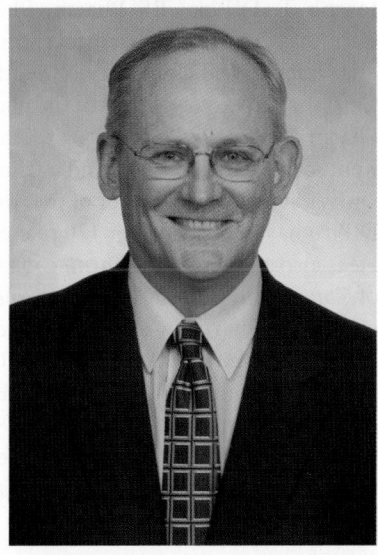

Patrick M. Malone, BS Pharm, PharmD, FASHP, is Professor and Associate Dean of Internal Affairs at The University of Findlay College of Pharmacy. Dr. Malone received his BS in Pharmacy from Albany College of Pharmacy and PharmD from the University of Michigan. He completed a clinical pharmacy residency at the Buffalo General Hospital, Drug Information Fellowship at the University of Nebraska Medical Center, and US West Fellowship in Academic Development and Technology at Creighton University. His practice and teaching have centered on drug information, and he is the first author for all four editions of *Drug Information—A Guide for Pharmacists*. Dr. Malone was also the drug information pharmacist at the XIII Winter Olympics. He has approximately 100 publications and numerous presentations and has held various offices in national organizations. He was the Director of the Web-Based Pharmacy Pathway at Creighton University Medical Center, from its initial establishment until after graduation of the first class. His hobby is building and flying radio-controlled aircraft.

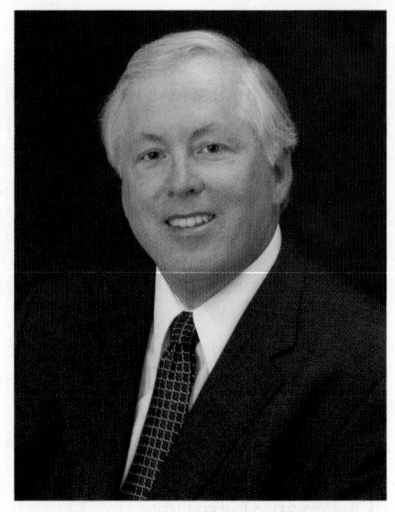

Jill M. Kolesar, BS Pharm, PharmD, BCPS, FCCP, is a Professor at the University of Wisconsin and the Director of the 3P Laboratory at the University of Wisconsin Carbone Comprehensive Cancer Center. She received a BS in pharmacy from the University of Wisconsin and a PharmD from the University of Texas. Dr. Kolesar also completed an oncology residency and fellowship at the University of Texas Health Science Center in San Antonio. Dr. Kolesar is the author of more than 100 peer reviewed publications and has received more than $1.2 million in external funding as a principal investigator. She holds two US and international patents for novel technologies invented in her laboratory and founded Helix Diagnostics based on this technology. She has served on the National Cancer Institute Central IRB, and is currently a member of the Pharmacology Taskforce, an advisory group to the Investigational Drug Steering Committee of the NCI. She also chairs the Lung Biology Subcommittee for the Thoracic Committee of the Eastern Cooperative Oncology Group. Dr. Kolesar received the Innovations in Teaching Award from AACP, and has served in multiple elected offices of national and international pharmacy organizations. Other books she coedits are *Top 300 Pharmacy Flash Cards*, *Pharmacogenomics: Applications to Patient Care* and *The Pharmacogenomics Handbook*. Dr. Kolesar loves to read, run, ski, and travel with her husband and five children. She has completed 2 marathons and 14 half-marathons.

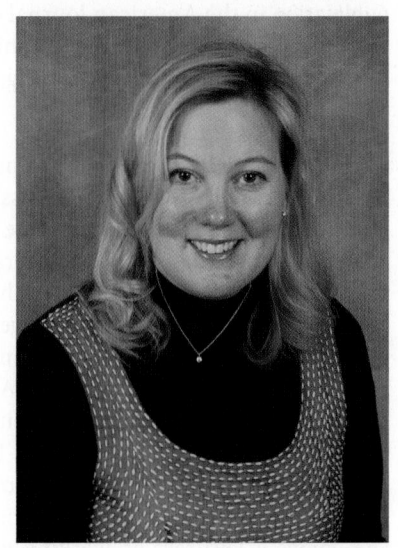

Joseph T. DiPiro, BS Pharm, PharmD, FCCP, is Executive Dean of the South Carolina College of Pharmacy, which is an integrated program of the Colleges of Pharmacy at the University of South Carolina and the Medical University of South Carolina. He received his BS in pharmacy from the University of Connecticut and PharmD from the University of Kentucky. He served a residency at the University of Kentucky Medical Center and a fellowship in Clinical Immunology at Johns Hopkins University. He is the Editor of the *American Journal of Pharmaceutical Education*. Dr. DiPiro has published over 120 refereed papers in academic and professional journals. He is also an editor for *Pharmacotherapy: A Pathophysiologic Approach*, and an author of *Concepts in Clinical Pharmacokinetics*. He was a President of the American College of Clinical Pharmacy and has served on the Research Institute Board of Trustees. In 2002, the American Association of Colleges of Pharmacy selected Dr. DiPiro for the Robert K. Chalmers Distinguished Educator Award. He has also received the Russell R. Miller Literature Award and the Education Award from the American College of Clinical Pharmacy, and the Award for Sustained Contributions to the Literature from the American Society of Health-System Pharmacists. He is an avid runner and has completed 15 marathons.

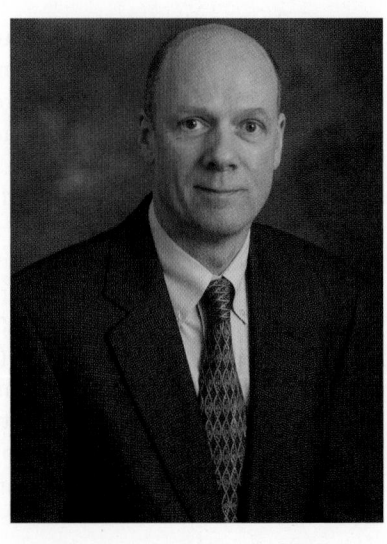

Jessica L. Adams, PharmD
Eshelman School of Pharmacy, University of North Carolina Chapel Hill, Chapel Hill, North Carolina
Chapter 87

Val Adams, PharmD, FCCP, BCCP
Associate Professor, University of Kentucky, Lexington, Kentucky
Chapter 90

Ronda L. Akins, PharmD
Associate Professor, Infectious Diseases, College of Pharmacy, University of Louisiana Monroe, Monroe, Louisiana; Gratis Assistant Professor, Department of Pediatrics and Internal Medicine, School of Medicine, Louisiana State University Health Sciences Center, Shreveport, Louisiana
Chapter 74

J. V. Anandan, PharmD
Pharmacy Specialist, Department of Pharmacy Services, Henry Ford Hospital; Adjunct Associate Professor, Eugene Appelbaum College of Pharmacy and Health Sciences, Wayne State University, Detroit Michigan
Chapter 78

David A. Apgar, PharmD
Assistant Professor, Department of Pharmacy Practice and Science, University of Arizona College of Pharmacy, Tucson, Arizona
Chapter 63

Justin Balko, PharmD, PhD
Research Fellow, Department of Medicine, Division of Hematology/Oncology, Vanderbilt University, Nashville, Tennessee
Chapter 90

Katie E. Barber, PharmD
PGYZ Infectious Diseases Specialty Resident, Detroit Medical Center, Detroit, Michigan
Chapter 74

Marianne Billeter, PharmD, BCPS
Director of Pharmacy, Ochsner Medical Center, New Orleans, Louisiana
Chapter 86

Christopher M. Bland, PharmD, BCPS
Critical Care Pharmacist/Infectious Disease Specialist, Dwight D. Eisenhower Army Medical Center, Augusta, Georgia
Chapter 82

P. Brandon Bookstaver, PharmD
Associate Professor, Department of Clinical Pharmacy and Outcomes Sciences, South Carolina College of Pharmacy, University of South Carolina, Columbia, South Carolina
Chapter 70

Jill S. Borchert, PharmD, BCPS, FCCP
Professor and Residency Program Director, Midwestern University Chicago College of Pharmacy, Downers Grove, Illinois
Chapter 60

Emily B. Borders, PharmD, BCOP
Assistant Professor, University of Oklahoma College of Pharmacy, Oklahoma City, Oklahoma
Chapter 91

Sheila Botts, PharmD, FCCP, BCPP
Clinical Pharmacy Specialist, Behavioral Health, Kaiser Permanente, Colorado, Hidden Lake Behavioral Health, Westminster, Colorado
Chapter 40

Bradley A. Boucher, PharmD, FCCP, FCCM
Professor of Clinical Pharmacy, Associate Professor, Department of Neurosurgery, University of Tennessee Health Science Center, Memphis, Tennessee
Chapter 13

Catherine A. Bourg, PharmD, BCPS
Clinical Assistant Professor University of Georgia College of Pharmacy, Athens, Georgia
Chapter 18

Evans Branch III, PharmD, CPh
Professor, Pharmacy Practice, College of Pharmacy, Florida Agricultural and Mechanical University, Miami, Florida
Chapter 80

Gretchen M. Brophy, PharmD, BCPS, FCCP, FCCM
Professor of Pharmacotherapy and Outcomes Science and Neurosurgery, Virginia Commonwealth University, Medical College of Virginia Campus, Richmond, Virginia
Chapter 32

Susan P. Bruce, PharmD, BCPS
Chair and Associate Professor, Pharmacy Practice, Northeast Ohio Medical University, Rootstown, Ohio
Chapter 57

Imad F. Btaiche, BS, PharmD, BCNSP
Professor and Associate Dean for Academic Affairs, School of Pharmacy, Lebanese American University, Byblos, Lebanon
Chapter 100

Karim Anton Calis, PharmD, MPH, FASHP, FCCP
Clinical Investigator, Eunice Kennedy Shriver National
Institute of Child Health and Human Development,
National Institutes of Health, Bethesda, Maryland;
Clinical Professor, University of Maryland School of
Pharmacy, Baltimore, Maryland; Clinical Professor,
Virginia Commonwealth University School of Pharmacy,
Richmond, Virginia
Chapters 45 and 46

Diane M. Cappelletty, RPh, PharmD
Department of Pharmacy Practice, University of Toledo
College of Pharmacy and Pharmaceutical Sciences,
Toledo, Ohio
Chapter 71

Marshall E. Cates, PharmD, BCPP, FASHP
Professor of Pharmacy Practice, Samford University
McWhorter School of Pharmacy, Birmingham, Alabama
Chapter 38

Larisa H. Cavallari, PharmD, BCPS, FCCP
Associate Professor, Department of Pharmacy Practice,
University of Illinois at Chicago, Chicago, Illinois
Chapter 7

Juliana Chan, PharmD
Clinical Associate Professor, Clinical Pharmacist—GI/
Hepatology and HCV Telemedicine, Departments of
Pharmacy Practice and Medicine, Colleges of Pharmacy
and Medicine, Sections of Hepatology and Digestive
Diseases & Nutrition, University of Illinois at Chicago,
Chicago, Illinois
Chapter 24

Sallie H. Charles, PMHNP-BC, MS, MBA
Clinical Practice Manager, Behavioral Health, Kaiser
Permanente, Denver, Colorado
Chapter 40

Judy T. Chen, PharmD, BCPS, CDE
Clinical Associate Professor of Pharmacy Practice, Purdue
University College of Pharmacy, Indianapolis, Indiana
Chapters 45 and 46

Marie A. Chisholm-Burns, PharmD, MPH, FCCP, FASHP
Dean and Professor, College of Pharmacy, University of
Tennessee, Memphis, Tennessee
Chapter 17

Kevin W. Cleveland, PharmD
Idaho State University College of Pharmacy, Department of
Pharmacy Practice and Administration, Pocatello, Idaho
Chapter 42

Amanda Corbett, PharmD, BCPS, FCCP, AAHIVE
Eshelman School of Pharmacy, University of North Carolina
at Chapel Hill, Chapel Hill, North Carolina
Chapter 87

Susan Cornell, BS, PharmD, CDE, FAPhA, FAADE
Associate Professor of Pharmacy Practice, Assistant Director
of Experiential Education, Midwestern University Chicago
College of Pharmacy, Downers Grove, Illinois
Chapter 43

Brian L. Crabtree, PharmD, BCPP
Professor and Chair, Department of Pharmacy Practice,
Eugene Applebaum College of Pharmacy and Health
Sciences, Wayne State University, Detroit, Michigan
Chapter 39

Nicole S. Culhane, PharmD, FCCP, BCPS
Director of Experiential Education, Associate Professor,
Clinical and Administrative Sciences, Notre Dame of
Maryland University, School of Pharmacy, Baltimore,
Maryland
Chapter 50

Clarence E. Curry Jr., PharmD
Associate Professor of Pharmacy Practice, Department of
Clinical and Administrative Pharmacy Sciences, College
of Pharmacy, Howard University, Washington, DC
Chapter 21

Devra K. Dang, PharmD, BCPS, CDE
Associate Clinical Professor, University of Connecticut
School of Pharmacy, Storrs, Connecticut
Chapters 45 and 46

Simon de Denus, BPharm, MSc(Pharm), PhD
Université de Montréal Beaulieu-Saucier Chair in
Pharmacogenomics, Researcher, Pharmacist, Montreal
Heart Institute; Associate Professor, Faculty of Pharmacy,
Université de Montréal, Montreal, Canada
Chapter 8

Robert J. DiDomenico, PharmD
Clinical Associate Professor, Department of Pharmacy
Practice, University of Illinois at Chicago, Chicago, Illinois
Chapter 7

Eric Dietrich, PharmD
Post Doctoral Fellow, Department of Pharmacotherapy and
Translational Research, University of Florida College of
Pharmacy, Gainesville, Florida
Chapter 58

Joseph T. DiPiro, PharmD, FCCP
Professor and Executive Dean, South Carolina College
of Pharmacy, University of South Carolina, Columbia,
Medical University of South Carolina, Charleston, South
Carolina
Chapter 77

John M. Dopp, PharmD, MS
Assistant Professor, School of Pharmacy, University of
Wisconsin-Madison, Madison, Wisconsin
Chapter 41

Julie B. Dumond, PharmD
Research Assistant Professor, Eshelman School of Pharmacy,
University of North Carolina at Chapel Hill, Chapel Hill,
North Carolina
Chapter 87

Megan J. Ehret, PharmD, MS, BCPP
Associate Professor, Department of Pharmacy Practice,
School of Pharmacy, University of Connecticut, Storrs,
Connecticut
Chapter 29

Clayton English, PharmD
Assistant Professor, Department of Pharmacy Practice,
Albany College of Pharmacy and Health Sciences,
Colchester, Vermont
Chapter 29

John Erramouspe, PharmD, MS
Professor, Pharmacy Practice and Administrative Sciences,
Idaho State University, Pocatello, Idaho
Chapter 42

Edward Faught, MD
Professor, Department of Neurology, Emory University,
Atlanta, Georgia
Chapter 31

Ema Ferreira, BPharm, MSc, PharmD, FCHSP
Pharmacist in Obstetrics and Gynecology, Clinical Associate
Professor, CHU Ste-Justine, Faculty of Pharmacy,
Université de Montréal, Montreal, Quebec, Canada
Chapter 47

Jack E. Fincham, PhD, RPh
Professor, University of Missouri-Kansas City, School
of Pharmacy, Division of Pharmacy Practice and
Administration, Kansas City, Missouri
Chapter 1

Steven Gabardi, PharmD, FCCP, BCPS
Abdominal Organ Transplant Clinical Specialist, Brigham
and Women's Hospital, Boston, Massachusetts; Assistant
Professor of Medicine, Harvard Medical School, Boston,
Massachusetts
Chapter 55

Angie L. Goeser-Iske, PharmD
Pharmacist, Integris Health, Oklahoma City, Oklahoma
Chapter 65

Maqual R. Graham, PharmD
Associate Professor of Pharmacy Practice and
Administration, University of Missouri-Kansas City
School of Pharmacy, Kansas City, Missouri
Chapter 102

Phyllis A. Grauer, PharmD
Clinical Assistant Professor, College of Pharmacy, Ohio State
University, Columbus, Ohio
Chapter 4

Erika L. Grigg, MD
Section of Gastroenterology, Georgia Health Sciences
University, Augusta, Georgia
Chapter 18

David R. P. Guay, PharmD
Professor Emeritus, Department of Experimental and
Clinical Pharmacology, College of Pharmacy, University
of Minnesota, Minneapolis, Minnesota
Chapter 53

John G. Gums, PharmD, FCCP
Professor of Pharmacy and Medicine, Director of
Clinical Research in Family Medicine, Associate Chair,
Department of Pharmacotherapy and Translational
Research, University of Florida, Gainesville, Florida
Chapter 58

Julie Haase, PharmD
Pharmacy Practice Resident, Creighton University Medical
Center, Omaha, Nebraska
Appendix E

Tracy M. Hagemann, PharmD, FCCP, FPPAG
Associate Professor, Clinical and Administrative Sciences,
University of Oklahoma College of Pharmacy, Oklahoma
City, Oklahoma
Chapter 68

Stuart T. Haines, PharmD, BCPS, BC-ADM
Professor, Department of Pharmacy Practice and Science,
University of Maryland School of Pharmacy, Baltimore,
Maryland; Clinical Pharmacy Specialist, West Palm Beach
VA Medical Center, West Palm Beach, Florida
Chapter 10

Kim Hawkins, MS, APRN-NP
Assistant Professor, Creighton University School of Nursing,
Omaha, Nebraska
Appendix E

Kathleen B. Haynes, PharmD
Clinical Coordinator, Bridges to Health, Community Health
Network, Indianapolis, Indiana
Chapter 48

Keith A. Hecht, PharmD, BCOP
Clinical Associate Professor of Pharmacy Practice, School
of Pharmacy, Southern Illinois University, Edwardsville,
Illinois
Chapter 97

Nancy Heideman, PharmD, BCPS
Clinical Specialist-Pediatrics, University of New Mexico
Hospital, Albuquerque, New Mexico
Chapter 95

Richard Heideman, MD
Professor of Pediatrics, University of New Mexico,
Albuquerque, New Mexico
Chapter 95

Brian A. Hemstreet, PharmD, BCPS
Associate Professor, Director, Pharmaceutical Care Learning
Center, Department of Clinical Pharmacy, University of
Colorado School of Pharmacy, Aurora, Colorado
Chapter 19

Elizabeth D. Hermsen, PharmD, MBA, BCPS-ID
Clinical Scientific Director, Cubist Pharmaceuticals,
Lexington, Massachusetts; Adjunct Associate Professor,
University of Nebraska Medical Center, College of
Pharmacy, Omaha, Nebraska
Chapter 76

Gerald Higa, PharmD
Professor, Schools of Pharmacy and Medicine, Mary Babb
Randolph Cancer Center, Morgantown, West Virginia
Chapter 89

Michelle L. Hilaire, PharmD, CDE, BCPS
Clinical Associate Professor of Pharmacy Practice,
University of Wyoming School of Pharmacy, Faculty
Pharmacist, Fort Collins Family Medicine Residencies,
Fort Collins, Colorado
Chapter 62

Jamie C. Holmes, PharmD
Assistant Professor, Department of Pharmacy Practice,
Rosalind Franklin University of Medicine and Science,
North Chicago, Illinois
Chapter 33

Marlon S. Honeywell, PharmD
Interim Associate Dean for Academic Affairs and Professor,
College of Pharmacy and Pharmaceutical Sciences, Florida
A&M University, Tallahassee, Florida
Chapter 80

Jaime R. Hornecker, PharmD, BCPS
Clinical Associate Professor of Pharmacy Practice,
University of Wyoming School of Pharmacy, Laramie,
Wyoming
Chapter 73

Melissa L. Hunter, PharmD
Drug Information Director, School of Pharmacy, University
of Wyoming, Laramie, Wyoming
Chapter 62

Jill Isaacs, MS, APRN-NP
Assistant Professor, Creighton University School of Nursing,
Omaha, Nebraska
Appendix E

Matthew K. Ito, PharmD, FCCP, FNLA, CLS
Professor, Department of Pharmacy Practice, Oregon State
University/Oregon Health and Science University College
of Pharmacy, Portland, Oregon
Chapter 12

Cherry W. Jackson, PharmD, BCPP, FASHP
Professor, Department of Pharmacy Practice, Auburn
University; Professor, Department of Psychiatric and
Behavioral Neurobiology, School of Medicine, University
of Alabama, Birmingham, Alabama
Chapter 38

Ziba Jalali
Assistant Professor, College of Medicine, University of
Nebraska Medical Center, Omaha, Nebraska
Chapter 76

Tommy Johnson, PharmD, BC-ADM, CDE, FAADE
Professor and Chair, Presbyterian College School of
Pharmacy, Clinton, South Carolina
Chapter 43

Mikael D. Jones, PharmD, BCPS
Clinical Associate Professor, Pharmacy Practice and Science,
College of Pharmacy, University of Kentucky, Lexington,
Kentucky
Chapter 61

Stephanie Kaiser, PharmD
Clinical Pharmacy Specialist, VA Medical Center, Danville,
Illinois
Chapter 5

Angela D.M. Kashuba, BScPhm, PharmD, DABCP
Associate Professor, Eshelman School of Pharmacy,
University of North Carolina at Chapel Hill, Chapel Hill,
North Carolina
Chapter 87

Michael D. Katz, PharmD
Professor and Director, International Education,
   Department of Pharmacy Practice and Science, College of
   Pharmacy, University of Arizona, Tucson, Arizona
Chapter 44

Deanna L. Kelly, PharmD, BCPP
Professor of Psychiatry, Director, Treatment Research
   Program, Maryland Psychiatric Research Center,
   University of Maryland School of Medicine, Baltimore,
   Maryland
Chapter 37

Jacqueline M. Klootwyk, PharmD, BCPS
Assistant Professor of Pharmacy Practice, Jefferson School
   of Pharmacy, Thomas Jefferson University, Philadelphia,
   Pennsylvania
Chapter 49

Emily Knezevich, PharmD, BCPS, CDE, RP
Associate Professor of Pharmacy Practice, School of
   Pharmacy and Health Professions, Creighton University,
   Omaha, Nebraska
Appendix E

Jon Knezevich, PharmD, BCPS
Assistant Professor of Pharmacy Practice, School of
   Pharmacy and Health Professions, Creighton University,
   Omaha, Nebraska
Appendix E

Julia M. Koehler, PharmD, FCCP
Associate Dean for Clinical Education and External
   Affiliations, Professor of Pharmacy Practice, Butler
   University College of Pharmacy and Health Sciences,
   Indianapolis, Indiana
Chapter 48

Michael D. Kraft, PharmD, BCNSP
Clinical Associate Professor, University of Michigan
   College of Pharmacy, Assistant Director—Education and
   Research, University of Michigan Health System, Ann
   Arbor, Michigan
Chapter 100

Sum Lam, PharmD
Associate Clinical Professor, Department of Clinical
   Pharmacy Practice, College of Pharmacy and Allied
   Health Professions, St. John's University, Queens,
   New York; Clinical Specialist in Geriatric Pharmacy,
   Divisions of Geriatric Medicine and Pharmacy, Winthrop
   University Hospital, Mineola, New York
Chapter 53

Rebecca M. T. Law, PharmD, BScPharm
Associate Professor, School of Pharmacy and Faculty of
   Medicine (Cross-Appointment: Discipline of Family
   Medicine), Memorial University of Newfoundland, St.
   John's, Newfoundland and Labrador, Canada
Chapter 64

Amber P. Lawson, PharmD, BCCP
Clinical Pharmacy Specialist, Hematology/Oncology,
   University of Kentucky Healthcare, Lexington, Kentucky
Chapter 98

Ellyn M. Lee, MD
Assistant Professor, Department of Medicine, Director
   of Palliative Medicine, University of Arizona, Tucson,
   Arizona
Chapter 2

Jeannie K. Lee, PharmD, BCPS
Assistant Professor, Department of Pharmacy Practice and
   Science, Assistant Professor, Department of Medicine,
   Colleges of Pharmacy and Medicine, University of
   Arizona; Clinical Pharmacy Specialist, Geriatrics,
   Southern Arizona VA Health Care System; Research
   Associate and Faculty, Arizona Center on Aging, Tucson,
   Arizona
Chapter 2

Mary Lee, PharmD, BCPS, FCCP
Professor of Pharmacy Practice, Chicago College of
   Pharmacy, Vice President and Chief Academic Officer,
   Midwestern University, Chicago, Illinois
Chapter 52

Russell E. Lewis, PharmD, FCCP, BCPS
Professor, University of Houston College of Pharmacy;
   Adjunct Professor, University of Texas M.D. Anderson
   Cancer Center, Houston, Texas
Chapter 84

Teresa V. Lewis, PharmD, BCPS
Assistant Professor, Department of Pharmacy, Clinical and
   Administrative Sciences, College of Pharmacy, University
   of Oklahoma Health Sciences Center, Oklahoma City,
   Oklahoma
Chapter 68

Cara Liday, PharmD, BCPS, CDE
Associate Professor, Department of Pharmacy Practice,
   College of Pharmacy, Idaho State University; Clinical
   Pharmacist, InterMountain Medical Clinic, Pocatello,
   Idaho
Chapter 51

Susanne E. Liewer, PharmD, BCOP
Clinical Pharmacy Specialist—Stem Cell Transplant,
    Nebraska Medical Center; Clinical Assistant Professor,
    College of Pharmacy, University of Nebraska Medical
    Center, Omaha, Nebraska
Chapter 97

Cameron C. Lindsey, PharmD, BC-ADM, CDE, BCACP
Professor of Pharmacy Practice and Administration,
    University of Missouri-Kansas City School of Pharmacy,
    Kansas City, Missouri
Chapter 102

Melissa Lipari, PharmD
Clinical Assistant Professor, Wayne State University Eugene
    Applebaum College of Pharmacy and Health Sciences;
    Clinical Pharmacy Specialist, Ambulatory Care, St. John
    Hospital and Medical Center, Detroit, Michigan
Chapter 20

Karl Madaras-Kelly, PharmD, MPH
Professor, Department of Pharmacy Practice, College of
    Pharmacy, Idaho State University, Boise, Idaho
Chapter 69

Mark A. Malesker, PharmD, FCCP, FCCP, FASHP, BCPS
Professor of Pharmacy Practice and Medicine, Creighton
    University, Omaha, Nebraska
Chapters 27 and 28

Michelle T. Martin, PharmD, BCPS, BCACP
Clinical Pharmacist, University of Illinois Medical Center
    at Chicago; Clinical Assistant Professor, University of
    Illinois at Chicago College of Pharmacy, Chicago, Illinois
Chapter 14

Spencer T. Martin, PharmD, BCPS
Clinical Pharmacy Manager, Cardiac Transplantation,
    Department of Pharmacy and Department of Advanced
    Cardiac Care, New York Presbyterian Hospital/Columbia
    Medical Center, New York City, New York
Chapter 55

Kathryn R. Matthias, PharmD, BCPS (AQ ID)
Assistant Professor, University of Arizona College of
    Pharmacy, University of Arizona Medical Center, Tucson,
    Arizona
Chapter 79

J. Russell May, PharmD, FASHP
Clinical Professor, Department of Clinical and
    Administrative Pharmacy, University of Georgia College
    of Pharmacy, Augusta, Georgia
Chapter 54

Joseph E. Mazur, PharmD, BCPS, BCNSP
Critical Care Clinical Specialist, Medical Intensive Care
    Unit; Clinical Associate Professor, South Carolina College
    of Pharmacy, Charleston, South Carolina
Chapter 77

Trevor McKibbin, PharmD, MS
Assistant Professor, Department of Clinical Pharmacy,
    College of Pharmacy, University of Tennessee, Memphis,
    Tennessee
Chapter 92

Patrick J. Medina, PharmD, BCOP
Associate Professor, College of Pharmacy, University of
    Oklahoma, Oklahoma City, Oklahoma
Chapter 91

Damian M. Mendoza, PharmD, CGP
Clinical Instructor in Pharmacy Practice and Science,
    University of Arizona College of Pharmacy; Clinical
    Pharmacy Specialist, Geriatrics, Southern Arizona VA
    Health Care System, Tucson, Arizona
Chapter 2

April D. Miller, PharmD, BCPS
Clinical Pharmacist, Critical Care Residency Program
    Director, Vidant Medical Center, Greenville, North
    Carolina
Chapter 70

Sarah J. Miller, PharmD, BCNSP
Professor, Department of Pharmacy Practice, University of
    Montana Skaggs School of Pharmacy; Pharmacy Clinical
    Coordinator, Saint Patrick Hospital, Missoula, Montana
Chapter 101

Beverly C. Mims, PharmD
Associate Professor of Pharmacy Practice, Howard
    University, College of Pharmacy, Clinical Pharmacist,
    Howard University Hospital, Washington, DC
Chapter 21

M. Jane Mohler, RN, MPH, PhD
Associate Professor, Section of Geriatrics, General and
    Palliative Medicine, University of Arizona, Tucson,
    Arizona
Chapter 2

Caroline Morin, BPharm, MSc
Associated Clinician, Université de Montreal Pharmacist,
    Centre Image, Obstetrics and Gynecology, CHU
    Ste-Justine, Montreal, Quebec, Canada
Chapter 47

Lee E. Morrow, MD, MSc
Associate Professor, Division of Pulmonary and Critical
Care Medicine, Nebraska and Western Iowa Veterans
Affairs Hospital and Creighton University School of
Medicine, Omaha, Nebraska
Chapters 27 and 28

Milap C. Nahata, PharmD, MS
Professor of Pharmacy, Pediatrics and Internal Medicine;
Chair, Division of Pharmacy Practice and Administration,
College of Pharmacy, Ohio State University; Associate
Director OSU Medical Center, Department of Pharmacy,
Columbus, Ohio
Chapter 3

Rocsanna Namdar, PharmD
Department of Clinical Pharmacy, University of Colorado,
Boulder, Colorado
Chapter 75

Melinda M. Neuhauser, PharmD, MPH
Clinical Pharmacy Specialist, Infectious Diseases, VA
Pharmacy Benefits Management Services, Hines, Illinois
Chapter 81

Douglas A. Newton, MD, MPH
Child and Adolescent Psychiatrist, Clinical Chief, Colorado
Permanente Medical Group, Denver, Colorado
Chapter 40

Tien M.H. Ng, PharmD, FCCP, BCPS AQ-C
University of Southern California, School of Pharmacy, Los
Angeles, California
Chapter 6

Kimberly J. Novak, PharmD, BCPS
Clinical Pharmacy Specialist, Pediatric Pulmonary Medicine,
Nationwide Children's Hospital; Clinical Assistant
Professor, Ohio State University College of Pharmacy,
Columbus, Ohio
Chapter 16

Edith A. Nutescu, PharmD, FCCP
Clinical Professor, Departments of Pharmacy Practice and
Administration, Center for Pharmacoeconomic Research,
Clinical Manager, Antithrombosis Clinic, University of
Illinois at Chicago, College of Pharmacy and Medical
Center, Chicago, Illinois
Chapter 10

Catherine M. Oliphant, PharmD
Associate Professor of Pharmacy Practice, College of
Pharmacy, Idaho State University, Meridan, Idaho
Chapter 69

Ali J. Olyaei, PharmD
Professor, Department of Medicine and Pharmacy Practice,
Oregon State University and Oregon Health and Sciences
University, Portland, Oregon
Chapter 55

Christine Karabin O'Neil, BS, PharmD, BCPS, CGP, FCCP
Professor of Pharmacy Practice, Division of Clinical, Social
and Administrative Sciences, Duquesne University, School
of Pharmacy, Pittsburgh, Pennsylvania
Chapter 34

Vinita B. Pai, PharmD, MS
Assistant Professor of Clinical Pharmacy, Ohio State
University, College of Pharmacy; Clinical Pharmacy
Specialist, Pediatric Blood and Marrow Transplant
Program, Nationwide Children's Hospital,
Columbus, Ohio
Chapter 3

David Parra, PharmD, FCCP, BCPS
Clinical Pharmacy Specialist in Cardiology, VA Medical
Center, West Palm Beach Florida; Clinical Associate
Professor, Department of Experimental and Clinical
Pharmacology, University of Minnesota College of
Pharmacy, Minneapolis, Minnesota
Chapter 5

Charles Peloquin, PharmD, FCCP
Professor, Emerging Pathogens Institute, University of
Florida, Gainesville, Florida
Chapter 75

Susan L. Pendland, MS, PharmD
Adjunct Associate Professor, University of Illinois at
Chicago, Chicago, Illinois; Clinical Staff Pharmacist, Saint
Joseph Berea Hospital, Berea, Kentucky
Chapter 81

Hanna Phan, PharmD, BCPS
Assistant Professor, Department of Pharmacy Practice and
Science, Assistant Professor, Department of Pediatrics,
Colleges of Pharmacy and Medicine, University of
Arizona; Clinical Pharmacy Specialist, Pediatric
Pulmonary Medicine, Arizona Respiratory Center,
University of Arizona Medical Center, Tucson, Arizona
Chapter 3

Trinh Pham, PharmD, BCOP
Associate Clinical Professor, University of Connecticut,
School of Pharmacy, Storrs, Connecticut
Chapter 93

Bradley G. Phillips, PharmD, FCCP, BCPS
Millikan-Revee Professor and Head, Department of Clinical
and Administrative Pharmacy, University of Georgia
College of Pharmacy, Athens, Georgia
Chapter 41

Beth Bryles Phillips, PharmD, FCCP, BCPS
Clinical Professor, University of Georgia College of
   Pharmacy; Director VAMC/UGA Ambulatory Care
   Residency Program, Athens, Georgia
Chapter 56

Amy M. Pick, PharmD, BCOP
Associate Professor of Pharmacy Practice, Creighton
   University School of Pharmacy and Health Professions,
   Omaha, Nebraska
Chapter 96

Melissa R. Pleva, PharmD, BCPS, BCNSP
Clinical Pharmacist and Adjunct Clinical Assistant
   Professor, University of Michigan Health System and
   College of Pharmacy, Ann Arbor, Michigan
Chapter 100

Frank Pucino Jr., PharmD, MPH
Clinical Investigator, National Institute of Arthritis and
   Musculoskeletal and Skin Diseases (NIAMS), National
   Institute of Diabetes and Digestive and Kidney Diseases
   (NIDDK); National Institutes of Health, Bethesda,
   Maryland
Chapters 45 and 46

Kelly R. Ragucci, PharmD, FCCP, BCPS, CDE
Professor and Assistant Dean, Clinical Pharmacy and
   Outcome Sciences, South Carolina College of Pharmacy,
   Medical University of South Carolina Campus,
   Charleston, South Carolina
Chapter 50

Gowtham A. Rao, MD, PhD, MPH
University of South Carolina School of Medicine, University
   of South Carolina, College of Pharmacy, William J.B.
   Dorn Veterans Affairs Medical Center, Columbia, South
   Carolina
Chapter 82

Évelyne Rey, MD, MSc
Professor, Department of Medicine and of Obstetrics and
   Gynecology, University of Montreal, CHU Sainte Justine
   Montreal, Quebec, Canada
Chapter 47

Anastasia Rivkin, BS, PharmD, BCPS
Associate Professor and Division Director of Pharmacy
   Practice, Arnold and Marie Schwartz College of Pharmacy
   and Health Sciences, Long Island University, Brooklyn,
   New York
Chapter 67

Leigh Ann Ross, PharmD, BCPS
Associate Dean for Clinical Affairs, Chair and Associate
   Professor, Department of Pharmacy Practice, University
   of Mississippi School of Pharmacy, Jackson, Mississippi
Chapter 35

Warren E. Rose, PharmD
Assistant Professor, Pharmacy Practice Division, University
   of Wisconsin School of Pharmacy, Madison, Wisconsin
Chapter 79

Brendan S. Ross, MD
Staff Physician, G.V. (Sonny) Montgomery Veterans Affairs
   Medical Center; Clinical Associate Professor, Department
   of Pharmacy Practice, University of Mississippi School of
   Pharmacy, Jackson, Mississippi
Chapter 35

John C. Rotschafer, PharmD, FCCP
Professor, College of Pharmacy, University of Minnesota,
   Minneapolis, Minnesota
Chapter 85

Heather M. Rouse, PharmD, BCPS
Clinical Pharmacy Specialist, Adult Critical Care, Penn State
   Milton S. Hershey Medical Center, Hershey, Pennsylvania
Chapter 23

Laurajo Ryan, PharmD, MSc, BCPS, CDE
Clinical Associate Professor, Department of Medicine,
   University of Texas at Austin College of Pharmacy,
   University of Texas Health Science Center,
   Pharmacotherapy Education Research Center, Austin,
   Texas
Chapter 22

Melody Ryan, PharmD, MPH
Associate Professor, Departments of Pharmacy Practice
   and Science and Neurology, University of Kentucky,
   Lexington, Kentucky
Chapter 30

Sarah L. Scarpace, PharmD, BCOP
Assistant Dean for Pharmacy Professional Affairs and
   Associate Professor, Pharmacy Practice, Albany College of
   Pharmacy and Health Sciences, Stratton Veterans' Affairs
   Medical Center, Albany, New York
Chapter 99

Lauren S. Schlesselman, MEd, PharmD
Assistant Clinical Professor and Director of Assessment
   and Accreditation, Department of Pharmacy Practice,
   University of Connecticut School of Pharmacy, Storrs,
   Connecticut
Chapter 83

Kristine S. Schonder, PharmD
Assistant Professor, Department of Pharmacy and
   Therapeutics, University of Pittsburgh School of
   Pharmacy, Pittsburgh, Pennsylvania
Chapter 26

Julie Sease, PharmD, BCPS, CDE
Associate Professor, Department of Pharmacy Practice, Presbyterian College School of Pharmacy, Clinton, South Carolina
Chapter 43

Roohollah Sharifi, MD
Section Head of Urology, Jesse Brown Veterans Administration Hospital, Chicago, Illinois
Chapter 52

Kayce Shealy, PharmD, BCPS
Assistant Professor of Pharmacy Practice, Presbyterian College School of Pharmacy, Clinton, South Carolina
Chapter 43

Bradley W. Shinn, PharmD
Associate Professor of Pharmacy Practice, University of Findlay College of Pharmacy, Findlay, Ohio
Chapter 76

Judith A. Smith, PharmD, BCOP, CPHQ, FCCP, FISOPP
Associate Professor, Department of Gynecologic Oncology and Reproductive Medicine, Division of Surgery, The University of Texas M.D. Anderson Cancer Center, Houston, Texas
Chapter 94

Philip H. Smith, MD, IAAAAI
Assistant Professor of Medicine, Georgia Health Sciences University, Augusta, Georgia
Chapter 54

Steven M. Smith, PharmD
Assistant Professor, Department of Clinical Pharmacy, School of Pharmacy, University of Colorado Denver, Aurora, Colorado
Chapter 58

Sarah A. Spinler, PharmD, FCCP, FAHA, FASHP, AACC, BCPC (AQ Cardiology)
Professor of Clinical Pharmacy, Philadelphia College of Pharmacy, University of the Sciences in Philadelphia, Philadelphia, Pennsylvania
Chapter 8

Mary K. Stamatakis, BS, PharmD
Associate Dean and Associate Professor, West Virginia University School of Pharmacy, Morgantown, West Virginia
Chapter 25

Robert J. Straka, PharmD, FCCP
Professor and Head, Experimental and Clinical Pharmacology Department, University of Minnesota College of Pharmacy, Minneapolis, Minnesota
Chapter 5

S. Scott Sutton, PharmD, BCPS
Associate Professor, South Carolina College of Pharmacy, University of South Carolina, Columbia, South Carolina
Chapter 82

Marc A. Sweeney, RPh, BSPharm, PharmD, MDiv
Professor and Dean, School of Pharmacy, Cedarville University, Cedarville, Ohio
Chapter 4

Robert K. Sylvester, PharmD
Professor, Department of Pharmacy Practice, College of Pharmacy, Nursing and Allied Sciences, North Dakota State University; Oncology Clinical Specialist, Sanford Health Medical Center, Fargo, North Dakota
Chapter 66

Eljim P. Tesoro, PharmD, BCPS
Clinical Pharmacist, Neurosciences ICU, Clinical Assistant Professor, College of Pharmacy, University of Illinois Medical Center at Chicago, Chicago, Illinois
Chapter 32

Christian J. Teter, PharmD, BCPP
Assistant Professor, Psychopharmacology, Department of Pharmacy Practice, College of Pharmacy, University of New England, Portland, Maine
Chapter 36

Janine E. Then, PharmD, BCPS
Unit-based Pharmacist, University of Pittsburgh Medical Center, Presbyterian-Shadyside Hospital, Pittsburgh, Pennsylvania
Chapter 23

Maria Miller Thurston, PharmD, BCPS
PGY-2 Ambulatory Care Resident, University of Georgia College of Pharmacy, Charlie Norwood Veterans Affairs Medical Center, Augusta, Georgia
Chapter 56

James E. Tisdale, PharmD, BCPS, FCCP, FAPhA, FAHA
Professor, College of Pharmacy, Purdue University; Adjunct Professor, School of Medicine, Indiana University, Indianapolis, Indiana
Chapter 9

Mary A. Ullman, PharmD
Pharmacist, Regions Hospital, St. Paul, Minnesota
Chapter 85

Elena M. Umland, PharmD
Associate Dean for Academic Affairs, Associate Professor of Pharmacy, Thomas Jefferson School of Pharmacy, Thomas Jefferson University, Philadelphia, Pennsylvania
Chapter 49

Heather L. VandenBussche, PharmD
Professor, Department of Pharmacy Practice, Ferris State University College of Pharmacy, Kalamazoo, Michigan
Chapter 72

Orly Vardeny, PharmD, MS
Assistant Professor, University of Wisconsin School of Pharmacy, Madison, Wisconsin
Chapter 6

Nicole D. Verkleeren, PharmD, BCPS
Clinical Pharmacy Specialist, Critical Care, Forbes Regional Hospital, Monroeville, Pennsylvania
Chapter 15

Mary L. Wagner, PharmD, MS
Associate Professor, Department of Pharmacy Practice and Administration, Ernest Mario School of Pharmacy, Rutgers, The State University of New Jersey, Piscataway, New Jersey
Chapter 33

Geoffrey C. Wall, PharmD, FCCP, BCPS, CGP
Professor of Clinical Sciences, Drake University College of Pharmacy and Health Sciences, Internal Medicine Clinical Pharmacist, Iowa Methodist Medical Center, Des Moines, Iowa
Chapter 59

Heidi J. Wehring, PharmD, BCPP
Assistant Professor, Department of Psychiatry, Maryland Psychiatric Research Center, University of Maryland School of Medicine, Washington, DC
Chapter 37

Elaine Weiner, MD
Assistant Professor, Department of Psychiatry, University of Maryland Medical School, Catonsville, Maryland
Chapter 37

Lydia E. Weisser, DO
Clinical Director, Mississippi State Hospital, Whitfield, Mississippi
Chapter 39

Timothy E. Welty, PharmD, MA, FCCP, BCPS
Professor and Chair, Department of Clinical Sciences, College of Pharmacy and Health Sciences, Drake University, Des Moines, Iowa
Chapter 31

Tara R. Whetsel, PharmD, BCACP
Clinical Associate Professor, West Virginia University School of Pharmacy, Morgantown, West Virginia
Chapter 15

Sheila Wilhelm, PharmD, BCPS
Clinical Assistant Professor, Wayne State University Eugene Applebaum College of Pharmacy and Health Sciences, Clinical Pharmacy Specialist, Internal Medicine, Harper University Hospital, Detroit, Michigan
Chapter 20

Lori Wilken, PharmD, CDE, AE-C
Clinical Pharmacist, University of Illinois Medical Center at Chicago; Clinical Assistant Professor, Ambulatory Care Pharmacy, University of Illinois at Chicago College of Pharmacy, Chicago, Illinois
Chapter 14

Amy Robbins Williams, PharmD, BCOP
Assistant Professor of Pharmacy Practice, Union University School of Pharmacy, Jackson, Tennessee
Chapter 88

Dianne Williams May, PharmD, BCPS
Campus Director for Pharmacy Practice Experiences, Clinical Associate Professor, Division of Experience Programs and Department of Clinical and Administrative Pharmacy, University of Georgia College of Pharmacy, Augusta, Georgia
Chapters 17 and 18

Susan R. Winkler, PharmD, FCCP, BCPS
Professor and Chair, Department of Pharmacy Practice, Midwestern University Chicago College of Pharmacy, Downers Grove, Illinois
Chapter 11

Ann K. Wittkowsky, PharmD, CACP, FASHP, FCCP
Clinical Professor, University of Washington School of Pharmacy, Director, Anticoagulation Services, University of Washington Medical Center, Seattle, Washington
Chapter 10

G. Christopher Wood, PharmD, FCCP
Associate Professor, Department of Clinical Pharmacy, University of Tennessee Health Science Center, College of Pharmacy, Memphis, Tennessee
Chapter 13

REVIEWERS

Rita R. Alloway, PharmD, FCCP
Research Professor, Director, Transplant Clinical Research, University of Cincinnati College of Medicine, Cincinnati, Ohio

Alexander K. Berg, PharmD, PhD
Clinical Pharmacology Fellow, Department of Molecular Pharmacology and Experimental Therapeutics, Mayo Clinic Rochester, Minnesota

Margaret T. Bowers, RN, MSN, FNP-BC, AACC
Assistant Professor, Duke University School of Nursing, Nurse Practitioner Duke Heart Failure Program, Durham, North Carolina

Jeffrey Bratberg, PharmD, BCPS
Clinical Associate Professor of Pharmacy Practice, URI College of Pharmacy, Kingston, Rhode Island; Adjunct Associate Professor of Medicine, Alpert Medical School of Brown University, Infectious Diseases Specialist, Roger Williams Medical Center, Providence, Rhode Island

Mary Brennan, DNP, ACNP-BC, GNP-BC, ANP, RN
Clinical Assistant Professor, New York University College of Nursing, Coordinator, Acute Care Nurse Practitioner Program, New York, New York

Denise Buonocore, MSN
Acute Care Nurse Practitioner HF Service, St. Vincent's Multispecialty Group, Bridgeport, Connecticut

Katie E. Cardone, PharmD, BCACP
Assistant Professor, Department of Pharmacy Practice, Albany College of Pharmacy and Health Sciences, Albany, New York

Elias B. Chahine, PharmD, BCPS
Assistant Professor of Pharmacy Practice, Department of Pharmacy Practice, Palm Beach Atlantic University, West Palm Beach, Florida; Clinical Pharmacist, Department of Pharmaceutical Services, JFK Medical Center, Atlantis, Florida

Amber N. Chiplinski, PharmD, BCPS
Clinical Assistant Professor, West Virginia University School of Pharmacy, Clinical Pharmacy Specialist, Internal Medicine Martinsburg Veterans Affairs Medical Center, Martinsburg, West Virginia

Jennifer Confer, PharmD, BCPS
Clinical Assistant Professor, West Virginia University School of Pharmacy, Critical Care Clinical Pharmacy Specialist, Cabell Huntington Hospital, Huntington, West Virginia

Bonnie A. Dadig, EdD, PA-C
Chair, Physician Assistant Department, Associate Professor College of Allied Health Sciences, Georgia Health Sciences University Augusta, Georgia

Lawrence W. Davidow, PhD, RPh
Directory, Pharmacy Skills Laboratory, University of Kansas School of Pharmacy, Lawrence, Kansas

David L. DeRemer, PharmD, BCOP
Clinical Assistant Professor, University of Georgia College of Pharmacy, Augusta, Georgia

Thomas Dowling, PharmD, PhD
Associate Professor of Pharmacy Practice, School of Pharmacy, University of Maryland, Baltimore, Maryland

David P. Elliott, PharmD, CGP, FASCP, FCCP, AGS
Professor and Associate Chair of Clinical Pharmacy, School of Pharmacy, West Virginia University, Charleston, West Virginia

Jingyang Fan, PharmD, BCPS
Clinical Associate Professor, Southern Illinois University Edwardsville, School of Pharmacy; Cardiovascular Clinical Pharmacist, Mercy Hospital, St. Louis, Missouri

Amanda Geist
Clinical Assistant Professor, Department of Clinical Pharmacy, West Virginia University School of Pharmacy, Charleston, West Virginia

Nancy S. Goldstein, DNP, ANP-BC, RN-C
The Johns Hopkins University School of Nursing, Baltimore, Maryland

Justine S. Gortney, PharmD, BCPS
Assistant Professor of Pharmacy Practice (Clinical) Eugene Applebaum College of Pharmacy and Health Sciences, Wayne State University, Detroit, Michigan, Clinical Pharmacy Specialist, Internal Medicine, Detroit Receiving Hospital, Detroit, Michigan

Erich J. Grant, MMS, PA-C, AAHIVS
Instructor, Department of Physician Assistant Studies, Wake Forest School of Medicine, Winston-Salem, North Carolina

Hillary Wall Grillo, PharmD
Adjunct Assistant Professor, Bernard J. Dunn School of Pharmacy, Shenandoah University Pharmacist, Winchester Medical Center, Winchester, Virginia

Nalo Hamilton, PhD, MSN, APRN-BC
Assistant Professor, UCLA School of Nursing, Los Angeles, California

Deborah Hass, PharmD, BCOP, BCPS
Assistant Professor, Midwestern University Chicago College of Pharmacy, Hematology/Oncology Clinical Pharmacist, Rush University Hospital, Chicago, Illinois

David Hawkins, PharmD
Professor and Dean, California Northstate College of Pharmacy, Rancho Cordova, California

Arthur J. Jacknowitz, PharmD
Professor and Distinguished Chair in Clinical Pharmacy, School of Pharmacy, West Virginia University, Morgantown, West Virginia

Jill T. Johnson, PharmD, BCPS
Associate Professor, Department of Pharmacy Practice, University of Arkansas for Medical Sciences College of Pharmacy, Little Rock, Arkansas

Mikael D. Jones, PharmD, BCPS
Clinical assistant Professor, Department of Pharmacy practice and Science, College of Pharmacy, University of Kentucky, Lexington, Kentucky

Lynn G. Kirkland, DNSc, WHNP, CNM
Assistant Professor, University of Tennessee Health Science Center at Memphis, College of Nursing, Memphis Obstetrics and Gynecological Association, PC, Memphis, Tennessee

Michael A. Mancano, PharmD
Clinical Professor, Interim Chair, Department of Pharmacy Practice, Temple University School of Pharmacy; Clinical Consultant, Pennsylvania Hospital, Philadelphia, Pennsylvania

Rupal Patel Mansukhani, PharmD
Clinical Assistant Professor, Ernest Mario School of Pharmacy, Rutgers University, Piscataway, New Jersey

Candis M. Morello, PharmD, CDE, FCSHP
Associate Professor of Clinical Pharmacy, Associate Dean for Student Affairs, University of California San Diego, Skaggs School of Pharmacy and Pharmaceutical Sciences, La Jolla, California; Clinical Pharmacist Specialist, Veterans Affairs San Diego Health, San Diego, California

Jadwiga Najib, BS, PharmD
Professor of Pharmacy Practice, Long Island University, Arnold and Marie Schwartz College of Pharmacy and Health Sciences, Brooklyn, New York; Clinical Pharmacist, St. Luke's/Roosevelt Hospital Center, New York, New York

Lisa M. Nissen, BPharm, PhD
Associate Professor, Quality Use of Medicines, School of Pharmacy, Deputy Director, Centre for Safe and Effective Prescribing, Pharmacy Australia Centre of Excellence, The University of Queensland, Brisbane, Australia

Stephen Orr, MD
Ophthalmologist, Spectrum Eye Care, Inc., Findlay, Ohio

Rolee Pathak, PharmD, BCPS
Clinical Pharmacist, St. Joseph's Regional Medical Center, Clinical Assistant Professor, Ernest Mario School of Pharmacy, Rutgers University; Clinical Coordinator, Englewood Hospital and Medical Center, Piscataway, New Jersey

Laura Perry
Assistant Professor of Pharmacy Practice, The University of Findlay College of Pharmacy, Findlay, Ohio

James Roch, PA-C, MPAS
Assistant Professor, Department of Physician Assistant Studies, Academic Coordinator, Midwestern University, Glendale, Arizona

Warren E. Rose, PharmD
Assistant Professor, Pharmacy Practice Division, University of Wisconsin School of Pharmacy, Madison, Wisconsin

Maha Saad, PharmD, CGP, BCPS
Assistant Clinical Professor, St. John's University, College of Pharmacy and Allied Health Professions, Queens, New York, and Clinical Coordinator, Long Island Jewish Medical Center, New Hyde Park, New York

JoAnne M. Saxe, RN, ANP-BC, MS, DNP
Health Sciences Clinical Professor, Department of Community Health Systems, School of Nursing, University of California, San Francisco, California

Denise Schentrup, DNP, ARNP-BC
Clinical Assistant Professor, Department of Women, Children and Family, College of Nursing, University of Florida, Gainesville, Florida

Lauren S. Schlesselman, MEd, PharmD
Assistant Clinical Professor, Department of Pharmacy Practice, University of Connecticut School of Pharmacy, Storrs, Connecticut

Bradley W. Shinn, PharmD
Associate Professor of Pharmacy Practice, The University of Findlay College of Pharmacy, Findlay, Ohio

Catherine N. Shull, PA-C, MPAS
Assistant Professor, Department of Physician Assistant
Studies, Wake Forest School of Medicine, Winston-Salem,
North Carolina

Douglas Slain, Pharm D, BCPS, FCCP
Associate Professor, Infectious Diseases Clinical Specialist,
West Virginia University, Morgantown, West Virginia

Jacqueline Jordan Spiegel, MS, PA-C
Associate Professor, College of Health Sciences, Director,
Clinical Skills and Simulation, Midwestern University,
Glendale, Arizona

Sneha Baxi Srivastava, PharmD
Chicago State University College of Pharmacy, Assistant
Professor of Pharmacy Practice, Chicago, Illinois

Javad Tafreshi, PharmD, BCPS, AQ Cardiology
Loma Linda University School of Pharmacy and Medical
Center, Loma Linda, California

Tanya Vadala, PharmD
Assistant Professor, Department of Pharmacy Practice,
Albany College of Pharmacy and Health Sciences, Albany,
New York

Lee C. Vermeulen, RPh, MS, FCCP
Director, UW Health Center for Clinical Knowledge
Management, Clinical Professor of Pharmacy, University
of Wisconsin, Madison, Wisconsin

Angie Veverka, PharmD, BCPS
Clinical Pharmacist, Internal Medicine, PGY1 Pharmacy
Residency Coordinator, Carolinas Medical Center,
Charlotte, North Carolina

Christine M. Werner, PA-C, PhD, RD
Associate Professor, Department of Physician Assistant
Education, Doisy College of Health Sciences, Saint Louis
University, St. Louis, Missouri

Thomas G. White, JD, MA, PA-C
Associate Professor, University of New England, Physician
Assistant Program, Portland, Maine

Jon P. Wietholter, PharmD, BCPS
Clinical Assistant Professor, West Virginia University School
of Pharmacy, Internal Medicine Clinical Pharmacist,
Cabell Huntington Hospital, Huntington, West Virginia

Monty Yoder, PharmD, BCPS
Clinical Specialist, Department of Pharmacy, Wake Forest
Baptist Health, Winston Salem, North Carolina

PREFACE

Pharmacotherapy Principles & Practice, a winner of the Medical Book Award from the American Medical Writers Association, has been well received and adopted by many pharmacy, nursing, and physician assistant schools. Chapters are written by content experts and reviewed critically by pharmacists, nurse practitioners, physician assistants, and physicians who are authorities in their fields. Written in a concise style that facilitates in-depth understanding of essential topics, the third edition meets the same high-quality expectations as previous editions.

Now more than ever, healthcare practitioners have a critical responsibility to their patients and society to deliver high-quality and cost-effective care. Development of these practice abilities requires an integration of knowledge, skills, attitudes, beliefs, and values that can be acquired only through a structured learning process that includes classroom work, independent study, mentorship, and ultimately, direct involvement in the care of patients in interprofessional settings. With its 102 chapters, *Pharmacotherapy Principles & Practice,* Third Edition, facilitates learning by using multiple teaching techniques and enhanced features. The textbook opens with an introductory chapter followed by chapters on pediatrics, geriatrics, and palliative care. The remainder of the book consists of 98 disease-based chapters that review disease etiology, epidemiology, pathophysiology, and clinical presentation, followed by clear therapeutic recommendations for drug selection, dosing, and patient monitoring.

Pharmacotherapy Principles & Practice is designed to meet classroom and independent study needs of today's learners in the health care professions. The following features were designed in collaboration with educational design specialists to enhance learning and retention:

- *Structured learning objectives* are included at the beginning of each chapter, with information in the text that corresponds to each learning objective identified by a vertical rule with a circle in the margin, allowing the reader to quickly find content related to each objective.

- *Key concepts related to patient assessment and treatment* are listed at the beginning of each chapter to help focus learning. Numbered icons are used throughout the chapter to identify content that develops these concepts.

- *Patient encounters* are distributed throughout each chapter to facilitate development of critical thinking skills and lend clinical relevance to the scientific foundation provided. This feature has been enhanced in the third edition.

- *Patient care and monitoring guidelines* are placed near the end of each chapter to assist students in their general approach to assessing, treating, and monitoring patients for therapeutic response and adverse events.

- *Up-to-date literature citations* for each chapter are provided to support treatment recommendations.

- *Tables, figures, text boxes, and algorithms* are used liberally to enhance understanding of pathophysiology, clinical presentation, drug selection, pharmacokinetics, and patient monitoring.

- *Medical abbreviations and their meanings* are placed at the end of each chapter to facilitate learning the accepted shorthand used in real-world healthcare settings.

- *A glossary of medical terms* is included as an appendix to the book; the first use of each glossary term in a chapter appears in bold colored font.

- *Self-assessment questions and answers for each chapter* are located in the Online Learning Center to facilitate self-evaluation of learning.

- *Laboratory values* are expressed as both conventional units and Systemè International (SI) units to facilitate learning by those in countries where these units of measure are the standard.

- *Appendices* contain: (1) conversion factors and anthropometrics; (2) common laboratory tests and their reference ranges; (3) common medical abbreviations; and (4) how to write a prescription.

The Online Learning Center at www.ChisholmPharmacotherapy.com provides self-assessment questions, a testing center that has the ability to grade and provide immediate feedback on the self-assessment questions as well as reporting capabilities, and other features designed to support learning.

A companion text, *Pharmacotherapy Principles and Practice Study Guide: A Case-Based Care Plan Approach,* is available to further enhance learning by guiding students through the process of applying knowledge of pharmacotherapy to specific patient cases. This study guide contains approximately 100 patient cases that correspond to chapters published in *Pharmacotherapy Principles & Practice.*

We acknowledge the commitment and dedication of the more than 182 contributing authors and more than 55 reviewers of the chapters contained in this text. A special thanks goes to the educators who have adopted this text in their courses. We also extend our thanks to McGraw-Hill Medical, especially Michael Weitz, Peter Boyle, and Laura Libretti, as well as the support teams at our individual universities for their dedication to this project.

The Editors
Third Edition, 2012

Part I

Basic Concepts of Pharmacotherapy Principles and Practices

1

Introduction

Jack E. Fincham

INTRODUCTION

Health professionals are given significant responsibilities in our healthcare system. These roles may be taken for granted by patients until a pharmacist, nurse practitioner, physician assistant, physician, or others perform assigned tasks that make a major impact on the lives of patients and patients' families in countless ways. The exemplary manner in which health professionals provide necessary care to patients is a hallmark of health professional practice and delivery of healthcare in the United States. Patients are thus well served, and fellow health professionals share knowledge and expertise specific to their profession. Despite this, many problems remain in the U.S. healthcare system; there were close to 50 million uninsured individuals in the United States in 2010, representing between 16% and 17% of the population.[1] This dramatic number of 50 million is but 10 million less than the entire population of either France or the United Kingdom. It is simply staggering in scope and has implications for the future collective health of the U.S. population. These figures are basically unchanged from the year 2009, except for the number of uninsured.

Countless other Americans are underinsured. They may have partial coverage, but for these Americans the high price of deductibles, copays, and monthly payments for insurance create an economic dilemma each time they seek care or pay premiums. According to the U.S. Centers for Medicare and Medicaid Services, National Health Expenditure data, well over $2.71 trillion was spent on healthcare in the United States during 2010, amounting to $8,327 per person, which amounts to 17% of the U.S. gross domestic product (GDP), some of it no doubt unnecessarily so.[1] By 2020, expenditures are projected to $4.64 trillion, which would be a projected $13,709 per person, 19% of the U.S. GDP. It is anticipated that with the enhanced focus on quality of the Patient Protection and Affordable Care Act, passed in 2009, that unnecessary expenditures and duplicative healthcare service may be reduced and lower the misspent money in parts of the health expenditures in the United States.

The use of medications in the healthcare system provides enormous help to many; lives are saved or enhanced, and lifespans are lengthened. Many other uses of medications lead to significant side effects, worsening states of health, and premature deaths. So how can we separate these disparate pictures of drug use outcomes? You, within your practices and within your healthcare workplace networks, can help to promote the former and diminish the latter. The authors of the chapters in this book have written informative, current, and superb chapters that can empower you to positively influence medication use.

DRUG USE IN THE HEALTHCARE SYSTEM

Spending on drugs, as a percentage of total healthcare, increased 5.3% in 2009 compared with the previous year.[2] Drivers for this significant increase include increases in available technologies, numbers of patients, prescriptions per patient, and number of seniors taking advantage of the Medicare Part D drug benefit.

Significant numbers of medications are used daily in the United States. Over one decade (1997 to 2007) prescriptions purchased zoomed from $2.2 billion to $3.8 billion.[3] The average number of prescriptions per capita in the United States rose from 8.9 in 1997 to 12.6 in 2007.[3] Problems occurring with drug use can include:

- Medication errors
- Suboptimal drug, dose, regimen, dosage form, and duration of use
- Unnecessary drug therapy
- Therapeutic duplication
- Drug–drug, drug–disease, drug–food, or drug–nutrient interactions
- Drug allergies
- Adverse drug effects, some of which are preventable

Clinicians are often called upon to identify, resolve, and prevent problems that occur due to undertreatment, overtreatment, or inappropriate treatment. Individuals can purchase medications through numerous outlets, including pharmacies, mail-order pharmacies, supermarkets, convenience stores, via the Internet, from physicians, from healthcare institutions, and through any number of additional outlets. Herbal remedies are also marketed and sold in numerous outlets. The monitoring of positive and negative outcomes of the use of drugs can be disjointed and incomplete. Clinicians and students in the health professions need to take ownership of these problems and improve patient outcomes resulting from drug use.

It is important to realize that, although clinicians are the gatekeepers for patients to obtain prescription drugs, patients can obtain prescription medications from numerous sources. Patients may also borrow from friends, relatives, or even casual acquaintances. In addition, patients obtain over-the counter (OTC) medications from physicians through prescriptions, on advice from pharmacists and other health professionals, through self-selection, or through the recommendations of friends or acquaintances. Through all of this, it must be recognized that there are both formal (structural) and informal (word-of-mouth) components at play. Health professionals may or may not be consulted regarding the use of medications, and in some cases they are unaware of the drugs patients are taking. In addition, herbal remedies or health supplements may be taken without the knowledge or input of a health professional.

External variables may greatly influence patients and their drug-taking behaviors. Coverage for prescribed drugs allows those with coverage to obtain medications with varying cost-sharing requirements. However, many do not have insurance coverage for drugs or other health-related needs. With Medicare Part D coverage for outpatient prescription medications, more elderly people have access to needed therapy than ever before.[4]

Self-Medication

Self-medication can be defined as a patient decision to consume a drug with or without the approval or direction of a health professional. Self-medication activities of patients have increased dramatically in the late 20th and early 21st centuries. Many factors affecting patients have fueled this increase. There are ever-increasing ways to purchase OTC medications. Many prescription items switched to OTC classification in the last 50 years, which has dramatically and significantly fueled the rapid expansion of OTC drug use. In addition, patients are increasingly comfortable with self-diagnosing and self-selection of OTC remedies. In many studies,[5] self-medication with nonprescribed therapies exceeds the use of prescription medications in the patient groups assessed.

Patients' use of self-selected products has the potential to provide enormous benefits.[6] Through the rational use of drugs, patients may avoid more costly therapies or expenditures for other professional services. Self-limiting conditions, and even some chronic health conditions (e.g., allergies and dermatologic conditions), if appropriately treated through patient self-medication, allow the patient to have a degree of autonomy in healthcare decisions.

Compliance Issues

Patient noncompliance with prescription regimens is one of the most understated problems in the healthcare system. Noncompliance has enormous ramifications for patients, caregivers, and health professionals. Noncompliance is a multifaceted problem with a need for interprofessional, multidisciplinary solutions. Interventions that are organizational (how clinics are structured), educational (patient counseling, supportive approach), and behavioral (impacting health beliefs and expectations) are necessary. Noncompliance leads to lack of disease control and a high discrepancy in how patients respond to therapies.[7] Identifying psychosocial interventions, which engage patients to self-manage their therapies, has proven efficacy.[7] Acknowledging barriers that people perceive in complying helps identify how to assist patients to overcome these distracters.[7] Compliant behavior can be enhanced through actions with the patients. Many times what is necessary is referral to specific clinicians for individualized treatment and monitoring to enhance compliance. The case histories provided in this text will allow you to follow what others have done in similar situations to optimally help patients succeed in improving compliance rates and positive health outcomes.

Drug Use by the Elderly

Various components of drug use in the elderly are worth noting. Problems with health literacy (i.e., understanding medical terminology and directions from providers) are more common among the elderly.[8] The burgeoning population of the elderly, coupled with their lack of health literacy, means that this issue will become even more problematic.[9]

Over the next decade, seniors will spend $1.8 trillion on prescription medications. Medicare proposals to provide a drug benefit for seniors have been suggested to cost $400 billion over a 10-year period. Thus the most elaborate current drug program will pay only 22% of seniors' drug costs. Enhanced use of pharmacoeconomic tenets to select appropriate therapy, while considering cost and therapeutic benefits for seniors and others, will become even more crucial.

Unnecessary drug therapy and overmedication are problems with drug use in the elderly. A joint effort by health professionals working together is the best approach to aiding seniors in achieving optimal drug therapy. Evaluation of all medications taken by seniors at each patient visit can help prevent polypharmacy from occurring.[10]

IMPACTING THE PROBLEMS OF DRUG USE

Medication Errors

There is no more glaring issue in medication use and monitoring than the need to reduce medication errors. Untold morbidity and mortality occur due to the many errors occurring in medication use. Studies have shown that reconciling the patient's medications, with coordination by caregivers, can reduce medication errors.[11] Current changes in how drugs are prescribed, such as electronic prescribing, barcode identification of patients, and electronic medication records, can all reduce medication errors.[12,13] As technologies are increasingly used, benefits will expand.

Incorporation of three key interventions (computerized physician order entry [CPOE], additional staffing, and bar coding) have been shown in an institutional setting to help reduce medication errors.[13] Being able to track drug order-ing, dispensing, and administration electronically has been shown to be cost effective in the long run.[14] Nurses and office staff have been proven a valuable resource for report-ing prescribing errors, especially with ongoing reminders to scrutinize orders.[15]

The Epidemic of Prescribed Drug Abuse

In 2009, approximately 7.0 million persons were current users of psychotherapeutic drugs taken nonmedically (2.8% of the U.S. population). This class of drugs is broadly described as those targeting the CNS, including drugs used to treat psychiatric disorders. These are the medications most commonly abused:

- Pain relievers: 5.3 million
- Tranquilizers: 2.0 million
- Stimulants: 1.3 million
- Sedatives: 0.4 million[16]

The most prominent group of abused drugs in the United States at present is prescription and OTC medications. These drugs now have more first-time abusers than most commonly thought of drugs of abuse, such as marijuana, and are now overtaking marijuana use as the first type of drugs abused. The main source for these drugs is the fam-ily medicine cabinet. Bond and colleagues[17] in describing a large-scale database study (National Poison Data System of the American Association of Poison Control Centers) from a 2001 to 2008 study note that prevention efforts have proved inadequate in the face of rising availability of prescription medications, particularly more dangerous medications such as particularly opioids, sedative-hypnotics, and cardiovascu-lar agents.[17] Abuse of prescription medications by adolescents is an ascending problem that all health professionals must address and work together to try to lessen in intensity.

HEALTHCARE REFORM

The potential for healthcare reform (Patient Protection and Affordable Care Act [PPACA]), passed by the U.S. Congress in 2009 to enhance patient outcomes and the quality of care provided to Americans, is very significant. The inclusion of health professionals in segments of the innovative medical homes and accountable care organizations will help physi-cians and primary care providers reach more patients need-ing care.[18]

Incorporation of primary care providers, clinics, and healthcare institutions will enable information sharing elec-tronically to better reduce errors, enhance outcomes, and help to save precious dollars in the healthcare system. Health professionals have already been shown to provide savings in pilot projects. An average savings of $1,595 per patient was achieved by 9 pharmacists working with 88 Medicaid patients in a pilot project sponsored by the Centers for Medi-care and Medicaid Services in a primary care setting.[19]

There are also covered preventive aspects enabled by the PPACA that include immunizations, screenings, and other offering at no charge as components of the PPACA. The pro-vision of these preventive activities by health professionals will serve patients long term very nicely and work to prevent costly care later on.

That discussion about the potential for healthcare reform to influence patient care and outcomes must be tempered by the view that things may change suddenly with legislation or U.S. Supreme Court decisions regarding the constitutional-ity of the legislation; also, states have been active in negating certain components or the entire legislation as it applies to them, and the outcomes of the elections of 2012 will certainly influence the eventual scope and form of the PPACA.

SUMMARY

Health professionals are at a crucial juncture as we face an uncertain, yet promising future. Technological advances, including electronic prescribing, may stem the tide of medication errors and inappropriate prescribing. These technological enhancements for physician order entry (via personal electronic devices, tablet devices, tablet computers, or through web access to pharmacies) have been imple-mented to reduce drug errors. Health professionals face daunting challenges in ensuring appropriate use of pharma-cotherapy. Sophisticated computer technology can further empower health professionals to play an ever-increasing and effective role in helping patients to practice safe and effec-tive use of prescribed medicine. Healthcare reform has the potential to have a dramatic impact on your practices in the healthcare system for the length of your careers.

This book is written by content experts in the material they cover. They are among the thought and practice forefront of delivery of healthcare services in the United States. The thorough analysis of common disease states, discussion of therapies to treat these conditions, and specific advice to pro-vide to patients to help them self-medicate when appropriate and safe to do so will help you immensely in your practices. The use of material in this text, which incorporates materials written by the finest minds in pharmacy practice and educa-tion, can enable you to play a crucial role in improving the drug use process for patients, providers, payers, and society. The purpose of this book is to help hone your skills so you can make a real improvement in the therapies you provide to your patients. As current and future clinicians, you can rely on the information laid out here to enhance your knowledge and allow you to assist your patients with the sound advice they expect. Use the text, case histories, and numerous examples detailed here to expand your therapeutic skills and to help you have a positive impact on your patients in the years to come.

You can help to reverse medication-related problems, improve outcomes of care both clinically and economically, and enable drug use to meet stated goals and objectives. This text provides a thorough analysis and summary of treatment options for commonly occurring diseases and the medica-tions or alternative therapies used to treat these conditions successfully.

REFERENCES

1. National Health Expenditures [Internet]. Washington, DC: U.S. Centers for Medicare and Medicaid Services; January 11, 2011 [cited 2011 Oct 10]. Available from: *https://www.cms.gov/NationalHealthExpendData/downloads/proj2010.pdf.*

2. National Health Expenditure Data Factsheet [Internet]. Washington, DC: U.S. Centers for Medicare and Medicaid Services, July 11, 2011 [cited 2011 Oct 10]. Available from: *www.cms.gov/NationalHealthExpendData/25_NHE_Fact_sheet.asp.*

3. Prescription Drug Trends, Fact Sheet (#3057-07) [Internet]. Washington, DC: Kaiser Family Foundation; September 2008 [cited 2011 Oct 10]. Available from: *http://kff.org/rxdrugs/upload/3057_07.pdf.*

4. Fincham JE. Pharmacy curricula and bellwether changes in payment for pharmacy practice services. Am J Pharm Educ 2005;69(3):392–393.

5. Johnson G, Helman C. Remedy or cure? Lay beliefs about over-the-counter medicines for coughs and colds. Br J Gen Pract 2004;54(499):98–102.

6. Hughes CM, McElnay JC, Fleming GF. Benefits and risks of self medication. Drug Saf 2001;24(14):1027–1037.

7. Vrijens B, Vincze G, Kristanto P, et al. Adherence to prescribed antihypertensive drug treatments: Longitudinal study of electronically compiled dosing histories. BMJ 2008;336(7653):1114–1117.

8. Williams A, Manias E, Walker R. Interventions to improve medication adherence in people with multiple chronic conditions: A systematic review. J Adv Nurs 2008;63(2):132–143.

9. Parker RM, Ratzan SC, Lurie N. Health literacy: A policy challenge for advancing high-quality health care. Health Aff 2003;22(4):147–153.

10. Hajjar ER, Cafiero AC, Hanlon JT. Polypharmacy in elderly patients. Am J Geriatr Pharmacother 2007;5:345–351.

11. Delate T, Chester EA, Stubbings TW, Barnes CA. Clinical outcomes of a home-based medication reconciliation program after discharge from a skilled nursing facility. Pharmacotherapy 2008;28:444–452.

12. Fincham JE. e-prescribing: The electronic transformation of medicine. Sudbury, MA: Jones and Bartlett, 2009.

13. Franklin BD, O'Grady K, Donyai P, et al. The impact of a closed-loop electronic prescribing and administration system on prescribing errors, administration errors and staff time: A before-and-after study. Qual Saf Health Care 2007;16:279–284.

14. Karnon J, McIntosh A, Dean J, et al. Modelling the expected net benefits of interventions to reduce the burden of medication errors. J Health Serv Res Policy 2008;13:85–91.

15. Kennedy AG, Littenberg B, Senders JW. Using nurses and office staff to report prescribing errors in primary care. Int J Qual Health Care 2008;20:238–245.

16. Topics in Brief: Prescription Drug Abuse [Internet]. Bethesda, MD: U.S. National Institute on Drug Abuse; May 2011 [cited 2011 Oct 10]. Available from: *http://www.drugabuse.gov/tib/prescription.html.*

17. Bond GR, Woodward RW, Ho M. The growing impact of pediatric pharmaceutical poisoning. J Pediatr 2012;160:266–270.

18. Smith M, Bates DW, Bodenheimer T, Cleary PD. Why pharmacists belong in the medical home. Health Aff 2010;29(5):906–913.

19. Smith M, Giuliano MR, Starkowski PP. In Connecticut: Improving patient medication management in primary care. Health Aff 2011;30(4):646–654.

2 Geriatrics

Jeannie K. Lee, Damian M. Mendoza,
M. Jane Mohler, and Ellyn M. Lee

LEARNING OBJECTIVES

● **Upon completion of the chapter, the reader will be able to:**

1. Explain the growth pattern of the elderly population.
2. Discuss age-related pharmacokinetic and pharmacodynamic changes.
3. Identify drug-related problems and associated morbidities commonly experienced by older adults.
4. Describe major components of geriatric assessment.
5. Recognize interprofessional patient care functions in various geriatric practice settings.

KEY CONCEPTS

❶ Population aging is an incontrovertible trend.

❷ Older Americans use considerably more healthcare services than younger Americans, and their healthcare needs are often complex.

❸ All four components of pharmacokinetics—absorption, distribution, metabolism, and excretion—are affected by aging; the most clinically important and consistent is the reduction of renal elimination of drugs.

❹ In general, the pharmacodynamic changes that occur in the elderly tend to increase their sensitivity to drug effects.

❺ Comorbidities and polypharmacy complicate elderly health status, particularly when polypharmacy includes inappropriate medications that lead to drug-related problems.

❻ Older adults are at greater risk for medication nonadherence due to the high prevalence of multiple comorbidities, including cognitive deficit, polypharmacy use, and financial barriers.

❼ The clinical approach to assessing older adults frequently goes beyond a traditional "history and physical" used in general internal medicine practice.

❽ Consideration of geriatric patients' vision, hearing, swallowing, cognition, motor impairment, and education and literacy levels during counseling and education can lead to enhanced medication adherence.

❾ Long-term care geriatric practices emphasize the interprofessional team approach.

The growth of the aging population and increasing lifespan require that healthcare professionals gain knowledge necessary to meeting the needs of this patient group. Despite the availability and benefit of numerous pharmacotherapies to treat their diseases, elderly patients commonly experience drug-related problems resulting in additional morbidities. Therefore, it is essential for clinicians serving older adults across all healthcare settings to understand the epidemiology of aging, age-related physiological changes, drug-related problems prevalent in the elderly, comprehensive geriatric assessment, and interprofessional approaches to geriatric care.

EPIDEMIOLOGY AND ETIOLOGY

As humans age, they are at increasingly elevated risk of disease, disability, and death primarily for three reasons: (a) genetic predisposition; (b) reduced immunological surveillance; and (c) the accumulated effects of physical, social, environmental, and behavioral exposures over the life course. Human relationships, social conditions, and networks interact with these accumulating exposures, and differences in time and place influence health outcomes by age cohort. Combined, these factors result in considerable variation by age in health states and healthcare requirements. All elders experience increasing vulnerability and **homeostenosis** as they age. Although resilient elders are able successfully to maintain high levels of physical and cognitive functioning, avoid chronic conditions, and remain socially engaged, others suffer functional decline, **frailty**, disability, or death. There is an urgent need for all clinicians to better understand the epidemiology of aging in order that healthcare needs of the elderly can be comprehensively addressed, and so that safe, quality services can be provided efficiently to optimize functioning and health-related quality of life for the aged.[1]

Sociodemographics

▶ *Population*

① *Population aging is an incontrovertible trend.* In 2010, 40.3 million U.S. residents were 65 years and older (13% of the total population), nearly 5.5 million people were 85 years or older (the "oldest-old"), and over 53,000 were centenarians.[2] The baby boomers (those born between 1946 and 1964) began turning 65 years in 2011; their numbers will double to 71.5 million in 2030, representing nearly 20% of the total U.S. population.[3] In 2010, there were a total of 22.9 million women and 17.4 million men (an average ratio of 100 women to 77.3 men) 65 years and older; this ratio widens as elders age. The oldest-old are projected to increase from 5.3 million in 2006 to nearly 21 million in 2050.[3] In addition, minority elder populations are projected to increase to 8.1 million in 2010 (20.1%), and up to 12.9 million in 2020 (23.6%), including disproportionate increases in Hispanics (254%); Asians and Pacific Islanders (208%); African Americans (147%); and Native Americans, Eskimos, and Aleuts (143%).[3] Surviving baby boomers will be proportionally more women, more racially diverse, better educated, and have more financial resources than were elders in previous generations.

▶ *Economics*

More elders are enjoying higher economic prosperity than ever before, with net worth increasing by nearly 80% for older Americans over the past 20 years. Still, major inequalities persist, with older blacks and those without high school diplomas reporting smaller economic gains and fewer financial resources.[4] Considerable disparities exist; the 2005 median net worth of households headed by whites 65 years and older was $226,900 compared with black elder household net worth of $37,800 (a sixfold difference).[4]

▶ *Education and Health Literacy*

By 2007, more than 75% of U.S. elders had graduated from high school, and nearly 20% had a bachelor's degree or higher. Still, substantial educational differences exist among racial and ethnic minorities. Whereas more than 80% of non-Hispanic white elders had high school degrees in 2007, only 72% of Asians, 58% of blacks, and 42% of Hispanic elders were graduates. Nearly 40% of people 75 years or older have low health literacy, more than any other age group.[4] Despite these limitations, the Pew Trust reports that more than 8 million Americans (22%) 65 years or older increasingly use the Internet,[5] and large healthcare plans such as the Veterans Administration are increasingly offering online health information to support this need. These advances in literacy are important because communication between healthcare providers and elders is vitally important in providing quality care, supporting self-care, and in negotiating the healthcare system.

Health Status

▶ *Life Expectancy*

Although Americans are living longer than ever before, an estimated average of 78.14 years overall in 2008, U.S. life expectancy lags behind that of many other industrialized nations.[6] There is nearly a 6-year gap between 2008 estimated life expectancy in men (75.29 years) and women (81.13 years).[6] Disparities in mortality persist, with estimated 2008 life expectancy in the white population nearly 5 years higher than that of the black population.[6] More than a third of U.S. deaths in 2000 were attributed to three risk behaviors: smoking, poor diet, and physical inactivity, accounting for nearly 35% of deaths. Currently, only 9% of Americans older than 65 years smoke; however, nearly 54% of men and 21% of women are former smokers.[7] Overweight elders 65 to 74 years of age increased from 57% to 73% in 2004 largely due to inactivity and a diet high in refined foods, saturated fats, and sugared beverages, and deficient in whole grains, fruits, vegetables, nuts, and seeds.[4] Despite the proven health benefits of regular physical activity, more than half of the older population is sedentary; 47% of those 65 to 74 years and 61% older than 75 years report no physical activity.[8]

The 2007 National Health Interview Survey indicated that 39% of non-Hispanic white elders reported "very good" or "excellent" health, compared with 29% of Hispanics and 24% of blacks.[9] Chronic diseases disproportionately affect older adults and are associated with disability, diminished quality of life, and increased costs for healthcare and long-term care. About 80% of older adults have at least one chronic condition, and 50% have at least two. The prevalence of certain chronic conditions differs by sex, with women reporting higher levels of arthritis (54% versus 43%), and men reporting higher levels of heart disease (37% versus 26%) and cancer (24% versus 19%).[5] Although many older Americans report multiple chronic health conditions, the rate of functional limitations among the elderly actually declined between 1992 and 2005 from 49% to 42%.[4] Among the 15 leading causes of death, age-adjusted death rates decreased significantly from 2004 to 2005 for the top three leading causes: heart disease (33%), cancer (22%), and stroke (8%), although chronic lower respiratory diseases, unintentional injuries, Alzheimer's disease, influenza and pneumonia, hypertension, and Parkinson's disease increased.[6] Figure 2–1 specifies the most common chronic conditions of elders, by sex. Frailty is a common biological syndrome in the elderly. Once frail, elders may rapidly progress toward failure to thrive and death. Only 3% to 7% of elders between the ages of 65 and 75 years are frail, increasing to more than 32% in those older than 90 years.[10]

▶ *Healthcare Utilization and Cost*

② *Older Americans use considerably more healthcare services than younger Americans, and their healthcare needs are often complex.* Although in 2005 hospital stays for those 65 years or older were half of what they had been in 1970 (5.5 versus 12.6 days), they accounted for more than 65% of hospitalizations overall, with longer lengths of stay corresponding to increasing age.[11] Nine persons per 1,000 aged 65 to 74 years lived in nursing homes in 2004, compared with 36 of 1,000 aged 75 to 84 years, and 139 of 1,000 aged 85 years or older[11]; as the aged live longer, more will require institutional care. After adjusting for inflation, healthcare costs increased significantly among older Americans from $8,644 in 1992 to $13,052 in 2004, three to five times greater than the cost for

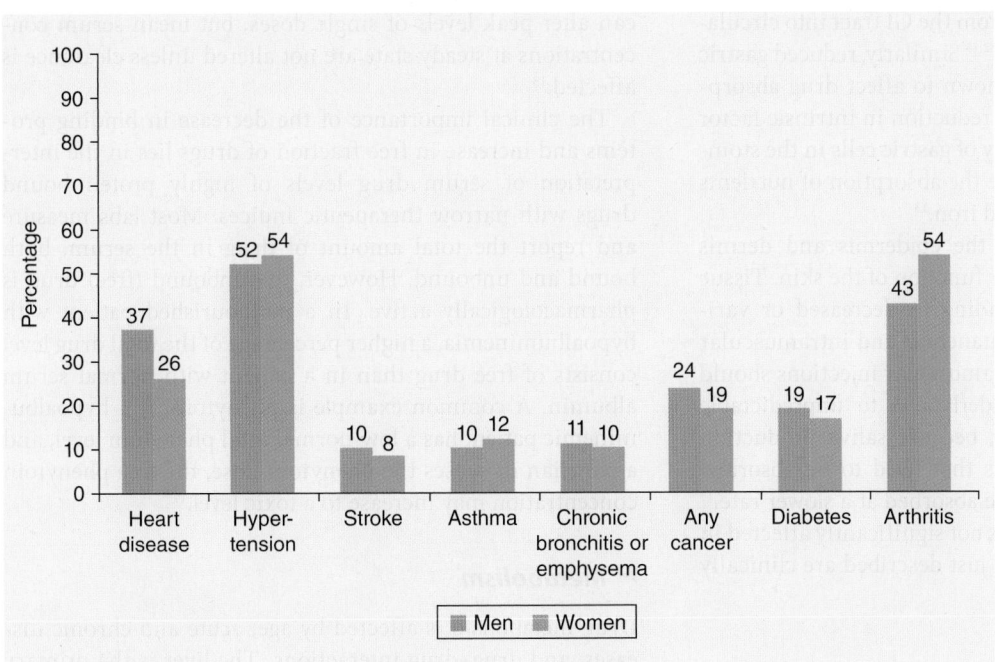

FIGURE 2–1. Percentage of people 65 years and older who reported having selected chronic conditions, by sex, 2005 to 2006. Note: Data are based on a 2-year average from 2005 to 2006. Reference population: These data refer to the civilian noninstitutionalized population. (From Centers for Disease Control and Prevention, National Center for Health Statistics, National Health Interview Survey.)

someone younger than 65 years. Medicare spending has grown nearly ninefold in the past 25 years, to more than $507 billion in 2008, and Medicare roles are expected to increase to $78 million by 2030.[5]

By knowing and applying the epidemiology of aging, clinicians can better understand the multiple points of potential pharmaceutical intervention to postpone disease, disability, and mortality, to avoid error, and to promote health, functioning, and health-related quality of life.

Patient Encounter, Part 1

RV is an 83-year-old woman who has lived in the United States for 62 years but speaks mostly Spanish. She finished 6th grade in Mexico and does not understand medical information. She presents to the Interprofessional Geriatric Clinic for a comprehensive medication review. Her chronic conditions include diabetes, stroke, hypertension, depression, seizure disorder, arthritis, insomnia, and glaucoma. RV uses 16 prescription medications for the described conditions including her eye drops; she also has five medications she "keeps on hand" for as-needed use. She is overweight and reports eating high amount of refined foods since she stopped cooking due to glaucoma. She watches TV most of the day and stays indoors; denies smoking or drinking alcohol.

What information is consistent with epidemiology of aging?

Which of RV's medical conditions are commonly found in older adults?

What additional information do you need before you review RV's medications and make recommendations?

AGE-RELATED CHANGES

In basic terms, pharmacokinetics is what the body does to the drug, and pharmacodynamics is what the drug does to the body. ❸ *All four components of pharmacokinetics—absorption, distribution, metabolism, and excretion—are affected by aging, the most clinically important and consistent is the reduction of renal elimination of drugs.*[12] As people age, they become more frail and are more likely to experience altered and variable drug pharmacokinetics and pharmacodynamics compared with younger people. Even though this alteration is influenced more by a patient's clinical state than their chronological age, the older patient is more likely to be malnourished and suffering from diseases that affect pharmacokinetics and pharmacodynamics.[13] For example, chronic uncontrolled diabetes has a greater impact on reducing renal function than age-related decline. Clinicians have the responsibility to use pharmacokinetic and pharmacodynamic principles to improve the care of elderly patients and avoid harmful side effects of the drugs used.

Pharmacokinetic Changes

▶ *Absorption*

Multiple changes occur throughout the GI tract with aging, but little evidence indicates that drug absorption is significantly altered. The changes include decreases in overall surface of the intestinal epithelium, gastric acid secretion, and splanchnic blood flow.[12] Peristalsis is weaker, and also gastric emptying is delayed. These changes slow absorption in the stomach, especially for enteric-coated and delayed-release preparations. Despite the decreased rate, the extent of absorption is not significantly altered. Delays in absorption may lead to a longer time required to achieve peak drug effects, but it does not significantly alter the amount of drug absorbed, and drug movement from the GI tract into circulation is not meaningfully altered.[12,13] Similarly, reduced gastric acid with aging has not been shown to affect drug absorption. Relative achlorhydria and reduction in intrinsic factor production are caused by atrophy of gastric cells in the stomach. These changes can decrease the absorption of nutrients such as vitamin B_{12}, calcium, and iron.[13]

Aging facilitates atrophy of the epidermis and dermis along with a reduction in barrier function of the skin. Tissue blood perfusion is reduced, leading to decreased or variable rates of transdermal, subcutaneous, and intramuscular drug absorption. Therefore, intramuscular injections should generally be avoided in the elderly due to unpredictable drug absorption.[12] Additionally, because saliva production decreases with age, medications that need to be absorbed rapidly by the buccal mucosa are absorbed at a slower rate.[13] Yet, for most drugs, absorption is not significantly affected in elderly patients and the changes just described are clinically inconsequential.[14]

▶ Distribution

Elderly patients can undergo significant structural changes in the body that alter drug distribution, half-life, and duration of action. Main factors that affect distribution of drugs in the body are changes in body fat and water and changes in protein binding. Lean body mass can decrease by as much as 12% to 19% through loss of skeletal muscle in the elderly. Thus, blood levels of drugs primarily distributed in muscle increase (e.g., digoxin), presenting a risk factor for overmedication.[13] A concern with frail elderly, having low muscle mass, is the risk of adverse effects when they receive higher doses per unit of body weight. While lean muscle mass decreases, adipose tissue can increase by 14% to 35% in the elderly (18% to 36% in men and 33% to 45% in women). Fat-soluble drugs have an increased volume of distribution (V_d), leading to higher tissue concentrations and prolonged duration of action. Greater V_d leads to an increased half-life and an increase in time required to reach a steady-state serum concentration. Examples of lipophilic drugs with increased V_d are diazepam (lipophilic benzodiazepine), amiodarone, and verapamil.[12,13]

Total body water decreases by about 10% to 15% by age 80. This lowers V_d of hydrophilic drugs leading to higher plasma drug concentrations than in younger adults when equal doses are used.[12,13] Toxic drug effects may be enhanced when dehydration occurs and when the extracellular space is reduced by diuretic use. Examples of commonly used hydrophilic drugs are aspirin, lithium, and ethanol. Elderly also experience a decline in gastric alcohol dehydrogenase, further increasing the peak effect of ethanol. Likewise, plasma albumin concentration decreases by 10% to 20%, although disease and malnutrition contribute more to this decrease than age alone.[12] In patients with an acute illness, rapid decreases in serum albumin can increase drug effects. Examples of highly protein-bound drugs include warfarin, phenytoin, and diazepam.[13] For most drugs these changes are not clinically important because the changes just cited

can alter peak levels of single doses, but mean serum concentrations at steady state are not altered unless clearance is affected.[13]

The clinical importance of the decrease in binding proteins and increase in free fraction of drugs lies in the interpretation of serum drug levels of highly protein-bound drugs with narrow therapeutic indices. Most labs measure and report the total amount of drug in the serum, both bound and unbound. However, the unbound (free) drug is pharmacologically active. In a malnourished patient with hypoalbuminemia, a higher percentage of the total drug level consists of free drug than in a patient with normal serum albumin. A common example is phenytoin. If a hypoalbuminemic patient has a low-normal total phenytoin level, and a clinician increases the phenytoin dose, the free phenytoin concentration may increase to a toxic level.[14]

▶ Metabolism

Drug metabolism is affected by age, acute and chronic diseases, and drug–drug interactions. The liver is the primary site of drug metabolism, which undergoes changes with age. Although there is not a consistent decline in the capacity of the liver to metabolize all drugs, older patients have decreased metabolism of many drugs.[12,14] There is also a decline with age in the liver's ability to recover from injury. Liver mass is reduced by 20% to 30% with advancing age, and hepatic blood flow is decreased by as much as 40%. These changes can drastically reduce the amount of drug delivered to the liver per unit of time, reduce its metabolism, and increase the elimination half-life.[13] Metabolic clearance of some drugs is decreased by 20% to 40% (e.g., amiodarone, amitriptyline, warfarin, and verapamil), but for others it is unchanged. Drugs with a low hepatic extraction are usually not affected by hepatic hemoperfusion.[13] Drugs that have high extraction ratios have significant first-pass metabolism, resulting in higher bioavailability for older adults. For example, the effect of morphine is increased due to a decrease in clearance by around 33%. Similar increases in bioavailability associated with reduced clearance can be seen with propranolol, levodopa, and hydroxymethylglutaryl coenzyme-A (HMG-CoA) reductase inhibitors (statins). Elderly patients may experience a similar clinical response to that of younger patients using lower doses.[13]

The effect of aging on liver enzymes (cytochrome P450 system, known as the CYP450 system) may lead to a decreased elimination rate of drugs that undergo oxidative phase I metabolism, but this is controversial.[13] Originally, it was thought that the CYP450 system was impaired in the elderly, leading to a decrease in drug clearance and an increase in serum half-life. Studies have not consistently confirmed this, and although there is an age-related increase in half-life of some drugs, it may be attributed to other factors such as changes in V_d. Thus variations in the CYP450 activity may not be due to aging but to lifestyle (e.g., smoking), illness, or drug interactions.[13,14] A patient's nutritional status plays a role in drug metabolism as well. Frail elderly have a more diminished drug metabolism than those with healthy body weight.[12]

Age does not have an effect on phase II hepatic metabolism, known as conjugation or glucuronidation, but conjugation is reduced with frailty. Temazepam and lorazepam are examples of drugs that undergo phase II metabolism.[13]

▶ Elimination

The most clinically important pharmacokinetic change in the elderly is the decrease in renal drug elimination.[12] As people age, renal blood flow, renal mass, glomerular filtration rate, filtration fraction, and tubular secretion decrease. After age 40, there is a decrease in the number of functional glomeruli, and renal blood flow declines by approximately 1% yearly. From age 25 to 85 years, average renal clearance declines by as much as 50% and is independent of the effects of disease.[12–14] Still, the impact of age on renal function is variable and not always a linear decline.[14] Longitudinal studies have suggested that a percentage (up to 33%) of elderly patients do not experience this age-related decline in renal function. Clinically significant effects of decreased renal clearance include prolonged drug half-life, increased serum drug level, and increased potential for **adverse drug reaction** (ADR).[12] Special attention should be given to renally eliminated drugs with a narrow therapeutic index (e.g., digoxin, aminoglycosides). Monitoring serum concentration and making appropriate dose adjustment for these agents can prevent serious ADR resulting from drug accumulation.[13] It is important to note that despite a dramatic decrease in renal function (creatinine clearance) with aging, serum creatinine may remain fairly unchanged and remain within normal limits. This is because elderly patients, especially the frail elderly, have decreased muscle mass resulting in less creatinine production for input into circulation.[12,13] Because chronic kidney disease can be overlooked if a clinician focuses only on the serum creatinine value, drugs can be dosed inappropriately.

For the reasons previously stated, creatinine clearance should always be calculated when starting or adjusting drugs in the elderly. Clearance measure using 24-hour urine collection is impractical, costly, and often done inaccurately. The Cockcroft-Gault equation is the most widely used formula for estimating renal function and adjusting drug doses. It incorporates serum creatinine, age, gender, and weight. See Chapter 25 (Table 25–2) for more details.

$$\text{Creatinine clearance} = \frac{(140 - \text{Age}) \times \text{Weight (kg)}}{\text{Serum creatinine} \times 72} \\ \times (0.85 \text{ if female})$$

when serum creatinine is expressed in mg/dL. Or:

$$\text{Creatinine clearance} = \frac{(140 - \text{Age}) \times \text{Weight (kg)} \times 1.23}{\text{Serum creatinine}} \\ \times (0.85 \text{ if female})$$

When serum creatinine is expressed in μmol/L.

This equation is also used by drug manufacturers to determine dosing guidelines. The Cockcroft-Gault equation provided the best balance between predictive ability and bias in a study that compared it with the Modification of Diet in Renal Disease (MDRD) and Jelliffe "bedside" clearance equations.[13] Understand that the predictive formulas can significantly overestimate actual renal function, especially in the chronically ill, debilitated elderly.

Pharmacodynamic Changes

Pharmacodynamics refers to the actions of a drug at its target site and the body's response to that drug. Pharmacodynamic changes associated with aging are not as well known as that of pharmacokinetics, but a better understanding of these effects can enhance the quality of medication prescribing. ❹ *In general, the pharmacodynamic changes that occur in the elderly tend to increase their sensitivity to drug effects.* Most pharmacodynamic changes in the elderly are associated with a progressive reduction in homeostatic mechanisms and changes in receptor properties. Although the end result of these changes is an increased sensitivity to the effects of many drugs, a decrease in response can also occur.[15] The changes in the receptor site include alterations in binding affinity of the drug, number or density of active receptors at the target organ, structural features, and postreceptor effects (biochemical processes/signal transmission). These include receptors in the adrenergic, cholinergic, and dopaminergic systems, as well as γ-*aminobutyric acid* (GABA) and opioid receptors.[12,13]

▶ Cardiovascular System

Decreased homeostatic mechanisms in older adults increase their susceptibility to orthostatic hypotension when taking drugs that affect the cardiovascular system and lower the arterial blood pressure. This is explained by a decrease in arterial compliance and baroreceptor reflex response, which limits their ability to compensate quickly for postural changes in blood pressure. It has been estimated that as many as 5% to 33% of the elderly experience drug-induced orthostasis. Examples of drugs other than typical antihypertensives that have a higher likelihood of causing orthostatic hypotension in geriatric patients are tricyclic antidepressants, antipsychotics, loop diuretics, direct vasodilators, and opioids.[12,13,15] Older patients have a decreased β-adrenergic receptor function, and they are less sensitive to β-agonists and β-adrenergic antagonists effects in the cardiovascular system and possibly in the lungs, but their response to α-agonists and antagonists is unchanged.[13,15] Increased hypotensive and heart rate response (to a lesser degree) to calcium channel blockers (e.g., verapamil) are reported. Increased risk of developing drug-induced QT prolongation and **torsade de pointes** is also present.[15] Therefore, clinicians must start medications at low doses and titrate slowly, closely monitoring the patient for any adverse response.

▶ Central Nervous System

Overall, geriatric patients exhibit a greater sensitivity to the effects of drugs that gain access to the CNS. In most cases, lower doses are required for adequate response, and patients have a higher incidence of adverse effects. For example, lower doses of opioids provide sufficient pain relief for older patients, whereas conventional doses can cause oversedation and respiratory depression.[12,13,15]

The blood–brain barrier becomes more permeable as people age; thus more medications can cross the barrier. Examples of problematic medications include benzodiazepines, antidepressants, neuroleptics, and antihistamines. There is a decrease in the number of cholinergic neurons as well as nicotinic and muscarinic receptors, decreased choline uptake from the periphery, and increased acetylcholinesterase.[13,15] The elderly have a decreased ability to compensate for these imbalances of the neurotransmitters, which can lead to movement and memory disorders. Older patients have an increased number of dopamine type 2 receptors, which makes them more susceptible to delirium from anticholinergic and dopaminergic drugs. At the same time, they have a reduced number of dopamine and dopaminergic neurons in the substantia nigra of the brain resulting in higher incidence of extrapyramidal symptoms from antidopaminergic medications (e.g., antipsychotics).[12,15]

▶ Fluids and Electrolytes

Fluid and electrolyte homeostatic mechanism is decreased in the geriatric population. The elderly experience more severe dehydration with equal amounts of fluid loss compared with younger adults. The multitude of factors involved include decreased thirst and cardiovascular reflexes, decreased fluid intake, decreased ability of the kidneys to concentrate urine, increased atrial natriuretic peptide, decreased aldosterone response to hyperkalemia, and decreased response to antidiuretic hormone. The result is an increased incidence of hyponatremia, hyperkalemia, and prerenal azotemia, especially when the patient is taking a thiazide or loop diuretic (e.g., hydrochlorothiazide, furosemide). Angiotensin-converting enzyme inhibitors have an increased potential to cause hyperkalemia and acute renal failure. Thus these agents need to be started low, titrated slowly, and monitored frequently.[12,15]

▶ Glucose Metabolism

An inverse relationship between glucose tolerance and age has been reported. This is likely due to a reduction in insulin secretion and sensitivity (greater insulin resistance). Consequently, there is an increased incidence of hypoglycemia when using sulfonylureas (e.g., glyburide, glipizide).[12] Due to an impaired autonomic nervous system, elderly patients may have a decreased response to, or awareness of, hypoglycemia (may not experience the sweating, palpitations, or tremors but instead will experience the neurological symptoms of syncope, ataxia, confusion, or seizures).

▶ Anticoagulants

The geriatric population is more sensitive to anticoagulant effects of warfarin compared with younger people. When similar plasma concentrations of warfarin are attained, there is greater inhibition of vitamin K–dependent clotting factors in older patients than in young. Overall, the risk of bleeding is increased in the elderly, and when overanticoagulated, the likelihood of morbidity and mortality is higher. This is further complicated by the presence of concomitant prescriptions/herbals/supplements, drug–drug interactions, nonadherence, confusion, and acute illness. Close monitoring of the international normalized ratio (INR) and screening for appropriate use is paramount. In contrast, there is no association between age and response to heparin.[12]

Patient Encounter, Part 2

RV's current chronic medications include (1) amlodipine 5 mg by mouth twice daily, (2) benazepril 20 mg by mouth every evening, (3) furosemide 40 mg by mouth every morning (patient takes irregularly), (4) fluoxetine 10 mg by mouth every evening, (5) glyburide 2 mg 1 tablet by mouth twice daily, (6) phenytoin 100 mg by mouth three times a day, (7) eszopiclone 3 mg by mouth at bedtime, (8) calcium (plus vitamin D) 600 mg by mouth twice daily, (9) oxycodone-acetaminophen 5–325 mg 1 to 2 tablets by mouth every 6 hours as needed for pain, (10) brimonidine 0.1% 1 drop in each eye twice daily, (11) brinzolamide 1% 1 drop in each eye twice daily, (12) timolol 0.5% 1 drop in each eye twice daily, (13) bimatoprost 0.3% 1 drop in each eye at bedtime, (14) serum tears 1 drop in each eye 4 times daily, (15) diphenhydramine 25 mg by mouth at bedtime, and (16) acetaminophen 500 mg by mouth 4 times daily as needed for pain. She has no known drug allergies.

RV's son (interpreter) states that one of her providers thought RV may need to double her phenytoin dose. She was recently hospitalized for dehydration and is recovering from "low kidney function."

VS: BP 98/60, P: 70 bpm, RR: 14, T: 38.4°C (101.1°F)
Ht: 5'2" (157 cm), Wt: 63 kg

Labs: Na 141 mEq/L (141 mmol/L), K 4.6 mEq/L (4.6 mmol/L), Cl 98 mEq/L (98 mmol/L), CO_2 25 mEq/L (25 mmol/L), BUN 55 mg/dL (19.6 mmol/L), creatinine 1.6 mg/dL (141 μmol/L), glucose 92 mg/dL (5.1 mmol/L), albumin 2.7 g/dL (27 g/L), HgbA1c 6.4% (0.064; 46 mmol/mol Hgb)

What is RV's estimated creatinine clearance?

How does phenytoin serum concentration react to RV's albumin level?

What steps should be taken prior to increasing phenytoin dose in this patient?

What potential drug-related problems does RV have?

DRUG-RELATED PROBLEMS

❺ *Comorbidities and polypharmacy complicate elderly health status, particularly when polypharmacy includes inappropriate medications that lead to drug-related problems.* It is reported that 28% of hospitalizations in older adults are due to medication-related problems including nonadherence and ADRs. Studies using the Beers criteria indicate that 14% to 40% of the frail elderly are prescribed at least one inappropriate drug, and unnecessary medication use was detected in 44% of older veterans at the time of hospital discharge.[16] Drug-related problems, including ADRs and therapeutic failure, lead to morbidity and mortality in nursing facilities and accrue healthcare cost of nearly $4 billion yearly.[17] Collaboration among interprofessional providers and older patients can ensure appropriate therapy, minimize adverse drug events, and maximize medication adherence.

Polypharmacy

Polypharmacy is defined as taking multiple medications concurrently (some report at least four and others at least five). Polypharmacy is prevalent in older adults who compose 14% of the U.S. population but receive 36.5% of all prescription drugs.[16] According to the Centers for Disease Control and Prevention, polypharmacy is the primary cause of drug-related adverse events in older adults. Medication use rises with age. An estimated 50% of the community-dwelling elderly take 5 or more medications, and 12% of them take 10 or more.[18] Also, common use of dietary supplements and herbal products in this population adds to polypharmacy. In nursing home settings, patients receiving nine or more chronic medications increased from 17% in 1997 to 27% in 2000.[16] Among various reasons for polypharmacy, an apparent one is a patient receiving multiple medications from different providers who treat the patient's comorbidities without coordinated care. Thus medication reconciliation will become increasingly important as the aging population continues to grow.

A recent review that analyzed studies aimed at reducing polypharmacy in elderly emphasized complete evaluation of all medications by healthcare providers at each patient visit to prevent polypharmacy.[19] Efforts should be made to reduce polypharmacy by discontinuing any medication without indication. However, clinicians should also understand that appropriate polypharmacy is indicated for older adults who have multiple diseases, and support should be provided for optimal adherence. Drug-related problems associated with polypharmacy can be identified by performing a comprehensive medication review during each patient encounter (see Patient Care and Monitoring box).

Inappropriate Prescribing

Inappropriate prescribing is defined as prescribing medications that cause a significant risk of an adverse event when there is an effective and safer alternative. It also includes prescribing a medication outside the bounds of accepted medical standards. The incidence of prescribing potentially inappropriate drugs to elderly patients has been reported to be as high as 12% in those living in the community and 40% in nursing home residents.[20,21] At times, medications are continued long after the initial indication has resolved. The clinician prescribing for older adults must understand the rate of adverse reactions and drug–drug interactions, the evidence available for using a specific medication, and patient use of over-the-counter (OTC) medications and herbal supplements.[20,22]

Screening tools have been developed to help the clinician identify potentially inappropriate drugs. The most utilized and well known is the Beers criteria,[23] first developed in 1991. It was most recently updated in 2012 by the American Geriatric Society using a systematic review of the evidence. It includes 53 medications or medication classes that are potentially inappropriate in elderly patients. The new Beers criteria are divided into three categories: (a) medications that should be avoided regardless of disease/condition, (b) medications to avoid in certain diseases/conditions, and (c) medications to use with caution.[23]

Some of the more common medications referred to in the Beers criteria[23] include the following:

- Tertiary Tricyclic Antidepressants (TCAs) like amitriptyline (strong anticholinergic and sedative properties)
- Benzodiazepines including diazepam (increased risk of falls, fractures, and cognitive impairment)
- First generation Antihistamines like diphenhydramine (confusion and sedation with a prolonged effect)
- Nonsteroidal anti-inflammatory drugs (NSAIDs) (increased potential to cause GI bleeding, exacerbate heart failure, and cause kidney injury
- Spironolactone greater than 25 mg/d (avoid in patients with heart failure or CrCl less than 30 mL/min due to increased hyperkalemia risk)

Examples of drug/disease combinations reported as potentially inappropriate are as follows:

- Strongly anticholinergic drugs in patients with bladder outlet obstruction or benign prostatic hyperplasia
- Metoclopramide and antipsychotics in patients with Parkinson's disease (worsening of symptoms) and antipsychotics in patients with dementia (increased risk of stroke and mortality)
- Benzodiazepines, anticholinergics, antispasmodics, and muscle relaxants with cognitive impairment

In 2008, a new screening tool of elderly patients' medicines was developed. The Screening Tool of Older People's Potentially Inappropriate Prescriptions (STOPP) tool, designed by 18 experts in geriatric pharmacotherapy, incorporates current clinical evidence to identify potentially inappropriate medications (PIMs) in older patients.[24] It is arranged according to relevant physiological system and incorporates commonly encountered instances of potentially inappropriate prescribing (drug–drug and drug–disease interactions, drugs increasing fall risk, and duplicate drug class prescriptions).[24]

Screening Tool to Alert Doctors to the Right Treatment (START) was designed to aid physicians in prescribing certain medications that have evidence of benefit in geriatric patients in selected clinical situations.[25,26] Whereas the STOPP criteria identify commission errors or inappropriately prescribed meds, the START criteria is a tool to identify omission errors. There is no convincing evidence that using the START/STOPP criteria reduces morbidity, mortality, or cost, but it can be used in a time-efficient manner to evaluate older patients' medications comprehensively. Its use can enhance clinical judgment in prescribing for older patients, thereby avoiding unnecessary and potentially harmful prescribing cascades.[24]

Examples of STOPP criteria[24] include:

- Cardiovascular system
  - Digoxin more than 125 mcg/day with impaired renal function
  - Diltiazem or verapamil with New York Heart Association class III or IV heart failure
- CNS
  - Tricyclic antidepressant with dementia
  - Prolonged use of first-generation antihistamines
- Urogenital system
  - Bladder antimuscarinic drugs with dementia

Examples of START criteria[25] include:

- Cardiovascular system
  - Warfarin in the presence of atrial fibrillation, where there is no contraindication
  - Angiotensin-converting enzyme inhibitor in chronic heart failure, where no contraindication exists
- Locomotor system
  - Bisphosphonate in patients taking glucocorticoids for more than 1 month
  - Calcium and vitamin D supplement in patients with known osteoporosis

Although the Beers criteria is commonly referred to in the literature and used in clinical practice, there is little evidence available reporting a tangible benefit to patients in terms of clinical outcomes, and all outcome studies are retrospective. Some studies have compared the performance of STOPP with that of the Beers criteria in detecting PIMs and adverse drug events causing hospital admission or emergency department visits. STOPP criteria identified a significantly higher proportion of patients requiring hospitalization as a result of PIM-related adverse events than Beers criteria in one study.[24] Another study found that of the adverse events that were avoidable and contributory to the hospitalization, the drugs involved were 2.8 times more likely to be on the STOPP list than the Beers list.[27]

As noted previously, the consequences of inappropriate prescribing are widespread and vary in severity. It is important to note that these medications are "potentially" inappropriate, and alternatives should be used or focused monitoring for adverse effects should be provided. Practical strategies for appropriate medication prescribing include establishing a partnership with patients and caregivers to enable them to understand and self-monitor their medication regimen. Providers should perform drug–drug and drug–disease interaction screening, and use time-limited trials to evaluate the benefits and risks of new regimens.[22]

Undertreatment

Much has been written about the consequences of overmedication and polypharmacy in the elderly. However, underutilization of medications is harmful in the elderly as well, resulting in reduced functioning and quality of life, and increased morbidity and mortality. There are instances when an indicated drug is truly contraindicated appropriately preventing its use, when a lower dose is indicated, or when prognoses dictate withholding of aggressive therapy. Outside of these scenarios, many elders still do not receive the therapeutic interventions that would provide benefit. This occurs for many reasons including the belief that treatment of the patient's primary problem is enough intervention, cost, concerns of nonadherence, fear of adverse effects and associated liability, starting low and slow and failing to increase to an appropriate dose, skepticism regarding secondary prevention for elders, or frank ageism. A study found evidence of underprescribing in 64% of older patients, and those on more than eight medications at the highest risk. Interestingly, the lack of proven beneficial therapy did not depend on age, race, sex, comorbidity, cognitive status, and dependence in activities of daily living.[28] Common categories of geriatric undertreatment are listed in Table 2–1.

Table 2–1	
Common Categories of Geriatric Undertreatment	
Therapy	**Concern**
Anticoagulation in patients with atrial fibrillation	Providers may be overly concerned with risk of bleeding or the risk of falls if anticoagulated
Malignant and nonmalignant pain complaints	Providers are often hesitant to prescribe opioids due to possible cognitive and bowel side effects, concerns about addiction; patients may often be hesitant to take opioids
Antihypertensive therapy	Providers may underestimate the benefit on stroke and cardiovascular events, and/or fail to add the second or third medication needed to attain control
β-Blocker treatment in heart failure	Providers are concerned about complications in high-risk patients despite the substantial evidence of mortality reduction
Statin treatment for hyperlipidemia	Providers may underestimate benefit or have high concern for adverse events
Treatment of osteopenia/osteoporosis in men and women at risk of fractures	Providers often fail to screen for bone mineral density and are therefore unaware to offer treatment

A reasoned clinical assessment strategy to weigh the potential benefit versus harm of the older patient's complete medication regimen is required. Once obvious contraindications have been dismissed, the patient's (a) goals and preferences, (b) prognosis, and (c) time until therapeutic benefit will be achieved should be taken into consideration to determine whether the therapy can meet treatment goals. Underprescribing can best be avoided by using careful clinical assessment strategies, improving adherence support, and increasing financial coverage of drugs.

Adverse Drug Reaction

ADR is defined by the World Health Organization as a reaction that is noxious and unintended, which occurs at dosages normally used in humans for prophylaxis, diagnosis, or therapy. (See the glossary for the American Society of Health-System Pharmacists' definition of an ADR.[29]) ADRs increase with polypharmacy use, and older adults commonly experience ADRs. In fact, ADRs are the most frequently occurring drug-related problem among elderly nursing home residents, and the yearly occurrence in outpatient elderly is noted to be 5% to 33%.[30]

Seven predictors of ADRs in older adults have been identified[30]: (a) taking more than four medications; (b) more than 14-day hospital stay; (c) having more than four active medical problems; (d) general medical unit admission versus geriatric ward; (e) alcohol use history; (f) lower Mini-Mental State Examination score (confusion, dementia); and (g) two to four new medications added during a hospitalization. Similarly, there are four predictors for severe ADRs experienced by the elderly[31]: (a) use of certain medications including diuretics, NSAIDs, antiplatelets, and digoxin; (b) number of drugs taken; (c) age; and (d) comorbidities. Suggested strategies to preventing ADRs in older adults are described in Table 2–2.[31] Particular caution must be taken when prescribing drugs that alter cognition in the elderly, including antiarrhythmics, antidepressants, antiemetics, antihistamines, anti-Parkinson's, antipsychotics, benzodiazepines, digoxin, histamine-2 receptor antagonists, NSAIDs, opioids, and skeletal muscle relaxants.[21]

One of the most damaging ADRs that frequently occur in older adults is medication-related falls. Falls are associated with a poor prognosis ranging from premature institutionalization to early death. Extrinsic factors for falling include taking certain medications or polypharmacy. A systematic review concluded that psychotropic medications including benzodiazepines, antidepressants, and antipsychotics have a strong association with increased risk of falls, whereas antiepileptics and antihypertensives have a weak association.[32] Comprehensive fall prevention strategies should always include medication simplification and modification to avoid or resolve ADRs.

Nonadherence

America's other drug problem is the term given to medication nonadherence by the National Council on Patient Information and Education.[33] Nonadherence to chronic pharmacotherapies is prevalent and escalates healthcare costs associated with worsening disease and increased hospitalization.[33] *Medication adherence* is a term used to describe a patient's medication-taking behavior, generally defined as the extent to which one adheres to an agreed regimen derived from collaboration with their healthcare provider. The word "adherence" is often preferred over "compliance" because medication compliance implies the patient passively complying to provider's medication orders with no attempts made at collaboration.[34]

❻ *Older adults are at greater risk for medication nonadherence due to high prevalence of multiple comorbidities, including cognitive deficit, polypharmacy use, and financial barriers.* Numerous barriers to optimal medication adherence exist and include patient's lack of understanding, provider's failure to educate, polypharmacy leading to complex regimen and inconvenience, treatment of asymptomatic conditions (such as hypertension and dyslipidemia), and cost of medications.[34] Factors influencing medication nonadherence are listed in Table 2–3.

Table 2–2

Strategies to Prevent Adverse Drug Reactions in Older Adults

- Evaluating comorbidities, frailty, and cognitive function
- Identifying caregivers to take responsibility for medication management
- Evaluating renal function and adjusting doses appropriately
- Monitoring drug effects
- Recognizing that clinical signs or symptoms can be an ADR
- Minimizing number of medications prescribed
- Adapting treatment to patient's life expectancy
- Realizing that self-medication and nonadherence are common and can induce ADRs

ADR, adverse drug reaction.

Adapted, with permission, from Merle L, Laroche ML, Dantoine T, et al. Predicting and preventing adverse drug reactions in the very old. Drugs Aging 2005;22(5):375–392.

Table 2–3

Factors Influencing Medication Nonadherence

Three or more chronic medical conditions	Living alone in the community
Five or more chronic medications	Recent hospital discharge
Three times or more per day dosing or 12 or more medication doses per day	Caregiver reliance
	Low health literacy
	Medication cost
Four or more medication changes in past 12 months	History of medication nonadherence
Three or more prescribers	
Significant cognitive or physical impairments	

Patient Encounter, Part 3

RV and her son are both willing to work with the new regimen after this comprehensive medication review. RV has been living with the son for more than 2 years after her stroke, but she is thinking about transitioning to a long-term care facility. Even though she is overweight, she has lost 5 kg in the last 6 months and developed a new coccyx ulcer. Today her pain score is 7/10.

What recommendations can be made about RV's medication regimen at this time?

If RV transitions to a long-term care facility, which quality indicators would be of concern?

Following is a list of six "how" questions to ask when assessing medication adherence[35]:

1. How do you take your medicines?
2. How do you organize your medicines to help you remember to take them?
3. How do you schedule your meal and medicine times?
4. How do you pay for your medicines?
5. How do you think the medicines are working for your conditions?
6. How many times in the last week/month have you missed your medicine?

Although no single intervention has found to improve adherence consistently, patient-centered multicomponent interventions such as combining education, convenience, and serial follow-up have resulted in a positive impact on medication adherence and associated health outcomes.[36] Future research needs include adherence studies evaluating belief-related variables, such as personal and cultural beliefs, in larger and more ethnically diverse samples of older populations.

GERIATRIC ASSESSMENT

The term *geriatric assessment* is used to describe the interprofessional team evaluation of the frail, complex elderly patient. Such a team may include but is not limited to a geriatrician, nurse, pharmacist, case manager/social worker, physical therapist, occupational therapist, speech therapist, psychologist, nutritionist, dentist, optometrist, and audiologist. Assessment may be performed in a centralized geriatric clinic or by a series of evaluations performed in separate settings after which the team may conduct an interprofessional case conference to discuss the patient's assessment and plan. For a healthy, active elderly patient, the assessment might require only two to three members of this team, with coordination of care provided by the patient's geriatrician.

Patient Interview

❼ *The clinical approach to assessing older adults frequently goes beyond a traditional "history and physical" used in general internal medicine practice.*[37] Functional status must be determined, which includes the activities of daily living (ADLs) and instrumental activities of daily living (IADLs). Refer to Table 2–4 for descriptions of ADLs and IADLs. Evidence of declining function in specific organ systems is sought. Of particular importance is cognitive assessment, which may require collateral history from family, friends, or other caregivers, and is important in determination of the patient's capacity to consent to medical treatment.[38] The mini-cog mental status examination,[39] shown in Figure 2–2, is a quick tool to assess patient's cognitive impairment. Commonly there is decreased visual acuity, hearing loss, dysphagia, and manual dexterity. Decreased skin integrity, if present, greatly increases risk for pressure ulcers. Sexual function is a sensitive but important area, and it should be specifically inquired about. Cardiac, renal, hepatic, and digestive insufficiencies can have significant implications for pharmacotherapy. Inadequate nutrition may lead to weight loss and impaired functioning at the cellular or organ level as discussed previously. See Table 2–5 for common problems experienced by older adults.

It is important to identify "geriatric syndromes" such as frailty, instability and falls, osteoporosis, insomnia, and incontinence that have an impact on quality of life and must be recognized. Common diseases present with atypical symptoms such as thyroid dysfunction and depression presenting as delirium. It is also important to assess for

---

Table 2–4

Activities of Daily Living and Instrumental Activities of Daily Living

ADLs			
Transfers	Dressing	Mobility	Eating
Bathing	Toileting	Grooming	

IADLs	
Using transportation	If still driving, assess driving ability (including cognitive function, medications that can impair driving ability, vision, neuromuscular conditions that may interfere with reaction time, ability to turn head) at the time of license renewal
Using the telephone	Check for emergency phone numbers located near the telephone
Management of finances	Assess the ability to balance checkbook and pay bills on time
Cooking	Check for safe operation of appliances and cooking tools as well as ability to prepare balanced meals
Housekeeping	Check for decline in cleanliness or neatness
Medication administration	Assess organization skills and adherence

ADL, activity of daily living; IADL, instrumental activity of daily living.

Three item recall
1. Ask the patient if you may test his or her memory.
2. Give the patient 3 words (e.g., apple, table, penny) to repeat and remember.
3. Have the patient repeat the 3 words from memory later (e.g., after the clock drawing test).

Clock drawing test
1. Have the patient draw the face of a clock, including numbers.
2. Instruct the patient to place the hands at a specific time, such as 11:10.

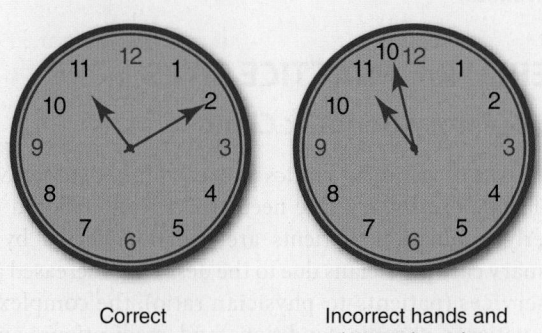

Correct   Incorrect hands and
                           inserted number

A positive dementia screen
1. Failure to remember all 3 words.
2. Failure to remember 1-2 words plus an abnormal clock drawing.

FIGURE 2–2. The mini-cog mental status examination. (Adapted from Borson S, Scanlan J, Brush M, Vitaliano P, Dokmak A. The mini-cog: A cognitive "vital signs" measure for dementia screening in multi-lingual elderly. Int J Geriatr Psychiatry 2000;15(11):1021–1027.)

caregiver stress and be aware of older patients' support systems. These may include family, friends, religious and social networks, as well as home health aides, homemakers, or sitters. Without such networks, the older adult may not be able to continue to live independently. Assessment of home safety

Table 2–5
The *Is* of Geriatrics: Common Problems in Older Adults

Immobility	Instability
Isolation	Intellectual impairment
Incontinence	Impotence
Infection	Immunodeficiency
Inanition (malnutrition)	Insomnia
Impaction	Iatrogenesis
Impaired senses	

Reprinted with permission from DiPiro JT, Talbert RL, Yee GC, et al. Pharmacotherapy: A Pathophysiologic Approach. 8th ed. New York, NY: McGraw-Hill, 2011.

is often necessary for the frail elderly. In addition, look for signs and symptoms of elder abuse, neglect, or exploitation. Health professionals are required to report suspicion of elder mistreatment to Adult Protective Services.[40]

Drug Therapy Monitoring

Geriatric patients often are frail, and they have multiple drugs, medical comorbidities, and prescribers. It is essential that there be a single individual, a pharmacist, nurse, or primary care physician, who oversees the patient's drug therapy. The providers need to be aware of the patient's Medicare Part C or D plan, and what type of coverage these plans afford. What is the copayment for generic, preferred, and nonpreferred drugs? Is the patient responsible for all drug costs during the Medicare "donut hole" period? (The first $2,250 of medication is partially subsidized, but the patient pays 100% of the next $2,850.[41]) Many Medicare patients, especially the socioeconomically challenged, have limited understanding of the complex Medicare drug benefit. This problem is compounded when the prescriber also does not understand the patient's insurance program.[42] Providers can assist patients by prescribing generic medication that are offered through retail pharmacy discount plans ($4 retail pharmacy programs do not bill insurance, so the cost of those medications are not counted toward the $2,250 benefit) and help patients apply for the medication assistance programs offered by drug manufacturers. Particularly challenging in the geriatric population is identifying the cause(s) of nonadherence to medical regimens. Providers assessing elderly patients' medication regimens should keep the following questions in mind:

- Are medications skipped or reduced due to cost?
- Can the patient benefit from sample drugs? Starting a patient on a free drug sample may increase patient costs in the long term because samples typically are newer, expensive drugs.[42]
- Is there an educational barrier such as low health literacy?
- Does the patient speak English but only read in another language?
- Can the patient see labels and written instructions?
- Does the patient have hearing problems? Patients might not admit they cannot hear instructions. Understanding instructions seems to be more about health literacy rather than a sensory problem.
- Can the patient manipulate pill bottles, syringes, inhalers, eye/ear drops?
- Has the patient's cognitive functioning worsened over time such that they can no longer follow the medication regimen?

Homeostenosis and comorbidities require more frequent monitoring for adverse effects: symptoms, abnormal laboratory results, drug interactions, and drug levels (see Table 2–6).

Table 2–6

Centers for Medicare and Medicaid Services Guidelines for Monitoring Medication Use

Drug	Monitoring
Acetaminophen (more than 3 g/day)	Hepatic function tests
Aminoglycosides	Serum creatinine, drug levels
Hypoglycemic agents	Blood glucose levels
Antiepileptic agents (older)	Drug levels
Angiotensin-converting enzyme inhibitors	Potassium level, serum creatinine
Antipsychotic agents	Extrapyramidal adverse effects
Appetite stimulants	Weight, appetite, blood clots
Digoxin	Serum creatinine, drug levels
Diuretic	Electrolyte levels, renal function
Erythropoiesis stimulants	Blood pressure, iron and ferritin levels, complete blood count
Fibrates	Hepatic function test, complete blood count
Iron	Iron and ferritin levels, complete blood count
Lithium	Drug levels
Niacin	Blood sugar levels, hepatic function tests
Statins	Hepatic function tests
Theophylline	Drug levels
Thyroid replacement	Thyroid function tests
Warfarin	Prothrombin time/international normalized ratio

Adapted from DiPiro JT, Talbert RL, Yee GC, et al. Pharmacotherapy: A Pathophysiologic Approach, 8th ed. New York, NY: McGraw-Hill, 2011.

Documentation

Clear, current, and correct medication lists must be available to patients and all individuals involved with their care. It is especially important for geriatric patients to bring their list, or preferably their medication containers, to each visit with medical providers. Medications taken may require verification with the pharmacist, caregivers, or family. Transitions in patient care, such as hospital to subacute nursing facility or home, are points of vulnerability for medication errors because medications may have been deleted or added.[43] It is now standard of care to conduct medication reconciliation upon hospital admission and discharge to ensure that the medication list is up to date.

Patient Education

Poor adherence in the geriatric age group could be related to inadequate patient education. "Ask me 3" cues the patient to ask three important questions of their providers to improve health literacy[44]:

1. What is my main problem?

2. What do I need to do?

3. Why is it important for me to do this?

The provider can assess patient grasp of medication instructions by asking the patient to repeat instructions initially and again in 3 minutes (teach-back method).

8 *Consideration of geriatric patients' vision, hearing, swallowing, cognition, motor impairment, and education and literacy levels during counseling and education can lead to enhanced medication adherence.* Specific routes of drug administration, such as metered-dose inhalers, ophthalmic/otic drops, and subcutaneous injections, may be difficult for older patients. More time needs to be spent in advising the patient and/or caregivers of potential ADRs and when to notify the provider about ADRs. (See Patient Care and Monitoring box for detailed information regarding patient education.)

GERIATRIC PRACTICE SITES

Ambulatory Geriatric Clinic

Ambulatory geriatric clinics are established to provide a multitude of primary care needs specifically tailored to the elderly population. Patients are usually referred by their primary care physicians due to the desire for increased access to services (patients-to-physician ratio), the complexity of the patient's chronic conditions and medications, and the need for specialized knowledge in geriatric treatment. It is common for the appearance of cognitive impairment to be the catalyst for a referral to such clinic. These clinics take advantage of the enhanced knowledge base gained from using multiple members of the healthcare team. Interprofessional geriatrics primary care teams can consist of one or more of the following: geriatrician, clinical pharmacist, nurses (registered nurse [RN], licensed practical nurse [LPN]), social worker, physical/occupational therapist, and dietician. The interprofessional team holds regular meetings to discuss patients and combine input on their care plans from each specialty area. The geriatrician assumes the overall care of the patient. This person has specialized training in treating the older population encompassing patient's physical, medical, emotional, and social needs. The clinical pharmacist assists in optimizing medication regimen by conducting comprehensive medication review, screening and resolving potential drug-related problems, and educating patients and caregivers about medications and monitoring parameters. Clinical pharmacists' effectiveness can be enhanced with the specialty certification in geriatrics. Nurses provide medical triage and day-to-day patient care activities such as obtaining vitals and providing wound care. Social workers are involved in various aspects from assessing mood and cognitive status of patients to obtaining placement in higher levels of care. Physical/occupational therapists are often involved in assessing the patient's functional status and the need for further therapy, and they help maintain a safe home environment. They provide adaptive equipments such as grab bars, raised toilet seat and shower bench for the bathroom, and cane or walker for ambulation. Nutritionists evaluate the patient's nutritional status and educate on proper diet and weight management. From these successful clinical strategies, specialty geriatric clinics have developed including a multidisciplinary geriatric oncology clinic[45] and a community-based memory clinic.[46]

Long-Term Care

Long-term care provides support for people who are dependent to varying degrees in ADLs and IADLs, numbering about 9 million people older than 65 years as of 2008.[47] Care is provided in the patient's home, in community settings such as adult care homes or assisted living facilities, as well as in nursing homes. Long-term care is expensive, typically several thousand dollars per month. Most care is provided at home by unpaid family members or friends. Medicare covers all or part of the cost of skilled nursing care for a limited period posthospitalization.[47,48] Medicare does not cover long-term care. Financing of long-term care comes from patients' and family savings and/or private long-term care insurance. When a patient's assets have been depleted, Medicaid provides basic nursing home care.[48] However, this care is heavily discounted, often resulting in economizing such as lower caregiver-to-patient ratios and higher number of patients per room. Nursing homes are highly regulated by state and federal government through the Center for Medicare and Medicaid Services.[47] Initial and continuing certification of the facility depends on periodic state and federal review of the facility. Auditors' ratings are available to consumers in an online Nursing Home Report Card.[49] **Quality indicators** are used by facility administrators and government overseers to identify problem areas, including the following[50]:

- Use of nine or more medications in single patient
- Prevalence of indwelling catheters
- Prevalence of antipsychotic, anxiolytic, and hypnotic use

Patient Care and Monitoring

1. Drug-related problems in the elderly patient can be identified by performing a comprehensive medication review.
2. Have the patient bring all of their medication bottles to the visit including:
   - Prescription medications
   - OTC drugs
   - Vitamin supplements
   - Herbal products
3. Identify the indication for all medications used by the patient.
4. Review medication doses to determine any underdose and/or overdose.
5. Screen for drug–drug, drug–disease, drug–vitamin/herbal, drug–food interactions.
6. Ensure that patient is not using any agents to which he or she has allergies or intolerances.
7. Assess medication adherence by single or combination methods (use combination methods whenever possible):
   - Self-report
   - Refill history
   - Tablet/capsule count
   - Demonstration of use for nonoral agents
8. Inquire about any adverse drug reactions experienced by the patient.
9. Identify untreated indication or undertreatment, including preventative therapy such as aspirin, calcium plus vitamin D, etc.
10. Assess vital signs including pain.
11. Evaluate laboratory findings to assess the following:
    - Renal function
    - Hepatic function
    - Therapeutic drug monitoring (e.g., digoxin, warfarin, phenytoin)
    - Therapeutic goals for chronic disease (e.g., HgbA1c, LDL-C)
12. Perform medication regimen tailoring when indicated:
    - Discontinue unnecessary medications/supplements/herbals
    - Simplify dosing times to minimize complex regimen
    - Tailor regimen to individual's daily routine to improve adherence
13. Recognize any physical or functional barriers that can be overcome, such as providing nonchild-resistant caps and tablet cutters.
14. Provide medication education and adherence aid:
    - Verbal and written information about medications and/or disease states in health literacy-sensitive manner
    - Specific product education for nonoral agents (e.g., inhalers, insulins, ophthalmic/otic drops, etc.)
    - Medication chart/list to include generic and brand names, indications, doses, directions for use, timing of doses, etc.
    - Information on medication storage, expiration date, and refill status
    - Medication organizer (e.g., pill box, blister packs) when indicated
    - List of future appointments
15. Promote self-monitoring and lifestyle modification:
    - Use of blood pressure monitoring device and glucose meter
    - Diet and exercise
    - Smoking cessation
    - Immunizations

- Use of physical restraints
- Prevalence of depression in patients without antidepressant therapy
- Clinical quality measures such as pressure ulcers
- Moderate daily pain or excruciating pain in residents

9 *Long-term care geriatric practices emphasize the inter-professional team approach.* The medical director leads regular meetings with all disciplines delivering care. These may include director of nursing, rehabilitation services (physical, occupation, and speech therapy), pharmacist, social worker, nutritionist, case manager, and psychologist. The pharmacist conducts a monthly drug review of each patient's medication list.[43] The physician is alerted to medication concerns and approves the patient's orders every 60 days. Such a team approach is vital to coordinate care for the typical frail, complex long-term care patient.

Abbreviations Introduced in This Chapter

ADL	Activities of daily living
ADR	Adverse drug reaction
GABA	Gamma aminobutyric acid
HgbA1c	HemoglobinA1c
IADL	Instrumental activities of daily living
INR	International normalized ratio
LDL-C	Low-density lipoprotein-cholesterol
MDRD	Modification of diet in renal disease
NSAID	Nonsteroidal anti-inflammatory drug
OTC	Over the counter
SSRI	Selective serotonin reuptake inhibitor
V_d	Volume of distribution

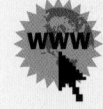 Self-assessment questions and answers are available at *http://www.mhpharmacotherapy.com/pp.html.*

REFERENCES

1. Institute of Medicine. Retooling for an Aging America: Building the Health Care Workforce. Washington, DC: National Academies Press, 2008.
2. U.S. Census Bureau. The 2010 Census Summary File 1 [Internet]. Washington, DC: U.S. Census Bureau; 2000 [updated 2010; cited 2011 Oct 20]. Available from: http://www.census.gov/prod/cen2010/briefs/c2010br-03.pdf.
3. U.S. Census Bureau. Population Division: Population Estimates [Internet]. Washington, DC: U.S. Census Bureau; May 26, 2000 [updated Dec 1, 2011; cited 2011 Oct 20]. Available from: http://www.census.gov/popest/.
4. Federal Interagency Forum on Aging-Related Statistics. Older Americans 2008: Key Indicators of Well-Being. Federal Interagency Forum on Aging-Related Statistics. Washington, DC: U.S. Government Printing Office, 2008.
5. Centers for Disease Control and Prevention and the Merck Company Foundation. The State of Aging and Health in America. Whitehouse Station, NJ: The Merck Company Foundation, 2007.
6. Kung HC, Hoyert DL, Xu JQ, Murphy SL. Deaths: Final Data for 2005, National Vital Statistics Reports. Vol 56, Report No. 10. Hyattsville, MD: National Center for Health Statistics, 2008.
7. U.S. Department of Health and Human Services. Health Consequences of Smoking: A Report of the Surgeon General [Internet]. Atlanta, GA: U.S. Department of Health and Human Services, Centers for Disease Control and Prevention, National Center for Chronic Disease Prevention and Health Promotion, Office on Smoking and Health; 2004 [cited 2011 Oct 20]. Available from: http://www.surgeongeneral.gov/library/Smokingconsequences/.
8. National Committee for Quality Assurance (NCQA). HEDIS 2008: Healthcare Effectiveness Data & Information Set. Vol. 2, Technical Specifications for Health Plans. Washington, DC: National Committee for Quality Assurance (NCQA), 2007.
9. Pleis JR, Lucas JW. Summary Health Statistics for U.S. Adults: National Health Interview Survey, 2007 [Vital Health Stat 10-240-2009]. Washington, DC: National Center for Health Statistics, 2009.
10. Ahmed N, Mandel R, Fain MJ. Frailty: An emerging geriatric syndrome. Am J Med 2007;120(9):748–753.
11. DeFrances CJ, Hall MJ. 2005 National Hospital Discharge Survey: Advance Data from Vital and Health Statistics [Report No. 385]. Hyattsville, MD: National Center for Health Statistics, 2007.
12. Turnmeim K. Drug therapy in the elderly. Exp Gerontol 2004;39:1731–1738.
13. Elliott DP. Pharmacokinetics and Pharmacodynamics in the Elderly. Pharmacotherapy Self-Assessment Program. 5th ed. Kansas City, KS: American College of Clinical Pharmacy, 2004:115–130.
14. Hilmer SN, McLachlan AJ, Le Couteur DG. Clinical pharmacology in the geriatric patient. Fundam Clin Pharmacol 2007;21(3):217–230.
15. Hutchison LC, O'Brien CE. Changes in pharmacokinetics and pharmacodynamics in the elderly patient. J Pharm Pract 2007;20(1):4–12.
16. Chutka DS, Takahashi PY, Hoel RW. Inappropriate medications for elderly patients. Mayo Clin Proc 2004;79:122–139.
17. Bootman JL, Harrison DL, Cox E. The health care cost of drug-related morbidity and mortality in nursing facilities. Arch Intern Med 1997;157:2089–2096.
18. Cannon KT, Choi MM, Zuniga MA. Potentially inappropriate medication use in elderly patients receiving home health care: A retrospective data analysis. Am J Geriatr Pharmacother 2006;4(2):134–143.
19. Hajjar ER, Cafiero AC, Hanlon JT. Polypharmacy in elderly patients. Am J Geriatr Pharmacother 2007;5:345–351.
20. Gallagher P, Barry P, O'Mahony D. Inappropriate prescribing in the elderly. J Clin Pharm Ther 2007;32:113–121.
21. Starner CI, Gray SL, Guay DR, et al. Geriatrics. In: DiPiro JT, Talbert RL, Yee GC, et al., eds. Pharmacotherapy: A Pathophysiologic Approach, 7th ed. New York, NY: McGraw-Hill, 2008:57–66.
22. Petrone K, Katz P. Approaches to appropriate drug prescribing for the older adult. Prim Care Clin Office Pract 2005;32:755–775.
23. The American Geriatrics Society 2012 Beers Criteria Update Expert Panel. American Geriatrics Society updated Beers Criteria for potentially inappropriate medication use in older adults. J Am Geriatr Soc 2012;60:616-631.
24. Gallagher P, O'Mahoney D. STOPP (Screening Tool of Older Persons' Potentially Inappropriate Prescriptions): Application to acutely ill elderly patients and comparison with Beer's criteria. Age Aging 2008;37:673–679.
25. Barry PJ, Gallagher P, Ryan C, et al. START (screening tool to alert doctors to the right treatment): an evidence based screening tool to detect prescribing omissions in elderly patients. Age Aging 2007;36:632–638.
26. Pyszka L, Seys Ranola TM, Milhans SM. Identification of inappropriate prescribing in geriatrics at a veterans affairs hospital using STOPP/START screening tools. Consult Pharm 2010;25:365–373.
27. Hamilton H, Gallagher P, Ryan C, et al. Potentially inappropriate medications defined by STOPP criteria and the risk of adverse drug events in older hospitalized patients. Arch Intern Med 2011;171(11):1013–1019.
28. American Geriatrics Society Clinical Practice Committee. The use of oral anticoagulants (warfarin) in older people. J Am Geriatr Soc 2002;50:1439.

29. American Society of Health-System Pharmacists. ASHP guidelines on adverse drug reaction monitoring and reporting. Am J Health Syst Pharm 1995;52:417–419.

30. Gurwitz JH, Field TS, Harrold LR, et al. Incidence and preventability of adverse drug events among older persons in the ambulatory setting. JAMA 2003;289:1107–1116.

31. Merle L, Laroche ML, Dantoine T, et al. Predicting and preventing adverse drug reactions in the very old. Drugs Aging 2005;22(5):375–392.

32. Hartikainen S, Lonnroos E, Louhivuori K. Medication as a risk factor for falls: Critical systematic review. J Gerontol Med Sci 2007;62A(10):1172–1181.

33. Sokol MC, McGuigan KA, Verbrugge RR, Epstein RS. Impact of medication adherence on hospitalization risk and healthcare cost. Med Care 2005;43:521–530.

34. Osterberg L, Blaschke T. Adherence to medication. N Engl J Med 2005;353:487–497.

35. MacLaughlin EJ, Raehl CL, TreadwayAK, et al. Assessing medication adherence in the elderly: Which tools to use in clinical practice? Drugs Aging 2005;22(3):231–255.

36. Lee JK, Grace KA, Taylor, AJ. Effect of a pharmacy care program on medication adherence and persistence, blood pressure, and low-density lipoprotein cholesterol: A randomized controlled trial. JAMA 2006;296:2563–2571.

37. Miller KE, Zylstra RG, Standridge JB. The geriatric patient: A systematic approach to maintaining health. Am Fam Physician 2000;61:1089–1104.

38. Appelbaum PS. Clinical practice. Assessment of patients' competence to consent to treatment. N Engl J Med 2007;357(18):1834–1840.

39. Borson S, Scanlan J, Brush M, Vitaliano P, Dokmak A. The mini-cog: A cognitive "vital signs" measure for dementia screening in multilingual elderly. Int J Geriatr Psychiatry 2000;15(11):1021–1027.

40. Armstrong J, Mitchell E. Comprehensive nursing assessment in the care of older people. Nurs Older People 2008;20(1):36–40.

41. Center for Medicare & Medicaid Service. Prescription Drug Coverage: Basic Information [Internet]. Washington, DC: Centers for Medicare & Medicaid Services 2008 [cited 2011 Oct 20]. Available from: http://www.medicare.gov/pdp-basic-information.asp/.

42. Piette JD, Heisler M. The relationship between older adults' knowledge of their drug coverage and medication cost problems. J Am Geriatr Soc 2006;54:91–96.

43. Levenson SA, Saffel DA. The consultant pharmacist and the physician in the nursing home: Roles, relationships, and a recipe for success. J Am Med Dir Assoc 2007;8:55–64.

44. National Patient Safety Foundation. Ask Me 3 [Internet]. Boston, MA: National Patient Safety Foundation; 2007 [updated 2009; cited 2011 Oct]. Available from: http://www.npsf.org/askme3/.

45. Lynch MP, Marcone D, Kagan SH. Developing a multidisciplinary geriatric oncology program in a community cancer center. Clin J Oncol Nurs 2004;11:929–933.

46. Grizzell M, Fairhurst A, Lyle S, Jolley D, Willmott S, Bawn S. Creating a community-based memory clinic for older people. Nurs Times 2006;102:32–34.

47. Centers for Medicare & Medicaid Services. Long Term Care [Internet]. Washington, DC: Centers for Medicare & Medicaid Services; 2007 [updated 2008; cited 2011 Oct]. Available from: http://www.medicare.gov/LongTermCare/Static/Home.asp/.

48. Gozalo PL, Miller SC, Intrator O, et al. Hospice effect on government expenditures among nursing home residents. Health Serv Res 2008;43(1):134–153.

49. Centers for Medicare & Medicaid Services. Nursing Home Compare [Internet]. Washington, DC: Centers for Medicare & Medicaid Services; 2008 [cited 2011 Oct]. Available from: http://www.medicare.gov/NHCompare/.

50. Hawes C, Mor V, Phillips CD, et al. The OBRA-87 nursing home regulations and implementation of the resident assessment instrument: Effects on process quality. J Am Geriatr Soc 1997;45:977–985.

3 Pediatrics

Hanna Phan, Vinita B. Pai, and Milap C. Nahata

LEARNING OBJECTIVES

● **Upon completion of the chapter, the reader will be able to:**

1. Define different age groups within the pediatric population.
2. Explain general pharmacokinetic and pharmacodynamic differences in pediatric versus adult patients.
3. Identify factors that affect selection of safe and effective drug therapy in pediatric patients.
4. Identify strategies for appropriate medication administration to infants and young children.
5. Apply pediatric pharmacotherapy concepts to make drug therapy recommendations, assess outcomes, and effectively communicate with patients and caregivers.

KEY CONCEPTS

❶ Despite the common misconception of pediatric patients as "smaller adults" where doses are scaled only for their smaller size, there are multiple factors to consider when selecting and providing drug therapy for patients in this specific population.

❷ Due to multiple differences including age-dependent development of organ function in pediatric patients, pharmacokinetics, efficacy, and safety of drugs within the pediatric population often differs from adults; thus pediatric dosing should not be calculated based on a single factor of difference.

❸ It is appropriate to use a drug off-label when no alternatives are available; however, clinicians should refer to published studies and case reports for available safety, efficacy, and dosing information.

❹ Medication errors among pediatric patients are possible due to differences in dose calculation and preparation; it is important to identify potential errors through careful review of orders, calculations, dispensing, and administration of drug therapy to infants and children.

❺ Comprehensive and clear parent/caregiver education improves medication adherence, safety, and therapeutic outcomes; thus caregiver education is essential because they are often responsible for the administration and monitoring of drug therapy in infants and young children.

INTRODUCTION

Pediatric clinical practice involves the care of infants, children, and adolescents with the goal of optimizing their health,

growth, and development toward adulthood. Clinicians serve as advocates for this unique and vulnerable patient population to optimize their well-being.

There is a continued need for pediatric healthcare resources, evidenced by the annual increase in the number of infants born in the United States.[1] Ambulatory care settings, such as the pediatrician office and emergency department, as well as hospitals, require the expertise of knowledgeable clinicians with pediatric experience. In fact, national data have noted the lack of appropriate services and supplies for pediatric patients at many institutions.[2] Pediatric care accounts for a considerable amount of total patient care annually. For example, patients younger than 15 years accounted for more than 20% of outpatient visits in the United States in 2008.[3] Among pediatric visits, more than half of the medications documented were new drug therapies with the majority being antibiotics.[4,5] ❶ *Despite the common misconception of pediatric patients as "smaller adults" where doses are scaled only for their smaller size, there are multiple factors to consider when selecting and providing drug therapy for patients in this specific population.* Pediatric patients significantly differ within their age groups and from adults regarding drug administration, psychosocial development, and organ function development, which affect the efficacy and safety of pharmacotherapy.

FUNDAMENTALS OF PEDIATRIC PATIENTS

Classification of Pediatric Patients

● Pediatric patients are those younger than 18 years, although some pediatric clinicians may care for patients up to age 21. Unlike an adult patient, whose age is commonly measured

Table 3–1

Pediatric Age Groups, Age Terminology, and Weight Classification

Age Group	Age
Neonate	Less than or equal to 28 days (4 weeks) of life
Infant	29 days to less than 12 months
Child	1–12 years
Adolescent	13–17 years (most common definition)

Age Terminology	Definition
Gestational age (GA)	Age from date of mother's first day of last menstrual period to date of birth
Full term	Describes infants born at 37-weeks gestation or greater
Premature	Describes infants born before 37-week gestation
Small for GA	Neonates with birth weight below the 10th percentile among neonates of the same GA
Large for GA	Neonates with birth weight above the 90th percentile among neonates of the same GA
Chronological or postnatal age	Age from birth to present, measured in days, weeks, months, or years
Corrected or adjusted age	May be used to describe the age of a premature child up to 3 years of age: Corrected age = Chronological age in months – [(40 – GA at birth in weeks) ÷ 4 weeks]. For example, if a former 29-week GA child is now 10 months old chronologically, his corrected age is approximately 7 months: 10 months – [(40–29 weeks) ÷ 4 weeks] = 7.25 months

Weight Classification	Definition
LBW infant	Premature infant with birth weight between 1,500 and 2,500 g
VLBW infant	Premature infant with birth weight 1,000 g to less than 1,500 g
ELBW infant	Premature infant with birth weight less than 1,000 g

GA, gestational age; LBW, low birth weight; VLBW, very low birth weight. ELBW, extremely low birth weight.

Based on defined terms in American Academy of Pediatrics, Committee on Fetus and Newborn. Age terminology during the perinatal period. Pediatrics 2004;114:1362–1364.

in years, a pediatric patient's age can be expressed in days, weeks, months, and years. Patients are classified based on age and may be further described based on other factors, including birth weight and prematurity status (Table 3–1).[6]

Growth and Development

Children are monitored for physical, motor, cognitive, and psychosocial development through clinical recognition of timely milestones during routine well-child visits. As a newborn continues to progress to infant, child, and adolescent stages, different variables are monitored to assess growth compared with the general population of similar age and size. Growth charts are used to plot head circumference, weight, length or stature, weight-for-length, and body mass index for a graphical representation of a child's growth compared with the general pediatric population. These markers of growth and development are both age- and gender-dependent; thus the use of the correct tool for measurement is important. For children younger than 2 years, one should use the World Health Organization growth standards (Fig. 3–1).[7] For children 2 years and older, the Centers for Disease Control and Prevention (CDC) Growth Charts (Fig. 3–2) are used.[8] These tools assess whether a child is meeting the appropriate physical growth milestones, thereby allowing identification of nutritional issues such as poor weight and height gain (e.g., failure to thrive).

Differences in Vital Signs

Normal values for heart rate and respiratory rate vary based on their age. Normal values for blood pressure vary based on gender and age for all pediatric patients, and also height percentile for patients older than 1 year. Normal values for blood pressure in pediatric patients can be found in various national guidelines and other pediatric diagnostic references.[9,10] In general, blood pressure increases with age, with average blood pressures of 70/50 in neonates, increasing throughout childhood to 110/65 in adolescents.[9,11] Heart rates are highest in neonates and infants, ranging from 85 to 205 beats per minute (bpm) and decrease with age, reaching adult rates (60 to 100 bpm) around 10 years of age. Respiratory rates are also higher in neonates and infants (30 to 60 breaths/minute), decreasing with age to adult rates around 15 years of age (12 to 16 breaths/minute).

Another vital sign commonly monitored in children by their caregivers is body temperature, especially when they seem "warm to the touch." The American Academy of Pediatrics (AAP) recommends rectal temperature measurement in children less than 4 years of age, using a digital thermometer. For children 4 years or older, axillary or oral temperature measurement is appropriate because the child is more able to cooperate when asked. Axillary thermometers can be used in children as young as 3 months but may be less accurate. Tympanic (otic) temperature readings are also used for all ages; however, these temperatures may be less accurate and can be affected by cerumen accumulation. Generally, rectal temperature is greater than oral temperature by 0.6°C (1°F), and oral temperature is 0.6°C (1°F) higher than axillary temperatures.[12] Low-grade fevers are considered those ranging from 37.8° to 39°C (100° to 102°F), with antipyretic treatment (e.g., acetaminophen)

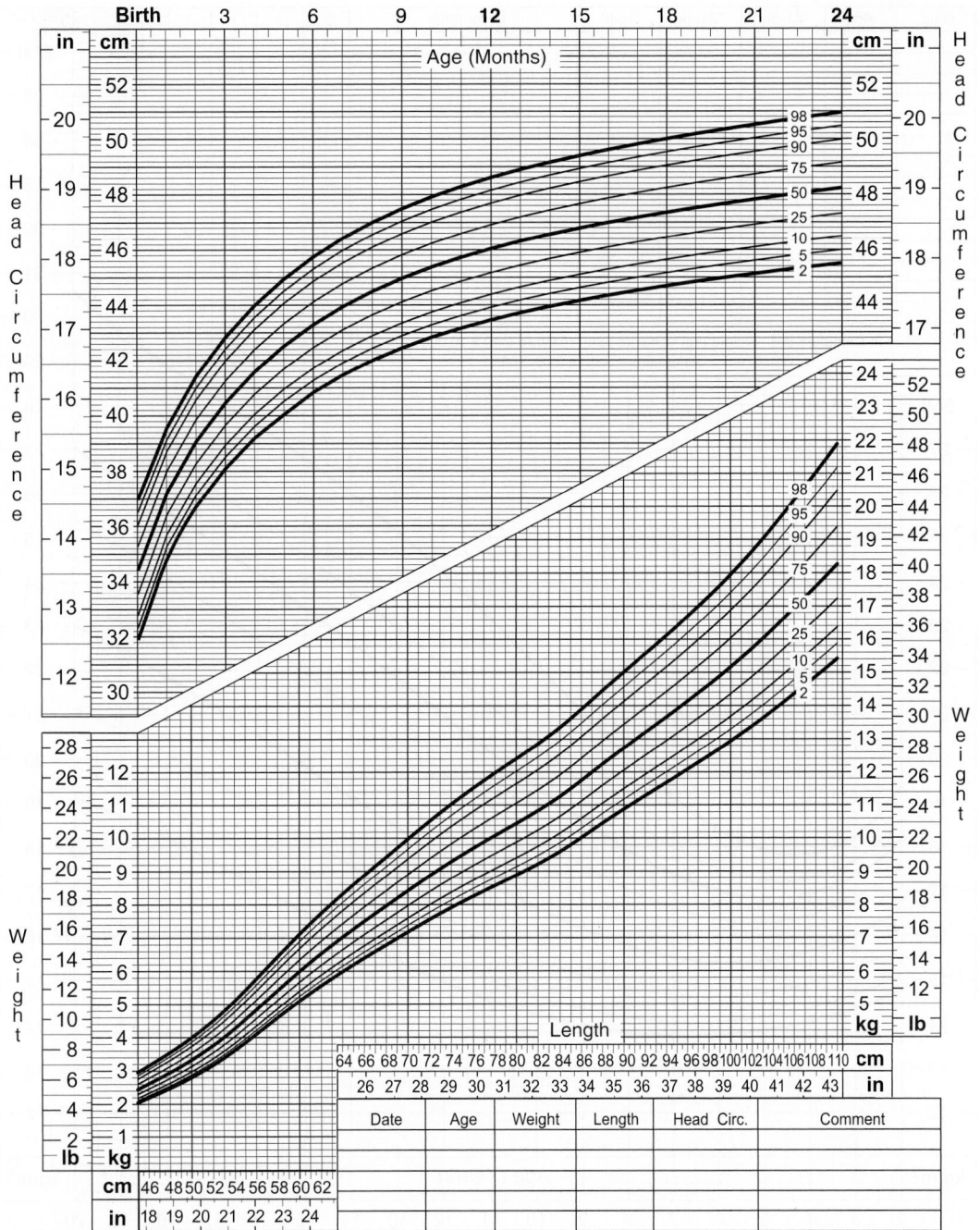

FIGURE 3–1. Example of WHO growth chart of girls, birth to 24 months: Head circumference-for-age and weight-for-length percentile, 2000. (From Centers for Disease Control and Prevention from the WHO Growth Standards. World Health Organization (WHO) Growth Standards, 2009 [updated September 9, 2010], *http://www.cdc.gov/growthcharts/who_charts.htm.*)

considered in cases of temperature greater than 38.3°C (101°F, any measurement route) accompanied by patient discomfort. Formal definition of fever, like other vital signs, is also age dependent, with a lower temperature threshold for neonates (38C° or 100.4°F) and infants (38.2°C or 100.7°F).[13,14]

Also sometimes considered as the fifth vital sign, pain assessment is more challenging to assess in neonate, infants,

and young children due to their inability to communicate symptoms. Indicators of possible pain include physiological changes such as increased heart rate, respiratory rate, and blood pressure, decreased oxygen saturation, as well as behavior changes such as prolonged, higher pitch crying and facial expressions.[15] Laboratory values also vary depending on age. Normal ranges are often noted by the laboratory facility on reported results.

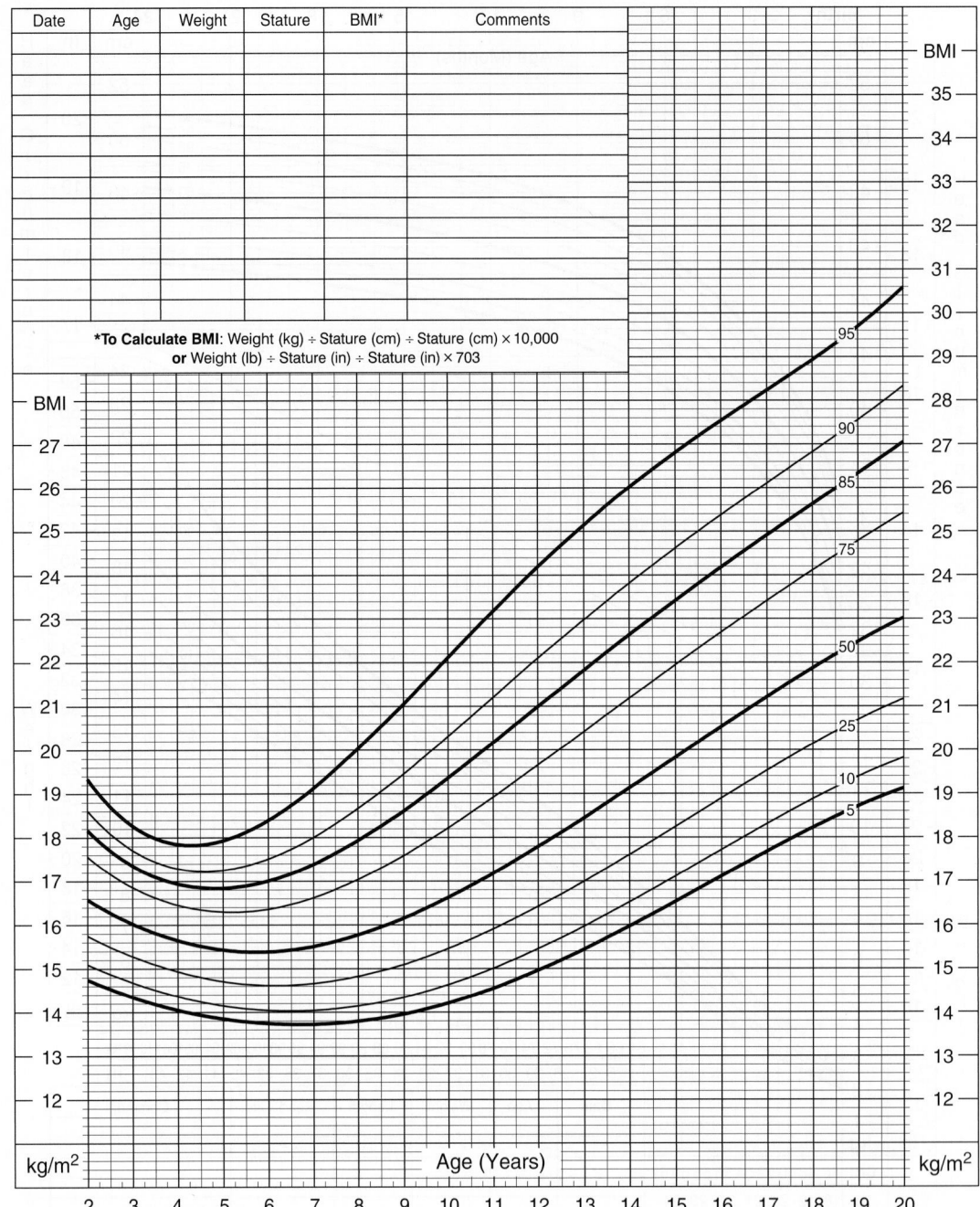

FIGURE 3–2. Example of CDC growth chart of boys, 2 to 20 years: Body mass index for age percentile, 2000. (From National Center for Health Statistics and National Center for Chronic Disease Prevention and Health Promotion. Center for Disease Control Growth Charts, 2000 [updated September 9, 2010], *http://www.cdc.gov/growthcharts*.)

Fluid Requirements

Fluid requirement and balance are important to monitor in pediatric patients, especially in premature neonates and infants. Maintenance fluid requirement can be calculated based on body surface area for patients greater than 10 kg with a range of 1,500 to 2,000 mL/m² per day. However, a weight-based method of determining normal maintenance fluid requirement for children is often used (Table 3–2).

Table 3–2

Maintenance Fluid Calculations by Body Weight

Patient Body Weight	Maintenance Fluid Requirement
Less than 10 kg	100 mL/kg/day
11–20 kg	1,000 mL + 50 mL/kg over 10 kg
More than 20 kg	1,500 mL + 20 mL/kg over 20 kg

Patient Encounter, Part 1

MM is a 36-week GA premature baby boy weighing 2,650 g, length 47 cm, born to a 21-year-old woman this morning. He requires maintenance IV fluids until his further assessment for total parenteral nutrition is complete.

What is MM's weight classification as a neonate?

Calculate MM's corrected age for MM 6 months from today.

How much maintenance fluid would you recommend for MM at birth?

EFFECTS OF PHARMACOKINETIC AND PHARMACODYNAMIC DIFFERENCES ON DRUG THERAPY

Drug selection strategy may be similar or different depending on age and disease state, as a result of differences in pathophysiology of certain diseases and pharmacokinetic and pharmacodynamic parameters among pediatric and adult patients. It is noteworthy that pediatric patients may require the use of different medications from those used in adults affected by certain diseases. For example, phenobarbital is commonly used for treatment of neonatal seizures but not often used for treatment of seizures in adults, due to differences in seizure etiology and availability of extensive data regarding its use in neonates compared with newer antiepileptic medications. There also exist commonalties between pediatric and adult patients, such as therapeutic serum drug concentrations required to treat certain diseases. For example, gentamicin peak and trough serum concentrations needed to treat gram-negative pneumonia are the same in children as in adults. The appropriate selection and dosing of drug therapy for a pediatric patient depends on a number of specific factors such as age, weight, height, disease being treated, comorbidities, developmental pharmacokinetics, and available drug dosage forms. Pediatric drug doses are often calculated based on body weight (e.g., mg/kg/dose) compared with uniform dosing for adult patients (e.g., mg/day or mg/dose) for adult patients. Thus, accurate weight should be available while prescribing or dispensing medications for this patient population. Pediatric doses may exceed adult doses by body weight for certain medications due to differences in pharmacokinetics and pharmacodynamics; hence, the use of pediatric drug dosing guides is recommended.

❷ *Due to multiple differences including age-dependent development of organ function in pediatric patients, pharmacokinetics, efficacy, and safety of drugs within the pediatric population often differs from adults; thus pediatric dosing should not be calculated based on a single factor of difference.* Equations proposed to calculate pediatric doses based on adjusted age or weight such as the Clark's, Fried's, or Young's rule should not be routinely used to calculate pediatric doses because they account for only one factor of difference, age or weight, and lack integration of the effect of growth and development on drug pharmacokinetics and pharmacodynamics in this population. For off-label medication dosing when no alternative treatment is available and limited dosage guidelines have been published, clinicians may choose to estimate a pediatric dose based on body surface area ratio.

Approximate pediatric dose = Adult dose
$$\times \text{[BSA (in m}^2) \div 1.73 \text{ m}^2]$$

Limitations for this dose-estimating approach include the need for the patient to be of normal height and weight for age, and lack of incorporation of exact pharmacokinetic differences regarding each medication.[16]

Absorption

- Oral absorption may be different in premature infants and neonates due to differences in gastric acid secretion and pancreatic and biliary function. Full-term neonates have a gastric pH of 6 to 8 at birth and pH 1 to 3 by 48 hours of age. Gastric acid output per kilogram is lower in premature infants and increases with age to adult levels by 6 months of age.[17,18] Low gastric acid secretion can result in increased serum concentrations of weak bases and acid-labile medications, such as penicillin, and decreased serum concentrations of weak acid medications, such as phenobarbital, due to increased ionization. Additionally, gastric emptying time and intestinal transit time are delayed in premature infants, increasing drug contact time with the GI mucosa and drug absorption.[19] Diseases such as gastroesophageal reflux, respiratory distress syndrome, and congenital heart disease may further delay gastric emptying time. Pancreatic exocrine and biliary function are also reduced in newborns, with about 50% less secretion of amylase and lipase than adults, reaching adult values as early as the end of the first year and as late as 5 years of age. Deficiency in pancreatic secretions and bile salts in newborns can result in decreased bioavailability of prodrug esters, such as erythromycin, which requires solubilization or intraluminal hydrolysis.[18] Due to limited data on oral bioavailability of medications in infants and children for newer agents, some drug dosing recommendations may be extrapolated from adult safety and efficacy studies and case reports.

- Topical or percutaneous absorption in neonates and infants is increased due to a thinner stratum corneum, increased cutaneous perfusion, and greater body surface-to-weight ratio. Hence, application of topical medications should be limited to the smallest amount possible. Increased percutaneous absorption can lead to high serum concentrations of topically applied drugs such as corticosteroids, lidocaine, or chlorhexidine, as well as inactive additives such as propylene glycol, potentially causing adverse effects.

- Intramuscular absorption in premature and full-term infants can be erratic due to variable perfusion, poor muscle contraction, and decreased muscle mass compared with older patients.[20] Intramuscular administration may be appropriate for some medications; however, use of this route of administration can be painful and is usually reserved when other routes are not accessible, e.g., for initial IV doses of ampicillin and gentamicin for neonatal sepsis.

Rectal absorption can also be erratic and is not a commonly recommended route of administration if there are other routes available (e.g., oral). This route is useful in cases of severe nausea and vomiting or status epilepticus. For medications that undergo extensive first-pass metabolism, bioavailability increases as the blood supply bypasses the liver from the lower rectum directly to the inferior vena cava.[20] Availability of rectal dosage forms varies, with acetaminophen suppositories and diazepam gel as examples of medications used by the rectal route in pediatric patients. Rectal use of oral medications or other dosage forms is based on limited studies and case reports.

Volume of Distribution

In pediatric patients, apparent volume of distribution (V_d) is normalized based on body weight and expressed as L/kg. Extracellular fluid and total body water per kilogram of body weight are increased in neonates and infants, resulting in higher V_d for water-soluble drugs such as aminoglycosides and decreases with age. Therefore, neonates and infants often require higher individualized doses by weight (mg/kg) than older children and adolescents to achieve the same therapeutic serum concentrations.[20-23] Neonates and infants have a lower normal range for serum albumin (2 to 4 g/dL, 20 to 40 g/L), reaching adult levels after 1 year of age. This affects highly protein-bound drugs such as phenytoin, resulting in lower total serum concentrations needed to achieve therapeutic unbound serum concentrations.[20]

Because premature neonates have lower body adipose composition compared with older children and adults, they have a decreased V_d for lipid-soluble drugs such as midazolam and require lower doses by body weight. Lipid-soluble drugs may also reach higher concentrations in the CNS due to an immature blood–brain barrier.[24]

Metabolism

Drug metabolism is slower at birth in full-term infants compared with adolescents and adults, with further delay in premature neonates. Phase 1 reactions and enzymes, such as oxidation and alcohol dehydrogenase, are impaired in premature neonates and infants and do not fully develop until later childhood or adolescence. Accordingly, the use of products containing ethanol or propylene glycol can result in increased toxicities, including respiratory depression, hyperosmolarity, metabolic acidosis, and seizures, and they should be avoided in neonates and infants. Cytochrome P450 isoenzymes (e.g., CYP2C9, CYP1A2) develop at various ages, ranging from a few months to 3 years of age, with delayed development in premature infants.[21]

Among phase 2 reactions, sulfate conjugation by sulfotransferases is well developed at birth in term infants.

Glucuronidation by the uridine diphosphate glucuronosyltransferases, in contrast, is immature in neonates and infants, requiring at least several months to develop to adult values at approximately 4 years of age. In neonates, this deficiency results in adverse effects including cyanosis, ash gray color of the skin, limp body tone, and hypotension, also known as "gray baby syndrome" with use of chloramphenicol.[25] Products containing benzyl alcohol or benzoic acid should be avoided in neonates due to immature glycine conjugation, resulting in accumulation of benzoic acid. This accumulation can lead to "gasping syndrome," which includes respiratory depression, metabolic acidosis, hypotension, seizures or convulsions, and gasping respirations.[26] Acetylation via N-acetyltransferase reaches adult maturation at around 1 year of life, but its impact is not well understood regarding neonatal drug therapy.[18] Thus, reduced dosing of medications undergoing hepatic metabolism may be required for full-term and premature neonates. Conversely, hepatic enzyme activity increases to nearly twice as much as adults at 6 months of age and may continue to be high through puberty, around 9 to 12 years of age.[20] These children may require higher doses per kilogram of body weight for hepatically metabolized medications. Common examples include antiepileptic medications such as phenytoin, carbamazepine, and valproic acid. This increase in metabolism slows to adult levels as the child goes through puberty into adulthood.[20]

Elimination

Renal drug clearance is reduced in infants and slowest in premature neonates, due to immature renal function, resulting in the need for longer dosing intervals for renally cleared medications, such as vancomycin, to prevent accumulation. Glomerular filtration rate (GFR) is lowest in premature neonates, increasing with age and peaking at 3 to 12 years of age, after which there is a gradual decline to approximate adult value. For example, vancomycin is often given every 18 to 24 hours in a low birth weight (LBW) premature neonate, every 6 hours in children with normal renal function, and every 8 to 12 hours in adult patients with normal renal function. Children with cystic fibrosis also present with greater renal clearance of drugs such as aminoglycosides, compared with children without the disease, requiring higher doses by weight and more frequent dosing intervals.[27]

Pediatric creatinine clearance (CrCl), an indicator of GFR, is normalized due to variable body size (mL/min/1.73 m²). The use of the Cockroft-Gault or Jelliffe equations for estimating CrCl in adults should not be used for evaluating patients younger than 18 years.[28,29] The Schwartz's equation is a common method of estimating pediatric CrCl for LBW infants up to 21 years of age (Fig. 3–3). This equation uses patient length (cm), serum creatinine (mg/dL), and a constant, k, which depends on age for all patients and also gender for those older than 2 years.[30] Because serum creatinine is a crude marker of GFR, the Schwarz equation, as with other estimation calculations, carries limitations including the potential for overestimating GFR in patients with moderate to severe

$$CrCl = \frac{kL}{SCr}$$

Age	k
Low birth weight less than 1 yr	0.33
Full term less than 1 yr	0.45
1–12 yr	0.55
13–21 yr (female)	0.55
13–21 yr (male)	0.70

k = Proportionality constant

L = Length in cm

SCr = Serum creatinine in mg/dL

CrCl = Creatinine clearance (or estimated glomerular

filtrate rate) in mL/min/1.73 m^2

FIGURE 3–3. Schwartz equation for estimation of creatinine clearance (CrCl) in pediatric patients 6 months to 21 years of age. (Schwartz GJ, Brion LP, Spitzer A. The use of plasma creatinine concentration for estimating glomerular filtration rate in infants, children, and adolescents. Pediatr Clin North Am 1987;34(3):571–590.)

renal insufficiency.[31,32] Urine output is also a parameter used to assess renal function in pediatric patients, with a urine output more than 1 to 2 mL/kg/h considered normal.

COMMON PEDIATRIC ILLNESSES

There may be similarities and differences in illnesses such as infections, asthma, allergic rhinitis, attention deficient hyperactivity disorder, diabetes, and seizure disorders between children and adults. These have been discussed throughout this textbook. The incidence of previously common childhood illness such as measles, mumps, and rubella has significantly decreased as a result of en masse vaccination of infants and children. The Advisory Committee on Immunization Practices (ACIP) within the CDC releases and updates child and adolescent immunization schedules every year. Patients' immunization records should be reviewed routinely for needed immunizations based on these schedules.[33] Most of the common illnesses in children leading to missed school and/or need for clinician consultation are ambulatory in nature; however, some complications may require hospitalization.

Presentation of common childhood illnesses may vary depending on age and development. Older children and adolescents are able to communicate symptoms verbally, making assessment and treatment easier, unlike infants and younger children who are less able to do so. In such cases, changes in vital signs, such as respiratory rate, heart rate, body temperature, and changes in oral intake, feeding pattern, and urine output, are used as indicators of potential illness. Parents may also note subjective items such as changes in mood (e.g., increased irritability or "fussiness").

Patient Encounter, Part 2

MM is now 7 weeks old (weight: 4.5 kg) and presents to the community pharmacy with a 2-day history of lethargy, poor oral intake, and fever. The pharmacist refers the child to seek medical attention at the emergency department. MM is admitted to the general pediatric ward for further assessment including a neonatal sepsis and meningitis rule-out. Blood samples, cerebral spinal fluid, and urine were collected for Gram stain and culture, still pending results. History of present illness reveals that his aunt who had a considerable flare-up of cold sores was babysitting him for the past week. He was empirically started on ampicillin 225 mg (50 mg/kg/dose) IV q 6 h, cefuroxime 225 mg IV q 6 h (50 mg/kg/dose), and acyclovir 90 mg IV q 8 h (20 mg/kg/dose). Given his poor oral intake on admission, the team requests addition of maintenance IV fluids and a nutrition consultation.

BB's Laboratory Values	Normal Ranges
WBC 18 × 10^3/μL	6–17 × 10^3/mm^3
(18 × 10^9/L)	(6–17 × 10^9/L)
Bands 7%	4–12%
Segs 36%	13–33%
Lymphs 51%	41–71%
Monocytes 6%	4–7%
Serum creatinine 0.5 mg/dL	Less than or equal to
(44.2 μmol/L)	0.6 mg/dL (53 μmol/L)

How much maintenance fluid would you recommend for MM now?

Because acyclovir can affect renal function, MM's creatinine clearance should be assessed. Using the most appropriate method, calculate a creatinine clearance for MM.

SPECIFIC CONSIDERATIONS IN DRUG THERAPY

In addition to differences in pharmacokinetics and pharmacodynamic parameters, other factors including dosage formulations, medication administration techniques, and parent/caregiver education should be considered when selecting drug therapy.

Off-Label Medication Use

Currently, there is a lack of pediatric dosing, safety, and efficacy information for more than 75% of drugs approved in adults.[34] Off-label use of medication is the use of a drug outside of its approved labeled indication. Such use is not considered improper or illegal; however, decision for use should be based on clinical judgment and in the best interest of the patient.[35] Off-label use occurs in both outpatient and inpatient settings. About 80% of hospitalized pediatric patients receive at least one off-label medication.[34] This includes the use of a medication in the treatment of illnesses not listed on the manufacturer's package insert, use outside the licensed age range, dosing outside those recommended, or use of a different route of administration.[36] Such off-label use in infants and children is frequently based on limited data. **❸** *It is appropriate to use a drug off-label when no alternatives are available; however, clinicians should refer to published studies and case reports for available safety, efficacy, and dosing information.* FDA regulatory changes, such as extended patent exclusivity, provide incentives for a pharmaceutical manufacturer to market new drugs for pediatric patients. However, such incentives are not available for generic drugs.

Routes of Administration and Drug Formulations

Depending on age, disease, and disease severity, different routes of administration may be considered. Use of rectal route of administration is reserved in cases where oral administration is not possible and IV route is not necessary. Topical administration is often used for treatment of dermatologic ailments. Transdermal routes are often not recommended, unless it is an approved indication such as the methylphenidate transdermal patch for treatment of attention deficit hyperactivity disorder. The injectable route of administration is used in patients with severe illnesses or when other routes of administration are not possible. As done with adult patients, IV compatibility and access should be evaluated when giving parenteral medications. Dilution of parenteral medications may be necessary to measure smaller doses for neonates. However, a higher concentration of parenteral medications may be necessary for patients with fluid restrictions such as premature infants and patients with cardiac anomalies and/or renal disease. Appropriate stability and diluent selection data should be obtained from the literature.

When oral drug therapy is needed, one must also consider the type of dosage form available. Children younger than 6 years are often not able to swallow oral tablets or capsules and may require oral liquid formulations. The child's ability to swallow a solid dosage form should be determined before selecting a drug product. Not all oral medications, especially those unapproved for use in infants and children, have a commercially available liquid dosage form. Use of a liquid formulation compounded from a solid oral dosage form is an option when data are available. Factors such as drug stability, suspendability, dose uniformity, and palatability should be considered when compounding a liquid formulation.[37] Commonly used suspending agents include methylcellulose and carboxymethylcellulose (e.g., Ora-Plus). Palatability of a liquid formulation can be enhanced by using simple syrup or OraSweet. If no dietary contraindications or interactions exist, doses can be mixed with food items such as pudding, fruit-flavored gelatin, chocolate syrup, applesauce, or other fruit puree immediately before administration of individual doses. Honey, although capable of masking unpleasant taste of medication, may contain spores of *Clostridium botulinum* and should not be given to infants younger than 1 year due to

increased risk for developing botulism. Most hospitals caring for pediatric patients compound formulations in their inpatient pharmacy. Limited accessibility to compounded oral liquids in community pharmacies poses a greater challenge. A list of community pharmacies with compounding capabilities should be maintained and provided to the parents and caregivers before discharge from the hospital.

Common Errors in Pediatric Drug Therapy

Prevention of errors in pediatric drug therapy begins with identification of possible sources. The error rate for medications is as high as 1 in 6.4 orders among hospitalized pediatric patients. Off-label use of medications increases risk of medication error and has been attributed to difference in frequency of errors compared with adults. One of the most common reasons for medication errors in this specialized population is incorrect dosing such as calculation error.[38] **❹** *Medication errors among pediatric patients are possible due to differences in dose calculation and preparation; it is important to identify potential errors through careful review of orders, calculations, dispensing, and administration of drug therapy to infants and children.* It is crucial to verify accurate weight, height, and age for dosing calculations and dispensing of prescriptions because pediatric patients are a vulnerable population for medication error. Consistent units of measurements in reporting patient weight (kg), height (cm), and age (weeks and years) should be used. Dosing units such as mg/kg, mcg/kg, mEq/kg, or units/kg should also be used accurately. Given the age-related differences in metabolism of additives such as propylene glycol and benzyl alcohol, careful consideration should be given to the active and inactive ingredients when selecting a formulation.

Decimal errors, including trailing zeroes (e.g., 1.0 mg misread as 10 mg) and missing leading zeroes (e.g., 0.5 mg misread as 5 mg) in drug dosing or body weight documentation are possible, resulting in several-fold overdosing. Strength or concentration of drug should also be clearly communicated by the clinician in prescription orders. Similarly, labels that look alike may lead to drug therapy errors (e.g., mistaking a vial of heparin for insulin when compounding parenteral solutions). Dosing errors of combination drug products can be prevented by using the right component for dose calculation (e.g., dose of sulfamethoxazole/trimethoprim is calculated based on the trimethoprim component).

Use of standardized concentrations and programmable infusion pumps, such as smart pumps with built-in libraries, is encouraged to minimize errors with parenteral medications, especially those for continuous infusions such as inotropes. Introduction of technological advances such as computer physician order entry (CPOE) systems with ability for dose range checks by weight for pediatric medication orders and the use of barcode technology for dispensing of medications have decreased medication errors.[39] Other technological advances for medication safety include the use of enhanced photoemission spectroscopy to scan small samples of compounded IV solutions of high-risk IV drugs for appropriate drug and concentration.[40]

Prevention of medication errors is a joint effort between healthcare professionals, patients, and parents/caregivers. Obtaining a complete medication history including over-the-counter (OTC) and complementary and alternative medicines (CAMs), simplification of medication regimen, clinician awareness for potential errors, and appropriate patient/parent/caregiver education on measurement and administration of medications are essential in preventing medication errors.

Complementary and Over-the-Counter Medication Use

Between 30% and 70% of children with a chronic illnesses (e.g., asthma, attention deficit hyperactivity disorder, autism, cancer) or disability use CAMs.[41] CAMs can include mind-body therapy (e.g., imagery, hypnosis), energy field therapies (e.g., acupuncture, acupressure), massage, antioxidants (e.g., vitamins C and E), herbs (e.g., St. John's wort, kava, ginger, valerian), prayer, immune modulators (e.g., echinacea), or other folk/home remedies. In a survey of pediatric medical staff, 65% of clinicians were aware of their patient's CAM use; however, communication between CAM providers and pediatric clinicians is rare (4%). Thus it is important to encourage communication about CAM use, including interdisciplinary discussion between CAM providers and pediatric healthcare providers.[42] It is critical to realize that there are limited data establishing efficacy of various CAM therapies in children.[41] For example, colic is a condition of unclear etiology in which an infant cries inconsolably for over a few hours in a 24-hour period, usually during the same time of day. Symptoms of excessive crying usually improve by the third month of life and often resolve by 9 months of age. No medication has been approved by the FDA for this condition. Some parents are advised by family and friends to use alternative treatments, such as gripe water, to treat colic. Gripe water is an oral solution containing a combination of ingredients such as chamomile and sodium bicarbonate, not regulated by the FDA. In addition, some gripe water products may contain alcohol, which is not recommended for infants due to their limited metabolism ability (i.e., alcohol dehydrogenase). Further, some CAM products (e.g., St. John's wort) can interact with prescription drugs and produce undesired outcomes. It is important to assess OTC product use in pediatric patients. For example, treatment of the common cold in children is similar to adults, including symptom control with adequate fluid intake, rest, use of saline nasal spray, and acetaminophen (10 to 15 mg/kg/ dose every 6 to 8 hours) or ibuprofen (4 to 10 mg/kg/dose every 8 hours) for relief of discomfort and fever. Other products such as a topical vapor rub or oral honey have demonstrated some potential for alleviation of symptoms such as cough, based on survey studies of parents for children of 2 years and older.[43,44] Unlike adults, symptomatic relief through the use of pharmacologic agents, such as OTC combination cold remedies, is not recommended for pediatric patients younger than 4 years. Currently, the FDA does not recommend the use of OTC cough and cold medications (e.g., diphenhydramine and dextromethorphan) in children younger than 2 years; however, the Consumer Healthcare Products Association, with the support of the FDA, has voluntarily changed product labeling of OTC cough and cold medications to state "do not use in children under 4 years of age." This is due to increased risk for adverse effects (e.g., excessive sedation, respiratory depression) and no documented benefit in relieving symptoms. It has also been noted that these medications may be less effective in children younger than 6 years compared with older children and adults.[45,46] Also noteworthy is the potential for medication error with use of OTC products in older children, such as cold medications containing diphenhydramine and acetaminophen. A parent/caregiver may inadvertently overdose a child on one active ingredient, such as acetaminophen, by administering acetaminophen suspension for fever and an acetaminophen-containing combination product for cold symptoms. The use of aspirin in patients younger than 18 years with viral infections is not recommended due to the risk of Reye's syndrome. While making an appropriate recommendation for an OTC product for a pediatric patient, the parent/caregiver should always be referred to their pediatrician for further advice and evaluation when severity of illness is a concern.

Clinicians should respect parents'/caregivers' beliefs in the use of CAM and OTC products and encourage open discussion with the intention of providing information regarding their risks and benefits to achieve desired health outcomes as well as optimize medication safety.

Medication Administration to Pediatric Patients and Caregiver Education

Considering the challenges in cooperation from infants and younger children, medication administration can become a difficult task for any parent or caregiver. One should also consider factors that may affect adherence to prescribed therapy including caregiver and/or patient's personal beliefs, socioeconomic limitation, and fear of adverse drug effects. One common factor to consider is ease of measurement and administration when selecting and dosing pediatric drug therapy. Clinicians should check concentrations of available products and round doses to a measurable amount. For example, if a patient were to receive an oral formulation, such as amoxicillin 400 mg/5 mL suspension, and the dose was calculated to be 4.9 mL, the dose should be rounded to 5 mL for ease of administration. Rounding the dose by 10% to the closest easily measurable amount is commonly practiced for most medications; however, drugs with narrow therapeutic indices are exceptions to this guideline.

The means or devices for measuring and administering medications by the caregivers should also be closely considered. Special measuring devices as well as clear and complete education about their use are essential. Oral syringes are accurate and offered at most community pharmacies for the measurement of oral liquid medications. Oral droppers that are included specifically with a medication may be appropriate for use in infants and young children. Medicine cups are not recommended for measuring doses for infants and young children due to the possible inaccuracy of measuring

Patient Encounter, Part 3

MM is now 36 months old, and his mother calls the clinic and tells you that her son is "just miserable" with a runny nose, cough, and a fever (axillary temperature) of 38.3°C (101°F). She wanted to know if she could use baby aspirin instead of the acetaminophen that does not seem to help. She also wanted to know which cough and cold preparation would be most appropriate for MM.

What additional information would you need to help MM and his mom?

What is your recommendation regarding use of aspirin for MM's fever?

What would you recommend for MM's cold symptoms?

outcomes; *thus caregiver education is essential because they are often responsible for administration and monitoring of drug therapy in infants and young children.* Information about the drug including appropriate and safe storage away from children, possible drug interactions, duration of therapy, importance of adherence, possible adverse effects, and expected therapeutic outcomes should be provided. Parent/caregiver education is important in both inpatient and outpatient care settings and should be reviewed at each point of care.

Because parents/caregivers are often sole providers of home care for ill children, it is important to demonstrate appropriate dose preparation and administration techniques to the caregivers before medication dispensing. First, a child should be calm for successful dose administration. Yet, calming a child is often a challenge during many methods of administration (e.g., otic, ophthalmic, rectal). Parents/caregivers should explain the process in a simple and understandable form to the child because this may decrease the child's potential anxiety. In addition, it is also recommended to distract younger children using a favorite item such as toy or to reward cooperative or "good" behavior during medication administration. Helpful tips regarding administration of selected dosage forms in pediatric patients are listed in Table 3–3.[47]

smaller doses. Household dining or measuring spoons are not accurate or consistent and should not be used for the administration of oral liquids.

⑤ *Comprehensive and clear parent/caregiver education improves medication adherence, safety, and therapeutic*

Table 3–3

Helpful Tips for Medication Administration for Selected Dosage Forms[47]

Dosage Form	Recommendations
Ophthalmic drops or ointment	• Wash hands thoroughly prior to administration • Position child laying down in supine position • Avoid contact of applicator tip to surfaces, including the eye • Drops should be placed in the pocket of the lower eyelid • Ointment strip should be placed along the pocket of the lower eyelid

Otic drops	• Wash hands thoroughly prior to administration
	• Position child laying down in prone position
	• Tilt head to expose treated ear, gently pull outer ear outward, then due to age-dependent change in angle of Eustachian tube:
	  • If child less than 3 years of age, gently pull downward and back; apply drops
	  • If child more than 3 years of age, gently pull upward and back; apply drops

Nasal drops	• Wash hands thoroughly prior to administration • Position child laying down in supine position • Slightly tilt head back; place drops in nostril(s) • Remain in position for appropriate distribution of medication
Rectal suppository	• Similar to adult administration; challenging route for administration • For younger patients (i.e., less than 3 years), a smaller finger (e.g., pinky finger) should be used to insert suppository
Metered-dose inhalers	• Use a spacer • For younger children, use one with a mask, be sure the mask is secured/placed closely up against the child's face, avoiding gaps between face and mask and creating a seal to ensure medication delivery • Child should take slow breaths in with each dose • Wait at least one minute between doses

Patient Encounter, Part 4

MM is now 4 years old, brought by his father to the pediatrician. He has a 4-day history of left ear pain, excessive crying, decreased appetite, and difficulty sleeping over the past 2 days. The child's temperature last night was 39ºC (102.2ºF) by electronic axial thermometer. The father gave the child several doses of ibuprofen, but the pain or temperature did not improve and none was given this morning. He has considerable recurrences of acute otitis media each year often treated with amoxicillin. He has had three episodes in the last 8 months, with the last episode treated 2 months ago using oral amoxicillin 90 mg/kg/day divided every 12 hours but developed a rash. He is also presenting with wheeze and cough. Dad states that he was recently diagnosed with asthma, but lost their prescription for his asthma medication and so never started it.

Home medications: Ibuprofen suspension (100 mg/5 mL) as needed for pain and fever.

PE:

General: crying, tugging on his left ear, coughing with wheeze

VS: T 39ºC (102.2ºF), BP 93/50 mm Hg, HR 115 bpm, RR 30 bpm, Wt 35 lb (16 kg), Ht 101.6 cm (40 in)

HEENT: Tympanic membranes erythematosus (L>R); left ear is bulging and nonmobile. Throat erythematous; nares patent.

Pulmonary: Wheeze bilaterally, no congestion noted

Diagnosis: (1) Acute otitis media, left ear and (2) newly diagnosed asthma, untreated

You and the pediatrician decide to start MM on oral cefdinir suspension (250 mg/5 mL) at 7 mg/kg/dose q 12 h for a total of 10 days and continue ibuprofen (100 mg/5 mL) at 10 mg/kg/dose every 6 to 8 hours as needed for fever or pain. In addition to treatment for acute otitis media, he needs treatment of asthma, so he is restarted on fluticasone HFA MDI 44 mcg 2 puffs twice a day with a spacer. MM's dad also asks about the use of an herbal supplement (from his traditional Eastern medicine herbalist) advertised for asthma because his brother-in-law uses it in addition to his prescribed asthma therapy.

Based on the information available, create a care plan for MM. The plan should include:

(a) Statement of the drug-related needs and/or problems,

(b) Patient-specific detailed therapeutic plan with specific dosing,

(c) Parent/caregiver education points, and

(d) Approach to Dad's inquiry about herbal supplement use for MM's asthma.

Accidental Ingestion in Pediatric Patients

Over 1.2 million accidental ingestions occurred in children younger than 6 years in 2001; these often occur in the home.[48] Ingested substances can vary, from household cleaning solutions to prescription and nonprescription medications. Medications account for the majority of fatalities involving accidental ingestions.[49] Management of accidental ingestions varies depending on the ingested substance, the amount, and the age and size of the child. Clinicians receiving calls regarding management of accidental ingestions should direct them to the local or regional poison control center for specific recommendations, which can be located through the American Association of Poison Control Centers (*www.aapcc.org*).

Inducing emesis is not recommended for suspected ingestions of acidic or alkaline substances. The American Academy of Clinical Toxicology and the AAP do not recommend the use of ipecac syrup because it can decrease effectiveness of activated charcoal treatment administered in the emergency department and compromise patient outcomes.[48] Use of activated charcoal is considered for treatment of patients in the emergency department with an intact airway who present soon after an ingestion of an adsorbable agent. The recommended dose of activated charcoal is 10 to 25 g/dose or 0.5 to 1 g/kg/dose for infants younger than 1 year, 25 to 50 g/dose or 0.5 to 1 g/kg/dose orally for children up to 12 years of age, and 25 to 100 g/dose for adolescents and adults.[50] Symptoms of toxicities from the substance ingested during hospitalization should be monitored. Parents/caregivers should continue monitoring at home following discharge.

Abbreviations Introduced in This Chapter

AAP	American Academy of Pediatrics
ACIP	Advisory Committee on Immunization Practices
bpm	Beats per minute
CAM	Complementary and alternative medicine
CDC	Centers for Disease Control and Prevention
CPOE	Computer physician order entry
CrCl	Creatinine clearance
ELBW	Extremely low birth weight

Patient Care and Monitoring

For all pediatric patients, review and consider the following to offer optimal drug therapy:

- Gestational age, postnatal age, and corrected age if the patient is a neonate
- Patient's demographic information including age, weight (and birth weight if a neonate), and gender
- Disease or illness for which treatment is needed
- Past medical history including comorbidities
- Medication history current and past (including OTC and complementary and alternative products)
- History of medication adherence
- Other concurrent medications
- Previous therapy failures
- Medication allergies and/or intolerances
- Patient and caregivers beliefs regarding illness, medication use
- Available routes of administration
  - Can the patient take medications orally?
  - If IV medication is needed, what types of IV accesses are available? For example, does the patient have a central or peripheral line?
  - Is intramuscular administration needed?
- Fluid status—Is the patient dehydrated, balanced, or edematous?
- Available data regarding safe and effective dosing of selected drug
- Verification of accurate dose calculation
  - Verify weight and dosing units (e.g., mg/kg/day, mg/kg/dose)
  - Is the dosing interval appropriate?

- Is the dose an easily measurable amount for the caregiver?
- Will the drug be administered at home and/or a daycare facility or school?
  - Does the parent/caregiver need additional documentation for medication administration at other locations?
  - Are additional supplies for medication administration at other locations needed?
- Educate parent/caregiver/patient regarding selected drug therapy including purpose, dose, administration, duration therapy, possible side effects, etc.
- Regular assessment of weight
  - Premature neonates and infants can change frequently, check weight daily
  - Depending on illness in older children, daily weight check may be necessary when admitted to hospital; it should be checked at every outpatient clinic visit
- Organ function
  - For drugs that undergo extensive hepatic metabolism and clearance, assess liver function at baseline and periodically (depending on severity of illness)
  - For drugs that undergo extensive renal elimination
    - Note changes in serum creatinine and urine output
    - Calculate creatinine clearance using Schwartz's or Traub–Johnson's equations
- Measure drug serum concentrations when appropriate
- Monitor clinical outcomes of pharmacotherapy
- Monitor, manage, and prevent adverse drug events
- Prevent drug–drug or drug–food interactions

GA	Gestational age
GFR	Glomerular filtration rate
HFA	Hydrofluoroalkane
LBW	Low birth weight
MDI	Metered-dose inhaler
OTC	Over-the-counter
V_d	Volume of distribution (apparent)
VLBW	Very low birth weight

Self-assessment questions and answers are available at *http://www.mhpharmacotherapy.com/pp.html.*

REFERENCES

1. Hamilton BE, Martin JA, Ventura SJ. Births: Preliminary data for 2007. National Vital Statistics Reports 57(12) [updated 2009 Mar 18; cited 2011 Sept 23]. Available at: *http://www.cdc.gov/nchs/data/nvsr/nvsr57/nvsr57_12.pdf.*
2. Committee on the Future of Emergency Care in the United States Health System, The Institute of Medicine. Emergency Care for Children, Growing Pains. Executive Summary [updated 2007; cited 2011 Sept 23]. Available at: *http://books.nap.edu/catalog/11655.html.*
3. Ambulatory and Hospital Care Statistics Branch of the Centers for Disease Control and Prevention's National Center for Health Statistics. National Hospital Ambulatory Medical Care Survey: 2008 Outpatient Department Summary Tables [updated 2011 Mar 7; cited 2011 Sept 23]. Available at: *http://www.cdc.gov/nchs/ahcd/web_tables.htm#2009.*
4. Cherry DK, Woodwell DA, Rechtsteiner EA. National Ambulatory Medical Care Survey: 2005 Summary. Adv Data 2007;387:1–39.
5. Centers for Disease Control and Prevention, National Center for Health Statistics. National Ambulatory Medical Care Survey (NAMCS)

and National Hospital Ambulatory Medical Care Survey (NHAMCS), Antibiotic Prescribing at Ambulatory Medical Care Visits for Colds per 10,000 Population United States, 2007–2008 [updated 2009; cited 2011 Sept 23]. Available from: *http://www.cdc.gov/nchs/data/ahcd/preliminary2008/table19.pdf*.

6. American Academy of Pediatrics, Committee on Fetus and Newborn. Age terminology during the perinatal period. Pediatrics 2004;114:1362–1364.

7. Centers for Disease Control and Prevention from the WHO Growth Standards. World Health Organization (WHO) Growth Standards, 2009 [updated 2010 Sept 9; cited 2011 Sept 23]. Available at: *http://www.cdc.gov/growthcharts/who_charts.htm*.

8. National Center for Health Statistics and National Center for Chronic Disease Prevention and Health Promotion. Center for Disease Control Growth Charts, 2000 [updated 2010 Sept 9; cited 2011 Sept 23]. Available at: *http://www.cdc.gov/growthcharts*.

9. National High Blood Pressure Education Program Working Group on High Blood Pressure in Children and Adolescents. The Fourth Report on the Diagnosis, Evaluation, and Treatment of High Blood Pressure in Children and Adolescents. NIH Publication No. 05-5268. Bethesda, MD: National Heart, Lung, and Blood Institute. Pediatrics 2004;114(2 Suppl 4th Report):555–576.

10. American Heart Association. Pediatric advanced life support provider manual. Dallas, TX: American Heart Association, 2006. 273 p.

11. Task Force on Blood Pressure Control in Children. Report of the Second Task Force on Blood Pressure Control in Children—1987. National Heart, Lung, and Blood Institute, Bethesda, Maryland. Pediatrics 1987;79(1):1–25.

12. American Academy of Pediatrics. Parenting Corner Q&A: What's the best way to take a child's temperature [updated 2012 Jan 9; cited 2012 Feb 5]. Available from: *http://www.healthychildren.org/English/health-issues/conditions/fever/pages/How-to-Take-a-Childs-Temperature.aspx*.

13. Baraff LJ, Bass JW, Fleisher GR, et al. Agency for Health Care Policy and Research. Practice guideline for the management of infants and children 0 to 36 months of age with fever without source. Ann Emerg Med 1993;22(7):1198–1210.

14. Sullivan JE, Farrar HC. Section on Clinical Pharmacology and Therapeutics and Committee on Drugs. Clinical report—Fever and antipyretic use in children. Pediatrics 2011;127(3):580–587.

15. Lawrence J, Alcock D, McGrath P, Kay J, MacMurray SB, Dulberg C. The development of a tool to assess neonatal pain. Neonatal Netw 1993;12(6):59–66.

16. Shirkey HC. Drug dosage for infants and children. JAMA 1965;193:443–446.

17. Boyle JT. Acid secretion from birth to adulthood. J Pediatr Gastroenterol Nutr 2003;37(Suppl 1):S12–16.

18. Alcorn J, Nakamura PJ. Pharmacokinetics in the newborn. Adv Drug Deliv Rev 2003;55:667–686.

19. Ramirez A, Wong WW, Shulman RJ. Factors regulating gastric emptying in preterm infants. J Pediatr 2006;149(4):475–479.

20. Soldin OP, Soldin SJ. Therapeutic drug monitoring in pediatric patients. Ther Drug Monit 2002;24(1):1–8.

21. Strolin Benedetti M, Baltes EL. Drug metabolism and disposition in children. Fundam Clin Pharmacol 2003;17(3):281–299.

22. Semchuk W, Shevchuk YM, Sankaran K, Wallace SM. Biol Neonate 1995;67(1):13–20.

23. Shevchuk YM, Taylor DM. Aminoglycoside volume of distribution in pediatric patients. DICP Ann Pharmacother 1990;24(3):273–276.

24. Blumer JL. Clinical pharmacology of midazolam in infants and children. Clin Pharmacokinet 1998;35(1):37–47.

25. Mulhall A, de Louvois J, Hurley R. Chloramphenicol toxicity in neonates: Its incidence and prevention. Br Med J (Clin Res Ed) 1983;287(6403):1424–1427.

26. Menon PA, Thach BT, Smith CH, et al. Benzyl alcohol toxicity in a neonatal intensive care unit. Incidence, symptomatology, and mortality. Am J Perinatol 1984;1(4):288–292.

27. Rey E, Tréluyer JM, Pons G. Drug disposition in cystic fibrosis. Clin Pharmacokinet 1998;35(4):313–329.

28. Cockroft DW, Gault MH. Prediction of creatinine clearance from serum creatinine. Nephron 1976;16:31–41.

29. Jelliffe RW. Creatinine clearance: Bedside estimate. Ann Intern Med 1973;79(4):604–605.

30. Schwartz GJ, Brion LP, Spitzer A. The use of plasma creatinine concentration for estimating glomerular filtration rate in infants, children, and adolescents. Pediatr Clin North Am 1987;34(3):571–590.

31. Seikaly MG, Browne R, Bajaj G, Arant BS Jr. Limitations to body length/serum creatinine ratio as an estimate of glomerular filtration in children. Pediatr Nephrol 1996;10(6):709–711.

32. Filler G, Lepage N. Should the Schwartz formula for estimation of GFR be replaced by cystatin C formula? Pediatr Nephrol 2003;18(10):981–985.

33. Advisory Committee on Immunization Practices (ACIP), Centers for Disease Control and Prevention. Child & Adolescent Immunization Schedules [updated 2012 Feb 1; cited 2012 Feb 5]. Available at: *http://www.cdc.gov/vaccines/recs/schedules/default.htm*.

34. Shah SS, Hall M, Goodman DM, et al. Off-label drug use in hospitalized children. Arch Pediatr Adolesc Med 2007;161(3):282–290.

35. American Academy of Pediatrics, Committee on Drugs. Uses of drugs not described in the package insert (off-label uses). Pediatrics 2002;110:181–183.

36. Conroy S. Unlicensed and off-label drug use: Issues and recommendations. Pediatr Drugs 2002;4:363–369.

37. Nahata MC, Pai VB. Pediatric Drug Formulations. 6th ed. Cincinnati, OH: Harvey Whitney Books, 2011. 385 p.

38. Stucky ER, American Academy of Pediatrics, Committee on Drugs and Committee on Hospital Care. Prevention of medication errors in the pediatric inpatient setting. Policy Statement. Pediatrics 2003;112(2):431–436.

39. Conroy S, Sweis D, Planner C, Yeung V, Collier J, Haines L, Wong IC. Interventions to reduce dosing errors in children: A systematic review of the literature. Drug Saf 2007;30(12):1111–1125.

40. Kaakeh Y, Phan H, DeSmet BD, et al. Enhanced photoemission spectroscopy for verification of high-risk I.V. medications. Am J Health Syst Pharm 2008;65(1):49–54.

41. Kemper KJ, Vohra S, Walls R; Task Force on Complementary and Alternative Medicine; Provisional Section on Complementary, Holistic, and Integrative Medicine, American Academy of Pediatrics. The use of complementary and alternative medicine in pediatrics. Pediatrics 2008;122(6):1374–1386.

42. Kundu A, Tassone RF, Jimenez N, Seidel K, Valentine JK, Pagel PS. Attitudes, patterns of recommendation, and communication of pediatric providers about complementary and alternative medicine in a large metropolitan children's hospital. Clin Pediatr (Phila) 2011;50(2):153–158.

43. Paul IM, Beiler J, McMonagle A, Shaffer ML, Duda L, Berlin CM Jr. Effect of honey, dextromethorphan, and no treatment on nocturnal cough and sleep quality for coughing children and their parents. Arch Pediatr Adolesc Med 2007;161(12):1140–1146.

44. Paul IM, Beiler JS, King TS, Clapp ER, Vallati J, Berlin CM Jr. Vapor rub, petrolatum, and no treatment for children with nocturnal cough and cold symptoms. Pediatrics 2010;126(6):1092–1099.

45. US Food and Drug Administration. Public Health Advisory: FDA recommends that over-the-counter (OTC) cough and cold products not be used for infants and children under 2 years of age [updated 2011 Dec 8; cited 2011 Sept]. Available at: *http://www.fda.gov/ForConsumers/ConsumerUpdates/ucm051137.htm*.

46. US Food and Drug Administration. FDA Statement Following CHPA's Announcement on Nonprescription Over-the-Counter Cough and Cold Medicines in Children [updated 2009 June 18; cited 2011 Sept 23]. Available at: *http://www.fda.gov/NewsEvents/Newsroom/PressAnnouncements/2008/ucm116964.htm*.

47. Buck ML, Hendrick AE. Pediatric Medication Education Text. 5th ed. American College of Clinical Pharmacy, 2009; Sec1: xvii–xxvii.

48. American Academy of Pediatrics Committee on Injury, Violence, and Poison Prevention. Poison treatment in the home. Pediatrics 2006;112(5):1182–1185.

49. Eldridge DL, Van Eyk J, Kornegay C. Pediatric toxicology. Emerg Med Clin North Am 2007;25(2):283–308.

50. Lapus RM. Activated charcoal for pediatric poisonings: The universal antidote? Curr Opin Pediatr 2007;19(2):216–222.

4 Palliative Care

Marc A. Sweeney and Phyllis A. Grauer

KEY CONCEPTS

❶ According to the World Health Organization (WHO), "Palliative care is defined as the active total care of patients whose disease is not responsive to curative treatment. The goal of palliative care is to achieve the best quality of life for patients and their families."

❷ The goals of palliative care include enhancing quality of life while maintaining or improving functionality.

❸ Palliative care is appropriate for all life-limiting diseases including cancer; chronic obstructive pulmonary disease; dementia, including Alzheimer's disease; Parkinson's disease; chronic cardiac disease; stroke, renal failure; hepatic failure; multiorgan failure; diabetes mellitus; etc.

❹ Following a complete assessment of the patient, developing a comprehensive therapeutic plan that uses the fewest number of medications to achieve the highest quality of life is essential.

❺ Palliative care is more than just pain management. It includes the treatment of symptoms resulting in the discomfort for the patient, which may include nausea and vomiting, agitation, anxiety, depression, delirium, dyspnea, anorexia and cachexia, constipation, diarrhea, pressure ulcers, and edema.

❻ Involving the patient, family, and caregivers in the development of the therapeutic plan demonstrates responsible palliative care.

❼ Positive therapeutic outcomes include resolution of symptoms while minimizing adverse drug events.

❽ Patient and caregiver education is vital to ensuring positive outcomes.

INTRODUCTION

❶ *According to the WHO, "Palliative care is an approach that improves the quality of life of patients and their families facing the problem associated with life-threatening illness, through the prevention and relief of suffering by means of early iden-tification and impeccable assessment and treatment of pain and other problems, physical, psychosocial and spiritual."* The goal of **palliative care** is to achieve the best **quality of life** for patients and their families.[1] "Palliate" literally means "to cloak." The WHO goal of achieving high quality of life depends on management of disease-related symptoms while honoring the patient's goals for care.[2] Palliative care is an approach to care focusing on patients and their families and the challenges they face associated with life-threatening illness.[3] The goal is to prevent and relieve suffering by means of early identification, assessment, and treatment of pain and other physical symptoms including associated psychosocial, emotional, and spiritual concerns.[1] The WHO goes on to state that the most effective palliative care is provided by a team of healthcare professionals. Palliative medicine is rapidly becoming a well-recognized medical specialty throughout the world.[4] This expanding specialty is much needed due to the increased number of patients with chronic, slowly debilitating diseases.[2]

The term *palliative care* is frequently used synonymously with hospice, and although hospice programs provide palliative care, palliative care has a much broader application. The goals for both types of care are similar; however, differences do exist. In the United States, hospice is defined by Medicare and other third-party payers as a medical or third-party benefit available to individuals who have less than or equal to 6 months life expectancy if the disease runs its typical course.[5] Hospice care guidelines and regulations are primarily defined by federal regulations. Palliative care outside of the umbrella of hospice care, in contrast, is not currently regulated and does not have the same reimbursement structure. Palliative care services may be provided at any point during the disease process and are not limited to the last 6 months of life; therefore, patients and families may receive benefits from palliative care services beginning at the time of diagnosis of a life-limiting illness. Palliative care, whether it is through a hospice program or a palliative care service, may be delivered to patients in all care settings including the hospital, outpatient clinic, extended-care facility, or at home.[6] Palliative medicine has become widely accepted as a specialty practice in medicine. Palliative care is not only a philosophy of patient care but a highly organized system to deliver care.[7] The foundation for providing quality palliative care centers around the active participation of an interdisciplinary group or team of professionals who work closely together to meet the goals of the patient and family. Palliative care team members include representatives from medicine, nursing, social work, pastoral or related counseling, pharmacy, nutrition, rehabilitation, and other professional disciplines. The involvement of multiple disciplines provides a holistic approach to the patient's care.

❷ *The goals of palliative care include enhancing quality of life while maintaining or improving functionality.*[7,8] Given this goal of patient care, palliative care should most logically be delivered to patients from the onset of any chronic, life-altering disease. Palliative care is not a new concept, in fact, it is one of the oldest approaches to patient care. Before many of our modern medical and therapeutic advancements were developed, curative treatments were not normally available.[9] Provision of comfort and addressing quality of life during illness was considered the mainstay for patient care. During the 20th century, advances in medical care, nutrition, public health, and trauma care resulted in fewer patient deaths attributed to acute illness or injury. Medical management shifted focus from comfort to a death-denying approach with prolonging life as the primary goal. With this shift in focus, palliative care became less of an emphasis until 1967 when the first modern hospice was established in London, England. Today the palliative care philosophy attempts to combine enhanced quality of life, compassionate care, and patient and family support with modern medical advances.

EPIDEMIOLOGY AND ETIOLOGY

Although the modern hospice model of care originated in England in 1967, the first hospice in the United States was founded in 1974. Since then, hospice acceptance and utilization has increased in the United States. The number of Medicare beneficiaries enrolled in hospice increased by 100% between 2000 and 2005.[10] Medicare spending for hospice care tripled during that same time period, reflecting a greater number of patients receiving the benefits of this type of care. The Medicare Hospice Benefit is now the fastest growing benefit in the Medicare program, representing 3% of Medicare costs.[11] Currently, approximately 5,000 hospice agencies care for patients across the United States. In 2009 approximately 69% of hospice patients were cared for in the home, and 83% of hospice patients were older than 65 years.[12] When the Medicare Hospice Benefit was introduced in 1982, most patients had a terminal diagnosis of cancer, representing more than 90% of beneficiaries.[13] According to the 2010 National Hospice and Palliative Care Organization (NHPCO) report, Facts and Figures on Hospice Care in America, 83% of patients are covered by the Medicare Hospice Benefit. Approximately 40% of patients receiving the Medicare Hospice Benefit have a cancer diagnosis, with the majority of hospice patients having other chronic or life-limiting diseases.[14] In 2009, the top four noncancer diagnoses for hospice admission were debility, heart disease, dementia, and lung disease. In 2009, NHPCO estimated that approximately 41.6% of all deaths in the United States were under the care of a hospice program. The median length of stay in hospice was 21 days, and the mean length of stay was 69 days. Unfortunately, also in 2009, approximately 34% of hospice patients died or were discharged within 7 days of admission to hospice care.[12] The underutilization of the hospice allowable eligibility benefit of 6 months prognosis results in less time for patients and families to benefit from the many services offered through hospice care.

According to a study published in 2007, hospice patients live 29 days longer than nonhospice patients, with the largest difference noted in chronic heart failure patients.[15] Lung cancer patients receiving early palliative care survived 23% longer than those with delayed palliative care, according to a 2010 study.[16] Early referrals to hospice appear to improve the overall care of the patient and offer prolonged survival in some patients. The integration of palliative care prior to the patient's eligibility for hospice care may prove to even further benefit the survival and quality of life and care of patients.

Because healthcare providers have an increasing recognition of the benefit of palliative care for patients with all life-limiting illness, increased integration of this model of care has extended to other disease states beyond cancer. Understanding differences and similarities in the pathophysiology of various disease states and their respective symptoms equips palliative care providers to develop appropriate individualized plans of care for patients that are disease state specific.

PATHOPHYSIOLOGY

In many respects, understanding the pathophysiology of multiple end-stage disease states is daunting, yet in palliative care, the emphasis is not so much on the disease state management as it is on the assessment and appropriate treatment of associated physical, psychological, social, and spiritual symptoms. Palliative care focuses on symptom management for patients with progressive life-limiting illnesses from diagnosis through death where the pathophysiological impact of disease on a patient's symptoms may vary greatly depending on the stage of a patient's illness. ❸ *Palliative care is appropriate for all life-limiting diseases including cancer; chronic obstructive pulmonary disease; dementia, including Alzheimer's disease; Parkinson's disease; chronic cardiac disease; stroke; renal failure; hepatic failure; multiorgan failure; diabetes mellitus; etc.*

For the purpose of this chapter, pathophysiology is not a primary focus. Rather, the philosophy of managing physical, psychological, social, and spiritual symptoms to maintain quality of life and prevent suffering is discussed within the context of progressively incurable illnesses. Although palliative care prior to the last several months before death may coexist with aggressive disease state management to extend life, as the patient approaches the end of life, philosophy and management generally moves away from those principles and concerns related to the disease state management of patients where prolonging life is the goal.

CLINICAL PRESENTATION AND DIAGNOSIS

Cancer

Palliative care is most commonly associated with patients who have cancer. Regardless of whether or not the cancer is curable, most patients have various degrees of physical, psychological, social, and spiritual symptoms that arise once a diagnosis is confirmed. The primary site of solid tumor and hematologic cancers associated with limited life include, but are not limited to, lung, bronchus, breast, colon, rectum, pancreas, prostate, ovaries, uterus, brain, esophagus, liver, kidneys, bladder, lymph system, bone marrow, and skin. The spread of cancer cells (metastases) to distant areas are associated with poorer prognosis. Once a cancer patient has failed curative and life-prolonging therapy, prognosis and disease trajectory is easier to determine than in patients with other life-limiting diseases. The change in focus from cure to symptom control becomes apparent and therefore more acceptable. Symptoms associated with cancer depend on both the primary tumor site and the location of metastatic spread.

Symptoms may also result from the effects of cancer treatments such as chemotherapy and radiation. (See Chaps. 88 to 99 for specific cancers and their treatments.)

End-Stage Heart Failure

Heart disease is the leading cause of death in the United States. Many forms of heart disease result in sudden death; however, the disease progression of heart failure is protracted yet unpredictable. Advanced heart failure (class III to IV or stage C or D) is characterized by persistent symptoms that limit activities of daily living despite optimal drug therapy. Common symptoms include fatigue, breathlessness, anxiety, fluid retention, and pain. In heart failure, standard medication management is intended to reduce the progression of cardiac remodeling and is considered disease modifying. However, as patients approach the final months of life, with the exception of cholesterol-lowering agents, these same cardiac medications are also palliative and should not be discontinued prematurely without cause (Fig. 4–1). Exacerbations of heart failure symptoms should be aggressively treated as long as the patient is responsive to therapy and wishes to receive treatment. In hospice, this can often be accomplished through medication manipulation in the patient's home without the need for hospitalization (see Chap. 6).

Chronic Obstructive Pulmonary Disease

Chronic obstructive pulmonary disease (COPD) has a prolonged and variable course. Patients with COPD have a high number of physician visits and hospital admissions. Palliative care treatment is directed at reducing symptoms, reducing the rate of decline in lung function, preventing and treating exacerbations, and maintaining quality of life. In end-stage COPD, bronchodilators and anti-inflammatory agents become less effective. As patients decline, their ability to use inhalers appropriately becomes more difficult.

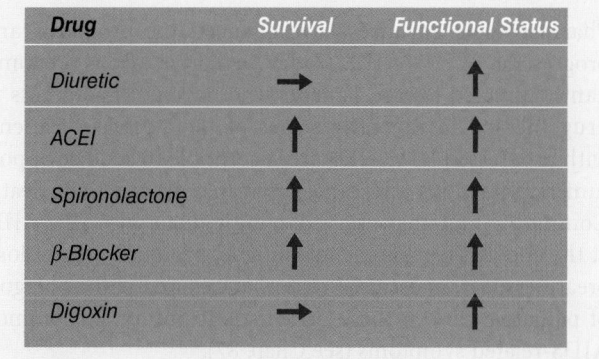

Drug	Survival	Functional Status
Diuretic	→	↑
ACEI	↑	↑
Spironolactone	↑	↑
β-Blocker	↑	↑
Digoxin	→	↑

FIGURE 4–1. Drugs, their use in Class III–IV heart failure, and their effects on survival, hospital admissions, and functional status. →, survival does not increase or decrease, but stays the same; ↑, survival increases. (Data from Strickland JM, Huskey AG. Palliative Care. Pharmacotherapy Self-Assessment Program, 5th ed. 2004:172.)

Utilizing a nebulizer to administer bronchodilators allows for more reliable drug delivery to the site of action. Symptoms of late-stage disease include wheezing, chronic sputum production, cough, frequent respiratory infections, dyspnea with exertion progressing to dyspnea at rest, fatigue, pain, hypoxia, and weight loss. Pulmonary hypertension may also occur and can lead to cor pulmonale or right-sided heart failure (see Chap. 15).

End-Stage Kidney Disease

Chronic kidney disease is progressive and leads to renal failure. In end-stage kidney disease, the only life-sustaining treatments are dialysis or renal transplant. Without treatment, kidney failure causes uremia, oliguria, hyperkalemia and other electrolyte disorders, fluid overload and hypertension unresponsive to treatment, anemia, hepatorenal syndrome, and uremic pericarditis. Symptoms associated with chronic kidney disease (stage 5) include fatigue, pruritus, nausea, vomiting, constipation, dysgeusia, muscle pain, agitation, and bleeding abnormalities. Palliative care in these patients includes the minimization of these symptoms; however, because many options for drug therapy will be cleared through the kidneys, agents should be chosen cautiously to avoid other complications (see Chap. 26).

End-Stage Liver Disease

Like kidney disease, the only treatment to prolong life in advanced liver disease is transplant. Patients with end-stage liver disease typically present with ascites, jaundice, pruritus, or encephalopathy, and frequently all four symptoms. Additionally, bleeding disorders are common, and associated esophageal or gastric varices bleeds are the cause of death in about one-third of those who die from liver disease. Palliative care in these patients focuses on the symptom management of end-stage liver disease complications.

Human Immunodeficiency Virus/Acquired Immune Deficiency Syndrome (HIV/AIDS)

Pharmacologic advances have changed the prognosis and progression of HIV/AIDS. Today, palliative care is predominantly directed toward patients who have not had access to drug therapy in the early stages of their disease. Patients with progressed HIV/AIDS are susceptible to acquire opportunistic infections and cancer that may hasten their death. Common symptoms observed in individuals with HIV/AIDS at the end of their life include fatigue, profound weight loss, breathlessness, nausea, GI disturbances, and pain. The goal of palliative care in these patients is to minimize common AIDS-related symptoms (see Chap. 87).

Stroke/Cerebral Vascular Accident

Stroke can be a result of hemorrhage or ischemia. The prognosis of patients who have had a cerebral vascular accident (CVA) is unpredictable and may be extended, resulting in caregiver fatigue. Approximately one-third of patients who have a stroke will die within 2 years. Patients with stroke deal with loss of physical and cognitive function, poststroke pain, and frequent depression. Incontinence, aphasia, dysphagia, and seizures are also common. Patients who have dysphagia have a high incidence of aspiration pneumonia, which often is the cause of death (see Chap. 11).

Parkinson's Disease

Parkinson's disease is a degenerative neurologic disease with a long chronic, progressive course evidenced by akinesia, rigidity, and tremor. The goal of therapy is to reduce symptoms and maintain or improve quality of life. Palliative care provides support to both the patient and caregiving system as patients become more disabled and as neuropsychiatric problems arise. Symptoms that frequently occur are skin infections and breakdown, constipation, pain, depression, hallucinations, and confusion. Individuals with Parkinson's disease often die from bronchial pneumonia due to dysphagia or complication from falls (see Chap. 33).

Amyotrophic Lateral Sclerosis (Lou Gehrig's Disease)

Amyotrophic lateral sclerosis (ALS) is a chronic neurodegenerative disorder characterized by progressive loss of motor neurons. The median survival is approximately 3 years from the onset of symptoms with less than 15% of patients surviving 10 years. Initially symptoms of ALS present as limb weakness, with other symptoms developing in no particular order including cramps, spasticity, pain, dysarthria, sialorrhea, fatigue, insomnia, depression, fear and anxiety, involuntary emotional expression disorder, constipation, aspiration, and laryngospasm. Many patients do not have cognitive impairment; however, one-fourth to one-half of patients with ALS may have associated frontal lobe dementia. Disease progression eventually involves all systems except sphincter control and eye movement. Unless the individual has long-term mechanical ventilation, the cause of death is typically respiratory failure.

Alzheimer's Disease and Other Dementia

Dementia is a progressive, nonreversible deterioration in cognitive function with associated behavioral dysfunction. Alzheimer's disease accounts for the majority of dementia cases; vascular, Parkinson's disease, dementia with Lewy body, and frontotemporal dementias are less prevalent. Drug therapy is targeted at slowing the progression of the cognitive symptoms and preserving the patient's function. As patients progress toward end-stage dementia, in addition to memory loss and personality and behavioral changes, they require assistance in basic activities of daily living such as feeding, dressing, and toileting. At this point they may not respond to their surroundings, may not communicate, or have impaired movements and dysphagia. Depression, agitation, delusions, compulsions, confusion, hallucinations, incontinence, and disruption of sleep/wake cycles are all common symptoms in end-stage dementias. Assessment of symptoms is challenging due to the cognitive impairment and frequent aphasia. Palliative care is not only directed toward the patient, but also emotional support is needed for those close to them (see Chap. 29).

Adult Failure to Thrive, Decline in Clinical Status, and Debility, Not Otherwise Specified

The diagnoses of "debility not otherwise specified", "adult failure to thrive" and "decline in clinical status" are used to describe unknown or ill-defined causes of morbidity. These conditions are most commonly seen in the frail and elderly who may not have one specific terminal illness but may have one or more chronic illnesses. In the absence of a specific known terminal illness, these patients often have poor appetite, loss of weight, increased fatigue, and a progressive functional decline. These individuals may be eligible for the services provided by the Medicare Hospice Benefit.

TREATMENT

④ *Following a complete assessment of the patient, developing a comprehensive therapeutic plan that utilizes the fewest number of medications to achieve the highest quality of life is essential.* Many times, one drug may provide relief for multiple symptoms, resulting in better patient care, lower costs, and a decreased number of medications. Cost-effective drug recommendations are essential for hospice agencies to control costs, given that Medicare and most other third-party payers reimburse hospice at a fixed per-diem rate. Avoiding polypharmacy will reduce the incidence of adverse drug events related to drug interactions, excessive side effects, and duplications of therapy. The following list of symptoms includes common symptoms observed in palliative and end-of-life care; however, it is not comprehensive. ⑤ *Palliative care is more than just pain management. It includes the treatment of symptoms resulting in the discomfort for the patient, which may include nausea and vomiting, agitation, anxiety, depression, delirium, dyspnea, anorexia and cachexia, constipation, diarrhea, pressure ulcers and edema.*

It should be noted that many drugs used for the treatment of symptoms in palliative and end-of-life care are often prescribed for unapproved uses, administered by unapproved routes or in dosages higher than that recommended by the package insert. This "off-label" use of medication is not unique to palliative care.

Anxiety

A comprehensive review of anxiety disorders may be found in Chapter 40.

▶ Palliative Care Considerations

- Anxiety is "a state of fearfulness, apprehension, worry, emotional discomfort, or uneasiness that results from an unknown internal stimulus, is excessive, or is otherwise inappropriate to a given situation."[17]

- Anxiety is closely related to fear, but fear has an identified cause or source of worry (e.g., fear of death). Fear may be more responsive to counseling than an anxiety state that the patient cannot attribute to a particular fearful stimulus. Anxiety disorders are the most prevalent class of mental disorders overall, so it is not surprising that anxiety is a common cause of distress at life's end.

In addition to anxiety disorders, a variety of conditions can cause, mimic, or exacerbate anxiety.[18,19] Delirium, particularly in its early stages, can easily be confused with anxiety. Physical complications of illness, especially dyspnea and undertreated pain, are common precipitants. Significant anxiety is present in most patients with advanced lung disease and is closely related to periods of oxygen desaturation. Medication side effects, especially akathisia from older antipsychotics and antiemetics (including and especially metoclopramide), can present as anxiety. Interpersonal, spiritual, or existential concerns can mimic and exacerbate anxiety. Patients with an anxious or dependent coping style are at high risk of anxiety as a complication of advanced illness. Short of making a diagnosis of a formal anxiety disorder, differentiating normal worry and apprehension from pathologic anxiety requires clinical judgment.

Behaviors indicative of pathological anxiety include intense worry or dread, physical distress (e.g., tension, jitteriness, or restlessness), maladaptive behaviors and diminished coping and inability to relax.

Pathological anxiety may be complicated by insomnia, depression, fatigue, GI upset, dyspnea, or dysphagia. Anxiety can also worsen these conditions if they are already present. Untreated anxiety may lead to numerous complications, including withdrawal from social support, poor coping, limited participation in palliative care treatment goals, and family distress. Reassess the patient for anxiety with any change in behavior or any change in the underlying medical condition. Search for probable etiologies, and assess for formal anxiety disorders or other contributing factors. Appropriate assessment of anxiety is key to its management.

▶ Nonpharmacologic Treatment in Palliative Care

Regardless of what treatment approach is chosen, the following principles apply. Ask questions and listen to patients' concerns and fears. Offer emotional support and reassurance when appropriate. Err on the side of treatment—be willing to palliate anxiety. Assess treatment response and side effects frequently. Aim to provide maximum resolution of anxiety and educate patients and families about anxiety and its treatments.

Psychotherapies can help in the management of anxiety, although the availability of trained therapists willing to make home visits, and limited stamina and attention span of seriously ill patients, typically make such therapies impractical in the hospice setting. Cognitive and behavioral therapies can be beneficial, including simple relaxation exercises or distraction strategies (i.e., focusing on something pleasurable or at least emotionally neutral). Encourage pastoral care visits, especially if spiritual and existential concerns predominate.

When an underlying cause of anxiety can be identified, treatment is initially aimed at the precipitating problem, with monitoring to see if anxiety improves or resolves as the underlying cause is addressed.

▶ *Pharmacotherapy in Palliative Care*

In most cases, management of pathological anxiety in the hospice setting involves pharmacologic therapies. Benzodiazepines are the gold standard for treatment; however, selective serotonin reuptake inhibitors (SSRIs), typical and atypical antipsychotics, and tricyclic antidepressants may also be appropriate based on the patient's life expectancy.[20] The primary goal of therapy for anxiety in hospice is patient comfort. Aim to prevent anxiety, not just treat it with as needed medications when it flares. Think of pain management as an analogy. As with all medications that act in the CNS, anxiolytics such as benzodiazepines should be dosed at the lower end of the dose range to prevent unnecessary sedation, particularly in the frail and elderly. However, recognize that standard or higher doses may be required. Avoid use of bupropion and psychostimulants for anxiety. Although effective for depression, they are ineffective for anxiety and may make anxiety worse. Many patients have difficulty swallowing as they approach the end of life. Lorazepam, alprazolam, and diazepam tablets are commonly crushed and placed under the tongue with a few drops of water if the liquid formulations are not readily available. Low-dose haloperidol is also used to treat anxiety in palliative care, particularly if delirium is present. Chapter 40 provides more detailed information on appropriate use of anxiolytic agents.

Delirium

▶ *Palliative Care Considerations*

Delirium is a very common disorder in hospice, occurring in more than 80% of terminally ill patients, most often in the last few days of life.[16] Potential causes of delirium in the hospice setting include, but are not limited to, medical illness, dehydration, hypoxia, sleep deprivation, metabolic disturbances, sepsis, side effects of drugs (particularly anticholinergic agents, benzodiazepines, opioids, corticosteroids, tricyclic antidepressants), urinary retention, urinary tract infection, constipation or impaction, uncontrolled pain, or alcohol or drug withdrawal.[21,22]

A classic symptom of delirium is clouding of consciousness. This can be manifested by an inability to either maintain or shift attention. Patients also have impaired cognitive functioning, which may or may not include memory disturbances. "Sundowning" is very common phenomenon at the end of life, especially in the presence of delirium. It presents as daytime sleepiness and nighttime agitation and restlessness. Another common characteristic is fluctuation in severity of delirium symptoms during the course of the day. This can even occur within the course of a single hour or also from day to day. Patients who exhibit agitation from

their delirium are easy to identify, but those who present as withdrawn and with diminished responsiveness ("quiet" delirium) are more difficult to diagnose. It is not uncommon for patients to exhibit both quiet and agitated delirium. Treatment is the same for both types of delirium. Delirium is difficult to distinguish from dementia. Delirium more commonly presents as a sudden onset (e.g., hours to days), with an altered level of consciousness and a clouded sensorium. However, dementia more commonly presents gradually and with an unimpaired level of consciousness.

▶ *Nonpharmacologic Treatment in Palliative Care*

Establishing a safe, soothing environment where there are familiar objects such as photographs and familiar music can be helpful to calm the patient. Minimizing risk of injury is important when the patient is agitated. Providing education to families and caregivers about the causes of delirium, signs and symptoms, and how to best manage it will help reduce their anxiety and distress when it occurs.

▶ *Pharmacotherapy in Palliative Care*

The most important initial step is to determine the goal of care. If possible, reverse the underlying cause of delirium to restore the patient to a meaningful cognitive status.[16,21] If the precipitating factors cannot be reversed, initiate therapy to treat the symptoms. Patients who are not agitated may not require any treatment other than comfort measures. If the patient is irreversibly delirious and agitated, drug therapy is generally indicated.

Antipsychotic (neuroleptic) drugs (conventional or atypical antipsychotics) are the drugs most commonly used to treat confusion and agitation associated with delirium. However, treatment of delirium with these drugs is an "off-label" indication. Atypical antipsychotics such as risperidone, olanzapine, quetiapine, ziprasidone, paliperidone, and aripiprazole account for a major portion of increasing medication costs in the geriatric population.[23]

Haloperidol, when given in doses less than 2 mg/day is well tolerated and nonsedating, and it is within the recommended dosing parameters for long-term care facilities. Doses greater than 4.5 mg/day are associated with increased incidence of extrapyramidal symptoms.[24] Cumulative doses of 35 mg or single IV doses greater than 20 mg have been associated with QTc prolongation.[25] When sedation is beneficial for terminal aggressive, agitated delirium, chlorpromazine is useful because it provides more sedation as compared with low-dose haloperidol. When patients are bedbound and in the final stages of life, orthostatic hypotension common with chlorpromazine is not a concern. Haloperidol and chlorpromazine are commonly given sublingually or rectally if swallowing becomes difficult, although these are not approved routes of administration. Haloperidol, but not chlorpromazine, can be given subcutaneously.[26]

Administering benzodiazepines alone in a patient with delirium can actually make the delirium and confusion worse, although it is sometimes helpful to add benzodiazepines along with antipsychotics if sedation is desired. Phenobarbital may also be used for this purpose.

Patient Encounter 1

LG is a 72-year-old male admitted to the hospital under the care of the palliative care team for management of uncontrolled symptoms. The patient has a primary diagnosis of prostate cancer with metastases to the bone and liver. LG has a past medical history that includes hypertension, chronic heart failure (CHF), and hypercholesterolemia. He is allergic to sulfa. The patient's chief complaint upon admission is pain, which he rates as a 7 on the pain scale (0–10), anxiety, depression, nausea and vomiting, and constipation. He describes his pain as an aching pain in the areas of his bone metastases. The pain increases with movement. He also has a constant deep pain in his right upper abdomen area but it is not as severe. LG is mostly bedbound due to pain.

VS: BP 124/88, RR 20, P 94, wt 61.4 kg (135 lb), ht 5'11" (180 cm)

Meds: Digoxin 0.125 mg by mouth daily; furosemide 40 mg by mouth daily; lisinopril 10 mg by mouth daily; spironolactone 25 mg by mouth daily; metoprolol XL 50 mg by mouth daily; simvastatin 40 mg by mouth daily; goserelin 10.8 mg subcutaneously every 3 months; zoledronic acid 4 mg IV every 4 weeks; hydrocodone/acetaminophen 5/325 1 to 2 tablets by mouth every 4 hours as needed; fentanyl patch 25 mcg/h; apply one patch every 72 hours; celecoxib 100 mg by mouth daily; multivitamin 1 tablet by mouth daily

What are the potential etiologies of the nausea and vomiting LG is experiencing?

What type of the pain is LG experiencing?

What questions would you ask LG during your assessment?

What potential drug–drug interactions may exist, and how would you monitor the patient for them?

What medications should be added, changed or discontinued?

List nonpharmacologic interventions that the practitioner should make to improve the care of LG.

Dyspnea

▶ Palliative Care Considerations

Dyspnea is described as an uncomfortable awareness of breathing. It is a subjective sensation, and patient self-report is the only reliable indicator. Respiratory rate or Po_1 often does not generally correlate with the feeling of breathlessness.[27] Respiratory effort and dyspnea are not the same. Patients may report substantial relief of dyspnea from opioids with no change in respiratory rate. The prevalence of dyspnea varies from 12% to 74% and tends to worsen in the last week of life in terminally ill cancer patients to between 50% and 70%. A thorough history and physical examination should

be taken and possible reversible causes of dyspnea should be identified and treated, if present.

▶ Nonpharmacologic Treatment in Palliative Care

Provide information and anticipate and proactively prepare the patient and family for worsening symptoms. Identify triggers that cause episodes of dyspnea and minimize them as much as possible. Educate patient and family regarding treatment of dyspnea, including the use of opioids and also benzodiazepines for dyspnea-associated anxiety. Prevent isolation and address spiritual issues that can worsen symptom. Encourage relaxation and minimize the need for exertion.

Reposition to comfort, usually to a more upright position or with the compromised lung down. Avoid strong odors, perfumes, and smoking in the patient's presence or in close proximity. Improve air circulation/quality: provide a draft, use fans, or open windows and adjust temperature/humidity with air conditioner or humidifier.

▶ Pharmacotherapy in Palliative Care

If no treatable causes can be identified or when treatments do not completely alleviate distressing symptoms, opioids are first-line agents for treating dyspnea.[28] Opioids suppress respiratory awareness, decrease response to hypoxia and hypercapnia, vasodilate, and have sedative properties. Low-dose opioids (e.g., starting oral dose of morphine ~5 mg) have been shown to be safe and effective in the treatment of dyspnea. Opioid doses should be titrated judiciously. Once an effective dose of an opioid has been established, converting to an extended-release preparation may simplify dosing. When using opioids, anticipate side effects and prevent constipation by initiating a stimulant laxative/stool softener combination.

Nebulized opioids for treatment of dyspnea are controversial. Study results have been inconsistent.[29,30] Nonrandomized studies, case reports, and chart reviews describe anecdotal improvement in dyspnea using nebulized opioids; however, several controlled studies using nebulized opioids have provided inconclusive or negative results. However, nebulized opioids may be an alternative in patients who are not able or willing to take an oral agent or cannot tolerate adverse effects of systemic administration.

Nebulized furosemide appears effective for dyspnea refractive to other conventional therapies.[31] The hypothesized mechanism of action of nebulized furosemide is its ability to enhance pulmonary stretch receptor activity, inhibition of chloride movement through the membrane of the epithelial cell, and its ability to increase the synthesis of bronchodilating prostaglandins.

Because anxiety can exacerbate dyspnea, benzodiazepines and antidepressants that have anxiolytic properties are frequently beneficial. Not all dyspnea is caused by low oxygen saturation. However, oxygen therapy is useful and beneficial for dyspnea if hypoxia is present.

For known etiologies of dyspnea, consider the following:

Bronchospasm or COPD exacerbation: Albuterol, ipratropium, and/or oral steroids are effective for symptoms management. Nebulized bronchodilators are more effective than using handheld inhalers in patients who are weak and have difficulty controlling their breathing.

- **Thick secretions**: If cough reflex is strong, loosen secretions by increasing fluid intake. Guaifenesin is used to thin secretions; however, its efficacy in the absence of hydration is controversial. Nebulized saline may also help loosen secretions. If the patient is unable to cough, hyoscyamine, glycopyrrolate, or scopolamine patch can effectively dry secretions.
- **Anxiety associated with dyspnea**: Consider benzodiazepines (e.g., lorazepam, diazepam).
- **Effusions**: Thoracentesis will be necessary.
- **Low hemoglobin**: Red blood cell transfusion (controversial) or erythropoietin (rarely used in hospice but might have a larger role in palliative care patients).
- **Infections**: Antibiotic therapy as appropriate.
- **Pulmonary emboli**: Anticoagulants for prevention and treatment or vena cava filter placement (rarely used in hospice but might have a larger role in palliative care patients).
- **Rales due to volume overload**: Reduction of fluid intake or diuretic therapy as appropriate.

Patient Encounter 2

NP is a 52-year-old male admitted to hospice with a primary diagnosis of chronic obstructive pulmonary disease (COPD). Other comorbidities include renal insufficiency, congestive heart failure, type 2 diabetes mellitus, hyperlipidemia, and hypothyroidism. The patient has no known drug allergies. NP has been hospitalized several times for respiratory failure and infections and no longer wants aggressive treatment. His appetite is poor and he is bedbound. NP's chief complaint is fatigue, shortness of breath, and edema.

VS: BP 90/50, RR 40, P 120, wt 76.4 kg (168 lb), ht 6'1" (185 cm)

Meds: fluticasone 500 mcg/salmeterol 50 mcg inhaled orally twice daily; tiotropium contents of 1 capsule (18 mcg) inhaled once daily; ipratropium bromide 18 mcg and albuterol 90 mcg aerosol oral inhaler 2 puffs every 2 hours as needed, insulin glargine 80 units subcutaneously daily, regular insulin administered on a sliding scale for fasting blood glucose more than 250 mg/dL; potassium chloride 10 mEq by mouth daily; furosemide 20 mg by mouth daily; levothyroxine 125 mcg daily; simvastatin 20 mg by mouth daily.

What potential interventions could the practitioner make to improve NP's care?

What medications could be added, changed, or discontinued?

What potential drug–drug interactions may exist? How would you monitor the patient for them?

Nausea and Vomiting

A comprehensive review of nausea and vomiting may be found in Chapter 20.

▶ Palliative Care Considerations

Up to 71% of palliative care patients will develop nausea and vomiting with ~40% experiencing these symptoms in the last 6 weeks of life. Chronic nausea can be defined as lasting longer than a week and without a well-identified or self-limiting cause such as chemotherapy, radiation, or infection.[32] Four major mechanisms are correlated with the stimulation of the vomiting center (**Fig. 4–2**). Potentially reversible causes of nausea and vomiting should not be overlooked. Causes of chronic nausea in end-of-life patients may include autonomic dysfunction, constipation, antibiotics, nonsteroidal anti-inflammatory drugs (NSAIDs), other drugs, infection, bowel obstruction, metabolic abnormalities (e.g., renal or hepatic failure, hypercalcemia), increased intracranial pressure, anxiety, radiation therapy, chemotherapy, or untreated pain.

▶ Nonpharmacologic Treatment in Palliative Care

Relaxation techniques may prove beneficial in some patients. Strong foods or odors should be avoided and, if possible, eliminate offending medications.

▶ Pharmacotherapy in Palliative Care

The clinical features of nausea and vomiting should guide the choice of antiemetics used (for a more comprehensive review, refer to Chap. 20). The following are examples of managing nausea and vomiting as it correlates with the etiology:

Chemoreceptor trigger zone (CTZ)-induced nausea and vomiting are caused by chemotherapeutic agents, bacterial toxins, metabolic products (e.g., uremia), and opioids. Dopamine (D_2), serotonin (5-HT), and neurokinin-1 are the primary neurotransmitters involved in this process. Therapy is based on blocking D_2 with D_2-antagonists including butyrophenones (e.g., haloperidol), phenothiazines, and metoclopramide.

Because of their receptor specificity, serotonin$_3$ (5-HT$_3$) antagonists such as ondansetron, granisetron, dolasetron, and palonosetron have limited usefulness in nausea and vomiting at the end of life.[33] They are typically indicated with emetogenic chemotherapy and up to 10 to 14 days posttreatment. Aprepitant is a neurokinin-1 antagonist that is also indicated for the treatment of nausea due to highly emetogenic chemotherapy in combination with a 5-HT$_3$ antagonist and corticosteroid. Aprepitant should not be used as a sole agent.

Cerebral cortex–induced nausea and vomiting can be caused by anxiety, taste, and smell, and also as a result of increased intracranial pressure. Corticosteroids are administered to decrease intracranial pressure due to tumor involvement. In addition to their usefulness in reducing intracranial pressure, corticosteroids have also been found to be effective in nonspecific nausea and vomiting. The mechanism of this

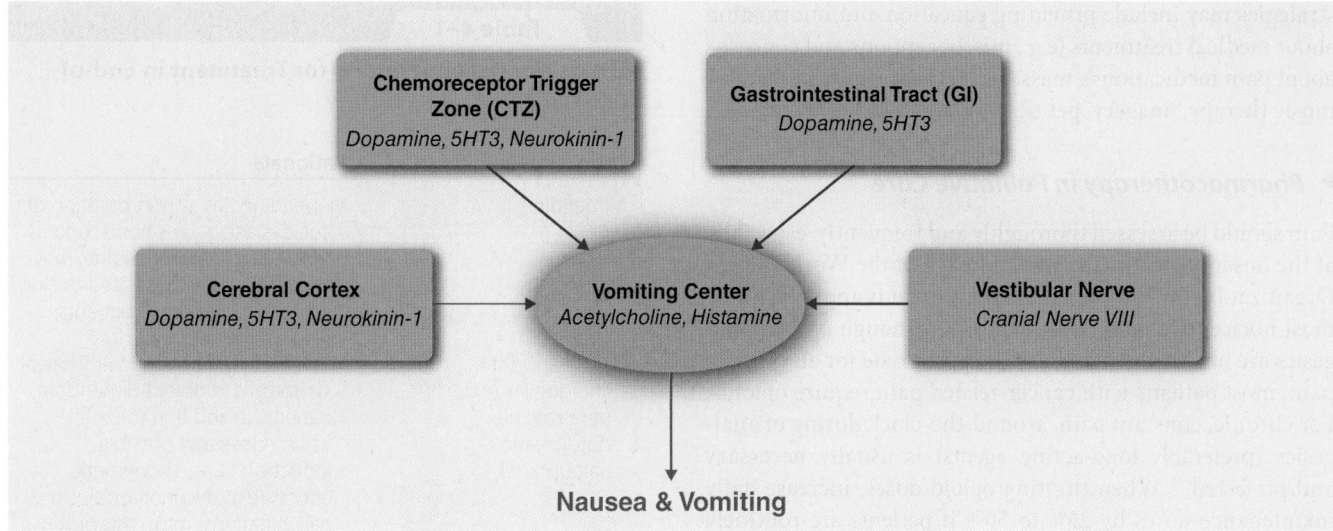

FIGURE 4–2. Mechanisms and associated neurotransmitters involved in nausea and vomiting.

action is unknown. Anxiolytics such as benzodiazepines are used to treat anxiety and "anticipatory" gustatory and olfactory stimulation.

Vestibular nausea and vomiting is triggered by motion. Opioids can sensitize the vestibular center resulting in movement-induced nausea. Ambulatory patients are more susceptible to vestibular nausea and vomiting then bedbound patients. Because histamine and acetylcholine are the predominant neurotransmitters here, antihistamines and anticholinergics are the drugs of choice in movement-induced nausea and vomiting.

GI tract stimulation occurs through vagal and sympathetic pathways. These pathways can be triggered by stimulation of either mechanoreceptors or chemoreceptors located in the gut. Gastric stasis, GI obstruction, drugs, metastatic disease, bacterial toxins, chemotherapeutic agents, and irradiation can lead to nausea and vomiting. Glossopharyngeal or vagus nerve stimulation in the pharynx by sputum, mucosal lesions, or infection (e.g., *Candida*) can also evoke nausea. The major neurotransmitters in the upper GI tract are D_2, acetylcholine, and 5-HT. Metoclopramide is a 5-HT_4 agonist and increases gastric motility above the jejunum, whereas anticholinergics decrease GI spasticity and motility in nausea induced by gut hyperactivity. In high doses, metoclopramide also acts as a 5-HT_3 antagonist.

Autonomic failure causes gastroparesis resulting in anorexia, nausea, early satiety, and constipation. Delayed gastric emptying is frequently observed in patients with diabetes mellitus, chronic renal failure, and neurological disorders. Malnutrition, cachexia, lung and pancreatic cancers, HIV, radiotherapy, and drugs such as opioids, anticholinergics, antidepressants, and vasodilators have been associated with autonomic failure and resulting chronic nausea, poor performance, tachycardia, and malnutrition. Evaluate underlying causes, including multiple drugs that may cause gastroparesis. If drug therapy is indicated, metoclopramide is effective in improving gastric emptying.

GI irritation can cause nausea and vomiting due to generalized gastritis, hiatal hernia, gastroesophageal reflux disease (GERD), or peptic ulcer disease. Histamine$_2$ (H_2) antagonists or proton pump inhibitors (PPIs) are considered the drugs of choice for ongoing gastritis.

Refractory cases of nausea and vomiting often require judiciously selected combinations of medications from different classes (e.g., various combinations of haloperidol, metoclopramide, diphenhydramine, lorazepam, and dexamethasone).

Pain

A comprehensive review of pain management may be found in Chapter 34.

▶ Palliative Care Considerations

According to the SUPPORT study, 74% to 95% of very ill or dying patients still experience uncontrolled pain.[34] Although existing drug therapy affords the opportunity to manage more than 90% of pain, many patients needlessly suffer.[48] Conducting a comprehensive pain assessment is key to choosing appropriate therapeutic interventions. Because pain is subjective, both physical and humanistic factors must be considered. Patients in an end-of-life setting must also be evaluated for anxiety, depression, delirium, and other neurological influences that may heighten a patient's awareness or response to pain.

▶ Nonpharmacologic Treatment in Palliative Care

Nonpharmacologic treatment is essential in chronic pain management. Physical, complementary, and cognitive behavioral interventions reduce the perception of pain and decrease the dose requirements of medications. Examples of such strategies may include providing education and information about medical treatments (e.g., misconceptions and concerns about pain medications), massage, ice, heat, physical therapy, music therapy, imagery, pet therapy, and psychotherapy.

▶ Pharmacotherapy in Palliative Care

Pain should be assessed thoroughly and frequently, especially at the onset of treatment. The approach of the World Health Organization (WHO) to pain management is appropriate for most nociceptive pain (see Chap. 34). Although opioid analgesics are not always necessary or appropriate for all types of pain, most patients with cancer-related pain require opioids. For chronic, constant pain, around-the-clock dosing of analgesics (preferably long-acting agents) is usually necessary and preferred.[35] When titrating opioid doses, increase daily maintenance doses by 25% to 50% if patients are routinely requiring three or more breakthrough doses per 24 hours as a result of around-the-clock maintenance dose failure. The around-the-clock maintenance doses should not be increased if breakthrough doses are used only for incident pain such as increased activity or dressing changes.

Fentanyl transdermal patches may be appropriate in some patients; however, many patients at the end of life experience fat and muscle wasting and dehydration, resulting in reduced and variable absorption. Fentanyl transdermal patches have a slow onset of action, contributing to difficulty in dose titration.

Only short-acting opioids should be used for breakthrough pain (e.g., immediate-release morphine, oxycodone, and hydromorphone are common examples). The dose of short-acting opioids for the treatment of breakthrough pain should be equal to 5% to 20% of the daily maintenance dose. Frequencies for breakthrough dosing should not exceed the following:

- **Oral:** Every 1 to 2 hours
- **Subcutaneous:** Every 20 to 30 minutes
- **IV:** Every 8 to 20 minutes

Monitor for and appropriately treat common side effects of opioids. Common side effects of opioids include constipation, nausea and vomiting, itching, and transient sedation. Because constipation occurs with all chronic opioid therapy, prevention is imperative. Stimulant laxatives (senna or bisacodyl) with or without a stool softener (docusate) are the drugs of choice for opioid-induced constipation. Myoclonus, delirium, hallucinations, and hyperalgesia are possible signs of opioid-induced neurotoxicity and require rotation to another opioid or dose reduction. Respiratory depression is uncommon with the appropriate opioid dose titration. However, if dangerous opioid-induced respiratory depression does occur, small doses (0.1 mg) of the μ receptor antagonist naloxone are appropriate and can be repeated as necessary. The goal is to increase respirations to a safe level while preventing the patient from experiencing a loss of pain control.

Drugs that should not be used for treatment of pain during end-of-life care are listed in Table 4–1.

Table 4–1
Drugs _Not_ Recommended for Treatment in End-of-Life Care

Drug	Rationale
Meperidine	Meperidine has a short duration of analgesia (e.g., 2–3 hours) and its metabolite, normeperidine, may accumulate with repeated dosing, especially in geriatric patients, resulting in neurotoxicity
Opioid agonist-antagonists (e.g., pentazocine, butorphanol, nalbuphine)	The risk of precipitating withdrawal symptoms in opioid-dependent patients in addition to their ceiling dose and possible induction of psychomimetic effects (e.g., dysphoria, delusions, hallucinations) make this group of analgesics inappropriate for use

Different types of pain may require specific types of analgesics or adjuvant medications. A few examples of types of pain other than nociceptive somatic pain that are commonly seen in patients with advanced illness are as follows.

Visceral pain (nociceptive pain that is caused by stretching or spasms of visceral organs such as the GI tract, liver, and pancreas) should be treated with the standard WHO step approach to pain, with the addition of anticholinergic agents or, if inflammation is associated with the pain, corticosteroids.

Bone pain (a common metastatic site of various cancers) is best treated with NSAIDs or corticosteroids in addition to standard opioid therapy.

Neuropathic pain (pain caused by damage to the afferent nociceptive fibers) can be managed with tricyclic antidepressants, antiepileptic drugs, tramadol, tapentadol or N-methyl-D-aspartate antagonists such as ketamine. Methadone is an opioid μ-agonist that has a role in neuropathic pain given its added N-methyl-D-aspartate antagonist activity.

Terminal Secretions

▶ Palliative Care Considerations

Terminal secretions, or death rattle, is the noise produced by the oscillatory movements of secretions in the upper airways in association with the inspiratory and expiratory phases of respiration.[36,37] As patients lose their ability to swallow and clear oral secretions, accumulation of mucus results in a rattling or gurgling sound produced by air passing through mucus in the lungs and air passages. The sound does not represent any discomfort for the patient. However, the sound is sometimes so distressing to the family that it should be treated. Terminal secretions are typically seen only in patients who are obtunded or are too weak to expectorate.

Drugs that decrease secretions are best initiated at the first sign of death rattle because they do not affect existing respiratory secretions. These agents have limited or no impact when the secretions are secondary to pneumonia or pulmonary congestion or edema.

▶ *Nonpharmacologic Treatment in Palliative Care*

Position the patient on his or her side or in a semiprone position to help facilitate drainage of secretions. If necessary, place the patient in the Trendelenburg position (lowering the head of the bed); this allows fluids to move into the oropharynx, facilitating an easy removal. Do not maintain this position for long because there is a risk of aspiration.

Oropharyngeal suctioning is another option but may be disturbing to both the patient and visitors. Fluid intake can also be decreased, as appropriate.

▶ *Pharmacotherapy in Palliative Care*

Anticholinergic drugs remain the standard of therapy for prevention and treatment of terminal secretions due to their ability to effectively dry secretions.[36-38] Drugs used for this indication are similar pharmacologically, and one can be selected by anticholinergic potency, onset of action, route of administration, alertness of patient, and cost. The most commonly used anticholinergic agents are atropine, hyoscyamine, scopolamine, and glycopyrrolate.

Anticholinergic side effects are common and include blurred vision, constipation, urinary retention, confusion, delirium, restlessness, hallucinations, dry mouth, and heart palpitations. Unlike the other anticholinergics, glycopyrrolate does not cross the blood–brain barrier and is associated with fewer CNS side effects. Glycopyrrolate is a potent drying agent when compared with others agents and has the potential to cause excessive dryness.[38]

Advanced Heart Failure

▶ *Palliative Care Considerations*

Heart failure symptoms at the end of life may include hypotension, volume overload, edema, and fatigue. Patients should be assessed to confirm symptoms are related to heart failure rather than other disease states to ensure appropriate treatment strategies.[39,40] The goals for advanced heart failure treatment will differ from traditional heart failure management. Drug therapy will be focused on symptom management rather than improving mortality. Prevention of cardiovascular disease through cholesterol reduction is no longer necessary at this point.

▶ *Nonpharmacologic Treatment in Palliative Care*

Patients should be maintained in a comfortable position with feet elevated to minimize lower leg fluid accumulation. Minimizing high-salt foods and limiting fluid intake can help reduce fluid accumulation associated with a failing heart. The patient should not overexert during physical activity.

At this stage in heart failure, comfort becomes the primary initiative.

▶ *Pharmacotherapy in Palliative Care*

As patients approach the end of life, it is difficult to determine when certain medications for heart failure should be dose reduced or discontinued. The following general principles may help serve as a guide. However, each individual's history, prognosis, and current condition should be evaluated to determine appropriateness.

If a patient becomes symptomatic due to hypotension, angiotensin-converting enzyme (ACE) inhibitor, angiotensin receptor blocker (ARB), and/or β-adrenergic blocker doses should be reduced or discontinued. For β-adrenergic blockers, in particular, this should be done gradually to avoid significant clinical deterioration. If volume overload occurs or persists while taking β-adrenergic blocker therapy, consider tapering off the medication. Likewise, for patients experiencing fatigue while taking a β-adrenergic blocking agent, consider tapering down the dose *only if* their heart rate does not increase with exertion. Consider discontinuing the ACE inhibitor (or the angiotensin receptor blocker) if the patient's renal function deteriorates (e.g., cardiorenal syndrome).

In patients with excessive fluid overload where sodium and water intake restrictions are not effective or not possible, consider increasing the dose of diuretic. However, vascular dehydration can occur in some patients with end-stage heart failure if the dose of diuretic is excessive.

Digoxin toxicity is common; therefore, patients should be carefully monitored and therapy adjusted or discontinued as appropriate. The symptoms of digoxin toxicity including complaints of anorexia, nausea and vomiting, visual disturbances, disorientation, confusion, or cardiac arrhythmias.

Hydroxymethylglutaryl coenzyme-A (HMG-CoA) reductase inhibitors (and other cholesterol-lowering medications) are likely to have a long-term effect rather than a palliative effect. If patients are eligible for hospice admission, consider discontinuing lipid lowering therapy.

Figure 4–1 provides a list of agents that improve functional status in advanced heart failure patients.

OUTCOME EVALUATION

6 *Involving the patient, family, and caregivers in the development of the therapeutic plan demonstrates responsible palliative care.* Before the implementation of drug therapy, the patient, family, and caregiver should be involved with the decision-making process. The practitioner should provide information about all reasonable options for care so that the patient, family and caregivers can collaborate with the healthcare team to meet their combined goals. **7** *Positive therapeutic outcomes include resolution of symptoms while minimizing adverse drug events.* When treating symptoms pharmacologically, adverse drug events must be avoided or minimized to prevent negative outcomes.

Patient Encounter 3

RD, a 73-year-old female, is admitted to the hospice inpatient unit with a complaint of fever, nausea and occasional vomiting, confusion, insomnia, and agitation. Her nausea started approximately 2 weeks ago and has progressively worsened. She has not had a bowel movement for 5 days. Her agitation and confusion began suddenly 2 days ago. The patient was admitted to hospice with a diagnosis of breast cancer with metastases to the brain, bone, liver, and lungs. RD also has a past medical history of osteoarthritis, hypertension, hypercholesterolemia, mild dementia, and frequent urinary tract infections. She has a Foley catheter in place. RD's family history is unknown. The patient's medical record states she is allergy to codeine.

Meds: Naproxen 500 mg every 6 hours as needed for osteoarthritis pain (started 4 weeks ago); enalapril 10 mg twice daily; simvastatin 40 mg by mouth daily; celecoxib 100 mg twice daily; acetaminophen 325 mg every 6 hours as needed for pain; morphine sustained-release tablets 15 mg every 12 hours, hydrocodone/acetaminophen 5/325 mg two tablets every 6 hours as needed for cancer pain; St. John's Wort (the patient takes as needed for depression)

What are potential causes of her nausea and vomiting and her confusion and agitation?

What potential drug–drug interactions and side effects exist in this patient?

What medications could be added, changed, and/or discontinued?

How does the patient's reported allergy to codeine impact potential treatment options?

Patient Care and Monitoring

Other symptoms that are commonly observed in palliative care that the practitioner should monitor:

- **Depression:** Patients may need to experience more immediate symptom relief than typical antidepressants may provide. Methylphenidate may be an appropriate option for treatment in patients with life expectancies less than 6 to 8 weeks.
- **Insomnia:** Many times patients experience insomnia due to a lack of appropriate symptom management. In addition to ensuring that all physical symptoms are controlled and that good sleep hygiene is practiced, addressing the emotional and spiritual concerns that patients frequently experience is critical for effectively managing insomnia.
- **Constipation:** Most patients experience constipation as a result of opioid use. Opioid-induced constipation requires management with a stimulant laxative such as senna or bisacodyl. Other causes of constipation include other drugs, including anticholinergic agents and calcium channel blockers, calcium, iron, and other dietary supplements, poor hydration, and immobility. Careful assessment of etiology is important before implementing treatment.
- **Diarrhea:** Patients experiencing fluid loss through excessive diarrhea need to be monitored for dehydration and electrolyte imbalance. Fluid replacement is typically the first line of therapy in addition to drug therapy to minimize the symptom. Overflow diarrhea from constipation or a bowel obstruction is often misdiagnosed and treated inappropriately, worsening the problem.
- **Dysphagia:** Difficulty swallowing is common in end-of-life patients and may necessitate that medications be given through alternative routes of administration. Knowledge of drug absorption and disposition when administered rectally, sublingually, and topically is key in good clinical decision making.

Patients with life-limiting diseases have emotional and spiritual issues that deserve attention by trained professionals. Addressing these concerns and providing support and coping skills can dramatically reduce the medication requirements for symptom control. Psychosocial and spiritual support is not only directed toward the patient in palliative care but also supports the family during the time of the illness and after the death of their loved one.

8 *Patient and caregiver education is vital to ensuring positive outcomes.* If the patient and caregiver are unaware of the purpose and goals for interventions used in palliative medicine, adherence to regimens will be hindered and outcomes will be compromised. Education regarding the role and value of the palliative care team will allow the patient and family to understand why palliative care is important to their overall quality of life. Patients will achieve the best possible outcomes when practitioners incorporate the interdisciplinary palliative care approach to care early in the disease progression of patients with life limiting illnesses.

Abbreviations Introduced in This Chapter

5-HT	5-Hydroxytriptophan (serotonin)
ACE	Angiotensin-converting enzyme
ALS	Amyotrophic lateral sclerosis
ARB	Angiotensin receptor blocker
CHF	Chronic heart failure
COPD	Chronic obstructive pulmonary disease
CTZ	Chemoreceptor trigger zone
CVA	Cerebrovascular accident
ESRD	End-stage renal disease
GERD	Gastroesophageal reflux disease

HMG-CoA	Hydroxymethylglutaryl coenzyme-A
NSAID	Nonsteroidal anti-inflammatory drug
PEG	Percutaneous endoscopic gastrostomy
PICC	Peripherally inserted central catheter
PPI	Proton pump inhibitors
SSRI	Selective serotonin reuptake inhibitor
WHO	World Health Organization

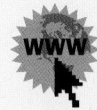 Self-assessment questions and answers are available at *http://www.mhpharmacotherapy. com/pp.html.*

REFERENCES

1. World Health Organization. WHO definition of palliative care. Geneva, Switzerland: World Health Organization [cited 2012 Feb 19]. Available from: *http://www.who.int/cancer/palliative/definition/en.*
2. Centers for Medicare & Medicaid Services. Medicare Hospice Benefits. Centers for Medicare and Medicaid Services. Washington, DC: Centers for Medicare and Medicaid Services, 2010 [cited 2012 Feb 19]. Available from: *http://www.medicare.gov/Publications/Pubs/pdf/02154.pdf*
3. National Consensus Project for Quality Palliative Care. Clinical Practice Guidelines for Quality Palliative Care, 2nd ed. Pittsburgh, PA: National Consensus Project for Quality Palliative Care, 2009 [cited 2011 Jan 7]. Available from: *http://nationalconsensusproject.org/ guideline.pdf*
4. Butterfield S. Growing specialty offers opportunity for hospitalists. ACPHospitalist. February 2009 [cited 2012 Feb 19]. Available from: *http://www.acphospitalist.org/archives/2009/02/cover.htm.*
5. Sepúlveda C, Marlin A, Yoshida T, Ullrich A. Palliative care: The World Health Organization's global perspective. J Pain Symptom Manage 2002;24:91.
6. Hill RR. Clinical pharmacy services in a home-based palliative care program. Am J Health Syst Pharm 2007;64:806–810.
7. Teno JM, Connor SR. Referring a patient and family to high-quality palliative care at the close of life: "We met a new personality . . . with this level of compassion and empathy." JAMA 2009;301:651.
8. Grauer P, Shuster J, Protus BM. Palliative Care Consultant, 3rd ed. Dubuque, IA: Kendall/Hunt Publishing, 2008.
9. Goldstein NE, Fischberg D. Update in palliative medicine. Ann Intern Med 2008;148:135–140.
10. Strickland JM, Huskey AG. Palliative Care. Pharmacotherapy Self-Assessment Program, 5th ed. 2004:191–218.
11. Hospice care. Health Letter. Cambridge, MA: Harvard Health Publications, July 2008.
12. Facts and Figures on Hospice Care in America: 2010. National Hospice and Palliative Care Organization, 2010.
13. Connor SR. Development of hospice and palliative care in the United States. Omega (Westport) 2007–08;56(1):89–99.
14. Xu J, Kochanek KD, Murphy SL, Tejada-Vera B. Deaths: Final Data for 2007; National Vital Statistics Reports 58(19). Hyattsville, MD: National Center for Health Statistics, 2010.
15. Connor SR, Pyenson B, Fitch K, Spence C, Iwasaki K. Comparing hospice and nonhospice patient survival among patients who die within a three year window. J Pain Symptom Manage 2007;33(3):238–246.
16. Ternel JS, Greer JA, Muzinkansky A, et al. Early palliative care for patients with metastatic non-small-cell lung cancer. N Engl J Med 2010;363(8):733–742.
17. Breitbart W, Alici Y. Agitation and delirium at the end of life "We can't manage him." JAMA 2008;300(24):2898–2910.
18. Stark D, Kiely M, Smith A, et al. Anxiety disorders in cancer patients: Their nature, associations, and relation to quality of life. J Clin Oncol 2002;20:3137.
19. Sarhill N, Walsh D, Nelson KA, et al. Assessment of delirium in advanced cancer: The use of the bedside confusion scale. Am J Hosp Palliat Care 2001;18:335.
20. Wilson KG, Chochinov, HM, Skirko MG, et al. Depression and anxiety disorders in palliative cancer care. J Pain Symptom Manage 2007;33:118–129.
21. Grauer PA, Shuster J, Protus BM. Palliative Care Consultant, 3rd ed. Dubuque, IA: Kendall-Hunt, 2008:29–31, 40–47, 78–85.
22. Shuster JL. Confusion, agitation, and delirium at the end-of-life. J Palliat Med 1998;1:177–186.
23. Katz IR. Optimizing atypical antipsychotic treatment strategies in the elderly. J Am Geriatr Soc 2004;52:272–277.
24. Lonergan E, Britton AM, Luxenberg J Antipsychotics for delirium. Cochrane Reviews [Internet]. 2009 Jan 21 [cited 2012 Mar 2]. Available from: *http://www2.cochrane.org/reviews/en/ab005594.html*
25. Haloperidol Monograph. Lexicomp Online. Hudson (OH): Lexi-Comp Inc. [cited 2012 Mar 2]. Available from: *http://www.crlonline.com/ crlsql/servlet/crlonline.*
26. Breitbart W, Marotta R, Platt MM, et al. A double-blind trial of haloperidol, chlorpromazine, and lorazepam in the treatment of delirium in hospitalized AIDS patients. Am J Psychiatry 1996;153:231–237.
27. Storey P, Knight CF. UNIPAC Four: Management of Selected Non-Pain Symptoms in the Terminally Ill, 2nd ed. New York, NY: Mary Ann Liebert, 2003:29–35.
28. Thomas JR, vonGunten CF. Management of dyspnea. J Support Oncol 2003;1:23–24.
29. Ferraresi V. Inhaled opioids for the treatment of dyspnea. Am J Health Syst Pharm 2005;62:319–320.
30. Emanuel LL, von Gunten CF, Ferris FD, HauserJM, eds. The Education for Physicians on End-of-life Care (EPEC) Curriculum. Module 10: Common Physical Symptoms. 2003:5–10.
31. Kohara H, Ueoka H, Aoe K, et al. Effect of nebulized furosemide in terminally ill cancer patients with dyspnea. J Pain Symptom Manage 2003;26:962–967.
32. Ferris FD, von Gunten CF, Emanuel LL. Ensuring competency in end-of-life care: Controlling symptoms. BMC Palliat Care 2002;1:5.
33. Vella-Brincat J, Macleod AD. Haloperidol in palliative care. Palliat Med 2004;18:195–201.
34. American Pain Society. Principles of Analgesic Use in the Treatment of Acute Pain and Cancer Pain, 5th ed. Glenview, IL: American Pain Society, 2003.
35. McCaffery M, Pasero C. Pain: Clinical Manual, 2nd ed. St. Louis, MO: Elsevier Mosby, 1999.
36. Morita T, Tsunoda J, Inone S, Chihara S. Risk factors for death rattle in terminally ill cancer patients: A prospective exploratory study. Palliat Med 2000;14:19–23.
37. Varkey B. Palliative care for end-stage lung disease patients. Clin Pulm Med 2003;10(5):269–277.
38. Hyson HC, Johnson AM, Jog MS. Sublingual atropine for sialorrhea secondary to parkinsonism: A pilot study. Mov Disorder 2002;17(6):1318–1320.
39. Hauptman PJ, Havranek EP. Integrating palliative care into heart failure care. Arch Intern Med 2005;165:374–378.
40. McPherson ML. Palliative Care and Appropriate Medication Use in End-Stage Heart Failure. Medscape Nurses. 2007 [cited 2012 Mar 2]. Available from: *http://www.medscape.com/viewarticle/556035.*

Part II

Disorders of Organ Systems

5 Hypertension

Robert J. Straka, David Parra, and
Stephanie Kaiser

LEARNING OBJECTIVES

Upon completion of the chapter, the reader will be able to:

1. Classify blood pressure (BP) levels and treatment goals.
2. Recognize underlying causes and contributing factors in the development of hypertension.
3. Describe the appropriate measurement of BP.
4. Recommend appropriate lifestyle modifications and pharmacotherapy for patients with hypertension.
5. Identify populations requiring special consideration when designing a treatment plan.
6. Construct an appropriate monitoring plan to assess hypertension treatment.

KEY CONCEPTS

① Hypertension is widely prevalent and significantly contributes to cardiovascular morbidity, mortality, and associated healthcare costs.

② The cause of hypertension is unknown in the majority of cases (primary hypertension), but for patients with secondary hypertension, specific causes can be identified.

③ Patients failing to achieve goal blood pressure (BP) despite adherence to optimal doses of three distinct antihypertensive agents (ideally, one being a diuretic) have resistant hypertension and should be evaluated for secondary causes of hypertension.

④ The pathophysiology of primary hypertension is heterogeneous but ultimately exerts its effects through the two primary determinants of BP: cardiac output (CO) and peripheral resistance (PR).

⑤ Appropriate technique in measuring BP is a vital component to the diagnosis and continued management of hypertension.

⑥ Drug selection for the management of patients with hypertension should be considered as adjunctive to nonpharmacologic approaches for BP lowering, and ultimately the attainment of target BP in many cases may be more important than the antihypertensive agent used.

⑦ Implementation of lifestyle modifications successfully lowers BP, often with results similar to those of therapy with a single antihypertensive agent.

⑧ An approach to selection of drugs for the treatment of patients with hypertension should be evidence based. Consideration should be given to the individual's comorbidities, co-prescribed medications, and practical patient-specific issues including costs.

⑨ Specific antihypertensive therapy is warranted for certain patients with comorbid conditions that may elevate their level of risk for cardiovascular disease (CVD).

⑩ The frequency of follow-up visits for patients with hypertension varies based on individual cases but is influenced by the severity of hypertension, comorbidities, and choice of agent selected.

INTRODUCTION

Despite efforts to promote awareness, treatment, and the means available to aggressively manage high blood pressure (BP), trends over the past 15 years demonstrate only modest improvements in its treatment and control. National and international organizations continually refine their recommendations of how clinicians should approach the management of patients with high BP, and although approaches vary to some degree, there are clear themes that emerge regardless of which national or international organization's algorithm is followed. The purpose of this chapter is to (a) provide a summary of key issues associated with the management of patients with hypertension, (b) discuss the basic approach to treating patients with hypertension and provide a functional summary of the currently prevailing themes of national guidelines, and (c) summarize salient pharmacotherapeutic issues essential for clinicians to consider when managing patients with hypertension.

Various algorithms recommend nonpharmacologic and pharmacologic management with the underlying theme that achievement of BP targets mitigate end-organ damage, leading to substantial reductions in stroke, myocardial infarction (MI), end-stage renal disease, and heart failure (HF). Although references to other algorithms are mentioned, this chapter focuses primarily on the American Heart Association (AHA) Scientific Statement on the treatment of hypertension in the prevention and management of ischemic heart disease,[1] the American College of Cardiology Foundation (ACCF)/AHA expert consensus document on hypertension in the elderly,[2] and the *Seventh Report of the Joint National Committee on Prevention, Detection, Evaluation and Treatment of High Blood Pressure*, more commonly referred to as the Joint National Committee Seventh Report (JNC 7) report.[3] Additional references to recommendations from other authoritative organizations are made when pertinent. It should be noted that an update of the JNC 7 report (JNC 8) is expected to be released in 2012.

The JNC 7 report describes four stages of BP classification and provides guidance on nonpharmacologic and pharmacologic approaches to managing patients with hypertension. The four stages of BP classification include normal, prehypertension, stage 1 hypertension, and stage 2 hypertension (Table 5–1). These stages are defined as such to connote a level of risk and thus the need for varying intensities of intervention with drug therapy (Fig. 5–1).[3] With the exception of individuals with "compelling indications," recommendations for drug therapy typically begin with one or two (in the case of stage 2) antihypertensive drugs as an initial step. Specific drug selection is guided by the presence of compelling indications—specific comorbid conditions. These compelling indications, such as HF, diabetes, and chronic kidney disease (CKD), represent specific conditions for which explicit evidence in the literature exists to document the utility of a particular agent or class of agents. Selection of drug therapy consequently involves an iterative process of considering multiple antihypertensive drugs as needed to achieve target BPs of less than 140/90 mm Hg for all patients, with more aggressive targets of less than 130/80 mm Hg for patients with diabetes or chronic (greater than 3 months) kidney disease (estimated glomerular filtration rate [GFR] less than 60 mL/min/1.73 m^2 [0.58 mL/s/m^2] or the presence of albuminuria [300 mg/day or 200 mg/g creatinine or 22.6 mg/mmol creatinine]).[3] In addition, the AHA scientific statement on the treatment of hypertension in the prevention and management of ischemic heart disease expands those in whom a lower BP target of less than 130/80 mm Hg should be pursued to include patients with known coronary artery disease or coronary artery disease risk equivalents (carotid artery disease, peripheral arterial disease, abdominal aortic aneurysm), or a 10-year Framingham risk score of greater than 10%. See Chapter 12, "Dyslipidemias." In patients with left ventricular dysfunction, additional BP lowering to a target of less than 120/80 mm Hg may also be considered.[1] However, in contrast, the ACCF/AHA expert consensus document on hypertension in the elderly (patients 65 years of age or older) considers an achieved systolic BP of 140 to 145 mm Hg acceptable, if tolerated, in patients 80 years or older, whereas in those younger than 80 an achieved systolic BP of less than 140 mm Hg is appropriate.[2]

Table 5–1

Classification of BP in Children, Adolescents, and Adults[a]

BP Classification	Adult SBP (mm Hg)	Adult DBP (mm Hg)	Children/Adolescents SBP or DBP Percentile[b]
Normal	Less than 120	and less than 80	Less than 90th
Prehypertension	120–139	or 80–89	90–95th or 120/80 mm Hg
Stage 1 hypertension	140–159	or 90–99	95–99th + 5 mm Hg[c]
Stage 2 hypertension	Greater than or equal to 160	Greater than or equal to 100	Greater than 99th + 5 mm Hg[d]

BP, blood pressure; DBP, diastolic blood pressure; SBP, systolic blood pressure.

[a]Defined as 18 years old or more.

[b]Tables contain the 50th, 90th, and 99th percentiles of SBP and DBP standards based on percentile height by age and sex, which is used to compare the child's measured BP on three separate occasions. The difference in BP of the 95th and 99th percentiles is 7 to 10 mm Hg, which requires an adjustment of 5 mm Hg to accurately categorize stage 1 or 2 hypertension. If the systolic and diastolic percentile categories are different, then classify hypertension by the higher BP value.

[c]Children and adolescents' stage 1 hypertension is classified by BP levels that range from the 95th percentile to 5 mm Hg above the 99th percentile.

[d]Children and adolescents' stage 2 hypertension is classified by BP levels that are greater than 5 mm Hg above the 99th percentile.

Adapted from Chobanian AV, Bakris GL, Black HR, et al. Seventh report of the Joint National Committee on Prevention, Detection, Evaluation, and Treatment of High Blood Pressure. Hypertension 2003;42:1206–1252.

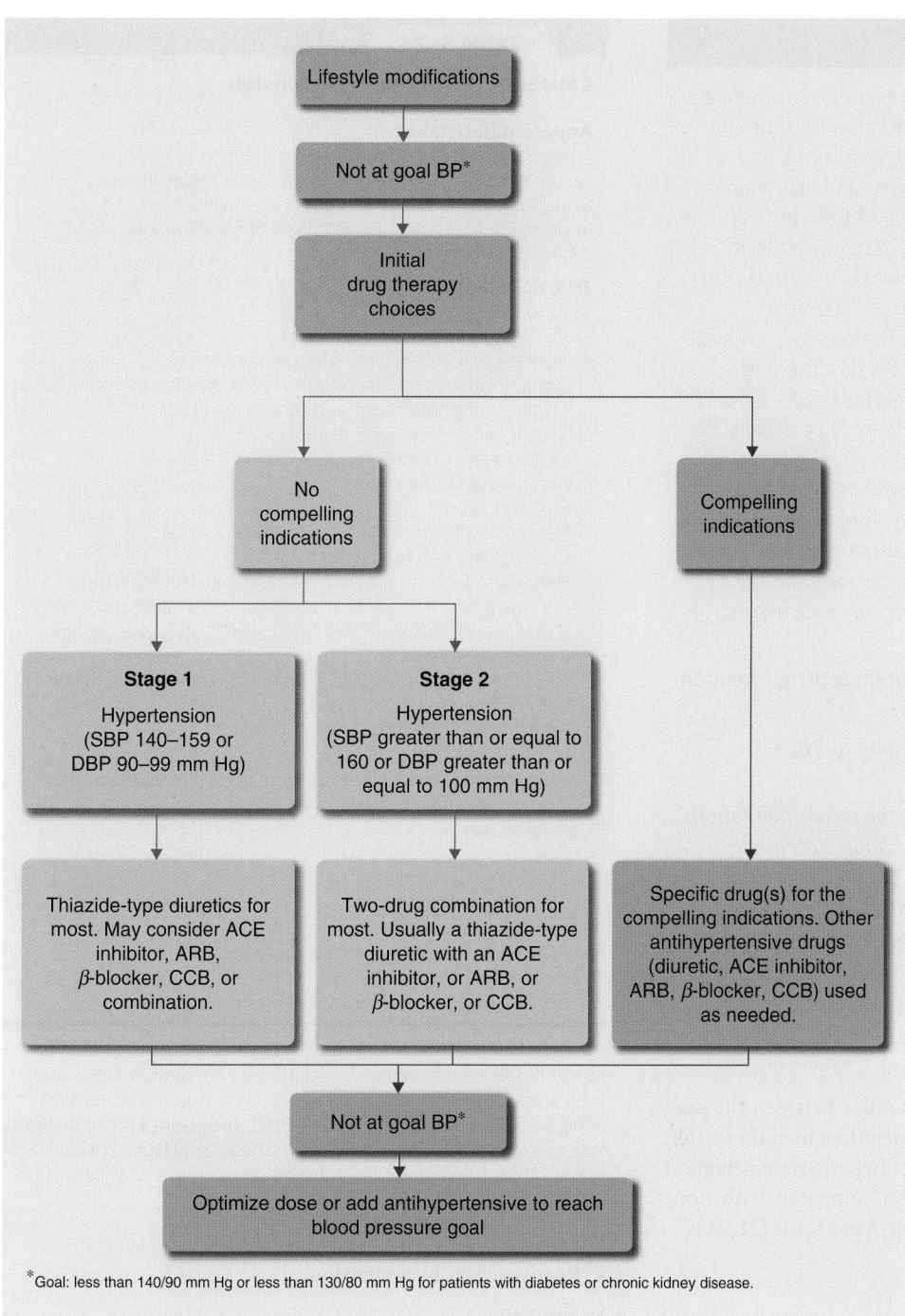

FIGURE 5–1. Algorithm for treatment of hypertension when patients are not at their goal BP. Compelling indications refer to specific indications where the selection of a particular antihypertensive drug class for a defined high-risk population is highly recommended. These recommendations are usually based on results from landmark randomized placebo-controlled outcome trials or consensus statements from clinical guidelines and are usually based on findings documenting superior outcomes in terms of morbidity and mortality. (ACE, angiotensin-converting enzyme; ARB, angiotensin receptor blocker; BP, blood pressure; CCB, calcium channel blocker; DBP, diastolic blood pressure; SBP, systolic blood pressure.) (From Chobanian AV, Bakris GL, Black HR, et al. Seventh report of the Joint National Committee on Prevention, Detection, Evaluation, and Treatment of High Blood Pressure. Hypertension 2003;42:1206–1252.)

EPIDEMIOLOGY

❶ *Hypertension is widely prevalent and significantly contributes to cardiovascular morbidity, mortality, and associated healthcare costs.* Worldwide prevalence of hypertension in 2000 was estimated to be 1 billion with a projected increase to over 1.5 billion by the year 2025.[4] Globally, 51% of all strokes and 45% of ischemic heart disease deaths are attributable to hypertension, and it is the leading risk factor for cause of death worldwide.[5] The prevalence of hypertension in the United States is among the highest in the world and estimated to include over 76 million individuals (1 in 3 adults 20 years of age or older), with an estimated $43.5 billion spent annually in direct and indirect costs. Furthermore, it is estimated that 29.7% of the U.S. population older than 20 years of age has prehypertension.[6] The prevalence of hypertension differs based on age, sex, and ethnicity. As individuals become older, their risk of systolic hypertension increases. Individuals 40 years of age who do not have hypertension are estimated to have a remaining lifetime risk of 90% of eventually developing hypertension. In the United States, hypertension is slightly more prevalent in men than

Patient Encounter 1

A 52-year-old African American man comes into your clinic with concerns about his BP. He arrived after his morning BP measurements at home were 154/96 mm Hg, and when repeated 160/100 mm Hg. Upon examination in your clinic, seated BP in the left arm is 144/86 mm Hg and 142/84 mm Hg in the right arm. You request that the patient return to your clinic in 1 week for a follow-up BP. His seated BPs in the left arm 1 week later were 148/84 mm Hg and 144/80 mm Hg. The patient's physical examination was unremarkable, but his past medical history was significant for dyslipidemia and depression. His previous cholesterol panel revealed a high-density lipoprotein of 52 mg/dL (1.34 mmol/L), triglyceride level of 180 mg/dL (2.03 mmol/L), and total cholesterol of 198 mg/dL (5.12 mmol/L). Calculated low-density lipoprotein level is 110 mg/dL (2.84 mmol/L). All other laboratory values were within normal limits. Of note, he does smoke one pack of cigarettes per day. Current medications include aspirin, simvastatin, and citalopram.

Based on the information above, what stage of hypertension does this patient have?

What is the patient's BP target according to JNC 7 guidelines?

What is the patient's BP target using the recommendations from the 2007 American Heart Association Statement on the treatment of hypertension in the prevention and management of ischemic heart disease?

What steps are involved in assuring that the patient's BP measurements are accurate?

Table 5–2

Causes of Resistant Hypertension

Apparent Resistance
Improper blood pressure measurement
Failure to receive or take antihypertensive medication
Inadequate doses (subtherapeutic)
Improper antihypertensive selection or combination
White coat effect

True Resistance
Secondary hypertension
Medication effects and interactions
  Nonsteroidal anti-inflammatory medications
  Sympathomimetics (decongestants, anorectics, and stimulants)
  Cocaine, amphetamines, and other illicit drugs
  Recent caffeine or nicotine intake
  Oral contraceptive hormones
  Adrenal steroid hormones
  Erythropoietin
  Natural licorice (including some chewing tobacco)
  Cyclosporine and tacrolimus
  Herbal products (ma huang, guarana, bitter orange, blue cohosh)
  Vascular endothelial growth factor inhibitors (bevacizumab, sorafenib, sunitinib)
  Neurologic and psychiatric agents (e.g., venlafaxine, modafinil)
  Volume overload
  Excess sodium intake
  Inadequate diuretic therapy
  Fluid retention from kidney disease or potent vasodilators (e.g., minoxidil)
Comorbidities
  Obesity
  Excess alcohol intake
  Chronic pain syndromes
  Intense vasoconstriction (arteritis)
  Anxiety-induced hyperventilation/panic attacks
Genetic variation
  Genetic differences in drug efficacy or metabolism

Adapted from Chobanian AV, Bakris GL, Black HR, et al. Seventh report of the Joint National Committee on Prevention, Detection, Evaluation, and Treatment of High Blood Pressure. Hypertension 2003;42:1206–1252; Izzo JL, Sica DA, Black HR, Council for High Blood Pressure Research (American Heart Association). Hypertension Primer, 4th ed. Philadelphia, PA: Lippincott Williams & Wilkins, 2008.

women before the age of 45 years, similar between the ages of 45 and 64 years, and higher in women than men thereafter. In addition, age-adjusted prevalence of hypertension is highest in non-Hispanic blacks (41.4%) when compared with non-Hispanic whites (28.1%) and Hispanic Americans (21.5%).[6]

ETIOLOGY

❷ *In most patients (greater than 90%), the cause of hypertension is unknown and referred to as primary hypertension as opposed to older nomenclature such as benign or essential hypertension.*[7] *However, in some patients there is an identifiable cause of hypertension, referred to as secondary hypertension. Common causes of secondary hypertension include*[1]:

- CKD
- Coarctation of the aorta
- Cushing's syndrome and other glucocorticoid excess states
- Drug induced/related (Table 5–2)
- Pheochromocytoma
- Primary aldosteronism and other mineralocorticoid excess states
- Renovascular hypertension
- Sleep apnea
- Thyroid or parathyroid disease

Identification of a secondary cause of hypertension is often not initially pursued unless suggested by routine clinical and laboratory evaluation of the patient or a failure to achieve BP control.

In addition to primary and secondary hypertension, the clinician may encounter what is referred to as resistant hypertension.[8] ❸ *Patients failing to achieve goal BP despite adherence to optimal doses of three antihypertensive agents of different classes (ideally, one being a diuretic) have resistant hypertension and should be evaluated for secondary causes of hypertension.* Several causes of resistant hypertension are listed in Table 5–2 and should be carefully considered in such patients.

PATHOPHYSIOLOGY

❹ *The pathophysiology of primary hypertension is heterogeneous but ultimately exerts its effects through the two primary determinants of BP:* cardiac output (CO) *and* peripheral resistance (PR). The processes influencing these two determinants are numerous and complex, and although the underlying cause of primary hypertension remains unknown, it is most likely multifactorial. An in-depth review of these mechanisms is beyond the scope of this text. See additional sources for more information on the pathophysiology behind the primary and secondary causes of hypertension.[7,9]

The development of primary hypertension can be summarized as an interplay between genetic and environmental factors and their subsequent interaction with multiple hypertensive mechanisms that can be classified as neural, renal, hormonal, and vascular. A brief description of these follows, but we remind you that no final common pathway has been identified, and as such, a single target for the treatment of primary hypertension remains elusive. Further complicating this is that different hemodynamic subsets and phenotypes of primary hypertension (e.g., diastolic hypertension in middle-aged persons, isolated systolic hypertension in the elderly, and obesity-related hypertension) may have different contributing mechanisms.[7]

Genetic Factors

Although multiple genetic polymorphisms have been associated with relatively small effects on hypertension including systolic blood pressure (SBP), diastolic blood pressure (DBP), and response to antihypertensive medications, replication of these findings in large populations are generally lacking. Consequently, the information available to date is far from being able to be used as a basis for any practical guidance for clinicians.[7] Nevertheless, it is estimated that up to 60% of the familial association of BP has a genetic basis,[10,11] and increasingly the genetic basis of variability in response to drug therapy continues to be pursued aggressively. Although progress related to understanding of drug response variability continues through utilizing novel approaches and large databases,[12] the status of these efforts and specific candidate gene approaches have yet to translate into any genetic-based guidance for clinicians seeking to use these tools when selecting and utilizing antihypertensive agents.[13]

Environmental Factors

As opposed to genetic factors, environmental factors contributing to hypertension are well characterized. Cigarette smoking (cigars and smokeless tobacco too) and caffeine cause transient increases in BP via norepinephrine release and, in the case of caffeine, by its antagonism of vasodilatory adenosine receptors.[14] Acute alcohol ingestion may have a variable effect (increased due to sympathetic nerve activity or lowering due to vasodilation), which is transient, whereas chronic heavy consumption of alcohol and binge drinking raises the risk of hypertension.[7,15] Many other environmental factors have been shown, or been proposed, to influence BP and, in some cases, contribute to the development of hypertension. Some of the more common ones include obesity, physical inactivity, fetal environment (e.g., maternal malnutrition, increased fetal exposure to maternal glucocorticoids), postnatal weight gain, potassium and magnesium depletion, vitamin D deficiency, and environmental toxins (e.g., lead).[7] Many of these environmental factors can and should be addressed by comprehensive dietary and lifestyle counseling by healthcare providers during patient encounters.

Neural Mechanisms

Overactivity of the sympathetic nervous system (SNS) in the early stages of primary hypertension manifests as increased heart rate, CO, and peripheral vasoconstriction. Despite this, it has been difficult to quantify the overall contribution of the SNS, and recent cardiovascular outcome trials have found that drugs targeting the SNS (α-adrenergic and β-adrenergic blockers) have not performed as well as other classes of drugs. Nevertheless, strategies aimed at targeting the SNS continue to be pursued with specific interest in invasive strategies aimed at severe refractory hypertension. These include baroreflex sensitization via implantation of a carotid sinus pacemaker and renal sympathetic denervation via catheter-based radiofrequency ablation.[7,16]

Renal Mechanisms

The contribution of sodium to the development of primary hypertension is related to excess sodium intake and/or abnormal sodium excretion by the kidneys. Proposed mechanisms supporting either of these are numerous and complex.[7] However, it is generally accepted that dietary salt is associated with increases in BP that can be lowered with reduction of sodium intake, particularly in individuals deemed salt sensitive.[3,17] Although variables such as ethnicity and level of hypertension play a role, some 30% to 50% of subjects may be salt sensitive. For example, 29% of the participants in the Dietary Approaches to Stop Hypertension (DASH)-Sodium trial were deemed to be salt sensitive and responded to reductions in salt intake.[17,18] In addition, there appears to be a threshold effect of sodium intake in the range of 50 to 100 mmol/day (1.2 to 2.4 g) and its impact on BP. The mean sodium intake per day is 175 mmol (4.1 g) for men and 120 mmol (2.7 g) for women in the United States, with the majority derived from processed foods.[3] Although population-wide based reduction in dietary sodium intake via global policies has been widely advocated as an approach to reduce hypertension and cardiovascular disease (CVD), it is not universally accepted, with calls for further scientific investigation into the matter.[19,20]

Hormonal Mechanisms

Since the discovery of renin over 100 years ago, the renin-angiotensin-aldosterone system (RAAS) has been extensively studied as a prime target or site of action for many effective antihypertensives.[21] Renin is produced and stored

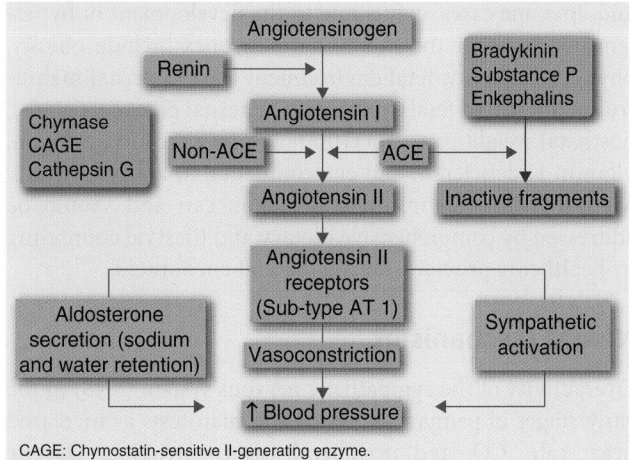

CAGE: Chymostatin-sensitive II-generating enzyme.

FIGURE 5–2. Diagram of the RAAS, a key system involved in the modulation of BP. The diagram depicts the pathways involved in the action of various antihypertensives including ACE inhibitors, ARBs, diuretics, and aldosterone antagonists. By inhibiting the action of angiotensin-converting enzymes, ACE inhibitors reduce both the formation of the vasoconstrictor angiotensin II and the degradation of vasodilating substances including bradykinin. ARBs primarily act through inhibition of the action of angiotensin II on the angiotensin-I receptors that modulate vasoconstriction. Aldosterone antagonists directly inhibit the actions of aldosterone; diuretics affect sodium and water retention at a renal level. (ACE, angiotensin-converting enzyme; ARB, angiotensin receptor blockers; AT1, angiotensin-1; BP, blood pressure; RAAS, renin-angiotensin aldosterone system.) (From Victor RG, Kaplan NM. Kaplan's Clinical Hypertension, 10th ed. Philadelphia, PA: Wollters Kluwer Lippincott Williams & Wilkins Health, 2010.)

in the juxtaglomerular cells of the kidney, and its release is stimulated by impaired renal perfusion, salt depletion, and β_1-adrenergic stimulation. The release of renin is the rate-limiting step in the eventual formation of angiotensin II, which is primarily responsible for the pressor effects mediated by the RAAS (Fig. 5–2[7]). The role of the RAAS in primary hypertension is supported by the presence of high levels of renin, suggesting the system is inappropriately activated. Proposed mechanisms behind this inappropriate activation include increased sympathetic drive, defective regulation of the RAAS (nonmodulation), and the existence of a subpopulation of ischemic nephrons that release excess renin.[7] However, there are also patients with primary hypertension and low levels of renin. This observation suggests that alternative mechanisms for hypertension unrelated to renin levels or activity may be in play, prompting renewed investigation into the use of plasma renin activity (PRA) measurements to guide antihypertensive therapy selection.[22–24] In fact, it has been demonstrated that patients with low PRA (less than 0.65 ng/mL/h [0.18 ng/L/s]) respond preferentially to diuretics, aldosterone antagonists, and calcium channel blockers, whereas those with higher PRA levels respond preferentially

to renin-mediated therapies such as β-blockers, angiotensin-converting enzyme (ACE) inhibitors, angiotensin receptor blockers (ARBs), and direct renin inhibitors.[25–27]

Vascular Mechanisms

Elevated peripheral arterial resistance is the hemodynamic hallmark of primary hypertension. The increase in peripheral resistance typically observed may be due to a reduction in the arterial lumen size as a result of vascular remodeling. This remodeling, or change in vascular tone, may be modulated by various endothelium-derived vasoactive substances, growth factors, and cytokines. This increase in arterial stiffness or reduced compliance results in the observed increase in systolic BP.[7]

Contributing Comorbidities

Several comorbidities have a high concurrence with the presence of hypertension leading to a higher risk of target organ damage, cardiovascular morbidity and mortality, and overall healthcare costs. Specifically, these include the presence of diabetes mellitus, dyslipidemia, obesity, and CKD. As such, the assessment of global cardiovascular risk in all patients with hypertension should be part of the management plan while also pursuing target BPs through nonpharmacologic and pharmacologic means. Regardless of the initiating process or processes leading to the development of hypertension, the ultimate goal is to reduce the risk of cardiovascular events and minimize target organ damage. This clearly requires the early identification of risk factors and treatment of patients with hypertension.

MEASUREMENT OF BLOOD PRESSURE

⑤ *Appropriate technique in measuring BP is a vital component to the diagnosis and continued management of hypertension.* Accurate measurement of a patient's BP identifies and controls for factors that may influence the variability in the measure. Failure to consider how each of these factors may influence BP measurement results in significant variation, leading to misclassification or inaccurate assessments of risk. Factors including body position, cuff size, device selection, auscultatory technique, and dietary intake prior to the clinic visit may contribute to such inaccuracies. Clinicians should instruct patients to avoid exercise, alcohol, caffeine, or nicotine consumption 30 minutes before BP measurement. Patients should be sitting comfortably with their back supported and arm free of constrictive clothing with legs uncrossed and feet flat on the floor for a minimum of 5 minutes before the first reading. Systolic and diastolic BP tend to increase when the cuff size is too small. Ideally, the cuff bladder should encircle at least 80% of the arm's circumference to ensure a more accurate measurement of BP.

Mercury sphygmomanometers are recommended for routine office measurements, but concerns of patient exposure and environmental contamination of mercury have fostered the development of other devices to measure BP.

Clinical Presentation and Diagnosis of Primary Hypertension

General

Age: Prevalence of hypertension is likely to be highest with middle-aged or older patients

Sex: In the United States, hypertension is slightly more prevalent in men than women before the age of 45 years, similar between the ages of 45 and 64 years, and higher in women than men thereafter

Symptoms

The patient with primary hypertension may be asymptomatic yet still have major CVD risk factors

Signs

Adult patients have an average of two or more BP readings (SBP and DBP) on two separate occasions indicating either:

	SBP (mm Hg)	DBP (mm Hg)
Normal	Less than 120	Less than 80
Prehypertension	120–139	or 80–89
Stage 1 hypertension	140–159	or 90–99
Stage 2 hypertension	Greater than or equal to 160	Greater than or equal to 100

Laboratory Tests (not necessarily indicative of hypertension but should be measured in patients with hypertension)

Fasting lipid panel:

- Low-density lipoprotein greater than 160 mg/dL (4.14 mmol/L)
- Total cholesterol greater than 240 mg/dL (6.21 mmol/L)
- HDL less than 40 mg/dL (1.03 mmol/L)
- Triglycerides greater than 200 mg/dL (2.26 mmol/L)

Fasting plasma glucose or hemoglobin A1c (does not need to be fasting):

- Impaired fasting glucose is 100–125 mg/dL (5.6–6.9 mmol/L)
- Diagnosis of diabetes with fasting glucose greater than or equal to 126 mg/dL (7.0 mmol/L) or a hemoglobin A1c

greater than or equal to 6.5% (0.065; 48 mmol/mol Hb) on two separate occasions, or a random plasma glucose reading of greater than or equal to 200 mg/L (11.1 mmol/L) with symptoms of diabetes

The following abnormal tests may indicate hypertension-related damage:

- Serum creatinine elevated (greater than 1.2 mg/dL [106 µmol/L])
- **Microalbuminuria,** which is diagnosed either from a 24-hour urine collection (20–200 mcg/min) or from elevated concentrations (30–300 mg/L) on at least two occasions. Use of the albumin-to-creatinine ratio (ACR) in a spot urine sample is becoming more common, and microalbuminuria is defined by this measure as 30–300 mg/g creatinine (3.4–33.9 mg/mmol creatinine)

Common Comorbidities and Factors Contributing to CV Risk

Diabetes mellitus

Metabolic syndrome

Insulin resistance

Dyslipidemia

Microalbuminuria/CKD

Family history

Central obesity

Physical inactivity

Tobacco use

Target Organ Damage

Heart (left ventricular hypertrophy, angina, prior myocardial infarction, prior coronary revascularization, HF)

Brain (stroke or transient ischemic attack, dementia)

CKD

Peripheral arterial disease

Retinopathy

However, there is no general consensus among healthcare providers as to an acceptable replacement for mercury sphygmomanometers.

To reduce deviations in BP measurement in the clinic, the patient and clinician should not talk during BP readings. The measurement arm is supported and positioned at heart level. If a mercury or aneroid device is used, then the palpatory method must be used first to estimate the SBP.[28] If an automated device is used, this is not necessary. After the patient's cuff is inflated above the systolic pressure, the mercury column should drop at a rate of 2 to 3 mm Hg/s. A stethoscope placed over the brachial artery in the antecubital fossa identifies the first and last

audible Korotkoff sounds, which should be taken as systolic and diastolic pressure, respectively. A minimum of two readings at least 1 minute apart are then averaged. If measurements vary by more than 5 mm Hg between the two readings, then one or two additional BP measurements are collected and the multiple readings averaged. BP classification is based on the average of two or more properly measured, seated BP readings on each of two or more office visits. Details and further recommendations for accurate measurement of BP in special populations can be reviewed in the American College of Cardiology (ACC)/AHA BP Measurement in Humans Statement for healthcare professionals.[28] Finally, the measurement of clinic or office BPs is poorly correlated with assessments of BP in other settings. Consequently, under select circumstances, clinicians are increasingly using 24-hour ambulatory BP monitoring devices and home BP monitors. These tools are useful in identifying patients with white coat hypertension or with elevations of BP during the night. They may also aid in the management of refractory hypertension with minor target organ damage, those with suspected autonomic neuropathy, those with hypotensive symptoms, and patients with large differences between home and clinic BP measurements. Benefits derived from alternative BP monitoring may be of greater prognostic significance than traditional office-based measurements.[28]

TREATMENT

Desired Outcomes

Hypertension management by nonpharmacologic and pharmacologic therapies has proven useful in reducing the risk of MI, HF, stroke, and kidney disease–associated morbidity and mortality. For every 20 mm Hg systolic or 10 mm Hg diastolic increase in BP above 115/75 mm Hg, there is a doubling of mortality for both ischemic heart disease and stroke.[29] The goal of BP management is to reduce the risk of CVD and target organ damage. Targeting a specific BP is actually a surrogate goal that has been associated with reductions in CVD and target organ damage.

General Approach to Treatment

❻ *Drug selection for the management of patients with hypertension should be considered as adjunctive to nonpharmacologic approaches for BP lowering, and ultimately the attainment of target BP in many cases may be more important than the antihypertensive agent used.* Previous clinical research has established the relative value of using individual antihypertensive drugs versus placebo to achieve reduction in morbidity and mortality by lowering BP. However, as newer antihypertensive agents are developed, it is difficult to justify the comparison of newer agents to placebo on ethical grounds. Consequently, contemporary large outcome-based multicenter trials have been designed to compare one specific agent-based therapy (along with options to add others) versus another agent-based therapy (along with options to add others of a different class). These attempts at "head-to-head" comparisons and meta-analyses of multidrug regimen trials have, in general, provided evidence supporting the position that the main benefits of pharmacologic therapy are related to the achievement of BP lowering and are generally largely independent of the selection of an individual drug regimen. Inherent in this position is the realization that nonpharmacologic approaches alone are rarely successful in attaining target BPs, and multidrug therapy (sometimes as many as three or more agents) is necessary for most patients with hypertension.[30] The JNC 7 focuses on utilizing BP levels in determining the threshold and target for treatment, and the European Society of Cardiology also incorporates total cardiovascular risk in determining thresholds for treatment. This approach results in a "flexible" definition of hypertension that depends on an individual's total cardiovascular risk.[8] Although acknowledging there are several approaches currently used to manage patients with hypertension, this chapter uses as its basis the AHA Scientific Statement on the treatment of hypertension in the prevention and management of ischemic heart disease, and the JNC 7 guidelines, while recognizing important recommendations in the ACCF/ AHA expert consensus document on hypertension in the elderly.

Nonpharmacologic Treatment: Lifestyle Modifications

Therapeutic lifestyle modifications consisting of nonpharmacologic approaches to BP reduction should be an active part of all treatment plans for patients with hypertension. The most widely studied interventions demonstrating effectiveness include:

- Weight reduction in overweight or obese individuals
- Adoption of a diet rich in potassium and calcium
- Dietary sodium restriction
- Physical activity
- Moderation of alcohol consumption

❼ *Implementation of these lifestyle modifications successfully lowers BP (Table 5–3), often with results similar to those of therapy with a single antihypertensive agent.*[31] Combinations of two or more lifestyle modifications can have even greater effects with BP lowering. BP lowering in overweight patients may be seen by a weight loss of as few as 4.5 kg (10 lb). The DASH trial demonstrated that a diet high in fruits, vegetables, and low-fat dairy products, along with a reduced intake of total and saturated fat, significantly reduced BP in as little as 8 weeks.[32] Sodium restriction in moderate amounts lowers BP, is generally well accepted, and is free of adverse effects, particularly in salt-sensitive individuals.[17,18] Restriction of sodium intake to 2.4 g (100 mmol) of elemental sodium (6 g of sodium chloride or 1 teaspoon of table salt) should be easily achievable in most patients simply by avoidance of highly salted processed foods.[33] Simple dietary advice and instructions on reading packaging labels should be introduced to the patient initially and assessed and reinforced at subsequent office visits. As is the case with weight loss, changes in physical activity do not need to be profound to have a significant effect on BP. It is generally accepted that 30 minutes of moderately intense aerobic activity (e.g., brisk walking) most days of the week will lower BP.[31] Although many patients can safely engage in moderately intense aerobic activity, individuals with known CVD, multiple risk factors with symptoms, or selected diabetic patients should undergo medical examination, possibly including exercise testing, prior to participation.[34,35] The acute effects of alcohol on BP are variable as previously described. Abstinence from alcohol in heavy drinkers leads to a reduction in BP.[36] In addition, alcohol also attenuates the effects of antihypertensive

Table 5–3		
Lifestyle Modifications to Manage Hypertension[a,3]		
Modification	**Recommendation**	**Approximate Systolic BP Reduction (Range)**
Weight reduction	Maintain normal body weight (body mass index: 18.5–24.9 kg/m²)	5–20 mm Hg/10 kg
Adopt DASH eating plan	Consume a diet rich in fruits, vegetables, and low-fat dairy products with a reduced content of saturated and total fat	8–14 mm Hg
Dietary sodium restriction	Reduce dietary sodium intake to no more than 100 mmol/day (2.4 g sodium or 6 g sodium chloride)	2–8 mm Hg
Physical activity	Engage in regular aerobic physical activity such as brisk walking (at least 30 min/day, most days of the week)	4–9 mm Hg
Moderation of alcohol consumption	Limit consumption to no more than 2 drinks (e.g., 24 oz [710 mL] beer, 10 oz [296 mL] wine, or 3 oz [89 mL] 80-proof whiskey) per day in most men and to no more than 1 drink per day in women and lighter weight persons	2–4 mm Hg

BP, blood pressure; DASH, Dietary Approaches to Stop Hypertension.

[a]For overall cardiovascular risk reduction, stop smoking. The effects of implementing these modifications are dose and time dependent and could be greater for some individuals.

therapy, which is mostly reversible within 1 to 2 weeks with moderation of intake.

In addition to their beneficial effects on lowering BP, lifestyle modifications also have a favorable effect on other risk factors such as dyslipidemia and insulin resistance, which are commonly encountered in the hypertensive population, and lifestyle modifications should be encouraged for this reason as well. Smoking cessation should also be encouraged for overall cardiovascular health despite its lack of chronic effects on BP.[37,38] Although lifestyle modifications have never been documented to reduce cardiovascular morbidity and mortality in patients with hypertension, they do effectively lower BP to some extent in most hypertensive patients. This may obviate the need for drug therapy in those with mild elevations in BP or minimize the doses or number of antihypertensive agents required in those with greater elevations in BP.

Pharmacologic Treatment

❽ *An approach to selection of drugs for the treatment of patients with hypertension should be evidence-based with considerations regarding the individual's coexisting disease states, co-prescribed medications, and practical patient-specific issues including cost.* The JNC 7 report and statements from other global organizations recommend drug therapy that is largely grounded in the best available evidence for superiority in outcomes—specifically morbidity and mortality.[1] The approach is often tempered with practical considerations related to competing options for specific comorbidities and issues regarding a patient's experience or tolerance for side effects and, in some cases, the cost of medications.

Although landmark trials such as the Antihypertensive and Lipid-Lowering Treatment to Prevent Heart Attack Trial (ALLHAT) have provided some objective basis for comparisons between initiating antihypertensive drug therapy with

one class of antihypertensives versus another, there is room for criticism of these studies.[30,39,40] Consequently, practical interpretations of their conclusions must always leave room for individualization based on clinical judgment. Overall, current clinical guidelines provide a reasonable basis for guiding the selection of drug classes for individuals based on their stage of hypertension, comorbidities, and special circumstances. The following section summarizes key features of specific drug classes and guideline recommendations for patients with hypertension. Finally, an overview of the specific oral antihypertensive drug classes in common use is summarized in Table 5–4.

Diuretics

Many authorities recognize the value of diuretics in the management of patients with hypertension. Among others, the basis for endorsement of diuretics for a variety of patient types includes their practical attributes (acquisition cost and availability as combination agents), extent of experience, and favorable outcomes in placebo-controlled trials.[1,3] These virtues are supported by results of studies such as ALLHAT.[30] This landmark double-blind study tested the hypothesis that newer antihypertensive agents would outperform thiazide-type diuretics when selected as initial drug therapy. After 4.9 years of follow-up in over 42,000 patients, the primary end point of fatal coronary heart disease and nonfatal MI was indistinguishable between chlorthalidone versus either amlodipine or lisinopril. A fourth arm examining doxazosin was terminated early based on a higher risk of HF for doxazosin compared with chlorthalidone.[65] In spite of these findings for the primary end point, differences in outcomes for select secondary end points demonstrated superiority of chlorthalidone over either of the two remaining comparison groups. These observations, along with perceived cost effectiveness (which was not specifically evaluated in this study), led the

Table 5–4

Commonly Used Oral Antihypertensive Drugs by Pharmacologic Class

Class	Drug Name and Usual Oral Dosage Range (mg/day)	Compelling Indications	Clinical Trials	Select Adverse Events	Comments[a]
Diuretic					
Thiazides	Chlorthalidone (Hygroton) 6.25–25 Indapamide (Lozol) 1.25–5 Hydrochlorothiazide 12.5–50 Metolazone (Zaroxolyn) 2.5–5	Heart failure stage A [chlorthalidone] High coronary disease risk [chlorthalidone] Diabetes [chlorthalidone] Stroke [perindopril + indapamide]	ALLHAT[30] PROGRESS[41] HYVET[42]	Hypokalemia and other electrolyte imbalances Negative effect on glucose and lipids	Chlorthalidone is about twice as potent as hydrochlorothiazide Thiazide diuretics are generally more effective antihypertensive agents than loop diuretics Not first-line agents in pregnancy, but probably safe per JNC 7 Monitor electrolytes (i.e., decreased serum potassium) and metabolic abnormalities (i.e., dyslipidemia, hyperglycemia) Use caution in patients with gout Contraindications include hypersensitivity, anuria, renal decompensation
Loops	Bumetanide (Bumex) 1–4 Furosemide (Lasix) 40–160 Torsemide (Demadex) 2.5–10				Monitor electrolytes (i.e., decreased potassium) and metabolic abnormalities (i.e., dyslipidemia, hyperglycemia) Use with caution in patients with gout Contraindications include hypersensitivity, anuria, acute renal insufficiency, hyperkalemia
Potassium-sparing aldosterone antagonists	Amiloride (Midamor) 5–20 Triamterene (Dyrenium) 50–200 Spironolactone (Aldactone) 25–100 Eplerenone (Inspra) 50–200	Heart failure [spironolactone] Heart failure post-MI [eplerenone]	RALES[43] EPHESUS[44]	Hyperkalemia Gynecomastia [spironolactone]	Potassium-sparing diuretics may enhance hyperkalemic effects of drug therapies (e.g., ACE inhibitor, aldosterone antagonist) Monitor electrolytes (i.e., decreased potassium) and metabolic abnormalities (i.e., dyslipidemias, hyperglycemia) Use with caution in patients with gout Contraindications include hypersensitivity, anuria, acute renal insufficiency, hyperkalemia Eplerenone contraindicated as an antihypertensive in patients with estimated creatinine clearance less than 50 mL/min (0.83 mL/s) or serum creatinine greater than 1.8 mg/dL (159 μmol/L) for women or 2 mg/dL (177 μmol/L) in men as well as type 2 diabetes mellitus with microalbuminuria. Also contraindicated in patients concomitantly receiving strong CYP3A4 inhibitors or a serum potassium greater than 5.5 mEq/L (5.5 mmol/L) at initiation
β-Blocker					
Cardioselective	Atenolol (Tenormin) 25–100 Bisoprolol (Zebeta) 2.5–10 Metoprolol tartrate (Lopressor) 100–200 Metoprolol succinate (Toprol XL) 50–100	Heart failure [metoprolol XL, carvedilol, bisoprolol] Heart failure post-MI [carvedilol] Post-MI [propranolol, β₁-antagonists]	MERIT-HF[45] COPERNICUS[46] CAPRICORN[47] BHAT[48] CIBIS-II[49]	Bradycardia Heart block Heart failure Hypotension/syncope Dyspnea, bronchospasm Fatigue, dizziness, lethargy, depression	Caution with heart rate less than 60 and respiratory disease Selectivity of β₁ agents is diminished at higher doses Abrupt discontinuation may cause rebound hypertension May mask signs/symptoms of hypoglycemia in diabetic patients

Class	Drug (brand) dose	Indications (trials)	Adverse effects	Contraindications/Cautions
Nonselective	Nadolol (Corgard) 40–120 Nebivolol (Bystolic) 2.5–40 Propranolol (Inderal) 40–160 Propranolol long-acting (Inderal LA, InnoPran XL) 60–180 Timolol (Blocadren) 20–40		Hyper/hypoglycemia, hyperkalemia, hyperlipidemia	Contraindicated in hypersensitivity, sinus node dysfunction or severe sinus bradycardia (in the absence of a pacemaker), heart block (greater than first-degree), cardiogenic shock, acute decompensated heart failure
Mixed α- and β-blocker	Carvedilol (Coreg) 25–100 Carvedilol CR (Coreg CR) 20–80 Labetalol (Trandate) 200–800	High coronary disease risk		

CCBA

Class	Drug (brand) dose	Indications (trials)	Adverse effects	Contraindications/Cautions
Nondihydropyridine	Diltiazem long-acting (Cardizem SR, Cardizem CD, others) 180–420 Verapamil sustained-release (Calan SR, Isoptin SR, Verelan) 120–360	High coronary disease risk [verapamil-trandolapril] INVEST[50] VALUE[40] ASCOT[39] Diabetes	Bradycardia, heart block [nondihydropyridines] Constipation [nondihydropyridines] Hypotension Peripheral edema, headache, flushing	Caution with heart rate less than 60 [verapamil, diltiazem] Use caution in concomitant use with β-blocker; may potentiate heart block Extended-release formulations are preferred for once- or twice-daily medication administration Contraindicated in hypersensitivity, sinus node dysfunction, or severe sinus bradycardia (in the absence of a pacemaker) [nondihydropyridines], heart block (greater than first degree) in the absence of a pacemaker [nondihydropyridines], atrial fibrillation/flutter associated with accessory bypass tract [nondihydropyridines], severe hypotension (systolic less than 90 mm Hg) [nondihydropyridines], severe left ventricular dysfunction [nondihydropyridines]
Dihydropyridines	Amlodipine (Norvasc) 2.5–10 Felodipine (Plendil) 5–20 Isradipine SR (DynaCirc SR) 2.5–10 Nicardipine SR (Cardene SR) 60–120 Nifedipine long-acting (Adalat CC, Procardia XL) 30–60 Nisoldipine (Sular) 10–40		Gingival hyperplasia [dihydropyridines] Reflex tachycardia [dihydropyridine]	
ACE Inhibitor	Benazepril (Lotensin) 20–80 Captopril (Capoten) 25–100 Enalapril (Vasotec) 2.5–40 Fosinopril (Monopril) 10–40 Lisinopril (Prinivil, Zestril) 10–40 Moexipril (Univasc) 7.5–30 Perindopril (Aceon) 4–8 Quinapril (Accupril) 10–40 Ramipril (Altace) 2.5–20 Trandolapril (Mavik) 1–4	Heart failure [enalapril] Heart failure post-MI [ramipril, trandolapril] Post-MI [captopril] High coronary disease risk [ramipril, perindopril] Diabetes [captopril] Chronic kidney disease [captopril, ramipril] Stroke [perindopril + indapamide] SOLVD[51] AIRE[52] TRACE[53] SAVE[54] HOPE[56] EUROPA[57] Captopril Trial[55] PROGRESS[41]	Cough Hyperkalemia Renal function deterioration Angioedema Hypotension/syncope	Monitor electrolytes (i.e., increased serum potassium) Monitor renal function with serum creatinine and blood urea nitrogen Initial dose may be reduced in renal impairment, the elderly, patients who are volume depleted or maintained on diuretic therapy Contraindicated in pregnancy and hypersensitivity, bilateral renal artery stenosis or unilateral renal artery stenosis in a solitary functional kidney, serum potassium greater than 5.5 mEq/L (5.5 mmol/L) that cannot be reduced
ARB	Candesartan (Atacand) 8–32 Eprosartan (Teveten) 400–800 Irbesartan (Avapro) 150–300 Losartan (Cozaar) 25–100 Olmesartan (Benicar) 20–40 Telmisartan (Micardis) 20–80 Valsartan (Diovan) 80–320	Heart failure [valsartan, candesartan] High coronary disease risk [losartan] Diabetes CKD [irbesartan, losartan] CHARM[58] LIFE[59] RENAAL[60] IDNT[61] IRMA-II[62] ValHeFT[63]	Hyperkalemia Renal function deterioration Angioedema Hypotension/syncope	Monitor electrolytes (i.e., increased serum potassium) Monitor renal function with serum creatinine and blood urea nitrogen Contraindicated in pregnancy and hypersensitivity

(Continued)

Table 5–4

Commonly Used Oral Antihypertensive Drugs by Pharmacologic Class (*Continued*)

Class	Drug Name and Usual Oral Dosage Range (mg/day)	Compelling Indications	Clinical Trials	Select Adverse Events	Comments[a]
Central α-2 Agonists	Methyldopa 250–1,000 Clonidine (Catapres) 0.1–0.8 Clonidine patch (Catapres TTS) 0.1–0.3 Guanabenz 4–32 Guanfacine 0.5–2	No recommendations at this time		Transient sedation initially Hepatotoxicity, hemolytic anemia, peripheral edema (methyldopa) Orthostatic hypotension (methyldopa, clonidine) Dry mouth, muscle weakness (clonidine)	First-line agent in pregnancy [methyldopa] Tolerance may occur 2–3 months after initiation of methyldopa; increase dose or add diuretic Contraindications include hypersensitivity, concurrent use of MAO inhibitor [methyldopa], hepatic disease [methyldopa]
α-1 Blockers	Doxazosin (Cardura) 1–16 Prazosin (Minipress) 2–20 Terazosin (Hytrin) 1–20	Benign prostatic hyperplasia		Syncope Dizziness Palpitations	Contraindicated in hypersensitivity
Direct Vasodilators	Isosorbide dinitrate 20 mg and hydralazine 37.5 (BiDil) 1–2 tablets three times a day Hydralazine (Apresoline) 25–100 Minoxidil (Loniten) 2.5–80	Heart failure [isosorbide dinitrate + hydralazine in African Americans]	A-HeFT[64]	Edema [minoxidil] Tachycardia Lupus-like syndrome [hydralazine]	Give minoxidil with diuretic and β-blocker Contraindicated in hypersensitivity, pheochromocytoma (minoxidil), acute closure glaucoma, head trauma or cerebral hemorrhage (isosorbide dinitrate + hydralazine)
Direct Renin Inhibitors	Aliskiren (Tekturna) 150–300	No recommendations at this time		Hyperkalemia Hypotension	Use caution in patients with severe renal impairment and in patients with deteriorating renal function or renal artery stenosis, both bi- and unilateral
Peripheral Sympathetic Inhibitors	Reserpine 0.05–0.25 Guanethidine 10–50 Guanadrel 10–75	No recommendations at this time		Mental depression Orthostatic hypotension Peripheral vascular disease Nasal congestion, fluid retention, peripheral edema Diarrhea, increased gastric secretion	Contraindications include hypersensitivity, peptic ulcer disease or ulcerative colitis [reserpine], history of mental depression or electroconvulsive therapy [reserpine], pheochromocytoma [guanethidine, guanadrel], concurrent use (within 1 week) of MAO inhibitor [guanethidine, guanadrel], heart failure exacerbation [guanethidine, guanadrel]

A-HeFT, African American Heart Failure Trial; ACE, angiotensin-converting enzyme; AIRE, Acute Infarction Ramipril Efficacy study; ALLHAT, Antihypertensive and Lipid-Lowering to Treatment Prevent Heart Attack Trial; ARB, angiotensin receptor blocker; ASCOT, Anglo-Scandinavian Cardiac Output Trial; BHAT, Beta-Blocker Heart Attack Trial; bpm, beats per minute; CAPRICORN, Carvedilol Post-Infarct Survival Control in Left Ventricular Dysfunction Trial; Captopril Trial; Collaborative Study Captopril Trial ("The Effect of Angiotensin-Converting Enzyme Inhibition on Diabetic Nephropathy"); CCBA, calcium channel blocker agent; CHARM, Candesartan in Heart Failure Assessment of Reduction in Morbidity and Mortality Trial; CIBIS-II, The Cardiac Insufficiency Bisoprolol Study II; CKD, chronic kidney disease; COPERNICUS, Carvedilol Prospective Randomized Cumulative Survival Trial; EPHESUS, Eplerenone Post-Acute Myocardial Infarction Heart Failure Efficacy and Survival Study; EUROPA, European Trial on Reduction of Cardiac Events with Perindopril in Stable Coronary Artery Disease Trial; HOPE, Heart Outcomes Prevention Evaluation Study; HYVET, Hypertension in the Very Elderly Trial; IDNT, Irbesartan Diabetic Nephropathy Trial; INVEST, International Verapamil-Trandolapril Study; IRMA-II, Irbesartan in Patients with Type 2 Diabetes and Microalbuminuria study; ISA, intrinsic sympathomimetic activity; JNC 7, Joint National Commission Seventh Report; LIFE, Losartan Intervention For Endpoint reduction in hypertension study; MAO, monoamine oxidase; MERIT-HF, Metoprolol CR/XL Randomized Intervention Trial in Congestive Heart Failure; MI, myocardial infarction; PROGRESS, Perindopril Protection Against Recurrent Stroke Study; RALES, Randomized Aldactone Evaluation Study; RENAAL, Reduction of Endpoints in NIDDM with the Angiotensin II Antagonist Losartan study; SAVE, Survival and Ventricular Enlargement trial; SOLVD, Studies of Left Ventricular Dysfunction; TRACE, Trandolapril Cardiac Evaluation; VALUE, Valsartan Antihypertensive Long-term Use Evaluation; ValHeFT, Veterans Affairs Cooperative I study.

[a]Comments listed are not intended to be inclusive of all adverse effects, monitoring parameters, cautions, or contraindications, and may vary by source.

authors of JNC 7 to endorse diuretics as initial drug therapy for most patients with hypertension. Nonetheless, substantial criticism of this trial has undermined the enthusiasm for diuretics as first-line therapy in the minds of some clinicians, as well as members of international guideline committees.[8] Criticism of the differential BPs achieved in the various treatment groups, the artificial construct guiding the use of add-on drugs to base therapy, and the overrepresentation of African Americans exhibiting select end points have weakened the interpretability of the authors' conclusions. Furthermore, other contemporary studies have also challenged the status of diuretics as ideal baseline choices for initial antihypertensive drug therapy for all patients.[39,40] This has refueled the debate over whether the means by which BP is lowered (drug selection) is more or less important than the extent and/or time taken to lower BP.[66] Furthermore, controversy has ignited as to whether the choice and dose of diuretic versus hydrochlorothiazide was partly responsible for the difference in study results, and it has raised the question whether chlorthalidone should be the preferred thiazide-type diuretic.[67] Nonetheless, diuretics remain supported by many as acceptable baseline initial therapy for hypertensive patients without compelling indications.

Key features of diuretics that must be kept in mind, along with evidence from outcome-based studies, include the diversity between the subtypes of diuretics and their corresponding diversity of pharmacologic actions. The four subtypes include thiazides, loop diuretics, potassium-sparing agents, and aldosterone antagonists. The latter will be discussed as a separate entity. Each subtype has clinically based properties that distinguish their roles in select patient populations. Thiazide diuretics are by far the most commonly prescribed subtype with the greatest number of outcome-based studies supporting their use. In the United States, hydrochlorothiazide and chlorthalidone represent the most commonly prescribed thiazide-type diuretics and have been the subject of most large outcome-based studies. Although subtle differences in pharmacokinetics between these agents exist, practical differences are limited to their relative diuretic potency. Chlorthalidone is considered approximately 1.5 to 2 times more potent than hydrochlorothiazide for BP reduction.[68] Several recent analyses have demonstrated the superiority of chlorthalidone over hydrochlorothiazide,[67,69] leading some national guidelines to give preference to chlorthalidone over hydrochlorothiazide.[70] Because the relationship between antihypertensive efficacy and metabolic/electrolyte-related side effects of thiazide diuretics is considered dose related, attention to this differential in potency may be important. Specifically, select metabolic effects (hyperlipidemic and hyperglycemic) and electrolyte-related effects (hypokalemic, hypomagnesemic, hyperuricemic, and hypercalcemic) seem to increase with higher doses. This has led to national guidelines recommending doses not exceed 25 mg/day for chlorthalidone or 50 mg/day for hydrochlorothiazide.[3] These metabolic effects may clearly complicate the management of higher risk patients with common comorbidities such as dyslipidemia or diabetes, or even those likely to be sensitive to the potassium- or magnesium-wasting effects of diuretics

(patients with dysrhythmias or those taking digoxin). Although rates of diabetes are higher following administration of thiazides, there is evidence that this can be greatly minimized by keeping potassium in the high normal range (i.e., above 4.0 mEq/L [4 mmol/L]).[71] Furthermore, whether the development of new-onset diabetes in association with thiazide diuretic is of clinical significance is in question because the large ALLHAT and the Systolic Hypertension in the Elderly Program (SHEP) trials showed no significant adverse cardiovascular events from new diuretic-associated diabetes, whereas a smaller trial did.[72] Nonetheless, clinicians should rarely approach the upper limits of these dosage ranges without careful assessment of their metabolic effects or potential to induce electrolyte disturbances. In this way, optimization of BP lowering potential may be achieved while minimizing potential adverse outcomes.

Another key feature of the thiazide-type diuretics is their limited efficacy in patients whose renal function, estimated by creatinine clearance, either approaches or is less than 30 mL/min (0.50 mL/s). In such cases, loop diuretics are regarded as superior to thiazide diuretics for lowering BP. Clinicians often fail to reevaluate the use of thiazide diuretics prescribed to individuals whose renal function has been declining with age and whose risk for the consequences of their metabolic effects such as increased uric acid and insulin resistance may be more significant.[2]

The loop diuretics, such as furosemide, bumetanide, torsemide, and ethacrynic acid, have a common site of action in the thick ascending limb of the loop of Henle.[73] Responsible for reabsorption of over 65% of the filtered sodium, their diuretic efficacy is clearly superior to that of the thiazides, potassium-sparing diuretics, and mineralocorticoids. Practically speaking, furosemide is the most common agent used as an alternative to thiazide-type agents for patients whose renal function has been compromised. With the exception of torsemide, which has a longer half-life, the loop diuretics should be administered twice daily versus once when utilized primarily for their antihypertensive (versus diuretic) effect. The most significant adverse effects related to loop diuretic use concern their potential for excessive diuresis leading to hyponatremia or hypotension. Additionally, hypokalemia, hypomagnesemia, and hypocalcemia may develop over time and contribute to the potential for cardiac arrhythmias. Overall relevance of drug–drug interactions and potential for aggravating select conditions (hyperglycemia, dyslipidemias, and hyperuricemia) should be routinely considered in the monitoring plan for those taking loop diuretics for extended periods of time.

Potassium-sparing diuretics that do not act through mineralocorticoid receptors include triamterene and amiloride. These agents are often prescribed with potassium-wasting diuretics in an attempt to mitigate the loss of potassium. When administered as a single entity or as one component of a combination product, these agents result in moderate diuresis. Potassium-sparing diuretics act on the late distal tubule and collecting duct, and thereby they have a limited ability to affect sodium reabsorption, which translates into modest diuresis. The most important adverse effects associated with these agents are their potential to contribute to hyperkalemia. This is especially relevant in the context of those patients receiving other agents with potassium-sparing properties, such as ACE inhibitors, ARBs, and potassium supplements, as well as nonsteroidal anti-inflammatory drugs (NSAIDs). It is also relevant in those with moderate to severe renal impairment.

Aldosterone Antagonists

Aldosterone antagonists such as spironolactone and eplerenone (Fig. 5–2) modulate vascular tone through a variety of mechanisms besides diuresis. Their potassium-sparing effects mediated through aldosterone antagonism complement the potassium-wasting effects of more potent diuretics such as thiazide or loop diuretics. Patients with resistant hypertension (with or without primary aldosteronism) experience significant BP reductions with the addition of low-dose spironolactone (12.5 to 50 mg/day) to diuretics, ACE inhibitors, and ARBs.[27,74,75] Although functional in this circumstance, it is important to recognize their potential to enhance the risk for hyperkalemia when used in conjunction with ACE inhibitors, ARBs, and direct renin inhibitors (DRIs). This is particularly relevant for individuals with comorbidities associated with reduced renal function or those receiving either potassium supplements, potassium-containing salt substitutes, or NSAIDs. The most commonly used potassium-sparing diuretic is spironolactone; however, eplerenone has been used with increasing frequency in patients with HF following acute myocardial infarction (AMI).[44] Although spironolactone is commonly associated with gynecomastia, eplerenone rarely causes this complication, presumably because of its greater specificity to block aldosterone while minimally affecting androgens and progesterone compared with spirinolactone.[76] The risk of hyperkalemia is also more commonly reported with patients on spironolactone.[77]

β-Blockers

Controversy surrounds the JNC 7 recommended role of β-blockers as first-line antihypertensive agents. For example, a meta-analysis by Lindholm et al demonstrated a higher risk of stroke in patients treated for primary hypertension with β-blockers compared with other antihypertensives.[78] Moreover, Messerli et al showed that β-blockers were ineffective in preventing coronary heart disease, cardiovascular mortality, and all-cause mortality compared with diuretics for elderly patients (60 years of age or older) treated for primary hypertension.[69] Consequently, current evidence suggests patients with uncomplicated hypertension may not benefit as much, if at all, from β-blocker therapy relative to other antihypertensives.[1] This may be in part due to their tendency to reduce central aortic pressure and cardiac afterload to a lesser degree relative to other agents.[79] It must be noted that all of these analyses were conducted with a limited number of β-blockers such as atenolol and metoprolol tartrate. Whether newer formulations such as metoprolol succinate or agents with unique properties such as carvedilol or nebivolol would be more efficacious in reducing morbidity and mortality is unknown. The drug with the most prominent difference in the increased risk of stroke among the three β-blocker subgroups is atenolol. The concern regarding β-blocker use in hypertensive patients without compelling indications is reflected in AHA's recommendations and the European Society of Cardiology's abandonment of β-blockers as first-line antihypertensive agents. However, the role of β-blockers in patients with specific select comorbidities is well established (Table 5–5). Specific outcome-based studies conducted in patients with comorbidities such as HF and recent MI have clearly demonstrated a benefit from β-blocker use.[80] Their hemodynamic effects and antiarrhythmic properties make them desirable agents for hypertensive patients who suffer from ischemic conditions including AMI.[73] When used judiciously in hypertensive patients with HF, β-blocker inhibition of neurohormonal-mediated cardiac remodeling reduces morbidity and mortality relative to standard HF therapies. The mechanisms through which β-blockers affect BP are complex but most certainly include their modulation of renin (Fig. 5–2), which appears to result in a reduction in CO and/or reduction in PR along with their negative inotropic/chronotropic actions.

The specific pharmacologic properties of β-blockers are varied and diverse. An understanding of these properties may assist in the selection of one agent over others given a

---

Table 5–5

Compelling Indications for Individual Drug Classes[3]

Compelling Indication	Recommended Drug Class						
	Diuretic	**Ald Ant**	**BB**	**CCBA**	**ACE-I**	**ARB**	**Dir Vaso**
Heart failure	X	X	X		X	X	X
Postmyocardial infarction		X	X		X		
High coronary disease risk	X		X	X	X		
Diabetes	X		X	X	X	X	
Chronic kidney disease					X	X	
Recurrent stroke prevention	X				X		

ACE-I, angiotensin-converting enzyme inhibitor; Ald Ant, aldosterone antagonist; ARB, angiotensin receptor blocker; BB, β-blocker; CCBA, calcium channel blocking agent; Dir Vaso, direct vasodilator.

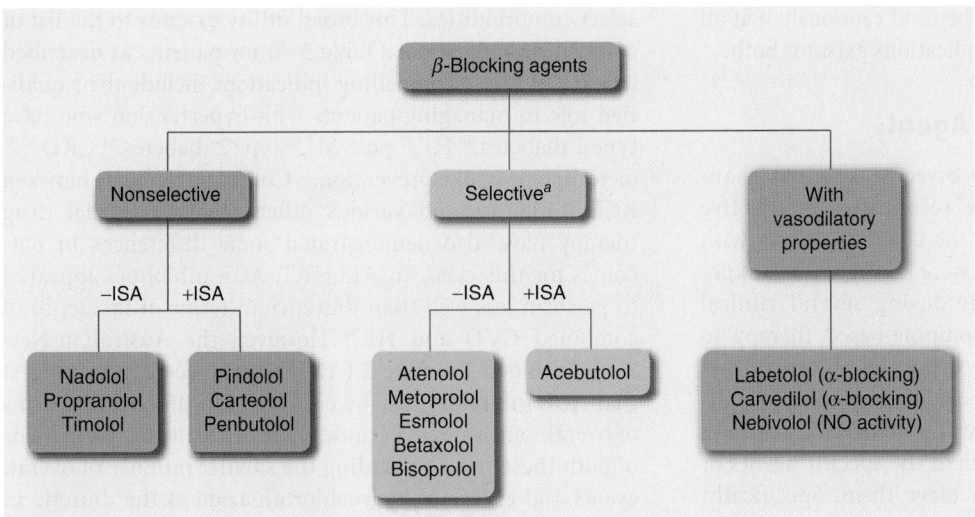

FIGURE 5–3. Flowchart listing various β-blocking agents separated by β-receptor activity and intrinsic sympathomimetic activity. ^{a}β-1 Cardioselective. (ISA, intrinsic sympathomimetic activity; NO, nitrous oxide.)

patient's specific condition(s). One of these properties is cardioselectivity—the property of some β-blockers that preferentially block β_1-receptor versus β_2-receptor. Another property exhibited by some β-blockers is membrane stabilization activity, which relates to the propensity of the β-blocker to possess some capacity for antiarrhythmic properties, in addition to β-receptor blocking properties. Some β-blockers (Fig. 5–3) possess properties referred to as intrinsic sympathomimetic activity (ISA).[6] β-Blockers possessing this property effectively block the β-receptor at higher circulating catecholamine levels, such as during exercise, while having modest β-blocking activity at times of lower catecholamine levels, such as at rest.[81]

When selecting a β-blocker, some of these properties may be of practical value. whereas others, such as membrane stabilization activity and ISA, are of theoretical interest only. Because neither membrane stabilization activity nor ISA has directly proven value in the clinical setting, they are not discussed further other than to point out that β-blockers with ISA are not recommended for use in the post-MI patient.[82] With regard to cardioselectivity, consider a patient with mild asthma, chronic obstructive pulmonary disease, or peripheral vascular disease (intermittent claudication). A β-blocker with relative cardioselectivity to block β_1-receptors may be more desirable in such a patient, whereas a nonselective β-blocker (Fig. 5–3) may be potentially disadvantageous. In such a patient, low doses of cardioselective β-blockers may achieve adequate blockade of β_1-receptors in the heart and kidneys while minimizing the undesirable effects of β_2-receptor blockade on the smooth muscle lining the bronchioles. In doing so, hypertension may be managed while avoiding complications of the coexisting reactive airway disease, which is mediated by β_2-receptor stimulation. Similarly, either because of a reduction in the β_2-mediated vascular blood flow or by enhanced unopposed α-agonist–mediated vasoconstriction, a patient with peripheral vascular disease (intermittent claudication) may experience a worsening of symptoms with use of a nonselective β-blocker (Fig. 5–3). It is important to remember that cardioselectivity

depends on dose, with diminished selectivity exhibited with higher doses.

A limited number of β-blockers also possess vasodilatory properties that are either mediated through α_1-receptor blockade (carvedilol, labetalol) or via L-arginine/nitric oxide-induced release from endothelial cells with subsequent increased nitric oxide bioavailability in the endothelium (nebivolol; Fig. 5–3). Reductions in PR through α_1-receptor mediated blockade or via L-arginine/nitric oxide-induced release, in addition to β-blockade, may benefit patients with hypertension. Such combinations should theoretically contribute to enhanced reductions in vascular tone. Nonetheless, there has been no proven evidence of superior outcomes from the use of β-blockers with vasodilatory properties through either means compared with those with only β-blocking activity.

The adverse effects of β-blockers logically follow their pharmacology. Initiating β-blockers to treat patients with hypertension may have the potential to precipitate bradycardia, various degrees of heart block, or signs and symptoms of HF. The latter is usually limited to those with a subclinical diagnosis and should be considered in the elderly or those with documented reductions in left ventricular function. Conversely, abrupt discontinuation of β-blockers has been cited as a precipitating factor in the development of ischemic syndromes, especially for those patients in whom β-blockers were used for extended periods of time, at higher doses, or who had underlying ischemic heart disease. In such cases, the dose of these agents should be reduced (tapered) over a period of several days to perhaps 1 or even 2 weeks depending on patient-related factors. β-Blocker use in diabetics is usually a complex decision requiring consideration of their consequential effects on insulin, glucose availability, and effects on blocking the signs and symptoms of hypoglycemia against their potential for morbidity/mortality benefits for select candidates with comorbidities such as HF with reduced systolic function. Lastly, β-blockers, particularly first-generation agents (i.e., those other than carvedilol, nebivolol) have a greater effect on glucose metabolism as well as other metabolic effects, and they should be used cautiously if at all with diuretics unless compelling indications exist for both.

Calcium Channel Blocking Agents

Exhibiting considerable interclass diversity, calcium channel blocking agents (CCBAs) are recognized as effective antihypertensives, particularly in the elderly. Patients with isolated systolic hypertension who were taking CCBAs experienced reduced CVD end points during several clinical trials. Two trials comparing amlodipine-based therapy to others furthered a theme of supporting the argument that regardless of the agents used, the evidence appears to indicate that the amount of BP lowering achieved may have more to do with event reduction than the specific agents or combinations of agents used to achieve them. Specifically, the Valsartan Antihypertensive Long-term Use Evaluation (VALUE) trial,[40] which compared valsartan-based therapy with amlodipine-based therapy in over 15,000 patients, and the Anglo-Scandinavian Cardiac Outcomes Trial-Blood Pressure Lowering Arm (ASCOT-BPLA) study,[39] which compared amlodipine-based therapy versus atenolol-based therapy in over 19,000 hypertensive patients, each failed to achieve their primary end point of composite cardiac mortality and morbidity. Yet cause-specific outcomes tended to favor the regimen affording the achievement of lower BPs—namely, the amlodipine-based therapy.

The diversity of pharmacologic properties among the subclasses of CCBAs is significant. A clinician's familiarity with these differences among subclasses helps categorize their expected effects on the cardiovascular system and potential risk of toxicities. Dihydropyridine CCBAs such as amlodipine are commonly associated with edema, especially when used at higher doses. Phenylalkylamine-verapamil and benzodiazepine-diltiazem are more commonly recognized for their electrophysiological effects, negative chronotropic effects, and negative inotropic effects. Many of these pharmacologic properties are exploited for their specific clinical utility. Given that verapamil and diltiazem (both are nondihydropyridine CCBAs) effectively block cardiac conduction through the atrioventricular node, their value in the management of patients with atrial fibrillation in addition to hypertension is obvious, whereas secondary to their negative inotropic effects, they should be avoided in patients with left ventricular systolic dysfunction. In contrast, the dihydropyridine subclass of agents has no utility in managing atrial dysrhythmias but may be used safely (exception being nifedipine) in patients with left ventricular systolic dysfunction. Similarly, all three subclasses of CCBAs possess some coronary vasodilating properties and hence may be used in select patients for the management of patients with angina, in addition to their antihypertensive benefits.

ACE Inhibitors

ACE inhibitors have been extensively studied for the treatment of hypertension, and outcome based trials generally support their use for a wide array of patients, especially with select comorbidities. This broad utility extends to the list of compelling indications (Table 5–5) for patients as described in JNC 7.[3] These compelling indications include their qualified role in managing patients with hypertension who have type 1 diabetes,[40] HF,[83] post-MI,[82] type 2 diabetes,[84] CKD,[85,86] or recurrent stroke prevention.[41] Comparative trials between ACE inhibitors and various other agents as initial drug therapy have also demonstrated some differences in outcomes for this class. In ALLHAT, ACE inhibitors appeared to perform less well than diuretics in terms of incidence of combined CVD and HF.[30] However, the Australian-New Zealand Blood Pressure-2 (ANBP2) trial seemed to suggest that ACE inhibitors may be equivalent to diuretics in terms of overall outcomes.[87] Because there are legitimate criticisms of both these trials (including the smaller number of overall events and choice of hydrochlorothiazide as the diuretic in ANBP2), it may only be safe to conclude that both diuretics and ACE inhibitors represent formidable agents as either first- or second-line hypertensive therapies that effectively achieve a target BP goal for most patients with or without comorbidities.

Although generally well tolerated, classic side effects associated with ACE inhibitors include their potential to cause hyperkalemia and a persistent dry cough. Modest elevations in serum potassium should be anticipated, particularly in patients with compromised renal function, those receiving concurrent NSAIDs, or those taking potassium supplementation or using a potassium-containing salt substitute. The elevations in potassium should be anticipated, if not prospectively considered, when starting or increasing the dose of an ACE inhibitor. Hyperkalemia is rarely a reason for discontinuation of therapy. Nonetheless, periodic monitoring of serum potassium is prudent for patients receiving ACE inhibitors. The dry cough associated with ACE inhibitors is thought to be caused by the accumulation of bradykinin resulting from a direct effect of inhibiting ACE. If a cough jeopardizes compliance with the agent, ARBs should be considered as possible alternative agents because there is less incidence of cough.

In general, the effects of ACE inhibitors on diminished renal function and potassium can be predicted given an understanding of their pharmacologic actions (Fig. 5–3). Inhibition of the generation of angiotensin II through ACE inhibition (or direct blockage of the angiotensin II receptor by angiotensin II receptor blockers) naturally would reduce the efferent renal artery tone, thereby changing the intraglomerular pressure. Although changes in the afferent renal artery tone also occur, the overall effects usually translate into a reduction in GFR, with resulting elevations of up to 30% in serum creatinine values.[86] It is important to recognize that such elevations in serum creatinine are not usually indications to discontinue use of the ACE inhibitor. Rather, possible dose reduction and continued monitoring for further increases in serum creatinine remains prudent. Alternatively, should elevations in serum creatinine exceed 30%, discontinuation is prudent until further evaluation can be made.

More rare forms of adverse effects of ACE inhibitors include blood dyscrasias, angioedema, and more serious effects on renal function. The latter include acute renal failure in those with preexisting kidney dysfunction, bilateral renal artery stenosis, or unilateral renal artery stenosis in a patient with one functioning kidney.

Angiotensin Receptor Blockers

ARBs are another key class of agents whose role in managing patients with hypertension has been further defined by recently completed studies. ARBs are inhibitors of the angiotensin-1 (AT1) receptors (Fig. 5–3). AT1 receptor stimulation evokes a pressor response via a host of accompanying effects on catecholamines, aldosterone, and thirst.[88] Consequently, inhibition of AT1 receptors directly prevents this pressor response and results in upregulation of the RAAS. Upregulation of the RAAS results in elevated levels of angiotensin II, which have the added effect of stimulating the angiotensin-2 (AT2) receptors. AT2-receptor stimulation is generally associated with antihypertensive activity; however, long-term effects of AT2-receptor stimulation that involve cellular growth and repair are relatively unknown. What is clear is that ARBs differ from ACE inhibitors in that the former causes upregulation of the RAAS, whereas the latter blocks the breakdown of bradykinin. The therapeutic relevance resulting from these pharmacologic differences has yet to be fully evaluated through long-term clinical comparative trials in hypertensive patients. However, data from other patient populations (HF, high-risk coronary artery disease patients) suggest the clinical benefits of ARBs are less robust than those of ACE inhibitors.[89,90] At this point, ARBs have emerged as an effective class of antihypertensives whose low incidence of side effects and demonstrated clinical role in patients with specific comorbidities have afforded them an attractive position in the antihypertensive armamentarium. Like ACE inhibitors, the antihypertensive effectiveness of ARBs is greatly enhanced by combining them with diuretics. Furthermore, they have proven their value as well-tolerated alternatives to ACE inhibitors for patients with CKD, diabetes mellitus, and post-AMI (Table 5–5). As of late, the addition of ARBs to standard therapy for patients with HF, including ACE inhibitors, have demonstrated additional incremental benefits for patients with systolic dysfunction[91] or diastolic dysfunction[88] or as alternatives to ACE inhibitors when ACE inhibitors are not tolerated.[92] Comparative studies with alternate (non-ACE inhibitors) antihypertensive regimens in patients with type 2 diabetes[88] and left ventricular hypertrophy[59] have demonstrated their usefulness as effective antihypertensives in these special populations. Studies (the Irbesartan Diabetic Nephropathy Trial [IDNT] and Reduction of Endpoints in NIDDM with the Angiotensin II Antagonist Losartan [RENAAL; NIDDM refers to noninsulin-dependent diabetes mellitus]) have demonstrated superiority of delaying progression toward renal dysfunction for ARBs relative to alternative antihypertensives in type 2 diabetics.[60,61,88] Although better tolerated than ACE inhibitors, ARBs have not been shown to demonstrate superiority of outcomes relative to ACE inhibitors. Like ACE inhibitors, patients may develop angioedema and, although estimates of cross-reactivity are reportedly modest

(less than 20%),[93] one should always exercise extreme caution when considering the use of an ARB in a patient with a known history of angioedema to an ACE inhibitor. This key observation, in addition to their relatively higher acquisition cost, has mitigated the growth of ARB use relative to ACE inhibitors.

Renin Inhibitors

Aliskiren is the first agent in the newest class of antihypertensive agents. Although similar to ACE inhibitors and ARBs in that it acts within the RAAS, it is unique in that it directly blocks renin, thereby reducing plasma renin activity and subsequently AT1 and AT2 with a resultant reduction in BP. This disruption of the negative feedback loop results in a compensatory increase in renin levels, the significance of which is not yet known. Aliskiren has been shown to be well tolerated and effective in reducing BP when used as monotherapy and in combination with hydrochlorothiazide or valsartan for patients with mild to moderate hypertension. However, long-term clinical trials evaluating efficacy and safety have yet to be completed, and thus the effects of aliskiren on morbidity and mortality are as yet unknown. Because of aliskiren's role in the RAAS, recommendations and precautions for monitoring serum potassium and kidney function should be similar to those of ACE inhibitors and ARBs.

α-Blockers

Generally, α_1-blockers are considered inferior agents and should not be used as monotherapy. The ALLHAT trial had an α_1-blocker arm that was discontinued early because doxazocin was associated with an increase in cardiovascular events.[30,65] α_1-Blockers may be considered as add-on therapy to other agents (i.e., fourth line) when hypertension is not adequately controlled. In addition, they may have a specific role in the antihypertensive regimen for elderly men with prostatism; however, their use is often curtailed by complaints of syncope, dizziness, or palpitations following the first dose and orthostatic hypotension with chronic use. The roles of doxazosin, terazosin, and prazosin in the management of patients with hypertension are limited due to the paucity of outcome data and the absence of a unique role for special populations or compelling indications from JNC 7.[3]

Central α₂-Agonists

Limited by their tendency to cause orthostasis, sedation, dry mouth, and vision disturbances, clonidine, methyldopa, guanfacine, and guanabenz represent rare choices in contemporary treatment of patients with hypertension. Their central α_2-adrenergic stimulation is thought to reduce sympathetic outflow and enhance parasympathetic activity, thereby reducing heart rate, CO, and total PR. Occasionally used for cases of resistant hypertension, these agents may have a role when other more conventional therapies appear ineffective. The availability of a transdermal clonidine patch applied once weekly may offer an alternative to hypertensive patients with adherence problems. Of particular importance is the issue of severe rebound hypertension when clonidine is abruptly discontinued. The dose of this agent should be tapered when discontinuation is considered. If the patient is also receiving concomitant β-blocker therapy, the β-blocker should be tapered to discontinuation, ideally several days before discontinuation of clonidine is initiated.

Other Agents

Direct vasodilators such as hydralazine and minoxidil represent additional alternative agents used for patients with resistant hypertension. Primarily acting to relax smooth muscles in arterioles and activate baroreceptors, their use in the absence of concurrently administered β-blockers and diuretics is uncommon. This is due to the need to offset their tendency to cause reflex tachycardia and fluid retention. Other, more rare adverse effects include hydralazine-induced lupus-like syndrome and hypertrichosis from minoxidil. Before using either of these agents, see additional literature describing the appropriate use and monitoring of these agents.[94,95] Although not commonly used, long-term nitrate administration has been shown in small short-term studies to lower BP, particularly in the elderly with elevated systolic pressure.[96,97] Finally, reserpine, although slow to act, represents another rarely used alternative agent for those who are recalcitrant to more standard therapy. This agent is a long-acting depleter of the catecholamine norepinephrine from sympathetic nerve endings and via blockade of norepinephrine transport into its storage granules that causes reduced sympathetic tone leading to reductions in PR. Reserpine's association with numerous side effects including gastric ulceration, depression, and sexual side effects has limited its perception as a useful agent, but in low doses it can be well tolerated. In fact, the SHEP trial demonstrated the BP-lowering effectiveness of low-dose reserpine (0.05 mg/day) when combined with a diuretic, with similar cardiopulmonary and psychosocial side effects between the treatment and placebo groups.[98] In addition, low-dose reserpine was also used as add-on therapy in the ALLHAT trial.[30] Two additional agents, guanethidine and guanadrel, act as postganglionic sympathetic inhibitors inhibiting the release of norepinephrine as well as depleting norepinephrine from these nerve terminals. However, these agents have little role in the management of hypertension because of significant adverse effects.

SPECIAL PATIENT POPULATIONS

Compelling Indications and Special Considerations

❾ *Specific antihypertensive therapy is warranted for certain patients with comorbid conditions that may elevate their level of risk for CVD.* Clinical conditions for which there is compelling evidence supporting one or more classes of drug therapy include[3]:

- Ischemic heart disease
- Heart failure
- Diabetes
- CKD
- Cerebrovascular disease

Compelling indications for specific drug therapies are summarized in Table 5–5.[3,99] In patients with hypertension and angina, β-blockers and long-acting CCBAs are indicated due to their antihypertensive and antianginal effects.[3,34] In addition, patients may benefit from the potential atherosclerotic plaque–stabilizing effects of amlodipine.[1] In patients at high risk of ischemic heart disease, such as diabetic patients with additional cardiovascular risk factors or chronic coronary artery or vascular disease, ACE inhibitors are particularly useful in reducing the risk of cardiovascular events regardless of whether the patient carries a concurrent diagnosis of hypertension.[3,56,57] In patients intolerant to an ACE inhibitor, an ARB may be substituted, given the findings of the recently completed Ongoing Telmisartan Alone and in Combination with Ramipril Global Endpoint Trial (ONTARGET).[90]

β-Blockers and ACE inhibitors are indicated for post-MI patients due to their proven reduction of cardiovascular morbidity and mortality in this population. Aldosterone antagonists are also indicated for the post-MI patient with reduced left ventricular systolic function and diabetes or signs and symptoms of HF.[3,82]

Patients with asymptomatic left ventricular systolic dysfunction and hypertension should be treated with β-blockers and ACE inhibitors. Those with HF secondary to left ventricular dysfunction and hypertension should be treated with drugs proven to also reduce the morbidity and mortality of HF, including β-blockers, ACE inhibitors, ARBs, or aldosterone antagonists, along with diuretics as needed for symptoms. In African Americans with HF and left ventricular systolic dysfunction, combination therapy with nitrates and hydralazine not only affords a morbidity and mortality benefit but may also be useful as antihypertensive therapy if needed.[64] The dihydropyridine CCBAs amlodipine or felodipine may be used in patients with HF and left ventricular systolic dysfunction for uncontrolled BP; however, they offer no beneficial effect on morbidity and mortality due to HF yet carry the expected risk of worsening edema.[83] For patients with HF and preserved ejection fraction, antihypertensive therapies that should be considered include diuretics, β-blockers, ACE inhibitors, ARBs, CCBAs (including nondihydropyridine agents), and others as needed to control BP.[3,83]

Patients with diabetes and hypertension should initially be treated with either ACE inhibitors, ARBs, β-blockers, diuretics, or CCBAs. There is a general consensus that therapy focused on RAAS inhibition by ACE inhibitors or ARBs may be optimal if the patient has additional cardiovascular risk factors such as left ventricular hypertrophy or CKD.[3,59]

In patients with CKD and hypertension, ACE inhibitors and ARBs are preferred, usually in combination with a diuretic.[85] ACE inhibitors in combination with a thiazide diuretic are also preferred in patients with a history of prior stroke or transient ischemic attack. This therapy reduces the risk of recurrent stroke, making it particularly attractive in these patients for BP control.[91]

There are several situations in the management of hypertension requiring special considerations including, but not limited to:

- Hypertensive crisis
- Elderly populations
- Isolated systolic hypertension
- Coronary artery disease
- Minority populations
- Pregnancy
- Pediatrics

Hypertensive crisis can be divided into hypertensive emergencies and hypertensive urgencies. A hypertensive emergency occurs when severe elevations in BP are accompanied by acute or life-threatening target organ damage such as AMI, unstable angina, encephalopathy, intracerebral hemorrhage, acute left ventricular failure with pulmonary edema, dissecting aortic aneurysm, rapidly progressive renal failure, accelerated malignant hypertension with papilledema, and eclampsia, among others. BP is generally greater than 220/140 mm Hg, although a hypertensive emergency can occur at lower levels, particularly in individuals without previous hypertension. The goal in a hypertensive emergency is to reduce mean arterial pressure by up to 25% to the range of 160/100 to 110 mm Hg in minutes to hours.[3,100] IV therapy is generally required and may consist of the agents listed in Table 5–6.[43] A hypertensive urgency is manifested as a severe elevation in BP without evidence of acute or life-threatening target organ damage. In these individuals, BP can usually be managed with orally administered short-acting medications (i.e., captopril, clonidine, or labetalol) and observation in the emergency department over several hours, with subsequent discharge on oral medications and follow-up in the outpatient setting within 24 hours.[3,99]

The treatment of elderly patients (65 years of age or older) with hypertension, as well as those with isolated systolic hypertension, should follow the same approach as with other populations with the exception that lower starting doses may be warranted to avoid symptoms. Special attention should be paid to postural hypotension. This should include a careful assessment of orthostatic symptoms, measurement of BP in the upright position upon standing for 1 to 3 minutes, and caution to avoid volume depletion and rapid titration of antihypertensive therapy.[3] The general recommended BP goal in uncomplicated hypertension in the elderly is less than 140/90 mm Hg. However, it is unclear whether the target SBP should be the same in those older than 80 years, and an achieved SBP of 140 to 145 mm Hg, if tolerated, can be acceptable, as well as attempts to avoid SBP of less than 130 mm Hg and a DBP of less than 65 mm Hg. A recently completed trial (HYVET) documented the benefits of antihypertensive therapy in patients older than 80 years because they experienced a significant reduction in all-cause mortality, fatal stroke, and HF when treated with a diuretic (indapamide) with or without an ACE inhibitor (Perindopril) to a target SBP of less than 150 mm Hg.[42] The BP achieved in the treated group was 144/78 mm Hg versus 161/84 mm Hg in those receiving placebo.[42] In individuals with isolated systolic hypertension, the optimal level of diastolic pressure is not known, and although treated patients who achieve diastolic pressures less than 60 to 70 mm Hg had poorer outcomes in a landmark trial, their cardiovascular event rate was still lower than those receiving placebo.[100]

In patients with coronary artery disease and hypertension, a recent AHA statement recommends a target BP of less than 130/80 mm Hg, with consideration given to less than 120/80 mm Hg if ventricular dysfunction is present. However, in patients with coronary artery disease and evidence of myocardial ischemia, caution is advised in inducing falls of DBP below 60 mm Hg if the patients also have diabetes mellitus or is older than 60 years. In patients with wide pulse pressures, lowering SBP may lead to very low DBP (less than 60 mm Hg), and the clinician must carefully assess for any untoward signs or symptoms.[1]

While the treatment approach of hypertension in minority populations is similar, special consideration should be paid to socioeconomic and lifestyle factors that may be important barriers to BP control. In addition, in patients of African origin, diminished BP responses have been seen with ACE inhibitors and ARBs compared with diuretics or calcium channel blockers.[3]

Hypertension in pregnancy is a major cause of maternal, fetal, and neonatal morbidity and mortality. There are many categories of hypertension in pregnancy; however, preexisting hypertension and preeclampsia are treated differently. The therapeutic selection of an oral antihypertensive agent (Table 5–7) in a pregnant patient with chronic hypertension is determined with regard to fetal safety. Therapeutic options for acute severe hypertension in preeclampsia may be reviewed in JNC 7.[3] Also refer to the American Society of Hypertension Position Article on Hypertension in Pregnancy for further information.[101]

Similar to the JNC 7 criteria (which has four stages for BP classification in adults), the measurement of three or more BPs in children and adolescents are compared with tables listing the 90th-, 95th-, and 99th-percentile BPs based on age, height, and gender that classify BP as normal, prehypertension, and stage 1 and stage 2 hypertension (Table 5–1).[102] The prevalence of hypertension in adolescent populations is increasing and associated with obesity, sedentary lifestyle, or a positive family history, which increases the risk of CVD. The clinician should be aware that secondary causes are common in adolescents with hypertension, and the identification and aggressive modification of risk factors with nonpharmacologic and pharmacologic interventions is par amount for risk reduction of target organ damage. The 2004 National High Blood Pressure Education Program (NHBPEP) Working Group Report on Hypertension in Children and Adolescents provides specific recommendations to modify and treat risk factors in this population of patients. In addition, the American Heart Association released a source in

Table 5–6

Parenteral Antihypertensive Agents for Hypertensive Emergency[a]

Drug	Dose Range	Onset of Action	Duration of Action	Adverse Effects[b]	Special Indications
Vasodilators					
Sodium nitroprusside	0.25–10 mcg/kg/min as IV infusion[c]	Immediate	1–2 minutes	Nausea, vomiting, muscle twitching, sweating, thiocyanate and cyanide intoxication	Most hypertensive emergencies; use with caution with high intracranial pressure or azotemia
Nicardipine hydrochloride	5–15 mg/h IV	5–10 minutes	15–30 minutes, may exceed 4 hours	Tachycardia, headache, flushing, local phlebitis	Most hypertensive emergencies except acute heart failure; use with caution with coronary ischemia
Fenoldopam mesylate	0.1–0.3 mcg/kg/min as IV infusion[c]	Less than 5 minutes	30 minutes	Tachycardia, headache, nausea, flushing	Most hypertensive emergencies; use with caution with glaucoma
Nitroglycerin	5–100 mcg/kg/min as IV infusion	2–5 minutes	5–10 minutes	Headache, vomiting, methemoglobinemia, tolerance with prolonged use	Coronary ischemia
Enalaprilat	1.25–5 mg every 6 hours IV	15–30 minutes	6–12 hours	Precipitous fall in pressure in high-renin states; variable response	Acute left ventricular failure; avoid in acute myocardial infarction
Hydralazine hydrochloride	10–20 mg IV 10–40 mg IM	10–20 minutes 20–30 minutes	1–4 hours IV 4–6 hours IM	Tachycardia, flushing, headache, vomiting, aggravation of angina	Eclampsia
Clevidipine	1–21 mg/h IV	2–4 minutes	5–15 minutes	Atrial fibrillation, fever, insomnia, nausea, headache, vomiting, postprocedural hemorrhage, acute renal failure, respiratory failure	Defective lipid metabolism (avoid use in these patients), severe aortic stenosis (avoid use)
Diazoxide	1–3 mg/kg or 50–100 mg every 5–15 minutes	2 minutes	3–12 hours	Hyperglycemia, sodium and water retention	Preeclampsia, eclampsia, impaired renal function
Furosemide	10–40 mg/h IV, maximum 80–160 mg/h IV	5 minutes	2 hours	Hypotension, electrolyte abnormalities, hearing impairment	Heart failure, fluid overload, adjunct therapy to vasodilators
Adrenergic Inhibitors					
Labetalol hydrochloride	20–80 mg IV bolus every 10 minutes	5–10 minutes	3–6 hours	Vomiting, scalp tingling, dizziness, bronchoconstriction, nausea, heart block, orthostatic hypotension	Most hypertensive emergencies except acute heart failure
Esmolol hydrochloride	250–500 mcg/kg/min IV bolus, then 50–100 mcg/kg/min by infusion; may repeat bolus after 5 minutes or increase infusion to 300 mcg/min	1–2 minutes	10–30 minutes	Hypotension, nausea, asthma, first-degree heart block, heart failure	Aortic dissection, perioperative
Phentolamine	5–15 mg IV bolus	1–2 minutes	10–30 minutes	Tachycardia flushing, headache	Catecholamine excess

IM, intramuscular.

[a]These doses may vary from those in the *Physicians' Desk Reference*.

[b]Hypotension may occur with all agents.

[c]Requires special delivery system.

Adapted from Saseen JJ, Maclaughlin EJ. Hypertension. In: DiPiro JT, Talbert RL, Yee GC, et al., eds. Pharmacotherapy: A Pathophysiologic Approach, 8th ed. New York, NY: McGraw-Hill, 2011:131, with permission.

Table 5–7

Treatment of Chronic Hypertension in Pregnancy[3]

Agent	Comments
Methyldopa	Preferred first-line therapy on the basis of long-term follow-up studies supporting safety after exposure in utero. Surveillance data do not support an association between drug and congenital defects when the mother took the drug early in the first trimester
Labetalol	Increasingly preferred to methyldopa because of reduced side effects. The agent does not seem to pose a risk to the fetus, except possibly in the first trimester
β-Blockers	Generally acceptable on the basis of limited data. Reports of intrauterine growth restriction with atenolol in the first and second trimesters
Clonidine	Limited data; no association between drug and congenital defects when the mother took the drug early in the first trimester, but number of exposures is small
Calcium channel antagonists	Limited data; nifedipine in the first trimester was not associated with increased rates of major birth defects, but animal data were associated with fetal hypoxemia and acidosis. This agent should probably be limited to mothers with severe hypertension
Diuretics	Not first-line agents; probably safe; available data suggest that throughout gestation, a diuretic is not associated with an increased risk of major fetal anomalies or adverse fetal-neonatal events
Angiotensin-converting enzyme inhibitors and angiotensin II receptor antagonists	Contraindicated; reported fetal toxicity and death

Patient Encounter 2

A 27-year-old white woman presents to your clinic with a diagnosis of hypertension. She is 5'3" (160 cm) and weighs 76 kg (167 lbs). She denies using tobacco or alcohol. Fasting laboratory values were significant for glucose of 160 mg/dL (8.9 mmol/L), serum creatinine of 1.1 mg/dL (97 μmol/L), hemoglobin A1c of 7.1% (0.071; 54 mmol/mol Hb), total cholesterol level of 212 mg/dL (5.48 mmol/L), triglyceride level of 200 mg/dL (2.26 mmol/L), and high-density lipoprotein level of 41 mg/dL (1.06 mmol/L). The calculated low-density lipoprotein level is 131 mg/dL (3.39 mmol/L). All other laboratory values are within normal limits. Urinalysis was unremarkable. The patient is in her second trimester of pregnancy. During the appointment, the patient states that she exercises two to three times a week for approximately 60 minutes. Because of her busy schedule, she admits that she eats a lot of microwave meals and canned soups. Her BP today in the clinic was 150/92 mm Hg with a pulse of 74 bpm. Her BP prior to pregnancy was 144/90 mm Hg.

What is the patient's target BP?

Based on the information presented, create a care plan for this patient's hypertension. This should include (a) goals of therapy, (b) a patient-specific therapeutic plan, and (c) a plan for appropriate monitoring to achieve goals and avoid adverse effects.

2008 guiding the role of ambulatory BP measurements in children and adolescents.[103] The *Nelson Textbook of Pediatrics* is also recommended for a comprehensive review of treatment of congenital and pediatric hypertension.[104]

PATIENT CARE AND MONITORING

⑩ *The frequency of follow-up visits for patients with hypertension varies based on individual cases but is influenced by the severity of hypertension, comorbidities, and choice of agent selected.* A recent analysis of the VALUE trial found that achieving BP control within 6 months reduced CV events compared with a longer time to achieve goal.[40] In addition, another analysis found that the more times a patient is below goal, the lower the risk.[8,105] These studies suggest there is an urgency to achieve and maintain BP control that may necessitate frequent assessment and adjustments (i.e., every 2 weeks). At a minimum, assessment of response to medications should be done at 1-month intervals.[1] In patients with stage 2 hypertension or those with comorbidities (e.g., diabetes, vascular disease, congestive HF, or CKD), shorter time frames of ≤2 weeks are more appropriate.[57] Once BP is controlled, annual or semiannual monitoring for changes in serum biochemistries such as serum creatinine or potassium are recommended.[1] However, for patients with congestive heart failure, CKD, or diabetes, more frequent monitoring is necessary to adequately control comorbid conditions. Another aspect to monitoring relates to the importance of medication adherence. Confirmation of continued use of antihypertensive medications should be considered in the routine monitoring of patients on numerous medications for hypertension. Evaluation of side effects, lab abnormalities, and/or progression to target organ damage should also be considered at appropriate intervals. Given the generally asymptomatic nature of hypertension, patient motivation to adhere to prescribed medications becomes a key tool in controlling hypertension.[1]

Given the chronic nature of hypertension, parsimony of medication regimens is a virtue of a good therapeutic plan.

Minimizing the number of medications a patient is required to take has the potential to enhance adherence and mitigate cost. Control of BP is often achieved by the use of two or even three or more BP-lowering medications.[106] Many combination products contain a diuretic as one of their active components. However, combination therapy may limit the ability of the clinician to titrate the dose of a specific agent. As such, the number of medications ("pill count") may often be reduced through the use of combination products. This inherently simplifies the number of medications and copays a patient may have to endure to achieve effective BP control. These practicalities, although obvious, go a long way to optimize adherence, another challenge to maximizing therapy effectiveness.

OUTCOME EVALUATION

- Short-term goals are to achieve reduction in BP safely through the iterative process of using pharmacologic therapy, along with nonpharmacologic therapy or lifestyle changes.

- Lifestyle changes should address other risk factors for CVD including obesity, physical inactivity, insulin resistance, dyslipidemia, smoking cessation, and others.

- Monitoring for efficacy, adverse events, and adherence to therapy is key to achieving the long-term goals of reducing the risk of morbidity and mortality associated with CVD.

Patient Encounter 3

A 62-year-old Hispanic man arrives at your clinic complaining of elevated BP despite being on metoprolol tartrate 100 mg twice daily, chlorthalidone 25 mg once daily, and amlodipine 10 mg daily. He states that he has been adherent with all medications and diet. He does not smoke. Past medical history is significant for hypertension and osteoarthritis. Physical examination was unremarkable. Laboratory values were significant for serum creatinine of 0.8 mg/dL (71 μmol/L), a potassium level of 3.6 mEq/L (3.6 mmol/L), total cholesterol of 220 mg/dL (5.69 mmol/L), HDL cholesterol of 35 mg/dL (0.91 mmol/L), triglyceride level of 150 mg/dL (1.70 mmol/L) and calculated LDL cholesterol of 155 mg/dL (4.01 mmol/L). The patient's seated BP in the left arm is 152/86 mm Hg and 150/82 mm Hg in the right arm. His pulse is 58 bpm. A plasma renin activity was drawn, and the result was 0.3 ng/mL/h (0.08 ng/L/s). An aldosterone level returned within normal limits at 5 ng/dL (139 pmol/L).

Based on the information provided, does the patient have resistant hypertension?

What is that patient's target BP using the recommendations from the 2007 American Heart Association Statement of the treatment of hypertension in the prevention and management of ischemic heart disease?

Based on the information presented, what pharmacological changes would you make to the patient's medications to reduce his BP closer to goal and reduce his overall cardiovascular risk?

Patient Care and Monitoring

1. Measure patient BP twice, at least 1 minute apart in a sitting position, and then average the readings to determine if BP is adequately controlled.

2. Conduct a medical history. Does the patient have any compelling indications? Is the patient pregnant?

3. Conduct a medication history (prescription, over-the-counter, and dietary supplements) to determine conditions or causes of hypertension. Does the patient take any medications, supplements, herbal products, or foods that may elevate SBP or DBP? Does the patient have drug allergies?

4. Review available laboratory tests to examine electrolyte balance and renal function.

5. Discuss lifestyle modifications that may reduce BP with the patient. Determine what nonpharmacologic approaches might be or have been helpful to the patient.

6. Evaluate the patient if pharmacologic treatment has reached the target BP goal. If the patient is at the goal, skip to step 9.

7. If patient is not at goal BP, assess efficacy, safety, and compliance of the antihypertensive regimen to determine if a dose increase or additional antihypertensive agent (step 8) is needed to achieve goal BP.

8. Select an agent to minimize adverse drug reactions and interactions when additional drug therapy is needed. Does the patient have prescription coverage or is the recommended agent in the formulary?

9. Open a dialogue to address patient concerns about hypertension and management of the condition.

10. Provide a plan to assess effectiveness and safety of therapy. Follow-up at monthly intervals or less until BP is achieved, otherwise semiannual or annual clinic visits to assess electrolyte balance and renal function once BP target is achieved. Presence of comorbidities (i.e., CKD) may require more frequent follow-up.

Abbreviations Introduced in This Chapter

ACC	American College of Cardiology
ACCF	American College of Cardiology Foundation
ACE	Angiotensin-converting enzyme
ACE-I	Angiotensin-converting enzyme inhibitor
ACR	Albumin-to-creatinine ratio
AHA	American Heart Association
A-HeFT	African American Heart Failure Trial
AIRE	Acute Infarction Ramipril Efficacy Study
Ald Ant	Aldosterone antagonist
ALLHAT	Antihypertensive and Lipid-Lowering Treatment to Prevent Heart Attack Trial
AMI	Acute myocardial infarction
ANBP2	Australian-New Zealand Blood Pressure-2 study
ARB	Angiotensin receptor blocker
ASCOT-BPLA	Anglo-Scandinavian Cardiac Outcomes Trial-Blood Pressure Lowering Arm study
AT1	Angiotensin-1
AT2	Angiotensin-2
BB	β-Blocker
BHAT	β-Blocker Heart Attack Trial
BP	Blood pressure
CAGE	Chymostatin-sensitive II-generating enzyme
CAPRICORN	Carvedilol Post-Infarct Survival Control in Left Ventricular Dysfunction Trial
Captopril Trial	Collaborative Study Captopril Trial ("The Effect of Angiotensin-Converting Enzyme Inhibition on Diabetic Nephropathy")
CCBA	Calcium channel blocker agent
CCB	Calcium channel blocker
CHARM	Candesartan in Heart Failure Assessment of Reduction in Morbidity and Mortality Trial
CIBIS-II	The Cardiac Insufficiency Bisoprolol Study II
CKD	Chronic kidney disease
CO	Cardiac output
COPERNICUS	Carvedilol Prospective Randomized Cumulative Survival Trial
CVD	Cardiovascular disease
DASH	Dietary Approaches to Stop Hypertension
DBP	Diastolic blood pressure
Dir Vaso	Direct vasodilator
DRI	Direct renin inhibitor
EPHESUS	Eplerenone Post-Acute Myocardial Infarction Heart Failure Efficacy and Survival Study
EUROPA	European Trial on Reduction of Cardiac Events with Perindopril in Stable Coronary Artery Disease Trial
GFR	Glomerular filtration rate
HF	Heart failure
HOPE	Heart Outcomes Prevention Evaluation Study
HYVET	Hypertension in the Very Elderly Trial
IDNT	Irbesartan Diabetic Nephropathy Trial
IM	Intramuscular
INVEST	International Verapamil-Trandolapril Study
IRMA-II	Irbesartan in Patients with Type 2 Diabetes and Microalbuminuria study

ISA	Intrinsic sympathomimetic activity
JNC 7	Joint National Committee Seventh Report
LIFE	Losartan Intervention For Endpoint reduction in hypertension study
MAO	Monoamine oxidase
MERIT-HF	Metoprolol CR/XL Randomised Intervention Trial in Congestive Heart Failure
MI	Myocardial infarction
NHBPEP	National High Blood Pressure Education Program
NIDDM	Noninsulin-dependent diabetes mellitus
NO	Nitric or nitrous oxide
NSAID	Nonsteroidal anti-inflammatory drug
ONTARGET	Ongoing Telmisartan Alone and in combination with Ramipril Global Endpoint Trial
PR	Peripheral resistance
PRA	Plasma rennin activity
PROGRESS	Perindopril Protection Against Recurrent Stroke Study
RAAS	Renin-angiotensin-aldosterone system
RALES	Randomized Aldactone Evaluation Study
RENAAL	Reduction of Endpoints in NIDDM with the Angiotensin II Antagonist Losartan study
SAVE	Survival and Ventricular Enlargement Trial
SBP	Systolic blood pressure
SHEP	Systolic Hypertension in the Elderly Program
SNS	Sympathetic nervous system
SOLVD	Studies of Left Ventricular Dysfunction
TRACE	Trandolapril Cardiac Evaluation
VALUE	Valsartan Antihypertensive Long-term Use Evaluation
ValHeFT	Veterans Affairs Cooperative I study

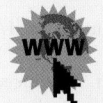 Self-assessment questions and answers are available at *http://www.mhpharmacotherapy.com/pp.html.*

REFERENCES

1. Rosendorff C, Black HR, Cannon CP, et al. Treatment of hypertension in the prevention and management of ischemic heart disease: A scientific statement from the American Heart Association Council for High Blood Pressure Research and the Councils on Clinical Cardiology and Epidemiology and Prevention. Circulation 2007;115(21): 2761–2788.

2. Aronow WS, Fleg JL, Pepine CJ, et al. ACCF/AHA 2011 expert consensus document on hypertension in the elderly: A report of the American College of Cardiology Foundation Task Force on Clinical Expert Consensus Documents. Circulation 2011;123(21):2434–2506.

3. Chobanian AV, Bakris GL, Black HR, et al. Seventh report of the Joint National Committee on Prevention, Detection, Evaluation, and Treatment of High Blood Pressure. Hypertension 2003;42(6): 1206–1252.

4. Kearney PM, Whelton M, Reynolds K, Muntner P, Whelton PK, He J. Global burden of hypertension: Analysis of worldwide data. Lancet. 2005;365(9455):217–223.

5. WHO. Global Health Risks: Mortality and burden of disease attributable to selected major risks, *http://www.who.int/healthinfo/global_burden_disease/GlobalHealthRisks_report_full.pdf*. Accessed September 30, 2011.

6. Roger VL, Go AS, Lloyd-Jones DM, et al. Heart disease and stroke statistics—2011 update: A report from the American Heart Association. Circulation 2011;123(4):e18–e209.

7. Victor RG, Kaplan NM. Kaplan's Clinical Hypertension, 10th ed. Philadelphia, PA: Wollters Kluwer Lippincott Williams & Wilkins Health, 2010.

8. Mancia G, De Backer G, Dominiczak A, et al. 2007 guidelines for the management of arterial hypertension: The Task Force for the Management of Arterial Hypertension of the European Society of Hypertension (ESH) and of the European Society of Cardiology (ESC). Eur Heart J 2007;28(12):1462–1536.

9. Izzo JL, Sica DA, Black HR, Council for High Blood Pressure Research (American Heart Association). Hypertension Primer, 4th ed. Philadelphia, PA: Lippincott Williams & Wilkins, 2008.

10. Dominiczak AF, Negrin DC, Clark JS, et al. Genes and hypertension: From gene mapping in experimental models to vascular gene transfer strategies. Hypertension 2000;35:164–172.

11. Kupper N, Willemsen G, Riese H, et al. Heritability of daytime ambulatory blood pressure in an extended twin design. Hypertension 2005;45(1):80–85.

12. Johnson AD, Newton-Cheh C, Chasman DI, et al. Association of hypertension drug target genes with blood pressure and hypertension in 86,588 individuals. Hypertension 2011;57(5):903–910.

13. FDA.gov. Table of pharmacogenomic biomarkers in drug labels. 2011. Available at *http://www.fda.gov/Drugs/ScienceResearch/ResearchAreas/Pharmacogenetics/ucm083378.htm*. Accessed October 17, 2011.

14. Grassi G, Seravalle G, Calhoun DA, et al. Mechanisms responsible for sympathetic activation by cigarette smoking in humans. Circulation 1994;90(1):248–253.

15. Kloner RA, Rezkalla SH. To drink or not to drink? That is the question. Circulation 2007;116(11):1306–1317.

16. Krum H, Schlaich M, Sobotka P, Scheffers I, Kroon AA, de Leeuw PW. Novel procedure- and device-based strategies in the management of systemic hypertension. Eur Heart J 2011;32(5):537–544.

17. Franco V, Oparil S. Salt sensitivity, a determinant of blood pressure, cardiovascular disease and survival. J Am Coll Nutr 2006;25(3 Suppl):247S–255S.

18. Obarzanek E, Proschan MA, Vollmer WM, et al. Individual blood pressure responses to changes in salt intake: Results from the DASH-Sodium trial. Hypertension 2003;42(4):459–467.

19. Alderman MH. Reducing dietary sodium: The case for caution. JAMA 2010;303(5):448–449.

20. Taylor RS, Ashton KE, Moxham T, Hooper L, Ebrahim S. Reduced dietary salt for the prevention of cardiovascular disease. Cochrane Database Syst Rev 2011(7):CD009217.

21. Phillips MI, Schmidt-Ott KM. The discovery of renin 100 years ago. News Physiol Sci 1999;14:271–274.

22. Egan BM, Basile JN, Rehman SU, et al. Plasma renin test-guided drug treatment algorithm for correcting patients with treated but uncontrolled hypertension: A randomized controlled trial. Am J Hypertens 2009;22(7):792–801.

23. Furberg CD. Renin-guided treatment of hypertension: Time for action. Am J Hypertens 2010;23(9):929–930.

24. Laragh J. Laragh's lessons in pathophysiology and clinical pearls for treating hypertension. Am J Hypertens 2001;14(1):84–89.

25. Buhler FR. Calcium antagonists as first-choice therapy for low-renin essential hypertension. Kidney Int 1989;36(2):295–305.

26. Stanton AV, Dicker P, O'Brien ET. Aliskiren monotherapy results in the greatest and the least blood pressure lowering in patients with high- and low-baseline PRA levels, respectively. Am J Hypertens 2009;22(9):954–957.

27. Vaclavik J, Sedlak R, Plachy M, et al. Addition of spironolactone in patients with resistant arterial hypertension (ASPIRANT): A randomized, double-blind, placebo-controlled trial. Hypertension 2011;57(6):1069–1075.

28. Pickering TG, Hall JE, Appel LJ, et al. Recommendations for blood pressure measurement in humans and experimental animals: Part 1: Blood pressure measurement in humans: A statement for professionals from the subcommittee of professional and public education of the American Heart Association Council on High Blood Pressure Research. Circulation 2005;111(5):697–716.

29. Lewington S, Clarke R, Qizilbash N, Peto R, Collins R. Age-specific relevance of usual blood pressure to vascular mortality: A meta-analysis of individual data for one million adults in 61 prospective studies. Lancet 2002;360(9349):1903–1913.

30. Major outcomes in high-risk hypertensive patients randomized to angiotensin-converting enzyme inhibitor or calcium channel blocker vs diuretic: The Antihypertensive and Lipid-Lowering Treatment to Prevent Heart Attack Trial (ALLHAT). JAMA 2002;288(23):2981–2997.

31. Whelton SP, Chin A, Xin X, He J. Effect of aerobic exercise on blood pressure: A meta-analysis of randomized, controlled trials. Ann Intern Med 2002;136(7):493–503.

32. Sacks FM, Svetkey LP, Vollmer WM, et al. Effects on blood pressure of reduced dietary sodium and the Dietary Approaches to Stop Hypertension (DASH) diet. DASH-Sodium Collaborative Research Group. N Engl J Med 2001;344(1):3–10.

33. Beard TC. The bread of the 21st century. Aust J Nutr Diet 1997;54:198–203.

34. Gibbons RJ, Abrams J, Chatterjee K, et al. ACC/AHA 2002 guideline update for the management of patients with chronic stable angina—summary article: A report of the American College of Cardiology/American Heart Association Task Force on practice guidelines (Committee on the Management of Patients with Chronic Stable Angina). J Am Coll Cardiol 2003;41(1):159–168.

35. Simmons-Morton DG. Exercise therapy. In: Izzo JL, Jr, Black HR, eds. Hypertension Primer: The Essentials of High Blood Pressure, 3rd ed. Philadelphia, PA: Lippincott Williams & Wilkins, 2003:388–389.

36. Xin X, He J, Frontini MG, Ogden LG, Motsamai OI, Whelton PK. Effects of alcohol reduction on blood pressure: A meta-analysis of randomized controlled trials. Hypertension 2001;38(5):1112–1117.

37. Omvik P. How smoking affects blood pressure. Blood Press 1996;5(2):71–77.

38. Primatesta P, Falaschetti E, Gupta S, Marmot MG, Poulter NR. Association between smoking and blood pressure: Evidence from the health survey for England. Hypertension 2001;37(2):187–193.

39. Dahlof B, Sever PS, Poulter NR, et al. Prevention of cardiovascular events with an antihypertensive regimen of amlodipine adding perindopril as required versus atenolol adding bendroflumethiazide as required, in the Anglo-Scandinavian Cardiac Outcomes Trial-Blood Pressure Lowering Arm (ASCOT-BPLA): A multicentre randomised controlled trial. Lancet 2005;366(9489):895–906.

40. Julius S, Kjeldsen SE, Weber M, et al. Outcomes in hypertensive patients at high cardiovascular risk treated with regimens based on valsartan or amlodipine: The VALUE randomised trial. Lancet 2004;363(9426):2022–2031.

41. Randomised trial of a perindopril-based blood-pressure-lowering regimen among 6,105 individuals with previous stroke or transient ischaemic attack. Lancet 2001;358(9287):1033–1041.

42. Beckett NS, Peters R, Fletcher AE, et al. Treatment of hypertension in patients 80 years of age or older. N Engl J Med 2008;358(18):1887–1898.

43. Pitt B, Zannad F, Remme WJ, et al. The effect of spironolactone on morbidity and mortality in patients with severe heart failure. Randomized Aldactone Evaluation Study Investigators. N Engl J Med 1999;341(10):709–717.

44. Pitt B, Remme W, Zannad F, et al. Eplerenone, a selective aldosterone blocker, in patients with left ventricular dysfunction after myocardial infarction. N Engl J Med 2003;348(14):1309–1321.

45. Effect of metoprolol CR/XL in chronic heart failure: Metoprolol CR/XL Randomised Intervention Trial in Congestive Heart Failure (MERIT-HF). Lancet 1999;353(9169):2001–2007.

46. Krum H, Roecker EB, Mohacsi P, et al. Effects of initiating carvedilol in patients with severe chronic heart failure: Results from the COPERNICUS Study. JAMA 2003;289(6):712–718.

47. Dargie HJ. Effect of carvedilol on outcome after myocardial infarction in patients with left-ventricular dysfunction: The CAPRICORN randomised trial. Lancet 2001;357(9266):1385–1390.

48. Lampert R, Ickovics JR, Viscoli CJ, Horwitz RI, Lee FA. Effects of propranolol on recovery of heart rate variability following acute myocardial infarction and relation to outcome in the Beta-Blocker Heart Attack Trial. Am J Cardiol 2003;91(2):137–142.

49. The Cardiac Insufficiency Bisoprolol Study II (CIBIS-II): A randomised trial. Lancet 1999;353(9146):9–13.

50. Pepine CJ, Handberg EM, Cooper-DeHoff RM, et al. A calcium antagonist vs a non-calcium antagonist hypertension treatment strategy for patients with coronary artery disease. The International Verapamil-Trandolapril Study (INVEST): A randomized controlled trial. JAMA. 2003;290(21):2805–2816.

51. Effect of enalapril on mortality and the development of heart failure in asymptomatic patients with reduced left ventricular ejection fractions. The SOLVD Investigattors. N Engl J Med 1992;327(10):685–691.

52. Effect of ramipril on mortality and morbidity of survivors of acute myocardial infarction with clinical evidence of heart failure. The Acute Infarction Ramipril Efficacy (AIRE) Study Investigators. Lancet 1993;342(8875):821–828.

53. Kober L, Torp-Pedersen C, Carlsen JE, et al. A clinical trial of the angiotensin-converting-enzyme inhibitor trandolapril in patients with left ventricular dysfunction after myocardial infarction. Trandolapril Cardiac Evaluation (TRACE) Study Group. N Engl J Med 1995;333(25):1670–1676.

54. Pfeffer MA, Braunwald E, Moye LA, et al. Effect of captopril on mortality and morbidity in patients with left ventricular dysfunction after myocardial infarction. Results of the survival and ventricular enlargement trial. The SAVE Investigators. N Engl J Med 1992;327(10):669–677.

55. Lewis EJ, Hunsicker LG, Bain RP, Rohde RD. The effect of angiotensin-converting-enzyme inhibition on diabetic nephropathy. The Collaborative Study Group. N Engl J Med 1993;329(20):1456–1462.

56. Yusuf S, Sleight P, Pogue J, et al. Effects of an angiotensin-converting-enzyme inhibitor, ramipril, on cardiovascular events in high-risk patients. The Heart Outcomes Prevention Evaluation Study Investigators. N Engl J Med 2000;342(3):145–153.

57. Fox KM. Efficacy of perindopril in reduction of cardiovascular events among patients with stable coronary artery disease: Randomised, double-blind, placebo-controlled, multicentre trial (the EUROPA study). Lancet 2003;362(9386):782–788.

58. Pfeffer MA, Swedberg K, Granger CB, et al. Effects of candesartan on mortality and morbidity in patients with chronic heart failure: The CHARM-Overall programme. Lancet 2003;362(9386):759–766.

59. Dahlof B, Devereux RB, Kjeldsen SE, et al. Cardiovascular morbidity and mortality in the Losartan Intervention For Endpoint reduction in hypertension study (LIFE): A randomised trial against atenolol. Lancet 2002;359(9311):995–1003.

60. Brenner BM, Cooper ME, de Zeeuw D, et al. Effects of losartan on renal and cardiovascular outcomes in patients with type 2 diabetes and nephropathy. N Engl J Med 2001;345(12):861–869.

61. Lewis EJ, Hunsicker LG, Clarke WR, et al. Renoprotective effect of the angiotensin-receptor antagonist irbesartan in patients with nephropathy due to type 2 diabetes. N Engl J Med 2001;345(12):851–860.

62. Parving HH, Lehnert H, Brochner-Mortensen J, Gomis R, Andersen S, Arner P. The effect of irbesartan on the development of diabetic nephropathy in patients with type 2 diabetes. N Engl J Med 2001;345(12):870–878.

63. Cohn JN, Tognoni G. A randomized trial of the angiotensin-receptor blocker valsartan in chronic heart failure. N Engl J Med 2001;345(23):1667–1675.

64. Taylor AL, Ziesche S, Yancy C, et al. Combination of isosorbide dinitrate and hydralazine in blacks with heart failure. N Engl J Med 2004;351(20):2049–2057.

65. Diuretic versus alpha-blocker as first-step antihypertensive therapy: Final results from the Antihypertensive and Lipid-Lowering Treatment to Prevent Heart Attack Trial (ALLHAT). Hypertension 2003;42(3):239–246.

66. Jamerson KA. Avoiding cardiovascular events in combination therapy in patients living with systolic hypertension. Paper presented at: American College of Cardiology Scientific Sessions; 2008; Chicago, IL.

67. Ernst ME, Carter BL, Goerdt CJ, et al. Comparative antihypertensive effects of hydrochlorothiazide and chlorthalidone on ambulatory and office blood pressure. Hypertension 2006;47(3):352–358.

68. Carter BL, Basile J. Development of diabetes with thiazide diuretics: The potassium issue. J Clin Hypertens (Greenwich) 2005;7(11):638–640.

69. Messerli FH, Grossman E, Goldbourt U. Are beta-blockers efficacious as first-line therapy for hypertension in the elderly? A systematic review. JAMA 1998;279(23):1903–1907.

70. NICE. Hypertension: NICE Clinical Guideline 127. 2011. *www.nice.org.uk/guidance/CG127.* Accessed September 30, 2011.

71. Zillich AJ, Garg J, Basu S, Bakris GL, Carter BL. Thiazide diuretics, potassium, and the development of diabetes: A quantitative review. Hypertension 2006;48(2):219–224.

72. Carter BL, Einhorn PT, Brands M, et al. Thiazide-induced dysglycemia: Call for research from a working group from the National Heart, Lung, and Blood Institute. Hypertension 2008;52(1):30–36.

73. Goodman LS, Brunton LL, Chabner B, Knollmann BC. Goodman & Gilman's Pharmacological Basis of Therapeutics, 12th ed. New York, NY: McGraw-Hill, 2011.

74. de Souza F, Muxfeldt E, Fiszman R, Salles G. Efficacy of spironolactone therapy in patients with true resistant hypertension. Hypertension 2010;55(1):147–152.

75. Nishizaka MK, Zaman MA, Calhoun DA. Efficacy of low-dose spironolactone in subjects with resistant hypertension. Am J Hypertens 2003;16(11 Pt 1):925–930.

76. Menard J. The 45-year story of the development of an anti-aldosterone more specific than spironolactone. Mol Cell Endocrinol 2004;217(1-2):45–52.

77. Sica DA. Pharmacokinetics and pharmacodynamics of mineralocorticoid blocking agents and their effects on potassium homeostasis. Heart Fail Rev 2005;10(1):23–29.

78. Lindholm LH, Carlberg B, Samuelsson O. Should beta blockers remain first choice in the treatment of primary hypertension? A meta-analysis. Lancet 2005;366(9496):1545–1553.

79. Williams B, Lacy PS, Thom SM, et al. Differential impact of blood pressure-lowering drugs on central aortic pressure and clinical outcomes: Principal results of the Conduit Artery Function Evaluation (CAFE) study. Circulation 2006;113(9):1213–1225.

80. Bangalore S, Messerli FH, Kostis JB, Pepine CJ. Cardiovascular protection using beta-blockers: A critical review of the evidence. J Am Coll Cardiol 2007;50(7):563–572.

81. Weber MA. The role of the new beta-blockers in treating cardiovascular disease. Am J Hypertens 2005;18(12 Pt 2):169S–176S.

82. Antman EM, Anbe DT, Armstrong PW, et al. ACC/AHA guidelines for the management of patients with ST-elevation myocardial infarction—executive summary: A report of the American College of Cardiology/American Heart Association Task Force on Practice Guidelines (Writing Committee to Revise the 1999 Guidelines for the Management of Patients With Acute Myocardial Infarction). Circulation 2004;110(5):588–636.

83. Hunt SA, Abraham WT, Chin MH, et al. ACC/AHA 2005 Guideline Update for the Diagnosis and Management of Chronic Heart Failure in the Adult—Summary Article: A Report of the American College of Cardiology/American Heart Association Task Force on Practice Guidelines (Writing Committee to Update the 2001 Guidelines for the Evaluation and Management of Heart Failure): Developed in collaboration with the American College of Chest Physicians and the International Society for Heart and Lung Transplantation: Endorsed by the Heart Rhythm Society. Circulation 2005;112(12):1825–1852.

84. Standards of medical care in diabetes. Diabetes Care 2005;28(Suppl 1):S4–S36.

85. K/DOQI clinical practice guidelines on hypertension and antihypertensive agents in chronic kidney disease. Am J Kidney Dis 2004;43(5 Suppl 1):S1–S290.

86. Bakris GL, Williams M, Dworkin L, et al. Preserving renal function in adults with hypertension and diabetes: A consensus approach. National Kidney Foundation Hypertension and Diabetes Executive Committees Working Group. Am J Kidney Dis 2000;36(3):646–661.

87. Wing LM, Reid CM, Ryan P, et al. A comparison of outcomes with angiotensin-converting-enzyme inhibitors and diuretics for hypertension in the elderly. N Engl J Med 2003;348(7):583–592.

88. Yusuf S, Pfeffer MA, Swedberg K, et al. Effects of candesartan in patients with chronic heart failure and preserved left-ventricular ejection fraction: The CHARM-Preserved Trial. Lancet 2003;362 (9386):777–781.

89. Ripley TL, Harrison D. The power to TRANSCEND. Lancet 2008; 372(9644):1128–1130.

90. Yusuf S, Teo K, Anderson C, et al. Effects of the angiotensin-receptor blocker telmisartan on cardiovascular events in high-risk patients intolerant to angiotensin-converting enzyme inhibitors: A randomised controlled trial. Lancet 2008;372(9644):1174–1183.

91. McMurray JJ, Ostergren J, Swedberg K, et al. Effects of candesartan in patients with chronic heart failure and reduced left-ventricular systolic function taking angiotensin-converting-enzyme inhibitors: The CHARM-Added trial. Lancet 2003;362(9386):767–771.

92. Granger CB, McMurray JJ, Yusuf S, et al. Effects of candesartan in patients with chronic heart failure and reduced left-ventricular systolic function intolerant to angiotensin-converting-enzyme inhibitors: The CHARM-Alternative trial. Lancet 2003;362(9386): 772–776.

93. Haymore BR, Yoon J, Mikita CP, Klote MM, DeZee KJ. Risk of angioedema with angiotensin receptor blockers in patients with prior angioedema associated with angiotensin-converting enzyme inhibitors: A meta-analysis. Ann Allergy Asthma Immunol 2008;101 (5):495–499.

94. Cohn JN, McInnes GT, Shepherd AM. Direct-acting vasodilators. J Clin Hypertens 2011;13(9):690–692.

95. Sica DA. Minoxidil: An underused vasodilator for resistant or severe hypertension. J Clin Hypertens 2004;6(5):283–287.

96. Pickering TG. Why don't we use nitrates to treat older hypertensive patients? J Clin Hypertens 2005;7(11):685–687, 690.

97. Simon G, Wittig VJ, Cohn JN. Transdermal nitroglycerin as a step 3 antihypertensive drug. Clin Pharmacol Ther 1986;40(1):42–45.

98. Prevention of stroke by antihypertensive drug treatment in older persons with isolated systolic hypertension. Final results of the Systolic Hypertension in the Elderly Program (SHEP). SHEP Cooperative Research Group. JAMA 1991;265(24):3255–3264.

99. DiPiro JT, Talbert RL, Yee GC, Matzke GR, Wells BG, Posey ML. Pharmacotherapy: A Pathophysiologic Approach, 8th ed. New York, NY: McGraw-Hill Medical, 2011.

100. Somes GW, Pahor M, Shorr RI, Cushman WC, Applegate WB. The role of diastolic blood pressure when treating isolated systolic hypertension. Arch Intern Med 1999;159(17):2004–2009.

101. Lindheimer MD, Taler SJ, Cunningham · FG. Hypertension in pregnancy. J Am Soc Hypertens 2008;2(6):484–494.

102. The fourth report on the diagnosis, evaluation, and treatment of high blood pressure in children and adolescents. Pediatrics 2004;114(2 Suppl 4th Report):555–576.

103. Urbina E, Alpert B, Flynn J, et al. Ambulatory blood pressure monitoring in children and adolescents: Recommendations for standard assessment: A scientific statement from the American Heart Association Atherosclerosis, Hypertension, and Obesity in Youth Committee of the council on cardiovascular disease in the young and the council for high blood pressure research. Hypertension 2008;52(3):433–451.

104. Kliegman R, Nelson WE. Nelson Textbook of Pediatrics, 18th ed. Philadelphia, PA: Saunders; 2007.

105. Weber MA, Julius S, Kjeldsen SE, et al. Blood pressure dependent and independent effects of antihypertensive treatment on clinical events in the VALUE Trial. Lancet 2004;363(9426):2049–2051.

106. Hansson L, Zanchetti A, Carruthers SG, et al. Effects of intensive blood-pressure lowering and low-dose aspirin in patients with hypertension: Principal results of the Hypertension Optimal Treatment (HOT) randomised trial. HOT Study Group. Lancet 1998;351(9118):1755–1762.

6 Heart Failure

Orly Vardeny and Tien M. H. Ng

KEY CONCEPTS

❶ The most common causes of heart failure are coronary artery disease (CAD), hypertension, and dilated cardiomyopathy.

❷ Development and progression of heart failure involves activation of neurohormonal pathways, including the sympathetic nervous system and the renin-angiotensin-aldosterone system (RAAS).

❸ The clinician must identify potential reversible causes of heart failure exacerbations, including prescription and nonprescription drug therapies, dietary indiscretions, and medication nonadherence.

❹ Symptoms of left-sided heart failure include dyspnea, orthopnea, and paroxysmal nocturnal dyspnea (PND), whereas symptoms of right-sided heart failure include fluid retention, GI bloating, and fatigue.

❺ General therapeutic management goals for chronic heart failure focus on preventing onset of clinical symptoms or reducing symptoms, preventing or reducing hospitalizations, slowing or preventing disease progression, improving quality of life, and prolonging patient survival.

❻ Nonpharmacologic treatment involves dietary modifications such as sodium and fluid restriction, risk factor reduction including smoking cessation, timely immunizations, and supervised regular physical activity.

❼ Diuretics are used for relief of acute symptoms of congestion and maintenance of euvolemia.

❽ Agents with proven benefits in improving symptoms, slowing disease progression, and improving survival in chronic heart failure target neurohormonal blockade; these include angiotensin-converting enzyme (ACE) inhibitors or angiotensin receptor blockers (ARBs), β-adrenergic blockers, and aldosterone antagonists.

❾ Combination therapy with hydralazine and isosorbide dinitrate is an appropriate substitute for angiotensin II antagonism in those unable to tolerate an ACE inhibitor or ARB or as add-on therapy in African Americans.

❿ Treatment of acute heart failure targets relief of congestion and optimization of cardiac output utilizing oral or IV diuretics, IV vasodilators, and when appropriate, inotropes. Current treatment strategies in acute heart failure target improving hemodynamics while preserving organ function.

Heart failure (HF) is defined as the inadequate ability of the heart to pump enough blood to meet the blood flow and metabolic demands of the body.[1] High-output HF is characterized by an inordinate increase in the body's metabolic demands that outpaces an increase in cardiac output (CO) of a generally normally functioning heart. More commonly, HF is a result of low CO secondary to impaired cardiac function. The term *heart failure* refers to low-output HF for the purposes of this chapter.

HF is a clinical syndrome characterized by a history of specific signs and symptoms related to congestion and hypoperfusion. Because HF can occur in the presence or absence of fluid overload, the term *heart failure* is preferred over the former term *congestive heart failure*. HF results from any structural or functional cardiac disorder that impairs the ability of the ventricle to fill with or eject blood.[1] Many disorders, such as those of the pericardium, epicardium, endocardium, or great vessels, may lead to HF, but most patients develop symptoms due to impairment in left ventricular (LV) myocardial function.

The term *acute heart failure* (AHF) is used to signify either an acute decompensation of a patient with a history of chronic HF or to refer to a patient presenting with new-onset HF symptoms. Terms commonly associated with HF, such as *cardiomyopathy* and *LV dysfunction,* are not equivalent to HF but describe possible structural or functional reasons for the development of HF.

EPIDEMIOLOGY AND ETIOLOGY

Epidemiology

HF is a major public health concern affecting approximately 6 million people in the United States. An additional 670,000 new cases are diagnosed each year. HF manifests most commonly in adults older than 60 years.[2] The growing prevalence of HF corresponds to (a) better treatment of patients with acute myocardial infarctions (MIs) who will survive to develop HF later in life, and (b) the increasing proportion of older adults due to the aging baby boomer population. The relative incidence of HF is lower in women compared with men, but there is a greater prevalence in women overall due to their longer life expectancy. Acute HF accounts for 12 to 15 million office visits per year and 6.5 million hospitalizations annually.[2] According to national registries, patients presenting with AHF are older (mean age: 75 years) and have numerous comorbidities such as coronary artery disease (CAD), renal insufficiency, and diabetes.[2]

Total estimated direct and indirect costs for managing both chronic and acute HF in the United States for 2009 was approximately $37 billion. Medications account for approximately 10% of that cost.[3] HF is the most common hospital discharge diagnosis for Medicare patients and the most costly diagnosis in this population.

The prognosis for patients hospitalized for AHF remains poor. Average hospital length of stay is estimated to be between 4 and 6 days, a number that has remained constant over the past decade.[3] The in-hospital mortality rate has been estimated at approximately 4%, but ranges from 2% to 20% depending on the report.[4] In-hospital mortality increases to an average of 10.6% in patients requiring an intensive care unit admission. Readmissions are also high, with up to 30% to 60% of patients readmitted within 6 months of their initial discharge date.[4] The 5-year mortality rate for chronic HF remains greater than 50%. Survival strongly correlates with severity of symptoms and functional capacity. Sudden cardiac death is the most common cause of death, occurring in approximately 40% of patients with HF.[2] Although therapies targeting the upregulated neurohormonal response contributing to the pathophysiology of HF have clearly impacted morbidity and mortality, long-term survival remains low.

Etiology

HF is the eventual outcome of numerous cardiac diseases or disorders (Table 6–1).[5] HF can be classified by the primary underlying etiology as ischemic or nonischemic, with 70% of HF related to ischemia. ❶ *The most common causes of HF are CAD, hypertension, and dilated cardiomyopathy.* CAD resulting in an acute MI and reduced ventricular function is a common presenting history. Nonischemic etiologies include hypertension, viral illness, thyroid disease, excessive alcohol use, illicit drug use, pregnancy-related heart disease, familial congenital disease, and valvular disorders such as mitral or tricuspid valve regurgitation or stenosis.

HF can also be classified based on the main component of the cardiac cycle leading to impaired ventricular function. A normal cardiac cycle depends on two components: systole and diastole. Expulsion of blood occurs during systole or contraction of the ventricles; diastole relates to filling of the ventricles. Ejection fraction (EF) is the fraction of the

---

Table 6–1
Causes of Heart Failure

Systolic Dysfunction (Decreased Contractility)
- Reduction in muscle mass (e.g., myocardial infarction)
- Dilated cardiomyopathies
- Ventricular hypertrophy
  - Pressure overload (e.g., systemic or pulmonary hypertension, aortic or pulmonic valve stenosis)
  - Volume overload (e.g., valvular regurgitation, shunts, high-output states)

Diastolic Dysfunction (Restriction in Ventricular Filling)
- Increased ventricular stiffness
- Ventricular hypertrophy (e.g., hypertrophic cardiomyopathy, pressure and/or volume overload)
- Infiltrative myocardial diseases (e.g., amyloidosis, sarcoidosis, endomyocardial fibrosis)
- Myocardial ischemia and infarction
- Mitral or tricuspid valve stenosis
- Pericardial disease (e.g., pericarditis, pericardial tamponade)

From Parker RB, Cavallari LH. Systolic heart failure. In: DiPiro JT, Talbert RL, Yee GC, et al., eds. Pharmacotherapy: A pathophysiologic approach, 8th ed. New York, NY: McGraw-Hill, 2011:138, with permission.

volume present at the end of diastole that is pushed into the aorta during systole. Abnormal ventricular filling (**diastolic dysfunction**) and/or ventricular contraction (**systolic dysfunction**) can result in a similar decrease in CO and cause HF symptoms. Most HF is associated with evidence of LV systolic dysfunction (evidenced by a reduced EF) with or without a component of diastolic dysfunction, which coexists in up to two-thirds of patients. Isolated diastolic dysfunction, occurring in approximately one-third of HF patients, is diagnosed when a patient exhibits impaired ventricular filling with or without accompanying HF symptoms but normal systolic function. Long-standing hypertension is the leading cause of diastolic dysfunction. Ventricular dysfunction can also involve either the left or right chamber of the heart or both. This has implications for symptomatology because right-sided failure manifests as systemic congestion, whereas left-sided failure results in pulmonary symptoms.

PATHOPHYSIOLOGY

A basic grasp of normal cardiac function sets the stage for understanding the pathophysiological processes leading to HF and selecting appropriate therapy for HF. CO is defined as the volume of blood ejected per unit of time (liters per minute) and is a major determinant of tissue perfusion. CO is the product of heart rate (HR) and stroke volume (SV): CO = HR × SV. The following sections describe how each parameter relates to CO.

HR is controlled by the autonomic nervous system, where sympathetic stimulation of β-adrenergic receptors results in an increase in HR and CO. SV is the volume of blood ejected with each systole. SV volume is determined by factors regulating **preload, afterload,** and contractility. Preload is a measure of ventricular filling pressure, or the volume of blood in the left ventricle (also known as LV end-diastolic volume). Preload is determined by venous return as well as atrial contraction. An increase in venous return to the left ventricle results in the stretch of cardiomyocyte sarcomeres (or contractile units) and a subsequent increase in the number of cross-bridges formed between actin and myosin myofilaments. This results in an increase in the force of contraction based on the **Frank-Starling mechanism.**[6] Afterload is the resistance to ventricular ejection and regulated by ejection impedance, wall tension, and regional wall geometry. Thus, elevated aortic and systemic pressures result in an increase in afterload and reduced SV. Contractility, also known as the **inotropic** state of the heart, is an intrinsic property of cardiac muscle incorporating fiber shortening and tension development. Contractility is influenced to a large degree by adrenergic nerve activity and circulating catecholamines such as epinephrine and norepinephrine.

Compensatory Mechanisms

In the setting of a sustained loss of myocardium, a number of mechanisms aid the heart when faced with an increased hemodynamic burden and reduced CO. They include the following: the Frank-Starling mechanism, tachycardia and increased afterload, and cardiac hypertrophy and remodeling (**Table 6–2**).[5,7]

▶ Preload and the Frank-Starling Mechanism

In the setting of a sudden decrease in CO, the natural response of the body is to decrease blood flow to the periphery to maintain perfusion to the vital organs such as the heart and brain. Therefore, renal perfusion is compromised due to both the decreased CO as well as the shunting of blood away from peripheral tissues. This results in activation

Table 6–2		
Beneficial and Detrimental Effects of the Compensatory Responses in Heart Failure		
Compensatory Response	**Beneficial Effects of Compensation**	**Detrimental Effects of Compensation**
Increased preload (through sodium and water retention)	Optimize stroke volume via Frank-Starling mechanism	Pulmonary and systemic congestion and edema formation Increased MVO_2
Vasoconstriction	Maintain blood pressure and perfusion in the face of reduced cardiac output	Increased MVO_2 Increased afterload decreases stroke volume and further activates the compensatory responses
Tachycardia and increased contractility (due to SNS activation)	Increase cardiac output	Increased MVO_2 Shortened diastolic filling time β_1-Receptor downregulation, decreased receptor sensitivity Precipitation of ventricular arrhythmias Increased risk of myocardial cell death
Ventricular hypertrophy and remodeling	Maintains cardiac output Reduces myocardial wall stress Decreases MVO_2	Diastolic dysfunction Systolic dysfunction Increased risk of myocardial cell death Increased risk of myocardial ischemia Increased arrhythmia risk

MVO_2, myocardial oxygen consumption; SNS, sympathetic nervous system.

of the renin-angiotensin-aldosterone system (RAAS). The decrease in renal perfusion is sensed by the juxtaglomerular cells of the kidneys leading to the release of renin and initiation of the cascade for production of angiotensin II. Angiotensin II stimulates the synthesis and release of aldosterone. Aldosterone in turn stimulates sodium and water retention in an attempt to increase intravascular volume and hence preload. In a healthy heart, a large increase in CO is usually accomplished with just a small change in preload. However, in a failing heart, alterations in the contractile filaments reduce the ability of cardiomyocytes to adapt to increases in preload. Thus, an increase in preload actually impairs contractile function in the failing heart and results in a further decrease in CO.

▶ *Tachycardia and Increased Afterload*

● Another mechanism to maintain CO when contractility is low is to increase HR. This is achieved through sympathetic nervous system (SNS) activation and the agonist effect of norepinephrine on β-adrenergic receptors in the heart. Sympathetic activation also enhances contractility by increasing cytosolic calcium concentrations. SV is relatively fixed in HF; thus HR becomes the major determinant of CO. Although this mechanism increases CO acutely, the **chronotropic** and inotropic responses to sympathetic activation increase myocardial oxygen demand, worsen underlying ischemia, contribute to proarrhythmia, and further impair both systolic and diastolic function.

Activation of both the RAAS and the SNS also contribute to vasoconstriction in an attempt to redistribute blood flow from peripheral organs such as the kidneys to coronary and cerebral circulation.[7] However, arterial vasoconstriction leads to impaired forward ejection of blood from the heart due to an increase in afterload. This results in a decrease in CO and continued stimulation of compensatory responses, creating a vicious cycle of neurohormonal activation.

▶ *Cardiac Hypertrophy and Remodeling*

Ventricular hypertrophy, an adaptive increase in ventricular muscle mass due to the growth of existing myocytes, occurs in response to an increased hemodynamic burden such as volume or pressure overload.[5] Hypertrophy can be concentric or eccentric. Concentric hypertrophy occurs in response to pressure overload such as in long-standing hypertension or pulmonary hypertension, whereas eccentric hypertrophy occurs after an acute MI. Eccentric hypertrophy involves an increase in myocyte size in a segmental fashion, as opposed to the global hypertrophy occurring in concentric hypertrophy. Although hypertrophy helps to reduce cardiac wall stress in the short term, continued hypertrophy accelerates myocyte cell death through an overall increase in myocardial oxygen demand.

Cardiac remodeling occurs as a compensatory adaptation to a change in wall stress and is largely regulated by neurohormonal activation, with angiotensin II and aldosterone being key stimuli.[7] The process entails changes in myocardial and extracellular matrix composition and function that results in both structural and functional alterations to the heart. In

HF, the changes in cardiac size, shape, and composition are pathological and detrimental to heart function. In addition to myocyte size and extracellular matrix changes, heart geometry shifts from an elliptical to a less efficient spherical shape. Even after remodeling occurs, the heart can maintain CO for many years. However, heart function will continue to deteriorate until progression to clinical HF. The timeline for remodeling varies depending on the cardiac insult. For example, in the setting of an acute MI, remodeling starts within a few days.[5] Chronic remodeling, however, is what progressively worsens HF, and therefore it is a major target of drug therapy.

Models of Heart Failure

Earlier models of HF focused on the hemodynamic consequences of volume overload from excess sodium and water retention, decreased CO secondary to impaired ventricular function, and vasoconstriction.[8] Congestion was a result of fluid backup due to inadequate pump function. Therefore, drug therapy was focused on relieving excess volume using diuretics, improving pump function with inotropic agents, and alleviating vasoconstriction with vasodilators. Although these agents improved HF symptoms, they did little to slow the progressive decline in cardiac function or to improve survival.

▶ *Neurohormonal Model*

❷ *Development and progression of HF involves activation of neurohormonal pathways including the sympathetic nervous system and the RAAS.* This model begins with an initial precipitating event or myocardial injury resulting in a decline in CO, followed by the compensatory mechanisms previously discussed. This includes activation of neurohormonal pathways with pathological consequences including the RAAS, SNS, endothelin, and vasopressin, and those with counterregulatory properties such as the natriuretic peptides and nitric oxide. This model currently guides our therapy for chronic HF in terms of preventing disease progression and mortality.

Angiotensin II Angiotensin II is a key neurohormone in the pathophysiology of HF. The vasoconstrictive effects of angiotensin II lead to an increase in systemic vascular resistance (SVR) and blood pressure. The resulting increase in afterload contributes to an increase in myocardial oxygen demand and opposes the desired increase in SV. In the kidneys, angiotensin II enhances renal function acutely by raising intraglomerular pressure through constriction of the efferent arterioles.[6] However, the increase in glomerular filtration pressure may be offset by a reduction in renal perfusion secondary to angiotensin II's influence over the release of other vasoactive neurohormones such as vasopressin and endothelin-1 (ET-1). Angiotensin II also potentiates the release of aldosterone from the adrenal glands and norepinephrine from adrenergic nerve terminals. Additionally, angiotensin II induces vascular hypertrophy and remodeling in both cardiac and renal cells. Clinical studies show that blocking the effects of the RAAS in HF is associated with improved cardiac function and prolonged survival. Thus, angiotensin-converting enzyme (ACE) inhibitors and angiotensin receptor blockers (ARBs) are the cornerstone of HF treatment.

Aldosterone Aldosterone's contribution to HF pathophysiology is also multifaceted. Renally, aldosterone causes sodium and water retention in an attempt to enhance intravascular volume and CO. This adaptive mechanism has deleterious consequences because excessive sodium and water retention worsen the already elevated ventricular filling pressures. Aldosterone also contributes to electrolyte abnormalities seen in HF patients. Hypokalemia and hypomagnesemia contribute to the increased risk of arrhythmias. In addition, evidence supports the role of aldosterone as an etiological factor for myocardial fibrosis and cardiac remodeling by causing increased extracellular matrix collagen deposition and cardiac fibrosis.[6] Aldosterone potentially contributes to disease progression via sympathetic potentiation and ventricular remodeling. In addition, the combination of these multiple effects is likely responsible for the increased risk of sudden cardiac death attributed to aldosterone. As elevated aldosterone concentrations have been associated with a poorer prognosis in HF, its blockade has become an important therapeutic target for improvement of long-term prognosis.

Norepinephrine Norepinephrine is a classic marker for SNS activation. It plays an adaptive role in the failing heart by stimulating HR and myocardial contractility to augment CO and by producing vasoconstriction to maintain organ perfusion. However, excess levels are directly cardiotoxic. In addition, sympathetic activation increases the risk for arrhythmias, ischemia, and myocyte cell death through increased myocardial workload and accelerated apoptosis (i.e., programmed cell death). Ventricular hypertrophy and remodeling are also influenced by norepinephrine.[8]

Plasma norepinephrine concentrations are elevated proportionally to HF severity, with highest levels correlating to the poorest prognosis. Several mechanisms relate to diminished responsiveness to catecholamines (e.g., norepinephrine) as cardiac function declines.[6] Adrenergic receptor desensitization and downregulation (decreased receptor number and postreceptor responses and signaling) occurs under sustained sympathetic stimulation. The desensitization contributes to further release of norepinephrine.[5] β-Adrenergic blocking agents, although intrinsically negatively inotropic, have become essential therapy for chronic HF.

Endothelin ET-1, one of the most potent physiological vasoconstrictors, is an important contributor to HF pathophysiology.[9] ET-1 binds to two G-protein coupled receptors, endothelin-A (ET-A) and endothelin-B (ET-B). ET-A receptors mediate vasoconstriction and are prevalent in vascular smooth muscle and cardiac cells. ET-B receptors are expressed on the endothelium and in vascular smooth muscle, and receptor stimulation mediates vasodilation. Levels of ET-1 correlate with HF functional class and mortality.

Arginine Vasopressin Higher vasopressin concentrations are linked to dilutional hyponatremia and a poor prognosis in HF. Vasopressin exerts its effects through vasopressin type 1a (V_{1a}) and vasopressin type 2 (V_2) receptors.[5,7] Vasopressin type 1a stimulation leads to vasoconstriction, whereas actions on the V_2 receptor cause free water retention through aquaporin channels in the collecting duct. Vasopressin increases preload, afterload, and myocardial oxygen demand in the failing heart.

Counterregulatory Hormones (Natriuretic Peptides, Bradykinin, and Nitric Oxide) Atrial natriuretic peptide (ANP) and B-type (formerly brain) natriuretic peptide (BNP) are endogenous neurohormones that regulate sodium and water balance. Natriuretic peptides decrease sodium reabsorption in the collecting duct of the kidney.[10] Natriuretic peptides also cause vasodilation through the cyclic guanosine monophosphate (cGMP) pathway. Atrial natriuretic peptide is synthesized and stored in the atria, while BNP is produced mainly in the ventricles. Release of ANP and BNP is stimulated by increased cardiac chamber wall stretch usually indicative of volume load. Higher concentrations of natriuretic peptides correlate with a more severe HF functional class and prognosis. BNP is sensitive to volume status; thus the plasma concentration can be used as a diagnostic marker in HF.[10]

Bradykinin is part of the kallikrein-kinin system, which shares a link to the RAAS through ACE. Bradykinin is a vasodilatory peptide that is released in response to a variety of stimuli, including neurohormonal and inflammatory mediators known to be activated in HF.[9] As a consequence, bradykinin levels are elevated in HF patients and thought to partially antagonize the vasoconstrictive peptides.

Nitric oxide, a vasodilatory hormone released by the endothelium, is found in higher concentrations in HF patients and provides two main benefits in HF: vasodilation and neurohormonal antagonism of endothelin.[9] Nitric oxide's production is affected by the enzyme inducible nitric oxide synthetase (iNOS), which is upregulated in the setting of HF, likely due to increased levels of angiotensin II, norepinephrine, and multiple cytokines. In HF, the physiological response to nitric oxide appears to be blunted, which contributes to the imbalance between vasoconstriction and vasodilation.

▶ Cardiorenal Model

There is growing evidence of a link between renal disease and HF.[8] Renal insufficiency is present in one-third of HF patients and is associated with a worse prognosis. In hospitalized HF patients, the presence of renal insufficiency is associated with longer lengths of stay, increased in-hospital morbidity and mortality, and detrimental neurohormonal alterations. Conversely, renal dysfunction is a common complication of HF or results from its treatment. Renal failure is also a common cause for HF decompensation.

▶ Proinflammatory Cytokines

Inflammatory cytokines have been implicated in the pathophysiology of HF.[9] Several proinflammatory (e.g., tumor necrosis factor [TNF]-α, interleukin-1, interleukin-6, and interferon-γ) and anti-inflammatory cytokines (e.g., interleukin-10) are overexpressed in the failing heart. The most is known about TNF-α, a pleiotropic cytokine that acts as a negative inotrope, stimulates cardiac cell apoptosis, uncouples β-adrenergic receptors from adenylyl cyclase, and is related to cardiac cachexia. The exact role of cytokines and inflammation in HF pathophysiology continues to be studied.

Precipitating and Exacerbating Factors in Heart Failure

HF patients exist in one of two clinical states. When a patient's volume status and symptoms are stable, their HF condition is said to be "compensated." In situations of volume overload or other worsening symptoms, the patient is considered "decompensated." Acute decompensation can be precipitated by numerous etiologies that can be grouped into cardiac, metabolic, or patient-related causes (Table 6–3).[5]

❸ *The clinician must identify potential reversible causes of HF exacerbations including prescription and nonprescription drug therapies, dietary indiscretions, and medication nonadherence.* Nonadherence with dietary restrictions or chronic HF medications deserves special attention because it is the most common cause of acute decompensation and can be prevented. As such, an accurate history regarding diet, food choices, and the patient's knowledge regarding sodium and fluid intake (including alcohol) is valuable in assessing dietary indiscretion. Nonadherence with medical recommendations such as laboratory and other appointment follow-up can also be indicative of nonadherence with diet or medications.

Table 6–3

Exacerbating or Precipitating Factors in Heart Failure

Cardiac	Metabolic	Patient-Related
Acute ischemia	Anemia	Dietary/fluid nonadherence
Arrhythmia	Hyperthyroidism/ thyrotoxicosis	HF therapy nonadherence
Endocarditis	Infection	Use of cardiotoxins (cocaine, chronic alcohol, amphetamines, sympathomimetics)
Myocarditis	Pregnancy	
Pulmonary embolus	Worsening renal function	
Uncontrolled hypertension		Offending medications (NSAIDs, COX-2 inhibitors, steroids, lithium, β-blockers, calcium channel blockers, antiarrhythmics, alcohol, thiazolidinediones)
Valvular disorders		

COX-2, cyclooxygenase-2; HF, heart failure; NSAID, nonsteroidal anti-inflammatory drug.

CLINICAL PRESENTATION AND DIAGNOSIS OF CHRONIC HEART FAILURE

In low-output HF, symptoms are generally related to either congestion behind the failing ventricle(s), or hypoperfusion (decreased tissue blood supply), or both. For example, a failing left ventricle causes fluid to back up in the lungs, and a patient with right ventricular failure would exhibit systemic symptoms of congestion. Congestion is the most common symptom in HF, followed by symptoms related to decreased perfusion to peripheral tissues including decreased renal output, mental confusion, and cold extremities. Activation of the compensatory mechanisms occurs in an effort to increase CO and preserve blood flow to vital organs. However, the increase in preload and afterload in the setting of a failing ventricle leads to elevated filling pressures and further impairment of cardiac function, which manifests as systemic and/or pulmonary congestion. It is important to remember that congestion develops behind the failing ventricle, caused by the inability of that ventricle to eject the blood that it receives from the atria and venous return. As such, signs and symptoms may be classified as left sided or right sided. **❹** *Symptoms of left-sided HF include dyspnea, orthopnea, and paroxysmal nocturnal dyspnea (PND), whereas symptoms of right-sided HF include fluid retention, GI bloating, and fatigue.* Although most patients initially have left ventricular failure (LVF; pulmonary congestion), the ventricles share a septal wall, and because LVF increases the workload of the right ventricle, both ventricles eventually fail and contribute to the HF syndrome. Because of the complex nature of this syndrome, it has become exceedingly more difficult to attribute a specific sign or symptom as caused by either right ventricular failure (RVF; systemic congestion) or LVF. Therefore, the numerous signs and symptoms associated with this disorder are collectively attributed to HF rather than to dysfunction of a specific ventricle.

General Signs and Symptoms

Hypoperfusion of skeletal muscles leads to fatigue, weakness, and exercise intolerance. Decreased perfusion of the central nervous system (CNS) is related to confusion, hallucinations, insomnia, and lethargy. Peripheral vasoconstriction due to SNS activity causes pallor, cool extremities, and cyanosis of the digits. Tachycardia is also common in these patients and may reflect increased SNS activity. Patients often exhibit polyuria and nocturia. Polyuria is a result of increased release of natriuretic peptides caused by volume overload. Nocturia occurs due to increased renal perfusion as a consequence of reduced SNS renal vasoconstrictive effects at night. In chronic severe HF, unintentional weight loss can occur that leads to a syndrome of cardiac cachexia. Cardiac cachexia can be defined as a nonedematous weight loss greater than 6% of the previous normal weight over a period of at least 6 months. HF prognosis worsens considerably once cardiac cachexia has been diagnosed, regardless of HF severity. This results from several factors including loss of appetite,

Clinical Presentation and Diagnosis of Chronic Heart Failure

General
Patient presentation may range from asymptomatic to cardiogenic shock.

Symptoms
- Dyspnea, particularly on exertion
- Orthopnea
- Shortness of breath (SOB)
- Paroxysmal nocturnal dyspnea
- Exercise intolerance
- Tachypnea
- Cough
- Fatigue
- Nocturia and/or polyuria
- Hemoptysis
- Abdominal pain
- Anorexia
- Nausea
- Bloating
- Ascites
- Mental status changes
- Weakness
- Lethargy

Signs
- Pulmonary rales
- Pulmonary edema
- S_3 gallop
- Pleural effusion
- Cheyne-Stokes respiration
- Tachycardia
- Cardiomegaly
- Peripheral edema (e.g., pedal edema, which is swelling of feet and ankles)
- Jugular venous distension (JVD)
- Hepatojugular reflux (HJR)
- Hepatomegaly
- Cyanosis of the digits
- Pallor or cool extremities

Laboratory Tests
- BNP greater than 100 pg/mL (greater than 100 ng/L or 28.9 pmol/L) or N-terminal proBNP (NT-proBNP) greater than 300 pg/mL (greater than 300 ng/L or greater than 35.4 pmol/L)
- Electrocardiogram (ECG): May be normal or could show numerous abnormalities including acute ST-T–wave changes from myocardial ischemia, atrial fibrillation, bradycardia, and LV hypertrophy.
- Serum creatinine: May be increased owing to hypoperfusion; preexisting renal dysfunction can contribute to volume overload.
- Complete blood count: Useful to determine if HF is due to reduced oxygen-carrying capacity.
- Chest x-ray: Useful for detection of cardiac enlargement, pulmonary edema, and pleural effusions.
- Echocardiogram: Used to assess LV size, valve function, pericardial effusion, wall motion abnormalities, and ejection fraction.

malabsorption due to GI edema, elevated metabolic rate, and elevated levels of norepinephrine and proinflammatory cytokines. Absorption of fats is especially affected, leading to deficiencies of fat-soluble vitamins.

Patients can experience a variety of symptoms related to buildup of fluid in the lungs. Dyspnea, or shortness of breath, can result from pulmonary congestion or systemic hypoperfusion due to LVF. Exertional dyspnea occurs when patients describe breathlessness induced by physical activity or a lower level of activity than previously known to cause breathlessness. Patients often state that activities such as stair climbing, carrying groceries, or walking a particular distance cause shortness of breath. Severity of HF is inversely proportional to the amount of activity required to produce dyspnea. In severe HF, dyspnea is present even at rest.

Orthopnea is dyspnea that is positional. Orthopnea is present if a patient is unable to breathe while lying flat on a bed (i.e., in the recumbent position). It manifests within minutes of a patient lying down and is relieved immediately when the patient sits upright. Patients can relieve orthopnea by elevating their head and shoulders with pillows. The practitioner should inquire as to the number of pillows needed to prevent dyspnea as a marker of worsening HF. PND occurs when patients awaken suddenly with a feeling of breathlessness and suffocation. PND is caused by increased venous return and mobilization of interstitial fluid from the extremities leading to alveolar edema, and it usually occurs within 1 to 4 hours of sleep. In contrast to orthopnea, PND is not relieved immediately by sitting upright and often takes up to 30 minutes for symptoms to subside.

Pulmonary congestion may also cause a nonproductive cough that occurs at night or with exertion. Cheyne-Stokes respiration, or periodic breathing, is also common in advanced HF. It is usually associated with low-output states and may be perceived by the patient as either severe dyspnea or transient cessation of breathing. In cases of pulmonary edema, the most severe form of pulmonary congestion, patients may produce a pink frothy sputum and experience extreme breathlessness and anxiety due to feelings of suffocation and drowning. If not treated aggressively, patients can become cyanotic and acidotic. Severe pulmonary edema can progress to respiratory failure, necessitating mechanical ventilation.

Systemic venous congestion results mainly from right ventricular failure. A clinically validated assessment of the jugular venous pressure (JVP) is performed by examining the right internal jugular vein for distention or elevation of the pulsation while reclining at a 45-degree angle. A JVP more than 4 cm above the sternal angle is indicative of elevated right atrial pressure. JVP may be normal at rest, but if application of pressure to the abdomen can elicit a sustained elevation of JVP, this is defined as hepatojugular reflux (HJR). A positive finding of HJR indicates hepatic congestion and results from displacement of volume from the abdomen into the jugular vein because the right atrium is unable to accept this additional blood. Hepatic congestion can cause abnormalities in liver function, which can be evident in liver function tests and/or clotting times. Development of hepatomegaly occurs infrequently and is caused by long-term systemic venous congestion. Intestinal or abdominal congestion can also be present, but it usually does not lead to characteristic signs unless overt ascites is evident. In advanced RVF, evidence of pulmonary hypertension may be present (e.g., right ventricular heave).

The most recognized finding of systemic congestion is peripheral edema. It usually occurs in dependent areas of the body, such as the ankles (pedal edema) for ambulatory patients or the sacral region for bedridden patients. Weight gain often precedes signs of overt peripheral edema. Therefore, it is crucial for patients to weigh themselves daily even in the absence of symptoms to assess fluid status.

Patients may complain of swelling of their feet and ankles, which can extend up to their calves or thighs. Abdominal congestion may cause a bloated feeling, abdominal pain, early satiety, nausea, anorexia, and constipation. Often patients may have difficulty fitting into their shoes or pants due to edema.

▶ Patient History

A thorough history is crucial to identify cardiac and noncardiac disorders or behaviors that may lead to or accelerate the development of HF. Past medical history, family history, and social history are important for identifying comorbid illnesses that are risk factors for the development of HF or underlying etiological factors. A complete medication history (including prescription and nonprescription drugs, herbal therapy, and vitamin supplements) should be obtained each time a patient is seen to evaluate adherence, to assess appropriateness of therapy, to eliminate drugs that may be harmful in HF (Table 6–4), and to determine additional monitoring requirements.[5] For newly diagnosed HF, previous use of chemotherapeutic agents as well as current or past use

Table 6–4
Drugs That May Precipitate or Exacerbate Heart Failure

Agents Causing Negative Inotropic Effect
Antiarrhythmics (e.g., disopyramide, flecainide, and others)
β-Blockers (e.g., propranolol, metoprolol, atenolol, and others)
Calcium channel blockers (e.g., verapamil and others)
Itraconazole
Terbinafine

Cardiotoxic Agents
Doxorubicin
Daunomycin
Cyclophosphamide

Agents Causing Sodium and Water Retention
Nonsteroidal anti-inflammatory drugs
COX-2 inhibitors
Glucocorticoids
Androgens
Estrogens
Salicylates (high dose)
Sodium-containing drugs (e.g., carbenicillin disodium, ticarcillin disodium)
Thiazolidinediones (e.g., pioglitazone)

COX-2, cyclooxygenase-2.

Adapted from Parker RB, Cavallari LH. Systolic heart failure. In: DiPiro JT, Talbert RL, Yee GC, et al., eds. Pharmacotherapy: A pathophysiologic approach, 8th ed. New York, NY: McGraw-Hill, 2011:137–172.

of alcohol and illicit drugs should be assessed. In addition, for patients with a known history of HF, questions related to symptomatology and exercise tolerance are essential for assessing any changes in clinical status that may warrant further evaluation or adjustment of the medication regimen.

Patient Encounter Part 1

DG is a 68-year-old man with a history of known coronary artery disease and type 2 diabetes mellitus who presents for a belated follow-up clinic visit (his last visit was 2 years ago). His most bothersome complaint is SOB at night when lying down flat; he has to sleep on three pillows to get adequate rest and sometimes even that does not help. Although he used to be able to walk a few blocks and two to three flights of stairs comfortably before getting breathless, he has had increasing symptoms and has now progressed to SOB with any walking and while cooking and getting dressed. He also notes his ankles are always swollen and his shoes no longer fit; therefore he only wears slippers. Additionally, his appetite is decreased, and he often feels bloated.

What information is suggestive of a diagnosis of HF?

What additional information do you need to know before creating a treatment plan for DG?

Heart Failure Classification

● There are two common systems for categorizing patients with HF. The New York Heart Association (NYHA) Functional Classification (FC) system is based on the patient's activity level and exercise tolerance. It divides patients into one of four classes, with functional class I patients exhibiting no symptoms or limitations of daily activities, and functional class IV patients who are symptomatic at rest (Table 6–5). The NYHA FC system reflects a subjective assessment by a healthcare provider and can change frequently over short periods of time. Functional class correlates poorly with EF; however, EF is one of the strongest predictors of prognosis. In general, anticipated survival declines in conjunction with a decline in functional ability.

The American College of Cardiology/American Heart Association (ACC/AHA) have proposed another system based on the development and progression of the disease. Instead of classifications, patients are placed into stages A through D (Table 6–5).[11] Because the staging system is related to development and progression of HF, it also proposes management strategies for each stage including

Table 6–5

New York Heart Association (NYHA) Functional Classification and American College of Cardiology/ American Heart Association (ACC/AHA) Staging

NYHA Functional Class	ACC/AHA Stage	Description
N/A	A	Patients at high risk for heart failure but without structural heart disease or symptoms of heart failure.
I	B	Patients with cardiac disease but without limitations of physical activity. Ordinary physical activity does not cause undue fatigue, dyspnea, or palpitation.
II	C	Patients with cardiac disease that results in slight limitations of physical activity. Ordinary physical activity results in fatigue, palpitations, dyspnea, or angina.
III	C	Patients with cardiac disease that results in marked limitation of physical activity. Although patients are comfortable at rest, less than ordinary activity will lead to symptoms.
IV	C, D	Patients with cardiac disease that results in an inability to carry on physical activity without discomfort. Symptoms of heart failure are present at rest. With any physical activity, increased discomfort is experienced. Stage D refers to end-stage heart failure patients.

risk factor modification. The staging system is meant to complement the NYHA FC system; however, patients can move between NYHA functional classes as symptoms improve with treatment, whereas HF staging does not allow for patients to move to a lower stage (e.g., patients cannot be categorized as stage C and move to stage B after treatment). Currently, patients are categorized based on both systems. Functional classification and staging are useful from a clinician's perspective, allowing for a longitudinal assessment of a patient's risk and progress, requirements for nonpharmacologic interventions, response to medications, and overall prognosis.

TREATMENT OF CHRONIC HEART FAILURE

Desired Therapeutic Outcomes

● There is no cure for HF. ⑤ *The general therapeutic management goals for chronic HF include preventing the onset of clinical symptoms or reducing symptoms, preventing or reducing hospitalizations, slowing progression of the disease, improving quality of life, and prolonging survival.* The ACC/AHA staging system described earlier provides a guide for application of these goals based on the clinical progression of HF for a given patient. The goals are additive as one moves from stage A to stage D.[1,11] For stage A, risk factor management is the primary goal. Stage B includes the addition of pharmacologic therapies known to slow the progression of the disease in an attempt to prevent the onset of clinical symptoms. Stage C involves the use of additional therapies aimed at controlling symptoms and decreasing morbidity. Finally, in stage D, the goals shift toward quality-of-life related issues. Only with aggressive management throughout all the stages of the disease will the ultimate goal of improving survival be realized. The attainment of these goals is based on designing a therapeutic approach that encompasses strategies aimed at control and treatment of contributing disorders, nonpharmacologic interventions, and optimal use of pharmacologic therapies.[12,13]

Control and Treatment of Contributing Disorders

All causes of HF must be investigated to determine the etiology of cardiac dysfunction in a given patient. Because the most common etiology of HF in the United States is ischemic heart disease, coronary angiography is warranted in most patients with a history suggestive of underlying CAD. Revascularization of those with significant CAD may help restore some cardiac function in patients with reversible ischemic defects. Aggressive control of hypertension, diabetes, and obesity is also essential because each of these conditions can cause further cardiac damage. Surgical repair of valvular disease or congenital malformations may be warranted if detected. Clinical HF partly depends on metabolic processes, so correction of imbalances such as thyroid disease, anemia,

Patient Encounter Part 2

DG's Medical History, Physical Examination, and Diagnostic Tests

PMH

Hypertension × 20 years

Type 2 diabetes mellitus × 15 years

Coronary artery disease × 10 years (MIs in 1999 and 2002)

Tobacco use

History of migraines × 40 years

Allergies

No known drug allergies

Meds

Verapamil SR 360 mg once daily

Nitroglycerin 0.4 mg sublingual (SL) as needed (last use yesterday after showering)

Glipizide 10 mg twice daily for diabetes

Pioglitazone 15 mg daily for diabetes

Ibuprofen 600 mg twice daily as needed for headaches

Vitamin B$_{12}$ once daily

Multivitamin daily

Aspirin 81 mg once daily

FH

Significant for early heart disease in father (MI at age 53)

SH

He is disabled from a previous accident; he is married, has three children, and runs his own business; he drinks three glasses of wine with dinner and smokes one to two packs of cigarettes per day.

PE

Blood pressure (BP) 146/70 mm Hg, pulse 60 bpm and regular, respiratory rate 16/minute, Ht 5'8" (173 cm), Wt 251 lb (114 kg), body mass index (BMI): 38.2 kg/m^2

Lungs are clear to auscultation with a prolonged expiratory phase; rales are present bilaterally

CV: Regular rate and rhythm with normal S$_1$ and S$_2$; there is an S$_3$ and a soft S$_4$ present; there is a 2/6 systolic ejection murmur heard best at the left lower sternal border; point of maximal impulse is within normal limits at the midclavicular line; there is no JVD

Abd: Soft, nontender, and bowel sounds are present; 2+ pitting edema of extremities extending to below the knees is observed

Chest x-ray: Bilateral pleural effusions and cardiomegaly

Echocardiogram: EF = 30% (0.30)

Laboratory Values

Hct: 41.1% (0.411)

WBC: 5.3 × 10^3/μL (5.3 × 10^9/L)

Sodium: 132 mEq/L (132 mmol/L)

Potassium: 3.2 mEq/L (3.2 mmol/L)

Bicarb: 30 mEq/L (30 mmol/L)

Chloride: 90 mEq/L (90 mmol/L)

Magnesium: 1.5 mEq/L (0.75 mmol/L)

Fasting blood glucose: 120 mg/dL (6.7 mmol/L)

Uric acid: 8 mg/dL (476 μmol/L)

Blood urea nitrogen (BUN): 40 mg/dL (14.3 mmol/L)

SCr: 0.8 mg/dL (71 μmol/L)

Alk Phos: 120 IU/L (2.0 μKat/L)

Aspartate aminotransferase: 100 IU/L (1.67 μKat/L)

What other laboratory or other diagnostic tests are required for the assessment of DG's condition?

How would you classify DG's NYHA functional class and ACC/AHA HF stage?

Identify exacerbating or precipitating factors that may worsen DG's HF.

What are your treatment goals for DG?

---

and nutritional deficiencies is required. Other more rare causes such as autoimmune disorders or acquired illnesses may have specific treatments. Identifying and discontinuing medications that can exacerbate HF is also an important intervention.

Nonpharmacologic Interventions

It is imperative that patients recognize the role of self-management in HF. ⑥ *Nonpharmacologic treatment involves dietary modifications such as sodium and fluid restriction, risk factor reduction including smoking cessation, timely immunizations, and supervised regular physical activity.*

Patient education regarding monitoring symptoms, dietary and medication adherence, exercise and physical fitness, risk factor reduction, and immunizations are important for the prevention of AHF exacerbations.

Patients should be encouraged to become involved in their own care through several avenues, the first of which is self-monitoring. Home monitoring should include daily assessment of weight and exercise tolerance. Daily weights should be done first thing in the morning upon arising and before any food intake to maintain consistency. Patients should record their weight daily in a journal and bring this log to each clinic or office visit. Changes in weight can indicate fluid retention and congestion prior to onset of peripheral or pulmonary symptoms. Individuals who have an increase of 2 to 3 pounds (0.91 to 1.36 kg) in a single day or 5 pounds (2.27 kg) over 5 days should alert their HF care provider. Some patients may be educated about self-adjusting diuretic doses based on daily weights. In addition to weight changes, a marked decline in exercise tolerance should also be reported to the HF care provider.

Nonadherence is an important issue because it relates to acute exacerbations of HF. Ensuring an understanding of the importance of each medication used to treat HF, proper administration, and potential adverse effects may improve adherence. Stressing the rationale for each medication is important, especially for NYHA FC I or ACC/AHA stage B patients who are asymptomatic yet started on drugs that may worsen symptoms initially. A clinician's involvement in emphasizing medication adherence, offering adherence suggestions such as optimal timing of medications or use of weekly pill containers, and providing intensive follow-up care has been shown to reduce AHF hospitalizations.

Dietary modifications in HF consist of initiation of an AHA step II diet as part of cardiac risk factor reduction, sodium restriction, and sometimes fluid restriction. Because sodium and water retention is a compensatory mechanism that contributes to volume overload in HF, salt and fluid restriction is often necessary to help avoid or minimize congestion. The normal American diet includes 3 to 6 g of sodium per day. Most patients with HF should limit salt intake to a maximum of 2 g/day. Patients should be educated to avoid cooking with salt and to limit intake of foods with high salt content, such as fried or processed food (lunch meats, soups, cheeses, salted snack foods, canned food, and some ethnic foods). Salt restriction can be challenging for many patients. The clinician should counsel to restrict salt slowly over time. Drastic dietary changes may lead to nonadherence due to an unpalatable diet. Substituting spices to flavor food is a useful recommendation. Salt substitutes should be used judiciously because many contain significant amounts of potassium that can increase the risk of hyperkalemia. Fluid restriction may not be necessary in many patients. When applicable, fluid intake is generally limited from all sources to less than 2 L/day.

Exercise, although discouraged when the patient is acutely decompensated to ease cardiac workload, is recommended when patients are stable. The heart is a muscle that requires activity to prevent atrophy. In addition, exercise improves peripheral muscle conditioning and efficiency, which may contribute to better exercise tolerance despite the low CO state. Regular low intensity, aerobic exercise that includes walking, swimming, or riding a bike is encouraged; heavy weight training is discouraged. The prescribed exercise regimen needs to be tailored to the individual's functional ability, and thus it is suggested that patients participate in cardiac rehabilitation programs, at least initially. It is important that patients not overexert themselves to fatigue or exertional dyspnea.

Modification of classic risk factors, such as tobacco and alcohol consumption, is important to minimize the potential for further aggravation of heart function. Data from observational studies suggest that patients with HF who smoke have a mortality rate 40% higher than those who do not consume tobacco products.[1] All HF patients who smoke should be counseled on the importance of tobacco cessation and offered a referral to a cessation program. Patients with an alcoholic cardiomyopathy should abstain from alcohol. Whether all patients with other forms of HF should abstain from any alcohol intake remains controversial. Proponents of moderation of alcohol base their rationale on the potential cardioprotective effects. However, opponents to any alcohol intake point out that alcohol is cardiotoxic and should be avoided.

In general, it is suggested that patients remain up to date on standard immunizations. Patients with HF should be counseled to receive yearly influenza vaccinations. Additionally, a pneumococcal vaccine is recommended.

Pharmacologic Treatment

In addition to determining therapeutic goals, the ACC/AHA staging system delineates specific therapy options based on disease progression.[1,11] For patients in stage A, every effort is made to minimize the impact of diseases that can injure the heart. Antihypertensive and lipid-lowering therapies should be utilized when appropriate to decrease the risk for stroke, MI, and HF. ACE inhibitors should be considered in high-risk vascular disease patients. For stage B patients, the goal is to prevent or slow disease progression by interfering with neurohormonal pathways that lead to cardiac damage and mediate pathological remodeling. The goal is to prevent the onset of HF symptoms. The backbone of therapy in these patients includes ACE inhibitors or ARBs and β-blockers. In stage C patients with symptomatic LV systolic dysfunction (EF less than 40% [0.40]), the goals focus on alleviating fluid retention, minimizing disability, slowing disease progression, and reducing long-term risk for hospitalizations and death. Treatment entails a strategy that combines diuretics to control intravascular fluid balance with neurohormonal antagonists to minimize the effects of the RAAS and SNS. Digoxin may be added to improve symptoms. If a patient continues to exhibit evidence of disease progression, other therapies can be used. In some cases, these include the combination of ACE inhibitors and ARBs, although the evidence for this option is limited. Another option is combination of hydralazine and isosorbide dinitrate in African American patients. Patients with advanced stage D disease are offered more modest goals, such as improvement in quality of life. Enhancing quality of life is often achieved at the expense of expected survival. Treatment options include mechanical support, transplantation, and continuous use of IV vasoactive therapies, in addition to maintaining an optimal regimen of chronic oral medications.

▶ Diuretics

Diuretics have been the mainstay for HF symptom management for many years. ❼ *Diuretics are used for relief of acute symptoms of congestion and maintenance of euvolemia.* These agents interfere with sodium retention by increasing urinary sodium and free water excretion. No prospective data exist on the effects of diuretics on patient outcomes.[14] Therefore, the primary rationale for the use of diuretic therapy is to maintain euvolemia in symptomatic or stages C and D HF. Diuretic therapy is recommended for all patients with clinical evidence of fluid overload.[15,16] In more mild HF, diuretics may be used on an as-needed basis. However, once the development of edema is persistent, regularly scheduled doses will be required.

Two types of diuretics are used for volume management in HF: thiazides and loop diuretics. Thiazide diuretics such as hydrochlorothiazide, chlorthalidone, and metolazone block sodium and chloride reabsorption in the distal convoluted tubule. Thiazides are weaker than loop diuretics in terms of effecting an increase in urine output and therefore are not utilized frequently as monotherapy in HF. They are optimally suited for patients with hypertension who have mild congestion. Additionally, the action of thiazides is limited in patients with renal insufficiency (creatinine clearance less than 30 mL/min [0.50 mL/s]) due to reduced secretion into their site of action. An exception is metolazone, which retains its potent action in patients with renal dysfunction. Metolazone is often used in combination with loop diuretics when patients exhibit diuretic resistance, defined as edema unresponsive to loop diuretics alone.

Loop diuretics are the most widely used diuretics in HF. These agents, including furosemide, bumetanide, and torsemide, exert their action at the thick ascending loop of Henle. Loop diuretics are not filtered through the glomerulus, but instead they undergo active transport into the tubular lumen via the organic acid pathway. As a result, drugs that compete for this active transport (e.g., probenecid and organic by-products of uremia) can lower efficacy of loop diuretics. Loop diuretics increase sodium and water excretion and induce a prostaglandin-mediated increase in renal blood flow that contributes to their natriuretic effect. Unlike thiazides, they retain their diuretic ability in patients with poor renal function. The various loop diuretics are equally effective when used at equipotent doses, although there are intrinsic differences in pharmacokinetics and pharmacodynamics (Table 6–6).[5] The choice of which loop diuretic to use and the route of administration depends on clinical factors such as the presence of intestinal edema and rapidity of the desired effect. Oral diuretic efficacy may vary based on differing bioavailability, which is almost complete for torsemide and bumetanide but averages only 50% for furosemide. Therefore, oral torsemide can be considered an alternative to the IV route of administration for patients who do not respond to oral furosemide in the setting of profound edema. The onset of effect is slightly delayed after oral administration but occurs within a few minutes with IV dosing. Consequently, bioequivalent doses of IV furosemide are half the oral dose, whereas bumetanide and torsemide IV doses are generally equivalent to the oral doses.

In patients with evidence of mild to moderate volume overload, diuretics should be initiated at a low dose and titrated to achieve a weight loss of up to 2 pounds (0.91 kg) per day. Patients with severe volume overload should

	Table 6–6		

Loop Diuretics Used in Heart Failure

	Furosemide	Bumetanide	Torsemide
Usual daily dose (oral)	20–160 mg	0.5–4 mg	10–80 mg
Ceiling dose:			
Normal renal function	80–160 mg	1–2 mg	20–40 mg
CrCL 20–50 mL/min (0.33–0.83 mL/s)	160 mg	2 mg	40 mg
CrCL less than 20 mL/min (0.33 mL/s)	400 mg	8–10 mg	100 mg
Bioavailability	10–100% (average 50%)	80–90%	80–100%
Affected by food	Yes	Yes	No
Half-life	0.3–3.4 hours	0.3–1.5 hours	3–4 hours

CrCL, creatinine clearance.

From Parker RB, Cavallari LH. Systolic heart failure. In: DiPiro JT, Talbert RL, Yee GC, et al., eds. Pharmacotherapy: A pathophysiologic approach, 8th ed. New York, NY: McGraw-Hill, 2011:152, with permission.

be managed in an inpatient setting. Once diuretic therapy is initiated, dosage adjustments are based on symptomatic improvement and daily body weight. Because body weight changes are a sensitive marker of fluid retention or loss, patients should continue to weigh themselves daily. Once a patient reaches a euvolemic state, diuretics may be cautiously tapered and then withdrawn in appropriate patients. In stable, educated, and adherent patients, another option is self-adjusted diuretic dosing. Based on daily body weight, patients may temporarily increase their diuretic regimen to reduce the incidence of overt edema. This also avoids overuse of diuretics and possible complications of overdiuresis such as hypotension, fatigue, and renal impairment.

The maximal response to diuretics is reduced in HF, creating a "ceiling dose" above which there is limited added benefit. This diuretic resistance is due to a compensatory increase in sodium reabsorption in the distal tubules, which decreases the effect of blocking sodium reabsorption in the loop of Henle.[17] In addition, there is a simultaneous increase in the reabsorption of sodium from the proximal tubule, allowing less to reach the site of action for loop diuretics. Apart from increasing diuretic doses, strategies to improve diuretic efficacy include increasing the frequency of dosing to two or three times daily, utilizing a continuous infusion of a loop diuretic, and/or combining a loop diuretic with a thiazide diuretic.[17,18] The latter strategy theoretically prevents sodium and water reabsorption at both the loop of Henle and the compensating distal convoluted tubule. Metolazone is used most often for this purpose because it retains its activity in settings of a low creatinine clearance. Metolazone can be dosed daily or as little as once weekly. This combination is usually maintained until the patient reaches his or her baseline weight. The clinician must use metolazone cautiously because its potent activity predisposes a patient to metabolic abnormalities as outlined next.

Diuretics cause numerous adverse effects and metabolic abnormalities, with severity linked to diuretic potency. A particularly worrisome adverse effect in the setting of HF is hypokalemia. Low serum potassium can predispose patients to arrhythmias and sudden death. Hypomagnesemia often occurs concomitantly with diuretic-induced hypokalemia, and therefore both should be assessed and replaced in patients needing correction of hypokalemia. Magnesium is an essential cofactor for movement of potassium intracellularly to restore body stores. Patients taking diuretics are also at risk for renal insufficiency due to overdiuresis and reflex activation of the renin-angiotensin system. The potential reduction in renal blood flow and glomerular pressure is amplified by concomitant use of ACE inhibitors or ARBs.

▶ Neurohormonal Blocking Agents

8 *Agents with proven benefits in improving symptoms, slowing disease progression, and improving survival in chronic HF target neurohormonal blockade. These include ACE inhibitors, ARBs, β-adrenergic blockers, and aldosterone antagonists.*

Angiotensin-Converting Enzyme Inhibitors ACE inhibitors are the cornerstone of treatment for HF. ACE inhibitors decrease neurohormonal activation by blocking the conversion of angiotensin I (AT_1) to angiotensin II (AT_2), a potent mediator of vasoconstriction and cardiac remodeling. The breakdown of bradykinin is also reduced. Bradykinin enhances the release of vasodilatory prostaglandins and histamines. These effects result in arterial and venous dilatation, and a decrease in myocardial workload through reduction of both preload and afterload. ACE inhibitors demonstrate favorable effects on cardiac hemodynamics, such as long-term increases in cardiac index (CI), stroke work index, and SV index, as well as significant reductions in LV filling pressure, SVR, mean arterial pressure, and HR.

There is extensive clinical experience with ACE inhibitors in systolic HF. Numerous clinical studies show ACE inhibitor therapy is associated with improvements in clinical symptoms, exercise tolerance, NYHA FC, LV size and function, and quality of life as compared with placebo.[18-21] ACE inhibitors significantly reduce hospitalization rates and mortality regardless of underlying disease severity or etiology. ACE inhibitors are also effective in preventing HF development in high-risk patients. Studies in acute MI patients show a reduction in new-onset HF and death with ACE inhibitors whether they are initiated early (within 36 hours) or started later. In addition, ACE inhibition decreases the risk of HF hospitalization and death in patients with asymptomatic LV dysfunction. The exact mechanisms for decreased HF progression and mortality are postulated to involve both the hemodynamic improvement and the inhibition of angiotensin II's growth promoting and remodeling effects. All patients with documented LV systolic dysfunction, regardless of existing HF symptoms, should receive ACE inhibitors unless a contraindication or intolerance is present.

There is no evidence to suggest that one ACE inhibitor is preferred over another. ACE inhibitors should be initiated using low doses and titrated up to target doses over several weeks depending on tolerability (adverse effects and blood pressure). The ACC/AHA 2005 guidelines advocate using the doses that were proven to decrease mortality in clinical trials as the target doses (Table 6–7).[1] If the target dose cannot be attained in a given patient, the highest tolerated dose should be used chronically. Although there is incremental benefit with higher doses of ACE inhibitors, it is accepted that lower doses provide substantial if not most of the effect.[22] Because ACE inhibitors are only one component of a mortality-reducing treatment plan in HF, targeting a high ACE inhibitor dose should be used cautiously to avoid a hypotensive effect that precludes starting a β-blocker or aldosterone antagonist.

Despite their clear benefits, ACE inhibitors are still underutilized in HF. One reason is undue concern or confusion regarding absolute versus relative contraindications for their use. Absolute contraindications include a history of angioedema, bilateral renal artery stenosis, and pregnancy. Relative contraindications include unilateral renal artery stenosis, renal insufficiency, hypotension, hyperkalemia, and cough. Relative contraindications provide a warning that close monitoring is required, but they do not necessarily preclude their use.

Clinicians are especially concerned about the use of ACE inhibitors in patients with renal insufficiency. It is important to recognize that ACE inhibitors can potentially contribute to the preservation or decline of renal function depending on the clinical scenario. Through preferential efferent arteriole vasodilation, ACE inhibitors can reduce intraglomerular pressure. Reduced glomerular pressures are renoprotective chronically; however, in situations of reduced or fixed renal blood flow, this leads to a reduction in filtration. In general, ACE inhibitors can be used in patients with serum creatinine less than 2.5 to 3 mg/dL (221 to 265 μmol/L). In HF, their addition can result in improved renal function through an increase in CO and renal perfusion. Although a small increase in serum creatinine (less than 0.5 mg/dL [44 μmol/L]) is possible with the addition of an ACE inhibitor, it is usually transient or becomes the patient's new serum creatinine baseline level. However, ACE inhibition can also worsen renal function because glomerular filtration is maintained in the setting of reduced CO through angiotensin II's constriction of the efferent arteriole. Patients most dependent on angiotensin II for maintenance of glomerular filtration pressure, and hence most susceptible to ACE inhibitor worsening of renal function, include those with hyponatremia, severely depressed LV function, or dehydration. The most common reason for creatinine elevation in a patient without a history of renal dysfunction is overdiuresis. Therefore, clinicians should consider decreasing or holding diuretic doses if an elevation in serum creatinine occurs concomitantly with a rise in blood urea nitrogen.

Hypotension occurs commonly at the initiation of therapy or with dosage increases but may happen anytime

Table 6–7

Dosing and Monitoring for Neurohormonal Blocking Agents

Drug	Initial Daily Dose	Target or Maximum Daily Dose	Monitoring
ACE Inhibitors[a]			
Captopril	6.25 mg 3 times	50 mg 3 times	BP
Enalapril	2.5 mg twice	10–20 mg twice	Electrolytes (K$^+$, BUN, SCr) at baseline, 2 weeks, and
Fosinopril	5–10 mg once	40 mg once	after dose titration, CBC periodically
Lisinopril	2.5–5 mg once	20–40 mg once	Adverse effects: cough, angioedema
Perindopril	2 mg once	8–16 mg once	
Quinapril	5 mg once	20 mg twice	
Ramipril	1.25–2.5 mg twice	5 mg twice	
Trandolapril	1 mg once	4 mg once	
Angiotensin Receptor Blockers[a]			
Candesartan	4–8 mg once	32 mg once	BP
Losartan	25–50 mg once	50–100 mg once	Electrolytes (K$^+$, BUN, SCr) at baseline, 2 weeks, and
Valsartan	20–40 mg once	160 mg twice	after dose titration, CBC periodically
			Adverse effects: cough, angioedema
Aldosterone Antagonists			
Spironolactone	12.5–25 mg once	25 mg once or twice	BP
Eplerenone	25 mg once	50 mg once	Electrolytes (K$^+$) at baseline and within 1 week of initiation and dose titration
			Adverse effects: gynecomastia or breast tenderness, menstrual changes, hirsutism
β-Blockers			
Bisoprolol	1.25 mg once	10 mg once	BP, HR baseline and after each dose titration, ECG
Carvedilol	3.125 mg twice	25 mg twice (50 mg twice for patients greater than 85 kg or 187 lbs)	Adverse effects: worsening HF symptoms (edema, SOB, fatigue), depression, sexual dysfunction
Metoprolol succinate	12.5–25 mg once	200 mg once	

[a]Use lower dose listed in patients with renal failure.

ACE, angiotensin-converting enzyme; BP, blood pressure; BUN, blood urea nitrate; CBC, complete blood cell count; ECG, electrocardiogram; HF, heart failure; HR, heart rate; K$^+$, potassium; SCr, serum creatinine; SOB, shortness of breath.

during therapy. Hypotension can manifest as dizziness, lightheadedness, presyncope, or syncope. The risk of hypotension due to possible volume depletion increases when ACE inhibitors are initiated or used concomitantly in patients on high diuretic doses. Therefore, in euvolemic patients, diuretic doses may often be decreased or withheld during ACE inhibitor dose titration. Initiating at a low dose and titrating slowly can also minimize hypotension. It may be advisable to initiate therapy with a short-acting ACE inhibitor, such as captopril, and subsequently switch to a longer-acting agent, such as lisinopril or enalapril, once the patient is stabilized.

Hyperkalemia results from reduced angiotensin II–stimulated aldosterone release. The risk of hyperkalemia with ACE inhibitors is also increased in HF due to a propensity for impaired renal function and additive effects with aldosterone antagonists. ACE inhibitor dose may need to be decreased or held if serum potassium increases above 5 mEq/L (5 mmol/L). Persistent hyperkalemia in the setting of renal insufficiency may preclude the use of an ACE inhibitor.

Cough is commonly seen with ACE inhibitors (5% to 15%) and may be related to accumulation of tissue bradykinins.[5]

It can be challenging to distinguish an ACE inhibitor–induced cough from cough caused by pulmonary congestion. A productive or wet cough usually signifies congestion, whereas a dry, hacking cough is more indicative of a drug-related etiology. If a cough is determined to be ACE inhibitor–induced, its severity should be evaluated before deciding on a course of action. If the cough is truly bothersome, a trial with a different ACE inhibitor or switching to an ARB is warranted.

Angiotensin Receptor Blockers Angiotensin receptor blockers (ARBs) selectively antagonize the effects of angiotensin II directly at the AT$_1$ receptor. AT$_1$ receptor stimulation is associated with vasoconstriction, release of aldosterone, and cellular growth promoting effects, whereas AT$_2$ stimulation causes vasodilation. By selectively blocking AT$_1$ but leaving AT$_2$ unaffected, ARBs block the detrimental AT$_1$ effects on cardiac function while allowing AT$_2$-mediated vasodilation and inhibition of ventricular remodeling. Angiotensin receptor blockers are considered an equally effective replacement for ACE inhibitors in patients who are intolerant or have a contraindication to an ACE inhibitor.

It was hoped that the more complete blockade of angiotensin II's AT_1 effects would confer greater long-term efficacy with ARBs compared with ACE inhibitors. However, prospective randomized trials suggest that the clinical efficacy of ARBs is similar to that of ACE inhibitors for reduction of hospitalizations for HF, sudden cardiac death, and all-cause mortality.[23-25] Despite poorer suppression of AT_2, comparable efficacy of ACE inhibitors may be due to the additional effects on the kallikrein-kinin system. Although ARBs produce hemodynamic and neurohormonal effects similar to those of ACE inhibitors, they are considered second-line therapy due to the overwhelming clinical trial experience with ACE inhibitors.

Because the mechanism for long-term benefit appears different for ACE inhibitors and ARBs, the combination has been studied for additive benefits. One study evaluated the addition of the ARB candesartan versus placebo in HF patients with systolic dysfunction intolerant to an ACE inhibitor, or systolic dysfunction currently on ACE inhibitor therapy, or patients with preserved systolic function.[25] Candesartan reduced the combined incidence of cardiovascular death and hospitalization for HF in all three groups; the greatest benefit was noted in those not on an ACE inhibitor. Candesartan significantly decreased mortality compared with placebo when all three groups were combined. Based on this study, the addition of an ARB to ACE inhibitor therapy can be considered in patients with evidence of disease progression despite optimal ACE inhibitor therapy, although this strategy is still undergoing investigation.[1] This study also demonstrates the importance of having some form of angiotensin II antagonism as part of a treatment regimen.

Angiotensin receptor blockers show similar tolerability to ACE inhibitors with regard to hypotension and hyperkalemia, but they are less likely to induce cough because ARBs do not cause an accumulation of bradykinin. Angiotensin receptor blockers can be considered in patients with ACE inhibitor–induced angioedema, but they should be initiated cautiously because cross-reactivity has been reported. Many of the other considerations for the use of ARBs are similar to those of ACE inhibitors, including the need for monitoring renal function, blood pressure, and potassium. Contraindications are similar to those of ACE inhibitors. In patients truly intolerant or contraindicated to ACE inhibitors or ARBs, the combination of hydralazine and isosorbide dinitrate should be considered.

Hydralazine and Isosorbide Dinitrate Complementary hemodynamic actions originally led to the combination of nitrates with hydralazine. Nitrates reduce preload by causing primarily venous vasodilation through activating guanylate cyclase and a subsequent increase in cGMP in vascular smooth muscle. Hydralazine reduces afterload through direct arterial smooth muscle relaxation via an unknown mechanism. More recently, nitric oxide has been implicated in modulating numerous pathophysiological processes in the failing heart including inflammation, cardiac remodeling, and oxidative damage. Supplementation of nitric oxide

via administration of nitrates has also been proposed as a mechanism for benefit from this combination therapy. The beneficial effect of an external nitric oxide source may be more apparent in the African American population, which appears to be predisposed to having an imbalance in nitric oxide production. In addition, hydralazine may reduce the development of nitrate tolerance when nitrates are given chronically.

The combination of hydralazine and isosorbide dinitrate was the first therapy shown to improve long-term survival in patients with systolic HF, but it has largely been supplanted by angiotensin II antagonist therapy (ACE inhibitors and ARBs).[26,27] Therefore, until recently, this combination therapy was reserved for patients intolerant to ACE inhibitors or ARBs secondary to renal impairment, angioedema, or hyperkalemia. New insight into the pathophysiological role of nitric oxide has reinvigorated research into this combination therapy.

The nitrate-hydralazine combination was first shown to improve survival compared with placebo.[26] Subsequently, the combination of isosorbide dinitrate 40 mg and hydralazine 75 mg, both given four times daily, was compared with the ACE inhibitor enalapril.[27] Enalapril produced a 28% greater decrease in mortality. Therefore, the combination is considered a third-line vasodilatory option for patients truly intolerant of ACE inhibitors and ARBs.

More recently, the value of adding the combination of isosorbide dinitrate 40 mg and hydralazine 75 mg three times daily to therapy including ACE inhibitors, β-blockers, digoxin, and diuretics was shown in a prospective randomized trial in African American patients.[28] ⑨ *Combination therapy with hydralazine and isosorbide dinitrate is an appropriate substitute for angiotensin II antagonism in those unable to tolerate an ACE inhibitor or ARB or as add-on therapy in African Americans.* The ACC/AHA HF guidelines now recommend considering the addition of isosorbide dinitrate and hydralazine in African Americans already on ACE inhibitors or ARBs.[1] Combination therapy with isosorbide dinitrate and hydralazine should be initiated and titrated as are other neurohormonal agents such as ACE inhibitors and β-blockers. Low doses are used to initiate therapy with subsequent titration of the dose toward target doses based on tolerability. Adverse effects such as hypotension and headache cause frequent discontinuations in patients taking this combination, and full doses often cannot be tolerated. Patients should be monitored for headache, hypotension, and tachycardia. Hydralazine is also associated with a dose-dependent risk for lupus.

The frequent dosing of isosorbide dinitrate (e.g., three to four times daily) is not conducive to patient adherence; therefore, a once-daily isosorbide mononitrate is commonly substituted for isosorbide dinitrate to simplify the dosing regimen. A nitrate-free interval is still required when using nitrates for HF.

β-Adrenergic Antagonists β-Adrenergic antagonists, or β-blockers, competitively block the influence of the SNS at β-adrenergic receptors. As recently as 15 to 20 years ago, β-adrenergic blockers were thought to be detrimental in HF due to their negative inotropic actions, which could potentially worsen symptoms and cause acute decompensations. Since then, the benefits of inhibiting the SNS have been recognized as far outweighing the acute negative inotropic effects. Chronic β-blockade reduces ventricular mass, improves ventricular shape, and reduces LV end-systolic and diastolic volumes.[6,8] β-Blockers also exhibit antiarrhythmic effects, slow or reverse catecholamine-induced ventricular remodeling, decrease myocyte death from catecholamine-induced necrosis or apoptosis, and prevent myocardial fetal gene expression. Consequently, β-blockers improve EF, reduce all-cause and HF-related hospitalizations, and decrease all-cause mortality in patients with systolic HF.[29-33]

The ACC/AHA recommends that β-blockers be initiated in all patients with NYHA FC I to IV or ACC/AHA stages B through D HF if clinically stable.[1] To date, only three β-blockers have been shown to reduce mortality in systolic HF including the selective β_1-antagonists bisoprolol and metoprolol succinate, and the nonselective β_1-, β_2-, and α_1-antagonist carvedilol.[29-33] The positive findings of β-blockers are not a class effect because bucindolol did not exhibit a beneficial effect on mortality when studied for HF, and there is limited information with propranolol and atenolol.

Although metoprolol and carvedilol are the most commonly used β-antagonists in HF, it is unknown whether one agent should be considered first line. To compare their relative effects on patient outcomes, one study compared immediate-release metoprolol tartrate to carvedilol in 3,000 patients with mild to severe HF.[33] Carvedilol lowered all-cause mortality significantly more than metoprolol tartrate. There are questions about the validity of using immediate-release metoprolol tartrate as the comparison agent, and the low average dose of metoprolol tartrate achieved in the study.

The key to utilizing β-blockers in systolic HF is initiation with low doses and slow titration to target doses over weeks to months. It is important that the β-blocker be initiated when a patient is clinically stable and euvolemic. Volume overload at the time of β-blocker initiation increases the risk for worsening symptoms. β-Blockade should begin with the lowest possible dose (Table 6–7), after which the dose may be doubled every 2 to 4 weeks depending on patient tolerability. β-Blockers may cause an acute decrease in left ventricular ejection fraction (LVEF) and short-term worsening of HF symptoms upon initiation and at each dosage titration. After each dose titration, if the patient experiences symptomatic hypotension, bradycardia, orthostasis, or worsening symptoms, further increases in dose should be withheld until the patient stabilizes. After stabilization, attempts to increase the dose should be reinstituted. If mild congestion ensues as a result of the β-blocker, an increase in diuretic dose may be warranted. If moderate or severe symptoms of congestion occur, a reduction in β-blocker dose should be considered along with an increase in diuretic dose. Dose titration should continue until target clinical trial doses are achieved (Table 6–7) or until limited by repeated hemodynamic or symptomatic intolerance. Patient education

regarding the possibility of acutely worsening symptoms but improved long-term function and survival is essential to ensure adherence.

Apart from possible clinical differences between the β-blockers approved for HF, selection of a β-blocker may also be affected by pharmacologic differences. Carvedilol exhibits a more pronounced blood pressure lowering effect, and thus causes more frequent dizziness and hypotension as a consequence of its β_1 and α_1-receptor blocking activities. Therefore, in patients predisposed to symptomatic hypotension, such as those with advanced LV dysfunction (LVEF less than 20% [0.20]) who normally exhibit low systolic blood pressures, metoprolol succinate may be the more desirable first-line β-blocker. In patients with uncontrolled hypertension, carvedilol may provide additional antihypertensive efficacy.

β-Blockers may be used by those with reactive airway disease or peripheral vascular disease but should be used with considerable caution or avoided if patients display active respiratory symptoms. Care must also be used in interpreting shortness of breath in these patients because the etiology could be either cardiac or pulmonary. A selective β_1-blocker such as metoprolol is a reasonable option for patients with reactive airway disease. The risk versus benefit of using any β-blocker in peripheral vascular disease must be weighed based on the severity of the peripheral disease, and a selective β_1-blocker is preferred.

Both metoprolol and carvedilol are metabolized by the liver through cytochrome P-450 (CYP450) 2D6 and undergo extensive first-pass metabolism. β-blockers should not be used in patients with severe hepatic failure. Bisoprolol is not as commonly used since it is not FDA approved for this use.

There is some debate regarding which class of agents should be initiated first in a patient with HF, namely ACE inhibitors or β-blockers. A recent study evaluated whether the order of initiation of these therapies affects all-cause mortality or hospitalization and found no difference but that more events occurred during the 6-month single-treatment phase part of the study.[34] These findings reinforce the importance of using both ACE inhibitors and β-blockers in the HF patient. As such, doses of the agent initiated first should not prohibit initiation of the second class of agents.

Aldosterone Antagonists Currently, the aldosterone antagonists available are spironolactone and eplerenone. Both agents are inhibitors of aldosterone that produce weak diuretic effects while sparing potassium concentrations. Eplerenone is selective for the mineralocorticoid receptor and hence does not exhibit the endocrine adverse effect profile commonly seen with spironolactone. The initial rationale for specifically targeting aldosterone for treatment of HF was based on the knowledge that ACE inhibitors do not suppress the chronic production and release of aldosterone. Aldosterone is a key pathological neurohormone that exerts multiple detrimental effects in HF. Similar to norepinephrine and angiotensin II, aldosterone levels are increased in HF and have been shown to correlate with disease severity and patient outcomes.

Each agent (spironolactone and eplerenone) has been studied in a defined population of patients with HF. One study established efficacy with low-dose spironolactone in NYHA FC III and IV HF patients in reducing HF hospitalizations, improving functional class, reducing sudden cardiac death, and improving all-cause mortality.[35] Another study investigated the use of eplerenone in patients within 14 days of MI and LVEF less than 40% (0.40).[36] Eplerenone was found to decrease mortality as well as cardiovascular death and related hospitalization, mainly due to reducing occurrence of sudden cardiac death. Based on these two studies, the ACC/AHA guidelines recommend the addition of spironolactone be considered in NYHA FC III and IV (ACC/AHA stages C and D) patients, and eplerenone in directly post-MI patients with evidence of LV dysfunction.[1] A more recent study investigated the use of eplerenone in NYHA FC II HF patients. Eplerenone reduced death from cardiovascular causes and hospitalizations due to HF.[37] It is likely that updated HF treatment guidelines will include the use of aldosterone antagonists in patients with mild to moderate HF symptoms and a reduced EF who are maximized on ACE inhibitors and β-blockers.

The major risk related to aldosterone antagonists is hyperkalemia. Therefore, the decision for use of these agents should balance the benefit of decreasing death and hospitalization from HF and the potential risks of life-threatening hyperkalemia. Before and within 1 week of initiating therapy, two parameters must be assessed: serum potassium and creatinine clearance (or serum creatinine). Aldosterone antagonists should not be initiated in patients with potassium concentrations greater than 5.5 mEq/L (5.5 mmol/L). Likewise, these agents should not be given when creatinine clearance is less than 30 mL/minute (0.50 mL/s) or serum creatinine is greater than 2.5 mg/dL (221 μmol/L).

In patients without contraindications, spironolactone is initiated at a dose of 12.5 to 25 mg daily, or occasionally on alternate days for patients with baseline renal insufficiency. Eplerenone is used at a dose of 25 mg daily, with the option to titrate up to 50 mg daily. Doses should be halved or switched to alternate-day dosing if creatinine clearance falls below 50 mL/min (0.83 mL/s). Potassium supplementation is often decreased or stopped after aldosterone antagonists are initiated, and patients should be counseled to avoid high-potassium foods. At any time after initiation of therapy, if potassium concentrations exceed 5.5 mEq/L (5.5 mmol/L), the dose of the aldosterone antagonist should be reduced or discontinued. In addition, worsening renal function dictates consideration for stopping the aldosterone antagonist. Other adverse effects observed mainly with spironolactone include gynecomastia for men and breast tenderness and menstrual irregularities for women. Gynecomastia leads to discontinuation in up to 10% of patients on spironolactone. Eplerenone is a CYP3 A4 substrate and should not be used concomitantly with strong inhibitors of 3A4.

▶ Digoxin

Digoxin has been used for several decades in the treatment of HF. Traditionally, it was considered useful for its positive inotropic effects, but more recently its benefits are thought to be related to neurohormonal modulation. Digoxin exerts positive inotropic effects through binding to sodium- and potassium-activated adenosine triphosphate (ATP) pumps, leading to increased intracellular sodium concentrations and subsequently more available intracellular calcium during systole. The mechanism of digoxin's neurohormonal blocking effect is less well understood but may be related to restoration of baroreceptor sensitivity and reduced central sympathetic outflow.[5]

The exact role of digoxin in therapy remains controversial largely due to disagreement on the risk versus benefit of routinely using this drug in patients with systolic HF. Digoxin was shown to decrease HF-related hospitalizations but did not decrease HF progression or improve survival.[38] Moreover, digoxin was associated with an increased risk for concentration-related toxicity and numerous adverse effects. Post hoc study analyses demonstrated a clear relationship between digoxin plasma concentration and outcomes. Concentrations below 1.2 ng/mL (1.5 nmol/L) were associated with no apparent adverse effect on survival, whereas higher concentrations increased the relative risk of mortality.[39,40]

Current recommendations are for the addition of digoxin for patients who remain symptomatic despite an optimal HF regimen consisting of an ACE inhibitor or ARB, β-blocker, and diuretic. In patients with concomitant atrial fibrillation, digoxin may be added to slow ventricular rate regardless of HF symptomatology.

Digoxin is initiated at a dose of 0.125 mg to 0.25 mg daily depending on age, renal function, weight, and risk for toxicity. The lower dose should be used if the patient satisfies any of the following criteria: older than 65 years, creatinine clearance less than 60 mL/min (1.0 mL/s), or ideal body weight less than 70 kg (154 lb). The 0.125-mg daily dose is adequate in most patients. Doses are halved or switched to alternate-day dosing in patients with moderate to severe renal failure. The desired concentration range for digoxin is 0.5 ng/mL to 1.2 ng/mL (0.6 nmol/L to 1.5 nmol/L), preferably with concentrations at or less than 0.8 ng/mL (1.0 nmol/L). Routine monitoring of serum drug concentrations is not required but recommended in those with changes in renal function, suspected toxicity, or after addition or subtraction of an interacting drug.

Digoxin toxicity may manifest as nonspecific findings such as fatigue or weakness and other CNS effects such as confusion, delirium, and psychosis. GI manifestations include nausea, vomiting, or anorexia, and visual disturbances may occur such as halos, photophobia, and color perception problems (red-green or yellow-green vision). Cardiac findings include numerous types of arrhythmias related to enhanced automaticity, slowed or accelerated conduction, or delayed after-depolarizations. These include ventricular tachycardia and fibrillation, atrioventricular nodal block, and sinus bradycardia. Risk of digoxin toxicity, in particular the cardiac manifestations, are increased with electrolyte disturbances such as hypokalemia, hypercalcemia, and hypomagnesemia. To reduce the proarrhythmic risk of digoxin, serum potassium and magnesium should be monitored closely and supplemented when appropriate to ensure adequate concentrations (potassium greater than 4.0 mEq/L [4.0 mmol/L] and magnesium greater than 2.0 mEq/L [1.0 mmol/L]). In patients with life-threatening toxicity due to cardiac or other findings, administration of digoxin-specific Fab antibody fragments usually reverses adverse effects within an hour in most cases.

▶ Calcium Channel Blockers

Treatment with nondihydropyridine calcium channel blockers (diltiazem and verapamil) may worsen HF and increase the risk of death in patients with advanced LV systolic dysfunction due to their negative inotropic effects. Conversely, dihydropyridine calcium channel blockers, although negative inotropes in vitro, do not appear to decrease contractility in vivo. Amlodipine and felodipine are the two most extensively studied dihydropyridine calcium channel blockers for systolic HF.[41,42] These two agents have not been shown to affect patient survival, either positively or negatively. As such, they are not routinely recommended as part of a standard HF regimen; however, amlodipine and felodipine can safely be used in HF patients to treat uncontrolled hypertension or angina once all other appropriate drugs are maximized.

▶ Antiplatelets and Anticoagulation

Patients with HF are at an increased risk of thromboembolic events secondary to a combination of hypercoagulability, relative stasis of blood, and endothelial dysfunction. However, the role of antiplatelets and anticoagulants remains debatable due to a lack of prospective clinical trials.

Aspirin is generally used in HF patients with an underlying ischemic etiology, a history of ischemic heart disease, or other compelling indications such as history of embolic stroke. Routine use in nonischemic cardiomyopathy patients is currently discouraged because of a lack of data supporting any long-term benefit, as well as the potential negative drug–drug interaction with ACE inhibitors and ARBs. If aspirin is indicated, the preference is to use a low dose (81 mg daily).[43]

Current consensus recommendations support the use of warfarin in patients with reduced LV systolic dysfunction and a compelling indication such as atrial fibrillation or prosthetic heart valves.[44] In addition, warfarin is empirically used in patients with echocardiographic evidence of a mural thrombus or severely depressed (LVEF less than 20% [0.20]) LV function.[45] However, there are limited data supporting the use of empirical warfarin based on echocardiographic findings. Patients with HF often have difficulty maintaining a therapeutic international normalized ratio (INR) due to fluctuating volume status and varying drug absorption. Therefore, the benefit of using warfarin should be evaluated in the context of the risk for bleeding.

▶ Complementary and Alternative Medications

Complementary and alternative medications (CAMs) are treatment strategies not commonly used in Western medicine and are considered nutrition supplements by the FDA. Some patients with HF use CAM for heart problems, weight loss,

Patient Encounter Part 3

Based on the information presented and your problem-based assessment, create a care plan for DG's HF. Your plan should include:

• Nonpharmacologic treatment options.
• Acute and chronic treatment plans to address DG's symptoms and prevent disease deterioration.
• Monitoring plan for acute and chronic treatments.

anxiety, and arthritis. Fish oils, n-3 polyunsaturated fatty acids, or w-3 fatty acids were recently studied for HF and found to mildly decrease cardiovascular admissions and mortality without significant adverse effects. Fish oils are more commonly used for the treatment of hypertriglyceridemia. Their mechanism in HF is incompletely understood but postulated to involve decreased membrane excitability (thus reducing arrhythmias), decreased inflammation and platelet aggregation, and favorable changes in autonomic tone. Hawthorn is another CAM studied in HF and shown to increase exercise capacity and reduce HF symptoms. Its benefits are thought to be due to flavonoids that increase force of contraction and cardiac output. The ACC/AHA guidelines do not currently advocate the use of fish oils and hawthorn for HF. It is important to counsel patients to remain on their other HF medications if they decide to initiate a CAM, and to let their healthcare providers know when starting a new supplement. As with any therapy, it is important to monitor for adverse events and therapeutic outcomes.

Heart Failure with Preserved Left Ventricular Ejection Fraction

It is now recognized that a significant number of patients exhibiting HF symptoms have normal systolic function or preserved LVEF (40% to 60% [0.40 to 0.60]). It is believed the primary defect in these patients is impaired ventricular relaxation and filling, commonly referred to as HF with preserved ejection fraction (HFpEF). HF with preserved EF is more prevalent in older women and closely associated with hypertension or diabetes and, to a lesser extent, CAD and atrial fibrillation.[46] Morbidity in HFpEF is comparable with those with depressed EF because both are characterized by frequent, repeated hospitalizations.[46] However, HFpEF appears to be associated with slightly lower mortality. The diagnosis is based on findings of typical signs and symptoms of HF, in conjunction with echocardiographic evidence of abnormal diastolic function, absence of significant LV chamber dilation, and no valvular disease.

Unlike systolic HF, few prospective trials have evaluated the safety and efficacy of various cardiac medications in patients with HFpEF. The PEP-CHF (Perindopril in Elderly People with Chronic Heart Failure) study was the first major randomized controlled trial to evaluate the use of an ACE inhibitor in patients with HFpEF.[47] The study did not find differences in mortality and hospitalizations between groups, but premature withdrawal of many patients after 1 year could have contributed to the neutral findings.[47] The Candesartan in Heart Failure Assessment of Reduction in Mortality and Morbidity (CHARM) study demonstrated that angiotensin receptor blockade with candesartan resulted in beneficial effects on HF morbidity in patients with preserved LVEF similar to those seen in depressed LV function.[25] However, the largest clinical trial in HFpEF, the I-PRESERVE (Irbesartan in Patients with Heart Failure and Preserved Ejection Fraction) study did not find a reduction in the primary composite outcome of death or hospitalizations.[48] In the absence of more landmark clinical studies, the current treatment approach for HFpEF is (a) correction or control of underlying etiologies (including optimal treatment of hypertension and CAD and maintenance of normal sinus rhythm); (b) reduction of cardiac filling pressures at rest and during exertion; and (c) increased diastolic filling time. Diuretics are frequently used to control congestion. Recent studies failed to show significant reductions in mortality or hospitalizations with the use of ARBs. β-Blockers and calcium channel blockers can theoretically improve ventricular relaxation through negative inotropic and chronotropic effects. Unlike in systolic HF, nondihydropyridine calcium channel blockers (diltiazem and verapamil) may be especially useful in improving diastolic function by limiting the availability of calcium that mediates contractility. A recent study did not find favorable effects with digoxin in patients with mild to moderate diastolic HF. Therefore, the role of digoxin for symptom management and HR control in these patients is not well established.

Special Populations and Patients with Concomitant Disorders

▶ Ethnic and Genetic Considerations

HF is more prevalent and associated with a worse prognosis in African Americans compared with the general population.[1] Unfortunately, deficiencies in disease prevention, detection, and access to treatment are well documented in minority populations. African Americans and other races are underrepresented in clinical trials, compromising the extrapolation of results from these studies to ethnic subpopulations. The influence of race on efficacy and safety of medications used in HF treatment has received additional attention with the advent of pharmacogenomics (the influence of genetics on drug response). The application of race and genetics to pharmacotherapeutic decision making for HF is in the early stages. However, these concepts are being applied to the use of hydralazine and isosorbide dinitrate in African American patients.[28] It is anticipated that further investigation will lead to better insight relating to the clinical applicability of genetic variations to drug responses.

▶ Peripartum Cardiomyopathy and Pregnancy

Peripartum cardiomyopathy (PPCM) is currently defined as clinical and echocardiographic evidence for new-onset HF occurring during pregnancy and up to 6 months after delivery, with other etiologies excluded. Although PPCM is not well understood, it manifests in pregnant women of all ages, but the risk is elevated in women older than 30 years.[49] The true incidence of idiopathic PPCM is debatable, with reported rates for peripartum HF at 1 case per 100 to 4,000 deliveries.[50] The leading hypothesis for PPCM pathogenesis is myocarditis caused by a viral infection or an abnormal immune response to pregnancy. HF may persist after delivery but can be reversible (with partial or full recovery of cardiac function) in many cases.[49]

The clinical presentation of peripartum HF is indistinguishable from that of other types of HF. Initial treatment is also similar, with the exception of ACE inhibitors and ARBs being contraindicated during the antepartum period. Treatment includes reducing preload by sodium restriction and diuretics, afterload reduction with vasodilators, and sometimes inotropic support with digoxin. Hydralazine is utilized frequently in pregnancy and classified as FDA pregnancy category C. Labetalol is used for acute parenteral control of blood pressure, but long-term β-blocker use corresponds with low birthweight infants. Management of the cardiomyopathy after delivery includes use of ACE inhibitors and β-blockers, although these treatment guidelines have been extrapolated from studies in patients with idiopathic dilated cardiomyopathy rather than specific trials in PPCM. Patients with PPCM also have a high rate of thromboembolism. Treatment options during pregnancy are limited to unfractionated heparin and low molecular weight heparin because warfarin is contraindicated. After delivery, anticoagulation is recommended in patients with LVEF less than 20% (0.20).[50]

Outcome Evaluation of Chronic Heart Failure

- The evaluation of therapy is influenced by the ability of treatment to successfully reduce symptoms, improve quality of life, decrease frequency of hospitalizations for acute HF, reduce disease progression, and prolong survival (Fig. 6–1).
- The major outcome parameters focus on (a) volume status, (b) exercise tolerance, (c) overall symptoms/quality of life, (d) adverse drug reactions, and (e) disease progression and cardiac function. Assess quality of life by evaluating patients' ability to continue their activities of daily living.
- Assess symptoms of HF such as dyspnea on exertion, orthopnea, weight gain, and edema, and abdominal manifestations such as nausea, bloating, and loss of appetite.
- If diuretic therapy is warranted, monitor for therapeutic response by assessing weight loss and improvement of fluid retention, as well as exercise tolerance and presence of fatigue.
- Once therapy for preventing disease progression is initiated, monitoring for symptomatic improvement continues.
- It is important to keep in mind that patients' symptoms of HF can worsen with β-blockers, and it may take weeks or months before patients notice improvement.

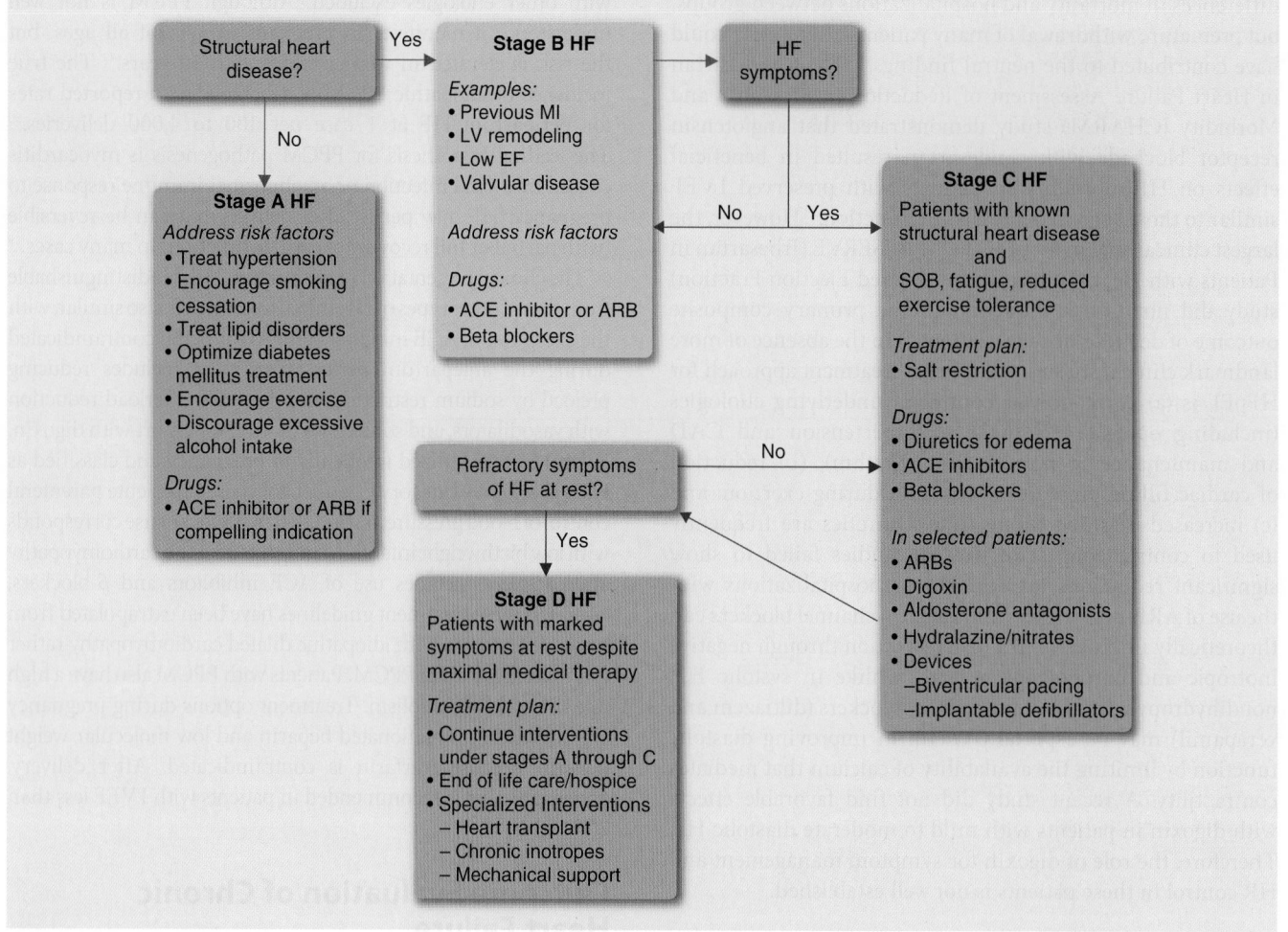

FIGURE 6–1. Treatment algorithm for chronic heart failure. (ACE, angiotensin-converting enzyme; ARB, angiotensin receptor blocker; EF, ejection fraction; HF, heart failure; LV, left ventricular; MI, myocardial infarction; SOB, shortness of breath.) Table 6–5 describes the staging of heart failure.

- Monitor blood pressure to evaluate for hypotension caused by drug therapy.

- To assess for prevention of disease progression, practitioners may utilize serial echocardiograms every 6 months to assess cardiac function and evaluate the effects of drug therapy.

- Occasional exercise testing is conducted to ascertain disease prognosis or suitability for heart transplant. Even though these tests can demonstrate improvement in heart function and therefore slowed disease progression, patient symptoms may not improve.

ACUTE AND ADVANCED HEART FAILURE

Clinical Presentation and Diagnosis of Acute Heart Failure

Patients with acute heart failure (AHF) present with symptoms of worsening fluid retention or decreasing exercise tolerance and fatigue (typically worsening of symptoms presented in the chronic HF clinical presentation text box). These symptoms reflect congestion behind the failing ventricle and/or hypoperfusion. Patients can be categorized into hemodynamic subsets based on assessment of physical signs and symptoms of congestion and/or hypoperfusion.[51] Patients can be described as "wet" or "dry" depending on volume status, as well as "warm" or "cool" based on adequacy of tissue perfusion. "Wet" refers to patients with volume/fluid overload (e.g., edema and jugular venous distention [JVD]), whereas "dry" refers to euvolemic patients. "Warm" refers to patients with adequate CO to perfuse peripheral tissues (and hence the skin will be warm to touch), whereas "cool" refers to patients with evidence of hypoperfusion (skin cool to touch with diminished pulses). Additionally, invasive hemodynamic monitoring can be used to provide objective data for assessing volume status (pulmonary capillary wedge pressure [PCWP]) and perfusion (CO). A CI below 2.2 L/min/m² is consistent with hypoperfusion and reduced contractility, and a PCWP above 18 mm Hg (2.4 kPa) correlates with congestion and an elevated preload. The four possible hemodynamic subsets a patient may fall into are "warm and dry," "warm and wet," "cool and dry," or "cool and wet."

Clinical Presentation of Acute Heart Failure

Subset I (Warm and Dry)

- Cardiac index (CI) *greater than* 2.2 L/min/m^2, pulmonary capillary wedge pressure (PCWP) *less than* 18 mm Hg (2.4 kPa)
- Patients considered well compensated and perfused, without evidence of congestion
- No immediate interventions necessary except optimizing oral medications and monitoring

Subset II (Warm and Wet)

- CI *greater than* 2.2 L/min/m^2, PCWP *greater than* or equal to 18 mm Hg (2.4 kPa)
- Patients adequately perfused and display signs and symptoms of congestion
- Main goal is to reduce preload (PCWP) carefully with loop diuretics and vasodilators

Subset III (Cool and Dry)

- CI *less than* 2.2 L/min/m^2, PCWP *less than* 18 mm Hg (2.4 kPa)
- Patients are inadequately perfused and not congested
- Hypoperfusion leads to increased mortality, elevating death rates fourfold compared with those who are adequately perfused
- Treatment focuses on increasing CO with positive inotropic agents and/or replacing intravascular fluids
- Fluid replacement must be performed cautiously because patients can rapidly become congested

Subset IV (Cool and Wet)

- CI *less than* 2.2 L/min/m^2, PCWP *greater than* 18 mm Hg (2.4 kPa)
- Patients are inadequately perfused and congested
- Classified as the most complicated clinical presentation of AHF with the worst prognosis
- Most challenging to treat; therapy targets alleviating signs and symptoms of congestion by increasing CI as well as reducing PCWP while maintaining adequate mean arterial pressure
- Treatment involves a delicate balance between diuretics, vasodilators, and inotropic agents
- Use of vasopressors is sometimes necessary to maintain blood pressure

Clinical Assessment and Diagnosis

▶ Precipitating Factors

❸ *It is important for the clinician to identify the cause(s) of AHF in order to maximize treatment efficacy and reduce future disease exacerbations. Cardiovascular, metabolic, and* lifestyle factors can all precipitate AHF. The most common precipitating factors for acute decompensation and how they contribute pathophysiologically are listed in Table 6–3.

▶ Laboratory Assessment

Routine laboratory testing of patients with AHF includes electrolytes and blood glucose, as well as serum creatinine and blood urea nitrogen to assess renal function. Complete blood cell count is measured to determine if anemia or infection is present. Creatine kinase and/or troponin concentrations are used to diagnose ischemia, and hepatic transaminases are measured to assess hepatic congestion. Thyroid function tests are measured to assess hyperthyroidism or hypothyroidism as causes of AHF. A urinalysis is attained in patients with an unknown history of renal disease to rule out nephrotic syndrome. Lastly, a toxicology screen is obtained in patients in whom the use of illicit drugs is suspected.

Assays measuring BNP and its degradation product NT-proBNP are being used with greater frequency in clinical practice.[10] B-type natriuretic peptide is synthesized, stored, and released from the ventricles in response to increased ventricular filling pressures. Hence plasma levels of BNP can be used as a marker for volume overload. The most widely accepted indication for BNP measurement is as an adjunctive aid for diagnosing a cardiac etiology for dyspnea.[10]

The current values for ruling out a cardiac etiology for dyspnea are a BNP less than 100 pg/mL (100 ng/L or 28.9 pmol/L) or an NT-proBNP less than 300 pg/mL (300 ng/L or 35.4 pmol/L). BNP measurements require cautious interpretation because numerous conditions can also elevate BNP concentrations. These include older age, renal dysfunction, pulmonary embolism, and chronic pulmonary disease. One group recommends age adjusted cut points for NT-proBNP as follows: 50 years old = 450 ng/mL, 50 to 75 years = 900 ng/mL, and greater than or equal to 75 years = 1800 ng/mL. Nesiritide, a recombinant BNP drug, has an identical structure to native BNP and will interfere with the commercial BNP assay, resulting in a falsely elevated level. Therefore, blood for BNP determination should be obtained 2 hours after the end of a nesiritide infusion, or alternatively the NT-proBNP assay should be utilized.

Other diagnostic tests should also be obtained in order to rule out precipitating factors (chest radiograph) and to evaluate cardiac function (electrocardiogram [ECG]).

Invasive hemodynamic monitoring in patients with HF entails placement of a right heart or pulmonary artery catheter (PAC). The catheter is inserted percutaneously through a central vein and advanced through the right side of the heart to the pulmonary artery. Inflation of a balloon proximal to the end port allows the catheter to "wedge," yielding the PCWP, which estimates pressures in the left ventricle during diastole. Additionally, CO can be estimated and SVR calculated (Table 6–8).

There are no universally accepted guidelines dictating when invasive monitoring in HF is required, and invasive monitoring has not been shown to improve mortality or reduce hospitalizations in high-risk patients. Nonetheless, the

Table 6–8	
Hemodynamic Monitoring: Normal Values	
Hemodynamic Variable	**Normal Value**
Central venous (right atrial) pressure, mean	Less than 5 mm Hg[a] (0.67 kPa)
Right ventricular pressure	25/0 mm Hg[a]
Pulmonary artery pressure	25/10 mm Hg[a]
Pulmonary artery pressure, mean	Less than 18 mm Hg[a] (2.4 kPa)
Pulmonary artery occlusion pressure, mean	Less than 12 mm Hg[a] (1.60 kPa)
Systemic arterial pressure	120/80 mm Hg[a]
Mean arterial pressure	90–120 mm Hg[a] (12.0–16.0 kPa)
Cardiac index	2.8–4.2 L/min/m^{2a}
Stroke volume index	30–65 mL/beat/m^{2a} (0.030–0.065 L·beat^{-1}·m^{-2})
Systemic vascular resistance	900–1.400 dyn·s·m^{-5} (90–140 MPa·s·m^{-3})
Pulmonary vascular resistance	150–250 dyn·s·m^{-5b} (15–25 MPa·s·m^{-3})
Arterial oxygen content	20 mL/dL[a] (200 mL/L)
Mixed venous oxygen content	15 mL/dL[a] (150 mL/L)
Arteriovenous oxygen content difference	3–5 mL/dL[a] (30–50 mL/L)

[a]1 mm Hg = 0.133 kPa; 1 mL/beat per square meter = 0.001 L·beat^{-1}·m^{-2}.

[b]1 dyn·s·m^{-5}= 0.1 MPa·s·m^{-3}; 1 mL/dL = 10 mL/L.

From Rodgers JE, Lee CR. Acute decompensated heart failure. In: DiPiro JT, Talbert RL, Yee GC, et al., eds. Pharmacotherapy: A pathophysiologic approach, 8th ed. New York, NY: McGraw-Hill, 2011:196, with permission.

use of a PAC remains an essential component of management and monitoring of patients in cardiogenic shock; however, the use of inotropic agents does not mandate invasive monitoring. Invasive hemodynamic monitoring is most commonly used to aid in the assessment of hemodynamics when there is disagreement between signs and symptoms and clinical response. In addition, invasive monitoring is helpful in guiding ongoing therapy for AHF. Invasive monitoring offers the advantage of immediate hemodynamic assessment of an intervention, allowing for prompt adjustments. Risks with PACs include infection, bleeding, thrombosis, catheter malfunction, and ventricular ectopy.

TREATMENT OF ACUTE HEART FAILURE

Desired Therapeutic Outcomes

The goals of therapy for AHF are to (a) correct the underlying precipitating factor(s); (b) relieve the patient's symptoms; (c) improve hemodynamics; (d) optimize a chronic oral medication regimen; and (e) educate the patient, reinforcing adherence to lifestyle modifications and the drug regimen. The ultimate goal for a patient hospitalized for AHF is the return to a compensated HF state and discharge to the outpatient setting on oral medications. Only through aggressive management to achieve all of these goals will a patient's prognosis be improved and future hospitalizations for acute decompensations be prevented.

Removal or control of precipitating factors is essential for an optimal response to pharmacologic therapy. Relief of symptoms should occur rapidly to minimize length of hospitalization. Although a rapid discharge from the hospital is desirable, a patient should not be discharged before ensuring that he or she is in a euvolemic, or nearly euvolemic, state with a body weight and functional capacity similar to before the acute decompensation. Oral agents such as β-blockers, ACE inhibitors or ARBs, and aldosterone antagonists should be initiated as soon as possible during the hospitalization. These chronic oral medications not only improve mortality and prevent readmissions, acutely they also contribute to improvement in hemodynamics. Patient education prior to discharge from the hospital is recommended to assist in minimizing adverse effects and nonadherence. Dissemination of written information, in addition to verbal information, is helpful for patient comprehension and retention. This can include therapy goals, lifestyle modifications, drug regimen, dosage information, and relevant adverse effects, as well as symptom and diary cards.

Pharmacologic Approaches to Treatment

⑩ *Treatment of AHF targets relief of congestion and optimization of CO utilizing oral or IV diuretics, IV vasodilators, and, when appropriate, inotropes, based on presenting hemodynamics. Current treatment strategies in AHF target improving hemodynamics while preserving organ function.* A specific treatment approach is formulated depending on the patient's symptoms (congestion versus hypoperfusion) and hemodynamic indices (CI and PCWP).[52,53] If the patient primarily exhibits signs and symptoms of congestion, treatment entails use of diuretics as first-line agents to decrease PCWP. Additionally, IV vasodilators are added to provide rapid relief of congestion and additional reductions in PCWP. By reducing congestion in the heart, cardiac contractile function may improve, which results in an increase in SV and CO, and hence perfusion to vital organs. The patient's presenting blood pressure can also help guide the clinician on choice of diuretic, vasodilator, or both. For the patient with a systolic blood pressure of 120 to 160 mm Hg in the setting of progressive worsening of chronic HF with pulmonary and systemic congestion, aggressive diuresis can be beneficial. In the patient with systolic blood pressure greater than 160 mm Hg and abrupt onset of pulmonary congestion, IV vasodilators may be indicated in addition to diuretics. For patients primarily displaying symptoms of hypoperfusion, treatment relies on use of agents that increase cardiac contractility, known as positive inotropes. Some patients display both symptoms of congestion as well as hypoperfusion and thus require use of combination therapies. One of the current challenges to the treatment of AHF is achieving hemodynamic improvement without adversely affecting organ function. In the case of inotropes, the increased contractility occurs at the expense of an

Table 6–9

IV Diuretics Used to Treat Heart Failure–Related Fluid Retention

	Onset of Action (minutes)	Duration of Action (hours)	Relative Potency	Intermittent Bolus Dosing (mg)	Continuous Infusion Dosing (bolus/infusion)
Furosemide	2–5	6	40	20–200+	20–40/2.5–10
Torsemide	Less than 10	6–12	20	10–100	20/2–5
Bumetanide	2–3	4–6	0.5	1–10	1–4/0.5–1
Ethacrynic acid	5–15	2–7		0.5–1 mg/kg per dose up to 100 mg/dose	

increase in cardiac workload and proarrhythmia. In addition, high-dose diuretic therapy is associated with worsened renal function and possibly neurohormonal activation.

▶ Diuretics

Loop diuretics, including furosemide, bumetanide, and torsemide, are the diuretics of choice in the management of AHF. Furosemide is the most commonly used agent. Diuretics decrease preload by functional venodilation within 5 to 15 minutes of administration and subsequently by an increase in sodium and water excretion. This provides rapid improvement in symptoms of pulmonary congestion. Diuretics reduce PCWP but do not increase CI like positive inotropes and arterial vasodilators. Patients who have significant volume overload often have impaired absorption of oral loop diuretics because of intestinal edema or altered transit time. Therefore, doses are usually administered via IV boluses or continuous IV infusions, given either at the same dose as the home oral dose for those taking diuretics regularly or at lower doses for diuretic-naive patients (Table 6–9). Higher doses may be required for patients with renal insufficiency due to decreased drug delivery to the site of action in the loop of Henle.

There is a paucity of clinical trial evidence comparing the benefit of diuretics with other therapies for symptom relief or long-term outcomes. Additionally, excessive preload reduction can lead to a decrease in CO resulting in reflex increase in sympathetic activation, renin release, and the expected consequences of vasoconstriction, tachycardia, and increased myocardial oxygen demand. Careful use of diuretics is recommended to avoid overdiuresis. Monitoring of serum electrolytes such as potassium, sodium, and magnesium is done frequently to identify and correct imbalances. Monitor serum creatinine and blood urea nitrogen daily at a minimum to assess volume depletion and renal function.

Occasionally, patients with HF do not respond to a diuretic, defined as failure to achieve a weight reduction of at least 0.5 kg (or negative net fluid balance of at least 500 mL) after several increasing bolus doses.[17]

Several strategies are used to overcome diuretic resistance. These include using larger oral doses, converting to IV dosing, or increasing the frequency of administration. A small study using low-dose continuous infusions of furosemide and torsemide have shown an increase in urine output compared with intermittent bolus dosing, but newer evidence suggests there may be little difference between intermittent bolus dosing and continuous infusion strategies on symptom relief at 72 hours.[54,55] Nonetheless, many regimens include a bolus dose followed by a maintenance infusion (Table 6–9).[56] Another useful strategy is to combine two diuretics with different sites of action within the nephron. The most common combination is the use of a loop diuretic with a thiazide diuretic such as metolazone. Combining diuretics should be used with caution due to an increased risk for cardiovascular collapse due to rapid intravascular volume depletion. Strict monitoring of electrolytes, vital signs, and fluid balance is warranted.

Finally, poor CO may contribute to diuretic resistance. In these patients, it may become necessary to add vasodilators or inotropes to enhance perfusion to the kidneys. Care must be taken because vasodilators can decrease renal blood flow despite increasing CO through dilation of central and peripheral vascular beds.

▶ Vasodilators

IV vasodilators cause a rapid decrease in arterial tone, resulting in a decrease in SVR and a subsequent increase in SV and CO. Additionally, vasodilators reduce ventricular filling pressures (PCWP) within 24 to 48 hours, reduce myocardial oxygen consumption, and decrease ventricular workload. Vasodilators are commonly used in patients presenting with AHF accompanied by moderate to severe congestion. This class includes nitroglycerin, nitroprusside, and nesiritide. Hemodynamic effects and dosages for these agents are included in Tables 6–10 and 6–11, respectively. Although vasodilators are generally safe and effective, identification of the proper patient for use is important to minimize the risk of significant hypotension. In addition, vasodilators are contraindicated in patients whose cardiac filling (and hence CO) depends on venous return or intravascular volume, as well as patients who present with shock.

Nitroglycerin Nitroglycerin acts as a source of nitric oxide, which induces smooth muscle relaxation in venous and arterial vascular beds. Nitroglycerin is primarily a venous vasodilator at lower doses, but it exerts potent arterial vasodilatory effects at higher doses. Thus, at lower doses, nitroglycerin causes decreases in preload (or filling pressures)

Table 6–10

Usual Hemodynamic Effects of Commonly Used IV Agents for Treatment of Acute or Severe Heart Failure

Drug	CO	PCWP	SVR	BP	HR
Diuretics	↑/↓/0	↓		↓	0
Nitroglycerin	↑	↓↓	↓	↓↓	↑/0
Nitroprusside	↑	↓↓↓	↓↓↓	↓↓↓	↑
Nesiritide	↑	↓↓	↓↓	↓↓	0
Dobutamine	↑↑	↓/0	↓/0	↓/0	↑↑
Milrinone	↑↑	↓↓	↓	↓	↑

BP, blood pressure; CO, cardiac output; HR, heart rate; PCWP, pulmonary capillary wedge pressure; SVR, systemic vascular resistance; ↑, increase; ↓, decrease; 0, no or little change.

Table 6–11

Usual Doses and Monitoring of Commonly Used Hemodynamic Medications

Drug	Dose	Monitoring Variables[a]
Dopamine	0.5–10 mcg/kg/min	BP, HR, urinary output and kidney function, ECG, extremity perfusion (higher doses only)
Dobutamine	2.5–20 mcg/kg/min	BP, HR, urinary output and function, ECG
Milrinone	0.375–0.75 mcg/kg/min	BP, HR, urinary output and function, ECG, changes in ischemic symptoms (e.g., chest pain), electrolytes
Nitroprusside	0.25–3 mcg/kg/min	BP, HR, liver and kidney function, blood cyanide and/or thiocyanate concentrations if toxicity suspected (nausea, vomiting, altered mental function)
Nitroglycerin	5–200+ mcg/kg/min	BP, HR, ECG, changes in ischemic symptoms
Nesiritide	Bolus: 2 mcg/kg; Infusion: 0.01 mcg/kg/min	BP, HR, urinary output and kidney function, blood BNP concentrations

[a]In addition to pulmonary capillary wedge pressure and cardiac output.

BNP, B-type natriuretic peptide; BP, blood pressure; ECG, electrocardiogram; HR, heart rate.

and improved coronary blood flow. At higher doses (greater than 100 mcg/min), additional reduction in preload is achieved, along with a decrease in afterload and subsequent increase in SV and CO. IV nitroglycerin is primarily used as a preload reducer for patients exhibiting pulmonary congestion or in combination with inotropes for congested patients with severely reduced CO.[52]

Continuous infusions of nitroglycerin should be initiated at a dose of 5 to 10 mcg/min and increased every 5 to 10 minutes until symptomatic or hemodynamic improvement. Effective doses range from 35 to 200 mcg/min. The most common adverse events reported are headache, dose-related hypotension, and tachycardia. A limitation to nitroglycerin's use is the development of tachyphylaxis, or tolerance to its effects, which can be evident within 12 hours after initiation of continuous infusion and necessitate additional titrations to higher doses.

Nitroprusside Nitroprusside, like nitroglycerin, causes the formation of nitric oxide and vascular smooth muscle relaxation. In contrast to nitroglycerin, nitroprusside is both a venous and arterial vasodilator regardless of dosage. Nitroprusside causes a pronounced decrease in PCWP, SVR, and blood pressure, with a modest increase in CO. Nitroprusside has been studied to a limited extent in AHF, and no studies have evaluated its effects on mortality.[52] Nitroprusside is initiated at 0.1 to 0.25 mcg/kg/min, followed by dose adjustments in 0.1 to 0.2 mcg/kg/min increments if necessary to achieve desired effect. Because of its rapid onset of action and metabolism, nitroprusside is administered as a continuous infusion that is easy to titrate and provides predictable hemodynamic effects. Nitroprusside requires strict monitoring of blood pressure and HR. Nitroprusside's use is limited in AHF due to recommended hemodynamic monitoring with an arterial line and mandatory intensive care unit admission at many institutions. Abrupt withdrawal of therapy should be avoided because rebound neurohormonal activation may occur. Therefore, the dose should be tapered slowly. Nitroprusside has the potential to cause cyanide and thiocyanate toxicity, especially in patients with hepatic and renal insufficiency, respectively. Toxicity is most common with use longer than 3 days and with higher doses. Nitroprusside should be avoided in patients with active ischemia because its powerful afterload-reducing effects within the myocardium can "steal" coronary blood flow from myocardial segments that are supplied by epicardial vessels with high-grade lesions.

Nesiritide B-type natriuretic peptide is an endogenous neurohormone that is synthesized and released from the ventricles in response to chamber wall stretch or increased filling pressures. Recombinant BNP, or nesiritide, is the newest compound developed for AHF. Nesiritide binds to guanylate cyclase receptors in vascular smooth muscle and endothelial cells, causing an increase in cGMP concentrations leading to vasodilation (venous and arterial) and natriuresis. Nesiritide also antagonizes the effects of the RAAS and endothelin. Nesiritide reduces PCWP, right atrial pressure, and SVR. Consequently, it also increases SV and CO without affecting heart rate. Continuous infusions result in sustained effects for 24 hours without tachyphylaxis, although experience with its use beyond 72 hours is limited.

Nesiritide has been shown to improve symptoms of dyspnea and fatigue. In a randomized clinical trial,[57] nesiritide was found to significantly decrease PCWP more than nitroglycerin and placebo over 3 hours. Nesiritide improved patients' self-reported dyspnea scores compared with placebo at 3 hours, but there was no difference compared with nitroglycerin. In the Acute Study of Clinical Effectiveness of Nesiritide in Decompensated Heart Failure,[58] nesiritide did not decrease death or rehospitalization for HF within 30 days. This is the largest prospective study in AHF to date, and it also shows that nesiritide does not worsen renal function or increase the risk for mortality, despite previous concerns regarding its association with elevations in serum creatinine.

Currently, nesiritide is indicated for patients with AHF exhibiting dyspnea at rest or with minimal activity. The recommended dose regimen is a bolus of 2 mcg/kg, followed by a continuous infusion for up to 24 hours of 0.01 mcg/kg/min. Because nesiritide's effects are predictable and sustained at the recommended dosage, titration of the infusion rate (maximum of 0.03 mcg/kg/min) is not commonly required nor is invasive hemodynamic monitoring. Nesiritide should be avoided in patients with systolic blood pressure less than 90 mm Hg. Although nesiritide's place in AHF therapy is not firmly defined, it can be used in combination with diuretics for patients presenting in moderate to severe decompensation, and it offers a unique mechanism of action. One potential disadvantage compared with other vasodilators is its longer half-life. If hypotension occurs, the effect can be prolonged (2 hours).

▶ Inotropic Agents

Currently available positive inotropic agents act via increasing intracellular cyclic adenosine monophosphate (cAMP) concentrations through different mechanisms. β-Agonists activate adenylate cyclase through stimulation of β-adrenergic receptors, which subsequently catalyzes the conversion of ATP to cAMP. In contrast, phosphodiesterase inhibitors reduce degradation of cAMP. The resulting elevation in cAMP levels leads to enhanced phospholipase activity, which then increases the rate and extent of calcium influx during systole, thereby enhancing contractility. Additionally, during diastole, cAMP promotes uptake of calcium by the sarcoplasmic reticulum, which improves cardiac relaxation. The inotropes approved for use in AHF are discussed in the following sections.

Dobutamine Dobutamine has historically been the inotrope of choice for AHF. As a synthetic catecholamine, it acts as an agonist mainly on β_1- and β_2-receptors and minimally on α_1-receptors. The resulting hemodynamic effects are due to both receptor- and reflex-mediated activities. These effects include increased contractility and HR through β_1- (and β_2-) receptors and vasodilation through a relatively greater effect on β_2- than α_1-receptors. Dobutamine can increase, decrease, or cause little change in mean arterial pressure depending on whether the resulting increase in CO is enough to offset the modest vasodilation. Although dobutamine has a half-life of approximately 2 minutes, its positive hemodynamic effects can be observed for several days to months after administration. The use of dobutamine is supported by several small studies documenting improved hemodynamics, but large-scale clinical trials in AHF are lacking.[59]

Dobutamine is initiated at a dose of 2.5 to 5 mcg/kg/min, which can be gradually titrated to 20 mcg/kg/min based on

clinical response. There are several practical considerations to dobutamine therapy in AHF. First, owing to its vasodilatory potential, monotherapy with dobutamine is reserved for patients with systolic blood pressures greater than 90 mm Hg. However, it is commonly used in combination with vasopressors in patients with lower systolic blood pressures. Second, due to downregulation of β_1-receptors or uncoupling of β_2-receptors from adenylate cyclase with prolonged exposure to dobutamine, attenuation of hemodynamic effects has been reported to occur as early as 48 hours after initiation of a continuous infusion, although tachyphylaxis is more evident with use spanning longer than 72 hours. Full sensitivity to dobutamine's effects can be restored 7 to 10 days after the drug is withdrawn. Third, many patients with AHF will be taking β-blockers chronically. Because of β-blockers' high affinity for β-receptors, the effectiveness of β-agonists such as dobutamine will be reduced. In patients on β-blocker therapy, it is recommended that consideration be given to the use of phosphodiesterase inhibitors such as milrinone, which do not depend on β-receptors for effect.[60,61] Although commonly practiced, use of high doses of dobutamine to overcome the β-blockade should be discouraged because this negates any of the protective benefits of the β-blocker.

Dopamine Dopamine is most commonly reserved for patients with low systolic blood pressures and those approaching cardiogenic shock. Dopamine exerts its effects through direct stimulation of adrenergic receptors, as well as release of norepinephrine from adrenergic nerve terminals. Dopamine produces hemodynamic effects that differ based on dosing. At lower doses, dopamine stimulates dopamine type 1 (D1) receptors and thus increases renal perfusion. Positive inotropic effects are more pronounced at doses of 3 to 10 mcg/kg/min. Cardiac index is increased due to increased SV and HR. At doses higher than 10 mcg/kg/min, chronotropic and α_1-mediated vasoconstriction effects are evident. This causes an increase in mean arterial pressure due to higher CI and SVR. The ultimate effect on cardiac hemodynamics will depend largely on the dosage prescribed and must be individually tailored to the patient's clinical status. Dopamine is generally associated with an increase in CO and blood pressure, with a concomitant increase in PCWP. Dopamine increases myocardial oxygen demand and may decrease coronary blood flow through vasoconstriction and increased wall tension. As with other inotropes, dopamine is associated with a risk for arrhythmias.

Phosphodiesterase Inhibitors Milrinone and inamrinone work by inhibiting phosphodiesterase III, the enzyme responsible for the breakdown of cAMP. The increase in cAMP levels leads to increased intracellular calcium concentrations and enhanced contractile force generation. Milrinone has replaced inamrinone as the phosphodiesterase inhibitor of choice due to the higher frequency of thrombocytopenia seen with inamrinone.

Milrinone has both positive inotropic and vasodilating properties and as such is referred to as an "inodilator." Its vasodilating activities are especially prominent on venous capacitance vessels and pulmonary vascular beds, although a reduction in arterial tone is also noted. IV administration results in an increase in SV and CO, and usually only minor changes in heart rate. Milrinone also lowers PCWP through venodilation. Routine use of milrinone during acute decompensations in NYHA FC II to IV heart failure is not recommended, and milrinone use remains limited to patients who require inotropic support.[62]

Dosing recommendations for milrinone include a loading dose of 50 mcg/kg, followed by an infusion beginning at 0.5 mcg/kg/min (range: 0.23 mcg/kg/min for patients with renal failure up to 0.75 mcg/kg/min). A loading dose is not necessary if immediate hemodynamic effects are not required or if patients have low systolic blood pressures (less than 90 mm Hg). Decreases in blood pressure during an infusion may necessitate dose reductions as well. Lower doses are also used in patients with renal insufficiency.

Milrinone is a good option for patients requiring an inotrope who are also chronically receiving β-blockers because the inotropic effects are achieved independent of β-adrenergic receptors. However, milrinone exhibits a long distribution and elimination half-life compared with β-agonists, thus requiring a loading dose when an immediate response is desired. Potential adverse effects include hypotension, arrhythmias, and, less commonly, thrombocytopenia. Additionally, milrinone has been associated with increased risk for death in some studies. Milrinone should not be used in patients in whom vasodilation is contraindicated.

Mechanical, Surgical, and Device Therapies

▶ Implantable Cardioverter Defibrillators

Implantable cardioverter defibrillators (ICDs) are the most effective modality for primary and secondary prevention of sudden cardiac death in patients with LV dysfunction. Studies universally demonstrate greater efficacy compared with antiarrhythmic therapy and a significant reduction in mortality compared with placebo.[63–65] Recent studies have expanded the eligible patient populations beyond classic indications, such as prior MI and nonsustained ventricular tachycardia or nonsuppressible ventricular tachycardia during an electrophysiological study. A clear advantage of implanting ICDs in all symptomatic patients with LVEF less than 35% (0.35) regardless of etiology or other cardiac parameters has been demonstrated.[65] Because ICD implantation and follow-up is associated with a significant economic burden, the cost effectiveness of widespread ICD use continues to be debated. Defining subgroups that would derive the greatest benefit and determining the optimal ICD configuration will aid in improving the potential costs compared with benefits.

▶ Cardiac Resynchronization Therapy

Dyssynchronous contraction, as a reflection of intra- and interventricular conduction delays between chambers of the heart, is common in advanced HF patients. Dyssynchrony contributes to diminished cardiac function and unfavorable myocardial energetics through altered filling times, valvular dysfunction, and wall motion defects. Cardiac resynchronization therapy (CRT) with biventricular pacing devices improves cardiac function, quality of life, and mortality in patients with NYHA FC III or IV heart failure, evidence of intraventricular conduction delay (QRS greater than 120 ms), depressed LV function (LVEF less than 35% [0.35]), and on an optimal pharmacologic regimen. A study also showed that the addition of an ICD to CRT with biventricular pacing further reduced hospitalizations and mortality.[66]

▶ Intraaortic Balloon Counterpulsation

Intraaortic balloon counterpulsation (IABC) or intraaortic balloon pumps (IABPs) are one of the most widely used mechanical circulatory assistance devices for patients with cardiac failure who do not respond to standard therapies. An IABP is placed percutaneously into the femoral artery and advanced to the high descending thoracic aorta. Once in position, the balloon is programmed to inflate during diastole and deflate during systole. Two main beneficial mechanisms are (a) inflation during diastole increases aortic pressure and perfusion of the coronary arteries, and (b) deflation just prior to the aortic valve opening reduces arterial impedance (afterload). As such, IABC increases myocardial oxygen supply and decreases oxygen demand. This device has many indications, including cardiogenic shock, high-risk unstable angina in conjunction with percutaneous interventions, preoperative stabilization of high-risk patients prior to surgery, and in patients who cannot be weaned from cardiopulmonary bypass. Possible complications include infection, bleeding, thrombosis, limb ischemia, and device malfunction. The device is typically useful for short-term therapy due to the invasiveness of the device, the need for limb immobilization, and the requirement for anticoagulation.

▶ Ventricular Assist Device

The ventricular assist device (VAD) is a surgically implanted pump that reduces or replaces the work of the right, left, or both ventricles. VADs are currently indicated for short-term support in patients refractory to pharmacologic therapies, as long-term bridge therapy (a temporary transition treatment) in patients awaiting cardiac transplant, or in some instances as the destination therapy (treatment for patients in lieu of cardiac transplant for those who are not appropriate candidates for transplantation).[1] The most common complications are infection and thromboembolism. Other adverse effects include bleeding, air embolism, device failure, and multiorgan failure.

▶ Surgical Therapy

Heart transplantation represents the final option for refractory end-stage HF patients who have exhausted medical and device therapies. Heart transplantation is not a cure but should be considered a trade between a life-threatening syndrome and the risks associated with the operation and long-term immunosuppression. Assessment of appropriate candidates includes comorbid illnesses, psychosocial behavior, available financial and social support, and patient willingness to adhere to lifelong therapy and close medical follow-up.[1] Overall, the transplant recipient's quality of life may be improved, but not all patients receive this benefit. Posttransplant survival continues to improve due to advances in immunosuppression, treatment and prevention of infection, and optimal management of patient comorbidities.

▶ Investigational Therapies

Clinical trials are currently investigating new agents for the treatment of AHF. These compounds offer unique mechanisms of action by targeting different neurohormonal receptors (vasopressin, endothelin, atrial natriuretic peptide, and adenosine) or through completely novel pharmacologic profiles (myosin ATPase agonists). Some agents or drug classes being studied include tolvaptan, a V_2-selective vasopressin antagonist; various ET-A selective and nonselective antagonists; and an adenosine-1 receptor agonist.

OUTCOME EVALUATION OF ACUTE HEART FAILURE

- Focus on (a) acute improvement of symptoms and hemodynamics due to IV therapies, (b) criteria for a safe discharge from the hospital, and (c) optimization of oral therapy.
- Initially, monitor patients for rapid relief of symptoms related to the chief complaint on admission. This includes improvement of dyspnea, oxygenation, fatigue, JVD, and other markers of congestion or distress.
- Monitor for adequate perfusion of vital organs through assessment of mental status, creatinine clearance, liver function tests, and a stable HR between 50 and 100 beats/min. Additionally, adequate skin and muscle blood perfusion and normal pH is desirable.
- Monitor changes in hemodynamic variables if available. CI should increase, with a goal to maintain it above 2.2 L/min/m². Pulmonary capillary wedge pressure should decrease in volume-overloaded patients to a goal of less than 18 mm Hg (2.4 kPa).

Patient Encounter Part 4

After 6 months, DG returns to the clinic complaining of extreme SOB with any activity, as well as at rest. He sleeps sitting up due to severe orthopnea, can only eat a few bites of a meal and then feels full and nauseous, and states he has gained 22 lb (10 kg) from his baseline weight. He is also profoundly dizzy when standing up from a chair and bending over. He states that he does not feel his furosemide therapy is working. He is admitted to the cardiology unit.

SH

DG admits to resuming smoking after quitting for 2 months; additionally, he has been eating out in restaurants more often in the past 2 weeks.

Meds

Lisinopril 10 mg once daily

Furosemide 80 mg twice daily

Glipizide 10 mg twice daily for diabetes

Metformin 1000 mg twice daily for diabetes

Nitroglycerin 0.4 mg sublingual (SL) as needed

Multivitamin daily

Aspirin 325 mg daily

VS: blood pressure 96/54 mm Hg, pulse 102 bpm and regular, respiratory rate 22/minute, temperature 37°C (98.6°F), Wt 271 lb (123 kg), BMI 41.2 kg/m²

Lungs: There are rales present bilaterally

CV: Regular rate and rhythm with normal S_1 and S_2; there is an S_3 and an S_4; a 4/6 systolic ejection murmur is present and heard best at the left lower sternal border; point of maximal impulse is displaced laterally; jugular veins are distended, JVP is 11 cm above sternal angle; a positive HJR is observed

Abd: Hard, tender, and bowel sounds are absent; 3+ pitting edema of extremities is observed

CXR: Bilateral pleural effusions and cardiomegaly

Echo: EF = 20% (0.20)

Pertinent labs

BNP 740 pg/mL (740 ng/L; 214 pmol/L), K: 4.2 mEq/L (4.2 mmol/L), BUN 64 mg/dL (23 mmol/L), SCr 2.4 mg/dL (212 μmol/L), Mg 1.8 mEq/L (0.90 mmol/L)

A pulmonary catheter is placed, revealing the following: PCWP 37 mm Hg (4.9 kPa); cardiac index 1.8 L/min/m²

What NYHA functional class, ACC/AHA stage, and hemodynamic subset is DG currently in?

What are your initial treatment goals?

What pharmacologic agents are appropriate to use at this time?

Identify a monitoring plan to assess for efficacy and toxicity of the recommended drug therapy.

Once DG's symptoms are improved, how would you optimize his oral medication therapy for HF?

Patient Care and Monitoring

1. Assess the severity and duration of the patient's symptoms including limitations in activity. Rule out potential exacerbating factors.

2. Obtain a thorough history of prescription, nonprescription, and herbal medication use. Is the patient taking any medications that can exacerbate HF?

3. Review available diagnostic information from the chest radiograph, ECG, and echocardiogram.

4. Review the patient's lifestyle habits including salt and alcohol intake, tobacco product use, and exercise routine.

5. If unknown, investigate the patient's underlying etiology of HF. Verify that comorbidities that lead to or worsen HF are optimally managed with appropriate drug therapy.

6. Educate the patient on lifestyle modifications such as salt restriction (maximum 2 to 4 g/day), fluid restriction if appropriate, limitation of alcohol, tobacco cessation, participation in a cardiac rehabilitation and exercise program, and proper immunizations such as the pneumococcal vaccine and yearly influenza vaccine.

7. Develop a treatment plan to alleviate symptoms and maintain euvolemia with diuretics. Daily weights to assess fluid retention are recommended.

8. Develop a medication regimen to slow the progression of HF with the use of neurohormonal blockers such as vasodilators (ACE inhibitors, ARBs, or hydralazine/isosorbide dinitrate), β-blockers, and aldosterone antagonists. Utilize digoxin if the patient remains symptomatic despite optimization of the therapies just described.

   • Is the patient at goal or maximally tolerated doses of vasodilator and β-blocker therapy?

   • Are aldosterone antagonists utilized in appropriate patients with proper electrolyte and renal function monitoring?

9. Stress the importance of adherence to the therapeutic regimen and lifestyle changes for maintenance of a compensated state and slowing of disease progression.

10. Evaluate the patient for presence of adverse drug reactions, drug allergies, and drug interactions.

11. Provide patient education with regard to disease state and drug therapy, and reinforce self-monitoring for symptoms of HF that necessitate follow-up with a healthcare practitioner.

• Closely monitor blood pressures and renal function while decreasing preload with diuretics and vasodilators.

• Ensure patients are euvolemic or nearly euvolemic prior to discharge.

• Because oral therapies can both improve symptoms and prolong survival, optimizing outpatient HF management is a priority when preparing a patient for hospital discharge. Ensure that the patient's regimen includes a vasodilator, β-blocker, a diuretic at an adequate dose to maintain euvolemia, and digoxin or aldosterone antagonist if indicated.

Abbreviations Introduced in This Chapter

ACC/AHA	American College of Cardiology/American Heart Association
ACE	Angiotensin-converting enzyme
AHF	Acute heart failure
ANP	Atrial natriuretic peptide
ARB	Angiotensin receptor blocker
AT_1	Angiotensin type 1
AT_2	Angiotensin type 2
ATP	Adenosine triphosphate
BMI	Body mass index
BNP	B-type natriuretic peptide
BP	Blood pressure
bpm	Beats per minute
BUN	Blood urea nitrogen
CAD	Coronary artery disease
CAM	Complementary and alternative medication
cAMP	Cyclic adenosine monophosphate
CBC	Complete blood cell count
cGMP	Cyclic guanosine monophosphate
CHARM	Candesartan in Heart Failure Assessment of Reduction in Mortality and Morbidity
CI	Cardiac index
CNS	Central nervous system
CO	Cardiac output
COX-2	Cyclooxygenase-2
CrCL	Creatinine clearance
CRT	Cardiac resynchronization therapy
CYP450	Cytochrome P-450 isoenzyme
D1	Dopamine receptor type 1
ECG	Electrocardiogram
EF	Ejection fraction
ET-1	Endothelin-1
ET-A	Endothelin-A
ET-B	Endothelin-B
HF	Heart failure
HFpEF	Heart failure with preserved ejection fraction

HJR	Hepatojugular reflux
HR	Heart rate
IABC	Intraaortic balloon counterpulsation
IABP	Intraaortic balloon pump
ICD	Implantable cardioverter defibrillator
iNOS	Inducible nitric oxide synthetase
INR	International normalized ratio
I-PRESERVE	Irbesartan in Patients with Heart Failure and Preserved Ejection Fraction
JVD	Jugular venous distention
JVP	Jugular venous pressure
K	Potassium
LV	Left ventricular
LVEF	Left ventricular ejection fraction
LVF	Left ventricular failure
MI	Myocardial infarction
MVO_2	Myocardial oxygen consumption
NSAID	Nonsteroidal anti-inflammatory drug
NT-proBNP	N-terminal proBNP
NYHA FC	New York Heart Association Functional Class
PAC	Pulmonary artery catheter
PCWP	Pulmonary capillary wedge pressure
PEP-CHF	Perindopril in Elderly People with Chronic Heart Failure
PND	Paroxysmal nocturnal dyspnea
PPCM	Peripartum cardiomyopathy
RAAS	Renin-angiotensin-aldosterone system
RVF	Right ventricular failure
SCr	Serum creatinine
SL	Sublingual
SNS	Sympathetic nervous system
SOB	Shortness of breath
SV	Stroke volume
SVR	Systemic vascular resistance
TNF-α	Tumor necrosis factor-α
V_{1a}	Vasopressin type 1a
V_2	Vasopressin type 2
VAD	Ventricular assist device

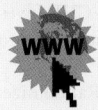 Self-assessment questions and answers are available at *http://www.mhpharmacotherapy.com/pp.html.*

REFERENCES

1. Hunt SA, Abraham WT, Chin MH, et al. 2009 Focused update incorporated into the ACC/AHA 2005 Guidelines for the Diagnosis and Management of Heart Failure in Adults A Report of the American College of Cardiology Foundation/American Heart Association Task Force on Practice Guidelines Developed in Collaboration with the International Society for Heart and Lung Transplantation. J Am Coll Cardiol 2009;53(15):e1–e90.
2. Centers for Disease Control and Prevention. Heart failure fact sheet, Available at: www.cdc.gov/cvh/library/fs_heart_failure.htm. Accessed January 5, 2012.
3. Nieminen MS, Harjola VP. Definition and epidemiology of acute heart failure syndromes. Am J Cardiol 2005;96(Suppl):5–10.
4. Bonow RO, Bennett S, Casey DE Jr, et al., for the Writing Committee to Develop Heart Failure Clinical Performance Measures. ACC/AHA clinical performance measures for adults with chronic heart failure: A report of the American College of Cardiology/American Heart Association Task Force on Performance Measures (Writing Committee to Develop Heart Failure Clinical Performance Measures) endorsed by the Heart Failure Society of America. J Am Coll Cardiol 2005;46(6):1144–1178.
5. Parker RB, Cavallari LH. Systolic heart failure. In: DiPiro JT, Talbert RL, Yee GC, et al., eds. *Pharmacotherapy: A pathophysiologic approach,* 8th ed. New York, NY: McGraw-Hill, 2011:137–172.
6. Jessup M, Brozena S. Heart failure. N Engl J Med 2003;348:2007–2018.
7. Schrier RW, Abraham WT. Hormones and hemodynamics in heart failure. N Engl J Med 1999;341(8):577–585.
8. Mann DL. Mechanisms and models in heart failure—A combinatorial approach. Circulation 1999;100:999–1008.
9. Mann DL. Inflammatory mediators and the failing heart—Past, present, and the foreseeable future. Circ Res 2002;91:988–998.
10. Silver MA, Maisel A, Yancy CW, et al. BNP Consensus Panel 2004: A clinical approach for the diagnostic, prognostic, screening, treatment monitoring, and therapeutic roles of natriuretic peptides in cardiovascular diseases. Congest Heart Fail 2004;10(5 Suppl 3):1–30.
11. Hunt SA, Baker DW, Chin MH, et al., for the Committee to Revise the 1995 Guidelines for the Evaluation and Management of Heart Failure. ACC/AHA guidelines for the evaluation and management of chronic heart failure in the adult: Executive summary: A report of the American College of Cardiology/American Heart Association Task Force on Practice Guidelines. (Committee to revise the 1995 Guidelines for the Evaluation and Management of Heart Failure). J Am Coll Cardiol 2001;38:2101–2113.
12. Consensus Recommendations for the Management of Chronic Heart Failure. Am J Cardiol 1999;83:1A–38A.
13. Heart Failure Society of America. Heart failure in patients with left ventricular systolic dysfunction. J Card Fail 2006;12(1):e38–e57.
14. Ng TMH, Carter O, Guillory GS, et al. High-impact articles related to the pharmacotherapeutic management of systolic heart failure. Pharmacotherapy 2004;24(11):1594–1633.
15. Brater DC. Diuretic therapy. N Engl J Med. 1998;339(6):387–395.
16. Brater DC. Diuretic therapy in congestive heart failure. Congest Heart Fail 2000;6(4):197–201.
17. De Bruyne LK. Mechanisms and management of diuretic resistance in congestive heart failure. Postgrad Med J 2003;79:268–271.
18. The CONSENSUS Trial Study Group. Effects of enalapril on mortality in severe congestive heart failure. N Engl J Med 1987;316:1429–1435.
19. The SOLVD Investigators. Effect of enalapril on survival in patients with reduced left ventricular ejection fractions and congestive heart failure. N Engl J Med 1991;325:293–302.
20. The SOLVD Investigators. Effect of enalapril on mortality and the development of heart failure in asymptomatic patients with reduced left ventricular ejection fractions. N Engl J Med 1992;327:685–691.
21. Pfeffer MA, Braunwald E, Move LA, et al. Effect of captopril on mortality and morbidity in patients with left ventricular dysfunction after myocardial infarction. Results of the Survival and Ventricular Enlargement Trial. N Engl J Med 1992;327:669–677.
22. Packer M, Wilson-Poole PA, Armstrong PW, et al. Comparative effects of low-and high doses of the angiotensin-converting enzyme inhibitor, lisinopril, or morbidity and mortality in chronic heart failure. Circulation 1999;100:2312–2318.
23. Pitt B, Poole-Wilson PA, Segal R et al., et al. on behalf of for the ELITE II Investigators. Effect of losartan compared with captopril on mortality in patients with symptomatic heart failure: Randomised trial—The Losartan Heart Failure Survival Study ELITE II. Lancet 2000;355:1582–1587.
24. Cohn JN, Tognoni G, for the Valsartan Heart Failure Trial Investigators. A randomized trial of the angiotensin-receptor blocker valsartan in chronic heart failure. N Engl J Med 2001;345:1667–1675.
25. Pfeffer MA, Swedberg K, Granger CB et al., for the CHARM Investigators and Committees. Effects of candesartan on mortality and morbidity in patients with chronic heart failure: The CHARM-Overall programme. Lancet 2003;362:759–766.

26. Cohn JN, Archibald DG, Ziesche S, et al. Effect of vasodilator therapy on mortality in chronic congestive heart failure. N Engl J Med 1986;314:1547–1552.

27. Cohn JN, Johnson G, Ziesche S, et al. A comparison of enalapril with hydralazine-isosorbide dinitrate in the treatment of chronic congestive heart failure. N Engl J Med 1991;325:303–310.

28. Taylor AL, Ziesche S, Yancy C, et al. Combination of isosorbide dinitrate and hydralazine in blacks with heart failure. N Engl J Med 2004;351(20):2049–2057.

29. Packer M, Bristow MR, Cohn JN, et al., for the U.S. Carvedilol Heart Failure Study Group. The effect of carvedilol on morbidity and mortality in patients with chronic heart failure. N Engl J Med1996;334: 1349–1355.

30. CIBIS-II Investigators and Committees. The cardiac insufficiency bisoprolol study II (CIBIS-II) a randomized trial. Lancet 1999;353: 9–13.

31. MERIT-HF Study Group. Effect of metoprolol CR/XL in chronic heart failure: Metoprolol CR/XL randomized intervention trial in congestive heart failure (MERIT-HF). Lancet 1999;353:2001–2007.

32. Packer M, Coats AJ, Fowler MB, et al., for the Carvedilol Prospective Randomized Cumulative Survival Study Group. N Engl J Med 2001;344(22):1651–1658.

33. Poole-Wilson PA, Swedberg K, Cleland JG, et al., for the COMET investigators. Comparison of carvedilol and metoprolol on clinical outcomes in patients with chronic heart failure in the Carvedilol or Metoprolol European Trial (COMET): Randomized controlled trial. Lancet 2003;362:7–13.

34. Funck-Brentano C, van Veldhuisen D, van de Ven L, et al. Influence of order and type of drug (bisoprolol vs. enalapril) on outcome and adverse events in patients with chronic heart failure: A post hoc analysis of the CIBIS-III trial. Eur J Heart Fail 2011;13:765–772.

35. Pitt B, Zannad F, Remme WJ, et al. The effect of spironolactone on morbidity and mortality in patients with severe heart failure. N Engl J Med 1999;341(10):709–717.

36. Pitt B, Williams G, Remme W, et al. Eplerenone, a selective aldosterone antagonist, in patients with left ventricular dysfunction after myocardial infarction (EPHESUS). N Engl J Med 2003;348(14):1309–1321.

37. Zannad F, McMurray JV, Krum H, et al. Eplerenone in patients with systolic heart failure and mild symptoms. N Engl J Med 2011;364(1):11–21.

38. The Digitalis Investigation Group. The effect of digoxin on mortality and morbidity in patients with heart failure. The Digitalis Investigation Group. N Engl J Med 1997;336:525–533.

39. Adams KF, Gheorghiade M, Uretsky BF, et al. Clinical benefits of low serum digoxin concentrations in heart failure. J Am Coll Cardiol 2002;39:946–953.

40. Rathore SS, Curtis JP, Wang Y, et al. Association of serum digoxin concentration and outcomes in patients with heart failure. JAMA 2003;289:871–878.

41. Packer M, O'Connor CH, Ghali JK, et al. Effect of amlodipine on morbidity and mortality in severe chronic heart failure. N Engl J Med 1996;335:1107–1114.

42. Cohn JN, Ziesche S, Smith R, et al. Effect of the calcium antagonist felodipine as supplementary vasodilator therapy in patients with chronic heart failure treated with enalapril. Circulation 1997;96:856–863.

43. Lip GY, Gibbs CR. Antiplatelet agents versus control or anticoagulation for heart failure in sinus rhythm: A Cochrane systematic review. Q J Med 2002;95:461–468.

44. Fuster V, Ryde'n LE, Asinger RW, et al., for the Committee to Develop Guidelines for the Management of Patients with Atrial Fibrillation. ACC/AHA/ESC guidelines for the management of patients with atrial fibrillation: A report of the American College of Cardiology/American Heart Association Task Force on Practice Guidelines and the European Society of Cardiology Committee for Practice Guidelines and Policy Conferences. (Committee to Develop Guidelines for the Management of Patients with Atrial Fibrillation). J Am Coll Cardiol 2001;38: 1266i–lxx.

45. Lip GY, Gibbs CR. Anticoagulation for heart failure in sinus rhythm: A Cochrane systematic review. Q J Med 2002;95:451–459.

46. Aurigenuna GP, Gaasch WH. Diastolic heart failure. N Engl J Med 2004;351(11):1097–1105.

47. Cleland JG, Tendera M, Adamus J, Freemantle N, Polonski L, Taylor J. The perindopril in elderly people with chronic heart failure (PEP-CHF) study. Eur Heart J 2006;27(19):2338–2345.

48. Massie BM, Carson PE, McMurray JJ, et al. Irbesartan in patients with heart failure and preserved ejection fraction. N Engl J Med 2008;359(23):2456–2467.

49. Pearson GD, Veille JC, Rahimtoola S, et al. Peripartum cardiomyopathy: National Heart, Lung, and Blood Institute and Office of Rare Diseases (National Institutes of Health) workshop recommendations and review. JAMA 2000;283(9):1183–1188.

50. Tidswell M. Peripartum cardiomyopathy. Crit Care Clin 2004;20: 777–788.

51. Stevenson LW. Tailored therapy to hemodynamic goals for advanced heart failure. Eur J Heart Fail 1999;1(3):251–257.

52. DiDomenico RJ, Park HY, Southworth MR, et al. Guidelines for acute decompensated heart failure treatment. Ann Pharmacother 2004;38(4):649–660.

53. Nohria A, Lewis E, Stevenson LW. Medical management of advanced heart failure. JAMA 2002;287:628–640.

54. Howard PA, Dunn MI. Severe heart failure in the elderly: Potential benefits of high-dose and continuous infusion diuretics. Drugs and Aging 2002;19:249–256.

55. Felker MG, Lee KL, Bull DA, et al. Diuretic strategies in patients with acute decompensated heart failure. N Engl J Med 2011;364:797–805.

56. Licata G, Pasquale PD, Parrinello G, et al. Effects of high-dose furosemide and small-volume hypertonic saline infusion in comparison with a high dose of furosemide as bolus in refractory congestive heart failure: Long term effects. Am Heart J 2003;145:459–466.

57. VMAC Investigators. Intravenous nesiritide versus nitroglycerin for treatment of decompensated congestive heart failure. JAMA 2002;287:1531–1540.

58. O'Connor CM, Starling RC, Hernandez, AF, et al. Effect of nesiritide in patients with acute decompensated heart failure. N Engl J Med 2011;365:32–43.

59. Felker GM, O'Connor CM. Inotropic therapy for heart failure: An evidence-based approach. Am Heart J 2001;142:393–401.

60. Stevenson LW. Clinical use of inotropic therapy for heart failure: Looking backward or forward? Part I: Inotropic infusions during hospitalizations. Circulation 2003;109:367–372.

61. Stevenson LW. Clinical use of inotropic therapy for heart failure: Looking backward or forward? Part II: Chronic inotropic therapy. Circulation 2003;108:492–497.

62. Cuffe MS, Califf RM, Adams KF, et al (for the OPTIME-CHF Investigators). Short-term intravenous milrinone for acute exacerbation of chronic heart failure. JAMA 2002;287:1541–1547.

63. Rose EA, Gelijns AC, Moskowitz AJ, et al., for the Randomized Evaluation of Mechanical Assistance for the Treatment of Congestive Heart Failure (REMATCH) Study Group. Long-term mechanical left ventricular assistance for end-stage heart failure. N Engl J Med 2001;345(20):1435–1443.

64. Abraham WT, Fisher WG, Smith AL, et al., for the MIRACLE Study Group. Cardiac resynchronization in chronic heart failure. N Engl J Med 2002;346(24):1845–1853.

65. Bardy GH, Lee KL, Mark DB, et al. Amiodarone or an implantable cardioverter-defibrillator for congestive heart failure. N Engl J Med 2005;352:225–237.

66. Abraham WT, Fisher WG, Smith AL, et al. Cardiac resynchronization in chronic heart failure. N Engl J Med 2002;346:1845–1853.

7 Ischemic Heart Disease

Larisa H. Cavallari and Robert J. DiDomenico

KEY CONCEPTS

❶ Ischemic heart disease results from an imbalance between myocardial oxygen demand and oxygen supply that is most often due to coronary atherosclerosis. Common clinical manifestations of ischemic heart disease include chronic stable angina and the acute coronary syndromes of unstable angina, non–ST-segment elevation myocardial infarction, and ST-segment elevation myocardial infarction.

❷ Early detection and aggressive modification of risk factors are the primary strategies for delaying ischemic heart disease progression and preventing ischemic heart disease–related events including death.

❸ Patients with chest pressure or heaviness that is provoked by activity and relieved with rest should be assessed for ischemic heart disease. Sharp pain is not a typical symptom of ischemic heart disease. Some patients may experience discomfort in the neck, jaw, shoulder, or arm rather than, or in addition to, the chest. Pain may be accompanied by nausea, vomiting, or diaphoresis.

❹ The major goals for the treatment of ischemic heart disease are to prevent acute coronary syndrome and death, alleviate acute symptoms of myocardial ischemia, prevent recurrent symptoms of myocardial ischemia, prevent disease progression, reduce complications, and avoid or minimize adverse treatment effects.

❺ Both 3-hydroxy-3-methylglutaryl coenzyme A reductase inhibitors (statins) and angiotensin-converting enzyme inhibitors are believed to provide vasculoprotective effects, and in addition to antiplatelet agents, they have been shown to reduce the risk of acute coronary events and death in patients with ischemic heart disease. Angiotensin receptor blockers may be used in patients who cannot tolerate angiotensin-converting enzyme inhibitors because of side effects (e.g., chronic cough). β-Blockers have been shown to decrease morbidity and improve survival in patients who have suffered a myocardial infarction.

❻ Antiplatelet therapy with aspirin should be considered for all patients without contraindications, particularly in patients with a history of myocardial infarction. Clopidogrel may be considered in patients with allergies or intolerance to aspirin. In some patients, combination antiplatelet therapy with aspirin and P2Y$_{12}$ inhibitor may be used.

❼ To control risk factors and prevent major adverse cardiac events, statin therapy should be considered in all patients with ischemic heart disease, particularly in those individuals with elevated low-density lipoprotein cholesterol. In the absence of contraindications, angiotensin-converting enzyme inhibitors are initiated in individuals with ischemic heart disease, diabetes mellitus, left ventricular dysfunction, or a history of myocardial infarction. Angiotensin receptor blockers may be used in patients who cannot tolerate angiotensin-converting enzyme inhibitors because of side effects.

❽ All patients with a history of angina should have sublingual nitroglycerin tablets or spray to relieve acute ischemic symptoms. Patients should be instructed to use one dose (tablet or spray) every 5 minutes until pain is relieved and to call 911 if pain is unimproved or worsens 5 minutes after the first dose.

9 β-Blockers are first-line therapy for preventing ischemic symptoms, particularly in patients with a history of myocardial infarction. Long-acting calcium channel blockers and long-acting nitrates may be added for refractory symptoms or substituted if a β-blocker is not tolerated.

10 Patients should be monitored to assess for drug effectiveness, adverse drug reactions, and potential drug–drug interactions. Patients should be assessed for adherence to their pharmacotherapeutic regimens and lifestyle modifications.

INTRODUCTION

Ischemic heart disease (IHD) is also called coronary heart disease (CHD) or coronary artery disease (CAD). The term *ischemic* refers to a decreased supply of oxygenated blood, in this case to the heart muscle. IHD is caused by the narrowing of one or more of the major coronary arteries that supply blood to the heart, most commonly by atherosclerotic plaques. Atherosclerotic plaques may impede coronary blood flow to the extent that cardiac tissue distal to the site of the coronary artery narrowing is deprived of sufficient oxygen in the face of increased oxygen demand. **1** *Ischemic heart disease results from an imbalance between myocardial oxygen supply and oxygen demand (Fig. 7–1). Common clinical manifestations of IHD include chronic stable angina and the acute coronary syndromes (ACS) of unstable angina, non–ST-segment elevation myocardial infarction (MI), and ST-segment elevation MI.*

Angina pectoris, or simply angina, is the most common symptom of IHD. Angina is discomfort in the chest that occurs when the blood supply to the myocardium is compromised. Chronic stable angina is defined as a chronic occurrence of chest discomfort due to transient myocardial ischemia with physical exertion or other conditions that increase oxygen demand. The primary focus of this chapter is on the management of chronic stable angina. However, some information is also provided related to ACS, given the overlap between the two disease states. The American College of Cardiology and the American Heart Association have jointly published practice guidelines for the management of patients with chronic stable angina. Refer to these guidelines for further information.[1,2]

EPIDEMIOLOGY AND ETIOLOGY

IHD affects over 16 million Americans and is the leading cause of death for both men and women in the United States.[3] The incidence of IHD is higher in middle-aged men compared with women. However, the rate of IHD increases two- to threefold in women after menopause. Chronic stable angina is the initial manifestation of IHD in about 50% of patients, whereas unstable angina or MI is the first sign of IHD in other patients. Chronic stable angina is associated with considerable patient morbidity, with many

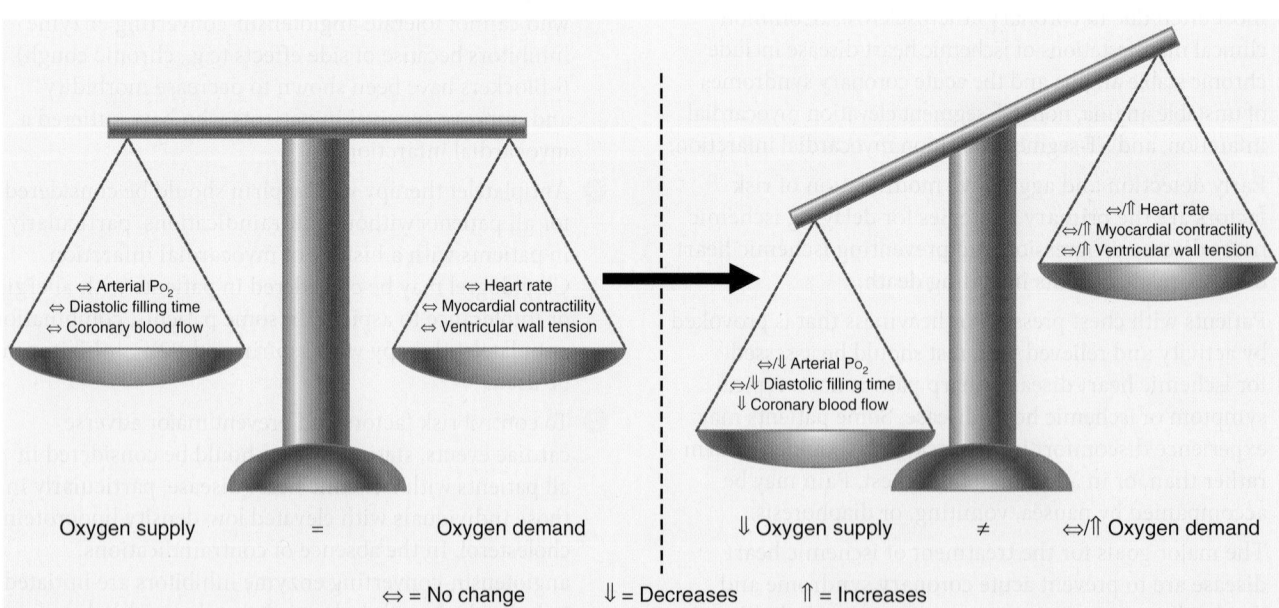

FIGURE 7–1. This illustration depicts the balance between myocardial oxygen supply and demand and the various factors that affect each. It should be noted that diastolic filling time is not an independent predictor of myocardial oxygen supply per se, but rather a determinant of coronary blood flow. On the left is myocardial oxygen supply and demand under normal circumstances. On the right is the mismatch between oxygen supply and demand in patients with ischemic heart disease. In patients without ischemic heart disease, coronary blood flow increases in response to increases in myocardial oxygen demand. However, in patients with ischemic heart disease, coronary blood flow cannot sufficiently increase (and may decrease) in response to increased oxygen demand resulting in angina. (Po₂, partial pressure of oxygen.)

affected patients eventually requiring hospitalization for ACS. In addition, chronic stable angina has a major negative impact on health-related quality of life. Thus, in patients with chronic stable angina, it is important to optimize pharmacotherapy to reduce symptoms, improve quality of life, slow disease progression, and prevent ACS.

Conditions Associated with Angina

Figure 7–2 shows the anatomy of the coronary arteries. The major epicardial coronary arteries are the left main, left anterior descending, left circumflex, and right coronary arteries.

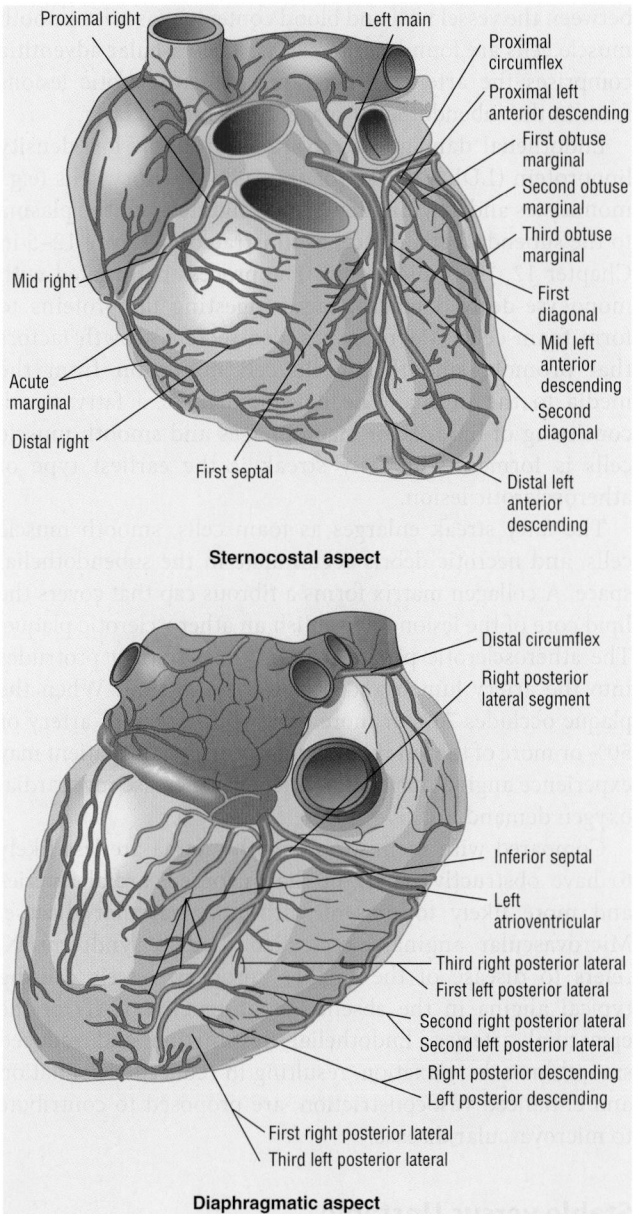

FIGURE 7–2. Coronary artery anatomy with sternocostal and diaphragmatic views. (Reproduced from Talbert RL. Ischemic heart disease. In: DiPiro JT, Talbert RL, Yee GC, et al, eds. *Pharmacotherapy: A pathophysiologic approach,* 6th ed. New York, NY: McGraw-Hill, 2005:263, with permission.)

Table 7–1	
Nonatherosclerotic Conditions That Can Cause Angina-Like Symptoms	
Organ System	**Condition**
Cardiac	Aortic dissection, aortic stenosis, coronary artery vasospasm, pericarditis, valvular heart disease, severe uncontrolled hypertension
Noncardiac	Anemia, anxiety disorders, carbon monoxide poisoning, chest wall trauma, cocaine use, esophageal reflux or spasm, generalized anxiety disorder, peptic ulcer, pleuritis, pneumonia, pneumothorax, pulmonary embolus, pulmonary hypertension, thyrotoxicosis

Atherosclerosis leading to obstructive lesions in one or more of the major coronary arteries or their principal branches is the major cause of angina. **Vasospasm** at the site of an atherosclerotic plaque may contribute to angina by further restricting blood supply to the distal myocardium. Less commonly, vasospasm in coronary arteries with no or minimal atherosclerotic disease can produce angina and even precipitate ACS. This type of vasospasm is referred to as variant or **Prinzmetal's angina**. Other nonatherosclerotic conditions that can cause angina-like symptoms are listed in Table 7–1. It is important to differentiate the etiology of chest discomfort because treatment varies depending on the underlying disease process.

Risk Factors

Factors that predispose an individual to IHD are listed in Table 7–2. Optimization of modifiable risk factors can significantly reduce the risk of MI.[4] Hypertension, diabetes, **dyslipidemia**, and cigarette smoking are associated with endothelial damage and dysfunction and contribute to

Table 7–2	
Major Risk Factors for Ischemic Heart Disease	
Modifiable	**Nonmodifiable**
Cigarette smoking Dyslipidemia • Elevated LDL or total cholesterol • Reduced HDL cholesterol Diabetes mellitus Hypertension Physical inactivity Obesity (body mass index greater than or equal to 30 kg/m²) Low daily fruit and vegetable consumption Alcohol overconsumption	Age 45 years or greater for men, age 55 years or greater for women Gender (men and postmenopausal women) Family history of premature cardiovascular disease, defined as cardiovascular disease in a male first-degree relative (i.e., father or brother) younger than 55 years old or a female first-degree relative (i.e., mother or sister) younger than 65 years

HDL, high-density lipoprotein; LDL, low-density lipoprotein.

atherosclerosis of the coronary arteries. The risk for IHD increases twofold for every 20 mm Hg increment in systolic blood pressure or 10 mm Hg increment in diastolic blood pressure and up to eightfold in the presence of diabetes.[3] Physical inactivity and obesity independently increase the risk for IHD, in addition to predisposing individuals to hypertension, dyslipidemia, and diabetes.

Patients with multiple risk factors, particularly those with diabetes, are at the greatest risk for IHD. Although alternative definitions exist, metabolic syndrome is generally considered as a constellation of common cardiovascular risk factors including hypertension, abdominal obesity, dyslipidemia, and insulin resistance. Metabolic syndrome increases the risk of developing IHD and related complications by twofold.[5] According to a joint statement from several large organizations, including the American Heart Association, patients must meet at least three of the following criteria for the diagnosis of metabolic syndrome:[5]

- Increased waist circumference (40 inches or greater or 102 cm or greater in men and 35 inches or greater or 89 cm or greater in women).
- Triglycerides of 150 mg/dL (1.70 mmol/L) or greater or active treatment to lower triglycerides.
- Low high-density lipoprotein (HDL) cholesterol (less than 40 mg/dL or 1.03 mmol/L in men and less than 50 mg/dL or 1.29 mmol/L in women) or active treatment to raise HDL cholesterol.
- Systolic blood pressure of 130 mm Hg or greater, diastolic blood pressure of 85 mm Hg or greater, or active treatment with antihypertensive therapy.
- Fasting blood glucose of 100 mg/dL (5.6 mmol/L) or greater or active treatment for diabetes.

❷ *Early detection and aggressive modification of risk factors are among the primary strategies for delaying IHD progression and preventing IHD-related events including death.*

PATHOPHYSIOLOGY

The determinants of oxygen supply and demand are shown in Figure 7–1. Increases in heart rate, cardiac contractility, and left ventricular wall tension increase the rate of myocardial oxygen consumption (MVO_2). Ventricular wall tension is a function of blood pressure, left ventricular end-diastolic volume, and ventricular wall thickness. Physical exertion increases MVO_2 and commonly precipitates symptoms of angina in patients with significant coronary atherosclerosis.

Reductions in coronary blood flow (secondary to atherosclerotic plaques, vasospasm, or thrombus formation) and arterial oxygen content (secondary to hypoxia) decrease myocardial oxygen supply. Because the coronary arteries fill during diastole, decreases in diastolic filling time (e.g., tachycardia) can also reduce coronary perfusion and myocardial oxygen supply. In chronic stable angina, atherosclerotic plaques are the most common cause of

coronary artery narrowing and reductions in coronary blood flow. In contrast, in ACS, disruption of an atherosclerotic plaque with subsequent thrombus (blood clot) formation causes abrupt reductions in coronary blood flow and oxygen supply. Anemia, carbon monoxide poisoning, and cyanotic congenital heart disease are examples of conditions that reduce the oxygen-carrying capacity of the blood, potentially causing ischemia in the face of adequate coronary perfusion.

Coronary Atherosclerosis

The normal arterial wall is illustrated in panel A of Figure 7–3. The intima consists of a layer of endothelial cells that line the lumen of the artery and form a selective barrier between the vessel wall and blood contents. Vascular smooth muscle cells are found in the media. The vascular adventitia comprises the artery's outer layer. Atherosclerotic lesions form in the subendothelial space in the intimal layer.

Endothelial damage and dysfunction allow low-density lipoprotein (LDL) cholesterol and inflammatory cells (e.g., monocytes and T lymphocytes) to migrate from the plasma to the subendothelial space, as illustrated in Figure 12–5 in Chapter 12, "Dyslipidemias." The process is initiated with monocyte-derived macrophages ingesting lipoproteins to form foam cells. Macrophages also secrete growth factors that promote smooth muscle cell migration from the media to the intima. The development of a fatty streak consisting of lipid-laden macrophages and smooth muscle cells is formed. The fatty streak is the earliest type of atherosclerotic lesion.

The fatty streak enlarges as foam cells, smooth muscle cells, and necrotic debris accumulate in the subendothelial space. A collagen matrix forms a fibrous cap that covers the lipid core of the lesion to establish an atherosclerotic plaque. The atherosclerotic plaque may progress until it protrudes into the artery lumen and impedes blood flow. When the plaque occludes 70% or more of a major coronary artery or 50% or more of the left main coronary artery, the patient may experience angina during activities that increase myocardial oxygen demand.

Compared with men, women with angina are less likely to have obstructive CAD of the major epicardial arteries and more likely to present with microvascular disease. Microvascular angina, also called cardiac syndrome X, refers to disease of the smaller coronary vessels causing typical angina in the absence of obstructive CAD of the epicardial arteries. Endothelial dysfunction and reduced smooth muscle relaxation, resulting in reduced vasodilation and enhanced vasoconstriction, are proposed to contribute to microvascular disease.[6]

Stable versus Unstable Atherosclerotic Plaques

The hallmark feature in the pathophysiology of chronic stable angina is an established atherosclerotic plaque in one or more of the major coronary arteries that impedes coronary

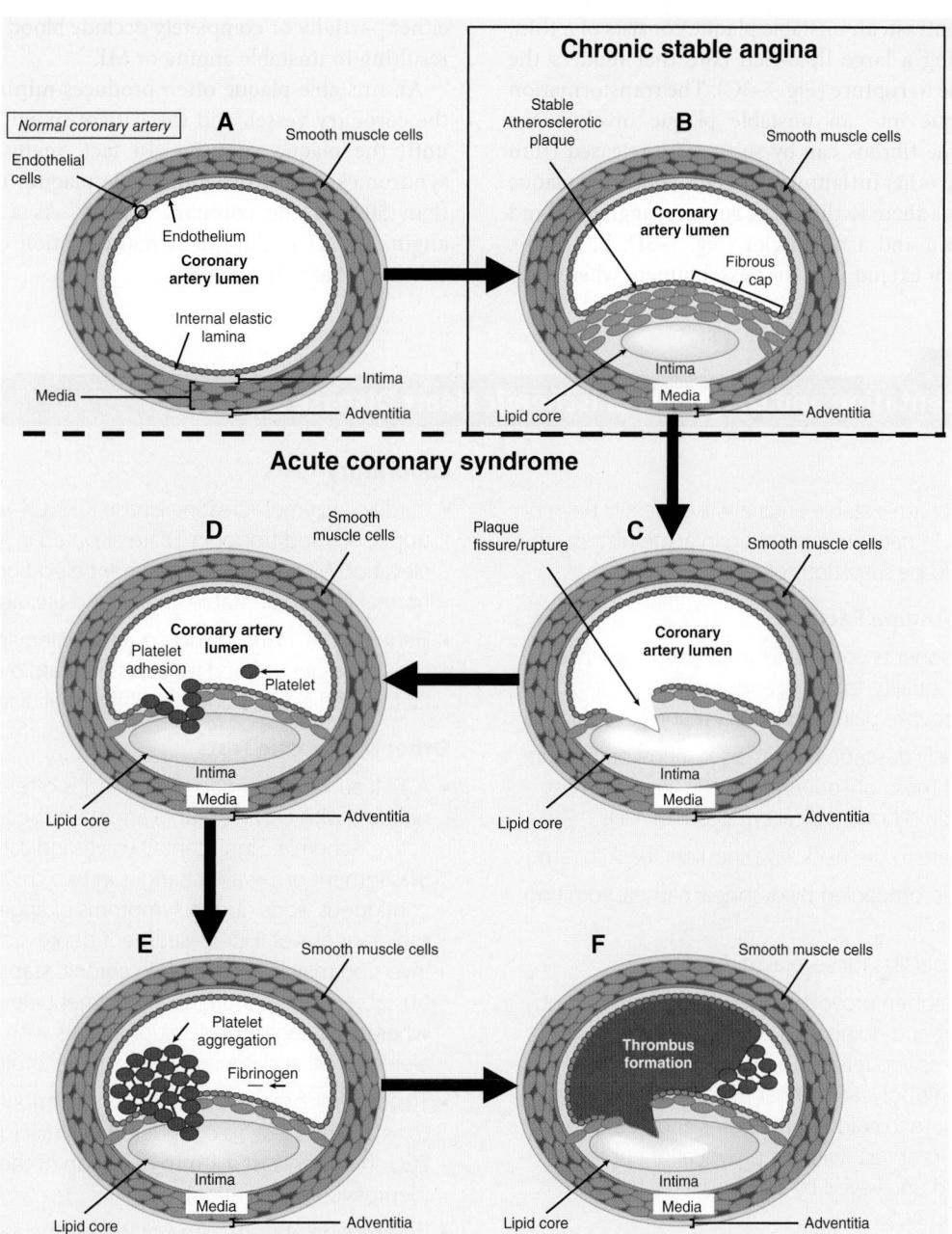

FIGURE 7–3. Pathophysiology of chronic stable angina versus acute coronary syndromes. Panel **A** depicts the cross-section of a normal coronary artery. Panel **B** depicts the cross-section of a coronary artery with a stable atherosclerotic plaque. Note that the lipid core is relatively small in size and the fibrous cap is made up of several layers of smooth muscle cells. Panel **C** depicts an unstable atherosclerotic plaque with a larger lipid core, and a thin fibrous cap composed of a single layer of smooth muscle cells with a fissure or rupture. Panel **D** depicts platelet adhesion in response to the fissured plaque. Platelet activation may ensue, leading to platelet aggregation as fibrinogen binds platelets to one another to form a mesh-like occlusion in the coronary lumen (Panel **E**). At this stage, patients may experience symptoms of acute coronary syndrome. If endogenous anticoagulant proteins fail to halt this process, platelet aggregation continues and fibrinogen is converted to fibrin, resulting in an occlusive thrombus (Panel **F**).

blood flow to the extent that myocardial oxygen supply can no longer meet increases in myocardial oxygen demand. In contrast, the hallmark feature in the pathophysiology of ACS is atherosclerotic plaque rupture with subsequent thrombus formation. Plaque rupture refers to fissuring of the fibrous cap and exposure of the plaque contents to

elements in the blood. Plaque composition, rather than the degree of coronary stenosis, determines the stability of the plaque and the likelihood of rupture and ACS. As depicted in Figure 7–3B, a stable lesion characteristic of chronic stable angina consists of a small lipid core surrounded by a thick fibrous cap that protects the lesion from the shear stress of blood flow. In contrast, an unstable plaque consists of a thin, weak cap covering a large lipid-rich core that renders the plaque vulnerable to rupture (Fig. 7–3C). The transformation of a stable plaque into an unstable plaque involves the degradation of the fibrous cap by substances released from macrophages and other inflammatory cells. Following plaque rupture, platelets adhere to the site of rupture, aggregate, and generate thrombin and a fibrin clot (Fig. 7–3D, E, and F). Coronary thrombi extend into the vessel lumen, where they either partially or completely occlude blood flow, potentially resulting in unstable angina or MI.

An unstable plaque often produces minimal occlusion of the coronary vessel, and the patient remains asymptomatic until the plaque ruptures. In fact, many acute coronary syndromes arise from vulnerable plaques that occlude less than 50% of the coronary lumen.[7] As a result, unstable angina or MI is the initial manifestation of IHD in about one-half of affected patients.

Clinical Presentation and Diagnosis of Ischemic Heart Disease

General

- Patients with chronic stable angina will generally be in no acute distress. In patients presenting in acute distress, the clinician should be suspicious of ACS.

Symptoms of Angina Pectoris

- The five components commonly used to characterize chest pain are quality, location, and duration of pain; factors that provoke pain; and factors that relieve pain.
- Patients typically describe pain as a sensation of pressure, heaviness, tightness, or squeezing in the anterior chest area. Sharp pain is not a typical symptom of IHD.
- Pain may radiate to the neck, jaw, shoulder, back, or arm.
- Pain may be accompanied by dyspnea, nausea, vomiting, or diaphoresis.
- Pain typically persists for several minutes.
- Symptoms are often provoked by exertion (e.g., walking, climbing stairs, and doing yard or housework) or emotional stress and relieved within minutes by rest or sublingual nitroglycerin. Other precipitating factors include exposure to cold temperatures and heavy meals. Pain that occurs at rest (without provocation) or that is prolonged and unrelieved by sublingual nitroglycerin is indicative of an ACS.
- Some patients, most commonly women and patients with diabetes, may present with atypical symptoms including indigestion, gastric fullness, back pain, and shortness of breath. Patients with diabetes and the elderly may experience associated symptoms, such as dyspnea, diaphoresis, nausea, fatigue, and dizziness, without having any of the classic chest pain symptoms.
- In some cases, ischemia may not produce any symptoms and is termed "silent ischemia."

Signs

- Findings on the physical examination are often normal in patients with chronic stable angina. However, during episodes of ischemia, patients may present with abnormal heart sounds, such as paradoxical splitting of the second heart sound, a third heart sound, or a loud fourth heart sound.

Laboratory Tests

- Cardiac enzymes (creatine kinase [CK], CK-MB fraction, troponin I, and troponin T) are elevated in MI (ST-segment elevation MI and non–ST-segment elevation MI), but normal in chronic stable angina and unstable angina.
- Hemoglobin, fasting glucose, and fasting lipid profile should be determined for assessing cardiovascular risk factors and establishing the differential diagnosis.

Other Diagnostic Tests

- A 12-lead ECG recorded during rest is often normal in patients with chronic stable angina in the absence of active ischemia. Significant Q waves indicate prior MI. ST-segment or T-wave changes in two or more contiguous leads during symptoms of angina support the diagnosis of IHD. ST-segment depression or T-wave inversion may be observed in chronic stable angina, unstable angina, and non–ST-segment elevation MI, whereas ST-segment elevation occurs with ST-segment elevation MI and Prinzmetal's (variant) angina.
- Treadmill or bicycle exercise ECG, commonly referred to as a "stress test," is considered positive for IHD if the ECG shows at least a 1-mm deviation of the ST-segment (depression or elevation).
- Wall motion abnormalities or left ventricular dilation with stress echocardiography are indicative of IHD.
- Stress myocardial perfusion imaging with the radionuclides technetium-99m sestamibi or thallium-201 allows for the identification of multivessel disease and assessment of myocardial viability.
- Coronary angiography detects the location and degree of coronary atherosclerosis and is used to evaluate the potential benefit from revascularization procedures. Stenosis of at least 70% of the diameter of at least one of the major epicardial arteries on coronary angiography is indicative of significant IHD.
- Coronary angiography may be normal in patients with microvascular angina.

Coronary Artery Vasospasm

Prinzmetal's or variant angina results from spasm (or vasoconstriction) of a coronary artery in the absence of significant atherosclerosis. Variant angina usually occurs at rest, especially in the early morning hours. Although vasospasm is generally transient, in some instances vasospasm may persist long enough to infarct the myocardium. Patients with variant angina are typically younger than those with chronic stable angina and often do not possess the classic risk factors for IHD. The cause of variant angina is unclear but appears to involve vagal withdrawal, endothelial dysfunction, and paradoxical response to agents that normally cause vasodilation. Precipitants of variant angina include cigarette smoking, cocaine or amphetamine use, hyperventilation, and exposure to cold temperatures. The management of variant angina differs from that of classic angina, and thus it is important to distinguish between the two.

CLINICAL PRESENTATION AND DIAGNOSIS

History

The evaluation of a patient with suspected IHD begins with a detailed history of symptoms. ❸ *The classic presentation of angina is described in the Clinical Presentation and Diagnosis box.* Chronic stable angina should be distinguished from unstable angina because the latter is associated with a greater risk for MI and death and requires more aggressive treatment. Because the pathophysiology of chronic stable angina is due primarily to increases in oxygen demand, rather than acute changes in oxygen supply, symptoms are typically reproducible when provoked by exertion, exercise, or stress. Specifically, a patient with angina secondary to significant coronary atherosclerosis generally experiences a similar pattern of chest, arm, or neck discomfort (i.e., same quality, location, and accompanying symptoms) with a similar level of exertion. The exception may be a patient with coronary artery vasospasm, in whom symptoms may be more variable and unpredictable. In contrast to chronic stable angina, ACS is due to an acute decrease in coronary blood flow leading to an insufficient oxygen supply. Consequently, ACS is marked by prolonged symptoms, symptoms that occur at rest, or an escalation in the frequency or severity of angina over a short period of time. The presentation of unstable angina is described in Table 7–3.[8]

The Canadian Cardiovascular Society Classification System

The Canadian Cardiovascular Society Classification System (Table 7–4) is commonly used to assess the degree of disability resulting from IHD.[9] Patients are categorized into one of four classes depending on the extent of activity that produces angina. Grouping patients according to this or a similar method is commonly used to assess changes in IHD severity over time and the effectiveness of pharmacologic therapy.

Table 7–3

Presentations of Acute Coronary Syndromes[8]

- Angina at rest that is prolonged in duration, usually lasting over 20 minutes.
- Angina of recent onset (within 2 months) that markedly limits usual activity.
- Angina that increases in severity (i.e., by Canadian Cardiovascular Society Classification System Class of one level or greater), frequency, or duration, or that occurs with less provocation over a short time period (i.e., within 2 months).

Table 7–4

The Canadian Cardiovascular Society Classification System of Angina

Class	Description
I	Able to perform ordinary physical activity (e.g., walking and climbing stairs) without symptoms. Strenuous, rapid, or prolonged exertion causes symptoms.
II	Symptoms slightly limit ordinary physical activity. Walking rapidly or for more than two blocks, climbing stairs rapidly, or climbing more than one flight of stairs causes symptoms.
III	Symptoms markedly limit ordinary physical activity. Walking less than two blocks or climbing one flight of stairs causes symptoms.
IV	Angina may occur at rest. Any physical activity causes symptoms.

Patient Encounter Part 1

DF is a 49-year-old African American man with a history of hypertension, diabetes, and dyslipidemia who presents to your clinic complaining of chest pain that occurred several times over the past few weeks. DF describes his chest pain as "a heaviness." He states that the discomfort first occurred while he was carrying groceries up to his third-floor apartment. Later, he experienced the same heavy sensation while raking leaves and again while carrying some boxes. The pain was located in the substernal area and radiated to his neck. The pain resolved after about 5 minutes of rest.

What information is suggestive of angina?

What tests would be beneficial in establishing a diagnosis?

What additional information do you need to create a treatment plan for this patient?

Physical Findings and Laboratory Analysis

A thorough medical history, physical examination, and laboratory analysis are necessary to ascertain cardiovascular risk factors and to exclude nonischemic and noncardiac conditions that could cause angina-like symptoms. Laboratory analyses should assess for glycemic control (i.e., fasting glucose, glycated hemoglobin), fasting lipids, hemoglobin, and organ function (i.e., blood urea nitrogen, creatinine, liver function tests, thyroid function tests). Additionally, serial measurements of cardiac enzymes (usually three measurements within 12 hours) are used to exclude the diagnosis of an acute MI. Cardiac findings on the physical examination are often normal in patients with chronic stable angina. However, findings such as carotid bruits or abnormal peripheral pulses would indicate atherosclerosis in other vessel systems and raise the suspicion for IHD.

Diagnostic Tests

A resting electrocardiogram (ECG) is indicated in all patients with angina-like symptoms. A 12-lead ECG should be done in patients with new or worsening symptoms of ischemia. Patients with characteristic chest discomfort, accompanied by ST-segment elevation in two or more contiguous leads, or a new bundle branch block, are diagnosed with an ST-segment elevation MI and are at the highest risk of death. These patients are treated as a medical emergency, often requiring percutaneous coronary interventions or pharmacologic therapies to achieve reperfusion of the occluded artery and restore blood flow to the myocardium. In patients without ST-segment elevation, troponin is the preferred biomarker to distinguish between unstable angina and non–ST-segment elevation MI in patients hospitalized for ACS.

"Stress" testing with either exercise or pharmacologic stressors increases myocardial oxygen demand and is commonly used to evaluate the patient with suspected IHD. Approximately 50% of patients with IHD who have a normal ECG at rest will develop ECG changes with exercise on a treadmill (most commonly) or bicycle ergometer. Dobutamine is a pharmacologic stressor used in patients who are unable to exercise. Dobutamine increases oxygen demand by stimulating the β_1-receptor, leading to increases in heart rate and contractility. Dobutamine is commonly used with echocardiography (referred to as dobutamine stress echocardiography) to identify stress-induced wall motion abnormalities indicative of coronary disease.

Adenosine, dipyridamole, dobutamine, or regadenoson are commonly combined with radionuclide myocardial perfusion imaging (nuclear imaging studies). Adenosine, dipyridamole, and regadenoson are coronary vasodilators that increase coronary blood flow in vessels free of disease but not in diseased vessels. An IV radioactive tracer is used to detect areas of the heart that receive less blood after adenosine, dipyridamole, or regadenoson administration, indicating a myocardial perfusion defect and coronary disease. Positive emission tomography is an alternative to conventional myocardial perfusion imaging that may be preferred in obese patients. This technique involves administration of a radioactive tracer that emits γ rays captured by a scanner to allow for assessment of myocardial perfusion and viability.

Coronary artery calcium scoring via computed tomography (CT), also known as electron beam CT (EBCT) or "ultrafast CT," may be performed as a noninvasive means to assess for CAD. Calcium deposits within the coronary arteries that are indicative of CAD are detected on CT. A calcium score is calculated, and the risk for IHD-related events is estimated.

Coronary angiography (also referred to as a cardiac catheterization or "cardiac cath") is considered the gold standard for the diagnosis of IHD. Coronary angiography is indicated when stress testing results are abnormal or symptoms of angina are poorly controlled. Angiography involves catheter insertion into either the femoral or radial artery and advancement into the aorta and into the coronary arteries. Contrast medium is injected through the catheter into the coronary arteries allowing visualization of the coronary anatomy by fluoroscopy and identification of significant lesions of the coronary arteries. Contrast medium must be used cautiously in patients with preexisting renal disease (especially in those with diabetes) to avoid contrast-induced nephropathy. Judicious hydration may be warranted to reduce the direct toxic effects of contrast medium. The use of low ionic contrast solutions may be used to prevent damage to the kidneys.

TREATMENT

Desired Outcomes

Once the diagnosis of IHD is established in a patient, the clinician should provide counseling on lifestyle modifications, institute appropriate pharmacologic therapy, and evaluate the need for surgical revascularization. Optimal medical therapy is essential for managing patients with IHD. ❹ *The major goals for the treatment of IHD are to:*

- *Prevent acute coronary syndrome and death*
- *Alleviate acute symptoms of myocardial ischemia*
- *Prevent recurrent symptoms of myocardial ischemia*
- *Prevent progression of the disease*
- *Reduce complications of IHD*
- *Avoid or minimize adverse treatment effects*

The treatment approach to address these goals is illustrated in Figure 7–4.

General Approach to Treatment

The primary strategies for preventing ACS and death are to:

- Aggressively modify cardiovascular risk factors
- Slow the progression of coronary atherosclerosis
- Stabilize existing atherosclerotic plaques

The treatment algorithm in Figure 7–5 summarizes the appropriate management of IHD. Risk factor modification is accomplished through lifestyle changes and pharmacologic therapy. ❺ *Both 3-hydroxy-3-methylglutaryl coenzyme A reductase inhibitors (HMG-CoA reductase inhibitors or*

Patient Encounter Part 2: Medical History, Physical Examination, and Diagnostic Tests

PMH

Hypertension, diagnosed 10 years ago

Diabetes, diagnosed 10 years ago

Dyslipidemia, diagnosed 8 years ago

Seasonal allergies, diagnosed ~25 years ago

Osteoarthritis

FH

Father with coronary artery disease, had a myocardial infarction at age 50 years

Two siblings each with coronary artery disease diagnosed in their 40s

Mother alive and well

SH

Quit smoking 5 years ago.

Denies alcohol or illicit drug use

No regular exercise program

Meds

- Amlodipine 5 mg PO once daily
- Metformin 500 mg PO twice daily
- Pravastatin 20 mg PO at bedtime (has not taken in several months)
- Desloratadine/pseudoephedrine 2.5 mg/120 mg PO twice daily
- Ibuprofen 400 mg twice daily as needed (uses most days)

Allergies: NKDA

PE

VS: Blood pressure = 164/90 mm Hg

Heart rate = 94 beats/min, respirations = 20

Temperature = 37°C (98.6°F)

Height = 5'10" (178 cm), weight = 360 lb (163.6 kg)

Cardiovascular: Regular rate and rhythm, normal S_1 and S_2, no S_3 or S_4; no murmurs, rubs, gallops

Lungs: Clear to auscultation and percussion

Abd: Nontender, nondistended, + bowel sounds

Ext: 1+ lower extremity edema to the ankles bilaterally

Labs

Fasting lipid profile: total cholesterol 196 mg/dL (5.07 mmol/L), HDL cholesterol 27 mg/dL (0.70 mmol/L), LDL cholesterol 127 mg/dL (3.28 mmol/L), triglycerides 211 mg/dL (2.38 mmol/L); fasting glucose 178 mg/dl (9.9 mmol/L); other labs within normal limits

Exercise treadmill test: Positive for ischemia

Identify DF's risk factors for ischemic heart disease.

How might DF's current drug regimen adversely affect his ischemic heart disease?

What therapeutic alternatives are available to manage DF's ischemic heart disease?

How does this patient's ancestry influence drug therapy decisions?

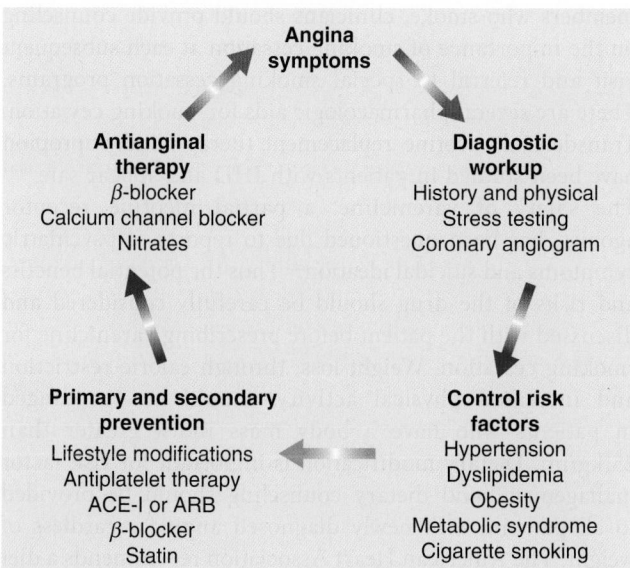

FIGURE 7–4. General treatment strategies for angina follow in clockwise fashion from the top center. (ACE-I, angiotensin-converting enzyme inhibitor; ARB, angiotensin receptor blocker.)

statins) and angiotensin-converting enzyme (ACE) inhibitors are believed to provide vasculoprotective effects (properties that are generally protective of the vasculature that may include anti-inflammatory effects, antiplatelet effects, improvement in endothelial function, and improvement in arterial compliance and tone), and, in addition to aspirin, have been shown to reduce the risk of acute coronary events as well as mortality in patients with IHD. In select patients with IHD (following hospitalization for ACS ± *percutaneous coronary intervention [PCI]* and/or following intracoronary stent placement), dual antiplatelet therapy with aspirin and a $P2Y_{12}$ antagonist has also been shown to reduce ischemic events. Angiotensin receptor blockers (ARBs) may be used in patients who cannot tolerate ACE inhibitors because of side effects (e.g., chronic cough). β-Blockers have been shown to decrease morbidity and improve survival in patients who have suffered an MI.

Therapies to alleviate and prevent angina are aimed at improving the balance between myocardial oxygen demand and supply. Because angina usually results from increased myocardial oxygen demand in the face of a relatively fixed reduction in oxygen supply, drug treatment is primarily aimed at reducing oxygen demand. Short-acting nitrates are indicated to acutely relieve angina. β-Blockers, calcium

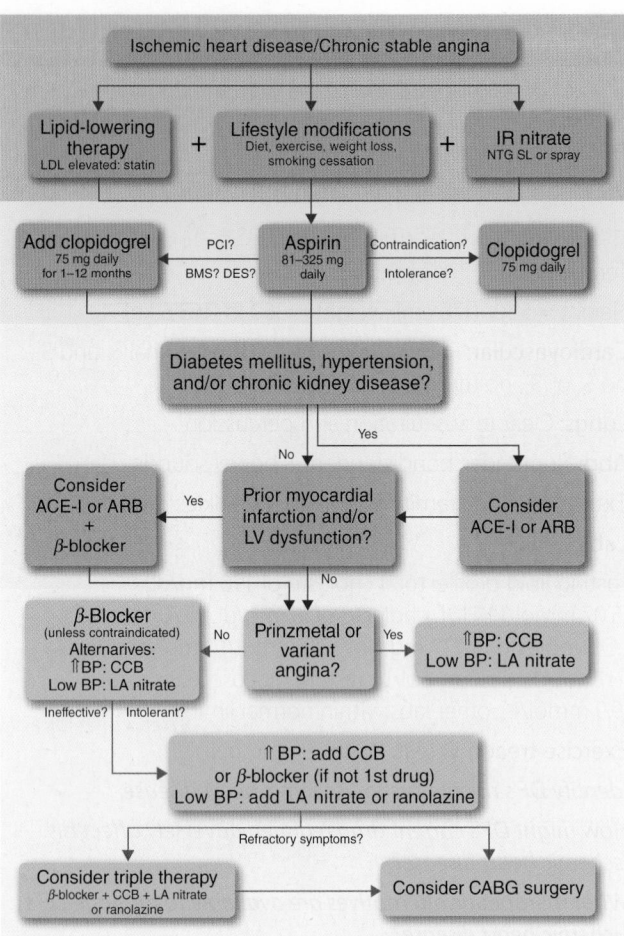

FIGURE 7–5. The treatment algorithm for ischemic heart disease. It begins at the top (blue section), which suggests risk factor modifications as the first treatment modality. Moving down to the green section, appropriate antiplatelet therapy is selected. The purple section identifies patients at high risk for major adverse cardiac events and suggests appropriate drug therapy to decrease cardiovascular risk. The yellow section at the bottom recommends appropriate antianginal therapy. *The minimum duration of clopidogrel therapy following intracoronary stent placement is as follows: at least 1 month for bare metal stents and at least 12 months for drug-eluting stents. (ACE-I, angiotensin-converting enzyme inhibitor; ARB, angiotensin receptor blocker; BMS, bare metal stent; BP, blood pressure; CABG, coronary artery bypass graft; CCB, calcium channel blocker; DES, drug-eluting stent; HR, heart rate; IR, immediate release; LA, long acting; LDL, low-density lipoprotein; LV, left ventricular; NTG, nitroglycerin; PCI, percutaneous coronary intervention; SL, sublingual.)

channel blockers (CCBs), and long-acting nitrates are traditionally used to reduce the frequency of angina and improve exercise tolerance. In most patients with IHD, the most effective treatments to improve myocardial oxygen supply are invasive mechanical interventions, PCI, and

coronary artery bypass graft (CABG) surgery, which are described later in the chapter in the section on interventional approaches. These interventional approaches are reserved for patients with symptoms despite optimal medical therapy and lifestyle modifications and those hospitalized for ACS.

Adverse treatment effects can be averted by avoiding drug interactions and the use of drugs that may have unfavorable effects on comorbid diseases. For example, β-blockers may exacerbate preexisting bronchospasm. β-Blockers are not absolutely contraindicated in bronchospastic disease but should be avoided in patients with poorly controlled symptoms. Although patients often require combination anti-anginal therapy, there is a potential pharmacodynamic drug interaction with the concurrent use of β-blockers and nondihydropyridine CCBs. Because both drug classes slow electrical conduction through the atrioventricular (AV) node, serious bradycardia or heart block may result with their concomitant use. Appropriate drug dosing and monitoring also reduces the risk for adverse treatment effects. Drugs should be initiated in low doses, with careful up-titration as necessary to control symptoms of angina and cardiovascular risk factors.

Lifestyle Modifications

Lifestyle modifications including smoking cessation, avoidance of secondhand smoke, dietary modifications, increased physical activity, and weight loss reduce cardiovascular risk factors, slow the progression of IHD, and decrease the risk for IHD-related complications. Cigarette smoking is the single most preventable cause of IHD and IHD-related death. Smoking may also attenuate the antianginal effects of drug therapy. The clinician should ascertain smoking status for the patient and family members on the patient's initial clinic visit. For patients and/or family members who smoke, clinicians should provide counseling on the importance of smoking cessation at each subsequent visit and referral to special smoking cessation programs. There are several pharmacologic aids for smoking cessation. Transdermal nicotine replacement therapy and bupropion have been studied in patients with IHD and appear safe.[10,11] The safety of varenicline, a partial nicotine receptor agonist, has been questioned due to reports of psychiatric symptoms and suicidal ideation.[12] Thus the potential benefits and risks of the drug should be carefully considered and discussed with the patient before prescribing varenicline for smoking cessation. Weight loss, through caloric restriction and increased physical activity, should be encouraged in patients who have a body mass index greater than 25 kg/m². Dietary modification is important for risk factor management, and dietary counseling should be provided to all patients with newly diagnosed angina regardless of weight. The American Heart Association recommends a diet that includes a variety of fruits, vegetables, grains, low-fat or nonfat dairy products, fish, legumes, poultry, and lean meats.[13] Fatty fish, such as salmon and herring, are high in ω-3 polyunsaturated fatty acids, which have been shown to reduce triglyceride concentrations at daily doses of 3 g or more, slow atherosclerotic plaque progression, and may have cardiovascular protective effects.[14] Specific dietary recommendations for patients with IHD should include the following:[2,13]

- Limit fat intake to less than 30% of total caloric consumption.
- Limit cholesterol intake to less than 200 mg/day.
- Limit consumption of saturated fat and trans unsaturated fat found in fatty meats, full-fat dairy products, and hydrogenated vegetable oils to less than 7% of total calories.
- Consume approximately 1 g of eicosapentaenoic acid (EPA) and docosahexaenoic acid (DHA) per day in the form of fatty fish or fish oil capsules.
- Consume at least six servings of grains, five servings of fruits and vegetables, and two servings of nonfat or low-fat dairy products per day.
- Consider plant stanol/sterols (2 g/day) and/or viscous fiber (over 10 g/day) to lower LDL cholesterol. It is recommended that patients with diabetes consume 14 g of fiber for every 1,000 kcal (4,200 kJ) consumed.
- Limit daily sodium intake to 2.4 g (6 g of salt) for blood pressure control.

Exercise facilitates both weight loss and blood pressure reduction. In addition, regular exercise improves functional capacity and symptoms in chronic stable angina.[1] Guidelines recommend moderate intensity aerobic activity, such as brisk walking, ideally for 30 to 60 minutes every day.[2] Medically supervised cardiac rehabilitation programs are recommended for high-risk patients.

Interventional Approaches

▶ *Percutaneous Coronary Intervention*

When optimal medical therapy fails (e.g., hospitalization for ACS) or if extensive coronary atherosclerosis is present, PCI is often performed to restore coronary blood flow and relieve symptoms. However, there is no reduction in major adverse cardiac events or mortality with PCI compared with optimal medical therapy alone in patients with stable IHD.[15] Thus optimal medical therapy is the preferred initial strategy for patients with stable IHD. Proceeding to PCI is appropriate for patients with one or more critical coronary stenoses (i.e., greater than 70% occlusion of the coronary lumen) detected during coronary angiography whose symptoms are unstable and/or persist despite optimal medical therapy. Several catheter-based interventions may be used during PCI, including:

- Percutaneous transluminal coronary angioplasty (PTCA)
- Intracoronary bare metal stent placement
- Intracoronary drug-eluting stent placement
- Rotational atherectomy

During PCI, a catheter is advanced into the blocked coronary artery, as described for cardiac catheterization. If PTCA (i.e., balloon angioplasty) is performed, a balloon at the end of the catheter is inflated inside the artery at the site of the critical stenosis. When inflated, this balloon catheter displaces the atherosclerotic plaque out of the lumen of the artery, restoring normal myocardial blood flow. Most PCI procedures involve the placement of a small mesh wire stent (similar in size and shape to the spring at the tip of a ballpoint pen) at the site of angioplasty. Coronary stenting involves use of a special balloon catheter containing the stent. When the balloon is inflated, the stent is deployed in the wall of the coronary artery, forming a sort of bridge or scaffold to maintain normal coronary blood flow. Either a bare metal stent or a drug-eluting stent may be used. Drug-eluting stents are impregnated with low concentrations of an antiproliferative drug (paclitaxel, everolimus, sirolimus, or zotarolimus), which is released locally over a period of weeks to inhibit **restenosis** or re-narrowing of the coronary artery after PCI. An observational study demonstrated a significant reduction in all-cause mortality over a 4.5-year interval among patients who received a drug-eluting stent compared to those with a bare metal stent.[16] Stents are thrombogenic, especially until they become endothelialized (covered in endothelial cells like a normal coronary artery). Dual antiplatelet therapy (discussed later) is required until the stent becomes endothelialized, generally a period of 6 to 12 months, and, in some cases indefinitely following stent placement to reduce the risk for stent thrombosis, MI, or death. Lastly, rotational atherectomy may be performed wherein a special catheter is used to essentially cut away the atherosclerotic plaque, restoring coronary blood flow.

▶ *Coronary Artery Bypass Graft Surgery*

As an alternative to PCI, CABG surgery, or open-heart surgery, may be performed if the patient is found to have extensive coronary atherosclerosis (generally greater than 70% occlusion of three or more coronary arteries) or is refractory to optimal medical treatment. In the former case, CABG surgery has been shown to reduce the need for revascularization, but not death, compared with PCI.[17] During CABG surgery, veins from the leg (i.e., saphenous veins) or arteries from the arm (i.e., radial artery) or chest wall (i.e., internal mammary arteries) are surgically removed. In the case of venous or radial artery conduits, one end of the removed blood vessel is attached to the aorta, and the other end is attached to the coronary artery distal to the atherosclerotic plaque. However, when internal mammary arteries are used, the distal end of the artery is detached from the chest wall and anastomosed to the coronary artery distal to the plaque. A median sternotomy, in which an incision the length of the sternum is made, is commonly required to gain access to the thoracic cavity and expose the heart. As the "new" blood vessels are being engrafted, the patient is typically placed on cardiopulmonary bypass (i.e., heart-lung machine) to maintain appropriate myocardial and systemic perfusion. Alternative surgical approaches for advanced IHD may be used in some settings including "off-pump" CABG (cardiopulmonary bypass is not required) and minimally invasive CABG (i.e., thorascopic surgery), although these techniques are not the norm. Because of the extremely invasive nature of this surgery, CABG surgery is generally reserved for patients with extensive coronary disease or as a treatment of last resort in patients with symptoms refractory to medical therapy.

Pharmacologic Therapy

▶ *Pharmacotherapy to Prevent Acute Coronary Syndromes and Death*

● **Control of Risk Factors** A major component of any IHD treatment plan, which is often underutilized, is control of modifiable risk factors, including dyslipidemia, hypertension, and diabetes. Treatment strategies for dyslipidemia and hypertension in the patient with IHD are summarized in the following paragraphs. Visit chapters in this textbook on the management of hypertension (Chapter 5) and dyslipidemias (Chapter 12) for further information.

Because lipoprotein metabolism and the pathophysiology of atherosclerosis are closely linked, treatment of dyslipidemias is critical for both primary and secondary prevention of IHD-related cardiac events. In 2004 the Adult Treatment Panel III of the National Cholesterol Education Program updated the guidelines for the management of dyslipidemia and recommended a LDL cholesterol goal of less than 100 mg/dL (2.59 mmol/L) for patients with documented IHD or IHD risk equivalents such as diabetes or other vascular disease.[18] Since the publication of these guidelines, new evidence from several primary and secondary prevention trials suggests there are additional clinical benefits from further reduction in LDL cholesterol (e.g., LDL cholesterol less than 70 mg/dL [1.81 mmol/L]).[19] In response to this evidence, more aggressive cholesterol-lowering goals were established for patients at *high risk* for developing IHD-related events, including those with diabetes or known ● cardiovascular disease. The following modifications were made to national treatment guidelines[19,20]:

- In addition to lifestyle modifications, statins or other LDL-lowering therapy are indicated for patients with cardiovascular disease, diabetes, and multiple cardiovascular risk factors, regardless of baseline LDL cholesterol.

- Intensity of LDL-lowering therapy should be sufficient to decrease LDL cholesterol by 30% to 40%.

- Goal LDL cholesterol in patients with known clinical cardiovascular disease, recent hospitalization for ACS, or diabetes plus one or more cardiovascular risk factors is less than 70 mg/dL (1.81 mmol/L).

Like dyslipidemia, hypertension is a major, modifiable risk factor for the development of IHD and related complications. Unfortunately, awareness, treatment, and

control of blood pressure are suboptimal.[4] Aggressive identification and control of hypertension is warranted in patients with IHD to minimize the risk of major adverse cardiac events. The American Heart Association recommends a goal blood pressure in patients with IHD of less than 130/80 mm Hg.[21] Because of their cardioprotective benefits, β-blockers and ACE inhibitors (or ARBs in ACE inhibitor–intolerant patients), either alone or in combination, are appropriate for most patients with both hypertension and IHD.

Antiplatelet Agents Platelets play a major role in the pathophysiology of ACS. Thromboxane is a potent platelet activator. Aspirin inhibits cyclooxygenase, an enzyme responsible for the production of thromboxane, thereby inhibiting platelet activation and aggregation. In patients with stable or unstable angina, aspirin has been consistently shown to reduce the risk of major adverse cardiac events, ● particularly MI.[22] ❻ *Antiplatelet therapy with aspirin should be considered for all patients without contraindications, particularly in patients with a history of myocardial infarction. Aspirin doses of 75 to 162 mg daily are recommended in patients with or at risk for IHD.[2,22] If aspirin is contraindicated (e.g., aspirin allergy) or is not tolerated by the patient, an alternative antiplatelet agent such as clopidogrel should be considered.*

Binding of adenosine diphosphate to the $P2Y_{12}$ receptors on platelets activates glycoprotein IIb/IIIa receptors leading to platelet aggregation and thrombus formation. ❻ *Inhibition of the $P2Y_{12}$ receptor with either a thienopyridine (ticlopidine, clopidogrel, prasugrel) or ticagrelor prevents platelet aggregation and is indicated in combination with aspirin in select patients with IHD.* Dual antiplatelet therapy with aspirin and a $P2Y_{12}$ inhibitor is recommended following hospitalization for ACS and/or PCI with stent placement to prevent ischemic events, although indications for specific drugs differ slightly (see later). Following stent placement, prolonged treatment with dual antiplatelet therapy (often greater than or equal to 12 months) is often necessary to prevent in-stent thrombosis prior to stent endothelialization. Historically, ticlopidine was the $P2Y_{12}$ inhibitor used in combination with aspirin. Clopidogrel, prasugrel, and ticagrelor have replaced ticlopidine due to the hematological toxicities (leucopenia) associated with ticlopidine and the growing body of evidence supporting the use of the other $P2Y_{12}$ inhibitors.

Clopidogrel is a prodrug that must be converted via a two-step process to its active thiol metabolite. The CYP2C19 enzyme is involved in both steps of the biotransformation. Individuals with reduced CYP2C19 activity, either from inherited deficiencies of CYP2C19 or use of CYP2C19 inhibitors (e.g., proton pump inhibitors), may produce less of the active thiol metabolite. These individuals are at increased risk for stent thrombosis and adverse cardiovascular events during clopidogrel treatment compared with those with "normal" CYP2C19 activity.[23] The clopidogrel labeling now warns of reduced effectiveness in CYP2C19 poor metabolizers. Poor metabolizers carry two dysfunctional *CYP2C19* gene alleles and may be identified through genotyping.

The *CYP2C19*2* and *CYP2C19*3* alleles are the most common alleles leading to reduced CYP2C19 activity.

Prasugrel is a thienopyridine that also requires biotransformation to its active metabolite. However, unlike clopidogrel, CYP2C19 deficiency does not appear to alter its effectiveness. Ticagrelor is a direct-acting P2Y$_{12}$ inhibitor that does not require biotransformation to exert its antiplatelet effects and is unaffected by CYP2C19 activity.[24] Thus prasugrel or ticagrelor may be suitable alternatives to clopidogrel, depending on the indication, when reduced CYP2C19 activity is suspected.

Antiproliferative drugs in drug-eluting stents delay endothelialization, and thus a longer period of dual antiplatelet therapy is recommended for drug-eluting stents compared with bare metal stents to prevent thrombosis. Guidelines advocate dual antiplatelet therapy for 12 months after stent placement.[25] The duration of dual antiplatelet therapy may be abbreviated in select patients with bare metal stents (i.e., high risk for bleeding, history of nonadherence, need for invasive procedures or major surgery), whereas some data support indefinite use of combination antiplatelet therapy following stent placement. Because of the risk for stent thrombosis with premature discontinuation of dual antiplatelet therapy, it is imperative for clinicians to educate patients on this risk and the need for continuation of combination antiplatelet therapy for the recommended duration.

Clopidogrel, prasugrel, and ticagrelor are all indicated in combination with aspirin for at least 1 year in patients with ACS who undergo PCI. Unlike prasugrel, both clopidogrel and ticagrelor are indicated in combination with aspirin in ACS patients regardless of whether PCI is performed. In this population, combination therapy with aspirin and either clopidogrel or ticagrelor more effectively reduces the risk of death, MI, and stroke compared with aspirin alone even in patients who were managed medically (e.g., in the absence of PCI).[26-28] When used in combination with aspirin in patients with ACS (with or without PCI), both prasugrel and ticagrelor may provide greater protection against cardiovascular events after stent placement compared with clopidogrel, but at the cost of an increased risk for bleeding.[28,29] For more information regarding the use of dual antiplatelet therapy in the setting of ACS, see Chapter 8.

Statins Statins are the preferred drugs to achieve LDL cholesterol goals based on their potency in lowering LDL cholesterol and efficacy in preventing cardiac events. Specifically, over the last decade, several studies in tens of thousands of patients have revealed that lowering cholesterol with statins is effective for both primary and secondary prevention of IHD-related events.[19] Statins shown to decrease morbidity and mortality associated with IHD include lovastatin, simvastatin, pravastatin, and atorvastatin. A meta-analysis showed the risk of major adverse cardiac events is reduced by 21% with the use of statins in patients at high risk for IHD-related events.[30]

Several studies have investigated whether statins possess pharmacologic properties in addition to their LDL cholesterol–lowering effect that may confer additional benefits in IHD.[31] These studies were prompted by evidence that patients with "normal" LDL cholesterol derived benefit from statins. Statins have been shown to modulate the following characteristics thought to stabilize atherosclerotic plaques and contribute to the cardiovascular risk reduction seen with these drugs:

- Shift LDL cholesterol particle size from predominantly small, dense, highly atherogenic particles to larger, less atherogenic particles.
- Improve endothelial function leading to more effective vasoactive response of the coronary arteries.
- Prevent or inhibit inflammation by lowering C-reactive protein and other inflammatory mediators thought to be involved in atherosclerosis.
- Possibly improve atherosclerotic plaque stability.

⑦ *In summary, to control risk factors and prevent major adverse cardiac events, statin therapy should be considered in all patients with ischemic heart disease, particularly in those with elevated low-density lipoprotein cholesterol or diabetes.* Statins are potent lipid-lowering agents, possess non–lipid-lowering effects that may provide additional benefit to patients with IHD, and have been shown to reduce morbidity and mortality in patients with IHD. Based on these benefits, statins are generally considered the drugs of choice in patients with dyslipidemias. Moreover, based on evidence that statins improve outcomes in patients with IHD and "normal" LDL cholesterol concentration, statins should be considered in all patients with IHD at high risk of major adverse cardiac events, regardless of baseline LDL cholesterol.

ACE Inhibitors and Angiotensin Receptor Blockers
Angiotensin II, a neurohormone produced primarily in the kidney, is a potent vasoconstrictor and stimulates the production of aldosterone. Together, angiotensin II and aldosterone increase blood pressure and sodium and water retention (increasing ventricular wall tension), cause endothelial dysfunction, promote blood clot formation, and cause myocardial fibrosis.

ACE inhibitors decrease angiotensin II production and have consistently been shown to decrease morbidity and mortality in patients with heart failure or a history of MI.[32,33] In addition, there is evidence that ACE inhibitors reduce the risk of vascular events in patients with chronic stable angina or risk factors for IHD.[34,35] Specifically, in nearly 10,000 patients with vascular disease (including IHD) or risk factors for vascular disease, such as diabetes, ramipril reduced the risk of death, acute MI, and stroke by 22% compared with placebo after an average of 5 years of treatment.[34] Similar results have been demonstrated with perindopril in patients with IHD.[35]

⑦ *In the absence of contraindications, ACE inhibitors should be considered in all patients with IHD, particularly those individuals who also have hypertension, diabetes mellitus, chronic kidney disease, left ventricular dysfunction, history of myocardial infarction, or any combination of these.*[2] *Additionally, ACE inhibitors should also be considered in patients at high risk for developing IHD based on findings from the studies summarized above. Angiotensin receptor blockers may be used in patients with indications for ACE inhibitors but who cannot tolerate them due to side effects (e.g., chronic cough). Angiotensin receptor blockers also* antagonize the effects of angiotensin II. In one large trial, valsartan was as effective as captopril at reducing morbidity and mortality in post-MI patients.[32] However, there are far more data supporting the use of ACE inhibitors in IHD. Therefore, ACE inhibitors should remain first line in patients with a history of MI, diabetes, chronic kidney disease, or left ventricular dysfunction. The ACE inhibitors and ARBs with indications for patients with or at risk for IHD or IHD-related complications are listed in Table 7–5.

Side effects with ACE inhibitors and ARBs include hyperkalemia, deterioration in renal function, and angioedema. Serum potassium increases are secondary to aldosterone inhibition and are more likely in the presence of preexisting renal impairment, diabetes, or concomitant therapy with nonsteroidal anti-inflammatory drugs (NSAIDs), potassium supplements, or potassium-sparing diuretics. Reductions in glomerular filtration may occur during ACE inhibitor or ARB initiation or up-titration due to inhibition of angiotensin II-mediated vasoconstriction of the efferent arteriole. This type of renal impairment is usually temporary and more common in patients with preexisting renal dysfunction or unilateral renal artery stenosis. Bilateral renal artery stenosis is a contraindication for ACE inhibitors and ARBs because of the risk for overt renal failure. Angioedema is a potentially life-threatening adverse effect that occurs in less than 1% of ACE inhibitor-treated white patients but up to 8% of African Americans. Angioedema may also occur with the administration of ARBs. Substitution of an ARB for an ACE inhibitor is appropriate for patients who develop a persistent cough with ACE inhibitor therapy because this cough is related to the accumulation of bradykinin secondary to ACE inhibition. Both ACE inhibitors and ARBs can cause fetal injury and death and are contraindicated in pregnancy.

▶ Nitroglycerin to Relieve Acute Symptoms

Short-acting nitrates are first-line treatment to terminate acute episodes of angina. ⑧ *All patients with a history of angina should have sublingual nitroglycerin tablets or spray to relieve acute ischemic symptoms.* Nitrates undergo biotransformation to nitric oxide. Nitric oxide activates smooth muscle guanylate cyclase, leading to increased intracellular concentrations of cyclic guanosine monophosphate, release of calcium from the muscle cell, and ultimately, to smooth muscle relaxation. Nitrates primarily cause venodilation, leading to reductions in preload. The resultant decrease in ventricular volume and wall tension leads to a reduction in myocardial oxygen demand. In higher doses, nitrates cause arterial dilation and reduce afterload and blood pressure. In addition to reducing oxygen demand, nitrates increase myocardial oxygen supply by dilating the epicardial coronary arteries and collateral vessels, as well as relieving vasospasm.

Short-acting nitrates are available in tablet and spray formulations for sublingual administration. Sublingual nitroglycerin tablets are well absorbed across the oral mucosa and produce an antianginal effect within 1 to 3 minutes and are less expensive than the spray. However, the spray is preferred for patients who have difficulty opening the tablet container or produce insufficient saliva for rapid dissolution of sublingual tablets. ⑧ *At the onset of an angina attack, a 0.3 to 0.4 mg dose of nitroglycerin (tablet or spray) should be administered sublingually, and repeated every 5 minutes up to three times or until symptoms resolve. Standing enhances venous pooling and may contribute to hypotension, dizziness, or lightheadedness. Sublingual nitroglycerin may be used to prevent effort-induced angina (i.e., angina that occurs with exertion). In this case, the patient should use sublingual nitroglycerin 2 to 5 minutes prior to an activity known to cause angina, with the effects persisting for approximately 30 minutes.* Isosorbide dinitrate, also available in a sublingual form, has a longer half-life with antianginal effects lasting up to 2 hours. The use of short-acting nitrates alone, without concomitant long-acting antianginal therapy, may be acceptable for patients who experience angina symptoms once every few days. However, for patients with more frequent attacks, long-acting antianginal therapy with β-blockers, CCBs, or long-acting nitrates is recommended.

The use of nitrates within 24 to 48 hours of a phosphodiesterase type 5 inhibitor (e.g. sildenafil, vardenafil, and tadalafil), commonly prescribed for erectile dysfunction,

---

Table 7–5

Doses of Angiotensin-Converting Enzyme Inhibitors and Angiotensin Receptor Blockers Indicated in Ischemic Heart Disease

Drug	Indications	Usual Dosage in IHD[a]
Angiotensin-converting enzyme inhibitors		
Captopril	HTN, HF, post-MI, diabetic nephropathy	6.25–50 mg 3 times daily
Enalapril	HTN, HF	2.5–40 mg daily in 1–2 divided doses
Fosinopril	HTN, HF	10–80 mg daily in 1–2 divided doses
Lisinopril	HTN, HF, post-MI	2.5–40 mg daily
Perindopril	HTN, IHD	4–8 mg daily
Quinapril	HTN, HF, post-MI	5–20 mg twice daily
Ramipril	HTN, high-risk for IHD, HF, post-MI	2.5–10 mg daily in 1–2 divided doses
Trandolapril	HTN, HF, post-MI	1–4 mg daily
Angiotensin receptor blockers		
Candesartan	HTN, HF	4–32 mg daily
Valsartan	HTN, HF, post-MI	80–320 mg daily in 1–2 divided doses
Telmisartan	HTN, high-risk for IHD	20–80 mg daily

HF, heart failure; HTN, hypertension; IHD, ischemic heart disease; MI, myocardial infarction.

[a]Reduce initial dose and gradually titrate upward as tolerated in renal impairment.

is contraindicated. Phosphodiesterase degrades cyclic guanosine monophosphate (cGMP), which is responsible for the vasodilatory effects of nitrates. Concomitant use of nitrates and phosphodiesterase type 5 inhibitors enhances cGMP-mediated vasodilation and can result in serious hypotension, decreased coronary perfusion, and even death.

- All patients with IHD should receive a prescription for sublingual nitrates and education regarding their use. Points to emphasize when counseling a patient on nitroglycerin use include:

  - The seated position is generally preferred when using nitroglycerin because the drug may cause dizziness.

  - Call 911 if symptoms are unimproved or worsen 5 minutes after the first dose.

  - Keep nitroglycerin tablets in the original glass container and close the cap tightly after use.

  - Nitroglycerin should not be stored in the same container as other medications because this may reduce nitroglycerin's effectiveness.

  - Repeated use of nitroglycerin is not harmful or addictive and does not result in any long-term side effects. Patients should not hesitate to use nitroglycerin whenever needed.

  - Nitroglycerin should not be used within 24 hours of taking sildenafil or vardenafil or within 48 hours of taking tadalafil because of the potential for life-threatening hypotension.

▶ *Pharmacotherapy to Prevent Recurrent Ischemic Symptoms*

- The overall goal of antianginal therapy is to allow patients with IHD to resume normal activities without symptoms of angina and to experience minimal to no adverse drug effects. The drugs traditionally used to prevent ischemic symptoms are β-blockers, CCBs, and nitrates. These drugs exert their antianginal effects by improving the balance between myocardial oxygen supply and demand, with specific effects listed in Table 7–6. β-Blockers, CCBs, and nitrates decrease the frequency of angina and delay the onset of angina during exercise. However, there is no evidence that any of these agents prevent ACS or improve survival in patients with chronic stable angina. Ranolazine, a newer molecular entity whose mechanism of action is unknown, is indicated for the treatment of chronic stable angina. Combination therapy with two or three antianginal drugs is often needed.

β-Blockers Stimulation of the β_1- and β_2-adrenergic receptors in the heart increases heart rate and cardiac contractility. β-Blockers antagonize β_1- and β_2-adrenergic receptors, reducing heart rate and cardiac contractility, and decreasing myocardial oxygen demand. β-Blockers may also reduce oxygen demand by lowering blood pressure and ventricular wall tension through inhibition of renin release from juxtaglomerular cells. By slowing heart rate, β-blockers prolong diastole, thus increasing coronary blood flow. However, with marked reductions in heart rate, β-blockers may actually increase ventricular wall tension. This is because

Table 7–6

Effects of Antianginal Medications on Myocardial Oxygen Demand and Supply

Antianginal Agent	Oxygen Demand			Oxygen Supply
	Heart Rate	Wall Tension	Cardiac Contractility	
β-Blockers	↓	↔ or ↑	↓	↔
Calcium channel blockers				
Verapamil, diltiazem	↓	↓	↓	↑
Dihydropyridines	↔ or ↑	↓	↓	↑
Nitrates	↑	↓	↔	↑
Ranolazine[a]	↔	↓	↔	↔

[a]The exact mechanism of the antiischemic effects of ranolazine is not known.

↓ decreases; ↔, no change; ↑, increases.

slower heart rates allow the ventricle more time to fill during diastole, leading to increased left ventricular volume, end diastolic pressure, and wall tension. However, the net effect of β-blockade is usually a reduction in myocardial oxygen demand. β-Blockers do not improve myocardial oxygen supply.

β-Blockers with intrinsic sympathomimetic activity (e.g., acebutolol, pindolol, and penbutolol) have partial β-agonist effects and cause lesser reductions in heart rate at rest. As a result, β-blockers with intrinsic sympathomimetic activity may produce lesser reductions in myocardial oxygen demand and should be avoided in patients with IHD. Other β-blockers appear equally effective at controlling symptoms of angina. The properties and recommended doses of various β-blockers used to prevent angina are summarized in Table 7–7. The frequency of dosing and drug cost should be taken into consideration when choosing a particular drug. Agents that can be dosed once or twice daily are preferred. Most β-blockers are available in inexpensive generic versions. β-Blockers should be initiated in doses at the lower end of the usual dosing range, with titration according to symptom and hemodynamic response. The β-blocker dose is commonly titrated to achieve the following:

- Resting heart rate between 55 and 60 beats/min.
- Maximum heart rate with exercise of 100 beats/min or less or 20 beats/min above the resting heart rate.

- ⑨ *β-Blockers are first-line therapy for preventing ischemic symptoms, particularly in patients with a history of myocardial infarction. In the absence of contraindications, β-blockers are the preferred antianginal therapy because of their potential cardioprotective effects.* Specifically, β-blockers possessing membrane stabilizing properties may prevent cardiac arrhythmias by decreasing the rate of spontaneous depolarization of ectopic pacemakers. Secondly, although the long-term effects of β-blockers on morbidity and mortality in patients with chronic stable angina are largely unknown,

Table 7–7

Properties and Dosing of β-Blockers in Ischemic Heart Disease

Drug	Receptor Affinity	Usual Dose Range	Dose Adjust in Hepatic Impairment	Dose Adjust in Renal Impairment
Atenolol	β_1-Selective	25–200 mg once daily	No	Yes
Betaxolol	β_1-Selective	5–20 mg once daily	No	Yes
Bisoprolol	β_1-Selective	2.5–10 mg once daily	Yes	Yes
Carvedilol	α_1, β_1, and β_2	3.125–25 mg twice daily	Avoid in severe impairment	No
Carvedilol phosphate	α_1, β_1, and β_2	10-80 mg once daily	Avoid in severe impairment	No
Labetalol	α_1, β_1, and β_2	100–400 mg twice daily	Yes	No
Metoprolol	β_1-Selective	50–200 mg twice daily (once daily for extended release)	Yes	No
Nadolol	β_1 and β_2	40–120 mg once daily	No	Yes
Propranolol	β_1 and β_2	20–120 mg twice daily (60–240 mg once daily for long-acting formulation)	Yes	No
Timolol	β_1 and β_2	10–20 mg twice daily	Yes	Yes

certain β-blockers have been shown to decrease the risk for reinfarction and improve survival in patients who have suffered an MI.[36,37] Specific β-blockers associated with mortality reductions in clinical trials include metoprolol, propranolol, and carvedilol. In a meta-analysis of 82 clinical trials investigating the use of β-blockers in patients following MI, the relative risk of death was reduced by 23% in patients treated with β-blockers compared with control subjects.[37] Long-term therapy (for at least 6 months) was associated with a greater mortality benefit compared with short-term β-blockade (6 weeks or less).

β-Blockers are contraindicated in patients with severe bradycardia (heart rate less than 50 beats/min) or AV conduction defects in the absence of a pacemaker. β-Blockers should be used with particular caution in combination with other agents that depress AV conduction (e.g., digoxin, verapamil, and diltiazem) because of the increased risk for bradycardia and heart block. Relative contraindications include asthma, bronchospastic disease, and severe depression. β_1-Selective blockers are preferred in patients with asthma or chronic obstructive pulmonary disease. However, selectivity is dose dependent, and β_1-selective agents may induce bronchospasm in higher doses.

There are several precautions to consider with the use of β-blockers in patients with diabetes or heart failure. All β-blockers may mask the tachycardia and tremor (but not sweating) that commonly accompany episodes of hypoglycemia in diabetes. In addition, nonselective β-blockers may alter glucose metabolism and slow recovery from hypoglycemia in insulin-dependent diabetes. β_1-Selective agents are preferred because they are less likely to prolong recovery from hypoglycemia. Importantly, β-blockers should not be avoided in patients with IHD and diabetes, particularly in patients with a history of MI who are at high risk for recurrent cardiovascular events. β-Blockers are negative inotropes (i.e., they decrease cardiac contractility). Cardiac contractility is impaired in patients with left ventricular dysfunction. Therefore, β-blockers may worsen symptoms of acute heart failure in patients with left

ventricular dysfunction (i.e., ejection fraction less than 40% [0.40]) and should be delayed until the patient has stabilized. β-blockers are indicated in patients with heart failure whose acute symptoms have resolved and who are euvolemic. Research has indicated that treatment with β-blockers is associated with a reduction in morbidity and mortality in this population. In particular, when used for the management of IHD in a patient with heart failure, β-blockers should be initiated in very low doses with slow up-titration to avoid worsening heart failure symptoms.

Other potential adverse effects from β-blockers include fatigue, sleep disturbances, malaise, depression, and sexual dysfunction. Abrupt β-blocker withdrawal may increase the frequency and severity of angina, possibly because of increased receptor sensitivity to catecholamines after long-term β-blockade. If the decision is made to stop β-blocker therapy, the dose should be tapered over several days to weeks to avoid exacerbating angina.

Calcium Channel Blockers Calcium channel blockers (CCBs) inhibit calcium entry into vascular smooth muscle and cardiac cells, resulting in the inhibition of the calcium-dependent process leading to muscle contraction. Inhibition of calcium entry into the vascular smooth muscle cells leads to systemic vasodilation and reductions in afterload. Inhibition of calcium entry into the cardiac cells leads to reductions in cardiac contractility. Thus CCBs reduce myocardial oxygen demand by lowering both wall tension (through reductions in afterload) and cardiac contractility. The nondihydropyridine CCBs, verapamil and diltiazem, further decrease myocardial oxygen demand by slowing cardiac sinoatrial and atrioventricular (AV) nodal conduction and lowering heart rate. Because of their negative chronotropic effects, verapamil and diltiazem are generally more effective antianginal agents than the dihydropyridine CCBs. In contrast, dihydropyridine CCBs, nifedipine in particular, inhibits calcium in the vasculature, and they are potent vasodilators that can cause baroreflex-mediated increases in sympathetic tone and heart rate.

In addition to decreasing myocardial oxygen demand, all CCBs increase myocardial oxygen supply by dilating coronary arteries, thus increasing coronary blood flow and relieving vasospasm.

In randomized controlled clinical trials, CCBs were as effective as β-blockers at preventing ischemic symptoms. ⑨ *Calcium channel blockers are recommended as alternative treatment in IHD when β-blockers are contraindicated or not tolerated. In addition, CCBs may be used in combination with β-blockers when initial treatment is unsuccessful.* The combination of a β-blocker and a dihydropyridine CCB may improve symptoms better than either drug used alone.[38] However, the combination of a β-blocker with either verapamil or diltiazem should be used with extreme caution because both drugs decrease AV nodal conduction, increasing the risk for severe bradycardia or AV block when used together. If combination therapy is warranted, a long-acting dihydropyridine CCB is preferred. β-Blockers will prevent reflex increases in sympathetic tone and heart rate with the use of CCBs with potent vasodilatory effects. For patients with variable and unpredictable occurrences of angina, indicating possible coronary vasospasm, CCBs may be more effective than β-blockers in preventing angina episodes. The dosing of CCBs in IHD is described in Table 7–8.

Verapamil and diltiazem are contraindicated in patients with bradycardia and preexisting conduction disease in the absence of a pacemaker. As previously noted, verapamil and diltiazem should be used with particular caution in combination with other drugs that depress AV nodal conduction (e.g., β-blockers and digoxin). Because of their negative inotropic effects, CCBs may cause or exacerbate heart failure in patients with preexisting left ventricular systolic dysfunction and should be avoided in this population. The exceptions are amlodipine and felodipine that have less negative inotropic effects compared with other CCBs and appear to be safe in patients with left ventricular

---

Table 7–8

Dosing of Calcium Channel Blockers in Ischemic Heart Disease

Drug	Usual Dose Range
Nondihydropyridines	
Diltiazem, extended release	120–360 mg once daily; consider dose adjustment in hepatic dysfunction
Verapamil, extended release	180–480 mg once daily; use initial dose of 120 mg in hepatic dysfunction
Dihydropyridines	
Amlodipine	5–10 mg once daily
Felodipine	5–10 mg once daily; use initial dose of 2.5 mg once daily in hepatic dysfunction
Nifedipine, extended release	30–90 mg once daily; dose adjust and monitor closely in hepatic dysfunction
Nicardipine	20–40 mg three times daily; dose twice daily in hepatic dysfunction and up-titrate slowly in both hepatic and renal dysfunction

---

Table 7–9

Nitrate Formulations and Dosing for Chronic Use

Formulation	Dose
Oral	
Nitroglycerin extended-release capsules	2.5 mg 3 times daily initially, with up-titration according to symptoms and tolerance; allow a 10- to 12-hour nitrate-free interval
Isosorbide dinitrate tablets	5–20 mg 2–3 times daily, with a daily nitrate-free interval of at least 14 hours (e.g., dose at 7 AM, noon, and 5 PM)
Isosorbide dinitrate slow-release capsules	40 mg 1–2 times daily, with a daily nitrate-free interval of at least 18 hours (e.g., dose at 8 AM and 2 PM)
Isosorbide mononitrate tablets	5–20 mg 2 times daily initially, with up-titration according to symptoms and tolerance; doses should be taken 7 hours apart (e.g., 8 AM and 3 PM)
Isosorbide mononitrate extended-release tablets	30–120 mg once daily
Transdermal	
Nitroglycerin extended-release film	0.2–0.8 mg/hour, on for 12–14 hours, off for 10–12 hours

---

systolic dysfunction.[39,40] Finally, there is some evidence that short-acting CCBs (particularly short-acting nifedipine and nicardipine) may increase the risk of cardiovascular events.[41] Therefore, short-acting agents should be avoided in the management of IHD.

Long-Acting Nitrates Nitrate products are available in both oral and transdermal formulations for chronic use. Commonly used products are listed in Table 7–9. All long-acting nitrate products produce effects within 30 to 60 minutes and are equally effective at preventing the recurrence of angina when used appropriately.

The major limitation of nitrate therapy is the development of tolerance with continuous use. The loss of antianginal effects may occur within the first 24 hours of continuous nitrate therapy. Although the cause of tolerance is unclear, several mechanisms have been proposed, including the generation of free radicals that degrade nitric oxide. The most effective method to avoid tolerance and maintain the antianginal efficacy of nitrates is to allow a daily nitrate-free interval of at least 8 to 12 hours. Nitrates do not provide protection from ischemia during the nitrate-free period. Therefore, the nitrate-free interval should occur when the patient is least likely to experience angina. Generally, angina is less common during the nighttime hours when the patient is sleeping and myocardial oxygen demand is reduced. Thus it is common to dose long-acting nitrates so that the nitrate-free interval begins in the evening. For example, isosorbide dinitrate is typically dosed on awakening and again 6 to 7 hours later.

Monotherapy with nitrates for the prevention of ischemia should generally be avoided for a couple of reasons. First, reflex increases in sympathetic activity and heart rate, with resultant increases in myocardial oxygen demand, may occur secondary to nitrate-induced venodilation. Second, patients are unprotected from ischemia during the nitrate-free interval. β-Blockers and CCBs are dosed to provide 24-hour protection from ischemia. ❾ *Treatment with long-acting nitrates should be added to baseline therapy with either a β-blocker or CCB or a combination of the two.* β-Blockers attenuate the increase in sympathetic tone and heart rate that occurs during nitrate therapy. In turn, nitrates attenuate the increase in wall tension during β-blocker therapy. As a result, the combination of β-blockers and nitrates is particularly effective at preventing angina and provides greater protection from ischemia than therapy with either agent alone. Monotherapy with nitrates may be appropriate in patients who have low blood pressure at baseline or who experience symptomatic hypotension with low doses of β-blockers or CCBs.

Common adverse effects of nitrates include postural hypotension, dizziness, flushing, and headache secondary to venodilation. Headache often resolves with continued therapy and may be treated with acetaminophen. Hypotension is generally of no serious consequence. However, in patients with hypertrophic obstructive cardiomyopathy or severe aortic valve stenosis, nitroglycerin may cause serious hypotension and syncope. Therefore, long-acting nitrates are relatively contraindicated in these conditions. Because life-threatening hypotension may occur with concomitant use of nitrates and phosphodiesterase type 5 inhibitors, nitrates should not be used within 24 hours of taking sildenafil or vardenafil or within 48 hours of taking tadalafil. Skin erythema and inflammation may occur with transdermal nitroglycerin administration and may be minimized by rotating the application site.

Ranolazine Ranolazine is an antiischemic agent indicated for the management of chronic angina. The mechanism of action is unclear, but it is believed to inhibit the late inward sodium current during the plateau phase of the cardiac action potential. Under ischemic conditions, excess sodium may enter the myocardial cell during systole. The resultant intracellular sodium overload leads to intracellular calcium accumulation (calcium overload) though a sodium/calcium exchange mechanism. Calcium overload results in increases in left ventricular wall tension and myocardial oxygen consumption. By reducing intracellular sodium concentrations in ischemic myocytes, ranolazine decreases intracellular calcium overload, left ventricular wall tension, and myocardial oxygen consumption.

In clinical trials, ranolazine reduced angina and increased exercise capacity when added to other antianginal therapy, with no effect on major cardiovascular events.[42,43] Ranolazine has minimal effects on heart rate or blood pressure; thus it may be an option in IHD patients with low baseline blood pressure or heart rate. Ranolazine is indicated as a first-line treatment for chronic stable angina. However, it is often reserved for patients with angina that is refractory to traditional antianginal medications due to its excessive cost and small risk for dose-related prolongation of the QT interval. When used at recommended doses, the mean prolongation of QT interval is minimal (2.6 ms).[42] However,

Table 7–10	
Contraindications and Precautions with Ranolazine	
Contraindications	**Precautions**
Liver cirrhosis increases ranolazine plasma concentrations by 30% to 80% resulting in increased risk for QT interval prolongation	Treatment with moderate CYP3A4 inhibitors including diltiazem, verapamil, grapefruit juice, erythromycin, and fluconazole increases ranolazine plasma concentrations (twofold with diltiazem and verapamil)
Treatment with potent CYP3A4 inhibitors, including ketoconazole, clarithromycin, and nelfinavir increases ranolazine concentrations (3.2-fold with ketoconazole)	Preexisting QT prolongation, history of torsades de pointes, or treatment with other QT-prolonging drugs
	Uncorrected hypokalemia
Treatment with CYP3A4 inducers including rifampin, phenobarbital, phenytoin, carbamazepine, and St. John's wart may significantly decrease the efficacy of ranolazine (by 95% with rifampin)	Treatment with a p-glycoprotein inhibitor, such as cyclosporine, may increase ranolazine absorption
	Ranolazine may increase bioavailability of p-glycoprotein substrates (increases digoxin plasma concentrations by 1.5-fold)
	Ranolazine may cause syncope; use caution when driving or operating machinery
	Ranolazine may cause reduced metabolism of CYP2D6 substrates
	Up to a 50% increase in ranolazine plasma concentration has been observed in renal impairment

the risk for QT interval prolongation is elevated in patients with hepatic impairment or taking other medications with the potential to prolong the QT interval. Ranolazine should be started at a dose of 500 mg twice daily and increased to 1000 mg twice daily if needed for symptom relief. Higher doses are poorly tolerated and should be avoided. Contraindications to ranolazine are shown in Table 7–10. Common adverse effects with ranolazine include dizziness, constipation, headache, and nausea. Syncope may occur infrequently. Ranolazine is a CYP3A4 substrate, weak CYP2D6 substrate, CYP2D6 inhibitor, and both an inhibitor and substrate of p-glycoprotein. Concomitant use of ranolazine with potent CYP3A4 inhibitors (e.g., ketoconazole, clarithromycin, and nelfinavir) or inducers (e.g., rifampin) is contraindicated. The use of ranolazine is contraindicated in patients with significant hepatic disease. The ranolazine dose should be limited to 500 mg twice daily when combined with moderate CYP3A4 inhibitors including diltiazem and verapamil. Ranolazine should be used cautiously with p-glycoprotein inhibitors (e.g., cyclosporine) and substrates (e.g., digoxin).

▶ *Pharmacotherapy with No Benefit or Potentially Harmful Effects*

Hormone Replacement Therapy Hormone replacement therapy (HRT) has favorable effects on lipoprotein cholesterol concentrations. Data from several observational studies suggested that HRT might reduce the risk of cardiovascular events in women with IHD. However, subsequent randomized controlled clinical trials failed to demonstrate a reduction in the risk for IHD or cardiovascular events with HRT in postmenopausal women.[44,45] In fact, HRT appeared to be harmful in this patient population, increasing the risk of thromboembolic events and breast cancer. Current guidelines recommend against the use of HRT to reduce cardiovascular risk.[1] Furthermore, the clinician should consider discontinuing HRT therapy in women who suffer an acute coronary event while receiving such therapy.

Antioxidants Oxidization of LDL-cholesterol is believed to play a significant role in the atherosclerotic process. The antioxidant vitamins, vitamin E, vitamin C, and β-carotene, protect LDL cholesterol from oxidation. Evidence from observational and animal studies suggests that an increased intake of antioxidant vitamins might inhibit the formation of atherosclerotic lesions and decrease the risk for cardiovascular events.[46] However, randomized prospective studies have not substantiated the findings from earlier studies and found no beneficial effect of vitamin E, vitamin C, or β-carotene on cardiovascular outcomes in patients with IHD or IHD risk factors.[47,48] Based on this evidence, current guidelines do not recommend supplementation with vitamin E or other antioxidants for the purpose of preventing cardiovascular events.

Folic Acid Elevated homocysteine concentrations have been associated with an increased risk for cardiovascular disease in both epidemiologic and clinical studies.[49] Although folic acid and vitamin B supplementation are effective at reducing homocysteine levels, neither treatment reduces cardiovascular events.[49] Based on available evidence, the use of folate or vitamin B supplementation for the prevention of cardiovascular events in patients with preexisting IHD or at risk for IHD is not recommended.

Herbal Supplements Herbal products are widely used for their purported cardiovascular benefits; examples of such products include danshen, dong quai, feverfew, garlic, hawthorn, and hellebore. However, strong evidence supporting their benefits in cardiovascular disease is generally lacking. Although small randomized controlled trials have shown benefits with some herbal supplements, the potential for drug interactions and the lack of product standardization limits the products' usefulness in clinical practice. Safety with herbal supplements in patients with IHD is a major concern. Numerous case reports of adverse cardiovascular events, including stroke, MI, and lethal cardiac arrhythmias with ephedra-based products (e.g., Ma huang), led the FDA to ban ephedra-containing products in 2004. However, other herbal supplements with potentially serious adverse cardiovascular effects remain easily accessible to the consumer. Some herbal supplements may interact with antiplatelet and antithrombotic therapy and increase bleeding risk. Dietary supplements purported to enhance sexual performance may contain phosphodiesterase-like chemicals and increase risk for serious hypotension with nitroglycerin. Other agents may reduce the effectiveness of antianginal medications, such

> ## Patient Encounter Part 3: Creating a Care Plan
>
> *Based on the information presented, create a specific plan for the management of DF's ischemic heart disease. Your plan should include (a) the goals of therapy, (b) specific nonpharmacologic and pharmacologic interventions to address these goals, and (c) a plan for follow-up to assess drug tolerance and whether the therapeutic goals have been achieved.*

as St. John's wart with ranolazine. Thus it is important to assess the use of herbal products in patients with IHD and to counsel patients about the potential for drug interactions and adverse events with herbal therapies.

Cyclooxygenase-2 Inhibitors and Nonsteroidal Anti-inflammatory Drugs Data suggest that cyclooxygenase-2 (COX-2) inhibitors and nonselective NSAIDs may increase the risk for MI and stroke.[50] The cardiovascular risk with COX-2 inhibitors and NSAIDs may be greatest in patients with a history of, or with risk factors for, cardiovascular disease. The COX-2 inhibitors rofecoxib and valdecoxib were withdrawn from the market in recent years because of safety concerns. The FDA requested the manufacturers of other COX-2 and nonselective NSAIDs (prescription and over-the-counter) to include information about the potential adverse cardiovascular effects of these drugs in their product labeling. The American Heart Association recommends that the use of COX-2 inhibitors be limited to low-dose, short-term therapy in patients for whom there is no appropriate alternative.[50] Patients with cardiovascular disease should consult a clinician before using over-the-counter NSAIDs.

SPECIAL POPULATIONS

Variant Angina

Vasospasm as the sole etiology of angina (Prinzmetal's or variant angina) is relatively uncommon. As a result, treatment options are not well studied. Nevertheless, based on the pharmacology of available drugs, several recommendations can be made. First, β-blockers should be avoided in patients with variant angina because of their potential to worsen vasospasm due to unopposed α-adrenergic receptor stimulation. In contrast, both CCBs and nitrates are effective in relieving vasospasm and are preferred in the management of variant angina. Nitrates have several limitations, outlined earlier, most notably, the need for an 8- to 12-hour nitrate-free interval. Therefore, the role of monotherapy with long-acting nitrates as prophylaxis for anginal attacks due to vasospasm is limited. However, immediate-release nitroglycerin is effective at terminating acute anginal attacks due to vasospasm. Therefore, all patients diagnosed with variant angina should be prescribed immediate-release nitroglycerin. CCBs are effective for monotherapy of variant angina. Because short-acting CCBs have been associated with increased risk of adverse cardiac events, they should be avoided.[41] Long-acting nitrates may be added to CCB therapy if needed.

Microvascular Angina

There are limited data on optimal therapy in patients with microvascular disease. Both ACE inhibitors and statins may produce beneficial effects on endothelial function and improve microvascular angina.[6] Short-acting nitrates remain the treatment of choice for relieving acute symptoms, although they may be less effective in microvascular disease. Similar to obstructive CAD, β-blockers are first line to control symptoms of angina in patients with microvascular disease and may be more effective than CCBs and long-acting nitrates in this setting.[6] Ranolazine may also produce favorable antianginal effects for patients with continued symptoms.

Elderly Patients with IHD

Elderly patients are more likely than younger patients to have other comorbidities that may influence drug selection for the treatment of angina. As a result, polypharmacy is more common in elderly patients, increasing the risk of drug–drug interactions, and perhaps decreasing medication adherence. Additionally, elderly patients are often more susceptible to adverse effects of antianginal therapies, particularly the negative chronotropic and inotropic effects of β-blockers and CCBs. Therefore, drugs should be initiated in low doses with close monitoring of elderly patients with IHD.

Acute Coronary Syndromes

The management of ACS is discussed in further detail in Chapter 8, "Acute Coronary Syndromes." It is important to educate patients with IHD on the signs of ACS and the steps to take if signs or symptoms occur. Importantly, patients should be instructed to seek emergent care if symptoms of angina last longer than 20 to 30 minutes, do not improve after 5 minutes of using sublingual nitroglycerin, or worsen after 5 minutes of using sublingual nitroglycerin. In patients with a history of ACS, it is crucial to select appropriate pharmacotherapy to prevent recurrent ACS and death. Appropriate pharmacotherapy for patients with a history of ACS includes aspirin (perhaps in combination with clopidogrel), ACE inhibitors or ARBs, β-blockers, and statins. In addition, determining appropriate goals and instituting appropriate therapy to meet the goals for cardiovascular risk factors (e.g., dyslipidemia, hypertension, and diabetes) is critical.

OUTCOME EVALUATION

Assessing for Drug Effectiveness and Safety

- ⑩ *Monitor symptoms of angina at baseline and at each clinic visit for patients with IHD to assess the effectiveness of antianginal therapy. In particular, assess the frequency and intensity of anginal symptoms.* Determining the frequency of sublingual nitroglycerin use is helpful in making this assessment. If angina is occurring with

increasing frequency or intensity, adjust antianginal therapy and refer the patient for additional diagnostic testing (e.g., coronary angiography) and possibly, coronary intervention (e.g., PCI or CABG surgery), if indicated.

- Assess the patient for IHD-related complications, such as heart failure. The presence of new comorbidities may indicate worsening IHD requiring additional workup or pharmacologic therapy.

- ⑩ *Routinely monitor hemodynamic parameters to assess drug tolerance. Assess blood pressure at baseline, after drug initiation and after dose titration. Blood pressure should be monitored periodically in patients treated with β-blockers, CCBs, nitrates, ACE inhibitors, and/or ARBs.*

- Blood pressure reduction may be particularly pronounced after initiation and dose titration of β-blockers that also possess α-blocking effects (e.g., labetalol and carvedilol).

- Because of the potential for postural hypotension, warn patients that dizziness, presyncope, and even syncope may result from abrupt changes in body position during initiation or up-titration of drugs with α-blocking effects.

- ⑩ *Closely monitor heart rate in patients treated with drugs that have negative chronotropic effects (e.g., β-blockers, verapamil, or diltiazem) or drugs that may cause reflex tachycardia (e.g., nitrates or dihydropyridine CCBs).*

- Treatment with β-blockers, verapamil, or diltiazem can usually be continued in patients with asymptomatic bradycardia. However, reduce or discontinue treatment with these agents in patients who develop symptomatic bradycardia or serious conduction abnormalities.

- Regularly assess control of existing risk factors and the presence of new risk factors for IHD. Routine screening for the presence of metabolic syndrome will help in assessing the control of known major risk factors and identifying new risk factors. If new risk factors are identified and/or the presence of metabolic syndrome is detected, modify the pharmacotherapy regimen, as discussed previously, to control these risk factors and lower the risk of IHD and IHD-related adverse events.

- ⑩ *In patients treated with ACE inhibitors and/or ARBs, routinely monitor renal function and potassium levels at baseline, after drug initiation and post dose titration, and periodically thereafter. This is particularly important when using these therapies in patients with preexisting renal impairment or diabetes because they may be more susceptible to these adverse events.*

Duration of Therapy

- Drugs that modify platelet activity, lipoprotein concentrations, and neurohormonal systems reduce the risk for coronary events and death. However, these therapies do not cure IHD.

- Treatment with antiplatelet (aspirin or clopidogrel), lipid-lowering, and neurohormonal-modifying therapy for IHD is generally lifelong. Similarly, antianginal therapy with a β-blocker, CCB, and/or nitrate is usually long term.

- A patient with severe symptoms managed with combination antianginal drugs who undergoes successful coronary revascularization may be able to reduce antianginal therapy. However, treatment with at least one agent that improves the balance between myocardial oxygen demand and supply is usually warranted.

Patient Care and Monitoring

1. Assess the patient's symptoms to determine whether the patient should be evaluated by a physician.
   - Determine the quality, location, and duration of pain.
   - Determine factors that provoke and relieve pain.
   - Are symptoms characteristic of angina?
2. Identify risk factors for IHD.
   - Are there any modifiable risk factors?
3. Obtain a thorough history of prescription drug, nonprescription drug, and herbal product use.
   - Is the patient taking any medications/supplements that may exacerbate angina or interact with antianginal drug therapy?
4. Educate the patient on lifestyle modifications to control risk factors for IHD.
5. Is the patient taking appropriate drug therapy to prevent ACS and death? If not, why?
6. Is the patient taking appropriate antianginal therapy? If not, why?
7. Develop a plan to assess effectiveness of antiischemic therapy after 1 to 2 weeks.
8. Evaluate the patient to assess for adverse drug reactions, drug intolerance, and drug interactions.
9. Stress the importance of adherence with the therapeutic regimen including lifestyle modifications.
10. Provide patient education regarding disease state, lifestyle modifications, and drug therapy:
    - What are the consequences of untreated IHD?
    - What lifestyle modifications should the patient follow?
    - When should the patient take his or her medications?
    - What potential adverse drug effects may occur?
    - Teach the patient how to monitor heart rate and blood pressure to assess tolerance to antianginal therapy.
    - Which drugs may interact with therapy or worsen IHD?
    - What should the patient do when chest pain or its equivalent occurs?
    - When should the patient seek emergent care?

Abbreviations Introduced in This Chapter

ACE	Angiotensin-converting enzyme
ACE-I	Angiotensin-converting enzyme inhibitor
ACS	Acute coronary syndrome
ARB	Angiotensin receptor blocker
AV	Atrioventricular
BMS	Bare metal stent
BP	Blood pressure
CABG	Coronary artery bypass graft
CAD	Coronary artery disease
CCB	Calcium channel blocker
cGMP	Cyclic guanosine monophosphate
CHD	Coronary heart disease
CK	Creatine kinase
CK-MB	Creatine kinase, MB fraction
COX-2	Cyclooxygenase-2
CT	Computed tomography
DES	Drug-eluting stent
DHA	Docosahexaenoic acid
EBCT	Electron beam computer tomography
ECG	Electrocardiogram
EPA	Eicosapentaenoic acid
HDL	High-density lipoprotein
HF	Heart failure
HMG-CoA	3-hydroxy-3-methylglutaryl coenzyme A
HR	Heart rate
HRT	Hormone replacement therapy
HTN	Hypertension
IHD	Ischemic heart disease
IR	Immediate release
LA	Long acting
LV	Left ventricular
LDL	Low-density lipoprotein
MI	Myocardial infarction
MVO_2	Myocardial oxygen consumption
NSAID	Nonsteroidal anti-inflammatory drug
NTG	Nitroglycerin
PCI	Percutaneous coronary intervention
Po_2	Partial pressure of oxygen
PTCA	Percutaneous transluminal coronary angioplasty
SL	Sublingual

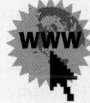 Self-assessment questions and answers are available at *http://www.mhpharmacotherapy.com/pp.html.*

REFERENCES

1. Gibbons RJ, Abrams J, Chatterjee K, et al. ACC/AHA 2002 guideline update for the management of patients with chronic stable angina— Summary article: A report of the American College of Cardiology/ American Heart Association Task Force on practice guidelines (Committee on the Management of Patients with Chronic Stable Angina). J Am Coll Cardiol 2003;41:159–168.

2. Fraker TD Jr, Fihn SD, Gibbons RJ, et al. 2007 chronic angina focused update of the ACC/AHA 2002 guidelines for the management of patients with chronic stable angina: A report of the American College of Cardiology/American Heart Association Task Force on Practice Guidelines Writing Group to develop the focused update of the 2002 guidelines for the management of patients with chronic stable angina. J Am Coll Cardiol 2007;50:2264–2274.

3. Roger VL, Go AS, Lloyd-Jones DM, et al. Heart disease and stroke statistics—2011 update: A report from the American Heart Association. Circulation 2011;123:e18–e209.

4. Chobanian AV, Bakris GL, Black HR, et al. Seventh report of the Joint National Committee on Prevention, Detection, Evaluation, and Treatment of High Blood Pressure. Hypertension 2003;42:1206–1252.

5. Alberti KG, Eckel RH, Grundy SM, et al. Harmonizing the metabolic syndrome: A joint interim statement of the International Diabetes Federation Task Force on Epidemiology and Prevention; National Heart, Lung, and Blood Institute; American Heart Association; World Heart Federation; International Atherosclerosis Society; and International Association for the Study of Obesity. Circulation 2009;120:1640–1645.

6. Lanza GA, Crea F. Primary coronary microvascular dysfunction: Clinical presentation, pathophysiology, and management. Circulation 2010;121:2317–2325.

7. Stone GW, Maehara A, Lansky AJ, et al. A prospective natural-history study of coronary atherosclerosis. N Engl J Med 2011;364:226–235.

8. Braunwald E, Jones RH, Mark DB, et al. Diagnosing and managing unstable angina. Agency for Health Care Policy and Research. Circulation 1994;90:613–622.

9. Sangareddi V, Chockalingam A, Gnanavelu G, et al. Canadian Cardiovascular Society classification of effort angina: An angiographic correlation. Coron Artery Dis 2004;15:111–114.

10. Tzivoni D, Keren A, Meyler S, et al. Cardiovascular safety of transdermal nicotine patches in patients with coronary artery disease who try to quit smoking. Cardiovasc Drugs Ther 1998;12:239–244.

11. Tonstad S, Farsang C, Klaene G, et al. Bupropion SR for smoking cessation in smokers with cardiovascular disease: A multicentre, randomised study. Eur Heart J 2003;24:946–955.

12. Kuehn BM. Varenicline gets stronger warnings about psychiatric problems, vehicle crashes. JAMA 2009;302:834.

13. Krauss RM, Eckel RH, Howard B, et al. AHA Dietary Guidelines: Revision 2000: A statement for healthcare professionals from the Nutrition Committee of the American Heart Association. Stroke 2000;31:2751–2766.

14. De Caterina R. n-3 fatty acids in cardiovascular disease. N Engl J Med 2011;364:2439–2450.

15. Boden WE, O'Rourke RA, Teo KK, et al. Impact of optimal medical therapy with or without percutaneous coronary intervention on long-term cardiovascular end points in patients with stable coronary artery disease (from the COURAGE Trial). Am J Cardiol 2009;104:1–4.

16. Shishehbor MH, Goel SS, Kapadia SR, et al. Long-term impact of drug-eluting stents versus bare-metal stents on all-cause mortality. J Am Coll Cardiol 2008;52:1041–1048.

17. Serruys PW, Morice MC, Kappetein AP, et al. Percutaneous coronary intervention versus coronary-artery bypass grafting for severe coronary artery disease. N Engl J Med 2009;360:961–972.

18. Executive Summary of The Third Report of The National Cholesterol Education Program (NCEP) Expert Panel on Detection, Evaluation, and Treatment of High Blood Cholesterol in Adults (Adult Treatment Panel III). JAMA 2001;285:2486–2497.

19. Grundy SM, Cleeman JI, Merz CN, et al. Implications of recent clinical trials for the National Cholesterol Education Program Adult Treatment Panel III guidelines. Circulation 2004;110:227–239.

20. Brunzell JD, Davidson M, Furberg CD, et al. Lipoprotein management in patients with cardiometabolic risk: Consensus conference report from the American Diabetes Association and the American College of Cardiology Foundation. J Am Coll Cardiol 2008;51:1512–1524.

21. Rosendorff C, Black HR, Cannon CP, et al. Treatment of hypertension in the prevention and management of ischemic heart disease: A scientific statement from the American Heart Association Council for High Blood Pressure Research and the Councils on Clinical Cardiology and Epidemiology and Prevention. Circulation 2007;115:2761–2788.

22. Patrono C, Baigent C, Hirsh J, Roth G. Antiplatelet drugs: American College of Chest Physicians Evidence-Based Clinical Practice Guidelines (8th Edition). Chest 2008;133:199S–233S.

23. Mega JL, Simon T, Collet JP, et al. Reduced-function CYP2C19 genotype and risk of adverse clinical outcomes among patients treated with clopidogrel predominantly for PCI: A meta-analysis. JAMA 2010;304:1821–1830.

24. Wallentin L, James S, Storey RF, et al. Effect of CYP2C19 and ABCB1 single nucleotide polymorphisms on outcomes of treatment with ticagrelor versus clopidogrel for acute coronary syndromes: A genetic substudy of the PLATO trial. Lancet 2010;376:1320–1328.

25. Kushner FG, Hand M, Smith SC Jr, et al. 2009 focused updates: ACC/AHA guidelines for the management of patients with ST-elevation myocardial infarction (updating the 2004 guideline and 2007 focused update) and ACC/AHA/SCAI guidelines on percutaneous coronary intervention (updating the 2005 guideline and 2007 focused update): A report of the American College of Cardiology Foundation/American Heart Association Task Force on Practice Guidelines. J Am Coll Cardiol 2009;54:2205–2241.

26. Yusuf S, Zhao F, Mehta SR, et al. Effects of clopidogrel in addition to aspirin in patients with acute coronary syndromes without ST-segment elevation. N Engl J Med 2001;345:494–502.

27. Chen ZM, Jiang LX, Chen YP, et al. Addition of clopidogrel to aspirin in 45,852 patients with acute myocardial infarction: Randomised placebo-controlled trial. Lancet 2005;366:1607–1621.

28. Wallentin L, Becker RC, Budaj A, et al. Ticagrelor versus clopidogrel in patients with acute coronary syndromes. N Engl J Med 2009;361:1045–1057.

29. Wiviott SD, Braunwald E, McCabe CH, et al. Prasugrel versus clopidogrel in patients with acute coronary syndromes. N Engl J Med 2007;357:2001–2015.

30. Baigent C, Keech A, Kearney PM, et al. Efficacy and safety of cholesterol-lowering treatment: Prospective meta-analysis of data from 90,056 participants in 14 randomised trials of statins. Lancet 2005;366:1267–1278.

31. Liao JK. Effects of statins on 3-hydroxy-3-methylglutaryl coenzyme a reductase inhibition beyond low-density lipoprotein cholesterol. Am J Cardiol 2005;96:24F–33F.

32. Pfeffer MA, McMurray JJ, Velazquez EJ, et al. Valsartan, captopril, or both in myocardial infarction complicated by heart failure, left ventricular dysfunction, or both. N Engl J Med 2003;349:1893–1906.

33. Rodrigues EJ, Eisenberg MJ, Pilote L. Effects of early and late administration of angiotensin-converting enzyme inhibitors on mortality after myocardial infarction. Am J Med 2003;115:473–479.

34. Yusuf S, Sleight P, Pogue J, et al. Effects of an angiotensin-converting-enzyme inhibitor, ramipril, on cardiovascular events in high-risk patients. The Heart Outcomes Prevention Evaluation Study Investigators. N Engl J Med 2000;342:145–153.

35. Fox KM. Efficacy of perindopril in reduction of cardiovascular events among patients with stable coronary artery disease: Randomised, double-blind, placebo-controlled, multicentre trial (the EUROPA study). Lancet 2003;362:782–788.

36. Kushner FG, Hand M, Smith SC Jr, et al. 2009 Focused Updates: ACC/AHA Guidelines for the Management of Patients with ST-Elevation Myocardial Infarction (updating the 2004 Guideline and 2007 Focused Update) and ACC/AHA/SCAI Guidelines on Percutaneous Coronary Intervention (updating the 2005 Guideline and 2007 Focused Update): A report of the American College of Cardiology Foundation/American Heart Association Task Force on Practice Guidelines. Circulation 2009;120:2271–2306.

37. Freemantle N, Cleland J, Young P, et al. β-Blockade after myocardial infarction: Systematic review and meta regression analysis. Br Med J 1999;318:1730–1737.

38. Leon MB, Rosing DR, Bonow RO, Epstein SE. Combination therapy with calcium-channel blockers and beta blockers for chronic stable angina pectoris. Am J Cardiol 1985;55:69B–80B.

39. Packer M, O'Connor CM, Ghali JK, et al. Effect of amlodipine on morbidity and mortality in severe chronic heart failure. Prospective Randomized Amlodipine Survival Evaluation Study Group. N Engl J Med 1996;335:1107–1114.

40. Cohn JN, Ziesche S, Smith R, et al. Effect of the calcium antagonist felodipine as supplementary vasodilator therapy in patients with chronic heart failure treated with enalapril: V-HeFT III. Vasodilator-Heart Failure Trial (V-HeFT) Study Group. Circulation 1997;96: 856–863.

41. Psaty BM, Smith NL, Siscovick DS, et al. Health outcomes associated with antihypertensive therapies used as first-line agents. A systematic review and meta-analysis. JAMA 1997;277:739–745.

42. Koren MJ, Crager MR, Sweeney M. Long-term safety of a novel antianginal agent in patients with severe chronic stable angina: the Ranolazine Open Label Experience (ROLE). J Am Coll Cardiol 2007;49:1027–1034.

43. Morrow DA, Scirica BM, Karwatowska-Prokopczuk E, et al. Effects of ranolazine on recurrent cardiovascular events in patients with non-ST-elevation acute coronary syndromes: The MERLIN-TIMI 36 randomized trial. JAMA 2007;297:1775–1783.

44. Hulley S, Grady D, Bush T, et al. Randomized trial of estrogen plus progestin for secondary prevention of coronary heart disease in postmenopausal women. Heart and Estrogen/progestin Replacement Study (HERS) Research Group. JAMA 1998;280:605–613.

45. Heiss G, Wallace R, Anderson GL, et al. Health risks and benefits 3 years after stopping randomized treatment with estrogen and progestin. JAMA 2008;299:1036–1045.

46. Bleys J, Miller ER 3rd, Pastor-Barriuso R, Appel LJ, Guallar E. Vitamin-mineral supplementation and the progression of atherosclerosis: A meta-analysis of randomized controlled trials. Am J Clin Nutr 2006;84:880–887; quiz 954–955.

47. Vivekananthan DP, Penn MS, Sapp SK, et al. Use of antioxidant vitamins for the prevention of cardiovascular disease: Meta-analysis of randomised trials. Lancet 2003;361:2017–2023.

48. Cook NR, Albert CM, Gaziano JM, et al. A randomized factorial trial of vitamins C and E and beta carotene in the secondary prevention of cardiovascular events in women: Results from the Women's Antioxidant Cardiovascular Study. Arch Intern Med 2007;167:1610–1618.

49. Marti-Carvajal AJ, Sola I, Lathyris D, Salanti G. Homocysteine lowering interventions for preventing cardiovascular events. Cochrane Database Syst Rev 2009:CD006612.

50. Bennett JS, Daugherty A, Herrington D, et al. The use of nonsteroidal anti-inflammatory drugs (NSAIDs): A science advisory from the American Heart Association. Circulation 2005;111:1713–1716.

8 Acute Coronary Syndromes

Sarah A. Spinler and Simon de Denus

● **Upon completion of the chapter, the reader will be able to:**

1. Define the role of atherosclerotic plaque, platelets, and the coagulation system in an acute coronary syndrome (ACS).

2. List key electrocardiogram (ECG) and clinical features identifying a patient with non-ST-segment elevation (NSTE) ACS who is at high risk of myocardial infarction (MI) or death.

3. Devise a pharmacotherapy treatment plan for a patient undergoing primary percutaneous coronary intervention (PCI) in ST-segment elevation (STE) MI and NSTE ACS given patient-specific data.

4. Compare and contrast the pharmacokinetics, antiplatelet effects, adverse effects, and drug–drug interactions between clopidogrel, prasugrel, and ticagrelor.

5. Devise a pharmacotherapy treatment plan for a patient with NSTE ACS given patient-specific data.

6. Develop a pharmacotherapy and risk-factor modification treatment plan for secondary prevention of coronary heart disease events in a patient following MI.

7. Identify the characteristics of patients who are ideal candidates for mineralocorticoid receptor antagonist therapy following MI.

8. Formulate a treatment and monitoring plan for a patient with STE MI or NSTE ACS.

9. List the quality performance measures of care for MI.

KEY CONCEPTS

❶ The cause of an acute coronary syndrome (ACS) is the rupture of an atherosclerotic plaque with subsequent platelet adherence, activation, and aggregation, and the activation of the clotting cascade. Ultimately, a clot forms composed of fibrin and platelets.

❷ The American College of Cardiology Foundation (ACCF), American Heart Association (AHA), and Society for Cardiovascular Angiography and Interventions (SCAI) recommend strategies, or guidelines, for ACS patient care for ST-segment elevation (STE) myocardial infarction (MI) and non-ST-segment elevation (NSTE) ACS, including guidelines for patients undergoing percutaneous coronary intervention (PCI).

❸ Patients with ischemic chest discomfort and suspected ACS are risk stratified based on a 12-lead electrocardiogram (ECG), past medical history, and results of the troponin and creatine kinase (CK) myocardial band (MB) tests. The diagnosis of myocardial infarction (MI) is confirmed based on the results of the CK MB and troponin biochemical marker tests.

❹ Early reperfusion therapy with primary PCI of the infarct artery is the recommended therapy for patients presenting with STE MI within 12 hours of symptom onset.

❺ The most recent PCI ACCF/AHA/SCAI clinical practice guidelines recommend coronary angiography with either PCI or coronary artery bypass graft (CABG) surgery revascularization as an early treatment (early invasive strategy) for patients with NSTE ACS at an elevated risk for death or MI, including those with a high risk score or patients with refractory angina, acute heart failure, other symptoms of cardiogenic shock, or arrhythmias.

❻ In addition to reperfusion therapy, other early pharmacotherapy that all patients with STE MI and without contraindications should receive within the first day of hospitalization, and preferably in the emergency department, are intranasal oxygen (if oxygen saturation is low), sublingual (SL) nitroglycerin (NTG), aspirin (ASA), a P2Y$_{12}$ inhibitor (clopidogrel, prasugrel, or ticagrelor depending on reperfusion strategy), and anticoagulation with bivalirudin, unfractionated heparin (UFH), or enoxaparin (agent dependent on reperfusion strategy). A glycoprotein (GP) IIb/IIIa inhibitor should be administered with UFH for patients undergoing primary PCI. IV β-blockers and IV NTG should be given in selected patients. Oral β-blockers should be initiated within the first day in patients without cardiogenic shock.

❼ In the absence of contraindications, all patients with NSTE ACS should be treated in the emergency department with intranasal oxygen (if oxygen saturation is low), SL NTG, ASA, and an anticoagulant, either UFH, enoxaparin, fondaparinux or bivalirudin. High-risk patients should proceed to early angiography and may receive a GP IIb/IIIa inhibitor. A $P2Y_{12}$ inhibitor (selection of agent and timing of initiation dependent upon selection of an interventional approach involving PCI or CABG surgery versus a noninterventional approach with medical management alone) should be administered to all patients. IV β-blockers and IV NTG should be given in selected patients. Oral β-blockers should be initiated within the first day in patients without cardiogenic shock.

❽ Secondary prevention guidelines from the ACCF/AHA suggest that following MI from either STE MI or NSTE ACS, all patients, in the absence of contraindications, should receive indefinite treatment with ASA, a β-blocker, and an angiotensin-converting enzyme (ACE) inhibitor for secondary prevention of death, stroke, or recurrent infarction. Most patients will receive a statin to reduce low-density lipoprotein cholesterol to less than 100 mg/dL (2.59 mmol/L) and ideally to less than 70 mg/dL (1.81 mmol/L). A $P2Y_{12}$ inhibitor should be continued for at least 12 months for patients undergoing PCI and for patients with NSTE ACS receiving a medical management strategy of treatment. Clopidogrel should be continued for at least 14 days in patients with STE MI not undergoing PCI. An angiotensin II receptor blocker and a mineralocorticoid receptor antagonist should be given to selected patients. For all patients with ACS, treatment and control of modifiable risk factors such as hypertension (HTN), dyslipidemia, obesity, smoking, and diabetes mellitus are essential.

❾ To determine the efficacy of nonpharmacologic treatments and pharmacotherapy, monitor patients for relief of ischemic discomfort, return of ECG changes to baseline, and absence or resolution of heart failure signs and symptoms. The most common adverse effects from pharmacotherapy of ACS are bleeding and hypotension.

INTRODUCTION

Cardiovascular disease (CVD) is the leading cause of death in the United States and one of the major causes of death worldwide. Acute coronary syndromes (ACSs), including unstable angina (UA) and myocardial infarction (MI), are a form of coronary heart disease (CHD) that comprises the most common cause of CVD death. **❶** *The cause of an ACS is primarily the rupture of an atherosclerotic plaque with subsequent platelet adherence, activation, and aggregation, and the activation of the clotting cascade. Ultimately, a clot*

forms composed of fibrin and platelets. **❷** *The American Heart Association (AHA) and the American College of Cardiology Foundation (ACCF) recommend strategies, or guidelines, for ACS patient care for ST-segment elevation (STE) and non-ST-segment elevation (NSTE) ACS. In collaboration with the Society for Cardiovascular Angiography and Interventions (SCAI), the ACCF and AHA issue joint guidelines for percutaneous coronary intervention (PCI), including PCI in the setting of ACS. These practice guidelines are based on a review of available clinical evidence, have graded recommendations based on evidence and expert opinion, and are updated periodically. These guidelines form the cornerstone for quality care of the ACS patient.*[2–8]

EPIDEMIOLOGY

Each year, more than 1.1 million Americans experience an ACS, and 150,000 die of an MI.[1] In the United States, more than 7 million living persons have survived an MI.[1]

CVDs are the leading cause of hospitalization in the United States, resulting in about 6.2 million hospital discharges per year. Each year, there are more than 1.3 million MIs, and one in six deaths is secondary to CHD.[1]

The proportion of patients with MI presenting with STE MI compared with NSTE MI decreased from approximately 80% in the early 1990s to 30% currently.[1] This may be secondary to the use of the more sensitive biomarker troponin (increasing the diagnosis of MI in the NSTE ACS group), greater use of antecedent revascularization procedures, decreased reinfarction from enhanced medical therapy after an initial event, or prevention of progression of unstable angina to MI through more effective anticoagulant and antiplatelet therapy.

According to data from the National Registry of Myocardial Infarction, in-hospital mortality has decreased by more than 20% during the past 20 years. Improvements in care that may have contributed to this mortality reduction include greater use of guideline-recommended drugs (e.g., aspirin [ASA], β-blockers, angiotensin-converting enzyme [ACE] inhibitors and angiotensin receptor blockers [ARBs], statins, clopidogrel); reductions in the median door-to-needle time for administering fibrinolytics and in the corresponding door-to-balloon time for primary PCI; and increased use of early coronary angiography and PCI for high-risk patients with NSTE ACS.[1]

In patients with STE MI, in-hospital death rates are approximately 3% in patients receiving primary PCI, 7% for patients who are treated with fibrinolytics and 16% for patients who do not receive reperfusion therapy. In patients with NSTE MI, in-hospital mortality is less than 5%. At 6 months and 1 year, mortality and reinfarction rates are similar between STE and NSTE MI.[9,10] Other than persistent ST-segment changes and troponin, other predictors of in-hospital mortality include older age, elevated serum creatinine, tachycardia, and heart failure (HF).[11]

CHD is the leading cause of premature, chronic disability in the United States. The risks of CHD events, such as death, recurrent MI, and stroke, are higher for patients with established CHD and a history of MI than for patients with no known CHD. The cost of CHD is high, with estimated direct and indirect costs of more than $177 billion.[10] The estimated cost of hospitalization for MI is $14,000, and the median length of hospital stay is 3.2 days.[12] Risk-standardized hospital mortality for MI as well as 30-day hospital readmission rates following MI and PCI are quality performance measures and Outcome of Care Measures that are publicly reportable by the Center for Medicare and Medicaid Services.[12] The Patient Protection and Affordable Care Act of 2010 links quality performance measures to hospital reimbursement.

ETIOLOGY

Endothelial dysfunction, inflammation, and the formation of fatty streaks contribute to the formation of atherosclerotic coronary artery plaques, the underlying cause of coronary artery disease (CAD).[13] ❶ *The predominant cause of ACS in more than 90% of patients is atheromatous plaque rupture, fissuring, or erosion of an unstable atherosclerotic plaque that* *occludes less than 50% of the coronary lumen prior to the event, rather than a more stable 70% to 90% stenosis of the coronary artery.*[14] Stable stenoses are characteristic of stable angina.

PATHOPHYSIOLOGY

Spectrum of ACSs

ACSs include all clinical syndromes compatible with acute MI resulting from an imbalance between myocardial oxygen demand and supply. In contrast to stable angina, an ACS results primarily from diminished myocardial blood flow secondary to an occlusive or partially occlusive coronary artery thrombus. ACSs are classified according to electrocardiogram (ECG) changes into STE MI or NSTE ACS (NSTE MI and UA) (Fig. 8–1).[15] An STE MI, formerly known as Q-wave or transmural MI, typically results in an injury that transects the thickness of the myocardial wall. Following an STE MI, pathological Q waves are frequently

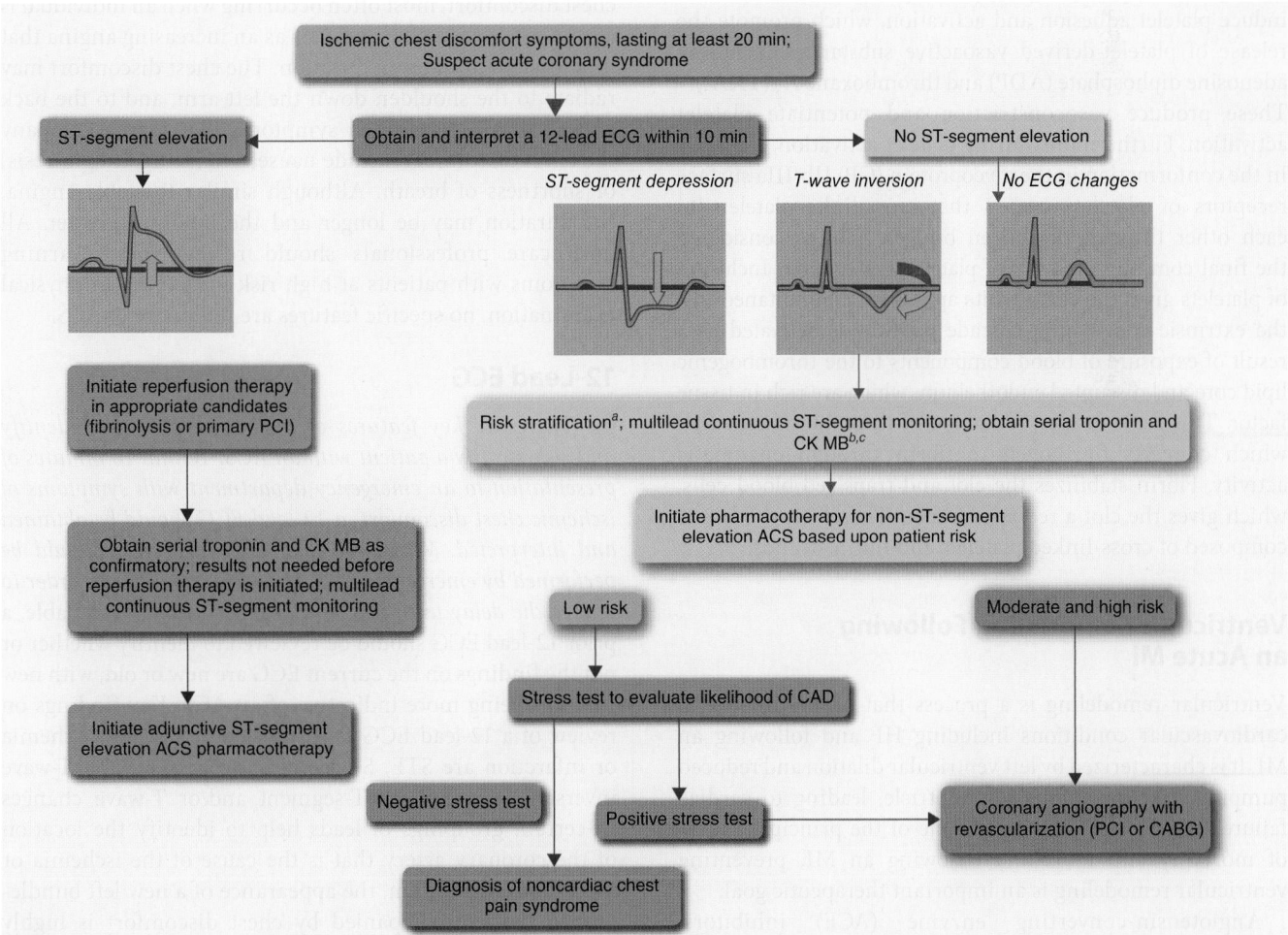

FIGURE 8–1. Evaluation of the acute coronary syndrome patient. *a*As described in Table 8–1. *b*"Positive": Above the myocardial infarction decision limit. *c*"Negative": Below the myocardial infarction decision limit. (ACS, acute coronary syndrome; CABG, coronary artery bypass graft; CAD, coronary artery disease; CK MB, creatine kinase myocardial band; ECG, electrocardiogram; PCI, percutaneous coronary intervention. Refer to Figure 9–2 for further details regarding ECG interpretation.) (Modified with permission from Spinler SA. Evolution of antithrombotic therapy used in acute coronary syndromes. In: Richardson MM, Chant C, Cheng JWM, et al., eds. Pharmacotherapy self-assessment program, 7th ed. Book 1: Cardiology. Lenexa, KS: American College of Clinical Pharmacy, 2010.)

seen on the ECG, indicating transmural MI, whereas such an ECG manifestation is seen less commonly in patients with NSTE MI.[5] Non-ST-segment elevation MI, formerly known as non-Q-wave or nontransmural MI, is limited to the subendocardial myocardium. Patients in this case do not usually develop a pathological Q wave on the ECG. Moreover, an NSTE MI is smaller and not as extensive as an STE MI. Non-ST-segment elevation MI differs from UA in that ischemia is severe enough to produce myocardial necrosis resulting in the release of a detectable amount of biomarkers, mainly troponins T or I, but also creatine kinase (CK) myocardial band (MB), from the necrotic myocytes in the bloodstream. The clinical significance of serum markers is discussed in greater detail in later sections of this chapter.

Plaque Rupture and Clot Formation

● Following plaque rupture, a clot (a partially or completely occlusive thrombus) forms on top of the ruptured plaque. The thrombogenic contents of the plaque are exposed to blood elements. Exposure of collagen and tissue factor induce platelet adhesion and activation, which promote the release of platelet-derived vasoactive substances including adenosine diphosphate (ADP) and thromboxane A_2 (TXA_2).[13] These produce vasoconstriction and potentiate platelet activation. Furthermore, during platelet activation, a change in the conformation in the glycoprotein (GP) IIb/IIIa surface receptors of platelets occurs that cross-links platelets to each other through fibrinogen bridges. This is considered the final common pathway of platelet aggregation. Inclusion of platelets gives the clot a white appearance. Simultaneously, the extrinsic coagulation cascade pathway is activated as a result of exposure of blood components to the thrombogenic lipid core and disrupted endothelium, which are rich in tissue factor. This leads to the production of thrombin (factor IIa), which converts fibrinogen to fibrin through enzymatic activity. Fibrin stabilizes the clot and traps red blood cells, which gives the clot a red appearance. Therefore, the clot is composed of cross-linked platelets and fibrin strands.[14,16]

Ventricular Remodeling Following an Acute MI

Ventricular remodeling is a process that occurs in several cardiovascular conditions including HF and following an MI. It is characterized by left ventricular dilation and reduced pumping function of the left ventricle, leading to cardiac failure.[17] Because HF represents one of the principal causes of mortality and morbidity following an MI, preventing ventricular remodeling is an important therapeutic goal.

Angiotensin-converting enzyme (ACE) inhibitors, angiotensin receptor blockers (ARBs), β-blockers, and mineralocorticoid receptor antagonists are all agents that slow down or reverse ventricular remodeling through inhibition of the renin-angiotensin aldosterone system and/or through improvement in hemodynamics (decreasing preload or afterload).[17] These agents also improve survival and are discussed in more detail in subsequent sections of this chapter.

Complications

This chapter focuses on management of the uncomplicated ACS patient. However, it is important for clinicians to recognize complications of MI because MI is associated with increased mortality. The most serious complication of MI is cardiogenic shock, occurring in approximately 5% to 6% of hospitalized patients presenting with STE MI.[18] Mortality in cardiogenic shock patients with MI is high, approaching 60%.[19] Other complications that may result from MI are HF, valvular dysfunction, bradycardia, heart block, pericarditis, stroke secondary to left ventricular thrombus embolization, venous thromboembolism, left ventricular free wall rupture, and ventricular and atrial tachyarrhythmias.[20] In fact, more than a quarter of MI patients die, presumably from ventricular fibrillation, prior to reaching the hospital.[1]

Symptoms and Physical Examination Findings

The classic symptom of an ACS is midline anterior anginal chest discomfort, most often occurring when an individual is at rest, as a severe new onset, or as an increasing angina that is at least 20 minutes in duration. The chest discomfort may radiate to the shoulder, down the left arm, and to the back or to the jaw. Associated symptoms that may accompany the chest discomfort include nausea, vomiting, diaphoresis, or shortness of breath. Although similar to stable angina, the duration may be longer and the intensity greater. All healthcare professionals should review these warning symptoms with patients at high risk for CHD. On physical examination, no specific features are indicative of ACS.

12-Lead ECG

❸ *There are key features of a 12-lead ECG that identify and risk-stratify a patient with an ACS. Within 10 minutes of presentation to an emergency department with symptoms of ischemic chest discomfort, a 12-lead ECG should be obtained and interpreted. When possible, a 12-lead ECG should be performed by emergency medical system providers in order to reduce the delay until myocardial reperfusion.* If available, a prior 12-lead ECG should be reviewed to identify whether or not the findings on the current ECG are new or old, with new findings being more indicative of an ACS. Key findings on review of a 12-lead ECG that indicate myocardial ischemia or infarction are STE, ST-segment depression, and T-wave inversion (Fig. 8–1).[15] ST-segment and/or T-wave changes in certain groupings of leads help to identify the location of the coronary artery that is the cause of the ischemia or infarction. In addition, the appearance of a new left bundle-branch block accompanied by chest discomfort is highly specific for acute MI. About one-half of patients diagnosed with MI present with STE on their ECG, with the remainder having ST-segment depression, T-wave inversion, or, in some instances, no ECG changes. Some parts of the heart are more "electrically silent" than others, and myocardial ischemia may not be detected on a surface ECG. Therefore, it is important to review findings from the ECG in conjunction

Clinical Presentation and Diagnosis of ACSs

General

- The patient is typically in acute distress and may develop or present with acute heart failure, cardiogenic shock, or cardiac arrest.

Symptoms

- The classic symptom of ACS is midline anterior chest discomfort. Accompanying symptoms may include arm, back, or jaw pain, nausea, vomiting, or shortness of breath.
- Patients less likely to present with classic symptoms include elderly patients, diabetic patients, and women.

Signs

- No signs are classic for ACS.
- Patients with ACS may present with signs of acute heart failure including jugular venous distention and an S_3 sound on auscultation.
- Patients may also present with arrhythmias and therefore may have tachycardia, bradycardia, or heart block.

Laboratory Tests

- Troponin I or T and CK-MB are measured at the time of first assessment and repeated at least once, 6 to 9 hours later to ascertain heart muscle damage, confirmatory for the diagnosis of infarction. For patients with non-ST-segment elevation ACS, an elevated troponin is diagnostic for MI, defining a NSTE MI. Patients presenting with suspected NSTE ACS who do not have an MI undergo further diagnostic testing to determine whether or not they have unstable angina or do not have ACS.
- Blood chemistry tests are performed with particular attention given to potassium and magnesium, which may affect heart rhythm.

- Serum creatinine is measured and creatinine clearance is used to identify patients who may need dosing adjustments for some medications, as well as those who are at high risk of morbidity and mortality.
- Baseline complete blood count (CBC) and coagulation tests (activated partial thromboplastin time [aPTT] and international normalized ratio [INR]) should be obtained because most patients will receive antithrombotic therapy that increases the risk for bleeding.
- Fasting lipid panel (optional).

Other Diagnostic Tests

- The 12-lead ECG is the first step in management. Patients are risk stratified into two groups: ST-segment elevation ACS and suspected non-ST-segment elevation ACS.
- High-risk ACS patients and those with recurrent chest discomfort will undergo coronary angiography via a left heart catheterization and injection of contrast dye into the coronary arteries to determine the presence and extent of coronary artery stenosis.
- During hospitalization, a measurement of left ventricular function, such as an echocardiogram, is performed to identify patients with low ejection fractions (less than 40%) who are at high risk of death following hospital discharge.
- Selected low-risk patients may undergo early stress testing.

With permission from Spinler SA, de Denus S. Acute coronary syndromes. In: DiPiro JT, Talbert RL, Yee GC, et al., eds. Pharmacotherapy: A Pathophysiologic Approach, 8th ed. New York, NY: McGraw-Hill, 2011:244.

with biochemical markers of myocardial necrosis, such as troponin I or T, and other risk factors for CHD to determine the patient's risk for experiencing a new MI or having other complications.

Biochemical Markers/Cardiac Enzymes

Biochemical markers of myocardial cell death are important for confirming the diagnosis of MI. ❸ *The diagnosis of MI is confirmed when the following conditions are met in a clinical setting consistent with myocardial ischemia: "Detection of a rise and/or fall of cardiac biomarkers (troponin preferred) with at least one value above the 99th percentile of the upper reference limit together with evidence of myocardial ischemia as recognized by at least one of the following: (a) symptoms of ischemia; (b) ECG changes of new ischemia or development of pathological Q waves; or (c) imaging evidence of new loss of viable myocardium or* new regional wall motion abnormality."[21] Typically, a blood sample is obtained once in the emergency department, then 6 to 9 hours later, and in patients at a high suspicion of MI but in whom previous measurements did not reveal elevations in biomarkers, 12 to 24 hours after. A single measurement of a biochemical marker is not adequate to exclude a diagnosis of MI, as up to 15% of values that were initially below the level of detection (a "negative" test) rise to the level of detection (a "positive" test) in subsequent hours. While troponins and CK-MB appear in the blood within 6 hours of infarction, troponins stay elevated for up to 10 days while CK-MB returns to normal values within 48 hours. Hence, traditionally, CK-MB was used to detect reinfarction. However, more recent data have suggested that troponins provide similar information to CK-MB in such a situation that has led to the use of troponins in this setting as well. Current guidelines suggest that, in patients in whom a recurrent MI is suspected, a cardiac biomarker should be immediately measured, followed by a second measurement 3 to 6 hours later. A recurrent MI is diagnosed when there is an increase of at least 20% in the second measurement of the biomarker, if this value exceeds the 99th percentile of the upper reference limit.[21]

Risk Stratification

Patient symptoms, past medical history, ECG, and biomarkers, particularly troponins, are utilized to stratify patients into low, medium, or high risk of death, MI, or likelihood of failing pharmacotherapy and needing urgent coronary angiography and PCI (Table 8–1). Initial treatment according to risk stratification is depicted in Figure 8–1.[4] Patients with STE MI are at the highest risk of death. Initial treatment of STE MI should proceed without evaluation of the troponins because these patients have a greater than 97% chance of having an MI subsequently diagnosed with biochemical markers. The ACCF/AHA define a target time to initiate reperfusion treatment as within 30 minutes of hospital presentation for fibrinolytics (e.g., streptokinase, alteplase, reteplase, and tenecteplase) and within 90 minutes or less from presentation for primary PCI.[8] The sooner the infarct-related coronary artery is opened for these patients, the lower their mortality and the greater the amount of myocardium that is preserved.[22,23] Although all patients should be evaluated

---

Table 8–1

Risk Stratification for Acute Coronary Syndromes[5]

TIMI Risk Score for NSTE ACSs

One point is assigned for each of the seven medical history and clinical presentation findings. The point total is calculated, and the patient is assigned a risk for experiencing the composite endpoint of death, myocardial infarction, or urgent need for revascularization as follows:

- Age 65 years or older
- Three or more CHD risk factors: smoking, hypercholesterolemia, hypertension, diabetes mellitus, family history of premature CHD death/events
- Known CAD (50% or greater stenosis of at least one major coronary artery on coronary angiogram)
- Aspirin use within the past 7 days
- Two or more episodes of chest discomfort within the past 24 hours
- ST-segment depression 0.5 mm or greater
- Positive biochemical marker for infarction

High-Risk	**Medium-Risk**	**Low-Risk**
TIMI Risk Score 5–7 points	TIMI Risk Score 3–4 points	TIMI Risk Score 0–2 points

TIMI Risk Score	**Mortality, MI, or Severe Recurrent Ischemia Requiring Urgent Target Vessel Revascularization**
0/1	4.7%
2	8.3%
3	13.2%
4	19.9%
5	26.2%
6/7	40.9%

GRACE Risk Factors for Increased Mortality and the Composite of Death or MI in ACS

Signs and symptoms of heart failure
Low systolic blood pressure
Elevated heart rate
Older age
Elevated serum creatinine
Baseline risk factors on clinical evaluation: cardiac arrest at admission, ST-segment deviation, elevated troponin
A high-risk patient is defined as a GRACE Risk Score more than 140 points.

ACS, acute coronary syndromes; CAD, coronary artery disease; CHD, coronary heart disease; GRACE, Global Registry of Acute Coronary Events; MI, myocardial infarction; NSTE, non-ST-segment elevation; TIMI, Thrombolysis in Myocardial Infarction.

An online calculator for the GRACE Risk Model is available at http://www.outcomes-umassmed.org/GRACE/acs_risk/acs_risk_content.html (Accessed December 1, 2011).

Reproduced from Spinler SA. Evolution of antithrombotic therapy used in acute coronary syndromes. In Richardson MM, Chessman KH, Chant C et al., eds. Pharmacotherapy Assessment Program, 7th ed. Book 1: Cardiology. Lenexa, KS: American College of Clinical Pharmacy, 2010:97–124. With permission from Spinler SA, de Denus S. Acute coronary syndromes. In: DiPiro JT, Talbert RL, Yee GC, et al., eds. Pharmacotherapy: A pathophysiologic approach, 8th ed. New York, NY: McGraw-Hill; 2011:246.

RR is a 65-year-old, 85-kg (187-lb) woman who developed chest heaviness/tightness at 10:15 hours while at her place of employment. Local paramedics were summoned and she was given three 0.4-mg sublingual nitroglycerin tablets by mouth, 325 mg ASA by mouth, and morphine 2-mg IV push without relief of chest discomfort. RR presented to the hospital at 11:00 hours. The hospital has a cardiac catheterization laboratory and primary PCI was selected as a treatment strategy for STE MI.

PMH: Hypertension (HTN) for 18 years; dyslipidemia for 6 years; transient ischemic attack 2 years ago

FH: Father with stroke at age 65; mother with HTN; no siblings

SH: Smoked one pack per day for 30 years, quit 6 years ago

Allergies: NKDA

Meds: Amlodipine 10 mg by mouth once daily; enalapril 5 mg by mouth once daily; ASA 325 mg by mouth once daily; simvastatin 20 mg by mouth once daily at bedtime

ROS: 10/10 chest discomfort/squeezing

PE:

HEENT: Normocephalic atraumatic

CV: Regular rate and rhythm S_1, S_2, $-S_3$, $-S_4$, no murmurs or rubs

VS: BP 110/70 mm Hg; HR 98 bpm; T 37°C (98.6°F)

Lungs: Clear to auscultation and percussion

Abd: Nontender, nondistended

GI: Normal bowel sounds

GU: Stool guaiac negative

Exts: No bruits, pulses 2+, femoral pulse present, good range of motion

Neuro: Alert and oriented × 3, cranial nerves intact

Labs: Sodium 138 mEq/L (138 mmol/L), potassium 4.2 mEq/L (4.2 mmol/L), chloride 105 mEq/L (105 mmol/L), bicarbonate 24 mEq/L (24 mmol/L), SCr 1.0 mg/dL (88 μmol/L), glucose 95 mg/dL (5.3 mmol/L), WBC 9.9 × 10³/mm³ (9.9 × 10⁹/L), hemoglobin 15.7 g/dL (157 g/L or 9.7 mmol/L), hematocrit 47% (0.47), platelets 220 × 10³/mm³ (220 × 10⁹/L), troponin I 1.8 ng/mL (1.8 mcg/L), oxygen saturation 99% (0.99) on room air

ECG: Normal sinus rhythm, PR 0.16 seconds, QRS 0.08 seconds, QTc 0.38 seconds, occasional polymorphic premature ventricular contractions, 3 mm ST-segment elevation anterior leads

CXR: No active disease

Echo: Anterior wall dyskinesis, LVEF 45% (0.45)

What information is suggestive of acute MI?

Are any complications of MI present?

Identify your acute treatment goals for RR.

What adjunctive pharmacotherapy should be administered to RR in the emergency department prior to proceeding to the cardiac catheterization laboratory?

What additional pharmacotherapy should be initiated on the first day of RR's hospitalization following successful PCI/intracoronary stenting?

for reperfusion therapy, not all patients may be eligible. Indications and contraindications for fibrinolytic therapy are described in the treatment section of this chapter. Less than 25% of hospitals in the United States are equipped to perform primary PCI. If patients are not eligible for reperfusion therapy, additional pharmacotherapy for STE patients should be initiated in the emergency department and the patient transferred to a coronary intensive care unit. The typical length of stay for a patient with uncomplicated STE MI is less than 4 days.[24]

Risk-stratification of the patient with NSTE ACS is more complex because in-hospital outcomes for this group of patients varies with reported rates of death of 0% to 12%, reinfarction rates of 0% to 3%, and recurrent severe ischemia rates of 5% to 20%.[22] Not all patients presenting with suspected NSTE ACS have CAD. Some eventually are diagnosed with nonischemic chest discomfort. In general, among NSTE patients, those with ST-segment depression (Fig. 8–1)[15] and/or elevated biomarkers are at higher risk of death or recurrent infarction.

TREATMENT

Desired Outcomes

Short-term desired outcomes in a patient with ACS are (a) early restoration of blood flow to the infarct-related artery to prevent infarct expansion (in the case of MI) or prevent complete occlusion and MI (in UA); (b) prevention of death and other MI complications; (c) prevention of coronary artery reocclusion; and as evidence of restoration of coronary artery blood flow; (d) relief of ischemic chest discomfort; and (e) resolution of ST-segment and T-wave changes on the ECG.

Long-term desired outcomes are control of cardiovascular (CV) risk factors, prevention of additional CV events, including reinfarction, stroke, and HF, and improvement in quality of life.

General Approach to Treatment

Selecting evidence-based therapies described in the ACCF/AHA guidelines for patients without contraindications result in lower mortality.[25–27] General treatment measures for all STE MI and high- and intermediate-risk NSTE ACS patients include admission to hospital, oxygen administration (if oxygen saturation is low, less than 90% [0.90]), continuous

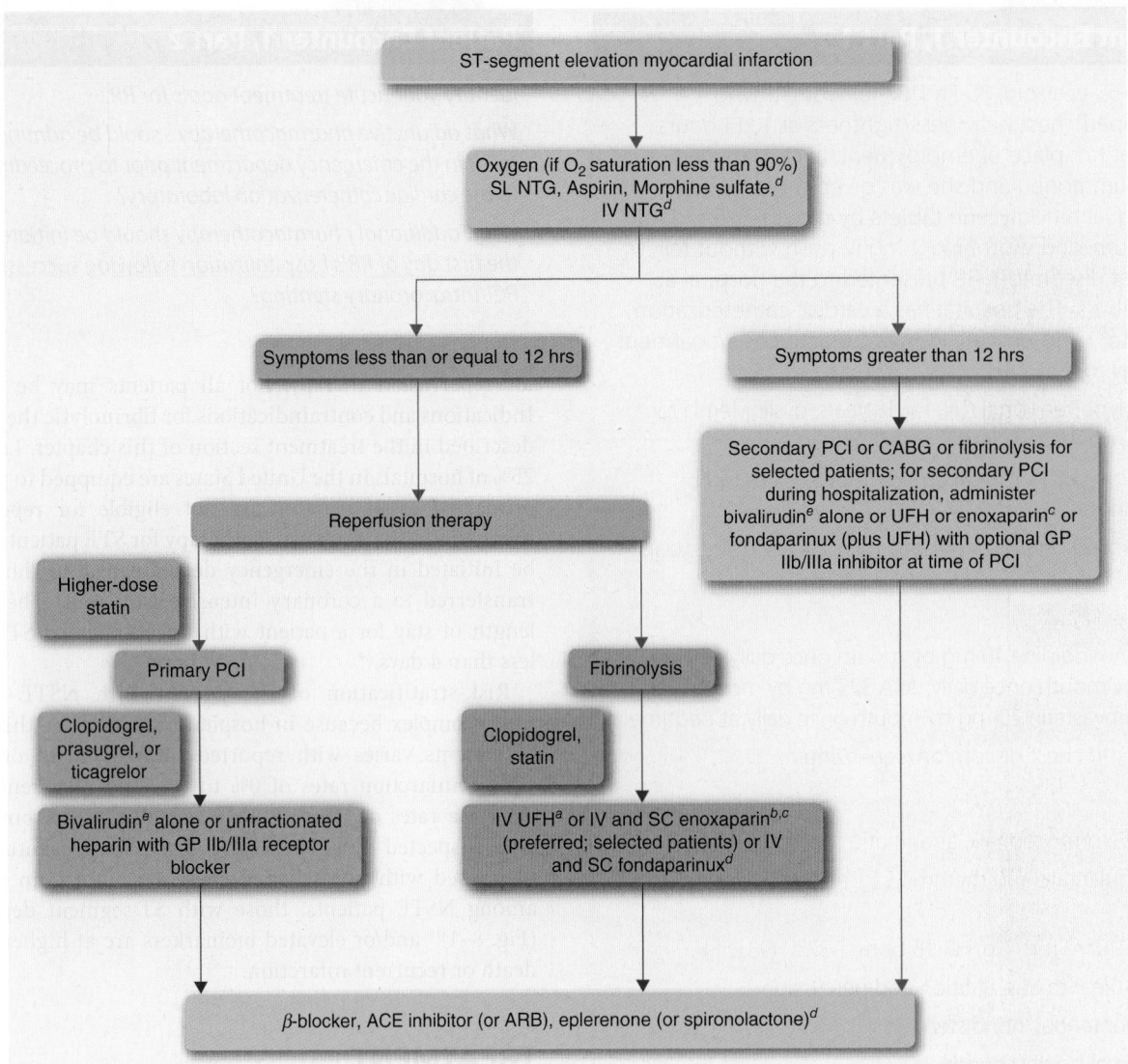

FIGURE 8–2. Initial pharmacotherapy for ST-segment elevation myocardial infarction. [a]For at least 48 hours. [b]See Table 8–2 for dosing and specific types of patients who should not receive enoxaparin. [c]For the duration of hospitalization, up to 8 days. [d]For selected patients, see Table 8–2. [e]If pretreated with UFH, stop UFH infusion for 30 minutes prior to administration of bivalirudin (bolus plus infusion). (ACE, angiotensin-converting enzyme; ARB, angiotensin receptor blocker; CABG, coronary artery bypass graft surgery; GP, glycoprotein; NTG, nitroglycerin; PCI, percutaneous coronary intervention; SC, subcutaneous; SL, sublingual; UFH, unfractionated heparin.) (Modified with permission from Spinler SA. Evolution of antithrombotic therapy used in acute coronary syndromes. In: Richardson MM, Chant C, Cheng JWM, et al., eds. Pharmacotherapy self-assessment program, 7th ed. Book 1: Cardiology. Lenexa, KS: American College of Clinical Pharmacy, 2010.)

multilead ST-segment monitoring for arrhythmias and ischemia, frequent measurement of vital signs, bed rest for 12 hours in hemodynamically stable patients, avoidance of the Valsalva maneuver (prescribe stool softeners routinely), and pain relief (Figs. 8–2 and 8–3).[2–8,28]

Because risk varies and resources are limited, it is important to triage and treat patients according to their risk category. Initial approaches to treatment of STE MI and NSTE ACS patients are outlined in Figure 8–1. Patients with STE are at high risk of death, and efforts to reestablish coronary perfusion, as well as adjunctive pharmacotherapy, should be initiated immediately.

Features identifying low-, moderate-, and high-risk NSTE ACS patients are described in Table 8–1.[29,30]

Nonpharmacologic Therapy

▶ Primary PCI for STE MIs

❹ Early reperfusion therapy with primary PCI of the infarct artery within 90 minutes from time of hospital presentation is the reperfusion treatment of choice for patients presenting with STE MI who present within 12 hours of symptom onset[3,8] (Fig. 8–2). For primary PCI, the patient is taken from the emergency department to the cardiac catheterization laboratory and undergoes coronary angiography with either balloon angioplasty or placement of a bare metal or drug-eluting intracoronary stent in the artery associated with the infarct. About 62% of patients with STE MI are treated with

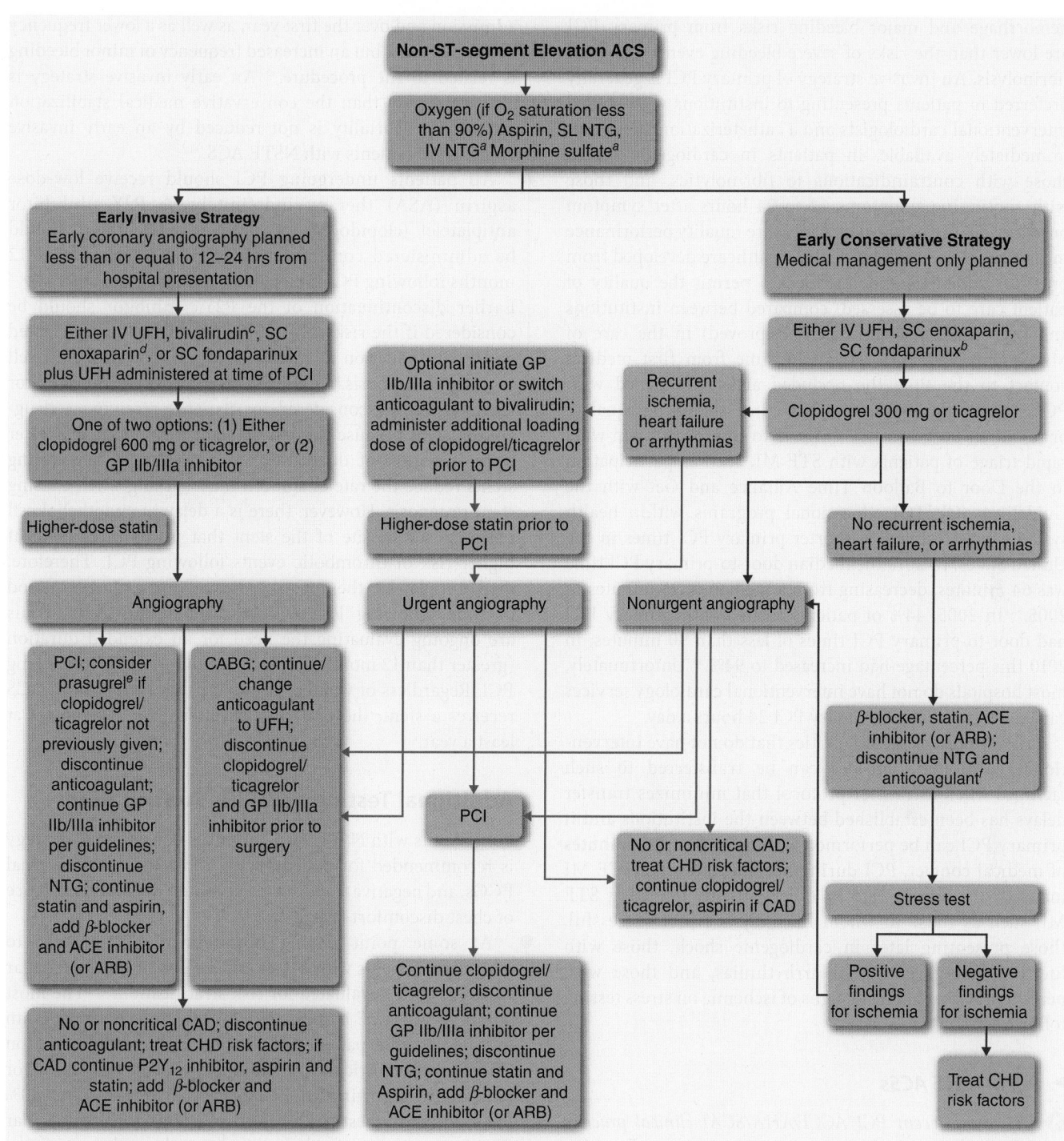

FIGURE 8–3. Initial pharmacotherapy for non-ST-segment elevation ACS. [a]For selected patients, see Table 8–2. [b]Preferred in patients at high risk for bleeding. [c]If pretreated with UFH, stop UFH infusion for 30 minutes prior to administration of bivalirudin bolus plus infusion. [d]May require IV supplemental dose of enoxaparin; see Table 8–2. [e]Do not use if prior history of stroke/transient ischemic attack (TIA), age older than 75 years, or body weight less than or equal to 60 kg. [f]SC enoxaparin or UFH can be continued at a lower dose for venous thromboembolism prophylaxis. (ACS, acute coronary syndrome; ACE, angiotensin-converting enzyme; ARB, angiotensin receptor blocker; CABG, coronary artery bypass graft; CAD, coronary artery disease; CHD, coronary heart disease; GP, glycoprotein; NTG, nitroglycerin; PCI, percutaneous coronary intervention; SC, subcutaneous; SL, sublingual; UFH, unfractionated heparin.)

primary PCI; 18% are treated with fibrinolytics. Results from a meta-analysis of trials comparing fibrinolysis with primary PCI indicate a lower mortality rate with primary PCI.[31] One reason for the superiority of primary PCI compared with

fibrinolysis is that more than 90% of occluded infarct-related coronary arteries are opened with primary PCI compared with fewer than 60% of coronary arteries opened with currently available fibrinolytics.[4,5] In addition, intracranial hemorrhage and major bleeding risks from primary PCI are lower than the risks of severe bleeding events following fibrinolysis. An invasive strategy of primary PCI is generally preferred in patients presenting to institutions with skilled interventional cardiologists and a catheterization laboratory immediately available, in patients in cardiogenic shock, those with contraindications to fibrinolytics, and those with continuing symptoms 12 to 24 hours after symptom onset.[8] A quality performance measure (quality performance measures are measures of quality healthcare developed from practice guidelines and intended to permit the quality of patient care to be assessed, compared between institutions and over time, and ultimately, improved) in the care of MI patients with STE MI is the time from first medical contact to the time the occluded artery is opened with PCI. This "door-to-primary PCI" time should be equal to or less than 90 minutes.[4,32] Efforts to improve system-wide rapid triage of patients with STE MI, such as participation in the Door to Balloon Time Alliance and Get with the Guidelines (GWTG) educational programs within health systems have resulted in shorter primary PCI times in the United States. In 2010 the median door-to-primary PCI time was 64 minutes, decreasing from a median of 96 minutes in 2005.[33] In 2005, 44% of patients treated with primary PCI had door-to-primary PCI times of less than 90 minutes; in 2010 this percentage had increased to 94%.[33] Unfortunately, most hospitals do not have interventional cardiology services capable of performing primary PCI 24 hours a day.

Patients presenting to facilities that do not have interventional cardiology services can be transferred to such facilities when a transfer protocol that minimizes transfer delays has been established between the institutions and if primary PCI can be performed within the first 120 minutes of medical contact. PCI during hospitalization for STE MI may also be appropriate in other patients following STE MI, such as those in whom fibrinolysis is not successful, those presenting later in cardiogenic shock, those with life-threatening ventricular arrhythmias, and those with persistent rest ischemia or signs of ischemia on stress testing following MI.[4,5]

▶ PCI in NSTE ACSs

⑤ *The most recent PCI ACCF/AHA/SCAI clinical practice guidelines recommend coronary angiography with either PCI or coronary artery bypass graft (CABG) surgery revascularization as an early treatment (early invasive strategy) for patients with NSTE ACS at an elevated risk for death or MI, including those with a high risk score (Table 8–1) or patients with refractory angina, acute HF, other symptoms of cardiogenic shock, or arrhythmias (Fig. 8–3).*[8] Several clinical trials support an "invasive" interventional strategy with early angiography and PCI or CABG versus a "conservative medical management" strategy, whereby coronary angiography with revascularization is reserved for patients with symptoms refractory to pharmacotherapy and patients with signs of ischemia on stress testing.[5,34] An early invasive approach results in a lower rate of refractory angina during hospital admission and over the first year, as well as a lower frequency of MI at 5 years, but an increased frequency of minor bleeding is related to the procedure.[35] An early invasive strategy is also less costly than the conservative medical stabilization approach.[34] Mortality is not reduced by an early invasive approach in patients with NSTE ACS.[34]

● All patients undergoing PCI should receive low-dose aspirin (ASA) therapy indefinitely. A $P2Y_{12}$ inhibitor antiplatelet (clopidogrel, prasugrel, or ticagrelor) should be administered concomitantly with ASA for at least 12 months following PCI for a patient with ACS (Table 8–2).[2–8] Earlier discontinuation of the $P2Y_{12}$ inhibitor should be considered if the risk of bleeding outweighs the anticipated benefit in reduction in risk of death, MI, or stroke as well as stent thrombosis.[8] A longer duration of $P2Y_{12}$ inhibitor therapy may be considered for patients receiving a drug-eluting stent because the risk of stent thrombosis is greater upon cessation of dual antiplatelet therapy.[8] Drug-eluting stents reduce the rate of smooth muscle cell growth causing stent restenosis. However, there is a delay in endothelial cell regrowth at the site of the stent that places the patient at higher risk of thrombotic events following PCI. Therefore, dual antiplatelet therapy is indicated for a longer period of time following PCI with a drug-eluting stent. Trials are ongoing evaluating the need for an extended duration (greater than 12 months) of $P2Y_{12}$ inhibitor therapy following PCI. Regardless of whether or not a patient with NSTE ACS receives a stent, the preferred duration $P2Y_{12}$ therapy is at least a year.[2]

Additional Testing and Risk Stratification

For patients with NSTE ACS, an initial conservative strategy is recommended for patients with a low risk score, normal ECGs, and negative troponin tests who are without recurrence of chest discomfort (Fig. 8–3).[6]

● At some point during hospitalization but prior to discharge, patients with MI should have their left ventricular function (LVF) evaluated for risk stratification.[4,32] The most common way LVF is measured is using an echocardiogram to calculate the patient's left ventricular ejection fraction (LVEF). Left ventricular function is the single best predictor of mortality following MI. Patients with LVEFs less than 40% (0.40) are at highest risk of death. Patients with ventricular fibrillation or sustained ventricular tachycardia occurring more than 2 days following MI and those with LVEF less than 30% (0.30; measured at least 1 month after STE MI and 3 months after coronary artery revascularization with either PCI or CABG) benefit from placement of an implantable cardioverter defibrillator (ICD).[36]

● Predischarge from the hospital, stress testing (Fig. 8–3) is indicated in patients with NSTE ACS where an initial conservative strategy is selected and for patients with STE MI where primary PCI was not performed and there has been no recurrent ischemia.[6,8] Following the stress test, patients deemed not at low risk should undergo left heart catheterization with coronary angiography and revascularization as indicated by the results.[6] Patients

Table 8-2

Evidence-Based Pharmacotherapy for ST-Segment Elevation Myocardial Infarction and Non-ST-Segment Elevation Acute Coronary Syndrome[2-8,46]

Drug	Clinical Condition and ACCF/AHA/ SCAI Guideline Recommendation[a]	Contraindications[b]	Dose and Duration of Therapy
Aspirin	STE MI, class I recommendation for all patients. NSTE ACS, class I recommendation for all patients.	Hypersensitivity, active bleeding, severe bleeding risk	160–325 mg orally once on hospital day 1. 75–162 mg once daily orally starting hospital day 2 and continued indefinitely in all patients. Limit dose to less than 100 mg if using ticagrelor.
Clopidogrel	NSTE ACS, class I recommendation added to aspirin. STE MI, class I recommendation added to aspirin. PCI in STE and NSTE ACS, class I recommendation. In patients with aspirin allergy, class I recommendation.	Hypersensitivity, active bleeding, severe bleeding risk	300 mg (class I recommendation) to 600 mg (class IIa recommendation) oral loading dose on hospital day 1 followed by a maintenance dose of 75 mg once daily starting on hospital day 2 in patients with NSTE ACS. 300 mg oral loading dose followed by 75 mg orally daily in patients receiving a fibrinolytic or who do not receive reperfusion therapy with a STE MI, avoid loading dose in patients 75 years or older. 600 mg (class I recommendation) loading dose before or when PCI performed (unless within 24 hours of fibrinolytic therapy, a dose of 300 mg should be given). Discontinue at least 5 days before CABG surgery if bleeding risk outweighs benefit (class I recommendation). Administer indefinitely in patients with aspirin allergy (class I recommendation). Continue for at least 12 months (class I recommendation) and possibly beyond 12 months (class IIb recommendation) in patients with ACS managed with PCI/stent. In patients with NSTE ACS treated medically, administer for 1 month and ideally for 1 year (class I recommendation). In patients receiving a fibrinolytic or who do not receive reperfusion therapy, administer for at least 14 days (class I recommendation) and up to 1 year (class IIa recommendation). Genetic testing might be considered to identify patients at high risk of poor response (class IIb recommendation). In these patients, an alternative P2Y$_{12}$ inhibitor might be considered (class IIb recommendation). The routine use of genetic testing is not recommended (class III recommendation).
Prasugrel	PCI in STE and NSTE ACS, added to aspirin, class I recommendation.	Active bleeding, prior stroke or TIA	Initiate in patients with known coronary artery anatomy only (so as to avoid use in patients needing CABG surgery; class I recommendation). Give no later than 1 hour after PCI. Patients who have history of prior stroke or TIA or are 75 years of age or more or weigh less than 60 kg (132 lb) have higher risk of bleeding and no added benefit compared with clopidogrel. 60 mg oral loading dose followed by 10 mg once daily for patients weighing 60 kg (132 lb) or more. 60-mg oral loading dose followed by 5 mg once daily in patients weighing less than 60 kg (132 lb) (based on limited data). Discontinue at least 7 days prior to CABG surgery if bleeding risk outweighs benefit (class I recommendation). Continue for at least 12 months (class I recommendation) and possibly beyond 12 months (class IIb recommendation) in patients with ACS managed with PCI/stent.

(Continued)

Table 8-2

Evidence-Based Pharmacotherapy for ST-Segment Elevation Myocardial Infarction and Non-ST-Segment Elevation Acute Coronary Syndrome[2–8,46] (Continued)

Drug	Clinical Condition and ACCF/AHA/SCAI Guideline Recommendation[a]	Contraindications[b]	Dose and Duration of Therapy
Ticagrelor	PCI in STE and NSTE ACS, added to aspirin, class I recommendation.	Active bleeding	180 mg (class I recommendation) oral loading dose in patients undergoing PCI, followed by 90 mg twice daily for at least 12 months (class I recommendation) and possibly beyond 12 months (class IIb recommendation) in patients with ACS managed with PCI/stent. Although not included in 2011 NSTE ACS guidelines, may also be used in medically managed patients with NTSE ACS. Current data are too limited to recommend use in patients with STE MI not undergoing primary PCI. Discontinue at least 5 days prior to CABG surgery if bleeding risk outweighs benefit (class I recommendation).
Unfractionated heparin	STE MI, class I recommendation in patients undergoing PCI and for those patients treated with fibrinolytics; class IIa recommendation for patients not treated with fibrinolytic therapy. NSTE ACS, class I recommendation in combination with antiplatelet therapy for conservative or invasive approach PCI, class I recommendation (NSTE ACS and STE MI).	Active bleeding, history of heparin-induced thrombocytopenia, severe bleeding risk, recent stroke	For STE MI with fibrinolytics, administer 60 Units/kg IV bolus (maximum 4000 Units) heparin followed by a constant IV infusion at 12 Units/kg/hr (maximum 1000 Units/hr). For STE MI primary PCI, administer 50–70 Units/kg IV bolus if a GP IIb/IIIa inhibitor planned; 70–100 Units/kg IV bolus if no GP IIb/IIIa inhibitor planned and supplement with IV bolus doses to maintain target ACT. For NSTE ACS, administer 60 Units/kg IV bolus (maximum 4000 Units) followed by a constant IV infusion at 12 Units/kg/hr (maximum 1000 Units/hr). Titrated to maintain an aPTT of 1.5 to 2.0 times control (approximately 50–70 seconds) for STE MI with fibrinolytics and for NSTE ACS. Titrated to ACT of 250–350 seconds for primary PCI without a concomitant GP IIb/IIIa inhibitor and 200–250 seconds in patients given a concomitant GP IIb/IIIa inhibitor. The first aPTT should be measured at 4–6 hours for NSTE ACS and STE ACS in patients not treated with fibrinolytics or undergoing primary PCI. The first aPTT should be measured at 3 hours in patients with STE ACS who are treated with fibrinolytics. Continue for 48 hours or until the end of PCI.
Enoxaparin	STE MI class I recommendation in patients receiving fibrinolytics and class IIa for patients not undergoing reperfusion therapy. NSTE ACS, class I recommendation in combination with aspirin for conservative or invasive approach. For PCI, class IIa recommendation as an alternative to UFH in patients with NSTE ACS. For primary PCI in STE MI, class IIb recommendation as an alternative to UFH.	Active bleeding, history of heparin-induced thrombocytopenia, severe bleeding risk, recent stroke, avoid enoxaparin if CrCl less than 15 mL/min (less than 0.25 mL/s), avoid if CABG surgery planned	Enoxaparin 1 mg/kg SC every 12 hours for patients with NSTE ACS (CrCl greater than or equal to 30 mL/min [greater than or equal to 0.50 mL/s]). Enoxaparin 1 mg/kg SC every 24 hours (CrCl 15–29 mL/min [0.25–0.49 mL/s]) for NSTE or STE MI. For all patients undergoing PCI following initiation of SC enoxaparin for NSTE ACS, a supplemental 0.3 mg/kg IV dose of enoxaparin should be administered at the time of PCI if the last dose of SC enoxaparin was given 8–12 hours prior to PCI or who received less than two therapeutic SC doses.

For patients with STE MI receiving fibrinolytics:

- Age less than 75 years: Administer enoxaparin 30 mg IV bolus followed immediately by 1 mg/kg.
  SC every 12 hours (first two doses administer maximum of 100 mg for patients weighing more than 100 kg).
- Age greater than or equal to 75 years: Administer enoxaparin 0.75 mg/kg SC every 12 hours (first two doses administer maximum of 75 mg for patients weighing more than 75 kg).

Continue throughout hospitalization or up to 8 days for STE MI.
Continue for 24–48 hours for NSTE ACS or until the end of PCI for NSTE MI.
Discontinue at least 12–24 hours after CABG surgery.

Drug	Dosing	Precautions/Contraindications	Recommendation
Bivalirudin	For NSTE ACS, administer 0.1 mg/kg IV bolus followed by 0.25 mg/kg/hr infusion. For PCI in NSTE ACS, administer a second bolus of 0.5 mg/kg IV and increase infusion rate to 1.75 mg/kg/hr. For PCI in STE MI, administer 0.75 mg/kg IV bolus followed by 1.75 mg/kg/hr infusion. If prior UFH given, discontinue UFH and wait 30 minutes before initiating bivalirudin. Dosage adjustment for renal failure: None required in the HORIZONS-AMI trial. Discontinue at end of PCI or continue at 0.25 mg/kg/hr if prolonged anticoagulation necessary. Lower bleeding rates are mitigated when administered with a glycoprotein IIb/IIIa inhibitor. Clopidogrel should be administered at least 6 hours before if a glycoprotein IIb/IIIa inhibitor is not used. Discontinue at least 3 hours prior to CABG surgery.	Active bleeding, severe bleeding risk	NSTE ACS class I recommendation for invasive strategy. PCI in STE MI (Class I recommendation).
Fondaparinux	For STE MI, 2.5 mg IV bolus followed by 2.5 mg SC once daily starting on hospital day 2. For NSTE ACS, 2.5 mg SC once daily. Continue until hospital discharge or up to 8 days. For PCI, give additional 85 Units/kg IV without and 60 Units/kg IV with GP IIb/IIIa inhibitor. Discontinue at least 24 hours prior to CABG surgery.	Active bleeding, severe bleeding risk, SCr greater than or equal to 3.0 mg/dL (greater than or equal to 265 μmol/L) or CrCl less than 30 mL/min (less than 0.50 mL/s)	STE MI class I recommendation receiving fibrinolytics and IIa for patients not undergoing reperfusion therapy. NSTE ACS class I recommendation for invasive or conservative approach. Class III as sole agent in PCI.
Fibrinolytic therapy	Streptokinase: 1.5 MU IV over 60 minutes. Alteplase: 15 mg IV bolus followed by 0.75 mg/kg IV over 30 minutes (maximum 50 mg) followed by 0.5 mg/kg (max 35 mg) over 60 minutes (maximum dose 100 mg). Reteplase: 10 Units IV × 2, 30 minutes apart. Tenecteplase: - Less than 60 kg (less than 132 lb), 30 mg IV bolus - 60–69.9 kg (132–153 lb), 35 mg IV bolus - 70–80 kg (154–176 lb), 40 mg IV bolus	Any prior intracranial hemorrhage, known structural cerebrovascular lesions, such as an arterial venous malformation, known intracranial malignant neoplasm, ischemic stroke within 3 months, active bleeding (excluding menses), significant closed head or facial trauma within 3 months	STE MI, class I recommendation for patients presenting within 12 hours following the onset of symptoms, class IIa in patients presenting between 12 and 24 hours following the onset of symptoms with continuing signs of ischemia. NSTE ACS, class III recommendation.

(Continued)

Table 8–2

Evidence-Based Pharmacotherapy for ST-Segment Elevation Myocardial Infarction and Non-ST-Segment Elevation Acute Coronary Syndrome[2–8,46] (Continued)

Drug	Clinical Condition and ACCF/AHA/ SCAI Guideline Recommendation[a]	Contraindications[b]	Dose and Duration of Therapy		Dosing adjustment for CKD
			Drug	**Dose**	
Glycoprotein IIb/IIIa receptor	NSTE ACS PCI, class I recommendation for abciximab, high-bolus dose tirofiban or double-bolus eptifibatide at the time of PCI in high-risk patients already receiving aspirin and not pretreated with a P2Y$_{12}$ inhibitor and not receiving bivalirudin as the anticoagulant; class IIa at the time of PCI for high-risk patients already receiving aspirin and pretreated with a P2Y$_{12}$ inhibitor; class IIb for upstream use in high-risk patients already receiving aspirin and pretreated with a P2Y$_{12}$ inhibitor and not receiving bivalirudin as the anticoagulant; class I for upstream use in addition to aspirin without P2Y$_{12}$ inhibitor pretreatment for moderate- to high-risk patients.	Active bleeding, thrombocytopenia, prior stroke, renal dialysis (eptifibatide)	Abciximab	0.25 mg/kg IV bolus followed by 0.125 mcg/kg/min (maximum 10 mcg/min) for 12 hours	None
			Eptifibatide	180 mcg/kg IV bolus × 2, 10 minutes apart with an infusion of 2 mcg/kg/min for 18–24 hours after PCI	Reduce maintenance infusion to 1 mcg/kg/min for CrCl less than 50 mL/min (less than 0.83 mL/s); contraindicated if patient dependent on dialysis. Patients weighing 121 kg (266 lb) or more should receive a maximum infusion rate of 22.6 mg per bolus and a maximum rate of 15 mg/hr
	NSTE ACS for patients not undergoing PCI (conservative medical management), class IIb recommendation. STE MI primary PCI, class IIa recommendation for abciximab, high-bolus dose tirofiban or double-bolus eptifibatide.		Tirofiban	25mcg/kg IV bolus followed by an infusion of 0.1 mcg/kg/min for up to 18 hours	Reduce maintenance infusion to 0.05 mcg/kg/min for patients with CrCl less than 30 mL/min (less than 0.05 mL/s)
Nitroglycerin	STE MI and NSTE ACS, class I recommendation in patients with ongoing ischemic discomfort, control of hypertension or management of pulmonary congestion.	Hypotension, sildenafil or vardenafil within 24 hours or tadalafil within 48 hours	0.4 mg SL, repeated every 5 minutes × 3 doses. 5 to 10 mcg/min IV infusion titrated up to 75–100 mcg/min until relief of symptoms or limiting side effects (headache) with a systolic blood pressure less than 90 mm Hg or more than 30% below starting mean arterial pressure levels if significant hypertension is present. Topical patches or oral nitrates are acceptable alternatives for patients without ongoing or refractory symptoms. Continue IV infusion for 24–48 hours.		

Drug Class	Indications/Recommendations	Contraindications	Dosing
β-Blockers[c]	STE MI and NSTE ACS, class I recommendation for oral β-blockers in all patients without contraindications in the first 24 hours, class IIa for IV β-blockers in hypertensive patients.	PR ECG segment greater than 0.24 seconds, second-degree or third-degree atrioventricular heart block, heart rate less than 60 beats/min, systolic blood pressure less than 90 mm Hg, shock, left ventricular failure with congestive heart failure, severe reactive airway disease	Target resting heart rate of 50–60 beats/min. Metoprolol 5 mg slow IV push (over 1–2 min), repeated every 5 min for a total of 15 mg followed in 1–2 hours by 25–50 mg orally every 6 hours; if a very conservative regimen is desired, initial doses can be reduced to 1–2 mg. Propranolol 0.5–1 mg IV dose followed in 1–2 hours by 40–80 mg orally every 6–8 hours. Atenolol 5 mg IV dose followed in 5 min by a second 5 mg IV dose for a total of 10 mg followed in 1–2 hours by 50–100 mg orally once daily. Alternatively, initial IV therapy can be omitted. Continue oral β-blocker indefinitely.
Calcium channel blockers	STE MI class IIa recommendation and NSTE ACS class I recommendation for patients with ongoing ischemia who are already taking adequate doses of nitrates and β-blockers or in patients with contraindications to or intolerance to β-blockers (diltiazem or verapamil preferred during initial presentation). NSTE ACS, class IIb recommendation for diltiazem for patients with AMI.	Pulmonary edema, evidence of left ventricular dysfunction, systolic blood pressure less than 100 mm Hg, PR ECG segment greater than 0.24 seconds second- or third-degree atrioventricular heart block for verapamil or diltiazem, pulse rate less than 60 beats/min for diltiazem or verapamil	Diltiazem 120–360 mg sustained release orally once daily. Verapamil 180–480 mg sustained release orally once daily. Amlodipine 5–10 mg orally once daily. Continue indefinitely if contraindication to oral β-blocker persists.

ACE inhibitors

NSTE ACS and STE MI, class I recommendation for patients with heart failure, left ventricular dysfunction and EF less than or equal to 40%, type 2 diabetes mellitus or CKD in the absence of contraindications. Consider in all patients with CAD (class I recommendation, class IIa in low-risk patients). Indicated indefinitely for all patients with EF less than 40% (class I recommendation).

Systolic blood pressure less than 100 mm Hg, history of intolerance to an ACE inhibitor, bilateral renal artery stenosis, serum potassium more than 5.5 mEq/L (greater than 5.5 mmol/L), acute renal failure, pregnancy

Drug	Initial Dose (mg)	Target Dose (mg)
Captopril	6.25–12.5	50 twice daily orally to 50 three times daily
Enalapril	2.5–5.0	10 twice daily orally
Lisinopril	2.5–5.0	10–20 once daily orally
Ramipril	1.25–2.5	5 twice daily or 10 once daily orally
Trandolapril	1.0	4 once daily orally

Continue indefinitely if contraindication to oral β-blocker persists.

Angiotensin receptor blockers

NSTE MI and STE MI, class I recommendation in patients with clinical signs of heart failure or left ventricular EF less than 40% and intolerant of an ACE inhibitor, class IIa recommendation in patients with clinical signs of heart failure or EF less than 40% and no documentation of ACE inhibitor intolerance. Class I in other ACE inhibitor–intolerant patients with hypertension.

Systolic blood pressure less than 100 mm Hg, bilateral renal artery stenosis, serum potassium more than 5.5 mEq/L (greater than 5.5 mmol/L), acute renal failure, pregnancy

Drug	Initial Dose (mg)	Target Dose (mg)
Candesartan	4–8	32 once daily orally
Valsartan	40	160 twice daily orally
Losartan	12.5–25	150 daily

Continue indefinitely.

(Continued)

Table 8–2

Evidence-Based Pharmacotherapy for ST-Segment Elevation Myocardial Infarction and Non-ST-Segment Elevation Acute Coronary Syndrome[2-8,46] (Continued)

Drug	Clinical Condition and ACCF/AHA/SCAI Guideline Recommendation[a]	Contraindications[b]	Dose and Duration of Therapy		
			Drug	Initial Dose (mg)	Maximum Dose (mg)
Aldosterone antagonists	NSTE MI and STE MI class I recommendation in patients with EF less than or equal to 40% and either diabetes mellitus or heart failure symptoms who are already receiving an ACE inhibitor.	Hypotension, hyperkalemia, serum potassium greater than 5.0 mEq/L (greater than 5 mmol/L), SCr greater than 2.5 mg/dL (221 μmol/L) and/or CrCl less than 30 mL/min (less than 0.50 mL/s)	Eplerenone	25	50 once daily orally
			Spironolactone	12.5	25–50 once daily orally
			Continue indefinitely.		
Morphine sulfate	STE and NSTE ACS, class I recommendation for patients whose symptoms are not relieved after three serial SL nitroglycerin tablets or whose symptoms recur with adequate antiischemic therapy.	Hypotension, respiratory depression, confusion, obtundation	2–4 mg IV bolus dose. May be repeated every 5–15 minutes as needed to relieve symptoms and maintain patient comfort.		

[a]Class I recommendations are conditions for which there is evidence and/or general agreement that a given procedure or treatment is useful and effective.

Class II recommendations are those conditions for which there is conflicting evidence and/or divergence of opinion about the usefulness/efficacy of a procedure or treatment. For Class IIa recommendations, the weight of the evidence/opinion is in favor of usefulness/efficacy. Class IIb recommendations are those for which usefulness/efficacy is less well established by evidence/opinion. Class III recommendations are those where the procedure or treatment is not useful and may be harmful.

[b]Allergy or prior intolerance contraindication for all categories of drugs listed in this chart.

[c]Choice of the specific agent is not as important as ensuring that appropriate candidates receive this therapy. If there are concerns about patient intolerance due to existing pulmonary disease, especially asthma, selection should favor a short-acting agent, such as metoprolol or the ultra short-acting agent, esmolol. Mild wheezing or a history of chronic obstructive pulmonary disease should prompt a trial of a short-acting agent at a reduced dose (e.g., 2.5 mg IV metoprolol, 12.5 mg oral metoprolol, or 25 mcg/kg/min esmolol as initial doses) rather than complete avoidance of β-blocker therapy.

ACCF, American College of Cardiology Foundation; ACE, angiotensin-converting enzyme inhibitor; AHA, American Heart Association; ACS, acute coronary syndrome; ACT, activated clotting time; AMI, acute myocardial infarction; aPTT, activated partial thromboplastin time; CABG, coronary artery bypass graft; CAD, coronary artery disease; CKD, chronic kidney disease; CrCl, Creatinine clearance; ECG, electrocardiogram; EF, ejection fraction; GP, glycoprotein; HORIZONS-AMI, Harmonizing Outcomes with Revascularization and Stents in Acute Myocardial Infarction; MI, myocardial infarction; NSTE, non-ST-segment elevation; PCI, percutaneous coronary intervention; SC, subcutaneous; SCAI, Society for Cardiac Angiography and Interventions; SCr, serum creatinine; SL, sublingual; STE, ST-segment elevation; TIA, transient ischemic attack; UFH, unfractionated heparin.

Reprinted with permission from Spinler SA. Evolution of antithrombotic therapy used in acute coronary syndromes. In: Richardson MM, Chessman KH, Chant C, Cheng JWM, Hemstreet BA, Hume AL, et al., eds. Pharmacotherapy Assessment Program, 7th ed. Cardiology. Lenexa, KS: American College of Clinical Pharmacy;2010, 97–124.

148

with NSTE ACS at low risk for recurrent CHD events following stress testing should be given ASA indefinitely and clopidogrel for a minimum of 1 month and ideally 12 months following hospital discharge in addition to other pharmacotherapy described later.[6] Patients with STE MI at low risk for recurrent CHD events should receive ASA indefinitely and clopidogrel for at least 14 days in addition to other pharmacotherapy described later (Fig. 8–2).[3]

Early Pharmacologic Therapy for STE MIs

Pharmacotherapy for early treatment of ACS is outlined in Fig. 8–2 and Table 8–2.[2–8] 6 *According to the ACCF/AHA STE MI practice guidelines, in addition to reperfusion therapy, other early pharmacotherapy that all patients with STE MI and without contraindications should receive within the first day of hospitalization, and preferably in the emergency department, are intranasal oxygen (if oxygen saturation is low), sublingual (SL) nitroglycerin (NTG), ASA, a P2Y$_{12}$ inhibitor (clopidogrel, prasugrel, or ticagrelor depending on reperfusion strategy), and anticoagulation with bivalirudin, unfractionated heparin (UFH), or enoxaparin (agent dependent on reperfusion strategy). A GP IIb/IIIa inhibitor should be administered with UFH for patients undergoing primary PCI. IV β-blockers and IV NTG should be given in selected patients. Oral β-blockers should be initiated within the first day in patients without cardiogenic shock*[2–4,8] Morphine is administered to patients with refractory angina as an analgesic and a venodilator that lowers preload. These agents should be administered early while the patient is still in the emergency department. Dosing and contraindications for SL and IV NTG, ASA, clopidogrel, β-blockers, anticoagulants, and fibrinolytics are listed in Table 8–2.[2–4,8]

▶ *Fibrinolytic Therapy*

Administration of a fibrinolytic agent is indicated in patients with STE MI who present to the hospital within 12 hours of the onset of chest discomfort, have at least a 1-mm STE in two or more contiguous ECG leads, and are not able to undergo primary PCI within 90 minutes of medical contact.[4] The mortality benefit of fibrinolysis is highest with early administration and diminishes after 12 hours. The use of fibrinolytics between 12 and 24 hours after symptom onset should be limited to patients with ongoing ischemia. Fibrinolytic therapy is preferred over primary PCI where there is no cardiac catheterization laboratory or there would be a delay in "door-to-primary PCI" of more than 90 minutes (of first medical contact) within the institution or 120 minutes (of first medical contact) if the patient is transferred. Indications and contraindications for fibrinolysis are listed in Table 8–3.[2] It is not necessary to obtain the results of biochemical markers before initiating fibrinolytic therapy. Because administration of fibrinolytics result in clot lysis, patients who are at high risk of major bleeding (including intracranial hemorrhage) presenting with an absolute contraindication should not receive fibrinolytic therapy; primary PCI is preferred. In patients who have a

Patient Encounter 2, Part 1

SD is a 66-year-old, 90-kg (198-lb) man who presents to the emergency department by ambulance complaining of 3 hours of continuous chest pressure that started while walking his dog. SD developed substernal chest pain about 15 minutes after walking. He stopped and rested but the chest pain did not resolve. He returned home and called 911. Local paramedics were summoned, and he was given three 0.4 mg sublingual nitroglycerin tablets by mouth, 325 mg ASA by mouth, and morphine 2 mg IV push without relief of chest discomfort. An early invasive strategy is selected.

PMH: HTN for 5 years; type 2 diabetes mellitus (DM) for 5 years; dyslipidemia for 2 years

FH: Father with myocardial infarction at age 75; mother and sister alive with type 2 DM

SH: Nonsmoker

Allergies: NKDA

Meds: Metformin 1,000 mg by mouth twice daily; ASA 325 mg by mouth once daily; lisinopril 20 mg by mouth once daily; simvastatin 20 mg by mouth once daily

ROS: 10/10 chest pressure/squeezing

PE:

HEENT: Normocephalic atraumatic

CV: Regular rate and rhythm S$_1$, S$_2$, –S$_3$, –S$_4$, no murmurs or rubs

VS: BP 150/92; HR 88 bpm; T 37°C (98.6°F)

Lungs: Clear to auscultation and percussion

Abd: Nontender, nondistended

GI: Normal bowel sounds

GU: Stool guaiac negative

Exts: No bruits, pulses 2+, femoral pulse present, good range of motion

Neuro: Alert and oriented × 3, cranial nerves intact

Labs: Sodium 136 mEq/L (136 mmol/L), potassium 4.0 mEq/L (4.0 mmol/L), chloride 105 mEq/L (105 mmol/L), bicarbonate 22 mEq/L (22 mmol/L), SCr 1.0 mg/dL (88 μmol/L), glucose 160 mg/dL (8.9 mmol/L), WBC 6.9 × 10³/mm³ (6.9 × 10⁹/L), hemoglobin 14.7 g/dL (147 g/L or 9.1 mmol/L), hematocrit 42% (0.42), platelets 320 × 10³/mm³ (320 × 10⁹/L), troponin I 1.0 ng/mL (1.0 mcg/L), oxygen saturation 99% (0.99) on room air

ECG: Normal sinus rhythm, PR 0.16 seconds, QRS 0.08 seconds, QT$_c$ 0.38 seconds, 1 mm ST-segment depression anterior leads

CXR: Normal

Echo: Anterior wall dyskinesis, LVEF 55% (0.55)

What type of ACS is this?

What information is suggestive of acute MI?

Table 8–3

Indications and Contraindications to Fibrinolytic Therapy per ACC/AHA Guidelines for Management of Patients with ST-Segment Elevation Myocardial Infarction[4]

Indications

1. Ischemic chest discomfort at least 20 minutes in duration but 12 hours or less since symptom onset
   and
   ST-segment elevation of at least 1 mm in height in two or more contiguous leads, or new or presumed new left bundle-branch block
2. Ongoing ischemic chest discomfort at least 20 minutes in duration 12–24 hours since symptom onset
   and
   ST-segment elevation of at least 1 mm in height in two or more contiguous leads

Absolute Contraindications

- Active internal bleeding (not including menses)
- Previous intracranial hemorrhage at any time; ischemic stroke within 3 months
- Known intracranial neoplasm
- Known structural vascular lesion (e.g., arteriovenous malformation)
- Suspected aortic dissection
- Significant closed head or facial trauma within 3 months

ACC, American College of Cardiology; AHA, American Heart Association

contraindication to fibrinolytics and PCI, or who do not have access to a facility that can perform PCIs, treatment with an anticoagulant (other than UFH) for up to 8 days can be administered.

In patients with symptoms lasting less than 6 hours, a more fibrin-specific agent such as alteplase, reteplase, or tenecteplase is preferred over a nonfibrin-specific agent such as streptokinase.[2] Fibrin-specific fibrinolytics open a greater percentage of infarcted arteries. In a large clinical trial, administration of alteplase reduced mortality by 1% (absolute reduction) and cost about $30,000 per year of life saved compared with streptokinase.[37] Two other trials compared alteplase with reteplase and alteplase with tenecteplase and found similar mortality between agents.[38,39] Therefore, alteplase, reteplase, or tenecteplase is acceptable as a first-line agent. Intracranial hemorrhage (ICH) and major bleeding are the most serious side effects of fibrinolytic agents. The risk of ICH is higher with fibrin-specific agents than with streptokinase.[22] However, the risk of systemic bleeding other than ICH is higher with streptokinase than with other more fibrin-specific agents and was higher with alteplase versus tenecteplase in one study.[22,37,39]

As mentioned previously, less than 20% of patients with STE MI receive fibrinolysis compared with more than 60% receiving primary PCI. However, 17% of eligible patients receive neither primary PCI nor fibrinolysis despite being eligible. The primary reason for lack of reperfusion therapy is that most patients present more than 12 hours after the time of symptom onset. The percentage of eligible patients who receive reperfusion therapy is a quality performance measure of care in patients with MI.[32] The "door-to-needle time," the time from hospital presentation to start of fibrinolytic therapy, is another quality performance measure.[32] The ACCF/AHA guidelines recommend a "door-to-needle time" of less than 30 minutes from the time of hospital presentation until start of fibrinolytic therapy.[4] The median administration time in the United States in 2006 was 29 minutes, with only 50% of patients meeting the quality performance target of less than 30 minutes.[40] All hospitals should have protocols addressing fibrinolysis eligibility, dosing, and monitoring.

▶ Aspirin

ASA is the preferred antiplatelet agent in the treatment of all ACS.[4,8] ASA administration to all patients who do not have contraindications to ASA therapy within 24 hours before or after hospital arrival is a quality performance measure for MI.[4,32] The antiplatelet effects of ASA are mediated by inhibiting the synthesis of thromboxane A_2 (TXA_2) through an irreversible inhibition of platelet cyclooxygenase-1. In patients undergoing PCI, ASA prevents acute thrombotic occlusion during the procedure. In patients receiving fibrinolytics, ASA reduces mortality, and its effects are additive to fibrinolysis alone.[4,41] Additionally, in patients undergoing PCI, ASA, in addition to a $P2Y_{12}$ inhibitor, reduces the risk of stent thrombosis.

In patients experiencing an ACS, an initial dose equal to or greater than 160 mg nonenteric ASA is necessary to achieve a rapid platelet inhibition.[42,43] Current guidelines for STE MI recommend an initial ASA dose of 162 to 325 mg (Table 8–2).[4] This first dose can be chewed in order to achieve high blood concentrations and platelet inhibition rapidly. Preferably, patients undergoing PCI not previously taking ASA should receive 325 mg nonenteric-coated ASA.[8] The notion of chewing ASA came from the use of an enteric-coated formulation of ASA in the Second International Study of Infarct Survival (ISIS-2) trial in order to break the enteric coating to ensure more rapid effect.[43] Current data suggest that although an initial dose 160 to 325 mg is required, long-term therapy with doses of 75 to 150 mg daily are as effective as higher doses, and therefore a daily maintenance dose of 75 to 162 mg is recommended in most patients to inhibit the 10% of the total platelet pool that is regenerated daily.[4,44-46] Because of increased bleeding risk in patients receiving ASA plus a $P2Y_{12}$ inhibitor compared with ASA alone, low-dose ASA (81 mg daily) is preferred following PCI.[8] In a large ($n = 25,086$) randomized trial, high-dose ASA, 300 to 325 mg daily, had similar frequency of CV death, MI, or stroke as well as major bleeding compared to low-dose ASA in the first 30 days following ACS presentation.[47] Minor bleeding and GI bleeding were less frequent with low-dose ASA. In this trial, patients undergoing PCI during hospitalization had a lower frequency of death, MI, or stroke, but major bleeding was increased with high-dose ASA.[48] In PLATO (the Study of Platelet Inhibition and Patient Outcomes), a randomized double-blind clinical trial comparing ticagrelor with clopidogrel in patients receiving ASA, a post hoc analysis suggested that maintenance doses of ASA above 100 mg daily reduced the effectiveness of ticagrelor.[49] Low-dose ASA should be continued indefinitely.[46]

Nonsteroidal anti-inflammatory agents other than ASA, as well as cyclooxygenase-2 (COX-2) selective anti-inflammatory agents, should be discontinued at the time of STE MI secondary to increased risk of death, reinfarction, HF, and myocardial rupture.[3]

The most frequent side effects of ASA are dyspepsia and nausea. Patients should be counseled about the risk of bleeding, especially GI bleeding, with ASA.

▶ Platelet P2Y₁₂ Inhibitors

Clopidogrel, prasugrel, and ticagrelor block a subtype of ADP receptor, the $P2Y_{12}$ receptor, on platelets, preventing the binding of ADP to the receptor and subsequent expression of platelet GP IIb/IIIa receptors, reducing platelet activation and aggregation. Both clopidogrel and prasugrel are thienopyridine and prodrugs that are converted to an active metabolite by a variety of cytochrome CYP450 isoenzymes (Table 8–4).[50–52]

Both of these agents bind irreversibly to $P2Y_{12}$ receptor. Ticagrelor, which is not a thienopyridine, is a reversible, noncompetitive $P2Y_{12}$ receptor inhibitor. Ticagrelor parent compound has antiplatelet effects and is also metabolized primarily by CYP3A to an active metabolite producing its antiplatelet effects.

Both prasugrel and ticagrelor are more potent ADP inhibitors than clopidogrel. Prasugrel has the fewest significant drug–drug interactions. The production of clopidogrel's active metabolite and consequently its antiplatelet effect is reduced by moderate and strong inhibitors of CYP2C19, whereas ticagrelor's concentration is reduced by strong inhibitors of CYP3A. Labeled drug interactions are described in Table 8–4. A more detailed discussion of the interaction between clopidogrel and proton pump inhibitors may be found in Chapter 7, "Ischemic Heart Disease."

A considerable amount of data support that genetic variations in the gene coding for *CYP2C19* significantly modulate the antiplatelet effects of clopidogrel. Specifically, carriers of reduced-function allele (i.e., *2 or *3) are not able to convert clopidogrel to its active metabolite to the extent of carriers of the wild-type allele. This results in decreased antiplatelet effects,[53] as well as higher rates of CV events, especially stent thrombosis and MI around the time of PCI.[54] Prasugrel is not as dependent on *CYP2C19* genotype for its conversion to the active metabolite and has a lower frequency of poor antiplatelet responsiveness.[55] Moreover, current data suggest the benefit of prasugrel compared with clopidogrel may only be apparent in carriers of these reduced function alleles,[55] whereas the benefits of ticagrelor over clopidogrel may be unrelated to *CYP2C19*.[56] Hence ticagrelor or prasugrel may be considered preferred agents in carriers of *CYP2C19* reduced function alleles.

Although the product labeling for clopidogrel suggests that genetic testing and alternative therapy should be selected

for patients that are *CYP2C19* poor metabolizers,[50] the most recent clinical practice guidelines of the ACCF/AHA/SCAI have not endorsed routine genotyping to guide the prescription of $P2Y_{12}$ inhibitors because no prospective randomized clinical study has demonstrated the benefit of such a genotype-based prescribing approach.[8]

Administration of a $P2Y_{12}$ receptor inhibitor, in addition to ASA, is recommended for all patients with STE MI.[2–4,8] For STE MI undergoing primary PCI, clopidogrel, prasugrel, or ticagrelor, in addition to ASA, should be administered to prevent subacute stent thrombosis and longer-term CV events (Table 8–2).[2,8] Although not FDA approved, a clopidogrel loading dose of 600 mg is recommended over administration of 300 mg for patients undergoing PCI. A systematic review and meta-analysis of randomized and nonrandomized trials in more than 25,000 patients demonstrated a reduction in CV ischemic events with a loading dose of 600 mg compared with 300 mg in patients undergoing PCI.[57]

In the most recent ACCF/AHA/SCAI PCI practice guidelines, no preference is given for one agent over the other. Nevertheless, clinical trials comparing these agents have highlighted distinct clinical differences between these antiplatelet agents.

A large randomized double-blind study demonstrated that, compared with clopidogrel, the addition of prasugrel to ASA for patients undergoing PCI in the setting of STE MI or NSTE ACS significantly reduced risk of CV death or MI by 19% (9.9% versus 12.1%), as well as MI and stent thrombosis, but increased the risk of major bleeding (not ICH) by 32% (2.4% versus 1.8%).[58] Patients with a history of prior stroke or transient ischemic attack (TIA) had an increased risk of ICH and no net clinical benefit from prasugrel, and the product label lists prior stroke or TIA as a contraindication to prasugrel.[51] Patients older than 75 years and those weighing less than 60 kg (132 lb) are at increased risk of bleeding with prasugrel compared with clopidogrel.[51] Two subgroups of patients do not have an increased bleeding risk with prasugrel compared with clopidogrel and have even greater benefit, namely patients undergoing primary PCI for STE MI and those patients with a history of diabetes mellitus (DM).[59,60]

PLATO compared ticagrelor with clopidogrel in patients receiving ASA and presenting with either STE MI or NSTE ACS and undergoing an intended interventional management strategy with PCI or conservative noninterventional management strategy with medical therapy alone. In this trial, ticagrelor significantly reduced the rate of CV death, MI, stroke, and stent thrombosis compared with clopidogrel.[61] Although no increase in study-defined major bleeding was noted with ticagrelor, the frequency of non-CABG major bleeding was increased compared with clopidogrel. As with the prasugrel trial previously described, several subgroups of patients enrolled in this trial had particular benefit with ticagrelor, including those with an intended invasive approach, those with an intended noninvasive approach, patients with STE MI primary PCI, and patients with DM.[62–65] Therefore, both of the more potent $P2Y_{12}$ inhibitors are more efficacious than clopidogrel but may also be associated with an increased risk of bleeding. No large randomized trial has directly

Table 8–4

Pharmacokinetics of Clopidogrel, Prasugrel, and Ticagrelor[50-52]

	Clopidogrel	Prasugrel	Ticagrelor
Pharmacologic class	Thienopyridine	Thienopyridine	Cyclopentyl triazolopyrimidine
ADP receptor binding	Irreversible	Irreversible	Reversible
Absorption and metabolism	Prodrug	Prodrug	Active moiety, bioavailability 36%
	Inactive metabolite SR266334 / Active metabolite R-130946	Active metabolite R-138727	Active metabolite AR-C124910XX approximately 30% to 40% activity of parent compound
	Metabolism to R-130946 is primarily by CYP2C19, with lesser contributions from CYP3A4, 2B6, and 1A2	Metabolism to R-138727 is primarily via CYP 3A4 and CYP 2B6	Metabolism is primarily via CYP 3A4/5
	Exposure to the active metabolite is affected by CYP 2C19 and possible ATP-binding cassette B1 (ABCB1) transporter (also called P-glycoprotein) polymorphisms	Exposure to the active metabolite is not affected by CYP 2C19 polymorphisms	Exposure to the active metabolite is not affected by CYP 2C19 polymorphisms
	Rapid conversion of the parent drug to active metabolite (mean time to peak plasma concentration of active metabolite approximately 1 hour)	Rapid conversion of the parent drug to active metabolite (median time to peak plasma concentration of active metabolite approximately 30 minutes)	Rapid conversion of the parent drug to active metabolite (median time to peak plasma concentration of active metabolite 2.5 hours)
Food effect	One report in healthy volunteers of bioavailability of inactive metabolite concentrations unaffected by food; one report in healthy volunteers of clopidogrel t_{max} delayed by 1.5 hours, C_{max} increased sixfold and bioavailability increased ninefold	Fasting administration preferred; C_{max} is reduced by 49% and t_{max} delayed 0.5–1.5 hours when administered with high-fat, high-calorie meal, although AUC is unaffected	May be taken with or without food; no effect on C_{max} and 21% increase in AUC when administered with high-fat, high-calorie meal. Decrease in C_{max} by 22% and no effect on AUC of active metabolite when administered with high-fat, high-calorie meal
Disposition	Linear pharmacokinetics at doses of 50–150 mg	Linear pharmacokinetics at doses up to 75 mg	Linear pharmacokinetics at doses up to 600 mg daily
Elimination	Elimination half-life of active metabolite is approximately 30 minutes after a 75-mg dose	Median elimination half-life of active metabolite approximately 7.4 hours	Median elimination half-life of the parent compound is approximately 7 hours and active metabolite approximately 9 hours
	Excretion is 50% urinary and 46% fecal	Excretion is primarily urinary (approximately 70%); fecal excretion less than 30%	Excretion is primarily metabolism (84%); fecal excretion 58%, urinary excretion 26%
Labeled drug interactions and suggested management of interaction	Enhanced bleeding with NSAIDS; avoid use	Enhanced bleeding with warfarin and NSAIDs, avoid use	Enhanced bleeding with warfarin and NSAIDs
	Enhanced bleeding with warfarin; monitor carefully for bleeding; target INR to 2.0–2.5 for most indications		Use aspirin doses less than or equal to 100 mg daily
	Avoid use with moderate or strong CYP2C19 inhibitors (e.g., omeprazole, esomeprazole, chloramphenicol, cimetidine, efavirenz, etravirine, felbamate, fluoxetine, fluconazole, fluvoxamine, isoniazid, oxcarbazepine, ketoconazole, voriconazole); select alternative noninteracting P2Y₁₂ inhibitor or alternative noninteracting drug		Avoid use with strong CYP3A inhibitors (atazanavir, clarithromycin, indinavir, itraconazole, nefazodone, nelfinavir, ketoconazole, ritonavir, saquinavir, telithromycin, voriconazole)
			Avoid use with potent CYP3A inducers (carbamazepine, dexamethasone, phenobarbital, phenytoin, rifampin)
			Avoid simvastatin and lovastatin doses more than 40 mg daily (ticagrelor inhibits CYP3A4 and increases statin concentration)
			Monitor digoxin serum concentrations with any change in ticagrelor dose (ticagrelor inhibits P-glycoprotein)

ADP, adenosine diphosphate; ATP, adenosine triphosphate; AUC, area under the curve; CYP, cytochrome P450; INR, international normalized ratio; NSAIDs, nonsteroidal anti-inflammatory drugs.

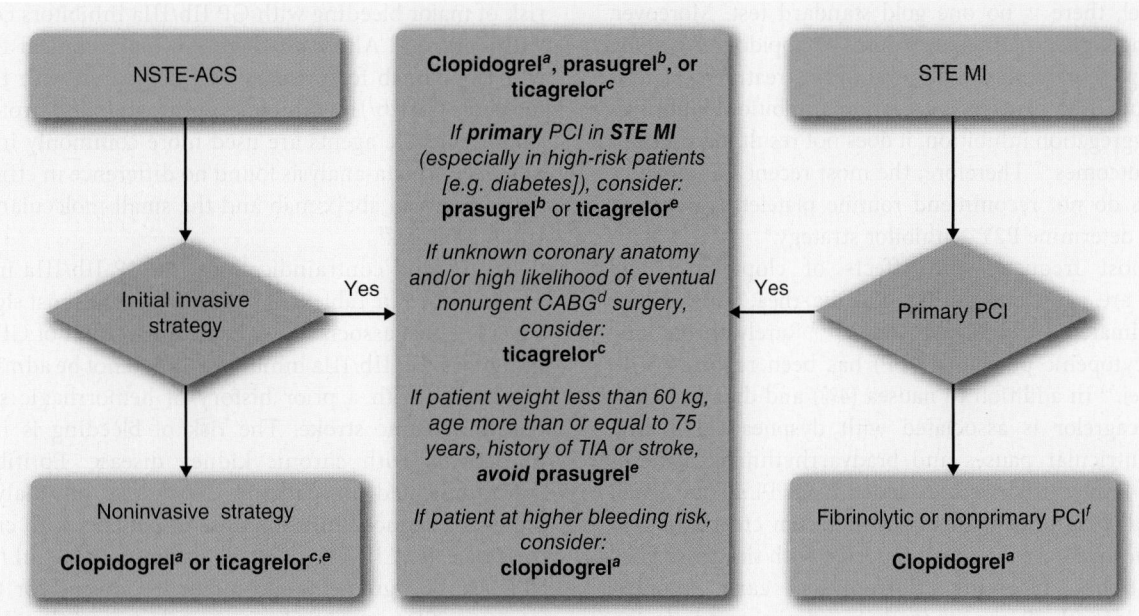

FIGURE 8–4. Proposed use of P2Y$_{12}$ inhibitors. [a]Do not use clopidogrel in patients with active pathological bleeding; consider alternative P2Y$_{12}$ receptor inhibitor if documented clopidogrel ineffectiveness (e.g., poor metabolism, stent thrombosis during clopidogrel therapy) or drug–drug interactions (e.g., avoid moderate and strong CYP2C19 inhibitors); clopidogrel should be held for at least 5 days before CABG surgery, if the surgery can be delayed. [b]Do not use prasugrel in patients with active pathological bleeding or a history of transient ischemic attack or stroke; if a patient subsequently goes on to receive CABG surgery, the drug should be held for at least 7 days if the surgery can be delayed. [c]Do not use ticagrelor in patients with active pathological bleeding or a history of intracranial hemorrhage, or in patients planned to undergo urgent CABG surgery; concomitant maintenance aspirin dose above 100 mg should be avoided; dose of ticagrelor should be held for 5 days before CABG surgery if the surgery can be delayed; when selecting this agent consider patient compliance (dosed twice daily), unique adverse effects (e.g., dyspnea), and potential drug–drug interactions (e.g., avoid strong CYP3A inhibitors/inducers). [d]Prior to diagnostic angiography, it is difficult to determine the likelihood that an individual patient will receive CABG surgery; notable variables that predict this occurrence include previous CABG, male gender, previous heart failure, presence of diabetes, previous percutaneous coronary intervention, among others. [e]Recommendation based on subgroup analysis. [f]At this time, there is insufficient data to support ticagrelor or prasugrel in the "fibrinolytic or nonprimary PCI" patient group. (ACS, acute coronary syndrome; CABG, coronary artery bypass surgery; MI, myocardial infarction; NSTE, non-ST-segment elevation; PCI, percutaneous coronary intervention; STE, ST-segment elevation; TIA, transient ischemic attack.) (Adapted from Crouch MA, Colucci VJ, Howard PA, Spinler SA. P2Y$_{12}$ receptor inhibitors: Integrating ticagrelor into the management of acute coronary syndrome. Ann Pharmacother 2011;45:1151–1156, with permission.)

compared ticagrelor and prasugrel. Figure 8–4 outlines the role of the newer P2Y$_{12}$ inhibitors in ACS compared with clopidogrel.[66]

Although a modest benefit of using a 7-day course of clopidogrel 150 mg compared to 75 mg daily has been suggested, it is also associated with a higher risk of major bleeding.[47] While mentioned in STE MI practice guidelines,[2,8] such a regimen is not used routinely in practice with the availability of the more potent agents, prasugrel and ticagrelor.

The recommended duration of P2Y$_{12}$ inhibitors for a patient undergoing PCI for ACS, either STE MI or NSTE ACS, is at least 12 months for patients receiving either a bare metal or a drug-eluting stent.[8] The benefit of prolonging treatment beyond 12 months is uncertain.[8] Nonadherence to P2Y$_{12}$ inhibitors is a major risk factor for stent thrombosis, and hence the likelihood of adherence to dual antiplatelet

therapy (ASA and a P2Y$_{12}$ inhibitor) should be assessed prior to angiography.[8] The use of a bare metal stent over a drug-eluting stent should be considered in patients who are anticipated to be nonadherent to 12 months of dual antiplatelet therapy.[8]

To minimize the risk of CV events, elective noncardiac surgery should be delayed to more than 4 to 6 weeks after angioplasty or bare metal stent implantation, or 12 months after drug-eluting stent implantation if the discontinuation of the P2Y$_{12}$ inhibitor is required.[8] If CABG surgery is planned, clopidogrel and ticagrelor should be withheld preferably for 5 days, and prasugrel at least 7 days, to reduce the risk of postoperative bleeding, unless the need for revascularization outweighs the bleeding risk.[8]

Although a variety of blood tests can assess functional platelet aggregation inhibition to P2Y$_{12}$ inhibitors, especially clopidogrel, there is no one gold standard test. Moreover, while using higher maintenance doses of clopidogrel (150 mg daily) in patients with a high level of on-treatment platelet aggregation (low platelet aggregation inhibition) improves platelet aggregation inhibition, it does not result in improved clinical outcomes.[67] Therefore, the most recent PCI practice guidelines do not recommend routine platelet aggregation testing to determine P2Y$_{12}$ inhibitor strategy.[8]

The most frequent side effects of clopidogrel and prasugrel are nausea, vomiting, and diarrhea, which occur in approximately 2% to 5% of patients.[50,51] Rarely, thrombotic thrombocytopenic purpura (TTP) has been reported with clopidogrel.[50] In addition to nausea (4%) and diarrhea (3%), use of ticagrelor is associated with dyspnea (14%) and, rarely, ventricular pauses and bradyarrhythmias. Patients at risk of bradycardia were excluded from PLATO.[52] Small nonclinically significant increases in serum creatinine and serum uric acid have also been reported with ticagrelor.[52]

In patients receiving fibrinolysis, early therapy with clopidogrel 75 mg once daily administered during hospitalization and up to 28 days (mean: 14 days) in patients with STE MI reduced mortality and reinfarction in patients treated with fibrinolytics without increasing the risk of major bleeding.[3,68,69] In adult patients younger than 75 years receiving fibrinolytics, the first dose of clopidogrel can be a 300-mg loading dose.[3,69] Although prasugrel and ticagrelor have been studied in the setting of PCI, no studies have evaluated their use when added to both ASA and a fibrinolytic.

Clopidogrel is currently the ACCF/AHA guideline-preferred P2Y$_{12}$ inhibitor added to ASA and should be continued for at least 14 days (and up to 1 year) for patients presenting with STE MI who do not undergo reperfusion therapy with either primary PCI or fibrinolysis.[3,68] However, recent subgroup analysis from PLATO suggests that ticagrelor may also be an option in medically managed patients with ACS because the frequency of CV death, MI, or stroke as well as mortality was lower in ticagrelor-treated patients compared with those receiving clopidogrel (Fig. 8–4).[62,66] Ticagrelor use was not associated with a higher bleeding rate compared with clopidogrel.[62]

▶ Glycoprotein IIb/IIIa Receptor Inhibitors

GP IIb/IIIa receptor inhibitors block the final common pathway of platelet aggregation, namely cross-linking of platelets by fibrinogen bridges between the GP IIb and IIIa receptors on the platelet surface. In patients with STE MI undergoing primary PCI who are treated with UFH, either abciximab (IV or intracoronary administration), eptifibatide or tirofiban may be administered.[8] Routine use of a GP IIb/IIIa receptor inhibitor is not recommended in patients who have received fibrinolytics or in those receiving bivalirudin secondary to increased bleeding risk. GP IIb/IIIa inhibitors should not be administered for medical management of the patient with STE MI who will not be undergoing PCI.[8] A meta-analysis of STE MI primary PCI trials demonstrated no reduction in mortality or 30-day reinfarction but increased

risk of major bleeding with GP IIb/IIIa inhibitors compared with control.[70] Although there are more clinical trial data with abciximab for primary PCI compared with the small molecule GP IIb/IIIa inhibitors eptifibatide and tirofiban, the small molecule agents are used more commonly in clinical practice. A meta-analysis found no difference in efficacy and safety between abciximab and the small molecular GP IIb/IIIa inhibitors.[71]

Dosing and contraindications for GP IIb/IIIa inhibitors are described in Table 8–2.[12] Bleeding is the most significant adverse effect associated with administration of GP IIb/IIIa inhibitors. GP IIb/IIIa inhibitors should not be administered to patients with a prior history of hemorrhagic stroke or recent ischemic stroke. The risk of bleeding is increased in patients with chronic kidney disease. Eptifibatide is contraindicated in patients dependent on dialysis and requires a reduced infusion dose in patients with creatinine clearance (CrCl) less than 50 mL/min (0.83 mL/s).[72] The STE MI PCI guideline-recommended dosing for tirofiban is not a FDA-approved regimen but one that has been studied in more contemporary clinical trials.[8,73] The dose of tirofiban should be halved in patients with CrCl less than 30 mL/min (0.50 mL/s).[74] No dosage adjustment for renal function is necessary for abciximab. An immune-mediated thrombocytopenia occurs in approximately 5% of patients with abciximab and less than 1% of patients receiving eptifibatide or tirofiban.[75]

▶ Anticoagulants

Options for anticoagulant therapy for patients with STE MI are outlined in Figure 8–2 and Table 8–2.[2–4,8] For patients undergoing primary PCI, either UFH or bivalirudin is preferred, whereas for fibrinolysis, enoxaparin is preferred.[2,3] For patients undergoing PCI, anticoagulation is discontinued immediately following the PCI procedures. In patients receiving enoxaparin plus a fibrinolytic, enoxaparin is continued for the duration of hospitalization, up to 8 days.[3] In patients who do not undergo reperfusion therapy, it is reasonable to administer anticoagulant therapy for up to 48 hours for UFH or for the duration of hospitalization for enoxaparin.[3,4]

Unfractionated heparin has been the traditional anticoagulant administered to patients with STE MI to prevent reocclusion of an infarct artery for more than 50 years. The results of a meta-analysis of more than 7,500 patients suggests that low molecular weight heparins (LMWHs) reduce both mortality and reinfarction compared with placebo in patients treated with fibrinolytics and ASA.[76] In a randomized open-label clinical trial of primary PCI for STE MI, bivalirudin, a direct thrombin inhibitor, significantly reduced the frequency of CV mortality by 45% (2.9% versus 5.1%) and all-cause mortality by 25% (5.9% versus 7.7%) at 3 years of follow-up while lowering the risk of in-hospital major bleeding events by 40% (4.9% versus 8.3%) compared with UFH plus a GP IIb/IIIa inhibitor (abciximab, eptifibatide, or tirofiban).[77,78] Therefore bivalirudin has similar or greater efficacy but better safety than UFH in the setting of primary PCI.

In patients with STE MI treated with fibrinolytics, enoxaparin, administered for a median of 7 days, has shown a reduction in the risk of death or non-fatal MI but increased bleeding risk compared with UFH administered for a median of 2 days in a large randomized clinical trial.[79] Enoxaparin dosing is adjusted for body weight and renal function, and when administered in combination with fibrinolysis, it has special dosing requirements for older patients and those weighing more than 100 kg (Table 8–2).

Besides bleeding, the most serious adverse effect of UFH and enoxaparin is heparin-induced thrombocytopenia. ACS registry data indicate, however, that the frequency of heparin-induced thrombocytopenia is rare (less than 0.5%).[80] Bivalirudin would be a preferred anticoagulant for patients with a history of heparin-induced thrombocytopenia undergoing PCI.[8]

▶ Nitrates

One SL NTG tablet should be administered every 5 minutes for up to three doses to relieve myocardial ischemia. If patients have been previously prescribed SL NTG and ischemic chest discomfort persists for more than 5 minutes after the first dose, the patient should be instructed to contact emergency medical services before self-administering subsequent doses to activate emergency care sooner. IV NTG should then be initiated in all patients with an ACS who have persistent ischemia, HF, or uncontrolled high blood pressure (BP) in the absence of contraindications.[4] IV NTG should be continued for approximately 24 hours after ischemia is relieved (Table 8–2). Nitrates promote the release of nitric oxide from the endothelium, which results in venous and arterial vasodilation. Venodilation lowers preload and myocardial oxygen demand. Arterial vasodilation may lower BP, thus reducing myocardial oxygen demand. Arterial vasodilation also relieves coronary artery vasospasm, dilating coronary arteries to improve myocardial blood flow and oxygenation. Although used to treat ACS, nitrates have been suggested to play a limited role in the treatment of ACS patients because two large randomized clinical trials failed to show a mortality benefit for IV nitrate therapy followed by oral nitrate therapy in acute MI.[81,82] The most significant adverse effects of nitrates are tachycardia, flushing, headache, and hypotension. Nitrate administration is contraindicated in patients who have received oral phosphodiesterase-5 inhibitors, such as sildenafil and vardenafil, within the past 24 hours, and tadalafil within the past 48 hours.[4]

▶ β-Blockers

A β-blocker should be administered early in the care of patients with STE MI and continued indefinitely. In ACS, the benefit of β-blockers results mainly from the competitive blockade of β_1-adrenergic receptors located on the myocardium. β_1-blockade produces a reduction in heart rate, myocardial contractility, and BP, decreasing myocardial oxygen demand. In addition, the reduction in heart rate increases diastolic time, thus improving ventricular filling and coronary artery perfusion. As a result of these effects, β-blockers reduce the risk for recurrent ischemia, infarct size, risk of reinfarction, and occurrence of ventricular arrhythmias in the hours and days following MI.

Landmark clinical trials have established the role of early β-blocker therapy in reducing MI mortality. Most of these trials were performed in the 1970s and 1980s before routine use of early reperfusion therapy.[83,84] However, data regarding the acute benefit of β-blockers in MI in the reperfusion era are derived mainly from a recently reported large clinical trial which suggests that although initiating IV followed by oral β-blockers early in the course of STE MI was associated with a lower risk of reinfarction or ventricular fibrillation, there may be an early risk of cardiogenic shock, especially in patients presenting with pulmonary congestion or systolic blood pressure less than 120 mm Hg.[85] Therefore, initiation of β-blockers, particularly when administered IV, should be limited to patients who are hemodynamically stable and who do not demonstrate any signs or symptoms of acute HF.[3] Careful assessment for signs of hypotension and HF should be performed following β-blocker initiation and prior to any dose titration. Patients already taking β-blockers can continue taking them.[3] The Joint Commission has retired the "Beta Blocker at Hospital Arrival" Core Measure and is no longer requiring hospital reporting of this measure.

The most serious side effects of β-blocker administration early in ACS are hypotension, acute HF, bradycardia, and heart block. Although initial acute administration of β-blockers is not appropriate for patients who present with acute HF, initiation of β-blockers may be attempted before hospital discharge in most patients following treatment of acute HF. β-blockers are continued indefinitely.[4]

▶ Calcium Channel Blockers

Calcium channel blockers in the setting of STE MI are used for relief of ischemic symptoms in patients who have certain contraindications to β-blockers. Current data suggest little benefit on clinical outcomes beyond symptom relief for calcium channel blockers in the setting of ACS.[4] Therefore, calcium channel blockers should be avoided in the acute management of all ACSs unless there is a clear symptomatic need or a contraindication to β-blockers. Agent selection is based on presenting heart rate and left ventricular dysfunction (diltiazem and verapamil are contraindicated in patients with bradycardia, heart block, or systolic HF). Nifedipine should be avoided because it has demonstrated reflex sympathetic activation, tachycardia, and worsened myocardial ischemia.[4] Dosing and contraindications are described in Table 8–2.

Early Pharmacotherapy for NSTE ACSs

In general, early pharmacotherapy of NSTE ACS (Fig. 8–3) is similar to that of STE MI. **7** *In the absence of contraindications,*

Patient Encounter 2, Part 2

Is reperfusion therapy with fibrinolysis indicated at this time for patient SD?

What adjunctive pharmacotherapy should be administered to SD in the emergency department?

What additional pharmacotherapy should be initiated on the first day of SD's hospitalization following successful reperfusion with PCI?

all patients with NSTE ACS should be treated in the emergency department with intranasal oxygen (if oxygen saturation is low), SL NTG, ASA, and an anticoagulant: UFH, enoxaparin, fondaparinux, or bivalirudin. High-risk patients should proceed to early angiography and may receive a GP IIb/IIIa inhibitor. A $P2Y_{12}$ inhibitor (selection of agent and timing of initiation dependent on selection of an interventional approach involving PCI or CABG surgery versus a noninterventional approach with medical management alone) should be administered to all patients. IV β-blockers and IV NTG should be given in selected patients. Oral β-blockers should be initiated within the first day in patients without cardiogenic shock.[5,6,8] Morphine is also administered to patients with refractory angina as described previously. These agents should be administered early while the patient is still in the emergency department. Fibrinolytic therapy is never administered. Dosing and contraindications for SL and IV NTG (for selected patients), ASA, $P2Y_{12}$ inhibitors, β-blockers, and anticoagulants are listed in Table 8–2.

▶ Fibrinolytic Therapy

Fibrinolytic therapy is not indicated in any patient with NSTE ACS because increased mortality has been reported with fibrinolytics compared with controls in clinical trials in which fibrinolytics have been administered to patients with NSTE ACS (patients with normal or ST-segment depression ECGs).

▶ Aspirin

ASA reduces the risk of death or developing MI by about 50% (compared with no antiplatelet therapy) in patients with NSTE ACS.[86] Therefore, ASA remains the cornerstone of early treatment for all ACS. Dosing of ASA for NSTE ACS is the same as that for STE MI (Table 8–2). Low-dose ASA is continued indefinitely.

▶ Anticoagulants

The choice of anticoagulant for a patient with NSTE ACS is guided by risk stratification and initial treatment strategy, either an early invasive approach with early coronary angiography and PCI or an early conservative strategy with angiography in selected patients guided by relief of symptoms and stress testing (Fig. 8–3). For patients treated by an early invasive strategy, UFH, enoxaparin, or bivalirudin should be administered.[6] In a large open-label, randomized clinical trial evaluating bivalirudin versus UFH or enoxaparin plus a GP IIb/IIIa inhibitor (abciximab, eptifibatide, or tirofiban) in moderate- and high-risk patients with NSTE ACS undergoing an early invasive strategy, bivalirudin demonstrated similar efficacy in preventing CV ischemic events but a lower bleeding rate.[87] Similarly, in a recent smaller randomized trial specifically comparing abciximab plus UFH with bivalirudin for patients with NSTE MI undergoing PCI, no differences in clinical outcomes but a lower bleeding risk with bivalirudin was observed.[88]

In patients in whom an initial conservative strategy is planned (i.e., they are not anticipated to receive angiography and revascularization), enoxaparin, UFH, or low-dose fondaparinux is recommended.[6] UFH and LMWH when added to ASA reduce the frequency of death or MI in patients presenting with NSTE ACS compared with control/placebo in patients primarily managed with a conservative strategy.[89,90] Compared with enoxaparin, fondaparinux showed similar ischemic outcomes with a lower bleeding rate in a large randomized trial of patients with NSTE ACS primarily managed with a conservative strategy.[91] For patients presenting with NSTE ACS in whom clinicians suspect a high risk for bleeding while receiving an anticoagulant, fondaparinux is the preferred anticoagulant recommended by the ACCF/AHA NSTE ACS guidelines.[6] Bivalirudin has not been studied for initial therapy in this setting. If fondaparinux is chosen for a patient initially receiving a conservative strategy who subsequently undergoes angiography and PCI, it should be administered in combination with UFH (and not as the sole anticoagulant) because the dose of fondaparinux studied appears too low to prevent thrombotic events during PCI.[6] Neither fondaparinux or bivalirudin are FDA approved for NSTE ACS despite being recommended by the ACCF/AHA NSTE ACS guidelines. Guideline-recommended dosing and contraindications are described in Table 8–2.

Therapy should be continued for at least 48 hours for UFH, until the patient is discharged from the hospital (or 8 days, whichever is shorter) for either enoxaparin or fondaparinux, and until the end of PCI or angiography procedure (or up to 72 hours following PCI) for bivalirudin.[2] UFH is the preferred anticoagulant following angiography in patients subsequently undergoing CABG during the same hospitalization because it has a short duration of action following discontinuation when the patient is proceeding to surgery.[7] Because enoxaparin is eliminated renally and patients with renal insufficiency generally have been excluded from clinical trials, some practice protocols recommend UFH for patients with CrCl rates of less than 30 mL/min (0.50 mL/s) based on total patient body weight using the Cockroft-Gault equation.[7] Although recommendations for dosing adjustment of enoxaparin in patients with CrCl between 10 and 30 mL/min (0.17 and 0.50 mL/s) are listed in the product manufacturer's label, the safety and efficacy of enoxaparin in this patient population remain vastly understudied. Administration of enoxaparin should be avoided in dialysis patients with ACS. It is unclear whether or not bivalirudin requires dose adjustment for patients with significant renal dysfunction. Although bivalirudin is eliminated renally, the duration of infusion in recent trials has been short (several hours only), and therefore the actual need for dosing adjustment is unlikely. Practice guidelines recommend manufacturer's suggesting dosing adjustment for patients with chronic kidney disease.[8] Patients with serum creatinine (SCr) greater than 3.0 mg/dL (265 μmol/L) were excluded from ACS trials with fondaparinux, and the product label states that fondaparinux is contraindicated in patients with CrCl less than 30 mL/min (0.50 mL/s) and in patients weighing less than 50 kg (110 lb).

UFH is monitored and the dose adjusted to a target activated partial thromboplastin time (aPTT), whereas enoxaparin is administered by a fixed actual body weight–based dose without routine monitoring of antifactor Xa levels. Some experts recommend antifactor Xa monitoring for LMWHs in patients with renal impairment during prolonged courses of administration of more than several days. No monitoring of coagulation is recommended for bivalirudin and fondaparinux.

▶ P2Y₁₂ Inhibitors

Figure 8–4 delineates the role of different P2Y₁₂ inhibitors in ACS. For patients with NSTE ACS where an initial invasive management strategy is selected, two initial options for dual antiplatelet therapy are described by the practice guidelines depending on choice of P2Y₁₂ inhibitor. In addition to ASA administered either prehospital or in the emergency department, either

1. Early use of clopidogrel[6] or ticagrelor[66] (in the emergency department), or

2. Double bolus dose eptifibatide or high-dose tirofiban administered at the time of PCI (bivalirudin should not be administered as the anticoagulant in this option)[6]

Subsequent antiplatelet therapy following PCI is selected based on the coronary anatomy at the time of angiography. For patients undergoing PCI initially treated with regimen 1 above, a GP IIb/IIIa inhibitor (abciximab, eptifibatide, or tirofiban) can be added and then clopidogrel continued with low-dose aspirin. For patients undergoing PCI initially treated with option 2, clopidogrel, prasugrel, or ticagrelor can be selected following PCI (within 1 hour following PCI) and the P2Y₁₂ inhibitor continued with low-dose ASA. In a subgroup of patients undergoing PCI enrolled in a large clinical trial evaluating clopidogrel versus placebo added to ASA in patients with NSTE ACS, clopidogrel reduced the frequency of death or MI by 30%.[92] In the large pivotal trials of prasugrel versus clopidogrel and ticagrelor versus clopidogrel (PLATO), no added benefit of the newer P2Y₁₂ inhibitors was observed in the subgroup of patients with NSTE ACS undergoing PCI.[58,61] Following PCI in ACS, dual oral antiplatelet therapy is continued for at least 12 months.[6]

For patients receiving an initial conservative treatment strategy, the 2011 ACCF/AHA NSTE ACS guidelines recommend early administration of clopidogrel (a 300-mg loading dose followed by 75 mg daily) in addition to ASA. The subgroup of medically managed patients in a large trial of clopidogrel in patients with NSTE ACS demonstrated a 20% reduction in the risk of CV death, MI, or stroke compared with aspirin alone, a benefit similar to that seen in patients undergoing PCI.[93] Ticagrelor is an alternative in medically managed patients as described in the section "Early Pharmacotherapy for STE MI."[62,66] Dual antiplatelet therapy is continued for at least 1 month and ideally for 1 year.

Specific dosing and contraindications of the P2Y₁₂ inhibitors are described in Table 8–2.

▶ Glycoprotein IIb/IIIa Receptor Inhibitors

The role of GP IIb/IIIa inhibitors in NSTE ACS is diminishing as P2Y₁₂ inhibitors are used earlier in therapy, and bivalirudin is selected more commonly as the anticoagulant in patients receiving an early intervention approach. See the preceding section (P2Y₁₂ inhibitors) that includes the selection and timing of GP IIb/IIIa inhibitors in patients with NSTE ACS undergoing PCI.[6,8] Routine administration of eptifibatide (added to aspirin and clopidogrel) prior to angiography and PCI (i.e., "upstream" use) in NSTE ACS does not reduce ischemic events and increases bleeding risk.[94] Therefore, the two antiplatelet initial therapy options, described in the previous section, are preferred.[6]

For low-risk patients where a conservative management strategy is selected, there is no role for routine GP IIb/IIIa inhibitors because the bleeding risk exceeds the benefit.[6] For patients in whom an initial conservative strategy was selected but who experience recurrent ischemia (chest discomfort and ECG changes), HF, or arrhythmias after initial medical therapy necessitating a change in strategy to angiography and revascularization, a GP IIb/IIIa inhibitor may be added to ASA and clopidogrel prior to the angiogram.[6]

Doses and contraindications to GP IIb/IIIa receptor inhibitors are described in Table 8–2.

▶ Nitrates

SL NTG followed by IV NTG should be administered to patients with NSTE ACS and ongoing ischemia, HF, or uncontrolled high BP (Table 8–2). The mechanism of action, dosing, contraindications, and adverse effects are the same as those described in the section on early pharmacologic therapy for STE MI. IV NTG is typically continued for approximately 24 hours following ischemia relief.

▶ β-Blockers

The use of β-blockers in NSTE ACS is similar to STE MI in that oral β-blockers should be initiated within 24 hours of hospital admission to all patients in the absence of contraindications. Benefits of β-blockers in this patient group are assumed to be similar to those seen in patients with STE MI. β-Blockers are continued indefinitely. The prescription of a β-blocker at hospital discharge used to be reported as a quality measure.

▶ Calcium Channel Blockers

As described in the previous section, calcium channel blockers should not be administered to most patients with ACS. Their role is a second-line treatment for patients with certain contraindications to β-blockers and those with continued ischemia despite β-blocker and nitrate therapy. Administration of amlodipine, diltiazem, or verapamil is preferred.[5]

Secondary Prevention Following MI

The long-term goals following MI are to (a) control modifiable CHD risk factors; (b) prevent the development of HF; (c) prevent recurrent MI and stroke; (d) prevent death, including sudden cardiac death; and (e) prevent stent thrombosis following PCI. Pharmacotherapy, which has been proven to decrease mortality, HF, reinfarction or stroke, and stent thrombosis, should be initiated prior to hospital discharge for secondary prevention. ❽ *Secondary prevention guidelines from the ACCF/AHA suggest that following MI, from either STE MI or NSTE ACS, all patients, in the absence of contraindications, should receive indefinite treatment with ASA, a β-blocker, and an angiotensin-converting enzyme (ACE) inhibitor for secondary prevention of death, stroke, or recurrent infarction.[46] Most patients will receive a statin to reduce low-density lipoprotein cholesterol to less than 100 mg/dL (2.59 mmol/L) and ideally to less than 70 mg/dL (1.81 mmol/L). A P2Y$_{12}$ inhibitor should be continued for at least 12 months for patients undergoing PCI and for patients with NSTE ACS receiving a medical management strategy of treatment.[3,6] Clopidogrel should be continued for at least 14 days in patients with STE MI not undergoing PCI.[8] An angiotensin II receptor blocker (ARB) and a mineralocorticoid receptor antagonist should be given to selected patients as discussed in greater detail later in the chapter.[46] For all patient with ACS, treatment and control of modifiable risk factors such as hypertension (HTN), dyslipidemia, obesity, smoking, and DM are essential.[46]* Dosing and contraindications are described in detail in Table 8–2. Benefits and adverse effects of long-term treatment with these medications are discussed in more detail later. Use of ICDs for the prevention of sudden cardiac death following MI in patients with diminished LVF and nonsustained ventricular arrhythmias is discussed in more detail in Chapter 9, "Arrhythmias."

▶ Aspirin

ASA decreases the risk of death, recurrent infarction, and stroke following MI. All patients should receive ASA indefinitely; those patients with a contraindication to ASA should receive clopidogrel.[46] The risk of major bleeding

from chronic ASA therapy is approximately 2% and is dose related. Higher doses of ASA, 160 to 325 mg, are not more effective than ASA doses of 75 to 81 mg but have higher rates of bleeding.[95] Therefore, chronic doses of ASA should not exceed 81 mg.[8,46]

▶ P2Y$_{12}$ Inhibitors

For patients with either STE MI or NSTE ACS, clopidogrel decreases the risk of CV events and stent thrombosis compared with placebo. Compared with clopidogrel, either prasugrel or ticagrelor lowers the risk of CV death, MI, or stroke by an additional 20% to 30% depending on the patient population studied. The frequency of stent thrombosis following PCI is also lower with prasugrel or ticagrelor compared with clopidogrel. However, the rate of non-CABG surgery-associated bleeding is higher with both prasugrel and ticagrelor compared with clopidogrel. The ACCF/AHA/SCAI PCI guidelines recommend that for patients with ACS, a P2Y$_{12}$ inhibitor should be continued for at least 12 months following PCI. For medically managed patients with STE MI, clopidogrel should be continued for at least 14 days and up to 1 year.[3] For medically managed NSTE ACS patients, clopidogrel should be continued at least 1 month and ideally up to 1 year.[6] Ticagrelor has also been studied for medical management of ACS and may be considered an option, although currently it is not a recommended therapy in ACCF/AHA guideline because these guidelines were published prior to the availability of ticagrelor in the United States.[62]

The combination of clopidogrel and aspirin increases the risk of major bleeding by approximately 50% and minor bleeding by approximately 40% but not fatal bleeding compared with a single agent alone.[96] Oral antiplatelet agents are the third leading cause of adverse drug reaction–associated hospital admissions after emergency department visits among seniors.[97] Therefore, patients should be counseled on the risks and sites of potential bleeding and should be told to seek medical care immediately if significant bleeding is noticed.

▶ β-Blockers, Nitrates, and Calcium Channel Blockers

Current treatment guidelines recommend that following an ACS, patients should receive a β-blocker indefinitely[3,6] whether they have residual symptoms of angina or not.[98] Overwhelming data support the use of β-blockers in patients with a previous MI. Currently, there are no data to support the superiority of one β-blocker over another in the absence of HF.

Although β-blockers should be avoided in patients with decompensated HF from left ventricular systolic dysfunction complicating an MI, clinical trial data suggest it is safe to initiate β-blockers prior to hospital discharge in these patients once HF symptoms have resolved.[99] These patients may actually benefit more than those without left ventricular dysfunction.[100] In patients who cannot tolerate or have a contraindication to a β-blocker, a calcium channel blocker can be used to prevent anginal symptoms but should not be used routinely in the absence of such symptoms.[4]

Finally, all patients should be prescribed short-acting sublingual NTG or lingual NTG spray to relieve any anginal symptoms when necessary and instructed on its use.[4,6] Chronic long-acting nitrate therapy has not been shown to reduce CHD events following MI. Therefore, IV NTG is not routinely followed by chronic, long-acting oral nitrate therapy in ACS patients who have undergone revascularization, unless the patient has chronic stable angina or significant coronary stenoses that were not revascularized.[101]

▶ ACE Inhibitors and ARBs

ACE inhibitors should be initiated in all patients following MI to reduce mortality, decrease reinfarction, and prevent the development of HF.[3,6,46] The benefit of ACE inhibitors in patients with MI most likely comes from their ability to prevent cardiac remodeling. The largest reduction in mortality is observed in patients with left ventricular dysfunction (low LVEF) or HF symptoms. Early initiation (within 24 hours) of an *oral* ACE inhibitor appears to be crucial during an acute MI because 40% of the 30-day survival benefit is observed during the first day, 45% from days 2 to 7, and approximately 15% from days 8 to 30.[102] However, current data do not support the early administration of IV ACE inhibitors in patients experiencing an MI because mortality may be increased.[103] Administration of ACE inhibitors should be continued indefinitely. Hypotension should be avoided because coronary artery filling may be compromised. Additional trials suggest that most patients with CAD, not just ACS or HF patients, benefit from ACE inhibitors. Therefore, ACE inhibitors should be considered in all patients following an ACS in the absence of a contraindication.

Many patients cannot tolerate chronic ACE inhibitor therapy secondary to adverse effects. The ARBs candesartan, valsartan, and losartan have been documented in trials to improve clinical outcomes in patients with HF.[104,105] Therefore, either an ACE inhibitor or candesartan, valsartan or losartan are acceptable choices for chronic therapy for patients who have a low LVEF and HF following MI.

Besides hypotension, the most frequent adverse reaction to an ACE inhibitor is cough, which may occur in up to 30% of patients. Patients with an ACE inhibitor cough and either clinical signs of HF or LVEF less than 40% (0.40) may be prescribed an ARB.[46] Other, less common but more serious adverse effects of ACE inhibitors and ARBs include acute renal failure, hyperkalemia, and angioedema.

▶ Mineralocorticoid Receptor Antagonists

To reduce mortality, administration of a mineralocorticoid receptor antagonist, either eplerenone or spironolactone, should be considered within the first 2 weeks following MI in all patients who are already receiving an ACE inhibitor (or ARB) and a β-blocker and have an LVEF equal to or less than 40% (0.40) and either HF symptoms or DM.[46] Aldosterone plays an important role in HF and in MI because it promotes vascular and myocardial fibrosis, endothelial dysfunction, HTN, left ventricular hypertrophy, sodium retention, potassium and magnesium loss, and arrhythmias. Mineralocorticoid receptor antagonists have been shown in experimental and human studies to attenuate these adverse effects.[106] Spironolactone decreases all-cause mortality in patients with stable severe HF.[107]

Eplerenone, like spironolactone, is an aldosterone antagonist that blocks the mineralocorticoid receptor. In contrast to spironolactone, eplerenone has no effect on the progesterone or androgen receptor, thereby minimizing the risk of gynecomastia, sexual dysfunction, and menstrual irregularities. In a large clinical trial,[108] eplerenone significantly reduced mortality as well as hospitalization for HF in post-MI patients with an LVEF less than 40% (0.40) and symptoms of HF at any time during hospitalization. Eplerenone has also been demonstrated to reduce mortality in patients with mild systolic HF.[109] The risk of hyperkalemia, however, was increased in both these studies. Therefore, patients with a SCr greater than 2.5 mg/dL (221 μmol/L) or CrCl less than 50 mL/min (0.83 mL/s) or serum potassium concentration of greater than 5.0 mmol/L (5.0 mEq/L) should not receive eplerenone (in addition to either an ACE inhibitor or ARB). Currently, there are no data to support that the more selective, more expensive eplerenone is superior to, or should be preferred to, the less expensive generic spironolactone unless a patient has experienced gynecomastia, breast pain, or impotence while receiving spironolactone. Finally, it should be noted that hyperkalemia is just as likely to appear with both of these agents, and it is more common in patients receiving concomitant ACE inhibitors.

▶ Lipid-Lowering Agents

Following MI, statins reduce total mortality, CV mortality, and stroke. According to the National Cholesterol Education Program (NCEP) Adult Treatment Panel recommendations, all patients with CAD should receive dietary counseling and pharmacologic therapy in order to reach a low-density lipoprotein (LDL) cholesterol of less than 100 mg/dL (2.59 mmol/L), with statins the preferred agents to lower LDL cholesterol.[110] Results from landmark clinical trials have unequivocally demonstrated the value of statins in secondary prevention following MI. A meta-analysis of randomized controlled clinical trials in almost 18,000 patients with recent ACS (less than 14 days) found that statin therapy reduces mortality by 19%, with benefits observed after approximately 4 months of treatment.[111] Although the primary effect of statins is to decrease LDL cholesterol, statins are believed to produce many non-lipid-lowering or "pleiotropic" effects such as anti-inflammatory and antithrombotic properties. Additional recommendations from the NCEP give an optional LDL cholesterol goal of less than 70 mg/dL (1.81 mmol/L).[112] The current evidence indicates that higher-dose statin therapy, such as atorvastatin 40 to 80 mg daily and rosuvastatin 10 to 20 mg daily, produces greater reduction in CV events such as MI, ischemic stroke, and revascularization than less intensive statin regimens (such as simvastatin 20 to 40 mg daily).[113] Moreover, the administration of high-dose statins prior to PCI may reduce the risk of periprocedural MI, and hence statins should be initiated as early as possible in ACS.[8]

A fibrate derivative, niacin, or fish oil may be considered in patients with an elevated non-high-density lipoprotein cholesterol level despite maximally tolerated statin therapy, although the benefits of this management strategy remain largely unproven.[46] In a large randomized trial of men with established CAD and low levels of high-density lipoprotein (HDL) cholesterol, the use of gemfibrozil (600 mg twice daily, alone and not added to a statin) significantly decreased the risk of nonfatal MI or death from coronary causes.[114] Studies with fenofibrate and niacin have produced less definitive results.[115,116]

▶ Other Modifiable Risk Factors

Smoking cessation, managing HTN, weight loss, exercise, and tight glucose control for patients with DM, in addition to treatment of dyslipidemia, are important treatments for secondary prevention of CHD events.[46] Referral to a comprehensive CV risk reduction program for cardiac rehabilitation is recommended.[46] The use of nicotine patches or gum, or of bupropion alone or in combination with nicotine patches, should be considered in appropriate patients.[3] HTN should be strictly controlled according to published guidelines.[46] Patients who are overweight should be educated on the importance of regular exercise, healthy eating habits, and reaching and maintaining an ideal weight. Moderate-intensity aerobic exercise for at least 30 minutes, 7 days per week (minimum 5 days per week) is recommended.[46] The goal body mass index is less than 25 kg/m². Finally, because patients with DM have up to a fourfold increased mortality risk compared with patients without DM, the importance of blood glucose control, as well as other CHD risk factor modifications, cannot be overstated.[46]

Patient Encounter 1, Part 3

Identify the long-term treatment goals for RR.

What additional pharmacotherapy should be initiated prior to hospital discharge?

Create a care plan for RR for hospital discharge that includes pharmacotherapy, desired treatment outcomes, and monitoring for efficacy and adverse effects.

Patient Encounter 2, Part 3

Patient SD undergoes coronary angiography and PCI with a drug-eluting stent placed for a 90% stenosis in his left anterior descending coronary artery on hospital day 1.

Identify the long-term treatment goals for SD.

What additional pharmacotherapy should be initiated prior to hospital discharge?

Create a care plan for SD for hospital discharge that includes pharmacotherapy, desired treatment outcomes, and monitoring for efficacy and adverse effects.

OUTCOME EVALUATION

- ⑨ *To determine the efficacy of nonpharmacologic and pharmacotherapy for both STE and NSTE ACS, monitor patients for (a) relief of ischemic discomfort; (b) return of ECG changes to baseline; and (c) absence or resolution of HF signs and symptoms.*

- Monitoring parameters for recognition and prevention of adverse effects from ACS pharmacotherapy are described in Table 8–5. ⑨ *In general, the most common adverse reactions from ACS therapies are hypotension and bleeding.* To treat for bleeding and hypotension, discontinue the offending agent(s) until symptoms resolve. Severe bleeding resulting in hypotension secondary to hypovolemia may require blood transfusion.

- Because poor medication adherence of secondary prevention medications following MI leads to worsened CV outcomes, patients should receive medication counseling (including counseling prior to hospital discharge) and be monitored for medication persistence.[8,117] Counseling should include assessment of health literacy level, assessment of barriers to adherence, assessment of access to medications, written and verbal instructions about the purpose of each medication, changes to previous medication regimen, optimal time to take each medication, new allergies or medication intolerances, need for timely prescription fill after discharge, anticipated duration of therapy, consequences of nonadherence, common and/or serious adverse reactions that may develop, drug–drug and drug–food interactions, and an assessment of instruction understanding).

- Process of care quality performance measures for MI endorsed by the AHA and Centers for Medicare and Medicaid Services are described in Table 8–6.[32,118]

Table 8–5

Therapeutic Drug Monitoring for Adverse Effects of Pharmacotherapy for Acute Coronary Syndromes

Drug	Adverse Effects	Monitoring
Aspirin	Dyspepsia, bleeding, gastritis	Clinical signs of bleeding[a]; GI upset; baseline CBC and platelet count; CBC platelet count every 6 months
Clopidogrel and prasugrel	Bleeding, diarrhea, rash, TTP (rare)	Clinical signs of bleeding[a]; baseline CBC and platelet count; CBC and platelet count every 6 months following hospital discharge
Ticagrelor	Bleeding, dyspnea, diarrhea, rash, elevated SCr, elevated serum uric acid	Clinical signs of bleeding[a]; baseline CBC and platelet count; CBC and platelet count every 6 months following hospital discharge
Unfractionated heparin	Bleeding, heparin-induced thrombocytopenia	Clinical signs of bleeding[a]; baseline aPTT, INR, CBC, and platelet count; aPTT every 6 hours until target then every 24 hours; daily CBC; platelet count every 2–3 days from days 4 to 14 until heparin is stopped (minimum, preferably every day)
Enoxaparin	Bleeding, heparin-induced thrombocytopenia	Clinical signs of bleeding[a]; baseline SCr, aPTT, INR, CBC, and platelet count; daily CBC, no routine platelet count monitoring unless recent UFH (less than 100 days) then baseline and within 24 hours; daily CBC and SCr
Fondaparinux	Bleeding	Clinical signs of bleeding[a]; baseline SCr, aPTT, INR, CBC, and platelet count; daily CBC and SCr
Bivalirudin	Bleeding	Clinical signs of bleeding[a]; baseline SCr, aPTT, INR, CBC, and platelet count
Fibrinolytics	Bleeding, especially intracranial hemorrhage	Clinical signs of bleeding[a]; baseline aPTT, INR, CBC, and platelet count; mental status every 2 hours for signs of intracranial hemorrhage; daily CBC
Glycoprotein IIb/IIIa receptor inhibitors	Bleeding, acute profound thrombocytopenia	Clinical signs of bleeding[a]; baseline SCr (for eptifibatide and tirofiban), CBC, and platelet count; platelet count at 4 hours after initiation; daily CBC (and SCr for eptifibatide and tirofiban)
IV nitrates	Hypotension, flushing, headache, tachycardia	BP and HR every 2 hours
β-Blockers	Hypotension, bradycardia, heart block, bronchospasm, acute heart failure, fatigue, depression, sexual dysfunction	BP, RR, HR, 12-lead ECG, and clinical signs of heart failure every 5 minutes during bolus IV dosing; BP, RR, HR, and clinical signs of heart failure every shift during oral administration during hospitalization, then BP and HR every 6 months following hospital discharge
Diltiazem and verapamil	Hypotension, bradycardia, heart block, heart failure, gingival hyperplasia	BP and HR every shift during oral administration during hospitalization, then every 6 months following hospital discharge; dental examination and teeth cleaning every 6 months
Amlodipine	Hypotension, dependent peripheral edema, gingival hyperplasia	BP every shift during oral administration during hospitalization, then every 6 months following hospital discharge; dental examination and teeth cleaning every 6 months
Angiotensin-converting enzyme (ACE) inhibitors and angiotensin receptor blockers (ARBs)	Hypotension, cough (with ACE inhibitors), hyperkalemia, prerenal azotemia, acute renal failure, angioedema (ACE inhibitors more so than ARBs)	BP every 4 hours × 3 for first dose, then every shift during oral administration during hospitalization, then once every 6 months following hospital discharge; baseline SCr and potassium; daily SCr and potassium while hospitalized, then every 6 months (or 1–2 weeks after each outpatient dose titration); closer monitoring required in selected patients using spironolactone or eplerenone or if renal insufficiency; counsel patient on throat, tongue, and facial swelling
Mineralocorticoid receptor antagonists	Hypotension, hyperkalemia, increased SCr	BP and HR every shift during oral administration during hospitalization, then once every 6 months; baseline SCr and serum potassium concentration; SCr and potassium at 48 hours, at 7 days, then monthly for 3 months, then every 3 months thereafter following hospital discharge
Morphine	Hypotension, respiratory depression	BP and RR 5 minutes after each bolus dose
Statins	GI upset, myopathy, hepatotoxicity	Liver function tests at baseline, at 6 weeks following initiation, and after titration to highest dose, then annually thereafter; counsel patient on myalgia; consider creatinine kinase at baseline if adding a fibrate or niacin

[a]Clinical signs of bleeding include bloody stools, melena, hematuria, hematemesis, bruising, and oozing from arterial or venous puncture sites.

ACE, angiotensin-converting enzyme; aPTT, activated partial thromboplastin time; ARB, angiotensin receptor blocker; BP, blood pressure; CBC, complete blood count; ECG, electrocardiogram; HR, heart rate; INR, international normalized ratio; RR, respiratory rate; SCr, serum creatinine, TTP, thrombotic thrombocytopenic purpura.

Table 8–6

Process of Care Quality Performance Measures for Myocardial Infarction[32,118]

- Median time to initial ECG (desired less than or equal to 10 minutes)[a]
- Aspirin at hospital arrival.[a,b]
- Fibrinolytic medication within 30 minutes of hospital arrival for STE MI ("door-to-needle" time)[a,b]
- Median time to fibrinolysis[a]
- PCI received within 90 minutes of hospital arrival for STE MI[a,b]
- Median time to transfer to another facility for PCI ("door in door out time" desired is less than or equal to 30 minutes)[a,b]
- Percentage of eligible patients with STE MI receiving reperfusion therapy with either fibrinolytics or PCI[b]
- Aspirin at hospital discharge[a,b]
- ACE Inhibitor or ARB for systolic dysfunction at hospital discharge[a,b]
- β-Blocker at hospital discharge[a,b]
- Smoking cessation advice/counseling[a,b]
- Statin at hospital discharge[b]
- Evaluation of LV function[b]
- Cardiac rehabilitation referral[b]

[a]2010 Center for Medicare and Medicaid Services process of care measures for myocardial infarction.

[b]American Heart Association 2008 myocardial infarction performance measure.

ACE, angiotensin-converting enzyme; ARB, angiotensin receptor blocker; ECG, electrocardiogram; LV, left ventricular; MI, myocardial infarction; PCI, percutaneous coronary intervention; STE, ST-segment elevation.

Patient Care and Monitoring

For patients in acute distress and ACS is suspected:

- Follow recommendations in Figures 8–1 and 8–2 and Table 8–2. Also incorporate into your plan the recommendations detailed below under "For patients diagnosed with ACS."

For patients diagnosed with ACS:

1. Review patient's medical record to determine indications for each medication.

2. Review patient's medical record to determine contraindications for each medication. For ASA, β-blockers, ACE inhibitors, and ARBs, document contraindications in patient's medical record.

3. Review doses of medications for appropriateness. Titration toward target doses of ACE inhibitors and β-blockers should be in progress. Evaluate if the dose of ASA may be reduced to less than 100 mg if no recent stent.

4. Interview the patient to assess health literacy, prescription medications, and complementary or alternative medication use.

5. Evaluate the patient's medical record and medication history, and conduct a patient interview to assess for the presence of drug allergies, adverse drug reactions, drug interactions, and medication adherence.

6. Educate the patient and evaluate their success with lifestyle modifications including smoking cessation, diet, weight loss, and exercise. For patients with DM, appropriate blood glucose control should be emphasized.

7. Provide patient education with regard to CAD, MI, indications for medications, and potential adverse effects and drug interactions.

   - What is CAD?
   - How can the progression of CAD and MI be prevented?
   - How does each medication benefit the patient?
   - Why is adherence important?
   - What potential adverse effects may occur?
   - What potential drug interactions may occur?
   - Warning signs to report to the physician or emergency medical services include chest squeezing, burning, or pain; jaw pain; pain radiation down the arm; bleeding; and loss of consciousness.
   - Dial 911 if there is no chest discomfort relief after one SL NTG tablet.
   - Important to train caregiver or relative to administer cardiopulmonary resuscitation (CPR).

8. Document smoking cessation counseling and patient receipt of discharge instructions in the patient's medical record.

Abbreviations Introduced in This Chapter

ABCB1	ATP-binding cassette B1
ACC	American College of Cardiology
ACCF	American College of Cardiology Foundation
ACE	Angiotensin-converting enzyme
ACS	Acute coronary syndrome
ACT	Activated clotting time
ADP	Adenosine diphosphate
AHA	American Heart Association
AMI	Acute myocardial infarction
aPTT	Activated partial thromboplastin time
ARB	Angiotensin receptor blocker
ASA	Aspirin
ATP	Adenosine triphosphate
AUC	Area under the curve
BP	Blood pressure
CABG	Coronary artery bypass graft (surgery)
CAD	Coronary artery disease
CBC	Complete blood count
CHD	Coronary heart disease
CK	Creatine kinase
CKD	Chronic kidney disease
COX-2	Cyclooxygenase-2
CPR	Cardiopulmonary resuscitation
CrCl	Creatinine clearance
CV	Cardiovascular
CVD	Cardiovascular disease
CYP	Cytochrome P450
DM	Diabetes mellitus
ECG	Electrocardiogram
EF	Ejection fraction
GP	Glycoprotein
GRACE	Global Registry of Acute Coronary Events
GWTG	Get With the Guidelines
HDL	High-density lipoprotein
HF	Heart failure
HORIZONS-AMI	Harmonizing Outcomes with Revascularization and Stents in Acute Myocardial Infarction
HR	Heart rate
HTN	Hypertension
ICD	Implantable cardioverter defibrillator
ICH	Intracranial hemorrhage
INR	International normalized ratio
ISIS-2	Second International Study of Infarct Survival
LDL	Low-density lipoprotein
LMWH	Low molecular weight heparin
LVEF	Left ventricular ejection fraction
LVF	Left ventricular function
MB	Myocardial band
MI	Myocardial infarction

NCEP	National Cholesterol Education Program
NSAID	Nonsteroidal anti-inflammatory drug
NSTE	Non-ST-segment elevation
NTG	Nitroglycerin
PCI	Percutaneous coronary intervention
PLATO	Study of Platelet Inhibition and Patient Outcomes
RR	Respiratory rate
SCAI	Society for Cardiovascular Angiography and Interventions
SCr	Serum creatinine
SC	Subcutaneous
SL	Sublingual
STE	ST-Segment elevation
TIA	Transient ischemic attack
TIMI	Thrombolysis in myocardial infarction
TTP	Thrombotic thrombocytopenia purpura
TXA_2	Thromboxane A_2
UA	Unstable angina
UFH	Unfractionated heparin

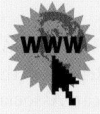 Self-assessment questions and answers are available at *http://www.mhpharmacotherapy. com/pp.html.*

REFERENCES

1. Roger L, Go AS, Lloyd-Jones DM, et al. Heart disease and stroke statistics—2011 update: A report from the American Heart Association. Circulation 2011;123:e18–e209.

2. Kushner FG, Hand M, Smith SC Jr, et al. American College of Cardiology Foundation/American Heart Association Task Force on Practice Guidelines. 2009 focused updates: ACCF/AHA guidelines for the management of patients with ST-elevation myocardial infarction (updating the 2004 guideline and 2007 focused update) and ACCF/AHA/SCAI guidelines on percutaneous coronary intervention (updating the 2005 guideline and 2007 focused update): A report of the American College of Cardiology Foundation/American Heart Association Task Force on Practice Guidelines. Circulation 2009;120:2271–2306. Erratum in: Circulation 2010;121:e257. Dosage error in article text.

3. Antman EM, Hand M, Armstrong PW, et al. 2007 Focused Update of the ACCF/AHA 2004 Guidelines for the Management of Patients with ST-Elevation Myocardial Infarction: A report of the American College of Cardiology/American Heart Association Task Force on Practice Guidelines: Developed in collaboration with the Canadian Cardiovascular Society endorsed by the American Academy of Family Physicians: 2007 Writing Group to Review New Evidence and Update the ACC/AHA 2004 Guidelines for the Management of Patients with ST-Elevation Myocardial Infarction, Writing on Behalf of the 2004 Writing Committee. Circulation 2008;117:296–329.

4. Antman EM, Anbe DT, Armstrong PW, et al. ACC/AHA guidelines for the management of patients with ST-elevation myocardial infarction—executive summary: A report of the American College of Cardiology/American Heart Association Task Force on Practice Guidelines (Writing Committee to Revise the 1999 Guidelines for the Management of Patients with Acute Myocardial Infarction). Circulation 2004;110:588–636.

5. Anderson JL, Adams CD, Antman EM, et al. ACC/AHA 2007 guidelines for the management of patients with unstable angina/non ST-elevation myocardial infarction: A report of the American College of

Cardiology/American Heart Association Task Force on Practice Guidelines (Writing Committee to Revise the 2002 Guidelines for the Management of Patients with Unstable Angina/Non ST-Elevation Myocardial Infarction): Developed in collaboration with the American College of Emergency Physicians, the Society for Cardiovascular Angiography and Interventions, and the Society of Thoracic Surgeons: Endorsed by the American Association of Cardiovascular and Pulmonary Rehabilitation and the Society for Academic Emergency Medicine. Circulation 2007;116:e148–e304.

6. Wright RS, Anderson JL, Adams CD, et al. 2011 ACCF/AHA focused update of the guidelines for the management of patients with unstable angina/non–ST-elevation myocardial infarction (updating the 2007 guideline): A report of the American College of Cardiology Foundation/American Heart Association Task Force on Practice Guidelines. Circulation 2011;123:2022–2060.

7. Anderson JL, Adams CD, Antman AM, et al. ACC/AHA 2007 guidelines for the management of patients with unstable angina/non ST-elevation myocardial infarction: A report of the American College of Cardiology/American Heart Association Task Force on Practice Guidelines (Writing Committee to Revise the 2002 Guidelines for the Management of Patients with Unstable Angina/Non ST-Elevation Myocardial Infarction): developed in collaboration with the American College of Emergency Physicians, the Society for Cardiovascular Angiography and Interventions, and the Society of Thoracic Surgeons: Endorsed by the American Association of Cardiovascular and Pulmonary Rehabilitation and the Society for Academic Emergency Medicine. Circulation 2007;116:e148-304. Erratum in: Circulation 2008;117(9):e180.

8. Levine GN, Bates ER, Blankeship JC, et al. 2011 ACCF/AHA/SCAI Guideline for Percutaneous Coronary Intervention: A Report of the American College of Cardiology Foundation/American Heart Association Task Force on Practice Guidelines and the Society for Cardiovascular Angiography and Interventions. Circulation 2011;124:e574–651. Erratum in: Circulation 2012;125:e412. Dosage error in article text.

9. Bassand JP, Agewall S, Bax J, et al. ESC Guidelines for the management of acute coronary syndromes in patients presenting without persistent ST-segment elevation: The task force for the management of acute coronary syndromes (ACS) in patients presenting without persistent ST-segment elevation of the European Society of Cardiology (ESC). Eur Heart J 2011;32:2999–3054.

10. Lloyd-Jones D, Adams RJ, Brown TM, et al. Executive summary: Heart disease and stroke statistics—2010 update: A report from the American Heart Association. Circulation 2010;121(7):948–954.

11. Chin CT, Chen AY, Wang TY, et al. Risk adjustment for in-hospital mortality of contemporary patients with acute myocardial infarction: The acute coronary treatment and intervention outcomes network (ACTION) registry-get with the guidelines (GWTG) acute myocardial infarction mortality model and risk score. Am Heart J 2011;161(1):113–122.e2.

12. U.S. Department of Health & Human Services. Calculation of 30-day Risk Standardized Mortality Rates and Rates of Readmission. Available at: http://hospitalcompare.hhs.gov/staticpages/for-professionals/ooc/calculation-of-30-day-risk.aspx. Accessed November 30, 2011.

13. Borissoff JI, Spronk HMH, ten Cate H. The hemostasis system as a modulator of atherosclerosis. N Engl J Med 2011;364:746–760.

14. Fuster V, Moreno PR, Fayad ZA, et al. Atherothrombosis and high-risk plaque: Part I: Evolving concepts. J Am Coll Cardiol 2005;46:937–954.

15. Spinler SA. Acute coronary syndromes. In: Dunsworth TS, Richardson MM, Cheng JWM, et al, eds. Pharmacotherapy self-assessment program. Book 1: Cardiology, 6th ed. Kansas City, KS: American College of Clinical Pharmacy, 2007:59–83.

16. Ruberg FL, Leopold JA, Loscalzo J. Atherothrombosis: Plaque instability and thrombogenesis. Prog Cardiovas Dis 2003;44:381–394.

17. Gajarsa JJ, Kloner RA. Left ventricular remodeling in the post-infarction heart: A review of cellular, molecular mechanisms, and therapeutic modalities. Heart Fail Rev 2011;16(1):13–21.

18. Goodman SG, Huang W, Yan AT, et al. The expanded Global Registry of Acute Coronary Events: Baseline characteristics, management practices and outcomes of patients with acute coronary syndromes. Am Heart J 2009;158:193–205.e5.

19. Fox KAA, Steg PG, Eagle KA, et al. Decline in rates of death and heart failure in acute coronary syndromes, 1999–2006. JAMA 2007;297:1892–1900.

20. Lavie CJ, Gersh BJ. Mechanical and electrical complications of acute myocardial infarction. Mayo Clin Proc 1990;65:709–730. Erratum in: Mayo Clin Proc 1990;65:1032.

21. Thygesen K, Alpert JS, White HD, et al. Universal definition of myocardial infarction. Circulation 2007;116:2634–2653.

22. Fibrinolytic Therapy Trialists' (FTT) Collaborative Group. Indications for fibrinolytic therapy in suspected myocardial infarction: Collaborative overview of early mortality and major morbidity results from all randomized trials of more than 1,000 patients. Lancet 1994;343:311–322.

23. Berger P, Ellis SG, Holmes DR Jr, et al. Relationship between delay in performing direct coronary angioplasty and early clinical outcome in patients with acute myocardial infarction: Results from the Global Use of Strategies to Open Occluded Arteries in Acute Coronary Syndromes (GUSTO-IIb) trial. Circulation 1999;100:14–20.

24. Steg PG, Goldberg RJ, Gore JM, et al. Baseline characteristics, management practices, and in-hospital outcomes of patients hospitalized with acute coronary syndromes in the Global Registry of Acute Coronary Events (GRACE). Am J Cardiol 2002;90:358–363.

25. Peterson ED, Roe MT, Muglund J, et al. Association between hospital process performance and outcomes among patients with acute coronary syndromes. JAMA 2006;295:1912–1920.

26. Eagle KA, Montoye CK, Riba AL, et al. Guideline-based standardized care is associated with substantially lower mortality in Medicare patients with acute myocardial infarction: the American College of Cardiology's Guidelines Applied in Practice (GAP) Projects in Michigan. J Am Coll Cardiol 2005;46:1242–1248.

27. Heidenreich PA, Lewis WR, LaBresh KA, et al. Hospital performance recognition with the Get with the Guidelines Program and mortality for acute myocardial infarction and heart failure. Am Heart J 2009;158:546–553.

28. Spinler SA. Evolution of antithrombotic therapy used in acute coronary syndromes. In: Richardson MM, Chessman KH, Chant C, Cheng JWM, et al., eds. Pharmacotherapy self-assessment program. Book 1: Cardiology, 7th ed. Lenexa, KS: American College of Clinical Pharmacy, 2010:97–124.

29. Antman EM, Cohen M, Bernink PJ, et al. The TIMI risk score for unstable angina/non-ST-segment-elevation MI: A method for prognostication and therapeutic decision-making. JAMA 2000;284:835–842.

30. Pieper KS, Gore JM, FitzGerald G, et al. Validity of a risk-prediction tool for hospital mortality: The Global Registry of Acute Coronary Events. Am Heart J 2009;157:1097–105.

31. Huynh T, Perron S, O'Loughlin J, et al. Comparison of primary percutaneous coronary intervention and fibrinolytic therapy in ST-segment-elevation myocardial infarction: Bayesian hierarchical meta-analyses of randomized controlled trials and observational studies. Circulation 2009;119:3101–3109.

32. Krumholz HM, Anderson JL, Bachelder BL, et al. ACC/AHA 2008 performance measures for adults with ST-elevation and non-ST-elevation myocardial infarction: A report of the American College of Cardiology/American Heart Association Task Force on Performance Measures (Writing Committee to Develop Performance Measures for ST-Elevation and Non-ST-Elevation Myocardial Infarction) Developed in Collaboration with the American Academy of Family Physicians and American College of Emergency Physicians Endorsed by the American Association of Cardiovascular and Pulmonary Rehabilitation, Society for Cardiovascular Angiography and Interventions, and Society of Hospital Medicine. J Am Coll Cardiol 2008;52:2046–2099.

33. Krumholz HM, Herrin J, Miller LE, et al. Improvements in door-to-balloon time in the United States, 2005 to 2010. Circulation 2011;124:1038–1045.

34. Hoenig MR, Aroney CN, Scott IA. Early invasive versus conservative strategies for unstable angina and non-ST elevation myocardial infarction in the stent era. Cochrane Database Syst Rev 2010;(3):CD004815.

35. Mahoney M, Jurkovitz CT, Chu H, et al. Cost and cost-effectiveness of an early invasive vs conservative strategy for the treatment of unstable angina and non-ST-segment elevation myocardial infarction. JAMA 2002;288:1851–1858.

36. Epstein AE, DiMarco JP, Ellenbogen KA, et al. ACC/AHA/HRS 2008 Guidelines for Device-Based Therapy of Cardiac Rhythm Abnormalities: A report of the American College of Cardiology/American Heart Association Task Force on Practice Guidelines (Writing Committee to Revise the ACC/AHA/NASPE 2002 Guideline Update for Implantation of Cardiac Pacemakers and Antiarrhythmia Devices) developed in collaboration with the American Association for Thoracic Surgery and Society of Thoracic Surgeons. J Am Coll Cardiol 2008;51(21):e1–e62.

37. Effectiveness of intravenous thrombolytic treatment in acute myocardial infarction. Gruppo Italiano per lo Studio della Streptochinasi nell'Infarto Miocardico (GISSI). Lancet 1896;1:397–402.

38. The Global Use of Strategies to Open Occluded Coronary Arteries (GUSTO III) Investigators. A comparison of reteplase with alteplase for acute myocardial infarction. N Engl J Med 1997;337:1118–1123.

39. Assessment of the Safety and Efficacy of a New Thrombolytic (ASSENT-2) Investigators. Single-bolus tenecteplase compared with front-loaded alteplase in acute myocardial infarction: The ASSENT-2 double-blind randomized trial. Lancet 2000;354:716–722.

40. Gibson CM, Pride YB, Frederick PD, et al. Trends in reperfusion strategies, door-to-needle and door-to-balloon times, and in-hospital mortality among patients with ST-segment elevation myocardial infarction enrolled in the National Registry of Myocardial Infarction from 1990 to 2006. Am Heart J 2008;156:1035–1044.

41. ISIS-2 (Second International Study of Infarct Survival) Collaborative Group. Randomised trial of intravenous streptokinase, oral aspirin, both, or neither among 17,187 cases of suspected acute myocardial infarction: ISIS-2. Lancet 1988;2:349–360.

42. Awtry EH, Loscalzo J. Aspirin. Circulation 2000;101:1206–1218.

43. ISIS-2 (Second International Study of Infarct Survival) Collaborative Group. Randomised trial of intravenous streptokinase, oral aspirin, both, or neither among 17,187 cases of suspected acute myocardial infarction: ISIS-2. Lancet 1988;2:349–360.

44. Campbell CL, Smyth S, Montalescot G, et al. Aspirin dose for the prevention of cardiovascular disease. JAMA 2007;297:2018–2024.

45. Antiplatelet Trialists' Collaboration. Collaborative meta-analysis of randomised trials of antiplatelet therapy for prevention of death, myocardial infarction, and stroke in high risk patients. Br Med J 2002;324:71–86.

46. Smith SC, Benjamin EJ, Bonow RO, et al. AHA/ACCF Secondary Prevention and Risk Reduction Therapy for Patients with Coronary and Other Atherosclerotic Vascular Disease: 2011 Update: A Guideline From the American Heart Association and American College of Cardiology Foundation Endorsed by the World Heart Federation and the Preventive Cardiovascular Nurses Association. J Am Coll Cardiol 2011;58:2432–2446.

47. CURRENT-OASIS 7 Investigators, Mehta SR, Bassand JP, Chrolavicius S, et al. Dose comparisons of clopidogrel and aspirin in acute coronary syndromes. N Engl J Med. 2010;363(10):930–042. Erratum in: N Engl J Med. 2010;363(16):1585.

48. Mehta SR, Tanguay JF, Eikelboom JW, et al. Double-dose versus standard-dose clopidogrel and high-dose versus low-dose aspirin in individuals undergoing percutaneous coronary intervention for acute coronary syndromes (CURRENT-OASIS 7): A randomised factorial trial. Lancet 2010;376:1233–1243.

49. Mahaffey KW, Wojdyla DM, Carroll K, et al. Ticagrelor compared with clopidogrel by geographic region in the Platelet Inhibition and Patient Outcomes (PLATO) trial. Circulation 2011;124:544–554.

50. Bristol-Myers Squibb/Sanofi Pharmaceuticals Partnership. Plavix (clopidogrel bisulphate tablets) [prescribing information], February 2011.

51. Eli Lilly and Company. Effient (prasugrel tablets) [prescribing information], September 27, 2011.

52. AstraZeneca. Brilinta (ticagrelor tablets) [prescribing information], July 11, 2011.

53. Mega JL Close SL, Wiviott SD, et al. Cytochrome P-450 polymorphisms and response to clopidogrel. N Engl J Med 2009;360:354–362.

54. Sofi F, Giusti B, Marcucci R, et al. Cytochrome P450 2C19*2 polymorphism and cardiovascular recurrences in patients taking clopidogrel: A meta-analysis. Pharmacogenomics J 2011;11:199–206.

55. Mega JL, Close SL, Wiviott SD, et al. Cytochrome P450 genetic polymorphisms and the response to prasugrel: Relationship to pharmacokinetic, pharmacodynamic, and clinical outcomes. Circulation 2009;119:2553–2560.

56. Wallentin L, James S, Storey RF, et al. Effect of CYP2C19 and ABCB1 single nucleotide polymorphisms on outcomes of treatment with ticagrelor versus clopidogrel for acute coronary syndromes: A genetic substudy of the PLATO trial. Lancet 2010;376:1320–1328.

57. Siller-Matula JM, Huber K, Christ G. Impact of clopidogrel loading dose on clinical outcome in patients undergoing percutaneous coronary intervention: A systematic review and meta-analysis. Heart 2011;97:98–105.

58. Wiviott SD, Braunwald E, McCabe CH, et al. Prasugrel versus clopidogrel in patients with acute coronary syndromes. N Engl J Med 2007;357;2001–2015.

59. Montalescot G, Wiviott SD, Braunwald E, et al. Prasugrel compared with clopidogrel in patients undergoing percutaneous coronary intervention for ST-elevation myocardial infarction (TRITON-TIMI 38): Double-blind, randomised controlled trial. Lancet 2009;373:723–731.

60. Wiviott SD, Braunwald E, Angiolillo DJ, et al. Greater clinical benefit of more intensive oral antiplatelet therapy with prasugrel in patients with diabetes mellitus in the trial to assess improvement in therapeutic outcomes by optimizing platelet inhibition with prasugrel-Thrombolysis in Myocardial Infarction 38. Circulation 2008;118:1626–1636.

61. Wallentin L, Becker RC, Budaj A, et al. Ticagrelor versus clopidogrel in patients with acute coronary syndromes. N Engl J Med 2009;361: 1045–1057.

62. James SK, Roe MT, Cannon CP, et al. Ticagrelor versus clopidogrel in patients with acute coronary syndromes intended for non-invasive management: Substudy from prospective randomised PLATelet inhibition and patient Outcomes (PLATO) trial. BMJ 2011;342:d3527.

63. James S, Angiolillo DJ, Cornel JH, et al; PLATO Study Group. Ticagrelor vs. clopidogrel in patients with acute coronary syndromes and diabetes: A substudy from the PLATelet inhibition and patient Outcomes (PLATO) trial. Eur Heart J 2010;31:3006–3016.

64. Steg PG, James S, Harrington RA, Ardissino D, et al; PLATO Study Group. Ticagrelor versus clopidogrel in patients with ST-elevation acute coronary syndromes intended for reperfusion with primary percutaneous coronary intervention: A Platelet Inhibition and Patient Outcomes (PLATO) trial subgroup analysis. Circulation 2010;122:2131–2141.

65. Cannon CP, Harrington RA, James S, et al. Comparison of ticagrelor with clopidogrel in patients with a planned invasive strategy for acute coronary syndromes (PLATO): A randomised double-blind study. Lancet 2010;375:283–293.

66. Crouch MA, Colucci VJ, Howard PA, Spinler SA. P2Y$_{12}$ receptor inhibitors: Integrating ticagrelor into the management of acute coronary syndrome. Ann Pharmacother 2011;45:1151–1156.

67. Price MJ, Berger PB, Teirstein PS, et al. Standard- vs high-dose clopidogrel based on platelet function testing after percutaneous coronary intervention: The GRAVITAS randomized trial. JAMA 2011;305:1097–1105. Erratum in: JAMA 2011;305:2174.

68. Chen ZM, Jiang XL, Chen YP, et al. Addition of clopidogrel to aspirin in 45,852 patients with acute myocardial infarction: Randomised placebo-controlled trial. Lancet 2005;366:1607–1621.

69. Sabatine MS, Cannon CP, Gibson CM, et al. Addition of clopidogrel to aspirin and fibrinolytic therapy for myocardial infarction with ST-segment elevation. N Engl J Med 2005;352:1179–1189.

70. De Luca G, Navarese E, Marino P. Risk profile and benefits from GP IIb-IIIa inhibitors among patients with ST-segment elevation

myocardial infarction treated with primary angioplasty: A meta-regression analysis of randomized trials. Eur Heart J 2009;30:2705–2713.

71. Gurm HS, Tamhane U, Meier P, et al. A comparison of abciximab and small-molecule glycoprotein IIb/IIIa inhibitors in patients undergoing primary percutaneous coronary intervention: A meta-analysis of contemporary randomized controlled trials. Circ Cardiovasc Interv 2009;2:230–236.

72. Merck & Co., Inc. Integrilin (eptifibatide) Injection [prescribing information], March 2011.

73. Juwana YB, Suryapranata H, Ottervanger JP, van 't Hof AW. Tirofiban for myocardial infarction. Expert Opin Pharmacother 2010;11:861–866.

74. Medicure Pharma, Inc. Aggrastat (tirofiban HCl) Injection Premixed [prescribing information], July 2008.

75. Dasgupta H, Blankenship JC, Wood C, et al. Thrombocytopenia complicating treatment with intravenous glycoprotein IIb/IIIa receptor inhibitors: A pooled analysis. Am Heart J 2000;140:206–211.

76. Eikelboom JW, Quinlan DJ, Mehta SR, et al. Unfractionated and low-molecular-weight heparin as adjuncts to thrombolysis in aspirin-treated patients with ST-elevation acute myocardial infarction: a meta-analysis of the randomized trials. Circulation 2005;112:3855–867.

77. Stone GW, Witzenbichler B, Guagliumi G, et al. Bivalirudin during primary PCI in acute myocardial infarction. N Engl J Med 2008;358:2218–2230.

78. Stone GW, Witzenbichler B, Guagliumi G, et al. Heparin plus a glycoprotein IIb/IIIa inhibitor versus bivalirudin monotherapy and paclitaxel-eluting stents versus bare-metal stents in acute myocardial infarction (HORIZONS-AMI): Final 3-year results from a multicentre, randomised controlled trial. Lancet 2011;377:2193–2204.

79. Antman EM, Morrow DA, McCabe CH, et al. Enoxaparin versus unfractionated heparin with fibrinolysis for ST-elevation myocardial infarction. N Engl J Med 2006;354:1477–1488.

80. Gore JM, Spencer FA, Gurfinkel EP, et al. Thrombocytopenia in patients with an acute coronary syndrome (from the Global Registry of Acute Coronary Events [GRACE]). Am J Cardiol 2009;103(2):175–180.

81. Gruppo Italiano per lo Studio della Sopravivenza nell'Infarcto Miocardico. GISSI-3: Effects of lisinopril and transdermal glyceryl trinitrate singly and together on 6-week mortality and ventricular function after acute myocardial infarction. Lancet 1994;343:1115–1122.

82. ISIS-4 (Fourth International Study of Infarct Survival [collaborative group]). ISIS-4: A randomised factorial trial assessing early oral captopril, oral mononitrate, and intravenous magnesium sulphate in 58,050 patients with suspected acute myocardial infarction. Lancet 1995;345:669–685.

83. First International Study of Infarct Survival Collaborative Group. Randomised trial of intravenous atenolol among 16,027 cases of suspected acute myocardial infarction: ISIS-1. Lancet 1986;2:57–661.

84. Metoprolol in acute myocardial infarction (MIAMI). A randomised placebo-controlled international trial. Eur Heart J 1985;6:199–226.

85. COMMIT (Clopidogrel and Metoprolol in Myocardial Infarction Trial [collaborative group]). Early intravenous then oral metoprolol in 45,852 patients with acute myocardial infarction: Randomised placebo-controlled trial. Lancet 2005;366:1622–1632.

86. Antiplatelet Trialists' Collaboration. Collaborative meta-analysis of randomised trials of antiplatelet therapy for prevention of death, myocardial infarction, and stroke in high risk patients. BMJ 2002;324:71–86.

87. Stone GW, McLaurin BT, Cox DA, et al. Bivalirudin for patients with acute coronary syndromes. N Engl J Med 2006;355:2203–2216.

88. Kastrati A, Neumann FJ, Schulz S, et al. Abciximab and heparin versus bivalirudin for non-ST-elevation myocardial infarction. N Engl J Med 2011;365:1980–1989.

89. Oler A, Whooley MA, Oler J, Grady D. Adding heparin to aspirin reduces the incidence of myocardial infarction and death in patients with unstable angina: A meta-analysis. JAMA 1996;276:811–815.

90. Fragmin During Instability in Coronary Artery Disease Study Group. Low-molecular-weight heparin during instability in coronary artery disease. Lancet 1996;347:561–568.

91. Yusuf S, Mehta SR, Chrolavicius S, et al. Effects of fondaparinux on mortality and reinfarction in patients with acute ST-segment elevation myocardial infarction: The OASIS-6 randomized trial. JAMA 2006;295:1519–1530.

92. Mehta SR, Yusuf S, Peters RJG, et al. Effects of pretreatment with clopidogrel and aspirin followed by long-term therapy in patients undergoing percutaneous coronary intervention: The PCI-CURE study. Lancet 2001;358:527–533.

93. Yusuf S, Zhao F, Meta SR, et al. Effects of clopidogrel in addition to aspirin in patients with acute coronary syndromes without ST-segment elevation. N Engl J Med 2001;345:494–502.

94. Giugliano RP, White JA, Bode C, et al. Early versus delayed, provisional eptifibatide in acute coronary syndromes. N Engl J Med 2009;360:2176–2190.

95. Serebruany VL, Steinhuble SR, Berger PB et al. Analysis of risk of bleeding complications after different doses of aspirin in 192,036 patients enrolled in 31 randomized controlled trials. Am J Cardiol 2005;95:1218–1222.

96. Serebruany VL, Malinin AI, Ferguson JJ, et al. Bleeding risks of combination vs. single antiplatelet therapy: A meta-analysis of 18 randomized trials comprising 129,314 patients. Fundam Clin Pharmacol 2008;22:315–321.

97. Budnitz DS, Lovegrove MC, Shehab N, Richards CL. Emergency hospitalizations for adverse drug events in older Americans. N Engl J Med 2011;365(21):2002–2012.

98. Freemantle N, Cleland J, Young P, et al. β-Blockade after myocardial infarction: Systematic review and meta regression analysis. Br Med J 1999;318:1730–1737.

99. Houghton T, Freemantle N, Cleland JG, et al. Are beta-blockers effective in patients who develop heart failure soon after myocardial infarction? A meta-regression analysis of randomised trials. Eur J Heart Fail 2000;2:333–340.

100. Dargie HJ. Effect of carvedilol on outcome after myocardial infarction in patients with left-ventricular dysfunction: The CAPRICORN randomised trial. Lancet 2001;357:1385–1390.

101. Gibbons RJ, Abrams J, Chatterjee K, et al. ACC/AHA 2002 guideline update for the management of patients with chronic stable angina: Summary article. A report of the American College of Cardiology/American Heart Association Task Force on Practice Guidelines (Committee on the Management of Patients with Chronic Stable Angina). J Am Coll Cardiol 2003;41:159–168.

102. ACE Inhibitor Myocardial Infarction Collaborative Group. Indications for ACE inhibitors in the early treatment of acute myocardial infarction: Systematic overview of individual data from 100,000 patients in randomized trials. Circulation 1998;97:2202–2212.

103. Swedberg K, Held P, Kjekshus J, et al. Effects of the early administration of enalapril on mortality in patients with acute myocardial infarction: Results of the Cooperative New Scandinavian Enalapril Survival Study II (CONSENSUS II). N Engl J Med 1992;327:678–684.

104. Pfeffer MA, McMurray JJV, Velazquez EJ, et al. Valsartan, captopril, or both in myocardial infarction complicated by heart failure, left ventricular dysfunction, or both. N Engl J Med 2003;349:1893–1906.

105. Granger CB, McMurray JV, Yusuf S, et al. Effects of candesartan in patients with chronic heart failure and reduced left-ventricular systolic function intolerant to angiotensin-converting-enzyme inhibitors: The CHARM-Alternative trial. Lancet 2004;362:772–776.

106. Makkar KM, Sanoski CA, Spinler SA. The role of angiotensin-converting enzyme inhibitors, angiotensin receptor blockers and aldosterone antagonists in the prevention of atrial and ventricular arrhythmias. Pharmacotherapy 2009;29:31–48.

107. Pitt B, Zannad F, Remme WJ, et al., for the Randomized Aldactone Evaluation Study Investigators. The effect of spironolactone on morbidity and mortality in patients with severe heart failure. N Engl J Med 1999;341:709–717.

108. Pitt B, Remme W, Zannad F, et al. Eplerenone, a selective aldosterone blocker in patients with left ventricular dysfunction after myocardial infarction. N Engl J Med 2003;348:1309–1321.

109. Zannad F, McMurray JJ, Krum H, et al. Eplerenone in patients with systolic heart failure and mild symptoms. N Engl J Med 2011;364:11–21.

110. Executive Summary of the Third Report of the National Cholesterol Education Program (NCEP) Expert Panel on Detection, Evaluation,

and Treatment of High Blood Cholesterol in Adults (Adult Treatment Panel III). JAMA 2001;285:2486–2497.

111. Hulten E, Jackson JL, Douglas K, et al. The effect of early, intensive statin therapy on acute coronary syndrome: A meta-analysis of randomized controlled trials. Arch Intern Med 2006;166:1814–1821.

112. Grundy SM, Cleeman JI, Bairey Merz, CN, et al., eds. Coordinating Committee of the National Cholesterol Education Program, Endorsed by the National Heart, Lung, and Blood Institute, American College of Cardiology Foundation, and American Heart Association. Implications of Recent Clinical Trials for the National Cholesterol Education Program Adult Treatment Panel III Guidelines. Circulation 2004;110:227–239.

113. Cholesterol Treatment Trialists' (CTT) Collaboration; Baigent C, Blackwell L. Efficacy and safety of more intensive lowering of LDL cholesterol: A meta-analysis of data from 170,000 participants in 26 randomised trials. Lancet 2010;376:1670–1681.

114. Rubins HB, Robins SJ, Collins D, et al. Gemfibrozil for the secondary prevention of coronary heart disease in men with low levels of high-density lipoprotein cholesterol. Veterans Affairs High-Density Lipoprotein Cholesterol Intervention Trial Study Group. N Engl J Med 1999;341:410–418.

115. The ACCORD Study Group. Effects of combination lipid therapy in type 2 diabetes mellitus. N Engl J Med 2010;362:1563–1564.

116. The AIM-HIGH Investigators, Boden WE, Probstfield JL, Anderson T, et al. Niacin in patients with low HDL cholesterol levels receiving intensive statin therapy. N Engl J Med 2011;365:2255–2267.

117. Ho PM, Spertus JA, Masoudi FA, et al. Impact of medication therapy discontinuation on mortality after myocardial infarction. Arch Intern Med 2006;166:1842–1847.

118. U.S. Department of Health & Human Services. Technical Appendix Hospital Process of Care Measure Set. List of Current Measures. Heart Attack (Acute Myocardial Infarction or AMI) and Chest Pain. Available at: http://www.hospitalcompare.hhs.gov/staticpages/for-professionals/poc/Technical-Appendix.aspx#POC3. Accessed November 30, 2011.

9 Arrhythmias

James E. Tisdale

● **Upon completion of the chapter, the reader will be able to:**

1. Describe the phases of the cardiac action potential, compare and contrast the cellular ionic changes corresponding to each phase, and explain the relationship between the cardiac action potential and the electrocardiogram (ECG).

2. Describe the modified Vaughan Williams classification of antiarrhythmic drugs, and compare and contrast the effects of available antiarrhythmic drugs on ventricular conduction velocity, refractory period, automaticity, and inhibition of ion flux through specific myocardial ion channels.

3. Compare and contrast the risk factors for and the features, mechanisms, etiologies, symptoms, and goals of therapy of (a) sinus bradycardia, (b) atrioventricular (AV) nodal blockade, (c) atrial fibrillation (AF), (d) paroxysmal supraventricular tachycardia (PSVT), (e) ventricular premature depolarizations (VPDs), (f) ventricular tachycardia (VT, including torsades de pointes), and (g) ventricular fibrillation (VF).

4. Compare and contrast appropriate nonpharmacologic and pharmacologic treatment options for sinus bradycardia and AV nodal blockade.

5. Compare and contrast the mechanisms of action of drugs used for ventricular rate control, conversion to sinus rhythm and maintenance of sinus rhythm in patients with AF, and explain the importance of anticoagulation for patients with AF.

6. Discuss nonpharmacologic methods for termination of PSVT, and compare and contrast the mechanisms of action of drugs used for acute termination of PSVT.

7. Compare and contrast the role of drug therapy versus nonpharmacologic therapy for long-term prevention of recurrence of PSVT.

8. Describe the role of drug therapy for management of asymptomatic and symptomatic VPDs.

9. Compare and contrast the mechanisms of action of drugs used for the treatment of acute episodes of VT (including torsades de pointes), and describe options and indications for nonpharmacologic treatment of VT and VF.

10. Design individualized drug therapy treatment plans for patients with (a) sinus bradycardia, (b) AV nodal blockade, (c) AF, (d) PSVT, (e) VPDs, (f) VT (including torsades de pointes), and (g) VF.

KEY CONCEPTS

❶ Cardiac arrhythmias may be caused by abnormal impulse formation (automaticity), abnormal impulse conduction (reentry), or both.

❷ Numerous drugs (β-blockers, diltiazem, verapamil, digoxin, dronedarone, and amiodarone) can cause bradyarrhythmias (sinus bradycardia and/or atrioventricular [AV] nodal blockade).

❸ Individualized goals of treatment for atrial fibrillation (AF) include (a) ventricular rate control with drugs that inhibit AV nodal conduction, (b) restoration of sinus rhythm

with direct current cardioversion or antiarrhythmic drugs (commonly referred to as "cardioversion" or "conversion to sinus rhythm"), (c) maintenance of sinus rhythm/reduction in the frequency of episodes, and (d) prevention of stroke.

❹ Antiarrhythmic drug therapy for maintenance of sinus rhythm/reduction in frequency of episodes of AF should be initiated only in patients in whom symptoms persist despite maximal tolerated doses of appropriate drugs for ventricular rate control.

❺ Most patients with AF require therapy with dabigatran or warfarin for stroke prevention; in some patients with no additional risk factors for stroke, anticoagulation may not be necessary.

⑥ Adenosine is the drug of choice for termination of paroxysmal supraventricular tachycardia.

⑦ Asymptomatic ventricular premature depolarizations (VPDs) should not be treated with antiarrhythmic drug therapy.

⑧ Implantable cardioverter defibrillators are more effective than antiarrhythmic drugs for reduction in the risk of sudden cardiac death due to ventricular tachycardia (VT) or ventricular fibrillation (VF).

⑨ The purpose of drug therapy for VF is facilitation of electrical defibrillation; in the absence of electrical defibrillation, drug therapy alone will not terminate VF.

⑩ Drugs with the potential to cause QT interval prolongation and torsades de pointes should be avoided or used with extreme caution in patients with other risk factors for torsades de pointes.

NORMAL AND ABNORMAL CARDIAC CONDUCTION AND ELECTROPHYSIOLOGY

The heart functions via both mechanical and electrical activity. The mechanical activity of the heart refers to atrial and ventricular contraction, the mechanism by which blood is delivered to tissues. When circulated blood returns to the heart via the venous circulation, the blood enters the right atrium. Right atrial contraction and changes in right ventricular pressure result in delivery of blood to the right ventricle through the tricuspid valve. Right ventricular contraction pumps blood through the pulmonic valve through the pulmonary arteries to the lungs, where the blood becomes oxygenated. The blood then flows through the pulmonary veins into the left atrium. Left atrial contraction and changes in left ventricular (LV) pressure result in delivery of blood through the mitral valve into the left ventricle. Contraction of the left ventricle results in pumping of blood through the aortic valve and to the tissues of the body.

The mechanical activity of the heart (contraction of the atria and ventricles) occurs as a result of the electrical activity of the heart. The heart possesses an intrinsic electrical conduction system (**Fig. 9–1**).[1] Normal myocardial contraction cannot occur without proper and normal function of the heart's electrical conduction system. Depolarization of the atria results in atrial contraction, and ventricular depolarization is followed by ventricular contraction. Malfunction of the heart's electrical conduction system may result in dysfunctional atrial and/or ventricular contraction and may reduce cardiac output.

The Cardiac Conduction System

Under normal circumstances, the sinoatrial (SA) node (also known as the sinus node), located in the upper portion of the right atrium, serves as the **pacemaker** of the heart and generates

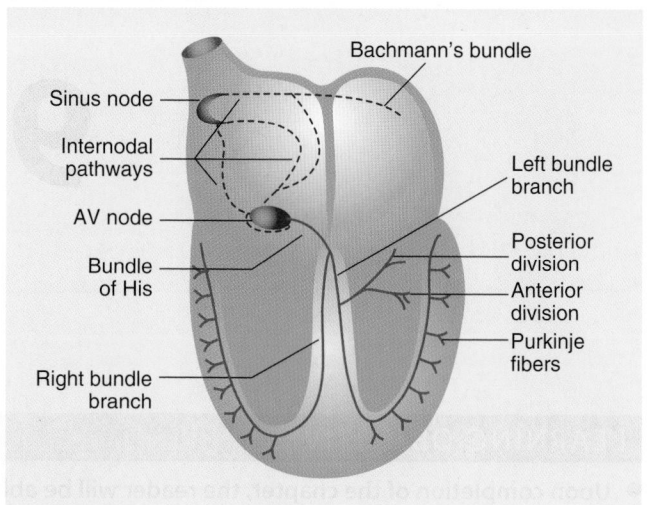

FIGURE 9–1. The cardiac conduction system. (AV, atrioventricular.)

the electrical impulses that subsequently result in atrial and **ventricular depolarization** (Fig. 9–1).[1] The SA node serves as the heart's dominant pacemaker because it has the greatest degree of **automaticity**, which is defined as the ability of a cardiac fiber or tissue to initiate depolarizations spontaneously. In adults at rest, the normal intrinsic depolarization rate of the SA node is 60 to 100 per minute. Other cardiac fibers also possess the property of automaticity, but normally the intrinsic depolarization rates are slower than that of the SA node. For example, the normal intrinsic depolarization rate of the atrioventricular (AV) node is 40 to 60 per minute; that of the ventricular tissue is 30 to 40 per minute. Therefore, because of greater automaticity, the SA node normally serves as the pacemaker of the heart. However, if the SA node fails to generate depolarizations at a rate faster than that of the AV node, the AV node may take over as the pacemaker. Similarly, if the SA node and AV node fail to generate depolarizations at a rate greater than 30 to 40 per minute, ventricular tissue may take over as the pacemaker.

Following initiation of the electrical impulse from the SA node, the impulse travels through the internodal pathways of the specialized atrial conduction system and Bachmann's bundle (Fig. 9–1).[1] The atrial conducting fibers do not traverse the entire breadth of the left and right atria; impulse conduction occurs across the internodal pathways, and when the impulse reaches the end of Bachmann's bundle, atrial depolarization spreads as a wave, conceptually similar to that which occurs upon throwing a pebble into water. As the impulse is conducted across the atria, each depolarized cell excites and depolarizes the surrounding connected cells, until both atria have been completely depolarized. Atrial contraction follows normal atrial depolarization.

Following atrial depolarization, impulses are conducted through the AV node, located in the lower right atrium (Fig. 9–1).[1] The impulse then enters the bundle of His and is conducted through the ventricular conduction system, consisting of the left and right bundle branches. The left ventricle requires a larger conduction system than the right ventricle due to its larger mass; therefore, the left bundle branch bifurcates into the left anterior and posterior divisions (also commonly known as "fascicles"). The bundle branches further divide into the Purkinje fibers through which impulse conduction results in ventricular depolarization, initiating ventricular contraction.

The Ventricular Action Potential

• The ventricular action potential is depicted in Figure 9–2. Cardiac myocyte resting membrane potential is usually −70 to −90 mV, due to the action of the sodium–potassium adenosine triphosphatase (ATPase) pump, which maintains relatively high extracellular sodium concentrations and relatively low extracellular potassium concentrations. During each action potential cycle, the potential of the membrane slowly increases to a threshold potential due to a slow influx of sodium into the cell, raising the threshold to −60 to −80 mV. When the membrane potential reaches this threshold, the fast sodium channels open, allowing sodium ions to rapidly enter the cell. This rapid influx of positive ions creates a vertical upstroke of the action potential, such that the potential reaches 20 to 30 mV. This is phase 0, which represents ventricular depolarization. At this point, the fast sodium channels become inactivated, and ventricular repolarization begins, consisting of phases 1 through 3 of the action potential. Phase 1 repolarization occurs primarily as a result of an efflux of potassium ions (Fig. 9–2). During phase 2, potassium ions continue to exit the cell, but the membrane potential is balanced by an influx of calcium and sodium ions, transported through slow calcium and slow sodium channels, resulting in a plateau. During phase 3, the efflux of potassium ions greatly exceeds calcium and sodium

influx, resulting in the major component of ventricular repolarization. During phase 4, sodium ions gradually enter the cell increasing the threshold again to −60 to −80 mV and initiating another action potential. An understanding of the ionic fluxes that are responsible for each phase of the action potential facilitates understanding of the effects of specific drugs on the action potential. For example, drugs that primarily inhibit ion flux through sodium channels influence phase 0 (ventricular depolarization), whereas drugs that primarily inhibit ion flux through potassium channels influence the repolarization phases, particularly phase 3.

The Electrocardiogram

The electrocardiogram (ECG) is a noninvasive means of measuring the electrical activity of the heart. The relationship between the ventricular action potential and the ECG is depicted in Figure 9–2. The P wave on the ECG represents atrial depolarization (atrial depolarization is not depicted in the action potential shown in Fig. 9–2, which shows only the
• ventricular action potential). Phase 0 of the action potential corresponds to the QRS complex; therefore, the QRS complex on the ECG is a noninvasive representation of ventricular depolarization. The T wave on the ECG corresponds to phase 3 ventricular repolarization. The interval from the beginning of the Q wave to the end of the T wave, known as the QT interval, is used as a noninvasive marker of ventricular repolarization time. Atrial repolarization is not visible on the ECG because it occurs during ventricular depolarization and is obscured by the QRS complex.

Several intervals and durations are routinely measured on the ECG. The PR interval represents the time of conduction of impulses from the atria to the ventricles through the

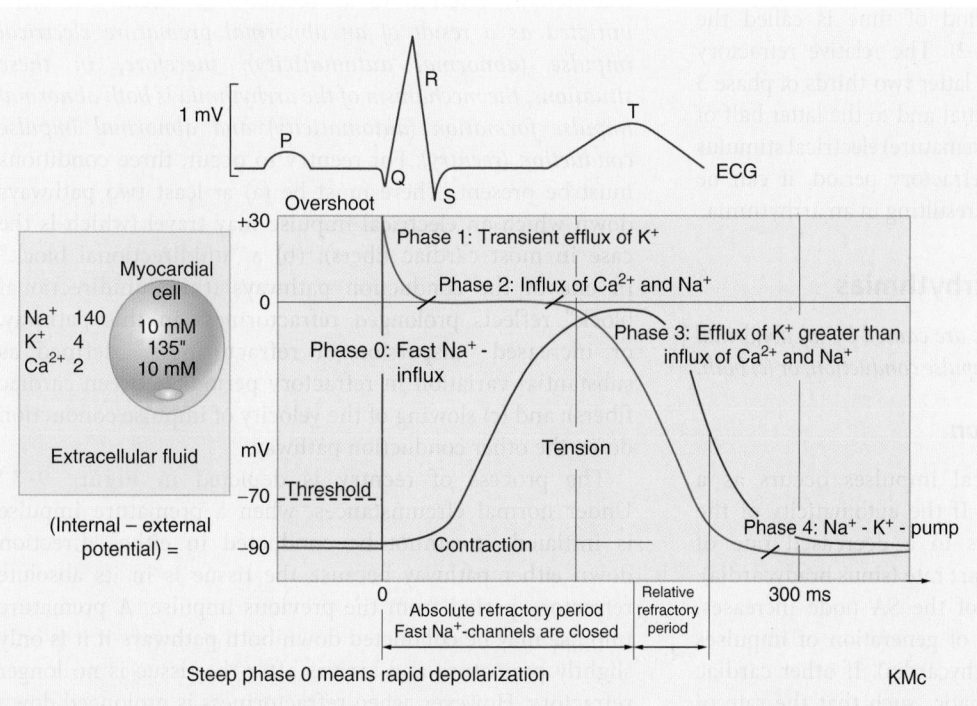

FIGURE 9–2. The ventricular action potential depicting the flow of specific ions responsible for each phase. The specific phases of the action potential that correspond to the absolute and relative refractory periods are portrayed, and the relationship between phases of the action potential and the electrocardiogram (ECG) are shown. (Ca, calcium; K, potassium; Na, sodium.)

AV node; the normal PR interval in adults is 0.12 to 0.2 seconds. The QRS duration represents the time required for ventricular depolarization, which is normally 0.08 to 0.12 seconds in adults. The QT interval, measuring 0.32 to 0.4 seconds, represents the time required for ventricular repolarization. The QT interval varies with heart rate—the faster the heart rate, the shorter the QT interval, and vice versa. Therefore, the QT interval is corrected for heart rate using Bazett's equation,[2] which is:

$$QT_c = \frac{QT}{\sqrt{RR}}$$

where QT_c is the QT interval corrected for heart rate, and RR is the interval from the onset of one QRS complex to the onset of the next QRS complex, measured in seconds (i.e., the heart rate, expressed in different terminology). The normal QT_c interval in adults is 0.36 to 0.47 seconds in men and 0.36 to 0.48 seconds in women.[3]

Refractory Periods

After an electrical impulse is initiated and conducted, there is a period of time during which cells and fibers cannot be depolarized again. This period of time is referred to as the absolute refractory period (Fig. 9–2) and corresponds to phases 1, 2, and approximately a third of phase 3 repolarization of the action potential. The absolute refractory period also corresponds to the period from the Q wave to approximately the first half of the T wave on the ECG (Fig. 9–2). During this period, if there is a premature stimulus for an electrical impulse, this impulse cannot be conducted because the tissue is absolutely refractory. However, there is a period of time following the absolute refractory period during which a premature electrical stimulus can be conducted and is often conducted abnormally. This period of time is called the relative refractory period (Fig. 9–2). The relative refractory period corresponds roughly to the latter two-thirds of phase 3 repolarization on the action potential and to the latter half of the T wave on the ECG. If a new (premature) electrical stimulus is initiated during the relative refractory period, it can be conducted abnormally, potentially resulting in an arrhythmia.

Mechanisms of Cardiac Arrhythmias

❶ *In general, cardiac arrhythmias are caused by (a) abnormal impulse formation, (b) abnormal impulse conduction, or (c) both.*

▶ Abnormal Impulse Initiation

Abnormal initiation of electrical impulses occurs as a result of abnormal automaticity. If the automaticity of the SA node decreases, this results in a decreased rate of impulse generation and a slow heart rate (sinus bradycardia). Conversely, if the automaticity of the SA node increases, this results in an increased rate of generation of impulses and a rapid heart rate (sinus tachycardia). If other cardiac fibers become abnormally automatic, such that the rate of

initiation of spontaneous impulses exceeds that of the SA node, or premature impulses are generated, other types of tachyarrhythmias may occur. Many cardiac fibers possess the capability for automaticity including the atrial tissue, the AV node, the Purkinje fibers, and the ventricular tissue. In addition, fibers with the capability of initiating and conducting electrical impulses are present in the pulmonary veins. Abnormal atrial automaticity may result in premature atrial contractions or may precipitate atrial tachycardia or atrial fibrillation (AF); abnormal AV nodal automaticity may result in "junctional tachycardia" (the AV node is also sometimes referred to as the AV junction). Abnormal automaticity in the ventricles may result in ventricular premature depolarizations (VPDs) or may precipitate ventricular tachycardia (VT) or ventricular fibrillation (VF). In addition, abnormal automaticity originating from the pulmonary veins is a precipitant of AF.

Automaticity of cardiac fibers is controlled in part by activity of the sympathetic and parasympathetic nervous systems. Enhanced activity of the sympathetic nervous system may result in increased automaticity of the SA node or other automatic cardiac fibers. Enhanced activity of the parasympathetic nervous system tends to suppress automaticity; conversely, inhibition of activity of the parasympathetic nervous system increases automaticity. Other factors may lead to abnormal increases in automaticity of extra-SA nodal tissues, including hypoxia, atrial or ventricular stretch (as might occur following long-standing hypertension or during and after the development of heart failure), and electrolyte abnormalities such as hypokalemia or hypomagnesemia.

▶ Abnormal Impulse Conduction

The mechanism of abnormal impulse conduction is traditionally referred to as reentry. ❶ *Reentry is often initiated as a result of an abnormal premature electrical impulse (abnormal automaticity); therefore, in these situations, the mechanism of the arrhythmia is both abnormal impulse formation (automaticity) and abnormal impulse conduction (reentry).* For reentry to occur, three conditions must be present. There must be (a) at least two pathways down which an electrical impulse may travel (which is the case in most cardiac fibers); (b) a "unidirectional block" in one of the conduction pathways (this "unidirectional block" reflects prolonged refractoriness in this pathway, or increased "dispersion of refractoriness," defined as substantial variation in refractory periods between cardiac fibers); and (c) slowing of the velocity of impulse conduction down the other conduction pathway.

The process of reentry is depicted in Figure 9–3.[4] Under normal circumstances, when a premature impulse is initiated, it cannot be conducted in either direction down either pathway because the tissue is in its absolute refractory period from the previous impulse. A premature impulse may be conducted down both pathways if it is only slightly premature and arrives after the tissue is no longer refractory. However, when refractoriness is prolonged down

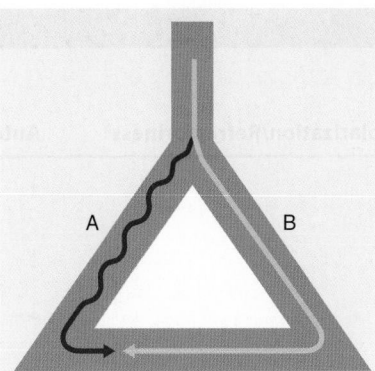

FIGURE 9–3. The process of initiation of reentry. There are two pathways for impulse conduction, slowed impulse conduction down pathway A and a longer refractory period in pathway B. A precisely timed premature impulse usually initiates reentry; the premature impulse cannot be conducted down pathway B because the tissue is still in the absolute refractory period from the previous, normal impulse. However, because of dispersion of refractoriness (i.e., different refractory periods down the two pathways), the impulse can be conducted down pathway A. Because conduction down pathway A is slowed, by the time the impulse reaches pathway B in a retrograde direction, the impulse can be conducted retrogradely up the pathway because the pathway is now beyond its refractory period from the previous impulse. This creates reentry, in which the impulse continuously and repeatedly travels in a circular fashion around the loop.

one of the pathways, a precisely timed premature beat may be conducted down one pathway but cannot be conducted in either direction in the pathway with prolonged refractoriness because the tissue is still in its absolute refractory period (Fig. 9–3).[4] When the third condition for reentry is present, that is, when the velocity of impulse conduction in one is slowed, the impulse traveling forward down the other pathway still cannot be conducted. However, because the impulse in one is traveling more slowly than normal, by the time it circles around and travels upward along the other pathway, sufficient time has passed so the pathway is no longer in its absolute refractory period, and now the impulse may travel upward in that pathway. In other words, the electrical impulse "reenters" a previously stimulated pathway in the reverse (retrograde) direction. This results in circular movement of electrical impulses; as the impulse travels in this circular fashion, it excites each cell around it, and if the impulse is traveling at a rate faster than the intrinsic rate of the SA node, a tachycardia occurs in the tissue in question. Reentry may occur in numerous tissues, including the atria, the AV node, and the ventricles.

Prolonged refractoriness and/or slowed impulse conduction velocity may be present in cardiac tissues for a variety of reasons. Myocardial ischemia may alter ventricular refractory periods or impulse conduction velocity, facilitating ventricular reentry. In patients with past myocardial infarction, the infarcted myocardium is dead and cannot conduct impulses. However, there is typically a border zone of tissue that is damaged and in which refractory periods and conduction velocity are often deranged, facilitating ventricular reentry. In patients with left atrial or LV hypertrophy as a result of long-standing hypertension, refractory periods and conduction velocity are often perturbed. In patients with heart failure due to LV dysfunction, ventricular refractoriness and conduction velocity are often altered due to LV hypertrophy, collagen deposition, and other anatomical and structural changes.

Vaughan Williams Classification of Antiarrhythmic Drugs

● The Vaughan Williams classification of antiarrhythmic drugs, first described in 1970[5] and subsequently further expanded,[6,7] is presented in Table 9–1. This classification is based on the effects of specific drugs on ventricular conduction velocity, repolarization/refractoriness, and automaticity. Class I drugs, which are the sodium channel blocking agents, primarily inhibit ventricular automaticity and slow conduction velocity. However, due to differences in the potency of the drugs to slow conduction velocity, the class I drugs are subdivided into class IA, IB, and IC. The class IC drugs have the greatest potency for slowing ventricular conduction, the class IA drugs have intermediate potency, and the class IB drugs have the lowest potency, with minimal effects on conduction velocity at normal heart rates. Class II drugs are the adrenergic β-receptor inhibitors (β-blockers), class III drugs are those that inhibit ventricular repolarization or prolong refractoriness, and class IV drugs are the calcium channel blockers (CCBs) diltiazem and verapamil.

The Vaughan Williams classification of antiarrhythmic drugs has been criticized for a number of reasons. The classification is based on the effects of drugs on normal, rather than diseased, myocardium. In addition, many of the drugs may be placed into more than one class. For example, the class IA drugs prolong repolarization/refractoriness, either via the parent drug[8,9] or an active metabolite,[10] and therefore they may also be placed in class III. Sotalol is also a β-blocker and therefore fits into class II. Amiodarone inhibits sodium and potassium conductance, is a noncompetitive inhibitor of β-receptors, and inhibits calcium channels, and therefore it may be placed into any of the four classes. For this reason, drugs within each class cannot be considered "interchangeable." Nonetheless, despite attempts to develop mechanism-based classifications that better distinguish the actions of antiarrhythmic drugs,[11] the Vaughan Williams classification continues to be widely used because of its simplicity and the fact that it is relatively easy to remember and understand.

CARDIAC ARRHYTHMIAS

In general, cardiac arrhythmias are classified into two broad categories: supraventricular (those occurring above the ventricles) and ventricular (those occurring in the ventricles).

Table 9–1

Vaughan Williams Classification of Antiarrhythmic Agents[a]

Class	Drug	Conduction Velocity[b]	Repolarization/Refractoriness[b]	Automaticity[b]
IA	Quinidine Procainamide Disopyramide	↓	↑	↓
IB	Lidocaine Mexiletine	0/↓	↓/0	↓
IC	Flecainide Propafenone	↓↓	0	↓

II	β-Blockers[c]
	    Acebutolol
	    Atenolol
	    Betaxolol
	    Bisoprolol
	    Carteolol
	    Carvedilol[d]
	    Esmolol
	    Labetalol[d]
	    Metoprolol
	    Nadolol
	    Nebivolol
	    Penbutolol
	    Pindolol
	    Propranolol
	    Timolol
		0	0	0

III	Amiodarone[e] Dofetilide Dronedarone[e] Ibutilide Sotalol	0	↑	0

IV	CCBs[c]
	    Diltiazem
	    Verapamil
		0	0	0

CCB, calcium channel blocker; ↑, increase/prolong; ↓, decrease; 0, no effect; 0/↓, does not change or may decrease: ↓/0, decreases or does not change.

[a]Adenosine and digoxin are agents used for the management of arrhythmias that do not fit into the Vaughan Williams classification.

[b]In ventricular tissue only; effects may differ in atria, sinus node, or atrioventricular node.

[c]Slow conduction, prolong refractory period, and reduce automaticity in sinoatrial node and AV node tissue but generally not in the ventricles.

[d]Combined α- and β-blockers.

[e]Amiodarone and dronedarone also slow conduction velocity and inhibit automaticity.

The names of specific arrhythmias are generally composed of two words; the first word indicates the location of the electrophysiological abnormality resulting in the arrhythmia (sinus, AV node, atrial, or ventricular), and the second word describes the arrhythmia in terms of whether it is abnormally slow (bradycardia) or fast (tachycardia), or the type of arrhythmia (block, fibrillation, or flutter).

SUPRAVENTRICULAR ARRHYTHMIAS
Sinus Bradycardia

Sinus bradycardia, an arrhythmia that originates in the SA node, is defined by a sinus rate less than 60 beats per minute (bpm).[12]

▶ Epidemiology and Etiology

Many individuals, particularly those who engage in regular vigorous exercise, have resting heart rates less than 60 bpm. For those individuals, sinus bradycardia is normal and healthy, and it does not require evaluation or treatment. However, some individuals may develop symptomatic sinus node dysfunction. In the absence of correctable underlying causes, idiopathic sinus node dysfunction is referred to as sick sinus syndrome[12] and occurs with greater frequency in association with advancing age. The prevalence of sick sinus syndrome is approximately 1 in 600 individuals older than 65 years.[12]

Sick sinus syndrome leading to sinus bradycardia may be caused by degenerative changes in the sinus node that occur

Clinical Presentation and Diagnosis of Sinus Bradycardia

Symptoms

- Many patients are asymptomatic, particularly those with normal resting heart rates less than 60 bpm as a result of physical fitness due to regular vigorous exercise
- Susceptible patients may develop symptoms, depending on the degree of heart rate lowering
- Symptoms of bradyarrhythmias include dizziness, fatigue, light-headedness, syncope, chest pain (in patients with underlying coronary artery disease [CAD]), and shortness of breath and other symptoms of heart failure (in patients with underlying left ventricular dysfunction)

Diagnosis

- Cannot be made on the basis of symptoms alone because the symptoms of all bradyarrhythmias are similar

- History of present illness, presenting symptoms, and 12-lead ECG that reveals sinus bradycardia
- Assess possible correctable etiologies, including myocardial ischemia, serum potassium concentration (for hyperkalemia), thyroid function tests (for hypothyroidism)
- Determine whether patient is taking any drugs known to cause sinus bradycardia. If the patient is currently taking digoxin, determine the serum digoxin concentration and ascertain whether it is supratherapeutic (greater than 2 ng/mL [2.6 nmol/L])

Table 9–2

Etiologies of Sinus Bradycardia[12,13]

Idiopathic ("sick sinus syndrome")
Myocardial ischemia
Carotid sinus hypersensitivity
Neurocardiac syncope
Electrolyte abnormalities: hypokalemia or hyperkalemia
Hypothyroidism
Hypothermia
Amyloidosis
Sarcoidosis
Systemic lupus erythematosus
Scleroderma
Sleep apnea
Drugs:

Adenosine	Fluoxetine
Amiodarone	Halothane
β-Blockers	Isradipine
Cisplatin	Ketamine
Citalopram	Neostigmine
Clonidine	Nicardipine
Cocaine	Nitroglycerin
Dexmedetomidine	Paclitaxel
Digoxin	Propafenone
Diltiazem	Propofol
Dipyridamole	Remifentanil
Disopyramide	Sotalol
Donepezil	Succinylcholine
Dronedarone	Thalidomide
Flecainide	Verapamil

with advancing age. ❷ *However, there are other possible etiologies of sinus bradycardia, including drugs* (Table 9–2).[13]

▶ Pathophysiology

Sick sinus syndrome leading to sinus bradycardia occurs as a result of fibrotic tissue in the SA node, which replaces normal SA node tissue.[12]

▶ Treatment

Desired Outcomes The desired outcomes of treatment are to restore normal heart rate and alleviate patient symptoms.

Pharmacologic Therapy Treatment of sinus bradycardia is only necessary in patients who become symptomatic. ❷ *If the patient is taking any medication(s) that may cause sinus bradycardia, the drug(s) should be discontinued whenever possible.* If the patient remains in sinus bradycardia after discontinuation of the drug(s) and after five half-lives of the drug(s) have elapsed, then the drugs(s) can usually be excluded as the etiology of the arrhythmia. In certain circumstances, however, discontinuation of the medication(s) may be undesirable, even if it may be the cause of symptomatic sinus bradycardia. For example, if the patient has a history of myocardial infarction or heart failure, discontinuation of a β-blocker may be necessary in the short term but undesirable in the long term because β-blockers have been shown to reduce mortality and prolong life in patients with those diseases, and the benefits of therapy with β-blockers outweigh the risks associated with sinus bradycardia. In these patients, clinicians and patients may elect to implant a permanent pacemaker to allow the patient to continue therapy with β-blockers.

Acute treatment of the symptomatic and/or hemodynamically unstable patient with sinus bradycardia includes administration of the anticholinergic drug atropine, which should be given in doses of 0.5 mg IV every 3 to 5 minutes. The maximum recommended total dose of atropine is 3 mg.[14] Atropine is generally used as a method of achieving acute symptom control while awaiting placement of a transcutaneous or transvenous pacemaker. Where necessary, transcutaneous pacing can be initiated during atropine administration. Atropine should be used cautiously in patients with myocardial ischemia or infarction because increasing heart rate and myocardial oxygen demand may aggravate ischemia or extend the infarct.[14]

In patients with hemodynamically unstable sinus bradycardia who do not respond to atropine, transcutaneous pacing may be initiated. In patients with hemodynamically unstable or severely symptomatic sinus bradycardia that is unresponsive to atropine and in whom temporary or **transvenous pacing** is not available or is ineffective, or while awaiting placement of a pacemaker, dopamine (2 to 10 mcg/kg/min, titrate to response), epinephrine (2 to 10 mcg/min, titrate to response), or isoproterenol (2 to 10 mcg/min, titrate to response) may be administered to increase heart rate.[14]

In patients with sinus bradycardia due to underlying correctable disorders (such as electrolyte abnormalities or hypothyroidism), management consists of correcting those disorders.

Nonpharmacologic Therapy Long-term management of patients with sick sinus syndrome requires implantation of a permanent pacemaker.[12]

▶ Outcome Evaluation

- Monitor the patient's heart rate and alleviation of symptoms.
- Monitor for adverse effects of medications such as atropine (dry mouth, mydriasis, urinary retention, and tachycardia).

AV Nodal Blockade

AV nodal blockade occurs when conduction of electrical impulses through the AV node is impaired to varying degrees. AV nodal blockade is classified into three categories. First-degree AV block is defined simply as prolongation of the PR interval to greater than 0.2 seconds. During first-degree AV block, all impulses initiated by the SA node that have resulted in atrial depolarization are conducted through the AV node; the abnormality is simply that the impulses are conducted more slowly than normal, resulting in prolongation of the PR interval.[15] Second-degree AV block is further distinguished into two types: **Mobitz type I** (also known as Wenckebach) and **Mobitz type II**. In both types of second-degree AV block, some of the impulses initiated by the SA node are not conducted through the AV node. This often occurs in a regular pattern; for example, every third or fourth impulse generated by the SA node may not be conducted. During third-degree AV block, which is also referred to as "complete heart block," none of the impulses generated by the SA node are conducted through the AV node. This results in "AV dissociation," during which the atria continue to depolarize normally as a result of normal impulses initiated by the SA node; however, the ventricles initiate their own depolarizations because no SA node–generated impulses are conducted to the ventricles. Therefore, on the ECG, there is no relationship between the P waves and the QRS complexes.

▶ Epidemiology and Etiology

The overall incidence of AV nodal blockade is unknown. AV nodal blockade may be caused by degenerative changes in

Table 9–3
Etiologies of AV Nodal Blockade[12,13,15]

Idiopathic degeneration of the AV node
Myocardial ischemia or infarction
Neurocardiac syncope
Carotid sinus hypersensitivity
Electrolyte abnormalities: hypokalemia or hyperkalemia
Hypothyroidism
Hypothermia
Infectious diseases: Chagas' disease or endocarditis
Amyloidosis
Sarcoidosis
Systemic lupus erythematosus
Scleroderma
Sleep apnea
Drugs:

Adenosine	Hydroxychloroquine
Amiodarone	Paclitaxel
β-Blockers	Phenylpropanolamine
Bupivacaine	Propafenone
Carbamazepine	Propofol
Chloroquine	Sotalol
Digoxin	Thioridazine
Diltiazem	Tricyclic antidepressants
Dronedarone	Verapamil
Flecainide	

AV, atrioventricular.

the AV node. ❷ *In addition, there are many other possible etiologies of AV nodal blockade including drugs* (**Table 9–3**).[12,13]

▶ Pathophysiology

First-degree AV nodal blockade occurs due to inhibition of conduction within the upper portion of the node.[15] Mobitz type I second-degree AV nodal blockade occurs as a result of inhibition of conduction further down within the node.[12,15] Mobitz type II second-degree AV nodal blockade is caused by inhibition of conduction within or below the level of the bundle of His.[12,15] Third-degree AV nodal blockade may be a result of inhibition of conduction either within the AV node or within the bundle of His or the His-Purkinje system.[12,15] AV block may occur as a result of age-related AV node degeneration.

▶ Treatment

Desired Outcomes The desired outcomes of treatment are to restore normal sinus rhythm and alleviate patient symptoms.

Pharmacologic Therapy Treatment of first-degree AV nodal blockade is rarely necessary because symptoms rarely occur. However, the ECGs of patients with first-degree AV nodal blockade should be monitored to assess the possibility of progression of first-degree AV nodal blockade to second- or third-degree block. Second- or third-degree AV nodal blockade requires treatment because bradycardia often results in symptoms. If the patient is taking any medication(s) that may cause AV nodal blockade, the drug(s) should be discontinued whenever possible. If the patient's rhythm still exhibits AV

Clinical Presentation and Diagnosis of AV Nodal Blockade

Symptoms

- First-degree AV nodal blockade is rarely symptomatic because it rarely results in bradycardia

- Second-degree AV nodal blockade may cause bradycardia because not all impulses generated by the SA node are conducted through the AV node to the ventricles

- In third-degree AV nodal blockade, or complete heart block, the heart rate is usually 30 to 40 bpm, resulting in symptoms

- Symptoms of bradyarrhythmias such as second- or third-degree AV block consist of dizziness, fatigue, light-headedness, syncope, chest pain (in patients with underlying CAD), and shortness of breath and other symptoms of heart failure (in patients with underlying left ventricular dysfunction)

Diagnosis

- Made on the basis of patient presentation, including history of present illness and presenting symptoms, as well as a 12-lead ECG that reveals AV nodal blockade

- Assess potentially correctable etiologies, including myocardial ischemia, serum potassium concentration (for hyperkalemia), and thyroid function tests (for hypothyroidism)

- Determine whether the patient is taking any drugs known to cause AV block

- If the patient is currently taking digoxin, determine the serum digoxin concentration and ascertain whether it is supratherapeutic (greater than 2 ng/mL [2.6 nmol/L])

nodal blockade after discontinuing the medication(s) and after five half-lives of the drug(s) have elapsed, then the drug(s) can usually be excluded as the etiology of the arrhythmia. However, in certain circumstances, discontinuation of a medication that is inducing AV nodal blockade may be undesirable. For example, if the patient has a history of myocardial infarction or heart failure, discontinuation of a β-blocker is undesirable because β-blockers have been shown to reduce mortality and prolong life in patients with those diseases, and the benefits of therapy with β-blockers outweigh the risks associated with AV nodal blockade. In these patients, clinicians and patients may elect to implant a permanent pacemaker in order to allow the patient to continue therapy with β-blockers.

Acute treatment of patients with second- or third-degree AV nodal blockade consists primarily of administration of atropine, which may be administered in the same doses as recommended for the management of sinus bradycardia. In patients with hemodynamically unstable or severely symptomatic AV nodal blockade that is unresponsive to atropine and in whom temporary or transvenous pacing is not available or is ineffective, epinephrine (2 to 10 mcg/min, titrate to response) and/or dopamine (2 to 10 mcg/kg/min) may be administered.[14]

In patients with second- or third-degree AV block due to underlying correctable disorders (such as electrolyte abnormalities or hypothyroidism), management consists of correcting those disorders.

Nonpharmacologic Therapy Long-term management of patients with second- or third-degree AV nodal blockade due to idiopathic degeneration of the AV node requires implantation of a permanent pacemaker.[12]

▶ Outcome Evaluation

- Monitor the patient for termination of AV nodal blockade and restoration of normal sinus rhythm, heart rate, and alleviation of symptoms.

- If atropine is administered, monitor the patient for adverse effects including dry mouth, mydriasis, urinary retention, and tachycardia.

Atrial Fibrillation

AF is the most common arrhythmia encountered in clinical practice. It is important for clinicians to understand AF because it is associated with substantial morbidity and mortality and because many strategies for drug therapy are available. Drugs used to treat AF often have a narrow therapeutic index and a broad adverse-effect profile.

▶ Epidemiology and Etiology

Approximately 2.2 million Americans have AF. The prevalence of AF increases with advancing age; roughly 8% of patients between the ages of 80 and 89 years have AF.[16] Similarly, the incidence of AF increases with age, and it occurs more commonly in men than in women.[16]

Etiologies of AF are presented in Table 9–4. The common feature of the majority of etiologies of AF is the development of left atrial hypertrophy. Hypertension may be the most important risk factor for development of AF. However, AF also occurs commonly in patients with CAD. In addition, heart failure is increasingly recognized as a cause of AF; approximately 25% to 30% of patients with New York Heart Association (NYHA) class III heart failure have AF,[17] and the arrhythmia is present in as many as 50% of patients with NYHA class IV heart failure.[18]

Drug-induced AF is relatively uncommon but has been reported (Table 9–4).[13] Acute ingestion of large amounts of alcohol may cause AF; this phenomenon has been referred to as the "holiday heart" syndrome.[19] In addition, recent reports have associated use of the bisphosphonate drugs zoledronic acid[20] and alendronate[21] with new-onset serious AF. The potential relationship between bisphosphonate use and new-onset AF requires further study.

Clinical Presentation and Diagnosis of AF

Symptoms

- Approximately 20% to 30% of patients with AF remain asymptomatic

- Symptoms typical of tachyarrhythmias such as AF include palpitations, dizziness, light-headedness, shortness of breath, chest pain (if underlying CAD is present), near-syncope, and syncope. Patients commonly complain of palpitations; often the complaint is "I can feel my heart beating fast" or "I can feel my heart fluttering" or "It feels like my heart is going to beat out of my chest"

- Other symptoms depend on the degree to which cardiac output is diminished, which in turn depends on the ventricular rate and the degree to which stroke volume is reduced by the rapidly beating heart

- In some patients, the first symptom of AF is stroke

Diagnosis

- Because the symptoms of all tachyarrhythmias depend on heart rate and are therefore essentially the same, the diagnosis depends on the presence of AF on the ECG

- AF is characterized on ECG by an absence of P waves, an undulating baseline that represents chaotic atrial electrical activity, and an irregularly irregular rhythm, meaning that the intervals between the R waves are irregular and there is no pattern to the irregularity

---

Table 9–4

Etiologies of AF[13,20,21,25]

Hypertension
Coronary artery disease
Heart failure
Diabetes
Hyperthyroidism
Rheumatic heart disease
Diseases of the heart valves:
    Mitral stenosis or regurgitation
    Mitral valve prolapse
Acute myocardial infarction
Pericarditis
Amyloidosis
Myocarditis
Pulmonary embolism
Idiopathic ("lone" AF)
Familial AF
Thoracic surgery:
    Coronary artery bypass graft surgery
    Pulmonary resection
    Thoracoabdominal esophagectomy
Drugs:
    Adenosine
    Albuterol
    Alcohol
    Alendronate
    Dobutamine
    Enoximone
    Ipratropium bromide
    Methylprednisolone
    Milrinone
    Mitoxantrone
    Paclitaxel
    Propafenone
    Theophylline
    Verapamil
    Zoledronic acid

AF, atrial fibrillation.

▶ Pathophysiology

❶ *AF may be caused by both abnormal impulse formation and abnormal impulse conduction.* Traditionally, AF was believed to be initiated by premature impulses initiated in the atria. However, it is now understood that in many patients AF is triggered by electrical impulses generated within the pulmonary veins.[22] These impulses initiate the process of reentry within the atria, and AF is believed to be sustained by multiple reentrant wavelets operating simultaneously within the atria. Some believe that, at least in some patients, the increased automaticity in the pulmonary veins may be the sole mechanism of AF and that the multiple reentrant wavelet hypothesis may be incorrect. However, the concept of multiple simultaneous reentrant wavelets remains the predominant hypothesis regarding the mechanism of AF.[23]

AF leads to electrical remodeling of the atria. Episodes of AF that are of longer duration and episodes that occur with increasing frequency result in progressive shortening of atrial refractory periods, further potentiating the reentrant circuits in the atria.[24] Therefore, it is often said that "atrial fibrillation begets atrial fibrillation"; that is, AF causes atrial electrophysiologic alterations that promote further AF.[23,24] AF is associated with chaotic, disorganized atrial electrical activity, resulting in no completed atrial depolarizations and therefore no atrial contraction.

A substantial amount of the atrial electrical activity occurring during AF may be conducted through the AV node into the ventricles, resulting in ventricular rates ranging from 100 to 200 bpm.

AF occurs in specific patterns: first detected, **paroxysmal,** persistent, or permanent (Fig. 9–4).[25] Patients with paroxysmal AF have episodes that begin suddenly and spontaneously, last minutes to hours, or rarely as long as 7 days, and terminate suddenly and spontaneously. Some patients with paroxysmal AF have episodes that do not terminate spontaneously; episodes that last greater than 7 days are termed persistent AF. Approximately 18% to 30% of patients with AF progress to the point of permanent AF; these patients are subsequently never in normal sinus rhythm but rather are always in AF.

AF is associated with substantial morbidity and mortality. This arrhythmia is associated with a risk of ischemic stroke of approximately 5% per year.[25] The risk of stroke is increased

Patient Encounter Part 1

DT is a 62-year-old man who presents to the emergency department (ED) complaining that he can "feel my heart beating fast." He states that this started several hours ago, and he waited to see if it would stop, but it has not. He also complains of feeling dizzy and nearly passing out. His pulse is irregularly irregular, with a rate of 130 bpm.

His physical examination is completely normal and no focal neurological deficits are observed.

What information is suggestive of AF?

What additional information do you need in order to develop a treatment plan?

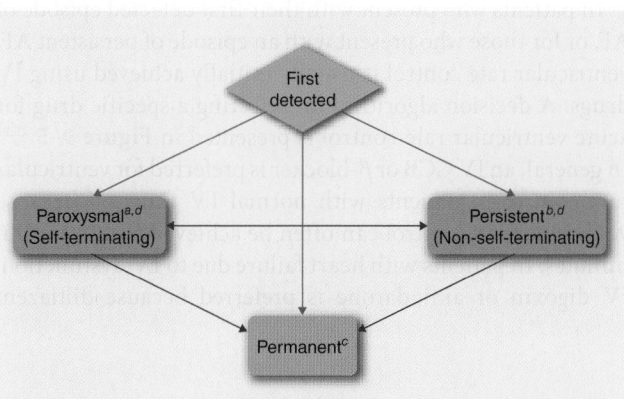

FIGURE 9-4. Patterns of atrial fibrillation. [a]Episodes that generally last 7 days or less (most less than 24 hours). [b]Episodes that usually last 7 days. [c]Cardioversion failed or not attempted. [d]Either paroxysmal or persistent atrial fibrillation may be recurrent. (From Fuster V, Rydén LE, Cannom DS, et al. 2011 ACCF/AHA/HRS focused updates incorporated into the ACC/AHA/ESC 2006 guidelines for the management of patients with atrial fibrillation: A report of the American College of Cardiology Foundation/American Heart Association Task Force on Practice Guidelines and the European Society of Cardiology Committee for Practice Guidelines. J Am Coll Cardiol 2011;57:e101–198.)

two- to sevenfold in patients with AF compared with patients without this arrhythmia.[25] AF is the cause of roughly one of every six strokes. During AF, atrial contraction is absent. Due to the fact that atrial contraction is responsible for approximately 30% of left ventricular filling, this blood that is not ejected from the left atrium to the left ventricle pools in the atrium, particularly in the left atrial appendage. Blood pooling facilitates the formation of a thrombus, which subsequently may travel through the mitral valve into the left ventricle and may be ejected during ventricular contraction. The thrombus then may travel through a carotid artery into the brain, resulting in an ischemic stroke.

AF may lead to the development of heart failure as a result of tachycardia-induced cardiomyopathy.[26] AF increases the risk of mortality approximately twofold compared with patients without AF[25]; the causes of death are likely stroke or heart failure.

▶ Treatment

● **Desired Outcomes** ❸ *The goals of individualized therapy for AF are (a) ventricular rate control, (b) termination of AF and restoration of sinus rhythm (commonly referred to as "cardioversion" or "conversion to sinus rhythm"), (c) maintenance of sinus rhythm, or reduction in the frequency of episodes of paroxysmal AF, and/or (d) prevention of stroke. These goals of therapy do not necessarily apply to all patients; the specific goal(s) that apply depend on the patient's AF pattern* (Table 9–5).

● **Hemodynamically Unstable AF** For patients who present with an episode of AF that is hemodynamically unstable, emergent conversion to sinus rhythm is necessary using **direct current cardioversion** (DCC). Hemodynamic instability may be defined as the presence of any one of the following[14]: (a) patient has acutely altered mental status, (b) hypotension (systolic blood pressure less than 90 mm Hg) or other signs of shock, (c) ischemic chest discomfort, and/or (d) acute heart failure.

● DCC is the process of administering a synchronized electrical shock to the chest. The purpose of DCC is to simultaneously depolarize all of the myocardial cells, resulting in interruption and termination of the multiple reentrant circuits and restoration of normal sinus rhythm. The recommended initial energy level for conversion of AF to sinus rhythm is 120 to 200 joules (J) for biphasic shocks or 200 J for monophasic shocks. If the DCC attempt is unsuccessful, the DCC energy should be increased in a stepwise fashion.[14]

Patient Encounter Part 2: Medical History, Physical Examination, and Diagnostic Tests

PMH: Hypertension × 15 years

Meds: Aspirin 81 mg once daily; hydrochlorothiazide 25 mg orally once daily; lisinopril 20 mg orally once daily

PE:

Ht 5 ft.10 in. (178 cm), wt 80 kg (176 lb), BP 100/60 mm Hg, P 130 bpm, RR 18/min; remainder of physical examination noncontributory

Labs: All within normal limits

CXR: No pulmonary edema

ECG: Atrial fibrillation

What is your assessment of DT's condition?

What are your treatment goals?

What pharmacologic or nonpharmacologic alternatives are available for each treatment goal?

Table 9-5			
Treatment Goals According to AF Pattern			
First Detected Episode	**Paroxysmal AF**	**Persistent AF**	**Permanent AF**
Ventricular rate control	Ventricular rate control	Ventricular rate control	Ventricular rate control
Stroke prevention	Stroke prevention	Stroke prevention	Stroke prevention
Conversion to sinus rhythm	Maintenance of sinus rhythm *if ventricular rate control is not sufficient to control symptoms*	Conversion to sinus rhythm	

AF, atrial fibrillation.

Delivery of the shock is synchronized to the ECG by the cardioverter machine, such that the electrical charge is not delivered during the latter portion of the T wave (i.e., the relative refractory period), to avoid delivering an electrical impulse that may be conducted abnormally, which may result in a life-threatening ventricular arrhythmia.

The remainder of this section is devoted to management of hemodynamically stable AF. The specific goals of therapy that apply to patients in each AF pattern are presented in Table 9-5.

▶ *Pharmacologic Therapy*

Ventricular Rate Control Ventricular rate control can be achieved by inhibiting the proportion of electrical impulses conducted from the atria to the ventricles through the AV node. Therefore, drugs that are effective for ventricular rate control are those that inhibit AV nodal impulse conduction: β-blockers, diltiazem, verapamil, digoxin, and amiodarone (Tables 9-6 and 9-7).

In patients who present with their first detected episode of AF, or for those who present with an episode of persistent AF, ventricular rate control is usually initially achieved using IV drugs. A decision algorithm for selecting a specific drug for acute ventricular rate control is presented in Figure 9-5.[25,27] In general, an IV CCB or β-blocker is preferred for ventricular rate control in patients with normal LV function because ventricular rate control can often be achieved within several minutes. In patients with heart failure due to LV dysfunction, IV digoxin or amiodarone is preferred because diltiazem

Table 9-6				
Drugs for Ventricular Rate Control in AF				
Drug	**Mechanism of Action**	**Loading Dose**	**Daily Dose**	**Drug Interactions**
Amiodarone	β-Blocker CCB	150 mg IV over 10 minutes	0.5–1 mg/min IV continuous infusion 200 mg orally once daily	Inhibits clearance of digoxin, warfarin, and other drugs
β-Blockers[a]	Inhibit AV nodal conduction by slowing AV nodal conduction and prolonging AV nodal refractoriness	Esmolol 500 mcg/kg IV over 1 minute Propranolol 0.15 mg/kg IV Metoprolol 2.5–5 mg IV × 2–3 doses	Esmolol 60–200 mcg/kg/min continuous IV infusion Propranolol 80–240 mg/day orally in divided doses Metoprolol 25–100 mg orally twice daily	
Diltiazem	Inhibits AV nodal conduction by slowing AV nodal conduction and prolonging AV nodal refractoriness	0.25 mg/kg IV load over 2 minutes. Additional 0.35 mg/kg in 15 minutes if needed	Continuous infusion of 5–15 mg/h 120–360 mg orally daily in divided doses	Inhibits elimination of cyclosporine
Verapamil	Inhibits AV nodal conduction by slowing AV nodal conduction and prolonging AV nodal refractoriness	0.075–0.15 mg/kg IV over 2 minutes. May repeat every 15–30 minutes to total dose of 20–30 mg	120–360 mg orally daily in divided doses	Inhibits digoxin elimination
Digoxin	Inhibits AV nodal conduction by (a) vagal stimulation by (b) directly slowing AV nodal conduction, and (c) prolonging AV nodal refractoriness	0.25 mg IV every 2 hours, up to 1.5 mg	0.125–0.375 mg orally once daily	Amiodarone, verapamil, inhibit digoxin elimination

AF, atrial fibrillation; AV, atrioventricular; CCB, calcium channel blocker.

[a]Although oral β-blockers are important agents for mortality reduction in patients with heart failure, IV β-blockers should be avoided due to the potential for heart failure exacerbation.

Table 9–7

Adverse Effects of Drugs Used to Treat Arrhythmias

Drug	Adverse Effects
Adenosine	Chest pain, flushing, shortness of breath, sinus bradycardia/AV block
Amiodarone	IV: Hypotension, sinus bradycardia
	Oral: Blue-gray skin discoloration, photosensitivity, corneal microdeposits, pulmonary fibrosis, hepatotoxicity, sinus bradycardia, hypo- or hyperthyroidism, peripheral neuropathy, weakness, AV block
Atropine	Tachycardia, urinary retention, blurred vision, dry mouth, mydriasis
Digoxin	Nausea, vomiting, anorexia, green-yellow halos around objects, ventricular arrhythmias
Diltiazem	Hypotension, sinus bradycardia, heart failure exacerbation, AV block
Dofetilide	Torsades de pointes
Dronedarone	Diarrhea, asthenia, nausea and vomiting, abdominal pain, bradycardia, GI distress, hepatotoxicity
Esmolol	Hypotension, sinus bradycardia, AV block, heart failure exacerbation
Flecainide	Dizziness, blurred vision, heart failure exacerbation
Ibutilide	Torsades de pointes
Metoprolol	Hypotension, sinus bradycardia, AV block, fatigue, heart failure exacerbation[a]
Mexiletine	Nausea, vomiting, GI distress, tremor, dizziness, fatigue, seizures (if dose too high)
Procainamide	Hypotension, torsades de pointes
Propafenone	Dizziness, blurred vision
Propranolol	Hypotension, bradycardia, AV block, heart failure exacerbation[a]
Sotalol	Sinus bradycardia, AV block, fatigue, torsades de pointes
Verapamil	Hypotension, heart failure exacerbation, bradycardia, AV block, constipation (oral)

AV, atrioventricular.

[a]Associated with IV administration, inappropriately high oral doses at initiation of therapy, or overly aggressive and rapid dose titration.

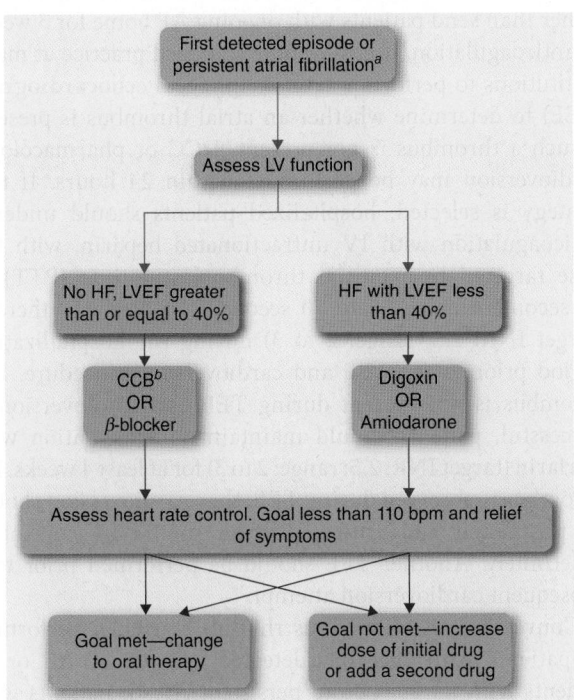

FIGURE 9–5. Decision algorithm for ventricular rate control using IV drug therapy for patients presenting with the first detected episode or an episode of persistent atrial fibrillation that is hemodynamically stable. [a]Drugs administered IV. [b]Diltiazem is generally preferred over verapamil because of a lower risk of severe hypotension. (β-Blocker, esmolol, metoprolol, or propranolol; bpm, beats per minute; CCB, calcium channel blocker [diltiazem or verapamil]; HF, heart failure; LV, left ventricular; LVEF, left ventricular ejection fraction; LVEF of 40% can also be expressed as 0.40.)

and verapamil are associated with negative inotropic effects and may exacerbate heart failure.[25,28] Similarly, although oral β-blockers are indicated in patients with heart failure due to LV dysfunction, IV β-blockers are generally avoided due to the potential for acutely exacerbating heart failure.

A decision strategy for long-term rate control with oral medications in patients with paroxysmal or permanent AF is presented in **Figure 9–6**.[25,27] In general, although digoxin is effective for ventricular rate control in patients at rest, it is less effective than CCBs or β-blockers for ventricular rate control in patients undergoing physical activity including activities of daily living. This is likely because activation of the sympathetic nervous system during exercise and activity overwhelms the stimulating effect of digoxin on the parasympathetic nervous system. Therefore, in patients with normal LV function, CCBs or β-blockers are preferred for long-term ventricular rate control. Diltiazem may be preferable to verapamil in older patients due to a lower incidence of constipation. However, in patients with heart failure, oral diltiazem and verapamil are contraindicated as a result of their negative inotropic activity and propensity to exacerbate heart failure. Therefore, the options in this population are β-blockers or digoxin. Most patients with heart failure should be receiving therapy with an oral β-blocker with the goal of achieving mortality risk reduction. In patients with heart failure who develop rapid AF while receiving therapy with β-blockers, digoxin should be administered for purposes of ventricular rate control. Fortunately, studies have found the combination of digoxin and β-blockers to be effective for ventricular rate control, likely as a result of β-blocker–induced attenuation of the inhibitory effects of the sympathetic nervous system on the efficacy of digoxin.

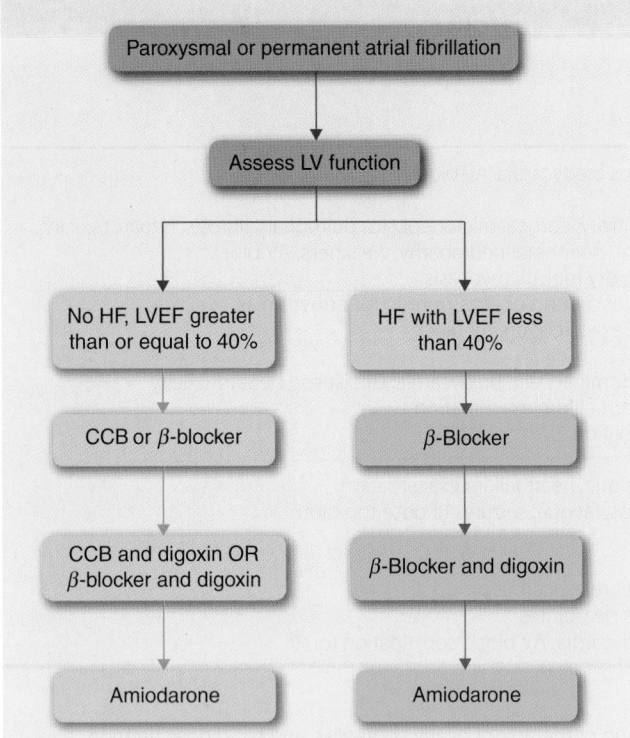

FIGURE 9–6. Decision algorithm for long-term ventricular rate control with oral drug therapy for patients with paroxysmal or permanent atrial fibrillation. With each therapy/dose change, assess heart rate control. Goal less than 100 bpm or reduction of heart rate by more than 20% with symptom relief. If goal is not met, move to next step in algorithm. (bpm, beats per minute; CCB, calcium channel blocker [diltiazem or verapamil]; HF, heart failure; LV, left ventricular function; LVEF, left ventricular ejection fraction; LVEF of 40% can also be expressed as 0.40.)

Conversion to Sinus Rhythm Termination of AF in hemodynamically stable patients may be performed using antiarrhythmic drug therapy or elective DCC. Drugs that may be used for conversion to sinus rhythm are presented in Table 9–8; these agents slow atrial conduction velocity and/or prolong refractoriness, facilitating interruption of reentrant circuits and restoration of sinus rhythm. DCC is generally more effective than drug therapy for conversion of AF to sinus rhythm. However, patients who undergo elective DCC must be sedated and/or anesthetized to avoid the discomfort associated with delivery of 120 to greater than or equal to 200 J of electricity to the chest. Therefore, it is important that patients scheduled to undergo elective DCC do not eat within approximately 8 to 12 hours of the procedure to avoid aspiration of stomach contents during the period of sedation/anesthesia. This often factors into the decision as to whether to use elective DCC or drug therapy for conversion of AF to sinus rhythm. If a patient presents with AF requiring nonemergent conversion to sinus rhythm, and the patient has eaten a meal that day, then pharmacologic

methods must be used for cardioversion on that day, or DCC must be postponed to the following day to allow for a period of fasting prior to the procedure.

A decision strategy for conversion of AF to sinus rhythm is presented in Figure 9–7.[25] The cardioversion decision strategy depends greatly on the duration of AF. If the AF episode began within 48 hours, conversion to sinus rhythm is safe and may be attempted with elective DCC or specific drug therapy (Fig. 9–7). However, if the duration of the AF episode is longer than 48 hours or if there is uncertainty regarding the duration of the episode, two strategies for conversion may be considered. Data indicate that a thrombus may form in the left atrium during AF episodes of 48 hours or longer; if an atrial thrombus is present, the process of conversion to sinus rhythm, whether with DCC or drugs, can dislodge the atrial thrombus, leading to embolization and a stroke. Therefore, in patients experiencing an AF episode of 48 hours or longer, conversion to sinus rhythm should be deferred unless it is known that an atrial thrombus is not present. In the past, common practice in patients with AF of greater than 48 hours duration was to anticoagulate with warfarin, maintaining a therapeutic **international normalized ratio** (INR) for 3 weeks, after which cardioversion may be performed. Patients were subsequently anticoagulated for a minimum of 4 weeks following the restoration of sinus rhythm. Today, rather than send patients with ongoing AF home for 3 weeks of anticoagulation, it has become standard practice at many institutions to perform a **transesophageal echocardiogram** (TEE) to determine whether an atrial thrombus is present; if such a thrombus is not present, DCC or pharmacologic cardioversion may be performed within 24 hours. If this strategy is selected, hospitalized patients should undergo anticoagulation with IV unfractionated heparin, with the dose targeted to a partial thromboplastin time (PTT) of 60 seconds (range: 50 to 70 seconds), or warfarin therapy (target INR: 2.5; range: 2 to 3) during the hospitalization period prior to the TEE and cardioversion procedure. If a thrombus is not present during TEE and cardioversion is successful, patients should maintain anticoagulation with warfarin (target INR: 2.5; range: 2 to 3) for at least 4 weeks. If a thrombus is observed during TEE, then cardioversion should be postponed and anticoagulation should be continued indefinitely. Another TEE should be performed prior to a subsequent cardioversion attempt.[29]

Conversion of AF to sinus rhythm is usually performed in patients with the first detected episode of AF or in patients with an episode of persistent AF. In patients with permanent AF, conversion to sinus rhythm is usually not attempted because cardioversion is unlikely to be successful, and in those rare patients in whom sinus rhythm is restored successfully, AF usually recurs shortly thereafter.

Maintenance of Sinus Rhythm/Reduction in the Frequency of Episodes of Paroxysmal AF In many patients, permanent maintenance of sinus rhythm following cardioversion is an unrealistic goal. Many, if not most, patients experience recurrence of AF after cardioversion. Similarly, in patients with paroxysmal AF, complete

Table 9–8

Drugs for Conversion of AF to Normal Sinus Rhythm

Treatment	Loading Dose	Maintenance Dose	Drug Interactions
Amiodarone	IV: 5–7 mg/kg over 30–60 minutes	1.2–1.8 g via continuous IV infusion over 24 hours	Inhibits elimination of digoxin and warfarin
	Oral (inpatient): 1.2–1.8 g per day in divided doses until 10 g total	200–400 mg once daily	
	Oral (outpatient): 600–800 mg daily in divided doses until 10 g total	200–400 mg once daily	
Dofetilide[a]		—	Cimetidine, hydrochlorothiazide, ketoconazole, medroxyprogesterone, promethazine, trimethoprim, verapamil (all inhibit dofetilide elimination)
Ibutilide	1 mg IV over 10 minutes, followed by a second 1 mg IV dose if necessary	—	—
Propafenone	600 mg single oral dose	—	—
Flecainide	200–300 mg single oral dose	—	—

AF, atrial fibrillation.

[a]Recommended initial dofetilide doses are:

Calculated creatinine clearance (mL/min):	Dose
Greater than 60	500 mcg twice daily
40–60	250 mcg twice daily
20–40	125 mcg twice daily
Less than 20	Contraindicated

Patients must be hospitalized for 3 days during initiation of therapy.

Calculated creatinine clearance of greater than 60, 40–60, 20–40, and less than 20 mL/min corresponds to greater than 1, 0.67–1, 0.33–0.67, and less than 0.33 mL/s, respectively.

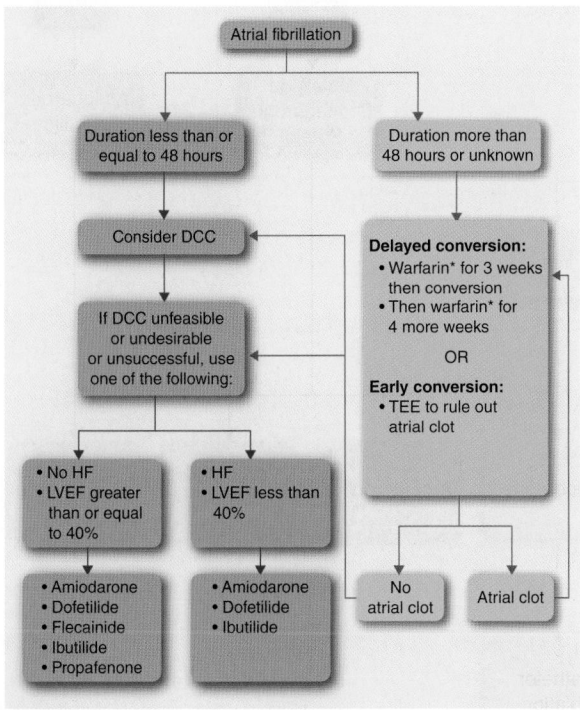

FIGURE 9–7. Decision algorithm for conversion of hemodynamically stable atrial fibrillation to normal sinus rhythm. (DCC, direct current cardioversion; HF, heart failure; LVEF, left ventricular ejection fraction; TEE, transesophageal echocardiogram; LVEF of 40% can also be expressed as 0.40.)
*International normalized ratio 2–3.

maintenance of sinus rhythm without recurrent episodes of AF is unrealistic. Therefore, a more realistic goal for many patients is not permanent maintenance of sinus rhythm, but rather reduction in the frequency of episodes of paroxysmal AF.

In recent years, numerous studies have been performed to determine whether drug therapy for maintenance of sinus rhythm is preferred to drug therapy for ventricular rate control.[30–34] In these studies, patients have been assigned randomly to receive therapy either with drugs for rate control or with drugs for rhythm control (Table 9–9). These studies have found no significant differences in mortality in patients who received rhythm control therapy versus those who received rate control therapy.[30–34] However, patients assigned to the rhythm control strategy were more likely to be hospitalized[30,32–34] and were more likely to experience adverse effects associated with drug therapy.[30,31]

❹ *Therefore, drug therapy for the purpose of maintaining sinus rhythm or reducing the frequency of episodes of AF should be initiated only in those patients with episodes of paroxysmal AF who continue to experience symptoms despite maximum tolerated doses of drugs for ventricular rate control.* A decision strategy for maintenance therapy of sinus rhythm is presented in Figure 9–8.[25,27] Drug therapy for maintenance of sinus rhythm and/or reduction in the frequency of episodes of paroxysmal AF should not be initiated in patients with underlying correctable causes of AF, such as hyperthyroidism; rather, the underlying cause of the arrhythmia should be corrected.

Table 9–9

Drugs for Maintenance of Sinus Rhythm/Reduction in the Frequency of Episodes of AF

Drug	Dose
Amiodarone	100–400 mg orally once daily
Dofetilide	As described in Table 9–8
Dronedarone	400 mg orally twice daily
Sotalol	80–160 mg orally twice daily
Propafenone	150–300 mg orally three times daily
Flecainide	100–150 mg orally three times daily

AF, atrial fibrillation.

● **Stroke Prevention** All patients with paroxysmal, persistent, or permanent AF should receive therapy for stroke prevention unless compelling contraindications exist. A decision strategy for assigning patients to receive anticoagulation for stroke prevention in AF is presented in Table 9–10.[29,35] ❺ *In general, most patients require therapy with dabigatran or warfarin; in some patients with no risk factors for stroke, anticoagulation may not be necessary.* For patients for whom oral anticoagulation is indicated (i.e., those with a CHADS$_2$ score of 1 or more), dabigatran 10 mg twice daily is suggested as preferable to warfarin titrated to an INR of 2.0–3.0.[29]

The landscape of anticoagulation for stroke prevention in AF has changed with the availability of dabigatran, the FDA approval of rivaroxaban in November 2011, and the potential FDA approval of apixaban. Dabigatran is a direct thrombin inhibitor that was approved by the FDA in October 2010 for stroke prevention in patients with nonvalvular AF. Dabigatran is now preferred over warfarin for the prevention of stroke and systemic embolism in patients with AF and risk factors for stroke and systemic embolization who do not have a prosthetic heart valve or hemodynamically significant heart valve disease.[29,36] Dabigatran should not be used in patients with severe kidney disease (creatinine clearance

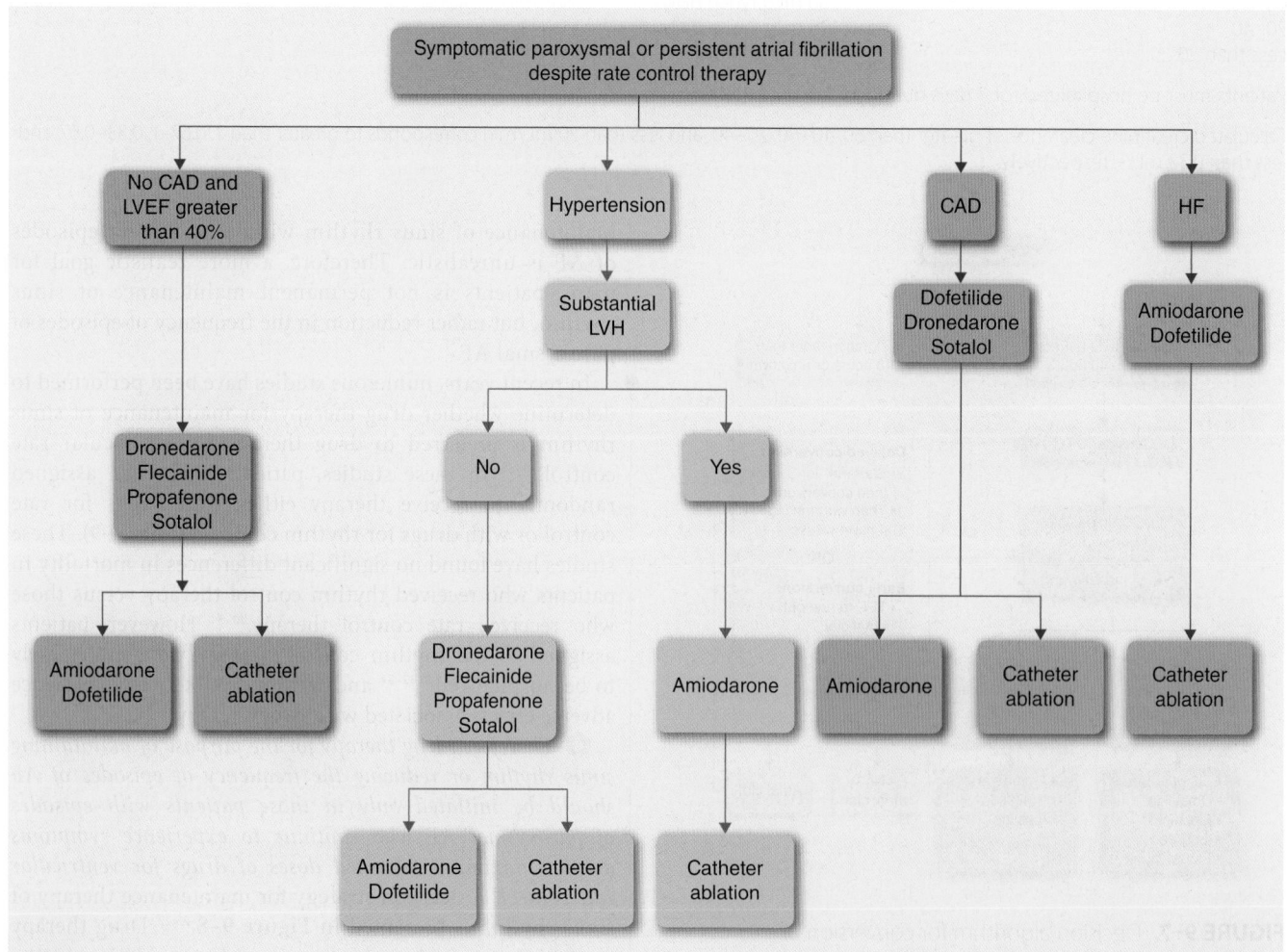

FIGURE 9–8. Decision algorithm for maintenance of sinus rhythm/reduction in the frequency of episodes of atrial fibrillation. (CAD, coronary artery disease; HF, heart failure; LVEF, left ventricular ejection fraction; LVH, left ventricular hypertrophy; LVEF of 40% can also be expressed as 0.40.)

Table 9–10

American College of Chest Physicians Recommendations for Stroke Prevention in AF[29,35]

CHADS$_2$ Score	Degree of Risk	Recommended Stroke Prevention Strategy
0	Low	Antithrombotic therapy is not recommended. For patients who choose antithrombotic therapy: aspirin 75–325 mg daily
Greater than or equal to 1	Moderate-High	Oral anticoagulation recommended; dabigatran preferred over warfarin (INR: 2–3)

CHADS$_2$ score calculated as follows:

Congestive heart failure	1 point
Hypertension	1 point
Age greater than or equal to 75 years	1 point
Diabetes mellitus	1 point
Stroke or TIA history	2 points

AF, atrial fibrillation; INR, international normalized ratio; TIA, transient ischemic attack.

under 15 mL/min [0.25 mL/s]) or advanced liver disease (impaired baseline clotting function).[36] The recommended dabigatran dose is 150 mg twice daily, except for patients with severe kidney disease (creatinine clearance: 15 to 30 mL/min [0.25 to 0.50 mL/s]), for whom the recommended dose is 75 mg twice daily. Advantages of dabigatran include the fact that INR monitoring is not required, and the drug's onset of action is rapid, eliminating the need for bridging with unfractionated or low molecular weight heparins.[37] In addition, there is a lower likelihood of drug interactions with dabigatran than with warfarin. However, dabigatran is a p-glycoprotein substrate, and therefore concomitant administration with p-glycoprotein inhibitors such as ketoconazole, amiodarone, and verapamil may result in increases in plasma dabigatran concentrations.[37] Similarly, concomitant administration of dabigatran with p-glycoprotein inducers such as rifampin may reduce plasma dabigatran concentrations.[37] Disadvantages of dabigatran include the fact that, in cases of dabigatran-associated bleeding, there is no antidote to reverse dabigatran's effects.

For patients for whom warfarin is preferred over dabigatran (such as those with severe kidney disease), specific genetic tests to guide the initiation of therapy have been approved by the FDA. These tests assess single nucleotide polymorphisms on the gene that encodes cytochrome P-450 2C19, the primary hepatic enzyme responsible for warfarin metabolism, and the gene *VKORC1*, which encodes vitamin K epoxide reductase, the enzyme that is inhibited by warfarin as its mechanism of anticoagulation. Some advocate that all patients in whom warfarin therapy is being initiated should undergo genetic testing to guide the initiation of therapy; patients with specific

polymorphisms of one or both of these genes may require adjustment of the initial warfarin dose to achieve adequate anticoagulation or avoid overanticoagulation and toxicity.[38] Genetic testing to guide the initiation of warfarin therapy has not yet become standard practice, and many have questioned the efficacy and cost effectiveness of incorporation of routine genetic testing into warfarin therapy. The role of genetic testing in selecting initial warfarin doses is likely to continue to evolve but at the present time appears to be limited.

Algorithms for estimating the initial dose of warfarin have been developed incorporating clinical and pharmacogenetic information.[39,40] One widely used algorithm, which provides warfarin dose computations with clinical data even if pharmacogenetic information is not obtainable, is available at http://www.warfarindosing.org.

Rivaroxaban, an oral factor Xa inhibitor, was approved by the FDA in November 2011 for stroke prevention in AF. Rivaroxaban was shown to be noninferior to warfarin for prevention of stroke or systemic embolism in patients with AF, and compared with warfarin, rivaroxaban was associated with a lower risk of intracranial and fatal bleeding.[41] Apixaban, an investigational oral factor Xa inhibitor, was shown to be superior to warfarin for prevention of stroke or systemic embolism in patients with AF, with lower bleeding risk.[42] At the time of the writing of this chapter, apixaban had not been approved by the FDA. The potential availability of these new anticoagulation options may markedly change the therapeutics of stroke prevention in AF in the future.

▶ *Outcome Evaluation*

- Monitor the patient to determine whether the goal of ventricular rate control is met: heart rate less than 110 bpm with relief of symptoms.

- Monitor ECG to assess continued presence of AF and to determine whether conversion to sinus rhythm has occurred.

- In patients receiving warfarin, monitor INR approximately monthly to make sure it is therapeutic (target: 2.5; range: 2 to 3).

- Monitor patients for adverse effects of specific drug therapy (Table 9–7). Monitor patients receiving warfarin or dabigatran for signs and symptoms of bruising or bleeding.

Patient Encounter Part 3: Creating a Care Plan

Based on the information presented, create a care plan for DT's acute AF episode and for long-term management of his AF.

Your plan should include (a) a statement of the drug-related needs and/or problems, (b) the goals of therapy, (c) a patient-specific detailed therapeutic plan, and (d) a plan for follow-up to determine whether the goals have been achieved and adverse effects avoided.

Paroxysmal Supraventricular Tachycardia

Paroxysmal supraventricular tachycardia (PSVT) is a term that refers to a number of arrhythmias that occur above the ventricles and require atrial or AV nodal tissue for initiation and maintenance.[43] The most common of these arrhythmias is known as AV reentrant tachycardia, in which the arrhythmia is caused by a reentrant circuit that involves the AV node or tissue adjacent to the AV node. Other types of PSVT include the relatively uncommon Wolff-Parkinson-White syndrome, which is caused by reentry through an accessory extra-AV nodal pathway. For the purposes of this section, the term *PSVT* refers to AV nodal reentrant tachycardia.

▶ Epidemiology and Etiology

Although PSVT can occur in patients experiencing myocardial ischemia or infarction, it often occurs in relatively young individuals with no history of cardiac disease. The overall incidence of PSVT is unknown.

▶ Pathophysiology

1 *Paroxysmal supraventricular tachycardia is caused by reentry that includes the AV node as a part of the reentrant circuit.* Typically, electrical impulses travel forward (antegrade) down the AV node and then travel back up the AV node (retrograde) in a repetitive circuit. In some patients, the retrograde conduction pathway of the reentrant circuit may exist in extra-AV nodal tissue adjacent to the AV node. One of these pathways usually conducts impulses rapidly while the other usually conducts impulses slowly. Most commonly, during PSVT the impulse conducts antegrade through the slow pathway and retrograde through the faster pathway; in approximately 10% of patients, the reentrant circuit is reversed.[43]

▶ Treatment

Desired Outcomes The desired outcomes for treatment are to terminate the arrhythmia, restore sinus rhythm, and prevent recurrence. Drug therapy is used to terminate the arrhythmia and restore sinus rhythm; nonpharmacologic measures are used to prevent recurrence.

Termination of PSVT Hemodynamically unstable PSVT should be treated with immediate synchronized DCC, using an initial energy level of 50 to 100 J; if the initial DCC attempt is unsuccessful, the shock energy should be increased in a stepwise fashion.[14]

The primary method of termination of hemodynamically stable PSVT is inhibition of impulse conduction and/or prolongation of the refractory period within the AV node. Because PSVT is propagated via a reentrant circuit involving the AV node, inhibition of conduction within the AV node interrupts and terminates the reentrant circuit.

Prior to initiation of drug therapy for termination of hemodynamically stable PSVT, some simple nonpharmacologic methods known as vagal maneuvers may be attempted.[14,44] Vagal maneuvers stimulate the activity of the parasympathetic nervous system, which inhibits AV nodal conduction, facilitating termination of the arrhythmia. Vagal maneuvers alone may terminate PSVT in up to 25% of cases.[14] Perhaps the simplest vagal maneuver is cough, which stimulates the vagus nerve. Instructing the patient to cough two or three times may successfully terminate the PSVT. Another vagal maneuver that may be attempted is carotid sinus massage; one of the carotid sinuses, located in the neck in the vicinity of the carotid arteries, may be gently massaged, stimulating vagal activity. Carotid sinus massage should not be performed in patients with a history of stroke or transient ischemic attack, or in those in whom carotid bruits may be heard on auscultation. The Valsalva maneuver, during which patients bear down against a closed glottis, may also be attempted.

If vagal maneuvers are unsuccessful, IV drug therapy should be initiated.[14,43,44] Drugs that may be used for termination of hemodynamically stable PSVT are presented in Table 9–11. A decision strategy for pharmacologic termination of hemodynamically stable PSVT is presented in Figure 9–9.[14,44]

Clinical Presentation and Diagnosis of PSVT

- May occur at any age, but most commonly during the fourth and fifth decades of life[44]
- Occurs more commonly in females than in males; approximately two-thirds of patients that experience PSVT are women[43]

Symptoms

- Symptoms typical of tachyarrhythmias such as PSVT include palpitations, dizziness, light-headedness, shortness of breath, chest pain (if underlying CAD is present), near-syncope, and syncope. Patients commonly complain of palpitations; often the complaint is "I can feel my heart beating fast" or "I can feel my heart fluttering" or "It feels like my heart is going to beat out of my chest"

- Other symptoms depend on the degree to which cardiac output is diminished, which in turn depends on the heart rate and the degree to which stroke volume is reduced by the rapidly beating heart

Diagnosis

- Because the symptoms of all tachyarrhythmias depend on heart rate and are therefore essentially the same, diagnosis depends on the presence of PSVT on the ECG, characterized by narrow QRS complexes (usually less than 0.12 seconds). P waves may or may not be visible, depending on the heart rate

- PSVT is a regular rhythm and occurs at rates ranging from 100 to 250 bpm

Table 9–11

Drugs for Termination of PSVT[14]

Drug	Mechanism	Dose	Drug Interactions
Adenosine	Direct AV nodal inhibition	6 mg IV rapid push followed by 20 mL saline flush. If no response in 1–2 minutes, 12 mg IV rapid push followed by 20-mL saline flush	Dipyridamole and carbamazepine accentuate response to adenosine
Diltiazem	Direct AV nodal inhibition	0.25 mg/kg IV over 2 minutes If insufficient response in 15 minutes, give second dose (0.35 mg/kg) IV over 2 minutes Maintenance infusion 5–15 mg/h	
Verapamil	Direct AV nodal inhibition	1. 2.5–5.0 mg IV over 2 minutes 2. May repeat as 5–10 mg IV every 15–30 minutes to total dose of 20–30 mg	
Digoxin	1. Vagal stimulation 2. Direct AV nodal inhibition	8–12 mcg/kg total loading dose, half of which should be administered over 5 minutes, with the remaining portion administered as 25% fractions at 4- to 8-hour intervals	Slow onset of action
β-Blockers	Direct AV nodal inhibition	Esmolol 500 mcg/kg IV over 1 minute then 50 mcg/kg/min continuous infusion. If inadequate response, give second loading dose of 500 mcg/kg and increase maintenance infusion to 100 mcg/kg/min. Increment dose increases in this manner as necessary to maximum infusion rate of 200 mcg/kg/min Propranolol 0.5–1.0 mg IV over 1 minute; repeat as necessary to a total dose of 0.1 mg/kg Metoprolol 5 mg IV over 1–2 minutes; repeat as necessary every 5 minutes to a total dose of 15 mg Atenolol 5 mg IV over 5 minutes; repeat 5 mg in 10 minutes if necessary	
Amiodarone	β-Blocker Calcium channel blocker	150 mg IV over 10 minutes; repeat if necessary. Follow with continuous infusion of 1 mg/min for 6 hours, followed by 0.5 mg/min. Total dose over 24 hours should not exceed 2.2 g	Inhibits elimination of digoxin and warfarin

AV, atrioventricular; PSVT, paroxysmal supraventricular tachycardia.

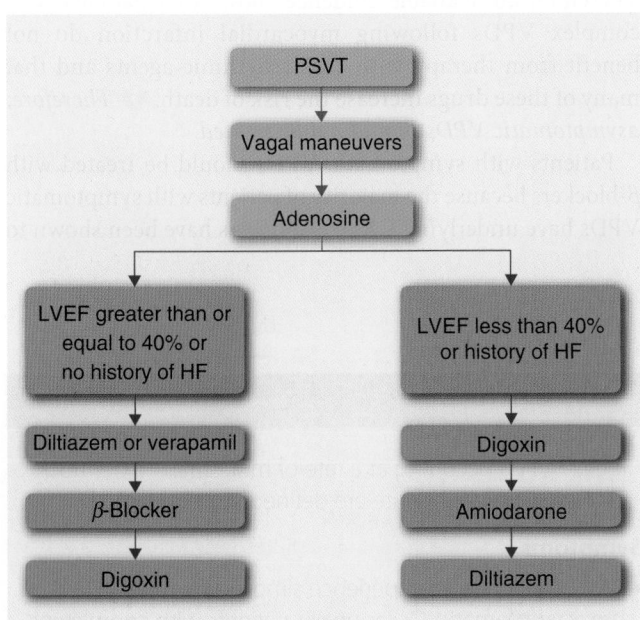

FIGURE 9–9. Decision algorithm for termination of PSVT. (HF, heart failure; LVEF, left ventricular ejection fraction; PSVT, paroxysmal supraventricular tachycardia; LVEF of 40% can also be expressed as 0.40.)

⑥ *Adenosine is the drug of choice for pharmacologic termination of PSVT and is successful in 90% to 95% of patients.* Adenosine inhibits conduction transiently and is associated with adverse effects (Table 9–7) including flushing, sinus bradycardia or AV nodal blockade, and bronchospasm in susceptible patients. In addition, adenosine may cause chest pain that mimics the discomfort of myocardial ischemia but is not actually associated with ischemia. The half-life of adenosine is approximately 10 seconds, due to deamination in the blood; therefore, in the vast majority of patients, adverse effects are of short duration.

If adenosine therapy is unsuccessful for termination of PSVT, subsequent choices of therapy depend on whether the patient has heart failure and/or a depressed left ventricular ejection fraction (LVEF).

Nonpharmacologic Therapy: Prevention of Recurrence

In the past, prevention of recurrence of PSVT was attempted using long-term oral therapy with drugs such as verapamil or digoxin. Unfortunately, oral therapy with these drugs was associated with relatively limited success. Currently, the treatment of choice for long-term prevention of recurrence of PSVT is **radiofrequency catheter ablation**. During this procedure, a catheter is introduced transvenously and directed to the right atrium under fluoroscopic guidance. The catheter is advanced to the AV node, and radiofrequency energy is delivered to ablate, or destroy, one of the pathways of the reentrant circuit. This procedure usually achieves a complete cure of PSVT and is associated with a relatively low risk of complications, and it therefore obviates the need for long-term antiarrhythmic drug therapy in this population.

▶ Outcome Evaluation

- Monitor patients for termination of PSVT and restoration of normal sinus rhythm.
- Monitor patients for adverse effects of adenosine or any other antiarrhythmic agents administered (Table 9–7).

VENTRICULAR ARRHYTHMIAS
Ventricular Premature Depolarizations

VPDs are ectopic electrical impulses originating in ventricular tissue, resulting in wide, misshapen, abnormal QRS complexes. VPDs are also commonly known by other terms, including premature ventricular contractions (PVCs), ventricular premature beats (VPBs), and ventricular premature contractions (VPCs).

▶ Epidemiology, Etiology, and Pathophysiology

VPDs occur with variable frequency, depending on underlying comorbid conditions. The prevalence of complex or frequent VPDs is approximately 33% and 12% in men with and without CAD, respectively[45]; in women, the prevalence of complex or frequent VPDs is 26% and 12% in those with and without CAD, respectively.[46] VPDs occur more commonly in patients with ischemic heart disease, a history of myocardial infarction, and heart failure due to LV dysfunction. They may also occur as a result of hypoxia, anemia, and following cardiac surgery.

❶ *VPDs occur as a result of abnormal ventricular automaticity due to enhanced activity of the sympathetic nervous system and altered electrophysiological characteristics of the heart during myocardial ischemia and following myocardial infarction.*

In patients with underlying CAD or a history of myocardial infarction, the presence of complex or frequent VPDs is associated with an increased risk of mortality due to sudden cardiac death.[47]

▶ Treatment

● Desired Outcomes The desired outcomes for treatment are to alleviate patient symptoms.

● Pharmacologic Therapy **❼** *Asymptomatic VPDs should not be treated with antiarrhythmic drug therapy.* Based on the knowledge that complex or frequent VPDs increase the risk of sudden cardiac death in patients with a history of myocardial infarction, the Cardiac Arrhythmia Suppression Trials (CAST I and II)[48,49] tested the hypothesis that suppression of asymptomatic VPDs with the drugs flecainide, encainide, or moricizine in patients with a relatively recent history of myocardial infarction would lead to a reduction in the incidence of sudden cardiac death. However, the results of the trial showed that not only did these antiarrhythmic agents not reduce the risk of sudden cardiac death, there was a significant *increase* in the risk of death in patients who received therapy with encainide or flecainide compared with those who received placebo.[48] During the continuation of the study with moricizine, a trend was found toward an increase in the incidence of death in the patients who received this antiarrhythmic drug as well.[49] A subsequent meta-analysis of studies of other Vaughan Williams class I agents, including quinidine, procainamide, and disopyramide, found that patients with complex VPDs who received these drugs following myocardial infarction were also at increased risk of death.[50] Therefore, all available evidence shows that patients with complex VPDs following myocardial infarction do not benefit from therapy with antiarrhythmic agents and that many of these drugs increase the risk of death. **❼** *Therefore, asymptomatic VPDs should not be treated.*

Patients with symptomatic VPDs should be treated with β-blockers because the majority of patients with symptomatic VPDs have underlying CAD. β-Blockers have been shown to

Clinical Presentation and Diagnosis of VPDs

- VPDs are usually categorized as simple or complex: simple VPDs are those that occur as infrequent, isolated single abnormal beats; complex VPDs are those that occur more frequently and/or in specific patterns
- Two consecutive VPDs are referred to as a couplet.[47] The term *bigeminy* refers to VPDs occurring with every other beat; *trigeminy* means VPDs occurring with every third beat; *quadrigeminy* means VPDs occurring every fourth

beat.[47] VPDs occurring at a rate of more than 10 per hour or 6 or more per minute are defined as frequent[47]

Symptoms
- Most patients who experience simple or complex VPDs are asymptomatic. Occasionally, patients with complex or frequent VPDs may experience symptoms of palpitations, light-headedness, fatigue, near-syncope, or syncope

reduce mortality in this population and have been shown to be effective for VPD suppression.[51]

▶ Outcome Evaluation

- Monitor patients for relief of symptoms.
- Monitor for adverse effects of β-blockers: reduced heart rate, decreased blood pressure, fatigue, masking of symptoms of hypoglycemia, glucose intolerance (in patients with diabetes), wheezing or shortness of breath (in patients with asthma or chronic obstructive pulmonary disease).

Ventricular Tachycardia

Ventricular tachycardia (VT) is a series of three or more consecutive VPDs at a rate greater than 100 bpm. VT is defined as nonsustained if it lasts less than 30 seconds and terminates spontaneously; sustained VT lasts greater than 30 seconds and does not terminate spontaneously but rather requires therapeutic intervention for termination.

▶ Epidemiology, Etiology, and Pathophysiology

Etiologies of VT are presented in Table 9–12. The incidence of VT is variable, depending on underlying comorbidities. Up to 20% of patients who experience acute myocardial infarction experience ventricular arrhythmias.[52] Approximately 2% to 4% of patients with myocardial infarction develop VT during the period of hospitalization.[51] Nonsustained VT occurs in 34% to 79% of patients with heart failure.[53] Other etiologies of VT include electrolyte abnormalities such as hypokalemia, hypoxia, and some drugs (Table 9–12).

❶ *Ventricular tachycardia is usually initiated by a precisely timed VPD, occurring during the relative refractory period, which provokes reentry within ventricular tissue.*

Sustained VT requires immediate intervention, because if untreated, the rhythm may cause sudden cardiac death via hemodynamic instability and the absence of a pulse (pulseless VT) or via degeneration of VT into VF.

Table 9–12

Etiologies of VT and VF

Coronary artery disease
Myocardial infarction
Heart failure
Electrolyte abnormalities: hypokalemia and hypomagnesemia
Drugs:

Adenosine	Propafenone
Amiodarone	Sotalol
Chlorpromazine	Terbutaline
Digoxin	Thioridazine
Disopyramide	Trazodone
Flecainide	Venlafaxine
Ibutilide	
Procainamide	

VF, ventricular fibrillation; VT, ventricular tachycardia.

Clinical Presentation and Diagnosis of VT

Symptoms

- As with other tachyarrhythmias, symptoms associated with VT depend primarily on heart rate and include palpitations, dizziness, light-headedness, shortness of breath, chest pain (if underlying CAD is present), near-syncope, and syncope
- Patients with nonsustained VT may be asymptomatic if the duration of the arrhythmia is sufficiently short. However, if the rate is sufficiently rapid, patients with nonsustained VT may experience symptoms
- Patients with sustained VT are usually symptomatic, provided that the rate is fast enough to provoke symptoms. Patients with rapid sustained VT may be hemodynamically unstable
- In some patients, sustained VT results in the absence of a pulse or may deteriorate to ventricular fibrillation, resulting in the syndrome of sudden cardiac death

Diagnosis

- Diagnosis of VT requires ECG confirmation of the arrhythmia
- VT is characterized by wide, misshapen QRS complexes, with the rate varying from 140 to 280 bpm
- In most patients with VT, the shape and appearance of the QRS complexes are consistent and similar, referred to as monomorphic VT. However, some patients experience polymorphic VT, in which the shape and appearance of the QRS complexes vary

▶ Treatment

Desired Outcomes The desired outcomes for treatment are to terminate the arrhythmia and restore sinus rhythm, and to prevent sudden cardiac death.

Pharmacologic Therapy Hemodynamically unstable VT should be terminated immediately using synchronized DCC beginning with 100 J (for monophasic shocks) and increasing subsequent shocks to 200, 300, and 360 J.[14] In the event that VT is present but the patient does not have a palpable pulse (and therefore no blood pressure), asynchronous defibrillation should be performed, at 360 J for monophasic waveforms and starting at 120 to 200 J for biphasic waveforms.[14]

Drugs used for the termination of hemodynamically stable VT are presented in Table 9–13. IV drug administration is required. A decision algorithm for management of hemodynamically stable VT is presented in Figure 9–10. The initial choice of drug depends on whether the patient has normal left ventricular function or heart failure due to left ventricular systolic dysfunction. If the patient has normal left ventricular function with no history of heart failure, the drug of choice is procainamide, followed by amiodarone

Table 9–13

Drugs for Termination of VT

Drug	Loading Dose	Maintenance Dose
Procainamide	20–50 mg/min continuous IV infusion until arrhythmia suppressed, hypotension occurs, QRS duration increases greater than 50%, or maximum dose of 17 mg/kg is reached	1–4 mg/min continuous IV infusion
Amiodarone	150 mg IV over 10 minutes. Repeat as needed if VT recurs.	1 mg/min continuous infusion for 6 hours, 0.5 mg/min for 18 hours

VT, ventricular tachycardia.

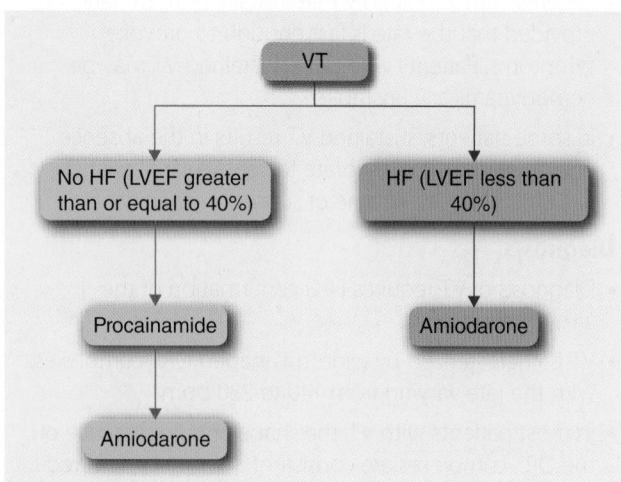

FIGURE 9–10. Decision algorithm for termination of hemodynamically stable ventricular tachycardia. (HF, heart failure; LVEF, left ventricular ejection fraction; VT, ventricular tachycardia; LVEF of 40% can also be expressed as 0.40.)

in refractory cases.[14] However, if the patient has heart failure associated with left ventricular systolic dysfunction, therapy with procainamide should be avoided due to the drug's negative inotropic effects and its propensity to cause hypotension and QT interval prolongation, for which patients with heart failure are at increased risk. Therefore, for patients with hemodynamically stable VT and concomitant heart failure due to left ventricular systolic dysfunction, treatment with IV amiodarone is recommended.[14]

Nonpharmacologic Therapy: Prevention of Sudden Cardiac Death ⑧ *In patients who have experienced VT and are at risk for sudden cardiac death, an implantable cardioverter-defibrillator (ICD) is the treatment of choice.*[54] An ICD is a device that provides internal electrical cardioversion of VT or defibrillation of VF; the ICD does not prevent the patient from developing the arrhythmia, but it reduces the risk that the patient will die of sudden cardiac death as a result of the arrhythmia. Whereas early versions of ICDs required a thoracotomy for implantation, these devices now may be implanted transvenously, similarly to pacemakers, markedly reducing the incidence of complications.

ICDs have been found to be significantly more effective than antiarrhythmic agents such as amiodarone or sotalol for reducing the risk of sudden cardiac death,[55,56] and they are the preferred therapy.[54] However, many patients with ICDs receive concurrent antiarrhythmic drug therapy to reduce the frequency with which patients experience the discomfort of shocks and to prolong battery life of the devices. Combined pharmacotherapy with amiodarone and a β-blocker is more effective than monotherapy with sotalol or β-blockers for reduction in the frequency of ICD shocks.[57]

▶ *Outcome Evaluation*

• Monitor patients for termination of VT and restoration of normal sinus rhythm.

• Monitor patients for adverse effects of antiarrhythmic drugs administered (Table 9–7).

Ventricular Fibrillation

VF is irregular, disorganized, chaotic electrical activity in the ventricles resulting in absence of ventricular depolarizations, and, consequently, lack of pulse, cardiac output, and blood pressure.

▶ *Epidemiology and Etiology*

Approximately 400,000 people die of sudden cardiac death annually in the United States. Although some of these deaths occur as a result of asystole, the majority occur as a result of primary VF or VT that degenerates into VF. Etiologies of VF are presented in Table 9–12 and are similar to those of VT.

▶ *Treatment*

Desired Outcomes The desired outcomes for treatment are to (a) terminate VF, (b) achieve return of spontaneous circulation, and (c) achieve patient survival to hospital admission (in those with out-of-hospital cardiac arrest) and to hospital discharge.

Pharmacologic and Nonpharmacologic Therapy VF is by definition hemodynamically unstable, due to the absence of a pulse and blood pressure. Initial management includes provision of basic life support, including calling for help and initiation of cardiopulmonary resuscitation (CPR).[14] Oxygen should be administered as soon as it is available. Most

Clinical Presentation and Diagnosis of VF

Symptoms

- VF results in immediate loss of pulse and blood pressure. Patients who are in the standing position at the onset of VF suddenly and immediately collapse to the ground

Diagnosis

- The absence of a pulse does not guarantee VF because the pulse may also be absent in patients with asystole, VT, or pulseless electrical activity
- Confirmation of the diagnosis with an ECG is necessary to determine appropriate treatment. ECG reveals no organized, recognizable QRS complexes. If treatment is not initiated within a few minutes, death will occur, or at best, resuscitation of the patient with permanent anoxic brain injury

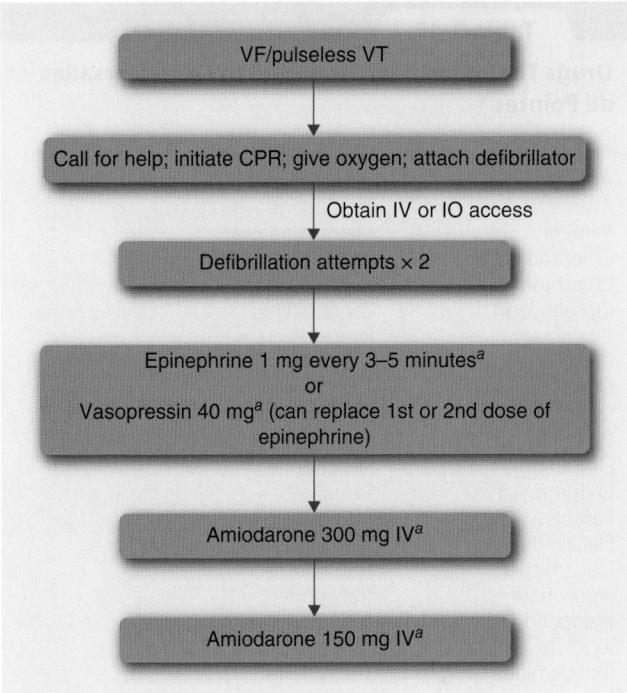

FIGURE 9–11. Decision algorithm for resuscitation of VF or pulseless VT. (CPR, cardiopulmonary resuscitation; IO, intraosseous; VF, ventricular fibrillation; VT, ventricular tachycardia). [a]Defibrillation attempt should be made after every dose of drug.

importantly, defibrillation should be performed as soon as possible. It is critically important to understand that the only means of successfully terminating VF and restoring sinus rhythm is electrical defibrillation. Defibrillation should be attempted using 360 J for monophasic defibrillators, and 120 to 200 J for biphasic shocks, after which CPR should be resumed immediately while the defibrillator charges; if the first shock was unsuccessful, subsequent defibrillation attempts should be performed at equivalent or higher energy doses.[14]

If VF persists following two defibrillation shocks, drug therapy may be administered. ⑨ *The purpose of drug administration for treatment of VF is to facilitate successful defibrillation. Drug therapy alone will not result in termination of VF.* Drugs used for facilitation of defibrillation in patients with VF are listed in **Table 9–14**. Drug administration should occur during CPR, before or after delivery of a defibrillation shock. The vasopressor agents epinephrine or vasopressin are administered initially because it has been shown that a critical factor in successful defibrillation is maintenance of coronary perfusion pressure, which is achieved via the vasoconstricting effects of these drugs. A decision algorithm for the treatment of VF is presented in **Figure 9–11**. Epinephrine and vasopressin are equally effective for facilitation of defibrillation leading

to survival to hospital admission in patients with out-of-hospital cardiac arrest due to VF. Amiodarone is effective for facilitation of defibrillation leading to survival to hospital admission in patients with VF.[58] Note that the amiodarone doses recommended for administration during a resuscitation attempt for VF (Table 9–14) are different than those recommended for administration for termination of VT (Table 9–13).

▶ *Outcome Evaluation*

- Monitor the patient for return of pulse and blood pressure, and for termination of VF and restoration of normal sinus rhythm.
- After successful resuscitation, monitor the patient for adverse effects of drugs administered (Table 9–7).

Torsades de Pointes

Torsades de pointes is a specific polymorphic VT associated with prolongation of the QT interval in the sinus beats that precede the arrhythmia.[59]

▶ *Epidemiology and Etiology*

The incidence of torsades de pointes in the population at large is unknown. The incidence of torsades de pointes associated with specific drugs ranges from less than 1% to as high as 8% to 10%, depending on dose and plasma

---

Table 9–14

Drugs for Facilitation of Defibrillation in Patients with VF

Drug	Dose
Epinephrine	1 mg IV every 3–5 minutes
Vasopressin	40 units IV single dose
Amiodarone	300 mg IV diluted in 20–30 mL D₅W. One subsequent dose of 150 mg IV may be administered

D₅W, 5% dextrose in water; VF, ventricular fibrillation.

Table 9–15

Drugs That Have Been Reported to Cause Torsades de Pointes[59]

Amiodarone	Levofloxacin
Amitriptyline	Levomethadyl
Arsenic	Methadone
Bepridil	Metoclopramide
Chloroquine	Moxifloxacin
Chlorpromazine	Ondansetron
Ciprofloxacin	Pentamidine
Citalopram	Pimozide
Clarithromycin	Procainamide
Disopyramide	Propafenone
Dofetilide	Quetiapine
Doxepin	Quinidine
Droperidol	Risperidone
Erythromycin	Sertraline
Famotidine	Sotalol
Flecainide	Tacrolimus
Fluconazole	Thioridazine
Fluoxetine	Trazodone
Haloperidol	Trimethoprim-sulfamethoxazole
Ibutilide	Voriconazole
Indapamide	Ziprasidone
Ketoconazole	

Table 9–16

Risk Factors for Drug-Induced Torsades de Pointes[59]

QT_c interval greater than 500 ms
Increase in QT_c interval by more than 60 ms compared with the pretreatment value
Female sex
Age greater than 65 years
Heart failure
Electrolyte abnormalities: hypokalemia, hypomagnesemia, hypocalcemia
Bradycardia
Elevated plasma concentrations of QT interval-prolonging drugs due to drug interactions or absence of dose adjustment for organ dysfunction
Rapid IV infusion of torsades-inducing drugs
Concomitant administration of more than one agent known to cause QT interval prolongation/torsades de pointes
Genetic predisposition
Previous history of drug-induced torsades de pointes

QT_c, corrected QT interval.

---

concentration of the drug and the presence of other risk factors for the arrhythmia.

Torsades de pointes may be inherited or acquired. Patients with specific genetic mutations may have an inherited long QT syndrome, in which the QT interval is prolonged, and these patients are at risk for torsades de pointes. Acquired torsades de pointes may be caused by numerous drugs (Table 9–15); the list of drugs known to cause torsades de pointes continues to expand.

▶ Pathophysiology

Torsades de pointes is caused by circumstances, often drugs, that lead to prolongation in the repolarization phase of the ventricular action potential (Fig. 9–2) manifested on the ECG by prolongation of the QT interval. Prolongation of ventricular repolarization occurs via inhibition of efflux of potassium through potassium channels; therefore, drugs that inhibit conductance through potassium channels may cause QT interval prolongation and torsades de pointes. ❶ *Prolongation of ventricular repolarization likely promotes the development of early ventricular afterdepolarizations during the relative refractory period, which may provoke reentry leading to torsades de pointes.*

❿ *Drug-induced torsades de pointes rarely occurs in patients without specific risk factors for the arrhythmia (Table 9–16). In* most cases, administration of a drug known to cause torsades de pointes is unlikely to cause the arrhythmia; however, the likelihood of the arrhythmia increases markedly in patients with concomitant risk factors.

The onset of torsades de pointes associated with oral drug therapy is somewhat variable and in some cases may be delayed; often, a patient can be taking a drug known to cause torsades de pointes for months or longer without problem until another risk factor for the arrhythmia becomes present, which then may trigger the arrhythmia.

In some patients, torsades de pointes may be of short duration and may terminate spontaneously. However, torsades de pointes may not terminate on its own, and if left untreated, it may degenerate into VF and result in sudden cardiac death.[59] Several drugs, including terfenadine, astemizole, and cisapride, have been withdrawn from the U.S. market as a result of causing deaths due to torsades de pointes.

▶ Treatment

Desired Outcomes The desired outcomes for treatment include (a) prevention of torsades de pointes, (b) termination of torsades de pointes, (c) prevention of recurrence, and (d) prevention of sudden cardiac death.

Pharmacologic and Nonpharmacologic Therapy ❿ *In patients with risk factors for torsades de pointes, drugs with the potential to cause QT interval prolongation and torsades de pointes should be avoided or used with extreme caution, and diligent QT interval monitoring should be performed.*

Management of drug-induced torsades de pointes includes discontinuation of the potentially causative agent. Patients with hemodynamically unstable torsades de pointes should undergo immediate synchronized DCC. In patients with hemodynamically stable torsades de pointes, electrolyte abnormalities such as hypokalemia, hypomagnesemia, or hypocalcemia should be corrected. Hemodynamically stable torsades de pointes is often treated with IV magnesium, irrespective of whether the patient is hypomagnesemic; magnesium has been shown to terminate torsades de pointes in normomagnesemic patients.[14] Magnesium may be administered IV in doses of 1 to 2 g, diluted in 50 to

Clinical Presentation and Diagnosis of Torsades de Pointes

Symptoms

- As with other tachyarrhythmias, symptoms associated with torsades de pointes depend primarily on heart rate and arrhythmia duration, and they include palpitations, dizziness, light-headedness, shortness of breath, chest pain (if underlying CAD is present), near-syncope, and syncope
- Torsades de pointes may be hemodynamically unstable if the rate is sufficiently rapid
- Like sustained monomorphic VT, torsades de pointes may result in the absence of a pulse or may rapidly degenerate into VF, resulting in the syndrome of sudden cardiac death

Diagnosis

- Diagnosis of torsades de pointes requires examination of the arrhythmia on ECG
- Torsades de pointes, or "twisting of the points," appears on ECG as apparent twisting of the wide QRS complexes around the isoelectric baseline
- The arrhythmia is associated with heart rates from 140 to 280 bpm
- Characteristic feature: a "long-short" initiating sequence that occurs as a result of a ventricular premature beat followed by a compensatory pause followed by the first beat of the torsades de pointes
- Episodes of torsades de pointes may self-terminate, with frequent recurrence

100 mL 5% dextrose in water (D_5W), administered over 5 to 10 minutes; doses may be repeated to a total of 12 g.

Alternatively, a continuous magnesium infusion may be initiated after the first bolus, at a rate of 0.5 to 1 g/h. Alternative treatments include transvenous insertion of a temporary pacemaker for overdrive pacing, which shortens the QT interval and may terminate torsades de pointes and reduce the risk of recurrence; or IV isoproterenol 2 to 10 mcg/min, to increase the heart rate and shorten the QT interval.

▶ Outcome Evaluation

- Monitor vital signs (heart rate and blood pressure).
- Monitor the ECG to determine the QT_c interval (maintain less than 470 ms in males and 480 ms in females)[60] and for the presence of torsades de pointes.
- Monitor serum potassium, magnesium, and calcium concentrations.
- Monitor for symptoms of tachycardia.

Patient Care and Monitoring

1. Perform a thorough medication history to determine whether the patient is receiving any prescription or nonprescription drugs that may cause or contribute to the development of an arrhythmia.

2. Evaluate the patient for the presence of drug-induced diseases, drug allergies, and drug interactions.

3. Determine and monitor the patient's serum electrolyte concentrations to determine the presence or absence of hypokalemia, hyperkalemia, hypomagnesemia, hypermagnesemia, or hypocalcemia.

4. Consider the patient's heart rate, blood pressure, and symptoms to determine whether he or she is hemodynamically stable or unstable.

5. Monitor the patient's 12-lead ECG or single rhythm strips to determine if an arrhythmia is present and to identify the specific arrhythmia, and evaluate and monitor the patient's symptoms.

6. Develop drug therapy treatment plans for management of the specific arrhythmia that the patient is experiencing: sinus bradycardia, AV nodal blockade, AF, PSVT, VPDs, VT (including torsades de pointes), or VF.

7. Develop specific drug therapy monitoring plans for the treatment plan implemented. Monitoring includes assessment of symptoms, ECG, adverse effects of drugs, and potential drug interactions.

8. In those receiving warfarin for AF, determine whether the patient's INR is therapeutic.

9. Provide information regarding safe and effective oral anticoagulation therapy:
   - Notify appropriate clinicians in the event of severe bruising, blood in urine or stool, or frequent nosebleeds.
   - Avoid radical changes in diet.
   - Avoid alcohol.
   - Do not take nonprescription medications or herbal/alternative/complementary medicines without notifying your physician, pharmacist, and/or healthcare team members.

10. Stress the importance of adherence to the therapeutic regimen.

11. Provide patient education regarding disease state and drug therapy.

Abbreviations Introduced in This Chapter

AF	Atrial fibrillation
ATPase	Adenosine triphosphatase
AV	Atrioventricular
bpm	Beats per minute
Ca	Calcium
CAD	Coronary artery disease
CAST	Cardiac Arrhythmia Suppression Trial
CCB	Calcium channel blocker
CPR	Cardiopulmonary resuscitation
DCC	Direct current cardioversion
D_5W	5% Dextrose in water
ECG	Electrocardiogram
ED	Emergency department
HF	Heart failure
ICD	Implantable cardioverter-defibrillator
INR	International normalized ratio
IO	Intraosseous
J	Joule
K	Potassium
LV	Left ventricular
LVEF	Left ventricular ejection fraction
LVH	Left ventricular hypertrophy
Na	Sodium
NYHA	New York Heart Association
PSVT	Paroxysmal supraventricular tachycardia
PTT	Partial thromboplastin time
PVC	Premature ventricular contraction
QT_c	Corrected QT interval
SA	Sinoatrial
TEE	Transesophageal echocardiogram
TIA	Transient ischemic attack
VPB	Ventricular premature beat
VPC	Ventricular premature contraction
VPD	Ventricular premature depolarization
VF	Ventricular fibrillation
VT	Ventricular tachycardia

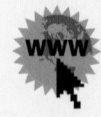 Self-assessment questions and answers are available at *http://www.mhpharmacotherapy.com/pp.html*.

REFERENCES

1. Cummins RO, ed. ACLS provider manual. Dallas, TX: American Heart Association, 2006.
2. Bazett HC. An analysis of time relationships of the electrocardiogram. Heart 1920;7:353–370.
3. Drew BJ, Ackerman MJ, Funk M, et al, on behalf of the American Heart Association Acute Cardiac Care Committee of the Council on Clinical Cardiology, the Council on Cardiovascular Nursing, and the American College of Cardiology Foundation. Prevention of torsades de pointes in hospital settings: A scientific statement from the American Heart Association and the American College of Cardiology Foundation. Circulation 2010;121:1047–1060.
4. Fogoros RN. Electrophysiologic testing, 4th ed. Malden, MA: Blackwell, 2006:17.
5. Vaughan Williams EM. Classification of anti-arrhythmic drugs. In: Sandoe E, Flensted-Jansen E, Olesen KH, eds. Symposium on Cardiac Arrhythmias. Sodertalje, Sweden: AB Astra, 1970:449–472.
6. Singh BN, Vaughan Williams EM. A third class of anti-arrhythmic action. Effects on atrial and ventricular intracellular potentials, and other pharmacological actions on cardiac muscle, of MJ 1999 and AH 3474. Br J Pharmacol 1970;39:675–687.
7. Singh BN, Vaughan Williams EM. A fourth class of anti-arrhythmic action? Effect of verapamil on ouabain toxicity, on atrial and ventricular intracellular potentials, and on other features of cardiac function. Cardiovasc Res 1972;6:109–119.
8. Snyders J, Knoth KM, Roberds SL, Tamkun MM. Time-, voltage-, and state-dependent block by quinidine of a cloned human cardiac potassium channel. Mol Pharmacol 1992;41:322–330.
9. Coraboeuf E, Deroubaix E, Escande D, Coulombe A. Comparative effects of three class I antiarrhythmic drugs on plateau and pacemaker currents of sheep cardiac Purkinje fibres. Cardiovasc Res 1988;22:375–384.
10. Komeichi K, Tohse N, Nakaya H, et al. Effects of N-acetylprocainamide and sotalol on ion currents in isolated guinea-pig ventricular myocytes. Eur J Pharmacol 1990;187:313–322.
11. Task Force of the Working Group on Arrhythmias of the European Society of Cardiology. The Sicilian gambit: A new approach to the classification of antiarrhythmic drugs based on their actions on arrhythmogenic mechanisms. Circulation 1991;84:1831–1851.
12. Mangrum JM, DiMarco JP. The evaluation and management of bradycardia. N Engl J Med 2000;342:703–709.
13. Tisdale JE. Supraventricular arrhythmias. In: Tisdale JE, Miller DA, eds. Drug-Induced Diseases: Prevention, Detection and Management, 2nd ed. Bethesda, MD: American Society of Health-System Pharmacists, 2010:445–484.
14. Neumar RW, Otto CW, Link MS, et al. Part 8: Adult advanced cardiovascular life support: 2010 American Heart Association Guidelines for Cardiopulmonary Resuscitation and Emergency Cardiovascular Care. Circulation 2010;122(Suppl 3):S729–S767.
15. Ufberg JW, Clark JS. Bradydysrhythmias and atrioventricular conduction blocks. Emerg Med Clin North Am 2006;24:1–9.
16. Kannel WB, Wolf PA, Benjamin EJ, Levy D. Prevalence, incidence, prognosis, and predisposing conditions for atrial fibrillation: Population-based estimates. Am J Cardiol 1998; 82:2N–9N.
17. Torp-Pedersen C, Moller M, Bloch-Thomsen PE, et al., for the Danish Investigations of Arrhythmia and Mortality on Dofetilide Study Group. Dofetilide in patients with congestive heart failure and left ventricular dysfunction. Danish Investigations of Arrhythmia and Mortality on Dofetilide Study Group. N Engl J Med 1999;341:857–865.
18. Maisel WH, Stevenson LW. Atrial fibrillation heart failure: Epidemiology, pathophysiology, and rationale for therapy. Am J Cardiol 2003;91:2D–8D.
19. Rich EC, Siebold C, Campion B. Alcohol-related acute atrial fibrillation. A case-control study and review of 40 patients. Arch Intern Med 1985;145:830–833.
20. Black DM, Delmas PD, Eastell R, et al. Once-yearly zoledronic acid for treatment of postmenopausal osteoporosis. N Engl J Med 2007;356:1809–1822.
21. Heckbert SR, Li G, Cummings SR, et al. Use of alendronate and risk of incident atrial fibrillation in women. Arch Intern Med 2008;168:826–831.
22. Haissaguerre M, Jais P, Shah DC, et al. Spontaneous initiation of atrial fibrillation by ectopic beats originating in the pulmonary veins. N Engl J Med 1998;339(10):659–666.
23. Cohen M, Naccarelli GV. Pathophysiology and disease progression of atrial fibrillation: Importance of achieving and maintaining sinus rhythm. J Cardiovasc Electrophysiol 2008;19:885–890.
24. Wijffels MC, Kirchhof CJ, Dorland R, Allessie MA. Atrial fibrillation begets atrial fibrillation. A study in awake chronically instrumented goats. Circulation 1995;92:1954–1968.

25. Fuster V, Rydén LE, Cannom DS, et al. 2011 ACCF/AHA/HRS focused updates incorporated into the ACC/AHA/ESC 2006 guidelines for the management of patients with atrial fibrillation: A report of the American College of Cardiology Foundation/American Heart Association Task Force on Practice Guidelines and the European Society of Cardiology Committee for Practice Guidelines. J Am Coll Cardiol 2011;57:e101–198.

26. Krahn AD, Manfreda J, Tate RB, et al. The natural history of atrial fibrillation: Incidence, risk factors, and prognosis in the Manitoba Follow-Up Study. Am J Med 1995;98:476–484.

27. Wann LS, Curtis AB, January CT, et al., writing on behalf of the 2006 ACC/AHA/ESC Guidelines for the Management of Patients with Atrial Fibrillation Writing Committee. 2011 ACCF/AHA/HRS focused update on the management of patients with atrial fibrillation (updating the 2006 guideline): A report of the American College of Cardiology Foundation/American Heart Association Task Force on Practice Guidelines. Circulation 2011;123:104–123.

28. Elkayam U, Shotan A, Mehra A, Ostrzega E. Calcium channel blockers in heart failure. J Am Coll Cardiol 1993;22(4 Suppl A):139A–144A.

29. You JJ, Singer DE, Howard PA, et al. Antithrombotic therapy for atrial fibrillation. Antithrombotic therapy and prevention of thrombosis, 9th ed: American College of Chest Physicians evidence-based clinical practice guidelines. Chest 2012;14(Suppl):e531S–e575S.

30. The Atrial Fibrillation Follow-up Investigation of Rhythm Management (AFFIRM) Investigators. A comparison of rate control and rhythm control in patients with atrial fibrillation. N Engl J Med 2002;347:1825–1833.

31. Van Gelder IC, Hagens VE, Bosker HA, et al., for the Rate Control versus Electrical Cardioversion for Persistent Atrial Fibrillation Study Group. A comparison of rate control and rhythm control in patients with recurrent persistent atrial fibrillation. N Engl J Med 2002;347:1834–1840.

32. Carlsson J, Miketic S, Windeler J, et al. Randomized trial of rate-control versus rhythm-control in persistent atrial fibrillation: The Strategies of Treatment of Atrial Fibrillation (STAF) study. J Am Coll Cardiol 2003;41:1690–1696.

33. Opolski G, Torbicki A, Kosior D, et al. Rhythm control versus rate control in patients with persistent atrial fibrillation. Results of the HOT CAFE Polish Study. Kardiol Pol 2003;59:1–16.

34. Roy D, Talajic M, Nattel S, et al. Rhythm control versus rate control for atrial fibrillation and heart failure. N Engl J Med 2008;358:2667–2677.

35. Gage BF, Waterman AD, Shannon W, Boechler M, Rich MW, Radford MJ. Validation of clinical classification schemes for predicting stroke: Results from the National Registry of Atrial Fibrillation. JAMA 2001;285:2864–2870.

36. Wann LS, Curtis AB, Ellenbogen KA, et al., writing on behalf of the 2006 ACC/AHA/ESC Guidelines for the Management of Patients with Atrial Fibrillation Writing Committee. 2011 ACCF/AHA/HRS focused update on the management of patients with atrial fibrillation (update on dabigatran): A report of the American College of Cardiology Foundation/American Heart Association Task Force on Practice Guidelines. J Am Coll Cardiol 2011;57:1330–1337.

37. Hankey GJ, Eikelboom JW. Dabigatran etexilate. A new oral thrombin inhibitor. Circulation 2011;123:1436–1450.

38. Johnson JA, Whirl-Carrilo M, Gage BF, et al. Clinical pharmacogenetics implementation consortium guidelines for CYP2C9 and VKORC1 genotypes and warfarin dosing. Clin Pharmacol Ther 2011;90:625–629.

39. Gage BF, Johnson JA, Deych E, et al. Use of pharmacogenetics and clinical factors to predict the therapeutic dose of warfarin. Clin Pharmacol Ther 2008;84:326–331.

40. International Warfarin Pharmacogenetics Consortium, Klein TE, Altman RB, Eriksson N, et al. Estimation of warfarin dose with clinical and pharmacogenetics data. N Engl J Med 2009;360:753–764.

41. Patel MR, Mahaffey KW, Garg J, et al. Rivaroxaban versus warfarin in nonvalvular atrial fibrillation. N Engl J Med 2011;365:883–891.

42. Granger CB, Alexander JH, McMurray JJV, et al., for the ARISTOTLE committee and investigators. Apixaban versus warfarin in patients with atrial fibrillation. N Engl J Med 2011;365:981–992.

43. Ganz LI, Friedman PL. Supraventricular tachycardia. N Engl J Med 1995;332:162–173.

44. Blomstrom-Lundqvist C, Scheinman MM, Aliot EM, et al., for the Writing Committee to Develop Guidelines for the Management of Patients with Supraventricular Arrhythmias. ACC/AHA/ESC guidelines for the management of patients with supraventricular arrhythmias—Executive summary: A report of the American College of Cardiology/American Heart Association Task Force on practice guidelines and the European Society of Cardiology Committee for Practice Guidelines (Writing Committee to Develop Guidelines for the Management of Patients with Supraventricular Arrhythmias). J Am Coll Cardiol 2003;42:1493–1531.

45. Bikkina M, Larson MG, Levy D. Prognostic implications of asymptomatic ventricular arrhythmias: The Framingham Heart Study. Am J Cardiol 1994;74:232–235.

46. Lown B, Wolf M. Approaches to sudden death from coronary heart disease. Circulation 1971;44:130–144.

47. Ruberman W, Weinblatt E, Goldberg JD, et al. Ventricular premature beats and mortality after myocardial infarction. N Engl J Med 1977;297:750–757.

48. Echt DS, Liebson PR, Mitchell LB, et al. Mortality and morbidity in patients receiving encainide, flecainide, or placebo. The Cardiac Arrhythmia Suppression Trial. N Engl J Med 1991;324:781–788.

49. The Cardiac Arrhythmia Suppression Trial II Investigators. Effect of the antiarrhythmic agent moricizine on survival after myocardial infarction. N Engl J Med 1992;327:227–233.

50. Teo KK, Yusuf S, Furberg CD. Effects of prophylactic antiarrhythmic drug therapy in acute myocardial infarction. An overview of results from randomized controlled trials. JAMA 1993;270:1589–1595.

51. Chandraratna PA. Comparison of acebutolol with propranolol, quinidine, and placebo: Results of three multicenter arrhythmia trials. Am Heart J 1985;109:1198–1204.

52. Al-Khatib SM, Stebbins AL, Califf RM, et al. Sustained ventricular arrhythmias and mortality among patients with acute myocardial infarction: Results from the GUSTO-III trial. Am Heart J 2003;145:515–521.

53. Stevenson WG, Ellison KE, Sweeney MO, et al. Management of arrhythmias in heart failure. Cardiol Rev 2002;10:8–14.

54. Epstein AE, DiMarco JP, Ellenbogen KA, et al. ACC/AHA/HRS 2008 Guidelines for Device-Based Therapy of Cardiac Rhythm Abnormalities: Executive summary: A report of the American College of Cardiology/American Heart Association Task Force on Practice Guidelines (Writing Committee to Revise the ACC/AHA/NASPE 2002 Guideline Update for Implantation of Cardiac Pacemakers and Antiarrhythmia Devices). Circulation 2008;117:2820–2840.

55. The Antiarrhythmics versus Implantable Defibrillators (AVID) Investigators. A comparison of antiarrhythmic-drug therapy with implantable defibrillators in patients resuscitated from near-fatal ventricular arrhythmias. N Engl J Med 1997;337:1576–1583.

56. Connolly SJ, Gent M, Roberts RS, et al. Canadian implantable defibrillator study (CIDS): A randomized trial of the implantable cardioverter defibrillator against amiodarone. Circulation 2000;101:1297–1302.

57. Connolly SJ, Dorian P, Roberts RS, et al. Comparison of β-blockers, amiodarone plus β-blockers, or sotalol for prevention of shocks from implantable cardioverter-defibrillators. The OPTIC study: A randomized trial. JAMA 2006;295:165–171.

58. Dorian P, Cass D, Schwartz B, et al. Amiodarone as compared with lidocaine for shock-resistant ventricular fibrillation. N Engl J Med 2002;346:884–890.

59. Tisdale JE. Ventricular arrhythmias. In: Tisdale JE, Miller DA, eds. Drug-Induced Diseases: Prevention, Detection and Management, 2nd ed. Bethesda, MD: American Society of Health-System Pharmacists, 2010:485–515.

60. Drew BJ, Ackerman MJ, Funk M, et al., on behalf of the American Heart Association Acute Cardiac Care Committee of the Council on Clinical Cardiology, the Council on Cardiovascular Nursing, and the American College of Cardiology Foundation. Prevention of torsade de pointes in hospital settings: A scientific statement from the American Heart Association and the American College of Cardiology Foundation. Circulation 2010;121:1047–1060.

10 Venous Thromboembolism

Edith A. Nutescu, Stuart T. Haines, and Ann K. Wittkowsky

LEARNING OBJECTIVES

● **Upon completion of the chapter, the reader will be able to:**

1. Identify risk factors and signs and symptoms of deep vein thrombosis (DVT) and pulmonary embolism (PE).

2. Describe the processes of hemostasis and thrombosis, including the role of the vascular endothelium, platelets, coagulation cascade, and thrombolytic proteins.

3. Determine a patient's relative risk (low, moderate, or high) of developing venous thrombosis.

4. Formulate an appropriate prevention strategy for a patient at risk for DVT.

5. State at least two potential advantages of newer anticoagulants (i.e., low molecular weight heparins, fondaparinux, oral direct thrombin inhibitors, and oral direct factor Xa inhibitors) over traditional anticoagulants (i.e., unfractionated heparin and warfarin).

6. Select and interpret laboratory test(s) to monitor antithrombotic drugs.

7. Identify factors that place a patient at high risk of bleeding while receiving antithrombotic drugs.

8. Manage a patient with an elevated international normalized ratio (INR) with or without bleeding.

9. Identify warfarin drug–drug and drug–food interactions.

10. Formulate an appropriate treatment plan for a patient who develops a DVT or PE, and develop a comprehensive education plan for a patient who is receiving an antithrombotic drug.

KEY CONCEPTS

❶ Antithrombotic therapies (thrombolytics and anticoagulants) require precise dosing and meticulous monitoring, as well as ongoing patient education. Well-organized anticoagulation management services improve the quality of patient care and reduce the overall cost.

❷ The risk of venous thromboembolism (VTE) is related to several identifiable factors including age, prior history of VTE, major surgery (particularly orthopedic procedures of the lower extremities), trauma, malignancy, pregnancy, estrogen use, and hypercoagulable states. These risks are additive.

❸ The symptoms of DVT or PE are nonspecific, and it is extremely difficult to distinguish VTE from other disorders on clinical signs alone. Therefore, objective tests are required to confirm or exclude the diagnosis.

❹ At the time of hospital admission, all patients should be evaluated for their risk of VTE, and strategies to prevent VTE appropriate for each patient's level of risk should

be routinely used. Prophylaxis should be continued throughout the period of risk.

❺ In the absence of contraindications, the treatment of VTE should initially include a rapid-acting anticoagulant (e.g., unfractionated heparin [UFH], low molecular weight heparin [LMWH], or fondaparinux) overlapped with warfarin for at least 5 days and until the patient's international normalized ratio (INR) is greater than 2 and stable. Anticoagulation therapy should be continued for a minimum of 3 months. However, the duration of anticoagulation therapy should be based on the patient's risk of VTE recurrence and major bleeding.

❻ Due to significant variability in interpatient response and changes in patient response over time, UFH requires close monitoring and periodic dose adjustment.

❼ Bleeding is the most common adverse effect associated with antithrombotic drugs. A patient's risk of major hemorrhage is related to the intensity and stability of therapy, age, concurrent drug use, history of GI bleeding, risk of falls or trauma, and recent surgery.

❽ Most patients with an uncomplicated deep vein thrombosis (DVT) can be managed safely at home.

❾ Warfarin has been the primary oral anticoagulant used in the United States for the past 60 years. Warfarin is the anticoagulant of choice when long-term or extended anticoagulation is required.

❿ Warfarin requires frequent laboratory monitoring to ensure optimal outcomes and minimize complications. Additionally, warfarin is prone to numerous clinically important drug–drug and drug–food interactions.

INTRODUCTION

Venous thromboembolism (VTE) is one of the most common cardiovascular disorders in the United States. VTE is manifested as deep vein thrombosis (DVT) and pulmonary embolism (PE) resulting from thrombus formation in the venous circulation (Fig. 10–1).[1] It is often provoked by prolonged immobility and vascular injury and most frequently seen in patients who have been hospitalized for a serious medical illness, trauma, or major surgery. VTE can also occur with little or no provocation in patients who have an underlying hypercoagulable disorder.

Although VTE may initially cause few or no symptoms, the first overt manifestation of the disease may be sudden death from PE, which can occur within minutes, before effective treatment can be given.[2] In addition to the symptoms produced by the acute event, there are long-term sequelae of VTE that can cause long-term pain and suffering. A history of VTE is a significant risk factor for recurrent thromboembolic events. The postthrombotic syndrome (PTS) is a complication of VTE that occurs due to damage to the vein caused by a blood clot and leads to development of symptomatic venous insufficiency such as chronic lower extremity swelling, pain, tenderness, skin discoloration, and ulceration.

The treatment of VTE is fraught with substantial risks.[3] ❶ *Antithrombotic therapies (thrombolytics and anticoagulants) require precise dosing and meticulous monitoring, as well as ongoing patient education.*[4,5] *Well-organized anticoagulation management services improve the quality of patient care and reduce the overall cost.* A systematic approach to drug therapy management substantially reduces these risks, but bleeding remains a common and serious complication.[5] Therefore, preventing VTE is paramount to improving outcomes. When VTE is suspected, a rapid and accurate diagnosis is critical to making appropriate treatment decisions. The optimal use of antithrombotic drugs requires not only an in-depth knowledge

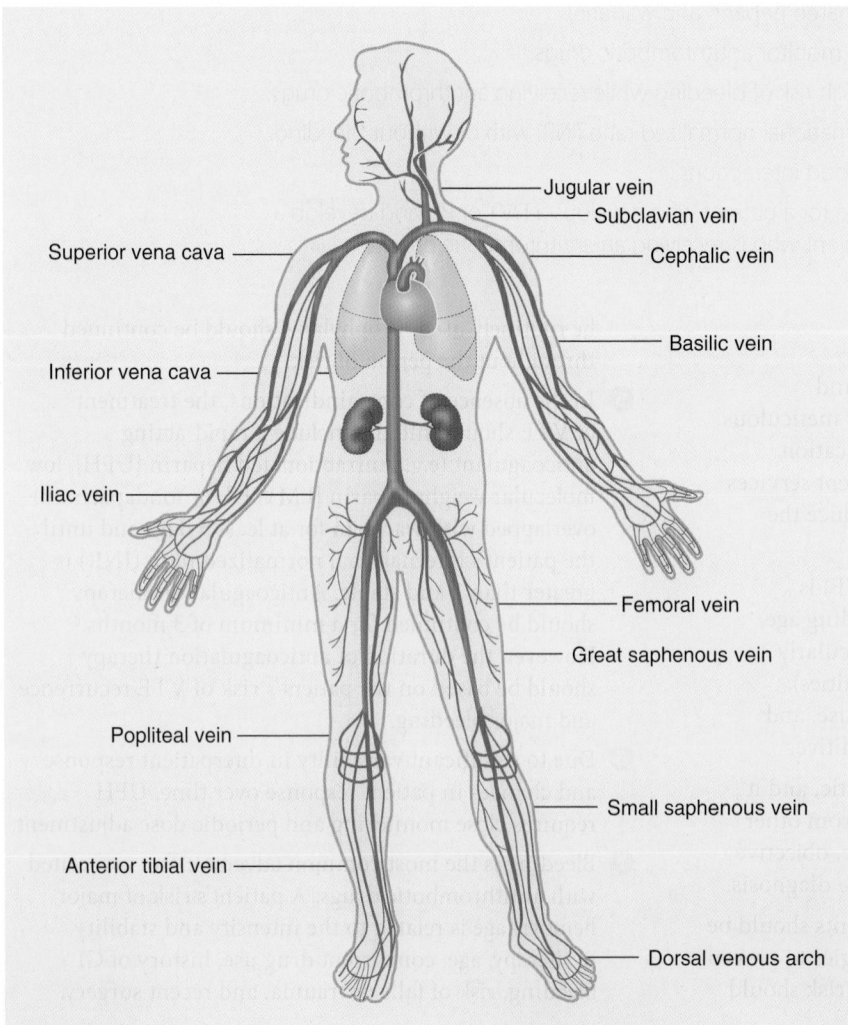

FIGURE 10–1. Venous circulation. (From Witt DM, Nutescu EA, Haines S. Venous thromboembolism. In: DiPiro JT, Talbert RL, Yee GC, et al., eds. Pharmacotherapy: A Pathophysiologic Approach, 8th ed. New York, NY: McGraw-Hill, 2011:312.)

of their pharmacology and pharmacokinetic properties but also a comprehensive approach to patient management.[6]

EPIDEMIOLOGY AND ETIOLOGY

The true incidence of VTE in the general population is unknown because many patients, perhaps more than 50%, have no overt symptoms or go undiagnosed.[7] An estimated 2 million people in the United States develop VTE each year, of whom 600,000 are hospitalized and 60,000 die. The estimated annual direct medical costs of managing the disease are well over $1 billion. The incidence of VTE nearly doubles in each decade of life over the age of 50 and is slightly higher in men. As the population ages, the total number of cases of DVT and PE continues to rise.[2]

❷ *The risk of VTE is related to several factors including age, prior history of VTE, major surgery (particularly orthopedic procedures of the lower extremities), trauma, malignancy, pregnancy, estrogen use, and hypercoagulable states* (Table 10–1).[2] VTE risk factors can be categorized in one of the three elements of Virchow's triad: stasis in blood flow, vascular endothelial injury, and inherited or acquired changes in blood constituents resulting in hypercoagulation states. These risk factors are additive, and some can be easily identified in clinical practice. A prior history of venous **thrombosis** is perhaps the strongest risk factor for recurrent VTE, presumably because of damage to venous valves and obstruction of blood flow caused by the initial event. Rapid blood flow has an inhibitory effect on thrombus formation, but a slow rate of flow reduces the clearance of activated clotting factors in the zone of injury and slows the influx of regulatory substances. Stasis tips the delicate balance of procoagulation and anticoagulation in favor of **thrombogenesis**. The rate of blood flow in the venous circulation, particularly in the deep veins of the lower extremities, is relatively slow. Valves in the deep veins of the legs, as well as contraction of the calf and thigh muscles, facilitate the flow of blood back to the heart and lungs. Damage to the venous valves and periods of prolonged immobility result in venous stasis. Vessel obstruction, either from a thrombus or external compression, promotes clot propagation. Numerous medical conditions and surgical procedures are associated with reduced venous blood flow and increase the risk of VTE. Greater than normal blood viscosity, seen in myeloproliferative disorders like polycythemia vera for example, may also contribute to slowed blood flow and thrombus formation.

A growing list of hereditary deficiencies, gene mutations, and acquired diseases have been linked to hypercoagulability (Table 10–1).[8] Activated protein C resistance is the most common genetic disorder leading to hypercoagulability, found in nearly 5% of individuals of northern European descent and in as many as 40% of those who experience an idiopathic DVT. Although these patients have normal plasma concentrations of protein C, they have a mutation on factor V that renders it resistant to degradation by

Table 10–1	
Risk Factors for VTE	
Risk Factor	**Example**
Age	Risk doubles with each decade after age 50
Prior history of VTE	Strongest known risk factor for DVT and PE
Venous stasis	Major medical illness (e.g., congestive heart failure)
	Major surgery (e.g., general anesthesia for greater than 30 minutes)
	Paralysis (e.g., due to stroke or spinal cord injury)
	Polycythemia vera
	Obesity
	Varicose veins
	Immobility (e.g., bedrest during hospital admission)
Vascular injury	Major orthopedic surgery (e.g., knee and hip replacement)
	Trauma (especially fractures of the pelvis, hip, or leg)
	Indwelling venous catheters
Hypercoagulable states	Malignancy, diagnosed or occult
	Activated protein C resistance/factor V Leiden
	Prothrombin (20210A) gene mutation
	Protein C deficiency
	Protein S deficiency
	AT deficiency
	Factor VIII excess (greater than 90th percentile)
	Factor XI excess (greater than 90th percentile)
	Antiphospholipid antibodies
	Dysfibrinogenemia
	PAI-I excess
	Pregnancy/postpartum
Drug therapy	Estrogen-containing oral contraceptive pills
	Estrogen replacement therapy
	SERMs
	HIT
	Chemotherapy

AT, antithrombin; DVT, deep vein thrombosis; HIT, heparin-induced thrombocytopenia; PAI-I, plasminogen activator inhibitor; PE, pulmonary embolism; SERMs, selective estrogen receptor modulators; VTE, venous thromboembolism.

activated protein C. This mutation is known as factor V Leiden, named after the city of Leiden, Holland, where the defect was initially reported. The prothrombin gene 20210A mutation is also a relatively common defect, occurring in as many as 3% of healthy individuals of southern European descent and 16% of those with an idiopathic DVT. Although less common, inherited deficiencies of the natural **anticoagulants** protein C, protein S, and antithrombin (AT) place patients at a high lifetime risk for VTE. Conversely, high concentrations of factors VIII, IX, and XI also increase the risk of VTE. Some patients have multiple genetic defects.

Acquired disorders of hypercoagulability include malignancy, antiphospholipid antibodies, estrogen use, and pregnancy.[2] The strong link between cancer and thrombosis has been recognized since the late 1800s.[9] Tumor cells secrete a number of procoagulant substances that activate the clotting cascade. Furthermore, patients with cancer often have suppressed levels of protein C, protein S, and AT. Antiphospholipid antibodies, commonly found in patients with autoimmune disorders such as systemic lupus erythematosus and inflammatory bowel disease, can cause venous and arterial thrombosis.[8] The antiphospholipid antibody syndrome is associated with repeated pregnancy loss. The precise mechanism by which these antibodies provoke thrombosis is unclear, but they activate the coagulation cascade and platelets, as well as inhibit the anticoagulant activity of proteins C and S. Estrogen-containing contraceptives, estrogen replacement therapy, and many of the selective estrogen receptor modulators (SERMs) increase the risk of venous thrombosis.[2,10,11] Although the mechanisms are not clearly understood, estrogens increase serum **clotting factor** concentrations and induce activated protein C resistance. Increased serum estrogen concentrations may explain, in part, the increased risk of VTE during pregnancy and the postpartum period.[11]

PATHOPHYSIOLOGY

Hemostasis, the arrest of bleeding following vascular injury, is essential to life.[12] Within the vascular system, blood remains in a fluid state, transporting oxygen, nutrients, plasma proteins, and waste. When a vessel is injured, a dynamic interplay between thrombogenic (activating) and antithrombotic (inhibiting) forces result in the local formation of a hemostatic plug that seals the vessel wall and prevents further blood loss (**Figs. 10–2, 10–3,** and **10–4**). A disruption of this delicate system of checks and balances may lead to inappropriate clot formation within the blood vessel that can obstruct blood flow or embolize to a distant vascular bed.

Under normal circumstances, the endothelial cells that line the inside of blood vessels maintain blood flow by producing a number of substances that inhibit platelet adherence, prevent the activation of the coagulation cascade, and facilitate **fibrinolysis**.[12] Vascular injury exposes the subendothelium (Fig. 10–3). Platelets readily adhere to the subendothelium, using glycoprotein (GP) Ib receptors found on their surfaces and facilitated by von Willebrand's factor (vWF). This causes platelets to become activated, releasing a number of procoagulant substances that stimulate circulating platelets to expose GP IIb and IIIa receptors and allow platelets to adhere to one another, resulting in platelet aggregation. The damaged vascular tissue releases tissue factor that activates the extrinsic pathway of the coagulation cascade (Fig. 10–4).

The **clotting cascade** is a stepwise series of enzymatic reactions that result in the formation of a fibrin mesh.[12] Clotting factors circulate in the blood in inactive forms. Once a precursor is activated by specific stimuli, it activates the next precursor in the sequence. The final steps in the cascade

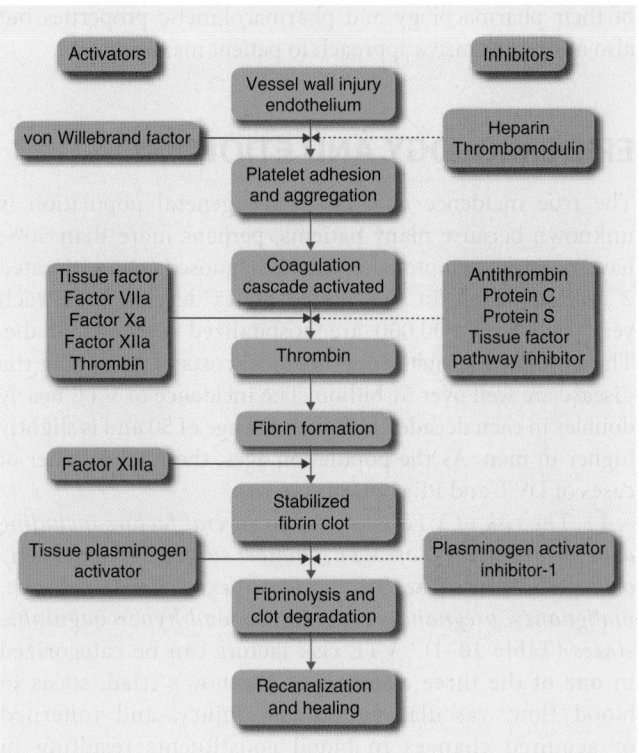

FIGURE 10–2. Hemostasis and thrombosis. (From Witt DM, Nutescu EA, Haines S. Venous thromboembolism. In: DiPiro JT, Talbert RL, Yee GC, et al., eds. Pharmacotherapy: A Pathophysiologic Approach, 8th ed. New York, NY: McGraw-Hill, 2011:314.)

are the conversion of **prothrombin** (factor II) to **thrombin** (factor IIa) and fibrinogen to **fibrin**. Thrombin plays a key role in the coagulation cascade; it is responsible not only for the production of fibrin, but also for the activation of factors V and VIII, creating a positive feedback loop that greatly accelerates the entire cascade. Thrombin also enhances platelet aggregation. Traditionally, the coagulation cascade has been divided into three distinct parts: the intrinsic, the extrinsic, and the common pathways (Fig. 10–4). This artificial division is misleading because there are numerous interactions between the three pathways.

A number of tempering mechanisms control coagulation (Fig. 10–2).[12] Without effective self-regulation, the coagulation cascade would proceed unabated until all the clotting factors and platelets are consumed. AT and heparin cofactor II (HCII) are circulating proteins that inhibit thrombin and factor Xa. The intact endothelium adjacent to the damaged tissue actively secretes several antithrombotic substances including heparan sulfate and thrombomodulin. Heparan sulfate exponentially accelerates AT and HCII activity. Protein C and its cofactor, protein S, are vitamin K–dependent anticoagulant proteins made in the liver. Activation of the clotting cascade activates protein C that, in turn, inhibits factor Va and VIIIa activity. Tissue factor pathway inhibitor (TFPI) inhibits the extrinsic coagulation pathway. When these self-regulatory mechanisms are

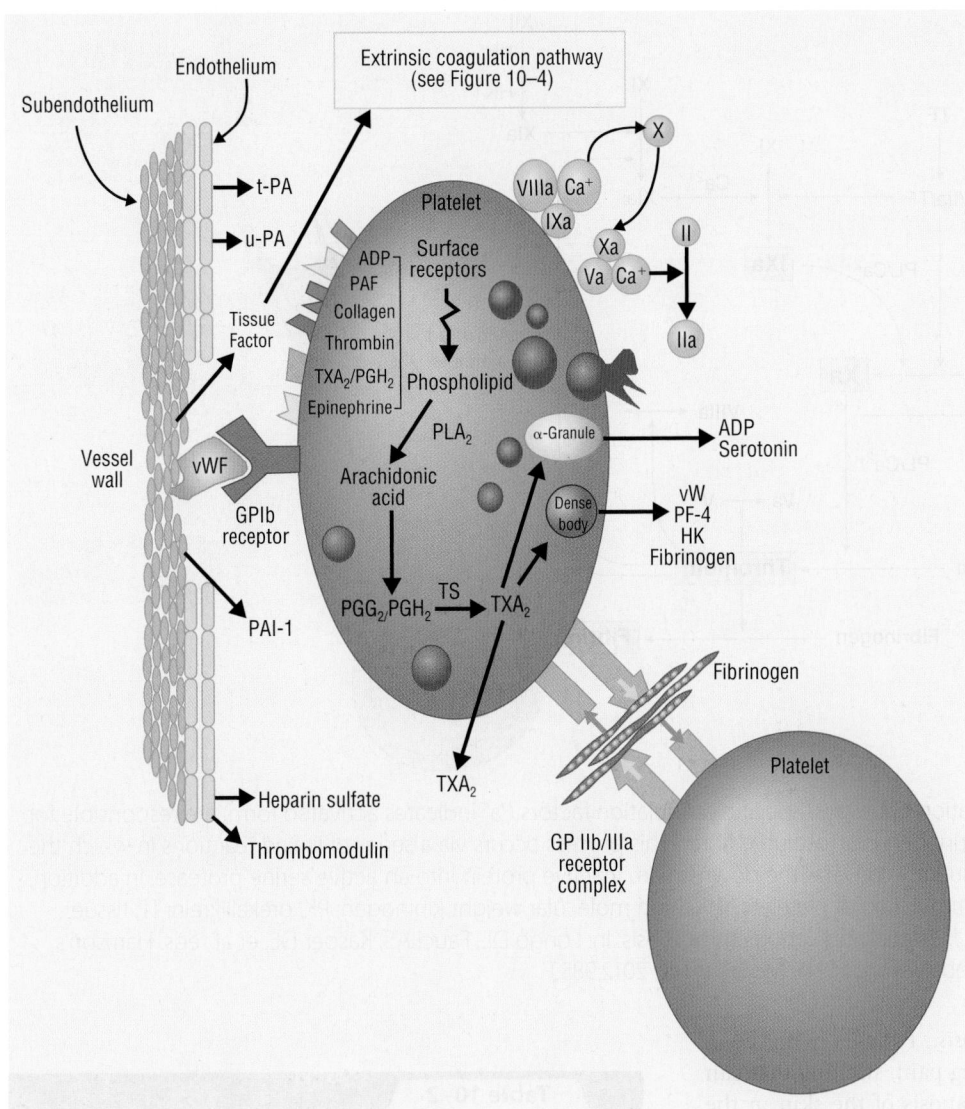

FIGURE 10–3. Vascular injury and thrombosis. (ADP, adenosine diphosphate; GP Ib, glycoprotein Ib; GP IIb/IIa, glycoprotein IIb/IIa; HK, high molecular weight kininogen; PAF, platelet activating factor-1; PAI-1, plasminogen activator inhibitor; PF-4, platelet factor-4; PGG/PGH, prostaglandins; PLA, phospholipase A; TS, thromboxane synthetase; TXA_2, thromboxane A_2; t-PA, tissue plasminogen activator; u-PA, urokinase plasminogen activator; vWF, von Willebrand's factor.) (From Witt DM, Nutescu EA, Haines S. Venous thromboembolism. In: DiPiro JT, Talbert RL, Yee GC, et al., eds. Pharmacotherapy: A Pathophysiologic Approach, 8th ed. New York, NY: McGraw-Hill, 2011:315.)

intact, the formation of the fibrin clot is limited to the zone of tissue injury. However, disruptions in the system often result in inappropriate localized or systemic clot formation.

The fibrinolytic protein plasmin degrades the fibrin mesh into soluble end products collectively known as fibrin split products or fibrin degradation products.[13] The fibrinolytic system is also under the control of a series of stimulatory and inhibitory substances. Tissue plasminogen activator (t-PA) and urokinase plasminogen activator (u-PA) convert plasminogen to plasmin. Plasminogen activator inhibitor (PAI)-1 inhibits the plasminogen activators and α_2-antiplasmin inhibits plasmin activity. Aberrations in the fibrinolytic system have also been linked to hypercoagulability.[13,14]

CLINICAL PRESENTATION AND DIAGNOSIS

Although a thrombus can form in any part of the venous circulation, most begin in the lower extremities. Once formed, a venous thrombus may behave in a combination of ways including (a) remain asymptomatic, (b) spontaneously lyse, (c) obstruct the venous circulation, (d) propagate into more proximal veins, (e) embolize, and/or (f) slowly incorporate into the endothelial layer of the vessel.[14] Most patients with VTE never develop symptoms.[2] However, even those who initially experience no symptoms may suffer long-term consequences, such as PTS and recurrent VTE.

Given that VTE can be debilitating or fatal, it is important to treat it quickly and aggressively.[15] However, because major bleeding induced by antithrombotic drugs can be equally harmful, it is important to avoid treatment when the diagnosis is not reasonably certain. Assessment of the patient's status should focus on the search for risk factors in the patient's medical history (Table 10–1).[16,17] Venous thrombosis is uncommon in the absence of risk factors, and the effects of these risks are additive. Indeed, if a patient has multiple risk factors, VTE should be strongly suspected even when the symptoms are very subtle.

❸ *The symptoms of DVT or PE are nonspecific, and it is extremely difficult to distinguish VTE from other disorders on clinical signs alone.*[16] *Therefore, objective tests are required*

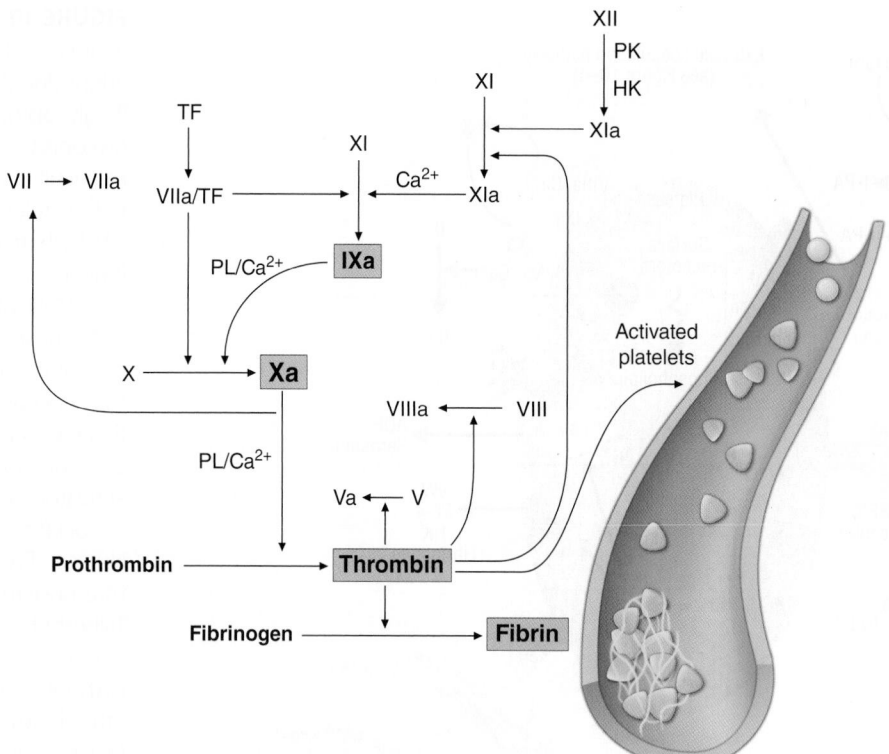

FIGURE 10–4. Summary of coagulation pathways. Specific coagulation factors ("a" indicates activated form) are responsible for the conversion of soluble plasma fibrinogen into insoluble fibrin. This process occurs via a series of linked reactions in which the enzymatically active product subsequently converts the downstream inactive protein into an active serine protease. In addition, the activation of thrombin leads to stimulation of platelets. (HK, high molecular weight kininogen; PK, prekallikrein; TF, tissue factor.) (From Freedman JE, Loscalzo J. Arterial and venous thrombosis. In: Longo DL, Fauci AS, Kasper DL, et al., eds. Harrison's Principles of Internal Medicine, 18th ed. New York, NY: McGraw-Hill, 2012:985.)

to confirm or exclude the diagnosis. Patients with DVT frequently present with unilateral leg pain, swelling that can persist after a night's sleep, and cyanosis of the skin in the affected leg. Similarly, PTS, a long-term complication of DVT caused by damage to the venous valves, produces chronic lower extremity swelling, pain, and tenderness that lead to skin discoloration and ulceration. To distinguish acute DVT from PTS and other possible diagnoses, a clinical prediction rule that incorporates signs, symptoms and risk factors can be used to categorize the patient as at a low, intermediate, or high probability of having acute DVT. This model, known as the Wells Criteria, is summarized in Table 10–2.[16] If the clinical probability of DVT is low, the D-dimer test can be used to confirm the patient does not have DVT. The D-dimer test is a quantitative measure of fibrin breakdown in the serum, and it is a marker of acute thrombotic activity. D-dimer assays are sensitive but not specific markers for VTE, so a negative D-dimer test can be used to rule out the diagnosis of DVT.

If the D-dimer test is positive in a low probability patient, or if the patient has a moderate or high probability of DVT, then an objective test is used to confirm the diagnosis of DVT. Contrast venography allows visualization of the entire venous system in the lower extremities. This radiographic contrast study is the most accurate and reliable method for the diagnosis of DVT and considered the gold standard in clinical trials.[18,19] However, venography is an expensive invasive procedure that is technically difficult to

Table 10–2

Clinical Model/Wells Criteria for Evaluating the Pretest Probability of Deep Vein Thrombosis[a]

Clinical Characteristic	Score
Active cancer (cancer treatment within previous 6 months or currently on palliative treatment)	+1
Paralysis, paresis, or recent plaster immobilization of the lower extremities	+1
Recently bedridden for 3 days or more, or major surgery within the previous 12 weeks requiring general or regional anesthesia	+1
Localized tenderness along the distribution of the deep venous system	+1
Entire leg swollen	+1
Calf swelling at least 3 cm larger than that on the asymptomatic side (measured 10 cm below tibial tuberosity)	+1
Pitting edema confined to the symptomatic leg	+1
Collateral superficial veins (nonvaricose)	+1
Previously documented deep vein thrombosis	+1
Alternative diagnosis at least as likely as deep vein thrombosis	–2

[a]Clinical probability of deep vein thrombosis: low, less than 0; moderate, 1–2; high, greater than 3. In patients with symptoms in both legs, the more symptomatic leg is used.

Clinical Presentation and Diagnosis of DVT

General

- VTE most commonly develops in patients with identifiable risk factors (Table 10–1) during or following a hospitalization. Many, perhaps most, patients have asymptomatic disease. Patients may die suddenly of PE.

Symptoms

- The patient may complain of leg swelling, pain, warmth, and/or skin discoloration. Symptoms are nonspecific, and objective testing must be performed to establish the diagnosis.

Signs

- The patient's superficial veins may be dilated and a "palpable cord" may be felt in the affected leg.

- The patient may experience unilateral leg edema with measurable difference in leg circumference, erythema, increase in warmth, and tenderness with palpation of calf muscles.

- The patient may experience pain in back of the knee or calf in the affected leg when the examiner dorsiflexes the foot while the knee is slightly bent (Homan's sign).

- Note: The physical examination signs can be unreliable. Homan's sign (a positive test is pain in the calf or popliteal region with dorsiflexion of the foot) can also be unreliable.

Clinical Probability

- Apply the Wells Criteria to determine the probability the patient's signs, symptoms and risk factors are the result of DVT (Table 10–2).

Laboratory Tests

- The initial laboratory evaluation should include CBC with differential, coagulation studies (such as prothrombin time [PT]/international normalized ratio [INR], activated partial thromboplastin time [aPTT]), serum chemistries with renal and liver function, and urinalysis.

- Serum concentrations of D-dimer, a by-product of thrombin generation, will be elevated in an acute event. A negative D-dimer in a patient with low clinical probability of DVT can be used to rule out DVT.

- The patient may have an elevated erythrocyte sedimentation rate (ESR) and white blood cell (WBC) count.

Diagnostic Tests

- Duplex ultrasonography is the most commonly used test to diagnose DVT. It is a noninvasive test that can measure the rate and direction of blood flow and visualize clot formation in proximal veins of the legs. It cannot reliably detect small blood clots in distal veins. Coupled with a careful clinical assessment, it can rule in or out (include or exclude) the diagnosis in most cases.

- Venography (also known as phlebography) is the gold standard for the diagnosis of DVT. However, it is an invasive test that involves injection of radiopaque contrast dye into a foot vein. It is expensive and can cause anaphylaxis and nephrotoxicity.

---

perform and evaluate. Severely ill patients may be unable to tolerate the procedure, and many develop hypotension and cardiac arrhythmias. Furthermore, the contrast material is irritating to vessel walls and toxic to the kidneys. For these reasons, noninvasive testing is preferred in clinical practice for the evaluation of patients with suspected DVT. The preferred test is duplex ultrasonography. See the Clinical Presentation and Diagnosis of DVT textbox for further information.

Symptomatic PE usually produces shortness of breath, tachypnea, and tachycardia.[16] Hemoptysis occurs in less than a third of patients. The most common subjective symptoms are dyspnea, pleuritic chest pain, apprehension (anxiety or a feeling of impending doom), and cough. The physical examination may reveal diminished breath sounds, crackles, wheezes, or a pleural friction rub during auscultation of the lungs. Cardiovascular collapse, characterized by cyanosis, shock, and oliguria, is an ominous sign.

Like DVT, the nonspecific nature of the signs and symptoms of PE requires further evaluation. Table 10–3 describes a validated prediction model that can be used to stratify patients into high, moderate, and low probability of PE.[16] In patients with a low clinical probability of PE,

the diagnosis of PE can be ruled out if D-dimer testing is negative. If D-dimer testing is positive, or if the patient has a moderate or high clinical probability of PE, diagnostic imaging studies should be performed. Pulmonary angiography allows the visualization of the pulmonary arteries. The diagnosis of VTE can be made if there is a persistent intraluminal filling defect observed on multiple x-ray films. However, as with DVT, a noninvasive test is preferred, such as computed tomography (CT) scans, magnetic resonance imaging (MRI), and ventilation/perfusion (V/Q) scans. See the Clinical Presentation and Diagnosis of PE textbox for further information.

PREVENTION

Given that VTE is often clinically silent and potentially fatal, prevention strategies have the greatest potential to improve patient outcomes.[2] To rely on the early diagnosis and treatment of VTE is unacceptable because many patients will die before treatment can be initiated. Furthermore, even clinically silent disease is associated with long-term morbidity from PTS and predisposes the patient to future thromboembolic events. Despite an immense body of literature that overwhelmingly

Clinical Presentation and Diagnosis of PE

General

- PE most commonly develops in patients with risk factors for VTE (Table 10–1) during or following a hospitalization. Although many patients will have symptoms of DVT prior to developing a PE, many do not. Patients may die suddenly before effective treatment can be initiated.

Symptoms

- The patient may complain of cough, chest pain, chest tightness, shortness of breath, wheezing, or palpitations.
- The patient may present with hemoptysis (spit or cough up blood).
- The patient may complain of dizziness or lightheadedness.
- Symptoms may be confused for a myocardial infarction or pneumonia, and objective testing must be performed to establish the diagnosis.

Signs

- The patient may have tachypnea (increased respiratory rate) and tachycardia (increased heart rate).
- The patient may appear diaphoretic (sweaty).
- The patient's neck veins may be distended reflecting increased jugular venous pressure.
- The examiner may hear diminished breath sounds, crackles, wheezes, or pleural friction rub, right ventricular S_3, or parasternal lift during auscultation of the lungs.
- In massive PE, the patient may appear cyanotic and hypotensive. In such cases, oxygen saturation by pulse oximetry or arterial blood gas will likely indicate the patient is hypoxic.

- In the worst cases, the patient may go into circulatory shock and die within minutes.

Clinical Probability

- Apply the Wells Criteria to determine the probability that the patient's signs, symptoms, and risk factors are the result of PE (Table 10–3).

Laboratory Tests

- Serum concentrations of D-dimer, a by-product of thrombin generation, will be elevated. A negative D-dimer in a patient with low clinical probability of PE can be used to rule out PE.
- The patient may have an elevated ESR and WBC count.
- The patient may have elevated serum LDH or AST (SGOT) with normal bilirubin.
- Serum troponin I and troponin T can be elevated in a large PE.

Diagnostic Tests

- A CT scan is the most commonly used test to diagnose PE, but some institutions still use a ventilation/perfusion (V/Q) scan. Spiral CT scans can detect emboli in the pulmonary arteries. A V/Q scan measures the distribution of blood and air flow in the lungs. When there is a large mismatch between blood and air flow in one area of the lung, there is a high probability the patient has a PE.
- Pulmonary angiography is the gold standard for diagnosis of PE. However, it is an invasive test that involves injection of radiopaque contrast dye into the pulmonary artery. The test is expensive and associated with a significant risk of mortality.

Table 10–3

Clinical Model/Wells Criteria for Evaluating the Pretest Probability of Pulmonary Embolism[a]

Clinical Characteristic	Score
Cancer	+1
Hemoptysis	+1
Previous PE or DVT	+1.5
Heart rate greater than 100 beats/min	+1.5
Recent surgery or immobilization	+1.5
Clinical signs of DVT	+3
Alternative diagnosis less likely than PE	+3

DVT, deep vein thrombosis; PE, pulmonary embolism.

[a]Clinical probability of PE: low, 0–1; moderate, 2–6; high, 7 or greater.

supports the widespread use of pharmacologic and nonpharmacologic strategies to prevent VTE, prophylaxis is underutilized in most hospitals. Even when prophylaxis is given, many patients receive prophylaxis that is less than optimal.

Educational programs and computerized clinical decision support systems have been shown to improve the appropriate use of VTE prevention methods.[2]

The goal of an effective VTE prophylaxis program is to identify all patients at risk, determine each patient's level of risk, and select and implement regimens that provide sufficient protection for the level of risk.[20] ❹ *At the time of hospital admission, all patients should be evaluated for their risk of VTE, and strategies to prevent VTE appropriate for each patient's level of risk should be routinely used. Prophylaxis should be continued throughout the period of risk.* The risk classification criteria and recommended prophylaxis strategies published by the American College of Chest Physicians (ACCP) Conference on Antithrombotic Therapy are widely used in North America (Table 10–4).[2] Several pharmacologic and nonpharmacologic methods are effective for preventing VTE, and these can be used alone or in combination. Nonpharmacologic methods improve venous blood flow by mechanical means; drug therapy prevents thrombus formation by inhibiting the coagulation cascade.

Table 10–4

Risk Classification and Consensus Guidelines for VTE Prevention

Level of Risk	Risk of VTE	Prevention Strategies
Low Minor surgery, in mobile patients Medical patients who are fully mobile	Less than 10%	Early and aggressive ambulation
Moderate Major surgery, and no clinical risk factors Acutely ill medical patients (e.g., myocardial infarction, ischemic stroke, heart failure exacerbation) at bed rest	10–40%	UFH 5,000 units SC every 8–12 hours Dalteparin 2,500–5,000 units SC every 24 hours Enoxaparin 40 mg SC every 24 hours Fondaparinux 2.5 mg SC every 24 hours Tinzaparin 3,500 units SC every 24 hours IPC[a]; GCS[a]
High Major lower extremity orthopedic surgery Hip fracture Major trauma	40–80%	Dalteparin 5,000 units SC every 24 hours Enoxaparin 30 mg SC every 12 hours or 40 mg SC every 24 hours Fondaparinux 2.5 mg SC every 24 hours Tinzaparin 75 units/kg SC every 24 hours Warfarin (target INR = 2–3) IPC[a]; GCS[a]

GCS, graduated compression stockings; INR, International Normalized Ratio; IPC, intermittent pneumatic compression; SC, subcutaneous; UFH, unfractionated heparin; VTE, venous thromboembolism.

[a]Mechanical methods of prophylaxis are used in patients at high risk of bleeding complications

From Geerts WH, Bergqvist D, Pineo GF, et al. Prevention of venous thromboembolism: American College of Chest Physicians Evidence-Based Clinical Practice Guidelines, 8th ed. Chest 2008;133:381S–453S

Nonpharmacologic Therapy

Ambulation as soon as possible following surgery lowers the incidence of VTE in low-risk patients.[2] Walking increases venous blood flow and promotes the flow of natural antithrombotic factors into the lower extremities. Although graduated compression stockings (GCS) can reduce the incidence of asymptomatic DVT in lower risk patients, they produce no significant reduction in mortality, symptomatic DVT, or PE.[2] Compared with anticoagulant drugs, GCS are relatively inexpensive and safe; however, in higher risk patients they are less effective than pharmacologic agents.[2] They are a good choice in low- to moderate-risk patients when pharmacologic interventions are contraindicated. When combined with pharmacologic interventions, GCS have an additive effect. However, some patients are unable to wear compression stockings because of the size or shape of their legs, and some patients may find them hot, confining, and uncomfortable.

Similar to GCS, intermittent pneumatic compression (IPC) devices increase the velocity of blood flow in the lower extremities.[2] These devices sequentially inflate a series of cuffs wrapped around the patient's legs from the ankles to the thighs and then deflate in 1- to 2-minute cycles. IPC has been shown to reduce the risk of VTE greater than 60% following general surgery, neurosurgery, and orthopedic surgery. Although IPC is safe to use in patients who have contraindications to pharmacologic therapies, it does have a few drawbacks: It is more expensive than GCS, it is a relatively cumbersome technique, some patients may have difficulty sleeping while using it, and some patients find the devices hot, sticky, and uncomfortable. To be effective, IPC needs to be used throughout the day. In practice, this is difficult to achieve, and special efforts should be made to ensure the devices are worn and operational for most of the day.

Inferior vena cava (IVC) filters, also known as Greenfield filters, provide short-term protection against PE in very high-risk patients by preventing the embolization of a thrombus formed in the lower extremities into the pulmonary circulation.[2] Insertion of a filter into the IVC is a minimally invasive procedure. Despite the widespread use of IVC filters, there are very limited data regarding their effectiveness and long-term safety. The evidence suggests that IVC filters, particularly in the absence of effective antithrombotic therapy, are thrombogenic themselves and increase the long-term risk of recurrent DVT and of filter thrombosis. In the only randomized clinical trial examining the short- and long-term effectiveness of the filters in patients with a documented proximal DVT, treatment with IVC filters reduced the risk of PE by more than 75% during the first 12 days following insertion.[21] However, this benefit was not sustained during 2 years of follow-up, and the long-term risk of recurrent DVT was nearly twofold higher in those who received a filter. Although IVC filters can reduce the short-term risk of PE in patients at highest risk, they should be reserved for patients in whom other prophylactic strategies cannot be used. To further reduce the long-term risk of VTE in association with IVC filters, pharmacologic prophylaxis is necessary in patients with IVC filters in place, and warfarin therapy should begin as soon as the patient is able to tolerate it.[2] Retrievable filters are preferred, which can be removed once pharmacologic prophylaxis can be safely administered or once the patient is no longer at risk for VTE.

Pharmacologic Therapy

Numerous randomized clinical trials have extensively evaluated pharmacologic strategies for VTE prophylaxis.[2] Appropriately selected drug therapies can dramatically reduce the incidence of VTE following hip replacement, knee replacement, general surgery, myocardial infarction, and ischemic stroke (Table 10–4). The choice of medication and dose to use for VTE prevention must be based on the patient's level of risk for thrombosis and bleeding complications, as well as the cost and availability of an adequate drug therapy monitoring system.

The ACCP Conference on Antithrombotic Therapy recommends against the use of aspirin as the primary method of VTE prophylaxis.[2] Antiplatelet drugs clearly reduce the risk of coronary artery and cerebrovascular events in patients with arterial disease, but aspirin produces a very modest reduction in VTE following orthopedic surgeries of the lower extremities. The relative contribution of venous stasis in the pathogenesis of venous thrombosis compared with that of platelets in arterial thrombosis likely explains the reason for this difference.

The most extensively studied drugs for the prevention of VTE are unfractionated heparin (UFH), the low molecular weight heparins (LMWHs; dalteparin, enoxaparin, and tinzaparin), fondaparinux, and warfarin.[2] The LMWHs and fondaparinux provide superior protection against VTE when compared with low-dose UFH after hip and knee replacement surgery and in other high-risk populations. Even so, UFH remains an effective, cost-conscious choice for moderate-risk patient populations, provided it is given in the appropriate dose (Table 10–4). Low-dose UFH (5,000 Units every 12 or 8 hours) given subcutaneously (SC) has been shown to reduce the risk of VTE significantly in patients undergoing a wide range of general surgical procedures as well as following a myocardial infarction or stroke. For patients who are hospitalized with an acute medical illness, the available evidence supports the use of UFH (5,000 Units every 12 or 8 hours), enoxaparin 40 mg SC daily, dalteparin 5,000 Units SC daily, or fondaparinux 2.5 mg SC daily.

For the prevention of VTE following hip and knee replacement surgery, the effectiveness of low-dose UFH is considerably lower. Adjusted-dose UFH therapy provided SC, which requires dose adjustments to maintain the aPTT at the high end of the normal range, may be used in the highest risk patient populations. However, adjusted-dose UFH has been studied in only a few relatively small clinical trials and requires frequent laboratory monitoring. The LMWHs and fondaparinux appear to provide a high degree of protection against VTE in most high-risk populations. The appropriate prophylactic dose for each LMWH product is indication specific (Table 10–4). There is no evidence that one LMWH is superior to another for the prevention of VTE. Fondaparinux

was significantly more effective than enoxaparin in several clinical trials that enrolled patients undergoing high-risk orthopedic procedures, but it has not been shown to reduce the incidence of symptomatic PE or mortality and has heightened the risk of bleeding. To provide optimal protection, some experts believe the LMWHs should be initiated prior to surgery.[2]

Warfarin is another commonly used option for the prevention of VTE following orthopedic surgeries of the lower extremities.[2] Warfarin appears to be as effective as the LMWHs for the prevention of symptomatic VTE events in the highest risk populations. When used to prevent VTE, the dose of warfarin must be adjusted to maintain an INR between 2 and 3. Oral administration and low drug cost give warfarin some advantages over the LMWHs and fondaparinux. However, warfarin does not achieve its full antithrombotic effect for several days and requires frequent monitoring and periodic dosage adjustments, making therapy cumbersome. Warfarin should only be used when a systematic patient monitoring system is available.

Patient Encounter 1

AL is a 61-year-old obese woman with a history of diverticulosis admitted to the hospital after a 2-day period of severe abdominal pain, fever, nausea, and constipation. She is diagnosed with peritonitis and started on antibiotic therapy.

PMH: Diverticulosis × 10 years; depression × 5 years; chronic knee pain × 3 years; hypertension × 2 years

FH: Nonsignificant

SH: Occasional alcohol use. Employed in county government. Lives at home with spouse and pets.

Home Meds: Aspirin 81 mg by mouth once daily; hydrochlorothiazide 25 mg by mouth once daily; bupropion XL 300 mg by mouth once daily

Allergies: NKDA

VS: BP 135/70 mm Hg, HR 72 bpm, RR 16, T 38.7°C (101.6°F), wt 90 kg (198 lb)

Labs: WBC 22.4 × 10³/mm³ (22.4 × 10⁹/L); estimated glomerular filtration rate (eGFR) = 80 mL/min/1.73 m² (0.77 mL/s/m²)

Hospital treatment: bowel rest with nothing by mouth; metronidazole 500 mg IV every 8 hours; ceftriaxone 1 g IV every 24 hours

Which risk factor(s) predispose AL to VTE?

What is AL's estimated risk for developing VTE?

Given AL's presentation and history, create an appropriate VTE prophylaxis plan including the pharmacologic agent, dose, route, and frequency of administration, duration of therapy, and monitoring parameters.

Patient Encounter 2

FA is a 64-year-old woman with a new diagnosis of squamous cell cancer of the tongue who is admitted to the hospital for extensive surgical resection of her tongue, feeding tube placement, and Port-a-Cath placement for future chemotherapy.

PMH: Dyslipidemia × 8 years; history of hip fracture 3 years ago with subsequent lower left extremity DVT, treated with LMWH and warfarin for 3 months

FH: Nonsignificant

SH: Smoked half a pack per day for 25 years; occasional alcohol use. Lives alone and expects to be discharged to a rehabilitation facility postoperatively before returning home.

Home meds: Simvastatin 40 mg by mouth daily; oxycodone 5–10 mg by mouth every 5 hours as needed for pain; docusate 250 mg by mouth twice daily

Allergies: NKDA

VS: BP 110/60 mm Hg, HR 55 bpm, RR 18, T 37.0°C (98.6°F), wt 127 kg (280 lb), BMI 40 kg/m²

Labs: All within normal limits; eGFR = 96 mL/min/1.73 m² (0.92 mL/s/m²)

Which risk factor(s) predispose FA to VTE?

How should postoperative VTE be prevented in FA?

How long should FA receive VTE prophylaxis?

What education about VTE prophylaxis should FA receive?

A new option for VTE prevention following hip and knee replacement surgery is rivaroxaban, an oral factor Xa inhibitor that recently was approved for this indication in the United States. This agent is given at a fixed dose of 10 mg once daily, without the need for routine laboratory monitoring and dosing adjustments (as with warfarin) and without the inconvenience of administration by injection (as with LMWH and fondaparinux). Compared with enoxaparin 40 mg SC once daily for VTE prevention in hip replacement, and to both enoxaparin 40 mg SC once daily and 30 mg SC twice daily in knee replacement, rivaroxaban was more effective in preventing postoperative VTE, with a similar rate of bleeding complications.[22] The role of this new agent has yet to be determined, but it may offer a convenient alternative to the agents that are currently recommended in evidence-based guidelines.[2]

The optimal duration for VTE prophylaxis is not well established.[2] Prophylaxis should be given throughout the period of risk. For general surgical procedures and medical conditions, once the patient is able to ambulate regularly and other risk factors are no longer present, prophylaxis can be discontinued. The risk of VTE in the first month following hospital discharge among patients who have undergone total knee replacement, total hip replacement, or hip fracture

repair is very high. Therefore, extended prophylaxis for 21 to 35 days following hospital discharge with an LMWH, fondaparinux, or warfarin is recommended.

TREATMENT

Desired Therapeutic Outcomes

The goal of VTE treatment is to prevent short- and long-term complications of the disease. In the short term (i.e., the first few days to 6 months), the aim of therapy is to prevent propagation or local extension of the clot, embolization, and death. In the long term (i.e., more than 6 months after the first event), the aim of therapy is to prevent complications, such as PTS, pulmonary hypertension, and recurrent VTE.[15,23]

General Treatment Principles

Anticoagulant drugs are considered the mainstay of therapy for patients with VTE, and the therapeutic strategies for DVT and PE are essentially identical.[15,23] ❺ *In the absence of contraindications, the treatment of VTE should initially include a rapid-acting anticoagulant (e.g., UFH, LMWH, or fondaparinux) overlapped with warfarin for at least 5 days and until the patient's INR is greater than 2. Anticoagulation therapy should be continued for a minimum of 3 months. However, the duration of anticoagulation therapy should be based on the patient's risk of VTE recurrence and major bleeding.* The treatment of VTE can be divided into acute, subacute, and chronic phases (Fig. 10–5).[23,24] The acute treatment phase of VTE is typically accomplished by administering a fast-acting parenteral anticoagulant (Table 10–5). The subacute and chronic phase treatments of VTE are usually accomplished using oral anticoagulant agents such as warfarin.[15,23] In certain populations, such as patients with cancer and women who are pregnant, the LMWHs are the preferred agents during subacute and chronic treatment phases.[15] In the last decade, several novel

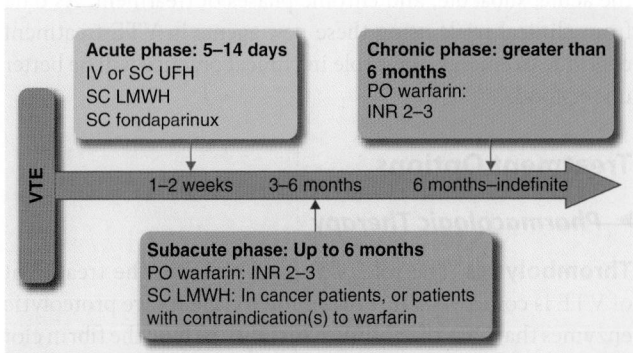

FIGURE 10–5. Treatment approach for patients with VTE. (INR, international normalized ratio; LMWH, low molecular weight heparin; PO, oral; SC, subcutaneous; UFH, unfractionated heparin; VTE, venous thromboembolism.) (From Nutescu EA. Emerging options in the treatment of venous thromboembolism. Am J Health Syst Pharm 2004;61:S12–S17.)

Table 10–5

Pharmacologic Options for the Initial Treatment of Acute VTE

UFH
IV administration:[a] use weight-based dosing nomogram (Table 10–7)
or
SC administration: 17,500 units (250 units/kg) given every
12 hours (an initial 5,000 unit IV bolus dose is recommended to obtain rapid anticoagulation)
Adjust subsequent doses to attain a goal aPTT based on the institution-specific therapeutic range
or
SC administration: 333 units/kg followed by 250 units/kg given every 12 hours (fixed-dose unmonitored dosing regimen)

LMWHs
Dalteparin: 200 units/kg SC once daily *or* 100 units/kg SC twice daily[b]
Enoxaparin: 1.5 mg/kg SC once daily *or* 1 mg/kg SC twice daily; if CrCl is less than 30 mL/min (0.50 mL/s): 1 mg/kg SC once daily
Tinzaparin: 175 units/kg SC once daily

Factor Xa Inhibitor
Fondaparinux:
    For body weight less than 50 kg (110 lb), use 5 mg SC once daily
    For body weight 50–100 kg (110–220 lb), use 7.5 mg SC once daily
    For body weight greater than 100 kg (220 lb), use 10 mg SC once daily

aPTT, activated partial thromboplastin time; CrCl, creatinine clearance; LMWHs, low–molecular weight heparins; SC, subcutaneous; UFH, unfractionated heparin; VTE, venous thromboembolism.

[a]IV administration preferred due to improved dosing precision.

[b]Not FDA-approved for treatment of VTE in noncancer patients.

From Kearon C, Kahn SR, Agnelli G, et al. Antithrombotic therapy for venous thromboembolic disease: American College of Chest Physicians Evidence-Based Clinical Practice Guidelines, 8th ed. Chest 2008;133:454S–545S.

Table 10–6

Thrombolysis for the Treatment of VTE

- Thrombolytic therapy should be reserved for patients who present with shock, hypotension, right ventricular injury, or massive DVT with limb gangrene
- Diagnosis must be objectively confirmed before initiating thrombolytic therapy
- Thrombolytic therapy is most effective when administered as soon as possible after PE diagnosis, but benefit may extend up to 14 days after symptom onset
- FDA-approved PE thrombolytic regimens:
  - Streptokinase 250,000 units IV bolus over 30 minutes followed by 100,000 units/h for 12–24 hours[a]
  - Urokinase 4,400 units/kg IV bolus over 10 minutes followed by 4,400 units/kg/h for 12–24 hours[a]
  - Alteplase (t-PA) 100 mg IV over 2 hours
- Non-FDA approved thrombolytic regimens:
  - Reteplase two 10-unit IV boluses given 30 minutes apart
  - Tenecteplase weight-adjusted IV bolus over 5 seconds (30–50 mg with a 5-mg step every 10 kg from less than 60 to greater than 90 kg)
- Factors that increase the risk of bleeding must be evaluated before thrombolytic therapy is initiated (i.e., recent surgery, trauma or internal bleeding, uncontrolled hypertension, recent stroke, or ICH)
- Baseline labs should include CBC and blood typing in case transfusion is needed
- UFH should not be used during thrombolytic therapy. Neither the aPTT nor any other anticoagulation parameter should be monitored during the thrombolytic infusion
- aPTT should be measured following the completion of thrombolytic therapy:
- If aPTT less than 2.5 times the control value, UFH infusion should be started and adjusted to maintain aPTT in therapeutic range
- If aPTT greater than 2.5 times the control value, remeasure every 2–4 hours and start UFH infusion when aPTT is less than 2.5
- Avoid phlebotomy, arterial puncture, and other invasive procedures during thrombolytic therapy to minimize the risk of bleeding

aPTT, activated partial thromboplastin time; CBC, complete blood count; DVT, deep vein thrombosis; ICH, intracranial hemorrhage; PE, pulmonary embolism; t-PA, tissue plasminogen activator; UFH, unfractionated heparin; VTE, venous thromboembolism.

[a]Two-hour infusions of streptokinase and urokinase are as effective and safe as alteplase.

anticoagulants, such as direct thrombin inhibitors (DTIs) and factor Xa inhibitors, have emerged as potential alternatives for the acute, subacute, and chronic phases of treatment. As data from clinical trials using these new agents in VTE treatment continue to emerge, their role in clinical practice will be better understood.[15,23]

Treatment Options

▶ Pharmacologic Therapy

Thrombolytics The role of thrombolysis in the treatment of VTE is controversial. Thrombolytic agents are proteolytic enzymes that have the ability to dissolve, or lyse, the fibrin clot (Table 10–6). Thrombolytics are administered systemically or directly into the thrombus using a catheter-directed infusion.[15] Compared with anticoagulants, thrombolytics restore venous patency more quickly; however, the bleeding risk associated with their use is significantly higher.[25] In patients with DVT, thrombolytics decrease short-term pain and swelling and prevent destruction of the venous valves. It is not clear if thrombolytics decrease the incidence and

severity of PTS. Clinical trials have failed to show any long-term benefits from the routine use of thrombolytics; therefore, their use in most patients is not recommended.[15,25] In a select group of high-risk patients with massive iliofemoral DVT who are at risk of limb gangrene, thrombolysis may be considered.[15]

In patients with acute PE, the use of thrombolytics provides short-term benefits such as restoring pulmonary artery patency and hemodynamic stability.[15,26] A meta-analysis of nine small randomized clinical trials showed a slightly lower risk of death or recurrent PE in patients treated with thrombolytics when compared with those treated with heparin alone. However, this small benefit was offset by a higher risk of major bleeding.[27] Streptokinase, urokinase, and t-PA are thrombolytics and have all been studied and are FDA approved in the treatment of PE. All three agents have comparable thrombolytic capacity, but t-PA has the potential advantage of a shorter infusion time. Reteplase and tenecteplase are not currently FDA approved for the treatment of PE but have also been studied. Reteplase is administered as two 10-Unit IV boluses given 30 minutes apart, and tenecteplase is given as a weight-adjusted IV bolus over 5 seconds (the dose range is 30 to 50 mg, administered in 5-mg step increments for every 10 kg of body weight, i.e., dose for less than 60 kg is 30 mg, greater than or equal to 60 kg to less than 70 kg is 35 mg, greater than or equal to 70 kg to less than 80 kg is 40 mg, greater than or equal to 80 kg to less than 90 kg is 45 mg, and greater than or equal to 90 kg is 50 mg; the total dose should not exceed 50 mg).[15,28] Given the relative lack of data to support their routine use, thrombolytics should be reserved for select high-risk circumstances (Table 10–6). Candidates for thrombolytic therapy are patients with acute massive embolism who are hemodynamically unstable (systolic blood pressure [SBP] less than 90 mm Hg) or with evidence of right ventricular injury (i.e., elevated troponins) and at low risk for bleeding.[15,28]

Unfractionated Heparin UFH has traditionally been the drug of choice for indications requiring a rapid anticoagulation including the acute treatment of VTE. Commercially available UFH preparations are derived from porcine intestinal mucosa or bovine lung. UFH is composed of a heterogeneous mixture of glycosaminoglycans with variable length, molecular weight, and pharmacologic properties. Unlike thrombolytics, UFH and other anticoagulants will not dissolve a formed clot but prevent its propagation and growth.[4,29] Heparin exerts its anticoagulant effect by augmenting the natural anticoagulant, AT. A specific pentasaccharide sequence on the heparin molecule binds to AT and causes a conformational change that greatly accelerates its activity (Fig. 10–6). This complex inhibits thrombin (factor IIa), as well as factors Xa, IXa, XIa, and XIIa. Thrombin and factor Xa are most sensitive to this inhibition and are inactivated in an equal 1:1 ratio. To inactivate thrombin, the UFH molecule needs to form a ternary complex by binding to both AT and thrombin. Only UFH molecules that are at least 18 saccharide units long are able to form this bridge between AT and thrombin. In contrast, inhibition of factor Xa does not require the formation of a ternary complex. UFH molecules as short as five saccharide units can catalyze the inactivation of factor Xa. Due to its nonspecific binding to cellular proteins, UFH has several limitations, including poor bioavailability when given SC and significant intra- and interpatient variability in anticoagulant response.[4,29]

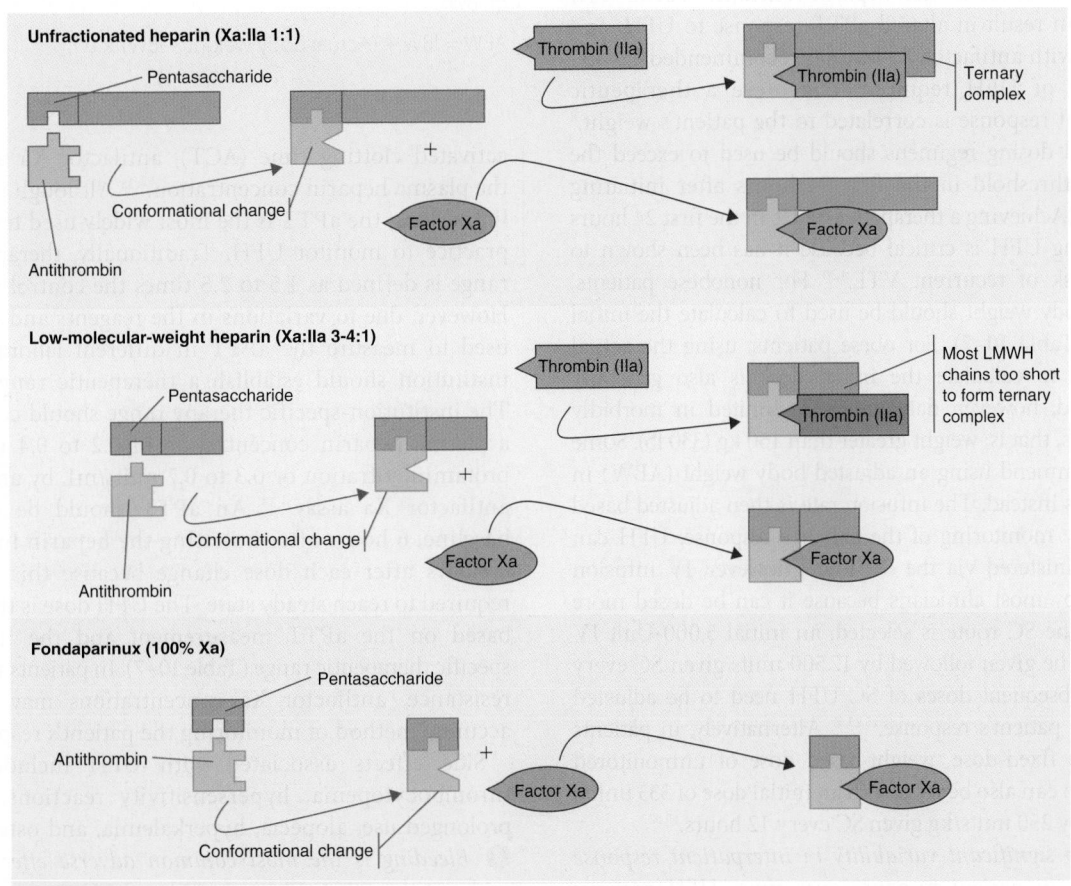

FIGURE 10–6. Mechanism of action of unfractionated heparin, low molecular weight heparin (LMWH), and fondaparinux. (From Witt DM, Nutescu EA, Haines S. Venous thromboembolism. In: DiPiro JT, Talbert RL, Yee GC, et al., eds. Pharmacotherapy: A Pathophysiologic Approach, 8th ed. New York, NY: McGraw-Hill, 2011:318.)

UFH can be administered via the IV or SC route.[4] When rapid anticoagulation is required, UFH should be administered IV and an initial bolus dose should be given. For the treatment of VTE, UFH is generally given as a continuous IV infusion. Intermittent IV bolus dosing is associated with a higher risk of bleeding and therefore not recommended. When given SC, the bioavailability of UFH ranges from 30% to 70%, depending on the dose given. Therefore, higher doses of UFH must be given if the SC route of administration is used. Onset of anticoagulation is delayed by 1 to 2 hours after the SC injection. Due to the risk of hematomas and erratic absorption, intramuscular (IM) administration is not recommended. The half-life of UFH is dose dependent and ranges from 30 to 90 minutes but may be significantly longer, up to 150 minutes, with high doses. UFH is eliminated by two mechanisms: (a) enzymatic degradation via a saturable zero-order process, and (b) renally via a first-order process. Lower UFH doses are primarily cleared via enzymatic processes, whereas higher doses are primarily renally eliminated. Clearance of UFH can be impaired in patients with renal and hepatic dysfunction. Patients with active thrombosis may require higher UFH doses due to a more rapid elimination or variations in the plasma concentrations of heparin-binding proteins. AT deficiency and elevated factor VIII levels are common in pregnant patients. AT deficiency has been linked to higher UFH dose requirements. The requirement of these higher UFH doses is termed *heparin resistance*. Factor VIII elevations can result in altered aPTT response to UFH, and monitoring with antifactor Xa levels is recommended.[4,29]

The dose of UFH required to achieve a therapeutic anticoagulant response is correlated to the patient's weight.[4] Weight-based dosing regimens should be used to exceed the therapeutic threshold in the first 24 hours after initiating treatment.[4,30] Achieving a therapeutic aPTT in the first 24 hours after initiating UFH is critical because it has been shown to lower the risk of recurrent VTE.[4,30] For nonobese patients, the actual body weight should be used to calculate the initial UFH dose (Table 10–7). For obese patients, using the actual body weight to calculate the initial dose is also generally recommended; however, data are more limited in morbidly obese patients, that is, weight greater than 150 kg (330 lb). Some experts recommend using an adjusted body weight (ABW) in these patients instead. The infusion rate is then adjusted based on laboratory monitoring of the patient's response. UFH can also be administered via the SC route; however, IV infusion is preferred by most clinicians because it can be dosed more precisely. If the SC route is selected, an initial 5,000-Unit IV bolus should be given followed by 17,500 units given SC every 12 hours. Subsequent doses of SC UFH need to be adjusted based on the patient's response.[15,23,31] Alternatively, in patients with DVT, a fixed-dose, weight-based dose of unmonitored UFH regimen can also be used with an initial dose of 333 units/kg followed by 250 units/kg given SC every 12 hours.[15,32]

6 *Due to significant variability in interpatient response and changes in patient response over time, UFH requires close monitoring and periodic dose adjustment.* The response to UFH can be monitored using a variety of laboratory tests including the aPTT, the whole blood clotting time,

Table 10–7

Weight-Based[a] Dosing for UFH Administered by Continuous IV Infusion for VTE

Initial Loading Dose	Initial Infusion Rate
80 units/kg (maximum = 10,000 units)	18 units/kg/h (maximum = 2,300 units/h)

aPTT (seconds)	Maintenance Infusion Rate Dose Adjustment
Less than 37 (or less than 12 seconds below institution-specific therapeutic range)	80 units/kg bolus then increase infusion by 4 units/kg/h
37–47 (or 1–12 seconds below institution-specific therapeutic range)	40 units/kg bolus then increase infusion by 2 units/kg/h
48–71 (within institution-specific therapeutic range)	No change
72–93 (or 1–22 seconds above institution-specific therapeutic range)	Decrease infusion by 2 units/kg/h
Greater than 93 (or greater than 22 seconds above institution-specific therapeutic range)	Hold infusion for 1 hour then decrease by 3 units/kg/h

aPTT, activated partial thromboplastin time; IBW, ideal body weight; UFH, unfractionated heparin. VTE, venous thromboembolism.

[a]Use actual body weight for all calculations. Adjusted body weight (ABW) may be used for morbidly obese patients (greater than 130% of IBW).

ABW = IBW + (Actual body weight − IBW) × 0.7.

activated clotting time (ACT), antifactor Xa activity, and the plasma heparin concentration.[4,33] Although it has several limitations, the aPTT is the most widely used test in clinical practice to monitor UFH. Traditionally, therapeutic aPTT range is defined as 1.5 to 2.5 times the control aPTT value. However, due to variations in the reagents and instruments used to measure the aPTT in different laboratories, each institution should establish a therapeutic range for UFH. The institution-specific therapy range should correlate with a plasma heparin concentration of 0.2 to 0.4 units/mL by protamine titration or 0.3 to 0.7 units/mL by an amidolytic antifactor Xa assay.[4,33] An aPTT should be obtained at baseline, 6 hours after initiating the heparin infusion, and 6 hours after each dose change because this is the time required to reach steady state. The UFH dose is then adjusted based on the aPTT measurement and the institutional-specific therapeutic range (Table 10–7). In patients with heparin resistance, antifactor Xa concentrations may be a more accurate method of monitoring the patient's response.[4,33]

Side effects associated with UFH include bleeding, thrombocytopenia, hypersensitivity reactions, and, with prolonged use, alopecia, hyperkalemia, and osteoporosis.[4,29] **7** *Bleeding is the most common adverse effect associated with antithrombotic drugs including UFH therapy. A patient's risk of major hemorrhage is related to the intensity and stability of therapy, age, concurrent drug use, history of GI bleeding, risk of falls or trauma, and recent surgery.* Several risk

---

Table 10–8

Risk Factors for Major Bleeding While Taking Anticoagulation Therapy

Anticoagulation intensity (e.g., INR greater than 5, aPTT greater than 120 seconds)
Initiation of therapy (first few days and weeks)
Unstable anticoagulation response
Age older than 65 years
Concurrent antiplatelet drug use
Concurrent nonsteroidal anti-inflammatory drug or aspirin use
History of GI bleeding
Recent surgery or trauma
High risk for fall/trauma
Heavy alcohol use
Renal failure
Cerebrovascular disease
Malignancy

aPTT, activated partial thromboplastin time; INR, international normalized ratio.

Table 10–9

Contraindications to Anticoagulation Therapy

General
Active bleeding
Hemophilia or other hemorrhagic tendencies
Severe liver disease with elevated baseline PT
Severe thrombocytopenia (platelet count less than $20 \times 10^3/mm^3$ [$20 \times 10^9/L$])
Malignant hypertension
Inability to meticulously supervise and monitor treatment

Product-Specific Contraindications
UFH
  Hypersensitivity to UFH
  History of HIT
LMWHs
  Hypersensitivity to LMWH, UFH, pork products, methylparaben, or propylparaben
  History of HIT or suspected HIT
Fondaparinux
  Hypersensitivity to fondaparinux
  Severe renal insufficiency (CrCl less than 30 mL/min) [0.50 mL/s])
  Body weight less than 50 kg (110 lb)
  Bacterial endocarditis
  Thrombocytopenia with a positive in vitro test for antiplatelet antibodies in the presence of fondaparinux
Lepirudin
  Hypersensitivity to hirudins
Argatroban
  Hypersensitivity to argatroban
Warfarin
  Hypersensitivity to warfarin
  Pregnancy
  History of warfarin-induced skin necrosis
  Inability to obtain follow-up PT/INR measurements
  Inappropriate medication use or lifestyle behaviors
Dabigatran
  Hypersensitivity to dabigatran
  Severe renal insufficiency (CrCl less than 15 mL/min [0.25 mL/s])
Rivaroxaban
  Hypersensitivity to rivaroxaban
  Severe renal insufficiency (CrCl less than 30 mL/min [0.50 mL/s] when used for VTE prevention)

CrCl, creatinine clearance; HIT, heparin-induced thrombocytopenia; INR, international normalized ratio; LMWHs, low molecular weight heparins; PT, prothrombin time; UFH, unfractionated heparin; VTE, venous thromboembolism.

---

factors can increase the risk of UFH-induced bleeding (Table 10–8). The risk of bleeding is related to the intensity of anticoagulation. Higher aPTT values are associated with an increased risk of bleeding. The risk of major bleeding is 1% to 5% during the first few days of treatment.[3] In addition to the aPTT, hemoglobin, hematocrit, and blood pressure should also be monitored. Concurrent use of UFH with other antithrombotic agents, such as thrombolytics and antiplatelet agents, also increases the risk of bleeding. Patients receiving UFH therapy should be closely monitored for signs and symptoms of bleeding, including epistaxis, hemoptysis, hematuria, hematochezia, melena, severe headache, and joint pain. If major bleeding occurs, UFH should be stopped immediately and the source of bleeding treated.[3,4] If necessary, use protamine sulfate to reverse the effects of UFH. The usual dose is 1 mg protamine sulfate per 100 units of UFH, up to a maximum of 50 mg, given as a slow IV infusion over 10 minutes. The effects of UFH are neutralized in 5 minutes, and the effects of protamine persist for 2 hours. If the bleeding is not controlled or the anticoagulant effect rebounds, repeated doses of protamine may be administered.[4]

Heparin-induced thrombocytopenia (HIT) is a very serious adverse effect associated with UFH use. Platelet counts should be monitored every 2 to 3 days during the course of UFH therapy.[4] HIT should be suspected if the platelet count drops by more than 50% from baseline or to below $120 \times 10^3/mm^3$ ($120 \times 10^9/L$). HIT should also be suspected if thrombosis occurs despite UFH use. Immediate discontinuation of all heparin-containing products including the use of LMWHs is in order. Alternative anticoagulation should be initiated. In patients with contraindications to anticoagulation therapy, UFH should not be administered (Table 10–9).

UFH is an FDA pregnancy category C drug and may be used to treat VTE during pregnancy. UFH should be used with caution in the peripartum period due to the risk of maternal hemorrhage. UFH is not secreted into the breast milk and is safe for use by women who wish to breast-feed.[11] For the treatment of VTE in children, the UFH dose is 50 units/kg bolus followed by an infusion of 20,000 units/m² per 24 hours. Alternatively, a loading dose of 75 units/kg followed by an infusion of 28 units/kg/h if younger than 12 months old and 20 units/kg/h if older than 1 year may be considered.[34]

Low Molecular Weight Heparins The LMWHs are smaller heparin fragments obtained by chemical or enzymatic depolymerization of UFH. LMWHs are heterogeneous mixtures of glycosaminoglycans, and each product has slightly different molecular weight distributions and pharmacologic properties.[4] Compared with UFH, LMWHs have improved pharmacodynamic and pharmacokinetic properties. They exhibit less binding to plasma and cellular proteins, resulting in a more predictable anticoagulant response. Consequently, routine monitoring of anticoagulation activity and dose adjustments are not required in most patients. LMWHs have longer plasma half-lives, allowing once- or twice-daily administration, improved SC bioavailability, and dose-independent renal clearance. In addition, LMWHs have a more favorable side-effect profile than UFH. They are also associated with a lower incidence of HIT and osteopenia. Three LMWHs are currently available in the United States: dalteparin, enoxaparin, and tinzaparin.[4,29]

Like UFH, LMWHs prevent the propagation and growth of formed thrombi. The anticoagulant effect is mediated through a specific pentasaccharide sequence that binds to AT. The primary difference in the pharmacologic activity of UFH and LMWH is their relative inhibition of thrombin (factor IIa) and factor Xa. Smaller heparin fragments cannot bind AT and thrombin simultaneously (Fig. 10–6). Due to their smaller chain length, LMWHs have relatively greater activity against factor Xa and inhibit thrombin to a lesser degree. The antifactor Xa-to-IIa activity ratio for the LMWHs ranges from 2:1 to 4:1. The SC bioavailability of the LMWHs is greater than 90%. The peak anticoagulant effect of the LMWHs is reached 3 to 5 hours after a SC dose. The elimination half-life is 3 to 6 hours and is agent specific. In patients with renal impairment, the half-life of LMWHs is prolonged.[4,29]

The dose of LMWHs for the treatment of VTE is determined based on the patient's weight and is administered SC once or twice daily (Table 10–5). Once-daily dosing of enoxaparin appears to be as effective as twice-daily dosing; however, some data suggest that twice-daily dosing may be more effective in patients who are obese or have cancer.[15,23,35] The dose of enoxaparin is expressed in milligrams, whereas the doses of dalteparin and tinzaparin are expressed in units of antifactor Xa activity. Due to their predictable anticoagulant effect, routine monitoring is not necessary in most patients.[4] LMWHs have been evaluated in a large number of randomized trials and have been shown to be at least as safe and effective as UFH for the treatment of VTE.[15,23] Indeed, the rate of mortality was lower in patients treated with a LMWH in clinical trials. This mortality benefit was primarily seen in patients with cancer.[31,36]

Prior to initiating treatment with a LMWH, baseline laboratory tests should include **prothrombin time** (PT)/INR, aPTT, CBC, and serum creatinine. Monitor the CBC with platelet count every 3 to 5 days during the first 2 weeks of therapy, and every 2 to 4 weeks with extended use.[4] Use LMWHs cautiously in patients with renal impairment due to the potential of drug accumulation and risk of bleeding. Specific dosing recommendations for patients with a creatinine clearance (CrCl) less than 30 mL/min (0.50 mL/s) are currently available for enoxaparin but are lacking for other agents of the class (Table 10–5). Higher mortality rate has been reported in elderly patients with renal dysfunction who were treated with the LMWH tinzaparin. Current guidelines recommend the use of UFH over LMWH in patients with severe renal dysfunction (CrCl less than 30 mL/min [0.50 mL/s]).[15,37]

⑧ *Most patients with an uncomplicated DVT can be managed safely at home.* LMWHs can be easily administered in the outpatient setting, thus enabling the treatment of VTE at home. Several large clinical trials have demonstrated the efficacy and safety of LMWHs for outpatient treatment of DVT.[15,20,31] Acceptance of this treatment approach has increased tremendously over the last several years among clinicians. Patients with DVT with normal vital signs, low bleeding risk, no other comorbid conditions requiring hospitalization, and who are stable may have anticoagulant initiated at home. Although the treatment of patients with PE in the outpatient setting is controversial, patients with submassive PE who are hemodynamically stable can be safely treated in the outpatient setting as well.[15,26] Patients considered for outpatient therapy must be reliable or have adequate caregiver support and must be able to strictly adhere to the prescribed treatment regimen and recommended follow-up visits. Close patient follow-up is critical to the success of any outpatient DVT treatment program. Home DVT treatment results in cost savings and improved patient satisfaction and quality of life.[20,37,38]

Laboratory methods of measuring a patient's response to LMWH may be warranted in certain situations.[4,39] Although controversial, measurement of antifactor Xa activity has been the most widely used method in clinical practice and is recommended by the College of American Pathologists.[39] Monitoring of antifactor Xa activity may be considered in adult patients who are morbidly obese (weight greater than 150 kg [330 lb] or body mass index [BMI] greater than 50 kg/m^2), weigh less than 50 kg (110 lb), or have significant renal impairment (CrCl less than 30 mL/min [0.50 mL/s]). Laboratory monitoring may also be useful in children and pregnant women. When monitoring antifactor Xa activity, the sample should be obtained approximately 4 hours after the SC dose is administered when peak concentration is anticipated. The therapeutic range for antifactor Xa activity has not been clearly defined, and there is a limited correlation between antifactor Xa activity and safety or efficacy.[39] For the treatment of VTE, an acceptable antifactor Xa activity range is 0.5 to 1 units/mL (0.5 to 1 kU/L) with twice-daily dosing. In patients treated with once-daily LMWH regimens, a target level between 1 and 2 units/mL (1 to 2 kU/L) is recommended by some experts.[4,15,35,39]

Similar to UFH, bleeding is the major complication associated with LMWHs. The frequency of major bleeding appears to be numerically lower with LMWHs than with UFH.[31] The incidence of major bleeding reported in clinical trials is less than 3%.[15] Minor bleeding, especially bruising at the injection site, occurs frequently. Protamine sulfate will partially reverse the anticoagulant effects of the LMWHs and should be administered in the event of major bleeding. Due to its limited binding to LMWH chains, protamine only neutralizes 60% of their antithrombotic activity. If the LMWH was administered within the previous 8 hours, give 1 mg protamine sulfate per 1 mg of enoxaparin or 100 antifactor Xa units of dalteparin or tinzaparin. If the bleeding is not controlled, give 0.5 mg of protamine sulfate for every antifactor Xa 100 units of LMWH. Give smaller protamine doses if more than 8 hours have lapsed since the last LMWH dose.[4]

The incidence of HIT is lower with LMWHs than with UFH. However, LMWHs cross-react with heparin antibodies in vitro and should not be given as an alternative anticoagulant in patients with a diagnosis or history of HIT. Monitor platelet counts every few days during the first 2 weeks and periodically thereafter.[4]

In patients undergoing spinal and epidural anesthesia or spinal puncture, spinal and epidural hematomas have been linked to the use of LMWHs. In patients with in-dwelling epidural catheters, concurrent use of LMWHs and all other agents that impact hemostasis should be avoided. When inserting and removing the in-dwelling epidural catheters, the timing of LMWH administration around catheter manipulation should be carefully coordinated. Catheter manipulation should only occur at minimal or trough anticoagulant levels.[4]

LMWHs are an excellent alternative to UFH for the treatment of VTE in pregnant women.[11] The LMWHs do not cross the placenta, and they are FDA pregnancy category B. Because the pharmacokinetics of LMWHs may change during pregnancy, monitor antifactor Xa activity every 4 to 6 weeks to make dose adjustments.[11,40] LMWHs have also been used to treat VTE in pediatric patients. Children younger than 1 year require higher doses (e.g., enoxaparin 1.5 mg/kg SC every 12 hours). Monitor antifactor Xa activity to guide dosing in children.[34]

Factor Xa Inhibitors Fondaparinux, the first agent in this class, is an indirect inhibitor of factor Xa and exerts its anticoagulant activity by accelerating AT. Fondaparinux contains the specific five-saccharide sequence found in UFH that is responsible for its pharmacologic activity. Due to its small size, fondaparinux exerts inhibitory activity specifically against factor Xa and has no effect on thrombin (factor IIa; Fig. 10–6).[29,41] Fondaparinux is currently the only agent of the class that is commercially available in the United States for the treatment of VTE. Idraparinux, rivaroxaban, and apixaban are antifactor Xa inhibitors that have completed or are currently undergoing phase 3 clinical trials for VTE treatment.[42] Rivaroxaban was recently approved by the FDA for VTE prevention after major orthopedic surgery and stroke prevention in atrial fibrillation. The efficacy and safety of rivaroxaban for VTE treatment has been demonstrated in two recently published trials, and an indication for VTE treatment is expected in the near future. Fondaparinux and idraparinux are administered SC; rivaroxaban and apixaban are administered orally. After SC administration, fondaparinux is completely absorbed, and peak plasma concentrations are reached within 2 to 3 hours.[41,42] After oral administration, rivaroxaban achieves peak plasma concentrations within 4 hours.[42]

As synthetic drugs (unlike UFH and the LMWHs), factor Xa inhibitors cannot transmit animal pathogens, are consistent from batch to batch, and are available in an unlimited supply. Other favorable attributes of factor Xa inhibitors include a predictable and linear dose–response relationship, rapid onset of activity, and long half-life.[29,41,42] Factor Xa inhibitors do not require routine coagulation monitoring or dose adjustments. Fondaparinux has a half-life of 17 to 21 hours, permitting

once- daily administration, but the anticoagulant effects of fondaparinux will persist for 2 to 4 days after stopping the drug. In patients with renal impairment, the anticoagulant effect persists even longer. Idraparinux has a significantly longer duration of activity and is being developed for once-weekly injection. The oral agents rivaroxaban and apixaban have half-lives ranging from 5 to 14 hours allowing once- or twice-daily administration.[41,42] Rivaroxaban has a relative oral bioavailability of 80% and dual excretion via both the biliary (28%) and renal (66%) routes, and it is metabolized via multiple CYP450 pathways as well as non-CYP-mediated hydrolysis. Metabolism is primarily mediated through CYP3A4/3A5, and to a lesser extent CYP2J2, indicating a concern for drug interactions with other CYP3A4 or P-glycoprotein (P-gp) substrates. Rivaroxaban use is contraindicated in patients with hepatic disease, including Child-Pugh class B and C, because it has been associated with coagulopathy and clinically relevant bleeding. Approximately two-thirds of rivaroxaban is excreted renally, and use in patients with decreased renal function has led to increases in rivaroxaban exposure. Therefore, rivaroxaban should be used with caution in patients with moderate renal dysfunction (CrCl 30 to 49 mL/min [0.50 to 0.82 mL/s]) and contraindicated in patients with severe renal impairment when used for VTE prevention (CrCl less than 30 mL/min [0.50 mL/s]).[42]

Neither fondaparinux nor idraparinux are metabolized in the liver and therefore have few drug interactions. However, concurrent use with other antithrombotic agents increases the risk of bleeding. Unlike the heparins, factor Xa inhibitors do not affect platelet function and do not react with the heparin platelet factor (PF)-4 antibodies seen in patients with HIT. Some centers use fondaparinux in patients with subacute HIT or a history of HIT who require anticoagulation therapy.[4,29,41]

Fondaparinux is as safe and effective as IV UFH for the treatment of PE and SC LMWH for DVT treatment.[43,44] The recommended dose for fondaparinux in the treatment of VTE is based on the patient's weight (Table 10–5). Fondaparinux is renally eliminated, and accumulation can occur in patients with renal dysfunction. Due to the lack of specific dosing guidelines, fondaparinux is contraindicated in patients with severe renal impairment (CrCl less than 30 mL/min [0.50 mL/s]). Baseline renal function should be measured and monitored closely during the course of therapy. Based on limited available data at this time, monitoring antifactor Xa activity to guide fondaparinux dosing is not recommended.[4,15,29]

As with other anticoagulants, the major side effect associated with fondaparinux is bleeding. Fondaparinux should be used with caution in elderly patients because their risk of bleeding is higher. Patients receiving fondaparinux should be carefully monitored for signs and symptoms of bleeding. A CBC should be obtained at baseline and monitored periodically to detect the possibility of occult bleeding. In the event of major bleeding, fresh-frozen plasma and factor concentrates should be given. In the case of a life-threatening bleed, recombinant factor VIIa may be considered, but this is a very costly option and it can also increase the risk of thrombosis. Fondaparinux is not reversed by protamine.[4,15,29,41]

Fondaparinux is pregnancy category B, but there are very limited data regarding its use during pregnancy. Use in pediatric patients has not been studied.[4,29,41]

DTIs Given that thrombin is the central mediator of coagulation and amplifies its own production, it is a natural target for pharmacologic intervention. DTIs bind thrombin and prevent interactions with their substrates (**Fig. 10–7**). Several injectable DTIs are approved for use in the United States including lepirudin, bivalirudin, argatroban, and desirudin. One oral DTI (dabigatran) is available in the United States, with several other oral DTIs also in development. These agents differ in terms of their chemical structure, molecular weight, and binding to the thrombin molecule. Potential advantages of DTIs include a targeted specificity for thrombin, the ability to inactivate clot-bound thrombin, and an absence of platelet interactions that can lead to HIT. Unlike heparins, DTIs do not require AT as a cofactor and do not bind to plasma proteins. Therefore, they produce a more predictable anticoagulant effect. DTIs are considered the drugs of choice for the treatment of VTE in patients with a diagnosis or history of HIT.[29,41,45]

The prototype of this class is hirudin, which was originally isolated from the salivary glands of the medicinal leech, *Hirudo medicinalis*. Hirudin itself is not commercially available, but recombinant technology has permitted production of hirudin derivatives, namely lepirudin and desirudin.[29,41,45] Lepirudin has a short half-life of approximately 40 minutes after IV administration and 120 minutes when given SC. Elimination of lepirudin is primarily renal; therefore, doses must be adjusted based on the patient's renal function. The dose should be monitored and adjusted to achieve an aPTT ratio of 1.5 to 2.5 times the baseline measurement. Lepirudin is currently approved for use in patients with HIT and related thrombosis. Up to 40% of patients treated with lepirudin develop antibodies to the drug.[29,41,45]

Bivalirudin, a smaller molecular weight DTI, is given by IV infusion. Bivalirudin has a shorter elimination half-life (approximately 25 minutes) than lepirudin and is only partially eliminated renally. Unlike lepirudin, bivalirudin is a reversible inhibitor of thrombin and provides transient antithrombotic activity. Patients with moderate or severe renal impairment (CrCl less than 60 mL/min [1.0 mL/s]) may require dose adjustment because clearance of bivalirudin is reduced by approximately 20% in these patients. Bivalirudin is approved for use in patients with unstable angina undergoing percutaneous transluminal coronary angioplasty. The ACT is used to monitor the anticoagulant effect of bivalirudin during percutaneous coronary intervention (PCI).[29,41,45]

Desirudin is a SC-administered DTI approved for VTE prevention after hip replacement surgery. Desirudin has an elimination half-life of 2 to 3 hours and typically dosed every 12 hours. It is primarily eliminated through the kidneys, so dose reduction is needed in patients with renal impairment. The aPTT should be used to measure desirudin's anticoagulant activity.[29,41,45]

Argatroban is a small synthetic molecule that binds reversibly to the active site of thrombin (Fig. 10–7). Argatroban is IV administered and has a 40- to 50-minute elimination half-life. The aPTT must be monitored to assess its anticoagulant activity. Argatroban is hepatically metabolized; therefore, dose reductions and careful monitoring are recommended in patients with hepatic dysfunction. Renal impairment has no influence on the elimination half-life or dosing of argatroban. Argatroban is approved for prevention and treatment of thrombosis in patients with HIT and in patients with HIT undergoing PCI.[29,41,45]

Small molecule DTIs have been structurally modified for oral administration. Several oral DTIs are in development, with one agent (dabigatran) currently approved in the United States for stroke prevention in patients with atrial fibrillation. Clinical trials have also been completed, and some are ongoing to investigate the efficacy and safety of dabigatran for the treatment of VTE. The potential advantages of oral DTIs include the ability to give them in fixed once- or twice-daily doses, without the need for routine coagulation monitoring, and a fast onset and offset of action, therefore offering more convenient anticoagulation options for patients and providers.[41,45–46]

Dabigatran, is a direct reversible, competitive inhibitor of thrombin and an oral prodrug of dabigatran etexilate. Dabigatran is converted to dabigatran etexilate by serum esterases that are independent of CYP450 pathways. Dabigatran has a half-life of 12 to 17 hours in healthy subjects and onset of effect of 2 hours. Dabigatran has an oral bioavailability of approximately 3% to 7% and requires an acidic environment for absorption. The prodrug is contained in small pellets coated with an acid core. These pellets are enclosed in a capsule shell. This specific capsule formulation improves the dissolution and absorption of the prodrug, independent of gastric pH. Therefore the capsules should not be broken, chewed, or opened

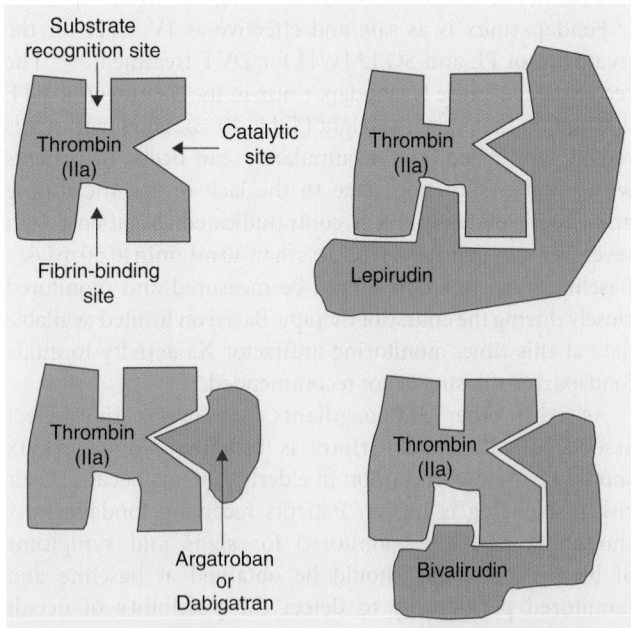

FIGURE 10–7. Mechanism of action of direct thrombin inhibitors. (From Witt DM, Nutescu EA, Haines S. Venous thromboembolism. In: DiPiro JT, Talbert RL, Yee GC, et al., eds. Pharmacotherapy: A Pathophysiologic Approach, 8th ed. New York, NY: McGraw-Hill, 2011:326.)

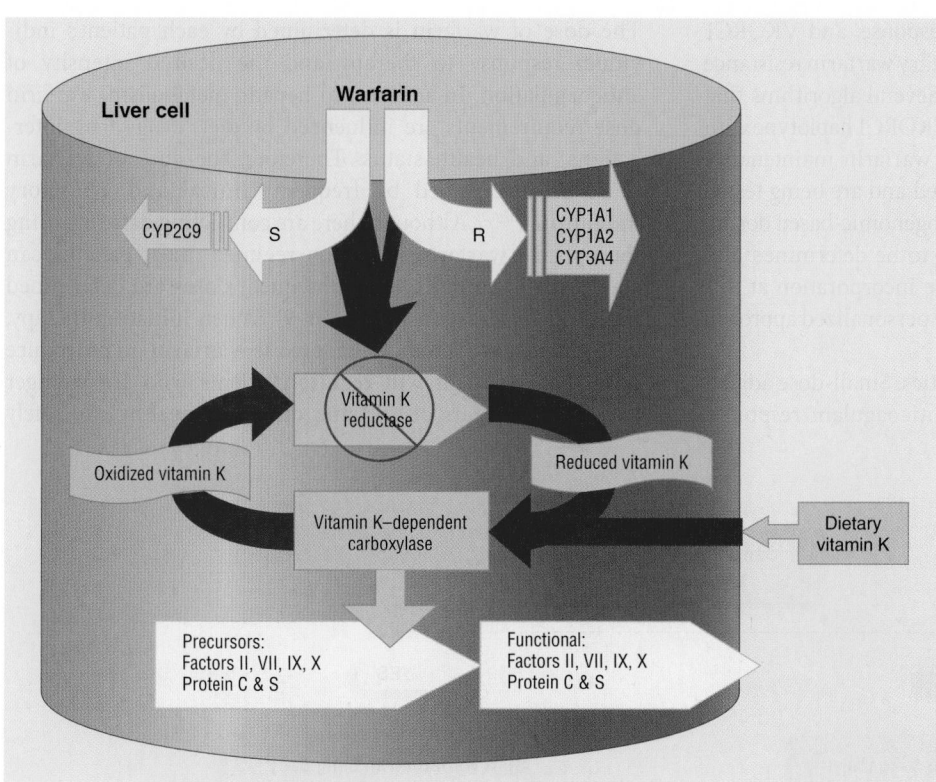

FIGURE 10–8. Pharmacologic activity and metabolism of warfarin. (CYP, cytochrome P-450 isoenzyme.) (From Witt DM, Nutescu EA, Haines S. Venous thromboembolism. In: DiPiro JT, Talbert RL, Yee GC, et al., eds. Pharmacotherapy: A Pathophysiologic Approach, 8th ed. New York, NY: McGraw-Hill, 2011:328.)

before administration. Dabigatran demonstrates 35% protein binding and is a substrate of the efflux transporter P-gp. Although the absence of CYP450 metabolism decreases potential for many drug interactions, coadministration with substrates, inhibitors, or inducers may affect the efficacy of dabigatran. Approximately 80% of dabigatran is eliminated in the urine, and a dose adjustment is recommended in patients with severe renal impairment (CrCl 15 to 30 mL/min [0.25 to 0.50 mL/s]). The use of dabigatran is contraindicated in patients with a CrCl less than 15 mL/min (0.25 mL/s).[41,46]

Contraindications to the use of DTIs and risk factors for bleeding are similar to those of other antithrombotic agents (Tables 10–8 and 10–9). Bleeding is the most common side effect reported with the use of DTIs. Concurrent use of DTIs with thrombolytics significantly increases bleeding complications. Currently, there are no known antidotes to reverse the effects of the DTIs. Fresh-frozen plasma, factor concentrates, or recombinant factor VIIa should be given in the event of a major bleed. DTIs can increase the PT/INR and can interfere with the accuracy of monitoring and dosing of warfarin therapy. Data on the use of DTIs in pregnancy and pediatric patients are very limited.[29,41,45]

Warfarin ❾ *Warfarin has been the primary oral anticoagulant used in the United States for the past 60 years. Warfarin is the anticoagulant of choice when long-term or extended anticoagulation is required.* Warfarin is FDA approved for the prevention and treatment of VTE, as well as the prevention of thromboembolic complications in patients with myocardial infarction, atrial fibrillation, and heart valve replacement. Although very effective, warfarin has a narrow

therapeutic index, requiring frequent dose adjustments and careful patient monitoring.[5,29]

Warfarin exerts its anticoagulant effect by inhibiting the production of the vitamin K–dependent coagulation factors II (prothrombin), VII, IX, and X, as well as the anticoagulant proteins C and S (Fig. 10–8). Warfarin has no effect on circulating coagulation factors that have been previously formed, and its full antithrombotic activity is delayed for 5 to 7 days, and potentially longer in slower metabolizers. This delay is related to half-lives of the clotting factors: 60 to 100 hours for factor II (prothrombin), 6 to 8 hours for factor VII, 20 to 30 hours for factor IX, and 24 to 40 hours for factor X. Proteins C and S, the natural anticoagulants, are inhibited more rapidly due to their shorter half-lives, 8 to 10 hours and 40 to 60 hours, respectively. Reductions in the concentration of natural anticoagulants before the clotting factors are depleted can lead to a paradoxical hypercoagulable state during the first few days of warfarin therapy. It is for this reason that patients with acute thrombosis should receive a fast-acting anticoagulant (heparin, LMWH, or fondaparinux) while transitioning to warfarin therapy.[5,20,29]

Warfarin is a racemic mixture of two isomers, the S and the R forms. The S-isomer is two to five times more potent than the R-isomer. Both isomers are extensively bound to albumin. The two isomers are metabolized in the liver via several isoenzymes including cytochrome P-450 (CYP) 1A2, 2C9, 2C19, 2C18, and 3A4 (Fig. 10–8). Hepatic metabolism of warfarin varies greatly among patients, leading to very large interpatient differences in dose requirements and genetic variations in these isoenzymes; specifically, polymorphisms in the CYP2C9*2, CYP2C9*3 genotype result in significantly lower warfarin dose requirement to achieve a therapeutic response, and VKORC1 haplotype mutations can result in hereditary warfarin resistance and increased warfarin requirements.[5] Several algorithms that incorporate CYP2C9 genotype and the VKORC1 haplotype with other patient characteristics to predict warfarin maintenance dosing requirements have been developed and are being tested in large populations. Whether pharmacogenomic-based dosing will improve clinical outcomes has yet to be determined and is not widely recommended for practice incorporation at this time, but it does hold promise for a more personalized approach to warfarin dosing.[5,47]

Warfarin does not follow linear kinetics. Small-dose adjustments can lead to large changes in anticoagulant response.

The dose of warfarin is determined by each patient's individual response to therapy and the desired intensity of anticoagulation. In addition to hepatic metabolism, warfarin dose requirements are influenced by diet, drug–drug interactions, and health status. Therefore, the dose of warfarin must be determined by frequent clinical and laboratory monitoring.[5,20,29] Although there are conflicting data regarding the optimal warfarin induction regimen, most patients can start with 5 mg daily, and subsequent doses are determined based on INR response (Fig. 10–9). When initiating therapy, it is difficult to predict the precise warfarin maintenance dose that a patient will require. Patients who are younger (less than 55 years of age) and otherwise healthy can safely

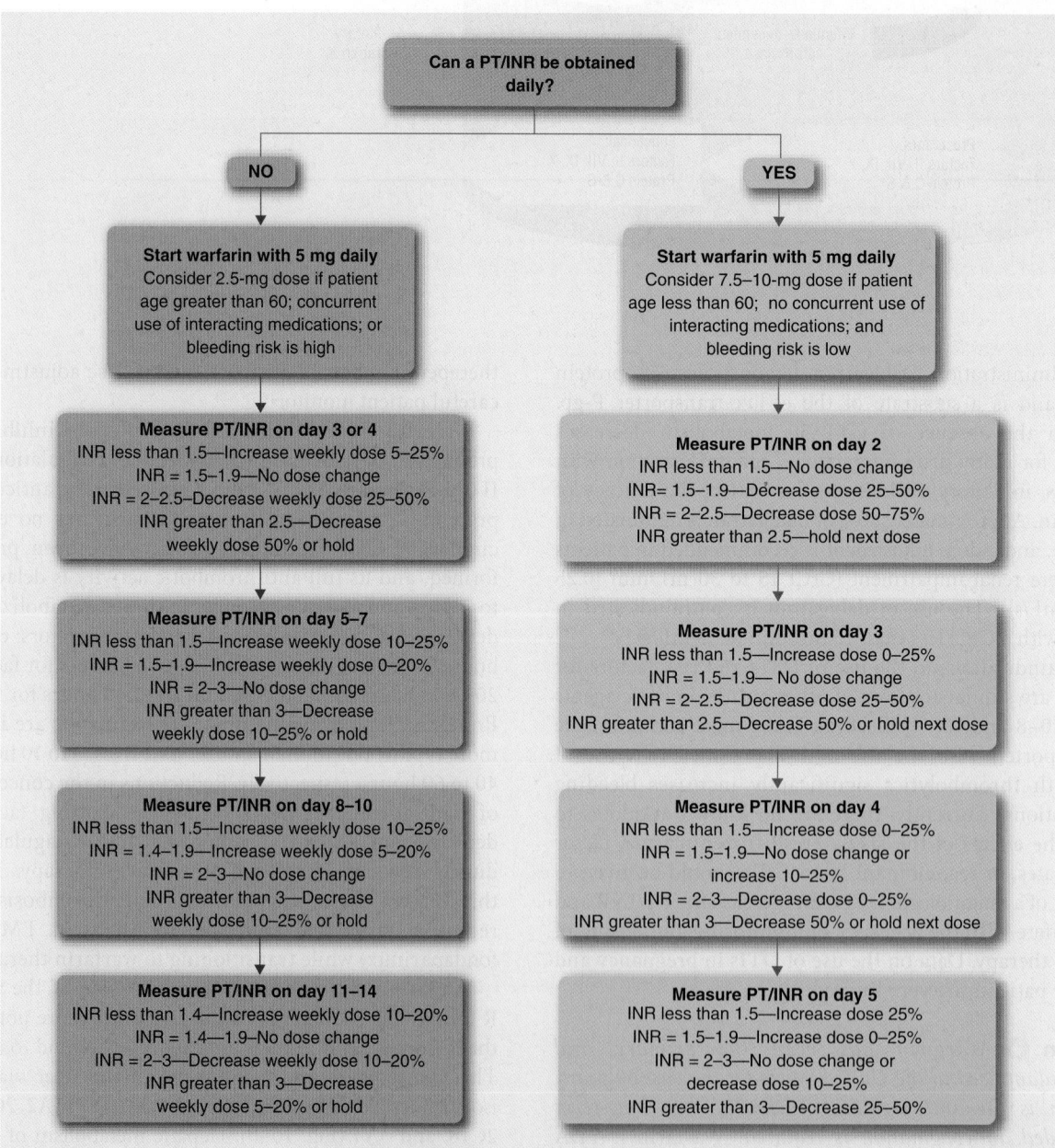

FIGURE 10–9. Initiation of warfarin therapy. (INR, international normalized ratio; PT, prothrombin time.) (From Witt DM, Nutescu EA, Haines S. Venous thromboembolism. In: DiPiro JT, Talbert RL, Yee GC, et al., eds. Pharmacotherapy: A Pathophysiologic Approach, 8th ed. New York, NY: McGraw-Hill, 2011:331.)

use higher warfarin "initiation" doses (e.g., 7.5 or 10 mg). A more conservative "initiation" dose (e.g., 5 mg or less) should be given to elderly patients (older than 75 years), patients with heart failure, liver disease, or poor nutritional status, and patients who are taking interacting medications or are at high risk of bleeding.[5,23] Loading doses of warfarin (e.g., 15 to 20 mg) are not recommended. These large doses can lead to the false impression that a therapeutic INR has been achieved in 2 to 3 days and lead to potential future overdosing.[5] Before initiating therapy, screen the patient for any contraindications to anticoagulation therapy and risk factors for major bleeding (Tables 10–8 and 10–9). In addition, conduct a thorough medication history including the use of prescription and nonprescription drugs, and any herbal supplements to detect interactions that may affect warfarin dosing requirements. In patients with acute VTE, a rapid-acting anticoagulant (UFH, LMWH, or fondaparinux) should be overlapped with warfarin for a minimum of 5 days and until the INR is greater than 2 and stable. This is important because the full antithrombotic effect will not be reached until 5 to 7 days or even longer after initiating warfarin therapy.[5,15] The typical maintenance dose of warfarin for most patients will be between 25 and 55 mg per week, although some patients require higher or lower doses. Adjustments in the maintenance warfarin dose should be determined based on the total weekly dose and by reducing or increasing the weekly dose by increments of 5% to 25%. When adjusting the maintenance dose, wait at least 7 days to ensure that a steady state has been attained on the new dose before checking the INR again. Checking the INR too soon can lead to inappropriate dose adjustments and unstable anticoagulation status.[5]

⑩ *Warfarin requires frequent laboratory monitoring to ensure optimal outcomes and minimize complications.* The PT is the most frequently used test to monitor warfarin's anticoagulant effect. The PT measures the biological activity of factors II, VII, and X. Due to wide variation in reagent sensitivity, different **thromboplastins** will result in different PT results, potentially leading to inappropriate dosing decisions.[5] To standardize result reporting, the World Health Organization (WHO) developed a reference thromboplastin and recommended the INR to monitor warfarin therapy. The INR corrects for the differences in thromboplastin reagents and uses the following formula: $INR = (PT^{Patient}/PT^{Control})^{ISI}$. The International Sensitivity Index (ISI) is a measure of the thromboplastin's responsiveness compared with the WHO reference.[5] The goal or target INR for each patient is based on the indication for warfarin therapy. For the treatment and prevention of VTE, the INR target is 2.5 with an acceptable range of 2 to 3. In certain high-risk patients (e.g., certain mechanical heart valves), a higher target INR of 3 with a range of 2.5 to 3.5 is recommended.[5] Before initiating warfarin therapy, a baseline PT/INR and CBC should be obtained. After initiating warfarin therapy, the INR should be monitored at least every 2 to 3 days during the first week of therapy. Once a stable response to therapy is achieved, INR monitoring is performed less frequently, weekly for the first 1 to 2 weeks, then every 2 weeks, and monthly thereafter.[5,48] At each encounter, the patient should be carefully questioned regarding any

factors that may influence the INR result. These factors include adherence to therapy, the use of interacting medications, consumption of vitamin K–rich foods, alcohol use, and general health status. Patients should also be questioned about symptoms related to bleeding and thromboembolic events. Warfarin dose adjustments should take into account not only the INR result but also patient-related factors that influence

---

Patient Encounter 3, Part 1

CR is a 47-year-old woman who presents to the emergency department complaining of chest pain, shortness of breath, and lightheadedness. The patient states that her symptoms started with some mild left calf pain approximately 5 days ago. She started feeling short of breath and experiencing chest pain last evening. She could not sleep, and her shortness of breath has gotten progressively worse in the last several hours. CR was hospitalized because she was suspected to have a PE.

PMH: Obesity × 12 years; chronic obstructive pulmonary disease

FH: Mother died of a stroke; paternal grandmother had clots in her legs

SH: The patient is a bus driver.

Current meds: Albuterol (salbutamol) metered-dose inhaler as needed; ortho-Tri-Cyclen Lo by mouth daily; echinacea one to two tablets by mouth daily as needed; multivitamin one tablet by mouth daily

Allergies: Shellfish, NKDA

PE:

VS: BP 104/64 mm Hg, HR 102 bpm, RR 20, T 38°C (100.4°F), wt 96 kg (211 lb), ht 65 in. (165 cm)

Labs: Within normal limits; eGFR 101 mL/min/1.73 m² (0.97 mL/s/m²)

Procedures/Tests

ECG: Normal sinus rhythm

CXR: Slightly enlarged heart

V/Q scan: High probability of PE

What symptoms are consistent with the diagnosis of PE in CR's case? What are the most likely etiologies for PE in this case?

What are appropriate initial and chronic treatment options for CR?

If UFH is chosen as the initial anticoagulation treatment option, what is the goal aPTT?

What is CR's goal INR for warfarin therapy?

How long should CR remain on anticoagulation therapy?

Given the list of medications CR took prior to hospitalization, should any of these medications be discontinued or changed? If changed, what alternative therapy would you recommend?

the result. Structured anticoagulation therapy management services (anticoagulation clinics) have been demonstrated to improve the efficacy and safety of warfarin therapy when compared with "usual" medical care.[5,48] Some patients engage in self-testing and self-management by using a point-of-care PT/INR device approved for home use. Highly motivated and well-trained patients are good candidates for self-testing or self-management.[5,48]

❼ *Similar to other anticoagulants, warfarin's primary side effect is bleeding.* Warfarin can unmask an existing lesion. The incidence of warfarin-related bleeding appears to be highest during the first few weeks of therapy. The annual incidence of major bleeding ranges from 1% to 10% depending on the

quality of warfarin therapy management. Bleeding in the GI tract is most common. Intracranial hemorrhage (ICH) is one of the most serious complications because it often causes severe disability and death. The intensity of anticoagulation therapy is related to bleeding risk. Higher INRs result in higher bleeding risk, and the risk of ICH increases when the INR exceeds 4.[3,5] Instability and wide fluctuations in the INR are also associated with higher bleeding risk. In cases of warfarin overdose or overanticoagulation, vitamin K may be used to reverse warfarin's effect (Fig. 10–10).[5] Vitamin K can be given by the IV or oral route; the SC route is not recommended. When given SC, vitamin K is erratically absorbed and frequently ineffective. The IV route

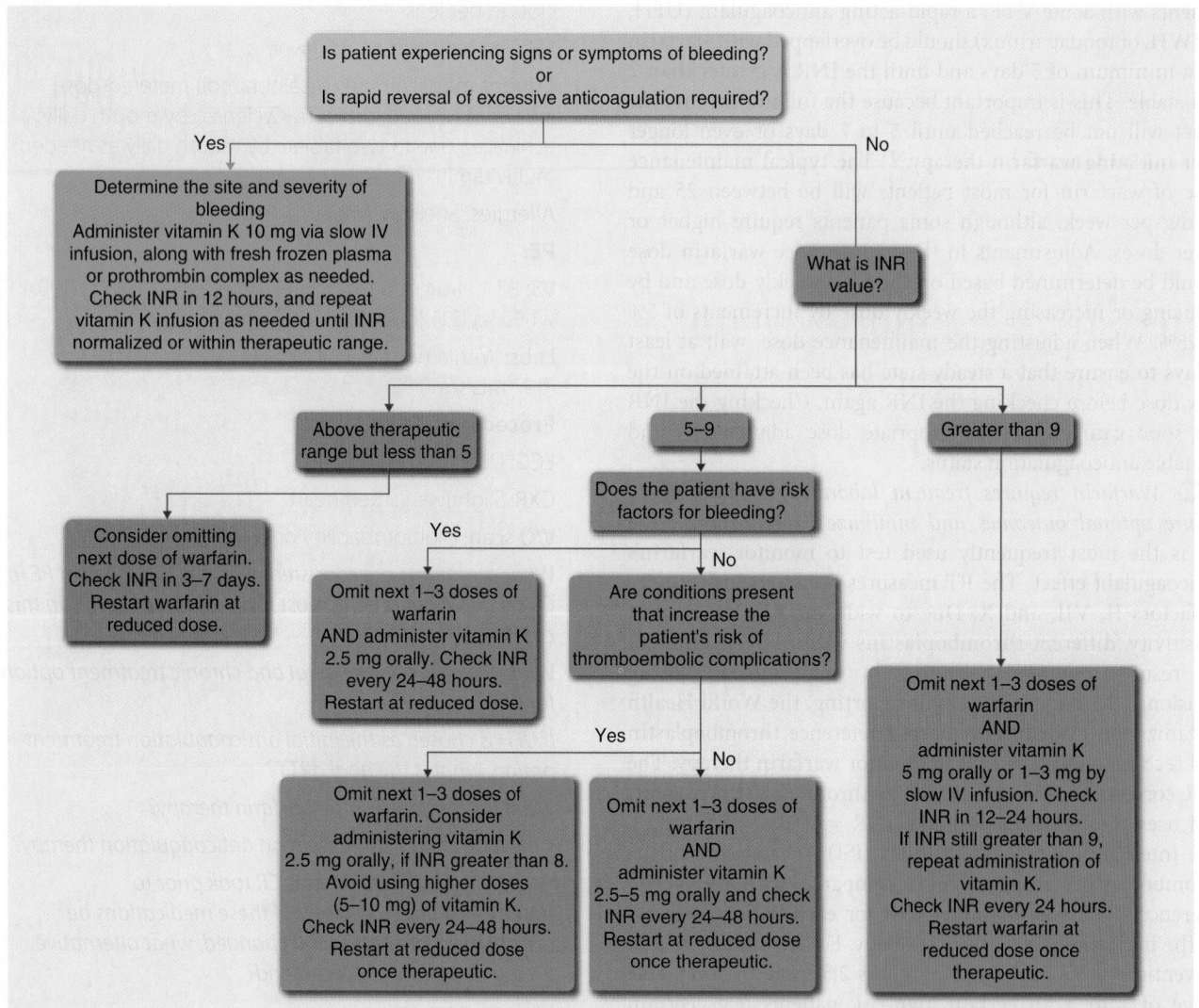

FIGURE 10–10. Management of an elevated INR in patients taking warfarin. Dose reductions should be made by determining the weekly warfarin dose and reducing the weekly dose by 10% to 25% based on the degree of INR elevation. Conditions that increase the risk of thromboembolic complications include history of hypercoagulability disorders (e.g., protein C or S deficiency, presence of antiphospholipid antibodies, antithrombin deficiency, or activated protein C resistance), arterial or venous thrombosis within the previous month, thromboembolism associated with malignancy, mechanical mitral valve in conjunction with atrial fibrillation, previous stroke, poor ventricular function, or coexisting mechanical aortic valve. (INR, international normalized ratio.) (From Witt DM, Nutescu EA, Haines S. Venous thromboembolism. In: DiPiro JT, Talbert RL, Yee GC, et al., eds. Pharmacotherapy: A Pathophysiologic Approach, 8th ed. New York, NY: McGraw-Hill, 2011:333.)

is reserved for cases of severe warfarin overdose (e.g., INR greater than 20) or major bleeding. Anaphylactoid reactions have been reported with rapid IV administration; therefore, slow infusion is recommended. An oral dose of vitamin K will reduce the INR within 24 hours. If the INR is still elevated after 24 hours, another dose of oral vitamin K can be given. The dose of vitamin K should be based on the INR elevation. A dose of 1 to 2.5 mg is sufficient when the INR is between 5 and 9, but 5 mg may be required for INRs greater than 9. Higher doses (e.g., 10 mg) can lead to prolonged warfarin resistance. In cases of life-threatening bleeding, fresh-frozen plasma or clotting factor concentrates should be administered, in addition to IV vitamin K. In patients in whom the INR is less than 9 and there is no active bleeding or imminent risk of bleeding, simply withholding warfarin until the INR decreases to within therapeutic range and reducing the weekly dose with more frequent monitoring is appropriate.[5]

Nonhemorrhagic side effects related to warfarin are rare but can be severe when they occur. Warfarin-induced skin necrosis presents as an eggplant-colored skin lesion or a maculopapular rash that can progress to necrotic gangrene. It usually manifests in fatty areas such as the abdomen, buttocks, and breasts. The incidence is less than 0.1%, and it generally appears during the first week of therapy. Patients with protein C or S deficiency or those who receive large loading doses of warfarin are at greatest risk.[5,11] The mechanism is thought to be due to imbalances between procoagulant and anticoagulant proteins early in the course of warfarin therapy. Warfarin-induced purple toe syndrome is another rare side effect; patients present with a purplish discoloration of their toes. If these side effects are suspected, warfarin therapy should be discontinued immediately and an alternative anticoagulant given. There is a theoretical risk that warfarin may cause accelerated bone loss with long-term use, but to date there is no evidence to support this concern. Warfarin is teratogenic and is FDA pregnancy category X. It should be avoided during pregnancy, and women of childbearing potential should be instructed to use an effective form of contraception. UFH and LMWH are the agents of choice for the treatment of VTE during pregnancy.[5,11]

🔟 Warfarin is prone to numerous clinically significant drug–drug and drug–food interactions (Tables 10–10, 10–11, and 10–12). Patients on warfarin should be questioned at every encounter to assess for any potential interactions with foods, drugs, herbal products, and nutritional supplements. When an interacting drug is initiated or discontinued, more frequent monitoring should be instituted. In addition, the dose of warfarin can be modified (increased or decreased) in anticipation of the expected impact on the INR.[5,49] Warfarin-related drug interactions can generally be divided into two major categories: pharmacokinetic and pharmacodynamic. Pharmacokinetic interactions are most commonly due to changes in hepatic metabolism or binding to plasma proteins. Drugs that affect the CYP2C9, CYP3A4, and CYP1A2 have the greatest impact on warfarin metabolism. Interactions that impact the metabolism of the S-isomer result in greater changes in the INR than interactions

affecting the R-isomer. Pharmacodynamic drug interactions enhance or diminish the anticoagulant effect of warfarin, increasing the risk of bleeding or clotting, but may not alter the INR.[5,49] There are increasing reports regarding dietary supplements, nutraceuticals, and vitamins that can interact with warfarin.[50] Patients on warfarin may experience changes in the INR due to fluctuating intake of dietary vitamin K. Patients should be instructed to maintain a consistent diet and avoid large fluctuations in vitamin K intake rather than strictly avoiding vitamin K–rich foods.[50]

Table 10–10

Clinically Significant Warfarin Drug Interactions

Increase Anticoagulation Effect (↑ INR)	Decrease Anticoagulation Effect (↓ INR)	Increase Bleeding Risk
Acetaminophen	Amobarbital	Argatroban
Alcohol binge	Butabarbital	Aspirin
Allopurinol	Carbamazepine	Clopidogrel
Amiodarone	Cholestyramine	Danaparoid
Cephalosporins (with MTP side chain)	Dicloxacillin	Dipyridamole
Chloral hydrate	Griseofulvin	LMWHs
Chloramphenicol	Nafcillin	Nonsteroidal anti-inflammatory drugs
Cimetidine	Phenobarbital	
Ciprofloxacin	Phenytoin	Ticlopidine
Clofibrate	Primidone	UFH
Danazol	Rifampin	
Disulfiram	Secobarbital	
Doxycycline	Sucralfate	
Erythromycin	Vitamin K	
Fenofibrate		
Fluconazole		
Fluorouracil		
Fluoxetine		
Fluvoxamine		
Gemfibrozil		
Influenza vaccine		
Isoniazid		
Itraconazole		
Lovastatin		
Metronidazole		
Miconazole		
Moxalactam		
Neomycin		
Norfloxacin		
Ofloxacin		
Omeprazole		
Phenylbutazone		
Piroxicam		
Propafenone		
Propoyxphene		
Quinidine		
Sertraline		
Sulfamethoxazole		
Sulfinpyrazone		
Tamoxifen		
Testosterone		
Vitamin E		
Zafirlukast		

INR, international normalized ratio; LMWHs, low molecular weight heparins; UFH, unfractionated heparin.

Table 10–11

Potential Warfarin Interactions With Herbal and Nutritional Products

Increased Anticoagulation Effect (Increase Bleeding Risk or ↑ INR)		Decreased Anticoagulation Effect (↓INR)
Arnica flower	Ginkgo	Coenzyme Q$_{10}$
Angelica root	Horse chestnut	Ginseng
Anise	Licorice root	Green tea
Asafoetida	Lovage root	St. John's wort
Bogbean	Meadowsweet	
Borage seed oil	Onion	
Bromelain	Papain	
Capsicum	Parsley	
Celery	Passionflower herb	
Chamomile	Poplar	
Clove	Quassia	
Danshen	Red clover	
Devil's claw	Rue	
Dong quai	Sweet clover	
Fenugreek	Turmeric	
Feverfew	Vitamin E	
Garlic	Willow bark	
Ginger		

INR, International Normalized Ratio.

Table 10–12

Vitamin K Content of Select Foods[a]

Very High (Greater Than 200 mcg)	High (100–200 mcg)	Medium (50–100 mcg)	Low (Less Than 50 mcg)
Brussels sprouts	Basil	Apple, green	Apple, red
Chickpea	Broccoli	Asparagus	Avocado
Collard greens	Canola oil	Cabbage	Beans
Coriander	Chive	Cauliflower	Breads and
Endive	Coleslaw	Mayonnaise	grains
Kale	Cucumber	Pistachios	Carrot
Lettuce, red	(unpeeled)	Squash,	Celery
leaf	Green onion/	summer	Cereal
Parsley	scallion		Coffee
Spinach	Lettuce,		Corn
Swiss chard	butterhead		Cucumber
Tea, black	Mustard greens		(peeled)
Tea, green	Soybean oil		Dairy
Turnip greens			products
Watercress			Eggs
			Fruit (varies)
			Lettuce, iceberg
			Meats, fish, poultry
			Pasta
			Peanuts
			Peas
			Potato
			Rice
			Tomato

[a]Approximate amount of vitamin K per 100 g (3.5 oz) serving.

Patient Encounter 3, Part 2

CR is discharged home on warfarin therapy. She was referred to a local area antithrombosis center for monitoring of her oral anticoagulation therapy and has been maintained on warfarin 6 mg daily for the last 3 months. The patient presents today for a routine visit for anticoagulation monitoring and her INR is 10.3. She reports that 6 days ago she was started on ciprofloxacin 500 mg by mouth twice daily, which was prescribed by her primary care physician for a urinary tract infection. In addition, the primary care physician told the patient that her thyroid gland was enlarged and ordered some lab tests to determine if she has a thyroid problem. The patient has not received the results. She also reports that her intake of vitamin K–rich foods (spinach, broccoli, and cabbage) has increased significantly over the last month because she is trying to lose weight. CR has no other complaints today and denies any signs or symptoms of bleeding.

What is the most likely explanation for the elevated INR in CR's case?

Should CR be given vitamin K? If yes, discuss the dose, route of administration, and an appropriate patient monitoring plan.

How will you manage CR's warfarin therapy? Outline a plan including specific dose changes, timing of monitoring, and patient education.

▶ Nonpharmacologic Therapy

Thrombectomy Most cases of VTE can be successfully treated with anticoagulation. In some cases, removal of the occluding thrombus by surgical intervention may be warranted. Surgical or mechanical thrombectomy can be considered in patients with massive iliofemoral DVT when there is a risk of limb gangrene due to venous occlusion. The procedure can be complicated by recurrence of thrombus formation. In patients who present with massive PE, pulmonary embolectomy can be performed in emergency cases when conservative measures have failed. Patients who are hemodynamically unstable and have a contraindication to thrombolysis are candidates for pulmonary embolectomy. Administer heparin by IV infusion to achieve a therapeutic aPTT during the operation and postoperatively. Thereafter, give warfarin for the usual recommended duration.[15,23,28]

Vena Cava Interruption Inferior vena cava (IVC) interruption is indicated in patients with PE who have a contraindication to anticoagulation therapy and in patients who have recurrent VTE while taking anticoagulation therapy.[15,23,28] IVC interruption is accomplished by inserting a filter through the internal jugular vein or femoral vein and advancing it into the IVC using ultrasound or fluoroscopic guidance. IVC filters reduce the short-term risk of PE, but this benefit is not sustained in the long term. The incidence of DVT at 1 year after IVC filter insertion is higher when compared with patients without filters. Survival after a PE is no different in patients with filters versus patients without filters.[21] Therefore, anticoagulation therapy should be resumed as soon as possible after filter insertion and continued as long as the filter is in place due to the high risk of DVT.[15] Temporary or removable filters are now increasingly used and are replacing the use of permanent filters.[15]

Compression Stockings PTS occurs in 20% to 50% of patients within 8 years after a DVT. Wearing GCS after a DVT reduces the risk of PTS by as much as 50%. Current guidelines recommend the use of GCS with an ankle pressure of 30 to 40 mm Hg for 2 years after a DVT. To be effective, GCS must fit properly. Traditionally, strict bed rest has been recommended after a DVT, but this approach has now been refuted, and patients should be encouraged to ambulate as tolerated.[15,20]

APPROACH TO TREATING PATIENTS WITH VTE

Once the diagnosis of VTE has been confirmed with an objective test, promptly start anticoagulation therapy in full therapeutic doses. If there is high clinical suspicion of VTE, anticoagulation therapy may be initiated while waiting for the results of diagnostic tests.[15] Initiate therapy with a rapid-acting anticoagulant such as UFH (given IV or SC), an LMWH (given SC), or fondaparinux (given SC) (Fig. 10–5 and Fig. 10–11). In patients with adequate renal function, the LMWHs and fondaparinux are preferred over UFH.[15] Recent evidence also supports the use of dabigatran and rivaroxaban in the acute and long-term treatment of DVT,[51,52] although neither agent is approved as of yet for this indication in the United States.

For the long-term treatment phase, an oral agent (i.e., warfarin), is the preferred approach. The novel oral agents (i.e., dabigatran, rivaroxaban) will provide more convenient alternatives to warfarin once approved and available for this indication. However, in patients with cancer, the LMWHs are recommended for the initial and subacute phase of treatment of VTE due to better efficacy in preventing recurrent thromboembolic events.[15] The efficacy and safety of dabigatran and rivaroxaban for the treatment of VTE in patients with cancer have not been evaluated in prospective clinical trials. When warfarin is used for treatment of VTE, it is important to initiate warfarin on the first day of therapy after the first dose of rapid-acting anticoagulant is given and overlap the two therapies for a minimum of 5 days. Warfarin should be dosed to achieve a goal INR range of 2 to 3. Once the INR is stable and above 2, the rapid acting anticoagulant should be discontinued.

Anticoagulation therapy is continued for a minimum of 3 months but should be given longer depending on the underlying etiology of the VTE and the patient's risk factors (Table 10–13).[15] Consider a thrombolytic only if the patient has a massive iliofemoral DVT and is at risk of limb gangrene. In patients with PE, consider a thrombolytic if the patient is hemodynamically unstable (i.e., SBP less than 90 mm Hg) or has evidence of right ventricular injury (i.e., elevated troponins).[28] If there is a contraindication to anticoagulation therapy or the patient has a recurrent event while taking an anticoagulant, a vena cava filter should be inserted. Encourage early ambulation as tolerated by the patient during the initial treatment phase.[15]

▶ *Outcome Evaluation*

- Achieve optimal outcomes by (a) preventing the occurrence of VTE in patients who are at risk, (b) administering effective treatments in a timely manner to patients who develop VTE, (c) preventing treatment-related complications, and (d) reducing the likelihood of long-term complications including recurrent events.

- Given that VTE is often clinically silent and potentially fatal, strategies to increase the widespread use of prophylaxis have the greatest potential to improve patient outcomes. Thus relying on the early diagnosis and treatment of VTE is unacceptable because many patients will die before treatment can be initiated.

- Effective VTE prophylaxis programs screen all patients admitted to hospital for VTE risk factors, determine each patient's level of risk, and select and implement prevention strategies that provide sufficient protection for the level of risk.

- Periodically evaluate patients who are receiving VTE prophylaxis for signs and symptoms of DVT, such as swelling, pain, warmth, and redness of lower extremities, and for PE, such as chest pain, shortness of breath, palpitations, and hemoptysis.

- Providing effective treatment in a timely manner is the primary goal for patients who develop VTE. Treat DVT and PE quickly and aggressively with effective doses of anticoagulant drugs.

- The short-term aim of therapy is to prevent propagation or local extension of the clot, embolization, and death.

- Regularly monitor patients for the development of new symptoms or worsening of existing symptoms.

- Anticoagulant drugs require precise dosing and meticulous monitoring. Closely monitor patients receiving anticoagulant therapy for signs and symptoms of bleeding including epistaxis, hemoptysis, hematuria, bright red blood per rectum, tarry stools, severe headache, and joint pain. If major bleeding occurs, stop therapy immediately and treat the source of bleeding. In addition, closely monitor patients for potential drug–drug and drug–food interactions and adherence with the prescribed regimen.

- The long-term goals of therapy are to prevent complications such as the PTS, pulmonary hypertension, and recurrent VTE.

- Encourage all patients who have had DVT to wear GCS.

- Continue long-term therapy (i.e., warfarin) for an appropriate duration based on the etiology of the initial clot and the presence of ongoing risk factors.

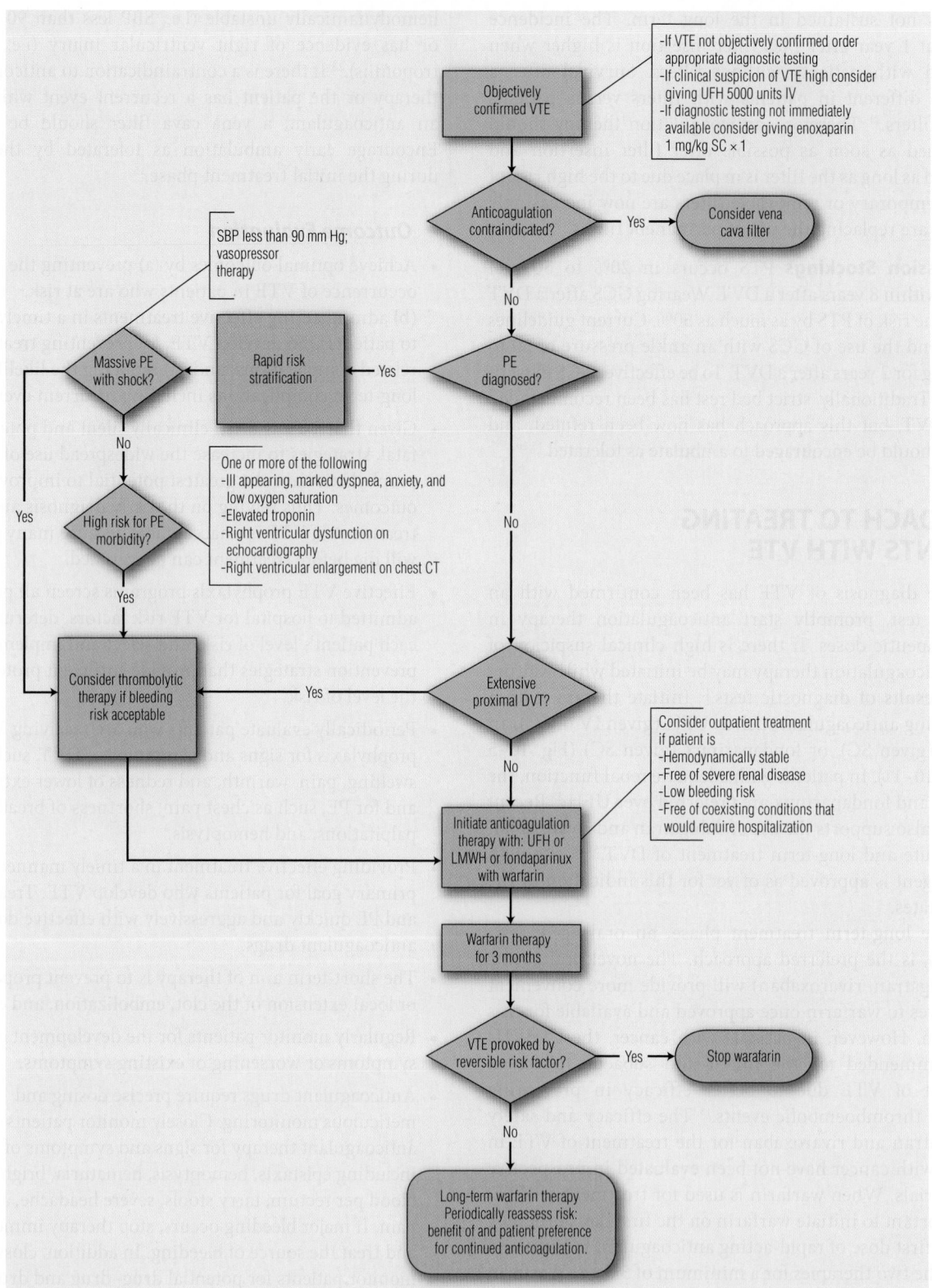

FIGURE 10–11. Treatment of VTE. (CT, computed tomography; DVT, deep vein thrombosis; LMWH, low molecular weight heparin; PE, pulmonary embolism; SBP, systolic blood pressure; SC, subcutaneous; UFH, unfractionated heparin; VTE, venous thromboembolism.) (From Witt DM, Nutescu EA, Haines S. Venous thromboembolism. In: DiPiro JT, Talbert RL, Yee GC, et al., eds. Pharmacotherapy: A Pathophysiologic Approach, 8th ed. New York, NY: McGraw-Hill, 2011:338.)

> ## Table 10–13

Duration of Anticoagulation Therapy for the Treatment of VTE

Patient Characteristics	Drug	Duration of Therapy (Months)	Comments
First episode of VTE secondary to a transient (reversible) risk factor	Warfarin	3	Recommendation applies to both proximal and calf vein thrombosis
First episode, unprovoked VTE	Warfarin	At least 3	After 3 months of therapy, evaluate patient for risk–benefit of long-term therapy
First episode, unprovoked proximal DVT or unprovoked PE		Long term	If risk for bleeding is low and good adherence to therapy and monitoring requirements are maintained
First episode of VTE and cancer	LMWH	6	LMWH is recommended over warfarin for the initial 6 months. Subsequent therapy (beyond the initial 6 months) until cancer is resolved is recommended with warfarin or LMWH
Second episode of unprovoked VTE	Warfarin	Long term	

DVT, deep vein thrombosis; LMWH, low molecular weight heparins; PE, pulmonary embolism; VTE, venous thromboembolism.

From Kearon C, Kahn SR, Agnelli G, et al. Antithrombotic therapy for venous thromboembolic disease: American College of Chest Physicians Evidence-Based Clinical Practice Guidelines, 8th ed. Chest 2008;133:454S–545S.

Patient Encounter 4, Part 1

LN is a 77-year-old woman who developed a DVT in her left leg 5 weeks following elective right hip replacement surgery. The patient was hospitalized for the past 2 days for acute DVT treatment and was discharged this morning. The plan is to continue treatment at home and for the patient to follow up with her primary physician in 2 weeks. The patient was instructed to get as much rest as possible, limiting her physical activity and elevating her leg most of the day. The patient was instructed to get the following prescriptions filled at her neighborhood pharmacy as soon as possible:

Fondaparinux 7.5 mg SC daily #14 refill 0

Warfarin 10 mg PO daily #30 refill 2

PMH: Hypertension; dyslipidemia; major depressive disorder; gastroesophageal reflux disorder (GERD)

FH: Father died of "old age"; mother died of cancer; brother (age 72) has hypertension and had myocardial infarction (age 66)

SH: The patient is a retired college professor (music theory)

Current meds: Lisinopril 20 mg/HCTZ 12.5 mg PO daily; amlodipine 5 mg PO daily; simvastatin 20 mg PO daily;

fluoxetine 20 mg PO daily; omeprazole 20 mg PO daily; aspirin 81 mg PO daily for stroke prevention

Allergies: Sulfa: rash

PE:

VS: BP 144/60 mm Hg, HR 88 bpm, RR 12, wt 66 kg (145 lb), ht 62 in. (157 cm), BMI = 26.5 kg/m^2

Labs: Within normal limits; except BUN = 21 mg/dL (7.5 mmol/L), SCr = 1.7 mg/dL (150 μmol/L), eGFR = 29 mL/min/1.73 m^2 (0.28 mL/s/m^2), PT = 17.8 seconds, and INR = 1.8

Is the prescribed treatment appropriate for LN?

What changes in LN's treatment plan should be recommended at this time to the prescribing physician?

What follow-up laboratory tests should be obtained, and when should they be obtained?

How long should LN remain on anticoagulation therapy?

Given the current list of medications that LN is taking, should any of these medications be discontinued or changed? If changed, what alternative therapy would you recommend?

Develop a patient education plan for LN including appropriate techniques for self-administering injectable anticoagulants.

Patient Encounter 4, Part 2

LN has been taking warfarin for the past 3 months. Over the past 8 weeks, her INR has been in her goal range and no changes in her warfarin dose have been made. LN states that she is currently taking warfarin 5 mg every day except 2.5 mg on Wednesdays and Saturdays. LN states she has had two nosebleeds in the past month and notices that she bruises more easily, but she has had no major bleeding episodes. Her DVT symptoms essentially resolved within the first month after her diagnosis, but she's noticed some mild pain and swelling in her left leg the past 2 weeks. LN states that she has been taking naproxen sodium 220 mg twice daily for her leg pain. Given that LN has been tolerating the treatment well and is able to obtain the necessary laboratory tests in a timely manner, her primary care physician has recommended that she continue warfarin therapy for another 6 months. LN is not very pleased about this recommendation because she finds it difficult to moderate her vitamin K intake ("I love Brussels sprouts!") and the frequent blood tests are annoying.

PE:

VS: BP 136/62 mm Hg, HR 74 bpm, wt 65 kg (142 lb), BMI = 26.2 kg/m²

Labs: CBC within normal limits; PT = 21.8 seconds, and INR = 3.1 (drawn this morning)

How should LN's recurrent symptoms (i.e., pain and swelling in left leg) be evaluated and addressed?

Outline a patient education plan to prevent and manage nosebleeds.

Is the current treatment plan appropriate? Outline a plan including specific medication changes, nonpharmacologic treatment recommendations, and a follow-up plan.

Assume that anticoagulation therapy is appropriate. Is LN a good candidate for dabigatran therapy? Justify your answer.

Patient Care and Monitoring

Day 1

1. It is critical to confirm the diagnosis of VTE
   - Clinical assessment: Look for risk factors for VTE
   - If DVT symptoms are present, obtain a venous ultrasound
   - If PE is suspected, obtain a V/Q or CT scan
   - D-dimer: This test may be a helpful adjunct to rule out VTE

2. Obtain baseline laboratory tests. These tests must be obtained prior to initiating anticoagulation therapy:
   - PT and calculated INR
   - aPTT or antifactor Xa activity
   - Serum creatinine, serum albumin, and blood urea nitrogen (BUN)
   - Liver function tests
   - Complete blood count (CBC) with platelets

3. Medications:
   - Screen the patient's medication profile including over-the-counter medications and herbal therapies used at home for potential drug–drug interactions with anticoagulation therapy
   - Initiate UFH, LMWH, or fondaparinux by injection (see Table 10–5 for dosing guidelines); [dabigatran and rivaroxaban will provide future therapeutic alternatives once approved by FDA for VTE treatment]
   - If warfarin will be used long term, start warfarin sodium orally every evening (see Fig. 10–9 for dosing guidelines)
   - Start pain medication if necessary (avoid nonsteroidal anti-inflammatory drugs)

4. Patient education:
   - Educate the patient regarding the purpose of therapy and importance of proper monitoring of anticoagulant drugs. Assist the patient to determine an appropriate provider for long-term monitoring of anticoagulation therapy.
   - If LMWH, fondaparinux, or UFH is selected for home treatment, teach the patient how to self-administer (if the patient or a family member is unwilling or unable to self-administer, visiting nurse services should be arranged). Initial injection should be administered in the medical office or hospital.
   - If warfarin is selected, inform patient about the effects of vitamin K–rich foods on warfarin therapy. Moderate intake (less than 500–1,000 mcg) of vitamin K is acceptable. Provide patient with written material regarding vitamin K content of foods.
   - If warfarin is selected, inform the patient about the potential drug–drug interactions, including over-the-counter medications and dietary supplements (Tables 10–10, 10–11, and 10–12). Instruct the patient to call the healthcare practitioner responsible for monitoring warfarin therapy before starting any new medications or dietary supplements.
   - Instruct the patient regarding nonpharmacologic strategies including elevation of the affected extremity and antiembolic exercises such as flexion/extension of the ankle (for lower extremity VTE) or hand squeezing/relaxation (for upper extremity VTE).

(Continued)

Patient Care and Monitoring (*Continued*)

5. Follow-up steps:

   • If LMWH, fondaparinux, or UFH is selected for home treatment, dispense to the patient a 5- to 7-day supply of prefilled LMWH or fondaparinux syringes in patient-specific dose.

   • If the patient is to be treated with IV UFH, measure aPTT or antifactor Xa activity 6 hours after initiating the IV infusion. Adjust dose if necessary (Table 10–7) and measure aPTT or antifactor Xa activity every 6 hours after each dose change until therapeutic. Measure aPTT or antifactor Xa activity daily thereafter.

   • Arrange for follow-up and long-term anticoagulation therapy management. Communicate with the patient's primary care physician and/or refer to a local antithrombosis service, if available. If the patient is to be treated primarily in the hospital, these arrangements can be made 1 to 2 days prior to hospital discharge.

6. Document all activities in medical record.

Day 2

1. If the patient is being treated with IV UFH, remeasure the aPTT or antifactor Xa activity, and adjust dose if necessary. If patient is being treated with LMWH, fondaparinux, or dabigatran, continue therapy.

2. Interview the patient to determine if there is worsening or new symptoms related to VTE. Ask the patient about overt bruising or bleeding, particularly at injection sites, as well as changes in stool or urine color.

3. Advise the patient to limit physical activity if pain persists and to elevate the extremity; increase activity as tolerated.

4. Document activities in medical record.

Days 3 to 5

1. If patient being treated with warfarin, measure PT/INR every 1 to 2 days.

2. Interview the patient to determine if there is worsening or new symptoms related to VTE. Inquire about and evaluate patient adherence to therapy. Ask the patient about overt bruising or bleeding, particularly at the injection site, as well as changes in stool or urine color. Advise the patient to limit physical activity if pain persists and to elevate the extremity; increase activity as tolerated.

3. If patient is being treated with warfarin, hold or adjust warfarin dose as necessary. If the patient is being treated with IV UFH, measure aPTT or antifactor Xa activity daily, and adjust dose if necessary. If the patient is being treated with an LMWH, fondaparinux, or dabigatran, continue therapy.

4. If patient is being treated with warfarin, reinforce previous patient education regarding potential drug–drug and drug–food interactions.

5. Document activities in medical record.

Days 6 to 8

1. Obtain CBC or platelet count. If patient is being treated with warfarin, measure PT/INR every 2 to 3 days.

2. Interview the patient to determine if there is worsening or new symptoms related to VTE. Inquire about and evaluate patient adherence to therapy. Ask the patient about overt bruising or bleeding, particularly at the injection site, as well as changes in stool or urine color. Advise the patient to limit physical activity if pain persists and to elevate the extremity; increase activity as tolerated.

3. If patient is being treated with warfarin, hold or adjust warfarin dose as necessary. Discontinue UFH, LMWH, or fondaparinux if INR is greater than 2 on two consecutive occasions.

4. If the patient is being treated with IV UFH and requires continued treatment, measure aPTT or antifactor Xa activity, and adjust dose if necessary.

5. If the patient is treated with UFH or LMWH and platelet count has dropped by greater than 50% from baseline or is less than 120×10^3 mm^3 (120×10^9/L), evaluate the patient for HIT.

6. Document activities in medical record.

Days 9 to 14

1. If patient is being treated with warfarin, measure PT/INR every 3 to 5 days.

2. Interview the patient to determine if there is worsening or new symptoms related to VTE. Inquire about and evaluate patient adherence to therapy. Ask the patient about overt bruising or bleeding, particularly at the injection site, as well as changes in stool or urine color. Advise the patient to elevate the extremity and increase activity as tolerated.

3. If patient is being treated with warfarin, hold or adjust warfarin dose as necessary. Discontinue UFH, LMWH, or fondaparinux if INR is greater than 2 on two consecutive occasions.

4. If the patient is being treated with IV UFH and requires continued treatment, measure aPTT or antifactor Xa activity, and adjust dose if necessary.

5. If the patient is being treated with UFH or LMWH, obtain CBC or platelet count. If the platelet count has dropped by more than 50% from baseline or is less than 120×10^3/mm^3 (120×10^9/L), evaluate the patient for HIT.

6. If patient is being treated with warfarin, reinforce previous patient education regarding vitamin K intake and potential drug–drug interactions.

7. Document activities in medical record.

(Continued)

Patient Care and Monitoring (*Continued*)

Days 15 to 90

1. Interview the patient to determine if there is worsening or new symptoms related to VTE. Inquire about and evaluate patient adherence to therapy. Ask the patient about overt bruising or bleeding as well as changes in stool or urine color. Encourage the patient to increase activity as tolerated.

2. If the patient is being treated with warfarin, measure PT/INR every 1 to 4 weeks based on the stability of the INR and patient's health status. Adjust warfarin dose as needed to maintain INR between 2 and 3.

3. If the patient is being treated with warfarin, reinforce previous patient education regarding vitamin K intake and potential drug–drug interactions with warfarin.

4. If patient is being treated with warfarin, consider restarting LMWH or fondaparinux if INR drops below 1.5.

5. Document activities in medical record.

Three Months and Beyond

1. Interview the patient to determine if there is worsening or new symptoms related to VTE. Inquire about and evaluate patient adherence to therapy. Ask the patient about overt bruising or bleeding as well as changes in stool or urine color.

2. Reevaluate the risks and benefits of continuing warfarin therapy. If unproved VTE, consider continuing therapy (see Table 10–13).

3. If patient is being treated with warfarin, measure PT/INR every 1 to 4 weeks based on the stability of the INR and patient's health status. Adjust warfarin dose as needed to maintain INR between 2 and 3. Consider reducing goal INR to 1.5 to 2 if patient is unable to obtain blood tests every 4 weeks.

3. If patient is being treated with warfarin, reinforce previous patient education regarding vitamin K intake and potential drug–drug interactions with warfarin.

4. Document activities in medical record.

Abbreviations Introduced in This Chapter

ABW	Adjusted body weight
ACCP	American College of Chest Physicians
ACT	Activated clotting time
ADP	Adenosine diphosphate
aPTT	Activated partial thromboplastin time
AT	Antithrombin
BMI	Body mass index
BUN	Blood urea nitrogen
CBC	Complete blood count
CrCl	Creatinine clearance
CT	Computed tomography
CYP	Cytochrome P-450 isoenzyme
DTI	Direct thrombin inhibitor
DVT	Deep vein thrombosis
eGFR	Estimated glomerular filtration rate
ESR	Erythrocyte sedimentation rate
GCS	Graduated compression stockings
GERD	Gastroesophageal reflux disorder
GP	Glycoprotein
HCII	Heparin cofactor II
HIT	Heparin-induced thrombocytopenia
HK	High molecular weight kininogen
IBW	Ideal body weight
ICH	Intracranial hemorrhage
IM	Intramuscular
INR	International normalized ratio
IPC	Intermittent pneumatic compression (device)
ISI	International Sensitivity Index
IVC	Inferior vena cava
LMWH	Low molecular weight heparin

MRI	Magnetic resonance imaging
PAF	Platelet activating factor
PAI-1	Plasminogen activator inhibitor-1
PCI	Percutaneous coronary intervention
PE	Pulmonary embolism
PF	Platelet factor
PF-4	Platelet factor-4
PGG/PGH	Prostaglandins
P-gp	P-glycoprotein
PK	Prekallikrein
PLA	Phospholipase A
PT	Prothrombin time
PTS	Post-thrombotic syndrome
SBP	Systolic blood pressure
SC	Subcutaneous
SERM	Selective estrogen receptor modulator
TF	Tissue factor
TFPI	Tissue factor pathway inhibitor
t-PA	Tissue plasminogen activator
TS	Thromboxane synthetase
TXA	Thromboxane A
UFH	Unfractionated heparin
u-PA	Urokinase plasminogen activator
V/Q	Ventilation/perfusion (scan)
VTE	Venous thromboembolism
vWF	von Willebrand's factor
WBC	White blood cell
WHO	World Health Organization

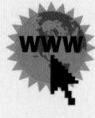 Self-assessment questions and answers are available at *http://www.mhpharmacotherapy.com/pp.html.*

REFERENCES

1. Turpie AGG, Chin BSP, Lip GYH. Venous thromboembolism: Pathophysiology, clinical features, and prevention. BMJ 2002;325:887–890.

2. Geerts WH, Bergqvist D, Pineo GF, et al. Prevention of venous thromboembolism: American College of Chest Physicians Evidence-Based Clinical Practice Guidelines, 8th ed. Chest 2008;133:381S–453S.

3. Schulman S, Beyth RJ, Kearon C, Levine MN; Hemorrhagic complications of anticoagulant and thrombolytic treatment: American College of Chest Physicians Evidence-Based Clinical Practice Guidelines, 8th ed. Chest 2008;133:257S–298S.

4. Hirsh J, Bauer KA, Donati MB, et al. Parenteral anticoagulants: American College of Chest Physicians Evidence-Based Clinical Practice Guidelines, 8th ed. Chest 2008;133:141S–159S.

5. Ansell J, Hirsh J, Hylek E, et al. Pharmacology and management of the vitamin K antagonists: American College of Chest Physicians Evidence-Based Clinical Practice Guidelines, 8th ed. Chest 2008;133:160S–198S.

6. Haines ST, Nutescu EA. Current and emerging treatment options for venous thrombosis: A case discussion. Am J Health Syst Pharm 2005;62:593–605.

7. Spencer FA, Emery C, Lessard D, et al. The Worcester venous thromboembolism study: A population-based study of the clinical epidemiology of venous thromboembolism. J General Intern Med 2006;21:722–727.

8. Johnson CM, Mureebe L, Silver D. Hypercoagulable states: A review. Vasc Endovascular Surg 2005;39:123–133.

9. Khorana AA. The NCCN Clinical Practice Guidelines on venous thromboembolic disease: Strategies for improving VTE prophylaxis in hospitalized cancer patients. Oncologist 2007;12:1361–1370.

10. Canonico M, Plu-Bureau G, Lowe GDO, Scarabin P-Y. Hormone replacement therapy and risk of venous thromboembolism in postmenopausal women: Systematic review and meta-analysis. BMJ 2008;336:1227–1231.

11. Bates SM, Greer IA, Pabinger I, Sofaer S, Hirsh J. American College of Chest Physicians. Venous thromboembolism, thrombophilia, antithrombotic therapy, and pregnancy: American College of Chest Physicians Evidence-Based Clinical Practice Guidelines, 8th ed. Chest 2008;133:844S–886S.

12. Aird WC. Coagulation. Crit Care Med 2005;33:S485–S487.

13. Cesarman-Maus G, Hajjar KA. Molecular mechanisms of fibrinolysis. Br J Haematol 2005;129:307–321.

14. Kearon C. Natural history of venous thromboembolism. Circulation 2003;107:I22–I30.

15. Kearon C, Kahn SR, Agnelli G, et al. Antithrombotic therapy for venous thromboembolic disease: American College of Chest Physicians Evidence-Based Clinical Practice Guidelines, 8th ed. Chest 2008;133:454S–545S.

16. Wells PS. Integrated strategies for the diagnosis of venous thromboembolism. J Thromb Haemost 2007;5(Suppl 1):41–50.

17. Sinert R, Foley M. Clinical assessment of the patient with a suspected pulmonary embolism. Ann Emerg Med 2008;52:76–79.

18. Kanne JP, Lalani TA. Role of computed tomography and magnetic resonance imaging for deep venous thrombosis and pulmonary embolism. Circulation 2004;109:I15–I21.

19. Zierler BK. Ultrasonography and diagnosis of venous thromboembolism. Circulation 2004;109:I9–I14.

20. Bates SM, Ginsberg JS. Clinical practice. Treatment of deep-vein thrombosis. N Engl J Med 2004;351:268–277.

21. Decousus H, Leizorovicz A, Parent F, et al. A clinical trial of vena caval filters in the prevention of pulmonary embolism in patients with proximal deep-vein thrombosis. N Engl J Med 1998;338: 409–415.

22. Mellilo SN, Scanlon JV, Exter BP, Steinberg M, Jarvis CI. Rivaroxaban for thromboprophylaxis in patients undergoing major orthopedic surgery. Ann Pharmacother 2010;44:1061–1071.

23. Buller HR, Sohne M, Middeldorp S. Treatment of venous thromboembolism. J Thromb Haemost 2005;3:1554–1560.

24. Nutescu EA. Emerging options in the treatment of venous thromboembolism. Am J Health Syst Pharm 2004;61:S12–S17.

25. Watson LI, Armon MP. Thrombolysis for acute deep vein thrombosis. Cochrane Database Syst Rev 2004:CD002783.

26. Tapson VF. Acute pulmonary embolism. N Engl J Med 2008;358: 1037–1052.

27. Agnelli G, Becattini C, Kirschstein T. Thrombolysis vs heparin in the treatment of pulmonary embolism: A clinical outcome-based meta-analysis. Arch Intern Med 2002;162:2537–2541.

28. Jaff MR, McMurtry MS, Archer SL, et.al. Management of massive and submassive pulmonary embolism, iliofemoral deep vein thrombosis, and chronic thromboembolic pulmonary hypertension: A scientific statement from the American Heart Association. Circulation. 2011;123(16):1788–1830.

29. Nutescu EA, Shapiro NL, Chevalier A, Amin AN. A pharmacologic overview of current and emerging anticoagulants. Cleve Clin J Med 2005;72(Suppl 1):S2–S6.

30. Raschke RA, Reilly BM, Guidry JR, et al. The weight-based heparin dosing nomogram compared with a "standard care" nomogram. Ann Intern Med 1993;119:874–881.

31. Segal JB, Streiff MB, Hofmann LV, et al. Management of venous thromboembolism: A systematic review for a practice guideline. Ann Intern Med 2007;146(3):211–222.

32. Kearon C, Ginsberg JS, Julian JA, et al. Comparison of fixed-dose weight-adjusted unfractionated heparin and low-molecular-weight heparin for acute treatment of venous thromboembolism. JAMA 2006;296(8):935–948.

33. Olson JD, Arkin CF, Brandt JT, et al. College of American Pathologists Conference XXXI on laboratory monitoring of anticoagulation therapy. Laboratory monitoring of unfractionated heparin therapy. Arch Pathol Lab Med 1998;122:782–788.

34. Monagle P, Chalmers E, Chan A, et al. Antithrombotic therapy in neonates and children: American College of Chest Physicians Evidence-Based Clinical Practice Guidelines, 8th ed. Chest 2008;133:887S–968S.

35. Nutescu EA, Wittkowsky AK, Dobesh PP, Hawkins DW, Dager WE. Choosing the appropriate antithrombotic agent for the prevention and treatment of VTE: A case-based approach. Ann Pharmacother 2006;40(9):1558–1571.

36. Akl EA, Rohilla S, Barba M, et al. Anticoagulation for the initial treatment of venous thromboembolism in patients with cancer. Cochrane Database Syst Rev 2008(1):CD006649.

37. Nutescu EA. Assessing, preventing, and treating venous thromboembolism: Evidence-based approaches. Am J Health Syst Pharm 2007;64 (11 Suppl 7):S5–S13.

38. Scarvelis D, Wells PS. Diagnosis and treatment of deep-vein thrombosis. CMAJ 2006;175(9):1087–1092.

39. Laposata M, Green D, Van Cott EM, et al. College of American Pathologists Conference XXXI on laboratory monitoring of anticoagulant therapy: The clinical use and laboratory monitoring of low-molecular-weight heparin, danaparoid, hirudin and related compounds, and argatroban. Arch Pathol Lab Med 1998;122:799–807.

40. Duhl AJ, Paidas MJ, Ural SH, et al., Pregnancy and Thrombosis Working Group. Antithrombotic therapy and pregnancy: Consensus report and recommendations for prevention and treatment of venous thromboembolism and adverse pregnancy outcomes. Am J Obstet Gynecol 2007;197(5):457.e1–e21.

41. Weitz J, Hirsh J, Samama MM. New antithrombotic drugs: American College of Chest Physicians Evidence-Based Clinical Practice Guidelines, 8th ed. Chest 2008;133:234S–256S.

42. Gulseth MP, Michaud J, Nutescu EA. Rivaroxaban: An oral direct inhibitor of factor Xa. Am J Health Syst Pharm 2008;65(16):1520–1529.

43. Buller HR, Davidson BL, Decousus H, et al. Subcutaneous fondaparinux versus intravenous unfractionated heparin in the initial treatment of pulmonary embolism. N Engl J Med 2003;349:1695–1702.

44. Buller HR, Davidson BL, Decousus H, et al. Fondaparinux or enoxaparin for the initial treatment of symptomatic deep venous thrombosis: A randomized trial. Ann Intern Med 2004;140:867–873.

45. Nutescu EA, Shapiro NL, Chevalier A. New anticoagulant agents: Direct thrombin inhibitors. Cardiol Clin 2008;26(2):169–187.

46. Nutescu E, Chuatrisorn I, Hellenbart E. Drug and dietary interactions of warfarin and novel oral anticoagulants: an update. J Thromb Thrombolysis. 2011;31(3):326–343.

47. Lenzini PA, Grice GR, Milligan PE, et al. Laboratory and clinical outcomes of pharmacogenetic vs. clinical protocols for warfarin initiation in orthopedic patients. J Thromb Haemost 2008;6(10):1655–1662.

48. Garcia DA, Witt DM, Hylek E, et al. Delivery of optimized anticoagulant therapy: Consensus statement from the Anticoagulation Forum. Ann Pharmacother 2008;42(7):979–988.

49. Holbrook AMMDPMF, Pereira JAM, Labiris RP, et al. Systematic overview of warfarin and its drug and food interactions. Arch Intern Med 2005;165:1095–1106.

50. Nutescu EA, Shapiro NL, Ibrahim S, West P. Warfarin and its interactions with foods, herbs and other dietary supplements. Expert Opin Drug Saf 2006;5(3):433–451.

51. Schulman S, Kearon C, Kakkar AK, et al; RE-COVER Study Group. Dabigatran versus warfarin in the treatment of acute venous thromboembolism. N Engl J Med 2009;361(24):2342–2352.

52. EINSTEIN Investigators, Bauersachs R, Berkowitz SD, Brenner B, et.al. Oral rivaroxaban for symptomatic venous thromboembolism. N Engl J Med 2010;363(26):2499–2510.

11 Stroke

Susan R. Winkler

LEARNING OBJECTIVES

● **Upon completion of the chapter, the reader will be able to:**

1. Differentiate the types of cerebrovascular disease including transient ischemic attack, ischemic stroke (cerebral infarction), and hemorrhagic stroke.

2. Identify modifiable and nonmodifiable risk factors associated with ischemic stroke and hemorrhagic stroke.

3. Explain the pathophysiology of ischemic stroke and hemorrhagic stroke.

4. Describe the clinical presentation of transient ischemic attack, ischemic stroke, and hemorrhagic stroke.

5. Evaluate the various treatment options for acute ischemic stroke.

6. Determine whether thrombolytic therapy is indicated in a patient with acute ischemic stroke.

7. Formulate strategies for primary and secondary prevention of acute ischemic stroke.

8. Evaluate treatment options for acute hemorrhagic stroke.

KEY CONCEPTS

① Ischemic stroke, which may be thrombotic or embolic, is the abrupt development of a focal neurological deficit that occurs due to inadequate blood supply to an area of the brain.

② Hemorrhagic stroke is a result of bleeding into the brain and other spaces within the CNS and includes subarachnoid hemorrhage (SAH), intracerebral hemorrhage (ICH), and subdural hematomas.

③ Transient ischemic attacks (TIAs) are a risk factor for acute ischemic stroke and precede acute ischemic stroke in approximately 15% of cases; therefore, preventive measures are the same for both TIA and ischemic stroke.

④ The long-term treatment goals for acute ischemic stroke include prevention of a recurrent stroke through reduction and modification of risk factors and by use of appropriate treatments.

⑤ All patients should have a brain computed tomography (CT) scan or magnetic resonance imaging (MRI) scan to differentiate an ischemic stroke from a hemorrhagic stroke because treatment differs and thrombolytic (fibrinolytic) therapy must be avoided until a hemorrhagic stroke is ruled out.

⑥ In carefully selected patients, alteplase should be given as soon as possible, preferably within 3 hours and not more than 4.5 hours after symptom onset.

⑦ Aspirin (ASA) therapy with an initial dose of 150 to 325 mg is recommended in most patients with acute ischemic stroke within 48 hours after stroke symptom onset.

⑧ Current stroke treatment guidelines recommend ASA, clopidogrel, or combination therapy with extended-release dipyridamole plus ASA as initial antiplatelet therapy for the secondary prevention of stroke.

⑨ Selection of the initial antiplatelet agent for secondary prevention of ischemic stroke should be individualized based on patient factors and cost. Clopidogrel and the combination of extended-release dipyridamole and ASA are preferred over ASA monotherapy.

⑩ There is no proven treatment for ICH. Management is based on neurointensive care treatment and prevention of complications.

EPIDEMIOLOGY

Cerebrovascular disease (CVD), or stroke, is the second most common cause of death worldwide and the fourth leading cause of death in the United States, declining from the third most common cause of death as a result of decades of progress in the treatment and prevention of CVD.[1] Approximately 795,000 strokes occur in the United States each year. New strokes account for 610,000 of this total; recurrent strokes account for the remaining 185,000 strokes each year. Stroke is the leading cause of long-term disability in adults, with 90% of survivors having residual deficits. Moderate to severe disability is seen in 70% of survivors. An estimated 15% to 30% of stroke survivors are permanently disabled, and 20% require institutional care at 3 months after the stroke. The American Heart Association estimates there are over 7 million survivors of stroke in the United States. The societal impact and economic burden is great, with total costs of $40.9 billion reported in the United States in 2007. Stroke mortality has declined due to improved recognition and treatment of risk factors; however, risk factor management is still inadequate. Stroke incidence increases with age, especially after age 55 years, resulting in an increased stroke incidence due to aging of the population.[2]

ETIOLOGY

Strokes can either be ischemic (88% of all strokes) or hemorrhagic (12% of all strokes). **Figure 11–1** provides a classification of stroke by mechanism. ❶ *Ischemic stroke, which may be thrombotic or embolic, is the abrupt development of a focal neurological deficit that occurs due to inadequate blood supply to an area of the brain.* A thrombotic occlusion occurs when a **thrombus** forms inside an artery in the brain. An embolic stroke typically occurs when a piece of thrombus,

originating either inside or outside of the cerebral vessels, breaks loose and is carried to the site of occlusion in the cerebral vessels. An extracerebral source of emboli is often the heart, leading to cardioembolic stroke.

❷ *Hemorrhagic stroke is a result of bleeding into the brain and other spaces within the CNS and includes subarachnoid hemorrhage (SAH), intracerebral hemorrhage (ICH), and subdural hematomas.* SAH results from sudden bleeding into the space between the inner layer and middle layer of the **meninges**, most often due to trauma or rupture of a cerebral aneurysm or arteriovenous malformation (AVM). ICH is bleeding directly into the brain parenchyma, often as a result of chronic uncontrolled hypertension. Subdural hematomas result from bleeding under the dura that covers the brain and most often occur as a result of head trauma.

CLASSIFICATION
Cerebral Ischemic Events

There are two main classifications of cerebral ischemic events: **transient ischemic attack** (TIA) and ischemic stroke (cerebral infarction). A TIA is a transient episode of neurological dysfunction caused by focal brain, spinal cord, or retinal ischemia without acute infarction. TIAs have a rapid onset and short duration, typically lasting less than 1 hour and often less than 30 minutes. The symptoms vary depending on the area of the brain affected; however, no deficit remains after the attack. The classic definition of TIA was based on symptom duration of less than 24 hours; symptoms lasting 24 hours or greater were categorized

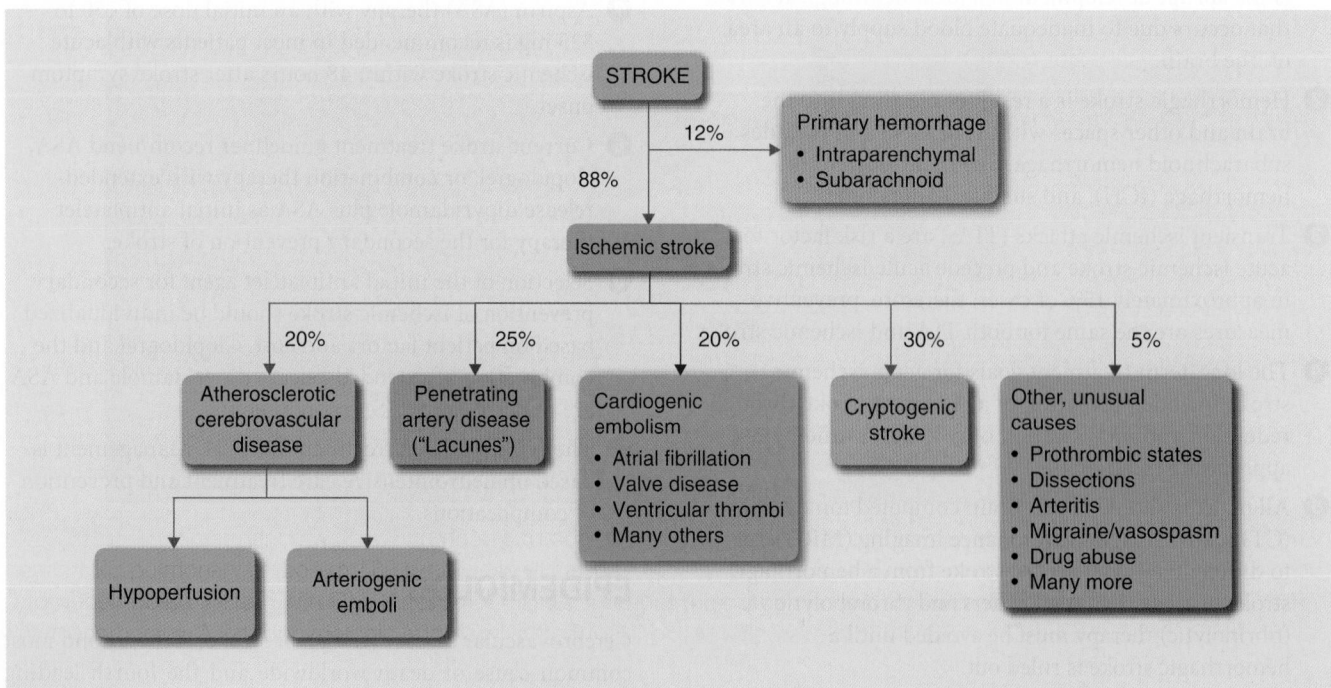

FIGURE 11–1. Classification of stroke. (From Fagan SC, Hess DC. Stroke. In: DiPiro JT, Talbert RL, Yee GC, et al., eds. Pharmacotherapy: A Pathophysiologic Approach, 8th ed. New York, NY: McGraw-Hill, 2011:354, with permission.)

as ischemic stroke. Improved neuroimaging techniques have revealed that clinical symptoms lasting greater than 1 hour are often ischemic stroke based on evidence of tissue infarction. Using the classic definition of TIA would potentially miscategorize the event in up to one-third of cases. For this reason, the definition of TIA has been changed to eliminate the focus on time and encourage prompt diagnosis and classification of the event.[3] ❸ *TIAs are a risk factor for acute ischemic stroke and precede acute ischemic stroke in approximately 15% of cases; therefore, preventive measures are the same for both TIA and ischemic stroke.[4]* Ischemic stroke is similar to a TIA; however, tissue injury and infarction are present, and in many patients, residual deficits remain after the event. A standardized tissue-based definition of cerebral infarction has been proposed as "cerebral infarction is defined as brain or retinal cell death due to prolonged ischemia."[5]

Hemorrhagic Events

A sudden severe headache, nausea and vomiting, and **photophobia** may be the first signs and symptoms of hemorrhagic stroke. Neck pain and **nuchal rigidity** may also be experienced at the time of the hemorrhage. Patients may complain the headache is "the worst headache of my life," especially if the cause is a SAH. It is important to note that a diagnosis of the type of stroke cannot be made solely on signs and symptoms because overlap occurs between the types of stroke.

Risk Factors

Assessment of risk factors for ischemic stroke as well as for hemorrhagic stroke is an important component of stroke prevention, diagnosis, and treatment of patients. A major goal in the long-term management of ischemic stroke involves primary prevention (prevention of the first stroke) and prevention of a recurrent stroke through the reduction and modification of risk factors. Risk factors for ischemic stroke can be divided into modifiable and nonmodifiable. Table 11–1 provides a list of risk factors for ischemic stroke. Every patient should have risk factors assessed and treated, if possible, because management of risk factors can decrease the occurrence and/or recurrence of stroke.[6,7]

Nonmodifiable risk factors for both types of stroke include age, gender, race/ethnicity, and genetic predisposition. Low birth weight is an additional risk factor for ischemic stroke. Ischemic stroke risk is increased in those older than 55 years of age, in men, and in African Americans, Hispanics, and Asian/Pacific Islanders. It is also increased in those with a family history of stroke. Modifiable risk factors include a number of treatable disease states and lifestyle factors that can greatly influence overall stroke risk. Hypertension is one of the major risk factors for both ischemic and hemorrhagic stroke. For ICH specifically, hypertension has been shown to increase risk by a factor of 3.68.[7,8] Other risk factors for hemorrhagic stroke include trauma, cigarette smoking,

Table 11–1

Nonmodifiable and Modifiable Risk Factors for Ischemic Stroke

Nonmodifiable Factors
- Age (greater than 55 years)
- Gender (males greater than females)
- Race and ethnicity (African American, Hispanic, or Asian/Pacific Islander)
- Genetic predisposition
- Low birth weight

Modifiable Factors
- Hypertension (single most important risk factor)
- Cardiac disease
  - Atrial fibrillation (most important and treatable cardiac cause of stroke)
  - Mitral stenosis
  - Mitral annular calcification
  - Left atrial enlargement
  - Structural abnormalities such as atrial-septal aneurysm
  - Acute MI
- Transient ischemic attacks or prior stroke (major independent risk factor)
- Diabetes (independent risk factor)
- Dyslipidemia
- Lifestyle factors
  - Cigarette smoking
  - Excessive alcohol use
  - Physical inactivity
  - Obesity
  - Diet
  - Cocaine and IV drug use
  - Low socioeconomic status
- Increased hematocrit
- Sickle cell disease
- Hyperhomocysteinemia (less well documented)
- Migraine (risk not clear)
- Asymptomatic carotid stenosis
- Oral contraceptive use (with estrogen content greater than 50 mcg)

MI, myocardial infarction.

cocaine use, heavy alcohol use, anticoagulant use, and cerebral aneurysm and AVM rupture.

PATHOPHYSIOLOGY
Ischemic Stroke

In ischemic stroke, there is an interruption of the blood supply to an area of the brain either due to thrombus formation or an embolism. Loss of cerebral blood flow results in tissue hypoperfusion, tissue hypoxia, and cell death. Thrombus formation usually starts with lipid deposits in the vessel wall that cause turbulent blood flow. This leads to vessel injury and vessel collagen becoming exposed to blood. This vessel injury initiates the platelet aggregation process due to the exposed subendothelium. Platelets release adenosine diphosphate (ADP), which causes platelet aggregation and consolidation of the platelet plug. Thromboxane A_2 is released, contributing to platelet aggregation and vasoconstriction. The vessel injury also activates the coagulation cascade, which leads to thrombin production. Thrombin converts fibrinogen to fibrin, leading to clot formation as fibrin molecules, platelets, and blood cells aggregate. Refer to Figures 7–3, 10–3, and 10–4 for a depiction of these processes.

After the initial event, secondary events occur at the cellular level that contribute to cell death. Regardless of the initiating event, the cellular processes that follow may be similar. Excitatory amino acids such as glutamate accumulate within the cells, causing intracellular calcium accumulation. Inflammation occurs and oxygen free radicals are formed resulting in the common pathway of cell death.

There is often a core of ischemia containing unsalvageable brain cells. Surrounding this core is an area termed the *ischemic penumbra*. In this area, cells are still salvageable; however, this is a time-sensitive endeavor. Without restoration of adequate perfusion, cell death continues throughout a larger area of the brain, ultimately leading to neurological deficits. No agents have been shown to be effective at providing neuroprotection at this time.

Hemorrhagic Stroke

The pathophysiology of hemorrhagic stroke is not as well studied as that of ischemic stroke; however, it is more complex than previously thought. Much of the process is related to the presence of blood in the brain tissue and/or surrounding spaces resulting in compression. The hematoma that forms may continue to grow and enlarge after the initial bleed, and early growth of the hematoma is associated with a poor outcome. Brain tissue swelling and injury is a result of inflammation caused by thrombin and other blood products. This can lead to increased intracranial pressure (ICP) and herniation.[9,10]

Patient Encounter Part 1

TK is a 73-year-old (72 kg [158.4 lb], 64" [163 cm]) White woman who presents to the emergency department with weakness in her right arm and leg and difficulty speaking. Her symptoms began approximately 2 1/2 hours ago during breakfast, prompting her daughter to call the paramedics. Her past medical history is significant for hypertension, dyslipidemia, migraine, and a previous stroke 7 years ago. Social history is significant for moderate alcohol use and cigarette smoking 1/2 pack per day for the past 50 years. Current medications include perindopril 4 mg once daily, simvastatin 40 mg daily, multivitamin tablet once daily, and sumatriptan 25 mg at the onset of migraine.

What signs and symptoms does TK have that are suggestive of stroke?

What nonmodifiable and modifiable risk factors does TK have for acute ischemic stroke?

Clinical Presentation and Diagnosis of Stroke

General

- The patient may not be able to reliably report the history owing to cognitive or language deficits. A reliable history may have to come from a family member or another witness.

Symptoms

- The patient may complain of weakness on one side of the body, inability to speak, loss of vision, vertigo, or falling. Stroke patients may complain of headache; however, with hemorrhagic stroke, the headache can be severe.

Signs

- Patients usually have multiple signs of neurologic dysfunction, and the specific deficits are determined by the area of the brain involved.
- Hemiparesis or monoparesis occur commonly, as does a hemisensory deficit.
- Patients with vertigo and double vision are likely to have posterior circulation involvement.
- Aphasia is seen commonly in patients with anterior circulation strokes.
- Patients may also suffer from dysarthria, visual field defects, and altered levels of consciousness.

Laboratory Tests

- There are no specific laboratory tests for stroke.

- Tests for hypercoagulable states, such as protein C deficiency and antiphospholipid antibody, should be done only when the cause of stroke cannot be determined based on the presence of well-known risk factors for stroke.

Other Diagnostic Tests

- A computed tomography (CT) scan of the head will reveal an area of hyperintensity (white) identifying that a hemorrhage has occurred. The CT scan will either be normal or hypointense (dark) in an area where an infarction has occurred. It may take 24 hours (and rarely longer) to reveal the area of infarction on a CT scan.
- Magnetic resonance imaging (MRI) of the head will reveal areas of ischemia earlier and with better resolution than a CT scan. Diffusion-weighted imaging can reveal an evolving infarct within minutes.
- Carotid Doppler studies will determine whether the patient has a high degree of stenosis in the carotid arteries supplying blood to the brain (extracranial disease).
- The electrocardiogram (ECG) will determine whether the patient has atrial fibrillation, which is a major risk factor for cardioembolic stroke.
- A transthoracic echocardiogram will identify whether there are heart valve abnormalities or problems with wall motion resulting in emboli to the brain.

DESIRED TREATMENT OUTCOMES

The short-term treatment goals for acute ischemic stroke include reducing secondary brain damage by reestablishing and maintaining adequate perfusion to marginally ischemic areas of the brain and protecting these areas from the effects of ischemia (i.e., neuroprotection). ❹ The long-term treatment goals for acute ischemic stroke include prevention of a recurrent stroke through reduction and modification of risk factors and by use of appropriate treatments.

Short-term treatment goals for hemorrhagic stroke include rapid neurointensive care treatment to maintain adequate oxygenation, breathing, and circulation. Management of increased ICP and blood pressure (BP) are important in the acute setting. Long-term management includes prevention of complications and prevention of a recurrent bleed and delayed cerebral ischemia.

Prevention of long-term disability and death related to the stroke are important regardless of stroke type.

GENERAL APPROACH TO TREATMENT

❺ All patients should have a brain computed tomography (CT) scan or magnetic resonance imaging (MRI) scan to differentiate an ischemic stroke from a hemorrhagic stroke because treatment differs and thrombolytic (fibrinolytic) therapy must be avoided until a hemorrhagic stroke is ruled out. A CT scan is the most important diagnostic test in patients with acute stroke. For those with an ischemic stroke, an evaluation should be done to determine the appropriateness of reperfusion therapy. In hemorrhagic stroke, a surgical evaluation should be completed to assess the need for surgical clipping of an aneurysm or other procedure to control the bleed and prevent rebleeding and other complications. Figure 11–2 provides an algorithm for the initial management of the acute stroke patient.

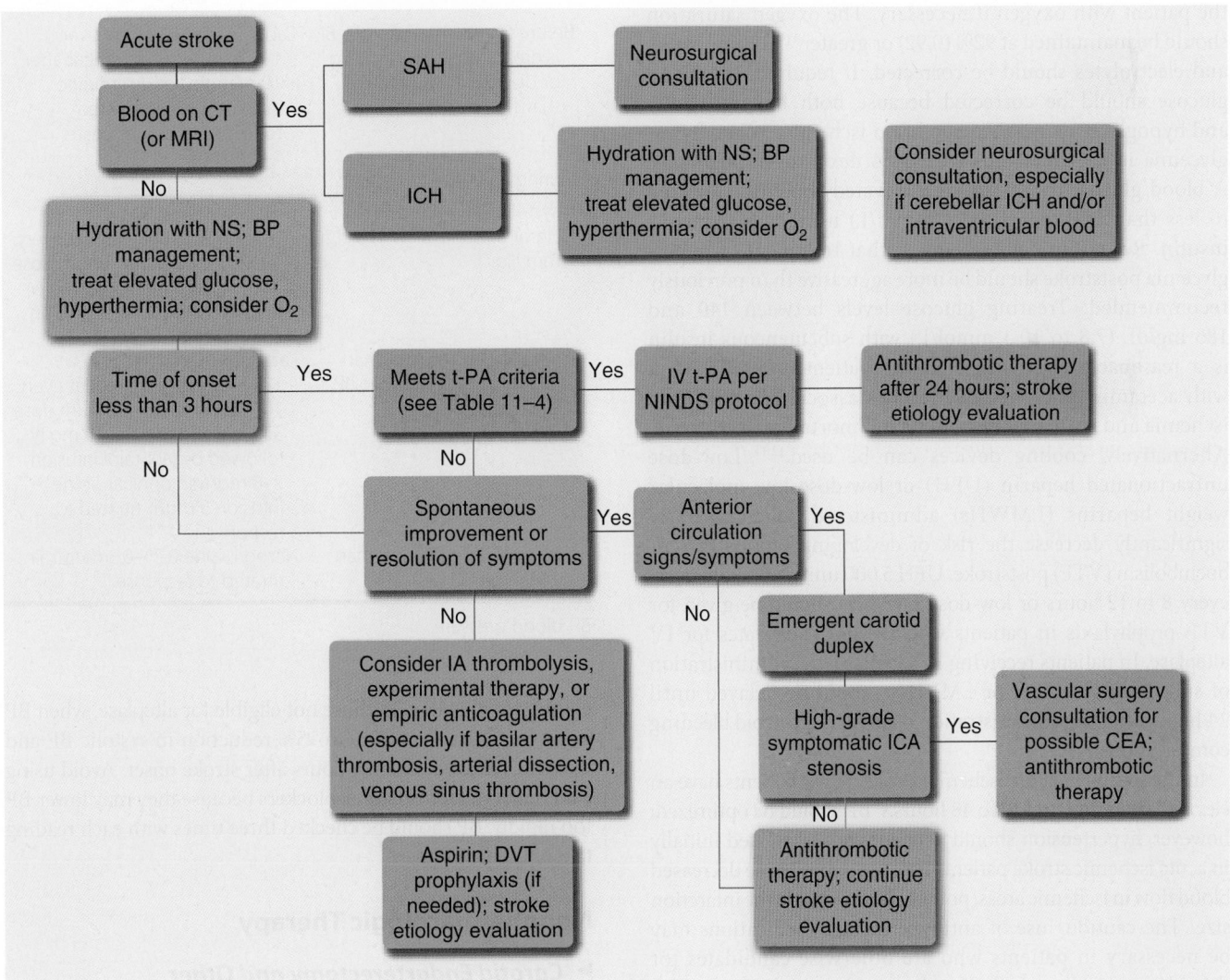

FIGURE 11–2. Acute stroke treatment algorithm. (BP, blood pressure; CEA, carotid endarterectomy; CT, computed tomography; DVT, deep vein thrombosis; IA, intraarterial; ICA, internal carotid artery; ICH, intracerebral hemorrhage; MRI, magnetic resonance imaging; NINDS, National Institute of Neurological Disorders and Stroke; NS, normal saline; SAH, subarachnoid hemorrhage; t-PA, tissue plasminogen activator.)

TREATMENT OF ACUTE ISCHEMIC STROKE

Acute ischemic stroke is a medical emergency. Identification of the time and manner of stroke onset is an important determinant in treatment. The time the patient was last without symptoms is used as the time of stroke onset. Because patients typically do not experience pain, determining the onset time can be difficult. It is also important to document risk factors and the previous functional status of the patient to assess current disability due to stroke.

Supportive Measures

Acute complications of ischemic stroke include cerebral edema, increased ICP, seizures, and hemorrhagic conversion. In the acute setting, supportive interventions and treatments to prevent acute complications should be initiated.

Tissue oxygenation should be maintained acutely. Measure the oxygen saturation using pulse oximetry and supplement the patient with oxygen if necessary. The oxygen saturation should be maintained at 92% (0.92) or greater.[11] Volume status and electrolytes should be corrected. If required, the blood glucose should be corrected because both hyperglycemia and hypoglycemia may worsen brain ischemia. When hypoglycemia is present, bolus with 50% dextrose immediately. A blood glucose that is severely elevated should be lowered to less than 200 mg/dL (11.1 mmol/L) using subcutaneous insulin. Recent guidelines suggest that treatment of hyperglycemia poststroke should be more aggressive than previously recommended. Treating glucose levels between 140 and 185 mg/dL (7.8 to 10.3 mmol/L) with subcutaneous insulin is a reasonable approach.[12,13] If the patient is febrile, treat with acetaminophen because fever is associated with brain ischemia and increased morbidity and mortality after stroke. Alternatively, cooling devices can be used.[12,14] Low-dose unfractionated heparin (UFH) or low-dose low molecular weight heparins (LMWHs) administered subcutaneously significantly decrease the risk of developing venous thromboembolism (VTE) poststroke. UFH 5,000 units subcutaneously every 8 to 12 hours or low-dose LMWHs should be given for VTE prophylaxis in patients who are not candidates for IV alteplase. In patients receiving IV alteplase, the administration of subcutaneous UFH or LMWHs should be delayed until 24 hours after the administration of alteplase to avoid bleeding complications.

In the setting of acute ischemic stroke, many patients have an elevated BP in the first 24 to 48 hours.[15] BP should be optimized; however, hypertension should generally not be treated initially in acute ischemic stroke patients because it may cause decreased blood flow in ischemic areas, potentially increasing the infarction size. The cautious use of antihypertensive medications may be necessary in patients who are otherwise candidates for thrombolytic therapy, including those with severely elevated BP (systolic BP greater than 220 mm Hg or diastolic BP greater than 120 mm Hg), and those with other medical disorders requiring immediate lowering of BP. Tables 11–2 and 11–3 provide recommendations on BP management in those eligible and not

---

Table 11–2

BP Recommendations for Ischemic Stroke (Not Eligible for Alteplase)

Systolic BP less than 220 mm Hg and diastolic BP less than 120 mm Hg	Observe unless other end-organ involvement
Systolic BP greater than 220 mm Hg or diastolic BP 121–140 mm Hg	Labetalol 10–20 mg IV over 1–2 minutes (may repeat every 10–20 minutes; maximum dose 300 mg) or nicardipine infusion 5 mg/h titrated to response
Diastolic BP greater than 140 mm Hg	Nitroprusside 0.25–0.3 mcg/kg/min titrated to response

BP, blood pressure.

Table 11–3

BP Recommendations for Ischemic Stroke (Eligible for Alteplase)

Before treatment: If systolic BP is greater than 185 mm Hg or diastolic BP is greater than 110 mm Hg	Labetalol 10–20 mg IV over 1–2 minutes (may repeat after 10 minutes) or nicardipine infusion 5 mg/h titrated to response or nitropaste 1–2 inches
During and after treatment:	
If systolic BP is 180–230 mm Hg or diastolic BP is 105–120 mm Hg	Labetalol 10 mg IV over 1–2 minutes (may repeat every 10–20 minutes; maximum dose 300 mg) or labetalol 10 mg IV followed by labetalol infusion 2–8 mg/min
If systolic BP is greater than 230 mm Hg or diastolic BP is 121–140 mm Hg	Labetalol 10 mg IV over 1–2 minutes (may repeat every 10–20 minutes; maximum dose 300 mg) or labetalol 10 mg IV followed by labetalol infusion 2–8 mg/min or nicardipine infusion 5 mg/h titrated to response
If diastolic BP is greater than 140 mm Hg	Nitroprusside 0.25–0.3 mcg/min titrated to response

BP, blood pressure.

---

eligible for alteplase. In those not eligible for alteplase, when BP is lowered, aim for a 10% to 15% reduction in systolic BP and diastolic BP in the first 24 hours after stroke onset. Avoid using sublingual calcium channel blockers because they may lower BP too rapidly. BP should be checked three times with each reading taken 5 minutes apart.

Nonpharmacologic Therapy

▶ Carotid Endarterectomy and Other Surgical Procedures

It is unknown whether carotid endarterectomy is of value when performed emergently after stroke, meaning within the first 24 hours after symptom onset.[12] Improvement after surgery has been shown in some patients with mild to moderate neurological deficits. In patients with more severe neurological deficits, the utility of carotid endarterectomy is unclear. Emergency bypass procedures and middle cerebral artery embolectomy are controversial. Due to the lack of proven efficacy of these procedures when performed emergently in acute ischemic stroke, they are not routinely recommended.

Thrombolytic Therapy

▶ Alteplase

● Alteplase (rt-PA; Activase) is an IV thrombolytic (fibrinolytic) that was approved for acute ischemic stroke treatment in 1996 based on the results of the National Institute of Neurological Disorders and Stroke (NINDS) rt-PA Stroke Trial.[16] The American Stroke Association guidelines include alteplase as the only FDA-approved acute treatment for ischemic stroke and strongly encourage early diagnosis and treatment of appropriate patients.[12] ⑥ *In carefully selected patients, alteplase should be given as soon as possible, preferably within 3 hours and not more than 4.5 hours after symptom onset.* Based on several assessment scales, patients treated with alteplase were 30% more likely to have minimal or no disability at 3 months compared with patients given placebo. Alteplase treatment resulted in an 11% to 13% absolute increase in patients with excellent outcomes at 3 months, independent of patient age, stroke subtype, stroke severity, or prior use of aspirin (ASA).[17] ICH within 36 hours after stroke onset occurred in 6.4% of those given alteplase versus 0.6% in those given placebo. There was no significant difference in mortality between the two groups at 3 months or 1 year. A dose of 0.9 mg/kg (maximum: 90 mg) is recommended; the first 10% is given as an IV bolus, and the remainder is infused over 1 hour. Table 11–4 details the inclusion and exclusion criteria for the administration of alteplase in acute ischemic stroke.

Subsequent studies that followed the NINDS trial protocol have supported alteplase use in acute ischemic stroke and have shown similar rates for both response and ICH occurrence. When the clinical trials are pooled, study results show that the sooner alteplase is given after the onset of stroke symptoms, the greater the benefit seen ● in neurological outcome.[18] Current guidelines recommend alteplase use within 3 hours after stroke onset in appropriate patients and further recommend that alteplase be started as soon as possible within this window of time.[17] A treatment effect between 3.0 and 4.5 hours was evaluated in the European Cooperative Acute Stroke Study III (ECASS III) trial.[19] In a second pooled analysis of the clinical trials that included the ECASS III trial, alteplase was shown to provide some benefit if administered within 4.5 hours of symptom onset.[20] A science advisory was published in 2009 updating the recommendations for alteplase use and extending the treatment window to 4.5 hours after stroke symptom onset.[21] Research trials to evaluate combination treatments and new thrombolytic agents are underway in an effort to improve outcomes after ischemic stroke.[22]

Antiplatelet agents, anticoagulants, and invasive procedures such as insertion of a central line or placement of a nasogastric tube should be avoided for 24 hours after the infusion of alteplase to prevent bleeding complications. Bladder catheterization should be avoided for 30 minutes postinfusion.

Efficacy is measured by the elimination of existing neurological deficits and the long-term improvement in neurological status and functioning based on neurological examinations and other outcome measures. Neurological examinations should be completed every 15 minutes during the infusion of alteplase, every 30 minutes for the first 6 hours after

---

Table 11–4

Inclusion and Exclusion Criteria for Alteplase Use in Acute Ischemic Stroke

Inclusion Criteria
- 18 years of age or older (more than 80 years old excluded from ECASS III trial)
- Clinical diagnosis of ischemic stroke causing a measurable neurological deficit
- Time of symptom onset well established to be less than 3 hours before treatment would begin; may extend timing to not more than 4.5 hours after symptom onset

Exclusion Criteria
- Evidence of intracranial hemorrhage on CT scan of the brain prior to treatment
- Minor or rapidly improving stroke symptoms
- Clinical presentation suggestive of SAH even with a normal head CT
- Active internal bleeding
- Known bleeding diathesis, including but not limited to (a) platelet count less than $100 \times 10^3/mm^3$ ($100 \times 10^9/L$); (b) heparin within 48 hours with an elevated aPTT; or (c) current oral anticoagulant use (e.g., warfarin) or recent use with an elevated PT (greater than 15 seconds) or INR (greater than 1.7)
- Intracranial surgery, serious head trauma, or previous stroke within 3 months
- Suspected aortic dissection associated with stroke
- Suspected subacute bacterial endocarditis or vasculitis
- History of GI or urinary tract hemorrhage within 21 days
- Major surgery or serious trauma within 14 days
- Recent arterial puncture at a noncompressible site
- Lumbar puncture within 7 days
- History of intracranial hemorrhage
- Known AVM or aneurysm
- Witnessed seizure at the same time as the onset of stroke symptoms occurred
- Recent acute MI
- SBP greater than 185 mm Hg or DBP greater than 110 mm Hg at the time of treatment, or patient requires aggressive treatment to reduce BP to within these limits
- Combination of previous stroke and diabetes mellitus (excluded from ECASS III trial)
- Oral anticoagulant use regardless of INR (excluded from ECASS III trial)

---

aPTT, activated partial thromboplastin time; AVM, arteriovenous malformation; CT, computed tomography; DBP, diastolic blood pressure; ECASS III, European Cooperative Acute Stroke Study III; INR, International Normalized Ratio; MI, myocardial infarction; PT, prothrombin time; SAH, subarachnoid hemorrhage; SBP, systolic blood pressure.

the infusion, and then every hour until 24 hours after alteplase administration. In the NINDS trial, neurological function was assessed 24 hours after the administration of alteplase using the National Institutes of Health Stroke Scale (NIHSS). This 42-point scale quantifies neurological deficits in patients who have had a stroke and is easily performed. At 3 months, the NIHSS and other neurological assessments were completed. Use of a standardized stroke scale such as the NIHSS is recommended at baseline and 24 hours after the administration of alteplase.

The major adverse effects of thrombolytic therapy are bleeding, including ICH and serious systemic bleeding. Mental status changes and a severe headache may indicate ICH. Signs of bleeding include easy bruising, hematemesis, guaiac-positive stools, black, tarry stools, hematoma formation, hematuria, bleeding gums, and nosebleeds. Angioedema is a potential side effect that may cause airway obstruction.

▶ Other Thrombolytics

Streptokinase and other thrombolytics, except alteplase, are not indicated for use in acute ischemic stroke. Three large randomized controlled trials evaluating streptokinase were stopped early due to a high incidence of hemorrhage in the streptokinase-treated patients.[23–25] Other thrombolytic agents, including tenecteplase, reteplase, desmoteplase, urokinase, and plasmin, are not recommended for treatment unless associated with a clinical trial. Although the results with these newer agents have been mixed, clinical trials are currently ongoing.[12,22]

▶ Intraarterial Thrombolytics

Intraarterial (IA) thrombolytics may improve outcomes in selected patients with acute ischemic stroke due to large-vessel occlusion. Patients in two clinical trials received pro-urokinase (r-pro UK) plus heparin or heparin alone within 6 hours of symptom onset.[26,27] Results from the first trial were not statistically significant but favored r-pro UK, whereas the results of the second trial showed a statistically significant benefit to r-pro UK. No difference in mortality was found, although the incidence of intracranial hemorrhage was greater in the r-pro UK plus heparin group versus heparin alone. Note that r-pro UK is not FDA-approved and not available for clinical use. A recent meta-analysis of five clinical trials evaluating IA thrombolytics found comparable results.[28] The treatment group was found to have a statistically significant benefit for either a good outcome or an excellent outcome. The incidence of intracranial hemorrhage was increased; however, no difference in mortality was observed. Interest in IA thrombolysis has continued as an option for patients who have contraindications to IV alteplase. It may be used in patients with middle cerebral artery occlusion within 6 hours of symptom onset. IA thrombolysis should be performed by qualified personnel and should not delay treatment with IV alteplase in eligible patients.[12]

Heparin

Full-dose IV UFH has been commonly used in acute stroke therapy; however, no adequately designed trials have been conducted to establish its efficacy and safety. Current acute ischemic stroke treatment guidelines do not recommend routine urgent full-dose anticoagulation with UFH due to the lack of a proven benefit in improving neurological function and the risk of intracranial bleeding.[12,17,29] Full-dose UFH may prevent early recurrent stroke in patients with large-vessel atherothrombosis or those thought to be at high risk of recurrent stroke (i.e., cardioembolic stroke); however, more study is required.

The major complications of heparin include conversion of the ischemic stroke into a hemorrhagic stroke, bleeding, and thrombocytopenia. The occurrence of severe headache and mental status changes may indicate ICH. Signs of bleeding mirror those listed for alteplase therapy. The hemoglobin, hematocrit, and platelet count should be obtained at least every 3 days to detect bleeding and thrombocytopenia.

LMWHs and Heparinoids

Full-dose LMWHs and heparinoids are not recommended in the treatment of acute ischemic stroke.[12,17,30] Studies with these agents have generally been negative, and no convincing evidence exists that these agents improve outcomes after ischemic stroke. An increased risk of bleeding complications and hemorrhagic transformation has been observed.

Antiplatelets

ASA in acute ischemic stroke was studied in two large randomized trials, the International Stroke Trial and the Chinese Acute Stroke Trial.[31,32] Patients who received ASA within 24 to 48 hours of the onset of acute ischemic stroke symptoms were less likely to suffer early recurrent stroke, death, and disability. ❼ *ASA therapy with an initial dose of 150 to 325 mg is recommended in most patients with acute ischemic stroke within 48 hours after stroke symptom onset.* The ASA dose may then be reduced to 50 to 100 mg daily to reduce bleeding complications.[17]

The administration of ASA should not replace other acute stroke treatments and should be delayed for 24 hours in those patients receiving alteplase. Clopidogrel either alone or in combination with ASA is not recommended in acute ischemic stroke. Glycoprotein IIb/IIIa receptor inhibitors are not recommended except in the setting of research.[12]

Ancrod

Ancrod is an investigational agent that acts to decrease plasma fibrinogen levels. Based on available clinical trials, ancrod appears to have a potential benefit when used within 3 hours of stroke symptom onset. A recent study using a 6-hour window after symptom onset found no difference in efficacy or mortality between the ancrod and placebo groups. Ancrod is not recommended for clinical use because efficacy and safety have not been definitively established.[12,33]

PREVENTION OF ACUTE ISCHEMIC STROKE

Primary Prevention

▶ Aspirin

The use of ASA in patients with no history of stroke or ischemic heart disease reduced the incidence of nonfatal myocardial infarction (MI) but not of stroke. The Women's Health Study evaluated over 39,000 women and found a benefit with ASA use in high-risk women 65 years and older.[34] Women with a history of hypertension, hyperlipidemia, diabetes, or a 10-year cardiovascular risk greater than or equal to 10% were found to have a reduced stroke risk. A recent meta-analysis found a higher risk of hemorrhagic stroke in men and a greater risk of major bleeding in both men and women.[35] Primary prevention guidelines recommend ASA for general cardiovascular prophylaxis (not specific to stroke) in men and women with a 10-year risk of cardiovascular events of 6% to 10% and in older women who are at high risk for stroke. The benefits must be weighed against the risk of major bleeding. Due to a lack of benefit observed in clinical trials, ASA is not recommended for primary prevention in patients with diabetes and asymptomatic peripheral arterial disease, or in those at low risk.[6]

▶ Diabetes

Diabetes has been shown to be an independent risk factor for stroke. Intensive glycemic control has not been shown to reduce stroke risk in either type 1 or type 2 diabetes mellitus. Aggressive control of blood pressure according to the Joint National Committee on the Prevention, Detection, Evaluation, and Treatment of High Blood Pressure (JNC 7) guidelines and management of dyslipidemia is recommended in individuals with diabetes.[6,36] Hypertension therapy that includes an angiotensin-converting enzyme inhibitor (ACE-I) or angiotensin receptor blocker (ARB) and the use of a statin are recommended to reduce stroke risk.

Patient Encounter Part 2

TK arrives in the emergency department 3 hours after the onset of her symptoms. In the emergency department, an IV line is placed, a physical and neurological examination is completed, and TK is moved to the stroke unit. A head CT scan is negative for hemorrhagic stroke. Her blood pressure on admission to the stroke unit is 194/110 mm Hg. TK denies other exclusions to IV alteplase. The neurologist is evaluating TK for alteplase administration.

Identify your acute treatment goals for TK.

Is TK a candidate for IV alteplase at this time?

What acute management would be appropriate for TK in the stroke unit?

▶ Dyslipidemia

Dyslipidemia has not previously been identified as an independent risk factor for stroke; however, recent studies have found a relationship between total cholesterol levels and stroke rate.[6] Statin use may reduce the incidence of a first stroke in high-risk patients (e.g., hypertension, coronary heart disease, or diabetes) including patients with normal lipid levels. Stroke risk was decreased by 27% to 32% overall in large clinical trials.[37,38] Patients with a history of MI, coronary artery disease (CAD), elevated lipid levels, diabetes, and other risk factors benefit from treatment with a lipid-lowering agent including patients with normal lipid levels.

▶ Hypertension

Hypertension is the most important and well-documented risk factor for stroke. Lowering BP in patients who are hypertensive has been shown to reduce the relative risk of stroke, both ischemic and hemorrhagic, by 35% to 44%.[39] All patients should have their BP monitored and controlled appropriately based on current guidelines for BP management. The BP goal is less than 140/90 mm Hg in the general population and less than 130/80 mm Hg when renal disease or diabetes is present.[36] Many patients require two or more drug therapies to achieve BP control. For the primary prevention of stroke, reduction in BP is the main goal because one antihypertensive agent has not been clearly shown to be more beneficial than any other.

▶ Smoking Cessation

The relationship between smoking and both ischemic and hemorrhagic stroke is clear. Smoking status should be assessed at every patient visit. Patients should be assisted and encouraged in smoking cessation as the stroke risk after cessation has been shown to decline over time. Effective treatment options are available including counseling, nicotine replacement products, and oral agents.

▶ Other Treatments

A number of other disease states and lifestyle factors should be addressed as primary prevention of stroke. Atrial fibrillation is an important and well-documented risk for stroke. See Chapter 9 for information on stroke prevention in atrial fibrillation. Asymptomatic carotid stenosis, cardiac disease, sickle cell disease, obesity, and physical inactivity are other risks that should be assessed and managed appropriately.

Secondary Prevention

▶ Nonpharmacologic Therapy

Carotid Endarterectomy The benefit of carotid endarterectomy for prevention of recurrent stroke has been studied in major clinical trials including a meta-analysis combining these clinical trials to evaluate 6,092 patients.[40] Carotid endarterectomy is recommended to prevent ipsilateral stroke in patients with symptomatic carotid artery stenosis of 70% or greater when the surgical risk is less than 6%.

In patients with symptomatic stenosis of 50% to 69%, a moderate reduction in risk is seen in clinical trials. In those patients with stenosis of 50% to 69% and a recent stroke, carotid endarterectomy is appropriate. In other patients, surgical risk factors and surgeon skill should be considered prior to surgery, and surgical risk should be less than 6%. Carotid endarterectomy is not beneficial for symptomatic carotid stenosis less than 50% and should not be considered in these patients.

Patients with asymptomatic carotid artery stenosis of 60% or more may benefit from carotid endarterectomy if surgical complication rates are low (less than 3%); however, this remains controversial. Recommendations suggest considering carotid endarterectomy in patients with carotid artery stenosis of 60% to 99% who are between 40 and 75 years of age if there is a 5-year life expectancy and the operative risks are low.[41]

Carotid Angioplasty Carotid angioplasty with stenting has evolved as a less invasive procedure with shorter recovery times for appropriate patients. Several trials have been completed comparing carotid angioplasty with stenting to carotid endarterectomy in symptomatic patients. A recent prospective randomized trial found no statistically significant difference in outcomes at 30 days and 4 years.[42] Carotid angioplasty with stenting is an alternative to carotid endarterectomy in high-risk surgical candidates with greater than 50% stenosis by angiography and greater than 70% stenosis by noninvasive imaging when performed by skilled clinicians.[43]

▶ *Pharmacologic Therapy*

Aspirin In a meta-analysis including 144,051 patients with previous MI, acute MI, previous TIA or stroke, or acute stroke, as well as others at high risk, ASA was found to decrease the risk of recurrent stroke by approximately 25%.[44] ASA decreases the risk of subsequent stroke by approximately 22% in both men and women with previous TIA or stroke.[44] Therefore, ASA is an option for initial therapy for secondary prevention of ischemic stroke. A wide range of doses have been used (30 to 1,500 mg/day); however, the FDA has approved doses of 50 to 325 mg for secondary ischemic stroke prevention. Current guidelines recommend varying ASA doses including ASA 50 to 100 mg daily and 50 to 325 mg daily.[17,43] Lower ASA doses are currently recommended to decrease the risk of bleeding complications associated with higher doses of ASA. Adverse effects of ASA include GI intolerance, GI bleeding, and hypersensitivity reactions.

Ticlopidine Ticlopidine is slightly more beneficial in secondary stroke prevention than ASA in men and women.[43] The usual recommended dosage is 250 mg orally twice daily. Ticlopidine is costly, and side effects include bone marrow suppression, rash, diarrhea, and an increased cholesterol level. Neutropenia is seen in approximately 2% of patients. Thrombotic thrombocytopenic purpura (TTP) occurs in 1 of every 2,000 to 4,000 patients treated with ticlopidine. Monitoring of the complete blood count (CBC) is required

every 2 weeks for the first 3 months of therapy. Due to the costly laboratory monitoring required and the adverse effect profile, ticlopidine is typically avoided clinically.

Clopidogrel Clopidogrel is slightly more effective than ASA and similar in efficacy to the combination of extended-release (ER) dipyridamole plus aspirin.[45,46] The usual dose is 75 mg orally taken once daily. Clopidogrel has a lower incidence of diarrhea and neutropenia than ticlopidine, and laboratory monitoring is not required. There have been 11 case reports of TTP occurring secondary to clopidogrel. Most occurred within the first 2 weeks of therapy; therefore, clinicians need to be aware of the potential for the development of TTP with clopidogrel. Proton pump inhibitors may decrease the effectiveness of clopidogrel. An H_2 blocker may be preferred in patients who require both acid suppression and clopidogrel.[47] Patients with a genetic variant of CYP2C19 classified as poor metabolizers may have a decrease in the active metabolite of clopidogrel.[48] Clopidogrel should be used as monotherapy for stroke prevention. It is an option for initial therapy for secondary prevention of ischemic stroke and considered first-line therapy in patients who also have peripheral arterial disease.

Extended-Release Dipyridamole Plus Aspirin Combination therapy with ER dipyridamole plus ASA was more effective than either treatment alone in the European Stroke Prevention Study 2 (ESPS 2).[49] Patients received either placebo, ASA 25 mg twice daily, ER dipyridamole 200 mg twice daily, or a combination of both agents. The risk reduction with ASA was 18.1% and 16.3% with ER dipyridamole, whereas the combination produced a 37% risk reduction. Headache and diarrhea were common adverse effects of dipyridamole; bleeding was more common in the treatment groups receiving ASA. This is the first study showing that combination antiplatelet therapy has additive effects over each agent alone. A trial comparing the combination of ER dipyridamole plus ASA to clopidogrel found no difference in outcomes; however, adverse events occurred more frequently in the combination of ER dipyridamole plus ASA group.[46] The currently available formulation is a combination product containing 25 mg ASA and 200 mg ER dipyridamole. This combination is an option for initial therapy, but is not appropriate for patients who are intolerant to ASA.

Current Clinical Trials Recent trials have been completed to evaluate other combinations of antiplatelet agents and to compare them against one another. In the Management of Atherothrombosis with Clopidogrel in High-risk Patients with Recent Transient Ischaemic Attack or Ischaemic Stroke (MATCH) trial, low-dose ASA plus clopidogrel combination therapy did not show a significant benefit in reducing recurrent stroke compared with clopidogrel alone.[50] This trial found that the addition of ASA to clopidogrel increased the risk of major bleeding. The Clopidogrel for High Atherothrombotic Risk and Ischemic Stabilization, Management, and Avoidance (CHARISMA) trial compared the combination of clopidogrel plus low-dose ASA to low-dose ASA alone in patients with cardiovascular disease or multiple risk factors.[51] The combination did not show a benefit over monotherapy in the prevention of cardiovascular events. An increased bleeding risk was observed in the stroke subgroup. The combination of ASA and clopidogrel is not recommended due to these concerns. The European/Australasian Stroke Prevention in Reversible Ischaemia Trial (ESPRIT) compared the combination of ASA and dipyridamole with ASA alone.[52] ASA was dosed between 30 and 325 mg daily and dipyridamole was dosed at 200 mg twice daily with 83% of patients using ER dipyridamole. This trial showed that the combination of ASA and dipyridamole was more effective at preventing recurrent stroke than ASA alone. In the Prevention Regimen for Effectively Avoiding Second Strokes (PRoFESS) trial, comparing the combination of ASA and ER dipyridamole to clopidogrel, neither agent was shown to be superior.[46]

Antiplatelet Therapy Summary ⑧ *Current stroke treatment guidelines recommend ASA, clopidogrel, or combination therapy with ER dipyridamole plus ASA as initial antiplatelet therapy for the secondary prevention of stroke.[17,43]* ⑨ *Initial choice of agent should be individualized based on patient factors and cost. Clopidogrel and the combination of ER dipyridamole and ASA are preferred over ASA monotherapy.* Therapeutic failure in this patient population is challenging because no data are available to guide a treatment decision. When a patient is on therapeutic doses of ASA, yet experiences a recurrent TIA or stroke, switching to either clopidogrel or the combination of ASA and ER dipyridamole is a reasonable option. If failure occurs on either clopidogrel or the combination of ASA and ER dipyridamole, switching to the alternate drug may be appropriate.

Warfarin Recent clinical trials have not found oral anticoagulation in those patients without atrial fibrillation or carotid stenosis to be better than antiplatelet therapy. In patients without atrial fibrillation, antiplatelet therapy is recommended over warfarin. Patients with atrial fibrillation and a previous TIA or stroke have the highest risk of recurrent stroke. Long-term anticoagulation with warfarin is effective and therefore recommended in the primary and secondary prevention of cardioembolic stroke.[17,43] The goal international normalized ratio (INR) for this indication is 2 to 3.

▶ Blood Pressure Management

Hypertension is an important risk factor for stroke; however, it had been unclear if lowering BP reduced the incidence of secondary ischemic stroke. In the Perindopril Protection Against Recurrent Stroke Study (PROGRESS), it was shown that BP reduction using the ACE-I perindopril alone resulted in a 28% reduction in recurrent stroke compared with placebo. With the addition of the diuretic indapamide to perindopril, a 43% reduction in stroke recurrence was seen.[53] This reduction in stroke incidence occurred even in patients who were not hypertensive. In patients with a previous history of TIA or stroke, the JNC 7 recommends a diuretic and an ACE-I.[36] Table 11–5 provides drug and dosing recommendations for the treatment of ischemic stroke.

▶ Other Recommendations

Management of diabetes and lipids based on treatment guidelines, cessation of smoking, increased physical activity, and reducing alcohol use in heavy drinkers are additional recommendations for management of patients with previous stroke or TIA.[43] Statin therapy is recommended in patients with previous stroke or TIA, regardless of history of coronary heart disease.

Table 11–5

Recommendations for Pharmacotherapy of Ischemic Stroke

	Primary Agents	Alternatives
Acute treatment	Alteplase 0.9 mg/kg IV (maximum dose 90 mg); 10% as IV bolus, remainder infused over 1 hour in selected patients within 3 hours of onset ASA 150–325 mg started within 48 hours of onset (may reduce dose to 50–100 mg daily after 48 hours)	Alteplase 0.9 mg/kg IV (maximum dose 90 mg); 10% as IV bolus, remainder infused over 1 hour in selected patients between 3 and 4.5 hours of onset Alteplase (various doses) intraarterially up to 6 hours after onset in selected patients
Secondary prevention	ASA 50–325 mg daily Clopidogrel 75 mg daily ASA 25 mg + ER dipyridamole 200 mg twice daily	Ticlopidine 250 mg twice daily
Cardioembolic	Warfarin (INR 2–3)	

All patients	ACE-I + diuretic or ARB; BP lowering:
	    Perindopril 2–8 mg daily
	    Indapamide 1.25–5 mg daily
	Statin therapy	

ACE-I, angiotensin-converting enzyme inhibitor; ARB, angiotensin receptor blocker; ASA, aspirin; BP, blood pressure; ER, extended-release; INR, International Normalized Ratio.

Patient Encounter Part 3

TK's blood pressure responds to the antihypertensive agent within 35 minutes and her current BP is 178/100 mm Hg. She is still experiencing weakness in the right arm and leg and difficulty speaking at times. The neurologist decides to administer IV alteplase because she is now 4 hours after the onset of symptoms and is being managed in the stroke unit.

What recommendations would you make regarding the administration of IV alteplase in TK?

What treatments would you recommend for TK at this time to reduce her risk of another stroke?

TREATMENT OF ACUTE HEMORRHAGIC STROKE

Supportive Measures

Acute hemorrhagic stroke is considered to be an acute medical emergency due to ICH, SAH, or subdural hematoma. Initially, patients experiencing a hemorrhagic stroke should be transported to a neurointensive care unit. ⑩ *There is no proven treatment for ICH. Management is based on neurointensive care treatment and prevention of complications.* Treatment should be provided to manage the needs of the critically ill patient including management of increased ICP, seizures, infections, and prevention of rebleeding and delayed cerebral ischemia. In those with severely depressed consciousness, rapid endotracheal intubation and mechanical ventilation may be necessary. BP is often elevated after hemorrhagic stroke; appropriate management is important to prevent rebleeding and expansion of the hematoma. Two trials in ICH patients have been completed evaluating early intensive BP management. Treatment guidelines have been updated to suggest that in patients with systolic BPs between 150 and 220 mm Hg, lowering the systolic BP to 140 mm Hg is a reasonable approach.[54] BP can be controlled with IV boluses of labetalol 10 to 80 mg every 10 minutes up to a maximum of 300 mg or with IV infusions of labetalol (0.5 to 2 mg/min) or nicardipine (5 to 15 mg/h). Deep vein thrombosis prophylaxis with intermittent compression stockings should be implemented early after admission. In those patients with SAH, once the aneurysm has been treated, heparin may be instituted. In ICH patients with lack of mobility after 1 to 4 days, heparin or LMWH may be started.[9,54]

Nonpharmacologic Therapy

Patients with hemorrhagic stroke are evaluated for surgical treatment of SAH and ICH. In SAH, either clipping of the aneurysm or coil embolization is recommended within 72 hours after the initial event to prevent rebleeding. Coil embolization, also called coiling, is a minimally invasive procedure in which a platinum coil is threaded into the aneurysm. The flexible coil fills up the space to block blood flow into the aneurysm thereby preventing rebleeding. Surgical removal of the hematoma in patients with ICH is controversial because trials have not consistently shown improved outcomes. Minimally invasive

clot removal techniques with or without thrombolytic therapy aspiration have been evaluated; however, these procedures are considered investigational because outcomes are not certain. Current guidelines note that surgical treatment of ICH is uncertain and is not recommended except in specific patient situations.[54]

Pharmacologic Therapy

▶ Calcium Antagonists

Oral nimodipine is recommended in SAH to prevent delayed cerebral ischemia. It is recommended to begin oral nimodipine promptly after the initial event, but no later than 96 hours following SAH. Delayed cerebral ischemia occurs 4 to 14 days after the initial aneurysm rupture and is a common cause of neurological deficits and death. A meta-analysis of 12 studies was conducted and concluded that oral nimodipine 60 mg every 4 hours for 21 days following aneurysmal SAH reduced the risk of a poor outcome and delayed cerebral ischemia.[55]

▶ Hemostatic Therapy

Recombinant factor VIIa has been shown to have a benefit in the treatment of ICH. The Recombinant Activated Factor VII Intracerebral Hemorrhage Trial compared doses of 40, 80, or 160 mcg/kg or placebo given as an IV infusion over 1 to 2 minutes within 4 hours after the onset of symptoms. Hematoma growth was decreased at 24 hours, mortality was decreased at 90 days, and overall functioning was increased at 90 days in the treatment group. An increased incidence of thromboembolic events was seen in the treatment group.[56] A recent phase 3 trial comparing 20 mcg/kg, 80 mcg/kg, and placebo showed that recombinant factor VIIa decreased growth of the hematoma, but did not improve survival or functional outcome. Intraventricular hemorrhage was more likely in the 80 mcg/kg group.[57] Current guidelines do not recommend treatment with recombinant factor VIIa due to an uncertain benefit and the increased risk of thromboembolic events. Further trials are warranted to determine specific patients that may benefit from therapy.[54]

OUTCOME EVALUATION

- Stroke outcomes are measured based on the neurological status and functioning of the patient after the acute event. The NIHSS is a measure of daily functioning and used to assess patient status following a stroke.

- Early rehabilitation can reduce functional impairment after a stroke. Recent stroke rehabilitation guidelines have been endorsed by the American Heart Association and the American Stroke Association. These guidelines recommend that patients receive care in a multidisciplinary setting or stroke unit, receive early assessment using the NIHSS, and recommend that rehabilitation is started as soon as possible after the stroke. Other recommendations include screening for dysphagia and aggressive secondary stroke prevention treatments.[58]

- Table 11–6 provides monitoring guidelines for the acute stroke patient.

Table 11–6

Monitoring the Stroke Patient

Treatment	Parameter(s)	Monitoring Frequency	Comments
Ischemic stroke			
Alteplase	BP	Every 15 minutes × 2 hours, every 0.5 hour × 6 hours, every 1 hour × 16 hours; then every shift	
	Neurologic function	Neurological exam every 15 minutes × 1 hour, every 0.5 hour × 6 hours, every 1 hour × 17 hours; NIHSS 24 hours after alteplase infusion and at discharge	
	Bleeding	Clinical signs of bleeding every 2 hours × 24 hours	
ASA	Bleeding Hb/Hct, platelets[a]	Daily	
Clopidogrel	Bleeding Hb/Hct, platelets[a]	Daily	
ASA/ER dipyridamole	Headache, bleeding Hb/Hct, platelets[a]	Daily	
Warfarin	Bleeding, INR, Hb/Hct[a]	INR daily × 3 days; weekly until stable; then monthly	
Hemorrhagic stroke			
	BP, neurologic function, ICP	Every 2 hours in ICU	May require treatments to lower BP to less than 180 mm Hg systolic
Nimodipine for SAH	BP, neurologic function, fluid status	Every 2 hours in ICU	

ASA, aspirin; BP, blood pressure; ER, extended-release; Hb, hemoglobin; Hct, hematocrit; ICP, intracranial pressure; ICU, intensive care unit; INR, International Normalized Ratio; NIHSS, National Institutes of Health Stroke Scale; SAH, subarachnoid hemorrhage.
[a]Hb/Hct and platelets should be monitored at baseline and every 6 months for ASA, clopidogrel, ASA/ER dipyridamole, and warfarin treatment.

Patient Care and Monitoring

1. Assess the patient's signs and symptoms including the time of symptom onset and the time of arrival in the emergency department.

2. Perform thorough neurological and physical examinations evaluating for potential causes of the stroke.

3. Perform a CT scan to rule out a hemorrhagic stroke prior to administering any treatment.

4. Evaluate the inclusion and exclusion criteria for thrombolytic therapy to determine appropriateness for the patient.

5. Transfer the patient to a stroke center if available and develop a plan for the acute management of the patient.

6. Determine the patient's risk factors for stroke.

7. Develop a plan for the long-term management of risk factors in order to prevent a recurrent stroke.

8. Educate the patient on appropriate lifestyle modifications that will reduce stroke risk.

9. Educate the patient on their medication regimen stressing the importance of adherence.

Abbreviations Introduced in This Chapter

ACE-I	Angiotensin-converting enzyme inhibitor
ADP	Adenosine diphosphate
aPTT	Activated partial thromboplastin time
ARB	Angiotensin receptor blocker
ASA	Aspirin
AVM	Arteriovenous malformation
BPH	Benign prostatic hypertrophy
BP	Blood pressure
CAD	Coronary artery disease
CBC	Complete blood count
CEA	Carotid endarterectomy
CHARISMA	Clopidogrel for High Atherothrombotic Risk and Ischemic Stabilization, Management, and Avoidance
CT	Computed tomography
CVD	Cerebrovascular disease
DBP	Diastolic blood pressure
DVT	Deep vein thrombosis
ECASS III	European Cooperative Acute Stroke Study III
ECG	Electrocardiogram
ER	Extended release
ESPRIT	European/Australasian Stroke Prevention in Reversible Ischaemia Trial

ESPS 2	European Stroke Prevention Study 2
Hb	Hemoglobin
Hct	Hematocrit
IA	Intraarterial
ICA	Internal carotid artery
ICH	Intracerebral hemorrhage
ICP	Intracranial pressure
ICU	Intensive care unit
INR	International normalized ratio
JNC 7	Joint National Committee on the Prevention, Detection, Evaluation, and Treatment of High Blood Pressure
LMWH	Low molecular weight heparin
MATCH	Management of Atherothrombosis with Clopidogrel in High-risk Patients with Recent Transient Ischaemic Attack or Ischaemic Stroke
MI	Myocardial infarction
MRI	Magnetic resonance imaging
NIHSS	National Institutes of Health Stroke Scale
NINDS	National Institute of Neurological Disorders and Stroke
NS	Normal saline
PRoFESS	Prevention Regimen for Effectively Avoiding Second Strokes
PROGRESS	Perindopril Protection Against Recurrent Stroke Study
PT	Prothrombin time
rt-PA	Alteplase
r-pro UK	Pro-urokinase
SAH	Subarachnoid hemorrhage
SBP	Systolic blood pressure
TIA	Transient ischemic attack
t-PA	Tissue plasminogen activator
TTP	Thrombotic thrombocytopenic purpura
UFH	Unfractionated heparin
VTE	Venous thromboembolism

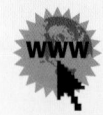 Self-assessment questions and answers are available at *http://www.mhpharmacotherapy. com/pp.html.*

REFERENCES

1. Towfight A, Saver JL. Stroke declines from third to fourth leading cause of death in the United States. Stroke 2011;42:2351–2355.
2. Roger VL, Go AS, Lloyd-Jones DM, et al.; on behalf of the American Heart Association Statistics Committee and Stroke Statistics Subcommittee. Heart disease and stroke statistics—2011 update: A report from the American Heart Association. Circulation 2011;123:e18–e209.
3. Easton JD, Saver JL, Albers GW, et al. Definition and evaluation of transient ischemic attack: A scientific statement for healthcare professionals from the American Heart Association/American Stroke Association Stroke Council; Council on Cardiovascular Surgery and Anesthesia; Council on Cardiovascular Radiology and Intervention; Council on Cardiovascular Nursing; and the Interdisciplinary Council on Peripheral Vascular Disease. Stroke 2009;40:2276–2293.
4. Hankey GJ. Impact of treatment of people with transient ischemic attack on stroke incidence and public health. Cerebrovasc Dis 1996;6(Suppl 1):26–33.
5. Saver JL. Proposal for a universal definition of cerebral infarction. Stroke 2008;39:3110–3115.
6. Goldstein LB, Bushnell CD, Adam R, et al.; on behalf of the American Heart Association Stroke Council, Council on Cardiovascular Nursing, Council on Epidemiology and Prevention, Council for High Blood Pressure Research, Council on Peripheral Vascular Disease, and Interdisciplinary Council on Quality of Care and Outcomes Research. Guidelines for the primary prevention of stroke: A guideline for healthcare professionals from the American Heart Association/American Stroke Association. Stroke 2011;42:517–584.
7. Grysiewicz RA, Thomas D, Pandey DK. Epidemiology of ischemic and hemorrhagic stroke: Incidence, prevalence, mortality and risk factors. Neurol Clin 2008;26:871-895.
8. Ariesen MJ, Claus SP, Rinkel GJE, Algra A. Risk factors for intracerebral hemorrhage in the general population: A systematic review. Stroke 2003;34:2060–2065.
9. Suarez JI, Tarr RW, Selman WR. Aneurysmal subarachnoid hemorrhage. N Engl J Med 2006;354:387–396.
10. Testai FD, Aiyagari V. Acute hemorrhagic stroke pathophysiology and medical interventions: Blood pressure control, management of anticoagulant-associated brain hemorrhage and general management principles. Neurol Clin 2008;26:963–985.
11. Treib J, Grauer MT, Woessner R, Morganthaler M. Treatment of stroke on an intensive stroke unit: A novel concept. Intensive Care Med 2000; 26:1598–1611.
12. Adams HP, del Zoppo G, Alberts MJ, et al. Guidelines for the early management of adults with ischemic stroke: A guideline from the American Heart Association/American Stroke Association Stroke Council, Clinical Cardiology Council, Cardiovascular Radiology and Intervention Council, and the Atherosclerotic Peripheral Vascular Disease and Quality of Care Outcomes in Research Interdisciplinary Working Groups. Stroke 2007;38:1655–1711.
13. Baker L, Juneja R, Bruno A. Management of hyperglycemia in acute ischemic stroke. Curr Treat Options Neurol 2011;13:616–628.
14. Kallmunzer B, Kollmar R. Temperature management in stroke—An unsolved, but important topic. Cerebrovasc Dis 2011;31:532–543.
15. Morfis L, Schwartz RS, Poulos R, Howes LG. Blood pressure changes in acute cerebral infarction and hemorrhage. Stroke 1997;28:141–145.
16. National Institute of Neurological Disorders and Stroke rt-PA Stroke Study Group. Tissue plasminogen activator for acute ischemic stroke. N Engl J Med 1995;333:1581–1587.
17. Albers GW, Amarenco P, Easton JD, Sacco RL, Teal P. Antithrombotic and thrombolytic therapy for ischemic stroke: American College of Chest Physicians evidence-based clinical practice guidelines. 8th ed. Chest 2008;133:630–669.
18. The ATLANTIS, ECASS, and NINDS rt-PA Study Group Investigators. Association of outcome with early stroke treatment: Pooled analysis of ATLANTIS, ECASS, and NINDS rt-PA stroke trials. Lancet 2004;363:768–774.
19. Hacke W, Kaste M, Bluhmke E, et al. Thrombolysis with alteplase 3 to 4.5 hours after acute ischemic stroke. N Engl J Med 2008;359(13):1317–1329.
20. Lees KR, Bluhmki E, von Kummer R, et al. Time to treatment with intravenous alteplase and outcome in stroke: An updated pooled analysis of ECASS, ATLANTIS, NINDS, and EPITHET trials. Lancet 2010;375:1695–1703.
21. del Zoppo GJ, Saver JL, Jauch ED, Adams HP Jr. Expansion of the time window for treatment of acute ischemic stroke with intravenous tissue plasminogen activator: A science advisory from the American Heart Association/American Stroke Association. Stroke 2009;40:2945–2948.
22. Barreto AD. Intravenous thrombolytics for ischemic stroke. Neurotherapeutics 2011;8:388–399.
23. Donnan GA, Davis SM, Chambers BR, et al. Streptokinase for acute ischemic stroke with relationship to time of administration: Australian Streptokinase (ASK) Trial Study Group. JAMA 1996;276:961–966.
24. Multicenter Acute Stroke Trial—Europe Study Group. Thrombolytic therapy with streptokinase in acute ischemic stroke. N Engl J Med 1996;335:145–150.

25. Multicentre Acute Stroke Trial—Italy (MAST-I) Group. Randomised controlled trial of streptokinase, aspirin, and combination of both in treatment of acute ischaemic stroke. Lancet 1995;346:1509–1514.

26. del Zoppo GJ, Higashida RT, Furlan AJ, et al. PROACT: A phase II randomized trial of recombinant pro-urokinase by direct arterial delivery in acute middle cerebral artery stroke. Stroke 1998;29:4–11.

27. Furlan A, Higashida R, Wechsler L, et al. Intra-arterial prourokinase for acute ischemic stroke. The PROACT II study: A randomized controlled trial. Prolyse in acute cerebral thromboembolism. JAMA 1999;282:2003–2011.

28. Lee M, Hong KS, Saver JL. Efficacy of intra-arterial fibrinolysis for acute ischemic stroke: Meta-analysis of randomized controlled trials. Stroke 2010;41:932-937.

29. Sandercock PA, Counsell C, Kamal AK. Anticoagulants for acute ischaemic stroke. Cochrane Database Syst Rev 2008;8(4):CD000024.

30. Sandercock PA, Counsell C, Tseng MC. Low-molecular-weight heparins or heparinoids versus standard unfractionated heparin for acute ischaemic stroke. Cochrane Database Syst Rev 2008;16(3):CD000119.

31. Chinese Acute Stroke Trial (CAST) Collaborative Group. CAST: A randomized, placebo-controlled trial of early aspirin use in 20,000 patients with acute ischemic stroke. Lancet 1997;349:1641–1649.

32. International Stroke Trial Collaborative Group. The International Stroke Trial (IST): A randomized trial of aspirin, subcutaneous heparin, both, or neither among 19,435 patients with acute ischemic stroke. Lancet 1997;349:1560–1581.

33. Levy DE, del Zoppo GJ, Demaerschalk BM, et al. Ancrod in acute ischemic stroke: Results of 500 subjects beginning treatment within 6 hours of stroke onset in the Ancrod Stroke Program. Stroke 2009;40:3796–3803.

34. Ridker PM, Cook NR, Lee IM, et al. A randomized trial of low-dose aspirin in the primary prevention of cardiovascular disease in women. N Engl J Med 2005;352:1293–1304.

35. Berger JS, Roncaglioni MC, Avanzini F, et al. Aspirin for the primary prevention of cardiovascular events in women and men: A sex-specific meta-analysis of randomized controlled trials. JAMA 2006;295:306–313.

36. Chobanian AV, Bakris GL, Black HR, et al. National Heart, Lung, and Blood Institute Joint National Committee on Prevention, Detection, Evaluation, and Treatment of High Blood Pressure; National High Blood Pressure Education Program Coordinating Committee. The seventh report of the Joint National Committee on Prevention, Detection, Evaluation, and Treatment of High Blood Pressure: The JNC 7 report. JAMA 2003;289:2560–2572.

37. Sever PS, Dahlof B, Poulter NR, et al.; ASCOT Investigators. Prevention of coronary and stroke events with atorvastatin in hypertensive patients who have average or lower-than-average cholesterol concentrations, in the Anglo-Scandinavian Cardiac Outcomes Trial-Lipid Lowering Arm (ASCOT-LLA): A multicentre randomised controlled trial. Lancet 2003;361:1149–1158.

38. Collins R, Armitage J, Parish S, et al. Heart Protection Study Collaborative Group. Effects of cholesterol-lowering with simvastatin on stroke and other major vascular events in 20536 people with cerebrovascular disease or other high-risk conditions. Lancet 2004;363:757–767.

39. Neal B, MacMahon S, Chapman N; Blood Pressure Lowering Treatment Trialists' Collaboration. Effects of ACE inhibitors, calcium antagonists, and other blood-pressure-lowering drugs: Results of prospectively designed overviews of randomized trials. Blood Pressure Lowering Treatment Trialists' Collaboration. Lancet 2000;356:1955–1964.

40. Rothwell PM, Eliasziw M, Fox AJ, et al.; for the Carotid Endarterectomy Trialists' Collaboration. Analysis of pooled data from the randomised controlled trials of endarterectomy for symptomatic carotid stenosis. Lancet 2003;361:107–116.

41. Chaturvedi A, Bruno A, Feasby T, et al. Carotid endarterectomy—An evidence-based review. Neurology 2005;65:794–801.

42. Brott TG, Hobson RW II, Howard G, et al. Crest investigators. Stenting versus endarterectomy for treatment of carotid-artery stenosis. N Engl J Med 2010;363:11–23.

43. Furie KL, Kasner SE, Adams RJ, et al.; on behalf of the American Heart Association Stroke Council, Council on Cardiovascular Nursing, Council on Clinical Cardiology, and Interdisciplinary Council on Quality of Care and Outcomes Research. Guidelines for the prevention of stroke in patients with stroke or transient ischemic attack: A guideline for healthcare professionals from the American Heart Association/American Stroke Association. Stroke 2011;42:227–276.

44. Collaborative meta-analysis of randomised trials of antiplatelet therapy for prevention of death, myocardial infarction, and stroke in high risk patients. BMJ 2002;324:71–86.

45. CAPRIE Steering Committee. A randomized, blinded, trial of clopidogrel versus aspirin in patients at risk of ischaemic events. Lancet 1996;348:1329–1339.

46. Sacco RL, Deiner HC, Yusuf S, et al.; PRoFESS Study Group. Aspirin and extended-release dipyridamole versus clopidogrel for recurrent stroke. N Engl J Med 2008;359:1238–1251.

47. Ho PM, Maddox TM, Wang L, et al. Risk of adverse outcomes associated with concomitant use of clopidogrel and proton pump inhibitors following acute coronary syndrome. JAMA 2009;301(9):937–944.

48. Mega JL, Close SL, Wiviott SD, et al. Cytochrome P-450 polymorphisms and response to clopidogrel. N Engl J Med 2009;360:354–362.

49. Diener HC, Cunha L, Forbes C, et al. European Stroke Prevention Study 2. Dipyridamole and acetylsalicylic acid in the secondary prevention of stroke. J Neurol Sci 1996;143:1–13.

50. Deiner HC, Bogousslavsky J, Brass LM, et al.; for the MATCH Investigators. Aspirin and clopidogrel compared with clopidogrel alone after recent ischaemic stroke or transient ischaemic attack in high-risk patients (MATCH): Randomised, double-blind, placebo-controlled trial. Lancet 2004;364:331–337.

51. Bhatt DL, Fox KA, Hacke W, et al.; CHARISMA Investigators. Clopidogrel and aspirin versus aspirin alone for the prevention of atherothrombotic events. N Engl J Med 2006;354(16):1706–1717.

52. The ESPRIT Study Group. Aspirin plus dipyridamole versus aspirin alone after cerebral ischaemia of arterial origin (ESPRIT): Randomized controlled trial. Lancet 2006;367:1665–1673.

53. PROGRESS Collaborative Group. Randomized trial of perindopril-based blood-pressure-lowering regimen among 6105 individuals with previous stroke or transient ischaemic attack. Lancet 2001;358:1033–1041.

54. Morgenstern LB, Hemphill JC 3rd, Anderson C, et al.; on behalf of the American Heart Association Stroke Council and Council on Cardiovascular Nursing. Guidelines for the management of spontaneous intracerebral hemorrhage: A guideline for healthcare professionals from the American Heart Association/American Stroke Association. Stroke 2010;41:1–22.

55. Dorhout Mees SM, Rinkel GJ, Feigin VL, et al. Calcium antagonists for aneurysmal subarachnoid haemorrhage. Cochrane Database Syst Rev 2007;3:CD000277.

56. Mayer SA, Brun NC, Begtrup K, et al., for the Recombinant Activated Factor VII Intracerebral Hemorrhage Trial Investigators. Recombinant activated factor VII for acute intracerebral hemorrhage. N Engl J Med 2005;352:777–785.

57. Mayer SA, Brun NC, Begtrup K. et al.; FAST Trial Investigators. Efficacy and safety of recombinant activated factor VII for acute intracerebral hemorrhage. N Engl J Med 2008;358:2127–2137.

58. Miller EL, Murray L, Richards L, et al.; on behalf of the American Heart Association Council on Cardiovascular Nursing and Stroke Council. Comprehensive overview of nursing and interdisciplinary rehabilitation care of the stroke patient: A scientific statement from the American Heart Association. Stroke 2010;41:2402–2448.

12 Dyslipidemias

Matthew K. Ito

LEARNING OBJECTIVES

● **Upon completion of the chapter, the reader will be able to:**

1. Identify the major components within each lipoprotein and their role in lipoprotein metabolism and the development of atherosclerosis.

2. Identify the common types of lipid disorders.

3. Determine a patient's coronary heart disease risk and corresponding treatment goals according to the National Cholesterol Education Program Adult Treatment Panel III guidelines.

4. Recommend appropriate therapeutic lifestyle changes (TLC) and pharmacotherapy interventions for patients with dyslipidemia.

5. Identify the diagnostic criteria and treatment strategies for metabolic syndrome.

6. Describe the components of a monitoring plan to assess effectiveness and adverse effects of pharmacotherapy for dyslipidemias.

7. Educate patients about the disease state, appropriate TLC, and drug therapy required for effective treatment.

KEY CONCEPTS

❶ The risk of atherosclerosis is directly related to increasing levels of serum cholesterol.

❷ The National Cholesterol Education Program (NCEP) Adult Treatment Panel III guidelines have set the "optimal" level for low-density lipoprotein (LDL) cholesterol for all adults as less than 100 mg/dL (2.59 mmol/L).

❸ The NCEP guidelines recommend that all adults older than 20 years should be screened at least every 5 years using a fasting blood sample to obtain a lipid profile.

❹ The benefits of lowering LDL cholesterol to as low as 70 mg/dL (1.81 mmol/L) have been demonstrated in clinical trials; however, the lowest level at which to treat LDL cholesterol where there are no further benefits in coronary heart disease (CHD) risk has not yet been determined.

❺ An adequate trial of therapeutic lifestyle changes (TLC) should be used in all patients, but pharmacotherapy should be instituted concurrently in higher-risk patients.

❻ Typically, 3-hydroxy-3-methylglutaryl coenzyme A (HMG-CoA) reductase inhibitors (or statins) are the medications of choice to treat high LDL cholesterol because of their: (1) ability to substantially reduce LDL cholesterol and reduce morbidity and mortality from atherosclerotic disease; (b) convenient once-daily dosing; and (c) low risk of side effects.

❼ Patients with metabolic syndrome have an additional lipid parameter that needs to be assessed, namely non–high-density lipoprotein (non-HDL) cholesterol (total cholesterol minus HDL cholesterol). The target for non-HDL cholesterol is less than the patient's LDL cholesterol target plus 30 mg/dL (0.78 mmol/L).

❽ After assessment and control of LDL cholesterol, patients with serum triglycerides of 200 to 499 mg/dL (2.26 to 5.64 mmol/L) should be assessed for atherogenic dyslipidemia (low HDL cholesterol and increased small-dense LDL particles) and metabolic syndrome.

❾ Combination drug therapy is an effective means to achieve greater reductions in LDL cholesterol (statin plus ezetimibe or bile acid resin, bile acid resin plus ezetimibe, or three-drug combinations) as well as raising HDL cholesterol and lowering serum triglycerides (statin plus niacin or fibrate).

❿ The evidence of reducing LDL cholesterol while substantially raising HDL cholesterol (statin plus niacin or fibrate) to reduce the risk of CHD-related events to a greater degree than statin monotherapy remains in question.

INTRODUCTION

① *The risk of atherosclerosis is directly related to increasing levels of serum cholesterol.* Hypercholesterolemia (elevation in serum cholesterol) and other abnormalities in serum lipids play a major role in plaque formation leading to coronary heart disease (CHD) as well as other forms of atherosclerosis, such as **carotid** and **peripheral artery disease** (atherosclerosis of the peripheral arteries). This predictive relationship has been demonstrated from large epidemiological, animal, and genetic studies.[1] CHD is the leading cause of death in both men and women in the United States and most industrialized nations. It is also the chief cause of premature, permanent disability in the U.S. workforce. Annually, approximately 785,000 Americans experience a new heart attack and 470,000 will have a recurrent event. The average age of a first heart attack is 66.5 years for American men and 70.3 years for women. According to a 2011 report, the direct and indirect cost of CHD to the U.S. economy in 2007 was almost $286.6 billion.[2] Clinical trials have consistently demonstrated that lowering serum cholesterol reduces atherosclerotic progression and mortality from CHD.

The development of CHD is a lifelong process. Except in rare cases of severely elevated serum cholesterol levels, years of poor dietary habits, sedentary lifestyle, and life-habit risk factors (e.g., smoking and obesity) contribute to the development of atherosclerosis.[3] Unfortunately, many individuals at risk for CHD do not receive lipid-modifying therapy or are not optimally treated. This chapter helps identify individuals at risk, assesses treatment goals based on the level of CHD risk, and implements optimal treatment strategies and monitoring plans.

PATHOPHYSIOLOGY

Cholesterol and Lipoprotein Metabolism

Cholesterol is an essential substance manufactured by most cells in the body. Cholesterol is used to maintain cell wall integrity and for the biosynthesis of **bile acids** and steroid hormones. Other major lipids in our body are triglycerides and phospholipids. Because cholesterol is a relatively water-insoluble molecule, it is unable to circulate through the blood alone. Cholesterol along with triglycerides and phospholipids are packaged in a large carrier protein called a lipoprotein (**Fig. 12–1**). Lipoproteins are water soluble, which allows transportation of the major lipids in the blood. These lipoproteins are spherical and vary in size (approximately 1,000 to 6 nm) and density (less than 0.94 to 1.21 g/mL) (**Table 12–1**). The amount of cholesterol and triglycerides vary by lipoprotein size. The major lipoproteins in descending size and ascending density are chylomicrons, very low-density lipoprotein (VLDL), intermediate-density lipoprotein (IDL), low-density lipoprotein (LDL), and high-density lipoprotein (HDL). When clinical laboratories measure and report serum total cholesterol, what they are measuring and reporting are the total cholesterol molecules in all the major lipoproteins. The estimated value of LDL cholesterol is found using the

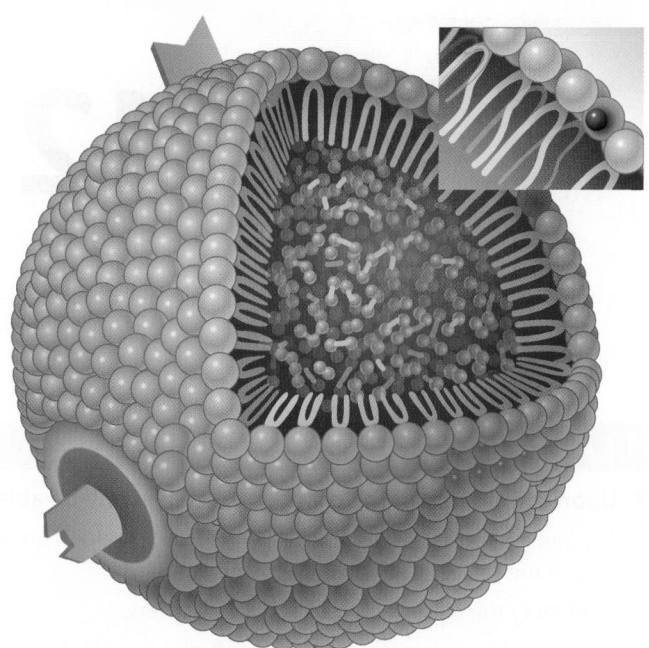

FIGURE 12–1. Lipoprotein structure. Lipoproteins are a diverse group of particles with varying size and density. They contain variable amounts of core cholesterol esters and triglycerides, and have varying numbers and types of surface apolipoproteins. The apolipoproteins function to direct the processing and removal of individual lipoprotein particles.

following equation (after fasting for 9 to 12 hours), which assumes the ratio of triglyceride to cholesterol molecules in VLDL is 5 to 1 molecules:

LDL cholesterol (mg/dL) = total cholesterol – (HDL cholesterol + triglycerides/5) using traditional units of mg/dL

Where triglycerides/5 = VLDL cholesterol

(To convert total, LDL, and HDL cholesterol to SI units: 1 mg/dL = 0.02586 mmol/L)

For example, if an individual's triglycerides = 250 mg/dL, HDL = 35 mg/dL, and total cholesterol = 240 mg/dL, then 155 mg/dL = 240 mg/dL – (35 mg/dL + 250 mg/dL/5).

If serum triglycerides are greater than 400 mg/dL (4.52 mmol/L), the normal ratio of triglycerides to cholesterol of 5:1 in VLDL is disrupted, chylomicrons are present, or the patient has type III hyperlipoproteinemia, this formula becomes inaccurate and LDL cholesterol must be directly measured.[3]

Each lipoprotein has various proteins called apolipoproteins (Apos) embedded on the surface (Fig. 12–1). These Apos serve four main purposes; they (a) are required for assembly and secretion of lipoproteins (such as Apos B-48 and B-100); (b) serve as major structural components of lipoproteins; (c) act as ligands (Apo B-100 and Apo E) for binding to receptors on cell surfaces (LDL receptors); and (d) can be cofactors (such as Apo C-II) for activation of enzymes

Table 12–1

Physical Characteristics of Lipoproteins

| Lipoprotein | Density Range (g/mL) | Size (nm) | Composition (%) | | Apolipoprotein |
			Cholesterol	Triglycerides	
Chylomicrons	Less than 0.95	100–1,000	3–7	85–95	A-I, A-II, A-IV, B-48, C-I, C-II, E
VLDL	Less than 1.006	40–50	20–30	50–65	B-100, C-I, C-II, C-III, E
IDL	1.006–1.019	25–30	40	20	B-100, E
LDL	1.019–1.063	20–25	51–58	4–8	B-100
HDL	1.063–1.21	6–10	18–25	2–7	A-I, A-II, C-I, C-II, C-III, E

HDL, high-density lipoprotein; IDL, intermediate-density lipoprotein; LDL, low-density lipoprotein; VLDL, very low-density lipoprotein.

(such as lipoprotein lipase [LPL]) involved in the breakdown of triglycerides from chylomicrons and VLDL.[4] Apos A-I and A-II are major structural proteins on the surface of HDL. Apo A-I interacts with adenosine triphosphate (ATP) binding cassette A1 and G1 to traffic cholesterol from extrahepatic tissue (such as the arterial wall) to immature or **nascent** HDL.

Cholesterol from the diet as well as from bile enters the small intestine, where it is emulsified by bile salts into **micelles** (**Fig. 12–2**). These micelles interact with the **duodenal** and **jejunal enterocyte** surfaces, and cholesterol is transported from the micelles into these cells by the Niemann-Pick C1 Like 1 (NPC1L1) transporter.[5] Some cholesterol and most

plant sterols, which are structurally similar to cholesterol, are exported back from the enterocyte into the intestinal lumen by the ATP-binding cassette (ABC) G5/G8 transporter. Cholesterol within enterocytes is esterified and packaged into chylomicrons along with triglycerides, phospholipids, and Apo B-48 as well as Apos C and E, which are then released into the **lymphatic** circulation. In the circulation, chylomicrons are converted to chylomicron remnants (through loss of triglycerides by the interaction of Apo C-II and LPL). During this process, chylomicrons also interact with HDL particles (**Fig. 12–3**) and exchange triglyceride and cholesterol content (facilitated by cholesterol ester transfer protein, or CETP), and

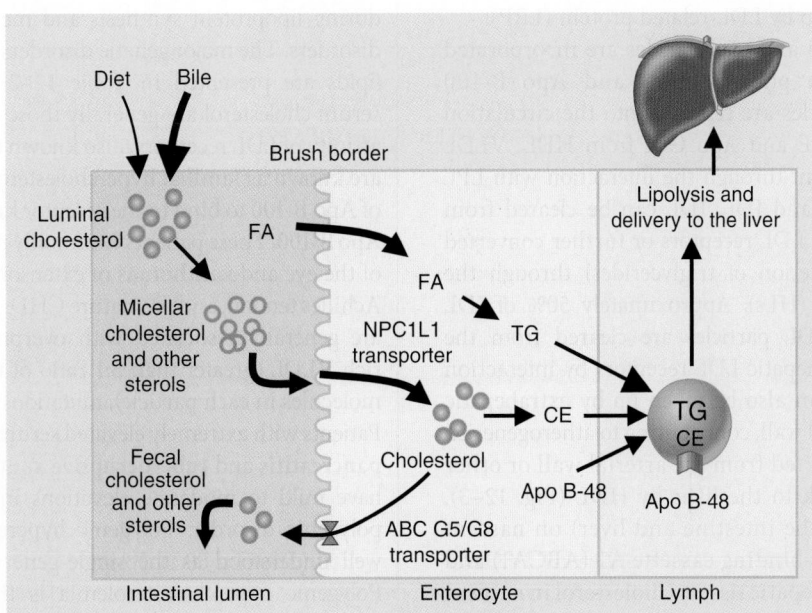

FIGURE 12–2. Intestinal cholesterol absorption and transport. Cholesterol from food and bile enter the gut lumen and are emulsified by bile acids into micelles. Micelles bind to the intestinal enterocytes, and cholesterol and other sterols are transported from the micelles into the enterocytes by a sterol transporter. Triglycerides synthesized by absorbed fatty acids, along with cholesterol and apolipoprotein B-48, are incorporated into chylomicrons. Chylomicrons are released into the lymphatic circulation and are converted to chylomicron remnants (through loss of triglyceride), and then taken up by the hepatic LDL receptor-related protein (LRP). (ABC G5/G8, ATP-binding cassette G5/G8; Apo, apolipoprotein; CE, cholesterol ester; FA, fatty acid; NPC1L1, Niemann-Pick C1 Like 1; TG, triglyceride.)

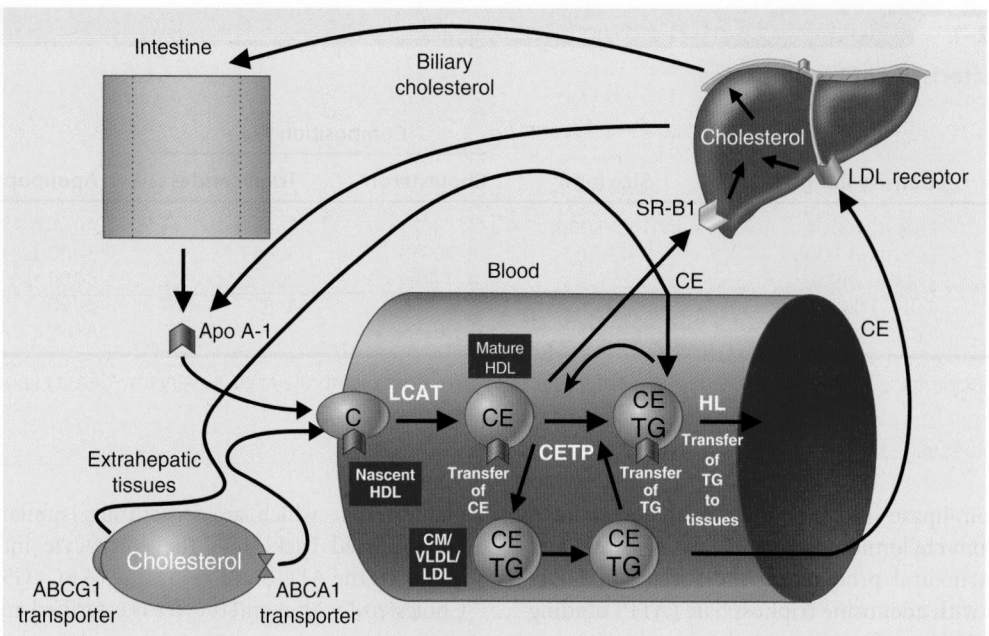

FIGURE 12–3. Reverse cholesterol transport. Cholesterol is transported from the arterial wall or other extrahepatic tissues back to the liver by HDL. Esterified cholesterol from HDL can be transferred to apolipoprotein B–containing particles in exchange for triglycerides. Cholesterol esters transferred from HDL to VLDL and LDL are taken up by hepatic LDL receptors or delivered back to extrahepatic tissue. (ABCA1, ATP-binding cassette A1; ABCG1, ATP-binding cassette G1; Apo, apolipoprotein; C, cholesterol; CE, cholesterol ester; CETP, cholesterol ester transfer protein; CM, chylomicrons; HDL, high-density lipoprotein; HL, hepatic lipase; LCAT, lecithin-cholesterol acyltransferase; LDL, low-density lipoprotein; SR-B1, scavenger receptors; TG, triglyceride; VLDL, very low-density lipoprotein.)

HDL particles acquire Apos A and C. Chylomicron remnant particles are then taken up by LDL-related protein (LRP).

In the liver, cholesterol and triglycerides are incorporated into VLDL along with phospholipids and Apo B-100 (Fig. 12–4). VLDL particles are released into the circulation where they acquire Apo E and Apo C-II from HDL. VLDL loses its triglyceride content through the interaction with LPL to form VLDL remnant and IDL. IDL can be cleared from the circulation by hepatic LDL receptors or further converted to LDL (by further depletion of triglycerides) through the action of hepatic lipases (HLs). Approximately 50% of IDL is converted to LDL. LDL particles are cleared from the circulation primarily by hepatic LDL receptors by interaction with Apo B-100. They can also be taken up by extrahepatic tissues or enter the arterial wall, contributing to atherogenesis.[6]

Cholesterol is transported from the arterial wall or other extrahepatic tissues back to the liver by HDL (Fig. 12–3). Apo A-I (derived from the intestine and liver) on nascent HDL interacts with ATP-binding cassette A1 (ABCA1) and G1 transporter on extrahepatic tissue. Cholesterol in nascent HDL is esterified by lecithin-cholesterol acyltransferase (LCAT) resulting in mature HDL. The esterified cholesterol can be transferred as noted previously to Apo B–containing particles in exchange for triglycerides. Triglyceride-rich HDL is hydrolyzed by HL, generating fatty acids and nascent HDL particles, or the mature HDL can bind to the scavenger receptors (SR-BI) on hepatocytes and transfer their cholesterol ester content for excretion in the bile.

A variety of genetic mutations occur in the steps just outlined during lipoprotein synthesis and metabolism that cause lipid disorders. The major genetic disorders and their effect on serum lipids are presented in Table 12–2. Disorders that increase serum cholesterol are generally those that affect the number or affinity of LDL receptors (also known as Apo B-E receptors) and are known as familial hypercholesterolemia (FH), or the ability of Apo B-100 to bind to the receptor known as familial defective Apo B-100. These patients commonly present with **corneal arcus** of the eye and **xanthomas** of extensor tendons of the hand and Achilles tendon, and premature CHD. Elevations in triglycerides are generally associated with overproduction of triglyceride-rich VLDL (greater than 5:1 ratio of triglyceride-to-cholesterol molecules in each particle), mutations in Apo E, or lack of LPL. Patients with extremely elevated serum triglycerides can develop **pancreatitis** and **tuberoeruptive xanthomas**. Most individuals have mild to moderate elevations in cholesterol caused by a polygenic disorder. Polygenic hypercholesterolemia is not as well understood as the single-gene disorders just discussed. Polygenic hypercholesterolemia is thought to be caused by various more subtle genetic defects as well as environmental factors such as diet and lack of physical activity.[3]

Pathophysiology of Clinical Atherosclerotic Disease

The most widely accepted theory of the process of atherosclerosis is that it is a low-grade inflammatory response

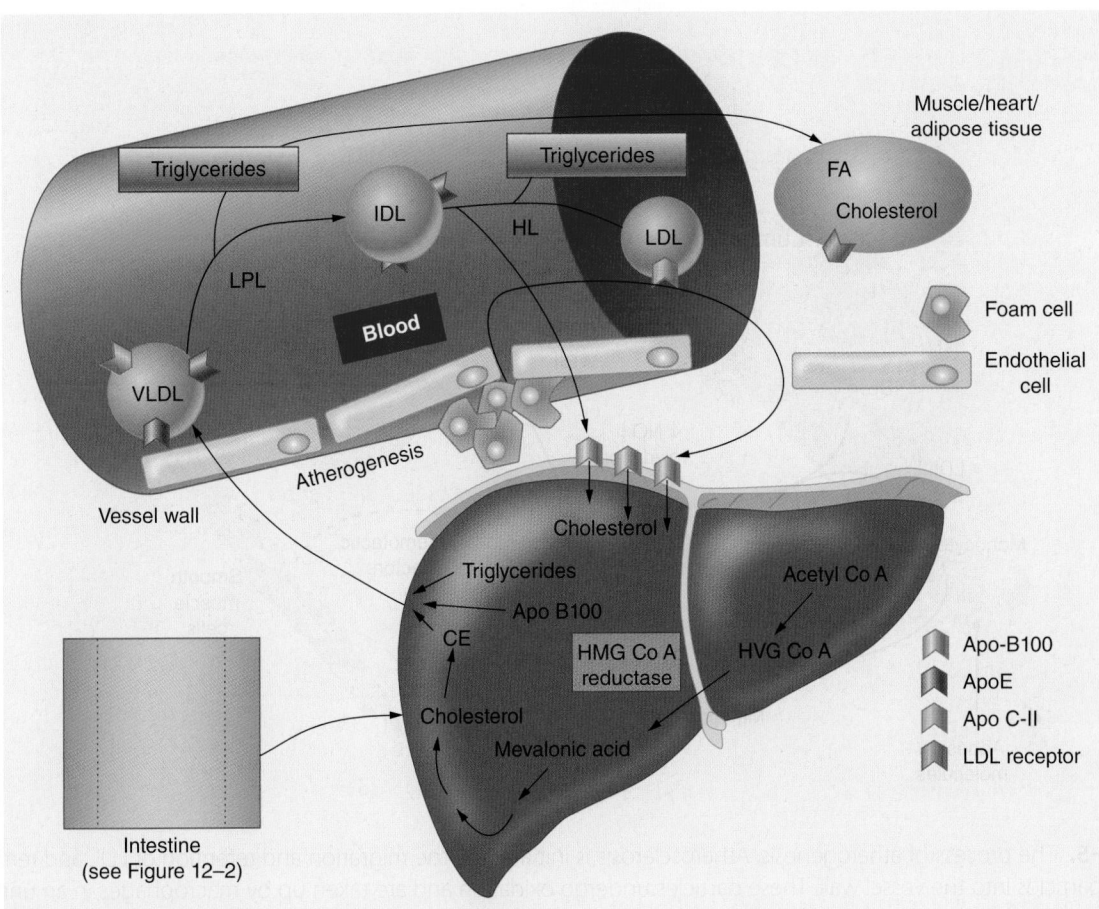

FIGURE 12–4. Endogenous lipoprotein metabolism. In liver cells, cholesterol and triglycerides are packaged into VLDL particles and exported into blood where VLDL is converted to IDL. Intermediate-density lipoprotein can be either cleared by hepatic LDL receptors or further metabolized to LDL. LDL can be cleared by hepatic LDL receptors or can enter the arterial wall, contributing to atherosclerosis. (Acetyl CoA, acetyl coenzyme A; Apo, apolipoprotein; CE, cholesterol ester; FA, fatty acid; HL, hepatic lipase; HMG-CoA, 3-hydroxy-3-methyglutaryl coenzyme A; IDL, intermediate-density lipoprotein; LDL, low-density lipoprotein; LPL, lipoprotein lipase; VLDL, very low-density lipoprotein.)

Table 12–2

Selected Characteristics of Primary Dyslipidemias

Disorder	Estimated Frequency	Metabolic Defect	Main Lipid Parameter
Familial hypercholesterolemia homozygous	1/1 million	LDL-receptor negative	LDL-C greater than 500 mg/dL (12.93 mmol/L)
Heterozygous	1/300–1/500	Reduction in LDL receptors	LDL-C 250–500 mg/dL (6.47–12.93 mmol/L)
Familial defective Apo B-100	1/1,000	Single nucleotide mutation	LDL-C 250–500 mg/L (6.47–12.93 mmol/L)
Polygenic hypercholesterolemia	Common	Metabolic and environmental	LDL-C 160–250 mg/dL (4.14–6.47 mmol/L)
Familial combined dyslipidemia	1/200–300	Overproduction of VLDL and/or LDL	LDL-C 250–350 mg/dL (6.47–9.05 mmol/L) TG 200–800 mg/dL (2.26–9.04 mmol/L)
Familial hyperapobetalipoproteinemia	5%	Increase Apo B production	Apo B greater than 125 mg/dL
Familial dysbetalipoproteinemia	0.5%	Apo E2/2 phenotype	LDL-C 300–600 mg/dL (7.76–15.52 mmol/L) TG 400–800 mg/dL (4.52–9.04 mmol/L
Familial hypertriglyceridemia			
Type IV	1/300	Unknown	TG 200–500 mg/dL (2.26–5.65 mmol/L)
Type V	1/205,000	Unknown	TG greater than 1000 mg/dL (11.3 mmol/L)
Hypoalphalipoproteinemia	3–5%	Defect in HDL catabolism	HDL-C less than 35 mg/dL (0.91 mmol/L)

Apo, apolipoprotein; C, cholesterol; HDL, high-density lipoprotein; LDL, low-density lipoprotein; TG, triglyceride; VLDL, very low-density lipoprotein.

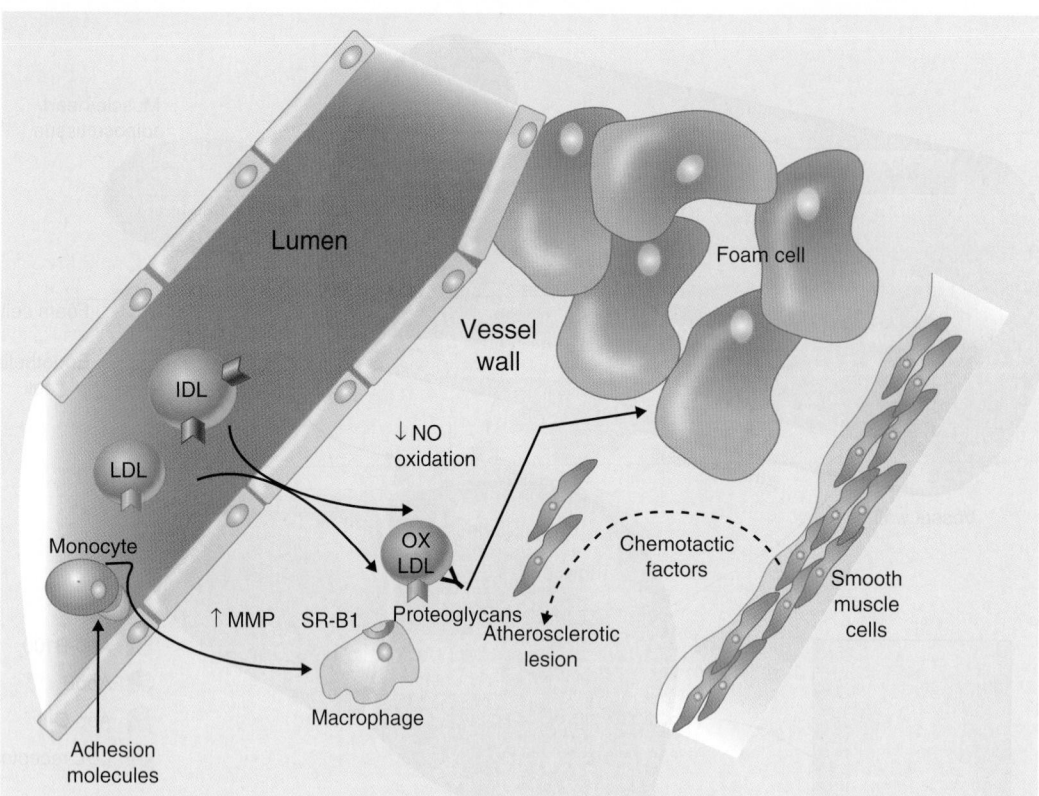

FIGURE 12–5. The process of atherogenesis. Atherosclerosis is initiated by the migration and retention of LDL and remnant lipoprotein particles into the vessel wall. These particles undergo oxidation and are taken up by macrophages in an unregulated fashion. The oxidized particles participate to induce endothelial cell dysfunction leading to a reduced ability of the endothelium to dilate the artery and cause a prothrombotic state. The unregulated uptake of cholesterol by macrophages leads to foam cell formation and the development of a blood clot–favoring fatty lipid core. The enlarging lipid core eventually causes an encroachment of the vessel lumen. Early in the process, smooth muscle cells are activated and recruited from the media to the intima, helping to produce a collagen matrix that covers the growing clot protecting it from circulating blood. Later, macrophages produce and secrete matrix metalloproteinases that degrade the collagen matrix, leading to unstable plaque that may cause a myocardial infarction. (IDL, intermediate-density lipoprotein; LDL, low-density lipoprotein; MMP, matrix metalloproteinases; NO, nitric oxide; SR-BI, scavenger receptors.)

due to injury of the vascular endothelium induced by lipoprotein retention and oxidation in the arterial wall.[6] The process begins when lipoproteins migrate between the **endothelial cells** into the arterial wall and bind to extracellular matrix molecules such as **proteoglycans** (Fig. 12–5). The initial lesion, known as a fatty streak, appears to form after accumulation of lipoproteins within the **intima**. After entering the intima, lipoproteins are then structurally modified by oxidation. Oxidized lipoproteins as well as other cytotoxic agents promote endothelial dysfunction by disturbing the production of vasoactive molecules such as **nitric oxide** that maintain vasomotor tone. Small, denser LDL particles migrate into the arterial wall more readily and are particularly susceptible to oxidation. The oxidized particles cause an increased expression of cell-adhesion molecules on vascular endothelial cells leading to recruitment of **monocytes** into the intima. The monocytes differentiate into **macrophages** and

express scavenger receptors, allowing enhanced uptake of these oxidized Apo B–containing lipoproteins. The macrophages continue to accumulate lipoproteins and ultimately develop into lipid-laden **foam cells**. Accumulation of foam cells leads to formation of a lipid-rich core, which marks the transition to a more complicated atherosclerotic plaque. Vascular wall remodeling leading to outward growth of the wall occurs to accommodate this lipid-rich core. Thus the vascular lumen is relatively well preserved, and generally the lesion would not be detected using traditional coronary angiographic techniques. Initially, smooth muscle cells migrate and proliferate from the **media** to the intima forming a protective fibrous cap that separates the potentially thrombogenic and necrotic lipid core from circulating blood. As the plaque matures, inflammatory cells secrete **matrix metalloproteinases** that degrade collagen and fibrin produced by smooth muscle cells that lead to a weakened fibrous cap. Ischemic events result when the fibrous

Clinical Presentation and Diagnosis

Lipid Panel

- Patients presenting with a total cholesterol level exceeding 200 mg/dL (5.17 mmol/L) or LDL cholesterol exceeding 100 mg/dL (2.59 mmol/L) should be evaluated for high cholesterol.

- Patients with serum triglycerides from 150 to 500 mg/dL (1.70 to 5.65 mmol/L) and serum HDL cholesterol less than 40 mg/dL (1.04 mmol/L) may have metabolic syndrome and need to be evaluated.

Physical Findings

- Patients with genetic disorders that cause a marked increase in serum LDL cholesterol (greater than 250 mg/dL [6.48 mmol/L]) may present with corneal arcus of the eye and xanthomas of extensor tendons of the hand and Achilles tendon.

- Patients with extremely elevated serum triglycerides (greater than 1,000 mg/dL [11.3 mmol/L]) can develop pancreatitis and tuberoeruptive xanthomas.

Indications for Lipid Panel

- All adults greater than 20 years of age should be screened at least every 5 years using a fasting blood sample to obtain a lipid profile (total cholesterol, LDL cholesterol, HDL cholesterol, and triglycerides). A fasting lipid profile is preferred so an accurate assessment of LDL cholesterol can be performed, and fasting will allow the clearance of triglycerides carried by chylomicrons from the circulation, allowing VLDL cholesterol to be determined.

- Children between 2 and 20 years old should be screened for high cholesterol if their parents have premature CHD or if one of their parents has a total cholesterol greater than 240 mg/dL (6.21 mmol/L). Early screening will help to identify children at highest risk of developing CHD in whom early education and dietary intervention is warranted.

Indications for Other Tests

- Conditions that may produce lipid abnormalities (such as those listed in Table 12–3) should be screened for using appropriate tests. If present, these conditions should be properly addressed.

---

cap of these unstable plaques rupture and produce an occlusive **thrombus**. In contrast, repeated wound healing secondary to less significant plaque disruption that causes no symptoms might produce a more stable plaque as a consequence of smooth muscle cell, collagen, and fibrin accumulation and a resolution of the lipid core.[6] These more stable plaques usually cause luminal encroachment (detected by traditional coronary angiographic techniques) and may produce **angina pectoris**. Unstable lesions usually outnumber the more stable plaques, thus accounting for most **acute coronary syndromes**. Evidence demonstrates that aggressive lipid lowering stabilizes these vulnerable lesions and restores endothelial function.[3,6,7]

TREATMENT

In the United States, prevention and treatment of CHD are based primarily on guidelines issued in 2001 by the National Cholesterol Education Program (NCEP) Expert Panel on Detection, Evaluation, and Treatment of High Blood Cholesterol in Adults (Adult Treatment Panel III [ATP III]).[3] The ATP IV guidelines are in development and will be available in 2012.[8] LDL cholesterol is the primary diagnostic and therapeutic target. ❷ *The NCEP ATP III guidelines have set the "optimal" level for LDL cholesterol for all adults as less than 100 mg/dL (2.59 mmol/L).* The NCEP panel issued an update in 2004 to the ATP III guidelines based on more recent clinical trial evidence.[9] The update outlines additional treatment options for certain patient populations, mainly those who are at very high risk of recurrent CHD events. These treatment options emphasize the benefits of diet, exercise, and weight control, and the use of 3-hydroxy-3-methylglutaryl coenzyme A (HMG-CoA) reductase inhibitors (or statins) as first-line drugs. If statins or other drugs used to treat hyperlipidemia are prescribed, doses that reduce LDL cholesterol by at least 30% to 40% should be recommended.[9] In addition, an LDL cholesterol goal of less than 70 mg/dL as a "therapeutic option" was recommended in very high-risk individuals defined as those who experienced an acute coronary syndrome or patients with established CHD plus either multiple major risk factors (especially diabetes), severe and poorly controlled risk factors (especially continued cigarette smoking), or multiple risk factors of the metabolic syndrome.

The American Heart Association and American College of Cardiology issued guidelines for secondary prevention in patients with established CHD based on the results of two additional trials published after the 2004 NCEP update.[10] These guidelines suggest it is reasonable to set an LDL cholesterol goal of less than 70 mg/dL (1.81 mmol/L) in all patients with CHD. If it is not possible to attain LDL cholesterol less than 70 mg/dL (1.81 mmol/L) due to a high baseline LDL cholesterol, it is generally possible to achieve an LDL cholesterol reduction of greater than 50% with more intensive LDL-lowering therapy, including combination drug therapy. Most recently, the National Lipid Association Expert Panel on FH published their recommendations for the management of FH patients. This report goes beyond previously published guidelines by providing specific clinical guidance for the primary care clinician and lipid specialist with the goal of improving care of patients with FH and reducing their elevated risk for CHD.[11]

Guidelines for Treatment

▶ Step 1: Patient Assessment

Determine lipoprotein profile after fasting for 9 to 12 hours. ❸ *The NCEP guidelines recommend that all adults older than 20 years should be screened at least every 5 years using a fasting blood sample to obtain a lipid profile (total cholesterol, LDL cholesterol, HDL cholesterol, and triglycerides).* A fasting lipid profile is preferred so an accurate assessment of LDL cholesterol can be performed. Fasting permits the clearance of triglycerides carried by chylomicrons from the circulation, thus allowing VLDL cholesterol to be determined. Children between 2 and 20 years old should be screened for high cholesterol if their parents have premature CHD or if one of their parents has a total cholesterol greater than 240 mg/dL (6.21 mmol/L).[3] Early screening will help identify children at highest risk of developing CHD, in whom early education and dietary intervention is warranted.

▶ Step 2: Rule Out Secondary Causes of Dyslipidemia

Certain drugs and diseases can cause abnormalities in serum lipids and should be evaluated (Table 12–3). Every effort should be made to correct or control underlying diseases such as hypothyroidism and diabetes. Concurrent medications known to induce lipid abnormalities should be evaluated for discontinuation prior to instituting long-term lipid-modifying therapy.[3]

▶ Step 3: Identify the Presence of Clinical Atherosclerotic Disease or Other Conditions That Confer High Risk for CHD Events

Individuals with established CHD, other clinical atherosclerotic disease (CAD), or diabetes have a greater than 20% risk over a 10-year period of developing CHD events.[3] The ATP III guidelines set the target LDL cholesterol level at less than 100 mg/dL (2.59 mmol/L) for high-risk patients who have a history of one or more of the following:

- Myocardial infarction (MI)
- Unstable angina
- Chronic stable angina
- Coronary interventions (coronary bypass, percutaneous transluminal coronary angioplasty, or stents)
- Peripheral arterial disease (claudication or ankle-brachial index less than 0.9)

Table 12–3

Secondary Conditions and Drugs That May Cause Hyperlipidemias

	↑LDL Cholesterol	↑Triglycerides	↓HDL Cholesterol
Other Conditions			
Diabetes		√	√
Hypothyroidism	√	√	
Obstructive liver disease/biliary cirrhosis	√		
Renal disease		√	
Nephrotic syndrome	√	√	
Chronic renal failure		√	
Hemodialysis patients		√	
Obesity		√	√
Drugs			
Estrogen		√	
Progestins	√		√
Protease inhibitors		√	√
Anabolic steroids	√		√
Corticosteroids	√	√	
Isotretinoin		√	
Cyclosporine	√		
Atypical antipsychotics		√	√
Thiazide diuretics	√	√	
β-Blockers		√	√

LDL, low-density lipoprotein; HDL, high-density lipoprotein.

- Symptomatic carotid artery disease (stroke or transient ischemic attack)
- Diabetes (types 1 and 2)
- Multiple risk factors with a Framingham calculated risk (Fig. 12–6) greater than 20%

❹ *The benefits of lowering LDL cholesterol to as low as 70 mg/dL (1.81 mmol/L) have been demonstrated in clinical trials.* Thus, in patients considered very high risk, an LDL cholesterol goal of less than 70 mg/dL (1.81 mmol/L) is a therapeutic option.[9,10] These individuals have established CAD or present with acute coronary syndromes. ❹ *The lowest level at which to treat LDL cholesterol where there are no further benefits in CHD risk has not yet been determined.*

▶ Step 4: Determine the Presence of Major Risk Factors According to ATP III

In individuals who do not have established CHD or CHD risk equivalent, the next step is to count major risk factors for CHD as presented in Table 12–4. These risk factors are considered independent predictors of CHD. HDL cholesterol

Men Estimate of 10-year risk for men					
(Framingham point scores)					

Age	Points
20–34	−9
35–39	−4
40–44	0
45–49	3
50–54	6
55–59	8
60–64	10
65–69	11
70–74	12
75–79	13

Total cholesterol	Points				
	Age 20–39	Age 40–49	Age 50–59	Age 60–69	Age 70–79
Less than 160	0	0	0	0	0
160–199	4	3	2	1	0
200–239	7	5	3	1	0
240–279	9	6	4	2	1
Greater than or equal to 280	11	8	5	3	1

	Points				
	Age 20–39	Age 40–49	Age 50–59	Age 60–69	Age 70–79
Nonsmoker	0	0	0	0	0
Smoker	8	5	3	1	1

HDL (mg/dL)	Points
Greater than or equal to 60	−1
50–59	0
40–49	1
Less than 40	2

Systolic BP (mm Hg)	If untreated	If treated
Less than 120	0	0
120–129	0	1
130–139	1	2
140–159	1	2
Greater than or equal to 160	2	3

Point total	10-year risk %
Less than 0	Less than 1
0	1
1	1
2	1
3	1
4	1
5	2
6	2
7	3
8	4
9	5
10	6
11	8
12	10
13	12
14	16
15	20
16	25
Greater than or equal to 17	Greater than or equal to 30

10-year risk _____ %

Women Estimate of 10-year risk for women					
(Framingham point scores)					

Age	Points
20–34	−7
35–39	−3
40–44	0
45–49	3
50–54	6
55–59	8
60–64	10
65–69	12
70–74	14
75–79	15

Total cholesterol	Points				
	Age 20–39	Age 40–49	Age 50–59	Age 60–69	Age 70–79
Less than 160	0	0	0	0	0
160–199	4	3	2	1	1
200–239	8	6	4	2	1
240–279	11	8	5	3	2
Greater than or equal to 280	13	10	7	4	2

	Points				
	Age 20–39	Age 40–49	Age 50–59	Age 60–69	Age 70–79
Nonsmoker	0	0	0	0	0
Smoker	9	7	4	2	1

HDL (mg/dL)	Points
Greater than or equal to 60	−1
50–59	0
40–49	1
Less than 40	2

Systolic BP (mmHg)	If untreated	If treated
Less than 120	0	0
120–129	1	3
130–139	2	4
140–159	3	5
Greater than or equal to 160	4	6

Point total	10-year risk %
Less than 9	Less than 1
9	1
10	1
11	1
12	1
13	2
14	2
15	3
16	4
17	5
18	6
19	8
20	11
21	14
22	17
23	22
24	27
Greater than or equal to 25	Greater than or equal to 30

10-year risk _____ %

FIGURE 12–6. Framingham Point Scale for estimating 10-year CHD risk. The Framingham score is used to determine a patient's CHD risk category when they are found to have two or more CHD risk factors (Table 12–4). This system assigns points to the following risk factors: age, total cholesterol level (in mg/dL), smoking status, HDL cholesterol level, and systolic blood pressure. The point total corresponds to the 10-year risk (%) of a CHD event (nonfatal myocardial infarction and coronary death), which serves as a basis for deciding how intensively to treat hypercholesterolemia and other risk factors. To calculate risk factor using the Framingham Point Scale, go to the following website: *http://www.nhlbi.nih.gov/guidelines/cholesterol/index.htm*. The Système International units for the corresponding conventional units in the Framingham Point Scale illustration include (a) total cholesterol (160 mg/dL = 4.14 mmol/L; 160–199 mg/dL = 4.14–5.15 mmol/L; 200–239 mg/dL = 5.17–6.18 mmol/L; 240–279 mg/dL = 6.21–7.21 mmol/L; 280 mg/dL = 7.24 mmol/L) and (b) HDL (60 mg/dL = 1.55 mmol/L; 50–59 mg/dL = 1.29–1.53 mmol/L; 40–49 mg/dL = 1.03–1.27 mmol/L; 40 mg/dL = 1.04 mmol/L). (BP, blood pressure; CHD, coronary heart disease; HDL, high-density lipoprotein.) (From *http://www.nhlbi.nih.gov/guidelines/cholesterol/index.htm*.)

Table 12–4

Risk Factors for Coronary Heart Disease According to ATP III

Risk Factor	Definition
Age (years)	Male greater than or equal to 45; female greater than or equal to 55
Family history of premature CHD events	Male first-degree relative at less than 55 years
	Female first-degree relative at less than 65 years
Hypertension	SBP greater than or equal to 140 mm Hg
	DBP greater than or equal to 90 mm Hg
HDL cholesterol	Less than 40 mg/dL (1.03 mmol/L)
Cigarette smoking	Within the past month

HDL cholesterol greater than or equal to 60 mg/dL (1.55 mmol/L) is considered a negative risk factor; thus subtract 1 risk factor from the total from above.

CHD, coronary heart disease; DBP, diastolic blood pressure; HDL, high-density lipoprotein; SBP, systolic blood pressure.

of greater than or equal to 60 mg/dL (1.55 mmol/L) is considered a negative risk factor and means one risk factor can be subtracted from the total count.[3]

▶ Step 5: If Two or More Risk Factors Are Present Without CHD or CHD Risk Equivalent, Assess 10-Year CHD Risk

Listed in Table 12–5 are the risk groups that require risk calculations using the Framingham scoring system.[3] Because individuals with two or more risk factors may carry a risk equivalent to individuals with established CHD, and therefore should be treated with the same intensity, a scoring system developed from the Framingham Coronary Heart Disease Study is used to estimate the 10-year risk of a

Table 12–5

CHD Risk Factors and Needed Risk Factors for Framingham Score Calculation

Risk Profile	10-Year Risk for CHD	Need for Framingham Calculation
Less than or equal to 1 risk factor	Less than 10%	No
Greater than or equal to 2 risk factors	0–10%	Yes
	10–20%	Yes
CAD or CAD risk equivalent	Greater than 20%	No
Very high risk	Much greater than 20%	No

CAD, clinical atherosclerotic disease; CHD, coronary heart disease.

nonfatal MI and CHD death (Fig. 12–6). This system assigns points to the following risk factors: age, total cholesterol level, smoking status, HDL cholesterol level, and systolic blood pressure. The score is used to determine a patient's risk category and the intensity of treatment to lower their LDL cholesterol. To calculate a Framingham score, visit the following website: *http://www.nhlbi.nih.gov/guidelines/cholesterol/index.htm.*

▶ Step 6: Determine Treatment Goals and Therapy

Treatment goals for LDL cholesterol and thresholds for the institution of therapeutic lifestyle changes (TLC) and pharmacotherapy is the next step (Table 12–6).

▶ Step 7: Initiate TLC If LDL Is Above Goal

TLC should be the first approach tried in all patients (Table 12–7).[3] ⑤ *An adequate trial of TLC should be used in all patients, but pharmacotherapy should be instituted concurrently in higher-risk patients (Table 12–6).* This includes dietary restrictions of cholesterol and saturated fats as well as regular exercise and weight reduction. In addition, therapeutic options to enhance LDL cholesterol lowering such as consumption of plant stanols/sterols (which competitively inhibit incorporation of cholesterol into micelles) and dietary fiber should be encouraged. These therapeutic options collectively may reduce LDL cholesterol by 20% to 25%. For a more detailed overview of lifestyle modifications, refer to the ATP III guidelines[3] and the American Heart Association's diet and lifestyle recommendations.[12]

▶ Step 8: Consider Adding Drug Therapy If LDL Is Above Threshold Level

Patients unable or unlikely to achieve their LDL cholesterol goals following a reasonable trial of TLC (typically 12 weeks for patients without CHD and sooner for those at high risk or with LDL cholesterol greater than 190 mg/dL [4.91 mmol/L] at baseline) are candidates for drug therapy (Table 12–6). ⑥ *Typically, statins are the medications of choice to treat high LDL cholesterol because of their (a) ability to substantially reduce LDL cholesterol and reduce morbidity and mortality from atherosclerotic disease, (b) convenient once-daily dosing, and (c) low risk of side effects.*

▶ Step 9: Identify Patients with the Metabolic Syndrome

Diagnosis of the metabolic syndrome is made when three or more of the following risk factors are present:[3,13]

- Waist circumference greater than or equal to 40 inches (102 cm) in men (35 inches [89 cm] in Asian men), or 35 inches (89 cm) in women (31 inches [79 cm] in Asian women)
- Triglycerides greater than or equal to 150 mg/dL (1.70 mmol/L) or on drug treatment for elevated triglycerides

---

Table 12–6

National Cholesterol Education Program (NCEP) Expert Panel on Detection, Evaluation, and Treatment of High Blood Cholesterol in Adults (Adult Treatment Panel III [ATP III]) Treatment Goals for LDL Cholesterol and Thresholds for Starting Therapeutic Lifestyle Changes and Pharmacotherapy

Risk Category	LDL Cholesterol Goal	Initiate Therapeutic Lifestyle Changes (TLC)	Consider Drug Therapy
High Risk CHD or CHD risk equivalents (10-year risk greater than 20%)	Less than 100 mg/dL (2.59 mmol/L)	Greater than or equal to 100 mg/dL (2.59 mmol/L)	Greater than or equal to 100 mg/dL (2.59 mmol/L)
Very-High Risk	Optional goal of less than 70 mg/dL[a] (1.81 mmol/L)		
Moderately-High Risk Greater than or equal to 2 risk factors (10-year risk 10–20%)	Less than 130 mg/dL (3.36 mmol/L) (Optional goal of less than 100 mg/dL[a] [2.59 mmol/L])	Greater than or equal to 130 mg/dL (3.36 mmol/L)	Greater than or equal to 130 mg/dL (3.36 mmol/L) (consider drug options if LDL cholesterol 100–129 mg/dL [2.59–3.34 mmol/L])
Moderate Risk Greater than or equal to 2 risk factors (10-year risk less than 10%)	Less than 130 mg/dL (3.36 mmol/L)	Greater than or equal to 130 mg/dL (3.36 mmol/L)	Greater than 160 mg/dL (4.14 mmol/L)
Low Risk	Less than 160 mg/dL (4.14 mmol/L)	Greater than or equal to 160 mg/dL (4.14 mmol/L)	Greater than or equal to 190 mg/dL (4.91 mmol/L) (consider drug options if LDL cholesterol 160–189 mg/dL [4.14–4.89 mmol/L])

[a]Optional goals indicated in the NCEP ATP III 2004 update of the guidelines.

CHD, coronary heart disease; LDL, low-density lipoprotein.

Table 12–7

Essential Components of Therapeutic Lifestyle Changes (TLC)

Component	Recommendation
LDL-raising nutrients	
Saturated fats	Total fat range should be 25–35% for most cases
Dietary cholesterol	Less than 7% of total calories and reduce intake of trans fatty acids
Therapeutic options for LDL-lowering plant stanols/sterols	Less than 200 mg/day 2 g/day
Increased viscous (soluble) fiber	10–25 g/day
Total calories	Adjust caloric intake to maintain desirable body weight and prevent weight gain
Physical activity	Include enough moderate exercise to expend at least 200 kcal (837 kJ)/day

LDL, low-density lipoprotein.

- HDL cholesterol less than 40 mg/dL (1.03 mmol/L) in men or 50 mg/dL (1.29 mmol/L) in women or on drug treatment for reduced HDL cholesterol

- Blood pressure greater than or equal to 130/85 mm Hg or on drug treatment for hypertension

- Fasting blood glucose greater than or equal to 100 mg/dL (5.6 mmol/L) or on drug treatment for elevated glucose

Patients with the metabolic syndrome are twice as likely to develop type 2 diabetes and four times more likely to develop CHD.[3,14] These individuals are usually insulin resistant, obese, have hypertension, are in a **prothrombotic state**, and have atherogenic dyslipidemia characterized by low HDL cholesterol and elevated triglycerides, and an increased proportion of their LDL particles are small and dense.[3]

NCEP ATP III identified the metabolic syndrome as an important target for further reducing CHD risk. Treatment of the metabolic syndrome starts with increased physical activity, weight reduction (which also enhances LDL cholesterol lowering and insulin sensitivity), and

---

Patient Encounter 1, part 1

RH is a 44-year-old man with a history of hypertension who was recently diagnosed with CHD after complaining of increasing chest discomfort while exercising. A drug-eluting stent was placed in the left anterior descending artery after his coronary angiography revealed 85% luminal narrowing. He presents to the clinic to follow up after his hospitalization for evaluation of his cholesterol. He denies having chest pain since the first incident of discomfort that precipitated his hospitalization. He indicates no history of myocardial infarction, stroke, or peripheral artery disease. He has no siblings, both parents are alive, and his mother had an MI when she was 47 years old and has elevated cholesterol. He is married with two children. He does not smoke and exercises regularly. He has been fasting for approximately 11 hours.

Can RH be evaluated today for his cholesterol?

Does an assessment of his risk factors for CHD need to be conducted?

What additional information do you need to know for the evaluation of RH?

---

moderation of ethanol use and carbohydrate intake, which effectively reduce many of the associated risk factors. Each of the risk factors should be addressed independently as appropriate, including treatment of hypertension and use of aspirin in CHD patients to reduce the prothrombotic state. ❼ *Patients with metabolic syndrome have an additional lipid parameter that needs to be assessed, namely non-HDL cholesterol (total cholesterol minus HDL cholesterol).*[3] *The target for non-HDL cholesterol is less than the patient's LDL cholesterol target plus 30 mg/dL (0.78 mmol/L).* ❽ *After assessment and control of LDL cholesterol, patients with serum triglycerides between 200 and 499 mg/dL (2.26 and 5.64 mmol/L) should be assessed for atherogenic dyslipidemia (low HDL cholesterol, increased small-dense LDL particles) and metabolic syndrome.* Non-HDL cholesterol estimates the cholesterol carried by all Apo B–containing lipoprotein particles. Thus non-HDL cholesterol represents the sum of LDL cholesterol, VLDL cholesterol, and other triglyceride-rich remnant particles. The non-HDL cholesterol goal is 30 mg/dL (0.78 mmol/L) higher than the LDL cholesterol goal. This is based on the premise that a VLDL cholesterol level less than or equal to 30 mg/dL (0.78 mmol/L) is normal. For example, the LDL cholesterol goal is less than 100 mg/dL (2.59 mmol/L) and the non-HDL cholesterol goal is less than 130 mg/dL (3.36 mmol/L) for a diabetic patient without a history of CHD. Two treatment approaches can be considered for achieving the non-HDL cholesterol goal: titrating existing LDL-lowering therapy or adding niacin or a fibrate to the LDL-lowering therapy.[3] See the chapters on ischemic heart disease and diabetes mellitus for further information regarding metabolic syndrome.

▶ **Step 10: Treatment of Elevated Triglycerides**

Patients with serum triglycerides exceeding 500 mg/dL (5.65 mmol/L) are at increased risk of pancreatitis, especially when levels exceed 1,000 mg/dL (11.3 mmol/L).[3] Reducing triglycerides in these individuals becomes the primary target for intervention. Reduction in fats, ethanol, and carbohydrates should be considered, and secondary causes (Table 12–3) should be assessed. Increase in exercise and weight loss if overweight should be encouraged. When pharmacotherapy is instituted, the goal is to reduce triglycerides to less than 150 mg/dL (1.70 mmol/L). Once triglycerides are less than 500 mg/dL (5.65 mmol/L) and the risk of pancreatitis is reduced, the primary focus of intervention should once again be on LDL cholesterol. As noted earlier, individuals with triglycerides between 200 and 499 mg/dL (2.26 and 5.64 mmol/L) have an increase in triglyceride-rich remnant lipoproteins and small-dense LDL particles. Non-HDL cholesterol should be a secondary target in these individuals. Niacin, fibrates, and ω-3 fatty acids are the most effective agents in patients with hypertriglyceridemia.[3]

Emerging and Life-Habit Risk Factors

In addition to the five major risks, the ATP III guidelines recognize other factors that contribute to CHD risk. These are classified as life-habit risk factors and emerging risk factors. Life-habit risk factors, consisting of obesity, physical inactivity, and an atherogenic diet, require direct intervention. For example, emerging risk factors are lipoprotein(a), prothrombotic/proinflammatory factors, lipoprotein-associated phospholipase A2 (Lp-PLA2), and C-reactive protein (CRP). CRP is a marker of low-level inflammation and appears to help predict CHD risk beyond LDL cholesterol and major CHD risk factors.[14] In a recent trial, rosuvastatin significantly reduced the incidence of major cardiovascular events in apparently healthy persons without hyperlipidemia (LDL cholesterol less than 130 mg/dL [3.36 mmol/L]) but with elevated high-sensitivity CRP levels.[15] These results will need to be considered by the ATP IV writing committee.[8] In some patients, emerging risk factors may be used to guide the intensity of risk-reduction therapy. Deciding when to consider emerging risk factors requires the use of clinical judgment. The National Lipid Association recently reviewed a number of these emerging risk factors and has offered some clinical guidance on their use.[16]

Pharmacotherapy

▶ **Statins (HMG-CoA Reductase Inhibitors)**

Statins are very effective LDL-lowering medications and are proven to reduce the risk of CHD, stroke, and death. Thus NCEP ATP III considers statins the preferred LDL-lowering medications. Data concerning the efficacy and safety of the statins now go back nearly 25 years. Statins are effective in reducing MIs, strokes, revascularization procedures,

Table 12–8

Effects of Lipid-Lowering Drugs on Serum Lipids at FDA-Approved Doses

Lipid-Lowering Drug	LDL Cholesterol	HDL Cholesterol	Triglycerides	Total Cholesterol
Statins				
Atorvastatin	−26% to −60%	+5% to +13%	−17% to −53%	−25% to −45%
Fluvastatin	−22% to −36%	+3% to +11%	−12% to −25%	−16% to −27%
Fluvastatin ER	−33% to −35%	+7% to +11%	−19% to −25%	−25%
Lovastatin	−21% to −42%	+2% to +10%	−6% to −27%	−16% to −34%
Lovastatin ER	−24% to −41%	+9% to +13%	−10% to −25%	−18% to −29%
Pitavastatin	−31% to.−45%	+1% to +8%	−13% to −22%	−23% to −31%
Pravastatin	−22% to −34%	+2% to +12%	−15% to −24%	−16% to −25%
Rosuvastatin	−45% to −63%	+8% to +14%	−10% to −35%	−33% to −46%
Simvastatin	−26% to −47%	+8% to +16%	−12% to −34%	−19% to −36%
Bile Acid Sequestrants				
Cholestyramine	−15% to −30%	+3% to +5%	May increase in patients with elevated triglycerides	−10% to −25%
Colesevelam	−15% to −18%	+3% to +5%		−70% to −10%
Colestipol	−15% to −30%	+3% to +5%		−10% to 25%
Cholesterol Absorption Inhibitor				
Ezetimibe	−18%	+1% to +2%	−7% to −9%	−12% to −13%
Nicotinic Acid				
Niacin ER	−5% to −17%	+14% to +26%	−11% to −38%	−3% to −12%
Niacin IR	−5% to −25%	+15% to +39%	−20% to −60%	−3% to −25%
Fibric Acid Derivatives				
Fenofibrate	−31% to +45%	+9% to +23%	−23% to −54%	−9% to −22%
Gemfibrozil	−30% to +30%	+10% to +30%	−20% to −60%	−2% to −16%
Combination Products				
Niacin ER and lovastatin	−30% to −42%	+20% to +30%	−32 to −44%	Not stated
Niacin ER and simvastatin[a]	−12% to −14%	+21% to +29%	−27% to −38%	−9% to −11%
Simvastatin and ezetimibe	−46% to −59%	+8% to +12%	−25% to −26%	−34% to −43%
Omega-3-Fatty Acids				
Lovaza	+45%	+9%	−44.9%	−9.7%

ER, extended-release; HDL, high-density lipoprotein; IR, immediate-release; LDL, low-density lipoprotein.

[a]% change relative to simvastatin 20 mg.

cardiovascular deaths, and, in some cases, total mortality. This effectiveness has been demonstrated in both genders, the elderly, patients with diabetes and hypertension, those with and without preexisting CHD, and following an acute coronary syndrome.[15–27] Statins inhibit conversion of HMG-CoA to L-mevalonic acid and subsequently cholesterol. Statins lower LDL cholesterol levels by approximately 25% to 62% (Table 12–8). A substantial reduction in LDL cholesterol occurs at the usual starting dose, and each doubling of the daily dose only produces an additional 6% average reduction (known as the "rule of 6"). This is important when considering dose escalation versus adding on an additional LDL-lowering drug. Statins are moderately effective at reducing triglycerides and modestly raise HDL cholesterol (Table 12–8). By inhibiting the synthesis of L-mevalonic acid, statins in turn inhibit other important by-products in the cholesterol biosynthetic pathway that affect intracellular transport, membrane trafficking, and gene transcription.[28] This may explain some of the cholesterol-independent benefits (so-called pleiotropic effects) of statins such as reducing lipoprotein oxidation, enhancing endothelial

synthesis of nitric oxide, and inhibiting thrombosis. These pleiotropic effects are thought to contribute to the rapid/ earlier benefits of statins on CHD risk while the decrease in serum lipids accounts for the slower late benefit.

Statins are well tolerated, with less than 4% of patients in clinical trials discontinuing therapy due to adverse side effects (Table 12–9). Elevations in liver function tests (LFTs) and myopathy, including rhabdomyolysis, are important adverse effects associated with the statins. Liver toxicity, defined as LFT elevations greater than three times the upper limit of normal, is reported in less than 2% of patients; however, the incidence is higher at higher doses, and the progression to liver failure is thought to be exceedingly rare. LFTs should be obtained at baseline and as clinically indicated thereafter. Annual monitoring of LFTs is usually sufficient. Myopathy, defined as muscle symptoms with creatine kinase (CK; or creatine phosphokinase [CPK]) 10 times the upper limit of normal, is reported to range from 0% to less than 0.5% for the currently marketed statins at FDA-approved doses. Rhabdomyolysis, defined as muscle symptoms with marked elevation in CK 10 times

Table 12-9

Formulation, Dosing, and Common Adverse Effects of Lipid-Lowering Drugs

Lipid-Lowering Drug	Dosage Forms	Usual Adult Maintenance Dose Range	Adverse Effects
Statins			
Atorvastatin	10-, 20-, 40-, 80-mg tablets	10–80 mg once daily (at any time of day). Dose adjustment in patients with renal dysfunction is not necessary	Most frequent side effects are constipation, abdominal pain, diarrhea, dyspepsia, and nausea. Statins should be discontinued promptly if serum transaminase levels (liver function tests) rise to three times upper limit of normal or if patient develops signs or symptoms of myopathy. Approximate equivalent doses of HMG-CoA reductase inhibitors are: atorvastatin 10 mg, fluvastatin 80 mg, lovastatin 40 mg, pitavastatin 2 mg, pravastatin 40 mg, simvastatin 20 mg, and rosuvastatin 5 mg
Fluvastatin	20-, 40- mg capsules; 80-mg extended-release tablets	20–40 mg/day as a single dose (evening) or 40 mg twice daily; 80 mg once daily (evening). Dose adjustments for mild to moderate renal impairment are not necessary	
Lovastatin	10-, 20-, 40-mg tablets	10 to 80 mg/day as a single dose (with evening meal) or divided twice daily with food. In patients with severe renal insufficiency (creatinine clearance less than 30 mL/min [0.5 mL/s]), dosage increases above 20 mg/day should be carefully considered and, if deemed necessary, implemented cautiously	
Lovastatin ER	20-, 30-, 60-mg tablets	20–60 mg/day as a single dose. In patients with severe renal insufficiency (creatinine clearance less than 30 mL/min [0.5 mL/s]), dosage increases above 20 mg/day should be carefully considered and, if deemed necessary, implemented cautiously	
Pravastatin	10-, 20-, 40-, 80-mg tablets	10 to 80 mg/day as a single dose at bedtime. In patients with a history of significant renal or hepatic dysfunction, a starting dose of 10 mg daily is recommended	
Pitavastatin	1-, 2-, 4-mg tablets	1–4 mg/day as a single dose can be taken with or without food, at any time of day. Moderate renal impairment (glomerular filtration rate 30–60 mL/min/1.73 m² [0.29 to 0.58 mL/s/m²]) and end-stage renal disease on hemodialysis: Starting dose of 1 mg once daily and maximum dose of 2 mg once daily	
Rosuvastatin	5-, 10-, 20-, 40 tablets	5–40 mg/day (at any time of day); 40 mg reserved for those who don't achieve LDL cholesterol goal on 20 mg. In patients with a history of significant renal or hepatic dysfunction, a starting dose of 10 mg daily is recommended	
Simvastatin	5-, 10-, 20-, 40-mg tablets	5 to 40 mg/day as a single dose in the evening, or divided. Recommended starting dose for patients at high risk of CHD is 40 mg/day. In patients with mild to moderate renal insufficiency dosage adjustment is not necessary. However, caution should be exercised in patients with severe renal insufficiency; such patients should be started at 5 mg/day and be closely monitored. Due to the increased risk of myopathy, including rhabdomyolysis, use of the 80-mg dose of simvastatin should be restricted to patients who have been taking simvastatin 80 mg chronically (e.g., for 12 months or more) without evidence of muscle toxicity. Because of an increased risk for myopathy in Chinese patients taking simvastatin 40 mg coadministered with lipid-modifying doses (greater than or equal to 1 g/day niacin) of niacin-containing products, caution should be used when treating Chinese patients with simvastatin doses exceeding 20 mg/day coadministered with lipid-modifying doses of niacin-containing products. Because the risk for myopathy is dose related, Chinese patients should not receive simvastatin 80 mg coadministered with lipid-modifying doses of niacin-containing products	

(Continued)

Table 12-9

Formulation, Dosing, and Common Adverse Effects of Lipid-Lowering Drugs (*Continued*)

Lipid-Lowering Drug	Dosage Forms	Usual Adult Maintenance Dose Range	Adverse Effects
Bile Acid Sequestrants			
Cholestyramine	4-g packets	4–24 g/day in two or more divided doses	Main side effects are nausea, constipation, bloating, and flatulence, although these may be less with colesevelam. Increasing fluid and dietary fiber intake may relieve constipation and bloating. Impair absorption of fat-soluble vitamins
Colesevelam	625-mg tablets	3,750–4,375 mg/day as a single dose or divided twice daily, with meals	
	3.75-g oral suspension packet	1 packet once a day with meals	
Colestipol	5-g packets	5–30 g/day as a single dose or divided	
	1-g tablets	2–16 g/day as a single dose or divided	
Cholesterol Absorption Inhibitors			
Ezetimibe	10-mg tablet	10 mg once daily. No dosage adjustment is necessary in patients with renal or mild hepatic insufficiency	The overall incidence of adverse events reported with ezetimibe alone was similar to that reported with placebo and generally similar between ezetimibe with a statin and statin alone. The frequency of increased transaminases was slightly higher in patients receiving ezetimibe plus a statin compared with those receiving statin monotherapy (1.3% vs. 0.4%).
Nicotinic Acid (Prescription products)			
Niacin ER (Niaspan)	500-, 750-, 1000-mg extended-release tablets	1000–2000 mg once daily at bedtime. Use with caution in patients with renal impairment	Side effects include flushing, itching, gastric distress, headache, hepatotoxicity, hyperglycemia, and hyperuricemia
Niacin IR (Niacor)	500-mg tablets	1–6 g/day in two to three divided doses. Do not exceed 6 g daily	
Fibric Acid Derivatives			
Fenofibrate	54-, 160-mg tablets[a]	54–160 mg/day; the dosage should be minimized in severe renal impairment	Most common side effects are nausea, diarrhea, abdominal pain, and rash. Increased risk of rhabdomyolysis when given with a statin. Fibric acids are associated with gallstones, myositis, and hepatitis
Gemfibrozil	600-mg tablets	1,200 mg/day in two doses, 30 minutes before meals; should be avoided in hepatic or severe renal impairment	
Combination Products			
Niacin ER and lovastatin	500 mg/20 mg, 750 mg/20 mg, 1000 mg/20 mg tablets	500 mg/20 mg to 2,000 mg/40 mg daily, at bedtime.	See previous entries for each drug (niacin ER and lovastatin)
Niacin ER and simvastatin	500 mg/20 mg, 500 mg/40 mg, 750 mg/20 mg, 1000 mg/20 mg, 1000 mg/40 mg	500 mg/20 mg to 2,000 mg/40 mg daily, at bedtime	See previous entries for each drug (niacin ER and simvastatin)

(Continued)

Table 12-9

Formulation, Dosing, and Common Adverse Effects of Lipid-Lowering Drugs (*Continued*)

Lipid-Lowering Drug	Dosage Forms	Usual Adult Maintenance Dose Range	Adverse Effects
Ezetimibe and simvastatin	10 mg/10 mg, 10 mg/20 mg, 10 mg/40 mg, 10 mg/80 mg	The dosage range is 10/10 mg/day through 10/40 mg/day. The recommended usual starting dose is 10/10 or 10/20 mg/day. Initiation of therapy with 10/10 mg/day may be considered for patients requiring less aggressive LDL cholesterol reductions. Due to the increased risk of myopathy, including rhabdomyolysis, use of the 10/80-mg dose of Vytorin should be restricted to patients who have been taking Vytorin 10/80 mg chronically (e.g., for 12 months or more) without evidence of muscle toxicity. Because of an increased risk for myopathy in Chinese patients taking simvastatin 40 mg coadministered with lipid-modifying doses (greater than or equal to 1 g/day niacin) of niacin-containing products, caution should be used when treating Chinese patients with Vytorin doses exceeding 10/20 mg/day coadministered with lipid-modifying doses (greater than or equal to 1 g/day niacin) of niacin-containing products. Because the risk for myopathy is dose-related, Chinese patients should not receive Vytorin 10/80 mg coadministered with lipid-modifying doses of niacin-containing products	See previous entries for each drug (ezetimibe and simvastatin)

CHD, coronary heart disease; ER, extended release; HMG-CoA, 3-hydroxy-3-methyglutaryl coenzyme A; IR, immediate-release; LDL, low-density lipoprotein.

[a]Dose strengths vary depending on brand.

the upper limit of normal with creatinine elevation usually associated with myoglobinuria and brown urine, is very rare.[29] The concern of statin-associated myopathy has increased since the voluntary removal of cerivastatin from the world market in 2001 because the reported rate of fatal rhabdomyolysis was 16 to 80 times higher than the rate for any other statin, and many of these cases were reported in patients treated with concomitant gemfibrozil.[30] The American College of Cardiology/American Heart Association/National Heart, Lung and Blood Institute published a clinical advisory with a focus on myopathy.[29] Listed here are the risks associated with statin-induced myopathy published in this report:

- Small body frame and frailty
- Multisystem disease (e.g., chronic renal insufficiency, especially due to diabetes)
- Multiple medications (see below)
- Perioperative periods
- Specific concomitant medications or consumptions (check specific statin package insert for warnings): fibrates (especially gemfibrozil, but other fibrates too), nicotinic acid (rarely), cyclosporine, azole antifungals such as itraconazole and ketoconazole, macrolide antibiotics such as erythromycin and clarithromycin, protease inhibitors used to treat Acquired Immunodeficiency Syndrome (AIDS), nefazodone (antidepressant), verapamil, amiodarone, large quantities of grapefruit juice (usually more than 1 quart [about

950 mL] per day), and alcohol abuse (independently predisposes to myopathy).

Baseline CK should be obtained in all patients prior to starting statin therapy. Follow-up CK should only be obtained in patients complaining of muscle pain, weakness, tenderness, or brown urine. Routine monitoring of CK is of little value in the absence of clinical signs or symptoms. Patient assessment for symptoms of myopathy should be done 6 to 12 weeks after starting therapy and at each visit. More frequent monitoring should be done in higher-risk individuals such as those just identified.

As mentioned earlier, statins inhibit production of other important by-products in the cholesterol biosynthesis pathway. Ubiquinone or coenzyme Q10 is an isoprenoid that plays a unique role in cellular electron transport and synthesizes energy. It is essential for the normal functioning of muscles. Statins have been shown to reduce blood levels of coenzyme Q10. The evidence of the value of supplementing coenzyme Q10 in patients experiencing statin-induced myopathy has been mainly anecdotal and is currently being evaluated in clinical trials.

Clinical trial data and several meta-analyses suggest that statins increase the risk of development of diabetes. The FDA recently added the warning of increased blood sugar and glycosylated hemoglobin (HbA1c) levels to the statin labels. The FDA continues to believe that the cardiovascular benefits of statins outweigh these small increased risks.

With the exception of pravastatin, which is mainly metabolized by isomerization in the gut to a relatively inactive

Patient Encounter 1, Part 2: Medical History, Physical Examination, and Diagnostic Tests

PMH: Hypertension for 9 years

FH: Father and mother both alive. Mother had MI at age 47.

SH: Works as a high school teacher and coaches the basketball team. He exercises regularly; drinks alcohol (2 to 3 beers) mainly on the weekends while watching sports on TV

Meds: Aspirin 325 mg once daily, clopidogrel 75 mg once daily, Verapamil SR 180 mg once daily

ROS: No chest pain, shortness of breath, or dizziness

PE:

VS: BP 142/86 mm Hg, pulse 71 beats per minute (bpm), respiratory rate 16 bpm, temperature 37°C (98.6°F), waist circumference 35 inches (89 cm)

CV: RRR, normal S_1, S_2; no murmurs, rubs, or gallops

Abd: Soft, nontender, nondistended; positive for bowel sounds, no hepatosplenomegaly or abdominal aortic aneurysm

Exts: Ankle-brachial index 1.1

Neck: No carotid and basilar bruits

EENT: Corneal arcus in both eyes

Labs: Total cholesterol 376 mg/dL (9.72 mmol/L), triglycerides 138 mg/dL (1.56 mmol/L), HDL cholesterol 42 mg/dL (1.09 mmol/L), LDL cholesterol 306 mg/dL (7.91 mmol/L), and glucose 98 mg/dL (5.4 mmol/L), all other labs within normal limits

Given this additional information, what is your assessment of RH's CHD risk?

What type of lipid disorder does RH have?

Identify your treatment goals for RH.

What nonpharmacologic and pharmacologic alternatives are available for RH?

Should RH's children be screened for high cholesterol and why?

Develop a care plan for RH.

metabolite, and pitavastatin, which primarily undergoes glucuronidation, the other statins undergo biotransformation by the cytochrome P-450 system. Therefore, drugs known to inhibit statin metabolism (e.g., cyclosporine A, erythromycin, gemfibrozil, protease inhibitors, ketoconazole, verapamil, rifampin, amiodarone) should be used cautiously or avoided. Medications such as cyclosporine A and gemfibrozil can inhibit drug transporters in the gut and liver, such as p-glycoprotein and organic anion-transporting polypeptide that can increase statin blood concentrations as well. The time until maximum effect on lipids for statins is generally 4 to 6 weeks.

▶ Cholesterol Absorption Inhibitors

Ezetimibe is the first drug in a new class of agents referred to as cholesterol absorption inhibitors. Ezetimibe blocks biliary and dietary cholesterol as well as phytosterol (plant sterol) absorption by interacting with the NPC1L1 transporter located in the brush border membrane of enterocytes (Fig. 12–2).[5] Ezetimibe inhibits 54% of all intestinal cholesterol absorption on average. By reducing the cholesterol content within chylomicrons delivered to the liver, ezetimibe reduces liver cholesterol stores, inducing an upregulation of LDL receptors resulting in a decrease in serum cholesterol. As a result, ezetimibe also induces a compensatory increase in cholesterol biosynthesis. Because statins inhibit cholesterol biosynthesis, the compensatory increase in cholesterol biosynthesis by ezetimibe can be blocked by combining ezetimibe with a statin.

Ezetimibe reduces LDL cholesterol by an average of 18% (Table 12–8). However, larger reductions can be seen in some individuals, presumably due to higher absorption of cholesterol. These individuals appear to have a blunted response to statin therapy. Ezetimibe lowers triglycerides by 7% to 9% and modestly increases HDL cholesterol.

Once absorbed, ezetimibe undergoes extensive glucuronidation in the intestinal wall to the active metabolite (ezetimibe glucuronide). Ezetimibe and the active metabolite are enterohepatically recirculated back to the site of action, which limits systemic exposure and may explain the low incidence of adverse effects (Table 12–9). Ezetimibe alone or with a statin is contraindicated in patients with active liver disease or unexplained persistent elevations in LFTs. Ezetimibe combined with simvastatin and simvastatin monotherapy were not associated with a reduction in carotid intima-media thickness in patients with heterozygous familial hypercholesterolemia.[31] The patients studied in this trial were well managed (80% were receiving statins prior to enrollment) and had "near normal" measurements of carotid intima-media thickness at baseline, which may explain the study findings. However, ezetimibe combined with simvastatin was associated with a reduced incidence of ischemic cardiovascular events in low-risk patients with mild to moderate asymptomatic aortic stenosis compared with placebo,[32] as well as reduced incidence of major atherosclerotic events in a wide range of patients with advanced chronic kidney disease.[33] Other clinical trials designed to determine ezetimibe's effects on CHD morbidity and mortality have not been completed. The time until maximum effect on lipids for ezetimibe is generally 2 weeks.

▶ Bile Acid Sequestrants

Cholestyramine, colestipol, and colesevelam are the bile acid-binding resins or sequestrants (BAS) currently available in the United States. Resins are highly charged molecules that bind to bile acids (which are produced from cholesterol) in the gut. The resin–bile acid complex is then excreted in the feces. The loss of bile causes a compensatory conversion of hepatic cholesterol to bile, reducing hepatocellular stores of cholesterol and resulting in an upregulation of LDL receptors to replenish hepatocellular stores, which then result in a decrease in serum cholesterol. Resins have been shown to reduce CHD events in patients without CHD.[34]

Resins are moderately effective in lowering LDL cholesterol but do not lower triglycerides (Table 12–8). Moreover, in patients with elevated triglycerides, the use of a resin may worsen the condition. This may be due to a compensatory increase in HMG-CoA reductase activity and results in an increase in assembly and secretion of VLDL. The increase in HMG-CoA reductase activity can be blocked with a statin, resulting in enhanced reductions in serum lipids (see section on combination therapy). Resins reduce LDL cholesterol from 15% to 30%, with a modest increase in HDL cholesterol (3% to 5%) (Table 12–8). Resins are most often used as adjuncts to statins in patients who require additional lowering of LDL cholesterol. Because these drugs are not absorbed, adverse effects are limited to the GI tract (Table 12–9). About 20% of patients taking cholestyramine or colestipol report constipation and symptoms such as flatulence and bloating. A large number of patients stop therapy because of this. Resins should be started at the lowest dose and escalated slowly over weeks to months as tolerated until the desired response is obtained. Patients should be instructed to prepare the powder formulations in 6 to 8 ounces (approximately 180 to 240 mL) of noncarbonated fluids, usually juice (enhances palatability) or water. Fluid intake should be increased to minimize constipation. Colesevelam is better tolerated with fewer GI side effects, although it is more expensive. All resins have the potential to prevent the absorption of other drugs such as digoxin, warfarin, thyroxine, thiazides, β-blockers, fat-soluble vitamins, and folic acid. Potential drug interactions can be avoided by taking a resin either 1 hour before or 4 hours after these other agents. Colesevelam appears less likely than the older agents to reduce drug absorption, but the manufacturer does recommend that colesevelam be dosed hours apart from other medications.[35] The time until maximum effect on lipids for resins is generally 2 to 4 weeks.

▶ Niacin

Niacin (vitamin B_3) has broad applications in the treatment of lipid disorders when used at higher doses than those used as a nutritional supplement. Niacin inhibits fatty acid release from adipose tissue and inhibits fatty acid and triglyceride production in liver cells. This results in an increased intracellular degradation of Apo B, and in turn, a reduction in the number of VLDL particles secreted (Fig. 12–4). The lower VLDL levels and the lower triglyceride content in these particles leads to an overall reduction in LDL cholesterol as well as a decrease in the number of small dense LDL particles. Niacin also reduces the uptake of HDL-Apo A1 particles and increases uptake of cholesterol esters by the liver, thus improving the efficiency of reverse cholesterol transport between HDL particles and vascular tissue (Fig. 12–4). Niacin is indicated for patients with elevated triglycerides, low HDL cholesterol, and elevated LDL cholesterol.[3]

Several different niacin formulations are available: niacin immediate-release (IR), niacin sustained-release (SR), and niacin extended-release (ER).[36,37] These formulations differ in terms of dissolution and absorption rates, metabolism, efficacy, and side effects. Limitations of niacin IR and SR are flushing and hepatotoxicity, respectively. These differences appear related to the dissolution and absorption rates of niacin formulations and their subsequent metabolism. Niacin IR is available by prescription (Niacor) as well as a dietary supplement which is not regulated by the FDA.[36] Currently, there are no FDA-approved niacin SR products; thus all SR products are available only as dietary supplements.[38]

Niacin IR is usually completely absorbed within 1 to 2 hours; thus it quickly saturates a high-affinity, low-capacity metabolic pathway, and most of the drug is metabolized by a second low-affinity, high-capacity system with metabolites associated with flushing.[38] Conversely, absorption of niacin SR may exceed 12 hours. Because niacin SR is absorbed over 12 or more hours, the high-affinity pathway metabolizes most of the drug, resulting in the production of metabolites associated with hepatotoxicity. Niacin ER was developed as a once-daily formulation to be taken at bedtime, with the goal of reducing the incidence of flushing without increasing the risk of hepatotoxicity. Niacin ER (Niaspan) is the only long-acting niacin product approved by the FDA for dyslipidemia. Niacin ER has an absorption rate of 8 to 12 hours, intermediate to niacin IR and SR, and therefore balances metabolism more evenly over the high-affinity, low-capacity pathway and the low-affinity, high-capacity pathway. Furthermore, taking niacin ER at bedtime can minimize the impact of flushing.

Niacin use is limited by cutaneous reactions such as flushing and pruritus of the face and body. The use of aspirin or a nonsteroidal anti-inflammatory drug (NSAID) 30 minutes prior to taking niacin can help alleviate these reactions because they are mediated by an increase in prostaglandin D2.[3] In addition, taking niacin with food and avoiding hot liquids or alcohol at the time niacin is taken is helpful in minimizing flushing and pruritus.

In general, niacin reduces LDL cholesterol from 5% to 25%, reduces triglycerides by 20% to 50%, and increases HDL cholesterol by 15% to 35% (Table 12–8). Niacin has been shown to reduce CHD events and total mortality,[39] as well as the progression of atherosclerosis when combined with a statin.[40] However, a recent trial that tested the effects of adding niacin ER to a statin (simvastatin) compared with statin alone in reducing long-term cardiovascular events in participants whose LDL cholesterol was controlled and who had a history of cardiovascular disease, low levels of HDL cholesterol, and high levels of triglycerides was stopped earlier than planned because no apparent benefits by adding niacin ER were found. Moreover, a small and unexplained increase in ischemic stroke in the niacin ER group was seen.[41] Another larger trial with a similar study design is currently underway and will help to adjudicate niacin's role in combination drug therapy.[42]

Niacin can raise uric acid levels, and in patients with diabetes can raise blood glucose levels. However, several clinical trials have shown that niacin can be used safely and effectively in patients with diabetes.[43] Due to the high cardiovascular risk of patients with diabetes, the benefits of improving the lipid profile appear to outweigh any adjustment in diabetic medication(s) that is needed.[44]

Niacin should be instituted at the lowest dose and gradually titrated to a maximum dose of 2 g daily for ER and SR products and no more than 6 g daily for IR products. FDA-approved niacin products are preferred because of product consistency. Moreover, niacin products labeled as "no flush" don't contain nicotinic acid and therefore have no therapeutic role in the treatment of lipid disorders.[36] The time until maximum effect on lipids for niacins is generally 3 to 5 weeks.

▶ Fibrates

The predominant effects of fibrates are a decrease in triglyceride levels by 20% to 50% and an increase in HDL cholesterol levels by 9% to 30% (Table 12–8). The effect on LDL cholesterol is less predictable. In patients with high triglycerides, however, LDL cholesterol may increase. Fibrates increase the size and reduce the density of LDL particles much like niacin. Fibrates are the most effective triglyceride-lowering drugs and are used primarily in patients with elevated triglycerides and low HDL cholesterol.

Fibrates work by reducing Apos B, C-III (an inhibitor of LPL), and E, and increasing Apos A-I and A-II through activation of peroxisome proliferator-activated receptor-alpha (PPAR-α), a nuclear receptor involved in cellular function. The changes in these Apos result in a reduction in triglyceride-rich lipoproteins (VLDL and IDL) and an increase in HDL.

Clinical trials of fibrate therapy in patients with elevated cholesterol and no history of CHD demonstrated a reduction in CHD incidence, although less than the reduction attained with statin therapy.[45] In addition, a large study of men with CHD, low HDL cholesterol, low LDL cholesterol, and elevated triglycerides demonstrated a 24% reduction in the risk of death from CHD, nonfatal MI, and stroke with gemfibrozil.[46] Fibrates may be appropriate in the prevention of CHD events for patients with established CHD, low HDL cholesterol, and triglycerides below 200 mg/dL (2.26 mmol/L). However, LDL-lowering therapy should be the primary target if LDL cholesterol is elevated. Evidence of a reduction in CHD risk among patients with established CHD has not been demonstrated with fenofibrate.

The fibric acid derivatives are generally well tolerated. The most common adverse effects include dyspepsia, abdominal pain, diarrhea, flatulence, rash, muscle pain, and fatigue (Table 12–9). Myopathy and rhabdomyolysis can occur, and the risk appears to increase with renal insufficiency or concurrent statin therapy. If a fibrate is used with a statin, fenofibrate is preferred because it appears to inhibit the glucuronidation of the statin hydroxy and moiety less than gemfibrozil, allowing greater renal clearance of the statins.[29,47] A CK level should be checked before therapy is started and if symptoms occur. Liver dysfunction has been reported, and LFTs should be monitored. Fibrates increase cholesterol in the bile and have caused gallbladder and bile duct disorders, such as cholelithiasis and cholecystitis. Unlike niacin, these agents do not increase glucose or uric acid levels. Fibrates are contraindicated in patients with gallbladder disease, liver dysfunction, or severe kidney dysfunction. The risk of bleeding is increased in patients taking both a fibrate and warfarin. The time until maximum effect on lipids is generally 2 weeks for fenofibrate and 3 to 4 weeks for gemfibrozil.

▶ Omega-3 Fatty Acids

Omega-3 fatty acids (eicosapentaenoic acid and docosahexaenoic acid), the predominant long-chain fatty acids in the oil of cold-water fish, lower triglycerides by as much as 45% when taken in large amounts (2 to 4 g). Omega-3 fatty acids may be useful for patients with high triglycerides despite diet and weight loss, alcohol restriction, and fibrate therapy. This effect may be modulated through PPAR-α and a reduction in Apo B-100 secretion. Omega-3 fatty acids reduce platelet aggregation and have antiarrhythmic properties, and therefore their use has been associated with a reduction in MI and sudden cardiac death, respectively.[48]

Prescription-grade omega-3 fatty acid ethyl esters are FDA approved at a dose of 4 g daily for the treatment of elevated triglycerides (greater than or equal to 500 mg/dL [greater than or equal to 5.65 mmol/L]). Use of high-quality ω-3 fatty acids free of contaminants such as mercury and organic pollutants should be encouraged when using these agents. Common side effects associated with ω-3 fatty acids are diarrhea and excess bleeding. Patients taking anticoagulant or antiplatelet agents should be monitored more closely when consuming these products because excessive amounts of ω-3 fatty acids (e.g., greater than 3 g daily) may lead to bleeding and may increase the risk of hemorrhagic stroke.

Combination Therapy

A large proportion of the U.S. population will not achieve their NCEP cholesterol targets for a variety of reasons.[49] These include inadequate patient adherence, adverse events, inadequate starting doses, lack of dose escalation, and lower treatment targets.[3,50] Moreover, patients with concomitant elevations in triglycerides and/or low levels of HDL cholesterol may need combination drug therapy to normalize their lipid profile. ⑨ *Combination drug therapy is an effective means to achieve greater reductions in LDL cholesterol (statin plus ezetimibe or bile acid resin, bile acid resin plus ezetimibe, or three-drug combinations) as well as raising HDL cholesterol and lowering serum triglycerides (statin plus niacin or fibrate).*

▶ Combination Therapy for Elevated LDL Cholesterol

For patients who do not achieve their LDL or non-HDL cholesterol goals with statin monotherapy and lifestyle modifications including those unable to tolerate high doses due to adverse effects, combination therapy may be appropriate. Resins or ezetimibe combine effectively with statins to augment LDL cholesterol reduction. When added to a statin, ezetimibe can reduce LDL cholesterol levels by an additional 18% to 21% or up to 65% total reduction with maximum doses of the more potent statins. Ezetimibe and simvastatin are available as a combination tablet (Vytorin) and indicated as adjunctive therapy to diet for the reduction of elevated total cholesterol, LDL cholesterol, Apo B, triglycerides, and non-HDL cholesterol, and to increase HDL cholesterol. The usual starting dose is 10 mg/20 mg, and the maximum dose is 10 mg/40 mg (Table 12–9). Adverse events are similar to those of each product taken separately; however, the percentage of patients with LFT elevations greater than three times normal is slightly higher than with a statin alone, and there appears to be a slightly higher risk of myopathy and rhabdomyolysis when statins and ezetimibe are combined. The time until maximum effect on lipids for this combination is generally 2 to 6 weeks.

A statin combined with a resin results in similar reductions in LDL cholesterol as those seen with ezetimibe. However, the magnitude of triglyceride reduction is less with a resin compared with ezetimibe, and this should be considered in patients with higher baseline triglyceride levels. In addition, GI-adverse events and potential drug interactions limit the utility of this combination.

Ezetimibe and a resin can also be combined. A study that assessed the effects of adding ezetimibe to ongoing resin therapy showed an additional 19% reduction in LDL cholesterol and an additional 14% reduction in triglycerides. This combination was well tolerated.[51]

Some patients, in particular those with genetic forms of hypercholesterolemia such as FH (Table 12–2), require three or more drugs to manage their disorder. Regimens using a statin, resin, and niacin were found to reduce LDL cholesterol up to 75%.[52] These early studies were conducted with lovastatin, so larger reductions would be expected with the more potent statins available today. It is recommended that patients with FH obtain a minimum of greater than or equal to 50% reduction in LDL cholesterol.[16]

▶ Combination Therapy for Elevated Cholesterol and Triglyceridemia With or Without Low HDL Cholesterol

Fibrates are the most effective triglyceride-lowering agents and also raise HDL cholesterol levels. Combination therapy with a fibrate, particularly gemfibrozil, and a statin has been found to increase the risk for myopathy. Of the 31 rhabdomyolysis deaths reported with cerivastatin use, 12 involved concomitant gemfibrozil.[30] Therefore, more frequent monitoring, thorough patient education, and consideration of factors that increase the risk as reviewed previously should be considered.

⑩ *The evidence of reducing LDL cholesterol while substantially raising HDL cholesterol (statin plus niacin or fibrate) to reduce the risk of CHD related events to a greater degree than statin monotherapy remains in question.* A recent trial randomized diabetes patients to simvastatin alone or simvastatin in combination with fenofibrate to determine if adding fenofibrate would further reduce CHD events. The

> ## Patient Encounter 2
>
> JR, a 58-year-old woman with a history of CHD, is obese (BMI: 32 kg/m²) and has been referred to you for a follow-up of her cholesterol. She is taking simvastatin 40 mg once daily in the evening for her cholesterol. Her blood glucose is 110 mg/dL (6.11 mmol/L). Her laboratory test results are within normal limits, except for her fasting lipid profile: total cholesterol 166 mg/dL (4.29 mmol/L), triglycerides 257 mg/dL (2.90 mmol/L), HDL cholesterol 46 mg/dL (1.19 mmol/L), LDL cholesterol 68 mg/dL (1.76 mmol/L), and non-HDL cholesterol 119 mg/dL (3.08 mmol/L).
>
> *What is your assessment of JR's cholesterol results?*
>
> *What diagnostic parameters does JR have for metabolic syndrome?*
>
> *Identify treatment goals for JR.*
>
> *Assess JR's risk for statin-induced side effects.*
>
> *Design a treatment plan for JR.*

combination of fenofibrate and simvastatin did not reduce the overall rate of fatal cardiovascular events, nonfatal myocardial infarction, or nonfatal stroke, as compared with simvastatin alone. However in a prespecified subgroup analysis, incremental benefits of adding a fenofibrate to simvastatin therapy were noted in patients with triglycerides greater than or equal to 204 mg/dL (greater than or equal to 2.31 mmol/L) and HDL cholesterol less than or equal to 34 mg/dL (less than or equal to 0.88 mmol/L).[53] Combining niacin with a statin augments the LDL-cholesterol lowering potential of niacin while enhancing both the HDL cholesterol–raising effects and triglyceride-lowering effects of the statin. A statin combined with niacin appears to offer greater benefits for reducing atherosclerosis progression compared with a statin alone.[37] As mentioned earlier, however, the incremental benefits on reducing CHD events remains in question.[41] Formulations combining ER niacin and lovastatin (Advicor) and ER niacin and simvastatin (Simcor) are available, and they are indicated for treatment of primary hypercholesterolemia and mixed dyslipidemia in patients treated with lovastatin or simvastatin who require further triglyceride lowering or HDL cholesterol raising and may benefit from having niacin added to their regimen. The combination is also indicated for patients treated with niacin who require further LDL-cholesterol lowering and may benefit from having lovastatin or simvastatin added to their regimen. The time until maximum effect on lipids for this combination is generally 3 to 6 weeks.

Niacin can be combined with a fibrate in patients with high elevations in serum triglycerides. The combination may increase the risk of myopathy compared with either agent alone.

Compared with monotherapy, combination therapy may reduce patient adherence through increased side effects and increased costs. When used appropriately and with proper precautions, however, they are effective in normalizing lipid abnormalities, particularly in patients who cannot tolerate adequate doses of statin therapy for more severe forms of dyslipidemia.

▶ Investigational Agents

Numerous investigational drugs are in development for the treatment of lipid disorders and the prevention of atherosclerosis. Many of these will likely be used in combination with currently available lipid-modulating drugs. The most promising is an antisense drug that significantly reduced Apo B-100 and LDL cholesterol.[54] Other agents in development include newer statins; bile acid transport inhibitors; phytostanol analogs; acyl coenzyme A: cholesterol acyltransferase (ACAT) inhibitors; squalene synthase inhibitors; CTEP inhibitors, proprotein convertase subtilisin/kexin type 9 (PCSK9), and newer PPAR-α, -γ, and -δ agonists, as well as dual PPAR-α/γ agonists.

These novel therapies will provide opportunities for developing different combination strategies to further reduce the risk of CHD even after adequate treatment with existing agents. Well-designed studies using noninvasive imaging technology and long-term follow-up periods are needed to ensure that there is a favorable risk-to-benefit ratio.

▶ Outcome Evaluation

- The successful outcome in cholesterol management is to reduce cholesterol and triglycerides below the NCEP ATP III goals in an effort to alter the natural course of atherosclerosis and decrease future cardiovascular events.

Patient Care and Monitoring

1. Assess the patient for the presence of CHD or other atherosclerosis disorders.

2. Assess major risk factors for CHD.

3. For patients without CHD or CHD risk equivalent, but two or more major CHD risk factors, perform the Framingham risk assessment.

4. Obtain fasting cholesterol profile and assess any abnormal lipid levels.

5. Obtain a thorough history of prescription, nonprescription, and natural drug product use. Determine what treatments for cholesterol the patient has used in the past (if any). Assess if the patient is taking any medications that may contribute to his or her abnormal lipid levels.

6. Assess concomitant diseases that may contribute to the patient's abnormal lipid levels.

7. Assess risk factors for metabolic syndrome.

8. Determine the treatment goal for LDL cholesterol based on the patient's CHD risk and non-HDL cholesterol goal if patient meets criteria for metabolic syndrome.

9. Educate all patients on therapeutic lifestyle changes (TLCs) and the importance of regular physical activity.

10. For patients exceeding their LDL cholesterol goal, initiate TLCs. Consider starting concurrent pharmacotherapy in patients in the high-risk or moderately high-risk categories. Pharmacotherapy should be initiated at a dose to reduce LDL cholesterol by 30% to 40% at a minimum. For patients with CHD who have an LDL cholesterol goal of less than 70 mg/dL, if it is not possible to attain this goal due to a high baseline LDL cholesterol, it is generally possible to achieve an LDL cholesterol reduction of greater than 50% with more intensive LDL-lowering therapy, including combination drug therapy.

11. For patients with familial hypercholesterolemia (FH), it is recommended that a greater than or equal to 50% reduction in LDL cholesterol be achieved.

12. Therapeutic lifestyle changes should be continued and intensified (consider adding plant sterols/stanols and increase fiber) after 6 weeks if not below LDL cholesterol target. For those patients above their LDL cholesterol target after adequate trial of TLC (12 to 18 weeks), pharmacotherapy should be strongly considered.

13. Institute appropriate pharmacotherapy based on lipid abnormality. Obtain appropriate baseline labs to monitor for adverse drug effects. Assess potential disease and drug interactions that may affect choice or intensity of pharmacotherapy.

14. Monitor response, safety, and adherence after a minimum of 4 to 6 weeks. Titrate therapy or add a second drug as needed.

15. Once the LDL cholesterol goal is achieved, assess non-HDL cholesterol in those with metabolic syndrome and intensify LDL-lowering therapy further or consider adding niacin or fibrate.

16. Provide patient education associated with CHD, hyperlipidemia, TLC, drug therapy, and therapy adherence.

17. Family screening is indicated if patient has FH.

- Use an adequate trial of TLC in all patients, but institute pharmacotherapy concurrently in higher-risk patients.

- When indicated, initiate drug therapy at a dose that will reduce LDL cholesterol in the range of 30% to 40%.

- Typically, statins are the medications of choice to treat high LDL cholesterol because of their ability to substantially reduce LDL cholesterol, ability to reduce morbidity and mortality from atherosclerotic disease, convenient once-daily dosing, and low risk of side effects.

- Use an individualized patient monitoring plan in an effort to minimize side effects, maintain treatment adherence, and achieve lipid goals.

Abbreviations Introduced in This Chapter

ABC	ATP-binding cassette
ABCA1	ATP-binding cassette A1
ABC G1	ATP-binding cassette G1
ABC G5/G8	ATP-binding cassette G5/G8
ACAT	Acyl coenzyme A: cholesterol acyltransferase
Acetyl CoA	Acetyl coenzyme A
AIDS	Acquired immunodeficiency syndrome
Apo	Apolipoprotein
ATP	Adenosine triphosphate
ATP III	Adult Treatment Panel III edition
BAS	Bile acid sequestrant
BP	Blood pressure
bpm	Beats per minute
C	Cholesterol
CAD	Clinical atherosclerotic disease
CE	Cholesterol ester
CETP	Cholesterol ester transfer protein
CHD	Coronary heart disease
CK	Creatine kinase
CM	Chylomicrons
CPK	Creatine phosphokinase
CRP	C-reactive protein
DBP	Diastolic blood pressure
ER	Extended-release
FA	Fatty acid
FH	Familial hypercholesterolemia
HbA1c	Glycosylated hemoglobin
HDL	High-density lipoprotein
HMG-CoA	3-hydroxy-3-methylglutaryl coenzyme A
HL	Hepatic lipase
IDL	Intermediate-density lipoprotein
IR	Immediate-release
LCAT	Lecithin-cholesterol acyltransferase
LDL	Low-density lipoprotein
LFT	Liver function test
LPL	Lipoprotein lipase
Lp-PLA2	Lipoprotein-associated phospholipase A2
LRP	LDL-related protein
MI	Myocardial infarction
MMP	Matrix metalloproteinase

NCEP	National Cholesterol Education Program
NO	Nitric oxide
NPC1L1	Niemann-Pick C1 Like 1
NSAID	Nonsteroidal anti-inflammatory drug
PPAR-α	Peroxisome proliferator-activated receptor-alpha
PCSK9	Proprotein convertase subtilisin/kexin 9
SBP	Systolic blood pressure
SR	Sustained-release
SR-BI	Scavenger receptors
TG	Triglyceride
TLC	Therapeutic lifestyle changes
VLDL	Very low-density lipoprotein

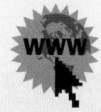 Self-assessment questions and answers are available at *http://www.mhpharmacotherapy. com/pp.html.*

REFERENCES

1. Kronmal RA, Cain KC, Ye Z, Omenn GS. Total serum cholesterol levels and mortality risk as a function of age. A report based on the Framingham data. Arch Intern Med 1993;153:1065–1073.

2. Roger VL, Go AS, Lloyd-Jones DM, et al. Heart disease and stroke statistics—2011 update: A report from the American Heart Association. Circulation 2011;123(4):e18–e209.

3. Third Report of the National Cholesterol Education Program (NCEP) Expert Panel on Detection, Evaluation, and Treatment of High Blood Cholesterol in Adults (Adult Treatment Panel III) Final Report. Circulation 2002;106 (25):3143–3421.

4. Genest J. Lipoprotein disorders and cardiovascular risk. J Inherit Metab Dis 2003;26:267–287.

5. Garcia-Calvo M, Lisnock J, Bull HG, et al. The target of ezetimibe is Niemann-Pick C1-Like 1 (NPC1L1). Proc Natl Acad Sci 2005;102(23): 8132–8137.

6. Libby P. Molecular basis of the acute coronary syndrome. Circulation 1995;91:2844–2850.

7. Brown BG, Zhao XQ, Chait A, et al. Simvastatin and niacin, antioxidant vitamins, or the combination for the prevention of coronary disease. N Engl J Med 2001;345:1583–1592.

8. National Heart Lung and Blood Institute. Detection, Evaluation, and Treatment of High Blood Cholesterol in Adults (Adult Treatment Panel IV). Available at *http://www.nhlbi.nih.gov/guidelines/cholesterol/atp4/ index.htm*. Accessed November 7, 2011.

9. Grundy SM, Cleeman JI, Bairey Merz CN, et al., for the Coordinating Committee of the National Cholesterol Education Program endorsed by the National Heart, Lung, and Blood Institute, American College of Cardiology Foundation, and American Heart Association. Update implications of recent clinical trials for the national cholesterol education program adult treatment panel III guidelines. Circulation 2004;110:227–239.

10. Smith SC Jr, Allen J, Blair SN, et al. AHA/ACC Guidelines for Secondary Prevention for Patients with Coronary and Other Atherosclerotic Vascular Disease: 2006 Update: Endorsed by the National Heart, Lung, and Blood Institute. Circulation 2006;113:2363–2372.

11. Goldberg AC, Hopkins PN, Toth PP, et al. Familial hypercholesterolemia: Screening, diagnosis and management of pediatric and adult patients: Clinical guidance from the National Lipid Association Expert Panel on Familial Hypercholesterolemia. J Clin Lipidol 2011;5(3):133–140.

12. Lichtenstein AH, Appel LJ, Brands M, et al. Diet and lifestyle recommendations revision 2006: A scientific statement from the American Heart Association Nutritional Committee. Circulation. 2006;114:82–96.

13. Grundy SM, Cleeman JI, Daniels SR, et al. Diagnosis and management of the metabolic syndrome: An American Heart Association/National

Heart, Lung, and Blood Institute scientific statement. Curr Opin Cardiol 2006;21:1–6.

14. Pearson TA, Mensah GA, Alexander RW, et al. Markers of inflammation and cardiovascular disease: Application to clinical and public health practice: A statement for healthcare professionals from the Centers for Disease Control and Prevention and the American Heart Association. Circulation 2003;107(3):499–511.

15. Ridker PM, Danielson E, Fonseca FA, et al. Rosuvastatin to prevent vascular events in men and women with elevated C-reactive protein. N Engl J Med 2008;359(21): 2195–2207.

16. Davidson MH, Ballantyne CM, Jacobson TA, et al. Clinical utility of inflammatory markers and advanced lipoprotein testing: Advice from an Expert Panel of Lipid Specialists. J Clin Lipidol 2011;5:338–367.

17. Shepherd J, Cobbe SM, Ford I, et al., for The West of Scotland Coronary Prevention Study Group. Prevention of coronary heart disease with pravastatin in men with hypercholesterolemia. N Engl J Med 1995;333:1301–1307.

18. Sever PS, Dahlof B, Poulter NR, et al. Prevention of coronary and stroke events with atorvastatin in hypertensive patients who have average or lower-than-average cholesterol concentrations, in the Anglo-Scandinavian Cardiac Outcomes Trial—Lipid-Lowering Arm (ASCOT-LLA): A multicentre randomised controlled trial. Lancet 2003;361:1149–1158.

19. The ALLHAT Officers and Coordinators for the ALLHAT Collaborative Research Group. Major outcomes in moderately hypercholesterolemia, hypertensive patients randomized to pravastatin vs usual care: The Antihypertensive and Lipid-Lowering Treatment to Prevent Heart Attack Trial (ALLHAT-LLT). JAMA 2002;288:2998–3007.

20. Calhoun HM, Betteridge DJ, Durrington PN, et al. Primary prevention of cardiovascular disease with atorvastatin in type 2 diabetes in the Collaborative Atorvastatin Diabetes Study (CARDS): Multicentre randomised placebo-controlled trial. Lancet 2004;364:685–696.

21. Scandinavian Simvastatin Survival Study Group. Randomised trial of cholesterol lowering in 4444 patients with coronary heart disease: The Scandinavian Simvastatin Survival Study (4S). Lancet 1994; 344:1383–1389.

22. Sacks FM, Pfeffer MA, Moye LA, et al., for the Cholesterol and Recurrent Events Trial Investigators. The effect of pravastatin on coronary events after myocardial infarction in patients with average cholesterol levels. Cholesterol and Recurrent Events Trial investigators. N Engl J Med 1996;335:1001–1009.

23. Heart Protection Study Collaborative Group. MRC/BHF Heart Protection Study of cholesterol lowering with simvastatin in 20,536 high-risk individuals: A randomized placebo-controlled trial. Lancet 2002;360(9326):7–22.

24. The Long-Term Intervention with Pravastatin in Ischemic Disease (LIPID) Study Group. Prevention of cardiovascular events and death with pravastatin in patients with coronary heart disease and a broad range of initial cholesterol levels. N Engl J Med 1998;399(19):1349–1357.

25. Cannon CP, Braunwald E, McCabe CH, et al. Intensive versus moderate lipid-lowering with statins after acute coronary syndromes. N Engl J Med 2004;350:1495–1504.

26. LaRosa JC, Grundy SM, Waters DD, et al. Treating to New Targets (TNT) Investigators. Intensive lipid lowering with atorvastatin in patients with stable coronary disease. N Engl J Med 2005;352:1425–1435.

27. Downs JR, Clearfield M, Weis S, et al., for the AFCAPS/TexCAPS Research Group. Primary prevention of acute coronary events with lovastatin in men and women with average cholesterol levels: Results of AFCAPS/TexCAPS. JAMA 1998;270:1615–1622.

28. Liao JK. Clinical implications for statin pleiotropy. Curr Opin Lipidol 2005;16(6):624–629.

29. Pasternak RC, Smith SC Jr, Bairey-Merz CN, et al. ACC/AHA/NHLBI clinical advisory on the use and safety of statins. J Am Coll Cardiol 2002;40:568–573.

30. Staffa JA, Chang J, Green L. Cerivastatin and reports of fatal rhabdomyolysis. New Engl J Med 2002;346(7):539–540.

31. Kastelein JJ, Akdim F, Stroes ES, et al. Simvastatin with or without ezetimibe in familial hypercholesterolemia. N Engl J Med 2008;358(14):1431–1443.

32. Rossebø AB, Pedersen TR, Boman K, et al. Intensive lipid lowering with simvastatin and ezetimibe in aortic stenosis. N Engl J Med 2008;359:1343–1356.

33. Baigent C, Landray MJ, Reith C, et al. The effects of lowering LDL cholesterol with simvastatin plus ezetimibe in patients with chronic kidney disease (Study of Heart and Renal Protection): A randomised placebo-controlled trial. Lancet 2011;377(9784):2181–2192.

34. The Lipid Research Clinics Coronary Primary Prevention Trial results. II. The relationship of reduction in incidence of coronary heart disease to cholesterol lowering. JAMA 1984;251:365–374.

35. Sankyo Pharma, Inc. Welchol [prescribing information]. Parsippany, NJ: Author. 2011.

36. Meyers CD, Carr MC, Park S, et al. Varying cost and free nicotinic acid content in over-the-counter niacin preparations for dyslipidemia. Ann Intern Med 2003;139:996–1002.

37. McKenney JM, Proctor JD, Harris S, et al. A comparison of the efficacy and toxic effects of sustained- vs immediate-release niacin in hypercholesterolemic patients. JAMA 1994;271:672–677.

38. Dunatchik AP, Ito MK, Dujovne CA. A systematic review on evidence of the effectiveness and safety of a wax-matrix niacin formulation J Clin Lipidol 2012;6:121–131.

39. Canner PL, Berge GK, Wender NK, et al. Fifteen-year mortality in Coronary Drug Project patients: Long-term benefit with niacin. J Am Coll Cardiol 1986;18:1245–1255.

40. Taylor AJ, Sullenberger LE, Lee HJ, et al. Arterial biology for the investigation of the treatment effects of reducing cholesterol (ARBITER) 2. A double-blind, placebo-controlled study of extended-release niacin on atherosclerosis progression in secondary prevention patients treated with statins. Circulation 2004;110:3512–3517.

41. AIM-HIGH Cholesterol Management Program. Available at http://www.aimhigh-heart.com/.

42. HPS2-Thrive. Available at http://www.thrivestudy.org/.

43. Bays HE, Dujovne CA, McGovern ME, et al. ADvicor versus Other Cholesterol-Modulating Agents Trial Evaluation. Comparison of once-daily, niacin extended-release/lovastatin with standard doses of atorvastatin and simvastatin (the ADvicor versus Other Cholesterol-Modulating Agents Trial Evaluation [ADVOCATE]). Am J Cardiol 2003;91(6):667–672.

44. Canner PL, Furberg CD, Terrin ML, et al. Benefits of niacin by glycemic status in patients with healed myocardial infarction (from the Coronary Drug Project). Am J Cardiol 2005;95:254–257.

45. Frick MH, Elo O, Haapa K, et al. Helsinki Heart Study: Primary prevention trial with gemfibrozil in middle aged men with dyslipidemia. Safety of treatment, changes in risk factors, and incidence of coronary heart disease. N Engl J Med 1987;317:1237–1245.

46. Robins SJ, Collins D, Wittes JT, et al., for the VA-HIT Study Group. Veterans Affairs High-Density Lipoprotein Intervention Trial. Relation of gemfibrozil treatment and lipid levels with major coronary events: VA-HIT: A randomized controlled trial. JAMA 2001;285(12):1585–1591.

47. Prueksaritanont T, Zhao JJ, Ma B, et al. Mechanistic studies on metabolic interactions between gemfibrozil and statins. J Pharmacol Exp Ther 2002;301(3):1042–1051.

48. Kris-Etherton PM Harris WS, Appel LJ, for the Nutrition Committee: Fish consumption, fish oil, omega-3 fatty acids, and cardiovascular disease. Circulation 2002;106:2747–2757.

49. Pearson TA, Laurora I, Chu H, et al. The lipid treatment assessment project (L-TAP): A multicenter survey to evaluate the percentages of dyslipidemic patients receiving lipid-lowering therapy and achieving low-density lipoprotein cholesterol goals. Arch Intern Med 2000;160:459–467.

50. Ito MK, Lin JC, Morreale AP, et al. Effect of pravastatin-to-simvastatin conversion on reducing low-density lipoprotein cholesterol. Am J Health Syst Pharm 2001;58:1734–1739.

51. Xydakis AM, Guyton JR, Chiou P, et al. Effectiveness and tolerability of ezetimibe add-on therapy to a bile acid resin-based regimen for hypercholesterolemia. Am J Cardiol 2004;94(6):795–797.

52. Leitersdorf E, Muratti EN, Eliav O, et al. Efficacy and safety of triple therapy (fluvastatin-bezafibrate-cholestyramine) for severe familial hypercholesterolemia. Am J Cardiol 1995;76:84A–88A.

53. The ACCORD Study Group. Effects of Combination Lipid Therapy in Type 2 Diabetes Mellitus. N Engl J Med 2010;362(17):1563–1574.

54. Ito MK. ISIS 301012 Gene therapy for hypercholesterolemia: Sense, antisense, or nonsense. Ann Pharmacother 2007;41:1669–1678.

13 Hypovolemic Shock

Bradley A. Boucher and G. Christopher Wood

KEY CONCEPTS

❶ Regardless of etiology, the most distinctive clinical manifestations of hypovolemic shock are arterial hypotension and metabolic acidosis. Metabolic acidosis is a consequence of an accumulation of lactic acid resulting from tissue hypoxia and anaerobic metabolism. If the decrease in arterial blood pressure (BP) is severe and protracted, such hypotension will inevitably lead to severe hypoperfusion and organ dysfunction.

❷ Hypovolemic shock occurs as a consequence of inadequate intravascular volume to meet the oxygen and metabolic needs of the body.

❸ Protracted tissue hypoxia sets in motion a downward spiral of events leading to organ dysfunction and eventual failure if untreated.

❹ The overarching goals in treating hypovolemic shock are to restore effective circulating blood volume, as well as managing its underlying cause, thereby reversing organ dysfunction and returning to homeostasis.

❺ Three major therapeutic options are available to clinicians for restoring circulating blood volume: crystalloids (electrolyte-based solutions), colloids (large molecular weight solutions), and blood products.

❻ In the absence of ongoing blood loss, administration of 2,000 to 4,000 mL (approximately 4 to 8 pints) of isotonic crystalloid normally reestablishes baseline vital signs in adult hypovolemic shock patients.

❼ Colloid solutions administered are primarily confined to the intravascular space, in contrast to isotonic crystalloid solutions that distribute throughout the extracellular fluid space.

❽ Blood products are indicated in adult hypovolemic shock patients who have sustained blood loss from hemorrhage exceeding 1,500 mL (approximately 3 pints).

❾ Vasopressors may be warranted as a temporary measure in patients with profound hypotension or evidence of organ dysfunction in the early stages of shock.

❿ Major treatment goals in hypovolemic shock following fluid resuscitation are as follows: arterial systolic blood pressure (SBP) greater than 90 mm Hg within 1 hour, organ dysfunction reversal, and normalization of laboratory measurements as rapidly as possible (less than 24 hours).

INTRODUCTION

The principal function of the circulatory system is to supply oxygen and vital metabolic compounds to cells throughout the body, as well as removal of metabolic waste products. Circulatory shock is a life-threatening condition whereby this principal function is compromised.[1] When circulatory shock is caused by a severe loss of blood volume or body water, it is called **hypovolemic shock**, which is the focus of this chapter. ❶ *Regardless of etiology, the most distinctive clinical manifestations of hypovolemic shock are arterial hypotension and* **metabolic acidosis**. *Metabolic acidosis is a consequence of an accumulation of lactic acid resulting from tissue hypoxia and anaerobic metabolism. If the decrease in arterial blood pressure (BP) is severe and protracted, such hypotension will inevitably lead to severe hypoperfusion and organ dysfunction.* Rapid and effective restoration of circulatory homeostasis through the use of fluids, pharmacologic agents, and/or blood products is imperative to prevent complications of untreated shock and ultimately death.

ETIOLOGY AND EPIDEMIOLOGY

Practitioners must have a good understanding of cardiovascular physiology to diagnose, treat, and monitor circulatory problems in critically ill patients. The interrelationships among the major hemodynamic variables are depicted in **Figure 13–1.**[2] These variables include arterial BP, cardiac output (CO), systemic vascular resistance (SVR), heart rate (HR), stroke volume (SV), left ventricular size, afterload,

myocardial contractility, and preload. Although an oversimplification, Figure 13–1 is beneficial in conceptualizing where the major abnormalities occur in patients with circulatory shock as well as predicting the body's compensatory responses.

Shock can be effectively categorized by etiology into four major types: hypovolemic, obstructive, cardiogenic, and distributive (**Table 13–1**).[1,3,4] As noted, all patients with shock have profound decreases in arterial BP. Understanding the primary cause of the circulatory abnormality in these respective shock states is invaluable to their management. Hypovolemic shock is caused by a loss of intravascular volume either by hemorrhage or fluid loss (e.g., dehydration). Obstructive shock is caused by an obstruction that directly compromises inflow or outflow of blood from the heart. Cardiogenic shock is caused by diminished myocardial contractility that results in decreased CO with an increase in SVR. Lastly, distributive shock is caused by a major decrease in SVR with an increase in CO. Differentiating between the underlying abnormality and the associated compensatory response is also essential in terms of treatment and monitoring. Hypovolemic shock is considered to be essentially a profound deficit in preload, defined as the volume in the ventricles at the end of diastole.

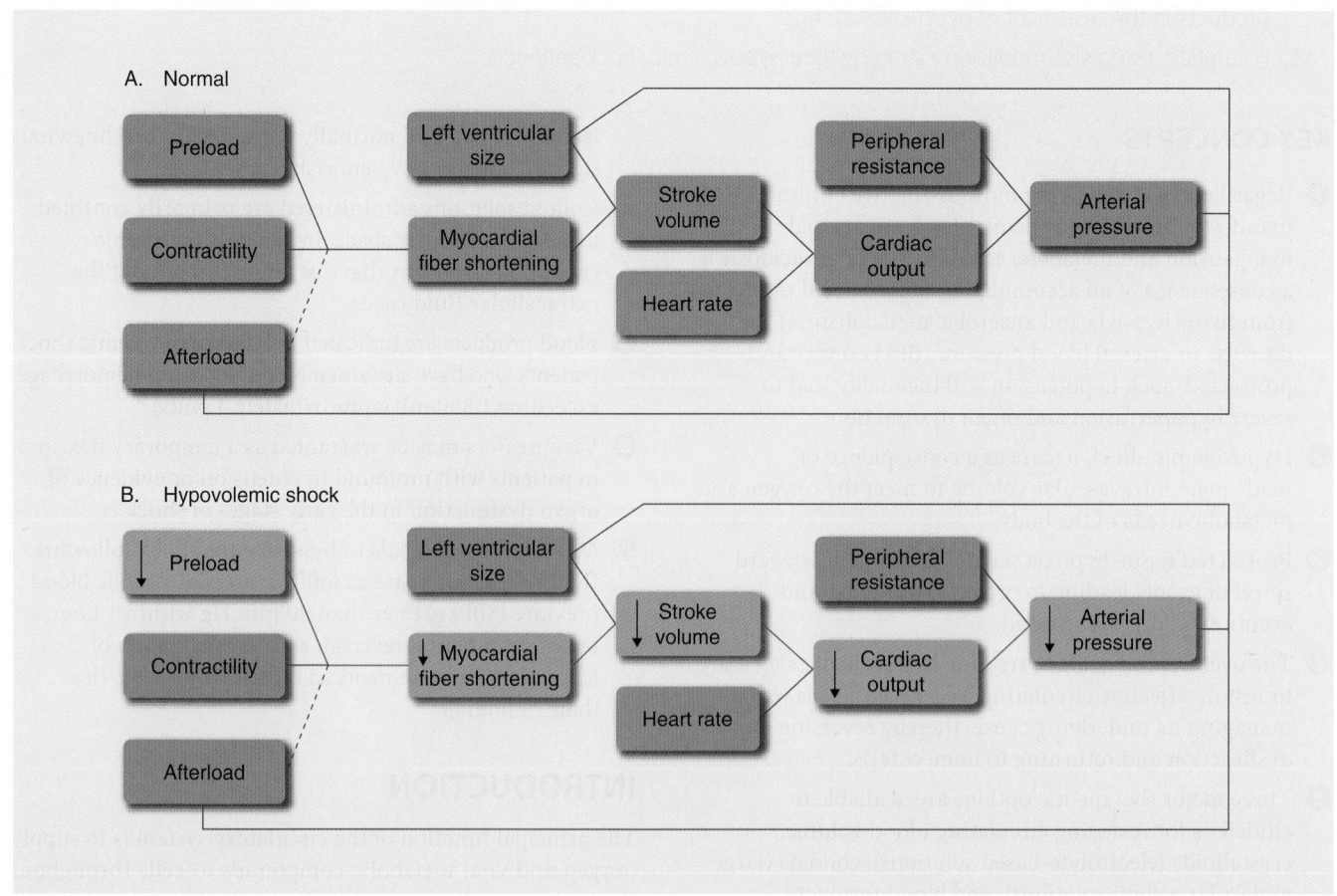

FIGURE 13–1. Hemodynamic relationships among key cardiovascular parameters (*A*). Solid lines represent a direct relationship; the broken line represents an inverse relationship. In *B*, the alterations typically observed in hypovolemic shock are highlighted with arrows depicting the likely direction of the alteration. (Panel A from Braunwald E. Regulation of the circulation. I. N Engl J Med 1974;290:1124–1129, with permission.)

Table 13-1

Major Shock Classifications and Selected Etiologies[1,3,4]

I. Hypovolemic

Hemorrhagic
   Trauma
   GI bleeding
   Abdominal aortic aneurysm

Nonhemorrhagic (dehydration)
   Vomiting
   Diarrhea
   Third spacing
   Burns
   Fistulae

II. Cardiogenic
   Myocardial infarction
   Septal wall rupture
   Acute mitral valve regurgitation
   Myocarditis
   Arrhythmias

III. Obstructive
   Pericardial tamponade
   Tension pneumothorax
   Pulmonary embolism
   Acute pulmonary hypertension
   Amniotic fluid embolism
   Aortic dissection

IV. Distributive
   Sepsis
   Anaphylactic
   Spinal cord injury
   Endocrinologic
   Pharmacologic

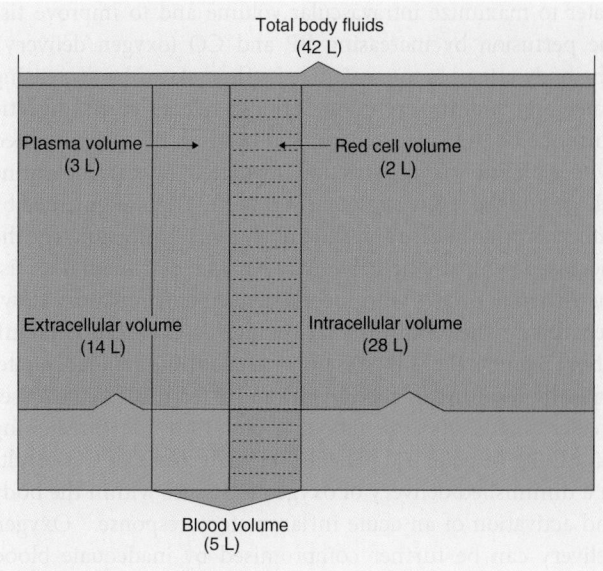

FIGURE 13-2. Distribution of body fluids showing the extracellular fluid volume, intracellular body fluid volume, and total body fluids in a 70-kg (154-lb) adult. Extracellular volume (ECV) comprises 14 L of total body fluid (42 L). Plasma volume makes up approximately 3 L of the 14 L of ECV. Intracellular volume accounts for the remaining 28 L of total body fluids with roughly 2 L located within the red blood cells. Blood volume (approximately 5 L) is also depicted and made up of primarily red blood cells and plasma. (From Guyton AC, Hall JE. Textbook of Medical Physiology, 8th ed. Philadelphia, PA: Saunders, 1991:275, with permission.)

Decreased preload results in subsequent decreases in SV, CO, and eventually, mean arterial pressure (MAP). As such, restoration of preload becomes an overriding goal in the management of hypovolemic shock.

The prognosis of shock patients depends on several variables including severity, duration, underlying etiology, preexisting organ dysfunction, and reversibility.[5] Data are not readily available on the incidence of hypovolemic shock, although hypovolemia due to hemorrhage is a major factor in 40% to 50% of trauma deaths annually.[6]

PATHOPHYSIOLOGY

The total amount of water in a typical 70-kg (154-lb) adult is approximately 42 L (Fig. 13–2). About 28 of the 42 L are inside the cells of the body (intracellular fluid); the remaining 14 L are in the extracellular fluid space (fluid outside of cells, i.e., interstitial fluid and plasma). Circulating blood volume for a normal adult is roughly 5 L (70 mL/kg) and is composed of 2 L of red blood cell fluid (intracellular) and 3 L of plasma (extracellular). ❷ *By definition, hypovolemic shock occurs as a consequence of inadequate intravascular volume to meet the oxygen and metabolic needs of the body.* Diminished intravascular volume can result from severe external or internal bleeding, profound fluid losses from GI sources such

as diarrhea or vomiting, or urinary losses such as diuretic use, diabetic ketoacidosis, or diabetes insipidus (Table 13–1).[1] Other sources of intravascular fluid loss can occur through damaged skin, as seen with burns, or via **capillary leak** into the interstitial space or peritoneal cavity, as seen with edema or ascites. This latter phenomenon is often referred to as **third spacing** because fluid accumulates in the interstitial space disproportionately to the intracellular and extracellular fluid spaces. Regional ischemia may also develop as blood flow is naturally shunted from organs such as the GI tract or the kidneys to more immediately vital organs such as the heart and brain.

Hypovolemic shock symptoms begin to occur with decreases in intravascular volume in excess of 750 to 1500 mL or 15% to 30% of the circulating blood volume (20 to 40 mL/kg in pediatric patients).[7] As previously stated, decreases in preload or ventricular end-diastolic volumes result in decreases in SV. Initially, CO may be partially maintained by compensatory tachycardia. Similarly, reflex increases in SVR and myocardial contractility may diminish arterial hypotension. Regardless, rapid losses (e.g., minutes) undoubtedly have more profound effects than losses over a longer period (e.g., hours). This neurohumoral response to hypovolemia is mediated by the sympathetic nervous system in an attempt to preserve perfusion to vital organs such as the heart and brain. Two major end points of this response are to conserve water to maximize intravascular volume and to improve tissue perfusion by increasing BP and CO (oxygen delivery). The body attempts to maximize its fluid status by decreasing water and sodium excretion through release of antidiuretic hormone (ADH), aldosterone, and cortisol. BP is maintained by peripheral vasoconstriction mediated by catecholamine release and the renin-angiotensin system.[1] CO is augmented by catecholamine release and fluid retention.[1,4] Unfortunately, the increased sympathetic drive may become detrimental as tissue ischemia occurs with inconsistent microcirculatory flow.[1] Regardless, when intravascular volume losses exceed 1,500 mL (about 3 pints), the compensatory mechanisms are inadequate, typically resulting in a fall in CO and arterial BP; acute losses greater than 2,000 mL (about 4 pints) are life threatening (35 mL/kg in pediatric patients).[8] The decrease in CO results in a diminished delivery of oxygen to tissues within the body and activation of an acute inflammatory response.[1,6] Oxygen delivery can be further compromised by inadequate blood hemoglobin levels due to hemorrhage and/or diminished hemoglobin saturation due to impaired ventilation. Decreased delivery of oxygen and other vital nutrients results in diminished production of the energy substrate, adenosine triphosphate (ATP). Lactic acid is then produced as a by-product of anaerobic metabolism within tissues throughout the body.[4] Hyperglycemia produced during the stress response from cortisol release is also a contributing factor in the development of lactic acidosis. Lactic acidosis indicates that inadequate tissue perfusion has occurred.[4] ❸ *Protracted tissue hypoxia sets in motion a downward spiral of events leading to organ dysfunction and eventual failure if untreated.* Table 13–2 describes the effects of shock on the body's major organs. Relative failure of

more than one organ, regardless of etiology, is referred to as the multiple organ dysfunction syndrome (MODS). Involvement of the heart is particularly devastating considering the central role it plays in oxygen delivery and the potential for myocardial dysfunction to perpetuate the shock state. Preexisting

---

Table 13–2

Shock Manifestations on Major Organs

Heart
- Myocardial ischemia
- Dysrhythmias

Brain
- Restlessness, confusion, obtundation
- Global cerebral ischemia

Liver
- Release of liver enzymes
- Biliary stasis

Lungs
- Pulmonary edema
- ARDS

Kidneys
- Oliguria
- Decreased glomerular filtration
- Acute kidney injury

GI tract
- Stress-related mucosal disease
- Bacterial translocation

Hematologic
- Thrombocytopenia
- Coagulopathies

ARDS, acute respiratory distress syndrome; GI, gastrointestinal.

Clinical Presentation and Diagnosis of Hypovolemic Shock

General

Patients will be in acute distress, although symptoms and signs will vary depending on the severity of the hypovolemia and whether the etiology is hemorrhagic versus nonhemorrhagic.

Symptoms
- Thirst
- Weakness
- Lightheadedness

Signs
- Hypotension, arterial systolic BP (SBP) less than 90 mm Hg or fall in SBP greater than 40 mm Hg
- Tachycardia
- Tachypnea
- Hypothermia
- Oliguria

- Dark, yellow-colored urine
- Skin color: pale to ashen; may be cyanotic in severe cases
- Skin temperature: cool to cold
- Mental status: confusion to coma
- Pulmonary artery (PA) catheter measurements: decreased CO, decreased SV, increased SVR, low pulmonary artery occlusion pressure (PAOP)

Laboratory Tests
- Hypernatremia
- Elevated serum creatinine (SCr)
- Elevated blood urea nitrogen
- Decreased hemoglobin/hematocrit (hemorrhagic hypovolemic shock)
- Hyperglycemia
- Increased serum lactate
- Decreased arterial pH

organ dysfunction and buildup of inflammatory mediators can also exacerbate the effects of hypovolemic shock to the point of irreversibility.[6] For example, acute or chronic heart failure can lead to pulmonary edema, further aggravating gas exchange in the lungs and ultimately tissue hypoxia. Another example is multiple organ dysfunction, which is frequently observed in trauma patients. Specifically, MODS develops in approximately 20% of trauma patients who require fluid resuscitation. Only about one-third of early-onset MODS is quickly reversible (within 48 hours) with proper fluid resuscitation. Thus it is imperative that hypovolemic shock be treated quickly to avoid MODS.[9]

TREATMENT

Desired Outcomes

④ *The overarching goals in treating hypovolemic shock are to restore effective circulating blood volume, as well as manage its underlying cause.* In achieving this goal, the downward spiral of events that can perpetuate severe or protracted hypovolemic shock is interrupted. This is accomplished through the delivery of adequate oxygen and metabolic substrates such as glucose and electrolytes to the tissues throughout the body that will optimally bring about a restoration of organ function and return to homeostasis. Evidence of the latter is a return to the patient's baseline vital signs, relative normalization of laboratory test results, and alleviation of the other signs and symptoms of hypovolemic shock previously discussed. Concurrent supportive therapies are also warranted to avoid exacerbation of organ dysfunction associated with the hypovolemic shock event.

General Approach to Therapy

Securing an adequate airway and ventilation is imperative in hypovolemic shock patients consistent with the airway, breathing, and circulation (ABCs) of life support. Any compromise in ventilation only accentuates the tissue hypoxia occurring secondary to inadequate perfusion. Thus early sedation with tracheal intubation and mechanical ventilation typically occurs at this stage of resuscitation (Fig. 13–3). IV access is also essential for administration of fluids and medications, and it can be accomplished through the placement of peripheral IV lines or catheterization with central venous lines if rapid or large volumes of resuscitative fluids are indicated. Although primarily facilitating fluid administration, the IV lines provide access for blood samples for obtaining appropriate laboratory tests. Placement of an arterial catheter is advantageous to allow for accurate and continual monitoring of BP, as well as arterial blood gas (ABG) sampling. A bladder catheter should be inserted for ongoing monitoring of urine output. Baseline laboratory tests that should be done immediately include complete blood cell count with differential, serum chemistry profile, liver enzymes, prothrombin and partial thromboplastin times, and serum lactate. A urinalysis and an ABG should also be obtained, and ongoing electrocardiogram (ECG) monitoring should be performed.

In addition to restoring circulating blood volume, it is necessary to prevent further losses from the vascular space. This is especially true with hemorrhagic hypovolemic shock where identifying the bleeding site and achievement of hemostasis are critical in the successful resuscitation of the patient. This frequently involves surgical treatment of hemorrhages.

Upon stabilization, placement of a pulmonary artery (PA) catheter may be indicated based on the need for more extensive cardiovascular monitoring than is available from non-invasive measurements such as vital signs, cardiac rhythm, and urine output.[10,11] Key measured parameters that can be obtained from a PA catheter are the pulmonary artery occlusion pressure (PAOP), which is a measure of left ventricular preload, and CO. From the CO values and simultaneous measurement of HR and BP, one can calculate the left ventricular SV and SVR.[11] Placement of a PA catheter should be reserved for patients at high risk of death due to the severity of shock or preexisting medical conditions such as heart failure.[12] Use of PA catheters in broad populations of critically ill patients is somewhat controversial because clinical trials have not shown consistent benefits with their use and may even be detrimental.[1,13] However, critically ill patients with a high severity of illness may have improved outcomes from PA catheter placement. It is not clear why this was seen, but it could be that more severely ill patients have less physiological reserve and less "room for error" and benefit from the therapeutic decisions that come from detailed PA catheter data.[14] An alternative to the PA catheter is placement of a central venous catheter that typically resides in the superior vena cava to monitor central venous pressure (CVP). Although central venous catheters are less expensive and more readily placed, they are not particularly accurate in monitoring effective fluid resuscitation.[11]

Patient Encounter Part 1

RW is a 45-year-old man admitted to the emergency department (ED) with nausea and vomiting for the past 12 hours. The patient's wife was concerned because the emesis contained large amounts of bright red blood. The patient cannot reliably communicate with the healthcare team because he is confused. The initial diagnosis by the ED team is hypovolemic shock. A physical examination is being performed and blood samples are being sent to the laboratory.

What type of hypovolemic shock does RW have and what is the cause?

What signs and symptoms would you expect to see in this patient with hypovolemic shock?

What laboratory abnormalities might be expected in this patient?

Describe the first nonpharmacologic steps in treating RW.

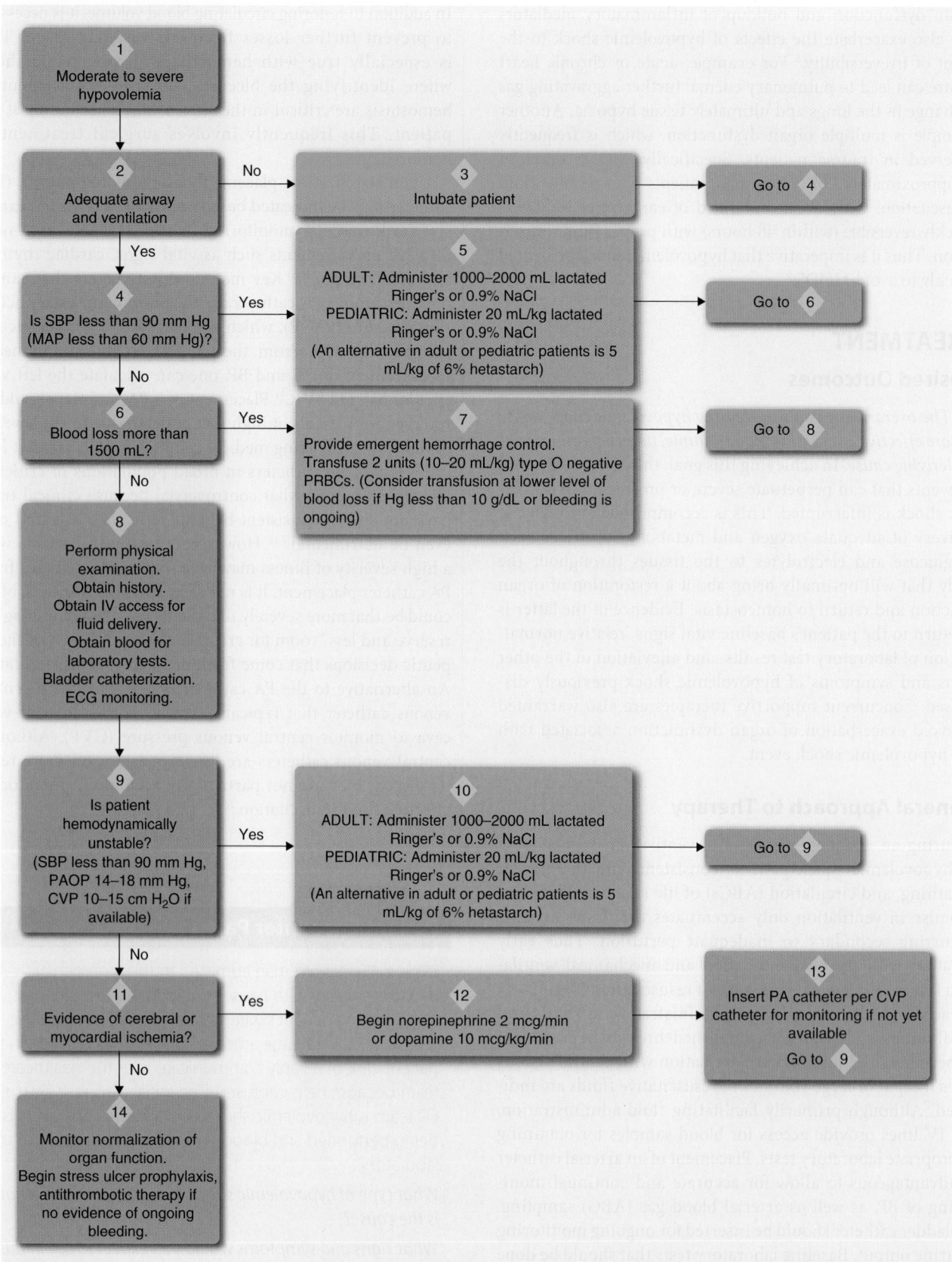

FIGURE 13–3. Treatment algorithm for the management of moderate to severe hypovolemia. (CVP, central venous pressure; ECG, electrocardiogram; MAP, mean arterial pressure; NaCl, sodium chloride or normal saline; PA, pulmonary artery; PAOP, pulmonary artery occlusion pressure; PRBCs, packed red blood cells; SBP, systolic blood pressure.) Hemoglobin concentration of 10 g/dL is equivalent to 100 g/L or 6.2 mmol/L.

▶ Fluid Therapy

The use of fluids is the cornerstone of managing all forms of shock including hypovolemic shock.[1] ⑤ *Three major therapeutic options are available to clinicians for restoring circulating blood volume:* **crystalloids** *(electrolyte-based solutions),* **colloids** *(large molecular weight solutions), and blood products.* Blood products are used only in instances involving hemorrhage (or severe preexisting anemia), thus leaving crystalloids and colloids as the mainstay of therapy in all types of hypovolemic shock, along with adjunctive **vasopressor** support. The aggressiveness of fluid resuscitation (rate and volume) is dictated by the severity of the hypovolemic shock and the underlying cause. Warming of all fluids to 37°C (98.6°F) prior to administration is an important consideration to prevent hypothermia, arrhythmias, and coagulopathy because they will have a negative impact on the success of the resuscitation effort.[15]

Crystalloids Conventional "balanced" crystalloids are fluids with (a) electrolyte composition that approximates plasma, such as lactated Ringer's (LR), or (b) a total calculated osmolality similar to that of plasma (280 to 295 mOsm/kg

or mmol/kg), such as 0.9% sodium chloride (also known as normal saline [NS] or 0.9% NaCl) (Table 13–3).[16] Thus conventional crystalloids distribute in normal proportions throughout the extracellular fluid space upon administration. In other words, expansion of the intravascular space only increases by roughly 200 to 250 mL for every liter of isotonic crystalloid fluid administered.[6] Hypertonic crystalloid solutions such as 3% NaCl or 7.5% NaCl have osmolalities substantially higher than plasma. The effect observed with these fluids is a relatively larger volume expansion of the intravascular space. By comparison with conventional crystalloids, administration of 250 mL of 7.5% sodium chloride results in an intravascular space increase of 500 mL.[6] This increase is a result of the fluid administered as well as osmotic drawing of intracellular fluid into the intravascular and interstitial spaces. This occurs because the hypertonic saline increases the osmolality of the intravascular and interstitial fluid compared with the intracellular fluid. Hypertonic saline also has the potential for decreasing the inflammatory response.[1] Despite these theoretical advantages, data are lacking demonstrating superiority of hypertonic crystalloid solutions compared with isotonic solutions.[17,18]

Table 13–3									
Composition of Common Resuscitation Fluids[16]									
Fluid	**Na (mEq/L)**[a]	**Cl (mEq/L)**[a]	**K (mEq/L)**[a]	**Mg (mEq/L)**[b]	**Ca (mEq/L)**[b]	**Lactate (mEq/L)**[a]	**Other**	**pH**	**Osmolality (mOsm/kg)**[c]
0.9% NaCl	154	154						5.0	308
3% NaCl	513	513						5.0	1,027
7.5% NaCl	1,283	1,283						5.0	2,567
Lactated Ringer's	130	109	4		3	28			
Hetastarch (Hextend)	143	124	3	0.9	5	28	Hetastarch 6 g/dL (60 g/L)	5.9	307
Hetastarch (Hespan)	154	154					Hetastarch 6 g/dL (60 g/L)	5.5	310
Pentastarch	154	154					Pentastarch 10 g/dL (100 g/L)	5.0	326
5% Albumin	130–160	130–160					Albumin 5 g/dL (50 g/L)	6.9	
25% Albumin	130–160	130–160					Albumin 25 g/dL (250 g/L)	6.9	
5% PPF	130–160	130–160	0.25				Plasma proteins 5 g/dL (50 g/L) (88% albumin)	7.0	
Dextran 40	154	154					Dextran 10 g/dL (100 g/L) (avg. molecular weight 40 kDa)		
Dextran 70	154	154					Dextran 6 g/dL (60 g/L) (avg. molecular weight 70 kDa)	5.5	308
Dextran 75	154	154					Dextran 6 g/dL (60 g/L) (avg. molecular weight 75 kDa)	5.5	308

avg., average; Ca, calcium; Cl, chloride; K, potassium; kDa, kilodalton; Mg, magnesium; Na, sodium; NaCl, sodium chloride or normal saline; PPF, plasma protein fraction.

[a]For these values, mEq/L = mmol/L (e.g., 154 mEq/L Na = 154 mmol/L).

[b]For these values, mEq/L × 0.5 = mmol/L (e.g., 0.9 mEq/L Mg = 0.45 mmol/L Mg).

[c]For this value, mOsm/kg = mmol/kg (e.g., 308 mOsm/kg = 308 mmol/kg).

Crystalloids are generally advocated as the initial resuscitation fluid in hypovolemic shock because of their availability, low cost, and equivalent outcomes compared with colloids.[10] A reasonable initial volume of an isotonic crystalloid (0.9% NaCl or LR) in adult patients is 1,000 to 2,000 mL (about 2 to 4 pints) administered over the first hour of therapy.[7] Ongoing external or internal bleeding requires more aggressive fluid resuscitation. ❻ *In the absence of ongoing blood loss, administration of 2,000 to 4,000 mL (about 4 to 8 pints) of isotonic crystalloid normally reestablishes baseline vital signs in adult hypovolemic shock patients.*[19] Selected populations, such as burn patients, may require more aggressive fluid resuscitation, while other patient subsets such as those with cardiogenic shock or heart failure may warrant less aggressive fluid administration to avoid overresuscitation.[20] In hemorrhagic shock patients, approximately three to four times the shed blood volume of isotonic crystalloids is needed for effective resuscitation.[20]

Side effects from crystalloids primarily involve fluid overload and electrolyte disturbances of sodium, potassium, and chloride.[1] Dilution of coagulation factors can also occur resulting in a dilutional coagulopathy.[6] Two clinically significant differences between LR and NS is that LR contains potassium and has a lower sodium content (130 vs. 154 mEq/L or mmol/L). Thus LR has a greater potential than NS to cause hyponatremia and/or hyperkalemia. Alternatively, NS can cause hypernatremia, hyperchloremia, metabolic acidosis, and hypokalemia. Based on the more physiological composition and buffering capacity of LR, and their respective side-effect profiles, LR is deemed in theory to be the superior resuscitative fluid compared with NS by some authorities.[21] However, improvements in outcome have not been documented.[22]

Colloids Understanding the effects of colloid administration on circulating blood volume necessitates a review of those physiological forces that determine fluid movement between capillaries and the interstitial space throughout the circulation (Fig. 13–4).[6,23] Relative hydrostatic pressure between the capillary lumen and the interstitial space is one of the major determinants of net fluid flow into or out of the circulation. The other major determinant is the relative colloid osmotic pressure between the two spaces. Administration of exogenous colloids results in an increase in the intravascular colloid osmotic pressure. The effects of colloids on intravascular volume are a consequence of their relatively large molecular size (greater than 30 kDa), limiting their passage across the capillary membrane in large amounts. Alternatively stated, colloids can be thought of as "sponges" drawing fluid into the intravascular space from the interstitial space. In the case of isosmotic colloids (5% albumin, 6% hetastarch, and dextran products), initial expansion of the intravascular space is essentially 65% to 75% of the volume of colloid administered, accounting for some "leakage" of the colloid from the intravascular space.[6] ❼ *Thus, in contrast to isotonic crystalloid solutions that distribute throughout the extracellular fluid space, the volume of iso-oncotic colloids administered remains relatively confined to the intravascular space.*

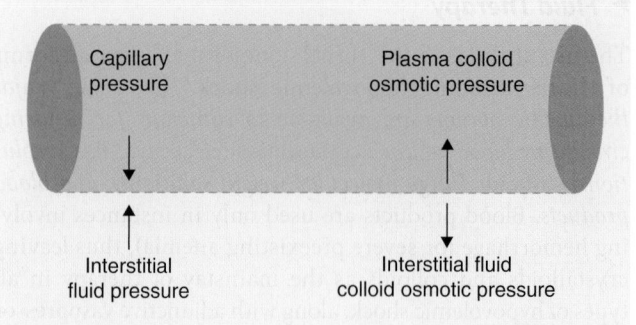

FIGURE 13–4. Operative forces at the capillary membrane tend to move fluid either outward or inward through the capillary membrane. In hypovolemic shock, one therapeutic strategy is the administration of colloids that can sustain and/or draw fluid from the interstitial space by increasing the plasma colloid osmotic pressure. (From Guyton AC, Hall JE. Textbook of Medical Physiology, 8th ed. Philadelphia, PA: Saunders, 1991:174, with permission.)

In the case of hyperoncotic solutions such as 25% albumin, fluid is pulled from the interstitial space into the vasculature, resulting in an increase in the intravascular volume that is much greater than the original volume of the 25% albumin that was administered. Although theoretically attractive, hyperoncotic solutions should not be used for hypovolemic shock because the expansion of the intravascular space is at the expense of depletion of the interstitial space. Exogenous colloids available in the United States include 5% albumin, 25% albumin, 5% plasma protein fraction (PPF), 6% hetastarch, 10% pentastarch, 10% dextran 40, 6% dextran 70, and 6% dextran 75 (Table 13–3). The first three products are derived from pooled human plasma. Hetastarch and pentastarch are semisynthetic hydroxyethyl starches derived from amylopectin. The dextran products are semisynthetic glucose polymers that vary in terms of the average molecular weight of the polymers. Superiority of one colloid solution over another has not been clearly established.[24]

For years within the critical care literature, a controversy known as the "colloid versus crystalloid debate" raged over the relative merits of the two types (colloid and crystalloid) of resuscitation fluids. At the center of the debate was what the goal of fluid resuscitation in shock should be: immediate expansion of the intravascular space with colloids versus expansion of the entire extracellular fluid space with crystalloids. A randomized controlled study involving 6,997 critically ill patients (Saline versus Albumin Fluid Evaluation [SAFE] study) demonstrated no difference in mortality between patients receiving saline versus albumin.[25] Largely in response to the SAFE trial, the FDA issued a notice to healthcare providers in May 2005 declaring albumin safe for use in most critically ill patients.[26] Burn, traumatic brain injury, and septic shock patients were excluded from the SAFE trial; however, based on previous data, there does not appear to be a clear-cut overall advantage for either crystalloids or colloids in these patient groups.[26] Thus, although the debate is not fully resolved, most clinicians today prefer using crystalloids based on their availability and inexpensive cost compared with colloids.[20,27]

Generally, the major adverse effects associated with colloids are fluid overload, dilutional coagulopathy, and anaphylactoid/anaphylactic reactions.[28] Although derived from pooled human plasma, there is no risk of disease transmission from commercially available albumin or PPF products because they are heated and sterilized by ultrafiltration prior to distribution. Because of direct effects on the coagulation system with the hydroxyethyl starch and dextran products, they should be used cautiously in hemorrhagic shock patients. This is another reason why crystalloids may be preferred in hemorrhagic shock. Furthermore, hetastarch can result in an increase in amylase not associated with pancreatitis. As such, the adverse-effect profiles of the various fluid types should also be considered when selecting a resuscitation fluid.

- **Blood Products** ⑧ *Blood products are indicated in hypovolemic shock patients who have sustained blood losses from hemorrhage exceeding 1,500 mL.* This, in fact, is the only setting in which freshly procured whole blood is administered. In virtually all other settings, blood products are given as the individual components of whole blood units, such as packed red blood cells (PRBCs), fresh-frozen plasma (FFP), platelets, cryoprecipitate, and concentrated coagulation factors.[29] This includes ongoing resuscitation of hemorrhagic shock when PRBCs can be transfused to increase oxygen-carrying capacity in concert with crystalloid solutions to increase blood volume. In patients with documented coagulopathies, FFP for global replacement of lost or diluted clotting factors, or platelets for patients with severe thrombocytopenia (less than 20 to 50 × 10³/mm³ or 20 to 50 × 10⁹/L]) should be administered.[30,31] Data suggests that increasing the ratio of FFP to PRBC units may be associated with improved mortality and a reduction in the number of PRBC transfusions in patients requiring multiple transfusions.[32,33] Type O negative blood or "universal donor blood" is given in emergent cases of hemorrhagic shock. Thereafter, blood that has been typed and cross-matched with the recipient's blood is given. The traditional threshold for PRBC transfusion in hypovolemic shock has been a serum hemoglobin of less than 10 g/dL (100 g/L or 6.2 mmol/L) and hematocrit less than 30% (0.30). However, for critically ill patients who have received appropriate fluid resuscitation and have no signs of ongoing bleeding, a more restrictive transfusion threshold of 7 g/dL (70 g/L or 4.34 mmol/L) appears to be safe.[34] Traditional risks from allogeneic blood product administration include hemolytic and nonhemolytic transfusion reactions and transmission of blood-borne infections in contaminated blood. However, recent large studies have also shown that transfusions are associated with higher mortality, possibly because of adverse immune and inflammatory effects.[29] Increased thromboembolic events and mortality have also been documented for patients receiving PRBCs stored longer than 28 days.[35] Thus administration of blood products should be restricted whenever possible and used as early as possible following donation. Due to blood shortages and associated risks with transfusions, there are ongoing research efforts concerning the development of red blood cell substitutes as a possible therapy alternative. Products that have reached clinical trials include perfluorocarbon emulsions and hemoglobin-based oxygen carriers (HBOCs).[36] These blood products have several advantages over PRBCs including greater availability (because donors are not needed), increased shelf life, absence of infectious risks, and no need for cross-matching. As such, red blood cell substitutes have the potential to serve as temporizing measures in hypovolemic shock patients until conventional red blood cell transfusions can be administered or in instances in which availability of donated PRBCs is extremely limited. Nonetheless, lack of adequate efficacy data and additional side effects associated with each of the respective red blood cell substitutes have precluded their approval in the United States at present.[36]

▶ Pharmacologic Therapy

Vasopressor Therapy *Vasopressor* is the term used to describe any pharmacologic agent that can induce arterial vasoconstriction through stimulation of the α_1-adrenergic receptors. ⑨ *Although replenishment of intravascular volume is undoubtedly the cornerstone of hypovolemic shock therapy, use of vasopressors may be warranted as a temporary measure in patients with profound hypotension or evidence of organ dysfunction in the early stages of shock.*[3,10] Vasopressors are typically used concurrently with fluid administration after the latter has not resulted in adequate restoration of blood pressure and/or tissue perfusion.[37] Table 13–4 lists those vasopressors used in the management of hypovolemic shock. Although vasopressor therapy may improve the hemodynamic

Table 13–4					
Vasopressor Drugs[1]					
Drug	Usual IV Dose	Adrenergic Effects			Potential to Cause Arrhythmias
		α	β₁	Dopaminergic	
Dopamine	10–30 mcg/kg/min[a]	+++	++	+++	+++
Norepinephrine	0.5–80 mcg/min	+++	++	0	++
Epinephrine	1–200 mcg/min	+	+++	0	+++
Phenylephrine	0.5–9 mcg/kg/min	+++	0	0	0

[a]Lower dosages of dopamine may not produce desired α_1-adrenergic (vasopressor) effects.

profile in shock patients, data are lacking that they improve mortality.[38] Furthermore, a recent study found that early use of vasopressors (i.e., phenylephrine, norepinephrine, dopamine, vasopressin) in the resuscitation of patients with hemorrhagic shock may actually be associated with increased mortality.[39] Regardless, data suggest that if vasopressors are used, norepinephrine may be preferable to dopamine secondary to increased incidence of arrhythmias associated with the latter agent in the treatment of shock patients.[40,41] Thus norepinephrine should be considered the first-line vasopressor therapy for these patients.[37] Epinephrine should be considered as a second-line vasopressor in patients with shock because of its association with tachyarrhythmias, impaired abdominal organ (splanchnic) circulation, and hypoglycemia.[37] Arginine vasopressin, although not a vasopressor per se, may be beneficial as an adjunctive therapy alone with vasopressors in refractory hemorrhage shock based on beneficial effects in other shock states.[37,42,43] In cases involving concurrent heart failure, an inotropic agent such as dobutamine may be needed, in addition to the use of a vasopressor.

Vasopressors are almost exclusively administered as continuous infusions because of their very short duration of action and the need for close titration of their dose-related effects. Starting doses should be at the lower end of the dosing range followed by rapid titration upward if needed to maintain adequate BP. Monitoring of end-organ function such as adequate urine output should also be used to monitor therapy. Once BP is restored, vasopressors should be weaned and discontinued as soon as possible to avoid any untoward events. The most significant systemic adverse events associated with vasopressors are excessive vasoconstriction resulting in decreased organ perfusion and potential to induce arrhythmias (Table 13–4). Central venous catheters should be used to minimize the risk of local tissue necrosis that can occur with extravasation of peripheral IV catheters.

Patient Encounter Part 2

PMH: "Stomach ulcers" and "reflux" per the wife

Meds: Omeprazole 40 mg PO daily, enteric-coated aspirin 81 mg PO daily

SH: "A six-pack of beer" every day per the wife

FH: Noncontributory

PE: Ht 5'9" (175 cm), Wt 90 kg (198 lb)

VS: 80/40 mm Hg, P 130, RR 22, T 35.0°C (95.0°F), urine output: none since catheterization 10 minutes ago

Neuro: Confused upon entering the ED. Now with recent loss of consciousness

Cardiovascular: Heart sounds and ECG normal except for tachycardia

Pulmonary: Normal breath sounds but undergoing tracheal intubation for mechanical ventilation

Abd: WNL

Extremities: Noncontributory

Pertinent labs: pH 7.20, $PaCO_2$ 50 mm Hg (6.65 kPa), PaO_2 70 mm Hg (9.31 kPa), Na 153 mEq/L (153 mmol/L), HCO_3 18 mEq/L (18 mmol/L), lactate 7.0 mg/dL (0.78 mmol/L), SCr 1.7 mg/dL (150 μmol/L), Hct 28% (0.28)

Describe treatment goals for RW in the next hour.

Describe treatment goals for RW in the next 24 hours.

Develop a pharmacologic and fluid therapy plan for initial therapy. Defend your selections compared with alternative agents.

Discuss the role in therapy for blood products, sodium bicarbonate, and recombinant factor VIIa in RW at this time.

Hemostatic Agents

The off-label use of the procoagulant **recombinant activated factor VII** (rFVIIa) as an adjunctive agent to treat uncontrolled hemorrhage has gained popularity in recent years. However, a phase 3 randomized study of rVIIa versus placebo in trauma patients with refractory hemorrhage demonstrated no differences in mortality despite a reduction in PRBC. transfusions.[44] Furthermore, the off-label use of rFVIIa has been criticized based on an increased risk of arterial thromboembolic events in patients, especially patients older than 65 years.[45,46] The optimal dose of rFVIIa in nonhemophilic patients is also unknown. In light of the uncertain efficacy, safety concerns, and its high acquisition costs, the use of rFVIIa cannot be advocated for patients with refractory hemorrhage. A promising alternative to rVIIa in patients with hemorrhagic shock is tranexamic acid, an antifibrinolytic. A recent study of tranexamic acid in trauma patients with or at risk of significant bleeding demonstrated a decrease in mortality compared with placebo.[47] As such, the use of antifibrinolytics such as tranexamic acid or ε-aminocaproic acid

appear in guidelines as adjunctive agents to consider in the management of bleeding trauma patients.[31]

Supportive Care Measures

Lactic acidosis, which typically accompanies hypovolemic shock as a consequence of tissue hypoxia, is best treated by reversal of the underlying cause. Administration of alkalizing agents such as sodium bicarbonate has not been demonstrated to have any beneficial effects and may actually worsen intracellular acidosis.[48] Because GI ischemia is a common complication of hypovolemic shock, prevention of stress-related mucosal disease should be instituted as soon as the patient is stabilized. The most common agents used for stress ulcer prophylaxis are the histamine$_2$-receptor antagonists and proton pump inhibitors. Prevention of thromboembolic events is another secondary consideration in hypovolemic shock patients. This can be accomplished with the use of external devices such as sequential compression devices and/ or antithrombotic therapy such as the low molecular weight

Patient Encounter Part 3

One hour after the initial fluid bolus, RW's vital signs are BP 85/50 mm Hg, P 120, RR 20, urine output: 15 mL in the past hour. Pertinent new labs: lactate 4.8 mg/dL (0.53 mmol/L). RW has regained consciousness but is weak and confused.

Assessment RW's condition compared with 1 hour ago.

Develop a plan for additional therapy, if any, that you recommend at this time.

Describe how RW's past medical history affects your investigation of his GI bleed etiology and subsequent therapeutic plan.

Outline a plan for monitoring RW over the next 24 hours.

heparin products or unfractionated heparin. Patients with adrenal insufficiency due to preexisting disease, glucocorticoid use, or critical illness may have refractory hypotension despite resuscitation. Such patients should receive appropriate glucocorticoid replacement therapy (e.g., hydrocortisone).

▶ **Outcome Evaluation**

⑩ *Successful treatment of hypovolemic shock is measured by the restoration of BP to baseline values and reversal of associated organ dysfunction.* The likelihood of a successful fluid resuscitation is directly related to the expediency of treatment. Therapy goals include:

- Arterial SBP greater than 90 mm Hg (MAP greater than 60 mm Hg) within 1 hour
- Organ dysfunction reversal evident by increased urine output to greater than 0.5 mL/kg/h (1.0 mL/kg/h in pediatrics), return of mental status to baseline, and normalization of skin color and temperature over the first 24 hours
- HR should begin to decrease reciprocally to increases in the intravascular volume within minutes to hours
- Normalization of laboratory measurements expected within hours to days following fluid resuscitation. Specifically, normalization of base deficit and serum lactate is recommended within 24 hours to potentially decrease mortality[49]
- Achievement of PAOP to a goal pressure of 14 to 18 mm Hg occurs (alternatively, CVP 8 to 15 mm Hg)

Patient Care and Monitoring

1. Does the patient have an adequate airway and ventilation (hemoglobin saturation greater than 92% [0.92])? If not, trained emergency personnel should consider performing tracheal intubation with initiation of mechanical ventilation.

2. Is there a detectable BP? If yes, obtain history, perform physical examination, obtain blood for baseline laboratory tests, and monitor ECG. If not, begin isotonic crystalloid fluid resuscitation immediately (see step 4).

3. Monitor the following serial laboratories for comparison to baseline values every 6 hours in the first 24 hours and daily thereafter until normalized: sodium, serum creatinine, blood urea nitrogen, serum lactate, glucose, bilirubin, hemoglobin, hematocrit, platelets, prothrombin time, partial thromboplastin time, ABGs, and pH.

4. Is the systolic BP less than 90 mm Hg (MAP less than 60 mm Hg)? If yes, start aggressive fluid therapy beginning with 1,000 to 2,000 mL lactated Ringer's over 1 hour in adults (20 mL/kg in pediatric patients). Monitor BP at least every 15 minutes (or continuously via an arterial catheter).

5. Is the patient bleeding? If yes, transfuse 5 to 10 mL/kg PRBCs. (Note: 1 unit PRBCs provides approximately 3% increase in hematocrit or 1 g/dL [10 g/L or 0.62 mmol/L] increase in hemoglobin.) Do not allow hemoglobin concentrations to fall below 7 g/dL (70 g/L or 4.34 mmol/L; hematocrit 20% [0.20]). Conventional acute goal hemoglobin concentration is 10 g/dL (100 g/L or 6.2 mmol/L; alternatively, hematocrit greater than or equal to 30% [0.30]). Provide emergent control of ongoing hemorrhaging.

6. Is there evidence of cerebral or myocardial ischemia? If yes, begin vasopressor therapy of dopamine 10 mcg/kg/min or norepinephrine 2 mcg/min. Titrate dosage every 5 minutes as needed. Wean and discontinue vasopressor as soon as the goal arterial BP has been achieved.

7. Has the goal arterial BP been achieved? If not, give additional fluid therapy hourly blending crystalloids and iso-oncotic colloids based on inadequate BP response.

8. Is the patient hemodynamically stable? If not, admit to the intensive care unit for ongoing treatment and monitoring. A PA catheter (or CVP catheter) should be inserted by trained medical personnel. Monitor PAOP to a goal pressure of 14 to 18 mm Hg and minimum cardiac index of 2.2 L/min/m² (alternatively CVP 8 to 15 cm H₂O).

9. Monitor normalization of organ function to baseline state including mental status, urine output to greater than 0.5 mL/kg/h (1 mL/kg/h in pediatric patients), normal skin color and temperature, and normalization of base deficit and/or lactate. Begin supportive care measures including stress ulcer prophylaxis and antithrombotic therapy if there is no evidence of ongoing bleeding.

10. Has the underlying cause of the hypovolemic shock been addressed to prevent its recurrence? If not, treat as necessary.

11. Is there any evidence of adverse events from the resuscitation therapies used such as fluid overload, electrolyte disturbances, transfusion reactions, and/or alterations in coagulation? If yes, manage the particular adverse event accordingly.

Abbreviations Introduced in This Chapter

ABCs	Airway, breathing, and circulation
ABG	Arterial blood gas
ADH	Antidiuretic hormone
ARDS	Acute respiratory distress syndrome
ATP	Adenosine triphosphate
BP	Blood pressure
Ca	Calcium
Cl	Chloride
CO	Cardiac output
CVP	Central venous pressure
ECG	Electrocardiogram
ECV	Extracellular volume
ED	Emergency department
FFP	Fresh-frozen plasma
HBOC	Hemoglobin-based oxygen carrier
Hct	Hematocrit
HR	Heart rate
K	Potassium
LR	Lactated Ringer's
MAP	Mean arterial pressure
Mg	Magnesium
MODS	Multiple organ dysfunction syndrome
Na	Sodium
NaCl	Sodium chloride, or normal saline
NS	Normal saline
PA	Pulmonary artery
PaO_2	Partial pressure of arterial oxygen
PAOP	Pulmonary artery occlusion pressure
$PaCO_2$	Partial pressure of arterial carbon dioxide
PPF	Plasma protein fraction
PRBCs	Packed red blood cells
rFVIIa	Recombinant activated factor VII
SAFE	Saline versus Albumin Fluid Evaluation
SBP	Systolic blood pressure
SCr	Serum creatinine
SV	Stroke volume
SVR	Systemic vascular resistance

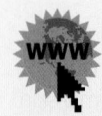 Self-assessment questions and answers are available at *http://www.mhpharmacotherapy.com/pp.html.*

REFERENCES

1. Todd RS, Turner KL, Moore FA. Shock: General. In: Gabrielli A, Lyon JA, Yu M, eds. Civetta, Taylor, & Kirby's Critical Care, 4th ed. Philadelphia, PA: Wolters Kluwer Lippincott Williams & Wilkins, 2009:813–834.
2. Braunwald E. Regulation of the circulation. I. N Engl J Med 1974;290(20):1124–1129.
3. Astiz ME. Pathophysiology cardiclassification of shock states. In: Fink MP, Abraham E, Vincent JL, Kochanek PM, eds. Textbook of Critical Care, 5th ed. Philadelphia, PA: Elsevier Saunders, 2005:897–910.
4. Jones AE, Kline JA. Shock. In: Marx JA, Hockberger RS, Walls RM, eds. Rosen's Emergency Medicine: Concepts and Clinical Practice, 6th ed. Philadelphia, PA: Mosby Elsevier, 2006:41–56.
5. Vallet B, Wiel E, Lebuffe G. Resuscitation from circulatory shock. In: Fink MP, Abraham E, Vincent JL, Kochanek PM, eds. Textbook of Critical Care, 5th ed. Philadelphia, PA: Elsevier Saunders; 2005:905–910.
6. Puyana JC. Resuscitation of hypovolemic shock. In: Fink MP, Abraham E, Vincent JL, Kochanek PM, eds. Textbook of Critical Care, 5th ed. Philadelphia, PA: Elsevier Saunders, 2006:1933–1943.
7. Cinat ME, Hoyt DB. Hemorrhagic shock. In: Gabrielli A, Lyon JA, Yu M, eds. Civetta, Taylor, & Kirby's Critical Care. Philadelphia, PA: Wolters Kluwer Lippincott Williams & Wilkins, 2009:893–923.
8. Harbrecht BG, Alarcon LH, Peitzman AB. Management of shock. In: Moore EE, Feliciano DV, Mattox KL, eds. Trauma, 5th ed. New York, NY: McGraw-Hill; 2004:201–226.
9. Ciesla DJ, Moore EE, Johnson JL, et al. Multiple organ dysfunction during resuscitation is not postinjury multiple organ failure. Arch Surg 2004;139(6):590–594.
10. Moore FA, McKinley BA, Moore EE. The next generation in shock resuscitation. Lancet 2004;363(9425):1988–1996.
11. Rhodes A, Grounds RM, Bennett ED. Hemodynamic monitoring. In: Fink MP, Abraham E, Vincent JL, Kochanek PM, eds. Textbook of Critical Care, 5th ed. Philadelphia, PA: Elsevier Saunders; 2005:735–739.
12. Practice guidelines for pulmonary artery catheterization: An updated report by the American Society of Anesthesiologists Task Force on Pulmonary Artery Catheterization. Anesthesiology 2003;99(4):988–1014.
13. Shah MR, Hasselblad V, Stevenson LW, et al. Impact of the pulmonary artery catheter in critically ill patients: Meta-analysis of randomized clinical trials. JAMA 2005;294(13):1664–1670.
14. Chittock DR, Dhingra VK, Ronco JJ, et al. Severity of illness and risk of death associated with pulmonary artery catheter use. Crit Care Med 2004;32(4):911–915.
15. Hoffman GL. Blood and blood components. In: Marx JA, Hockberger RS, Walls RM, eds. Rosen's Emergency Medicine Concepts and Clinical Practice, 6th ed. Philadelphia, PA: Mosby Elsevier, 2006:56–61.
16. Zaloga GP, Kirby RR, Bernards WC, Layon AJ. Fluids and electrolytes. In: Civetta JM, Taylor RW, Kirby RR, eds. Critical Care, 3rd ed. New York, NY: Lippincott-Raven; 1997:413–441.
17. Bauer M, Kortgen A, Hartog C, et al. Isotonic and hypertonic crystalloid solutions in the critically ill. Best Pract Res Clin Anaesthesiol 2009;23(2):173–181.
18. Bunn F, Roberts I, Tasker R, Akpa E. Hypertonic versus near isotonic crystalloid for fluid resuscitation in critically ill patients. Cochrane Database Syst Rev 2004(3):CD002045.
19. Mullins RJ. Management of shock. In: Mattox KL, Feliciano DV, Moore EE, eds. Trauma. New York, NY: McGraw-Hill, 2000:195–232.
20. Shafi S, Kauder DR. Fluid resuscitation and blood replacement in patients with polytrauma. Clin Orthop Relat Res 2004(422):37–42.
21. Todd SR, Malinoski D, Muller PJ, Schreiber MA. Lactated Ringer's is superior to normal saline in the resuscitation of uncontrolled hemorrhagic shock. J Trauma 2007;62(3):636–639.
22. Moore FA, McKinley BA, Moore EE, et al. Inflammation and the host response to injury, a large-scale collaborative project: patient-oriented research core—Standard operating procedures for clinical care. III. Guidelines for shock resuscitation. J Trauma 2006;61(1):82–89.
23. Guyton AC, Hall JE. Textbook of Medical Physiology, 10th ed. Philadelphia, PA: Saunders, 2000.
24. Bunn F, Trivedi D, Ashraf S. Colloid solutions for fluid resuscitation. Cochrane Database Syst Rev 2011(3):CD001319.
25. Finfer S, Bellomo R, Boyce N, et al. A comparison of albumin and saline for fluid resuscitation in the intensive care unit. N Engl J Med 2004;350(22):2247–2256.
26. Safety of albumin administration in critically ill patients [Internet]. Rockville, MD: U.S. Food and Drug Administration; 2005 [cited July 20, 2011]. Available at: *http://www.fda.gov/BiologicsBloodVaccines/SafetyAvailability/BloodSafety/ucm095539.htm.*
27. Perel P, Roberts I. Colloids versus crystalloids for fluid resuscitation in critically ill patients. Cochrane Database Syst Rev 2007(4):CD000567.
28. Barron ME, Wilkes MM, Navickis RJ. A systematic review of the comparative safety of colloids. Arch Surg 2004;139(5):552–563.

29. Boucher BA, Hannon TJ. Blood management: A primer for clinicians. Pharmacotherapy 2007;27(10):1394–1411.

30. Kelley DM. Hypovolemic shock: An overview. Crit Care Nurs Q 2005; 28(1):2–19.

31. Rossaint R, Bouillon B, Cerny V, et al. Management of bleeding following major trauma: An updated European guideline. Crit Care 2010;14(2):R52.

32. Maegele M, Lefering R, Paffrath T, et al. Red-blood-cell to plasma ratios transfused during massive transfusion are associated with mortality in severe multiple injury: A retrospective analysis from the Trauma Registry of the Deutsche Gesellschaft fur Unfallchirurgie. Vox Sang 2008;95(2):112–119.

33. Wafaisade A, Maegele M, Lefering R, et al. High plasma to red blood cell ratios are associated with lower mortality rates in patients receiving multiple transfusion (4</=red blood cell units<10) during acute trauma resuscitation. J Trauma 2011;70(1):81–88.

34. Napolitano LM, Kurek S, Luchette FA, et al. Clinical practice guideline: Red blood cell transfusion in adult trauma and critical care. Crit Care Med 2009;37(12):3124–3157.

35. Spinella PC, Carroll CL, Staff I, et al. Duration of red blood cell storage is associated with increased incidence of deep vein thrombosis and in hospital mortality in patients with traumatic injuries. Crit Care 2009;13(5):R151.

36. Stollings JL, Oyen LJ. Oxygen therapeutics: Oxygen delivery without blood. Pharmacotherapy 2006;26(10):1453–1464.

37. Hollenberg SM. Vasoactive drugs in circulatory shock. Am J Respir Crit Care Med 2011;183(7):847–855.

38. Havel C, Arrich J, Losert H, et al. Vasopressors for hypotensive shock. Cochrane Database Syst Rev 2011;5:CD003709.

39. Sperry JL, Minei JP, Frankel HL, et al. Early use of vasopressors after injury: Caution before constriction. J Trauma 2008;64(1):9–14.

40. De Backer D, Biston P, Devriendt J, et al. Comparison of dopamine and norepinephrine in the treatment of shock. N Engl J Med 2010;362(9):779–789.

41. Patel GP, Grahe JS, Sperry M, et al. Efficacy and safety of dopamine versus norepinephrine in the management of septic shock. Shock 2010;33(4):375–380.

42. Rajani RR, Ball CG, Feliciano DV, Vercruysse GA. Vasopressin in hemorrhagic shock: Review article. Am Surg 2009;75(12):1207–1212.

43. Russell JA, Walley KR, Singer J, et al. Vasopressin versus norepinephrine infusion in patients with septic shock. N Engl J Med 2008; 358(9):877–887.

44. Hauser CJ, Boffard K, Dutton R, et al. Results of the CONTROL trial: efficacy and safety of recombinant activated factor VII in the management of refractory traumatic hemorrhage. J Trauma 2010;69(3): 489–500.

45. Levi M, Levy JH, Andersen HF, Truloff D. Safety of recombinant activated factor VII in randomized clinical trials. N Engl J Med 2010; 363(19):1791–1800.

46. O'Connell KA, Wood JJ, Wise RP, et al. Thromboembolic adverse events after use of recombinant human coagulation factor VIIa. JAMA 2006;295(3):293–298.

47. Shakur H, Roberts I, Bautista R, et al. Effects of tranexamic acid on death, vascular occlusive events, and blood transfusion in trauma patients with significant haemorrhage (CRASH-2): A randomised, placebo-controlled trial. Lancet 2010;376(9734):23–32.

48. Boyd JH, Walley KR. Is there a role for sodium bicarbonate in treating lactic acidosis from shock? Curr Opin Crit Care 2008;14(4):379–383.

49. Tisherman SA, Barie P, Bokhari F, et al. Clinical practice guideline: Endpoints of resuscitation. J Trauma 2004;57(4):898–912.

14 Asthma

Lori Wilken and Michelle T. Martin

LEARNING OBJECTIVES

● Upon completion of the chapter, the reader will be able to:

1. Discuss the economic and health burden caused by asthma.
2. Explain the pathophysiology of asthma.
3. Describe the clinical presentation of acute and chronic asthma.
4. Identify factors that affect asthma severity.
5. Identify the goals of asthma management.
6. Classify asthma severity based on impairment due to asthma and future risk for negative outcomes due to asthma.
7. Recommend environmental control strategies for patients with identified allergies.
8. Educate patients on the use of inhaled drug delivery devices, peak flow meters, and asthma education plans.
9. Develop a therapeutic plan for patients with chronic asthma that maximizes patient response while minimizing adverse drug events and other drug-related problems.
10. Evaluate current asthma control and make therapeutic changes when necessary.
11. Develop a therapeutic plan for treating patients with acute asthma.

KEY CONCEPTS

❶ Asthma is a complex disease that presents in a heterogeneous manner.

❷ Asthma is the most prevalent chronic disease of childhood, and it causes significant morbidity and mortality in both adults and children.

❸ Asthma is characterized by inflammation, airway hyperresponsiveness (AHR), and airway obstruction.

❹ In chronic asthma, initial classification of asthma severity is based on current disease impairment and future risk.

❺ Direct airway administration of asthma medications through inhalation is the most efficient route, and it minimizes systemic adverse effects.

❻ Short-acting-inhaled β_2-agonists are the most effective agents for reversing acute airway obstruction caused by bronchoconstriction and are the drugs of choice for treating acute asthma and symptoms of chronic asthma.

❼ Inhaled corticosteroids (ICS) are the preferred therapy for all forms of persistent asthma in all age groups.

❽ The intensity of pharmacotherapy for chronic asthma is based on disease severity for initial therapy and level of control for subsequent therapies.

❾ In acute asthma, early and appropriate intensification of therapy is important to resolve the exacerbation and prevent relapse and future severe airflow obstruction.

INTRODUCTION

In 2011, the Global Strategy for Asthma Management and Prevention, Global Initiative for Asthma (GINA) defines asthma as "a chronic inflammatory disorder of the airways, involving airway hyperresponsiveness that leads to widespread and variable episodes of reversible airway obstruction." This airway obstruction results in wheezing, breathlessness, chest tightness, and coughing, particularly at night or early in the morning.[1]

❶ *Asthma is a complex disease that presents in a heterogeneous manner.* Severity of chronic disease ranges from mild intermittent symptoms to a severe and disabling disease if left untreated. Despite variances in the underlying severity of chronic asthma, all patients with asthma are at risk of acute severe disease. The National Heart, Lung, and Blood Institute (NHLBI) National Asthma Education and Prevention Program (NAEPP) Expert Panel Report-3 (EPR-3) *Guidelines for the Diagnosis and Management of Asthma*[2] and GINA emphasize the importance of treating underlying airway inflammation to control asthma and reduce asthma-associated risks.

EPIDEMIOLOGY AND ETIOLOGY

❷ *Asthma is the most prevalent chronic disease of childhood, and it causes significant morbidity and mortality in both adults and children.*[3] It is estimated that 235 million adults and children worldwide have asthma.[4] The diagnosis of asthma increased from 2001 to 2009. In 2009, non-Hispanic blacks had the highest asthma rate of all racial groups, with 1 in 9 adults and 1 in 6 children having asthma. Puerto Ricans are twice as likely to be diagnosed with asthma and have the highest asthma rate among the Latino population.[5] Nine deaths related to asthma occurred each day in the United States during 2007.[3]

Asthma is also a significant economic burden in the United States, with an estimated direct cost of $14.8 billion in 2009. Prescription medications are the single largest direct medical expenditure and account for 71% of direct medical costs.[6] Costs increase with disease severity, and it has been suggested that less than 20% of asthma patients account for more than 80% of direct medical expenditures.[7]

Asthma results from a complex interaction of genetic and environmental factors, but the underlying cause is not well understood. The onset of asthma occurs early in life for most patients. There appears to be an inherited component because the presence of asthma in a parent is a strong risk factor for development of asthma in a child. This risk increases when a family history of atopy is also present. The presence of atopy is a strong prognostic factor for continued asthma as an adult. Furthermore, the severity of early childhood asthma is a predictor of adult asthma severity.[8]

Environmental exposure also appears to be an important factor in the etiology of asthma. Patients with occupational asthma develop the disease late in life upon exposure to specific allergens in the workplace. Exposure to secondhand smoke after birth increases the risk of childhood asthma.[9] Adult-onset asthma may be related to atopy, nasal polyps, aspirin sensitivity, occupational exposure, or a recurrence of childhood asthma.

PATHOPHYSIOLOGY

❸ *Asthma is characterized by inflammation, airway hyperresponsiveness (AHR), and airway obstruction.* Inhaled antigens induce a type 2 T-helper CD4+ (T$_H$2) response. Antigens are taken up by antigen-presenting cells, and presentation of antigens to T-lymphocytes causes activation of the T$_H$2 type response. This leads to B-cell production of antigen-specific immunoglobulin E (IgE) as well as proinflammatory cytokines and chemokines that recruit and activate eosinophils, neutrophils, and alveolar macrophages.[10,11]

Further exposure to the antigen results in cross-linking of cell-bound IgE in mast cells and basophils, causing the release of preformed inflammatory mediators such as histamine or generation of new inflammatory mediators such as leukotriene C$_4$, and prostaglandins.[12] Activation and degranulation of mast cells and basophils result in an early-phase response involving acute bronchoconstriction that lasts approximately 1 hour after allergen exposure.[10]

In the late-phase response, activated airway cells release inflammatory cytokines and chemokines, thereby recruiting more inflammatory cells into the lungs. The late-phase response occurs 4 to 6 hours after the initial allergen challenge and results in a less intense bronchoconstriction as well as increased AHR and airway inflammation.[10]

Airway Inflammation and Hyperresponsiveness

Although the symptoms of asthma are intermittent, airway inflammation is chronic.[11] Considerable variations in the pattern of inflammation may exist, resulting in phenotypic differences.[1,2] T-lymphocytes release cytokines that coordinate eosinophilic infiltration and IgE production by B-lymphocytes.[13] Mast cells, eosinophils, macrophages, neutrophils, fibroblasts, and airway smooth muscle cells are also activated in asthma. Mast cells infiltrate airway smooth muscle and bronchial epithelium and may cause mucous gland hyperplasia. Proinflammatory mediators generated during mast cell degranulation propagate the inflammatory response and contribute to AHR and airway remodeling.[14]

AHR is the exaggerated ability of the airways to narrow in response to a variety of stimuli. AHR is a characteristic feature of asthma and is related to airway inflammation and structural changes in the airways.[1,2] Clinically, AHR manifests as increased variability of airway function. AHR is evaluated clinically using a methacholine or histamine bronchoprovocation test.[15]

Airway Obstruction

Symptoms of airway obstruction include chest tightness, cough, and wheezing. Airway obstruction can be caused by multiple factors including airway smooth muscle constriction, airway edema, mucus hypersecretion, and airway remodeling. Airway smooth muscle tone is maintained by an interaction between sympathetic, parasympathetic, and nonadrenergic mechanisms. Acute bronchoconstriction usually results from mediators such as histamine, cysteinyl leukotrienes, prostaglandins, and tryptase released or generated during degranulation of mast cells and basophils.[1,2] Inflammatory mediators such as histamine, leukotrienes, and bradykinin increase microvascular permeability leading to mucosal edema, which causes the airways to become more rigid and limits airflow.[16] These changes exaggerate the consequences of acute bronchoconstriction. In patients with asthma, there is an increased number and volume of mucous glands, with increased mucus secretion.[17] Extensive mucus plugging may be a cause of persistent airway obstruction in acute severe attacks.

Although airway obstruction in asthma is generally reversible, some patients with asthma have an irreversible or fixed obstruction. *Airway remodeling* is the term used to describe the process that produces the structural airway changes leading to this fixed obstruction; it is characterized by airway epithelial damage, subepithelial **fibrosis,** airway smooth muscle **hypertrophy,** increased mucus production, and increased vascularity of the airways.[2,16] These changes increase airflow obstruction and airway responsiveness and may decrease patient responsiveness to therapy.[1,2]

CLINICAL PRESENTATION AND DIAGNOSIS

Please see the accompanying text box for the clinical presentation and diagnosis of asthma. The diagnosis of asthma is based on a detailed medical history, a physical examination of the upper respiratory tract and skin, and spirometry. The clinician determines if episodic symptoms of airflow obstruction are present, whether airflow obstruction is at least partially reversible, and that alternative diagnoses are excluded.[1,2] Spirometry is required for diagnosing asthma in patients older than 5 years because the medical history and physical examination are not reliable for characterizing the status of lung impairment or excluding other diagnoses.[1,2]

▶ Chronic Asthma

Chronic asthma is classified as either: (a) intermittent asthma or (b) persistent asthma that may be categorized as mild, moderate, or severe. Initial assessment of severity is made at the time of diagnosis, and initial therapy is based on this assessment. Table 14–1 describes the categories of asthma severity in patients younger than 12 years. The assessment of severity is similar in older patients. However, in patients

Clinical Presentation and Diagnosis of Asthma

General
- Asthma severity ranges from normal pulmonary function with symptoms only during acute exacerbations to significantly decreased pulmonary function with continuous symptoms.
- Acute asthma can present rapidly (within 3 to 6 hours), but it is more common for deterioration to occur over a longer period, even days or weeks. Acute asthma can be a life-threatening event, and severity does not necessarily correspond to severity of the chronic disease.
- The patient's family history, social history, precipitating factors, history of exacerbations, development of symptoms, and treatments are important components of an asthma diagnosis.

Symptoms
- Patients usually complain of wheezing, shortness of breath, coughing (usually worse at night), and chest tightness.
- Patients may be anxious and agitated. In acute severe asthma, patients may be unable to communicate in complete sentences.
- Mental status changes may indicate impending respiratory failure.
- The presence of precipitating factors worsens symptoms.
- Symptoms usually have a pattern.

Signs
- Vital signs may reflect tachypnea and tachycardia.
- On inspection, there may be hyperexpansion of the thorax and use of accessory muscles.
- Auscultation of the lungs may detect end-expiratory wheezes in mild exacerbations or wheezing throughout inspiration and expiration in severe exacerbations.

- Bradycardia and absence of wheezing may indicate impending respiratory failure.
- In acute asthma, patients may also present with pulsus paradoxus, diaphoresis, and cyanosis.

Laboratory tests
- Spirometry demonstrates reversible airway obstruction with an FEV_1/FVC less than 80% and either: (a) an increase in FEV_1 of 12% or 200 mL after receiving a bronchodilator, or (b) an increase of 10% in the predicted FEV_1 after receiving a bronchodilator.
- Spirometry may be normal if the patient is not symptomatic.
- Elevated immunoglobulin E (IgE) levels may be present.
- Some patients will have positive skin test or radioallergosorbent test (RAST) to allergens.

Other Diagnostic Tests
- Arterial blood gases (to evaluate Pco_2) should be obtained for patients in severe distress, suspected hypoventilation, or when PEF or FEV_1 is 30% or less after initial treatment.
- A complete blood count with differential should be obtained in patients with fever or purulent sputum.
- Serum electrolytes should be obtained because frequent β_2-agonist administration decreases serum potassium, magnesium, and phosphate.

Other Diagnostic Tests
- Pulmonary function tests
- Pulse oximetry
- Chest x-ray when pneumonia is suspected

Table 14–1

Classification of Asthma Severity in Patients 0 to 11 Years Old[a]

Components of Severity		Intermittent	Persistent		
			Mild	Moderate	Severe
Impairment	Symptoms	2 days/week or less	More than 2 days/week but not daily	Daily	Throughout the day
	Nighttime awakenings				
	Ages 0–4	0	1–2 times/month	3–4 times/month	More than 1 time/week
	Ages 5–11	2 times/month or less	3–4 times/month	More than 1 time/week but not nightly	Often 7 nights/week
	SABA use for symptoms (not prevention of EIB)	2 days/week or less	More than 2 days/week but not more than 1 time/day	Daily	Several times/day
	Interference with normal activity	None	Minor limitation	Some limitation	Extremely limited
	Lung function[b] ages 5–11	FEV_1 more than 80%, FEV_1/FVC more than 85%	FEV_1 more than 80%, FEV_1/FVC more than 80%	FEV_1 60–80%, FEV_1/FVC 75–80%	FEV_1 less than 60%, FEV_1/FVC less than 75%
Risk	Exacerbations requiring systemic (oral) corticosteroids				
	Ages 0–4	0–1/year	2 or more exacerbations in 6 months, 4 or more wheezing episodes/year lasting for more than 1 day *and* risk factors for persistent asthma		
	Ages 5–11	0–1/year	2/year or more ————————————————————→		
	Recommended step for initiating treatment	Step 1	Step 2	Step 3, and consider short course of oral corticosteroids	

SABA, short-acting β_2-agonist; EIB, exercise-induced bronchospasm.

[a]From NHLBI National Asthma Education and Prevention Program, Expert Panel Report-3. Guidelines for the diagnosis and management of asthma. NIH Publication No. 07-4051. Bethesda, MD: U.S. Department of Health and Human Services, 2007, *http://www.nhlbi.nih.gov/guidelines/asthma*. See *http://www.nhlbi.nih.gov/guidelines/asthma/asthgdln.pdf* for adults and children 12 years of age and older.

[b]Normal FEV_1/FVC: ages 8–19 = 85%; ages 20–39 = 80%; ages 40–59 = 75%; ages 60–80 = 70%.

12 years of age and older, it is recommended to initiate treatment in severe persistent asthma at step 4 or 5 (instead of step 3 in children younger than 12 years).

❹ *In chronic asthma, initial classification of asthma severity is based on current disease impairment and future risk.* The term *impairment* refers to the frequency and severity of symptoms, use of short-acting β_2-agonists (SABA) for quick relief of symptoms, pulmonary function, and impact on normal activity and quality of life. *Risk* refers to the potential for future severe exacerbations and asthma-related death, progressive loss of lung function (adults) or reduced lung growth (children), and the occurrence of drug-related adverse effects.

▶ *Acute Asthma*

In acute asthma, the severity of an exacerbation does not depend on the classification of the patient's chronic asthma because even patients with intermittent asthma can have life-threatening acute exacerbations. Severity at the time of the evaluation can be estimated by signs and symptoms or presenting peak expiratory flow (PEF) or forced expiratory volume in 1 second (FEV_1). The exacerbation is considered *mild* if the patient is only having dyspnea with activity and the PEF is at least 70% of the personal best value, *moderate* if the dyspnea

limits activity and the PEF is 40% to 69% of the personal best, and *severe* with PEF less than 40% and dyspnea interferes with conversation or occurs at rest. When the patient is not able to speak and the personal best PEF is less than 25% of the personal best predicted value, it is a *life-threatening* exacerbation.

TREATMENT OF ASTHMA

Desired Outcomes

▶ *Chronic Asthma*

Therapy for chronic asthma is directed at maintaining long-term control of asthma using the least amount of medications and minimizing adverse effects.[1,2] Treatment goals are to: (a) prevent chronic and troublesome symptoms, (b) require infrequent use (2 or fewer days/week) of SABA for quick relief of symptoms, (c) maintain normal or near-normal pulmonary function, (d) maintain normal activity levels, (e) meet patients' and families' expectations of satisfaction with asthma care, (f) prevent exacerbations of asthma and the need for emergency department visits or hospitalizations, (g) prevent progressive loss of lung function, and (h) provide optimal pharmacotherapy with minimal or no adverse effects.

Patient Encounter 1

JB is a 26-year-old woman with moderate persistent asthma. She has concerns about her asthma control. The temperature is getting colder outside, and cold weather has always been a trigger for her asthma. She also states that strong odors are a trigger. She is taking her asthma medications properly and without complaints. She recently saw the allergist, and her skin testing was positive for dust and molds. She uses an air purifier and a humidifier in her bedroom. She uses a cleaning service and leaves her home when it is being cleaned. She does not wear perfume and does wear a coat and hat in the wintertime.

What educational points may help with her asthma triggers?

What immunizations are recommended for her if she has not had any since childhood?

▶ Acute Asthma

Acute or worsening asthma can be a life-threatening situation and requires rapid assessment and appropriate intensification of therapy. Mortality associated with asthma exacerbations is usually related to inappropriate assessment of the severity of the exacerbation resulting in insufficient treatment or referral for medical care.[18] The goals of therapy are to: (a) correct significant **hypoxemia**, (b) reverse airflow obstruction rapidly, and (c) reduce the likelihood of exacerbation relapse or recurrence of severe airflow obstruction in the future.[1,2]

Nonpharmacologic Therapy

Nonpharmacologic therapy is incorporated into each step of asthma care, and patient education occurs at all points where healthcare professionals interact with patients. Patient education begins at the time of diagnosis and is tailored to meet individual patient needs. Some components of asthma education involve asthma trigger avoidance, proper administration of inhaled medications, and asthma self-management.

▶ Factors Associated with Worsening Asthma Control

Major triggers that may worsen asthma control include pollen, mold, dust mites, cockroaches, pet dander, air pollution, cold air, exercise, strong odors, emotions, tobacco smoke, certain medications, illicit drug use, sulfite-containing foods and beverages, and comorbid conditions (e.g., allergic rhinitis, sinusitis, upper respiratory infections, gastroesophageal reflux disease, obesity, obstructive sleep apnea, allergic broncho-pulmonary aspergillosis, and hormonal changes).

▶ Trigger Avoidance

Education on identifying and controlling asthma triggers is critical to providing adequate asthma treatment.[1,2] Environmental controls to reduce the allergen load in the patient's home may reduce asthma symptoms, school absences because of asthma, and unscheduled clinic and emergency visits for asthma.[19] Various informational resources are available on controlling or avoiding asthma triggers.[20,21]

Exercise is one of the most common precipitants of asthma symptoms. Shortness of breath, wheezing, or chest tightness usually occur during or shortly after vigorous exercise, peak 5 to 10 minutes after stopping the activity, and resolve within 20 to 30 minutes. Warming up prior to exercise and covering the mouth and nose with a scarf or mask during cold weather may prevent exercise-induced asthma. Pretreatment with a SABA 5 minutes prior to exercise is the treatment of choice and will protect against bronchospasm for 2 to 3 hours.[2] Regular treatment with an inhaled corticosteroid (ICS) also prevents bronchospasm associated with exercise.

A yearly influenza vaccine is recommended for patients 6 months and older with asthma to decrease the risk of complications from influenza.[22] The pneumococcal vaccine may decrease the risk of invasive pneumococcal disease in patients with asthma and is recommended as a one-time immunization before the age of 65 years and again after age 65.[23] In patients older than 11 years, providing a booster vaccine to protect against pertussis is becoming standard practice. The varicella vaccine is also highly recommended.[2]

Nonselective β-blockers, such as carvedilol, labetalol, nadolol, pindolol, propranolol, and timolol (including those in ophthalmic preparations) may worsen asthma control.

Patient Encounter 2

AJ is a 3-year-old girl seen today by the pediatrician. She has been diagnosed with intermittent asthma based on her symptoms. She is not symptomatic today, but a prescription for albuterol is provided to be used as needed for wheezing and worsening asthma symptoms.

What is the best way to deliver the medication for this patient's asthma?

What education is required for the method of medication delivery that you would recommend?

If AJ requires an inhaled corticosteroid in 6 weeks, what are the options for delivering it?

Describe the education that you would provide to AJ's parents about using an inhaled corticosteroid.

What is the best way to deliver asthma medication when AJ is 8 years old?

What education is required for the method of medication delivery you would recommend for an 8-year-old patient?

These agents are avoided in patients with asthma unless the benefits of therapy outweigh the risks.[2] In patients with asthma requiring β-blocker therapy, a β_1-selective agent such as metoprolol or atenolol is the best option. Because selectivity is dose related, the lowest effective dose is used.

Patients with aspirin-sensitive asthma are usually adults and often present with the triad of rhinitis, nasal polyps, and asthma. In these patients, acute asthma may occur within minutes of receiving aspirin or nonsteroidal anti-inflammatory drugs (NSAIDs). These patients are counseled against using NSAIDs.[2] Although acetaminophen is generally safe, doses larger than 1 g may cause acute asthmatic reactions in some patients.[24]

Pharmacologic Therapy

Treatment of chronic asthma involves avoidance of triggers known to precipitate or worsen asthma and use of long-term control and quick-relief medications. Long-term control medications include ICS, inhaled long-acting β_2-agonists (LABAs), oral theophylline, oral leukotriene receptor antagonists (LTRAs), and omalizumab. In patients with severe asthma, systemic corticosteroids may be used as a long-term control medication. Quick-relief medications include SABAs, anticholinergics, and short bursts of systemic corticosteroids.

▶ Drug Delivery Devices

⑤ *Direct airway administration of asthma medications through inhalation is the most efficient route and minimizes systemic adverse effects.* Inhaled asthma medications are available in metered-dose inhalers (MDIs), dry powder inhalers (DPIs), and nebulized solutions. Selection of the appropriate inhalation device depends on patient characteristics and medication availability (Table 14–2).

Poor inhaler technique results in increased oropharyngeal deposition of the drug, leading to decreased efficacy and increased adverse effects. Figure 14–1 describes the steps for appropriate use of MDIs. Because MDIs are challenging to use correctly, use of valved-holding chambers (VHCs) is recommended with MDIs to decrease the need for coordination of actuation with inhalation, decrease oropharyngeal deposition, and increase pulmonary drug delivery.[25,26]

▶ β_2-Adrenergic Agonists

β_2-Agonists relax airway smooth muscle by directly stimulating β_2-adrenergic receptors in the airway.[27] They also increase mucociliary clearance and stabilize mast cell membranes. The early-phase response to antigen in an asthma exacerbation is blocked by pretreatment with inhaled SABAs. Short-acting β_2-agonists have significantly better

---

Table 14–2

Age Recommendations and Features of Inhalation Devices.[2]

Device Type	Recommended Age	Advantages	Disadvantages
Metered-dose inhaler (MDI)	5 years of age and older	• Newer inhalers have a dose counter • Delivery of medication in less than 2 min • Portable, durable • Lower medication dose needed vs. nebulization	• Older inhalers do not have a dose counter • Technique/coordination may be difficult • Propellant may taste bad or irritate the airways
MDI plus valved-holding chamber (VHC)	If less than 4 years old, use VHC with mask; If 4 years of age or older, use VHC	• VHC enhances MDI technique • VHC decreases topical side effects of ICS • Albuterol MDI with VHC is as effective as nebulization for asthma exacerbation	• Bulky • Lack of coverage by some insurance plans • Limited testing of MDIs with various VHC, leading to unpredictable results • Potential for increased systemic side effects with inhaled corticosteroids (ICS)
Jet nebulizer	Any age, preferably infants or elderly	• No coordination required • Oxygen may be delivered simultaneously with medications	• Requires 5–15 minutes to deliver medication • Limited number of medications available for nebulization • Not portable (most require electricity)
Ultrasonic nebulizer	Any age; preferably infants or elderly	• Typically more portable than jet nebulizer • Faster delivery of medications than jet nebulizer	• Heat generated from nebulizer breaks down suspensions for nebulization • Do not use with budesonide suspension for nebulization
Dry powder inhaler (DPI)	Aerolizer 5 years of age and older; Diskus 4 years of age and older; Flexhaler 6 years of age and older; Twisthaler age 12 years and older	• Easy to use; has dose counter • Sweet taste • Quick delivery of medication	• Limited product stability 30–45 days after opening • Optimal delivery of medication in children less than 4 years old is not feasible because high inspiratory volume is needed • Amount of lactose filler is insufficient to cause concern in lactose intolerance

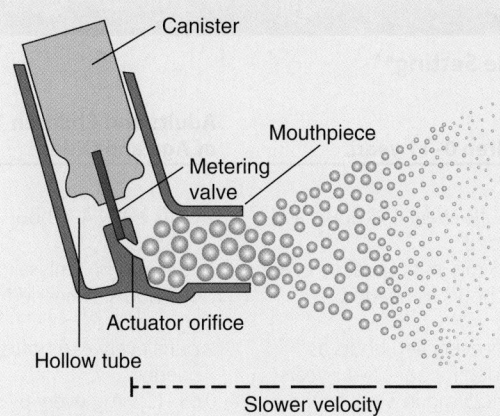

1. Remove the cap and shake the inhaler well.
2. Exhale all air away from the inhaler.
3. Place the mouthpiece into the mouth with lips closed tightly around the inhaler.
4. To deliver a dose, press down on the canister **one time** while inhaling a slow steady breath. A puff or mist of medication is sprayed out of the inhaler into the mouth.
5. Hold your breath for 10 seconds.
6. Exhale.
7. Wait 1 minute if the dose is to be repeated.
8. Recap the inhaler when you are finished.
9. Rinse your mouth with water if the medication is an inhaled corticosteroid.

Comments

- Prime the MDI the first time it is used or if it has not been used in 10 days. Prime the inhaler by spraying 4 sprays into the air.
- For patients who cannot hold their breath for 10 seconds, instruct them to hold their breath as long as possible.
- Do not immerse the canister of medication in water at any time.
- If a counter is not available on the inhaler, the patient should tally the number of puffs used to determine when the inhaler is empty.

FIGURE 14–1. Proper Use of a Metered-Dose Inhaler (MDI). Inhaler image reprinted with permission from Kelly HW, Sorkness CA. Asthma. In: DiPiro JT, Talbert RL, Yee GC, et al, eds. Pharmacotherapy: A Pathophysiologic Approach, 8th ed. New York: McGraw-Hill, 2011. Figure 33-4, 448

bronchodilating activity in acute asthma than theophylline or anticholinergic agents.

Adverse effects of β_2-agonists include tachycardia, tremor, and hypokalemia, which are usually not troublesome with inhaled dosage forms. Oral β_2-agonists have increased adverse effects and are not used in the treatment of asthma. Inhaled β_2-agonists are classified as either short- or long-acting based on duration of action.

Short-Acting Inhaled β_2-Agonists ⑥ *Inhaled SABAs are the most effective agents for reversing acute airway obstruction caused by bronchoconstriction and are the drugs of choice for treating acute asthma and symptoms of chronic asthma* as well as preventing exercise-induced bronchospasm.[1] Inhaled SABAs have an onset of action of less than 5 minutes and a duration of action of 4 to 6 hours. Using an MDI with a spacer is quicker and at least as effective as administration by nebulization.

Albuterol (known as salbutamol outside the United States), the most commonly used inhaled SABA, is available as an MDI and solution for nebulization. Levalbuterol, the pure R-enantiomer of albuterol (and referred to as R-salbutamol outside the United States), is available as an MDI and solution for nebulization. Levalbuterol has similar efficacy to albuterol and is purported to have fewer side effects; however, clinical trials have not demonstrated this benefit.[28]

Doses for SABAs are provided in Table 14–3. During an asthma exacerbation, the usual SABA doses are doubled and the regimen changes from as needed to scheduled use. Scheduled chronic daily dosing of SABAs is not recommended for two reasons. First, the need to use an inhaled SABA is one key indicator of uncontrolled asthma. Therefore, patients are educated to record SABA use. Second,

scheduled SABA use decreases the duration of bronchodilation provided by the SABA.

Long-Acting Inhaled β_2-Agonists Salmeterol and formoterol are LABAs that provide up to 12 hours of bronchodilation after a single dose. Because of the long duration of bronchodilation, these agents are useful for patients experiencing nocturnal symptoms. Salmeterol is a partial agonist with an onset of action of approximately 30 minutes. Formoterol is a full agonist that has an onset of action similar to that of albuterol, but it is not currently approved for the treatment of acute bronchospasm.

LABAs are indicated for chronic treatment of asthma as add-on therapy for patients not controlled on low to medium doses of ICS. Adding an LABA is at least as effective in improving symptoms and decreasing asthma exacerbations as doubling the dose of an ICS or adding an LTRA to ICS.[29] Adding an LABA to ICS therapy also reduces the amount of ICS necessary for asthma control.

Although both formoterol and salmeterol are effective as add-on therapy for moderate persistent asthma, neither agent should be used as monotherapy for chronic asthma. There may be an increased risk of severe asthma exacerbations and asthma-related deaths when LABAs are used alone.[30] The labeling for all drugs containing LABAs includes a black box warning against their use without an ICS. The risk of increased severe asthma exacerbations does not appear to be increased in adults receiving both an LABA and ICS.[31]

Salmeterol and formoterol are available in fixed-ratio combination products containing fluticasone, budesonide, or mometasone. Combination products may increase adherence because of the need for fewer inhalers and inhalations.

Table 14–3

Usual Dosages for Quick-Relief Medications for Asthma in Home Setting[a,b]

Medications	Dosage Form	Children 0–11 years	Adults and Children 12 Years of Age and Older
Inhaled SABA			
Albuterol	HFA (MDI) 90 mcg/puff, 200 puffs/canister	1–2 puffs every 4–6 hours as needed	2 puffs every 4–6 hours as needed
Albuterol	Nebulizer solution 0.63 mg/3 mL, 1.25 mg/3 mL, 2.5 mg/3 mL, 5 mg/mL (0.5%)	0.63–5 mg in 3 mL saline every 4–6 hours as needed	1.25–5 mg in 3 mL saline every 4–8 hours as needed
Levalbuterol	HFA (MDI) 45 mcg/puff, 200 puffs/canister	2 puffs every 4–6 hours as needed for ages 5–11 years	2 puffs every 4–6 hours as needed
Levalbuterol	Nebulizer solution 0.31 mg/3 mL, 0.63 mg/3 mL, 1.25 mg/0.5 mL, 1.25 mg/3 mL	0.31–1.25 mg in 3 mL every 6–8 hours as needed	0.63–1.25 mg every 6–8 hours as needed
Systemic Corticosteroids			
Methylprednisolone	2, 4, 6, 8, 16, 32 mg oral tablets	40–60 mg/day by mouth as single or 2 divided doses for 3–10 days	40–60 mg/day by mouth as single or 2 divided doses for 3–10 days
Prednisolone	5 mg oral tablets; 5 mg/5 mL and 15 mg/5 mL oral liquid	1–2 mg/kg/day, (maximum 60 mg/day) for 3–10 days	40–60 mg/day by mouth as single or 2 divided doses for 3–10 days
Prednisone	1, 2.5, 5, 10, 20, 50 mg oral tablets; 5 mg/mL and 5 mg/5 mL oral liquid	1–2 mg/kg/day, (maximum 60 mg/day) for 3–10 days	40–60 mg/day by mouth as single or 2 divided doses for 3–10 days

HFA, hydrofluoroalkane; IM, intramuscular; MDI, metered-dose inhaler; N/A, safety and efficacy not established; SABA, short-acting β_2-agonist.

[a]Dosages are provided for products that have been approved by the U.S. FDA or have sufficient clinical trial safety and efficacy data in the appropriate age ranges to support their use.

[b]Doses are increased in the hospital/emergency department setting.

However, they offer less flexibility in dosage adjustment of individual ingredients if that is necessary. Doses used for long-term control of chronic asthma are provided in Table 14–4.

▶ Corticosteroids

Corticosteroids are the most potent anti-inflammatory agents available for the treatment of asthma and are available in inhaled, oral, and injectable dosage forms. They decrease airway inflammation, attenuate AHR, and minimize mucus production and secretion. Corticosteroids also improve the response to β_2-agonists.

Inhaled Corticosteroids ❼ *ICS are the preferred therapy for all forms of persistent asthma in all age groups.*[1,2] ICS are more effective than LTRA and theophylline in improving lung function and preventing emergency department visits and hospitalizations due to asthma exacerbations.[1,2] The primary advantage of using ICS compared with systemic corticosteroids is the targeted drug delivery to the lungs, which decreases the risk of systemic adverse effects. Product selection is based on preference for dosage form, delivery device, and cost.

All ICS are equally effective if given in equipotent doses (Table 14–5).[32] ICS have a flat dose–response curve; doubling the dose has a limited additional effect on asthma control.[33] The ICS are more effective when given twice daily rather than once daily.[32] Cigarette smoking decreases the response to ICS, and smokers require higher doses of ICS than nonsmokers.[34] Although some beneficial effect is seen within 12 hours of administration of an ICS, 2 weeks of therapy is necessary

Patient Encounter 3

SR is a 25-year-old man with a past medical history of human immunodeficiency virus (HIV), asthma, and migraines. Until recently, his asthma was controlled with as-needed albuterol. Four weeks ago he was seen in clinic with worsening migraine headaches and was started on medication for migraine prophylaxis. He had an asthma exacerbation 2 weeks ago and was started on a medium-dose inhaled corticosteroid. Today he has complaints of weight gain and a "puffy face." His medication regimen includes:

Ritonavir 100 mg daily
Darunavir 400 mg 2 tablets by mouth daily
Raltegravir 400 mg by mouth twice daily
Propranolol 20 mg by mouth twice daily
Ibuprofen 200 mg 2 capsules by mouth every 8 hours as needed for headache
Acetaminophen 325 mg 2 tablets by mouth every 4 hours as needed for headache
Fluticasone 110 mcg 2 puffs twice daily
Albuterol 90 mcg 2 puffs every 6 hours as needed for shortness of breath

Which of his medications is most likely worsening his asthma control?

Which of the medications are interacting and causing the weight gain and "puffy face"?

What would be an appropriate alternative asthma regimen?

Table 14–4

Usual Doses of Long-Term Control Medications in Asthma[a]

Medication	Dosage Form	Ages 0–11 Years	Adult and Children Greater Than or Equal to 12 Years of Age
Inhaled Corticosteroids (see Table 14–5)			
Long-Acting β₂-Agonists			
Salmeterol	DPI 50 mcg/blister	Ages 0–4 years: N/A Ages 5–11 years: Contents of one blister every 12 hours	Contents of one blister every 12 hours
Formoterol	DPI 12 mcg/capsule	Ages 0–4 years: N/A Ages 5–11 years: Contents of one capsule every 12 hours	Contents of one capsule every 12 hours
Leukotriene Modifiers			
Montelukast	4 mg or 5 mg chewable tablets 4 mg granule packets 10 mg tablet	Ages 1–5 years: 4 mg at bedtime Ages 6–11 years: 5 mg at bedtime	Ages 12–14 years: 5 mg at bedtime Ages 15 and older: 10 mg at bedtime
Zafirlukast	10 or 20 mg tablets	Ages 0–6 years: N/A Ages 7–11 years: 10 mg twice daily	20 mg tablet twice daily
Zileuton	600 mg extended-release tablet 600 mg tablet	N/A N/A	1200 mg twice daily after meals 600 mg 4 times daily
Methylxanthines			
Theophylline	100, 200, 300, 400, 450, 600 mg extended-release tablets; 80 mg/15mL solution and elixir; liquids, sustained-release tablets and capsules	Ages less than 1 year: [0.2 (age in weeks) + 5] × body weight in kg (in divided doses/day)[b] Ages 1–11 years (less than 45 kg): Starting dose 12–14 mg/kg/day (max 300 mg/day) × 3 days, increase to 16 mg/kg/day (max 400 mg/day) × 3 days, then increase to 20 mg/kg/day (max 600 mg/day) Ages 1–11 years (45 kg or greater): Starting dose 300 mg/day (in divided doses) × 3 days, titrate up 400 mg/day × 3 days, then titrate up to usual maximum of 600 mg/day	Starting dose 300 mg/day (in divided doses or daily depending on product) × 3 days, titrate up 400 mg/day × 3 days, then titrate up to usual maximum of 600 mg/day; monitor serum levels
Immunomodulator			
Omalizumab	SC injection, 150 mg/1.2 mL after reconstitution with 1.4 mL sterile water for injection	N/A	150–375 mg SC every 2–4 weeks, depending on body weight and pretreatment serum IgE level. See dosing chart.[c]

DPI, dry powder inhaler; IgE, immunoglobulin E; N/A, safety and efficacy not established; SC, subcutaneously.

[a]Dosages are provided for products that have been approved by the U.S. FDA or have sufficient clinical trial safety and efficacy data in the appropriate age ranges to support their use.

[b]See guidelines for premature infants.

[c]*http://www.gene.com/gene/products/information/pdf/xolair-prescribing.pdf.*

to see significant clinical effects. Longer treatment may be necessary to realize the full effects on airway inflammation.

For most delivery devices, the majority of the drug is deposited in the mouth and throat and swallowed. Local adverse effects of ICS include oral candidiasis, cough, and dysphonia. The incidence of local adverse effects can be reduced by using a VHC and by having the patient rinse the mouth with water and expectorate after using the ICS. Decreasing the dose reduces the incidence of hoarseness.

Systemic absorption occurs via the pulmonary and oral routes. Systemic adverse effects are dose dependent and rare with low to medium doses. However, high-dose ICS have been associated with adrenal suppression, decreased bone mineral density, skin thinning, cataracts, and easy bruising.[2] Nonprogressive growth suppression in children occurs primarily in the first month of treatment and is reported with low- and medium-dose ICS.[35,36] A significant drug interaction causing Cushing's syndrome and adrenal insufficiency occurs when potent inhibitors of CYP3A4 (ritonavir, itraconazole, ketoconazole) are administered with high doses of ICS.[32]

Considerable variability in response to ICS exists, with up to 40% of patients not responding to ICS. This lack of response may be related to a functional glucocorticoid-induced

Table 14–5

Estimated Comparative Daily Dosages for Inhaled Corticosteroids for Asthma[2,32]

Medication	Low Daily Dose		Medium Daily Dose		High Daily Dose	
	Ages 0–11 Years	Ages 12 Years or More	Ages 0–11 Years	Ages 12 Years or More	Ages 0–11 Years	Ages 12 Years or More
Beclomethasone HFA (MDI) 40 or 80 mcg/puff	40 mcg, 1–2 puffs twice daily or 80 mcg, 1 puff twice daily[a]	40 mcg, 1–3 puffs twice daily or 80 mcg, 1 puff twice daily	40 mcg, 3–4 puffs twice daily or 80 mcg, 2 puffs twice daily[a]	40 mcg, more than 3 puffs twice daily or 80 mcg, 3 puffs twice daily	80 mcg, more than 2 puffs twice daily[a]	80 mcg, more than 3 puffs twice daily
Budesonide DPI 90 or 180 mcg/inhalation	90 mcg, 1–2 inhalations twice daily or 180 mcg, 1 inhalation twice daily[a]	90 mcg, 1–3 inhalations twice daily or 180 mcg, 1 inhalation twice daily	90 mcg, 3 inhalations twice daily or 180 mcg, 2 inhalations twice daily[a]	180 mcg, 2–3 inhalations twice daily	180 mcg, more than 2 inhalations twice daily[a]	180 mcg, more than 3 inhalations twice daily
Budesonide inhalation suspension for nebulization 0.25 mg/2 mL, 0.5 mg/2 mL, 1 mg/2 mL	Ages 0–4: 0.25 mg once or twice daily; Ages 5–11: 0.25 mg twice daily or 0.5 mg once daily	N/A	Ages 0–4: 0.25–0.5 mg twice daily; Ages 5–11: 0.5 mg twice daily	N/A	Ages 0–4: more than 0.5 mg twice daily; Ages 5–11: 1 mg twice daily	N/A
Ciclesonide HFA 80, 160 mcg/puff	80 mcg, 1 puff once or twice daily or 160 mcg, 1 puff daily[b]	80 mcg, 1–2 puffs once or twice daily or 160 mcg, 1 puff once or twice daily	80 mcg, more than 1–2 puffs twice daily or 160 mcg, 1 puff twice daily[b]	80 mcg, 3–4 puffs twice daily or 160 mcg, 2 puffs twice daily	80 mcg, more than 2 puffs twice daily or 160 mcg, more than 1 puff twice daily[b]	80 mcg, more than 4 puffs twice daily or 160 mcg, more than 2 puffs twice daily
Flunisolide HFA 80 mcg/puff	80 mcg, 1 puff twice daily[a]	80 mcg, 2 puffs twice daily	80 mcg, 2 puffs twice daily[a]	80 mcg, 3–4 puffs twice daily	80 mcg, 3–4 puffs twice daily[a]	80 mcg, more than 4 puffs twice daily
Fluticasone HFA (MDI) 44, 110, or 220 mcg/puff	44 mcg, 1–2 puffs twice daily	44 mcg, 1–3 puffs twice daily or 110 mcg, 1 puff twice daily	44 mcg, 3–4 puffs twice daily or 110 mcg, 1 puff twice daily	44 mcg, 4–5 puffs twice daily or 110 mcg, 2 puffs twice daily or 220 mcg, 1 puff twice daily	44 mcg, more than 4 puffs twice daily or 110 mcg, more than 1 puff twice daily or 220 mcg, 1 puff twice daily	110 mcg, more than 2 puffs twice daily or 220 mcg, more than 1 puff twice daily
Fluticasone DPI 50, 100, or 250 mcg/inhalation	50 mcg, 1–2 inhalations twice daily or 100 mcg, 1 inhalation twice daily[a]	50 mcg, 1–3 inhalations twice daily or 100 mcg, 1 inhalation twice daily	50 mcg, 3–4 inhalations twice daily or 100 mcg, 2 inhalations twice daily[a]	50 mcg, 4 inhalations twice daily or 100 mcg, 2 inhalations twice daily or 250 mcg, 1 inhalation twice daily	100 mcg, more than 2 inhalations twice daily[a]	250 mcg, more than 1 inhalation twice daily
Mometasone DPI 110, 220 mcg/inhalation	110 mcg, 1 inhalation daily[c]	220 mcg, 1 inhalation daily	110 mcg, 1–2 inhalations twice daily or 220 mcg, 1 inhalation twice daily[c]	220 mcg, 1 inhalation twice daily or 2 inhalations daily	110 mcg, more than 2 inhalations twice daily or 220 mcg, more than 1 inhalation twice daily[c]	110 mcg, more than 2 inhalations twice daily or 220 mcg, more than 1–2 inhalations twice daily
Combined ICS/LABA						
Fluticasone/Salmeterol DPI 100/50 mcg, 250/50 mcg, 500/50 mcg; HFA (MDI) 45/21 mcg, 115/21 mcg, 230/21 mcg	100/50 mcg, 1 inhalation twice daily[d]	100/50 mcg, 1 inhalation twice daily or 45/21 mcg, 2 puffs twice daily	100/50 mcg, 1 inhalation twice daily[d]	250/50 mcg, 1 inhalation twice daily or 115/21 mcg, 2 puffs twice daily	100/50 mcg, 1 inhalation twice daily[d]	500/50 mcg, 1 inhalation twice daily or 230/21 mcg, 2 puffs twice daily

(Continued)

Table 14–5						

Estimated Comparative Daily Dosages for Inhaled Corticosteroids for Asthma[2,32] (*Continued*)

Medication	Low Daily Dose		Medium Daily Dose		High Daily Dose	
	Ages 0–11 Years	Ages 12 Years or More	Ages 0–11 Years	Ages 12 Years or More	Ages 0–11 Years	Ages 12 Years or More
Budesonide/Formoterol HFA (MDI) 80/4.5 mcg, 160/4.5 mcg	N/A[b]	80/4.5 mcg, 1 puff twice daily	N/A[b]	80/4.5 mcg, 2 puffs twice daily or 160/4.5 mcg, 1 puff twice daily	N/A[b]	160/4.5 mcg, 2 puffs twice daily
Mometasone/Formoterol 100/5 mcg, 200/5 mcg	N/A[b]	100/5 mcg, 1 puff twice daily	N/A[b]	100/5 mcg, 2 puffs twice daily or 200/5 mcg, 1 puff twice daily	N/A[b]	200/5 mcg, 2 puffs twice daily

DPI, dry powder inhaler; HFA, hydrofluoroalkane; ICS, inhaled corticosteroid; LABA, long-acting β_2-agonist; MDI, metered-dose inhaler, N/A, safety and efficacy not established.

[a]N/A in children 0–4 years of age.

[b]Not yet FDA approved in children 0–11 years of age.

[c]Doses based on clinical trials. FDA approved in children ages 4–11 years at maximum dose of 110 mcg daily.

[d]Doses based on clinical trials. A maximum of fluticasone/salmeterol 100/50 mcg, 1 inhalation twice daily is approved in children ages 4–11 years without specification of low, medium, or high dosage.

transcript 1 gene (*GLCCI1*) variant in some patients with asthma.[37] Future directions in pharmacogenomics will assist with individualized asthma treatment algorithms.

Systemic Corticosteroids Prednisone, prednisolone, and methylprednisolone are systemic corticosteroids used in asthma treatment. These medications are the cornerstone of treatment for acute asthma not responding to an SABA.[1,2] Recommended doses for systemic corticosteroids are included in Table 14–3.

The onset of action for systemic corticosteroids is 4 to 12 hours. For this reason, systemic corticosteroids are started early in the course of acute exacerbations. The oral route is preferred in acute asthma; there is no evidence that IV corticosteroid administration is more effective. Therapy with systemic corticosteroids is continued until the PEF is 70% or more of the personal best measurement and asthma symptoms are resolved. The duration of therapy usually ranges from 3 to 10 days. Tapering the corticosteroid dose in patients receiving short bursts (up to 10 days) is usually not necessary because any adrenal suppression is transient and rapidly reversible.[2]

Because of serious potential adverse effects, systemic corticosteroids are avoided as long-term controller medication for asthma, if possible. Systemic corticosteroids are only used in patients who have failed other therapies, including immunomodulators. If systemic therapy is necessary, once-daily or every-other-day therapy is used with repeated attempts to decrease the dose or discontinue the drug.

▶ *Anticholinergics*

Two anticholinergic medications are available: ipratropium bromide and tiotropium bromide. Anticholinergic agents act by inhibiting the effects of acetylcholine on muscarinic receptors in the airways and protecting against cholinergic-mediated bronchoconstriction.[27] The bronchodilating effects are not as effective as SABAs in asthma.

Ipratropium bromide (Atrovent) is available as an MDI and solution for nebulization. Its onset of action is approximately 30 minutes, and the duration of action is 4 to 8 hours. The addition of ipratropium bromide to SABAs during a moderate to severe asthma exacerbation improves pulmonary function and decreases hospitalization rates in both adult and pediatric patients.[38] Combining an SABA with ipratropium is only indicated in the emergency department setting. There is no evidence to support continued use of ipratropium during hospitalization or for chronic asthma treatment.[2]

Tiotropium bromide (Spiriva) is a long-acting inhaled anticholinergic available in a DPI; it has an onset of action of approximately 30 minutes and duration of action longer than 24 hours. There is increasing evidence supporting its use as a long-term controller medication in patients with uncontrolled asthma already taking an ICS.[39,40]

Anticholinergic drugs may cause bothersome adverse effects such as blurred vision, dry mouth, and urinary retention. Increased cardiovascular events have been reported for ipratropium but not tiotropium.[41,42]

▶ *Leukotriene Receptor Antagonists*

The LTRAs are anti-inflammatory medications that either inhibit 5-lipoxygenase (zileuton) or competitively antagonize the effects of leukotriene D_4 (montelukast and zafirlukast). These agents improve FEV_1 and decrease asthma symptoms, SABA use, and asthma exacerbations. Although these agents offer the convenience of oral administration, they are significantly less effective than low ICS doses.[2,43] Combining an LTRA with an ICS or LABA is not as effective as an ICS plus an LABA.[2] LTRA are beneficial for asthma patients with allergic rhinitis or aspirin sensitivity. See Table 14–4 for dosing.

Montelukast (Singulair) is generally well tolerated with minimal need for monitoring and few drug interactions. Zileuton (Zyflo) and zafirlukast (Accolate) are not commonly used because of the risk of hepatotoxicity. Both zileuton and zafirlukast require liver function monitoring at baseline and every 3 months for the first year of use and then periodically thereafter. Zileuton and zafirlukast are metabolized through the CYP 2C9 hepatic pathway and have significant drug interactions. All three agents have reports of neuropsychiatric events, such as sleep disorders, aggressive behavior, and suicidal thoughts that need to be monitored.

▶ Methylxanthines

Theophylline has anti-inflammatory properties and causes bronchodilation by inhibiting phosphodiesterase and antagonizing adenosine.[44] Its use is limited because of inferior efficacy as a long-term controller medication compared with ICS, a narrow therapeutic index with potentially life-threatening toxicity, and multiple clinically important drug interactions.

Theophylline is primarily metabolized by CYP1A2 and CYP3A4 and is involved in a large number of disease and drug interactions. Theophylline exhibits nonlinear pharmacokinetics; therefore, serum concentration changes due to dosage adjustments, drug interactions, and hepatic function may not always be predictable.

Target serum theophylline concentrations are 5 to 15 mg/L (28 to 83 μmol/L); an increased risk of adverse effects outweighs the increased bronchodilation in most patients above 15 mg/L (83 μmol/L).[44] Headache, nausea, vomiting, and insomnia may occur at serum concentrations less than 20 mg/L (111 μmol/L) but are rare when the dose is started low and increased slowly. See Table 14–4 for dosing. More serious adverse effects can occur at higher concentrations (e.g., cardiac arrhythmias, seizures, and death).

▶ Immunomodulators

Omalizumab (Xolair) is a recombinant humanized monoclonal anti-IgE antibody that inhibits binding of IgE to receptors on mast cells and basophils, resulting in inhibition of inflammatory mediator release and attenuation of the early- and late-phase allergic response. Omalizumab is indicated for treatment of patients with moderate to severe persistent asthma whose asthma is not controlled by ICS and who have a positive skin test or in vitro reactivity to aeroallergens. Omalizumab significantly decreases ICS use, reduces the number and length of exacerbations, and increases asthma-related quality of life.[45]

Omalizumab is given as a subcutaneous injection every 2 to 4 weeks in the office or clinic. The initial dose is based on the patient's weight and baseline total serum IgE concentration (see Table 14–4). Subsequent IgE levels are not monitored.

The most common adverse effects are injection site reactions and include bruising, redness, pain, stinging,

---

Patient Encounter 4

CE is a 52-year-old woman with severe persistent asthma since she was a child, allergic rhinitis, and gastroesophageal reflux disease (GERD). She is currently taking budesonide/formoterol 160/4.5 mcg, 2 puffs twice daily, montelukast 10 mg by mouth at bedtime, fluticasone 50 mcg/actuation 2 sprays in each nostril daily, omeprazole 20 mg by mouth daily, and prednisone 40 mg daily for 3 to 5 days every other month for asthma exacerbations. Her IgE level is 100 IU/mL (100 kIU/L) and her weight is 150 pounds (68 kg). She tested positive for allergies to pollens and dust mites.

The physician plans to start omalizumab. Do you agree with this plan?

What is the appropriate dose, route of administration, and frequency for this medication?

If omalizumab therapy is initiated, what information should be provided to the patient?

Outline a monitoring plan for omalizumab for an adult patient with asthma.

---

itching, and burning. Anaphylactic reactions are rare but may occur at any time after medication administration. Monitoring the patient for an anaphylactic reaction for 2 hours after medication administration is recommended for the first 3 months; thereafter, monitoring time can be reduced to 30 minutes.[46] It is also important to issue a prescription for and provide patient education on the use of subcutaneous epinephrine for an anaphylactic reaction from omalizumab.

Treatment of Chronic Asthma

❽ *The intensity of pharmacotherapy for chronic asthma is based on disease severity for initial therapy and level of control for subsequent therapies.* The least amount of medications necessary to meet the goals of asthma therapy is used.[2]

The first step in asthma management is evaluating the patient's asthma severity and control (refer to Table 14–1 for descriptions of asthma severity). Pharmacologic treatment is initiated based on the recommendations for stepwise therapy (Fig. 14–2). The EPR-3 separates treatment recommendations into three categories based on patient age: (a) children younger than 5 years, (b) children between the ages of 5 and 11 years, and (c) individuals 12 years and older. Therapeutic plans must be individualized.

▶ Intermittent Asthma

Patients with intermittent asthma only need SABAs. This classification of asthma includes patients with exercise-induced bronchospasm (EIB), seasonal asthma, or asthma symptoms associated with infrequent trigger exposure. Patients pretreat with an SABA prior to exposure to a known trigger, such as exercise.

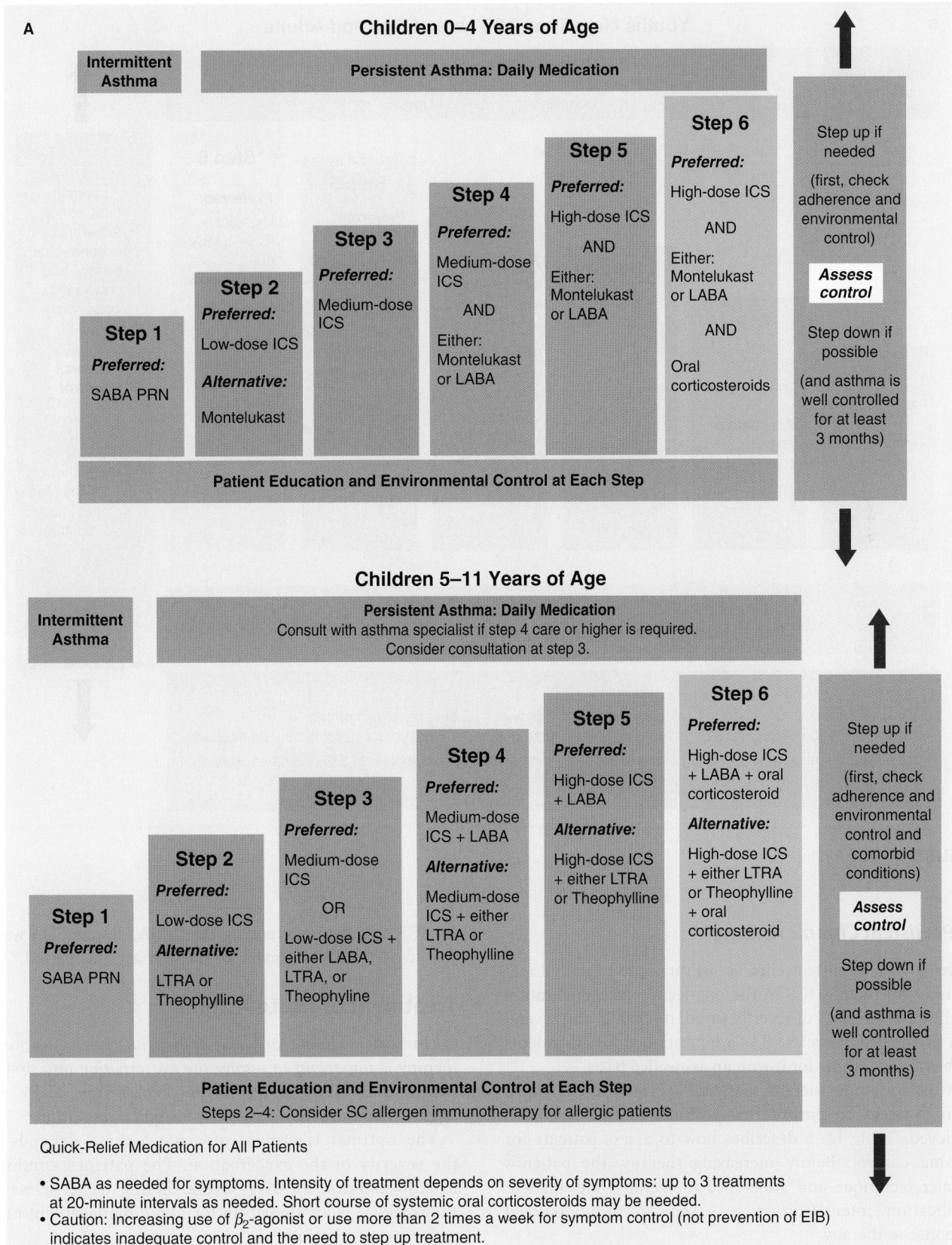

FIGURE 14–2. Stepwise approach for managing asthma in (**A**) children and (**B**) adults. (ICS, inhaled corticosteroid; LABA, long-acting β-agonist; LTRA, leukotriene receptor antagonist; PRN, as needed; SABA, short-acting β₂-agonist; SC, subcutaneous.)

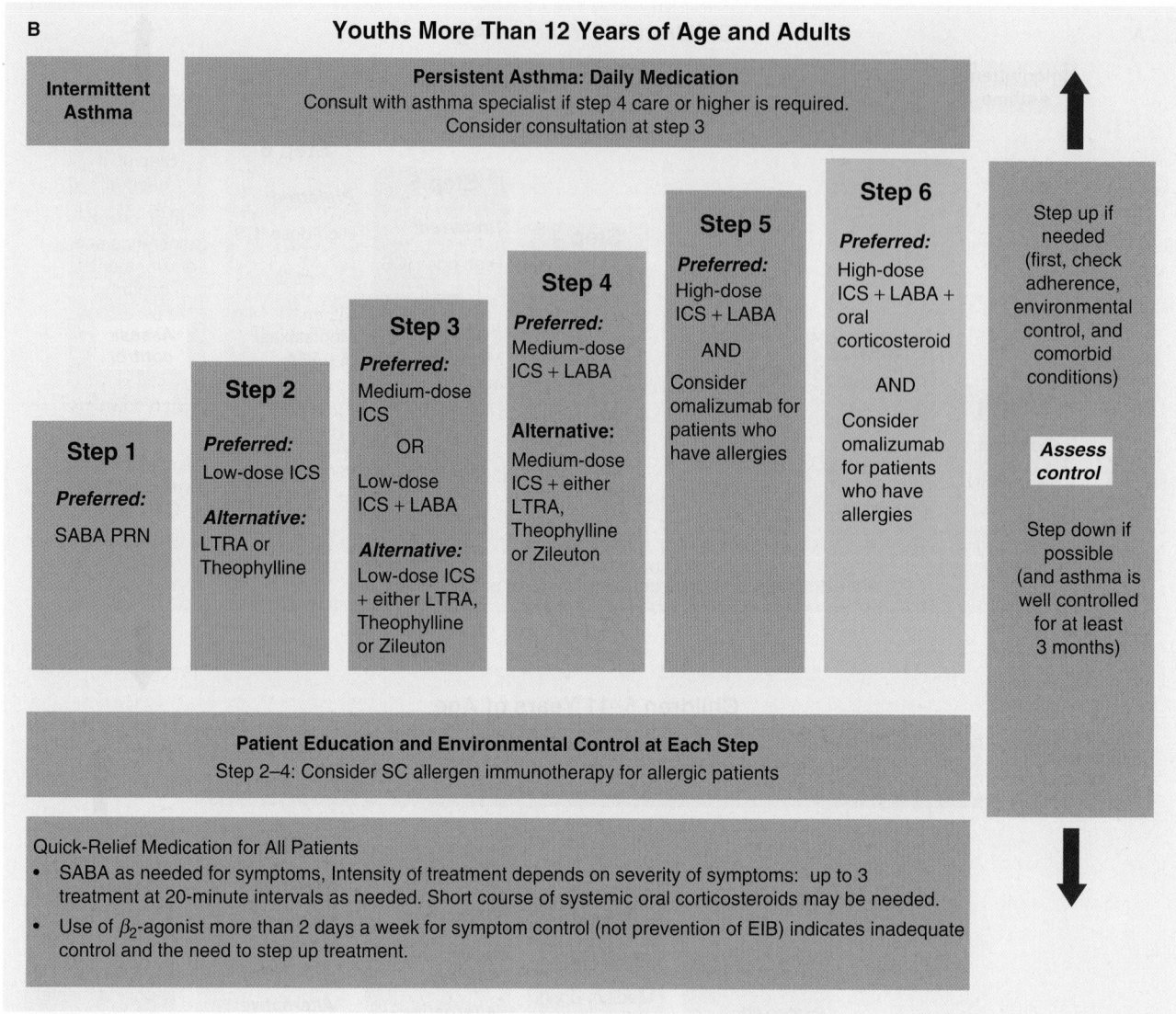

FIGURE 14–2. *(Continued)*

▶ *Persistent Chronic Asthma*

Patients with persistent chronic asthma require daily long-term control therapy. ICS are the long-term control medication of choice at all levels of severity (mild, moderate, and severe) and in all age groups.[2] SABAs are prescribed for all patients with chronic asthma for use on an as-needed basis.

After initiating therapy, patients are monitored within 2 to 6 weeks to ensure that asthma control has been achieved. Table 14–6 describes how to assess patients for asthma control. Before increasing therapy, the patient's inhaler technique and adherence to therapy is evaluated. Medication intensification is based on individualized response to therapy.[29]

Patients with controlled asthma are monitored at 1- to 6-month intervals to ensure that control is maintained. A gradual stepdown in long-term controller therapy is attempted once control has been maintained for at least 3 months. Controversy exists about how to taper long-term controller medication. Current literature supports decreasing the ICS dose before removing the LABA, despite FDA warnings to use LABA treatment for the shortest time period.[47]

Treatment of Acute Asthma

⑨ *In acute asthma, early and appropriate intensification of therapy is important to resolve the exacerbation and prevent relapse and future severe airflow obstruction.* Early and aggressive treatment is necessary for quick resolution.[48]

The optimal treatment of acute asthma depends on the severity of the exacerbation. The patient's condition usually deteriorates over several hours, days, or weeks. Figure 14–3 is an algorithm for home management of an asthma exacerbation.

Based on the initial response to SABA therapy, the severity of the exacerbation is assessed, and treatment is appropriately intensified. Patients deteriorating quickly or not responding to quick-relief medications should go to the emergency department for assessment and treatment of the asthma exacerbation. Figure 14–4 provides a treatment

Table 14–6

Assessing Asthma Control and Adjusting Therapy Based on Age[1]

Components of Control	Well Controlled			Not Well Controlled			Very Poorly Controlled		
	Ages 0–4	Ages 5–11	12 Years or More	Ages 0–4	Ages 5–11	12 Years or More	Ages 0–4	Ages 5–11	12 Years or More
Impairment — Symptoms	2 days/week or less but not more than once each day	2 days/week or less	2 days/week or less	More than 2 days/week or multiple times on 2 days/week or less	More than 2 days/week	More than 2 days/week	Throughout the day →		
Nighttime awakenings	1 time/month or less	1 time/month or less	2 times/month or less	More than 1 time/month	2 times/week or more	1–3 times/week	More than 1 time/week	2 times/week or more	4 times/week or more
SABA use for symptoms (not EIB prevention)	2 days/week or less →			More than 2 days/week →			Several times per day →		
Interference with normal activity	None →			Some limitation →			Extremely limited →		
FEV₁ or PEFR	N/A	More than 80%	More than 80% predicted/personal best	N/A	60–80%	60–80% predicted/personal best	N/A	Less than 60%	Less than 60% predicted/personal best
FEV₁/FVC	N/A	More than 80%	More than 80%	N/A	75–80%	60–80%	N/A	Less than 75%	Less than 60%
Questionnaires: ATAQ / ACQ / ACT	N/A	N/A	0 / 0.75 or less[a] / 20 or more	N/A	N/A	1–2 / 1.5 or more / 16–19	N/A	N/A	3–4 / N/A / 15 or less
Risk — Exacerbations requiring oral systemic corticosteroids	0–1/year. Consider severity and interval since last exacerbation	0–1/year. Consider severity and interval since last exacerbation	0–1/year. Consider severity and interval since last exacerbation	2–3/year	2/year or more	2/year or more	More than 3/year	2/year or more	2/year or more
Reduction in lung growth or progressive loss of lung function	N/A	Requires long-term follow-up	Requires long-term follow-up	N/A	Requires long-term follow-up	Requires long-term follow-up	N/A	Requires long-term follow-up	Requires long-term follow-up
Treatment-related ADRs	Medication side effects can vary in intensity from none to very troublesome and worrisome. The level of intensity does not correlate with specific levels of control but should be considered in the overall assessment of risk.								
Recommended action for treatment. See Figure 14–4 for treatment steps.	Maintain current step. Follow-up every 1–6 months. Consider step down if well controlled at 3 months.			Step up 1 step. Reevaluate in 2–6 weeks. If ADRs, consider alternative treatment options.			Consider short course of systemic (oral) corticosteroids. Step up 1–2 steps. Reevaluate in 2 weeks. If ADRs, consider alternative treatment options.		

[a]ACQ values of 0.76–1.4 are indeterminate regarding well-controlled asthma.

ACT, Asthma Control Test; ACQ, Asthma Control Questionnaire; ATAQ, Asthma Therapy Assessment Questionnaire; ADR, adverse drug reaction; EIB, exercise-induced bronchospasm; FEV₁, forced expiratory volume in 1 second; FVC, forced vital capacity; N/A, safety and efficacy not established; PEFR, peak expiratory flow rate; SABA, short-acting β_2-agonist.

Patient Encounter 5

TM is a 6-year-old boy seen in the emergency department for an asthma exacerbation. He has not seen the doctor in over 1 year, and his parents ran out of refills for his asthma medications. He was previously prescribed budesonide 90 mcg, 1 inhalation twice daily and levalbuterol 2 puffs every 4 hours as needed for shortness of breath. His weight today is 50 pounds (23 kg). The physician makes the diagnosis of a moderate asthma exacerbation.

What medication regimen would you recommend for TM while in the emergency department?

The patient's asthma improves, and he is ready to be discharged home from the emergency department. His mother informs you that she is not able to afford the asthma medication. His insurance provider has albuterol, fluticasone, and mometasone on its formulary. Based on this information, what medication regimen would you recommend upon discharge from the emergency department?

Provide the patient and his mother with a written asthma action plan. The parent refuses to monitor peak flow readings.

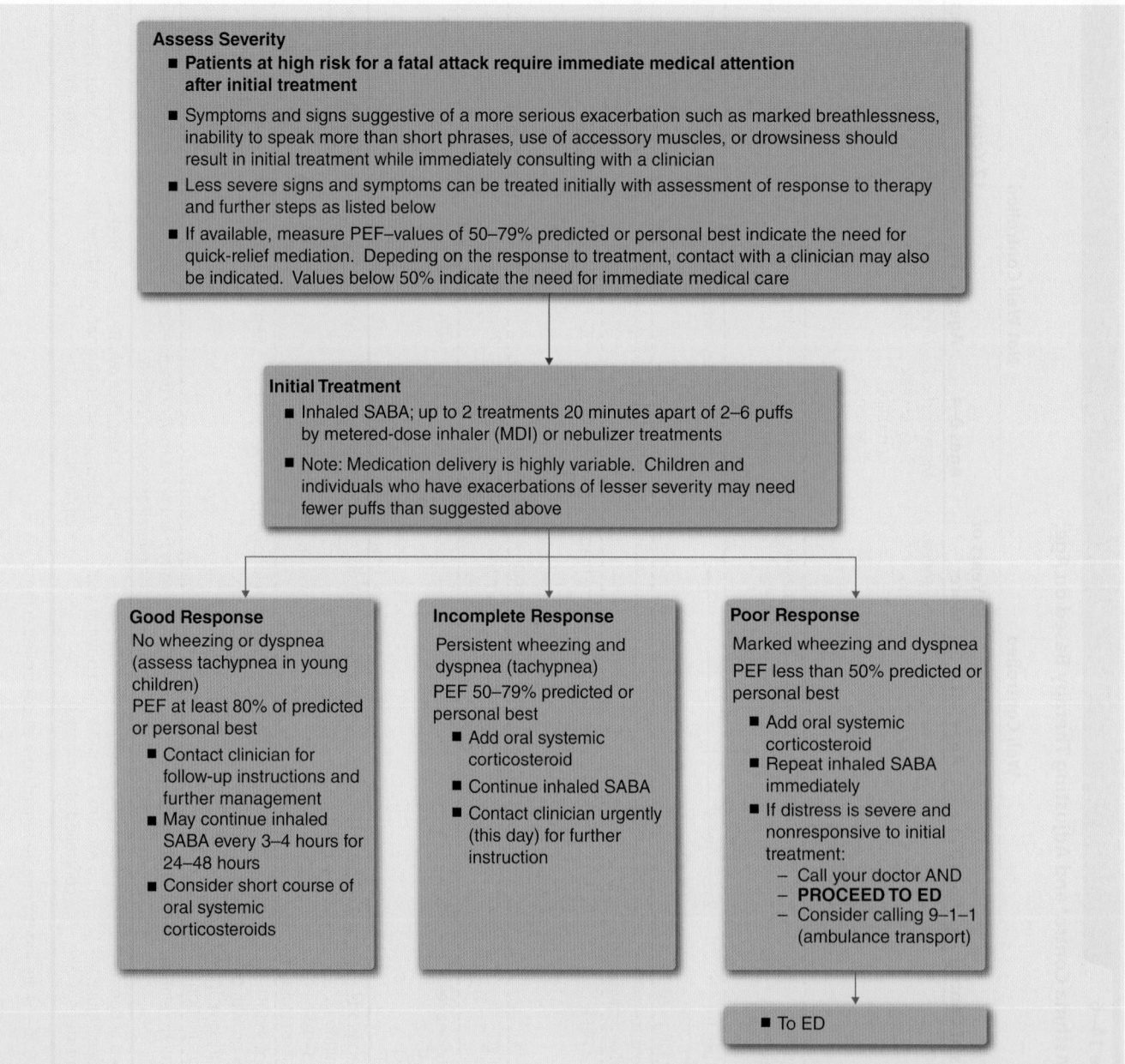

FIGURE 14-3. Management of asthma exacerbations: home treatment. (ED, emergency department; MDI, metered-dose inhaler; PEF, peak expiratory flow; SABA, short-acting β_2-agonist; SC, subcutaneous.) (From NHLBI National Asthma Education and Prevention Program, Expert Panel Report-3. Guidelines for the diagnosis and management of asthma. NIH Publication No. 07-4051. Bethesda, MD: U.S. Department of Health and Human Services, 2007, *http://www.nhlbi.nih.gov/guidelines/asthma*.)

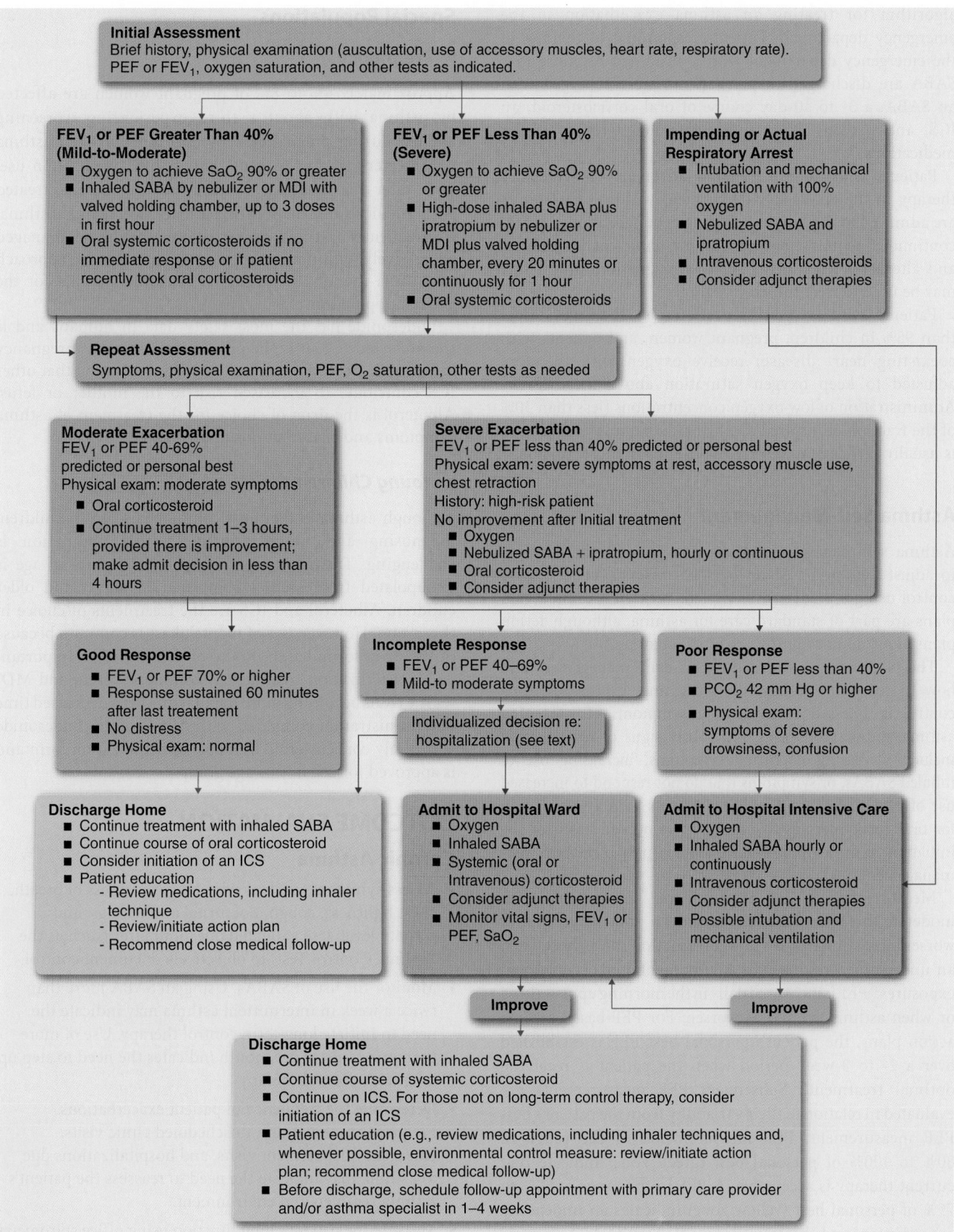

Initial Assessment
Brief history, physical examination (auscultation, use of accessory muscles, heart rate, respiratory rate). PEF or FEV₁, oxygen saturation, and other tests as indicated.

FEV₁ or PEF Greater Than 40% (Mild-to-Moderate)
- Oxygen to achieve SaO₂ 90% or greater
- Inhaled SABA by nebulizer or MDI with valved holding chamber, up to 3 doses in first hour
- Oral systemic corticosteroids if no immediate response or if patient recently took oral corticosteroids

FEV₁ or PEF Less Than 40% (Severe)
- Oxygen to achieve SaO₂ 90% or greater
- High-dose inhaled SABA plus ipratropium by nebulizer or MDI plus valved holding chamber, every 20 minutes or continuously for 1 hour
- Oral systemic corticosteroids

Impending or Actual Respiratory Arrest
- Intubation and mechanical ventilation with 100% oxygen
- Nebulized SABA and ipratropium
- Intravenous corticosteroids
- Consider adjunct therapies

Repeat Assessment
Symptoms, physical examination, PEF, O₂ saturation, other tests as needed

Moderate Exacerbation
FEV₁ or PEF 40-69%
predicted or personal best
Physical exam: moderate symptoms
- Oral corticosteroid
- Continue treatment 1–3 hours, provided there is improvement; make admit decision in less than 4 hours

Severe Exacerbation
FEV₁ or PEF less than 40% predicted or personal best
Physical exam: severe symptoms at rest, accessory muscle use, chest retraction
History: high-risk patient
No improvement after Initial treatment
- Oxygen
- Nebulized SABA + ipratropium, hourly or continuous
- Oral corticosteroid
- Consider adjunct therapies

Good Response
- FEV₁ or PEF 70% or higher
- Response sustained 60 minutes after last treatement
- No distress
- Physical exam: normal

Incomplete Response
- FEV₁ or PEF 40–69%
- Mild-to moderate symptoms

Individualized decision re: hospitalization (see text)

Poor Response
- FEV₁ or PEF less than 40%
- PCO₂ 42 mm Hg or higher
- Physical exam: symptoms of severe drowsiness, confusion

Discharge Home
- Continue treatment with inhaled SABA
- Continue course of oral corticosteroid
- Consider initiation of an ICS
- Patient education
  - Review medications, including inhaler technique
  - Review/initiate action plan
  - Recommend close medical follow-up

Admit to Hospital Ward
- Oxygen
- Inhaled SABA
- Systemic (oral or Intravenous) corticosteroid
- Consider adjunct therapies
- Monitor vital signs, FEV₁ or PEF, SaO₂

Admit to Hospital Intensive Care
- Oxygen
- Inhaled SABA hourly or continuously
- Intravenous corticosteroid
- Consider adjunct therapies
- Possible intubation and mechanical ventilation

Improve

Improve

Discharge Home
- Continue treatment with inhaled SABA
- Continue course of systemic corticosteroid
- Continue on ICS. For those not on long-term control therapy, consider initiation of an ICS
- Patient education (e.g., review medications, including inhaler techniques and, whenever possible, environmental control measure: review/initiate action plan; recommend close medical follow-up)
- Before discharge, schedule follow-up appointment with primary care provider and/or asthma specialist in 1–4 weeks

FIGURE 14–4. Management of asthma exacerbations: emergency department and hospital-based care. (FEV₁, forced expiratory volume in 1 second; ICS, inhaled corticosteroid; MDI, metered-dose inhaler, Pco₂, partial arterial pressure of carbon dioxide; PEF, peak expiratory flow; SABA, short-acting β₂-agonist; Sao₂, oxygen saturation.) (From Ref. 2.)

algorithm for treating an asthma exacerbation in the emergency department. Patients responding to therapy in the emergency department with a sustained response to a SABA are discharged home. Patients are discharged with an SABA, a 3- to 10-day course of oral corticosteroid, an ICS, and perhaps other appropriate long-term controller medications.

Patients who do not respond adequately to intensive therapy in the emergency department within 3 to 4 hours are admitted to the hospital. During hospitalization, oxygen, continuous nebulization of SABA, systemic corticosteroids, and alternative treatments such as magnesium and heliox may be used to treat the exacerbation.

Patients with oxygen saturation less than 90% (less than 95% in children, pregnant women, and patients with coexisting heart disease) receive oxygen with the dose adjusted to keep oxygen saturation above these levels. Administration of low oxygen concentrations (less than 30% of the fraction of inspired air) by nasal cannula or facemask is usually sufficient to reverse hypoxemia in most patients.

Asthma Self-Management

Asthma self-management plans give patients the freedom to adjust therapy based on personal assessment of disease control using a predetermined plan. Written asthma action plans are part of standard care for asthma, although action plans alone do not improve asthma outcomes.[49]

The plan includes instructions on daily management and how to recognize and handle worsening asthma.[2] Asthma control is assessed by evaluating symptoms of worsening asthma and/or monitoring PEF. Early signs of deterioration include increasing nocturnal symptoms, increasing use of inhaled SABAs, or symptoms that do not respond to increased use of inhaled SABAs. Providing patients with a prescription for oral corticosteroids to use on an as-needed basis for the initiation of an asthma exacerbation is part of asthma self-management.

Measurement of PEF is considered for patients with moderate to severe persistent asthma, a poor perception of worsening asthma or airflow obstruction, and those with an unexplained response to environmental or occupational exposures.[2] PEF is measured daily in the morning upon waking or when asthma symptoms worsen. For PEF-based asthma action plans, the patient's personal best PEF is established over a 2- to 3-week period when the patient is receiving optimal treatment.[2] Subsequent PEF measurements are evaluated in relation to their variability from the patient's best PEF measurement. PEF measurements in the range of 80% to 100% of personal best (green zone) indicate that current therapy is acceptable. A PEF in the range of 50% to 79% of personal best (yellow zone) indicates an impending exacerbation, and therapy is intensified with SABA therapy, possibly oral corticosteroids, and a call to the physician. A PEF less than 50% (red zone) signals a medical alert; patients use their SABA immediately, take oral corticosteroids, and go to the emergency department.

Special Populations

▶ Pregnancy

Approximately 4% to 8% of pregnant women are affected by asthma with about a third experiencing worsening asthma during pregnancy.[50] Because uncontrolled asthma is a greater risk to the fetus than asthma medication use, it is safer for pregnant women to have asthma treated with medications than to experience worsening asthma. Consequently, asthma exacerbations should be managed aggressively with pharmacotherapy. The stepwise approach to asthma therapy in pregnancy is similar to that for the general population.

Budesonide has the most safety data in humans and is the preferred ICS; it is the only ICS classified as pregnancy category B. However, there are no data indicating that other ICS contribute to increased risk to the mother or fetus. Albuterol is the drug of choice for the treatment of asthma symptoms and exacerbations in pregnancy.

▶ Young Children

Although asthma is the most common disease in children, diagnosing and monitoring it in this population is challenging. Treatment in children 0 to 4 years of age is extrapolated from studies completed in adults and older children. Albuterol and ICS are the treatments of choice in this group. However, use of montelukast is common because of the drug formulation. Route of delivery is an important issue. Nebulization treatment is commonly used, and MDI with VHC is becoming more popular due to its decreased time of administration compared with nebulization. Budesonide is the only corticosteroid available in nebulization form and is approved for use in this age group.[51]

OUTCOME EVALUATION

Chronic Asthma

- Assess symptoms such as wheezing, shortness of breath, chest tightness, cough, nocturnal awakenings, and activity level. Use validated questionnaires (such as the Asthma Control Test) to objectively document control.

- Monitor the use of SABAs. Using an SABA more than twice a week in intermittent asthma may indicate the need to initiate long-term control therapy. Use of more than one canister per month indicates the need to step up long-term control therapy.

- Determine the frequency of patient exacerbations. Frequent exacerbations, unscheduled clinic visits, emergency department visits, and hospitalizations due to asthma may indicate the need to reassess the patient's asthma regimen and environment.

- Measure the patient's lung function using office spirometry at each clinic visit for patients older than 5 years.

- Identify environmental factors triggering asthma exacerbations and provide trigger avoidance recommendations.

Patient Care and Monitoring

Chronic Asthma

1. Ask about patient (or caregiver) goals and satisfaction with asthma control.

2. Assess asthma control with a validated questionnaire (Asthma Control Test, Asthma Therapy Assessment Questionnaire, or Asthma Control Questionnaire).

3. Evaluate the number of asthma exacerbations since the last clinic visit, including emergency department visits and/or oral corticosteroid use.

4. Measure spirometry at each clinical visit in patients older than 5 years.

5. Evaluate medication issues, including side effects, adherence, cost, and any patient concerns.

6. Review proper use of inhalers, including indication, technique, and determining when to get a refill.

7. Provide an updated asthma action plan with medication changes at least yearly.

8. Review environmental asthma triggers and avoidance plans.

9. Update immunizations.

10. Check spirometry yearly.

11. Schedule follow-up physician visits depending on asthma control (2 weeks to 6 months).

Acute Asthma

1. Assess for wheezing, chest tightness, and shortness of breath.

2. Obtain and evaluate peak flow measurement.

3. Assess severity of dyspnea (i.e., it occurs only with activity, it limits activity, it occurs at rest and interferes with conversation, or the patient is too dyspneic to speak).

4. Evaluate response to SABA.

5. Check respiratory rate.

6. Obtain oxygenation saturation.

7. Assess use of accessory muscles in infants.

8. Perform other tests as appropriate: arterial blood gases, serum electrolytes, chest radiography, and electrocardiogram.

9. Review previous need for emergency department and hospital management for asthma exacerbations.

10. Plan for patient and family response to asthma exacerbations.

11. Provide education about proper inhaler technique, indication and proper use of medications, and self-titration of medications with worsening asthma.

12. Educate about environmental triggers.

13. Provide a follow-up appointment with the primary care physician within 1 to 4 weeks.

- Perform medication reconciliation to identify discrepancies in medications prescribed and used by the patient and to determine drug and disease state interactions.

- Assess the patient's inhaler technique at every visit and always ensure proper technique before stepping up therapy.

- Determine adherence to long-term controller medications. Assess the patient's understanding of the indication for long-term controller medication and identify adverse events, cost issues, and need for refills.

- Review and update the patient's asthma action plan and provide the patient with a written copy of the plan.

- Update the patient's immunization status and provide an annual influenza vaccination.

Acute Asthma

In addition to the outcomes measured for chronic asthma, acute asthma monitoring also includes the following:

- Measure PEF and assess asthma symptoms. The goal PEF measurement is 70% of the patient's personal best peak flow after the first three doses of an inhaled SABA and improved asthma symptoms. Spirometry is not usually conducted in the emergency department.

- Measure oxygenation using pulse oximetry and provide oxygen via nasal cannula if needed. The goal oxygen saturation is greater than 90% in adults and greater than 95% in children, pregnant women, and patients with coexisting cardiovascular disease.

- Obtain a Pco_2 measurement via arterial blood gases in patients with severe asthma exacerbations. An increased Pco_2 indicates the potential for respiratory failure.

- Monitor serum potassium for hypokalemia upon admission and periodically throughout the admission in patients receiving high-dose or continuous nebulization of SABA.

Abbreviations Introduced in This Chapter

AHR	Airway hyperresponsiveness
CFC	Chlorofluorocarbon
CYP	Cytochrome P-450 isoenzyme
DPI	Dry powder inhaler
EPR-3	Expert Panel Report-3
FEV$_1$	Forced expiratory volume in 1 second
FVC	Forced vital capacity
HFA	Hydrofluoroalkane

ICS   Inhaled corticosteroid
IgE   Immunoglobulin E
LABA   Long-acting β_2-agonist
MDI   Metered-dose inhaler
NAEPP   National Asthma Education and Prevention Program
NHLBI   National Heart, Lung, and Blood Institute
NSAID   Nonsteroidal anti-inflammatory drug
Pao_2 Partial arterial pressure of oxygen
Pco_2 Partial arterial pressure of carbon dioxide
PEF   Peak expiratory flow
SABA   Short-acting β_2-agonist
T_H2 Type 2 T-helper CD4+ cell

> **WWW**
>
> Self-assessment questions and answers are available at *http://www.mhpharmacotherapy.com/pp.html.*

REFERENCES

1. Global strategy for asthma management and prevention 2010 (update) [Internet]. Available at *http://www.ginasthma.org/pdf/GINA_Report_2010.pdf.*
2. NHLBI National Asthma Education and Prevention Program, Expert Panel Report-3 [Internet]. Guidelines for the diagnosis and management of asthma. NIH Publication No. 07-4051. Bethesda, MD: U.S. Department of Health and Human Services, 2007. Available at *http://www.nhlbi.nih.gov/guidelines/asthma.*
3. CDC Vital Signs. Asthma in the US growing every year. May 2011 [Internet]. Available at *http://www.cdc.gov/VitalSigns/Asthma/index.html.*
4. World Health Organization. Asthma fact sheet No. 307. May 2011. Available from *http://www.who.int/mediacentre/factsheets/fs307/en/index.html.*
5. Pruitt K. Luchando por el Aire: The Burden of Asthma on Hispanics. Disparities in Health series. Available at *http://www.lungusa.org/lung-disease/disparities-reports/burden-of-asthma-on-hispanics/.*
6. Barnett SBL, Nurmagambetov TA. Control of asthma in the United States: 2002–2007. J Allergy Clin Immunol 2011;127:145–152.
7. Weiss KB, Sullivan SD. The health economics of asthma and rhinitis. I. Assessing the economic impact. J Allergy Clin Immunol 2001;107:3–8.
8. Reed CE. The natural history of asthma. J Allergy Clin Immunol 2006;110:543–548.
9. U.S. Department of Health and Human Services. Children and secondhand smoke exposure. Excerpts from the health consequences of involuntary exposure to tobacco smoke: A report of the Surgeon General. Atlanta, GA: U.S. Department of Health and Human Services, Centers for Disease Control and Prevention, Coordinating Center for Health Promotion, National Center for Chronic Disease Prevention and Health Promotion, Office on Smoking and Health, 2007. Available at *http://www.cdc.gov/tobacco.*
10. Busse WW, Lemanske RF Jr. Advances in immunology: Asthma. N Engl J Med 2001;344:350–362.
11. Larché M, Robinson DS, Kay AB. The role of T lymphocytes in the pathogenesis of asthma. J Allergy Clin Immunol 2003;111:450–463.
12. Robinson DS. The role of mast cells in asthma: Induction of airway hyperresponsiveness by interaction with smooth muscle? J Allergy Clin Immunol 2004;114:58–65.
13. Cohn L, Elias JA, Chupp GL. Asthma: Mechanisms of disease persistence and progression. Annu Rev Immunol 2004;22:789–815.
14. Bradding P, Walls AF, Holgate ST. The role of the mast cell in the pathophysiology of asthma. J Allergy Clin Immunol 2006;117:1277–1284.
15. Birnbaum S, Barreiro TJ. Methacholine challenge testing; identifying its diagnostic role, testing, coding, and reimbursement. Available at *http://chestjournal.chestpubs.org/content/131/6/1932.full.html.*
16. Lemanske RF Jr, Busse WW. Asthma. J Allergy Clin Immunol 2003;111:S502–S519.
17. Beckett PA, Howarth PH. Pharmacotherapy and airway remodeling in asthma? Thorax 2003;58:163–174.
18. Rodrigo GJ, Rodrigo C, Hall JB. Acute asthma in adults: A review. Chest 2004;125:1081–1102.
19. O'Connor GT. Allergen avoidance in asthma: What do we do now? J Allergy Clin Immunol 2005;116:26–30.
20. Asthma and Allergy Foundation of America. Tips to control indoor allergens. Available at *http://www.aafa.org/display.cfm?id=9&sub=18&cont=533.*
21. Respiratory Health Association of Metropolitan Chicago. What you need to know about … asthma and triggers. Available at *http://www.lungchicago.org/site/files/487/54229/419920/573653/Asthma_and_Triggers.pdf.*
22. Centers for Disease Control and Prevention. Flu and people with asthma. Available at *http://www.cdc.gov/flu/asthma/.*
23. Centers for Disease Control and Prevention. Updated recommendations for prevention of invasive pneumococcal disease among adults using the 23-valent pneumococcal polysaccharide vaccine (PPSV23). MMWR 2010;59(34):1102–1106.
24. Eneli I, Sadri K, Camargo C, et al. Acetaminophen and the risk of asth-ma: The epidemiologic and pathophysiologic evidence. Chest 2005;127:604–612.
25. Dolovich MB, Ahrens RC, Hess DR, et al. Device selection and outcomes of aerosol therapy: Evidence-based guidelines. Chest 2005;127:335–371.
26. Rubin BK. Pediatric aerosol therapy; new devices and new drugs. Respir Care 2011;56(9):1411–1421.
27. Proskocil BJ, Fryer AD. β_2-agonist and anticholinergic drugs in the treatment of lung disease. Proc Am Thorac Soc 2005;2:305–310,
28. Kelly HW. Levalbuterol for asthma: A better treatment? Curr Allergy Asthma Rep 2007;7:310–314.
29. Lemanske RF, Mauger DT, Sorkness CA. Step-up therapy for children with uncontrolled asthma receiving inhaled corticosteroids. N Engl J Med 2010;362:975–985.
30. Nelson HS, Weiss ST, Bleeker ER, et al, and the Smart Study Group. The salmeterol multicenter asthma research trial: A comparison of usual pharmacotherapy for asthma or usual pharmacotherapy plus salmeterol. Chest 2006;129:15–26.
31. Bateman E, Neslon H, Bousquet J, et al. Meta-analysis: Effects of adding salmeterol to inhaled corticosteroids on serious asthma-related events. Ann Intern Med 2008;149:33–42.
32. Kelly HW. Comparison of inhaled corticosteroids: An update. Ann Pharmacother 2009;43:519–527.
33. Kelly HW. Inhaled corticosteroid dosing: Doubling for nothing? J Allergy Clin Immunol 2011; 128:278–281.
34. Tomlinson JEM, McMahon AD, Chaudhuri R, et al. Efficacy of low and high dose inhaled corticosteroid in smokers versus non-smokers with mild asthma. Thorax 2005;60:282–287.
35. Martinez FD, Chinchilli VM, Morgan WJ. Use of beclomethasone dipropionate as rescue treatment for children with mild persistent asthma (TREXA): A randomized, double-blind, placebo-controlled trial. Lancet 2011;377:650–657.
36. Guilbert TW, Morgan WJ, Zeiger RS, et al. Long-term inhaled corticosteroids in preschool children at high risk for asthma. N Engl J Med 2006;354:1985–1997.
37. Tantisira KG, Lasky-Su J, Harada M. Genomewide association between GLCCI1 and response to glucocorticoid therapy in asthma. N Engl J Med 2011;365:1173–1183.
38. Rodrigo GJ, Castro-Rodrigo JA. Anticholinergics in the treatment of children and adults with acute asthma: A systematic review with meta-analysis. Thorax 2005;60:740–746.
39. Peters SP, Kunselman SJ, Icitovic N, et al. Tiotropium bromide step-up therapy for adults with uncontrolled asthma. N Engl J Med 2010;363:1715–1726.
40. Kerstjens HAM, Disse B, Schroder-Babo W, et al. Tiotropium improves lung function in patients with severe uncontrolled asthma: A randomized controlled trial. J Allergy Clin Immunol 2011;128:308–314.

41. Ogale SS, Lee TL, Au DH, et al. Cardiovascular events associated with ipratropium bromide in COPD. Chest 2010;137:13–19.

42. Celli B, Decramer M, Leimer I, et al. Cardiovascular safety of tiotropium in patients with COPD. Chest 2010;137:20–30.

43. Sorkness CA, Lemanske RF Jr, Mauger DT, et al. Long-term comparison of 3 controller regiments for mild-moderate persistent childhood asthma: The pediatric asthma controller trial. J Allergy Clin Immunol 2007;119:64–72.

44. Barnes PJ. Theophylline. New perspective on an old drug. Am J Respir Crit Care Med 2003;167:813–818.

45. Busse WW, Morgan WJ, Gergen PJ. Randomized trial of omalizumab (Anti-IgE) for asthma in inner-city children. N Engl J Med 2011;364: 1005–1015.

46. Kim HL, Leigh R, Becker A. Omalizumab: Practical considerations regarding the risk of anaphylaxis. Allergy Asthma Clin Immunol 2010; 6:32–41.

47. Rogers L, Reibman J. Stepping down asthma treatment: How and when. Curr Opin Pulm Med 2012;18(1):70–75.

48. Camargo CA Jr. Rachelefsky G, Schatz M. Managing asthma exacerbations in the emergency department: Summary of the National Asthma Education and Prevention Program Expert Panel Report 3 guidelines for the management of asthma exacerbations. Proc Am Thorac Soc 2009;6(4):357–366.

49. Agrawal SK, Singh M, Mathew JL, et al. Efficacy of an individualized written home-management plan in the control of moderate persistent asthma: A randomized, controlled trial. Acta Pediatr 2005;94:1742–1746.

50. American College of Obstetricians and Gynecologists (ACOG). Asthma in pregnancy. ACOG practice bulletin no. 90. Washington, DC: American College of Obstetricians and Gynecologists, February 2008.

51. James J. Safety of budesonide inhalation suspension in infants aged six to twelve months with mild to moderate persistent asthma or recurrent wheeze. Pediatrics 2006;118:S41.

15 Chronic Obstructive Pulmonary Disease

Tara R. Whetsel and Nicole D. Verkleeren

LEARNING OBJECTIVES

● **Upon completion of the chapter, the reader will be able to:**

1. Describe the pathophysiology of chronic obstructive pulmonary disease (COPD).

2. Identify signs and symptoms of COPD.

3. List the treatment goals for a patient with COPD.

4. Design an appropriate COPD treatment regimen based on patient-specific data.

5. Develop a monitoring plan to assess effectiveness and adverse effects of pharmacotherapy for COPD.

6. Formulate an appropriate education plan for a patient with COPD.

KEY CONCEPTS

❶ Inflammation plays a key role in the pathophysiology of chronic obstructive pulmonary disease (COPD), but it differs from that seen in asthma; therefore, the use of and response to anti-inflammatory medications are different.

❷ An integrated approach of health maintenance (e.g., smoking cessation), drug therapy, and supplemental therapy (e.g., oxygen and pulmonary rehabilitation) should be used in a stepwise manner. Symptom severity and risk of COPD exacerbations can be used to guide therapy decisions.

❸ Smoking cessation slows the rate of decline in pulmonary function in patients with COPD.

❹ Bronchodilators are the mainstay of treatment for symptomatic COPD. They reduce symptoms and improve exercise tolerance and quality of life.

❺ Inhaled corticosteroids are recommended for patients with severe and very severe COPD and frequent exacerbations that are not adequately controlled by long-acting bronchodilators.

❻ Antibiotics should be used in patients with COPD exacerbations who: (a) have all three cardinal symptoms (increased dyspnea, increased sputum volume, and increased purulence); (b) have increased sputum purulence and one other cardinal symptom; or (c) experience a severe exacerbation requiring mechanical ventilation.

INTRODUCTION

Chronic obstructive pulmonary disease (COPD) is a progressive disease characterized by airflow limitation that is not fully reversible. It is caused by exposure to noxious particles or gases, most commonly cigarette smoke. It is a major cause of morbidity and mortality and a leading cause of disability in the United States.

Previous definitions of COPD included chronic bronchitis and emphysema. Chronic bronchitis is defined clinically as a chronic productive cough for at least 3 months in each of two consecutive years in a patient in whom other causes have been excluded.[1] Chronic bronchitis can exist in patients with normal spirometry and may precede the development of COPD. Emphysema is defined pathologically as destruction of alveoli.[1] The major risk factor for both conditions is cigarette smoking, and many patients share characteristics of each condition. Therefore, guidelines have moved away from using these subsets and instead focus on chronic airflow limitation.

The Global Initiative for Chronic Obstructive Lung Disease (GOLD) is an expert panel of health professionals who have developed a consensus document with recommendations for the diagnosis and care of patients with COPD.[1] The online document is updated annually and is commonly referred to as the GOLD guidelines. Major revisions were released in January 2012. The American College of Physicians (ACP), American College of Chest Physicians (ACCP), American Thoracic Society (ATS), and European Respiratory Society (ERS) have jointly published guidelines for the diagnosis

305

and management of stable COPD.[2] The GOLD guidelines are more comprehensive and include recommendations for managing exacerbations and comorbidities, whereas the ACP guidelines provide a more thorough review of major clinical trials impacting recommendations.

EPIDEMIOLOGY AND ETIOLOGY

In 2008, 13.1 million U.S. adults 18 years of age and older were estimated to have COPD.[3] The true prevalence is larger; COPD is underdiagnosed because many patients have few or no symptoms in the early stages.

COPD is the third leading cause of death in the United States; in 2007, 124,477 adults died from the disease.[3] In 2010, COPD was estimated to cost the United States $49.9 billion, with direct medical costs accounting for $29.5 billion of the total.[3] Morbidity, mortality, and costs are all expected to increase; by 2030, it is expected to be the fourth leading cause of death worldwide.[1]

Exposures and host factors play a role in the development of COPD. Cigarette smoking is the leading cause of COPD and accounts for 80% to 90% of cases in developed countries.[4] Environmental tobacco smoke (i.e., secondhand smoke) may increase the risk of COPD.[1] Occupational exposure to dusts and chemicals (vapors, irritants, and fumes) also plays a role. Environmental air pollution has been implicated as an etiologic factor, but its exact role is unclear. Not all smokers develop clinically significant COPD, which suggests that genetic susceptibility plays a role. The best documented genetic factor is a rare hereditary deficiency of α_1-antitrypsin (AAT). Severe deficiency of this enzyme results in premature and accelerated development of emphysema. Asthma and airway hyperresponsiveness have been identified as risk factors, but how they influence the development of COPD is unknown. Failure to reach maximal lung function, due to recurrent infections or exposure to tobacco smoke during childhood, may also increase the risk of COPD.

PATHOPHYSIOLOGY

COPD is characterized by pathologic changes in the central airways, peripheral airways, lung parenchyma, and pulmonary vasculature. Chronic inflammation in the lung from repeated exposure to noxious particles and gases is primarily responsible for these changes.[1] An imbalance between proteinases and antiproteinases in the lung and oxidative stress are also thought to be important in the pathogenesis of COPD. These processes may be a result of ongoing inflammation or may arise from environmental (e.g., oxidants in cigarette smoke) or genetic (e.g., AAT deficiency) factors (Fig. 15–1).[1] In addition to these destructive processes, chronic inflammation and exposure to noxious particles and gases disrupts or impairs the normal protective and repair mechanisms.

Inflammation is present in the lungs of all smokers. It is unclear why only 15% to 20% of smokers develop

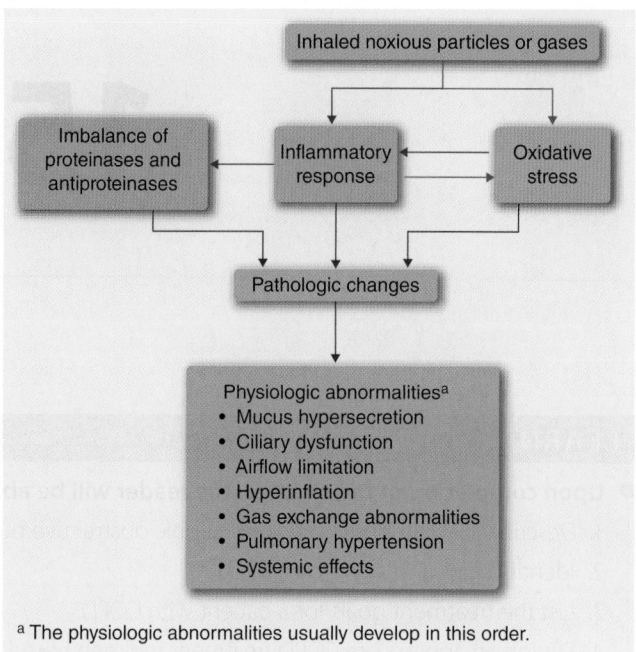

FIGURE 15–1. Pathophysiology of COPD.

COPD, but susceptible individuals appear to have an exaggerated inflammatory response.[5] ❶ *The inflammation of COPD differs from that seen in asthma, so the use of and response to anti-inflammatory medications are different.* The inflammation of asthma is mainly mediated through eosinophils and mast cells. In COPD, the primary inflammatory cells include neutrophils, macrophages, and CD8[+] T lymphocytes.[6] Eosinophils may be increased in some patients, particularly during exacerbations. Activated inflammatory cells release a variety of mediators, most notably leukotriene B$_4$, interleukin-8, and tumor necrosis factor-α (TNF-α) Various proteinases, such as elastase, cathepsin G, and proteinase-3, are secreted by activated neutrophils. These mediators and proteinases are capable of sustaining inflammation and damaging lung structures.

Proteinases and antiproteinases are part of the normal protective and repair mechanisms in the lungs. The imbalance of proteinase–antiproteinase activity in COPD is a result of either increased production or activity of destructive proteinases or inactivation or reduced production of protective antiproteinases. AAT (an antiproteinase) inhibits trypsin, elastase, and several other proteolytic enzymes. Deficiency of AAT results in unopposed proteinase activity, which promotes destruction of alveolar walls and lung parenchyma, leading to emphysema.

Markers of oxidative stress (e.g., hydrogen peroxide, nitric oxide, and 8-isoprostane) have been found in the epithelial fluid, breath, and urine of cigarette smokers and patients with COPD.[1] Increased oxidative stress contributes to COPD in a variety of ways. Oxidants (e.g., reactive oxygen species, superoxide, and nitric oxide) can react with and damage a variety of molecules leading to cell dysfunction and damage to the lung extracellular matrix. Oxidative stress promotes inflammation and contributes to the proteinase–antiproteinase imbalance by reducing antiproteinase activity. In addition, oxidants constrict airway smooth muscle, contributing to reversible airway narrowing.

In the central airways (the trachea, bronchi, and bronchioles greater than 2 to 4 mm in internal diameter), inflammatory cells and mediators stimulate mucus-secreting gland hyperplasia and mucus hypersecretion. Mucus hypersecretion and ciliary dysfunction lead to chronic cough and sputum production. The major site of airflow obstruction is the peripheral airways (small bronchi and bronchioles with an internal diameter less than 2 mm). Three mechanisms are postulated to be involved in the narrowing of these small airways.[5] First, airways may be blocked by inflammatory exudates and mucus hypersecretion. Second, loss of elasticity and destruction of alveolar attachments leads to loss of support and closure of small airways during expiration. Third, infiltration of inflammatory cells, increased smooth muscle tissue, and fibrosis cause thickening of airway walls. Of these three mechanisms, the structural changes in the airway walls are the most important cause of fixed airflow obstruction.

As airflow obstruction worsens, the rate of lung emptying is slowed and the interval between inspirations does not allow expiration to the relaxation volume of the lungs. This leads to pulmonary hyperinflation, which initially only occurs during exercise but later is also seen at rest. Hyperinflation contributes to the discomfort associated with airflow obstruction by flattening the diaphragm and placing it at a mechanical disadvantage.

In advanced COPD, airflow obstruction, damaged bronchioles and alveoli, and pulmonary vascular abnormalities lead to impaired gas exchange. This results in hypoxemia and eventually hypercapnia. Hypoxemia is initially present only during exercise but occurs at rest as the disease progresses. Inequality in the ventilation-to-perfusion ratio (V_A/Q) is the major mechanism behind hypoxemia in COPD. As hypoxemia worsens, the body may compensate by increasing the production of erythrocytes in an attempt to increase oxygen delivery to tissues.

Pulmonary hypertension develops late in the course of COPD, usually after the development of severe hypoxemia. It is the most common cardiovascular complication of COPD and can result in cor pulmonale, or right-sided heart failure. Hypoxemia plays the primary role in the development of pulmonary hypertension by causing vasoconstriction of the pulmonary arteries and promoting vessel wall remodeling. Destruction of the pulmonary capillary bed by emphysema further contributes by increasing the pressure required to perfuse the pulmonary vascular bed. Cor pulmonale is associated with venous stasis and thrombosis that may result in pulmonary embolism. Another important systemic effect is the progressive loss of skeletal muscle mass, which contributes to exercise limitations and declining health status. These extrapulmonary effects may contribute to disease severity and should not be overlooked.

CLINICAL PRESENTATION AND DIAGNOSIS

See text box on the next page for the clinical presentation of COPD.

Diagnosis

A suspected diagnosis of COPD should be based on the patient's symptoms and history of exposure to risk factors. Spirometry is required to confirm the diagnosis, using the ratio of forced expiratory volume in 1 second (FEV_1) to forced vital capacity (FVC). A postbronchodilator FEV_1/FVC ratio less than 70% confirms airflow limitation that is not fully reversible.[1,2] Spirometry results can further be used to classify severity of airflow limitation (Table 15–1). Full pulmonary function tests (PFTs) with lung volumes and diffusion capacity and arterial blood gases (ABGs) are not necessary to establish the diagnosis or severity of COPD.

Table 15–1	
GOLD Classification of Severity of Airflow Limitation in Patients with FEV_1/FVC Less Than 70%	
Classification	**Postbronchodilator FEV_1**
GOLD 1: Mild	80% predicted or greater
GOLD 2: Moderate	50–79% predicted
GOLD 3: Severe	30–49% predicted
GOLD 4: Very severe	Less than 30% predicted

FEV_1, forced expiratory volume in 1 second; FVC, forced vital capacity; GOLD, Global Initiative for Chronic Obstructive Lung Disease.

From GOLD Science Committee. Global strategy for the diagnosis, management, and prevention of chronic obstructive pulmonary disease, revised 2011, *www.goldcopd.com.*

Patient Encounter, Part 1

MB, a 58-year-old woman with a medical history of osteoarthritis, presents to the clinic complaining of shortness of breath and cough that began 3 or 4 years ago. Her symptoms have gradually worsened over the past year. She is only able to walk one flight of stairs without getting short of breath. In the morning she has a cough associated with yellowish phlegm production. She is a current smoker of about one and a half packs of cigarettes a day and has done so for the last 38 years. She drinks on average one beer a day. She denies any recreational drug use. She does not have any significant occupational exposures to dust, gases, or fumes.

What information is suggestive of COPD?

What risk factors does she have for COPD?

What additional information do you need to create a treatment plan for this patient?

Clinical Presentation of COPD

General

- Patients with COPD are asymptomatic initially. The disease is usually not diagnosed until declining lung function leads to significant symptoms and prompts patients to seek medical care.

Symptoms

- The onset of symptoms is variable and does not correlate well with severity of airflow limitation measured by FEV_1.[1]
- Initial symptoms include chronic cough (for more than 3 months) that may be intermittent at first, chronic sputum production, and dyspnea on exertion.
- As COPD progresses, dyspnea at rest develops and the ability to perform activities of daily living declines.

Signs

- Observation of the patient may reveal use of accessory muscles of respiration (manifested as paradoxical movements of the chest and abdomen, in a seesaw-type motion), pursed-lips breathing, and hyperinflation of the chest with increased anterior–posterior diameter ("barrel chest").
- On lung auscultation, patients may have distant breath sounds, wheezing, a prolonged expiratory phase, and rhonchi.

- In advanced COPD, signs of hypoxemia may include cyanosis and tachycardia.
- Signs of cor pulmonale include increased pulmonic component of the second heart sound, jugular venous distention (JVD), lower extremity edema, and hepatomegaly.

Laboratory Tests

- Hematocrit may be elevated and may exceed 55% (0.55) (polycythemia).
- Pulse oximetry should be obtained in patients with an FEV_1 less than 35% predicted or signs or symptoms suggestive of cor pulmonale or respiratory failure.[1] If oxygen saturation is less than 92%, ABGs should be assessed. COPD patients characteristically exhibit normal or increased arterial carbon dioxide tension ($Paco_2$) and decreased arterial oxygen tension (Pao_2).
- An AAT level should be obtained in younger patients (less than 45 years old) presenting with COPD signs and symptoms, especially if there is a strong family history of emphysema.

It is important to distinguish COPD from asthma because treatment and prognosis differ. Differentiating factors include age of onset, smoking history, triggers, occupational history, and degree of reversibility measured by pre- and postbronchodilator spirometry. In some patients, a clear distinction between asthma and COPD is not possible. Management of these patients should be similar to that of asthma. Bronchiectasis, cystic fibrosis, obliterative bronchiolitis, congestive heart failure, and tuberculosis are other possible differential diagnoses that are usually easier to distinguish from COPD. Chest radiography or high-resolution computed tomography (CT) along with patient presentation help rule out these other lung diseases.

TREATMENT

Desired Outcomes

The goals of COPD management include: (a) smoking cessation, (b) reducing symptoms, (c) improving exercise tolerance, (d) minimizing the rate of decline in lung function, (e) maintaining or improving the quality of life, (f) preventing and treating exacerbations, and (g) limiting complications.

General Approach to Treatment

❷ *An integrated approach of health maintenance (e.g., smoking cessation), drug therapy, and supplemental therapy (e.g., oxygen and pulmonary rehabilitation) should be used in a stepwise manner. Symptom severity and risk of COPD exacerbations can be used to guide therapy decisions* (Table 15–2). **Figure 15–2** provides an overview of the management of stable COPD.

Nonpharmacologic Therapy

▶ Smoking Cessation

❸ *Smoking cessation slows the rate of decline in pulmonary function in patients with COPD.*[7,8] Stopping smoking can also reduce cough and sputum production and decrease airway reactivity. Therefore, it is a critical part of any treatment plan for patients with COPD. Unfortunately, achieving and maintaining cessation is a major challenge. A clinical practice guideline from the U.S. Public Health Service recommends a specific action plan depending on the current smoking status and desire to quit (**Fig. 15–3**).[9] Brief interventions are effective and can increase cessation rates significantly. The five As and the five Rs can be used to guide brief interventions (**Table 15–3**).

Table 15–2

Assessment of Symptoms and Future Risk of Exacerbations

Patient Category[a]	Characteristics	Spirometric Classification	Exacerbations Per Year	mMRC Grade	CAT Score
A	Low risk, fewer symptoms	GOLD 1 or 2	0–1	0–1	Less than 10
B	Low risk, more symptoms	GOLD 1 or 2	0–1	2 or more	10 or more
C	High risk, fewer symptoms	GOLD 3 or 4	2 or more	0–1	Less than 10
D	High risk, more symptoms	GOLD 3 or 4	2 or more	2 or more	10 or more

mMRC, modified Medical Research Council Questionnaire; CAT, COPD Assessment Test; GOLD, Global Initiative for Chronic Obstructive Lung Disease.

[a]When assessing risk, choose the highest risk according to spirometric classification or exacerbations per year. For symptom assessment, use mMRC or CAT; CAT is preferred because it provides a more comprehensive assessment. It is unnecessary to use both mMRC and CAT.

From GOLD Science Committee. Global strategy for the diagnosis, management, and prevention of chronic obstructive pulmonary disease, revised 2011, *www.goldcopd.com.*

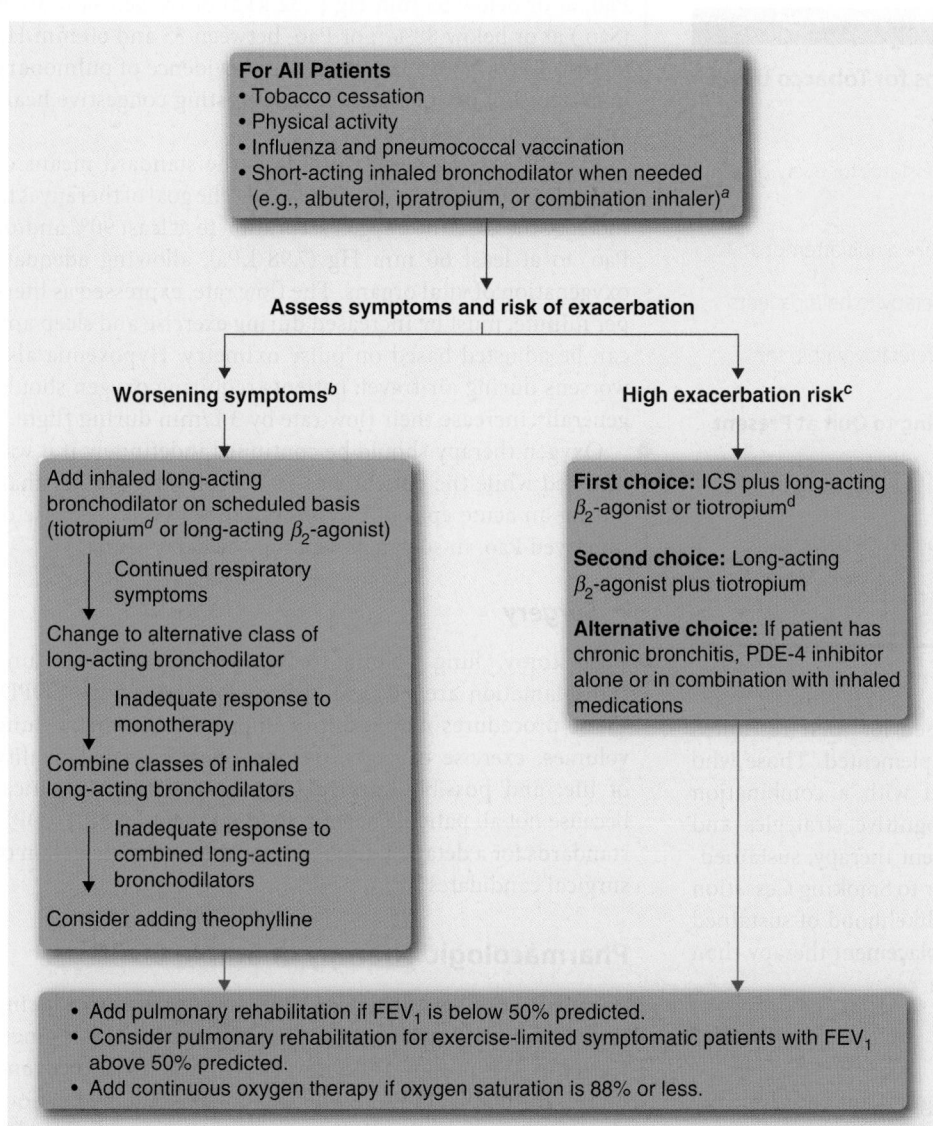

For All Patients
- Tobacco cessation
- Physical activity
- Influenza and pneumococcal vaccination
- Short-acting inhaled bronchodilator when needed (e.g., albuterol, ipratropium, or combination inhaler)[a]

Assess symptoms and risk of exacerbation

Worsening symptoms[b]

Add inhaled long-acting bronchodilator on scheduled basis (tiotropium[d] or long-acting β_2-agonist)

Continued respiratory symptoms

Change to alternative class of long-acting bronchodilator

Inadequate response to monotherapy

Combine classes of inhaled long-acting bronchodilators

Inadequate response to combined long-acting bronchodilators

Consider adding theophylline

High exacerbation risk[c]

First choice: ICS plus long-acting β_2-agonist or tiotropium[d]

Second choice: Long-acting β_2-agonist plus tiotropium

Alternative choice: If patient has chronic bronchitis, PDE-4 inhibitor alone or in combination with inhaled medications

- Add pulmonary rehabilitation if FEV$_1$ is below 50% predicted.
- Consider pulmonary rehabilitation for exercise-limited symptomatic patients with FEV$_1$ above 50% predicted.
- Add continuous oxygen therapy if oxygen saturation is 88% or less.

FIGURE 15–2. Treatment Algorithm for Stable COPD.[1,2] (ICS, inhaled corticosteroid; PDE-4, phosphodiesterase-4; FEV$_1$, forced expiratory volume in 1 second.) [a]GOLD patient category A. [b]GOLD patient category B. [c]GOLD patient category C or D. [d]Albuterol should be used as rescue therapy for patients treated with tiotropium.

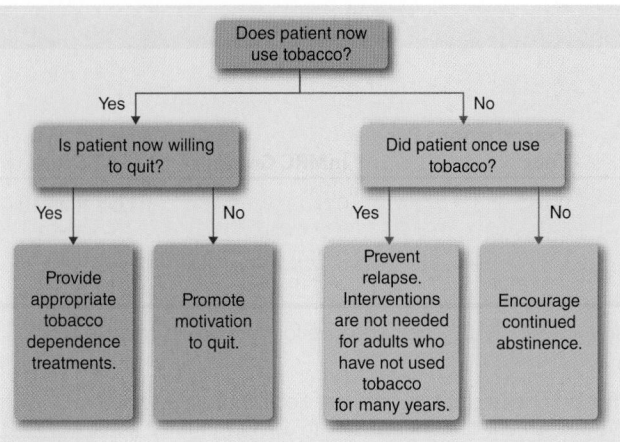

FIGURE 15–3. Algorithm for routine assessment of tobacco use status. (From Fiore MC, Jaén CR, Baker TB, et al. Treating tobacco use and dependence. Clinical Practice Guideline. U.S. Department of Health and Human Services, 2008, *www. surgeongeneral.gov/tobacco/treating_tobacco_use08.pdf*.)

Table 15–3

Components of Brief Interventions for Tobacco Users

The 5 As for Brief Intervention

Ask: Identify and document tobacco-use status for every patient at every visit

Advise: Urge every tobacco user to quit

Assess: Is the tobacco user willing to make a quit attempt at this time?

Assist: Use counseling and pharmacotherapy to help patients willing to make a quit attempt

Arrange: Schedule follow-up contact, preferably within the first week after the quit date

The 5 Rs to Motivate Smokers Unwilling to Quit at Present

Relevance: Tailor advice and discussion to each smoker

Risks: Help the patient identify potential negative consequences of tobacco use

Rewards: Help the patient identify the potential benefits of quitting

Roadblocks: Help the patient identify barriers to quitting

Repetition: Repeat the motivational message at every visit

All tobacco users should be assessed for their readiness to quit and appropriate strategies implemented. Those who are ready to quit should be treated with a combination of counseling on behavioral and cognitive strategies and pharmacotherapy (nicotine replacement therapy, sustained-release bupropion, or varenicline; refer to Smoking Cessation in Chap. 36). In COPD patients, the likelihood of sustained abstinence is higher with nicotine replacement therapy than that with sustained-release bupropion.[10]

▶ *Pulmonary Rehabilitation*

Pulmonary rehabilitation results in significant and clinically meaningful improvements in dyspnea, exercise capacity, health status, and healthcare utilization.[11] It should be prescribed for symptomatic patients with an FEV_1 less than 50% predicted.[2] Clinicians may consider pulmonary rehabilitation for symptomatic patients with an FEV_1 above 50% predicted, but evidence of benefit is less clear. A comprehensive pulmonary rehabilitation program should include exercise training, smoking cessation, nutrition counseling, and education.

Rehabilitation programs may be conducted in the inpatient, outpatient (most common), or home setting. The minimum length of an effective program is 6 weeks; the longer the program, the more sustained the results.[1,11] It is important for patients to continue with a home exercise program to maintain the benefits gained from the pulmonary rehabilitation program.

▶ *Long-Term Oxygen Therapy*

Long-term administration of oxygen (more than 15 hours/day) to patients with chronic respiratory failure has been shown to reduce mortality and improve quality of life.[1,2] Oxygen therapy should be initiated in stable patients with COPD who have severe resting hypoxemia as determined by Pao_2 at or below 55 mm Hg (7.32 kPa) or oxygen saturation (Sao_2) at or below 88%[1,2]; or Pao_2 between 55 and 60 mm Hg (7.32 to 7.98 kPa) or Sao_2 of 89% and evidence of pulmonary hypertension, peripheral edema suggesting congestive heart failure, or polycythemia.[1]

The dual-prong nasal cannula is the standard means of delivering continuous flow of oxygen. The goal of therapy is to increase the baseline oxygen saturation to at least 90% and/or Pao_2 to at least 60 mm Hg (7.98 kPa), allowing adequate oxygenation of vital organs. The flow rate, expressed as liters per minute, must be increased during exercise and sleep and can be adjusted based on pulse oximetry. Hypoxemia also worsens during air travel; patients requiring oxygen should generally increase their flow rate by 3 L/min during flight.[1]

Oxygen therapy should be continued indefinitely if it was initiated while the patient was in a stable state (rather than during an acute episode). Withdrawal of oxygen because of improved Pao_2 in such a patient may be detrimental.

▶ *Surgery*

Bullectomy, lung volume reduction surgery, and lung transplantation are surgical options for very severe COPD. These procedures may result in improved spirometry, lung volumes, exercise capacity, dyspnea, health-related quality of life, and possibly survival. Patient selection is critical because not all patients benefit. Refer to the ATS/ERS COPD standards for a detailed discussion of appropriate selection of surgical candidates.[12]

Pharmacologic Therapy of Stable COPD

The medications available for COPD are effective for reducing or relieving symptoms, improving exercise tolerance, reducing the number and severity of exacerbations, and improving quality of life. Evidence showing that medications slow the rate of decline in lung function is inconclusive.[1,2]

▶ *Bronchodilators*

4 *Bronchodilators are the mainstay of treatment for symptomatic COPD. They reduce symptoms and improve exercise tolerance and quality of life.*[1] They can be used as needed for symptoms or on a scheduled basis to prevent or reduce symptoms. Bronchodilator drugs commonly used in COPD include β_2-agonists, anticholinergics, and theophylline. The choice depends on availability, individual response, side-effect profile, and preferences. The inhaled route is preferred, but attention must be paid to proper inhaler technique training. Long-acting bronchodilators are more expensive than short-acting bronchodilators but are superior on important clinical outcomes, including frequency of exacerbations, degree of dyspnea, and health-related quality of life.[1,13] Monotherapy with long-acting bronchodilators is preferred; combination therapy may be appropriate in symptomatic patients with an FEV_1 less than 60% predicted, although it is unclear when combination therapy provides added benefit.[2]

β_2-Agonists β_2-Agonists cause airway smooth muscle relaxation by stimulating adenyl cyclase to increase the formation of cyclic adenosine monophosphate (cAMP). They may also improve mucociliary transport. β_2-Agonists are available in inhalation, oral, and parenteral dosage forms; the inhalation route is preferred because of fewer adverse effects.

These drugs are also available in short-acting and long-acting formulations (Table 15–4). The short-acting β_2-agonists include albuterol (known as salbutamol outside the United States), levalbuterol (known as R-salbutamol outside the United States), and terbutaline. They are used as "rescue" therapy for acute symptom relief. Most COPD patients need continuous bronchodilator therapy on a scheduled basis every day. For these patients, short-acting β_2-agonists are inconvenient because of the need for frequent dosing. In addition, short-acting β_2-agonists have been associated with a slight, but statistically significant, loss of effectiveness when used regularly longer than 3 months (tachyphylaxis).[14]

Long-acting β_2-agonists include salmeterol, formoterol, arformoterol, and indacaterol. Salmeterol is a partial agonist with a slower onset of action than short-acting β_2-agonists. Formoterol is a more complete agonist and has an onset of action similar to that of albuterol. Arformoterol is the (R,R)-isomer of formoterol; both are available for nebulization, providing an alternative for patients with poor inhaler technique. Indacaterol is a partial agonist with a fast onset of action similar to that of albuterol. Full agonists (formoterol and arformoterol) produce greater response at full receptor capacity than partial agonists (salmeterol and indacaterol). Bronchodilator effects of long-acting β_2-agonists last at least 12 hours except for indacaterol, which has a 24-hour duration of action. The U.S. FDA approved indacaterol at a lower dose (75 mcg) than that used in other countries. The effect of this lower dose on the rate of exacerbations is unknown. Formoterol and salmeterol decrease COPD exacerbations and improve exercise tolerance, dyspnea,

and quality of life.[13] Patients treated with long-acting β_2-agonists should also have a short-acting β_2-agonist such as albuterol available for as-needed use ("rescue" medication).

Adverse effects of both long- and short-acting β_2-agonists are dose related and include palpitations, tachycardia, hypokalemia, and tremor. Sleep disturbance may also occur and appears to be worse with higher doses of inhaled long-acting β_2-agonists. Increasing doses beyond those clinically recommended is without benefit and could be associated with increased adverse effects. Patients should be advised to avoid excessive use of short-acting β_2-agonists while being treated with long-acting β_2-agonists.

Anticholinergics Ipratropium and tiotropium are inhaled anticholinergic medications commonly used for COPD. They produce bronchodilation by competitively blocking muscarinic receptors in bronchial smooth muscle. They may also decrease mucus secretion, although this effect is variable. Tiotropium dissociates from receptors extremely slowly, resulting in a half-life longer than 36 hours, allowing for once-daily dosing. Ipratropium has an elimination half-life of about 2 hours, necessitating dosing every 6 to 8 hours.

Tiotropium significantly decreases exacerbations and related hospitalizations, reduces symptoms, and improves quality of life compared with placebo or ipratropium.[15] When added to other respiratory medications for COPD, tiotropium reduces the rate of exacerbations, increases the time to first exacerbation, improves dyspnea, and reduces the incidence of respiratory failure compared with placebo.[16] Tiotropium may be more effective than salmeterol for reducing exacerbations in patients with moderate to very severe COPD.[17] Other comparative studies and meta-analyses have found little to no differences among long-acting bronchodilators.[1,2] Patients using tiotropium as maintenance therapy should be prescribed albuterol as their rescue therapy. The combination of ipratropium and tiotropium is not recommended because of the risks of excessive anticholinergic effects.

Inhaled anticholinergics are well tolerated with the most common adverse effect being dry mouth. Occasional metallic taste has also been reported with ipratropium. Other anticholinergic adverse effects include constipation, tachycardia, blurred vision, and precipitation of narrow-angle glaucoma symptoms. Urinary retention could be a problem, especially for those with concurrent bladder outlet obstruction. Earlier studies suggested that inhaled anticholinergics may increase the risk of myocardial infarction and cardiovascular death in patients with COPD.[18,19] More recent large trials of tiotropium have found no increased cardiovascular risk.[16,17]

Methylxanthines Theophylline is a nonspecific phosphodiesterase inhibitor that increases intracellular cAMP within airway smooth muscle resulting in bronchodilation. It has a modest bronchodilator effect in patients with COPD, and its use is limited due to a narrow therapeutic index, multiple drug interactions, and adverse effects. Theophylline should be reserved for patients who cannot use inhaled medications or who remain symptomatic despite appropriate use of inhaled bronchodilators.

Table 15–4

Maintenance Medications for COPD

	Medication	Onset	Peak	Duration	Usual Dose
Short-Acting β₂-Agonists	Albuterol[a]				
	Nebulization	5–15 minutes	0.5–2 hours	2–6 hours	2.5 mg every 6–8 hours (max: 30 mg/day)
	Inhalation	5–15 minutes	0.5–2 hours	2–6 hours	MDI (90 mcg/puff) 1–2 puffs every 4–6 hours (max: 1,080 mcg/day)
	Oral	7–30 minutes	2–3 hours	4–6 hours ER: 8–12 hours	2–4 mg 3–4 times a day ER: 4–8 mg every 12 hours (max: 32 mg/day)
	Levalbuterol				
	Nebulization	10–20 minutes	1.5 hours	5–8 hours	0.63–1.25 mg 3 times/day, 6–8 hours apart (max: 3.75 mg/day)
	Inhalation	5–10 minutes	1–1.5 hours	3–6 hours	MDI (45 mcg/puff) 1–2 puffs every 4–6 hours (max: 540 mcg/day)
	Terbutaline				
	Oral	0.5–2 hours	1–3 hours	6–8 hours	2.5–5 mg 3 times/day, 6 hours apart[b] (max: 15 mg/day)
Long-Acting β₂-Agonists	Formoterol				
	Inhalation	1–3 minutes	1–3 hours	12 hours	Powder (12 mcg/inhalation) 1 inhalation every 12 hours (max: 24 mcg/day)
	Nebulization	1–3 minutes	1–3 hours	12 hours	20 mcg every 12 hours (max: 40 mcg/day)
	Salmeterol				
	Inhalation	10 minutes to 2 hours	2–5 hours	12 hours	Powder (50 mcg/inhalation) 1 inhalation every 12 hours (max: 100 mcg/day)
	Indacaterol				
	Inhalation	5 minutes	1–4 hours	24 hours	Powder (75 mcg/inhalation) 1 inhalation every 24 hours (max: 75 mcg/day)
	Arformoterol				
	Nebulization	7–20 minutes	1–3 hours	12 hours	15 mcg every 12 hours (max: 30 mcg/day)
Short-Acting Anticholinergic	Ipratropium				
	Nebulization	1–30 minutes	1.5–2 hours	4–6 hours	500 mcg every 6–8 hours (max: 2,000 mcg/day)
	Inhalation	1–30 minutes	1.5–2 hours	4–6 hours	MDI (18 mcg/puff) 2 puffs 4 times/day (max: 216 mcg/day)
Long-Acting Anticholinergic	Tiotropium				
	Inhalation	30 minutes	1–4 hours	24 hours	Powder (18 mcg/inhalation) 1 inhalation every 24 hours (max: 18 mcg/day)[c]
Methylxanthine	Theophylline				
	Oral	0.5–2 hours	Up to 24 hours, depending on formulation	6–24 hours	400–600 mg/day divided every 6–24 hours based on formulation (max: 800 mg/day) Adjust dose to serum concentrations of 5–15 mcg/mL (5–15 mg/L; 28–83 μmol/L)
Phosphodiesterase-4 Inhibitor	Roflumilast				
	Oral	4 weeks	—	—	500 mcg daily[d]
Inhaled Corticosteroids	Beclomethasone	1–7 days	1–4 weeks		MDI (40, 80 mcg/puff) 40–160 mcg twice a day (max: 640 mcg/day)
	Budesonide	1–7 days	1–2 weeks		Powder (90, 180 mcg/inhalation) 180–360 mcg twice a day (max: 1,440 mcg/day)
	Ciclesonide	1–7 days	1–4 weeks		MDI (80, 160 mcg/puff) 80–320 mcg 1 or 2 times/day (max: 640 mcg/day)

(Continued)

Table 15–4

Maintenance Medications for COPD (*Continued*)

Medication	Onset	Peak	Duration	Usual Dose
Fluticasone	1–7 days	1–2 weeks		MDI (44, 110, 220 mcg/puff) 88–440 mcg twice a day (max: 1,760 mcg/day) Powder (50, 100, 250 mcg/inhalation) 100–1000 mcg twice a day (max: 2,000 mcg/day)
Mometasone	1–7 days	1–2 weeks		Powder (110, 220 mcg/inhalation) 220–440 mcg 1 or 2 times/day (max: 880 mcg/day)

In elderly patients, start with the lowest recommended dose and increase as necessary.

ER, extended-release; MDI, metered-dose inhaler.

[a]Albuterol is known as salbutamol outside the United States.

[b]Not recommended if creatinine clearance (CrCl) less than or equal to 10 mL/min (0.17 mL/s); for CrCl 11–50 mL/min (0.18–0.83 mL/s), reduce dose by 50%.

[c]Patients with reduced activity in the CYP2D6 pathway (poor metabolizers [PMs]) have higher plasma concentrations than those with normal activity (extensive metabolizers [EMs]); PMs may require lower doses and should be monitored closely for adverse effects.

[d]Not recommended in patients with moderate or severe hepatic impairment.

Theophylline's bronchodilatory effects depend on achieving adequate serum concentrations, and therapeutic drug monitoring is needed to optimize therapy because of wide interpatient variability. If theophylline is used, serum concentrations in the range of 5 to 15 mcg/mL (5 to 15 mg/L; 28 to 83 μmol/L) provide adequate clinical response with a greater margin of safety than the traditionally recommended range of 10 to 20 mcg/mL (10 to 20 mg/L; 55 to 111 μmol/L). The most common adverse effects include heartburn, restlessness, insomnia, irritability, tachycardia, and tremor. Dose-related adverse effects include nausea and vomiting, seizures, and arrhythmias.

Tobacco smoke contains chemicals that induce the cytochrome P-450 isoenzymes 1A1, 1A2, and 2E1. Theophylline is metabolized by 1A2 and 2E1, and therefore smoking leads to increased clearance and subsequently decreased plasma levels of the drug.[20] Because most patients with COPD are current or past smokers, it is important to assess current tobacco use and adjust the theophylline dose as required based on altered plasma theophylline levels if tobacco use changes.

▶ Corticosteroids

Inhaled corticosteroids improve symptoms, lung function, quality of life, and exacerbation rates in patients with an FEV_1 less than 60%.[1,2] They do not appear to modify the rate of decline in pulmonary function or improve mortality.[1,21] Inhaled corticosteroids are recommended for patients with severe and very severe COPD and frequent exacerbations that are not adequately controlled by long-acting bronchodilators.[1] Monotherapy with inhaled corticosteroids is less effective than when combined with a long-acting β_2-agonist and is therefore not recommended.[1] Combination inhaler devices

(Advair [fluticasone/salmeterol], Symbicort [budesonide/formoterol], and Dulera [mometasone/formoterol]) are convenient and ensure patients receive both medications.

The most common adverse effects from inhaled corticosteroids include oropharyngeal candidiasis and hoarse voice. These can be minimized by rinsing the mouth after use and by using a spacer device with metered-dose inhalers (MDIs). Increased bruising, decreased bone density, and increased incidence of pneumonia have also been reported; the clinical importance of these effects remains uncertain.[1,2,21] Upon discontinuation of inhaled corticosteroids, some patients may experience deterioration in lung function and an increase in dyspnea and mild exacerbations.[22]

Long-term use of oral corticosteroids should be avoided due to an unfavorable risk-to-benefit ratio. The steroid myopathy that can result from long-term use of oral corticosteroids weakens muscles, further decreasing the respiratory drive in patients with advanced disease.

▶ Phosphodiesterase-4 Inhibitors

Phosphodiesterase (PDE)-4 inhibitors are believed to reduce inflammation by inhibiting the breakdown of cAMP. They do not cause direct bronchodilation. Roflumilast is an oral PDE-4 inhibitor approved for prevention of COPD exacerbations in patients with severe COPD associated with chronic bronchitis and a history of exacerbations. Roflumilast has more frequent adverse events than inhaled treatment options and only a modest benefit in lung function and exacerbation rate.[1,23] Common adverse effects include diarrhea, weight loss, nausea, headache, insomnia, decreased appetite, and abdominal pain; neuropsychiatric effects such as anxiety and depression have also been reported.

Roflumilast is an option in select patients who are not adequately controlled by long-acting bronchodilators.[1]

▶ Combination Therapy

For patients who remain symptomatic on monotherapy, a combination of bronchodilators can be used.[1,2] Combining albuterol plus ipratropium, a long-acting β_2-agonist plus theophylline, or a long-acting β_2-agonist plus tiotropium, produces a greater change in spirometry than either drug alone.[1,24,25] Administering a long-acting β_2-agonist plus ipratropium leads to fewer exacerbations than either drug alone.[26] Some studies have found an increase in adverse events without added benefit when combinations of bronchodilators are used.

Triple therapy with inhaled corticosteroid, long-acting β_2-agonist, and tiotropium is commonly used. Triple therapy appears to improve lung function and quality of life but may not further reduce exacerbations or dyspnea.[27-29] Further studies are needed to determine if the benefits of triple therapy outweigh the increased risk of adverse effects and added cost.

Potential benefits and risks of any combination therapy should be considered on a case-by-case basis. Patients should be monitored closely and therapy should be changed if the combination is not more effective.

▶ Immunizations

Serious illness and death in COPD patients can be reduced by about 50% with annual influenza vaccination. The optimal time for vaccination is usually from early October through mid-November. A onetime pneumococcal polysaccharide vaccine should be administered to all adults with COPD. Patients older than 65 years should be revaccinated if it has been more than 5 years since initial vaccination and they were younger than 65 years at the time.

▶ a_1-Antitrypsin Augmentation Therapy

The ATS and the ERS have published standards for the diagnosis and management of individuals with AAT deficiency.[30] They recommend IV augmentation therapy for individuals with AAT deficiency and moderate airflow obstruction (FEV_1 35% to 60% predicted). In these patients, augmentation therapy appears to reduce overall mortality and slow the decline in FEV_1, although large randomized controlled trials have not been conducted.

Augmentation therapy consists of weekly transfusions of pooled human AAT with the goal of maintaining adequate plasma levels of the enzyme. The benefits of augmentation therapy are unclear in patients with severe (FEV_1 less than 35% predicted) or mild (FEV_1 greater than 60% predicted) airflow obstruction. Augmentation therapy is not recommended for individuals with AAT deficiency who do not have lung disease.

▶ Other Pharmacologic Therapies

Leukotriene modifiers (e.g., zafirlukast and montelukast) have not been adequately evaluated in COPD patients and are not recommended for routine use. Small short-term studies showed improvement in pulmonary function, dyspnea, and quality of life when leukotriene modifiers were added to inhaled bronchodilator therapy.[31] Additional long-term studies are needed to clarify their role.

N-acetylcysteine has antioxidant and mucolytic activity, which makes it a promising agent for COPD treatment, but clinical trials have produced conflicting results. One of the largest trials found N-acetylcysteine to be ineffective in reducing the decline in lung function and preventing exacerbations.[32] Routine use cannot be recommended at this time.

A recent trial found that prophylactic treatment with daily azithromycin significantly reduced the incidence of acute exacerbations in select subgroups of COPD patients; however, the risks of microbial resistance associated with long-term antibiotic use should be further studied before continuous prophylactic use of antibiotics can be recommended.[33]

Antitussives are contraindicated because cough has an important protective role. Opioids may be effective for dyspnea in advanced disease but may have serious adverse effects; they may be used to manage symptoms in terminal patients.

Traditionally, β-blockers have been used sparingly, if at all, in patients with COPD due to concerns of worsening dyspnea. An observational study in 2010 suggested that β-blockers may improve outcomes in patients with COPD.[34] More studies are needed before β-blockers can be recommended for COPD, but they appear to be safe and thus can be used to treat comorbidities when needed.[35] Selective β_1-blockers should be used, and patients should be monitored for worsening symptoms.

Therapy of COPD Exacerbations

An exacerbation is acute worsening of the patient's symptoms from his or her usual stable state that is beyond normal day-to-day variations; an exacerbation warrants a change in medications. Common symptoms are worsening of dyspnea, increased sputum production, and change in sputum color. The most common causes of an exacerbation are respiratory infection and air pollution, but the cause cannot be identified in about one-third of severe exacerbations.[1]

Treatment depends on the symptoms and severity of the exacerbation. Mild exacerbations can often be treated at home with short-acting inhaled bronchodilators with or without oral corticosteroids. Antibiotics are indicated when there are specific signs of airway infection (e.g., change in color of sputum and/or increased sputum production or dyspnea) or when mechanical ventilation is needed. Moderate to severe exacerbations require management in the emergency department or hospital. Management should consist of controlled oxygen therapy, bronchodilators, oral or IV corticosteroids, antibiotics if indicated, and consideration of mechanical ventilation (noninvasive or invasive).

▶ Bronchodilators

Albuterol is the preferred bronchodilator for treatment of acute exacerbations because of its rapid onset of action. Ipratropium can be added to allow for lower doses of albuterol,

Patient Encounter, Part 2: The Medical History, Physical Examination, and Diagnostic Tests

PMH: Osteoarthritis for 6 years

SH: Unemployed; married with three children

FH: Diabetes and colon cancer in mother; COPD and heart disease in sister; schizophrenia in brother

Meds: Aspirin 81 mg daily, calcium carbonate 500 mg plus vitamin D 400 IU 1 tablet twice daily, albuterol MDI 1 to 2 puffs every 4 to 6 hours as needed; naproxen 500 mg 1 tablet twice daily

ROS: (–) fever, chills, or night sweats; (–) skin rash; (–) nasal congestion, drainage; (–) chest pain, paroxysmal nocturnal dyspnea, orthopnea; (+) shortness of breath, cough with yellowish phlegm; (–) wheezing; (–) hemoptysis; (–) heartburn, reflux symptoms, N/V/D, change in appetite, change in bowel habits; (+) joint pain in knee; (–) pedal edema

PE:

VS: BP 128/78 mm Hg, P 76 bpm, RR 20/min, T 35.8°C (96.4°F), Wt 60 kg (132 lb), Ht 64 in. (163 cm), BMI 22.7 kg/m²

HEENT: EOMI; mucosal membranes are moist; no evidence of JVD; no palpably enlarged cervical lymph nodes

Lungs: Clear breath sounds; expiratory phase is very diminished; no wheezes, rhonchi, or crackles

CV: RRR, normal S_1, S_2; no murmur, gallop, or rub

Abd: Soft, nontender, audible bowel sounds, no hepatosplenomegaly

Ext: No cyanosis, edema, or finger clubbing

Pulmonary Function Tests

	Prebronchodilator		Postbronchodilator	
	Actual	% Predicted	Actual	% Predicted
FVC (L)	2.76	85%	2.83	87%
FEV_1(L)	1.21	48%	1.11	44%
FEV_1/FVC (%)			39%	

CXR: Upper lobe bullous emphysema with hyperexpansion bilaterally

COPD Assessment Test score: 19

Given this additional information, what is your assessment of the patient's condition?

What are the treatment goals for this patient?

What nonpharmacologic and pharmacologic alternatives are feasible for this patient?

Develop a treatment plan for this patient.

---

thus reducing dose-dependent adverse effects such as tachycardia and tremor. Delivery can be accomplished through MDI and spacer or nebulizer. The nebulizer route is preferred in patients with severe dyspnea and/or cough that would limit delivery of medication through an MDI with spacer. If response is inadequate, theophylline can be considered; however, clinical evidence supporting its use is lacking.

▶ Oral Corticosteroids

● Systemic corticosteroids shorten the recovery time, help to restore lung function more quickly, and reduce the risk of early relapse.[36] The GOLD guidelines recommend oral prednisolone 30 to 40 mg/day for 10 to 14 days. Shorter courses (7 days or fewer) may be as effective, but further studies are needed.[37] Prolonged treatment and/or higher doses do not result in greater efficacy and increase the risk of adverse effects. If inhaled corticosteroids are part of the patient's usual treatment regimen, they should be continued during systemic therapy.

▶ Antibiotics

The role of antibiotics in treating COPD exacerbation is evolving, and evidence suggests that subsets of patients may ● benefit from antibiotic treatment. ❻ *Antibiotics should be used in patients with COPD exacerbations who: (a) have all three cardinal symptoms (increased dyspnea, increased sputum* *volume, and increased purulence); (b) have increased sputum purulence and one other cardinal symptom; or (c) experience a severe exacerbation requiring mechanical ventilation.*[1]

The predominant bacterial organisms in patients with mild exacerbations are *Streptococcus pneumoniae, Haemophilus influenzae,* and *Moraxella catarrhalis.* In patients with more severe underlying COPD, other bacteria such as enteric gram-negative bacilli (*Escherichia coli, Klebsiella pneumoniae,* and *Enterobacter cloacae*) and *Pseudomonas aeruginosa* may be more common. Selection of empirical antibiotic therapy should be based on the most likely organism(s) thought to be responsible for the infection and on local resistance patterns. A risk stratification approach has been advocated to help guide antibiotic selection.[1,12,38] This approach is based on risk factors found to be predictive of treatment failure or early relapse. Patients at risk for poor outcome are candidates for more aggressive initial antibiotic treatment. Table 15–5 provides recommended antibiotic treatment based on this risk stratification approach.[1,12,38] ● Antibiotic treatment for most patients should be maintained for 5 to 10 days. Exacerbations due to certain infecting organisms (*P. aeruginosa, E. cloacae,* and methicillin-resistant *Staphylococcus aureus*), although not common, require more lengthy courses of therapy (21 to 42 days).

If there is worsening clinical status or inadequate clinical response in 48 to 72 hours, reevaluate the patient, consider sputum Gram stain and culture if not already obtained, and

Table 15-5

Recommended Antibiotic Therapy in Acute Exacerbations of COPD

Patient Characteristics	Likely Pathogens	Recommended Antibiotics[a,b]
Mild Exacerbation Without Risk Factors for Poor Outcome		
Not requiring hospitalization Less than three exacerbations per year No comorbid illness FEV$_1$ greater than 50% predicted No recent antibiotic therapy	*Streptococcus pneumoniae* *Haemophilus influenzae* *Moraxella catarrhalis* *Chlamydia pneumoniae* Viruses	*Oral First-Line Therapy:* β-Lactam (high-dose amoxicillin)[c] β-Lactam/β-lactamase inhibitor (amoxicillin-clavulanate) Tetracycline Trimethoprim/sulfamethoxazole *Alternative Oral Therapy:* Macrolides (azithromycin, clarithromycin) Second- or third-generation cephalosporins (cefuroxime, cefpodoxime, cefdinir, cefprozil) *IV Therapy:* Not recommended
Moderate Exacerbation With Risk Factors for Poor Outcome		
FEV$_1$ less than 50% predicted Comorbid diseases Three or more exacerbations per year Antibiotic therapy in the previous 3 months	Above organisms *plus:* Resistant pneumococci (β-lactamase producing, penicillin-resistant), *Escherichia coli, Proteus* spp, *Enterobacter* spp, *Klebsiella pneumoniae*	*Oral First-Line Therapy:* β-Lactam/β-lactamase inhibitor (amoxicillin-clavulanate) *Alternative Oral Therapy:* Fluoroquinolone with enhanced pneumococcal activity (levofloxacin, gemifloxacin, moxifloxacin) *IV Therapy:* β-lactam/β-lactamase inhibitor (ampicillin–sulbactam) Second- or third-generation cephalosporin (cefuroxime, ceftriaxone) Fluoroquinolone with enhanced pneumococcal activity (levofloxacin, moxifloxacin)
Severe Exacerbation With Risk Factors for *Pseudomonas aeruginosa*		
Recent hospitalization Four or more courses of antibiotics in the last year Very severe COPD (GOLD 4) Previous isolation of *P. aeruginosa*	Above organisms *plus:* P. aeruginosa	*Oral First-Line Therapy:* Antipseudomonal fluoroquinolone (ciprofloxacin, high-dose levofloxacin) *IV Therapy:* Antipseudomonal β-lactamase-resistant penicillin (piperacillin-tazobactam) Third- or fourth-generation cephalosporin with antipseudomonal activity (ceftazidime, cefepime) Antipseudomonal fluoroquinolone (ciprofloxacin, high-dose levofloxacin)

COPD, chronic obstructive pulmonary disease; FEV$_1$, forced expiratory volume in 1 second.

[a]Antibiotics are indicated for patients with COPD exacerbations who: (a) have all three cardinal symptoms (increased dyspnea, increased sputum volume, and increased purulence); (b) have increased sputum purulence and one other cardinal symptom; or (c) experience a severe exacerbation requiring mechanical ventilation.

[b]Antibiotic choices should take into consideration local resistance patterns.

[c]High-dose amoxicillin is recommended due to the prevalence of penicillin-resistant *S. pneumoniae*.

adjust antimicrobial therapy. If Gram stain and culture results are available, narrow the antibiotic therapy according to cultured organism(s) and sensitivities. If no cultures have been obtained, or cultures remain negative, consider additional antibiotics and/or change to antibiotics with a broader spectrum of activity.

▶ Oxygen

The goal of oxygen therapy is to maintain Pao$_2$ above 60 mm Hg (7.98 kPa) or Sao$_2$ above 90% to prevent tissue hypoxia and preserve cellular oxygenation.[12] The GOLD guidelines recommend a target Sao$_2$ of 88% to 92%.[1] Increasing the Pao$_2$ much further confers little added benefit and may increase the risk of CO$_2$ retention, which may lead to respiratory acidosis. ABGs should be obtained after 30 to 60 minutes to assess for hypercapnia and acidosis.

In advanced COPD, caution should be used because overly aggressive administration of oxygen to patients with chronic hypercapnia may result in respiratory depression and respiratory failure. In these patients, mild hypoxemia, rather than CO$_2$ accumulation, triggers their drive to breathe.

▶ Assisted Ventilation

Mechanical ventilation can be administered as invasive (through an endotracheal tube) or noninvasive (by nasal or facial mask). Noninvasive mechanical ventilation (NIV) is preferred whenever possible. It improves signs and symptoms, decreases the length of hospital stay, and most importantly, reduces mortality.[1] Appropriate patients to consider for NIV include those with at least one of the following characteristics: (a) severe dyspnea with clinical signs suggestive of respiratory muscle fatigue such as use of accessory muscles and paradoxical abdominal motion; (b) respiratory acidosis (arterial pH at or below 7.35 and/or $Paco_2$ at or above 45 mm Hg [5.99 kPa]).[1] Invasive mechanical ventilation should be used in patients with more severe symptoms and in those failing NIV.

OUTCOME EVALUATION

- Monitor the patient for improvement in symptoms (dyspnea, cough, sputum production, exercise tolerance, sleep disturbance, and fatigue).

- Changes in FEV_1 should not be the main outcome assessed. FEV_1 changes are weakly related to symptoms, exacerbations, and health-related quality of life (outcomes that are important to patients). There is no evidence to support routine periodic spirometry after initiation of therapy.[2] The GOLD guidelines recommend annual spirometry to assess decline in lung function.[1]

Patient Care and Monitoring

1. Assess the patient's symptoms and history of exposure to risk factors. For new patients, obtain a detailed medical history including:
   - Medical conditions, especially history of respiratory disorders
   - Immunization status (pneumococcal and influenza)
   - Family history of COPD or other chronic respiratory disease
   - History of exacerbations or previous hospitalizations for respiratory disorders
   - Impact of disease on the patient's life, including limitation of activity, missed work, and feelings of depression or anxiety

2. Obtain spirometry measurements to assess airflow limitation and aid in severity classification and treatment decisions. Measure oxygen saturation in patients with an FEV_1 less than 35% predicted or signs or symptoms suggestive of cor pulmonale or respiratory failure. If oxygen saturation is less than 92%, ABGs should be assessed.

3. Obtain a thorough history of prescription, nonprescription, and dietary supplement use. Assess inhaler technique and adherence to the medication regimen. Ask the patient about effectiveness of medications at controlling symptoms and adverse effects.

4. Ask current tobacco users about daily quantity, past quit attempts, and current readiness to quit.

5. Design a therapeutic plan including lifestyle modifications (e.g., smoking cessation) and optimal drug therapy. Consider need for pulmonary rehabilitation, oxygen therapy, and/or surgery.

6. Provide patient education about the disease state and therapeutic plan:
   - What COPD is, and what its natural course is like
   - Smoking cessation counseling
   - Role of regular exercise and healthy eating
   - How and when to take medications; importance of adherence to the medication plan; adverse effects and how to minimize them
   - Signs and symptoms of an exacerbation and what to do if one occurs
   - Advanced directives and end-of-life issues for patients with more severe disease

7. Determine the follow-up period based on patient status and needs (typically 3 to 6 months).

8. Follow-up visits should include:
   - Assessment of tobacco use and/or quit attempts
   - Assessment of change in symptoms. Suggested questions for assessing whether a patient has had a symptomatic response to treatment include[1]:
     ✓ Have you noticed a difference since starting this treatment?
     ✓ If you are better: Are you less breathless? Can you do more? Can you sleep better? Describe what difference it has made to you.
     ✓ Is that change worthwhile to you?
   - Review of drug therapy (dosages, adherence, inhaler technique, effectiveness, adverse effects, and drug interactions)
   - Evaluation of exacerbation frequency, severity, and likely causes

9. Perform spirometry at least annually to assess disease progression.

10. Provide annual influenza vaccination.

11. Assess inhaler technique at every visit. Have the patient demonstrate proper use of each device using a placebo inhaler or personal inhaler. Proper use of these devices is critical for therapeutic success.

Table 15–6

Medical Research Council Dyspnea Scale

Grade	Modified Grade	Statement About Perceived Breathlessness[a]
1	0	"I only get breathless with strenuous activity"
2	1	"I get short of breath when hurrying on the level or up a slight hill"
3	2	"I walk slower than people of the same age on the level because of breathlessness or I have to stop for breath after a mile or so on the level at my own pace"
4	3	"I stop for breath after walking 100 yards (91 m) or after a few minutes on the level"
5	4	"I am too breathless to leave the house or I get breathless while dressing"

[a]The last statement to which the patient answers "yes" is his or her grade.

- The Medical Research Council dyspnea scale can be used to monitor physical limitation due to breathlessness (Table 15–6). The scale is simple to administer and correlates well with scores of health status.[39]

- The COPD Assessment Test (CAT) is an eight-item questionnaire that can be used every 2 to 3 months to assess for trends and changes in symptoms and disease impact on daily life.[1] It can be accessed at www.catestonline.org.

- Assess quality of life using the St. George's Respiratory Questionnaire, which has been validated and is specific for COPD patients.[40]

- Monitor theophylline levels with goal serum concentrations in the range of 5 to 15 mcg/mL (5 to 15 mg/L; 28 to 83 μmol/L). Trough levels should be obtained 1 to 2 weeks after initiation of treatment and after any dosage adjustment. Routine levels are not necessary unless toxicity is suspected or disease has worsened.

Abbreviations Introduced in This Chapter

AAT	α_1-Antitrypsin
ABG	Arterial blood gas
ATS	American Thoracic Society
cAMP	Cyclic adenosine monophosphate
COPD	Chronic obstructive pulmonary disease
ERS	European Respiratory Society
FEV$_1$	Forced expiratory volume in 1 second
FVC	Forced vital capacity
GOLD	Global Initiative for Chronic Obstructive Lung Disease
MDI	Metered-dose inhaler
MMRC	Modified Medical Research Council
NIV	Noninvasive mechanical ventilation

Paco$_2$	Partial pressure of arterial carbon dioxide
Pao$_2$	Partial pressure of arterial oxygen
PDE-4	Phosphodiesterase-4
PFTs	Pulmonary function tests
Sao$_2$	Arterial oxygen saturation
TNF-α	Tumor necrosis factor-α
V_A/Q	Ventilation-to-perfusion ratio

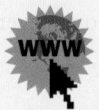

Self-assessment questions and answers are available at *http://www.mhpharmacotherapy.com/pp.html.*

REFERENCES

1. GOLD Science Committee. Global strategy for the diagnosis, management, and prevention of chronic obstructive pulmonary disease, revised 2011, *www.goldcopd.com.*

2. Qaseem A, Wilt TJ, Weinberger, et al. Diagnosis and management of stable chronic obstructive pulmonary disease: A clinical practice guideline update from the American College of Physicians, American College of Chest Physicians, American Thoracic Society, and European Respiratory Society. Ann Intern Med 2011;155:179–191.

3. American Lung Association. Chronic Obstructive Pulmonary Disease (COPD) Fact Sheet, February 2011, *www.lungusa.org.*

4. Altose MD. Approaches to slowing the progression of COPD. Curr Opin Pulm Med 2003;9:125–130.

5. Hogg JC. Pathophysiology of airflow limitation in chronic obstructive pulmonary disease. Lancet 2004;364:709–721.

6. Cosio MG, Saetta M, Agusti A. Immunologic aspects of chronic obstructive pulmonary disease. N Engl J Med 2009;360:2445–2454.

7. Anthonisen NR, Connett JE, Murray RP. Smoking and lung function of the lung health study participants after 11 years. Am J Respir Crit Care Med 2002;166:675–679.

8. Scanlon PD, Connett JE, Waller LA, et al. Smoking cessation and lung function in mild-to-moderate chronic obstructive pulmonary disease. The Lung Health Study. Am J Respir Crit Care Med 2000;161:381–390.

9. Fiore MC, Jaén CR, Baker TB, et al. Treating tobacco use and dependence. Clinical Practice Guideline. U.S. Department of Health and Human Services, 2008, *www.surgeongeneral.gov/tobacco/treating_tobacco_use08.pdf.*

10. Strassmann R, Bausch B, Spaar A, et al. Smoking cessation interventions in COPD: A network meta-analysis of randomised trials. Eur Respir J 2009;34:634–640.

11. Casaburi R, ZuWallack R. Pulmonary rehabilitation for management of chronic obstructive pulmonary disease. N Engl J Med 2009;360: 1329–1335.

12. American Thoracic Society/European Respiratory Society Task Force. Standards for the diagnosis and management of patients with COPD, v.1.2. New York, NY: American Thoracic Society, 2004, *www.thoracic.org/go/copd.*

13. Tashkin DP, Fabbri LM. Long-acting beta-agonists in the management of chronic obstructive pulmonary disease: current and future agents. Respir Res 2010;11:149, *http://respiratory-research.com/content/11/1/149.*

14. Rennard SI, Serby CW, Ghafouri M, et al. Extended therapy with ipratropium is associated with improved lung function in patients with COPD. A retrospective analysis of data from seven clinical trials. Chest 1996;110:62–70.

15. Barr RG, Bourbeau J, Camargo CA. Tiotropium for stable chronic obstructive pulmonary disease. Cochrane Database Syst Rev 2005: CD002876.

16. Tashkin DP, Celli B, Senn S, et al. A 4-year trial of tiotropium in chronic obstructive pulmonary disease. N Engl J Med 2008;359:1543–1554.

17. Vogelmeier C, Hederer B, Glaab T, et al. Tiotropium versus salmeterol for the prevention of exacerbations of COPD. N Engl J Med 2011;364:1093–1103.
18. Singh S, Loke YK, Furberg CD. Inhaled anticholinergics and risk of major adverse cardiovascular events in patients with chronic obstructive pulmonary disease. JAMA 2008;300:1439–1450.
19. Lee TA, Pickard AS, Au DH, et al. Risk for death associated with medications for recently diagnosed chronic obstructive pulmonary disease. Ann Intern Med 2008;149:380–390.
20. Zevin S, Benowitz NL. Drug interactions with tobacco smoking. An update. Clin Pharmacokinet 1999;36:425–438.
21. Calverley PMA, Anderson JA, Celli B, et al. Salmeterol and fluticasone propionate and survival in chronic obstructive pulmonary disease. N Engl J Med 2007;356:775–789.
22. Wouters EF, Postma DS, Fokkens B, et al. Withdrawal of fluticasone propionate from combined salmeterol/fluticasone treatment in patients with COPD causes immediate and sustained disease deterioration: A randomised controlled trial. Thorax 2005;60:480–487.
23. Fabbri LM, Calverley PMA, Izquierdo-Alonso JL, et al. Roflumilast in moderate-to-severe chronic obstructive pulmonary disease treated with long-acting bronchodilators: Two randomized clinical trials. Lancet 2009;374:695–703.
24. Tashkin DP, Pearle J, Iezzoni D, Varghese ST. Formoterol and tiotropium compared with tiotropium alone for treatment of COPD. COPD 2009;6:17–25.
25. van Noord JA, Aumann JL, Janssens E, et al. Comparison of tiotropium once daily, formoterol twice daily and both combined once daily in patients with COPD. Eur Respir J 2005;26:214–222.
26. van Noord JA, de Munck DRAJ, Bantje TA, et al. Long-term treatment of chronic obstructive pulmonary disease with salmeterol and the additive effect of ipratropium. Eur Respir J 2000;15:878–885.
27. Welte T, Miravitlles M, Hernandez P, et al. Efficacy and tolerability of budesonide/formoterol added to tiotropium in patients with chronic obstructive pulmonary disease. Am J Respir Crit Care Med 2009;180:741–750.
28. Aaron SD, Vandemheen KL, Fergusson D, et al. Tiotropium in combination with placebo, salmeterol, or fluticasone-salmeterol for treatment of chronic obstructive pulmonary disease: A randomized trial. Ann Intern Med 2007;146:545–555.
29. Karner C, Cates CJ. Combination inhaled steroid and long-acting beta$_2$-agonist in addition to tiotropium versus tiotropium or combination alone for chronic obstructive pulmonary disease. Cochrane Database Syst Rev 2011:CD008532.
30. Alpha-1 Antitrypsin Deficiency Task Force. American Thoracic Society/European Respiratory Society statement: Standards for the diagnosis and management of individuals with alpha-1 antitrypsin deficiency. Am J Respir Crit Care Med 2003;168:818–900.
31. Usery JB, Self TH, Muthiah MP, Finch CK. Potential role of leukotriene modifiers in the treatment of chronic obstructive pulmonary disease. Pharmacotherapy 2008;28:1183–1187.
32. Decramer M, Rutten-van Molken M, Dekhuijzen PNR, et al. Effects of N-acetylcysteine on outcomes in chronic obstructive pulmonary disease (Bronchitis Randomized on NAD Cost-Utility Study, BRONCUS): A randomised placebo-controlled trial. Lancet 2005;365:1552–1560.
33. Albert RK, Connett J, Bailey WC, et al. Azithromycin for prevention of exacerbations of COPD. N Engl J Med 2011;365:689–698.
34. Rutten FH, Zuithoff NPA, Hak E, et al. Beta-blockers may reduce mortality and risk of exacerbations in patients with chronic obstructive pulmonary disease. Arch Intern Med 2010;170:880–887.
35. Salpeter S, Ormiston T, Salpeter E. Cardioselective beta-blockers for chronic obstructive pulmonary disease. Cochrane Database Syst Rev 2005:CD003566.
36. Walters JAE, Gibson PG, Wood-Baker R, et al. Systemic corticosteroids for acute exacerbations of chronic obstructive pulmonary disease. Cochrane Database Syst Rev 2009:CD001288.
37. Walters JAE, Wang W, Morley C, et al. Different durations of corticosteroid therapy for exacerbations of chronic obstructive pulmonary disease. Cochrane Database Syst Rev 2011:CD006897.
38. Sethi S, Murphy TF. Acute exacerbations of chronic bronchitis: New developments concerning microbiology and pathophysiology—Impact on approaches to risk stratification and therapy. Infect Dis Clin North Am 2004;18:861–882.
39. Bestall JC, Paul EA, Garrod R, et al. Usefulness of the Medical Research Council (MRC) dyspnoea scale as a measure of disability in patients with chronic obstructive pulmonary disease. Thorax 1999;54:581–586.
40. Jones PW, Quirk FH, Baveystock GM, Littlejohns P. A self-complete measure of health status for chronic airflow limitation. The St. George's Respiratory Questionnaire. Am Rev Respir Dis 1992;145:1321–1327.

16 Cystic Fibrosis

Kimberly J. Novak

KEY CONCEPTS

① In cystic fibrosis (CF), the CF transmembrane regulator (CFTR) chloride channel is dysfunctional and usually results in decreased chloride secretion and increased sodium absorption, leading to altered viscosity of fluid excreted by the exocrine glands and mucosal obstruction.

② Pulmonary disease is characterized by thick mucus secretions, impaired mucus clearance, chronic airway infection and colonization, obstruction, and an exaggerated neutrophil-dominated inflammatory response.

③ Maximizing nutritional status through pancreatic enzyme replacement and vitamin and nutritional supplements is necessary for normal growth and development and for maintaining long-term lung function.

④ Airway clearance therapy is a necessary routine for all CF patients to clear secretions and control infection.

⑤ Antibiotic therapy is indicated in three distinct situations over the course of CF: (a) early eradication and delay of colonization, (b) suppression of bacterial growth once colonization occurs, and (c) reduction of bacterial load in acute overgrowth.

⑥ Antibiotic selection is based on periodic culture and sensitivity data, typically covering all organisms identified during the preceding year. If no culture data

are available, empirical antibiotics should cover the most likely organisms for the patient's age group.

⑦ Antibiotic regimens in severe CF exacerbations usually include an IV antipseudomonal β-lactam plus an aminoglycoside.

⑧ CF patients have larger volumes of distribution for many antibiotics due to an increased ratio of lean body mass to total body mass and lower fat stores. CF patients also have an enhanced total body clearance, although the exact mechanism has not been determined.

⑨ Titration of pancreatic enzyme doses is based on control of steatorrhea, stool output, and abdominal symptoms.

⑩ Because CF-related diabetes results from insulin insufficiency, exogenous insulin replacement is usually required.

INTRODUCTION

Cystic fibrosis (CF) is an inherited multiorgan system disorder affecting children and, increasingly, adults. It is the most common life-shortening genetic disease among whites and the major cause of severe chronic lung disease and pancreatic insufficiency in children. Disease generally manifests as mucosal obstruction of exocrine glands caused by defective ion transport within epithelial cells. Due to the array of affected organ systems and complicated medical therapies, appropriate CF treatment necessitates multidisciplinary team collaboration.

EPIDEMIOLOGY AND ETIOLOGY

In the United States, CF most commonly occurs in whites, ranging from 1 in 1,900 to 3,700 individuals. CF is less common in Hispanics (1 in 9,000), African Americans (1 in 15,000), and Asian Americans (1 in 32,000).[1] CF is inherited as an autosomal recessive trait, and approximately 1 in 25 whites are heterozygous carriers. Offspring of a carrier couple (each parent being heterozygous) have a 1 in 4 chance of having the disease (homozygous), a 1 in 2 chance of being a carrier (heterozygous), and a 1 in 4 chance of receiving no trait. The gene mutation is found on the long arm of chromosome 7 and encodes for the CF transmembrane regulator (CFTR) protein, which functions as a chloride channel to transport water and electrolytes. Over 1,800 mutations have been described in the CF gene; however, the ΔF508 mutation is the most common and is present in 70% to 90% of CF patients in the United States.[2–4]

PATHOPHYSIOLOGY

● CF is a disease of exocrine gland epithelial cells where CFTR expression is prevalent. Normally, these cells transport chloride through CFTR chloride channels with sodium and water accompanying this flux across the cell membrane (Fig. 16–1). CFTR is regulated by protein kinases in response to varying levels of the intracellular second messenger cyclic-3′,5′-adenosine monophosphate (cAMP). CFTR also downregulates the epithelial sodium channel and regulates calcium-activated chloride and potassium channels, and it may function in exocytosis and formation of plasma membrane molecular complexes and proteins important in inflammatory responses.[3] ❶ *In CF, the CFTR chloride channel is dysfunctional and usually results in decreased chloride secretion and increased sodium absorption, leading to altered viscosity of fluid excreted by the exocrine glands and mucosal obstruction.*

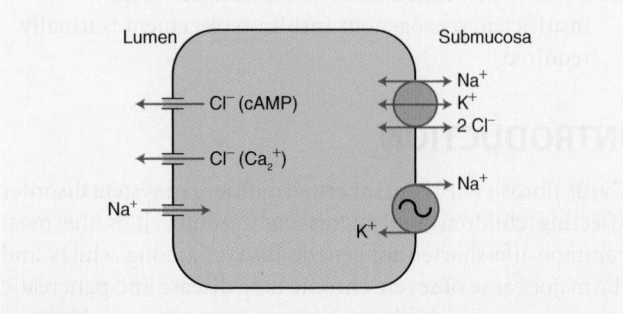

FIGURE 16–1. Electrolyte transport in the airway epithelial cell. (Ca, calcium; cAMP, cyclic-3′, 5′-adenosine monophosphate; Cl, chloride; Na, sodium; K potassium.) (From Milavetz G, Smith JJ. Cystic fibrosis. In: DiPiro JT, Talbert RL, Yee GC, et al., eds. Pharmacotherapy: A Pathophysiologic Approach, 7th ed. New York, NY: McGraw-Hill, 2008:536.)

Pulmonary System

Chronic lung disease is a hallmark of CF, leading to death in 90% of patients. ❷ *Pulmonary disease is characterized by thick mucus secretions, impaired mucus clearance, chronic airway infection and colonization, obstruction, and an exaggerated neutrophil-dominated inflammatory response.*[5] This process leads to air trapping, atelectasis, mucus plugging, bronchiectasis, cystic lesions, pulmonary hypertension, and eventual respiratory failure. In the U.S. CF population, pulmonary function declines approximately 2% per year, as measured by forced expiratory volume in 1 second (FEV$_1$). An individual's rate of decline varies depending on severity of CFTR dysfunction and comorbidities.[1] Sinusitis and nasal polyps are also common, and microbial colonization is similar to that of the lungs.

Bacterial pathogens are often acquired in age-dependent sequence, and prevalence is tracked in the Cystic Fibrosis Foundation Patient Registry. Early infection is most often caused by *Staphylococcus aureus* and nontypeable *Haemophilus influenza*. *Pseudomonas aeruginosa* infection is the most significant CF pathogen among all age groups. *P. aeruginosa* expresses extracellular toxins that perpetuate lung inflammation. Mucoid strains of *P. aeruginosa* produce an alginate biofilm layer that interferes with antibiotic penetration. Other organisms identified later in the disease course include *Stenotrophomonas maltophilia*, *Achromobacter (Alcaligenes) xylosoxidans*, *Burkholderia cepacia*, fungi including *Candida* and *Aspergillus* species, and nontuberculous mycobacteria among others.[1] Cultured organisms may represent initial infection, chronic colonization, or microbial overgrowth in an acute exacerbation.

Gastrointestinal System

GI involvement often presents as meconium ileus, small bowel obstruction shortly after birth due to abnormally thick meconium. Older CF patients may similarly develop distal intestinal obstruction syndrome (DIOS) due to fecal impaction in the terminal ileum and cecum.

Maldigestion due to pancreatic enzyme insufficiency is present in 85% to 90% of CF patients.[6,7] Thick pancreatic secretions and cellular debris obstruct pancreatic ducts and lead to fibrosis. Volume and concentration of pancreatic enzymes and bicarbonate are reduced, leading to maldigestion of fat and protein and subsequent malabsorption of fat-soluble vitamins (A, D, E, and K). Symptoms include abdominal distention, steatorrhea, flatulence, and malnourishment despite voracious intake. Maldigestion is progressive and may develop later in a previously pancreatic-sufficient patient. Other complications may include GI reflux, dysmotility, salivary dysfunction, intussusception, volvulus, atresia, rectal prolapse, and complications related to corrective surgery for meconium ileus.[7]

Hepatobiliary disease occurs due to bile duct obstruction from abnormal bile composition and flow. Hepatomegaly, splenomegaly, and cholecystitis may be present. Hepatic steatosis may be present due to effects of malnutrition.

Progression from cholestasis (impaired bile flow) to portal fibrosis and to focal and multilobar cirrhosis, esophageal varices, and portal hypertension takes several years. Many patients are compensated and asymptomatic but may be susceptible to acute decompensation in the event of extrinsic hepatic insult from viruses, medications, or other factors.[8]

Endocrine System

CF-related diabetes (CFRD) occurs in approximately 20% of adolescents and 40% to 50% of adults, disproportionally affecting women. Although it shares characteristics of both type 1 and type 2 diabetes mellitus, CFRD is categorized separately. Reduced functional pancreatic islet cells and increased islet amyloid deposition results in insulin insufficiency, the primary cause of CFRD. Insulin secretion is delayed in response to glucose challenge, and absolute insulin secretion over time is reduced. Some insulin resistance may also be present in CFRD and may fluctuate in relation to infection and inflammation.[9]

Postprandial hyperglycemia is common, but because some basal insulin secretion is maintained, fasting hyperglycemia is less severe and ketosis is rare.[6] Diet, acute and chronic infection, and corticosteroid use lead to fluctuations in glucose tolerance over time.[9] CFRD is associated with greater nutritional failure, increased pulmonary disease, and earlier mortality. Pulmonary function decline and nutritional consequences associated with progressive CFRD may overshadow risks of long-term macrovascular and microvascular disease.

Reproductive System

CF patients often experience delayed puberty. In females, menarche occurs 18 months later than average; menstrual irregularity is common, and fertility is reduced due to increased cervical mucus viscosity. Due to increasing life expectancy, pregnancy is becoming more common; however, outcomes depend on prepartum nutritional and pulmonary status. Almost all males with CF are azoospermic due to congenital absence of the vas deferens with resultant obstruction; however, conception still occurs occasionally. Conception can also occur through application of assisted reproductive technologies.[10]

Musculoskeletal System

Several factors contribute to development of bone disease in CF: (a) malabsorption of vitamins D and K and calcium, (b) poor nutrition and decreased body mass, (c) physical inactivity, (d) corticosteroid therapy, and (e) delayed puberty. Chronic pulmonary infection, through release of inflammatory cytokines, can increase bone resorption and decrease formation. Osteopenia, osteoporosis, pathological fractures, and kyphosis can occur.[11] Episodic or chronic arthritis and hypertrophic pulmonary osteoarthropathy may occur due to immune complex formation in response to chronic inflammation.[12] Digital clubbing is commonly observed and is a marker for hypoxia.

Hematological System

Anemia may be present due to impaired erythropoietin regulation, nutritional factors (vitamin E and iron malabsorption), or chronic inflammation. Increased cytokine production can lead to shortened red blood cell survival, reduced erythropoietin response, and impaired mobilization of iron stores. Additionally, with chronic hypoxia, normal hemoglobin and hematocrit values may represent relative anemia.[13] Increased red blood cell production is a physiological response to hypoxia; however, this response may be blunted in CF and may result in symptoms of anemia despite normal lab values.

Abnormal bleeding or clotting may also be observed as a result of vitamin K malabsorption, antibiotic-associated depletion of GI flora and vitamin K synthesis, reduced coagulation factor synthesis due to liver disease, and/or a procoagulant state due to inflammation.

Integumentary System

Sweat contains abnormally high concentrations of sodium and chloride due to impaired reabsorption within the sweat duct from loss of CFTR channels. Patients are usually asymptomatic (other than a characteristic salty taste to the skin).[3] In rare instances such as hot weather or excessive sweating during physical activity, patients may become dehydrated and experience symptoms of hyponatremia (nausea, headache, lethargy, and confusion).

CLINICAL PRESENTATION AND DIAGNOSIS

See the text box on the next page for the clinical presentation of CF.

Diagnosis

Diagnosis of CF is based on two separate elevated sweat chloride concentrations of 60 mEq/L (60 mmol/L) or greater obtained through pilocarpine iontophoresis (the "sweat test"). Genetic testing (CFTR mutation analysis) may be performed to confirm the diagnosis, screen in utero, or detect carrier status. More than 70% of diagnoses are made by 12 months of age, and almost all are made by age 12. CF is a component of required newborn screening panels in all U.S. states in an effort to identify patients prior to symptom development, initiate early intervention with CF therapies, and improve long-term outcomes.[14] A positive newborn screen for CF is not diagnostic (due to false-positive results among CF carriers), nor does a negative screen universally exclude the diagnosis. All "positive screens" are referred to a CF care center for sweat chloride test and genetic evaluation.

Clinical Course and Prognosis

Life expectancy has greatly increased from a predicted survival of 16 years of age in 1970 to more than 40 years for

Clinical Presentation of CF

General

- CF is usually diagnosed in neonates (meconium ileus at birth or newborn screening) or during early childhood. Some patients may present later in life due to less severe symptoms or misdiagnosis.

Symptoms

- Pulmonary: Chronic cough, sputum production, decreased exercise tolerance, and recurrent respiratory tract infections (pneumonia and sinusitis). Acute infection may be marked by increased cough, changes in sputum (darker and thicker), hemoptysis, dyspnea, and fever.
- GI: Numerous large, foul-smelling loose stools (steatorrhea), flatulence, and abdominal pain. Intestinal obstruction may present as abdominal pain and distention and/or decreased bowel movements.
- Nutritional: Poor weight gain, voracious appetite, and hunger. Dry skin, skin rash, and visual disturbances may be noted in vitamin deficiency.
- CFRD: Weight loss, increased thirst, and more frequent urination.

Signs

- Obstructive airway disease: tachypnea, dyspnea, cyanosis, wheezes, crackles, sternal retractions, digital clubbing, and barrel chest.
- Failure to thrive: Despite apparent adequate caloric intake, children may be below age-based normal in both height and weight, and adults may be near/below ideal body weight or have a low BMI.
- Salty taste to the skin.
- Hepatobiliary disease: Asymptomatic or evidenced by hepatomegaly, splenomegaly, or prolonged bleeding.
- Recurrent pancreatitis (usually in pancreatic-sufficient patients): Episodic epigastric abdominal pain, persistent vomiting, and fever.

Laboratory Tests

- WBC with an associated increase in polymorphonuclear (PMN) leukocytes and bands may occur in acute pulmonary infection; however, infection may occur without these laboratory abnormalities.
- Maldigestion: Decreased serum levels of fat-soluble vitamins (A, D, E, and K). Decreased vitamin K levels may result in elevated prothrombin time (PT) and international normalized ratio (INR).
- Glucose intolerance: Blood glucose between 140 and 199 mg/dL (7.8 to 11.0 mmol/L) 2 hours after an oral glucose-tolerance test.
- CFRD: Blood glucose 200 mg/dL (11.1 mmol/L) or higher 2 hours after an oral glucose-tolerance test or fasting hyperglycemia (fasting blood glucose 126 mg/dL (7.0 mmol/L) or more regardless of the postglucose challenge level).
- Hepatobiliary disease: Serum aspartate aminotransferase, alanine aminotransferase, alkaline phosphatase, γ-glutamyltransferase, and bilirubin may be elevated.

Other Tests

- Microbial cultures (sputum, throat, bronchoalveolar lavage, or sinus): Isolation of *P. aeruginosa*, *S. aureus*, *S. maltophilia*, and other CF-related organisms.
- PFTs: Decreased FEV_1, decreased forced vital capacity (FVC), and increased residual volume. Values are typically lower during acute pulmonary exacerbations.
- Chest x-ray or chest CT scan: Infiltrates, atelectasis, bronchiectasis, and mucus plugging.
- Abdominal x-ray or CT scan: If present, intestinal obstruction may be manifested as meconium ileus, DIOS, or intussusception. Rectal prolapse may be noted on physical examination.
- Maldigestion: Elevated fecal fat content, reduced fecal pancreatic elastase-1 (less than or equal to 200 mcg/g of feces).

---

patients born in the 1990s.[6] The average age of patients in the Cystic Fibrosis Foundation Registry is now more than 16 years, and 47% of CF patients in the 2010 Registry annual report are over 18 years old with the oldest age 78.[14]

Clinical course varies among patients because of multiple genetic mutations and heterogeneous profile of the ΔF508 mutation. Some patients develop severe lung disease early in childhood and reach end-stage disease by adolescence, whereas others maintain near-normal lung function into adulthood. Newly diagnosed adults tend to present with chronic respiratory symptoms but usually have milder lung disease, less frequent *Pseudomonas* infection, and less severe pancreatic insufficiency.[6]

TREATMENT

Desired Outcomes

Therapeutic outcomes in CF care relate to chronic and acute treatment goals. With chronic management, the primary goals are to delay disease progression and optimize quality of life. ❸ *Maximizing nutritional status through pancreatic enzyme replacement and vitamin and nutritional supplements is necessary for normal growth and development and for maintaining long-term lung function.* Reduction of airway inflammation and infection and aggressive preventive therapies minimize acute pulmonary exacerbations and delay pulmonary decline. In pulmonary exacerbations, therapy is

Patient Encounter, Part 1

TJ is a 2-month-old male infant being seen at the cystic fibrosis center due to an abnormal newborn screen. Sweat chloride testing is performed on bilateral thighs with results reported as follows:

Sample 1: Sweat chloride 120 mEq/L (120 mmol/L)

Sample 2: Sweat chloride 138 mEq/L (138 mmol/L)

Upon parental interview, TJ is a voracious eater and has six to eight loose stools per day. He is entirely breastfed and has just regained his birth weight of 3.1 kg. Parents also report that he passed his meconium in the newborn nursery on his second day of life and that he arches and cries after most feeds. TJ has been otherwise healthy.

What information is consistent with a diagnosis of cystic fibrosis (CF)?

What are the next steps in the CF diagnostic process for TJ?

TJ's parents are overwhelmed with his diagnosis of CF and are very worried about his life expectancy. How would you explain his prognosis?

directed toward reducing acute airway inflammation and obstruction through more aggressive airway clearance and antibiotic therapy with a goal of returning lung function to pre-exacerbation levels or greater.

Nonpharmacologic Therapy

▶ Airway Clearance Therapy

④ Airway clearance therapy is a necessary routine for all CF patients to clear secretions and control infection, even at diagnosis prior to becoming symptomatic. Waiting until development of a first pneumonia or daily symptoms delays benefits and may facilitate a faster pulmonary decline. The traditional form of chest physiotherapy (CPT) is known as percussion and postural drainage. Areas of the patient's chest, sides, and back are rapidly "clapped" by hand in different patient positions, followed by cough or forced expiration to mobilize secretions. Patients may also be taught autogenic drainage, which consists of deep breathing exercises followed by forced cough.

Several airway clearance devices are also available. Flutter valve devices use oscillating positive expiratory pressure (OPEP) to cause vibratory airflow obstruction and an internal percussive effect to mobilize secretions. Intrapulmonary percussive ventilation (IPV) provides continuous oscillating pressures during inhalation and exhalation. High-frequency chest compression (HFCC) with an inflatable vest that provides external oscillation is most commonly used. Vest therapy is often preferred because patients can perform therapy independently from an early age.[6,15]

If performed appropriately, airway clearance techniques provide similar efficacy, so choice should be based on patient preference and adherence. Effective cough and expectoration of mucus are essential for good clearance technique. Airway clearance therapy is typically performed once or twice daily for maintenance care and is increased to three or four times per day for acute exacerbations.

▶ Nutrition

Most CF patients have increased caloric needs due to increased energy expenditure through increased work of breathing, increased basal metabolism, and maldigestion. Prevention of malnutrition requires early patient-specific nutritional intervention. Caloric requirements to promote age-appropriate weight gain or maintenance are typically 110% to 200% of the recommended daily allowance (RDA) for age, gender, and size and increase as disease progresses.[16]

Nutrition in malnourished patients consists of baseline required calories plus additional calories for weight gain. Even with aggressive diet and oral supplements, the caloric requirement may not be achieved, and placement of a **gastrostomy** or **jejunostomy** tube to support nighttime supplemental feeds may be necessary.[6] Patients with refractory malabsorption, CFRD, and/or tube feedings have unique caloric needs. Collaboration with dieticians specially trained in CF nutrition is essential.

Pharmacologic Therapy

▶ Pulmonary System

Airway clearance therapy is usually accompanied by bronchodilator treatment (albuterol [known as salbutamol outside the United States] by nebulizer or metered-dose inhaler) to stimulate mucociliary clearance and prevent bronchospasm associated with therapy (Table 16–1).

A mucolytic agent is administered subsequently to reduce sputum viscosity and enhance clearance. Dornase alfa (Pulmozyme) is a recombinant human (rh) DNase that selectively cleaves extracellular DNA released during neutrophil degradation in viscous CF sputum. Nebulization of dornase alfa 2.5 mg once or twice daily improves daily pulmonary symptoms and function, reduces pulmonary exacerbations, and improves quality of life.[17]

Hypertonic saline for inhalation (Hyper-Sal) 7% or 3.5% is often used as an add-on mucolytic agent via osmotic effects or for sputum induction. It must be preceded by a bronchodilator due to a greater incidence of bronchospasm and may not be tolerated by some patients.[18] N-acetylcysteine is another mucolytic agent, but its unpleasant odor and taste limit patient acceptance.[6]

Many patients with CF also have reactive airways or concurrent asthma and benefit from long-acting β_2-agonists.[6] Patients with recurrent wheezing or dyspnea who have demonstrated improvement with albuterol (salbutamol) should be considered for maintenance asthma therapy, as should patients with bronchodilator-responsive pulmonary

Table 16–1		
Common Pulmonary Medications in CF		
Medication	**Pediatric Dose**	**Adult Dose**
Albuterol (salbutamol)	2.5 mg nebulized with chest physiotherapy 2 to 4 times daily; alternatively, two puffs via metered-dose inhaler may be substituted	2.5 mg nebulized with chest physiotherapy 2 to 4 times daily; alternatively, two puffs via metered-dose inhaler may be substituted
Dornase alfa	2.5 mg nebulized once or twice daily	2.5 mg nebulized once or twice daily
Hypertonic saline 7%, 3.5%, or 3%	4 mL nebulized 1–4 times/day	4 mL nebulized 1–4 times/day
Azithromycin	Body weight 25–39 kg: 250 mg on Mondays, Wednesdays, and Fridays	Body weight 40 kg or more: 500 mg on Mondays, Wednesdays, and Fridays
Ibuprofen[a]	20–30 mg/kg/dose given twice daily	20–30 mg/kg/dose given twice daily
Ivacaftor[b]	150 mg every 12 hours	150 mg every 12 hours

[a]Adjusted to achieve peak plasma concentrations of 50 to 100 mcg/mL (243 to 485 μmol/L). Maintain chronic dosing with same dosage form and manufacturer. Note that therapy is not always continued into adulthood.

[b]Dose may require adjustment in patients with moderate or severe hepatic impairment and/or when coadministered with moderate or strong CYP3A inhibitors.

function tests (PFTs). Inhaled corticosteroids may attenuate reactive airways and reduce airway inflammation in some patients; however, clear benefit in CF has not been established.[1,19] Drug delivery to the site of inflammation is limited by mucus plugging, which may limit efficacy. Patients on asthma therapies should administer these medications after airway clearance to optimize drug delivery. Montelukast, antihistamines, and/or intranasal steroids are sometimes used for CF patients with allergic or rhinosinusitis symptoms.

Long-term systemic corticosteroids reduce airway inflammation and improve lung function. However, beneficial effects diminish upon discontinuation, and concern for long-term adverse effects limits use as maintenance therapy.[19] In clinical practice, systemic corticosteroids may be used short term in acute exacerbations or for treatment of allergic response to *Aspergillus* colonization (allergic bronchopulmonary aspergillosis, or ABPA); however, dose and duration of therapy should be minimized.[1,20]

High-dose ibuprofen targeting peak concentrations of 50 to 100 mcg/mL (243 to 485 μmol/L) has been shown to slow progression of disease, particularly in children 5 to 13 years of age with mild lung disease (FEV1 greater than 60% [0.60]). At high doses, ibuprofen inhibits the lipoxygenase pathway, reducing neutrophil migration and function as well as release of lysosomal enzymes. At lower concentrations achieved with analgesic dosing, neutrophil migration increases, potentially increasing inflammation.[21,22] A dose of 20 to 30 mg/kg given twice daily is usually needed to attain target levels, but interpatient variability necessitates serum concentration monitoring.[21] Due to monitoring requirements and concerns regarding long-term safety and tolerability, only a few CF centers prescribe high-dose ibuprofen.[1,19]

Azithromycin is a macrolide antibiotic commonly used in CF as an anti-inflammatory agent to improve overall lung function, although long-term clinical safety and efficacy data are lacking. Proposed mechanisms include interference with

Pseudomonas alginate biofilm production, bactericidal activity during stationary *Pseudomonas* growth, neutrophil inhibition, interleukin-8 reduction, and reduction in sputum viscosity.[23,24] Due to its long tissue half-life, azithromycin is typically dosed 3 days per week (Monday, Wednesday, and Friday) at 500 mg for patients weighing at least 40 kg and 250 mg for patients weighing 25 to 39 kg. Alternatively, patients may take 500 or 250 mg either daily or only Monday through Friday, based on the same weight parameters. Patients should have a screening acid-fast bacillus sputum culture prior to initiation and then every 6 months due to risk for selection of macrolide-resistant nontuberculous mycobacteria (a contraindication to chronic azithromycin therapy).[19]

Antibiotic Therapy

⑤ *Antibiotic therapy is used in three distinct clinical settings within the course of CF: (a) eradication and delay of colonization in early lung disease, (b) suppression of bacterial growth once colonization is present, and (c) reduction of bacterial load in acute exacerbations in an attempt to return lung function to pre-exacerbation levels or greater.*[1] ⑥ *Antibiotic selection is based on periodic culture and sensitivity data, typically covering all organisms identified during the preceding year. If no culture data are available, empirical antibiotics should cover the most likely organisms for the patient's age group.* Due to altered pharmacokinetics and microorganism resistance, dose optimization is key (Table 16–2).

Severity of pulmonary symptoms also guides antibiotic selection. For recent-onset or mild symptoms, patients may be treated with outpatient oral and inhaled antibiotics for 14 to 21 days. Oral fluoroquinolones are a mainstay for *P. aeruginosa* treatment in CF, even in children. Despite concerns regarding cartilage and tendon toxicity in young animals, clinical practice has not shown an increased risk in human children.[25] To prevent development of resistance and promote synergy,

Table 16–2
Selected Antibiotic Dosing in CF[a]

Antibiotic	Pediatric Dose (mg/kg/day)	Adult Maximum Daily Dose	Interval (hours)
Intravenous			
Tobramycin, gentamicin[b]	10	None	8–24
Amikacin[b]	30	None	8–24
Ceftazidime	150–200	6–8 g	6–8
Cefepime	150	6 g	8
Piperacillin–tazobactam[c]	400	16 g	6
Ticarcillin–clavulanate[c]	400–600	12–18 g	4–6
Meropenem	120	6 g	8
Imipenem–cilastatin[c]	100	2 g	6
Aztreonam	200	8 g	6
Ciprofloxacin	30	1.2 g	8–12
Levofloxacin	10–20	750 mg	12–24
Nafcillin	200	12 g	4–6
Vancomycin[b]	60	None	6–12
Linezolid	30	1.2 g	8–12
Colistin	5–8	480 mg	8
Chloramphenicol[b]	60–80	4 g	6
Oral			
Amoxicillin ± clavulanic acid[c]	45–90	4 g	12
Dicloxacillin	100	2 g	6
Cephalexin	50–100	4 g	6–8
Trimethoprim–sulfamethoxazole[d]	10–20	1,280 mg	6–12
Clindamycin	30	1.8 g	6–8
Ciprofloxacin	40	2 g	12
Levofloxacin	10–20	750 mg	12–24
Minocycline[e]	4	200 mg	12
Linezolid	30	1.2 g	8–12
Inhaled			
Tobramycin	160–600 mg/day	600 mg	12
Aztreonam lysine	225 mg/day	225 mg	8
Colistin	75–150 mg/day	300 mg	12

[a]All doses assume normal renal and hepatic function. Consult a specialized drug reference for dosage adjustment if function is impaired. Dose and/or interval may require adjustment.

[b]Empirical starting doses only. Adjust dose per therapeutic drug monitoring.

[c]Dose based on β-lactam component.

[d]Dose based on trimethoprim component.

[e]Children older than 8 years.

inhaled tobramycin, aztreonam, or colistin is usually added for double coverage.[1,26] Methicillin-sensitive *S. aureus* (MSSA) may be treated with oral amoxicillin–clavulanic acid, dicloxacillin, first- or second-generation cephalosporins, trimethoprim–sulfamethoxazole, clindamycin, doxycycline, or minocycline, depending on sensitivity. Likewise, methicillin-resistant *S. aureus* (MRSA) may be treated with oral trimethoprim–sulfamethoxazole, clindamycin, doxycycline, minocycline, or linezolid. *H. influenzae* often produces β-lactamases but can usually be treated with amoxicillin–clavulanic acid, a cephalosporin, or trimethoprim–sulfamethoxazole.

Oral trimethoprim–sulfamethoxazole or minocycline may be used to treat *S. maltophilia*.

For severe infections or patients failing outpatient therapy, IV antibiotic therapy is prescribed for 2 to 3 weeks as inpatient therapy. Depending on the availability of home health services, some patients may be discharged to finish their course or even receive their entire course at home. ❼ *Typical regimens for severe infections include an antipseudomonal β-lactam plus an aminoglycoside for added synergy and delay of resistance development.*[1,26,27] Cephalosporins tend to be better tolerated and offer the benefit of less frequent administration. Extended-spectrum penicillins have been associated with a higher incidence of allergy. Aztreonam offers the added benefit of little cross-reactivity in penicillin- or cephalosporin-allergic patients; however, it has no gram-positive coverage. Meropenem should be reserved for organisms resistant to all other antibiotics to minimize development of resistance in the carbapenem drug class.

Tobramycin IV is generally the first-line aminoglycoside. Isolates are usually resistant to gentamicin, and amikacin is reserved for tobramycin-resistant strains. Pharmacokinetic goals are listed in Table 16–3. Higher peak serum concentrations are targeted to maximize efficacy, whereas lower serum trough levels are targeted to reduce risk of toxicity. Some centers use once-daily dosing (tobramycin 10 to 15 mg/kg/day or amikacin 35 mg/kg/day) targeting higher peaks and lower troughs. Because aminoglycosides exhibit concentration-dependent killing, once-daily dosing may optimize this effect. However, time below the minimum inhibitory concentration (MIC) is prolonged with once-daily administration in children, possibly leading to loss of synergy for a substantial portion of the dosing interval. Due to a shorter half-life, once-daily dosing is not always optimal for younger children. However, it may be a reasonable option for some children, adolescents, and adults in whom the time below the MIC can be minimized. Long-term studies are needed to examine the efficacy and resistance patterns associated with once-daily aminoglycosides in the CF population.[1,26,27]

Most other serious gram-negative infections are also treated with combination therapy. *S. maltophilia* is highly resistant and most often treated with trimethoprim–sulfamethoxazole or ticarcillin–clavulanate. *A. xylosoxidans* and *B. cepacia* may have minimal therapeutic options. A fluoroquinolone may be substituted for an aminoglycoside based on sensitivity data or presence of renal dysfunction and/or ototoxicity. Due to excellent bioavailability, fluoroquinolones, trimethoprim–sulfamethoxazole, doxycycline, minocycline, and linezolid should be used orally for most patients. Due to toxicity risk, colistin IV and chloramphenicol IV are reserved for life-threatening highly resistant infections.

Inpatient treatment of MRSA can consist of IV vancomycin or oral agents as previously described, depending on the severity of infection and concomitant organisms. Vancomycin IV may also be converted to oral stepdown therapy upon discharge.

Table 16–3

Pharmacokinetic Goals in Cystic Fibrosis

Antibiotic	Traditional Units of Measurement		SI Units of Measurement	
	Goal Peak[a] (mcg/mL)	Goal Trough[b] (mcg/mL)	Goal Peak[a] (μmol/L)	Goal Trough[b] (μmol/L)
Tobramycin, gentamicin	10–12[c]	Less than 1.5[c]	21–26[c]	Less than 3.2[c]
	20–30[d]	Less than 1[d]	42–63[d]	Less than 2.1[d]
Amikacin	30–40[c]	Less than 5[c]	51–68[c]	Less than 8.6[c]
	60–90[d]	Less than 3[d]	103–154[d]	Less than 5.1[d]
Vancomycin	–[e]	15–20	–[e]	10–14

Note: Values reported in mcg/mL are numerically equivalent to mg/L.

[a]Peaks calculated 30 minutes after end of infusion for aminoglycosides.

[b]Troughs calculated immediately prior to the time the dose is due.

[c]Goals refer to traditional dosing (every 8 or 12 hours). Higher peaks may be targeted with corresponding lower trough concentrations for aminoglycosides based on center practice.

[d]Goals refer to once-daily (high-dose extended interval) dosing.

[e]Not routinely measured.

Chronic or rotating inhaled antibiotic maintenance therapy may be used to suppress *P. aeruginosa* colonization; however, long-term systemic antibiotics are not recommended due to emergence of resistance.[1] Inhaled tobramycin (TOBI) is typically administered to patients 6 years of age and older in alternating 28-day cycles of 300 mg nebulized twice daily, followed by a 28-day washout period to minimize development of resistance. Long-term cyclical administration improves pulmonary function, decreases microbial burden, and reduces hospitalization for IV therapy.[28,29] Due to minimal systemic absorption, pharmacokinetic monitoring is not necessary with normal renal function. Lower doses of nebulized tobramycin solution for injection have been used in younger children, and *Pseudomonas* eradication studies used 300 mg twice daily in children as young as 6 months.[30]

Aztreonam lysine for inhalation (Cayston) is approved for *P. aeruginosa* suppression in 28-day on/off cycles for CF patients 6 years of age and older. A dose of 75 mg three times daily is given via the Altera nebulizer system, a novel high-efficiency drug delivery device.[31,32] Both aztreonam lysine and its drug-specific nebulizer system are currently only available through a specialty mail-order pharmacy access program.

Nebulized colistin using the IV formulation may be an option in patients with tobramycin-resistant strains or intolerance to inhaled tobramycin or aztreonam lysine. Pretreatment with albuterol is necessary due to increased risk of bronchoconstriction.[1,6]

Selection of inhaled antibiotics is based on culture data and patient preference. Alternating inhaled antibiotic regimens are sometimes used in patients with more advanced lung disease. Inhaled antibiotics are typically stopped during acute exacerbations requiring IV therapy because drug delivery is reduced with increased sputum production, and concomitant use of IV aminoglycosides may increase risk of toxicity.[26]

Pharmacokinetic Considerations

8 *CF patients have larger volumes of distribution for many antibiotics due to an increased ratio of lean body mass to total body mass and lower fat stores. CF patients also have enhanced total body clearance, although the exact mechanism has not been determined.* Increased renal clearance, increased glomerular filtration rate, decreased protein binding, increased tubular secretion, decreased tubular reabsorption, extrarenal elimination, and increased metabolism have all been proposed.

Because of these pharmacokinetic changes, higher doses of aminoglycosides are needed to achieve target serum levels and promote adequate tissue penetration. Higher doses of β-lactam antibiotics are also needed to achieve and sustain levels above the MIC. Trimethoprim–sulfamethoxazole displays enhanced renal clearance and hepatic metabolism in the CF population. Fluoroquinolones and vancomycin have fewer pharmacokinetic deviations; however, higher doses are typically needed to attain inhibitory serum and tissue concentrations against CF pathogens.[33]

Although most CF patients have shorter drug half-lives and larger volumes of distribution than non-CF patients, some patients exhibit decreased renal clearance. Concomitant use of nephrotoxic medications, presence of diabetic nephropathy, history of transplantation (immunosuppressant use and/or procedural hypoxic injury), age-related decline in renal function in adult patients, and cumulative lifetime exposure to aminoglycosides decrease clearance. Evaluation of previous pharmacokinetic parameters and trends, along with incorporation of new health information, is key to appropriate dosing.

Gastrointestinal System

● Pancreatic enzyme replacement is the mainstay of GI therapy. Enzyme products available in the United States (Table 16–4) are formulated as capsules containing enteric-coated microspheres or microtablets that escape inactivation of enzymes by gastric acid and promote dissolution in the more alkaline duodenum. Capsules may be opened and the microbeads swallowed with food (for infants and young children), as long as they are not chewed or mixed with alkaline or hot foods (which denature enzymes). Although different products may contain similar enzyme ratios, they are not bioequivalent and cannot be interchanged.[6,34] Due to an ongoing mandated FDA approval process, product availability has been evolving in recent years.

● Pancreatic enzymes are initiated at 500 to 1,000 units/kg/meal of lipase component (because fats are the most difficult components to digest) with half-doses given for snacks. Enzymes should be taken at the beginning or divided throughout the meal and must be given with any fat-containing snack. Infants are typically started at 1,500 to 2,500 units of lipase per 120 mL of formula or breast milk and may require division of capsule contents via visual estimation to obtain appropriate doses. Pancreatic enzymes cannot be placed in formula bottles due to inability to pass consistently through the nipple slit. Instead, enzyme microbeads are placed on a small dot of infant applesauce (or moistened infant rice cereal) and administered via infant spoon with subsequent nursing or bottle-feeding to facilitate swallowing. The oral mucosa must be examined afterward to ensure that all enzymes are swallowed, because remnant microbeads can cause oral erosions (ulcers).

❾ *Titration of pancreatic enzyme doses is based on control of steatorrhea, stool output, and abdominal symptoms.* Infants should have no more than three to four stools per day, whereas older patients should have no more than two to three (children) or one to two (adolescents/adults) well-formed stools per day. Doses are titrated at 2- to 3-week intervals in increments of 150 to 250 units of lipase/kg/meal (or the next easily administered capsule or half-capsule) up to 2,500 units/kg/meal. Higher doses should be used cautiously due to risk of fibrosing colonopathy.[6,7,34] Patients responding poorly to maximal doses of one product may benefit from changing to another product[6] and/or addition of a histamine H_2-receptor antagonist or proton pump inhibitor. Acid suppression may boost the effective enzyme dose, if duodenal pH is not alkaline enough to neutralize residual gastric acid and dissolve enteric coating. Acid suppression also treats concomitant gastroesophageal reflux disease.[6,7,34]

● Fat-soluble vitamin supplementation is usually required in pancreatic insufficiency. Specially formulated products for CF patients (AquADEKs, SourceCF, and Vitamax) are usually sufficient to attain normal serum vitamin levels at a dose of 1 mL daily for infants, one tablet daily for younger children, and one tablet/capsule twice daily for teenagers and adults. Additional supplementation may be needed in uncontrolled malabsorption or for replacement of severe vitamin deficiency.[6,34] Appetite stimulants such as cyproheptadine may be an option for promoting nutrition and weight gain, but efficacy has not been established.

Ursodiol at 20 mg/kg/day in two divided doses may slow progression of liver disease. It improves bile flow and may displace toxic bile acids that accumulate in a cholestatic liver, stimulate bicarbonate secretion into the bile, offer a cytoprotective effect, and reduce elevated liver enzymes.[6,8]

Treatment of DIOS consists of enteral administration of polyethylene glycol (PEG) electrolyte solutions. Enemas may also be used to facilitate stool clearance, and severe presentations may require surgical resection. IV fluids are often required to correct dehydration due to vomiting or decreased oral intake. Reevaluation of enzyme adherence and dosing is essential to prevent recurrence, and some patients may require daily PEG administration (MiraLAX).[6]

Table 16–4

Common Pancreatic Enzyme Replacement Products

Trade Name[a]	Lipase (Units)	Amylase (Units)	Protease (Units)
Creon 3,000	3,000	15,000	9,500
Creon 6,000	6,000	30,000	19,000
Creon 12,000	12,000	60,000	38,000
Creon 24,000	24,000	120,000	76,000
Pancreaze MT 4	4,200	17,500	10,000
Pancreaze MT 10	10,500	43,750	25,000
Pancreaze MT 16	16,800	70,000	40,000
Pancreaze MT 20	21,000	61,000	37,000
Zenpep 3,000	3,000	16,000	10,000
Zenpep 5,000	5,000	27,000	17,000
Zenpep 10,000	10,000	55,000	34,000
Zenpep 15,000	15,000	82,000	51,000
Zenpep 20,000	20,000	109,000	68,000
Zenpep 25,000	25,000	136,000	85,500

[a]The number after a trade name refers to the number of thousands of units of lipase contained per dosage form.

Patient Encounter, Part 2

TJ's parents have received CF disease state education and have met the multidisciplinary CF team. Additional laboratory testing has been sent to confirm the CF genotype. The team would like to initiate first-line CF therapies at this time because TJ displays symptoms of pancreatic insufficiency as outlined in Part 1. TJ weighs 3.1 kg and is 52 cm long.

Given this information, what is your assessment of TJ's nutritional status?

What are the treatment goals for this patient?

What nonpharmacologic therapy should be initiated?

What pharmacologic therapy should be initiated?

▶ Endocrine System

Patients with mild CFRD may be managed with carbohydrate modification if nutritional status is optimal. However, most patients present with poor nutrition and weight loss and require more aggressive treatment. ⑩ *Because CFRD results from insulin insufficiency, exogenous insulin replacement is usually required.* Many patients can be successfully managed by meal coverage with short- or rapid-acting insulin (regular, lispro, or aspart) dosed per carbohydrate counting. Patients with fasting hyperglycemia or patients receiving nighttime tube feedings typically also require longer-acting basal insulin. Regular home glucose monitoring is essential to appropriate therapy. Oral antidiabetic agents have not been studied adequately in CFRD, and routine use is not recommended.[6,9]

▶ Musculoskeletal System

CF patients with low bone mineral density and low serum vitamin D levels may improve bone health through supplemental vitamin D analogs beyond those found in standard CF vitamins. For ergocalciferol (or cholecalciferol), a minimum of 400 IU and 800 IU should be taken daily by infants and patients older than 1 year of age, respectively.[11,34] Total weekly or biweekly doses of 12,000 IU for children younger than 5 years of age and 50,000 IU for patients 5 years of age and older may be required to achieve target vitamin D concentrations. Supplemental calcium should be provided if 1,300 to 1,500 mg of elemental calcium intake cannot be achieved through diet.[11,34]

Antiresorptive agents (oral or IV bisphosphonates) may be used to treat adult CF patients with osteoporosis. Remaining upright daily for 30 minutes after dosing may be difficult for patients needing to perform airway clearance therapy, so products offering less frequent dosing should be considered. Gastroesophageal reflux or cirrhosis-associated esophageal varices may complicate therapy and increase the risk of erosive esophagitis. Pamidronate 30 mg IV every 3 months has increased bone mineral density in adult CF patients, and studies using IV bisphosphonates in children with CF are underway.[11] Androgen replacement in male CF patients with documented hypogonadism may benefit bone health in some patients.[11]

Short courses of nonsteroidal anti-inflammatory drugs (NSAIDs) can be used to treat CF-related arthritis and hypertrophic pulmonary osteoarthropathy.[6] The impact on neutrophil recruitment in the lung with long-term NSAID therapy at lower analgesic doses is unknown.

▶ Innovative Therapeutic Directions

Development of new therapies has extended the CF lifespan over the past several decades. Since the discovery of the CF gene and the CFTR protein defect, research has focused on gene therapy to restore normal CFTR function through DNA transfer. Newer research efforts focus on gene mutation-specific pharmacologic approaches

---

Patient Encounter, Part 3

TJ is now 9 months old (weight: 8.5 kg) and presents to a routine CF clinic appointment. His parents report that TJ has had a cough productive of yellow sputum for the past week and an intermittent low-grade fever of 101.1°F (38.4°C). Also, TJ is not eating as well as he usually does and has been sleeping more. The following vital signs are noted by clinic staff: RR 45/min, T 101.3°F (38.5°C), oxygen saturation 94% (0.94). Review of TJ's throat cultures since diagnosis reveals the following organisms: *H. influenzae* (β-lactamase positive), *P. aeruginosa* (sensitive to ceftazidime, cefepime, piperacillin/tazobactam, ticarcillin–clavulanate, aztreonam, meropenem, ciprofloxacin, levofloxacin, and tobramycin; resistant to amikacin and gentamicin), and *S. maltophilia* (sensitive to trimethoprim–sulfamethoxazole, minocycline, and ticarcillin–clavulanate; resistant to ceftazidime, meropenem, and levofloxacin). TJ has no known drug allergies.

Based on the information available, design an antibiotic regimen for outpatient therapy of TJ's first pulmonary exacerbation.

What antibiotic(s) and dose(s) would you recommend for inpatient therapy?

Develop a monitoring plan to assess antibiotic response.

---

to correct or modulate dysfunctional CFTR protein on a gene-specific basis (VX-770, VX-809, ataluren).[14] Additional research is being conducted with inhaled antibiotics (tobramycin powder for inhalation, liposomal amikacin), anti-inflammatory therapies, antipseudomonal vaccines, and exogenous cationic antimicrobial peptides to mimic those found naturally in the lung.[1]

In January 2012, the FDA approved ivacaftor (Kalydeco, formerly VX-770) as the first CFTR potentiator for treatment of CF patients 6 years and older who have at least one G551D CFTR gene mutation (present in approximately 4% of the CF population in the United States). Ivacaftor treatment (added to standard CF care) is associated with improved lung function (approximately 10% increase in FEV_1), decreased pulmonary exacerbations, weight gain, and increased quality of life.[35] Ivacaftor tablets are dosed at 150 mg orally every 12 hours with fat-containing food. Therapy is generally well tolerated, although elevated liver enzymes have been reported and should be monitored quarterly in the first year of therapy. Additional CFTR potentiators targeting other CFTR gene mutations are currently under investigation.

OUTCOME EVALUATION

Pulmonary System

- Monitor for changes in pulmonary symptoms (cough, sputum production, respiratory rate, and oxygen saturation). Symptoms should improve with antibiotics

Patient Care and Monitoring

1. Perform a thorough history of prescription, nonprescription, and alternative medications. Assess adherence, including timing of inhaled medications with respect to airway clearance therapies and timing of enzymes and insulin with regard to meals. Is the patient taking medications not prescribed by the CF center team?

2. Is the patient on all appropriate maintenance medications? Are medications at the appropriate doses for weight and/or age? If the patient is admitted, are maintenance medications ordered?

3. Evaluate the medication regimen for drug interactions, adverse reactions, and allergies.

4. Assess pulmonary symptoms. Review the incidence and quality of cough, dyspnea, respiratory rate, sputum production, and fever. Are the patient's PFTs decreased? Is there an oxygen requirement?

5. Review culture and sensitivity history over the last 1 to 2 years. What antibiotics were used in the past, and did the patient appear to respond better to a particular regimen? Is the patient currently on antibiotics, and if so, are the symptoms improving? Recommend an appropriate antibiotic regimen based on culture and sensitivity data.

6. Review the pharmacokinetic history. Are there likely changes in clearance since the last antibiotic course? Will the patient be discharged home on IV antibiotics? Can the IV regimen be simplified or made more convenient for home administration? Recommend appropriate doses based on the patient's clearance and an appropriate but convenient schedule.

7. Perform pharmacokinetic adjustments as necessary. Recommend a monitoring plan for the antibiotic course. Are any other laboratory tests necessary? Are signs of toxicity present?

8. Assess nutritional status. Is the patient gaining or maintaining weight according to age? Are any oral supplements or tube feedings being used?

9. Assess GI symptoms. What is the quantity and quality of bowel movements? Does the patient have bloating, flatulence, or abdominal pain?

10. Assess quality-of-life measures such as physical, psychological, and social well-being.

11. Understand that CF therapy is complicated, and recommend regimens that ease care burden.

12. Educate the patient and family, stressing importance of adherence to the regimen.

and aggressive airway clearance therapy. PFTs should be markedly increased after 1 week and trend back to pre-exacerbation levels after 2 weeks of therapy. If improvement lags, 3 weeks of therapy may be needed.

- For IV antimicrobial therapy, obtain serum drug levels for aminoglycosides and/or vancomycin and perform pharmacokinetic analysis. Adjust the dose, if needed, according to the parameters in Table 16–3. Obtain follow-up trough levels and serum creatinine at weekly intervals or sooner if renal function is unstable. Hearing tests may be scheduled yearly or per patient preference.

Gastrointestinal System

- Monitor short- and long-term nutritional status through evaluation of height, weight, and body mass index (BMI). Ideally, parameters should be near the normals (50th percentile) for non-CF patients.

- Evaluate the patient's stool patterns. Steatorrhea indicates suboptimal enzyme replacement or noncompliance. Infants should have two to three well-formed stools daily, whereas older children and adults may have one or two stools daily.

- Monitor efficacy of vitamin supplementation through yearly serum vitamin levels. Obtain levels more frequently if treating a deficiency.

Endocrine System

- Monitor blood glucose several times daily in patients with CFRD or those taking systemic corticosteroids. Follow A1C levels on an outpatient basis to assess long-term glucose control. Levels may be falsely low in CF due to a shorter red blood cell half-life.

Abbreviations Introduced in This Chapter

ABPA	Allergic bronchopulmonary aspergillosis
BMI	Body mass index
cAMP	Cyclic 3′,5′-adenosine monophosphate
CF	Cystic fibrosis
CFRD	Cystic fibrosis-related diabetes
CFTR	Cystic fibrosis transmembrane regulator
CPT	Chest physiotherapy
DIOS	Distal intestinal obstruction syndrome
ESBL	Extended-spectrum β-lactamase
FEV1	Forced expiratory volume in 1 second
FVC	Forced vital capacity
HFCC	High-frequency chest compression
INR	International normalized ratio
IPV	Intrapulmonary percussive ventilation
MIC	Minimum inhibitory concentration
MRSA	Methicillin-resistant *Staphylococcus aureus*
MSSA	Methicillin-sensitive *S. aureus*
NSAID	Nonsteroidal anti-inflammatory drug
OPEP	Oscillating positive expiratory pressure

PEG   Polyethylene glycol
PFT   Pulmonary function test
PMN   Polymorphonuclear
PT   Prothrombin time
RDA   Recommended daily allowance

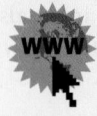 Self-assessment questions and answers are available at *http://www.mhpharmacotherapy. com/pp.html*.

REFERENCES

1. Gibson RL, Burns JL, Ramsey BW. State of the art: Pathophysiology and management of pulmonary infections in cystic fibrosis. Am J Respir Crit Care Med 2003;168:918–951.
2. Cystic fibrosis mutation database [Internet]. Available at: http://www.genet.sickkids.on.ca/StatisticsPage.html. Updated April 25, 2011. Accessed September 23, 2011.
3. Rowe SM, Miller SM, Sorscher EJ. Mechanisms of disease: Cystic fibrosis. N Engl J Med 2005;352:1992–2001.
4. Davis PB. Cystic fibrosis since 1938. Am J Respir Crit Care Med. 2006;173(5):475–482.
5. Conese M, Copreni E, Di Gioia S, et al. Neutrophil recruitment and airway epithelial cell involvement in chronic cystic fibrosis lung disease. J Cyst Fibros 2003;2:129–135.
6. Yankaskas JR, Marshall BC, Sufian JD, et al. Cystic fibrosis adult care consensus conference report. Chest 2004;125:1S–39S.
7. Littlewood JM, Wolfe SP. Control of malabsorption in cystic fibrosis. Paediatr Drugs 2000;2:205–222.
8. Debray D, Deirdre K, Houwen R, et al. Best practice guideline for the diagnosis and management of cystic fibrosis-associated liver disease. J Cyst Fibros 2011;10(2):S29–S36.
9. Moran A, Brunzell C, Cohen RC, et al. Clinical care guidelines for cystic fibrosis related diabetes. Diabetes Care 2010;33(12):2697–2708.
10. Sueblinvong V, Whittaker LA. Fertility and pregnancy: Common concerns of the aging cystic fibrosis population. Clin Chest Med 2007;28(2):433–443.
11. Aris RM, Merkel PA, Bachrach LK, et al. Consensus statement: Guide to bone health and disease in cystic fibrosis. J Clin Endocrinol Metab 2005;90:1888–1896.
12. Botton E, Saraux A, Laselve H, et al. Muscular manifestations in cystic fibrosis. Joint Bone Spine 2003;70:327–335.
13. O'Conner TM, McGrath DS, Short C, et al. Subclinical anaemia of chronic disease in adult patients with cystic fibrosis. J Cyst Fibros 2002;1:31–34.
14. Cystic Fibrosis Foundation. Cystic fibrosis foundation patient registry annual report 2010. Bethesda, MD: Cystic Fibrosis Foundation, 2011.
15. Lester MK, Flume PA. Airway-clearance therapy guidelines and implementation. Respir Care 2009;54(6):733–753.
16. Stallings VA, Stark LJ, Robinson KA, et al. Evidence-based practice recommendations for nutrition-related management of children and adults with cystic fibrosis and pancreatic insufficiency: Results of a systematic review. J Am Diet Assoc 2008;108:832–839.
17. Fuchs HJ, Borowitz DS, Christiansen DH, et al. Effect of aerosolized recombinant human DNase on exacerbations of respiratory symptoms and on pulmonary function in patients with cystic fibrosis. N Engl J Med 1994;331:637–642.
18. Elkins MR, Robinson M, Rose BR, et al. A controlled trial of long-term inhaled hypertonic saline in patients with cystic fibrosis. N Engl J Med 2006;354:229–240.
19. Prescott WA, Johnson CE. Antiinflammatory therapies for cystic fibrosis: Past, present, and future. Pharmacotherapy 2005;25(4):555–573.
20. Nichols DP, Konstan MW, Chmiel JF. Anti-inflammatory therapies for cystic fibrosis-related lung disease. Clinic Rev Allerg Immunol 2008;35:135–156.
21. Konstan MW, Byard PJ, Hoppel CL, Davis PB. Effect of high-dose ibuprofen in patients with cystic fibrosis. N Engl J Med 1995;332:848–854.
22. Konstan MW, Krenicky JE, Finney MR, et al. Effect of ibuprofen on neutrophil migration in vivo in cystic fibrosis and healthy subjects. J Pharmacol Exp Ther 2003;306:1086–1091.
23. Equi A Balfour-Lynn IM, Bush A, Rosenthal AB. Long term azithromycin in children with cystic fibrosis: A randomized, placebo-controlled crossover trial. Lancet 2002;360:978–984.
24. Saiman L, Marshall BC, Mayer-Hamblett N, et al. Azithromycin in patients with cystic fibrosis chronically infected with pseudomonas aeruginosa: A randomized controlled trial. JAMA 2003;290:1749–1756.
25. Yee CL, Duffy C, Gerbino PG, et al. Tendon or joint disorders in children after treatment with fluoroquinolones or azithromycin. Pediatr Infect Dis J 2002;21:525–529.
26. Kirkby S, Novak K, McCoy K. Update on antibiotics for infection control in cystic fibrosis. Expert Rev Anti Infect Ther 2009;7(8):967–980.
27. Flume PA, Mogayzel PJ, Robinson KA, et al. Cystic fibrosis pulmonary guidelines: Treatment of pulmonary exacerbations. Am J Respir Crit Care Med 2009;180(9):802–808.
28. Ramsey BW, Pepe MS, Quan JM, et al. Intermittent administration of inhaled tobramycin in patients with cystic fibrosis. N Engl J Med 1999; 340:23–30.
29. Flume PA, O'Sullivan BP, Robinson KA, et al. Cystic fibrosis pulmonary guidelines: Chronic medications for maintenance of lung health. Am J Respir Crit Care Med 2007;176(10):957–969.
30. Ratjen F, Munck A, Kho P, Angyalosi G. Treatment of early *Pseudomonas aeruginosa* infection in patients with cystic fibrosis: The ELITE trial. Thorax 2010;65(4):289–291.
31. McCoy KS, Quittner AL, Oermann CM, et al. Inhaled aztreonam lysine for chronic airway *Pseudomonas aeruginosa* in cystic fibrosis. Am J Respir Crit Care Med 2008;178(9):921–928.
32. Kirkby S, Novak K, McCoy. Aztreonam (for inhalation solution) for the treatment of chronic lung infections in patients with cystic fibrosis: An evidence based review. Core Evidence 2011;6:59–66.
33. Touw DJ, Vinks AA, Mouton JW, Horrevorts AM. Pharmacokinetic optimisation of antibacterial treatment in patients with cystic fibrosis: Current practice and suggestions for future directions. Clin Pharmacokinet 1998;35:437–459.
34. Borowitz D, Baker RD, Stallings V. Consensus report on nutrition for pediatric patients with cystic fibrosis. J Pediatr Gastroenterol Nutr 2002; 35(3):246–259.
35. Ramsey BW, Davies J, McElvaney NG, et al. A CFTR potentiator in patients with cystic fibrosis and the G551D mutation. N Engl J Med 2001; 365:1663–1672.

17 Gastroesophageal Reflux Disease

Dianne Williams May and Marie A. Chisholm-Burns

● **Upon completion of the chapter, the reader will be able to:**

1. Explain the underlying causes of gastroesophageal reflux disease (GERD).

2. Differentiate among typical, atypical, and complicated symptoms of GERD.

3. Determine which diagnostic tests should be recommended based on the patient's clinical presentation.

4. Identify the desired therapeutic outcomes for patients with GERD.

5. Recommend appropriate lifestyle modifications and pharmacotherapy interventions for patients with GERD.

6. Discuss other nonpharmacologic interventions that may be appropriate for patients with GERD.

7. Formulate a monitoring plan to assess the effectiveness and safety of pharmacotherapy for GERD.

8. Educate patients on appropriate lifestyle modifications and drug therapy issues including compliance, adverse effects, and drug interactions.

KEY CONCEPTS

❶ Esophageal gastroesophageal reflux disease (GERD) syndromes can be divided into two distinct categories: (a) symptomatic esophageal syndromes and (b) syndromes associated with esophageal tissue injury.

❷ Patients with GERD may display symptoms described as: (a) typical, (b) atypical, or (c) complicated.

❸ Patients presenting with uncomplicated typical symptoms of reflux (heartburn and regurgitation) do not usually require invasive esophageal evaluation.

❹ The goals of treatment of GERD are to alleviate symptoms, decrease the frequency of recurrent disease, promote healing of mucosal injury, and prevent complications.

❺ Treatment for GERD involves one or more of the following modalities: (a) patient-specific lifestyle changes and patient-directed therapy, (b) pharmacologic intervention primarily with acid-suppressing agents, (c) antireflux surgery, or (d) endoscopic therapies.

❻ Acid-suppressing therapy is the mainstay of GERD treatment and should be considered for anyone not responding to lifestyle changes and patient-directed therapy after 2 weeks.

❼ Antireflux surgery or endoscopic therapies offer an alternative treatment for refractory GERD or when pharmacologic management is undesirable.

❽ Many patients with GERD experience relapse if medication is withdrawn, and long-term maintenance treatment may be required in these patients.

❾ Patient medication profiles should be reviewed for drugs that may aggravate GERD.

INTRODUCTION

Gastroesophageal reflux disease (GERD) is defined as troublesome symptoms and/or complications caused by refluxing the stomach contents into the esophagus.[1,2] The key is that these troublesome symptoms adversely affect the well-being of the patient.[2] ❶ *Esophageal GERD syndromes can be divided into two distinct categories: (a) symptomatic esophageal syndromes and (b) syndromes associated with esophageal tissue injury.*[2] Symptomatic (or symptom-based) esophageal syndrome is associated with severe reflux symptoms with normal endoscopic findings. Syndromes associated with esophageal tissue injury include erosive esophagitis, strictures, Barrett's esophagus, and esophageal adenocarcinoma. Erosive esophagitis occurs when the esophagus is repeatedly exposed to refluxed material for prolonged periods. The inflammation that occurs progresses to erosions of the squamous epithelium.

Barrett's esophagus is a complication of GERD, characterized by replacement of the normal squamous epithelial lining of the esophagus by specialized columnar-type epithelium. Barrett's esophagus is more likely to occur in patients with a long history (years) of reflux and may be a risk factor for developing adenocarcinoma of the esophagus because of this change in the epithelial lining. The risk of progression to high-grade dysplasia or adenocarcinoma remains controversial but can be a source of psychological stress for those with Barrett's esophagus.

Certain extraesophageal syndromes have an association with GERD and manifest as symptoms occurring outside the esophagus. Chronic cough, laryngitis, and asthma have the strongest association with GERD. Reflux chest pain syndrome may also occur with chest pain often being indistinguishable from cardiac chest pain. With all of these extraesophageal or "atypical" manifestations, other causes must be ruled out before considering a diagnosis of GERD.

EPIDEMIOLOGY AND ETIOLOGY

GERD is prevalent in patients of all ages and appears to be increasing in both adults and children. It is estimated that 14% to 20% of adults in the United States are affected.[3] Although mortality associated with GERD is rare, symptoms can significantly decrease quality of life. The true prevalence and incidence of GERD are unknown because: (a) many patients do not seek medical treatment, (b) symptoms do not always correlate well with disease severity, and (c) there is no standard method for diagnosing the disease. There does not appear to be a major gender difference in incidence except for its association with pregnancy. Gender is an important factor in the development of Barrett's esophagus, which occurs more frequently in males.

PATHOPHYSIOLOGY

The retrograde movement of acid or other noxious substances from the stomach into the esophagus is a major factor in the development of GERD.[4] Commonly, gastroesophageal reflux is associated with defective lower esophageal sphincter (LES) pressure or function. Problems with other normal mucosal defense mechanisms such as anatomic factors, esophageal clearance, mucosal resistance, gastric emptying, epidermal growth factor, and salivary buffering may also contribute to the development of GERD. Other factors that may promote esophageal damage upon reflux into the esophagus include gastric acid, pepsin, bile acids, and pancreatic enzymes. Therapeutic regimens for GERD are designed to maximize normal mucosal defense mechanisms and attenuate these other factors that contribute to the disease.

Lower Esophageal Sphincter Pressure

The LES is a manometrically defined zone of the distal esophagus with an elevated basal resting pressure. The sphincter is normally in a tonic, contracted state, preventing the reflux of gastric material from the stomach. It relaxes on swallowing to permit the free passage of food into the stomach.

Mechanisms by which defective LES pressure may cause gastroesophageal reflux are threefold. First, and probably most important, reflux may occur after spontaneous transient LES relaxations that are not associated with swallowing.[5] Esophageal distention, vomiting, belching, and retching can cause relaxation of the LES. Transient decreases in sphincter pressure are responsible for approximately 40% of the reflux episodes in patients with GERD.[5]

Second, reflux may occur after transient increases in intra-abdominal pressure (stress reflux).[4] An increase in intra-abdominal pressure such as that occurring during straining, bending over, or a Valsalva maneuver may overcome a weak LES, and thus may lead to reflux.

Third, the LES may be atonic, thus permitting free reflux. Although transient relaxations are more likely to occur when there is normal LES pressure, the latter two mechanisms are more likely when the LES pressure is decreased by such factors as fatty foods, gastric distention, or smoking. Certain foods and medications may worsen esophageal reflux by decreasing LES pressure or by irritating the esophageal mucosa (Table 17–1).[6,7]

Table 17–1

Foods and Medications That May Worsen GERD Symptoms

Decreased LES Pressure

Foods

Fatty meal/fried foods	Coffee, caffeinated drinks
Carminatives (e.g., peppermint)	Garlic
	Onions
Chocolate	Chili peppers

Medications

Anticholinergics	Ethanol
Barbiturates	Isoproterenol
Benzodiazepines	Narcotics (e.g., morphine)
Caffeine	Nicotine
Dihydropyridine calcium channel blockers	Nitrates
Dopamine	Phentolamine
	Progesterone
Estrogen	Theophylline

Direct Irritants to the Esophageal Mucosa

Foods

Spicy foods	Tomatoes
Citrus fruits, orange juice	Coffee, carbonated beverages

Medications

Bisphosphonates	NSAIDs
Aspirin	Quinidine
Iron	Potassium chloride

GERD, gastroesophageal reflux disease; LES, lower esophageal sphincter; NSAIDs, nonsteroidal anti-inflammatory drugs.

Adapted from Williams DB, Schade RR. Gastroesophageal reflux disease. In: DiPiro JT, Talbert RL, Yee GC, et al., eds. Pharmacotherapy: A Pathophysiologic Approach, 8th ed. New York, NY: McGraw-Hill, 2011:550, with permission.

Anatomic Factors

Disruption of the normal anatomic barriers by a hiatal hernia was once thought to be a primary etiology of gastroesophageal reflux and esophagitis. Currently, the presence of a hiatal hernia is generally considered to be a separate entity that may or may not be associated with reflux.

Esophageal Clearance

Many patients with GERD produce normal amounts of acid, but the acid produced spends too much time in contact with the esophageal mucosa. The contact time depends on the rate at which the esophagus clears the noxious material, as well as the frequency of reflux. The esophagus is cleared by primary peristalsis in response to swallowing or by secondary peristalsis in response to esophageal distention and gravitational effects.

Swallowing contributes to esophageal clearance by increasing salivary flow. Saliva contains bicarbonate that buffers the residual gastric material on the surface of the esophagus. The production of saliva decreases with increasing age, making it more difficult to maintain a neutral intraesophageal pH. Therefore, esophageal damage due to reflux occurs more often in the elderly and patients with Sjögren's syndrome or xerostomia. Swallowing is also decreased during sleep, which contributes to nocturnal GERD in some patients.

Mucosal Resistance

The esophageal mucosa and submucosa consist of mucus-secreting glands that contain bicarbonate. Bicarbonate moving from the blood to the lumen can neutralize acidic refluxate in the esophagus. A decrease in this normal defense mechanism can potentially lead to erosions in the esophagus. When the mucosa is repeatedly exposed to the refluxate in GERD, or if there is a defect in the normal mucosal defenses, hydrogen ions diffuse into the mucosa, leading to the cellular acidification and necrosis that ultimately cause esophagitis.

Gastric Emptying and Increased Abdominal Pressure

Gastric volume is related to the amount of material ingested, rate of gastric secretion, rate of gastric emptying, and amount and frequency of duodenal reflux into the stomach. Delayed gastric emptying can lead to increased gastric volume and can contribute to reflux by increasing intragastric pressure. Factors that increase gastric volume and/or decrease gastric emptying, such as smoking and high-fat meals, are often associated with gastroesophageal reflux. This partially explains the prevalence of postprandial gastroesophageal reflux. Obesity has been linked to GERD because of increased abdominal pressure. Morbidly obese patients may also have more transient LES relaxations, incompetent LES, and impaired esophageal motility.[5]

Composition of Refluxate

The composition, pH, and volume of the refluxate are other factors associated with gastroesophageal reflux. Duodenogastric reflux esophagitis, or "alkaline esophagitis," refers to esophagitis induced by the reflux of bilious and pancreatic fluid. Although bile acids have both a direct irritant effect on the esophageal mucosa and an indirect effect of increasing hydrogen ion permeability of the mucosa, symptoms are more often related to acid reflux than to bile reflux. The percentage of time that esophageal pH is below 4 is greater for patients with severe disease.

The pathophysiology of GERD is a complex process. It is difficult to determine which occurs first: gastroesophageal reflux leading to defective peristalsis with delayed clearing or an incompetent LES pressure leading to gastroesophageal reflux. Understanding factors associated with the development of GERD is essential to providing effective treatment (Fig. 17–1).

CLINICAL PRESENTATION AND DIAGNOSIS

❷ *Patients with GERD may display symptoms described as: (a) typical, (b) atypical, or (c) complicated* (see Clinical Presentation box on next page).

Diagnosis of GERD

The most useful tool in the diagnosis of GERD is the clinical history, including both the presenting symptoms and associated risk factors. ❸ *Patients presenting with*

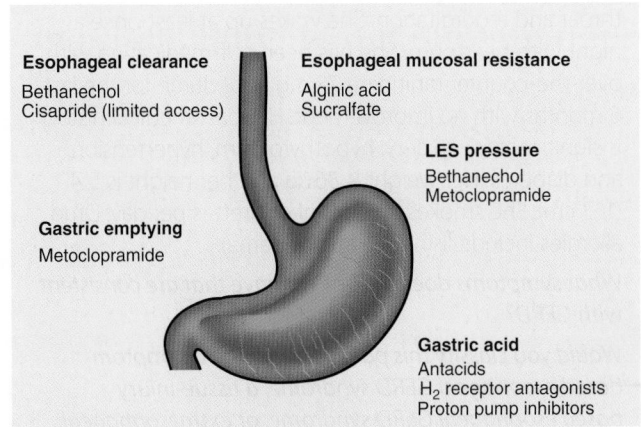

FIGURE 17–1. Therapeutic interventions in the management of gastroesophageal reflux disease. Pharmacologic interventions are targeted at improving defense mechanisms or decreasing aggressive factors. (LES, lower esophageal sphincter.) (Adapted with permission from Williams DB, Schade RR. Gastroesophageal reflux disease. In: DiPiro JT, Talbert RL, Yee GC, et al., eds. Pharmacotherapy: A Pathophysiologic Approach, 8th ed. New York, NY: McGraw-Hill, 2008:553.)

Clinical Presentation of GERD

Typical Symptoms

- Heartburn is the hallmark symptom and is described as a substantial sensation of warmth or burning rising up from the abdomen that may radiate to the neck. It may be waxing and waning in character.
- Regurgitation.
- Symptoms may be worse after a fatty meal, when bending over, or when lying in a recumbent position.[1]
- Hypersalivation and belching.

Atypical Symptoms

- Asthma, chronic cough, hoarseness, pharyngitis, chest pain, and dental erosions.
- It is important to distinguish GERD symptoms from those of other diseases.

Complicated Symptoms

- Continual pain, dysphagia (difficulty swallowing), odynophagia (painful swallowing), bleeding, unexplained weight loss, unexplained anemia, and choking.
- These symptoms may be indicative of complications of GERD such as Barrett's esophagus, esophageal strictures, or esophageal cancer.

Patient Encounter, Part 1

JM is a 58-year-old African American woman who comes to your clinic with a 1-year history "severe burning" in her throat and regurgitation. She wakes up at least once a night with heartburn. She has been self-medicating with over-the-counter ranitidine 75 mg at bedtime for the last 6 months with no improvement. Her past medical history is significant for anxiety, hypothyroidism, hypertension, and diabetes. Her weight is 86 kg and her height is 5′4″ (163 cm). She smokes 2 packs of cigarettes per day. Drug allergies include lisinopril (angioedema).

What symptoms does the patient have that are consistent with GERD?

Would you classify this patient as having a symptom-based esophageal GERD syndrome, a tissue-injury based esophageal GERD syndrome, or extraesophageal syndrome? Explain.

Which risk factors does she have that may worsen her GERD symptoms?

uncomplicated, typical symptoms of reflux (heartburn and regurgitation) do not usually require invasive esophageal evaluation. These patients generally benefit from a trial of patient-specific lifestyle modifications and empiric acid-suppressing therapy.[2] A clinical diagnosis of GERD is assumed in

those responding to appropriate therapy. Further diagnostic testing is indicated to: (a) avert misdiagnosis, (b) identify complications, and (c) evaluate empiric treatment failures.

Endoscopy with biopsy is the preferred diagnostic test for assessing the mucosa for esophagitis, Barrett's esophagus, and esophageal adenocarcinoma. It should also be performed in patients with troublesome dysphagia, unexplained weight loss, epigastric mass, or patients with esophageal GERD syndrome who have not responded to an empiric trial of twice-daily proton pump inhibitor (PPI) therapy.[2] Previous data suggested that long-standing symptomatic GERD is a possible risk factor for developing Barrett's esophagus, and consequently, esophageal adenocarcinoma.[8] Unfortunately, the presence of Barrett's esophagus may not correlate well with reflux symptoms. This may explain why endoscopic screening for esophageal adenocarcinoma in patients with severe long-standing symptoms has not been as successful as expected.[9]

Patients with esophageal GERD syndromes who have failed twice-daily PPI therapy and have normal findings on endoscopy may benefit from manometry. Manometry helps to localize the LES for ambulatory pH monitoring, evaluates peristaltic function in patients considering surgery, and identifies possible motor disorders.[2]

In patients with normal endoscopic and manometry findings who are still symptomatic despite appropriate treatment, esophageal pH monitoring may be useful. There are various methods that may be used including ambulatory impedance pH, catheter pH, or wireless pH monitoring. These tests can objectively prove that symptoms are reflux related.[2] **Impedance pH monitoring** allows reflux episodes to be characterized as acid or nonacid.[10] This method may be useful in patients with refractory symptoms. Wireless pH monitoring can record data for up to 48 hours and therefore may be more sensitive than catheter studies for detecting esophageal acid exposure.[2] For best results, PPI therapy should be withheld for 7 days prior to ambulatory impedance pH, catheter pH, or wireless pH monitoring.[2]

TREATMENT

Desired Outcomes

4 *The goals of treatment of GERD are to alleviate symptoms, decrease the frequency of recurrent disease, promote healing of mucosal injury, and prevent complications.* Inadequate treatment and consequent long-term acid exposure may lead to complications such as Barrett's esophagus and possibly esophageal adenocarcinoma.[2]

General Approach to Treatment

5 *Treatment for GERD involves one or more of the following modalities: (a) lifestyle changes and patient-directed therapy, (b) pharmacologic intervention primarily with acid-suppressing agents, (c) antireflux surgery, or (d) endoscopic therapies.* The first therapeutic option used depends on the patient's condition (i.e., frequency of symptoms, degree of esophagitis, and presence of complications; Table 17–2).

Table 17–2

Therapeutic Approach to GERD in Adults

Patient Presentation	Recommended Treatment Regimen	Comments

Intermittent, mild heartburn	A. Individualized lifestyle modifications
	PLUS
	B. Antacids
	• Magnesium/aluminum hydroxide 30 mL after meals and at bedtime as needed
	• Antacid/alginic acid (Gaviscon) 2 tablets or 15 mL after meals and at bedtime
	AND/OR
	C. Patient-directed therapy
	• OTC H₂RAs (each taken up to twice daily)
	   Cimetidine 200 mg
	   Famotidine 10 mg
	   Nizatidine 75 mg
	   Ranitidine 75 mg
	OR
	• OTC PPI (taken once daily)
	   Omeprazole 20 mg
	   Omeprazole 20 mg/sodium bicarbonate 1100 mg
	   Lansoprazole 15 mg
		• If symptoms are unrelieved with lifestyle changes and OTC after 2 weeks, begin therapy with a standard dose acid-suppressing agent
		• Aluminum-containing antacids may accumulate in renal failure.
		• Calcium-containing antacids may need to be decreased in patients with CrCl less than 25 mL/min (0.42 mL/s) (based on serum calcium level)
		• In general, give 50% of H_2RA dose with CrCl less than 50 mL/min (0.83 mL/s)

Symptomatic GERD	A. Individualized lifestyle modifications
	PLUS
	B. Standard dose acid-suppressing therapy
	• H₂RAs (taken twice daily) for 6–12 weeks
	   Cimetidine 800 mg
	   Famotidine 20 mg
	   Nizatidine 150 mg
	   Ranitidine 150 mg
	OR
	• PPIs (taken once daily) for 4–8 weeks; increase to twice daily in patients with inadequate symptom response to once daily therapy.
	   Dexlansoprazole 30 mg
	   Esomeprazole 20 mg
	   Lansoprazole 15–30 mg
	   Omeprazole 20 mg
	   Pantoprazole 40 mg
	   Rabeprazole 20 mg
		• For typical symptoms, treat empirically with standard doses of acid-suppressing therapy
		• Mild GERD may be treated effectively with H₂RAs. Patients with moderate to severe symptoms should receive a PPI as initial therapy. If symptoms are relieved, treat recurrences on an as-needed basis
		• If symptoms recur frequently, consider maintenance therapy with the lowest effective dose

Healing of erosive esophagitis or treatment of moderate to severe symptoms or complications	A. Individualized lifestyle modifications
	PLUS
	B. PPIs (taken once or twice daily) for 4–16 weeks
	   Dexlansoprazole 60 mg
	   Esomeprazole 20–40 mg
	   Lansoprazole 30 mg
	   Omeprazole 20 mg
	   Rabeprazole 20 mg
	   Pantoprazole 40 mg
		• For extraesophageal symptoms, give a trial of a PPI or H₂RA. Reflux chest syndrome: Start with twice-daily PPI
		• If symptoms are relieved, consider maintenance therapy
		• PPIs are the most effective maintenance therapy in patients with extraesophageal symptoms, complicated symptoms, or erosive disease
		• Patients not responding to acid-suppressing therapy, including those with persistent extraesophageal symptoms, may be candidates for antireflux surgery

CrCl, creatinine clearance; GERD, gastroesophageal reflux disease; H₂RA, histamine₂-receptor antagonist; PPI, proton pump inhibitor.

Adapted from Williams DB, Schade RR. Gastroesophageal reflux disease. In: DiPiro JT, Talbert RL, Yee GC, et al., eds. Pharmacotherapy: A Pathophysiologic Approach, 8th ed. New York, NY: McGraw-Hill, 2011:555, with permission.

6 *Acid-suppressing therapy is the mainstay of GERD treatment and should be considered for anyone not responding to patient-specific lifestyle changes and patient-directed therapy after 2 weeks.* The PPIs provide the greatest relief of symptoms and highest rates of healing, especially in patients with erosive disease or moderate to severe symptoms.

Maintenance therapy is generally necessary to control symptoms and prevent complications. GERD refractory to

Patient Encounter, Part 2: Medical History, Physical Examination, and Diagnostic Tests

PMH: Type 2 diabetes mellitus since age 45 (well controlled); hypertension for 20 years (well controlled)

FH: Noncontributory

SH: Works as a teacher in an elementary school; lives at home with husband and teenage daughter

Meds: Metformin 500 mg orally twice daily; hydrochlorothiazide 12.5 mg orally once daily; amlodipine 10 mg orally once daily, levothyroxine 0.025 mg once daily, and lorazepam 0.5 mg at bedtime

ROS: (+) Heartburn, regurgitation; (–) chest pain, nausea, vomiting, diarrhea, weight loss, change in appetite, shortness of breath or cough, difficulty or painful swallowing

PE:

VS: BP 128/76 mm Hg, P 79 bpm, RR 16 breaths/min, T 37°C (98.6°F)

CV: RRR, normal S_1, S_2; no murmurs, rubs, or gallops

Abd: Soft, nontender, nondistended; (+) bowel sounds, (–) hepatosplenomegaly, heme (–) stool

Given this additional information, are there any other factors that could be contributing to her GERD symptoms?

Should patient-directed therapy with over-the-counter ranitidine 75 mg at bedtime be continued? Explain.

What nonpharmacologic and pharmacologic changes would you recommend for her GERD therapy?

JM returns to your clinic after her second 8-week course of lansoprazole 30 mg once daily because her symptoms still have not improved. What would you recommend next for this patient?

When would further diagnostic testing be indicated?

adequate acid suppression is rare. In these cases, the diagnosis should be confirmed through further diagnostic tests before long-term, high-dose therapy or antireflux surgery or endoscopic therapies are considered.

Nonpharmacologic Therapy

Nonpharmacologic treatment of GERD includes patient-specific lifestyle modifications, antireflux surgery, or endoscopic therapies.

▶ Lifestyle Modifications

Although most patients do not respond to lifestyle changes alone, the importance of maintaining these changes throughout the course of GERD therapy should be discussed. The most beneficial lifestyle changes include: (a) losing weight if overweight or obese, and (b) elevating the head of the bed if symptoms are worse when recumbent. Elevating the head

of the bed about 6 to 10 in. (15 to 25 cm) with a foam wedge (not just elevating the head with pillows) decreases nocturnal esophageal acid contact time and should be recommended.

Other lifestyle modifications should be considered based on the circumstances of the individual patient. These include: (a) eating smaller meals and avoiding meals 3 hours before sleeping, (b) avoiding foods or medications that exacerbate GERD, (c) smoking cessation, and (d) avoiding alcohol.

Patient medications and food histories should be evaluated to identify potential factors that may exacerbate GERD symptoms (see Table 17–1). Patients should be monitored closely for symptoms when medications known to worsen GERD are started.

▶ Antireflux Surgery and Endoscopic Therapies

7 *Antireflux surgery or endoscopic therapies offer alternative treatments for refractory GERD or when pharmacologic management is undesirable.* Surgical intervention is a viable alternative for selected patients with well-documented GERD.[2] The goal of surgery is to reestablish the antireflux barrier, to position the LES within the abdomen where it is under positive (intra-abdominal) pressure, and to close any associated hiatal defect. It should be considered in patients who: (a) fail to respond to or are intolerant to pharmacologic treatment, (b) opt for surgery despite successful treatment because of lifestyle considerations, (c) have complications of GERD, or (d) have extraesophageal manifestations.[2,11]

Three main endoscopic approaches for the management of GERD are available: (a) application of radiofrequency energy to the LES area, (b) endoscopic suturing to produce a plication, and (c) endoscopic injection of bulking agents, or implantation of a bioprosthesis into the lower esophageal sphincter zone.[12] These cannot currently be recommended for routine use in patients with esophageal GERD syndromes.[2]

Pharmacologic Therapy

▶ Antacids and Antacid–Alginic Acid Products

Antacids are an appropriate component of treating mild GERD because they are effective for immediate, symptomatic relief. They are often used concurrently with other acid-suppressing therapies. Common antacids include magnesium hydroxide/aluminum hydroxide combination products (e.g., Mylanta, Maalox) and those containing calcium carbonate, such as Tums.

An antacid product combined with alginic acid (Gaviscon) is not a potent neutralizing agent but forms a highly viscous solution that floats on the surface of the gastric contents. This viscous solution serves as a protective barrier for the esophagus against reflux of gastric contents.

Dosage recommendations for antacids vary and range from hourly dosing to administration on an as-needed basis. In general, antacids have a short duration of action, which requires frequent administration throughout the day to provide continuous acid neutralization.

Antacids also have clinically significant drug interactions with ferrous sulfate, isoniazid, sulfonylureas, and quinolone antibiotics. Antacid–drug interactions are influenced by antacid composition, dose, dosage schedule, and formulation.

▶ Histamine$_2$-Receptor Antagonists

The histamine$_2$-receptor antagonists (H$_2$RAs)—cimetidine, famotidine, nizatidine, and ranitidine—decrease acid secretion by inhibiting the histamine$_2$-receptors in gastric parietal cells. When given in divided doses, they are effective for patients with mild to moderate GERD.[1] Standard doses provide symptomatic improvement in about 60% of patients after 12 weeks of therapy.[1] Healing rates per endoscopy tend to be lower (50%).[1] Response to the H$_2$RAs depends on the severity of disease, the dosage regimen used, and the duration of therapy.

For symptomatic relief of mild GERD, low-dose, nonprescription H$_2$RAs may be beneficial. For patients not responding to patient-directed therapy with over-the-counter (OTC) agents after 2 weeks, standard-dose acid-suppressing therapy is warranted. Although higher doses of H$_2$RAs may provide greater symptomatic and endoscopic healing rates, limited information exists regarding their safety, and they can be less effective and more costly than once-daily PPIs.

Because all H$_2$RAs have similar efficacy, selection should be based on differences in dosage regimen, safety profile, and cost. In general, H$_2$RAs are well tolerated. Patients should be monitored for adverse effects and potential drug interactions. Cimetidine has the most drug interactions.

▶ Proton Pump Inhibitors

The PPIs—esomeprazole, lansoprazole, omeprazole, pantoprazole, rabeprazole, and dexlansoprazole—block gastric acid secretion by inhibiting gastric H$^+$/K$^+$-adenosine triphosphatase in gastric parietal cells. This produces a profound, long-lasting antisecretory effect capable of maintaining the gastric pH above 4, even during acid surges seen postprandially.

The PPIs are superior to H$_2$RAs in patients with moderate to severe GERD. This includes not only patients with erosive esophagitis or complicated symptoms (Barrett's esophagus or strictures) but also those with symptomatic esophageal syndromes. Symptomatic relief is seen in approximately 83% of patients, and healing rates at 8 weeks as judged by endoscopy are 78%.[1]

A PPI should be given empirically to patients with troublesome symptoms of GERD. If the standard once-daily course of therapy is not effective in eliminating symptoms, then empiric therapy with twice-daily dosing should be given. Patients not responding to twice-daily PPI therapy should be considered treatment failures, and further diagnostic evaluation should be performed.[2] Evidence does not support using higher than normal doses of PPIs in patients with Barrett's esophagus with the sole intent of reducing the risk of progression to dysplasia or cancer.[13] The risks and benefits of long-term PPI therapy in patients with Barrett's esophagus should be considered.

Comparable daily doses of PPIs are omeprazole 20 mg = esomeprazole 20 mg = lansoprazole 30 mg = dexlansoprazole 30 mg = rabeprazole 20 mg = pantoprazole 40 mg. The PPIs degrade in acidic environments and are therefore formulated in delayed-release capsules or tablets.[14] Lansoprazole, esomeprazole, and omeprazole contain enteric-coated (pH-sensitive) granules in a capsule form. For patients unable to swallow the capsule, pediatric patients, or those with a nasogastric tube, the contents of the capsule can be mixed in applesauce or placed in orange juice.[15] The acidic juices help maintain the integrity of the enteric-coated pellets until they reach the small intestine.[15] Esomeprazole pellets can be mixed with water prior to delivery through a nasogastric tube.[15] Lansoprazole is also available in a delayed-release orally disintegrating tablet. Esomeprazole and omeprazole are available in a delayed-release oral suspension powder packet.

Omeprazole is also available in an immediate-release formulation combined with sodium bicarbonate (Zegerid). The proposed benefit of this combination product is fast onset of action and increase in pH by the sodium bicarbonate, which helps prevent degradation of omeprazole in the stomach. Sodium bicarbonate may also stimulate gastrin production, which may activate the proton pumps and optimize the effectiveness of omeprazole.

Patients taking pantoprazole or rabeprazole should be instructed not to crush, chew, or split the delayed-release tablets. Pantoprazole and esomeprazole are available in IV formulations that offer an alternative route for patients unable to take oral medications. The IV product is not more effective than the oral forms and is significantly more expensive.

Patients should be instructed to take their PPI in the morning, 30 to 60 minutes before breakfast to maximize efficacy, because these agents inhibit only actively secreting proton pumps. Although usually given prior to breakfast, patients with nighttime symptoms may benefit from taking their PPI prior to the evening meal.[1] If a second dose is needed, it should be administered before the evening meal and not at bedtime.[1] Regardless of the time of day, PPIs should be given prior to a meal to gain the most benefit. The exception to this is the immediate-release omeprazole–sodium bicarbonate combination product, which can be given at bedtime.

All PPIs can decrease the absorption of drugs (e.g., ketoconazole) that require an acidic environment to be absorbed. All PPIs are metabolized by the cytochrome P-450 system to some extent. Omeprazole and lansoprazole are metabolized by CYP2C19 enzymes. Concerns have been raised about PPIs used concurrently with clopidogrel, a prodrug that must be converted to its active form by CYP2C19. Inhibition of CYP2C19 by PPIs has been suggested to decrease the effectiveness of clopidogrel and increase the risk of cardiac events. A recent consensus report found little evidence to suggest cardiovascular harm when PPIs were used concurrently with clopidogrel.[16] Omeprazole is the most likely PPI to cause problems in patients on clopidogrel, and the FDA has identified this agent as the only one of concern. Patients who are slow metabolizers or the slow biotransformer phenotype for clopidogrel require further study. The consensus report recommended PPIs due to superior efficacy in patients with a history of upper GI bleeding or with multiple risk factors for GI bleeding who require antiplatelet therapy.[16] Risk factors for GI bleeding include a history of bleeding or other complication of peptic ulcer disease; advanced age; use of anticoagulants, corticosteroids, or nonsteroidal anti-inflammatory drugs (NSAIDs); and presence of *Helicobacter pylori*.[16] Consider an H_2RA for patients at lower risk of GI bleeding.

No interactions with lansoprazole, pantoprazole, or rabeprazole have been seen with CYP2C19 substrates such as diazepam, warfarin, or phenytoin.[17] Esomeprazole does not appear to interact with warfarin or phenytoin. Pantoprazole is metabolized by a cytosolic sulfotransferase and therefore less likely to have significant drug interactions than other PPIs. Although generally not of major concern, omeprazole may inhibit the metabolism of warfarin, diazepam, and phenytoin. Drug interactions with omeprazole are of particular concern in patients who are considered "slow metabolizers," approximately 3% of the white population. Unfortunately, it is unclear which patients have the polymorphic gene variation that makes them slow metabolizers. Alternatively, patients who are considered rapid metabolizers, which is most common in the Asian population (12% to 20%), may not respond as well as those who are considered slow metabolizers.[18] This genetic variation among patients may alter the effect of PPIs due to the ability of their enzyme system to metabolize the drug.[18] Esomeprazole is metabolized more by CYP3A4 enzymes and may be affected less by the patient's genotype.[19]

The PPIs are generally well tolerated. The most common side effects are headache, diarrhea, constipation, and abdominal pain. Potential concerns about long-term use of PPIs include development of hypergastrinemia, enteric infections, vitamin B_{12} deficiency, or hypomagnesemia. Prolonged hypergastrinemia associated with PPI use causing enterochromaffin-like cell hyperplasia or carcinoid tumors has not been convincingly proven.[20] Enteric infections, including *Clostridium difficile*, may be caused by numerous factors (e.g., age, antibiotic use, contact with infected healthcare worker, crowding, and immunosuppression). Therefore, the role PPIs may play in the development of these infections is speculative. PPIs may inhibit the secretion of intrinsic factor by the parietal cells, which may lead to decreased absorption of vitamin B_{12} with subsequent deficiency. There is little evidence to support clinical relevance to this finding. Although hypomagnesemia is a rare side effect of PPI therapy, it can potentially be life threatening. Higher doses and long-term use (more than 1 year) are most likely to be associated with hypomagnesemia.

Conflicting data are available regarding the risk of fractures in patients taking concomitant PPI therapy.[21] A recent FDA advisory warned of the potential risk for osteoporosis and fractures in patients taking long-term PPI therapy (more than 1 year) or high-dose PPI therapy.[21] The advisory was revised 10 months later to remove the fracture risk warning on the OTC PPIs because fractures with short-term low-dose PPI are unlikely.[22] Another study showed that fracture risk with PPI use was only significant in those who also had other risk factors for fracture or osteoporosis.[23] Because the data are conflicting, patients with clear indications should receive PPI therapy. Routine bone density studies or calcium supplementation are not warranted based on PPI use alone.[2]

Because all PPIs have similar efficacy, selection of the specific agent should be based on factors such as differences in dosage regimen, safety profile, and cost.

▶ *Prokinetic Agents*

The prokinetic agents include metoclopramide and bethanechol. The inferior efficacy and adverse effect profiles of metoclopramide and bethanechol limit their use in the treatment of GERD, and they are not recommended.

▶ *Mucosal Protectants*

Sucralfate, a nonabsorbable aluminum salt of sucrose octasulfate, has very limited value in the treatment of GERD and is not recommended.

Combination Therapy

Two agents of different therapeutic classes should not be used routinely. Only modest improvements have been shown when a prokinetic agent is combined with a standard dose of an H_2RA. Therefore, patients not responding to standard H_2RA doses should be switched to a PPI instead of adding a prokinetic agent. Monotherapy with a PPI is not only more effective, but it also improves compliance with once-daily dosing and is ultimately more cost effective.

The addition of an H_2RA at bedtime to PPI therapy has been suggested to decrease nocturnal acid breakthrough. Although there may be an immediate effect to control symptoms and keep the pH greater than 4, tachyphylaxis may quickly develop. If H_2RAs are used at night, it may be preferable to only use them as needed to provide a "drug holiday" that may lessen the occurrence of tachyphylaxis.[24] There is no evidence supporting the addition of a nocturnal dose of an H_2RA to twice-daily PPI therapy.[2] Immediate-release omeprazole–sodium bicarbonate has been shown to decrease nocturnal acid exposure compared with pantoprazole administered daily with the evening meal and lansoprazole administered at bedtime. Although more studies are needed, immediate-release omeprazole may offer an effective option for controlling nocturnal acid exposure and symptoms over the addition of an H_2RA.

Maintenance Therapy

⑧ *Many patients with GERD experience relapse if medication is withdrawn, and long-term maintenance treatment may be required in these patients.*[1] Candidates for maintenance therapy include patients whose symptoms return once therapy is discontinued or decreased, patients with a history of esophagitis healed by PPIs, patients with complications such as Barrett's esophagus or strictures, and perhaps patients with atypical symptoms. In some patients, the dose of acid-suppressing therapy may be titrated to the lowest dose that controls symptoms.[2]

The goal of maintenance therapy is to improve quality of life by controlling symptoms and preventing complications. Acid suppressing therapy should be reduced to the lowest dose that controls symptoms and routinely evaluated to determine if long-term therapy is indicated. This is especially true in light of more recent safety concerns with long-term PPI use.

The H$_2$RAs may be effective maintenance therapy for patients with mild disease. The PPIs are first choice for maintenance treatment of moderate to severe GERD. A short course of "on-demand" therapy may be appropriate in patients with symptomatic esophageal syndromes without esophagitis when symptom control is the primary outcome of interest.[2] Antacids have the fastest onset and may be used in combination with an H$_2$RA or PPI for on-demand symptom relief.

Although patients with a history of esophagitis and/or complications generally require long-term maintenance therapy with a PPI, the dose should be titrated down to the lowest effective dose to provide adequate symptom control.[2] Long-term use of higher PPI doses is not indicated unless the patient has complicated symptoms, has erosive esophagitis per endoscopy, or has had further diagnostic evaluation to determine degree and frequency of acid exposure. Antireflux surgery and endoscopic therapies may be viable alternatives to long-term drug use for maintenance therapy in selected patients.

Special Population Considerations

▶ Patients with Extraesophageal GERD

GERD therapy has not been shown to be beneficial in treating extraesophageal symptoms in patients without concomitant typical GERD symptoms.[2] Other causes should be ruled out before attributing the symptoms to GERD. Chronic cough, laryngitis, and asthma have established associations with GERD.[2] In patients presenting with extraesophageal GERD syndromes such as laryngitis or asthma, treatment with twice-daily PPI therapy for 2 months is probably warranted when there is a concomitant esophageal GERD syndrome.[2] Patients with suspected reflux chest pain syndrome should receive twice-daily PPI therapy for 4 weeks after cardiac causes have been excluded. Manometry and pH or impedance pH monitoring should be considered in patients who do not respond to PPI therapy.[2]

Maintenance therapy is generally indicated in patients with extraesophageal GERD syndromes and concomitant esophageal GERD syndromes but not with reflux chest pain syndrome alone.[2]

▶ Pediatric Patients with GERD

Generally, gastroesophageal reflux (GER) is a normal physiologic process occurring several times per day with no clinical consequence. As with adults, GERD is present when symptoms become troublesome or if complications are present.[25]

Regurgitation is common in pediatric patients and usually described as the effortless and nonprojectile passage of refluxed gastric contents into the pharynx or mouth. This is also known as spitting-up or the "happy spitter," which may occur daily in as many as 50% of infants younger than 3 months.[25] Reflux episodes are common during transient LES relaxations not related to swallowing.[25] This is due to developmental immaturity of the LES. Other causes include impaired luminal clearance of gastric acid and type of infant formula. Patients with neurologic impairment, obesity, repaired esophageal atresia, congenital esophageal disease, cystic fibrosis, hiatal hernia, repaired achalasia, lung transplant, or family history are at a higher risk for developing GERD.[25]

Uncomplicated GERD usually resolves by 12 to 18 months of life and responds to supportive therapy, including dietary adjustments such as smaller meals, more frequent feedings, or thickened infant formula. Postural management (e.g., positioning the infant in an upright position, especially after meals) may also be helpful. If lifestyle modifications are not effective, medical therapy may be indicated. Acid suppression with either an H$_2$RA or PPI is the mainstay of pharmacologic therapy.[25] Monotherapy with an H$_2$RA is commonly used; ranitidine 2 to 4 mg/kg/day IV (or 4 to 8 mg/kg/day orally) is effective in neonates and pediatric patients. However, chronic use may lead to tachyphylaxis.

The use of PPIs in pediatric patients has increased significantly. Safety and effectiveness of lansoprazole has been shown for pediatric patients 1 to 17 years old for short-term treatment of symptomatic GERD and erosive esophagitis.[26] Studies in adolescents (12 to 17 years old) demonstrated pharmacokinetics similar to those seen in adults.[26] The recommended dose is 15 mg once daily for children weighing 30 kg or less and 30 mg once daily for those weighing more than 30 kg. The approved GERD dose of omeprazole in children 12 to 17 years old is 20 mg to 40 mg and 10 mg to 20 mg in patients 1 to 11 years old. Although not approved in pediatric patients younger than 1 year, omeprazole 1 mg/kg/day (given once or twice daily) has been used for esophagitis. The long-term safety of prolonged use in children is unknown, and therefore clinicians must carefully weigh risk versus benefit.[25]

▶ Elderly Patients with GERD

Older individuals have decreased host defense mechanisms such as slowed gastric emptying and decreased saliva production. These patients often do not seek medical attention because they believe their symptoms are part of the normal aging process. PPIs are the most useful option in this population because they have superior efficacy and are dosed once daily. In addition, there are fewer drug–drug and drug–disease state interactions compared with H$_2$RAs and metoclopramide. Elderly patients may be sensitive to the CNS effects of metoclopramide and H$_2$RAs.

▶ Patients with Refractory GERD

Refractory GERD may be present in patients not responding to 4 to 8 weeks of twice-daily PPI therapy. Compliance and timing of medication should always be assessed prior to deciding that a patient is refractory to acid-suppressing therapy. Endoscopy is indicated to determine if underlying pathology exists. In addition, patients with esophagitis may have a genotype that renders the PPIs less effective.[17] Patients with normal endoscopy should undergo further testing with ambulatory pH monitoring or impedance monitoring to identify acid and nonacid reflux episodes, respectively.[17] Patients not responding to PPI therapy may in fact have nonacid reflux approximately 20% to 30% of the time.[10] Consideration may be made to switch to an alternative PPI, due to variability of patient responses, before increasing to twice-daily PPI in patients not responding to once-daily PPI therapy. Up to 20% of patients on twice-daily PPI therapy with continued symptoms have nonacid reflux.[27,28] Non-reflux-related esophageal causes may include dysmotility syndromes such as achalasia or scleroderma, or eosinophilic esophagitis.[29]

Patient Encounter, Part 3: Monitoring for Safety and Efficacy

JM returns to your clinic for her annual follow-up appointment. Her GERD symptoms are now well controlled, and she is receiving maintenance therapy with lansoprazole 30 mg every morning. She is worried that she may develop a bone fracture if she continues her proton pump inhibitor, but her symptoms return when she tries to stop it. She wants to know if she should start a calcium supplement to prevent fractures.

What would you tell this patient about taking calcium supplements as a prophylactic measure to prevent fractures due to PPI use?

Based on the information presented, how should you monitor the patient for safety and efficacy outcomes?

OUTCOME EVALUATION

- Monitor for symptom relief and the presence of complicated symptoms.
- Record the frequency and severity of symptoms by interviewing the patient after 4 to 8 weeks of acid-suppressing therapy. Continued symptoms may indicate the need for long-term maintenance therapy.
- Monitor for adverse drug reactions, drug–drug interactions, and adherence.

- Educate patients about symptoms that suggest the presence of complications requiring immediate medical attention, such as dysphagia or odynophagia.
- Refer patients who present with atypical symptoms to their physician for further diagnostic evaluation.
- Reassess the need for chronic PPI therapy.
- ❾ *Review patient profiles for drugs that may aggravate GERD.*

Patient Care and Monitoring

1. Assess symptoms to determine if further diagnostic evaluation is necessary. Does the patient have complications?
2. Perform a thorough medication history by evaluating nonprescription, prescription, and dietary supplement products.
3. Determine what treatments have been helpful in the past.
4. Instruct patient to avoid foods that aggravate GERD symptoms.
5. Educate patient on lifestyle modifications.
6. Review the results of diagnostic tests.
7. Recommend appropriate therapy and develop a plan to assess effectiveness. Patients should receive 4 to 8 weeks of empiric acid-suppressing therapy. Patients who fail to respond should be assessed for compliance and proper medication administration. Twice-daily PPI therapy should be considered in patients not responding to once-daily therapy.

8. Evaluate for adverse drug reactions, drug allergies, and drug interactions.
9. Stress the importance of adherence.
10. Determine if long-term maintenance treatment is necessary.
11. Assess improvement in quality-of-life measures.
12. Provide patient education on disease, lifestyle modifications, and drug therapy:
    - What causes GERD and what are things to avoid?
    - What are possible complications?
    - When should medications be taken?
    - What potential adverse effects may occur?
    - Which drugs may interact with their therapy?
    - What warning signs should be reported to the physician?

Abbreviations Introduced in This Chapter

GER	Gastroesophageal reflux
GERD	Gastroesophageal reflux disease
H_2RA	Histamine$_2$-receptor antagonist
LES	Lower esophageal sphincter
NSAID	Nonsteroidal anti-inflammatory drug
PPI	Proton pump inhibitor

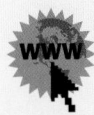 Self-assessment questions and answers are available at *http://www.mhpharmacotherapy.com/pp.html.*

REFERENCES

1. DeVault KR, Castell DO. Updated guidelines for the diagnosis and treatment of gastroesophageal reflux disease. Am J Gastroenterol 2005;100:190–200.

2. AGA Institute Medical Position Panel. American Gastroenterological Association Medical Position Statement on the management of gastroesophageal reflux disease. Gastroenterology 2008;135:1383–1391.

3. Camilleri M, Dubois D, Coulie B, et al. Prevalence and socioeconomic impact of functional gastrointestinal disorders in the United States: Results from the U.S. Upper Gastrointestinal Study. Clin Gastroenterol Hepatol 2005;3:543–552.

4. Boeckxstaens GEE. Review article: The pathophysiology of gastro-oesophageal reflux disease. Aliment Pharmacol Ther 2007;26:149–160.

5. Herbella FA, Patti MG. Gastroesophageal reflux disease: From pathophysiology to treatment. World J Gastroenterol 2010;16(30):3745–3749.

6. Williams DB, Schade RR. Gastroesophageal reflux disease. In: DiPiro JT, Talbert RL, Yee GC, et al., eds. Pharmacotherapy: A Pathophysiologic Approach, 8th ed. New York, NY: McGraw-Hill, 2008:556.

7. Kahrilas PJ. Gastroesophageal reflux disease. N Engl J Med 2008;359:1700–1707.

8. Lagergren J, Bergstrom R, Lindgren A, et al. Symptomatic gastroesophageal reflux as a risk factor for esophageal adenocarcinoma. N Engl J Med 1999;340:825–831.

9. Nason KS, Wichienkuer PP, Awais O, et al. Gastroesophageal reflux disease symptom severity, proton pump inhibitor use, and esophageal carcinogenesis. Arch Surg 2011;146:851–858.

10. Karamonolis G, Sifrim D. Developments in pathogenesis and diagnosis of gastroesophageal reflux disease. Curr Opin Gastroenterol 2007;23(4):428–433.

11. Stefanidis D, Hope WW, Kohn GP, et al. Guidelines for surgical treatment of gastroesophageal reflux disease (GERD). Practice/Clinical Guidelines published on 2/2010 by the Society of American Gastrointestinal and Endoscopic Surgeons (SAGES) [Internet]. Available from: *http://www.sages.org/publication/id/22/.*

12. AGA Institute Medical Position Statement on the use of endoscopic therapy for gastroesophageal reflux disease. Gastroenterology 2006;131: 1313–1314.

13. American Gastroenterological Association. Medical position statement of the management of Barrett's esophagus. Gastroenterology 2011;140: 1084–1091.

14. Horn J. The proton-pump inhibitors: Similarities and differences. Clin Ther 2000;22:266–280.

15. Williams NT. Medication administration through enteral feeding tubes. Am J Health Syst Pharm 2008;65:2347–2357.

16. Abraham NS, Hlatky MA, Antman EM, et al. ACCF/ACG/AHA 2010 Expert consensus document on the concomitant use of proton pump inhibitors and thienopyridines: A focused update of the ACCF/ACG/AHA 2008 expert consensus document on reducing the gastrointestinal risks of antiplatelet therapy and NSAID use: A report of the American College of Cardiology Foundation Task Force on expert consensus documents. Circulation 2010;122:2619–2633.

17. Welage LS, Berardi RR. Evaluation of omeprazole, lansoprazole, pantoprazole, and rabeprazole in the treatment of acid-related disorders. J Am Pharm Assoc 2000;40:52–62.

18. Richter JE. How to manage refractory gastroesophageal reflux disease. Nat Clin Pract Gastroenterol Hepatol 2007;4(12):658–664.

19. Schwab M, Klotz U, Hofmann U, et al. Esomeprazole-induced healing of gastroesophageal reflux disease is unrelated to the genotype of CYP2C19: Evidence from clinical and pharmacokinetic data. Clin Pharmacol Ther 2005;78:627–634.

20. Thomson ABR, Sauve MD, Kassam N, Kamitakahara H. Safety of the long-term use of proton pump inhibitors. World J Gastroenterol 2010;16(19):2323–2330.

21. FDA Drug Safety Communication [Internet]. Possible increased risk of fractures of the hip, wrist, and spine with the use of proton pump inhibitors [cited 2010 May 25]. Available from: *www.fda.gov.*

22. FDA Drug Safety Communication [Internet]. Possible increased risk of fractures of the hip, wrist, and spine with the use of proton pump inhibitors. Available from: *www.fda.gov.* Updated March 23, 2011.

23. Corley DA, Kubo A, Zhao W, Quesenberry C. Proton pump inhibitors and histamine-2 receptor antagonists are associated with hip fractures among at-risk patents. Gastroenterology 2010;139:93–101.

24. Fackler WK, Ours T, Vaezi M, Richter J. Long-term effect of H2RA therapy on nocturnal gastric acid breakthrough. Gastroenterology 2002;122:625–632.

25. Vandenplas Y, Rudolph CE, Di Lorenz C, et al. Pediatric gastroesophageal reflux clinical practice guidelines: Joint recommendations of the North American Society for Pediatric Gastroenterology, Hepatology, and Nutrition (NASPGHAN) and the European Society for Pediatric Gastroenterology, Hepatology, and Nutrition (ESPGHAN). J Pediatr Gastroenterol Nutr 2009;49:498–547.

26. Prevacid (Lansoprazole) [package insert]. Deerfield, IL: Takeda Pharmaceuticals America, 2011.

27. Zerbib F, Roman S, Ropert A, et al. Esophageal pH-impedance monitoring and symptom analysis in GERD: A study in patients on and off therapy. Am J Gastroenterol 2006;101:1956–1963.

28. Mainie I, Tutuian R, Shay S, et al. Acid and non-acid reflux in patients with persistent symptoms despite acid suppressive therapy: A multicenter study using ambulatory impedance-pH monitoring. Gut 2006; 55:1398–1402.

29. Dellon ES, Shaheen NJ. Persistent reflux symptoms in the proton pump inhibitor era: The changing face of gastroesophageal reflux disease. Gastroenterology 2010;139:7–13.

18 Peptic Ulcer Disease

Catherine A. Bourg, Erika L. Grigg,
and Dianne Williams May

LEARNING OBJECTIVES

Upon completion of the chapter, the reader will be able to:

1. Recognize differences between ulcers induced by *Helicobacter pylori*, nonsteroidal anti-inflammatory drugs (NSAIDs), and stress-related mucosal damage (SRMD) in terms of risk factors, pathogenesis, signs and symptoms, clinical course, and prognosis.

2. Identify desired therapeutic outcomes for patients with *H. pylori*–associated ulcers and NSAID-induced ulcers.

3. Identify factors that guide selection of an *H. pylori* eradication regimen and improve adherence with these regimens.

4. Determine the appropriate management for a patient taking a nonselective NSAID who is at high risk for ulcer-related GI complications (e.g., GI bleed) or who develops an ulcer.

5. Devise an algorithm for the evaluation and treatment of a patient with signs and symptoms suggestive of an *H. pylori*–associated or NSAID-induced ulcer.

6. Given patient-specific information and the prescribed drug treatment regimen, formulate a monitoring plan for a patient who is receiving drug therapy either to eradicate *H. pylori* or to treat an active NSAID-induced ulcer or GI complication.

KEY CONCEPTS

❶ Patients with peptic ulcer disease (PUD) should avoid exposure to factors known to worsen the disease, exacerbate symptoms, or lead to ulcer recurrence (e.g., NSAID use, alcohol consumption, or cigarette smoking).

❷ Reliance on conventional antiulcer drug therapy as an alternative to *Helicobacter pylori* eradication is inappropriate because it is associated with a higher incidence of ulcer recurrence and ulcer-related complications.

❸ Eradication therapy with a proton pump inhibitor (PPI)–based three-drug regimen should be considered for all patients who test positive for *H. pylori* and have an active ulcer or a documented history of either an ulcer or ulcer-related complication. Different antibiotics should be used if a second course of *H. pylori* eradication therapy is required.

❹ In patients at risk for NSAID-induced ulcers, PPIs at standard doses reduce the risk of both gastric and duodenal ulcers as effectively as misoprostol and more effectively than histamine$_2$-receptor antagonists (H$_2$RAs).

❺ Selective cyclooxygenase (COX)-2 inhibitors are no more effective than the combination of a PPI and a nonselective NSAID in reducing the incidence of ulcers and are associated with a greater incidence of cardiovascular (CV) events (e.g., ischemic stroke).

❻ Indications for stress ulcer prophylaxis include major trauma or surgery, severe head trauma, multiple organ failure, burns covering more than 25% to 30% of body, severe sepsis, shock, mechanical ventilation, coagulopathy, and high-dose corticosteroid use.

❼ Low-dose maintenance therapy with a PPI or H$_2$RA is only indicated in patients with severe complications secondary to PUD such as gastric outlet obstruction or patients who need to be on long-term NSAIDs or high-dose corticosteroids and are at high risk for bleeding.

INTRODUCTION

Peptic ulcer disease (PUD) refers to a defect in the gastric or duodenal mucosal wall that extends through the **muscularis mucosa** into the deeper layers of the submucosa.[1] PUD is a significant cause of morbidity and is associated with substantial healthcare costs. Over the past several decades, the prevalence of PUD has declined due to the discovery of *Helicobacter pylori* and effective acid-suppressing medications. Although there are many etiologies of PUD (Table 18–1), the three most common causes are (a) *H. pylori* infection, (b) use of NSAIDs,

---

Table 18–1

Etiologies of Peptic Ulcer Disease

Helicobacter Pylori-Positive Infection	NSAID-Induced PUD
Viral infections (e.g., CMV or HSV, especially in immunocompromised patients)	Tumors (cancer, lymphoma, primary, or metastatic)
Stress related mucosal damage	Cameron ulcer (ulcer within a hiatal hernia where the hernia passes the diaphragmatic hiatus)
Acid hypersecretory state (e.g., ZES)	Radiation damage
Anastomotic site ulcer	Idiopathic
Chemotherapy	Vascular insufficiency

CMV, cytomegalovirus; HSV, herpes simplex virus; NSAID, nonsteroidal anti-inflammatory drug; PUD, peptic ulcer disease; ZES, Zollinger–Ellison syndrome.

---

or, less commonly, (c) stress-related mucosal damage (SRMD).

Complications of PUD include GI bleeding, perforation, and obstruction. Complications of untreated or undiagnosed *H. pylori* infection include gastric cancer and PUD. This chapter focuses mainly on strategies to optimize pharmacotherapy for patients with PUD related to *H. pylori* or NSAID therapy. Stress ulcer prophylaxis (SUP) is an issue seen in hospitalized patients and is also discussed briefly.

EPIDEMIOLOGY AND ETIOLOGY

The prevalence of *H. pylori* has decreased over the past few decades, probably due to improved sanitary conditions; however, *H. pylori* infection remains a public health issue in developing countries.[2,3] The prevalence of *H. pylori* in the United States and Canada is about 30%, whereas the global prevalence is greater than 50%. Factors that influence the incidence and prevalence of *H. pylori* include age, ethnicity, sex, geography, and socioeconomic status. Unfortunately, there is no vaccine available for *H. pylori* because the exact source of the infection is not yet known.[3]

In the United States, PUD affects approximately 4.5 million people annually with lifetime prevalence estimated to be 11% to 14% in men and 8% to 11% in women. PUD costs an estimated $5.65 billion per year including hospitalizations, outpatient care, and work loss expenditures, not including medication costs.[4] Despite the widespread use of conventional and effective antiulcer therapy, ulcers frequently recur.[2] *H. pylori* infection and NSAID use account for most cases of PUD. Although hospitalizations related to PUD have decreased over the past 2 decades, the incidence of PUD-related complications such as bleeding and perforation remains unchanged.[2]

In general, ulcers related to *H. pylori* infection more commonly affect the duodenum, whereas ulcers related to NSAIDs more frequently affect the stomach (Fig. 18–1). However, ulcers may be found in either location from either cause. Gastric ulcers (GUs) may occur anywhere in the stomach; duodenal ulcers (DUs) tend to occur most often in the duodenal bulb. The epigastric pain associated with a DU typically occurs during the fasting state or at night and

is often relieved by food, whereas pain from a GU is usually aggravated by food intake.[5] Malignancy is more commonly found with GU than DU.[1]

Helicobacter Pylori

Helicobacter pylori causes gastritis in all infected patients. However, only a small proportion (less than 10%) of patients actually develops symptomatic PUD. In 2005, Warren and Marshall received the Nobel Prize for recognizing *H. pylori* eradication as a cure for PUD.[6]

H. pylori is usually contracted in the first few years of life and tends to persist indefinitely unless treated. The infection normally resides in the stomach and is transmitted via the fecal–oral route or through ingestion of fecal-contaminated water or food. Prevalence varies greatly throughout the world, increasing with older age and with lower socioeconomic

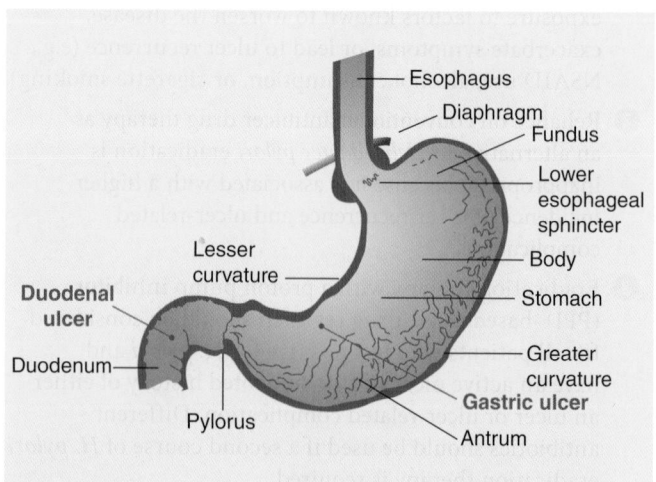

FIGURE 18–1. Anatomic structure of the stomach and duodenum and most common locations of gastric and duodenal ulcers (From Berardi R, Fugit R. Peptic ulcer disease. In: DiPiro JT; Talbert RA; Yee GC, et al., eds. Pharmacotherapy: A Pathophysiologic Approach, 8th ed. New York, NY: McGraw-Hill, 2011:563–585.)

status during childhood.[7] Infection with *H. pylori* is more common in developing countries because of the presence of contaminated food and water.

Nonsteroidal Anti-inflammatory Drugs

NSAIDs are one of the most widely used classes of medications in the United States, particularly in the elderly. The odds of GI bleeding are increased by five- to sixfold in patients taking NSAIDs. Up to 4% of NSAID users have a serious ulcer-related complication, accounting for up to 100,000 hospitalizations and more than 20,000 deaths in the United States per year.[2] Chronic NSAID ingestion leads to symptoms of nausea and dyspepsia in nearly half of patients. Peptic ulceration occurs in up to 30% of patients who use NSAIDs (including aspirin) chronically, with GI bleeding or perforation occurring in 1.5% of patients who develop an ulcer.[2]

Risk factors for NSAID-induced peptic ulcers and complications are presented in Table 18–2. Important principles to consider when estimating the risk for developing PUD in a patient taking an NSAID include the following: (a) risk factors are generally additive, (b) some risk factors (e.g., corticosteroid therapy) are not independent risk factors for ulceration but increase PUD risk substantially when combined with NSAID therapy, and (c) many of the risk factors postulated to increase PUD risk in a patient taking an NSAID (e.g., rheumatoid arthritis, tobacco smoking, and alcohol consumption) remain unproven and thus should not generally be considered independent risk factors for NSAID-induced ulceration.[8] Whether *H. pylori* infection is a risk factor for NSAID-induced ulcers remains controversial; however, *H. pylori* and NSAIDs act independently to increase ulcer risk and ulcer-related bleeding and also appear to have synergistic effects.[9]

Stress-Related Mucosal Damage

SRMD occurs most frequently in critically ill patients and is due to compromised mesenteric perfusion resulting in mucosal defects.[5] Although the etiology of stress ulceration is multifactorial, there are two necessary conditions: gastric mucosal ischemia and intraluminal acid.[10] SRMD usually develops within the first few hours after a major trauma or serious illness. The ulcers are usually superficial; however SRMD may also penetrate into the submucosa and result in significant GI bleeding.[10]

Physiologically stressful situations that lead to SRMD include sepsis, organ failure, prolonged mechanical ventilation, thermal injury, trauma, and surgery. The utility of stress ulcer prophylaxis (SUP) has been well described in a certain subset of critically ill patients, and guidelines have been published (Table 18–3).[11] Proton pump inhibitors (PPIs) and H_2RAs are the drugs of choice for SUP.

Zollinger–Ellison Syndrome

Zollinger–Ellison syndrome (ZES) is caused by a gastrin-producing tumor called a gastrinoma. This results in a state of gastric acid hypersecretion in which patients develop diarrhea and malabsorption. Ulcers tend to be numerous and have a high risk of perforation and bleeding.[5] Radiographic and endoscopic procedures are used to localize and stage the tumor. High-dose oral PPI therapy is the treatment of choice for ZES and may be used long term in patients when the tumor cannot be identified or fully resected.[5] Patients without hepatic metastases should undergo surgical resection of tumor.

Other Causative Factors

Cigarette smoking is associated with a higher prevalence of ulcers in patients infected with *H. pylori*; however, it does

---

Table 18–2

Established Risk Factors for Ulcers and GI Complications Related to NSAID Use

Age over 60 years
Concomitant anticoagulant use
Preexisting coagulopathy (elevated INR or thrombocytopenia)
Concomitant corticosteroid or selective serotonin reuptake inhibitor therapy
Previous PUD or PUD complications (bleeding/perforation)
CV disease and other comorbid conditions
Multiple NSAID use (e.g., low-dose aspirin in conjunction with another NSAID)
Duration of NSAID use (greater than 1 month)
High-dose NSAID use
NSAID-related dyspepsia
Cigarette smokers

CV, cardiovascular; INR, international normalized ratio; NSAID, nonsteroidal anti-inflammatory drug; PUD, peptic ulcer disease.

Table 18–3

ASHP Guidelines on Appropriate Indications for SUP in ICU patients (1999)

Mechanical ventilation for longer than 48 hours
Coagulopathy or hepatic failure (platelet count less than $50 \times 10^3/mm^3$ (50×10^9/L), INR greater than 1.5, or aPTT less than two times control)
History of GI ulceration or bleeding within 1 year of admission
Head trauma or Glasgow Coma Score of 10 or less (or inability to obey simple commands)
Thermal injuries to more than 35% of body surface area
Multiple traumas (injury severity score of 16 or greater)
Partial hepatectomy
Transplant patients in the ICU perioperatively
Spinal cord injuries
Two of the following risk factors: sepsis, ICU stay for more than 1 week, occult bleeding lasting 6 or more days, and use of high-dose corticosteroids (more than 250 mg/day of hydrocortisone or equivalent)

ASHP, American Society of Health-System Pharmacists; SUP, stress ulcer prophylaxis; ICU, intensive care unit; INR, international normalized ratio; aPTT, activated partial thromboplastin time.

not seem to increase the risk of recurrence once *H. pylori* has been eradicated.[2] The exact mechanisms for the detrimental effects of smoking on the gastric mucosa are unclear but may involve increased pepsin secretion, duodenogastric reflux of bile salts, elevated levels of free radicals, and reduced bicarbonate and prostaglandin (PG) production.[12] It is unknown whether nicotine or one of the other ingredients found in cigarettes is responsible for these deleterious effects.

Until the discovery of *H. pylori*, psychological stress was considered one of the primary causes of PUD. Although psychosocial factors such as life stress, baseline personality patterns, and depression may influence PUD prevalence, a clear causal relationship has not been demonstrated.[2]

Dietary factors such as coffee, tea, cola, alcohol, and a spicy diet may cause dyspepsia but have not been shown independently to increase PUD risk. Although caffeine increases gastric acid secretion and alcohol ingestion causes acute gastritis, there is no conclusive evidence that either of these substances is an independent risk factor for PUD.[2]

PATHOPHYSIOLOGY

Ulcer formation is the net result of a lack of homeostasis between factors within the GI tract responsible for the breakdown of food (e.g., gastric acid and pepsin) and factors that promote mucosal defense and repair (e.g., bicarbonate, mucus secretion, and PGs).

Gastric Acid and Pepsin

Hydrochloric acid and pepsin are the primary substances that cause gastric mucosal damage in PUD. Three different stimuli (e.g., histamine, acetylcholine, and gastrin) are responsible for acid secretion through their interactions with the histaminic, cholinergic, and gastrin receptors on the surface of parietal cells. Gastric acid output occurs in two stages: (a) basal acid output, which reflects the baseline output of acid during the fasting state, and (b) maximal acid output, which occurs in response to meals. Basal acid secretion follows a circadian cycle and is modulated by the effects of acetylcholine and histamine acting on the parietal cell.[13]

Food can cause gastric acid secretion in two ways. In the cephalic phase of acid secretion, the vagus nerve stimulates acid secretion in response to the sight, smell, or taste of food. In both the gastric and intestinal phases of acid secretion, the physical distention caused by food induces gastrin secretion resulting in acid production. After stimulation by histamine, acetylcholine, and gastrin, acid is secreted by the H^+-K^+-ATPase (proton) pump, located on the luminal side of parietal cells. Acid secretion in PUD is usually normal or slightly elevated. NSAID ingestion usually does not affect acid secretion, whereas *H. pylori* infection usually leads to a slight increase in acid output. This is in contrast to ZES, in which acid secretion is substantially elevated.[13]

Pepsinogen released from chief cells in the body of the stomach is converted to pepsin in the presence of an acidic environment and plays a key role in the initiation of protein digestion, proteolysis of collagen, and as a signal for the release of other digestive enzymes such as gastrin and cholecystokinin.[14] The proteolytic activity of pepsin appears to influence ulcer formation.

Mucosal Defense and Repair

Several defense and repair mechanisms are responsible for preventing mucosal damage and subsequent ulcer formation. The mucus/phospholipid and bicarbonate barrier, through its buffering action, is the primary source of defense for the gastric epithelial surface against gastric acid.[2] It allows an acidic environment to be maintained in the lumen but a near neutral pH to be maintained on the epithelial lining. This lining has a number of protective mechanisms responsible for the repair of damaged cells, production of defense mechanisms, and the promotion of epithelial growth.

PGs inhibit gastric acid secretion and have numerous mucosal protective effects, including stimulation of mucus, bicarbonate, and phospholipid production. They also increase mucosal blood flow and stimulate epithelial cell regeneration.[2] Damage to the mucosal defense system is the primary method by which *H. pylori* or NSAIDs cause peptic ulcers.

▶ *Helicobacter Pylori*

H. pylori, a gram-negative microaerophilic S-shaped rod, is found on the surface of the gastric epithelium and has a number of adaptive functions to allow it to live within the acidic environment of the stomach. *H. pylori* colonization does not necessarily reflect an active infection because the organism can attach itself to the gastric epithelium without invading cells. The motility provided by the flagella allows the organism to penetrate the mucous gel barrier and cause an acute infection in the epithelial cells.[7] The organism is able to survive in the acidic environment of the stomach via production of urease, an enzyme that hydrolyzes urea (found in gastric juice) into carbon dioxide and ammonia.[7] Cellular invasion by *H. pylori* is necessary for an active infection. In addition to PUD, *H. pylori* infection may also result in gastric cancer (0.1% to 3%) and gastric mucosa-associated lymphoid-tissue (MALT) lymphoma (less than 0.01%).[7]

A number of host and pathogenic factors contribute to the ability of *H. pylori* to cause gastroduodenal mucosal injury including (a) direct mucosal damage, (b) alterations to host inflammatory responses, and (c) hypergastrinemia leading to a state of elevated acid secretion. *H. pylori* isolated from patients with PUD carry a high virulence that include a strong adhesive property and increased production of potentially toxic enzymes.[5] The complex interplay between bacterial virulence factors and an enhanced inflammatory response results in a chronic *H. pylori* infection that increases acid production and reduces various host protective factors.

Nonsteroidal Anti-inflammatory Drugs

Nonselective NSAIDs (those that inhibit both COX-1 and COX-2) cause gastric mucosal damage by two primary mechanisms: direct or topical irritation of the gastric epithelium and systemic inhibition of endogenous mucosal PG synthesis. COX-2 NSAIDs have been shown to reduce, but not eliminate the risk of PUD and its complications.[5]

Direct irritation of the mucosal lining by NSAIDs occurs because NSAIDs are weak acids. Less acidic agents, such as nonacetylated salicylates, may confer decreased GI toxicity.[15] Although the direct irritant effects of NSAIDs play a contributory role in the development of NSAID-induced gastritis, this mechanism generally plays a minor role in the evolution of NSAID-induced PUD.

The systemic effects of NSAIDs are the primary cause of PUD. COX is the rate-limiting enzyme in the PG synthesis pathway (Fig. 18–2). Inhibition of PG production is the primary therapeutic effect of NSAIDs. COX is responsible for the conversion of arachidonic acid to PGs such as PGG_2 and PGH_2. COX-1 is routinely found in body tissues that produce PGs for normal physiological maintenance. In contrast, COX-2 is an inducible enzyme that is expressed during states in which cytokines and inflammatory mediators are elevated (e.g., fever and pain). Inhibition of the COX-1 isoenzyme decreases production of endogenous PGs, particularly PGE_1, PGE_2, and PGI_2. Administration of NSAIDs parenterally (e.g., ketorolac) and rectally (e.g., indomethacin) is associated with an incidence of PUD similar to that with oral NSAIDs. Topical NSAIDs (e.g., diclofenac) would be unlikely to cause PUD given the very low serum concentrations that are achieved with this route of administration compared with that observed with oral therapy.

PGs are important factors in gastric healing and protection. Inhibition of PG production by NSAIDs compromises these important protective mechanisms. Finally, the antiplatelet effects of NSAIDs may worsen bleeding complications associated with PUD.

CLINICAL PRESENTATION AND DIAGNOSIS

Clinical Presentation

See text box on next page for the clinical presentation of PUD. Dyspepsia refers to upper abdominal discomfort and is found in 10% to 40% of the general population. PUD is found in 5% to 15% of patients with dyspepsia. Patients with new onset dyspepsia who are older than 50 years and patients of any age with alarming features should undergo an upper endoscopy to evaluate for PUD.[1,16,17]

Patients with dyspepsia who are younger than 50 to 55 years and do not have alarming features should be tested for *H. pylori* and treated if positive.[1,16,18] NSAIDs should also be stopped if possible. Patients who test negative for *H. pylori* should be offered a trial (4 to 8 weeks) of acid suppression or they can proceed with endoscopy evaluation. Upper endoscopy should be performed in any patient who has persistent dyspepsia symptoms despite a trial of acid suppressive therapy.[1]

PUD can be classified as uncomplicated or complicated. Complicated disease implies GI bleeding, obstruction, or perforation. Hemorrhage is the most common complication of PUD and may occur when an ulcer erodes the wall of a gastric or duodenal artery. GI bleeding may be occult or may present as melena or hematemesis. Bleeding occurs in approximately 15% of PUD patients and is more common in patients older than 60 years, particularly those who ingest NSAIDs.[19] Up to 20% of patients who develop a PUD-related hemorrhage do not have prior symptoms. Mortality associated with PUD remains 5% to 10% despite advances in medical and endoscopic therapies.[19] Endoscopic therapy achieves successful hemostasis in 90% of patients; however, rebleeding may occur in 10% to 30% of high-risk patients even after successful initial treatment.[20]

Perforation, another complication of PUD, requires emergent surgical intervention. These patients should not undergo endoscopy.

Gastric outlet obstruction occurs in approximately 2% of PUD patients and is usually caused by ulcer-related inflammation or scar formation. Patients typically present with early satiety after meals, nausea, vomiting, abdominal pain, and weight loss. Ulcer healing with conventional acid suppressive therapy, cessation of NSAID use, and treatment of *H. pylori* infection

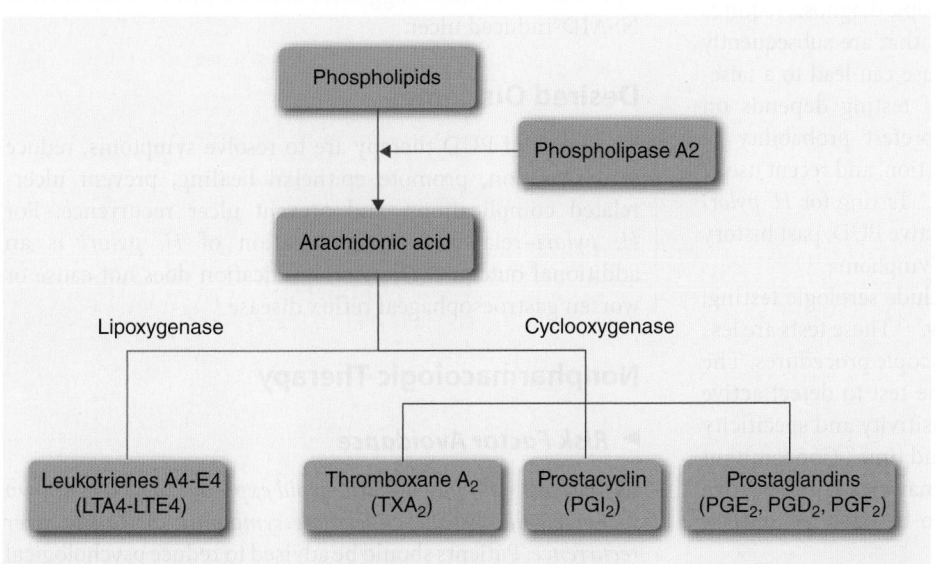

FIGURE 18–2. The arachidonic acid pathway.

Clinical Presentation of PUD

Symptoms

- Mild epigastric pain that may be described as burning, gnawing, or aching in character.
- Abdominal pain may be described as burning or a feeling of discomfort.
- Some patients report nocturnal pain.
- The severity of pain often fluctuates.
- The intensity of pain can vary widely (e.g., from dull to sharp).
- DU pain occurs 1 to 3 hours after meals and may be relieved by food ingestion.
- GU pain occurs immediately after meals and is often aggravated by food.
- Patients may also complain of heartburn, belching, bloating, nausea, or vomiting.

Signs

- Weight loss may be associated with nausea and vomiting.
- Complications such as bleeding, perforation, or obstruction may occur.
- Alarm signs and symptoms include family history of upper GI malignancy, unintentional weight loss, overt GI bleeding, iron deficiency anemia, progressive dysphagia or odynophagia, early satiety, persistent vomiting, prior history of esophagogastric malignancy, palpable mass, or lymphadenopathy.

if indicated is the primary treatment, but if unsuccessful, endoscopic therapy with balloon dilation is required.[1]

Diagnosis

Diagnostic tests for the presence of *H. pylori* can be either endoscopic or nonendoscopic.[7,18] Endoscopic diagnosis requires the extraction of gastric tissue samples that are subsequently tested for *H. pylori*.[18] Recent antibiotic use can lead to a false-negative biopsy result. The choice of testing depends on availability, cost, clinical situation, pretest probability of infection, population prevalence of infection, and recent use of antisecretory treatment and antibiotics.[3] Testing for *H. pylori* infection is indicated in patients with active PUD, past history of documented PUD, or gastric MALT lymphoma.[18]

Nonendoscopic testing methods include serologic testing, urea breath test, and stool antigen assay.[7,18] These tests are less invasive and less expensive than endoscopic procedures. The urea breath test is usually the first-line test to detect active *H. pylori* infection because it has a sensitivity and specificity greater than 95% and a short turnaround time.[7] Concomitant acid-suppressive or antibiotic therapy may give false-negative results.[7] The urea breath test can also be used to confirm eradication of *H. pylori* infection.[7]

Office-based serologic testing provides a quick assessment (within 15 minutes) of an exposure to *H. pylori*, but this method is not able to determine active versus previously treated *H. pylori* infection because patients can remain seropositive for years after eradication. In addition, it is less sensitive and specific than the urea breath test.[7] Serologic testing is recommended and considered diagnostic in patients with a bleeding ulcer, gastric atrophy, MALT lymphoma, and recent or current antibiotic or acid-suppressing therapy.[21]

Stool antigen assays can be useful for the initial diagnosis or to confirm *H. pylori* eradication, and they are affected less by concomitant medication use.[7] The sensitivity and specificity of the stool antigen assay is greater than 95%.[7] The use of antimicrobial agents within 4 weeks, PPIs within 2 weeks, and H_2RAs within 24 hours of testing can suppress the infection, reduce the sensitivity of testing, and should be avoided.[7]

Endoscopic testing is an invasive and expensive way to test for *H. pylori*, but it is indicated in patients older than 50 years with new symptoms of dyspepsia or any patient with alarming features.[1,16,18] *H. pylori* is difficult to culture because the organism grows slowly and requires specialized culture media and a controlled microaerophilic environment.[22] Rapid urease testing is inexpensive, but its sensitivity is reduced in the posttreatment setting.[18]

Radiologic and/or endoscopic procedures are usually required to document the presence of ulcers. However, the cost and complexity of testing has led to the promotion of early empiric treatment strategy for patients at low risk for PUD-related sequelae (e.g., malignancy). An empiric treatment strategy is appropriate for symptomatic patients younger than 50 to 55 years without alarming features or evidence of PUD complications.[7,16,18]

TREATMENT

The treatment selected for PUD depends on the etiology of the ulcer, whether the ulcer is new or recurrent, and whether complications have occurred. Figure 18–3 shows an algorithm for the evaluation and treatment of a patient with signs and symptoms suggestive of an *H. pylori*–associated or NSAID-induced ulcer.

Desired Outcomes

The goals of PUD therapy are to resolve symptoms, reduce acid secretion, promote epithelial healing, prevent ulcer-related complications, and prevent ulcer recurrence. For *H. pylori*–related PUD, eradication of *H. pylori* is an additional outcome. *H. pylori* eradication does not cause or worsen gastroesophageal reflux disease.[3]

Nonpharmacologic Therapy

▶ Risk Factor Avoidance

❶ *Patients with PUD should avoid exposure to factors known to worsen the disease, exacerbate symptoms, or lead to ulcer recurrence.* Patients should be advised to reduce psychological

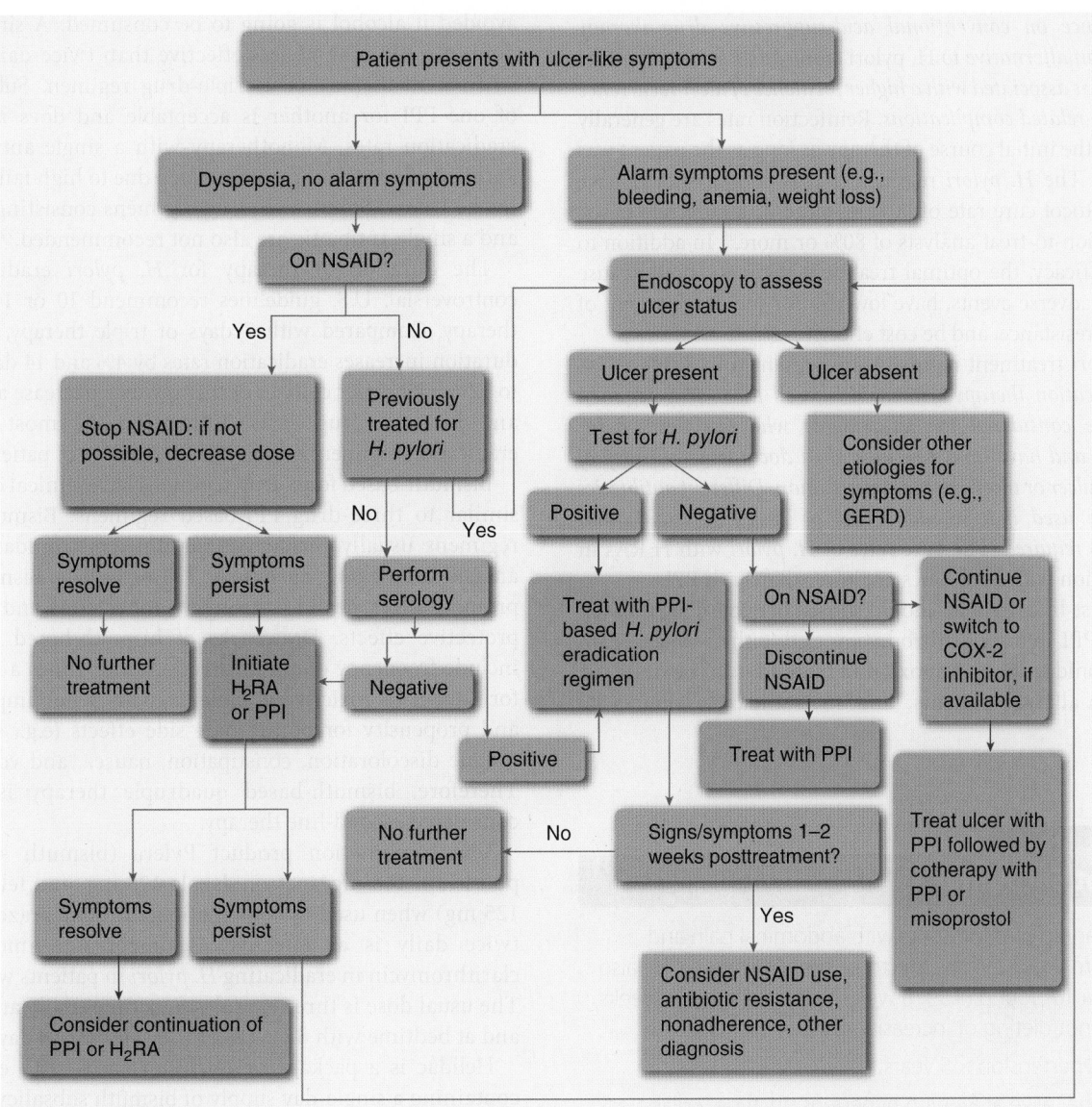

FIGURE 18–3. Approach to the patient presenting with ulcer-like symptoms. (GERD, gastroesophageal reflux disease. (HP, *Helicobacter pylori*; H$_2$RA, histamine$_2$-receptor antagonist; NSAID, nonsteroidal anti-inflammatory drug; PPI, proton pump inhibitor.) (From Berardi R, Fugit R. Peptic ulcer disease. In: DiPiro JT; Talbert RA; Yee GC, et al., eds. Pharmacotherapy: A Pathophysiologic Approach, 8th ed. New York, NY: McGraw-Hill, 2011:563–585.)

stress and avoid cigarette smoking, alcohol consumption, and NSAID or aspirin use. Patients who require chronic NSAID therapy (e.g., for rheumatoid arthritis) may be given prophylaxis with misoprostol or a PPI (see section on prevention of NSAID-induced ulcers).

▶ *Surgery*

The high success rates of medical therapies have reduced the number of surgical procedures performed. Elective surgeries performed for PUD have decreased by more than 70% since the 1980s mainly due to *H. pylori* eradication.[23] For this reason, surgical interventions are generally reserved for complicated or refractory PUD.[9] Definitive surgical procedures to treat PUD usually involve some type of **vagotomy** (to block further acid secretion) with or without partial **gastrectomy**.[9]

Complications are rare but can include dumping syndrome, bile reflux, diarrhea, malabsorption, and gastric atony.[9]

For patients with acute GI bleeding, endoscopic hemostasis can be achieved using contact thermal therapy, mechanical therapy using clips, or epinephrine injection followed by either thermal or mechanical therapy.[19] **Angiography** with embolization of bleeding lesions can be used if the bleeding cannot be stopped endoscopically and the patient is either high risk for surgery or not a surgical candidate.[24]

Pharmacologic Therapy

▶ *Treatment of* H. pylori–*Associated Ulcers*

● The primary goal of *H. pylori* therapy is to completely eradicate the organism using an effective antibiotic-containing regimen.

❷ *Reliance on conventional acid-suppressive drug therapy alone as an alternative to* H. pylori *eradication is inappropriate because it is associated with a higher incidence of ulcer recurrence and ulcer-related complications.* Reinfection rates are generally low after the initial course of therapy as long as the patient was adherent. The *H. pylori* regimen that is chosen should have a per-protocol cure rate of 90% or more or a cure rate based on intention-to-treat analysis of 80% or more.[18] In addition to proven efficacy, the optimal treatment regimen should cause minimal adverse events, have low risk for the development of bacterial resistance, and be cost effective.[7,18]

H. pylori treatment regimens are presented in Table 18–4. **❸** *Eradication therapy with a PPI-based three-drug regimen should be considered for all patients who test positive for* H. pylori *and have an active ulcer or a documented history of either an ulcer or ulcer-related complication. Different antibiotics should be used if a second course of* H. pylori *eradication therapy is required.* The cure rates of *H. pylori* with H$_2$RAs in combination with antibiotics are lower than with PPIs.

The first-line regimen should consist of triple drug therapy with a PPI plus clarithromycin and either amoxicillin or metronidazole.[7,25] Amoxicillin should not be used in penicillin-allergic patients, and metronidazole should be

avoided if alcohol is going to be consumed. A single daily dose of a PPI may be less effective than twice-daily dosing when used as part of a triple-drug regimen. Substitution of one PPI for another is acceptable and does not affect eradication rates. Monotherapy with a single antibiotic or antiulcer agent is not recommended due to high failure rates. In the United States, two-drug regimens consisting of a PPI and a single antibiotic are also not recommended.[22]

The duration of therapy for *H. pylori* eradication is controversial. U.S. guidelines recommend 10 or 14 days of therapy. Compared with 7 days of triple therapy, a 10-day duration increases eradication rates by 4% and 14 days by 5% to 12%.[21,25] Longer courses of therapy may decrease adherence and increase drug costs; ultimately, the most effective eradication regimens still fail in 10% to 20% of patients.[5]

Bismuth-based four-drug regimens have clinical cure rates similar to three-drug PPI-based regimens. Bismuth-based regimens usually include tetracycline, metronidazole, and an acid suppressing agent (e.g., PPI or H$_2$RA). Bismuth salts promote ulcer healing through antibacterial and mucosal protective effects. Drawbacks of bismuth-based regimens include frequency of administration (four times a day), risk for salicylate toxicity in patients with renal impairment, and propensity for bothersome side effects (e.g., stool and tongue discoloration, constipation, nausea, and vomiting).[5] Therefore, bismuth-based quadruple therapy is usually considered second-line therapy.

The combination product Pylera (bismuth subcitrate potassium 140 mg, metronidazole 125 mg, and tetracycline 125 mg) when used in combination with omeprazole 20 mg twice daily is as effective as omeprazole–amoxicillin–clarithromycin in eradicating *H. pylori* in patients with DU.[22] The usual dose is three capsules four times daily after meals and at bedtime with 8 oz. (237 mL) water for 10 days.

Helidac is a package of 14 blister cards with each card containing a single-day supply of bismuth subsalicylate (two 262.4-mg chewable tablets four times daily), metronidazole (250-mg tablet four times daily), and tetracycline (500-mg capsule four times daily). Unlike Pylera, Helidac is not a combination product; all three medications must be taken four times daily for 14 days in combination with an H$_2$RA rather than a PPI. However, cure rates are less with H$_2$RA than with PPI and therefore not preferred.[7] A 10-day course of Pylera or a 14-day course of Helidac are substantially more expensive than the costs of their individual generic and nonprescription components.

Patients may remain infected with *H. pylori* after the initial course of therapy because of reinfection, nonadherence, or antimicrobial resistance. Factors associated with decreased adherence include polypharmacy, need for frequent drug administration or long treatment duration, and use of drugs that may cause intolerable side effects. Potential adverse drug effects include taste disturbances (clarithromycin and metronidazole), nausea, vomiting, abdominal pain, and diarrhea. Superinfections with oral thrush or vaginal candidiasis can occur. Alcohol should be avoided during treatment with metronidazole or tinidazole due to the potential for a disulfiram-like reaction with alcohol use.[22]

Patient Encounter 1

A 62-year-old man presents with abdominal pain and heartburn that occur two to three times per week. He also reports a 10-pound (4.5-kg) weight loss in the last 6 weeks, despite not dieting or increasing physical activity.

PMH: Hypertension × 5 years

FH: Mother alive at 84 with hypertension, type 2 diabetes; father deceased at 68 following MI

SH: Smokes 1/2 pack per day; 2 alcoholic beverages 3 times per week; no illicit drug use

Allergies: NKDA

Meds: Lisinopril/hydrochlorothiazide 20/25 mg daily, acetaminophen 500 mg as needed for headache

Based on this patient's clinical presentation, what is the most appropriate course of action to establish a diagnosis?

The patient receives a diagnosis of H. pylori *infection based on the diagnostic method recommended. What eradication therapy would you recommend?*

The patient completes a course of eradication therapy, and 3 months later he presents with similar dyspeptic symptoms. H. pylori *recurrence is confirmed with a urea breath test. Discuss possible reasons for treatment failure in this patient.*

What regimen would you recommend for salvage eradication therapy?

Table 18–4

Drug Regimens to Eradicate *Helicobacter Pylori*[a,b]

Treatment Regimen	Cure Rates[b]
Three Drugs	
Clarithromycin 500 mg + metronidazole 500 mg (or tinidazole 500mg) + omeprazole 20 mg, each given two times a day	Good to excellent
Clarithromycin 500 mg + amoxicillin 1 g + lansoprazole 30 mg, each given two times a day	Good to excellent
Four Drugs	
Helidac (bismuth subsalicylate 525 mg + metronidazole 250 mg + tetracycline 500 mg, each given four times a day) + H$_2$RA (conventional healing dose)[c]	Good
Bismuth subsalicylate 525 mg four times a day + metronidazole 250 mg four times a day + amoxicillin 1 g twice daily + PPI twice daily[d]	Good
Pylera (bismuth subcitrate potassium 140 mg + metronidazole 125 mg + tetracycline 125 mg) 3 capsules two times a day + omeprazole 20 mg two times a day × 10 days	Good to excellent
Rescue Therapy	
Bismuth subsalicylate 525 mg + metronidazole 500 mg + tetracycline 500 mg, each given four times a day + omeprazole 20 mg two times a day[d]	Good to excellent
Amoxicillin 1 g + rifabutin 150 mg + pantoprazole 40 mg, each given two times a day[e]	Good to excellent
Amoxicillin 1 g + levofloxacin 250 mg + pantoprazole 40 mg, each given two times a day[e]	Good to excellent
Sequential Therapy	
Days 1–5: Amoxicillin 1 g + PPI, each given twice daily	Good to excellent
Days 6–10: Clarithromycin 500 mg + metronidazole 500 mg (or tinidazole 500 mg) + PPI, each given twice daily	

[a]Regimens are based on efficacy for a 14-day treatment duration unless otherwise noted.

[b]Based on cure rates of 80% to 90% = good; and greater than 90% = excellent.

[c]Although commercially available, regimens containing H$_2$RAs are not preferred.

[d]Duration of therapy is 7 to 10 days.

[e]Given for 10 to 14 days.

H$_2$RA, histamine-2 receptor antagonist; PPI, proton pump inhibitor.

Preexisting antimicrobial resistance accounts for up to 70% of all treatment failures and is most often related to metronidazole or clarithromycin. Metronidazole-resistant strains are more prevalent in Asia (85%) than North America (40%).[22] Clarithromycin resistance rates are approximately 10% in the United States. Primary resistance to amoxicillin and tetracycline remains low in both the United States and Europe.[22] Culture and sensitivity studies are not routinely performed with *H. pylori* infection unless a patient has already failed two different treatment regimens.[7,18,21]

Initiation of a second *H. pylori* treatment regimen after failure of initial treatment is usually associated with a lower success rate. Reasons for failure are often the same as those reported with failure of the initial regimen. In these situations, quadruple therapy for 14 days is generally required, and metronidazole or clarithromycin should be replaced by another antibiotic if either one of these agents was used in the initial regimen.[22] If both clarithromycin and metronidazole were used as initial therapy, a regimen consisting of amoxicillin 1 g twice daily, levofloxacin 250 mg twice daily, and a PPI twice daily may be used for 10 to 14 days.[26] Another salvage therapy consisting of a PPI twice daily, amoxicillin 1 g twice daily, and rifabutin 300 mg once daily for 10 to 14 days resulted in eradication rates greater than 80%.[5,27,28]

There is no standard third-line therapy for *H. pylori* treatment. If the patient was adherent with initial treatment, then culture and sensitivity testing should be completed in order to select an antimicrobial regimen with adequate sensitivities.[5,21] Sequential therapy is a possible alternative 10-day regimen that may also be used to treat *H. pylori* infection and consists of using different combinations of antibiotics for 5 days each in addition to a PPI twice daily. Eradication rates are reported between 84% and 93%.[29]

Confirmation of *H. pylori* infection eradication is recommended in patients with a history of *H. pylori*–associated ulcer, MALT lymphoma, those who have undergone resection for early gastric cancer, and patients whose symptoms persist after *H. pylori* treatment for dyspepsia.[7] Eradication may be confirmed by either a urea breath test or stool antigen testing. Eradication may also be confirmed on endoscopy; however, this should only be done when endoscopy is required because this method is more expensive and invasive.[7]

▶ *Treatment of NSAID-Induced Ulcers*

● Treatment recommendations to heal NSAID-induced ulcers or provide maintenance therapy in patients receiving NSAIDS are shown in Table 18–5. Choice of regimen depends on whether NSAID use is to be continued. NSAIDs should

---

Table 18–5

Oral Drug Regimens to Heal Peptic Ulcers or Maintain Ulcer Healing in the Absence of Antibiotic Therapy

Drug	DU or GU Healing (mg/day)	Maintenance of DU or GU Healing (mg/day)
Mucosal Protectant		
Sucralfate	1 g four times a day	1 g four times a day
	2 g two times a day	1–2 g two times a day
H₂-Receptor Antagonists		
Cimetidine	300 mg four times a day	400–800 mg daily
	400 mg two times a day	
	800 mg at bedtime	
Famotidine	20 mg two times a day	20–40 mg daily
	40 mg at bedtime	
Nizatidine	150 mg two times a day	150–300 mg daily
	300 mg at bedtime	
Ranitidine	150 mg two times a day	150–300 mg daily
	300 mg at bedtime	
Proton Pump Inhibitors		
Dexlansoprazole	30–60 mg daily	30–60 mg daily
Esomeprazole	20–40 mg daily	20–40 mg daily
Lansoprazole	15–30 mg daily	15–30 mg daily
Omeprazole	20–40 mg daily	20–40 mg daily
Pantoprazole	40 mg daily	40 mg daily
Rabeprazole	20 mg daily	20 mg daily

DU, duodenal ulcer; GU, gastric ulcer.

Patient Encounter 2

A 68-year-old woman presents with reports of dark, tarry stools for 3 days. She denies coffee-ground emesis or recent weight loss but reports occasional abdominal pain.

PMH: Hypertension × 10 years, type 2 diabetes × 5 years, dyslipidemia × 5 years, osteoarthritis × 3 years

FH: Parents deceased; mother with stroke at age 82, father with MI at age 74; one sister alive at 74 with hypertension, type 2 diabetes, and dyslipidemia

SH: Denies tobacco or illicit drug use; two glasses of red wine at card club on Saturdays

Allergies: NKDA

Meds: Lisinopril 40 mg daily, amlodipine 5 mg daily, metformin 1,000 mg twice daily, glipizide 10 mg twice daily, simvastatin 40 mg daily, diclofenac 75 mg twice daily, aspirin 81 mg daily, Tums Extra Strength as needed for dyspeptic symptoms

Other: An endoscopy is performed and reveals a duodenal ulcer that is negative for *H. pylori*.

What risk factors does this patient have for GI complications related to NSAID use?

Make a recommendation for treatment of this patient's ulcer.

Discuss the use of prophylactic therapy in this patient after the treatment course is completed.

---

be discontinued if possible and replaced with alternatives (e.g., acetaminophen), when possible. For patients who cannot discontinue NSAID therapy, PPIs, H₂RAs, or sucralfate are effective for ulcer healing and to prevent further recurrences.[5] PPIs are usually preferred because they provide more rapid relief of symptoms, have the strongest acid suppression, and heal ulcers more quickly than H₂RAs or sucralfate.[5] Standard doses of H₂RAs effectively heal DUs but are minimally effective in GUs. In ulcers larger than 5 mm, the rate of ulcer healing may be as low as 25% after 8 weeks of therapy with an H₂RA.[9] A PPI provides equivalent efficacy with treatment duration of only 4 weeks. PPI therapy should only be continued for longer than 4 weeks if an ulcer is confirmed to still be present or if the patient develops severe complications from PUD.

▶ Prevention of NSAID-Induced Ulcers

Prophylactic regimens against PUD are often required in patients on long-term NSAID or aspirin therapy for osteoarthritis (OA), rheumatoid arthritis (RA), or cardioprotection.[30] Misoprostol, H₂RAs, PPIs, and COX-2 selective inhibitors have been evaluated in controlled trials to reduce the risk of NSAID-induced PUD. ❹ *In patients at risk for NSAID-induced ulcers, PPIs at standard doses reduce the risk of both gastric and DU as effectively as misoprostol and more effectively than H₂RAs.* In addition, PPIs are generally better tolerated than misoprostol.

Although acute GI bleeding is the most serious adverse outcome of NSAID therapy, few studies have compared PUD prophylaxis strategies using this outcome measure due to the low frequency with which bleeding occurs in NSAID users, the small size of most prophylaxis studies, and their short duration.[30]

Misoprostol Misoprostol is a synthetic PGE1 analog that exogenously replaces PG stores. It is indicated for reducing the risk of NSAID-induced GUs in patients at high risk of complications from GUs (e.g., the elderly and patients with concomitant debilitating disease), as well as patients at high risk of developing gastric ulceration, such as patients with a history of ulcers. Misoprostol at 200 mcg four times a day reduces ulcer complications by inhibiting acid secretion and promoting mucosal defense.[9] Misoprostol use is limited by a high frequency of bothersome GI effects such as abdominal pain, flatulence, and diarrhea, and it is contraindicated in pregnancy due to potential abortifacient effects. Arthrotec is a combination product that contains diclofenac (either 50 or 75 mg) and misoprostol 200 mcg in a single tablet. Misoprostol is indicated for patients at high risk for NSAID-induced ulceration, and it has been found to be superior to H$_2$RAs for the prevention of NSAID-induced ulcers.

H$_2$-Receptor Antagonists The efficacy of H$_2$RAs (e.g., famotidine 40 mg daily) in preventing NSAID-related ulcers varies.[31] DUs appear to respond better than GUs (the most frequent type of ulcer-associated with NSAIDs). Higher doses of H$_2$RAs (e.g., famotidine 40 mg twice daily) may reduce the risk of NSAID-induced GUs and DUs, but results from clinical trials are variable.

Duexis, a prescription combination product containing ibuprofen 800 mg and famotidine 26.6 mg, is indicated for the relief of signs and symptoms of RA and OA and to decrease the risk of developing upper GI ulcers. The recommended dosage is one tablet by mouth three times daily. Clinical trials evaluating this agent are 6 months or less in duration and primarily evaluated patients younger than 65 years with no ulcer history.[32]

Proton Pump Inhibitors PPI therapy is more effective than H$_2$RAs in reducing the risk of nonselective NSAID-related GUs and DUs. PPIs are as effective as misoprostol but better tolerated. All PPIs are effective when used in standard doses. In patients who experience a PUD-related bleeding event while taking aspirin but who require continued aspirin therapy, the addition of a PPI reduces the incidence of recurrent GI bleeding.[5] Prevacid NapraPAC provides naproxen (either 250, 375, or 500 mg) and lansoprazole 15 mg in individual blister packages.

COX-2 Selective Inhibitors With the availability of NSAIDs with COX-2 selectivity, clinicians postulated that these agents would avoid the need to add an additional prophylactic agent in patients with PUD risk factors. ❺ *However, selective COX-2 inhibitors are no more effective than the combination of a PPI and a nonselective NSAID in reducing the incidence of ulcers and are associated with a greater incidence of CV events (e.g., ischemic stroke).*[5] Celecoxib is the only agent in this class that remains on the market; its postulated improved GI safety when compared with nonselective NSAIDs has not

been established.[33] Controlled studies also demonstrate that celecoxib is no better than the combination of diclofenac and omeprazole.[34]

Longer term studies evaluating the CV risks associated with use of COX-2 inhibitors found a higher incidence of CV mortality compared with traditional NSAIDs.[35,36] This prompted the withdrawal of both rofecoxib and valdecoxib from the market and the inclusion of a black box warning in the celecoxib package insert.[37] Given the CV risk of the COX-2 inhibitors, a nonselective NSAID and a PPI is recommended instead of celecoxib in patients at high risk for NSAID-related PUD.[5,38]

Sucralfate This drug is a negatively charged, nonabsorbable agent that forms a complex by binding with positively charged proteins in exudates, forming a viscous, paste-like adhesive substance that protects the ulcerated area of the gastric mucosa against gastric acid, pepsin, and bile salts.[9,15] Limitations of sucralfate include the need for multiple daily dosing, large tablet size, and interaction with a number of other medications (e.g., digoxin and fluoroquinolones).

Adverse effects of sucralfate include constipation, nausea, metallic taste, and the possibility for aluminum toxicity in patients with renal failure. Sucralfate is effective in the treatment of NSAID-related ulcers when the NSAID will be stopped, but it is not recommended for NSAID-related ulcer prophylaxis.

▶ *Prevention of Stress-Related Mucosal Damage*

Prevention of stress ulcers involves maintaining hemodynamic stability to maximize mesenteric perfusion and pharmacologic suppression of gastric acid production. SUP is only indicated in intensive care unit (ICU) patients with certain risk factors.[11] ❻ *Indications for stress ulcer prophylaxis include major trauma, major surgery, severe head trauma, multiple organ failure, burns covering more than 25% to 30% of body, severe sepsis, shock, mechanical ventilation, coagulopathy, and high-dose steroid use.*[39] The clinician must weigh the risks and benefits of using acid suppression, especially PPIs, in low-risk patients. PPIs and H$_2$RAs are the drugs of choice for SUP; however, antacids and sucralfate may be acceptable options in some patients.

▶ *Long-Term Maintenance of Ulcer Healing*

❼ *Low-dose maintenance therapy with a PPI or H$_2$RA is only indicated* in patients with severe complications secondary to PUD such as gastric outlet obstruction or patients who need to be on long-term NSAIDs or high-dose corticosteroids and are at high risk for bleeding. Drug regimens and doses for PUD treatment and maintenance are presented in Table 18–5.

▶ *Treatment of GI Bleeding*

The immediate priorities in treating patients with a bleeding peptic ulcer are to achieve IV access, correct fluid losses, and restore hemodynamic stability. Insertion of a nasogastric tube is helpful in initial patient assessment, but the absence of bloody or coffee-ground material does not definitively

Patient Encounter 3

A 45-year-old man is brought to the surgical ICU after emergency surgery for a ruptured appendix. The physician would like him to remain NPO (nothing by mouth, except for medications) for at least a couple of days until he improves clinically and can sit up in bed.

PMH: Hypertension × 10 years, type 2 diabetes × 5 years

FH: Father with type 2 diabetes

SH: Smokes 1 pack per day; no alcohol use; no illicit drug use

Allergies: NKDA

Meds: Lisinopril/hydrochlorothiazide 20/25 mg daily, metformin 500 mg twice daily, ibuprofen 800 mg alternating with oxycodone 5 mg /acetaminophen 325 mg 2 tablets every 8 hours for surgical site pain

Based on this patient's clinical presentation, is he a candidate for stress ulcer prophylaxis?

What pharmacologic therapy would you recommend for this patient?

Two days later, the patient is transferred to a general medicine floor and begins a regular diet that is well tolerated. Ibuprofen has been discontinued, and he is alternating between oxycodone/acetaminophen and acetaminophen alone to relieve incision site pain. He is sitting up in bed and feeling much better. Is this patient still a candidate for stress ulcer prophylaxis?

Patient Encounter 4

A 64-year-old man presents to the emergency department complaining of vomiting blood and having black, tarry stools for the past 24 hours. He has never had a prior similar episode, and he denies any abdominal pain or unintentional weight loss.

PMH: Hypertension × 5 years, gout × 2 years

Allergies: NKDA

SH: Smokes 1 pack per day; drinks 6 to 12 beers per day; no illicit drug use

FH: Father died at 75 from heart disease (MI); mother died at 82 from a stroke

Meds: Metoprolol 50 mg twice daily, allopurinol 100 mg daily, NSAIDs (ibuprofen, naproxen) for gout flares as needed

PE:

VS: BP 72/46, P 132, RR 22, T 37.3°C (99.2°F)

Gen: Slightly confused, obese male

CV: Tachycardic, regular, no murmurs

Resp: Tachypneic, clear bilaterally

Abd: Soft, obese, nontender, nondistended, hypoactive bowel sounds

Rect: Melena, no pain, normal sphincter tone

What are the most important initial steps in the management of this patient?

After the patient is stabilized, what should be done next?

An EGD shows a 2-cm duodenal ulcer with an adherent clot in the duodenal bulb. The clot is removed and shows a visible vessel. The lesion in injected with epinephrine, and three clips are placed successfully to control the bleeding. What additional management steps should be taken for this patient? How would you identify the etiology of his ulcer?

rule out ongoing or recurrent bleeding; about 15% of patients without bloody nasogastric tube output have a high-risk lesion at endoscopy.[19]

Patients should be started on IV PPI therapy because optimal platelet aggregation, partially inhibited fibrinolysis, and better clot stabilization on the ulcer are achieved when the gastric pH is greater than 6.[20] IV PPI therapy should be continued for 72 hours because most rebleeding occurs during this time followed by oral PPI. Three-day PPI infusion therapy has been shown to be as effective as twice-daily IV PPI therapy.[20]

▶ *Treatment of Refractory Ulcers*

Refractory ulcers are defined as ulcers that fail to heal despite 8 to 12 weeks of acid suppressive therapy.[1] The presence of refractory ulcers requires a thorough assessment, including evaluation of medication adherence, extensive counseling and questioning regarding recent over-the-counter and prescription medication use, and testing for *H. pylori* using a different method than previously done if testing was negative. Changing from H_2RA therapy to a PPI should be considered.[15] Other considerations include esophagogastroduodenoscopy (EGD) with biopsy of the ulcer to exclude malignancy, *H. pylori* testing (if not done initially), serum gastrin measurement to exclude ZES, and gastric acid

studies. Increasing the starting dose of PPI therapy may heal up to 90% of refractory ulcers after 8 weeks of therapy.[15]

OUTCOME EVALUATION[15]

- Obtain a baseline complete blood count (CBC). Recheck the CBC if the patient exhibits alarm signs or symptoms.
- Obtain a baseline serum creatinine measurement. Calculate the estimated creatinine clearance and adjust the dose of H_2RAs and sucralfate if needed.
- Obtain a history of symptoms from the patient. Monitor for improvements in pain symptoms (e.g., epigastric or abdominal pain) daily.
- Monitor the patient for the development of any alarm signs and symptoms.

Patient Care and Monitoring

General Recommendations: *H. pylori*–Associated and NSAID-Induced Ulcers

1. Assess the severity of signs and symptoms. Identify the presence of any alarm signs and symptoms.

2. Educate the patient on monitoring for alarm signs and symptoms.

3. Obtain a history of prescription medication, over-the-counter medication, and dietary supplement use.

4. Encourage lifestyle modifications such as reducing tobacco use and ethanol ingestion and decreasing psychological stress.

5. Determine the appropriate duration for acid-suppressive therapy.

6. Define the current impact of PUD on the patient's quality of life and the improvement in these outcomes sought with drug therapy.

7. Evaluate current drug therapy for potential adverse drug reactions and drug interactions.

H. pylori–Associated Ulcers

1. Recommend an appropriate drug regimen that will eradicate the organism.

2. Identify the patient's drug allergies and avoid drug classes a patient is allergic to.

3. Educate patients on specific adverse drug effects, particularly with metronidazole (avoidance of alcohol), bismuth (change in stool color), and clarithromycin (taste disturbance).

4. Assess the potential for drug interactions, particularly in patients taking regimens containing metronidazole, clarithromycin, and/or cimetidine.

5. Recommend different antibiotics if this treatment regimen is a result of failure of a prior *H. pylori* regimen.

6. Educate the patient on the importance of adherence to eradication therapy.

NSAID-Associated Ulcers

1. Assess for risk factors for NSAID ulcers and recommend an appropriate strategy to reduce ulcer risk.

2. Monitor for signs and symptoms of complications associated with NSAID-related ulceration.

3. Recommend an appropriate treatment regimen to heal the ulcer.

4. Assess and counsel patients on potential adverse drug events and drug interactions.

5. Inform patients who are receiving prophylactic therapy on the importance of its use, potential adverse drug events, and the possible alarm symptoms associated with PUD.

- Recommend a follow-up visit if signs and symptoms worsen at any time or do not improve within the defined treatment period.

- Assess for potential drug interactions whenever there is a change in the patient's medications.

- Educate the patient on the importance of adhering to the *H. pylori* eradication regimen.

- Monitor the patient for complications related to antibiotic therapy (e.g., diarrhea or oral thrush) during and after completion of *H. pylori* eradication therapy.

- Recommend follow-up care if the patient's signs and symptoms do not improve after completion of *H. pylori* eradication therapy.

Abbreviations Introduced in This Chapter

COX	Cyclooxygenase
CV	Cardiovascular
DU	Duodenal ulcer
EGD	Esophagogastroduodenoscopy
GU	Gastric ulcer
H_2RA	Histamine-2 receptor antagonist

INR	International normalized ratio
MALT	Mucosa-associated lymphoid tissue
NSAID	Nonsteroidal anti-inflammatory drug
PG	Prostaglandin
PPI	Proton pump inhibitor
PUD	Peptic ulcer disease
SRMD	Stress-related mucosal damage
SUP	Stress ulcer prophylaxis
ZES	Zollinger–Ellison syndrome

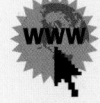 Self-assessment questions and answers are available at *http://www.mhpharmacotherapy.com/pp.html*.

REFERENCES

1. Banerjee S, Cash BD, Dominitz JA, et al. The role of endoscopy in the management of patients with peptic ulcer disease. Gastrointest Endosc 2010;71:663–668.

2. Vakil N. Peptic ulcer disease. In: Feldman M, Friedman LW, Brandt L, eds. Sleisenger and Fordtran's Gastrointestinal and Liver Disease, 9th ed. Philadelphia, PA: Saunders, 2010:861–868.

3. Hunt RH, Xiao SD, Megraud F, et al. World Gastroenterology Organisation Global Guideline: *Helicobacter pylori* in developing countries. J Clin Gastroenterol 2011;45:383–388.

4. Sonnenberg A, Everhart JE. Health impact of peptic ulcer in the United States. Am J Gastroenterol 1997;92:614–620.

5. Malfertheiner P, Chan F, McColl K. Peptic ulcer disease. Lancet 2009;374:1449–1461.

6. Warren JR, Marshall BJ. Unidentified curved bacilli on gastric epithelium in active chronic gastritis. Lancet 1983;1:1273–1275.

7. McColl KE. *Helicobacter pylori* infection. N Engl J Med 2010;362:1597–1604.

8. Chan FK, Graham DY. Review article: Prevention of non-steroidal anti-inflammatory drug gastrointestinal complications—Review and recommendations based on risk assessment. Aliment Pharmacol Ther 2004;19:1051–1061.

9. Chan FK, Lau JY. Treatment of peptic ulcer disease. In: Feldman M, Friedman LW, Brandt L, eds. Sleisenger and Fordtran's Gastrointestinal and Liver Disease, 9th ed. Philadelphia, PA: Saunders, 2010:869–886.

10. Stollman N, Metz DC. Pathophysiology and prophylaxis of stress ulcer in intensive care unit patients. J Crit Care 2005;20:35–45.

11. American Society of Health-System Pharmacists: ASHP Therapeutic Guidelines on Stress Ulcer Prophylaxis. Am J Health Syst Pharm 1999;56:347–379.

12. Wu WK, Cho CH. The pharmacological actions of nicotine on the gastrointestinal tract. J Pharmacol Sci 2004;94:348–358.

13. Schubert ML, Kaunitz JD. Gastric secretion. In: Feldman M, Friedman LW, Brandt L, eds. Sleisenger and Fordtran's Gastrointestinal and Liver Disease, 9th ed. Philadelphia, PA: Saunders, 2010:817–832.

14. Semrin MG, Russo MA. Anatomy, Histology, Embryology, and Developmental anomalies of the stomach and duodenum. In: Feldman M, Friedman LW, Brandt L, eds. Sleisenger and Fordtran's Gastrointestinal and Liver Disease, 9th ed. Philadelphia, PA: Saunders, 2010: 773–788.

15. Berardi R, Fugit R. Peptic ulcer disease. In: DiPiro JT; Talbert RA; Yee GC, et al., eds. Pharmacotherapy: A Pathophysiologic Approach, 8th ed. New York, NY: McGraw-Hill, 2011:563–585.

16. American Gastroenterological Association Medical Position Statement: Evaluation of dyspepsia. Gastroenterology 2005;129:1753–1755.

17. Ikenberry SO, Harrison ME, Lichtenstein D, et al. The role of endoscopy in dyspepsia. Gastrointest Endosc 2007;66:1071–1075.

18. Chey WD, Wong BCY. American College of Gastroenterology Guideline on the Management of *Helicobacter pylori* Infection. Am J Gastroenterol 2007;102:1808–1825.

19. Gralnek IM, Barkun AN, Bardou M. Management of acute bleeding from a peptic ulcer. N Engl J Med 2008;359:928–937.

20. Songür Y, Balkarli A, Acartürk G, Senol A. Comparison of infusion or low-dose proton pump inhibitor treatments in upper gastrointestinal system bleeding. Eur J Intern Med 2011;22:200–204.

21. Malfertheiner P, Megraud F, O'Morain C, et al. The European Helicobacter Study Group (EHSG). Current concepts in the management of *Helicobacter pylori* infection: The Maastricht III Consensus Report. Gut 2007;56:772–781.

22. Peura DA, Crowe SE. *Helicobacter pylori*. In: Feldman M, Friedman LW, Brandt L, eds. Sleisenger and Fordtran's Gastrointestinal and Liver Disease, 9th ed. Philadelphia, PA: Saunders, 2010:833–844.

23. Bertleff MJ, Lange JF. Perforated peptic ulcer disease: A review of history and treatment. Dig Surg 2010;27:161–169.

24. Wong TCI, Wong KT, Chiu PWY, et al. A comparison of angiographic embolization with surgery after failed endoscopic hemostasis to bleeding peptic ulcers. Gastrointest Endosc 2011;73:900–908.

25. Fuccio L, Minardi ME, Zagari RM, et al. Meta-analysis: Duration of first-line proton-pump inhibitor based triple therapy for *Helicobacter pylori* eradication. Ann Intern Med 2007;147:553–562.

26. Jodlowski TZ, Lam S, Ashby CR. Emerging therapies for the treatment of *Helicobacter pylori* infections. Ann Pharmacother 2008;42:1621–1639.

27. Qasim A, Sebastian S, Thornton O, et al. Rifabutin- and furazolidone-based *Helicobacter pylori* eradication therapies after failure of standard first- and second-line eradication attempts in dyspepsia patients. Aliment Pharmacol Ther 2005;21:91–96.

28. Jafri NS, Hornung CA, Howden CW. Meta-analysis: Sequential therapy appears superior to standard therapy for *Helicobacter pylori* infection in patients naive to treatment. Ann Intern Med 2008;148:923–931.

29. Gisbert JP, Pajares JM. *Helicobacter pylori* "rescue" regimen when proton pump inhibitor-based triple therapies fail. Aliment Pharmacol Ther 2002;16:1047–1057.

30. Targownik LE, Metge CJ, Leung S, Chateau DG. The relative efficacies of gastroprotective strategies in chronic users of nonsteroidal anti-inflammatory drugs. Gastroenterology 2008;134:937–944.

31. Agrawal NM, Campbell DR, Safdi MA, et al. Superiority of lansoprazole vs ranitidine in healing nonsteroidal anti-inflammatory drug-associated gastric ulcers: Results of a double-blind, randomized, multicenter study. NSAID-associated gastric ulcer study group. Arch Intern Med 2000;160:1455–1461.

32. Duexis (ibuprofen/famotidine) [product information]. Northbrook, IL: Horizon Pharma USA, April 2011.

33. Silverstein FE, Faich G, Goldstein JL, et al. Gastrointestinal toxicity with celecoxib vs nonsteroidal anti-inflammatory drugs for osteoarthritis and rheumatoid arthritis: The CLASS study: A randomized controlled trial. Celecoxib long-term arthritis safety study. JAMA 2000;284:1247–1255.

34. Chan FK, Hung LC, Suen BY, et al. Celecoxib versus diclofenac and omeprazole in reducing the risk of recurrent ulcer bleeding in patients with arthritis. N Engl J Med 2002;347:2104–2110.

35. Nussmeier NA, Whelton AA, Brown MT, et al. Complications of the COX-2 inhibitors parecoxib and valdecoxib after cardiac surgery. N Engl J Med 2005;352:1081–1091.

36. Bresalier RS, Sandler RS, Quan H, et al. Cardiovascular events associated with rofecoxib in a colorectal adenoma chemoprevention trial. N Engl J Med 2005;352:1092–1102.

37. FDA Alert: Information for Healthcare Professionals: Celecoxib (marketed as Celebrex) [Internet] (cited 2005 April 7). Available from: *http://www.fda.gov/Drugs/DrugSafety/PostmarketDrugSafetyInformationforPatientsandProviders/ucm124655.htm*.

38. Chan FK, Abraham NS, Scheiman JM, et al. Management of patients on nonsteroidal anti-inflammatory drugs: A clinical practice recommendation from the first international working party on gastrointestinal and cardiovascular effects of nonsteroidal anti-inflammatory effects and anti-platelet agents. Am J Gastroenterol 2008;103:2908–2918.

39. Grube RA, May B. Stress ulcer prophylaxis in hospitalized patients not in intensive care units. Am J Health Syst Pharmacy 2007;64:1396–1400.

19 Inflammatory Bowel Disease

Brian A. Hemstreet

LEARNING OBJECTIVES

● **Upon completion of the chapter, the reader will be able to:**

1. Characterize the pathophysiologic mechanisms underlying inflammatory bowel disease (IBD).

2. Recognize the signs and symptoms of IBD, including major differences between ulcerative colitis (UC) and Crohn's disease (CD).

3. Identify appropriate therapeutic outcomes for patients with IBD.

4. Describe pharmacologic treatment options for patients with acute or chronic symptoms of UC and CD.

5. Create a patient-specific drug treatment plan based on symptoms, severity, and location of UC or CD.

6. Recommend appropriate monitoring parameters and patient education for drug treatments for IBD.

KEY CONCEPTS

❶ Inflammatory bowel disease (IBD) includes both ulcerative colitis (UC) and Crohn's disease (CD) and is associated with chronic inflammation of various areas of the GI tract.

❷ Differentiation of UC and CD is based on signs and symptoms as well as characteristic endoscopic findings including the extent, pattern, and depth of inflammation.

❸ Patients may manifest extraintestinal symptoms of IBD, such as arthritis, primary sclerosing cholangitis, erythema nodosum, and pyoderma gangrenosum, among others.

❹ Major treatment goals for patients with IBD include alleviation of signs and symptoms, induction of remission, suppression of inflammation during acute episodes, and maintenance of remission thereafter.

❺ When designing a drug regimen for treatment of IBD, several factors should be considered, including the patient's symptoms, medical history, current medication use, drug allergies, and location and severity of disease.

❻ Antidiarrheal medications that reduce GI motility, such as loperamide, diphenoxylate/atropine, and codeine, should be avoided in patients with active IBD due to the risk of precipitating acute colonic dilation (toxic megacolon).

❼ Treatment of acute episodes of UC is dictated by the severity and extent of disease, and first-line therapy of mild to moderate disease involves oral or topical aminosalicylate derivatives.

❽ Maintenance of remission of UC may be achieved with oral or topical aminosalicylates. Immunosuppressants such as azathioprine, 6-mercaptopurine (6-MP), or infliximab can be used for unresponsive patients or those who develop corticosteroid dependency.

❾ Treatment of active mild to moderate CD involves use of oral budesonide or oral or topical aminosalicylate derivatives, whereas moderate to severe disease may require systemic corticosteroid or anti-tumor necrosis factor (anti-TNF) antibody therapy.

❿ Maintenance of remission of CD may be achieved with immunosuppressants (azathioprine, 6-MP, or methotrexate), biologic agents (infliximab, adalimumab, certolizumab pegol, or natalizumab), and less frequently with oral or topical aminosalicylate derivatives.

INTRODUCTION

❶ *Inflammatory bowel disease (IBD) encompasses both Crohn's disease (CD) and ulcerative colitis (UC). Both disorders are associated with chronic inflammation of various regions within the GI tract.* Differences exist between UC and CD with regard to the regions of the GI tract that may be affected as well as in the distribution and depth of inflammation. Some patients with IBD may also have inflammation involving organs other than the GI tract, known as extraintestinal manifestations. Symptoms of IBD are associated with significant morbidity, reduction in quality of life, and substantial costs to the healthcare system. For purposes of this chapter, references made to IBD include both UC and CD. Significant differences between UC and CD are discussed separately when applicable.

EPIDEMIOLOGY

IBD is most common in Western countries such as the United States and Northern Europe. The age of initial presentation of IBD is bimodal, with patients typically diagnosed between the ages of 20 to 40 or 60 to 80 years. The incidence and prevalence of UC in the United States are reported as 9 to 12 cases per 100,000 and 205 to 240 cases per 100,000.[1-6] The incidence and prevalence of CD is reported as 6 to 8 cases per 100,000 and 100 to 200 cases per 100,000.[6] Peak incidence of UC occurs between the ages of 15 and 30 years.[6]

Men and women are approximately equally affected by IBD in Western countries.[6] In general, whites are affected more often than blacks, and persons of Jewish descent also have higher reported incidences of IBD. One of the greatest risk factors for development of IBD is a positive family history of the disease. The incidence of IBD is 10 to 40 times greater in patients with a first-degree relative who has IBD compared with the general population.[4,5,7] A positive family history may be more of a contributing factor for development of CD than UC.[7-9]

ETIOLOGY

The exact cause of IBD is not fully understood. Processes thought to be involved in its development include genetic predisposition, dysregulation of the inflammatory response within the GI tract, or perhaps environmental or antigenic factors.[3,4] The fact that a positive family history is a strong predictor of IBD supports the theory that genetic predisposition may be responsible in many cases. Many potential candidate genes have been identified. An example is a gene found on chromosome 16 that encodes for nucleotide oligomerization domain 2 (NOD2).[6] NOD2 is a cytoplasmic protein expressed in macrophages, monocytes, and gut epithelial cells thought to be involved in recognition and degradation of bacterial products by the gut wall. Less is known about genetic alterations that may predispose patients to UC, but UC may share common genetic features with CD.

An alteration in the inflammatory response regulated by intestinal epithelial cells may also contribute to development of IBD. This may involve inappropriate processing of antigens presented to the GI epithelial cells.[3,4,10,11] The inflammatory response in IBD may actually be directed at bacteria that normally colonize the GI tract. Products derived from these bacteria may translocate across the mucosal layer of the GI tract and interact with various cells involved in immunologic recognition. The result is T-cell stimulation, excess production of proinflammatory cytokines, and persistent inflammation within the GI tract.

The intestinal mucosa of patients with CD has a preponderance of CD4+ type 1 helper T cells (Th1), whereas patients with UC have more CD4+ lymphocytes with atypical type 2

helper T cells (Th2).[10] Likewise, drugs such as nonsteroidal anti-inflammatory drugs (NSAIDs) that disrupt the integrity of the GI mucosa may facilitate mucosal entry of intestinal antigens and lead to disease flares in patients with IBD.[12]

The role of antigens derived from dietary intake in the development of IBD is less well defined. There is some speculation that ingestion of large quantities of refined carbohydrates or margarine leads to higher rates of CD. Use of oral contraceptives has been associated with increased development of IBD in some cohort studies, but a strong causal relationship has not been proven.[6,8] Isotretinoin use has also been associated with the development of IBD.

Lastly, positive smoking status has been shown to have protective effects in UC, leading to reductions in disease severity.[6] The opposite is true in CD because smoking may lead to increases in symptoms or worsening of the disease.[6,10]

PATHOPHYSIOLOGY

Ulcerative Colitis

The inflammatory response in UC is propagated by atypical type 2 helper T cells that produce proinflammatory cytokines such as interleukin (IL)-1, IL-6, and tumor necrosis factor-alfa (TNF-α).[8] As discussed previously, a genetic predisposition to UC may partially explain the development of excessive colonic and rectal inflammation. The finding of positive perinuclear antineutrophil cytoplasmic antibodies (pANCA) in association with the human leukocyte antigen (HLA)-DR2 allele in a large percentage of patients with UC supports this theory.[13]

The potential role of environmental factors in development of UC implies that the immune response is directed against an unknown antigen. The findings that development and severity of UC are reduced in patients who smoke, or in those with appendectomies, may support the theory that these factors may somehow modify either the genetic component or phenotypic response to immunologic stimuli.[3,12]

The inflammatory process within the GI tract is limited to the colon and rectum in patients with UC (Fig. 19–1). Most patients with UC have involvement of the rectum (*proctitis*) or both the rectum and the sigmoid colon (proctosigmoiditis). Inflammation involving the entire colon is referred to as *pancolitis* or extensive disease. Left-sided (distal) disease, defined as inflammation extending from the rectum to the splenic flexure, occurs in 30% to 40% of patients.[12] A small number of cases of UC involve mild inflammation of the terminal ileum, referred to as "backwash ileitis."

The pattern of inflammation in UC is continuous and confluent throughout the affected areas of the GI tract. The inflammation is also superficial and does not typically extend below the submucosal layer of the GI tract (Fig. 19–2). Ulceration or erosion of the GI mucosa may be present and varies with disease severity. The formation of *crypt abscesses* within the mucosal layers of the GI tract is characteristic of UC and may help to distinguish it from CD. Severe inflammation may also result in areas of hypertrophied GI mucosa, which may manifest as *pseudopolyps* within the

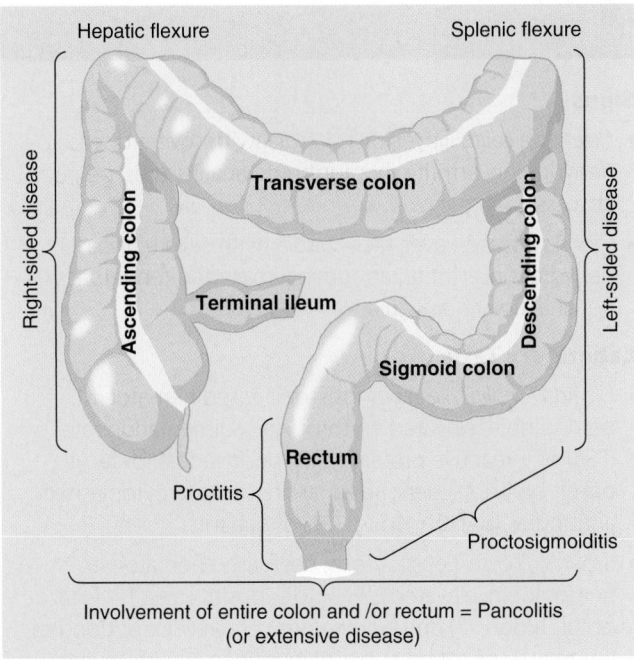

FIGURE 19–1. Major GI landmarks and disease distribution in inflammatory bowel disease.

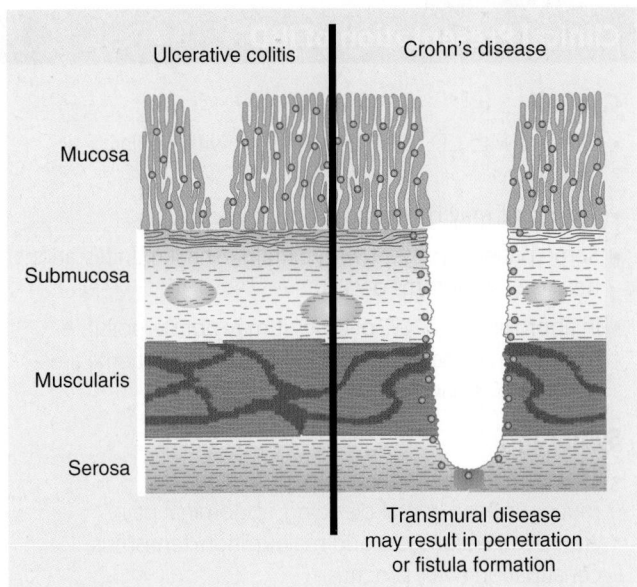

Transmural disease may result in penetration or fistula formation

FIGURE 19–2. Depth of disease penetration in ulcerative colitis and Crohn's disease.

colon.[13] The inflammatory response may progress in severity, leading to mucosal friability and significant GI bleeding.

Crohn's Disease

As with UC, the immune activation seen in CD involves the release of many proinflammatory cytokines. Cytokines thought to play major roles in CD are derived from T-helper type 1 cells and include interferon-γ, TNF-α, and IL-1, IL-6, IL-8, and IL-12. TNF-α is a major contributor to the inflammatory process seen in CD. Its physiologic effects include activation of macrophages, procoagulant effects in the vascular endothelium, and increases in production of matrix metalloproteinases in mucosal cells.[13–15] Excessive production of both interferon-γ and TNF-α may account for the excessive clinical evidence of granulomatous disease in patients with CD.[11] TNF-α is also thought to induce production of nuclear factor $\kappa\beta$, which stimulates further production of TNF-α and other proinflammatory cytokines.[3,15]

The role of an immune response directed against endogenous bacteria as the initiating factor is more evident in CD, as evidenced by the apparent strong T-helper 1 activation against bacteria seen in animal models of this disease. The role of dietary antigens in the development of CD compared with UC is also another potential initiating factor. Excess ingestion of refined sugars or margarine may be higher in patients who develop CD.[8]

The distribution of inflammation in CD differs from that seen in UC because any part of the entire GI tract may be affected in CD. The small intestine is the site most commonly involved. Within the small intestine, the terminal ileum and cecum are almost always affected. Approximately 20% of patients have isolated colonic involvement, whereas inflammation proximal

to the small intestine is almost never seen without the presence of small or large intestinal disease.[13]

In contrast to UC, the pattern of inflammation in CD is described as discontinuous. Areas of inflammation are intermixed with areas of normal GI mucosa, resulting in characteristic "skip lesions." Superficial **aphthous ulcers** may also develop in the GI mucosa. These ulcers may coalesce into larger linear ulcers, resulting in fissure formation as they increase in depth, giving rise to the characteristic "cobblestone" pattern observed upon examination of the mucosa.

Furthermore, the inflammation may be **transmural**, penetrating to the muscularis or serosal layers of the GI tract (**Fig. 19–2**). The propensity for transmural involvement may lead to serious complications of CD such as **strictures**, **fistulae**, abscesses, and perforation.[13] Although rectal inflammation is typically less common in CD than UC, several types of perianal lesions may be observed in patients with CD. These include skin tags, hemorrhoids, fissures, anal ulcers, abscesses, and fistulae.[14]

CLINICAL PRESENTATION AND DIAGNOSIS

❷ *Differentiation between UC and CD is based on signs and symptoms as well as characteristic endoscopic findings, including the extent, pattern, and depth of inflammation (see Clinical Presentation box).*

Extraintestinal Manifestations and Complications of IBD

❸ *Patients may manifest signs and symptoms of disease in areas outside the GI tract. These extraintestinal manifestations may occur in various body regions.*[5,13] Painful joint complications

Clinical Presentation of IBD

General

- Patients with CD or UC may present with similar symptoms.
- The onset may be insidious and subacute.
- Some patients present with extraintestinal manifestations before GI symptoms occur.
- In approximately 10% of cases it may not be possible to distinguish between UC and CD. These patients are described as having "indeterminate colitis."

Symptoms

- *Ulcerative colitis*: Diarrhea (bloody, watery, or mucopurulent), rectal bleeding, abdominal pain/cramping, weight loss and malnutrition, tenesmus, constipation (with proctitis)
- *Crohn's disease*: Diarrhea (less bloody than UC), rectal bleeding (less than UC), abdominal pain/cramping, weight loss and malnutrition (more common than UC), fatigue/malaise

Signs

- *Ulcerative colitis*: Fever, tachycardia (with severe disease), dehydration, arthritis, hemorrhoids, anal fissures, perirectal abscesses
- *Crohn's disease:* Fever, tachycardia (with severe disease), dehydration, arthritis, abdominal mass and tenderness, perianal fissure or fistula

Laboratory Tests

- *Ulcerative colitis*: Leukocytosis, decreased hematocrit/hemoglobin, elevated erythrocyte sedimentation rate (ESR) or C-reactive protein (CRP), positive test for fecal occult blood, (+) perinuclear antineutrophil cytoplasmic antibodies (pANCA; up to 70% of patients)
- *Crohn's disease*: Leukocytosis, decreased hematocrit/hemoglobin, elevated ESR or CRP, positive test for fecal occult blood, (+) anti–*Saccharomyces cerevisiae* antibodies (up to 50% of patients), hypoalbuminemia with severe disease

associated with IBD include sacroiliitis and ankylosing spondylitis. Ocular involvement with episcleritis, uveitis, or iritis may manifest as blurred vision, eye pain, and photophobia. Associated skin findings include pyoderma gangrenosum (involving papules and vesicles that develop into painful ulcerations) and erythema nodosum (red nodules of varying size typically found on the lower extremities). Nephrolithiasis may also develop at a higher rate in patients with IBD. Oxalate stones are more common in CD, and uric acid–containing stones are more common in UC.[13]

Liver and biliary manifestations of IBD include an increased incidence of gallstone formation in patients with CD and development of sclerosing cholangitis or cholangiocarcinoma in patients with UC. Patients with UC are also at increased risk for development of colorectal cancer and should undergo periodic cancer screening. Ongoing inflammation due to active IBD may induce a hypercoagulable state, resulting in higher rates of both arterial and venous thromboembolism. Likewise, inflammation and recurrent blood loss may result in the development of chronic anemia. Patients with IBD also have higher rates of osteopenia, osteoporosis, and fractures, which are most strongly associated with use of corticosteroids.[16] Patients with IBD are also at risk for developing thromboembolic disease, such as deep vein thrombosis and pulmonary embolism.

A serious complication of UC is toxic megacolon, defined as dilation of the transverse colon of greater than 6 cm (2.4 in.). Patients with toxic megacolon typically manifest systemic signs of severe inflammation such as fever, tachycardia, and abdominal distention.[3,13] Surgical intervention, including colonic resection, may be necessary to acutely manage toxic megacolon.

Formation of strictures, abscesses, fistulae, and obstructions in patients with CD is possible. Patients with CD may develop significant weight loss or nutritional deficiencies secondary to malabsorption of nutrients in the small intestine, or as a consequence of multiple small- or large-bowel resections. Common nutritional deficiencies encountered in IBD include vitamin B_{12}, fat-soluble vitamins, zinc, folate, and iron. Malabsorption in children with CD may contribute to significant reductions in growth and development.

Diagnosis

Because patients often present with nonspecific GI symptoms, initial diagnostic evaluation includes methods to characterize the disease and rule out other potential etiologies. This may include stool cultures to examine for infectious causes of diarrhea.

Endoscopic approaches are typically used and may include colonoscopy, proctosigmoidoscopy, or possibly upper GI endoscopy in patients with suspected CD. Endoscopy is useful for determining the disease distribution, pattern and depth of inflammation, and to obtain mucosal biopsy specimens. Supplemental information from imaging procedures, such as computed tomography, abdominal x-ray, abdominal ultrasound, or intestinal barium studies may provide evidence of complications such as obstruction, abscess, perforation, or colonic dilation.[3]

After the diagnosis is made, the information derived from diagnostic testing and the patient's medical history and symptoms are used to gauge disease severity. The severity of

Patient Encounter 1, Part 1

A 32-year-old white man presents to the emergency department with complaints of crampy abdominal pain and 6 to 7 loose stools per day. He describes intermittent blood in the stool and states that these symptoms have been present for 3 days. He also reports malaise, fatigue, fever, and excessive thirst. He denies any sick contacts. He denies vomiting and has been using nonprescription loperamide for the last 36 hours to treat diarrhea. He consumes alcohol socially and does not use tobacco. He is admitted to the general medicine floor for management of his symptoms.

What other pertinent pieces of history would be beneficial to obtain from this patient regarding potential contributing factors or causes?

How would your classify the severity of this patient's IBD based on the information presented?

What additional information would you obtain prior to recommending drug therapy?

active UC is generally classified as mild, moderate, severe, or fulminant.[1] Mild UC typically involves up to four bloody or watery stools per day without systemic signs of toxicity or elevation of erythrocyte sedimentation rate (ESR). Moderate disease is classified as more than four stools per day with evidence of systemic toxicity. Severe disease is considered more than six stools per day and evidence of anemia, tachycardia, or an elevated ESR or C-reactive protein (CRP). Lastly, fulminant UC may present as more than 10 stools per day with continuous bleeding, signs of systemic toxicity, abdominal distention or tenderness, colonic dilation, or a requirement for blood transfusion.

A similar classification scheme is used to gauge the severity of active CD.[2] Patients with mild to moderate CD are typically ambulatory and have no evidence of dehydration; systemic toxicity; loss of body weight; or abdominal tenderness, mass, or obstruction. Moderate to severe disease is considered in patients who fail to respond to treatment for mild to moderate disease or those with fever, weight loss, abdominal pain or tenderness, vomiting, intestinal obstruction, or significant anemia. Severe to fulminant CD is classified as the presence of persistent symptoms or evidence of systemic toxicity despite outpatient corticosteroid treatment, or the presence of cachexia, rebound tenderness, intestinal obstruction, or abscess.

TREATMENT

Desired Outcomes

Pharmacologic interventions for IBD are designed to target the underlying inflammatory response. Treatment goals involve both management of active disease and prevention of disease relapse. ❹ *Major treatment goals include alleviation of signs and symptoms and suppression of inflammation during acute* episodes and maintenance of remission thereafter. Addressing active IBD in a timely and appropriate manner may prevent major complications such as perforation and may reduce the need for hospitalization or surgical intervention.

Once control of active disease is obtained, treatment regimens are designed to achieve the following long-term goals: (a) maintenance of remission and prevention of disease relapse, (b) improvement in the patient's quality of life, (c) prevention of surgical intervention or hospitalization, (d) management of extraintestinal manifestations, (e) prevention of malnutrition, and (f) prevention of treatment-associated adverse effects.

General Approach to Treatment

❺ *When designing a drug regimen for treatment of IBD, several factors should be considered, including the patient's symptoms; medical history; current medication use; drug allergies; and extent, location, and severity of disease.* A thorough patient history may also help to identify a family history of IBD or potential exacerbating factors, such as tobacco or NSAID use.

Nonpharmacologic Therapy

No specific dietary restrictions are recommended for patients with IBD, but avoidance of high-residue foods in patients with strictures may help to prevent obstruction. Avoidance of excess fat in the diet may be preferred as well. Nutritional strategies in patients with long-standing IBD may include use of vitamin and mineral supplementation. Administration of vitamin B_{12}, folic acid, fat-soluble vitamins, and iron may be needed to prevent or treat deficiencies. In severe cases, enteral or parenteral nutrition may be needed to achieve adequate caloric intake.

Patients with IBD, particularly those with CD, are also at risk for bone loss. This may be a function of malabsorption or an effect of repeated courses of corticosteroids.[16] Risk factors for osteoporosis should be determined, and baseline bone density measurement may be considered.[16] Vitamin D and calcium supplementation should be used in all patients receiving long-term corticosteroids. Oral bisphosphonate therapy may also be considered in patients receiving prolonged courses of corticosteroids or in those with osteopenia or osteoporosis.

Surgical intervention is a potential treatment option in patients with complications such as fistulae or abscesses, or in patients with medically refractory disease. UC is curable with performance of a total colectomy. Patients with UC may opt to have a colectomy to reduce the chance of developing colorectal cancer. Patients with CD may have affected areas of intestine resected. Unfortunately, CD may recur following surgical resection. Repeated surgeries may lead to significant malabsorption of nutrients and drugs consistent with development of short-bowel syndrome.

Pharmacologic Therapy

Several pharmacologic classes are available for the acute treatment and maintenance therapy of IBD. Because there may be differences in the underlying disease process, distribution, and severity between CD and UC, response rates to drugs in the same pharmacologic class may differ between these two diseases. Therefore, initial selection of an appropriate agent for patients with active IBD should be designed to deliver maximum efficacy while minimizing toxicity. Response rates to individual classes of medications for both UC and CD are discussed within the specific treatment section for each disease.

▶ Symptomatic Interventions

Patients with active IBD often have severe abdominal pain and diarrhea. Medications used to manage these types of symptoms may have adverse consequences in patients with active IBD. ❻ *Antidiarrheal medications that reduce GI motility such as loperamide, diphenoxylate/atropine, and codeine should be avoided in patients with active IBD due to the risk of precipitating acute colonic dilation (toxic megacolon).*[13] Drugs with anticholinergic properties, such as hyoscyamine and dicyclomine, are often used to treat intestinal spasm and pain, but these drugs may also reduce GI motility and should generally be avoided in active IBD.

Patients who have had multiple intestinal resections due to CD may have diarrhea related to the inability to reabsorb bile salts. Cholestyramine has been demonstrated to improve diarrheal symptoms in this population.[14] NSAIDs should be avoided for pain management due to their ability to worsen IBD symptoms. Opioid analgesics should be used with caution because they may significantly reduce GI motility.

▶ Aminosalicylates

The aminosalicylates are among the most commonly used drugs for inducing and maintaining remission in patients with IBD (Table 19–1). These drugs are designed to deliver 5-aminosalicylate (5-ASA, mesalamine) to areas of inflammation within the GI tract. Although the mechanism of mesalamine is not fully understood, it appears to have favorable anti-inflammatory effects. The delivery of mesalamine to the affected sites is accomplished by either linking mesalamine to a carrier molecule or altering the formulation to release drug in response to changes in intestinal pH. Topical suppositories and enemas are designed to deliver mesalamine directly to the distal colon and rectum.[7,17-20]

The prototypical aminosalicylate is sulfasalazine, which is composed of mesalamine linked by a diazo bond to the carrier molecule sulfapyridine. This linkage prevents premature absorption of mesalamine in the small intestine. Once sulfasalazine is delivered to the colon, bacterial degradation of the diazo bond frees mesalamine from sulfapyridine. Sulfapyridine is then absorbed and excreted renally while mesalamine acts locally within the GI tract.

Newer mesalamine products utilize nonsulfapyridine methods for drug delivery. Olsalazine uses two mesalamine molecules linked together, whereas balsalazide uses the inert carrier molecule 4-aminobenzoyl-β-alanine. Both drugs use a diazo bond similar to sulfasalazine. Other mesalamine formulations are pH-dependent formulations that release mesalamine at various points throughout the GI tract. The newest mesalamine products include Lialda, a multimatrix (MMX) formulation with a pH-sensitive coat that releases in the terminal ileum, allowing for once-daily dosing.[17] Enteric-coated mesalamine granules that also use a polymer matrix for extended release (Apriso) are also able to be given in a once-daily fashion.

Sulfasalazine is associated with various adverse effects, most of which are thought to be due to the sulfapyridine component. Common adverse effects that may be dose related

Table 19–1

Aminosalicylates for Treatment of IBD

Drug	Trade Names	Formulation	Strengths	Daily Dosage Range (g)	Site of Action
Sulfasalazine	Azulfidine Azulfidine Entabs	Immediate-release or enteric-coated tablets	500 mg	2–6	Colon
	Sulfazine Sulfazine EC	Suspension	250 mg/5mL		
Mesalamine	Rowasa	Enema	4 g/60 mL	4	Distal left colon and rectum
	Asacol Asacol-HD	Delayed-release resin tablet	400 mg, 800 mg	1.6–4.8	Distal ileum and colon
	Canasa	Rectal suppository	1,000 mg	1	Rectum
	Pentasa	Microgranule controlled-release capsule	250 mg 500 mg	2–4 2–4	Small bowel Colon
	Lialda	MMX formulated pH-dependent polymer film coated tablet	1.2 g	1.2–4.8	Terminal ileum and colon
	Apriso	Enteric-coated granules in polymer matrix	375 mg	1.5	Colon
Olsalazine	Dipentum	Delayed-release capsule	250 mg	1–3	Colon
Balsalazide	Colazal	Delayed-release capsule	750 mg	2–6.75	Colon

MMX, multimatrix.

include headache, dyspepsia, nausea, vomiting, and fatigue.[20-22] Idiosyncratic effects include bone marrow suppression, reduction in sperm counts in males, hepatitis, and pulmonitis. Hypersensitivity reactions may occur in patients allergic to sulfonamide-containing medications. Patients who are genetically slow acetylators may be more prone to adverse effects.

The use of nonsulfapyridine-based aminosalicylates has led to greater tolerability. Although the adverse effects are similar to those of sulfasalazine, they occur at a much lower rate. Olsalazine, in particular, is associated with a higher incidence of secretory diarrhea. These agents can also be used safely in patients with a reported sulfonamide allergy. They are more expensive than sulfasalazine products that are available generically.

▶ Corticosteroids

Corticosteroids have potent anti-inflammatory properties and are used in active IBD to suppress inflammation rapidly. They may be administered systemically or delivered locally to the site of action by altering the drug formulation (Table 19–2). Because these drugs usually improve symptoms and disease severity rapidly, they should be restricted to short-term management of active disease. Long-term use of systemic corticosteroids is associated with significant adverse effects, including cataracts, skin atrophy, hypertension, hyperglycemia, adrenal suppression, osteoporosis, increased risk of infection, and delayed growth in children, among others.[20-22]

Budesonide is a high-potency glucocorticoid used in CD that has low systemic bioavailability when administered orally.[23] The formulation releases budesonide in the terminal ileum for treatment of disease involving the ileum or ascending colon. Due to its reduced bioavailability, budesonide may prevent some long-term adverse effects in patients who have steroid-dependent IBD.[22,23]

▶ Immunosuppressants

Agents targeting the excessive immune response or cytokines involved in IBD are potential treatment options (Table 19–3). Azathioprine and its active metabolite 6-mercaptopurine (6-MP) are inhibitors of purine biosynthesis and reduce IBD-associated GI inflammation. They are most useful for maintaining remission of IBD or reducing the need for long-term use of corticosteroids.[22,24] Use in active disease is limited by their slow onset of action, which may be as long as 3 to 12 months. Adverse effects associated with azathioprine and 6-MP include hypersensitivity reactions resulting in pancreatitis, fever, rash, hepatitis, and leukopenia.[21,22,24] Patients should be tested for activity of thiopurine methyltransferase (TPMT), the major enzyme responsible for metabolism of azathioprine prior to use. Deficiency or reduced activity of TPMT may result in toxicity from azathioprine and 6-MP.

Methotrexate is a folate antagonist used primarily for maintaining remission of CD. It may be administered orally, subcutaneously, or IV and may result in a steroid-sparing effect in patients with steroid-dependent disease.[6,22]

Table 19–2
Corticosteroids for Treatment of IBD

Drug	Trade Names	Daily Dose
Prednisone	Generic	20–60 mg orally
Prednisolone	Generic	20–60 mg orally
Budesonide	Entocort EC	Induction: 9 mg orally Maintenance: 6 mg orally
Methylprednisolone	Medrol (orally) Solu-Medrol (IV)	15–60 mg orally or IV
Hydrocortisone	Solu-Cortef	300 mg IV in three divided doses
	Cortenema	100 mg rectally at bedtime
	Cortifoam	90 mg rectally once or twice daily
	Anucort-HC 25 mg	25–50 mg rectally twice daily
	Proctocort 30 mg	25–50 mg rectally twice daily

Table 19–3
Immunosuppressant and Biologic Agents for Treatment of IBD

Drug	Trade Name(s)	Dose
Azathioprine	Imuran, Azasan	1.5–2.5 mg/kg/day orally
6-Mercaptopurine	Purinethol	1.5–2.5 mg/kg/day orally
Methotrexate	Trexall	15–25 mg weekly (IM/SC/orally)
Cyclosporine	Sandimmune	4 mg/kg/day IV continuous infusion
Infliximab	Remicade	Induction: 5 mg/kg IV at 0, 2, and 6 weeks; 10 mg/kg per dose IV for nonresponders Maintenance: 5 mg/kg IV every 8 weeks
Adalimumab	Humira	Induction: 160 mg SC day 1 (given as four 40-mg injections in 1 day or as two 40-mg injections per day for 2 consecutive days), then 80 mg SC 2 weeks later (day 15) Maintenance: 40 mg SC every other week, starting on day 29 of therapy
Certolizumab	Cimzia	Induction: 400 mg SC initially, then 400 mg SC at 2 and 4 weeks Maintenance: 400 mg SC every 4 weeks if initial response
Natalizumab	Tysabri	Induction/maintenance: 300 mg IV every 4 weeks

IM, intramuscular; PEG, polyethylene glycol.

Long-term methotrexate use may result in serious adverse effects, including hepatotoxicity, pulmonary fibrosis, and bone marrow suppression.

Cyclosporine is a cyclic polypeptide immunosuppressant typically used to prevent organ rejection in transplant patients. Its use is restricted to patients with fulminant or refractory symptoms in patients with active IBD. Significant toxicities associated with cyclosporine are nephrotoxicity, risk of infection, seizures, hypertension, and liver function test abnormalities.[1,22]

▶ Biologic Agents

Several biologic agents targeting TNF-α are used for the treatment of IBD (Table 19–3). Reduction in TNF-α activity is associated with improvement in the underlying inflammatory process. Infliximab is the prototypical agent and is used in both UC and CD, whereas the other agents are approved for use only in CD. Due to its chimeric structure (i.e., 75% human, 25% mouse), antibodies to infliximab may develop, resulting in loss of efficacy over time. Newer biologic agents are humanized and have a lower propensity for antibody development.[25]

Disadvantages of anti-TNF biologic therapy include the need for parenteral administration, significant drug cost, and the potential for serious adverse effects. Adverse effects may include infusion-related reactions such as fever, chest pain, hypotension, and dyspnea. Antibodies may develop to infliximab over time that may reduce its efficacy and predispose patients to development of infusion-related adverse effects. All of the TNF-α inhibitors have also been associated with reactivation of serious infections, particularly intracellular pathogens such as tuberculosis, as well as hepatitis B.[15,21] These agents should not be used in patients with current infections, and patients should be screened for latent tuberculosis and viral hepatitis prior to initiating therapy. Exacerbation of heart failure is also a potential adverse effect, and biologic agents should be avoided in patients with advanced or decompensated heart failure.[15,20,21] The anti-TNF-α biologics also carry a risk of developing lymphoma, including a rare form known as hepatosplenic T-cell lymphoma. The risk appears to be highest in younger male patients and those using concomitant azathioprine or 6-MP. Therefore, this potential risk should be considered in patients who meet these criteria.

Natalizumab is a humanized monoclonal antibody that antagonizes integrin heterodimers, prevents α_4-mediated leukocyte adhesion to adhesion molecules, and prevents migration across the endothelium.[26] It has been associated with development of progressive multifocal leukoencephalopathy, and its use is restricted to patients with CD who have failed other

---

Patient Encounter 1, Part 2: Medical History and Physical Examination

PMH: Type 1 diabetes, appendectomy at age 25, seasonal allergies

FH: Both parents alive; father has history of MI and type 2 DM. Mother has a history of hypothyroidism; brother with type 1 DM

SH: Works as an electrical engineer; social alcohol use and no tobacco use

Allergies: Penicillin (rash)

Meds: Loperamide orally as needed, insulin glargine 25 units at bedtime; insulin aspart with meals based on correction factor, fluticasone nasal spray once daily, cetirizine 10 mg as needed

ROS: (+) Diarrhea, abdominal pain, fatigue, fever, thirst

PE:

VS: BP 120/75 mm Hg, P 110 bpm, RR 17/min, T 38.3°C (100.9°F)

CV: Tachycardia with normal rhythm. No murmurs, rubs, or gallops

HEENT: Dry mucous membranes

Skin: Dry with evidence of tenting

Abd: Soft, nondistended, moderate diffuse tenderness, (+) bowel sounds, (–) hepatosplenomegaly, (–) masses, heme (+) stool

MS: 5/5 strength in upper and lower extremities; normal ROM

Labs: Sodium 132 mEq/L (132 mmol/L), potassium 2.8 mEq/L (2.8 mmol/L), chloride 99 mEq/L (99 mmol/L), bicarbonate 28 mEq/L (28 mmol/L), BUN 27 mg/dL (9.6 mmol/L), serum creatinine 1.4 mg/dL (124 μmol/L), serum glucose 180 mg/dL (10.0 mmol/L) albumin 4.2 g/dL (42 g/L), ALT 25 IU/L (0.42 μkat/L), AST 23 IU/L (0.38 μkat/L), ESR 110 mm/h, CRP 0.9 mg/dL (9 mg/L), A1C 7.8% (0.078; 62 mmol/mol hemoglobin), hemoglobin 10 g/dL (100 g/L or 6.2 mmol/L), hematocrit 31%, (0.31), WBC count 17.0 × 10³/mm³ (17.0 × 10⁹/L), platelets 420 × 10³/mm³ (420 × 10⁹/L), Urinalysis: 2+ protein; (–) ketones; SG = 1.025, (–) bacteria; (–) WBCs

Abdominal x-ray: (–) obstruction, free-air, or colonic dilation

Colonoscopy: Diffuse superficial inflammation extending to the hepatic flexure with evidence of recent bleeding, (–) polyps or strictures, biopsy taken

Path: Evidence of crypt abscesses and PMN infiltration

How is this additional information helpful in determining disease type and severity?

What factors should you consider in choosing appropriate therapy for this patient?

What treatment options would you consider at this time?

therapies. Natalizumab should not be used concomitantly with immunosuppressants or TNF-α inhibitors, and use requires enrollment in the manufacturer's prescribing program.

▶ Other Agents

Antibiotics have been studied based on the rationale that they may interrupt the inflammatory response directed against endogenous bacterial flora. Metronidazole and ciprofloxacin have been the two most widely studied agents.[1,2,27] Metronidazole may benefit some patients with pouchitis (inflammation of surgically created intestinal pouches) and patients with CD who have had ileal resection or have perianal fistulas. Ciprofloxacin has shown some efficacy in refractory active CD. Both drugs may cause diarrhea, and long-term use of metronidazole is associated with the development of peripheral neuropathy.

Because smoking is associated with reduced symptoms of UC, nicotine has been studied as a potential treatment option. However, results have been mixed; transdermal nicotine may result in some improvement in mild to moderate UC symptoms and may be more effective in patients who are ex-smokers.[1,28] Daily doses between 15 and 25 mg appear to be most effective.

Probiotics such as *Lactobacillus acidophilus* or *Bifidobacterium* have been used with the rationale that modification of the host flora may alter the inflammatory response. There are minimal data to support use of probiotics in CD.[2] In patients with UC, the probiotic preparation VSL#3 demonstrated efficacy in reducing recurrence of pouchitis in patients with ileal pouch anal anastomosis and may prevent relapse in mild to moderate disease.[1,29]

Treatment of UC

Drug and dosing guidelines based on disease severity and location are presented in Table 19–4.

▶ Mild to Moderate Active UC

❼ *Treatment of acute episodes of UC is dictated by the severity and extent of disease, and first-line therapy of mild to moderate disease involves oral or topical aminosalicylate*

Table 19–4

Treatment Recommendations for UC

Disease Severity and Location	Active Disease	Maintenance of Remission
Mild Disease		
Proctitis	Mesalamine suppository 1 g rectally daily	May reduce suppository frequency to 1 g 3 times/week
Left-sided disease	Mesalamine enema 1 g rectally daily, *or* Mesalamine 2.4–4.8 g/day or sulfasalazine 4–6 g/day orally	May reduce enema frequency to 1 g every other day, *or* taper to mesalamine 1.6–2.4 g/day or sulfasalazine 2–4 g/day orally
Extensive disease	Mesalamine 2.4–4.8 g/day or sulfasalazine 4–6 g/day orally	Taper to mesalamine 1.6–2.4 g/day or sulfasalazine 2–4 g/day orally
Moderate Disease		
Proctitis	Mesalamine suppository 1 g rectally daily; If no response to mesalamine: • Prednisone 40–60 mg/day orally	May reduce suppository frequency to 1 g 3 times/week; taper prednisone as soon as possible; Consider adding azathioprine or 6-MP 1.5–2.5 mg/kg/day orally
Left-sided disease	Mesalamine enema 1 g rectally at bedtime daily, *or* mesalamine 2.4–4.8 g/day or sulfasalazine 4–6 g/day orally May combine enema and oral therapies	May reduce enema frequency to 1 g 3 times/week if symptoms permit May reduce dose of oral agents if symptoms permit; consider adding azathioprine or 6-MP 1.5–2.5 mg/kg/day orally
Extensive disease	Mesalamine 2.4–4.8 g/day or sulfasalazine 4–6 g/day orally; If no response to mesalamine or sulfasalazine: • Prednisone 40–60 mg/day orally; *or* • Infliximab 5 mg/kg IV at weeks 0, 2, and 6	Taper mesalamine to 1.6–2.4 g/day or sulfasalazine 2–4 g/day orally; If prednisone or infliximab were required: • Taper prednisone as soon as possible; • Give infliximab 5 mg/kg IV every 8 weeks Consider adding azathioprine or 6-MP 1.5–2.5 mg/kg/day orally
Severe or Fulminant Disease	Hydrocortisone 300 mg IV daily (or equivalent) × 7 days, *or* Infliximab 5 mg/kg IV at weeks 0, 2, and 6 If no response to IV corticosteroids or infliximab: • Cyclosporine 4 mg/kg/day IV	Change to oral corticosteroid and taper as soon as possible Restart oral mesalamine or sulfasalazine May continue infliximab at maintenance doses of 5 mg/kg every 8 weeks

6-MP, 6-mercaptopurine.

derivatives. Topical suppositories and retention enemas are preferred for active distal UC (left-sided disease and proctitis) because they deliver mesalamine directly to the site of inflammation. Topical mesalamine is superior to both topical corticosteroids and oral aminosalicylates for inducing remission in active mild to moderate UC.[1,30–33] Enemas are appropriate for patients with left-sided disease because the medication will reach the splenic flexure. Suppositories deliver mesalamine up to approximately 20 cm and are most appropriate for treating proctitis.[6,7,30]

Topical mesalamine products provide a more rapid response than oral preparations. Improvement in symptoms may be seen in as little as 2 days, but up to 4 weeks of treatment may be necessary for maximal response. Oral and topical mesalamine preparations may be used together to provide maximal effect. Oral mesalamine may also be used for patients who are unwilling or unable to use topical preparations.[30–32]

Topical corticosteroids are typically reserved for patients who do not respond to topical mesalamine.[1,22] Patients should be properly educated regarding appropriate use of topical products. This includes proper administration and adequate retention of topical mesalamine products in order to maximize efficacy.

For patients with more extensive disease extending proximal to the splenic flexure, oral sulfasalazine or any of the newer oral mesalamine products is considered first-line therapy.[1,6] Doses should provide 4 to 6 g of sulfasalazine or 2.4 g of mesalamine or equvalent.[6] Although little differences in efficacy exist between mesalamine products, sulfasalazine and olsalazine have a higher incidence of adverse effects.[17] Use of the once-daily formulations of mesalamine may improve patient adherence.[17] Induction of remission may require 4 to 8 weeks of therapy at appropriate treatment doses.

Oral corticosteroids may be used for patients who are unresponsive to sulfasalazine or mesalamine. Prednisone doses of 40 to 60 mg/day (or equivalent) are recommended.[1,22] Azathioprine or 6-MP is used for patients unresponsive to corticosteroids or those who become steroid dependent. Infliximab 5 mg/kg may also be used for patients who are unresponsive to conventional oral therapies and may reduce the need for colectomy after 3 months of treatment. Infliximab may also be used in patients who are refractory to or dependent on corticosteroids.[33]

▶ Severe or Fulminant UC

Patients with severe UC symptoms require hospitalization for management of their disease. If the patient is unresponsive to oral or topical mesalamine and oral corticosteroids, a course of IV corticosteroids should be initiated.[1] Hydrocortisone 300 mg/day given in three divided doses or methylprednisolone 60 mg daily for 7 to 10 days are the preferred therapies.[1,22]

Infliximab 5 mg/kg is also an option for severe UC. Cyclosporine 2 to 4 mg/kg/day given as a continuous IV infusion should be reserved for patients unresponsive to 7 to 10 days of IV corticosteroid therapy.

Patients with fulminant disease are treated similarly, although infliximab is not indicated for this population.

Patients with fulminant UC should be assessed for signs of significant systemic toxicity or colonic dilation, which may require earlier surgical intervention.

▶ Maintenance of Remission in UC

Unfortunately, up to 50% of patients receiving oral therapies and up to 70% of untreated patients relapse within 1 year after achieving remission.[34] For this reason, patients may require maintenance drug therapy indefinitely to preserve remission.

❽ *Maintenance of remission of UC may be achieved with oral or topical aminosalicylates.* In patients with proctitis, mesalamine suppositories 1 g daily may prevent relapse in up to 90% of patients.[1,7,30] Mesalamine enemas are appropriate for left-sided disease and may often be dosed two to three times weekly. Oral mesalamine at lower doses (e.g., 1.2 to 1.6 g/day) may be combined with topical therapies to maintain remission. Topical or oral corticosteroids are not effective for maintaining remission of distal UC and should be avoided.

Oral sulfasalazine or mesalamine is effective in maintaining remission in patients with more extensive disease.[1,6] Lower daily doses (e.g., 2 to 4 g sulfasalazine or 2 to 2.4 g mesalamine) may be used for disease maintenance. As with distal UC, oral corticosteroids are not effective for maintaining remission and should be avoided due to the high incidence of adverse effects.

❽ *Immunosuppressants such as azathioprine, 6-MP, or infliximab can be used for unresponsive patients or those who develop corticosteroid dependency.* Remission may be maintained in up to 58% of patients after 5 years of treatment.[1,6,24] Intermittent infliximab dosing (5 mg/kg IV every 8 weeks) may be used to maintain disease remission and reduce the need for corticosteroids in patients with

---

Patient Encounter 2

A 47-year-old African American woman presents to the clinic for follow-up management of CD. She has disease in the jejunum, ileum, and ascending colon that was diagnosed 12 months ago. She takes Pentasa 1,000 mg four times per day. She reports 2–3 loose stools/day on 5–6 days per week with intermittent blood and abdominal pain. This is interfering with her daily activities and ability to work and socialize. Her medical history is also significant for GERD and dyslipidemia, for which she takes omeprazole and atorvastatin. She reports an allergy to shellfish (hives).

How would you assess this patient's disease control and current drug therapy?

What treatment options are available?

How would you educate this patient on her drug therapy for IBD, including any changes you would consider making to her current therapy?

CHAPTER 19 | INFLAMMATORY BOWEL DISEASE

Table 19–5		
Treatment Recommendations for CD		
Disease Location and Severity	**Active Disease**	**Maintenance of Remission**
Mild Disease		
Ileal or ileocolonic	Mesalamine 3.2–4.8 g/day or sulfasalazine 4–6 g/day orally	Taper mesalamine 1.6–2.4 g/day or sulfasalazine 2–4 g/day orally
Ileal ± ascending colon	Budesonide 9 mg daily orally for up to 8 weeks	Taper budesonide to 6 mg daily for up to 3 months
Perianal	Mesalamine 2.4–4.8 g/day or sulfasalazine 4–6 g/day orally May add metronidazole 10–20 mg/kg/day or ciprofloxacin 1 g daily	Taper mesalamine to 1.6–2.4 g/day or sulfasalazine 2–4 g/day orally
Moderate Disease	Same treatment as for mild disease but may consider: • Infliximab *or* adalimumab *or* certolizumab (see Table 19–3 for dosage regimens) *or* • Prednisone 40–60 mg/day orally, *or* • Budesonide 9 mg/day orally for up to 8 weeks • Consider natalizumab if no response to prior therapies	Continue aminosalicylate at maintenance dose; If loss of response to infliximab, consider adalimumab Taper prednisone as soon as possible; Taper budesonide to 6 mg daily for 3 months Consider adding azathioprine or 6-MP 1.5–2.5 mg/kg/day orally or methotrexate 12.5–25 mg orally or IM/SC once weekly
	If fistulizing disease, consider: • Infliximab, adalimumab, or certolizumab pegol	Consider natalizumab if no response to previous therapies
Severe or Fulminant Disease	Hydrocortisone 300 mg IV daily (or equivalent) × 7 days, *or* Infliximab (severe or fistulizing disease) 5 mg/kg IV at 0, 2, and 6 weeks • Adalimumab or certolizumab *or* • Consider natalizumab if no response to prior therapies Consider cyclosporine 4 mg/kg/day for refractory disease	Taper corticosteroid as soon as possible May continue infliximab, adalimumab, certolizumab, or natalizumab (see Table 19–3 for dosage regimens) Consider adding azathioprine or 6-MP 1.5–2.5 mg/kg/day orally or methotrexate 12.5–25 mg orally or IM/SC weekly

6-MP, 6-mercaptopurine; IM, intramuscular; SC, subcutaneous.

moderate to severe UC. Colectomy is an option for patients with progressive disease who cannot be maintained on drug therapy alone.

▶ Treatment of CD

Drug and dosing guidelines based on disease severity and location are presented in Table 19–5.

▶ Mild to Moderate Active CD

9 *Induction of remission of mild to moderate active CD may be accomplished with oral budesonide or possibly aminosalicylates.* Budesonide 9 mg orally once daily for up to 8 weeks may be used for mild to moderate active CD in patients with involvement of the terminal ileum or ascending colon, with success expected in 50% to 69% of patients.[6,22,23,35] Because the formulation releases budesonide in the terminal ileum, it is not effective in reaching sites distal to the ascending colon.[24,36] Conventional oral corticosteroids such as prednisone and methylprednisolone may also be used and may be slightly more effective than budesonide for inducing remission, but they carry a higher risk of adverse effects.[6]

Mesalamine products have demonstrated minimal efficacy but may be tried in patients with ileal, ileocolonic, or colonic CD.[2,6,36] These drugs are typically better tolerated

than sulfasalazine at full treatment doses. Induction of remission may require up to 16 weeks of treatment at full doses.[35] Sulfasalazine 4 to 6 g/day is most effective for patients with active colonic or ileocolonic involvement, with response rates of approximately 50%.[2,5,35]

Metronidazole or ciprofloxacin can be used in patients who do not respond to budesonide or oral aminosalicylates. Response rates of up to 50% are reported, but data are conflicting, and these agents should generally not be considered first-line therapy.[2,6,27]

▶ Moderate to Severe Active CD

9 *Patients with moderate to severe active CD may be treated with oral corticosteroids (e.g., prednisone 40 to 60 mg daily) or budesonide (moderate activity), or anti-TNF antibody therapies (infliximab, adalimumab, or certolizumab pegol) (moderate to severe activity).*[2,6] Budesonide 9 mg orally once daily may be used for moderately active CD involving the terminal ileum or ascending colon. All anti-TNF-α therapies are effective in inducing closure and cessation of drainage in patients with fistulae.[6]

Infliximab is an effective alternative to corticosteroid therapy for patients with moderate to severe CD including patients with fistulizing or perianal disease.[14,23,35] The recommended regimen for induction of remission is infliximab 5 mg/kg at weeks 0, 2, and 6; it is effective in inducing remission in approximately 80% of patients at 8 weeks. Complete closure of existing enterocutaneous fistulae occurs in approximately 50% of patients.[14,23,35]

Adalimumab is effective in moderate to severe active CD and used preferably in patients with diminished response to infliximab. The approved adult dose of 160 mg on day 1, 80 mg at 2 weeks, and 40 mg at day 29 resulted in a remission rate of 36% at 4 weeks.[6,16]

Certolizumab is also effective, with a dose of 400 mg subcutaneously initially, and then at 2 and 4 weeks resulting in a clinical response rate of 37% at 6 weeks.[15,22] Natalizumab 300 mg IV every 4 weeks has been reported to induce remission in up to 37% of patients at 10 weeks, which was similar to placebo.[6,16,32]

For patients with simple perianal fistulae, antibiotics (metronidazole or ciprofloxacin), infliximab, adalimumab, and certolizumab pegol are appropriate treatment options. Complex perianal fistulae are those associated with multiple openings, abscess, stricture, or penetration into the vaginal wall. These types of perianal fistulae may require surgical intervention but may also be amenable to treatment with antibiotics, infliximab, azathioprine, or 6-MP.[2,6,16,15,22]

▶ *Severe to Fulminant Active CD*

Most patients with severe to fulminant CD require hospitalization for appropriate treatment. Patients should be assessed for possible surgical intervention if abdominal distention, masses, abscess, or obstruction are present. Daily IV doses of corticosteroids equivalent to prednisone 40 to 60 mg are recommended as initial therapy to rapidly suppress severe inflammation.

If there are no contraindications, infliximab 5 mg/kg followed by 5 mg/kg at weeks 2 and 6 may be used for severe active CD. There is no evidence that infliximab is either safe or effective for fulminant disease. Adalimumab or certolizumab are also options for patients with severe CD, particularly those who have lost response to infliximab or those who are nonresponsive to traditional therapies. Natalizumab can be used for severe CD but is reserved for patients failing other available therapies, including TNF-α inhibitors.

Adjunctive therapy with fluid and electrolyte replacement should be initiated. Nutritional support with enteral or parenteral nutrition may be indicated for patients unable to eat for more than 5 to 7 days.[2] Some evidence suggests that enteral nutrition provides anti-inflammatory effects in patients with active CD.[36,37]

Limited evidence indicates that cyclosporine, or possibly tacrolimus, may be effective as salvage therapy for patients who fail IV corticosteroid therapy.[2,6,22] Surgical intervention may ultimately be necessary for medically refractory disease.

▶ *Maintenance of Remission in CD*

Patients with CD are at high risk for disease relapse after induction of remission. Within 2 years, up to 80% of patients experience a relapse; therefore, most patients should be evaluated for indefinite maintenance therapy.

🔟 Maintenance of remission of CD may be achieved with immunosuppressants (azathioprine, 6-MP, or methotrexate), biologic agents (infliximab, adalimumab, certolizumab pegol, or natalizumab), and less frequently with oral or topical aminosalicylate derivatives.

In contrast to their use in UC, sulfasalazine and the newer aminosalicylates are marginally effective in preventing CD relapse in patients with medically induced remission, with success rates of only 10% to 20% at 1 year.[6,34] Despite not being recommended as first-line therapy, aminosalicylates are routinely used to maintain remission of CD. Some evidence suggests that aminosalicylates may prevent or delay disease recurrence in patients with surgically induced remisson.[2,34]

Several other treatment options exist for maintaining remission that may also reduce the need for corticosteroids. Infliximab has been shown to maintain remission in 46% of patients compared with 23% of those treated with placebo over a 54-week period.[15,22,32] Adalimumab 40 mg subcutaneously given every other week has been shown to maintain remission in up to 36% of patients at 56 weeks of treatment.[15,38] Certolizumab 400 mg IV every 4 weeks has also been effective in maintaining remission in up to 61% of patients at 26 weeks.[15,32] Patients with a baseline CRP of greater than 1 mg/dL (10 mg/L) may have a more favorable response. Natalizumab may also be used for maintenance in patients unresponsive to anti-TNF-α agents. Up to 40% of patients may maintain remission at 15 months.[15,32]

Azathioprine and 6-MP in oral doses up to 2.5 mg/kg/day have been shown to maintain remission in 45% of patients for up to 5 years.[2,6,22,24,29] These drugs may be used to prevent disease recurrence after surgically induced remission. Methotrexate in doses ranging from 12.5 to 25 mg once weekly given orally, intramuscularly, or subcutaneously has resulted in remission rates of up to 52% at 3 years.[6,29,34] Corticosteroids, although effective for inducing remission rapidly, are not effective for maintenance therapy and are associated with significant adverse effects with long-term use. Therefore, systemic or topical corticosteroids should not be used for maintaining remission in patients with IBD. Unfortunately up to 50% of patients treated acutely with corticosteroids become dependent on them to prevent symptoms.[2]

In place of conventional corticosteroids, budesonide 6 mg orally once daily may be used for up to 3 months after remission induction for mild to moderate CD or in patients dependent on corticosteroids, although budesonide's efficacy is questionable when extended to this duration.[6]

Treatment of IBD in Special Populations (Table 19–6)

▶ *Elderly Patients*

Approximately 8% to 20% of patients with UC and 7% to 26% of patients with CD are elderly at initial diagnosis.[38] In general, IBD presents similarly in elderly patients compared with younger individuals. Elderly patients may have more comorbid diseases, some of which may make the diagnosis of IBD more difficult. Such conditions include ischemic colitis,

Table 19–6

Dosing Considerations of IBD Therapies in Special Populations

Therapy	Pediatric Patients	Elderly Patients	Pregnancy[44–46]
Sulfasalazine	Age more than 2 years: 40–60 mg/kg/day in 3–6 divided doses; 30 mg/kg/day in 3–6 divided doses for maintenance	No specific changes	Category B Administer folic acid 2 mg daily during prenatal period and pregnancy
Mesalamine	No specific changes; Balsalazide indicated for age more than 5 years	No specific changes	Category B (Olsalazine Category C) Generally considered safe and effective
Corticosteroids	No specific changes	No specific changes Elderly patients at high risk for osteoporosis	Older agents not rated Budesonide category C Generally considered safe and effective
TNF-α inhibitors	Infliximab indicated for pediatric patients: 5 mg/kg at 0, 2, and 6 weeks, then every 8 weeks Adalimumab has been used at doses of 80 mg SC day 0, then 40 mg SC every other week	Avoid in patients with heart failure Elderly patients at higher risk for infections	Category B Pregnancy registry for adalimumab via manufacturer
Natalizumab	Dose of 3 mg/kg IV at 0, 4, and 8 weeks reported; data are lacking in children	No specific changes	Category C Report pregnancy to manufacturer's pregnancy registry
Azathioprine 6-Mercaptopurine	1.5–2 mg/kg/day to start	No specific changes	Category D Accepted as safe Avoid initiating during pregnancy, but continue if patient is already receiving when pregnant
Methotrexate	17 mg/m² orally/SC/IM	No specific changes	Category X Contraindicated
Cyclosporine	No specific changes	No specific changes	Category C Use only in refractory patients
Metronidazole	30–50 mg/kg/day divided every 6 hours	No specific changes	Category B Use short courses if possible
Ciprofloxacin	Avoid use	Adjust dose for CrCl less than 50 mL/min (0.83 mL/s)	Category C Consider other alternatives

CrCl, creatinine clearance; IM, intramuscular; SC, subcutaneously.

diverticular disease, and microscopic colitis. Increased age is also associated with a higher incidence of adenomatous polyps, but the onset of IBD at an advanced age does not appear to increase the risk of developing colorectal cancer. Elderly patients may also use more medications, particularly NSAIDs, which may induce or exacerbate colitis.

Treatment of elderly patients with IBD is similar to that for younger patients, but special consideration should be given to some of the medications used. Corticosteroids may worsen diabetes, hypertension, heart failure, or osteoporosis. The TNF-α inhibitors should be used cautiously in patients with heart failure and should be avoided in New York Heart Association class III or IV disease. Lastly, elderly patients requiring major surgical interventions may be at higher risk for surgical complications or may not meet eligibility criteria for surgery because of comorbid conditions, age-related organ dysfunction, or reduced functional status.

► Children and Adolescents

CD occurs in approximately 4.56 per 100,000 pediatric patients, and UC occurs in about 2.14 cases per 100,000.[39]

A major issue in children with IBD is the risk of growth failure secondary to inadequate nutritional intake and corticosteroid therapy. Failure to thrive may be an initial presentation of IBD in this population. Aggressive nutritional interventions may be required to facilitate adequate caloric intake. Chronic corticosteroid therapy may also be associated with reductions in growth and bone demineralization. Exploration of using lower doses in patients who are corticosteroid dependent may result in fewer problems with altered height velocity.[40] Guidelines for management of acute severe UC in children have recently been published and favor use of methylprednisolone as first-line therapy, with calcineurin inhibitors or infliximab used for unresponsive patients.[41]

The aminosalicylates, azathioprine, 6-MP, and infliximab are all viable options for treatment and maintenance of IBD in pediatric patients. Infliximab is approved for use in the United States for patients 6 to 17 years of age with moderate to severe active CD. Use of immunosuppressive therapy or infliximab may help reduce overall corticosteroid exposure. Adalimumab is approved for use in patients 4 years of age or older with juvenile rheumatoid arthritis. Limited recent information suggests that adalimumab may be effective in pediatric patients with CD.[42,43] Certolizumab and natalizumab are only FDA approved for use in adult patients with IBD; data in children are limited.[44]

▶ *Pregnant Women*

Inducing and maintaining remission of IBD prior to conception is the optimal approach in women planning to become pregnant. Active IBD may result in prematurity and low birth weight. Thus pregnant women with IBD should be monitored closely, particularly during the third trimester.[45–47]

Patients do not need to discontinue drug therapy for IBD once they become pregnant, but certain adjustments may be required.[45–47] The aminosalicylates are considered safe to use in pregnancy, but sulfasalazine is associated with folate malabsorption. Because pregnancy results in a higher folate requirement, pregnant patients treated with sulfasalazine should be supplemented with folic acid 1 mg orally twice daily.[45]

As with nonpregnant patients, corticosteroids may be used for treatment of active disease but not for maintenance of remission. Generally, corticosteroids confer no additional risk on the mother or fetus and are generally well tolerated. Both azathioprine and 6-MP have been used successfully in pregnant patients and appear to carry minimal risk, despite carrying an FDA pregnancy category D rating.[46] Infliximab, adalimumab, and certolizumab are all FDA category B drugs and appear to carry minimal risk in pregnant patients.[47] Little is known about excretion of these drugs in breast milk, so benefit versus risk should be considered if they are used during nursing. Natalizumab is a pregnancy category C drug and should be used only when other therapies have been exhausted.

Methotrexate is a known abortifacient and carries an FDA category X pregnancy rating. Thus, it is contraindicated during pregnancy. Metronidazole carries a theoretical risk of mutagenicity in humans, but short courses are safe during pregnancy. Prolonged use of metronidazole should be avoided in pregnant patients due to lack of safety data supporting its use.[45] Ciprofloxacin should be avoided in pregnant women. First-trimester use of the antidiarrheal diphenoxylate has been associated with fetal malformations and should be avoided.

Patient Care and Monitoring

1. Evaluate the patient's symptoms to determine if they are consistent with UC or CD. Determine whether the patient has evidence of extraintestinal manifestations or GI complications related to IBD. Identify any psychosocial problems related to the presence of IBD.

2. If the patient is presenting with an exacerbation of preexisting IBD, determine if the symptoms are similar in type and severity to the patient's previous episodes.

3. Assess the patient's medical history for pertinent drug allergies, tobacco use, and current prescription and nonprescription drug therapies. Determine if any of the medications could exacerbate IBD. If applicable, inquire about adherence or recent changes to the patient's current IBD drug regimen.

4. Use available diagnostic laboratory, endoscopic, and imaging data to gauge the extent and severity of the patient's disease.

5. Construct a drug treatment plan based on the disease severity and location. Identify potential contraindications or financial barriers to drug therapy. Inquire if the patient has an aversion to or inability to properly use certain drug formulations that you may wish to recommend, such as topical (rectal) products.

6. Assess whether the patient will require maintenance therapy after remission induction. If so, identify the treatment duration. Decide when the patient should receive follow-up care.

7. Outline parameters to evaluate the efficacy and toxicity of the drug regimen you are recommending.

Determine whether the patient will need preventive drug therapy or diagnostic testing to prevent or screen for potential drug-related toxicities.

8. Educate the patient on proper use of drug therapy, including when to expect symptom improvement after initiation of treatment and which signs or symptoms to report that might be related to adverse drug effects.

9. Provide patient education on the proper use of aminosalicylate medications and assess regularly for adherence. Include the following:

   • Proper use of suppositories and enemas

   • The appropriate number of tablets or capsules to take per day. Reinforce that tablets and capsules are delayed release and should not be crushed, opened, or chewed.

   • Appropriate dose titration, particularly with oral sulfasalazine

   • The time frame the patient can expect improvement based on drug dose and disease severity

   • Signs or symptoms of potential adverse effects

10. Once remission is achieved, evaluate the patient's drug regimen to determine if dose reductions or changes in frequency of administration are required. Reinforce the need for adherence to drug therapy in order to maximize effectiveness.

11. Educate patients about their disease state. Refer patients to available support groups or IBD organizational resources if they are having difficulty in coping with their disease.

OUTCOME EVALUATION

- Monitor for improvement of symptoms in patients with active IBD, such as reduction in the number of daily stools, abdominal pain, fever, and heart rate.

- For patients in remission, assure that proper maintenance doses of medications are used and educate the patient to seek medical attention if symptoms recur or worsen.

- Evaluate patients receiving systemic corticosteroid therapy for improvement in symptoms and opportunities to taper or discontinue corticosteroid therapy. For patients using more than 5 mg daily of prednisone for more than 2 months or for steroid-dependent patients consider the following:

  - Central bone mineral density testing to evaluate the need for preventive or therapeutic bisphosphonate therapy;

  - Periodic monitoring of blood glucose, lipids, and blood pressure;

  - Evaluation for evidence of cushingoid features or signs or symptoms of infection.

- When considering treatment with azathioprine or 6-MP, obtain baseline complete blood count (CBC), liver function tests, and TPMT activity. These tests, except TPMT, should be monitored closely (every 2 to 4 weeks) at the start of therapy and then approximately every 3 months during maintenance therapy.

- With azathioprine and 6-MP, monitor for hypersensitivity reactions including severe skin rashes and pancreatitis. Educate the patient regarding signs and symptoms of pancreatitis (nausea, vomiting, and abdominal pain).

- Prior to initiating methotrexate therapy, obtain CBC, serum creatinine, liver function tests, chest x-ray, and pregnancy test (if female). Monitor blood counts weekly for 1 month, then monthly thereafter.

- Prior to initiating infliximab, adalimumab, or certolizumab, obtain a tuberculin skin test to rule out latent tuberculosis, monitor for signs and symptoms of tuberculosis, and measure viral hepatitis serologies. Also monitor patients with a prior history of hepatitis B virus infection for signs of liver disease, such as jaundice. Assure that patients do not have a clinically significant systemic infection or New York Heart Association class III or IV heart failure.

- In patients receiving infliximab, monitor for infusion-related reactions such as hypotension, dyspnea, fever, chills, or chest pain when administering IV doses.

- In patients with fistulae, monitor at every infliximab, adalimumab, or certolizumab dosing interval for evidence of fistula closure and overall reduction in the number of fistulae.

- Obtain a magnetic resonance imaging procedure prior to initiation of natalizumab therapy. Monitor patients for signs of progressive multifocal leukoencephalopathy such as mental status changes, signs of liver disease (e.g., jaundice), and hypersensitivity reactions following administration.

Abbreviations Introduced in This Chapter

5-ASA	5-Aminosalicylate
6-MP	6-Mercaptopurine
CD	Crohn's disease
CRP	C-reactive protein
ESR	Erythrocyte sedimentation rate
HLA	Human leukocyte antigen
IBD	Inflammatory bowel disease
IL	Interleukin
NOD2	Nucleotide oligomerization domain 2
NSAID	Nonsteroidal anti-inflammatory drug
pANCA	Perinuclear antineutrophil cytoplasmic antibodies
PPAR-γ	Peroxisome proliferator activated receptor-γ
PR	Per rectum
TNF-α	Tumor necrosis factor-α
TPMT	Thiopurine methyltransferase
UC	Ulcerative colitis

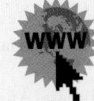

Self-assessment questions and answers are available at *http://www.mhpharmacotherapy. com/pp.html.*

REFERENCES

1. Kornbluth A, Sachar DB. Ulcerative practice guidelines in adults: American College of Gastroenterology, Practice Parameters Committee. Am J Gastroenterol 2010;105:501–523.

2. Lichtenstein GR, Hanauer SB, Sandborn WJ. The Practice Parameters Committee of the American College of Gastroenterology. Management of Crohn's disease in adults. Am J Gastroenterol 2009;104:465–483.

3. Schirbel A, Fiocchi C. Inflammatory bowel disease: Established and evolving considerations on its etiopathogenesis and therapy. J Dig Dis 2010;11:266–276.

4. Lakatos PL, Fischer S, Lakatos L, Gal I, Papp J. Current concept on the pathogenesis of inflammatory bowel disease-crosstalk between genetic and microbial factors: Pathogenic bacteria and altered bacterial sensing or changes in mucosal integrity take "toll." World J Gastroenterol 2006;12(12):1829–1841.

5. Gismera CS, Aladrén BS. Inflammatory bowel diseases: A disease(s) of modern times? Is incidence still increasing? World J Gastroenterol 2008;14(36):5491–5498.

6. Talley NJ, Abreu MT, Anchkar JP, et al. An evidenced based systematic review on medical therapies for inflammatory bowel disease. Am J Gastroenterol 2011;106:S2–S25.

7. Regueiro M, Loftus, EV, Steinhart H, Cohen RD. Clinical guidelines for the medical management of left-sided ulcerative colitis and ulcerative proctitis: Summary statement. Inflamm Bowel Dis 2006;12:972–978.

8. Sandler RS, Eisen GM. Epidemiology of inflammatory bowel disease. In: Kirsner JB, ed. Inflammatory Bowel Diseases. Philadelphia, PA: Saunders, 2000:89–112.

9. Achkara JP, Duerr R. The expanding universe of inflammatory bowel disease genetics. Curr Opin Gastroenterol 2008;24:429–434.

10. Podolsky DK. Inflammatory bowel disease. N Engl J Med 2002;347: 417–429.

11. MacDonald TT, DiSabatino A, Gordon JN. Immunopathogenesis of Crohn's disease. JPEN J Parenter Enteral Nutr 2005;29(4):S118–S125.

12. Cipolla G, Crema F, Sacco S, et al. Nonsteroidal anti-inflammatory drugs and inflammatory bowel disease: Current perspectives. Pharmacol Res 2002;46:1–6.

13. Judge TA, Lichtenstein GR. Inflammatory bowel disease. In: Current Diagnosis & Treatment in Gastroenterology, 2nd ed. [Internet]. Available from: *http://online.statref.com/document.aspx?fxid=23&docid=72.*

14. American Gastroenterological Association. AGA technical review on perianal Crohn's disease. Gastroenterology 2003;125:1508–1530.

15. Ford AC, Sandborn WJ, Khan KJ, et al. Efficacy of biological therapies in inflammatory bowel disease: Systematic review and meta-analysis. Am J Gastroenterol 2011;106:644–659.

16. American Gastroenterological Association. AGA technical review on osteoporosis in gastrointestinal diseases. Gastroenterology 2003;124:795–841.

17. Ng SC, Kamm MA. Review article: New drug formulations, chemical entities and therapeutic approaches for the management of ulcerative colitis. Aliment Pharmacol Ther 2008;28:815–829.

18. Sandborn WJ, Hanauer SB. Systematic review: The pharmacokinetic profiles of oral mesalamine formulations and mesalazine pro-drugs used in the management of ulcerative colitis. Aliment Pharmacol Ther 2003;17:29–42.

19. Sandborn WJ. Rational selection of oral 5-aminosalicylate formulations and prodrugs for the treatment of ulcerative colitis [editorial]. Am J Gastroenterol 2002;97(12):2939–2941.

20. Navarro F, Hanauer SB. Treatment of inflammatory bowel disease: Safety and tolerability issues. Am J Gastroenterol 2003;98(12 Suppl):S18–S23.

21. Pascal J, Valérie P, Felley C, et al. Drug safety in Crohn's disease therapy. Digestion 2007;76:161–168.

22. American Gastroenterological Association Institute. Technical review on corticosteroids, immunomodulators, and infliximab in inflammatory bowel disease. Gastroenterology 2006;130:940–987.

23. Hofer KN. Oral budesonide in the management of Crohn's disease. Ann Pharmacother 2003;37:1457–1464.

24. Fraser AG, Orchard TR, Jewell DP. The efficacy of azathioprine for the treatment of inflammatory bowel disease: A 30 year review. Gut 2002;50:485–489.

25. Tracey D, Klareskog L, Sasso EH, Salfeld JG, Tak PP. Tumor necrosis factor antagonist mechanism of action: A comprehensive review. Pharmacol Ther 2008;117:244–279.

26. Stefanelli T, Malesci A, De La Rue SA, Danese S. Anti-adhesion molecule therapies in inflammatory bowel disease: Touch and go. Autoimmun Rev 2008;7: 364–369.

27. Khan KJ, Ullman TA, Ford AC, et al. Antibiotic therapy in inflammatory bowel disease: A systematic review and meta-analysis. Am J Gastroenterol 2011;106:661–673.

28. Nikfar S, Ehteshami-Ashar S, Rahimi R, Abdollahi M. Systematic review and meta-analysis of the efficacy and tolerability of nicotine preparations in active ulcerative colitis. Clin Ther 2010;32: 2304–2315.

29. Williams NT. Probiotics. Am J Health Syst Pharm 2010;67:449–458.

30. Marshall JK, Irvine EJ. Putting rectal 5-aminosalicylic acid in its place: The role in distal ulcerative colitis. Am J Gastroenterol 2000;95: 1628–1636.

31. Cohen RD, Woseth DM, Thisted RA, Hanauer SB. A meta-analysis and overview of the literature on treatment options for left-sided ulcerative colitis and ulcerative proctitis. Am J Gastroenterol 2000;95:1263–1276.

32. Brain O, Travis SPL. Therapy of ulcerative colitis: State of the art. Curr Opin Gastroenterol 2008;24:469–474.

33. Willert RP, Lawrance IC. Use of infliximab in the prevention and delay of colectomy in severe steroid dependant and refractory ulcerative colitis. World J Gastroenterol 2008;14(16):2544–2549.

34. Sandborn WJ, Feagan BG, Lichtenstein GR. Medical management of mild to moderate Crohn's disease: Evidence-based treatment algorithms for induction and maintenance of remission. Drugs 2007;67(17): 2511–2537.

35. Griffiths AM. Enteral nutrition in the management of Crohn's disease. JPEN J Parenter Enteral Nutr 2005;29(4 Suppl):S108–S117.

36. Sanderson IR, Croft NM. The anti-inflammatory effects of enteral nutrition. JPEN J Parenter Enteral Nutr 2005;29(4 Suppl):S134–S140.

37. Robertson DJ, Grimm IS. Inflammatory bowel disease in the elderly. Gastroenterol Clin North Am 2001;30:409–426.

38. Kim SC, Ferry GD. Inflammatory bowel diseases in pediatric and adolescent patients: Clinical, therapeutic, and psychosocial considerations. Gastroenterology 2004;126:1550–1560.

39. Navarro FA, Hanauer SB, Kirschner BS. Effect of long-term low-dose prednisone on height velocity and disease activity in pediatric and adolescent patients with Crohn's disease. J Pediatr Gastroenterol Nutr 2007;45:312–318.

40. Turner D, Travis SP, Griffiths AM, et al. Consensus for managing acute severe ulcerative colitis in children: A systematic review and joint statement from ECCP, ESPGHAN, and the Porto IBD Working group of ASPGHAN. Am J Gastroenterol 2011;106:574–588.

41. Noe JD, Pfefferkorn M. Short-term response to adalimumab in childhood inflammatory bowel disease. Inflamm Bowel Dis 2008;14: 1683–1687.

42. Wyneski MJ, Green A, Kay M, et al. Safety and efficacy of adalimumab in pediatric patients with Crohn disease. J Pediatr Gastroenterol Nutr 2008;47:19–25.

43. Hyams JS, Wilson DC, Thomas A, et al. Natalizumab therapy for moderate to severe Crohn disease in adolescents. J Pediatr Gastroenterol Nutr 2007;44:185–191.

44. Steinlauf AF, Present DH. Medical management of the pregnant patient with inflammatory bowel disease. Gastroenterol Clin North Am 2004;33:361–385.

45. Ferrero S, Ragni N. Inflammatory bowel disease: Management issues during pregnancy. Arch Gynecol Obstet 2004;270:79–85.

46. Dubinsky M, Abraham B, Mahadevan U. Management of the pregnant IBD patient. Inflamm Bowel Dis 2008;14:1736–1750.

20 Nausea and Vomiting

Sheila Wilhelm and Melissa Lipari

LEARNING OBJECTIVES

● **Upon completion of the chapter, the reader will be able to:**

1. Identify several causes of nausea and vomiting.

2. Describe the pathophysiologic mechanisms of nausea and vomiting.

3. Identify the three stages of nausea and vomiting.

4. Distinguish between simple and complex nausea and vomiting.

5. Create goals for treating nausea and vomiting.

6. Recommend a treatment regimen for a patient with nausea and vomiting associated with cancer chemotherapy, surgery, pregnancy, or motion sickness.

7. Outline a monitoring plan to evaluate the treatment outcomes for nausea and vomiting.

KEY CONCEPTS

❶ Nausea and vomiting are symptoms that can be due to a number of different causes.

❷ To treat nausea and vomiting most effectively, it is important to first identify the underlying cause of the symptoms.

❸ Nonpharmacologic approaches to treating nausea and vomiting include dietary, physical, and psychological changes.

❹ For prevention of acute chemotherapy-induced nausea and vomiting (CINV) for patients receiving moderately or highly emetogenic chemotherapy, a combination of antiemetics with different mechanisms of action is recommended.

❺ Droperidol or a 5-hydroxytryptamine (serotonin) type 3 (5-HT_3) receptor antagonist should be administered at the end of surgery to patients at high risk for developing postoperative nausea and vomiting (PONV).

❻ Nausea and vomiting affect the majority of pregnant women; the teratogenic potential of the therapy is the primary consideration in drug selection.

❼ Because the vestibular system is replete with muscarinic type cholinergic and histaminic (H_1) receptors, anticholinergics and antihistamines are the most commonly used pharmacologic agents to prevent and treat motion sickness.

INTRODUCTION

Nausea and vomiting are due to complex interactions of the gastrointestinal (GI) system, the vestibular system, and various portions of the brain. Nausea and vomiting have a variety of causes that can be simple or complex. Preventing and treating nausea and vomiting require pharmacologic and nonpharmacologic measures tailored to individual patients and situations.

ETIOLOGY AND EPIDEMIOLOGY

● ❶ *Nausea and vomiting are symptoms that can be due to a number of different causes.* Various disorders of the GI, cardiac, neurologic, and endocrine systems can lead to nausea and vomiting (Table 20–1).[1-3] Cancer chemotherapy agents are rated according to their emetogenic potential, and antiemetic therapy is prescribed based on these ratings. Due to potentially severe nausea and vomiting, some patients are unable to complete their chemotherapy treatment regimen. Radiation therapy can induce nausea and vomiting, especially when it is used to treat abdominal malignancies.[4]

Oral contraceptives, hormone therapy, oral hypoglycemic agents, anticonvulsants, and opioids are other common therapies that can cause nausea and vomiting.[1,5] Some medications, such as digoxin and theophylline, cause nausea and vomiting in a dose-related fashion. Nausea and vomiting may indicate higher than desired drug concentrations. Ethanol and other toxins also cause nausea and vomiting.

Table 20–1

Causes of Nausea and Vomiting

GI or Intraperitoneal	Cardiac	Neurologic	Other Causes	Therapy Induced	Endocrine/Metabolic
Obstructing disorders	Cardiomyopathy	Motion sickness	Bulimia and	Cancer	Pregnancy (morning
Pyloric obstruction	Myocardial	Labyrinthitis	anorexia	chemotherapy	sickness and
Small bowel obstruction	infarction	Head trauma	nervosa	Antibiotics	hyperemesis
Colonic obstruction	Congestive heart	Migraine headache	Cyclic vomiting	Cardiac	gravidarum)
Achalasia	failure	Increased intracranial	syndrome	antiarrhythmics	Renal disease (uremia)
Superior mesenteric artery		pressure		Digoxin	Diabetes (ketoacidosis)
syndrome		Intracranial		Oral hypoglycemics	Thyroid and
Enteric infections		hemorrhage		Oral contraceptives	parathyroid disease
Inflammatory bowel		Meningitis		Theophylline	Adrenal insufficiency
diseases		Hydrocephalus		Opioids	Electrolyte abnormalities
Pancreatitis		Psychogenic		Anticonvulsants	(hyponatremia,
Appendicitis		Depression		Radiation therapy	hypercalcemia)
Cholecystitis		Self-induced		Ethanol	
Biliary colic		Anticipatory		Toxins	
Gastroparesis		Rumination		Operative	
Postvagotomy syndrome				procedures	
Intestinal pseudo-					
obstruction					
Functional dyspepsia					
Gastroesophageal reflux					
Peptic ulcer disease					
Hepatitis					
Peritonitis					
Gastric malignancy					
Liver failure					

Postoperative nausea and vomiting (PONV) occurs in 30% of surgical patients overall and in up to 70% of high-risk patients.[6,7] This can be due to severing or disturbing the vagus nerve leading to gastric motility abnormalities. Additional risk factors for PONV include female gender, history of motion sickness or PONV, nonsmoking status, and use of opioids in the postoperative period.[7–9] The choice of anesthetic agents and the duration of surgery may also contribute to PONV.[6,7,9]

Pregnancy-associated nausea and vomiting is common, affecting 70% to 85% of pregnant women, especially early in pregnancy.[10] Approximately one-half of pregnant women experience nausea and vomiting of pregnancy (NVP), one-quarter experience nausea alone, and one-quarter are not affected.[10] In 0.5% to 2% of pregnancies, this can lead to hyperemesis gravidarum, a potentially life-threatening condition of prolonged nausea, vomiting, and consequently, malnutrition.[10]

PATHOPHYSIOLOGY

Nausea and vomiting consist of three stages: nausea, retching, and vomiting. Nausea is the subjective feeling of a need to vomit.[1,5] It is often accompanied by autonomic symptoms such as pallor, tachycardia, diaphoresis, and salivation. Retching, which follows nausea, consists of diaphragm, abdominal wall, and chest wall contractions and spasmodic breathing against a closed glottis.[1] Retching can occur without vomiting, but this stage produces the pressure gradient needed for vomiting, although no gastric contents are expelled. Vomiting, or emesis, is a reflexive, rapid, and forceful oral expulsion of upper GI contents due to powerful and sustained contractions in the abdominal and thoracic musculature.[1] Vomiting, like nausea, can be accompanied by autonomic symptoms.

Regurgitation, unlike vomiting, is a passive process without involvement of the abdominal wall and diaphragm wherein gastric or esophageal contents move into the mouth.[1] In patients with gastroesophageal reflux disease (GERD), one hallmark symptom is acid regurgitation.

Various areas in the brain and the GI tract are stimulated when the body is exposed to noxious stimuli (e.g., toxins), GI irritants (e.g., infectious agents), or chemotherapy. These areas include the chemoreceptor trigger zone (CTZ) in the area postrema of the fourth ventricle of the brain, the vestibular system, visceral afferents from the GI tract, and the cerebral cortex.[2,3,5] These in turn stimulate regions of the reticular areas of the medulla within the brainstem. This area is the central vomiting center, the area of the brainstem that coordinates the impulses sent to the salivation center, respiratory center, and the pharyngeal, GI, and abdominal muscles that lead to vomiting (Fig. 20–1).[11]

The CTZ, located outside the blood–brain barrier, is exposed to cerebrospinal fluid and blood.[2,3] Therefore, it is easily stimulated by uremia, acidosis, and the circulation of toxins such as chemotherapeutic agents. The CTZ has many 5-hydroxytryptamine (serotonin) type 3 (5-HT_3), neurokinin-1 (NK_1), and dopamine (D_2) receptors.[2,12] Visceral vagal nerve fibers are rich in 5-HT_3 receptors. They respond to GI distention, mucosal irritation, and infection.

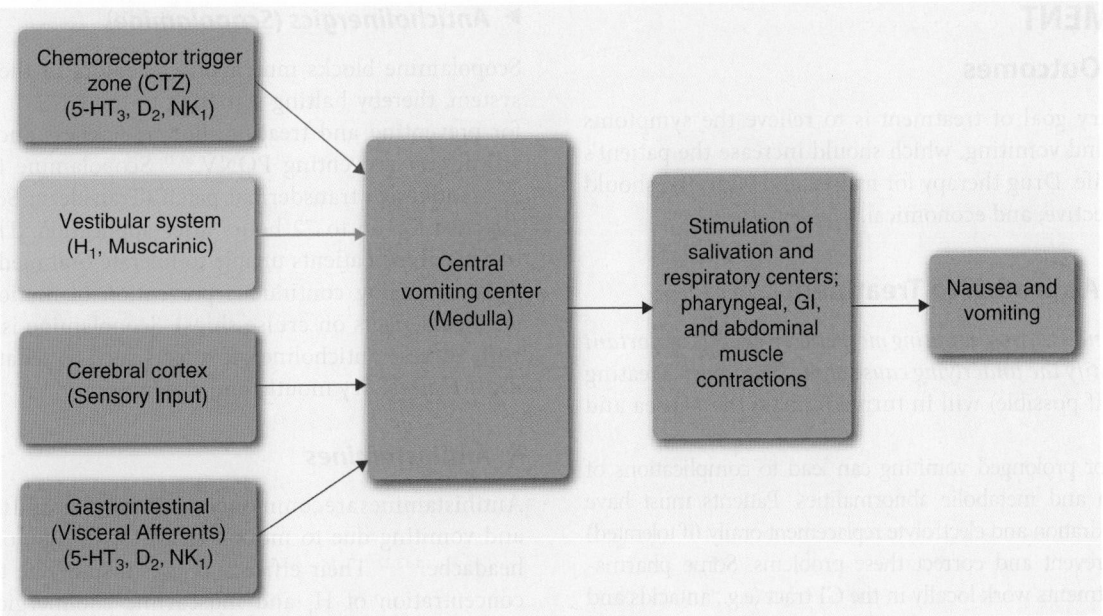

FIGURE 20–1. Physiologic pathways that result in nausea and vomiting. (5-HT$_3$, serotonin type 3 receptor; D$_2$, dopamine type 2 receptor; H$_1$, histamine type 1 receptor, NK$_1$, neurokinin-1.) (From ASHP Therapeutic Guidelines on the Pharmacologic Management of Nausea and Vomiting in Adult and Pediatric Patients Receiving Chemotherapy or Radiation Therapy or Undergoing Surgery. Am J Health Syst Pharm 1999;56:729–764.)

Motion sickness is caused by stimulation of the vestibular system.[13] This area contains many histaminic (H$_1$) and muscarinic cholinergic receptors. The higher brain (i.e., cerebral cortex) is affected by sensory input such as sights, smells, or emotions that can lead to vomiting. This area is involved in anticipatory nausea and vomiting associated with chemotherapy.

Nausea and vomiting can be classified as either simple or complex.[14] Simple nausea and vomiting occurs occasionally and is either self-limiting or relieved by minimal therapy. It does not have detrimental effects on hydration status, electrolyte balance, or weight because it is short lived.

Alternatively, complex nausea and vomiting requires more aggressive therapy because electrolyte imbalances, dehydration, and weight loss may occur. Unlike simple nausea and vomiting, complex nausea and vomiting can be caused by exposure to noxious agents.

CLINICAL PRESENTATION AND DIAGNOSIS

Refer to the box below for the clinical presentation and diagnosis of nausea and vomiting.

Clinical Presentation and Diagnosis of Nausea and Vomiting

Symptoms
- Patients with nausea often complain of autonomic symptoms such as diaphoresis, general disinterest in surroundings, pallor, faintness, and salivation.

Signs
- With complex and prolonged nausea and vomiting, patients may show signs of malnourishment, weight loss, and dehydration (dry mucous membranes, skin tenting, tachycardia, and lack of axillary moisture).

Laboratory Tests
- Dehydration, electrolyte imbalances, and acid–base disturbances may be evident in complex and prolonged nausea and vomiting.

- Dehydration is suggested by elevated blood urea nitrogen (BUN) and serum creatinine (SCr) concentrations, especially with a BUN-to-SCr ratio of 20:1 or greater (for results reported in mg/dL).
- Calculated fractional excretion of sodium (FeNa) less than 1% in patients with compromised baseline renal function and less than 0.2% in patients with normal baseline renal function indicates dehydration and reduced renal perfusion.
- Low serum chloride and elevated serum bicarbonate levels indicate metabolic alkalosis.
- Arterial blood gases with a normal or elevated pH indicates metabolic alkalosis that may or may not be compensated.
- Hypokalemia may occur from GI potassium losses and intracellular potassium shifts to compensate for alkalosis.

TREATMENT

Desired Outcomes

● The primary goal of treatment is to relieve the symptoms of nausea and vomiting, which should increase the patient's quality of life. Drug therapy for nausea and vomiting should be safe, effective, and economical.

General Approach to Treatment

❷ *To treat nausea and vomiting most effectively, it is important to first identify the underlying cause of the symptoms.* Treating the cause (if possible) will in turn eliminate the nausea and vomiting.

Profuse or prolonged vomiting can lead to complications of dehydration and metabolic abnormalities. Patients must have adequate hydration and electrolyte replacement orally (if tolerated) or IV to prevent and correct these problems. Some pharmacologic treatments work locally in the GI tract (e.g., antacids and prokinetic agents), whereas others work in the central nervous system (CNS) (e.g., antihistamines and anticholinergics).[1]

Nonpharmacologic Therapy

A variety of effective pharmacologic treatments exist for nausea and vomiting, but they all have unwanted adverse treatment effects. For this reason, nonpharmacologic treatment options may be considered in selected patients.

Nonpharmacologic options are desirable for treating NVP due to concern for teratogenic effects with drug therapies. When treating PONV, the nonpharmacologic approach is appealing to minimize additive CNS depression with antiemetics and anesthetic agents. ❸ *Nonpharmacologic approaches to treating nausea and vomiting include dietary, physical, and psychological changes.*

Dietary approaches are the cornerstone of treatment for NVP.[15] They are included in treatment guidelines even though there is little evidence to support their effectiveness.[10] Recommendations include eating frequent small meals; avoiding spicy or fatty foods; eating high-protein snacks; and eating bland or dry foods the first thing in the morning.[10,15] Women who have higher protein portions in their diet may experience less severe NVP.[16] The use of ginger was effective in NVP in some studies.[17] In addition to dietary changes, women taking a multivitamin at the time of conception may be less likely to seek medical attention for NVP.[10]

Acupressure and electro-acupoint stimulation of the P6 (Neiguan) point on the inside of the wrist seem safe and cost effective; however, efficacy data in the treatment of NVP, PONV, and motion sickness are conflicting.[10,18,19] Hypnosis and psychotherapy are also safe during pregnancy and in situations where adverse drug effects and interactions are a concern.

Pharmacologic Therapy

Table 20–2 contains the names, usual dosages, and common adverse effects of the pharmacologic treatments for nausea and vomiting.[1,4,7,14]

▶ *Anticholinergics (Scopolamine)*

Scopolamine blocks muscarinic receptors in the vestibular system, thereby halting signaling to the CNS. It is effective for preventing and treating motion sickness and has some efficacy in preventing PONV.[20,21] Scopolamine is available as an adhesive transdermal patch (Transderm Scop) that is effective for up to 72 hours after application. This may be beneficial for patients unable to tolerate oral medications or those requiring continuous prevention of motion sickness (e.g., passengers on cruise ships). Scopolamine is associated with adverse anticholinergic effects such as sedation, visual disturbances, dry mouth, and dizziness.

▶ *Antihistamines*

Antihistamines are commonly used to prevent and treat nausea and vomiting due to motion sickness, vertigo, or migraine headache.[1,13,22] Their efficacy is presumably due to the high concentration of H_1 and muscarinic cholinergic receptors within the vestibular system. Similarly to scopolamine, antihistamines such as diphenhydramine and meclizine cause undesired effects including drowsiness and blurred vision. Cetirizine and fexofenadine, two second-generation antihistamines without CNS depressant properties, were found to be ineffective for treating motion sickness, perhaps because they lack CNS effects.[22]

Some antihistamines such as diphenhydramine, dimenhydrinate, and meclizine are available without a prescription, making self-treatment convenient for patients. Antihistamines are available in a variety of dosage forms, including oral capsules, tablets, and liquids. Liquid formulations are convenient for children or adults who are unable to swallow solid dosage forms.

▶ *Dopamine Antagonists*

Stimulation of D_2 receptors in the CTZ leads to nausea and vomiting (Fig. 20–1). Phenothiazine antiemetics act primarily via a central antidopaminergic mechanism in the CTZ.[1] Phenothiazines commonly used to treat nausea and vomiting include promethazine, prochlorperazine, chlorpromazine, and thiethylperazine. They are available as oral solids and liquids, rectal suppositories, and parenteral formulations. This permits effective use of phenothiazines in a variety of settings including treatment of severe motion sickness or vertigo, gastritis or gastroenteritis, NVP, PONV, or chemotherapy-induced nausea and vomiting (CINV).[4,6,7,10,23–25]

Phenothiazines may cause sedation, orthostatic hypotension, and **extrapyramidal symptoms (EPS)** such as dystonia (involuntary muscle contractions), tardive dyskinesia (irreversible and permanent involuntary movements), and akathisia (motor restlessness or anxiety).[1,26] Chronic phenothiazine use has been associated with EPS, but single doses have also caused these effects.[27]

Droperidol, a butyrophenone, is another centrally acting antidopaminergic agent effective for preventing PONV and treating opioid-induced nausea and vomiting.[1,6] It may also be used for treating CINV for patients who are intolerant

Table 20–2

Antiemetic Agents: Doses for Adults and Children and Adverse Effects

Drug	Adult Dosing	Pediatric Dosing	Adverse Effects[a]
Anticholinergics			
Scopolamine (Transderm Scop)	TD: 1.5-mg patch applied every 72 hours as needed	N/A	Most common: Dry mouth, drowsiness, impaired eye accommodation Rare: Disorientation, memory disturbances, dizziness, hallucinations
Antihistamines			
Cyclizine (Marezine)	Orally: 50 mg every 4–6 hours as needed	Orally, 6–11 years: 25 mg every 6-8 hours as needed (maximum: 3 tablets/day)	Most common: Sedation, dry mouth, constipation
Dimenhydrinate (Dramamine)	Orally: 50–100 mg every 4–6 hours as needed	Orally, 2–6 years: 12.5–25 mg every 6–8 hours Orally, 6–12 years 25–50 mg every 6–8 hours	Less common: Confusion, blurred vision, urinary retention
Diphenhydramine (Benadryl)	Orally: 25–50 mg every 4–6 hours IV/IM: 10–50 mg every 2–4 hours as needed	Orally/IV/IM: 2–6 years: 6.25 mg every 4–6 hours, max 37.5 mg/day; 6–12 years: 12.5–25 mg every 4–6 hours, max 150 mg/day	
Hydroxyzine (Atarax, Vistaril)	Orally/IV/IM: 25–100 mg every 4–6 hours as needed	Orally: 0.6 mg/kg IM: 0.5–1 mg/kg	
Meclizine (Bonine, Antivert)	Orally: 12.5–25 mg every 12–24 hours as needed	Orally: 12 years or older: Use adult dose	
Phenothiazines			
Chlorpromazine (Thorazine)	Orally: 10–25 mg every 4–6 hours as needed IV/IM: 25–50 mg every 4–6 hours as needed	Orally, 6 months and older: 0.5 mg/kg every 4–6 hours as needed IV/IM: 6 months and older: 0.5–1 mg/kg every 6–8 hours; max dose less than 5 years: 40 mg/day; max for 5–12 years: 75 mg/day	Most common: Sedation, lethargy, skin sensitization Less common: Cardiovascular effects, extrapyramidal effects, cholestatic jaundice, hyperprolactinemia
Prochlorperazine (Compazine)	Orally: 5–10 mg 3–4 times a day as needed Supp: 25 mg twice daily as needed IV/IM 2.5–10 mg every 3–4 hours as needed	Orally: over 2 years and more than 9 kg: 0.4 mg/kg/day or 10 mg/m² daily in 2–3 divided doses; Max daily dose: 9–13 kg, 7.5 mg; 13.1–17 kg, 10 mg; 17.1–37 kg, 15 mg Supp: See PO dosing IM: over 2 years and more than 9 kg: 0.13 mg/kg	
Promethazine (Phenergan)	Orally/IM/IV/Supp: 12.5–25 mg every 4–6 hours as needed	Orally/IM/IV/Supp: 2 years and older: 0.25–0.5 mg/kg or 7.5–15 mg/m² 4–6 times daily; maximum 25 mg/dose	
Butyrophenones			
Droperidol (Inapsine)[b]	IM/IV: 0.625–2.5 mg every 4–6 hours as needed	IM/IV: 2–12 years: 0.05–0.1 mg/kg (max 2.5 mg) every 4–6 hours as needed	Most common: Sedation, hypotension, tachycardia
Haloperidol (Haldol)	Orally, IM/IV: 0.5–5 mg every 12 hours as needed	N/A	Less common: Extrapyramidal effects, dizziness, increase in blood pressure, chills, hallucinations
Benzamides			
Domperidone (Motilium)[c]	Orally: 10–20 mg every 4–8 hours as needed Supp: 30–60 mg every 4–8 hours as needed	Orally: 0.2–0.4 mg/kg every 4–8 hours as needed for CINV prophylaxis Supp: Max daily dose based on weight: 10–15 kg, 30 mg; 15.5–25 kg, 60 mg; 25.5–35 kg, 90 mg; 35.5–45 kg, 120 mg	Most common: Sedation, restlessness, diarrhea (metoclopramide), agitation, CNS depression
Metoclopramide (Reglan)[d]	PONV: 10–20 mg PO/IV/IM 10 minutes prior to anesthesia CINV Prophylaxis: 1–2 mg/kg PO/IV every 2–4 hours	N/A	Less common: Extrapyramidal effects (more frequent with higher doses), hypotension, neuroleptic syndrome, supraventricular tachycardia (with IV administration)

(Continued)

Table 20–2

Antiemetic Agents: Doses for Adults and Children and Adverse Effects (*Continued*)

Drug	Adult Dosing	Pediatric Dosing	Adverse Effects[a]
Trimethobenzamide (Tigan)	Orally: 300 mg 3–4 times a day as needed IM: 200 mg 2–4 times a day as needed	Orally: 15–20 mg/kg/day divided into 3–4 doses Not recommended	
Corticosteroids			
Dexamethasone (Decadron)	*CINV*: 12–20 mg orally/IV day 1, then 8–12 mg PO/IV daily *PONV*: 4–5 mg orally/IV at induction of anesthesia	*CINV*: 10 mg/m² prior to chemotherapy then 5 mg/m²	Most common: GI upset, anxiety, insomnia
Methylprednisolone (Solu-Medrol)	125–500 mg orally/IV every 6 hours for total of 4 doses	N/A	Less common: Hyperglycemia, facial flushing, euphoria, perineal itching or burning (with dexamethasone, probably secondary to vehicle and rate of injection)
Cannabinoids			
Dronabinol (Marinol)	Orally: 5–15 mg/m² every 2–4 hours as needed	Use adult dose, use with caution and adjust dose based on response	Most common: Drowsiness, euphoria, somnolence, vasodilation, vision difficulties, abnormal thinking, dysphoria
Nabilone (Cesamet)	Orally: 1–2 mg 2–3 times a day as needed	N/A	Less common: Diarrhea, flushing, tremor, myalgia
Benzodiazepines			
Lorazepam (Ativan)	Orally/IV: 0.5–2 mg prior to chemotherapy	Orally/IV: 2–15 years old: 0.05 mg/kg (up to 2 mg) prior to chemotherapy	Most common: Sedation, amnesia
Alprazolam (Xanax)	Orally: 0.5–2 mg 3 times a day prior to chemotherapy	N/A	Rare: Respiratory depression, ataxia, blurred vision, hallucinations, paradoxical reactions (weeping, emotional reactions)
Serotonin Antagonists			
Dolasetron (Anzemet)	*CINV*: 1.8 mg/kg or 100 mg IV/po before chemotherapy; *PONV*: 12.5 mg IV 15 minutes before end of anesthesia or at onset of N/V *or* 100 mg PO within 2 hours before surgery	*CINV*, 2–16 years: 1.8 mg/kg IV/po (maximum 100 mg) *PONV*: 0.35 mg/kg IV (maximum 12.5 mg) OR 1.2 mg/kg PO (maximum 100 mg) within 2 hours before surgery	Most common: Headache, asymptomatic prolongation of electrocardiographic interval
Granisetron (Kytril)	*CINV*: 10 mcg/kg IV prior to chemotherapy; or 1 mg orally 1 hour before chemotherapy and 1 mg 12 hours after the first dose, or 2 mg 1 hour before chemotherapy *PONV*: 1 mg IV before induction of anesthesia OR immediately before reversal of anesthesia, OR at onset of N/V	*CINV*: 2–16 years: Use adult dosing IV or PO regimen *PONV*: Not recommended for pediatric patients	Less common: Constipation, asthenia, somnolence, diarrhea, fever, tremor or twitching, ataxia, lightheadedness, dizziness, nervousness, thirst, muscle pain, warm or flushing sensation on IV administration
Granisetron (Sancuso)	*CINV*: 1 patch 24–48 hours before chemotherapy; may be worn for up to 7 days (delivers 3.1 mg granisetron per 24 hours)	N/A	Rare: Transient elevations in hepatic transaminases
Ondansetron (Zofran)ᵉ	*CINV*: orally: 24 mg prior to chemotherapy as a single dose, *or* 8 mg prior to chemotherapy; repeat every 12 hours.	*CINV*: orally: 4–11 years: 4 mg 30 minutes prior to chemotherapy, repeat at 4 and 8 hours and every 8 hours for 1–2 days after chemotherapy completion	Granisetron may be degraded by direct sunlight or exposure to sunlamps. Patients should be advised to cover the patch application site (e.g., with clothing) if there is a risk of exposure to sunlight or sunlamps during use and for 10 days after removal

(Continued)

Table 20–2

Antiemetic Agents: Doses for Adults and Children and Adverse Effects (*Continued*)

Drug	Adult Dosing	Pediatric Dosing	Adverse Effects[a]
	IV: 8–12 mg IV 30 minutes prior to chemotherapy, *or* 0.15 mg/kg 3 times a day beginning prior to chemotherapy *PONV:* 4 mg IV/IM before anesthesia induction or at onset of N/V; 16 mg orally once given 1 hour before anesthesia induction	IV: over 6 months: 0.15 mg/kg 3 times a day beginning prior to chemotherapy *PONV:* 1 month–12 years: 4 mg IV/IM before anesthesia induction for over 40 kg and 0.1 mg/kg IV for under 40 kg Oral recommendations not available	
Palonosetron (Aloxi)	*CINV:* 0.25 mg IV 30 minutes before chemotherapy; 0.5 mg orally 1 hour before chemotherapy *PONV:* 0.075 mg IV before anesthesia induction	N/A	
Neurokinin-1 Antagonist Aprepitant (Emend)	*CINV:* 150 mg IV (fosaprepitant) 30 minutes before chemotherapy on first day of chemotherapy only; or 125 mg orally on day 1, 1 hour prior to chemotherapy followed by 80 mg on days 2 and 3 *PONV:* 40 mg orally 3 hours prior to anesthesia induction	N/A	Most common: Fatigue, hiccups Less common: Dizziness, headache, insomnia Rare: Transient elevations in hepatic transaminases

CINV, chemotherapy-induced nausea and vomiting; IM, intramuscularly; Inj, injectable dosage form for IV or IM use; N/A, not available; PONV, postoperative nausea and vomiting; TD, transdermal; Supp, rectal suppository.

[a]Most common, greater than 10%; less common, 1% to 10%; rare, less than 1%. On the basis of U.S. FDA-approved labeling and generalized to drug class.

[b]See text for warnings.

[c]Not available in the United States.

[d]Reduce dose by half if creatinine clearance is less than 40 mL/min (0.67 mL/s).

[e]Daily dose not to exceed 8 mg in severe hepatic impairment (Child-Pugh score 10 or more).

to serotonin receptor antagonists and corticosteroids.[4] Its adverse effects include sedation, agitation, and restlessness. In addition, droperidol carries a U.S. FDA black box warning regarding the potential for QT interval prolongation and cardiac arrhythmias that may result in torsades de pointes and sudden cardiac death.[28] Droperidol should not be used in patients with a prolonged QT interval or in those who are at risk for developing a prolonged QT interval (e.g., heart failure, electrolyte abnormalities, or concurrently taking other medications that may prolong the QT interval).[28] A 12-lead ECG is recommended prior to treatment with droperidol.

Haloperidol is another butyrophenone with some antiemetic effects at low doses (0.5 to 2 mg).[7] It has been explored as an alternative to droperidol.[29]

Both metoclopramide and domperidone (not available in the United States) act as D_2 receptor antagonists centrally in the CTZ and peripherally in the GI tract.[1,30] They also display cholinergic activity, which increases lower esophageal sphincter tone and promotes gastric motility. Because metoclopramide and domperidone have both antiemetic and prokinetic effects, both are used for a variety of disorders including PONV, CINV, NVP, gastroparesis, GERD, and migraine headaches.[1,4,6,10,31,32] Metoclopramide is available in injectable, oral solid, and oral liquid dosage forms, allowing for its use in both hospitalized and ambulatory patients. Other substituted benzamides include trimethobenzamide and benzquinamide.

Metoclopramide crosses the blood–brain barrier and has centrally mediated adverse effects. Young children and the elderly are especially susceptible to these effects, which include somnolence, reduced mental acuity, anxiety, depression, and EPS (akathisia, dystonia, and tardive dyskinesia).[33] The overall incidence of adverse effects is estimated to be 10% to 20%.[1]

Domperidone minimally crosses the blood–brain barrier and is less likely to cause the centrally mediated adverse effects seen with metoclopramide.[1,33] It should not be used for patients with underlying long QT interval or for those on other medications that prolong the QT interval. Both metoclopramide and domperidone can cause hyperprolactinemia, galactorrhea, and gynecomastia.

▶ Corticosteroids

Corticosteroids, especially dexamethasone and methylprednisolone, are used alone or in combination with other antiemetics for preventing and treating PONV, CINV, or radiation-induced nausea and vomiting.[4,7,12,34] They are administered either orally or IV. Their efficacy is thought to be due to the release of 5-HT, reduction in the permeability of the blood–brain barrier, and reduction of inflammation.[35] Common adverse effects with short-term use include GI upset, anxiety, insomnia, and hyperglycemia.[4] Because their use is generally of short duration, long-term adverse effects (e.g., reduction in bone mineral density, corticosteroid-related diabetes, and cataracts) are not usually seen.

▶ Cannabinoids

Cannabinoids have antiemetic activity when used alone or in combination with other antiemetics.[36] Dronabinol and nabilone are commercially available oral formulations used for preventing and treating refractory CINV.[4,36] Cannabinoids are thought to exert their antiemetic effect centrally, although the exact mechanism of action is unknown.[36] Sedation, euphoria, hypotension, ataxia, dizziness, and vision difficulties can occur with cannabinoids.

▶ Benzodiazepines

Benzodiazepines, especially lorazepam, are used to prevent and treat CINV.[4,12,34] Lorazepam is thought to prevent input from the cerebral cortex and limbic system from reaching the central vomiting center in the brainstem.[11] Sedation and amnesia are common side effects. Respiratory depression can occur with high doses or when other central depressants such as alcohol are combined with benzodiazepines.

▶ Serotonin Antagonists

Serotonin is a monoamine neurotransmitter synthesized in neurons in the CNS and in enterochromaffin cells of the GI tract. Chemotherapeutic agents release 5-HT, which is a predominant mediator in nausea and vomiting.[37] This increase in 5-HT concentrations stimulates the visceral vagal nerve fibers and CTZ, thereby triggering nausea and vomiting.[2] Selective 5-HT$_3$ receptor antagonists (ondansetron, granisetron, dolasetron, and palonosetron) are available to prevent and treat nausea and vomiting due to stimulation of these receptors, especially for prevention and treatment of CINV and PONV.[4,6,7,9,12,34,37] These agents are well tolerated; the most common adverse effects are headache, somnolence, diarrhea, and constipation.[4]

Palonosetron is the first 5-HT$_3$ antagonist to be approved for prevention of both acute and delayed CINV.[4] Compared with the other 5-HT$_3$ antagonists, palonosetron has a longer serum half-life (40 hours compared with 4 to 9 hours) and a higher receptor-binding affinity, which may contribute to its efficacy in preventing delayed CINV.[38] Palonosetron combined with dexamethasone is the 5-HT$_3$ antagonist of choice for prevention of CINV due to moderately emetogenic chemotherapy.[4]

▶ Neurokinin-1 Receptor Antagonists

Neurokinin-1 (NK-1) receptors are found on vagal afferents in the GI tract, as well as in the brain.[39] Substance P is a neurokinin neurotransmitter that binds to NK-1 receptors and is believed to mediate both acute and delayed nausea and vomiting. Aprepitant is the first NK-1 receptor antagonist antiemetic drug.[40] Aprepitant is effective for preventing acute and delayed CINV when used with a 5-HT$_3$ antagonist and a corticosteroid.[4,40,41] It is also effective for the prevention of PONV.[7,42] Aprepitant has numerous drug interactions because it is an inhibitor and substrate of the CYP 3A4 metabolic pathway, which is involved in the metabolism of many drugs.[43]

Chemotherapy-Induced Nausea and Vomiting

CINV is classified as: (a) acute (occurring within 24 hours after receiving chemotherapy), (b) delayed (occurring more than 24 hours after receiving chemotherapy), or (c) anticipatory (occurring prior to chemotherapy in patients who experienced acute or delayed nausea and vomiting with previous courses).[4,34] Risk factors for CINV include poor emetic control with prior chemotherapy, female gender, low chronic alcohol intake, and younger age.[34] Chemotherapeutic agents are classified according to their emetogenic potential (Table 20–3), which aids in predicting CINV.[4,12,44] Risk factors that are useful in predicting anticipatory nausea and vomiting include poor prior control of CINV and a history of motion sickness or NVP.[4]

❹ *For prevention of acute CINV for patients receiving moderately or highly emetogenic chemotherapy, a combination of antiemetics with different mechanisms of action is recommended* (Table 20–4).[4,12,34] Patients receiving chemotherapeutic agents with low emetogenic potential should receive a corticosteroid as CINV prophylaxis, and those receiving chemotherapy with minimal emetogenic risk do not require prophylaxis.

Delayed nausea and vomiting is more difficult to prevent and treat. It occurs most often with cisplatin- and cyclophosphamide-based regimens, especially if delayed nausea and vomiting occurred with previous courses of chemotherapy.[4,34] Patients at greatest risk are those who previously had poorly controlled acute CINV.[4]

Antiemetics can be administered either IV or orally for CINV, depending on patient characteristics such as ability to take oral medications, dosage form availability, and cost.[4] The IV and oral routes are equally effective.

Patients undergoing chemotherapy should have antiemetics available to treat breakthrough nausea and vomiting even if prophylactic antiemetics were given.[4,34] A variety of antiemetics may be used, including lorazepam, dexamethasone, methylprednisolone, prochlorperazine,

Table 20–3

Emetogenicity of Chemotherapeutic Agents

Minimal Emetogenic Potential (Less Than 10% Risk)[a]	Moderate Emetogenic Potential (30%–90% Risk)
Bevacizumab	Azacitidine
Bleomycin	Alemtuzumab
Busulfan	Bendamustine
Cetuximab	Carboplatin
Chlorambucil	Clofarabine
2-Chlorodeoxyadenosine	Cyclophosphamide
Erlotinib	less than 1,500 mg/m²
Fludarabine	Cytarabine greater than
Hydroxyurea	1,000 mg/m²
Pralatrexate	Daunorubicin[b]
Rituximab	Doxorubicin[b]
Vinblastine	Epirubicin[b]
Vincristine	Idarubicin[b]
Vinorelbine	Ifosfamide
	Irinotecan
	Oxaliplatin

Low Emetogenic Potential (10%–30% Risk)	High Emetogenic Potential (Greater Than 90% Risk)
Bortezomib	Carmustine
Cabazitaxel	Cisplatin
Catumaxomab	Cyclophosphamide
Cytarabine 1 g/m² or less	1,500 mg/m² or more
Docetaxel	Dactinomycin
Doxorubicin liposome injection	Dacarbazine
Etoposide	Lomustine
Fluorouracil	Mechlorethamine
Gemcitabine	Pentostatin
Methotrexate	Streptozotocin
Mitomycin	
Mitoxantrone	
Paclitaxel	
Panitumumab	
Pemetrexed	
Temsirolimus	
Topotecan	
Trastuzumab	

[a]"% risk" is the incidence of emesis without the administration of antiemetics.

[b]Anthracyclines when combined with cyclophosphamide are considered high emetic risk.

From Refs. 4, 12, 34.

promethazine, metoclopramide, 5-HT₃ antagonists, and dronabinol. If breakthrough CINV occurs, it may be best treated with an antiemetic with a mechanism of action that differs from the medications already administered.

The best strategy for preventing anticipatory nausea and vomiting is to prevent acute and delayed CINV by using the most effective antiemetic regimens recommended based on the emetogenic potential of the chemotherapy and patient factors. CINV should be aggressively prevented with the first cycle of therapy rather than waiting to assess patient response to less effective regimens. If anticipatory nausea and vomiting occurs, benzodiazepines and behavioral therapy such as relaxation techniques are the recommended approaches.[4,12]

Patient Encounter 1

A 45-year-old woman with a diagnosis of refractory non-Hodgkin's lymphoma has received chemotherapy in the past and is about to undergo her first round of chemotherapy with cytarabine 1 g/m². She is concerned about experiencing nausea and vomiting after treatment because this has been an issue with previous treatments. She often experienced nausea and vomiting both before receiving chemotherapeutic agents and afterward on the day of therapy.

Past medical history: Hypertension, dyslipidemia × 2 years

Social history: Does not smoke; occasional alcohol use

Family history: Hypertension, diabetes mellitus type 2

Current medications: Lisinopril 20 mg daily, simvastatin 20 mg daily

Vital signs: Blood pressure 132/82, Heart rate 80 bpm, Temperature 98.6°F (37.0°C)

Labs: Serum creatinine 0.9 mg/dL (80 μmol/L), total cholesterol 161 mg/dL (4.16 mmol/L), LDL 96 mg/dL (2.48 mmol/L), HDL 47 mg/dL (1.22 mmol/L), triglycerides 89 mg/dL (1.01 mmol/L)

What types of CINV does this patient experience?

What is the emetogenic potential of this patient's new chemotherapy regimen?

What nonpharmacologic and pharmacologic options are available for this woman?

Postoperative Nausea and Vomiting

PONV is a common complication of surgery and can lead to delayed discharge and unanticipated hospitalization.[6] The overall incidence of PONV for all surgeries and patient populations is 25% to 30%, but PONV can occur in 70% to 80% of high-risk patients.[6,7,9] Risk factors for PONV include patient factors (female sex, nonsmoking status, and history of PONV or motion sickness), anesthetic factors (use of volatile anesthetics, nitrous oxide, or intraoperative or postoperative opioids), and surgical factors (duration and type of surgery).[6–9]

The first step in preventing PONV is reducing baseline risk factors when appropriate.[6,7] For example, the incidence of PONV may be less with regional anesthesia than general anesthesia, and nonsteroidal anti-inflammatory drugs may cause less PONV than opioid analgesics.

⑤ *Droperidol or a 5-HT₃ receptor antagonist should be administered at the end of surgery to patients at high risk for developing PONV.*[1,6,9] Dexamethasone is also effective when given as a single dose prior to induction of anesthesia.[6] Anticholinergics and antihistamines are also effective for preventing PONV.[6]

Aprepitant, an NK-1 receptor antagonist, prevents PONV; however, it does not appear to be more effective than other

---

Table 20–4

Recommended Drug Regimens for Prevention of CINV Based on Emetogenic Risk

Emetogenic Risk	Acute CINV (Day 1)	Delayed CINV (Days 2–4)
Minimal	None	None
Low	Dexamethasone	None
Moderate	Palonosetron[a] + dexamethasone	Dexamethasone (days 2 and 3)
	Alternative regimen: Any 5-HT$_3$ antagonist + aprepitant[b] + dexamethasone	Aprepitant (days 2 and 3)
High (includes AC regimens)	Any 5-HT$_3$ antagonist + dexamethasone + aprepitant[b]	Aprepitant (days 2 and 3) + dexamethasone (days 2–3 or days 2-4)

AC, anthracycline (daunorubicin, doxorubicin, epirubicin, or idarubicin) plus cyclophosphamide; CINV, chemotherapy-induced nausea and vomiting.

[a]If palonosetron is not available, may substitute a first generation 5-HT$_3$ antagonist, preferably granisetron or ondansetron.

[b]If fosaprepitant 150 mg IV is substituted for oral aprepitant on day 1, subsequent aprepitant doses on days 2 and 3 are not required.

From Refs. 4, 12, 34.

---

agents and is costly.[7] Conversely, metoclopramide, ginger, and cannabinoids have been shown to be of limited utility for PONV and are not recommended.[7]

Combinations of antiemetics are recommended to prevent PONV for high-risk patients.[7] Droperidol plus a 5-HT$_3$ antagonist or dexamethasone plus a 5-HT$_3$ antagonist are effective combinations.[7]

If PONV occurs despite appropriate prophylaxis, it should be treated with an antiemetic from a pharmacologic class not already administered.[7,9] If no prophylaxis was used, a low-dose 5-HT$_3$ antagonist should be used.[7,9]

Nausea and Vomiting of Pregnancy

⑥ *Nausea and vomiting affects most pregnant women; the teratogenic potential of the therapy is the primary consideration in drug selection.*[10] Risks and benefits of any therapy must be weighed by the healthcare professional and the patient.

Nonpharmacologic therapy such as dietary, physical, and behavioral approaches should be considered first.[10,15] Pyridoxine (vitamin B$_6$) 10 to 25 mg three to four times daily alone or in combination with an antihistamine such as doxylamine is often used for NVP.[10,15-17] This combination was previously marketed as Bendectin or Debendox but was withdrawn due to concerns over possible teratogenic effects, although the literature did not support this claim.[45] Pyridoxine is well tolerated, but doxylamine and other antihistamines commonly cause drowsiness.

For more severe NVP, promethazine, metoclopramide, and trimethobenzamide may be effective and have not been associated with teratogenic effects.[10,15] Ondansetron, which is pregnancy category B, has been used to treat severe NVP. Animal data do not indicate a safety concern in pregnancy, but safety and efficacy data in humans for NVP are sparse.

In rare instances (0.5–2% of pregnancies), NVP progresses to hyperemesis gravidarum.[10] Treatment may require the use of enteral or parenteral nutrition if weight loss is present. A corticosteroid such as methylprednisolone may be considered. Methylprednisolone is associated with oral clefts in the fetus when used during the first trimester. Therefore, corticosteroids should be reserved as a last resort and should be avoided during the first 10 weeks of gestation.[10,15,45]

Motion Sickness and Vestibular Disturbances

Nausea and vomiting can be caused by disturbances of the vestibular system in the inner ear.[13,46] Vestibular disturbances can result from infection, traumatic injury, neoplasm, and motion. Patients may experience dizziness and vertigo in addition to nausea and vomiting. If a patient is susceptible to motion sickness, some general preventive measures include minimizing exposure to movement, restricting visual activity, ensuring adequate ventilation, reducing the magnitude of movement, and taking part in distracting activities.[13]

⑦ *Because the vestibular system is replete with muscarinic-type cholinergic and histaminic (H$_1$) receptors, anticholinergics*

Patient Encounter 2

A 27-year-old healthy woman seeks your advice. She is 10 weeks pregnant and complains of constant nausea, frequent vomiting, and weight loss. She does not smoke or drink alcohol. She was not taking prenatal vitamins prior to her pregnancy.

What type of nausea and vomiting is this patient experiencing?

What are some nonpharmacologic and pharmacologic treatment options that may help prevent and treat this patient's nausea and vomiting?

Should this patient seek additional medical attention for her current symptoms?

Patient Encounter 3

A 54-year-old man who presents to your practice is planning a road trip for a family vacation. His past medical history includes benign prostatic hypertrophy and hypertension treated with dutasteride and lisinopril, respectively. He has experienced nausea and vomiting during long car rides in the past and is seeking your advice.

What recommendations for nonpharmacologic interventions would you give this patient to help prevent motion sickness?

What are the pharmacologic options for this patient to prevent or treat nausea and vomiting?

What potential adverse effects would you counsel this patient about?

and antihistamines are the most commonly used pharmacologic agents to prevent and treat motion sickness. Oral medications should be taken prior to motion exposure to allow time for adequate absorption. Once nausea and vomiting due to motion sickness occur, oral medication absorption may be unreliable, making the therapies ineffective. Scopolamine, the anticholinergic medication used for motion sickness, is available as a transdermal patch, which may be helpful for patients who cannot tolerate oral medications or who require treatment for a prolonged period.[20] Drowsiness and reduced mental acuity are the most bothersome side effects of antihistamines and anticholinergics. Visual disturbances, dry mouth, and urinary retention can also occur.

OUTCOME EVALUATION

- The symptoms of simple nausea and vomiting are self-limited or can be relieved with minimal treatment. Monitor patients for adequate oral intake and alleviation of nausea and vomiting.
- Patients with complex nausea and vomiting may have malnourishment, dehydration, and electrolyte abnormalities.
- Monitor patients for adequate oral intake. If the patient has weight loss, assess whether enteral or parenteral nutrition is needed.
- Assess for dry mucous membranes, skin tenting, tachycardia, and lack of axillary moisture to determine if dehydration is present.
- Obtain blood urea nitrogen (BUN), serum creatinine (SCr), calculated fractional excretion of sodium (FeNa), serum electrolytes, and arterial blood gases.
- Ask patients to rate the severity of nausea.
- Monitor the number and volume of vomiting episodes.
- Ask patients about adverse effects to the antiemetics used. Use this information to assess efficacy and tailor the patient's antiemetic regimen.

Patient Care and Monitoring

1. Identify the underlying cause of the nausea and vomiting and eliminate it if possible. Counsel the patient to avoid known triggers.

2. Assess the patient to determine whether the nausea and vomiting is simple or complex and whether patient-directed therapy is appropriate.

3. Obtain a thorough patient history including the prescription, nonprescription, and herbal medications being used. Identify any substances that may be causing or worsening nausea and vomiting. Determine which treatments for nausea and vomiting have been used in the past and their degree of efficacy.

4. Develop a treatment plan with the patient and other healthcare professionals if appropriate. Choose therapeutic options based on the underlying cause of nausea and vomiting, duration and severity of symptoms, comorbid conditions, medication allergies, presence of contraindications, risk of drug–drug interactions, and treatment adverse-effect profiles.

5. Use the oral route of administration if the patient has mild nausea with minimal or no vomiting. Seek an alternative route (e.g., transdermal, rectal suppository, or parenteral) if the patient is unable to retain oral medications due to vomiting.

6. Educate the patient about nonpharmacologic measures such as stimulus avoidance, dietary changes, acupressure or acupuncture, and psychotherapy.

7. To assess efficacy, ask the patient whether he or she is still experiencing nausea or vomiting while using the therapy. Assess whether treatment failure is due to inappropriate medication use or the need for additional or different treatments and proceed accordingly.

8. Assess adverse effects by asking the patient what he or she has experienced. Patient observation or examination is also useful for diagnosing adverse effects such as EPS.

9. Provide patient education regarding causes of nausea and vomiting, avoidance of triggers, potential complications, therapeutic options, medication adverse effects, and when to seek medical attention.

Abbreviations Introduced in This Chapter

ASCO	American Society of Clinical Oncology
BUN	Blood urea nitrogen
CINV	Chemotherapy-induced nausea and vomiting
CNS	Central nervous system
CTZ	Chemoreceptor trigger zone
D_2	Dopamine type 2 receptor
EPS	Extrapyramidal symptoms

FeNa   Fractional excretion of sodium
GERD   Gastroesophageal reflux disease
GI   Gastrointestinal
H_1 Histamine type 1 receptor
$5-HT_3$ 5-Hydroxytryptamine (serotonin) type 3 receptors
NK_1 Neurokinin type 1 receptors
NVP   Nausea and vomiting of pregnancy
PONV   Postoperative nausea and vomiting
SCr   Serum creatinine

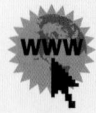 Self-assessment questions and answers are available at *http://www.mhpharmacotherapy.com/pp.html.*

REFERENCES

1. Quigley EM, Hasler WL, Parkman HP. AGA technical review on nausea and vomiting. Gastroenterology 2001;120:263–286.
2. Kearney DJ. Approach to the patient with gastrointestinal disorders. In: Friedman SL, McQuaid KR, Grendell JH, eds. Current Diagnosis and Treatment in Gastroenterology, 2nd ed. New York, NY: McGraw-Hill, 2003:1–33.
3. Proctor DD. Approach to the patient with gastrointestinal disease. In: Goldman L, Ausiello D, Arend W, et al., eds. Cecil Medicine: Expert Consult (Cecil Textbook of Medicine), 23rd ed. Philadelphia, PA: Saunders, 2007.
4. Basch E, Prestrud AA, Hesketh PJ, et al. Antiemetics: American Society of Clinical Oncology clinical practice guideline update. J Clin Oncol 2011;29:4189–4198.
5. Chepyala P, Olden KW. Nausea and vomiting. Curr Treat Options Gastroenterol 2008;11:135–144.
6. Gan TJ, Meyer T, Apfel CC, et al. Consensus guidelines for managing postoperative nausea and vomiting. Anesth Analg 2003;97:62–71.
7. Gan TJ, Meyer TA, Apfel CC, et al. Society for Ambulatory Anesthesia guidelines for the management of postoperative nausea and vomiting. Anesth Analg 2007;105:1615–1628.
8. Apfel CC, Laara E, Koivuranta M, Greim CA, Roewer N. A simplified risk score for predicting postoperative nausea and vomiting: Conclusions from cross-validations between two centers. Anesthesiology 1999;91:693–700.
9. Wilhelm SM, Dehoorne-Smith ML, Kale-Pradhan PB. Prevention of postoperative nausea and vomiting. Ann Pharmacother 2007;41:68–78.
10. ACOG (American College of Obstetrics and Gynecology) Practice Bulletin: Nausea and vomiting of pregnancy. Obstet Gynecol 2004;103:803–814.
11. ASHP Therapeutic Guidelines on the Pharmacologic Management of Nausea and Vomiting in Adult and Pediatric Patients Receiving Chemotherapy or Radiation Therapy or Undergoing Surgery. Am J Health Syst Pharm 1999;56:729–764.
12. Hesketh PJ. Chemotherapy-induced nausea and vomiting. N Engl J Med 2008;358:2482–2494.
13. Shupak A, Gordon CR. Motion sickness: Advances in pathogenesis, prediction, prevention, and treatment. Aviat Space Environ Med 2006;77:1213–1223.
14. DiPiro CV, Ignoffo RJ. Nausea and vomiting. In: DiPiro JT, Talbert RL, Yee GC, Matzke GR, Wells BG, Posey LM, eds. Pharmacotherapy: A Pathophysiologic Approach, 8th ed. New York, NY: McGraw-Hill, 2011:607–619.
15. Badell ML, Ramin SM, Smith JA. Treatment options for nausea and vomiting during pregnancy. Pharmacotherapy 2006;26:1273–1287.
16. Ebrahimi N, Maltepe C, Einarson A. Optimal management of nausea and vomiting of pregnancy. Int J Womens Health 2010;2:241–248.
17. Niebyl JR. Clinical practice. Nausea and vomiting in pregnancy. N Engl J Med 2010;363:1544–1550.
18. Miller KE, Muth ER. Efficacy of acupressure and acustimulation bands for the prevention of motion sickness. Aviat Space Environ Med 2004;75:227–234.
19. Lee A, Done ML. Stimulation of the wrist acupuncture point P6 for preventing postoperative nausea and vomiting. Cochrane Database Syst Rev 2004:CD003281.
20. Spinks AB, Wasiak J, Villanueva EV, Bernath V. Scopolamine (hyoscine) for preventing and treating motion sickness. Cochrane Database Syst Rev 2007:CD002851.
21. Apfel CC, Zhang K, George E, et al. Transdermal scopolamine for the prevention of postoperative nausea and vomiting: A systematic review and meta-analysis. Clin Ther 2010;32:1987–2002.
22. Cheung BS, Heskin R, Hofer KD. Failure of cetirizine and fexofenadine to prevent motion sickness. Ann Pharmacother 2003;37:173–177.
23. Bles W, Bos JE, Kruit H. Motion sickness. Curr Opin Neurol 2000;13:19–25.
24. Ernst AA, Weiss SJ, Park S, Takakuwa KM, Diercks DB. Prochlorperazine versus promethazine for uncomplicated nausea and vomiting in the emergency department: A randomized, double-blind clinical trial. Ann Emerg Med 2000;36:89–94.
25. Habib AS, Gan TJ. The effectiveness of rescue antiemetics after failure of prophylaxis with ondansetron or droperidol: A preliminary report. J Clin Anesth 2005;17:62–65.
26. Olsen JC, Keng JA, Clark JA. Frequency of adverse reactions to prochlorperazine in the ED. Am J Emerg Med 2000;18:609–611.
27. Collins RW, Jones JB, Walthall JD, et al. Intravenous administration of prochlorperazine by 15-minute infusion versus 2-minute bolus does not affect the incidence of akathisia: A prospective, randomized, controlled trial. Ann Emerg Med 2001;38:491–496.
28. MedWatch 2001 [Internet]. Safety information summaries: Inapsine (Droperidol). Available from: *http://www.fda.gov/Safety/MedWatch/SafetyInformation/SafetyAlertsforHumanMedicalProducts/ucm173778.htm.*
29. Rosow CE, Haspel KL, Smith SE, Grecu L, Bittner EA. Haloperidol versus ondansetron for prophylaxis of postoperative nausea and vomiting. Anesth Analg 2008;106:1407–1409.
30. Masaoka T, Tack J. Gastroparesis: Current concepts and management. Gut Liver 2009;3:166–173.
31. Bsat FA, Hoffman DE, Seubert DE. Comparison of three outpatient regimens in the management of nausea and vomiting in pregnancy. J Perinatol 2003;23:531–535.
32. Colman I, Brown MD, Innes GD, Grafstein E, Roberts TE, Rowe BH. Parenteral metoclopramide for acute migraine: Meta-analysis of randomised controlled trials. BMJ 2004;329:1369–1373.
33. Patterson D, Abell T, Rothstein R, Koch K, Barnett J. A double-blind multicenter comparison of domperidone and metoclopramide in the treatment of diabetic patients with symptoms of gastroparesis. Am J Gastroenterol 1999;94:1230–1234.
34. Lohr L. Chemotherapy-induced nausea and vomiting. Cancer J 2008;14:85–93.
35. Minami M, Endo T, Hirafuji M, et al. Pharmacological aspects of anticancer drug-induced emesis with emphasis on serotonin release and vagal nerve activity. Pharmacol Ther 2003;99:149–165.
36. Davis M, Maida V, Daeninck P, Pergolizzi J. The emerging role of cannabinoid neuromodulators in symptom management. Support Care Cancer 2007;15:63–71.
37. Trigg ME, Higa GM. Chemotherapy-induced nausea and vomiting: antiemetic trials that impacted clinical practice. J Oncol Pharm Pract 2010;16:233–244.
38. Gralla R, Lichinitser M, Van Der Vegt S, et al. Palonosetron improves prevention of chemotherapy-induced nausea and vomiting following moderately emetogenic chemotherapy: Results of a double-blind randomized phase III trial comparing single doses of palonosetron with ondansetron. Ann Oncol 2003;14:1570–1577.
39. Massaro AM, Lenz KL. Aprepitant: A novel antiemetic for chemotherapy-induced nausea and vomiting. Ann Pharmacother 2005;39:77–85.
40. Warr DG, Hesketh PJ, Gralla RJ, et al. Efficacy and tolerability of aprepitant for the prevention of chemotherapy-induced nausea and

vomiting in patients with breast cancer after moderately emetogenic chemotherapy. J Clin Oncol 2005;23:2822–2830.

41. Hesketh PJ, Grunberg SM, Gralla RJ, et al. The oral neurokinin-1 antagonist aprepitant for the prevention of chemotherapy-induced nausea and vomiting: A multinational, randomized, double-blind, placebo-controlled trial in patients receiving high-dose cisplatin—the Aprepitant Protocol 052 Study Group. J Clin Oncol 2003;21:4112–4119.

42. Golembiewski J, Tokumaru S. Pharmacological prophylaxis and management of adult postoperative/postdischarge nausea and vomiting. J Perianesth Nurs 2006;21:385–397.

43. Ruhlmann CH, Herrstedt J. Safety evaluation of aprepitant for the prevention of chemotherapy-induced nausea and vomiting. Expert Opin Drug Saf 2011;10:449–462.

44. Hesketh PJ, Kris MG, Grunberg SM, et al. Proposal for classifying the acute emetogenicity of cancer chemotherapy. J Clin Oncol 1997;15:103–109.

45. Lane CA. Nausea and vomiting of pregnancy: A tailored approach to treatment. Clin Obstet Gynecol 2007;50:100–111.

46. Zajonc TP, Roland PS. Vertigo and motion sickness. Part I: Vestibular anatomy and physiology. Ear Nose Throat J 2005;84:581–584.

21

Constipation, Diarrhea, and Irritable Bowel Syndrome

Beverly C. Mims and Clarence E. Curry Jr.

LEARNING OBJECTIVES

● **Upon completion of the chapter, the reader will be able to:**

1. Identify the causes of constipation.

2. Compare the features of functional constipation with those of irritable bowel syndrome (IBS) with constipation (IBS-C).

3. Recommend general and dietary modifications and therapeutic interventions for the treatment of functional constipation.

4. Distinguish between acute and chronic diarrhea.

5. Compare and contrast diarrhea caused by different infectious agents.

6. Explain how medication use can lead to diarrhea.

7. Discuss nonpharmacologic strategies for treating diarrhea.

8. Identify the signs and symptoms of IBS.

9. Contrast IBS with diarrhea (IBS-D) and IBS with constipation (IBS-C).

10. Discuss the goals of IBS treatment.

11. Evaluate the effectiveness of principal pharmaceutical therapies for IBS.

KEY CONCEPTS

❶ Constipation is defined in many ways, and it is important to know what is meant when the term is used.

❷ Functional constipation exists when criteria are fulfilled for at least 3 months with symptom onset at least 6 months before diagnosis.

❸ General and dietary modifications should be employed prior to the use of laxatives in most instances of constipation.

❹ Oral laxatives comprise the primary pharmacologic intervention for relief of constipation.

❺ When diarrhea is severe and oral intake is limited, dehydration can occur, particularly in the elderly and infants.

❻ The primary treatment of acute diarrhea includes fluid and electrolyte replacement, dietary modifications, and drug therapy.

❼ Irritable bowel syndrome (IBS) is generally described as a functional disorder rather than a distinct disease entity.

❽ IBS symptoms typically cluster around two main types: IBS with diarrhea and IBS with constipation.

❾ Diagnosis of IBS is made by symptom-based criteria and the exclusion of organic disease.

❿ The principal goal of IBS treatment is to reduce or control symptoms.

CONSTIPATION

❶ *Constipation is defined in many ways, and it is important to know what is meant when the term is used.* Constipation, when not associated with symptoms of irritable bowel syndrome (IBS), can be defined as a heterogeneous disorder characterized by disorganized passage of feces resulting in infrequent stools, difficult passage of stools, or both.[1] It may be described as difficulty in passing stool with too much effort, unproductive urges, too small amount of stool, too hard consistency of stool, painful elimination of stool, or a feeling of incomplete evacuation. The existence of some or all of these symptoms suggests the presence of constipation when the frequency of elimination of feces is limited to less than two times weekly or when more than 3 days have passed without elimination of stool.[1] ❷ *Functional constipation exists when symptoms last for at least 3 months with onset at least 6 months prior to diagnosis.*[2]

EPIDEMIOLOGY AND ETIOLOGY

Constipation is a common complaint of patients seeking medical attention, and about one-third of patients with constipation seek medical treatment. Constipation occurs in approximately 20% of the population.[3] Approximately 2.5 million physician visits and 90,000 hospitalizations per year in the United States are due to constipation.[4,5] Many medications and some disease states are associated with constipation. Constipation is associated with high socioeconomic costs and has considerable quality-of-life ramifications.[6]

Elderly patients, nonwhites, women, and those of lower educational and socioeconomic levels are more likely to report being constipated. Constipation in children can occur because of a change in the usual diet or fluid intake, a deviation from usual toileting routines such as during vacations, avoidance of bowel movements because of pain associated with having a stool, or due to the use of medications. Children who are diagnosed with severe constipation at a young age are likely to continue to suffer through puberty.

PATHOPHYSIOLOGY

Constipation can be due to primary and secondary causes (Table 21–1). Primary or idiopathic constipation is categorized as normal-transit constipation, slow-transit constipation, and dyssynergic defecation. In the normal-transit type, colonic motility is unchanged and patients tend to experience hard stools despite normal movements. In the slow-transit type, motility is decreased leading to infrequent, harder, drier stools. In dyssynergic defecation (also known as pelvic floor dysfunction), patients have lost the ability to relax the anal sphincter while coordinating muscle contractions of the pelvic floor. Some causes of secondary constipation are listed in Table 21–1.

Table 21–1

Causes of Constipation

Primary Causes

Normal-transit constipation (includes idiopathic or functional disorders)
Slow-transit constipation (includes motility disorders)
Defecatory or rectal evacuation disorders (e.g., Hirschsprung's disease, pelvic floor dyssynergia)

Secondary Causes (Selected)

Endocrine/metabolic conditions (diabetes mellitus, hypothyroidism, hypercalcemia)
GI conditions (IBS, diverticulitis, hemorrhoids)
Neurogenic conditions (brain trauma, spinal cord injury, cerebrovascular accident, Parkinson's disease)
Psychogenic (postponing the urge to defecate, psychiatric conditions)
Medications (analgesics, anticholinergics, calcium channel blockers, clonidine, diuretics, phenothiazines, tricyclic antidepressants, iron supplements, calcium- and aluminum-containing antacids)
Miscellaneous (immobility, poor diet, laxative abuse, hormonal disturbances)

Constipation affects about 50% of pregnant women. Progesterone levels may be responsible in part for slowing digestion. Reabsorption mechanisms may affect colon water during pregnancy leading to harder stools and more difficult bowel movements. Intake of iron supplements may also contribute to constipation during pregnancy.

CLINICAL PRESENTATION AND DIAGNOSIS

Refer to the box below for the clinical presentation of constipation.

Diagnosis

A complete history should be obtained so that the patient's symptoms can be evaluated and the diagnosis of functional constipation confirmed. The diagnosis of functional

---

Clinical Presentation of Constipation

Symptoms

- Functional constipation (constipation occurring in the absence of a demonstrated pathologic condition) involves the presence of at least two of the following symptoms: straining, lumpy or hard stools, sensation of incomplete evacuation, sensation of anorectal obstruction or blockage, need for manual maneuvers to facilitate defecation, and/or infrequent bowel movements (fewer than three per week).
- Other complaints may include painful or difficult defecation, bloating, and absence of loose stools.
- Alarm (or red flag) symptoms include worsening of constipation, blood in the stools, weight loss, fever, anorexia, nausea, and vomiting.
- The patient should seek medical attention when symptoms are severe, last longer than 3 weeks, are disabling, when alarm symptoms occur, or whenever a significant change in usual bowel habits occurs.

Laboratory Tests (to Identify Secondary Causes)

- Thyroid function tests; abnormal thyroid hormone levels may suggest hypothyroidism, which may be associated with constipation.
- Serum calcium; either increased or decreased serum calcium levels may be associated with constipation.
- Glucose; increased blood glucose may indicate diabetes mellitus, which may be associated with constipation.
- Serum electrolytes; dehydration may be associated with constipation.
- Urinalysis may also indicate dehydration, if present.
- Complete blood count (CBC); anemia may be due to cancer or another systemic disorder accompanied by constipation.

constipation is suggested by the presence of two or more of the following criteria: (a) straining, (b) hard or lumpy stools, (c) sensation of incomplete evacuation, (d) sensation of anorectal blockage/obstruction, (e) need for manual maneuvers, or (f) fewer than three defecations per week for at least 25% of defecations. The symptoms must have been present for the last 3 months with onset at least 6 months prior to diagnosis. In addition, the criteria for meeting the diagnosis of IBS are not met.[2]

Dietary habits should be evaluated; patients should be encouraged to maintain adequate fiber intake and hydration. Evaluation of psychosocial status is recommended. Constipation may occur in patients who are depressed or in psychosocial distress. A complete family history should be obtained, particularly as it relates to inflammatory bowel disease and colon cancer. A full record of prescription and over-the-counter medications is mandatory to identify drug-related causes of constipation.

In most cases, there is no underlying cause of constipation, and the physical examination and rectal examination are normal. **Endoscopic evaluation** is required in patients who have weight loss, rectal bleeding, or anemia with constipation. These examinations can be used to exclude the presence of cancer or strictures, especially in patients older than 50 years. Endoscopic evaluation is appropriate in patients without alarm symptoms and those younger than 50 years. However, all adults older than 50 years who present with new-onset constipation should undergo endoscopic evaluation to rule out malignancy.[7]

TREATMENT

Desired Outcomes

In patients with constipation, the principal goals are to: (a) identify and treat secondary causes, (b) relieve symptoms, and (c) restore normal bowel function.

Nonpharmacologic Therapy

❸ *General and dietary modifications should be employed prior to the use of laxatives in most instances of constipation.* Treatment of constipation depends on the characteristics and severity of symptoms. Intake of dietary fiber increases fecal bulk by promoting movement of water into the feces and bacterial proliferation. Increasing fiber intake to 20 to 35 g/day may help improve symptoms. Foods high in fiber include beans, whole grains, bran cereals, fresh fruits, and vegetables such as asparagus, brussels sprouts, cabbage, and carrots. Persons with constipation should avoid excessively processed low-fiber foods such as luncheon meats, hot dogs, certain cheeses, and ice cream.

Adequate fluid intake is also important; patients should be encouraged to drink when thirsty. The thirst mechanism changes with age; maintenance of a daily intake diary may assist patients who need to be reminded to drink fluids.

Walking and other aerobic exercises help to tone the muscles of the lower abdominal area, which promotes propulsion in the bowel. Constipation is a frequent complaint of sedentary persons.

Each day most persons experience a strong peristaltic wave known as the gastrocolic reflex. A bowel movement usually follows. When the urge to have a bowel movement occurs, it should not be ignored. Some people put off having a stool for various reasons, which may lead to more difficulty in passing stool. Time should be planned daily to attempt having a stool. A busy lifestyle should not be allowed to interfere with normal bowel function.

In patients with pelvic floor dysfunction, biofeedback electromyography provides retraining for sensation and control of the rectal floor.[8] Laxatives are employed to extend the treatment of constipation. The recommended route of administration depends on individual patient needs.

Pharmacologic Therapy

❹ *Oral laxatives are the primary pharmacologic intervention for relief of constipation* (Table 21–2). There are several different drug classes, as described next.

▶ Bulk Producers

These agents are either naturally derived (psyllium), semisynthetic (polycarbophil), or synthetic (methylcellulose). They act by swelling in intestinal fluid, forming a gel that aids in fecal elimination and promoting peristalsis. They may cause flatulence (which is less common with methylcellulose) and abdominal cramping. Bulk-forming laxatives must be taken with sufficient water (8 oz or 240 mL/dose) to avoid becoming lodged in the esophagus and producing obstruction or worsening constipation. Hypersensitivity reactions may occur and rarely may be manifested as an anaphylactic reaction.

▶ Hyperosmotics

These products cause water to enter the lumen of the colon. Lactulose, sorbitol, and glycerin are osmolar sugars. Polyethylene glycol 3350 with electrolytes is most useful for acute complete bowel evacuation prior to GI examination. Polyethylene glycol 3350 without electrolytes is useful in patients who are experiencing acute constipation or who have had inadequate response to other agents.[9] Lactulose causes acidification of the contents of the colon, increases water content of the gut, and softens the stool. Glycerin causes local irritation and possesses hyperosmotic action. Osmotic agents may cause flatulence, abdominal cramping, and bloating.

Sorbitol and glycerin may be administered rectally for treatment of constipation. Rectal discomfort and irritation may occur when administered rectally. Glucose levels should be monitored in diabetic patients who ingest oral sorbitol.

▶ Lubricants

Lubricant laxatives work by coating the stool, which allows it to be expelled more easily. The oily film covering the stool also keeps the stool from losing its water to intestinal

Table 21–2

Dosage Recommendations for Laxatives and Cathartics

Agent	Adults and Children Ages 12 and Over	Children Ages 6–11 Years
Agents That Cause Softening of Feces in 1–3 Days		
Bulk-forming agents/osmotic laxatives		
Methylcellulose	4–6 g/day	0.45–1.5 g po per dose up to 3 g/day
Polycarbophil	4–6 g po daily	On advice of practitioner
Psyllium	Varies with product	On advice of practitioner
Emollients		
Docusate sodium	50–360 mg po daily	50–100 mg po daily
Docusate calcium	50–360 mg po daily	On advice of practitioner
Docusate potassium	100–300 mg po daily	100 mg po daily
Lactulose	15–30 mL po daily	7.5 mL (5 g) po daily
Sorbitol	30–50 g/day po daily	2 mL/kg (as 70% solution) po daily
Mineral oil	15–30 mL po daily	5–15 mL po daily
Agents That Result in Soft or Semifluid Stool in 6–12 Hours		
Bisacodyl (oral)	5–15 mg po	5–10 mg (0.3 mg/kg) po
Senna	Dose varies with formulation	6–25 mg po once or twice daily
Agents That Cause Watery Evacuation in 1–6 Hours		
Magnesium citrate[a]	120–300 mL po	100–150 mL po
Magnesium hydroxide[a]	30–60 mL po (15–30 mL of concentrate po)	2.5–5 mL po up to 4 times
Magnesium sulfate[a]	10–30 g po	5–10 g po
Bisacodyl (suppository)	10 mg rectally	5 mg rectally (1/2 suppository)
Polyethylene glycol–electrolyte preparations	Up to 4 L po	Safety and efficacy not established

po, orally.

[a]Magnesium can accumulate in renal dysfunction.

Adapted from Powell PH, Fleming VH. Diarrhea, constipation and irritable bowel syndrome. In: DiPiro JT, Talbert RL, Yee GC, et al., eds., Pharmacotherapy: A Pathophysiologic Approach, 8th ed. New York, NY: McGraw-Hill, 2011:621–638, with permission.

reabsorption processes. Mineral oil (liquid petrolatum) is a nonprescription heavy oil that should be used with caution, if at all, because it can be aspirated into the lungs and cause lipoid pneumonia when ingested orally. This is of particular concern in the young or the elderly. It may also interfere with the absorption of fat-soluble vitamins.

▶ Stimulant Laxatives

Diphenylmethane derivatives (e.g., bisacodyl) and anthra-quinones (e.g., senna) have a selective action on the nerve plexus of intestinal smooth muscle leading to enhanced motility. Enteric-coated bisacodyl tablets should be swallowed whole to avoid gastric irritation and vomiting. Ingestion should be avoided within 1 to 2 hours of antacids, H_2-receptor antagonists, proton pump inhibitors, and milk. Bisacodyl rectal suppository and enema products are available. The onset of effect is rapid but the effects can be harsh (cramping), depending on the dose taken. Castor oil is another member of this class that is used less frequently. Castor oil is classified as pregnancy category X. It is associated with uterine contractions and rupture. The use of castor oil in breast-feeding is considered as "possibly unsafe."

▶ Emollients

Also known as surfactants and stool softeners, emollients (e.g., salts of docusate) act by increasing the surface-wetting action on the stool leading to a softening effect. They reduce friction and make the stool easier to pass. These agents are not recommended for treating constipation of long duration.

▶ Saline Agents

Salts of sodium, magnesium, and phosphate pull water into the lumen of the intestines resulting in increased enteral pressure. Magnesium and phosphate may accumulate in patients with renal dysfunction. Principal concerns with sodium phosphate derivative use include dehydration, hypernatremia, hyperphosphatemia, acidosis, hypocalcemia, and worsening renal function. Patients with congestive heart failure and renal dysfunction should be advised to avoid these agents. Nonprescription oral sodium phosphate solutions were voluntarily recalled by the manufacturer because of the risk of acute phosphate nephropathy. Prescription oral phosphate products contain a black box warning about use in high-risk patients.

▶ Lubiprostone

Lubiprostone (Amitiza), a bicyclic acid oral agent, is approved for treatment of chronic idiopathic constipation in adults. It has not been studied in children. Lubiprostone acts locally on intestinal chloride channels and increases intestinal fluid secretion, resulting in increased intestinal motility and thereby increasing the passage of stool.[9]

Lubiprostone is contraindicated in patients with a history of mechanical GI obstruction and should not be used in patients suspected of having GI obstruction. Safety has not been established in pregnant women; animal studies indicated the potential to cause fetal loss. Women who could become pregnant should have a negative pregnancy test result prior to beginning therapy with lubiprostone. Patients receiving lubiprostone who become pregnant should be advised of the potential harm to the fetus (pregnancy category C).

Patients who experience adverse effects of dyspnea, nausea, and diarrhea should report them to their prescribers. Other adverse effects include abdominal distention, abdominal pain, flatulence, vomiting, and loose stools. Nausea is a prominent adverse effect and may be minimized by taking lubiprostone with food.

The recommended dose of lubiprostone is 24 mcg orally twice daily with food and water. The capsule should be swallowed whole; it should not be chewed or broken apart. Studies evaluated lubiprostone use for no longer than 4 weeks. Patients should be assessed periodically for the need to continue therapy. Lubiprostone has not been studied in children or patients with renal or hepatic dysfunction.[10]

▶ Methylnaltrexone Bromide

Methylnaltrexone bromide (Relistor) is indicated for opioid-induced constipation in patients with advanced illness, receiving palliative care, and who have experienced insufficient response to laxative therapy. It is a selective antagonist of opioid binding at the mu-receptor. It has limited ability to cross the blood–brain barrier and causes laxation in patients with opioid-induced constipation without reducing the analgesic effects of opioids or inducing opioid withdrawal.

Methylnaltrexone bromide is administered subcutaneously no more than once daily or every other day dosages based on body weight. Patients weighing 38 to 62 kg should receive 8 mg, patients weighing 62 to 114 kg should receive 12 mg, and patients who weigh more than 114 kg should receive 0.15 mg/kg (rounded up to the nearest 0.1 mL of volume). In patients with renal impairment (creatinine clearance less than 30 mL/min [0.5 mL/s]), the dose should be reduced by 50%. Dosing in dialysis-dependent patients has not been studied. No dosage adjustment is necessary in patients with mild to moderate hepatic impairment (Child-Pugh class A and B). Dosage in patients with severe hepatic impairment has not been studied.

Pregnancy adverse effects of methylnaltrexone were not observed in animal experiments. No well-controlled and adequate studies exist in pregnant women (pregnancy category B).

The most common side effects are abdominal pain and cramping, flatulence, nausea, dizziness, hyperhidrosis, and diarrhea. Additional adverse effects are body temperature increase, muscle spasm, and syncope. Methylnaltrexone is contraindicated in patients with known or suspected GI obstruction.

▶ Alvimopan

Alvimopan (Entereg) is an opioid receptor antagonist that blocks opioid binding at the mu-receptor. It selectively binds to mu-receptors in the GI tract and antagonizes the peripheral effects of opioids on GI secretion and motility. Early experience suggests that it does not affect opioid analgesic effects or induce opioid withdrawal syndromes.

Alvimopan may be administered only by hospitals that are enrolled in the ENTEREG Access Support and Education (E.A.S.E.) Program. Alvimopan is limited to the short-term inpatient use (no more than 15 doses). Hospital staff education programs must be conducted. Hospitals may contact the E.A.S.E. program at 1-866-423-6567.

E.A.S.E. program trained hospital staff may administer the initial dose of alvimopan 15 mg orally 30 minutes to 5 hours prior to surgery with or without food. The maintenance dose is 12 mg by mouth twice daily beginning the day after surgery for a maximum of 7 days or until the patient is discharged. The maximum total therapy must not exceed 15 doses. Alvimopan is not dispensed to patients who have been discharged from the hospital.

Alvimopan is contraindicated in patients who have taken treatment doses of opioids for more than 7 consecutive days immediately prior to alvimopan administration because these patients may be more sensitive to GI side effects. The effects of alvimopan were reportedly affected by the use of opioid analgesics.

Adverse effects associated with alvimopan include hypokalemia, dyspepsia, urinary retention, anemia, and back pain. An increased incidence of myocardial infarction was observed in one 12-month alvimopan study.

▶ Treatment Recommendations

Slow-transit constipation can be treated with chronic administration of hyperosmotic laxatives. Senna, bisacodyl, and other stimulants should be used only when the others fail to deliver the desired effect.

Laxatives may provide appropriate relief when constipation occurs during the postpartum period, when not breast-feeding, and in immobile patients. Patients who are not constipated but who need to avoid straining (e.g., patients with hemorrhoids, hernia, or myocardial infarction) may benefit from stool softeners or mild laxatives such as polyethylene glycol 3350.

Laxatives should not be given to children younger than 6 years unless prescribed by a physician. Because children may not be able to describe their symptoms well, they should be evaluated by a healthcare provider before being given a laxative. Treating secondary causes may resolve the constipation without the use of laxatives. As in adults, children benefit from a healthy balanced diet, adequate fluid, and regular exercise.

Because many elderly persons experience constipation, laxative use is sometimes viewed as a normal part of daily life. However, oral ingestion of mineral oil can be a special hazard in bedridden elderly persons because it can lead to pneumonia through inhalation of oil droplets into the lungs. Lactulose may be a better choice in this situation. Regular use of any laxative that affects fluid and electrolytes may result in significant unwanted adverse effects.

Bulk producers are commonly used during pregnancy. Stool softeners (pregnancy category C) are probably safe to use at any time during a pregnancy because they are poorly absorbed. Lactulose and magnesium products are classified as pregnancy category B. No human studies are available concerning use of lactulose in pregnant women. Magnesium-based antacids are not classified according to pregnancy categories and are associated with low-risk and minimal absorption in pregnant women. Long-term use of magnesium citrate should be avoided (pregnancy category B).

To avoid constipation, pregnant women should be advised to eat regular meals that are balanced among fruits, vegetables, and whole grains; maintain adequate water intake; and get appropriate exercise.

Patients with the following conditions should use laxatives only under the supervision of a healthcare provider: (a) colostomy; (b) diabetes mellitus (some laxatives contain large amounts of sugars such as dextrose, galactose, and/or sucrose); (c) heart disease (some products contain sodium); (d) kidney disease; and (e) swallowing difficulty (bulk-formers may produce esophageal obstruction).

OUTCOME EVALUATION

- Ask the patient about the absence or improvement in symptoms to determine whether laxative therapy is effective. Patients should have an increase in stool frequency to three or more well-formed stools per week. Patients should report the absence of prolonged defecation time or the absence of the need for excessive straining.

- When acute overuse or chronic misuse of saline or stimulant laxatives is suspected, it may be necessary to check for electrolyte disturbances (e.g., hypokalemia, hypernatremia, hyperphosphatemia, or hypocalcemia).

- Some laxatives (e.g., bulk producers) contain significant amounts of sodium or sugar and may be unsuitable for salt-restricted or diabetic patients. Monitoring of fluid retention (edema) and blood pressure changes are indicated in patients on sodium-restricted diets. Glucose monitoring may be required in diabetic patients as needed with chronic use. Use of low-sodium or sugar-free products may be indicated.

- Saline laxatives containing magnesium, potassium, or phosphates should be used cautiously in persons with reduced kidney function. Monitor appropriate serum electrolyte concentrations in patients with unstable renal function evidenced by changing serum creatinine or creatinine clearance.

DIARRHEA

Diarrhea is a symptom of an underlying problem, not a disease. It is characterized by increased stool frequency (usually more than three times daily), stool weight, liquidity, and decreased consistency of stools compared with a patient's usual pattern. Acute diarrhea is defined as diarrhea lasting for 14 days or less. Diarrhea lasting more than 30 days is called chronic diarrhea. Illness of 15 to 30 days is referred to as persistent diarrhea.[11]

EPIDEMIOLOGY AND ETIOLOGY

Most cases of diarrhea in adults are mild and resolve quickly. Infants and children (especially younger than 3 years) are highly susceptible to the dehydrating effect of diarrhea, and its occurrence in this age group should be taken seriously.

Acute Diarrhea

Acute diarrhea has many possible causes, but infection is the most common. Infectious diarrhea occurs because of food and water contamination via the fecal–oral route. Viruses are the cause in a large proportion of cases. Likely viral suspects include Rotavirus, Norwalk, and adenovirus. Patients usually exhibit sudden low-grade fever, vomiting, and watery stools. Some practitioners use the terms *acute diarrhea* and *acute gastroenteritis* interchangeably. However, they are not synonymous because diarrheal events do not invariably produce enteritis or involve the stomach.

Bacterial precipitants in many other cases include *Escherichia coli, Salmonella* species, *Shigella* species, *Vibrio cholerae,* and *Clostridium difficile.* The term *dysentery* describes some of these bacterial infections when associated with serious occurrences of bloody diarrhea. Additionally, acute diarrheal conditions can be prompted by parasites and protozoa such as *Entamoeba histolytica, Microsporidium, Giardia lamblia,* and *Cryptosporidium parvum.* Most of these infectious agents can cause traveler's diarrhea, a common malady afflicting travelers worldwide. It usually occurs during or just after travel following the ingestion of fecally contaminated food or water. It has an abrupt onset but usually subsides within 2 to 3 days.

Noninfectious causes of acute diarrhea include drugs and toxins (Table 21–3), laxative abuse, food intolerance, IBS, inflammatory bowel disease, ischemic bowel disease, lactase deficiency, Whipple's disease, pernicious anemia, diabetes mellitus, malabsorption, fecal impaction, diverticulosis, and celiac sprue.

Lactose intolerance is responsible for many cases of acute diarrhea, especially in patients of African descent, Asians, and Native Americans. Possible food-related causes include fat substitutes, dairy products, and products containing nonabsorbable carbohydrates.

The diarrhea of IBS is sudden and perhaps watery but likely loose, usually accompanied by urgency, bloating, and abdominal pain occurring upon arising in the morning or immediately following a meal. Inflammatory bowel disease is typically associated with the sudden onset of bloody diarrhea accompanied by urgency, crampy abdominal pain, and fever. Patients who experience bowel ischemia may develop bloody diarrhea, particularly if they progress to shock.

Chronic Diarrhea

Chronic diarrhea lasts 4 weeks or more. Most cases result from functional or inflammatory bowel disorders, endocrine disorders, malabsorption syndromes, and drugs (including laxative abuse). In chronic diarrhea, daily watery stools may not occur. Diarrhea may be either intermittent or persistent.

PATHOPHYSIOLOGY

During normal processes, approximately 9 L (about 2.4 gallons) of fluid traverse the GI tract daily. Of this amount, 2 L represent gastric juice, 1 L is saliva, 1 L is bile, 2 L are pancreatic juice, 1 L is intestinal secretions, and 2 L are ingested. Of these 9 L of fluid presented to the intestine, only about 150 to 200 mL remain in the stool after reabsorptive processes occur.

Any event that leads to a significant increase in the amount of fluid retained in the stool may result in diarrhea. Large-stool diarrhea often signifies small intestinal involvement, whereas small-stool diarrhea usually originates in the colon. Diarrhea may be classified according to pathophysiologic mechanisms that include osmotic, secretory, inflammatory, and altered motility.

Osmotic diarrhea results from the intake of unabsorbable but water-soluble solutes in the intestinal lumen leading to water retention. Common causes include lactose intolerance and ingestion of magnesium-containing antacids.

Secretory diarrhea results in an increase in the net movement (secretion) of ions into the intestinal lumen leading to an increase in intraluminal fluid. Medications, hormones, and toxins may be responsible for secretory activity.

Inflammatory (or exudative) diarrhea results from changes to the intestinal mucosa that damage absorption processes and lead to an increase in proteins and other products in the intestinal lumen with fluid retention. The presence of blood or fecal leukocytes in the stool is indicative of an inflammatory process. The diarrhea of inflammatory bowel disease (e.g., ulcerative colitis) is inflammatory in nature.

Increased motility results in decreased contact between ingested food and drink and the intestinal mucosa, leading to reduced reabsorption and increased fluid in the stool. Diarrhea resulting from altered motility is often established after other mechanisms have been excluded. IBS-related diarrhea is due to altered motility.

Although diarrhea can often be attributed to a specific mechanism, some patients develop diarrhea due to overlapping mechanisms. For example, malabsorption syndromes

Table 21–3

Selected Drugs and Substances That May Cause Acute Diarrhea

Drugs

Antibiotics	Hydralazine	Metformin	Sorbitol
Colchicine	Laxatives	Misoprostol	Theophylline
Digitalis	Mannitol	Quinidine	Thyroid products

Dietary Supplements

St. John's wort	Echinacea	Ginseng	Aloe vera

Poisons

Arsenic	Cadmium	Mercury	Monosodium glutamate

and traveler's diarrhea are associated with both secretory and osmotic diarrhea.

Drug-induced diarrhea can occur by several mechanisms. First, water can be drawn into the intestinal lumen osmotically. Second, the intestinal bacterial ecosystem can be upset leading to the emergence of invasive pathologic organisms triggering secretory and inflammatory processes. Saline laxatives are an example of the first mechanism, and many antibiotics act by the second. A third way is through altered motility as may occur with tegaserod maleate. Other drugs such as procainamide or colchicine produce diarrhea through undetermined mechanisms. Discontinuation of the offending drug may be the only measure needed to ameliorate the diarrhea.

CLINICAL PRESENTATION AND DIAGNOSIS

Refer to the box below for the clinical presentation of diarrhea.

Diagnosis

Patients with diarrhea should be questioned about the onset of symptoms, recent travel, diet, source of water, and medication use. Other important considerations include duration and severity of the diarrhea along with an accounting of the presence of associated abdominal pain or vomiting, blood in the stool, stool consistency, stool appearance, stool frequency, and weight loss. Although most cases of diarrhea are self-limited, infants, children, elderly persons, and immunocompromised patients are at risk for increased morbidity.

Findings on physical examination can assist in determining hydration status and disease severity. The presence of blood in the stool suggests an invasive organism, an inflammatory process, or perhaps a neoplasm. Large-volume stools suggest a small-intestinal disorder, whereas small-volume stools suggest a colon or rectal disorder. Patients with prolonged or severe symptoms may require colonoscopic evaluation to identify the underlying cause.

Treatment

Most healthy adults with diarrhea do not develop significant dehydration or other complications and can be treated symptomatically by self-medication. ❺ *When diarrhea is severe and oral intake is limited, dehydration can occur, particularly in the elderly and infants. Other complications*

Clinical Presentation of Diarrhea

Signs and Symptoms of Acute Diarrhea

- Patients with acute diarrhea have the abrupt onset of loose, watery, or semiformed stools.
- Abdominal cramps and tenderness, rectal urgency, nausea, bloating, and fever may be present.
- The disorder is generally self limited, lasting 3 to 4 days even without treatment.
- Patients with acute infectious diarrhea from invasive organisms also have bloody stools and severe abdominal pain.

Laboratory Tests in Acute Diarrhea

- Stool cultures can help identify infectious causes. Cultures are subject to time delay. New methodology using real-time polymerase chain reaction shortens the reporting time.
- Stool may also be analyzed for mucus, fat, osmolality, fecal leukocytes, and pH. The presence of mucus suggests colonic involvement. Fat in the stool may be due to a malabsorption disorder. Fecal leukocytes can be found in inflammatory diarrheas including infections and caused by invasive bacteria (e.g., *E. coli*, and *Shigella* and *Campylobacter* species). Stool pH (normally greater than 6) is decreased by bacterial fermentation processes.
- Stool volume and electrolytes can be assessed in large-volume watery stools to determine whether the diarrhea is osmotic or secretory.

- CBC and blood chemistries may be helpful in patients whose symptoms persist. The presence of anemia, leukocytosis, or neutropenia may provide further clues to the underlying cause.

Signs and Symptoms of Chronic Diarrhea

- In patients with chronic diarrhea, symptoms may be severe or mild. Weight loss can be demonstrated, and weakness may be present.
- Dehydration may be manifested by decreased urination, dark-colored urine, dry mucous membranes, increased thirst, and tachycardia.

Laboratory Tests in Chronic Diarrhea

- All of the tests described for acute diarrhea would be used to establish a diagnosis of chronic diarrhea because the differential diagnosis is more complicated. The data obtained can help categorize the diarrhea as watery, inflammatory, or fatty, narrowing the focus on a primary disorder.
- Colonoscopy allows visualization and biopsy of the colon and is preferred if blood has been found in the stool or if the patient has acquired immune deficiency syndrome.

of diarrhea resulting from fluid loss include electrolyte disturbances, metabolic acidosis, and cardiovascular collapse.

Children are more susceptible to dehydration (particularly when vomiting occurs) and may require medical attention early in their course, especially if younger than 3 years. Physician intervention is also necessary for elderly patients who are sensitive to fluid loss and electrolyte changes due to concurrent chronic illness.

Patients should undergo medical evaluation in the following circumstances: (a) moderate to severe abdominal tenderness, distention, or cramping; (b) bloody stools; (c) evidence of dehydration (e.g., thirst, dry mouth, fatigue, dark-colored urine, infrequent urination, reduced urine, dry skin, lack of skin elasticity, rapid pulse, rapid breathing, muscle cramps, muscle weakness, sunken eyes, or lightheadedness); (d) high fever (greater than or equal to 38.3°C or 101°F); (e) evidence of weight loss greater than 5% of total body weight; and (f) diarrhea that lasts longer than 48 hours.

Desired Outcomes

The goals of treatment for diarrhea are to relieve symptoms, maintain hydration, treat the underlying cause(s), and maintain nutrition. ❻ *The primary treatment of acute diarrhea includes fluid and electrolyte replacement, dietary modifications, and drug therapy.*

Nonpharmacologic Therapy

▶ Fluid and Electrolytes

Fluid replacement is not a treatment to relieve diarrhea but rather an attempt to restore fluid balance. In many parts of the world where diarrheal states are frequent and severe, fluid replacement is accomplished using **oral rehydration solution** (ORS), a measured mixture of water, salts, and glucose. The solution recognized by the World Health Organization consists of 75 mEq/L (75 mmol/L) sodium, 75 mmol/L glucose, 65 mEq/L (65 mmol/L) chloride, 20 mEq/L (20 mmol/L) potassium, and 10 mEq/L (3.3 mmol/L) citrate, having a total osmolarity of 245 mOsm/L. A simple solution can be prepared from 1 L water mixed with eight teaspoonfuls of sugar and one teaspoonful of table salt. Some commercial products include Pedialyte, Rehydralyte, and CeraLyte.

Consistent intake of water (perhaps by slowly sipping), along with eating as tolerated, should restore lost fluids and salt for typical diarrhea sufferers. Patients may also replace lost fluid by drinking flat soft drinks such as ginger ale, tea, fruit juice, broth, or soup. Although sports drinks may be used to treat dehydration, caution should be exercised so they are not viewed as a casual panacea. Severe diarrhea may require use of parenteral solutions, and parenteral products should be used if patients are vomiting or unconscious.[12]

▶ Dietary Modifications

Once an acute diarrheal situation ensues, patients typically eat less as they become focused on the diarrhea. Both children and adults should attempt to maintain nutrition. Food provides nutrients and fluid volume that help replace what is lost. However, food-related fluid may not be enough to compensate for diarrheal losses. Some foods may be inappropriate if they irritate the GI tract or if they are implicated as the cause of the diarrhea. Patients with chronic diarrhea may find that increasing bulk in the diet may help (e.g., rice, bananas, whole wheat, and bran).

Pharmacologic Therapy

The goal of drug therapy is to control symptoms, enabling the patient to continue with as normal a routine as possible while avoiding complications (Table 21–4). Most infectious diarrheas are self limited or curable with anti-infective agents.

Table 21–4		
Pharmacotherapy for Diarrhea		
Drug	**Usual Oral Dose**	**Type of Diarrhea**
Attapulgite	Adults: 1,200–1,500 mg after each loose stool. Maximum: 9,000 mg in 24 hours Children 6–12 years: 750 mg after each loose stool. Maximum: 4,500 mg in 24 hours	Acute and chronic
Calcium polycarbophil	Adults: 1,000 mg 4 times daily or after each loose stool, not to exceed 12 tablets/day Children 6–12 years: 500 mg 3 times daily Children 3–6 years: 500 mg twice daily	Chronic
Loperamide	Adults: 4 mg initially, then 2 mg after each subsequent loose stool. Maximum: 16 mg in 24 hours Children maximum doses: Age 2–5: 3 mg Age 6–8: 3 mg Age 8–12: 6 mg	Acute and chronic
Diphenoxylate/ atropine	Adults: Two tablets (5 mg) initially, then one tablet every 3–4 hours, not to exceed 20 mg in 24 hours Children 2–12 years: Oral solution (avoid tablets) 0.3–0.4 mg/kg/day in divided doses. Do not administer to children younger than 2 years	Acute and chronic
Bismuth subsalicylate	Adults: 30 mL (regular strength) or 2 tablets, repeated every 30–60 minutes as needed. Maximum: 8 doses daily Children: Consumers should speak with a physician before giving to children under 12 years of age	Traveler's and nonspecific acute diarrhea

▶ Adsorbents and Bulk Agents

Attapulgite adsorbs excess fluid in the stool with few adverse effects. Formulations of attapulgite are available in Canada but not generally within the United States. Calcium polycarbophil is a hydrophilic polyacrylic resin (widely available in the United States) that also works as an adsorbent, binding about 60 times its weight in water and leading to the formation of a gel that enhances stool formation. Neither attapulgite nor polycarbophil is systemically absorbed. Calcium polycarbophil is effective in reducing fluid in the stool. However, caution must be exercised because it can also adsorb nutrients and other medications, thereby reducing their benefits. Its administration should be separated from other oral medications by 2 to 3 hours. Psyllium and methylcellulose products may also be used to reduce fluid in the stool and relieve chronic diarrhea.

▶ Antiperistaltic (Antimotility) Agents

Antiperistaltic drugs prolong intestinal transit time, thereby reducing the amount of fluid lost in the stool. The two drugs in this category are loperamide HCl (available over-the-counter as Imodium A–D and generically) and diphenoxylate HCl with atropine sulfate (available by prescription as Lomotil and generically). The atropine is included only as an abuse deterrent; when taken in large doses, the unpleasant anticholinergic effects of atropine negate the euphoric effect of diphenoxylate. Both loperamide and diphenoxylate are effective in relieving symptoms of acute noninfectious diarrhea and are safe for most patients experiencing chronic diarrhea. These products should be discontinued in patients whose diarrhea worsens despite therapy.

▶ Antisecretory Agents

Bismuth subsalicylate (BSS) is thought to have antisecretory and antimicrobial effects and is used to treat acute diarrhea. Although it passes largely unchanged through the GI tract, the salicylate portion is absorbed in the stomach and small intestine. For this reason, BSS should not be given to people who are allergic to salicylates, including aspirin. Caution should be exercised with regard to the total dose given to patients taking salicylates for other reasons to avoid salicylism. Patients taking BSS should be informed that their stool will turn black.

Octreotide is an antisecretory agent that has been used for severe secretory diarrhea associated with cancer chemotherapy, human immunodeficiency virus, diabetes, gastric resection, and GI tumors. It is administered as a subcutaneous or IV bolus injection in an initial dose of 50 mcg three times daily to assess the patient's tolerance to GI adverse effects. Biweekly serum levels of insulinlike growth factor (IGF)-1 or somatomedin C can be used as a guide to dose titration. Possible adverse effects include nausea, bloating, pain at the injection site, and gallstones (with prolonged therapy).

▶ Probiotics

Probiotics are dietary supplements containing bacteria that may promote health by enhancing the normal microflora of the GI tract while resisting colonization by potential pathogens. Probiotics can stimulate the immune response and suppress the inflammatory response. Yogurt can provide relief from diarrhea due to lactose intolerance. It supports digestion of lactose because the bacteria used to make yogurt produce lactase and digest the lactose before it reaches the colon. The *Lactobacillus acidophilus* in yogurt, cottage cheese, and acidophilus milk improve digestion of lactose and may prevent or relieve diarrhea related to lactose deficiency and milk intake. Although lactase is not a probiotic, lactase tablets may also be used to prevent diarrhea in susceptible patients.

▶ Antiinfectives

Empiric antibiotic therapy is an appropriate approach to traveler's diarrhea. Eradication of the causal microbe depends on the etiologic agent and its antibiotic sensitivity. Most cases of traveler's diarrhea and other community-acquired infections result from enterotoxigenic (ETEC) or enteropathogenic *Escherichia coli* (EPEC). Routine stool cultures do not identify these strains; primary empiric antibiotic choices include fluoroquinolones such as ciprofloxacin or levofloxacin. Azithromycin may be a feasible option when fluoroquinolone resistance is encountered. Rifaximin is another agent that can effectively treat traveler's diarrhea (see additional discussion of rifaximin in the irritable bowel syndrome section).

Patient Encounter 2

DT, a 48-year-old woman, lives in a rural community and works as an elementary school bus driver. She presents to the clinic complaining of fatigue, nausea, vomiting, episodes of mild abdominal pain, and frequent watery stools for the past 2 days. Her lips appear chapped, and she also states that she has been thirstier than usual and her saliva has been thick and sticky. She also states that her heart was racing after her evening walk the night before, which was atypical for her. She had been feeling tired over the past few days when workmen repairing her home's septic system occupied much of her time. Her husband took her temperature before bringing her to the clinic and said the reading was 100°F (37.8°C). She is otherwise healthy and reports no known allergies or medical conditions; she takes a multivitamin daily.

Assess the likelihood that DT's diarrhea is due to an invasive microorganism.

Identify which of her symptoms suggest the presence of dehydration.

Discuss potential treatment measures for this woman.

Although most cases of infectious diarrhea resolve with therapy, routine antibiotic use may contribute to antimicrobial resistance. Empiric treatment should be considered for other acute infectious diarrhea including those caused by nonhospital-acquired invasive organisms such as *Campylobacter*, *Salmonella*, and *Shigella* organisms producing moderate to severe fever, tenesmus, and bloody stools. Shiga toxin-producing *Escherichia coli* (STEC) O157 should not be treated with quinolones, trimethoprim-sulfamethoxazole, or antimotility agents.[13]

OUTCOME EVALUATION

- Monitor the patient with diarrhea from the point of first contact until symptoms resolve, keeping in mind that most episodes are self-limiting.
- Question the patient to determine whether symptom resolution occurs within 48 to 72 hours in acute diarrhea.
- Monitor for the maintenance of hydration, particularly when symptoms continue for more than 48 hours.

Patient Care and Monitoring for Diarrhea

1. Assess the patient's symptoms to determine if patient-directed therapy is appropriate or whether the patient should be evaluated by a physician. Determine the type of symptoms, severity, frequency, and exacerbating factors. Remember to inquire about recent foreign travel.

2. Determine if the patient is dehydrated.

3. Determine whether the patient has a history of disease that might be associated with diarrhea.

4. Obtain a thorough current history of prescription, nonprescription, and dietary supplement use. Remember to review the current therapy as a potential cause of diarrhea.

5. Determine if any diarrhea treatments have been attempted, including home remedies.

6. Medical referral is advised if the patient is pregnant, breast-feeding, younger than 3 or older than 70 years, or has multiple medical conditions.

7. If home care is recommended, provide clear instructions about how to proceed if symptoms do not improve or new symptoms emerge.

8. Discuss the importance of maintaining nutrition by modifying the diet.

9. Educate the patient about: (a) the causes of acute and chronic diarrhea, (b) the possible complications of diarrhea, (c) the goals of treatment for diarrhea, (d) the antidiarrheal medication used to manage acute or chronic diarrhea, and (e) if appropriate, the circumstances when antibiotics are used to treat diarrhea.

Look for increasing thirst, decreased urination, dark-colored urine, dry mucous membranes, and rapid heartbeat as suggestive of dehydration, especially when nausea and vomiting have been present.

- Monitor for symptom control in patients with chronic diarrhea.
- When antibiotics are used, monitor for completion of the course of therapy.

IRRITABLE BOWEL SYNDROME

IBS is a disorder of the GI tract that interferes with the normal functions of the colon. At various points in the past, IBS has been referred to as mucous colitis, spastic colon, irritable colon, or nervous stomach. ❼ *IBS is generally described as a functional disorder rather than a disease per se. A functional disorder involves symptoms that cannot be attributed to a specific injury, infection, or other physical problem. A functional disorder occurs because of altered physiologic processes rather than structural or biochemical defects and may be subject to nervous system influence.*

IBS is associated with frequent fluctuation in symptoms, loss of productivity, and decreased quality of life. Although IBS has been referred to as functional bowel disease, true functional bowel disease may be more indicative of widespread GI involvement including (but not limited to) the colon.

EPIDEMIOLOGY AND ETIOLOGY

IBS is one of the most common disorders seen in primary care and the most common reason for referral to gastroenterologists. Although between 15% and 20% of Americans suffer from IBS, only about one-quarter of those affected seek medical attention. The associated costs to society are estimated to be billions of dollars,[14] and the recurrent nature of IBS contributes to these costs through missed workdays, inattention on the job, and high consumption of health services.

In the United States, IBS affects women about twice as often as men. However, this may reflect a woman's tendency to seek medical care more often than a man. IBS can occur at any age but is most common between 20 and 50 years; onset beyond age 60 is rare. However, prevalence for older adults is the same as for young persons. Prevalence is similar in whites and African Americans but may be lower in people of Hispanic origin. A genetic link is unproven, but IBS seems more common in certain families.

There is a strong association between emotional distress and IBS. Psychosocial trauma (e.g., a history of abuse, recent death of a close relative or friend, or divorce) is more likely to be found in patients presenting with IBS than in the general population. An increased prevalence of psychiatric disorders such as anxiety, depression, personality disorders, and somatization (psychological distress expressed as physical symptoms) occurs among adult patients with IBS. Alcohol consumption and smoking have not been shown to be risk factors for developing IBS.[15] However, alcohol use can worsen symptoms in affected persons.

Some people show first evidence of IBS after contracting gastroenteritis (sometimes referred to as postinfectious IBS). This has led to speculation about whether infection heightens GI tract susceptibility. Women with IBS may have symptoms triggered by menstrual periods.

PATHOPHYSIOLOGY

Enteric nerves control intestinal smooth muscle action and are connected to the brain by the autonomic nervous system. IBS is thought to result from dysregulation of this "brain–gut axis." The enteric nervous system is composed of two ganglionated plexuses that control gut innervation: the submucous plexus (Meissner's plexus) and the myenteric plexus (Auerbach's plexus). The enteric nervous system and the CNS are interconnected and interdependent. A number of neurochemicals mediate their function, including serotonin (5-hydroxytryptamine or 5-HT), acetylcholine, substance P, and nitric oxide, among others.

Serotonin is of great importance because the GI tract contains the largest amounts in the body. Two 5-HT receptor subtypes, $5-HT_3$ and $5-HT_4$, are involved in gut motility, visceral sensitivity, and gut secretion. The $5-HT_3$ receptors slow colonic transit and increase fluid absorption, whereas $5-HT_4$ receptor stimulation results in accelerated colonic transit.

Although no single pathologic defect has been found to account for the pattern of exacerbations and remissions seen in IBS, CNS abnormalities, dysmotility, visceral hypersensitivity, and a number of other factors have been implicated.[16]

The passage of fluids into and out of the colon is regulated by epithelial cells. In IBS, the colonic lining (epithelium) appears to work properly. However, increased movement of the contents in the colon can overwhelm its absorptive capacity. Disturbed intestinal motility appears to be a central feature of IBS, which leads to altered stool consistency. Studies suggest that the colon of IBS sufferers is abnormally sensitive to normal stimuli.[17] This enhanced visceral sensitivity manifests as pain, especially related to gut distention.

IBS activity may be affected by the immune system. Some IBS patients have been found to have antibodies that may indicate food hypersensitivity that might be involved in symptom production.[18] Specifically, sensitivity has been demonstrated to common foods such as wheat, beef, pork, soy, and eggs. Recent evidence suggest that an immune component may be involved in IBS patients who experience bloating and dysmotility-like dyspepsia and that gender specificity exists.[19]

CLINICAL PRESENTATION AND DIAGNOSIS

Refer to the box on the next page for the clinical presentation of IBS.

Diagnosis

❾ *The diagnosis of IBS is made by symptom-based criteria and the exclusion of organic disease.* IBS is diagnosed by obtaining a careful and thorough history to identify symptoms characteristic of the disorder. It is equally important to distinguish among IBS and conditions having similar symptoms. Patients should be questioned about the character of their stools. This should include questions about frequency, consistency, color, and size. Moreover, because of the functional nature of IBS, a patient may present with symptoms of upper GI problems such as gastroesophageal reflux disease or with excessive flatulence. Patients should also be questioned about diet to determine whether symptoms seem to occur in relationship to meals or specifically after consumption of certain dietary products.

Barium enema, sigmoidoscopy, or colonoscopy may be indicated in the presence of red flag symptoms (fever, weight loss, bleeding, and anemia, possibly accompanied by persistent severe pain), which often point to a potentially serious non-IBS problem. A barium enema may identify polyps, diverticulosis, tumors, or other abnormalities that might be responsible for the symptoms. In addition, exaggerated haustral contractions may be noted with barium enema. Such contractions impede stool movement and contribute to constipation. Flexible sigmoidoscopy can be performed to identify obstruction in the rectum and lower colon, whereas colonoscopy can evaluate the entire colon for organic disease.

IBS diagnosis has long been symptom based. Manning defined the first widely used practical criteria: (a) abdominal pain relieved by defecation with either (i) looser stools with pain onset, or (ii) frequent stools with pain onset; (b) abdominal distention; (c) mucus in the stool; and (d) sensation of incomplete evacuation.[14,20]

The Rome III criteria are the most current diagnostic criteria and can also be applied clinically.[2] They presume the absence of a structural or biochemical explanation for the symptoms. The Rome III criteria define IBS as occurring when symptoms of recurrent abdominal pain or discomfort exist for at least 3 days/month in the last 3 months associated with two or more of the following: (a) improvement with defecation, (b) onset associated with a change in the frequency of stool, and/or (c) onset associated with a change in the form (appearance) of stool. These criteria should be fulfilled for the previous 3 months with symptom onset at least 6 months prior to diagnosis. IBS is unlikely if symptom onset occurs in old age, the disorder has a steady but aggressive course, or the patient experiences frequent awakening because of symptoms.

TREATMENT

General Approach to Treatment

❿ *The principal goal of IBS treatment is to reduce or control symptoms.* The treatment strategy is based on: (a) the prevailing symptoms and their severity, (b) the degree of functional impairment, and (c) the presence of psychological

Clinical Presentation of IBS

Symptoms

- Patients report a history of abdominal pain or discomfort that is relieved with defecation. Symptom onset is associated with change in frequency or appearance of stool. Some persons experience hard, dry stools, whereas others experience loose or watery stools. Some stools may be small and pellet-like in appearance; others may be narrow and pencil-like.

- ❽ *Symptoms can typically be categorized as either IBS with diarrhea (IBS-D) or IBS with constipation (IBS-C). Patients with IBS-D usually report more than three loose or watery stools daily. Those with IBS-C usually have fewer than three bowel movements per week; stools are typically hard and lumpy and accompanied by straining. However, stool frequency may be normal in many cases. The Rome III diagnostic criteria (see Diagnosis) place more emphasis on stool form unlike Rome II, which emphasized frequency.*

- Although many patients fit into one of these subtypes, some patients report alternating episodes of diarrhea and constipation (irritable bowel syndrome with constipation and diarrhea [IBS-M], where M represents mixed).

- Other common symptoms include: (a) feelings of incomplete evacuation, (b) abdominal fullness, (c) bloating, (d) flatulence, (e) passage of clear or white mucus with a stool, and (f) occasional fecal incontinence.

- Periods of normal stools and bowel function are punctuated by episodes of sudden symptoms.

- Symptoms are often exacerbated by stress.

- Left lower quadrant abdominal pain is often brought on or made worse by eating. Passage of stool or flatus may provide some relief.

- IBS-C can often be distinguished from functional constipation primarily by the presence of abdominal pain and discomfort. Although pain and discomfort may be present in some patients with functional constipation, it is an expected feature of IBS.

- Patients with IBS may experience comorbidities outside the GI tract such as fibromyalgia, sleep disturbances, headaches, dyspareunia, and temporomandibular joint syndrome.

Signs

- The physical examination is often normal in IBS.

- The patient may appear to be anxious.

- Palpation of the abdomen may reveal left lower quadrant tenderness, which may indicate a tender sigmoid colon.

- Abdominal distention may be present in some cases.

- The following "red flag" or alarm features are *not* associated with IBS and may indicate inflammatory bowel disease, cancer, or other disorders: fever, weight loss, bleeding, and anemia, which may be accompanied by persistent severe pain.

Laboratory Tests

- In most cases, laboratory testing reveals no abnormalities in IBS, but certain tests can be used to identify other causes for the patient's symptoms.

- CBC may identify anemia, which may suggest blood loss and an organic source for GI symptoms.

- Serum electrolytes and chemistries may indicate metabolic causes of symptoms.

- Thyroid-stimulating hormone (TSH) should be ordered when thyroid dysfunction is suspected. Hypothyroidism may be responsible for constipation and related symptoms.

- Stool testing for ova and parasites may identify *C. difficile* and amoebae as possible causes of diarrhea rather than IBS.

- Fecal leukocytes can be found in inflammatory diarrhea, especially when due to invasive microorganisms.

- A positive stool guaiac test indicating blood in the GI tract does not support a diagnosis of IBS.

- An elevated erythrocyte sedimentation rate is consistent with a systemic inflammatory process such as inflammatory bowel disease rather than IBS.

- Testing for lactase deficiency can confirm the presence of lactose intolerance, which may explain the symptoms.

---

components. A standard treatment regimen is not possible because of the heterogeneous nature of the IBS patient population. Patients suffering from IBS can benefit from clinician support and reassurance, because specific pathology is unlikely to be found.

Nonpharmacologic Therapy

▶ *Diet and Other General Modifications*

Dietary modification is a standard therapeutic modality. Food hypersensitivities and adverse effects are thought to occur widely in IBS patients, especially those with IBS with diarrhea subtype. Elimination diets are the most commonly used strategy, usually focusing on milk and dairy products, fructose and sorbitol, wheat, and beef. Flatulence may be controlled by reducing gas-causing foods such as beans, celery, onions, prunes, bananas, carrots, and raisins. Response to elimination diets varies widely, but they may be useful in individual patients. Care must be taken to avoid creating nutritional deficits while attempting to eliminate an offending food.

Probiotics may also be an option for some patients with IBS. *Bifidobacterium infantis* is one product used for its effect in

Patient Encounter 3, Part 1

A recently divorced 33-year-old African American woman presents to the clinic complaining of headaches, sleep disturbances, cramping abdominal pain, bloating, excessive flatulence, and loose watery stools. When asked to show where her abdomen hurts, she specifically points to both her lower left and lower right abdomen. She indicates that the pain seems to lessen after a bowel movement. Further, she states the symptoms have become worse over the last month, alternating between episodes of watery stools and hard, dry stools that make it difficult to defecate. During some weeks, her diarrheal episodes cause her to call in sick to work. During other weeks, she can go a couple of days without a single bowel movement. She recently canceled a trip to California with friends because she was worried about her body "acting up." She was diagnosed with fibromyalgia 7 months ago and reports that her deceased mother (7 years ago) had irritable bowel syndrome. Her doctor started nortriptyline to treat fibromyalgia. She states that the nortriptyline has helped but not eliminated her joint and muscle pain.

Identify symptoms characteristic of IBS in this patient.

Discuss how this patient fits within the typical epidemiologic profile of patients with IBS.

Patient Encounter 3, Part 2

Upon further questioning, the patient recalls experiencing similar symptoms 7 years ago when her mother lost her battle to lung cancer. She never sought medical attention because her symptoms slowly subsided within a few weeks after her mother's funeral. She is a full-time pharmacy technician and recently started studying for the PCAT, which she plans to take in a couple of months. Her diet consists mostly of frozen dinners and fast food to fit her busy lifestyle.

PMH: Insomnia, headaches, fibromyalgia

FH: Mother had IBS (unspecified type)

SH: Smokes occasionally (during times of stress) and has a glass of wine with dinner.

Meds:

Nortriptyline 25 mg by mouth three times daily for fibromyalgia

Edluar 10 mg one sublingually at bedtime as needed for insomnia

Ibuprofen 600 mg by mouth every 6 hours as needed for headache

Loperamide 2 mg by mouth as needed for diarrhea

Docusate sodium 100 mg by mouth as needed for constipation

Allergies: Penicillin (rash, hives, and difficulty breathing after taking amoxicillin at the age of 9).

PE:

General: Well nourished; somewhat anxious and nervous when speaking.

VS: BP 129/82 mmHg; Pulse 85 bpm; RR 18 breaths/min; Temperature 97.4°F (36.3°C); Height 5′4″ (163 cm); Weight 104 lbs (47.3 kg)

Integ: Nails are chewed up; skin appears dry and scaly

HEENT: PERRLA, EOMI

Ext: Normal, no swelling

Chest: Clear to A and P bilaterally

CV: RRR

Abd: (+) BS, tender LLQ and LRQ

Rectal: No abnormalities, negative stool guaiac test.

Which of this patient's findings are indicative of IBS?

Propose a comprehensive treatment approach to IBS in this patient. Where appropriate, consider the presence and influence of comorbidities.

---

constipation, diarrhea, gaseousness, bloating, and abdominal discomfort. Reportedly, it is not associated with significant untoward effects.[21] The usual dose is one 4-mg capsule daily.

▶ Psychological Treatments

Psychotherapy focused on reducing the influence of the CNS on the gut has been studied. Cognitive behavioral therapy (CBT), dynamic psychotherapy, relaxation therapy, and hypnotherapy have been reported to be effective in some patients. However, psychological approaches are not considered replacements for usual care.[22]

Pharmacologic Therapy

▶ Botanicals

Peppermint oil is widely advocated; it acts as an antispasmodic agent due to its ability to relax GI smooth muscle. However, it also relaxes the lower esophageal sphincter, which could allow reflux of gastric contents into the esophagus. The usual dose is 1 to 2 enteric-coated capsules containing 0.2 mL of peppermint oil two to three times daily.

Matricaria recutita, known as German chamomile, is also purported to have antispasmodic properties. It is taken most often as a tea up to four times a day. Benzodiazepine, alcohol, and warfarin users should be cautioned against taking this product because it can cause drowsiness, and it contains

coumarin derivatives.[23] Primrose oil is used by some patients, but evidence of effectiveness is lacking.

▶ Antispasmodics

Antispasmodic agents such as dicyclomine or hyoscyamine have been among the most frequently used medications for treating abdominal pain in patients with IBS (Table 21–5). Side effects include blurred vision, constipation, urinary retention, and (rarely) psychosis. Although their effectiveness remains unconfirmed, these drugs may deserve a trial in patients with intermittent postprandial pain.[14,20]

▶ Antidepressants

Tricyclic antidepressants (TCAs) such as amitriptyline and doxepin have been used with some success in the treatment of IBS-related pain (Table 21–5). They modulate pain principally through their effect on neurotransmitter reuptake, especially norepinephrine and serotonin. Their helpfulness in functional GI disorders seems independent of mood-altering effects normally associated with these agents. Low-dose TCAs (e.g., amitriptyline, desipramine, or doxepin 10 to 25 mg daily) may help patients with IBS who predominantly experience diarrhea or pain.

Table 21–5
Common Pharmacologic Treatments for IBS

Generic (Brand) Name	Dose
Antispasmodics	
Dicyclomine (Bentyl)	10–20 mg po every 4–6 hours as needed
Hyoscyamine (Levsin)	0.125–0.25 po mg or sublingually every 4 hours as needed
Propantheline bromide (Pro-Banthine)	15 mg po 3 times a day (before meals) and 30 mg at bedtime
Clidinium bromide plus chlordiazepoxide HCl (Librax)	5–10 mg po 3–4 times a day
Hyoscyamine, scopolamine, atropine, phenobarbital (Donnatal)	1–2 tablets po 3–4 times daily
Tricyclic Antidepressants (TCAs)	**In IBS with Diarrhea:**
Amitriptyline	50–150 mg po daily
Doxepin	10–150 mg po daily
Selective Serotonin-Reuptake Inhibitors	**In IBS with Constipation:**
Paroxetine (others can be used)	10–40 mg po daily
Bulk-Forming Laxatives	
Psyllium (Metamucil)	2.5–4 g po daily
Methylcellulose (Citrucel)	4–6 g po daily
Antimotility Agents	
Loperamide (Imodium A/D)	4 mg po; then 2 mg po after each loose stool; daily maximum: 16 mg
5-HT$_3$ Receptor Antagonist	
Alosetron (Lotronex)[a]	1 mg po daily
5-HT$_4$ Receptor Agonist	
Tegaserod maleate (Zelnorm)[b]	6 mg po twice daily

[a]Withdrawn from general use; available only under special circumstances.

[b]Withdrawn from general use; available only as emergency treatment.

The selective serotonin-reuptake inhibitors (SSRIs) paroxetine, fluoxetine, and sertraline are potentially useful due to the significant effect of serotonin in the gut. SSRIs principally act on 5-HT$_1$ or 5-HT$_2$ receptors, but they can also have some effect on gut-predominant 5-HT$_3$ and 5-HT$_4$ receptors, perhaps reducing visceral hypersensitivity. They may be beneficial for patients with IBS-C or when the patient presents with IBS complicated by a mood disorder.[24] Serotonin–norepinephrine reuptake inhibitors may offer some benefit in IBS patients who also have depression or anxiety accompanied by significant pain.

▶ Bulk Producers

Bulk producers may improve stool passage in IBS-C but are unlikely to have a favorable effect on pain or global IBS symptoms.[24] Psyllium may increase flatulence, which may worsen discomfort in some patients. Methylcellulose products are less likely to increase gas production. Although fiber-based supplements are more likely to be useful in IBS-C, these products may be dose adjusted in diarrhea to increase stool consistency. Other laxative products might be used in IBS-C, but most are less desirable than bulking agents due to the potential for unwanted effects.

▶ Antimotility Agents

Loperamide stimulates enteric nervous system receptors, inhibiting peristalsis and fluid secretion. It improves stool consistency and reduces the number of stools.[24] Consequently, it is most useful in patients who have diarrhea as a prominent symptom. However, it does not lessen abdominal pain and can occasionally aggravate the pain.

▶ Alosetron

Stimulation of 5-HT$_3$ receptors triggers hypersensitivity and hyperactivity of the large intestine. Alosetron (Lotronex), a selective 5-HT$_3$ antagonist, blocks these receptors and is used to treat women with severe IBS-D. Eligible patients should have frequent and severe abdominal pain, frequent bowel urgency or incontinence, and restricted daily activities. Alosetron has been shown to improve overall symptoms and quality of life. Alosetron can cause constipation in some patients.

Because alosetron has been associated with ischemic colitis, it can be prescribed only under strict guidelines, including signing of a consent form by both patient and physician. Patients selected for therapy should exhibit severe chronic IBS symptoms and should have failed to respond to conventional therapy.

▶ Tegaserod Maleate

Tegaserod maleate (Zelnorm) stimulates 5-HT$_4$ receptors in the GI tract, thereby increasing intestinal secretion, peristalsis, and small bowel transit. It also reduces sensitivity related to abdominal distention. It has been shown to be more effective than placebo in improving global IBS symptoms and altered bowel habits in IBS-C.[24] However, because of a higher risk of heart attack, stroke, and unstable angina (heart/chest pain) in patients treated with tegaserod maleate, the drug has been withdrawn from the market. The FDA can authorize use of tegaserod maleate for emergency situations only. The FDA must also authorize the drug to be shipped.

▶ *Rifaximin*

Rifaximin (Xifaxan) is a semisynthetic antibiotic with very low systemic absorption. It is believed that bacterial overgrowth plays a role in some IBS patients and that some antibiotics might be helpful. Rifaximin's lack of absorption reduces the likelihood of adverse effects, and its good antibacterial activity coupled with low microbial resistance make it a promising agent for a segment of the IBS population.[25] However, it did not carry FDA-approved labeling for this indication at the time of this writing.

OUTCOME EVALUATION

- Because symptoms vary in intensity and among patients, a specific drug therapy may not lead to equivalent symptom abatement in different patients.

- Monitor for adequate relief of symptoms. Patients whose pain does not respond to drug therapy may have a psychological comorbid condition and may require psychiatric intervention.

- Specifically, monitor for relief of pain if present initially. Monitor patients with symptoms of constipation or diarrhea for frequency, appearance, and size of stools in relationship to their normal characteristics. As stools normalize, associated symptoms such as bloating and abdominal distention should resolve.

- For IBS-C patients taking bulk producers, monitor for relief of constipation. Hard stools should become softer within 72 hours. IBS-M patients may gain relief with these agents as well.

- Monitor antidepressant therapy for relief of lower abdominal pain.

- Antispasmodics may provide limited relief of crampy abdominal pain.

- Assess 5-HT$_4$ receptor agonists (tegaserod) for relief of crampy abdominal pain and bloating.

- Evaluate 5-HT$_3$ receptor antagonists (alosetron) for relief of abdominal pain and fecal incontinence.

- Antimotility agents should be expected to reduce stool frequency and control diarrhea.

- Monitor complete blood cell count, serum electrolytes and chemistries, stool guaiac, and erythrocyte

Patient Care and Monitoring for IBS

1. Assess symptoms to determine if patient-directed therapy is appropriate or whether physician evaluation is needed.

2. Determine the type, severity, and frequency of symptoms and possible exacerbating factors.

3. Listen attentively to the patient's complaints and reassure the patient to allay fears about invasive disease.

4. Obtain a thorough current history of prescription, nonprescription, and dietary supplement use.

5. Determine if any IBS treatments have been attempted and how effective they have been.

6. Determine whether the patient has received educational intervention about IBS, health promotion, and symptom prevention measures.

7. Provide patient education about IBS symptoms, lifestyle modifications, and drug therapy for IBS:

   - Explain how to use medications relative to symptom intensity.
   - If taking alosetron, determine nonadherence with special use requirements.
   - Describe potential adverse effects.
   - List drugs that may interact with the therapy.
   - Discuss what to do if red flag symptoms occur.

sedimentation rate yearly for changes that might signal an overlapping organic problem.

- Refer any patient presenting with red flag signs for medical evaluation.

Abbreviations Introduced in This Chapter

BSS	Bismuth subsalicylate
CBT	Cognitive behavioral therapy
EPEC	Enteropathogenic *Escherichia coli*
ETEC	Enterotoxigenic *E. coli*
FGID	Functional gastrointestinal disorder
IBS	Irritable bowel syndrome
IBS-C	Irritable bowel syndrome with constipation
IBS-D	Irritable bowel syndrome with diarrhea
IBS-M	Irritable bowel syndrome with constipation and diarrhea (mixed)
ORS	Oral rehydration solution
TCA	Tricyclic antidepressant

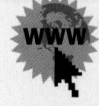 Self-assessment questions and answers are available at *http://www.mhpharmacotherapy. com/pp.html.*

REFERENCES

1. Brandt L, Schoenfeld P, Prather C, et al. American College of Gastroenterology Functional Gastrointestinal Disorders Task Force. An evidence based approach to the management of chronic constipation in North America. Am J Gastroenterol 2005;100:S1–S21.

2. Drossman DA. The functional gastrointestinal disorders and the Rome III process. Gastroenterology 2006;130:1377–1390.

3. Locke GR, Pemberton JH, Phillips SF. American Gastroenterological Association medical position statement on constipation. Gastroenterology 2000;119:1766–1778.

4. Irvine EJ, Ferrazzi S, Pare P. Health-related quality of life in functional GI disorders: Focus on constipation and resource utilization. Am J Gastroenterol 1998;97:1986–1993.

5. Sonnenberg A, Koch TR. Physician visits in the United States for constipation: 1958 to 1986. Dig Dis Sci 1989;34:606–611.

6. Drossman DA, Li Z, Andruzzi E, et al. US householder survey of functional gastrointestinal disorders: Prevalence, sociodemography, and health impact. Dig Dis Sci 1993;38:1569–1580.

7. Longstreth GF, Thompson WG, Chey WD. Functional bowel disorders. Gastroenterology 2006;130:1480–1491.

8. Heymen S, Scarlett Y, Jones K, et al. Randomized, controlled trial shows biofeedback to be superior to alternative treatments for patients with pelvic floor dyssynergia-type constipation. Dis Colon Rectum 2007;50(4):428–441.

9. Lembo A, Camilleri M. Chronic constipation. N Engl J Med 2003;349:1360–1368.

10. Amitiza [package insert]. Bethesda, MD: Sucampo Pharmaceuticals, 2006.

11. Gadewar S, Fasano A. Current concepts in the evaluation, diagnosis and management of acute infectious diarrhea. Curr Opin Pharmacol 2005;5(6):559–565.

12. Pawlowski SW, Warren CA, Guerrant R. Diagnosis and treatment of acute or persistent diarrhea. Gastroenterology 2009;136:1874–1886.

13. Thielman NM, Guerrant RL. Acute infectious diarrhea. N Engl J Med 2004;350:38–47.

14. Changa JY, Talley NJ. An update on irritable bowel syndrome: From diagnosis to emerging therapies Curr Opin Gastroenterol 2011; 27:72–78.

15. Cremonini F, Talley NJ. Irritable bowel syndrome: Epidemiology, natural history, health care seeking, and emerging risk factors. Gastroenterol Clin North Am 2005;34:189–204.

16. Gunnarsson J, Simén M. Peripheral factors in the pathophysiology of irritable bowel syndrome. Dig Liver Dis 2009;41(1):788–793.

17. Schwetz I, Bradesi S, Mayer EA. The pathophysiology of irritable bowel syndrome. Minerva Med 2004;95:418–426.

18. Atkinson W, Sheldon TA, Shaath N, et al. Food elimination based on IgG antibodies in irritable bowel syndrome: A randomised controlled trial. Gut 2004;53:1459–1464.

19. Cremon C, Gargano L, Morselli-Labate AM, et al. Mucosal immune activation in irritable bowel syndrome: Gender-dependence and association with digestive symptoms. Am J Gastroenterol 2009;104(2):401–403.

20. Thoua NM, Murray CD. Motility and functional bowel disease: Irritable bowel syndrome. Gastroenterology 2011;39(4):214–217.

21. O'Mahony L, McCarthy J, Kelly P, et al. *Lactobacillus and Bifidobacterium* in irritable bowel syndrome: Symptom responses and relationship to cytokine profiles. Gastroenterology 2005;128:541–551.

22. Zijdenbos IL, de Wit NJ, van der Heijden GJ, et al. Psychological treatments for the management of irritable bowel syndrome. Cochrane Database Syst Rev 2009:CD006442.

23. Miller LG. Herbal medicinals: Selected clinical considerations focusing on known or potential drug-herb interactions. Arch Intern Med 1998;158:2200–2211.

24. Schoenfeld P. Efficacy of current drug therapies in irritable bowel syndrome: What works and does not work. Gastroenterol Clin North Am 2005;34:319–335.

25. Drossman DA. Rifaximin for treatment of irritable bowel syndrome. Gastroenterol Hepatol 2011;7(3):180–181.

REFERENCES

1. Brandt LJ, Schoenfeld P, Prather C, et al. American College of Gastroenterology Functional Gastrointestinal Disorders Task Force. An evidence-based approach to the management of chronic constipation in North America. Am J Gastroenterol 2005;100:1–S21.

2. Drossman DA. The functional gastrointestinal disorders and the Rome III process. Gastroenterology 2006;130:1377–1390.

3. Locke GR, Pemberton JH, Phillips SF. American Gastroenterological Association medical position statement on constipation. Gastroenterology 2000;119:1761–1778.

4. Irvine EJ, Ferrazzi S, Pare P. Health-related quality of life in functional GI disorders: focus on constipation and resource utilization. Am J Gastroenterol 2002;97:1986–1993.

5. Sonnenberg A, Koch TR. Physician visits in the United States for constipation: 1958 to 1986. Dig Dis Sci 1989;34:606–611.

6. Pare P, Ferrazzi S, Thompson WG, et al. An epidemiological survey of constipation in Canada: definitions, rates, demographics, and predictors of health care seeking. Am J Gastroenterol 2001;96:3130–3137.

7. Higgins PD, Johanson JF. Epidemiology of constipation in North America: a systematic review. Am J Gastroenterol 2004;99:750–759.

8. Heymen S, Scarlett Y, Jones K, et al. Randomized, controlled trial shows biofeedback to be superior to alternative treatments for patients with pelvic floor dyssynergia-type constipation. Dis Colon Rectum 2007;50:428–441.

9. Lembo A, Camilleri M. Chronic constipation. N Engl J Med 2003;349:1360–1368.

10. Ashraf W, Park F, Lof J, Quigley EM. An examination of the reliability of reported stool frequency in the diagnosis of idiopathic constipation. Am J Gastroenterol 1996;91:26–32.

11. Lembo A, Camilleri M. Current concepts in the evaluation, diagnosis and management of non-infectious diarrhea. Curr Opin Pharmacol 2008;8:636–642.

12. Thielman NM, Guerrant RL. Acute infectious diarrhea. N Engl J Med 2004;350:38–47.

13. DuPont HL, Hornick RB. An update on traveler's diarrhea: diagnosis, treatment, and prevention. Curr Opin Gastroenterol 2011;27:272–278.

14. Cremonini F, Talley NJ. Irritable bowel syndrome: epidemiology, natural history, health care seeking and emerging risk factors. Gastroenterol Clin North Am 2005;34:189–204.

15. Quigley EM, Abdel-Hamid H, Barbara G, et al. A global perspective on irritable bowel syndrome: a consensus statement of the World Gastroenterology Organisation Summit Task Force on irritable bowel syndrome. J Clin Gastroenterol 2012;46:356–366.

16. Grundmann O, Yoon SL. Irritable bowel syndrome: epidemiology, diagnosis and treatment: an update for health-care practitioners. J Gastroenterol Hepatol 2010;25:691–699.

17. Camilleri M, Chang L. Challenges to the therapeutic pipeline for irritable bowel syndrome: end points and regulatory hurdles. Gastroenterology 2008;135:1877–1891.

18. Quartero AO, Meineche-Schmidt V, Muris J, et al. Bulking agents, antispasmodic and antidepressant medication for the treatment of irritable bowel syndrome. Cochrane Database Syst Rev 2005;CD003460.

19. Mayer EA. Clinical practice. Irritable bowel syndrome. N Engl J Med 2008;358:1692–1699.

20. Schoenfeld P. Efficacy of current drug therapies in irritable bowel syndrome: what works and does not work. Gastroenterol Clin North Am 2005;34:319–335.

21. Drossman DA. Do the various treatments of irritable bowel syndrome. Gastrointestinal Hepatol 2013;7:380–381.

22 Portal Hypertension and Cirrhosis

Laurajo Ryan

KEY CONCEPTS

❶ Portal hypertension is the precipitating factor for many of the complications of cirrhosis. Lowering portal pressure can reduce the complications of cirrhosis and decrease morbidity and mortality.

❷ Chronic excessive ethanol intake causes progressive liver damage primarily because both ethanol and its metabolic products are direct hepatotoxins.

❸ Cirrhosis is irreversible; treatments are directed at limiting disease progression and minimizing complications.

❹ Nonselective β-blockers are first-line treatment for preventing variceal bleeding; they vasoconstrict the splanchnic bed through multiple mechanisms.

❺ The goals of treating ascites are to minimize acute discomfort, reequilibrate ascitic fluid, and prevent spontaneous bacterial peritonitis (SBP). Treatment should modify the underlying disease pathology; without directed therapy, fluid will rapidly reaccumulate.

❻ Cirrhosis is a high aldosterone state; spironolactone is a direct aldosterone antagonist and the primary treatment for ascites.

❼ Acute variceal hemorrhage is an emergency. It is crucial to control bleeding, decrease risk of rebleeding, and prevent SBP.

❽ Long-term antibiotic prophylaxis for SBP decreases mortality in patients with a history of SBP or low-protein ascites plus one of the following: serum creatinine (SCr) 1.5 mg/dL (133 μmol/L) or greater, blood urea nitrogen (BUN) 25 mg/dL (8.9 mmol/L) or greater, serum sodium 130 mEq/L (130 mmol/L) or less, or Child–Pugh score of at least 9, with bilirubin of at least 3 mg/dL (51.3 μmol/L).

❾ Lactulose is the foundation of pharmacotherapy to prevent and treat hepatic encephalopathy (HE). It binds ammonia in its ionic form in the gut and facilitates its excretion.

INTRODUCTION

Cirrhosis is the progressive replacement of normal hepatic cells with fibrous scar tissue. This scarring is accompanied by the loss of viable hepatocytes, which are the functional cells of the liver. ❶ *Cirrhosis is irreversible and leads to portal hypertension, which is in turn responsible for many of the complications of advanced liver disease. Cirrhotic complications include (but are not limited to) ascites, spontaneous bacterial peritonitis (SBP), hepatic encephalopathy (HE), hepatorenal syndrome (HRS), and variceal bleeding.*[1]

EPIDEMIOLOGY AND ETIOLOGY

Cirrhosis is the result of long-term insult to the liver; damage is typically not evident clinically until the fourth decade of life. Chronic liver disease and cirrhosis combined were the 12th leading cause of death in the United States in 2007. In patients between the ages of 25 and 64 years, damage from excessive alcohol use accounted for over one-half of the deaths.[2] Alcoholic liver disease and viral hepatitis C are the most common causes of cirrhosis in the United States, whereas hepatitis B accounts for the majority of cases worldwide.[3] Once cirrhosis is diagnosed, the disease progression is similar, regardless of the initial insult to the liver.

Estimates vary, but alcoholic cirrhosis can develop with as little as 2 to 3 drinks per day in women and 3 to 4 drinks per day in men, although 5 to 8 drinks per day is more typical.[4] A standard drink (14 g of ethanol) is equivalent to 1.5 oz (45 mL) of hard liquor, 5 oz (150 mL) of wine, or a 12-oz (360-mL) beer. With equivalent alcohol intake; women usually develop cirrhosis more quickly than men. Differences in alcohol metabolism may account for this gender disparity; women metabolize less alcohol in the GI tract; this allows delivery of more ethanol (which is directly hepatotoxic) to the liver.[5] Genetic factors also play a role in alcoholic liver disease; some people progress to cirrhosis with much less cumulative alcohol intake than that of a typical cirrhotic patient (either fewer drinks per day or faster disease development), whereas others do not develop the disease even with more excessive intake.

Infection with one or more strains of viral hepatitis causes acute, potentially reversible, hepatic inflammation, whereas chronic infection with hepatitis B or C can lead to cirrhosis. Hepatitis B and C are common in IV drug users (direct blood transmission) or sexual contact (common route of hepatitis B transmission). Many cases of hepatitis C are idiopathic.[6] See Chapter 24, "Viral Hepatitis," for a complete discussion of infectious hepatitis.

Between 30% and 40% of patients with cirrhosis can be expected to experience a variceal bleed at some point in their disease.[7] Variceal bleeding carries a remarkably high mortality rate; 6-week mortality is as high as 30% in patients with advanced disease. Mortality correlates with disease severity; risk factors include poor liver function, large varices, and red signs (wales) on endoscopic examination.[8] More than two-thirds of patients who survive the first incidence of variceal bleeding experience a repeat episode.

Development of ascites in cirrhotic patients is a particularly ominous marker; 2-year mortality after initial presentation with ascites is approximately 50%.[9] In addition to the high mortality rate, cirrhosis carries an enormous economic and social burden from hospitalizations, lost wages, and decreased productivity, not to mention the emotional strain of the disease on both patients and families.

Determining the specific cause of cirrhosis requires examination of both physical presentation and a thorough past medical history. An accurate social history is particularly important because few factors in the physical or laboratory examination indicate disease etiology. Identifying the cause of cirrhosis is imperative; disease etiology can affect treatment decisions and therapeutic options.

PATHOPHYSIOLOGY

Portal Hypertension and Cirrhosis

The portal vein is the primary vessel leading into the liver; it receives deoxygenated venous blood from the splanchnic bed (intestines, stomach, pancreas, and spleen) (**Fig. 22–1**). Portal flow accounts for approximately 75% of blood delivered to the liver (approximately 1 to 1.5 L/min in noncirrhotics). The hepatic artery provides the remaining 25% in the form of oxygenated blood from the abdominal aorta. Normal portal vein pressure is 5 to 10 mm Hg; this maintains liver blood flow of approximately 1 L/min. **Portal hypertension** occurs when portal pressure exceeds 10 to 12 mm Hg.[10]

Portal hypertension is a consequence of increased resistance to blood flow through the portal vein. This is often a result of restructuring of intrahepatic tissue (sinusoidal damage) but may also be caused by presinusoidal (prehepatic) injury such as portal vein occlusion from trauma, malignancy, or thrombosis. The third (and least common) cause of portal hypertension is outflow obstruction of the hepatic vein. Hepatic vein obstruction is considered posthepatic; normal liver structure is maintained. This chapter focuses on portal hypertension caused by intrahepatic damage from cirrhosis.

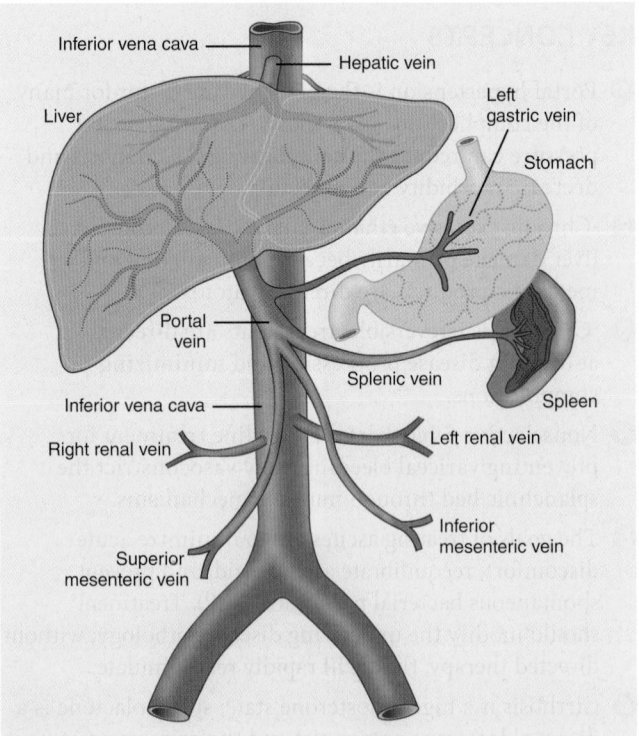

FIGURE 22–1. The portal venous system. (From Sease JM. Portal hypertension and cirrhosis. In: DiPiro JT, Talbert RL, Yee GC, et al., eds. Pharmacotherapy: A Pathophysiologic Approach, 8th ed. New York, NY: McGraw-Hill, 2011:640, with permission.)

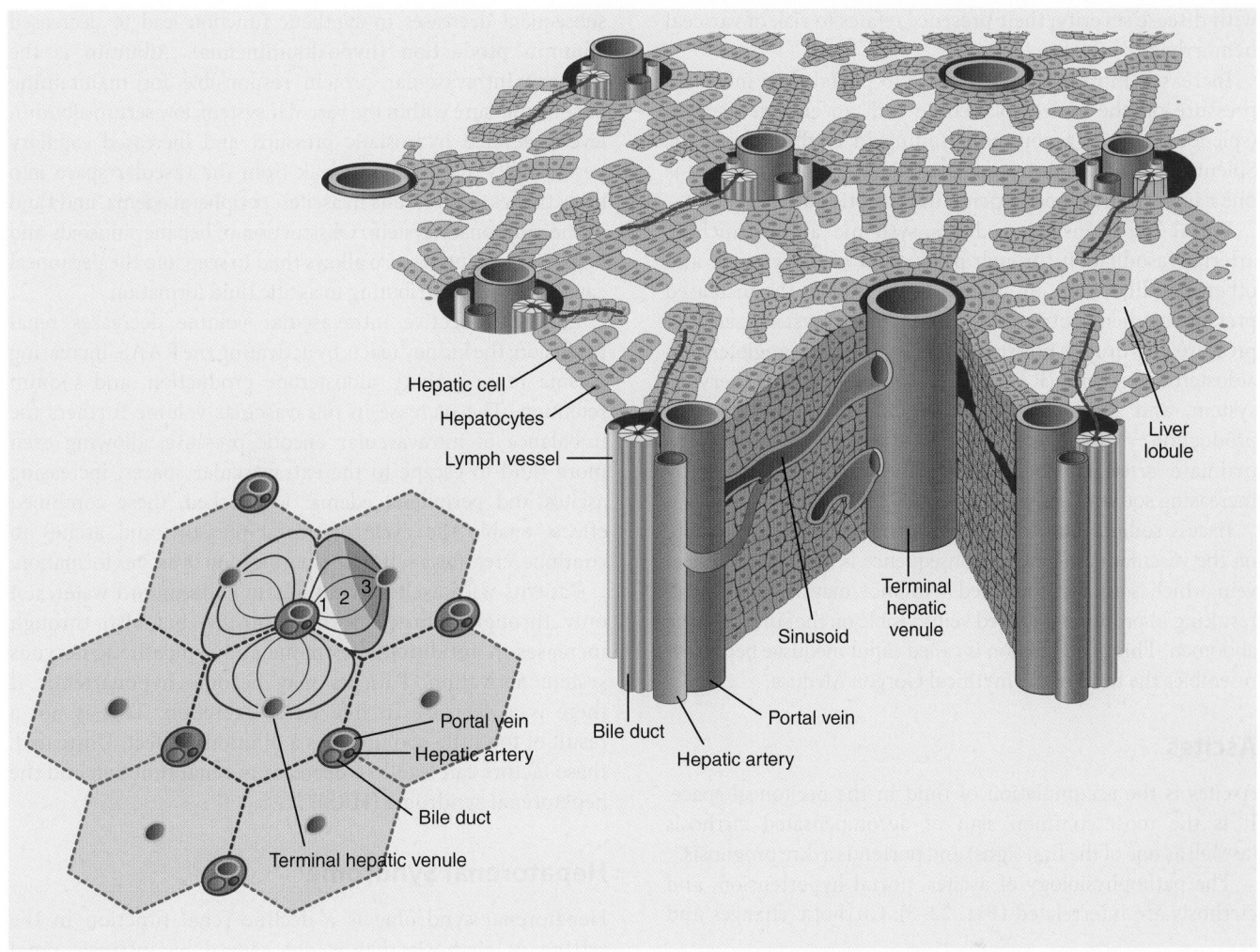

FIGURE 22–2. Relationship of sinusoids to hepatocytes and the venous system. (From Sease JM. Portal hypertension and cirrhosis. In: DiPiro JT, Talbert RL, Yee GC, et al., eds. *Pharmacotherapy: A Pathophysiologic Approach*, 8th ed. New York, NY: McGraw-Hill, 2011:641, with permission.)

Sinusoidal damage from cirrhosis is the most common cause of portal hypertension. The sinusoids are porous vessels within the liver that surround radiating rows of hepatocytes, the functional cells of the liver (Fig. 22–2). Sinusoids transport systemic blood, which contains ingested substances (e.g., food, drugs, and toxins) to the hepatocytes. The liver processes the nutrients (carbohydrates, proteins, lipids, vitamins, and minerals) for either immediate use or storage, while drugs and toxins are broken down through a variety of metabolic processes.

Progressive destruction of hepatocytes and an increase in fibroblasts and connective tissue surrounding the hepatocytes culminate in cirrhosis. Fibrosis and regenerative nodules of scar tissue modify the basic architecture of the liver, disrupting hepatic blood flow and normal liver function.

Reduced hepatic blood flow can significantly alter normal metabolic processes and decrease protein synthesis within the liver. Hepatic processing of drugs is reduced, resulting in higher drug concentrations and extended half-life of drugs normally eliminated through first-pass metabolism. Decreased hepatic metabolism can also reduce or delay prodrug activation, which can result in therapeutic failure. The liver also processes metabolic waste products for excretion. In cirrhosis, bilirubin (from the enzymatic breakdown of heme) can accumulate; this causes jaundice (yellowing of the skin), scleral icterus (yellowing of the sclera), and tea-colored urine (urinary bilirubin excreted as urobilinogen).

Changes in steroid hormone production, conversion, and handling are prominent features of cirrhosis. These changes can result in decreased libido, gynecomastia (development of breast tissue in men), testicular atrophy, and features of feminization in men. Another effect of changes in sex hormone metabolism is development of spider angiomata (nevi), which are vascular lesions found mainly on the trunk. The lesions have a central arteriole (body) surrounded by radiating "legs." When blanched, the lesions fill from the center body outward toward the legs. Spider angiomata are not specific to cirrhosis, but the number and size do correlate with disease severity; their presence relates to risk of variceal hemorrhage.[11]

Increased intrahepatic resistance to portal flow increases pressure on the entire splanchnic bed; an enlarged spleen (splenomegaly) is a common finding in cirrhotic patients. Splenic platelet sequestration secondary to splenomegaly is one cause of thrombocytopenia in cirrhotic patients.

Portal hypertension mediates systemic and splanchnic arterial vasodilation through production of nitric oxide and other vasodilators in an attempt to counteract the increased pressure gradient. Nitric oxide causes a fall in systemic arterial pressure; this drop in pressure activates the renin–angiotensin–aldosterone system (RAAS) and the sympathetic nervous system, and increases antidiuretic hormone (vasopressin) production.[12] These systems are activated in an attempt to maintain arterial blood pressure and renal blood flow by increasing sodium and water retention.

Excess sodium and water retention put increased pressure on the vascular system. One consequence is that the umbilical vein, which is usually eradicated in infancy, may become patent, resulting in prominent dilated veins visible on the surface of the abdomen. This phenomenon is called caput medusae because it resembles the head of the mythical Gorgon Medusa.

Ascites

Ascites is the accumulation of fluid in the peritoneal space. It is the most common sign of decompensated cirrhosis (as well as one of the first signs) and portends a dire prognosis.[13]

The pathophysiology of ascites, portal hypertension, and cirrhosis are interrelated (Fig. 22–3). Cirrhotic changes and

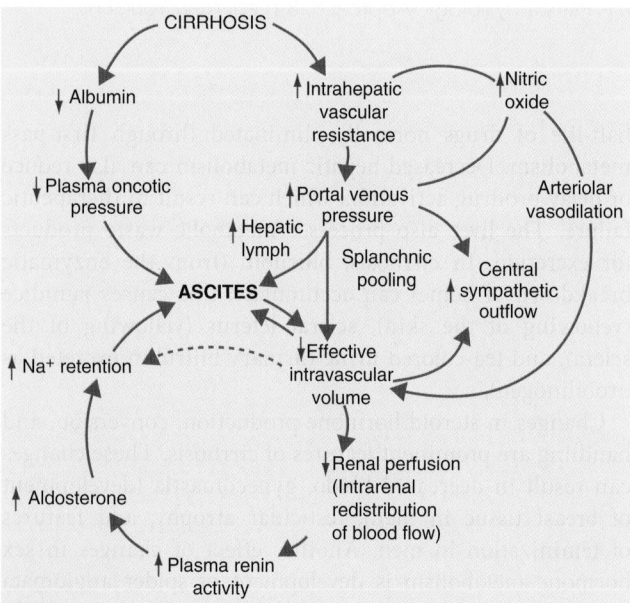

FIGURE 22–3. Factors involved in the development of ascites. (From Chung RT, Podolsky DK. Cirrhosis and its complications. In: Kasper DL, Braunwald E, Fauci AS, et al., eds. Harrison's Principles of Internal Medicine, 17th ed. New York, NY: McGraw-Hill, 2005:1858–1869, with permission.)

subsequent decreases in synthetic function lead to decreased albumin production (hypoalbuminemia). Albumin is the primary intravascular protein responsible for maintaining oncotic pressure within the vascular system; low serum albumin levels, elevated hydrostatic pressure, and increased capillary permeability allow fluid to leak from the vascular space into body tissues. This results in ascites, peripheral edema, and fluid in the pulmonary system. Obstruction of hepatic sinusoids and hepatic lymph nodes also allows fluid to seep into the peritoneal cavity, further contributing to ascitic fluid formation.

Lowered effective intravascular volume decreases renal perfusion; the kidney reacts by activating the RAAS, increasing plasma renin activity, aldosterone production, and sodium retention. The increase in intravascular volume furthers the imbalance of intravascular oncotic pressure, allowing even more fluid to escape to the extravascular spaces, increasing ascites and peripheral edema. Unchecked, these combined effects enable the cycle of portal pressure and ascites to continue, creating a self-perpetuating loop of ascites formation.

Patients with ascites avidly retain sodium and water, not only through aldosterone mechanisms, but also through increases in antidiuretic hormone and sympathetic nervous system activation. Patients may become hyponatremic if there is a decrease in free water excretion. This is not a result of too little sodium; it is a dilutional effect. Untreated, these factors can lead to a decrease in renal function and the hepatorenal syndrome (HRS).[4,12]

Hepatorenal Syndrome

Hepatorenal syndrome is a decline renal function in the setting of cirrhosis that is not caused by intrinsic renal disease. Type 1 HRS is characterized by rapid deterioration of renal function (acute kidney injury [AKI]) in the presence of decompensated cirrhosis that is not reversible with volume repletion. Untreated it is rapidly fatal with a 50% mortality rate at 14 days. Renal artery vasoconstriction (stimulated by the sympathetic nervous system) and decreased mean arterial pressure (mediated by nitric oxide) decrease renal perfusion and precipitate renal failure. The kidneys attempt to counteract this drop in renal perfusion through RAAS activation. Production of renin stimulates a cascade that causes fluid retention and peripheral vasoconstriction in an attempt to increase renal blood flow. Prostaglandin E_2 and prostacyclin production are increased to stimulate renal vasodilation. HRS develops when these mechanisms are overwhelmed and renal perfusion drops acutely. SBP is often a trigger for HRS, and nonsteroidal anti-inflammatory drugs (NSAIDs) precipitate HRS by inhibiting prostaglandins. Type 2 HRS has similar pathophysiology to type1 HRS but is characterized by a less acute decline in renal function.

The traditional renal function monitoring parameters of SCr and blood urea nitrogen (BUN) tend to be low in cirrhotic patients secondary to reduced muscle mass and decreased hepatic urea production, respectively. Because of this, even minor changes in these parameters should be monitored closely; seemingly small changes may represent large changes in renal function.

Varices

The splanchnic system drains venous blood from the GI tract to the liver. In portal hypertension, there is increased resistance to drainage from the originating organ, so collateral vessels (varices) develop in the esophagus, stomach, and rectum to compensate for the increased blood volume. Varices divert blood meant for hepatic circulation back to the systemic circulation, decreasing clearance of medications and potential toxins through loss of first-pass metabolism. Varices are weak superficial vessels; any additional increase in pressure can cause them to rupture and bleed.[14]

Spontaneous Bacterial Peritonitis

SBP is an acute bacterial infection of peritoneal (ascitic) fluid in the absence of intra-abdominal infection or intestinal perforation. Estimated SBP prevalence in patients with ascites ranges from 10% to 30%.[15] The peritoneal cavity is usually a sterile space. One proposed mechanism of bacterial contamination is translocation of intestinal bacteria to mesenteric lymph nodes, which then seed the ascitic fluid.[16] Bacterial translocation correlates with the delay in intestinal transit time and increased intestinal wall permeability observed in cirrhotic patients. Another possible mechanism is the hematogenous spread of bacteria into the peritoneal space.[17] Low protein (less than 1 g/dL [10 g/L]) ascites is also associated with increased rates of SBP; presumably low protein is correlated to low antibacterial activity.

Enteric gram-negative aerobes are the most common bacteria isolated from ascitic fluid, usually *Escherichia coli* or *Klebsiella pneumoniae*. *Streptococcus pneumoniae* is the most common gram-positive pathogen associated with SBP.[18] Once a bacterial pathogen has been identified, the antimicrobial spectrum can be narrowed; SBP is rarely polymicrobial.

Hepatic Encephalopathy

Numerous factors, many of them poorly understood, are involved in the development of HE. In severe hepatic disease, systemic circulation bypasses the liver; so many substances normally metabolized by the liver remain in the systemic circulation and accumulate. In excess, these metabolic by-products, especially nitrogenous waste, cause alterations in CNS functioning.[19]

Ammonia (NH_3) is just one of the toxins implicated in HE. It is a metabolic by-product of protein catabolism; it is also generated by bacteria in the GI tract. In a normally functioning liver, hepatocytes degrade ammonia to form urea, which is renally excreted. In cirrhosis, the conversion to urea is retarded and ammonia accumulates, resulting in encephalopathy. Patients with HE commonly have elevated serum ammonia concentrations, but ammonia levels do not correlate with the degree of CNS impairment.[19] Decreased urea formation is evident on laboratory assessments as decreased BUN, but BUN levels do not correlate with the degree of HE.

High levels of false neurotransmitters (aromatic amino acids, γ-aminobutyric acid, and endogenous benzodiazepines) have also been implicated in HE. These substances bind to both the γ-aminobutyric acid and benzodiazepine receptors and act as agonists at the active receptor sites.[19]

Decreased cognition, confusion, and changes in behavior combined with physical signs such as asterixis (characteristic flapping of hands upon extension of arms with wrist flexion) indicate HE. Patients with previously stable cirrhosis who develop acute encephalopathy often have an identifiable precipitating event that can account for the increased production and/or decreased elimination of toxins. Infections, variceal hemorrhage, renal insufficiency, electrolyte abnormalities, and increased dietary protein have all been associated with acute development of HE. Acute HE triggers can often be treated, reversing encephalopathy. Changes of a more chronic, insidious nature are more difficult to treat; patients rarely recover from chronic HE.

Bleeding Diathesis and Synthetic Failure

Coagulopathies signal end-stage liver disease. The liver manufactures procoagulation and anticoagulant factors essential for blood clotting and maintenance of blood homeostasis. In advanced disease, the liver is unable to synthesize these proteins, resulting in extended clotting times (e.g., prothrombin time) and bleeding irregularities.[20]

Thrombocytopenia is another coagulation abnormality seen in advanced liver disease. This is a result of decreased platelet production in the bone marrow (triggered by a lack of thrombopoietin stimulation by the liver) as well as the splenic sequestration of formed platelets.

Macrocytic anemia occurs because of decreased intake, metabolism, and storage of folate and vitamin B_{12}. Individuals who continue to drink exacerbate blood abnormalities further; ethanol is toxic to bone marrow.

Alcoholic Liver Disease

The course of alcoholic liver disease moves through several distinct phases from fatty liver to alcoholic hepatitis and finally cirrhosis. Metabolism of large amounts of ethanol shifts hepatic metabolic processes away from oxidation and toward reduction. These changes in metabolism account for the fatty liver, hypertriglyceridemia, and acidemia observed in alcoholic liver disease. Fatty liver and alcoholic hepatitis may be reversible with cessation of alcohol intake. The scarring of cirrhosis is permanent, but maintaining abstinence from alcohol can decrease complications and slow progression to end-stage liver disease.[21] Continuing to drink alcohol speeds the advancement of liver dysfunction and cirrhotic complications.

Ethanol metabolism begins prior to absorption; alcohol dehydrogenase (ADH) in the gastric mucosa oxidizes a portion of ingested alcohol to acetaldehyde. The remaining alcohol is rapidly absorbed from the GI tract, and because it is highly lipid soluble, it enters the body tissues quite easily. ❷ *ADH oxidizes ethanol in body tissues, primarily the liver, causing inflammation and fibrosis.*[22] High ethanol levels saturate the ADH enzyme system. When ADH is overwhelmed, the microsomal ethanol oxidizing system takes over the detoxification process. This system is an inducible cytochrome P-450 (CYP 450) enzyme system; it participates in phase 1 metabolism and like ADH, produces acetaldehyde as its end product.[23] Acetaldehyde exerts direct toxic effects on the liver by damaging hepatocytes, inducing fibrosis, and directly coupling to proteins, interfering with their intended actions.

Less Common Causes of Cirrhosis

Genetics and metabolic risk factors mediate other less common causes of cirrhosis. These diseases vary widely in prevalence, disease progression, and treatment options.

Primary biliary cirrhosis is characterized by progressive inflammatory destruction of the bile ducts. This immune-mediated inflammation of the intrahepatic bile ducts causes remodeling and scarring, resulting in retention of bile in the liver, hepatocellular damage, and cirrhosis. The number of patients affected with primary biliary cirrhosis is difficult to estimate because it is often asymptomatic and people may be diagnosed incidentally during a routine healthcare visit.

Nonalcoholic fatty liver disease (NAFLD) begins with asymptomatic fatty liver but can progress to cirrhosis. NAFLD is a diagnosis of exclusion; viral, genetic, or environmental causes must be eliminated prior to making this diagnosis. NAFLD is directly related to numerous metabolic abnormalities. Risk factors include diabetes mellitus, dyslipidemia, obesity, insulin resistance, and other conditions associated with increased hepatic fat.[24]

Hereditary hemochromatosis is an autosomal recessive disease that causes increased intestinal iron absorption and subsequent deposition in hepatic, cardiac, and pancreatic tissue. Hepatic iron overload results in fibrosis, hepatic scarring, cirrhosis, and hepatocellular carcinoma. Repeated blood transfusions can also cause hemochromatosis, but this mechanism rarely leads to cirrhosis.

Wilson's disease is an autosomal recessive disease that leads to cirrhosis through protein abnormalities. The protein responsible for facilitating copper excretion in the bile is faulty, so copper accumulates in hepatic tissue. High copper levels are toxic to hepatocytes. Fibrosis and cirrhosis may develop in untreated patients. Patients with Wilson's disease usually present with symptoms of liver and/or neurologic disease while still in their teens.

A third autosomal recessive genetic disease is α_1-antitrypsin deficiency. Abnormalities in the α_1-antitrypsin protein impair its secretion from the liver. α_1-Antitrypsin deficiency causes cirrhosis in children as well as adults; adults usually have concomitant pulmonary disease such as chronic obstructive pulmonary disease.

CLINICAL PRESENTATION AND DIAGNOSIS

See the clinical presentation text box on the next page for the symptoms, signs, and laboratory abnormalities associated with cirrhosis.

Diagnosis of Cirrhosis

In some cases, cirrhosis is diagnosed incidentally before the patient develops symptoms or acute complications, but many patients have decompensated cirrhosis at initial presentation. Patients may present with variceal bleeding, ascites, SBP, or HE. At diagnosis, patients may have some, all, or none of the laboratory abnormalities and/or signs and symptoms that are associated with cirrhosis (see clinical presentation text box).[25]

Liver biopsy is the only way to definitively diagnose cirrhosis, but this is often deferred in lieu of a presumptive diagnosis. Ultrasound and computed tomography are used routinely to evaluate cirrhosis; a small nodular liver with increased echogenicity is consistent with cirrhosis. The modified Child–Pugh and Model for End-Stage Liver Disease (MELD) classification systems (Table 22–1) are used to classify disease severity and evaluate the need for transplantation.

Patients with ascites or known varices are presumed to have portal hypertension. Direct measurements of portal

Table 22–1

Child–Pugh and MELD Classifications for Determining Severity of Liver Damage

Child–Pugh Classification[a]

Variable	1 Point	2 Points	3 Points
Bilirubin (mg/dL) (μmol/L)	Less than 2	2–3	Greater than 3
	Less than 34	34–51	Greater than 51
Albumin (g/dL) (g/L)	Greater than 3.5	2.8–3.5	Less than 2.8
	Greater than 35	28–35	Less than 28
Prothrombin time (seconds prolonged) or	1–3	4–6	Greater than 6
INR	Less than 1.8	1.8–2.3	Greater than 2.3
Ascites	None	Slight	Moderate
Encephalopathy	None	Grade 1–2	Grade 3–4

MELD Classification

The formula for the MELD score is 3.8 × Ln(bilirubin [mg/dL]) + 11.2 × Ln(INR) + 9.6 × Ln(creatinine [mg/dL]) + 6.4 × (etiology: 0 if cholestatic or alcoholic, 1 otherwise).
Using SI units, the MELD score is 3.8 × Ln(bilirubin [μmol/L]/17.1) + 11.2 × Ln(INR) + 9.6 × Ln(creatinine [μmol/L]/88.4) + 6.4 × (etiology: 0 if cholestatic or alcoholic, 1 otherwise).

INR, international normalized ratio; MELD, Model for End-Stage Liver Disease; Ln, natural logarithm.

[a]Class A: 1 to 6 total points; B: 7 to 9 points; C: 10 to 15 points.

From Lucey MR, Brown KA, Everson GT, et al. Minimal criteria for placement of adults on the liver transplant waiting list: A report of a national conference organized by the American Society of Transplant Physicians and the American Association for the Study of Liver Diseases. Liver Transpl Surg 1997;3:628–637; and Kamath PS, Wiesner RH, Malinchoc M, et al. A model to predict survival in patients with end-stage liver disease. Hepatology 2001;33:464–470.

Clinical Presentation of Cirrhosis and Complications of Portal Hypertension

General

- Most signs and symptoms are specific to the complication the patient is experiencing at the time of presentation.

Symptoms

- Patients with cirrhosis may be asymptomatic until acute complications develop.
- Nonspecific symptoms may include anorexia, fatigue, weakness, and changes in libido and sleep patterns.
- Patients may experience easy bruising and may bleed from minor injuries.
- Pruritus may be present, particularly with biliary involvement.
- Patients with ascites may complain of abdominal pain, nausea, increasing tightness and fullness in the abdomen, shortness of breath, and early satiety.
- Hemorrhage from esophageal or gastric varices may be associated with melena, pallor, fatigue, and weakness from blood loss. Patients often present with nausea, vomiting, and hematemesis because blood in the GI tract is nauseating. Bleeding from rectal varices may present as **hematochezia**.
- In patients with bleeding varices, digestion of swallowed blood represents a high protein load; this causes nausea and can precipitate symptoms of HE.
- In patients with HE, neurologic changes can be overwhelming or so subtle that they are not clinically apparent except during a targeted clinical evaluation.
- Patients with HE may complain of disruption of sleep patterns and day-to-night inversion; patients have delayed bedtime and wake times, which may progress to complete inversion of the normal diurnal cycle.
- If SBP occurs, symptoms of infection may include fever, chills, abdominal pain, and mental status changes.

Signs

- Nonspecific signs on physical examination include jaundice, scleral icterus, tea-colored urine, bruising, hepatomegaly, splenomegaly, spider angiomata, caput medusae, palmar erythema, gynecomastia, and testicular atrophy.
- Ascites can be detected by increased abdominal girth accompanied by shifting dullness and a fluid wave.
- Signs of variceal bleeding depend on the degree of blood loss and abruptness of onset. Rapid and massive blood loss is more likely to result in hemodynamic instability than slow, steady bleeding. Signs of acute bleeding may include pallor, hypotension, tachycardia, mental status changes, and hematemesis.
- Markers of hepatic encephalopathy (HE) include decreased cognition, confusion, changes in behavior, and asterixis.
- Patients with SBP may present with fever, painful tympanic abdomen, and changes in mental status.
- Decreases in clotting factors may manifest as abnormal bruising and bleeding.

- Dupuytren's contracture is a contraction of the palmar fascia that usually affects the fourth and fifth digits. It is not specific to cirrhosis and can also be seen in repetitive use injuries.

Laboratory Abnormalities

- Hepatocellular damage manifests as elevated alanine aminotransferase (ALT) and aspartate aminotransferase (AST). The degree of transaminase elevation does not correlate with the remaining functional metabolic capacity of the liver. An AST level twofold higher than ALT suggests alcoholic liver damage.
- Elevated alkaline phosphatase is nonspecific and may correlate with liver or bone disease; it tends to be elevated in biliary tract disease.
- γ-Glutamyl transferase (GGT) is specific to the bile ducts, and in conjunction with an elevated alkaline phosphatase, it suggests hepatic disease. Extremely elevated GGT levels further indicate obstructive biliary disease. GGT is also elevated in individuals who drink three or more alcoholic drinks daily.
- Increased total, direct, and indirect bilirubin concentrations indicate defects in transport, conjugation, or excretion of bilirubin.
- Lactate dehydrogenase (LDH) is a nonspecific marker of hepatocyte damage; a disproportionate elevation of LDH indicates ischemic injury.
- Thrombocytopenia may occur because of decreased platelet production and splenic platelet sequestration.
- Anemia (decreased hemoglobin and hematocrit) occurs as a result of variceal bleeding, decreased erythrocyte production, and hypersplenism.
- Elevated prothrombin time (PT) and international normalized ratio (INR) are coagulation derangements that indicate loss of synthetic capacity in the liver and correlate with functional loss of hepatocytes.
- Decreased serum albumin and total protein occur in chronic liver damage due to loss of synthetic capacity within the liver.
- The serum albumin-to-ascites gradient is 1.1 g/dL (11 g/L) or greater caused by portal hypertension.
- Increased blood ammonia concentration is characteristic of HE, but levels do not correlate well with the degree of impairment.
- Increased serum creatinine signaling a decline in renal function may be seen with hepatorenal syndrome.
- Signs and symptoms of SBP in a patient with cirrhosis and ascites should prompt a diagnostic paracentesis (Fig. 22–5). In SBP, there is decreased total serum protein, elevated white blood cell count (with left shift), and the ascitic fluid contains at least 250 cells/mm³ (250×10^6/L) neutrophils. Bacterial culture of ascitic fluid may be positive, but lack of growth does not exclude the diagnosis.

pressure require invasive procedures and increase the risk of bleeding; this is usually deferred in lieu of presumptive therapy.

Diagnosis of Ascites

In obese patients or those with only small amounts of fluid accumulation, ultrasound evaluation may be necessary to detect ascites. Analysis of ascitic fluid obtained during **paracentesis** provides diagnostic clues to the etiology of the ascites. Diagnostic evaluation should include cell count with differential, albumin, total protein, Gram stain, and bacterial cultures. In patients without an established diagnosis of liver disease, the serum ascites-albumin gradient (SAAG) is used to determine if the ascites is caused by portal hypertension.[21] SAAG compares serum albumin concentration to ascitic fluid albumin concentration:

$$Alb_{serum} - Alb_{ascites} = SAAG$$

A value of 1.1 g/dL (11 g/L) or greater identifies portal hypertension as the cause of the ascites with 97% sensitivity.[21] In portal hypertension, the ascitic fluid is low in albumin; this balances the oncotic pressure gradient with the hydrostatic pressure gradient of portal hypertension. The differential diagnoses for SAAG values less than 1.1 g/dL (11 g/L) include peritoneal carcinoma, peritoneal infection (tuberculosis, fungal, or cytomegalovirus), and nephrotic syndrome. Serum albumin measurements should be made at the time of paracentesis for an accurate comparison.[21]

TREATMENT OF PORTAL HYPERTENSION, CIRRHOSIS, AND COMPLICATIONS

Desired Outcomes

Recognizing and treating the cause of cirrhosis is paramount. ❸ *Cirrhosis is irreversible; treatments are directed at limiting disease progression and minimizing complications.* The immediate treatment goals are to stabilize acute complications such as variceal bleeding and prevent SBP. Once life-threatening conditions have stabilized, the focus shifts to preventing complications and further liver damage. Preventing complications involves both primary and secondary prophylaxis. To determine appropriate prophylactic therapy, a careful analysis of patient characteristics and disease history is mandatory. The sections that follow concentrate on treatment and prevention of cirrhotic complications.

Nonpharmacologic Therapy

Lifestyle modifications can limit disease complications and slow further liver damage. Avoiding additional hepatic insult is critical for successful cirrhosis treatment. The only proven treatment for alcoholic liver disease is immediate cessation of alcohol use. Patients with cirrhosis from causes other than alcohol also benefit from avoiding alcohol;

Patient Encounter Part 1

LT is a 49-year-old woman who is brought to the emergency department by her husband. This evening when he returned home from work, he found LT asleep in the living room. He attempted to wake her up, but she was "out of it," so he brought her for medical attention.

Chief complaint: Not obtained; minimal response to stimuli

HPI: Husband states that LT had complained of weakness and fatigue for approximately 2 days

PMH: Four pregnancies, four live births; skull fracture 4 years ago secondary to a fall, type 2 diabetes (diet controlled)

PSH: Cesarean section, tubal ligation

SH: Married, lives with her brother, her husband, and their four children; works as a bartender; drinks "socially" per husband; no tobacco or illicit drug use

FH: Mother with osteoporosis, hypothyroidism, depression, and hypertension; father's medical history is unknown; two brothers with type 2 diabetes

Outpatient meds: No prescriptions; OTC acetaminophen for frequent headaches

ROS: (+) weakness and fatigue per husband

PE:

VS: BP 77/31 mm Hg, P 118 bpm, T 99.1°F (37.3°C), RR 22 breaths/min, oxygen saturation 96% (0.96) on room air, height 61" (155 cm), weight 68 kg, BMI 28.3 kg/m²

HEENT: PERRL, EOMI, (+) scleral icterus, mild jaundice

CV: Tachycardic; RR; no murmurs, rubs, or gallops

Chest: CTA bilaterally, no crackles or wheezes

Abd: Soft, nontender, slightly distended abdomen, normal bowel sounds, mild hepatosplenomegaly, possible small ascites

Ext: 2+ pedal pulses, mild to moderate pitting edema

Based on the current information, what is the most likely cause of her mental status changes?

What signs and symptoms does this patient have that are consistent with cirrhosis?

What risk factors does she have for cirrhosis?

---

regardless of the etiology, all cirrhotic patients should abstain from alcohol to prevent further liver damage.

Patients with ascites require dietary sodium restriction. Intake should be limited to less than 800 mg sodium (2 g sodium chloride) per day. More stringent restriction may cause faster mobilization of ascitic fluid, but adherence to such strict limits is very difficult. Ascites usually responds well to sodium restriction accompanied by diuretic therapy.[13,21] A spot urine sodium-to-potassium ratio greater than 1 indicates nonadherence to dietary sodium goals.

Medication use must be monitored carefully for potential hepatotoxicity. Hepatically metabolized medications have the potential to accumulate in patients with liver disease. Little guidance is available on drug dosing in hepatic impairment because these patients have historically been excluded from drug trials. Daily acetaminophen use should not exceed 2 g. Dietary supplements, herbal remedies, and nutraceuticals have not been well studied in hepatic impairment and cannot be recommended.

In patients with variceal bleeding, nasogastric (NG) suction reduces the risk of aspirating stomach contents. Aspiration pneumonia is a major cause of death in patients with variceal bleeding. NG suction can also decrease vomiting by removing blood from the GI tract during acute episodes of variceal bleeding; blood in the GI tract is very nauseating.

Endoscopic band ligation (application of a stricture around the varix) is used to stop acutely bleeding varices. Band ligation has replaced sclerotherapy (injection of a caustic substance into the varix) as the preferred endoscopic treatment and is effective in stopping acute variceal bleeding in up to 90% of patients.[26] It is the standard of care for secondary prophylaxis of repeat bleeding in patients with a history of either esophageal or gastric variceal bleeding. Band ligation is best used in conjunction with pharmacologic treatment.[27–29]

Balloon tamponade involves the application of direct pressure to the area of bleeding with an inflatable balloon attached to an NG tube. It is an option when drug therapy and band ligation fail to stop variceal bleeding. Balloon tamponade is used only for rescue therapy. Once the direct pressure of the balloon is removed, rebleeding often occurs, so balloon tamponade is only a temporary measure prior to more definitive treatment such as shunting.[10]

During episodes of acute HE, temporary protein restriction to decrease ammonia production can be a useful adjuvant to pharmacologic therapy. Long-term protein restriction in cirrhotic patients is not recommended. Cirrhotic patients are already in a nutritionally deficient state, and prolonged protein restriction will exacerbate the problem.[19]

Hepatitis A and B vaccination is recommended in patients with cirrhosis to prevent additional liver damage from an acute viral infection.[30] Pneumococcal and influenza vaccination may also be appropriate and can reduce hospitalizations.

Shunts are long-term solutions to decrease elevated portal pressure. Shunts divert blood flow through or around the diseased liver, depending on the location and type of shunt employed. Transjugular intrahepatic portosystemic shunts (TIPS) create a communication pathway between the intrahepatic portal vein and the hepatic vein. TIPS procedures have an advantage over surgically inserted shunts because they are placed through the vascular system rather than through more invasive surgical procedures, but they still carry a risk of bleeding and infection. TIPS placement is associated with improvement in HRS but also with an increased incidence of HE.[31] HE associated with TIPS placement results from decreased detoxification of nitrogenous waste products because the shunt allows blood to evade metabolic processing.

Pharmacologic Therapy

Drug therapy targeted to reduce portal hypertension and cirrhosis can alleviate symptoms and prevent complications but cannot reverse cirrhosis.

▶ *Portal Hypertension*

④ *Nonselective β-blockers such as propranolol and nadolol are first-line treatments to reduce portal hypertension.* They reduce bleeding and decrease mortality in patients with known varices. Use of β-blockers for primary prevention of variceal formation is controversial.

Only nonselective β-blockers (those that block both β_1 and β_2 receptors) reduce bleeding complications in patients with known varices. Blockade of β_1 receptors reduces cardiac output and splanchnic blood flow. β_2-Adrenergic blockade prevents β_2-receptor–mediated splanchnic vasodilation while allowing unopposed α-adrenergic effects; this enhances vasoconstriction of the systemic and splanchnic vascular beds. The combination of β_1 and β_2 blockade makes the nonselective β-blockers preferable to cardioselective agents (those blocking primarily β_1 receptors) in treating portal hypertension.[1,27,32,33] Although cardioselective β-blockers do lose their cardioselectivity at higher doses, most patients with cirrhosis cannot tolerate the high doses.

Because β-blockers decrease blood pressure and heart rate, they should be started at low doses to increase tolerability; cirrhotic patients often already have low blood pressure and heart rate. Propranolol is hepatically metabolized; initial concentration, half-life, and pharmacologic effects are prolonged in portal hypertension. A reasonable starting dose of propranolol is 10 mg once or twice daily.

Doses should be titrated as tolerated with the goal of decreasing heart rate by 25% or to approximately 55 to 60 bpm.[10,27] Heart rate is not an accurate predictor of portal pressure reduction, but it is the acknowledged surrogate marker for effectiveness because there are no other acceptable alternatives.

Nitrates have been suggested for patients who do not achieve therapeutic goals (heart rate reduction) with β-blocker therapy alone. Nitrates (e.g., isosorbide mononitrate), both alone and in combination with β-blockers, show enhanced reduction of portal pressure in clinical trials; however, there is an increase in mortality when nitrates are used alone. Patients treated with the combination of nonselective β-blockers and nitrates have significantly more adverse events compared with β-blocker monotherapy.[34,35] Current evidence only supports use of the combination to prevent rebleeding, not for primary prophylaxis. Unfortunately, β-blockers either alone or in combination may be intolerable for many patients with cirrhosis.

▶ *Ascites*

⑤ *The goals of treating ascites are to minimize acute discomfort, reequilibrate ascitic fluid, and prevent SBP. Treatment should modify underlying disease pathology; without directed therapy, fluid will rapidly reaccumulate.*

Acute discomfort from ascites may be ameliorated by therapeutic paracentesis. Often the removal of just 1 to 2 L of ascitic fluid provides relief from pain and fullness. For large volume "taps" (5 L or more), volume resuscitation should be provided with 6 to 8 g of IV albumin per liter of fluid removed. Albumin 25% should be used because it has one-fifth the volume of the 5% product. Large-volume paracentesis without albumin administration is known to precipitate HRS through decreased perfusion. If less than 5 L of fluid is removed in a hemodynamically stable patient, albumin use is not warranted.[21]

▶ Diuretics

Diuretics are usually required in addition to sodium restriction (see Nonpharmacologic Therapy). ❻ *Cirrhosis is a high aldosterone state; spironolactone is an aldosterone antagonist and counteracts the effects of activation of the RAAS. Spironolactone with or without furosemide forms the basis of pharmacologic therapy for ascites.* In hepatic disease, not only is aldosterone production increased, but its half-life is prolonged because of decreased hepatic metabolism. Spironolactone also conserves potassium that would otherwise be excreted because of elevated aldosterone levels.

Spironolactone is typically used with a loop diuretic (e.g., furosemide) for more potent diuresis. A ratio of 40 mg furosemide (the most commonly used loop diuretic) to each 100 mg spironolactone can usually maintain serum potassium concentrations within the normal range. Therapy is commonly initiated with oral spironolactone 100 mg and furosemide 40 mg/day.

Doses should be titrated at intervals no more frequent than every 2 to 3 days. Because spironolactone is used for its antialdosterone effects, higher doses (up to 400 mg/day) are used compared with doses used to treat hypertension. If intolerable side effects such as painful gynecomastia occur with spironolactone, other potassium-sparing diuretics may be used, but clinical trials have not shown equivalent efficacy.[21]

The maximum ascitic fluid that can be removed through diuresis is approximately 0.5 L/day.[21] Because ascites equilibrates with vascular fluid at a much slower rate than does peripheral edema, aggressive diuresis is associated with intravascular volume depletion rather than depletion of peritoneal fluid. Aggressive diuresis should be avoided unless patients have concomitant peripheral edema. Patients with peripheral edema in addition to ascites may require increasing furosemide doses until euvolemia is achieved; IV diuretics are often necessary.[21] Diuretic therapy in cirrhosis is typically lifelong.

▶ Varices

Variceal bleeding is common in cirrhotic patients; it accounts for up to 10% of all cases of upper GI hemorrhage. ❼ *During acute variceal hemorrhage, it is crucial to control bleeding,*

Patient Encounter, Part 2

Laboratory results for LT showed the following:

Sodium 126 mEq/L (126 mmol/L)	Albumin 2.3 g/dL (23g/L)
Potassium 2.9 mEq/L (2.9 mmol/L)	Total bilirubin 1.9 mg/dL (32.5 μmol/L)
Chloride 97 mEq/L (97 mmol/L)	Alk phos 213 IU/L (3.55 μkat/L)
Bicarbonate 18 mEq/L (18 mmol/L)	AST 137 IU/L (2.28 μkat/L)
BUN 12 mg/dL (4.3 mmol/L)	ALT 66 IU/L (1.10 μkat/L)
SCr 0.8 mg/dL (71 μmol/L)	INR 1.4
Glucose 114 mg/dL (6.3 mmol/L)	PT 19 seconds
Hemoglobin 7.6 g/dL (76 g/L; 4.7 mmol/L)	GGT 163 IU/L (2.72 μkat/L)
Hematocrit 23% (0.23)	LDH 187 IU/L (3.12 μkat/L)
WBC 5.4 × 10³/mm³ (5.4 × 10⁹/L)	Serum NH₃ 72 mcg/dL (42 μmol/L)
Platelets 109 × 10³/mm³ (109 × 10⁹/L)	Blood alcohol undetectable

Which laboratory values suggest a diagnosis of cirrhosis?

What is the likely cause of LT's mental status change? Are there other conditions that may have contributed to the mental status change?

What is a likely trigger for LT's mental status change?

How does this relate to her complaints of weakness and fatigue?

ALT, alanine aminotransferase; AST, aspartate aminotransferase; GGT, γ-glutamyl transferase; INR, international normalized ratio; IU, international units; LDH, lactate dehydrogenase; PT, prothrombin time.

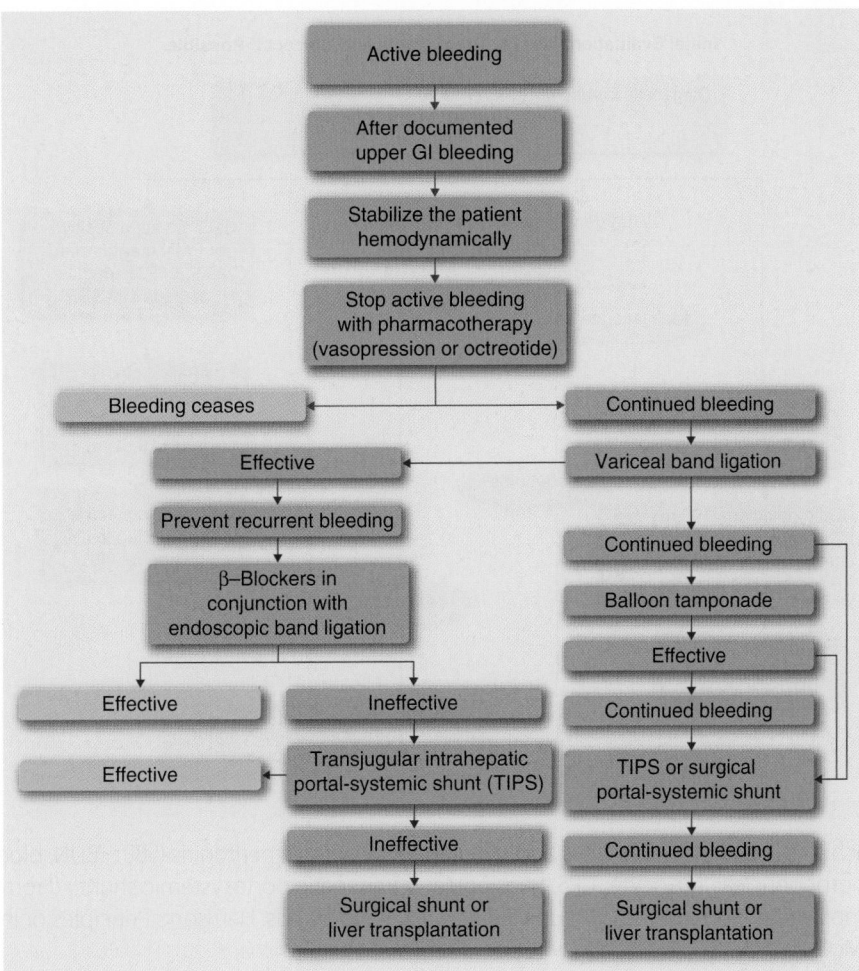

FIGURE 22–4. Treatment algorithm for active GI bleeding resulting from portal hypertension. (Adapted from Schiano TD, Bodenheimer HC. Complications of chronic liver disease. In: Friedman SL, McQuaid KR, Grendell JH, eds. Current Diagnosis and Treatment in Gastroenterology, 2nd ed. New York, NY: McGraw-Hill, 2003:649, with permission).

prevent rebleeding, and avoid acute complications such as SBP. Acute mortality is approximately 20%, with 1-year mortality greater than 60% in patients with very elevated portal pressure; patients must be treated aggressively.[8] A treatment algorithm for acute variceal bleeding is depicted in **Figure 22–4**.

Octreotide is a synthetic somatostatin analog; it causes selective vasoconstriction of the splanchnic bed, decreasing portal venous pressure with few serious side effects. The recommended octreotide dose is a 50- to 100-mcg IV loading dose followed by a 25 to 50 mcg/h continuous IV infusion. Therapy should continue for at least 24 to 72 hours after bleeding has stopped. Some clinicians continue octreotide for a full 5 days because this is the time frame during which the risk of rebleeding is highest. Octreotide combined with endoscopic therapy results in decreased rebleeding rates and transfusion needs when compared with endoscopic treatment alone.[28]

▶ *Spontaneous Bacterial Peritonitis*

Prophylactic antibiotic therapy is recommended during acute variceal bleeding to prevent SBP; this is typically initiated with a third-generation cephalosporin (1 g IV ceftriaxone daily) or a fluoroquinolone (norfloxacin 400 mg orally twice daily, ciprofloxacin 500 mg orally twice daily, or ciprofloxacin 400 mg IV twice daily) for 7 days. If the patient is actively bleeding, consider IV instead of oral therapy. Avoid fluoroquinolone therapy in patients who have used this drug class for long-term prophylaxis; they may have developed fluoroquinolone resistance. Prophylactic antibiotic therapy reduces in-hospital infections and mortality in patients hospitalized for variceal bleeding.[34]

If SBP is suspected, empiric antibiotic therapy should be initiated with a broad-spectrum antiinfective agent after ascitic fluid collection, pending cultures and susceptibilities (**Fig. 22–5**).[36,37] In the setting of presumed infection, delaying treatment while awaiting laboratory confirmation is inappropriate and may result in death. The initial antibiotic should be an IV third-generation cephalosporin (e.g., cefotaxime 2 g every 8 hours, ceftriaxone 1 g every 24 hours), an IV extended-spectrum penicillin (e.g., piperacillin-tazobactam 3.375 g every 6 hours or 4.5 g every 8 hours), or an IV fluoroquinolone (e.g., ciprofloxacin 400 mg IV every 12 hours; only if the patient has not received long-term prophylaxis with

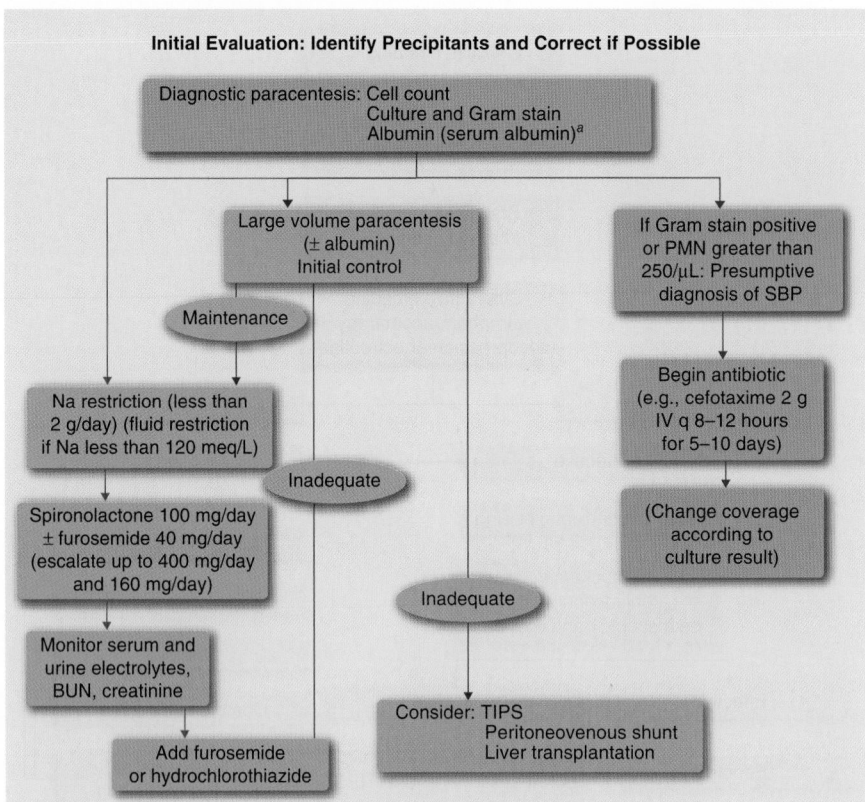

FIGURE 22–5. Approach to the patient with ascites and spontaneous bacterial peritonitis (SBP). (BUN, blood urea nitrogen; Na, sodium; PMN polymorphonuclear leukocyte; TIPS, transjugular intrahepatic portosystemic shunt.) (From Chung RT, Podolsky DK. Cirrhosis and its complications. In: Kasper DL, Braunwald E, Fauci AS, et al., eds. Harrison's Principles of Internal Medicine, 17th ed. New York, NY: McGraw-Hill, 2005:1858–1869, with permission.)

^{a}If PMN is greater than 250/μL(250 ×106/L) but culture is negative (culture-negative neutrocytic ascites), begin empiric antibiotics and retap after 48 hours. If culture is positive but PMN less than 250/μL (250 × 10⁶/L), treat as if PMN greater than 250/μL (250 × 10⁶/L) (presumed SBP). If polymicrobial infection exists, exclude SBP.

a fluoroquinolone). These agents cover the most common gram-negative and gram-positive agents implicated in SBP. Third-generation cephalosporins are usually recommended as first-line therapy. Local resistance patterns must be taken into account when choosing empiric antibiotic therapy. Once a bacterial pathogen has been identified, coverage may be narrowed to an agent that is highly active against that particular organism. SBP is rarely polymicrobial.

SBP has been identified as a cause of HRS. The risk of renal failure is reduced with IV albumin therapy, dosed at 1.5 g/kg of body weight initially, followed by 1 g/kg of body weight on day 3 of SBP therapy.[38]

❽ *Long-term antibiotic prophylaxis for SBP decreases mortality and is recommended in patients with a history of SBP or low-protein ascites (ascitic fluid albumin less than 1.5 g/dL [15 g/L]) plus one of the following: SCr 1.5 mg/dL (133 μmol/L) or greater, BUN ≥25 mg/dL (8.9 mmol/L) or greater, serum sodium 130 mEq/L (130 mmol/L) or less, or Child–Pugh score of at least 9, with bilirubin of at least 3 mg/ dL (51.3 μmol/L).* Recommended oral regimens include one trimethoprim–sulfamethoxazole double-strength tablet daily, norfloxacin 400 mg daily, or ciprofloxacin 750 mg daily.[18]

▶ *Encephalopathy*

Lactulose ❾ *Lactulose is the foundation of pharmacologic therapy to prevent and treat HE. It is a nondigestible synthetic disaccharide laxative that is hydrolyzed in the gut to an osmotically active compound that draws water into the colon and stimulates defecation.* Lactulose lowers colonic pH, which favors the conversion of ammonia (NH_3) to ammonium (NH_4^+).[39] Ammonium is ionic and cannot cross back from the gut into systemic circulation; it is eliminated in the feces. Lactulose is usually initiated at 15 to 30 mL two to three times per day and titrated to a therapeutic goal of two to four soft bowel movements daily.[19,40,41]

Antibiotic Therapy Rifaximin is a nonabsorbable antibiotic that is used extensively in Europe as first-line therapy for HE. Rifaximin decreases urease-producing gut bacteria, which decreases ammonia production. Rifaximin therapy has been shown to be both efficacious and well tolerated, but its expense in the United States (it is only licensed for HE prophylaxis, not treatment) may be prohibitive for long-term use. The rifaximin dose is 550 mg twice daily given with lactulose. At this dose it costs approximately 10-fold more

Patient Encounter, Part 3

While in the ED, LT was given 3 units of packed red blood cells and ceftriaxone 1 g IV. She was taken for an endoscopy, but she did not have any actively bleeding varices. She developed mild itching, and the antibiotic was discontinued. About 6 hours later LT is awake and oriented. When her husband is out of the room, she does admit to heavy alcohol use. She also states that she has had dark tarry stools for about a week, and 3 days prior to admission she began vomiting. She states that the emesis "looked like coffee grounds."

What pharmacologic and nonpharmacologic interventions are needed to prevent progression of cirrhosis and future decompensation?

Patient Encounter, Part 4

The next day, LT's mental status declines; she becomes somnolent and irritable. On physical examination her abdomen is tender to mild palpation.

VS: BP 98/70 mm Hg, P 102 bpm, T 101.9°F (38.8°C), RR 18 breaths/min, oxygen saturation 98% (0.98) on room air.

The medical resident suspects SBP and orders a paracentesis. The ascitic fluid shows PMN 300 cells/µL (300 × 10^6/L), gram stain negative, SAAG 1.4 g/dL (14 g/L).

What is the implication of the ascitic fluid findings?

Should you wait for the culture results to be sure there is actually an infection before starting antibiotics?

If antibiotics are indicated, what drug(s) and regimen(s) would you recommend?

What additional treatment should she receive?

If SBP is not treated appropriately, what are potential clinical consequences?

Is LT a candidate for long-term antibiotic prophylaxis?

What are the feasible options for long-term antibiotic prophylaxis?

than lactulose. Another commonly used regimen is 400 mg every 8 hours for 5 to 10 days.

Metronidazole and neomycin have also been used to treat hepatic encephalopathy but are not generally recommended because of toxicity; metronidazole is associated with peripheral neuropathy with prolonged use, and although neomycin is classified as a nonabsorbable antibiotic, patients with cirrhosis have detectable plasma concentrations. This is thought to be due to decreased integrity of the intestinal mucosa and may lead to nephrotoxicity. Neomycin should not be used.

Flumazenil Evidence for false transmitters as the cause of encephalopathy is demonstrated by the fact that administration of flumazenil (a benzodiazepine antagonist) has resulted in functional improvement. Unfortunately, long-term benefit has not been shown, and because flumazenil can only be administered parenterally, it is not an appropriate choice for clinical use. Flumazenil use is limited to the research setting.

Hepatorenal Syndrome

HRS is a life-threatening complication of cirrhosis. Targeted treatment increases central venous system volume. Peripheral vasoconstriction redistributes fluid from the periphery to the venous system; fluid is retained in the vascular space by administering albumin (to increase oncotic pressure). The ultimate goal is to increase renal perfusion.

A common regimen involves giving albumin 1 g/kg on day 1, followed by 20 to 40 g on subsequent treatment days. This regimen is used in combination with midodrine (an α-agonist) and octreotide. Midodrine is typically initiated at 7.5 mg orally three times daily, and octreotide is administered subcutaneously (as opposed to IV during variceal bleeding) 100 mcg three times daily. Both drugs can be titrated as tolerated to achieve increases in mean arterial pressure of 15 mm Hg or greater.

Terlipressin, a vasopressin analog available in Europe, has been used with success in patients with HRS, but it is not currently available in the United States.

▶ *Coagulation Abnormalities*

Vitamin K is essential to produce active coagulation factors in the liver. Elevated clotting time resulting from decreased protein synthesis is indistinguishable from that produced by low vitamin K levels secondary to malnutrition or poor intestinal absorption. When given subcutaneously (10 mg for 3 days), Vitamin K$_1$ (phytonadione) can replete stores and establish if coagulation abnormalities are secondary to decreased synthetic function alone. It is unusual to completely reverse clotting abnormalities, but most patients experience a decrease in international normalized ratio (INR), conferring a decreased risk of bleeding. Because cirrhotic patients may have decreased bile production resulting in decreased absorption of fat-soluble vitamins, phytonadione should be given subcutaneously instead of orally to ensure absorption.

OUTCOME EVALUATION

- Reevaluate the pharmacotherapy regimen at each visit to assess adherence, effectiveness, adverse events, and need for drug titration.

- Determine adherence to lifestyle changes such as cessation of ethanol intake and avoidance of over-the-counter medications (particularly NSAIDs and acetaminophen) and herbal remedies that may exacerbate complications of cirrhosis.

- Assess the effectiveness of β-blocker therapy by measuring heart rate. Heart rate reduction of 25% from baseline or to 55 to 60 bpm is desirable. Ask the patient specific, directed questions regarding adverse effects of β-blockers; inquire about symptoms of orthostatic hypotension (e.g., lightheadedness, dizziness, or fainting).

- Evaluate effectiveness of diuretic therapy with regard to ascitic fluid accumulation and development of peripheral edema. Ask the patient directed questions regarding abdominal girth, fullness, tenderness, and pain. Weigh the patient at each visit, and ask the patient to keep a weight diary. Assess for peripheral edema at each visit.

- Assess dietary sodium intake by patient food recall. Measure dietary sodium adherence using spot urine sodium-to-potassium ratio. Assess for appropriate sodium excretion.

- Obtain complete blood count and prothrombin time (PT)/INR to assess for anemia, thrombocytopenia, or coagulopathy. Ask about bruising, bleeding, hematemesis, hematochezia, and melena to assess for bleeding.

- Review biopsy reports and laboratory data. Hepatic transaminases and blood ammonia levels do not correlate well with disease progression, but increased coagulation times are markers of loss of synthetic function.

- Evaluate for signs and symptoms of HE. Mental status changes may be subtle; questioning family members or caregivers about confusion or personality changes may reveal mild HE even if the patient is unaware of deficits.

- In patients taking lactulose therapy, titrate the dose to achieve two to four soft bowel movements daily.

Patient Care and Monitoring

1. Obtain a complete history of alcohol intake and hepatotoxic drug use, including over-the-counter products and dietary supplements.

2. At each encounter, ask the patient specific questions about adherence to prescribed therapy, dietary restrictions, and cessation of alcohol intake.

3. At each visit, evaluate the pharmacotherapy regimen for appropriate drug choice and dose, nonprescription drug use, adverse effects, and use of potentially hepatotoxic medications.

4. Question the patient about adverse effects because hepatically metabolized medications may accumulate and cause adverse effects.

5. Consider antibiotic prophylaxis for SBP in patients with low-protein ascites or prior SBP.

6. Conduct a review of systems and physical examination at each visit to determine if the patient has had progression of complications.

7. Ask specific questions about bleeding, bruising, and fatigue. There is a direct link between loss of synthetic function and disease progression.

8. Refer the patient to substance abuse counseling for education about alcohol cessation if appropriate.

9. Provide education regarding dietary sodium restriction at each visit; consider referral to a dietician if appropriate.

Abbreviations Introduced in This Chapter

ADH	Alcohol dehydrogenase
ALT	Alanine aminotransferase
AST	Aspartate aminotransferase
BUN	Blood urea nitrogen
CYP450	Cytochrome P-450 isoenzyme
GGT	γ-Glutamyl transpeptidase
HE	Hepatic encephalopathy
HRS	Hepatorenal syndrome
INR	International normalized ratio
LDH	Lactate dehydrogenase
MELD	Model for End-Stage Liver Disease
NAFLD	Nonalcoholic fatty liver disease
NG	Nasogastric
NH_3	Ammonia
NH_4^+	Ammonium
NSAID	Nonsteroidal anti-inflammatory drug
PT	Prothrombin time
RAAS	Renin-angiotensin-aldosterone system
SAAG	Serum ascites-albumin gradient
SBP	Spontaneous bacterial peritonitis
TIPS	Transjugular intrahepatic portosystemic shunt

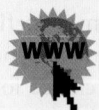 Self-assessment questions and answers are available at *http://www.mhpharmacotherapy. com/pp.html.*

REFERENCES

1. Lubel JS, Angus PW. Modern management of portal hypertension. Int Med J 2005;35:45–49.
2. Jiaquan X, Kochanek MA, Murphy SL, Tejada-Vera B. Deaths: Final data for 2007 [Internet]. Centers for Disease Control and Prevention Web site. Available from: *http://www.cdc.gov/nchs/fastats/liverdis. htm.*
3. National Digestive Diseases Information Clearinghouse. Cirrhosis of the liver. NIH Publication No. 04-1134. Bethesda, MD: Author, 2003.
4. Rehm J, Taylor B, Mohapatra S, et al. Alcohol as a risk factor for liver cirrhosis: A systematic review and meta-analysis. Drug Alcohol Rev 2010;29;437–445.
5. Soldin OP, Mattison DR. Sex differences in pharmacokinetics and pharmacodynamics. Clin Pharmacokinet 2009;48:143–157.
6. Te HS, Jensen DM. Epidemiology of hepatitis B and C viruses: A global overview. Clin Liver Dis 2010;14:1–21.
7. Sharma P, Kumar A, Sharma BC, Sarin SK. Early identification of haemodynamic response to pharmacotherapy is essential for primary prophylaxis of variceal bleeding in patients with 'high-risk' varices. Aliment Pharmacol Ther 2009; 30:48–60.
8. Garcia-Tsao G, Bosch J. Management of varices and variceal hemorrhage in cirrhosis. N Engl J Med 2010;362:823–832.

9. Krige JEJ, Beckingham IJ. ABC of diseases of liver, pancreas, and biliary system: Portal hypertension 2: Ascites, encephalopathy, and other conditions. BMJ 2001;322:416–418.

10. DeFranchis R. Updating consensus in portal hypertension: Report of the Baveno III workshop on definitions, methodology and therapeutic strategies in portal hypertension. J Hepatol 2000;33:846–852.

11. Berzigotti A, Gilabert R, Abraldes JG, et al. Noninvasive prediction of clinically significant portal hypertension and esophageal varices in patients with compensated liver cirrhosis. Am J Gastroenterol 2008;103:1159–1167.

12. Afzelius P, Bazeghi N, Bie P, et al. Circulating nitric oxide products do not solely reflect nitric oxide release in cirrhosis and portal hypertension. Liver Int 2011;31:1381–1387.

13. Gines P, Cardena A, Arroyo V, Rodes J. Management of cirrhosis and ascites. N Engl J Med 2004;350:1646–1654.

14. Garcia-Tsao G, Sanyal AJ, Grace ND, et al. AASLD practice guidelines: Prevention and management of gastroesophageal varices and variceal hemorrhage in cirrhosis. Hepatology 2007;46:922–938.

15. Rimola A, Garcia-Tsao G, Navasa M, et al. Diagnosis, treatment and prophylaxis of spontaneous bacterial peritonitis: A consensus document. J Hepatol 2000;32:142–145.

16. Steed H, Macfarlane GT, Blackett KL, et al. Bacterial translocation in cirrhosis is not caused by an abnormal small bowel gut microbiota. FEMS Immunol Med Microbiol 2011;63:346–354.

17. Such J, Frances R, Munoz C, et al. Detection and identification of bacterial DNA in patients with cirrhosis and culture-negative, nonneutrocytic ascites. Hepatology 2002;36:135–141.

18. Runyon BA. American Association for the Study of Liver Diseases (AASLD) practice guideline: Management of adult patients with ascites due to cirrhosis: An update. Hepatology 2009;49:2087–2107.

19. Blei AT, Cordoba J. The Practice Parameters Committee of the American College of Gastroenterology. Hepatic encephalopathy practice guidelines. Am J Gastroenterol 2001;96:1968–1976.

20. Armando Tripodi A, Primignani M, Chantarangkul V, et al. An imbalance of pro- vs anti-coagulation factors in plasma from patients with cirrhosis. Gastroenterol 2009;137:2105–2111.

21. Runyon BA. American Association for the Study of Liver Diseases (AASLD) practice guideline: Management of adult patients with ascites due to cirrhosis. Hepatology 2004;39:841–856.

22. Devanshi S, Haber PS, Syn W, et al. Pathogenesis of alcohol-induced liver disease: Classical concepts and recent advances. J Gastroenterol Hepatol 2011;26:1088–1105.

23. Sakaguchi S, Takahashi S, Sasaki T et al. Progression of alcoholic and non-alcoholic steatohepatitis: Common metabolic aspects of innate immune system and oxidative stress. Drug Metab Pharmacokinet 2011;26:30–46.

24. Chitturi S, Abeygunasekera S, Farrell GC, et al. NASH and insulin resistance: Insulin hypersecretion and specific association with the insulin resistance syndrome. Hepatology 2002;35:373–379.

25. Bravo A, Sheth S, Chopra S. Liver biopsy. N Engl J Med 2001;344:495–500.

26. Runyon BA, Montano A, Akrivadis E, et al. The serum ascites albumin gradient is superior to the exudate-transudate concept in the differential diagnosis of ascites. Ann Intern Med 1992;117:215–220.

27. Sharara AI, Rockey DC. Gastroesophageal variceal hemorrhage. N Engl J Med 2001;345:669–681.

28. Grace ND, American College of Gastroenterology Practice Parameters Committee. Diagnosis and treatment of gastrointestinal bleeding secondary to portal hypertension. Am J Gastroenterol 1997;92:1081–1091.

29. Lo GH, Lai KH, Cheng JS, et al. Endoscopic variceal ligation plus nadolol and sucralfate compared with ligation alone for the prevention of variceal rebleeding: A prospective, randomized trial. Hepatology 2000;32:461–465.

30. De La Pena J, Brullet E, Sanchez-Hernandez E, et al. Variceal ligation plus nadolol compared with ligation for prophylaxis of variceal rebleeding: A multicenter trial. Hepatology 2005;41:572–578.

31. Centers for Disease Control and Prevention. Sexually transmitted diseases treatment guidelines 2002. MMWR Recomm Rep 2002;51(RR-6):1–78.

32. Boyer TD, Haskal ZJ. American Association for the Study of Liver Diseases (AASLD) practice guideline: The role of transjugular intrahepatic portosystemic shunt in the management of portal hypertension. Hepatology 2005;41:386–401.

33. Pagliaro L, D'Amico G, Sorensen TI, et al. Prevention of first bleeding in cirrhosis. A meta-analysis of randomized trials of nonsurgical treatment. Ann Intern Med 1992;117:59–70.

34. Merkel C, Sacerdoti D, Bolognesi M, et al. Hemodynamic evaluation of the addition of isosorbide-5-mononitrate to nadolol in cirrhotic patients with insufficient response to the beta-blocker alone. Hepatology 1997;26:34–39.

35. Gournay J, Masliah C, Martin T, et al. Isosorbide mononitrate and propranolol compared with propranolol alone for the prevention of variceal rebleeding. Hepatology 2000;6:1239–1245.

36. Such J, Runyon BA. Spontaneous bacterial peritonitis. Clin Infect Dis 1998;27:669–674.

37. Soares-Weiser K, Brezis M, Tur-Kaspa R, et al. Antibiotic prophylaxis of bacterial infections in cirrhotic inpatients: A meta-analysis of randomized controlled trials. Scand J Gastroenterol 2003;38:193–200.

38. Sort P, Navasa M, Arroyo V, et al. Effect of intravenous albumin on renal impairment and mortality in patients with cirrhosis and spontaneous bacterial peritonitis. N Engl J Med 1999;341:403–409.

39. Pasricha PJ. Treatment of disorders of bowel motility and water flux; antiemetics; agents used in biliary and pancreatic disease. In: Brunton LL, LAZO JS, Parker KL, eds. Goodman & Gilman's The Pharmacologic Basis of Therapeutics, 11th ed. New York, NY: McGraw-Hill, 2005:1335–1358.

40. Mortensen PB. The effect of oral-administered lactulose on colonic nitrogen metabolism and excretion. Hepatology 1992;16:1350–1356.

41. Mortensen PB, Holtug K, Bonnen H, Clausen MR. The degradation of amino acids, proteins, and blood to short-chain fatty acids in colon is prevented by lactulose. Gastroenterology 1990;98:353–360.

23 Pancreatitis

Janine E. Then and Heather M. Rouse

LEARNING OBJECTIVES

● **Upon completion of the chapter, the reader will be able to:**

1. Describe the pathophysiology of acute and chronic pancreatitis.

2. Differentiate acute from chronic pancreatitis.

3. Discuss the clinical implications of pancreatic fluid collections, pancreatic abscess, and pancreatic necrosis in acute pancreatitis.

4. Formulate care plans for managing acute pancreatitis.

5. Identify pharmacologic and nonpharmacologic means of preventing repeat episodes of chronic pancreatitis.

6. Choose appropriate pancreatic enzyme supplementation for patients with chronic pancreatitis.

KEY CONCEPTS

① The most common causes of acute and chronic pancreatitis in adults are ethanol abuse and biliary stones.

② Pancreatic necrosis occurs within the first 2 weeks of acute pancreatitis and develops in 10% to 20% of patients with acute pancreatitis.

③ Therapy of acute pancreatitis is primarily supportive unless a specific etiology is identified. Supportive therapy involves fluid repletion, nutrition support, and analgesia.

④ Medications aimed at decreasing pancreatic enzyme release, nasogastric suction, and anticholinergic medications have not shown benefit in the treatment of acute pancreatitis.

⑤ Long-term sequelae of chronic pancreatitis include dietary malabsorption, impaired glucose tolerance, cholangitis, and potential addiction to opioid analgesics.

⑥ Treatment of chronic pancreatitis is aimed at removing the cause (ethanol abuse, cigarette smoking, or biliary stones), providing analgesia, supplementing with pancreatic enzyme preparations, and implementing dietary restrictions.

INTRODUCTION

The pancreas is a gland in the abdomen lying in the curvature of the stomach as it empties into the duodenum. The pancreas functions primarily as an exocrine gland, although it also has endocrine function. The exocrine cells of the pancreas are called **acinar cells** that produce and store various digestive enzymes that mix with a bicarbonate-rich solution released from duct cells to produce pancreatic juice. This pancreatic juice is released through the **ampulla of Vater** into the duodenum to aid in the digestive process as well as buffer acidic fluid released from the stomach (**Fig. 23–1**).[1]

These enzymes are produced and stored as inactive proenzymes within **zymogen** granules to prevent autolysis and digestion of the pancreas. The zymogen granules are also responsible for enzyme transport to the pancreatic duct. Amylase and lipase are released from the zymogen granules in the active form, whereas the proteolytic enzymes are activated in the duodenum by enterokinase. Enterokinase triggers the conversion of trypsinogen to the active protease **trypsin**, which then activates the other proenzymes to their active enzymes. The pancreas contains a trypsin inhibitor to prevent autolysis.

ACUTE PANCREATITIS

EPIDEMIOLOGY AND ETIOLOGY

① *In the Western Hemisphere, acute pancreatitis is caused mainly by ethanol use/abuse and gallstones (cholelithiasis).* Ethanol use accounts for about 30% of acute pancreatitis cases and gallstones about 30% to 40% of cases. Other common causes of acute pancreatitis include hypertriglyceridemia,

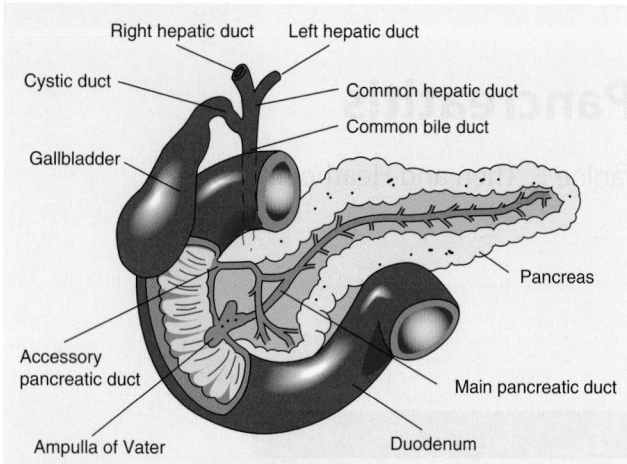

FIGURE 23–1. Anatomical structure of the pancreas and biliary tract. (From Bolesta S, Montgomery PA. Pancreatitis. In: DiPiro JT, Talbert RL, Yee GC, et al., eds. Pharmacotherapy: A Pathophysiologic Approach, 8th ed. New York, NY: McGraw-Hill, 2011; Figure 46–1, with permission.)

endoscopic retrograde cholangiopancreatography (ERCP), pregnancy, and autodigestion due to early activation of pancreatic enzymes. Numerous medications have also been implicated as causes of acute pancreatitis, but other causes should be ruled out before discontinuing a medication indefinitely (Table 23–1).[2]

PATHOPHYSIOLOGY

Ethanol abuse may cause precipitation of pancreatic enzymes in the ducts of the pancreas, leading to chronic inflammation

Table 23–1

Selected Medications Associated with Acute Pancreatitis

Definite Association	Probable Association
5-Aminosalicylic acid	Angiotensin-converting enzyme
Asparaginase	inhibitors
Azathioprine	HMG-CoA reductase inhibitors
Corticosteroids	Cimetidine
Didanosine	Cisplatin
Estrogens	Clozapine
Furosemide	Ethacrynic acid
6-Mercaptopurine	Indinavir
Cytarabine	Interferon α-2b
Pentamidine	Lamivudine
Sulfonamides	NSAIDs
Sulindac	Propofol
Tigecycline	Salicylates
Valproic acid/salts	Thiazide diuretics
	Zalcitabine

Adapted from Bolesta S, Montgomery PA. Pancreatitis. In: DiPiro JT, Talbert RL, Yee GC, et al., eds. Pharmacotherapy: A Pathophysiologic Approach, 8th ed. New York, NY: McGraw-Hill, 2011; Table 46–2, with permission.

and fibrosis resulting in loss of exocrine function. Ethanol itself may be directly toxic to the pancreatic cells and may lead to an upregulation of enzymes that produce toxic metabolites leading to further damage.[3] Gallstones can obstruct the ampulla of Vater causing pancreatic enzymes or bile to move in a retrograde fashion into the pancreas. This retrograde movement may be responsible for pancreatic autolysis.[1]

Autolysis of the pancreas can occur when zymogens are activated in the pancreas before being released into the duodenum. Acute pancreatitis can result from the initial injury to the zymogen-producing cells, which is followed by neutrophil, lymphocyte, and macrophage invasion of the pancreas and further activation of enzymes within the pancreas. This cascade of events is destructive to the pancreas and harmful to the patient.

Acute pancreatitis can progress to several distinct consequences. Acute peripancreatic fluid collections are located in or around the pancreas. They form within the first 4 weeks of acute pancreatitis and are not walled off. They are usually sterile but can become infected or hemorrhagic. Acute peripancreatic fluid collections are expected to resolve spontaneously and intervention may introduce infection.[4]

Pancreatic pseudocysts are formed at least 4 weeks after the start of acute pancreatitis and are walled-off collections of tissue, pancreatic enzymes, and blood. Many pancreatic pseudocysts resolve spontaneously, but some require surgical or percutaneous drainage. Rupture of a pancreatic pseudocyst is the most serious complication and can lead to peritonitis and GI bleeding.[4]

Pancreatic necrosis is a diffuse inflammation of the pancreas containing both necrotic tissue and fluid that over time undergoes liquefaction. Necrosis is due to pancreatic enzyme damage to the pancreatic tissue. ❷ *Pancreatic necrosis occurs within the first 2 weeks of acute pancreatitis and develops in 10% to 20% of patients with acute pancreatitis.* Infected necrotic fluid collections occur in 16% to 47% of patients, usually due to bacteria normally present in the GI tract. These organisms include *Escherichia coli*, Enterobacteriaceae, *Staphylococcus aureus*, viridans group streptococci, and anaerobes. Disseminated infection may result from pancreatic necrosis.[4,5]

Walled-off pancreatic necrosis, or pancreatic abscess, is pancreatic necrosis that is surrounded by granulation tissue and occurs weeks after acute pancreatitis. Pancreatic abscess is usually less life threatening than pancreatic necrosis and can be managed with percutaneous drainage, ideally after the third or fourth week to allow demarcation.[4]

CLINICAL PRESENTATION AND DIAGNOSIS

Patients with acute pancreatitis may develop many severe local and systemic complications. Multiorgan failure is a poor prognostic indicator. Early aggressive care should be sought for those presenting with more severe disease.

Disease severity can be predicted in many ways. The Ranson criteria, Glasgow severity scoring system, Acute

Symptoms

- Sudden upper abdominal pain is the most common presenting symptom. Pain can be due to intestinal immobility or chemical peritonitis induced by pancreatic enzymes.
- Pain and abdominal distention may also be due to local complications such as fluid collection, necrosis, or abscess in the pancreas.
- Pain may radiate to the back, and ecchymoses may be present in the flank and periumbilical areas.
- Nausea and vomiting are other common symptoms.

Signs

- Tachycardia, hypotension, fever, and abdominal distention may be present.
- There may be a positive Cullen's sign (bluish discoloration of the periumbilical skin indicating blood in the peritoneum).
- After 2 to 3 days of acute hemorrhagic pancreatitis, there may be a positive Turner's sign (local areas of bruising and induration of the skin near the umbilicus due to extravasation of blood).

Laboratory Tests

- The serum amylase may be elevated to greater than three times the upper limit of normal within the first 12 hours of the onset of acute pancreatitis. The degree of elevation does not correlate with the severity of disease.
- As acute pancreatitis progresses, serum lipase becomes elevated.
- Other possible laboratory abnormalities include elevated WBC count, hyperglycemia, hypocalcemia, hyperbilirubinemia, elevated serum lactate dehydrogenase (LDH), and hypertriglyceridemia.

Physiology and Chronic Health Evaluation II (APACHE II), and sequential organ failure assessment (SOFA) have all been used to predict mortality. A Ranson or Glasgow score of 3 or greater or an APACHE II score of 8 or greater is predictive of severe acute pancreatitis and may signal the need for treatment in an intensive care unit.[6]

DIAGNOSIS

Diagnosis of acute pancreatitis is based on the patient's history, signs and symptoms, and laboratory values. The history can identify risk factors for acute pancreatitis including alcohol abuse and medications. A serum lipase greater than three times the normal limit supports the diagnosis. The serum lipase has greater sensitivity and specificity for acute pancreatitis than does the serum amylase. The serum amylase is also elevated early in the disease process but may return

to normal prior to hospital presentation in some patients.[7] Serum lipase remains elevated for days after the onset of the acute event. Elevated hepatic enzymes may indicate gallstone pancreatitis, and triglycerides should be checked to rule out hypertriglyceridemia as the cause of pancreatitis.[6,7]

Abdominal ultrasound is able to identify gallstones and sludge in the common bile duct but is limited in its sensitivity. Computed tomography (CT) may be more useful in staging pancreatitis or identifying complications. Magnetic resonance imaging (MRI) and magnetic resonance cholangiopancreatography (MRCP) are more costly options that can be used to evaluate severity and pancreatic abnormalities.[6,7]

TREATMENT

Desired Outcomes

The goals of treatment for acute pancreatitis include: (a) resolution of nausea, vomiting, abdominal pain, and fever; (b) ability to tolerate oral intake; (c) normalization of serum amylase, lipase, and white blood cell (WBC) count; and (d) resolution of abscess, pseudocyst, or fluid collection as measured by CT scan.

Nonpharmacologic Therapy

Many medications can precipitate an attack of acute pancreatitis. If a medication is determined to be the cause of acute pancreatitis, it should be discontinued and an alternative therapy should be considered. If the medication is deemed clinically necessary, it is appropriate to rechallenge if there is not strong evidence that pancreatitis was due to the medication.[2]

3 *Therapy of acute pancreatitis is primarily supportive unless a specific etiology is identified (Fig. 23–2). Supportive therapy involves fluid repletion, nutrition support, and analgesia.* Patients with acute pancreatitis are administered IV fluids to maintain hydration and blood pressure. Fluids may be given in the form of crystalloids (e.g., 0.9% sodium chloride for infusion) or colloids (e.g., hetastarch or albumin for infusion). The rate and amount of fluids administered should

JR is a 45-year-old man who presents to the emergency department with a 2-day history of nausea and vomiting. He also complains of abdominal pain that is unrelieved and persistent. He has not eaten in the past 2 days because food exacerbates the pain. Upon examination, his abdomen is found to be distended.

What information about the patient presentation is consistent with acute pancreatitis?

What tests may be helpful in the diagnosis of acute pancreatitis?

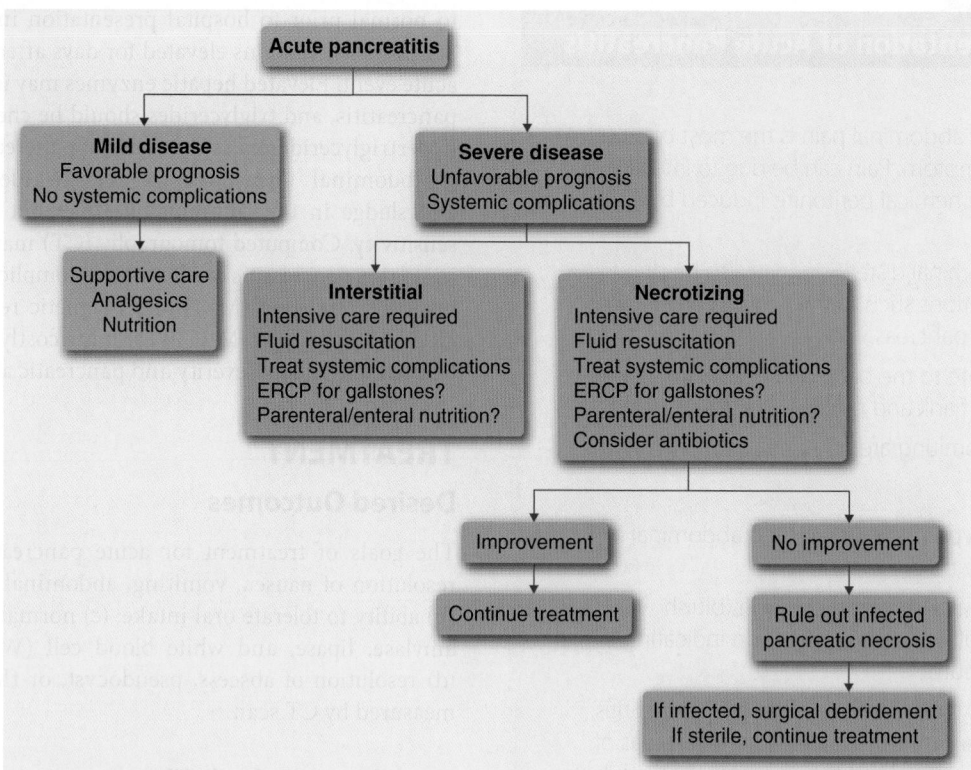

FIGURE 23–2. Algorithm for evaluation and treatment of acute pancreatitis. (ERCP, endoscopic retrograde cholangiopancreatography.) (From Bolesta S, Montgomery PA. Pancreatitis. In: DiPiro JT, Talbert RL, Yee GC, et al., eds. Pharmacotherapy: A Pathophysiologic Approach, 8th ed. New York, NY: McGraw-Hill, 2011; Figure 46–3, with permission.)

be based on vital signs and urine output. Assessment of fluid requirements should be more frequent for patients with concomitant cardiac, renal, and liver disease.[6] An increase in hematocrit as a marker of dehydration is a poor prognostic sign.[5,8] Electrolytes such as potassium and magnesium may be added to the infusions if necessary. Hyperglycemia can be managed with insulin-containing IV infusions.

It is common practice to discontinue oral feedings during an attack of acute pancreatitis. In fact, this practice does not prevent further damage because the secretion of trypsin is reduced during acute pancreatitis.[5] In mild to moderate pancreatitis, the patient's diet should be advanced based on resolution of nausea, vomiting, and pain. In severe pancreatitis, enteral nutrition should be started as early as possible and may include nasogastric or nasojejunal feedings. Nasojejunal tube feedings feed the patient beyond the ampulla of Vater, minimizing stimulation of the pancreas. Early use of enteral nutrition has been shown to decrease surgical interventions and infectious complications. In severe pancreatitis, enteral nutrition can be supplemented with total parenteral nutrition to maintain adequate nutrition.[5,7,9]

If pancreatic necrosis or abscesses are present, surgical or interventional procedures should be considered. CT-guided percutaneous drainage may be used to drain abscesses or as a bridge to surgery. Endoscopic necrosectomy and open

necrosectomy may be required and may involve repeat procedures until all of the necrotic tissue is removed.[7] An ERCP may be used early in the course of treatment if there are retained bile duct stones or signs of cholangitis. Delayed intervention with ERCP may be indicated if symptoms resolve.[7]

Pharmacologic Therapy

▶ *Analgesics*

Meperidine has historically been the most popular analgesic in acute pancreatitis because it is purported to cause less spasm and resulting pain in the sphincter of Oddi than other opioids. However, the importance of this has not been confirmed in clinical studies. As a result, patients with acute pancreatitis should be given the most effective analgesic. Hydromorphone, morphine, and fentanyl are reasonable alternatives to meperidine and may be more desirable due to other adverse effects associated with meperidine. Refer to Chapter 34 on pain management for guidance in selecting an analgesic dose.

▶ *Antibiotics*

Empiric antibiotics are not indicated if the patient has mild disease or a noninfectious etiology of acute pancreatitis. Antibiotics have not been shown to prevent the formation of

Patient Encounter 1, Part 2

PMH: Hypertension, hypercholesterolemia

Allergies: Penicillin (anaphylaxis)

FH: Father—MI at 48 years of age, CHF, COPD; mother—osteoporosis, breast cancer, gallstones

SH: History of heaving drinking but stopped 12 years ago when his first child was born; no tobacco; no recreational drugs

Meds: Enalapril, atorvastatin, and an over-the-counter "stomach pill"

ROS: Positive for sharp RUQ abdominal pain that radiates to the right shoulder and back, nausea, vomiting; negative for substernal chest pain

PE:

VS: BP 105/60 seated, 90/50 standing, P 120 bpm, RR 22 breaths/min, T 37.9°C (100.2°F), pain score 9/10, wt 91 kg (200 lb), ht 6'1" (185 cm)

CV: Regular rate and rhythm, no murmurs

Abd: Distended, (+) rebound tenderness, (+) bowel sounds, (+) guarding

Labs: Amylase 90 IU/L (1.5 μkat/L), lipase 1250 IU/L (20.8 μkat/L), WBC 15.8 × 10³/mm³ (15.8 ×10⁹/L), Hgb 10.9 g/dL (109 g/L, 6.77 mmol/L), Hct 30% (0.30), platelets 250 × 10³/mm³ (250 × 10⁹/L), BUN 19 mg/dL (6.8 mmol/L), SCr 1.2 mg/dL (106 μmol/L), glucose 220 mg/dL (12.2 mmol/L), AST 520 IU/L (8.67 μkat/L), ALT 480 IU/L (8.00 μkat/L), LDH 1,050 IU/L (17.50 μkat/L)

Abdominal x-ray and ultrasound: Pending

What is your assessment of this patient given the above findings?

What additional information is needed at this point?

What treatment(s) would you initiate?

pancreatic abscess or necrosis when given early in the course of acute pancreatitis.

In pancreatic necrosis, 40% to 70% of patients have infected necrotic tissue. Multiple studies have found no clear mortality benefit with the use of prophylactic antibiotics in necrotizing pancreatitis. However, antibiotics may be appropriate in patients with multiorgan failure or in those with suspected infection. The use of prophylactic antibiotics may lead to more resistant infections or a change in the infecting flora to gram-positive or fungal organisms. As such, the decision to use antibiotics is highly individualized. Consideration should be given to discontinuing antibiotics if no source of infection is confirmed. Selected IV antibiotic regimens are shown in Table 23–2. If necrosis is confirmed, antibiotics are insufficient as sole therapy; surgical debridement is necessary for cure.[5,7,10]

Broad-spectrum antibiotics with activity against enteric gram-negative bacilli are appropriate. It is often difficult to narrow the spectrum of activity of the antibiotic choice because the infections are usually polymicrobial. As such, patients may receive long courses of broad-spectrum antibiotics such as meropenem and may develop superinfections due to resistant bacteria. Antifungal agents such as fluconazole may be considered if peritonitis or GI perforation develops due to the presence of fungi such as *Candida albicans* in the GI tract.[11]

▶ Ineffective Therapies

Several pharmacologic therapies have been proven to be ineffective in reducing morbidity or mortality from the disease. ❹ *Ineffective therapies include reducing pancreatic secretion by administering somatostatin or atropine, reducing gastric acidity and decreasing pancreatic secretion with histamine$_2$-receptor antagonists, probiotics, and immunomodulation.* Nasogastric suction has only been effective in patients with ileus or persistent vomiting.[6,7]

OUTCOME EVALUATION

- Monitor hydration status closely. Administer fluids using crystalloids or colloids, and replete electrolytes as necessary.
- Provide patients with analgesia and monitor pain severity using validated scales.
- Initiate nutrition support as early as possible. Enteral nutrition is preferred, but parenteral nutrition may be considered if enteral nutrition is not tolerated.
- Monitor patients with moderate to severe pancreatitis in an intensive care setting where frequent monitoring of vital signs can be provided.
- Continually assess patients for signs of infection including fever, leukocytosis, and other signs of sepsis.

Table 23–2

Selected IV Antimicrobial Regimens for Pancreatic Necrosis

Drug	Usual Dose^a	Notes
Meropenem	1 g every 8 hours	Risk of superinfection
Piperacillin/tazobactam	3.375 g every 6 hours	Avoid if allergic to penicillin
Cefepime + metronidazole	2 g every 12 hours + 500 mg every 6 hours	Will not cover enterococci
Aztreonam + vancomycin + metronidazole	1 g every 8 hours + 15 mg/kg every 8–12 hours + 500 mg every 6 hours	Option for penicillin-allergic patients

^{a}Doses must be adjusted for the degree of renal impairment.

CHRONIC PANCREATITIS

EPIDEMIOLOGY AND ETIOLOGY

The incidence of chronic pancreatitis (CP) ranges from 3.5 to 10 per 100,000 population. ❶ *The most common cause of chronic pancreatitis in adults in Western countries is ethanol abuse.* Other causes of CP include genetic predisposition, obstructive disease (secondary to ductal strictures or pseudocysts), autoimmune pancreatitis, abnormal cystic fibrosis transmembrane conductance regulator (CFTR) function as seen in cystic fibrosis (CF) patients, tropical pancreatitis, and idiopathic pancreatitis.[3,12,13] More recently, cigarette smoking was identified as an independent risk factor for CP.[14]

PATHOPHYSIOLOGY

Chronic pancreatitis is an inflammatory process that occurs over time leading to impaired endocrine and exocrine function secondary to diffuse scarring and fibrosis.[12,13] There are multiple hypotheses to the pathogenesis of ethanol-induced pancreatitis including: (a) precipitation of secreted pancreatic proteins within small pancreatic ducts leading to acinar atrophy and fibrosis, (b) disruption of acinar cells leading to early activation of digestive enzymes and autodigestive pancreatic injury, and (c) oxidative pancreatic stress caused by toxic metabolites of ethanol.[12]

❺ *Long-term sequelae of chronic pancreatitis include dietary malabsorption, impaired glucose tolerance, cholangitis, and potential addiction to opioid analgesics.* As patients lose exocrine function of the pancreas, they have a decreased ability to absorb lipids and protein ingested with normal dietary intake. Weight loss from nutritional malabsorption is a common symptom of CP. Fatty- or protein-containing stools are also common; carbohydrate absorption is usually unaffected. Even though patients with CP have decreased ability to absorb lipid from the GI tract, they do not appear to have a higher incidence of fat-soluble vitamin deficiency.[12,15]

CLINICAL PRESENTATION AND DIAGNOSIS

The symptoms, signs, and laboratory abnormalities associated with CP are shown in the accompanying text box. Pancreatic biopsy with histologic examination is the gold standard for diagnosis for CP, but it is rarely performed. In the absence of histology, abdominal ultrasound, CT, MRCP, or ERCP can assist in the diagnosis.[3,12]

Patient Encounter 1, Part 3

JR has now been hospitalized for 10 days with continued pain and food intolerance. This morning his WBC count is elevated at $21.2 \times 10^3/mm^3$ ($21.2 \times 10^9/L$), and he has a temperature of 38.7°C (101.6°F). He is hypotensive with a MAP of 60 mm Hg, and his HR is 115 bpm. His respiratory rate is 28 breaths/min and his SCr is 2.0 mg/dL (177 μmol/L). A CT scan demonstrates pancreatic necrosis, and antibiotics are started. His APACHE II score is calculated to be 13.

Based on his APACHE II score of 13, should JR be considered for transfer to the intensive care unit?

Which microorganisms should empiric antibiotics cover?

What antimicrobials would be appropriate to initiate at this time?

Besides antibiotics, what other pharmacologic treatments may need to be optimized?

Clinical Presentation of Chronic Pancreatitis

General

- The presentation of chronic pancreatitis can be similar to that of acute pancreatitis.

Symptoms

- Pain is the most common symptom, and it typically starts in the epigastrium and may radiate to the back or scapula. Pain can be sharp or dull, and it may be relieved by leaning forward or sitting upright. The pain is not relieved by antacids and can be provoked by ethanol ingestion or a fatty meal.
- The pain may be associated with nausea and vomiting, causing patients to avoid food.
- Weight loss can result from chronic fat and protein malabsorption.

Signs

- Steatorrhea (due to fat malabsorption), malnutrition, and glucose intolerance are often present in advanced CP.[3,13]
- GI bleeding can result from erosion of intestinal blood vessels by pancreatic enzymes or as a result of thrombosis.
- Chronic obstruction of the common bile duct by the inflamed pancreas can cause icterus, cholangitis, and biliary cirrhosis.

Laboratory Tests

- Glucose intolerance may occur because of chronic destruction of the endocrine function of the pancreas.
- Serum amylase and lipase concentrations may be normal to slightly elevated in CP, and they are not particularly useful in the diagnosis of CP.[12,13]
- The serum bilirubin or alkaline phosphatase may be elevated due to inflammation near the common bile duct.

TREATMENT

Desired Outcomes

The goals of pharmacotherapy for CP include: (a) relief of acute and chronic abdominal pain, (b) correction of dietary malabsorption with exogenous pancreatic enzymes, and (c) treatment of endocrine insufficiency and associated diabetes.[12]

Nonpharmacologic Therapy

Lifestyle modifications are an important part of the therapy for CP. ❻ *Avoidance of ethanol, cigarette smoking, and fatty meals can decrease the pain of chronic pancreatitis.* There is evidence that alcohol and cigarette abstainers have slower disease progression and better response to pain therapy than nonabstainers.[3,12,14] Patients should also be advised to consume a diet consisting of frequent small low-fat meals (less than 20 g fat/day) or one with medium-chain triglycerides where absorption requires only minimal amounts of pancreatic enzymes.[12,13,16]

Many surgical procedures have been employed to reduce the inflammation or remove the strictures that cause pain in CP. However, most procedures (e.g., nerve blocks) have not been studied in clinical trials and carry a high risk of morbidity and mortality.[12]

Pharmacologic Therapy

▶ Analgesics

❻ *Pain management is an important component of therapy and similar to that of acute pancreatitis.* Nonopioid analgesics (e.g., acetaminophen, nonsteroidal anti-inflammatory drugs [NSAIDs]) are preferred, but the severe and persistent nature of the pain often requires opioid therapy. Patients can require chronic doses of opioid analgesics, with a resulting risk of addiction.[13,17] Patients should also be assessed for neuropathic pain and treated accordingly (e.g., tricyclic antidepressants, pregabalin).[17,18] Refer to Chapter 34 on pain management for guidance in selecting an analgesic dose.

▶ Pancreatic Enzymes

Pancreatic enzyme supplementation is indicated in symptomatic patients with steatorrhea. The goal is to deliver exogenous enzyme to the duodenum without causing further GI side effects, risking noncompliance due to the large number of dosage units required, or causing undue medication expense.[16,19] ❻ *Supplementation with pancreatic enzymes may reduce the pain and fatty diarrhea associated with chronic pancreatitis* (Table 23–3). Common pancreatic enzyme supplements (PESs) contain lipase, amylase, and protease in varying proportions. The half-life of endogenous lipase is based on the presence of its substrates (i.e., triglycerides), and therefore dietary fat restriction should be reconsidered when pancreatic enzyme replacement is used.[16]

PESs were previously exempt from the Food, Cosmetic and Drug Act of 1938 and therefore did not require FDA approval

Table 23–3				
Frequently Used Pancreatic Enzyme Preparations				
		Enzyme Content (Units)[a]		
Product	**Dosage Form**	**Lipase**	**Amylase**	**Protease**
Creon-6	Microsphere	6,000	30,000	19,000
Creon-12	Microsphere	12,000	60,000	38,000
Creon-24	Microsphere	24,000	76,000	120,000
Pancreaze-4	Microtablet	4,200	17,500	10,000
Pancreaze-10	Microtablet	10,500	43,750	25,000
Pancreaze-16	Microtablet	16,800	70,000	40,000
Pancreaze-21	Microtablet	21,000	61,000	37,000
Pancrelipase	Beads	5,000	27,000	17,000
Zenpep-3	Beads	3,000	16,000	10,000
Zenpep-5	Beads	5,000	27,000	17,000
Zenpep-10	Beads	10,000	55,000	34,000
Zenpep-15	Beads	15,000	82,000	51,000
Zenpep-20	Beads	20,000	109,000	68,000

[a]All listed products are supplied as capsules with delayed-release, enteric-coated delivery systems. All products are porcine derived.

prior to marketing. In the past, PESs were available in a variety of formulations including microsphere, microcapsule, enteric-coated, and non–enteric-coated products. These PES were considered to be effective, but treatment failures sometimes occurred when patients switched to a different unapproved product. This prompted the FDA to review the various products; the agency found large differences in clinical response between the products. In 2004, the FDA required all PESs to gain new drug application (NDA) approval by April 2010.[20]

There are currently three FDA-approved PESs in the United States (Table 23–3). Each product is enteric coated and releases enzymes in the alkaline environment (pH 5.5) of the duodenum, thus minimizing enzyme destruction in the stomach. Enteric-coated PESs require fewer daily dosage units than their non–enteric-coated predecessors. However, in patients with delayed gastric emptying, the efficacy of the enteric-coated PES may be decreased due to the early activation of the lipase enzymes. Addition of an H_2-blocker or proton pump inhibitor will decrease the acidity in the stomach, thereby enhancing delivery of the PES to the site of action.[16]

Pancreatic enzyme supplements should be taken immediately prior to meals and snacks to aid in the digestion and absorption of food. Dosing is based on body weight, clinical symptoms, and stool fat content. A normal starting dose is 500 units/kg/meal of lipase with half of the mealtime dose administered with snacks. Doses of lipase more than 10,000 units/kg/day should be used with caution because they may be associated with colonic stricture and fibrosis. Capsules may be opened; however, the contents of the capsule should not be crushed or chewed.

▶ Other Therapies

In patients with autoimmune pancreatitis, prednisolone 30 to 40 mg/day tapered over a 3-month period may provide

Patient Encounter 2

KS is a 53-year-old woman who presents to the emergency department complaining of a chronic dull pain in her abdomen for several months that is no longer relieved with over-the-counter analgesics. She has also had light-colored liquid stools for the past month and has lost 10 pounds because of decreased appetite.

PMH: Hypothyroidism, depression, recurrent acute pancreatitis

SH: Consumes a six-pack of beer/day and has a 35 pack–year history of cigarette smoking

Meds: Citalopram 20 mg daily, levothyroxine 50 mcg every morning, recent use of ibuprofen 400 mg every 4 hours without pain relief

ROS: (+) for RUQ abdominal pain that radiates to her back, decreased appetite, 10-lb (4.5-kg) weight loss and fatty diarrhea for the past month. (–) for chest pain or shortness of breath.

PE:

VS: BP 125/79 mm Hg, HR 75 bpm, RR 15 breaths/ min, T 37.1°C (98.8°F), weight 63.2 kg (139 lb), height 5'4" (163 cm)

CV: Regular rate and rhythm, no murmurs noted

Abd: Distended, (+) rebound tenderness, (+) bowel sounds

Labs: Amylase 50 IU/L (0.83 μkat/L) , lipase 100 IU/L (1.7 μkat/L); BUN 19 mg/dL (6.8 mmol/L), SCr 0.75 mg/dL (66 μmol/L), glucose 248 mg/dL (13.8 mmol/L), AST 32 IU/L (0.53 μkat/L), ALT 29 IU/L (0.48 μkat/L)

CT scan abdomen: Diffuse pancreatic scarring and calcifications

What signs and symptoms are consistent with chronic pancreatitis?

Why are the serum amylase and lipase normal?

What lifestyle modifications would you recommend for this patient?

What, if any, treatment regimens would you initiate, and how would you monitor their effects?

Patient Care and Monitoring

1. Determine whether ethanol is a contributing causative factor. If so, reinforce counseling on the need for abstinence and provide appropriate resources to maintain abstinence (e.g., professional counseling, Alcoholics Anonymous).

2. Obtain a thorough history of prescription, nonprescription, and dietary supplement use to identify products that may exacerbate chronic pancreatitis.

3. Refer the patient for nutritional counseling if there is decreased caloric intake and weight loss. Compare actual body weight to ideal body weight.

4. Make a plan for analgesia, in conjunction with a pain management service if possible, to control and prevent pain. Recommend an analgesic with ease of dosing and minimal side effects, realizing that patients with chronic pancreatitis may require large doses of opioids.

5. Pancreatic enzyme supplementation should be initiated in patients with steatorrhea. Doses should start at 500 units/kg/meal of lipase with half of the dose administered with snacks.

6. Develop a plan for reassessing pancreatic enzyme supplementation and analgesia on an outpatient basis.

7. Assess improvement in quality-of-life measures such as physical, psychological, and social functioning and well-being.

rapid relief of symptoms. Antioxidants such as methionine, ascorbic acid, and selenium may reduce the number of painful days per month in patients with CP.[3]

OUTCOME EVALUATION

- Monitor pain control and adjust analgesics accordingly.
- Encourage lifestyle modifications such as abstinence from ethanol and cigarettes.
- Counsel patients to monitor for weight gain or loss and fatty stool output as a marker of malabsorption.
- Educate patients that adherence with dietary pancreatic enzyme supplementation is key to improved outcomes.[13,16,19]

Abbreviations Introduced in This Chapter

APACHE II	Acute Physiology and Chronic Health Evaluation II
CF	Cystic fibrosis
CFTR	Cystic fibrosis transmembrane conductance regulator
CP	Chronic pancreatitis
CT	Computed tomography
ERCP	Endoscopic retrograde cholangiopancreatography
MAP	Mean arterial pressure
MRCP	Magnetic resonance cholangiopancreatography
PES	Pancreatic enzyme supplement
RUQ	Right upper quadrant
SOFA	Sequential organ failure assessment

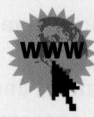 Self-assessment questions and answers are available at *http://www.mhpharmacotherapy. com/pp.html.*

REFERENCES

1. Hegyi P, Pandol S, Venglovecz V, Rakonczay Z Jr. The acinar-ductal tango in the pathogenesis of acute pancreatitis. Gut 2011;60: 544–552.

2. Nitsche CJ, Jamieson N, Lerch MM, Mayerle JV. Drug induced pancreatitis. Best Pract Res Clin Gastroenterol 2010;24:143–155.

3. Braganza JM, Lee SH, McCloy RF, McMahon MJ. Chronic pancreatitis. Lancet 2011;377:1184–1197.

4. Brun A, Agarwal N, Pitchumoni CS. Fluid collections in and around the pancreas in acute pancreatitis. J Clin Gastroenterol 2011;45:614–625.

5. Talukdar R, Vege SS. Early management of severe acute pancreatitis. Curr Gastroenterol Rep 2011;13:123–130.

6. Pezzilli R, Zerbi A, Di Carlo V, Bassi C, Delle Fave GF. Practical guidelines for acute pancreatitis. Pancreatology 2010;10:523–535.

7. Schneider L, Buchler MW, Werner J. Acute pancreatitis with an emphasis on infection. Infect Dis Clin North Am 2010;24:921–941.

8. Brisinda G, Vanella S, Crocco A, et al. Severe acute pancreatitis: Advances and insights in assessment of severity and management. Eur J Gastroenterol Hepatol 2011;23:541–551.

9. Quan H, Wang X, Guo C. A meta-analysis of enteral nutrition and total parenteral nutrition in patients with acute pancreatitis. Gastroenterol Res Pract 2011; article ID 698248.

10. Nicholson LJ. Acute pancreatitis: Should we use antibiotics? Curr Gastroenterol Rep 2011;13:336–343.

11. Trikudanathan G, Navaneethan U, Vege SS. Intra-abdominal fungal infections complicating acute pancreatitis: A review. Am J Gastroenterol 2011;106:1188–1192.

12. Witt H, Apte MV, Keim V, Wilson JS. Chronic pancreatitis: Challenges and advances in pathogenesis, genetics, diagnosis and therapy. Gastroenterology 2007;132:1557–1573.

13. Steer ML, Waxman I, Freedman S. Chronic pancreatitis. N Engl J Med 1995;332:1482–1490.

14. Yadav D, Whitcomb DC. The role of alcohol and smoking in pancreatitis. Nat Rev Gastroenterol Hepatol 2010;7:131–145.

15. Beglinger C. Relevant aspects of physiology in chronic pancreatitis. Digest Dis 1992;10:326–329.

16. Domínquez-Muñoz JE. Pancreatic exocrine insufficiency: Diagnosis and treatment. J Gastroenterol Hepatol 2011;26(Suppl 2):12–16.

17. Puylaert M, Kapural L, Van Zundert J, et al. Pain in chronic pancreatitis. Pain Practice 2011;11(5):492–505.

18. Olesen SS, Bouwense SA, Wilder-Smith OH, Van Goor H, Drewes AM. Pregabalin reduces pain in patients with chronic pancreatitis in a randomized, controlled trial. Gastroenterology 2011;141:536–543.

19. Brown A, Hughes M, Tenner S, Banks PA. Does pancreatic enzyme supplementation reduce pain in patients with chronic pancreatitis: A meta-analysis. Am J Gastroenterol 1997;92:2032–2035.

20. Giuliano CA, Dehoorne-Smith ML, Kale-Pradhan PB. Pancreatic enzyme products: Digesting the changes. Ann Pharmacother 2011;45: 658–666.

24 Viral Hepatitis

Juliana Chan

LEARNING OBJECTIVES

● **Upon completion of the chapter, the reader will be able to:**

1. Differentiate the five types of viral hepatitides by their epidemiology, etiology, pathophysiology, clinical presentation, and natural history.

2. Identify modes of transmission and risk factors among the major types of viral hepatitis.

3. Evaluate hepatic serologies to understand how the type of hepatitis is diagnosed.

4. Create treatment goals for a patient infected with viral hepatitis.

5. Recommend appropriate pharmacotherapy for prevention of viral hepatitis.

6. Develop a pharmaceutical care plan for treatment of chronic viral hepatitis.

7. Formulate a monitoring plan to assess adverse effects of pharmacotherapy for viral hepatitis.

KEY CONCEPTS

❶ Prevention and treatment of viral hepatitis may prevent progression to chronic hepatitis, cirrhosis, end-stage liver disease, and hepatocellular carcinoma.

❷ Acute viral hepatitis is primarily managed with supportive care.

❸ Good personal hygiene and proper disposal of sanitary waste are required to prevent fecal–oral transmission of the hepatitis A and E virus.

❹ Individuals may minimize the risk of acquiring both hepatitis B and C infection by avoiding contaminated blood products and not partaking in high-risk behavior such as illicit IV drug use.

❺ Persons at high risk of acquiring viral hepatitis A, B, or C infection should be vaccinated with the hepatitis A and/or B vaccine to prevent complications of liver disease.

❻ A vaccine that combines both inactivated hepatitis A and recombinant hepatitis B (Twinrix) is approved for immunizing individuals older than 18 years with indications for both hepatitis A and B vaccines.

❼ The drug of choice for chronic hepatitis B depends on the patient's past medical history, alanine aminotransferase (ALT) level, hepatitis B virus (HBV) DNA level, hepatitis B envelope antigen (HBeAg) status,

severity of liver disease, and history of previous HBV therapy.

❽ Treatment for chronic hepatitis C depends on the patient's past medical history, previous hepatitis C virus (HCV) treatment history, severity of liver disease, and HCV genotype.

INTRODUCTION

The most common types of viral hepatitis include hepatitis A (HAV), B (HBV), C (HCV), D (HDV), and E (HEV). Acute hepatitis may be associated with all five types of hepatitis and rarely exceeds 6 months in duration. Chronic hepatitis (disease lasting longer than 6 months) is usually associated with hepatitis B, C, and D. ❶ *Chronic viral hepatitis may lead to the development of cirrhosis and may result in end-stage liver disease (ESLD) and hepatocellular carcinoma (HCC).* Complications of ESLD include ascites, edema, hepatic encephalopathy, infections (e.g., spontaneous bacterial peritonitis), hepatorenal syndrome, and esophageal varices. *Therefore, prevention and treatment of viral hepatitis may prevent ESLD and HCC.*

Viral hepatitis may occur at any age and is the most common cause of liver disease in the world. The true prevalence and incidence may be underreported because most patients are asymptomatic. The epidemiology, etiology, and pathogenesis vary depending on the type of hepatitis and are considered separately below.

EPIDEMIOLOGY AND ETIOLOGY

Hepatitis A

Hepatitis A (HAV) affects 1.4 million people yearly worldwide.[1] The prevalence is highest in underdeveloped countries including Africa, parts of South America, the Middle East, and Southeast Asia. Australia, parts of western and northern Europe, Japan, and the United States have a lower prevalence. This is primarily due to vaccination programs, but outbreaks may still occur, as evidenced in 2003 by a food outbreak in Pennsylvania and in 2009 with international adoptees from countries known to have high or intermediate endemicity.[2,3] The number of infections and hospitalizations due to acute HAV infection annually have decreased markedly since the introduction of the HAV vaccine in 1996.[4,5]

HAV is primarily detected in contaminated feces and infects people via the fecal–oral route.[5] Outbreaks occur primarily in areas of poor sanitation.[1,5] Individuals at greatest risk of acquiring HAV are listed in Table 24–1.[5] Approximately 50% of the reported cases have no identifiable risk factors.[5]

To date, there are no documented cases of chronic hepatitis A.[1,5] Death associated with HAV is rare and mostly associated with fulminant hepatitis, with which approximately 100 people die annually.[5]

Table 24–1

Risk Factors for Acquiring Viral Hepatitis

Hepatitis A
International travelers to endemic areas (e.g., Africa, Asia, and parts of South America)
Sexual contact with infected persons (e.g., men having sex with other men)
Shellfish infected with HAV (e.g., raw oysters)
Daycare centers or household contacts with people infected with HAV
Healthcare workers
IV drug users using unsterilized needles
Workers involved with nonhuman primates
Food service handlers
Patients with clotting factor disorders
Individuals residing in healthcare institutions

Hepatitis B and D
Men having sex with other men
Individuals with multiple heterosexual partners
IV drug users using unsterilized needles
Recipients of blood products
Household contacts with acute hepatitis B with open cuts
Healthcare providers in contact with contaminated needles
Patients undergoing dialysis

Hepatitis C
Recipients of blood products
Healthcare providers in contact with infected needles
Individuals having multiple sexual partners
Perinatal transmission (less than 5%)
Unprofessional body piercing and tattooing

Hepatitis E
International travelers to endemic areas (e.g., parts of Asia, Africa, and Mexico)
Ingesting foods and drinks contaminated with bodily waste

Hepatitis B

Hepatitis B is a bloodborne infection affecting approximately 2 billion people worldwide.[6] About 350 million people have chronic hepatitis B (CHB) infection that may lead to cirrhosis and complications of ESLD.[6] Annually, an estimated 1 million deaths are associated with hepatitis B.[6] Despite having an effective vaccine against HBV, more than 300,000 newly diagnosed infections emerge each year. Less than 1% of individuals in North America and western Europe are chronically infected compared with 8% to 10% in developing areas such as Southeast Asia.[6]

The highest concentration of the HBV is found in blood and serous fluids. The primary modes of transmission are either by blood or body fluids through perinatal, sexual, or percutaneous exposure (Table 24–1).[7] Infants born to mothers who are infected with actively replicating HBV have a 90% risk of becoming chronic HBV carriers.[8–10] Approximately 33% of the reported cases have no identifiable risk factors.[7]

Hepatitis C

More than 170 million people are infected with hepatitis C worldwide, and it is estimated that 3.2 million have the disease in the United States.[11,12] The prevalence is higher among non-Hispanic blacks than non-Hispanic whites, and men are more likely to be infected than women.[13] Additionally, genotypes are geographically specific. For example, genotype 1 is common in the United States, whereas genotype 4 is common in the Middle East.[12] Approximately 75% with HCV in the United States have genotype 1, and about 14% and 5% have genotypes 2 and 3, respectively.[11] Genotype does not indicate disease severity or clinical outcomes but is used to determine the duration of therapy and the likelihood of therapeutic response.[13]

IV drug users using contaminated paraphernalia are responsible for about 60% of HCV transmissions (Table 24–1).[12] Because of the routine screening of blood products, the risk of HCV transmission via blood transfusion is very low (0.004% to 0.0004% per unit transfused).[12,14] Approximately 10% of individuals with HCV have no identifiable risk factors.[14]

Hepatitis D

Hepatitis D affects approximately 15 million people worldwide.[15] Parts of Asia, including Indonesia and Vietnam, have the lowest prevalence of HDV despite having a high prevalence of HBV infections.[15] Areas with the highest prevalence of HDV include the Middle East, parts of Africa, Western and Central Asia, parts of South America, and the South Pacific islands.[15]

Eight genotypes associated with HDV have been identified, with genotype 1 the most prevalent.[15] Genotype 1 primarily affects individuals residing in North America, Europe, the Middle East, and East Asia. Individuals residing in Japan and Taiwan are mostly diagnosed with genotype 2. Patients in northern parts of South America are mostly infected with genotype 3.[15]

Patient Encounter, Part 1

AB is a 29-year-old black woman who is at the doctor's office for a yearly check-up. Her only complaint is fatigue for 6 months. She was in Mexico vacationing 2 months ago. She states that she got sick for about a week while on the trip, but by the time she returned home she was getting better so did not seek medical treatment.

PMH: Rosacea, joint pain, mild depression, hypertension

PSH: Caesarean section 2 years ago (required a blood transfusion) and at age 5 had fractured ribs from falling out of a tree.

FH: Mother with osteoporosis; father alive and well. Has one brother with diabetes. Married with a 2-year-old daughter and 3-year-old son.

SH: She is in a monogamous relationship. Has never smoked tobacco. Used illicit drugs at age 15. Drinks alcohol socially. Had one tattoo placed unprofessionally. Employed as a secretary at a law firm.

Meds: Multivitamin daily, atenolol 100 mg daily, calcium with vitamin D twice daily, St. John's wort, birth control pills

ROS: Complains of irritability and insomnia; no nausea, vomiting, diarrhea, abdominal pain, or anorexia; never experienced an episode of jaundice, pale stools, or tea-colored urine

PE:

VS: BP 132/86 mm Hg, P 80 bpm, RR 20/minute, T 37.0°C (98.6°F), wt 70 kg (154 lb), ht 5'9" (175 cm)

Abd: Soft, nontender, normal liver span; no hepatosplenomegaly, no ascites.

The remainder of the examination was within normal limits.

Labs:

- Sodium 141 mEq/L (141 mmol/L), potassium 4.1 mEq/L (4.1 mmol/L), chloride 99 mEq/L (99 mmol/L), CO_2 21 mEq/L (21 mmol/L), BUN 20 mg/dL (7.1 mmol/L), serum creatinine 1.2 mg/dL (106 μmol/L), glucose 122 mg/dL (6.8 mmol/L)

- Hemoglobin 13.1 g/dL (131 g/L or 8.13mmol/L), hematocrit 38% (0.38), WBC $5.1 \times 10^3/mm^3$ (5.1×10^9/L), platelets $135 \times 10^3/mm^3$ (135×10^9/L)

- AST 69 IU/L (1.15 μkat/L), ALT 92 IU/L (1.53 μkat/L)

- Total bilirubin 1.0 mg/dL (17.1 μmol/L), albumin 3.7 g/dL (37 g/L), alkaline phosphatase 164 IU/L (2.73 μkat/L), TSH 1.3 μIU/mL (1.3 mIU/L)

- Anti-HAV IgM (−), anti-HAV IgG (+), anti-HBs (−), HBsAg (−), HBeAg (−), anti-HBc IgG (−), anti-HBc IgM (−), anti-HBe (−), anti-HCV (+), genotype 1a; HCV RNA 751,230 IU/mL (751,230 kIU/L)

- Liver biopsy: Mild inflammation and moderate fibrosis (grade 1, stage 2 disease) consistent with chronic hepatitis C

What information is suggestive of viral hepatitis?

What risk factors does she have for viral hepatitis?

What additional information do you need before creating a treatment plan for this patient?

The most likely modes of transmitting HDV are similar to those of HBV, including IV drug use with unsterilized needles and administration of contaminated blood products (Table 24–1). Sexual and perinatal transmissions are rare for HDV.[15]

Hepatitis E

Hepatitis E is found worldwide, but acute cases occur primarily in Central and Southeast Asia, the Middle East, North Africa, and Mexico.[16] Hepatitis E affects industrialized as well as underdeveloped countries. In the United States, up to 30% of the people may test positive for the HEV compared with 70% in developing countries.[17] The HEV is primarily transmitted by the fecal–oral route via fecally contaminated water.[16,17]

PATHOPHYSIOLOGY

Hepatitis A

Hepatitis A is a nonenveloped single-stranded RNA virus classified as the *Hepatovirus* genus under the Picornaviridae family.[1,4] The primary host for the HAV is humans, with hepatic cells as the main site for viral replication. As part of the viral degradation process, the HAV is released into the biliary system causing elevated concentrations of the virus in the feces.[18] Hepatitis A infections are usually self-limiting and do not lead to chronic disease; they may rarely result in fulminant hepatitis.[1,18]

Hepatitis B

The hepatitis B virus (also known as the Dane particle) belongs to the Hepadnaviridae family.[9] It is a partially double-stranded DNA virus with a phospholipid layer containing hepatitis B surface antigen (HBsAg) that surrounds the nucleocapsid. The nucleocapsid contains the core protein that produces hepatitis B core antigen (HBcAg), which is undetectable in the serum. Hepatocellular injury from HBV is thought to be due to a cytotoxic immune reaction that occurs when HBcAg is expressed on the surface of the hepatic cells. Fortunately, antibodies against hepatitis B core antigen (anti-HBc) are measurable in the blood, where anti-HBc to immunoglobulin M (IgM) indicates active infection and anti-HBc to IgG relates to either chronic infection or possible immunity against HBV.

Viral replication occurs when the hepatitis B envelope antigen (HBeAg) is present and circulating in the blood. The serum HBV DNA concentration is a measure of viral infectivity and quantifies viral replication. Once the hepatitis B infection resolves, antibodies against the hepatitis B envelope (anti-HBe) and antibodies against hepatitis B surface antigen (anti-HBs) develop, and HBV DNA levels become undetectable. However, if these antibodies do not develop, the likelihood of developing CHB increases. This depends primarily on the host's immune system at the time of the infection. In immunocompetent individuals, the disease resolves spontaneously and does not lead to further complications. In immunocompromised persons, the HBV is less likely to be eradicated, thus causing persistent infection. This often leads to hepatic cell damage and inflammation that may lead to cirrhosis and hepatocellular carcinoma.[19]

Chronic HBV occurs in less than 5% of those who are older than 5 years, whereas the rate is more than 90% in infants born to mothers infected with HBV.[7] Approximately 90% of adults infected with the HBV develop anti-HBs, which results in lifelong immunity. About 30% of adults with initial symptoms of HBV present with jaundice or fatigue, and about 0.5% exhibit fulminant hepatitis.[7] Cirrhosis and HCC are the two major complications associated with CHB hepatitis B infections.[19]

Hepatitis C

Hepatitis C, first known as non-A, non-B hepatitis, is a bloodborne infection caused by a single-stranded RNA virus belonging to the Flaviviridae family and the *Hepacivirus* genus.[14] There are 11 genotypes (numbered 1 to 11) and more than 90 subtypes (genotypes 1a, 1b, 2a, 3b, etc.) that are unique to hepatitis C.[11]

Antibodies against HCV (anti-HCV) in the blood indicate infection. If the infection persists for more than 6 months and viral replication is confirmed by HCV RNA levels, the person has chronic hepatitis C.

Only 10% to 15% of patients have acute hepatitis C that resolves without any further complication. In more than 70% of cases, hepatitis C develops into a chronic disease that is asymptomatic in about 60% to 80% of patients.[11,14] Chronic disease may be due to an ineffective host immune system, with cytotoxic T lymphocytes being unable to eradicate the HCV, thereby allowing persistent damage to hepatic cells. Therefore, individuals who are

immunocompromised are less likely to eradicate the virus. Risk factors for developing hepatic fibrosis include obesity, diabetes, heavy alcohol use, male sex, and acquiring HCV when older than 40 years.[20]

Approximately 70% of chronic cases progress to mild, moderate, or severe hepatitis. Cirrhosis and its complications occur in 15% to 20% of patients infected with HCV. In 10% to 20% of cases, 20 to 40 years may elapse between the time of exposure and the development of cirrhosis. Once cirrhosis is confirmed, the rate of developing HCC increases by 1% to 4% per year.

Hepatitis D

The hepatitis D virus (originally called delta hepatitis) belongs to the genus *Delta virus* of the Deltaviridae family.[15] The HDV virion is a defective single-stranded circular RNA virus that requires the presence of HBV for HDV viral replication. This is because the HDV antigen (HDVAg) is coated by the HBsAg.[15] The mechanism of hepatic damage is undetermined, but it is known that replication of HDV cannot occur without HBV present causing either coinfection (both hepatitis B and D infection occurring simultaneously) or superinfection (acquiring HDV after having long-standing disease with HBV).[15]

Hepatitis E

Hepatitis E is a nonenveloped single-stranded messenger RNA virus of the Hepevirus genus.[17] The HEV is similar to HAV in that the virus is found in contaminated feces, thus infecting people via the fecal–oral route. High HEV levels in the bile often prompt viral shedding in the feces. Hepatitis E infections are usually self-limiting and rarely result in hepatic complications. Chronic hepatitis E occurs rarely and is more likely to occur in immunocompromised individuals such as patients with human immunodeficiency virus (HIV) or posttransplant recipients.[16]

CLINICAL PRESENTATION AND DIAGNOSIS

See text box below for the clinical presentation of viral hepatitis.

Clinical Presentation of Viral Hepatitis

Symptoms
- Most patients infected with any type of viral hepatitis have no symptoms.
- Symptomatic patients may experience a flu-like syndrome, fevers, fatigue/malaise, anorexia, nausea, vomiting, diarrhea, dark urine, pale-appearing stools, pruritus, and abdominal pain.

Signs
- Jaundice may be evident in the whites of the eyes (scleral icterus) or skin.

- An enlarged liver (hepatomegaly) and spleen (splenomegaly) may be present.
- In fulminant hepatitis with hepatic encephalopathy, patients may have **asterixis** and coma.
- In rare instances, extrahepatic symptoms may develop: arthritis, postcervical lymphadenopathy, palmar erythema, cryoglobulinemia, and vasculitis.

Laboratory Tests
- See Table 24–2.

Diagnosis of Viral Hepatitis

Diagnosing viral hepatitis may be difficult because most infected individuals are asymptomatic.[5,7,14] Because symptoms cannot identify the specific type of hepatitis, laboratory serologies must be obtained (Table 24–2). In addition, liver function tests may aid in assessing the extent of cholestatic and hepatocellular injury. However, the definitive test to determine the amount of damage and inflammation of hepatic cells is a **liver biopsy**.

▶ *Hepatitis A*

The diagnosis of hepatitis A is made by detecting immuno-globulin antibodies to the capsid proteins of the HAV. The presence of IgM anti-HAV in the serum indicates an acute infection. IgM appears approximately 3 weeks after exposure and becomes undetectable within 6 months. In contrast, IgG anti-HAV appears in the serum at approximately the same time IgM anti-HAV develops but indicates protection and lifelong immunity against hepatitis A.[1]

Table 24–2			

Interpretation of Viral Hepatitis Serology Panels

Type	Laboratory Test	Result	Interpretation of Panel
Hepatitis A	IgM anti-HAV IgG anti-HAV	Negative Negative	Susceptible to infection
	IgM anti-HAV	Positive	Acutely infected
	IgG anti-HAV	Positive	Immune due to either natural infection or HAV vaccine
Hepatitis B[a]	HBsAg Anti-HBc Anti-HBs	Negative Negative Negative	Susceptible to infection
	HBsAg Anti-HBc Anti-HBs	Negative Positive Positive	Immune due to natural infection
	HBsAg Anti-HBc Anti-HBs	Negative Negative Positive	Immune due to hepatitis B vaccination
	HBsAg Anti-HBc IgM anti-HBc Anti-HBs	Positive Positive Positive Negative	Acutely infected
	HBsAg Anti-HBc IgM anti-HBc Anti-HBs	Positive Positive Negative Negative	Chronically infected
	HBsAg Anti-HBc Anti-HBs	Negative Positive Negative	Four interpretations possible: (a) Resolved infection (most common); (b) false-positive anti-HBc, thus susceptible; (c) low-level chronic infection; (d) resolving acute infection
Hepatitis C	Anti-HCV	Negative	Susceptible to infection
	Anti-HCV	Positive	Acutely or chronically infected
Hepatitis D[b]	IgM anti-HDV HDVAg HBsAg HBeAg Anti-HBc	Positive Positive Positive Positive Positive	Acute HBV-HDV coinfection
Hepatitis E	IgM anti-HEV IgG anti-HEV	Negative Negative	Susceptible to infection
	IgM anti-HEV	Positive	Acutely infected
	IgG anti-HEV	Positive	Immune due to natural infection

Anti-HAV, hepatitis A antibody; anti-HBc, hepatitis B core antibody; anti-HBs, hepatitis B surface antibody; HBsAg, hepatitis B surface antigen; anti-HCV, hepatitis C antibody; anti-HDV, hepatitis D antibody; anti-HEV, hepatitis E antibody; HAV, hepatitis A virus; HBV, hepatitis B virus; HDV, hepatitis D virus; HDVAg, hepatitis D antigen; IgG, immunoglobulin G; IgM, immunoglobulin M.

[a]Centers for Disease Control and Prevention. Hepatology [Internet]. Available at: *http://www.cdc.gov/hepatitis/HBV/PDFs/SerologicChartv8.pdf*.

[b]Hepatitis D should be suspected in those who have HBsAg positivity. Hepatitis D may present as either coinfection where both HDV and HBV serologies appear simultaneously, whereas for superinfection, HBV has been present for some time and later HDV develops.

▶ *Hepatitis B*

Hepatitis B is diagnosed when HBsAg is detectable in the serum. The nucleocapsid of the HBsAg contains the core protein that produces HBcAg, which is undetectable in the serum. The presence of antibodies against HBcAg to IgM indicates active infection. Anti-HBc to IgG relates to either chronic infection or possible immunity against HBV.[6,7]

In most cases, HBeAg is detected in the blood indicating active viral replication. Measurement of HBV DNA is used to determine viral infectivity and quantify viral replication. Once the hepatitis B infection resolves, antibodies to HBeAg (anti-HBe) develop, indicating viral replication has ceased, and eventually anti-HBs develop. Patients may develop antibodies to HBeAg and still have active viral replication because of a mutation in the HBV.[9] Therefore, chronic hepatitis B infections may be differentiated as either HBeAg-positive or HBeAg-negative.[9,10]

▶ *Hepatitis C*

Hepatitis C is diagnosed by testing for anti-HCV in the serum and confirmed by the presence of HCV RNA. HCV RNA levels quantify viral replication and are used to determine if antiviral treatment for HCV is effective. Once an infection has been confirmed, an HCV genotype should be obtained to determine the likelihood of response to antiviral therapy and the duration of treatment required.[11,14]

▶ *Hepatitis D*

Hepatitis D infection requires the presence of HBV for HDV viral replication. Measuring HDV RNA levels in the serum by polymerase chain reaction (PCR) confirms the presence of the HDV and is the most accurate diagnostic test. The presence of IgM antibodies to HDV Ag (IgM anti-HD) indicates active disease, and IgG anti-HD also becomes detectable if the infection does not resolve spontaneously. HDV antibodies do not confer immunity.[15]

▶ *Hepatitis E*

The diagnosis of hepatitis E is based on the presence of anti-HEV antibodies (IgM anti-HEV). IgG anti-HEV emerges when the acute phase of the HEV infection resolves.[16] A blood test for hepatitis E RNA levels is available, but its use is currently limited to clinical trials.

PREVENTION AND TREATMENT OF VIRAL HEPATITIS

Desired Outcomes

General desired outcomes for treating hepatitis are to (a) prevent the spread of the disease, (b) prevent and treat symptoms, (c) suppress viral replication, (d) normalize hepatic aminotransferases, (e) improve histology on liver biopsy, and (f) decrease morbidity and mortality by preventing cirrhosis, HCC, and ESLD.

For hepatitis B, additional treatment goals include (a) seroconversion or loss of HBsAg, (b) seroconversion or loss of HBeAg, and (c) achieving undetectable HBV DNA levels. An additional goal for chronic hepatitis C is achieving undetectable HCV RNA 6 months after hepatitis C therapy by achieving a sustained virologic response (SVR).

General Approach

Managing viral hepatitis involves both prevention and treatment. Prevention of hepatitis A and B (and indirectly for hepatitis D) can be achieved with immune globulin or vaccines. ❷ *Acute viral hepatitis is primarily managed with supportive care.* Mild to moderate symptoms rarely require hospitalization, but admission is recommended in individuals experiencing significant nausea, vomiting, diarrhea, and encephalopathy. Liver transplantation may be required in rare instances if fulminant hepatitis develops. Treatment is available for chronic liver disease (HBV, HCV, and HDV) to prevent ESLD and ultimately HCC.

Hepatitis A Prevention

❸ *Good personal hygiene and proper disposal of sanitary waste are required to prevent fecal–oral transmission of the HAV.*[1,5] This includes frequent hand washing with soap and water after using the bathroom and prior to eating meals. Drinking bottled water and avoiding fruits, vegetables, and raw shellfish harvested from sewage-contaminated water in areas where HAV is most endemic also minimizes the risk of becoming infected with hepatitis A.

Individuals at high risk of acquiring hepatitis A (Table 24–1) should receive either serum immune globulin or the hepatitis A vaccine, depending on their personal circumstances, as described below.[5,21]

▶ *Immune Globulin*

Immune globulin (IG) is a solution containing antibodies from sterilized pooled human plasma that provides passive immunization against various infectious diseases, including hepatitis A.[5] IG is available for either IV (IGIV) or intramuscular (IGIM) administration, but only IGIM is used for prevention of hepatitis A. IGIM does not confer lifelong immunity, but it is effective in providing pre- and postexposure prophylaxis against HAV.[5]

IGIM should be injected into a deltoid or gluteal muscle. It does not affect the immune response of inactivated vaccines, oral polio virus, or yellow fever vaccine. The administration of live vaccines (e.g., measles, mumps, rubella [MMR] vaccine) concomitantly with IGIM may decrease the immune response significantly; thus MMR and varicella vaccines should be delayed for at least 3 and 5 months, respectively, after IGIM has been administered. Additionally, IGIM should not be given within 2 weeks of the MMR administration or within 3 weeks of the varicella vaccine to maximize the efficacy of the immunization.[5]

Preexposure Prophylaxis Preexposure prophylaxis with IGIM is indicated for individuals at high risk of acquiring the HAV who (a) are younger than 12 months, (b) elect not to receive the hepatitis A vaccine, or (c) cannot receive the hepatitis A vaccine (e.g., because of allergy to the components alum or 2-phenoxyethanol). Because active vaccine immunity takes several weeks to develop, travelers who are older than 40 years, are immunocompromised, or have chronic liver disease or other chronic medical conditions who plan to depart for endemic areas within 2 weeks *and* have not received the hepatitis A vaccine should receive IGIM. If the duration of travel is less than 3 months, these individuals should receive a dose of IGIM 0.02 mL/kg and hepatitis A vaccine at the same time but administered at different injection sites.[5,21]

If travel duration is expected to be greater than 2 months, IGIM at a dose of 0.06 mL/kg should be administered to provide immunity up to 5 months. If protection against HAV is required beyond 5 months, readministration of IGIM is recommended.[5,21]

Postexposure Prophylaxis Individuals in contact with people infected with acute HAV (including household and sexual partners), staff and children from daycare facilities, and food handlers of restaurant establishments may be candidates for postexposure prophylaxis. IGIM is preferred in individuals who are younger than 12 months or older than 40 years of age, immunocompromised, diagnosed with chronic liver disease, or have contraindications to the hepatitis A vaccine.[5,21]

The risk of infection may be decreased by 90% if IGIM 0.02 mL/kg is given within 2 weeks of being exposed to the HAV. IGIM may still be beneficial if given more than 2 weeks after exposure to a known case of HAV because it may decrease the severity of hepatic damage.[5,21]

▶ Hepatitis A Vaccine

Persons at risk of acquiring HAV should receive the hepatitis A vaccine when appropriate. The vaccine is effective in providing pre- and postexposure prophylaxis against clinical hepatitis A infections when given in two injections 6 months apart (referred to as months 0 and 6).[5,21] Two inactivated hepatitis A vaccines, HAVRIX and VAQTA, are available in the United States. These vaccines are considered interchangeable, and doses depend on age (Table 24–3).[5]

Efficacy is defined by measuring antibody response with the modified enzyme immunoassay. Protective levels are considered to be greater than 20 mIU/mL (20 IU/L) for HAVRIX and greater than 10 mIU/mL (10 IU/L) for VAQTA. After administration of the first dose of vaccine, 94% to 100% of adults and 97% to 100% of children and adolescents develop protective antibody concentrations. All recipients older than 2 years receiving the second dose at month 6 have 100% antibody coverage; therefore, postvaccination measurement of antibody response is not required.[5]

For preexposure prophylaxis, the hepatitis A vaccine is recommended for travelers to endemic hepatitis A countries. It should be administered to healthy international travelers 40 years of age and younger regardless of the scheduled dates for departure. This recommendation does not apply to adults older than 40 years, the immunocompromised, or those with chronic medical conditions with or without chronic liver disease. Individuals who plan to depart to an endemic country in less than 2 weeks should receive both the hepatitis A vaccine and IGIM (0.02 mL/kg).[21]

For postexposure prophylaxis, the hepatitis A vaccine is effective in preventing clinical infection in healthy individuals between 12 months and 40 years of age when administered within 14 days after exposure.[21] Individuals outside these age ranges or with significant comorbid conditions should receive IGIM for postexposure prophylaxis rather than the hepatitis A vaccine because this population has not been studied.[21]

The hepatitis A vaccine may provide effective immunity for 8 years in adults and children. Kinetic models have theorized that immunity may last longer than 20 years, but this has not been confirmed in clinical trials.[5] The most common and often self-limiting adverse effects in adults include injection site reactions (e.g., tenderness, pain, and warmth), headaches within 5 days after vaccination, and fatigue. Infants and children may have feeding disturbances. Local reactions may be minimized by using an appropriate

---

Table 24–3

Recommended Intramuscular Doses of Hepatitis A Vaccines

Product	Recipient Age (years)	Dose	Volume (mL)	No. of Doses	Schedule (months)
VAQTA	1–18	25 units	0.5	2	0, 6–18
	19 or more	50 units	1	2	0, 6
HAVRIX	1–18	720 ELISA units	0.5	2	0, 6–12
	19 or more	1,440 ELISA units	1	2	0, 6–12

ELISA, enzyme-linked immunosorbent assay.

From Chan J. Viral hepatitis. Pharmacotherapy Self-Assessment Program, 5th ed. Kansas City, MO: American College of Clinical Pharmacy, 2005:1, 4, with permission.

needle length based on the person's age and size and by administering intramuscularly in the deltoid muscle. Hepatitis A vaccine given during pregnancy has not been evaluated in clinical trials. Because both brands of vaccine are made from inactivated HAV, the risk of developing fetal complications should be minimal.[5]

Hepatitis B Prevention

④ *Individuals may minimize their risk of acquiring the hepatitis B infection by avoiding contaminated blood products or participating in high-risk behavior such as IV drug use.* In addition, those at high risk of acquiring the HBV (Table 24–1) should be vaccinated with the hepatitis B vaccine.[7] Screening pregnant women for hepatitis B and providing universal hepatitis B vaccinations to all newborns is effective in preventing hepatitis B infections.[22] In some cases, postexposure prophylaxis with hepatitis B immune globulin (HBIG) may be recommended to prevent the development of acute infection and complications associated with HBV.

▶ Hepatitis B Immune Globulin

Hepatitis B immune globulin (HBIG) is a sterile solution containing antibodies prepared from pooled human plasma that has a high concentration of anti-HBs. HBIG provides passive immunization for postexposure prophylaxis against HBV. A single dose of HBIG 0.06 mL/kg is effective in preventing chronic hepatitis B infections in adults.[7] Similar to IGIM, HBIG should only be administered intramuscularly.

The most common side effects of HBIG include erythema at the injection site, headaches, myalgia, fatigue, urticaria, nausea, and vomiting. Serious adverse effects are rare and may include liver function test abnormalities,

arthralgias, and anaphylactic reactions. HBIG should be used with caution in individuals who have experienced hypersensitivity reactions to immune globulin or those who have immunoglobulin A deficiency. Similar to IGIM, concomitant administration of HBIG and live vaccines should be avoided because the efficacy of the immunization may decrease significantly.

▶ Hepatitis B Vaccine

The two hepatitis B vaccines available in the United States are Recombivax HB and Engerix-B. These vaccines are produced with recombinant DNA technology by inserting the gene for HBsAg into the plasmid that is synthesized by *Saccharomyces cerevisiae* cells. ⑤ *Persons at high risk (Table 24–1) of acquiring the hepatitis B virus should be vaccinated with the hepatitis B vaccine at months 0, 1, and 6.* The hepatitis B vaccine dose depends on the person's age (Table 24–4).

In addition to preexposure prophylaxis, the hepatitis B vaccine is indicated after exposure to prevent CHB. Adults acutely exposed to blood containing HBsAg from an accidental needlestick, sexual contacts, or IV drug use should receive the hepatitis B vaccine with or without HBIG, preferably within 24 hours of exposure based on the source of exposure and the vaccination status of the exposed person (Table 24–5).[7] Postexposure prophylaxis for perinatal exposure depends on several factors including maternal HBsAg status and the newborn's weight.[22] For mothers who are HBsAg-positive, newborns should be immunized within 12 to 24 hours after birth with the hepatitis B vaccine and HBIG 0.5 mL. If the mother is HBsAg-negative, the newborn should receive only the hepatitis B vaccine (Table 24–6).

For optimal response, the hepatitis B vaccine should be administered intramuscularly (into the anterolateral thigh region in neonates and infants and into the deltoid region in older children and adults) and not IV or intradermally.

		Dose (mcg)	Volume (mL)	No. of Doses	Schedule (months)
Table 24–4					
Recommended Intramuscular Dosing Regimens for Hepatitis B Vaccines					
Product	**Patient Categories**				
Recombivax HB	0–19 years of age	5	0.5	3	0, 1, 6
	11–15 years of age[a]	10	1	2	1, 4–6
	20 years of age or older	10	1	3	0, 1, 6
	Hemodialysis[b] younger than 20 years of age	5	0.5	3	0, 1, 6
	Hemodialysis 20 years of age or older	40	1	3	0, 1, 6
Engerix-B	0–19 years of age	10	0.5	3	0, 1, 6
	20 years of age or older	20	1	3	0, 1, 6
	Hemodialysis[b] younger than 20 years of age	10	0.5	3	0, 1, 6
	Hemodialysis 20 years of age or older	40[c]	2	4	0, 1, 2, 6

[a]Adolescents 11 through 15 years of age may receive either the 5-mcg three-dose pediatric formulation or a 10-mcg two-dose regimen using the adult formulation.

[b]Higher doses might be more immunogenic, but no specific recommendations have been made.

[c]Two 1.0-mL doses administered at one site.

Modified from Chan J. Viral hepatitis. In: Pharmacotherapy Self-Assessment Program, 5th ed. Kansas City, MO: American College of Clinical Pharmacy, 2005:1, 8, with permission.

Table 24–5

Recommendations for Prophylaxis After Nonoccupational Exposure to the Hepatitis B Virus

Exposed Person's Vaccination Status	Treatment to Administer If Serology Test of Source Person Is:	
	HBsAg-Positive	Unknown HBsAg Status
Unvaccinated	HBIG × 1 and initiate HB vaccine series	Initiate HB vaccine series
Previously vaccinated[a]	Administer HB vaccine booster dose	No treatment

HB, hepatitis B; HBsAg, hepatitis B surface antigen; HBIG, hepatitis B immune globulin.

[a]A person who has written documentation of a complete hepatitis B vaccine series and did not receive postvaccination testing.

Table 24–6

Recommendations for Hepatitis B Prophylaxis to Prevent Perinatal Transmission

Treatment	Mother's HBsAg Status		
	Positive	Negative	Unknown
HBIG[a]	Given within 12 hours of birth	None	Test HBsAg. If positive, give within 7 days; if negative, give none
AND			
Hepatitis B vaccine[b]			
Dose 1	Within 12 hours of birth	Based on infant's weight[c]	Within 12 hours of birth
Dose 2	At month 1–2	At month 1–2	At month 1–2
Dose 3[d]	At month 6	At month 6–18	At month 6

[a]0.5 mL intramuscularly in a different site from vaccine.

[b]See Table 24–4 for appropriate hepatitis B vaccine dose.

[c]Full-term infants who are medically stable and weigh 2,000 g or more born to HBsAg-negative mothers should receive the hepatitis B vaccine before hospital discharge. Preterm infants weighing less than 2,000 g born to HBsAg-negative mothers should receive the first dose of hepatitis B vaccine 1 month after birth or at hospital discharge.

[d]The final dose in the vaccine series should not be administered before age 24 weeks (164 days).

From Mast EE, Margolis HS, Fiore AE, et al. A comprehensive immunization strategy to eliminate transmission of hepatitis B virus infection in the United States: Recommendations of the Advisory Committee on Immunization Practices (ACIP) part 1: Immunization of infants, children, and adolescents. MMWR Recomm Rep 2005; 54(RR-16):1–31.

The vaccine should not be given in the gluteal region because it may result in lower rates of immunity.[7,22]

The hepatitis B vaccine is effective when antibody concentrations are greater than 10 mIU/mL (10 IU/L). Because most people completing the vaccination series obtain adequate antibody levels, postvaccination testing is not routinely recommended. The immunogenicity rate in healthy adults younger than 40 years is greater than 90% at completion of the three-dose hepatitis B immunization series.[7,22] Effective immunity may last for more than 20 years in healthy individuals. However, patients with poor immune systems may have an anamnestic response and may require titers to be checked periodically with booster doses given.[7,22]

The most frequent adverse effects are local reactions at the injection site (pain, tenderness, erythema, swelling, and pruritus), fever, headaches, dizziness, and irritability. Anaphylaxis, a serum sickness–like hypersensitivity syndrome, chronic fatigue syndrome, and neurologic diseases (leukoencephalitis,

optic neuritis, and transverse myelitis) have been reported rarely.[7] Hepatitis B vaccine is not contraindicated during pregnancy.[7]

▶ *Hepatitis A and B Combination Vaccine*

6 *A vaccine that combines both inactivated hepatitis A and recombinant hepatitis B (Twinrix) is approved for immunizing individuals older than 18 years with indications for both hepatitis A and B vaccines.*[7,23] A 1-mL dose of Twinrix contains the antigenic components of not less than 720 enzyme-linked immunosorbent assay (ELISA) units of HAVRIX and 20 mcg of recombinant HBsAg protein of Engerix-B and should be administered at months 0, 1, and 6. Twinrix may also be given at day 0, 7, 21 to 31, and the fourth dose at month 12.[23] Antibody seroconversion for hepatitis A and B was greater than 98% in adult volunteers tested 1 month after a three-dose vaccine series and with similar antibody protection with the four-dose series.[7,23] The side-effect profile of Twinrix is similar to giving each vaccine separately.

Chronic Hepatitis B Treatment

According to the American Association for the Study of Liver Diseases (AASLD) guidelines, patients with HBeAg-positive CHB (also known as wild-type CHB) with persistently elevated ALT (more than two times the upper limit of normal) and elevated HBV DNA levels greater than 20,000 IU/mL (20,000 kIU/L) require treatment to delay progression to cirrhosis and prevent the development of ESLD.[24] Similar treatment criteria apply to patients infected with HBeAg-negative CHB (also known as precore mutant or promoter mutant) with the exception of HBV DNA levels; therapy should be initiated when viral levels are greater than 2,000 IU/mL (2,000 kIU/L).[24]

The treatment endpoints for HBeAg-positive patients are different from those who are HBeAg-negative because the latter disease does not allow for HBeAg seroconversion. Thus an undetectable HBV DNA level, not seroconversion, is considered a treatment endpoint. Additionally, the ideal treatment should induce a biochemical response (decrease or normalize ALT levels) and histological response (decrease liver biopsy scores).[24] HBeAg-negative HBV infections are more likely to develop liver fibrosis and may require lifelong treatment because undetectable HBV DNA levels are difficult to achieve.

❼ *The drug of choice for CHB depends on the patient's past medical history, ALT, HBV DNA level, HBeAg status, severity of liver disease, and history of previous HBV therapy.* The safety and efficacy profile of the medication and the likelihood of developing drug resistance should also be considered. There are seven approved agents for the treatment of HBV: two interferons and five nucleoside/nucleotide analogs.

Entecavir and tenofovir are recommended as first line due to profound HBV DNA suppression and minimal resistance.[24] Pegylated interferon-α_{2a} is also considered a first-line agent for patients with compensated liver disease because it lacks drug resistance. Pegylated interferon has replaced unmodified interferon because the pegylated form may be given subcutaneously once weekly rather than three times weekly.

Adefovir is second line to tenofovir because the drug is less potent in suppressing hepatitis B viral replication in treatment-naive patients. Lamivudine is no longer recommended as first-line therapy due to a high rate of resistance.[24,25] Patients currently on adefovir or lamivudine and responding to treatment should continue with the regimen. However, if there is inadequate virologic response or drug resistance develops, adding another hepatitis B antiretroviral agent or switching to a more potent drug should be considered. The role of telbivudine in HBV therapy is limited due to its intermediate rate of resistance.[24] Each therapeutic agent is described briefly in the sections that follow.

▶ Interferon and Pegylated Interferon

Interferon-α_{2b} and pegylated interferon-α_{2a} are the only interferon therapies approved for treatment of chronic hepatitis B. Pegylated interferon is interferon attached to a polyethylene glycol molecule that increases the half-life of the drug, thereby allowing once-weekly dosing versus thrice-weekly administration of unmodified interferon. Unlike other antiretroviral treatments, interferon therapy is effective in suppressing, and in some cases ceasing, viral replication without inducing resistance.[24] Approximately a third of HBeAg-positive patients achieved HBeAg seroconversion after 48 weeks of pegylated interferon therapy[24,25] Patients with HBeAg-negative hepatitis B may require at least 48 weeks of pegylated interferon to attain undetectable HBV DNA levels[26] Factors in achieving a greater chance of HBeAg seroconversion include low baseline HBV DNA concentrations, high pretreatment ALT levels, and high histological activity.[24,26]

Pegylated interferon is well tolerated with similar or better efficacy than unmodified interferon; thus it is recommended over unmodified interferon for the treatment of CHB.[24] The approved dose of pegylated interferon-α_{2a} (Pegasys) for HBeAg-positive CHB is 180 mcg subcutaneously once weekly for 48 weeks. The same dose of pegylated interferon is recommended for HBeAg-negative CHB; however, the duration of therapy may be greater than 48 weeks to increase sustained responses.[24]

Even though the advantages of interferon or pegylated interferon include a finite duration of treatment, lack of resistance, and possible HBsAg loss or seroconversion (development of anti-HBs), there are several significant disadvantages. These include the need for subcutaneous injections and a pronounced adverse-effect profile that may require dosage reductions or treatment discontinuation. Refer to the subsequent section on hepatitis C for the type and management of pegylated interferon adverse effects. Approximately 35% of patients develop an ALT flare when treated with interferon. An increase in ALT has been associated with a positive response, but it may lead to hepatic decompensation, which can be fatal. Therefore, only patients with compensated liver disease and stable medical comorbidities should be considered for treatment with pegylated interferon.

▶ *Entecavir*

Entecavir (Baraclude) is a guanosine nucleoside analog that is highly effective in suppressing HBV DNA polymerase. Entecavir is approved for HBeAg-positive, HBeAg-negative, and lamivudine-resistant CHB.[24–26] Resistance rates are low (1% to 2%) in patients treated with entecavir for up to 5 years in lamivudine-naive individuals. For patients previously treated with lamivudine and switched to entecavir, the resistance rate is approximately 50% at 5 years.[24,25]

The dose of entecavir is 0.5 mg once daily for patients with compensated liver disease and naive to lamivudine therapy. Higher doses of entecavir at 1 mg once daily are recommended for lamivudine or telbivudine resistance or decompensated liver disease. Entecavir should be given on an empty stomach. Dosage adjustments are required in patients with renal dysfunction. The side-effect profile for entecavir is similar to lamivudine and adefovir dipivoxil. Patients treated with entecavir should be monitored for signs and symptoms of lactic acidosis and severe hepatomegaly with steatosis because some cases have been fatal.

The labeling for entecavir contains a black box warning stating that monotherapy should not be recommended for patients coinfected with HIV and HBV because there is a greater potential for developing resistance to HIV antiretroviral agents. Therefore, patients coinfected with HIV and HBV should only receive entecavir if highly active antiretroviral therapy (HAART) therapy is also prescribed.

▶ Tenofovir Disoproxil Fumarate

Tenofovir disoproxil fumarate (Viread) is an acyclic adenine nucleotide reverse transcriptase inhibitor that is similar in structure to adefovir dipivoxil. Tenofovir inhibits HIV and hepatitis B viral replication and is indicated for HBeAg-positive and HBeAg-negative CHB and HIV when prescribed with other HAART therapies.

Tenofovir is preferred over adefovir for CHB infections because of greater effectiveness in inhibiting viral replication and lack of resistance at week 72.[25] Patients who developed resistance to lamivudine, entecavir, or adefovir may benefit from tenofovir.[24,25]

The dose of tenofovir is 300 mg orally once daily taken on an empty stomach. Dose adjustments are required in patients with renal dysfunction because tenofovir is primarily renally excreted. Tenofovir is well tolerated with adverse effects similar to adefovir and other hepatitis B oral agents. Several case reports have implicated tenofovir in causing nephrotoxicity and Fanconi's syndrome.[24,26] Decreased bone mineral density and osteomalacia have been reported in HIV patients undergoing tenofovir treatment. It would be prudent to monitor for creatinine clearance, phosphate levels, liver function tests, and bone mineral density prior to initiating treatment and during the course of therapy. Patients should also be monitored for signs and symptoms of lactic acidosis and severe hepatomegaly with steatosis because some cases have been fatal. Hepatic function should be carefully monitored if treatment is to be discontinued because severe acute exacerbations of hepatitis have been reported.

▶ Adefovir Dipivoxil

Adefovir dipivoxil (Hepsera) is a prodrug of adefovir, an adenosine nucleotide analog that inhibits DNA polymerase. Adefovir dipivoxil is indicated for CHB in patients older than 12 years. Resistance to adefovir dipivoxil is minimal for the first few years of treatment but increases to approximately 30% after 5 years of therapy.[24] Because adefovir and tenofovir are structurally similar, there is a high likelihood of developing cross-resistance when switching from adefovir to tenofovir. HIV resistance may develop if adefovir dipivoxil is given as monotherapy; therefore, it is recommended to test individuals to ensure they are not HIV positive.

The dose of adefovir dipivoxil is 10 mg once daily taken with or without food. The most common side effects include asthenia, abdominal pain, diarrhea, dyspepsia, headaches, nausea, and flatulence. Adefovir dipivoxil is also associated with nephrotoxicity. Serum creatinine monitoring is recommended at baseline and every 3 months to detect renal tubular injury.[24] The dose must be reduced in patients with renal insufficiency. Monitor for signs and symptoms of lactic acidosis and severe hepatomegaly with steatosis because some cases have been fatal. Hepatic function should be carefully monitored if treatment is discontinued because severe acute exacerbations of hepatitis have been reported.

▶ Lamivudine

Lamivudine (Epivir-HBV) is an oral synthetic cytosine nucleoside analog having antiviral effects against HIV and hepatitis B virus. Lamivudine is effective in suppressing hepatitis B viral replication, normalizing ALT levels, and improving liver histology. Patients may have a similar or a superior response in achieving these end points when compared with interferon or pegylated interferon. Prolonged lamivudine therapy (up to 5 years) may be needed to sustain seroconversion, but this leads to lamivudine resistance as high as 60% to 70% at 5 years.[25,26] Due to the high rate of resistance, lamivudine is no longer recommended as first-line therapy for CHB.[24]

The adult dose of lamivudine is 100 mg orally once daily for treatment of CHB without HIV coinfections. Lamivudine at 3 mg/kg once daily up to a maximum dose of 100 mg is approved for pediatric patients (2 to 17 years of age). It may be taken with or without food. The dose must be adjusted in patients with renal dysfunction. Prior to prescribing lamivudine for CHB, it is important to confirm that the individual is not infected with HIV because treating with lamivudine alone for HIV will result in resistance.

Adverse effects are minimal and include fatigue, diarrhea, nausea, vomiting, and headaches. ALT levels should be monitored carefully because a two- to threefold increase may be observed. ALT should be monitored closely when therapy is discontinued because increased levels may indicate a flare in disease activity leading to liver failure. Similar to the other oral antihepatitis B agents, signs and symptoms of lactic acidosis and severe hepatomegaly should be monitored.

▶ Telbivudine

Telbivudine (Tyzeka) is an L-nucleoside analog that inhibits HBV replication. It is indicated for patients 16 years or older with HBeAg-positive or HBeAg-negative CHB with compensated liver disease. Telbivudine offers a slightly more effective reduction in HBV DNA levels and normalization of aminotransferases than lamivudine. Telbivudine resistance is lower than with lamivudine, but rates are significant with continued treatment; therefore, this drug is not highly recommended for hepatitis B infections.[24] Telbivudine may be considered if there is adefovir or tenofovir resistance.

The dose of telbivudine is 600 mg orally once daily with or without food. Dosage adjustments are required in patients with renal dysfunction. Adverse effects are similar to other HBV oral agents including lactic acidosis and severe hepatomegaly. Patients should also be monitored for signs and symptoms of myopathy characterized by elevated creatine kinase levels and muscle weakness.[27] Peripheral neuropathy has also occurred, mostly in patients who were treated concomitantly with pegylated interferon.[24,26] ALT and AST levels may become elevated while on treatment at rates similar to lamivudine. Telbivudine is not recommended for use in patients coinfected with HIV and HBV because HIV drug resistance may develop with telbivudine monotherapy.

Hepatitis C Prevention

The risk factors for hepatitis C and hepatitis B are quite similar; thus the risk of acquiring HCV is minimized by avoiding contaminated blood products and high-risk behaviors such as sharing needles among IV drug users. The risk of HCV transmission through a blood transfusion is 1 in 2 million. No vaccines are available for preventing hepatitis C, but several are under development.[28] High-risk individuals (Table 24–1) should be tested for HCV because most patients will be asymptomatic and unaware they are infected.[14]

Chronic Hepatitis C Treatment

Individuals with confirmed chronic hepatitis C should be evaluated for treatment to prevent the development of cirrhosis, liver cancer, and ESLD.[29-31] The primary goal of HCV treatment is to achieve a sustained virologic response (SVR). Several other virological responses have been defined to determine if HCV treatment should be continued or discontinued. An undetectable HCV RNA level at week 4 of therapy is called a rapid virologic response (RVR), and an undetectable level at week 12 is an early virologic response (EVR). RVR is an important time point used in response-guided therapy (RGT) to determine the duration of HCV therapy, whereas an EVR is an indicator to discontinue treatment if the HCV RNA is still detectable. Additional goals of therapy include normalizing hepatic aminotransferases and improving liver histology.

8 *Treatment for chronic hepatitis C depends on the patient's past medical history, previous HCV treatment history, severity of liver disease, and HCV genotype.* The most important predictor of response to therapy is the hepatitis C genotype. Individuals with genotype 2 or 3 achieve a higher SVR than patients with genotype 1.[29,30] The genotype also determines the duration of therapy.

Interferon-α_{2a} (Roferon A), interferon-α_{2b} (Intron-A), and interferon alfacon-1 (Infergen) were first approved for chronic hepatitis C but are no longer recommended because less than 10% of patients with genotype 1 and about 30% with genotype 2 or 3 achieve a SVR.[29] Pegylated interferon-α_{2a} (Pegasys) and pegylated interferon-α_{2b} (PEG-Intron) were later introduced in the early 2000s for the treatment of hepatitis C. Pegylated interferons have an extended half-life that allows for once-weekly administration. The SVR to pegylated interferon alone (25% to 40%) can be increased by adding ribavirin, a synthetic guanosine analog that inhibits viral polymerase (45% to 55%). Based on the second National Institutes of Health (NIH) 2002 Consensus Development Conference, pegylated interferon plus ribavirin is the regimen of choice for chronic hepatitis C.[29] The recommended treatment duration is 24 weeks for genotypes 2 and 3 and 48 weeks for genotype 1.[29]

Boceprevir and telaprevir are protease inhibitors that belong to a new class of drugs known as direct-acting antivirals (DAAs). They are approved for the treatment of HCV genotype 1 disease and must be coadministered with pegylated interferon and ribavirin. Pegylated interferon, ribavirin, and the two DAAs are discussed further in the sections that follow.

▶ *Pegylated Interferon and Ribavirin*

Pegylated interferon-α_{2a} and pegylated interferon-α_{2b} are indicated for chronic hepatitis C infections. The recommended dose of pegylated interferon-α_{2a} (Pegasys) is 180 mcg once weekly, and the adult dose of pegylated interferon-α_{2b} (PEG-Intron) is 1.5 mcg/kg/week, both administered subcutaneously. Patients with renal impairment (creatinine clearance less than 50 mL/min [0.83 mL/s]) should have the dose of pegylated interferon modified.

The dose of ribavirin is weight based according to genotype (Table 24–7). Doses higher than the recommended 15 mg/kg may be considered to increase the chance of SVR.[30,31] The ribavirin dose must be adjusted in patients with creatinine clearance less than 50 mL/min (0.83 mL/s).

Most patients treated with pegylated interferon experience flulike symptoms (fevers, chills, rigors, and myalgias). These symptoms may be mild to moderate in severity and usually occur with the first injection and diminish with continued treatment. Flulike symptoms may be minimized by premedication with acetaminophen or nonsteroidal anti-inflammatory drugs. Patients may also self-administer pegylated interferon prior to bedtime so they can sleep through the symptoms.

Psychiatric adverse effects occur frequently and may include irritability, depression, and, rarely, suicidal ideation. Patients developing mild to moderate psychiatric symptoms may require antidepressants or anxiolytics. Those with severe symptoms including suicidal ideation should discontinue treatment immediately.[29,30]

Patient Encounter, Part 2: Creating a Care Plan

Based on the information presented, create a care plan for this patient's hepatitis. Your plan should include:

(a) a statement of the drug-related needs and/or problems;

(b) the goals of therapy;

(c) a patient-specific detailed therapeutic plan;

(d) a follow-up plan to determine whether the goals have been achieved; and

(e) a follow-up plan to identify potential adverse effects of therapy.

Table 24–7

Dosing Recommendation for Pegylated Interferon and Ribavirin[1] for Chronic Hepatitis C

Genotype 1 disease; creatinine clearance (CrCl) greater than 50 mL/min (0.83 mL/s)

Dose and Duration of Therapy	Pegylated interferon-a_{2a} (Pegasys)	Pegylated interferon-a_{2b} (PEGINTRON)
Pegylated interferon (weekly dose)	180 mcg[2]	1.5 mcg/kg
Ribavirin (in 2 divided daily doses)	1000 mg if less than or equal to 75 kg[2]	800 mg if less than or equal to 65 kg
	1200 mg if more than 75 kg[2]	1000 mg if more than 65–85 kg
		1200 mg if more than 85–105 kg
		1400 mg if more than 105 kg
Planned duration	Response guided therapy	Response guided therapy

Genotype 2/3 disease; CrCl greater than 50 mL/min (0.83 mL/s)

Dose and Duration of Therapy	Pegylated interferon-a_{2a} (Pegasys)	Pegylated interferon-a_{2b} (PEGINTRON)
Pegylated interferon (weekly dose)	180 mcg[2]	1.5 mcg/kg
Ribavirin (in 2 divided daily doses)	800 mg[2]	800 mg
Planned duration	24 weeks	24 weeks

Dose adjustment of pegylated interferon and ribavirin based on CrCl.

CrCl	Pegylated interferon-a_{2a} (Pegasys)	Pegylated interferon-a_{2b} (PEGINTRON)	Ribavirin (Copegus)[3]
30–50 mL/min (0.50–0.83 mL/s)	180 mcg	reduce by 25%	Alternating doses: 200 mg and 400 mg every other day
Less than 30 mL/min (0.50 mL/s)	135 mcg	reduce by 50%	200 mg daily
Hemodialysis	135 mcg	reduce by 50%	200 mg daily

[1]Generic ribavirin may be used instead of proprietary products (Copegus, Rebetol).

[2]Doses of pegylated interferon and ribavirin must be renally adjusted base on CrCl.

[3]These dosing recommendations reflect the package labeling for Copegus; labeling for Rebetol states that it should not be used in patients with CrCl below 50 mL/min (0.83 mL/s).

Up to 35% of patients treated with pegylated interferon and ribavirin require either a dosage reduction or drug discontinuation due to the hematologic complications of thrombocytopenia, neutropenia, or anemia.[32,33] A decrease in platelet count of 25% to 30% usually occurs within 6 to 8 weeks after initiation of treatment. The pegylated interferon dose should either be reduced or discontinued if the platelet count declines significantly or symptoms of bruising and bleeding are present. Neutropenia associated with pegylated interferon plus ribavirin therapy may be more pronounced when boceprevir is also administered. Neutropenia usually occurs within the first 2 weeks after initiating treatment, with the WBC count and ANC levels stabilizing by week 4 or 6. Neutropenia is reversible upon discontinuing the medications. Granulocyte colony-stimulating factor has been used as an adjunctive therapy for neutropenia.[29,30]

Ribavirin causes a dose-related hemolytic anemia.[34] Patients treated with pegylated interferon and ribavirin with or without DAAs may require dosage reductions when hemoglobin levels decrease to less than 10.5 g/dL (105 g/L or 6.52 mmol/L) or when intolerable symptoms such as shortness of breath or severe fatigue develop. Reducing the dose of ribavirin and blood transfusions may be necessary in rare cases when hemoglobin levels fall below 8.5 g/dL (85 g/L or 5.28 mmol/L) when being treated with DAAs. If warranted, epoetin alfa or darbepoetin may be used as adjunctive therapy for anemia.[29,30]

Because ribavirin can be teratogenic and embryocidal, all women of childbearing age and men who are able to father a child must use two forms of contraception with hepatitis C therapy and for 6 months after treatment.[30]

Adherence to therapy is an important factor in increasing and maintaining SVR. Patients who were adherent with pegylated interferon and ribavirin therapy (taking more than 80% of doses for more than 80% of the treatment duration) had an SVR of 52%, whereas those who were not adherent had an SVR of 44%.[35]

► Boceprevir

Boceprevir (Victrelis) is a protease inhibitor that inhibits HCV viral replication in patients with genotype 1 disease.[30,31] Boceprevir is indicated for adult naive or previously treated patients with compensated liver disease who failed previous treatment with interferon or pegylated interferon plus ribavirin. Monotherapy is not recommended because of drug resistance; therefore, it must be coadministered with pegylated interferon and ribavirin.[30,31,36] The SVR rate with boceprevir triple therapy is 63% to 66% compared with the pegylated interferon plus ribavirin SVR of about 50%.[31] In addition to the possible adverse effects of pegylated interferon and ribavirin, patients receiving triple therapy have a higher incidence of anemia and neutropenia.[30,31] Complete blood counts with differential should be obtained at baseline and at least every 4 weeks during therapy. Dysgeusia, skin rash, itching, and dry skin were also more common with boceprevir.

The dose of boceprevir is 800 mg (four 200-mg capsules) three times a day with food in combination with pegylated interferon and ribavirin. Using a "lead-in" phase, pegylated interferon and ribavirin are given in recommended doses for 4 weeks, and boceprevir is added during week 5.[31] The duration of therapy is based on the patient's viral load at weeks 8, 12, and 24, known as response-guided therapy (RGT). If the HCV RNA level is greater than 100 IU/mL (100 kIU/L) at week 12 or continues to be detectable at week 24, all three medications are to be discontinued.

▶ Telaprevir

Telaprevir (Incivek) is a protease inhibitor that inhibits HCV replication. It is indicated for hepatitis C genotype 1 disease in treatment-naive patients or those who failed prior pegylated interferon plus ribavirin treatment. Telaprevir must be administered as a triple therapy with pegylated interferon and ribavirin to reduce the likelihood of drug resistance.[36] The SVR rates with telaprevir, pegylated interferon, and ribavirin range from 72% to 79%.[29,31]

The most common side effects of telaprevir are anemia, skin rash and pruritus, nausea, diarrhea, and anorectal discomfort. The dose of telaprevir is 750 mg (two 375-mg tablets) three times a day with food in combination with pegylated

interferon and ribavirin. The meal taken with telaprevir must contain at least 20 g of fat and must be ingested within 30 minutes prior to each dose to increase systemic absorption.[30] Telaprevir is administered with pegylated interferon and ribavirin from day 1 up to week 12 if the HCV RNA level is undetectable at week 4.

Boceprevir and telaprevir are potent CYP3A4 inhibitors; therefore, serum concentrations of concomitantly administered drugs may be elevated, prolonging their therapeutic and adverse effects. Therefore a thorough medication history including prescription, over-the-counter, and dietary and herbal supplements must be obtained prior to prescribing DAAs.

Hepatitis D Prevention and Treatment

Hepatitis D infection is possible only if the patient is also infected with HBV; therefore, hepatitis B vaccination can indirectly prevent hepatitis D infections. The recommended treatment for HDV is pegylated interferon for 48 to 72 weeks.[15] First-line oral agents for treating HBV infections (e.g., tenofovir) may be considered in patients coinfected with HDV and HBV if HBV DNA levels are high. Monotherapy with nucleoside/nucleotide analogs is ineffective in reducing HDV DNA levels but may decrease hepatitis B viral loads.[15]

Hepatitis E Prevention and Treatment

Because hepatitis E is transmitted via the fecal–oral route, good personal hygiene and proper disposal of sanitary waste are the most effective ways to prevent viral acquisition. There are no commercial vaccines available to prevent hepatitis E; however, a recombinant hepatitis E vaccine undergoing Phase II/III study has produced promising preliminary results.[16,37]

● OUTCOME EVALUATION

Monitoring for efficacy in patients treated for chronic hepatitis B or C includes evaluating aminotransferase levels and hepatitis B or C viral levels.

Hepatitis B

- Obtain an ALT at baseline and then every 3 to 6 months during hepatitis B treatment.
- Monitor HBV DNA levels every 3 to 6 months to determine treatment response in patients with CHB undergoing HBV therapy.
- Monitor HBeAg and anti-HBe every 6 months to determine if seroconversion to anti-HBe occurred or HBeAg was lost in patients with HBeAg-positive CHB.[24,25]
- Monitor HBsAg every 6 to 12 months to determine if HBsAg was lost or anti-HBs developed in patients with HBeAg-negative chronic hepatitis B with persistently undetectable serum HBV DNA levels.[24,25]
- Reevaluate the patient at month 6 and either switch or add a more potent hepatitis B antiviral agent to the

---

Patient Encounter, Part 3

The patient received treatment for hepatitis C for 4 weeks, and the following laboratory results have just been obtained:

- Sodium 138 mEq/L (138 mmol/L), potassium 4.0 mEq/L (4.0 mmol/L), chloride 98 mEq/L (98 mmol/L), CO_2 19 mEq/L (19 mmol/L), BUN 21 mg/dL (7.5 mmol/L), serum creatinine 1.0 mg/dL (88 μmol/L), glucose 103 mg/dL (5.7 mmol/L)
- Hemoglobin 10.1 g/dL (101 g/L or 6.3 mmol/L), hematocrit 30.3% (0.303), WBC $2.2 \times 10^3/mm^3$ ($2.2 \times 10^9/L$), platelets $104 \times 10^3/mm^3$ ($104 \times 10^9/L$), ANC $0.92 \times 10^3/mm^3$ ($0.92 \times 10^9/L$)
- AST 41 IU/L (0.68 μkat/L), ALT 32 IU/L (0.53 μkat/L)
- Total bilirubin 1.0 mg/dL (17.1 μmol/L), albumin 3.6 g/dL (36 g/L), alkaline phosphatase 168 IU/L (2.8 μkat/L)
- HCV RNA level: 530 IU/mL (530 kIU/L)

What questions should you ask the patient?

What action should you take to treat any complaints the patient may have?

What action should you take based on the patient's week 4 HCV RNA level?

current hepatitis B regimen if the HBV DNA level has not decreased by 2 logs at 6 months of therapy.[24]

- Continue treatment in patients with HBeAg-positive CHB until HBeAg seroconversion has been attained along with undetectable HBV DNA levels. Once anti-HBe appears, complete an additional 6 months of hepatitis B therapy.[24]

- Continue treatment in patients with HBeAg-negative CHB until HBsAg is lost.[24]

- Monitor all patients closely for hepatitis flare and viral relapse when discontinuing hepatitis B therapy.

- Obtain a CBC with differential every 4 weeks and thyroid-stimulating hormone (TSH) and fasting lipid panel every 12 weeks in patients receiving pegylated interferon therapy for hepatitis B.[24]

- For patients receiving tenofovir or adefovir, monitor serum creatinine for nephrotoxicity at baseline and every 12 weeks.

- For patients taking telbivudine, monitor creatine kinase at baseline and periodically (e.g., every 12 weeks) because muscle weakness and myopathy have occurred.[24,26]

Hepatitis C

- Sustained virologic response (SVR) is defined as having an undetectable HCV RNA level at 6 months posttreatment; this is the ultimate goal of HCV therapy and indicates a cure.[29,31]

- Rapid virologic response (RVR) is defined as having an undetectable HCV RNA level at week 4 of treatment; this is an important time point to determine the duration of therapy with DAAs.

- Extended rapid virologic response (eRVR) is having undetectable HCV RNA level at week 4 and week 12 of treatment; this is a time point to determine if HCV treatment should be continued beyond 12 weeks.

- End of treatment response (ETR or EOT) is defined as having undetectable HCV RNA levels at the end of treatment.

- Response-guided therapy (RGT) is an approach used to determine the duration of therapy based on HCV RNA levels when treated with DAA agents.[31]

- Biochemical response is defined as normalization of ALT; monitor ALT levels every 4 weeks.

- Histologic response is defined as improving inflammation and fibrosis as documented by liver biopsy scores.

- Check the HCV RNA level at week 12 of therapy to determine the effectiveness of pegylated interferon and ribavirin. Discontinue treatment if the HCV RNA has not decreased by at least 2 logs or become undetectable by week 12.

- For patients with genotype 1 HCV: If the HCV RNA level is undetectable at week 12 of pegylated interferon and ribavirin therapy, continue treatment for at least another

36 weeks (48 weeks total). Obtain an HCV RNA level to determine ETR of the 48-week treatment, and repeat at 6 months posttherapy to determine SVR. This does not apply to DAAs.

- For patients treated with pegylated interferon and ribavirin with genotypes 2 and 3 HCV: Check the HCV RNA level at week 12. If HCV RNA is undetectable, continue treatment for a total of 24 weeks. Repeat the HCV RNA 24 weeks after completion of therapy to determine SVR.

- In patients receiving treatment with pegylated interferon with or without ribavirin, monitor the WBC, ANC, platelets, and hemoglobin levels either weekly or biweekly during the first month of therapy and monthly thereafter if stable.

Patient Encounter, Part 4

The patient has now been treated for a total of 12 weeks and the HCV RNA level is less than 12 IU/mL (12 kIU/L) at weeks 8 and 12

What action should you take based on the week 12 HCV RNA level?

What other information should you counsel the patient about in addition to the side effects associated with the hepatitis C therapy?

Patient Encounter, Part 5

AB's husband was recently tested for viral hepatitis and found to be positive for hepatitis B. His only past medical history is mild depression. He has not had any surgeries. He is not taking any medications, over-the-counter drugs, or dietary supplements.

All labs are normal except for the following:

- AST 69 IU/L (1.15 μkat/L), ALT 92 IU/L (1.53 μkat/L)
- Anti-HAV IgM (−), anti-HAV IgG (−), anti-HBs (−), HBsAg (+), HBeAg (−), anti-HBcIgG (+), anti-HBcIgM (−), anti-HBe (−), anti-HCV (−), HCV RNA less than 615 IU/mL (less than 615 kIU/L), HBV DNA 1,478,015 IU/mL (1,478,015 kIU/L).

Based on the information presented:

(a) create a detailed therapeutic care plan for the patient;

(b) discuss adverse effects to monitor;

(c) discuss a follow-up plan to determine whether the treatment goals have been achieved.

Patient Care and Monitoring

1. Evaluate the patient for risk factors for acquiring viral hepatitis (Table 24–1).
2. Educate patients to avoid hepatotoxic agents (e.g., some dietary supplements).
3. Educate patients to avoid consuming any alcohol if viral hepatitis has been diagnosed.
4. Determine if the patient has been vaccinated against hepatitis A and B. If not, then vaccinate accordingly (Tables 24–3 and 24–4).
5. Obtain a thorough past medical history focusing on psychiatric disorders, cardiac disorders, endocrine disease, and renal insufficiency.
6. If available, review the liver biopsy report to determine the severity of liver damage and assess the need for chronic hepatitis B or C treatment.
7. Assess for adverse effects in patients with hepatitis B or C.
8. Encourage medication compliance with viral hepatitis treatments to increase the SVR.
9. Encourage patients to drink at least 8 glasses of water daily to prevent dehydration.
10. Educate all women of childbearing age and men who are able to father a child to use two forms of contraception during and for 6 months after ribavirin therapy.
11. Provide patient education:
    - How to prevent viral hepatitis transmission
    - Who should be vaccinated against hepatitis A and B
    - Importance of taking all medications daily at scheduled times
    - Adverse effects of hepatitis B and C medications
    - How to self-administer pegylated interferon injections correctly
    - Importance of appropriate disposal of used injection needles

- Monitor TSH and fasting lipid panel every 12 weeks while on hepatitis C treatment.
- Monitor serum creatinine in patients receiving ribavirin to detect renal insufficiency that may result in ribavirin accumulation and toxicity (e.g., hemolytic anemia).

Abbreviations Introduced in This Chapter

ALT	Alanine aminotransferase
ANC	Absolute neutrophil count
Anti-HAV	Hepatitis A virus antibody
Anti-HBc	Hepatitis B core antibody
Anti-HBe	Hepatitis B envelope antibody
Anti-HBs	Hepatitis B surface antibody
Anti-HCV	Hepatitis C antibody
Anti-HDV	Hepatitis D antibody
Anti-HEV	Hepatitis E antibody
AST	Aspartate aminotransferase
CHB	Chronic hepatitis B infection
CrCl	Creatinine clearance
DAA	Direct acting antiretroviral
ETR	End of treatment response
ESLD	End-stage liver disease
eRVR	Extended rapid virologic response
EVR	Early virologic response
HAV	Hepatitis A virus
HBcAg	Hepatitis B core antigen
HBeAg	Hepatitis B envelope antigen
HBIG	Hepatitis B immunoglobulin
HBsAg	Hepatitis B surface antigen
HBV	Hepatitis B virus
HBV DNA	Hepatitis B deoxyribonucleic acid
HCV	Hepatitis C virus
HCV RNA	Hepatitis C virus ribonucleic acid
HDV	Hepatitis D virus
HDVAg	Hepatitis D antigen
HDV RNA	Hepatitis D virus ribonucleic acid
HEV	Hepatitis E virus
IgG	Immunoglobulin G
IgG anti-HD	IgG antibodies to hepatitis D virus antigen
IgM	Immunoglobulin M
IgM anti-HD	IgM antibodies to hepatitis D virus antigen
IG	Immune globulin
IGIM	Immune globulin for intramuscular administration
IGIV	Immune globulin for IV administration
MMR	Measles, mumps, rubella vaccine
PCR	Polymerase chain reaction
RVR	Rapid virologic response
SVR	Sustained virologic response

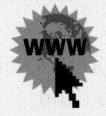 Self-assessment questions and answers are available at *http://www.mhpharmacotherapy.com/pp.html*.

REFERENCES

1. World Health Organization. Department of Communicable Disease Surveillance and Response. WHO/CDS/CSR/EDC/2000.7 [Internet]. Available at: *http://www.who.int/csr/disease/hepatitis/whocdscsredc2007/en/index.html.* Accessed September 1, 2011.

2. Centers for Disease Control and Prevention (CDC). Hepatitis A outbreak associated with green onions at a restaurant—Monaca, Pennsylvania, 2003. MMWR Morb Mortal Wkly Rep 2003;52(47):1155–1157.

3. Centers for Disease Control and Prevention (CDC). Updated Recommendations from the Advisory Committee on Immunization Practices (ACIP) for Use of Hepatitis A Vaccine in Close Contacts of Newly Arriving International Adoptees. MMWR Morb Mortal Wkly Rep 2009;58(36):1006–1007.

4. Daniels D, Grytdal S, Wasley A. Surveillance for acute viral hepatitis—United States, 2007. MMWR Surveill Summ 2009;58(3):1–27.

5. Advisory Committee on Immunization Practices (ACIP), Fiore AE, Wasley A, Bell BP. Prevention of hepatitis A through active or passive immunization: Recommendations of the Advisory Committee on Immunization Practices (ACIP). MMWR Recomm Rep 2006;55 (RR-7):1–23.

6. Keystone JS, Hershey JH. The underestimated risk of hepatitis A and hepatitis B: Benefits of an accelerated vaccination schedule. Int J Infect Dis 2008;12:3–11.

7. Mast EE, Weinbaum CM, Fiore AE, et al. A comprehensive immunization strategy to eliminate transmission of hepatitis B virus infection in the U.S.: Recommendations of the Advisory Committee on Immunization Practices (ACIP) Part II: Immunization of adults. MMWR Recomm Rep 2006;55(RR-16):1–33.

8. Centers for Disease Control (CDC). Prevention of perinatal transmission of hepatitis B virus: Prenatal screening of all pregnant women for hepatitis B surface antigen. MMWR Morb Mortal Wkly Rep 1988;37:341–346, 351.

9. Hadziyannis SJ. Natural history of chronic hepatitis B in Euro-Mediterranean and African Countries. J Hepatol 2011;55(1):183–191.

10. Chen CJ, Yang HI. Natural history of chronic hepatitis B revealed. J Gastroenterol Hepatol 2011;26(4):628–638.

11. World Health Organization. Department of Communicable Disease Surveillance and Response. WHO/CDS/CSR/LYO/2003. Hepatitis C [Internet]. Available at: *http://www.who.int/csr/disease/hepatitis/whocdscsrlyo2003/en/index.html.* Accessed August 21, 2011.

12. Centers for Disease Control and Prevention. Hepatitis C FAQs for Health Professionals [Internet]. Available at: *http://www.cdc.gov/hepatitis/HCV/HCVfaq.htm#.* Accessed August 21, 2011.

13. Missiha SB, Ostrowski M, Heathcote EJ. Disease progression in chronic hepatitis C: Modifiable and nonmodifiable factors. Gastroenterology 2008;134(6):1699–1714.

14. Centers for Disease Control and Prevention. Recommendations for prevention and control of hepatitis C virus (HCV) infection and HCV-related chronic disease. MMWR Recomm Rep 1998;47(RR-19):1–39.

15. Hughes SA, Wedemeyer H, Harrison PM. Hepatitis delta virus. Lancet 2011;378:73–85.

16. Teshale EH, Hu DJ, Holmberg SD. The two faces of hepatitis E virus. Clin Infect Dis 2010;51(3):328–334.

17. Meng XJ. Recent advances in hepatitis E virus. J Viral Hepat 2010;17(3):153–161.

18. Martin A, Lemon SM. Hepatitis A Virus: From discovery to vaccines. Hepatology 2006;43(2 Suppl 1):S164–S172.

19. Chisari FV, Isogawa M, Wieland SF. Pathogenesis of hepatitis B virus infection. Pathol Biol 2010;58(4):258–266.

20. Poynard T, Afdhal NH. Perspectives on fibrosis progression in hepatitis C: An à la carte approach to risk factors and staging of fibrosis. Antivir Ther 2010;15(3):281–291.

21. Centers for Disease Control and Prevention (CDC). Update: Prevention of hepatitis A after exposure to hepatitis A virus and in international travelers. Updated recommendations of the Advisory Committee on Immunization Practices (ACIP). MMWR Morb Mortal Wkly Rep 2007;56(41):1080–1084.

22. Mast EE, Margolis HS, Fiore AE, et al. A comprehensive immunization strategy to eliminate transmission of hepatitis B virus infection in the United States: Recommendations of the Advisory Committee on Immunization Practices (ACIP) Part 1: Immunization of infants, children, and adolescents. MMWR Recomm Rep 2005;54 (RR-16):1–31.

23. Notice to Readers: FDA Approval of an Alternate Dosing Schedule for a Combined Hepatitis A and B Vaccine (Twinrix). MMWR Recomm Rep 2007;56(40):1057.

24. Lok AS, McMahon BJ. Chronic hepatitis B: Update 2009. Hepatology 2009:1–36 [Internet]. Available at: *http://www.aasld.org/practiceguidelines/documents/bookmarked%20practice%20guidelines/chronic_hep_b_update_2009%208_24_2009.pdf.* Accessed August 30, 2011.

25. Rijckborst V, Sonneveld MJ, Janssen HL. Review article: Chronic hepatitis B—anti-viral or immunomodulatory therapy? Aliment Pharmacol Ther 2011;33(5):501–513.

26. Hongthanakorn C, Lok AS. New pharmacologic therapies in chronic hepatitis B. Gastroenterol Clin North Am 2010;39(3):659–680.

27. Lai CL, Gane E, Liaw YF, Hsu CW, et al. Telbivudine versus lamivudine in patients with chronic hepatitis B. N Engl J Med 2007;357: 2576–2588.

28. Yu CI, Chiang BL. A new insight into hepatitis C vaccine development. J Biomed Biotechnol 2010;2010:548280.

29. Ghany MG, Strader DB, Thomas DL, Seeff LB. Diagnosis, management, and treatment of hepatitis C: An update. Hepatology 2009;49: 1335–1374.

30. Chan J. Treatment of chronic hepatitis C: The new standard of care for the future. Formulary 2011;46:314–338.

31. Ghany MG, Nelson DR, Strader DB, et al. An update on treatment of genotype 1 chronic hepatitis C virus infection: 2011 practice guideline by the American Association for the Study of Liver Diseases. Hepatology 2011 54(4):1433–1444.

32. Sulkowski MS, Cooper C, Hunyady B, et al. Management of adverse effects of Peg-IFN and ribavirin therapy for hepatitis C. Nat Rev Gastroenterol Hepatol 2011;8(4):212–223.

33. Negro F. Adverse effects of drugs in the treatment of viral hepatitis. Best Pract Res Clin Gastroenterol 2010;24(2):183–192.

34. McHutchison JG, Manns MP, Brown RS Jr, et al. Strategies for managing anemia in hepatitis C patients undergoing antiviral therapy. Am J Gastroenterol 2007;102:880–889.

35. McHutchison JG, Manns M, Patel K, et al. Adherence to combination therapy enhances sustained response in genotype-1-infected patients with chronic hepatitis C. Gastroenterology 2002;123:1061–1069.

36. Rong L, Dahari H, Ribeiro RM, Perelson AS. Rapid emergence of protease inhibitor resistance in hepatitis C virus. Sci Transl Med 2010;2(30):30ra32.

37. Shrestha MP, Scott RM, Joshi DM, et al. Safety and efficacy of a recombinant hepatitis E vaccine. N Engl J Med 2007;356:895–903.

25 Acute Kidney Injury

Mary K. Stamatakis

LEARNING OBJECTIVES

● **Upon completion of the chapter, the reader will be able to:**

1. Assess a patient's kidney function based on clinical presentation, laboratory results, and urinary indices.

2. Identify pharmacotherapeutic outcomes and endpoints of therapy in a patient with acute kidney injury (AKI).

3. Apply knowledge of the pathophysiology of AKI to the development of a treatment plan.

4. Design a diuretic regimen based on the pharmacokinetic and pharmacodynamic characteristics of the drug.

5. Select pharmacotherapy to treat complications associated with AKI.

6. Develop strategies to minimize the occurrence of AKI.

7. Monitor and evaluate the safety and efficacy of the therapeutic plan.

KEY CONCEPTS

❶ Equations to estimate creatinine clearance (CrCl) that incorporate a single serum creatinine concentration (e.g., Cockcroft-Gault) typically overestimate kidney function.

❷ There is currently no drug therapy that hastens patient recovery in AKI, decreases length of hospitalization, or improves survival.

❸ Loop diuretics are the diuretics of choice for the management of volume overload in AKI.

❹ There is no indication for the use of low-dose dopamine in the treatment of AKI.

❺ Identifying patients at risk for development of AKI and implementing preventive methods to decrease its occurrence or severity is critical.

Acute kidney injury (AKI) is a potentially life-threatening clinical syndrome that occurs primarily in hospitalized patients and frequently complicates the course of the critically ill. It is characterized by a rapid decrease in **glomerular filtration rate** (GFR) and the resultant accumulation of nitrogenous waste products (e.g., creatinine and urea nitrogen), with or without a decrease in urine output. The term *acute renal failure* (ARF) has largely been replaced by AKI in recent years because AKI more completely encompasses the entire spectrum of acute injury to the

kidney, from mild changes in kidney function to end-stage kidney disease requiring renal replacement therapy (RRT). Furthermore, the definition of ARF has been inconsistent in the literature, and a recent survey showed more than 30 different definitions in the literature.[1] Efforts to standardize the definition of ARF has led to a change in terminology to AKI as well as the development of a consensus definition and severity staging for AKI.[2]

The first consensus definition/classification for AKI was the *RIFLE* classification system, which categorizes patients into groups based on their change in serum creatinine or GFR from baseline, or decreased urine output.[3] The categories of kidney dysfunction in the *RIFLE* classification include patients at risk (R), those with kidney injury (I), and those with kidney failure (F). Two additional categories of clinical outcomes are sustained loss (L), which requires RRT for at least 4 weeks; and end stage (E), which necessitates RRT for at least 3 months. Patients are assigned a class based on their indicator with the greatest severity. The complete schematic for the RIFLE classification system is depicted in **Figure 25–1**.

Subsequent to the development of the *RIFLE* criteria, the Acute Kidney Injury Network (AKIN) has adopted and further modified the *RIFLE* definition and staging for AKI. This system uses three stages (stages 1 to 3) and includes an absolute increase in serum creatinine of 0.3 mg/dL (27 μmol/L) or greater in stage 1. This highlights the importance that even small increases in serum creatinine concentration can be associated with high morbidity and

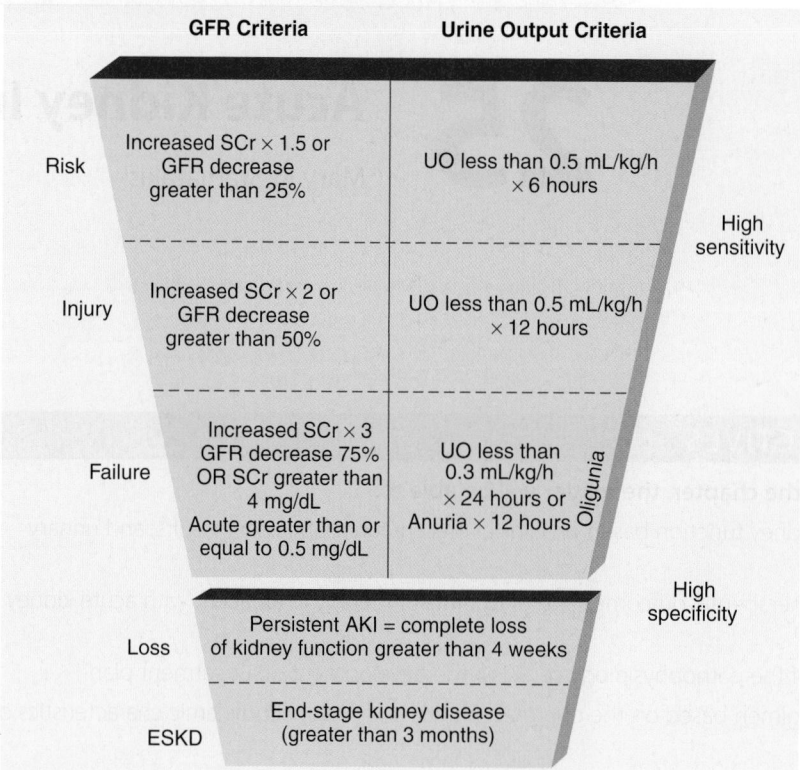

FIGURE 25–1. Algorithm for classification of acute kidney injury. The classification system includes separate criteria for creatinine and urine output. A patient can fulfill the criteria through changes in serum creatinine or changes in urine output, or both. The criteria that lead to the worst possible classification should be used. Note that the F component of RIFLE (Risk of renal dysfunction, Injury to the kidney, Failure of kidney function, Loss of kidney function, and End-stage kidney disease) is present even if the increase in SCr is under threefold as long as the new SCr is greater than 4 mg/dL (350 μmol/L) in the setting of an acute increase of at least 0.5 mg/dL (44 μmol/L). The designation RIFLE-FC should be used in this case to denote "acute-on-chronic" disease. Similarly, when the RIFLE-F classification is achieved by urine output criteria, a designation of RIFLE-FO should be used to denote oliguria. The shape of the figure denotes the fact that more patients (high sensitivity) will be included in the mild category, including some without actually having renal failure (less specificity). In contrast, at the bottom of the figure the criteria are strict and therefore specific, but some patients will be missed. (AKI, acute kidney injury; GFR, glomerular filtration rate; SCr, serum creatinine concentration; UO, urine output.) (From Bellomo R, Ronco C, Kellum, et al.; the ADQI Workgroup. Acute renal failure—definition, outcome measures, animal models, and information technology needs: The Second International Consensus Conference of the Acute Dialysis Quality Initiative (ADQI) Group. Crit Care 2004;8:R204–R212.)

mortality, and early detection is critical. It also includes a time constraint of 48 hours for diagnosis and categorizes all patients receiving RRT into stage 3, regardless of the length of RRT.[4] The AKIN three-stage classification of AKI is shown in Table 25–1.

EPIDEMIOLOGY AND ETIOLOGY

Approximately 5% to 7% of all hospitalized patients develop AKI. AKI is 5 to 10 times more prevalent in the hospital setting than in the community setting.[5] About 5% to 20% of critically ill patients develop AKI,[5] and 30% to 40% of survivors progress to chronic kidney disease.[6] Despite improvements in the medical care of individuals with AKI, mortality generally exceeds 50%.[7]

PATHOPHYSIOLOGY

There are typically three categories of AKI: prerenal, intrinsic, and postrenal AKI. The pathophysiologic mechanisms differ for each of the categories.

Prerenal AKI

Prerenal AKI is characterized by reduced blood delivery to the kidney. A common cause is intravascular volume depletion due to conditions such as hemorrhage, dehydration, or GI fluid losses. Early restoration of volume replacement can prevent progression and improve recovery because no structural damage to the kidney has occurred.[8] Conditions of reduced cardiac output (e.g., congestive heart failure [CHF] or myocardial infarction)

Table 25–1

AKIN Classification/Staging System for AKI

Stage	Absolute Serum Creatinine Increase from Baseline	Percentage Serum Creatinine Increase from Baseline	Urine Output	Need for Renal Replacement Therapy
1	Greater than or equal to 0.3 mg/dL (27 μmol/L)	150–200% (1.5–2-fold)	Less than 0.5 ml/kg per hour for more than 6 hours	No
2	—	200–300% (2–3-fold)	Less than 0.5 ml/kg per hour for more than 12 hours	No
3	Greater than or equal to 4 mg/dL (354 μmol/L) with an acute increase of at least 0.5 mg/dL (44 μmol/L)	300% or greater (greater than 3-fold)	Less than 0.3 ml/kg for 24 hours or anuria for 12 hours	Need for renal replacement therapy indicates stage 3 regardless of serum creatinine or urine output

Based on the Acute Injury Network Classification/staging system for AKI.[4] Only one of the three criteria needs to be met in order to qualify for the higher stage. Change in serum creatinine or urine output must occur within 48 hours.

---

and hypotension can also reduce renal blood flow, resulting in decreased glomerular perfusion and prerenal AKI. With a mild to moderate decrease in renal blood flow, intraglomerular pressure is maintained by dilation of afferent arterioles (arteries supplying blood to the glomerulus), constriction of efferent arterioles (arteries removing blood from the glomerulus), and redistribution of renal blood flow to the oxygen-sensitive renal medulla. Drugs may cause a functional AKI when these adaptive mechanisms are compromised. Nonsteroidal anti-inflammatory drugs (NSAIDs) impair prostaglandin-mediated dilation of afferent arterioles. Angiotensin-converting enzyme (ACE) inhibitors and angiotensin receptor blockers (ARBs) inhibit angiotensin II–mediated efferent arteriole vasoconstriction and cause prerenal AKI in 6% to 38% of treated patients.[9] Cyclosporine and tacrolimus, particularly in high doses, are potent renal vasoconstrictors. All of these agents can reduce intraglomerular pressure, with a resultant decrease in GFR. Prompt discontinuation of the offending drug can often return kidney function to normal. Other causes of prerenal AKI are renovascular obstruction (e.g., renal artery stenosis), hyperviscosity syndromes (e.g., multiple myeloma), or systemic vasoconstriction (e.g., hepatorenal syndrome). Prerenal AKI occurs in approximately 10% to 25% of patients diagnosed with AKI.

Intrinsic AKI

Intrinsic renal failure is caused by diseases that can affect the integrity of the tubules, glomerulus, interstitium, or blood vessels. Damage is within the kidney; changes in kidney structure can be seen on microscopy.[10] **Acute tubular necrosis** (ATN) is a term that is often used synonymously with intrinsic renal failure, but it relates more specifically to a pathophysiologic condition that results from toxic (e.g., aminoglycosides, contrast agents, or amphotericin B) or ischemic insult to the kidney only. ATN results in necrosis of the proximal tubule epithelium and basement membrane, decreased glomerular capillary permeability, and back leak of glomerular filtrate into the venous circulation.[11] ATN

accounts for 50% of all cases of AKI.[9] Glomerular, interstitial, and blood vessel diseases may also lead to intrinsic AKI but occur with a much lower incidence. Examples include glomerulonephritis, systemic lupus erythematosus, interstitial nephritis, and vasculitis. In addition, prerenal AKI can progress to intrinsic AKI if the underlying condition is not promptly corrected.[10]

Postrenal AKI

Postrenal AKI is due to obstruction of urinary outflow. Causes include benign prostatic hypertrophy, pelvic tumors, and precipitation of renal calculi.[10] Rapid resolution of postrenal AKI without structural damage to the kidney can occur if the underlying obstruction is corrected. Postrenal AKI accounts for less than 10% of cases of AKI.

ASSESSMENT OF KIDNEY FUNCTION

The most common measure of overall kidney function is GFR. It is defined as the volume of plasma filtered across the glomerulus per unit time and correlates well with the filtration, secretion, reabsorption, endocrine, and metabolic functions of the kidney. In addition to aiding in the diagnosis and assessment of the severity of AKI, an accurate estimate of GFR can assist in proper dosing of drugs that undergo renal elimination. In an individual with normal kidney function, GFR ranges from approximately 90 to 120 mL/min (1.5 to 2.0 mL/s). Because GFR is difficult to measure directly, it is routinely estimated by determining the renal clearance of a substance that is filtered at the glomerulus and does not undergo significant tubular reabsorption or secretion. Creatinine is an endogenous substance that is a normal by-product of muscle metabolism. Ninety percent of creatinine is eliminated by glomerular filtration; tubular secretion is responsible for the remaining 10%.

Direct measurement of **creatinine clearance** (CrCl) requires collection of urine over an extended time interval (usually 24 hours) with measurement of urine volume, urine

---

Table 25–2

Equations for Estimation of CrCl

Urine Collection Method

$$CrCl \ (mL/min) = \frac{(Ucr)(V)}{(SCr)(T)}$$

Ucr = urine creatinine concentration, mg/dL
V = volume of urine, mL
SCr = serum creatinine concentration, mg/dL
T = time of urine collection, minute
(Note: Time equals 1,440 minutes for a 24-hour collection)

Cockcroft–Gault Equation for Adults[11]

$$CrCl \ (mL/min) = \frac{(140 - Age) \times (BW)}{(SCr) \times 72} \ (\times \ 0.85 \ if \ women)$$

Age, years
BW = actual body weight, kg^a
SCr = serum creatinine concentration, mg/dL

Jelliffe Equation for Changing Renal Function[14]

Males
$E^{SS} = IBW \ [(29.3 - 0.203 \ (age)]$
$E^{SS}_{corr} = E^{SS} \ [1.035 - 0.0337 \ (SCr)]$
$E = E^{SS}_{corr} - \dfrac{[4 \times IBW \times (SCr_2 - SCr_1)]}{\Delta t}$
$CrCl \ (mL/min/1.73 \ m^2) = E/[(14.4)(SCr)]$

Females
$E^{SS} = IBW \ [25.1 - 0.175 \ (age)]$
$E^{SS}_{corr} = E^{SS} \ [1.035 - 0.0337 \ (SCr)]$
$E = E^{SS}_{corr} - \dfrac{[4 \times IBW \times (SCr_2 - SCr_1)]}{\Delta t}$
$CrCl \ (mL/min/1.73 \ m^2) = E/[(14.4)(SCr)]$

E^{SS} = steady-state creatinine excretion
Δt = time in days between measurement of SCr_1 and SCr_2
IBW = ideal body weight, kg

Age, years

E^{SS}_{corr} = corrected steady-state creatinine excretion
SCr_1 = first serum creatinine concentration
SCr_2 = second serum creatinine concentration

E = creatinine excretion

---

^{a}Typically substituted with ideal body weight, or adjusted body weight when body weight is significantly greater (i.e., greater than 130%) than ideal body weight: Adjusted body weight = Ideal body weight + 0.25 (Actual body weight − Ideal body weight).

CrCl, creatinine clearance. For conversion of mg/dL to µmol/L creatinine multiply by 88.4.

---

creatinine concentration, and serum creatinine concentration (SCr; Table 25–2). Although 24-hour urine collections have been used to measure CrCl in clinical practice, difficulty in collection of accurate 24-hour specimens renders this method time consuming and error prone. Collection intervals as short as 8 hours have yielded estimates similar to those obtained with 24-hour collections in several studies, and they may minimize overcollection or undercollection of urine that can occur with a 24-hour collection.

Because kidney function can fluctuate significantly during AKI, this method may also underestimate or overestimate kidney function depending on whether AKI is worsening or resolving.

Numerous equations have been developed for a quick bedside estimate of CrCl or GFR. They incorporate patient-specific variables such as SCr, body weight, age, and gender. One of the most widely used equations is the Cockcroft-Gault equation (Table 25–2).[11] It is generally considered acceptable in individuals whose renal function is relatively constant, as defined as a daily change in serum creatinine of less than 10% to 15% within 24 hours. ❶ *Equations to estimate creatinine clearance (CrCl) that incorporate a single serum creatinine concentration such as the Cockcroft-Gault equation typically overestimate kidney function.*[12] A 10% to 15% overestimation of CrCl occurs due to secretion of creatinine into the tubules, particularly at lower GFRs, where the contribution of creatinine secretion can become significant.

In instances where kidney function is fluctuating, several equations (Jelliffe, Brater, Chiou) have been developed to assess unstable kidney function.[13-15] These equations estimate CrCl by considering the change in serum creatinine over a specified time period (Table 25–2, Jelliffe equation). Although they are more mathematically difficult to calculate, they take into consideration a change in serum creatinine compared with an equation that only includes a single creatinine concentration. It should be noted that these methods have not been validated, and drug dosage adjustments based on CrCl estimates from these formulas in patients with AKI have not been evaluated. Calculations of CrCl in AKI must be viewed as best estimates under variable conditions, and ongoing patient monitoring is necessary to avoid drug toxicity.

Estimating CrCl is only one part of evaluating a patient's overall kidney function. Other factors, such as symptomatology, laboratory test results, urinary indices, and results of diagnostic procedures, will aid in the diagnosis and assessment of the severity of disease. By monitoring SCr on a routine basis, it can be estimated whether kidney function is improving or worsening. Kidney function can also be evaluated based on urine output. Oliguria and anuria are defined as urine outputs of less than 400 mL and 50 mL over 24 hours, respectively. Patients with reduced urine output often have an increased mortality and may represent a more severe form of AKI. Nonoliguric AKI is defined as a urine output of greater than 400 mL/day. It may still represent severe AKI but is associated with better patient outcomes.[16]

Clinical Presentation and Diagnosis of AKI

While some clinical and laboratory findings assist in the general diagnosis of AKI, others are used to differentiate among prerenal, intrinsic, and postrenal AKI. For example, patients with prerenal AKI typically demonstrate enhanced sodium reabsorption, which is reflected by a low urine sodium concentration and a low fractional excretion of sodium. Urine is typically more concentrated with prerenal AKI, and there is a higher urine osmolality and urine-to-plasma creatinine ratio compared with intrinsic and postrenal AKI.

Signs and Symptoms of Uremia

- Peripheral edema
- Weight gain
- Nausea/vomiting/diarrhea/anorexia
- Mental status changes
- Fatigue
- Shortness of breath
- Pruritus
- Volume depletion (prerenal AKI)
- Weight loss (prerenal AKI)
- Anuria alternating with polyuria (postrenal AKI)
- Colicky abdominal pain radiating from flank to groin (postrenal AKI)

Physical Examination Findings

- Hypertension
- Jugular venous distention (JVD)
- Pulmonary edema
- Rales
- Asterixis
- Pericardial or pleural friction rub
- Hypotension/orthostatic hypotension (prerenal AKI)
- Rash (acute interstitial nephritis)
- Bladder distention (postrenal bladder outlet obstruction)
- Prostatic enlargement (postrenal AKI)

Laboratory Tests

- Elevated SCr (normal range approximately 0.6 to 1.2 mg/dL [53 to 106 μmol/L])
- Elevated BUN concentration (normal range approximately 8 to 25 mg/dL [2.9 to 8.9 mmol/L])
- Decreased CrCl (normal range: 90 to 120 mL/min [1.5 to 2.0 mL/s])
- BUN-to-creatinine ratio greater than 20:1 for units of mg/dL (prerenal AKI); less than 20:1 for units of mg/dL (intrinsic or postrenal AKI)
- Hyperkalemia
- Metabolic acidosis

Urinalysis

- Sediment
  - Scant or bland (prerenal or postrenal AKI)
  - Brown, muddy granular casts (highly indicative of ATN)
  - Proteinuria (glomerulonephritis or allergic interstitial nephritis)
  - Eosinophiluria (acute interstitial nephritis)
  - Hematuria/red blood cell casts (glomerular disease or bleeding in urinary tract)
  - WBCs or casts (acute interstitial nephritis or severe pyelonephritis)

Urinary Indices	Prerenal AKI	Intrinsic and Postrenal AKI
Urine osmolality (concentration of solutes in the urine in mOsm/kg or mmol/kg)	Greater than 500	Less than 350
Urine sodium concentration (mEq/L or mmol/L)	Less than 20	Greater than 40
Specific gravity	Greater than 1.020	Less than 1.015
Urine-to-plasma creatinine ratio	Greater than 40:1	Less than 20:1
Fractional excretion of sodium (FENa)	Less than 1%	Greater than 1%

$$\text{Fractional excretion of sodium (FENa)} = 100 \times \frac{\text{Urinary sodium concentration} \times \text{Plasma creatinine concentration}}{\text{Plasma sodium concentration} \times \text{Plasma creatinine concentration}}$$

FENa is a measure of the percentage of sodium excreted by the kidney. A FENa less than 1% may indicate prerenal AKI because it represents the response of the kidney to decreased renal perfusion by decreasing sodium excretion. Loop diuretics such as furosemide enhance sodium excretion and increase FENa, confounding the interpretation of the test.

Common Diagnostic Procedures

- Urinary catheterization (insertion of a catheter into a patient's bladder; an increase in urine output may occur with postrenal obstruction)
- Renal ultrasound (uses sound waves to assess size, position, and abnormalities of the kidney; dilatation of the urinary tract can be seen with postrenal AKI)
- Renal angiography (administration of IV contrast dye to assess the vasculature of the kidney)
- Retrograde pyelography (injection of contrast dye into the ureters to assess the kidney and collection system)
- Kidney biopsy (collection of a tissue sample of the kidney for the purpose of microscopic evaluation; may aid in the diagnosis of glomerular and interstitial diseases)

TREATMENT

Desired Outcomes

A primary goal in the care of patients with AKI is ameliorating any identifiable underlying causes of AKI such as hypovolemia, nephrotoxic drug administration, or ureter obstruction. Prerenal and postrenal AKI can be reversed if the underlying problem is promptly identified and corrected, whereas treatment of intrinsic renal failure is more supportive in nature. ❷ *There is no evidence that drug therapy hastens patient recovery in AKI, decreases length of hospitalization, or improves survival.* Therefore, options are limited to supportive therapy, such as fluid, electrolyte, and nutritional support, RRT, and treatment of nonrenal complications such as sepsis and GI bleeding while regeneration of the renal epithelium occurs. In addition, prevention of adverse drug reactions by discontinuing nephrotoxic drugs or adjustment of drug dosages based on the patient's renal function is desired.

Pharmacologic Therapy

▶ *Loop Diuretics*

There is significant controversy over the role of loop diuretics in the treatment of AKI. Theoretical benefits of loop diuretics in hastening recovery of renal function include decreased tubular oxygen requirements of the kidney, increased resistance to ischemia, increased urine flow rates that reduce intraluminal obstruction and filtrate back leak, and renal vasodilation. Theoretically, these effects could lead to increased urine output, decreased need for dialysis, improved renal recovery, and ultimately, increased survival. However, there are conflicting reports in the literature over the efficacy of loop diuretics. Most studies demonstrate an improvement in urine output but with no effect on survival or need for dialysis. There are some reports that loop diuretics may worsen kidney function.[17] This may be due in part to excessive preload reduction that results in renal vasoconstriction. Thus loop diuretics are limited to instances of volume overload and edema, and they are not intended to hasten renal recovery or improve survival.

Loop diuretics (furosemide, bumetanide, torsemide, and ethacrynic acid) are all equally effective when given in equivalent doses. Therefore, selection is based on the side-effect profile, cost, and pharmacokinetics of the agents. The incidence of ototoxicity is significantly higher with ethacrynic acid compared with the other loop diuretics; therefore, its use is limited to patients who are allergic to the sulfa component in the other loop diuretics.[18] Although ototoxicity is a well-established side effect of furosemide, its incidence may be greater when administered by the IV route at a rate exceeding 4 mg/min. Torsemide has not been reported to cause ototoxicity.

There are several pharmacokinetic differences between loop diuretics. Fifty percent of a dose of furosemide is excreted unchanged by the kidney with the remainder undergoing glucuronide conjugation in the kidney.[19] In contrast, liver metabolism accounts for 50% and 80% of the elimination of bumetanide and torsemide, respectively.[19] Thus patients with AKI may have a prolonged half-life of furosemide. The bioavailability of both torsemide and

---

Patient Encounter, Part I

JD is a 65-year-old woman who presents to the clinic for follow-up evaluation of her type 2 diabetes and dyslipidemia. She also has a past medical history of stage 2 chronic kidney disease with proteinuria, hypothyroidism, gout, hypertension, allergic rhinitis, and chronic back pain. She reports having nausea, vomiting, and a low-grade fever last week. Her grandson had similar symptoms, and she did not seek treatment. Her fever resolved with ibuprofen, but she still feels weak and nauseated. She states that she feels like she is "holding on to water." Her weight is usually about 135 pounds (61 kg), and she now weighs 140 lbs (64 kg). Upon preliminary examination, she was found to have 2+ pitting edema, elevated blood pressure, and crackles on auscultation.

Meds:

Fexofenadine 180 mg orally once daily

Valsartan 160 mg orally once daily

Hydrochlorothiazide 25 mg orally once daily

Atorvastatin 10 mg orally daily

Metformin 500 mg orally twice daily

Glipizide 5 mg orally daily

Metoprolol 25 mg orally twice daily

Allopurinol 300 mg orally daily

Levothyroxine 25 mcg orally daily

Acetaminophen 500 mg 1 to 2 tablets orally every 6 hours as needed

Ibuprofen 400 to 800 mg as needed for arthritis pain and fever

What signs and symptoms suggest AKI?

What risk factors does she have for developing AKI?

What additional laboratory and physical examination information do you need to fully assess the patient?

What questions would you ask her regarding her pharmacotherapy?

bumetanide is higher than for furosemide. The IV-to-oral ratio for bumetanide and torsemide is 1:1, bioavailability of oral furosemide is approximately 50%, with a reported range of 10% to 100%.[20]

Furosemide and bumetanide are both available in generic formulations and generally less expensive than torsemide.

The pharmacodynamic characteristics of loop diuretics are similar when equivalent doses are administered. Because loop diuretics exert their effect from the luminal (urinary) side of the tubule, urinary excretion correlates with diuretic response. Substances that interfere with the organic acid pathway, such as endogenous organic acids that accumulate in renal disease, competitively inhibit secretion of loop diuretics into the lumen of the tubules. Therefore, large doses of loop diuretics may be required to ensure that adequate drug reaches the nephron lumen. In addition, loop diuretics have a ceiling effect where maximal natriuresis occurs.[19,21] Thus very large doses of furosemide (e.g., 1 g) are generally not considered necessary and may unnecessarily increase the risk of ototoxicity.

Several adaptive mechanisms by the kidney limit effectiveness of loop diuretic therapy. Postdiuretic sodium retention occurs as the concentration of diuretic in the loop of Henle decreases. This effect can be minimized by decreasing the dosage interval (i.e., dosing more frequently) or by administering a continuous infusion.[22] In patients with a CrCl of 25 mL/min (0.42 mL/s) or higher, furosemide at a dose of 10 mg/h would be a reasonable starting dose.[19] A starting dose of 20 mg/h would be reasonable in patients with a CrCl less than 25 mL/min (0.42 mL/s).[19] With a continuous infusion, a loading dose is recommended. Continuous infusion loop diuretics may be easier to titrate than bolus dosing, requires less nursing administration time, and may lead to fewer adverse reactions.

Prolonged administration of loop diuretics can lead to a second type of diuretic resistance. Enhanced delivery of sodium to the distal tubule can result in hypertrophy of distal convoluted cells.[19] Subsequently, increased sodium chloride absorption occurs in the distal tubule that diminishes the effect of the loop diuretic on sodium excretion. Addition of a distal convoluted tubule diuretic, such as metolazone or hydrochlorothiazide, to a loop diuretic can result in a synergistic increase in urine output. There are no data to support the efficacy of one distal convoluted tubule diuretic over another. The common practice of administering the distal convoluted tubule diuretic 30 to 60 minutes prior to the loop diuretic has not been studied, although this practice may first inhibit sodium reabsorption at the distal convoluted tubule before it is inundated with sodium from the loop of Henle.

A usual starting dose of IV furosemide for the treatment of AKI is 40 mg (**Fig. 25–2**). Reasonable starting doses for bumetanide and torsemide are 1 mg and 20 mg, respectively.[19] Efficacy of diuretic administration can be determined by comparison of a patient's hourly fluid balance. Other methods to minimize volume overload, such as fluid restriction and concentration of IV medications, should be initiated as needed. If urine output does not increase to about 1 mL/kg/h, the dosage can be increased to a maximum of 160 to 200 mg of furosemide or its equivalent (Fig. 25–2).[20] Dosing frequency is based on the patient's response, the ability to restrict sodium intake, and the duration of action of the diuretic. Other methods to improve diuresis can be initiated sequentially, such as (a) shortening the dosage interval, (b) adding hydrochlorothiazide or metolazone, and (c) switching to a continuous infusion loop diuretic. A loading dose should be administered prior to both initiating a continuous infusion and increasing the infusion rate. When high doses of loop diuretics are administered, especially in combination with distal convoluted tubule diuretics, the hemodynamic and fluid status of the patient should be monitored every shift, and the electrolyte status of the patient should be monitored at least daily to prevent profound diuresis and electrolyte abnormalities, such as hypokalemia. Patients will not benefit from switching from one loop diuretic to another because of the similarity in mechanisms of action.

▶ Other Diuretics

Thiazide diuretics, when used as single agents, are generally not effective for fluid removal. Mannitol is also not recommended for the treatment of volume overload associated with AKI. Mannitol is removed by the body by glomerular filtration. In patients with renal dysfunction, mannitol excretion is decreased, resulting in expanded blood volume and hyperosmolality. Potassium-sparing diuretics, which inhibit sodium reabsorption in the distal nephron and collecting duct, are not sufficiently effective in removing fluid. In addition, they increase the risk of hyperkalemia in patients already at risk. ❸ *Thus loop diuretics are the diuretics of choice for the management of volume overload in AKI.*

▶ Dopamine

Low-dose dopamine (LDD), in doses ranging from 0.5 to 3 mcg/kg/min, predominantly stimulates dopamine-1 receptors, leading to renal vascular vasodilation and increased renal blood flow. Although this effect has been substantiated in healthy euvolemic individuals with normal kidney function, a lack of efficacy data exists in patients with AKI. The most comprehensive study evaluating efficacy of LDD, the Australian and New Zealand Intensive Care Society (ANZICS) Clinical Trials Group study, did not find that LDD alters peak SCr, need for RRT, duration of stay in the intensive care unit, or survival to discharge compared with placebo.[23] A meta-analysis was performed on all published human trials that used LDD in the prevention or treatment of AKI.[24] A total of 61 studies were identified that randomized more than 3,300 patients to LDD or placebo. Results reveal no significant difference between the treatment and control groups for mortality, requirement for RRT, or adverse effects. Based on the results of the ANZICS trial, the lack of conclusive evidence in many earlier studies, and several meta-analyses, ❹ *there is no indication for the use of LDD in the treatment of AKI.*

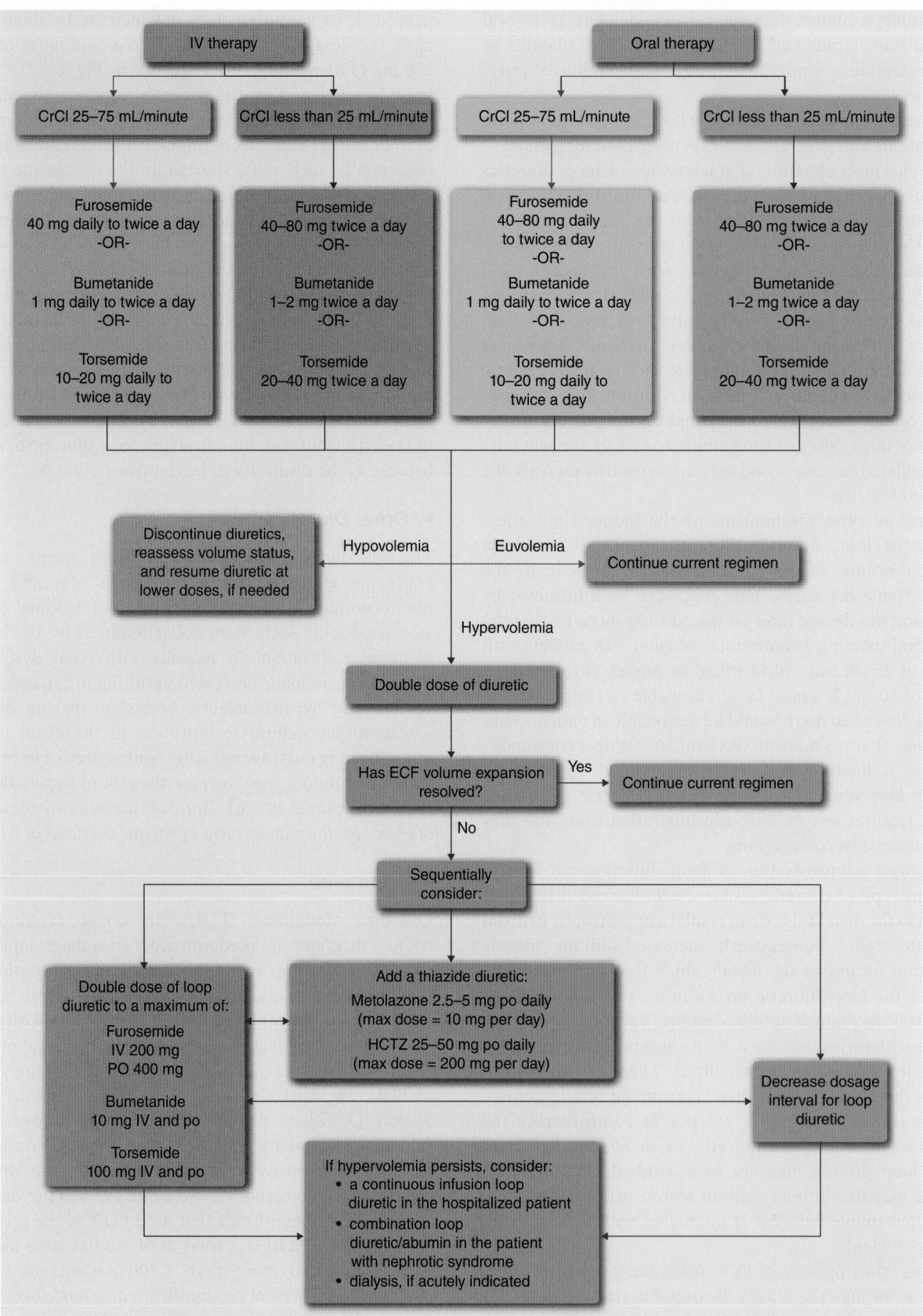

FIGURE 25–2. Algorithm for treatment of extracellular fluid expansion. (CrCl, creatinine clearance; ECF, extracellular fluid; HCTZ, hydrochlorothiazide; po, oral.)

▶ Fenoldopam

Fenoldopam is a selective dopamine-1 receptor agonist that is approved for short-term management of severe hypertension. Because it does not stimulate dopamine-2, α-adrenergic, and β-adrenergic receptors, fenoldopam causes vasodilation in the renal vasculature with potentially fewer nonrenal effects than dopamine. In normotensive individuals with normal kidney function, IV fenoldopam increases renal blood flow without lowering systemic blood pressure. A prospective randomized study comparing fenoldopam to placebo in early ATN did not find a difference in need for dialysis or mortality.[25] A second prospective randomized study in septic patients did find less of an increase in SCr in the fenoldopam group compared with placebo but no difference in survival or need for RRT.[26]

Nonpharmacologic Treatment

▶ Renal Replacement Therapy

RRT may be necessary in patients with established AKI to treat volume overload that is unresponsive to diuretics, to minimize the accumulation of nitrogenous waste products, and to correct electrolyte and acid–base abnormalities while renal function recovers. There is wide variation in practice on indications for RRT, timing of initiation/discontinuation of RRT, intensity of treatment, and optimal type of RRT,

and well-controlled studies are needed to guide treatment. Absolute indications for dialysis usually include:

- BUN greater than 100 mg/dL (35.7 mmol/L)
- Potassium greater than 6 mEq/L (6 mmol/L)
- Magnesium greater than 9.7 mg/dL (4 mmol/L)
- Metabolic acidosis with a pH less than 7.15
- Diuretic-resistant fluid overload.[27]

A BUN greater than 76 mg/dL (27.1 mmol/L) is a relative indicator for RRT. Approximately 5% to 30% of patients with AKI treated with dialysis will not have recovery of their renal function and will need to remain on long-term dialysis. This may be due in part to underlying illnesses because AKI is often seen in the setting of multiorgan failure.

The two types of dialysis modalities commonly used in AKI are intermittent hemodialysis (IHD) and continuous renal replacement therapy (CRRT). IHD is a higher efficiency form of dialysis that is provided for several hours a day at a variable frequency (usually daily or three to five times per week) at a higher blood flow rate. CRRT is a pump-driven form of dialysis that provides slow fluid and solute removal on a continuous 24-hour basis. The primary advantage of CRRT is hemodynamic stability and better volume control, particularly in patients who are unable to tolerate rapid fluid removal. The primary disadvantages associated with CRRT are continuous nursing requirements, continuous

---

Patient Encounter, Part 2

PMH:

Type 2 diabetes mellitus for 10 years (labs from 3 months ago: HgA1c = 7.4% [0.074; 57 mmol/mol hemoglobin], SCr = 0.9 mg/dL [80 μmol/L])

Dyslipidemia for 10 years

Hypothyroidism for 15 years

Hypertension for 10 years

Gout

Allergic rhinitis

Episodic back pain secondary to a motor vehicle accident

FH: Father with history of type 2 diabetes and chronic kidney disease; mother with history of hypertension

SH: No smoking, no alcohol use

PE:

VS: BP 165/95, pulse 85 bpm, RR 22/min, temperature 37.6°C, weight 62 kg, ht 5'7" (170 cm)

Chest: Basilar crackles, inspiratory wheezes

CV: RRR, S_1, S_2 normal

MS/Ext: 2 + pitting edema

Urinalysis: Color, yellow; character, hazy; glucose (–); ketones (–); specific gravity 1.010; pH 5; (+) protein; no bacteria; nitrite (–); blood (–); osmolality 325 mOsm/kg (325 mmol/kg); urinary sodium 77 mEq/L (77 mmol/L); creatinine 25 mg/dL (2.21 mmol/L)

Laboratory values: Sodium 136 mEq/L (136 mmol/L), potassium 4.2 mEq/L (4.2 mmol/L), chloride 105 mEq/L (105 mmol/L), bicarbonate 22 mEq/L (22 mmol/L), BUN 32 mg/dL (11.4 mmol/L), SCr 1.8 mg/dL (159 μmol/L), magnesium 1.6 mg/dL (0.66 mmol/L), glucose 120 mg/dL (6.7 mmol/L), WBC 6.9×10^3 (6.9×10^9/L), hemoglobin 14.4 g/dL (144 g/L; 8.94 mmol/L), and hematocrit 42% (0.42).

Interview information: Patient takes all of her medications as prescribed. She checks her fasting glucose each morning. It ranges from 110 to 125 mg/dL (6.1 to 6.9 mmol/L). She takes acetaminophen about three or four times a day for back pain. She recently started taking ibuprofen 3 weeks ago because her neighbor told her it was better for pain. She takes it about two or three times a day.

Given this additional information, what is your assessment of the patient's condition?

Identify your treatment goals for the patient.

anticoagulation, frequent clotting of the dialyzer, patient immobility, and increased cost. There is no conclusive evidence that one type of dialysis is preferred to another in terms of mortality and recovery of renal function. Thus selection of CRRT over IHD is often governed by the critical illness of the patient and by the comfort level of the institution with one particular type of dialysis. Mortality in critically ill patients receiving CRRT is 40% to 53%.[28,29]

Studies are underway to identify new markers for early detection of AKI (e.g., cystatin C, neutrophil gelatinase-associated lipocalin, N-acetyl-β-d-glucosaminidase, kidney injury molecule-1) that can assist not only in the early diagnosis of AKI, but also to guide decisions on when to initiate RRT.[30]

▶ Supportive Therapy

Supportive therapy in AKI includes adequate nutrition, correction of electrolyte and acid–base abnormalities (particularly hyperkalemia and metabolic acidosis), fluid management, and correction of any hematologic abnormalities. Because AKI is often associated with multiorgan failure, treatment includes the medical management of infections, cardiovascular and GI conditions, and respiratory failure. Finally, all drugs should be reviewed and dosage adjustments made based on an estimate of the patient's GFR.

PREVENTION OF ACUTE RENAL FAILURE

Avoidance

● The best preventive measure for AKI, especially in individuals at high risk, is to avoid medications that are known to precipitate AKI. Nephrotoxicity is a significant side effect of aminoglycosides, ACE inhibitors, angiotensin receptor antagonists, amphotericin B, NSAIDs, cyclosporine, tacrolimus, and radiographic contrast agents.[8] Unfortunately, an effective, nonnephrotoxic alternative may not always be appropriate for a given patient, and the risks and benefits of selecting a drug with nephrotoxic potential must be considered. For example, serious gram-negative infections may require double antibiotic coverage, and based on culture and sensitivity reports, aminoglycoside therapy may be necessary. In cases such as this, other measures to reduce the risk of AKI should be instituted. ❺ *Thus identifying patients at high risk for development of AKI and implementing preventive methods to decrease its occurrence or severity is critical.*

● Drug-Induced ARF

▶ Aminoglycosides

Aminoglycosides (gentamicin, tobramycin, and amikacin) causes nonoliguric intrinsic AKI in about 10% to 25% of treated patients.[31] Injury is due to binding of aminoglycosides to proximal tubular cells in the renal cortex, and subsequent cellular uptake and cell death. In addition, aminoglycosides cause renal vasoconstriction and mesangial contraction.[32] In clinical practice, all aminoglycosides have comparable nephrotoxicity; thus similar precautions should be used for all of the agents. High cumulative drug exposure increases the incidence of aminoglycoside-induced AKI. Additional risk factors include a prolonged course of aminoglycoside therapy (typically after 7 to 10 days of therapy), preexisting chronic kidney disease, increased age, and concurrent administration with other nephrotoxic drugs. Alternative antibiotics should be considered in individuals with AKI or those who are at a high risk for developing AKI, although resistance of some strains of gram-negative organisms to other antibiotics may necessitate their use.

Methods to minimize drug exposure with conventional (multiple doses per day) dosing include maintaining trough concentrations less than 2 mcg/mL (2 mg/L; 4.2 μmol/L) for gentamicin and tobramycin and less than 10 mcg/mL (10 mg/L; 17.1 μmol/L) for amikacin, minimizing length of therapy, and avoiding repeated courses of aminoglycosides. Concurrent exposure to other nephrotoxic medications and dehydration may also worsen AKI. There is conflicting evidence as to whether the combination of vancomycin and an aminoglycoside has a higher incidence of AKI than aminoglycoside therapy alone. Aminoglycoside-induced AKI is usually reversible upon drug discontinuation; however, dialysis may be needed in some individuals while kidney function improves.

Another method to minimize toxicity is with extended-interval dosing (e.g., once daily). The goal of extended-interval dosing is to provide greater efficacy against the microorganism with a lower incidence of nephrotoxicity. Aminoglycosides demonstrate concentration-dependent killing and a prolonged postantibiotic effect.[31] The mechanism by which extended-interval aminoglycoside dosing reduces the incidence of nephrotoxicity is by providing high transient concentrations of drug that saturate proximal tubule uptake sites. Once saturated, the remaining aminoglycoside molecules pass through the proximal tubule and are excreted in the urine.[33] Thus less drug is available for cellular uptake during a 24-hour period. A consistent finding in studies is that extended-interval aminoglycoside dosing is as effective as conventional dosing and is not more nephrotoxic, and in some studies it is less nephrotoxic than conventional dosing. Aminoglycosides can also cause hearing loss and/or vestibular toxicity, although the incidence of ototoxicity appears to be similar with extended-dosing and conventional dosing. Prolonged exposure to the drug, repeated courses of therapy, and concurrent use of other ototoxic drugs increase toxicity. Extended-interval dosing is not recommended in patients with preexisting kidney disease, conditions where high concentrations are not needed (e.g., urinary tract infections), hyperdynamic patients that may demonstrate increased drug clearance (e.g., burn patients), and others where you would suspect altered pharmacokinetics or increased risk of ototoxicity.

● ▶ Amphotericin B

The reported incidence of amphotericin B–induced AKI varies widely in the literature, from about 30% to as high as 80% of patients treated with the conventional desoxycholate formulation.[34] Nephrotoxicity is due to renal arterial vasoconstriction and distal renal tubule cell damage. Risk factors for development of AKI include high daily dosage, large cumulative dose (greater than 2 to 3 g), preexisting kidney dysfunction, dehydration, and concomitant use of other nephrotoxic drugs. Tubular abnormalities manifesting as hypomagnesemia and hypokalemia often occur within the first 2 weeks of treatment, followed by the overt development of AKI. Three lipid-based formulations of amphotericin B have been developed in an attempt to improve efficacy and limit toxicity, particularly nephrotoxicity: amphotericin B lipid complex, amphotericin B colloidal dispersion, and liposomal amphotericin B. The range of nephrotoxicity reported is 15% to 25% for these formulations. The mechanism for decreased nephrotoxicity has not been completely elucidated, but it is thought to be due to preferential delivery of amphotericin B to the site of infection, with less of an affinity for the kidney.[35] Costs for liposomal formulations is significantly higher than the convention formulation; thus lipid-based formulations are typically recommended for individuals with risk factors for AKI. Administration of IV normal saline may also attenuate nephrotoxicity associated with amphotericin B.

Whether there are significant differences in nephrotoxicity between the three lipid-based formulations remains unclear. In a recent meta-analysis of eight studies evaluating the nephrotoxicity of liposomal amphotericin B compared with amphotericin B lipid complex, nephrotoxicity was generally similar.[36] However, large prospective studies comparing the incidence of nephrotoxicity between liposomal formulations are needed to ascertain differences in nephrotoxicity.

► *Radiocontrast Agents*

Intravascular radiographic contrast agents are administered during radiologic studies and carry with them the well-documented risk of AKI. Patients at risk for developing AKI include patients with chronic kidney disease, diabetic nephropathy, dehydration, and higher doses of contrast dye.[37] Contrast agents are water-soluble, triiodinated, benzoic acid salts that cause an osmotic diuresis due to their osmolality, which exceeds that of plasma. The mechanism of nephrotoxicity is not fully understood; however, direct tubular toxicity, renal ischemia, and tubular obstruction have been implicated.[38] Diatrizoate and iothalamate are ionic contrast agents. Iohexol, iopamidol, ioversol, and iopromide represent nonionic agents. The incidence of nephrotoxicity with ionic and nonionic agents is similar in patients at low risk for developing AKI; however, in high-risk patients, nephrotoxicity is significantly greater when ionic contrast agents are used. In diabetic patients with chronic kidney disease and a SCr greater than 1.5 mg/dL (133 μmol/L), nephrotoxicity occurred in 33.3% and 47.7% of patients receiving nonionic and ionic contrast agents, respectively.[39] The cost of nonionic agents is approximately 10-fold higher, which may limit their routine use in all patients undergoing radiographic studies.

Therapeutic measures that have been used to decrease the incidence of contrast-induced nephropathy include extracellular volume expansion, minimization of the amount of contrast administered, and treatment with oral acetylcysteine. Theophylline, fenoldopam, loop diuretics, mannitol, dopamine, and calcium antagonists have no effect or may worsen AKI.

The most effective therapeutic maneuver to decrease the incidence of contrast-induced nephropathy is extracellular volume expansion.[40] Several studies have compared the efficacy of isotonic sodium chloride (0.9%) to half normal saline (0.45%) or to oral hydration.[41,42] Isotonic fluid is superior to hypotonic fluid in prevention of nephropathy. A common regimen is IV isotonic sodium chloride (1 mL/kg of body weight/hour) administered for 12 hours before and 12 hours after the procedure. Fluid should be administered cautiously to patients with CHF, left ventricular dysfunction, and significant renal dysfunction. Recent evidence suggests that hydration, plus sodium bicarbonate to alkalize renal tubule fluid, may reduce free radical formation and lead to less oxidant damage, although studies have been conflicting.[43,44] Most studies investigating sodium bicarbonate hydration administered therapy at a rate of 3 mL/kg/h (154 mEq/L [154 mmol/L]) for 1 hour before the procedure, and 1 mL/kg/h during and 6-hour postcontrast. A large randomized clinical trial that provides definitive conclusions is needed.

Minimizing the quantity of contrast media administered may be beneficial in preventing nephropathy. Some studies, but not all, have directly associated dose of contrast media with nephrotoxicity. Avoidance of contrast dye by using alternative diagnostic procedures should be considered in high-risk patients but may not always be feasible. In addition, avoidance of multiple contrast studies in a short time period will allow renal function to return to normal between procedures.

Because production of reactive oxygen species has been implicated in the pathophysiology of contrast-induced AKI, prophylactic administration of the antioxidant acetylcysteine has been investigated. An oral dose of 600 mg twice daily the day before and the day of the procedure decreased the incidence of AKI in one small study, although patient outcomes such as mortality and length of hospitalization were not evaluated.[45] Since then, more than 30 additional studies evaluating the efficacy of oral acetylcysteine have been conducted, with mixed results. In addition, a series of meta-analyses have also analyzed the results of the studies with varying conclusions. The studies were varied in terms of study population, sample size, definition of contrast nephropathy, type of contrast agent used, hydration, and formulation of acetylcysteine administered, thus making collective interpretation of the results difficult. It is routinely used in many hospitals due to its low cost and safe side-effect profile at low oral doses, although data are not conclusive that it prevents development of AKI or alters patient outcomes such as mortality, need for dialysis, and length of hospitalization. The recommended dose of acetylcysteine is 600 to 1,200 mg orally every 12 hours, with the first dose administered prior to the contrast procedure and three doses postexposure. It is noted that acetylcysteine is not considered a replacement for adequate hydration, which remains the standard of care for prevention of contrast nephropathy.

▶ *Cyclosporine and Tacrolimus*

Cyclosporine and tacrolimus are calcineurin inhibitors that are administered as part of immunosuppressive regimens in kidney, liver, heart, lung, and bone marrow transplant recipients. In addition, they are used in autoimmune disorders such as psoriasis and multiple sclerosis. The pathophysiologic mechanism for AKI is renal vascular vasoconstriction.[46] It often occurs within the first 6 to 12 months of treatment and can be reversible with dose reduction or drug discontinuation. Risk factors include high dose, elevated trough blood concentrations, increased age, and concomitant therapy with other nephrotoxic drugs.[46] Cyclosporine and tacrolimus are extensively metabolized by the liver through the cytochrome P450 3A4 pathway, and drugs that inhibit their metabolism (e.g., erythromycin, clarithromycin, fluconazole, ketoconazole, verapamil, diltiazem, and nicardipine) can precipitate AKI. Because AKI is dose dependent, careful monitoring of cyclosporine or tacrolimus trough concentrations can minimize its occurrence; however, AKI can still occur with normal or low blood concentrations. In addition, there is some evidence that calcium channel blockers have a renoprotective effect through dilation of the afferent arterioles and are often used preferentially as antihypertensive agents in kidney transplant recipients.

It is often difficult to differentiate AKI from acute rejection in the kidney transplant recipient because both conditions may present with similar symptoms and physical examination findings. However, fever and graft tenderness are more likely to occur with rejection, whereas neurotoxicity is more likely to occur with cyclosporine or tacrolimus toxicity. Kidney biopsy is often needed to confirm the diagnosis of rejection.

▶ *ACE Inhibitors and ARBs*

In instances of decreased renal blood flow (e.g., kidney disease, renal artery stenosis), production of angiotensin II increases, resulting in efferent arteriole vasoconstriction and maintenance of glomerular capillary pressure and GFR. ACE inhibitors or ARB result in a decrease in angiotensin II synthesis, thereby dilating efferent arterioles and decreasing glomerular capillary pressure and GFR.[33] When initiating therapy with an ACE inhibitor or ARB, a modest increase in SCr should be anticipated within the first week of starting therapy due to the drug's mechanism of action.[33] However, large increases (greater than a 30% increase in SCr above baseline) that do not plateau after several weeks of therapy is indicative of AKI, and the drug should be discontinued.[33] Risk factors for developing AKI are preexisting renal dysfunction, severe atherosclerotic renal artery stenosis, volume depletion, and severe CHF. Discontinuation of the drug usually results in the return of renal function to baseline. Initiating therapy with low doses of a short-acting agent such as captopril is recommended for patients at risk of developing AKI. If tolerated, patients can later be converted to a longer-acting agent.

▶ *Nonsteroidal Anti-inflammatory Drugs*

NSAIDs (e.g., ibuprofen, naproxen, sulindac) can likewise cause prerenal AKI through inhibition of prostaglandin-mediated renal vasodilation. Risk factors are similar to those of ACE inhibitors and ARBs. Additional risk factors include hepatic disease with ascites, systemic lupus erythematosus, and advanced age. The onset is often within days of initiating therapy, and patients typically present with oliguria. It is usually reversible with drug discontinuation. Agents that preferentially inhibit cyclooxygenase-2 pose a similar risk as traditional nonselective NSAIDs.[33]

▶ *Other Drugs*

Other drugs that are commonly implicated in causing AKI include acyclovir, adefovir, carboplatin, cidofovir, cisplatin, foscarnet, ganciclovir, indinavir, methotrexate, pentamidine, ritonavir, sulfinpyrazone, and tenofovir.[47] A list of drugs that commonly cause AKI and their mechanism is found in Table 25–3.

Table 25–3

Drugs Implicated in Causing Acute Kidney Injury by Mechanism for Commonly Prescribed Drugs

Prerenal AKI (Hemodynamic mediated)	• Angiotensin-converting enzyme inhibitors • Angiotensin receptor blockers • Nonsteroidal anti-inflammatory drugs • Cyclosporine • Tacrolimus
Intrarenal Acute tubular necrosis	• Aminoglycosides • Amphotericin B • Cisplatin and carboplatin
Acute interstitial nephritis	• β-Lactam antibiotics • Fluoroquinolones • Thiazide diuretics • Loop diuretics • Allopurinol • Sulfonamides • Nonsteroidal anti-inflammatory drugs • Rifampin
Postrenal AKI (nephrolithiasis)	• Acyclovir • Methotrexate • Indinavir

---

Patient Encounter, Part 3

JD is admitted to the hospital for AKI. Based on the information available, create a care plan for this patient's AKI and provide overall recommendations for her drug therapy. The plan should include (a) a statement of the drug related needs and/or problems, (b) a patient-specific detailed therapeutic plan, and (c) monitoring parameters to assess efficacy and safety.

OUTCOME EVALUATION

Goals of therapy are to maintain a state of euvolemia with good urine output (at least 1 mL/kg/h), to return serum creatinine to baseline, and to correct electrolyte and acid-base abnormalities. In addition, appropriate drug dosages based on kidney function and avoidance of nephrotoxic drugs are goals of therapy. Assess vital signs, weight, fluid intake, urine output, BUN, creatinine, and electrolytes daily in the unstable patient.

DRUG DOSING CONSIDERATIONS IN AKI

Determining the optimal dose of drugs in AKI is challenging. A variety of factor influence drug dosing, such as (1) alterations in drug pharmacokinetics that occur during AKI, (2) difficulties in accurately quantifying kidney function in AKI, (3) the influence of intermittent or continuous RRT on drug clearance, and (4) challenges in interpreting information from the literature and applying it to a specific patient. Table 25-4 provides a more complete list of different considerations when dosing medications in patients with AKI.

For drugs with a narrow therapeutic window, serum drug concentration monitoring may be available to guide drug dosing. If drug monitoring is not available, conservative dosing based on an estimated creatinine clearance is recommended, with frequent reassessment of kidney function and evaluation of the patient's status to assess efficacy and adverse effects of the patient's therapy. Selection of a drug with hepatic elimination rather than renal excretion is a reasonable alternative, if possible.

DRUG DOSING CONSIDERATIONS IN CRRT

Hemodialysis removes solutes from the body by diffusion, where substances move from the higher concentration in the blood to the lower concentration in the dialysis solution, across a semipermeable membrane. Poor size of the membrane governs drug removal. For low flux membranes, drugs with a molecular weight less than 1,000 Da are removed. With high flux membranes that have larger poor sizes, drugs in the range of 10,000 to 20,000 Da can be removed. Because the dialysis solution moves in a countercurrent direction to blood flow through the dialysis membrane, the concentration gradient is maximized.

With hemofiltration, water moves across a hemofiltration membrane due to hydrostatic pressure into the ultrafiltrate compartment and drags along dissolved solute through a process known as convection. Because no dialysis solution is pumped through the dialyzer, diffusion does not occur. Larger molecules are removed up to the molecular weight cutoff of the hemofilters, usually about 40,000 Da.

There are primarily three types of CRRT commonly used in AKI, based on these principles of hemodialysis and hemofiltration: continuous venovenous hemofiltration (CVVH), continuous venovenous hemodialysis (CVVHD), and continuous venovenous hemodiafiltration (CVVFDF).

Table 25-4

Drug Dosing Considerations in AKI

Alteration in drug pharmacokinetics	• Increase in volume of distribution due to fluid retention may occur • Reduction in excretion of both drugs and metabolites eliminated by the kidney • Nonrenal clearance of some drugs may be reduced
Difficulty in quantifying an accurate assessment of kidney function in AKI	• Cockcroft-Gault and MDRD equations not meant for AKI population; equations are based on a single SCr • SCr as a marker for kidney function influenced by non-renal factors (such as nutritional status and liver function) • Equations to estimate kidney function in cases of changing kidney function have not been well studied
AKI patients undergoing dialysis	• Different types of dialysis modalities results in differences in drug removal (e.g., IHD vs. CRRT) • Differences in intensity of dialysis dose may affect drug removal (eg, length of dialysis treatment, blood and dialysate flow rate) • Populations studied in literature are likely to be different than the specific patient being treated (e.g., different types of dialysis, length of treatment).
Textbook dosing and literature recommendations	• Studies in patients with AKI are sparse • Many drug information recommendations on dosing are based on the manufacturer's original pharmacokinetics information, often in patients with chronic kidney disease • Most drug dosing guidelines were developed prior to standardization of SCr measurements between labs; thus today's SCr measurements are 5–10% higher than those reported prior to 2010[49] • There is a growing body of support for incorporation of the MDRD equation in future pharmacokinetic studies and to guide drug dosing, although use of this equation is limited to chronic kidney disease

MDRD = Modification of Diet in Renal Disease Equation.

In these procedures, drug removal is governed by either diffusion (CVVHD), convection (CVVH), or a combination of the two (CVVHDF).

In additional to molecular weight, there are three additional characteristics of a drug that governs removal during dialysis: percentage of drug eliminated by the kidney, volume of distribution, and protein binding. Removal during CRRT is greater when renal clearance accounts for 30% or more of total body clearance of the drug, volume of distribution is less than 1 L/kg, and protein binding is less than 50% because dialysis cannot remove protein-bound drugs.[48] Other factors that affect drug clearance with CRRT include type of CRRT (i.e., CVVH, CVVHD); characteristics of the dialysis membrane; and blood, ultrafiltrate, and dialysis flow rates. In general, drug removal is greatest with CVVHDF, followed by CVVH and then IHD.[49]

Drug information references may provide general drug dosing recommendations in CRRT; however, they must be interpreted cautiously due to the variability in CRRT techniques used.

Mathematical models can be used to calculate drug dosages based on the patient's residual renal clearance and dialysis clearance compared with clearance in a patient with normal kidney function. In addition, plasma concentrations should be used to guide treatment if available. Close monitoring of the patient's clinical response is critical.

Patient Care and Monitoring

1. Assess kidney function by evaluating a patient's signs and symptoms, laboratory test results, and urinary indices. Calculate a patient's CrCl to evaluate the severity of kidney disease.

2. Obtain a thorough and accurate drug history including the use of nonprescription drugs such as NSAIDs.

3. Evaluate a patient's current drug regimen to:

   - Determine if drug therapy may be contributing to AKI. Consider not only drugs that can directly cause AKI (e.g., aminoglycosides, amphotericin B, NSAIDs, cyclosporine, tacrolimus, ACE inhibitors, and ARBs) but also drugs that can predispose a patient to nephrotoxicity or prerenal AKI (i.e., diuretics and antihypertensive agents).

   - Determine if any drugs need to be discontinued, or alternative drugs selected, to prevent worsening of renal function.

   - Adjust drug dosages based on the patient's CrCl or evidence of adverse drug reactions or interactions.

4. Develop a plan to provide symptomatic care of complications associated with AKI, such as diuretic therapy to treat volume overload. Monitor the patient's weight, urine output, electrolytes (such as potassium), and blood pressure to assess efficacy of the diuretic regimen.

Abbreviations Introduced in This Chapter

ACE	Angiotensin-converting enzyme
AKI	Acute kidney injury
ANZICS	Australian and New Zealand Intensive Care Society
ARB	Angiotensin receptor blocker
ARF	Acute renal failure
ATN	Acute tubular necrosis
BW	Body weight
BUN	Blood urea nitrogen
CHF	Congestive heart failure
CrCl	Creatinine clearance
CRRT	Continuous renal replacement therapy
DM	Diabetes mellitus
FENa	Fractional excretion of sodium
GFR	Glomerular filtration rate
IBW	Ideal body weight
IHD	Intermittent hemodialysis
JVD	Jugular venous distention
LDD	Low-dose dopamine
MDRD	Modification of Diet in Renal Disease
NSAIDs	Nonsteroidal anti-inflammatory drugs
PGE_2	Prostaglandin E_2
RRT	Renal replacement therapy
SCr	Serum creatinine concentration

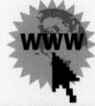 Self-assessment questions and answers are available at *http://www.mhpharmacotherapy. com/pp.html.*

REFERENCES

1. Bellomo R, Kellum JA, Ronco C. Defining and classifying acute renal failure: from advocacy to consensus and validation of the RIFLE criteria. Intensive Care Med 2007;33:409–413.
2. Bellomo R, Ronco C, Kellum, et al.; the ADQI Workgroup. Acute renal failure—definition, outcome measures, animal models, and information technology needs: The Second International Consensus Conference of the Acute Dialysis Quality Initiative (ADQI) Group. Crit Care 2004;8:R204–R212.
3. Kellum JA. Acute kidney injury. Crit Care Med 2008;36:S141–S145.
4. Mehta RL, Kellum JA, Shah SV, et al. Acute Kidney Injury Network: Report of an initiative to improve outcomes in acute kidney injury. Crit Care 2007;11:R31.
5. Yong K, Dogra G, Boudville N, Pinder M, Lim W. Acute kidney injury: Controversies revisited. Int J Nephrol 2011:762634.
6. Goldber R, Dennen P. Long-term outcomes of acute kidney injury. Adv Chronic Kidney Dis 2008;15:297–307.
7. Ympa YP, Sakr Y, Reinhart K, et al. Has mortality from acute renal failure decreased? A systematic review of the literature. Am J Med 2005;118:827–832.
8. Himmelfarb J, Joannidis M, Molitoris B, et al. Evaluation and initial management of acute kidney injury. Clin J Am Soc Nephrol 2008;3:962–967.
9. Lameire N, van Biesen W, Vanholder R. Acute renal failure. Lancet 2005;365:417–430.

10. Bellomo R. Defining, quantifying, and classifying acute renal failure. Crit Care Clin 2005;21:223–237.
11. Cockroft DW, Gault MH. Prediction of creatinine clearance from serum creatinine. Nephron 1976;16:31–41.
12. Bouchard J, Macedo E, Soroko S, et al. Comparison of methods for estimating glomerular filtration rate in critically ill patients with acute kidney injury. Nephrol Dial Transplant 2010;25:102–107.
13. Brater DC. Drug Use in Renal Disease. Balgowlah, Australia: ADIS Health Science Press, 1983:22–56.
14. Jelliffe R. Estimation of creatinine clearance in patients with unstable renal function, without a urine specimen. Am J Nephrol 2002;22:320–324.
15. Chiou WL, Hou FH. A new simple rapid method to monitor renal function based on pharmacokinetic considerations of endogenous creatinine. Res Commun Chem Pathol Pharmacol 1975;10:315–330.
16. Bellomo R, Kellum JA, Ronco C. Defining acute renal failure: Physiologic principles. Intensive Care Med 2004;30:33–37.
17. Bagshaw SM, Bellomo R, Kellum JA. Oliguria, volume overload, and loop diuretics. Crit Care Med 2008;36:S172–S178.
18. Molnar J, Somber JC. The clinical pharmacology of ethacrynic acid. Am J Ther 2009;16:86–92.
19. Brater DC. Update in diuretic therapy: Clinical pharmacology. Semin Nephrol 2011;31:483–494.
20. Wargo KA, Banta WM. A comprehensive review of the loop diuretics: Should furosemide be first line? Ann Pharmacother 2009;43:1836–1847.
21. Ho KM, Sheridan DJ. Meta-analysis of furosemide to prevent or treat acute renal failure. BMJ 2006;333:420–423.
22. Asare K. Management of loop diuretic resistance in the intensive care unit. Am J Health Syst Pharm 2009;66:1635–1640.
23. Bellomo R, Chapman M, Finfer S, et al. Low-dose dopamine in patients with early renal dysfunction: A placebo-controlled randomized trial. Australian and New Zealand Intensive Care Society (ANZICS) Clinical Trials Group. Lancet 2000;356:2139–2143.
24. Friedrich JO, Adhikari N, Herridge MS, et al. Meta-analysis: Low-dose dopamine increases urine output but does not prevent renal dysfunction or death. Ann Intern Med 2005;142:510–524.
25. Tumlin JA, Finkel KW, Murray PT, et al. Fenoldopam mesylate in early acute tubular necrosis: A randomized, double-blind, placebo-controlled clinical trial. Am J Kidney Dis 2005;46:26–34.
26. Morelli A, Ricci Z, Bellomo R, et al. Prophylactic fenoldopam for renal protection in sepsis. A randomized, double-blind, placebo-controlled pilot study. Crit Care Med 2005;33:2451–2456.
27. Gibney N, Burdmann EA, Bunchman T, et al. Timing of initiation and discontinuation of renal replacement therapy in AKI: Unanswered key questions. Clin J Am Soc Nephrol 2008;3:876–880.
28. Bellomo R, Cass A, Cole L, et al. The RENAL Replacement Therapy Study Investigators. N Engl J Med 2009;361:1627–1638.
29. Palevsky PM, Hongyuan J, O'Connor TZ, et al. The VA/NIH Acute Renal Failure Trial Network. N Engl J Med 2008;359:7–20.
30. Cruz DN, de Geus HR, Bagshaw SM. Biomarker strategies to predict need for renal replacement therapy in acute kidney injury. Semin Dial 2011:24:124–131.
31. Pagkalis S, Mantadakis E, Mavros MN, Ammari C, Falagas ME. Pharmacological considerations for the proper clinical use of aminoglycosides. Drugs 2011;71:2277–2294.
32. Lopez-Novoa JM, Quiros Y, Vicente L, Morales AI, Lopez-Hernandez J. New insights into the mechanism of aminoglycoside nephrotoxicity: An integrative point of view. Kidney Int 2011;79:33–45.
33. Pannu N, Nadim M. An overview of drug-induced acute kidney injury. Crit Care Med 2008;36:S216–S223.
34. Sadfar A, Ma J, Saliba F, et al. Drug-induced nephrotoxicity caused by amphotericin B lipid complex and liposomal amphotericin B. Medicine 2010;89:236–244.
35. Saliba F, Dupont B. Renal impairment and amphotericin B formulations in patients with invasive fungal infections. Med Mycol 2008;46:97–112.
36. Moen MD, Lyseng-Williamson KA, Scott LJ. Liposomal amphotericin B: A review of its use as empirical therapy in febrile neutropenia and in the treatment of invasive fungal infections. Drugs 2009;69:361–392.
37. Weisbord SD, Palevsky PM. Radiocontrast-induced acute renal failure. J Intensive Care Med 2005;20:63–75.
38. McCullough PA, Soman SS. Contrast-induced nephropathy. Crit Care Clin 2005;21:261–280.
39. Rudnick MR, Goldfarb S, Wexler L, et al. Nephrotoxicity of ionic and nonionic contrast media in 1196 patients: A randomized trial. Kidney Int 1995;47:254–261.
40. Solomon R, Werner C, Mann D, et al. Effects of saline, mannitol, and furosemide on acute decreases in renal function by radiocontrast agents. N Engl J Med 1994;331:1416–1420.
41. Mueller C, Buerkle G, Buettner HJ, et al. Prevention of contrast media-associated nephropathy: Randomized comparison of 2 hydration regimens in 1620 patients undergoing coronary angioplasty. Arch Int Med 2002;162:329–336.
42. Trivedi HS, Moore H, Nasr S, et al. A randomized prospective trial to assess the role of saline hydration on the development of contrast nephrotoxicity. Nephron 2003;93:C29–C34.
43. Briguori C, Airoldi F, D'Andrea D, et al. Renal insufficiency following Contrast Media Administration Trial (REMEDIAL). A randomized comparison of three preventative strategies. Circulation 2007;115:1211–1217.
44. Brar SS, Shen AY, Jorgensen MB, et al. Sodium bicarbonate vs sodium chloride for the prevention of contrast medium-induced nephropathy in patients undergoing coronary angiography. JAMA 2008;300:1038–1046.
45. Tepel M, Van der Giet M, Schwarzfeld C, et al. Prevention of radiographic contrast agent-induced reduction in renal function by acetylcysteine. N Engl J Med 2000;343:180–184.
46. De Mattos AM, Olyaei AJ, Bennett WM. Nephrotoxicity of immunosuppressive drugs: Long-term consequences and challenges for the future. Am J Kidney Dis 2000;35:333–346.
47. Izzedine H, Launay-Vacher V, Deray G. Antiviral drug-induced nephropathy. Am J Kidney Dis 2005;45:804–817.
48. Susla GM. The impact of continuous renal replacement therapy on drug therapy. Clin Pharmacol Ther 2009;86:562–565.
49. Pea F. Viale P, Pavan F, Furlanut M. Pharmacokinetic considerations for antimicrobial therapy in patients receiving replacement therapy. Clin Pharmacokinet 2007;46:997–1038.

26 Chronic and End-Stage Renal Disease

Kristine S. Schonder

LEARNING OBJECTIVES

● **Upon completion of the chapter, the reader will be able to:**

1. List the risk factors for development and progression of chronic kidney disease (CKD).

2. Explain the mechanisms associated with progression of CKD.

3. Outline the desired outcomes for treatment of CKD.

4. Develop a therapeutic approach to slow progression of CKD including lifestyle modifications and pharmacologic therapies.

5. Identify specific consequences associated with CKD.

6. Design an appropriate therapeutic approach for specific consequences associated with CKD.

7. Recommend an appropriate monitoring plan to assess the effectiveness of pharmacotherapy for CKD and specific consequences.

8. Educate patients with CKD about the disease state, the specific consequences, lifestyle modifications, and pharmacologic therapies used for treatment of CKD.

KEY CONCEPTS

❶ **Chronic kidney disease** (CKD) is defined by a staging system based on glomerular filtration rate (GFR) level, which also accounts for evidence of kidney damage in the absence of changes in GFR, as in stage 1 CKD.

❷ CKD is a progressive disease that eventually leads to kidney failure (end-stage kidney disease [ESKD]).

❸ Early detection and treatment of CKD are fundamental factors in minimizing morbidity and mortality associated with CKD.

❹ Declining kidney function disrupts the homeostasis of the systems regulated by the kidney, leading to fluid and electrolyte imbalances, anemia, and metabolic bone disease.

❺ Angiotensin-converting enzyme inhibitors (ACE-Is) and angiotensin II receptor blockers decrease protein excretion and are the drugs of choice for hypertension in patients with CKD.

❻ The most common complication of CKD is anemia, which is caused by a decline in erythropoietin production by the kidneys and can lead to cardiovascular disease (CVD).

❼ Bone and mineral metabolism disorders stem from disruptions in calcium, phosphorus, and vitamin D homeostasis through the interaction with the parathyroid hormone.

❽ The management of **secondary hyperparathyroidism** (sHPT) involves correction of serum calcium and phosphorus levels, and decreasing parathyroid hormone secretion.

❾ Patient education and planning for **dialysis** should begin at stage 4 CKD, before ESKD is reached, to allow for time to establish appropriate access for dialysis.

❿ Dialysis involves the removal of metabolic waste products and excess fluids and electrolytes by **diffusion** and **ultrafiltration** from the bloodstream across a semipermeable membrane into an external dialysate solution.

The kidney is made up of approximately 2 million **nephrons** that are responsible for filtering, reabsorbing, and excreting solutes and water. As the number of functioning nephrons declines, the primary functions of the kidney that are affected include:

- Production and secretion of **erythropoietin**
- Activation of vitamin D
- Regulation of fluid and electrolyte balance
- Regulation of acid–base balance

Chronic kidney disease (CKD), also known as chronic kidney insufficiency, progressive kidney disease, or nephropathy, is defined as the presence of kidney damage or decreased **glomerular filtration rate** (GFR) for 3 months or more.[1] Generally, CKD is a progressive decline in kidney function (a decline in the number of functioning nephrons) that occurs over a period of several months to years. A decline in kidney function that occurs more rapidly, over a period of days to weeks, is known as acute kidney injury (AKI), which is discussed in Chapter 25. The decline in kidney function in CKD is often irreversible. Therefore, measures to treat CKD are aimed at slowing the progression to end-stage kidney disease (ESKD).

EPIDEMIOLOGY AND ETIOLOGY

❶ *The National Kidney Foundation (NKF) developed a classification system for CKD (Table 26–1).[1] The staging system defines the stages of CKD based on GFR level but also accounts for evidence of kidney damage in the absence of changes in GFR, as in stage 1 CKD.* The GFR is calculated using the abbreviated IDMS-traceable Modification of Diet in Renal Disease study equation[2]:

GFR = 175 × (SCr)$^{-1.154}$ × (age)$^{-0.203}$ × (0.742 if female) × (1.21 if African American) for serum **creatinine** expressed in mg/dL (serum creatinine expressed in µmol/L must first be divided by 88.4 to convert to mg/dL to calculate accurate eGFR by this equation)

Alternatively, GFR can be calculated using the Chronic Kidney Disease Epidemiology Collaboration equation (CKD-EPI):[3]

GFR = 141 × min(SCr/κ, 1)$^{\alpha}$ × max(SCr/κ, 1)$^{-1.209}$ × 0.993^{Age} × 1.018 [if female] × 1.159 [if African American], where κ is 0.7 for females and 0.9 for males, α is −0.329 for females and −0.411 for males, min indicates the minimum of SCr/κ or 1, max indicates the maximum of SCr/κ or 1, and SCr is expressed in mg/dL dL (serum creatinine expressed in µmol/L should first be divided by 88.4 to convert to mg/dL to calculate accurate eGFR by this equation).

The CKD-EPI formula provides better estimates than the MDRD at higher GFRs and may be preferred for determining GFR in earlier stages of CKD.

The United States Renal Data System (USRDS), using data from the National Health and Nutrition Examination Survey (NHANES), estimates the prevalence of CKD in the United States is 15.1%, corresponding to nearly 31 million people.[4] This number is increased from 12.8% reported with the previous NHANES report from 1988 to 1994,[4] which is attributed to the increased prevalence of diabetes and hypertension, and the aging population.[5]

❷ *CKD is a progressive disease that eventually leads to ESKD.* The prevalence of ESKD has increased more than fivefold since 1980 to more than 570,000 people in 2009 with over 116,000 new cases of ESKD diagnosed in 2009.[4] The prevalence of ESKD is related to ethnicity, affecting 3.5 times more African Americans and 1.9 times more Native Americans as whites.[4] This is likely because these ethnicities have increased risk and prevalence of the causes of CKD, including diabetes mellitus (DM) and hypertension, and other vascular diseases.[1] The incidence of CKD is greatly influenced by the patient's access to medical care.

Because of the progressive nature of CKD, determination of risk factors for CKD is difficult. Risk factors identified for CKD are classified into three categories (Table 26–2):

- **Susceptibility factors**, which are associated with an increased risk of developing CKD but are not directly proven to cause CKD. These factors are generally not modifiable by pharmacologic therapy or lifestyle modifications.

- **Initiation factors**, which directly cause CKD. These factors are modifiable by pharmacologic therapy.

Table 26–1

NKF-K/DOQI Classification for CKD

State	GFR (mL/min/1.73 m²)^b
1	90^a or higher
2	60–89, or kidney damage
3	30–59
4	15–29
5	Less than 15 (includes patients on dialysis)

GFR, glomerular filtration rate; NKF-K/DOQI, National Kidney Foundation-Dialysis Outcome Quality Initiative.

^{a}CKD can be present with a normal or near normal GFR if other markers of kidney disease are present such as proteinuria, hematuria, biopsy results showing kidney damage, or anatomical abnormalities (e.g., cysts).

^{b}To convert of SI units of mL/s/m², multiply by 0.00963.

Table 26–2

Risk Factors Associated with CKD

Susceptibility
- Advanced age
- Reduced kidney mass
- Low birth weight
- Racial/ethnic minority
- Family history of kidney disease
- Low income or education
- Systemic inflammation
- Dyslipidemia

Initiation
- Diabetes mellitus
- Hypertension
- Autoimmune disease
- Polycystic kidney disease
- Drug toxicity
- Urinary tract abnormalities (infections, obstruction, stones)

Progression
- Hyperglycemia: Poor blood glucose control (in patients with diabetes)
- Hypertension: Elevated blood pressure
- Proteinuria
- Tobacco smoking

- **Progression factors**, which result in a faster decline in kidney function and cause worsening of CKD. These factors may also be modified by pharmacologic therapy or lifestyle modifications to slow the progression of CKD.

Susceptibility Factors

Susceptibility factors can be readily used to develop screening programs for CKD. For example, older patients, those with low kidney mass or birth weight, and those with a family history of kidney disease should be routinely screened for CKD. Minority and low socioeconomic communities may be targets for more widespread CKD screening programs. Other factors, such as hyperlipidemia, are not directly proven to cause CKD but can be modified by drug therapies.

▶ Hyperlipidemia

Patients with CKD have a higher prevalence of dyslipidemia compared with the general population. More than 81% of patients with a GFR less than 60 mL/min/1.73 m² (0.58 mL/s/m²) had hyperlipidemia.[4] The dyslipidemia in CKD is manifested primarily as elevated triglycerides and lipoprotein(a) levels, and decreased high-density lipoprotein cholesterol (HDL-C) levels. Total cholesterol and low-density lipoprotein cholesterol (LDL-C) levels generally remain within normal limits.[6] Kidney disease alters lipid metabolism, allowing lipoproteins to remain in circulation longer.[6] In contrast, patients with nephrotic syndrome, which is characterized by urine protein rates that exceed 3 g/24 hours, often have elevated total cholesterol and LDL-C. It is hypothesized that nephrotic syndrome is associated with increased hepatic lipid production and decreased LDL-receptor activity.[7] Dyslipidemia can promote kidney injury and subsequent progression of CKD. Endothelial dysfunction results from inflammation and monocyte activation, whereas deposition of lipids results in glomerulosclerosis and glomerular mesangium dysfunction.[6]

Initiation Factors

The three most common causes of CKD in the United States are DM, hypertension, and **glomerulonephritis**. Together these account for about 75% of the cases of CKD (37% for diabetes, 24% for hypertension, and 14% for glomerulonephritis).[4] These are discussed in further detail below.

▶ Diabetes

DM is the most common cause of CKD, causing 38% of all ESKD, which is an increase from 18% in 1985.[4] The risk of developing diabetic kidney disease (DKD) associated with DM is closely linked to hyperglycemia and is similar for both type 1 and type 2. The prevalence of **microalbuminuria** is 25% to 40% in patients with type 1 DM after 15 to 25 years[8] and 43% in patients with type 2 DM.[9]

▶ Hypertension

The second most common cause of CKD is hypertension.[4] It is more difficult to determine the true risk of developing CKD in patients with hypertension because the two are so closely linked, with CKD also being a cause of hypertension. The prevalence of hypertension is correlated with the degree of kidney dysfunction (decreased GFR) with 40% of patients with CKD stage 1, 55% of patients with CKD stage 2, and over 81% of patients with CKD stage 3 presenting with hypertension.[4] The risk of developing ESKD increases with the degree of hypertension and is linked to both systolic and diastolic blood pressure.[10]

▶ Glomerulonephritis

The term *glomerulonephritis* includes many specific diseases that can affect glomerular function. These include such diseases as IgA nephropathy, Wegener's granulomatosis, and glomerulonephritis associated with systemic lupus erythematosus and streptococcal disease, among many others. The etiologic and pathophysiologic features of glomerular diseases vary with the specific disease, making it difficult to extrapolate the risk for progression of CKD in patients affected by glomerular diseases. Certain glomerular diseases are known to rapidly progress to ESKD; others progress more slowly or may be reversible.

Progression Factors

Progression factors can be used as predictors of CKD. The most important predictors of CKD include **proteinuria**, elevated blood pressure, hyperglycemia, and tobacco smoking.

▶ Proteinuria

The presence of protein in the urine is a marker of glomerular and tubular dysfunction. The degree of proteinuria correlates with the risk for progression of CKD.[11] The effects of proteinuria appear to be worse with milder stages of CKD. Compared with patients with no proteinuria, proteinuric patients with stage 3 CKD are 15 times more likely to double serum creatinine; patients with stage 4 CKD are 8 times more likely to double serum creatinine.[11] The mechanisms by which proteinuria potentiates CKD are discussed later. Microalbuminuria (30 to 300 mg albumin excreted per day) is also linked with vascular injury and increased cardiovascular mortality.[9]

▶ Elevated Blood Pressure

Systemic blood pressure correlates with glomerular pressure, and elevations in both systemic blood pressure and glomerular pressure contribute to glomerular damage. The rate of GFR decline is related to elevated systolic blood pressure and mean arterial pressure. The decline in GFR is estimated to be 14 mL/min per year (0.23 mL/s per year) with a sustained systolic blood pressure of 180 mm Hg. Conversely, the decline in GFR decreases to 2 mL/min per year (0.03 mL/s per year) with a systolic blood pressure of 135 mm Hg.[12]

▶ *Elevated Blood Glucose*

The reaction between glucose and protein in the blood produces advanced glycation end products (AGEs), which are metabolized in the proximal tubules. Hyperglycemia increases the synthesis of AGEs in patients with diabetes. Accumulation of AGEs affects glomerular, tubular, and vascular function in the kidney. AGEs are known to affect the activity of podocytes, the epithelial cells responsible for filtering blood, in the glomerulus, which contributes to proteinuria, which, in turn, damages tubules.[13]

▶ *Tobacco Smoking*

Smoking is also an independent and dose-dependent risk factor for development of CKD and microalbuminuria, and progression to ESKD.[14,15] The risk is more pronounced in men compared with women (odds ratio [OR]: 2.4), independent of other risk factors.[15] The risk of developing CKD increases with the dose (greater than 20 cigarettes per day, OR: 1.51), duration (greater than 40 years, OR: 1.45), and cumulative consumption (greater than 30 pack-years, OR: 1.52).[16]

The effects of smoking on the kidney are multifactorial and occur in both healthy individuals and those with CKD.

Smoking induces endothelial dysfunction and atherosclerosis systemically and in the glomerulus.[14] These effects are related to nicotine and other components of cigarette smoking, including tar and smoke.[14]

PATHOPHYSIOLOGY

A number of factors can cause initial damage to the kidney. The resulting sequelae, however, follow a common pathway that promotes progression of CKD and results in irreversible damage leading to ESKD (Fig. 26–1).

The initial damage to the kidney can result from any of the initiation factors listed in Table 26–2. Regardless of the cause, however, the damage results in a decrease in the number of functioning nephrons. The remaining nephrons hypertrophy to increase glomerular filtration and tubular function, both reabsorption and secretion, in an attempt to compensate for the loss of kidney function. Initially, these adaptive changes preserve many of the clinical parameters of kidney function, including creatinine and electrolyte excretion. However, as time progresses, angiotensin II is required to maintain the hyperfiltration state of the functioning nephrons. Angiotensin II is a potent vasoconstrictor of both the afferent

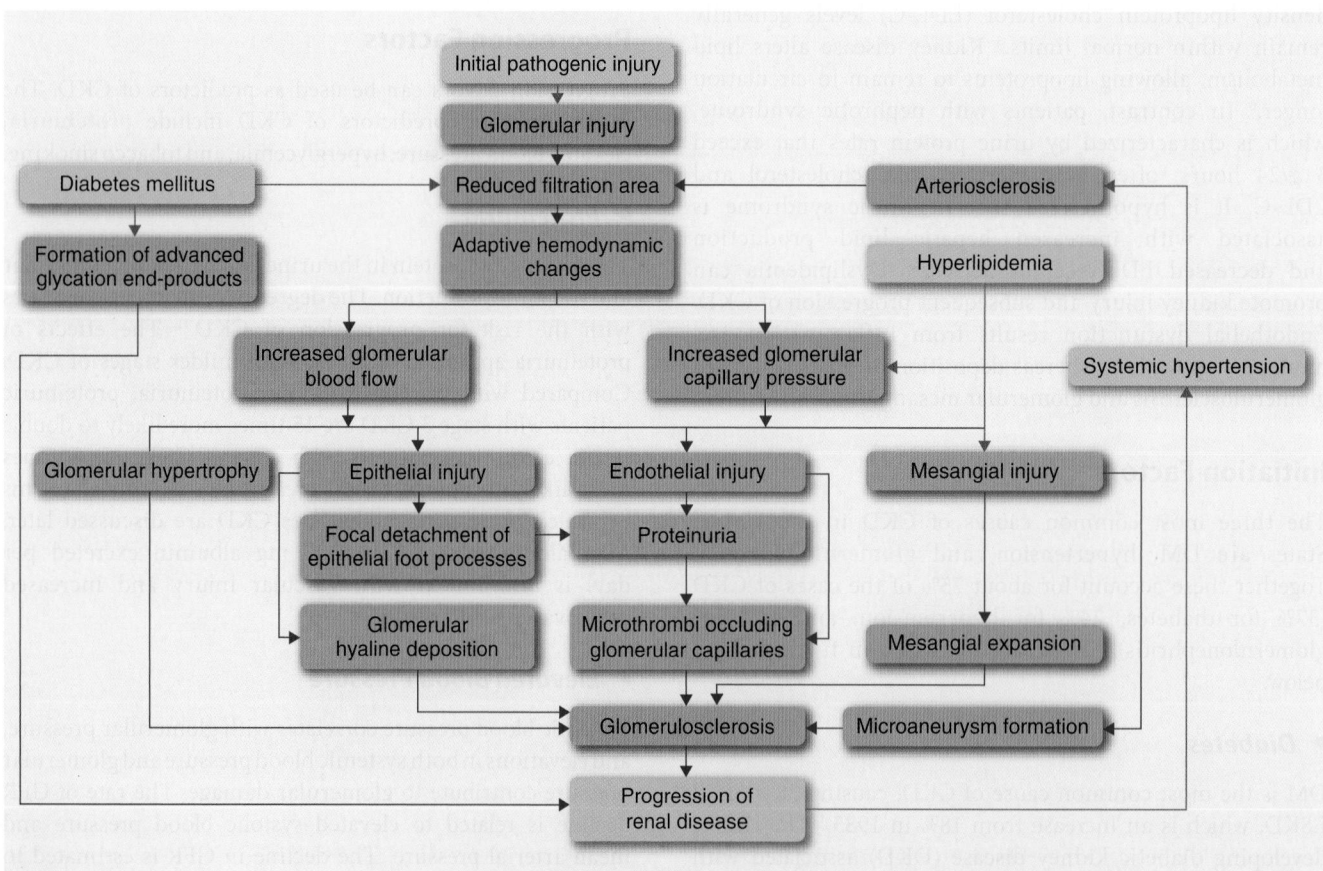

FIGURE 26–1. Proposed mechanisms for progression of kidney disease. (From Derebail VK, Kshirsagar AV, Joy MS. Chronic kidney disease: Progression-modifying therapies. In: DiPiro JT, Talbert RL, Yee GC, et al., eds. Pharmacotherapy: A Pathophysiologic Approach, 8th ed. New York, NY: McGraw-Hill, 2011:771, with permission.)

and efferent arterioles but has a preferential effect to constrict the efferent arteriole, thereby increasing the pressure in the glomerular capillaries. Increased glomerular capillary pressure expands the pores in the glomerular basement membrane, altering the size-selective barrier and allowing proteins to be filtered through the glomerulus.[17]

Protein excretion through the nephron, or proteinuria, increases nephron loss through various complex mechanisms. Filtered proteins are reabsorbed in the renal tubules, which activates the tubular cells to produce inflammatory and vasoactive cytokines and triggers complement activation.[16] These cytokines cause interstitial damage and scarring in the renal tubules, leading to damage and loss of more nephrons. Ultimately, the process leads to progressive loss of nephrons to the point where the number of remaining functioning nephrons is too small to maintain clinical stability, and kidney function declines.

ASSESSMENT

Because CKD often presents without symptoms, assessment for CKD relies on appropriate screening strategies in all patients with risk factors for developing CKD (Table 26–2). Evaluation for CKD and the subsequent treatment strategies depend on the diagnosis, comorbid conditions, severity and complications of disease, and risk factors for the progression of CKD. ❸ *Early treatment of CKD and the associated complications of CKD are the most important factors to decrease morbidity and mortality associated with CKD.* However, the probability of patients not diagnosed with CKD to have an assessment of serum creatinine (SCr) is 0.77, whereas the probability of having an assessment of urine protein excretion was only 0.1.[4] Screening for CKD should be performed in all people with an increased risk for developing CKD including patients with DM, hypertension, genitourinary abnormalities, autoimmune disease, increased age, or a family history of kidney disease. The assessment for CKD should include measurement of SCr, urinalysis, blood pressure, serum electrolytes, and/or imaging studies.

The primary marker of structural kidney damage is proteinuria, even in patients with normal GFR. Clinically significant proteinuria is defined as urinary protein excretion greater than 300 mg/day or greater than 20 mcg/min in a timed urine collection. Significant proteinuria can also be determined by a spot urine dipstick greater than 30 mg/dL (300 mg/L) or a urine protein/creatinine ratio greater than 200 mg/g (22.6 mg/mmol creatinine).[1] Microalbuminuria is defined as 30 to 300 mg of albumin excreted in the urine per day or a urine albumin-to-creatinine ratio of 30 to 300 mg/g (3.4 to 34 mg/mmol creatinine).[1] The NKF recommends routine assessment of proteinuria to detect CKD. A urine dipstick positive for the presence of protein warrants quantification of proteinuria. Patients with a urine protein-to-creatinine ratio greater than 200 mg/g (22.6 mg/mmol creatinine) or urine albumin-to-creatinine ratio greater than 30 mg/g (3.4 mg/mmol creatinine) should undergo diagnostic evaluation; patients with values below

these levels should be reevaluated routinely.[1] Assessment of microalbuminuria is particularly important in patients with DM. Screening for microalbuminuria should be performed 5 years after the diagnosis of type 1 DM and at the time of diagnosis of type 2 DM.[18]

Other markers for structural kidney damage that can be used in place of proteinuria include abnormalities in urinary sediment, such as hematuria, or abnormalities in imaging studies or kidney biopsy.[1]

Complications

❹ *The decline in kidney function is associated with a number of complications, which are discussed later in the chapter, including:*

- *Hypertension*
- *Fluid and electrolyte disorders*
- *Anemia*
- *Metabolic bone disease*

TREATMENT

Desired Outcomes

The primary goal is to slow and prevent the progression of CKD. This requires early identification of patients at risk for CKD to initiate interventions early in the course of the disease.

Nonpharmacologic Therapy

▶ *Nutritional Management*

Reduction in dietary protein intake has been shown to slow the progression of kidney disease.[18] However, protein restriction must be balanced with the risk of malnutrition in patients with CKD. Patients with a GFR less than 25 mL/min/1.73 m^2 (0.24 mL/s/m^2) received the most benefit from protein restriction[19]; therefore, patients with a GFR above this level should not restrict protein intake. The NKF recommends that patients who have a GFR less than 25 mL/min/1.73 m^2 (0.24 mL/s/m^2) who are not receiving dialysis, however, should restrict protein intake to 0.6 g/kg/day. If patients are not able to maintain adequate dietary energy intake, protein intake may be increased up to 0.75 g/kg/day.[19] Malnutrition is common in patients with ESKD for various reasons, including decreased appetite, hypercatabolism, and nutrient losses through dialysis. For this reason, patients receiving dialysis should maintain protein intake of 1.2 g/kg/day to 1.3 g/kg/day.

Protein intake can have unique contributions to kidney damage in patients with DM. Dietary protein, particularly protein from animal sources, produces AGEs, which are an important cause of kidney damage in patients with DM.[12] The NKF recommends that patients with DM with CKD stages 1 to 4 should limit protein intake to 0.8 g/kg/day to reduce proteinuria and stabilize kidney function.[19]

Clinical Presentation and Diagnosis of CKD

General

The development of CKD is usually subtle in onset, often with no noticeable symptoms.

Symptoms

Stages 1 and 2 CKD are generally asymptomatic.

Stages 3 and 4 CKD may be associated with minimal symptoms.

Stage 5 CKD can be associated with pruritus, dysgeusia, nausea, vomiting, constipation, muscle pain, fatigue, and bleeding abnormalities.

Signs

Cardiovascular: Worsening hypertension, edema, dyslipidemia, left ventricular hypertrophy, electrocardiographic changes and chronic heart failure.

Musculoskeletal: Cramping.

Neuropsychiatric: Depression, anxiety, impaired mental cognition.

GI: Gastroesophageal reflux disease, GI bleeding, and abdominal distention.

Genitourinary: Changes in urine volume and consistency, "foaming" of urine (indicative of proteinuria), and sexual dysfunction.

Laboratory Tests

Stages 1 and 2 CKD: Increased blood urea nitrogen (BUN) and serum creatinine (SCr) and decreased GFR.

Stages 3, 4, and 5 CKD: Increased BUN and SCr; decreased GFR.

Advanced stages: Increased potassium, phosphorus, and magnesium; decreased bicarbonate (metabolic acidosis); calcium levels are generally low in earlier stages of CKD and may be elevated in stage 5 CKD, secondary to the use of calcium-containing phosphate binders.

Decreased albumin, if inadequate nutrition intake in advanced stages.

Decreased red blood cell (RBC) count, hemoglobin (Hgb) and hematocrit (Hct); iron metabolism may also be altered (iron level, total iron binding capacity [TIBC], serum ferritin level, and transferrin saturation [TSAT]). Erythropoietin levels are not routinely monitored and are generally normal to low. Urine positive for albumin or protein.

Increased parathyroid hormone (PTH) level; decreased vitamin D levels (stages 4 or 5 CKD).

Stool may be Hemoccult-positive if GI bleeding occurs from uremia.

Other Diagnostic Tests

Structural abnormalities of kidney may be present on diagnostic examinations.

Pharmacologic Therapy

▶ Intensive Blood Glucose Control (for Patients with Diabetes)

The target glycated hemoglobin level (HbA1c) should be less than 7.0% (0.07; 53 mmol/mol Hgb) for patients with DM to decrease the incidence of proteinuria and albuminuria in patients with and without documented DKD.[18] This generally involves intensive insulin therapy for type 1 DM or insulin-dependent type 2 DM with administration of insulin three or more times daily to maintain preprandial blood glucose levels between 70 and 120 g/dL (3.9 to 6.7 mmol/L) and postprandial blood glucose levels less than 180 g/dL (10.0 mmol/L). This strategy has been proven to be effective in delaying the development and progression of DKD in patients with type 1[21] and type 2 DM.[18] A decrease in HbA1c levels by 0.9% (0.009; 10 mmol/mol Hgb) has been shown to decrease the relative risk for microalbuminuria by 30% in patients with type 2 DM.[20] Oral hypoglycemic agents can also be used in non-insulin-dependent type 2 DM to maintain similar blood glucose levels.

▶ Optimal Blood Pressure Control

Reductions in blood pressure are associated with a decrease in proteinuria, leading to a decrease in the rate of progression of kidney disease. The NKF recommends a goal blood pressure of less than 130/80 mm Hg in patients with stages 1 through 4 CKD.[21]

In patients with stage 5 CKD who are receiving hemodialysis, cardiovascular mortality is affected by blood pressure levels both before and after hemodialysis.[22] Elevated blood pressure levels after hemodialysis increases cardiovascular risk. Both systolic blood pressure greater than 180 mm Hg and diastolic blood pressure greater than 90 mm Hg are independently associated with an increased risk of cardiovascular mortality (relative risk: 1.96 and 1.73, respectively).[22] Likewise, low blood pressure levels either before or after hemodialysis are also associated with increased cardiovascular mortality. A systolic blood pressure less than 110 mm Hg before hemodialysis is associated with a fourfold increase in cardiovascular mortality; the same blood pressure at the end of hemodialysis is associated with a 2.62 relative risk.[22] Therefore, the NKF recommends achieving a goal blood pressure less than 140/90 mm Hg before hemodialysis and less than 130/80 mm Hg after hemodialysis.[23] These goals are controversial, however; one study demonstrated an increased risk of mortality for patients who achieved the target blood pressure recommended by the guidelines (hazards ratio: 1.9).[24] Newer evidence suggests that blood pressure on nonhemodialysis days may be a more appropriate measure.

Because hypertension and kidney dysfunction are linked, blood pressure control can be more difficult to attain in patients with CKD compared with patients with normal kidney function. All antihypertensive agents have similar effects on reducing blood pressure. However, three or more agents are generally required to achieve the blood pressure goal of less than 130/80 mm Hg in CKD patients.[21] Timing of blood pressure medications may also be important. A recent study suggested that administration of at least one antihypertensive medication at bedtime decreased cardiovascular risk by 14% in patients with CKD compared with taking all antihypertensive medications in the morning.[25]

▶ Reduction in Proteinuria

Reduction of proteinuria within the first year of therapy predicts long-term renal and cardiovascular prognosis.[26] The ability of antihypertensive agents to reduce protein excretion differs. Angiotensin-converting enzyme inhibitors (ACEIs) and angiotensin receptor blockers (ARBs) decrease glomerular capillary pressure and volume because of their effects on angiotensin II. This, in turn, reduces the amount of protein filtered through the glomerulus, independent of the reduction in blood pressure,[26] which ultimately decreases the progression of CKD. ❺ *The ability of ACEIs and ARBs to reduce proteinuria is greater than that of other antihypertensives, up to 35% to 40%,[26] making ACEIs and ARBs the antihypertensive agents of choice for all patients with CKD, unless contraindicated.* All patients with documented proteinuria should receive an ACE-I or ARB, regardless of blood pressure.[26] Because diabetes is associated with an early onset of microalbuminuria, all patients with diabetes should also receive an ACE-I or ARB, regardless of blood pressure.[26] When initiating ACE-I or ARB therapy, the dose should be titrated to the maximum tolerated dose, even if the blood pressure is less than 130/80 mm Hg. **Figure 26–2** depicts an algorithm for the treatment of hypertension in patients with CKD. Combining ACE-Is and ARBs should be done with caution. Some studies have demonstrated that combination therapy leads to greater reductions in protein excretion with the combination,[27] whereas others have demonstrated worsening of progression of CKD.[28]

The nondihydropyridine calcium channel blockers (CCBs) have been shown to also decrease protein excretion in patients with and without diabetes,[29] but the reduction in proteinuria appears to be related to the reductions in blood pressure. The maximal effect of nondihydropyridine CCBs on proteinuria is seen with a blood pressure reduction to less than 130/80 mm Hg, and no additional benefit is seen with increased doses.

Dihydropyridine CCBs, however, do not have the same effects on protein excretion. In fact, dihydropyridine CCBs worsen protein excretion, despite similar reductions in blood pressure as nondihydropyridine CCBs.[29]

Other Interventions to Limit Progression of CKD

▶ Hyperlipidemia Treatment

Hyperlipidemia plays a role in the development of cardiovascular disease (CVD) in patients with CKD. The primary goal of treatment of dyslipidemias is to decrease the risk of atherosclerotic CVD. A secondary goal in patients with CKD is to reduce proteinuria and decline in kidney function. Treatment of hyperlipidemia in patients with CKD has been demonstrated to increase GFR by 1 mL/min per year (0.016 mL/s per year) of treatment with antihyperlipidemic agents.[6]

The NKF suggests that CKD should be classified as a coronary heart disease (CHD) risk equivalent and the goal LDL-C level should be below 100 mg/dL (2.59 mmol/L) in all patients with CKD.[23,30] The most frequently used agents for the treatment of dyslipidemias in patients with CKD are the 3-hydroxy-3-methylglutaryl coenzyme A (HMG-CoA) reductase inhibitors ("statins") and the fibric acid derivatives. However, other treatments have been studied in patients with CKD and should be considered if first-line therapies are contraindicated.

▶ Smoking Cessation

Although the effects of smoking on the development and progression of CKD are well established, as discussed previously, the effect of smoking cessation on CKD progression has not been studied. Data are emerging that suggest that smoking cessation may be a practical approach to slow the progression of CKD. Smoking cessation has been shown to reduce the risk of myocardial infarction by 50% to 70%, regardless of previous nicotine exposure.[31] However, smoking cessation does not reverse existing kidney dysfunction in former smokers.

▶ Anemia Treatment

Anemia decreases oxygen delivery to the renal tubules, promoting the release of inflammatory and vasoactive cytokines, which contribute to the progression of CKD. Treatment of anemia in patients with CKD reduces the cardiovascular effects of anemia and has been demonstrated to decrease morbidity and mortality by as much as 20%.[32] Studies have demonstrated that treatment of anemia may slow the progression of CKD.[33] The management of anemia is discussed later.

Outcome Evaluation

Monitor SCr and potassium levels and blood pressure within 1 week after initiating ACE-I or ARB therapy. Discontinue the medication and switch to another agent if a sudden increase

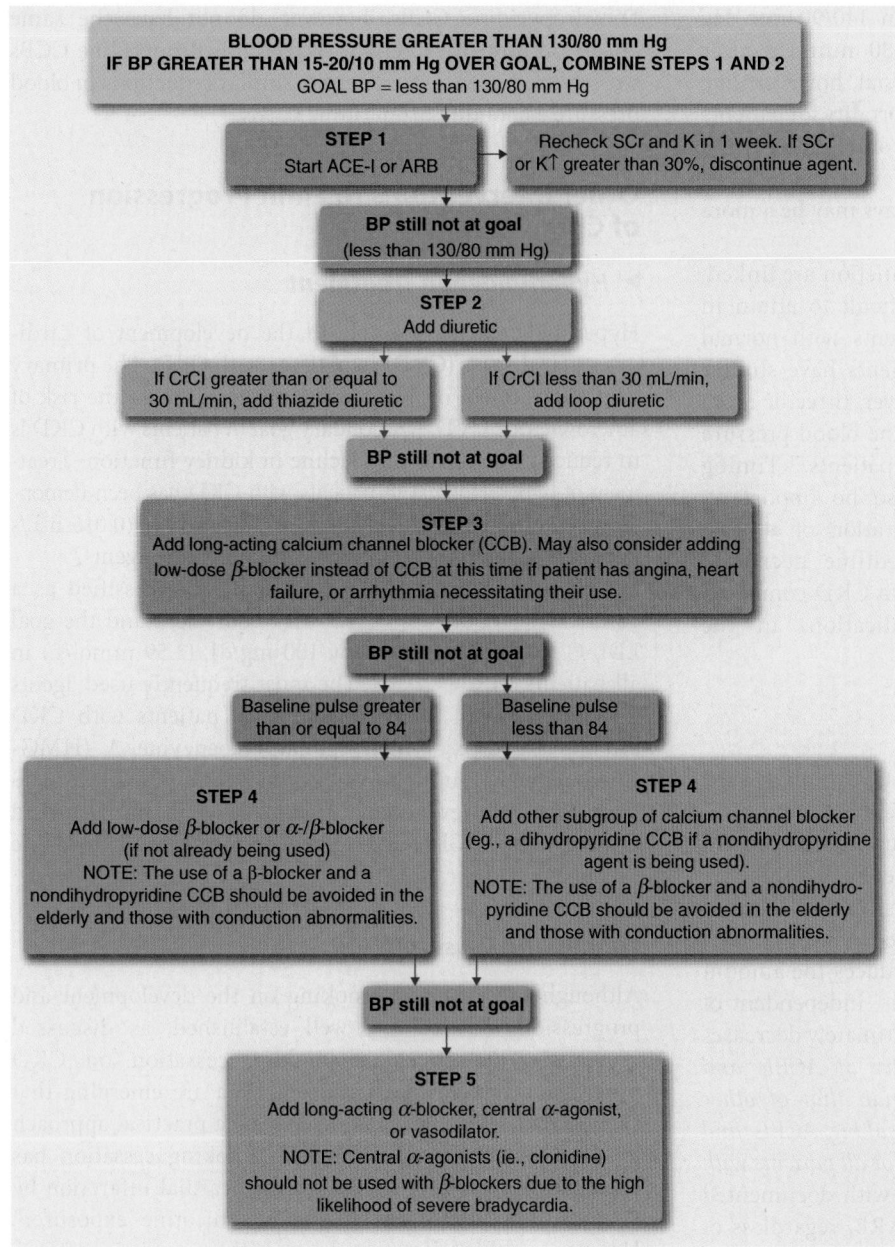

FIGURE 26–2. Hypertension management algorithm for patients with CKD. Dosage adjustments should be made every 2 to 4 weeks as needed. The dose of one agent should be maximized before another is added. (ACE-I, angiotensin-converting enzyme inhibitor; ARB, angiotensin receptor blocker; BP, blood pressure; CAD, coronary artery disease; CCB, calcium channel blocker; CHF, congestive heart failure; MI, myocardial infarction; UP:Cr, urinary protein-to-creatinine ratio.) (From Derebail VK, Kshirsagar AV, Joy MS. Chronic kidney disease: Progression-modifying therapies. In: DiPiro JT, Talbert RL, Yee GC, et al., eds. Pharmacotherapy: A Pathophysiologic Approach, 8th ed. New York, NY: McGraw-Hill, 2011:775, with permission.)

in SCr greater than 30% occurs, hyperkalemia develops, or the patient becomes hypotensive. Titrate the dose of the ACE-I or ARB every 1 to 3 months to the maximum tolerable dose. If blood pressure is not reduced to less than 130/80 mm Hg, add another agent to the regimen. Refer the patient to a nephrologist to manage complications associated with CKD. As CKD progresses to stage 4, begin discussion to prepare the patient for renal replacement therapy (RRT).

CONSEQUENCES OF CKD AND ESKD

Impaired Sodium and Water Homeostasis

Sodium and water balance are primarily regulated by the kidney. Reductions in the number of functioning nephrons decrease glomerular filtration and subsequent reabsorption of sodium and water, leading to edema.

▶ Pathophysiology

Sodium and water balance can be maintained despite wide variations in intake with normal kidney function. The fractional excretion of sodium (FE_{Na}) is approximately 1% to 3% with normal kidney function, allowing sodium balance to be maintained with a sodium intake of 120 to 150 mEq (120 to 150 mmol) per day. Urine osmolality can range from 50 to 1,200 mOsm/kg (50 to 1,200 mmol/kg) with normal kidney function, allowing for water balance to be maintained with a wide range of fluid intake. As the number of functioning nephrons decreases, the remaining nephrons increase sodium excretion, and FE_{Na} may increase up to 10% to 20%.[34] This produces an osmotic diuresis that impairs the ability of the kidneys to concentrate and dilute urine, and the urine becomes fixed at an osmolality close to that of the plasma, approximately 300 mOsm/kg (300 mmol/kg).

Patient Encounter 1

A 58-year-old African American man presents to the clinic for a routine checkup. He has been watching his diet closely and losing weight to control his blood sugars but has been unable to get his blood pressure under control.

PMH: Diabetes mellitus, diagnosed 3 years ago; hypertension, diagnosed 10 years ago.

SH: He is unemployed; he denies smoking but drinks alcohol two to three times weekly; he denies illicit drug use.

Meds: Hydrochlorothiazide 25 mg orally daily; amlodipine 10 mg orally daily; glipizide-metformin 5 mg/500 mg orally twice daily.

ROS: Unremarkable.

PE:

VS: BP 168/102 mm Hg; P 85 bpm; T 98.8°F (37.1°C); ht 6'1" (185 cm); wt 215 lb (97.7 kg)

CV: RRR, normal S_1, S_2; no murmurs, rubs or gallops; lungs clear

Abd: Obese; no organomegaly, bruits or tenderness, (+) bowel sounds; heme (−) stool

Exts: Trace pedal edema bilaterally; decreased sensation in feet to light touch; no lesions

Labs (Fasting): Sodium 139 mEq/L (139 mmol/L); potassium 3.9 mEq/L (3.9 mmol/L); chloride 101 mEq/L (101 mmol/L); carbon dioxide 25 mEq/L (25 mmol/L); blood urea nitrogen (BUN) 28 mg/dL (10.0 mmol/L); serum creatinine (SCr) 1.8 mg/dL (159 μmol/L); glucose 102 mg/dL 5.7 mmol/L); total cholesterol 187 mg/dL (4.84 mmol/L); low-density lipoprotein cholesterol (LDL-C) 120 mg/dL (3.10 mmol/L); high-density lipoprotein cholesterol (HDL-C) 42 mg/dL (1.09 mmol/L); triglycerides 125 mg/dL (1.41 mmol/L); hemoglobin$_{A1c}$ (Hb$_{A1c}$) 6.9% (0.069; 52 mmol/mol Hgb); urine microalbumin 150 mg/dL (1.5 g/L)

What risk factors does the patient have for the development of CKD?

What signs and symptoms are consistent with CKD?

How would you classify his CKD?

What lifestyle modifications would you recommend for this patient with CKD?

What pharmacologic alternatives are available for this patient for treatment of CKD?

The inability of the kidney to concentrate the urine results in nocturia in patients with CKD, usually presenting as early as stage 3 CKD.

As the number of functioning nephrons continues to decline, the sodium load overwhelms the remaining nephrons and total sodium excretion is decreased, despite the increase in sodium excretion by the functioning nephrons. Sodium retention increases thirst and also causes fluid retention that increases intravascular volume and raises systemic blood pressure. Severe volume overload can lead to pulmonary edema.

▶ Treatment

Nonpharmacologic Therapy The kidney is unable to adjust to abrupt changes in sodium intake in patients with severe CKD. Therefore, patients should be advised to refrain from adding salt to their diet but should not restrict sodium intake. Changes in sodium intake should occur slowly over a period of several days to allow adequate time for the kidney to adjust urinary sodium content. Sodium restriction produces a negative sodium balance, which causes fluid excretion to restore sodium balance. The resulting volume contraction can decrease perfusion of the kidney and hasten the decline in GFR. Saline-containing IV solutions should be used cautiously in patients with CKD because the salt load may precipitate volume overload.

Fluid restriction is generally unnecessary as long as sodium intake is controlled. The thirst mechanism remains intact in

Clinical Presentation and Diagnosis of Impaired Sodium and Water Homeostasis

General

Alterations in sodium and water balance in CKD manifests as increased edema.

Symptoms

Nocturia can present in stage 3 CKD.

Edema generally presents in stage 4 CKD or later.

Signs

Cardiovascular: Worsening hypertension, edema.

Genitourinary: Change in urine volume and consistency.

Laboratory Tests

Increased blood pressure.

Sodium levels remain within the normal range.

Urine osmolality is generally fixed at 300 mOsm/kg (300 mmol/kg).

CKD to maintain total body water and plasma osmolality near normal levels. Fluid intake should be maintained at the rate of urine output to replace urine losses, usually fixed at approximately 2 L/day as urine concentrating ability is lost. Significant increases in free water intake orally or

IV can precipitate volume overload and hyponatremia. Patients with stage 5 CKD require RRT to maintain normal volume status. Fluid intake is often limited in patients receiving hemodialysis to prevent fluid overload between dialysis sessions.

● **Pharmacologic Therapy** Diuretic therapy is often necessary to prevent volume overload in patients with CKD in those who still produce urine. Loop diuretics are most frequently used to increase sodium and water excretion. Thiazide diuretics are ineffective when used alone in patients with a GFR less than 30 mL/min/1.73 m^2 (0.29 mL/s/m^2).[21] As CKD progresses, higher doses, as much as 80 to 1,000 mg/day of furosemide, or continuous infusion of loop diuretics may be needed, or combination therapy with loop and thiazide diuretics to increase sodium and water excretion.[21]

▶ *Outcome Evaluation*

● Monitor edema after initiation of diuretic therapy. Monitor fluid intake to ensure obligatory losses are being met and avoid dehydration. If adequate diuresis is not attained with a single agent, consider combination therapy with another diuretic.

Impaired Potassium Homeostasis

Potassium balance is also primarily regulated by the kidney via the distal tubular cells. Reduction in the number of functioning nephrons decreases the overall tubular secretion of potassium, leading to hyperkalemia. Hyperkalemia is estimated to affect more than 50% of patients with stage 5 CKD.[35]

▶ *Pathophysiology*

The distal tubules secrete 90% to 95% of the daily dietary intake of potassium. The fractional excretion of potassium (FE$_K$) is approximately 25% with normal kidney function.[36] The GI tract excretes the remaining 5% to 10% of dietary potassium intake. Following a large potassium load, extracellular potassium is shifted intracellularly to maintain stable extracellular levels.

As the number of functioning nephrons decreases, both the distal tubular secretion and GI excretion are increased in the functioning nephrons because of aldosterone stimulation. Functioning nephrons increase FE$_K$ up to 100% and GI excretion increases as much as 30% to 70% in CKD,[37] as a result of aldosterone secretion in response to increased potassium levels.[37] This maintains serum potassium concentrations within the normal range through stages 1 to 4 CKD. Hyperkalemia begins to develop when GFR falls below 20% of normal, when the number of functioning nephrons and renal potassium secretion is so low that the capacity of the GI tract to excrete potassium has been exceeded.[37]

● Medications can increase the risk of hyperkalemia in patients with CKD, including ACE-I and ARBs, used for the treatment of proteinuria and hypertension. Potassium-sparing

---

Clinical Presentation and Diagnosis of Hyperkalemia

General

Hyperkalemia is generally asymptomatic in patients with CKD until serum potassium levels are greater than 5.5 mEq/L (5.5 mmol/L), when cardiac abnormalities present.

Symptoms

Mild hyperkalemia is generally not associated with overt symptoms.

Symptoms generally appear in stage 4 or 5 CKD, such as muscle weakness, fatigue, nausea, and paresthesias.

Signs

Cardiovascular: ECG changes (peaked T waves, widened QRS complex, loss of P wave).

Laboratory Tests

Increased serum potassium levels.

---

diuretics, used for the treatment of edema and chronic heart failure, can also exacerbate the development of hyperkalemia, and they should be used with caution in patients with stage 3 CKD or higher.

▶ *Treatment*

Nonpharmacologic Therapy Patients with CKD should
● avoid abrupt increases in dietary intake of potassium because the kidney is unable to increase potassium excretion with an acute potassium load, particularly in latter stages of the disease. Hyperkalemia resulting from an acute increase in
● potassium intake can be more severe and prolonged. Patients who develop hyperkalemia should restrict dietary intake of potassium to 50 to 80 mEq (50 to 80 mmol) per day. Potassium concentrations can also be altered in the dialysate for patients receiving hemodialysis and peritoneal dialysis to manage hyperkalemia. Because GI excretion of potassium plays a large role in potassium homeostasis in patients with stage 5 CKD, a good bowel regimen is essential to minimize constipation, which can occur in 40% of patients receiving
● hemodialysis.[36] Severe hyperkalemia is most effectively managed by hemodialysis.

● **Pharmacologic Therapy** Patients with acute hyperkalemia usually require other therapies to manage hyperkalemia until dialysis can be initiated. Patients who present with hyperkalemia-induced cardiac abnormalities, which manifest as peaked T waves, a widened QRS complex, or loss of P waves, should receive calcium gluconate or chloride (1 g IV) to reverse the cardiac effects. Temporary measures can be employed to shift extracellular potassium into the intracellular compartment to stabilize cellular membrane effects of excessive serum potassium levels. Such measures include the use of regular insulin (5 to 10 units IV) and dextrose (5% to 50% IV), or nebulized albuterol (salbutamol) (10 to 20 mg). Sodium bicarbonate should not be used to shift extracellular potassium intracellularly in patients with CKD unless severe metabolic acidosis (pH less than 7.2) is present. These measures will decrease serum potassium levels within 30 to 60 minutes after treatment, but potassium must still be removed from the body. Shifting potassium to the intracellular compartment, however, decreases potassium removal by dialysis. Often, multiple dialysis sessions are required to remove potassium that is redistributed from the intracellular space back into the serum.

Sodium polystyrene sulfonate (SPS, 15 to 30 g orally or rectally), a sodium–potassium exchange resin, promotes potassium excretion from the GI tract. The onset of action is within 2 hours after administration of SPS, but the maximum effect on potassium levels may not be seen for up to 6 hours, which limits the utility in patients with severe hyperkalemia. Of note, loop diuretics are often used to decrease potassium levels in patients with normal or mildly decreased kidney function, but they are not useful in patients with stage 5 CKD to decrease potassium concentrations. Fludrocortisone is a mineralocorticoid that mimics the effects of aldosterone and increases potassium excretion in the distal tubules and through the GI tract. However, fludrocortisone causes significant sodium and water retention, which exacerbates edema and hypertension, and it may not be tolerated by many CKD patients.

▶ Outcome Evaluation

Monitor ECG continuously in patients with cardiac abnormalities until serum potassium levels drop below 5 mEq/L (5 mmol/L) or cardiac abnormalities resolve. Evaluate serum potassium and glucose levels within 1 hour in patients who receive insulin and dextrose therapy. Evaluate serum potassium levels within 2 to 4 hours after treatment with SPS or diuretics. Repeat doses of diuretics or SPS if necessary until serum potassium levels fall below 5 mEq/L (5 mmol/L). Monitor blood pressure and serum potassium levels in 1 week in patients who receive fludrocortisone.

Anemia of CKD

The progenitor cells of the kidney produce 90% of the hormone erythropoietin (EPO), which stimulates red blood cell (RBC) production. ❻ *Reduction in the number of functioning nephrons decreases renal production of EPO, which is the primary cause of anemia in patients with CKD. The development of anemia of CKD results in decreased oxygen delivery and utilization, leading to increased cardiac output and left ventricular hypertrophy (LVH), which increase the cardiovascular risk and mortality in patients with CKD.*

▶ Epidemiology and Etiology

Current Kidney Disease Improving Global Outcomes (KDIGO) guidelines define anemia as a hemoglobin (Hgb) level less than 13 g/dL (130 g/L or 8.06 mmol/L) in males and less than 12 g/dL (120 g/L or 7.45 mmol/L) in females.[38] A number of factors can contribute to the development of anemia including deficiencies in vitamin B_{12} or folate, hemolysis, bleeding, or bone marrow suppression. Many of these can be detected by alterations in RBC indices, which should be included in the evaluation for anemia. A complete blood cell count is also helpful in evaluating anemia to determine overall bone marrow function.

The prevalence of anemia correlates with the degree of kidney dysfunction. More than 26% of patients with a GFR greater than 60 mL/min/1.73 m² (0.58 mL/s/m²) are estimated to have Hgb levels less than 12 g/dL (120 g/L or 7.45 mmol/L), and the number increases to 75% in patients with a GFR less than 15 mL/min/1.73 m² (0.14 mL/s/m²).[39] The risk of developing anemia also increases as GFR declines, doubling for patients with stage 3 CKD, increasing to 3.8-fold in patients with stage 4 CKD, and to 10.5-fold for patients with stage 5 CKD, compared with stages 1 and 2 CKD.[39]

▶ Pathophysiology

The primary cause of anemia in patients with CKD is a decrease in EPO production. With normal kidney function, as Hgb, hematocrit (Hct), and tissue oxygenation decrease, the plasma concentration of EPO increases exponentially. As the number of functioning nephrons decrease, EPO production also decreases. Thus, as Hgb, Hct, and tissue oxygenation decrease in patients with CKD, plasma EPO levels remain constant within the normal range but low relative to the degree of hypoxia present. The result is a normochromic, normocytic anemia.

Several other factors also contribute to the development of anemia in patients with CKD. Uremia, the accumulation of toxins that results from declining kidney function, decreases the lifespan of RBCs from a normal of 120 days to as low as 60 days in patients with stage 5 CKD. Iron deficiency and blood loss from regular laboratory testing and hemodialysis also contribute to the development of anemia in patients with CKD.

However, as CKD progress, adaptive mechanisms develop that protect the body from the decreased oxygen-carrying capacity associated with lower Hgb levels. As oxygen saturation decreases with lower Hgb levels, the affinity of 2,3-diphosphoglycerate (2,3-DPG) for Hgb is increased, allowing oxygen to more readily dissociate from Hgb at the tissue site. Acidosis and uremia also contribute to the increased affinity of 2,3-DPG, increasing oxygen delivery to tissues to minimize the potential for hypoxemia.[40]

▶ Treatment

General Approach to Therapy Studies have demonstrated that initiation of treatment for anemia before stage 5 CKD decreases mortality in patients with ESKD receiving dialysis, particularly in the elderly.[41] The treatment of anemia can decrease morbidity, increase exercise capacity and tolerance, and slow the progression of CKD if target Hgb levels are achieved.[42]

Clinical Presentation and Diagnosis of Anemia of CKD

General

Anemia of CKD generally presents with fatigue and decreased quality of life.

Symptoms

Anemia of CKD is associated with symptoms of cold intolerance, shortness of breath, and decreased exercise capacity.

Signs

Cardiovascular: Left ventricular hypertrophy, ECG changes, congestive heart failure.

Neurologic: Impaired mental cognition.

Genitourinary: Sexual dysfunction.

Laboratory Tests

Decreased RBC count, Hgb, and Hct.

Decreased serum iron level, TIBC, serum ferritin, and TSAT.

Patients with CKD should be evaluated for anemia when the GFR falls below 60 mL/min (1.0 mL/s) or if the SCr rises above 2 mg/dL (20 g/L or 177 mmol/L). An anemia workup should be performed if the Hgb is less than 13 g/dL (130 g/L or 8.06 mmol/L) in males or less than 12 g/dL (120 g/L or 7.45 mmol/L) in females. The workup for anemia should rule out other potential causes for anemia (see Chapter 66). Abnormalities found during the anemia workup should be corrected before initiating erythropoiesis-stimulating agents (ESAs), particularly iron deficiency, because iron is

an essential component of RBC production. If Hgb is below 10 g/dL (100 g/L or 6.21 mmol/L) when all other causes of anemia have been corrected, EPO deficiency should be assumed. EPO levels are not routinely measured and have little clinical significance in monitoring progression and treatment of anemia in patients with CKD.

Generally, treatment for anemia of CKD requires a combination of iron supplementation and ESAs. The goals for iron supplementation are:

- Serum ferritin levels greater than 500 ng/mL (500 mcg/L; 1,123 pmol/L)

- Transferrin saturation (TSAT): greater than 30% (0.3).[38]

ESAs may be considered if Hgb levels remain persistently low to improve symptoms of anemia. In patients not receiving dialysis, the decision to initiate ESAs should be based on the rate of Hgb decline, prior response to anemia treatment, risks associated with ESAs and the patient's symptoms. The KDIGO guidelines recommend considering to initiate ESAs when Hgb is less than 10 g/dL (100 g/L or 6.2 mmol/L) in patients not receiving dialysis.[38] In patients receiving dialysis, most clinicians initiate ESAs when Hgb is less than 9 g/dL (90 g/L or 5.58 mmol/L). However, the target for Hgb is unclear because use of ESAs to increase Hgb levels beyond 12 g/dL (120 g/L or 7.44 mmol/L) is associated with increased mortality.[43]

The approach to the management of anemia of CKD with iron supplementation and ESAs is illustrated in **Figure 26–3**.

Nonpharmacologic Therapy Approximately 1 to 2 mg of iron is absorbed daily from the diet. This small amount is generally not adequate to preserve adequate iron stores to promote RBC production. RBC transfusions have been used in the past as the primary means to maintain Hgb and Hct levels in patients with anemia of CKD. This treatment

---

Patient Encounter 2, Part 1

A 43-year-old white man with a history of IgA nephropathy presents to your clinic for a routine checkup. He complains of getting fatigued easily at work. He works as a mechanic and finds himself not able to keep up with the job as much as he had in the past. He notes that he feels winded when he walks even short distances.

Current meds: Atenolol 100 mg orally daily; lisinopril 20 mg orally daily; furosemide 20 mg orally daily.

ROS: Skin pale in color; fatigue daily throughout the day with minimal exertion; otherwise unremarkable.

PE:

VS: BP 132/82 mm Hg; P 88 bpm; T 97.2°F (36.2°C); ht 5′11″ (180 cm); wt 215 lb (97.7 kg)

CV: RRR, normal S_1, S_2

Abd: Obese; no organomegaly, bruits or tenderness; (+) bowel sounds; heme (−) stool

Ext: 1+ pedal edema bilaterally

Labs: Sodium 141 mEq/L (141 mmol/L); potassium 4.9 mEq/L 4.9 mmol/L); chloride 99 mEq/L (99 mmol/L); carbon dioxide 19 mEq/L (19 mmol/L); BUN 42 mg/dL (15.0 mmol/L); Scr 3.2 mg/dL (283 μmol/L); glucose 78 mg/dL (4.3 mmol/L); white blood cell (WBC) count 5.6×10^3 cells/mm³ (5.6×10^9/L); red blood cell (RBC) count 2.7×10^6 cells/mm³ (2.7×10^{12}/L); hemoglobin (Hgb) 8.1 g/dL (81 g/L; 5.03 mmol/L); hematocrit 24% (0.24); platelets 325×10^3 cells/mm³ (325×10^9/L)

What signs and symptoms are consistent with anemia of CKD?

What additional information could you request to determine other causes of anemia in this patient?

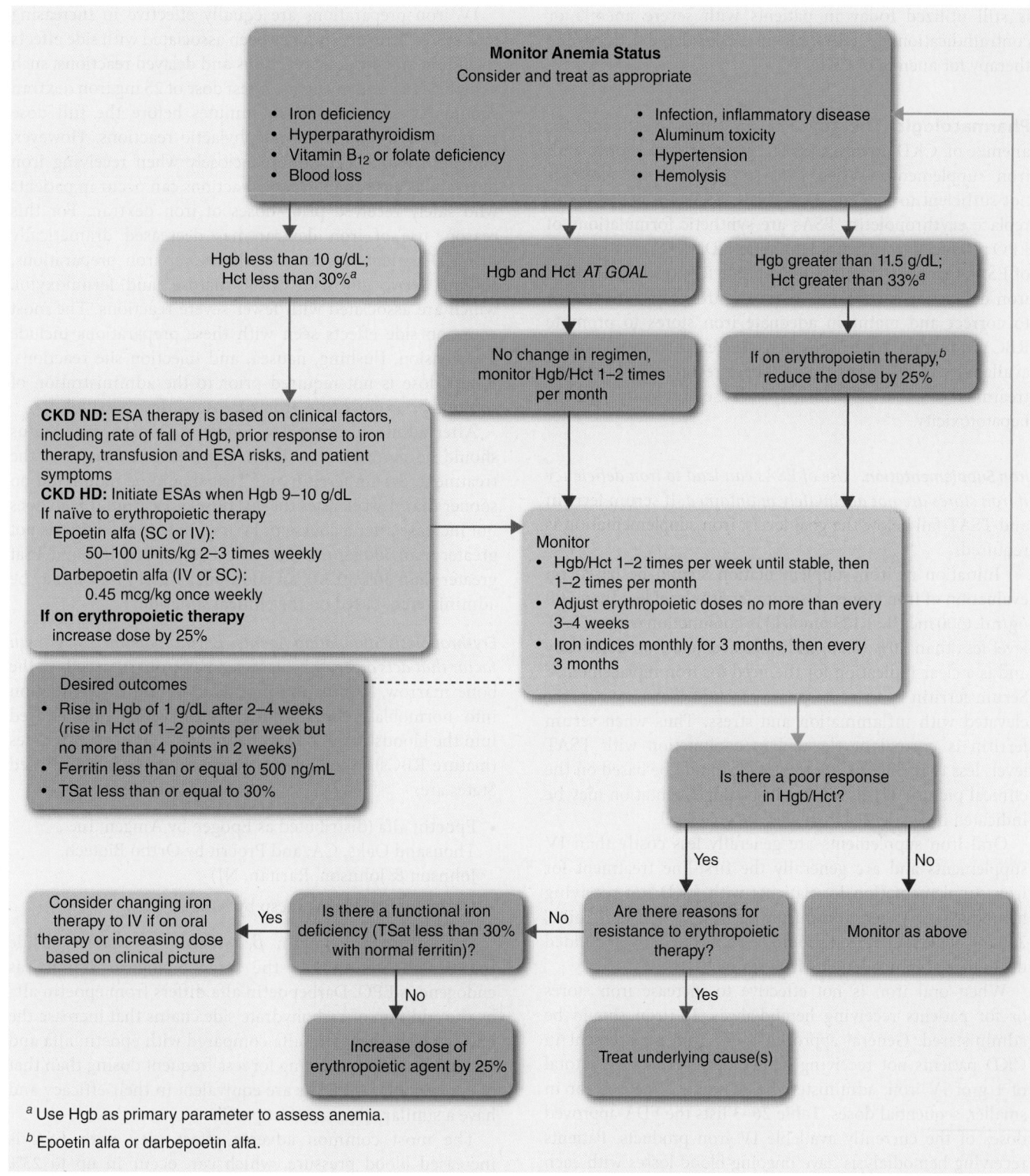

FIGURE 26–3. Algorithm for erythropoietic-stimulating agent therapy in the management of anemia of CKD. (CKD HD, chronic kidney disease receiving hemodialysis; CKD ND, chronic kidney disease not receiving dialysis; ESA, erythropoiesis-stimulating agent; Hb, hemoglobin; SC, subcutaneous; TSAT, transferrin saturation.) (Adapted from Hudson JQ. Chronic kidney disease: Management of complications. In: DiPiro JT, Talbert RL, Yee GC, et al., eds. Pharmacotherapy: A Pathophysiologic Approach, 8th ed. New York, NY: McGraw-Hill, 2011:800, with permission.)

is still utilized today in patients with severe anemia or contraindications to ESAs, but it is considered a third-line therapy for anemia of CKD.

Pharmacologic Therapy The first-line treatment for anemia of CKD involves replacement of iron stores with iron supplements. When iron supplementation alone is not sufficient to increase Hgb levels, ESAs are necessary to replace erythropoietin. ESAs are synthetic formulations of EPO produced by recombinant human DNA technology. Use of ESAs increases the iron demand for RBC production and iron deficiency is common, requiring iron supplementation to correct and maintain adequate iron stores to promote RBC production. Androgens were used extensively before the availability of ESAs but are no longer recommended for the treatment of anemia[38] primarily because of toxicity, namely, hepatotoxicity.

Iron Supplementation. Use of ESAs can lead to iron deficiency if iron stores are not adequately maintained. If serum ferritin and TSAT fall below the goal levels, iron supplementation is required.

Initiation of iron supplementation should be based on evaluation of iron stores. A serum ferritin level less than 500 ng/mL (500 mcg/L; 1,123 pmol/L) in conjunction with a TSAT level less than 30% (0.30) indicates absolute iron deficiency and is a clear indication for the need for iron replacement.[38] Serum ferritin is an acute phase reactant that may become elevated with inflammation and stress. Thus when serum ferritin is normal or elevated in conjunction with TSAT levels less than 30% (0.30), treatment should be based on the clinical picture of the patient. Iron supplementation may be indicated if Hgb levels are below the goal level.

Oral iron supplements are generally less costly than IV supplements and are generally the first-line treatment for iron supplementation for patients with CKD not receiving hemodialysis. When administering iron by the oral route, 200 mg of elemental iron should be delivered daily in divided doses to maintain adequate iron stores.[38]

When oral iron is not effective to increase iron stores or for patients receiving hemodialysis, IV iron should be administered. General approach to IV iron replacement in CKD patients not receiving hemodialysis is to give a total of 1 g of IV iron, administered as a single large dose or in smaller, sequential doses. Table 26–3 lists the FDA-approved doses of the currently available IV iron products. Patients receiving hemodialysis have ongoing blood losses with each hemodialysis session, which can lead to iron losses of 1–2 g per year.[38] For hemodialysis, IV iron may be administered in 1 g doses periodically based on routine surveillance of iron stores. An alternative method to administer IV iron is to give smaller maintenance doses of iron weekly or with each dialysis session (e.g., iron dextran or iron sucrose 20 to 100 mg/week; sodium ferric gluconate 62.5 to 125 mg/week). The latter approach of giving smaller maintenance doses may result in lower cumulative doses of iron and lower doses of ESAs.[38]

IV iron preparations are equally effective in increasing iron stores. Iron dextran has been associated with side effects including anaphylactic reactions and delayed reactions, such as arthralgias and myalgias. A test dose of 25 mg iron dextran should be administered 30 minutes before the full dose to monitor for potential anaphylactic reactions. However, patients should be monitored closely when receiving iron dextran because anaphylactic reactions can occur in patients who safely received prior doses of iron dextran. For this reason, use of iron dextran has decreased dramatically in CKD patients in favor of the newer iron preparations, sodium ferric gluconate, iron sucrose, and ferumoxytol, which are associated with fewer severe reactions. The most common side effects seen with these preparations include hypotension, flushing, nausea, and injection site reactions. A test dose is not required prior to the administration of sodium ferric gluconate, iron sucrose, or ferumoxytol.

After administering a 1-g course of IV iron, iron status should be monitored to determine the effectiveness of the treatment. Serum ferritin and TSat should be monitored no sooner than 1 week after the last dose of IV iron. If Hgb does not increase after a course of IV iron or serum ferritin is not greater than 500 ng/mL (500 mcg/L; 1,123 pmol/L) and TSat greater than 30% (0.30), an additional 1 g of IV iron may be administered, based on the clinical situation.

Erythropoiesis-Stimulating Agents. Erythropoietin is a growth factor that acts on erythroblasts formed from stem cells in the bone marrow, stimulating proliferation and differentiation into normoblasts, then reticulocytes, which are released into the bloodstream to eventually mature into erythrocytes (mature RBCs). The ESAs currently available in the United States are:

- Epoetin alfa (distributed as Epogen by Amgen, Inc., Thousand Oaks, CA; and Procrit by Ortho Biotech, Johnson & Johnson, Raritan, NJ)
- Darbepoetin alfa (Aranesp by Amgen, Inc.)

Epoetin α and epoetin β, which is available outside the United States, have the same biological activity as endogenous EPO. Darbepoetin alfa differs from epoetin alfa by the addition of carbohydrate side chains that increase the half-life of darbepoetin alfa compared with epoetin alfa and endogenous EPO, allowing for less frequent dosing than that of epoetin alfa. All ESAs are equivalent in their efficacy and have a similar adverse-effect profile.

The most common adverse effect seen with ESA is increased blood pressure, which can occur in up to 23% of patients.[36] Antihypertensive agents may be required to control blood pressure in patients receiving ESAs. Caution should be used when initiating an ESA in patients with very high blood pressures (greater than 180/100 mm Hg). If blood pressures are refractory to antihypertensive agents, ESAs may need to be withheld. Darbepoetin has also been reported to increase the risk of strokes in patients with CKD.[44]

Subcutaneous (SC) administration of ESA produces a more predictable and sustained response than IV administration, and it is therefore the preferred route of administration for

Table 26–3

IV Iron Products

Iron Formulation (Product)	FDA-approved Indications	FDA-Approved Dosing	Warnings	Dose Ranges[a]	How Supplied
Iron dextran (INFeD, Dexferrum)	Patients with iron deficiency in whom oral iron is unsatisfactory	IV push: 100 mg over 2 minutes (25 mg test dose required)	Black box (risk of anaphylactic reactions)	25–1,000 mg	2-mL vials containing 50 mg elemental iron per mL
Ferric gluconate (Ferrlecit)	Adult and pediatric HD patients age 6 years and older receiving ESA therapy	IV push (adult): 125 mg over 10 minutes; IV infusion (adult): 125 mg in 100 mL of 0.9% NaCl over 60 minutes; IV infusion (pediatric): 1.5 mg/kg in 25 mL of 0.9% NaCl over 60 minutes; maximum dose 125 mg	General	6.25–1,000 mg	5-mL ampules containing 62.5 mg elemental iron (12.5 mg/mL)
Iron sucrose (Venofer)	HD patients with CKD receiving ESA therapy	IV push: 100 mg over 2–5 minutes; IV infusion: 100 mg in maximum of 100 mL of 0.9% NaCl over 15 minutes	General	25–1,000 mg	5-mL single-dose vials containing 100 mg elemental iron (20 mg/mL)
	Nondialysis-CKD patients receiving or not receiving ESA therapy	IV push: 200 mg over 2–5 minutes on five different occasions within 14-day period			
	PD patients receiving ESA therapy	IV infusion: 2 infusions 14 days apart, of 300 mg in maximum of 250 mL of 0.9% NaCl over 1.5 hour, followed by 1 infusion 14 days later, of 400 mg in maximum of 250 mL of 0.9% NaCl over 2.5 hours			
Ferumoxytol (Feraheme)	Adults with iron-deficiency anemia associated with CKD	IV: 510 mg (17 mL) as a single dose, followed by a second 510-mg dose 3–8 days after the initial dose (rate of 1 mL or 30 mg/second)	General	510 mg	17 mL vials containing 510 mg (0 mg/mL)

CKD, chronic kidney disease; ESA, erythropoietin-stimulating agent; HD, hemodialysis; PD, peritoneal dialysis.

[a]Small dosing ranges (e.g., 25 to 100 mg/week) generally used for maintenance regimens. Larger doses (e.g., 1 g) should be administered in divided doses.

both agents. IV administration is often utilized in patients who have established IV access or are receiving hemodialysis. Starting doses of ESAs depend on the patient's Hgb level, the target Hgb level, the rate of Hgb increase, and clinical circumstances.[38] The initial increase in Hgb should be 1 to 2 g/dL (10 to 20 g/L or 0.62 to 1.24 mmol/L) per month. The recommended starting dose of epoetin alfa is 50 to 100 units/kg/dose administered SC or IV two to three times weekly; the starting dose of darbepoetin alfa is 0.45 mcg/kg administered SC or IV once weekly (Table 26–4).

When prescribing ESAs, clinicians should not attempt to target "normal" Hgb levels (i.e., greater than 13 g/dL [130 g/L or 8.07 mmol/L] in males; greater than 12 g/dL [120 g/L or 7.45 mmol/L] in females). Several clinical trials have demonstrated that targeting Hgb levels greater

than 13 g/dL (130 g/L or 8.07 mmol/L) resulted in more cardiovascular complications or death, compared with target Hgb levels less than 11 g/dL (110 g/L or 6.83 mmol/L), with little or no benefit on the quality of life.[43,45] Although not completely understood, the increased mortality is postulated to result from increased blood viscosity, which can trigger platelet activity, and hemoconcentration, which occurs when large amounts of fluid are removed during hemodialysis.[45] A third mechanism may relate to relative unphysiological concentrations of EPO that are achieved with intermittent dosing of ESAs, which may promote inflammation or thrombosis.[45]

Further studies are needed to evaluate the appropriate target level for Hgb. Nonetheless, based on these findings, the U.S. FDA recommended addition of a black box warning

Table 26–4

Estimated Starting Doses of Darbepoetin Alfa Based on Previous Epoetin Alfa Dose

Previous Epoetin Alfa Dose (units/week)	Weekly Darbepoetin Alfa Dose (mcg/week)
Less than 2,500	6.25
2,500–4,999	12.5
5,000–10,999	25
11,000–17,999	40
18,000–33,999	60
34,000–59,999	100
60,000–89,999	150
90,000 or more	200

to the product information for all ESAs indicating the maximum target Hgb should not exceed 11 g/dL (110 g/L or 6.83 mmol/L) for patients who are receiving ESAs.

▶ Outcome Evaluation

● Evaluate Hgb every 1 to 2 weeks when ESA therapy is initiated or the dose is adjusted to ensure Hgb does not exceed 11.5 g/dL (115 g/L or 7.13 mmol/L).[38] Once a stable Hgb is attained, evaluate Hgb every 2 to 4 weeks thereafter. While the patient is receiving ESA therapy, monitor iron stores monthly in patients who are not receiving iron supplements or every 3 months in patients who are receiving iron supplements. When the goal Hgb is reached, monitor iron stores every 3 months. Serum ferritin and TSat should be monitored no sooner than 1 week after the last dose of IV iron is administered.

Patient Encounter 2, Part 2

The patient returns to your clinic in 1 week and states that his symptoms have not changed. He is asking about the results of his laboratory studies.

Labs: WBC 6.1 × 10³ cells/mm³ (6.1 × 10⁹/L); RBC 2.6 × 10⁶ cells/mm³ (2.6 × 10¹²/L); Hgb 8.1 g/dL (81 g/L; 5.03 mmol/L); hematocrit 25% (0.25); mean corpuscular volume (MCV) 82 fL; mean corpuscular hemoglobin concentration (MCHC) 34 g/dL (340 g/L); platelets 315 × 10³ cells/mm³ (315 × 10⁹/L); iron 29 mcg/dL (5.2 μmol/L); total iron binding capacity (TIBC) 487 mcg/dL (87.2 μmol/L); ferritin 68 ng/mL (68 mcg/L); transferrin saturation (TSAT) 12% (0.12); stool guaiac negative × 3

What treatment would you recommend for this patient for treatment of anemia?

How would you evaluate the effectiveness of treatment of anemia?

CKD-Mineral and Bone Disorder and Secondary Hyperparathyroidism

▶ Epidemiology and Etiology

Increases in parathyroid hormone (PTH) occur early as kidney function begins to decline. The actions of PTH on bone turnover lead to CKD-mineral and bone disorders (CKD-MBD). As many as 75% to 100% of patients with stage 3 CKD have CKD-MBD.[46] The type of bone disease can vary based on the degree of bone turnover. High bone turnover is the most common cause of bone abnormalities in patients with CKD, present in as many as 75% of patients receiving dialysis,[46] and it is generally mediated by high levels of PTH. Adynamic bone disease, characterized by low bone turnover, is less common, although the prevalence appears to be increasing,[46] which may be related to more aggressive treatment of hyperparathyroidism. The development of CKD-MBD can dramatically affect morbidity in patients with CKD.

▶ Pathophysiology

As kidney function declines in patients with CKD, decreased phosphorus excretion disrupts the balance of calcium and phosphorus homeostasis. Decreased vitamin D activation in the kidney also decreases calcium absorption from the GI tract. Fibroblast growth factor 23 (FGF-23) is a hormone produced by osteocytes and osteoblasts that is stimulated by increased phosphate and calcitriol. In CKD, elevated phosphate concentrations increase expression of FGF-23, which downregulates vitamin D activation in the kidney.[47] Each of these stimulates the parathyroid glands. **❼** *The parathyroid glands release PTH in response to decreased serum calcium and increased serum phosphorus levels. The actions of PTH include the following*:

- Increasing calcium resorption from bone
- Increasing calcium reabsorption from the proximal tubules in the kidney
- Decreasing phosphorus reabsorption in the proximal tubules in the kidney
- Stimulating activation of vitamin D by 1-α-hydroxylase to calcitriol (1,25-dihydroxyvitmin D_3) to promote calcium absorption in the GI tract and increased calcium mobilization from bone

All of these actions are directed at increasing serum calcium levels and decreasing serum phosphorus levels, although the activity of calcitriol also increases phosphorus absorption in the GI tract and mobilization from the bone, which can worsen hyperphosphatemia. Calcitriol also decreases PTH levels through a negative feedback loop. These measures are sufficient to correct serum calcium levels in the earlier stages of CKD.

As kidney function continues to decline and the GFR falls less than 30 mL/min/1.73 m² (0.29 mL/s/m²), phosphorus excretion continues to decrease and calcitriol production decreases,[48] causing PTH levels to begin to rise significantly, leading to **secondary hyperparathyroidism** (sHPT).

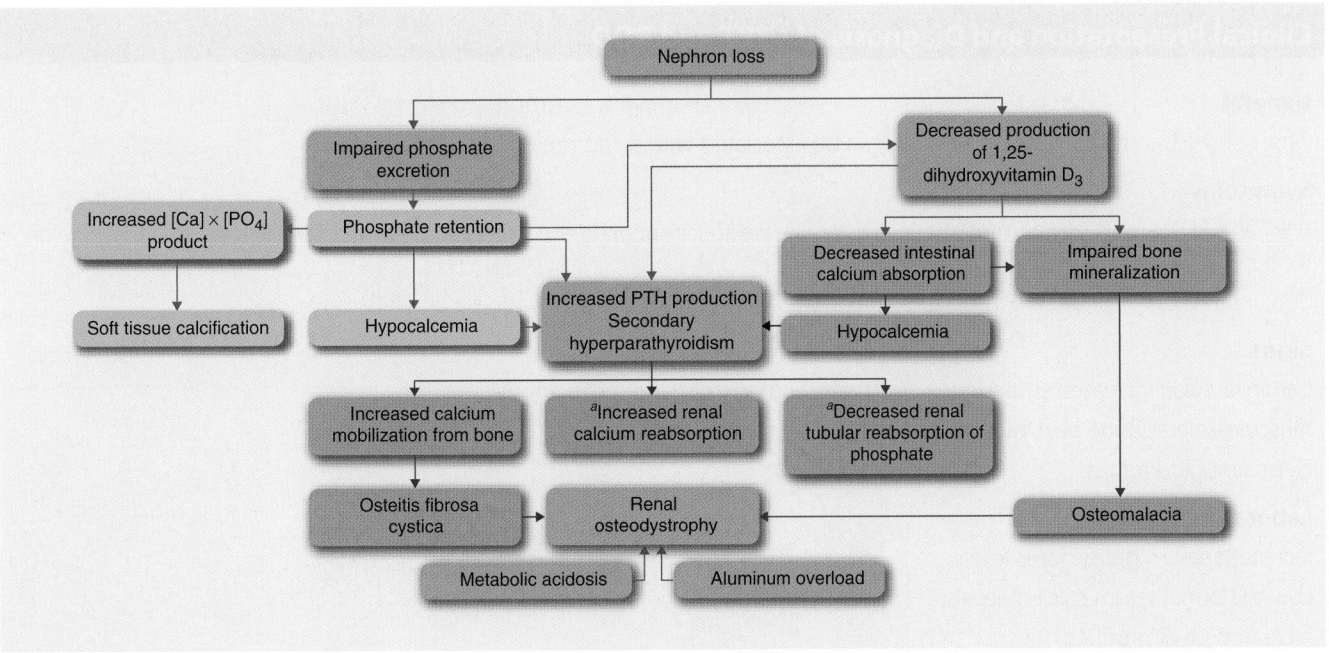

FIGURE 26–4. Pathogenesis of CKD-MBD and **renal osteodystrophy**. *a*These adaptations are lost as kidney failure progresses. (From Hudson JQ. Chronic kidney disease: Management of complications. In: DiPiro JT, Talbert RL, Yee GC, et al., eds. Pharmacotherapy: A Pathophysiologic Approach, 8th ed. New York, NY: McGraw-Hill, 2011:790, with permission.)

The excessive production of PTH leads to hyperplasia of the parathyroid glands, which decreases the sensitivity of the parathyroid glands to serum calcium levels and calcitriol feedback, further promoting sHPT.

The most dramatic consequence of sHPT is alterations in bone turnover and the development of **renal osteodystrophy** (ROD). Other complications of CKD can also promote ROD. Metabolic acidosis decreases bone formation by reducing hydroxyapatite solubility, inhibiting osteoblast activity, stimulating osteoclast activity, and reducing the sensitivity of the parathyroid gland to serum calcium levels.[49] Excessive aluminum levels cause aluminum uptake into bone in place of calcium, weakening the bone structure. The pathogenesis of sHPT and CKD-MBD are depicted in **Figure 26–4**.

▶ Treatment

General Approach ⑧ *Diagnosis and management of bone disease in CKD is based on corrected serum levels of calcium and phosphorus, and intact PTH levels (iPTH).*[50] In general, calcium, phosphorus, and PTH levels should be maintained in the normal range for all stages of CKD. For patients receiving dialysis, it is often difficult to achieve normal serum levels for these parameters. Attempts should be made to maintain calcium and phosphorus levels as close to normal as possible, but levels slightly above the normal range are acceptable in most cases. Target ranges for the various parameters are listed in **Table 26–5**.

The primary target for treatment is control of serum phosphorus levels because this is the initial parameter that disrupts homeostasis. However, serum phosphorus can be difficult to control, particularly in the latter stages of CKD. Management of sHPT often requires supplemental treatment with vitamin D analogs or cinacalcet in addition to phosphorus management.

Nonpharmacologic Therapy The first-line treatment for the management of hyperphosphatemia is dietary phosphorus restriction to 800 to 1,000 mg/day in patients with stage 3 CKD or higher who have phosphorus levels at the upper limit of the normal range or elevated iPTH levels.[50,51] Foods high in phosphorus are also high in protein, which can make it difficult to restrict phosphorus intake while maintaining adequate protein intake to avoid malnutrition. Hemodialysis and peritoneal dialysis can remove up to 2 to 3 g of phosphorus per week. However, this is insufficient to control hyperphosphatemia, and pharmacologic therapy is necessary in addition to dialysis treatment.

Other nonpharmacologic strategies to manage sHPT and CKD-MBD include restriction of aluminum exposure and parathyroidectomy. Chronic ingestion of aluminum-containing antacids and other aluminum-containing products should be avoided in patients with stage 4 CKD or higher (GFR less than 30 mL/min/1.73 m² [0.29 mL/s/m²]) because of the risk of aluminum toxicity and potential uptake into the bone. Purification techniques for dialysate solutions also minimize the risk of exposure to aluminum.

Parathyroidectomy is a treatment of last resort for sHPT, but should be considered in patients with persistently elevated iPTH levels above 800 pg/mL (800 ng/L; 85.6 pmol/L) that is refractory to medical therapy to lower serum calcium and/or phosphorus levels.[50] A portion or all of the parathyroid tissue may be removed, and in some cases

Clinical Presentation and Diagnosis of sHPT and ROD

General

Onset of sHPT and ROD is subtle and may not be associated with symptoms.

Symptoms

sHPT and ROD are usually asymptomatic in early disease. Calcification in the joints can be associated with decreased range of motion.

Conjunctival calcifications are associated with a gritty sensation in the eyes, redness, and inflammation.

Signs

Cardiovascular: Increased stroke index, heart rate, and diastolic and mean arterial pressures.

Musculoskeletal: Bone pain, muscle weakness.

Dermatologic: Pruritus.

Laboratory Tests

Increased serum phosphorus levels.

Low to normal serum calcium levels.

Increased Ca–P product.

Increased PTH levels.

Decreased vitamin D levels.

Diagnostic Tests

Radiographic studies show calcium–phosphate deposits in joints and/or cardiovascular system.

Bone biopsy of the iliac crest.

a portion of the parathyroid tissue may be transplanted into another site, usually the forearm for easy surgical access. After parathyroidectomy, serum calcium levels can decrease dramatically due to the low levels of PTH after the parathyroid tissue is removed, which decreases intestinal calcium absorption and bone resorption. Therefore, serum ionized calcium levels should be monitored frequently (every 4 to 6 hours for the first 48 to 72 hours) in patients receiving a parathyroidectomy. Calcium supplementation is usually necessary, administered IV initially, then orally (with vitamin D supplementation) once normal calcium levels are attained for several weeks to months after the procedure.

Table 26–5

Target Levels for Calcium, Phosphorus, and Intact PTH

Parameter	Guideline	Stage 3–4 CKD	Stage 5 CKD	Stage 5 CKD on dialysis
Corrected Calcium	KDOQI (2003)	"Normal"	8.4–9.5 mg/dL (2.1–2.38 mmol/L)	8.4–9.5 mg/dL (2.1–2.38 mmol/L)
	KDIGO (2009)	"Normal"	"Normal"	"Normal"
Phosphorus	KDOQI	2.7–4.6 mg/dL (0.87–1.49 mmol/L)	3.5–5 mg/dL (1.13–1.62 mmol/L)	3.5–5 mg/dL (1.13–1.62 mmol/L)
	KDIGO	"Normal"	"Normal"	"Near normal"
Ca–P Product	KDOQI	Less than 55 mg²/dL² (less than 4.44 mmol²/L²)	Less than 55 mg²/dL² (less than 4.44 mmol²/L²)	Less than 55 mg²/dL² (less than 4.44 mmol²/L²)
	KDIGO	Not recommended to use this parameter	Not recommended to use this parameter	Not recommended to use this parameter
Intact PTH	KDOQI	35–70 pg/mL[a] (3.7–7.5 pmol/L)	70–100 pg/mL (7.5–10.7 pmol/L)	150–300 pg/mL (16.0–32.1 pmol/L)
	KDIGO	"Normal"	"Normal"	2–9 times normal

PTH, parathyroid hormone; CKD, chronic kidney disease; KDOQI, Kidney Disease Outcomes Quality Initiative; KDIGO, Kidney Disease: Improving Global Outcomes; Ca–P, calcium–phosphorus product.

[a]Units of pg/mL are equivalent to ng/L

Pharmacologic Therapy

● *Phosphate-Binding Agents.* When serum phosphorus levels cannot be controlled by restriction of dietary intake, phosphate-binding agents are used to bind dietary phosphate in the GI tract to form an insoluble complex that is excreted in the feces. Phosphorus absorption is decreased, thereby decreasing serum phosphorus levels. The drugs used for binding dietary phosphate are listed in Table 26–6. These agents should be administered with each meal and can be tailored to the amount of phosphorus that is typically ingested during each meal. For example, patients can take a smaller dose with smaller meals or snacks, and a larger dose with larger meals. Although phosphate binders are not FDA approved for patients with CKD who are not receiving dialysis, they are used clinically when phosphorus levels are elevated, regardless of the stage of CKD.

Calcium-based phosphate binders, including calcium carbonate and calcium acetate, are effective in decreasing serum phosphate levels, as well as in increasing serum calcium levels. Calcium acetate binds more phosphorus than the carbonate salt, making it a more potent agent for binding dietary phosphate. Calcium citrate is usually not used as a phosphate-binding agent because the citrate salt can increase aluminum absorption. The calcium-containing phosphate binders also aid in the correction of metabolic acidosis, another complication of kidney failure. Calcium-based phosphate binders should not be used if serum calcium levels are near the upper end of the normal range or are elevated, if arterial calcifications are present, or if the patient

● has adynamic bone disease.[50] The dose of calcium-based phosphate binders should not provide more than 1,500 mg of elemental calcium per day, and the total elemental calcium intake per day should not exceed 2,000 mg including medication and dietary intake.[51] The most common adverse effects of calcium-containing phosphate binders are constipation and hypercalcemia.

Aluminum- and magnesium-containing phosphate-binding agents are not recommended for chronic use in patients with CKD to avoid aluminum and magnesium accumulation.

● Aluminum-containing agents may be used for a short course of therapy (less than 4 weeks) if phosphorus levels are significantly elevated greater than 7 mg/dL (2.26 mmol/L), but should be replaced by other phosphate-binding agents after no more than 4 weeks. Excessive aluminum levels lead to aluminum intoxication, causing neurotoxicity that can manifest as encephalopathy or dementia, bone disease, and anemia. In addition to the risk of magnesium accumulation, the use of magnesium-containing agents is also limited by the GI side effects, primarily diarrhea.

● Phosphate-binding agents that do not contain calcium, magnesium, or aluminum include sevelamer hydrochloride, sevelamer carbonate, and lanthanum carbonate. These agents are particularly useful in patients with hyperphosphatemia who have elevated serum calcium levels or who have vascular or soft tissue calcifications. Sevelamer is a cationic polymer that is not systemically absorbed and binds to phosphate in the GI tract, and it prevents absorption and promotes

excretion of phosphate through the GI tract via the feces. Sevelamer has an added benefit of reducing LDL-C by up to 30% and increasing HDL-C levels.[51] The most common side effects of sevelamer are GI complaints including nausea, constipation, and diarrhea. The cost of sevelamer is significantly higher compared with calcium-containing phosphate binders, which often makes sevelamer a second-line agent for controlling phosphorus levels. However, recent studies have demonstrated that sevelamer may decrease mortality in patients receiving hemodialysis compared with calcium-containing phosphate binders, primarily by decreasing the occurrence of calcifications in the coronary arteries.[50] Sevelamer carbonate may have added benefit to aid in the correction of metabolic acidosis.

Lanthanum is a naturally occurring trivalent rare earth element (atomic number 57). Lanthanum carbonate quickly dissociates in the acidic environment of the stomach, where the lanthanum ion binds to dietary phosphorus, forming an insoluble compound that is excreted in the feces. Lanthanum has been shown to be as effective as other phosphate binders and may improve bone turnover, compared with calcium-containing products.[50] Side effects of lanthanum include nausea, peripheral edema, and myalgias.

Vitamin D Therapy. Exogenous vitamin D compounds that mimic the activity of calcitriol act directly on the parathyroid gland to decrease PTH secretion. This is particularly useful when reduction of serum phosphorus levels does not sufficiently reduce PTH levels. The most active form of vitamin D is calcitriol (1,25-dihydroxyvitamin D). The effects of calcitriol are mediated by upregulation of the vitamin D receptor in the parathyroid gland, which decreases parathyroid gland hyperplasia and PTH synthesis and secretion.

● Vitamin D supplementation (Table 26–7) can be used to lower serum PTH levels in patients with CKD. Ergocalciferol and cholecalciferol have been shown to be effective in lowering PTH secretion in patients with stage 3 CKD.[52] However, as CKD progresses to stages 4 and 5, the kidney loses the ability to produce 1α-hydroxylase, which is responsible for renal activation of vitamin D. In these later stages of CKD, activated vitamin D analogs must be used to decrease PTH secretion. Calcitriol (1,25-dihydroxyvitamin D_3, Rocaltrol by Roche Laboratories, Inc., Nutley, NJ, and Calcijex by Abbott Laboratories, North Chicago, IL). This analog has the same biologic activity as endogenous calcitriol. Doxercalciferol (1-α-hydroxyvitamin D_2) is another vitamin D analog that is hydroxylated in the liver to 1,25-dihydroxyvitamin D_2, which has the same biologic activity as calcitriol. Both calcitriol and doxercalciferol upregulate vitamin D receptors in the intestines, which increases calcium and phosphorus absorption, increasing the risk of hypercalcemia and hyperphosphatemia. It is important that serum calcium and phosphorus levels are within the normal range for the stage of CKD prior to starting either of these therapies. Paricalcitol (19-nor-1,25-dihydroxyvitamin D_2, Zemplar by Abbott Laboratories, North Chicago, IL) is a vitamin D analog that has equal efficacy to calcitriol but may cause

Table 26–6

Phosphate-Binding Agents Used in the Treatment of Hyperphosphatemia in CKD

Compound	Trade Name	Dosage Form	Compound Content (mg)	Elemental Calcium Content (mg)	Starting Dose	Comments
Calcium carbonate (40% elemental calcium)	Tums	Chewable tablet	500, 750, 1,000; 1,250	200, 300, 400, 500	0.5–1 g (elemental calcium) three times a day with meals	First-line agent; dissolution characteristics and phosphorus-binding effect may vary from product to product; try to limit daily intake of elemental calcium to 1,500 mg/day
	Oscal-500	Tablet	1,250	500		
	Caltrate 600	Tablet	1,500	600		
	Nephro Calci	Tablet	1,500	600		
	LiquiCal	Liquid gelcap	1,200	480		
	Calci-Chew	Chewable tablet	1,250	500		Approximately 39 mg phosphorus bound per 1 g calcium carbonate
Calcium acetate (25% elemental calcium)	Phos-Lo	Tablet	667	167	0.5–1 g (elemental calcium) three times a day with meals	First-line agent; comparable efficacy to calcium carbonate with one-half the dose of elemental calcium; do not exceed 1,500 mg elemental calcium intake per day
	Phoslyra	Suspension	667/5 mL			Approximately 45 mg phosphorus bound per 1 g calcium acetate
						By prescription only
Sevelamer HCl	Renagel	Tablet	400, 800	—	800 mg three times a day with meals	First-line agent; lowers LDL-C
Sevelamer carbonate	Renvela	Tablet	800			More expensive than calcium products; preferred in patients at risk for extraskeletal calcification
						May require large doses to control phosphorus levels
Lanthanum	Fosrenol	Chewable tablet	250, 500	—	750–1,500 mg three times a day with meals	Second-line agent; more expensive than calcium products; preferred in patients at risk for extraskeletal calcification
						Most patients require 1,500–3,000 mg/day to control phosphorus
Aluminum hydroxide	AlternaGEL	Suspension	600 mg/5 mL	—	300–600 mg three times a day with meals	Third-line agents; do not use concurrently with citrate-containing products
	Amphojel	Tablet	300, 600			
	Alu-Cap, Alu-Tab	Suspension Capsule, Tablet	320 mg/5 mL 400			Reserve for short-term use (4 weeks) in patients with hyperphosphatemia not responding to other binders
Aluminum carbonate	Basaljel	Tablet, capsule	500	—	450–500 mg three times a day with meals	Same as for aluminum hydroxide
		Suspension	400 mg/5 mL			
Magnesium carbonate	Mag-Carb	Capsule	70	—	70 mg three times a day with meals	Third-line agent; diarrhea common; monitor serum magnesium
Magnesium hydroxide	Milk of magnesia	Tablet Suspension	300, 600 400 mg/5 mL, 800 mg/5 mL	—	300–400 mg three times a day with meals	Same as for magnesium carbonate
Magnesium carbonate/ calcium carbonate	MagneBind 400	Tablet	400 mg (elemental magnesium)	80	400 mg three times a day with meals	Same as for calcium carbonate and magnesium carbonate

LDL-C, low-density lipoprotein cholesterol

Table 26–7

Available Treatments for Secondary Hyperparathyroidism

Generic Name	Trade Name	Dosage Range	Dosage Forms	Frequency of Administration
Vitamin D precursor				
Ergocalciferol	Vitamin D$_2$	400–50,000 IU	PO	Daily (doses of 400–2000 IU)
Cholecalciferol	Vitamin D$_3$			Weekly or monthly for higher doses (50,000 IU)
Active vitamin D				
Calcitriol	Calcijex	0.5–5 mcg	IV	Three times per week
	Rocaltrol	0.25–5 mcg	PO	Daily, every other day, or three times per week
Vitamin D analogs				
Paricalcitol	Zemplar	1–4 mcg	PO	Daily or three times per week
		2.5–15 mcg	IV	Three times per week
Doxercalciferol	Hectorol	5–20 mcg	PO	Daily or three times per week
		2–8 mcg	IV	Three times per week
Calcimimetics				
Cinacalcet	Sensipar	30–180 mg	PO	Daily

less hypercalcemia. Alfacalcidol (1-α-hydroxyvitamin D$_3$), falecalcitriol, and 22-oxacalcitriol (maxacalcitol) are only available outside the United States.

It is important to monitor vitamin D therapy aggressively to assure that PTH levels are not oversuppressed. Oversuppression of PTH levels can induce adynamic bone disease, which manifests as decreased osteoblast and osteoclast activity, decreased bone formation, and low bone turnover.

● **Calcimimetics** Cinacalcet is a calcimimetic that increases the sensitivity of receptors on the parathyroid gland to serum calcium levels to reduce PTH secretion. In addition to lowering PTH levels, cinacalcet has been shown to reduce serum calcium levels by approximately 5% and serum

phosphorus levels by 2.6% to 8.4%.[53] This makes cinacalcet beneficial to use in patients with elevated PTH levels who have an increased calcium or phosphorus levels or cannot use vitamin D therapy. Because the effects of cinacalcet on PTH can reduce serum calcium levels and result in hypocalcemia, cinacalcet should not be used if serum calcium levels are below 8.4 mg/dL (2.1 mmol/L). Cinacalcet should also be used with caution in patients with seizure disorders because low serum calcium levels can lower the seizure threshold.[53]

● **Reversal of Metabolic Acidosis** Studies have demonstrated that reversal of metabolic acidosis can improve bone disease associated with CKD.[49] Serum bicarbonate levels should be maintained at 22 mEq/L (22 mmol/L) in patients

Patient Encounter 3

A 62 year-old African American woman with a history of type 2 diabetes mellitus presents to your clinic for a routine follow-up. She has no complaints at this time.

Current meds: Pioglitazone 30 mg orally daily; glipizide 5 mg orally twice daily; fosinopril 40 mg orally daily; amlodipine 10 mg orally daily; furosemide 60 mg orally daily; ferrous sulfate 325 mg orally three times daily

ROS: Unremarkable.

PE:

VS: BP 142/92 mm Hg; P 72 bpm; T 98.4°F (36.9°C); ht 5′4″ (163 cm); wt 164 lb (74.5 kg)

CV: RRR, normal S$_1$, S$_2$

Abd: Obese; no organomegaly, bruits, tenderness; (+) bowel sounds; heme (−) stool

Ext: 2+ edema bilaterally; lesion on L foot appears to be healing slowly; decreased sensation in LE

Labs: Sodium 143 mEq/L (143 mmol/L); potassium 5.1 mEq/L (5.1 mmol/L); chloride 101 mEq/L (101 mmol/L); carbon dioxide 17 mEq/L (17 mmol/L); BUN 38 mg/dL (13.6 mmol/L urea); SCr 2.4 mg/dL (212 μmol/L); glucose 156 mg/dL (8.7 mmol/L); calcium 8.4 mg/dL 2.1 mmol/L); phosphate 7.9 mg/dL (2.55 mmol/L); albumin 3.2 g/dL (32 g/L); intact parathyroid hormone (iPTH) 478 pg/mL (478 ng/L; 51.1 pmol/L); WBC 4.8 × 10^3 cells/mm^3 (4.8 × 10^9/L); RBC 3.7 × 10^6 cells/mm^3 (3.7 × 10^{12}/L); Hgb 10.4 g/dL (104 g/L; 6.46 mmol/L); Hct 31% (0.31); platelets 350 × 10^3 cells/mm^3 (350 × 10^9/L)

What signs are consistent with secondary hyperparathyroidism (sHPT)?

What treatment would you recommend for sHPT?

with bone disease associated with CKD.[51] The treatment of metabolic acidosis is described later.

▶ Outcome Evaluation

● Monitor serum calcium and phosphorus levels regularly in patients receiving phosphate-binding agents. When initiating therapy, monitor serum levels every 1 to 4 weeks, depending on the severity of hyperphosphatemia. Titrate doses of phosphate binders to achieve the target levels of serum calcium and phosphorus and iPTH (Table 26–5). Once target levels are achieved, monitor serum calcium and phosphorus levels every 1 to 3 months. Monitor intact PTH levels monthly while initiating vitamin D therapy, then every 3 months once stable iPTH levels are achieved. When starting or increasing the dose of cinacalcet, monitor serum calcium and phosphorus levels within 1 week; iPTH levels should be monitored within 1 to 4 weeks. Once target levels are achieved, decrease monitoring to every 3 months.

Metabolic Acidosis

▶ Epidemiology and Etiology

Approximately 80% of patients with a GFR less than 20 to 30 mL/min/1.73 m² (0.19 to 0.29 mL/s/m²) develop metabolic acidosis.[49] Metabolic acidosis can increase protein catabolism and decrease albumin synthesis, which promote muscle wasting and alter bone metabolism. Other consequences associated with metabolic acidosis in CKD include worsening cardiac disease, impaired glucose tolerance, altered growth hormone and thyroid function, and inflammation.[49]

▶ Pathophysiology

The kidney plays a key role in the management of acid–base homeostasis in the body by regulating excretion of hydrogen ions. With normal kidney function, bicarbonate that is freely filtered through the glomerulus is completely reabsorbed via the renal tubules. Hydrogen ions are generated at a rate of 1 mEq/kg (1 mmol/kg) per day during metabolism of ingested food and are excreted at the same rate by the kidney via buffers in the urine created by ammonia generation and phosphate excretion. As a result, the pH of body fluids is maintained within a very narrow range.

As kidney function declines, bicarbonate reabsorption is maintained, but hydrogen excretion is decreased because the ability of the kidney to generate ammonia is impaired. The positive hydrogen balance leads to metabolic acidosis, which is characterized by a serum bicarbonate level of 15 to 20 mEq/L (15 to 20 mmol/L), resulting in a pH less than 7.35. This picture is generally seen when the GFR declines below 20 to 30 mL/min/1.73 m² (0.19 to 0.29 mL/s/m²).[49]

▶ Treatment

● Serum electrolytes should be monitored in patients with CKD for the development of metabolic acidosis. Metabolic acidosis in patients with CKD is generally characterized by

an elevated anion gap greater than 17 mEq/L (17 mmol/L), due to the accumulation of phosphate, sulfate, and other organic anions.

Nonpharmacologic Therapy Treatment of metabolic acidosis in CKD requires pharmacologic therapy. Other disorders that may contribute to metabolic acidosis should also be addressed. Altering bicarbonate levels in the dialysate fluid in patients receiving dialysis may assist with the treatment of metabolic acidosis, although pharmacologic therapy may still be required.

● **Pharmacologic Therapy** Pharmacologic therapy with sodium bicarbonate or citrate/citric acid preparations may be needed in patients with stage 3 CKD or higher to replenish body stores of bicarbonate. Calcium carbonate and calcium acetate, used to bind phosphorus in sHPT, also aid in increasing serum bicarbonate levels, in conjunction with other agents.

Sodium bicarbonate tablets are administered in increments of 325- and 650-mg tablets. A 650-mg tablet of sodium bicarbonate contains 7.7 mEq (7.7 mmol) each of sodium and bicarbonate. Sodium retention associated with sodium bicarbonate can cause volume overload, which can exacerbate hypertension and chronic heart failure. Patient tolerability of sodium bicarbonate is low because of carbon dioxide production in the GI tract that occurs during dissolution.

Solutions that contain sodium citrate/citric acid (Shohl's solution and Bicitra) provide 1 mEq/L (1 mmol/L) each of sodium and bicarbonate. Polycitra is a sodium/potassium citrate solution that provides 2 mEq/L (2 mmol/L) of bicarbonate but contains 1 mEq/L (1 mmol/L) each of sodium and potassium, which can promote hyperkalemia in patients with severe CKD. The citrate portion of these preparations is metabolized in the liver to bicarbonate; the citric acid portion is metabolized to CO_2 and water, increasing tolerability compared with sodium bicarbonate. Sodium retention is also decreased with these preparations. However, these products are liquid preparations, which may not be palatable to some patients. Citrate can also promote aluminum intoxication by augmenting aluminum absorption in the GI tract.

● When determining the dose of bicarbonate replacement, the goal for therapy is to achieve a normal serum bicarbonate level of 24 mEq/L (24 mmol/L). The dose is usually determined by calculating the base deficit: [0.5 L/kg × (body weight)] × [(normal CO_2) – (measured CO_2)]. Because of the risk of volume overload resulting from the sodium load administered with bicarbonate replacement, the total base deficit should be administered over several days. Once the goal serum bicarbonate level is attained, a maintenance dose of bicarbonate is necessary and should be titrated to maintain serum bicarbonate levels.

▶ Outcome Evaluation

● Monitor serum electrolytes and arterial blood gases regularly. Correct metabolic acidosis slowly to prevent the development of metabolic alkalosis or other electrolyte abnormalities.

Other Therapeutic Considerations in CKD

▶ Uremic Bleeding

Uremia can lead to a number of alterations in clotting ability, resulting in hemorrhage. Bleeding complications associated with CKD include ecchymoses, prolonged bleeding from mucous membranes and puncture sites used for blood collection and hemodialysis, GI bleeding, intramuscular bleeding, and others. Most bleeding complications associated with CKD are mild. However, serious bleeding events including GI bleeds and intracranial hemorrhage can occur.

Pathophysiology Uremia alters a number of mechanisms that contribute to bleeding. Platelet function and aggregation are altered through decreased production of thromboxane.[54] Platelet–vessel wall interactions are also altered in patients with uremia because of decreased activity of von Willebrand's factor[54] and are exacerbated by anemia in CKD patients. With a normal RBC count in the plasma, platelets skim the surface of the endothelial tissue in the blood vessels. In patients with anemia, RBC count is decreased and platelets circulate closer to the center of the vessels, which decreases the interaction with the vessel wall. The risk of bleeding is increased in patients receiving hemodialysis. Medications administered to prevent or treat clotting during hemodialysis or in vascular access sites, including heparin, warfarin, aspirin, and clopidogrel, exacerbate the risk of bleeding in these patients.

Treatment

Nonpharmacologic Therapy. The incidence and severity of bleeding associated with uremia has decreased since dialysis has become the mainstay of treatment for ESKD. Dialysis initiation improves platelet function and reduces bleeding time.[54] Improved care of the patient with ESKD, with anemia treatment and improvement in nutritional status, are also likely contributors to decreased uremic bleeding.

Pharmacologic Therapy. Treatments used to decrease bleeding time in patients with uremic bleeding include cryoprecipitate, which contains various components important in platelet aggregation and clotting, such as von Willebrand's factor and fibrinogen. Cryoprecipitate decreases bleeding time within 1 hour in 50% of patients. However, cost and the risk of infection have limited the use of cryoprecipitate.

Desmopressin (DDAVP) increases the release of factor VIII (von Willebrand's factor) from endothelial tissue in the vessel wall. Bleeding time is promptly reduced, within 1 hour of administration, and is sustained for 4 to 8 hours.[54] Doses used for uremic bleeding are 0.3 to 0.4 mcg/kg IV over 20 to 30 minutes, 0.3 mcg/kg subcutaneously, or 2 to 3 mcg/kg intranasally. Repeated doses can cause tachyphylaxis by depleting stores of von Willebrand's factor. Side effects of DDAVP include flushing, dizziness, and headache.

Estrogens have also been used to decrease bleeding time. The onset of action is slower than that of DDAVP, but more sustained, and it depends on the route of administration. IV doses of 0.6 mg/kg/day for 4 to 5 days decreases bleeding time within 6 hours of administration, and produces an effect that lasts up to 2 weeks after stopping therapy. The onset of action with oral doses of 50 mg/kg daily is within 2 days of treatment and is sustained for 4 to 5 days after stopping therapy. Transdermal patches providing 50 to 100 mcg/day have also been shown to be effective in decreasing bleeding time.[54] Side effects of estrogen use include hot flashes in both females and males, fluid retention, and hypertension.

▶ Pruritus

Pruritus can affect 25% to 86% of patients with advanced stages of CKD, and it is not related to the cause of kidney failure.[55] Pruritus can be significant and has been linked to mortality in patients receiving hemodialysis.[55]

Pathophysiology The cause of pruritus is unknown, although several mechanisms have been proposed. Vitamin A is known to accumulate in the skin and serum of patients with CKD, but a definite correlation with pruritus has not been established. Histamine may also play a role in the development of pruritus, which may be linked to mast cell proliferation in patients receiving hemodialysis. Hyperparathyroidism has also been suggested as a contributor to pruritus, despite the fact that serum PTH levels do not correlate with itching. Accumulation of divalent ions, specifically magnesium and aluminum, may also play a role in pruritus in patients with CKD. Other theories that have been proposed include inadequate dialysis, dry skin, peripheral neuropathy, calcium-phosphate deposits, and opiate accumulation.[55]

Treatment

Nonpharmacologic Therapy. Pruritus associated with CKD is difficult to alleviate. It is important to evaluate other potential dermatologic causes of pruritus to maximize the potential for relief. Adequate dialysis is generally the first line of treatment in patients with pruritus. However, this has not been shown to decrease the incidence of pruritus significantly. Maintaining proper nutritional intake, especially with regard to dietary phosphorus and protein intake, may lessen the degree or occurrence of pruritus. Patients who do not attain relief from other measures may benefit from ultraviolet B phototherapy.

Pharmacologic Therapy. Topical emollients have been used as treatment for pruritus in patients with dry skin, but they are often not effective in relieving pruritus associated with CKD. Antihistamines, such as hydroxyzine 25 to 50 mg or diphenhydramine 25 to 50 mg orally or IV, are used as first-line oral agents used to treat pruritus. Cholestyramine has also been used at doses of 5 g twice daily. Oral activated charcoal has also been used in doses of 1 to 1.5 g four times daily with some demonstrated efficacy. Gabapentin has also been shown to be effective, but it must be used with caution in patients with CKD to minimize risk of neurotoxicity. Other therapies that are often used in combination with other agents include oral serotonin reuptake inhibitors, ondansetron, and naloxone and topical capsaicin. Each has been reported to have efficacy in the treatment of pruritus associated with CKD.[55]

Vitamin Replacement

Water-soluble vitamins removed by hemodialysis (HD) contribute to malnutrition and vitamin deficiency syndromes. Patients receiving HD often require replacement of water-soluble vitamins to prevent adverse effects. The vitamins that may require replacement are ascorbic acid, thiamine, biotin, folic acid, riboflavin, and pyridoxine. Patients receiving HD should receive a multivitamin B complex with vitamin C supplement, but they should not take supplements that include fat-soluble vitamins, such as vitamins A, E, or K, which can accumulate in patients with kidney failure.

RENAL REPLACEMENT THERAPY

Patients who progress to ESKD require RRT. The modalities that are used for RRT are dialysis, including HD and peritoneal dialysis (PD), and kidney transplantation. The United States Renal Data Service (USRDS) reported that the number of patients with ESKD was 613,432, with 116,395 new cases diagnosed in 2009.[4] Kidney transplantation is the preferred method of RRT, owing to improved patient survival. The 3-year survival of patients with ESKD is 81% for kidney transplantation, compared with only 50% for dialysis.[4] However, organ availability limits the number of patients who can receive a kidney transplant. Only 2% of patients with newly diagnosed ESKD receive kidney transplants each year.[4] Therefore, the most common form of RRT is dialysis, accounting for 70% of all patients with ESKD.[4] The principles and complications associated with dialysis are discussed later. Chapter 55 discusses the principles of kidney transplantation.

Indications for Dialysis

9 *Planning for dialysis should begin when GFR falls less than 30 mL/min/1.73 m² (0.29 mL/s/m²) (stage 4 CKD),[1] when progression to ESKD is inevitable, to allow time to educate the patient and family on the treatment modalities and establish the appropriate access for the modality of choice.* Ideally, initiation of dialysis should be done at a point when the patient is ready to undergo treatment, rather than when the patient is in emergent need of dialysis.

Initiation of dialysis depends on the patient's clinical status and not based on laboratory values. Symptoms that may indicate the need for dialysis include persistent anorexia, nausea, vomiting, fatigue, and pruritus. Other criteria that indicate the need for dialysis include declining nutritional status, declining serum albumin levels, uncontrolled hypertension, and volume overload, which may manifest as chronic heart failure, and electrolyte abnormalities, particularly hyperkalemia. **Blood urea nitrogen** (BUN) and SCr levels may be used as a guide for the initiation of dialysis, but they should not be the absolute indicator. Dialysis is initiated in most patients

---

Table 26–8

Advantages and Disadvantages of Hemodialysis

Advantages
1. Higher solute clearance allows intermittent treatment
2. Parameters of adequacy of dialysis are better defined and therefore underdialysis can be detected early
3. The technique's failure rate is low
4. Even though intermittent heparinization is required, hemostasis parameters are better corrected with hemodialysis than peritoneal dialysis
5. In-center hemodialysis enables closer monitoring of the patient

Disadvantages
1. Requires multiple visits each week to the hemodialysis center, which translates into loss of control by the patient
2. Dysequilibrium, dialysis, hypotension, and muscle cramps are common. May require months before patient adjusts to hemodialysis
3. Infections in hemodialysis patients may be related to the choice of membranes; the complement-activating membranes are more deleterious
4. Vascular access is frequently associated with infection and thrombosis
5. Decline of residual renal function is more rapid compared with peritoneal dialysis

From Sowinski KM, Churchwell MD. Hemodialysis and peritoneal dialysis. In: DiPiro JT, Talbert RL, Yee GC, et al., eds. Pharmacotherapy: A Pathophysiologic Approach, 8th ed. New York, NY: McGraw-Hill, 2011:O338, with permission.

---

when the GFR falls below 15 mL/min/1.73 m² (0.14 mL/s/m²).[1] Patients should determine which modality of dialysis to use based on their own preferences. Advantages and disadvantages of hemodialysis and peritoneal dialysis are listed in Tables 26–8 and 26–9, respectively.

The goals of dialysis are to remove toxic metabolites to decrease uremic symptoms, correct electrolyte abnormalities, restore acid–base status, and maintain volume status to ultimately improve quality of life and decrease the morbidity and mortality associated with ESKD.

Hemodialysis

Hemodialysis is the most common method of RRT, initiated in 91% of patients with newly diagnosed ESKD each year, with a total of 370,264 patients receiving HD in 2009.[4] Home HD is becoming increasingly more popular, but most patients continue to receive HD from a dialysis center.

▶ Principles of Hemodialysis

10 *Hemodialysis involves the exposure of blood to a semipermeable membrane (dialyzer) against which a physiologic solution (dialysate) is flowing (Fig. 26–5).* The dialyzer is composed of thousands of capillary fibers made up of the semipermeable membrane, which are enclosed in the dialyzer, to increase the surface area of blood exposure to maximize the efficiency of removing substances. The

Table 26–9

Advantages and Disadvantages of Peritoneal Dialysis

Advantages

1. More hemodynamic stability (blood pressure) due to slow ultrafiltration rate
2. Increased clearance of larger solutes, which may explain good clinical status in spite of lower urea clearance
3. Better preservation of residual renal function
4. Convenient intraperitoneal route of administration of drugs such as antibiotics and insulin
5. Suitable for elderly and very young patients who may not tolerate hemodialysis well
6. Freedom from the "machine" gives the patient a sense of independence (for continuous ambulatory peritoneal dialysis)
7. Less blood loss and iron deficiency, resulting in easier management of anemia or reduced requirements for erythropoietin and parenteral iron
8. No systemic heparinization requirement
9. Subcutaneous versus IV erythropoietin or darbepoetin is usual, which may reduce overall doses and be more physiologic

Disadvantages

1. Protein and amino acid losses through the peritoneum and reduced appetite owing to continuous glucose load and sense of abdominal fullness predispose to malnutrition
2. Risk of peritonitis
3. Catheter malfunction, and exit site and tunnel infection
4. Inadequate ultrafiltration and solute dialysis in patients with a large body size, unless large volumes and frequent exchanges are employed
5. Patient burnout and high rate of technique failure
6. Risk of obesity with excessive glucose absorption
7. Mechanical problems such as hernias, dialysate leaks, hemorrhoids, or back pain may occur
8. Extensive abdominal surgery may preclude peritoneal dialysis
9. No convenient access for IV iron administration

From Sowinski KM, Churchwell MD. Hemodialysis and peritoneal dialysis. In: DiPiro JT, Talbert RL, Yee GC, et al., eds. Pharmacotherapy: A Pathophysiologic Approach, 8th ed. New York, NY: McGraw-Hill, 2011:O339, with permission.

dialysate is composed of purified water and electrolytes, and it is run through the dialyzer countercurrent to the blood on the other side of the semipermeable membrane. The process allows for the removal of several substances from the bloodstream, including water, urea, creatinine, electrolytes, uremic toxins, and drugs. Sterilization is not required for dialysate because the membrane prevents bacteria from entering into the bloodstream. However, if the membrane ruptures during hemodialysis, infection becomes a major concern for the patient.

Three types of membranes used for dialysis are classified by the size of the pores and the ability to remove solutes from the bloodstream:

- Conventional (standard) membranes have small pores, which limit solute removal to relatively small molecules, such as creatinine and urea.
- High-efficiency membranes also have small pores but have a higher surface area that increases removal of small molecules, such as water, urea, and creatinine from the blood.
- High-flux membranes have larger pores that allow for the removal of substances with higher molecular-weight, including some drugs, such as vancomycin, than conventional membranes.

Three primary processes are utilized for the removal of substances from the blood:

- Diffusion is the movement of a solute across the dialyzer membrane from an area of higher concentration (usually the blood) to a lower concentration (usually the dialysate). This process is the primary means for small molecules, such as electrolytes, to be removed from the bloodstream. At times, solutes can be added to the dialysate that are diffused into the bloodstream. Changing the composition of the dialysate allows for control of the amount of electrolytes that are being removed.

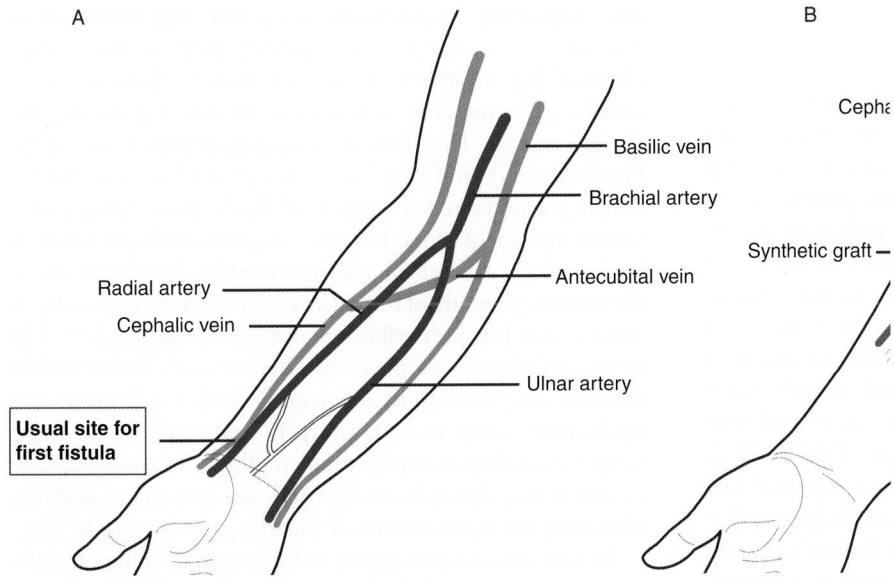

A

- Basilic vein
- Brachial artery
- Antecubital vein
- Radial artery
- Cephalic vein
- Ulnar artery

Usual site for first fistula

B

Cepha

Synthetic graft

FIGURE 26–5. In hemodialysis, the patient's blood is pumped to the dialyzer at a rate of 300 to 600 mL/min. An anticoagulant (usually heparin) is administered to prevent clotting in the dialyzer. The dialysate is pumped at the rate of 500 to 1,000 mL/min through the dialyzer countercurrent to the flow of blood. The rate of fluid removal from the patient is controlled by adjusting the pressure in the dialysate compartment. (From Foote EF, Manley HJ. Hemodialysis and peritoneal dialysis. In: DiPiro JT, Talbert RL, Yee GC, et al., eds. Pharmacotherapy: A Pathophysiologic Approach, 7th ed. New York, NY: McGraw-Hill, 2008:O106, with permission.)

Patient Encounter 4, Part 1

A 52 year-old white woman with a history of polycystic kidney disease (PCKD) presents to the clinic with complaints that she "feels awful." She hasn't felt like eating for several weeks and has lost 10 lb (4.51 kg) in the last 6 months.

Current medications: Valsartan 80 mg orally daily; atenolol 100 mg orally daily; furosemide 120 mg orally daily; sevelamer 800 mg orally three times a day; calcitriol 0.25 mcg orally daily; sodium bicarbonate 1,300 mg orally twice daily.

ROS: Lethargic female in mild distress.

PE:

VS: BP 190/118 mm Hg; P 88 bpm; T 98.6°F (37.0°C); ht 5′6″ (168 cm); wt 127 lb (57.7 kg)

CV: RRR, normal S_1, S_2, S_4 present; (+) pericardial friction rub

Ext: 4+ bilateral lower extremity edema present to midcalf line

Labs: Sodium 141 mEq/L (141 mmol/L); potassium 5.9 mEq/L (5.9 mmol/L); chloride 103 mEq/L (103 mmol/L); carbon dioxide 17 mEq/L (17 mmol/L); BUN 75 mg/dL (26.8 mmol/L); SCr 3.5 mg/dL (309 μmol/L); glucose 67 mg/dL (3.7 mmol/L); calcium 8.9 mg/dL (2.23 mmol/L); phosphate 6.2 mg/dL (2.00 mmol/L); iPTH 429 pg/mL (429 ng/L; 45.9 pmol/L); WBC 6.1×10^3 cells/mm^3 (6.1×10^9/L); RBC 3.5×10^6 cells/mm^3 (3.5×10^{12}/L); Hgb 11.4 g/dL (114 g/L; 7.08 mmol/L); Hct 35% (0.35); platelets 327×10^3 cells/mm^3 (327×10^9/L)

What indications does the patient have for dialysis?

What alternatives for renal replacement therapy exist for the patient?

What are the advantages and disadvantages of each modality for renal replacement?

- **Ultrafiltration** is the movement of solvent (plasma water) across the dialyzer membrane by applying hydrostatic or osmotic pressure, and it is the primary means for removing water from the bloodstream. Changing the hydrostatic pressure applied to the dialyzer or the osmotic concentration of the dialysate allows for control of the amount of water being removed.

- **Convection** is the movement of dissolved solutes across the dialyzer membrane by "dragging" the solutes along a pressure gradient with a fluid transport and is the primary means for larger molecules to be removed from the bloodstream, such as urea. Changing the pore size of the dialyzer membrane alters the efficiency of convection and allows for control of the amount of water removed in relation to the amount of solute being removed.

▶ Vascular Access

Long-term permanent access to the bloodstream is a key component of HD. There are three primary techniques used to obtain permanent vascular access in patients receiving HD: arteriovenous fistulas (AVFs), arteriovenous grafts (AVGs) and catheters. An AVF is the preferred access method because it has the longest survival rate and the fewest complications.[56] An AVF is made by creating an anastomosis between an artery and a vein, usually in the forearm of the nondominant arm (Fig. 26–6). An AVG results in a similar access site but uses a synthetic graft, usually made of polytetrafluoroethylene, to connect the artery and vein in the forearm (Fig. 26–6). The advantages of the AVG is that it is able to be used within 2 to 3 weeks, compared with 2 to 3 months for an AVF. However, AVGs are complicated by stenosis, thrombosis, and infections, which lead to a shorter survival time of the graft. Double-lumen venous catheters,

placed in the femoral, subclavian, or jugular vein, are often used as temporary access while waiting for the AVF or AVG to mature. The catheters are tunneled beneath the skin to an exit site to reduce the risk of infection. Venous catheters can also be used as permanent access in patients in whom arteriovenous access cannot be established.

▶ Complications of Hemodialysis

Complications associated with HD include hypotension, muscle cramping, thrombosis, and infection.

Hypotension Hypotension is the most common complication seen during hemodialysis. It has been reported to occur with approximately 10% to 30% of dialysis sessions but may be as frequent as 50% of sessions in some patients.[57]

Pathophysiology. Hypotension associated with hemodialysis manifests as a symptomatic sudden drop of more than 30 mm Hg in mean arterial or systolic pressure or a systolic pressure drop to less than 90 mm Hg during the dialysis session. The primary cause is fluid removal from the bloodstream. Ultrafiltration removes fluid from the plasma, which promotes redistribution of fluids from extracellular spaces into the plasma. However, decreased serum albumin levels and removal of solutes from the bloodstream decrease the osmotic pressure of the plasma relative to the extracellular spaces, slowing redistribution during hemodialysis.[58] The decreased plasma volume causes hypotension. Other factors that can contribute to hypotension include antihypertensive medications prior to HD, a target "dry weight" (the target weight after HD session is complete) that is too low, diastolic or autonomic dysfunction, low dialysate calcium or sodium, high dialysate temperature, or ingesting meals prior to HD.

Risk factors that may increase the potential for hypotension include elderly age, diabetes, autonomic neuropathy, uremia,

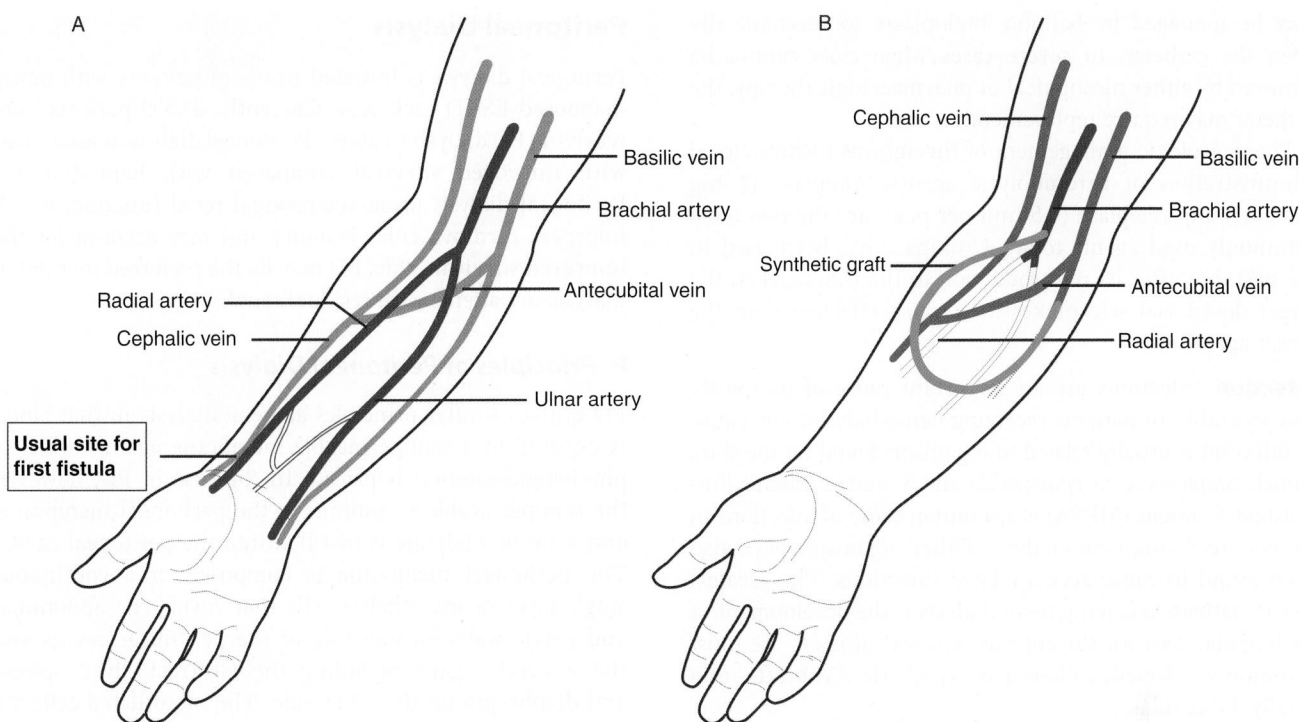

FIGURE 26–6. The predominant types of vascular access for chronic dialysis patients are (A) the arteriovenous fistula and (B) the synthetic arteriovenous forearm graft. The first primary arteriovenous fistula is usually created by the surgical anastomosis of the cephalic vein with the radial artery. The flow of blood from the higher-pressure arterial system results in hypertrophy of the vein. The most common AV graft (depicted in green) is between the brachial artery and the basilic or cephalic vein. The flow of blood may be diminished in the radial and ulnar arteries because it preferentially flows into the low pressure graft. (From Foote EF, Manley HJ. Hemodialysis and peritoneal dialysis. In: DiPiro JT, Talbert RL, Yee GC, et al., eds. Pharmacotherapy: A Pathophysiologic Approach, 7th ed. New York, NY: McGraw-Hill, 2008:O106, with permission.)

and cardiac disease.[57] The symptoms associated with hypotension during dialysis include dizziness, nausea, vomiting, sweating, and chest pain.

Treatment. Nonpharmacologic management of acute hypotension that occurs during dialysis involves placing the patient in the Trendelenburg position (with the head lower than the feet), decreasing the ultrafiltration rate, and cooling the dialysate. Pharmacologic management of acute hypotension during dialysis includes administration of normal saline (100 to 200 mL), hypertonic saline (23.4%, 10 to 20 mL), or mannitol (12.5 g) to restore intravascular volume.

Preventive measures for patients who may be prone to hypotension include accurate determination of the "dry weight" and maintaining a constant ultrafiltration rate. Midodrine is an α-adrenergic agonist that is effective in reducing hypotension in patients with autonomic dysfunction that is taken with each dialysis session or as chronic therapy. Midodrine can be administered at doses of 2.5 to 10 mg prior to HD or 5 mg twice daily for chronic hypotension. Side effects of midodrine include pruritus and paresthesias.

Hypotension may be related to alterations in levocarnitine levels during dialysis. Patients who have low levels of levocarnitine may benefit from supplementation. Levocarnitine is administered as doses of 20 mg/kg IV at the end of each dialysis session. However, levocarnitine should not be used as a first-line agent for the treatment of hypotension because of the significant cost associated with the treatment. Other preventive measures that have not been well studied include caffeine, sertraline, or fludrocortisone.

Muscle Cramps Muscle cramps can occur with up to 20% of dialysis sessions.[59] The cause is often related to excessive ultrafiltration, which causes hypoperfusion of the muscles. Other contributing factors to the development of muscle cramps include hypotension and electrolyte and acid–base imbalances that occur during hemodialysis sessions.

Treatment. Nonpharmacologic treatments of muscle cramping that occurs during hemodialysis include decreasing the ultrafiltration rate and accurately determining the "dry weight." Pharmacologic measures include vitamin E, which is administered at doses of 400 IU daily. Other options that are not as well studied include oxazepam and prazosin.

Thrombosis Thrombosis associated with hemodialysis most commonly occurs in patients with venous catheter access for dialysis and is a common cause of catheter failure. However, thrombosis can occur in synthetic grafts and less frequently in AV fistulas.

Nonpharmacologic management of thrombosis in a hemodialysis catheter involves saline flushes. Smaller clots may be managed by balloon angioplasty to mechanically open the catheter. In severe cases when clots cannot be removed by either mechanical or pharmacologic therapy, the catheter may require replacement.

Pharmacologic management of thrombosis includes local administration of thrombolytic agents. Alteplase (2 mg per port) and reteplase (0.5 unit per port) are the two most commonly used agents today. Urokinase has been used in the past, but after its reintroduction to the U.S. market, the larger dosed vial size makes it less cost effective than the newer agents.

Infection Infections are an important cause of morbidity and mortality in patients receiving hemodialysis. The cause of infection is usually related to organisms found on the skin, namely *Staphylococcus epidermidis* and *S. aureus*. Methicillin-resistant *S. aureus* (MRSA) is a common cause of infections in patients receiving hemodialysis. Other organisms have also been found to cause access-related infections. The greatest risk to patients receiving hemodialysis is the development of bacteremia. As with thrombosis, venous catheters are most commonly infected, followed by synthetic AV grafts, and finally AV fistulas.

Blood cultures should be obtained for any patient receiving hemodialysis who develops a fever. Nonpharmacologic management of infections involves preventive measures with sterile technique, proper disinfection, and minimizing the use and duration of venous catheters for hemodialysis access.

Pharmacologic management of infections should cover the gram-positive organisms that most frequently cause access-related infections. Patients who have positive blood cultures should receive treatment tailored to the organism isolated. Preventive measures for access-related infections include mupirocin at the exit site and povidone-iodine ointment. The recommendations of the NKF for treatment of infections associated with hemodialysis are listed in Table 26–10.

Peritoneal Dialysis

Peritoneal dialysis is initiated in 6% of patients with newly diagnosed ESKD each year. Currently, 27,559 patients were receiving PD dialysis in 2009.[4] Peritoneal dialysis is associated with improved survival compared with hemodialysis.[4] Peritoneal dialysis preserves residual renal function, which improves cardiovascular stability and may account for the improved survival. Thus PD may be the preferred method of dialysis in patients with residual renal function.[60]

▶ Principles of Peritoneal Dialysis

PD utilizes similar principles as hemodialysis in that blood is exposed to a semipermeable membrane against which a physiologic solution is placed. In the case of PD, however, the semipermeable membrane is the peritoneal membrane, and a sterile dialysate is instilled into the peritoneal cavity. The peritoneal membrane is composed of a continuous single layer of mesothelial cells that covers the abdominal and pelvic walls on one side of the peritoneal cavity, and the visceral organs including the GI tract, liver, spleen, and diaphragm on the other side. The mesothelial cells are covered by microvilli that increase the surface area of the peritoneal membrane to approximate body surface area (1 to 2 m²). Blood vessels that supply the abdominal organs, muscle, and mesentery serve as the blood component of the system.

The gaps between the mesothelial cells allow for large solutes to pass through into the bloodstream. Both the interstitium and endothelial cells of the blood vessels provide resistance to limit the solute size that is removed from the blood. Diffusion is the most important component of solute transport in PD, which is enhanced by the large surface area and volume of dialysate, as well as contact time with the peritoneal membrane. Ultrafiltration is achieved in PD by

Table 26–10
Management of Hemodialysis Access Infections

AV Fistula	Treat as subacute bacterial endocarditis for 6 weeks
	Initial antibiotic choice should always cover gram-positive organisms (e.g., vancomycin 20 mg/kg IV with serum concentration monitoring or cefazolin 20 mg/kg IV three times per week)
	Gram-negative coverage is indicated for patients with diabetes, HIV infection, prosthetic valves, or those receiving immunosuppressive agents (gentamicin 2 mg/kg IV with serum concentration monitoring)
Synthetic Grafts (AVG)	
Local infection	Empiric antibiotic coverage for gram-positive, gram-negative, and *Enterococcus* (e.g., gentamicin plus vancomycin, then individualize after culture results become available); continue for 2–4 weeks
Extensive infection	Antibiotics as above plus total resection
Access less than 1-month old	Antibiotics as above plus removal of the graft
Tunneled Cuffed Catheters (Internal Jugular, Subclavian)	
Infection localized to catheter exit site	No drainage: topical antibiotics (e.g., mupirocin ointment)
	Drainage present: Gram-positive coverage (e.g., cefazolin 20 mg/kg IV three times a week)
Bacteremia with or without systemic signs or symptoms	Gram-positive coverage as above
	If stable and asymptomatic, change catheter and provide culture-specific antibiotic coverage for a minimum of 3 weeks

AV, arteriovenous.

Patient Encounter 4, Part 2

The patient returns to the dialysis clinic 6 months later for her scheduled hemodialysis session. Two hours into the session, she begins to complain of dizziness and lightheadedness.

PE:

VS: BP 98/58 mm Hg (was 146/94 mm Hg at the start of hemodialysis); P 100 bpm; T 96.7° F (35.9° C); wt 118 lb (53.6 kg)

CV: RRR, normal S_1, S_2

What are the potential causes of her hypotension?

What are the treatment alternatives for hypotension in this patient?

What are potential alternatives to avoid hypotension in future dialysis sessions?

creating an osmotic pressure gradient between the dialysate and the blood. Traditionally, glucose has been used to create the osmotic gradient, but the solutions are not biocompatible with the peritoneal membrane, resulting in cytotoxicity of the cells. More recently, polymeric glucose derivatives such as icodextrin have been used to create a colloid-driven osmosis that results in ultrafiltration and convection of solute removal.

In PD, prewarmed dialysate is instilled into the peritoneal cavity where it "dwells" for a specified length of time (usually one to several hours, depending on the type of PD) to adequately clear metabolic waste products and excess fluids and electrolytes. At the end of the dwell time, the dialysate is drained and replaced with fresh dialysate. The continuous nature of PD provides for a more physiologic removal of waste products from the bloodstream, which mimics endogenous kidney function by decreasing the fluctuations seen in serum concentrations of the waste products. Similarly, water is removed at a more constant rate, lessening the fluctuations in intravascular fluid balance and providing for more hemodynamic stability.

Several types of PD are used:

- Continuous ambulatory peritoneal dialysis (CAPD) is the most common. The patient exchanges 1 to 3 L of dialysate every 4 to 6 hours throughout the day with a longer dwell time overnight.

- Automated peritoneal dialysis (APD) procedures involve the use of a cycler machine that performs sequential exchanges overnight while the patient is sleeping.

- Continuous cycling PD (CCPD) performs three to five exchanges throughout the night. The final exchange remains in the peritoneal cavity to dwell for the duration of the day.

- Nightly intermittent PD (NIPD) performs six to eight exchanges throughout the night. The final exchange of dialysate is drained in the morning, and the peritoneal cavity remains empty throughout the day.

- Nocturnal tidal PD (NTPD) is similar to NIPD, with the exception that only a portion of the dialysate is exchanged throughout the night. The final exchange is drained in the morning, and the peritoneal cavity remains empty throughout the day.

▶ Peritoneal Access

Access to the peritoneal cavity requires placement of an indwelling catheter with the distal end of the catheter resting in the peritoneal cavity. The central portion of the catheter is generally tunneled under the abdominal wall and subcutaneous tissue where it is held in place by cuffs that provide stability and mechanical support to the catheter. The proximal portion of the catheter exits the abdomen near the umbilicus (**Fig. 26–7**). Several types of indwelling catheters are available; the most common is the Tenckhoff catheter. Placement and handling of the catheter during PD exchanges requires a sterile environment to minimize the risk of infectious complications.

▶ Complications of Peritoneal Dialysis

Complications associated with PD include mechanical problems related to the PD catheter, metabolic problems associated with the components of the dialysate fluid, damage to the peritoneal membrane, and infections (**Table 26–11**). Strategies to manage infectious complications of PD are discussed below.

Peritonitis Peritonitis is a leading cause of morbidity in PD patients, which often leads to loss of the catheter and subsequent change to HD as the treatment modality. However,

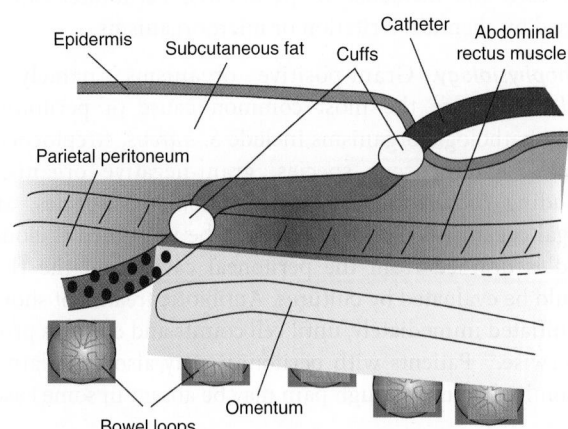

FIGURE 26–7. Diagram of the placement of a peritoneal dialysis catheter through the abdominal wall into the peritoneal cavity. (From Foote EF, Manley HJ. Hemodialysis and peritoneal dialysis. In: DiPiro JT, Talbert RL, Yee GC, et al., eds. Pharmacotherapy: A Pathophysiologic Approach, 7th ed. New York, NY: McGraw-Hill, 2008:O110, with permission.)

Table 26–11

Common Complications During Peritoneal Dialysis

Mechanical Complications
Kinking in catheter
Catheter migration
Catheter adherence to peritoneal tissue
Excessive movement of catheter at exit site

Peritoneal Damage
Alterations in permeability of the peritoneal membrane
Sclerosis of the peritoneal membrane

Pain
Impingement of the catheter tip on visceral organs
Instillation pain
• Rapid inflow of dialysate
• Acidic pH of dialysate
• Chemical irritation from dialysate additives (e.g., antibiotics)
• Low dialysate temperature

Infections
Peritonitis
Exit-site infections
Tunnel infections

Metabolic Complications
Exacerbation of diabetes mellitus from glucose load
Fluid overload
• Exacerbation of chronic heart failure
• Edema
• Pulmonary congestion
Electrolyte abnormalities
Malnutrition
• Albumin and amino acid loss
• Muscle wasting
• Increased adipose tissue
• Fibrin formation in dialysate

---

recent advances with connectors used during instillation and drainage of dialysate and delivery systems have dramatically decreased the incidence of peritonitis. Peritonitis can be caused by chemical irritation or microorganisms.

Pathophysiology. Gram-positive organisms, namely *S. epidermidis*, are the most common cause of peritonitis. Other pathologic organisms include *S. aureus*, streptococcal species, enterococcus species, gram-negative organisms including *Escherichia coli* and *Pseudomonas* species, and fungal organisms. Peritonitis should be presumed if cloudy fluid is drained from the peritoneal cavity and the fluid should be evaluated by cultures. Antibiotic treatment should be initiated immediately, until cell counts and cultures prove otherwise.[61] Patients with peritonitis may also complain of abdominal pain, although pain may be absent in some cases.

Treatment. The International Society of Peritoneal Dialysis (ISPD) revised the recommendations for the treatment of PD-related infections in 2010.[61] Drug selection for empirical treatment of peritonitis should cover both gram-positive and gram-negative organisms specific to the dialysis center and be based on the protocols and sensitivity patterns of organisms known to cause peritonitis, as well as the history

of infections in the patient. First-generation cephalosporins, such as cefazolin, or vancomycin are recommended for empirical coverage of gram-positive organisms. Appropriate coverage for gram-negative organisms includes third- or fourth-generation cephalosporins, such as ceftazidime or cefepime, or aminoglycosides. Alternatives for gram-negative coverage include oral fluoroquinolones. An example of an appropriate empiric treatment for peritonitis includes cefazolin in combination with ceftazidime, cefepime, or an aminoglycoside. If the patient has a cephalosporin allergy, vancomycin in combination with an aminoglycoside is an alternative empirical treatment.[61] It should be noted that aminoglycosides can decrease residual renal function in patients receiving peritoneal dialysis.

The preferred route of administration is intraperitoneal (IP) rather than IV to achieve maximum concentrations at the site of infection. Antibiotics can be administered IP intermittently as a single large dose in one exchange per day or continuously as multiple smaller doses with each exchange. Intermittent administration requires at least 6 hours of dwell time in the peritoneal cavity to allow for adequate systemic absorption and provides adequate levels to cover the 24-hour period. However, continuous administration is better suited for PD modalities that require more frequent exchanges (less than 6-hour dwell time). See the ISPD guidelines for dosing recommendations for IP antibiotics in CAPD and automated PD patients.[61] The dose of the antibiotics should be increased by 25% for patients with residual kidney function who are able to produce more than 100 mL urine output per day.

Once the organism has been identified and sensitivities are known, drug selection should be adjusted to reflect the susceptibilities of the organism. Streptococcal, staphylococcal, and enterococcal species sensitive to β-lactam antibiotics should be treated with continuous IP dosing to increase efficacy and minimize resistance.[61] Peritonitis caused by *S. aureus* or *P. aeruginosa* are often associated with catheter-related infections, which are difficult to treat and often require removal of the catheter. Rifampin 600 mg orally daily (in a single or divided dose) may be added to IP vancomycin for the treatment of methicillin-resistant *S. aureus* (MRSA) but should be limited to duration of 1 week to minimize the development of resistance. Two antibiotics are required for treatment of *P. aeruginosa* peritonitis.[61] If multiple organisms are cultured, treatment should cover all of the organisms, including anaerobic organisms, and the patient should be evaluated for other intra-abdominal pathologies.[61]

Peritonitis caused by fungal organisms is associated with mortality in 25% of patients,[61] which can be reduced by removing the catheter after fungal organisms are identified. Empirical treatment should include IP amphotericin B and flucytosine.[61] Although IP amphotericin administration is associated with chemical irritation and pain, penetration of amphotericin into the peritoneal cavity is poor with IV administration. Fluconazole, voriconazole, or caspofungin may be suitable alternatives, depending on culture results.

Catheter-Related Infections Catheter-related infections generally occur at the exit site or the portion of the catheter that is tunneled in the subcutaneous tissue. Previous infections increase the risk and incidence of catheter-related infections.

Pathophysiology. The major pathologic organisms responsible for causing catheter-related infections are *S. aureus* and *P. aeruginosa*. These organisms also cause the most serious catheter-related infections. *S. epidermidis* is found in less than 20% of catheter-related infections. Other organisms include diphtheroids, anaerobic bacteria, *Legionella*, and fungi.[61]

Exit-site infections present with purulent drainage at the site. Erythema may or may not be present with an exit-site infection. Tunnel infections are generally an extension of the exit-site infection and rarely occur alone. Symptoms of a tunnel infection may include tenderness, edema, and erythema over the tunnel pathway but are often asymptomatic. Ultrasound can be used to detect tunnel infections in asymptomatic patients. Exit-site infections caused by *S. aureus* and *P. aeruginosa* often spread to tunnel infections and are the most common causes of catheter-infection–related peritonitis.

Treatment. Exit-site infections may be treated immediately with empiric coverage, or treatment may be delayed until cultures return. Empiric treatment of catheter-related infections should cover *S. aureus*. Coverage for *P. aeruginosa* should also be included if the patient has a history of infections with this organism.[61] Cultures and sensitivity testing are particularly important in tailoring antibiotic therapy for catheter-related infections to ensure eradication of the organism and prevent recurrence or related peritonitis.

Less severe infections may be treated with topical antibiotic cream, although this practice is controversial. Oral antibiotics are also effective for treatment of catheter-related infections. Empiric or routine use of vancomycin for gram-positive infections should be avoided unless the infection is caused by MRSA. Rifampin may be added to therapy for severe infections or slowly resolving *S. aureus* infections, but monotherapy is not recommended.[61] Oral fluoroquinolones are used as first-line agents to treat *P. aeruginosa*, which can be difficult to treat and require prolonged treatment. If the infection is slow to resolve or if it recurs, IP ceftazidime or a second agent should be added.[61] Treatment of catheter-related infections should be continued until the exit site appears normal with no erythema or drainage. Generally, at least 2 weeks of therapy or longer are required to ensure complete eradication of the organism and prevent future recurrence, which is common with *S. aureus*

Patient Care and Monitoring

1. Assess the patient to determine if the patient should be evaluated for CKD. Does the patient have any risk factors for CKD?

2. Review any available laboratory data to determine the staging of CKD.

3. Obtain a thorough medical and medication history from the patient. Does the patient have any concomitant diseases such as diabetes or hypertension that should be treated to prevent the progression of CKD?

4. Determine if an ACE-I or ARB is appropriate for the patient. Does the patient have proteinuria?

5. Develop a plan to assess and optimize treatment of CKD.

6. Determine if the patient requires medical treatment for electrolyte imbalances. Does the patient have edema? Does the patient have an arrhythmia?

7. Educate the patient on dietary changes to manage electrolyte imbalances associated with CKD.

8. Assess the patient for the presence of anemia. Do the laboratory tests suggest the patient requires medical treatment?

9. Develop a plan to assess and optimize treatment for anemia.

10. Determine if the patient requires medical intervention to prevent the development of or treatment for sHPT.

11. Develop a plan to assess and optimize treatment for sHPT.

12. Establish if the patient requires RRT.

13. Evaluate the patient for complications associated with dialysis. Does the patient develop hypotension or cramps during hemodialysis? Does the patient have symptoms consistent with peritonitis or a catheter infection?

14. Develop a plan to assess and optimize treatment for complications associated with dialysis.

15. Stress the importance of adherence with the treatments for CKD and associated complications including lifestyle modifications and medications. Recommend a therapeutic regimen that is easy for the patient to accomplish.

16. Provide patient education with regard to CKD and the associated complications, lifestyle modifications, and drug therapy:
    - What causes CKD and what things to avoid.
    - Possible complications of CKD and symptoms associated with the complications.
    - When to take medications.
    - What potential adverse effects may occur.
    - Which drugs may interact with therapy.
    - Warning signs to report to the physician (edema, irregular heartbeat, fatigue, unusual bleeding).

and *P. aeruginosa*. Infections that do not resolve may require replacement of the PD catheter. Catheter-related infections that present in conjunction with or progress to peritonitis with the same organism require removal of the PD catheter until the peritonitis is resolved.[61]

Prophylaxis of Peritonitis and Catheter-Related Infections Prevention of peritonitis and catheter-related infections starts when the catheter is placed. The exit site should be properly cared for until it is well healed before it can be used for PD. Patients should receive proper instructions for care of the catheter during this time period, which can last up to 2 weeks. Patients should also be instructed on the proper techniques to use for dialysate exchanges to minimize the risk of infections during exchanges, which is the most common cause of peritonitis.

Intranasal *S. aureus* increases the risk of *S. aureus* exit-site infections, tunnel infections, peritonitis, and subsequent catheter loss.[61] Several measures have been used to decrease the risk of peritonitis caused by *S. aureus*, including mupirocin cream applied daily around the exit site, intranasal mupirocin cream twice daily for 5 days each month, or rifampin 300 mg orally twice daily for 5 days, repeated every 3 months.[61] Mupirocin use is preferred over rifampin to prevent the development of resistance to rifampin, although mupirocin resistance has also been reported.[61] Other measures that have been used to decrease both *S. aureus* and *P. aeruginosa* infections include gentamicin cream applied twice daily and ciprofloxacin otic solution applied daily to the exit site.[61]

Outcome Evaluation Clinical improvement should be seen within 48 hours of initiating treatment for peritonitis or catheter-related infections. Perform daily inspections of peritoneal fluid or the exit site to determine clinical improvement. Peritoneal fluid should become clear with improvement of peritonitis and erythema, and discharge should remit with improvement of catheter-related infections. If no improvement is seen within 48 hours, obtain additional cultures and cell counts to determine the appropriate alterations in therapy.

Abbreviations Introduced in This Chapter

2,3-DPG	2,3-Diphosphoglycerate
ACE-I	Angiotensin-converting enzyme inhibitor
AGE	Advanced glycation end-product
AKI	Acute kidney injury
APD	Automated peritoneal dialysis
ARB	Angiotensin receptor blocker
AVF	Arteriovenous fistula
AVG	Arteriovenous graft
BUN	Blood urea nitrogen
Ca–P	Calcium–phosphorus product
CAPD	Continuous ambulatory peritoneal dialysis
CCPD	Continuous cycling peritoneal dialysis
CHD	Coronary heart disease
CKD	Chronic kidney disease
CKD-EPI	Chronic Kidney Disease Epidemiology Collaboration equation
CKD-MBD	Chronic kidney disease mineral and bone disease
CVD	Cardiovascular disease
DDAVP	Desmopressin
DKD	Diabetic kidney disease
DM	Diabetes mellitus
ECG	Electrocardiogram
EPO	Erythropoietin
ESA	Erythropoiesis-stimulating agent
FE_K	Fractional excretion of potassium
FE_{Na}	Fractional excretion of sodium
GFR	Glomerular filtration rate
HbA1c	Hemoglobin$_{a1c}$
Hct	Hematocrit
HD	Hemodialysis
HDL-C	High-density lipoprotein cholesterol
Hgb	Hemoglobin
HMG-CoA	3-Hydroxy-3-methylglutaryl coenzyme A
IP	Intraperitoneal
iPTH	Intact parathyroid hormone
ISPD	International Society of Peritoneal Dialysis
KDIGO	Kidney Disease: Improving Global Outcomes
LDL-C	Low-density lipoprotein cholesterol
LVH	Left ventricular hypertrophy
MCHC	Mean corpuscular hemoglobin concentration
MCV	Mean corpuscular volume
MDRD	Modification of Diet in Renal Disease (study)
MRSA	Methicillin-resistant *Staphylococcus aureus*
NIPD	Nightly intermittent peritoneal dialysis
NKF	National Kidney Foundation
NKF-K/DOQI	National Kidney Foundation-Dialysis Outcome Quality Initiative
NTPD	Nocturnal tidal peritoneal dialysis
PD	Peritoneal dialysis
PTH	Parathyroid hormone
RBC	Red blood cell
ROD	Renal osteodystrophy
RRT	Renal replacement therapy
SC	Subcutaneous
SCr	Serum creatinine
sHPT	Secondary hyperparathyroidism
SPS	Sodium polystyrene sulfonate
TIBC	Total iron binding capacity
TSAT	Transferrin saturation
USRDS	United States Renal Data Service

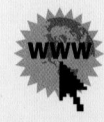 Self-assessment questions and answers are available at *http://www.mhpharmacotherapy.com/pp.html*.

REFERENCES

1. National Kidney Foundation. K/DOQI clinical practice guidelines for chronic kidney disease: Evaluation, classification and stratification. Am J Kidney Dis 2002;39 (Suppl 1):S1–S266.
2. Levey AS, Coresh J, Breene T, et al. Using standardized serum creatinine values in the Modification of Diet in Renal Disease Study equation for estimating the glomerular filtration rate. Ann Intern Med 2006;145(4):247–254.
3. Levey AS, Stevens LA, Schmid SH, et al. A new equation to estimate glomerular filtration rate. Ann Intern Med. 2009;150(9):604–612.
4. U.S. Renal Data System (USRDS). Annual Data Report: Atlas of Chronic Kidney Disease and End-Stage Renal Disease in the United States. Bethesda, MD: National Institutes of Health, National Institute of Diabetes and Digestive and Kidney Diseases, 2011.
5. Coresh J, Selvin E, Stevens LA, et al. Prevalence of chronic kidney disease in the United States. JAMA 2007;298(17):2038–2047.
6. Attman PO, Samuelsson O. Dyslipidemia of kidney disease. Curr Opin Lipidol 2009;20(4):293–299.
7. Tsimihodimos V, Dounousi E, Siamopoulos KC. Dyslipidemia in chronic kidney disease: An approach to pathogenesis and treatment. Am J Nephrol 2008;28(6):958–973.
8. Steinke JM. The natural progression of kidney injury in young type 1 diabetic patients. Curr Diab Rep 2009;9(6):473–479.
9. Kalaitzidis R, Bakris G. Pathogenesis and treatment of microalbuminuria in patients with diabetes: The road ahead. J Clin Hypertens 2009;11(11):636–643.
10. Udani SM, Koyner JL. Effect of blood pressure lowering on markers of kidney disease progression. Curr Hypertens Rep 2009;11(5):368–374.
11. Hemmelgarn BR, Manns, BJ, Lloyd A, et al. Relation between kidney function, proteinuria, and adverse outcomes. JAMA 2010;303(5):423–429.
12. Bakris GL. A practical approach to achieving recommended blood pressure goals in diabetic patients. Arch Int Med 2001;161:2661–2667.
13. D.Agati V, Schmidt AM. RAGE and the pathogenesis of chronic kidney disease. Nat Rev Nephrol 2010;6:352–360.
15. Mercado C, Jaimes EA. Cigarette smoking as a risk factor for atherosclerosis and renal disease: novel pathogenic insights. Curr Hypertens Rep 2007;9:66–72.
16. Jones-Burton C, Seliger SL, Scherer RW, et al. Cigarette smoking and incident chronic kidney disease: A systematic review. Am J Nephrol 2007;27:342–351.
17. López-Novoa J, Martínez-Salgado C, Rodríguez-Peña AB, Hernández FJL. Common pathophysiological mechanisms of chronic kidney disease: Therapeutic perspectives. Pharmacol Ther 2010;128(1):61–81.
18. National Kidney Foundation. KDOQI clinical practice guidelines and clinical practice recommendations for diabetes and chronic kidney disease. Am J Kidney Dis 2007;49(2 Suppl 2):S12–S154.
19. National Kidney Foundation. K/DOQI clinical practice guidelines for nutrition in chronic renal failure. Am J Kidney Dis 2000;35(6 Suppl 2):S1–S140.
20. United Kingdom Prospective Diabetes Study (UKPDS) Group. Intensive blood-glucose control with sulfonylureas or insulin compared with conventional treatment and risk of complications in patients with type 2 diabetes. Lancet 1998;352:837–853.
21. National Kidney Foundation. K/DOQI clinical practice guidelines on hypertension and antihypertensive agents in chronic kidney disease. Am J Kidney Dis 2004;43(Suppl 1):S1–S290.
22. Zager PG, Nikolic J, Brown RH, et al. "U" curve association of blood pressure and mortality in hemodialysis patients. Kidney Int 1998;54:561–569.
23. National Kidney Foundation. K/DOQI clinical practice guidelines for cardiovascular disease in dialysis patients. Am J Kidney Dis. 2005;45(Suppl 4):S1–S153.
24. Tentori F, Hunt WC, Rohrscheib M, et al. Which targets in clinical practice guidelines are associated with improved survival in a large dialysis organization? J Am Soc Nephrol 2007;18:2377–2384.
25. Hermida RC, Ayala DE, Mojón A, Fernández JR. Bedtime dosing of antihypertensive medications reduces cardiovascular risk in CKD. J Am Soc Nephrol 2011;22(12):2313–2321.
26. Bakris GL. Slowing nephropathy progression: Focus on proteinuria reduction. Clin J Am Soc Nephrol. 2008;3 (Suppl):S3–10.
27. Acri M, Erdem Y. Dual blockade of the renin-angiotensin system for cardiorenal protection: An update. Am J Kidney Dis 2009;53(2):332–345.
28. Mann JFE, Schmieder RE, McQueen M, et al. Renal outcomes with telmisartan, ramipril, or both, in people at high vascular risk (the ONTARGET study): A multicenter, randomized, double-blind, controlled trial. Lancet 2008;372:547–553.
29. Kalaitzidis RG, Bakris GL. Should proteinuria reduction be the criterion for antihypertensive drug selection for patients with kidney disease? Curr Opin Nephrol 2009;18:386–391.
30. National Kidney Foundation. K/DOQI clinical practice guidelines for managing dyslipidemias in chronic kidney disease. Am J Kidney Dis 2003;41(Suppl 3):S1–S92.
31. Stack AF, Murthy BVR. Cigarette use and cardiovascular risk in chronic kidney disease: An unappreciated modifiable lifestyle risk factor. Sem Dial 2010;23(3):298–305.
32. Tsakiris D. Morbidity and mortality reduction associated with the use of erythropoietin. Nephron 2000;85(Suppl 1):2–8.
33. Rossert J, Fouqueray B, Boffa JJ. Anemia management and the delay of chronic renal failure progression. J Am Soc Nephrol 2003;14:S173–S177.
34. Shemin D, Dworkin LD. Sodium balance in renal failure. Curr Opin Nephrol Hyperten 1997;6(2):128–132.
35. Gennari FJ, Segal AS. Hyperkalemia: An adaptive response in chronic renal insufficiency. Kidney Int 2002;62:1–9.
36. Ahmed J, Weisberg LS. Hyperkalemia in dialysis patients. Semin Dial 2001;14(5):348–356.
37. Musso CG. Potassium metabolism in patients with chronic kidney disease (CKD), part I: Patients not on dialysis (stages 3–4). Int Urol Nephrol 2004;36:465–468.
38. Kidney Disease: Improving Global Outcomes. KDIGO clinical practice guideline for anemia in chronic kidney disease. Kidney Int Suppl 2012;2(4):279–335.
39. McClellan W, Aronoff SL, Bolton WK, et al. The prevalence of anemia in patients with chronic kidney disease. Curr Med Res Opin 2004;20(9):1501–1510.
40. Hertig A, Ferrer-Marin F. Correction of anaemia on dialysis: Did we forget physiology? Nephrol Dial Transplant 2011;26(4):1120–1122.
41. Xue JL, St. Peter WL, Ebben JP, et al. Anemia treatment in the pre-ESRD period and associated mortality in elderly patients. Am J Kidney Dis 2002;40(6):1153–1161.
42. Hudson JQ, Schonder KS. Advances in anemia management in chronic kidney disease. J Pharm Pract 2002;15(6):437–455.
43. Drueke TB, Loctelli F, Clyne N, et al. Normalization of hemoglobin level in patients with chronic kidney disease and anemia. N Engl J Med 2006;335(20):2071–2084.
44. Pfeffer MA, Burdmann EA, Chen CY, et al. A trial of darbepoetin alfa in type 2 diabetes and chronic kidney disease. N Engl J Med 2009;361(21):2019–2032.
45. Singh AK. What is causing the mortality in treating the anemia of chronic kidney disease: Erythropoietin dose or hemoglobin level? Curr Opin Nephrol Hypertens 2010;19(5):420–424.
46. de Francisco ALM. Secondary hyperparathyroidism: Review of the disease and its treatment. Clin Ther 2004;26(12):1976–1993.
47. Cunningham J, Locatelli F, Rodriguez M. Secondary hyperparathyroidism: Pathogenesis, disease progression, and therapeutic options. Clin J Am Soc Nephrol 2011;6(4):913–921.
48. Saliba W, El-Haddad B. Secondary hyperparathyroidism: Pathophysiology and treatment. J Am Board Fam Med 2009;22(5):574–581.
49. Kraut JA, Kurtz I. Metabolic acidosis of CKD: Diagnosis, clinical characteristics and treatment. Am J Kidney Dis 2005;45:978–993.
50. KDIGO clinical practice guideline for the diagnosis, evaluation, prevention, and treatment of chronic kidney disease-mineral and bone disorder (CKD-MBD). Kidney Int 2009;76 (Suppl 113):S1–130.

51. National Kidney Foundation. K/DOQI clinical practice guidelines for bone metabolism and disease in chronic kidney disease. Am J Kidney Dis 2003;42(Suppl 3):S1–S202.

52. Al-Aly A, Qazi RA, González EA, et al. Changes in serum 25-hydroxyvitamin D and plasma intact PTH levels following treatment with ergocalciferol in patients with CKD. Am J Kidney Dis 2007;50(1):59–68.

53. Byrnes CA, Shepler BM. Cinacalcet: A new treatment for secondary hyperparathyroidism in patients receiving hemodialysis. Pharmacotherapy 2005;25(5):709–716.

54. Hedges SJ, Dehoney SB, Jooper JS, et al. Evidence-based treatment recommendations for uremic bleeding. Nat Clin Pract Nephrol 2007;3:138–153.

55. Manenti L, Tansinda P, Vaglio A. Uraemic pruritus: Clinical characteristics, pathophysiology and treatment. Drugs 2009;69(3):251–263.

56. National Kidney Foundation. K/DOQI clinical practice guidelines for vascular access: Update 2000. Am J Kidney Dis. 2001;37(1 Suppl 1):S137–S180.

57. Davenport A. Intradialytic complications during hemodialysis. Hemodial Int 2006;10(2):162–167.

58. Rosner MH. Hemodialysis for the non-nephrologist. S Med J 2005;98(8):785–791.

59. Himmelfarb J. Hemodialysis complications. Am J Kidney Dis 2005;45(6):1122–1131.

60. van den Berg R, Cnossen TT, Konings CJAM, Kooman JP, van der Sande FM, Leunissen KML. Different treatment options in peritoneal dialysis. Nephrol Dial Transplant Plus 2008;1(Suppl 4):14–17.

61. Li PKT, Szeto CC, Piraino B, et al. ISPD guidelines/recommendations: Peritoneal dialysis-related infections recommendations: 2010 update. Perit Dial Int 2010;30(4):393–423.

27 Fluids and Electrolytes

Mark A. Malesker and Lee E. Morrow

LEARNING OBJECTIVES

● **Upon completion of the chapter, the reader will be able to:**

1. Estimate the volumes of various body fluid compartments.
2. Calculate the daily maintenance fluid requirement for patients given their weight, and gender.
3. Differentiate among currently available fluids for volume resuscitation.
4. Identify the electrolytes primarily found in the extracellular and intracellular fluid compartments.
5. Describe the unique relationship between serum sodium concentration and total body water (TBW).
6. Review the etiology, clinical presentation, and management for disorders of sodium, potassium, calcium, phosphorus, and magnesium.

KEY CONCEPTS

❶ Total body water (TBW) is approximately 50% of lean body weight in normal females and 60% of lean body weight in males. For clinical purposes, most clinicians generalize that total body water accounts for 60% of lean body weight in adults, regardless of gender. TBW is composed of the intracellular fluid (two-thirds of TBW) and the extracellular fluid (one-third of TBW). The extracellular fluid is made up of two major fluid subcompartments: the interstitial fluid and the intravascular fluid.

❷ Therapeutic fluids include crystalloid and colloid solutions. The most commonly used crystalloids include normal saline, dextrose/half-normal saline, hypertonic saline, and lactated Ringer's solution. Examples of colloids include albumin, the dextrans, hetastarch, and fresh-frozen plasma (FFP).

❸ The calculated serum osmolality helps determine deviations in TBW content.

❹ Concentrated electrolytes (potassium chloride [KCl], potassium phosphate, and sodium chloride [NaCl] greater than 0.9%) should not be stored in patient care areas as a patient safety measure.

❺ Hyponatremia is the most common electrolyte disorder in hospitalized patients and is defined as a serum sodium concentration below 136 mEq/L (136 mmol/L).

❻ IV potassium infusions running at rates of greater than 10 mEq/h (10 mmol/h) require cardiac monitoring.

❼ Calcium gluconate is the preferred peripherally infused calcium supplement because it is less irritating to the veins. Calcium chloride (CaCl) must be infused via a central line.

❽ Severe hypophosphatemia can result in impaired diaphragmatic contractility and acute respiratory failure.

❾ Serum magnesium concentrations do not correlate well with total body magnesium stores. For this reason, magnesium supplementation is often given empirically to critically ill patients.

BODY FLUID COMPARTMENTS

A thorough understanding of the fundamentals of fluid and electrolyte homeostasis is essential given the frequency with which clinical disturbances are seen and the profound effects these disturbances can have on various aspects of patient care. However, the interplay of body fluids, serum electrolytes, and clinical monitoring is complex, and a thorough command of these issues is a challenging task even for advanced practitioners.[1] Practitioners must be familiar with the key concepts of body compartment volumes, calculation of daily fluid requirements, and the various types of fluid available for replacement. The management of disorders of sodium, potassium, calcium, phosphorus, and magnesium integrates these concepts with issues of dose recognition and patient safety.

The most fundamental concept to grasp is an assessment of total body water (TBW), which is directly related to body weight. ❶ *TBW constitutes approximately 50% of lean body weight in healthy females and 60% of lean body weight in males.*

For clinical purposes, most clinicians generalize that total body water accounts for 60% of lean body weight in adults, regardless of gender. The percentage of TBW decreases as body fat increases and/or with age (75% to 85% of body weight is water for newborns). Unless the patient is obese (body weight greater than 120% of ideal body weight [IBW]), clinicians typically use a patient's actual body weight when calculating TBW.[2] In obese patients, it is customary to estimate TBW using lean body weight or IBW as calculated by the Devine–Devine method: males' lean body weight = 50 kg + (2.3 kg/in. × [height in inches − 60]) and females' lean body weight = 45.5 kg + (2.3 kg/in. × [height in inches − 60]).[3-5] Note that 1 kg is equivalent to 2.2 lb, 1 in. is equivalent to 2.54 cm, and 1 L of water weighs 1 kg (2.2 lb).

The intracellular fluid (ICF) represents the water contained within cells and is rich in electrolytes such as potassium, magnesium, phosphates, and proteins. ❶ *The ICF is approximately two-thirds of TBW regardless of gender.* For a 70-kg person, this would mean that the TBW is 42 L and the ICF is approximately 28 L. Note that ICF represents approximately 40% of total body weight.

The extracellular fluid (ECF) is the fluid outside the cell and is rich in sodium, chloride, and bicarbonate. ❶ *The ECF is approximately one-third of TBW (14 L in a 70-kg person) and is subdivided into two compartments: the interstitial fluid and the intravascular fluid.* The interstitial fluid represents the fluid occupying the spaces between cells and is about 25% of TBW (10.5 L in a 70-kg person). The intravascular fluid (also known as plasma) represents the fluid within the blood vessels and is about 8% of TBW (3.4 L in a 70-kg person). Because the exact percentages are cumbersome to recall, many clinicians accept that the ECF represents roughly 20% of body weight (regardless of gender) with 15% in the interstitial space and 5% in the intravascular space.[6] Note that serum electrolytes are routinely measured from the ECF.

The transcellular fluid includes the viscous components of the peritoneum, pleural space, and pericardium, as well as the cerebrospinal fluid, joint space fluid, and the GI digestive juices. Although the transcellular fluid normally accounts for about 1% of TBW, this amount can increase significantly during various illnesses favoring fluid collection in one of these spaces (e.g., pleural effusions or ascites in the peritoneum). The accumulation of fluid in the transcellular space is often referred to as "third spacing." To review the calculations of the body fluid compartments in a representative patient, see Patient Encounter 1.

Fluid balance is assessed by several means each of which has its limitations. Blood pressure (BP) measurements estimate fluid status relative to the amount of blood volume pumped by the heart but are affected by cardiac function and vascular pliability. Patients with significant volume deficiency may appear hypotensive, but this is a late finding that may require greater than 20% of TBW to be lost. Patients with significant volume excess may appear edematous; however, third spacing may hide this finding until late in the course as well. The physical examination can indicate the presence of fluid deficits (dry mucous membranes) and fluid excess (peripheral edema, coarse breath sounds). More invasive assessments would include the use of an arterial catheter, a pulmonary artery catheter to measure left ventricular function and fluid status, and a central venous catheter that measures fluid status and right ventricular function. However, the correlation between these measured pressures and their associated volume is an area of debate.

To maintain fluid balance, the total amount of fluid gained throughout the day (input, or "ins") must equal the total amount of fluid lost (output, or "outs"). Although most forms of the body's input and output can be measured, several cannot. For a normal adult on an average diet, ingested fluids are easily measured and average 1,400 mL/day. Other fluid inputs, such as those from ingested foods and the water by-product of oxidation, are not directly measurable. Fluid outputs such as urinary and stool losses are also easily measured and referred to as sensible losses. Other sources of fluid loss, such as evaporation of fluid through the skin and/or lungs, are not readily measured and are called insensible losses. Table 27–1 shows the estimated ins and outs (I&Os) for a healthy 68-kg (150-lb) man.[6] The measurable I&Os are routinely measured in hospitalized patients and are used to estimate total fluid balance for each 24-hour period. It is important to realize that in hospitalized patients, multiple other forms of fluid loss must be considered. These include losses from enteric suctioning (most commonly, nasogastric [NG] tubes), from surgical drains (e.g., chest tubes, nephrostomy tubes, and pancreatic drains), via fistulous tracts, and enhanced evaporative losses (burns and fever).

TBW depletion (often referred to as "dehydration") is typically a gradual, chronic problem. Because TBW depletion represents a loss of hypotonic fluid (proportionally more water is lost than sodium) from all body compartments, a primary disturbance of osmolality is usually seen. The signs and symptoms of TBW depletion include CNS disturbances

---

Patient Encounter 1: Body Fluid Compartments

Calculate the total body water, ICF, and ECF in a 80-kg male.

Table 27–1

Approximate I&Os for a Healthy 68-kg (150-lb) Man

Input	mL/day	Output	mL/day
Ingested fluid[a]	1,400	Urine[a]	1,500
Fluid in food	850	Skin losses	500
Water of oxidation	350	Respiratory tract losses	400
		Stool	200
Total	2,600	Total	2,600

[a]Readily quantifiable.

Table 27–2

Useful Calculations for the Estimation of Patient Maintenance Fluid Requirements

Neonate (1–10 kg) = 100 mL/kg
Child (10–20 kg) = 1,000 mL + 50 mL for each kilogram greater than 10
Adult (greater than 20 kg) = 1,500 mL + 20 mL for each kilogram greater than 20

(mental status changes, seizures, and coma), excessive thirst, dry mucous membranes, decreased skin turgor, elevated serum sodium, increased plasma osmolality, concentrated urine, and acute weight loss. Common causes of TBW depletion include insufficient oral intake, excessive insensible losses, diabetes insipidus, excessive osmotic diuresis, and impaired renal concentrating mechanisms. Elderly long-term care residents are frequently admitted to the acute care hospital with TBW depletion secondary to lack of adequate oral intake, often with concurrent excessive insensible losses.

The volume of fluid required to correct TBW depletion equals the basal fluid requirement plus ongoing exceptional losses plus the fluid deficit. Basal daily fluid requirements are calculated using the formulas in Table 27–2. For an adult, this represents 1,500 mL/day for the first 20 kg of body weight plus 20 mL/day for each additional kilogram. The volume of replacement fluids required for a given patient (the fluid deficit) can be estimated by the acute weight change in the patient (1 kg = 1 L of fluid). Because the precise weight change is not typically known, it is often calculated as follows: fluid deficit = normal TBW − present TBW. Normal TBW is estimated based on the patient's height using the formulas in Table 27–2, and the present TBW is estimated based on the patient's current body weight. The choice of fluids used for replacement is guided by the presence of concurrent electrolyte abnormalities. The adequacy of replacement is guided by each patient's objective response to fluid replacement (improved skin turgor, adequate urine output, normalization of heart rate, BP, etc.).

Once TBW has been restored, the volume of "maintenance" fluid equals the basal fluid requirement plus ongoing exceptional losses. If the pathophysiologic process leading to TBW depletion has not been identified and corrected (or accounted for in the calculation of maintenance fluid requirements), TBW depletion will quickly recur. To review the concepts involved in the calculation of replacement fluids for a representative patient, see Patient Encounter 2.

Patient Encounter 2: Fluid Requirements

Calculate the daily fluid requirement for a 85-kg adult male.

Compared with TBW depletion, ECF depletion tends to occur acutely. In this setting, rapid and aggressive fluid replacement is required to maintain adequate organ perfusion. Because ECF depletion is generally due to the loss of isotonic fluid (proportional losses of sodium and water), major disturbances of plasma osmolality are not common. ECF depletion manifests clinically as signs and symptoms associated with decreased tissue perfusion: dizziness, orthostasis, tachycardia, decreased urine output, increased hematocrit, decreased central venous pressure, and/or hypovolemic shock. Common causes of ECF depletion include external fluid losses (burns, hemorrhage, diuresis, GI losses, and adrenal insufficiency) and third spacing of fluids (septic shock, anaphylactic shock, or abdominal ascites).

In clinical practice, the most commonly encountered problem is depletion of TBW and ECF. Accordingly, the fluid resuscitation strategy should address both of these compartments. As these compartments are repleted, serum electrolytes must be monitored closely as discussed in subsequent sections of this chapter.

THERAPEUTIC FLUIDS

Crystalloids

❷ *Therapeutic IV fluids include crystalloid solutions, colloidal solutions, and oxygen-carrying resuscitation solutions.* Crystalloids are composed of water and electrolytes, all of which pass freely through semipermeable membranes and remain in the intravascular space for shorter periods of time. As such, these solutions are very useful for correcting electrolyte imbalances but result in smaller hemodynamic changes for a given unit of volume.

Crystalloids can be classified further according to their tonicity. Isotonic solutions (i.e., normal saline or 0.9% sodium chloride [NaCl]) have a tonicity equal to that of the ICF (approximately 310 mEq/L or 310 mmol/L) and do not shift the distribution of water between the ECF and the ICF. Because hypertonic solutions (i.e., hypertonic saline or 3% NaCl) have greater tonicity than the ICF (greater than 376 mEq/L or 376 mmol/L), they draw water from the ICF into the ECF. In contrast, hypotonic solutions (i.e., 0.45% NaCl) have less tonicity than the ICF (less than 250 mEq/L or 250 mmol/L) leading to osmotic pressure gradient that favors shifts of water from the ECF into the ICF. The tonicity, electrolyte content, and glucose content of selected fluids are shown in Table 27–3.

The tonicity of crystalloid solutions is directly related to their sodium concentration. The most commonly used crystalloids include normal saline, dextrose/half-normal saline, hypertonic saline, and lactated Ringer's solution. Excessive administration of any fluid replacement therapy, regardless of tonicity, can lead to fluid overload, particularly in patients with cardiac or renal insufficiency. Glucose is often added to hypotonic crystalloids in amounts than result in isotonic fluids (D_5W, D5½NS, and D5¼NS). These solutions are often used as maintenance fluids to provide basal amounts of calories and water.

Table 27–3

Electrolyte and Dextrose Content of Selected Crystalloid Fluids

IV Solution	Osmolarity (mOsm)	Dextrose) (g/L) mmol/L	Sodium (mEq/L) mmol/L	Potassium (mEq/L) mmol/L	Calcium (mEq/L) mmol/L	Chloride (mEq/L) mmol/L	Lactate (mEq/L) mmol/L
D5%	250	50 / 2.78					
D10%	505	100 / 5.55					
0.9% NaCl	308		154			154	
0.45% NaCl	154		77			77	
3% NaCl	1,025		512			512	
D5% and 0.45% NaCl	405	50 / 2.78	77			77	
D5% and 0.2% NaCl	329	50 / 2.78	34			34	
Ringer's injection	310		147	4	5 / 2.5	156	
Lactated Ringer's solution	274		130	4	3 / 1.5	109	28
Lactated Ringer's solution and D5%	525	50 / 2.78	130	4	3 / 1.5	109	28

D, dextrose; NaCl, sodium chloride.

▶ Normal Saline (0.9% NaCl or NS)

● Normal saline is an isotonic fluid composed of water, sodium, and chloride. It provides primarily ECF replacement and can be used for virtually any cause of TBW depletion. Common uses of normal saline include perioperative fluid administration; volume resuscitation of shock, hemorrhage, or burn patients; fluid challenges in hypotensive or oliguric patients; and hyponatremia. Normal saline can also be used to treat metabolic alkalosis (also known as contraction alkalosis).

▶ Half-Normal Saline (0.45% NaCl or ½ NS)

● Half-normal saline is a hypotonic fluid that provides free water in relative excess when compared with the sodium concentration. This crystalloid is typically used to treat patients who are hypertonic due to primary depletion of the ECF. Because half-normal saline is hypotonic, serum sodium must be closely monitored during administration.

▶ 5% Dextrose/Half-Normal Saline (D5 ½ NS)

● D5 ½ NS is a hypotonic fluid that is commonly used as a maintenance fluid. This crystalloid is typically used once fluids deficits have been corrected with normal saline or lactated Ringer's solution. Because half-normal saline is hypotonic, serum sodium must be closely monitored during administration.

▶ Hypertonic Saline (3% NaCl)

● Hypertonic saline is obviously hypertonic and provides a significant sodium load to the intravascular space. This solution is used very infrequently given the potential to cause significant shifts in the water balance between the ECF and the ICF. It is typically used to treat patients with severe hyponatremia who have symptoms attributable to low serum sodium. Hypertonic saline in concentrations of 7.5% to 23.4% has been used to acutely lower intracranial pressure in the setting of traumatic brain injury and stroke. The literature is inconsistent for the appropriate hypertonic concentration, dosing, timing of replacement, and goals for use in this population. Serum sodium and neurologic status must be very closely monitored whenever given.

▶ Ringer's Lactate

● This isotonic volume expander contains sodium, potassium, chloride, and lactate in concentrations that approximate the fluid and electrolyte composition of the blood. Ringer's lactate (also known as "lactated Ringer," or LR) provides ECF replacement and is most often used in the perioperative setting and for patients with lower GI fluid losses, burns, or dehydration. The lactate component of LR works as a buffer to increase the pH. Accordingly, large volumes of LR may cause iatrogenic metabolic alkalosis. Because patients with significant liver disease are unable to metabolize lactate sufficiently, LR administration in this population may lead to accumulation of lactate with iatrogenic lactic acidosis.

▶ *5% Dextrose in Water (D₅W)*

D$_5$W solution is a combination of free water and dextrose that provides a modest amount of calories but no electrolytes. Although it is technically isotonic, it acts as a hypotonic solution in the body. It is commonly used to treat severe hypernatremia. D5W is also used in small volumes (100 mL) to dilute many IV medications or at a low infusion rate (10 to 15 mL/h) to "keep the vein open" (KVO) for IV medications.

Colloids

In contrast to crystalloids, colloids do not dissolve into a true solution and therefore do not pass readily across semipermeable membranes. As such, colloids effectively remain in the intravascular space and increase the oncotic pressure of the plasma. This effectively shifts fluid from the interstitial compartment to the intravascular compartment. In clinical practice, these theoretical benefits are generally short lived (given metabolism of colloidal proteins/sugars), and for most patients there is little therapeutic advantage of colloids over crystalloids or vice versa. Examples of colloids include 5% albumin, 25% albumin, the dextrans, hetastarch, and fresh-frozen plasma (FFP). Because each of these agents contains a substance (proteins and complex sugars) that will ultimately be metabolized, the oncotic agent will be ultimately lost and only the remaining hypotonic fluid delivery agent will remain. As such, use of large volumes of colloidal agents is more likely to induce fluid overload compared with crystalloids. Although smaller volumes of colloids have equal efficacy as larger volumes of crystalloids, they generally must be infused more slowly. Often the net result is that the time to clinical benefit is the same regardless of which class of fluid is utilized. For example, 500 mL of normal saline is required to increase the systolic BP to the same degree as seen with approximately 250 mL of 5% albumin; however, the normal saline can be administered twice as fast.

▶ *Albumin*

Albumin is a protein derived from fractionating human plasma. Because albumin infusion is expensive and may be associated with adverse events, it should be used for acute volume expansion and *not* as a supplemental source of protein calories. Historically, albumin was used indiscriminately in the intensive care unit until anecdotal publications suggested that albumin may cause immunosuppression. However, the recently completed Saline Versus Albumin Fluid Evaluation (SAFE) trial randomized nearly 7,000 hypovolemic patients to either albumin or normal saline therapy and found that the mortality for those who received albumin was the same as for those who received normal saline.[7] A subsequent post hoc analysis reported that patients with traumatic brain injury had higher mortality rates when given

albumin for fluid resuscitation. These conflicting findings highlight the controversy and confusion surrounding the use of human albumin versus normal saline therapy for resuscitation of critically ill patients.[8-10] Albumin combined with furosemide has been demonstrated to improve fluid balance, oxygenation, and hemodynamics in the subset of patients with acute lung injury who have low serum protein.[11]

Recent events have resulted in an albumin shortage in the United States with ongoing allocation of all albumin products. In brief, albumin is obtained as a by-product of routine intravenous immunoglobulin (IVIG) processing. As a result, the albumin supply is driven by the amount of plasma fractioning for IVIG. Increased efficiency of the IVIG collection techniques and decreased IVIG consumption has led to an unintended shortage of albumin available for use. Based on this limited availability, health systems and hospitals have had to define the appropriate albumin indications for their patients and ration albumin accordingly. Evidence-based indications for albumin include plasmapheresis/apheresis, large-volume paracentesis (greater than 4 L removed), hypotension in hemodialysis, and the need for aggressive diuresis in hypoalbuminemic hypotensive patients. Inappropriate uses of albumin include nutritional supplementation, impending hepatorenal syndrome, pancreatitis, alteration of drug pharmacokinetics, or acute normovolemic hemodilution in surgery. Practitioners can keep up with medication shortages by checking the American Society of Health-System Pharmacists (ASHP) website (*www.ashp.org*).

▶ *Hetastarch and Dextran*

While albumin is the most commonly used colloid, the other available products are not without their own risks and benefits. Hetastarch (various manufacturers) and Voluven contain 6% starch and 0.9% NaCl. These products have no oxygen-carrying capacity and are administered intravenously as plasma expanders. Limitations of these products include acquisition cost, hypersensitivity reactions, and bleeding. Dosing should be reduced in the presence of renal dysfunction. There is evidence to suggest that Voluven can be administered safely in a larger volume (4 L versus 1 L of hetastarch) for volume expansion to minimize the need for albumin. Hextend is a comparable plasma expander that contains 6% hetastarch in lactated electrolyte solution. Low molecular weight dextran (various manufacturers) and high molecular weight dextran (various manufacturers) are polysaccharide plasma expanders. Anaphylactic reactions and prolonged bleeding times have limited the use of these products. Potential mechanisms of colloid solution-induced bleeding include platelet inhibition or possible dilution of clotting factors via infusion of a large-volume colloid solution. Although FFP has been used as a volume expander in cases of excessive blood loss (surgery or trauma) and to prevent bleeding in the presence of abnormal coagulation studies, it is now rarely used for volume expansion given risks of anaphylaxis, potential for viral transmission, and increased nosocomial infection rates.

Fluid Management Strategies

Classic indications for IV fluid include maintenance of BP, restoring the ICF volume, replacing ongoing renal or insensible losses when oral intake is inadequate, and the need for glucose as a fuel for the brain.[12] Although large volumes of fluid are given during the resuscitation of most trauma patients, a recent analysis reported uncertainty about the use of early large-volume fluid replacement in patients with active bleeding, calling into question our understanding of the need for fluids in various patient populations.[13]

When determining the appropriate fluid to be utilized, it is important to first determine the type of fluid problem (TBW versus ECF depletion), and start therapy accordingly. For patients demonstrating signs of impaired tissue perfusion, the immediate therapeutic goal is to increase the intravascular volume and restore tissue perfusion. The standard therapy is normal saline given at 150 to 500 mL/h (for adult patients) until perfusion is optimized. Although LR is a therapeutic alternative, lactic acidosis may arise with massive or prolonged infusions. LR has less chloride content versus normal saline (109 mEq/L [109 mmol/L] versus 154 mEq/L [154 mmol/L]) and has the advantage of use when large volumes of normal saline produce acidosis during fluid resuscitation. In severe cases, a colloid or blood transfusion may be indicated to increase oncotic pressure within the vascular space. Once euvolemia is achieved, patients may be switched to a more hypotonic maintenance solution (0.45% NaCl) at a rate that delivers estimated daily needs.

The clinical scenario and the severity of the volume abnormality dictate monitoring parameters during fluid replacement therapy. These may include the subjective sense of thirst, mental status, skin turgor, orthostatic vital signs, pulse rate, weight changes, blood chemistries, fluid input and output, central venous pressure, pulmonary capillary wedge pressure, and cardiac output. Fluid replacement requires particular caution in patient populations at risk of fluid overload, such as those with renal failure, cardiac failure, hepatic failure, or the elderly. Other complications of parenteral fluid therapy include IV site infiltration, infection, phlebitis, thrombophlebitis, and extravasation.

In summary, common settings for fluid resuscitation include hypovolemic patients (e.g., sepsis or pneumonia), hypervolemic patients (e.g., congestive heart failure [CHF], cirrhosis, or renal failure), euvolemic patients who are unable to take oral fluids in proportion to insensible losses (e.g., the perioperative period), and patients with electrolyte abnormalities (see below).

ELECTROLYTES

Normally, the number of anions (negatively charged ions) and cations (positively charged ions) in each fluid compartment are equal. Cell membranes play the critical role of maintaining distinct ICF and ECF spaces, which are biochemically distinct. Serum electrolyte measurements reflect the stores of ECF electrolytes rather than that of ICF electrolytes. Table 27–4 lists the chief cations and anions along with their normal

concentrations in the ECF and ICF. The principal cations are sodium, potassium, calcium, and magnesium; the key anions are chloride, bicarbonate, and phosphate. In the ECF, sodium is the most common cation and chloride is the most abundant anion; in the ICF, potassium is the primary cation and phosphate is the main anion. Normal serum electrolyte values are listed in Table 27–5.

Osmolality is a measure of the number of osmotically active particles per unit of solution, independent of the weight or nature of the particle. Equimolar concentrations of all substances in the undissociated state exert the same osmotic pressure. Although the normal serum osmolality is 280 to 300 mOsm/kg (280 to 300 mmol/kg), multiple scenarios exist where this value becomes markedly abnormal. ❸ *The calculated serum osmolality helps determine deviations in TBW content.* As such, it is often useful to calculate the serum osmolality as follows:

Table 27–4

Normal Cation and Anion Concentrations in the ECF and ICF

Ion Species	ECF Plasma (mEq/L or mmol/L)	ECF Interstitial Fluid (mEq/L or mmol/L)	Ion Species	ICF mEq/L or mmol/L
Cations			Cations	
Na⁺	142	144	K⁺	135
K⁺	4	4	Mg²⁺	43
Ca²⁺	5	2.5		
Mg²⁺	3	1.5		
Total	154	152	Total	178
Anions			Anions	
Cl⁻	103	114	PO₄²⁻	90
HCO₃⁻	27	30	Protein	70
PO₄²⁻	2	2	SO₄²⁻	18
SO₄²⁻	1	1		
Organic acid	5	5		
Protein	16	0		
Total	154	152	Total	178

ECF, extracellular fluid; ICF, intracellular fluid.

Table 27–5

Normal Ranges for Serum Electrolyte Concentrations

Sodium	136–145 mEq/L or 136–145 mmol/L
Potassium	3.5–5.0 mEq/L or 3.5–5.0 mmol/L
Chloride	98–106 mEq/L or 98–106 mmol/L
Bicarbonate	21–30 mEq/L or 21–30 mmol/L
Magnesium	1.4–2.2 mEq/L or 0.7–1.1 mmol/L
Calcium:	
Total	4.4–5.2 mEq/L (9–10.5 mg/dL) or 2.2–2.6 mmol/L
Ionized	2.2–2.8 mEq/L (4.5–5.6 mg/dL) or 1.1–1.4 mmol/L
Phosphorus	3–4.5 mg/dL (1.0–1.4 mmol/L)

- Serum **osmolality** (mOsm/kg) =
  2 (Na mEq/L) + (glucose [mg/dL])/18 +
  (BUN [mg/dL])/2.8.

  Serum osmolality using SI units (mmol/kg) =
  2 (Na mmol/L) + (glucose mmol/L) +
  (BUN mmol/L)

Because the body regulates water to maintain osmolality, deviations in serum osmolality are used to estimate TBW stores. Water moves freely across all cell membranes, making serum osmolality an accurate reflection of the osmolality within all body compartments. An increase in osmolality is equated with a loss of water greater than the loss of solute (TBW depletion). A decrease in serum osmolality is seen when water is retained in excess of solute (CHF or hepatic cirrhosis). The difference between the measured serum osmolality and the calculated serum osmolality, using the equation just stated, is referred to as the **osmolar gap**. Under normal circumstances the osmolar gap should be 10 mOsm/kg or less. An increased osmolar gap suggests the presence of a small osmotically active agent and is most commonly seen with the ingestion of alcohols (ethanol, methanol, ethylene glycol, or isopropyl alcohol) or medications such as mannitol or lorazepam. Patient Encounter 3 illustrates the utility of serum osmolality in a clinical setting.

Many of the electrolyte disturbances discussed in the remainder of this chapter represent medical emergencies that call for aggressive interventions including the use of concentrated electrolytes. It is very difficult to immediately reverse the effects of concentrated electrolytes when they are administered improperly, and these solutions are a frequent source of medical errors with significant potential for patient harm. ❹ *As such, The Joint Commission recommends that concentrated electrolyte solutions (KCl, potassium phosphate, and NaCl greater than 0.9%) be removed from patient care areas.* Hospitals should keep concentrated electrolytes in patient care areas only when patient safety necessitates their immediate use and precautions are used to prevent inadvertent administration. Collaborative cooperation among pharmacists, nurses, and physicians is essential. In addition,

The Joint Commission recommends standardizing and limiting the number of drug concentrations available in each institution and the use of ready-to-administer dosage forms so as to further reduce the risk of medication errors and improve outcomes.[14]

Sodium

The body's normal daily sodium requirement is 1.0 to 1.5 mEq/kg (1.0 to 1.5 mmol/kg) (80 to 130 mEq, which is 80 to 130 mmol) to maintain a normal serum sodium concentration of 136 to 145 mEq/L (136 to 145 mmol/L).[15] Sodium is the predominant cation of the ECF and largely determines ECF volume. Sodium is also the primary factor in establishing the osmotic pressure relationship between the ICF and ECF. All body fluids are in osmotic equilibrium, and changes in serum sodium concentration are associated with shifts of water into and out of body fluid

- compartments. When sodium is added to the intravascular fluid compartment, fluid is pulled intravascularly from the interstitial fluid and the ICF until osmotic balance is restored. As such, a patient's measured sodium concentration should *not* be viewed as an index of sodium need because this parameter reflects the balance between total body sodium content and TBW. Disturbances in the sodium concentration most often represent disturbances of TBW. Sodium imbalances cannot be properly assessed without first assessing body fluid status.

❺ *Hyponatremia is* the most common electrolyte disorder in *hospitalized patients and defined as a serum sodium concentration below 136 mEq/L (136 mmol/L).* Clinical signs and symptoms appear at concentrations below 120 mEq/L (120 mmol/L) and typically consist of irritability, mental slowing, unstable gait/falls fatigue, headache, and nausea. With profound hyponatremia (less than 110 mEq/L [110 mmol/L]), confusion, seizures, stupor/coma, and respiratory arrest may be seen. Because therapy is also influenced by volume status, hyponatremia is further defined as (a) hypertonic hyponatremia, (b) hypotonic hyponatremia with an increased ECF volume, (c) hypotonic hyponatremia with a normal ECF volume, and (d) hypotonic hyponatremia with a decreased ECF volume.[16]

- Hypertonic hyponatremia is usually associated with significant hyperglycemia. Glucose is an osmotically active agent that leads to an increase in TBW with little change in total body sodium. For every 60 mg/dL (3.3 mmol/L) increase in serum glucose above 200 mg/dL (11.1 mmol/L), the sodium concentration is expected to decrease by approximately 1 mEq/L
- (1 mmol/L). Appropriate treatment of the hyperglycemia will return the serum sodium concentration to normal.[15]

Hypotonic hyponatremia with an increase in ECF (hypervolemic hyponatremia) is also known as dilutional hyponatremia. In this scenario, patients have an excess of total body sodium and TBW; however, the excess in TBW is greater than the excess in total body sodium. Common causes include CHF, hepatic cirrhosis, and nephrotic syndrome. Treatment includes sodium and fluid restriction in conjunction with treatment of the underlying disorder—for example, salt and

---

Patient Encounter 3: Calculate the Plasma Osmolality

A 50-year-old homeless man is brought to the emergency department staggering and smelling like beer. Rapid respiration, tachycardia, and a BP of 90/60 mm Hg were noted. The sodium is 142 mEq/L (142 mmol/L), potassium 3.6 mEq/L (3.6 mmol/L), chloride 100 mEq/L (100 mmol/L), bicarbonate 12 mEq/L (12 mmol/L), glucose 180 mg/dL (10.0 mmol/L), and BUN 28 mg/dL (10.0 mmol/L). The measured osmolarity is 360 mOsm/kg (360 mmol/kg).

Calculate the osmolality.

Calculate the osmolar gap.

What is the likely cause of an increased gap in this patient?

water restrictions are used in the setting of CHF along with loop diuretics, angiotensin-converting enzyme inhibitors, and spironolactone.[15]

In hypotonic hyponatremia with a normal ECF volume (euvolemic hyponatremia), patients have an excess of TBW with relatively normal sodium content. In essence, there is a presence of excess free water. This is most frequently seen in patients with the syndrome of inappropriate antidiuretic hormone secretion (SIADH). Common causes of SIADH include carcinomas (e.g., lung or pancreas), pulmonary disorders (e.g., pneumonias or tuberculosis), CNS disorders (e.g., meningitis, stroke, tumor, or trauma), and medications (e.g., sulfonylureas, antineoplastic agents, barbiturates, morphine, antipsychotics, tricyclic antidepressants, nonsteroidal anti-inflammatory agents, selective serotonin reuptake inhibitors, dopamine agonists, and general anesthetics). These medications stimulate the release of antidiuretic hormone (ADH) from the pituitary gland resulting in water retention and dilution of the body's sodium stores.

Short-term treatment of euvolemic hyponatremia includes fluid restriction, isotonic normal saline, hypertonic saline, or conivaptan. Initial treatment generally consists of fluid restriction alone. Hypertonic saline is used only when the sodium concentration is less than 110 mEq/L (110 mmol/L) and/or severe symptoms (e.g., seizures) are present. Given the limitations associated with these treatment strategies (unpredictable therapeutic effects and side effects), the arginine vasopressin antagonist conivaptan (Vaprisol, Astellas Pharma) was developed for short-term treatment of euvolemic hyponatremia. While conivaptan can also be used to manage hypervolemic hyponatremia in hospitalized patients, it should not be used for hypovolemic hyponatremia. Conivaptan is dosed 20 mg IV over 30 minutes, followed by a 20-mg continuous infusion over 24 hours for up to 4 days. The initial formulation of conivaptan contained propylene glycol and was associated with infusion site reactions. The revised formulation is better tolerated.

Long-term treatment options for euvolemic hyponatremia include fluid restriction, demeclocycline, loop diuretics, saline, lithium, urea, and tolvaptan. Demeclocycline (available as generic) is dosed at 600 to 1,200 mg/day, takes days before clinical effect is realized, and can cause nephrotoxicity. Lithium (various generics) also has a slow onset of action and is limited by CNS side effects, GI disturbances and cardiotoxicity. Furosemide (various generics) or other loop diuretics allow relaxation of fluid restriction but can cause significant volume depletion and electrolyte disturbances, and it has the potential for ototoxicity. No specific USP formulation exists for urea and poor palatability, and side effects limits it use. Tolvaptan (Samsca [Otsuka]) is an oral alternative to IV conivaptan. This product is indicated for treatment of clinically significant hypervolemic and euvolemic hyponatremia (sodium less than 125 mEq/L [less than 125 mmol/L]) or less marked hyponatremia that is symptomatic and has resisted correction with fluid restriction. Patients with CHF, cirrhosis, and SIADH would be candidates for long-term use. Tolvaptan has a boxed warning for

initiation of treatment in a hospital setting because of the need for close sodium monitoring. The initial dose is 15 mg orally daily and may be titrated up to a max of 60 mg. Concurrent use with potent CYP 3A4 inhibitors should be avoided: ketoconazole (available as generic), clarithromycin (available as generic), ritonavir (Norvir, Abbott), diltiazem (available as generic), verapamil (available as generic), fluconazole (available as generic), and grapefruit juice.

In hypotonic hyponatremia with a decreased ECF volume (hypovolemic hyponatremia), patients usually have a deficit of both total body sodium and TBW, but the sodium deficit exceeds the TBW deficit. Common causes include diuretic use, profuse sweating, wound drainage, burns, GI losses (vomiting or diarrhea), hypoadrenalism (low cortisol and low aldosterone), and renal tubular acidosis. Treatment includes the administration of sodium to correct the sodium deficit and water to correct the TBW deficit. The sodium deficit can be calculated with the following equation[2]:

Sodium deficit (mEq or mmol) = (TBW [in liters]) (desired Na$^+$ concentration [mEq/L or mmol/L] − current Na$^+$ concentration).

Although both water and sodium are required in this instance, sodium needs to be provided in excess of water to fully correct this abnormality. As such, hypertonic saline (3% NaCl) is often used. One can estimate the change in serum sodium concentration after 1 L of 3% NaCl infusion using the following equation[16]:

Change in serum Na$^+$ (mEq/L or mmol/L) = (infusate Na$^+$ − serum Na$^+$)/(TBW + 1).

In this formula, TBW is increased by 1 to account for the addition of the liter of 3% NaCl. Patient Encounters 4 and 5 illustrate the concepts of calculating and correcting the sodium deficit.

Depending on the severity of the hyponatremia and acuity of onset, 0.9%, 3%, or 5% NaCl can be utilized. Most patients can be adequately managed with normal saline rehydration, which is generally the safest agent. Hypertonic

Patient Encounter 4: Calculation of Sodium Deficit

Calculate the sodium deficit for an 80-kg male with a serum sodium of 123 mEq/L (123 mmol/L).

Patient Encounter 5: Estimate the Anticipated Change in Serum Sodium

Estimate the anticipated change in serum sodium concentration after the infusion of 1 L of 3% NaCl in an 80-kg male with a serum sodium of 123 mEq/L (123 mmol/L).

saline (3% or 5% NaCl) is generally reserved for patients with severe hyponatremia (less than 120 mEq/L [120 mmol/L]) accompanied by coma, seizures, or high urinary sodium losses. Roughly one-third of the sodium deficit can be replaced over the first 12 hours as long as the replacement rate is less than 0.5 mEq/h (0.5 mmol/h). The remaining two-thirds of the deficit can be administered over the ensuing days. Overly aggressive correction of symptomatic hyponatremia (greater than 12 mEq/L [12 mmol/L] per day) can result in central pontine myelinolysis.[17] Given the potential for irreversible neurologic damage if untreated or if improperly treated, acute hyponatremia is an urgent condition that should be promptly treated with careful attention to monitoring serial sodium values and adjusting therapeutic infusions accordingly.[18]

Hypernatremia is a serum sodium concentration greater than 145 mEq/L (145 mmol/L) and can occur in the absence of a sodium deficit (pure water loss) or in its presence (hypotonic fluid loss).[19] The signs and symptoms of hypernatremia manifest with a serum sodium concentration greater than 160 mEq/L (160 mmol/L) and are usually the same as those found in TBW depletion: thirst, mental slowing, and dry mucous membranes. Signs and symptoms become more profound as hypernatremia worsens, with the patient eventually demonstrating confusion, hallucinations, acute weight loss, decreased skin turgor, intracranial bleeding, and/or coma. Many coexisting disorders and medications may complicate the diagnosis.

The classic causes of hypernatremia are associated with TBW depletion. These include dehydration from loss of hypotonic fluid from the respiratory tract or skin, decreased water intake, osmotic diuresis (e.g., mannitol, available as generic), and diabetes insipidus (e.g., decreased ADH; phenytoin, available as generic; lithium, available as generic). Hypernatremia in hospitalized patients occurs secondary to inappropriate fluid management in patients at risk for increased free water losses and impaired thirst or restricted water intake.[20] Iatrogenic hypernatremia is occasionally caused by the administration of excessive hypertonic saline. Treatment of hypernatremia includes calculation of the TBW deficit followed by the administration of hypotonic fluids as previously described. The fluid volume should be replaced over 48 to 72 hours depending on the severity of symptoms and the degree of hypertonicity.[21] For asymptomatic patients, the rate of correction should not exceed 0.5 mEq/L/h (0.5 mmol/L/h). One rule of thumb is to replace half the calculated TBW deficit over 12 to 24 hours and the other half of the deficit over the next 24 to 48 hours.[2,19] Excessively rapid correction of hypernatremia may lead to cerebral edema and death. Patient Encounters 6 and 7 reinforce the concepts of calculating TBW deficit and expected changes in serum sodium concentration with therapy.

Potassium

The body's normal daily potassium requirement is 0.5 to 1 mEq/kg (0.5 to 1 mmol/kg) or 40 to 80 mEq (40 to 80 mmol) to maintain a serum potassium concentration of

---

Patient Encounter 6: Calculate Water Deficit

Calculate the water deficit in an 80-kg male with a serum sodium of 154 mEq/L (154 mmol/L).

Patient Encounter 7: Calculate the Anticipated Change in Serum Sodium

Calculate the anticipated change in serum sodium concentration after IV infusion of 1 L of 5% dextrose in a 80 kg male with a serum sodium of 156 mEq/L (156 mmol/L).

3.5 to 5 mEq/L (3.5 to 5 mmol/L). Potassium is the most abundant cation in the ICF, balancing the sodium contained in the ECF and maintaining electroneutrality of bodily fluids. Because the majority of potassium is intracellular, serum potassium concentration is not a good measure of total body potassium; however, clinical manifestations of potassium disorders correlate well with serum potassium. The acid–base balance of the body affects serum potassium concentrations: hyperkalemia is routinely seen in patients with decreased pH (acidosis). Potassium regulation is primarily under the control of the kidneys with excess dietary potassium being excreted in the urine. Although mild abnormalities of serum potassium are considered a nuisance, severe hyperkalemia or hypokalemia can be life threatening.[22–24]

Hypokalemia (serum potassium less than 3.5 mEq/L [3.5 mmol/L]) is a common clinical problem. While generally asymptomatic, signs and symptoms of hypokalemia include cramps, muscle weakness, polyuria, electrocardiogram (ECG) changes (flattened T waves and presence of U waves), and cardiac arrhythmias (bradycardia, heart block, atrial flutter, premature ventricular contractions, and ventricular fibrillation). Causes of hypokalemia include GI losses (vomiting, diarrhea, or NG tube suction), renal losses (high aldosterone and low magnesium), inadequate potassium intake (in IV fluids or oral), or alkalosis. Many medications can precipitate hypokalemia. β_2-agonists (e.g., albuterol, available as generic) and insulin (multiple product formulations) lower potassium via cellular redistribution. The use of loop diuretics (furosemide [Lasix], also available as generic), thiazide diuretics (hydrochlorothiazide, available as generic), high-dose antibiotics (penicillin, available as generic), and corticosteroids (prednisone, available as generic) cause renal potassium wasting. In addition, amphotericin B (available as generic), cisplatin (available as generic), and foscarnet (available as generic) can also produce hypokalemia secondary to depletion of magnesium. Hypomagnesemia diminishes intracellular potassium concentration and produces potassium wasting. Given the potential for significant morbidity and mortality, serum potassium concentrations should be monitored closely for patients with known (or suspected) hypokalemia.[2,24,25] Hypokalemia is a risk factor for digitalis toxicity.

Table 27–6

Potassium Content in Various Potassium Salt Preparations

Potassium Salt	mEq/g (mmol/L)
Potassium gluconate[a]	4.3
Potassium citrate[a]	9.8
Potassium bicarbonate[a]	10.0
Potassium acetate[a]	10.2
Potassium chloride[b]	13.4

[a]Favored for hypokalemia and concurrent acidosis.

[b]Favored for hypokalemia and concurrent alkalosis.

Each 1 mEq/L (1 mmol/L) fall in serum potassium (i.e., from 4 to 3 mEq/L [4 to 3 mmol/L]) represents a loss of approximately 200 mEq (200 mmol) of potassium in the adult. However, when the serum potassium is below 3 mEq/L (3 mmol/L), each 1 mEq/L (1 mmol/L) fall in serum potassium represents a 200 to 400 mEq (200 to 400 mmol) reduction in serum concentration in the adult patient. Potassium repletion should be guided by close monitoring of serial serum concentrations instead of using empirically chosen amounts. Of the five potassium salts available, potassium acetate (10.2 mEq/K$^+$/g or 10.2 mmol/K$^+$/g) and KCl (13.4 mEq/K$^+$/g or 13.4 mmol/K$^+$/g) are the most commonly used forms. When hypokalemia occurs in the setting of alkalosis, KCl is the preferred agent; in acidosis, potassium should be provided in the form of acetate, citrate, bicarbonate, or gluconate salt. Table 27–6 outlines the potassium content of each potassium salt preparation, and Table 27–7 lists each of the oral potassium replacement products. Potassium acetate and chloride are available for IV infusions as premixed solutions. The usual dose of these agents is 10 to 20 mEq (10 to 20 mmol) diluted in 100 mL of normal saline.[2,25,26]

Table 27–7

Oral Potassium Replacement Products

Product	Salt	Strength[a]
Extended/controlled-release tablets	Chloride	8 mEq (600 mg) 10 mEq (750 mg) 15 mEq (1,125 mg) 20 mEq (1,500 mg)
Effervescent tablets	Chloride and bicarbonate	10 mEq 20 mEq 25 mEq 50 mEq
Liquid	Chloride	20 mEq/15 mL (10%) 40 mEq/15 mL (20%)
Powder packets	Chloride	20 mEq 25 mEq

[a]For potassium, 1 mEq = 1 mmol.

Moderate hypokalemia is defined as a serum potassium of 2.5 to 3.5 mEq/L (2.5 to 3.5 mmol/L) without ECG changes. In this setting, potassium replacement can usually be given orally at a dose of 40 to 120 mEq/day (40 to 120 mmol/day). Anecdotally, oral potassium supplementation (see Table 27–7) is often more effective in repleting moderate hypokalemia. For patients with an ongoing source of potassium loss, chronic replacement therapy should be considered. The potassium deficit is a rough approximation of the amount of potassium needed to be replaced and can be estimated as follows:

Potassium deficit (mEq or mmol/L) = (4.0 − current serum potassium) × 100

Severe hypokalemia is defined as a serum potassium less than 2.5 mEq/L (2.5 mmol/L) or hypokalemia of any magnitude that is associated with ECG changes (e.g., flattening of T wave or elevation of U wave) and cardiac arrhythmias. In these situations, IV replacement should be initiated urgently. ⑥ *Potassium infusion at rates exceeding 10 mEq/h (10 mmol/h) requires cardiac monitoring given the potential for cardiac arrhythmias.* Although the maximally concentrated solution for potassium replacement is 80 mEq/L (80 mmol/L), the maximum infusion rate is 40 mEq/h (40 mmol/h) and must be administered via a central line. Table 27–8 outlines current IV potassium replacement guidelines.

Caution must be exercised when repleting potassium with IV agents given possible vein irritation and/or thrombophlebitis. The risk of these complications is minimized by using less concentrated solutions and by giving infusions via central access if possible. Administration of potassium in vehicles containing glucose is discouraged because glucose facilitates the intracellular movement of potassium. Posttherapy improvements in serum potassium may be transient, and continuous monitoring is required. Patients with low serum magnesium will have exaggerated potassium losses from the kidneys and GI tract leading to refractory hypokalemia. In this situation, the magnesium deficit must be corrected in order to successfully treat the concurrent potassium deficiency. In the hypokalemic patient

Table 27–8

Recommended Potassium Dosage/Infusion Rate

Clinical Scenario	Maximum Infusion Rate[a]	Maximum Concentration[a]	Maximum 24-Hour Dose[a]
K$^+$ greater than 2.5 mEq/L *and* No ECG changes of hypokalemia	10 mEq/h	40 mEq/L	200 mEq
K$^+$ less than 2.5 mEq/L *or* ECG changes of hypokalemia	40 mEq/h	80 mEq/L	400 mEq

[a]For potassium, 1 mEq = 1 mmol.

with concurrent acidosis, potassium is often given as the acetate salt, given that acetate is metabolized to bicarbonate. In the patient with depleted phosphorus and potassium, therapy with potassium phosphate is the natural choice.[22,27,28]

Hyperkalemia is defined as a serum potassium concentration greater than 5 mEq/L (5 mmol/L). Manifestations of hyperkalemia include muscle weakness, paresthesias, hypotension, ECG changes (e.g., peaked T waves, shortened QT intervals, and wide QRS complexes), cardiac arrhythmias, and a decreased pH. Causes of hyperkalemia fall into three broad categories: (a) increased potassium intake, (b) decreased potassium excretion, and (c) potassium release from the intracellular space.

Increased potassium intake results from excessive dietary potassium (salt substitutes), excess potassium in IV fluids, and other select medications (potassium-sparing diuretics, cyclosporine [available as generic], angiotensin-converting enzyme inhibitors, nonsteroidal anti-inflammatory agents, pentamidine [available as generic], unfractionated heparin, and low molecular weight heparins). Decreased potassium excretion results from acute renal failure, chronic renal failure, or Addison's disease. Excess potassium release from cells results from tissue breakdown (surgery, trauma, hemolysis, or rhabdomyolysis), blood transfusions, and metabolic acidosis.

In addition to discontinuing all potassium supplements, potassium-sparing medications, and potassium-rich salt substitutes, management of hyperkalemia addresses three concurrent strategies: (a) agents to antagonize the proarrhythmic effects of hyperkalemia, (b) agents to drive potassium into the intracellular space and acutely lower the serum potassium, and (c) agents that will definitively (but more gradually) lower the total body potassium content.[29] If the serum potassium concentration is greater than 7 mEq/L (7 mmol/L) and/or ECG changes are present, IV calcium is provided to stabilize the myocardium. Depending on the acuity of the situation, 1 g of calcium chloride (13.5 mEq or 6.75 mmol) is administered by direct injection or diluted in 50 mL of D_5W and delivered IV over 15 minutes. Clinical effects are seen within 1 to 2 minutes of infusion and persist for 10 to 30 minutes. Repeat doses may be administered as necessary. Because most patients with clinically significant hyperkalemia receive multiple boluses of calcium directed by ECG findings, iatrogenic hypercalcemia is a potential complication of hyperkalemia treatment. As such, total calcium concentration is commonly checked with each potassium concentration measurement. Ionized calcium measurements should be obtained in patients who have comorbid conditions that would lead to inconsistency between total serum calcium and free calcium (abnormal albumin, protein, or immunoglobulin concentrations).

Dextrose and insulin (with or without sodium bicarbonate) are typically given at the time of calcium therapy in order to redistribute potassium into the intracellular space. Dextrose 50% (25 g in 50 mL) can be given by slow IV push over 5 minutes or dextrose 10% with 20 units of regular insulin can be given by continuous IV infusion over 1 to 2 hours. The onset of action for this combination is 30 minutes; the duration of clinical effects is 2 to 6 hours. High-dose inhaled β_2-agonists (e.g., albuterol, available as generic) may also be used to acutely drive potassium into the intracellular space.

It is critically important to recognize that the treatments of hyperkalemia discussed thus far are transient, temporizing measures. They are intended to provide time to institute definitive therapy aimed at removing excess potassium from the body. Agents that increase potassium excretion from the body include sodium polystyrene sulfonate (Kayexalate, available as generic), loop diuretics, and hemodialysis or hemofiltration (used only in patients with renal failure). Sodium polystyrene sulfonate can be given orally, via NG tube, or as a rectal retention enema and is dosed at 15 to 60 g in four divided doses per day. In September 2009, MedWatch issued a safety alert that cases of colonic necrosis and other serious GI-adverse events (bleeding, ischemic colitis, perforation) had been reported in association with Kayexalate use. The majority of these cases reported the concurrent use of sorbitol. Concurrent administration of sorbitol is no longer recommended. Medication safety alerts are available at *www.fda.gov/MedWatch*.

Calcium

More than 99% of total body calcium is found in bone; the remaining less than 1% is in the ECF and ICF. Calcium plays a critical role in the transmission of nerve impulses, skeletal muscle contraction, myocardial contractions, maintenance of normal cellular permeability, and the formation of bones and teeth. There is a reciprocal relationship between the serum calcium concentration (normally 8.6 to 10.2 mg/dL [2.15 to 2.55 mmol/L]) and the serum phosphate concentration that is regulated by a complex interaction between parathyroid hormone, vitamin D, and calcitonin. About one-half of the serum calcium is bound to plasma proteins; the other half is free ionized calcium. Given that the serum calcium has significant protein binding, the serum calcium measurement must be corrected in patients who have low albumin concentrations (the major serum protein). The most commonly used formula adds 0.8 mg/dL (0.2 mmol/L) of calcium for each gram of albumin deficiency as follows:

Corrected [Ca mg/dL] = Measured [Ca mg/dL] + [0.8 × (4−measured albumin g/dL)][30–32]

Corrected [Ca mmol/L] = Measured [Ca mmol/L] + [0.02 × (40−measured albumin g/L)]

Hypocalcemia is caused by inadequate intake (vitamin deficiency, poor dietary calcium sources, alcoholism) or excessive losses (hypoparathyroidism, renal failure, alkalosis, pancreatitis). Clinical manifestations of hypocalcemia are seen with total serum concentrations less than 6.5 mg/dL (1.63 mmol/L) or an ionized calcium less than 1.12 mmol/L and include tetany, circumoral tingling, muscle spasms, hypoactive reflexes, anxiety, hallucinations, hypotension, myocardial infarction, seizures, lethargy, stupor, and Trousseau's sign or Chvostek's sign.[24,33] **Trousseau's sign is** elicited by inflating a BP cuff on the patient's upper arm, whereby hypocalcemic patients will experience tetany of the wrist and hand as evidenced by thumb adduction, wrist flexion, and metacarpophalangeal joint flexion. **Chvostek's sign** is elicited by tapping on the proximal distribution of the facial nerve (adjacent to the ear). This will produce a brief spasm of the upper lip, eye, nose, or face in hypocalcemic patients. Ionized calcium concentrations are typically used to assess calcium status in the critically ill patient.

Causes of hypocalcemia include hypoparathyroidism, hypomagnesemia, alcoholism, hyperphosphatemia, blood product infusion (due to chelation by the citrate buffers), chronic renal failure, vitamin D deficiency, acute pancreatitis, alkalosis, and hypoalbuminemia. In the setting of hypocalcemia, magnesium concentration should be checked and corrected if low. Given that hypocalcemia may be caused by hypomagnesemia, clinicians should be aware that the serum calcium concentrations may not normalize until serum magnesium is replaced. Medications that cause hypocalcemia include phosphate replacement products, loop diuretics, phenytoin (Dilantin, available as generic), phenobarbital (available as generic), corticosteroids, aminoglycoside antibiotics, and acetazolamide (available as generic).[34-36]

Oral calcium replacement products include calcium carbonate (Os-Cal [GlaxoSmithKline] and various generics; Tums [GlaxoSmithKline] and various generics) and calcium citrate (Citracal [Mission Bayer] and various generics). IV calcium replacement products include calcium gluconate and calcium chloride (both products available as generic). ❼ *Calcium gluconate is preferred for peripheral use because it is less irritating to the veins; it may also be given intramuscularly.* Each 10 mL of a 10% calcium gluconate solution provides 90 mg (4.5 mEq or 2.25 mmol) of elemental calcium. ❼ *Calcium chloride is associated with more venous irritation and extravasation and is generally reserved for administration via central line.* Each 10 mL of a 10% calcium chloride solution contains 270 mg (13.5 mEq or 6.75 mmol) of elemental calcium. IV calcium products are given as a slow push or added to 500 to 1,000 mL of 0.9% normal saline for slow infusion.[33,36] In addition to hypocalcemia, IV calcium may also be used for massive blood transfusions, calcium channel blocker overdose, and emergent hyperkalemia and hypermagnesemia.

For acute symptomatic hypocalcemia, 200 to 300 mg of elemental calcium is administered IV and repeated until symptoms are fully controlled. This is achieved by infusing 1 g of calcium chloride or 2 to 3 g of calcium gluconate at a rate no faster than 30 to 60 mg of elemental calcium per minute. More rapid administration is associated with hypotension, bradycardia, or cardiac asystole. Total calcium concentration is commonly monitored in critically ill patients. Under normal circumstances, about half of calcium is loosely bound to serum proteins while the other half is free. Total calcium concentration measures bound and free calcium. Ionized calcium measures free calcium only. Under usual circumstances, a normal calcium concentration implies a normal free ionized calcium concentration. Ionized calcium should be obtained in patients with comorbid conditions that would lead to inconsistency between total calcium and free serum calcium (abnormal albumin, protein, or immunoglobulin concentrations). For chronic asymptomatic hypocalcemia, oral calcium supplements are given at doses of 2 to 4 g/day of elemental calcium. Many patients with calcium deficiency have concurrent vitamin D deficiency that must also be corrected in order to restore calcium homeostasis.[2,33,37]

Hypercalcemia is defined as a calcium concentration greater than 10.2 mg/dL (2.55 mmol/L). It may be categorized as mild if total serum calcium is 10.3 to 12 mg/dL (2.58 to 3.00 mmol/L), moderate if total serum calcium is 12.1 to 13 mg/dL (3.03 to 3.25 mmol/L), or severe when serum concentration is greater than 13 mg/dL (3.25 mmol/L). Causes of hypercalcemia include hyperparathyroidism, malignancy, Paget's disease, Addison's disease, granulomatous diseases (e.g., tuberculosis, sarcoidosis, or histoplasmosis), hyperthyroidism, immobilization, multiple bony fractures, acidosis, and milk-alkali syndrome. Multiple medications cause hypercalcemia and include thiazide diuretics, estrogens, lithium (available as generic), tamoxifen (Nolvadex, available as generic), vitamin A, vitamin D, and calcium supplements.[2,33,36,37]

Because the severity of symptoms and the absolute serum concentration are poorly correlated in some patients, institution of therapy should be dictated by the clinical scenario. All patients with hypercalcemia should be treated with aggressive rehydration: normal saline at 200 to 300 mL/h is a routine initial fluid prescription. For patients with mild hypercalcemia, hydration alone may provide adequate therapy. The moderate and severe forms of hypercalcemia are more likely to have significant manifestations and require prompt initiation of additional therapy. These patients may present with anorexia, confusion, and/or cardiac manifestations (bradycardia and arrhythmias with ECG changes). Total calcium concentrations greater than 13 mg/dL (3.25 mmol/L) are particularly worrisome because these concentrations can unexpectedly precipitate acute renal failure, ventricular arrhythmias, and sudden death.

Once fluid administration has repleted the ECF, forced diuresis (with associated calcium loss) can be initiated with a loop diuretic. For this approach to be successful, normal kidney function is required. In renal failure patients, the alternative therapy is emergent hemodialysis. Other treatment options include bisphosphonates (zoledronic acid [Zometa, Novartis], pamidronate [Aredia, available as generic]), hydrocortisone (available as generic), calcitonin, and gallium. Given their efficacy and favorable side-effect profile, bisphosphonates are typically the agents of choice. Table 27–9 outlines the treatment options for hypercalcemia including time to onset of effect, duration of effect, and efficacy.[2,33,34,37]

Phosphorus

Phosphorus is primarily found in the bone (80% to 85%) and ICF (15% to 20%): the remaining less than 1% is found in the

Table 27–9

Selected Treatment Options for the Management of Hypercalcemia

Therapy	Dose	Onset	Duration	Efficacy[a]
Normal saline	3–6 L/day	Hours	Hours	1–2 mg/dL (0.25–0.50 mmol/L)
Furosemide (Lasix, available as generic)	80–160 mg/day	Hours	Hours	1–2 mg/dL (0.25–0.50 mmol/L)
Hydrocortisone (available as generic)	200 mg/day	Hours	Days	Mild/unpredictable
Calcitonin (Miacalcin, Novartis)	4–8 units/kg	Hours	Hours	1–2 mg/dL (0.25–0.50 mmol/L)
Pamidronate (Aredia, available as generic)	30–90 mg/week	Days	1–4 weeks	1–5 mg/dL(0.25–1.25 mmol/L)
Zoledronic acid (Zometa, Novartis)	4–8 mg	Days	Weeks	1–5 mg/dL (0.25–1.25 mmol/L
Gallium (Ganite, Genta Inc.)	200 mg/m^2	Days	Days–weeks	1–5 mg/dL (0.25–1.25 mmol/L)

[a]Expected decrease in serum Ca^{2+}.

ECF. Note that phosphorus is the major anion within the cells. Given this distribution, serum phosphate concentration does not accurately reflect total body phosphorus stores. Phosphorus is expressed in milligrams (mg) or millimoles (mmol), not as milliequivalents (mEq). Because phosphorus is the source of phosphate for adenosine triphosphate (ATP) and phospholipid synthesis, manifestations of phosphorus imbalance are variable.

Dietary intake, parathyroid hormone levels, and renal function are the major determinants of the serum phosphorus concentration, which is normally 2.7 to 4.5 mg/dL (0.87 to 1.45 mmol/L).[2,33,39,40] Hypophosphatemia is defined by a serum phosphorus concentration less than 2.5 mg/dL (0.81 mmol/L); severe hypophosphatemia occurs when the phosphorus concentration is less than 1 mg/dL (0.32 mmol/L). Hypophosphatemia can be caused by increased distribution to the ICF (hyperglycemia, insulin therapy, or malnourishment), decreased absorption (starvation, excessive use of phosphorus-binding antacids, vitamin D deficiency, diarrhea, or laxative abuse) or increased renal loss (diuretic use, diabetic ketoacidosis, alcohol abuse, hyperparathyroidism, or burns).[35,37] ❽ *Severe hypophosphatemia can result in impaired diaphragmatic contractility and acute respiratory failure.* Medications that cause hypophosphatemia include diuretics (acetazolamide [Diamox, available as generic], furosemide [Lasix, available as generic], hydrochlorothiazide [HydroDIURIL, available as generic]), sucralfate (Carafate, available as generic), corticosteroids, cisplatin (available as generic), antacids (aluminum carbonate, calcium carbonate, and magnesium oxide [antacids all available as generic]), foscarnet (available as generic), phenytoin (Dilantin, available as generic), phenobarbital (available as generic), and phosphate binders (sevelamer [Renvela, Genzyme Corp.], and calcium acetate [PhosLo, available as generic]).

Signs and symptoms of hypophosphatemia include paresthesias, muscle weakness, myalgias, bone pain, anorexia, nausea, vomiting, red blood cell breakdown (hemolysis), acute respiratory failure, seizures, and coma.[37,41] For mild hypophosphatemia, patients should be encouraged to eat a high-phosphorus diet including eggs, nuts, whole grains, meat, fish, poultry, and milk products. For moderate hypophosphatemia (1 to 2.5 mg/dL, 0.32 to 0.81 mmol/L), oral supplementation of 1.5 to 2 g/day (30 to 60 mmol/day) is usually adequate. Diarrhea may be a dose-limiting side effect with oral phosphate replacement products.

Injectable phosphate products are reserved for patients with severe hypophosphatemia or those in the intensive care unit.[42] The available agents are provided as sodium or potassium salts; however, unless concurrent hypokalemia is present, sodium phosphate is usually used. Empirically, for a mild serum phosphorus deficiency (2.3 to 3.0 mg/dL, 0.74 to 0.97 mmol/L), the corresponding IV phosphorus dose is 0.32 mmol/kg; for a moderate deficiency of serum phosphorus 1.6 to 2.2 mg/dL (0.52 to 0.71 mmol/L), the replacement dose is 0.64 mmol/kg; and the dose is 1 mmol/kg when the serum phosphorus is less than 1.5 mg/dL (0.48 mmol/L).[36] IV phosphorus preparations are usually infused over 4 to 12 hours. Table 27–10 compares the available phosphate replacement products.

Table 27–10

Phosphate Replacement Products

Product	Route	mgPO$_4^-$	mmolPO$_4^-$	mEq (mmol) Na$^+$	mEq (mmol) K$^+$
Potassium phosphate (KPO$_4$/mL), available as generic	IV	94	3	0	4.4
Sodium phosphate (NaPO$_4$/mL), available as generic	IV	94	3	4	0
Phos-NaK packets	Oral	250	8	7.2	7
K-Phos Neutral Tablets, Beach	Oral	250	8	13.1	1.4
Uro-KP-Neutral tablets, Star	Oral	250	8	10.9	1.27

Hyperphosphatemia is defined by a serum phosphorus concentration greater than 4.5 mg/dL (1.45 mmol/L). The manifestations of hyperphosphatemia are similar to findings of hypocalcemia (see earlier), and include paresthesias, ECG changes (prolonged QT interval and prolonged ST segment), and metastatic calcifications. Causes of hyperphosphatemia include impaired phosphorus excretion (hypoparathyroidism or renal failure), redistribution of phosphorus to the ECF (acid–base imbalance, rhabdomyolysis, muscle necrosis, or tumor lysis during chemotherapy), and increased phosphorus intake (various medications).[37] Medications that can cause hyperphosphatemia include enemas containing phosphorus (e.g., Fleet, Fleet), laxatives containing phosphate or phosphorus, parenteral or oral supplements (e.g., K-Phos Neutral, Beach), vitamin D supplements, and the bisphosphonates (e.g., pamidronate, various manufacturers).[43]

Hyperphosphatemia is generally benign and rarely needs aggressive therapy. Dietary restriction of phosphate and protein is effective for most minor elevations. Phosphate binders such as aluminum-based antacids, calcium carbonate, calcium acetate (PhosLo, available as generic), sevelamer (Renvela, Genzyme), and lanthanum carbonate (Fosrenol, Shire) may be necessary for some patients (typically those with chronic renal failure).[49] If patients exhibit findings of hypocalcemia (tetany), IV calcium should be administered empirically.

Magnesium

The body's normal daily magnesium requirement is 300 to 350 mg/day to maintain a serum magnesium concentration of 1.5 to 2.4 mEq/L (0.75 to 1.20 mmol/L). Because magnesium is the second most abundant ICF cation, serum concentrations are a relatively poor measure of total body stores. Magnesium catalyzes and/or activates more than 300 enzymes, provides neuromuscular stability, and is involved in myocardial contraction. Magnesium is generally not part of standard chemistry panels and therefore must be ordered separately.[2,33,43–45]

Hypomagnesemia is defined as a serum magnesium less than 1.5 mEq/L (0.75 mmol/L) and is most frequently seen in the intensive care and postoperative settings. Hypomagnesemia results from inadequate intake (alcoholism, dietary restriction, or inadequate magnesium in total parenteral nutrition [TPN]), inadequate absorption (steatorrhea, cancer, malabsorption syndromes, or excess calcium or phosphorus in the GI tract), excessive GI loss of magnesium (diarrhea, laxative abuse, NG tube suctioning, or acute pancreatitis), or excessive urinary loss of magnesium (primary hyperaldosteronism, certain medications, diabetic ketoacidosis, and renal disorders). Hypomagnesemia often occurs in the setting of hypokalemia and hypocalcemia. Clinicians should evaluate the magnesium concentration in these patients and correct if low. In order for calcium and potassium concentrations to normalize, magnesium supplementation is often required. Medications that potentially can cause hypomagnesemia include aminoglycoside antibiotics, amphotericin B (available as generic), cisplatin (available as generic), insulin, cyclosporine (available as generic), loop diuretics, and thiazide diuretics There is also a strong correlation between hypokalemia and hypomagnesemia.[37,38,43,46] Clinicians should be alerted that the long-term use of proton pump inhibitors may be associated with unexplained hypomagnesemia, with subsequent hypokalemia or hypocalcemia.

The findings of hypomagnesemia include muscle weakness, cramps, agitation, confusion, tremor, seizures, ECG changes (increased PR interval, prolonged QRS complex, and increased QT interval), findings of hypocalcemia (see earlier), refractory hypokalemia (see earlier), metabolic alkalosis, and digoxin toxicity.[43,47,48]

Asymptomatic mild magnesium deficiencies (1.0 to 1.5 mEq/L) (0.50 to 0.75 mmol/L) can be managed with increased oral intake of magnesium-containing foods or with oral supplementation. Magnesium oxide (Mag-Ox, Blaine Pharmaceuticals and various manufacturers) 400-mg tablets contain 241 mg (20 mEq or 10 mmol) of magnesium, and magnesium chloride hexahydrate tablets (Slow-Mag, Purdue) contains 64 mg of elemental magnesium. Diarrhea is often a dose-limiting side effect of oral supplementation. Severely deficient patients (less than 1.0 mEq/L) (0.50 mmol/L) and all deficient critically ill patients should be managed with IV magnesium sulfate. Ten milliliters of a 10% magnesium sulfate solution contains 1 g of magnesium, which is equivalent to 98 mg (8.12 mEq or 4.06 mmol) of elemental magnesium. IV magnesium supplementation may also be used in the setting of status asthmaticus, premature labor, and torsade de pointes. Magnesium concentrations need to be monitored closely in these patients. ❾ *Because magnesium concentration does not correlate well with total body magnesium stores, magnesium is often administered empirically to critically ill patients.*[2,33]

The most common causes of hypermagnesemia are renal failure, often in conjunction with magnesium-containing medications (cathartics, antacids, or magnesium supplements), and lithium therapy (available as generic). Hypermagnesemia is defined as a serum magnesium concentration greater than 2.4 mEq/L (1.20 mmol/L). Mild hypermagnesemia is present if the serum magnesium concentration is between 2.5 and 4 mEq/L (1.25 to 2.00 mmol/L) and manifests as nausea, vomiting, cutaneous vasodilation, and bradycardia. Moderate hypermagnesemia is present if the serum magnesium concentration is between 4 and 12 mEq/L (2 to 6 mmol/L) and may manifest with hyporeflexia, weakness, somnolence, hypotension, and ECG changes (increased QRS interval). Severe hypermagnesemia is present if the serum magnesium concentration is greater than 13 mEq/L (6.5 mmol/L) and can manifest as muscle paralysis, complete heart block, asystole, respiratory failure, refractory hypotension, and death.[2,50]

All patients with hypermagnesemia should have all magnesium supplements or magnesium-containing medications discontinued.[2,33] Iatrogenic hypermagnesemia has been observed after IV magnesium therapy for refractory asthma or preeclampsia. Mild hypermagnesemia and moderate hypermagnesemia without cardiac findings can be treated with normal saline infusion and furosemide therapy (assuming the patient has normal renal function). Moderate hypermagnesemia with cardiac irritability and severe hypermagnesemia require concurrent IV calcium gluconate to reverse the neuromuscular and cardiovascular effects. Calcium gluconate given at typical doses of 1 to 2 g IV will have transient effects and can be repeated as clinically indicated. Hemodialysis may be necessary for those with severely compromised renal function.

Patient Encounter 8: Putting It All Together

DM, a 77-year-old male nursing home resident, is admitted to the hospital with a 3-day history of altered mental status. The patient was unable to give a history or review of systems. On physical examination, the vital signs revealed a BP of 100/60 mm Hg, pulse 110 beats per minute, respirations 14 per minute, and a temperature of 38.3°C (101°F). Rales and dullness to percussion were noted at the posterior right base. The cardiac examination was significant for tachycardia. No edema was present. Laboratory studies included sodium 160 mEq/L (160 mmol/L), potassium 4.6 mEq/L (4.6 mmol/L), chloride 120 mEq/L (120 mmol/L), bicarbonate 30 mEq/L (30 mmol/L), glucose 104 mg/dL (5.8 mmol/L), BUN 34 mg/dL (12.1 mmol/L), and creatinine 2.2 mg/dL (194 µmol/L). The CBC was within normal limits. Chest x-ray indicated a right lower lobe pneumonia. The patient is 5 ft 10 in. (178 cm) tall and currently weighs 72.7 kg (160 lb). His normal weight is 77.3 kg (170 lb).

What are the likely causes for the increased sodium concentration in this patient?

Calculate the TBW, ICF, and ECF for this patient.

Calculate DM's fluid deficit if one is present.

In the next 24 hours, the medical team wants to replace 50% of the fluid deficit plus an extra 240 mL to account for increased insensible losses in addition to the patient's maintenance needs. Using the equation (1,500 mL + 20 mL for each kilogram greater than 20 kg), calculate the rate of fluid administration for the total fluids needed in this 24-hour period and over the next 48 hours.

Calculate DM's daily maintenance fluids.

Calculate DM's fluid administration rate for the first 24 hours (hospital day 1).

Calculate DM's fluids for the subsequent 48 hours (hospital days 2 and 3) if the goal is to replete the remaining fluid deficit during that time.

What type of fluid should be used to treat DM's fluid disorder?

CONCLUSION

Because disturbances in fluid balance are routinely encountered in clinical medicine, it is essential to have a thorough understanding of body fluid compartments and the therapeutic use of fluids. Similarly, disturbances in serum sodium, potassium, calcium, phosphorus, and magnesium are ubiquitous and must be mastered by all clinicians. Dysregulation of fluid and/or electrolyte status has serious implications regarding the concepts of drug absorption, volumes of distribution, and toxicity. Similarly, many medications can disrupt fluid and/or electrolyte balance as an unintended consequence.

Abbreviations Introduced in This Chapter

ADH	Antidiuretic hormone
ASHP	American Society of Health-System Pharmacists
ATP	Adenosine triphosphate
BP	Blood pressure
BUN	Blood urea nitrogen
Ca^{++}	Calcium
CHF	Congestive heart failure
Cl	Chloride
D5W	Dextrose 5% water
ECF	Extracellular fluid
ECG	Electrocardiogram
FFP	Fresh-frozen plasma
IBW	Ideal body weight
ICF	Intracellular fluid
IVIG	Intravenous immune globulin
I&Os	Ins and outs
JCAHO	Joint Commission on Accreditation of Healthcare Organizations
K^+	Potassium
KPO^4	Potassium phosphate
KVO	Keep the vein open
LR	Lactated Ringer's (solution)
Mg^{++}	Magnesium
Na^+	Sodium
NaCl	Sodium chloride
NaPO4	Sodium phosphate
NG	Nasogastric
NS	Normal saline
SI	Standardized international units
SIADH	Syndrome of inappropriate antidiuretic hormone secretion
TBW	Total body water
TPN	Total parenteral nutrition

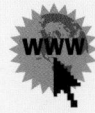

Self-assessment questions and answers are available at *http://www.mhpharmacotherapy.com/pp.html*.

REFERENCES

1. Faber MD, Kupin WL, Heilig CW, Narins RG. Common fluid–electrolyte and acid–base problems in the intensive care unit: Selected issues. Semin Nephrol 1994;14:8–22.

2. Kraft MD, Btaiche IF, Sacks GS, Kudsk KA. Treatment of electrolyte disorders in adult patients in the intensive care unit. Am J Health Syst Pharm 2005;62:1663–1682.

3. Faubel S, Topf J. The Fluid Electrolyte and Acid–Base Companion. San Diego, CA: Alert and Oriented Publishing, 1999.

4. Chenevey B. Overview of fluids and electrolytes. Nurs Clin North Am 1987;22:749–759.

5. Devine BJ. Gentamicin therapy. Drug Intell Clin Pharm 1974;7:650–655.

6. Rose BD, Post TW. Clinical Physiology of Acid–Base and Electrolyte Disorders. New York, NY: McGraw Hill, 2001.

7. The SAFE Study Investigators. A comparison of albumin and saline for fluid resuscitation in the intensive care unit. N Engl J Med 2004;350:2247–2256.

8. The Albumin Reviewers (Alderson P, Bunn F, Lefebvre C, Li Wan Po A, Li L, Roberts I, Schlerhout G). Human albumin solution for resuscitation and volume expansion in critically ill patients. Cochrane Database Syst Rev 2004:CD001208.

9. Vincent JL, Gerlach H. Fluid resuscitation in severe sepsis and septic shock: An evidence based review. Crit Care Med 2004;32(Suppl):S451–S454.

10. Weil MH, Tang W. Albumin versus crystalloid solutions for the critically ill and injured. Crit Care Med 2004;32:2154–2155.

11. Martiin GS, Mangialardi RJ, Wheeler AP, et al. Albumin and furosemide therapy in hypoproteinemic patients with acute lung injury. Crit Care Med 2002;30:2175–2182.

12. Shafiee MAS, Bohn D, Hoorn EJ, Halperin ML. How to select optimal maintenance intravenous therapy. QJ Med 2003;96:601–610.

13. Kwan I, Bunn F, Roberts I, on behalf of the WHO Pre-Hospital Trauma Care Steering Committee. Timing and volume of fluid administration for patients with bleeding. Cochrane Database Syst Rev 2003:CD002245.

14. The Joint Commission [Internet]. Oakbrook Terrace (IL): The Joint Commission; c2012 [updated 2012 Feb 1; cited 2012 Feb 2]. Available from: http://www.jointcommission.org

15. Kumar S, Berl T. Sodium. Lancet 1998;352:220–228.

16. Adrigoue H, Madias NE. Hyponatremia. N Engl J Med 2000;342:1581–1589.

17. Sterns RH. The treatment of hyponatremia: First, do no harm. Am J Med 1990;88:557–560.

18. Cluitmans FHM, Meinders AE. Management of severe hyponatremia: Rapid or slow correction? Am J Med 1990;88:161–166.

19. Adrogue HJ, Madias NE. Hypernatremia. N Engl J Med 2000;342:1493–1499.

20. Palevsky PM, Bhagrath R, Greenberg A. Hypernatremia in hospitalized patients. Ann Intern Med 1996;124:197–203.

21. Kang SK, Kim W, Oh MS. Pathogenesis and treatment of hypernatremia. Nephron 2002;92(Suppl 1):14–17.

22. Mandal AK. Hypokalemia and hyperkalemia. Med Clin North Am 1997;81:611–639.

23. Halperin ML. Potassium. Lancet 1998;352:135–140.

24. Body JJ, Bouillon R. Emergencies of calcium homeostasis. Rev Endocr Metab Disord 2003;4:167–175.

25. Gennari FJ. Hypokalemia. N Engl J Med 1998;339:451–458.

26. Hamil RJ, Robinson LM, Wexler HR, Moote C. Efficacy and safety of potassium infusion therapy in hypokalemic critically ill patients. Crit Care Med 1991;19:694–699.

27. Kruge JA, Carlson RW. Rapid correction of hypokalemia using concentrated intravenous potassium chloride infusions. Arch Intern Med 1990;150:613–617.

28. Cohn JN, Kowey PR, Whelton PK, Prisant M. New guidelines for potassium replacement in clinical practice. Arch Intern Med 2000;160:2429–2436.

29. Williams ME. Hyperkalemia. Crit Care Clin 1991;7:155–174.

30. Carroll MF, Schade DS. A practical approach to hypercalcemia. Am Fam Physician 2003;67:1959–1966.

31. Bushinsky DA, Monk RD. Calcium. Lancet 1998;352:305–311.

32. Zaloga GP. Hypocalcemia in critically ill patients. Crit Care Med 1992;20:251–262.

33. Metheny NM. Fluid and Electrolyte Balance: Nursing Considerations, 4th ed. New York, NY: Lippincott, 2000.

34. Davidson TG. Conventional treatment of hypercalcemia of malignancy. Am J Health-Syst Pharm 2001;58(Suppl 3):S8–S15.

35. Weisinger JR, Bellorin-Font E. Magnesium and phosphorous. Lancet 1998;352:391–396.

36. Brown KA, Dickerson RN, Morgan LM, Alexander KH, Minard G, Brown RO. A new graduated regimen for phosphorous replacement in patients receiving nutritional support. J Parenteral Enteral Nutr 2006;30:209–214.

37. Just the Facts: Fluids and Electrolytes. Philadelphia, PA: Lippincott Williams & Wilkins, 2005.

38. Bilezikian JP. Clinical review 51. Management of hypercalcemia. J Clin Endocrinol Metab 1993;77:1445–1449.

39. Knochel JP. The pathophysiology and clinical characteristics of severe hypophosphatemia. Arch Intern Med 1977;137:203–220.

40. Stoff JS. Phosphate homeostasis and hypophosphatemia. Am J Med. 1982;72:489–495.

41. Aubier M, Murciano D, Lecocguic Y, et al. Effect of hypophosphatemia on diaphragmatic contractility in patients with acute respiratory failure. N Engl J Med 1985;313:420–424.

42. Perreault MM, Ostron NI, Tiemey MG. Efficacy and safety of intravenous phosphate replacement in critically ill patients. Ann Pharmacother 1997;31:683–688.

43. Kee JL, Paulanka BJ, Purnell LD. Fluids and Electrolytes with Clinical Applications. A Programmed Approach, 7th ed. Clifton Park, NY: Delmar Learning, 2000.

44. Oster JR, Epstein M. Management of magnesium depletion. Am J Nephrol 1988;8:349–354.

45. Al-Ghamdi SMG, Cameron EC, Sutton AL. Magnesium deficiency: Pathophysiologic and clinical overview. Am J Kidney Dis 1994;24:737–752.

46. Salem M, Munoz R, Chernow B. Hypomagnesemia in critical illness: A common and clinically important problem. Crit Care Clin 1991;7:225–252.

47. Zalman SA. Hypomagnesemia. J Am Soc Nephrol 1999:10:1616–1622.

48. Dube L, Granry JC. The therapeutic use of magnesium in anesthesiology, intensive care and emergency medicine: A review. Can J Anesth 2003;50:732–746.

49. Schucker JJ, Ward KE. Hyperphosphatemia and phosphate buffers. Am J Health-Syst Pharm 2005;62:2355–2361.

50. Van Hook JW. Hypermagnesemia. Crit Care Clin 1991;7:215–223.

28 Acid–Base Disturbances

Lee E. Morrow and Mark A. Malesker

LEARNING OBJECTIVES

● **Upon completion of the chapter, the reader will be able to:**

1. Compare and contrast the four primary acid–base disturbances within the human body.

2. Apply simple formulas in a systematic manner to determine the etiology of simple acid–base disturbances and the adequacy of compensation.

3. Integrate the supplemental concepts of the anion gap and the excess gap to further assess for complex acid–base disturbances.

4. Discuss the most common clinical causes for each primary acid–base abnormality.

5. Describe the potential clinical complications of altered acid–base homeostasis.

6. Propose an appropriate treatment plan for patients with deranged acid–base physiology.

KEY CONCEPTS

❶ Acid–base homeostasis is tightly regulated by the complex, but predictable, interactions of the kidneys, the lungs, and various buffer systems. The kidneys control serum bicarbonate (HCO_3^-) concentration through the excretion or reabsorption of filtered HCO_3^-, the excretion of metabolic acids, and synthesis of new HCO_3^-. The lungs control the arterial carbon dioxide (CO_2) concentration through changes in the depth and/or rate of respiration.

❷ Respiratory acidosis and alkalosis result from primary disturbances in the arterial CO_2 concentration. Metabolic compensation of respiratory disturbances is a slow process, requiring days for the serum HCO_3^- to reach the steady state.

❸ Respiratory acidosis is caused by respiratory insufficiency resulting in an increased arterial CO_2 concentration. The compensation for respiratory acidosis (if present for prolonged periods) is an increase in serum HCO_3^-.

❹ Respiratory alkalosis is caused by hyperventilation resulting in a decreased arterial CO_2 concentration. The compensation for respiratory alkalosis (if present for prolonged periods) is a decrease in serum HCO_3^-.

❺ Metabolic acidosis and alkalosis result from primary disturbances in the serum HCO_3^- concentration. Respiratory compensation of metabolic disturbances begins within minutes and is complete within 12 hours.

❻ Metabolic acidosis is characterized by a decrease in serum HCO_3^-. The anion gap is used to narrow the differential diagnosis because metabolic acidosis may be caused by addition of acids (increased anion gap) or loss of HCO_3^- (normal anion gap). The compensation for metabolic acidosis is an increase in ventilation with a decrease in arterial CO_2.

❼ Metabolic alkalosis is characterized by an increase in serum HCO_3^-. This disorder requires loss of fluid that is low in HCO_3^- from the body or addition of HCO_3^- to the body. The compensation for metabolic alkalosis is a decrease in ventilation with an increase in arterial CO_2.

❽ Arterial blood gases, serum electrolytes, physical examination findings, the clinical history, and the patient's recent medications must be reviewed in order to establish the etiology of a given acid–base disturbance.

❾ It is critical to treat the underlying causative process to effectively resolve most observed acid–base disorders. However, supportive treatment of the pH and electrolytes is often needed until the underlying disease state is improved.

Given its reputation for complexity and the need to memorize innumerable formulas, acid–base analysis intimidates many healthcare providers. In reality, acid–base disorders always obey well-defined biochemical and physiological principles. The pH determines a patient's acid–base status and an assessment of the bicarbonate (HCO_3^-)

and arterial carbon dioxide ($Paco_2$) values identifies the underlying process. Rigorous use of a systematic approach to arterial blood gases increases the likelihood that derangements in acid–base physiology are recognized and correctly interpreted. This chapter outlines a clinically useful approach to acid–base abnormalities and then applies this approach in a series of increasingly complex clinical scenarios.

Disturbances of acid–base equilibrium occur in a wide variety of illnesses and are among the most frequently encountered disorders in critical care medicine. The importance of a thorough command of this content cannot be overstated given that acid–base disorders are remarkably common and may result in significant morbidity and mortality. Although severe derangements may affect virtually any organ system, the most serious clinical effects are cardiovascular (arrhythmias and impaired contractility), neurologic (coma and seizures), pulmonary (dyspnea, impaired oxygen delivery, respiratory fatigue, and respiratory failure), and/or renal (hypokalemia). Changes in acid–base status also affect multiple aspects of pharmacokinetics (clearance and protein binding) and pharmacodynamics.

ACID–BASE HOMEOSTASIS

Acid–base homeostasis is responsible for maintaining blood hydrogen ion concentration [H^+] near normal despite the daily acidic and/or alkaline loads derived from the intake and metabolism of foods. Acid–base status is traditionally represented in terms of pH, the negative logarithm of [H^+]. Because [H^+] is equal to 24 times the ratio of $Paco_2$ to HCO_3^-, the pH can be altered by a change in either the bicarbonate concentration or the dissolved carbon dioxide. A critically important concept is that [H^+] depends only on the *ratio* of $Paco_2$ to HCO_3^- and not the absolute amount of either. As such, a normal $Paco_2$ or HCO_3^- alone does not guarantee that the pH will be normal. Conversely, a normal pH does not imply that either the $Paco_2$ or HCO_3^- will be normal.[1]

❶ *Acid–base homeostasis is tightly regulated by the complex, but predictable, interactions of the kidneys, the lungs, and various buffer systems. The kidneys control serum bicarbonate (HCO_3^-) concentration through the excretion or reabsorption of filtered HCO_3^-, the excretion of metabolic acids, and synthesis of new HCO_3^-. The lungs control arterial carbon dioxide (CO_2) concentrations through changes in the depth and/or rate of respiration.* The net result is tight regulation of the blood pH by these three distinct mechanisms working in harmony: extracellular bicarbonate and intracellular protein buffering systems; pulmonary regulation of $Paco_2$, effectively allowing carbonic acid to be eliminated by the lungs as CO_2; and renal reclamation or excretion of HCO_3^- and excretion of acids such as ammonium.

Because the kidneys excrete less than 1% of the estimated 13,000 mEq (13,000 mmol) of H^+ ions generated in an average day, renal failure can be present for prolonged periods before life-threatening imbalances occur. Conversely, cessation of breathing for minutes results in profound acid–base disturbances.[1]

The best way to assess a patient's acid–base status is to review the results of an arterial blood gas (ABG) specimen.

Blood gas analyzers directly measure the pH and $Paco_2$, while the HCO_3^- value is calculated using the Henderson-Hasselbalch equation. A more direct measure of serum HCO_3^- is obtained by measuring the total venous carbon dioxide (tCO_2). Because dissolved carbon dioxide is almost exclusively in the form of HCO_3^-, tCO_2 is essentially equivalent to the measured serum HCO_3^- concentration. This value (HCO_3^-) is routinely reported on basic chemistry panels. In the remainder of this chapter, the pH and $Paco_2$ values should be assumed to come from an ABG while HCO_3^- values should be considered to be measured serum concentrations.

BASIC PATHOPHYSIOLOGY

● Under normal circumstances, the arterial pH is tightly regulated between 7.35 and 7.45. **Acidemia** is an abnormally low arterial blood pH (less than 7.35) while acidosis is a pathologic process that acidifies body fluids. Similarly, **alkalemia** is an abnormally high arterial blood pH (greater than 7.45) while **alkalosis** is a pathologic process that alkalinizes body fluids. As such, although a patient can simultaneously have acidosis *and* alkalosis, the end result will be acidemia *or* alkalemia.

Changes in the arterial pH are driven by changes in the $Paco_2$ and/or the serum HCO_3^-. Carbon dioxide is a volatile acid regulated by the depth and rate of respiration. Because CO_2 can be either "blown off" or "retained" by the respiratory system, it is referred to as being under respiratory control. ❷ *Respiratory acidosis and alkalosis result from primary disturbances in the arterial CO_2 concentration. Metabolic compensation of respiratory disturbances is a slow process, often requiring days for the serum HCO_3^- to reach the steady state.* ❸ *Respiratory acidosis is caused by respiratory insufficiency resulting in an increased arterial CO_2 concentration. The compensation for respiratory acidosis (if present for prolonged periods) is an increase in serum HCO_3^-.* ❹ *Respiratory alkalosis is caused by hyperventilation resulting in a decreased arterial CO_2 concentration. The compensation for respiratory alkalosis (if present for prolonged periods) is a decrease in serum HCO_3^-.*

A respiratory acid–base disorder is a pH disturbance caused by pathologic alterations of the respiratory system or its CNS control. Such an alteration may result in the accumulation of $Paco_2$ beyond normal limits (greater than 45 mm Hg or 6.0 kPa), a situation termed *respiratory acidosis*, or it may result in the loss of $Paco_2$ beyond normal limits (less than 35 mm Hg or 4.7 kPa), a condition termed *respiratory alkalosis*. Variations in respiratory rate and/or depth allow the lungs to achieve changes in the $Paco_2$ very quickly (within minutes).

Bicarbonate is a base regulated by renal metabolism via the enzyme carbonic anhydrase. As such, bicarbonate is often referred to as being under metabolic control. ❺ *Metabolic acidosis and alkalosis result from primary disturbances in the serum HCO_3^- concentration. Respiratory compensation of metabolic disturbances begins within minutes and is complete within 12 hours.* ❻ *Metabolic acidosis is characterized by a* *decrease in serum HCO_3^-. The anion gap is used to narrow the differential diagnosis because metabolic acidosis may be caused by addition of acids (increased anion gap) or loss of HCO_3^- (normal anion gap). The compensation for metabolic acidosis is an increase in ventilation with a decrease in arterial CO_2.* ❼ *Metabolic alkalosis is characterized by an increase in serum HCO_3^-. This disorder requires loss of fluid that is low in HCO_3^- from the body or addition of HCO_3^- to the body. The compensation for metabolic alkalosis is a decrease in ventilation with an increase in arterial CO_2.*

A metabolic acid–base disorder is a pH disturbance caused by derangement of the pathways responsible for maintaining a normal HCO_3^- concentration. This may result in a pathologic accumulation of HCO_3^- (greater than 26 mEq/L or mmol/L), a condition termed *metabolic alkalosis*, or it may result in the loss of HCO_3^- beyond normal (less than 22 mEq/L or mmol/L), a condition termed *metabolic acidosis*. In contrast to the lungs' rapid effects on CO_2, the kidneys change the HCO_3^- very slowly (hours to days).

Respiratory and metabolic derangements can occur in isolation or in combination. If a patient has an isolated primary acid–base disorder that is not accompanied by another primary acid–base disorder, a **simple (uncomplicated) disorder** is present. The most common clinical disturbances are simple acid–base disorders. If two or three primary acid–base disorders are simultaneously present, the patient has a **mixed (complicated) disorder**. More complex clinical situations lead to mixed acid–base disturbances. Because CO_2 is a volatile acid, it can rapidly be changed by the respiratory system. If a respiratory acid–base disturbance is present for minutes to hours, it is considered an **acute disorder**, while if it is present for days or longer it is considered a **chronic disorder**. By definition, the metabolic machinery that regulates HCO_3^- results in slow changes, and all metabolic disorders are chronic.

Changes that follow the primary disorder and attempt to restore the blood pH to normal are referred to as compensatory changes. It should be stressed that compensation never normalizes the pH. Because all metabolic acid–base disorders are chronic and the normal respiratory system can quickly alter the $Paco_2$, essentially all metabolic disorders are accompanied by some degree of respiratory compensation.[2,3] Similarly, chronic respiratory acid–base disorders are typically accompanied by attempts at metabolic compensation.[4,5] However, with acute respiratory acid–base disorders there is insufficient time for the metabolic pathways to compensate significantly.[6] As such, acute respiratory derangements are essentially uncompensated.

The amount of compensation (metabolic or respiratory) can be reliably predicted based on the degree of derangement in the primary disorder. **Table 28–1** outlines the simple acid–base disorders and provides formulas for calculating the expected compensatory responses.[7] Although it is not mandatory to memorize these formulas in order to interpret acid–base problems, they can be helpful tools. If the measured values differ markedly from the calculated values (the measured serum HCO_3^- is greater than 2 mEq/L [2 mmol/L] from the calculated value or the measured $Paco_2$ is more than

Table 28–1			
The Six Simple Acid–Base Disorders			
Type of Disorder	**pH**	**$Paco_2$[a]**	**HCO_3^-**
1. Metabolic acidosis	↓	Decreased[b] $Paco_2 = (1.5 \times HCO_3^-) + 8$	Decreased[c]
2. Metabolic alkalosis	↑	Increased[b] $Paco_2 = (0.9 \times HCO_3^-) + 15$	Increased[c]
3. Acute respiratory acidosis	↓	Increased[c]	Approximately normal $\Delta HCO_3^- = 0.1 \times \Delta Paco_2$[a]
4. Chronic respiratory acidosis	↓	Increased[c]	Increased[d] $\Delta HCO_3^- = 0.35 \times \Delta Paco_2$[a]
5. Acute respiratory alkalosis	↑	Decreased[c]	Approximately normal $\Delta HCO_3^- = 0.2 \times \Delta Paco_2$[a]
6. Chronic respiratory alkalosis	↓	Decreased[c]	Decreased[d] $\Delta HCO_3 = 0.4 \times \Delta Paco_2$[a]

[a]$Paco_2$ in mm Hg.
[b]Respiratory compensation: If inappropriate, see Table 28–2.
[c]Primary disorder.
[d]Metabolic compensation: If inappropriate, see Table 28–2

Table 28–2		
Diagnosis of Concurrent Acid–Base Disturbances When Compensation Is Inappropriate		
Primary Acid–Base Disturbance	**Assessment of Compensation**	**Concurrent Acid–Base Disturbance**
Metabolic acidosis	$Paco_2$ too low[a]	Respiratory alkalosis
	$Paco_2$ too high[a]	Respiratory acidosis
Metabolic alkalosis	$Paco_2$ too low[a]	Respiratory alkalosis
	$Paco_2$ too high[a]	Respiratory acidosis
Respiratory acidosis	HCO_3^- too low[b]	Metabolic acidosis
	HCO_3^- too high[b]	Metabolic alkalosis
Respiratory alkalosis	HCO_3^- too low[b]	Metabolic acidosis
	HCO_3^- too high[b]	Metabolic alkalosis

[a]Measured $Paco_2$ more than 4 mm Hg from the calculated value.
[b]Measured HCO_3^- more than 2 mEq/L (mmol/L) from the calculated value.

4 mm Hg [0.5 kPa] from the calculated value), a second acid–base disorder is present as outlined in **Table 28–2**.

APPLICATION OF BASIC PATHOPHYSIOLOGY

When given an ABG for interpretation, it is essential to use an approach that is focused yet comprehensive.[8] An algorithm illustrating this concept is shown in **Figure 28–1**.

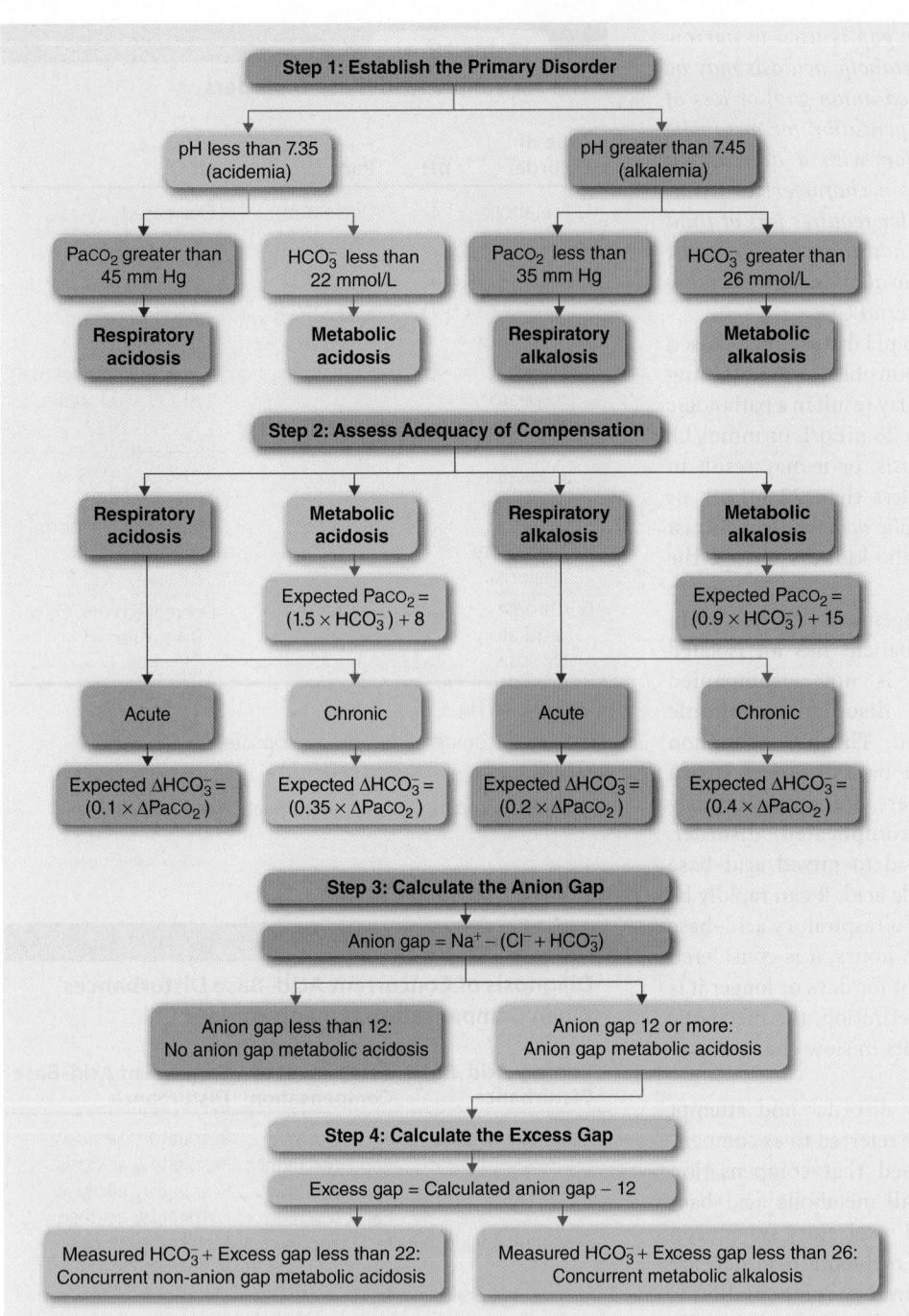

FIGURE 28–1. An algorithmic approach to acid–base disorders. Normal values: pH 7.35 to 7.45, $Paco_2$ 35 to 45 mm Hg (4.7 to 6.0 kPa), HCO_3^- 22 to 26 mEq/L (mmol/L), anion gap less than 12 mEq/L (mmol/L). Note that $Paco_2$ should be in millimeters of mercury to use the equations in the figure. (Cl^-, chloride ion; HCO_3^-, bicarbonate; Na^+, sodium ion; $Paco_2$, partial pressure of arterial carbon dioxide.)

Using this algorithm, Step 1 is to identify all abnormalities in the pH, $Paco_2$, and/or HCO_3^- and then decide which abnormal values are primary and which are compensatory. This is best done by initially looking at the pH. Whichever side of 7.40 the pH is on, the process that caused it to shift to that side is the primary abnormality. If the arterial pH is lower than 7.40 (acidemia), an elevated $Paco_2$ (greater than 45 mm Hg or 6.0 kPa, **respiratory acidosis**) or a lowered HCO_3^- (less than 22 mEq/L or mmol/L, **metabolic acidosis**) would be the primary abnormality. If the arterial pH is higher than 7.40 (alkalemia), a decreased Paco2 (less than 35 or 4.7 kPa, **respiratory alkalosis**) or an increased HCO_3^-

(greater than 25 mEq/L or mmol/L, **metabolic alkalosis**) would be the primary abnormality. Once the primary disorder is established, step 2 is to apply the formulas from Table 28–1 to assess whether compensation is appropriate and to look for concurrent processes.[7]

An alternative to a diagnostic algorithm is use of a graphic nomogram.[9] Nomograms are plots of the pH, $Paco_2$, and HCO_3^- that allow the user to rapidly determine whether arterial blood gas values are consistent with one of the six simple primary acid–base disturbances. Although nomograms are commonly used to identify acid–base disturbances in clinical practice, only individuals who

Patient Encounters 1 Through 5: Application of Basic Pathophysiology

Case Study 1

An unconscious 57-year-old man is brought to the emergency department by his wife who was unable to awaken him when she returned home from work. She discloses that he is on disability and has been taking "lots of pain pills" for his chronic low back pain. The initial ABG has a pH of 7.20, a Pa_{CO_2} of 65 mm Hg (8.6 kPa), and an HCO_3^- of 27 mEq/L (mmol/L).

What is the primary acid–base disorder?

Has compensation occurred?

Given the clinical history, what is the most likely explanation for the ABG findings?

Case Study 2

The next patient is a 69-year-old woman whose ongoing habit of smoking two packs of unfiltered cigarettes each day has led to advanced emphysema and the need for chronic oxygen therapy. During a routine office visit an ABG is checked to satisfy her insurance company's requirements to certify her supplemental oxygen prescription. Her blood gas sample has a pH of 7.34, a Pa_{CO_2} of 65 mm Hg (8.6 kPa), and an HCO_3^- of 33 mEq/L (mmol/L).

What is the primary acid–base disorder?

Has compensation occurred?

Given the clinical history, what is the most likely explanation for the ABG findings?

Case Study 3

Now consider an otherwise healthy 80-year-old retired librarian. She has grown increasingly agitated because her pension check is late and the bank's customer service representatives have been unable to assist her. She is boisterous, breathless, and convinced the tingling in her lips is due to a stroke. Her ABG shows a pH of 7.50, a Pa_{CO_2} of 25 mm Hg (3.3 kPa), and an HCO_3^- of 21 mEq/L (mmol/L).

What is the primary acid–base disorder?

Has compensation occurred?

Given the clinical history, what is the most likely explanation for the ABG findings?

Case Study 4

This 55-year-old man has a history of viral myocarditis with cardiomyopathy: his subsequent chronic congestive heart failure requires daily furosemide therapy. When he presented to the emergency department with increasing dyspnea, an ABG was drawn and shows the following: pH of 7.50, a Pa_{CO_2} of 50 mm Hg (6.7 kPa), and an HCO_3^- of 40 mEq/L (mmol/L).

What is the primary acid–base disorder?

Has compensation occurred?

Given the clinical history, what is the most likely explanation for the ABG findings?

Case Study 5

The final patient in this section is a 44-year-old man with chronic renal insufficiency who has suffered from gastroenteritis with refractory diarrhea for the past 72 hours. His ABG shows a pH of 7.20, a Pa_{CO_2} of 20 mm Hg (2.7 kPa), and an HCO_3^- of 8 mEq/L (mmol/L).

What is the primary acid–base disorder?

Has compensation occurred?

Given the clinical history, what is the most likely explanation for the ABG findings?

---

fully comprehend the fundamental concepts of acid–base assessment should use these tools. Also, appreciate that nomograms have limited utility when dealing with complex acid–base derangements.

Acid–base disturbances are always manifestations of underlying clinical disorders. It is useful to specifically define the primary acid–base abnormality because each disorder is caused by a limited number of disease processes. Establishing the specific disease process responsible for the observed acid–base disorder is clinically important because treatment of a given disorder will only be accomplished by correcting the underlying disease process.

ADVANCED PATHOPHYSIOLOGY

The concepts in this section are used to further expand on steps 3 and 4 of the diagnostic algorithm shown in Figure 28–1. Under normal circumstances the serum is in the isoelectric state. This means that the positively charged entities reported in a standard chemistry panel (cations: sodium and potassium) should be exactly balanced by the negatively charged entities (anions: chloride and bicarbonate). However, this relationship is consistently incorrect because the measured cations are higher than the measured anions by 10 to 12 mEq/L (mmol/L). This discrepancy results from the presence of unmeasured anions (e.g., circulating proteins, phosphates, and sulfates). This apparent difference in charges, the serum **anion gap**, is calculated as follows:

$$\text{Anion gap} = Na^+ - (Cl^- + HCO_3^-).$$

Because the serum potassium content is relatively small and is very tightly regulated, it is generally omitted from the calculation.[10]

It is important to realize that the serum HCO_3^- concentration may be affected by the presence of unmeasured endogenous acids (lactic acid or ketoacids). Bicarbonate will attempt to buffer these acids, resulting in a 1 mEq (1 mmol) loss of serum HCO_3^- for each 1 mEq (1 mmol) of acid titrated. Because the cation side of the equation is not affected by this transaction, the loss of serum HCO_3^- results in an increase in

Table 28–3

Mnemonics for the Differential Diagnoses of Metabolic Acidosis

Elevated Anion Gap[a]	Normal Anion Gap[a]
M—Methanol, metformin	U—Ureteral diversion
U—Uremia	S—Saline infusion
D—Diabetic (or alcoholic) ketoacidosis	E—Exogenous acid
P—Paraldehyde, phenformin	D—Diarrhea
I—Isoniazid, iron	C—Carbonic anhydrase inhibitors
L—Lactic acidosis	A—Adrenal insufficiency
E—Ethylene glycol, ethanol	R—Renal tubular acidosis
S—Salicylates	

[a]Anion gap = serum sodium concentration – (serum chloride concentration + serum bicarbonate concentration). Under normal circumstances, the anion gap should be 10 mEq/L (mmol/L) or less.

the calculated anion gap. Identification of an increased anion gap is very important because a limited number of clinical scenarios lead to this unique acid–base disorder. A mnemonic to recall the differential diagnosis for an anion gap acidosis is shown in Table 28–3. The concept of the increased anion gap is applied later in Patient Encounters 6 through 10.

Step 3 in Figure 28–1 suggests that any time an ABG is analyzed it is wise to concurrently inspect the serum chemistry values and to calculate the anion gap. The body does not generate an anion gap to compensate for a primary disorder. As such, if the calculated anion gap exceeds 12 mEq/L (mmol/L) there is a primary metabolic acidosis regardless of the pH or the serum HCO_3^- concentration. The anion gap may be artificially lowered by decreased serum albumin, multiple myeloma, lithium intoxication, or a profound increase in the serum potassium, calcium, or magnesium.[11]

Step 4 in Figure 28–1 shows how calculation of the anion gap also facilitates determination of the **excess gap** or the degree to which the calculated anion gap exceeds the normal anion gap. The excess gap is calculated as follows:

Excess gap = anion gap − 12 = $[Na^+ - (Cl^- + HCO_3^-)]$ − 12.

The excess gap represents the amount of HCO_3^- that has been lost due to buffering unmeasured cations. The excess gap can be added back to the measured HCO_3^- to determine what the patient's HCO_3^- would be if these endogenous acids were not present. This is a very valuable tool that can be used in narrowing the differential diagnosis of certain acid–base disorders as well as in uncovering occult or mixed acid–base disorders.

In summary, the approach to assessment of acid–base status involves four key steps as outlined in Figure 28–1: step 1 = initial inspection of the pH, $Paco_2$, and HCO_3^-; step 2 = assessment of the adequacy of compensation; step 3 = calculation of the anion gap; and step 4 = calculation of the excess gap.

ETIOLOGY AND TREATMENT

⑧ *Arterial blood gases, serum electrolytes, physical examination findings, the clinical history, and the patient's recent medications must be reviewed in order to establish the etiology of a given acid–base disturbance.* Tables 28–3 through 28–7 outline the most commonly encountered causes for each of the primary acid–base disorders. The therapeutic approach to each of these acid–base derangements should emphasize a search for the cause, as opposed to immediate attempts to normalize the pH.

⑨ *It is critical to treat the underlying causative process to effectively resolve most observed acid–base disorders. However, supportive treatment of the pH and electrolytes is often needed until the underlying disease state is improved.*[12,13]

All patients with significant disturbances in their acid–base status require continuous cardiovascular and hemodynamic monitoring. Because frequent assessment of the patient's response to treatment is critical, an arterial line is often placed to minimize patient discomfort with serial ABG collections. If the anion gap was initially abnormal, serial chemistries should be followed to ensure that the anion gap resolves with treatment. Specific treatment decisions depend on the underlying pathophysiologic state (e.g., dialysis for renal failure, insulin for diabetic ketoacidosis, or improving tissue perfusion and oxygenation for lactic acidosis).

Metabolic Acidosis

Metabolic acidosis is characterized by a reduced arterial pH, a primary decrease in the HCO_3^- concentration, and a compensatory reduction in the $Paco_2$. The etiologies of metabolic acidosis are divided into those that lead to an increase in the anion gap and those associated with a normal anion gap and are listed in Table 28–4. Although there are numerous mnemonics to recall the differential diagnosis of the metabolic acidosis, two simple ones are shown in Table 28–3. High anion gap metabolic acidosis is most frequently caused by lactic acidosis, ketoacidosis, and/or renal failure. Although there is considerable variation, the largest anion gaps are caused by ketoacidosis, lactic acidosis, and methanol or ethylene glycol ingestion.[14]

Symptoms of metabolic acidosis are attributable to changes in cardiovascular, musculoskeletal, neurologic, or pulmonary functioning. Respiratory compensation requires marked increases in minute ventilation and may lead to dyspnea, respiratory fatigue, and respiratory failure. Acidemia predisposes to ventricular arrhythmias and reduces cardiac contractility, each of which can result in pulmonary edema and/or systemic hypotension.[15] Neurologic symptoms range from lethargy to coma and are usually proportional to the severity of the pH derangement. Chronic metabolic acidosis leads to a variety of musculoskeletal problems including impaired growth, rickets, osteomalacia, or osteopenia. These changes are believed to be caused by the release of calcium and phosphate during bone buffering of excess H^+ ions.

As previously discussed, in anion gap metabolic acidosis, the isoelectric state is maintained because unmeasured

Patient Encounters 6 through 10: Application of Advanced Pathophysiology

Case Study 6

A 21-year-old college student presents to the emergency department after ingesting an entire bottle of aspirin tablets as a suicide gesture. The presenting labs show a pH of 7.50, a $Paco_2$ of 20 mm Hg (2.7 kPa), an HCO_3^- of 16 mEq/L (mmol/L), a sodium concentration of 140 mEq/L (mmol/L), and a chloride level of 103 mEq/L (mmol/L).

What is the primary acid–base disorder?

Is there a mixed disorder?

Given the clinical history, what is the most likely explanation for the ABG findings?

Case Study 7

A 51-year-old homeless man is brought to the emergency department by police for medical clearance before taking him to the city jail. They were called for reports of a "profoundly intoxicated" man who was vomiting off an overpass onto passing vehicles below. Shortly after arrival he has an episode of bloody emesis with witnessed aspiration and respiratory distress. He is urgently intubated and transferred to the intensive care unit where his blood work shows a pH of 7.50, a $Paco_2$ of 20 mm Hg (2.7 kPa), an HCO_3^- of 15 mEq/L (mmol/L), a sodium concentration of 145 mEq/L (mmol/L), and a chloride level of 100 mEq/L (mmol/L).

What is the primary acid–base disorder?

Is there a mixed disorder?

Given the clinical history, what is the most likely explanation for the ABG findings?

Case Study 8

A 19-year-old diabetic woman is brought in by rescue squad after her friends found her unresponsive on the couch. They report that she has had several days of "stomach flu" with stomach cramps and frequent bouts of emesis. Given her limited oral intake, she stopped using her insulin pump a couple days ago. When they brought her soup today, they immediately called 911 given her unconsciousness and slow, shallow breaths. The blood work drawn prior to

urgent intubation shows a pH of 7.09, a $Paco_2$ of 50 mm Hg (6.7 kPa), an HCO_3^- of 15 mEq/L (mmol/L), a sodium concentration of 145 mEq/L (mmol/L), and a chloride level of 100 mEq/L (mmol/L).

What is the primary acid–base disorder?

Is there a mixed disorder?

Given the clinical history, what is the most likely explanation for the ABG findings?

Case Study 9

A 63-year-old man with end-stage renal disease underwent urgent laparotomy for intestinal obstruction: widely disseminated colon cancer was discovered intraoperatively. Given his poor prognosis and multiple comorbidities he is now refusing hemodialysis. Given steady deterioration in his mental status, an ABG and chemistries are obtained and show pH of 7.40, $Paco_2$ of 40 mm Hg (5.3 kPa), HCO_3^- of 24 mEq/L (mmol/L), sodium concentration of 145 mEq/L (mmol/L), and chloride level of 100 mEq/L (mmol/L).

What is the primary acid–base disorder?

Is there a mixed disorder?

Given the clinical history, what is the most likely explanation for the ABG findings?

Case Study 10

The final patient is a 37-year-old man who was admitted 8 hours ago for diabetic ketoacidosis. With appropriate therapy his hyperglycemia has improved and the serum ketones are improving. Because he continues to feel poorly, repeat blood work is ordered. Studies show a pH of 7.15, a $Paco_2$ of 15 mm Hg (2.0 kPa), an HCO_3^- of 5 mEq/L (mmol/L), a sodium concentration of 140 mEq/L (mmol/L), and a chloride level of 110 mEq/L (mmol/L).

What is the primary acid–base disorder?

Is there a mixed disorder?

Given the clinical history, what is the most likely explanation for the ABG findings?

---

anions are present. With a *normal* anion gap metabolic acidosis, the isoelectric state is maintained by an increase in the measured chloride. Because of this, normal anion gap metabolic acidosis is often referred to as hyperchloremic acidosis.

In patients with a normal anion gap metabolic acidosis, it is often helpful to calculate the urine anion gap (UAG).[16] The UAG is calculated as follows:

$$UAG = (Urine\ Na^+ + Urine\ K^+) - Urine\ Cl^-.$$

The normal UAG ranges from 0 to 5 mEq/L (mmol/L) and represents the presence of unmeasured urinary anions. In smetabolic acidosis, the excretion of NH_4^+ and concurrent Cl^- should increase markedly if renal acidification is intact. This results in UAG values from −20 to −50 mEq/L (mmol/L). This occurs because the urinary Cl^- concentration now markedly exceeds the urinary Na^+ and K^+ concentrations. Diagnoses consistent with an excessively negative UAG include proximal (type 2) renal tubular acidosis, diarrhea, or administration of acetazolamide or hydrochloric acid (HCl).

Table 28–4

Common Causes of Metabolic Acidosis

Elevated Anion Gap[a]	Normal Anion Gap[a]
Intoxications	Bowel fistula
Methanol	Diarrhea
Ethylene glycol	Dilutional acidosis
Salicylates	Drugs
Paraldehyde	Acetazolamide[b]
Isoniazid	Ammonium chloride[b]
Ketoacidosis	Amphotericin B[b]
Diabetic	Arginine
Ethanol	hydrochloride[c]
Starvation	Cholestyramine[b]
Lactic acidosis	Hydrochloric acid[b]
Carbon monoxide poisoning	Lithium[b]
Drugs	Parenteral nutrition[b]
IV lorazepam (due to vehicle)[c]	Topiramate[b]
Metformin[b]	Zonisamide[b]
Nitroprusside (due to cyanide	Lead poisoning
accumulation)[b]	Renal tubular acidosis
Nucleoside reverse	Surgical drains
transcriptase inhibitors[b]	Ureteral diversion
Propofol[c]	Villous adenomas (some)
Seizures	
Severe hypoxemia	
Shock	
Renal failure	

[a]Anion gap = serum sodium concentration – (serum chloride concentration + serum bicarbonate concentration). Under normal circumstances, the anion gap should be 10 mEq/L (mmol/L) or less.

[b]May be observed with therapeutic doses or overdoses.

[c]Typically observed only with overdoses.

Excessively positive values of the UAG suggest a distal (type 1) renal tubular acidosis.

In order to effectively treat metabolic acidosis, the *causative process* must be identified and treated.[17] The precise role of adjunctive therapy with sodium bicarbonate ($NaHCO_3$) is not universally agreed upon. However, most practitioners accept that $NaHCO_3$ is indicated when renal dysfunction precludes adequate regeneration of HCO_3^- or when severe acidemia (pH less than 7.10) is present. The metabolic acidosis seen with lactic acidosis and ketoacidosis generally resolves with therapy targeted at the underlying cause, and $NaHCO_3$ may be unnecessary regardless of the pH. The metabolic acidosis of renal failure, renal tubular acidosis, or intoxication with ethylene glycol, methanol, or salicylates is much more likely to require $NaHCO_3$ therapy.

If $NaHCO_3$ is used, the plasma HCO_3^- should not be corrected entirely. Instead, aim at increasing HCO_3^- above an absolute value of 10 mEq/L (10 mmol/L). The total HCO_3^- deficit can be calculated from the current bicarbonate concentration ($HCO_{3\,corr}^-$), the desired bicarbonate concentration ($HCO_{3\,post}^-$), and the body weight (in kilograms) as follows:

$$HCO_3^- \text{ deficit} = [(2.4/HCO_{3\,corr}^-) + 0.4] \times \text{weight}$$
$$\times (HCO_{3\,corr}^- - HCO_{3\,post}^-).$$

No more than half of the calculated HCO_3^- deficit should be given initially to avoid volume overload, hypernatremia, hyperosmolarity, overshoot alkalemia, hypocalcemia and/or hypokalemia. The calculated HCO_3^- deficit reflects only the present situation and does not account for ongoing H^+ production and HCO_3^- loss. When giving HCO_3^- therapy, serial blood gases are needed to monitor therapy.

Another option for patients with severe acidemia is tromethamine (THAM).[18] This inert amino alcohol buffers acids and CO_2 through its amine ($-NH_2$) moiety:

$$THAM-NH_2 + H^+ = THAM-NH_3^+$$

$$THAM-NH_2 + H_2O + CO_2 = THAM-NH_3^+ + HCO_3^-$$

Protonated THAM (with Cl^- or HCO_3^-) is excreted in the urine at a rate that is slightly higher than creatinine clearance. As such, THAM augments the buffering capacity of the blood without generating excess CO_2. THAM is less effective in patients with renal failure, and toxicities may include hyperkalemia, hypoglycemia, and possible respiratory depression. THAM is particularly useful in patients with volume overload because it does not contain sodium.

THAM is often administered as an empiric dose of 18 g (150 mEq [150 mmol]) in 500 mL water via slow IV infusion. Additional infusions are given as dictated by the severity and progression of acidosis.

Chronic metabolic acidosis can successfully be managed using potassium citrate/citric acid (Polycitra-K, Cytra-K) or sodium citrate/citric acid (Bicitra, Oracit).

Metabolic Alkalosis

Metabolic alkalosis is characterized by an increased arterial pH, a primary increase in the HCO_3^- concentration, and a compensatory increase in the $Paco_2$. Patients will always hypoventilate to compensate for metabolic alkalosis—even if it results in profound hypoxemia. For a metabolic alkalosis to persist, there must concurrently be a process that elevates serum HCO_3^- concentration (gastric or renal loss of acids) and another that impairs renal HCO_3^- excretion (hypovolemia, hypokalemia, or mineralocorticoid excess). The etiologies of metabolic alkalosis are listed in Table 28–5.

Patients with metabolic alkalosis rarely have symptoms attributable to alkalemia. Rather, complaints are usually related to volume depletion (muscle cramps, positional dizziness, weakness) or to hypokalemia (muscle weakness, polyuria, polydipsia).

In order to effectively treat metabolic alkalosis, the *causative process* must be identified and treated. The major causes of metabolic alkalosis are often readily apparent after carefully reviewing the patient's history and medication list. In hospitalized patients, always look for administration of compounds such as citrate in blood products and acetate in parenteral nutrition that can raise the HCO_3^- concentration. If the etiology of the metabolic alkalosis is still unclear, measurement of the urinary chloride may be useful. Some processes leading to metabolic alkalosis (vomiting, nasogastric suction losses, factitious diarrhea) will have low urinary

Table 28–5

Common Causes of Metabolic Alkalosis

Urine Cl⁻ Less Than 10 mEq/L (Less Than 10 mmol/L)	Urine Cl⁻ Greater Than 10 mEq/L (Greater Than 10 mmol/L)

Alkali administration
  IV bicarbonate therapy
  Oral alkali therapy
Parenteral nutrition with acetate
"Contraction alkalosis"
  postdiuretic use
Decreased chloride intake
Loss of gastric acid
  Vomiting
  Nasogastric suction
Posthypercapnia
Villous adenomas (some)
	Drugs[a]
	  Corticosteroid therapy
	  Diuretics
	Hypokalemia
	Mineralocorticoid excess
	  Hyperaldosteronism
	  Bartter's syndrome
	  Cushing's syndrome

[a]May be observed with therapeutic doses or overdoses.

Cl⁻ concentrations (less than 25 mEq/L or mmol/L) and are likely to respond to administration of saline. Other causes (diuretics, hypokalemia, and mineralocorticoid excess) will have higher urinary Cl⁻ concentrations (greater than 40 mEq/L or mmol/L) and are less likely to correct with saline infusion.

In general, contributing factors such as diuretics, nasogastric suction, and corticosteroids should be discontinued if possible. Any fluid deficits should be treated with IV normal saline. Again, patients with metabolic alkalosis and high urine Cl⁻ (while relatively uncommon) are generally resistant to saline loading. Potassium supplementation should always be given if it is also deficient.

In patients with mild or moderate alkalosis who require ongoing diuresis but have rising HCO_3^- concentrations, the carbonic anhydrase inhibitor acetazolamide can be used to reduce the HCO_3^- concentration. Acetazolamide is typically dosed at 250 mg every 6 to 12 hours as needed to maintain the pH in a clinically acceptable range. This agent results in gradual changes in the serum HCO_3^- and is not used to acutely correct a patient's acid–base status. If alkalosis is profound and potentially life threatening (due to seizures or ventricular tachyarrhythmias), hemodialysis or transient HCl infusion can be considered. The hydrogen ion deficit (in milliequivalents or millimoles) can be estimated from the current bicarbonate concentration ($HCO_{3\,curr}^-$), the desired bicarbonate concentration ($HCO_{3\,post}^-$), and the body weight (in kilograms) as follows:

$$H^+ \text{ deficit} = 0.4 \times \text{weight} \times (HCO_{3\,curr}^- - HCO_{3\,post}^-).$$

After estimating the H⁺ deficit, 0.1 to 0.2 N hydrochloric acid (HCl) is infused at 20 to 50 mEq/h (mmol/h) into a central vein. Arterial pH must be monitored at least hourly and the infusion stopped as soon as clinically feasible. Ammonium chloride and arginine hydrochloride, agents that result in the formation of HCl, are not commonly prescribed because they may lead to significant toxicity. Ammonium chloride may

cause accumulation of ammonia leading to encephalopathy while arginine hydrochloride can induce life-threatening hyperkalemia through unclear mechanisms.

Respiratory Acidosis

Respiratory acidosis is characterized by a reduced arterial pH, a primary increase in the arterial $Paco_2$ and, when present for sufficient time, a compensatory rise in the HCO_3^- concentration. Because increased CO_2 is a potent respiratory stimulus, respiratory acidosis represents ventilatory failure or impaired central control of ventilation as opposed to an increase in CO_2 production. As such, most patients will have hypoxemia in addition to hypercapnia. The most common etiologies of respiratory acidosis are listed in Table 28–6.

Severe, acute respiratory acidosis produces a variety of neurologic abnormalities. Initially these include headache, blurred vision, restlessness, and anxiety. These may progress to tremors, asterixis, somnolence, and/or delirium. If untreated, terminal manifestations include peripheral vasodilation leading to hypotension and cardiac arrhythmias. Chronic respiratory acidosis is typically associated with cor pulmonale and peripheral edema.

In order to effectively treat respiratory acidosis, the *causative process* must be identified and treated. If a cause is identified, specific therapy should be started. This may

Table 28–6

Common Causes of Respiratory Acidosis

CNS disease
  Brainstem lesions
  Central sleep apnea
  Infection
  Intracranial hypertension
  Trauma
  Tumor
  Vascular
Drugs[a]
  Aminoglycosides
  Anesthetics
  β-Blockers
  Botulism toxin
  Hypnotics
  Narcotics
  Neuromuscular blocking agents
  Organophosphates
  Sedatives
Neuromuscular disease
  Guillain-Barré syndrome
  Muscular dystrophy
  Myasthenia gravis
  Polymyositis
Pulmonary disease
  Lower airway obstruction
    Chronic obstructive
      pulmonary disease
  Foreign body
  Status asthmaticus
	Pneumonia
	Pneumonitis
	Pulmonary edema
	Restrictive lung disease
	  Ascites
	  Chest wall disorder
	  Fibrothorax
	  Kyphoscoliosis
	  Obesity
	  Pleural effusion
	  Pneumoconiosis
	  Pneumothorax
	  Progressive systemic
	    sclerosis
	  Pulmonary fibrosis
	  Spinal arthritis
	Smoke inhalation
	Upper airway obstruction
	  Foreign body
	  Laryngospasm
	  Obstructive sleep apnea
	Others
	  Abdominal distention
	  Altered metabolic rate
	  Congestive heart failure
	  Hypokalemia
	  Hypothyroidism
	  Inadequate mechanical
	    ventilation

[a]May be observed with therapeutic doses or overdoses.

include naloxone for opiate-induced hypoventilation or bronchodilator therapy for acute bronchospasm. Because respiratory acidosis represents ventilatory failure, an increase in alveolar ventilation is required. This can often be achieved by controlling the underlying disease (e.g., bronchodilators and corticosteroids in asthma) and/or physically augmenting ventilation.

Although their precise role and mechanisms of action are unclear, agents such as medroxyprogesterone, theophylline, and doxapram stimulate respiration and have been used to treat mild to moderate respiratory acidosis. Moderate or severe respiratory acidosis requires assisted ventilation. This can be provided to spontaneously breathing patients via bilevel positive airway pressure (BiPAP) delivered via a tight-fitting mask or by intubation followed by mechanical ventilation. In mechanically ventilated patients, respiratory acidosis is treated by increasing the minute ventilation. This is achieved by increasing the respiratory rate and/or tidal volume.

As with the treatment of metabolic acidosis, the role of $NaHCO_3$ therapy is not well defined for respiratory acidosis. Realize that administration of $NaHCO_3$ can paradoxically result in increased CO_2 generation ($HCO_3^- + H^+ \rightarrow H_2CO_3 + CO_2$) and worsened acidemia. Careful monitoring of the pH is required if $NaHCO_3$ therapy is started for this indication. The use of tromethamine in respiratory acidosis (see Metabolic Acidosis section earlier) has unproven safety and benefit.

The goals of therapy in patients with chronic respiratory acidosis are to maintain oxygenation and to improve alveolar ventilation if possible. Because of the presence of renal compensation it is usually not necessary to treat the pH, even in patients with severe hypercapnia. Although the specific treatment varies with the underlying disease, excessive oxygen and sedatives should be avoided because they can worsen CO_2 retention.

Respiratory Alkalosis

Respiratory alkalosis is characterized by an increased arterial pH, a primary decrease in the arterial $Paco_2$ and, when present for sufficient time, a compensatory fall in the HCO_3^- concentration. Respiratory alkalosis represents hyperventilation and is remarkably common. The most common etiologies of respiratory alkalosis are listed in Table 28–7 and range from benign (anxiety) to life threatening (pulmonary embolism). Some causes of hyperventilation and respiratory acidosis are remarkably common (hypoxemia or anemia).

The symptoms produced by respiratory alkalosis result from increased irritability of the central and peripheral nervous systems. These include light-headedness, altered consciousness, distal extremity paresthesias, circumoral paresthesia, cramps, carpopedal spasms, and syncope. Various supraventricular and ventricular cardiac arrhythmias may occur in extreme cases, particularly in critically ill patients. An additional finding in many patients with severe respiratory alkalosis is hypophosphatemia, reflecting a shift

Table 28–7

Common Causes of Respiratory Alkalosis

CNS disease	Pulmonary disease
Infection	Early restrictive lung disease
Trauma	Infection
Tumor	Pneumothorax
Vascular	Pulmonary edema
Drug or toxin induced[a]	Pulmonary embolism
Catecholamines	Tissue hypoxia
Doxapram	Burn injury
Methylphenidate	Excessive mechanical
Methylxanthines	ventilation
Nicotine	Fever
Progesterone	Hepatic failure
Salicylates	Hypoxemia
Psychiatric disease	Pain
Anxiety	Postmetabolic acidosis
Hyperventilation	Pregnancy
Hysteria	Severe anemia
Panic disorder	Thyrotoxicosis

[a]May be observed with therapeutic doses or overdoses.

of phosphate from the extracellular space into the cells. Chronic respiratory alkalosis is generally asymptomatic.

It is imperative to identify serious causes of respiratory alkalosis and institute effective treatment. In spontaneously breathing patients, respiratory alkalosis is typically only mild or moderate in severity and no specific therapy is indicated. Severe alkalosis generally represents respiratory acidosis imposed on metabolic alkalosis and may improve with sedation or rebreathing maneuvers (rebreathing mask, paper bag). Patients receiving mechanical ventilation are treated with reduced minute ventilation achieved by decreasing the respiratory rate and/or tidal volume. If the alkalosis persists in the ventilated patient, high-level sedation or paralysis is effective.

SUMMARY

Acid–base disturbances are common clinical problems that are not difficult to analyze if approached in a consistent manner. The pH, $Paco_2$, and HCO_3^- should be inspected to identify all abnormal values. This should lead to an assessment of which deviations represent the primary abnormality and which represent compensatory changes. The serum electrolytes should always be used to calculate the anion gap. In cases in which the anion gap is increased, the excess anion gap should be added back to the measured HCO_3^-. The anion gap and the excess gap are useful tools that can identify hidden disorders. This rigorous assessment of the patient's acid–base status, incorporated with the available clinical data, increases the likelihood that the clinician will successfully determine the cause of each identified disorder. Although supportive therapy is often required for profound acid–base disturbances, definitive therapy must target the underlying process that has led to the observed derangements.

Patient Care and Monitoring

1. Every patient with a suspected acid–base disturbance should have an arterial blood gas and a serum chemistry panel drawn concurrently. The results of these tests should be reviewed using a systematic approach to ensure proper interpretation.

2. What is the primary disorder? Has compensation occurred?

3. Is the anion gap excessively large? If so, does calculation of the excess gap identify another acid–base disorder?

4. Continuous cardiovascular and hemodynamic monitoring should be used for significant pH disturbances because the most serious sequelae of acid–base disorders include electrolyte abnormalities, cardiac dysrhythmias, and systemic hypotension.

5. All acid–base abnormalities result from underlying disease processes. Definitive therapy for these disturbances requires treatment of the illness that has disrupted the pH equilibrium.

6. Review each patient's history, physical examination, and current medication list for clues regarding potential causes of the observed acid–base disorder.

7. Serial arterial blood gases and serum chemistries should be compared because every patient's acid–base status is continuously changing based on the underlying disease state and any therapy initiated.

Abbreviations Introduced in This Chapter

ABG	Arterial blood gas
BiPAP	Bilevel positive airway pressure
Cl^-	Chloride ion
CO_2	Carbon dioxide
Δ(delta)	Change
H^+	Hydrogen ion
HCl	Hydrochloric acid
HCO_3^-	Bicarbonate
$HCO_{3\,curr}^-$	Current bicarbonate
$HCO_{3\,post}^-$	Posttherapy bicarbonate
Hg	Mercury
K^+	Potassium ion
Na^+	Sodium ion
$NaHCO_3$	Sodium bicarbonate
NH_2	Terminal amine group
NH_4^+	Ammonium
pH	Logarithm of the hydrogen ion concentration
$Paco_2$	Partial pressure of arterial carbon dioxide
tCO_2	Total venous carbon dioxide
THAM	Tromethamine
UAG	Urine anion gap

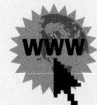 Self-assessment questions and answers are available at *http://www.mhpharmacotherapy.com/pp.html.*

REFERENCES

1. Rose BD, Post TW. Clinical Physiology of Acid–Base and Electrolyte Disorders, 5th ed. New York, NY: McGraw-Hill, 2001:299.
2. Schlichtig R, Grogono A, Severinghaus J. Human $Paco_2$ and standard base excess for compensation of acid–base imbalances. Crit Care Med 1998;26:1173–1179.
3. Pierce NF, Fedson DS, Brigham KL, et al. The ventilatory response to acute base deficit in humans. Time course during development and correction of metabolic acidosis. Ann Intern Med 1970;72:633–640.
4. Javaheri S, Kazemi H. Metabolic alkalosis and hypoventilation in humans. Am Rev Respir Dis 1987;136:1011–1016.
5. Polak A, Haynie GD, Hays RM, Schwartz WB. Effects of chronic hypercapnia on electrolyte and acid–base equilibrium. J Clin Invest 1961;40:1223–1237.
6. Gennari FJ, Goldstein MB, Schwartz WB. The nature of the renal adaptation to chronic hypocapnia. J Clin Invest 1972;51:1722–1730.
7. van Yperselle de Striho C, Brasseur L, de Coninck JD. The "carbon dioxide response curve" for chronic hypercapnia in man. N Engl J Med 1966;275:117–122.
8. Haber RJ. A practical approach to acid–base disorders. West J Med 1991;155:146–151.
9. Arbus GS. An in-vivo acid–base nomogram for clinical use. Can Med Assoc J 1973;109:291–293.
10 Narins R. Clinical Disorders of Fluid and Electrolyte Metabolism, 5th ed. New York, NY: McGraw-Hill, 1994:778.
11. Goodkin DA, Gollapudi GK, Narins RG. The role of the anion gap in detecting and managing mixed metabolic acid–base disorders. Clin Endocrinol Metab 1984;13:333–349.
12. Adrogué HJ, Madias NE. Management of life-threatening acid–base disorders. First of two parts. N Engl J Med 1998;338:26–34.
13. Adrogué HJ, Madias NE. Management of life-threatening acid–base disorders. Second of two parts. N Engl J Med 1998;338:107–111.
14. Abelow B. Understanding Acid–Base. Baltimore, MD: Williams & Wilkins, 1998:229.
15. Kearns T, Wolfson A. Metabolic acidosis. Emerg Med Clin North Am 1989;7:823–835.
16. Batlle DC, Hizon M, Cohen E, Gutterman C, Gupta R. The use of the urinary anion gap in the diagnosis of hyperchloremic metabolic acidosis. N Engl J Med 1988;318:594–599.
17. Hood FL, Tannen RL. Protection of acid–base balance by pH regulation of acid production. N Engl J Med 1998;339:819–826.
18. Chernow B, ed. The Pharmacologic Approach to the Critically Ill Patient, 3rd ed. Baltimore, MD: Williams & Wilkins, 1994:965.

29 Alzheimer's Disease

Megan J. Ehret and Clayton English

LEARNING OBJECTIVES

● **Upon completion of the chapter, the reader will be able to:**

1. Describe the epidemiology of Alzheimer's disease (AD) and its effects on society.

2. Describe the pathophysiology, including genetic and environmental factors that may be associated with the disease.

3. Detail the clinical presentation of the typical patient with AD.

4. Describe the clinical course of the disease and typical patient outcomes.

5. Describe how nonpharmacologic therapy is combined with pharmacologic therapy for patients with AD.

6. Recognize and recommend treatment options for disease-specific symptoms as well as behavioral/noncognitive symptoms associated with the disease.

7. Develop an alternative treatment plan for patients with AD.

8. Educate patients and/or caregivers about the expected outcomes for patients with AD, and provide contact information for support/advocacy agencies.

KEY CONCEPTS

❶ Alzheimer's disease (AD) is characterized by progressive cognitive decline including memory loss, disorientation, and impaired judgment and learning.

❷ Pathologic hallmarks of the disease in the brain include *neurofibrillary tangles* and *neuritic plaques (senile plaques)* made up of various proteins that result in a shortage of the neurotransmitter acetylcholine.

❸ The diagnosis of AD is established following an extensive history and physical examination, and by ruling out other potential causes of dementia.

❹ Treatment is focused on delaying disease progression and preservation of functioning as long as possible.

❺ The current gold standard of treatment for cognitive symptoms includes pharmacologic management with a cholinesterase inhibitor and/or an *N*-methyl-D-aspartate (NMDA) receptor antagonist.

❻ Future therapies for AD may be based on disease-modifying therapies.

❼ Treatment of behavioral symptoms should begin with nonpharmacologic treatments but may also include antipsychotic agents and/or antidepressants.

❽ Therapeutic response in AD is genotype specific, depending on the genes associated with pathogenesis and/or genes responsible for drug metabolism.

❶ *Alzheimer's disease (AD) is a nonreversible, progressive dementia manifested by gradual deterioration in cognition and behavioral disturbances.* It is primarily diagnosed by exclusion of other potential causes for dementias. There is no single symptom unique to AD; therefore, diagnosis relies on a thorough patient history. The exact pathophysiologic mechanism underlying AD is not entirely known, although certain genetic and environmental factors may be associated with the disease. There is currently no cure for AD; however, drug treatment can slow symptom progression over time.

Family members of AD patients are profoundly affected by the increased dependence of their loved ones as the disease progresses. Referral to an advocacy organization, such as the Alzheimer's Association, can provide early education and social support of both the patient and family. The Alzheimer's Association has developed a list of common warning signs (Table 29–1).[1]

EPIDEMIOLOGY AND ETIOLOGY

● AD is the most common type of dementia, affecting an estimated 5.4 million Americans in 2011. It represents the sixth leading cause of death across all age groups in the United States, and it is the fifth leading cause of death for individuals 65 years of age and older.[2] Various classifications of dementia include dementia of the Alzheimer's type, vascular dementia, and dementia due to human

Table 29–1
Ten Warning Signs of AD
1. Memory loss that disrupts daily life.
2. Challenges in planning or solving problems.
3. Difficulty completing familiar tasks at home, at work, or at leisure.
4. Confusion with time or place.
5. Trouble understanding visual images and spatial relationships.
6. New problems with words in speaking or writing.
7. Misplacing things and losing the ability to retrace steps.
8. Decreased or poor judgment.
9. Withdrawal from work or social activities.
10. Changes in mood or personality.

From Alzheimer's Association [Internet]. Cited 2011 Oct 10. Available from: *http://www.alz.org/alzheimers_disease_10_signs_of_alzheimers. asp*, with permission.

immunodeficiency virus (HIV) disease, head trauma, Parkinson's disease, Huntington's disease, Pick's disease, or Creutzfeldt-Jakob disease.[3] This chapter addresses only dementia of the Alzheimer's type.

The prevalence of AD increases with age. Of those affected, 6% were 65 to 74 years of age, 45% were between 75 and 84 years of age, and 45% were persons older than 85 years.[2] It is projected that by the year 2050, there will be a threefold increase in prevalence yielding potentially 11 to 16 million AD patients due to a population increase in persons older than 65 years.[2] Additionally, the cost to society will continually increase, as total spending for AD is projected to increase from $183 billion in 2011 to over $1 trillion in 2050.[2] Furthermore, the costs paid by Medicare and Medicaid for AD in 2050 will have increased from 2010 by more than 600% and 400%, respectively.[4] The severity of AD also correlates with increasing age and is classified as mild, moderate, or severe. Other risk factors associated with AD besides age include family history, female gender, and vascular risk factors such as diabetes, hypertension, heart disease, and current smoking.[5] However, it is unknown how other factors such as environment contribute and interact with the genetic predisposition for AD.

The mean survival time of persons with AD is reported to be approximately 6 years from the onset of symptoms until death. However, age at diagnosis, severity of AD, and other medical conditions affect survival time.[6] Although AD does not directly cause death, it is associated with an increase in various risk factors that often contribute to death, such as senility, sepsis, stroke, pneumonia, dehydration, and decubitus ulcers.

The exact etiology of AD is unknown; however, it has been suggested that genetic factors may contribute to errors in protein synthesis resulting in the formation of abnormal proteins involved in the pathogenesis of AD.[7] Early onset, which is defined as AD prior to age 60, accounts for approximately 1% of all AD. This type is usually familial and follows an autosomal dominant pattern in approximately 50% of cases of early-onset AD. Mutations in three genes, presenilin

1 on chromosome 14, amyloid precursor protein (APP) on chromosome 21, and presenilin 2 on chromosome 1, lead to an increase in the accumulation of amyloid beta (Aβ) in the brain, resulting in oxidative stress, neuronal destruction, and the clinical syndrome of AD.[8,9]

The genetic basis for the more common late-onset AD appears more complex. Genetic susceptibility is more sporadic, and it may be more dependent on environmental factors.[7] The apolipoprotein E (apo E) gene on chromosome 19 has been identified as a strong risk factor for late-onset AD. There are three variants of apo E; however, carriers of two or more of the apo E4 allele have an earlier onset of AD (approximately 6 years earlier) compared with noncarriers.[7] Only 50% of AD patients have the apo E4 allele, thus indicating it is only a susceptibility marker.

PATHOPHYSIOLOGY

② *The pathologic hallmarks of the disease in the brain include neurofibrillary tangles and neuritic plaques made up of various proteins, which result in a shortage of the neurotransmitter acetylcholine (Ach).* These are primarily located in brain regions involved in learning, memory, and emotional behaviors such as the cerebral cortex, hippocampus, basal forebrain, and amygdala.[10]

Tangles

Neurofibrillary tangles are intracellular and consist of abnormally phosphorylated tau (τ) protein, which is involved in microtubule assembly. Tangles interfere with neuronal function, resulting in cell damage, and their presence has been correlated with the severity of dementia.[11] Unfortunately, these tangles are insoluble even after the cell dies, and they cannot be removed once established. The neurons that provide most of the cholinergic innervation to the cortex are most prominently affected.[12] Therefore, prevention is the key to targeted therapy of these tangles.

Plaques

Neuritic or senile plaques are extracellular protein deposits of fibrils and amorphous aggregates of β-amyloid protein.[10] This formed protein is central to the pathogenesis of AD. The β-amyloid protein is present in a nontoxic, soluble form in human brains. In AD, conformational changes occur that render it insoluble and cause it to deposit into amorphous diffuse plaques associated with dystrophic neuritis.[13] Over time, these deposits become compacted into plaques, and the β-amyloid protein becomes fibrillar and neurotoxic. Inflammation occurs secondary to clusters of astrocytes and microglia surrounding these plaques.

Acetylcholine

The neurotransmitter Ach is responsible for transmitting messages between certain nerve cells in the brain. In AD, the plaques and tangles damage these pathways, leading to a shortage of Ach, resulting in learning and memory impairment.[14] The loss of Ach activity correlates with the severity of AD. The basis of pharmacologic treatment of AD has been to improve cholinergic neurotransmission in the brain. Acetylcholinesterase is the enzyme that degrades Ach in the synaptic cleft. Blocking this enzyme leads to an increased level of Ach with a goal of stabilizing neurotransmission.[14]

Glutamate

Glutamate is the primary excitatory neurotransmitter in the CNS; it is involved in memory, learning, and neuronal plasticity. It acts by providing information from one brain area to another and affects cognition through facilitation of connections with cholinergic neurons in the cerebral cortex and basal forebrain.[15] In AD, one type of glutamate receptor, N-methyl-D-aspartate (NMDA), is less prevalent than normal. There also appears to be overactivation of unregulated glutamate signaling. This results in a rise in calcium ions that induces secondary cascades, which lead to neuronal death and an increased production of APP.[14] The increased production of APP is associated with higher rates of plaque development and hyperphosphorylation of τ protein.[15]

Cholesterol

Increased cholesterol concentrations have been associated with AD. The cholesterol increases β-amyloid protein synthesis, which can lead to plaque formation.[14] Also, the apo E4 allele is thought to be involved in cholesterol metabolism and is associated with higher cholesterol levels.[14]

Estrogen

Estrogen appears to have properties that protect against memory loss associated with normal aging. It has been suggested that estrogen may block β-amyloid protein production and even trigger nerve growth in cholinergic nerve terminals.[16] Estrogen is also an antioxidant and helps prevent oxidative cell damage.[16] It is important to note, however, that the Women's Health Initiative Memory Study reported that hormone replacement with either estrogen alone or estrogen plus medroxyprogesterone resulted in negative effects on memory.[17]

CLINICAL PRESENTATION AND DIAGNOSIS

❸ *Diagnosing AD relies on a thorough medical and psychological history, mental status testing, and laboratory data to exclude other possible causes of dementia.* There are no biological markers other than those pathophysiological changes found at autopsy that can confirm AD, although the development of in vivo plaque detection methods may change this.

AD is a progressive disease that, over time, affects multiple areas of cognition. The symptoms of AD can be divided into cognitive symptoms, noncognitive symptoms, and functional symptoms for assessment and treatment purposes.

The National Institute on Aging and the Alzheimer's Association workgroup recently revised the 1984 criteria for AD dementia. The group defined all-cause dementia, probable AD dementia, possible AD dementia, and probable or possible AD dementia with evidence of the AD pathophysiological process. The routine use of AD biomarker tests for routine diagnostic purposes is not advocated at this time. These tests are reserved for research purposes. See Tables 29–2, 29–3, and 29–4 for full criteria.[18]

Clinical Presentation and Diagnosis of Alzheimer's Disease

General

The diagnosis of AD relies on thorough mental status testing and neuropsychological tests, medical and psychiatric history, neurological examination, interview of caregivers and family members, and laboratory and imaging data to support the diagnosis and exclude other causes.

Signs and Symptoms

- Cognitive: memory loss, problems with language, disorientation to time and place, poor or decreased judgment, problems with learning and abstract thinking, misplacing things
- Noncognitive: Changes in mood or behavior, changes in personality, or loss of initiative
- Functional: Difficulty performing familiar tasks

Laboratory Tests

- MRI or CT is used to measure changes in brain size and volume and rule out stroke, brain tumor, or cerebral edema.
- Tests to exclude possible causes of dementia include a depression screen, vitamin B_{12} deficiency, thyroid function tests (thyroid-stimulating hormone and free triiodothyronine and thyroxine), complete blood count, and chemistry panel.[21]
- Other diagnostic tests to consider for differential diagnosis: erythrocyte sedimentation rate, urinalysis, toxicology, chest x-ray, heavy metal screen, HIV testing, CSF examination, electroencephalography, and neuropsychological tests such as the Folstein Mini Mental Status Examination.

Table 29–2

Criteria for All-Cause Dementia: Core Clinical Criteria

Cognitive or behavioral (neuropsychiatric) symptoms that:

1. Interfere with the ability to function at work or at usual activities
2. Represent a decline from previous levels of functioning and performing
3. Are not explained by delirium or major psychiatric disorder
4. Is detected and diagnosed through a combination of:
   a. History taking from the patient and a knowledgeable informant
   b. Objective cognitive assessment
5. Involves a minimum of two of the following domains:
   a. Impaired ability to acquire and remember new information
   b. Impaired reasoning and handling of complex tasks; poor judgment
   c. Impaired visuospatial abilities
   d. Impaired language functions
   e. Changes in personality, behavior, or comportment

From McKhann GM, Knopman DS, Chertkow H, et al. The diagnosis of dementia due to Alzheimer's disease: Recommendations from the National Institute on Aging and the Alzheimer's Association Workgroup. Alzheimers Dement 2011;7:263–269, with permission.

Table 29–3

Probable AD Dementia: Core Clinical Criteria

1. Meets criteria for dementia and has the following characteristics:
   a. Insidious onset
   b. Clear-cut history of worsening of cognition by report or observation
   c. Initial and most prominent cognitive deficits are evident on history and examination in one of the following categories:
      (i) Amnestic presentation: deficits include impairment in learning and recall of recently learned information; should be evidence of cognitive dysfunction in at least one other cognitive function
      (ii) Nonamnestic presentation: language, visuospatial, or executive dysfunction presentation; deficits in other cognitive domains should be present
2. Should not be applied when there is evidence of:
   a. Substantial concomitant cerebrovascular disease
   b. Core features of dementia with Lewy bodies other than dementia itself
   c. Prominent features of behavioral variant frontotemporal dementia
   d. Prominent features of semantic or nonfluent/agrammatic variant primary progressive aphasia
   e. Another concurrent, active neurologic disease, or nonneurologic medical comorbidity or use of medication that could have a substantial effect on cognition

From McKhann GM, Knopman DS, Chertkow H, et al. The diagnosis of dementia due to Alzheimer's disease: Recommendations from the National Institute on Aging and the Alzheimer's Association Workgroup. Alzheimers Dement 2011;7:263–269, with permission.

Table 29–4

Possible AD Dementia: Core Clinical Criteria

Diagnosis made in either of the following circumstances:

1. Atypical course: Meets the core clinical criteria in terms of the nature of the cognitive deficits for AD dementia but either has a sudden onset of cognitive impairments or demonstrates insufficient historical detail or objective cognitive documentation of progressive decline
2. Etiologically mixed presentation: Meets all core clinical criteria for all-cause dementia but has evidence of:
   a Concomitant cerebrovascular disease
   b Features of dementia with Lewy bodies other than the dementia itself
   c Another neurologic disease or a nonneurologic medical comorbidity or medication use that could have a substantial effect on cognition

From McKhann GM, Knopman DS, Chertkow H, et al. The diagnosis of dementia due to Alzheimer's disease: Recommendations from the National Institute on Aging and the Alzheimer's Association Workgroup. Alzheimers Dement 2011;7:263–269, with permission.

TREATMENT

Desired and Expected Outcomes

Although there are currently four agents approved for the treatment of AD, none of these agents are curative or are known to directly reverse the disease process.

❹ *Consequently, the primary desired outcome of treatment of AD is to symptomatically treat the cognitive symptoms of the patient and preserve the patient's functioning for as long as possible.* Secondary goals include treating psychiatric and behavioral symptoms that may occur during the course of the disease.

General Approach to Treatment

❺ *The current gold standard of treatment for cognitive symptoms includes pharmacologic management with a **cholinesterase (ChE) inhibitor** and/or an **NMDA antagonist.*** Donepezil, rivastigmine, and galantamine are three ChEs used for cognitive symptoms. The first ChE approved for AD was tacrine; however, it is currently no longer available on the U.S. market. The use of tacrine was limited in practice due to its propensity for hepatotoxicity, difficult titration schedule, four times daily dosing, poor bioavailability, and troublesome incidence of nausea, diarrhea, and urinary incontinence. The only NMDA antagonist is memantine. Psychiatric and behavioral symptoms that occur during the course of the disease should be treated as they occur.

Essential elements in the treatment of AD include education, communication, and planning with the family/caregiver of the patient. Treatment options, legal and financial decisions, and course of the illness need to be discussed with the patient and family members. In this

Table 29–5

Basic Principles in the Management of Patients With AD

- Using a gentle, calm approach to the patient
- Giving reassurance when needed
- Empathizing with the patient's concerns
- Using distraction and redirection
- Maintaining daily routines
- Providing a safe environment
- Providing daytime activities
- Avoiding overstimulation
- Using familiar decorative items in the living area
- Bringing abrupt declines in function and the appearance of new symptoms to professional attention

Table 29–6

Treatment Algorithm for Cognitive Symptoms of AD

1. Patient diagnosed with AD
2. Assess all comorbid medical disorders and drug therapies that may affect cognition
3. Rule out comorbid depression
4. Evaluate for pharmacotherapy based on illness stage
   a Mild AD: Cholinesterase inhibitor
   b Moderate to severe AD: Cholinesterase inhibitor, memantine, or combination cholinesterase inhibitor and memantine
5. Deteriorating Mini Mental Status Exam (MMSE) score greater than 2–4 points after 1 year: Change to a different cholinesterase inhibitor
6. Stable MMSE: Continue regimen

regard, the clinician's emphasis should be on helping to maintain a therapeutic living environment while minimizing the burden of care resulting from the disease.

Nonpharmacologic Treatment

Treatment of AD involves both pharmacologic and non-pharmacologic methods. Upon the initial diagnosis, the patient and family should be counseled on the course of the illness, prognosis, available treatments, legal decisions, and quality-of-life issues. The life of a patient with AD must become progressively more simple and structured as the disease progresses, and the caregiver must learn to keep requests and demands on the patient simple. Basic principles in the treatment of patients with AD are shown in Table 29–5.

Conventional Pharmacologic Treatment for Cognitive Symptoms

▶ ChE Inhibitors (Donepezil, Rivastigmine, and Galantamine)

The ChE inhibitors all have the indication for the treatment of dementia of the Alzheimer's type. Guidelines for the treatment of AD recommend the use of ChE inhibitors as a valuable treatment for AD and the use of memantine for moderate to severe AD.[19–21] Few head-to-head studies comparing the ChE Inhibitors exist. The few available trials conclude no major difference in clinical outcomes, so the decision to use one ChE over another should be based on differences in mechanisms of action, adverse reactions, and titration schedules.[22]

Treatment should begin as early as possible in patients with a diagnosis of AD.[23] Table 29–6 provides a recommended treatment algorithm for AD. Patients should be switched to another ChE inhibitor from their initial ChE inhibitor if they show an initial lack of efficacy, initially respond to treatment but lose clinical benefit, or experience

safety/tolerability issues. This switch should not be attempted until the patient has been on a maximally tolerated dose for a period of 3 to 6 months. The switch should also be based on realistic expectations of the patient and/or caregiver.[24] ChE inhibitor therapy should be discontinued in patients who experience poor tolerance or adherence, who show a lack of clinical improvement after 6 months at optimal dosing, who have failed attempts at monotherapy with at least two agents or combination therapy, who continue to deteriorate at the pretreatment rate, who demonstrate dramatic clinical deterioration following initiation of treatment, or who deteriorate to the point where there is no significant effect on quality of life. Patients with a Mini Mental Status Exam (MMSE) score less than 10 may also benefit from discontinuation of medication; however, this has not been substantially proven in clinical studies.[25]

Donepezil

Donepezil is a piperidine ChE inhibitor that reversibly and noncompetitively inhibits centrally active acetylcholinesterase.[26] Donepezil is approved for the treatment of mild to moderate AD. A dose of 10 mg/day has demonstrated efficacy in patients with either mild to moderate or moderate to severe forms of AD. A 23-mg dose of donepezil is also approved for patients with moderate to severe disease. The 23-mg dose showed a small improvement in cognitive symptoms over 10 mg/day; however, there was no improvement on overall patient functioning, and there was a higher incidence of adverse effects with the 23-mg dose.[27] Table 29–7 describes the dosing strategies for all of the approved agents for AD. The most frequent adverse effects are mild to moderate gastrointestinal symptoms. Others include headache, dizziness, syncope, bradycardia, and muscle weakness. Table 29–8 compares their major side effects.[26,28–31]

Only a small number of drug interactions have been reported with donepezil. In vitro studies show a low rate of

Table 29–7				
Dosing Strategies for Cognitive Agents				
	Donepezil (Aricept)	**Rivastigmine (Exelon)**	**Galantamine (Razadyne)**	**Memantine (Namenda)**[a]
Starting dose	5 mg daily	1.5 mg 2 × daily or 4.6 mg/24 h applied daily (patch)	4 mg 2 × daily or 8 mg daily	5 mg daily or 7 mg daily (ER formulation)
Maintenance dose	5–23 mg daily	3–6 mg 2 × daily or 9.5 mg/24 h applied daily (patch)	8–12 mg 2 × daily or 16–24 mg daily	10 mg 2 × daily or 28 mg daily (ER formulation)
Time between dose adjustments	4–6 weeks between 5 and 10 mg increment; 3 months between 10 and 23 mg increment	2 weeks for oral and 4 weeks for patch	4 weeks	1 week
Dosage adjustments for renal or hepatic impairment	None	None	Do not exceed 16 mg for moderately impaired hepatic or renal function; do not administer in severe renal or hepatic impairment	Caution should be taken in patients with severe hepatic impairment

[a]Memantine XR is currently approved, but a launch date is unknown.

From Refs. 33, 35–38.

binding of donepezil to cytochrome P450 (CYP)3A4 or 2D6. Whether donepezil has the potential for enzyme induction is not known. Monitoring for possible increased peripheral side effects is advised when adding a CYP2D6 or 3A3/4 inhibitor to donepezil treatment. Also, inducers of CYP2D6 and 3A4 could increase the rate of elimination of donepezil.[26]

Rivastigmine

Rivastigmine, which is approved for the treatment of mild to moderate dementia of AD, has central activity for both the acetylcholinesterase and butyrylcholinesterase enzymes.[28] Acetylcholinesterase is found in two forms:

Table 29–8						
Adverse Effects for Currently Approved Medications for Alzheimer's Disease*						
Adverse Event	**Donepezil 5–10 mg/day (%) (n = 747)**	**Donepezil 23 mg/day (%) (n = 963)**	**Rivastigmine 6–12 mg/day (%) (n = 1,189)**	**Galantamine IR 16–24 mg/day (%) (n = 1,040)**	**Memantine IR 5–20 mg/day (%) (n = 940)**	**Memantine XR 28 mg/day (%) (n= 341)**
Nausea	11	12	47	24	NR	NR
Vomiting	5	9	31	13	3	2
Diarrhea	10	8	19	9	NR	5
Headache	10	4	17	8	6	6
Dizziness	8	5	21	9	7	5
Muscle cramps	6	NR	NR	NR	NR	NR
Insomnia	9	3	9	5	NR	NR
Fatigue	5	2	9	5	2	3
Anorexia	4	5	17	9	NR	NR
Depression	3	NR	6	7	NR	3
Abnormal dreams	3	NR	NR	NR	NR	NR
Weight decrease	3	5	3	7	NR	NR
Abdominal pain	NR	NR	13	5	NR	2
Rhinitis	NR	NR	4	4	NR	NR

NR, not reported.

*Caution is urged in making comparisons between drugs based on these data because different clinical trials often collect adverse event data using different methodologies.

From Refs. 33, 35–38.

globular 4 and globular 1. In postmortem studies, globular 4 is significantly depleted, whereas globular 1 is still abundant. Thus blocking metabolism of globular 1 may lead to higher concentrations of Ach. Rivastigmine has higher activity at globular 1 than at globular 4. Theoretically, this may be advantageous because rivastigmine prevents the degradation of Ach via the acetylcholinesterase globular 1 over the course of the disease as compared with the other ChE inhibitors.

The dual inhibition of acetylcholinesterase and butyrylcholinesterase may lead to broader efficacy. As acetylcholinesterase activity decreases with disease progression, the acetylcholinesterase-selective agents may lose their effect, whereas the dual inhibitors may still be effective due to the added inhibition of butyrylcholinesterase. However, this has not been demonstrated clinically.

Rivastigmine, in addition to the oral formulation, is also available in a patch formulation. When switching from the oral formulation to the patch, if the patient is taking less than 6 mg/day of oral, then the 4.6 mg/24 h patch is recommended. If the patient is taking 6 to 12 mg/day of oral, then the 9.5 mg/24 h patch is recommended. The first patch should be applied on the day following the last oral dose.[28]

Cholinergic side effects are common with rivastigmine, but they are usually well tolerated if the recommended dosing schedule is followed. If side effects cause intolerance, several doses can be held, then dosing can be restarted at the same or next lower dose. Drugs that induce or inhibit CYP450 metabolism are not expected to alter the metabolism of rivastigmine.[28]

Galantamine

Galantamine, which is approved for the treatment of mild to moderate dementia of AD, is a ChE inhibitor, which elevates Ach in the cerebral cortex by slowing the degradation of Ach.[29] It also modulates the nicotinic Ach receptors to increase Ach release from surviving presynaptic nerve terminals. In addition, it may increase glutamate and serotonin levels. The clinical benefit of action of these additional neurotransmitters is unknown.

CYP3A4 and 2D6 are the major enzymes involved in the metabolism of galantamine. Pharmacokinetic studies with inhibitors of this system have resulted in increased galantamine concentrations or reductions in clearance. Similarly to donepezil, if inhibitors are given concurrently with galantamine, monitoring for increased cholinergic side effects should be done.[29]

NMDA Receptor Antagonist

Memantine is a noncompetitive antagonist of the NMDA type of glutamate receptors, which are located ubiquitously throughout the brain. It regulates activity throughout the brain by controlling the amount of calcium that enters the nerve cell, a process essential for establishing an environment required for information storage. Overstimulation of the NMDA receptor by excessive glutamate allows too much calcium into the cell, disrupting information processing. Blocking NMDA receptors with memantine may protect neurons from the effects of excessive glutamate without disrupting normal neurotransmission.[30,31]

Memantine is indicated for the treatment of moderate to severe dementia of the Alzheimer's type. It can be given as a monotherapy or in combination with ChE inhibitors. Memantine is not indicated for mild AD, and currently there is a lack of evidence to use it in mild AD.[32] An extended-release formulation of memantine is approved for once-daily administration, although the launch date of the product is currently unknown.[31] The higher dose of memantine extended release (28 mg) has not been compared with the immediate-release formulation; thus it is unknown if the 28 mg/day dose of memantine is more effective than the traditional 20 mg/day maximum. Adverse reactions associated with memantine include constipation, confusion, dizziness, headache, coughing, and hypertension. Extra monitoring should be done if memantine is given concurrently with a ChE inhibitor.

In vitro studies have shown that memantine produces minimal inhibition of CYP450 enzymes CYP1A2, 2A6, 2C9, 2D6, 2E1, and 3A4. These data indicate that no pharmacokinetic interactions with drugs metabolized by these enzymes should be expected.[30,31]

Future Therapies

6 *Future therapies for AD may be based on disease-modifying therapies.* Current investigations involving the amyloid hypothesis are reviewing various compounds in the secondary prevention of AD. Mechanisms by which these compounds are thought to work include[8]:

- Decreasing the production of Aβ
- Stimulation of clearance of Aβ formed

Patient Encounter, Part 1

A woman presents at the clinic with her 70-year-old mother, KE, complaining that her mother's memory is not getting better. The woman complains that her mother is continuing to forget things, including paying the bills and taking out the trash. Six months ago KE was started on donepezil 5 mg daily, which the daughter administers. The woman asks if there is anything else her mother could take to help her memory.

What counseling points about Alzheimer's disease would you provide to the daughter?

Where would you recommend the daughter find more information about Alzheimer's disease?

How would you address the daughter's question regarding the pharmacologic management of her mother's Alzheimer's disease?

- Prevention of aggregation of Aβ into amyloid plaques
- Prevention of neuronal damage by limiting inflammation and neurotoxicity caused by Aβ

Currently, bapineuzumab (AAB-001; Janssen/Elan/Pfizer), a humanized monoclonal antibody targeting the Aβ, is in phase 3 clinical trials for the treatment of AD.[33]

Nonconventional Pharmacologic Treatment

Many other nonconventional treatments have been used as adjunctive treatments during the course of AD. Vitamin E was previously recommended for use as an adjunctive treatment because of its antioxidant properties, but a meta-analysis suggested that high doses (greater than 400 IU/day) should be avoided due to an increased all-cause mortality.[34] Currently, vitamin E is not recommended for the treatment of AD.[20] Estrogen has been investigated for use in AD, but as mentioned previously, it was associated with an increased risk of dementia. Nonsteroidal anti-inflammatory drugs (NSAIDs) have also been investigated. There is a lack of convincing data supporting efficacy, and significant adverse effects (gastritis and GI bleeds) are associated with their use, so they are not recommended for general use in the treatment or prevention of AD at this time.[35] Statins (3-hydroxy-3-methylglutaryl-CoA reductase inhibitors) should be reserved for those patients who have other indications for their use.[36] Ginkgo biloba has also been studied, and until this product has a more standardized manufacturing process and its long-term safety and efficacy are established, it should be recommended with caution.[37] The medical food caprylidene (AC-1202, Axona) is an approved medical food for the dietary management of metabolic processes associated with mild to moderate AD.[38] Reduced metabolic processing of glucose in neurons has been associated with AD. Ketone bodies can potentially be used as an alternative energy source for AD patients with reduced neuronal glucose metabolism.[38] Caprylidene is a medium chain triglyceride that is converted by the liver into the ketone body β-hydroxybutyrate (BHB). BHB crosses the blood–brain barrier and can be utilized by neurons as a potential energy source to generate ATP and increase pools of acetylcholine. Caprylidene is available only by prescription and is supplied in 40-g powder packets. One packet can be mixed with 4 to 8 ounces of liquid (~120 to 240 mL) and dosed once daily after a meal. The most common side effects are mild GI disturbances including nausea, diarrhea, flatulence, and dyspepsia.[39]

Treatment of Behavioral Symptoms

❼ *Treatment of behavioral symptoms should begin with nonpharmacologic treatments but may also include antipsychotic agents and/or antidepressants.* Nonpharmacologic recommendations for treatment include[40]:

- Music
- Videotapes of family members
- Audiotapes of the voices of caregivers

- Walking and light exercise
- Sensory stimulation and relaxation

Antipsychotics are frequently used in the management of neuropsychiatric symptoms associated with AD. A recent meta-analysis concluded that only 17% to 18% of dementia patients demonstrated treatment response to atypical antipsychotics.[41] A double-blind placebo-controlled trial of olanzapine, quetiapine, or risperidone for the treatment of psychosis, aggression, or agitation in patients with AD concluded that adverse effects offset the advantages in the efficacy of atypical antipsychotics.[42]

In April 2005, the FDA issued a statement requesting black-box warnings on all atypical antipsychotics stating that elderly people with dementia-related psychosis treated with an atypical antipsychotic are at an increased risk of death compared with those treated with placebo. Of a total of 17 placebo-controlled trials investigating olanzapine, aripiprazole, quetiapine, and risperidone in elderly demented patients with behavioral disorders, 15 showed a numerical increase in mortality in the drug-treated group compared with the placebo-treated groups (1.6 to 1.7 times increased risk of death). Specific causes for these deaths were heart-related events (heart failure and sudden death) and infections (mostly pneumonia).

The atypical antipsychotics are not currently approved for the treatment of elderly patients with dementia-related psychosis. Therefore, it is important to individually assess and balance the risk versus benefit of antipsychotic use in this population.

Depressive symptoms occur in as many as 50% of patients with AD and can be difficult to differentiate from symptoms of dementia, so symptoms of depression should be documented for several weeks prior to initiating therapy for depression with AD.[20] The selective serotonin reuptake inhibitors (SSRIs) are most commonly used based on their side-effect profile and evidence of efficacy.[20] Indications for the use of antidepressants include depression characterized by poor appetite, insomnia, hopelessness, anhedonia, withdrawal, suicidal thoughts, and agitation. A recent trial has suggested a lack of benefit of sertraline and mirtazapine compared with placebo and an increased risk of adverse effects with them.[43]

Other miscellaneous therapies for AD include benzodiazepines for anxiety, agitation, and aggression. However, their routine use is not advised.[20] Additionally, benzodiazepines have been associated with an increase in falls leading to the potential for hip fractures in the elderly.[44] Mood stabilizer anticonvulsants, carbamazepine, valproic acid, or gabapentin may be used as alternatives, but the current evidence is conflicting.[45] Buspirone has shown benefit in treating agitation and aggression in a limited number of patients with minimal adverse effects.[46,47] In open-label and controlled studies, selegiline decreased anxiety, depression, and agitation.[48,49] Finally, trazodone has been shown to decrease insomnia, agitation, and dysphoria, and it has been used to treat sundowning in AD patients. Table 29–9 provides dosing strategies for the noncognitive symptoms of AD.[50]

Table 29–9

Medications Used in Noncognitive Symptoms of Dementia

Drugs	Starting Dose (mg)	Maintenance Dose in Dementia (mg/day)	Dosing Adjustment for Hepatic Impairment (mg)	Dosing Adjustment for Renal Impairment (mg)	Target Symptoms
Antipsychotics					
Haloperidol	0.25	1–3	None needed	None needed	Psychosis: hallucinations, delusions, suspiciousness
Olanzapine	2.5	5–10	None needed	None needed	Disruptive behaviors: agitation, aggression
Quetiapine	25	100–300	Lower starting dose and longer titration schedule to effective dose based on response and tolerability	None needed	
Risperidone	0.25	0.75–2	Lower starting dose and longer titration schedule to effective dose based on response and tolerability	Lower starting dose and longer titration schedule to effective dose based on response and tolerability	
Ziprasidone	20	40–160	None needed	None needed	
Antidepressants					
Citalopram	10	10–20	20 mg/day maximum; may increase only in nonresponsive patients	Mild to moderate impairment: none needed	Depression: poor appetite, insomnia, hopelessness, anhedonia, withdrawal, suicidal thoughts, agitation, anxiety
Escitalopram	5	20–40	10 mg/day maximum	Mild to moderate impairment: none needed	
Fluoxetine	5	10–40	A lower dose or less frequent schedule is recommended	None needed	
Paroxetine	10	10–40	10 mg/day; may increase by 10 mg/day at intervals of at least 1 week	10 mg/day; may increase by 10 mg/day at intervals of at least 1 week	
Sertraline	25	75–100	Lower or less frequent doses should be used	None needed	
Venlafaxine	25	75–225	Decrease usual dose by ≥50%	Decrease usual dose by 25% to 50%	
Trazodone	25	75–150	None needed	None needed	
Anticonvulsants					
Carbamazepine	100	200–600	Should not be used in aggravated liver dysfunction or active liver disease	None needed	Agitation or aggression
Valproic acid	125	500–1000	Should not be administered	None needed	

Adapted from Slattum PW, Swerdlow PH, Massey-Hill A. Alzheimer's disease. In: Dipiro JT, Talbert RL, Yee GC, et al, eds. Pharmacotherapy: A Pathophysiologic Approach. 8th ed. New York, NY: McGraw-Hill; 2011:947–961, with permission.

Patient Encounter, Part 2

KE returns to the clinic in 6 months. She has been receiving 10 mg/day of donepezil. Her memory symptoms have slowed in their decline, but recently KE has been agitated at bedtime, talking to her deceased husband. The daughter is particularly concerned about the symptoms and wants to know what she could do to treat them. Her medical record is as follows:

PMH:

- Diabetes mellitus since age 55; it was well controlled until last year when it worsened because of increased confusion about when to take her medication
- Hypertension treated for 20 years and well controlled; has been hypotensive on a few occasions recently during physicals

FH: Father died of myocardial infarction at age 76; mother died of breast cancer at age 79

SH: Lives with daughter; denies drinking alcohol or smoking

Medications:

- Hydrochlorothiazide 25 mg orally once daily
- Losartan 50 mg orally twice daily
- Metformin 1,000 mg orally twice daily
- Donepezil 10 mg daily

ROS: (+) weight loss of 5.5 kg (12 lb); (−) N/V/D, change in appetite, heartburn, chest pain, or shortness of breath

PE:

VS: BP 128/62 mm Hg supine, P 77 beats/min, RR 15/min, T 37°C (98.6°F)

Gen: Poorly groomed, thin woman looks stated age

Neuro: Folstein Mini Mental Status Exam score 18/30; disoriented to month, date, and day of week, clinic name and floor; poor registration with impaired attention and short-term memory; good language skills but problems with commands

CT scan: Mild to moderate generalized cerebral atrophy

What do you recommend with regard to her current donepezil treatment?

What nonpharmacologic and pharmacologic interventions could be recommended for the agitation and psychosis?

GENOMICS

8 *Therapeutic response in AD is genotype specific, depending on the genes associated with pathogenesis and/or genes responsible for drug metabolism.* Recent investigations have demonstrated that the therapeutic response in AD is genotype specific, depending on genes associated with AD pathogenesis and/or genes responsible for drug metabolism. Apo E-4/4 carriers tend to show a faster disease progression and a poorer therapeutic response to all available treatments than any other polymorphic variants associated with AD. CYP450 enzyme extensive and intermediate metabolizers are the best responders to pharmacotherapy, while poor and ultrarapid metabolizers are the worst responders. The pharmacogenetic response in AD may depend on the interaction of genes involved in drug metabolism and the genes associated with AD pathogenesis.[51]

OUTCOME EVALUATION

- The success of therapy is measured by the degree to which the care plan decreases the pretreatment deterioration rate, preserves the patients' functioning, and treats psychiatric and behavioral symptoms. The primary outcome measure is thus subjective information from the patient and the caregiver, although the MMSE can be a helpful tool. There are no physical examination or laboratory parameters that are used to evaluate the success of therapy.

- Once a tolerated agent is found, continue that therapy until poor tolerance or poor adherence occurs, no clinical improvement is seen with 3 to 6 months of optimal dosing, or the pretreatment deterioration rate continues.

- Inform the patient and the caregiver that the treatments available for AD are not curative but may slow the rate of deterioration.

- Treat behavioral and psychiatric issues as they arise. Consider the patient's choices of nonpharmacologic and pharmacologic options before recommending a treatment.

- Discontinue the pharmacologic treatments periodically to reevaluate the need for continued treatment.

- Develop a plan to assess the effectiveness of the ChE inhibitor in slowing the deterioration of cognitive functioning after an appropriate interval (3 to 6 months).

- Assess improvement in quality-of-life measures such as ability to function independently and for slowing of memory deterioration.

Patient Encounter, Part 3

KE returns to the clinic for follow-up 1 year later. Her daughter states her memory is slowly getting worse. Her current MMSE is 16/30. The addition of olanzapine 2.5 mg at bedtime helped with the agitation. Her daughter would like to know if there are any other choices to help treat her mom.

What changes to KE's current medications would you recommend?

- Evaluate the patient for the presence of adverse drug reactions, drug allergies, and drug interactions at appropriate intervals.
- Continue to be a resource for the patient and caregiver throughout the long course of the disease.

CONCLUSION

AD is a progressive deterioration of cognitive abilities, and patients are likely to have behavioral disturbances and personality changes in the later stages of the disease. In an effort to help prepare patients and their caregivers for the inevitable, the Alzheimer's Association has developed ten quick tips on "Living with Alzheimer's disease" (Table 29–10).[52] The Alzheimer's Association can provide many resources as well as facilitate contacts with other organizations. Contact the association at:

Alzheimer's Association
Contact Center: 1-800-272-3900
TDD access: 1.312.335.8882
Website: www.alz.org
E-mail: info@alz.org
National office: 225 N. Michigan Ave., Fl. 17
Chicago, IL 60601–7633

Table 29–10

Living with AD: Ten Quick Tips

1. Carry with you a book of important notes and photos
2. Enroll in Alzheimer's Association Safe Return
3. Be open to accepting help from others
4. Keep doing the things you most enjoy
5. Talk to others who have AD
6. Find ways to laugh as often as you can
7. Maintain your physical health
8. Take steps to make your home safe
9. Extend the time you can live safely in your home with help from your family and friends
10. Put plans in place now for your future

From Alzheimer's Association [Internet]. If you have Alzheimer's disease [cited 2011 Oct 10]. Available from: *www.alz.org/national/documents/brochure_ifyouhave_earlystage.pdf*, with permission.

Patient Care and Monitoring

1. Assess the frequency and duration of the patient's cognitive and noncognitive symptoms. Could the patient be depressed?

2. Review any available diagnostic data from the medical and psychiatric history including interviews from family, neuropsychologic testing, and other labs.

3. Obtain a thorough history of prescription, nonprescription, and natural drug product use. Is the patient taking any medications that could contribute to cognitive changes in the elderly?

4. Educate both the patient and caregivers about lifestyle modification and refer them to support when needed.

5. Monitor pharmacotherapy initiation. Is it titrated correctly?

6. Develop a plan to monitor cognitive response to treatment over time.

7. Routinely assess medication adherence.

8. Educate patient and caregivers on what to expect from pharmacotherapy.

9. Regularly evaluate the patient for the presence of adverse drug reactions, drug allergies, and drug–drug and drug–disease interactions.

10. Be a resource and give continuous support to the patient and caregivers throughout the long course of the disease.

Abbreviations Introduced in This Chapter

Ach	Acetylcholine
Aβ	Amyloid beta
AD	Alzheimer's disease
apo E	Apolipoprotein E
APP	Amyloid precursor protein
βHB	β-Hydroxybutyrate
ChE	Cholinesterase
CYP	Cytochrome P450
MMSE	Mini Mental Status Examination
NMDA	N-Methyl-D-aspartate
NSAID	Nonsteroidal anti-inflammatory drug
SSRI	Selective serotonin reuptake inhibitor
τ	Tau protein

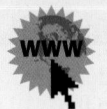 Self-assessment questions and answers are available at *http://www.mhpharmacotherapy.com/pp.html.*

REFERENCES

1. Alzheimer's Association [Internet], [cited 2011 Oct 10]. Available from: *http://www.alz.org/alzheimers_disease_10_signs_of_alzheimers.asp.*

2. Hebert LE, Scherr PA, Bienias JL, et al. Alzheimer disease in the U.S. population: Prevalence estimates using the 2000 census. Arch Neurol 2003;60:1119–1122.

3. American Psychiatric Association. Diagnostic and Statistical Manual of Mental Disorders. 4th ed. Text revision. Washington, DC: American Psychiatric Association; 2000:147–154.

4. Report of the Lewin Group to the Alzheimer's Association [Internet], [cited 2011 Oct 10]. *Available from: www.alz.org/tractory.*

5. Luchsinger JA, Reitz C, Honig LS, et al. Aggregation of vascular risk factors and risk of incident Alzheimer disease. Neurology 2005;65:545–551.

6. Ganguli M, Dodge HH, Shen C, et al. Alzheimer disease and mortality. Arch Neurol 2005;62:779–784.

7. Kamboh MI. Molecular genetics of late-onset Alzheimer's disease. Ann Hum Genet 2004;68:381–404.

8. van Marum RJ. Current and future therapy in Alzheimer's disease. Fundam Clin Pharmacol 2008;22:265–274.

9. Holmes C. Genotype and phenotype in Alzheimer's disease. Br J Psychiatry 2002;180:131–134.

10. Mattson MP. Pathways towards and away from Alzheimer's disease. Nature 2004;430:631–639.

11. DeKosky ST. Pathology and pathways of Alzheimer's disease with an update on new developments in treatment. J Am Geriatr Soc 2003;51:S314–S320.

12. Munoz DG, Feldman H. Causes of Alzheimer's disease. Can Med Assoc J 2000;162:65–72.

13. Yankner BA, Lu T. Amyloid beta-protein toxicity and the pathogenesis of Alzheimer's disease. J Biol Chem 2009;284:4755–4759.

14. Pietrzik C, Behl C. Concepts for the treatment of Alzheimer's disease: Molecular mechanisms and clinical application. Int J Exp Pathol 2005;86:173–185.

15. Sze C, Bi H, Kleinschmidt-DeMasters BK, et al. N-Methyl-D-aspartate receptor subunit proteins and their phosphorylation status are altered selectively in Alzheimer's disease. J Neurol Sci 2001;182:151–159.

16. Gonzalez C, Diaz F, Alonso A. Neuroprotective effects of estrogens: cross-talk between estrogen and intracellular insulin signaling. Infect Disord Drug Targets 2008;8:65–67.

17. Shumaker SA, Legault C, Kuller L, et al. Conjugated equine estrogens and incidence of probable dementia and mild cognitive impairment in postmenopausal women (Women's Health Initiative Memory Study). JAMA 2004;291:2947–2958.

18. McKhann GM, Knopman DS, Chertkow H, et al. The diagnosis of dementia due to Alzheimer's disease: Recommendations from the National Institute on Aging and the Alzheimer's Association Work-group. Alzheimers Dement 2011;7:263–269.

19. Doody RS, Stevens JC, Beck C, et al. Practice parameter: Management of dementia (an evidence-based review). Neurology 2001;56:1154–1166.

20. APA Working Group on Alzheimer's Disease and other Dementias; Rabins PV, Blacker D, et al. American Psychiatric Association practice guideline for the treatment of patients with Alzheimer's disease and other dementias. 2nd ed. Am J Psychiatry 2007;164:5–56.

21. Small GW, Rabins PV, Barry PP, et al. Diagnosis and treatment of Alzheimer's disease and related disorders: Consensus statement of the American Association for Geriatric Psychiatry, the Alzheimer's Association, and the American Geriatrics Society. JAMA 1997;278:1363–1371.

22. Birks J. Cholinesterase inhibitors for Alzheimer's disease. Cochrane Database Syst Rev 2006:CD005593.

23. Hogan DB, Bailey P, Black S, et al. Diagnosis and treatment of dementia: 5. Nonpharmacologic and pharmacologic therapy for mild to moderate dementia. CMAJ 2008;179:1019–1026.

24. Gauthier S, Emre M, Farlow MR, et al. Strategies for continued successful treatment of Alzheimer's disease: Switching cholinesterase inhibitors. Curr Med Res Opin 2003;19(8):707–714.

25. Swanwick GR, Lawlor BA. Initiating and monitoring cholinesterase inhibitor treatment for Alzheimer's disease. Int J Geriatr Psych 1999;14:244–248.

26. Eisai. Aricept (donepezil hydrochloride) [product information]. Teaneck, NJ: Author, 2010.

27. Farlow MR, Salloway S, Atriot PN, et al. Effectiveness and tolerability of high dose (23mg/d) versus standard-dose (10mg/d) donepezil in moderate to severe Alzheimer's disease: A 24-week, randomized, double-blind study. Clin Ther 2010;32:1234–1251.

28. Novartis. Exelon (rivastigmine tartrate) [product information]. East Hanover, NJ: Author, 2008.

29. Ortho-McNeil Neurologics. Razadyne ER/Razadyne (galantamine hydrobromide) [product information]. Titusville, NJ: Author, 2011.

30. Forest Pharmaceutica, Inc. Namenda (memantine hydrochloride) [product information]. St. Louis, MO: Author, 2007.

31. Forest Pharmaceutica, Inc. Namenda XR (memantine hydrochloride) extended release [product information]. St. Louis, MO: Author, 2010.

32. Schneider LS, Dogerman KS, Higgins JP, et al. Lack of evidence for the efficacy of memantine in mild Alzheimer's disease. Arch Neurol 2011;68:991–998.

33. Kerchner GA, Boxer AL. Bapineuzumab. Expert Opin Biol Ther 2010;10:1121–1130.

34. Miller ER, Pastor-Barriuso R, Dalal D, et al. Meta-analysis: High-dosage vitamin E supplementation may increase all-cause mortality. Ann Intern Med 2005;142:37–46.

35. Aisen PS, Schafer KA, Grundman M, et al. Effects of rofecoxib or naproxen versus placebo on Alzheimer's disease progression. JAMA 2003;289:2819–2826.

36. Cooper JL. Dietary lipids in the etiology of Alzheimer's disease. Drugs Aging 2003;20:399–418.

37. Dekosky ST, Williamson JD, Fitzpatrick AL, et al. Ginkgo biloba for prevention of dementia: a randomized controlled trial. JAMA 2008;300:2253–2262.

38. Shan RC. Medical foods for Alzheimer's disease. Drugs Aging 2011;28:421–428.

39. Accera. Axona (caprylidene) [product information]. Bloomfield, CO: Author, 2011.

40. Cummings J. Drug therapy: Alzheimer's disease. N Engl J Med 2004;351:56–67.

41. Schneider LS, Dagerman K, Insel PS. Efficacy and adverse effects of atypical antipsychotics for dementia. Meta-analysis of randomized, placebo-controlled trials. Am J Geriatr Psychiatry 2006;14:191–210.

42. Schneider LS, Tariot PN, Dagerman KS, et al. Effectiveness of atypical antipsychotic drugs in patients with Alzheimer's disease. N Engl J Med 2006;355:1525–1538.

43. Banerjee S, Hellier J, Dewey M, et al. Sertraline or mirtazapine for depression in dementia (HTA-SADD): a randomized, multicentre, double-blind, placebo-controlled trial. Lancet 2011;378:403–411.

44. Allain H, Bentue-Ferrer D, Polard E, et al. Postural instability and consequent falls and hip fractures associated with use of hypnotics in the elderly: a comparative review. Drugs Aging 2005;22:749–765.

45. Passmore MJ, Gardner DM, Polak Y, et al. Alternatives to atypical antipsychotics for the management of dementia-related agitation. Drugs Aging 2008;25:381–398.

46. Sakuye KM, Camp CJ, Ford PA. Effects of buspirone on agitation associated with dementia. Am J Geriatr Psychol 1993;1:82–84.

47. Hermann N, Eryavec G. Buspirone in the management of agitation and aggression associated with dementia. Am J Geriatr Psychol 1993;1:249–253.

48. Tariot PN, Cohen RM, Sunderland T, et al. L-deprenyl in Alzheimer's disease. Arch Gen Psychol 1987;44:427–433.

49. Schneider LS, Pollock VE, Zemansky MF, et al. A pilot study of low dose L-deprenyl in Alzheimer's disease. J Geriatr Psychol Neurol 1991;4:143–148.

50. Slattum PW, Swerdlow PH, Massey-Hill A. Alzheimer's disease. In: Dipiro JT, Talbert RL, Yee GC, et al, eds. Pharmacotherapy: A Pathophysiologic Approach. 8th ed. New York, NY: McGraw-Hill; 2011:947–961.

51. Cacabelos R. Pharmacogenomics and therapeutic prospects in dementia. Eur Arch Psychiatry Clin Neurosci 2008;258:28–47.

52. Alzheimer's Association. If you have Alzheimer's disease [Internet], [cited 2011 Oct 10]. Available from: *www.alz.org/national/documents/brochure_ifyouhave_earlystage.pdf.*

30 Multiple Sclerosis

Melody Ryan

LEARNING OBJECTIVES

● **Upon completion of the chapter, the reader will be able to:**

1. Identify risk factors for multiple sclerosis (MS).

2. Describe pathophysiologic findings of MS.

3. Distinguish between the forms of MS based on patient presentation and course of disease.

4. Compare and contrast MS disease-modifying treatment choices for a specific patient.

5. Determine appropriate symptomatic treatment choices and develop a detailed therapeutic plan for a specific patient.

6. Develop a monitoring plan for a patient placed on specific medications.

KEY CONCEPTS

❶ Multiple sclerosis (MS) symptoms depend on the location of lesions within the central nervous system (CNS).

❷ MS has four clinical patterns: relapsing remitting, secondary progressive, primary progressive, and progressive relapsing.

❸ The McDonald criteria, using clinical examination in combination with magnetic resonance imaging (MRI) data, facilitates earlier diagnosis and thus earlier treatment initiation.

❹ Acute relapses are treated with corticosteroids to speed recovery.

❺ Disease-modifying therapies decrease the number of relapses, prevent permanent neurologic damage, and prevent disability.

❻ Symptomatic treatment minimizes the impact of MS on quality of life.

❼ Dose–response curves have been observed with the β-interferons.

❽ There is no consensus on the best medication for initial therapy.

❾ Mitoxantrone and natalizumab should be reserved for patients with rapidly advancing disease who have failed other therapies.

❿ MS patients must be treated with agents specific for upper motor neuron **spasticity**.

M ultiple sclerosis (MS) is an inflammatory disease of the CNS, variable in symptoms and presentation. *Multiple* describes the number of CNS lesions, and *sclerosis* refers to the demyelinated lesions, today called plaques.

EPIDEMIOLOGY AND ETIOLOGY

Epidemiology

● Approximately 400,000 Americans have MS.[1] Diagnosis usually occurs between the ages of 20 and 50. Twice as many women as men develop MS.[1] Whites and people of northern European heritage are more likely to have MS.[2] Risk factors for MS include family history of MS, autoimmune diseases, or migraine; personal history of autoimmune diseases or migraine; and, in women, smoking and exposure to second-hand smoke. Prevalence decreases with decrease in latitude.[2]

Etiology

▶ *Inheritance Theory*

MS probably has a genetic component, likely carried in the human leukocyte antigen chromosomal region. Family members of MS patients have a 5% risk; monozygotic twins have a concordance rate of 25% to 30%.[2] A straightforward inheritance pattern cannot fully explain the etiology of MS because only a small proportion of patients report a family member with MS.

▶ *Environment Theory*

Currently, human herpes virus 6, herpes zoster virus, or Epstein-Barr virus are thought to be possible infectious etiologic agents.[3] Infection with these viruses cannot fully explain MS because there is a high rate of seropositivity in the population, but MS is much less common. Another theory involves decreased sunlight exposure. Lower serum concentrations of 25-hydroxyvitamin D are associated with higher rates of MS diagnosis.[2]

PATHOPHYSIOLOGY

While the causative agent of MS is unclear, the result is the development of an autoimmune disorder with areas of CNS inflammation and degeneration.

Inflammation

An unknown antigen presented by the major histocompatibility complex (MHC) class II molecules causes T cells to become autoreactive (Fig. 30–1). Autoreactive T cells enter lymphatic tissues to expand. Upon a signal involving sphingosine-1-phosphate, T cells reenter the circulation.[4] Once activated, T cells penetrate the blood–brain barrier by attachment to upregulated adhesion molecules and production of matrix metalloproteinases (MMP) that cause blood–brain barrier breakdown. In the CNS, T cells come into contact with antigen-presenting cells (APCs) and proliferate. The T-helper cells differentiate into proinflammatory T-helper-1 cells (Th1 cells) and anti-inflammatory T-helper-2 cells (Th2 cells).[4] Th1 cells secrete cytokines that enhance macrophage and microglial cells that attack myelin.[4]

B cells cross previously damaged sections of the blood–brain barrier to arrive in the CNS, an area normally free of B cells. Autoreactive T cells trigger B cells to form myelin autoantibodies. B-cell antibodies also initiate the complement cascade, causing myelin degradation.[4] These inflammatory processes probably cause relapses.[4] All current MS therapies are targeted toward preventing or slowing the inflammatory processes.

Degeneration

Axonal injury and transection disrupts nerve signals completely. Growing evidence suggests cytotoxic T cells cause axonal injury as early as 2 weeks after diagnosis and throughout the disease.[4] Axonal loss is likely responsible for MS progression.[4]

CLINICAL PRESENTATION, CLINICAL COURSE, AND DIAGNOSIS

Clinical Course

② *MS has four clinical patterns: relapsing remitting, secondary progressive, primary progressive, and progressive relapsing* (Fig. 30–2). Relapsing remitting MS develops into secondary

Table 30–1
Clinical Rating Scales Used in MS
EDSS
Rates functional systems from 0 (normal) to 10 (death due to MS) Emphasis is on ambulation over other symptoms
MSFC
Three-part tool rating ambulation, limb function, and cognitive function Composite score is compared with standardized population Correlates better with MRI data than EDSS

MS, multiple sclerosis; EDSS, Expanded Disability Status Scale; MSFC, multiple sclerosis functional composite.

From Refs. 12 and 13.

progressive MS in 50% of patients within 10 years and in 75% within 25 years of diagnosis.[1] Rating scales are used clinically (Table 30–1). MS reduces overall life expectancy by 10 years.[14] Suicide is disproportionately high in MS patients, causing 15% of MS-related deaths.[15]

Diagnosis

MS diagnostic criteria were revised in 2010 (Fig. 30–3).[16] Diagnosis of relapsing remitting MS requires plaque dissemination in time and space. Previously, diagnosis relied on clinical examination. **③** *The McDonald criteria, which uses the clinical examination in combination with magnetic resonance imaging (MRI) data, facilitates earlier diagnosis and thus earlier treatment initiation.* Primary progressive MS diagnosis requires 1 year of disease progression and two of the following: evidence for dissemination in space on MRI of the brain, evidence for dissemination in space on MRI in the spinal cord based on two or more T2-weighted lesions, and positive cerebrospinal fluid (CSF) (oligoclonal immunoglobulin G bands or elevated immunoglobulin G index).[16]

TREATMENT

Desired Outcomes and General Approach to Treatment

The goal of treatment is preventing permanent neurologic damage. There are three general approaches to treatment. **④** *First, acute relapses are treated with corticosteroids to speed recovery.* **⑤** *Second, disease-modifying therapies decrease the number of relapses, prevent permanent neurologic damage, and prevent disability.* **⑥** *Third, symptomatic treatments minimize the impact of MS on quality of life.*

Pharmacologic Treatment

▶ *Treatment of Acute Relapses*

The mechanism of action of corticosteroids is unclear but may involve:

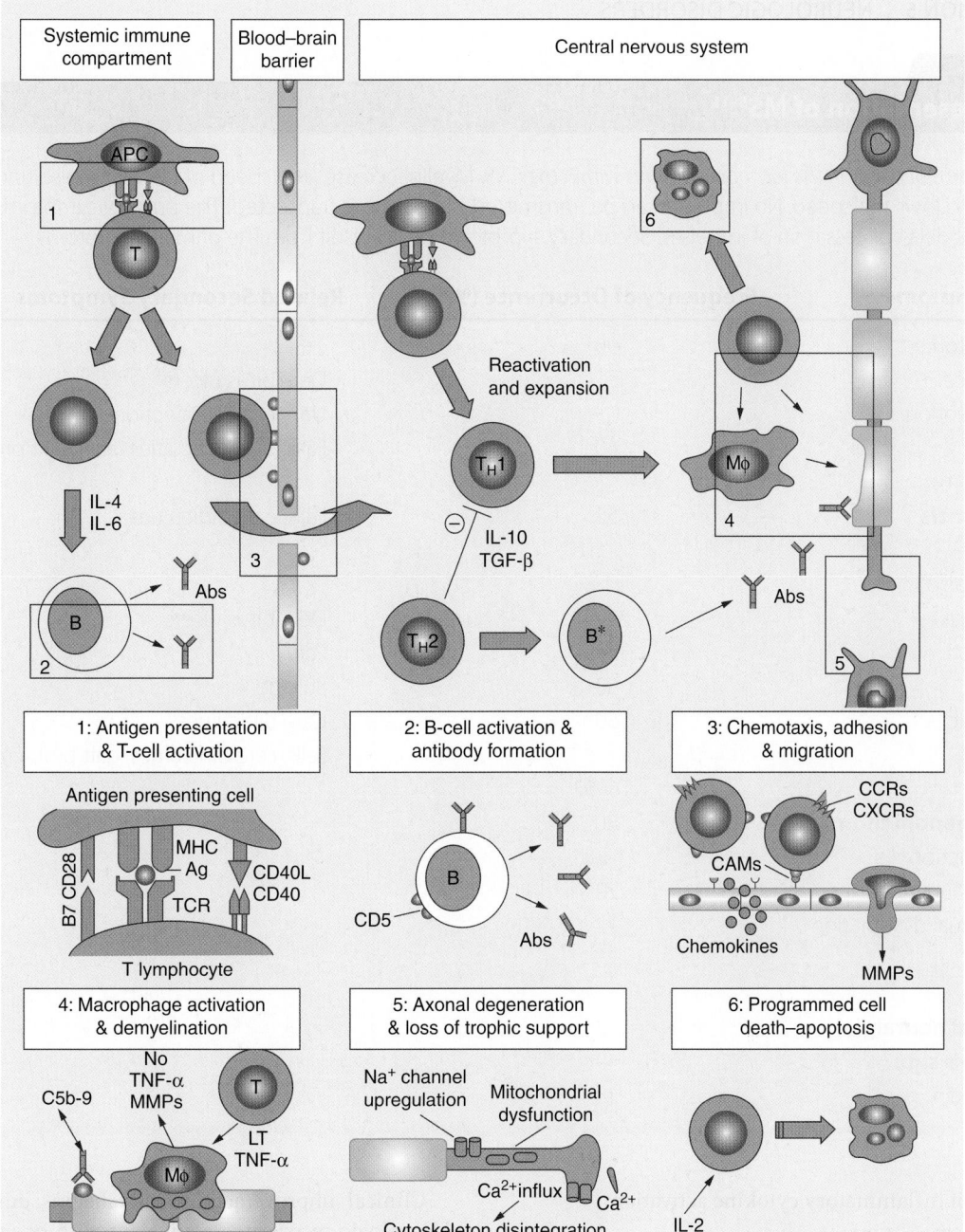

FIGURE 30–1. Autoimmune theory of the pathogenesis of multiple sclerosis (MS). In MS, the immunogenic cells tend to be more myelin-reactive, and these T-cells produce cytokines mimicking a Th1-mediated proinflammatory reaction. T-helper cells (CD4+) appear to be key initiators of myelin destruction in MS. These autoreactive CD4+ cells, especially of the T-helper cells type 1 (Th1) subtype, are active in the periphery, perhaps following a viral infection, and express adhesion molecules on their surfaces that allow them to attach and roll along the endothelial cells that constitute the blood–brain barrier. For this reaction to occur, costimulation and MHC along with an antigen on an APC (macrophage, dendrite cell, B cell) must be present. The activated T cells also produce MMP that help to create openings in the blood–brain barrier, allowing entry of the activated T cells past the blood–brain barrier and into the CNS. Once inside the CNS, the T cells produce proinflammatory cytokines, especially interleukins (ILs) 1, 2, 12, 17, and 23, tumor necrosis factor (TNF)-α, and interferon (INF)-γ, which further create openings in the blood–brain barrier, allowing entry of B cells, complement, macrophages, and antibodies. The T cells also interact within the CNS with the resident microglia, astrocytes, and macrophages, further enhancing production of proinflammatory cytokines and other potential mediators of CNS damage, including reactive oxygen intermediates and nitric oxide. The role of modulating, or downregulating, cytokines such as IL-4, IL-5, IL-10, and transforming growth factor (TGF)-β also has been described. These cytokines are the products of CD4+, CD8+, and Th1 cells. New pathogenic mechanisms involve, but are not limited to, receptor-ligand–mediated T-cell entry via choroid plexus (CCR6-CCL20 axis), coupling of key receptor-ligands for inhibition of myelination/demyelination (LINGO-1/NOGO66/p75, or TROY complex, Jagged-Notch signaling). (AG, antigens; APC, antigen-presenting cell; DC, dendrite cell; IgG, immunoglobulin G; Mφ, macrophage; NA+, sodium ion; MMP, matrix metalloproteinases; MHC, major histocompatibility complex; OPC, oligodendrocyte precursor cell; VLA, very late antigen; VCAM, vascular cell adhesion molecule.) (From Bainbridge JL, Corboy JR. Multiple sclerosis. In: DiPiro JT, Talbert RL, Yee GC, et al, eds. Pharmacotherapy: A Pathophysiologic Approach. 8th ed. New York, NY: McGraw-Hill; 2011:963–978.)

Clinical Presentation of MS[5-11]

❶ *MS symptoms depend on the location of lesions within the CNS.* Myelin increases the speed of nerve impulse transmission; demyelination slows the speed. No impulses can be transmitted if the axon is transected. The primary symptoms of MS are caused by this delay or cessation of impulses. Secondary symptoms of MS result from the primary symptoms.

Primary Symptoms	Frequency of Occurrence (%)	Related Secondary Symptoms
Urinary symptoms	90	
Incontinence		Decubitus ulcers
Urinary retention		Urinary tract infections
Spasticity	60	Falls, care difficulties, pain, gait problems
Visual symptoms		
Optic neuritis	55	Falls, care difficulties
Diplopia		
Bowel symptoms		
Incontinence	29–51	Decubitus ulcers
Constipation	35–54	Pain
Depression	50	Suicide
Cognitive deficits	50	Care difficulties
Weakness		Falls, care difficulties, gait problems
Fatigue	76–92	
Uhthoff's phenomenon	80	
Sexual dysfunction		
Erectile dysfunction	70	
Female sexual dysfunction	72	
Tremor	25	
Pain		
Trigeminal neuralgia	2	
Lhermitte's sign	9	
Dysesthetic pain	18	

- Prevention of inflammatory cytokine activation
- Inhibition of T- and B-cell activation
- Prevention of immune cells from entering the CNS
- Increased regulatory T-cell activity that controls autoimmune T-cell formation[17,18]

IV adrenocorticotropic hormone, IV methylprednisolone, or oral prednisone hasten functional recovery.[19] Traditionally, IV methylprednisolone was used because an optic neuritis study demonstrated reduced recurrence with IV methylprednisolone but not oral prednisone.[20] More recent studies show equal efficacy of equivalent doses of IV and oral dosage forms, and oral dosing avoids discomfort, inconvenience, and expense of IV therapy.[21]

Adverse Effects The most common adverse effects are GI upset, insomnia, and mood swings.[22]

Dosing and Administration Methylprednisolone is given 1 g/day IV as one dose or in divided doses for 3 to 5 days. Oral prednisone 1,250 mg/day given every other day for five doses provides an equivalent dose.

Clinical improvement usually begins during treatment. Neurologic recovery is equivalent with or without a subsequent oral prednisone taper.[23]

▶ *Outcome Evaluation*

- Monitor for symptom improvement
- Educate regarding adverse effects

Disease-Modifying Therapies

Seven agents are indicated for MS: subcutaneous interferon β-1a (Rebif); intramuscular interferon β-1a (Avonex); interferon β-1b (Betaseron, Extavia); glatiramer acetate (Copaxone); mitoxantrone (Novantrone); natalizumab (Tysabri); and fingolimod (Gilenya). Generally, these immunomodulators reduce annualized relapse rates 30% to 70%.[24-26]

▶ *β-Interferons*

Pharmacology and Mechanism of Action The mechanism of action of β-interferons is unknown. The following properties are thought to be important:

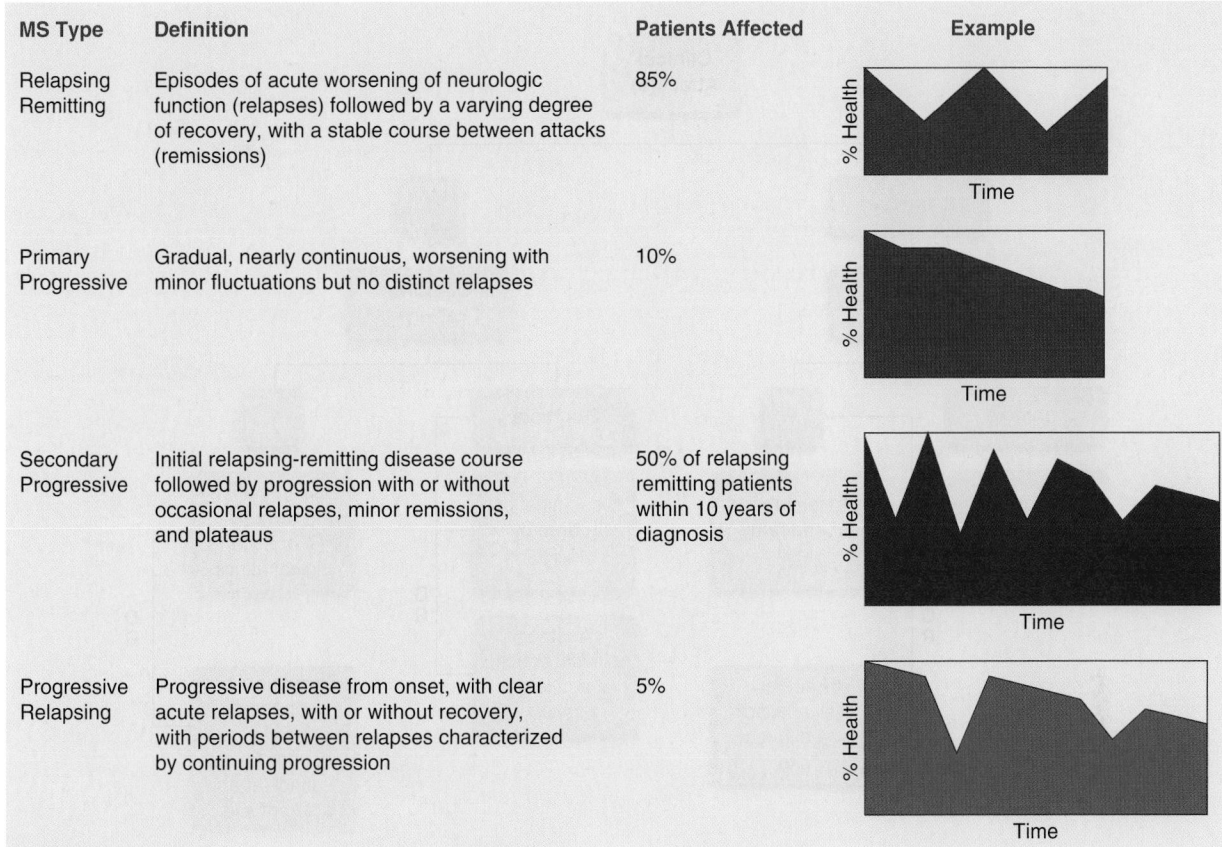

MS Type	Definition	Patients Affected	Example
Relapsing Remitting	Episodes of acute worsening of neurologic function (relapses) followed by a varying degree of recovery, with a stable course between attacks (remissions)	85%	
Primary Progressive	Gradual, nearly continuous, worsening with minor fluctuations but no distinct relapses	10%	
Secondary Progressive	Initial relapsing-remitting disease course followed by progression with or without occasional relapses, minor remissions, and plateaus	50% of relapsing remitting patients within 10 years of diagnosis	
Progressive Relapsing	Progressive disease from onset, with clear acute relapses, with or without recovery, with periods between relapses characterized by continuing progression	5%	

FIGURE 30–2. Comparison of clinical course of MS by type.

Patient Encounter, Part 1

SN is a 30-year-old white woman who visits the emergency department today with complaints of weakness and tingling in her right arm that developed over several hours. She has never experienced symptoms like this previously. She has been generally healthy but has experienced occasional migraine headaches since puberty. She has recently moved to your area to work at the university. Before that, she lived in Minnesota her entire life.

What information is suggestive of multiple sclerosis (MS)?

What risk factors does she have for MS?

What additional information or testing would assist in making the diagnosis of MS?

What treatment could be provided to SN for the current acute event?

- Decrease in T-cell activation, decreasing cytokine secretion, and preserving myelin
- Prevention of upregulation of adhesion molecules on activated T cells, limiting the number of T cells that can get into the brain

- Suppression of MMPs, maintaining the integrity of the blood–brain barrier
- Decrease in microglial proliferation, preserving myelin
- Promotion of formation of Th2 cells rather than Th1 cells, decreasing inflammation
- Inhibition of viruses, important if MS has a viral etiology[27]

▶ *Efficacy*

Patients with Relapsing Remitting MS β-Interferons reduce relapses by about one-third, compared with placebo.[28] Early treatment after a first clinical attack delayed time to a second attack by 9 to 13 months compared with placebo[29,30] and was associated with a lower incidence of developing clinically definite MS compared with delaying treatment.[31,32]

Patients with Secondary Progressive MS Who Experience Relapses β-Interferons have mixed results for slowing disease progression in secondary progressive MS. Treatment is most likely to be effective if clinical relapses or MRI signs of inflammatory activity are present.[33]

Adverse Effects Adverse effects are common with β-interferons (Table 30–2). Flu-like symptoms include fever, fatigue, muscle aches, malaise, and chills. Symptoms begin a few hours postinjection and dissipate within 8 to 24 hours.[34] Injection site reactions range from redness to necrosis. There

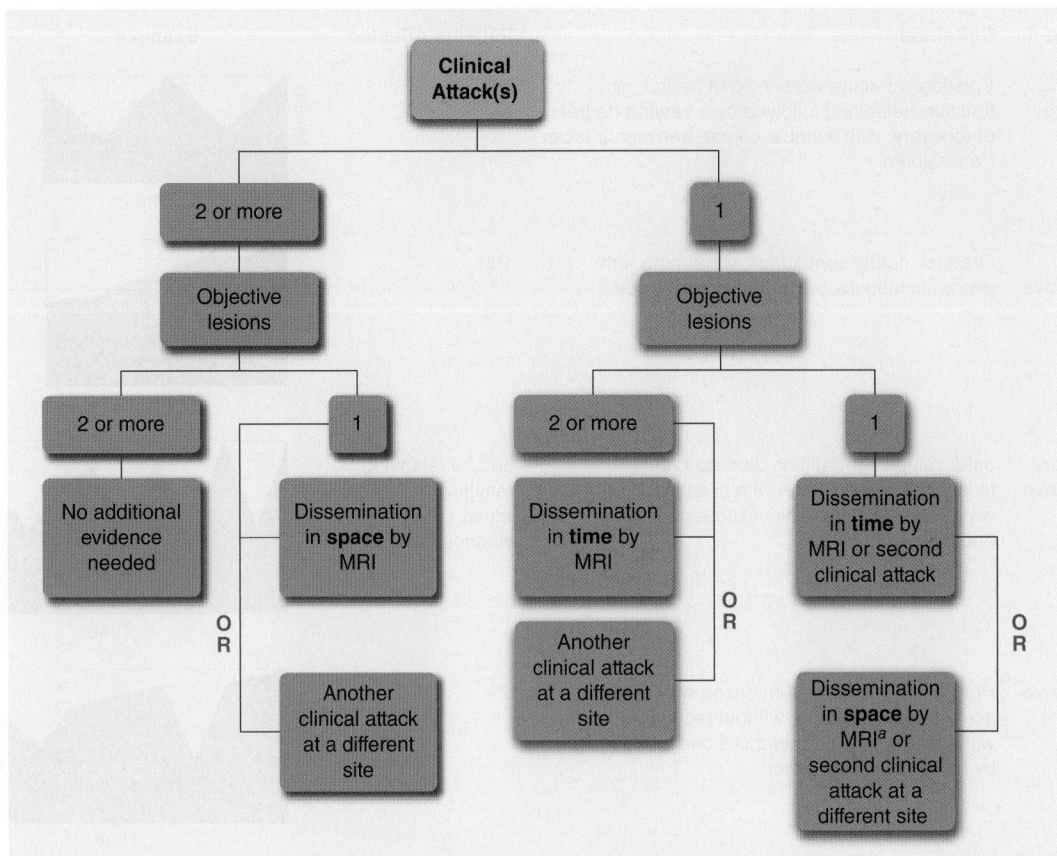

FIGURE 30–3. McDonald diagnostic criteria for MS.[16] An attack is defined as a patient-reported or objectively observed event typical of an acute inflammatory demyelinating event in the CNS with a duration of at least 24 hours in the absence of fever or infection. Magnetic resonance imaging (MRI) evidence of dissemination over time is a new T2-weighted lesion after the initial clinical event or the simultaneous presence of asymptomatic gadolinium-enhancing and nonenhancing lesions at any time.

[a]Dissemination in space by MRI evidence of one or more T2-weighted lesions in at least two of the following areas: periventricular, juxtacortical, infratentorial, spinal cord.

are preventive and treatment measures for these reactions (Table 30–3). Periodic laboratory monitoring for adverse effects is recommended (Table 30–4). At the threshold laboratory values (Table 30–3), interferon should be suspended. When values normalize, interferon may be resumed with gradual dose increases and careful monitoring.[34] The α- and γ-interferons are associated with depression. Up to 50% of MS patients experience depression, even without β-interferon treatment.[9] Because of conflicting data, it is difficult to determine the role of β-interferons in depression.[9]

Tests for Responsiveness Antibodies to β-interferons can reduce clinical benefit.[37] **Neutralizing antibodies** develop 18 to 24 months after initiation. Neutralizing antibodies can form against any β-interferon and are cross-reactive, but frequency and route of administration affect development: 28% to 47% for subcutaneous interferon β-1b; 12% to 28% for subcutaneous interferon β-1a; and 2% to 6% for intramuscular interferon β-1a.[37]

Issues surround neutralizing antibodies: standardization of the assay, testing recommendations, and treatment recommendations for positive tests.[37] Neutralizing antibodies may disappear even during continued treatment.[37]

β-interferons induce the expression of interferon-responsive genes such as myxovirus-resistance-protein A (MxA). Lack of expression to MxA testing is associated with MS relapses.[38]

Dosing and Administration Dose, frequency, and route of administration differ among the β-interferon products (Table 30–2). ❼ *Dose–response curves have been observed with the β-interferons.* However, it is unknown if the total weekly dose or the frequency of administration is more important.[33]

▶ **Glatiramer Acetate**

Pharmacology and Mechanism of Action The mechanism of action of glatiramer acetate is unknown; the following properties have been observed:

- Binds to MHC class II, blocking the activation of T cells
- Activates Th2 cells, preventing inflammation
- Activated Th2 cells secrete brain-derived neurotrophic factor, which may be neuroprotective.[27]

Efficacy Glatiramer acetate reduces relapses by 28% each year compared with placebo. Additionally, relapses occur later compared with placebo (322 versus 219 days).[39]

Table 30–2				
Comparison of Disease-Modifying Therapies				
Drug	**Dose**	**Route**	**Frequency**	**Selected Adverse Effects**
Interferon β-1a (Avonex)	30 mcg	IM	Weekly	Flu-like symptoms 61% Anemia 8%
Interferon β-1a (Rebif)	44 mcg	SQ	3 × per week	Flu-like symptoms 28% Injection site reactions 66% Leukopenia 22% Increased aspartate aminotransferase/alanine transaminase 17–27%
Interferon β-1b (Betaseron, Extavia)	0.25 mg	SQ	Every other day	Flu-like symptoms 60–76% Injection site reactions 50–85% Asthenia 49% Menstrual disorder 17% Leukopenia 10–16% Increased aspartate aminotransferase/alanine transaminase 4–19%
Glatiramer acetate (Copaxone)	20 mg	SQ	Daily	Injection site reaction 90% Systemic reaction 15%
Mitoxantrone (Novantrone)	12 mg/m² up to 140 mg/m² (maximum lifetime dose)	IV	Every 3 months	Nausea 76% Arrhythmia 3–18% Cardiotoxicity Alopecia 61% Menstrual disorders 61% Urinary tract infection 32% Amenorrhea 25% Leukopenia 19% γ-Glutamyl transpeptidase increase 15%
Natalizumab (Tysabri)	300 mg	IV	Every 4 weeks	Headache 38% Fatigue 27% Arthralgia 19% Urinary tract infection 20% Hypersensitivity reaction less than 1% Progressive multifocal leukoencephalopathy 0.13%
Fingolimod (Gilenya)	0.5 mg	PO	Daily	Headache 25% Increased aspartate aminotransferase/alanine transaminase 14% Influenza viral infections 13% Diarrhea 12% Cough 10% Bradycardia 4% Lymphopenia 4%

From Refs. 19, 25, 26, 34, 35, 36.

Adverse Effects Patients report injection site reactions (Table 30–2). Icing the injection site pre- and postinjection and/or topical anesthetics improve these reactions. Systemic reactions involve flushing, chest tightness, palpitations, anxiety, and shortness of breath. This reaction usually occurs within 30 minutes of the injection; recurrence is infrequent. Doses may be reduced by 75% for the week following the reaction, then increased by 25% per week to the full dose.[35]

▶ Issues with Self-Injected Disease-Modifying Therapies

Adherence Adherence to injectable medications is a significant problem, with no significant difference in discontinuation rates between products (17%–41%). Reasons for discontinuation are adverse effects and lack of efficacy. Realistic therapy expectations, higher educational levels, and higher self-efficacy improve adherence rates; depression and cognitive problems lower adherence.[40,41]

● **Choosing Therapy** ⑧ *There is no consensus on the best medication for initial therapy.* Comparative β-interferon trials indicate better efficacy with more frequent and/or higher dosing.[33] This consideration must be balanced with neutralizing antibody development, patient acceptance, and tolerance. Head-to-head trials between β-interferons and glatiramer acetate demonstrated similar efficacy and tolerability.[42,43]

Patient Education Refer to Table 30–5 for patient education for self-injection.

Table 30–3

Prevention or Treatment Strategies for β-Interferon Adverse Effects

Flu-Like Symptoms	Injection Site Reaction	Laboratory Abnormalities[a]
Inject dose in the evening	Bring medication to room temperature	Hemoglobin less than 9.4 g/dL (94 g/L or 5.8 mmol/L)
Begin at ¼–½ dose for 2 weeks of treatment; then increase to a full dose	Ice injection site before and after injection	White blood cells less than 3×10^3/mm^3 (less than 3×10^9/L)
Use ibuprofen 200 mg before and 6 and 12 hours after injection	Rotate injection sites	Absolute neutrophil count less than 1.5×10^3/mm^3 (less than 1.5×10^9/L)
Alternatives to ibuprofen include acetaminophen, prednisone taper, and pentoxifylline	Inject in areas with more subcutaneous fat (buttocks or abdomen)	Platelets less than 75×10^3/mm^3 (less than 75×10^9/L)
	Use an autoinjection device	Bilirubin more than 2.5 × baseline
	If severe, use hydrocortisone 1% cream on the site	AST/ALT more than 5 × baseline
	If necrotic: temporarily discontinue; consult dermatologist; do not use topical corticosteroids	Alkaline phosphatase more than 5 × baseline

ALT, alanine aminotransferase; AST, aspartate aminotransferase.

[a]At these threshold values, β-interferon should be temporarily discontinued and laboratory values monitored.

From Refs. 34 and 35.

Table 30–4

Monitoring Disease-Modifying Therapies

Therapy	Tests	Frequency
β-Interferons (Avonex, Betaseron, Rebif)	CBC, bilirubin, electrolytes, AST, ALT, γ-glutamyl transferase, alkaline phosphatase	Baseline, 1, 3, and 6 months; then every 3 months
	Thyroid function tests	Baseline and every 6 months in patients with a history of thyroid dysfunction
	EDSS, MSFC, neurologic history and examination	Every 3 months during the first year of therapy; then every 6 months
Glatiramer acetate (Copaxone)	EDSS, MSFC, neurologic history and examination	Every 3 months during the first year of therapy; then every 6 months
Mitoxantrone (Novantrone)	CBC, bilirubin, AST, ALT, alkaline phosphatase, pregnancy test	Before each infusion
	ECG	Baseline and prior to each infusion
	Echocardiogram or MUGA scan	Baseline; prior to each infusion, and yearly after stopping mitoxantrone
	EDSS, MSFC, neurologic history and examination	Every 3 months during the first year of therapy; then every 6 months
Natalizumab (Tysabri)	EDSS, MSFC, neurologic history and examination	Baseline; every 3 months during the first year of therapy; then every 6 months
	HIV, CBC, AST, ALT, MRI	Baseline; repeat MRI at 6 months; then yearly
	MRI, CSF examination for JC virus	At onset of new neurologic symptoms not suggestive of MS
	Preinfusion patient checklist	Prior to every infusion
	Status report and reauthorization questionnaire	Every 6 months
Fingolimod (Gilenya)	EDSS, MSFC, neurologic history and examination	Every 3 months during the first year of therapy; then every 6 months
	Varicella zoster immunity evaluation and/or vaccination and FEV$_1$ (full pulmonary function testing if patient has history of asthma or COPD)	Baseline
	CBC, ALT, AST	Baseline and every 6 months
	Pulse and blood pressure	Baseline; observe in clinical area for 6 hours after initial dose with periodic monitoring
	Ophthalmology evaluation	Baseline; 4 months; then as needed
	Dermatologic evaluation	Baseline; then as needed

ALT, alanine aminotransferase; AST, aspartate aminotransferase; CBC, complete blood count; COPD, chronic obstructive pulmonary disease; CSF, cerebrospinal fluid; EDSS, Expanded Disability Status Scale; FEV$_1$, forced expiratory volume in 1 second; HIV, human immunodeficiency virus; MRI, magnetic resonance imaging; MS, multiple sclerosis; MSFC, Multiple Sclerosis Functional Composite; MUGA, multiple-gated acquisition.

Table 30–5
Patient Education for Self-Injection

Keep all nonrefrigerated supplies together and out of the reach of children and pets
If refrigerated, allow medication to warm to room temperature
Wash hands thoroughly
Choose injection site, rotating among sites
Ice area to be injected for no more than 15 minutes, if desired
Clean injection site thoroughly with alcohol or soap and water
Administer injection
Ice injection site for no more than 15 minutes after injection, if desired

▶ Mitoxantrone

Pharmacology and Mechanism of Action Mitoxantrone is an anthracenedione antineoplastic indicated for MS. The mechanisms of action thought to be important for MS include:

- Causes apoptosis in T and APCs, preventing initial T-cell activation
- Inhibits DNA and RNA synthesis, decreasing proliferation of T cells, B cells, and macrophages
- Decreases cytokine release, preventing inflammation
- Inhibits macrophages, preventing myelin degradation[44]

Efficacy Mitoxantrone is indicated for secondary progressive MS, progressive relapsing MS, and for patients with worsening relapsing remitting MS. It reduces the relapse rate and attack-related MRI outcome measures. ❾ *Because of its potential for significant toxicities, mitoxantrone is reserved for patients with rapidly advancing disease who have failed other therapies.*[19]

Adverse Effects Adverse effects are seen regularly in patients given mitoxantrone (Table 30–2). Bluish discoloration of the sclera and the urine lasts 24 hours postinfusion.[36] Transient leukopenia and neutropenia are common.[49] Patients taking mitoxantrone should not receive live virus vaccines; other vaccines should be held for 4 to 6 weeks after a mitoxantrone dose.[36] Amenorrhea may be permanent.[36]

Cardiotoxicity is a serious adverse effect; reduction in left ventricular ejection fraction is not related to dose, sex, or age.[36,45] Mitoxantrone should not be used in patients with baseline cardiomyopathy, even if asymptomatic. Cyclooxygenase-2 inhibitors should be avoided in patients receiving mitoxantrone because of a potential for worsening cardiac toxicity.[36] The maximum lifetime dose of mitoxantrone is 140 mg/m^2.

Acute myelogenous leukemia occurred in 0.07% of mitoxantrone-treated patients, appearing within 2 to 4 years of initiating mitoxantrone and responsive to standard therapy.[36]

Dosing and Administration Mitoxantrone is infused intravenously over 30 minutes to reduce the chance of cardiotoxicity.[36] Mitoxantrone is administered every 3 months, if cardiac function and laboratory values are normal (Table 30–4).

▶ Natalizumab

Pharmacology and Mechanism of Action Natalizumab is a α_4-integrin antagonist indicated for relapsing forms of MS. Its postulated mechanism of action follows:

- Binds to $\alpha_4\beta_1$ and $\alpha_4\beta_7$ integrins, preventing lymphocytes migration into the CNS and inflammation
- Inhibits binding of α_4-positive leukocytes to fibronectin and osteopontin, decreasing the activation of leukocytes already within the CNS[26]

Efficacy Treatment with natalizumab reduced relapses by 68% at 1 year and disability by 42% at 2 years compared with placebo.[26]

Adverse Effects Adverse effects of natalizumab include infection, arthralgia, headache, and fatigue (Table 30–2).[26] Hypersensitivity reactions have been observed; symptoms may include itching, dizziness, fever, rash, hypotension, dyspnea, chest pain, and anaphylaxis, usually within 2 hours of administration. If these symptoms occur, natalizumab is discontinued. An infusion reaction consisting of headache, dizziness, fatigue, nausea, sweats, and rigors may occur within 2 hours of dosing.[46] Histamine 1 and 2 receptor blockers can be used to prevent these symptoms, and discontinuation is not required. A much more serious, but rare, adverse effect is progressive multifocal leukoencephalopathy (PML). PML, caused by the JC polyomavirus virus, is rapidly progressive and usually results in death or permanent disability. Due to this risk, natalizumab is distributed through a restricted program. ❾ These concerns lead to the recommendation that *natalizumab be reserved for patients with rapidly advancing disease who have failed other therapies.* Specific recommendations are to avoid in immunocompromised patients; carefully assess for immune compromise in patients previously treated with immunosuppression, radiation therapy, or chemotherapy; and to carefully monitor patients.[47] Between 2006 and 2010, 31 new cases of natalizumab PML were reported.[48] Risk of PML increases with increased infusions.[48] Vigilance is paramount because PML can mimic symptoms associated with MS.[49]

Antinatalizumab antibodies develop in 9% to 12% of patients. If patients are persistently antibody positive, relapse rates and disability increase; antibody development is also associated with hypersensitivity reactions.[50]

Dosing and Administration Natalizumab should be used as monotherapy.[47] Natalizumab is administered 300 mg in 100 mL normal saline over a 1-hour IV infusion every 4 weeks. Few patients have been treated for more than 3 years with natalizumab.

▶ Fingolimod

Pharmacology and Mechanism of Action Fingolimod, indicated for relapsing forms of MS, is a sphingosine 1-phosphate receptor modulator. It retains T cells in lymphoid tissues, thus depleting peripheral blood and CNS lymphocytes.[51]

Efficacy Treatment with fingolimod reduced the annualized relapse rate to 0.18 compared with 0.40 for placebo.[25]

Adverse Effects Fingolimod is generally well-tolerated (Table 30–2), but it has serious adverse effects. Fingolimod reduces circulating lymphocytes by about 75%; thus infections and malignancies are concerns.[25,52] Sphingosine 1-phosphate receptors elsewhere in the body are associated with first-dose bradycardia, macular edema, and reduced forced vital capacity.[53] With the exception of bradycardia, these effects persist for 2 months after medication discontinuation due to the long half-life of fingolimod.[54]

Dosing and Administration Fingolimod is given 0.5 mg orally once daily.

▶ Outcome Evaluation

- Assess periodically for symptom changes.
- In β-interferon-treated patients with frequent relapses, testing for neutralizing antibodies and/or MxA gene expression may assist in choosing therapy.
- Monitor for medication-specific adverse effects (Tables 30–2 and 30–4).
- Assess adherence with all components of therapy regularly.

▶ Symptomatic Therapies

The symptoms most unique to MS are fatigue, spasticity, impaired ambulation, and pseudobulbar affect. Other important symptoms such as urinary incontinence, pain, depression, cognitive impairment, and sexual dysfunction are discussed only briefly (refer to other chapters).

Fatigue There are nonpharmacologic and pharmacologic strategies for decreasing the impact of fatigue on the lifestyle of MS patients (Table 30–6). Pharmacologic management of fatigue includes amantadine or stimulants; however, evidence of efficacy from randomized controlled trials is limited.

Spasticity Spasticity treatment goals are patient specific. For ambulatory patients, reducing spasticity may improve mobility. For bed-bound patients, treating spasticity may relieve pain and facilitate care. Physical therapy is a nonpharmacologic treatment for spasticity.[5]

MS patients usually have upper motor neuron spasticity that cannot be treated with muscle relaxants (e.g., carisoprodol). ❿ *MS patients must be treated with agents specific for upper motor neuron spasticity (Table 30–7).*[5] MS spasticity is classified as focal or generalized. If the spasticity involves only one muscle group, it is focal and may benefit from botulinum toxin administration.[5] Systemic medications are used for generalized spasticity. No clear conclusion can be reached regarding the efficacy superiority of one agent; medication selection is based on adverse effects (see Table 30–7).[5]

Patient Encounter, Part 2

PMH: Migraine headaches

FH: No history of MS. Both parents and one sister alive and well.

SH: Faculty member in Psychology Department. Single. She does not smoke or use illicit drugs. She does have two to four drinks per week of alcohol.

Allergies: NKDA

Medications: Zolmitriptan 5 mg by mouth as needed for headache. May repeat once in 2 hours, if needed.

ROS: (–) N/V/D, HA, SOB, chest pain, cough

PE:

VS: 126/74, P 70, RR 18, T 38°C (100.4°F)

Skin: warm, dry

HEENT: NC/AT, PERRLA, TMs intact

CV: RRR, normal S_1 and S_2, no m/r/g

Chest: CTA

Abd: Soft, NT/ND

Neuro: A & O × 3; CN II-XII intact, end point nystagmus on lateral gaze bilaterally

Motor: mild weakness in right arm, poor finger-to-nose left upper extremity

LABS: WNL

Imaging: T-2 weighted MRI shows a gadolinium-enhancing T2-weighted lesion in the left corona radiate (periventricular region), five nonenhancing T2-weighted white matter lesions scattered near the cortex (juxtacortical region), and one nonenhancing T2-weighted lesion in the white matter tracts of the left medial cerebellum (infratentorial region).

Given this additional information, what is your assessment of SN's condition?

Identify your treatment goals for this patient.

What pharmacologic alternatives are available for SN?

What counseling points will you give SN for administration of your chosen therapy?

Impaired Ambulation Gait abnormalities decrease walking speed and endurance and lead to use of assistive devices. An extended-release form of dalfampridine is indicated for improvement in walking ability. This potassium channel blocker probably prolongs the action potential and improves conduction in demyelinated neurons.[58] Not all patients respond to therapy, but in responders, times to complete a 25-foot (7.6-m) timed walk decrease about 25%.[59] Urinary tract infections, insomnia, dizziness, headache, nausea, asthenia, back pain, and balance disorder all occur relatively frequently with extended-release dalfampridine.[58] Seizures are an uncommon adverse effect; patients with preexisting seizure disorders should not receive extended-release dalfampridine.[58]

Table 30–6

Pharmacologic and Nonpharmacologic Treatments for Fatigue

Nonpharmacologic	Pharmacologic	Renal Dosing
Appropriate rest-to-activity ratio Use of assistive devices to conserve energy	*First-line therapy:* Amantadine 100 mg orally every morning and early afternoon	CrCl 30–50 mL/min (0.50–0.84 mL/s): 100 mg/day CrCl 15–29 mL/min (0.25–0.49 mL/s): 100 mg every other day CrCl less than 15 mL/min (less than 0.25 mL/s): 200 mg every 7 days
Environmental modifications to make activities more energy efficient Cooling strategies to avoid fatigue caused by elevations in core body temperature due to heat, exercise-related exertion, and fever Regular aerobic exercise, geared to the person's ability, to promote cardiovascular health, strength, improved mood, and reduce fatigue Progressive resistance training of lower limb muscles Stress management techniques	*Second-line therapy:* Methylphenidate 10–20 mg every morning and noon	

CrCl, creatinine clearance.

From Refs. 6, 55, 56.

● **Pseudobulbar Affect** Ten percent of patients with MS develop pseudobulbar affect, characterized by inappropriate laughing or crying.[60] These outbursts can cause patients to become socially isolated. Dextromethorphan prevents the release of excitatory neurotransmitters. Low-dose quinidine blocks first-pass metabolism of dextromethorphan and increases serum concentrations. A 49% decrease in inappropriate emotional episodes was seen with treatment.[60]

● **Other Symptoms** Two types of urinary tract symptoms are commonly seen in MS: incomplete bladder emptying and incontinence. Dyscoordination of the external urethral sphincter and detrusor activity causes incomplete bladder emptying.[8] Most patients with this condition require urinary catheterization.[8] Incontinence is usually caused by neurogenic detrusor overactivity. First-line treatments are anticholinergics such as oxybutynin or tolterodine.

● Bowel symptoms in MS patients include fecal incontinence and constipation. Fecal incontinence is difficult to treat; a regular schedule for emptying the bowel with laxative suppositories or enemas may be helpful. Alternatively, antidiarrheal medications such as loperamide can be used.[8]

Table 30–7

Comparison of Antispasticity Agents

Place in Therapy	Medication	Mechanism of Action	Dose
First line	Baclofen	Pre- and postsynaptic γ-aminobutyric acid β-receptor blocker	5 mg orally 3 × daily; increase by 5 mg/dose every 3 days to a maximum of 80 mg/day *Renal dysfunction:* Dose reduction may be necessary
	Tizanidine	Centrally acting a_2-receptor agonist	4 mg orally daily; increase by 2–4 mg 3–4 × daily to a maximum of 36 mg/day *Hepatic and renal dysfunction:* Dose reduction may be necessary
Second line	Dantrolene	Direct inhibitor of muscle contraction by decreasing the release of calcium from skeletal muscle sarcoplasmic reticulum	25 mg orally daily; increase to 25 mg 3–4 × daily; then increase by 25 mg every 4–7 days to a maximum of 400 mg/day
	Diazepam	γ-Aminobutyric acid agonist	2–10 mg orally 3–4 × daily *Cirrhosis:* Reduce dose by 50%
Third-line	Intrathecal baclofen	Pre- and postsynaptic γ-aminobutyric acid β-receptor blocker	Titrated individually; usual range: 62–749 mcg/day
Focal spasticity	Botulinum toxin	Prevents release of acetylcholine in the neuromuscular junction	Individualized

Data from Refs. 5 and 57.

Patient Encounter, Part 3

SN begins therapy with interferon β-1b subcutaneously every other day. She does very well with no relapses and minimal adverse effects for 2 years. Then, within the course of 6 months, she experiences two relapses. Her MRI shows several new lesions, and her neurologist orders a neutralizing antibody titer. The laboratory reports the titer as "high" with 160 neutralizing units/mL. SN also complains of fatigue that worsens throughout the day to the point that she says she is unable to get off the couch in the evenings and frequently skips her evening meal.

How will you respond to the neutralizing antibody titer?

What nonpharmacologic and pharmacologic treatments can you recommend for SN's fatigue?

Pain occurs in up to 86% of patients. Pain may be neuropathic, related to spasticity, related to treatment, or unrelated to MS. Correct pain type classification is necessary for effective treatment.[9]

Desipramine and sertraline are efficacious for MS-related depression.[9] Discontinuation of β-interferon treatment may be considered.

Patient Care and Monitoring

1. Once diagnosed, work with the patient to select therapy, considering:
   - Route of administration
   - Frequency of administration
   - Adverse-effect profile and other concerns (e.g., neutralizing antibodies and concomitant depression)

2. Obtain the required baseline laboratory studies (Table 30–6).

3. Educate the patient regarding self-injection (Table 30–5).

4. Assess the patient for symptomatic treatment needs.

5. Initiate needed symptomatic treatments.

6. Refer the patient to the National MS Society for information, newsletters, and local support groups (www.nmss.org).

7. Instruct the patient to contact the clinician for any sudden symptom changes that suggest a relapse.

8. Monitor the patient for efficacy and adverse effects of disease-modifying and symptomatic therapies every 3 months for the first year and every 6 months thereafter and as required for selected therapy (Table 30–6).

9. Treat any relapses with methylprednisolone IV or prednisone orally.

Cognitive impairment and memory dysfunction can be troublesome, affecting 40% to 60% of patients. Treatment with β-interferon or acetylcholinesterase inhibitors has demonstrated improvement.[61]

Phosphodiesterase type 5 inhibitors are effective for MS-induced erectile dysfunction.[8] In women, vaginal dryness or dyspareunia may respond to lubricating jellies.

▶ *Outcome Evaluation*

- Assess for improvement/recurrence of symptoms.
- Monitor for adverse effects of medications.
- Monitor for adherence.

Abbreviations Introduced in This Chapter

Abs	Autoantibodies
ALT	Alanine aminotransferase
APC	Antigen-presenting cell
AST	Aspartate aminotransferase
CAM	Cellular adhesion molecule
CNS	Central nervous system
CSF	Cerebrospinal fluid
EDSS	Expanded Disability Status Scale
HHV-6	Human herpes virus 6
IL	Interleukin
LT	Lymphotoxin
MHC	Major histocompatibility complex
MMP	Matrix metalloproteinase
MS	Multiple sclerosis
MSFC	Multiple Sclerosis Functional Composite
MUGA	Multiple-gated acquisition
MxA	Myxovirus-resistance-protein A
NO	Nitric oxide
PML	Progressive multifocal leukoencephalopathy
TCR	T-cell receptor
TGF	Transforming growth factor
Th1	T-helper-1 cells
Th2	T-helper-2 cells
TNF	Tumor necrosis factor

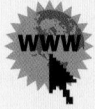 Self-assessment questions and answers are available at *http://www.mhpharmacotherapy.com/pp.html.*

REFERENCES

1. National Multiple Sclerosis Society. Multiple sclerosis: just the facts [Internet]: 2011 [cited August 10, 2011]. Available from: *http://www.nationalmssociety.org/about-multiple-sclerosis/index.aspx.*

2. Ramagopalan SV, Dobson R, Meier UC, Giovannoni G. Multiple sclerosis: risk factors, prodromes, and potential causal pathways. Lancet Neurol 2010;9:727–739.

3. Kang JH, Sheu JJ, Kao S, Lin HC. Increased risk of multiple sclerosis following herpes zoster: A nationwide, population-based study. J Infect Dis 2011;402:188–192.

4. Aktas O, Kieseier B, Hartung HP. Neuroprotection, regeneration and immunomodulation: Broadening the therapeutic repertoire in multiple sclerosis. Trends Neurosci 2010;33:140–152.

5. Hasselkorn JK, Balsdon RC, Fry WD, et al. Overview of spasticity management in multiple sclerosis. Evidence-based management strategies for spasticity treatment in multiple sclerosis. J Spinal Cord Med 2005;28:167–199.

6. Lapierre Y, Hum S. Treating fatigue. Int MS J 2007;14:64–71.

7. Andersson KE, Pehrson R. CNS involvement in overactive bladder: Pathophysiology and opportunities for pharmacological intervention. Drugs 2003;63: 2595–2611.

8. DasGupta R, Fowler CJ. Bladder, bowel and sexual dysfunction in multiple sclerosis: Management strategies. Drugs 2003;63:153–166.

9. Goldman Consensus Group. The Goldman Consensus statement on depression in multiple sclerosis. Mult Scler 2005;11:328–337.

10. Pittock SJ, McClelland BL, Mayr WT, et al. Prevalence of tremor in multiple sclerosis and associated disability in the Olmsted County population. Mov Disord 2004;19:1482–1485.

11. Pollmann W, Feneberg W. Current management of pain associated with multiple sclerosis. CNS Drugs 2008; 22:291–324.

12. Rudick RA, Cutter G, Reingold S. The Multiple Sclerosis Functional Composite: A new clinical outcome measure for multiple sclerosis trials. Mult Scler 2002;8:359–365.

13. Kurtzke JF. Rating neurologic impairment in multiple sclerosis: An expanded disability status scale (EDSS). Neurology 1983;33:1444–1452.

14. Bronnum-Hansen H, Koch-Henriksen N, Stenager E. Trend in survival and cause of death in Danish patients with multiple sclerosis. Brain 2004;127:844–850.

15. Sadovnick AD, Eisen K, Ebers GC, Paty DW. Cause of death in patients attending multiple sclerosis clinics. Neurology 1991;41:1193–1196.

16. Polman CH, Reingold SC, Banwell B, et al. Diagnostic criteria for multiple sclerosis: 2010 revisions to the McDonald criteria. Ann Neurol 2011;69:292–302.

17. Sloka JS, Stefanelli M. The mechanism of action of methylprednisolone in the treatment of multiple sclerosis. Mult Scler 2005;11:425–432.

18. Xu L, Xu Z, Xu M. Glucocorticoid treatment restores the impaired suppressive function of regulatory T cells in patients with relapsing-remitting multiple sclerosis. Clin Exper Immunol 2009;158:26–30.

19. Goodin DS, Frohman EM, Garmany GP, et al. Disease modifying therapies in multiple sclerosis: Report of the Therapeutics and Technology Assessment Subcommittee of the American Academy of Neurology and the MS Council for Clinical Practice Guidelines. Neurology 2002;58:169–178.

20. Beck RW, Cleary PA, Anderson MM, et al. A randomized, controlled trial of corticosteroids in the treatment of acute optic neuritis. The Optic Neuritis Study Group. N Engl J Med 1992;326:581–588.

21. Burton JM, O'Connor PW, Hohol M, Beyene J. Oral versus intravenous steroids for treatment of relapses in multiple sclerosis. Cochrane Database of Syst Rev 2009:CD006921.

22. Filippini G, Brusaferri F, Sibley WA, et al. Corticosteroids or ACTH for acute exacerbations in multiple sclerosis (review). *Cochrane Database Syst Rev* 2004:D001331.

23. Perumal JS, Caon C, Hreha S, et al. Oral prednisone taper following intravenous steroids fails to improve disability or recovery from relapses in multiple sclerosis. Eur J Neurol 2008;15:677–680.

24. Medical Advisory Board of the National Multiple Sclerosis Society, Changing Therapy Consensus Statement Taskforce. Changing therapy in relapsing multiple sclerosis: Considerations and recommendations of a task force of the National Multiple Sclerosis Society [Internet] [cited August 12, 2011]. Available from: *http://www.nationalmssociety.org/for-professionals/healthcare-professionals/publications/expert-opinion-papers/index.aspx.*

25. Kappos L, Radue EW, O'Connor P, et al. A placebo-controlled trial of oral fingolimod in relapsing multiple sclerosis. N Engl J Med 2010;362: 387–401.

26. Polman CH, O'Connor PW, Havrdova E, et al. A randomized, placebo-controlled trial of natalizumab for relapsing multiple sclerosis. N Engl J Med 2006;354; 899–910.

27. Graber JJ, McGraw CA, Kimbrough D, Dhib-Jalbut S. Overlapping and distinct *mechanisms of action of multiple sclerosis therapies.* Clin Neurol Neurosurg 2010;112:583–591.

28. Rudick RA, Goelz SE. Beta-interferon for multiple sclerosis. Exp Cell Res 2011;317:1301–1311.

29. Jacobs LD, Beck RW, Simon JH, et al. Intramuscular interferon beta-1a therapy initiated during a first demyelinating event in multiple sclerosis. N Engl J Med 2000;343:898–904.

30. Comi G, Filippi M, Barkhof F, et al. Effect of early interferon treatment on conversion to definite multiple sclerosis: A randomized study. Lancet 2001;357:1576–1582.

31. CHAMPIONS Study Group. IM interferon β-1a delays definite multiple sclerosis 5 years after a first demyelinating event. Neurology 2006;66:678–684.

32. Kappos L, Freedman MS, Polman CH, et al. Effect of early versus delayed interferon beta-1b treatment on disability after a first clinical event suggestive of multiple sclerosis: A 3-year follow-up analysis of the BENEFIT study. Lancet 2007;370:389–397.

33. Multiple Sclerosis Therapy Consensus Group. Escalating immunotherapy of multiple sclerosis: New aspects and practical application. J Neurol 2004;251:1329–1339.

34. Moses H, Brandes DW. Managing adverse effects of disease-modifying agents used for treatment of multiple sclerosis. Curr Med Res Opin 2008;24:2679–2690.

35. Galetta SL, Markowitz C. U.S. FDA-approved disease-modifying treatments for multiple sclerosis: Review of adverse effect profiles. CNS Drugs 2005;29:239–252.

36. Cohen BA, Mikol DD. Mitoxantrone treatment of multiple sclerosis: Safety considerations. Neurology 2004;63:S28–S32.

37. Polman CH, Bertolotto A, Deisenhammer F, et al. Recommendations for clinical use of data on neutralizing antibodies to interferon-beta therapy in multiple sclerosis. Lancet Neurol 2010;9:740–750.

38. Malucchi S, Gilli F, Caldano M, et al. Predictive markers for response to interferon therapy in patients with multiple sclerosis. Neurology 2008;70:1119–1127.

39. Boneschi FM, Rovaris M, Johnson KP, et al. Effects of glatiramer acetate on relapse rate and accumulated disability in multiple sclerosis: Meta-analysis of three double-blind, randomized, placebo-controlled clinical trials. Mult Scler 2003;9:349–355.

40. Daugherty KK, Butler JS, Mattingly M, Ryan M. Factors leading patients to discontinue multiple sclerosis therapies. J Am Pharm Assoc 2005;45:371–375.

41. Caon C, Saunders C, Smrtka J, et al. Injectable disease-modifying therapy for relapsing-remitting multiple sclerosis: a review of adherence data. J Neurosci Nurs 2010;42:S5–S9.

42. Mikol DD, Barkhof F, Chang P, et al. Comparison of subcutaneous interferon beta-1a with glatiramer acetate in patients with relapsing multiple sclerosis (the REbif vs. Glatiramer Acetate in Relapsing MS Disease [REGARD] study): a multicentre, randomized, parallel, open-label trial. Lancet Neurol 2008;7:903–914.

43. 250 µg or 500 µg interferon beta-1b versus 20 mg glatiramer acetate in relapsing-remitting multiple sclerosis: A prospective, randomized, multicentre study. Lancet Neurol 2009;8:880–897.

44. Chofflon M. Mechanisms of action for treatments in multiple sclerosis: Does a heterogeneous disease demand and multi-targeted therapeutic approach? Biodrugs 2005;19:299–308.

45. Kingwell E, Koch M, Leung B, et al. Cardiotoxicity and other adverse events associated with mitoxantrone treatment for MS. Neurology 2010;74:1822–1826.

46. Foley J. Recommendations for the selection, treatment, and management of patients utilizing natalizumab therapy for multiple sclerosis. Am J Manag Care 2010;16:S178–S183.

47. Kappos L, Bates D, Hartung HP, et al. Natalizumab treatment for multiple sclerosis: Recommendations for patient selection and monitoring. Lancet Neurol 2007;6:431–441.

48. Food and Drug Administration. Risk of progressive multifocal leukoencephalopathy (PML) with the use of Tysabri (natalizumab) [Internet] 2010 [cited August 15, 2011]. Available from: *http://www.fda.gov/Drugs/DrugSafety/PostmarketDrugSafetyInformationforPatientsandProviders/ucm199872.htm.*

49. Clifford DB, DeLuca A, Simpson DM, et al. Natalizumab-associated progressive multifocal leukoencephalopathy in patients with multiple sclerosis: Lessons from 28 cases. Lancet Neurol 2010;9:438–446.

50. Calabresi PA, Giovannoni G, Confavreux C, et al. The incidence and significance of anti-natalizumab antibodies: Results from AFFIRM and SENTINEL. Neurology 2007;69:1391–1403.

51. FTY720 (fingolimod) in multiple sclerosis: Therapeutic effects in the immune and the central nervous system. British J Pharmacol 2009;158:1173–1182.

52. O'Connor P, Comi G, Montalban X, et al. Oral fingolimod (FTY720) in multiple sclerosis: Two-year results of a phase II extension study. Neurology 2009;72:73–79.

53. Cohen JA, Barkhof F, Comi G, et al. Oral fingolimod or intramuscular interferon for relapsing multiple sclerosis. N Engl J Med 2010;362:402–415.

54. Kovarik JM, Hartmann S, Bartlett M, et al. Oral-intravenous crossover study of fingolimod pharmacokinetics, lymphocyte responses and cardiac effects. Biopharm Drug Dispos 2007;28:97–104.

55. Lee D, Newell R, Ziegler L, Topping A. Treatment of fatigue in multiple sclerosis: A systematic review of the literature. Int J Nurs Pract 2008;14:81–93.

56. Dodd K, Taylor N, Shields N, et al. Progressive resistance training did not improve walking but can improve muscle performance, quality of life and fatigue in adults with multiple sclerosis: a randomized controlled trial. Mult Scler 2011;17:1362–1374.

57. Shakespeare DT, Boggild M, Young C. Anti-spasticity agents for multiple sclerosis. The Cochrane Database of Systematic Reviews 2003:CD001332.

58. Chwieduk CM, Keating GM. Dalfampridine extended release in multiple sclerosis. CNS Drugs 2010;24:883–891.

59. Goodman AD, Brown TR, Edwards KR, et al. A phase 3 trial of extended release oral dalfampridine in multiple sclerosis. Ann Neurol 2010;68:494–502.

60. Pioro EP, Brooks BR, Cummings J, et al. Dextromethorphan plus ultra low-dose quinidine reduces pseudobulbar affect. Ann Neurol 2010;68: 693–702.

61. Christodoulou C, Melville P, Scherl WF, et al. Effect of donepezil on memory and cognition in multiple sclerosis. J Neurol Sci 2006;245:127–136.

31 Epilepsy

Timothy E. Welty and Edward Faught

LEARNING OBJECTIVES

1. Describe the epidemiology and social impact of epilepsy.
2. Define terminology related to epilepsy, including seizure, convulsion, and epilepsy.
3. Describe the basic pathophysiology of seizures.
4. Describe the basic pathophysiology of epilepsy.
5. Differentiate and classify seizure types when provided a description of the clinical presentation of the seizure and electroencephalogram.
6. Identify key therapeutic decision points in the treatment of epilepsy.
7. Establish therapeutic goals for pharmacotherapy in a patient with epilepsy.
8. Discuss nonpharmacologic treatments for epilepsy.
9. Recommend an appropriate pharmacotherapeutic regimen for the treatment of epilepsy.
10. Select appropriate monitoring parameters for a pharmacotherapeutic regimen for epilepsy.
11. Devise a plan for switching a patient from one antiepileptic regimen to a different regimen.
12. Recognize complications of pharmacotherapy for epilepsy.
13. Analyze potential drug interactions with antiepileptic drugs (AEDs).
14. Determine when and how to discontinue AED therapy.
15. Educate a patient or caregiver on epilepsy and pharmacotherapy for this disorder.

KEY CONCEPTS

❶ A distinction between convulsions, a single seizure, pseudoseizure, and epilepsy should be made in patients presenting with possible seizures.

❷ Selection of appropriate pharmacotherapy depends on distinguishing, identifying, and understanding different seizure types.

❸ Prior to starting pharmacologic therapy, it is essential to determine the risk of having a subsequent seizure.

❹ Mechanisms of action, effectiveness for specific seizure types, common adverse effects, and potential for drug interactions are key elements in selecting a medication for individual patients.

❺ Antiepileptic drug (AED) therapy should usually be initiated carefully using a titration schedule to minimize adverse events.

❻ Changes in AED regimens should be done in a stepwise fashion, keeping in mind drug interactions that may be present and may necessitate dosage changes in concomitant drugs.

❼ Discontinuation of AEDs should be done gradually, only after the patient has been seizure-free for 2 to 5 years, and with careful consideration of factors predictive of seizure recurrence.

❽ Children and women with epilepsy have unique problems related to the use of AEDs.

❾ Older adults have the highest incidence of newly diagnosed epilepsy and face unique challenges in treatment.

❿ Patients receiving AEDs for seizures should have regular monitoring for seizure frequency, seizure patterns, acute adverse effects, chronic adverse effects, and possible drug interactions.

EPIDEMIOLOGY, SOCIAL IMPACT, AND ETIOLOGY

Epidemiology

Epilepsy is a disorder that afflicts approximately 2 million individuals in the United States, with an age-adjusted prevalence of approximately 4 to 7 cases/1,000 persons.[1] The incidence of epilepsy in the United States is estimated at 35 to 75 cases/100,000 persons per year.[2,3] In developing countries, the incidence is higher at 100 to 190 cases/100,000 persons per year, possibly related to poor health care and prenatal care, increased risk of neurologic trauma, and increased rates of infections. About 8% of the U.S. population will experience a seizure during their lifetime. New-onset seizures occur most frequently in infants younger than 1 year of age and in adults after age 55.[4] However, the largest number of patients suffering from epilepsy are between the ages of 15 and 64 years.

Social Impact

Epilepsy is a disorder with a profound impact on a patient's life. All states limit driving for individuals who have recently had a seizure with impaired consciousness, and restrictions vary from state to state.[5] Patients who live in communities without adequate public transportation face major impediments to simple activities of life such as purchasing groceries or getting to a job. Education is also problematic for patients with epilepsy.[6,7] Fifty percent of patients with epilepsy complain of cognitive difficulties and believe their seizures interfere with learning. Transportation and educational difficulties combine with persistent seizures to cause patients with epilepsy to be unemployed or underemployed. Thus this group of patients faces multiple financial difficulties and often do not have health insurance.

Finally, patients with epilepsy often depend on caregivers to assist with medications, transportation, and ensuring the patient's safety. Caregivers should be informed of the patient's medical needs and how to assist should a seizure occur.

Etiology

For nearly 80% of patients with epilepsy, the underlying etiology is unknown.[8] The most common recognized causes of epilepsy are head trauma and stroke. Developmental and genetic defects cause about 5% of cases of epilepsy. CNS tumors, CNS infections, and neurodegenerative diseases are other common causes. Human immunodeficiency virus infection or neurocysticercosis infection, primarily occurring in Latin America, are also important causes.

Isolated seizures that are not epilepsy can be caused by stroke, CNS trauma, CNS infections, metabolic disturbances (e.g., hyponatremia, hypoglycemia), and hypoxia. If these underlying causes of seizures are not corrected, they may lead to the development of epilepsy. Medications can also cause seizures. Some drugs that are commonly associated with seizures include tramadol, bupropion, theophylline, some antidepressants, some antipsychotics, amphetamines, cocaine, imipenem, lithium, excessive doses of penicillins or cephalosporins, and sympathomimetics or stimulants.

PATHOPHYSIOLOGY

Seizures

Regardless of the underlying etiology, all seizures involve a sudden electrical disturbance of the cerebral cortex. A population of neurons fires rapidly and repetitively for seconds to minutes. Cortical electrical discharges become excessively rapid, rhythmic, and synchronous. This phenomenon is presumably related to an excess of excitatory neurotransmitter action, a failure of inhibitory neurotransmitter action, or a combination of the two. In the individual patient, it is usually impossible to identify which neurochemical factors are responsible.

Neurotransmitters

The major excitatory neurotransmitter in the cerebral cortex is glutamate.[9] When glutamate is released from a presynaptic neuron, it attaches to one of several receptor types on the postsynaptic neuron. The result is opening of membrane channels to allow sodium or calcium to flow into the postsynaptic neuron, depolarizing it and transmitting the excitatory signal.[10] Many antiepileptic drugs (e.g., phenytoin, carbamazepine, lamotrigine) work by interfering with this mechanism, either by blocking the release of glutamate or by blocking the sodium or calcium channels, thus preventing excessive excitation.[11] These drugs typically do not block normal neuronal signaling, only the excessively rapid firing characteristic of a seizure. For this reason, they do not usually affect normal brain function.

The major inhibitory neurotransmitter in the cerebral cortex is *γ-aminobutyric acid* (GABA). It attaches to neuronal membranes and opens chloride channels. When chloride flows into the neuron, it becomes hyperpolarized and less excitable. This mechanism is probably critical for shutting off seizure activity by controlling the excessive neuronal firing. Some antiepileptic drugs (AEDs), primarily barbiturates and benzodiazepines, work by enhancing the action of GABA.

Cortical function is modulated by many other neurotransmitters. However, their role in the pathophysiology of epilepsy and in the action of AEDs is not well understood.

Neuronal Mechanisms

Seizures originate in a group of neurons that do not have normal electrical behavior.[12] Presumably, this is due to an underlying imbalance of neurotransmitter function as described earlier. At the level of the individual neuron, firing is excessively prolonged and repetitive. Instead of firing a single action potential, these neurons stay depolarized too long, firing a train of many action potentials. This long, abnormal depolarization is called a *paroxysmal depolarizing shift (PDS)*.

The excessive electrical discharges can spread to other neurons, either adjacent ones or distant ones connected by fiber tracts. The seizure thus spreads to other areas of the brain, recruiting them into the uncontrolled firing pattern.

The neurons involved may not be abnormal themselves but are diverted from their normal functioning to participate in the wildly excessive discharges. The degree of spread and the location of brain areas involved determine the clinical manifestations of the seizure.

Nearly all seizures stop spontaneously because brain inhibitory mechanisms become strong enough to shut off the abnormal excitation.

Epilepsy

Epilepsy is the tendency to have recurrent, unprovoked seizures. This implies that there is a permanent change in cortical function that renders neurons more likely to participate in a seizure discharge. This process is called epileptogenesis, and the exact way in which it occurs is not known. A process thought to be similar to epileptogenesis in humans occurs after prolonged, intermittent electrical stimulation of animal brains and is known as kindling. Epilepsy may develop days, months, or many years after an insult to the cortex. It may be that an originally small group of abnormal neurons causes adjacent or connected neurons to gradually become abnormal as well, by bombarding them over time with frequent, repeated electrical impulses. When the network of abnormal neurons becomes sufficiently large, it becomes capable of sustaining an excessive firing pattern for at least several seconds: a seizure. This hyperexcitable network of neurons is then the seizure focus.

If the change in cortical electrical characteristics is permanent, why do seizures not occur all the time? This is probably because the occurrence of an individual seizure depends on an interplay of environmental and internal brain factors that intermittently result in loss of the normal mechanisms that control abnormal neuronal firing. Some common factors are sleep loss and fatigue, but it is impossible to determine what sets off a particular seizure in most patients.

In some patients, epilepsy worsens over time, with the seizures becoming more frequent as patients grow older. This does not occur in most patients with epilepsy. In those so affected, it is possible that the seizures themselves may cause some damage to the cortex; loss of neurons, especially inhibitory neurons, has been demonstrated in tissue from seizure foci. Other changes occur in brain areas affected by seizures: reorganization of connections between groups of neurons may strengthen excitatory connections and weaken inhibitory connections, making the occurrence of future seizures more likely. Additionally, epilepsy is associated with an increased mortality rate.[13] For these reasons, an argument can be made for controlling epileptic seizures with medications as early as possible. This may reduce the possibility of permanent changes in brain function, although this hypothesis is unproven.

Genetic Factors

Patients with seizures may be concerned that their children or other family members will inherit epilepsy. This fear is usually unfounded. Patients with acquired causes of seizures, such as head trauma or stroke, will not transmit the problem. There is a group of patients, however, who apparently have epilepsy on a genetic basis. Most of these individuals have primary generalized epilepsy.[14,15] Usually these patients develop seizures during childhood. However, the hereditary tendency is not strong. Complex inheritance patterns are usually seen, indicating the likely involvement of several abnormal genes or other factors for seizures to be seen in offspring. Most patients can be reassured that their children and siblings are unlikely to develop epilepsy. Increasing numbers of epilepsy syndromes are being identified as being of genetic origin, and once the specific genes are identified, it may be possible to target drug therapies toward individual biochemical defects.

SEIZURE CLASSIFICATION AND PRESENTATION

General Principles

Careful diagnosis and identification of seizure types is essential to proper treatment of epilepsy. Numerous schemes and descriptions of seizures exist, but the International League Against Epilepsy (ILAE) has established the currently accepted standard for classifying epileptic seizures (Fig. 31–1) and epilepsies or epilepsy syndromes (Table 31–1).[16,17] Classification of epileptic seizures is based on electroencephalographic (EEG) findings combined with the clinical findings or semiology of the seizure events. Clinical presentations of seizures vary widely depending on the region and amount of brain involved in the seizure.

Primary Generalized Seizures

If the entire cerebral cortex is involved in the seizure from the onset of the seizure, the seizure is classified as primary generalized. The following are types of primary generalized seizures:

- Tonic-clonic: Characterized by a sudden loss of consciousness accompanied by tonic extension and rhythmic clonic contractions of all major muscle groups. The duration of the seizure is usually 1 to 3 minutes. These seizures are often described as "grand mal."

- Absence: Characterized by sudden and brief (i.e., several seconds in duration) losses of consciousness without muscle movements. These seizures are often described as daydreaming or blanking-out episodes. A common term for these seizures is "petit mal."

- Myoclonic: Characterized by single and very brief jerks of all major muscle groups. Patients with these seizures may not lose consciousness due to the seizure lasting less than 3 to 4 seconds. Patients may describe these seizures as shoulder shrugs or spinal chills. Myoclonic seizures may cluster and build into a generalized tonic-clonic seizure.

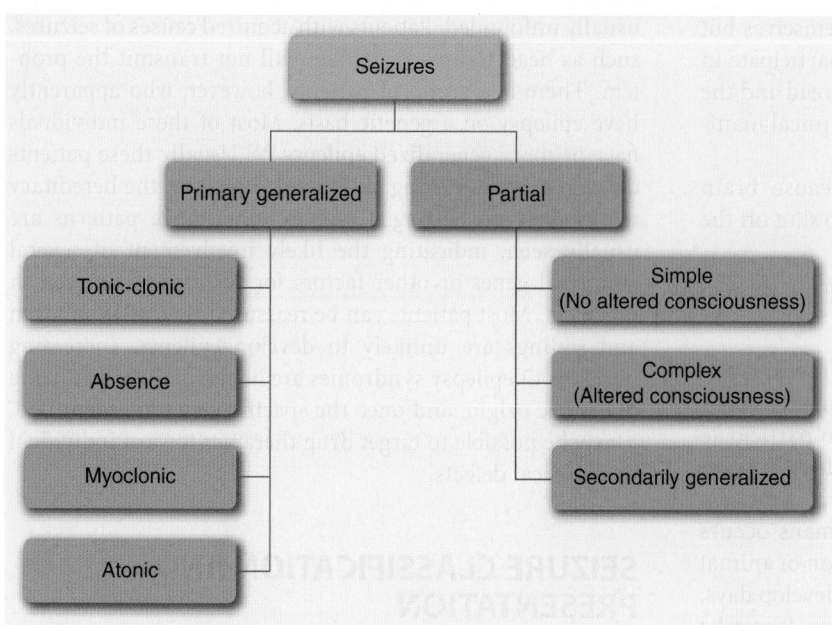

FIGURE 31–1. ILAE classification of epileptic seizures (1981). (From Commission on Classification and Terminology of the International League Against Epilepsy. Proposal for revised clinical and electroencephalographic classification of epileptic seizures. Epilepsia 1981;22:489–501.)

- **Atonic:** Characterized by loss of consciousness and muscle tone. No muscle movements are typically noted, and the patient falls if not lying down or sitting in a chair. These seizures may be described as "falling out."

Partial Seizures

When the seizure begins in a localized area of the brain, it is defined as partial. There are three types of partial seizures in the current classification system (Fig. 31–1):

Table 31–1

ILAE Classification Scheme for Epilepsies and Epilepsy Syndromes

I. Localization-related (focal, local, partial) epilepsies and epileptic syndromes
   A. Idiopathic with age-related onset
      1. Benign childhood epilepsy with centrotemporal spikes
      2. Childhood epilepsy with occipital paroxysms
   B. Symptomatic
II. Generalized epilepsies and epileptic syndromes
   A. Idiopathic and age-related onset
      1. Benign neonatal epilepsy
      2. Childhood absence epilepsy (pyknolepsy)
      3. Juvenile myoclonic epilepsy (impulsive petit mal)
      4. Juvenile absence epilepsy with generalized tonic-clonic seizure on awakening
   B. Secondary (idiopathic or symptomatic)
      1. West's syndrome (infantile spasms)
      2. Lennox-Gastaut syndrome
   C. Symptomatic
      1. Nonspecific etiology (early myoclonic encephalopathy)
      2. Specific syndromes (epileptic seizures that may complicate many diseases, e.g., Ramsay-Hunt syndrome, Unverricht's disease)

Data from Commission on Classification and Terminology of the International League Against Epilepsy. Proposal for revised classification of epilepsies and epileptic syndromes. Epilepsia 1989;30:389–399.

- **Simple:** The patient has a sensation or uncontrolled muscle movement of a portion of their body without an alteration in consciousness. The type of sensation or movement depends on the location of seizure in the brain.
- **Complex:** Although the seizure is localized in a specific area of the brain, like a simple partial seizure, there is an alteration in the patient's level of consciousness.
- **Secondarily generalized:** The seizure starts as a simple or complex partial seizure and spreads to the entire brain. Patients may report a warning or aura, and these are actually the start of the seizure.

Epilepsy Syndromes

Classification of epilepsies and epilepsy syndromes is helpful in determining appropriate pharmacotherapy. This classification scheme is based on the type of seizures a patient has and an attempt to identify the etiology of the epilepsy or epilepsy syndrome:

- **Idiopathic epilepsies:** These syndromes are thought to be due to genetic alterations, but the underlying etiology is not identified. Neurologic functions are completely normal apart from the occurrence of seizures.
- **Symptomatic epilepsies:** There is an identifiable cause for the seizures, such as trauma or hypoxia.
- **Cryptogenic epilepsies:** In these epilepsies the seizures are the result of an underlying neurologic disorder that is often ill defined. Neurologic functions are often abnormal or developmentally delayed in patients with cryptogenic epilepsies.

A complete description of a patient's epilepsy should include the seizure type with the epilepsy or syndrome type (e.g., idiopathic, symptomatic, cryptogenic).

Commonly encountered epilepsy syndromes are:

- **Juvenile myoclonic epilepsy (JME):** A primary generalized epilepsy syndrome that usually starts in the early to middle teenage years and has a strong familial component. Patients have myoclonic jerks and tonic-clonic seizures and may also have absence seizures.

- **Lennox-Gastaut syndrome (LGS):** Patients with this syndrome have cognitive dysfunction and mental retardation. Their seizures usually consist of a combination of tonic-clonic, absence, atonic, and myoclonic seizures.

- **Mesial temporal lobe epilepsy (MTLE):** A type of epilepsy that consists of partial seizures arising from the mesial temporal lobe of the brain. Often this type of epilepsy is associated with an anatomical change described as hippocampal sclerosis. Patients with this type of epilepsy often have excellent surgical outcomes.

- **Infantile spasms:** A seizure syndrome in infants younger than 1 year of age. It is characterized by a specific EEG pattern and spasms or jitters. Another name is West's syndrome. Infants with infantile spasms often develop other seizure types and epilepsies later in life.

Other Classifications

The ILAE is proposing a new classification system that improves the description of the seizure type and epilepsy.[18,19] The proposed scheme revolves around five axes:

- Axis 1: Description of the seizure event
- Axis 2: Epileptic seizure type or types
- Axis 3: Any syndrome type
- Axis 4: Etiology when known
- Axis 5: Degree of impairment by the epilepsy

This classification system is undergoing final review and should become the standard in the near future.

DIAGNOSIS

Determining a correct and accurate diagnosis is essential to any consideration of pharmacotherapy. ❶ *A distinction between convulsions, a single seizure, pseudoseizure, and epilepsy should be made in patients presenting with possible seizures.* Numerous other disorders, including convulsions,

Clinical Presentation and Diagnosis of Epilepsy

General

Typically, healthcare providers are not able to observe a patient's seizures, and for most types of seizures the patient has no memory of the event. It is important to obtain a careful history from the patient and any individuals who witness the seizures.

Common Descriptions of Seizures

The clinical presentation of seizures varies from patient to patient depending on the portion of brain involved in the seizure. Events tend to be stereotypical for an individual patient.

Patients who experience seizures may complain of paroxysmal spells of

- Blanking-out spells, lapses in memory, periods of altered consciousness
- Warnings or auras consisting of various sensations or automatic, uncontrolled movements
- Daydreaming
- Jerks, shoulder shrugs, sudden chills of spine
- Falling out

Associated Symptoms

- Incontinence, usually of urine
- Tongue biting
- Traumatic injuries, usually associated with falling during a seizure

Diagnosis

Description of events: The patient and any witnesses to the seizures should be carefully interviewed to obtain a full and complete description of typical seizures.

Neurologic examination: Usually, the neurologic physical examination is completely normal. Any neurologic deficits identified should be fully investigated because seizures do not usually cause permanent, detectable neurologic deficits.

Electroencephalogram (EEG): A routine EEG can be helpful if epileptiform discharges are seen. However, the EEG may be normal between seizures, and most routine EEGs are not performed during a seizure. Maneuvers such as sleep deprivation, photic stimulation, hyperventilation, or prolonged monitoring can help expose EEG changes consistent with epilepsy.

Neuroimaging (preferably an MRI of the brain): Imaging of the brain is important to rule out obvious causes of seizures such as stroke or tumors. An MRI scan is also helpful in detecting mesial temporal sclerosis, a finding often associated with mesial temporal epilepsy and predictive of positive surgical outcomes.

Video EEG monitoring: A procedure consisting of continuous video monitoring of the patient with a simultaneous EEG. Usually a patient is monitored in the hospital for 4 to 5 days. This procedure is used to determine if the patient is truly having seizures, to determine the specific type of seizures the patient is having, and to localize the area of the brain that is the origin of the seizures.

syncope, psychogenic nonepileptic events (i.e., pseudoseizures), anxiety attacks, cardiac arrhythmias, hypoglycemia, transient ischemic attacks, tics, and complicated migraine headaches, are often mistaken for seizures by patients and caregivers. Seizures are typically brief spells, lasting no more than 5 minutes. However, seizures can be prolonged and can last for ≥15 minutes. In this situation the patient is in status epilepticus and requires immediate medical attention.

A proper diagnostic workup of a patient presenting with seizures should include the following elements:

• Thorough neurologic examination
• EEG
• Laboratory tests (complete blood count [CBC], liver function tests [LFTs], serum chemistry)
• Neuroimaging (preferably magnetic resonance imaging [MRI]).

In patients with epilepsy these laboratory findings may be normal. Many of the tests are done to rule out other causes of seizures (e.g., infection, electrolyte imbalance). Often the EEG appears normal between seizures.[20] Sleep deprivation, photic stimulation, prolonged (more than 20 minutes) EEG recording, and 24-hour EEG monitoring with video correlation can be done in an attempt to capture seizure or seizure-like activity on the EEG.

TREATMENT

Desired Outcomes

The ultimate outcome goal for any patient with epilepsy is elimination of all seizures without any adverse effects of the treatment. An effective treatment plan would allow the patient to pursue a normal lifestyle with complete control of seizures. Specifically, the treatment should enable the patient to drive, perform well in school, hold a reasonable job, and function effectively in the family and community. However, due to the intractability of the seizures or sensitivity to AEDs, many patients are not able to achieve these outcomes. In these cases, the goal of therapy is to provide a tolerable balance between reduced seizure severity and/or frequency and medication adverse effects, enabling the individual to have a lifestyle as nearly normal as possible.

General Approach to Treatment

Once it is concluded that the patient has seizures, the type of seizure and epilepsy syndrome, if any, must be determined. ❷ *Selection of appropriate pharmacotherapy depends on distinguishing, identifying, and understanding different seizure types.* Without an accurate classification of the seizure type, it is possible to select a medication that is ineffective or even harmful to the patient.

❸ *Prior to starting pharmacologic therapy, it is essential to determine the risk of having a subsequent seizure.* If there is an underlying treatable cause, such as hyponatremia or a CNS infection, the risks of another seizure and the

development of epilepsy are very small. In these cases, the only necessary pharmacotherapy is to correct the underlying problem and possibly short-term use of an AED. Risk factors for repeated seizures in patients without an underlying disorder include:

• Structural CNS lesion
• Abnormal EEG
• Partial seizure type
• Positive family history
• Postictal motor paralysis[21]

If no risk factors are present, the risk of another seizure is 10% to 15%. However, if two or more risk factors are present, the risk of another seizure is 100%.

When sufficient evidence is available to determine the patient has seizures and is at risk for another seizure, pharmacotherapy is usually started (**Fig. 31–2**). The patient should be in agreement with the plan, be willing to take the medication, and be able to monitor seizure frequency and adverse drug effects. ❹ *Mechanisms of action, effectiveness for specific seizure types, common adverse effects, and potential for drug interactions are key elements in selecting a medication for individual patients.* Other patient factors such as gender, concomitant drugs, age, economic factors, and lifestyle also need to be considered.

Nonpharmacologic Therapy

Several nonpharmacologic treatments for epilepsy are available. For some patients, surgery is the treatment approach with the greatest probability of eliminating seizures.[22] The most common surgical approach for epilepsy is temporal lobectomy. When the seizure focus can be localized and it is in a region of the brain that is not too close to critical areas, such as those responsible for speech or muscle control, surgical removal of the focus can result in 80% to 90% of patients becoming seizure free. According to a National Institutes of Health Consensus Conference, three criteria should be met for patients to be candidates for surgery.[23] These criteria are (a) a definite diagnosis of epilepsy, (b) failure of adequate drug therapies, and (c) definition of the electroclinical syndrome (i.e., localization of the seizure focus in the brain). Other surgical procedures that are less likely to make a patient seizure free include corpus callosotomy and extratemporal lesion removal.

Vagal nerve stimulation is another nonpharmacologic approach to treating all types of seizures.[24] In this treatment, a unit that generates an intermittent electrical current is placed under the skin in the chest. A wire is tunneled under the skin to the left vagus nerve in the neck. The unit generates a small electrical current that stimulates the vagus nerve. Additional stimulations can be initiated by the patient swiping a magnet over the device located in the chest. This treatment approach is essentially equivalent to starting a new medication with regard to efficacy. Approximately 25% to 50% of patients who have a vagal nerve stimulator placed will experience at least a 50% reduction in seizure frequency.

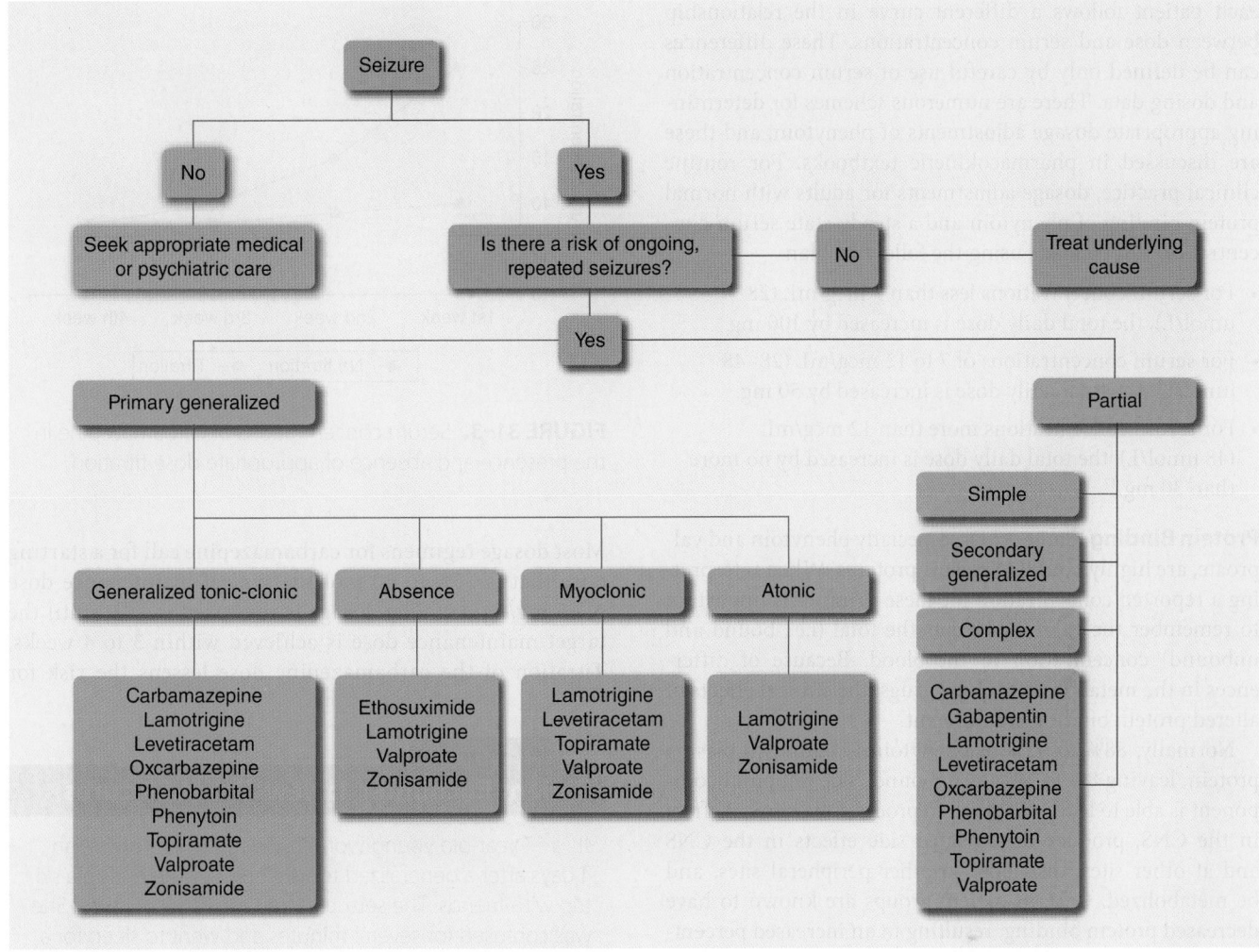

FIGURE 31–2. Treatment algorithm for management of seizure disorders.

However, fewer than 10% become seizure free. Adverse effects include hoarseness, swallowing difficulties, tingling or vibration in the neck, infection or bleeding due to surgery, and, rarely, laryngeal spasms. Vagal nerve stimulation is usually reserved for patients who do not respond to several drugs and are not surgical candidates.

One of the oldest nonpharmacologic treatments is the ketogenic diet.[25] Modern use of the diet was started in the 1920s. This diet produces a keto-acidotic state through the elimination of nearly all carbohydrates. To initiate the diet, patients undergo 24 to 48 hours of fasting until ketones are detected in the urine. The diet consisting of dietary fats (e.g., butter, heavy cream, fatty meats) and protein with no added sugar is started. Daily urinalysis for ketones is performed to ensure the patient remains in ketosis. Any inadvertent consumption of sugar results in the diet needing to be reinitiated. Pharmacists have an important role in maintaining the diet, by determining the sugar or carbohydrate content of medications the patient is taking. This diet is typically used only in children with difficult-to-control seizures. In certain patients the diet can be extremely effective, resulting in complete seizure control and reduction of AEDs. However, it is

hard to maintain a ketotic state, and palatability of the diet is a concern. Additionally, there are concerns about growth retardation in children and hypercholesterolemia with prolonged use of the diet.

Pharmacologic Therapy

▶ Special Considerations

Use of AEDs presents some unique challenges, some of which relate to their pharmacokinetic properties, which need to be clearly understood.[26]

Michaelis-Menten Metabolism Phenytoin metabolism is capacity limited. Michaelis-Menten metabolism or Michaelis-Menten pharmacokinetics occurs when the maximum capacity of hepatic enzymes to metabolize the drug is reached within the normal dosage range. The clinical significance is that small changes in doses result in disproportionate and large changes in serum concentrations. The patient is at risk of sudden toxicity if too large a dose increase is made, or a breakthrough seizure may occur if too large a reduction in dose is made. Due to individual differences in metabolism, each patient follows a different curve in the relationship between dose and serum concentrations. These differences can be defined only by careful use of serum concentration and dosing data. There are numerous schemes for determining appropriate dosage adjustments of phenytoin, and these are discussed in pharmacokinetic textbooks. For routine clinical practice, dosage adjustments for adults with normal protein binding of phenytoin and a steady-state serum concentration can be made using the following plan:

- For serum concentrations less than 7 mcg/mL (28 μmol/L), the total daily dose is increased by 100 mg.

- For serum concentrations of 7 to 12 mcg/mL (28–48 μmol/L), the total daily dose is increased by 50 mg.

- For serum concentrations more than 12 mcg/mL (48 μmol/L), the total daily dose is increased by no more than 30 mg.[27]

Protein Binding Some AEDs, especially phenytoin and valproate, are highly bound to plasma proteins. When interpreting a reported concentration for these drugs, it is important to remember the value represents the total (i.e., bound and unbound) concentration in the blood. Because of differences in the metabolism of these drugs, the clinical effects of altered protein binding are different.

Normally, 88% to 92% of phenytoin is bound to plasma protein, leaving 8% to 12% as unbound. The unbound component is able to leave the blood to produce the clinical effect in the CNS, produce dose-related side effects in the CNS and at other sites, distribute to other peripheral sites, and be metabolized. Certain patient groups are known to have decreased protein binding, resulting in an increased percentage of drug that is unbound. These patient groups include:

- Those with kidney failure
- Those with hypoalbuminemia
- Neonates
- Pregnant women
- Those taking multiple highly protein-bound drugs
- Patients in critical care

Due to the Michaelis-Menten metabolism of phenytoin, alterations in its protein binding will result in increased severity of dose-related adverse effects. In patients with suspected changes in protein binding, it is useful to measure unbound phenytoin concentrations.

When valproate protein binding is altered, the risk for severe dose-related adverse effects is much less compared with phenytoin. Michaelis-Menten metabolism is not a factor with valproate, so hepatic enzymes are able to efficiently metabolize the additional unbound portion.

Autoinduction Carbamazepine is a potent inducer of hepatic microsomal enzymes. Not only does it increase the rate of metabolism for many other drugs, it increases the rate of its own metabolism. Hepatic enzymes become maximally induced over several weeks, necessitating a small initial dose of carbamazepine that is increased over time to compensate for the enzyme induction (Fig. 31–3).

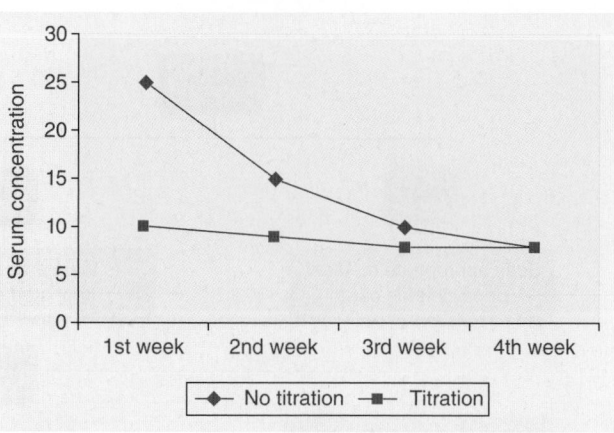

FIGURE 31–3. Serum concentrations of carbamazepine in the presence and absence of appropriate dose titration.

Most dosage regimens for carbamazepine call for a starting dose that is 25% to 30% of the typical maintenance dose of 15 mg/kg/day. The dosage is increased weekly until the target maintenance dose is achieved within 3 to 4 weeks. Titration of the carbamazepine dose lessens the risk for

Patient Encounter 1: New-Onset Seizures

JL, a 17-year-old young woman, is seen by her physician 4 days after a generalized tonic-clonic seizure during a ski trip with friends. The seizure lasted for 1 to 2 minutes. She was confused for several minutes and went to sleep for a few hours after the seizure.

Her physical examination is completely normal, and no focal neurologic deficits were observed. An MRI was ordered and reported as normal. An EEG shows generalized 3- to 4-Hz spike waves.

What additional information is needed to make a decision about pharmacotherapy?

How should this information be used to make choices concerning AED therapy?

During the visit she mentions several previous episodes of brief jerks in the early morning. These started a couple of years ago and now occur 2 to 3 days of the week.

Is pharmacotherapy indicated?

If it is indicated, what drug should be used and how should it be started?

What adverse effects are important to monitor?

Three months later she is doing well. She reports no generalized tonic-clonic seizures and jerks on only a few days a month.

What adjustments in pharmacotherapy should be made at this point?

Is it possible for her to discontinue AED therapy at some time in the future?

severe dose-related adverse effects when carbamazepine is first started.

▶ *Drug Selection and Seizure Type*

The key to selecting effective pharmacotherapy is to base the decision on the seizure type. Several consensus treatment guidelines from the Scottish Intercollegiate Guidelines Network (SIGN), the National Institute for Clinical Excellence in the United Kingdom (NICE), the American Academy of Neurology (AAN), and ILAE all use determination of seizure type as the basis for selection of pharmacotherapy (Table 31–2).[28-30] While the guidelines make recommendations for specific drugs to be used in certain seizure types, the consensus recommendations use only

data available from the medical literature. In many cases, a recommendation is not made because there are no published data on which to make an evidence-based decision. Therefore, a drug may not currently be recommended for a seizure type simply because it has not been studied for that seizure type. Absence of a recommendation should not be taken to mean the drug is ineffective for a specific seizure type. For example, according to the AAN Practice Parameter, topiramate is useful as monotherapy for primary generalized tonic-clonic seizures, and there is insufficient evidence to make any recommendation regarding gabapentin, lamotrigine, oxcarbazepine, tiagabine, levetiracetam, or zonisamide.[31]

Outside of the evidence-based guidelines, other pharmacologic treatments are commonly used or avoided. For

Table 31–2

Evidence-Based Guidelines for Initial Monotherapy Treatment of Epilepsy

Seizure Type	AAN	SIGN	NICE	ILAE
Primary generalized tonic-clonic	Carbamazepine[a] Lamotrigine[a] Oxcarbazepine[a] Phenobarbital[a] Phenytoin[a] Topiramate[a] Valproate[a]	Lamotrigine Valproate	Carbamazepine Lamotrigine Topiramate Valproate *Second-line:* Clobazam Levetiracetam Oxcarbazepine	*Adults:* Carbamazepine[c] Lamotrigine[c] Oxcarbazepine[c] Phenobarbital[c] Phenytoin[c] Topiramate Valproate[c] *Children:* Carbamazepine[c] Phenobarbital[c] Topiramate[c] Valproate[c]
Absence	Lamotrigine (children)	Ethosuximide Lamotrigine Valproate	Ethosuximide Lamotrigine Valproate *Second-line:* Clobazam Clonazepam Topiramate	*Children:* Ethosuximide[c] Lamotrigine[c] Valproate[c]
Myoclonic	Not mentioned	Lamotrigine Valproate	Valproate Topiramate (children with severe myoclonic epilepsy of infancy) *Second-line:* Clobazam Clonazepam Lamotrigine Levetiracetam Piracetam[b] Topiramate	Clonazepam[d] Lamotrigine[d] Levetiracetam[d] Topiramate[d] Valproate[d] Zonisamide[d]
Tonic	Not mentioned	Not mentioned	Lamotrigine Valproate *Second-line:* Clobazam Clonazepam Levetiracetam Topiramate	Not mentioned

(Continued)

Table 31–2

Evidence-Based Guidelines for Initial Monotherapy Treatment of Epilepsy *(Continued)*

Seizure Type	AAN	SIGN	NICE	ILAE

Atonic	Not mentioned	Not mentioned	Lamotrigine
			Valproate
			Second-line:
			  Clobazam
			  Clonazepam
			  Levetiracetam
			  Topiramate
				Not mentioned

Partial with or without secondary generalization	Carbamazepine
	Gabapentin
	Lamotrigine
	Oxcarbazepine
	Phenobarbital
	Phenytoin
	Topiramate
	Valproate
		Phenytoin
		Carbamazepine
		Valproate
		Lamotrigine
		Oxcarbazepine
			Carbamazepine
			Lamotrigine
			Oxcarbazepine
			Valproate
			Topiramate
			Second-line:
			  Clobazam
			  Gabapentin
			  Levetiracetam
			  Phenytoin
			  Tiagabine
				Adults:
				  Carbamazepine[e]
				  Phenytoin[e]
				  Valproate[e]
				  Gabapentin[c]
				  Lamotrigine[c]
				  Oxcarbazepine[c]
				  Phenobarbital[c]
				  Topiramate[c]
				  Vigabatrin[c]
				Children:
				  Oxcarbazepine[e]
				  Carbamazepine[c]
				  Phenobarbital[c]
				  Phenytoin[c]
				  Topiramate[c]
				  Valproate[c]
				  Lamotrigine[c]
				  Vigabatrin[c]
				Elderly:
				  Lamotrigine[e]
				  Gabapentin[e]
				  Carbamazepine[c]
				  Topiramate[c]
				  Valproate[c]

AAN, American Academy of Neurology; ILAE, International League Against Epilepsy; NICE, National Institute for Clinical Excellence in the United Kingdom; SIGN, Scottish Intercollegiate Guidelines Network.

[a]Based on data from newly diagnosed epilepsy patients of multiple seizure types.

[b]Not currently available in the United States.

[c]Possibly effective.

[d]Probably effective.

[e]Proven effective.

Data from Refs. 27–30.

initial treatment of absence seizures, ethosuximide and valproate are commonly used. Zonisamide may be also used for the initial treatment of absence and myoclonic seizures. In absence and myoclonic seizures, carbamazepine, oxcarbazepine, gabapentin, tiagabine, and pregabalin should be avoided because they have been associated with an exacerbation of these types of seizures.

⑤ *Antiepileptic drug therapy should usually be initiated carefully using a titration schedule to minimize adverse events.* Usually a moderate target dose is chosen until the patient's response can be further evaluated in the clinic. If seizures continue, the dose should be increased gradually until the patient becomes seizure free or adverse effects appear. For some drugs like lamotrigine, specific titration guidelines are established by the manufacturer.

Refractory seizure (i.e., unresponsive to at least two first-line AEDs) treatment is somewhat different. Combinations of drugs are not addressed by guidelines but may be useful in patients with difficult to control primary generalized seizures. All AEDs, except ethosuximide, are effective in combination therapy for partial seizures.

▶ *Complications of Pharmacotherapy*

● Adverse effects of AEDs are frequently dose limiting or can cause a drug to be discontinued. Two types of adverse effects occur with AEDs: serum concentration-related and idiosyncratic (Table 31–3). Concentration-related adverse effects happen with increasing frequency and severity as the dose or serum concentration of a drug is increased. For many AEDs,

Table 31-3

Characteristics of Common AEDs

Drug	Mechanism of Action	Dose	Pharmacokinetic Parameters	Usual Serum Concentration Range	Dose-Related Adverse Effects	Idiosyncratic Adverse Effects
Carbamazepine (Tegretol, Tegretol XR, Carbatrol, generic)	Fast sodium channel inactivation	*Loading dose:* Not recommended due to excessive dose-related toxicity *Maintenance dose:* Titrate dosage to target over 3–4 weeks Adults: 10–20 mg/kg/day as a divided dose Children: 20–30 mg/kg/day as a divided dose	*Half-life:* 10–25 hours with chronic dosing *Apparent volume of distribution:* 0.8–1.9 L/kg *Protein binding:* 67–81% *Primary elimination route:* Hepatic	4–12 mcg/mL (17–51 μmol/L)	Diplopia, drowsiness, nausea, sedation	Aplastic anemia, hyponatremia, leucopenia, osteoporosis, rash
Clobazam (Onfi)	Enhance GABA	Weight less than 30 kg, start 5 mg/day, titrate to 20 mg/day in 2 divided doses Weight more than 30 kg start 10 mg/day, titrate to 40 mg/day in 2 divided doses	*Half-life:* 10–50 hours *Apparent volume of distribution:* ~0.9 L/kg *Protein binding:* ~90% *Primary elimination route:* Hepatic; metabolized to active metabolite that is further metabolized by CYP 2C19	Not established	Sedation somnolence lethargy pyrexia irritability drooling aggression	
Clonazepam (Klonopin, generic)	Enhance GABA activity	*Loading dose:* Not recommended due to increased adverse effects *Maintenance dose:* Initiate at 0.5 mg 1–3 times daily, titrate dose to effectiveness, usually 3–5 mg daily in 2 or 3 divided doses	*Half-life:* 30–40 hours *Apparent volume of distribution:* 3.2 L/kg *Protein binding:* 47–80% *Primary elimination route:* Hepatic	Not established	Ataxia, memory impairment, sedation, slowed thinking	
Ethosuximide (Zarontin, generic)	Modulate calcium channels	*Loading dose:* Not recommended due to increased adverse effects *Maintenance dose:* Initiate at 250 mg twice daily and titrate to 500–1,000 mg twice daily	*Half-life:* 60 hours *Apparent volume of distribution:* 0.6–0.7 L/kg *Protein binding:* None *Primary elimination route:* Hepatic	40–100 mcg/mL (283–708 μmol/L)	Ataxia, sedation	Hepatotoxicity, neutropenia, rash

(Continued)

567

Table 31-3

Characteristics of Common AEDs (Continued)

Drug	Mechanism of Action	Dose	Pharmacokinetic Parameters	Usual Serum Concentration Range	Dose-Related Adverse Effects	Idiosyncratic Adverse Effects
Felbamate (Felbatol)	Inhibit glutamate activity	*Loading dose:* Not recommended due to increased adverse effects *Maintenance dose:* 1,200–3,600 mg/day in 3 or 4 divided doses	*Half-life:* Monotherapy: 20 hours Concurrent enzyme inducers: 11–16 hours *Apparent volume of distribution:* 0.7–0.8 L/kg *Protein binding:* 25–35% *Primary elimination route:* Hepatic	Not established	Anxiety, insomnia, nausea	Anorexia, aplastic anemia, headache, hepatotoxicity, weight loss
Gabapentin (Neurontin, generic)	Modulate calcium channels and enhance GABA activity	*Loading dose:* Not recommended due to short half-life *Maintenance dose:* 900–3,600 mg/day in 3 or 4 divided doses (doses up to 10,000 mg/day have been tolerated)	*Half-life:* 5–7 hours (proportional to creatinine clearance) *Apparent volume of distribution:* 0.6–0.8 L/kg *Protein binding:* less than 10% *Primary elimination route:* Renal	Not established	Drowsiness, sedation	Peripheral edema, weight gain
Lacosamide (Vimpat)	Slow sodium channel inactivation; modulate collapsin response; mediator protein-2	*Loading dose:* Data unavailable *Maintenance dose:* 200–400 mg/day; Start at 100 mg/day in 2 divided doses and titrate upward according to response	*Half-life:* Approximately 13 hours *Volume of distribution:* 0.6 L/kg *Protein binding:* Less than 15% *Primary elimination route:* 40% renal 60% hepatic	Not established	Ataxia, dizziness, diplopia, headache, nausea, vomiting	PR interval prolongation
Lamotrigine (Lamictal, Lamictal XR, generic)	Fast sodium channel inactivation	*Loading dose:* Not recommended due to increased risk of rash *Maintenance dose:* 150–800 mg/day in 2 or 3 divided doses. Doses should be initiated and titrated according to the manufacturer's recommendations to reduce the risk of rash	*Half-life:* Monotherapy: 24 hours Concurrent enzyme inducers: 12–15 hours Concurrent enzyme inhibitors: 55–60 hours *Apparent volume of distribution:* 1.1 L/kg *Protein binding:* 55% *Primary elimination route:* Hepatic	Not established	Ataxia, drowsiness, headache, insomnia, sedation	Rash

Drug	Mechanism	Dose	Pharmacokinetics	Therapeutic level	Common adverse effects	Other adverse effects
Levetiracetam (Keppra, Keppra XR, generic)	Modulate synaptic vesicle protein	*Loading dose:* Not recommended due to excessive adverse effects *Maintenance dose:* 1,000–3,000 mg/day. Start at 1,000 mg/day and titrated upward as indicated by response	*Half-life:* 6–8 hours *Apparent volume of distribution:* 0.5–0.7 L/kg *Protein binding:* Less than 10% *Primary elimination route:* 70% renal 30% hepatic	Not established	Somnolence, dizziness	Depression
Oxcarbazepine (Trileptal, generic)	Fast sodium channel inactivation	*Loading dose:* Not recommended due to excessive adverse effects *Maintenance dose:* 600–1,200 mg/day. Start at 300 mg twice daily and titrated upward as indicated by response	*Half-life:* Parent drug Approximately 2 hours; 10-monohydroxy Metabolite Approximately 9 hours *Apparent volume of distribution:* 0.5–0.7 L/kg *Protein binding:* 40% *Primary elimination route:* Hepatic	Not established	Diplopia, dizziness, somnolence	Hyponatremia, 25–30% cross sensitivity in patients with hypersensitivity to carbamazepine
Phenobarbital (Luminal, generic)	Fast sodium channel inactivation	*Loading dose:* 10–20 mg/kg as single or divided IV infusion or orally in divided doses over 24–48 hours *Maintenance dose:* Adults: 1–4 mg/kg/day as a single or divided dose Children: 3–6 mg/kg/day as divided dose Neonates: 1–3 mg/kg/day as divided dose	*Half-life:* Adults: 49–120 hours; Children: 37–73 hours; Neonates: approximately 115 hours *Volume of distribution:* 0.7–1 L/kg *Protein binding:* Approximately 50% *Primary elimination route:* Hepatic	15–40 mcg/mL (65–172 μmol/L)	Ataxia, drowsiness, sedation	Attention deficit, cognitive impairment, hyperactivity, osteoporosis, passive-aggressive behavior

(Continued)

Table 31–3

Characteristics of Common AEDs (Continued)

Drug	Mechanism of Action	Dose	Pharmacokinetic Parameters	Usual Serum Concentration Range	Dose-Related Adverse Effects	Idiosyncratic Adverse Effects
Phenytoin (Dilantin, generic)	Fast sodium channel inactivation	*Loading dose:* Adults: 15–20 mg/kg single IV dose or divided oral dose Infants younger than 3 months: 10–15 mg/kg single IV dose Neonates: 15–20 mg/kg single IV dose *Maintenance dose:* Adults: 5–7 mg/kg/day, as single or divided dose Children: 6–15 mg/kg/day, as divided dose Neonates: 3–8 mg/kg/day, as divided dose	*Half-life:* Follows capacity-limited or Michaelis-Menten pharmacokinetics. Half-life increases as the dose and serum concentration increases. *Volume of distribution:* Adults: 0.7 L/kg Children: 0.8 L/kg Neonates: 1.2 L/kg *Protein binding:* Adults, children: 88–92% Neonates: 65% *Primary elimination route:* Hepatic	10–20 mcg/mL (40–79 μmol/L) total concentration 1–2 mcg/mL (4–8 μmol/L) unbound concentration	Ataxia, diplopia, drowsiness, sedation	Anemia, gingival hyperplasia, hirsutism, lymphadenopathy, osteoporosis, rash
Pregabalin (Lyrica)	Modulate calcium channels	*Loading dose:* Not recommended due to increased adverse effects *Maintenance dose:* Initiate at 150 mg/day in 2 or 3 divided doses and titrate to a maximum dose of 600 mg/day	*Half-life:* 6.3 hours, proportional to creatinine clearance *Apparent volume of distribution:* 0.5 L/kg *Protein binding:* Negligible *Primary elimination route:* Renal	Not established	Ataxia, blurred vision, dizziness, dry mouth, somnolence	Edema, weight gain
Rufinamide (Banzel)	Unknown, may enhance inactivation of sodium channels	*Loading dose:* Data unavailable *Maintenance dose:* Children: 45 mg/kg/day or 3,200 mg/day; start at 10 mg/kg/day in 2 divided doses and titrate upward according to response Adults: 3,200 mg/day; start at 400–800 mg/day in 2 divided doses and titrate upward according to response	*Half-life:* 6–10 hours *Apparent volume of distribution:* Approximately 0.7 L/kg, varies with dose *Protein binding:* 34% (27% to albumin) *Primary elimination route:* Hepatic	Not established	Dizziness, fatigue, headache, nausea, somnolence, vomiting	

Drug	Mechanism of action	Dosing	Pharmacokinetics	Therapeutic range	Adverse effects
Tiagabine (Gabitril, generic)	Enhance GABA activity	*Loading dose:* Not recommended due to excessive adverse effects *Maintenance dose:* 32–56 mg/day in 4 divided doses. Doses should be titrated upward over 6 weeks, starting at 4 mg/day	*Half-life:* Monotherapy: 7–9 hours Concurrent enzyme inducers: 2.5–4.5 hours *Apparent volume of distribution:* 0.6–0.8 L/kg *Protein binding:* 96% *Primary elimination route:* Hepatic	Not established	Dizziness, somnolence, irritability, slowed thinking
Topiramate (Topamax, generic)	Fast sodium channel inactivation, inhibit glutamate activity, enhance GABA activity	*Loading dose:* Not recommended due to excessive adverse effects *Maintenance dose:* 100–400 mg/day in 2 or 3 divided doses. Doses should be started at 25–50 mg/day and gradually titrated upward over 3–6 weeks to avoid excessive adverse effects	*Half-life:* Monotherapy: 21 hours Concurrent enzyme inducers: 11–16 hours *Apparent volume of distribution:* 0.55–0.8 L/kg *Protein binding:* 13–17% *Primary elimination route:* 60% renal 40% hepatic	Not established	Ataxia, dizziness, drowsiness, slowed thinking Acute glaucoma, metabolic acidosis, oligohidrosis, paresthesia, renal calculi, weight loss
Valproic acid/ divalproex sodium (Depakene, Depakote, Depakote ER, generic)	Fast sodium channel inactivation	*Loading dose:* 20–40 mg/kg *Maintenance dose:* Adults: 15–45 mg/kg/day in 2–4 divided doses Children: 5–60 mg/kg/day in 2–4 divided doses	*Half-life:* Adults: 8–15 hours Children: 4–15 hours Infants younger than 2 months: 65 hours *Volume of distribution:* 0.1–0.5 L/kg *Protein binding:* 90% (decreases with increasing serum concentrations) *Primary elimination route:* Hepatic	50–100 mcg/mL (346–693 µmol/L). Children may require concentrations up to 150 mcg/mL (1,040 µmol/L)	Drowsiness, nausea, sedation, tremor Hepatotoxicity, osteoporosis, pancreatitis, weight gain

(Continued)

Table 31-3

Characteristics of Common AEDs (Continued)

Drug	Mechanism of Action	Dose	Pharmacokinetic Parameters	Usual Serum Concentration Range	Dose-Related Adverse Effects	Idiosyncratic Adverse Effects
Vigabatrin (Sabril)	Inhibits GABA transaminase	*Children:* 1 month–2 years: 50 mg/kg/day in 2 divided doses *Adults:* Initiate at 1,000 mg/day in 2 divided doses, titrate up to 3,000 mg/day *Renal failure:* CrCl 50–80 mL/min, decrease dose by 25%; CrCl 30–50 mL/min, decrease dose by 50%; CrCl 10–30 mL/min, decrease dose by 75%	*Half-life:* 7.5 hours, proportional to creatinine clearance *Volume of distribution:* 1.1 L/kg *Protein binding:* negligible *Primary route of elimination:* Renal	Not established	Convulsion, dizziness, headache, nasopharyngitis, somnolence, weight gain	Vision loss and blindness
Zonisamide (Zonegran, generic)	Modulate sodium and calcium channels	*Loading dose:* Not recommended due to excessive adverse effects *Maintenance dose:* 100–600 mg/day; start at 100 mg/day and titrated upward as indicated by response	*Half-life:* Approximately 63 hours *Apparent volume of distribution:* 1.45 L/kg *Protein binding:* 40% *Primary elimination route:* Hepatic	Not established	Dizziness, somnolence	Metabolic acidosis, oligohidrosis, paresthesia, renal calculi

GABA, γ-aminobutyric acid.

Data from Refs. 25, 35, 38.

common concentration-related adverse effects include sedation, ataxia, and diplopia. These adverse effects should be carefully considered and used as one of the AED selection criteria. For example, if a patient has a job that requires mental alertness, it is best to choose an AED that is less likely to cause sedation (e.g., lamotrigine).

Idiosyncratic adverse effects are not dose or concentration related and will almost always result in the AED being discontinued. Rash, hepatotoxicity, and hematological toxicities are the most common idiosyncratic reactions seen with AED. Because many of these adverse effects are life threatening or potentially life threatening, the AED should be discontinued immediately when the reaction is observed. Carbamazepine, phenytoin, phenobarbital, valproate, lamotrigine, oxcarbazepine, and felbamate are most likely to cause these types of reactions. Many of these reactions are thought to occur primarily on an immunological basis, which raises the possibility of cross-reactivity. This is especially true for carbamazepine, phenytoin, phenobarbital, and oxcarbazepine, where 15% to 25% of patients who have an idiosyncratic reaction to one drug will have a similar reaction to the other drugs.

▶ Chronic Adverse Effects

Because AEDs are administered for long periods of time, adverse effects due to prolonged drug exposure are of concern. Some chronic adverse effects associated with AEDs include peripheral neuropathy and cerebellar atrophy. Other chronic adverse effects are extensions of acute adverse effects, for example, weight gain.

One chronic adverse effect that is of concern is osteoporosis.[32,33] Carbamazepine, phenytoin, phenobarbital, oxcarbazepine, and valproate have all been shown to decrease bone mineral density, even after only 6 months of treatment. Data on the relationship between other AEDs and osteoporosis are not currently available. Multiple studies have shown the risk of osteoporosis due to chronic AED use to be similar to the risk with chronic use of glucocorticosteroids. Patients taking carbamazepine, oxcarbazepine, phenytoin, phenobarbital, or valproate more than 6 months should take supplemental

calcium and vitamin D. Additionally, routine monitoring for osteoporosis should be performed every 2 years, and patients should be instructed on ways to protect themselves from fractures.

▶ Practical Issues

Comorbid Disease States Patients with epilepsy often have comorbid disease states. Disorders such as chronic headaches and asthma are frequent problems. For patients who also have asthma, care must be taken to identify drug interactions between AEDs and medications used for asthma. These interactions necessitate close monitoring for changes in efficacy or increased toxicity, and dosage changes of other drugs may be necessary when an AED is added or removed. Patients with chronic headaches need special attention in the selection of an AED. Agents known to prevent headache (e.g., valproate and topiramate) may be preferred among several choices, and agents associated with increased headaches (e.g., lamotrigine and felbamate) may be a secondary or tertiary alternative.

Depression is a common problem in patients with epilepsy, with approximately 30% having symptoms of major depression at some point.[34] Patients with epilepsy should be routinely assessed for signs of depression, and treatment should be initiated if necessary. Certain AEDs may exacerbate depression, for example, levetiracetam and phenytoin. Other AEDs (e.g., lamotrigine, carbamazepine, oxcarbazepine) may be useful in treating depression. Changes in mood can be precipitated by the addition or discontinuation of an AED. If treatment for depression is necessary, caution should be exercised in choosing an agent that does not increase seizure frequency and does not interact with AEDs.

Switching Drugs Changing from one AED to another can be a complex process. If the first drug is stopped too abruptly, breakthrough seizures may occur. ❻ *Changes in AED regimens should be done in a stepwise fashion, keeping in mind drug interactions that may be present and may necessitate dosage changes in concomitant drugs.* Typically the new drug is started at a low initial dose and gradually increased over several weeks. Once the new drug is at a minimally effective dose, the drug to be discontinued is gradually tapered while the dose of the new drug continues to be increased to the target dose. During a transition between drugs, patients should be cautioned about the possibility of increased seizures or adverse reactions.

Stopping Therapy Epilepsy is generally considered to be a lifelong disorder that requires ongoing treatment. However, many patients who are seizure free may desire to discontinue their medications.[35] Patients who become seizure free following surgery for their epilepsy may have medications slowly tapered starting 1 to 2 years after their surgery. Many patients will choose to stay on at least one medication, following successful surgery, to ensure they remain seizure free. ❼ *Discontinuation of AEDs should be done gradually, only after the patient has been seizure free for 2 to 5 years and with careful consideration of factors predictive of seizure recurrence.*[36] They are:

Patient Encounter 2: Managing Chronic Adverse Reactions

PL, a 41-year-old man with complex partial seizures, has been treated with carbamazepine 800 mg/day for 20 years. His seizures are well controlled on this regimen, and he works as a dental equipment sales representative. He expresses concern about taking the carbamazepine for so long.

What chronic adverse effects are important to monitor in this patient?

How should monitoring for these adverse effects be done?

What measures can be taken to prevent these adverse effects?

- No seizures for 2 to 5 years
- Normal neurologic examination
- Normal intelligence quotient
- Single type of partial or generalized seizure
- Normal EEG with treatment

Individuals who fulfill all of these criteria have a 61% chance of remaining seizure free after AEDs are discontinued. Additionally, there is a direct relationship between the duration of seizure freedom while taking medications and the chance of being seizure free after medications are withdrawn. Withdrawal of AEDs is done slowly, usually with a tapering dose over at least 1 to 3 months.

▶ Dosing

Dosing of AEDs is determined by general guidelines and response of the patient. Serum concentrations may be helpful in benchmarking a specific response. Therapeutic ranges that are often quoted are broad guidelines for dosing but should never replace careful evaluation of the patient's response. It is not unusual for a patient to be well managed with serum concentrations or doses outside the typical ranges.

▶ Drug Interactions

AEDs are associated with many different drug interactions.[37-39] These interactions are primarily in relation to absorption, metabolism, and protein binding. Tube feedings and antacids are known to reduce the absorption of phenytoin and carbamazepine. Phenytoin, carbamazepine, and phenobarbital are potent inducers of various CYP 450 isoenzymes, increasing the clearance of other drugs metabolized through these pathways (Table 31–4). In contrast, valproate is a CYP 450 and UDP-glucuronosyltransferase (UGT) isoenzyme inhibitor and reduces the clearance of some drugs. Phenytoin and valproate are highly protein bound and can be displaced when taken concurrently with other highly protein-bound drugs. For example, when phenytoin and valproate are taken together, there may be increased dose-related adverse effects within several hours of dosing. This can be avoided by staggering doses or giving smaller doses more frequently during the day. Whenever a change in a medication regimen occurs, drug interactions should be considered and appropriate adjustments in dose of AEDs made.

▶ Special Populations

⑧ *Children and women with epilepsy have unique problems related to the use of AEDs.* In children, developmental changes occur rapidly, and metabolic rates are greater than those seen in adults. When treating a child, it is imperative to control seizures as quickly as possible to avoid interference with development of the brain and cognition. AED doses are increased rapidly, and frequent changes in the regimen are made to maximize control of seizures. Due to the rapid metabolic rates seen in children, doses of AEDs are typically higher on a milligram per kilogram basis compared with

---

Table 31–4

Cytochrome P450 and AED Interactions

Enzyme	Substrate	Common Inducers	Common Inhibitors
CYP 1A2	Carbamazepine	Carbamazepine Phenytoin Phenobarbital Rifampin	Cimetidine Ciprofloxacin Erythromycin Clarithromycin
CYP 2C9	Phenobarbital[a] Phenytoin[a] Carbamazepine Valproate	Carbamazepine Phenytoin Phenobarbital Rifampin	Amiodarone Cimetidine Fluconazole Valproate
CYP 2C19	Phenobarbital Phenytoin Valproate Lacosamide		Felbamate Ticlopidine Topiramate Zonisamide
CYP 2D6	Zonisamide	Carbamazepine	
CYP 3A4	Carbamazepine[a] Tiagabine[a] Zonisamide[a]	Carbamazepine Phenytoin Phenobarbital Rifampin	Amiodarone Erythromycin Propoxyphene Ketoconazole
Uridine diphosphate glucuronyl-transferase	Lamotrigine[a] Carbamazepine Valproate	Lamotrigine Phenobarbital Phenytoin Hormonal contraceptives	Valproate

[a]Primary route of metabolism.

Data from Refs. 37–39.

Patient Encounter 3: Pregnancy

MA is a 28-year-old woman who comes with her husband to clinic. They would like to start a family and have several questions regarding AEDs and pregnancy. She is currently taking lamotrigine 400 mg/day for complex partial seizures. Her seizures are well controlled, except for two seizures in the last year when she missed doses due to not getting refills on time. Otherwise she is in good health.

What is the risk of birth defects if she gets pregnant while taking AEDs?

What can be done to limit the risk of birth defects?

What AEDs should generally be avoided in women of childbearing potential?

How should lamotrigine be managed when she becomes pregnant and after delivery?

adults, and serum concentrations are used more extensively to help ensure an adequate trial of a drug has been given.

For women, the treatment of epilepsy poses challenges, including teratogenicity, interactions between AEDs and hormonal contraceptives, and reduced fertility.[40,41] Recommendations for managing women of childbearing potential and who are pregnant have been developed (Table 31–5). Several AEDs have been implicated in causing both minor and serious birth defects.[42] Of special concern are neural tube defects (e.g., spina bifida, microcephaly, anencephaly) associated most commonly with valproate and possibly carbamazepine. Additionally, valproate has been associated with impaired cognitive development in children born to women taking valproate during pregnancy. Use of valproate is not absolutely contraindicated in women who may become pregnant, but it is appropriate to use alternative AEDs, if possible, in women of childbearing potential. All women of childbearing potential who have epilepsy should take 1 to 4 mg daily of supplemental folic acid to reduce the risk of these defects. Many AEDs are excreted in breast milk.

However, infants were exposed to higher concentrations of AED in utero, so it is unclear if drugs in breast milk are harmful to the child. Decisions about breast-feeding should be made on an individual basis.

As noted earlier, many of the AEDs induce hepatic microsomal enzyme systems and thus reduce the effectiveness of hormonal contraceptives. Women taking AEDs that may reduce the effectiveness of hormonal contraceptives should be encouraged to also use other forms of birth control. In contrast to these interactions, hormonal contraceptives induce glucuronidation of lamotrigine and valproate. Oral contraceptives that cycle hormones cause reductions in serum concentrations of lamotrigine or valproate during days of the cycle when hormones are taken; serum concentrations increase during days when hormones are not taken. Due to induction or inhibition of sex hormone metabolism and changes in binding of hormones to sex hormone binding globulin, some AEDs may reduce fertility. For example, valproate has been associated with a drug-induced polycystic ovarian syndrome. Women who experience difficulties with fertility should seek the advice of healthcare professionals with expertise in fertility.

❾ *Older adults have the highest incidence of newly diagnosed epilepsy and face unique challenges in treatment.* The highest incidence of seizures and epilepsy is in individuals older than 65 years. Cerebrovascular disease, tumors, trauma, and neurodegenerative diseases are the primary causes of epilepsy in this age group. Diagnosis of epilepsy in older adults is often difficult. This is due to the subtle symptoms of seizures in the elderly, their often compromised memory, and the fact that many elderly live alone. Carbamazepine, lamotrigine, and gabapentin have been studied in this age group, and all are effective in controlling seizures.[43-45] Fewer adverse events occur with lamotrigine and gabapentin. Elderly patients are more sensitive to adverse events, so smaller doses tend to be used in this age group.

Table 31–5

Management of AEDs During Pregnancy

Give supplemental folic acid 1–4 mg daily to all women of childbearing potential
Use monotherapy whenever possible
Use lowest doses that control seizures
Continue pharmacotherapy that best controls seizures prior to pregnancy
Monitor AED serum concentrations at start of pregnancy and monthly thereafter
Adjust AED doses to maintain baseline serum concentrations
Administer supplemental vitamin K during eighth month of pregnancy to women receiving enzyme-inducing AEDs
Monitor postpartum AED serum concentrations to guide adjustments of drug doses

Patient Encounter 4: Seizures in Older Adults

SB is a 78-year-old woman with a recent onset of spells where she is briefly confused. Her daughter has observed some of these episodes and reports that her mother has no memory of these events. During the spells she is unable to talk, and she has no memory of the episodes. SB has a history of hypertension and a minor stroke several years ago. Her MRI is consistent with an old stroke and her EEG is reported as normal.

Should pharmacotherapy be started in this patient?

If pharmacotherapy is started, what AED is preferable?

How should the efficacy and toxicity be monitored in this patient?

OUTCOME EVALUATION

❿ *Patients receiving AEDs for seizures should have regular monitoring for seizure frequency, seizure patterns, acute adverse effects, chronic adverse effects, and possible drug interactions.*

Efficacy

- Seizure counts are the only reasonable and standard way to evaluate the efficacy of treatment.

- Encourage patients to keep a seizure calendar that notes the time and day a seizure occurs and the type of seizure. Compare seizure counts on a monthly basis to determine the level of seizure control.

Toxicity

- Monitor acute toxicity of AEDs at every clinic visit.

Patient Care and Monitoring

1. *Monitor the patient's seizure frequency and characteristics.* The only objective measure of efficacy for AEDs is a count of seizure frequency. Ask patients to keep seizure calendars, noting the numbers and types of seizures that occur, and have them bring the calendars to clinic at every visit for analysis and documentation of seizure frequency.

2. *Monitor for acute and chronic adverse effects of AED.* Acute adverse effects are best detected by a thorough neurologic examination at clinic visits. Instruct patients to report sedation, ataxia, rash, or other problems immediately. Monitor for chronic adverse effects, including a loss of bone mineral density, which should be measured every 2 years in patients taking phenytoin, phenobarbital, carbamazepine, and valproate.

3. *Monitor for comorbid disease states at each clinic visit.* Evaluate for depression at every clinic visit. Monitor comorbid disease states when a change in AED therapy is made.

4. *Take measures to ensure compliance with medications and access to care.* Compliance with medication regimens is a common problem for patients with epilepsy. Ask patients at every visit how they are taking their medications and whether they miss any doses. Identify barriers to care such as financial issues or transportation problems.

5. *Instruct patients, family members, and caregivers on first aid for seizures.* First aid for seizures consists primarily of keeping patients from hurting themselves. They should be placed on the floor, if possible, and their head cushioned. First responders to a seizure should never attempt to restrain the patient or force an item into their mouth. If a seizure lasts more than 5 to 10 minutes, emergency medical assistance should be called.

- Question patients about common adverse effects of the AEDs they are receiving. Weigh the impact of acute adverse effects against the extent of seizure control achieved from a treatment regimen. If it is determined the adverse effects negatively impact the patient more than the extent of seizure control benefits the patient, adjust the therapeutic regimen. Continuously monitor chronic adverse effects of AEDs.

Abbreviations Introduced in This Chapter

AAN	American Academy of Neurology
AED	Antiepileptic drug
CNS	Central Nervous System
EEG	Electroencephalograph
GABA	Gamma-aminobutyric acid
ILAE	International League Against Epilepsy
JME	Juvenile myoclonic epilepsy
LFTs	Liver function tests
LGS	Lennox-Gastaut syndrome
MRI	Magnetic resonance imaging
MTLE	Mesial temporal lobe epilepsy
NICE	National Institute for Clinical Excellence in the United Kingdom
PDS	Paroxysmal depolarizing shift
SIGN	Scottish Intercollegiate Guidelines Network

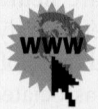 Self-assessment questions and answers are available at *http://www.mhpharmacotherapy. com/pp.html.*

REFERENCES

1. Hauser WA, Kurland LT. The epidemiology of epilepsy in Rochester, Minnesota, 1935 through 1967. Epilepsia 1975;16:143–161.
2. Annegers JF, Hauswer WA, Eleveback LR. Remission of seizures and relapse in patients with epilepsy. Epilepsia 1979;20:729–737.
3. Shamansky SL, Glaser GH. Socioeconomic characteristics of childhood seizure disorders in the New Haven area: An epidemiologic study. Epilepsia 1979;20:457–474.
4. Jallon P, Samdja D, Cabre P, et al. Epileptic seizures epilepsy and risk factors: Experiences with an investigation in Martinique. Epimart Group. Rev Neurol (Paris) 1998;154:408–411.
5. Epilepsy Foundation. Driver information by state [Internet], [cited 2011 Oct 10]. Available from: *http://www.epilepsyfoundation.org/living/ wellness/transportation/drivinglaws.etm.*
6. Elger CE, Helmstaedter C, Kurthen M. Chronic epilepsy and cognition. Lancet Neurol 2004;3(11):663–672.
7. Epilepsy Foundation. Education [Internet], [cited 2011 Oct 10]. Available from: *http://www.epilepsyfoundation.org/answerplace/Social/ education/.*
8. Jallon P, Loiseau P, Loiseau J. Newly diagnosed unprovoked epileptic seizures: Presentation at diagnosis in the CAROLE study. Epilepsia 2001;42:464–475.
9. Najm I, Möddel G, Janigro D. Mechanisms of epileptogenesis and experimental models of seizures. In: Wyllie E, ed. The Treatment of Epilepsy. 4th ed. Philadelphia, PA: Lippincott Williams & Wilkins; 2006.

10. Jones SW. Basic cellular neurophysiology. In: Wyllie E, ed. The Treatment of Epilepsy. 4th ed. Philadelphia, PA: Lippincott Williams & Wilkins; 2006.

11. Czapinski P, Blaszczyk B, Czuczwar SJ. Mechanisms of action of antiepileptic drugs. Curr Top Med Chem 2005;5(1):3–14.

12. Abrous DN, Koehl M, Le Moal M. Adult neurogenesis: From precursors to network and physiology. Physiology 2005;85(2):523–569.

13. Gaitatzis A, Sander JW. The mortality of epilepsy revisited. Epileptic Disord 2004;6:3–13.

14. Panayiotopoulos CP. Idiopathic generalized epilepsies: A review and modern approach. Epilepsia 2005;46(Suppl 9):1–6.

15. Wong M. Advances in the pathophysiology of developmental epilepsies. Semin Pediatr Neurol 2005;12:72–87.

16. Commission on Classification and Terminology of the International League Against Epilepsy. Proposal for revised clinical and electroencephalographic classification of epileptic seizures. Epilepsia 1981;22:489–501.

17. Commission on Classification and Terminology of the International League Against Epilepsy. Proposal for revised classification of epilepsies and epileptic syndromes. Epilepsia 1989;30:389–399.

18. Fisher RS, van Emde Boas W, Blume W, et al. Epileptic seizures and epilepsy: Definitions proposed by the International League Against Epilepsy (ILAE) and the International Bureau for Epilepsy (IBE). Epilepsia 2005;46(4):470–472.

19. Engel J Jr. A proposed diagnostic scheme for people with epileptic seizures and with epilepsy: Report of the ILAE Task Force on Classification and Terminology. Epilepsia 2001;42:796–803.

20. Smith SJ. EEG in the diagnosis, classification, and management of patients with epilepsy. J Neurol Neurosurg Psychiatry 2005;76(Suppl 2):ii2–ii7.

21. Hauser WA, Rich SS, Annegers JF, et al. Seizure recurrence after a first unprovoked seizure: An extended follow-up. Neurology 1990;40:1163–1170.

22. Lachhwani DK, Wyllie E. Outcome and complications of epilepsy surgery. In: Wyllie E, ed. The Treatment of Epilepsy. 4th ed. Philadelphia, PA: Lippincott Williams & Wilkins; 2006.

23. National Institute of Neurological Disorders and Stroke. Surgical treatment of epilepsy. Proceedings of a Consensus Conference. March 19–21, 1990. Epilepsy Res 1992;5(Suppl):1–250.

24. Wheless JW. Vagus nerve stimulation therapy. In: Wyllie E, ed. The Treatment of Epilepsy. 4th ed. Philadelphia, PA: Lippincott Williams & Wilkins; 2006.

25. Nordli DR, DeVivo DC. The ketogenic diet. In: Wyllie E, ed. The Treatment of Epilepsy. 4th ed. Philadelphia, PA: Lippincott Williams & Wilkins; 2006.

26. Perruca E. An introduction to antiepileptic drugs. Epilepsia 2005;46(Suppl 4):31–37.

27. Privitera MD. Clinical rules for phenytoin dosing. Ann Pharmacother 1993;27(10):1169–1173.

28. Scottish Intercollegiate Guidelines Network. Diagnosis and management of epilepsy in adults [Internet], [cited 2011 Oct 10]. Available from: *http://www.sign.ac.uk/pdf/sign70.pdf*.

29. National Institute for Clinical Excellence. The epilepsies: The diagnosis and management of the epilepsies in children and adults in primary and secondary care [Internet], [cited 2011 Oct 10]. Available from: *http://www.guidance.nice.org.uk/CG20*.

30. French JA, Kanner AM, Bautista J, et al. Efficacy and tolerability of the new antiepileptic drugs I: Treatment of new onset epilepsy report of the Therapeutics and Technology Assessment Subcommittee and Quality Standards Subcommittee of the American Academy of Neurology and the American Epilepsy Society. Neurology 2005;62:1252–1260.

31. French JA, Kanner AM, Bautista J, et.al. Efficacy and tolerability of the new antiepileptic drugs II: Treatment of refractory epilepsy report of the Therapeutics and Technology Assessment Subcommittee and Quality Standards Subcommittee of the American Academy of Neurology and the American Epilepsy Society. Neurology 2005;62:1261–1273.

32. Vestergaard P. Epilepsy, osteoporosis and fracture risk—A meta-analysis. Acta Neurol Scand 2005;112:227–286.

33. Koppel BS, Harden CL, Nikolov BG, Labar DR. An analysis of lifetime fractures in women with epilepsy. Acta Neurol Scand 2005;111(4):225–228.

34. Harden CL, Goldstein MA. Mood disorders in patients with epilepsy: Epidemiology and management. CNS Drugs 2002;16:291–302.

35. Schmidt D, Loscher W. Uncontrolled epilepsy following discontinuation of antiepileptic drugs in seizure-free patients: A review of current clinical experience. Acta Neurol Scand 2005;111(5):291–300.

36. Tsur VG, O'Dell C, Shinnar S. Initiation and discontinuation of antiepileptic drugs. In: Wyllie E, ed. The Treatment of Epilepsy. 4th ed. Philadelphia, PA: Lippincott Williams & Wilkins; 2006.

37. Perucea E. Clinically relevant drug interactions with antiepileptic drugs. Br J Clin Pharmacol 2006;61(3):246–255.

38. Bailer M. The pharmacokinetics and interactions of new antiepileptic drugs: An overview. Their Drug Monit 2005;27(6):722–726.

39. Anderson GD. Pharmacogenetic and enzyme induction/inhibition properties of antiepileptic drugs. Neurology 2004;63(10 Suppl 4):53–58.

40. Crawford P. Best practice guidelines for the management of women with epilepsy. Epilepsia 2005;46(Suppl 9):117–124.

41. Foldvary-Schaefer N, Morrel MJ. Epilepsy in women: The biological basis for the female experience. Cleve Clin J Med 2004;71(Suppl 2):S1–S8.

42. Artama M, Auvinen A, Raudaskoski T, et al. Antiepileptic drug use of women with epilepsy and congenital malformations in offspring. Neurology 2005;64(11):1874–1878.

43. Brodie MJ. Overstall, PW, Giorgi L. Multicentre, double-blind, randomized, comparison between lamotrigine and carbamazepine in elderly patients with newly diagnosed epilepsy. Epilepsy Res 1999;37:81–87.

44. Rowan AJ, Ramsay RE, Collins JF, et.al. New onset geriatric epilepsy, a randomized study of gabapentin, lamotrigine, and carbamazepine. Neurology 2005;64:1868–1873.

45. Saetre E, Peruccad, E, Isojärvi J, et.al. An international multicenter randomized double-blind controlled trial of lamotrigine and sustained-release carbamazepine in the treatment of newly diagnosed epilepsy in the elderly. Epilepsia 2007;48:1292–1302.

32

Status Epilepticus

Gretchen M. Brophy and Eljim P. Tesoro

LEARNING OBJECTIVES

● **Upon completion of the chapter, the reader will be able to:**

1. Describe the pathophysiology of status epilepticus.

2. Explain the urgency of diagnosis and treatment of status epilepticus.

3 Recognize the signs and symptoms of status epilepticus.

4. Identify the treatment options available for termination of status epilepticus.

5. Formulate an initial treatment strategy for a patient in generalized convulsive status epilepticus.

6. Compare the pharmacotherapeutic options for refractory status epilepticus.

7. Describe adverse drug events associated with the pharmacotherapy of status epilepticus.

8. Recommend monitoring parameters for a patient in status epilepticus.

KEY CONCEPTS

❶ Status epilepticus is a neurologic emergency that can lead to permanent brain damage or death.

❷ Status epilepticus can be practically defined as continuous seizure activity lasting more than 5 minutes or two or more seizures without complete recovery of consciousness.

❸ It is important to evaluate possible etiologies of status epilepticus and treat underlying causes to obtain timely and optimal seizure control. A thorough history along with laboratory and diagnostic testing should be conducted.

❹ The goal of therapy is to terminate physical and electroencephalographic evidence of seizures, prevent their recurrence, and minimize adverse drug events.

❺ The first-line treatment for status epilepticus is IV benzodiazepines (emergent therapy). Lorazepam is currently considered the first-line agent by most clinicians.

❻ Urgent therapy with antiepileptic drugs (AEDs) should be used to prevent seizure recurrence. IV phenytoin (or fosphenytoin), valproate sodium, and phenobarbital are options after benzodiazepines.

❼ Seizure activity that does not respond to benzodiazepines (emergent therapy) and antiepileptics (urgent therapy) or persists beyond 30 to 60 minutes in duration can be considered refractory status epilepticus.

❽ Midazolam, propofol, and pentobarbital infusions are commonly used for refractory status epilepticus, but intensive monitoring and supportive care are required.

❶ *Status epilepticus (SE) is a neurologic emergency that can lead to permanent brain damage or death.* ❷ *SE can be practically defined as continuous seizure activity lasting more than 5 minutes or two or more seizures without complete recovery of consciousness.*[1] Refractory status epilepticus (RSE) can be defined as seizure activity that does not respond to first-line (emergent) or second-line (urgent) antiepileptic therapy.[2]

SE can present as nonconvulsive status epilepticus (NCSE) or generalized convulsive status epilepticus (GCSE). NCSE is characterized by a persistent state of impaired consciousness without clinical seizure activity. For patients with NCSE, electroencephalography (EEG) is essential for diagnosis. GCSE is characterized by full-body motor seizures and involves the entire brain. This chapter focuses on GCSE, the most common type of SE, which is associated with the greatest risk of neurologic and physical damage.

EPIDEMIOLOGY AND ETIOLOGY

There are an estimated 150,000 cases of SE each year in the United States, with approximately 55,000 associated deaths, and an estimated annual direct cost for inpatient admissions of $4 billion.[3,4] Status epilepticus occurs more frequently in African Americans, children, and the elderly.

❸ *It is important to evaluate possible etiologies of SE to obtain timely and optimal seizure control.* The causes of SE

Patient Encounter 1, Part 1

SR is a 56-year-old woman with a history of hypertension, diabetes, and arthritis who was admitted with a traumatic subdural hematoma after sustaining a fall down a flight of stairs in her home. She underwent surgery to evacuate the hematoma and is currently recovering in the ICU. Her nurse reports that a few minutes ago SR was alert and awake, but now she is unarousable and is having jerky, convulsive movements on both sides of her body. Her diagnosis is status epilepticus.

Ht 165 cm (5'5"); Wt 100 kg (220 lbs)

What initial assessments should be performed?

What are some possible etiologies for her seizure?

What interventions need to be performed at this time?

can be categorized as acute or chronic. Acute changes that cause SE include metabolic disturbances (e.g., hyponatremia, hypernatremia, hyperkalemia, hypocalcemia, hypomagnesemia, hypoglycemia); central nervous system (CNS) disorders, infections, or injuries; hypoxia; and drug toxicity (e.g., theophylline, isoniazid, cyclosporine, cocaine). Chronic processes that cause SE include preexisting epilepsy, chronic alcohol abuse (withdrawal seizures), CNS tumors, and strokes.[2] In patients with epilepsy, the common causes of SE are anticonvulsant withdrawal or subtherapeutic anticonvulsant levels. Patients with SE due to chronic processes generally respond well to antiepileptic drug therapy.

PATHOPHYSIOLOGY

Status epilepticus occurs when the brain fails to stop an isolated seizure. The exact reason for this failure is unknown and probably involves multiple mechanisms. A seizure is likely to occur due to a mismatch of excitatory and inhibitory neurotransmitters in the brain. The primary excitatory neurotransmitter is glutamate. Glutamate stimulates postsynaptic N-methyl-D-aspartate (NMDA) receptors, causing an influx of calcium into the cells and depolarization of the neuron. Sustained depolarization may maintain SE, eventually causing neuronal injury and death.[5] The primary inhibitory neurotransmitter, γ-aminobutyric acid (GABA), opposes the excitatory response by stimulating $GABA_A$ receptors, enhancing chloride inhibitory currents, producing hyperpolarization, and inhibiting the postsynaptic cell membrane. The inhibitory ability of GABA diminishes as the duration of seizures increases, perhaps due to a mechanistic shift in the functional properties of the $GABA_A$ receptors that causes a decrease in response to GABA-receptor agonists.[6] Seizures lasting more than 30 minutes can cause injury and neuronal loss in the hippocampal, cortical, and thalamic regions. These neurologic sequelae are related to the excessive electrical activity and alterations in cerebral metabolic

demand. The clinical impact of the $GABA_A$-receptor changes on treatment response and the worsening degree of neuronal injury with prolongation of seizure activity necessitates rapid control of SE.

Several systemic changes occur in two phases during the course of SE. Phase I occurs during the first 30 minutes of seizure activity, and phase II occurs after 30 to 60 minutes of seizure activity.[7]

Phase I

During phase I, each seizure causes a sharp increase in autonomic activity with elevated epinephrine, norepinephrine, and steroid plasma concentrations, resulting in hypertension, tachycardia, hyperglycemia, hyperthermia, sweating, and salivation. Cerebral blood flow is also increased to preserve the oxygen supply to the brain during this period of high metabolic demand. Increases in sympathetic and parasympathetic stimulation with muscle hypoxia can lead to ventricular arrhythmias, severe acidosis, and rhabdomyolysis, which could then lead to hypotension, shock, hyperkalemia, and acute tubular necrosis.

Phase II

After approximately 30 to 60 minutes of continuous seizure activity, phase II begins with loss of cerebral autoregulation, decreased cerebral blood flow, increased intracranial pressure, and systemic hypotension. Metabolic demand is still high; however, the body is no longer able to compensate.

The systemic changes that may occur include hypoglycemia, hyperthermia, respiratory failure, hypoxia, respiratory and metabolic acidosis, hyperkalemia, hyponatremia, and uremia. It is important to note that motor activity may not be clinically evident during prolonged seizures, but the electrical activity may still exist. This is referred to as nonconvulsive or subclinical seizure activity and needs to be recognized and treated aggressively.

CLINICAL PRESENTATION AND DIAGNOSIS

History

③ *When a patient presents with seizures, a thorough history is needed to determine the type and duration of the seizure activity. This will help guide therapy and identify which laboratory and diagnostic tests need to be conducted. A firm diagnosis of SE can be made when a patient with a history of repeated seizures and impaired consciousness has a seizure witnessed by a healthcare professional. However, emergent treatment should not be delayed if seizure activity is suspected based on reports provided by the patient's family or emergency response personnel.*

Physical Examination

Once seizures are controlled, a neurologic examination should be conducted to evaluate the level of consciousness

Clinical Presentation of Status Epilepticus

General

The patient may present with or without clinically noticeable seizure activity.

Symptoms

- Impaired consciousness ranging from lethargy to coma
- Disorientation after cessation of GCSE
- Pain from associated injuries (e.g., tongue lacerations, dislocated shoulder, head trauma, facial trauma)

Signs

Phase I:	Phase II (>30 minutes of SE):
Generalized convulsions	Respiratory failure with pulmonary edema
Hypertension, tachycardia	
Fever and sweating	Cardiac failure (arrhythmias, shock)
Muscle contractions, spasms	
Respiratory compromise	Hypotension
Incontinence	Hyperthermia
	Rhabdomyolysis and multiorgan failure

Laboratory Tests

- Hyperglycemia (phase I) and hypoglycemia (phase II) can occur
- Hyponatremia, hypernatremia, hyperkalemia, hypocalcemia, hypomagnesemia, and hypoglycemia can cause SE
- The WBC count may slightly increase
- Abnormal ABGs due to hypoxia and respiratory or metabolic acidosis
- Elevated serum creatinine will be present in renal failure patients
- Myoglobinuria can occur in patients with continuous seizures

Diagnostic Tests

EEG to confirm seizure activity

CT or MRI may reveal mass lesions or hemorrhage

---

will resolve soon after the seizure is terminated. A loss of bowel or bladder function, respiratory compromise, and **nystagmus** may also be observed. When seizure activity is sustained for more than approximately 30 to 60 minutes, muscle contractions may no longer be visible, but the patient remains in SE. Twitching of the face, hands, or feet may be seen in these comatose patients with prolonged seizures. As motor signs diminish, an EEG will be necessary to diagnosis SE.

Laboratory Parameters

3 *It is important to obtain a serum chemistry profile to help identify possible underlying causes of SE.* Abnormalities that can cause seizures include hypoglycemia, hypo- or hypernatremia, hypomagnesemia, and hypocalcemia; patients with renal and liver failure are at high risk as well. In a febrile patient with an elevated white blood cell (WBC) count, an active infection should be ruled out or treated appropriately. Cultures from the blood, cerebrospinal fluid (CSF), respiratory tract, and urine should be obtained once the seizures are controlled. Computed tomography (CT) or magnetic resonance imaging (MRI) can be done to rule out CNS abscesses, bleeding, or tumors, all of which may be a source of seizure activity. A blood alcohol level and urine toxicology screen for drugs of abuse should also be conducted to determine if alcohol withdrawal, illicit drug use, or a drug overdose could be the underlying cause of SE. Also, drug levels should be obtained in a drug overdose situation to rule out toxicity as a cause of SE. **3** *Knowing the source of SE will help guide the initial antiepileptic therapy and increase the probability of halting seizure activity.*

In patients with epilepsy who use AEDs, a baseline serum concentration may be useful to determine if the drug concentration is below the desired range and if a loading dose is needed. Albumin levels, renal function tests, and liver function tests can also be used when assessing antiepileptic therapy.

Hypoxia and respiratory or metabolic acidosis are common in patients with SE. Therefore, pulse oximetry and arterial blood gas (ABG) measurements are used to assess respiratory status and determine if airway protection or supplemental oxygen is needed. Metabolic acidosis typically corrects on its own after clinical seizure activity stops, so pharmacologic treatment is not required.

(coma, lethargy, or somnolence), motor function and reflexes (rhythmic contractions, rigidity, spasms, or posturing), and pupillary response. A physical examination to identify secondary injuries from SE should also be conducted.

Clinical Symptoms

Patients with SE usually present with generalized, convulsive tonic-clonic seizure activity. They may also be hypertensive, tachycardic, febrile, and diaphoretic; however, these symptoms

Diagnostic Tests

The only way to determine if a comatose patient has SE is by EEG. Continuous EEG monitoring should be used in patients who remain unconscious after initial antiepileptic treatment and for those who receive long-acting paralytic agents or require prolonged therapy for RSE. Treatment should never be delayed while awaiting EEG results. An electrocardiogram (ECG) should be obtained to rule out cardiac dysfunction when hypotension or an abnormal heart rate is observed.

Patient Encounter 1, Part 2

Physical examination and a review of her chart and recent laboratory studies reveal the following additional information about SR:

PE:

VS: blood pressure 178/92 mm Hg, pulse 109 bpm, respiratory rate 26 breaths/min, temperature 39.0°C (102.2°F)

CNS: Unresponsive, unarousable

CV: Sinus tachycardia; normal S_1, S_2; no murmurs, rubs, gallops

Pulm: Tachypneic; oxygen saturation 88% (0.88) on room air; no rhonchi, wheezes, rales

Abd: Deferred

Exts: Rhythmic tonic-clonic movements of all extremities

GU: Incontinent of urine and stool

HEENT: Persistent upward gaze

Medications

Phenytoin 100 mg IV q 8 h
Famotidine 20 mg IV q 12 h
Metoprolol 50 mg PO q 12 h
Insulin glargine 25 U SQ at bedtime
Insulin aspart 5 U SQ with meals
Acetaminophen/hydrocodone 325 mg/5 mg tablet PO q 4 h as needed for pain
Morphine 2 mg IVP q 2 h as needed for pain

Labs

Sodium 135 mEq/L (135 mmol/L)
Potassium 4.1 mEq/L (4.1 mmol/L)
Phenytoin 8.7 mcg/mL (35 μmol/L)
Albumin 3.5 g/dL (35 g/L)
Chloride 105 mEq/L (105 mmol/L)
Carbon dioxide 12 mEq/L (12 mmol/L)
Blood urea nitrogen 10 mg/dL (3.6 mmol/L)
Serum creatinine 0.9 mg/dL (80 μmol/L)
Glucose 54 mg/dL (3.0 mmol/L)
WBC 15 × 10³/mm³ (15 × 10⁹/L)
Hemoglobin 9.6 g/dL (96 g/L or 5.96 mmol/L)
Hematocrit 28% (0.28 volume fraction)
Platelets 235 × 10³/mm³ (235 × 10⁹/L)
Prothrombin time 12 seconds
International normalized ratio 1.1
Activated partial thromboplastin time 28 seconds

What is your assessment of the cause of this patient's condition?

Identify your goals of therapy for this patient.

What therapies must be instituted next?

TREATMENT

Desired Outcomes

④ *The goal of therapy is to terminate physical and electroencephalographic evidence of seizures, prevent their recurrence, and minimize adverse drug events.* Poor outcomes have been associated with longer duration of SE or the development of refractory SE.[8] Complications of SE should also be treated.

General Approach

● The initial approach to SE involves first removing the patient from harmful surroundings and ensuring a safe airway to prevent respiratory collapse or aspiration. A benzodiazepine is the first medication administered (emergent therapy) because benzodiazepines are the drugs of choice to stop acute seizure activity, followed by the initiation of an AED (urgent therapy) for continued suppression of seizures. Medications are typically given IV for immediate onset of action, but if no IV access is available, select medications may be given rectally, intramuscularly (IM), buccally, or nasally. Once the seizures stop, clinicians must identify and treat any underlying cause of the seizures, such as toxins, hypoglycemia, or brain injury. Patients with known seizure disorders should be evaluated for abrupt cessation of their medications or for history of noncompliance.

Nonpharmacologic Treatment

Nondrug interventions include administration of oxygen or intubation for mechanical ventilation in cases of hypoxia or body cooling for febrile seizures. Specialists in neurology or epileptology should be consulted as appropriate. Admission to an intensive care unit (ICU) allows appropriate monitoring during the seizure and postictal period.

Pharmacologic Treatment

▶ Initial Treatment

All patients suspected of having hypoglycemia-induced SE should receive IV dextrose. In patients with a history of alcohol abuse, IV thiamine 100 mg should be given prior to the administration of any dextrose-containing solutions to prevent encephalopathy.

▶ Benzodiazepines

⑤ *Initial or emergent drug therapy begins with the administration of an IV benzodiazepine, a class of agents that is highly effective in aborting seizure activity.*[9,10] IV bolus doses of diazepam, lorazepam, and midazolam have all been used in SE because of their rapid effects on GABA receptors in the CNS. Lorazepam is now considered the first-line agent by most clinicians. When treating patients on chronic benzodiazepine therapy, clinicians should consider using higher doses to overcome the effects of tolerance. Diazepam and lorazepam should be diluted with normal saline in a 1:1 ratio before parenteral administration via peripheral veins to avoid venous irritation from the propylene glycol diluent in the formulation.

Diazepam Extremely lipophilic, diazepam penetrates quickly into the CNS but rapidly redistributes out into the body fat and muscle. This results in a faster decline in CNS levels and early recurrence of seizures. It is dosed at 5 to 10 mg (or 0.15 mg/kg) and infused no faster than 5 mg/min. Repeated doses can be given every 5 minutes until seizure activity stops or toxicities are seen (e.g., respiratory depression). Diazepam can also be administered as a rectal suppository, making it possible for nonmedical personnel to provide rapid therapy for seizures that develop at home or in public areas.[11] The adult dose is 10 mg given rectally, and this dose may be repeated once if necessary. Diazepam is erratically absorbed via the IM route; therefore, IM administration is not recommended.

Lorazepam Less lipophilic than diazepam, lorazepam has a longer redistribution half-life, resulting in longer duration of action and a decrease in the need for repeated doses. Both lorazepam and diazepam are effective in stopping seizures,[12] but lorazepam is currently the preferred agent due to a longer duration of action. Lorazepam is given as a single IV dose of 0.1 mg/kg (up to 4 mg/dose) with a maximum rate of infusion of 2 mg/min. It can be redosed every 5 to 10 minutes (up to a maximum cumulative dose of 8 mg) until seizure activity stops or side effects such as respiratory depression occur. IM administration is not preferred due to slow and unpredictable absorption.

Midazolam Midazolam is water soluble and can be administered IM,[13] buccally,[14,15] and nasally.[16,17] At physiologic pH, it becomes more lipophilic and can diffuse into the CNS. Compared with diazepam and lorazepam, it has fewer effects on the respiratory and cardiovascular systems. Its short half-life requires that it be redosed frequently or administered as a continuous IV infusion. Midazolam is given at a dose of 0.2 mg/kg IM as a single dose, up to a maximum dose of 10 mg. The liquid or injectable formulation can be given buccally or intranasally (0.3 mg/kg) in pediatric patients.

Patient Encounter 2, Part 1

DB is a 26-year-old man admitted for intractable headaches for the last 4 weeks. He does not take any medications and has no allergies to medications. The CT scan of his head reveals a large right frontal lobe mass. While the nurse is taking his vital signs, he becomes confused and then unarousable with jerky movements in all of his extremities. His diagnosis is status epilepticus.

VS: blood pressure 102/65 mm Hg, pulse 112 beats/min, respiratory rate 23 breaths/min, temperature 37.0°C (98.6°F), Wt 85 kg (187 lb), Ht 173 cm (5'8")

What is the most likely cause of this patient's SE?

What possible treatment options exist at this time?

How would you optimize this patient's outcome?

Nasal administration in SE can be hindered by rapid breathing and increased nasal secretions. A recent study in adults and children showed that IM midazolam was as safe and effective as IV lorazepam for prehospital administration for seizure cessation.[17]

▶ Anticonvulsants

⑥ *Once the first dose of benzodiazepine is given, an AED such as phenytoin (or fosphenytoin), valproate sodium, or phenobarbital should be started to prevent further seizures from occurring (urgent therapy).* AEDs must not be given as first-line therapy because they are infused relatively slowly to avoid adverse effects, delaying their onset of action. If the underlying cause of the seizures has been corrected (e.g., hypoglycemia) and seizure activity has ceased, an AED may not be necessary. This may be reasonable when patients are completely alert and oriented or if an EEG confirms absence of ongoing seizure activity.

Once the loading dose of the AED is administered, it is important to initiate maintenance doses to ensure that therapeutic levels are sustained. Chronic and idiosyncratic side effects as well as potential drug interactions should be considered if the patient will continue AED therapy indefinitely. All drugs should be adjusted for any hepatic or renal disease states. Table 32–1 summarizes the drug doses used in SE, and Table 32–2 provides an example of an algorithm for the treatment of patients in SE.

Phenytoin The most widely used AED for the urgent treatment of SE is phenytoin, which is available in its original form or as a prodrug, fosphenytoin, which is described later. Phenytoin is administered IV as a loading dose (for patients previously not on phenytoin) of 15 to 20 mg/kg. The loading dose must be modified in patients taking phenytoin who have subtherapeutic levels in order to avoid toxic serum concentrations. The loading dose is infused no faster than 50 mg/min due to potential risks of hypotension or arrhythmias. Continuous monitoring of ECG and blood pressure is recommended. Maintenance dosing can be started 12 hours after the loading dose. Phenytoin should not be infused with other medications because of stability concerns (it is soluble in propylene glycol and compatible only in 0.9% sodium chloride solutions). It should not be given via the IM route due to its alkaline nature. Extravasation of the drug can cause local tissue discoloration, edema, pain, and sometimes necrosis (purple glove syndrome). Oral loading is not recommended in SE due to the limitations of single-dose absorption (i.e., doses greater than approximately 400 mg are not fully absorbed) and delayed peak concentrations when given by this route.

Fosphenytoin Fosphenytoin is a water-soluble, phosphoester prodrug that is rapidly converted to phenytoin in the body. It is compatible with most IV solutions. It is dosed in phenytoin equivalents (PEs), and it can be infused three times as fast as phenytoin, up to 150 mg PE/min. The loading dose for patients not taking phenytoin is 15 to 20 mg

Table 32-1

Parenteral Medications Used in Status Epilepticus in Adults

Drug Name (Brand Name)	Loading Dose and RSE Maintenance Dose (If Applicable)	Administration Rate	Therapeutic Level	Side Effects	Comments
Diazepam (Valium)	0.15 mg/kg (up to 10 mg/dose)	5 mg/min (IVP)	N/A	Hypotension, respiratory depression	Rapid redistribution rate; can be given rectally
Lorazepam (Ativan)	0.1 mg/kg (up to 4 mg/dose)	2 mg/min (IVP)	N/A	Hypotension, respiratory depression	May be longer-acting than diazepam
Midazolam (Versed)	0.2 mg/kg IM up to 10 mg/dose RSE: 0.2 mg/kg (2 mg/min) IV then 0.05–2 mg/kg/h		N/A	Sedation, respiratory depression	Can also be given buccally, intranasally; expensive
Phenytoin (Dilantin)	15–20 mg/kg	Up to 50 mg/min	10–20 mcg/mL (40–79.2 μmol/L)	Arrhythmias, hypotension,	Hypotension, especially in elderly
Fosphenytoin (Cerebyx)	15–20 mg PE/kg	Up to 150 mg PE/min	10–20 mcg/mL of phenytoin (40–79.2 μmol/L)	Paresthesias, hypotension	Less CV side effects than phenytoin
Phenobarbital (Luminal)	15–20 mg/kg	50–100 mg/min	15–40 mcg/mL (65–172 μmol/L)	Hypotension, sedation, respiratory depression	Long acting
Valproate sodium (Depacon)	15–20 mg/kg (up to 40 mg/kg)	3–6 mg/kg/min	50–150 mcg/mL (347–1039 μmol/L)		Less CV side effects than phenytoin
Propofol (Diprivan)	1–2 mg/kg RSE: 30–250 mcg/kg/min	Approximately 40 mg q 10 s	N/A (typically titrated to EEG)	Hypotension, respiratory depression	Requires mechanical intubation; high lipid load (increased calories); propofol-related infusion syndrome
Pentobarbital (Nembutal)	10–15 mg/kg RSE: 0.5 – 4 mg/kg/h	Up to 50 mg/min	10–20 mcg/mL (44–89 μmol/L) (typically titrated to EEG)	Hypotension, respiratory depression, cardiac depression, infection, ileus	Requires mechanical intubation, vasopressors, hemodynamic monitoring

CV, cardiovascular; EEG, electroencephalogram; IM, intramuscular; IVP, intravenous push; N/A, not applicable; PE, phenytoin equivalents.

PE/kg. Although it has fewer cardiovascular side effects than phenytoin, clinicians should still continuously monitor blood pressure, ECG, and heart rate. Maintenance doses are begun 12 hours after the loading dose. A common side effect is paresthesias, especially around the lips and groin, which typically resolve within a few minutes and should not necessitate stopping the infusion. If a postload serum level is desired, it should be obtained 2 hours after an IV load. Generic fosphenytoin is now available, so increased expense is no longer an issue.

Phenobarbital If phenytoin or fosphenytoin fails to prevent seizure recurrence, phenobarbital can be considered. However, emerging evidence suggests that phenobarbital may not be effective if SE persists after giving benzodiazepines and phenytoin. This may be due to the progressive resistance of the $GABA_A$ receptor, where barbiturates also act.[18] It is dosed as an IV load of 15 to 20 mg/kg with a maximum rate of administration of 100 mg/min. Adverse reactions of phenobarbital include sedation, hypotension, and respiratory depression; therefore, patients who receive a rapid

IV loading dose of phenobarbital should have hemodynamic monitoring and be mechanically ventilated if at high risk of respiratory compromise. Its long half-life makes it a popular agent for both acute treatment and chronic maintenance therapy or as adjunct therapy to prevent withdrawal seizures when weaning refractory SE patients off pentobarbital continuous infusions.

Valproate Sodium Although valproate sodium is not FDA approved for SE, its IV use has been documented in various types of SE including generalized tonic-clonic, myoclonic, and nonconvulsive SE.[19] One study comparing it with phenytoin found similar efficacy (80% cessation of seizure activity) but with less cardiopulmonary side effects.[20] Additional studies also support its use for urgent therapy,[21,22] especially in patients who are not intubated and/or are allergic to phenytoin and phenobarbital.[23] Valproate sodium can be loaded IV at 15 to 20 mg/kg and infused at a rate of up to 6 mg/kg/min. Higher doses (up to 30 to 40 mg/kg) have also been used to attain serum levels of 100 to 150 mcg/mL (693 to 1039 μmol/L) in less responsive cases of SE.[24]

Table 32–2

Algorithm for Treatment of Status Epilepticus in Adults

Time (minutes)	Assessment/Monitoring	Treatment
0	Vital signs (HR, RR, BP, T) Assess airway Monitor cardiac function (ECG) Pulse oximeter Check blood glucose Check laboratory tests: complete blood count, serum chemistries, liver function tests, arterial blood gas, blood cultures, serum anticonvulsant levels, urine drug/alcohol screen	Stabilize airway (intubate if necessary) Administer oxygen Secure IV access and start fluids Give IV thiamine (100 mg), then IV dextrose (50 mL of 50% solution) if hypoglycemic
0–10	Vital signs Physical examination Patient history including medications (prescription, OTC, and herbals)	Lorazepam 0.1 mg/kg (maximum 4 mg) IVP at 2 mg/min (may repeat in 5–10 minutes to maximum of 8 mg if no response) If no IV access, can give: diazepam 10 mg PR (may repeat in 10 minutes if no response); midazolam 0.2 mg/kg IM (maximum 10 mg; may repeat in 10 minutes if no response) AED may not be necessary if underlying cause is corrected and seizures have ceased
10–20	Vital signs Review laboratory results and correct any underlying abnormalities CT scan (if seizures controlled)	Phenytoin 15–20 mg/kg IV at a maximum rate of 50 mg/min (or fosphenytoin 15–20 mg PE/kg IV at a maximum rate of 150 mg/min) In patients allergic to phenytoin, give valproate sodium 20 mg/kg IV at a maximum rate of 6 mg/kg/min Treat for possible infection
20–30	Vital signs Consult neurologist/epileptologist Consider admission to ICU Consider EEG	If seizures continue: additional phenytoin bolus 5–10 mg/kg (or fosphenytoin 5–10 mg PE/kg) or start phenobarbital at 20 mg/kg IV at a maximum rate of 100 mg/min or start valproate sodium 20 mg/kg IV at a maximum rate of 6 mg/kg/min in patients who are not intubated
Greater than 30–60 *refractory status epilepticus*	Vital signs Transfer to ICU Obtain EEG Consider MRI when controlled	Midazolam 0.2 mg/kg IV bolus followed by 0.05–2 mg/kg/h CI *or* propofol 1 mg/kg bolus followed by 30–250 mcg/kg/min CI *or* pentobarbital 10–15 mg/kg bolus over 1–2 hours followed by 0.5–4 mg/kg/h Consider intubation and/or vasopressor support if needed Optimize AED levels: repeat boluses of phenobarbital 10 mg/kg *or* valproate sodium 20 mg/kg at 6 mg/kg/min max

BP, blood pressure; CI, continuous infusion; CT, computed tomography; ECG, electrocardiogram; EEG, electroencephalography; HR, heart rate; ICU, intensive care unit; IVP, intravenous push; OTC, over the counter; MRI, magnetic resonance imaging; PE, phenytoin equivalents; PR, per rectum; RR, respiratory rate; T, temperature.

Treatment of Refractory Status Epilepticus

⑦ *Seizure activity that does not respond to benzodiazepines (emergent therapy) and antiepileptics (urgent therapy) or persists beyond 30 to 60 minutes in duration can be considered RSE.*[25] RSE can occur in up to 30% of patients with SE and has a mortality rate approaching 50%. Patients in RSE are unlikely to return to their baseline state, even if the seizures are eventually controlled. As RSE progresses, clinical signs may become subtle, and in certain patients, an EEG is required to detect ongoing seizure activity. ❶ *Even SE patients without clinical signs of seizing are at risk for brain damage or even death.*

The optimal therapy for RSE has not been determined.[26] Clinicians must aggressively investigate and treat possible causes including infection, tumors, drugs or toxins, metabolic disorders, liver failure, or fever. In general, patients with RSE are managed in an ICU where hemodynamic and respiratory support are available and frequent monitoring

Patient Encounter 2, Part 2

Over the next hour, DB is treated with your recommendations for emergent and urgent treatment as above. His jerky movements have stopped, but he remains comatose. His breathing is shallow and slow, and his oxygen saturation is 90% (0.90).

VS: blood pressure 101/72 mm Hg, pulse 98 beats/min, respiratory rate 10 breaths/min, temperature 37.0°C (98.6°F)

What is your assessment of the patient's condition at this time?

What recommendations for further drug therapy would you make?

How would you optimize his outcome?

can be performed. Continuous EEG monitoring is essential to document cessation of seizure activity and should not be delayed. Any AEDs initiated before treatment for RSE should be continued and their serum levels optimized to minimize any breakthrough or withdrawal seizures. ❽ *Treatment of RSE typically consists of intensive monitoring, supportive care, and a continuous IV infusion of midazolam, propofol, or pentobarbital to suppress all clinical and EEG evidence of seizures.*[27] These agents are typically titrated to achieve "burst suppression" on the EEG, although no strong evidence exists to support this as the universal goal. Patients should be intubated and mechanically ventilated before initiating these treatment strategies for RSE. Consultation with a neurologist or epileptologist is highly recommended in these cases.

▶ Midazolam

A loading dose of 0.2 mg/kg IV (repeated up to a maximum of 2 mg/kg) followed by a continuous infusion of 0.05 to 2 mg/kg/h is recommended in RSE.[28,29] The dose must be adjusted during prolonged infusions, especially in patients with renal impairment, because the active metabolite can accumulate.[30] Breakthrough seizures are common with midazolam infusions and usually respond to a bolus and a 20% increase in the infusion rate. Despite this, tachyphylaxis can occur, and the patient should be switched to another agent if seizures continue.

▶ Propofol

The anesthetic agent propofol can be started with loading doses of 1 to 2 mg/kg repeated every 3 to 5 minutes until a clinical response is achieved, after which the infusion can be initiated at 30 to 60 mcg/kg/min. Propofol can cause hypotension, especially with loading doses; therefore, some clinicians avoid loading doses and go directly to continuous infusion propofol and rapidly titrate it to effect. Long-term, high-dose (>80 mcg/kg/min) propofol infusions are associated with rhabdomyolysis, acidosis, and cardiac arrhythmias (propofol-related infusion syndrome), especially in children.[31,32] Propofol has a very short serum half-life and should be tapered off slowly to avoid withdrawal seizures. High-dose propofol infusions can also provide a considerable amount of calories (1 kcal/mL) over time, so other sources of nutrition may have to be adjusted accordingly.

▶ Pentobarbital

Barbiturate infusions have been reported to be highly successful in treating RSE,[33] but their side effects are considerable. They can cause significant hypotension, myocardial and respiratory depression, ileus, and infection (especially gram-positive organisms). As a result, patients require mechanical ventilation and invasive hemodynamic monitoring. In addition, they also often require IV vasopressor therapy and total parenteral nutrition while undergoing "barbiturate coma." However, barbiturates are beneficial in decreasing elevated intracranial pressure (ICP).

Pentobarbital is commonly loaded at a dose of 10 to 15 mg/kg over 1 to 2 hours, followed by a continuous infusion of 0.5 to 4 mg/kg/h. Therapy can be tapered off after 12 to 24 hours of seizure control as evident on EEG.[34] One meta-analysis reported a lower incidence of treatment failure with pentobarbital (3%) when compared with midazolam (21%) or propofol (20%), although the risk of hypotension requiring vasopressor therapy was higher with pentobarbital.[33] This relative efficacy for pentobarbital must be considered together with its complications when determining which agent to use. Patients who fail midazolam and/or propofol infusions should be switched over to pentobarbital therapy.

▶ Levetiracetam

Although not FDA-approved for SE, levetiracetam is a newer AED that does not have the significant cardiopulmonary, hepatic, and sedative side effects seen with the other agents; nor does it have potentially harmful drug interactions. Both IV[35] and oral[36] formulations have been used in RSE patients as add-on therapy with some success, although it is unclear if levetiracetam would be effective as a single agent in these cases.[37] Loading doses of up to 2000 mg over 15 to 30 minutes in the critically ill have been documented with very little toxicity noted.[38]

▶ Other Agents

Ketamine,[39] topiramate, and inhaled anesthetics have also been used to treat RSE. Ketamine is an NMDA receptor antagonist that has been given orally[40] and IV[41] for RSE in children. Topiramate is an oral AED with multiple mechanisms of action that may have some benefit in RSE. The oral dose in adults ranges from 300 to 1600 mg/day.[42] Children have also been administered topiramate at a starting dose of 2 to 3 mg/kg/day and titrated to a maintenance dose of 5 to 6 mg/kg/day.[43] Topiramate can induce metabolic acidosis, which should be monitored carefully. The inhaled anesthetics, desflurane and isoflurane,[44] are normally delivered in an operating room, and they require special equipment for administration in an ICU. One of the newest agents that have been used in RSE is lacosamide, an enhancer of slow inhibition of sodium channels with limited drug interactions.[45] It has been used both orally[46] and IV[47] in the setting of refractory partial SE. Future studies are needed to determine the place of these agents in therapy.

Special Populations

Certain patient populations require special considerations due to their altered metabolism, unique volume of distribution, or increased risk for side effects.[48] Although many of these patients are excluded from clinical trials in SE, the standard algorithm for SE still applies in terms of immediate care, assessment, and drugs (see Table 32–2).

▶ Pediatrics

The treatment approach of SE in children is similar to that in adults with a few exceptions (Table 32–3). The doses are also weight based but are typically higher than those used in adults due to higher clearance by the liver. It may be

Table 32–3

Drugs Used in Pediatric Status Epilepticus

Drug	Dose	Comments
Diazepam (Valium injection, Diastat rectal gel)	IV: 0.2–0.3 mg/kg over 2–5 minutes	Maximum dose in children less than 5 years: 5 mg
		Maximum dose in children greater than 5 years: 15 mg
	PR: 2–5 years: 0.5 mg/kg 6–11 years: 0.3 mg/kg More than 12 years: 0.2 mg/kg	A second rectal dose can be given 4–12 hours after the first dose if necessary
Lorazepam (Ativan)	0.05–0.1 mg/kg IV over 2–4 minutes	May redose twice in 10–15 minutes if necessary
Midazolam (Versed)	0.2 mg/kg IV bolus followed by 0.05–0.6 mg/kg/h continuous infusion	Bolus dose may also be given intranasally, buccally, or intramuscularly
Phenytoin (Dilantin)	15–20 mg/kg IV at 1–3 mg/kg/min *max*	
Fosphenytoin (Cerebyx)	15–20 mg PE/kg IV at 3 mg/kg/min *max*	
Phenobarbital (Luminal)	15–20 mg/kg IV at 100 mg/min *max*	
Valproate sodium (Depacon)	15–20 mg/kg IV at 1.5–3 mg/kg/min	May have fewer cardiovascular side effects than other agents
Propofol (Diprivan)		Not recommended due to adverse events (e.g., propofol-related infusion syndrome)
Pentobarbital (Nembutal)	10–15 mg/kg IV over 1–2 hours followed by continuous infusion at 1 mg/kg/h	Titrated to EEG

PR, per rectum; EEG, electroencephalograph; PE phenytoin equivalent.

difficult to rapidly obtain IV access in children, so alternative routes of drug administration have been studied, including intranasal, buccal, rectal, and IM. Early administration of benzodiazepines and reduced time to hospital admission are important factors in decreasing the incidence of prolonged seizures.[49]

▶ Geriatrics

The elderly are prone to injury and toxicity from multiple concomitant disease states and polypharmacy. Seizures in the elderly can easily arise from metabolic disorders, drug interactions, or even incorrect dosing of medications in patients with impaired renal and hepatic function and decreased protein binding. Clinicians treating elderly patients with SE should investigate drug- and disease state–induced causes because treating these etiologies alone may terminate seizures. Acute treatment with benzodiazepines and AEDs is no different in the elderly, but they may have more pronounced reactions to these medications in terms of their sedative and cardiorespiratory side effects. Phenytoin and fosphenytoin loading doses should be carefully calculated in the elderly because their weights may be overestimated, and they may not tolerate high doses. They should also be infused at slower rates to minimize hypotension and arrhythmias. Phenobarbital may cause respiratory depression earlier in the elderly, especially once benzodiazepines are administered. Clinicians should consider using smaller doses and evaluate for renal and hepatic insufficiency if repeated doses are to be given.

▶ Pregnancy

The main concern in the treatment of pregnant females in SE is the safety of the fetus that is at risk of hypoxia during periods of prolonged seizures. Although many of the agents used in SE are teratogenic, clinicians should still use them as acute measures to stop the seizures and consider alternative agents as maintenance therapy.[50] The volume of distribution and clearance of many drugs are typically increased during pregnancy, which should be considered when calculating doses.

OUTCOME EVALUATION

❹ *The success of treatment is measured by the early termination of seizures without adverse drug effects or brain injury.* Therefore, start pharmacologic treatment as soon as possible.

- First-line (emergent) treatment for SE should halt seizure activity within minutes of administration.

- In patients who are unarousable following treatment, confirm termination of seizures with an EEG.

- Perform a physical examination and evaluation of the patient's laboratory results to help determine if the cause or complications of seizure activity are being appropriately treated.

- Once seizure activity has ceased and the patient has stabilized, review the patient's therapeutic regimen.

- Evaluate and monitor serum trough concentrations of AEDs with defined target ranges to determine patient-specific therapeutic goals.

- Treat known causes of SE and simplify therapy.

- In patients with RSE on multiple AEDs, slowly decrease the dose of one drug at a time while continuing to evaluate the patient for seizure activity.

- Base the titration schedule on the half-life of the drug and individual patient response.

- Optimize treatment using the fewest medications to prevent seizure recurrence without causing adverse drug reactions.

- Continue to monitor AED serum trough concentrations approximately every 3 to 5 days until the AEDs have reached steady-state concentrations.

- Give additional loading doses or hold doses as needed to maintain target trough concentrations.

- Monitor the patient for signs of drug toxicity and seizures until drug concentrations have stabilized.

- Closely evaluate medication profiles, and change drugs or doses to minimize any drug interactions, if possible.

Patient Care and Monitoring

1. Obtain a seizure history from the patient or family members, including precipitating factors and duration of seizure activity.

2. Identify and correct the underlying cause of the seizures, if possible. Does the patient have any laboratory abnormalities? Is there a positive toxicology screen for alcohol or drugs?

3. Obtain a thorough history of nonprescription, prescription, and alternative drug or herbal use. Determine adherence with the medication regimen and whether barriers to care exist. Does the patient have the financial ability and transportation to obtain the prescriptions?

4. Assess the AED serum concentration and adjust therapy as needed for agents with a defined therapeutic range (e.g., phenytoin, carbamazepine, valproic acid, and phenobarbital). Drug levels can also be used to determine adherence to medication regimens for agents that do not have defined ranges. Monitoring free phenytoin concentrations is recommended in critically ill patients with hypoalbuminemia.[51]

5. Evaluate the patient for adverse drug reactions, IV site extravasation, and allergic reactions. What alternative AEDs should be used if a drug allergy is identified?

6. Determine whether there are any drug interactions with the patient's current or home medication regimens. Do you need to adjust the dose of any medications for toxic or subtherapeutic concentrations from the drug interaction?

7. Maintain adequate cardiovascular support, nutrition, and electrolyte and glucose serum concentrations to prevent recurrence of seizure activity.

8. Continue to evaluate the patient for seizure activity and adjust therapy as needed to control seizures and optimize quality of life.

Abbreviations Introduced in This Chapter

ABG	Arterial blood gas
AED	Antiepileptic drug
CSF	Cerebrospinal fluid
CT	Computed tomography
ECG	Electrocardiogram
EEG	Electroencephalography
GABA	γ-Aminobutyric acid
GCSE	Generalized convulsive status epilepticus
ICP	Intracranial pressure
ICU	Intensive care unit
IM	Intramuscular
MRI	Magnetic resonance imaging
NCSE	Nonconvulsive status epilepticus
NMDA	*N*-methyl-D-aspartate
PE	Phenytoin equivalent
RSE	Refractory status epilepticus
SE	Status epilepticus
WBC	White blood cell

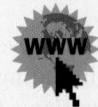 Self-assessment questions and answers are available at *http://www.mhpharmacotherapy. com/pp.html.*

REFERENCES

1. Lowenstein DH, Bleck T, Macdonald RL. It's time to revise the definition of status epilepticus. Epilepsia 1999;40:120–122.
2. Lowenstein DH, Alldredge BK. Status epilepticus. N Engl J Med 1998;338:970–976.
3. DeLorenzo RJ, Pellock JM, Towne AR, Boggs JG. Epidemiology of status epilepticus. J Clin Neurophysiol 1995;12:316–325.
4. Penberthy LT, Towne A, Garnett LK, Perlin JB, DeLorenzo RJ. Estimating the economic burden of status epilepticus to the health care system. Seizure 2005;14:46–51.
5. Wu YW, Shek DW, Garcia PA, Zhao S, Johnston SC. Incidence and mortality of generalized convulsive status epilepticus in California. Neurology 2002;58:1070–1076.
6. Chen JW, Naylor DE, Wasterlain CG. Advances in the pathophysiology of status epilepticus. Acta Neurol Scand Suppl 2007;186:7–15.
7. Huff JS, Fountain NB. Pathophysiology and definitions of seizures and status epilepticus. Emerg Med Clin North Am 2011;29:1–13.
8. Legriel S, Azoulay E, Resche-Rigon M, et al. Functional outcome after convulsive status epilepticus. Crit Care Med 2010;38:2295–2303.
9. Treiman DM, Meyers PD, Walton NY, et al. A comparison of four treatments for generalized convulsive status epilepticus. Veterans Affairs Status Epilepticus Cooperative Study Group. N Engl J Med 1998;339:792–798.
10. Alldredge BK, Gelb AM, Isaacs SM, et al. A comparison of lorazepam, diazepam, and placebo for the treatment of out-of-hospital status epilepticus. N Engl J Med 2001;345:631–637.
11. Fitzgerald BJ, Okos AJ, Miller JW. Treatment of out-of-hospital status epilepticus with diazepam rectal gel. Seizure 2003;12:52–55.
12. Cock HR, Schapira AH. A comparison of lorazepam and diazepam as initial therapy in convulsive status epilepticus. QJM 2002;95:225–231.
13. Towne AR, DeLorenzo RJ. Use of intramuscular midazolam for status epilepticus. J Emerg Med 1999;17:323–328.

14. Scott RC, Besag FM, Boyd SG, Berry D, Neville BG. Buccal absorption of midazolam: Pharmacokinetics and EEG pharmacodynamics. Epilepsia 1998;39:290–294.

15. Kutlu NO, Dogrul M, Yakinci C, Soylu H. Buccal midazolam for treatment of prolonged seizures in children. Brain Dev 2003;25:275–278.

16. Knoester PD, Jonker DM, Van Der Hoeven RT, et al. Pharmacokinetics and pharmacodynamics of midazolam administered as a concentrated intranasal spray. A study in healthy volunteers. Br J Clin Pharmacol 2002;53:501–507.

17. Silbergleit R, Durkalski V, Lowenstein D, et al., for the NETT Investigators. Intramuscular versus intravenous therapy for prehospital status epilepticus. N Engl J Med 2012;366:591–600.

18. Mazarati AM, Baldwin RA, Sankar R, Wasterlain CG. Time-dependent decrease in the effectiveness of antiepileptic drugs during the course of self-sustaining status epilepticus. Brain Res 1998;814:179–185.

19. Limdi NA, Shimpi AV, Faught E, Gomez CR, Burneo JG. Efficacy of rapid IV administration of valproic acid for status epilepticus. Neurology 2005;64:353–355.

20. Agarwal P, Kumar N, Chandra R, Gupta G, Antony AR, Garg N. Randomized study of intravenous valproate and phenytoin in status epilepticus. Seizure 2007;16:527–532.

21. Misra UK, Kalita J, Patel R. Sodium valproate vs phenytoin in status epilepticus: A pilot study. Neurology 2006;67:340–342.

22. Gilad R, Izkovitz N, Dabby R, et al. Treatment of status epilepticus and acute repetitive seizures with I.V. valproic acid vs phenytoin. Acta Neurol Scand 2008;118:296–300.

23. Alvarez V, Januel JM, Burnand B, Rossetti AO. Second-line status epilepticus treatment: Comparison of phenytoin, valproate, and levetiracetam. Epilepsia 2011;52:1292–1296.

24. Uberall MA, Trollmann R, Wunsiedler U, Wenzel D. Intravenous valproate in pediatric epilepsy patients with refractory status epilepticus. Neurology 2000;54:2188–2189.

25. Mayer SA, Claassen J, Lokin J, Mendelsohn F, Dennis LJ, Fitzsimmons BF. Refractory status epilepticus: Frequency, risk factors, and impact on outcome. Arch Neurol 2002;59:205–210.

26. Holtkamp M. Treatment strategies for refractory status epilepticus. Curr Opin Crit Care 2011;17:94–100.

27. Shorvon S. Super-refractory status epilepticus: An approach to therapy in this difficult clinical situation. Epilepsia 2011;52 (Suppl 8):53–56.

28. Claassen J, Hirsch LJ, Emerson RG, Bates JE, Thompson TB, Mayer SA. Continuous EEG monitoring and midazolam infusion for refractory nonconvulsive status epilepticus. Neurology 2001;57:1036–1042.

29. Ulvi H, Yoldas T, Mungen B, Yigiter R. Continuous infusion of midazolam in the treatment of refractory generalized convulsive status epilepticus. Neurol Sci 2002;23:177–182.

30. Naritoku DK, Sinha S. Prolongation of midazolam half-life after sustained infusion for status epilepticus. Neurology 2000;54:1366–1368.

31. Kang TM. Propofol infusion syndrome in critically ill patients. Ann Pharmacother 2002;36:1453–1456.

32. Iyer VN, Hoel R, Rabinstein AA. Propofol infusion syndrome in patients with refractory status epilepticus: An 11-year clinical experience. Crit Care Med 2009;37:3024–3030.

33. Claassen J, Hirsch LJ, Emerson RG, Mayer SA. Treatment of refractory status epilepticus with pentobarbital, propofol, or midazolam: A systematic review. Epilepsia 2002;43:146–153.

34. Krishnamurthy KB, Drislane FW. Depth of EEG suppression and outcome in barbiturate anesthetic treatment for refractory status epilepticus. Epilepsia 1999;40:759–762.

35. Moddel G, Bunten S, Dobis C, et al. Intravenous levetiracetam: A new treatment alternative for refractory status epilepticus. J Neurol Neurosurg Psychiatry 2009;80:689–692.

36. Patel NC, Landan IR, Levin J, Szaflarski J, Wilner AN. The use of levetiracetam in refractory status epilepticus. Seizure 2006;15:137–141.

37. Knake S, Gruener J, Hattemer K, et al. Intravenous levetiracetam in the treatment of benzodiazepine refractory status epilepticus. J Neurol Neurosurg Psychiatry 2008;79:588–589.

38. Ruegg S, Naegelin Y, Hardmeier M, Winkler DT, Marsch S, Fuhr P. Intravenous levetiracetam: Treatment experience with the first 50 critically ill patients. Epilepsy Behav 2008;12:477–480.

39. Borris DJ, Bertram EH, Kapur J. Ketamine controls prolonged status epilepticus. Epilepsy Res 2000;42:117–122.

40. Mewasingh LD, Sekhara T, Aeby A, Christiaens FJ, Dan B. Oral ketamine in paediatric non-convulsive status epilepticus. Seizure 2003;12:483–489.

41. Sheth RD, Gidal BE. Refractory status epilepticus: Response to ketamine. Neurology 1998;51:1765–1766.

42. Towne AR, Garnett LK, Waterhouse EJ, Morton LD, DeLorenzo RJ. The use of topiramate in refractory status epilepticus. Neurology 2003;60:332–334.

43. Kahriman M, Minecan D, Kutluay E, Selwa L, Beydoun A. Efficacy of topiramate in children with refractory status epilepticus. Epilepsia 2003;44:1353–1356.

44. Mirsattari SM, Sharpe MD, Young GB. Treatment of refractory status epilepticus with inhalational anesthetic agents isoflurane and desflurane. Arch Neurol 2004;61:1254–1259.

45. Kellinghaus C, Berning S, Immisch I, et al. Intravenous lacosamide for treatment of status epilepticus. Acta Neurol Scand 2011;123:137–141.

46. Tilz C, Resch R, Hofer T, Eggers C. Successful treatment for refractory convulsive status epilepticus by non-parenteral lacosamide. Epilepsia 2010;51:316–317.

47. Goodwin H, Hinson HE, Shermock KM, Karanjia N, Lewin JJ 3rd. The use of lacosamide in refractory status epilepticus. Neurocrit Care 2011;14:348–353.

48. Leppik IE. Treatment of epilepsy in 3 specialized populations. Am J Manag Care 2001;7:S221–S226.

49. Chin RF, Neville BG, Peckham C, Wade A, Bedford H, Scott RC. Treatment of community-onset, childhood convulsive status epilepticus: A prospective, population-based study. Lancet Neurol 2008;7:696–703.

50. Molgaard-Nielsen D, Hviid A. Newer-generation antiepileptic drugs and the risk of major birth defects. JAMA 2011;305:1996–2002.

51. Tesoro EP, Brophy GM. Pharmacological management of seizures and status epilepticus in critically ill patients. J Pharm Pract 2010;23:441–454.

33 Parkinson's Disease

Mary L. Wagner and Jamie C. Holmes

LEARNING OBJECTIVES

● **Upon completion of the chapter, the reader will be able to:**

1. Describe the pathophysiology of Parkinson's disease (PD) related to neurotransmitter involvement and targets for drug therapy in the brain.

2. Recognize the cardinal motor symptoms of PD and determine a patient's clinical status and disease progression based on the Unified Parkinson's Disease Rating Scale (UPDRS).

3. For a patient initiating therapy for PD, recommend appropriate drug therapy and construct patient-specific treatment goals.

4. Recognize and recommend appropriate treatment for nonmotor symptoms.

5. Formulate a plan to minimize patient "off-time" and maximize "on-time" including timing, dosage, and frequency of medications.

6. Recognize and treat various motor complications that develop as PD progresses.

7. Construct appropriate patient counseling regarding medications and lifestyle modifications for a patient with PD.

8. Develop a monitoring plan to assess effectiveness and adverse effects of treatment.

KEY CONCEPTS

❶ Parkinson's disease (PD) is a slow, progressive neurodegenerative disease of the extrapyramidal motor system that features classic motor symptoms of tremor, rigidity, akinesia/bradykinesia, and postural/gait instability (TRAP).

❷ The most useful diagnostic tool is the clinical history, including both presenting symptoms and associated risk factors. The Unified Parkinson's Disease Rating Scale (UPDRS) is used to define the degree of disability.

❸ The goals of treatment are to maintain patient independence, activities of daily living (ADLs), and quality of life (QOL) by alleviating the patient's symptoms, minimizing the development of response fluctuations, and limiting medication-related adverse effects.

❹ The treatment of PD is categorized into three types: (1) lifestyle changes, nutrition, and exercise; (2) pharmacologic intervention, primarily with drugs that enhance dopamine concentrations; and (3) surgical treatments for those who fail pharmacologic interventions.

❺ Drug therapy is aimed at enhancing dopaminergic activity in the substantia nigra. The best time to initiate dopaminergic therapy is controversial and patient specific.

❻ Medication schedules should be individualized. The doses are divided throughout the day to maximize **on time** and minimize **off time.**

❼ The treatment of nonmotor symptoms should be based on whether they are worse during an off state or potentially related to other neurotransmitter dysfunction.

❽ As the disease progresses, most patients develop response fluctuations. Treatment is based on optimizing the pharmacokinetic and pharmacodynamic properties of PD medications.

❾ Patient monitoring should involve a regular systematic evaluation of efficacy and adverse events, referral to appropriate specialists, and patient education.

Parkinson's disease (PD) is a slow, progressive neurodegenerative disease of the extrapyramidal motor system. Dopamine neurons in the substantia nigra are primarily affected, and degeneration of these neurons causes a disruption in the ability to generate body movements. Cardinal features of PD include tremor at rest, rigidity, akinesia/bradykinesia, and postural instability. There is no cure, and treatment is aimed at controlling symptoms and slowing disease progression.

EPIDEMIOLOGY AND ETIOLOGY

PD affects approximately 1 million Americans, with a lifetime risk of developing the disease of 1.5%. The median age of onset is 60 years of age, but about 10% of people with PD are younger than 45 years. There is an estimated mortality ratio of 2:1 in PD, and the average duration of time from diagnosis to death is about 15 years. About 15% of patients with PD have a first-degree relative with the disease.[1,2]

The etiology of neuron degeneration in PD remains unknown, but aging has been implicated as a primary risk factor. Other explanations for cell death may include oxidative stress, mitochondrial dysfunction, increased concentrations of excitotoxic amino acids and inflammatory cytokines, immune system disorders, trophic factor deficiency, signal-mediated apoptosis, and environmental toxins. Genetic mutations such as those in *LRRK2* have been linked to the disease.[2,3] Genetic factors contributing to the development of PD may include mutations in several genes, including glucocerebrosidase, leucine-rich repeat kinase, and *PTEN*-induced putative kinase.[1] These mutations may predict early versus late onset of the disease. It is not certain if genetic mutations alone contribute to the development of PD or if this risk factor is greater when combined with aging, environmental toxins, and oxidative stress, glutamate excitotoxicity, mitochondrial dysfunction, neuroinflammation, and apoptosis.[2] Conditions that may promote oxidative stress include increased monoamine oxidase-B metabolism or decreased glutathione clearance of free radicals.[1-5]

In PD there is a loss of pigmented cells in the substantia nigra that make and store dopamine. When patients are diagnosed, they have lost 50% to 60% of their dopamine neurons in the substantia nigra, and the remaining neurons beyond the substantia nigra in the basal ganglia, spinal cord, and neurocortex may not function well. Neurons have lost about 80% of their activity in the striatum at the onset of PD.

There may be cortical Lewy bodies along with Lewy neurites seen in microscopic samples from the basal ganglia, cortex, brainstem, spinal cord, sympathetic ganglia, cardiac plexus, and GI system that may explain some of the nonmotor symptoms of PD.[2,4,5]

PATHOPHYSIOLOGY

The extrapyramidal motor system controls muscle movement through pathways and nerve tracts that connect the cerebral cortex, basal ganglia, thalamus, cerebellum, reticular formation, and spinal neurons. Patients with PD lose dopamine neurons in the substantia nigra, which is located in the midbrain within the brainstem. The substantia nigra sends nerve fibers up to the corpus striatum, which is part of the basal ganglia in the cerebrum. The corpus striatum is made up of the caudate nucleus and the lentiform nuclei that consist of the pallidum (globus pallidus) and putamen (Fig. 33–1). As dopamine neurons die, dopamine-relayed messages cannot communicate to other motor centers of the brain, and patients develop motor symptoms. A variety of neurotransmitters are active in the basal ganglia including acetylcholine, histamine, glutamate, serotonin, dopamine, norepinephrine, epinephrine, γ-aminobutyric acid (GABA), enkephalins, substance P, and adenosine. Some of these neurotransmitters also decrease in concentration as other brain regions degenerate, resulting in degeneration of norepinephrine neurons in the locus ceruleus and acetylcholine neurons in the nucleus basalis, as well as selected neurons of the dorsal motor nucleus of the vagus, spinal cord, and peripheral autonomic system. Decreases in these neurotransmitters may explain some of the nonmotor symptoms of PD.[2,5,6] For example, loss of dopamine and norepinephrine neurons in the limbic system is associated with depression and anxiety.[7] Loss of acetylcholine, dopamine, norepinephrine, and serotonin, in the substantia nigra, locus coeruleus,

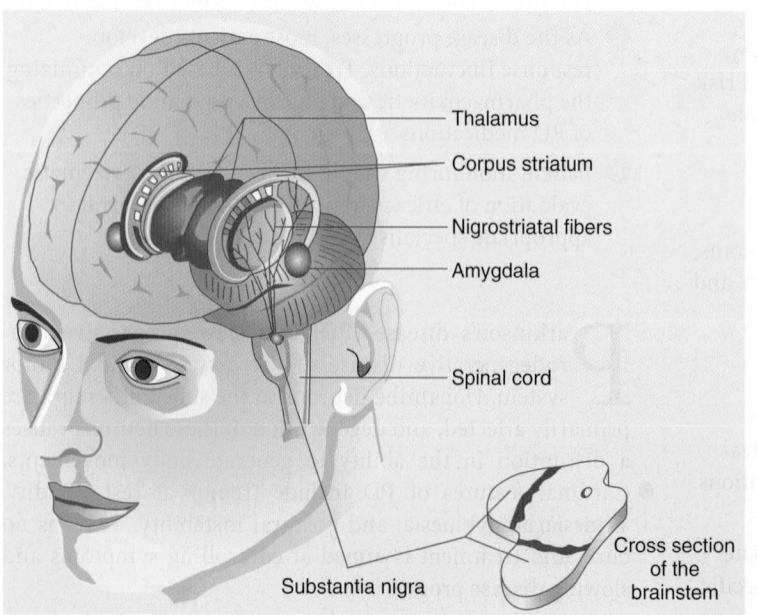

FIGURE 33–1. Anatomy of the extrapyramidal system. The extrapyramidal motor system controls muscle movement through a system of pathways and nerve tracts that connect the cerebral cortex, basal ganglia, thalamus, cerebellum, reticular formation, and spinal neurons. Patients with PD have a loss of dopamine neurons in the substantia nigra in the brainstem that leads to depletion of dopamine in the corpus striatum. The corpus striatum is made up of the caudate nucleus and the lentiform nuclei that are made up of the putamen and the globus pallidus.

Thalamus

Corpus striatum

Nigrostriatal fibers

Amygdala

Spinal cord

Substantia nigra

Cross section of the brainstem

Clinical Presentation of PD

Patients with PD display both motor and nonmotor symptoms. The nonmotor symptoms may precede the motor symptoms.

Motor Symptoms (mnemonic TRAP)

T = Tremor at rest ("pill rolling")

R = Rigidity (stiffness and cogwheel rigidity)

A = Akinesia or bradykinesia

P = Postural instability and gait abnormalities

Nonmotor Symptoms (mnemonic SOAP)

S = Sleep disturbances (insomnia, rapid eye movement sleep behavioral disorder, restless legs syndrome [RLS])

O = Other miscellaneous symptoms (problems with nausea, fatigue, speech, pain, **dysesthesias**, vision, seborrhea)

A = Autonomic symptoms (drooling, constipation, sexual dysfunction, urinary problems, sweating, orthostatic hypotension, dysphagia)

P = Psychological symptoms (anxiety, psychosis, cognitive impairment, depression)

Response Fluctuations (mnemonic MAD)

M = Motor fluctuations (delayed peak, wearing off, random off, freezing)

A = Akathisia

D = Dyskinesias (e.g., chorea, dystonia, diphasic dyskinesia)

Patient Encounter, Part 1: Initial Visit—Medical History

GR, a 60-year-old woman with a 5-year history of PD, comes in for an initial visit at the movement disorder clinic to assess worsening symptoms. She was last seen 6 months ago by her family doctor where her UPDRS score was 35 (while on), and no changes were needed in her medications other than adding a stool softener and fiber laxative for constipation. Since her last visit, she has noticed increased stiffness, slowness, and progression of tremor in both hands instead of one. She tends to have off periods that make it difficult for her to make dinner. She denies any postural problems or falls. She reports some improvement in bowel movements.

Identify this patient's motor and nonmotor symptoms of PD.

What additional information would you collect before creating this patient's treatment plan?

nucleus raphe, and limbic system is associated with cognitive impairment.[7]

Based on patient symptoms, the disease may begin in the autonomic system, olfactory system, or vagus nerve in the lower brainstem and then spread to the upper brainstem and cerebral hemisphere affecting dopamine pathways later in the course of disease progression.[2] It is essential to rule out drug-induced PD before providing treatment because most cases are reversible. Offending agents include drugs that deplete dopamine such as antipsychotics, metoclopramide, and some antiemetics. Treatment includes removal of the offending agent.[8]

CLINICAL PRESENTATION AND DIAGNOSIS

Motor Symptoms

❶ *Parkinson's disease (PD) is a slow, progressive neurodegenerative disease of the extrapyramidal motor system that features classic motor symptoms of tremor, rigidity, akinesia/bradykinesia, and postural/gait instability (TRAP).*

A thorough patient history and detailed description of symptom onset is essential in making an accurate diagnosis of PD. The onset is gradual and presents with impairment of movement that may go unnoticed. The tremor of PD occurs during rest and disappears with purposeful movement. The hand tremor can appear as if the patient is rolling a pill between their fingers. Patients usually describe rigidity as stiffness. Muscles display uniform resistance on examination and seem to be in a constant state of increased tone. Cogwheel rigidity is found when the examiner extends or flexes the patient's extremities and feels as if they are rhythmically hitting a series of teeth on the rim of a wheel. Bradykinesia is noted when there is hesitancy in movement initiation, slowness in movement performance, or rapid fatiguing during movement. Patients may have a decrease in automatic movements, such as eye blinking, hypomimia, or a decrease in arm swing while walking. Postural instability is a result of the loss of reflexes necessary to maintain balance when ambulating and stooped posture. Patients may report feeling unsteady. Gait abnormalities may be evidenced by slow shuffling, leg dragging, festination, propulsion, retropulsion, or freezing. Rigidity and bradykinesia may make handwriting difficult as evidenced by micrographia.[2,9–13]

Nonmotor Symptoms

Nonmotor symptoms associated with PD commonly include sleep disturbances, autonomic impairment in the form of sexual dysfunction or constipation, psychological disturbances such as anxiety or depression, and many miscellaneous symptoms such as anosmia or sensory disturbances. Nonmotor symptoms may be a result of PD itself or medications. Nonmotor symptoms may precede the onset of motor symptoms by many years.[2,6,9,14–20]

Speech problems may manifest as hypophonia, slurring, monotone speech, rapid speech, or stammering. Visual problems such as difficulty reading, double vision, perceptual changes, decreased blink, burning eyes, or itchy eyes are the result of impaired function of the muscles that move the eyeball and decreased retinal dopamine.[2,6,9,10,14]

Because the autonomic system is disturbed in patients with PD, orthostatic hypotension, GI, urinary, sexual, and dermatologic symptoms are common. Patients with orthostatic hypotension may experience dizziness, lightheadedness, fainting upon standing, or fall-related injuries. GI symptoms include constipation and dysphagia due to a slowing of the automatic pattern of contraction and relaxation of the throat muscles. Swallowing difficulties may lead to weight loss, sialorrhea, and aspiration.[14,16] Genitourinary symptoms include incontinence, urgency, and frequency. Symptoms may worsen at night, causing nocturia. Sexual dysfunction includes decreased libido or inability to achieve orgasm in both sexes and erectile or ejaculatory dysfunction in men. Skin symptoms include sweating and intolerance to temperature changes.[2,6,9,14,16]

Psychological symptoms may occur during the natural course of PD, during symptom exacerbation, or as adverse effects from medications. These symptoms may include psychosis, dementia, impaired cognitive function, depression, and anxiety. Psychosis occurs in nearly 30% of PD patients and is exhibited as vivid dreams, hallucinations (usually visual), paranoia, and delusions. Hallucinations may be more common when the patient is in dim light, falling asleep, or upon awakening. Dementia occurs in 20% to 44% of patients. Major depressive disorder occurs in 40% to 50% of PD patients and is likely due to abnormalities in the pathways of the neurotransmitters dopamine and serotonin. Some features of PD, such as the decreased facial expression and bradykinesia, may make the diagnosis of depression more difficult. Anxiety may present as panic attacks, phobia, or generalized anxiety. Anxiety was noted in 66% of patients with motor fluctuations and is often comorbid with depression.[2,7,14,17-19] Psychosis is rarely found in untreated patients with PD and can subsequently present a difficult clinical situation when treated patients experience symptoms such as psychosis. It is likely that this phenomena results from a complex interaction of neurotransmitters, pathology, hypersensitivity to dopamine receptors, as well as changes in other neurotransmitters and brain pathways.[14,17]

Sleep disorders may occur commonly. Patients have abnormal polysomnogram findings ranging from decreases in slow-wave sleep, total sleep time, and sleep efficiency. Disturbances may include excessive daytime sleepiness, insomnia, and abnormal sleep events, such as REM behavior disorder (RBD). Possible etiologies include disease progression, sleep-related motor symptoms, depression, and poor sleep hygiene. Medications such as amantadine and selegiline may worsen insomnia, and dopamine agonists may contribute to somnolence. The loss of neuronal functioning in various pathways related to sleep may contribute to sleep problems in PD patients.[9,14,15]

Motor Complications

Motor complications occur with disease progression, as the patient's dopamine reserves are depleted, and as a complication of treatment, mainly with levodopa. Motor complications include delayed peak response, early and unpredictable "wearing off," freezing, and dyskinesias. Dyskinesias include chorea and dystonia. Risk factors for developing motor complications include younger age at diagnosis, high dosage of levodopa, and longer duration and severity of disease. Wearing off can be visualized by imagining the therapeutic window of levodopa narrowing over time. The therapeutic window is defined as the minimum effective concentration of levodopa required to control PD symptoms ("on" without dyskinesia) and the maximum concentration before experiencing side effects from too much levodopa ("on" with dyskinesia). Early in the disease, plasma concentrations following doses of levodopa are supplemented by the brain's supply of dopamine. Thus, although the plasma half-life of levodopa is 1.5 to 2 hours, the therapeutic effect lasts about 5 hours, and the patient experiences no dyskinesias. As the disease progresses, the therapeutic window narrows, and each dose of levodopa acts unpredictably, with the therapeutic effect lasting only 2 to 3 hours and dyskinesias occurring during the on state.[5,20,21]

2 *The most useful diagnostic tool is the clinical history, including both presenting symptoms and associated risk factors. The Unified Parkinson's Disease Rating Scale (UPDRS) is used to define the degree of disability.*

The patient's degree of disability should be evaluated by using the UPDRS, which has six parts. This clinician-rated scale combines patient history and a physical examination that is performed bilaterally because symptoms may initially appear asymmetric. It evaluates mentation, behavior, mood, ADLs, motor symptoms, and complications of therapy. It also includes the modified Hoehn and Yahr stage of disease and Schwab and England ADL.[22] The modified Hoehn and Yahr staging scale defines eight stages of PD ranging from asymptomatic to wheelchair or bedbound. A copy of the examination can be obtained at *http://www.mdvu.org/library/ratingscales/pd/updrs.pdf.*

TREATMENT
Desired Outcomes

3 *The goals of treatment are to maintain patient independence, activities of daily living (ADLs), and quality of life (QOL) by alleviating the patient's symptoms, minimizing the development of response fluctuations, and limiting medication-related adverse effects.*

General Approach to Treatment

4 *The treatment of PD is categorized into three types: (1) lifestyle changes, nutrition, and exercise; (2) pharmacologic intervention, primarily with drugs that enhance dopamine concentrations; and (3) surgical treatments for those who fail pharmacologic interventions.*

Initial treatment depends largely on the patient's age, risk of adverse effects, degree of physical impairment, and readiness to initiate therapy. The 2002 American Academy of Neurology guidelines[23] and 2006 European National Institute for Health and Clinical Excellence guidelines suggest that symptomatic

Patient Encounter, Part 2: Initial Visit—Physical Examination and Diagnostic Tests

Chief complaint: Increased tremor, stiffness, and slowness

PMH: Constipation >10 years

SH: Retired. Lives with husband and has no children. Drinks a glass of wine a few times per month. Denies smoking.

Meds:

Carbidopa/levodopa 25 mg/100 mg orally at 7 AM, noon, and 7 PM

Docusate sodium 100 mg 2 caps at bedtime

Psyllium unflavored (Metamucil) 1 rounded teaspoon in 8 oz (~240 mL) of juice three times daily

ROS: (–) agitation, depression, or psychosis; (–) N/V/D, HA, dizziness, or pain

PE:

Gen: Flat affect, looks older than stated age, slow, shuffling gait

VS: BP: sitting 125/80 mm Hg, standing 110/80 mm Hg (with no orthostatic symptoms); P 65 bpm, RR 18/min, weight 59 kg (130 lb), height 165 cm (65 inches)

HEENT: Decreased eye blinking and facial expression, CN II-XII intact, PERRLA, TMs intact

CV: RRR, normal S_1, S_2; no murmurs, rubs, gallop

Abd: Soft, nontender, nondistended; (+) bowel sounds, no hepatosplenomegaly

Skin: Normal

Exts: Mild tremor in both hands and feet. Cogwheel rigidity bilateral elbows, no edema

Neuro: Slow, shuffling gait, sensory function intact, normal muscle strength, normal reflexes, alert, mental status exam normal

Rating Scales:

Mini Mental Status Exam (MMSE) = Normal 30/30

Handwriting sample micrographia

UPDRS = 45 while "on"

Labs: Normal metabolic profile and CBC

Given this additional information, what is your assessment of the patient's condition?

Identify treatment goals for the patient.

Describe nonpharmacologic and pharmacologic treatments that are available for the patient.

---

treatment should be delayed until the patient experiences functional disability.[24] Some data, however, suggest that earlier treatment may delay the progression of disease, possibly by normalizing basal ganglia physiology that supports compensatory mechanisms, limiting the neurotoxic changes that occur as dopamine neurons diminish. In support of this, some note that progression of symptoms occurs most rapidly around the time of diagnosis and in early PD, whereas progression of symptoms slows later in the disease.[25,26] Although patients receiving rasagiline early in treatment, or potentially other dopamine medications with longer half-lives, may have better outcomes, the studies have design flaws and inconsistent results.[11,13] Until current clinical practice guidelines are revised, one must consider the pros and cons of delaying pharmacotherapy or starting medications early.[23]

Nonpharmacologic Therapy

► Lifestyle Modifications

Nonpharmacologic therapy including education, support, and lifestyle modifications such as exercise should be started early and continued throughout treatment for PD. These treatments may improve ADLs, gait, balance, and mental health. The most common interventions include maintaining good nutrition, physical condition, and social interactions.[1,27] The multidisciplinary care approach is ideal. Patients should maintain regular visits with their optometrist/ophthalmologist and dentist. PD medications decrease saliva flow, increasing the risk of dental caries.

Dietary modifications improve constipation, nausea, erratic drug absorption, and minimize the risk of aspiration and weight loss. Dieticians help with meal selection, increasing calories, and suggestions for protein intake to maximize medication absorption. Speech therapy may improve swallowing, articulation, and the force of speech.

Physical therapy may improve a patient's strength, activity, and reduce fall risk. An exercise program and activity during the day should minimize daytime sleepiness, possibly improving sleep at night, and may be neuroprotective.[1,28] Occupational therapists provide information about adaptive equipment for the home, specialized clothing, and personal training that can maximize independence, safety, and ADLs. They can help evaluate driving ability, improve handwriting, and train patients to use communication software.

Social workers help patients and families handle disease progression and arrange for special community assistance programs. Family counseling may help patients engage in family activities and minimize family conflicts.

Surgery

Surgical treatment, for patients with inadequate control of motor symptoms despite medical treatment, may decrease symptoms by 40% to 75%. Symptoms of imbalance, akinesia, speech impairment, and freezing do not improve with surgery. Deep-brain stimulation, the surgery of choice, involves electrical stimulation of the globus pallidus and subthalamic nucleus.[2,29,30]

Pharmacologic Therapy

❺ *Drug therapy is aimed at enhancing dopaminergic activity in the substantia nigra. The best time to initiate dopaminergic therapy is controversial and patient specific.* Medications help minimize motor symptoms, improve QOL and ADLs, but they are not curative (Table 33–1).[1,2,31-33] PD patients with optimal treatment still have greater mortality and morbidity than the general population.[1]

❻ *Choice of pharmacologic agent should be individualized based on patient-specific parameters, and dose frequency should be scheduled based on individual response to maximize "on" and minimize "off" time.*

Pharmacologic options for PD include anticholinergics, amantadine, monoamine oxidase type B inhibitors (MAO-B), dopamine agonists, levodopa/carbidopa, and catechol-*O*-methyltransferase (COMT) inhibitors. Because most pharmacologic treatments in PD aim to avoid degeneration of the dopaminergic nigrostriatal pathway, it is essential to understand how all drugs may affect dopamine concentrations (Fig. 33–1). The American Academy of Neurology and the Movement Disorder Society determined that it is reasonable to start treatment with either levodopa, a dopamine precursor, or a dopamine agonist.[10-14]

Choice of agent varies based on clinical experience and patient preference. Starting with a dopamine agonist rather

---

Table 33–1

Dosing of Medications to Treat PD

Generic Name (Trade Name)	Dosing
Levodopa with carbidopa (Sinemet)	Start with (Sinemet) ½ tab (100 mg LD, 25 mg CD) twice daily for 1 week, then ½ tab three times daily; then increase by ½ tab daily every week; usual MD is 300–2,000 mg daily; because the duration of LD is 2–3 hours, patients may require doses q 2 h
(Parcopa with phenylalanine)	Rapid-dissolving LD dosed as with Sinemet
(Sinemet CR)	Start with 1 tab (100 mg LD, 25 mg CD) 2–3 times daily; as symptoms increase, use 200 mg LD tab 2–4 times daily; usual MD is 200–2,200 mg daily
(Duodopa orphan drug on fast track for approval)	Portable pump that continuously delivers LD 20 mg/mL and carbidopa 5 mg/mL via a duodenal tube
Apomorphine (Apokyn)	Start an antiemetic for 3 days; then give apomorphine 2 mg SC injection (1 mg if outpatient) while monitoring blood pressure; then increase by 1–2 mg every ≥2 hours; usual MD is 2–6 mg 3–5 times daily for off periods. Reduce initial dose to 1 mg SC in mild to moderate renal failure.
Bromocriptine (Parlodel)	Start with 1.25 mg daily at bedtime, then 1.25 mg twice daily; on week 2, increase to 2.5 mg twice daily, then increase by 2.5 mg daily every 2–4 weeks up to 15–45 mg daily divided 2–3 times daily. Dosing adjustments may be necessary with hepatic impairment.
Pramipexole (Mirapex)	Start with 0.125 mg three times daily; increase about weekly by 0.375–0.75 mg/day to an MD of 0.5–1.5 mg three times daily; dosage reduction needed in patients with creatinine clearance less than 60 mL/min (1 mL/s).
(Mirapex ER)	Start with 0.375 mg once daily; may increase up to 0.75 mg/day after a minimum of 5 days. Dose may then be increased in increments of 0.75 mg/day no more frequently than every 5–7 days. Maximum recommended dose is 4.5 mg/day.
Ropinirole (Requip)	Start with 0.25 mg three times daily; increase about weekly by 0.75–1.5 mg daily to a MD dose of 3–8 mg three times daily.
(Requip XL)	Start with 2 mg once daily for 1–2 weeks, increase by 2 mg/day in 1-week intervals; maximum dose is 24 mg/day. When switching from immediate-release form, use dose closest to the total daily dose.
Selegiline (Eldepryl)	Start with 5 mg in the morning; if symptoms continue, add 5 mg at noon; 5 mg daily may be as clinically effective as 10 mg daily with fewer side effects.
(Zelapar with phenylalanine)	Start with 1.25 mg every morning before breakfast; if symptoms continue after 6 weeks, increase dose to 2.5 mg every morning. Avoid food or liquid for 5 minutes before or after the dose.
Rasagiline (Azilect)	Start with 0.5 mg daily. If symptoms continue, increase to 1 mg daily. Patients with mild hepatic impairment (Child-Pugh score 5–6) should be given the dose of 0.5 mg/day as plasma concentration may increase up to twofold. Do not use in moderate to severe liver disease (Child-Pugh score greater than 7) because plasma concentration may exceed sevenfold.
Tolcapone (Tasmar)	Start with 100 mg with first Sinemet dose once daily; if symptoms continue, increase to 2 and then 3 times daily, then to 200 mg each dose; usual MD is 100–200 mg 3 times daily. Do not use in patients with active liver disease or SGPT/ALT or SGOT/AST greater than the upper limit of normal.
Entacapone (Comtan)	200-mg tab with each Sinemet dose up to 8 tabs daily; usual MD is 200 mg 3–4 times daily. Decrease dose by 50% with hepatic impairment because C_{max} may double.
CD/LD/Entacapone (Stalevo)	Usual MD is 300–1,600 mg LD daily; the largest strength tab contains 150 mg LD and 200-mg entacapone; patients requiring larger LD doses will need additional LD medication; titrate as with LD
Amantadine (Symmetrel)	Start with 100 mg daily at breakfast; after 1 week, add 100 mg daily, decrease dose as creatinine clearance decreases less than 80 mL/min (1.3 mL/s); usual MD is 200–300 mg daily with last dose in afternoons.

Ach, acetylcholine; CD, carbidopa; COMT, catechol-*O*-methyltransferase; D1, a class of dopamine receptors that includes D_1, and D_5 subtypes; D2, a class of dopamine receptors that includes D_2, D_3, and D_4 subtypes; DA, dopamine; LD, levodopa; MAO, monoamine oxidase; MD, maintenance dose; NMDA, *N*-methyl-D-aspartate.

From Refs. 1, 2, 31–33.

than levodopa may help to delay the onset of dyskinesias and the on and off fluctuations seen with long-term levodopa use. However, initiating therapy with a dopamine agonist instead of levodopa/carbidopa may result in less motor benefit and greater risk of hallucinations or somnolence. Levodopa results in greater motor improvement and should be used as initial therapy in the elderly (older than 75 years) and in those with cognitive impairment.[26] There is no preference for using controlled-release over immediate-release levodopa as initial therapy. There are insufficient data to recommend initiating treatment with both levodopa and a dopamine agonist. Initiating treatment with anticholinergic medications, amantadine, or MAO-B inhibitors is only for patients who have mild symptoms because they are not as effective as dopamine agonists.[1,2,10–14,31–33]

Medications should be started at the lowest dose and increased gradually based on symptoms (Table 33–1). Adjust dose timing, frequency, or both based on the patient's report of "on" time duration and wearing off symptoms. Consider more frequent dosing or long-acting formulations when available. Dyskinesias related to dopamine concentrations can be managed by decreasing the dose, frequency, or use of medications that may enhance dopamine concentrations.

▶ Anticholinergics

Anticholinergics (Ach) block acetylcholine, decreasing the acetylcholine to dopamine concentration ratio. They minimize resting tremor and drooling, but they are not as effective as other agents in controlling rigidity, bradykinesia, and gait problems. Anticholinergics should be discontinued gradually to avoid withdrawal effects or worsening of symptoms. Side effects of anticholinergics include dry mouth, blurred vision, constipation, cognitive impairment, hallucinations, urinary retention, orthostatic hypotension, temperature sensitivity, and sedation. They are usually avoided or used with caution in patients older than 70 years because of an increased risk of cognitive impairment.[1,2,9,31,32] Use of anticholinergics is associated with an increased incidence of amyloid plaques and neurofibrillary tangles in patients with PD that may translate to an increased risk of Alzheimer's disease.[34] Anticholinergics decrease gastric motility, which may decrease levodopa drug absorption.[27]

▶ Amantadine

Amantadine is a *N*-methyl-D-aspartate (NMDA)-receptor antagonist that blocks glutamate transmission, promotes dopamine release, and blocks acetylcholine. It improves PD symptoms in mildly affected patients and has reduced dyskinesias.[21] Amantadine may minimize or delay the development of motor complications because levodopa's pulsatile stimulation of dopamine receptors is associated with NMDA receptor changes and resultant motor complications. Patients who develop tolerance to amantadine's effects may benefit from a drug holiday. When stopping amantadine, it should be gradually discontinued to minimize potential withdrawal effects. Side effects include nausea, dizziness, livedo reticularis (purple mottling of the skin), peripheral edema, orthostatic hypotension, hallucinations, restlessness, and anticholinergic

effects. Its stimulant action may worsen insomnia, so amantadine should not be dosed in the evening. It should be avoided in the elderly who cannot tolerate its anticholinergic effects.[31,32,35] It should be used cautiously with memantine because there may be an increased risk of psychosis and prolonged QT interval.[27,36]

▶ MAO-B Inhibitors

Selegiline and rasagiline selectively and irreversibly block MAO-B metabolism of dopamine in the brain. They may provide a mild symptomatic benefit for patients who choose to delay dopaminergic medications, and they reduce off time when added to therapy.[10–13,37] Combining selegiline or rasagiline with levodopa in early treatment may delay motor complications.[21,25,37]

Both rasagiline and selegiline are thought to be neuroprotective; however, there is no evidence to fully validate neuroprotection by any agent in PD patients to date. In two large blinded, randomized, controlled trials evaluating rasagiline 1 mg and 2 mg in early PD, significant UPDRS change was inconsistent between studies and cannot be used to support the neuroprotection theories.[38]

Selegiline is available in a patch formulation that is used in patients with depression but not PD. The orally disintegrating tablet formulation avoids first-pass metabolism that improves bioavailability and decreases serum concentrations of its amphetamine metabolite. Side effects of selegiline are minimal but include nausea, confusion, hallucinations, headache, jitteriness, and orthostatic hypotension. The amphetamine-like metabolite may improve fatigue but cause insomnia. Thus selegiline should not be dosed in the late afternoon or evening. Doses are limited to 10 mg daily in divided doses because MAO-B selectivity may be lost at higher doses increasing the risk of adverse effects and drug interactions. Selegiline may interact with serotonergic agents, increasing the risk of serotonin syndrome[1,25–27]

Rasagiline is less likely to cause insomnia because it is not metabolized to amphetamines. Side effects are primarily GI with no increased risk of vasoreactive or psychiatric effects. The approved labeling of rasagiline states that restriction of tyramine-containing foods is not ordinarily required at recommended dosages, but eating certain foods with extremely high levels of tyramine and exceeding recommend dosing of rasagiline may increase the risk of hypertensive crisis. The manufacturer of rasagiline also recommends that serotonergic agents be avoided, and extra monitoring is required if they are prescribed together.[37]

Dyskinesias can be minimized by decreasing the levodopa dose when adding either of these agents. Patients should avoid or use these medications cautiously with narcotic analgesics, antidepressants, or sympathomimetic amines (cold and weight loss products). Rasagiline is metabolized by the CYP1A2 pathway; thus drugs that inhibit CYP1A2 (e.g., ciprofloxacin or cimetidine) increase rasagiline concentrations, and inducers (e.g., omeprazole) may reduce rasagiline concentrations. Rasagiline does not induce or inhibit enzymes in the P450 system. Selegiline is metabolized by

CYP2B6 and CYP3A4. It does not inhibit P450 enzymes, but CYP3A4 inducers (e.g., phenytoin and carbamazepine) could reduce selegiline concentrations.[1,27,31-33]

Safinamide is an investigational MAO-B inhibitor and a dopamine reuptake inhibitor.[39]

▶ Dopamine Agonists

Dopamine agonists bind to postsynaptic dopamine receptors. They are useful as initial therapy because they can delay starting levodopa and can decrease the risk of developing motor fluctuations by two- to threefold during the first 4 to 5 years of treatment. Eventually, they inadequately control the patient's symptoms, and levodopa needs to be started. In advanced disease, they can be added to levodopa because their longer duration of action can minimize fluctuations in dopamine blood concentrations, decrease off time, improve wearing-off symptoms, allow a reduction in levodopa dose, and improve ADLs.[1,2,10,12,40] The 2010 Scottish Intercollegiate Guidelines Network suggests using dopamine agonists in early PD.[33]

Dopamine agonists include the ergot derivatives (bromocriptine) and the nonergot derivatives (rotigotine, pramipexole, ropinirole, and apomorphine). Generally, all are equally effective. There are five subtypes of dopamine receptors that are divided into two classes called D1 (D_1 and D_5 subtypes) and D2 (D_2, D_3, and D_4 subtypes). Receptor selectivity may result in subtle differences between the products. Rotigotine, a once-daily skin patch, minimizes pulsatile dopaminergic stimulation; however, it contains sodium metabisulfite, that may cause allergic-type reactions in people allergic to sulfites. Rotigotine was withdrawn in the United states due to stability problems in 2008, but it was reformulated to prevent crystallization and remarketed in 2012. If patients fail one dopamine agonist, another can be tried. Although not well established, it appears that bromocriptine 30 mg, ropinirole 15 mg, and pramipexole 4.5 mg are equivalent, and this relationship can be a guide when switching agents.[1,26,31,32,35]

Common side effects include nausea, vomiting, sedation (highest with apomorphine), pedal edema, orthostatic hypotension (highest with pramipexole and cabergoline), and psychiatric effects that are greater than with levodopa (nightmares, confusion, and hallucinations). Ergot side effects are uncommon but include painful reddish discoloration of the skin over the shins and pleuropulmonary, retroperitoneal, and cardiac fibrosis.[1,31,32,35] Patients with PD are commonly affected with impulse control disorders (ICDs). Dopamine agonists may cause changes in the striatum, possibly enhancing sensitivity to risky behavior such as gambling or compulsive shopping. Reducing or eliminating the agonist usually resolves these problems.[41]

Excessive daytime sleepiness can be caused by dopamine agonists and may occur in 50% of patients with PD. Dopamine agonist–induced sleep attacks can be very dangerous if the patient is performing an activity that requires mental alertness such as driving. However, using agents such as modafinil to promote wakefulness remains controversial.[42]

All dopamine agonists are metabolized by the liver except pramipexole, which is eliminated unchanged in the urine by active tubular secretion, and it requires dose reduction when creatinine clearance is less than 60 mL/min (1 mL/s). Drug interactions may occur if it is given concurrently with other agents that are eliminated by active tubular secretion, such as verapamil and cimetidine. Ropinirole is metabolized by cytochrome P450 oxidation in the liver and subject to drug–drug interactions with drugs that induce (i.e., smoking) or inhibit (i.e., ciprofloxacin, fluvoxamine, and mexiletine) CYP1A2.[31,32,35]

Apomorphine is approved for acute off episodes in patients with advanced stages of PD when rapid rescue therapy is needed. It requires premedication with an antiemetic because it causes nausea and vomiting.[31,32,35]

Phase III studies are currently underway for partial dopamine agonist pardoprunox (SLV308) in the treatment of patients with early PD.[43]

▶ Levodopa/Carbidopa

Although levodopa, a dopamine precursor, is the most effective agent for PD, when to initiate therapy remains controversial. Patients experience a 40% to 50% improvement in motor function with levodopa versus 30% with dopamine agonists.[1,2,26] However, some feel it best to delay starting treatment with levodopa because approximately 70% of patients experience motor complications within 6 years. Others start sooner because it may normalize basal ganglia dysfunction. In support of this idea, patients from the pre-levodopa era who delayed starting levodopa until it became available developed dyskinesias sooner than modern era patients.[1,20,26,31,32]

Levodopa is absorbed in the small intestine and peaks in the plasma in 30 to 120 minutes. Excess stomach acid, food, or anticholinergic medications delay gastric emptying time and decrease the amount of levodopa absorbed. Antacids decrease stomach acidity and improve levodopa absorption. Levodopa absorption requires active transport by a large neutral amino acid transporter protein (Fig. 33–2). Levodopa competes with other amino acids, such as those contained in food, for this transport mechanism. Thus, in advanced disease, avoidance of protein-rich meals in relationship to levodopa doses may be helpful. Levodopa also binds to iron supplements, and administration of iron products should be spaced by at least 2 hours from the levodopa dose.[1,26,31,32]

The controlled-release (CR) formulation (labeled as sustained release or extended release depending on brand) is more slowly absorbed and longer acting than immediate-release tablets. With these dosage forms the total daily dose should be increased by 30% because it is not as bioavailable as the immediate-release levodopa/carbidopa. The CR formulation has a delayed onset (45 to 60 minutes) compared with the standard formulation (15 to 30 minutes). Thus patients may also need to take immediate-release tablets or even a liquid formulation when they want a quicker onset of effect, such as with the first morning dose.[1,26,31,32]

Converting patients from oral formulations to enteral or duodenal levodopa administration reduces motor fluctuations and improves UPDRS scores over oral formulations. The levodopa/carbidopa combination can be administered directly to the duodenum via small tube and is marketed

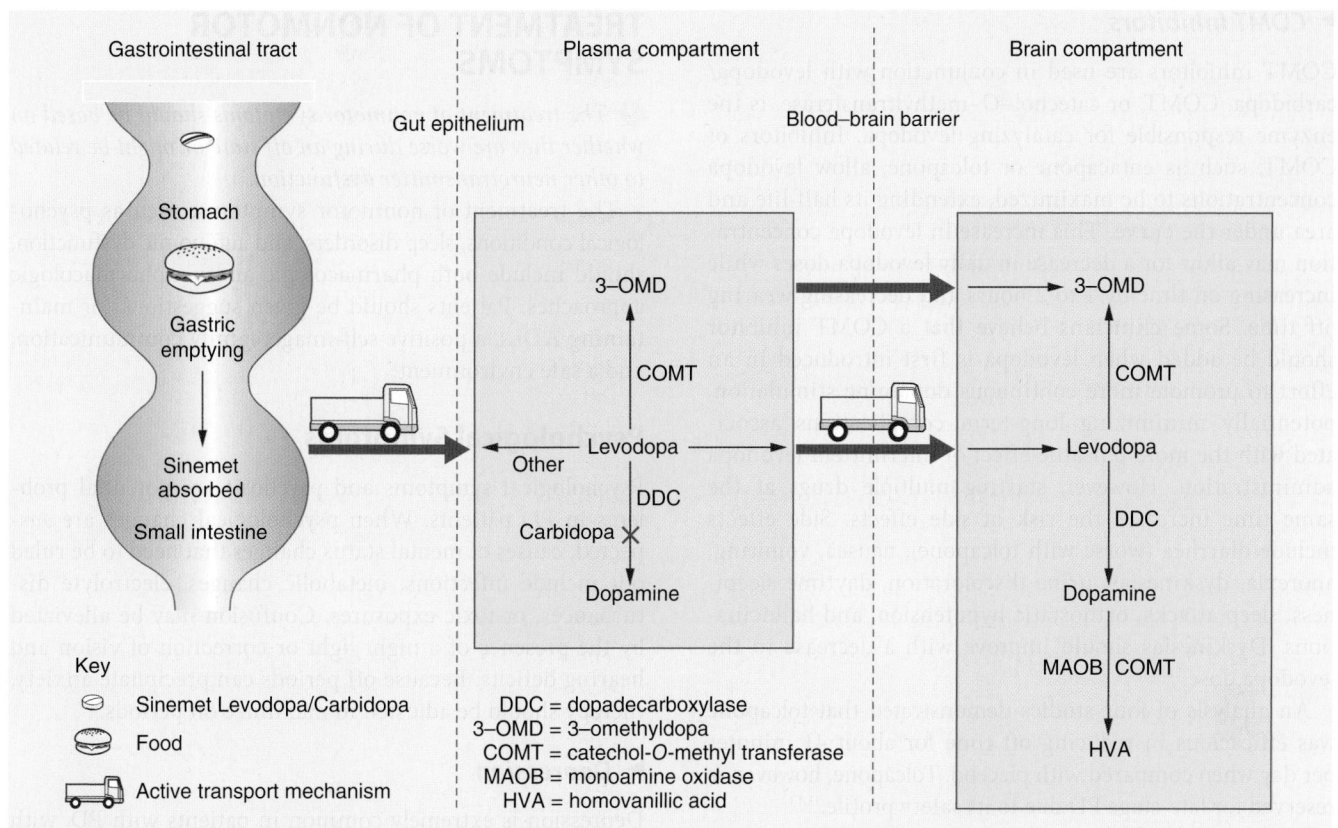

FIGURE 33–2. Levodopa absorption and metabolism. Levodopa is absorbed in the small intestine and distributed into the plasma and brain compartments by an active transport mechanism. Levodopa is metabolized by dopa decarboxylase, monoamine oxidase, and catechol-*O*-methyltransferase. Carbidopa does not cross the blood–brain barrier. Large neutral amino acids in food compete with levodopa for intestinal absorption (transport across gut endothelium to plasma). They also compete for transport into the brain (plasma compartment to brain compartment). Food and anticholinergics delay gastric emptying resulting in levodopa degradation in the stomach and a decreased amount of levodopa absorbed. If the interaction becomes a problem, administer levodopa 30 minutes before or 60 minutes after meals.

under the trade name Duodopa in the European Union, Norway, Switzerland, and Canada. It is indicated for patients with advanced levodopa-responsive PD with severe motor fluctuations and hyper/dyskinesia when available combinations of PD medications are unsatisfactory. A positive clinical response to Duodopa administered via a temporary nasoduodenal tube is required before a permanent tube is inserted. This delivery system allows direct absorption of the medication through the GI tract, and the dose and frequency of administration is determined by a programmable pump. The patient wears a small cassette outside of the body.[39] This system is currently undergoing phase III trials in the United States.

Additional formulations of levodopa in development include a long-acting formulation, IPX066, a levodopa prodrug, XP21279, and an effervescent levodopa prodrug formulation, melevodopa.[39]

Levodopa is usually administered as a combination product with carbidopa, a dopa-decarboxylase inhibitor, which decreases the peripheral conversion of levodopa to dopamine. Carbidopa does not cross the blood–brain barrier and does not interfere with levodopa conversion in the brain. Concomitant administration of carbidopa and levodopa allows for lower

levodopa doses and minimizes levodopa peripheral side effects such as nausea, vomiting, anorexia, and hypotension. Generally 75 to 100 mg daily of carbidopa is required to adequately block peripheral dopa-decarboxylase. Higher doses of carbidopa may reduce nausea related to initiating levodopa.[1,26,31,32]

Initial levodopa side effects include orthostatic hypotension, dizziness, anorexia, nausea, vomiting, and discoloration of urine/sweat. Most of these effects can be minimized by taking levodopa with food and using a slow dose titration. Side effects that develop later in therapy include dyskinesias, sleep attacks, impulse control disorders, and psychiatric effects (confusion, hallucinations, nightmares, and altered behavior). Dyskinesias caused by adding other PD drugs to levodopa may be improved by decreasing the levodopa dose.[1,26,31,32]

Levodopa commonly causes end of dose wearing off periods, and medication adjustments may ameliorate this phenomenon. Patients with severe dyskinesias and off periods may achieve more constant blood concentrations (lower peak and higher trough concentrations) by taking a liquid formulation of levodopa with carbidopa. Levodopa solution is available in a 1 mg/mL concentration, which allows patients to take a precisely adjusted dose more frequently when needed.[26,31,32,44]

▶ COMT Inhibitors

● COMT inhibitors are used in conjunction with levodopa/carbidopa. COMT, or catechol–O–methyltransferase, is the enzyme responsible for catalyzing levodopa. Inhibitors of COMT, such as entacapone or tolcapone, allow levodopa concentrations to be maximized, extending its half-life and area under the curve. This increase in levodopa concentration may allow for a decrease in daily levodopa doses while increasing on time by 1 to 2 hours and decreasing wearing off time. Some clinicians believe that a COMT inhibitor should be added when levodopa is first introduced in an effort to promote more continuous dopamine stimulation, potentially minimizing long-term complications associated with the more pulsatile effect of intermittent levodopa administration. However, starting multiple drugs at the same time increases the risk of side effects. Side effects include diarrhea (worse with tolcapone), nausea, vomiting, anorexia, dyskinesias, urine discoloration, daytime sleepiness, sleep attacks, orthostatic hypotension, and hallucinations. Dyskinesias should improve with a decrease in the levodopa dose.[26,31,32]

An analysis of four studies demonstrated that tolcapone was efficacious in reducing off time for about 41 minutes per day when compared with placebo. Tolcapone, however, is reserved for late-stage PD due to its safety profile.[11,13]

● Tolcapone should be used only in patients who cannot take or do not respond to entacapone due to its hepatic safety profile. Serum liver function tests should be monitored at baseline, then every 2 to 4 weeks for 6 months, and then periodically for the remainder of therapy. Patients who fail to show symptomatic benefit after 3 weeks should discontinue tolcapone.[26,31–33]

▶ Adenosine-2 Antagonists

The adenosine-2 antagonist receptors are currently being explored as a nondopaminergic therapy for the treatment of PD. They are proposed to facilitate intrastriatal GABA release, reducing striatopallidal neuronal over activity and restoring balance within the basal ganglia. Currently, several compounds are in development, and the drug preladenant has reached phase II trials.[39]

▶ Herbs and Supplements

There is very little support for using creatine, gingko, ginseng, green tea, ginger, yohimbine, or St. John's wort in patients with PD. Melatonin and valerian may improve insomnia, but there are insufficient data in PD patients.

Patients should eat a balanced diet and take a multi-vitamin with minerals, but there is generally no need to supplement with specific vitamins. Metabolism of levodopa may elevate homocysteine concentrations. Administering levodopa with a COMT inhibitor may minimize the increase in homocysteine, and patients may have a greater requirement for B vitamins than patients not receiving levodopa. Excess pyridoxine (vitamin B_6) may decrease the effect of levodopa, so limit doses to less than 50 mg per day.[45,46]

TREATMENT OF NONMOTOR SYMPTOMS

❼ *The treatment of nonmotor symptoms should be based on whether they are worse during an off state or might be related to other neurotransmitter dysfunction.*

The treatment of nonmotor symptoms, such as psychological conditions, sleep disorders, and autonomic dysfunction, should include both pharmacologic and nonpharmacologic approaches. Patients should be given suggestions for maintaining ADLs, a positive self-image, family communication, and a safe environment.

Psychological Symptoms

Psychological symptoms and psychosis are potential problems in PD patients. When psychological changes are suspected, causes of mental status changes that need to be ruled out include infections, metabolic changes, electrolyte disturbances, or toxic exposures. Confusion may be alleviated by the presence of a night light or correction of vision and hearing deficits. Because off periods can precipitate anxiety, therapy should be adjusted to maximize on periods.

▶ Depression

Depression is extremely common in patients with PD, with some estimating that ≥40% of patients may have coexisting depression. Experts believe that depression often precedes PD. Brain catecholamine changes and serotonin dysregula-
● tion contribute to depression associated with PD. Although the body of evidence supports efficacy of tricyclic antidepressants in patients with both depression and PD, the adverse effect profile of these agents limits its use. Alternatively, selective serotonin reuptake inhibitors may be considered. Pramipexole may also improve depression.[18] Although maximizing on time may help, drug therapy is usually required. Antidepressants may also be useful for the maintenance of anxiety disorders. Electroconvulsive therapy in depressed patients who fail medications should be considered.[2,6,7,9,14,17]

▶ Dementia

Dementia occurs in approximately 80% of patients with PD 20 years after disease diagnosis, and it can significantly impair a patient's quality of life. A decrease in cholinergic neurotransmission is implicated in dementia associated with PD. Patients with dementia and PD have an increased risk for falls compared with patients without dementia. Patients must be assessed carefully for fall risk, and appropriate safety measures should be in place to ensure fall prevention. Atypical antipsychotics can be used, but they carry a Boxed Warning for increased risk of death in elderly patients with dementia, and they can worsen symptoms of PD.
● Cholinesterase inhibitor drugs may be effective. The efficacy of memantine in this patient population is unclear.[2,14,17–19]

▶ Psychosis

Low-efficacy PD medications should be gradually decreased
● and stopped in patients with psychosis. If reducing PD

medication compromises motor control or does not improve psychosis, low-dose quetiapine (12.5 to 200 mg) at bedtime may improve psychosis. However, it should be used with caution due to long-term metabolic side effects. Clozapine is also recommended but requires stringent monitoring.[2,14,17–19]

Sleep Problems

Sleep problems and fatigue are common in PD and may be due to medications, uncontrolled PD symptoms, or other causes such as nocturia, depression, RBD, or restless legs syndrome (RLS). Disorders of wakefulness such as sleep attacks may also affect adequate and restful sleep. Patients may benefit from instruction on good sleep hygiene, improvement in nighttime PD symptoms, or cognitive behavioral therapy.[6,14,15]

Ongoing studies have indicated that the nonergot dopamine agonist rotigotine may improve early morning motor function and overall quality of sleep.[47]

Amantadine and selegiline may worsen insomnia, selegiline and tricyclic antidepressants may worsen REM sleep, and some antidepressants and antipsychotics may worsen RLS. Ramelteon may improve circadian sleep disorders (study in progress). Melatonin may improve patient perception of sleep, but this has not been validated using objective measures of sleep. Levodopa/carbidopa reduces nighttime periodic leg movements, but data regarding nonergot dopamine agonists are lacking in patients with PD. When iron is used for RLS, it may decrease the absorption of levodopa and increase constipation. A nighttime dose of a COMT inhibitor may help RLS.[2,6,15]

Autonomic and Other Problems

Drooling may be accompanied by speech problems and dysphagia. Anticholinergics, botulinum toxin injections, and sublingual atropine can decrease drooling. Speech therapists can perform swallowing studies to assess the risk of aspiration, and nutritionists can optimize diet. Patients at high risk of aspiration or poor nutrition may require placement of a percutaneous endoscopic gastrostomy tube. Nausea improves if patients take their PD medications with meals, and pharmacologic therapy (e.g., domperidone [or trimethobenzamide]) can also help. Sexual dysfunction or urinary problems may require further evaluation. Adjustment of PD therapy to increase on time, removal of drugs that decrease sexual response, and pharmacologic therapy (e.g., sildenafil) may help treat sexual dysfunction. Studies of sexual dysfunction in women with PD are lacking. Patients with urinary frequency may find a bedside urinal and a decrease in evening fluid intake helpful. Improvement in PD symptom control can improve urinary frequency, but worsening symptoms may require catheterization or pharmacologic measures (e.g., oxybutynin, tolterodine, propantheline, imipramine, hyoscyamine, or nocturnal intranasal desmopressin). Anticholinergic drugs can cause urinary retention and constipation. Constipation can be improved by increased fluid intake, a fiber-rich diet, and physical activity.

Patients should generally avoid cathartic laxatives and use stool softeners, osmotic or bulk-forming laxatives, glycerin suppositories, or enemas. Dyskinesia-related sweating may respond to PD therapy adjustment or β-blockers. Orthostasis may respond to the removal of offending drugs (e.g., tricyclic antidepressants, PD medications, alcohol, and antihypertensives) increasing carbidopa doses, addition of salt or fluids to the diet, compression stockings, fludrocortisone, indomethacin, or midodrine. Seborrhea usually responds to over-the-counter dandruff shampoos or topical steroids.[2,6,9,16]

Treatment of Response Fluctuations

8 *As the disease progresses, most patients develop response fluctuations. Treatment is based on optimizing the pharmacokinetic and pharmacodynamic properties of PD medications.*

Treatment includes adjusting or adding medications to maximize the patient's on time, minimize the time on with dyskinesia, and minimize off time (Table 33–2). Use various dosage plans to minimize suboptimal or delayed peak levodopa concentrations by adding longer acting medications to minimize wearing-off periods, adding or adjusting medications to stop an unpredicted off period, and providing treatments that decrease freezing episodes. It also involves adjusting or adding medications to decrease chorea, dystonia, diphasic dyskinesias, or akathisia. Patients should schedule activities when they are on. Patients can also keep an extra dose of medication with them when they are away from home in case their medication wears off.[2,6,11,13,21]

Patient Encounter, Part 3: First Follow-up Visit 3 Months Later

GR comes in for a follow-up visit with complaints of agitation and visual hallucinations. At her last visit 3 months ago, ropinirole was added. Since then, she reports improvement in her ability to get out of bed in the morning. She feels that she has less tremor and stiffness throughout the day. She has no off periods. However, her husband reports that GR has become increasingly frustrated and agitated, and sometimes she claims to see faces in the shadows at night. She also reports vivid dreams. She seems very suspicious of her husband at times and has had an increased interest in Internet shopping, which her husband says is a new behavior. She is more physically active with improved PD symptoms. She is taking polyethylene glycol one time per week with five to seven bowel movements per week.

UPDRS 35 (on)

Create a problem list and provide an assessment of each problem.

Considering the goals of therapy, treatment options, and your assessment of each of the problems, create a care plan for each problem.

Management of Motor Complications in Advanced PD

I. Motor fluctuations

A. Suboptimal or delayed peak response
 1. Take Sinemet on an empty stomach
 2. Decrease dietary protein and fat around the dose that is delayed
 3. Use rapid-dissolving tablet (Parcopa), crush Sinemet, or make liquid Sinemet
 4. Substitute standard Sinemet for some of the Sinemet CR
 5. Minimize constipation
 6. Withdraw drugs with anticholinergic properties
 7. Add intermittent subcutaneous apomorphine

B. Optimal peak but early wearing off
 1. Decrease dose and increase frequency of standard Sinemet
 2. Substitute Sinemet CR for some of the standard Sinemet
 3. Add other PD medications (dopamine agonist, MAO-B inhibitor, amantadine, or COMT inhibitor)

C. Optimal peak but unpredictable offs
 1. Adjust time of medications with meals and avoid high-protein meals or redistribute the amount of protein in diet
 2. Substitute or add rapid-dissolving tablet form or liquid form of Sinemet
 3. Add COMT inhibitor
 4. Add or try a different dopamine agonist
 5. Consider continuous infusion of levodopa (Duodopa), apomorphine, or lisuride
 6. Deep-brain stimulation procedure

D. Freezing
 1. Gait modifications (use visual cues such as walkover lines, tapping, rhythmic commands, rocking; use rolling walker)
 2. Difficult to treat, so adjust current medication up or down based on other PD symptoms
  a. On freezing, reduce dopamine medications, inject botulinum toxin
  b. Off freezing, increase Sinemet dose or add dopamine agonists
 3. Treat anxiety if present

II. Dyskinesias

A. Chorea
 1. Evaluate the value of adjunctive PD medications
 2. Decrease risk by lowering Sinemet dose when adding other PD medications
 3. Adjust levodopa formulation, dose, or frequency
 4. Add amantadine
 5. Add propranolol, fluoxetine, buspirone, or clozapine
 6. Deep-brain stimulation

B. Off period dystonia in the early morning (e.g., foot cramping)
 1. Add Sinemet CR or dopamine agonist at bedtime if having nighttime offs
 2. Morning Sinemet dose should be immediate-release with or without CR
 3. Selective denervation with botulinum toxin
 4. Add lithium or baclofen

C. Diphasic dyskinesia
 1. Avoid controlled-release preparations; consider liquid Sinemet
 2. Add dopamine agonist, amantadine, or COMT inhibitor
 3. Increase Sinemet dose and frequency
 4. Deep-brain stimulation

III. Akathisia

 1. Benzodiazepine
 2. Propranolol
 3. Dopamine agonists
 4. Gabapentin

COMT, catechol-O-methyltransferase.
From Refs. 2, 11, 20, 21.

OUTCOME EVALUATION

⑨ *Patient monitoring should involve a regular systematic evaluation of efficacy and adverse events, referral to appropriate specialists, and patient education.*

Evaluate the clinical outcomes of treatment over time by assessing the change in the UPDRS from baseline and over time. Patients should record daily the amount of on and off time in a diary to guide medication adjustment. A variety of scales can be used to assess QOL, depression, anxiety, and sleep disorders. PD cannot be cured, but treatment is aimed at decreasing symptoms and improving ADLs and QOL.

Patient Encounter, Part 4: Second Follow-up Visit 3 Months Later

GR, a 61-year-old woman with PD, comes in for a follow-up visit with no new complaints. At her last visit 3 months ago, ropinirole was removed, and her daily Sinemet dose was increased to cover the afternoon off period that had previously been treated with ropinirole. Since then, her symptoms have improved, and she is able to prepare dinner. She denies any auditory or visual hallucinations or vivid dreams. Her husband says that she is less agitated, suspicious, and has stopped Internet shopping. She has joined an exercise class at the senior center. She continues to have five to seven bowel movements per week.

UPDRS 35 (on)

Medications

Sinemet 25/100 7 AM, 11:30 AM, 4 PM, 9 PM

Docusate sodium 100 mg 2 caps at bedtime

Psyllium unflavored (Metamucil) 1 rounded teaspoon in 8 oz (~240 mL) of juice three times daily

Polyethylene glycol (MiraLAX) 17 g/scoop. 1 scoop in 4 to 8 oz (~120 to 240 mL) of liquid, 1 to 2 times per week as needed for constipation.

If GR's psychosis had continued and was determined to be a nonmotor symptom of PD rather than an adverse effect of her dopaminergic therapy, what options might you consider?

How would you counsel a patient who has been on PD medications and is initiating an atypical antipsychotic such as quetiapine?

Were therapeutic goals achieved in GR after discontinuation of her dopamine agonist and adjustment of her carbidopa/levodopa?

If a patient was unable to speak due to disease progression, what would be the advantages and disadvantages of having a significant other communicate for the patient?

Patient Care and Monitoring

1. Determine type of symptoms, frequency, and exacerbating factors. Assess for PD treatment-related complications. Assess the patient's symptoms to determine if therapy should be adjusted or maintained, or if referral for more extensive evaluation is needed.

2. Review any available diagnostic data to determine status, motor ability, dyskinesias, and nonmotor symptoms.

3. Obtain a thorough history of prescription, nonprescription, and complementary/alternative medication use. Determine what treatments have been helpful to the patient in the past. Is the patient taking any medications that may increase PD symptoms?

4. Educate the patient about lifestyle modifications that will improve symptoms and sustain independence.

5. Determine whether the patient is taking the appropriate dose of PD medication to maximize on time and minimize adverse effects. If not, why?

6. Determine if polytherapy treatment is necessary and/or adequate.

7. Assess improvement in QOL measures.

8. Evaluate the patient for the presence of drug adverse reactions, allergies, and interactions.

9. Recommend a therapeutic regimen that is easy for the patient to follow. Educate the patient on how to use medications, and allow the patient to adjust medications for fluctuations in response.

10. Educate patient regarding PD, including lifestyle modifications and drug therapy, including:

    • When and how to take medications

    • The potential adverse effects that may occur

    • Which drugs may interact with therapy (give patient a list)

    • Warning signs to report to the physician

    • Where the patient can obtain further information such as books and websites (e.g., *http://www.apdaparkinson.org; http://www.parkinson.org*.)

11. Refer patient to a local PD support group to obtain educational materials as well as empathy and social support from fellow PD patients. Support groups that include patients with advanced disease may upset patients with early disease; therefore, the advantages and disadvantages of attending should be explained to the patient.

Abbreviations Introduced in This Chapter

ADLs   Activities of daily living
COMT   Catechol-*O*-methyltransferase
CR   Controlled-release
DIP   Drug-induced Parkinsonism
GABA   *γ*-Aminobutyric acid
GI   Gastrointestinal
MAO   Monoamine oxidase
NMDA   *N*-Methyl-D-aspartate
PD   Parkinson's disease
QOL   Quality of life
RBD   Rapid eye movement sleep behavior disorder
RLS   Restless legs syndrome
UPDRS   Unified Parkinson's Disease Rating Scale

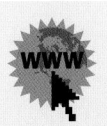

Self-assessment questions and answers are available at *http://www.mhpharmacotherapy. com/pp.html.*

REFERENCES

1. Nutt JG, Wooten GF. Diagnosis and initial management of Parkinson's disease. N Engl J Med 2005;353:1021–1027.

2. Lees AJ, Hardy J, Revesz T. Parkinson's disease. Lancet 2009;373(9680): 2055–2066. Review. Erratum in: Lancet 2009;374(9691):684.

3. Tanner CM, Ross GW, Jewell SA, et al. Occupation and risk of parkinsonism: a multicenter case-control study. Arch Neurol 2009; 66(9):1106–1113.

4. Suchowersky O, Gronseth G, Perlmutter J, et al; Quality Standards Subcommittee of the American Academy of Neurology. Practice parameter: neuroprotective strategies and alternative therapies for Parkinson disease (an evidence-based review): Report of the Quality Standards Subcommittee of the American Academy of Neurology. Neurology 2006;66:976–982. Erratum in: Neurology 2006;67(2):299.

5. Goetz CG. Hypokinetic Movement Disorders in Textbook of Clinical Neurology [Internet]. 3rd ed. Philadelphia, PA: Saunders; 2007:Chap.16 [cited 2011 Oct 10]. Available from: *http://www.mdconsult.com.*

6. Truong DD, Bhidayasiri R, Wolters E. Management of non-motor symptoms in advanced Parkinson disease. J Neurol Sci 2008;266:216–228.

7. Blonder LX, Slevin JT. Emotional dysfunction in Parkinson's disease. Behav Neuro 2011;24(3):201–217.

8. Susatia F, Fernandez HH. Drug-induced parkinsonism. Curr Treat Options Neurol 2009;11(3):162–169.

9. Weiner WJ, Shulman LM, Lang AE. Parkinson's Disease: A Complete Guide for Patients and Families. 2nd ed. Baltimore, MD: John Hopkins University Press; 2006.

10. Horstink M, Tolosa E, Bonuccelli U, et al; European Federation of Neurological Societies; Movement Disorder Society-European Section. Review of the therapeutic management of Parkinson's disease. Report of a joint task force of the European Federation of Neurological Societies and the Movement Disorder Society-European Section. Part I: early (uncomplicated) Parkinson's disease. Eur J Neurol 2006;13(11):1170–1185.

11. Horstink M, Tolosa E, Bonuccelli U, et al; European Federation of Neurological Societies; Movement Disorder Society-European Section. Review of the therapeutic management of Parkinson's disease. Report of a joint task force of the European Federation of Neurological Societies (EFNS) and the Movement Disorder Society-European Section (MDS-ES). Part II: late (complicated) Parkinson's disease. Eur J Neurol 2006;13(11):1186–1202.

12. Oertel WH, Berardelli A, Bloem BR. Early (uncomplicated) Parkinson's disease. In: Gilhus NE, Barnes MP, Brainin M, eds. European Handbook of Neurological Management. Vol. 1. 2nd ed. Blackwell, 2011:217–236.

13. Oertel WH, Berardelli A, Bloem BR. Late (uncomplicated) Parkinson's disease. In: Gilhus NE, Barnes MP, Brainin M, eds. European Handbook of Neurological Management. Vol. 1. 2nd ed. Blackwell, 2011:237–267.

14. Zesiewicz TA, Sullivan KL, Arnulf I, et al; Quality Standards Subcommittee of the American Academy of Neurology. Practice parameter: treatment of nonmotor symptoms of Parkinson disease: report of the Quality Standards Subcommittee of the American Academy of Neurology. Neurology 2010;74(11):924–931.

15. Jahan I, Hauser RA, Sullivan KL, et al. Sleep disorders in Parkinson's disease. Neuropsychiatr Dis Treat 2009;5:535–540.

16. Dewey RB. Autonomic dysfunction in Parkinson's disease. Neurol Clin 2004;22:S127–S140.

17. Aarsland D, Marsh L, Schrag A. Neuropsychiatric symptoms in Parkinson's disease. Mov Disord 2009;24:15:2175–2186.

18. Bakay S, Bechet S, Barjona A, et al. Dementia in Parkinson's disease: Risk factors, diagnosis and treatment. Rev Med Liege 2011;66(2):75–81.

19. Burn DJ. The treatment of cognitive impairment associated with Parkinson's disease. Brain Pathol 2010;20(3):672–678.

20. Bhidayasiri R, Truong DD. Motor complications in Parkinson disease: Clinical manifestations and management. J Neurol Sci 2008;266:204–215.

21. Gottwald MD, Aminoff MJ. Therapies for dopaminergic-induced dyskinesias in Parkinson disease. Ann Neurol 2011;69(6):919–927.

22. Fahn S, Elton R; Members of the UPDRS Development Committee. In: Fahn S, Marsden CD, Calne DB, Goldstein M, eds. Recent Developments in Parkinson's Disease. Vol. 2. Florham Park, NJ: Macmillan Health Care Information; 1987:153–163, 293–304.

23. Miyasaki JM, Martin W, Suchowersky O, et al. Practice parameter: Initiation of treatment for Parkinson's disease: An evidence-based review. Report of the Quality Standards Subcommittee of the American Academy of Neurology. Neurology 2002;58:11–17.

24. National Collaborating Centre for Chronic Conditions. Parkinson's disease: National Clinical Guideline for Management in Primary and Secondary Care [Internet]. London, UK: Royal College of Physicians; 2006 [cited 2011 Oct 10]. Available from: *http://www.ncbi.nlm.nih.gov/books/NBK48513/.*

25. Clarke CE, Patel S, Ives N, et al. Should treatment for Parkinson's disease start immediately on diagnosis or delayed until functional disability develops? Mov Disord 2011;26(7):1187–1193.

26. Olanow CW, Stern MB, Sethi K. The scientific and clinical basis for the treatment of Parkinson's disease. Neurology 2009;72(21 Suppl 4):S1–S136.

27. Jost WH, Bruck C. Drug interactions in the treatment of Parkinson's disease. J Neurol 2002;249(Suppl 3):S24–S29.

28. Keus SHJ, Bloem BR, Hendriks EJM, et al. Evidence-based analysis of physical therapy in Parkinson's disease with recommendations for practice and research. Mov Disord 2007;22:451–460.

29. Esselink RA, de Bie RM, de Haan RJ, et al. Unilateral pallidotomy versus bilateral subthalamic nucleus stimulation in PD: A randomized trial. Neurology 2004;62(2):201–207.

30. Weaver FM, Follett K, Stern M, et al. CSP 468 Study Group. Bilateral deep brain stimulation vs best medical therapy for patients with advanced Parkinson disease: A randomized controlled trial. JAMA 2009;301(1):63–73.

31. Chen JJ, Swope DM. Pharmacotherapy for Parkinson's disease. Pharmacotherapy 2007;27(12 Pt2):S161–S173.

32. Anonymous. Treatment guidelines from the medical letter. Drugs Parkinson's Dis 2011;9(101):1–6.

33. Scottish Intercollegiate Guidelines Network (SIGN). Diagnosis and pharmacological management of Parkinson's disease. A national clinical guideline [Internet]. Edinburgh, UK: Scottish Intercollegiate Guidelines Network (SIGN); 2010 Jan. 61 p. (SIGN publication; no. 113), [cited 2011 Oct 10]. Available from: *www.sign.ac.uk/pdf/sign113.pdf.*

34. Perry EK, Kilford L, Lees AJ, et al. Increased Alzheimer's pathology in Parkinson's disease related to antimuscarinic drugs. Ann Neurol 2003;54:235–238.

35. Olanow CW, Watts RI, Koller WC. An algorithm (decision tree) for the management of Parkinson's diseases: Treatment-guidelines. Neurology 2001;56(Suppl 5):S1–S88.

36. Factor SA, Molho ES, Brown DL. Acute delirium after withdrawal of amantadine in Parkinson's disease. Neurology 1998;50:1456–1458.

37. Fernandez HH, Chen JJ. Monoamine oxidase-B inhibition in the treatment of Parkinson's disease. Pharmacotherapy 2007;27(12 Pt 2):S174–S185.

38. Ahlskog JE, Uitti RJ. Rasagiline, Parkinson neuroprotection, and delayed-start trials: Still no satisfaction? Neurology 2010;74(14):1143–1148.

39. Hickey P, Stacy M. Available and emerging treatments for Parkinson's disease: A review. Drug Des Devel Ther 2011;5:241–254.

40. Hauser RA. Early pharmacologic treatment in Parkinson's disease. Am J Manag Care 2010;(16 Suppl Implications):S100–S107.

41. Voon V, Gao J, Brezing C, et al. Dopamine agonists and risk: impulse control disorders in Parkinson's disease. Brain 2011;134(Pt 5):1438–1446.

42. Knie B, Mitra MT, Logishetty K, Chaudhuri KR. Excessive daytime sleepiness in patients with Parkinson's disease. CNS Drugs 2011;25(3):203–212.

43. Sampaio C, Bronzova J, Hauser RA, et al. Pardoprunox in early Parkinson's disease: Results from 2 large, randomized double-blind trials. Mov Disord 2011;26(8):1464–1476.

44. Pappert EJ, Goetz CG, Niederman F, et al. Liquid levodopa/carbidopa produces significant improvement in motor function without dyskinesia exacerbation. Neurology 1996;47:1493–1495.

45. Rogers JD, Sanchez-Saffon A, et al. Elevated plasma homocysteine levels in patients treated with levodopa: Association with vascular disease. Arch Neurol 2003;60:59–64.

46. Miller JW, Selhub J, Nadeau MR, et al. Effect of L-dopa on plasma homocysteine in PD patients' relationship to B-vitamin status. Neurology 2003;60:1125–1129.

47. Trenkwalder C, Kies B, Rudzinska M, et al; Recover Study Group. Rotigotine effects on early morning motor function and sleep in Parkinson's disease: a double-blind, randomized, placebo-controlled study (RECOVER). Mov Disord 2011;26(1):90–99.

34 Pain Management

Christine Karabin O'Neil

LEARNING OBJECTIVES

● **Upon completion of the chapter, the reader will be able to:**

1. Identify characteristics of the types of pain: nociceptive, inflammatory, neuropathic, and functional.

2. Explain the mechanisms involved in pain transmission.

3. Select an appropriate method of pain assessment.

4. Recommend an appropriate choice of analgesic, dose, and monitoring plan for a patient based on type and severity of pain and other patient-specific parameters.

5. Perform calculations involving equianalgesic doses, conversion of one opioid to another, rescue doses, and conversion to a continuous infusion.

6. Educate patients and caregivers about effective pain management, dealing with chronic pain, and the use of nonpharmacologic measures.

KEY CONCEPTS

❶ Pain is an unpleasant, subjective experience that is the net effect of a complex interaction of the ascending and descending neurons involving biochemical, physiologic, psychological, and neocortical processes.

❷ Following initial assessment of pain, reassessment should be done as needed based on medication choice and the clinical situation.

❸ Effective treatment involves an evaluation of the cause, duration, and intensity of the pain and selection of an appropriate treatment modality for the pain situation.

❹ Whenever possible, the least potent oral analgesic should be selected.

❺ Equianalgesic doses should be used when converting from one opioid to another.

Pain is defined by the International Association for the Study of Pain (IASP) as "an unpleasant sensory and emotional experience associated with actual or potential tissue damage, or described in terms of such damage."[1] ❶ *Pain is an unpleasant subjective experience that is the net effect of a complex interaction of the ascending and descending neurons involving biochemical, physiologic, psychological, and neocortical processes.* Pain can affect all areas of a person's life including sleep, thought, emotion, and activities of daily living. Because there are no reliable objective markers for

pain, the patient is the only person who can describe the intensity and quality of their pain.

Pain is the most common symptom prompting patients to seek medical attention and is reported by more than 80% of individuals who visit their primary care provider.[2] Despite the frequency of pain symptoms, individuals often do not obtain satisfactory relief of pain. This has led to initiatives in healthcare to make pain the fifth vital sign, thus making pain assessment equal in importance to obtaining a patient's temperature, pulse, blood pressure, and respiratory rate.

EPIDEMIOLOGY AND ETIOLOGY

Prevalence of Pain

Most people experience pain at some time in their lives, and pain is a symptom of a variety of diseases. For some, pain might be mild to moderate, intermittent, easily managed, and have minimal effect on daily activities. For others, pain might be chronic, severe, or disabling, all consuming, and treatment resistant. Thus identifying the exact prevalence of pain is a difficult task. According to the American Pain Foundation, more than 76 million people in the United States suffer from chronic pain, and an additional 25 million experience acute pain from injury or surgery.[2] About 26% of the adults, mostly women and the elderly, experience chronic pain such as back pain, headache, and joint pain.

Prevalence rates for a variety of different types of pain have been described. Approximately one-fourth of U.S. adults reported having low back pain lasting at least 1 day in the past 3 months.[3] Migraine affects more than 28 million Americans, and 78% of Americans experience a tension headache during their lifetime.[4] Pain resulting from fibromyalgia affects 10 million Americans.[5] Pain ranges in prevalence from 14% to 100% among cancer patients. Cancer is commonly associated with both acute and chronic pain, and about 50% to 70% of those in active treatment will experience significant pain.[6]

The prevalence of neuropathic pain is unknown because of the lack of epidemiologic studies. Current estimates suggest that approximately 1.5% of the population in the United States might be affected by neuropathic pain.[7] However, this figure is probably an underestimate and will likely increase due to the increase in disorders associated with neuropathic pain in the ever-growing older population. Approximately 25% to 50% of all pain clinic visits are related to neuropathic pain.[8] Central neuropathic pain is estimated to occur in 2% to 8% of all stroke patients.[9]

The elderly, defined as people 65 years and older, bear a significant burden of pain, and pain continues to be under-recognized and undertreated in this population. The prevalence of pain in people older than 60 years is twice that in those younger than 60 years.[10] Studies suggest that 25% to 50% of community-dwelling elderly suffer pain. Pain is quite common among nursing home residents. It is estimated that pain in 45% to 80% of nursing home patients contributes to functional impairment and a decreased quality of life.[11]

The financial impact of pain is considered to be significant. Low back pain alone was responsible for direct medical costs of more than $26 billion annually in 1998 and as much as $50 billion per year in indirect costs.[12] The American Productivity Audit of the U.S. workforce, conducted from 2001 to 2002, revealed that the cost of lost productivity due to arthritis, back pain, headache, and other musculoskeletal pain was approximately $61.2 billion per year.[13]

Undertreatment of Pain

Despite the growing emphasis on pain management, pain often remains undertreated and continues to be a problem in hospitals, long-term care facilities, and the community. In one series of reports, 50% of seriously ill hospitalized patients reported pain; however, 15% were dissatisfied with pain control, and some remained in pain after hospitalization.[14,15]

Misconceptions about pain management, both from patients and healthcare providers, are among the most common causes of analgesic failure. Some clinicians might be hesitant to treat pain because either they do not believe the patient's reports of pain or feel the patient is exaggerating symptoms in order to obtain medications. Inadequate clinical knowledge of available pain management strategies, including pharmacologic, nonpharmacologic, and alternative therapy options, also often leads to suboptimal pain management. In one survey, approximately three-fourths of physicians cited low competence in pain assessment as the major barrier to effective pain management.[16] Concerns about opiate misuse, abuse, and diversion also contribute to less than optimal pain management and cause providers to exercise caution

when prescribing opiates for pain. Misunderstandings about the terms addiction, physical dependence, tolerance, and pseudoaddiction are additional obstacles to optimal pain management.

Patients might present barriers to pain management by not reporting pain symptoms because of fear of becoming addicted or because of cultural beliefs. Elderly patients might not report pain for a variety of reasons including belief that pain is something they must live with, fear of consequences (e.g., hospitalization, loss of independence), or fear that the pain might be forecasting impending illness, inability to understand terminology used by healthcare providers, or a belief that showing pain is unacceptable behavior.

PATHOPHYSIOLOGY

Types of Pain

Several distinct types of pain have been described, for example, nociceptive, inflammatory, neuropathic, and functional.[17] Nociceptive pain is a transient pain in response to a noxious stimulus at nociceptors that are located in cutaneous tissue, bone, muscle, connective tissue, vessels, and viscera. Nociceptors are classified as thermal, chemical, or mechanical. The nociceptive system extends from the receptors in the periphery to the spinal cord, brainstem, to the cerebral cortex where pain sensation is perceived. This system is a key physiologic function that prevents further tissue damage due to the body's autonomic withdrawal reflex. When tissue damage occurs despite the nociceptive defense system, inflammatory pain ensues. The body now changes focus from protecting against painful stimuli to protecting the injured tissue. The inflammatory response contributes to pain hypersensitivity that serves to prevent contact or movement of the injured part until healing is complete, thus reducing further damage.

Neuropathic pain is defined as spontaneous pain and hypersensitivity to pain associated with damage to or pathologic changes in the peripheral nervous system as in painful diabetic peripheral neuropathy (DPN), adult immune deficiency syndrome (AIDS), polyneuropathy, postherpetic neuralgia (PHN), or in the CNS, which occurs with spinal cord injury, multiple sclerosis, and stroke. Functional pain, a relatively newer concept, is pain sensitivity due to an abnormal processing or functioning of the CNS in response to normal stimuli. Several conditions considered to have this abnormal sensitivity or hyperresponsiveness include fibromyalgia and irritable bowel syndrome.

Mechanisms of Pain

▶ Pain Transmission

The mechanisms of nociceptive pain are well defined and provide a foundation for the understanding of other types of pain.[18] Following nociceptor stimulation, tissue injury causes the release of substances (bradykinin, serotonin, potassium, histamine, prostaglandins, and substance P) that might further sensitize and/or activate nociceptors. Nociceptor activation produces action potentials (transduction) that are transmitted along myelinated Aδ-fibers and unmyelinated C-fibers to the spinal cord. The Aδ-fibers are responsible for first, fast, sharp pain and release excitatory amino acids that activate α-amino-3-hydroxy-5-methylisoxazole-4-propionic acid (AMPA) receptors in the dorsal horn. The C-fibers produce second pain, which is described as dull, aching, burning, and diffuse. These nerve fibers synapse in the dorsal horn of the spinal cord, where several neurotransmitters are released including glutamate, substance P, and calcitonin gene-related peptide. Transmission of pain signals continues along the spinal cord to the thalamus, which serves as the pain relay center, and eventually to the cortical regions of the brain where pain is perceived.

▶ Pain Modulation

Modulation of pain (inhibition of nociceptive impulses) can occur by a number of processes. Based on the gate-control theory, pain modulation might occur at the level of the dorsal horn.[19] Because the brain can process only a limited number of signals at one time, other sensory stimuli at nociceptors might alter pain perception. This theory supports the effectiveness of counterirritants and transcutaneous electrical nerve stimulation (TENS) in pain management. Pain modulation can occur through several other complex processes. The endogenous opiate system consists of endorphins (enkephalins, dynorphins, and β-endorphins) that interact with μ-, δ-, and κ-receptors throughout the CNS to inhibit pain impulses and alter perception. The CNS also includes inhibitory descending pathways from the brain that can attenuate pain transmission in the dorsal horn. Neurotransmitters involved in this descending system include endogenous opioids, serotonin, norepinephrine, γ-aminobutyric acid (GABA), and neurotensin. The perception of pain involves not only nociceptive stimulation but physiologic and emotional input that contributes to the perception of pain. Consequently, cognitive behavioral treatments such as distraction, relaxation, and guided imagery can reduce pain perception by altering pain processing in the cortex.

▶ Peripheral Sensitization, Central Sensitization, and Windup

Under normal conditions, a balance generally exists between excitatory and inhibitory neurotransmission. Changes in this balance can occur both peripherally and centrally, resulting in exaggerated responses and sensitization, such as that observed in inflammatory, neuropathic, or functional chronic pain. Pain in these settings might occur spontaneously without any stimulus or might be evoked by a stimulus. Evoked pain might arise from a stimulus that normally does not cause pain (allodynia) such as a light touch in neuropathic pain. Hyperalgesia, an exaggerated and/or prolonged pain response to a stimulus that normally causes pain, can also occur as a result of increased sensitivity in the CNS.

During normal pain transmission, the AMPA receptors are activated, but the N-methyl-D-aspartate (NMDA)

receptor is blocked by magnesium.[16] Repeated nerve depolarization causes release of the magnesium block, allowing the influx of calcium and sodium, and results in excessive excitability and amplification of signals. Continued input from C-fibers and subsequent increases in substance P and glutamate causes the activation of the NMDA receptor, a process referred to as windup. Windup increases the number and responsiveness of neurons in the dorsal horn irrespective of the input from the periphery. Recruitment of neurons not normally involved in pain transmission or spread occurs, leading to allodynia, hyperalgesia, and spread to uninjured tissues.[20] The windup phenomenon supports the observation that untreated acute pain can lead to chronic pain and the belief that pain processes are plastic and not static.

CLINICAL PRESENTATION AND DIAGNOSIS

Classification of Pain

Pain has always been described as a symptom. However, recent advances in the understanding of neural mechanisms have demonstrated that unrelieved pain might lead to changes in the nervous system known as neural plasticity. Because these changes reflect a process that influences a physiologic response, pain, particularly chronic pain, might be considered a disease unto itself.

Pain can be divided into two broad categories: acute and chronic pain. Acute pain is also referred to as adaptive pain because it serves to protect the individual from further injury or promote healing.[17] However, chronic pain has been called maladaptive, a pathologic function of the nervous system or pain as a disease.

▶ Acute Pain

Acute pain is pain that occurs as a result of injury or surgery and is usually self-limited, subsiding when the injury heals. Untreated acute pain can produce physiologic symptoms including tachypnea, tachycardia, and increased sympathetic nervous system activity, such as pallor, diaphoresis, and pupil dilation. Furthermore, poorly treated pain can cause psychological stress and compromise the immune system due to the release of endogenous corticosteroids. Somatic acute pain arises from injury to skin, bone, joint, muscle, and connective tissue, and it is generally localized to the site of injury. Visceral pain involves injury to nerves on internal organs (e.g., intestines, liver) and can present as diffuse, poorly differentiated, and often referred pain. Acute pain should be treated aggressively, even before the diagnosis is established, except in conditions of head or abdominal injury where pain might assist in the differential diagnosis.

▶ Chronic Pain

Chronic pain persists beyond the expected normal time for healing and serves no useful physiologic purpose. Chronic pain might be nociceptive, inflammatory, neuropathic, or functional in origin; however, all forms share some common characteristics. Chronic pain can be intermittent or persistent, or both. Physiologic responses observed in acute pain are often absent in chronic pain; however, other symptoms might predominate. The four main effects of chronic pain include (a) effects on the physical function, (b) psychological changes, (c) social consequences, and (d) societal consequences. Effects of chronic pain on physical function include impaired activities of daily living and sleep disturbances. Psychological components of chronic pain might include depression, anxiety, anger, and loss of self-esteem. As a result of physical and psychological changes, social consequences might ensue, such as changes in relationships with friends and family, intimacy, and isolation. On a societal level, chronic pain contributes to increased healthcare costs, disability, and lost productivity. Management of chronic pain should be multimodal and might involve cognitive interventions, physical manipulations, pharmacologic agents, surgical intervention, and regional or spinal anesthesia.

Chronic Malignant Pain Chronic malignant pain is associated with a progressive disease that is usually life threatening such as cancer, AIDS, progressive neurologic diseases, end-stage organ failure, and dementia.[21] The goal is pain alleviation and prevention, often through a systematic and stepwise approach. Tolerance, dependence, and addiction are often not a concern due to the terminal nature of the illness.

Chronic Nonmalignant Pain Pain not associated with a life-threatening disease and lasting more than 6 months beyond the healing period is referred to as chronic nonmalignant pain. Pain associated with low back pain, osteoarthritis, previous bone fractures, peripheral vascular disease, genitourinary infection, rheumatoid arthritis, and coronary heart disease is considered nonmalignant. The numerous causes of this type of chronic pain make treatment complex and involves a multidisciplinary approach. Treatment is initially conservative but might involve the use of more potent analgesics including opiates in psychologically healthy patients.[22]

Neuropathic Pain Neuropathic pain is considered to be a type of chronic nonmalignant pain involving disease of the central and peripheral nervous systems. Neuropathic pain might be broadly categorized as peripheral or central in nature. Examples of neuropathic pain include PHN, which is pain associated with acute herpetic neuralgia or an acute shingles outbreak. Peripheral or polyneuropathic pain is associated with the distal polyneuropathies of diabetes, human immunodeficiency virus (HIV), and chemotherapeutic agents. Types of central pain include central stroke pain, trigeminal neuralgia, and a complex of syndromes known as complex regional pain syndrome (CRPS). CRPS includes both reflex sympathetic dystrophy and causalgia, both of which are neuropathic pain associated with abnormal functioning of the autonomic nervous system. One of the newest categories of neuropathic pain is neuropathic low back pain.

The symptoms of neuropathic pain are characterized as tingling, burning, shooting, stabbing, electric shock–like quality, or radiating pain. The patient might describe either

---

Clinical Presentation and Diagnosis of Pain Management

General

Patients may be in acute distress (acute pain) or have no signs or symptoms of suffering (chronic pain).

Symptoms

Pain is described based on the following characteristics: onset, duration, location, quality, severity, and intensity. Other symptoms may include anxiety, depression, fatigue, anger, fear, and insomnia.

Signs

Acute pain may cause hypertension, tachycardia, diaphoresis, mydriasis, and pallor.

Diagnosis

The patient is the only person who can describe the intensity and quality of their pain. There are no laboratory tests that can diagnose pain.

---

a constant dull throbbing or burning pain, or an intermittent pain that is stabbing or shooting. Damage to the peripheral nerves might frequently be referred to the body region innervated by those nerves.

Pain Assessment

Effective pain management begins with a thorough and accurate assessment of the patient. Even though pain is a common presenting complaint, lack of regular assessment and reassessment of pain remains a problem and contributes to the undertreatment of pain.[23]

▶ Pain Assessment Guidelines/Regulations for Specific Practice Settings

Screening for pain should be a part of a routine assessment, which has led several organizations such as the Veterans Health Administration (VHA) and the American Pain Society (APS) to declare pain as the fifth vital sign. Many states have adopted a bill of rights for patients in pain. In 2001, the Joint Commission on Accreditation of Health Care Organizations (JCAHO) incorporated pain as the fifth vital sign in its accreditation standards.[24] According to the JCAHO, patients have a right to appropriate assessment and management of their pain and education regarding their pain. ❷ *Following initial assessment of pain, reassessment should be done as needed based on medication choice and the clinical situation.*

▶ Methods of Pain Assessment

A patient-oriented approach to pain is essential, and methods do not differ greatly from those used in other medical conditions. A comprehensive history (medical, family, and psychological) and physical are necessary to evaluate under-lying disease processes for the source of pain and other factors contributing to the pain.[20] A thorough assessment of the characteristics of the pain should be completed, including questions about the pain (onset, duration, location, quality, severity, and intensity), pain relief efforts, and efficacy and side effects of current and past treatments for pain. A common mnemonic for pain assessment is PQRST (Palliative/precipitating, Quality, Radiation, Severity, and Time).[25] Some clinicians have suggested the addition of U ("you") to this mnemonic.[26] During the pain interview, the impact of the pain on the patient's functional status, behavior, and psychological states should also be assessed. Evaluation of psychological status is especially important in patients with chronic pain because depression and affective disorders might be common comorbid conditions. A history of drug and alcohol use should be elicited due to the potential for addiction in patients who might require opiates or other pain medications with a potential for abuse. Other conditions, such as renal or hepatic dysfunction, diabetes, and conditions that affect bowel function, can influence therapy choices and goals. A discussion of the patient's expectations and goals with respect to pain management (level of pain relief, functional status, and quality of life) should also be part of any pain interview.

▶ Pain Assessment Tools

Pain, particularly acute pain, might be accompanied by physiologic signs and symptoms, but there are no reliable objective markers for pain. Many tools have been designed for assessing the severity of pain including rating scales and multidimensional pain assessment tools.

Rating scales provide a simple way to classify the intensity of pain, and they should be selected based on the patient's ability to communicate (Fig. 34–1).[27] Numeric scales are widely used and ask patients to rate their pain on a scale of 0 to 10, with 0 indicating no pain and 10 being the worst pain possible. Using this type of scale, 1 to 3 is considered mild pain, 4 to 6 is moderate pain, and 7 to 10 is severe pain. The visual analog scale (VAS) is similar to the numerical scale in that it requires patients to place a mark on a 10-cm line where one end is no pain, and the worst possible pain is on the other end. For patients who have difficulty assigning a number to their pain, a categorical scale might be an option to communicate the intensity of the pain experience. Examples of this include a simple descriptive list of words and the Wong-Baker FACES of Pain Rating Scale.[28]

Multidimensional assessment tools obtain information about the pain and impact on quality of life, but they are often more time consuming to complete. Examples of these types of tools include the Initial Pain Assessment Tool, Brief Pain Inventory, McGill Pain Questionnaire, the Neuropathic Pain Scale, and the Oswestry Disability Index.[29–33]

▶ Pain Assessment in Challenging Populations

Children   Pain interviews can be conducted with children as young as 3 or 4 years of age; however, communication might be limited by vocabulary.[34] Terms familiar to children such

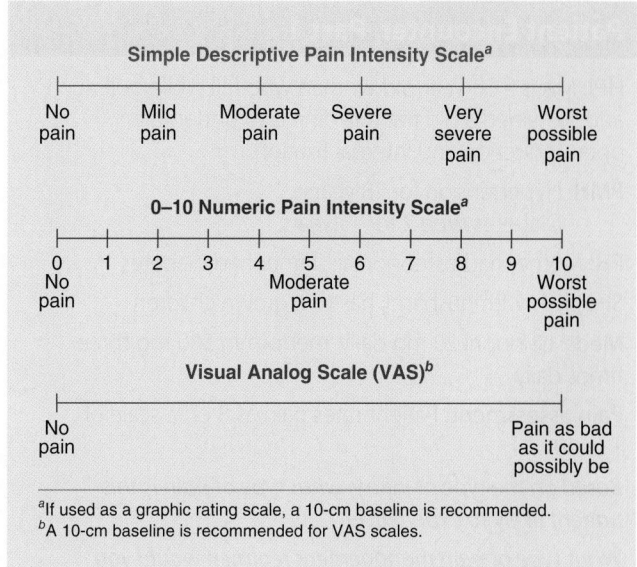

FIGURE 34–1. Pain rating scales. (From U.S. Department of Health and Human Services, Agency for Health Care Policy and Research. Clinical practice guideline, cancer pain management. Rockville, MD: AHCPR; 1994 [cited 2011 Oct 10]. Available from: *http://www.ncbi.nlm.nih.gov/books/bookres. fcgi/hstat6/f37_capcf4.gif.*)

as *hurt, owie,* or *boo boo* might be used to describe pain. The VAS is best used with children older than 7 years. Other scales based on numbers of objects (e.g., pokers chips), increasing color intensity, or faces of pain might be helpful for children between 4 and 7 years of age. In children younger than 3 to 4 years, behavioral or physiologic measures, such as pulse or respiratory rate, might be more appropriate. Pain assessment in newborns and infants relies on behavioral observation for such clues as vocalizations (crying and fussing), facial expressions, body movements (flailing of limbs and pulling legs in), withdrawal, and change in eating and sleeping habits.[35] Preschool children experiencing pain might become clingy, lose motor and verbal skills, and start to deny pain because treatment might be linked to discomfort or punishment. School-age children might exhibit aggressiveness, nightmares, anxiety, and withdrawal when in pain; adolescents might respond to pain with oppositional behavior and depression.

Elderly   Most of the previously discussed pain scales can be used in older persons who are cognitively intact or with mild dementia. The pain thermometer and FACES of pain have been studied in older persons. In persons with moderate to severe dementia or those who are nonverbal, observation of pain behaviors, such as guarding or grimacing, provides an alternative for pain assessment. The Pain Assessment in Advanced Dementia (PAINAD) tool might be used to quantify signs of pain and involves observing the older adult for 15 minutes for breathing, negative vocalizations, facial expression, body language, and consolability.[36] Regardless of which pain assessment tool is used, the practitioner should first determine if the patient understands the concept of the scale to ensure reliability of the instrument.

Patient Encounter, Part 1

HPI: MA is a 68-year-old woman who fell while golfing and sustained a hip fracture. She is to undergo an open-reduction and internal fixation.

PMH: Hypertension for 18 years
Diabetes type 2 for 13 years

FH: Mother had osteoporosis; father had diabetes

SH: Lives with husband; has two grown children

Meds: Lisinopril 20 mg daily, metformin 500 mg three times daily

Pain assessment: Patient rates pain as 8 on a scale of 1 to 10

Based on the type of injury, what type of pain is this patient likely to experience?

What type of pain management regimen would you recommend in the postoperative period? Explain your answer.

TREATMENT

General Approach to Treatment

❸ *Effective treatment involves an evaluation of the cause, duration, and intensity of the pain, and selection of an appropriate treatment modality for the pain situation.* Depending on the type of pain, treatment might involve pharmacologic and nonpharmacologic therapy or both. General principles for the pharmacologic management of pain are listed in the section "Patient Care and Monitoring." Two common approaches to the selection of treatment are based on severity of pain and the mechanism responsible for the pain (Fig. 34–2). Clinical practice guidelines for pain management are available from the APS, the Agency for Healthcare Research and Quality (AHRQ), the American Geriatrics Society (AGS), and the American Society of Anesthesiologists (ASA).

▶ Selection of Agent Based on Severity of Pain

❹ *Whenever possible, the least potent oral analgesic should be selected.* Guidelines for the selection of therapeutic agents based on pain intensity are derived from the World Health Organization (WHO) analgesic ladder for the management of cancer pain (Table 34–1).[37] Mild to moderate pain is generally treated with nonopioid analgesics. Combinations of medium-potency opioids and acetaminophen (APAP) or nonsteroidal anti-inflammatory drugs (NSAIDs) are often used for moderate pain. Potent opioids are recommended for severe pain. Throughout this progression, adjuvant medications are added, as needed, to manage side effects and to augment analgesia. While these guidelines can be useful for initial therapy, the clinical situation (type of pain), cost and pharmacokinetic profile of available drugs, and patient-specific factors (age, concomitant illnesses, previous response, and other medications) must also be considered. Pain medications might also be used in the absence of pain

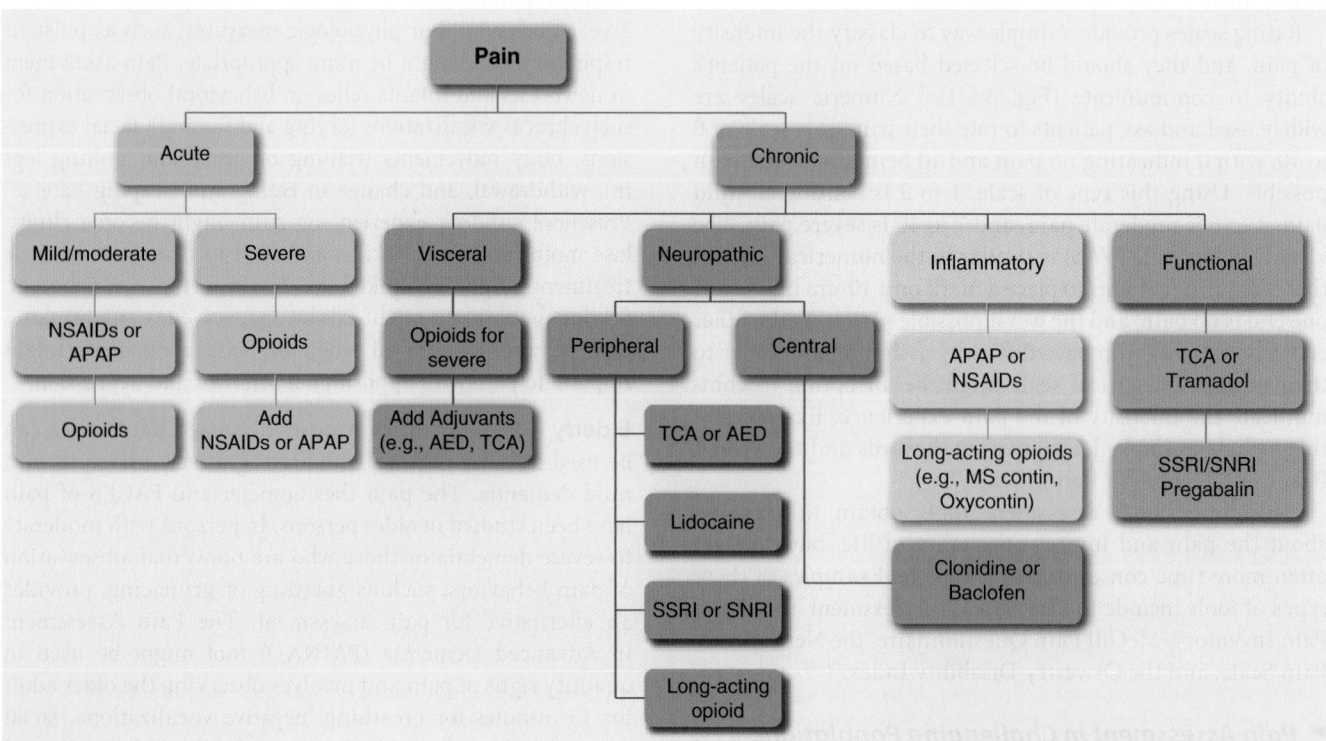

FIGURE 34–2. Pain algorithm. (AED, antiepileptic drugs; APAP, acetaminophen; MS, morphine sulfate; NSAIDs, nonsteroidal anti-inflammatory drugs; SNRI, serotonin norepinephrine reuptake inhibitors; SSRI, selective serotonin reuptake inhibitors; TCA, tricyclic antidepressants.)

Table 34–1

Selection of Analgesics Based on Intensity of Pain

Pain Intensity	Corresponding Numerical Rating	WHO Therapeutic Recommendations	Examples of Initial Therapy	Comments
Mild	1–3/10	Nonopioid analgesic; regular scheduled dosing	Acetaminophen 1,000 mg q 6 h; ibuprofen 600 mg q 6 h	Consider adding an adjunct or using an alternate regimen if pain is not reduced in 1–2 days
Moderate	4–6/10	Add an opioid to the nonopioid for moderate pain; regular scheduled dosing	Acetaminophen 325 mg + codeine 60 mg q 4 h; acetaminophen 325 mg + oxycodone 5 mg q 4 h	Consider step-up therapy if pain is not relieved by two or more different drugs
Severe	7–10/10	Switch to a high-potency opioid; regular scheduled dosing	Morphine 10 mg q 4 h; or hydromorphone 4 mg q 4 h	

Data from Ref. 37, 39, 45.

in anticipation of a painful event such as surgery to minimize peripheral and central sensitization.

▶ Mechanistic Approach to Therapy

Current analgesic therapy is aimed at controlling or blunting pain symptoms. However, diverse mechanisms contributing to the various types of pain continue to be further elucidated. An understanding of these new mechanisms of pain transmission might lead to improvement in pain management as pharmacologic management of pain becomes more mechanism specific. Use of NSAIDs for inflammatory types of pain is an example of a mechanistic approach. Because several mechanisms of pain often coexist, a polypharmacy approach seems rational to target each mechanism.

Two current foci in pain management are to identify the mechanisms that are responsible for pain hypersensitivity and to prevent this initial hypersensitivity. Therefore, the goal of pain therapy is to reduce peripheral sensitization and subsequent central stimulation and amplification associated with windup, spread, and central sensitization.[17]

Nonpharmacologic Therapy

Nonpharmacologic therapies (psychological interventions and physical therapy) might be used in both acute and chronic pain. Psychological interventions can reduce pain as well as the anxiety, depression, fear, and anger associated with pain. Psychological interventions helpful in management of acute pain are imagery (picturing oneself in a safe, peaceful place) and distraction (listening to music or focusing on breathing). Chronic pain patients might benefit from relaxation, biofeedback, cognitive behavioral therapy, psychotherapy, support groups, and spiritual counseling. Biofeedback teaches patients to control physiologic responses to pain and has been effective in headache and chronic low back pain. Cognitive therapy encourages patients to monitor their perceptions of pain, reducing stress and negativism.

Psychotherapy is very useful for patients with chronic pain; it can also assist in the treatment of psychiatric comorbidities and help patients deal with terminal illness.[38] The patient should be educated about what to expect regarding pain and its treatment, whether pain is acute pain (e.g., preoperative explanations of expected postsurgical pain) or chronic (e.g., patient and family education in hospice care).

Physical therapy is an essential part of many types of pain situations. Treatment modalities include heat, cold, water, ultrasound therapy, TENS, massage, and therapeutic exercise. Heat and cold therapy are utilized in a variety of musculoskeletal conditions (muscle spasms, low back pain, fibromyalgia, sprains, and strains). Heating modalities include local hot packs, paraffin wrap, hydrotherapy, and deep-heating methods (ultrasound). Cold treatments might be delivered via cold packs, ice massage, cold water immersion, or coolant sprays. TENS therapy is based on the theory that electrical stimulation of a nerve in a particular area can block pain impulses originating from that area. TENS is also believed to release endogenous endorphins and enkephalins. Massage therapy is used to relieve muscle tension and stiffness and is also felt to increase endogenous endorphins. Therapeutic exercise improves not only strength, endurance, and range of motion but also provides cardiovascular, psychological, and other health benefits.

Pharmacologic Therapy

▶ Nonopioid Analgesics

Acetaminophen   APAP, an analgesic and antipyretic, is often selected as initial therapy for mild to moderate pain and is considered first line in several pain situations such as low back pain and osteoarthritis.[39] Mechanistically, APAP is believed to inhibit prostaglandin synthesis in the CNS and block pain impulses in the periphery. APAP is well tolerated at usual doses and has few clinically significant drug interactions except causing increased hypoprothrombinemic response to warfarin in patients receiving APAP doses of more than 2,000 mg/day. The maximum recommended dose for patients with normal renal and hepatic function is 4,000 mg/day. Hepatotoxicity has been reported with excessive use and overdose, and the risk of this adverse effect increases in those with hepatitis or chronic alcohol use, as well as those who binge drink or are in a fasting state. Regular chronic use of APAP has been associated with chronic renal failure, but reports are conflicting. For these reasons, the maximum dose should be reduced by 50% to 75% in patients with renal dysfunction or hepatic disease and in those who engage in excessive alcohol use. Due to concerns about increasing rates of acetaminophen toxicity, the FDA commissioned a working group within the Center for Drug Evaluation and Research to recommend interventions to reduce APAP induced liver toxicity. An assembly of three advisory panels reviewed the report of the working group and endorsed the following three recommendations including a reduction of the maximum daily dose from 4 g to possibly 3,250 mg daily, a reduction in acetaminophen dose to 325 mg in prescription narcotic-acetaminophen combinations, and a reduction of the maximum single nonprescription dose from 1 g to 650 mg, thus relegating the 500-mg dosage strength to prescription status.[40]

Aspirin and Other Salicylates Aspirin, nonacetylated salicylates, and other NSAIDs have analgesic, antipyretic, and anti-inflammatory actions. These agents inhibit cyclooxygenase (COX-1 and COX-2) enzymes, thereby preventing prostaglandin synthesis, which results in reduced nociceptor sensitization and an increased pain threshold. NSAIDs are the preferred agents for mild to moderate pain in situations that are mediated by prostaglandins (rheumatoid arthritis, menstrual cramps, and postsurgical pain) and in the management of pain from bony metastasis, but they are of minimal use in neuropathic pain.

Aspirin is effective for mild to moderate pain; however, the risk of GI irritation and bleeding limits frequent use of this drug for pain management. Direct effects of aspirin on the GI mucosa and irreversible platelet inhibition contribute to this risk, which can occur even at low doses. Hypersensitivity reactions are also possible and might occur in 25% of patients with coexisting asthma, nasal polyps, or chronic urticaria. Of additional concern is the potential for cross-sensitivity of other NSAIDs in this group of patients. Nonacetylated salicylates (choline magnesium salicylate and sodium salicylate) have a reduced risk of GI effects and platelet inhibition and might be used in aspirin-sensitive patients. Diflunisal, a salicylic acid derivative, is associated with fewer GI complaints compared with aspirin, but platelet inhibition does increase the risk of GI bleeding.

Nonsteroidal Anti-inflammatory Drugs NSAIDs provide analgesia equal to or better than that of aspirin or APAP combined with codeine, and they are very effective for inflammatory pain and pain associated with bone metastasis.[18] These agents are classified by their chemical structures (fenamates, acetic acids, propionic acids, pyranocarboxylic acids, pyrrolizine carboxylic acids, and COX-2 inhibitors). Although only some members of this class have approval for treatment of pain, it is likely that all of them have similar analgesic effects.

All members of this class appear to be equally effective, but there is great intrapatient variability in response. After an adequate trial of 2 to 3 weeks with a particular oral agent, it is reasonable to switch to another member of the class. Ketorolac and ibuprofen are available in parenteral and oral dosage forms; unlike other NSAIDs, ketorolac's duration of use is limited to 5 days. NSAIDs demonstrate a flat-dose response curve, with higher doses producing no greater efficacy than moderate doses but resulting in an increased incidence of adverse effects (GI irritation, hepatic dysfunction, renal insufficiency, platelet inhibition, sodium retention, and CNS dysfunction).

Patients at increased risk of NSAID-induced GI adverse effects (e.g., dyspepsia, peptic ulcer formation, and bleeding) include the elderly, those with peptic ulcer disease, coagulopathy, and patients receiving high doses of concurrent corticosteroids. Nephrotoxicity is more common in the elderly, patients with creatinine clearance values less than 50 mL/min (0.84 mL/s), and those with volume depletion or on diuretic therapy. NSAIDs should be used with caution in patients with reduced cardiac output due to sodium retention and in patients receiving antihypertensives, warfarin, and lithium.

NSAIDs are classified as nonselective (they inhibit COX-1 and COX-2) or selective (inhibit only COX-2) based on degree of COX inhibition. COX-2 inhibition is responsible for anti-inflammatory effects, whereas COX-1 inhibition contributes to increased GI and renal toxicity associated with nonselective agents. Because the antiplatelet effect of nonselective NSAIDs is reversible, concurrent use might reduce the cardioprotective effect of aspirin due to competitive inhibition of COX-1. For this reason, administration of aspirin prior to the NSAID is recommended.[41] The cardiovascular safety of the COX-2 inhibitors has been questioned due to increased risk of myocardial infarction (MI) and stroke noted in several trials.[42-44] The FDA Committees on Arthritis and Drug Safety and Risk Management convened in February 2005 to evaluate the published studies and manufacturer information about the cardiovascular-adverse events associated with COX-2 inhibitors. As a follow-up to the committee's recommendations, the FDA took regulatory action in April 2005 announcing that the increased risk of cardiovascular events was likely a class effect of NSAIDs. A Boxed Warning highlighting the potential for increased risk of cardiovascular events and GI bleeding is now required for all prescription nonselective NSAIDs and celecoxib. Stronger warnings about these adverse events are also required on nonprescription NSAIDs. As a result of the data and subsequent events, two members of this class, rofecoxib and valdecoxib, were withdrawn from the market. Future COX-2 inhibitors and nonselective NSAIDs will likely have to undergo cardiovascular safety studies before receiving FDA approval. When a NSAID is needed in a patient with cardiovascular risk, the benefits of therapy must outweigh the risks, and the lowest effective dose of the NSAID is recommended.[45]

▶ Opioid Analgesics

Opioids are considered the agents of choice for the treatment of severe acute pain and moderate to severe pain associated with cancer.[46] For chronic pain, their use was once highly controversial; however, use of opioids in chronic pain is now gaining acceptance.[47] Opioids are classified by their activity at the receptor site, usual pain intensity treated, and duration of action (short acting versus long acting).

Selection and Dosing   The opioids exert their analgesic efficacy by stimulating opioid receptors (μ, κ, and δ) in the CNS. There is a wide variety of potencies among the opioids, with some used for moderate pain (codeine, hydrocodone, tramadol, and partial agonists) and others reserved for severe pain (morphine and hydromorphone). Pure agonists (morphine) bind to μ-receptors to produce analgesia that increases with dose without a ceiling effect. Pure agonists are divided into three chemical classes: phenanthrenes or morphine-like, phenyl piperidine or meperidine-like, and diphenyl heptane or methadone-like. Partial agonists/antagonists (butorphanol, pentazocine, and nalbuphine) partially stimulate the μ-receptor and antagonize the κ-receptors. This activity results in reduced analgesic efficacy with a ceiling dose, reduced side effects at the μ-receptor, psychotomimetic side effects due to κ-receptor antagonism, and possible withdrawal symptoms in patients who are dependent on pure agonists.

Selection of the agent and route depend on individual patient-related factors including severity of pain, individual perceptions, weight, age, opioid tolerance, and concomitant disease (renal or hepatic dysfunction). Because pure agonists are pharmacologically similar, choice of agent might be also guided by pharmacokinetic parameters and other drug characteristics. Hepatic impairment can decrease the metabolism of most opioids, particularly methadone, meperidine, and pentazocine. Furthermore, the clearance of meperidine and morphine and their metabolites is reduced in renal dysfunction.

Table 34–2 provides a summary of opiate options, but several drugs warrant further discussion. Normeperidine, the active metabolite of meperidine, can produce tremors, myoclonus, delirium, and seizures. Due to the potential for accumulation of normeperidine, meperidine should not be used in the elderly, those with renal impairment, in patients using patient-controlled analgesia (PCA) devices, or for more than 1 to 2 days of intermittent dosing. Methadone is unique among the opiates because it has several mechanisms (μ-agonist, NMDA-receptor antagonist, and inhibition of reuptake of serotonin and norepinephrine) that make it an interesting choice for chronic pain. The long-half of methadone (30 hours) permits extended dosing intervals; however, the potential for accumulation with repeated dosing often results in challenging dose conversion. Tramadol is a synthetic opioid with a dual mechanism of action (μ-agonist and inhibition of serotonin and norepinephrine reuptake) and efficacy and safety similar to that of equianalgesic doses of codeine plus APAP. Tramadol has been evaluated in several types of neuropathic pain and might have a role in the treatment of chronic pain. Tramadol is associated with an increased risk of seizures in patients with a seizure disorder, those at risk for seizures, and those taking medications that can lower the seizure threshold. Doses greater than 500 mg have also been associated with seizures. The use of tramadol with other serotonergic drugs (e.g., selective serotonin

reuptake inhibitors [SSRIs]) might precipitate serotonin syndrome. Although originally thought not to be habit forming, dependence can occur with tramadol.

About 70% of individuals will experience significant analgesia from 10 mg/70 kg of body weight of IV morphine or its equivalent.[18] For severe pain in opiate-naive patients, a usual starting dose is 5 to 10 mg of morphine every 4 hours. In the initial stages of severe pain, medication should be given around the clock. Rescue doses should be made available for breakthrough pain in doses equivalent to 10% to 20% of the total daily opioid requirement and administered every 2 to 6 hours if needed. Alternatively, one-sixth of the total daily dose or one-third of the 12-hourly dose might be used. Scheduled doses should be titrated based on the degree of pain. One method involves adjustment of the maintenance dose based on the total 24-hour rescue dose requirement. Alternatively, utilizing dose escalation, doses could be increased by 50% to 100% or 30% to 50% of the current dose, for those in severe and moderate pain, respectively. Once pain relief is achieved, and if treatment is necessary for more than a few days, conversion to a controlled-release or long-acting opioid should be made with an equal amount of agent. Several sustained-release products are available containing morphine, oxycodone, and fentanyl. Some clinicians will reduce the total daily dose of the long-acting dosage form by 25% when initiating a sustained-release product to reduce the likelihood of oversedation. The dose of a pure agonist is limited only by tolerability to side effects. Tolerance might

Table 34–2

Equianalgesic Doses of Selected Opioids

Opioid (Brand Name)	Parenteral (mg)	Oral (mg)
Mild to Moderate Pain		
Codeine (generic, various)	120	200
Hydrocodone (Vicodin, Lorcet)	N/A	30
Oxycodone (OxyContin, OxyFAST, Oxy IR)	N/A	20
Meperidine (Demerol)	100	400
Moderate to Severe Pain		
Morphine (Roxanol, MS Contin, Kadian, Avinza)	10	30
Hydromorphone (Dilaudid)	1.5	7.5
Oxymorphone (Opana, Opana SR, Numorphan)	1	N/A
Levorphanol (Levo-Dromoran)	2	4
Fentanyl (Duragesic)	0.1–0.2	N/A[a]
Methadone (Dolophine)	10[b]	3–5[b]

Dose Equianalgesic to 10 mg of Parenteral Morphine (mg)

[a]Transdermal: 100 mcg/h = 2–4 mg/h of IV morphine.

[b]Dosage calculations when converting from morphine to methadone are not linear. The equianalgesic dose of methadone will decrease progressively as the morphine equivalents increase (Table 34–4).

Data from Refs. 26, 45, 49, 51.

develop to analgesic effects, necessitating increasing doses to achieve the same level of pain relief. Physical dependence will also occur with the long-term use of opioids. However, addiction or psychological dependence is unlikely in legitimate pain patients unless there are predisposing risk factors. Pain patients who are undertreated might appear to be drug seeking (pseudoaddiction); however, effective pain management resolves the behaviors. When opioids are used for chronic pain, use of informed consent for chronic opioid therapy, medication management agreements, or pain contracts might be appropriate to monitor the use (prescribing and dispensing) of controlled substances.

Opioids are administered by a variety of routes, including oral (tablet and liquid), sublingual, rectal, transdermal, transmucosal, IV, subcutaneous, and intraspinal. Although the oral and transdermal routes are most common, the method of administration is based on patient needs (severity of pain) and characteristics (swallowing difficulty and preference). Oral opioids have an onset of effect of 45 minutes, so IV or subcutaneous administration might be preferred if more rapid relief is desired. Intramuscular (IM) injections are not recommended because of pain at the injection site and wide fluctuations in drug absorption and peak plasma concentrations achieved. More invasive routes of administration such as PCA and intraspinal (epidural and intrathecal) are primarily used postoperatively but might also be used in refractory chronic pain situations. PCA delivers a self-administered dose via an infusion pump with a preprogrammed dose, minimum dosing interval, and a maximum hourly dose. Morphine, fentanyl, and hydromorphone are commonly administered via PCA pumps by the IV route but less frequently by the subcutaneous or epidural route.

Epidural analgesia is frequently used for lower extremity procedures and pain (e.g., knee surgery, labor pain, and some abdominal procedures). Intermittent bolus or continuous infusion of preservative-free opioids (morphine, hydromorphone, or fentanyl) and local anesthetics (bupivacaine) might be used for epidural analgesia. Opiates given by this route might cause pruritus that is relieved by naloxone. Adverse effects including respiratory depression, hypotension, and urinary retention might occur. When epidural routes are used in narcotic-dependent patients, systemic analgesics must also be used to prevent withdrawal because the opioid is not absorbed and remains in the epidural space. Doses of opioids used in epidural analgesia are 10 times less than IV doses, and intrathecal doses are 10 times less than epidural doses (i.e., 10 mg of IV morphine is equivalent to 1 mg epidural morphine and 0.1 mg of intrathecally administered morphine).[45]

Combination Analgesics Combinations of opioids and nonopioids often result in enhanced analgesia and lower dose of each. Combination analgesics are frequently used in moderate pain. However, in severe pain, the nonopioid component reaches maximum dosage, and thus the usefulness of nonopioids in this situation is limited. Additionally, the combination products are short acting and often not suitable for chronic therapy. Single agents offer greater dosing flexibility than combination products.

Opioid Allergy True narcotic allergies are rare and should not be confused with pruritus associated with opiate use. Cross-sensitivity between morphine-like, meperidine-like, and methadone-like agents is unlikely. Therefore, when an individual is allergic to one drug in a chemical class of opioids, it is reasonable to select an agent in another chemical class. For the purpose of drug selection in patients with allergies, mixed agonists/antagonists should be treated as morphine-like agents.

Tapering of Opioids Tapering of opioids might be necessary once the painful situation has resolved in patients receiving doses greater than 160 mg/day of oral morphine (or the equivalent) or in those with prolonged opioid use. In these situations the dose should be reduced by 15% to 20% each day to avoid withdrawal symptoms.

Managing Opioid Side Effects and Drug Interactions
Side effects common to all opioids include sedation, hallucinations, constipation, nausea and vomiting, urinary retention, myoclonus, and respiratory depression. Table 34–3 shows management strategies for side effects. In terms of medication management, the most frequent are sedation, nausea, and constipation. Sedation and nausea are common when initiating therapy and when increasing doses. Nausea

Table 34–3
Managing Opioid Side Effects

Adverse Effects	Drug Treatment/Management
Excessive sedation	Reduce dose by 25% or increase dosing interval
Constipation	Casanthranol-docusate 1 cap at bedtime or twice daily; senna 1–2 tabs at bedtime or twice daily; bisacodyl 5–10 mg daily plus docusate 100 mg twice daily
Nausea and vomiting	Prevention: Hydroxyzine 25–100 mg (PO/IM) every 4–6 hours as needed; diphenhydramine 25–50 mg (PO/IM) q 6 h as needed; ondansetron 4 mg IV or 16 mg PO
	Treatment: Prochlorperazine 5–10 mg (PO/IM) q 3–4 h as needed or 25 mg PR twice daily; ondansetron 4–8 mg IV q 8 h as needed
Gastroparesis	Metoclopramide 10 mg (PO/IV) q 6–8 h
Vertigo	Meclizine 12.5–25 mg PO q 6 h as needed
Urticaria/itching	Hydroxyzine 25–100 mg (PO/IM) q 4–6 h as needed; diphenhydramine 25–50 mg (PO/IM) q 6 h as needed
Respiratory depression	Mild: Reduce dose by 25%
	Moderate to severe: Naloxone 0.4–2 mg IV q 2–3 min (up to 10 mg) for complete reversal; 0.1–0.2 mg IV q 2–3 min until desired reversal for partial reversal; may need to repeat in 1–2 hours depending on narcotic half-life
CNS irritability	Discontinue opioid; treat with benzodiazepine

IM, intramuscular; PO, orally; PR, per rectum.

Data from Refs. 27, 45, 49.

can be prevented with a centrally acting antiemetic. Sedation usually improves with continued therapy but might become intractable at high doses, and stimulants such as methylphenidate might be needed. Respiratory depression is a serious adverse effect and usually occurs after acute administration in opioid-naive patients. Tolerance to respiratory depression develops rapidly with repeated doses, and respiratory depression is rarely a clinically significant problem in pain patients even those with respiratory impairment. Constipation is a significant adverse effect to which tolerance does develop, and prophylaxis with stimulant laxatives (e.g., senna or bisacodyl) and stool softeners such as docusate is recommended.

Codeine, hydrocodone, morphine, methadone, and oxycodone are substrates of the cytochrome P450 (CYP) enzyme: CYP2D6.[48] Inhibition of CYP2D6 results in decreased analgesia of codeine and hydrocodone due to decreased conversion to the active metabolites (e.g., morphine and hydromorphone, respectively) and increased effects of morphine, methadone, and oxycodone. Methadone is also a substrate of CYP3A4, and its metabolism is increased by phenytoin and decreased by cimetidine. CNS depressants might potentiate the sedative effects of opiates.

Opioid Rotation   Opioid rotation is the switch from one opioid to another to achieve a better balance between analgesia and treatment-limiting adverse effects. This practice is often used when escalating doses (more than 1 g morphine/day) become ineffective. In some settings, opioid rotation is used routinely to prevent the development of analgesic tolerance.[49]

Equianalgesic Dosing of Opioid Analgesics   Conversion from one dosage form to another or from one opioid to another might be necessary in situations such as ineffective pain control, emergence of side effects, change in patient status, and in formulary restrictions. ❺ *Equianalgesic doses should be used when converting from one opioid to another.* Clinicians should be familiar with the equianalgesic dosing and conversion strategies to avoid analgesic failure. Equianalgesic tables serve as a guide for selection of the dosage of the new opioid, but they have limitations because they are often based on single-dose studies and clinical observations.[50] Opioid potency is compared using a reference standard of 10 mg parenteral morphine. Switching from one dosage form to another of the same opioid (i.e., IV to oral) is relatively simple. The current total daily dose is calculated and the total of the new dosage form is determined using a ratio of the equianalgesic doses. This result is then adjusted based on the usual dosing frequency of the new form. When converting to a sustained-release form of the same opioid, dosage may be reduced by 25% to avoid initial sedation; however, the specific product literature should also be consulted.

The first step in an opioid rotation is to calculate the patient's total daily dose of opioid based on the regularly scheduled dose and the total amount of rescue dose needed in 24 hours. This total is then converted to morphine-dosing equivalents using equianalgesic doses (Table 34–2). The total daily morphine dose is then used to calculate the daily dose of the new opioid using dosing equivalents from an equianalgesic table. Because cross-tolerance may not be complete between opioids, some references suggest that the calculated equianalgesic dose be reduced by 25% to 50%.[50] If the opioid switch is due to uncontrolled pain, a dosage reduction may not be needed. The calculated equianalgesic dose may need to be reduced more in the medically frail and when converting to methadone.[51,52] Methadone appears to be much more potent than once believed, and morphine-to-methadone ratios vary according to the total dose of morphine taken at the time of making the conversion to methadone (Table 34–4).[53,54] Conversion to methadone is a complex process, and several different strategies have been proposed including a switch of the entire dose in 1 day or a gradual conversion over 3 days.

▶ Adjuvant Agents for Chronic Pain

The role of NSAIDs and opioids in chronic nonmalignant pain has been discussed; however, a review of adjuvant agents

---

Patient Encounter, Part 2

Following surgery MA was placed on morphine patient-controlled analgesia (PCA). She has been using 80 mg of morphine/24 hours with adequate pain control; however, she has developed redness and itching on her neck that was believed to be due to the morphine.

Current medications: Morphine PCA, lisinopril 20 mg daily, metformin 500 mg three times daily, Lovenox 30 mg subcutaneously daily, until ambulating. She will be discharged to a skilled nursing facility for rehabilitation therapy.

The physician would like to convert her to a combination preparation of oxycodone and APAP.

What dosing regimen would you suggest?

Recommend a monitoring plan for this patient.

How would you assess pain response?

The patient is concerned about the redness and itching she developed while on morphine. What other interventions or education may be necessary at this time?

Table 34–4

Methadone Dose Conversions

Total Daily Dose of Oral Morphine	Morphine:Methadone Factor
Less than 100 mg	3:1
	3 mg morphine:1 mg methadone
101–300 mg	5:1
301–600 mg	10:1
601–800 mg	12:1
801–1,000 mg	15:1
More than 1,000 mg	20:1

Data from Ripamonti C, Bianchi M. The use of methadone for cancer pain. Hematol Oncol Clin North Am 2002;16:543–555.

Patient Encounter, Part 3

MA was discharged to a skilled nursing facility and is receiving physical therapy and occupational therapy 6 days each week.

Current medications: Lisinopril 20 mg daily; metformin 500 mg three times daily; Lovenox 30 mg subcutaneously daily, until ambulating; hydrocodone/acetaminophen 5/325 mg q 6 h as needed for pain.

Pain Assessment: Patient reports pain of 7 out of 10; worse with movement.

Physical therapy notes indicate patient is unable to complete therapy goals due to complaints of pain.

Based on this information, what would you recommend as the consultant pharmacist to optimize pain control?

Table 34–5

Selected Adjuvant Analgesics and Suggested Dosing

Agent	Dosing Guidelines	FDA-Approved Indication
Amitriptyline (Elavil)	10–25 mg at bedtime with weekly increments to a target dose of 25–150 mg of amitriptyline or an equivalent dose of another TCA	
Duloxetine (Cymbalta)	DPN: 60 mg daily Fibromyalgia: 30 mg daily, may be increased by 30 mg increments to a maximum of 120 mg daily	DPN, fibromyalgia
Gabapentin (Neurontin)	Initially, 300 mg three times a day up to a maximum of 3,600 mg daily, in divided doses[a]	PHN
Pregabalin (Lyrica)	DPN: Initially, 50 mg three times a day; may be increased to 100 mg three times a day within 1 week based on efficacy and tolerability[a] PHN: Initially 75 mg twice a day or 50 mg three times a day; may be increased to 100 mg three times a day within 1 week based on efficacy and tolerability[a] Fibromyalgia: Initially 75 mg twice a day, increase to 300 mg daily over 7 days	DPN, PHN, and fibromyalgia
Lidocaine 5% (Lidoderm patch)	Up to 3 patches may be applied directly over the painful site once daily; patches are applied using a regimen of 12 hours on and 12 hours off	PHN

DPN, diabetic peripheral neuropathy; PHN, postherpetic neuralgia; TCA, tricyclic antidepressant.

[a]Dosing for creatinine clearance of ≥60 mL/min (1.0 mL/s).

Data from Refs. 54–58.

for chronic pain, particularly neuropathic pain, is warranted. Adjuvant analgesics are drugs that have indications other than pain but are useful as monotherapy or in combination with nonopioids and opioids. Common adjuvants include antiepileptic drugs (AEDs), antidepressants, antiarrhythmic drugs, local anesthetics, topical agents (e.g., capsaicin), and a variety of other drugs (e.g., NMDA antagonists, clonidine, and muscle relaxants).

There is little consensus on the optimal management of neuropathic pain because much of the evidence for treatment effectiveness consists of anecdotal reports or poorly designed trials. Published guidelines have been suggested for the general management of neuropathic pain.[55] Suggestions for first-line therapy include gabapentin or pregabalin, transdermal lidocaine, or tricyclic antidepressants (TCAs) (Table 34–5).[55-59] Newer antidepressants, such as the SSRIs, have fewer side effects but appear to be less effective than the TCAs for neuropathic pain. However, serotonin-norepinephrine reuptake inhibitors (SNRIs), (e.g., duloxetine and venlafaxine) have been used successfully for painful DPN. A stepwise approach is suggested for managing the patient with neuropathic pain beginning with the least invasiv, effective therapeutic choice and proceeding to the rational use of multiple drug regimens. To guide the choice of pharmacologic agents, patients might be identified as candidates for AEDs, TCAs, or opioids based on the presence of peripheral or central nerve pain and description of symptoms (Fig. 34–2). Choice of agent might also depend on dosing frequency and comorbidities. Data on combination therapy are lacking, and the use of combined treatment is empirical based on the additive therapeutic benefit. Scheduled medication regimens instead of "as-needed" dosing should be used when treating chronic pain, and the effectiveness of therapy should be reassessed regularly. If patients are managed on a multiple drug regimen and changes are indicated, changing only one drug at a time is suggested. Topical agents (e.g., capsaicin) might be added to a regimen to reduce the oral medication load, particularly if adverse effects are a problem or if pain is not relieved.

▶ Complementary and Alternative Medicine

Complementary and alternative medicine (CAM) is a term used to encompass a variety of therapies (e.g., acupuncture, chiropractic, botanical, and nonbotanical dietary supplements, and homeopathy). Painful conditions are among the most common reasons individuals seek relief from CAM. In a recent survey, neck pain, joint pain, arthritis, and headache were among the top 10 reasons for use of CAM, and low back pain ranked the number-one reason for CAM therapies. Of the CAM therapies, chiropractic and acupuncture are the most accepted and used modalities. A variety of dietary supplements have been suggested for painful conditions such as S-adenosylmethionine (SAM-e), ginger, fish oil, feverfew, γ-linoleic acid, glucosamine, and chondroitin. Of these, glucosamine and chondroitin are the most popular and have the most evidence supporting their efficacy. Glucosamine in doses of 1,500 mg/day has been shown to be effective in reducing the pain of osteoarthritis by fostering repair of cartilage, and it is recommended by the Osteoarthritis Research Society International (OARSI).[39]

OUTCOME EVALUATION

Individualize the treatment goals at the beginning of treatment. Use information obtained during the pain interview to create goals that are consistent with the patient's expectations. Prevention, reduction, and/or elimination of pain are important goals for the treatment of acute pain. With chronic pain, elimination of pain might not be possible, and goals might focus on improvement or maintenance of functional capacity and quality of life. Thus, for example, pain goals might include "pain scale less than 3," or "be able to play a game with grandchildren," or "be able to knit again." Assess patients periodically, depending on the method of analgesia and pain condition, for achievement of pain goals. Evaluate the patient for the presence of adverse drug reactions, drug allergies, and drug interactions.

Abbreviations Introduced in This Chapter

AED	Antiepileptic drug
AGS	American Geriatrics Society
AHRQ	Agency for Healthcare Research and Quality
AMPA	α-amino-3-hydroxy-5-methylisoxazole-4-propionic acid
APAP	Acetaminophen
APS	American Pain Society
ASA	American Society of Anesthesiologists
CAM	Complementary and alternative medicine
CHF	Congestive heart failure
COX	Cyclooxygenase
CRPS	Complex regional pain syndrome
CYP	Cytochrome P450 enzyme
DPN	Cytochrome P450 enzyme
GABA	γ-Aminobutyric acid
HIV	Human immunodeficiency virus
HTN	Hypertension
IASP	International Association for the Study of Pain
IM	Intramuscular
JCAHO	Joint Commission on Accreditation of Healthcare Organizations
MI	Myocardial infarction
NMDA	N-methyl-D-aspartate
NSAID	Nonsteroidal anti-inflammatory drug
OARSI	Osteoarthritis Research Society International
PAINAD	Pain Assessment in Advanced Dementia (tool)
PCA	Patient-controlled analgesia
PHN	Postherpetic neuralgia
PQRST	Palliative/precipitating, Quality, Radiation, Severity, and Time
SAM-e	S-adenosylmethionine
SNRI	Serotonin-norepinephrine reuptake inhibitor
SSRI	Selective serotonin reuptake inhibitor
TCA	Tricyclic antidepressant
TENS	Transcutaneous electrical nerve stimulation
VAS	Visual analog scale
VHA	Veterans Health Administration
WHO	World Health Organization

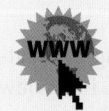 Self-assessment questions and answers are available at *http://www.mhpharmacotherapy.com/pp.html.*

REFERENCES

1. International Association for the Study of Pain. IASP Taxonomy [Internet], [cited 2011 Oct 10]. Available from: *http://www.iasp-pain.org/AM/Template.cfm?Section=Pain_Defi...isplay.cfm&ContentID=1728.*

2. American Pain Foundation. Pain Facts and Figures [Internet], [cited 2011 Oct 10]. Available from: *http://www.painfoundation.org/media/resources/pain-facts-figures.html.*

3. Deyo RA, Mirza SK, Martin BL. Back pain prevalence and visit rates: Estimates from U.S. national surveys, 2002. Spine 2006;31:2724–2727.

4. National Headache Foundation. Common headache conditions: Migraine and tension-type headache [Internet], [cited 2011 Oct 10]. Available from: *http://www.headaches.org/educational_modules/np_modules/p1_1a.html.*

5. National Fibromyalgia Association. Prevalence [Internet], [cited 2011 Oct 10]. Available from: *http://www.fmaware.org/site/PageServera6cc.html?pagename=fibromyalgia_affected.*

6. Christo PJ, Mazloomdoost D. Cancer pain and analgesia. Ann N Y Acad Sci 2008;1138:278–298.

7. Dieleman JP, Kerklaan J, Huygen FJ, et al. Incidence rates and treatment of neuropathic pain conditions in the general population. Pain 2008;137:681–688.

8. Wallace MS. Diagnosis and treatment of neuropathic pain. Curr Opin Anaesthesiol 2005;18:548–554.

9. Sadosky A, McDermott AM, Brandenburg NA, Strauss M. A review of the epidemiology of painful diabetic peripheral neuropathy, postherpetic neuralgia, and less commonly studied neuropathic pain conditions. Pain Pract 2008;8:45–56.

10. American Geriatrics Society Panel on the Pharmacological Management of Persistent Pain in Older Persons. Pharmacological management of persistent pain in older persons. J Am Geriatr Soc 2009;57:1331–1346.

11. Ferrell BA. The management of pain in long-term care. Clin J Pain 2004;20:240–243.

12. Luo X, Pietrobon R, Sun SX, et al. Estimates and patterns of direct health care expenditures among individuals with back pain in the United States. Spine 2004;29:79–86.

13. Stewart WF, Ricci JA, Chee E, et al. Lost productivity time and cost due to common pain conditions in the US workforce. JAMA 2003;290:2443–2454.

14. Desbiens NA, Wu AW, Broste SK, et al. Pain and satisfaction with pain control in seriously ill hospitalized adults: Findings from the SUPPORT research investigations. Crit Care Med 1996;24:1953–1961.

15. Desbiens NA, Wu AW. Pain and suffering in seriously ill hospitalized patients. J Am Geriatr Soc 2000;48:S183–S186.

16. Von Roenn JH, Cleeland CS, Gonin R, et al. Physician attitudes and practice in cancer pain management. A survey from the Eastern Cooperative Oncology Group. Ann Intern Med 1993;119:121–126.

17. Woolf CJ. Pain: moving from symptom control toward mechanism-specific pharmacologic management. Ann Intern Med 2004;140:441–451.

18. Reisner L, Koo PJS. Pain and its management. In: Koda-Kimble MA, Young LY, Kradjan WA, et al, eds. Applied Therapeutics: The Clinical Use of Drugs. 8th ed. Philadelphia, PA: Lippincott Williams & Wilkins; 2005:9-1–9-40.

19. Renn CL, Doresy SG. The physiology and processing of pain. A review. AACN Clin Issues 2005;16:277–290.

20. Heinricher MM, Tavares I, Leith JL, Lumb BM. Descending control of nociception: Specificity, recruitment and plasticity. Brain Res Rev 2009;60:214–225.

21. Ashburn MA, Lipman AG. Pain in society. In: Lipman AG, ed. Pain Management for Primary Care Clinicians. Bethesda, MD: American Society of Health-System Pharmacists; 2004:1–12.

22. Noble M, Tregear SJ, Treadwell JR, Schoelles K. Long-term opioid therapy for chronic noncancer pain: A systematic review and meta-analysis of efficacy and safety. J Pain Symptom Manage 2008;35:214–228.

23. Curtiss CP, McKee AL. Assessment of the person with pain. In: Lipman AG, ed. Pain Management for Primary Care Clinicians. Bethesda, MD: American Society of Health-System Pharmacists; 2004:27–42.

24. Joint Commission on Accreditation of Healthcare Organizations. Pain assessment and management: An organizational approach. Oakbrook Terrace, IL: JCAHO; 2000:1–6.

25. Twycross RG. Pain and analgesics. Curr Med Res Opin 1978;5:497–505.

26. Gammaitoni AR, Fine P, Alvarez N, et al. Clinical application of opioid equianalgesic data. Clin J Pain 2003;19:286–297.

27. U.S. Department of Health and Human Services, Agency for Health Care Policy and Research. Clinical practice guideline, cancer pain management. Rockville, MD: AHCPR, 1994 [Internet], [cited 2011 Oct 10]. Available from: *http://www.ncbi.nlm.nih.gov/books/bookres.fcgi/hstat6/f37_capcf4.gif.*

28. Wong D, Baker C. Pain in children: Comparison of assessment scales. Pediatr Nurs 1988;14:9–17.

29. Brief Pain Inventory [Internet], [cited 2011 Oct 10]. Available from: *http://www.mdanderson.org/education-and-research/departments-programs-and-labs/departments-and-divisions/symptom-research/symptom-assessment-tools/bpilong.pdf.*

30. Initial Pain Assessment Tool [Internet], [cited 2011 Oct 10]. Available from: *http://www.partnersagainstpain.com/printouts/A7012AF4.pdf.*

31. Melzack R. The McGill Pain Questionnaire. From description to measurement. Anesthesiology 2005;103:199–202.

32. Galer BS, Jensen MP. Development and preliminary validation of a pain measure specific to neuropathic pain: The Neuropathic Pain Scale. Neurology 1997;48:332–338.

33. Oswestry Disability Index [Internet], [cited 2011 Oct 10]. Available from: *http://thepainsource.com/wp-content/uploads/2010/12/Oswestry-Disability-Questionnaire.pdf.*

34. American Academy of Pediatrics. Committee on Psychosocial Aspects of Child and Family Health; Task Force on Pain in Infant, Children, and Adolescents. The assessment and management of acute pain in infants, children, and adolescents. Pediatrics 2001;108:793–797.

35. Mathew PJ, Mathew JL. Assessment and management of pain in infants. Postgrad Med J 2003;79:438–443.

36. Warden V, Hurley AC, Volicer L. Development and psychometric evaluation of the Pain Assessment in Advanced Dementia (PAINAD) scale. J Am Med Dir Assoc 2003;4:9–15.

37. World Health Organization. WHO's pain ladder [Internet], [cited 2011 Oct 10]. Available from: *http://www.who.int/cancer/palliative/painladder/en/.*

38. Gallagher RM. Rational integration of pharmacologic, behavioral, and rehabilitation strategies in the treatment of chronic pain. Am J Phys Med Rehabil 2005;84(suppl):S64–S76.

39. Zhang W, Moskowitz RW, Nuki G, et al. OARSI recommendations for the management of hip and knee osteoarthritis, Part II: OARSI evidence-based, expert consensus guidelines. Osteoarthritis Cartilage 2008;16:137–162.

40. The Acetaminophen Hepatotoxicity Working Group. 2009 Joint Meeting of the Drug Safety and Risk Management Advisory Committee with the Anesthetic and Life Support Drugs Advisory Committee and the Nonprescription Drugs Advisory Committee [Internet], [cited 2011 Oct 10]. Available from: *http://www.fda.gov/downloads/AdvisoryCommittees/CommitteesMeetingMaterials/Drugs/DrugSafetyandRiskManagementAdvisoryCommittee/ucm161518.pdf.*

41. Kurth T, Glynn RJ, Walker AM, et al. Inhibition of clinical benefits of aspirin on first myocardial infarction by nonsteroidal anti-inflammatory drugs. Circulation 2003;108:1191–1195.

42. Rahme E, Nedjar H. Risks and benefits of COX-2 inhibitors vs non-selective NSAIDs: Does their cardiovascular risk exceed their gastrointestinal benefits? A retrospective cohort study. Rheumatology (Oxford) 2007;46:435–438.

43. Naesdal J, Brown K. NSAID-associated adverse effects and acid control aids to prevent them. A review of current treatment options. Drug Saf 2006;29:119–132.

44. Farkouh ME, Greenberg BP. An evidence-based review of the cardiovascular risks of nonsteroidal anti-inflammatory drugs. Am J Cardiol 2009;103:1227–1237.

45. Moore RA, Derry S, McQuay HJ. Cyclo-oxygenase 2-selective inhibitors and nonsteroidal anti-inflammatory drugs: Balancing gastrointestinal and cardiovascular risk. BMC Musculoskelet Disord 2007;8:73.

46. American Pain Society. Principles of Analgesic Use in the Treatment of Acute Pain and Cancer Pain. 5th ed. Glenview, IL: American Pain Society; 2003:13–41.

47. Ballantyne JC, Mao J. Opioid analgesia: Perspectives on right use and utility. Pain Physician 2007;10:479–491.

48. Armstrong SC, Wynn GH, Sandson NB. Pharmacokinetic drug interactions of synthetic opiate analgesics. Psychosomatics 2009;50: 169–176.

49. Cleary JF. The pharmacologic management of cancer pain. J Palliat Med 2007;10:1369–1394.

50. Pereira J, Lawlor P, Vigrano A, et al. Equianalgesic dose ratios for opioids: A critical review and proposals for long-term dosing. J Pain Symptom Manage 2001;22:672–687.

51. Ripamonti C, Groff L, Brunelli C, et al. Switching from morphine to oral methadone in treating cancer pain: What is the equianalgesic dose ratio? J Clin Oncol 1998;16:3216–3221.

52. Mancini I, Lossignol D, Body JJ. Opioid switch to oral methadone in cancer pain. Curr Opin Oncol 2000;12:308–313.

53. Ripamonti C, Bianchi M. The use of methadone for cancer pain. Hematol Oncol Clin North Am 2002;16:543–555.

54. Gazelle G, Fine PG. Fast fact and concepts #75. Methadone for the treatment of pain. End-of-life Physician Education Resource Center [Internet], [cited 2011 Oct 10]. Available from: *http://www.eperc.mcw.edu/EPERC/FastFactsIndex/ff_075.htm.*

55. Gilron I, Watson CP, Cahill CM, Moulin DE. Neuropathic pain: A practical guide for the clinician. CMAJ 2006;175:265–275.

56. Finnerup NB, Otto M, McQuay HJ, et al. Algorithm for neuropathic pain treatment: An evidence based proposal. Pain 2005;118: 289–305.

57. Freynhagen R, Bennett MI. Diagnosis and management of neuropathic pain. BMJ 2009;339:b3002.

58. Zin CS, Nissen LM, Smith MT, et al. An update on the pharmacological management of post-herpetic neuralgia and painful diabetic neuropathy. CNS Drugs 2008;22:417–442.

59. Dworkin RH, O'Connor AB, Backonja M, et al. Pharmacologic management of neuropathic pain: Evidence-based recommendations. Pain 2007; 132:237–251.

35 Headache

Leigh Ann Ross and Brendan S. Ross

LEARNING OBJECTIVES

● **Upon completion of the chapter, the reader will be able to:**

1. Differentiate types of headache syndromes based on clinical features.

2. Recommend nonpharmacologic measures for headache treatment and prevention.

3. Determine when the pharmacologic treatment of headache is indicated.

4. Construct individualized treatment regimens for the acute and chronic management of headache syndromes.

5. Monitor headache treatment to ensure its safety, tolerability, and efficacy.

KEY CONCEPTS

❶ Headache may be a primary condition or a secondary one arising from an underlying medical disorder.

❷ Most primary headache syndromes are benign and can be classified as migraine, tension-type, or cluster.

❸ Tension-type headache is the most prevalent and can be episodic or chronic.

❹ Migraine headache can be further classified as with or without aura.

❺ The short-term goal of headache treatment is pain relief; the long-term goal is preventing recurrence.

❻ The pharmacologic treatment of headache should be provided promptly to improve response to therapy.

❼ Several clinical markers, so-called red flags, have been identified that warrant urgent physician referral and further diagnostic evaluation.

❽ Prophylactic treatment is indicated if headaches are frequent, severe, or require the use of pain relievers two or more times per week.

❾ Treatment regimens should be individualized: based on the pattern of occurrence, response to therapy, medication tolerability, and comorbid medical conditions.

INTRODUCTION

Headache is a common medical complaint associated with significant quality of life and economic issues. ❶ *Even when persistent or recurrent, headaches are usually a benign primary condition; secondary headaches are caused by an* underlying medical disorder and may be medical emergencies. Primary headache syndromes are the focus of this chapter. Patients may seek headache care from multiple providers. All clinicians should be familiar with the various types of headache, clinical indicators suggesting the need for urgent medical attention or specialist referral, and nonpharmacologic and pharmacologic options for treatment. ❷ *The International Headache Society (IHS) classifies primary headaches as migraine, tension-type, or cluster and other trigeminal autonomic cephalalgias.*[1] Tension-type headaches (TTHs) are more common than migraine, and both are more common in women than men. Cluster headache is a much less common chronic headache syndrome that affects predominantly men.

EPIDEMIOLOGY OF HEADACHE DISORDERS

Migraine Headache

Migraine is a primary headache disorder that is estimated to affect 10% to 15% of adults in the United States.[2] Less than one-half of headaches meeting the diagnostic criteria for migraine are appropriately diagnosed. Migraine runs in families, and its prevalence depends on age and gender. In children younger than 12 years of age, migraines are more prevalent in males. At puberty, this prevalence shifts markedly to women. This change in gender distribution is thought to be due to the hormonal changes of menarche.[3] Onset typically occurs between the ages of 10 and 30 years, but the prevalence is greatest between the ages of 35 to 45 years.[4] Migraines can significantly impact function; more than one-half of patients report symptoms necessitating bed rest during an attack.

Migraines are the leading cause of employee absenteeism and decreased workplace productivity.[5]

Tension-Type Headache

❸ *TTH is the most common primary headache disorder and can be further divided into episodic or chronic.* TTHs are underrepresented in clinical practice because most patients do not present for care.[6] The term *TTH* is used to describe all headache syndromes in which sensitization to pericranial nociception, noxious stimuli, is the most significant factor in the pathogenesis of pain. The 1-year prevalence of TTH in the United States ranges from 30% to 90%.[6] Such headaches are more common in adult females. Environmental factors, as opposed to genetic predisposition, play a central role in the development of TTH. The mean frequency of attacks is 3 days per month in episodic disorders; chronic TTH is defined as 15 or more attacks in a 1-month period.[7] The estimated prevalence of chronic TTH is less than 5%.[6] Some researchers believe that chronic TTH represents a continuum of headache severity with migraine headache.[8] When severe headaches are difficult to differentiate clinically, treatment should initially target TTH.

Cluster Headache and Other Trigeminal Autonomic Cephalalgias

Cluster headache disorders are the most uncommon and severe primary headache syndromes.[9] The estimated point prevalence is less than 0.5% to 1%. Unlike migraine and TTH, cluster headaches are more frequently found in men. Onset most commonly occurs prior to age 30 years.[6] A genetic predisposition is apparent, although affected individuals often provide the additional history of tobacco use and alcohol abuse.[6] Attacks consist of debilitating, unilateral head pains that occur in series lasting up to months at a time but remit over months to years between occurrences. In rare instances, cluster headache can be a chronic disorder without remission.[4]

ETIOLOGY AND PATHOPHYSIOLOGY OF HEADACHE DISORDERS

Migraine Headache

The exact mechanism by which migraines produce headache remains obscure, but the belief that only vascular changes are responsible for the pain is no longer accepted.[10] The vascular hypothesis suggested that intracerebral vasoconstriction led to neural ischemia, which was followed by reflex extracranial vasodilation and pain. Negative neuroimaging evidence for such vascular changes and the effectiveness of medications with no vascular properties make this contention untenable.[6] A neuronal etiology has emerged as the leading mechanism for the development of migraine pain.[11] It is believed that depressed neuronal electrical activity spreads across the brain, producing transitory neural dysfunction.[12] Headache pain is likely due to compensatory overactivity in the trigeminovascular system of the brain. Activation of trigeminal sensory nerves leads to the release of vasoactive neuropeptides (e.g., calcitonin gene-related peptide [CGRP], neurokinin A, substance P) that produce a sterile inflammatory response around vascular structures in the brain, provoking the sensation of pain.[11] Continued sensitization of CNS sensory neurons can potentiate and intensify headache pain as an attack progresses.[12] Bioamine pathways projecting from the brainstem regulate activity within the trigeminovascular system. The pathogenesis of migraine is most likely due to an imbalance in the modulation of nociception and blood vessel tone by serotonergic and noradrenergic neurons.[13]

Tension-Type Headache

The pathophysiologic mechanisms producing TTHs are not clearly understood and are likely multifactorial. However, central sensitization to peripheral nociceptive input arising from the pericranial myofascia is the leading hypothesis. The belief that sustained muscle contraction is solely responsible for generating the pain cannot be supported. Muscle tenderness is prominent in this syndrome, but it only reflects a heightened sensitivity to pain. TTH pain is believed to arise by disturbances in the muscles and tissues of the head being misinterpreted due to disordered CNS pain processing.[14] Repetitive pain transmission from peripheral structures may be responsible for the evolution from episodic to chronic TTH.[15]

Clinical Presentation and Diagnosis of Migraine Without Aura

Patients experiencing "migraine without aura" may display the following headache symptoms and characteristics:

Two or more of the following are present:

1. Pain interrupts or worsens with physical activity

2. Unilateral pain

3. Pulsating pain

4. Moderate to severe pain intensity

Two or more of the following are present during headache:

1. Nausea

2. Vomiting

3. **Photophobia**

4. **Phonophobia**

5. **Osmophobia**

Duration: 4 to 72 hours (treated or not treated)

Criteria for diagnosis: Five or more attacks fulfilling above criteria are necessary

Laboratory assessments that may be helpful in excluding medical comorbidities: Complete blood count (CBC), chemistry panel, thyroid function tests (TFTs), erythrocyte sedimentation rate (ESR)

Clinical Presentation and Diagnosis of Migraine With Aura

Patients experiencing "migraine with aura" may display the following headache symptoms and characteristics:

One or more of the following present with no motor weakness:

1. Visual symptoms (positive and/or negative; reversible)
2. Sensory symptoms (positive and/or negative; reversible)
3. Dysphasic speech (reversible)
4. Moderate or severe pain intensity

Two or more of the following:

1. Homonymous visual symptoms and/or unilateral sensory symptoms
2. One aura symptom develops at least 5 minutes prior and/or a second aura symptom develops in 5 minutes or more after headache starts
3. Duration of each symptom 5 to 60 minutes

Criteria for diagnosis: Two or more attacks fulfilling above criteria are necessary

Clinical Presentation and Diagnosis of Cluster Headache

Patients experiencing "cluster headache" may display the following headache symptoms and characteristics:

1. Unilateral pain
2. Orbital, supraorbital, or temporal pain
3. Sharp and stabbing pain

One or more of the following present:

1. Conjunctival injection and/or lacrimation
2. Nasal congestion and/or rhinorrhea
3. Eyelid edema

Duration of pain: 2 seconds to 10 minutes

Frequency of attacks: One or more per day more than half of the time

Criteria for diagnosis: 20 or more attacks fulfilling above criteria are necessary

Clinical Presentation and Diagnosis of Tension-Type Headache

Patients experiencing TTH may display the following headache symptoms and characteristics:

Two or more of the following present:

1. Bilateral pain
2. Nonpulsating pain
3. Mild or moderate pain intensity

Both of the following:

1. No nausea or vomiting (anorexia possible)
2. Either photophobia or phonophobia (not both)

Duration: 30 minutes to 7 days

Criteria for diagnosis: 10 or more attacks fulfilling above criteria occurring on average less than 1 day per month are necessary

Cluster Headache and Other Trigeminal Autonomic Cephalalgias

Cluster headache is one of a group of disorders referred to as trigeminal autonomic cephalalgias.[16] This autonomic nervous system dysfunction is characterized by sympathetic underactivity coupled with parasympathetic activation. Similar to migraine, the pain of a cluster headache is believed to be the result of vasoactive neuropeptide release and neurogenic inflammation. The exact cause of trigeminal activation in this intermittently manifest syndrome is unclear.[9] One hypothesis is that hypothalamic dysfunction, occasioned by diurnal or seasonal changes in neurohumoral balance, are responsible for headache periodicity.[6] Serotonin affects neuronal activity in the hypothalamus and trigeminal system and may play a role in the pathophysiology of cluster headache. The precipitation of cluster headache by high-altitude exposure also implicates hypoxemia in the pathogenesis of trigeminal autonomic cephalalgias.[17]

CLINICAL PRESENTATION OF HEADACHES

Migraine Headache

Migraine presents as a recurrent headache that is severe enough to interfere with daily functioning. ❹ *Migraine headaches are classified as migraine with aura and migraine without aura.*[6] The correlative terms of "classic" and "common" migraine are no longer used. Aura is defined as a transient focal neurologic symptom that can be positive or negative and can occur prior to or during an attack.[18] Examples of positive symptoms include the visual perception of flickering lights, spots, or wavy lines; the partial loss of vision, called a scotoma, is considered a negative finding. The IHS outlines diagnostic criteria that differentiate migraine with and without aura. The pain of a migraine headache is typically described as moderate to severe, throbbing, unilateral, and retroorbital in location.[6] The pain can be accompanied by nausea, sensitivity to light and sound, and difficulty concentrating.[19] Migraines can be triggered by hormonal, emotional, or environmental factors. Menstrual migraines, headaches precipitated by stress or sleep disorders, and pain due to exposures to noxious odors or extremes of weather are well recognized. Untreated migraines can last from 4 to 72 hours. Migraines occurring 15 or more days per month for a 3-month period or longer, without the overuse of analgesic medications, are classified as chronic migraines.[6] Severe and debilitating migraine pain lasting more than 72 hours is termed status migrainosus.[19] Even in the absence of neurologic focality, brain imaging is mandated in patients with frequent, severe, and prolonged attacks or attacks that are atypical for a migraine patient's stereotyped presentation.[20]

Tension-Type Headache

TTH pain differs from migraine pain in that it is usually reported to be mild to moderate in severity, nonpulsating, and bilateral.[6] The pain is described by sufferers as a band-like tightness or pressure around the head. No transient neurologic deficits are noted, and systemic symptoms are rare.[4] TTHs infrequently disrupt normal activity. Muscle tenderness in the frontotemporal and parietooccipital regions is a common finding on physical examination.[4] Neuroimaging and laboratory testing are unrevealing, and such tests are usually unnecessary if the presentation and clinical history is classic for TTHs.

Cluster Headache

Pain associated with cluster headache differs from migraine and TTH in that it is severe, intermittent, and short in duration.[6] Headaches typically occur at night, but attacks may occur multiple times per day.[9] The pain is usually unilateral, but, unlike migraine, it is not described as pulsatile.[6] Aura is not a feature, and pain intensity peaks early after onset, although it may persist for hours.[6] The headache is described as explosive and excruciating. A constellation of

features, ascribed to parasympathetic overactivity, can be seen, such as ipsilateral conjunctival injection and lacrimation, rhinorrhea, and sweating.[9] Cluster headache patients tend to become excited and restless during attacks, rather than seeking quiet and solitude as in migraine.[16]

TREATMENT OF HEADACHE DISORDERS

Desired Outcomes

⑤ *The short-term treatment goal of migraine is to achieve rapid pain relief to allow the patient to resume normal activities.*[21] The long-term goal of therapy is to prevent headache recurrences and to diminish headache severity. Similarly, the goal of TTH care is to lessen headache pain, whereas the long-term goal is to avoid analgesic overuse and dependence.[22] The short-term therapeutic goal in cluster headache is to achieve rapid pain relief. Prophylactic therapy may be necessary to obtain the intermediate-term outcome of reducing the frequency and severity of headaches within a periodic cluster series, as well as to achieve the long-term goal of delaying or eliminating recurrent periods.[23]

General Approach to Treatment

The most important goal of acute headache management is pain relief. First-line pharmacologic agents include nonsteroidal and opiate analgesics, and serotonin-receptor agonists (triptans).[24] Despite the availability of targeted prescription therapies, most headache patients rely on over-the-counter (OTC) products for pain relief and so are not treated adequately.[25] **⑥** *Pharmacologic treatment of acute headache should be started early to abort the intensification of pain and to improve response to therapy.* The long-term management of headache syndromes focuses on lifestyle modification and other nonpharmacologic therapeutic options; if headaches are severe and frequent, then prophylactic pharmacologic therapy is needed.[26] **⑦** *Several clinical markers, so-called red flags, have been identified that warrant urgent physician referral and further diagnostic evaluation* (Table 35–1).

Patient Encounter, Part 1

A 48-year-old man complains of "almost daily" headaches that make it difficult to work. He describes his pain as dull, bilateral, and steady, "like a tight cap." His headaches are not associated with visual changes or GI distress. Previously, his pain had responded to OTC analgesics. Lately, he has had to take acetaminophen or aspirin in combination with daily caffeine to obtain relief.

What type of headache is the patient most likely experiencing?

What characteristics of the headache support this diagnosis?

What are possible causes or triggers of headache in this patient?

What additional information is needed to formulate a treatment plan?

Table 35–1

Headache "Red Flags" Indicating Need for Urgent Medical Evaluation

New-onset sudden and/or severe pain
Onset after 40 years of age
Stereotyped pain pattern worsens
Systemic signs (e.g., fever, weight loss, or accelerated hypertension)
Focal neurologic symptoms (i.e., other than typical visual or sensory aura)
Papilledema
Cough-, exertion-, or Valsalva-triggered headache
Pregnancy or postpartum state
Patients with cancer, human immunodeficiency virus (HIV), and other infectious and immunodeficiency disorders
Seizures

CHAPTER 35 | HEADACHE   625

Nonpharmacologic Therapy

The successful management of headache disorders depends on comprehensive patient education. Recording headache frequency, duration, and severity in a "headache diary" provides beneficial information for the patient regarding headache precipitants and useful insights for the clinician selecting appropriate management strategies.[27] To prevent future occurrences, exposure to headache triggers (Table 35–2) should be limited. In the acute setting, environmental control can lessen the severity of an attack, so patients may benefit from resting in a dark, quiet area.[28] Behavioral interventions, such as biofeedback, relaxation therapy, and cognitive-behavioral training, are effective and can be recommended for headache prevention.[17] Headache sufferers may also benefit from stress management training.[17] Acupuncture has yielded inconsistent benefits in clinical trials.[22] Although the response is variable, headache patients should be advised to moderate alcohol use and curtail tobacco abuse.[23] Emotional distress may compound headache pain through the outward displacement of inner conflicts: somatization. Psychological interventions

┌─ Table 35–2 ─┐

Table 35–2

Migraine Triggers

Behavioral:
Fatigue
Menstruation or menopause
Sleep excess or deficit
Stress
Vigorous physical activity

Environmental:
Flickering lights
High altitude
Loud noises
Strong smells
Tobacco smoke
Weather changes

Food:
Alcohol
Caffeine intake or withdrawal
Chocolate
Citrus fruits, bananas, figs, raisins
Dairy products
Fermented or pickled products

Food containing:
Monosodium glutamate (MSG): Asian food, seasoned salt
Nitrites: processed meats
Saccharin/aspartame: diet soda or diet food
Sulfites: shrimp
Tyramine: cheese, wine, organ meats
Yeast: breads

Medications:
Cimetidine
Estrogen or oral contraceptives
Indomethacin
Nifedipine
Nitrates
Reserpine
Theophylline
Withdrawal due to overuse of analgesics, benzodiazepines, decongestants, or ergotamines

Patient Encounter, Part 2: Medical History, Physical Examination, and Diagnostic Tests

PMH: Hypertension (HTN); gastroesophageal reflux disease (GERD); dyslipidemia

FH: Father living, age 77 years: HTN, diabetes mellitus; mother living, age 72 years: "sinus" headaches; two sisters in good health

SH: Recently divorced; general contractor; smoker; "social" alcohol intake (one to two beers per day, more on weekends), four to six cups of coffee per day

Meds: Hydrochlorothiazide/triamterene 50/25 mg orally per day; esomeprazole 20 mg orally twice daily; rosuvastatin 20 mg orally once daily; naproxen 220 mg, two tablets orally twice daily as needed for headache, or OTC headache "powders"

ROS: Headache, moderate intensity, no sensitivity to light or sound; no dizziness; no chest pain or palpitations; no shortness of breath with exertion; pyrosis without dysphagia; no weakness or joint discomfort

PE:

VS: BP 154/72, P 85, RR 18, T 37.0°C (98.6°F) oral

HEENT: No papilledema, neck tender without stiffness, bitemporal muscle tenderness

CV: RRR, normal S1, S2, S4 gallop, no MR

Chest: CTA

Abd: Benign, bowel sounds positive

Neuro: Nonfocal

Labs: CBC and chemistry panel within normal limits

What is your assessment of this patient's condition?

What medical comorbidities or drug therapies may be contributing to his distress?

Identify treatment goals for this patient.

What nonpharmacologic options are needed at present, and what options are appropriate in the long term?

What pharmacologic therapy would you recommend in the acute setting?

Does this patient require long-term pharmacologic prophylaxis against recurrent headaches?

are urged in such instances and should be considered in all headache sufferers resistant to standard medication treatments.[29] All such nonpharmacologic therapies may be useful in augmenting pharmacologic response.

Pharmacologic Therapy

▶ Migraine

Analgesics, such as nonsteroidal anti-inflammatory drugs (NSAIDs) and acetaminophen, with or without an opioid, are the initial pharmacologic option for the acute management of migraine headache. If these analgesics prove to be ineffective, then migraine-specific medications, such as triptans, are administered.[30] Early, abortive treatment should be the rule. If the orally administered route is selected for medication administration, then larger doses than otherwise required to produce pain relief may need to be provided, due to the enteric stasis and poor drug absorption accompanying migraine attacks.[20] Intranasal, parenteral, and rectal administration can circumvent this complication.

Clinical trial evidence supports many NSAID medications in the acute treatment of migraines with and without aura.[30] Acetaminophen alone or in proprietary combinations with aspirin, opioids, caffeine, or the barbiturate butalbital is also effective.[28] Although deemed to have a benign adverse effect profile on gastric mucosal integrity and renal blood flow, overwhelming clinical experience supports the observation that the overuse of acetaminophen may lead to tolerance or dependence clinically manifested as acute withdrawal headaches.[31] These so-called "rebound" headaches are the result of poor attention to prevention therapies and thus the chronic use of daily short-acting analgesics.[32] Proprietary fixed-dose combinations of anti-inflammatories with oral triptans may facilitate proper care.

The triptans are considered specific therapies in that they target the pathophysiology underlying migraine.[33] They abort headache through beneficial effects on neuronal imbalances.[11] Triptans inhibit neurotransmission in the trigeminal complex and activate serotonin 1B/1D pathways in the brainstem, which modulate nociception. They also decrease the release of vasoactive neuropeptides leading to vascular reactivity and pain.[34] The triptans are available in intranasal, subcutaneous, and oral dosage forms. The available agents differ in their dosing and pharmacokinetic properties, but all are effective treatments to abort or diminish migraine headache (Table 35–3).[43] Patient responses can be variable; if a patient does not respond to one agent, then another is selected before a patient is prematurely labeled as triptan-unresponsive.[44] The initial severity of headache correlates with symptomatic response; thus administration should be prompt. Relief is usually experienced within 2 to 4 hours. Treatment delay may lead to decreased analgesia through the development of refractory central pain sensitization. Efficacy tends to be dose related, although adverse effects are less so.[45] These medications are well tolerated; the most common side effects are dizziness, a sensation of warmth, chest fullness, and nausea. Rarely, ischemic vascular events may be precipitated by the potential vasoconstrictive nature of these drugs.[34] An initial dose under direct practitioner supervision is indicated for patients at increased cardiovascular risk. Triptans are avoided in patients with migraine associated with neurologic focality, a history of previous stroke, poorly controlled hypertension, or unstable angina. Triptans are relatively contraindicated for routine use in pregnancy.[30] Triptans should not be used with concurrent ergotamine administration.[34]

Ergotamine derivatives produce salutary effects on serotonin receptors similar to triptans. They also impact adrenergic and dopaminergic receptors. Ergotamine tartrate and dihydroergotamine (DHE) are the most commonly used agents.[20] The latter is not available in an oral dosage form. Analgesic onset is within 4 hours, although additional dosing is required if an

Table 35–3

Comparison of Serotonin Receptor Agonists (Triptans)

Medication (Brand Name)	Dosage Forms	Strength (mg)	Usual Dosage (mg)	May Repeat in (hours)	Potential Drug Interactions
Almotriptan (Axert)	Oral tablets	6.25 12.5	6.25–12.5		Ergot derivatives
Eletriptan (Relpax)	Oral tablets	20 40	20–40		Substrate: CYP 3A4, CYP 2D6; ergot derivatives
Frovatriptan (Frova)	Oral tablets	2.5	2.5	2	Substrate: CYP 1A2; ergot derivatives
Naratriptan (Amerge)	Oral tablets	1 2.5	2.5	4	Substrate: CYP (various); ergot derivatives
Rizatriptan (Maxalt and Maxalt MLT)	Oral tablets	5	5–10	2	Ergot derivatives
	Disintegrating tablets	10			MAO-A inhibitors
Sumatriptan (Imitrex)	Subcutaneous injection	6	6	1	Ergot derivatives
	Oral tablets	25, 50, 100	50	2	MAO-A inhibitors
Sumatriptan/naproxen sodium (Treximet)	Nasal spray	5, 20	5–20	2	
	Oral tablets	85/500	85/500	12	
Zolmitriptan (Zomig and Zomig-ZMT)	Oral tablets	2.5, 5	2.5	2	Substrate: CYP 1A2;
	Disintegrating tablets	5	5	2	Ergot derivatives
	Nasal spray				MAO-A inhibitors

CYP, cytochrome P450 enzyme; MAO-A, monoamine oxidase type A.

Data from Refs. 35–42.

acceptable response is not achieved. When dosed parenterally, these drugs are usually provided with an antiemetic, due to their potential to worsen the nausea associated with migraine. Metoclopramide and chlorpromazine are the drugs of choice in such instances. Intranasal DHE can be self-administered to abort an attack.[20] The outpatient use of subcutaneous ergotamines is limited by the lack of a prefilled syringe form. The same cautions associated with triptan use are also applicable to ergot use in patients at risk for vascular events.

The choice of initial therapy for acute migraine attacks is a subject of debate among specialists.[46] Some believe that nonspecific analgesics should be used first-line, whereas others believe migraine-specific drugs should be the choice for patients with severe pain or a history of significant disability.[47] A stepped-care approach within attacks from less to more specific drugs is usually recommended. Once a history of headache refractory to common analgesics is established, triptans should be used as initial therapy. In patients who present to the hospital with intractable pain, IV metoclopramide supplemented with DHE may be needed. Oral medications in this setting are not used because nausea and vomiting limit their bioavailability. Migraine patients with frequent and severe attacks are candidates for prophylactic treatment.

▶ Tension-Type Headache

Most individuals who experience episodic TTHs will not seek medical attention.[22] Instead, they will find relief with the use of widely available OTC analgesics. Acetaminophen products and NSAIDs are commonly utilized. An individual patient may benefit from topical analgesics (e.g., ice packs) or physical manipulation (e.g., massage) during an acute attack, but the evidence supporting nonpharmacologic therapies is inconsistent.[6] Relaxation techniques can often reduce headache frequency and severity. When pain is unrelieved, prescription-strength NSAID use is required, or the combination of acetaminophen with an opioid analgesic may be necessary. The frequent use of these more potent analgesics should be limited, so that the development of dependency is prevented. Use for more than 2 days per week suggests the need for prophylactic therapy.[48] In sufferers who do not seek medical attention but rely on the frequent use of unprescribed analgesics, medication-overuse headache (MOH) may supervene. This secondary syndrome of chronic daily headaches requires physician referral to desensitize patient-initiated analgesic tolerance and dependence; weaning analgesics through the use of tricyclic antidepressant (TCA) coprescribing is usually helpful.[49]

▶ Cluster Headache

Cluster headache responds to many of the treatment modalities used in acute migraine; however, initial prophylactic therapy is required to limit the frequency of recurrent headaches within a periodic series. A therapy specific to cluster headaches is the administration of high-flow-rate oxygen: 100% at 5 to 10 L/min by nonrebreather face mask for approximately 15 minutes.[50] If the pain is not aborted, retreatment is indicated. No long-term side effects are seen with short-term

oxygen use. If oxygen therapy is not wholly effective, then drugs are useful adjunctive therapy. Drug therapy is also used when supplemental oxygen is not readily available. The triptan class is safe and effective. Intranasal or subcutaneous sumatriptan has demonstrated efficacy in decreasing cluster headache pain.[51] Oral triptans are also effective, but their delayed onset of action may limit their applicability in acute cluster headache treatment.[52] Cluster headache is rapid in onset and achieves peak intensity quickly, but it can be of short duration. Oral agents may have utility in limiting the recurrence of cluster attacks. Intranasal, intramuscular, or IV ergotamine agents are an alternative to triptan use.[6] Repeated dosing may break a cluster series. For those patients in whom triptans and ergotamine derivatives are contraindicated due to ischemic vascular disease, octreotide may be helpful to relieve pain.[53] Octreotide is a somatostatin analogue that has a short half-life and may be administered subcutaneously. Unlike the other abortive agents, it has no vasoconstrictive effects; the most prominent treatment emergent adverse effect is GI upset. Glucocorticoids, provided IV and later tapered orally, are effective when cluster headache attacks are not satisfactorily controlled.[9]

Pharmacologic Therapy for Headache Prophylaxis

8 *Prophylaxis for headache disorders is indicated if headaches are frequent or severe, if significant disability occurs, or if pain-relieving medications are used two or more times per week.*

▶ Migraine Prophylaxis

Migraine headaches that are severe, frequent, or lead to significant disability require long-term medication therapy. Prophylactic therapy is also recommended for migraines associated with neurologic focality because it may prevent permanent disability. Although multiple medication classes have garnered FDA labeling for migraine prevention, there is no consensus on the best initial therapy (Table 35–4). **9** *The choice of pharmacologic agent is individually tailored to patient tolerability and medical comorbidities.*

The β-blockers propranolol and timolol are FDA approved for migraine prophylaxis, but others in the class are also as effective.[57] Cautious dosage titration is advised for those patients who do not have other indications for β-blocker use. Rizatriptan interacts with propranolol, and thus dosages must be downward titrated, or another triptan should be chosen for abortive therapy.[44] Comorbid reactive airway disease is a relative contraindication to β-blocker prophylaxis, and patients with cardiac conduction disturbances should be closely monitored. Calcium channel antagonists are often used when patients cannot tolerate β-blockers. They are purported to beneficially impact aura as well as pain. The different calcium-blocker drugs are variably effective, and none carries an FDA indication. Moreover, even in responsive patients, tachyphylaxis may develop. Renin-angiotensin

Table 35–4

Medications for Prophylaxis of Migraines

Medication (Brand Name)	Usual Dosage (mg/day)	Main Adverse Effects
Antiepileptics:		
Gabapentin (Neurontin)	1,200–2,400	Paresthesias, dizziness, fatigue, nausea
Lamotrigine (Lamictal)	50–200	
Topiramate[a] (Topamax)	50–200	
Valproic acid (Depakene)	500–1,500	
Divalproex sodium[a] (Depakote)	500–1,500	
β-Blockers:		
Atenolol (Tenormin)	50–200	
Metoprolol (Lopressor)	50–200	Fatigue, exercise intolerance
Nadolol (Corgard)	20–160	
Propranolol[a] (Inderal)	80–240	
Timolol[a] (Blocadren)	20–30	
Calcium channel blockers:		
Amlodipine (Norvasc)	2.5–10	
Verapamil (Calan)	120–320	Constipation
Tricyclic antidepressants:		
Amitriptyline (Elavil)	10–150	
Nortriptyline (Pamelor)	10–150	Weight gain, dry mouth, sedation
Ergot alkaloids:		
Ergotamine tartrate (Cafergot)	1	
Methysergide (Sansert)	2–6	
Others:		
Hormones (various)	Varies per agent	
Muscle relaxants (various)	Varies per agent	
Trazodone (Desyrel)	25–150	

[a]FDA approved for migraine prophylaxis.

Data from Refs. 54–56.

antagonists have also been noted to decrease headache frequency and severity in migraine sufferers.[58] Consensus recommendations for hypertension treatment often advocate multidrug regimens to achieve tight control.[59] Combination therapies with the antihypertensive agents noted earlier are ideal combinations for migraine patients.

Low-dose amitriptyline or other TCAs are of proven efficacy in migraine prevention.[27] Due to sedation, these medications are commonly administered at night. The use of later generation tricyclic medications (e.g., nortriptyline) or heterocyclic compounds (e.g., trazodone) decreases the dose-limiting adverse effects of TCAs, especially those attributable to their anticholinergic properties (e.g., dry mouth, constipation, and urinary retention). Whether the various selective serotonin reuptake inhibitors (SSRIs) can yield consistent efficacy in the majority of migraineurs is questionable.[21] Although they affect serotonin balance in the brain, their utility may be derived from their beneficial impact on mood and anxiety, rather than through serotonergic effects on migraine generation. Concurrent TCA and triptan administration may rarely precipitate the serotonin syndrome, a

serious and potentially life-threatening drug–drug interaction that presents clinically with confusion, GI upset, symptomatic blood pressure (BP) changes, and muscle rigidity.[20]

The antiepileptics valproic acid and topiramate are approved for migraine prophylaxis. Gabapentin and lamotrigine are anecdotally reported to be efficacious as well. In patients whose migraine headaches are believed to be related to trigeminal neuralgia, carbamazepine is used as prevention for both disorders. The precise mechanism of benefit of these agents is unclear, but enhancement of γ-aminobutyric acid (GABA) neuroinhibition and modulation of the neuroexcitatory amino acid glutamate is likely.[60] Divalproex sodium doses are gradually titrated to 1,000 mg/day; topiramate is titrated to a maximum of 100 mg twice per day. At these doses, serum drug level monitoring is infrequently needed. These medications are as effective as propranolol at reducing the frequency and severity of migraines and are preferred for prevention in patients intolerant to β-blockers.[61] Topiramate is especially useful in metabolic syndrome, diabetes, and dyslipidemic patients because it is unlikely to lead to the weight gain often seen with valproic acid. Patients prescribed topiramate should be advised to stay well hydrated to prevent dysgeusia, disordered taste, and, more seriously, hyperthermia.

Methysergide is an ergotamine derivative that impacts central serotonin balance. Inflammatory fibrosis is a rare but serious, adverse reaction associated with the prolonged use of methysergide. Retroperitoneal fibrosis, pulmonary fibrosis, or fibrosis in cardiac tissue can occur. These conditions may resolve upon drug withdrawal, but cardiac valvular damage can be irreversible. Some experts believe it is the best choice for refractory migraine with frequent attacks, but due to its significant adverse effect profile, it is not marketed in the United States.[62]

▶ **Tension-Type Headache Prophylaxis**

The prevention of chronic TTHs uses the same pharmacologic strategies as for migraine prophylaxis. TCAs are a mainstay of chronic therapy. The efficacy of serotonergic agonists remains in question. Although there is little need for muscle relaxants (e.g., methocarbamol) in the treatment of acute TTH, they are often provided as a preventive intervention.[6] Combination prophylactic therapies may be needed to wean patients from daily analgesic abuse. Stress reduction techniques may be particularly effective in this setting. The injection of botulinum toxin into cranial muscles has demonstrated prophylactic efficacy for severe TTHs.[49]

▶ **Cluster Headache Prophylaxis**

The calcium channel blocker verapamil is the mainstay of cluster attack prevention and chronic prophylaxis.[6] Within an attack period, it is dosed at 240 to 360 mg/day. Higher doses may be necessary to stave off recurrent cluster periods. Beneficial effects may be appreciated after 1 week of treatment, but 4 to 6 weeks is usually needed. Adverse effects include smooth muscle relaxation with the subsequent exacerbation of gastroesophageal reflux and the development of constipation. Caution should be exercised in patients with myocardial disease because verapamil is an inotropic and chronotropic cardiac suppressant. Pharmacokinetic drug–drug interactions must be considered, as verapamil is a potent inhibitor of oxidative metabolism through cytochrome P450 (CYP) enzyme 3A4. Eletriptan is a CYP 3A4 substrate and should not be administered concurrently with verapamil.[44] Lithium is another effective therapy to reduce headache frequency in a cluster series and to limit recurrences.[9] The dose administered should be individualized to achieve a low serum concentration (0.4–0.8 mEq/L [mmol/L]). Dose adjustments in the setting of renal disease or congestive heart failure are required.[6] Lithium is contraindicated in patients concurrently prescribed thiazide diuretics and angiotensin-converting enzyme inhibitors (ACEIs) or angiotensin receptor blockers (ARBs). Patient persistence with long-term lithium therapy may be hindered by the emergence of tremor, GI distress, and lethargy. Verapamil and lithium doses can be lowered when used in combination with ergotamine. If possible, bedtime dosing is recommended, given the nocturnal predilection of cluster headache attacks.[16]

SPECIAL POPULATIONS

Migraine Headache in Children and Adolescents

Migraine headaches are common in children, and their prevalence increases in the adolescent years.[2,3] The diagnosis and evaluation of headaches is especially difficult in children, given their decreased ability to articulate symptoms. Treatment presents another challenge to the practitioner because medications used for headache management in adults have not been fully evaluated for efficacy and safety in children. Consensus panel recommendations identify ibuprofen as effective and acetaminophen as probably effective in the acute treatment of headache in patients older than 6 years.[26] Aspirin use is avoided due to the risk of precipitating Reye's syndrome. Antiemetic therapy can be used alone or in combination with analgesics; promethazine is usually prescribed, as it is less prone to cause extrapyramidal reactions than other antiemetics. For adolescents older than 12, triptans are effective and are beneficial for abortive migraine therapy.[26] Medication prophylaxis for migraines in children and adolescents is understudied. The data are conflicting, and no consensus recommendation for the use of preventive drug therapy exists.[26] Nonpharmacologic interventions and trigger identification and avoidance are advised.

Pregnancy

Headaches are more common in women than in men. Fluctuations in estrogen levels are believed to account for this gender discrepancy.[63] Hence headaches are common in pregnancy. TTHs predominate; migraine attacks may increase in frequency, but more usually they decrease during pregnancy.[64] Recommendations for headache care during pregnancy are based on a limited evidence base and largely anecdotal. Because headaches are not associated with fetal harm, reflexive pharmacologic therapy should be avoided and drug treatment choices considered carefully. Standard nonpharmacologic therapies are often sufficient. Acetaminophen is safe for the pregnant woman and her fetus.[65] NSAIDs are avoided late in the third trimester to prevent detrimental prostaglandin alterations leading to premature ductus arteriosus closure. Opioids are second-line agents and should not to be used chronically because they can lead to dependence in the mother and to acute withdrawal in the infant after birth. Centrally acting antiemetic agents are safe and may be useful as adjunctive agents. Corticosteroids may be needed for intractable headache relief. Prednisone and methylprednisone are preferred, as they are metabolized in the placenta and do not expose the fetus. In pregnant women with migraine, vasoconstrictive agents such as triptans are relatively contraindicated, even though maternal registry data reveal little teratogenicity.[66] Ergot compounds are strictly avoided because they may precipitate uterine contractions and placental ischemia leading to hypoxemia in the fetus. Migraine prophylaxis is considered cautiously because β-blockers and calcium-channel antagonists may lead to maternal hypotension and diminished placental blood flow or fetal bradycardia. Antiepileptic drug use in this setting has not been sufficiently studied to allow definitive recommendations.

Some headache disorders are specific to the pregnant state. These include postprocedure headache and those associated with preeclampsia. The former are the result of dural puncture with cerebrospinal fluid (CSF) leak after spinal anesthesia and generally respond to bed rest in the supine position.[67] The latter are seen in the third trimester accompanied by the clinical triad of hypertension, edema, and proteinuria. Preeclamptic headache is believed to result from alterations in cerebral blood flow.[68] Headaches experienced in preeclamptic women herald eclampsia, and urgent delivery is indicated.[69] Antihypertensives are administered to prevent intracranial hemorrhage, and prophylactic anticonvulsants are provided to prevent eclamptic seizures.

Patient Care and Monitoring

9 *Treatment regimens for headache disorders should be individualized: based on headache type, pattern of occurrence, response to therapy, medication tolerability, and comorbid medical conditions.*

1. Assess the patient complaint to yield a detailed description of the headache and to determine if immediate referral for emergency or specialist care is necessary.

2. Obtain a complete medical and social history to identify any potential drug–disease interactions or social factors that may influence treatment choices.

3. Obtain a family medical history, focusing on headache or mental health disorders in first-degree relatives.

4. Complete a review of systems and physical examination to identify causes or complications of headache.

5. Identify medication allergies, and obtain a thorough history of nonprescription and prescription drug use to identify potential drug–drug interactions that may

arise when selecting acute and prophylactic headache treatment.

6. Determine the type of headache disorder and rule out acute complications.

7. Recommend appropriate pharmacologic therapy to abort headache based on type, patient characteristics, current medication profile, and comorbid conditions.

8. Educate the patient on the administration, maximum dosage, and anticipated adverse effects of the prescribed medication, and advise the patient when to seek emergency medical attention.

9. Recommend appropriate nonpharmacologic therapy to abort headache and to prevent headache recurrence.

10. Determine if the patient is a candidate for prophylactic pharmacologic therapy, and if not, instruct the patient to keep a headache diary to assess therapeutic response.

Abbreviations Introduced in This Chapter

ACEI	Angiotensin-converting enzyme inhibitor
AMI	Acute myocardial infarction
ARB	Angiotensin receptor blocker
CCU	Coronary care unit
CGRP	Calcitonin gene-related peptide
CHF	Congestive heart failure
CSF	Cerebrospinal fluid
CT	Computed tomography
CTA	Clear to auscultation
CYP	Cytochrome P450 isoenzyme system
DHE	Dihydroergotamine
ESR	Erythrocyte sedimentation rate
GABA	γ-Aminobutyric acid
GERD	Gastroesophageal reflux disease
IHS	International Headache Society
MAO-A	Monoamine oxidase type A
MOH	Medication overuse headache
MRG	Murmur, rub, gallop
NSAID	Nonsteroidal anti-inflammatory drug
OTC	Over the counter
RR	Respiratory rate
SNRI	Serotonin-norepinephrine reuptake inhibitor
SSRI	Selective serotonin reuptake inhibitors
TCA	Tricyclic antidepressant
TTH	Tension-type headache

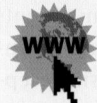 Self-assessment questions and answers are available at *http://www.mhpharmacotherapy.com/pp.html.*

REFERENCES

1. The International Classification of Headache Disorders. 2nd ed. Headache Classification Subcommittee of the International Headache Society. Cephalalgia 2004;24 (Suppl 1):9.
2. Lipton RB, Stewart WF, Diamond S, et al. Prevalence and burden of migraine in the United States: Data from the American Migraine Study II. Headache 2001;41:646–657.
3. Loder E. Menstrual migraine: Timing is everything. Neurology 2004;63:202.
4. Headache Classification Committee of the International Headache Society. The international classification of headache disorders. 2nd ed. Cephalalgia 2004;24(Suppl 1):1–160.
5. Hu XH, Markson LE, Lipton RB, et al. Burden of migraine in the United States. Arch Intern Med 1999;159:813–818.
6. Silberstein SD, Lipton RB, Goadsby PJ. Headache in Clinical Practice. London, UK: Martin Dunitz; 2002:21–33,69–128.
7. Lipton RB, Bigal ME, Steiner MB, et al. Classification of primary headaches. Neurology 2004;63:427–435.
8. Ruoff G, Urban G. Treatment of primary headache: Episodic tension-type headache. In: Standards of Care for Headache Diagnosis and Treatment. Chicago, IL: National Headache Foundation; 2004: 53–58.
9. Bahra A, May A, Goadsby PJ. Cluster headache: A prospective clinical study with diagnostic implications. Neurology 2002;58:354–361.

10. Goadsby PJ, Lipton RB, Ferrari MD. Migraine—current understanding and treatment. N Engl J Med 2002;346:257–270.

11. Hargreaves RJ, Shepheard SL. Pathophysiology of migraine: New insights. Can J Neurol Sci 1999;26(Suppl 3):S12–S19.

12. Edvinsson L. On migraine pathophysiology. In: Edvinsson OL, ed. Migraine and Headache Pathophysiology. London, UK: Martin Dunitz; 1999:3–15.

13. MacGregor EA, Brandes J, Eikermann A. Migraine prevalence and treatment patterns: The global migraine and zolmitriptan evaluation survey. Headache 2003;43:19–26.

14. Jenson R. Pathophysiological mechanisms of tension-type headache: A review of epidemiological and experimental studies. Cephalalgia 1999;19:602–621.

15. Dodick PW. Chronic daily headache. N Engl J Med 2006;354(2): 158–165.

16. Matharu MS, Boees CJ, Goadsby PJ. Management of trigeminal autonomic cephalalgias and hemicrania continua. Drugs 2003;63: 1637–1677.

17. King DS, Wofford MR. Headache Disorders. In: DiPiro JT, Talbert RL, Yee GC, et al., eds. Pharmacotherapy: A Pathophysiologic Approach. 7th ed. New York, NY: McGraw-Hill; 2008:1105–1121.

18. Silberstein SD. Migraine. Lancet 2004;363:381–391.

19. Solomon S. Migraine variants. Curr Pain Headache Rep 2001;5: 165–169.

20. Silberstein SD. Practice parameter: Evidence-based guidelines for migraine headache (an evidence-based review). Neurology 2000;55:754–763.

21. Silberstein SD, Goadsby PJ, Lipton RB. Management of migraine: An algorithmic approach. Neurology 2000;55(Suppl 2):S46–S52.

22. Mueller L. Tension-type, the forgotten headache. Postgrad Med 2002;111:25–50.

23. Biondi D, Mendes P. Treatment of primary headache: Cluster headache. In: Standards of Care for Headache Diagnosis and Treatment. Chicago, IL: National Headache Foundation; 2004:59–72.

24. Peters M, Abu-Saad HH, Vydelingum V, et al. Migraine and chronic daily headache management: A qualitative study of patients' perceptions. Scand J Caring Sci 2004;18:294–303.

25. Wenzel RG, Schommer JC, Marks TG. Morbidity and medication preferences of individuals with headache presenting to a community pharmacy. Headache 2004;44:90–94.

26. Lewis D, Ashwal S, Hershey A, et al. Practice parameter: Pharmacological treatment of migraine headache in children and adolescents. Report of the American Academy of Neurology Quality Standards Subcommittee and the Practice Committee of the Child Neurology Society. Neurology 2004;63:2215–2224.

27. Silberstein SD, Goadsby PJ. Migraine: Preventive treatment. Cephalalgia 2002;22:491–512.

28. Snow V, Weiss K, Wall EM, Mottur-Pilson C. Pharmacologic management of acute attacks of migraine and prevention of migraine headache. Ann Intern Med 2002;137:840–849.

29. Rollnik JD, Karst M, Piepenbrock S, et al. Gender differences in coping with tension-type headaches. Eur Neurol 2003;50:73–77.

30. del Rio MS, Silberstein SD. How to pick optimal acute treatment for migraine headache. Curr Pain Headache Rep 2001;5:170–178.

31. Lipton RB, Stewart WF, Ryan RE, et al. Efficacy and safety of acetaminophen, aspirin, and caffeine in alleviating migraine headache pain: Three double-blind, randomized, placebo-controlled trials. Arch Neurol 1998;55:210–217.

32. Relja G, Granato A, Antonello RM, Zorzon M. Headache induced by chronic substance use: Analysis of medication overused and minimum dose required to induce headache. Headache 2004;44:148–153.

33. Goldstein J, Silberstein SD, Saper JR, et al. Acetaminophen, aspirin, and caffeine versus sumatriptan succinate in the early treatment of migraine: Results from the ASSET trial. Headache 2005;45(8): 973–982.

34. Ferrari MD. Migraine. Lancet 1998;351:1043–1051.

35. Axert [package insert]. Raritan, NJ: Ortho-McNeil Neurologics; 2009.

36. Relpax [package insert]. New York, NY: Pfizer Inc.; 2011.

37. Frova [package insert]. Chadds Ford, PA: Endo Pharmaceuticals Inc.; 2007.

38. Amerge [package insert]. Research Triangle Park, NC: GlaxoSmithKline; 2010.

39. Maxalt [package insert]. Whitehouse Station, NJ: Merck & Co.; 2011.

40. Imitrex [package insert]. Research Triangle Park, NC: GlaxoSmithKline; 2010.

41. Zomig [package insert]. Wilmington, DE: AstraZeneca Pharmaceuticals; 2008.

42. Treximet [package insert]. Research Triangle Park, NC: GlaxoSmithKline; 2011.

43. Ferrari MD, Roon KI, Lipton RB, Goadsby PJ. Oral triptans (serotonin 5-HT1B/1D agonists) in acute migraine treatment: A meta-analysis of 53 trials. Lancet 2001;358:1558–1575.

44. Pringsheim T, Gawel M. Triptans: Are they all the same? Curr Pain Headache Rep 2002;6:140–146.

45. Deleu D, Hanssens Y. Current and emerging second-generation triptans in acute migraine therapy: A comparative review. J Clin Pharmacol 2000;40:687–700.

46. Dahlof CGH. Current concepts of migraine and its treatment. Neurology 1999;14:67–77.

47. Pascual J, Cabarrocas X. Within-patient early versus delayed treatment of migraine attacks with almotriptan: The sooner the better. Headache 2002;42:28–31.

48. Lipton RB, Stewart WF, Stone AM, et al. Stratified care vs step care strategies for migraine: The Disability in Strategies of Care (DISC) Study: A randomized trial. JAMA 2000;284:2599–2606.

49. Jenson R, Olesen J. Tension-type headache: An update on mechanisms and treatment. Curr Opin Neurol 2000;13:285–289.

50. Rozen TD. High oxygen flow rates for cluster headache. Neurology 2004;63(3):593.

51. Gobel H, Lindner V, Heinz A, et al. Acute therapy for cluster headache with sumatriptan: Findings of a one-year long-term study. Neurology 1998;51:430–435.

52. Bahra A, Gawel MJ, Hardebo JE, et al. Oral zolmitriptan is effective in the acute treatment of cluster headache. Neurology 2000;54: 291–296.

53. Goadsby PJ. New targets in the acute treatment of headache. Curr Opin Neurol 2005;18:283–288.

54. Topamax [package insert]. Titusville, NJ: Janssen Pharmaceuticals; 2009.

55. Depakote [package insert]. North Chicago, IL: Abbott Laboratories; 2009.

56. Inderal [package insert]. Philadelphia, PA: Wyeth Pharmaceuticals; 2011.

57. Linde K, Rossnagel K. Propranolol for migraine prophylaxis. Cochrane Database Syst Rev 2004;2:CD003225.

58. Tronvik E, Stovener LJ, Helde G, et al. Prophylactic treatment of migraine with angiotensin II receptor blocker: A randomized, controlled trial. JAMA 2003;289:65–69.

59. Joint National Committee on Prevention, Detection, Evaluation, and Treatment of High Blood Pressure. The Seventh Report of the Joint National Committee on Prevention, Detection, Evaluation, and Treatment of High Blood Pressure: The JNC 7 Report. JAMA 2003;289:2560–2572.

60. Cutrer FM. Antiepileptic drugs: How they work in headache. Headache 2001;41(Suppl):S3–S10.

61. Bigal ME, Krymchantowski AV, Rapoport AM. New developments in migraine prophylaxis. Expert Opin Pharmacother 2003;4: 433–443.

62. Silberstein SD. Methysergide. Cephalalgia 1998;18:421–435.

63. Winner P, Rothner AD, Saper J, Nett R. A randomized double-blind, placebo-controlled study of sumatriptan nasal spray in the treatment of acute migraine in adolescents. Pediatrics 2000;106: 989–997.

64. Maggioni F, Alessi C, Maggino T, Zanchin G. Headache during pregnancy. Cephalalgia 1997;17:765–769.

65. Scharff L, Marcus DA, Turk DC. Headache during pregnancy and in the postpartum: A prospective study. Headache 1997;37: 203–210.

66. Lipton RB, Baggish JS, Stewart WF, et al. Efficacy and safety of acetaminophen in the treatment of migraine: Results of a randomized, double-blind, placebo-controlled, population-based study. Arch Intern Med 2000;160:3486–3492.

67. Olesen C, Steffensen FH, Sorensen HT, et al. Pregnancy outcome following prescription for sumatriptan. Headache 2000;40:20–24.

68. Evans RW, Armon C, Frohman EM, Goodin DS. Assessment: Prevention of post-lumbar puncture headaches. Report of the Therapeutics and Technology Assessment Subcommittee of the American Academy of Neurology. Neurology 2000;55:909–914.

69. Belfort MA, Saade GR, Grunewald C, et al. Association of cerebral perfusion pressure with headache in women with pre-eclampsia. Br J Obstet Gynaecol 1999;106:814–821.

36 Substance-Related Disorders

Christian J. Teter

LEARNING OBJECTIVES

● **Upon completion of the chapter, the reader will be able to:**

1. Identify the prevalence of abuse for commonly used substances (i.e., alcohol, opioids, central nervous system [CNS] stimulants, and nicotine) in the U.S. population.

2. Explain the commonalities of action of abused substances on the reward system in the brain.

3. Identify the typical signs and symptoms of intoxication and withdrawal associated with the use of alcohol, opioids, CNS stimulants, and nicotine.

4. Determine the appropriate treatment measures to produce a desired outcome after episodes of intoxication and withdrawal.

5. Determine when a patient meets criteria for substance dependence.

6. Choose specific pharmacotherapeutic options based on patient-specific factors.

7. Recommend a comprehensive medication treatment and monitoring program to help maintain recovery and prevent relapse to substance abuse.

KEY CONCEPTS

❶ Pharmacotherapy has been shown to have a role in treatment of some substance-related disorders, including intoxication, withdrawal, and long-term relapse prevention. These substances include alcohol, opioids, CNS stimulants, and nicotine.

❷ Virtually all abused substances appear to activate the same brain reward pathway, which is highlighted by dopaminergic neurotransmission arising in the ventral tegmental area and projecting to the nucleus accumbens and prefrontal cortex.

❸ Although activation of the reward pathways explains the pleasurable sensations associated with acute substance use, chronic use of abused substances, which may result in addiction and withdrawal, may be related to neuroadaptive effects occurring within the brain.

❹ Individuals with a pattern of chronic use of commonly abused substances should be assessed to determine if they meet the *Diagnostic and Statistical Manual*, fourth edition, text revision, criteria for substance dependence or withdrawal.

❺ The treatment goals for acute intoxication of ethanol, CNS stimulants, and opioids include (a) management of psychological and psychiatric manifestations of intoxication, such as aggression, hostility, and psychosis and (b) management of medical manifestations of intoxication, such as respiratory depression, hyperthermia, hypertension, cardiac arrhythmias, and stroke.

❻ The treatment goals for withdrawal from ethanol, CNS stimulants, and opioids include (a) a determination if pharmacologic treatment of withdrawal symptoms is necessary, (b) management of other medical manifestations, and (c) referral to the appropriate program for long-term substance abuse treatment.

❼ A multimodal and comprehensive approach is usually preferred when treating individuals with substance use disorders given the heterogeneous nature of addiction. Pharmacologic treatment is always adjunctive to psychosocial therapy.

❽ Certain pharmacologic agents have been shown to be helpful for long-term maintenance in patients with substance dependence. Typically, these medications exert their effects by one of the following theorized mechanisms: (a) drug substitution therapy with an agonist, (b) blocking drug effects with an antagonist, and (c) miscellaneous relapse prevention medications with indirect mechanisms of action.

❾ A major component of successful treatment of addiction is to continue monitoring the use of medications and to identify a mechanism for long-term support of sobriety that might be appropriate, such as

Alcoholics Anonymous (AA) or recovery programs for professionals such as doctors, nurses, or pharmacists.

⑩ Clinicians must be familiar with "essential" resources, many of which are in the public domain.

Substance abuse and dependence are highly prevalent problems in the United States and worldwide. In the United States, the use of all substances of abuse has undergone a series of periodic cycles of societal tolerance or condemnation. As an example, cocaine was first isolated from coca leaves in 1860 by a chemistry graduate student in Germany. Its use was advocated by many in the medical establishment until around the mid-1890s when it became evident that chronic use of cocaine might be addictive in some individuals and could be associated with deleterious physiologic effects. Its use decreased after restriction of prescribing and dispensing of cocaine in the early 20th century, but it continued to be abused by a small segment of the population. Unfortunately, in the 1980s, a smokeable formulation of cocaine (i.e., crack) became available, and cocaine use again became an epidemic. This historically cyclic nature of substance abuse is common to many substances of abuse.

① *Pharmacotherapy has been shown to have a role in treatment of some substance-related disorders, including intoxication, withdrawal, and/or long-term relapse prevention. These substances include alcohol, opioids, central nervous system (CNS) stimulants, and nicotine. This chapter focuses on efficacious pharmacotherapy for these common substance-related disorders.* Although many more substances can be and have been abused, these drugs are among the most popular and are treatable with medication.

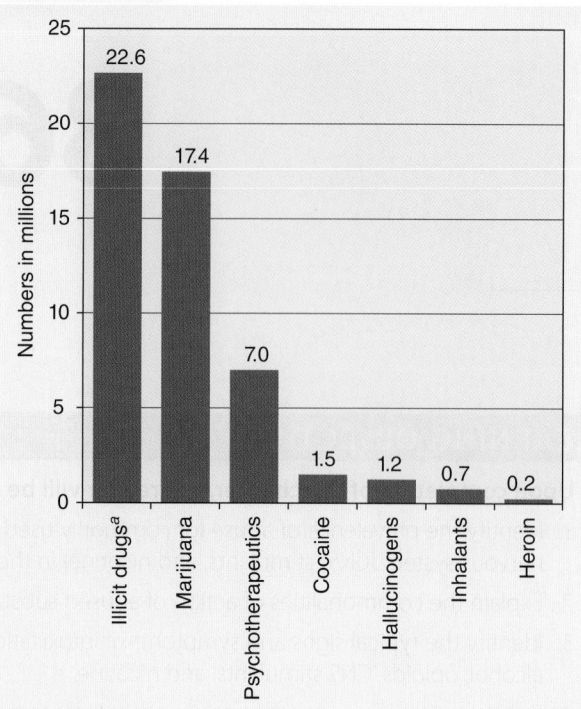

FIGURE 36–1. Past-month illicit drug use among the U.S. population in 2010. *ᵃIllicit drug use includes a wide variety of substances such as marijuana or hashish, cocaine (including crack), heroin, hallucinogens, inhalants, or prescription-type psychotherapeutics used nonmedically. (Data from Substance Abuse and Mental Health Services Administration (SAMHSA). Results from the 2010 National Survey on Drug Use and Health: Summary of National Findings, NSDUH Series H-41, HHS Publication No. (SMA) 11-4658. Rockville, MD: Substance Abuse and Mental Health Services Administration; 2011.)*

EPIDEMIOLOGY

In the United States, the federal government annually conducts the National Survey on Drug Use and Health (NSDUH) using a representative sample of persons who are 12 years of age or older to determine the prevalence of licit and illicit drug use.[1] In 2010, more than half (51.8%; 131.3 million) of Americans reported being a current (i.e., past month) alcohol drinker; about one quarter (23.1%; 58.6 million) reported binge drinking (i.e., 5+ drinks) at least once in the 30 days before the survey; and heavy drinking (i.e., binge drinking on 5+ occasions in past 30 days) was reported by 6.7% (16.9 million) of Americans in 2010. In 2010, approximately one-quarter (27.4%; 69.6 million Americans) were current users of tobacco products, with young adults aged 18 to 25 reporting the highest rates of current tobacco product use (40.8%). Regarding illicit drug use, 8.9% of the U.S. population (22.6 million) reported current illicit drug use, with nonmedical psychotherapeutics being second only to marijuana (Fig. 36–1). In 2010, there were 3.0 million illicit drug initiates, with marijuana being the first drug in a majority of cases (61.8%). However, approximately one-quarter (26.2%) nonmedically used a psychotherapeutic as their first illicit drug (i.e., 17.3% with pain relievers, 4.6%

with tranquilizers, 2.5% with stimulants, and 1.9% with sedatives).[1] The results of NSDUH (a gold-standard, national U.S. survey) indicate that substance use is wide ranging; peaks in the age range of 18 to 25 years; and consists of a significant number of individuals reporting the nonmedical use of prescription medications, which is a relatively new and growing public health concern.

PATHOPHYSIOLOGY

Reward Pathway

② *Virtually all abused substances appear to activate the same brain reward pathway, which is highlighted by dopaminergic neurotransmission arising in the ventral tegmental area (VTA) and projecting to the nucleus accumbens (NA) and prefrontal cortex (PFC).*

Figure 36–2 shows a depiction of the mesocorticolimbic dopamine pathway. Key components are dopamine (DA) projections from the VTA to the NA and to the PFC.[2,3] It appears clear from many studies, using a variety of

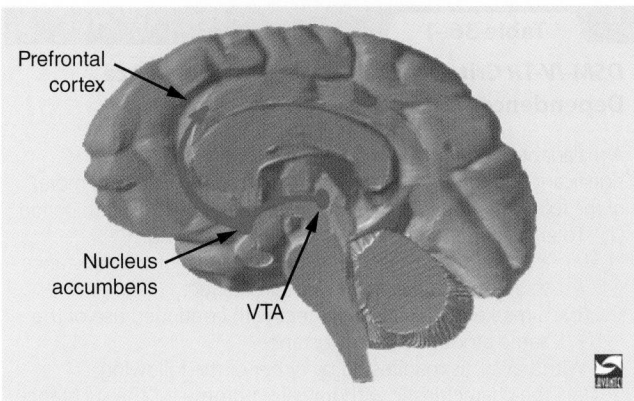

FIGURE 36–2. The mesocorticolimbic dopaminergic pathway (i.e., the "reward pathway"). VTA, ventral tegmental area. (Data from The Neurobiology of Drug Addiction [Internet]. Available at: *http://www.drugabuse.gov/pubs/teaching/Teaching2/Teaching.html.*)

techniques, that this mesolimbic DA system is involved in natural rewards and drug reinforcement[4]; however, there is also evidence that dopamine-independent reinforcement exists.[5] In any case, abused drugs generally produce pleasant effects that are desired by the user. The initial hedonic experiences secondary to use of drugs appear to be primarily attributable to their ability to activate the primary reward circuits in the brain. These same reward circuits operate under normal circumstances to reinforce certain activities that promote survival, such as food and water, social affiliation, or sexual activity. However, these systems appear to be disrupted after drug use in susceptible individuals.

However, although most individuals will experience pleasant effects, not everyone abuses these drugs, and not everyone who abuses them becomes dependent on them. Why some persons abuse drugs while most people do not is a complex area of research. It appears that genetic, environmental, and cultural factors may all interact to predispose some individuals to substance abuse and subsequent dependence.

Neuronal Adaptation

❸ *Although activation of the reward pathways explains the pleasurable sensations associated with acute substance use, chronic use of abused substances, which may result in addiction and withdrawal, may be related to neuroadaptive effects occurring within the brain.*

A recent review by two of the preeminent researchers in the addiction sciences thoroughly describes the addiction cycle moving past the acute rewarding effects of substances of abuse and into other important processes.[5] In their review, they describe three phases of the addiction cycle: (a) binge/intoxication, (b) withdrawal/negative affect, and (c) preoccupation/anticipation. The first phase of binge/intoxication refers to the acute rewarding effects of drugs of abuse and the corresponding CNS circuitry. However, chronic use of substances leads to alterations in the brain and associated symptoms. For example, in phase 2 proposed

by Koob and Volkow, chronic drug exposure leads to neuroadaptations such as decreased activity in the brain circuits involved in the acute rewarding phase. More specifically, chronic use of drugs of abuse appears to cause a generalized decrease in DA neurotransmission, probably in response to the intermittent increases in DA induced by the frequent use of these drugs. Additionally, with chronic drug use, release of corticotropin-releasing factor (CRF) is increased, indicating an activation of central stress pathways. In phase 3 of the framework, other neurotransmitter systems (i.e., beyond DA) are postulated to be involved. For example, elevated CRF, norepinephrine, and glutamate may exist in the "extended amygdala" during prolonged abstinence. Perhaps these changes lead to a long-term need to use substances to relieve unpleasant symptoms, such as stress.[5] Multiple factors are associated with an increased risk of relapse, including the availability of the abused drug, an increase in psychological stressors, and a triggering of conditioning factors (cues) such as seeing a white powder or going to a location where drugs were often previously used or obtained. These factors may be acting to trigger residual adaptive changes (e.g., elevated glutamatergic activity) that occurred in the brain during the period of drug addiction.

OVERALL THEORY OF USE OF PHARMACOLOGIC AGENTS TO TREAT SUBSTANCE-RELATED DISORDERS

Unfortunately, unlike some medical diseases, substance dependence cannot be cured with medications alone. However, we can sometimes alleviate the effects of drug intoxication, attenuate the adverse effects of withdrawal, or use agents that may somewhat decrease craving for and relapse to abused substances. For example, the pleasurable and intoxicating effects of opioids appear to be caused by their action as agonists on μ-receptors of the opioid neurotransmitter system. Competitive μ-opioid antagonists such as naloxone and naltrexone acutely reverse many of the effects of opioids. To date, we do not have specific antagonists for most other abused substances, so rapid pharmacologic reversal of intoxication is usually not possible. Similarly, reversal of withdrawal syndromes caused by abused substances is not always possible. One pharmacologic solution for reversing a drug withdrawal syndrome, most commonly used by substance dependent individuals, is to readminister the drug that caused the physiologic dependence. The more commonly used treatment method is to administer a medication that has some cross-dependence with the abused drug but also has fewer of the reinforcing effects and a more predictable pharmacokinetic profile. A good example is the use of benzodiazepines for the withdrawal of ethanol. Although benzodiazepines can cause dependence, they are rated as less desirable than ethanol by substance abusers, cause fewer of the long-term adverse health effects of ethanol, and are easier to manage medically. Regarding longer term dependence, an example is maintaining an opioid-addicted individual on a regimen of medically managed, orally administered opioids (referred to as substitution therapy) compared with more dangerous illicit opioid use. Regardless of the specific pharmacotherapy chosen for each symptom presentation, medications should always be used as adjuncts to a comprehensive psychosocial approach.

CLINICAL PRESENTATION AND DIAGNOSIS

❹ *Individuals with a pattern of chronic use of commonly abused substances should be assessed to determine if they meet the* Diagnostic and Statistical Manual, *fourth edition, text revision (DSM-IV-TR) criteria for substance dependence or withdrawal.*[6] Criteria are not defined for each separate abused substance; rather, a pattern of behavior common to the abuse or dependence of all drugs of abuse is established. The criteria for abuse indicate an established pattern of using a substance that has resulted in undesirable family, job, or legal consequences, such as recurrent instances of neglecting school, work, or family responsibilities, or being arrested for driving under the influence. However, abuse becomes dependence when tolerance to the drug, withdrawal from the drug, or an inability to discontinue use of the drug is apparent. Most notably, in cases of addiction, there is a loss of control over its use or the use has become compulsive. The criteria for substance dependence from the *DSM-IV-TR* are listed in Table 36–1.[6]

In addition to formal diagnostic criteria, a variety of standardized instruments are available to screen for and assess the various stages of substance use and its consequences,

---

Table 36–1

DSM-IV-TR Criteria for Diagnosis of Substance Dependence

A maladaptive pattern of substance use, leading to clinically significant impairment or distress, as manifested by three (or more) of the following, occurring at any time in the same 12-month period:
(1) Tolerance, as defined by either of the following:
  (a) a need for markedly increased amounts of the substance to achieve intoxication or desired effect
  (b) a markedly diminished effect with continued use of the same amount of the substance
(2) Withdrawal, as manifested by either of the following:
  (a) the characteristic withdrawal syndrome for the substance
  (b) the same (or a closely related) substance is taken to relieve or avoid withdrawal symptoms
(3) The substance is often taken in larger amounts or over a longer period than was intended
(4) There is a persistent desire or unsuccessful efforts to cut down or control substance use
(5) A great deal of time is spent in obtaining the substance (e.g., visiting multiple doctors or driving long distances), using the substance (e.g., chain-smoking), or recovering from its effects
(6) Important social, occupational, or recreational activities are given up or reduced because of substance use
(7) The substance use is continued despite knowledge of having a persistent or recurrent physical or psychological problem that is likely to have been caused or exacerbated by the substance (e.g., current cocaine use despite recognition of cocaine-induced depression, or continued drinking despite recognition that an ulcer was made worse by alcohol consumption)
Specify if:
• With physiologic dependence: Evidence of tolerance or withdrawal (i.e., either Item 1 or 2 is present)
• Without physiologic dependence: No evidence of tolerance or withdrawal (i.e., neither Item 1 nor 2 is present)

Data from American Psychiatric Association. Diagnostic and Statistical Manual of Mental Disorders. 4th ed, text rev. Washington, DC: American Psychiatric Association; 2000; with permission.

Patient Encounter 1

GC, a 43-year-old man with a history of diabetes, presents to your clinic for follow-up evaluation of his diabetes. You notice that he admits to drinking a pint of Scotch whiskey per day despite his unstable diabetes. He states that his drinking has "crept up" on him over the years and that he finds a pint to be "just the right amount." When you question him about his drinking, he says it is not a problem because he can still "mountain bike with the best of them." He does, however, admit his wife is concerned with his drinking. The only times his drinking bothers him are when he is too hung over to mountain bike on the Saturday morning group rides (patient notes that riding is his favorite part of the day) and when he occasionally "messes up his sugar control" because he is intoxicated. Other than that, GC truly feels that his drinking is under his control.

What information would suggest this patient might be alcohol dependent?

Are there any standardized instruments that you can recommend to assess the impact of drinking on the patient's overall functioning?

---

such as withdrawal symptoms and functional impairment (see Table 36–2).[7-10] Some instruments are specific to a particular substance (e.g., Clinical Institute Withdrawal Assessment Scale for Alcohol—Revised [CIWA-Ar]), and others cover a wide range of substances. For example, the Addiction Severity Index (ASI) is a gold-standard instrument that assesses seven problem areas associated with substance use, such as medical status and psychiatric status, in addition to measures of alcohol and drug use.[8]

Intoxication Signs and Symptoms

Intoxication caused by most substances of abuse is described in the *DSM-IV* as clinically significant, **maladaptive** behavioral, physiologic, or psychological changes to the user. These changes are seen during or shortly after use of the substance. Euphoria or the experience of a pleasurable sensation are common effects of most drugs of abuse.[11] Other signs and symptoms are specific to the particular drug or class of drugs

Table 36–2

Commonly Used Instruments for Substance Use Disorders

Instrument	Purpose	Values and Interpretation
Addiction Severity Index (ASI) Assessment tool (past 30 days or lifetime) for various substances	Semi-structured interview that addresses seven problem areas: medical status, employment and support, alcohol use, drug use, legal status, family and social status, and psychiatric status Questions include frequency, duration, and severity of problems	Patient and interviewer ratings included Interviewer severity ratings of the "need for additional treatment" + composite scores to measure problem severity Scoring completed by a technician or computerized scoring and interpretation Composite score normative data from a nationally representative sample of treatment programs is available for those seeking to compare a patient's ASI data with national data (available at *http://www.tresearch.org*); otherwise, comparisons with previous (e.g., baseline) composite scores are useful
Alcohol Use Disorders Identification Test (AUDIT)	Evaluates quantity and frequency of drinking; physiologic dependence on alcohol; and harmful use	10 items (scores 0–40) Score of 8 or above identifies heavy drinkers and those with alcohol use disorders
Screening tool	Clinician administered	"Zones" of interventions based on scores
CAGE C = Cut down A = Angry or annoyed G = Guilty E = Eye opener Screening tool	Clinician or self-administered Used to identify the presence of problematic drinking No training is necessary	Four items Score of 2 or more is positive and suggests problem drinking Positive screen prompts the need for further assessment
Clinical Institute for Withdrawal Assessment–Alcohol, Revised (CIWA-Ar) Assessment tool	Gold standard alcohol withdrawal assessment; used as part of symptom-triggered approach Clinician administered	10 items; maximum score = 67 Less than 10: mild withdrawal; likely does not require medication 10–18: moderate withdrawal Greater than 18: severe withdrawal Monitor scores over time; lower score implies less withdrawal severity; higher scores (e.g., 8 to 10 or greater, depending on institutional protocols or co-occurring conditions) indicate need for medication
Clinical Opiate Withdrawal Scale (COWS) Assessment tool	Used to follow the course of withdrawal symptoms and the effectiveness of medication regimens Clinician administered	11 items; scoring is 0 (asymptomatic) to 4 or 5 (severely symptomatic); scale for each item based on intensity of signs and symptoms Total score (sum of all 11 items): 5–12: Mild 13–24: Moderate 25–36: Moderately severe Greater than 36: Severe withdrawal Monitor scores over time (lower score implies less opioid withdrawal severity); higher scores (i.e., scores of 5 or greater represent increasing levels of withdrawal symptoms) may indicate the need for medication, although no standard cut-off exists for this indication
Fagerstrom Test for Nicotine Dependence	Assesses extent of nicotine tolerance, dependence, and craving; contains six questions (tolerance, withdrawal symptoms, and craving); higher scores may predict greater difficulty in quitting	Total scoring for dependence: 0–2: Very low 3–4: Low 5: Moderate 6–7: High 8–10: Very high

Data from Refs. 7–10.

Table 36–3

Signs and Symptoms of Drug Intoxication for Select Substances

Drug	Behavioral Effects	Physiologic Effects
Ethanol	Changes in mood and behavior, inappropriate aggressive or sexual behavior, giddiness or verbally loud, impaired judgment; possibly progressing to somnolence and coma as the blood level increases	At blood levels of 0.02–0.1% (20–100 mg/dL or 4.34–21.7 mmol/L): Euphoria, feeling of well-being, disinhibition, slight impairment (e.g., reaction time) At blood levels from 0.1% to 0.2% (100–200 mg/dL or 21.7–43.4 mmol/L): Significant impairment (e.g., balance, speech, vision and hearing, reaction times), dysphoria At blood levels from 0.2% to 0.3% (200–300 mg/dL or 43.4–65.1 mmol/L): Marked ataxia, mental confusion, and possible nausea and vomiting At blood levels from 0.3% to 0.4% (300–400 mg/dL or 65.1–86.8 mmol/L): Severe dysarthria, amnesia, hypothermia At blood levels greater than 0.4% (400 mg/dL or 86.8 mmol/L): Alcoholic coma, decreased respiration or respiratory arrest; aspiration of gastric contents or airway obstruction caused by flaccid tongue, drop in blood pressure and body temperature
Opioids	Drowsiness or sedation, slurred speech, impaired memory and attention, psychomotor retardation	Nausea and vomiting, respiratory depression (dose-related), stupor, coma, constipation very common in chronic users, itching, miosis (pinpoint pupils), hypothermia, bradycardia
CNS stimulants	Initially, most prominent effect is elated mood, hypervigilance, anxiety or panic, impairment of judgment, violence to others or self, paranoia or psychosis with delusions and hallucinations (hallucinations are generally tactile or auditory, rarely visual), an increase in motor activity, compulsive or stereotyped behavior (e.g., skin picking)	Neurologic: Pupillary dilation, headache, tremor, hyperreflexia, muscle twitching, flushing, hyperthermia or cold sweats, seizures, coma Cardiovascular: Increased pulse and blood pressure, peripheral vasoconstriction, arrhythmias, myocardial infarction, cerebral hemorrhage GI: Nausea and vomiting, weight loss Neuromuscular: Rhabdomyolysis, possibly resulting in renal failure, muscular weakness, dyskinesias

CNS, central nervous system; GI, gastrointestinal.

Data from Refs. 6, 12–15.

involved. Table 36–3 lists the psychological/behavioral and physiologic effects of intoxication with ethanol, opioids, and CNS stimulants.[6,12-15]

Withdrawal Signs and Symptoms

Although most abused drugs can cause some degree of physiologic dependence, the severity of withdrawal varies considerably among these drugs. Table 36–4 lists the common withdrawal symptoms seen upon abstinence from drug use.[6,12-16] It is typical that withdrawal symptoms appear opposite to the acute effects of drug use. For example, although alcohol is a CNS depressant, many of the signs and symptoms of withdrawal signify a hyper-alert physiologic response.

TREATMENT OF INTOXICATION SYNDROMES

⑤ *The treatment goals for acute intoxication of ethanol, CNS stimulants, and opioids include (a) management of psychological/ psychiatric manifestations of intoxication, such as aggression, hostility, and psychosis and (b) management of medical manifestations of intoxication, such as respiratory depression, hyperthermia, hypertension, cardiac arrhythmias, and stroke.* In all cases of intoxication associated with a substance use disorder (abuse or dependence), referral to and participation in substance abuse treatment after acute treatment for intoxication is desirable.

Patient Encounter 2

CD, a 27-year-old woman, was admitted to the cardiology unit from the emergency department (ED) after she called 911 claiming that she had severe chest pain and that her heart was racing. Upon arrival in the ED, it was noted that her blood pressure was slightly elevated at 143/92 mm Hg and that she was diaphoretic. She was in otherwise good physical condition with no previous cardiac history. After a urine toxicology screen was positive for cocaine, she admitted that she had snorted several large lines of cocaine before having the chest pain. She said she almost never uses cocaine, but that it helps her chronic depression (diagnosed at age 19 years), which has worsened since she lost her job approximately 3 weeks ago. The treatment plan is to address the patient's stimulant use and major depressive disorder (MDD) after the cardiac issues are resolved.

What are the possible physical signs and symptoms of CD's cocaine use that are consistent with cocaine intoxication?

What is the most appropriate pharmacotherapy for this patient's acute condition?

What is the most appropriate long-term pharmacotherapy for this patient?

Table 36–4

Signs and Symptoms of Drug Withdrawal for Select Substances

Drug	Timeline	Symptoms
Ethanol	As ethanol level decreases (especially after last drink):	
	Early symptoms	Tremor, nausea and vomiting, tachycardia (greater than 110 bpm), hypertension (greater than 140/90 mm Hg), headache, vivid dreams, insomnia
	Peak at 24 hours	Convulsions (usually one or two of grand mal type but can be numerous and possibly fatal)
	72 to 96 hours	Delirium tremens
	Onset at any time	Hallucinations, usually visual
Opioids	For shorter acting opioids (e.g., heroin, morphine, hydrocodone, oxycodone) withdrawal may begin within 6–24 hours after the last dose and last for about 1 week; with longer acting opioids (e.g., methadone) it may take up to 2–4 days for withdrawal to emerge, and it will last longer	GI: Nausea and vomiting, diarrhea, and dehydration Neurologic or psychological: Irritability, restlessness, yawning, tremulousness, and twitching Cardiovascular: Increase in heart rate and blood pressure Musculoskeletal: Chills, increased body temperature, piloerection, and rhinorrhea Ocular: Lacrimation and dilated pupils
Nicotine	Begins within 24 hours of cessation of use; may persist	The severity of symptoms reflects the degree and duration of nicotine use; symptoms include anxiety, irritability, frustration, anger, craving, difficulty concentrating, decreased heart rate, and increased appetite
CNS stimulants	Immediately after binge	Stimulant craving, accompanied by intense dysphoria, depression, anxiety, and agitation
	Within 1–4 hours	Desire for sleep, dysphoria continues
	Days 3–4	Hypersomnia, increased appetite, craving may dissipate slightly but returns strongly later

CNS, central nervous system; GI, gastrointestinal.

Data from Refs. 6, 12–16.

Alcohol Intoxication

Most cases of mild to moderate intoxication with alcohol, as well as cases in which blood alcohol concentrations (BACs) are at the lower limits of legal intoxication, do not require formal treatment. Such intoxications are characterized by **mood lability**, loud or inappropriate behavior, slurred speech, incoordination, or an unsteady gait. Providing a safe environment and supportive reassurance until the effects of alcohol have worn off is sufficient in most cases. At more severe levels of intoxication, confusion, stupor, coma, and death may be observed. As shown in Table 36–3, in nontolerant individuals, confusion, impaired consciousness, and vomiting are observed at BACs of 200 to 300 mg/dL (0.2% to 0.3% or 43.4 to 65.1 mmol/L); stupor and coma are seen with BACs exceeding 300 to 400 mg/dL (0.3% to 0.4% or 65.1 to 86.8 mmol/L). Death may occur at levels of 400 mg/dL (0.4% or 86.8 mmol/L) or higher from cardiac arrhythmias or respiratory depression. Thus, the most important physiologic goal of treating high levels of intoxication is maintaining cardiopulmonary functioning, including the prevention of aspiration. Accordingly, vital signs must be monitored regularly. Serial BACs at least hourly are strongly recommended, and patients should not be allowed to leave the treatment setting on their own while legally intoxicated (greater than or equal to 80 mg/dL [0.08% or 17.4 mmol/L]). Initially, BACs may continue to rise if gastrointestinal (GI) absorption is still occurring. Otherwise, the BAC generally decreases at a rate of 15 to 20 mg/dL (0.015% to 0.02% or 3.3 to 4.3 mmol/L) per hour. Although more tolerant individuals may not show the same level of symptoms for a given BAC as nontolerant individuals, behavioral tolerance and tolerance for vital physiologic functions may differ. Thus, alcoholic patients who are awake and alert at a BAC greater than or equal to 400 mg/dL (0.4% or 86.8 mmol/L) may still be at risk for cardiopulmonary instability and collapse.

Other causes of confusion, stupor, or coma must be ruled out because alcohol-intoxicated individuals commonly combine alcohol with other substances, sustain head and other injuries, and have vitamin deficiencies and electrolyte abnormalities. If consciousness is impaired, then thiamine should be given intravenously (IV) or intramuscularly (IM) at 100 mg/day for at least 3 days. If hypoglycemia is suspected, then thiamine administration should precede administration of glucose-containing fluids to prevent precipitation of an acute **Wernicke's encephalopathy**. Thiamine administration will be discussed in further detail below in the Alcohol Withdrawal section. Patients may also develop adverse interactions between alcohol and medications that have been prescribed including disulfiram. See Table 36–5 for a listing of drug–drug interactions with abused substances.[17,18]

Table 36–5

Clinically Relevant Drug Interactions With Abused Drugs or Medications Used to Treat Substance Use Disorders

Drug	Interacting Drug	Type of Interaction and Appropriate Action
Amphetamines (including dextro- and methamphetamine)	MAOIs (phenelzine, selegiline, tranylcypromine, possibly linezolid)	Pharmacodynamic interaction resulting in an increase in blood pressure; possibly resulting in a hypertensive emergency or stroke; **AVOID** this drug combination
	Sodium bicarbonate	Sodium bicarbonate increases renal tubular reabsorption of amphetamine, resulting in a prolonged amphetamine elimination half-life; closely monitor this combination
Bupropion	MAOIs	Neurotoxicity; **AVOID** this drug combination
	Substances that lower seizure threshold	Alcohol (*withdrawal*); **AVOID** bupropion use in patients at risk for experiencing alcohol withdrawal
Buprenorphine	Atazanavir	Combination of buprenorphine + atazanavir (without ritonavir) results in both lower atazanavir levels and greater buprenorphine exposure; **AVOID** this bidirection-interacting drug combination
	Conivaptan	Conivaptan is a potent inhibitor of CYP3A4, and the manufacturer recommends that its use be **avoided** with medications metabolized by CYP3A4
	CYP3A4 inhibitors (in addition to the specific medications listed above)	May raise buprenorphine levels; monitor for greater than expected buprenorphine effects
Cigarette smoking	Clozapine and olanzapine	Cigarette smoking induces CYP1A2, increasing the metabolism of clozapine; may need to increase usual clozapine dose when a patient begins to smoke or decrease clozapine dose if smoking is stopped or nicotine replacement is used instead of smoking
	Theophylline	Theophylline is also a CYP1A2 substrate; may need to increase the usual theophylline dose when a patient begins to smoke or decrease the theophylline dose if smoking is stopped or nicotine replacement is used instead of smoking
Disulfiram	Alcohol-containing solutions (variety of medications)	Disulfiram reaction; **AVOID** this combination
	Metronidazole	The combination of disulfiram and metronidazole has lead to CNS effects (e.g., psychosis); **AVOID** this combination
	Benzodiazepines (including alprazolam, chlordiazepoxide, diazepam, flurazepam, triazolam)	Disulfiram (weakly) inhibits CYP enzymes 1A2, 2C9, and 3A4; many benzodiazepines are metabolized via these pathways; lorazepam, temazepam, and oxazepam are primarily conjugated to inactive products and are reasonable alternatives Otherwise, if benzodiazepines are combined with disulfiram, the pharmacologic effect may be greater than expected, and the dose of benzodiazepine may need to be lowered
	Cocaine	Disulfiram decreases the clearance of cocaine from the body; may see increased or prolonged cocaine effects with this combination
	Phenytoin	Disulfiram decreases the metabolism of phenytoin, resulting in higher phenytoin levels; dose of phenytoin will need to be reduced; because phenytoin undergoes nonlinear metabolism, it is difficult to predict the magnitude of increase in blood levels that could be seen; it is best to avoid this interaction if possible
Ethanol (alcohol)	Acetaminophen	Chronic ethanol use increases the risk of hepatotoxicity when acetaminophen is used in high doses
	Bupropion	Abrupt *discontinuation* of alcohol with continued bupropion use may lower seizure threshold; this combination should be **avoided** in those at risk for seizure activity (e.g., alcoholics with co-occurring depressive symptoms)
	Cefamandole, cefoperazone, cefotetan, and moxalactam, metronidazole	A disulfiram-type reaction may occur when these anti-infectives are combined with alcohol; the reaction includes flushing, diaphoresis, tachycardia, headache, and increases in blood pressure; **avoid** alcohol if these drugs are used
	Cycloserine	Neurotoxicity (specifically seizure risk) may be enhanced with the combination of alcohol and cycloserine; **AVOID** combination
	Didanosine	The risk for pancreatitis may be increased with the combination of alcohol and didanosine; **AVOID** combination
	Methotrexate	Hepatotoxicity is a higher risk when methotrexate is given to those who chronically drink large amounts of alcohol; **avoid** methotrexate in this group if possible; otherwise monitor LFTs

(Continued)

Table 36–5

Clinically Relevant Drug Interactions With Abused Drugs or Medications Used to Treat Substance Use Disorders (*Continued*)

Drug	Interacting Drug	Type of Interaction and Appropriate Action
	MAOIs	Ethanol **DOES NOT** interact with MAOIs; however, tyramine may be a component of some aged alcoholic drinks, such as red wines or tap beers; if a reaction occurs, hypertension and a pounding headache are the most likely symptoms; usually white wine is tolerable (in moderation) and most widely available domestic canned beers do not contain significant amounts of tyramine
	Tapentadol	The combination of alcohol and *extended-release* tapentadol may result in increased maximum serum concentrations of tapentadol; **AVOID** this drug combination
Methadone	Carbamazepine	Carbamazepine is a potent inducer of CYP3A4 and methadone is primarily metabolized via CYP3A4; if carbamazepine is added to a drug regimen containing methadone, the methadone dose will probably need to be adjusted upward to avoid withdrawal
	Conivaptan	Conivaptan is a potent inhibitor of CYP3A4, and the manufacturer recommends that its use be **avoided** in medications metabolized by CYP3A4
	CYP3A4 inhibitors (in addition to the specific medications listed)	Methadone serum concentrations may be increased when combined with potent CYP3A4 inhibitors; adjustment of methadone dose should be based on clinical judgment, but a decrease of dose may be necessary
	Didanosine	Methadone decreases the amount of didanosine that is orally absorbed; therapeutic monitoring of didanosine effects are recommended, and doses may need to be increased
	Efavirenz	This HIV drug is a CYP3A4 inducer; efavirenz decreases methadone blood levels and has precipitated withdrawal in opioid-dependent individuals; may need to increase methadone dose
	MAOIs	Potential serotonin syndrome when MAOIs are combined with methadone; transdermal selegiline lists co-treatment with methadone as a **CONTRAINDICATION**
	Nevirapine	Nevirapine is an HIV drug that is a CYP3A4 inducer; in a small sample, nevirapine caused a 50% reduction in methadone blood levels, resulting in complaints of methadone withdrawal symptoms in patients receiving methadone maintenance; may need to increase methadone dose in patients who have nevirapine added to their drug regimen
	QTc-prolonging drugs or medications	Medications that prolong the QT interval (e.g., ziprasidone) should be **AVOIDED** with methadone co-administration when possible because of potential additive QT-prolonging effects
	Stavudine	Methadone decreases the amount of stavudine (a reverse transcriptase inhibitor) by about 25%. Although this may not be clinically significant in some cases, the clinician should be aware of the possibility of this interaction
	St. John's wort	This herbal remedy may induce CYP3A4; the certainty of an interaction probably rests on the specific preparation being used, but caution dictates that this herbal product should be avoided in those receiving methadone treatment; withdrawal symptoms have been noted in patients taking methadone maintenance who have added St. John's wort to their drug regimen
	Tamoxifen	Methadone may inhibit the formation of important active tamoxifen metabolites (e.g., endoxifen), and therapeutic monitoring is recommended
	Zidovudine	Methadone increases the blood level of this anti-HIV drug, probably via methadone inhibition of both metabolic and renal clearance of zidovudine; may need to decrease zidovudine dose to avoid toxicity

CYP, cytochrome P450 isoenzyme; LFT, liver function test; MAOI, monoamine oxidase inhibitor.

Data from Refs. 17 and 18.

Behaviorally, patients may insist on driving, become physically aggressive and agitated, or otherwise become a danger to themselves or others. Indeed, most suicidal behaviors among alcohol-dependent individuals occur while they are intoxicated. In such cases, the desired outcomes are appropriate management of medical problems, prevention of harmful behaviors, and stabilization of mood. Antipsychotics may lower the seizure threshold and are best avoided. However, in some instances, agitation may require treatment with haloperidol such as 5 to 10 mg by mouth every 2 to 4 hours or 5 mg either IV or IM every 1 to 2 hours. Sedation with benzodiazepines has been used in some cases, but the risk of respiratory depression when mixed with the alcohol already in the patient's system can be dangerous if not fatal.

There are no available medications that can fully reverse the effects of alcohol intoxication. Caffeine and other stimulants can induce arousal and alertness, but they are less effective at reversing poor judgment and motor incoordination, which are vital for complex tasks such as driving. Thus, stimulants are neither indicated nor considered a viable option to make driving safe.

Opioid Intoxication

The word *opioid* is used in this chapter to refer to the overall class of medications and substances that exert their mechanism of action through the body's opioid system. Opioids encompass a wide range of substances, including naturally occurring (e.g., morphine) and synthetic (e.g., oxycodone) substances.

Patients who are acutely intoxicated with an opioid usually present with miosis, euphoria, slow breathing, slow heart rate, low blood pressure, and constipation. Seizures may occur with certain agents, such as meperidine (Demerol). It is critically important to monitor patients carefully to avoid cardiac and respiratory depression and death from an excessive dose of opioids. One strategy is to reverse the intoxication by using naloxone (Narcan) 0.4 to 2 mg IV every 2 to 3 minutes up to 10 mg. Alternatively, the IM or subcutaneous (SC) route may be used if an IV access is not available. Because naloxone is shorter acting than most abused opioids, it may need to be readministered at periodic intervals; otherwise, patients could lapse into cardiopulmonary arrest after a symptom-free interval of reversed intoxication. In addition, naloxone can induce withdrawal symptoms in opioid-dependent patients, so patients may awaken feeling quite distressed and agitated. The other critical issue is to secure the airway and breathing. In some cases, intubation and manual or mechanical ventilation might be required to avoid oxygen desaturation leading to brain hypoxia or anoxia that may cause brain damage or death.

Stimulant (Cocaine and Amphetamines) Intoxication

The desired outcomes of stimulant intoxication are appropriate management of medical and psychiatric problems. Medical problems include hyperthermia, hypertension, cardiac arrhythmias, stroke, and seizures. Some medical problems are related to route of administration such as nosebleeds with intranasal administration and infections with IV administration. Psychiatric effects include anxiety, irritability and aggression, and psychosis.

Notably, stimulant intoxication is the only stimulant use disorder for which specific pharmacotherapy has been shown to be effective. Current guidelines from the American Heart Association indicate that acute use of β-blockers may lead to worsening cocaine-related chest pain (caused by coronary vasoconstriction) and hypertension secondary to unopposed alpha activity; they are not recommended for acute use. Recommended medication options in the acute setting include benzodiazepines, aspirin, nitroglycerin, nitroprusside, and phentolamine.[19]

Cocaine is short acting, and a single dose of a benzodiazepine sedative–hypnotic may be sufficient treatment for anxiety reactions. Depending on the half-life of the benzodiazepine, one or more sequential doses may be required for longer acting amphetamine intoxication. Antipsychotics are indicated when psychosis is present, and the psychosis usually responds quite rapidly in the absence of other co-occurring psychiatric disorders.

TREATMENT OF WITHDRAWAL SYNDROMES

⑥ *The treatment goals for withdrawal from ethanol, CNS stimulants, and opioids include (a) a determination if pharmacologic treatment of withdrawal symptoms is necessary, (b) management of other medical manifestations, and (c) referral to the appropriate program for long-term substance abuse treatment.* The desired outcomes in the treatment of withdrawal syndromes are to ensure patient safety, comfort, and successful transition from treatment of withdrawal to treatment of dependence. Referral to specialized treatment for substance dependence is strongly recommended after treatment for withdrawal syndromes because treatment of withdrawal is not sufficient treatment to prevent relapse to problematic substance use. Achieving a drug-free state by detoxification and then rehabilitation with a focus on total abstinence is the ideal outcome.

Alcohol Withdrawal

There are four different alcohol withdrawal syndromes, which differ in terms of their pharmacologic treatment and need for hospitalization.

▶ *Uncomplicated Alcohol Withdrawal*

This is the most commonly observed syndrome, and as the name denotes, is not complicated by seizures, delirium tremens (DTs), or hallucinosis. Symptoms are typically rated using a validated scale such as the CIWA-Ar (Table 36–2). The recommended CIWA-Ar threshold score for treating uncomplicated alcohol withdrawal with medications on an outpatient basis is between 8 and 10. For patients who score greater than or equal to 15, inpatient treatment should be strongly considered. Patients who score 20 or higher on the CIWA-Ar should always be treated with medications. The risks of not treating high-scoring patients with medications are seizures and DTs, and those with a prior history of seizures or DTs have an increased risk for subsequent episodes. Therefore, when a history of seizures or DTs is positive, the lower threshold of 8 is recommended, and hospitalization is safer than outpatient detoxification. There is some evidence for "kindling" during successive episodes of alcohol withdrawal, such that symptom severity and complications increase with additional withdrawal episodes. Thus, it may be advisable to use medications when the CIWA-Ar score is in the 8 to 10 range.

Benzodiazepines are the treatment of choice for uncomplicated alcohol withdrawal.[10,12] Some of the anticonvulsants have also been used to treat uncomplicated withdrawal (particularly carbamazepine and sodium valproate). Although anticonvulsants provide an alternative to benzodiazepines, they are not as well studied and are less commonly used. The most commonly used benzodiazepines are lorazepam, oxazepam, diazepam, and chlordiazepoxide. They differ in three major ways: (a) their pharmacokinetic properties, (b) the available routes for their administration, and (c) the rapidity of their onset of action due to the rate of GI absorption and rate of crossing the blood–brain barrier.

Benzodiazepines can be administered using a symptom-triggered approach when withdrawal signs and symptoms are already present. [20] In this approach, medication is administered every hour when the CIWA-Ar is greater than or equal to eight. For the shorter acting agents, oxazepam (15 to 60 mg orally) or lorazepam (1 to 4 mg orally), the CIWA-Ar is repeated hourly after each administration during the first 24 hours until the patient is comfortably sedated. Because of their short half-life, dosing of lorazepam or oxazepam on subsequent days may be needed, and the risk of seizures may possibly (although not definitively proven) be higher. For the longer acting agents, chlordiazepoxide and diazepam, the symptom-triggered approach is used in combination with another technique known as loading. With the loading technique, chlordiazepoxide at doses of 50 to 100 mg or diazepam (10 to 20 mg) is administered orally at 1-hour intervals during the first 24 hours until the patient is comfortably sedated and the CIWA-Ar score is lower than 4. Then loading is stopped, and for the next 24 hours, the benzodiazepine is used as needed only if the CIWA-Ar score is greater than or equal to eight, although the long half-lives of these drugs and their active metabolites usually provide a natural taper without further drug administration. The loading technique is especially useful in the hospital, where patients can be medically monitored throughout the day.

In contrast to chlordiazepoxide and diazepam, lorazepam and oxazepam are not metabolized into active compounds in the liver. Instead, they are excreted by the kidneys after glucuronidation. This is important because many alcohol-dependent patients have compromised liver function. Therefore, when treatment is initiated before the results of blood tests for liver function are known, as is often the case in outpatient clinics, lorazepam and oxazepam may be preferred. Patients with liver disease may still be treated with diazepam or chlordiazepoxide but at lower doses. This can be accommodated with the loading technique, although hourly dosing with 5 mg of diazepam or 25 mg of chlordiazepoxide may be sufficient.

Oxazepam is available in oral form only, so it is useful only for uncomplicated withdrawal. Other benzodiazepines are available in injectable form and are further described below. Diazepam is more lipophilic than lorazepam, chlordiazepoxide,

and oxazepam, resulting in quicker GI absorption and passage across the blood–brain barrier, which makes it valuable in an inpatient setting, especially to prevent seizures. However, a faster onset of action may be associated with feeling high (i.e., "euphoria"), which can be a treatment disadvantage.

The American Psychiatric Association (APA) Guidelines recommend that thiamine be given routinely to patients being treated for moderate to severe alcohol use disorders to treat or prevent adverse neurologic symptoms.[12] However, according to a recent Cochrane Review, there are inadequate data from randomized controlled trials regarding the most efficacious thiamine dose, frequency, and route of administration to prevent or treat Wernicke's encephalopathy associated with alcohol use disorders.[21] The APA Guidelines recommend thiamine 50 to 100 mg per day given IV or IM, although some guidelines recommend higher doses.[22] Regardless of the dose chosen, it is particularly important that administration of thiamine (essential for proper energy utilization by the CNS) precedes administration of any glucose-containing IV fluids, which can help prevent an acute exacerbation of Wernicke's encephalopathy.

▶ Alcohol Withdrawal Seizures

Alcohol withdrawal seizures are a medical emergency and should be treated in an inpatient setting. Withdrawal seizures are usually few in number and generalized. The occurrence of focal seizures or status epilepticus may suggest another etiology. Management consists of keeping the airway open and preventing self-injury during convulsions. Benzodiazepines are the treatment of choice. IV diazepam 5 to 10 mg is preferred to terminate a seizure in progress if IV access is available. The dose may be repeated in 5 minutes if seizures persist. Alternatively, lorazepam 4 mg may be given IM followed by insertion of an IV line when convulsive movements have subsided. In the event of a recurrent seizure, lorazepam 2 mg IV may be administered if the patient already received IM lorazepam. IM use of diazepam or chlordiazepoxide should be avoided because of erratic absorption that complicates the timing of subsequent doses and can result in delayed oversedation. IV benzodiazepines may depress respiration, so they should be administered only when and where advanced cardiopulmonary support is readily available. When the patient becomes conscious enough to take medication orally, then treatment may continue using the loading procedure for diazepam or the symptom-triggered technique for lorazepam as described above. Electrolyte imbalances can contribute to seizures and should be corrected if they exist. For example, it may be advisable to administer magnesium in addition to benzodiazepine treatment.

▶ Alcohol Withdrawal Delirium (Delirium Tremens)

Delirium tremens is another medical emergency that requires hospitalization in order to prevent mortality. Parenterally administered benzodiazepines are the treatment of choice.[23] DTs are characterized by hallucinations, delirium, severe agitation, fever, elevations of blood pressure and heart rate, and possible cardiac arrhythmias. A sample regimen consists of diazepam 5 mg IV (at 2.5 mg/min) every 5 to 10 minutes until "light somnolence" is achieved, referring to a tendency to fall asleep without stimulation or a light stage of sleep from which the patient is easily awakened. If the first two doses of diazepam are not effective, then 10 mg IV every 5 to 10 minutes can be administered for the third and fourth doses. If still not effective, then up to 20 mg IV may be used thereafter. When a state of light somnolence is induced, then it should be maintained with diazepam 5 to 20 mg IV every 1 hour as needed. Similarly, lorazepam 1 to 4 mg IV every 5 to 10 minutes or lorazepam 1 to 4 mg IM every 30 to 60 minutes may be given to achieve light somnolence, which is then maintained by similar doses every hour as needed. The antipsychotic haloperidol is given only for severe agitation that is unresponsive to benzodiazepine therapy. The evidence does not support the use of an antipsychotic as a single agent.[23] Furthermore, newer generation antipsychotic agents have not been studied yet for the treatment of DTs. Lastly, thiamine should be given according to the same guidelines described above.

▶ *Alcohol Hallucinosis*

Alcohol hallucinosis refers to hallucinations that occur during a clear sensorium, which distinguishes it from DTs, during which hallucinations are associated with a reduced clarity of awareness of the environment. Alcohol hallucinosis is generally treated with oral antipsychotics at usual therapeutic dosages for psychosis.

Opioid Withdrawal

Although it is rare to die from opioid withdrawal per se, underlying medical complications (e.g., hypertension) and recent myocardial infarction increase the risk of complications and death. Therefore, it is important to manage and stabilize any medical issues (e.g., uncontrolled blood pressure, diabetes) and then determine if hospitalization is appropriate. Patients with underlying medical problems should be evaluated for possible triage to an inpatient detoxification program to be followed up with substance abuse treatment in either the inpatient or outpatient setting. Rapid referral for substance abuse treatment will help "seize the moment" and introduce patients to the concept of recovery while they still vividly remember the negative consequences from using substances. Withdrawal from opioids is commonly described by patients as resembling "a bad case of the flu," and symptoms include nausea; vomiting; diarrhea; anxiety; headaches; mydriasis; rhinorrhea; lacrimation; muscle, bone, and joint pain; piloerection; yawning; fever; increased heart rate; and hypertension.

The use of clinical withdrawal scales, such as Clinical Opiate Withdrawal Scale (COWS), provides high interrater reliability and clinical utility because it is an objective measurement of withdrawal severity. The full items contained in the COWS instrument (*along with many other substance use disorder [SUD] instruments*) can be obtained free-of-charge from the Substance Abuse and Mental Health Services Administration (SAMHSA).[9] Furthermore, a brief overview

is provided in Table 36–2. The baseline score helps to make the decision to treat pharmacologically or to observe. As the scores become higher, the indication for either opioid substitution or a "symptoms-based approach" may be indicated. In severe withdrawal, either buprenorphine (i.e., partial μ-opioid agonist) or methadone (i.e., full μ-opioid agonist) are recommended for detoxification. Methadone is the gold-standard full μ-agonist, but under current U.S. law, methadone detoxification requires referral to a federally approved methadone detoxification program. The two possible options for the treatment of opioid withdrawal in regular clinical settings are opioid substitution with buprenorphine and symptomatic treatment, which is discussed in the following paragraphs.

▶ *Opioid Substitution*

Treatment with a μ-opioid agonist is accomplished with either buprenorphine or methadone. Methadone can be used for opioid detoxification and long-term relapse prevention. However, in the United States, this can be done only at a federally approved opioid treatment program (OTP). Because this drug cannot legally be used for opioid detoxification by general clinicians, methadone detoxification regimens are not covered here because they are readily available elsewhere.

Buprenorphine is a partial agonist at the μ-opioid receptors that can be used sublingually. It is available in three formulations in the United States, two of which are indicated for the treatment of addiction. Buprenorphine plus naloxone (Suboxone) in ratio of 4:1 (2 mg:0.5 mg or 8 mg:2 mg) is the recommended formulation unless the patient is pregnant or hypersensitive to naloxone, in which case buprenorphine without naloxone (Subutex) is recommended. Naloxone was added to the Suboxone formulation to secure Food and Drug Administration (FDA) approval in the United States. Because naloxone is poorly absorbed when used sublingually but blocks opioid receptors if injected, this combination is designed to minimize diversion of the drug to the street for IV use. Only 10% of buprenorphine is bioavailable if it is swallowed, but 50% is bioavailable via the sublingual route.

To initiate a buprenorphine induction, a patient has to be experiencing moderate or severe withdrawal, and the last opioid use should be at least 12 to 24 hours earlier, depending on the half-life of the particular opioid (the longer the half-life, the longer a clinician should wait before initiating buprenorphine induction). The score on the COWS should be greater than or equal to 5 (i.e., suggesting some level of opioid withdrawal); otherwise, buprenorphine likely will induce withdrawal because it has high affinity for μ-receptors, and it will displace any other full μ-opioid agonist that is present. When withdrawal is established, buprenorphine can be initiated, and protocols such as the example provided in Table 36–6 can be used to titrate the dosing and administration.[9] When a final dose is established, there are generally two treatment approaches, depending on many factors (e.g., patient preference). A maintenance dose can be prescribed or the dose can be tapered down gradually to zero within 1 to 2 weeks (a 25% reduction per day is a general rule of thumb).

Table 36-6

Sample Regimen*a* for Buprenorphine Induction Treatment of Opioid Withdrawal and Long-Term Relapse Prevention

Day	Buprenorphine Oral Dosage
1	2 mg every 2 hours (maximum, 8 mg on first day)
2	Start with total dose of day 1 with additional 2–4 mg every 2 hours (maximum, 16 mg)
3+	Start with total dose of day 2, with additional 2–4 mg every 2 hours (maximum, 32 mg)
4–5	Maintain on dose required to alleviate withdrawal symptoms*b*

*a*For withdrawal from any long-acting opioid.

*b*Patient will likely be transitioned to long-term maintenance dose indefinitely.

Data from Center for Substance Abuse Treatment. Clinical Guidelines for the Use of Buprenorphine in the Treatment of Opioid Addiction. Treatment Improvement Protocol (TIP) Series 40. DHHS Publication no. (SMA) 04–3939. Rockville, MD: Substance Abuse and Mental Health Services Administration; 2004.

▶ Symptoms-Based Treatment

Symptomatic treatment focuses on minimizing the withdrawal symptoms to help patients be as comfortable as possible. Symptom-specific medications, as shown in Table 36–7, are often used as adjunct medication with opioid substitution.[9,12] Clonidine is one of the primary non-opioid medications used during withdrawal to decrease the excessive noradrenergic symptoms (e.g., sweating) of opioid withdrawal. However, the use of clonidine requires close monitoring of blood pressure; it should be held if systolic blood pressure is below 90 mm Hg or diastolic blood pressure is below 60 mm Hg. Compared with opioid substitution, clonidine does not help other withdrawal symptoms, such as craving or distress.[12]

Table 36-7

A "Symptoms-Based" Treatment Approach for Opioid Withdrawal

The following medications are used for symptoms that cause distress. This approach includes the use of any single or a combination of two or more of the following agents, depending on the symptoms reported:
1. Insomnia: Diphenhydramine 50–100 mg, trazodone 75–200 mg, or hydroxyzine 25–50 mg at bedtime
2. Headache, muscle aches, and pain: Acetaminophen 500 mg–1 g every 6 hours, ibuprofen 600 mg by mouth every 8 hours, or naproxen 600 mg by mouth every 12 hours
3. Noradrenergic hyperactivity: Clonidine (Catapres) 0.1–0.2 mg every 6–8 hours; maximum dosage not to exceed 1.2 mg in 24 hours
4. Abdominal cramps: Dicyclomine 10–20 mg every 6 hours
5. Constipation: Milk of magnesia at 30 mL daily
6. Diarrhea: Bismuth subcarbonate 30 mL can be given every 2 to 3 hours

Data from Refs. 9 and 12.

▶ General Patient Guidelines for Outpatient Opioid Detoxification

When treating opioid withdrawal with pharmacologic agents, patient safety is the highest priority. The first step is to educate patients about the course of withdrawal. Symptoms peak at around 5 to 7 days and may last up to 2 weeks, depending on the half-life of the opioid that was being used before detoxification. Patients also should be advised regarding the side effects of the drugs used to detoxify. For instance, clonidine causes dizziness from low blood pressure, sedation (which may impair driving or operating heavy machinery), and dry mouth. There is also an overdose potential if clonidine is mixed with opioids or other CNS sedatives or antihypertensives. The risk of these adverse events needs to be balanced with potential benefits. The side effects of buprenorphine include constipation, sedation, and headaches. It should also be noted that there is a potential for serious overdose when buprenorphine is mixed with benzodiazepines or other sedative–hypnotics. The risk of developing physiologic tolerance to buprenorphine is high if it is used for prolonged periods. In this case, buprenorphine should be slowly tapered to discontinuation. However, withdrawal from buprenorphine is easier and less severe than withdrawal from a pure agonist, such as methadone.

Successful transition from treatment of withdrawal to treatment of opioid dependence in a rehabilitation setting is the most important challenge for a clinician. Patients often think that all they need is detoxification, but this is not the case because a successful outcome is tied to successful rehabilitation and acquiring recovery skills after detoxification. This goal can be accomplished by either achieving detoxification on site during rehabilitation or by quick and seamless transition of the patient from detoxification to a rehabilitation program. The more time that elapses between the two modalities, the greater the likelihood of treatment failure and return to drug use.

Central Nervous System Stimulant (Cocaine, Amphetamines) Withdrawal

Cocaine and amphetamine withdrawal are grouped together because their symptom profiles as described in *DSM-IV-TR*[6] are identical, and the physiologic basis of their withdrawal syndromes involves the DA neurotransmitter system. Stimulants of this group also include methylphenidate but not nicotine and caffeine, which have different neurophysiologic mechanisms of action. Although neurophysiologic alterations underlie the syndrome of stimulant withdrawal, its symptoms are manifested psychologically for the most part as a depressed or dysphoric mood. Consequently, the major adverse complication of stimulant withdrawal is profound depression with suicidal thoughts, and the major goal of treatment is to prevent suicide. Therefore, unless suicidality warrants hospitalization, stimulant withdrawal can be treated on an outpatient basis with psychological support and reassurance with an emphasis on patient safety. A number of medications have been studied to alleviate symptoms of stimulant withdrawal and the intense craving that may accompany it, but inconsistent results across controlled trials preclude any recommendations for their routine use. Patients with stimulant use disorders should be referred for substance abuse treatment because of the high risk for continued use either during or immediately following stimulant withdrawal.

Treatment referral (after intoxication or withdrawal): Overall, intoxication or withdrawal with any of the substances discussed above is evidence of substance abuse and is strongly suggestive of substance dependence. In all cases, it is important to strongly emphasize to the patient that this is an issue that needs to be addressed and that treatment may be beneficial depending on how frequent and severe the intoxication or withdrawal symptoms present.

GENERAL APPROACH TO THE TREATMENT OF SUBSTANCE DEPENDENCE

❼ *A multimodal and comprehensive approach is usually preferred when treating individuals with substance use disorders given the heterogeneous nature of addiction. Pharmacologic treatment is always adjunctive to psychosocial therapy.* The overall goals in recovery from addiction are the same for all substances, and they consist of the following components:[12]

- Assessment includes (a) patient history (e.g., past and present substance use, including the effect of substance use on the patient's functioning), (b) medical and psychiatric history and examination, (c) treatments and associated outcomes, (d) family and social history, (e) alcohol and drug testing (e.g., urine drug testing), (f) laboratory tests (e.g., liver function tests), and (g) corroborating evidence

- Psychiatric management: includes (a) motivating the patient to change, (b) establishing a therapeutic alliance, (c) ensuring patient safety and monitoring clinical status, (d) managing intoxication and withdrawal, (e) monitoring and ensuring treatment adherence, (f) preventing relapse, (g) educating patients, and (h) reducing negative consequences of substance use

- Treatment:
  - Pharmacotherapy: intoxication, withdrawal, long-term maintenance
  - Psychosocial: examples include cognitive-behavioral therapies (CBTs), motivational enhancement therapy (MET), behavioral therapies

- Treatment plan: patient specific (i.e., individualized) aims and outcomes of treatment

- Treatment setting: least restrictive while maintaining patient safety

Using the above steps, the overarching aims (i.e., outcomes) that are desired include:

- Achieve abstinence or reduce substance use
- Reduce negative consequences associated with use
- Reduction in the frequency or severity of relapse to substance use
- Improve psychological and social functioning

It is important to remember that mere treatment of withdrawal is not sufficient treatment of *DSM-IV-TR* dependence and that medications are always adjunctive to psychosocial therapy. Comorbid psychiatric conditions such as anxiety, depression, insomnia, pain, and continued smoking should be addressed. All of these conditions increase the risk of relapse to use of drugs. Additionally, although complete abstinence may be desirable in many patients, decreasing substance use and negative consequences may be sufficient in certain cases. The latter concept is also known as "harm reduction." For example, if a patient relapses to alcohol consumption, at least ensure the patient is not driving and is in a safe environment.

Nonpharmacologic Therapy

Although pharmacologic agents may help prevent relapse, psychotherapy should be the core therapeutic intervention. Psychotherapy encompasses widely different approaches. However, they typically address one or more of the following tasks:

- Motivation enhancement to stop or reduce drug use
- Coping skills education
- Providing alternative reinforcement
- Managing painful affect
- Enhancing social support and interpersonal functioning

There are many examples of psychosocial approaches, and a thorough review of these approaches is beyond the scope of this chapter and are available elsewhere.[12] However, a few of the commonly used techniques are CBT, MET, and behavioral therapies (e.g., community reinforcement).

Pharmacologic Therapy

▶ *Maintenance Treatment*

❽ *Certain pharmacologic agents have been shown to be helpful for long-term maintenance in patients with substance dependence. Typically, these medications exert their effects by one of the following theorized mechanisms: (a) drug substitution therapy with an agonist, (b) blocking drug effects with an antagonist, and (c) miscellaneous relapse prevention medications with indirect mechanisms of action.* Medications from each of these categories are discussed in greater detail in the following paragraphs for alcohol, opioid, stimulant, and nicotine dependence.

▶ *Alcohol Dependence*

Currently, the three FDA-approved medications that are indicated to treat alcohol dependence are disulfiram, naltrexone (oral and depot), and acamprosate. Among the three agents, naltrexone and acamprosate are generally considered first-line agents as evidence by their "grade A" efficacy rating in the seminal paper by Garbutt et al.[24] However, in motivated patients, disulfiram is another reasonable option.[25]

Disulfiram First marketed in the United States in the 1950s, disulfiram works by irreversibly blocking the enzyme aldehyde dehydrogenase (ALDH), a step in the metabolism of alcohol. The result of inhibiting ALDH is increased blood levels of the toxic metabolite acetaldehyde. As levels of acetaldehyde increase, the patient experiences decreased blood pressure, increased heart rate, chest pain, palpitations, dizziness, flushing, sweating, weakness, nausea and vomiting, headache, shortness of breath, blurred vision, and syncope. These effects are commonly referred to as the disulfiram–ethanol reaction. Their severity increases with the amount of alcohol that is consumed, and they may warrant emergency treatment. Psychologically, disulfiram works through aversion, and drinking is avoided to prevent the aversive disulfiram–ethanol reaction. The efficacy of disulfiram has always been found to be directly dependent on medication adherence,[26] and more recent reports advocate that disulfiram can be highly effective when procedures for enhancing adherence are used, such as supervised administration.[25]

The usual starting dose of disulfiram is 250 mg/day orally (appropriate to be started at 500 mg/day for the first 1 to 2 weeks), and the range is 125 to 500 mg/day. Compared with 250 mg/day, the larger dose is recommended if a patient does not experience a disulfiram–ethanol reaction after alcohol consumption, and the smaller dose is given when intolerable side effects are experienced at higher doses. Dosing begins only after the BAC is zero (usually 12 to 24 hours after the last drink) and after the patient understands the consequences of the disulfiram–ethanol reaction.

Disulfiram is contraindicated in patients who have cardiovascular or cerebrovascular disease or in combination with antihypertensive medications because the cardiovascular effects of the disulfiram–alcohol reaction could be fatal in such patients. The most common side effects are rash, drowsiness, a metallic or garlic-like taste, and headache. If drowsiness occurs, the dose may be lowered or given at night. Other less common but concerning adverse effects include neuropathies and hepatoxicity. Given the serious nature of these adverse effects, baseline and periodic monitoring is recommended. If serum levels of alanine aminotransferase (ALT) or aspartate aminotransferase (AST) are greater than three times the upper limit of normal values, then disulfiram should be withheld and the tests repeated every 1 to 2 weeks until they are normal. When liver function tests (LFTs) return to the normal range, they may be repeated every 1 to 6 months. It is advisable to follow LFTs and clinical symptoms until resolution has been confirmed.[27] Although elevated LFTs may signal disulfiram-induced hepatotoxicity, it is also likely the patient was nonadherent to treatment and resumed drinking, ultimately leading to hepatotoxicity. Another uncommon side effect of disulfiram is psychosis, which has been reported in doses exceeding 500 mg/day, especially in predisposed patients. This may be related to disulfiram's ability to inhibit dopamine β-hydroxylase, resulting in increased dopamine activity. Nevertheless, alcohol-dependent patients with schizophrenia and other co-occurring mental disorders have received disulfiram at usual therapeutic doses without difficulties.[28]

Drug Interactions. The disulfiram–ethanol interaction is described above and is the intended interaction that serves as disulfiram's mechanism of action. Depending on the dose of disulfiram, sensitivity to disulfiram, amount of alcohol consumed, and metabolism, patients may be at risk for an adverse interaction with alcohol for 2 to 14 days after stopping disulfiram (5 days on average) and should be warned accordingly. See Table 36–5 for additional relevant interactions that occur with disulfiram (particularly with metronidazole).

Naltrexone Naltrexone is a competitive opioid antagonist that decreases alcohol intake in both animals and humans. There is evidence that it works by decreasing both craving for alcohol and alcohol-induced euphoria (i.e., reduces positive reinforcement associated with drinking). Numerous controlled trials and meta-analyses have demonstrated that naltrexone is more efficacious than placebo for a variety of drinking measures.[12] For example, one meta-analysis that included more than 20 controlled trials demonstrated naltrexone significantly decreased risk of relapse compared with placebo.[29] Reported predictors of naltrexone efficacy include a family history of alcoholism, genetic differences in opioid alleles, drinking problems at an early age, and high levels of craving.[12,30] In a landmark study assessing the efficacy of behavioral treatment, medication management, and their combinations for the treatment of alcohol dependence, naltrexone was associated with high rates of percent days abstinence.[31] The trial design was very complex, and the details of the study are beyond the scope of this chapter. However, an oversimplification of the findings suggests that naltrexone was effective (e.g., percent days abstinent), but acamprosate (discussed in greater detail below) was not associated with any treatment advantage.[31]

Naltrexone is available in both oral and sustained-release injections. The usual therapeutic dose of oral naltrexone is 50 mg/day, with a range from 25 to 100 mg. The 25-mg dose is commonly given initially as a test dose to minimize side effects, especially nausea, and then increased to 50 mg/day as tolerated. Adherence to daily doses of naltrexone strongly affects drinking outcomes. Therefore, a sustained-release IM injection of naltrexone, designed to be given once monthly, has been marketed. A 380-mg monthly injection of naltrexone (Vivitrol) resulted in a significantly greater reduction in heavy drinking days compared with placebo injection.[32]

The most common side effects are GI complaints, headache, insomnia, and nervousness. Injectable naltrexone is also associated with injection site pain or reactions. Because naltrexone can precipitate withdrawal in patients dependent on opioids, the first dose should be withheld for 7 to 10 days after the last use of opioids and given only when the urine drug screen result for opioids is negative. Also, naltrexone can be hepatotoxic, albeit typically not at oral doses less than 250 mg/day or at the recommended injectable dose of 380 mg per month. Nevertheless, baseline and periodic monitoring of LFTs is recommended.

It is important for patients to carry a pocket warning card or wear a warning bracelet because, in the event that emergency treatment is needed, they will be insensitive to opioid analgesia unless usually toxic doses are administered. Patients need to be warned of the potential for an opioid overdose under two different conditions. First, dosing with opioids to reverse opioid insensitivity (i.e., naltrexone's competitive blockade of opioid receptors) requires very high doses of opioids that can cause respiratory depression and death. Second, chronic antagonist therapy with naltrexone may cause patients to become hypersensitive to opioid drugs after stopping naltrexone, thereby facilitating respiratory depression and death when opioids are used.

Drug Interactions. Naltrexone can block the effects of opioid receptor agonists, rendering them therapeutically ineffective. Given that opioid agonists are a mainstay of pain management, alternative pain treatment options (e.g., conscious sedation) may be required in a patient receiving naltrexone maintenance for alcoholism.

Acamprosate Acamprosate appears to be a glutamatergic antagonist and may also have GABA-ergic effects.[3] Alcohol use acutely inhibits glutamatergic function and chronically causes upregulation of glutamate receptors. During alcohol withdrawal and postacute alcohol withdrawal, increased activity of the glutamate system is caused by upregulation of receptors and the absence of alcohol-related inhibition. Thus, it has been postulated that acamprosate may restore the glutamate/GABA imbalance that occurs after chronic alcohol dependence (e.g., reduces negative reinforcement associated with postacute withdrawal and craving).

Generally, trials assessing the efficacy of acamprosate have shown mixed results. However, this may be partly attributable to differences in research methodologies, such as varying levels of abstinence required in trials before acamprosate initiation.[12] Notably, in the landmark Combining Medications and Behavioral Interventions for Alcoholism (COMBINE) study described earlier, acamprosate appeared to offer no treatment advantage,[31] but a relatively recent meta-analysis of randomized control trials suggests that it is more efficacious than placebo.[33] Another recent meta-analysis suggests that acamprosate may be more effective at maintaining abstinence, but naltrexone may more effectively prevent full relapse to heavy drinking in non-abstinent individuals.[34] Despite the availability of mixed findings (and study methodologies) in the literature, there appears to be sufficient evidence that acamprosate is more effective than placebo, although differences may be modest.

The therapeutic dose of acamprosate is 666 mg orally three times daily, and it is supplied as a 333-mg tablet. It is not metabolized by the liver and is excreted unchanged by the kidneys. Consequently, it is contraindicated in patients with severe renal impairment (creatinine clearance less than or equal to 30 mL/min [0.50 mL/sec]), and a dose reduction is necessary when the creatinine clearance is between 30 and 50 mL/min (0.50 and 0.83 mL/sec). The most common side effects are GI and include nausea and diarrhea. CNS adverse effects include insomnia, anxiety, and depressive symptoms.

Medication Selection Please refer to Table 36–8 for patient-specific factors that can be used to guide medication

Table 36–8

Alcohol Use Disorder Medication Decision Grid

Pretreatment Indicator	Acamprosate (Campral)	Disulfiram (Antabuse)	Oral Naltrexone (ReVia)	Injectable Naltrexone (Vivitrol)
Renal failure	X	A	A	A
Significant liver disease	A	C	C	C
Coronary artery disease	A	C	A	A
Chronic pain	A	A	C	C
Current opioid use	A	A	X	X
Psychosis	A	C	A	A
Unwilling or unable to sustain total abstinence	A	X	A	A
Risk factors for poor medication adherence	C	C	C	A
Diabetes	A	C	A	A
Obesity that precludes IM injection	A	A	A	X
Family history of AUDs	A	A	+	+
Bleeding or other coagulation disorders	A	A	A	C
High level of craving	A	A	+	+
Opioid dependence in remission	A	A	+	+
History of postacute withdrawal syndrome	+	A	+	A
Cognitive impairment	A	X	A	A

+ = particularly appropriate; A = appropriate to use; C = use with caution; X = contraindicated.

AUD, alcohol use disorder; IM, intramuscular.

Data from Center for Substance Abuse Treatment. Incorporating Alcohol Pharmacotherapies into Medical Practice. Treatment Improvement Protocol (TIP) Series 49. HHS Publication No. (SMA) 09-4380. Rockville, MD: Substance Abuse and Mental Health Services Administration; 2009.

management for alcohol dependence.[27] Given the lack of universally accepted treatment algorithms for the treatment of alcohol dependence, this table may help guide medication selection.

▶ Opioid Dependence

After the conclusion of withdrawal, some patients still do not feel their usual selves for a long time and may relapse to using opioids again, just to "feel normal." Long-term use of opioids results in changes in the brain, and the brain might not readily return to its prior homeostasis. Because the goal of treatment is to encourage stability, both in the body and in the patient's life, if an individual is not successful in tapering off of opioids because of a reemergence of severe withdrawal or a return to opioid use, then maintenance treatment should be considered.

Opioid Agonists The time-honored opioid agonist treatment for opioid dependence is methadone maintenance. However, methadone maintenance can be provided only in federally approved OTPs, which is beyond the scope of this chapter. The other first-line agent, which will be the focus of this chapter, is buprenorphine maintenance.

The more widely available office-based opioid treatment (OBOT) exclusively uses buprenorphine, a partial μ-agonist.[9] The effective maintenance dose of buprenorphine (+/− naloxone) is usually between 8 and 16 mg/day, with maximum reported efficacy at 64 mg/day. Patients receiving buprenorphine maintenance should sign a treatment contract requiring full compliance, financial responsibility for treatment, adherence to office policies, respectful behavior to staff, and agreement to provide random urine samples for drug screens, and patients should bring their bottles for pill counts at every visit. In the event of failure of OBOT, the alternative to buprenorphine maintenance is a referral to an OTP for methadone administration. Under the provisions of the Drug Addiction Treatment Act of 2000, physicians may prescribe buprenorphine (Suboxone or Subutex) in their office if they meet the predetermined requirements (e.g., training) and become qualified providers. When these criteria are met, they obtain an "X" on their Drug Enforcement Administration (DEA) number.[9]

Although there are no treatment algorithms to guide medication selection, there are protocols for some medications that assist with dosing and titration. For example, the extensive buprenorphine treatment protocol available from SAMHSA provides guidelines on how to dose buprenorphine from induction to maintenance treatment.[9] Furthermore, findings from a recent Cochrane meta-analysis indicate that methadone may offer an advantage over buprenorphine for select treatment outcomes (e.g., retention in treatment).[35] Therefore, there may be circumstances for which methadone remains the best medication option.

▶ Stimulant Dependence

There are no proven pharmacotherapies for treatment of CNS stimulant dependence at this time. However, the APA Practice Guidelines mention three medications as possible treatment options for CNS stimulant dependence when combined with psychosocial approaches (i.e., after psychosocial approaches alone have failed). These medications include topiramate, disulfiram, and modafinil. For example, disulfiram shows some promise in randomized, controlled trials possibly due to its inhibition of the dopamine β-hydroxylase enzyme that converts DA to NE in the brain. The resulting increase in DA levels may counter the DA deficiency state that is believed to underlie cocaine withdrawal and craving.[12]

▶ Tobacco Cessation

Nonpharmacologic Behavioral treatment delivered by a variety of clinicians (e.g., physician, psychologist, nurse, pharmacist, and dentist) increases abstinence rates. The five As should be applied by all clinicians.[16]

- Ask if they smoke.
- Advise to quit.
- Assess motivation for change.
- Assist if willing to change.
- Arrange for follow-up.

Smoking cessation counseling should be provided to all smokers, and those interested should be assisted to achieve cessation. Furthermore, it is now a standard of practice for clinicians to screen for smoking and provide all smokers with brief advice and assistance with appropriate medications to quit or provide referral to specialized services when needed.

Pharmacologic According to the seminal tobacco use clinical practice guideline,[16] there are seven first-line medications available to treat nicotine use disorders. Table 36–9 provides product-specific overviews and recommendations, such as dosing, for each of these medications.[36]

Table 36–9

First-Line Medications for Treatment of Nicotine Dependence

Medication	Dosing and Administration	Adverse Effects

Nicotine patch (7, 14, and 21 mg)	One patch per day on a hairless area of body between the waist and neck; rotate patch site
	More than or equal to 10 cigarettes/day: 21 mg × 4 weeks, 14 mg × 2–4 weeks, 7 mg × 2–4 weeks
	Less than 10 cigarettes /day: 14 mg × 4 weeks, 7 mg × 4 weeks
	Duration: 8–12 weeks
		Local skin reactions, insomnia, vivid dreams, headache
		May apply hydrocortisone or triamcinolone to ameliorate skin reactions
		Warnings and Precautions:
		  Pregnancy category D
		  CV risks: Recent (less than 2 weeks) MI, arrhythmias, unstable angina

Nicotine gum (2 or 4 mg)	One piece every 1–2 hours (maximum, 24 pieces/day); chew and "park"
	Use 2-mg dose if 25 cigarettes/day or less and the 4-mg dose if 25 cigarettes/day or more or chewing tobacco
	Do not eat or drink (except water) 15 minutes before or during use
	Duration: 12 weeks (or as needed)
		Sore mouth, hiccups, stomachache, dyspepsia, insomnia
		Avoid chewing (i.e., should "park" the gum in cheek) and limit swallowing excess saliva to avoid GI problems
		Warnings and Precautions:
		  Pregnancy category D
		  CV risks: Recent (less than 2 weeks) MI, arrhythmias, unstable angina

Nicotine lozenge (2 or 4 mg)	Use 2-mg dose for first cigarette 30 minutes or more after waking or 4-mg dose for first cigarette less than 30 minutes after waking
	Weeks 1–6: 1 every 1–2 h; weeks 7–9: 1 every 2–4 h, weeks 10–12: 1 every 4–8 h
	Do not eat or drink 15 minutes before or during use
	Maximum is 20 lozenges per day; use one lozenge at a time
	Duration: 3 to 6 months
		Hiccups, cough, heartburn, nausea, headache, insomnia
		Avoid chewing (i.e., should "park" the lozenge in cheek) and limit swallowing excess saliva to avoid GI problems
		Warnings and Precautions:
		  Pregnancy category (not evaluated)
		  CV risks: Recent (less than 2 weeks) MI, arrhythmias, unstable angina

Nicotine nasal spray (0.5 mg delivered to each nostril)	One "dose" = 1 squirt/nostril
	1 to 2 doses/h (8–40 doses per day; maximum, 5 doses/h)
	Do not inhale
	Duration: 3 to 6 months; taper (see dependence risk)
		Nasal irritation, nasal congestion, changes in smell
		Warnings and Precautions:
		  Pregnancy category D
		  CV risks: Recent (less than 2 weeks) MI, arrhythmias, unstable angina
		Avoid in persons with reactive airway disease
		Dependence (risk is higher)

Nicotine inhaler (4 mg in each cartridge)	Use 6–16 cartridges per day
	Inhale (i.e., "puff") 80 times/cartridge
	Do not eat or drink 15 minutes before or during use; puff lightly and do not inhale into lungs (avoid coughing); avoid cold temperatures
	Duration: Up to 6 months; taper
		Mouth and throat irritation (improves with use), cough, rhinitis, sneezing, headache
		Warnings and Precautions:
		  Pregnancy category D
		  CV risks: Recent (less than 2 weeks) MI, arrhythmias, unstable angina

Bupropion	Initial dosing: 150 mg once daily × 3 days Maintenance dosing: 150 mg twice daily Should initiate at least 1 week before target quit date; efficacy of maintenance at 300 mg/day has been shown up to 6 months May be combined with NRT	U.S. Boxed Warning(s): Serious neuropsychiatric events (e.g., mood disturbances) when used for smoking cessation
Varenicline	Initial dosing: Days 1–3: 0.5 mg once daily Days 4–7: 0.5 mg twice daily Maintenance dosing: Day 8 and after: 1 mg twice daily Renal dosing (CrCl less than 30 mL/min [less than 0.50 mL/s]): Requires lower doses; 0.5 mg once daily with a maximum of 0.5 mg twice daily Initiate varenicline at least 1 week before target quit date or begin varenicline dosing and then quit smoking between days 8 and 35	CNS: Insomnia, headache, abnormal dreams GI: Dose-related nausea U.S. Boxed Warning: Serious neuropsychiatric events (depression, suicidal thoughts, and suicide) have been reported with varenicline use

CNS, central nervous system; CrCl, creatinine clearance; CV, cardiovascular; GI, gastrointestinal; NRT, nicotine replacement therapy; MI, myocardial infarction.

Data from Teter CJ. Substance Use Disorders. 2012 Board Certified Psychiatric Pharmacist (BCPP) Examination Review and Recertification Course. Lincoln, NE: College of Psychiatric & Neurologic Pharmacists; 2012.

Symptomatic detoxification and maintenance for nicotine dependence is achieved with any single or combination of the currently available nicotine replacement therapies (NRTs).[16] Similar to opioid agonists, these nicotine replacement therapies act as substitution therapy using a safer alternative. NRT is generally considered safe with one notable exception: Given the pregnancy category D assigned to NRT, the decision to use NRT for pregnant women must be made on a case-by-case basis. According to the clinical practice guidelines, pregnant smokers should be encouraged to quit smoking without the use of medication.[16] Given there are various NRT products that are efficacious at treating tobacco dependence, the choice of specific NRT depends on other factors, such as patient preference.[12]

First-line non-nicotine medications that have proven beneficial for treating nicotine dependence are bupropion and varenicline. The sustained-release form of the antidepressant bupropion was approved by the FDA with a new brand name (Zyban) for the treatment of tobacco dependence. Bupropion blocks reuptake of DA and NE, and it appears that one of its metabolites is a nicotinic antagonist.[3] These mechanisms may help explain how bupropion acts to reduce nicotine reinforcement, withdrawal, and craving.

The FDA has approved varenicline (Chantix), which is a $\alpha_4\beta_2$ nicotinic acetylcholine (nACh) partial agonist.[3] Varenicline decreases withdrawal and craving and prevents reinforcing effects of nicotine if the patient relapses and is at least as effective as bupropion in clinical trials. Caution must be taken with both bupropion and varenicline because both have been associated with severe psychiatric disturbances when used for smoking cessation.[37-38]

As shown in Table 36–10, various NRTs, bupropion, and varenicline increase abstinence rates at 6 months relative to placebo.[16] Furthermore, combining the nicotine patch with ad libitum nicotine gum provides the highest likelihood of abstinence at 6 months. The single agent (i.e., monotherapy) with the highest odds of maintaining abstinence is varenicline (2 mg/day dose).

OUTCOME EVALUATION

❾ *A major component of successful treatment of addiction is to continue monitoring the use of medications and to identify a mechanism for long-term support of sobriety that might be appropriate for a specific individual such as AA, or recovery programs for professionals such as doctors, nurses, or pharmacists.*

To determine immediate treatment outcomes for patients with intoxication and withdrawal syndromes, evaluate parameters such as blood pressure, heart rate, respirations, and body temperature, as well as mental state. Choose from a number of validated and standardized rating scales to monitor the responsiveness of withdrawal syndromes to medical treatment. To determine the overall effectiveness

Table 36–10		
Six-Month Post-Quit Abstinence Rates and Associated Odds Ratios[a]		
Medication	**Abstinence Rate (%)**	**Odds Ratio (95% CI)**
Placebo	13.8	1.0
NRTs		
Nicotine gum (6–14 weeks)	19.0	1.5 (1.2–1.7)
Nicotine patch (6–14 weeks)	23.4	1.9 (1.7–2.2)
Nicotine gum (more than 14 weeks)	26.1	2.2 (1.5–3.2)
Nicotine patch (more than 14 weeks)	23.7	1.9 (1.7–2.3)
Non-NRTs		
Bupropion SR	24.2	2.0 (1.8–2.2)
Varenicline (1 mg/day)	25.4	2.1 (1.5–3.0)
Varenicline (2 mg/day)	33.2	3.1 (2.5–3.8)
Combination Strategies		
Patch (more than 14 weeks) + ad lib gum or spray	36.5	3.6 (2.5–5.2)
Patch + bupropion SR	28.9	2.5 (1.9–3.4)

[a]Meta-analysis; 83 studies included.

CI, confidence interval; NRT, nicotine replacement therapy; SR, sustained release.

Data from Refs. 16 and 36.

of your health system for the treatment of substance abuse and dependence, you could monitor outcomes using sentinel events such as the rates of cardiopulmonary arrest, seizures, discharges against medical advice, patient violence, and use of physical restraints. The ultimate goal should be to enable the transition of patients to formal substance abuse treatment when indicated.

Important outcome indicators to evaluate postintoxication and/or postwithdrawal treatment can be divided into three major groups: decreased consumption of substances, decreased problems associated with substance use, and improved psychosocial functioning. When complete abstinence has not been achieved, quantify the consumption of substances using quantity–frequency measures, rates of abstinence, and time to first relapse as determined by interviews and self-report and by biological markers such as urine and blood tests. The Addiction Severity Index (see Table 36–2) is a gold-standard instrument that can be used to assess alcohol and drug-related problems in various domains and provides a more comprehensive picture of the substance user's life.

❿ *Clinicians must be familiar with "essential" resources, many of which are in the public domain.* Table 36–11 provides a list of these resources along with their website address. These websites provide information useful for clinical management, research, teaching, and policy development purposes.

Table 36–11

Essential Substance Use Disorder Treatment Resources[a]

Source	Website	Example Highlight
American Psychiatric Association (APA)	www.psych.org	Practice Guidelines (*evidence-based treatment recommendations*)
American Society of Addiction Medicine (ASAM)	www.asam.org	Principles of Addiction Medicine (*gold-standard addiction textbook*)
National Institute on Alcohol Abuse and Alcoholism (NIAAA)	www.niaaa.nih.gov	Alcohol Research & Health (*peer-reviewed journal*)
National Institute on Drug Abuse (NIDA)	www.drugabuse.gov	Education Resources (*downloadable teaching slides; see Fig. 36–2 for an example*)
Substance Abuse and Mental Health Services Administration (SAMHSA)	www.samhsa.gov	National Survey on Drug Use and Health (NSDUH) (*national, representative alcohol and drug use survey*)
		Treatment Improvement Protocols (TIPs) (*evidence-based treatment recommendations*)

[a]There is a great deal of information from these resources that is available in the public domain and may be used without permission. For example, the Treatment Improvement Protocols are comprehensive documents that can be accessed (free of charge) via the internet.

Patient Care and Monitoring

1. By evaluating the patient's history and symptoms, determine if substance intoxication, or withdrawal are likely.

2. If drug intoxication is the likely scenario:
   - Conduct a physical examination and measure blood pressure, heart and respiratory rate, and body temperature.
   - In most cases, management of intoxication is supportive. The most important goal is to maintain cardiopulmonary function. If consciousness is impaired, obtain blood chemistries and administer thiamine (100 to 250 mg) followed by IV glucose. Thiamine must be administered before glucose.
   - Cocaine or stimulant intoxication may require administration of a small dose of a short-acting benzodiazepine (e.g., lorazepam 1 to 2 mg) for agitation or severe anxiety. Avoid β-blocker monotherapy because of unopposed alpha adrenergic activity. If hyperthermia is present, initiate cooling measures.
   - Observe the patient until the intoxication has resolved (if alcohol, the BAC should be less than 80 mg/dL [0.08% or 17.4 mmol/L]) for the patient's safety and the safety of others. Encourage the patient to consider treatment for substance abuse, especially if this is not the first episode of intoxication.

3. If substance withdrawal is the likely scenario:
   - Determine from which substance or substances the patient is withdrawing.
   - Conduct a physical examination to help determine if medical problems are present.
   - Select the appropriate standardized withdrawal severity instrument to determine the degree of drug withdrawal and to help guide medication use and dosing. Refer to the correct scoring procedure for each instrument.
   - More severe symptoms, such as alcohol withdrawal seizures and DTs, should be treated in the inpatient setting with benzodiazepines. These conditions can be fatal if left untreated.
   - Withdrawal from opioids and CNS stimulants is uncomfortable but unlikely to be fatal unless the patient has underlying medical problems.

4. Withdrawal from nicotine is treated in the outpatient setting. Symptomatic detoxification from nicotine is achieved with any single or combination of NRTs. Additional non-nicotine first-line medications, such as bupropion or varenicline, may be helpful to reduce craving and various other withdrawal symptoms.

5. The overall goals in recovery from addiction are the same for all substances and include improved coping skills and relapse prevention.
   - To achieve long-term recovery, consider medication management as an adjunct to psychosocial approaches. The combination of medication and psychosocial support provides the greatest likelihood of recovery for many individuals who struggle with substance-related disorders.

Abbreviations Introduced in This Chapter

AA	Alcoholics Anonymous
ALDH	Aldehyde dehydrogenase
ALT	Alanine aminotransferase
ASI	Addiction Severity Index
AST	Aspartate aminotransferase
AUDIT	Alcohol Use Disorders Identification Test
BAC	Blood alcohol concentration
CBT	Cognitive-behavioral therapy
CIWA-Ar	Clinical Institute Withdrawal Assessment for Alcohol—Revised
CNS	Central Nervous System
COWS	Clinical Opiate Withdrawal Scale
CRF	Corticotropin-releasing factor
DA	Dopamine
DEA	Drug Enforcement Administration
DSM-IV-TR	*Diagnostic and Statistical Manual of Mental Disorders,* 4th ed, text revision
DTs	Delirium tremens
ED	Emergency department
GABA	γ-aminobutyric acid
5-HT	Serotonin
IM	Intramuscular
IV	Intravenous
LFT	Liver function test
MET	Motivational enhancement therapy
NA	Nucleus accumbens
nACh	Nicotinic acetylcholine
NE	Norepinephrine
NMDA	*N*-Methyl-D-aspartate
NRT	Nicotine replacement therapy
NSDUH	National Survey on Drug Use and Health
OBOT	Office-Based Opioid Treatment
OTP	Opioid Treatment Program
PFC	Prefrontal cortex
SAMHSA	Substance Abuse and Mental Health Services Administration
SC	Subcutaneous
SUD	Substance use disorder
VTA	Ventral tegmental area

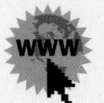

Self-assessment questions and answers are available at *http://www.mhpharmacotherapy.com/pp.html.*

ACKNOWLEDGMENTS

The author and editors wish to acknowledge and thank Dr. Sally K. Guthrie, the primary author of this chapter in the first and second editions of this book; Dr. Kirk J. Brower and Dr. Maher Karam-Hage, co-authors of this chapter in the first edtion; and Dr. Theadia L. Carey, a co-author of this chapter in the second edition.

REFERENCES

1. Substance Abuse and Mental Health Services Administration (SAMHSA). Results from the 2010 National Survey on Drug Use and Health: Summary of National Findings, NSDUH Series H-41, HHS Publication No. (SMA) 11-4658. Rockville, MD: Substance Abuse and Mental Health Services Administration, 2011.
2. The Neurobiology of Drug Addiction [Internet]. Bethesda (MD): The National Institute on Drug Abuse [accessed 2011 Oct 25]. Available at: *http://www.drugabuse.gov/pubs/teaching/Teaching2/Teaching.html.*
3. Stahl SM. Stahl's Essential Psychopharmacology: Neuroscientific Basis and Practical Applications. 3rd ed. New York: Cambridge University Press; 2008.
4. Dobrin CV, Roberts DCS. The anatomy of addiction. In: Ries RK, Fiellin DA, Miller SC, Saitz R, eds. Principles of Addiction Medicine, 4th ed. Philadelphia, PA: Lippincott Williams & Wilkins, 2009:27–38.
5. Koob GF, Volkow ND. Neurocircuitry of addiction. Neuropsychopharmacology 2010;35:217–238.
6. American Psychiatric Association. Diagnostic and Statistical Manual of Mental Disorders. 4th ed, text rev. Washington, DC: American Psychiatric Association, 2000:191–296.
7. Rush AJ, First MB, Blacker D, eds. Handbook of Psychiatric Measures. 2nd ed. Arlington, VA: American Psychiatric Publishing; 2008.
8. Addiction Severity Index (ASI) [Internet]. Philadelphia (PA): Treatment Research Institute [last accessed and cited 2011 Oct 25]. Available at: *http://www.tresearch.org.*
9. Center for Substance Abuse Treatment. Clinical Guidelines for the Use of Buprenorphine in the Treatment of Opioid Addiction. Treatment Improvement Protocol (TIP) Series 40. DHHS Publication no. (SMA) 04–3939. Rockville, MD: Substance Abuse and Mental Health Services Administration; 2004.
10. Center for Substance Abuse Treatment. Detoxification and Substance Abuse Treatment. Treatment Improvement Protocol (TIP) Series 45. DHHS Publication No. (SMA) 06-4131. Rockville, MD: Substance Abuse and Mental Health Services Administration; 2006.
11. Volkow ND, Li T-K. Drug addiction: The neurobiology of behavior gone awry. In: Ries RK, Fiellin DA, Miller SC, Saitz R, eds. Principles of Addiction Medicine. 4th ed. Philadelphia, PA: Lippincott Williams & Wilkins; 2009:3–12.
12. American Psychiatric Association. Practice Guideline for the Treatment of Patients with Substance Use Disorders, 2nd ed. Arlington, VA: American Psychiatric Association, 2006.
13. Mayo-Smith MF. Management of alcohol intoxication and withdrawal. In: Ries RK, Fiellin DA, Miller SC, Saitz R, eds. Principles of Addiction Medicine. 4th ed. Philadelphia, PA: Lippincott Williams & Wilkins; PA 2009:559–572.
14. Tetrault JM, O'Connor PG. Management of opioid intoxication and withdrawal. In: Ries RK, Fiellin DA, Miller SC, Saitz R, eds. Principles of Addiction Medicine. 4th ed. Philadelphia, PA: Lippincott Williams & Wilkins; 2009:589–606.
15. Wilkins JN, Danovitch I, Gorelick DA. Management of stimulant, hallucinogen, marijuana, phencyclidine, and club drug intoxication and withdrawal. In: Ries RK, Fiellin DA, Miller SC, Saitz R, eds. Principles of Addiction Medicine. 4th ed. Philadelphia, PA: Lippincott Williams & Wilkins; 2009:607–628.
16. Fiore MC, Jaén CR, Baker TB, et al. Treating tobacco use and dependence: 2008 Update. Clinical Practice Guideline. Rockville, MD: U.S. Department of Health and Human Services. Public Health Service, 2008.
17. Lexi-Comp Online [Internet]. Hudson, OH: Lexi-Comp; 2011 [accessed October 11, 2011 from institutional university access database].
18. Clinical Pharmacology [Internet]. Tampa (FL): Elsevier/Gold Standard; 2011 [accessed October 11, 2011 from institutional university access database].
19. McCord J, Jneid H, Hollander JE, et al. Management of cocaine-associated chest pain and myocardial infarction: A scientific statement from the American Heart Association Acute Cardiac Care Committee of the Council on Clinical Cardiology. Circulation 2008;117:1897–1907.
20. Daeppen JB, Gache P, Landry U, et al. Symptom-triggered vs fixed-schedule doses of benzodiazepine for alcohol withdrawal: A randomized treatment trial. Arch Intern Med 2002;162:1117–1121.

21. Day E, Bentham P, Callaghan R, et al. Thiamine for Wernicke-Korsakoff syndrome in people at risk from alcohol abuse. Cochrane Database Syst Rev 2004;(1):CD004033.

22. Lingford-Hughes AR, Welch S, Nutt DJ. Evidence-based guidelines for the pharmacological management of substance misuse, addiction and comorbidity: Recommendations from the British Association for Psychopharmacology. J Psychopharmacol 2004;18:293–335.

23. Mayo-Smith MF, Beecher LH, Fischer TL, et al. Management of alcohol withdrawal delirium. An evidence-based practice guideline. Arch Intern Med 2004;164:1405–1412.

24. Garbutt JC, West SL, Carey TS, et al. Pharmacological treatment of alcohol dependence: a review of the evidence. JAMA 1999; 281: 1318–1325.

25. Fuller RK, Gordis E. Does disulfiram have a role in alcoholism treatment today? Addiction 2004;99:21–24.

26. Fuller RK, Branchey L, Brightwell DR, et al. Disulfiram treatment of alcoholism. A Veterans Administration cooperative study. JAMA 1986;256:1449–1455.

27. Center for Substance Abuse Treatment. Incorporating Alcohol Pharmacotherapies into Medical Practice. Treatment Improvement Protocol (TIP) Series 49. HHS Publication No. (SMA) 09-4380. Rockville, MD: Substance Abuse and Mental Health Services Administration; 2009.

28. Petrakis IL, Poling J, Levinson C, et al. Naltrexone and disulfiram in patients with alcohol dependence and comorbid psychiatric disorders. Biol Psychiatry 2005;57:1128–1137.

29. Srisurapanont M, Jarusuraisin N. Naltrexone for the treatment of alcoholism: A meta-analysis of randomized controlled trials. Int J Neuropsychopharmacol 2005;8:267–280.

30. Rubio G, Ponce G, Rodriguez-Jimenez R, et al. Clinical predictors of response to naltrexone in alcoholic patients: Who benefits most from treatment with naltrexone? Alcohol and Alcoholism 2005;40:227–233.

31. Anton R, O'Malley SS, Ciraulo DA, et al, for the COMBINE Study Research Group. Combined pharmacotherapies and behavioral interventions for alcohol dependence. The COMBINE Study: A randomized controlled trial. JAMA 2006;295:2003–2017.

32. Garbutt JC, Kranzler HR, O'Malley SS, et al. Efficacy and tolerability of long-acting injectable naltrexone for alcohol dependence: A randomized controlled trial. JAMA 2005;293:1617–1625.

33. Mann K, Lehert P, Morgan MY. The efficacy of acamprosate in the maintenance of abstinence in alcohol-dependent individuals: Results of a meta-analysis. Alcohol Clin Exp Res 2004;28:51–63.

34. Rösner S, Leucht S, Ehert P, Soyka M. Acamprosate supports abstinence, naltrexone prevents excessive drinking: Evidence from a meta-analysis with unreported outcomes. J Psychopharmacol 2008;22:11–23.

35. Mattick RP, Kimber J, Breen C, Davoli M. Buprenorphine maintenance versus placebo or methadone maintenance for opioid dependence. Cochrane Database Syst Rev 2008;(3):CD002207.

36. Teter CJ. Substance Use Disorders. 2012 Board Certified Psychiatric Pharmacist (BCPP) Examination Review and Recertification Course. Lincoln, NE: College of Psychiatric & Neurologic Pharmacists, 2012.

37. U.S. Food and Drug Administration. Drug Safety Newsletter Volume 2, Number 1, 2009.

38. U.S. Food and Drug Administration [Internet]. Varenicline (marketed as Chantix) Information [accessed October 11, 2011]. Available from: *http://www.fda.gov/Drugs/DrugSafety/ PostmarketDrugSafetyInformationforPatientsandProviders/ ucm106540.htm.*

37

Schizophrenia

Deanna L. Kelly, Elaine Weiner, and
Heidi J. Wehring

LEARNING OBJECTIVES

● **Upon completion of the chapter, the reader will be able to:**

1. Recognize the signs and symptoms of schizophrenia and be able to distinguish among positive, negative, and cognitive symptoms of the illness.

2. Explain the pathophysiologic mechanisms that are thought to underlie schizophrenia.

3. Identify the treatment goals for a patient with schizophrenia.

4. Recommend appropriate antipsychotic medications based on patient-specific data.

5. Compare the side effect profiles of individual antipsychotics.

6. Educate patients and families about schizophrenia, treatments, and the importance of adherence to antipsychotic treatment.

7. Describe the components of a monitoring plan to assess the effectiveness and safety of antipsychotic medications.

KEY CONCEPTS

① A diagnosis of schizophrenia is made clinically because there are no psychological assessments, brain imaging, or laboratory examinations that confirm the diagnosis.

② Patients presenting with odd behaviors, illogical thought processes, bizarre beliefs, and hallucinations should be assessed for schizophrenia.

③ The goals of treatment are to reduce symptomatology, decrease psychotic relapses, and improve patient functioning and social outcomes.

④ The cornerstone of treatment is antipsychotic medications. Because most patients with schizophrenia relapse when not medicated, long-term treatment is usually necessary.

⑤ Psychosocial support is needed to help improve functional outcomes.

⑥ Compared with the older antipsychotics (first-generation antipsychotics [FGAs], typical antipsychotics), the more recently developed second-generation antipsychotics (SGAs, atypical antipsychotics) are associated with a lower risk of motor side effects (tremor, stiffness, restlessness, and dyskinesia); may offer greater benefits for affective, negative, and cognitive symptoms; and may prolong the time to psychotic relapse.

⑦ SGAs as a class are heterogeneous with regard to side effect profiles. Many SGAs carry an increased risk for weight gain and for the development of glucose and lipid abnormalities; therefore, careful monitoring is essential.

⑧ Education of the patient and family regarding the benefits and risks of antipsychotic medications and the importance of adherence to their therapeutic regimen must be integrated into pharmacologic management.

In most cases, schizophrenia is a devastating, chronically debilitating disorder. Conceptually, it may be thought of as a clinical syndrome, comprising several disease entities that manifest with psychotic symptoms, including hallucinations, delusions, and disordered thinking. Commonly, these more flagrant symptoms are accompanied by more insidious ones, including cognitive impairment (abnormalities in thinking, reasoning, attention, memory, and perception), impaired insight and judgment, loss of motivation (avolition), loss of emotional range (restricted affect), and a decrease in spontaneous speech (poverty of speech). The latter three symptoms are termed negative symptoms and collectively are frequently called the deficit syndrome. Cognitive impairments and negative symptoms account for much of the poor social and functional outcomes observed in schizophrenia. Schizophrenia is the fourth leading cause of disability among adults and is associated with substantially lower rates of employment, marriage, and independent living compared with population norms. However, earlier diagnosis and treatment, as well as advances in research and newer

Patient Encounter, Part 1

KH is a 24-year-old single woman with an approximately 1-year history of paranoia, continuously hearing voices of "spirits" advising her daily activities, and social withdrawal. KH withdrew from college 2 years ago after having difficulty concentrating, and she was employed up until 6 months ago as a cashier at a local fast food restaurant. She eventually left her job because of missing too many shifts secondary to her beliefs that others could read her mind. KH lives with her parents, who have become increasingly worried about her throughout the past year. When she lost her job, she began to "go downhill fast," her father says. She is spending more and more time in her room, which she says is the only place in the house where she feels comfortable. The voices, which she calls "spirits," have been advising her that she needs to limit time outside her room. She also has stopped doing activities she used to enjoy, such as listening to music and going to movies. She states she "doesn't really miss" doing these things. KH has also become irritable and complains she is sleeping poorly. When her mother asked that she leave her room to join the family for dinner, KH recently became angry and so agitated that she threw a vase at her mother. Although her parents are supportive, they are worried about her symptoms and frustrated about her recent behavior and withdrawal.

What diagnoses are suggested by this presentation?

What additional information would help to clarify the diagnosis?

treatment developments, have led to better outcomes for people who have this complex and challenging illness.

EPIDEMIOLOGY AND ETIOLOGY

One percent of the world's population suffers from schizophrenia, and symptoms usually first present in late adolescence or early adulthood.[1] Although equally prevalent between the genders, symptoms generally appear earlier in men, and men have a younger age at first hospitalization (15 to 24 years) compared with women (25 to 34 years).

The etiology of schizophrenia remains largely unknown, although the evidence strongly supports a genetic basis for the disorder. First-degree relatives of patients with schizophrenia carry a 10% risk of developing the disorder. When both parents have the diagnosis, the risk to their offspring is 40%. For monozygotic twins, the likelihood of one twin developing the illness if the other twin has schizophrenia is about 50%. Many genes have been weakly associated with the development of schizophrenia; however, no clear association exists for any one gene. There is probably no single "schizophrenia gene," but research continues in the hopes of more fully exploring candidate genes, loci, and copy number variants.[2] Environmental stimuli or triggers along with genetic liability may contribute to the expression of the illness. Some data suggest intrauterine exposure to viral or bacterial infections may be a risk factor; however, more research is needed.

PATHOPHYSIOLOGY

The oldest theory associated with the pathophysiology of schizophrenia is the dopamine hypothesis, which proposes that psychosis is caused by excessive dopamine in the brain. This hypothesis dates from the late 1950s after the discovery that chlorpromazine, the first antipsychotic, acted as a postsynaptic dopamineantagonist. Drugs that cause an increase in dopamine (e.g., cocaine and amphetamines) increase psychotic symptoms, and drugs that decrease dopamine (e.g., all current antipsychotic medications) decrease psychotic symptoms. However, data over the past several decades revealed a more complicated picture with both hyperdopaminergic and hypodopaminergic brain regions in schizophrenia. Hypodopaminergic activity observed in the prefrontal lobe is thought to relate to the core negative symptoms associated with schizophrenia. Thus, a more modern reworking of the dopamine hypothesis is the "dysregulation hypothesis," which takes these findings into account.[3] It is possible, however, that the dopamine abnormalities hypothesized to underlie the etiology of schizophrenia may represent compensatory changes that occur secondary to other pathophysiologic abnormalities intrinsic to the illness. Other neurotransmitter systems have also been implicated in schizophrenia. Some investigators have suggested that a combined dysfunction of the dopamine and glutamate transmitter systems may better explain the disorder.[4] In particular, it is hypothesized that glutamate, possibly through malfunctioning N-methyl-D-aspartate (NMDA) receptors, impacts dopaminergic activity in brain areas such as the mesolimbic and mesocortical pathways. NMDA antagonists such as phencyclidine (PCP) and ketamine can elicit a state resembling psychotic symptoms of schizophrenia, including positive, negative, and cognitive symptoms. There has also been a great deal of speculation regarding a role for serotonin receptor antagonism in antipsychotic efficacy[5] because many second-generation antipsychotics (SGAs) are active at serotonin receptors. Serotonin receptor binding may be important to drug action, possibly by modulating dopamine activity in mesocortical pathways. However, a compelling pathophysiologic theory relating to dopamine and serotonin receptor affinities does not yet exist. It is important to note that to date, antipsychotics without any primary or secondary dopamine-modulating properties have been ineffective for the treatment of positive symptoms of schizophrenia.

CLINICAL PRESENTATION AND DIAGNOSIS

People with schizophrenia may appear uncooperative, suspicious, hostile, anxious, or aggressive because of their misinterpretation of reality. They may have poor

Clinical Presentation of Schizophrenia

General

Schizophrenia is a chronic disorder of thought and affect, causing a significant disturbance in the individual's ability to function vocationally and interpersonally. The onset of symptoms in most cases is insidious, usually preceded by a prodromal phase characterized by gradual social withdrawal, diminished interests, changes in appearance and hygiene, changes in cognition, and bizarre or odd behaviors. Despite the tendency of the media to portray a stereotype, the clinical presentation of a person with schizophrenia is extremely varied. Hallmark symptoms include psychotic symptoms, negative symptoms, and cognitive impairments that last for at least 6 months.

Symptoms

Psychotic symptoms: These symptoms are sometimes called positive symptoms because they are "added on to" a person's normal experience. They may include hallucinations (distortions or exaggeration of perception), delusions (fixed false beliefs), and thought disorder (illogical thought and speech). Hallucinations, most frequently auditory, can also be visual, olfactory, gustatory, and tactile. Auditory hallucinations may be experienced as voices or as thoughts that feel distinct from the person's own thoughts. The content of the hallucinations is variable, but often they are threatening or commanding (e.g., commanding the person to perform a particular action). Patients may feel compelled to perform the commanded task or may experience much anxiety when they do not. Delusions frequently involve fixed false beliefs despite invalidating evidence and may be bizarre in nature. Often they have

paranoid themes, which may make the patient suspicious of others. The characteristic thought disorder of schizophrenia includes loosening of associations, tangentiality, thought blocking, concreteness, circumstantiality, and perseveration. Thinking and speech may be incomprehensible and illogical. Subtle disturbances in associative thinking may develop years before disorganized thinking (formal thought disorder).

Negative symptoms: So called because they are qualities "taken away" from the personality, include impoverished speech and thinking, lack of social drive, flatness of emotional expression, and apathy. Although quite ubiquitous, these symptoms are difficult to evaluate because they occur in a continuum with normality and can be attributable to secondary causes, including medication side effects, mood disorder, environmental understimulation, or demoralization. When caused by schizophrenia itself, they are termed *primary negative symptoms or deficit symptoms.* The best strategy for differentiating primary from secondary negative symptoms is to observe for their persistence over time despite efforts at resolving the other causes. Approximately 10% to 15% of people with schizophrenia may present primarily with negative symptoms; these people may be referred to as having a deficit syndrome.

Cognitive symptoms: Neuropsychological research shows that patients with schizophrenia show abnormalities in the areas of attention, processing speed, verbal and visual memory, working memory, and problem solving. There is a loss of, on average, 1 standard deviation of pre-illness IQ, with the average IQ between 80 and 84.

hygiene and appear unkempt because both psychotic and depressive symptoms may lead to impaired self-care. Sleep and appetite are often disturbed. People with schizophrenia often have difficulty living independently and forming close relationships with others. Additionally, they have problems initiating or maintaining employment. Comorbid medical disorders, such as type 2 diabetes and chronic obstructive pulmonary disease, are prevalent in people with schizophrenia because of sedentary lifestyles, poor dietary habits, obesity, or cigarette smoking. Approximately 60% of people with schizophrenia smoke, and approximately 50% use drugs and alcohol, rates much higher than the general population.[6]

❶ *A diagnosis of schizophrenia is made clinically because there are no psychological assessments, brain imaging, or laboratory examinations that confirm the diagnosis.*

Although biological markers are being investigated, currently the diagnosis is made by ruling out other causes of psychosis and meeting specified diagnostic criteria that are based on symptoms and functioning. A family

history of psychiatric disorders is helpful in supporting the diagnosis. The commonly accepted diagnostic criteria for schizophrenia are from the *Diagnostic and Statistical Manual of Mental Disorders*, fourth edition, text revision (*DSM-IV-TR*)[7] (Table 37–1).

❷ *Patients presenting with odd behaviors, illogical thought processes, bizarre beliefs, and hallucinations should be assessed for schizophrenia.*

A person presenting with an initial episode of psychosis requires a comprehensive assessment and careful diagnosis because psychosis is not pathognomonic for schizophrenia. Often, people present with a short history of psychopathology and cannot recall historical information accurately. This lack of information, along with frequent comorbid substance abuse, medical illnesses, and psychosocial stressors, often confounds the diagnosis. Patients presenting with psychotic symptoms, particularly those in their initial episode, should have a thorough medical and laboratory evaluation (electrolytes, blood urea nitrogen, serum creatinine, urinalysis, liver and thyroid function profile, syphilis serology, serum

---

Table 37–1

Diagnostic Criteria for Schizophrenia

A. *Characteristic symptoms:* Two (or more) of the following, each present for a significant portion of time during a 1-month period (or less if successfully treated):[a]
   - Delusions
   - Hallucinations
   - Disorganized speech (e.g., frequent derailment or incoherence)
   - Grossly disorganized or catatonic behavior
   - Negative symptoms (e.g., flat affect, alogia, avolition)
B. *Social or occupational dysfunction:* For a significant portion of the time since the onset of the disturbance, one or more major areas of functioning such as work, interpersonal relations, or self-care are markedly below the level achieved before onset (or when onset is in childhood or adolescence, failure to achieve the expected level of interpersonal, academic, or occupational achievement)
C. *Duration:* Continuous signs of disturbance persist for at least 6 months. This 6-month period must include at least 1 month of symptoms (or less if successfully treated) that meets criterion A (i.e., active-phase symptoms) and may include periods of prodromal or residual symptoms. During these prodromal or residual periods, the signs of disturbance may be manifested by only negative symptoms or by two or more symptoms listed in category A present in an attenuated form (e.g., odd beliefs, unusual perceptual experiences)
D. *Ruling out other disorders:*
   - Schizoaffective and mood disorder exclusion: Schizoaffective disorder and mood disorder with psychotic features have been ruled out because either (a) no major depressive, manic, or mixed episodes have occurred concurrently with the active-phase symptoms or (b) if mood episodes have occurred during active-phase symptoms, their total duration has been brief relative to the duration of the active and residual periods
   - Substance and general medical condition exclusion: The disturbance is not attributable to the direct physiologic effects of a substance (e.g., drug of abuse or medication) or a general medical condition
   - Pervasive developmental disorder: If the patient has a history of autistic disorder or another pervasive developmental disorder, the additional diagnosis of schizophrenia is made only if prominent delusions or hallucinations are also present for at least 1 month (or less if successfully treated)

[a]Only one symptom from category A is required if delusions are bizarre or hallucinations consist of a voice maintaining a running commentary on the person's behavior or thoughts or two or more voices conversing.

Adapted from American Psychiatric Association. Diagnostic and Statistical Manual of Mental Disorders. 4th ed, text rev. Washington, DC: American Psychiatric Association; 2000.

---

pregnancy test, and urine toxicology), including a careful review of systems and a physical examination, including a neurologic evaluation. At the minimum, in accordance with the American Psychiatric Association (APA) Practice Guidelines[8] and the Expert Consensus Guideline Series for Schizophrenia,[9] patients with psychosis should have a medical workup at the time of admission to rule out other diagnoses or contributing factors.

COURSE AND PROGNOSIS

The onset of psychosis, whether insidious or acute, is marked by difficulties for patients, families, and clinicians. Patients may keep symptoms hidden from family and friends; they may also isolate themselves from social support networks. The gradual development of psychosis and the frequent misunderstanding of symptoms generally lead to a substantial time period between symptom onset and diagnosis and treatment. Recent data suggest that people treated early in their illness may have a better prognosis. Therefore, the first challenge of optimal therapy is to move treatment initiation closer to the onset of psychosis.

Although the course of schizophrenia is variable, the long-term prognosis for independent function is often poor. The course of illness is marked by intermittent acute psychotic episodes with a downward decline in psychosocial functioning. Over time, a patient may become more withdrawn, bizarre, and nonfunctional. Many of the more dramatic and acute symptoms fade with time, but severe residual symptoms may persist. Family and friends often find this illness difficult to interpret and understand. Involvement with the law is fairly common for misdemeanors such as vagrancy, loitering, and disturbing the peace. The overall life expectancy is shortened primarily because of suicide, accidents, and the inability of self-care. The lifetime risk of suicide for people with schizophrenia is 5% to 10%.[10] Persistent compliance with a tolerable drug regimen improves prognosis, although relapse without medication exceeds 50% annually.

TREATMENT

Desired Outcomes

❸ *The goals of treatment are to reduce symptomatology and psychotic relapses and to improve functional and social outcomes.*[9] Patients should receive, as early in their course as possible, comprehensive treatment designed to achieve functional outcomes. Although in the past, the primary treatment goal was to decrease positive symptoms and the associated hostile and aggressive behaviors, newer approaches to treatment have a wider focus, including positive, negative, depressive, and anxious symptoms, as well as preserving cognition. Combativeness, hostility, sleep

Patient Encounter, Part 2

Past Psychiatric History: KH has not had any extensive psychiatric treatment. When she withdrew from college 2 years ago, she cited concentration difficulties as the main factor. However, when referred for a psychological evaluation, she did not follow through with the referral.

Past Medical History: She has no history of medical illness, head trauma, or seizure disorder. KH is 160 cm (63 in) tall and weighs 66 kg (145 lb). Toxicology screen results are negative for alcohol and drugs of abuse.

Social History: KH grew up in a middle class family, completed high school, and entered college. Initially, she was very involved in coursework, but she withdrew 2 years ago citing concentration difficulties. Her GPA dropped dramatically from her first to her third year of college. KH periodically drinks alcohol and smokes marijuana, by her estimation, once a month. She has never been diagnosed with any substance use disorder. KH has held several part time jobs from the ages of 18 to 23 years, the last of which was as a cashier at a fast food restaurant. She has no health insurance.

Family History: KH's grandfather had an alcohol problem, and her great uncle has a history of depression. KH's mother and aunt both have type 2 diabetes.

Mental Status Exam

Appearance: Appears somewhat disheveled, dressed in dirty clothes, and hair looks like it has not been washed or brushed for several days. No abnormal movements. Poor eye contact

Speech: Quiet and somewhat monotonous
Mood: Nervous
Affect: Guarded and mildly anxious with restricted range
Thought content: She is an adequate historian but with a tendency to leave out detail. Hears the voices of "spirits" daily, which give her advice, and she feels like others can read her thoughts. KH denies suicidal or homicidal thoughts.
Thought processes: Vague and sometimes illogical
Cognition: Grossly intact
Insight and judgment: Impaired at this time. She does not feel like anything is wrong with her, and does not recognize that some of her recent behaviors are inappropriate (throwing vase) or that her experiences may be symptoms (paranoia, hallucinations, etc.) of an illness

Given this additional information, how has your differential diagnosis changed?

What are the goals of acute treatment?

What medications would you recommend as first-line options for KH, and why?

disturbances, appetite, and hallucinations may be some of the first symptoms to improve. Improvements in negative symptoms, cognitive functioning, social skills, and judgment generally require a longer period to improve.

General Approach to Treatment

Over the past few years, partial recovery and remission have become an increasingly prominent paradigm for treatment of schizophrenia. A range of interventions must be incorporated into long-term treatment strategies, including pharmacologic interventions and psychosocial therapies. Current treatment planning is increasingly focused on functional outcomes by providing treatment and recovery-oriented services to people with schizophrenia. Also, implementation of evidence-based practice, whereby new information from the published literature gets incorporated into clinicians' prescribing behavior, has led to the use of interventions that promote a remission or recovery attitude.[10–12] Moreover, recent attempts have been made to address and measure patient satisfaction with treatments and instill hope and optimism in order to empower patients. Unfortunately, despite these advances and recent treatment improvements, long-term outcomes currently remain poor, and many patients fail to receive comprehensive care.

❹ *The cornerstone of treatment is antipsychotic medications. Because most patients with schizophrenia relapse when not medicated, long-term treatment is usually necessary.* Because early detection and intervention in schizophrenia is important for maximizing outcomes, treatment with antipsychotic medications should begin as soon as psychotic symptoms are recognized. Antipsychotic medications are the cornerstone of therapy for people with schizophrenia, and most patients are on lifelong therapy because nonadherence and discontinuation of antipsychotics are associated with high relapse rates. If other symptoms are present such as depression and anxiety, these symptoms should also be aggressively treated. Additionally, psychosocial treatments should be used concomitantly to improve patient outcomes.

Nonpharmacologic Therapy

❺ *Psychosocial support is needed to help improve functional outcomes.* Only 30% of patients respond robustly to antipsychotics, another 30% respond partially, and another 30% have a minimal response. Responding patients often continue to have residual symptoms such as amotivation, isolation, and impaired social functioning, thus limiting their participation in social, vocational, and educational endeavors. Psychosocial interventions are based on the premise that increased psychosocial functioning will lead to improvements in subjective feelings of self-esteem and life satisfaction. A few of the best-supported and most promising approaches to psychosocial rehabilitation are social skills training (SST), cognitive-behavioral therapy (CBT), and cognitive remediation (CR). These treatments are mainly used as targeted treatments for social and cognitive impairments and as adjuncts to pharmacotherapy for psychotic symptoms.[13] Most psychosocial studies have been carried out in the United Kingdom, and findings are not yet widely used in the United States. Nonetheless, there are substantial data to support that family education and vocational support help to improve long-term functional outcomes. In addition, Assertive Community Treatment (ACT), programming designed to provide direct service provision and high frequency of patient contact by a multidisciplinary team, has been found to reduce hospitalizations and homelessness in persons with schizophrenia.[13]

Pharmacologic Therapy

Generally, along with antipsychotic medications, adjunctive medications should be used when necessary for specific symptoms or comorbid diagnoses. Because each schizophrenic patient presents differently, each treatment regimen should be individually tailored. For years, only first-generation antipsychotics (FGAs; typical antipsychotics) were available, but since 1990, nine new antipsychotics have been marketed in the United States. These agents, known as SGAs (atypical antipsychotics), include risperidone (Risperdal), olanzapine (Zyprexa), quetiapine (Seroquel), ziprasidone (Geodon), aripiprazole (Abilify), paliperidone (Invega), iloperidone (Fanapt), asenapine (Saphris), lurasidone (Latuda), and clozapine (Clozaril). Clozapine, the prototype of this class of medications, is reserved as second-line therapy because of its unusual side effect profile (see below).

❻ *Compared with the older FGAs, the more recently developed SGAs are associated with a lower risk of motor side effects (tremor, stiffness, restlessness, and dyskinesia); may offer greater benefits for affective, negative, and cognitive symptoms; and may prolong the time to psychotic relapse.*

Since the introduction of SGAs, the use of FGAs has progressively decreased, and the current market share for FGAs in treatment of schizophrenia is less than 10%. This decline occurred because of the touted lower side effect profile and other benefits of SGAs in several domains of illness. Early comparative studies used high-dose, high-potency FGAs such as haloperidol and concluded that SGAs were more effective in some domains. More recently, a large multisite clinical trial (n = more than 1,400 patients) examined the effectiveness of SGAs relative to a midpotency FGA, perphenazine (the Clinical Antipsychotics Trials of Intervention Effectiveness; CATIE trial). Findings were that FGAs may be as effective as SGAs when using the primary endpoint of time to discontinuation of medication.[14] Thus, although these results suggest that midpotency FGAs may be similar in efficacy to SGAs, the CATIE trial had several limitations, and other evidence suggests SGAs may be more effective in some illness domains, such as relapse prevention, affective and negative symptoms, and cognitive function. The SGAs have historically been much more expensive than the FGAs; however risperidone, olanzapine,

and clozapine are now available in generic formulations, and other SGAs will lose patent protection in the next 5 years. In conclusion, when selecting among the various agents, the risk-to-benefit profile becomes fundamental, and all the antipsychotics are associated with somewhat different side effect profiles.

Second-Generation (Atypical) Antipsychotics

Although the FGAs exert most of their effects through dopamine-receptor blockade at the dopamine$_2$ (D$_2$) receptor, the SGAs may work through a more complicated mechanism. The SGAs have greater affinity for serotonin receptors than for dopamine receptors. Despite being heterogeneous with regard to receptor binding, the overall efficacy among the SGAs is similar.[14] Recent comparative data among SGAs and FGAs (lower doses) have reported that overall efficacy is similar between groups, which suggests a reevaluation of the place of FGAs in therapy is needed.[14] Only clozapine, however, has demonstrated superior efficacy for some patients (see Treatment-Resistant Patients). An important distinction of the SGAs as a class is their lower propensity to cause extrapyramidal symptoms (EPS) and tardive dyskinesia (TD). The annual risk of TD is considered to be less than 1.5% per year in adults (younger than 54 years old) taking SGAs compared to approximately a 5% per year risk in those taking FGAs.[15] Pharmacologic profiles and side effect profiles, however, are very different among the agents.

❼ *The SGAs as a class are heterogeneous with regard to side effect profiles. Many SGAs carry an increased risk for weight gain and for the development of glucose and lipid abnormalities; therefore, careful monitoring is essential.* Table 37–2 lists the SGA agents, recommended dosing, and dosage forms available. Table 37–3 lists the side effect profiles of the SGAs and haloperidol.

▶ Risperidone

Risperidone, a benzisoxazole derivative, was the first SGA to be marketed after the release of clozapine and was the initial first-line oral SGA to become available generically. It has high binding affinity to both serotonin 2$_A$ (5-HT$_{2A}$) and D$_2$ receptors and binds to α_1 and α_2 receptors, with very little blockade of cholinergic receptors.[16] Multicenter registry trials found 6 to 16 mg of risperidone at least equal in efficacy to haloperidol (20 mg), but 6 mg of risperidone produced EPS at a rate no different than placebo.[17] Risperidone is also approved for relapse prevention and is associated with significantly lower relapse rates than long-term haloperidol treatment.[18] At clinically effective doses (less than or equal to 6 mg/day), EPSs are low, although higher doses are clearly associated with a greater incidence of EPS. Risperidone is associated with serum prolactin elevations that are similar to or greater than those seen with the FGAs. Elevated prolactin levels can, but do not always, lead to clinical symptoms such as hormonal problems (e.g., amenorrhea, galactorrhea, and gynecomastia) or sexual dysfunction. Risperidone is associated with mild

Table 37–2

Second-Generation (Atypical) Antipsychotics

Second-Generation Antipsychotic	Usual Target Dose (mg/day)	Maximal Dose Likely to Be Beneficial (mg/day)	Available Dosage Forms
Aripiprazole (Abilify)	15–30	30	• 2-, 5-, 10-, 15-, 20-, and 30-mg tablets • 1-mg/mL oral solution • 10- and 15-mg discmelt orally disintegrating tablets • IM 9.75 mg/1.3 mL
Asenapine (Saphris)	10	10–20	• 5- and 10-mg sublingual tablets
Clozapine (Clozaril, also available generically)	400	500–800	• 12.5-, 25-, 50-, 100-, and 200-mg tablets • FazaClo (orally disintegrating tablets) 12.5, 25, and 100 mg
Iloperidone (Fanapt)	12–24	24	• 1-, 2-, 4-, 6-, 8-, 10-, 12-mg tablets
Lurasidone (Latuda)	40–80	80	• 40- and 80-mg tablets
Olanzapine (Zyprexa)	15–20	30–40[a]	• 2.5-, 5-, 7.5-, 10-, 15-, and 20-mg tablets • Zyprexa Zydis (orally disintegrating tablets) 5, 10, 15, and 20 mg • IM 10 mg vial (after reconstitution, ~5 mg/mL) • Zyprexa Relprevv 210-, 300-, and 405-mg/vial powder for suspension long-acting injection
Paliperidone (Invega)	6	6–12	• 1.5-, 3-, 6-, and 9-mg tablets • Invega sustenna 39-, 78-, 117-, 156-, 234-mg prefilled syringes
Quetiapine (Seroquel)	300–800	800	• 25-, 50-, 100-, 200-, 300-, and 400-mg tablets • Seroquel XR (extended-release tablets) 50, 150, 200, 300, and 400 mg
Risperidone (Risperdal, also available generically)	3–6	6–8	• 0.25-, 0.5-, 1-, 2-, 3-, and 4-mg tablets • 1 mg/mL (30 mL) solution • Risperdal M-tab (orally disintegrating tablets) 0.5, 1, 2, 3, and 4 mg • Risperdal Consta long-acting injectable 12.5-, 25-, 37.5-, and 50-mg vial/kit
Ziprasidone (Geodon)	100–120	160–240[a]	• 20-, 40-, 60-, and 80-mg capsules • IM 20 mg/mL

[a]Outside product labeling guidelines.

IM, intramuscular.

Table 37–3

Comparative Side Effects Among the SGAs and Haloperidol

Side Effect	Cloz	Risp[a]	Olan	Quet	Zip	Aripip	Iloper	Asen	Luras	Hal
Anticholinergic side effects	+++	±	++ (Higher doses)	+	±	±	±	+	±	±
EPS at clinical doses	+	+	±	±	±	±	+	+	+	++
Dose-dependent EPS	0	++	+	0	+	±	+	+	+	+++
Orthostatic hypotension	+++	++	+	++	+	+	++	+	+	++
Prolactin elevation	0	+++	+	±	+	0	+	±	±	+
QTc prolongation	+	±	±	+	+	±	+	±	±	±
Sedation	+++	+	+	++	+	+	++	+	+	+
Seizures	++	±	±	±	±	±	±	±	±	±
Weight gain	+++	++	+++	++	+	+	+	+	+	±
Glucose dysregulation	++	+	++	+	±	±	±	±	±	±
Lipid abnormalities	+++	+	+++	++	±	±	±	±	±	±

Cloz, clozapine; Risp, risperidone; Olan, olanzapine; Quet, quetiapine; Zip, ziprasidone; Aripip, aripiprazole; Iloper, iloperidone; Asen, asenapine; Luras, lurasidone; Hal, haloperidol.

[a]Side effects similar for paliperidone.

0, absent; ±, minimal; +, mild or low risk; ++, moderate; +++, severe; EPS, extrapyramidal side effects; SGA, second-generation antipsychotic.

to moderate weight gain, and mild elevations in lipid and glucose may occur. However, patients chronically treated with other antipsychotics such as olanzapine may experience a decline in cholesterol and triglyceride levels when changed to risperidone monotherapy.[14]

▶ Olanzapine

Olanzapine has greater affinity for 5-HT$_{2A}$ than for D$_2$ receptors. In addition, the compound has affinity at the binding sites of D$_4$, D$_3$, 5-HT$_3$, 5-HT$_6$, α_1-adrenergic, muscarinic$_{1-5}$ (M$_{1-5}$), and histamine$_1$ (H$_1$) receptors.[19]

Olanzapine has recently become available in generic form. Multicenter clinical trials have reported that the effectiveness of olanzapine is at least equal to that of haloperidol for the treatment of positive symptoms[20,21] and equal or superior to haloperidol for the treatment of negative symptoms. The premarketing clinical trials reported no significant differences in efficacy among dosage groups. However, the higher dose range appeared to offer the greatest benefits for both positive and negative symptoms when compared with haloperidol (20 mg). In one study, olanzapine (16.3 mg/day) was superior to haloperidol (16.4 mg/day) for the treatment of negative symptoms,[20] but another study found that 13.2 mg olanzapine was superior for both positive and negative symptoms compared with 11.8 mg haloperidol.[21] Among the first-line agents, olanzapine is associated with the longest time to treatment discontinuation,[14] a finding that suggests that olanzapine may somewhat differ from the other SGAs in effectiveness. Olanzapine has a low rate of EPS and causes slight, transient prolactin elevations. Clinically significant weight gain occurs with olanzapine across the dosage range. The degree of weight gain is similar to that seen with clozapine and greater than that observed with the other SGAs. Olanzapine is also associated with hypertriglyceridemia, increased fasting glucose, and new-onset type 2 diabetes (i.e., metabolic syndrome), and among the first-line SGAs, it is associated with the greatest elevations in these metabolic parameters.[14]

▶ Quetiapine

Structurally quetiapine is related to clozapine and olanzapine. Quetiapine has high affinity for $5\text{-}HT_{2A}$ receptors and lower affinity for D_2 and D_1 receptors. This drug has some affinity for α_1, α_2, and H_1 receptors, and very little for muscarinic receptors. The efficacy of quetiapine for psychosis was established in two controlled trials, which found that maximum benefits occurred at 300 mg/day or greater.[22,23] The most effective doses of quetiapine may be higher than 500 mg/day. Quetiapine may have beneficial effects for anxious and depressive symptoms. Because of its low D_2 occupancy, motor side effects and prolactin elevations are usually not seen with quetiapine. Orthostasis occurred in 4% of subjects in clinical trials. Sedation may occur but is generally transient. Mild weight gain and minor elevations in triglycerides can occur. The use of agents that can prolong the QT interval corrected for heart rate (QTc interval) should be avoided during quetiapine treatment, and quetiapine should not be used in circumstances that may increase risk of torsades de pointes (congenital long QT syndrome, arrhythmia, hypokalemia, or hypomagnesemia).

▶ Ziprasidone

Ziprasidone was developed specifically to block D_2 receptors but also bind with even greater affinity to central $5\text{-}HT_{2A}$ receptors. As a result, ziprasidone has a binding affinity ratio of 11:1 for $5\text{-}HT_{2A}$:D_2 receptors. Ziprasidone also has a relatively high affinity for $5\text{-}HT_{2C}$, $5\text{-}HT_{1D}$, α_1-adrenergic, and D_1 receptors.[24] Several short-term, placebo-controlled,

premarketing clinical trials led to the recommended dose range of 40 to 160 mg/day with food,[25] but current practice suggests that efficacy may be greater at doses over 200 mg/day. Liability for EPS, weight gain, and lipid elevations were very low in the clinical trials. Ziprasidone is associated with some prolongation of the QTc interval in adults. However, drug overdose data and studies of pharmacokinetic interactions have thus far shown little evidence that significant QTc prolongation occurs. Use caution, however, when using medications affecting ziprasidone metabolism or when prescribed along with other medications known to prolong QTc. Please see the Pharmacokinetics section of this chapter for further discussion. Caution should also be used when prescribing ziprasidone in situations that have increased risk for prolongation of QTc including comorbid diabetes, electrolyte disturbances (e.g., low serum sodium and potassium concentrations), heavy alcohol consumption, female gender, and congenital QTc disorder.

▶ Aripiprazole

Aripiprazole was formulated to function as a potential dopamine modulator, with both antagonist and agonist activity at the D_2 receptor. It is the first D_2 partial agonist available for the treatment of schizophrenia. This antipsychotic functions as an antagonist in a hyperdopaminergic state and as an agonist when in a hypodopaminergic state. Aripiprazole is also a partial agonist at $5\text{-}HT_{1A}$ receptors, an antagonist at $5\text{-}HT_{2A}$ receptors, and also has affinity for D_3 receptors. Additionally, it has a moderate affinity for α_1 and H_1 receptors with no appreciable affinity for the M_1 receptor.[26] In short- and long-term studies, aripiprazole has been shown to improve positive and negative symptoms of schizophrenia compared with placebo.[27] The recommended starting dose is 10 to 15 mg/day. No titration is required because the starting dose is an effective dose. The recommended dosing range is 10 to 30 mg/day; doses greater than 30 mg have not been systematically evaluated. Doses should be adjusted in persons who are CYP2D6-poor metabolizers by starting with one-half the usual dose and then adjusting to clinical efficacy, and by giving one-quarter the usual dose if given concomitantly with a CYP3A4 inhibitor. Side effects are low with sedation, nausea, and vomiting occurring most frequently. Elevations in weight, lipids, and glucose are generally negligible, and because of its partial dopamine receptor agonism, it does not usually cause elevations in prolactin. In fact, patients switched to aripiprazole from other antipsychotic agents may experience decreases in prolactin levels.

▶ Paliperidone

Paliperidone is the separately marketed 9-hydroxy metabolite of risperidone. The effects of risperidone and paliperidone in the body are expected to be similar because the effects of risperidone are thought to be a result of both the parent drug and the 9-hydroxy metabolite. The neurotransmitter receptor binding affinity is also similar between the two agents, with paliperidone having a greater affinity at $5\text{-}HT_{2A}$ compared with D_2 receptors. Unlike many other antipsychotic medications, paliperidone is mostly excreted unchanged. Patients may be told to expect to see the shell of the tablet in the stool because it does not dissolve in the digestive tract. Short- and long-term studies have established the efficacy of paliperidone compared with placebo.[28] For adults with schizophrenia, the recommended oral dose is 6 mg every morning. No dose titration is required; however, if needed, the dose can be adjusted at 5-day intervals to doses of 3 to 12 mg once daily. Side effects of paliperidone are expected to be similar to those of risperidone, including the potential for dose-related EPS and prolactin elevation.[29]

▶ Iloperidone

Iloperidone is indicated for acute treatment of adults with schizophrenia. Iloperidone exhibits high affinity for $5HT_{2a}$ and dopamine D_2 and D_3 receptors and acts as an antagonist at these receptors, as well as the $5HT_{1a}$ and norepinephrine α_1/α_{2c} receptors. Efficacy for short-term treatment of schizophrenia has been established for positive and negative symptoms of schizophrenia.[30] Doses must be titrated because of the risk of orthostatic hypotension and start at 1 mg twice daily, titrating daily up to the recommended dose of 12 to 24 mg (total daily dose). The maximum dose recommendation is 24 mg total daily dose (12 mg twice daily). Dosing should be reduced by half in persons who are poor metabolizers at CYP2D6. Iloperidone has the potential to prolong the QT interval, so clinicians should consider using other drugs first. Common adverse reactions include dizziness, dry mouth, fatigue, orthostatic hypotension, tachycardia, and weight gain. Dizziness, tachycardia, and weight gain were at least two times as common with higher dose (20 to 24 mg total daily dose) iloperidone compared with lower doses (10 to 16 mg total daily dose) in clinical trials.[31]

▶ Asenapine

Asenapine is indicated for the acute treatment of schizophrenia in adults. Its mechanism of action is thought to be associated with antagonistic activity at $5HT_{2a}$ and D_2 receptors. Asenapine also exhibits a high affinity for other serotonergic and dopaminergic receptors, as well as α_1- and α_2-adrenergic receptors and H_1-receptors. Asenapine's efficacy for short-term and maintenance treatment of schizophrenia has been established.[31] The recommended starting and target dose for the treatment of symptoms of schizophrenia is 5 mg sublingually twice a day, which is lower than the maximum dose recommended for bipolar disorder. Tablets must be placed under the tongue and allowed to dissolve completely; the tablets should not be chewed or swallowed. Patients should refrain from drinking or eating for 10 minutes after administration. In controlled trials, no added benefit was seen with doses above 10 mg twice daily, but there was an increase in adverse effects. Adverse effects commonly seen with asenapine may include somnolence, dizziness, and akathisia. Somnolence is the most commonly occurring side effect. Asenapine has shown little effect on metabolic parameters and weight change. Recently, labeling for asenapine was modified to alert clinicians regarding the occurrence of hypersensitivity reactions, including anaphylaxis and angioedema.[31]

▶ Lurasidone

Lurasidone is indicated for the treatment of adults with schizophrenia. Lurasidone's effectiveness for longer term use (greater than 6 weeks) has not yet been established, so healthcare professionals prescribing lurasidone for extended periods of time should periodically evaluate long-term usefulness for each individual patient. Lurasidone's mechanism of action, like most SGA, is thought to be D_2 and $5HT_{2A}$ receptors. Lurasidone also has moderate affinity as antagonist at α_{2C} and is a partial agonist at $5HT_{1A}$ and antagonist at α_{2A}-receptors. Lurasidone's efficacy for the short-term treatment of acute schizophrenia has been established. Prescribing information recommends starting lurasidone at a dose of 40-mg tablet once daily, and initial dose titration is not required. The maximum recommended dose of lurasidone is 80 mg once daily; doses greater than 80 mg/day do not appear to add great benefit, and may be associated with an increase in certain side effects. Lurasidone should be taken with food. Adverse reactions reported in at least 5% of patients (and at least twice the placebo rate) include somnolence, akathisia, nausea, parkinsonism, and agitation. Lurasidone has shown only small effect on weight, and minimal changes in other metabolic parameters.[31]

Patient Encounter, Part 3

KH is hospitalized and prescribed risperidone, titrated to 6 mg/day. After 6 weeks, her sleep pattern has normalized, her irritability and agitation have decreased, she is less preoccupied by the feeling that others can read her thoughts, and her auditory hallucinations of the "spirits" have decreased significantly, so that she is able to ignore them and no longer follows their advice. She is discharged from the hospital and returns home with her parents. Unfortunately, KH misses her first follow-up appointment at the outpatient clinic, and she is not seen again until 2 months after discharge. When she comes in for this appointment, it is apparent that KH is having trouble. She's pacing around the room, stating that she is so restless that she cannot sit still, which started happening a few days ago. Apparently, KH started skipping doses of risperidone last month, after another patient told her it could "mess with my reproduction." Her symptoms started getting worse last week, and her mother, after finding out about the skipped doses, made KH start doubling the prescribed dose of risperidone. It is thought that she's been taking 12 mg of risperidone for the past 5 days.

How would a clinician address KH's ideas that risperidone could "mess with her reproduction?"

What is the basis for this information told to her by another patient?

What side effect is KH currently experiencing, and why?

First-Generation (Typical) Antipsychotics

The FGAs are high-affinity D_2-receptor antagonists. During chronic treatment, these agents block 65% to 80% of D_2 receptors in the striatum and block dopamine receptors in the other dopamine tracts in the brain as well.[32] Clinical response is generally associated with 60% D_2-receptor blockade, but 70% and 80% are associated with hyperprolactinemia and EPS, respectively. This group of antipsychotics was widely used from the 1950s to the 1990s, when the SGAs began to replace these agents as first-line therapy.

Dosages for these agents are frequently given as chlorpromazine equivalent dosages, which are defined as the dosage of any of the FGAs equipotent with 100 mg of chlorpromazine. The target dose recommendation for acute psychosis is 400 to 600 chlorpromazine equivalents unless the patient's history indicates that this dose may result in intolerable side effects. Generally, maintenance therapy should provide a dose of 300 to 600 chlorpromazine equivalents for maximum efficacy. Information on dosing and available dosage forms is provided in Table 37–4. All FGAs are equally efficacious in groups of patients when used in equipotent doses. However, individual variation does occur, such that a patient may not respond equally to each antipsychotic. Selection of a particular antipsychotic should be based on patient variables, such as the need to avoid certain side effects or drug–drug interactions or previous patient or family history of response.

▶ Decanoates

Long-acting, depot preparations are available for two FGAs (fluphenazine decanoate and haloperidol decanoate) in the United States. These compounds are esterified antipsychotics formulated in sesame seed oil for deep intramuscular (IM) injection. Because these are long-acting preparations, patients should be exposed to the oral form of the drug first to ensure tolerability. With initial dosing of haloperidol decanoate, oral supplementation may temporarily be necessary because the drug accumulates over many weeks, not reaching steady state until 4 to 5 dosing intervals have elapsed. The pharmacokinetic profiles of the depot agents are useful parameters for strategic dosing. Patients may be dosed with fluphenazine decanoate on a 1- to 3-week interval, but haloperidol decanoate is usually dosed once a month. Conversion from oral to depot and maintenance dosing recommendations are shown in Table 37–5. Based on these recommendations, a reasonable estimate is that 12.5 mg (0.5 mL) of fluphenazine decanoate given every 2 weeks is approximately equivalent to 10 mg/day of fluphenazine orally. A maintenance haloperidol decanoate dose of 150 mg every 4 weeks is approximately equivalent to 10 mg/day of oral haloperidol. Initial decanoate injections should be preceded by a small test dose.

Side Effects of the First-Generation Antipsychotics

The FGAs are associated with a host of side effects that largely differ between high- and low-potency agents. In general, the low-potency agents are less likely to cause EPS than the high-potency agents. Of note, lower equivalent doses and midpotency agents may be associated with less EPS than once believed and similar to SGAs in clinical trials.[14]

The FGAs are associated with EPS, including akathisia (motor or subjective restlessness), dystonia (muscle spasm), and pseudoparkinsonism (akinesia, tremor, and rigidity). These fairly common motor side effects are caused by dopamine antagonism in the nigrostriatal pathways. Akathisia is the most frequently occurring motor side effect, with approximately 20% to 40% of people treated with FGA drugs experiencing it. Roughly half of the cases of akathisia present within 1 month of antipsychotic initiation, although the onset of akathisia many times may be within 5 to 10 days after the first dose or increase in dosage. Younger people

Table 37–4

First-Generation (Typical) Antipsychotics[a]

Class	Agent (Brand Name)	Dosage Range (mg/day)	Chlorpromazine Equivalents (mg)	Available Formulations
Butyrophenone	Haloperidol (Haldol)	5–30	2	T, LC, I
Dibenzoxazepine	Loxapine (Loxitane)	25–100	10	C
Diphenylbutylpiperidine	Pimozide (Orap)	1–10	1–2	T
Indole	Molindone (Moban)	25–100	10	T
Phenothiazines	Chlorpromazine (Thorazine)	300–800	100	T, LC, I, R
	Fluphenazine (Prolixin)	2–40	2	T, L, I
	Perphenazine (Trilafon)	8–64	10	T, LC
	Thioridazine (Mellaril)	300–800	100	T, LC
	Trifluoperazine (Stelazine)	15–30	5	T
Thioxanthenes	Thiothixene (Navane)	5–40	4	C

[a]Low-potency antipsychotics include thioridazine, mesoridazine, and chlorpromazine. High-potency antipsychotics include haloperidol, fluphenazine, thiothixene, and pimozide.

C, capsule; C-SR, controlled or sustained release; I, injection; L, liquid solution, elixir, or suspension; LC, liquid concentrate, R, rectal suppository; T, tablet.

Table 37–5

Antipsychotic Dosing of Long-Acting Preparations

Drug	Starting Dose	Maintenance Dose	Comments
Haloperidol decanoate	20 × oral haloperidol daily dose; in the elderly use 10–15 × oral haloperidol daily dose Generally 100–450 mg/mo Initial dose should not exceed 100 mg regardless of previous dose requirements (if more than 100 mg, give 3–7 days apart)	10–15 × oral haloperidol daily dose, generally 50–300 mg/mo	With initial dosing, oral supplementation may temporarily be necessary; deep IM injection generally with 21-gauge needle; maximum volume per injection site should not exceed 3 mL Available in 50 and 100 mg/mL (5-mL vials and 1-mL ampules)
Fluphenazine decanoate	1.2 × oral fluphenazine daily dose; generally 12.5–mg/2–3 weeks	Based on starting dose and clinical response Generally 12.5–25 mg dosed at 2–4-wk intervals (may be up to 6 weeks in some cases)	Can be administered IM or SC; 21-gauge needle, must be dry Should not exceed 100 mg; when dosing above 50 mg, should increase in increments of 12.5 mg Available in 25 mg/mL (5-mL vials)
Olanzapine (Zyprexa Relprevv)	To target oral 10 mg/day dose: Either 210 mg/2 wk or 405 mg/4 wk during first 8 wk To target oral 15 mg/day dose: 300 mg/2 wk for first 8 wk To target 20 mg/day oral dose: 300 mg/2 wk	To target oral 10 mg/day dose: after 8 wk, give 150 mg/2 wk or 300 mg/4 wk To target oral 15 mg/day dose: after 8 wk, 210 mg/2 wk or 405 mg/4 wk To target 20 mg/day oral dose: continue with 300 mg/2 wk	Gluteal injection, 19-gauge needle Do not confuse with rapid-acting IM injection Must reconstitute with included diluent Measure amount to inject from vial (there will be remaining suspension in vial) 3-hour observation period; patient must be accompanied to destination No refrigeration needed
Paliperidone (Invega Sustenna)	Initiate with 234 mg on day 1 and 156 mg 1 wk later, both in deltoid muscle	Recommended monthly maintenance dose is 117 mg (range, 39–234 mg)	First two doses must be given in the deltoid muscle; after that, monthly doses given in either the deltoid or gluteal muscle; available as 39-, 78-, 117-, 156-, and 234-mg prefilled syringes
Risperidone long-acting injection (Risperdal Consta)	25 mg every 2 wk	25–50 mg every 2 wk	Previous antipsychotics should be continued for 3 wk after initial dose of risperidone long-acting injection Recommended to establish tolerability with oral risperidone prior to initiation of long-acting injection Available in 12.5-, 25-, 37.5-, and 50-mg vial/kit; must use needle supplied with kit, administer IM

IM, intramuscular; SC, subcutaneous.

and those taking high doses of high-potency antipsychotics are at greater risk for the development of akathisia. Acute dystonic reactions are abrupt in onset and are usually seen within 24 to 96 hours after a first dose or increase in dosage. Characteristic signs and symptoms include abnormal positioning or spasm of the muscles of the head, neck, limbs, or trunk. Dystonia may occur in 10% to 20% of patients. There is higher risk for dystonia in young male patients and those taking high-potency FGAs. Pseudoparkinsonism resembles idiopathic Parkinson's disease, and features may be present in up to 30% to 60% of people treated with FGAs. The onset of symptoms is usually seen within 1 to 2 weeks after initiation of dosing or a dose increase. Risk factors include older age, female gender, high doses, and possibly those with depressive symptoms.[33]

Tardive dyskinesia is a movement disorder characterized by abnormal choreiform (rapid, objectively purposeless, irregular, and spontaneous movement) and athetoid (slow and irregular) movements occurring late in onset in relation to initiation of antipsychotic therapy. This adverse effect usually develops over several months or after at least 3 months of cumulative exposure to antipsychotic medications. The severity of TD can range from mild and barely noticeable to severe, with interference with ambulation. TD may stigmatize persons taking antipsychotics if symptoms are visible to others. The estimated average prevalence of TD is 20% with a range of 13% to 36%. The incidence of new cases per treatment year with FGAs is approximately 5%.[34] TD is reversible in one-third to half of cases with the cessation of the antipsychotic.[35] When the antipsychotic is tapered or discontinued, there is typically an initial worsening of abnormal movements. Risk factors for TD include older age; longer duration of antipsychotic treatment; and presence of EPS, substance abuse, and mood disorders. SGAs carry a lower risk of TD than FGAs. A pooled analysis of studies indicated that new-onset TD incidence was 0.8% per year with SGA treatment versus 5.4% per year for FGAs.[15] A more recent review of studies published from 2004 to

Table 37–6

Side Effects of First-Generation Antipsychotics

	EPS	Sedation	Anticholinergic Side Effects	Cardiovascular Side Effects	Seizure Effects/QTc Prolongation
Chlorpromazine	++	++++	+++	++++	++
Thioridazine	++	++++	++++	++++	+++
Loxapine	+++	+++	++	+++	+
Trifluoperazine	+++	++	++	++	+
Molindone	++	+	++	++	+
Perphenazine	+++	++	++	++	+
Thiothixene	+++	++	++	++	+
Fluphenazine	++++	++	++	++	+
Haloperidol	++++	+	+	+	+

+, very low; ++, low; +++, moderate; ++++, high; EPS, extrapyramidal side effects.

2008 reported a smaller difference in incidence of TD between agents at 3.9% for SGAs and 5.5% for FGAs.[36]

Neuroleptic malignant syndrome (NMS), a life-threatening emergency characterized by severe muscular rigidity, autonomic instability, and altered consciousness, can occur uncommonly with all the FGAs and may also occur with SGAs. Rapid dose escalation, the use of high-potency FGAs at higher doses, and younger patients are associated with a higher risk of NMS. When NMS is diagnosed or suspected, antipsychotics should be discontinued and supportive and symptomatic treatment begun (e.g., antipyretics, cooling blanket, intravenous fluids, oxygen, monitoring of liver enzymes, and complete blood cell count). Dopamine agonists (e.g., bromocriptine) should be considered in moderate to severe cases.

Additionally, dermatologic side effects, photosensitivity, and cataracts may occur with the phenothiazine agents. Sedation is mediated by H_1-receptor antagonism; anticholinergic side effects (constipation, blurred vision, dry mouth, and urinary retention) are caused from M_1-receptor antagonism; and α_1-receptor blockade is associated with orthostatic hypotension and tachycardia (Table 37–6). QTc prolongation may occur with the lower potency FGAs, and thioridazine has a black box warning for QTc prolongation.

Treatment Guidelines and Algorithms

Because of the plethora of choices and the rising costs of SGAs, algorithms and treatment and consensus guidelines have been developed for the treatment of schizophrenia. One widely accepted algorithm in the United States was developed as part of the Texas Implementation of Medication Algorithms (TIMA). A national panel of experts developed this algorithm, most recently updated in 2006.[37] Algorithms go beyond guidelines, providing a framework for clinical decision making at critical decision points. According to the TIMA schizophrenia algorithm, the SGAs (except clozapine) should be used as first-line treatment. The choice of SGA is guided by consideration of the side effect profiles and the clinical characteristics of the patient. Treatment with a given drug should be continued for 4 to 6 weeks to assess

response. If only partial response or nonresponse is noted, a trial of a second SGA should be initiated (Fig. 37–1). Other similar guidelines include the APA Practice Guidelines for schizophrenia,[8] the Expert Consensus Guideline Series,[9] and the 2009 Schizophrenia Patient Outcomes Research Team (PORT) Treatment Recommendations.[38] In contrast to the TIMA guidelines, the PORT recommends either the use of FGAs or SGAs as first-line therapy.

Treatment Adherence

Medication nonadherence in schizophrenia is common and often associated with symptom relapse.[39] Estimates of nonadherence to antipsychotics range from approximately 24% to 88% with a mean of approximately 50%. Subjects who are nonadherent have approximately a fourfold greater risk of a relapse than those who are adherent. Adherence to antipsychotic regimens is problematic for many reasons. Neurocognitive deficits and paranoid symptoms may hamper adherence, and identification of nonadherence by caretakers and providers can be challenging. Frequently, there is no obvious connection between nonadherence and symptom exacerbation because there may be no immediate consequences of missing a dose, and patients may relapse suddenly after several weeks or months of nonadherence. The antipsychotic side effects such as EPS, weight gain, and sexual dysfunction are also a major contributing factor to treatment nonadherence. Several other factors associated with nonadherence include delusions, substance abuse, and deficit symptoms.[40] For patients who have relapsed several times because of nonadherence, have a history of dangerous behavior, or risk a significant loss of social or vocational gains when relapsed, treatment with long-acting formulations should be encouraged. Risperidone, paliperidone, and olanzapine are all available as long-acting formulations (Table 37–5).

Special Populations

▶ Dosing in Renal and Hepatic Impairment

See Table 37–7 for dosing guidance on specific antipsychotic medications.

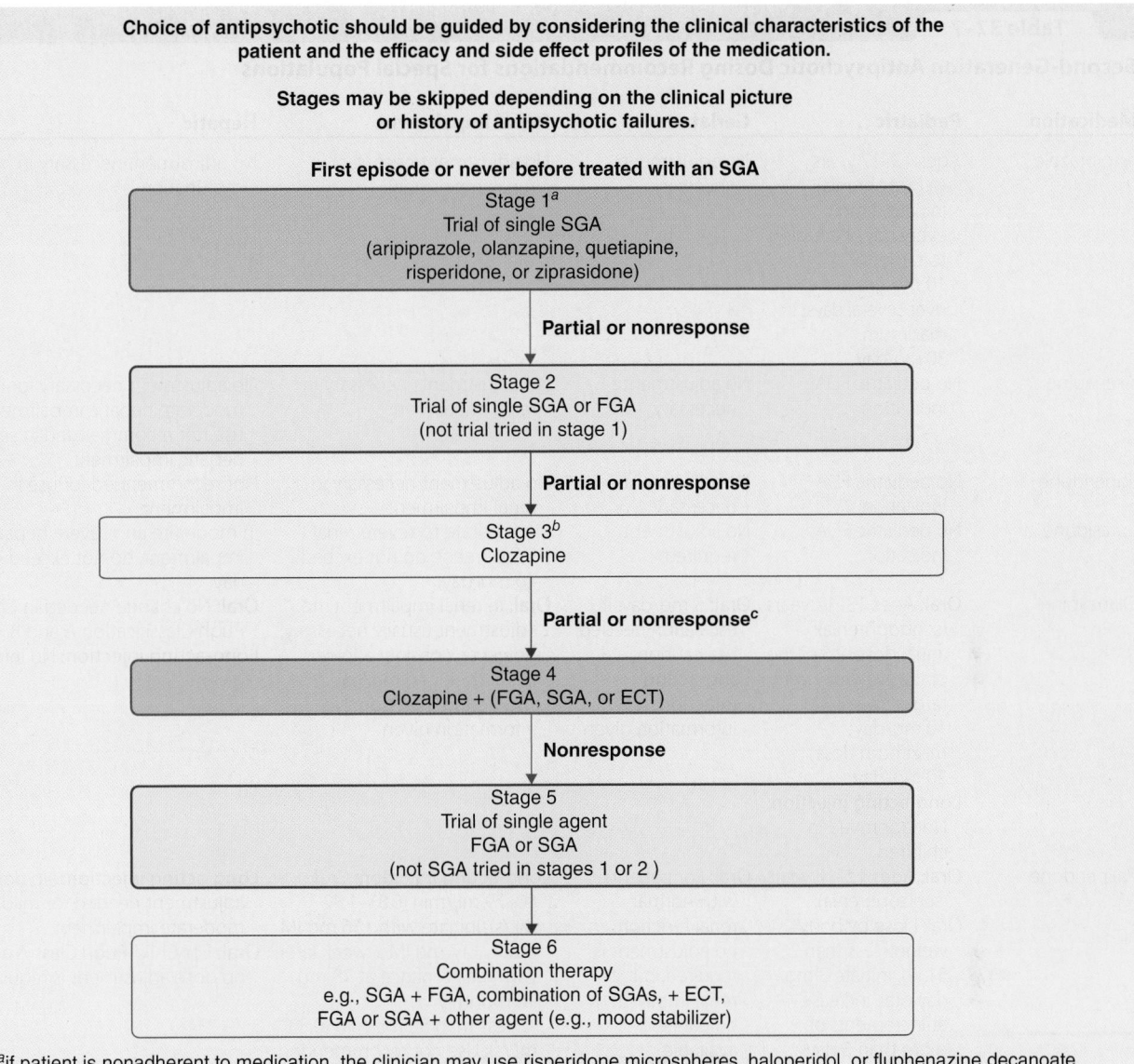

Choice of antipsychotic should be guided by considering the clinical characteristics of the patient and the efficacy and side effect profiles of the medication.

Stages may be skipped depending on the clinical picture or history of antipsychotic failures.

First episode or never before treated with an SGA

Stage 1[a]
Trial of single SGA
(aripiprazole, olanzapine, quetiapine, risperidone, or ziprasidone)

Partial or nonresponse

Stage 2
Trial of single SGA or FGA
(not trial tried in stage 1)

Partial or nonresponse

Stage 3[b]
Clozapine

Partial or nonresponse[c]

Stage 4
Clozapine + (FGA, SGA, or ECT)

Nonresponse

Stage 5
Trial of single agent
FGA or SGA
(not SGA tried in stages 1 or 2)

Stage 6
Combination therapy
e.g., SGA + FGA, combination of SGAs, + ECT,
FGA or SGA + other agent (e.g., mood stabilizer)

[a]if patient is nonadherent to medication, the clinician may use risperidone microspheres, haloperidol, or fluphenazine decanoate at any stage, but should carefully assess side effects.
[b]May consider earlier trial of clozapine if history of recurrent suicidality, violence, comorbid substance abuse, or persistent positive symptoms >2 years. If persistent positive symptoms >5 years, clozapine trial independent of number of preceding trials.
[c]Evaluate patient for other underlying or concomitant factors; consider adding cognitive behavioral therapy and other psychosocial interventions.

FIGURE 37–1. Texas Implementation of Medication Algorithms (TIMA) algorithm for antipsychotic treatment in schizophrenia. Choice of antipsychotic should be guided by considering the clinical characteristics of the patient and the efficacy and side effect profiles of the medication. Any stage may be skipped depending on the clinical picture or history of antipsychotic failures. (ECT, electroconvulsive therapy; FGA, first-generation antipsychotic; SGA, second-generation antipsychotic.) (Adapted from the Texas Department of State Health Services.)

▶ Children and Adolescents

Epidemiologic data show that 10% to 30% of patients with schizophrenia develop their first psychotic symptoms before their 18th birthday. The diagnosis of schizophrenia in children and adolescents is often difficult to make, and the differential diagnosis includes pervasive developmental disorders, attention-deficit hyperactivity disorder, and language or communication disorders. The existence of prominent hallucinations or delusions, however, helps make the diagnosis because they are not a prominent part of the other disorders. Fifty-four percent to 90% of patients developing schizophrenia before age 18 years have premorbid abnormalities such as withdrawal, odd traits, and isolation.[41]

Treatment for psychotic children and adolescents ideally involves an intensive and comprehensive program with a highly structured environment that includes special education and psychoeducation. Day treatment, hospitalization, or long-term residential treatment may be necessary. Pharmacologic treatment is indicated if psychotic symptoms

Table 37–7

Second-Generation Antipsychotic Dosing Recommendations for Special Populations

Medication	Pediatric	Geriatric	Renal Impairment	Hepatic
Aripiprazole	Ages 13–17 years (schizophrenia): Initiate 2 mg every day, increasing to target of 10 mg gradually over several days; maximum, 30 mg/day	No adjustment necessary	No adjustment necessary in renal impairment	No adjustment necessary in hepatic dysfunction
Asenapine	No pediatric FDA indication	No adjustment necessary	No adjustments necessary in renal impairment	No adjustment necessary for mild to moderate hepatic impairment, but use not recommended in severe hepatic impairment
Iloperidone	No pediatric FDA indication	No adjustment necessary	No adjustment necessary in renal impairment	Not recommended for use in hepatic impairment
Lurasidone	No pediatric FDA indication	No adjustment required	In moderate to severe renal impairment, do not exceed 40 mg/day	In moderate and severe hepatic impairment, do not exceed 40 mg/day
Olanzapine	**Oral:** Ages 13–17 years (schizophrenia): Initial dose, 2.5–5 mg orally every day with target dose of 10 mg/day; maximum dose, 20 mg/day **Long-acting injection:** Not approved in children	**Oral:** 5 mg/day, if escalation needed use caution **Long-acting injection:** No information given	**Oral:** In renal impairment, no adjustment usually necessary; however, consider a lower initial dose of 5 mg/day **Long-acting injection:** No information given	**Oral:** No change needed in Childs Pugh Classification A and B **Long-acting injection:** No information given
Paliperidone	**Oral:** Ages 12–17 years (schizophrenia): Oral: Dose by body weight: less than 51 kg, initiate 3 mg/day oral, increase at increments of more than 5 days; maximum, 6 mg/day At least 51 kg/day, initiate at 3 mg/day, increase at increments of more than 5 days, maximum of 12 mg/day	**Oral:** For patients with normal renal function, no adjustment is required, but if renal impairment guidance is available	**Long-acting injection:** CrCl 50–79 mL/min (0.83–1.32 mL/s); initiate with 156 mg IM day 1, 117 mg IM 1 week later, with maintenance at 78 mg IM monthly CrCl less than 50 mL/min (0.83 mL/s): Use not recommended **Oral:** CrCl 50–79 mL/min (0.83–1.32 mL/s): 3 mg once daily initiation, maximum 6 mg/day CrCl between 10 and 49 mL/min (0.17–0.82 mL/s): 1.5 mg once daily initiation; maximum, 3 mg/day CrCl less than 10 mL/min (0.17 mL/s): Use is not recommended	**Long-acting injection:** No dosage adjustment needed for mild or moderate impairment **Oral:** For Child-Pugh Class A and B, no dose adjustment is required
Quetiapine	**Regular-release tablets ONLY:** Indicated for schizophrenia (ages 13–17 years): Initiate 50 mg/day on day 1; may increase to 400 mg gradually by day 5 administered as 2–3 doses; recommended 400–800 mg/day; maximum, 800 mg/day	**Regular-release tablets:** Slower dose escalation and a lower target dose **Extended-release tablets:** Initiate at 50 mg/day and increase at 50-mg/day increments based on response or tolerance	No dosing recommendations for renal dysfunction	**Regular-release tablets:** Initiate at 25 mg/day, increasing daily in amounts of 25–50 mg/day to effective dose **Extended-release tablets:** Should be initiated with 50 mg/day, increasing in 50-mg/day increments

(Continued)

Table 37–7

Second-Generation Antipsychotic Dosing Recommendations for Special Populations *(Continued)*

Medication	Pediatric	Geriatric	Renal Impairment	Hepatic
Risperidone	Oral: Pediatric ages 13 years and older (schizophrenia): Initiate at 0.5 mg orally daily, adjusting at intervals of at least 24 hours and in increments of 0.5–1 mg/day as tolerated Recommended target dose, 3 mg/day	Long-acting IM: Initial dose, 25 mg IM every 2 wk with a 3-week oral crossover Oral: Initiate at 0.5 mg twice daily; may increase by 0.5 mg twice daily, increases above 1.5 mg twice daily done at intervals of at least 1 week	Long-acting IM: Patients with renal impairment should receive titrated doses of oral risperidone before initiation of IM (more detail in prescribing information) Oral: Recommended initial dose in severe renal impairment, 0.5 mg twice daily; dose may be increased by 0.5 mg twice daily, but increases above 1.5 mg twice daily should be done at intervals of at least 1 week	Long-acting IM: Titrate with oral risperidone (see renal dosing) Oral: Recommended initiation in severe hepatic impairment (see renal dosing)
Ziprasidone	No pediatric indication	No official adjustment recommended	Oral doses: No adjustment necessary for mild to moderate renal impairment IM doses: Use with caution because of cyclodextrin sodium excipient	No adjustment necessary for mild to moderate hepatic impairment

CrCl, creatinine clearance; FDA, Food and Drug Administration; IM, intramuscular.

cause significant impairments or interfere with other interventions. Children and adolescents are more vulnerable to EPS, particularly dystonias, than are adults. Because of concerns about EPS and TD, it has been recommended that pharmacotherapy in children and adolescents should be initiated with SGAs. Aripiprazole, risperidone, quetiapine, and paliperidone are indicated by the Food and Drug Administration (FDA) for the treatment of schizophrenia in varying ages of pediatric populations. Recommended initiation and target dosing is lower for adolescents than adults.

Agents with significant sedation and anticholinergic side effects are not preferred because they can cause attention difficulties and cognitive dulling that may interfere with optimal school performance. Compared with adults, children and adolescents tend to gain more weight when taking these agents. Young patients should be started on lower doses than adults and should be titrated at a slower rate. Side effects should be monitored closely during initiation and throughout maintenance therapy. Informed consent, addressing the rationale for treatment and potential risks and benefits of therapy, should be obtained from the parents or guardians before treatment with any antipsychotic medication, and assent should be obtained from the child as well.

▶ Elderly

Psychotic symptoms in late life (after 65 years of age) are generally a result of an ongoing chronic illness carried over from younger life; however, a small percentage of patients develop psychotic symptoms de novo, defined as late-life schizophrenia. However, other illnesses presenting with psychotic symptoms are common in this population; approximately one-third of patients with Alzheimer's disease, Parkinson's disease,

and vascular dementia experience psychotic symptoms. The majority of data for antipsychotic use in the elderly comes from experience treating these other disease states.

Antipsychotics can be safe and effective for the treatment of psychosis in the elderly, if used at lower doses than those commonly used in younger adults. Older adults are particularly vulnerable to the side effects of the FGAs. Parkinsonian symptoms reportedly occur in more than 50% of all elderly patients receiving these agents, and the cumulative annual incidence of TD in middle-aged and elderly patients is greater than 25%. With the SGAs, the risk of TD appears to be approximately 4%. However, these numbers are based on limited data, and future investigations are likely to yield more specific information regarding TD risk with the SGAs.[42] The likelihood of reversing this potentially debilitating condition diminishes with age.

Orthostasis, estimated to occur in 5% to 30% of geriatric patients, is a major contributing factor to falls that often leads to fractures, injuries, and loss of independence. Low-potency antipsychotics and clozapine are more likely to cause significant drops in orthostatic blood pressure. Antipsychotics may cause or worsen anticholinergic effects, including constipation, dry mouth, urinary retention, and cognitive impairment. Cognitive impairment may lead to decreased independence, and a more rapid decline in cognitive functioning may occur in the elderly treated with antipsychotics than in the younger adult population. As a result of data showing a statistically significant increase in mortality rate in elderly dementia patients who are treated with SGAs, a warning was added in 2005, and this warning was extended to include all antipsychotics, FGA and SGA, as of 2008, when the results of two epidemiological studies suggested that the risk for FGA was comparable to or higher than those for SGA. Because all antipsychotics now carry a warning, patients and families should be informed of this risk before treatment with these agents in patients with dementia. Dosing in the elderly is initiated lower, and titration is slower than in younger adults. Maximum doses are often half of adult doses. See Table 37–7 for specific dosing information for certain antipsychotics.

▶ Dually Diagnosed Patients

The prevalence of substance dependence and abuse among persons with schizophrenia is significantly higher than in the general population. Estimates of the proportion of schizophrenic patients abusing alcohol and/or illicit drugs range from 40% to 60%.[43] The most common drugs of abuse are cannabis, cocaine, and alcohol. Unfortunately, substance use often worsens the course and complicates the treatment of schizophrenia. Dually diagnosed patients are more likely to be nonadherent with treatment. Characteristically, they have a poorer response rate to the FGAs, have more severe psychosis, and have higher rates of relapse and rehospitalization than patients who are not abusing substances. EPS may occur more frequently in substance-abusing patients, and alcohol use is a risk factor for developing TD. A growing body of literature indicates that the SGAs are effective in this population, and some studies have shown a reduction in the use of drugs and alcohol with the SGAs.[44]

▶ Treatment-Resistant Patients

For approximately 20% to 30% of people with schizophrenia, drug treatment is ineffective. A standard definition of treatment resistance is persistent positive symptoms despite treatment with at least two different antipsychotics given at adequate doses (a dose equivalent to at least 600 mg of chlorpromazine) for an adequate duration (4 to 6 weeks). In addition, patients must have a moderately severe illness as defined by rating instruments, and have a persistence of illness for at least 5 years.[45] These patients are often highly symptomatic and require extensive periods of hospital care.

Clozapine To date, clozapine remains the only drug with proven and superior efficacy in treatment-resistant patients, and it is currently the only drug approved for treatment-resistant schizophrenia. Studies have shown a response of approximately 30% to 50% in treatment-resistant patients. Clinical trials have consistently found clozapine superior to traditional antipsychotics for treatment-refractory patients, and it is efficacious even after nonresponse to other SGAs and in partially responsive patients. It is often effective even in those who have had a poor response to other medication for years. Recent studies have demonstrated that it has a beneficial effect for aggression and suicidality, which led to the FDA approval for the treatment of suicidal behavior in people with psychosis.[46]

To date, it has not been elucidated what pharmacologic properties of clozapine contribute to its superior efficacy. Clozapine has a low affinity for D_2 receptors, blocks D_1 receptors, and is a 5-HT$_{2A}$ antagonist. Its unsurpassed efficacy suggests that there is a neuropharmacologic effect associated with clozapine that to date is unique to this agent.

Clozapine's use is limited by its association with the rare but life-threatening risk of agranulocytosis. Other side effects include seizures, as well as common unpleasant side effects, including sedation, enuresis, anticholinergic effects, weight gain, and hypersalivation. The long-term hematologic monitoring (see monitoring section) required for prevention of agranulocytosis can be a barrier for both patients and care providers. The optimal plasma level of clozapine is a minimum trough level of 300 to 350 ng/mL (300 to 350 mcg/L or 0.92 to 1.07 μmol/L or 918 to 1,071 nmol/L), usually corresponding to a daily dose of 200 to 400 mg, although dosage must be individualized. According to published guidelines and recommendations, clozapine should be considered after two failed antipsychotic trials but may be considered sooner if the individual patient situation warrants.[37]

Other Strategies Approximately 30% of patients treated with clozapine will not respond, and another 30% will have only a partial response to the drug. Treatment options with other medications are limited after clozapine nonresponse. For these patients, the best evidence points to augmentation using an FGA, SGA, or electroconvulsive therapy (ECT). The only available data support the combination of clozapine with risperidone, clozapine with lamotrigine, or clozapine with aripiprazole; however, controlled trial results are mixed. Other potential strategies include combining antipsychotics with mood stabilizers (e.g., lithium, valproate, and topiramate) or antidepressants (mirtazapine).[37]

▶ Acutely Psychotic Patients

Psychiatric emergencies occur in a variety of settings, including emergency departments, psychiatric units, medical facilities, and outpatient settings. Although verbal interventions are recommended as initial interventions, most psychiatric emergencies require both pharmacologic and psychological interventions. Often, the psychiatrist must make decisions based on limited information and history. IM formulations are available for a number of FGAs and three SGAs (aripiprazole, ziprasidone, and olanzapine). These formulations are safe and effective in treating patients with acute psychosis. These SGAs are now recommended as first-line therapy in agitated schizophrenia patients; however, IM lorazepam with or without concomitant oral (tablets, liquid, or disintegrating tablets) SGAs are also used. Concomitant olanzapine and benzodiazepines may cause orthostasis. High doses of FGAs, termed *rapid neuroleptization*, is no longer recommended.

▶ Pregnancy and Lactation

When to use antipsychotics in pregnancy and during lactation remains a complicated decision based on a careful analysis of risks and benefits. Women with schizophrenia, even those who are unmedicated, have a significantly greater risk for stillbirth, infant death, preterm delivery, low infant birth weight, and infants who are small for gestational age. A labeling change for antipsychotic medications has been implemented by the FDA in order to address the potential risk for EPS and symptoms of withdrawal in newborns whose mothers were treated with antipsychotics in the third trimester of pregnancy. Symptoms may include agitation, abnormal muscle tone, tremor (increased or decreased), sleepiness, and difficulty in breathing or feeding, and they may last for hours to days after delivery. In some newborns, symptoms do not require specific treatment, but in other situations, longer hospital stays may be required.

Women who experience a relapse in psychotic symptoms during pregnancy are at the greatest risk for birth complications.[47] Because risks related to psychotic relapse may be more detrimental than antipsychotic treatment to both the mother and baby, antipsychotics are often continued during this period. Women treated with antipsychotics who become pregnant should not discontinue use of these agents without consulting their healthcare professionals.

Essentially all antipsychotic medications pass through the placenta. Both FGAs and SGAs may be associated with an increased risk of neonatal complications. High-potency FGAs are associated with a low risk for congenital abnormalities; however, limb defects and dyskinesias have been reported.[48] Low-potency phenothiazine antipsychotics may increase the risk of congenital abnormalities when used in the first trimester. According to the relevant literature published to date, there appears to be little risk associated with the first-line SGAs.[49] Long-term neurobehavioral studies of children

exposed to SGAs in utero have not yet been done, however, and certain FGA agents may be preferred in drug-naïve pregnant patients because of a larger reproductive safety profile and cumulative exposure data. If pregnancy occurs during antipsychotic treatment, however, continuation of previous therapy should be considered preferential. On the basis of available data, generalization is impossible, and each case and specific antipsychotic should be weighed on an individual basis. Although SGAs are excreted in breast milk, most case reports have reported a low frequency of deleterious effects on the infant. Women taking SGAs may have enhanced fertility compared with women taking FGAs because the SGAs (except risperidone and paliperidone) are less likely to cause prolactin elevations leading to anovulation. Therefore, careful discussion with patients, including education about birth control, must occur.

Pharmacokinetics

Pharmacokinetic and pharmacodynamic issues are not generally a major concern with antipsychotic treatment; however, additive side effects may occur with combined treatment, and a few clinically significant drug interactions are notable (Table 37–8). In addition, cigarette smoking can cause significant interactions with the metabolism of certain antipsychotics by induction of CYP1A2 (clozapine, olanzapine). All of the antipsychotics are highly protein bound; however, protein-binding interactions are generally not clinically significant. Absorption of most antipsychotics is not affected by food, with the exception of lurasidone and ziprasidone. The mean maximum concentration of

Table 37–8

Metabolism and Drug Interactions With Antipsychotics

Antipsychotic	Major CYP450 Metabolic Enzyme	Other CYP450 Metabolic Pathways	Increase Antipsychotic Concentrations	Decrease Antipsychotic Concentrations
Aripiprazole	3A3/4	2D6	Fluvoxamine, ketoconazole	Carbamazepine
Asenapine	Glucuronidation by UGT1A4 and CYP 1A2	3A4, 2D6	Fluvoxamine	
Clozapine	1A2	3A3/4, 2D6, 2C19	Fluvoxamine, ciprofloxacin, paroxetine	Cigarette smoking
Haloperidol	2D6, 3A3/4		Fluvoxamine, fluoxetine, ketoconazole	Carbamazepine
Iloperidone	2D6, 3A4		Ketoconazole, fluoxetine, paroxetine	
Lurasidone	3A4		Ketoconazole, diltiazem	Rifampin
Olanzapine	1A2	2D6	Fluvoxamine, ciprofloxacin, paroxetine	Cigarette smoking
Paliperidone	2D6, 3A4 (in vitro, but limited role in vivo)		Divalproex sodium, paroxetine	Carbamazepine (via increased renal elimination)
Perphenazine	2D6		Fluvoxamine, fluoxetine, paroxetine	
Quetiapine	3A3/4	2D6	Fluvoxamine, ketoconazole	Carbamazepine
Risperidone	2D6	3A3/4	Fluoxetine, paroxetine	Carbamazepine
Thioridazine	2D6	1A2	Fluvoxamine	Cigarette smoking
Ziprasidone	3A3/4		Fluvoxamine, ketoconazole	Carbamazepine

CYP450, cytochrome P-450 isoenzyme.

lurasidone increases threefold when administered with food, and ziprasidone's absorption is increased by 60% to 70% when given with meals.

All antipsychotics are, at least to some extent, metabolized by hepatic microsomal enzymes to water-soluble compounds that are excreted by the kidneys. Table 37–8 lists the primary metabolic enzymes and some potential drug interactions for the antipsychotic medications. Clinicians should assess the clinical impact of the addition or discontinuation of these drugs in individual patients and should make appropriate adjustments when necessary. Unlike the other antipsychotics, ziprasidone is mostly metabolized by aldehyde oxidase, a metabolic system independent of the CYP450 system. Paliperidone, the 9-hydroxy metabolite of risperidone, is mostly excreted unchanged in the urine, although up to one-third may be metabolized. Another recent discovery in metabolism of antipsychotics and their distribution involves the transmembrane energy-dependent efflux transporter, P-glycoprotein. This may limit the ability of a number of drugs to penetrate the blood–brain barrier and therefore impact pharmacologic activity in the brain.[50] Antipsychotics currently known to use this pathway include perphenazine, haloperidol, fluphenazine, quetiapine, risperidone, and olanzapine.[51]

Because of its propensity to cause prolongation of the QTc interval, the use of ziprasidone with other agents that prolong the QTc interval should be avoided. These other agents include, but are not limited to, antiarrhythmic medications such as quinidine and sotalol, certain FGAs (chlorpromazine, droperidol, mesoridazine, pimozide, and thioridazine), and certain antibiotics (e.g., gatifloxacin, halofantrine, mefloquine, moxifloxacin, and pentamidine). Ziprasidone has not been shown to have clinically significant drug interactions with the CYP4503A3/4 inhibitors regarding increasing the QTc; however, higher doses, especially given with inhibitors of CYP4503A3/4 (e.g., ketoconazole and erythromycin), should be used cautiously. The use of quetiapine with other agents that prolong the QTc interval should also be avoided. Clinicians should also be vigilant to avoid pharmacodynamic interactions with any of the antipsychotics involving additive side effects from combination therapies. Side effects that may be worsened with combination therapies include sedation, hypotension, anticholinergic symptoms, and weight gain or metabolic abnormalities.

Adjunct Pharmacologic Treatments

The judicious use of pharmacologic therapies other than antipsychotics is often necessary in the treatment of patients with schizophrenia. Concomitant medications may be indicated for the treatment of motor side effects, anxiety, depression, mood elevation, and possibly refractory psychotic symptoms. Anticholinergic medications (e.g., benztropine, 1 to 2 mg two times daily; trihexyphenidyl, 1 to 3 mg three times daily; and diphenhydramine, 25 to 50 mg two times daily) are used to effectively treat EPS, thereby improving the tolerability of these medications. They may be prescribed prophylactically with high-D_2-binding agents or in patients at risk for EPS or for treatment of EPS. Beta-blockers (e.g., propranolol 30 to 120 mg/day) are sometimes effective for

patients who develop akathisia. In some situations, such as on an inpatient unit, the concomitant use of benzodiazepines (e.g., lorazepam 1 to 3 mg/day) with the SGAs may be necessary for agitation and insomnia.

Antidepressants may be useful for patients with depressive symptoms. Because suicide and depression are linked, aggressive treatment is necessary when depression is present. The selective serotonin reuptake inhibitors (SSRIs) are the preferred agents, but may inhibit the CYP450 enzymes, thus raising plasma concentrations of clozapine, olanzapine, and haloperidol. The mood stabilizers, such as lithium and the anticonvulsants, have long been used adjunctively with the antipsychotics to treat the affective component of schizoaffective disorder. Last, much research is currently underway to develop better treatments for primary negative symptoms and cognitive impairment; however, no approved treatments are yet available.

OUTCOME EVALUATION

Patient Education

8 *Education of the patient and family regarding the benefits and risks of antipsychotic medications and the importance of adherence to their therapeutic regimens must be integrated into pharmacologic management.* Meetings for purposes of medication management offer an opportunity to provide some education on the general illness. Discuss the nature and course of schizophrenia and be prepared to accept that the patient might have a different understanding of the nature of his or her illness. Key points to cover include:

- Involve families in the education and treatment plans because family psychoeducation may decrease relapse, improve symptomatology, and enhance psychosocial and family outcomes.[52]
- Be clear that there is no cure for schizophrenia and that medications only help to decrease the symptoms.
- Explain common and rare but dangerous side effects.
- Stress the importance of medication and treatment adherence for improving long-term outcomes in schizophrenia.

Symptom Monitoring

Develop a good working alliance with the patient. In the absence of a solid therapeutic foundation, patients are frequently reluctant to share their psychotic experiences. When a solid working relationship and some knowledge of the patient's psychotic experiences exist, perform a more structured interview. Many assessments are available to objectively rate positive and negative symptoms, level of function, and life satisfaction. The most commonly used scales include:

- Positive and Negative Symptom Scale (PANSS)
- Brief Psychiatric Rating Scale (BPRS)
- Clinical Global Impression (CGI) Scale

Using these scales on a regular basis, particularly when switching medications or changing doses, is a more reliable means of monitoring for improvement. Certainly, symptom assessments cannot capture the full range of possible improvements a patient may experience, but they can be useful in deciding whether a medication is having substantial benefit.

Side Effect Monitoring

❼ *Regularly monitor patients for side effects and overall health status while taking antipsychotic medications.*[53,54] Perform orthostatic blood pressure measurements before initiating antipsychotics and throughout treatment. Ask about impaired menstruation, libido, and sexual performance regularly. Encourage patients to have annual eye examinations because several antipsychotic medications have been associated with the premature development of cataracts. Check body weight, fasting glucose, glycated hemoglobin, and lipid profile at baseline, at 4 months after initiation of medication, and then yearly.[55] For patients at higher risk of developing diabetes and those who gain weight, check body weight more often (Table 37–9). Encourage patients to act proactively against weight gain through healthier eating and exercise. Perform baseline electrocardiography for patients with preexisting cardiovascular disease or risk for arrhythmia. With clozapine therapy, there is a risk for the development of agranulocytosis, which is greatest in the first 6 months of treatment. Current guidelines require the monitoring of white blood cell counts before drug dispensing (Table 37–10).

Table 37–9

Monitoring Protocol for Patients on Second-Generation Antipsychotics

	Baseline	4 Weeks	8 Weeks	12 Weeks	Quarterly	Annually	Every 5 Years
Personal or family history[a]	X					X	
Weight	X	X	X	X	X		
Waist circumference	X					X	
Blood pressure	X			X		X	
Fasting plasma glucose	X			X		X	
Fasting plasma lipids	X			X			X

[a]Of obesity, diabetes, dyslipidemia, hypertension, or cardiovascular disease.

Data from Love RC, Mackowick M, Carpenter D, Burks EJ. Expert consensus-based medication-use evaluation criteria for atypical antipsychotic drugs. Am J Health Syst Pharm 2003;60:2455–2470.[56]

Table 37–10

Monitoring of White Blood Cell Count and Absolute Neutrophil Count During Clozapine Treatment

	Hematologic Values[a]	Frequency of WBC and ANC Monitoring
Before clozapine initiation	Recommended levels: WBC ≥3.5 × 10³/mm³ (3.5 × 10⁹/L) and ANC ≥2 × 10³/mm³ (2 × 10⁹/L) No history of a **myeloproliferative disorder** or clozapine-induced agranulocytosis	
Initiation to 6 months	WBC ≥3.5 × 10³/mm³ (3.5 × 10⁹/L) and ANC ≥2 × 10³/mm³ (2 × 10⁹/L)	Weekly for 6 months
6–12 months	WBC ≥3.5 × 10³/mm³ (3.5 × 10⁹/L) and ANC ≥2 × 10³/mm³ (2 × 10⁹/L)	Every 2 weeks for 6 months
After 12 months of therapy	WBC ≥3.5 × 10³/mm³ (3.5 × 10⁹/L) and ANC ≥2 × 10³/mm³ (2 × 10⁹/L)	Every 4 weeks
Whenever clozapine is discontinued		Weekly for at least 4 weeks from day of discontinuation
Mild leukopenia or granulocytopenia	WBC value lies between 3 × 10³/mm³ (3 × 10⁹/L) and 3.5 × 10³/mm³ (3.5 × 10⁹/L) or ANC lies between 1.5 × 10³/mm³ (1.5 × 10⁹/L) and 2 × 10³/mm³ (2 × 10⁹/L)	Twice weekly until returned to recommended levels
Moderate leukopenia or granulocytopenia	WBC value lies between 2 × 10³/mm³ (2 × 10⁹/L) and 3 × 10³/mm³ (3 × 10⁹/L) or ANC value lies between 1 × 10³/mm³ (1 × 10⁹/L) and 1.5 × 10³/mm³ (1.5 × 10⁹/L)	Interrupt therapy; monitor daily until WBC >3 × 10³/mm³ (3 × 10⁹/L) and ANC >1.5 × 10³/mm³ (1.5 × 10⁹/L); then twice weekly until back to recommended levels
Severe leukopenia or granulocytopenia or agranulocytosis	WBC <2 × 10³/mm³ (2 × 10⁹/L) or ANC <1 × 10³/mm³ (1 × 10⁹/L) ANC ≤0.5 × 10³/mm³ (0.5 × 10⁹/L) (agranulocytosis)	Discontinue treatment and do not rechallenge; monitor daily until WBC > 3 × 10³/mm³ (3 × 10⁹/L) and ANC > 1.5 × 10³/mm³ (1.5 × 10⁹/L); then twice weekly until back to recommended levels

[a]3.5 × 10³/mm³ = 3.5 × 10⁹/L; 3 × 10³/mm³ = 3 × 10⁹/L; 2 × 10³/mm³ = 2 × 10⁹/L; 1.5 × 10³/mm³ = 1.5 × 10⁹/L; 1 × 10³/mm³ = 1 × 10⁹/L; 0.5 × 10³/mm³ = 0.5 × 10⁹/L.

ANC, absolute neutrophil count; WBC, white blood cell count.

Commonly used rating scales to monitor for EPS include the Simpson Angus Scale (SAS) and the Extrapyramidal Symptom Rating Scale (ESRS). Akathisia is commonly monitored by the Barnes Akathisia Scale (BAS). The emergence of dyskinesias (writhing or involuntary movements) could represent the emergence of TD. Monitor for TD at least annually, and if FGAs are used, patients should be evaluated at each visit. The most commonly used instrument to measure these symptoms is the Abnormal Involuntary Movement Scale (AIMS).

Patient Encounter, Part 4

KH is restarted on risperidone 6 mg/day. She is seen weekly to monitor for EPS or akathisia. After 18 months of treatment, however, KH has gained 20 lb (9.1 kg). In addition, she and her clinician began noticing slight mouth movements that could have been associated with preliminary TD movements. KH became unwilling to continue risperidone, and with her history of nonadherence in the past, discussed different treatment options with her healthcare providers. She recently started treatment with aripiprazole and was stabilized at 10 mg/day 2 weeks ago. She started volunteering at the local library restocking book shelves 5 hours a week and continues to live with her parents. She hopes to return to college someday and to increase her interactions with family and make friends.

Based on the information above, create a care plan for this patient's treatment. Your plan should include (a) a statement of the drug-related concerns or problems, (b) the goals of therapy, and (c) a plan for monitoring and follow-up to determine whether the goals have been achieved and adverse effects minimized.

Patient Care and Monitoring

1. Assess the patient's symptoms, review the patient and family history, and obtain initial medical evaluation to rule out other causes of psychosis.

2. Periodically review patient data for consistency with diagnostic criteria, and regularly monitor changes in symptomatology.

3. Obtain a thorough history of prescription medication use, and determine what treatments have been helpful in the past, which treatments the patient is currently receiving, and previous side effects experienced.

4. Determine whether the patient is taking an appropriate antipsychotic drug and dose and whether the patient has other symptoms that may need to be treated.

5. Educate the patient and the family, if possible, about the disease state, medication treatments, possible side effects, and goals of treatment.

6. Develop a plan to assess the effectiveness of the current treatment regimen. Also, consider alternative treatments if current treatment is ineffective.

7. Encourage a healthy lifestyle, including eliminating or decreasing substance abuse and cigarette use, as well as appropriate nutritional counseling and exercise suggestions.

8. Determine the role of psychosocial treatments.

9. Evaluate the patient for the presence of adverse drug reactions, drug interactions, and allergies.

10. Monitor the appropriate laboratory measures to prevent or minimize metabolic abnormalities and other side effects.

11. Stress the importance of adherence with the treatment regimen and maintaining treatment even if the patient is feeling well.

Abbreviations Introduced in This Chapter

5-HT	Serotonin
ACT	Assertive Community Treatment
AIMS	Abnormal Involuntary Movement Scale
ANC	Absolute neutrophil count
BAS	Barnes Akathisia Scale
BPRS	Brief Psychiatric Rating Scale
CATIE	Clinical Antipsychotics Trials of Intervention Effectiveness
CBT	Cognitive-behavioral therapy
CGI	Clinical Global Impression Scale
CR	Cognitive remediation
CYP450	Cytochrome P-450 isoenzyme
D	Dopamine
DSM-IV-TR	*Diagnostic and Statistical Manual of Mental Disorders*, 4th edition, text revision
ECT	Electroconvulsive therapy
EPS	Extrapyramidal side effects
ESRS	Extrapyramidal Symptom Rating Scale
FGA	First-generation antipsychotic
H	Histamine
IM	Intramuscular
M	Muscarinic
NMDA	N-methyl-D-aspartate
NMS	Neuroleptic malignant syndrome
PCP	Phencyclidine
PANSS	Positive and Negative Symptom Scale
PORT	Schizophrenia Patient Research Outcomes Team
QTc	Corrected QT interval
SAS	Simpson Angus Scale
SGA	Second-generation antipsychotic
SNP	Single nucleotide polymorphism
SSRI	Selective serotonin reuptake inhibitor
SST	Social skills training
TD	Tardive dyskinesia
TIMA	Texas Implementation of Medication Algorithms
WBC	White blood cell

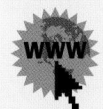 Self-assessment questions and answers are available at *http://www.mhpharmacotherapy. com/pp.html.*

REFERENCES

1. Schultz SK, Andreasen NC. Schizophrenia. Lancet 1999;353(9162):1425–1430.
2. Kim Y, Zerwas S, Trace SE, Sullivan PF. Schizophrenia genetics: Where next? Schizophr Bull 2011;37(3):456–463.
3. Abi-Dargham A. Do we still believe in the dopamine hypothesis? New data bring new evidence. Int J Neuropsychopharmacol 2004;7 (Suppl 1):S1–S5.
4. Javitt DC. Glutamate and schizophrenia: phencyclidine, N-methyl-D-aspartate receptors, and dopamine-glutamate interactions. Int Rev Neurobiol 2007;78:69–108.
5. Meltzer HY, Massey BW. The role of serotonin receptors in the action of atypical antipsychotic drugs. Curr Opin Pharmacol 2011;11(1):59–67.
6. Goff DC, Cather C, Evins AE, et al. Medical morbidity and mortality in schizophrenia: guidelines for psychiatrists. J Clin Psychiatry 2005;66(2):183–194.
7. American Psychiatric Association. Diagnostic and Statistical Manual of Mental Disorders. 4th ed, text rev. Washington, DC: American Psychiatric Association; 2000.
8. American Psychiatric Association. Practice guidelines for the treatment of patients with schizophrenia. Am J Psychiatry 2004;161 (2 Suppl):1–56.
9. The expert consensus guideline series: Treatment of schizophrenia. J Clin Psychiatry 1996;57(Suppl 12B):31.
10. Hor K, Taylor M. Suicide and schizophrenia: A systematic review of rates and risk factors. J Psychopharmacol 2010;24(4 Suppl):81–90.
11. Casey DE. Long-term treatment goals: Enhancing healthy outcomes. CNS Spectr 2003;8(11 Suppl 2):26–28.
12. Resnick SG, Fontana A, Lehman AF, Rosenheck RA. An empirical conceptualization of the recovery orientation. Schizophr Res 2005;75(1):119–128.
13. Dixon LB, Dickerson F, Bellack AS, et al. The 2009 Schizophrenia PORT Psychosocial Treatment Recommendations and Summary Statements. Schizophr Bull 2010;36(1):48-70.
14. Lieberman JA, Stroup TS, McEvoy JP, et al. For the Clinical Antipsychotic Trials of Intervention Effectiveness (CATIE) Investigators. Effectiveness of antipsychotic drugs in people with chronic schizophrenia. N Engl J Med 2005;353(12):1209–1223.
15. Correll CU, Leucht S, Kane JM. Lower risk for tardive dyskinesia associated with second-generation antipsychotics: A systematic review of 1-year studies. Am J Psychiatry 2004;161(3):414–425.
16. Schotte A, Janssen PFM, Gommeren W, et al. Risperidone compared with new and reference antipsychotic drugs: In vitro and in vivo receptor binding. Psychopharmacology 1996;124(1–2):57–73.
17. Marder SR, Meibach RC. Risperidone in the treatment of schizophrenia. Am J Psychiatry 1994;151(6):825–835.
18. Csernansky JG, Mahmoud R, Brenner R, Risperidone-USA-79 Study Group. A comparison of risperidone and haloperidol for the prevention of relapse in patients with schizophrenia. N Engl J Med 2002;346(1):16–22.
19. Richelson E. Receptor pharmacology of neuroleptics: Relation to clinical effects. J Clin Psychiatry 1999;60(Suppl 10):5–14.
20. Beasley CM, Tollefson G, Tran P, et al. Olanzapine versus placebo and haloperidol: Acute phase results of the North American double-blind olanzapine trial. Neuropsychopharmacology 1996;14(2):111–123.
21. Tollefson GD, Beasley CM, Tran PV, et al. Olanzapine versus haloperidol in the treatment of schizophrenia and schizoaffective and schizophreniform disorders: Results of an international collaborative trial. Am J Psychiatry 1997;154(4):457–465.
22. Arvanitis LA, Miller BG, the Seroquel Trial 13 Study Group. Multiple fixed doses of Seroquel (quetiapine) in patients with acute exacerbation of schizophrenia: A comparison with haloperidol and placebo. Biol Psychiatry 1997;42(4):233–246.
23. Small JG, Hirsch SR, Arvenitis LA, et al. Quetiapine in patients with schizophrenia: A high- and low-dose double-blind comparison with placebo. Arch Gen Psychiatry 1997;54(6):549–557.
24. Seeger TF, Seymour PA, Schmidt AW, et al. Ziprasidone (CP-88,059): A new antipsychotic with combined dopamine and serotonin receptor antagonist activity. J Pharmacol Exp Ther 1995;275(1):101–113.
25. Daniel DG, Zimbroff DL, Potkin SG, et al. Ziprasidone 80 mg/day and 160 mg/day in the acute exacerbation of schizophrenia and schizoaffective disorder: A 6-week placebo-controlled trial. Neuropsychopharmacology 1999;20(5):491–505.

26. Shapiro DA, Renock S, Arrington E, et al. Aripiprazole, a novel atypical antipsychotic drug with a unique and robust pharmacology. Neuropsychopharmacology 2003;28(8):1400–1411.

27. Stip E, Tourjman V. Aripiprazole in schizophrenia and schizoaffective disorder: A review. Clin Ther 2010;32(Suppl 1):S3–S20.

28. Fowler JA, Bettinger TL, Argo TR. Paliperidone extended-release tablets for the acute and maintenance treatment of schizophrenia. Clin Ther 2008;30(2):231–248.

29. Dolder C, Nelson M, Deyo Z. Paliperidone for schizophrenia. Am J Health Syst Pharm 2008;65(5):403–413.

30. Arif SA, Mitchell MM. Iloperidone: A new drug for the treatment of schizophrenia. Am J Health-Syst Pharm 2011;68:301–308.

31. Citrome L. Iloperidone, asenapine, and lurasidone: A brief overview of 3 new second generation antipsychotics. Postgrad Med 2011;123(2):153–162.

32. Kapur S, Seeman P. Does fast dissociation from the dopamine d(2) receptor explain the action of atypical antipsychotics? A new hypothesis. Am J Psychiatry 2001;158(3):360–369.

33. Wirshing WC. Movement disorders associated with neuroleptic treatment. J Clin Psychiatry 2001;62(Suppl 21):15–18.

34. Margolese HC, Chouinard G, Kolivakis TT, et al. Tardive dyskinesia in the era of typical and atypical antipsychotics. Part 2: Incidence and management strategies in patients with schizophrenia. Can J Psychiatry 2005;50(11):703–714.

35. van Harten PN, Tenback DE. Tardive dyskinesia: Clinical presentation and treatment. Int Rev Neurobiol 2011;98:187–210.

36. Correll CU, Schenk EM. Tardive dyskinesia and new antipsychotics. Curr Opin Psychiatry 2008;21:151–156.

37. Moore TA, Buchanan RW, Buckley PF, et al. The Texas Medication Algorithm Project antipsychotic algorithm for schizophrenia: 2006 update. J Clin Psychiatry 2007;68(11):1751–1762.

38. Buchanan RW, Kreyenbuhl J, Kelly DL, et al. The 2009 schizophrenia PORT psychopharmacological treatment recommendations and summary statements. Schizophr Bull 2010;36(1):71–93.

39. Byerly MJ, Nakonezny PA, Lescouflair E. Antipsychotic medication adherence in schizophrenia. Psychiatr Clin North Am 2007;30(3):437–452.

40. Ascher-Svanum H, Zhu B, Faries D, et al. A prospective study of risk factors for nonadherence with antipsychotic medication in the treatment of schizophrenia. J Clin Psychiatry 2006;67(7):1114–1123.

41. Remschmidt H. Early-onset schizophrenia as a progressive-deteriorating developmental disorder: Evidence from child psychiatry. J Neural Transm 2002;109:101–117.

42. Jeste DV, Caligiuri MP, Paulsen JS, et al. Risk of tardive dyskinesia in older patients. A prospective longitudinal study of 266 outpatients. Arch Gen Psychiatry 1995;52:756–765.

43. Lubman DI, King JA, Castle DJ. Treating comorbid substance use disorders in schizophrenia. Int Rev Psychiatry 2010;22(2):191–201.

44. Wobrock T, Soyka M. Wobrock T, Soyka M. Pharmacotherapy of schizophrenia with comorbid substance use disorder: Reviewing the evidence and clinical research. Prog Neuropsychopharmacol Biol Psychiatry 2008;32(6):1375–1385.

45. Conley RR, Kelly DL. Management of treatment resistance in schizophrenia. Biol Psychiatry 2001;50(11):898–911.

46. Meltzer HY. Suicide in schizophrenia, clozapine and adoption of evidence-based medicine. J Clin Psychiatry 2005;60(Suppl 12):47–50.

47. Nilsson E, Hultman CM, Cnattinguis S, et al. Schizophrenia and offspring's risk for adverse pregnancy outcomes and infant death. Br J Psychiatry 2008;193:311–315.

48. Diav-Citrin O, Schechtman S, Ornoy S, et al. Safety of haloperidol and penfluridol in pregnancy: A multicenter, prospective, controlled study. J Clin Psychiatry 2005;66(3):317–322.

49. Gentile S. Antipsychotic therapy during early and late pregnancy. A systematic review. Schizophr Bull 2010;36(3):518–544.

50. Wang JS, Taylor R, Ruan Y, et al. Olanzapine penetration into brain is greater in transgenic Abcb1a P-glycoprotein-deficient mice and FVB1 (wild type) animals. Neuropsychopharmacology 2004;29(3):551–557.

51. Sandson NB, Armstrong SC, Cozza KL. An overview of psychotropic drug-drug interactions. Psychosomatics 2005;46(5):464–494.

52. Murray-Swank AB, Dixon L. Family psychoeducation as evidence-based practice. CNS Spect 2004;9(12):905–912.

53. Marder SR, Essock SM, Miller AL, et al. The Mount Sinai conference on the pharmacotherapy of schizophrenia. Schizophr Bull 2002;28(1):5–16.

54. Marder SR, Essock SM, Miller AL, et al. Physical health monitoring of patients with schizophrenia. Am J Psychiatry 2004;161(8):1334–1349.

55. American Diabetes Association, American Psychiatric Association, American Association of Clinical Endocrinologists, North American Association for the Study of Obesity. Consensus development conference on antipsychotic drugs and obesity and diabetes. Diabetes Care 2004;27(2):596–601.

56. Love RC, Mackowick M, Carpenter D, Burks EJ. Expert consensus-based medication-use evaluation criteria for atypical antipsychotic drugs. Am J Health Syst Pharm 2003;60:2455–2470.

38 Major Depressive Disorder

Cherry W. Jackson and Marshall E. Cates

LEARNING OBJECTIVES

● **Upon completion of the chapter, the reader will be able to:**

1. Explain the etiology and pathophysiology of major depressive disorder (MDD).

2. Identify symptoms and clinical features of MDD.

3. Differentiate antidepressants according to pharmacologic properties, adverse effect profiles, pharmacokinetic profiles, drug interaction profiles, and dosing features.

4. Predict adverse effect profiles of antidepressants based on pharmacology.

5. State the goals of pharmacotherapy in MDD.

6. Educate patients and caregivers on the proper use of antidepressants.

KEY CONCEPTS

❶ Classic views as to the cause of major depressive disorder (MDD) focus on the monoamine neurotransmitters norepinephrine (NE); serotonin (5-HT); and to a lesser extent, dopamine (DA) in terms of both synaptic concentrations and receptor functioning.

❷ It is not uncommon for a patient to experience only a single major depressive episode, but most patients with MDD experience multiple episodes.

❸ One extremely important goal in the treatment of MDD is the prevention of suicide attempts.

❹ Sexual dysfunction, common and challenging to manage, often leads to noncompliance with serotonergic medications.

❺ Each antidepressant has a response rate of approximately 60% to 80%, and no antidepressant medication or class has been reliably shown to be more efficacious than another.

❻ It is widely accepted that approximately 2 to 4 weeks of treatment is required before improvement is seen in emotional symptoms of depression, such as sadness and anhedonia. Furthermore, as long as 6 to 8 weeks of treatment may be required to see the full effects of antidepressant therapy.

❼ Because the typical major depressive episode lasts 6 months or longer, if antidepressant therapy is interrupted for any reason after the acute phase of treatment, the patient may relapse into the depressive episode. When treating the first depressive episode, antidepressants must be given for an additional 4 to 9 months in the continuation phase for the purpose of preventing relapse.

❽ Pediatric patients and young adults should be observed closely for suicidality, worsened depression, agitation, irritability, and unusual changes in behavior, especially during the initial few months of therapy and at times of dosage changes. Furthermore, families and caregivers should be advised to monitor patients for such symptoms.

❾ Lack of patient understanding concerning optimal antidepressant drug therapy frequently leads to partial compliance or noncompliance with therapy; thus, the primary purpose of antidepressant counseling is to enhance compliance and improve outcomes.

> My spirit is broken, my days are cut short, the grave awaits me.
>
> —*Job 17:1*

Contrary to popular belief, major depression is not a fleeting "bad day," is not the result of personal weaknesses or character flaws, and does not respond to volitional efforts simply to feel better. Major depressive disorder (MDD) is a serious medical condition with a biological foundation, and it responds to biological and psychological treatments. Individuals with MDD experience significant and pervasive symptoms that can affect mood, thinking, physical health, work, and relationships. Unfortunately, suicide is often the result of MDD that has not been diagnosed and treated adequately.

Patient Encounter, Part 1

LM, a 40-year-old white woman, presents to the inpatient psychiatric service after being referred from the mental health center. She is admitted secondary to stress over the holidays resulting in exacerbation of long-standing psychiatric illness. She complains of depressed mood, difficulty falling asleep, middle of the night awakening, early morning awakening, poor energy, poor concentration, recent weight loss of 15 lb (6.8 kg) over a 6-week period, nervousness, and frequent thoughts of death.

What information is suggestive of MDD?

What medical or psychiatric issues could be contributing to her symptoms?

Does she have risk factors for depression?

What additional information do you need to know before creating a treatment plan for this patient?

The past 2 decades have seen improvements in the screening, diagnosis, and treatment of MDD. The willingness of general practitioners to involve themselves in the identification and treatment of MDD is noteworthy. To that end, antidepressants have become some of the most commonly prescribed drugs, and they account for 10 of the top 200 prescription drugs dispensed in the United States.[1] Inadequate treatment remains a serious concern.[2]

EPIDEMIOLOGY AND ETIOLOGY

Major depressive disorder is quite common; lifetime and 12-month prevalence estimates are 13.2% and 5.2%, respectively.[2] Women are approximately twice as likely as men to experience MDD.[2] The average age at onset is the midtwenties.[3] Interestingly, MDD appears to occur earlier in life in people born in more recent decades.[2] Most patients with MDD also have comorbid psychiatric disorders, especially anxiety disorders and substance use disorders.[2]

According to the World Health Organization (WHO), depression is the leading cause of disability (based on years lived with disability) and the fourth leading contributor to the global burden of disease (based on disability-adjusted life years).[4]

PATHOPHYSIOLOGY

The exact cause of MDD remains unknown, but it is probably multifactorial. Biological, psychological, and social theories abound, and many practitioners suggest that the development of depression often is predicated on the complex synthesis of genetic predisposition, psychological stressors, and biological pathophysiology. At present, there are currently no accepted unifying theories that explain these various factors adequately.

Genetics

First-degree relatives of MDD patients are about three times more likely to develop MDD compared with first-degree relatives of normal control individuals. Adoption studies and twin studies reveal that the familial aggregation of MDD is due to genetic influences.[5]

Life Stress

Depression can occur in the absence of major life stressors, and conversely, major life stressors do not invariably cause depression. Nevertheless, there is an undeniable association between life stressors and depression, and there appears to be a significant interaction between life stressors and genetic liability in causing depression.[6] Although acute stressors may precipitate depression, chronic stressors have a longer risk period, cause longer episodes, and are more likely to lead to **relapse** and **recurrence**.[6]

Monoamine Neurotransmitter and Receptor Hypotheses

① *Classic views as to the cause of MDD focus on the monoamine neurotransmitters norepinephrine (NE); serotonin (5-HT); and to a lesser extent, dopamine (DA) in terms of both synaptic concentrations and receptor functioning.* The monoamine hypothesis asserts that depression is attributable to a deficiency of monoamine neurotransmitters. The major supporting evidence for this hypothesis is that existing antidepressants increase synaptic monoamine concentrations through various mechanisms (see Pharmacologic Therapy). One argument against the monoamine hypothesis is that depressed patients do not consistently exhibit decreased monoamine concentrations. In addition, monoamine levels are altered within hours of the initiation of antidepressant therapy, but there is a latency period of weeks before the actual antidepressant effect is typically evident.[7–9]

The neurotransmitter receptor hypothesis suggests that depression is related to abnormal functioning of neurotransmitter receptors. In this model, antidepressants presumably exert therapeutic effects by altering receptor sensitivity. In fact, chronic administration of antidepressants has been shown to cause desensitization, or down-regulation, of β-adrenergic receptors and various 5-HT receptors. Importantly, the time required for changes in receptor sensitivity corresponds to the onset of antidepressant effects.[7–9]

Such models of the pathophysiology of depression are assuredly an oversimplification. Depression probably involves a complex dysregulation of monoamine systems, and these systems in turn modulate and are modulated by other neurobiological systems.[10]

Other Neurobiological Hypotheses

Various other pathophysiologic hypotheses have been proposed. These hypotheses include the role of nonmonoamine

Clinical Presentation of Major Depressive Disorder

Patients typically present with a combination of emotional, physical, and cognitive symptoms:

- Emotional
  - Sadness
  - Anhedonia
  - Pessimism
  - Feeling of emptiness
  - Irritability
  - Anxiety
  - Worthlessness
  - Thoughts of death or suicidal ideation
- Physical
  - Disturbed sleep
  - Change in appetite or weight
  - Psychomotor changes
  - Decreased energy
  - Fatigue
  - Bodily aches and pain

- Cognitive
  - Impaired concentration
  - Indecisiveness
  - Poor memory

Occasionally, severely depressed patients also will present with psychotic symptoms:

- Hallucinations
- Delusions

Some patients present with "atypical features" of depression:

- Reactive mood (i.e., mood improves in response to positive events)
- Significant increase in appetite/weight gain
- Hypersomnia
- Heavy feelings in arms or legs
- Sensitivity to interpersonal rejection

---

neurotransmitters (e.g., glutamate and γ-aminobutyric acid), neuroendocrine systems (e.g., the hypothalamic–pituitary–adrenal axis), neurosteroids (e.g., allopregnanolone), neuronal plasticity (e.g., brain-derived neurotrophic factor),[11] messenger cascades, and gene expression.[12]

CLINICAL PRESENTATION AND DIAGNOSIS

The diagnosis of a major depressive episode requires the presence of a certain number of depressive symptoms (five) for a minimum specified duration (2 weeks) that cause clinically significant effects (Table 38–1).[3]

HINT: To remember the nine diagnostic symptoms for a major depressive episode, learn the following mnemonic: Depression = SIG E CAPS (depression equals sleep, interest, guilt, energy, concentration, appetite, psychomotor, suicide).

In turn, the diagnosis of MDD is based on the presence of one or more major depressive episodes during a person's lifetime.[3]

Differential Diagnosis

Major depressive episodes also occur in patients with bipolar disorder. Persons with bipolar disorder also experience manic, hypomanic, or mixed episodes (see Chapter 39) during the course of their illness, but persons with MDD do not.[3]

The presence of a significant medical disorder can produce depressive symptoms via either psychological or

Table 38–1

Diagnostic Criteria for Major Depressive Episode

At least five of the following symptoms have been present during the same 2-week period and represent a change from previous functioning:
- Depressed mood[a]
- Markedly diminished interest or pleasure in usual activities[a]
- Increase or decrease in appetite or weight
- Increase or decrease in amount of sleep
- Increase or decrease in psychomotor activity
- Fatigue or loss of energy
- Feelings of worthlessness or guilt
- Diminished ability to think, concentrate, or make decisions
- Recurrent thoughts of death, suicidal ideation, or suicide attempt

The symptoms cause clinically significant distress or impairment in functioning
The symptoms are not due to the direct physiologic effects of a substance or medical condition

[a]One of these two symptoms must be present.

Data from American Psychiatric Association. Diagnostic and Statistical Manual of Mental Disorders. 4th ed, text revision. Washington, DC: American Psychiatric Association; 2000:356.

physiologic mechanisms. Examples include hypothyroidism, neoplasms, anemia, infections, electrolyte disturbances, folate deficiency, cardiovascular diseases, neurologic disorders, and many others.[9] Various psychiatric conditions, such as substance use disorders and anxiety disorders, have been associated with depression as well.[9] The use of central nervous system (CNS) depressants, such as benzodiazepines and narcotics, is associated with an increased propensity for depression.[13] Drugs that reportedly cause depressive symptoms or depressive-like side effects include corticosteroids, contraceptives, gonadotropin-releasing hormone agonists, interferon-α, interleukin-2, mefloquine, isotretinoin, propranolol, and sotalol.[14]

Dysthymia is a condition that must be differentiated from MDD. Many of the symptoms of dysthymia are similar to those of MDD, but in dysthymia, the symptoms are chronic and milder. Symptoms of dysthymia must be present for at least 2 years and may include sleep and appetite disturbances, a loss of energy, a lack of interest in things that would usually be enjoyable, and poor self-image. Patients with dysthymia often have family members with a history of depression or dysthymia. It occurs more frequently in women, and patients with dysthymia are more likely to develop major depression than the general population.[3]

COURSE AND PROGNOSIS

● Symptoms of a major depressive episode usually develop over days to weeks, but mild depressive and anxiety symptoms may last for weeks to months before the onset of the full syndrome. Left untreated, major depressive episodes typically last 6 months or more, but a minority of patients experience chronic episodes that last at least 2 years. Approximately two-thirds of patients recover fully from major depressive episodes and return to normal mood and full functioning, but the other one-third have only partial remission.[3]

The course of MDD varies markedly from patient to patient. ❷ *It is not uncommon for a patient to experience only a single major depressive episode, but most patients with MDD experience multiple episodes.* Some patients experience isolated episodes separated by many years, others have clusters of episodes, and still others have more frequent episodes as they age. Some experience seasonal affective disorder (SAD) in which symptoms occur certain times of the year, usually in the winter. The number of prior episodes predicts the likelihood of developing subsequent episodes. A patient experiencing a third major depressive episode has about a 90% chance of having a fourth one. MDD is associated with a high mortality rate because about 15% of patients ultimately commit suicide.[3]

TREATMENT
Desired Outcomes

● The goals of therapy for depressed patients are the resolution of depressive symptoms, a return to euthymia, and prevention of relapse and recurrence of depressive symptoms. ❸ *One extremely important goal in the treatment of MDD is the prevention of suicide attempts.* Other desired outcomes include improvement of the patient's quality of life, normalization of functioning in areas such as work and relationships, avoidance or minimization of adverse effects, and reduction of health care costs.[15]

Patient Encounter, Part 2: Medical History, Physical Examination, and Diagnostic Tests

The workup on LM reveals:

PMH: She has multiple medical problems, including insulin-dependent diabetes mellitus, hypertension, congestive heart failure, hypothyroidism, endometrial cancer by history, status post hysterectomy, and obesity. She is followed by a local internist.

PPH: Patient has multiple psychiatric hospitalizations with the last being 2 years before this admission. She has a diagnosis of major depressive episode (MDE).

FH: Mother with diabetes mellitus and MDD; father is alive and well with no medical problems; brother is a recovered alcoholic.

SH: Worked for a mortgage company, but job ended 2 months ago. For the past several months, she has been drinking three to four beers per night. She denies smoking cigarettes and using illicit substances.

Current Meds: Sertraline 100 mg/day, trazodone 150 mg at bedtime, nicardipine 20 mg four times daily, furosemide 100 mg/day, albuterol inhaler 2 puffs every 6 hours, levothyroxine 0.05 mg every morning, Novulin 70/30 56 units in the morning and 15 units in the evening.

ROS: Decreased energy; decreased sleep; decreased concentration; nervousness; all others noncontributory

PE:

Ht: 5 ft, 3 in (160 cm); wt, 83 kg (183 lb); weight loss of 6.8 kg (15 lb) over past 6 weeks

MSE: Depressed mood; decreased concentration; nervousness; positive suicidal ideation without plan

Labs: Within normal limits

Given this additional information, what is your assessment of the patient's condition?

Identify your treatment goals for the patient.

What nonpharmacologic and pharmacologic alternatives are available for this patient?

Nonpharmacologic Therapy

Interpersonal therapy and cognitive-behavioral therapy are psychotherapies that have well-documented efficacy for the treatment of MDD. Psychotherapy alone is an initial treatment option for mild to moderate depression, and it may be useful when combined with pharmacotherapy in the treatment of more severe cases. The combination of psychotherapy and pharmacotherapy can be more effective than either treatment modality alone in severe or recurrent MDD. It may be especially helpful for patients with significant psychosocial stressors, interpersonal difficulties, or comorbid personality disorders.[16]

Electroconvulsive therapy (ECT) is a highly efficacious treatment for MDD. The **response** rate is about 80% to 90%, and it exceeds 50% for patients who have failed pharmacotherapy.[16,17] ECT may be particularly beneficial for MDD that is complicated by psychotic features, severe suicidality, refusal to eat, pregnancy, or contraindication or nonresponse to pharmacotherapy.[16,17] Around 6 to 12 treatments are typically necessary with response occurring in 10 to 14 days. When ECT is discontinued, antidepressants are initiated to help maintain the response. ECT is typically a very safe treatment alternative, but various cautions do exist. Side effects include confusion and retrograde and anterograde amnesia.[16]

Light therapy is an alternative treatment for depression associated with seasonal (e.g., winter) exacerbations. Side effects include eye strain, headache, insomnia, and hypomania.[16,17] Potentially vulnerable patients, such as those with photosensitivity or a history of skin cancer, should be evaluated carefully before therapy.[16,17]

Vagus nerve stimulation (VNS), which was approved by the Food and Drug Administration (FDA) in 2005, may be used for adult patients with treatment-resistant depression. A pulse generator is surgically implanted under the skin of the left chest, and an electrical lead connects the generator to the left vagus nerve. Stimulation of this nerve sends signals to the brain. This therapy is used along with traditional therapies such as pharmacotherapy and ECT.[18] Adverse effects of VNS include alterations in patients' voice, coughing, pharyngitis, sore throat, hoarseness, headache, nausea, vomiting, dyspnea, and paresthesias.[18]

Transcranial magnetic stimulation is a noninvasive and well-tolerated procedure that is FDA approved for use after one failed trial of an antidepressant.[19] Some data suggest that physical exercise may reduce depressive symptoms, but well-controlled studies are needed to document efficacy.[20]

Pharmacologic Therapy

Each antidepressant has its unique blend of characteristics, and in fact, even individual drugs within the same class have important differences.[21] Table 38–2 demonstrates the differing pharmacologic properties of the antidepressant medications,[7–9] and Table 38–3 delineates the results of those pharmacologic actions.[7,8] Monoamine oxidase inhibitors (MAOIs) inhibit the enzyme responsible for the intraneuronal breakdown of 5-HT, NE, and DA. There are two main forms of MAO, MAO-A and MAO-B; inhibition of MAO-A impacts the breakdown of 5-HT, epinephrine, and NE, and MAO-B is primarily involved in the inhibition of dopamine and phenethylamine. Dietary restrictions are necessary for MAO-A but not usually for MAO-B inhibitors. The tricyclic antidepressants (TCAs) possess both 5-HT (serotonin) reuptake inhibition (SRI) and NE reuptake inhibition (NRI) properties but unfortunately also block the so-called "dirty receptors," including α_1-adrenergic, histamine-1, and muscarinic cholinergic receptors, which contribute to side effects but not efficacy. The selective serotonin reuptake inhibitors (SSRIs) are classified as such because SRI is the predominant effect. Bupropion is an NE and DA reuptake inhibitor (NDRI). Venlafaxine, desvenlafaxine, and duloxetine are 5-HT and NE reuptake inhibitors (SNRIs)

Table 38–2

Primary Pharmacologic Actions of Antidepressants[a]

Action	MAOIs	TCAs	SSRIs	Bupropion	SNRIs	Vilazodone	Trazodone	Nefazodone	Mirtazapine
Monoamine oxidase inhibition	X								
Serotonin reuptake inhibition		X	X		X	X	X	X	
Norepinephrine reuptake inhibition		X		X	X				
Dopamine reuptake inhibition				X					
α_2-Adrenergic receptor blockade									X
Serotonin$_{2A}$ receptor blockade							X	X	X
Serotonin$_{2C}$ receptor blockade							X	X	X
Serotonin$_3$ receptor blockade									X
α_1-Adrenergic receptor blockade		X					X	X	
Histamine-1 receptor blockade		X					X		X
Muscarinic cholinergic receptor blockade		X							
Serotonin$_{1A}$ receptor partial agonist						X			

[a]See text for discussion of more secondary pharmacologic actions.

MAOI, monoamine oxidase inhibitor; SNRI, serotonin norepinephrine reuptake inhibitor; SSRI, selective serotonin reuptake inhibitor; TCA, tricyclic antidepressant.

Data from Refs. 7–9.

Table 38–3	
Efficacy and Adverse Effect Profiles Based on Pharmacology	
Pharmacologic Action	**Result**
SRI	Antidepressant and antianxiety efficacy (via interaction of 5-HT at 5-HT$_{1A}$ receptors)
	Anxiety, insomnia, sexual dysfunction (via interaction of 5-HT at 5-HT$_{2A}$ receptors)
	Anxiety, anorexia (via interaction of 5-HT at 5-HT$_{2C}$ receptors)
	Nausea, GI problems (via interaction of 5-HT at 5-HT$_3$ receptors)
NRI	Antidepressant efficacy
	Tremor, tachycardia, sweating, jitteriness, increased blood pressure
Dopamine reuptake inhibition	Antidepressant efficacy
	Euphoria, psychomotor activation, aggravation of psychosis
α_2-Adrenergic receptor blockade	Increase in serotonergic and noradrenergic activity—see actions of SRI and NRI above
Serotonin$_{1A}$ partial agonism	Antianxiety, antidepressant augmentation, decreased blood pressure, decreased heart rate
Serotonin$_{2A}$ receptor blockade	Antianxiety efficacy
	Increased REM sleep; decreased sexual dysfunction
Serotonin$_{2C}$ receptor blockade	Antianxiety efficacy
	Increased appetite or weight gain
Serotonin$_3$ receptor blockade	Antinauseant, decreased GI problems
α_1-Adrenergic receptor blockade	Orthostatic hypotension, dizziness, reflex tachycardia
Histamine-1 receptor blockade	Sedation, weight gain
Muscarinic cholinergic receptor blockade	Dry mouth, blurred vision, constipation, urinary hesitancy, sinus tachycardia, memory problems

GI, gastrointestinal; NRI, norepinephrine reuptake inhibition; REM, rapid eye movement; SRI, serotonin reuptake inhibition.

Data from Refs. 7 and 8.

but are also weak inhibitors of DA reuptake. Compared with venlafaxine and desvenlafaxine, which have primarily SRI activity, duloxetine has more balanced SRI and NRI activities and has a higher affinity for the reuptake sites. Nefazodone and trazodone are 5-HT antagonists/reuptake inhibitors. Their SRI activity is not as pronounced as that of the SSRIs, but they potently block 5-HT$_{2A}$ receptors, which allow more 5-HT to interact at postsynaptic 5-HT$_{1A}$ sites. In addition, trazodone blocks histaminergic and α-adrenergic receptors, and nefazodone possesses weak NRI and α-adrenergic blocking properties. Vilazodone is a combination of an SRI and a partial agonist at the 5-HT$_{1A}$ receptor. Partial agonist activity at the 5-HT$_{1A}$ receptor is thought to reduce negative feedback on endogenous serotonin receptors which is thought to improve the medications antidepressant effect. [22] Finally, mirtazapine is a noradrenergic and specific serotonergic antidepressant. It blocks presynaptic α_2 receptors, both autoreceptors on noradrenergic neurons and heteroreceptors on serotonergic neurons, with resulting increases in NE and 5-HT synaptic concentrations, respectively. Mirtazapine also blocks various postsynaptic serotonergic receptors and histamine-1 receptors.[7-9]

▶ *Complementary and Alternative Treatments*

• St. John's wort (*Hypericum perforatum*) is a herbal medication that has shown some efficacy in mild to moderate depression but minimal efficacy for moderate to severe depression.[20] It has some mild MAO-inhibiting properties. Many patients believe that herbal medications, being "natural" products, are devoid of adverse effects and drug interactions; however,

St. John's wort can cause gastrointestinal (GI) irritation, headache, fatigue, and nervousness,[17] and it triggers drug interactions through induction of CYP3A4 enzymes, as well as other potential mechanisms.[22] The safety and efficacy of St. John's wort combined with standard antidepressant medications remains unknown.[16]

S-adenosyl methionine (SAM-e) is a naturally occurring compound that tends to be lower in people with major depression. Treatment with SAM-e increases blood levels of both S-adenosyl methionine and hydroxyindoleacetic acid. It is sold as a nutritional supplement and lacks the standardization of medications that are FDA approved.[20]

Low folate levels have been associated with a greater risk of depression or with a lack of response to antidepressants. Because folic acid prevents neural tube defects in pregnancy and causes few to no adverse effects, it can be used in doses of 0.4 to 1 mg/day to improve the efficacy of antidepressants.[20]

Omega-3 fatty acids (eicosapentaenoic acid, docosahexaenoic acid, or both) have been used adjunctively for major depression. Doses typically at the lower end of 1 to 9 g/day appear useful for the treatment of major depression, but more study needs to be completed to establish their role.[20]

▶ *Adverse Effects*

• The important adverse effects of the various antidepressants are often a function of their underlying pharmacologic profiles[7,8] (Table 38–3). The TCAs cause problematic sedative, anticholinergic, and cardiovascular adverse effects owing to their interaction with "dirty receptors." Although these adverse effects generally are considered to be common and bothersome, they can be quite serious in some cases. For example, constipation in its extreme form can lead to paralytic ileus. The tertiary amines (e.g., amitriptyline, imipramine) are more sedative and anticholinergic than the secondary amines (e.g., desipramine, nortriptyline). The TCAs have a quinidine-like effect on the heart, which makes them quite toxic on overdose. The average lethal dose in a young adult is only 30 mg/kg, which is typically less than a 1 month's supply.[7,9,21,23]

The adverse effect profile of the SSRIs includes sexual dysfunction (e.g., delayed or absent orgasms), CNS stimulation (e.g., nervousness and insomnia), and GI disturbances (e.g., nausea and diarrhea).[7,9,21,23] ❹ *Sexual dysfunction, common and challenging to manage, often leads to noncompliance.*[24] Various strategies to deal with antidepressant-induced sexual dysfunction include waiting for symptoms to subside, reducing the dosage, permitting periodic "drug holidays," prescribing adjunctive therapy, and switching antidepressants.[25] However, waiting for symptoms to subside usually does not work because sexual dysfunction may very well persist throughout the duration of therapy. Reducing the dose and using drug holidays may weaken the antidepressant effects. Thus, clinicians often prescribe adjunctive therapy such as dopaminergic drugs (e.g., bupropion or amantadine), 5-HT$_2$ antagonists (e.g., cyproheptadine or nefazodone), and phosphodiesterase inhibitors (e.g., sildenafil) or simply switch to antidepressants with less likelihood of causing these effects, such as bupropion, mirtazapine, or nefazodone, which may rarely cause liver failure.[24,25]

Bupropion causes insomnia, nightmares, decreased appetite, anxiety, and tremors, but the most concerning adverse effect is seizures. Because of the risk for seizures, patients with a CNS lesion, history of seizures, head trauma, or bulimia should not receive the drug. The daily dose of bupropion should not exceed 450 mg/day (immediate release and extended release), and any single dose of the immediate-release formulation should not exceed 150 mg. The maximum dose of sustained release is 200 mg twice daily. Occurrences of insomnia and/or nightmares often respond to moving the last daily dose from bedtime to late afternoon.[7,9,21,23]

The adverse effects of the SNRIs are similar to those of the SSRIs. Nausea can be particularly troublesome with venlafaxine and desvenlafaxine, which sometimes necessitates using lower starting dosages than usual and giving the medication with food. A dose-related elevation in blood pressure can occur at higher doses, probably owing to the NRI effects. Blood pressure monitoring should be conducted for patients receiving venlafaxine and desvenlafaxine therapy. As a rule, duloxetine should not be prescribed to patients with extensive alcohol use or evidence of chronic liver disease owing to the potential for hepatic injury.[9,21,26,27]

Trazodone routinely causes sedation, which is why it is used far more often as an adjunct with other antidepressants for sleep than as an antidepressant. Priapism is a rare but serious adverse effect in men who take trazodone. In addition, orthostatic hypotension and dizziness are more common with trazodone than with nefazodone because the latter agent has a weaker effect at α-adrenergic receptors and also has a balancing of adrenergic effects owing to weak NRI activity. Unfortunately, nefazodone has been associated with development of hepatotoxicity, which has led to a black-box warning and a great reduction in its use. It has been discontinued in some countries.[7,9,21,23]

Mirtazapine can cause sedation and weight gain by virtue of blocking histamine-1 receptors. Despite being partially a serotonergic drug, it rarely causes serotonergic-related adverse effects because it blocks the various postsynaptic 5-HT receptors. Although it carries a bolded warning for neutropenia owing to a handful of cases reported during clinical trials, it is questionable whether neutropenia is any more problematic with this agent than other antidepressants.[9,21,23]

The relative incidences of adverse effects among some of the newer antidepressant agents are shown in Table 38–4.[9,13,28]

Table 38–4

Relative Incidence of Adverse Effects of Various Newer Antidepressants

Drug	Sedation	Activation	Weight Gain	Weight Loss	GI Upset	Sexual Dysfunction
Bupropion	+	++++	+	++	+++	+
Citalopram	+	+	+	+	++++	++++
Desvenlafaxine	++	+++	+	+	++++	++++
Fluoxetine	+	++++	+	+	++++	++++
Mirtazapine	+++	+	++	+	+	+
Nefazodone	++	+	+	+	++	+
Paroxetine	++	++	+	+	++++	++++
Sertraline	+	+++	+	+	++++	++++
Venlafaxine	++	+++	+	+	++++	++++
Vilazodone	+	+	+	+	++++	+

+, minimal; ++, low; +++, moderate; ++++, high; GI, gastrointestinal.

Data from Refs. 9, 13, and 28.

Table 38–5

Pharmacokinetic Parameters of Newer Antidepressants

Drug	Protein Binding (%)	Elimination Half-Life (hours)	Active Metabolite(s)
Bupropion	84	10–21	Yes
Citalopram	80	33	Yes
Desvenlafaxine	30	7.5	No
Duloxetine	90	9–19	No
Escitalopram	56	27–32	No
Fluoxetine	94	4–6 days with chronic dosing; 4–16 days (active metabolite)	Yes
Fluvoxamine	77	15–26	No
Mirtazapine	85	20–40	No
Nefazodone	99	2–4	Yes
Paroxetine	95	21	No
Selegiline	99	1.2–2	Yes
Sertraline	98	27	Yes
Venlafaxine	27	5	Yes
Vilazodone	99	25	No

Data from Refs. 9 and 29.

▶ Pharmacokinetic Parameters

Pharmacokinetic parameters of the newer antidepressants are shown in Table 38–5.[9,29] Several antidepressants are not highly protein bound, and the most notable of these are venlafaxine and desvenlafaxine. The elimination half-lives of nefazodone and venlafaxine are relatively short compared with those of the other agents. Conversely, fluoxetine has a very long half-life (i.e., 5 to 9 days) with chronic dosing, and its active metabolite (norfluoxetine) has an even longer half-life. Owing to the extremely long half-life of fluoxetine and its active metabolite, a 5-week washout of fluoxetine is required before starting an MAOI. A 2-week washout is generally considered sufficient for other SSRIs. Sertraline and citalopram are the other SSRIs with active metabolites, but these metabolites (desmethylsertraline and desmethylcitalopram, respectively) are only about one-eighth as potent as the parent compounds in terms of SRI activity.

▶ Drug Interactions

The major drug interactions of the antidepressants are shown in Table 38–6.[9,22,30] The usual pharmacodynamic drug interactions involve the "dirty receptors" blocked by some antidepressants. Hence, TCAs especially can cause significant additive effects with drugs that cause sedation, hypotension, or anticholinergic effects. Similarly, trazodone and mirtazapine can interact with other drugs that cause hypotensive and sedative effects, respectively. By far, the most concerning pharmacodynamic interactions are hypertensive crisis and 5-HT syndrome, which are both potentially life threatening when they occur. Hypertensive crisis is characterized by sharply elevated blood pressure, occipital headache, stiff or sore neck, nausea, vomiting, and sweating. It may result during MAOI therapy if the patient takes a sympathomimetic drug, such as ephedrine, pseudoephedrine, phenylephrine, or phenylpropanolamine

Table 38–6

Drug Interactions of Antidepressants[a]

Antidepressants	Type of Interaction	Examples of Interacting Drugs
TCAs, trazodone, mirtazapine	Pharmacodynamic—additive sedation	Benzodiazepines, alcohol, antihistamines
TCAs, trazodone	Pharmacodynamic—additive hypotensive effects	Prazosin, antipsychotics
TCAs	Pharmacodynamic—additive anticholinergic effects	Phenothiazines, benztropine
TCAs	Pharmacodynamic—additive cardiac toxicity	Thioridazine, quinidine
TCAs	Pharmacodynamic—decreased antihypertensive effect	Guanethidine, clonidine, methyldopa
Bupropion	Pharmacodynamic—increased seizure risk	TCAs, phenothiazines
MAOIs	Pharmacodynamic—hypertensive crisis	Tyramine-rich foods, sympathomimetics
MAOIs, TCAs, SSRIs, SNRIs, SARIs	Pharmacodynamic—5-HT syndrome	Serotonergic antidepressants, meperidine, dextromethorphan, tramadol
Fluvoxamine	Pharmacokinetic—CYP1A2 inhibition	TCAs, clozapine, theophylline
Fluoxetine, fluvoxamine, sertraline	Pharmacokinetic—CYP2C inhibition	TCAs, phenytoin, warfarin, tolbutamide
Fluoxetine, paroxetine, duloxetine, sertraline, bupropion	Pharmacokinetic—CYP2D6 inhibition	TCAs, haloperidol, risperidone, codeine, propranolol, propafenone
Nefazodone, fluoxetine, fluvoxamine	Pharmacokinetic—CYP3A4 inhibition	TCAs, alprazolam, verapamil, carbamazepine, lovastatin

[a]Not an all-inclusive list.

5-HT, serotonin; MAOI, monoamine oxidase inhibitor; SARI, serotonin antagonist and reuptake inhibitor; SNRI, serotonin and norepinephrine reuptake inhibitor; SSRI, selective serotonin reuptake inhibitor; TCA, tricyclic antidepressant.

Data from Refs. 9, 22, and 30.

or stimulants such as amphetamines or methylphenidate or if the patient consumes foods rich in tyramine, such as tap beers, aged cheeses, fava beans, yeast extracts, liver, dry sausage, sauerkraut, or tofu.[23] There are extensive lists of foods and drinks that are permitted and not permitted during therapy with MAOIs, and these always should be provided to patients. Because many over-the-counter products contain sympathomimetics, patients always should be told to consult with their clinician and/or pharmacist before using these drugs. 5-HT syndrome is characterized by confusion, restlessness, fever, abnormal muscle movements, hyperreflexia, sweating, diarrhea, and shivering.[31] It may result when a serotonergic agent is added to any serotonergic antidepressant, but the MAOIs are strongly associated with severe cases of 5-HT syndrome.[31] 5-HT syndrome is complicated by (a) an unawareness by clinicians of the diagnosis[31] and (b) the fact that many implicated drugs are not obviously serotonergic in nature, such as dextromethorphan, meperidine, tramadol, linezolid, and triptans.

Several antidepressants, including most of the SSRIs, bupropion, nefazodone, and duloxetine, are known to inhibit various cytochrome P450 isoenzymes, thereby elevating plasma levels of substrates for those isoenzymes and thus potentially leading to increased adverse effects or toxicity. The propensity to cause these drug interactions will vary with the particular antidepressant and the precise isoenzyme[9,22,30] (Table 38–6).

▶ Dosing

Dosing is summarized in Table 38–7.[13,16,17,20,29,32] The extended-release formulations of venlafaxine and bupropion allow for once-daily dosing. The delayed-release capsule of fluoxetine can be given once weekly, which can be started 7 days after the last regular-release capsule or tablet. Selegiline is available as a transdermal patch, and a dose of 6 mg/24 hours can be used without the usual dietary restrictions associated with MAOI use, although patients on the higher doses (9 and 12 mg/24 hours) should follow the usual dietary restrictions. Liquid dosage forms and disintegrating tablets of various antidepressants are ideal for patients who have difficulty swallowing tablets or capsules and those who otherwise may attempt to "cheek" their medication.

The starting dose is the usual therapeutic dose for most of the SSRIs, desvenlafaxine, duloxetine, and mirtazapine, but there is usually need for at least some upward titration of venlafaxine, vilazodone, bupropion, and nefazodone. A particular disadvantage of TCAs is that the customary way of dosing them involves meticulous upward titration from a small starting dose to a wide usual therapeutic dosage range. On the contrary, one advantage of some TCAs is that plasma levels may be used to help guide dosing, especially for those that have well-defined therapeutic plasma level ranges, including nortriptyline (50 to 150 ng/mL or mcg/L, or 190 to 570 nmol/L), desipramine (100 to 160 ng/mL or mcg/L, or

375 to 600 nmol/L), amitriptyline (75 to 175 ng/mL or mcg/L, 270 to 631 nmol/L), and imipramine (200 to 300 ng/mL or mcg/L, or 714 to 1,071 nmol/L).[28]

▶ Efficacy of Pharmacotherapy

⑤ *Each antidepressant has a response rate of approximately 60% to 80%, and no antidepressant medication or class has been reliably shown to be more efficacious than another.*[7,21] MAOIs may be the most effective therapy for atypical depression, but MAOI use continues to wane because of problematic adverse effects, dietary and drug restrictions, and the possibility of fatal drug interactions.[21,28] There is some evidence that dual-action antidepressants, such as TCAs and SNRIs, may be more effective for inpatients with severe depression than are the single-action drugs such as SSRIs,[21,28] but the more general assertion that multiple mechanisms of action confer efficacy advantages is quite controversial.[33]

▶ Selection of Medication

Figure 38–1 depicts a well-known algorithm for the pharmacologic treatment of nonpsychotic MDD—the Texas Medication Algorithm Project.[34] Notable aspects of this algorithm include the preferential use of newer antidepressants in the earlier stages of treatment and sequential trials of antidepressant monotherapy prior to the use of combination therapy (see Managing Partial Response or Nonresponse). It has been shown that patients undergoing treatment guided by this algorithm fared better than those who received treatment not guided by the algorithm during a 1-year period, as measured by clinician-rated symptoms, self-reported symptoms, and overall mental functioning.[35] Antipsychotic medication should be combined with antidepressant medication in cases of depression with psychotic features.[16]

Various factors must be taken into account when selecting antidepressant therapy for a particular patient. The most reliable predictor of response is the patient's history of response (e.g., efficacy, side effects, and overall satisfaction) to antidepressants. To a lesser extent, the history of a first-degree relative's response to antidepressants may be used to predict a patient's response. Adverse effect profiles should be considered because compliance is influenced greatly by tolerability. In this regard, a frank discussion should occur with the patient in order to determine which adverse effects are acceptable and which are not and how to deal with side effects (e.g., using chewing gum, hard candy, or ice chips for dry mouth). The clinician must be careful to contemplate potential drug–drug interactions and disease-state interactions. For instance, a patient with seizure disorder would be an inappropriate candidate for bupropion therapy. The presence of comorbid psychiatric conditions can help the clinician to determine the best antidepressant to choose for a patient. For example, an SSRI can treat both MDD and panic disorder, obviating the need for separate

Table 38-7

Dosing of Antidepressants in Adult Patients

Generic Name	Brand Name	Generic	Initial Dose (mg/day)	Usual Dosing Range (mg/day)	Usual Dosage Schedule	Renal Dosing Adjustment	Hepatic Dosing Adjustment[d]
MAOIs							
Phenelzine	Nardil	No	15–30	15–90	Twice daily	None	None
Selegiline	Emsam	No	6	6–12	Once daily	None	None
Tranylcypromine	Parnate	No	10–20	30–60	Twice daily	None	None
TCAs and Tetracyclics							
Amitriptyline	Elavil[a]	Yes	25–50	100–300	Once daily	Nondialyzable	Use with caution
Amoxapine	Asendin[a]	Yes	25–50	100–400	Once to twice daily	None	None
Clomipramine	Anafranil	Yes	25	100–250	Once daily	Use with caution	None
Desipramine	Nortriptyline	Yes	25–50	100–300	Once daily	None	Use with caution
Doxepin	Sinequan[a]	Yes	25–50	100–300	Once daily	Use with caution	Use a lower dose
Imipramine	Tofranil	Yes	25–50	100–300	Once daily	Use with caution	None
Maprotiline	Ludiomil[a]	Yes	50–75	100–225	Once to twice daily	None	None
Nortriptyline	Pamelor	Yes	25	50–150	Once daily	Use with caution	Use a lower dose
Protriptyline	Vivactil	No	5–10	15–60	Once daily	Use with caution	Use with caution
Trimipramine	Surmontil	No	25–50	100–300	Once daily	Use with caution	Use with caution
SSRIs							
Citalopram	Celexa	Yes	20	20–40[b]	Once daily	No adjustment for clcr greater than 20; for clcr less than 20, use with caution	20 mg/day maximum; may increase to 40 mg in nonresponders
Escitalopram	Lexapro	Yes	10	10–20	Once daily	No adjustment for clcr greater than 20; for clcr less than 20, use with caution	10 mg/day
Fluoxetine	Prozac	Yes	10–20	20–80	Once daily	None	Use lower or less frequent dosing
	Prozac weekly	Yes	90	90	Once weekly	None	Use lower or less frequent dosing
Fluvoxamine	Luvox	Yes	50	50–300	Twice daily	None	Reduce dose
	Luvox CR	No	100	100–300	Once daily	None	Reduce dose
Paroxetine	Paxil	Yes	10–20	20–50	Once daily	In ClCr less than 30, 10 mg/day increase weekly to a dose of 40 mg/day	Severe impairment, 10 mg daily; increase weekly to dose of 40 mg/day
	Paxil CR	Yes	12.5–25	25–62.5	Once daily	In ClCr less than 30, 12.5 mg daily increase weekly daily, to a dose of 50 mg/day	Severe impairment, 12.5 mg daily, increase weekly to dose of 40 mg/day
Sertraline	Zoloft	Yes	25–50	50–200	Once daily	None	Use a lower dose
NDRI							
Bupropion	Wellbutrin	Yes	150–200	300–450[c]	Twice to thrice daily	Consider lower dose	75 mg/day
	Wellbutrin SR	Yes	150	300–400[c]	Twice daily	Consider lower dose	100 mg/day or 150 mg every other day
	Wellbutrin XL	Yes	150	300–450[c]	Once daily	Consider lower dose	150 mg every other day
SNRIs							
Desvenlafaxine	Pristiq	No	50	50–100	Once daily	ClCr 30–50 50 mg maximum daily, ClCr 50 mg every other day	50 mg/day, 100 mg/day maximum
Duloxetine	Cymbalta	Yes	40–60	40–60	Once to twice daily	Use lower dose, not recommended For ClCr less than 30	Not recommended
Venlafaxine	Effexor	Yes	37.5–75	75–225	Once daily	Reduce dose 25%–50%	Reduce dose by 50%
	Effexor XR	Yes	37.5–75	75–225	Once daily	Reduce dose 25%–50%	Reduce dose by 50%

(Continued)

Table 38–7

Dosing of Antidepressants in Adult Patients *(Continued)*

Generic Name	Brand Name	Generic	Initial Dose Range (mg/day)	Usual Dosing Range (mg/day)	Usual Dosage Schedule	Renal Dosing Adjustment	Hepatic Dosing Adjustment[d]
SARIs							
Nefazodone	Serzone[a]	Yes	100–200	300–600	Twice daily	Use with caution	Discontinue if ALT/AST is more than 3 times normal
Trazodone	Desyrel[a]	Yes	50–150	200–600	Twice daily	Use with caution	Use with caution
	Olpetro	No	150	150–375	Daily	Use with caution	Use with caution
NaSSA							
Mirtazapine	Remeron	Yes	15	15–45	Once daily	ClCr less than 40, 30% decreased clearance	Clearance decreased by 30%
						ClCr less than 10, 50% decreased clearance	Clearance decreased by 30%
SRI/5-HT$_{2A}$							
Vilazodone	Viibryd	No	10	40	Once daily	None	Use with caution

[a]Brand no longer available in the United States.

[b]Maximum dose is 40 mg/day.

[c]Upper limit of this range is the maximum dose.

[d]All creatinine clearances (ClCrs) are stated in terms of milliliters per minute.

ALT, alanine aminotransferase; AST, aspartate aminotransferase; MAOI, monoamine oxidase inhibitor; NaSSA, noradrenergic and specific serotonergic antidepressant; NDRI, norepinephrine and dopamine reuptake inhibitor; SARI, serotonin antagonist and reuptake inhibitor; SNRI, serotonin and norepinephrine reuptake inhibitor; SSRI, selective serotonin reuptake inhibitor; SRI/5-HT$_{2A}$, partial agonist-serotonin reuptake inhibitor/serotonin$_{2A}$ partial agonist; TCA, tricyclic antidepressant.

Data from Refs. 13, 16, 17, 20, 22, 29, and 32.

medication therapy. Fluvoxamine, an SSRI, is marketed for obsessive compulsive disorder, although it also treats depression. The patient must be willing and able to comply with dosing schedules (e.g., upward titration of TCAs or twice-daily dosing of nefazodone) and special instructions (e.g., dietary restrictions with MAOI therapy) associated with certain antidepressants. Another patient-specific factor is the potential for accidental or intentional overdosing because certain antidepressants (e.g., TCAs) are quite toxic and potentially lethal in overdose situations. Finally, the patient should be able to comfortably afford the chosen medication or else compliance is at risk.[21]

Time Course of Response

Unfortunately, the antidepressants do not produce a clinical response immediately. Improvement in physical symptoms, such as sleep, appetite, and energy, can occur within the first week or so of treatment. Although a recent meta-analysis suggests earlier effects of antidepressant treatment,[36] ⑥ *it is widely accepted that approximately 2 to 4 weeks of treatment is required before improvement is seen in emotional symptoms of depression, such as sadness and anhedonia. Furthermore, as long as 6 to 8 weeks of treatment may be required to see the full effects of antidepressant therapy.*[7,21,23]

Managing Partial Response or Nonresponse

Approximately one-third of patients with MDD do not respond satisfactorily to their first antidepressant medication.[37] In such cases, the clinician must evaluate the adequacy of antidepressant therapy, including dosage, duration, and patient compliance.[17] Treatment reappraisal should also include verification of the patient's diagnosis and reconsideration of clinical factors that could be impeding successful therapy, such as concurrent medical conditions (e.g., thyroid disorder), comorbid psychiatric conditions (e.g., alcohol abuse), and psychosocial issues (e.g., marital stress).[16]

A series of reports from the Sequenced Treatment Alternatives to Relieve Depression (STAR*D) trial revealed that remission is associated with a better overall prognosis for patients than is improvement alone. STAR*D also established that in patients with a greater level of resistance, clinicians are less likely to push the patient to achieve remission, and in addition, those patients with the greatest levels of resistance had the highest rates of relapse. In these cases, STAR*D established some successful treatment recommendations.[37]

For patients who have experienced a partial response, extending the medication trial and/or using higher doses within the recommended dosage range of the antidepressant may be helpful.[16] Another option is to use augmentation

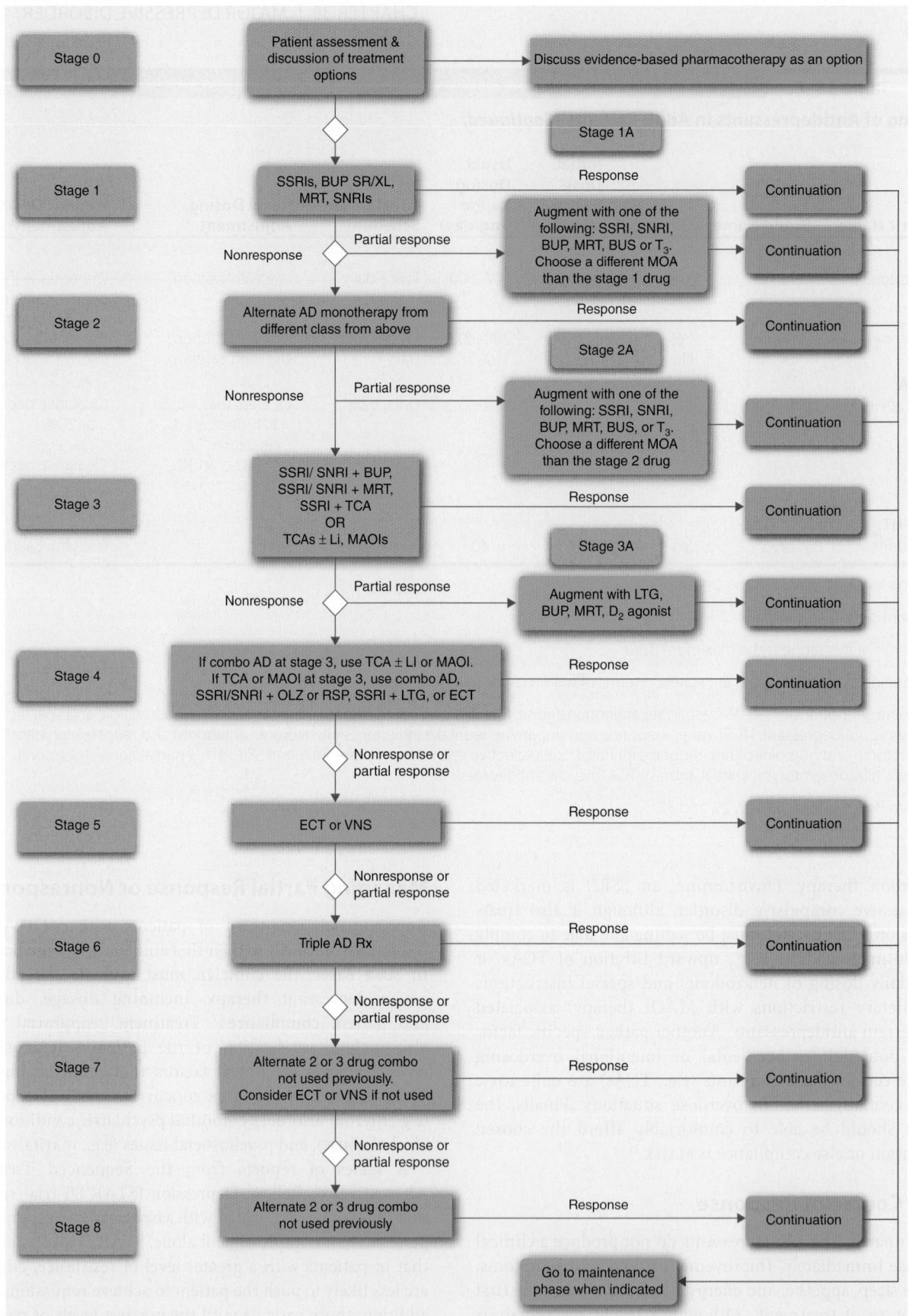

FIGURE 38–1. Strategies for the treatment of nonpsychotic major depression. (AD, antidepressant; BUP, bupropion; BUS, buspirone; ECT, electroconvulsive therapy; Li, lithium; T_3, liothyronine; LTG, lamotrigine; MAOI, monoamine oxidase inhibitor; MOA, mechanism of action; MRT, mirtazapine; OLZ, olanzapine; RSP, risperidone; Rx, prescription; SNRI, serotonin and norepinephrine reuptake inhibitor; SSRI, selective serotonin reuptake inhibitor; SSRI, selective serotonin reuptake inhibitor; TCA, tricyclic antidepressant; VNS, vagus nerve stimulation.) (Redrawn with permission from the Texas Medication Algorithm Project.[34])

therapy, that is, adding another medication that generally is not used as an antidepressant.[38] Augmenting agents with clear efficacy include lithium, buspirone, and triiodothyronine.[39] Aripiprazole and the extended-release formulation of quetiapine, second-generation antipsychotics, were recently approved by the FDA for augmenting partial response to antidepressants. Whereas efficacy has been suggested for dopaminergic drugs (e.g., pramipexole) and psychostimulants (e.g., methylphenidate), various other medications such as anticonvulsants (e.g., valproic acid), modafinil, and estrogen have anecdotal evidence to support their use as augmenting agents.[39] A third option is to make use of combination therapy, whereby another antidepressant, typically from a different pharmacologic class, is added to the first antidepressant medication. Examples include combining bupropion and SSRIs and combining TCAs and SSRIs.[39,40]

Switching to a different antidepressant is a common strategy for patients who have had no response to initial antidepressant therapy but also is acceptable in cases of partial response.[16] Relative to augmentation or combination, advantages of switching include improved compliance, decreased costs, and less concern over drug–drug interactions. Disadvantages include loss of time ("reset the clock") and loss of any improvement seen with the initial drug.[40] When switching from one antidepressant to another, clinicians may choose to stay within the same class (e.g., sertraline to fluoxetine) or go outside of the class (e.g., paroxetine to venlafaxine).[38,40] The olanzapine–fluoxetine combination medication Symbyax has been approved for treatment-resistant depression.[20]

Nonpharmacologic interventions in cases of treatment nonresponse include adding or changing to psychotherapy or initiating ECT.[16]

Duration of Therapy

Treatment of MDD can be conceptualized as a series of three phases: acute, continuation, and maintenance[7,8,16] (Fig. 38–2). During a major depressive episode, a clinician will initiate antidepressant therapy for the purpose of attaining **remission** of symptoms. This acute phase of treatment typically lasts 6 to 12 weeks. ❼ *Because the typical major depressive episode lasts 6 months or longer, if antidepressant therapy is interrupted for any reason after the acute phase, the patient may relapse into the depressive episode. When treating the first depressive episode, antidepressants must be given for an additional 4 to 9 months in the continuation phase for the purpose of preventing relapse.* Maintenance treatment takes place after the normal course of a major depressive episode to prevent recurrence, which is the development of future episodes. This phase can last for years, if not for a lifetime. Although all patients who have a major depressive episode should receive both acute and continuation treatment, not all of them will require maintenance treatment. The reason for this is because not all patients experience multiple major depressive episodes, and even in many cases in which they do, many years may separate the episodes. Therefore, the clinician must consider various factors in determining whether an individual patient requires maintenance treatment. A major factor is the number of prior episodes experienced by the patient. As discussed earlier, the more episodes experienced, the more likely future episodes will occur. This has led many clinicians to adopt the "three strikes and you're on" approach, whereby a patient with a history of three or more major depressive episodes is given lifelong maintenance treatment because of the very high (i.e., 90%) chance of experiencing additional episodes. Other factors to consider are the severity of previous episodes, especially if suicide attempts were made or psychotic features were present, and patient preference.[16] In general, the dose of the antidepressant required in the acute phase of treatment should be sustained during the continuation and maintenance phases.[16]

Discontinuation of Therapy

When the clinician and patient are ready to attempt discontinuation of therapy, whether at the end of the continuation phase or during the maintenance phase, it is best to do so via gradual taper of the antidepressant. This is done for two reasons. First, almost all antidepressants can

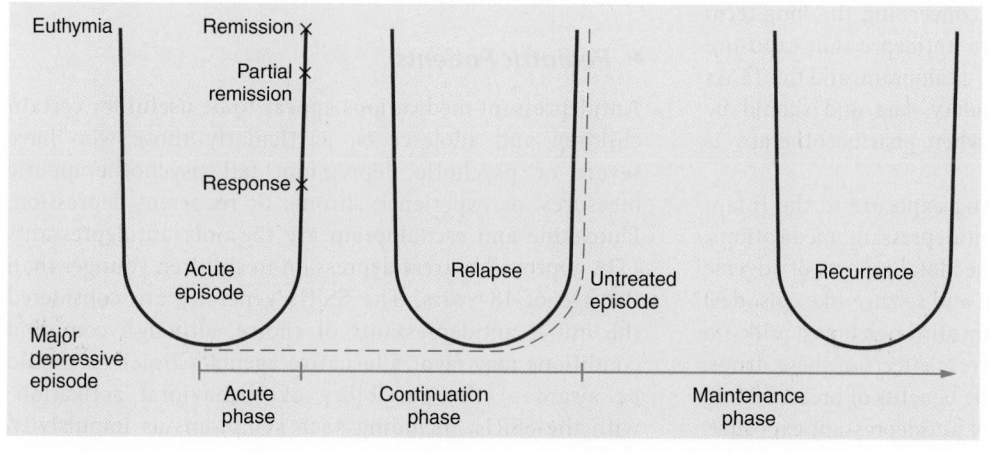

FIGURE 38–2. The course of depression and phases of treatment. (From Refs. 7 and 8).

produce withdrawal syndromes if discontinued abruptly or tapered too rapidly, especially antidepressants with shorter half-lives (e.g., venlafaxine, paroxetine, and fluvoxamine).[17] These withdrawal syndromes can cause sleep disturbances, anxiety, fatigue, mood changes, malaise, GI disturbances, and a host of other symptoms[17] and often are confused with depressive relapse or recurrence.[16] In general, a tapering schedule involving a small dosage decrement (e.g., paroxetine 5 mg) every 3 to 5 days should prevent significant withdrawal symptoms.[17] Second, depressive symptoms may return on taper or discontinuation of the antidepressant. If antidepressant therapy is discontinued abruptly and depressive symptoms return weeks later, then the lag time to onset of action must be observed when the antidepressant is restarted ("reset the clock"); however, if gradual tapering is carried out, then early signs of depression can be countered with a return to the original dosage and a potentially quicker response.[16] Depending on the patient's illness and the clinical circumstances, tapering of the antidepressant can be extended for weeks or even months because of the concern over relapse or recurrence.

Special Considerations

▶ Pregnant or Breastfeeding Patients

It is a common misconception that pregnancy protects against depression. Depression actually is quite common in pregnancy, especially for women with a history of recurrent depression. Both maternal and fetal well-being must be considered when weighing the benefits and risks of using antidepressant therapy during pregnancy. The prescribing information for paroxetine was changed to reflect the findings of epidemiological studies showing an increased risk of congenital malformations, particularly atrial and ventricular septal defects, in infants born to women taking the drug during the first trimester of pregnancy.[41] Sertraline and citalopram have also been associated with causing septal heart defects when taken during the first trimester. In addition, the incidence of having a baby with a septal heart defect was four times higher for mothers taking more than one SSRI in the first trimester.[42] Antidepressants have been reported occasionally to cause perinatal sequelae, such as poor neonatal adaptation, respiratory distress, feeding problems, and jitteriness.[43] Data concerning the long-term neurobehavioral effects of in utero antidepressant exposure remain quite limited.[43] Fluoxetine, citalopram, and the TCAs have the greatest reproductive safety data and should be considered first-line treatments when pharmacotherapy is indicated.[43]

There will be at least some drug exposure to the infant from nursing mothers taking antidepressant medications. Although there have been rare anecdotal reports of adverse effects (i.e., respiratory depression and seizure-like episodes) in infants exposed to antidepressants through breast milk, no rigorous study has confirmed adverse effects of these drugs, and it is generally accepted that the benefits of breastfeeding outweigh the risks to the infant of antidepressant exposure.

However, the decision needs to be made on an individual basis.[44]

▶ Geriatric Patients

It is generally agreed that depression in older adults is underrecognized and undertreated.[45] Although not uncommon in community samples, MDD is particularly prevalent among those living in long-term care facilities.[15,45] Barriers to recognition of geriatric depression include the tendency toward "masked" presentations, that is, complaints of physical symptoms (e.g., pain and GI problems) instead of mood symptoms, the frequent presence of medical illnesses, and the overlap of mood and cognitive symptoms with those of dementia.[15,45] Age-related pharmacokinetic and pharmacodynamic changes cause geriatric patients to be more sensitive to the effects of antidepressant medications.[15] Thus, lower starting doses of antidepressants with slow upward titrations as tolerated are recommended for geriatric patients.[13,16,45] The SSRIs are chosen frequently to treat geriatric depression because of their overall favorable adverse effect profiles and low toxicity; most TCAs are avoided owing to problematic anticholinergic, cardiovascular, and sedative properties.[45] Desipramine and nortriptyline are two TCAs that are more tolerable in terms of these adverse effects and thus may be used in geriatric depression.[45] Other newer antidepressants, such as bupropion, venlafaxine, nefazodone, and mirtazapine, are alternatives for the treatment of geriatric patients as well.[45]

▶ Pediatric Patients

Antidepressant medications appear to be useful for certain children and adolescents, particularly those who have severe or psychotic depression, fail psychotherapeutic measures, or experience chronic or recurrent depression. Fluoxetine and escitalopram are the only antidepressants FDA approved to treat depression in children younger than the age of 18 years. The SSRIs generally are considered the initial antidepressants of choice, although comorbid conditions may favor alternative agents. Clinicians should be aware of the possibility of "behavioral activation" with the SSRIs, including such symptoms as impulsivity,

Table 38–8

Patient Counseling

Counseling Point	Clinical Rationale
Mechanism of action—The medication works by affecting certain chemicals in the brain	Patient may feel that depression is a character weakness or personality flaw instead of a biological disorder
Lack of addiction potential—Although the medication affects certain chemicals in the brain, it is not addicting	Patient may worry that because the antidepressant is psychoactive, it must be addicting
Need for routine use—The medication will only work if it is taken as prescribed every day	Patient may try taking the medication on an as-needed basis
Delayed onset of action—It may take several weeks to see significant improvement in symptoms	Patient may prematurely discontinue therapy before the onset of beneficial effects
Prolonged duration of therapy—The medication should be taken for at least 6–12 months; do not discontinue it without consulting with the prescriber	Patient may prematurely discontinue therapy after symptoms have remitted, which could lead to relapse or recurrence
Adverse effects—Mention common and expected adverse effects as well as what to do if they occur	Patient may be more likely to discontinue therapy and distrust the prescriber if adverse effects occur without forewarning
Avoidance of alcohol and CNS depressants—Use of alcohol or other CNS depressants could cause worsened depression and additive adverse effects with the medicine	Patient may be unaware of the possible consequences of drinking alcohol or taking other drugs with antidepressants
Risk of suicidality—Be alert to symptoms of worsening depression and suicidality	Patient may become suicidal or have suicidal thinking while taking the antidepressant

CNS, central nervous system.

From Refs. 28 and 49.

silliness, daring conduct, and agitation.[46] Desipramine should be used with caution in this population because of several reports of sudden death, and a baseline and follow-up electrocardiography may be warranted when this medication is used to treat pediatric patients.[9]

The FDA has warned that antidepressants increase the risk of suicidality (i.e., suicidal thinking and behavior) in children and young adults. A large analysis of clinical trials revealed that the risk of such events was 4% for antidepressant medications versus 2% for placebo, although no completed suicides occurred in the trials. Because of this increased risk, antidepressants have black-box warnings concerning the matter, and patient medication guides are required to be distributed with each prescription or refill of antidepressant medications. **❽** *Pediatric patients and young adults should be observed closely for suicidality, worsened depression, agitation, irritability, and unusual changes in behavior, especially during the initial few months of therapy and at times of dosage changes. Furthermore, families and caregivers should be advised to monitor patients for such symptoms.*[47]

▶ Suicidal Patients

The FDA has determined that in addition to children and adolescents, there is an increased risk of suicidality in patients between the ages of 18 and 24 years, with no increased risk after the age of 24 years. Similar monitoring for suicidality and clinical worsening that is mandated for pediatric patients should also be followed for young adult patients.[48]

Clinicians should bear in mind the toxic potential for the various antidepressant medications when patients already have or develop suicidality. Whereas the TCAs and MAOIs have narrow therapeutic indices, the SSRIs, SNRIs, nefazodone, and mirtazapine have wide therapeutic indices.[21]

Patient Counseling

Major counseling points and the clinical rationales behind them are outlined in Table 38–8.[28,49] **❾** *Lack of patient understanding concerning optimal antidepressant drug therapy frequently leads to partial compliance or noncompliance with therapy; thus, the primary purpose of antidepressant counseling is to enhance compliance and improve outcomes.*[49]

OUTCOME EVALUATION

- Review the patient's medication profile to ensure that there are no potential or actual pharmacotherapy problems related to dosing, disease-state precautions or contraindications, drug–drug interactions, or unnecessary therapeutic duplication.

- Verify the extent of compliance with pharmacotherapy.

- Assess the response to pharmacotherapy, especially with regard to suicidality and symptoms that cause significant subjective distress and/or functional impairment.

- Determine whether the patient is experiencing any adverse effects of pharmacotherapy. Although general questioning (e.g., "Are you having any side effects?") may reveal some problems with therapy, it is better to use direct questioning concerning adverse effects that are most common and/or most problematic (e.g., "Have you noticed any change in your sexual functioning?").

- Provide counseling to enhance patient understanding of MDD and its pharmacotherapy.

Patient Care and Monitoring

1. Assess the patient's severity of symptoms to determine if self-care is appropriate or whether a psychiatrist should evaluate the patient.

2. Obtain a thorough history of prescription, nonprescription, natural, and illicit drug use. Rule out medications or medical disorders that may cause or mimic depressive symptoms.

3. Review the *Diagnostic and Statistical Manual of Mental Disorders*, 4th edition, text revision (*DSM-IV-TR*) criteria to determine an appropriate diagnosis.

4. Determine appropriate pharmacologic and psychological treatments (e.g., cognitive-behavioral therapy), including what has been helpful to the patient in the past.

5. Educate the patient and/or caretaker about the disease state, lifestyle modifications, and medication therapy.

   - What risk factors are present that could contribute to depression?
   - What lifestyle modifications could be made to improve the condition (e.g., exercise)?
   - How the medication should be taken?
   - What potential adverse effects may occur?
   - Which drugs may interact with their therapy?
   - Warning signs and prevention of suicidal and/or homicidal ideation.

6. Develop a plan to assess effectiveness of pharmacologic therapy after 4 weeks of being on a clinically effective dose.

7. Evaluate the patient for the presence of adverse drug reactions, drug allergies, and drug interactions.

8. Assess improvement in quality-of-life measures such as physical, psychological, and social functioning and well-being.

9. If the patient does not respond, determine if the patient is taking the appropriate medication and dose.

10. Recommend changes in therapy if the patient does not respond.

11. Assess the need for long-term maintenance therapy.

Abbreviations Introduced in This Chapter

DA	Dopamine
DRI	Dopamine reuptake inhibitor
DSM-IV-TR	*Diagnostic and Statistical Manual of Mental Disorders*, 4th ed, text revision
ECT	Electroconvulsive therapy
GI	Gastrointestinal
5-HT	Serotonin
MAOI	Monoamine oxidase inhibitor
MDD	Major depressive disorder
NaSSA	Noradrenergic and specific serotonergic antidepressant
NDRI	Norepinephrine and dopamine reuptake inhibitor
NE	Norepinephrine
NRI	Norepinephrine reuptake inhibitor
SAD	Seasonal affective disorder
SARI	Serotonin antagonist and reuptake inhibitor
SI	Suicidal ideation
SNRI	Serotonin and norepinephrine reuptake inhibitor
SRI	Serotonin reuptake inhibition
SSRI	Selective serotonin reuptake inhibitor
STAR*D	Sequenced Treatment Alternatives to Relieve Depression
TCA	Tricyclic antidepressant
VNS	Vagus nerve stimulation
WHO	World Health Organization

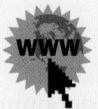 Self-assessment questions and answers are available at *http://www.mhpharmacotherapy.com/pp.html.*

REFERENCES

1. Top 200 drugs [online]. 2010. [cited 2011 Oct 10]. Available from: *http://wwwpharmacytimes.com/publications/issue/2010/May2010/RxFocusTopDrugs-0510.* Accessed September 15, *2011.*

2. Hasin DS, Goodwin RD, Stinson FS, et al. Epidemiology of major depressive disorder. Arch Gen Psychiatry 2005;62:1097–1106.

3. American Psychiatric Association. Diagnostic and Statistical Manual of Mental Disorders. 4th ed, text revision. Washington, DC: American Psychiatric Association; 2000:356.

4. World Health Organization. Depression [online]. [cited 2011 Oct 10]. Available from: *http://www.who.int/mental_health/management/depression/definition/en/print.html.* Accessed October 1, 2011.

5. Levinson DF. The genetics of depression: A review. Biol Psychiatry 2006;60:84–92.

6. Muscatell KA, Slavich GM, Monroe SM, et al. Stressful life events, chronic difficulties, and the symptoms of clinical depression. J Nerv Ment Dis 2009;197:154-160.

7. Boland RJ, Keller MB. Antidepressants. In: Tasman A, Kay J, Lieberman JA, eds. Psychiatry. 3rd ed. Hoboken; NJ: Wiley; 2008:292–334.

8. Stahl SM. Essential Psychopharmacology: Neuroscientific Basis and Practical Applications. 3rd ed. New York: Cambridge University Press; 2008:135–295.

9. Teter CJ, Kando JC, Wells BG. Depressive disorders. In: DiPiro JT, Talbert RL, Yee GC, et al, eds. Pharmacotherapy: A Pathophysiologic Approach. 8th ed. New York: McGraw-Hill; 2011:1173–1190.

10. Belmaker RH, Agam G. Major depressive disorder. New Engl J Med 2008;358:55–68.

11. Krishnan V, Nestler EJ. The molecular neurobiology of depression. Nature 2008; 455:894–902.

12. Maletic V, Robinson M, Oakes T. Neurobiology of depression: An integrated view of key findings. Int J Clin Pract 2007;61:2030–2040.

13. Narasimhan M, Raynor JD, Jones AB. Depression in the medically ill: diagnostic and therapeutic implications. Curr Psychiatry Rep 2008;10:272–279.

14. Patten SB, Barbui C. Drug-induced depression: A systematic review to inform clinical practice. Psychother Psychosom 2004;73:207–215.

15. Raj A. Depression in the elderly. Tailoring medical therapy to their special needs. Postgrad Med 2004;115:26–28, 37–42.

16. Kaiser Permanente Care Management Institute. Depression Clinical Practice Guidelines Oakland (CA). Kaiser Permanente Care Management Institute; 2006;1–196.

17. Trivedi M, Fava M, Marangell LB. Use of treatment algorithms for depression. J Clin Psychiatry 2006;67:1458–1465.

18. VNS therapy system [online]. [cited 2011 Oct 10]. Available from: *http://www.fda.gov/cdrh/mda/docs/p970003s050.html*. Accessed September 18, 2011.

19. George MS, Post RM. Daily left prefrontal repetitive transcranial magnetic stimulation for acute treatment of medication resistant depression. Am J Psychiatry 2011;168:356–364.

20. Practice guideline for the treatment of patients with major depressive disorder [online]. 3rd ed. [cited 2011 Oct 10]. Available from: *http://www.psych.org/guidelines/mdd2010*. Accessed October 2, 2011.

21. Sussman N, Thase ME. Selecting a first-line antidepressant: New analysis. Primary Psychiatry 2009;16:19–22.

22. Forest Pharmaceuticals, Inc. Manufacturer's Information. St. Louis, MO: Viibryd; 2011.

23. Schellander R, Donnerer J. Antidepressants: Clinically relevant drug interactions to be considered. Int J Exp Clin Pharmacol 2010;86:203–215.

24. Cassano P, Fava M. Tolerability issues during long-term treatment with antidepressants. Ann Clin Psychiatry 2004;16:15–25.

25. Kennedy SH, Rizvi S. Sexual dysfunction, depression, and the impact of antidepressants. J Clin Psychopharmacol 2009;29:157–164.

26. Westanmo AD, Gayken J, Haight R. Duloxetine: A balanced and selective norepinephrine- and serotonin-reuptake inhibitor. Am J Health-Syst Pharm 2005;62:2481–2490.

27. Eli Lilly and Company. Prozac: Manufacturer's information. Indianapolis, IN, 2007.

28. Stimmel GL. Mood disorders. In: Helms RA, Quan DJ, eds. Textbook of Therapeutics: Drug and Disease Management. 8th ed. Philadelphia, PA: Lippincott Williams & Wilkins, 2006:1416–1431.

29. Clinical pharmacology [online]. [cited 2011 Oct 10]. Available from: *http://cpip.gsm.com*. Accessed September 8, 2011.

30. Devane CL. Antidepressant-drug interactions are potentially but rarely significant. Neuropsychopharmacology 2006;31:1594–1604.

31. Boyer EW, Shannon M. The serotonin syndrome. N Engl J Med 2005;352:1112–1120.

32. To SE, Zepf RA, Woods AG. The symptoms, neurobiology, and current pharmacological treatment of depression. J Neurosci Nurs 2005;37:102–107.

33. Burke WJ. Selective versus multi-transmitter antidepressants: Are two mechanisms better than one? J Clin Psychiatry 2004;65(Suppl 4):37–45.

34. Texas Medication Algorithm Project—nonpsychotic depression algorithm [online]. [cited 2011 Oct 10]. Available from: *http://www.dshs.state.tx.us/mhprograms/disclaimer.shtm*. Accessed November 28, 2011.

35. Trivedi MH, Rush AJ, Crismon ML, et al. Clinical results for patients with major depressive disorder in the Texas Medication Algorithm Project. Arch Gen Psychiatry 2004;61:669–680.

36. Posternak MA, Zimmerman M. Is there a delay in the antidepressant effect? A meta-analysis. J Clin Psychiatry 2005;66:148–158.

37. Rush JA. STAR*D: What have we learned? Am J Psychiatry 2007;164:201–204.

38. Klein N, Sacher J, Wallner H, et al. Therapy of treatment resistant depression: Focus on the management of TRD with atypical antipsychotics. CNS Spectr 2004;9:823–832.

39. McIntyre J, Moral MA. Augmentation in treatment-resistant depression. Drugs Future 2006;31:1069–1072.

40. Thase ME. Management of patients with treatment-resistant depression. J Clin Psychiatry 2008;69(3):e08.

41. FDA public health advisory—paroxetine [online]. [cited 2011 Oct 10]. Available from: *http://www.fda.gov/cder/drug/advisory/paroxetine200512.htm*. Accessed September 25, 2011.

42. Pedersen LH, Henriksen TB, Vestergaard M, et al. Selective serotonin reuptake inhibitors in pregnancy and congenital malformations: Population based cohort study. BMJ 2009;339:b3569.

43. Cohen LS, Nonacs R, Viguera AC, Reminick A. Diagnosis and treatment of depression during pregnancy. CNS Spectr 2004;9:209–216.

44. Gentile S. The use of contemporary antidepressants during breastfeeding: A proposal for a specific safety index. Drug Safety 2007;30:107–121.

45. Mukai Y, Rajesh R, Tampi MD. Treatment of depression in the elderly: A review of the recent literature on the efficacy of single-versus dual-action antidepressants. Clin Ther 2009;31:945–961.

46. Ryan ND. Treatment of depression in children and adolescents. Lancet 2005;366:933–940.

47. FDA public health advisory—suicidality in children and adolescents being treated with antidepressant medications [online]. [cited 2011 Oct 10]. Available from: *http://www.fda.gov/cder/drug/antidepressants/SSRIPHA200410.htm*. Accessed September 25, 2011.

48. FDA public health advisory—antidepressant use in children, adolescents and adults [online]. [cited 2011 Oct 10]. Available from: *http://www.fda.gov/Drugs/DrugSafety/InformationbyDrugClass/UCM096273*. Accessed September 30, 2011.

49. Bollini P, Pampallona S, Kupelnick B, et al. Improving compliance in depression: A systematic review of narrative reviews. J Clin Pharm Ther 2006;31:253–260.

39

Bipolar Disorder

Brian L. Crabtree and Lydia E. Weisser

KEY CONCEPTS

❶ Patients presenting with depressive or elevated mood features and a history of abnormal or unusual mood swings should be assessed for bipolar disorder.

❷ The diagnosis of bipolar disorder is made based on clinical presentation, a careful diagnostic interview, and a review of the history. There are no laboratory examinations, brain imaging studies, or other procedures that confirm the diagnosis.

❸ Goals of treatment are to reduce symptoms, induce remission, prevent relapse, improve patient functioning, and minimize adverse effects of drug therapy.

❹ Psychotherapy improves functional outcomes and may help treat or prevent mood episodes.

❺ The primary treatment modality for manic episodes is mood stabilizing agents or antipsychotic drugs, often in combination.

❻ The primary treatment for depressive episodes in bipolar disorder is mood stabilizing agents or certain antipsychotic drugs, sometimes combined with antidepressant drugs.

❼ The primary treatment for relapse prevention is mood stabilizing agents, often combined with antipsychotic drugs.

❽ Education of the patient regarding benefits and risks of drug therapy and the importance of adherence to treatment must be integrated into pharmacologic management.

INTRODUCTION

Bipolar disorder is a mood disorder characterized by one or more episodes of mania or **hypomania**, often with a history of one or more major depressive episodes.[1] It is a chronic illness with relapses and improvements or remissions. Mood episodes can be manic, depressed, or mixed. They can be separated by long periods of stability or can cycle rapidly. They occur with or without psychosis. Disability and other consequences (e.g., increased risk of suicide) of bipolar

Chief Complaint: "My family doctor made me come here. I'm not crazy."

History of Present Illness:

Roger is a 28-year-old attorney with a local law firm. He presents somewhat reluctantly after being told by his supervisor that he needed to seek help for some unusual behavior. Roger initially presented to his family physician, who performed a physical examination and some screening to include CBC, metabolic profile, thyroid function, and ECG. All results were unremarkable. He was then referred to a psychiatric clinician for further evaluation.

Roger is an unmarried, well-nourished, well-developed white man appearing his stated age. He is wearing a suit and is well-groomed; however, his speech is somewhat rapid, and you find it difficult to interrupt him to get him to answer your questions. He paces around your office while speaking and is quite distractible. Roger says he has been experiencing decreased sleep, getting only 2 or 3 hours per night without feeling fatigued the next day. In fact, he says he feels, "more energetic than ever." His appetite is decreased, and he has lost about 10 lb (4.5 kg) over the past few weeks. He has been working hard on a project for the firm and, to his annoyance, his boss and coworkers told him his work is less than up to standard and full of mistakes. He admits to some recent financial problems as well.

What diagnoses are suggested by this patient's presentation?

What additional information is needed to clarify the diagnosis?

disorder can be devastating to patients and their families. Correct diagnosis and treatment are essential as early as possible in the course of the illness to prevent complications and maximize response to treatment.

EPIDEMIOLOGY AND ETIOLOGY

Epidemiology

Bipolar disorders are categorized into bipolar I disorder, bipolar II disorder, and bipolar disorder not otherwise specified (NOS). Bipolar I disorder is characterized by one or more manic or **mixed mood episodes**. Bipolar II disorder is characterized by one or more major depressive episodes and at least one hypomanic episode. Hypomania is an abnormally and persistently elevated, expansive, or irritable mood but not of sufficient severity to cause significant impairment in social or occupational function and does not require hospitalization. The lifetime prevalence of bipolar I disorder is estimated to be between 0.3% and 2.4%. The lifetime prevalence of bipolar II disorder ranges from 0.2% to 5%. When including the entire spectrum of bipolar disorder diagnoses, the lifetime prevalence is between 3% and 6.5%.[1]

Bipolar I disorder affects men and women equally. Bipolar II is more common in women. Rapid cycling and mixed mood episodes occur more often in women. In all, 78% to 85% of individuals with bipolar disorder report having another *Diagnostic and Statistical Manual*, 4th edition, text revision (*DSM-IV-TR*), diagnosis during their lifetime. The most common comorbid conditions include anxiety, substance abuse, and impulse control disorders. Nonpsychiatric medical comorbidities are also common.[2]

The mean age of onset of bipolar disorder is 20 years, although onset may occur in early childhood to the mid-40s.[1] If the onset of symptoms occurs after age 60, the condition is probably secondary to medical causes. An early onset of bipolar disorder is associated with greater comorbidities, more mood episodes, a greater proportion of days depressed, and greater lifetime risk of suicide attempts compared with bipolar disorder with a later onset. Substance abuse and anxiety disorders are more common in patients with an early onset. Patients with bipolar disorder also have higher rates of suicidal thinking, suicide attempts, and completed suicides than the general population.

Etiology

The precise etiology is unknown. Thought to be genetically based, bipolar disorder is influenced by a variety of factors that may enhance gene expression. These include trauma, environmental factors, anatomical abnormalities, exposure to chemicals or drugs, and others.[3-5] Neurochemical abnormalities in bipolar disorder may be caused by these factors, which are discussed further in the pathophysiology section.

PATHOPHYSIOLOGY

Neurochemical

The pathophysiology remains incompletely understood. Imaging techniques such as positron emission tomography (PET) scans and functional magnetic resonance imaging (fMRI) are being used to elucidate the cause. Research in the 1970s focused on neurotransmitters such as norepinephrine (NE), dopamine (DA), and serotonin. One hypothesis was that bipolar disorder is caused by an imbalance of cholinergic and catecholaminergic neuronal activity. Serotonin (5-HT) has been suggested to modulate catecholamine activity. Dysregulation of this relationship could cause a mood disturbance. Early theories included that an elevation of NE and DA caused mania and a reduction caused depression, but these theories are now considered overly simplistic.[3] Other neurotransmitters are involved and interact with multiple neurochemical and neuroanatomic mechanisms and pathways.[6] The pathophysiology has also been hypothesized from the mechanisms of action of lithium and other mood stabilizers. Lithium, valproate, and carbamazepine all have similar effects on neuronal growth that are reversible by inositol, supporting the hypothesis that bipolar disorder is related to inositol disturbance.[7] Evidence has shown that brain-derived neurotrophic factor (BDNF) may also play a role in bipolar disorder. Serum BDNF is low in mania and improves with response to treatment.[8]

Genetic

Results of family and twin studies suggest a genetic basis for bipolar disorder.[4] The lifetime risk of bipolar disorder in relatives of a bipolar patient is 40% to 70% for a monozygotic twin and 5% to 10% for another first-degree relative.

CLINICAL PRESENTATION AND DIAGNOSIS

Diagnosis of Bipolar Disorder

1 *Patients presenting with depressive or elevated mood features and a history of abnormal or unusual mood swings should be assessed for bipolar disorder.* Bipolar disorder is categorized into four subtypes: bipolar I (periods of major depressive, manic, and/or mixed episodes); bipolar II (periods of major depression and hypomania), cyclothymic disorder (periods of hypomanic episodes and depressive episodes that do not meet all criteria for diagnosis of a major depressive episode), and bipolar disorder NOS. The defining feature of bipolar disorders is one or more manic or hypomanic episodes in addition to depressive episodes that are not caused by a medical condition, substance abuse, or other psychiatric disorder.[1]

Initial and subsequent episodes of bipolar disorder are mostly depressive.[9] Studies that followed patients with bipolar disorder over an average of about 13 years show that bipolar I patients spend about 32% of weeks with depressive symptoms compared with 9% of weeks with manic or hypomanic symptoms.[10] Patients with bipolar II disorder spend 50% of weeks symptomatic for depression and only 1% with hypomanic symptoms.[11] Because patients may present with depression and spend more time depressed than with mood elevation, bipolar disorder is often misdiagnosed or underdiagnosed. It is helpful to use a screening tool such as the mood disorder questionnaire.[12]

DSM-IV-TR criteria for the diagnosis of bipolar disorder are summarized in Table 39–1.

Patient Encounter, Part 2: Medical History, Physical Examination, and Laboratory Examination

Your interview reveals the following information:

Past Medical History: No known medical problems except a history of mildly elevated blood pressure, controlled by hydrochlorothiazide 25 mg/day. One episode of gonorrhea in his early 20s.

Past Psychiatric History: Noncontributory

Family History: Parents alive and well. A paternal uncle committed suicide several years ago. A maternal aunt has history of alcohol, opiate, and benzodiazepine abuse. The patient's paternal grandfather reportedly had episodes of "moodiness" and bizarre behavior at times but was never treated. Two sisters in good health, although older sister has been treated for depression in the past.

Social History: The patient is bisexual with a history of multiple casual partners of both genders whom he meets at parties and bars. He graduated from college with honors and a degree in political science. He subsequently graduated from law school and has worked at his current job for 1 year. He began work at one law firm immediately upon graduation but was terminated because of frequent absences. He quit his previous job because he "wants to rise to the top" of his field as quickly as possible and thought his current firm was more prestigious. He lives alone but has an active sexual life and enjoys gambling at casinos. He reports a similar episode in college when he felt naturally energetic and, on a dare, jumped on a plane to go to Washington to tell the president some of his ideas about Homeland Security.

Substance Use History: Denies use of tobacco products; cocaine; hallucinogens; intravenous drugs; amphetamines; and overuse of prescription medications, such as opiates and benzodiazepines. However, he admits to smoking marijuana "to calm myself down" at times and tends to binge drink on the weekend when at casinos or at parties. He also drinks several mixed drinks each night to help get to sleep. He drinks one cup of coffee each morning and denies use of vitamins and herbal supplements.

Medications: Hydrochlorothiazide 25 mg po daily.

ROS: Increased energy, racing thoughts, decreased need for sleep, decreased appetite.

PE:

VS: BP 135/80, P 90, RR 20, T 98.6°F (37.0°C)

HEENT: PERRLA. Extraocular movements intact. Nares patent. Ear canals patent and eardrums easily visualized. Neck supple without JVD, bruits, or adenopathy. Thyroid smooth, symmetric, and nontender.

CV: Regular rate and rhythm without murmurs, gallops, or rubs.

Abd: Soft, nontender, no organomegaly or masses. Positive bowel sounds.

Exts: Without clubbing, cyanosis, or edema. Peripheral pulses full and equal bilaterally.

CN: II–XII intact.

Labs: Urine drug screen + for THC. HIV negative

Considering this additional information, what is the most likely diagnosis?

What are the key pieces of information leading you to this conclusion?

Table 39–1

Evaluation and Diagnostic Criteria of Mood Episodes

Diagnostic workup depends on clinical presentation and findings		• Mental status examination • Psychiatric, medical, and medication history • Physical and neurologic examination • Basic laboratory tests: CBC, blood chemistry screen, thyroid function, urinalysis, urine drug screen • Psychological testing • Brain imaging: MRI and fMRI; alternative: CT, PET • Lumbar puncture • Electroencephalogram
Diagnosis episode	Impairment of functioning or need for hospitalization[a]	*DSM-IV-TR* criteria[b]
Major depressive	Yes	Greater than or equal to 2-week period of either depressed mood or loss of interest or pleasure in normal activities, associated with at least five of the following symptoms: • Depressed, sad mood (adults); can be irritable mood in children • Decreased interest and pleasure in normal activities • Decreased appetite, weight loss • Insomnia or hypersomnia • Psychomotor retardation or agitation • Decreased energy or fatigue • Feelings of guilt or worthlessness • Impaired concentration and decision making • Suicidal thoughts or attempts
Manic	Yes	Greater than or equal to 1-week period of abnormal and persistent elevated mood (expansive or irritable), associated with at least three of the following symptoms (four if the mood is only irritable): • Inflated self-esteem (grandiosity) • Racing thoughts (FOI) • Distractible (poor attention) • Increased activity (either socially, at work, or sexually) or increased motor activity or agitation • Excessive involvement in activities that are pleasurable but have a high risk for serious consequences (buying sprees, sexual indiscretions, poor judgment in business ventures)
Hypomanic	No	At least 4 days of abnormal and persistent elevated mood (expansive or irritable); associated with at least three of the following symptoms (four if the mood is only irritable): • Inflated self-esteem (grandiosity) • Decreased need for sleep • Increased talking (pressure of speech) • Racing thoughts (FOI) • Increased activity (either socially, at work, or sexually) or increased motor activity or agitation • Excessive involvement in activities that are pleasurable but have a high risk for serious consequences (buying sprees, sexual indiscretions, poor judgment in business ventures)
Mixed	Yes	Criteria for both a major depressive episode and manic episode (except for duration) occur nearly every day for at least a 1-week period
Rapid cycling	Yes	More than three major depressive or manic episodes (manic, mixed, or hypomanic) in 12 months

[a]Impairment in social or occupational functioning; need for hospitalization because of potential self-harm, harm to others, or psychotic symptoms.

[b]The disorder is not caused by a medical condition (e.g., hypothyroidism) or substance-induced disorder (e.g., antidepressant treatment, medications, electroconvulsive therapy).

Data from American Psychiatric Association. Diagnostic and Statistical Manual of Mental Disorders. 4th ed, text rev. Washington, DC: American Psychiatric Press; 2000 and Drayton SJ. Bipolar disorder. In: DiPiro JT, Talbert RL, Yee GC, Matzke GR, Wells BG, Posey LM, eds. Pharmacotherapy: A Pathophysiologic Approach. 8th ed. New York, NY: McGraw-Hill. 2010; 1191–1208. With permission.

▶ Bipolar I Disorder

● The diagnosis of bipolar I disorder requires at least one episode of mania for at least 1 week or longer with a persistently elevated, expansive, or irritable mood with related symptoms of decreased need for sleep, excessive energy, racing thoughts, a propensity to be involved in high-risk activities, and excessive talkativeness.[1] Bipolar I depression can be misdiagnosed as major depressive disorder (MDD); therefore, it is essential to rule out past episodes of hypomania or mania. If bipolar depression is mistaken for MDD and the patient is treated with antidepressants, it can precipitate a manic episode or induce rapid cycling of depression and mania.

▶ Bipolar II Disorder

● The distinguishing feature of bipolar II disorder is depression with past hypomanic episodes that often are not recalled by the individual as being unusual. Irritability and anger episodes are also common. There cannot have been a prior full-manic episode.[1]

▶ Cyclothymic Disorder

● Cyclothymic disorder is a chronic mood disturbance generally lasting at least 2 years (1 year in children and adolescents) and characterized by mood swings that include periods of hypomania and depressive symptoms. Hypomanic symptoms include inflated self-esteem or **grandiosity** (nondelusional), decreased need for sleep, pressure of speech, **flight of ideas (FOI)**, distractibility, and increased involvement in goal-directed activities, not causing severe impairment in social or occupational functioning or requiring hospitalization. Psychotic features are not present in cyclothymic disorder.[1]

▶ Suicide

Patients with bipolar disorder have a high risk of suicide. Factors that increase that risk are early age at disease onset, high number of depressive episodes, comorbid alcohol abuse, personal history of antidepressant-induced mania, and family history of suicidal behavior. About one-third of individuals

❶ Clinical Presentation and Diagnosis

General

The patient may present in a hypomanic, manic, depressed, or mixed state and may or may not be in acute distress.

Symptoms

Mood and Affect:

- Mood elevation
- Expansive mood
- Irritable mood
- Depression
- Hopelessness
- Suicidality

Physical and Behavioral:

- Agitation
- Impulsivity
- Aggression
- Rapid, pressured speech
- Decreased need for sleep
- Insomnia (sometimes for days or weeks)
- Hypersexuality
- Increased physical energy
- Inflated self-esteem, boasting, grandiosity
- Heightened interest in pleasurable activities with a high risk of negative consequences (e.g., spending sprees, promiscuity)
- Fatigue
- Hypersomnia

Thought Processes, Content, and Perceptions:

- Racing thoughts, FOI, distractibility
- Delusions of grandeur, ideas of reference, persecution, wealth, religion

Psychosocial

- Substance use
- Disrupted relationships
- Job loss

Laboratory and Other Diagnostic Assessments

❷ *There are no objective laboratory tests or procedures to diagnose bipolar disorder, but such testing can be done to rule out other medical diagnoses.*

- Urinalysis, urine toxicology, thyroid function, and white blood cell count in elderly patients to rule out urinary tract infection
- Mood disorder questionnaire, completed by the patient, asks about common symptoms of bipolar disorder, problems caused by the symptoms, and family history in a "yes" or "no" answer format. It is then scored by the clinician

Suicidality risk is increased in the presence of:

- Substance abuse
- Prior suicide attempts and lethality of attempts
- Access to a means of suicide
- Command hallucinations or psychosis
- Severe anxiety
- Family history of attempted or completed suicide

Data from Refs. 1, 3, and 16.

with bipolar disorder report a previous suicide attempt.[13] One of five suicide attempts is fatal in contrast to one of 10 to one of 20 in the general population.

▶ Differential Diagnosis

Schizophrenia and bipolar disorder share certain symptoms, including psychosis in some patients. The prominence of mood symptoms and the history of mood episodes distinguish bipolar disorder and schizophrenia. In addition, the psychosis of schizophrenia occurs in the absence of prominent mood symptoms.

Schizoaffective disorder may also be considered when developing a differential diagnosis for bipolar disorder. Schizoaffective disorder is characterized by an uninterrupted period of illness during which there is either a major depressive episode, a manic episode, or a mixed episode concurrent with symptoms that meet criterion A for schizophrenia (e.g., delusions, hallucinations, disorganized speech, grossly disorganized or catatonic behavior, and/or negative symptoms such as affective flattening, alogia, or avolition). The major depressive episode must include depressed mood. During the same period of illness, there have been delusions or hallucinations for at least 2 weeks in the absence of prominent mood symptoms. Schizoaffective Disorder may be of two different types. The bipolar type includes a manic or mixed episode or a manic or mixed episode and major depressive episodes. The depressive type includes only major depressive episodes.[1]

Personality disorders are inflexible and maladaptive patterns of behavior that deviate markedly from expectations of society beginning in adolescence or early adulthood.[1] Personality disorders and bipolar disorder may be comorbid, and patients with personality disorders may have mood symptoms. The two diagnoses are distinguished by the predominance of mood symptoms and the episodic course of bipolar disorder in contrast to the stability and persistence of the behavioral patterns of personality disorders.

▶ Comorbid Psychiatric and Medical Conditions

Lifetime prevalence rates of psychiatric comorbidity with bipolar disorder are up to 58%.[14] Comorbidities, especially substance abuse, make establishing a definitive diagnosis more difficult and complicate the treatment. Comorbidities also place the patient at risk for a poorer outcome, high rates of suicidality, onset of depression, and higher costs of treatment.[2,13] Psychiatric comorbidities include:

- Personality disorders
- Alcohol and substance abuse or dependence
- Anxiety disorders
- Panic disorder
- Obsessive-compulsive disorder
- Social phobia
- Eating disorders
- Attention-deficit hyperactivity disorder

Medical comorbidities include:

- Migraine
- Multiple sclerosis
- Cushing's syndrome
- Brain tumor
- Head trauma

TREATMENT

Desired Outcomes

❸ Goals of treatment are to reduce symptoms, induce remission, prevent relapse, improve patient functioning, and minimize adverse effects of drug therapy.

General Approach to Treatment

Treatment guidelines for manic and depressive episodes of bipolar disorder are included in Table 39–2.

Although not all patients achieve remission, this is a goal of treatment. The mainstay of drug therapy has been mood-stabilizing drug but new research based on multiple-treatments meta-analysis indicates antipsychotic drugs, both first-generation antipsychotics (FGAs) and second-generation antipsychotics (SGAs), may be more effective for acute mania.[15] Antipsychotic drugs may be used as monotherapy or adjunctively with mood-stabilizing drugs. A person entering treatment for a first mood episode in bipolar disorder must have a complete assessment and careful diagnosis to rule out nonpsychiatric causes. A variety of conditions can cause similar symptoms (Table 39–3). Because early and accurate diagnosis is essential to maximizing response to treatment, pharmacologic and nonpharmacologic therapy should begin as soon as possible. Treatment is often lifelong. Comorbid conditions should also be addressed aggressively.

▶ Suicidality Risk

Patients should be assessed for their potential for violence and harm to others. Friends or family can be asked to remove from home guns, caustic chemicals, medications, and objects that patients might use to harm themselves or others. Risk factors for suicide include severity of depression, feelings of

---

Patient Encounter, Part 3: Creating a Care Plan

Based on all information presented, create a care plan for this patient's bipolar disorder. Your plan should include (a) a statement of the drug-related needs or problems, (b) the goals of therapy, (c) a patient-specific therapeutic plan, and (d) a plan for follow-up to assess therapeutic response and adverse effects.

Table 39–2

Guidelines for the Acute Treatment of Mood Episodes in Patients With Bipolar I Disorder

Acute Manic or Mixed Episode	Acute Depressive Episode
General guidelines	General guidelines
Assess for secondary causes of mania or mixed states (e.g., alcohol or drug use)	Assess for secondary causes of depression (e.g., alcohol or drug use)
Taper off antidepressants, stimulants, and caffeine if possible	Taper off antipsychotics, benzodiazepines or sedative-hypnotic agents if possible
Treat substance abuse	Treat substance abuse
Encourage good nutrition (with regular protein and essential fatty acid intake), exercise, adequate sleep, stress reduction, and psychosocial therapy	Encourage good nutrition (with regular protein and essential fatty acid intake), exercise, adequate sleep, stress reduction, and psychosocial therapy
Optimize the dose of mood stabilizing medication(s) before adding on benzodiazepines; if psychotic features are present, add on antipsychotic; ECT used for severe or treatment-resistant manic/mixed episodes or features	Optimize the dose of mood stabilizing medication(s) before adding on lithium lamotrigine, or antidepressant (e.g., bupropion or an SSRI); if psychotic features are present, add on antipsychotic; ECT used for severe or treatment-resistant depressive episodes or for psychotic catatonia

Hypomania	Mania	Mild to Moderate Depressive Episode	Severe Depressive Episode
First, optimize current mood stabilizer or initiate mood-stabilizing medication: lithium,[a] valproate,[a] or carbamazepine.[a] Consider adding a benzodiazepine (lorazepam or clonazepam) for short-term adjunctive treatment of agitation or insomnia if needed	First, two- or three-drug combinations: lithium or valproate plus a benzodiazepine (lorazepam or clonazepam) for short-term adjunctive treatment of agitation or insomnia; lorazepam is recommended for catatonia. If psychosis is present, initiate atypical antipsychotic in combination with above	First, initiate and/or optimize mood-stabilizing medication: lithium[a] or lamotrigine[b]	First, two- or three-drug combinations: lithium[a] or lamotrigine[b] plus an antidepressant[c]; lithium plus lamotrigine. If psychosis is present, initiate atypical antipsychotic in combination with above
Alternative medication treatment options: carbamazepine[a]; If patient does not respond or tolerate, consider atypical antipsychotic (e.g., olanzapine, quetiapine, risperidone) or oxcarbazepine	Alternative medication treatment options: carbamazepine[a]; If patient does not respond or tolerate, consider oxcarbazepine	Alternative anticonvulsants: valproate,[a] carbamazepine,[a] or oxcarbazepine	Alternative anticonvulsants: valproate;[a] carbamazepine,[a] or oxcarbazepine. Second, if response is inadequate, consider adding an atypical antipsychotic (quetiapine). Third, if response is inadequate, consider a three-drug combination:
Second, if response is inadequate, consider a two-drug combination: • Lithium[a] plus an anticonvulsant or an atypical antipsychotic • Anticonvulsant plus an anticonvulsant or atypical antipsychotic	Second, if response is inadequate, consider a three-drug combination: • Lithium[a] plus an anticonvulsant plus an atypical antipsychotic • Anticonvulsant plus an anticonvulsant plus an atypical antipsychotic Third, if response is inadequate consider ECT for mania with psychosis or catatonia[a]; or add clozapine for treatment-refractory illness		• Lamotrigine[b] plus an anticonvulsant plus an antidepressant • Lamotrigine[b] plus lithium[a] plus an antidepressant Fourth, if response is inadequate, consider ECT for treatment-refractory illness and depression with psychosis or catatonia[d]

ECT, electroconvulsive therapy; MAOI, manoamine oxidase inhibitor, SNRI, serotonin-norepinephrine reuptake inhibitor; SSRI, selective serotonin reuptake inhibitor; TCA, tricyclic antidepressant.

[a]Use standard therapeutic serum concentration ranges if clinically indicated; if partial response or breakthrough episode, adjust dose to achieve higher serum concentrations without causing intolerable adverse effects; valproate is preferred over lithium for mixed episodes and rapid cycling; lithium and/or lamotrigine is preferred over valproate for bipolar depression.

[b]Lamotrigine is not approved for the acute treatment of depression, and the dose must be started low and slowly titrated to decrease adverse effects if used for maintenance therapy of bipolar I disorder. A drug interaction and a severe dermatologic rash can occur when lamotrigine is combined with valproate (i.e., lamotrigine doses must be halved from standard dosing titration).

[c]Antidepressant monotherapy is not recommended for bipolar depression. Bupropion, SSRIs (e.g., citalopram, escitalopram, or sertraline), and SNRIs (e.g., venlafaxine) have shown good efficacy and fewer adverse effects in the treatment of unipolar depression; MAOIs and TCAs have more adverse effects (e.g., weight gain) and can have a higher risk of causing antidepressant-induced mania; fluoxetine, fluvoxamine, nefazodone, and paroxetine inhibit liver metabolism and should be used with caution in patients on concomitant medications that require cytochrome P450 clearance; paroxetine and venlafaxine have a higher risk for a discontinuation syndrome.

[d]ECT is used for severe mania or depression during pregnancy and for mixed episodes; prior to treatment, anticonvulsants, lithium, benzodiazepines should be tapered off to maximize therapy and minimize adverse effects.

Data from Refs. 32, 47 (with permission), 48, and 49.

Table 39–3

Secondary Causes of Mania

General Medical Conditions

Alzheimer's disease
Cerebral infarction
Cerebral tumors
Closed head injury
Cushing's syndrome
Hemodialysis
Hepatic encephalopathy
Huntington's disease
Hyperthyroidism
Ictal or postictal mania
Multiple sclerosis
Neurosyphilis
Systemic lupus erythematosus
Vitamin B deficiency

Medications

Corticosteroids
Diltiazem
Levodopa
Oral contraceptives
Zidovudine

Illicit Substances

Anabolic steroids
Hallucinogens
Stimulants (cocaine, amphetamines)

Data from Ref. 16.

hopelessness, comorbid personality disorder, and a history of a previous suicide attempt.[13]

▶ Nonpharmacologic Therapy

❹ *Interpersonal, family, or group psychotherapy with a qualified therapist or clinician assists individuals with bipolar disorder to improve functional outcomes and may help treat or prevent mood episodes,* establish and maintain a daily routine and sleep schedule, and improve interpersonal relationships.[17,18]

Cognitive-behavioral therapy (CBT) is a type of psychotherapy that combines cognitive and behavioral theories. It stresses the importance of recognizing patterns of cognition (thought) and how thoughts influence subsequent feelings and behaviors. Other people, situations, and events external to the individual are not seen as the sources of thoughts and behaviors. With CBT, patients are taught self-management skills to change their negative thoughts even if external circumstances do not change.

Electroconvulsive therapy (ECT) is the application of prescribed electrical impulses to the brain for the treatment of severe depression, mixed states, psychotic depression, and treatment refractory mania. It also may be used in pregnant

women who cannot take carbamazepine, lithium, or divalproex (DVP).

Psychoeducation for patients, their families, and groups regarding the chronicity of bipolar disorders and self-management through sleep hygiene, nutrition, exercise, stress reduction, and abstinence from alcohol or drugs is critical to the success of supporting the individual in managing bipolar disorder. The development of a crisis intervention plan is essential.

The following websites provide additional information:

- National Association of Cognitive Behavioral Therapists—*http://www.nacbt.org/*
- National Alliance on Mental Illness—*http://www.nami.org/*
- National Institutes for Mental Health, Bipolar Disorder—*http://nimh.nih.gov/health/topics/bipolar-disorder/index.shtml*

▶ Pharmacologic Therapy

❺ *Pharmacotherapy is the primary treatment modality of acute and maintenance treatment of bipolar disorder.* Mood-stabilizing drugs are first-line treatments and include lithium, DVP, carbamazepine, and lamotrigine. The SGAs, including risperidone, olanzapine, quetiapine, ziprasidone, aripiprazole, and asenapine, are also approved for treatment of acute mania. Lithium, lamotrigine, aripiprazole, olanzapine, and quetiapine are approved for maintenance therapy. Quetiapine's maintenance therapy indication is adjunctive with lithium or DVP. Drugs used with less research support and without Food and Drug Administration (FDA) approval include topiramate and oxcarbazepine. Benzodiazepines are used adjunctively for mania.

❻ *Mood-stabilizing drugs are the primary treatment for bipolar depression.* Among antipsychotic drugs, quetiapine as monotherapy and olanzapine in combination with fluoxetine are approved for bipolar depression. Antidepressants can be used but along with a mood stabilizing agent to reduce risk of a mood switch to mania and after the patient has failed to respond adequately to optimal mood stabilizing therapy. Evidence of efficacy of antidepressant drugs in bipolar depression is considered less robust than evidence for mood-stabilizing drugs quetiapine, and the olanzapine–fluoxetine combination.[19,20] Combinations of two mood-stabilizing drugs or a mood-stabilizing drug and either an antipsychotic or antidepressant drug are common, especially in acute mood episodes.

❼ *Mood-stabilizing drugs are considered the primary pharmacotherapy for relapse prevention, and they are often combined with antipsychotic drugs.* Aripiprazole, olanzapine, and quetiapine are approved for maintenance therapy.

Table 39–4 includes a summary of current drug therapy for bipolar disorder. An algorithm for treatment of bipolar mania is shown in Table 39–2.

▶ Mood-Stabilizing Drugs

The optimal mood-stabilizing drug would be effective in treatment of acute mania and acute bipolar depression and in prevention of manic relapse and bipolar depression relapse. All currently approved mood-stabilizing drugs have demonstrated efficacy over placebo for one or more of these

Table 39–4

Product Formulation, Dose, and Clinical Use of Agents Used in the Treatment of Bipolar Disorder

Generic Name	Brand Names	Formulations	Dosages	Clinical Use	Dosage Adjustment in Renal or Hepatic Impairment
Lithium salts					
FDA approved in bipolar disorder					
Lithium carbonate	Lithobid	ER tablets: 300 mg	900–2400 mg/day once daily or in 2–4 divided doses, preferably with meals. There is wide variation in the dosage needed to achieve therapeutic response and 12-hour serum lithium concentration (i.e., 0.6–1.2 mEq/L (mmol/L) for maintenance therapy and 1.0–1.5 mEq/L (mmol/L) for acute mood episodes taken 12 hours after last dose). Single daily dosing is effective and causes fewer renal effects	Monotherapy or in combination with other drugs for the acute treatment of mania and for maintenance treatment	Reduce starting dosage by at least 50% in renal impairment
	Generic	ER tablets: 450 mg			
	Generic	ER tablets: 300 mg			
	Generic	Tablet: 300 mg			
	Generic	Capsules: 150, 300, 600 mg			
Lithium citrate	Generic	300 mg (8 mmol)/5 mL			
Anticonvulsants					
FDA approved for use in bipolar disorder					
Carbamazepine	Equetro (only the Equetro brand is FDA approved for bipolar disorder)	Capsules: 100 mg, 200 mg, 300 mg SR; may open capsule but do not crush or chew beads; take with food	Start at 100–200 mg bid; increase by 200 mg every 3–4 days to 200–1,800 mg/day in 2–4 divided doses. Target serum concentration is 4–12 mcg/mL (17–51 μmol/L)	Monotherapy or in combination with other drugs for the acute treatment of mania or mixed episodes for bipolar I disorder	Reduce starting dosage by at least half or avoid in hepatic impairment
	Tegretol, generic	Tablets: 200 mg			
	Tegretol XR	Chewable tablet: 100 mg			
		Suspension: 100 mg/5 mL			
	Carbatrol	ER tablets: 100, 200, 400 mg			
		ER capsules: 100, 200, 300 mg			
Divalproex sodium	Depakote, generic	Enteric-coated, delayed-release tablets: 125, 250, 500 mg	750–3,000 mg/day (20–60 mg/kg per day) in 2–3 divided doses for delayed-release divalproex or valproic acid	Monotherapy or in combination with other drugs for the acute treatment of mania. Although commonly used for relapse prevention, maintenance treatment is not FDA approved	Reduce starting dosage by half or avoid in hepatic impairment
	Depakote ER	Sprinkles: 125 mg	ER divalproex may be given once daily.		
		ER tablets: 250, 500 mg	A loading dose of 20–30 mg/kg per day can be given, then 20 mg/kg per day and titrated to a serum		
Valproic acid	Depakene, generic	Capsules: 250 mg	concentration of 50–125 mcg/mL (347–866 μmol/L)		
Valproic acid syrup	Depakene, generic	250 mg/5 mL			
Lamotrigine	Lamictal, generic	Tablets: 25, 100, 150, 200 mg	50–400 mg/day in divided doses. Dosage should be slowly increased by following prescribing information. If divalproex is added to lamotrigine, the lamotrigine dosage should be reduced by half	Monotherapy or in combination with other drugs for maintenance treatment	
		Chewable tablets: 2, 5, 25 mg			
	Lamictal XR (not FDA approved for bipolar disorder)	Orally disintegrating tablets: 25, 50, 100, 200 mg			
		ER tablets: 25, 50, 100, 200 mg			

(Continued)

Table 39–4

Product Formulation, Dose, and Clinical Use of Agents Used in the Treatment of Bipolar Disorder (Continued)

Generic Name	Brand Names	Formulations	Dosages	Clinical Use	Dosage Adjustment in Renal or Hepatic Impairment
Anticonvulsants and Other Drugs Not FDA Approved for Use in Bipolar Disorder					
Clonazepam	Klonopin, generic	Tablets: 0.5, 1, 2 mg Wafers: 0.125, 0.25, 0.5, 1, 2 mg	0.5–20 mg/day in divided doses or one dose at bedtime Dosage should be slowly adjusted up and down according to response and adverse effects	Use in combination with other drugs for the acute treatment of mania or mixed episodes	
Lorazepam	Ativan, generic	Tablets: 0.5, 1, 2 mg Oral solution: 2 mg/mL Injection: 2, 4 mg/mL	2–10 mg/day in divided doses or one dose at bedtime Dosage should be slowly adjusted up and down according to response and adverse effects		
Oxcarbazepine	Trileptal, generic	Tablets: 150, 300, 600 mg Suspension: 300 mg/5 mL	300–1200 mg/day in two divided doses Doses should be slowly adjusted up and down according to response and adverse effects (e.g., 150–300 mg twice daily and increase by 300–600 mg/day at weekly intervals)	May cause fewer adverse drug–drug interactions than carbamazepine, but causes more gastrointestinal side effects and hyponatremia. Evidence is limited regarding efficacy	
Atypical Antipsychotics FDA approved for bipolar disorder					
Aripiprazole	Abilify Abilify Discmelt	Tablets: 2, 5, 10, 15, 20, 30 mg Oral solution: 5 mg/5 mL Tablets, orally disintegrating: 10, 15 mg	10–30 mg/day once daily	Use as monotherapy or in combination with lithium or valproate for the acute treatment of mania or mixed states for bipolar I disorder and prevention of manic relapse	
Asenapine	Saphris	Sublingual tablets: 5, 10 mg	5–20 mg/day in two divided doses. Must be held under the tongue until dissolved completely, not chewed or swallowed, with no food or liquid for 10 minutes after administering	Use as monotherapy or in combination with lithium or valproate for the acute treatment of mania or mixed states of bipolar I disorder	
Olanzapine Olanzapine/ Fluoxetine combination (OFC)	Zyprexa, generic Zyprexa Zydis Symbyax	Tablets: 2.5, 5, 7.5, 10, 15, 20 mg Tablets, orally disintegrating: 5, 10, 15, 20 mg Capsules: 3/25, 6/25, 6/50, 12/25, 12/50 mg	5–20 mg/day in 1 or 2 doses	Used as monotherapy or in combination with lithium or valproate for acute treatment of mania or mixed states for bipolar I disorder and prevention of manic relapse. Used in combination with fluoxetine (OFC) for treatment of bipolar depression	
Quetiapine	Seroquel Seroquel XR	Tablets: 25, 50, 100, 200, 300, 400 mg ER tablets: 50, 150, 200, 300, 400 mg	50–800 mg/day in divided doses or once daily when stabilized	Used as monotherapy or in combination with lithium or divalproex for acute treatment of mania, mixed states for bipolar I disorder, and depression of bipolar I and bipolar II disorder. Used adjunctively with lithium or divalproex for relapse prevention of bipolar mania and depression	
Risperidone	Risperdal, generic Risperdal M-Tabs Risperdal Consta	Tablets: 0.25, 0.5, 1, 2, 3, 4 mg Oral solution: 1 mg/mL Tablets, orally disintegrating: 0.5, 1, 2, 3, 4 mg Long-acting injectable: 12.5, 25, 37.5, 50 mg	0.5 – 6 mg/day in 1 or 2 doses	Used as monotherapy or adjunctively with lithium or divalproex for acute mania or mixed episodes of bipolar I disorder	
Ziprasidone	Geodon	Capsules: 20, 40, 60, 80 mg	40–160 mg/day in divided doses	Used as monotherapy or adjunctively with lithium or divalproex for acute mania or mixed episodes of bipolar I disorder	

DVP, divalproex; ER, extended release; FDA, Food and Drug Administration; SR, sustained release.

Data from Ref. 15, 26, 28–32, and 36–38.

areas, but there are differences among them with regard to specific patient populations. The choice of treatment is dictated by individual patient characteristics and history. Few studies have compared mood-stabilizing drugs with each other in systematic clinical trials. Effect sizes across placebo-controlled trials of individual agents are generally similar. Lithium and DVP are first-choice drugs for the classic presentation of bipolar disorder. Treatment of childhood bipolar disorder is less well researched. Lithium is FDA approved in children and adolescents as young as age 12 years. Among the antipsychotic drugs, aripiprazole, olanzapine, quetiapine, and risperidone are FDA approved in children and adolescents as young as age 10 years. Treatment of bipolar disorder during pregnancy and during breastfeeding is a challenge because of the risks of drug exposure in utero and transmission of drugs via breast milk.

Lithium Lithium was the first approved mood-stabilizing drug. It remains a first-line agent and sets the standard for efficacy against which other drugs are usually measured. It has antimanic efficacy, prevents bipolar disorder relapse, and has more modest efficacy for acute bipolar depression. One of the oldest drugs used for psychiatric illness, research continues to strongly support its use and place in therapy.[21] In most studies, lithium's efficacy is equivalent to that of anticonvulsant mood stabilizers and SGAs, although recent data regarding antipsychotic drugs make a conclusive statement about lithium's efficacy less clear.[15] It is most effective for patients with few previous episodes, symptom-free interepisode remission, and a family history of bipolar disorder with good response to lithium. Increasing evidence suggests genetic phenotypes that are more responsive to lithium.[22] However, patients with rapid cycling bipolar disorder are less responsive to lithium than to other mood-stabilizing drugs such as DVP.[23] Additionally, its efficacy for bipolar depression is less robust than for mania.[19] It may also be less effective in patients with mixed mood episodes (symptoms of mania and depression occurring simultaneously) and in mania secondary to nonpsychiatric illness.

Evidence shows lithium's effect on suicidal behavior is superior to that of other mood-stabilizing drugs.[24] Lithium reduces the risk of deliberate self-harm or suicide by about 70%.

Mechanism of Action. Lithium's pharmacologic mechanism of action is not well understood and involves multiple effects. Possibilities include altered ion transport, effects on neurotransmitter signaling, blocking adenyl cyclase systems, effects on inositol, neuroprotection or increased BDNF, and inhibition of second messenger systems.[25]

Dosing and Monitoring. Lithium is usually initiated at a dosage of 600 to 900 mg/day. Although it is most commonly given in a divided dosage, once-daily dosing is acceptable, especially with sustained-release formulations. Once-daily dosing can improve patient adherence and reduce some side effects. Lithium has a narrow therapeutic index, meaning the toxic dosage is not much greater than the therapeutic dosage. Lithium requires regular serum concentration monitoring as a guide to dosage titration and to minimize adverse effects.

At least weekly monitoring is recommended until the patient is stabilized; then the frequency can be decreased. Well-maintained patients who tolerate lithium without difficulty can be monitored by serum concentration as infrequently as twice yearly. The dosage is titrated to achieve a serum lithium concentration of 0.6 to 1.4 mEq/L (mmol/L). Higher serum concentrations are usually required to treat an acute episode than to prevent relapse. Serum lithium maintained above 0.8 mEq/L (mmol/L) may be more effective at preventing relapse, however, than lower serum concentrations. The suggested therapeutic serum concentration range is based on a 12-hour postdose sample collection, usually a morning trough in patients taking more than one dose per day. At least 2 weeks at a suggested therapeutic serum concentration is required for an adequate trial of lithium. Table 39–5 shows pharmacokinetic parameters and desired serum concentrations of mood-stabilizing drugs used for bipolar disorder. It is common for lithium to be combined with other mood-stabilizing drugs or antipsychotic drugs to achieve more complete remission of symptoms.

Adverse Effects. The most common adverse effects are gastrointestinal (GI) upset, tremor, and polyuria,[26] which are dose related. Nausea, dyspepsia, and diarrhea can be minimized by coadministration with food, use of the sustained-release formulation, and giving smaller doses more frequently to reduce the amount of drug in the GI tract at a given time. Tremor is present in up to 50% of patients. In addition to the approaches above, low-dose β-blocker therapy, such as propranolol 20 to 60 mg/day, often reduces the tremor.

Lithium impairs the kidney's ability to concentrate urine because of its inhibitory effect on vasopressin. This causes an increase in urine volume and urinary frequency and a consequent increase in thirst. Polyuria and polydipsia occur in up to 70% of patients. A severe form of polyuria, when urine volume exceeds 3 L/day, is known as lithium-induced nephrogenic diabetes insipidus. It can be treated with hydrochlorothiazide or amiloride. If the former is used, the lithium dosage should be reduced by 33% to 50% to account for the drug–drug interaction that could increase serum lithium concentrations and cause toxicity. Long-term lithium therapy has been associated with structural kidney changes, such as glomerular sclerosis or tubular atrophy. Once-daily dosing of lithium is less likely to cause renal adverse effects than divided-daily dosing.

Lithium is concentrated in the thyroid gland and can impair thyroid hormone synthesis. Although goiter is uncommon, as many as 30% of patients develop at least transiently elevated thyroid-stimulating hormone values. Lithium-induced hypothyroidism is not usually an indication to discontinue the drug. Patients can be supplemented with levothyroxine if continuation of lithium is desired.[26]

Other common adverse effects include poor concentration, acneiform rash, alopecia, worsening of psoriasis, weight gain, metallic taste, and impaired glucose regulation. Lithium causes a flattening of the T wave of the electrocardiogram (ECG), which is generally considered benign and not clinically significant. Less commonly, it can cause or worsen

Table 39–5

Pharmacokinetics and Therapeutic Serum Concentrations of Lithium and Anticonvulsants Used in the Treatment of Bipolar Disorder

	Lithium	Carbamazepine	Oxcarbazepine	Divalproex (DVP) Sodium/Valproic Acid (VPA)	Lamotrigine
Gastrointestinal Absorption					
Regular release	Rapid: 95%–100% within 1–6 hours	Slow and erratic: 85%–90%	Slow and complete: 100%	Rapid and complete (VPA)	Rapid: 98%
Syrup, suspension, solution	Faster rate of absorption: 100%	Faster rate of absorption	Unknown	Faster rate of absorption than tablets	NA
ER/enteric-coated tablets	Delayed absorption: 60%–90%	Delayed absorption: 89% of the suspension; and less than regular-release tablets	NA	Delayed absorption with delayed-release tablets; valproate is rapidly converted to VPA in the intestine and then is rapidly and almost completely absorbed from the GI tract. ER bioavailability is approximately 15% less than delayed release	Delayed absorption but not significantly different from regular release
Delay in absorption by food	Yes	No; reports of increased rate of absorption with fatty meals (ER capsule)	No	Yes; food slows the rate of absorption but not the extent for DVP	Bioavailability not affected by food
Time to reach peak serum concentrations	0.5–3 hours (regular-release) 4–12 hours (ER) 0.25–1 hour (oral solution)	4–5 hours (regular-release); 1.5 hours (suspension); 3–12 hours (ER tablets); 4.1–7.7 hours (ER capsules); higher peak concentrations with chewable tablets	4.5 hours (range of 3–13 hours)	1–4 hours (VPA) 3–5 hours (DVP single dose) 7–14 hours (DVP ER multiple dosing)	1–4 hours (regular release), 4–6 hours (ER)
Distribution					
Volume of distribution	Initial: 0.3–0.4 L/kg Steady state: 0.7–1 L/kg	0.6–2 L/kg (adults)	10-monohydroxy metabolite: 49 L/kg	11 L/1.73 m² (total valproate); 92 L/1.73 m² (free valproate)	0.9–1.3 L/kg
Crosses the placenta	Yes; pregnancy risk category: D Risk of cardiac defects: 0.1%–0.5%	Yes; pregnancy risk category: D	Yes; pregnancy risk category: C	Yes; pregnancy risk category: D Risk of neural tube defects: 1%–5%	Yes; pregnancy risk category: C
Crosses into breast milk	Yes; 35%–50% of mother's serum concentration; breastfeeding not recommended	Yes; ratio of concentration in breast milk to plasma is 0.4 for drug and 0.5 for epoxide metabolite; considered compatible with breastfeeding	Yes; both drug and active metabolite; breastfeeding not recommended	Yes; considered compatible with breastfeeding	Yes; breastfeeding not recommended
Protein binding	No	75%–90%	40% of active metabolite	80%–90% (dose dependent)	55%
Renal clearance	Yes; 10–40 mL/min with 90%–98% of dose excreted in urine; 80% of lithium that is filtered by the renal glomeruli is reabsorbed	Yes; 1%–3% excreted unchanged in urine	Yes; 95% excreted in the urine; less than 1% excreted unchanged	Yes; 30%–50% excreted as glucuronide conjugate; less than 3% excreted unchanged	Yes; 94% excreted as glucuronide conjugate

(Continued)

Table 39–5

Pharmacokinetics and Therapeutic Serum Concentrations of Lithium and Anticonvulsants Used in the Treatment of Bipolar Disorder (*Continued*)

Metabolism

Hepatic metabolism	No	Yes; oxidation and hydroxylation; induces liver enzymes to increase its own metabolism and metabolism of other drugs	Yes; oxidation and conjugation	Yes; oxidation and glucuronide conjugation	Yes; glucuronic acid conjugation induces its own metabolism in normal volunteers
Metabolites	No	Yes; 10, 11–epoxide (active)	Yes; 10-monohydroxy metabolite (active)	Yes (not active)	No
Kinetics	First-order	First-order after initial enzyme induction phase	First-order	First-order	First-order
Half-life (t₁/₂)	18-27 hours (adult); greater than 36 hours (elderly or patients with renal impairment)	Half-life decreases over time due to autoinduction: 25–65 hours (initial) 12–17 hours (adult multiple dosing) 8–14 hours (children multiple dosing)	2 hours (parent) 9 hours (metabolite)	5–20 hours (adults)	25 hours; increases to 59 hours with concomitant VPA therapy

Cytochrome P-450 (CYP450) isoenzyme

CYP450 substrate	No	2C8 and 3A3/4	Unknown	2C19	Unknown
CYP450 inhibitor	No	No	2C19	2C9, 2D6, and 3A3/4	Unknown
CYP450 inducer	No	1A2, 2C9/10, and 3A3/4	3A3/4	No	Unknown

Therapeutic Serum/Plasma Concentrations

	1–1.5 mEq/L (mmol/L): for adult, acute mania 0.4–0.6 mEq/L (mmol/L): for elderly or medically ill patients 0.6–1.2 mEq/L (mmol/L): for adult, maintenance; ranges based on 12-hour postdose sample collection	4–12 mcg/mL (17–51 µmol/L): for adult, acute mania and maintenance 4–8 mcg/mL (17–34 µmol/L): for elderly or medically ill	No established therapeutic range; 12–30 mcg/mL (47–118 µmol/L) for 10-hydroxy metabolite based on epilepsy trials	50–125 mcg/mL (347–866 µmol/L): adult, acute mania and maintenance 40–75 mcg/mL (277–520 µmol/L): elderly or medically ill	No established therapeutic range: 4–20 mcg/mL (16–80 µmol/L) based on epilepsy trials

ER, extended release; GI, gastrointestinal; NA, not applicable.

Data from Refs. 26 and 28–31.

arrhythmias. Cardiology consultation is recommended for patients with preexisting cardiac disease who are candidates for lithium therapy. A benign leukocytosis is also common.[26]

Lithium and other mood-stabilizing drugs require baseline and routine laboratory monitoring to help determine medical appropriateness for initiation of therapy and monitoring of potential adverse effects. Guidelines for such monitoring are outlined in Table 39–6.

Acute lithium toxicity, which can occur at serum concentrations over 2 mEq/L (mmol/L), can be severe and life threatening, necessitating emergency medical treatment.

Symptoms include worsening of GI distress to include severe vomiting and diarrhea; deterioration in motor coordination, including a coarse tremor, ataxia, and dysarthria; and impaired cognition. In its most severe form, seizures, cardiac arrhythmias, coma, and kidney damage have been reported. Treatment includes discontinuation of lithium, IV fluids to correct fluid and electrolyte imbalance, and osmotic diuresis or hemodialysis. In case of overdose, gastric lavage is indicated. Clinical symptoms can continue well after the serum concentration is lowered because clearance from the central nervous system (CNS) is slower than from the serum. Factors

Table 39-6

Guidelines for Baseline and Routine Laboratory Tests and Monitoring for Agents Used in the Treatment of Bipolar Disorder

	Baseline: Physical Examination and General Chemistry[a]	Hematologic Tests[b]		Metabolic Tests[c]		Liver Function Tests[d]		Renal Function Tests[e]		Thyroid Function Tests[f]		Serum Electrolytes[g]		Dermatologic[h]	
	Baseline	Baseline	6–12 Months	Baseline	6–12 Months	Baseline	6–12 Months	Baseline	6–12 Months	Baseline	6–12 Months	Baseline	6–12 Months	Baseline	3–6 Months
Atypical antipsychotics[i]	X			X	X										
Carbamazepine[j]	X	X	X			X	X	X				X	X	X	X
Lamotrigine[k]	X													X	X
Lithium[l]	X	X	X	X				X	X	X	X	X	X		
Oxcarbazepine[m]	X											X	X		
Valproate[n]	X	X	X	X	X	X	X							X	

[a]Screen for drug abuse and serum pregnancy.

[b]CBC with differential and platelets.

[c]Fasting glucose, serum lipids, weight.

[d]Lactate dehydrogenase, aspartate aminotransferase, alanine aminotransferase, total bilirubin, alkaline phosphatase.

[e]Serum creatinine, blood urea nitrogen, urinalysis, urine osmolality, specific gravity.

[f]Triiodothyronine, total thyroxine, thyroxine uptake, and thyroid-stimulating hormone.

[g]Serum sodium.

[h]Rashes, hair thinning, alopecia.

[i]Atypical antipsychotic: Monitor for increased appetite with weight gain (primarily in patients with initial low or normal body mass index); monitor closely if rapid or significant weight gain occurs during early therapy; cases of hyperlipidemia and diabetes reported.

[j]Carbamazepine: Manufacturer recommends CBC and platelets (and possibly reticulocyte counts and serum iron) at baseline, and that subsequent monitoring be individualized by the clinician (e.g., CBC, platelet counts, and liver function tests every 2 weeks during the first 2 months of treatment, then every 3 months if normal). Monitor more closely if patient exhibits hematologic or hepatic abnormalities or if the patient is receiving a myelotoxic drug; discontinue if platelets are less than $100,000/mm^3$, if WBC is less than $3,000/mm^3$ or if there is evidence of bone marrow suppression or liver dysfunction. Serum electrolyte levels should be monitored in the elderly or those at risk for hyponatremia. Carbamazepine interferes with some pregnancy tests.

[k]Lamotrigine: If renal or hepatic impairment, monitor closely and adjust dosage according to manufacturer's guidelines. Serious dermatologic reactions have occurred within 2 to 8 weeks of initiating treatment and are more likely to occur in patients receiving concomitant valproate, with rapid dose escalation, or using doses exceeding the recommended titration schedule.

[l]Lithium: Obtain baseline ECG for patients older than 40 years or if pre-existing cardiac disease (benign, reversible T-wave depression can occur). Renal function tests should be obtained every 2 to 3 months during the first 6 months, then every 6 to 12 months; if impaired renal function, monitor 24-hour urine volume and creatinine every 3 months; if urine volume more than 3 L/day, monitor urinalysis, osmolality, and specific gravity every 3 months. Thyroid function tests should be obtained once or twice during the first 6 months, then every 6 to 12 months; monitor for signs and symptoms of hypothyroidism; if supplemental thyroid therapy is required, monitor thyroid function tests and adjust thyroid dose every 1 to 2 months until thyroid function indices are within normal range, then monitor every 3 to 6 months.

[m]Oxcarbazepine: Hyponatremia (serum sodium concentrations less than 125 mEq/L) has been reported and occurs more frequently during the first 3 months of therapy; serum sodium concentrations should be monitored in patients receiving drugs that lower serum sodium concentrations (e.g., diuretics or drugs that cause inappropriate antidiuretic hormone secretion) or in patients with symptoms of hyponatremia (e.g., confusion, headache, lethargy, and malaise). Hypersensitivity reactions have occurred in approximately 25% to 30% of patients with a history of carbamazepine hypersensitivity and requires immediate discontinuation.

[n]Valproate: Weight gain reported in patients with low or normal body mass index. Monitor platelets and liver function during first 3 to 6 months if evidence of increased bruising or bleeding. Monitor closely if patients exhibit hematologic or hepatic abnormalities or in patients receiving drugs that affect coagulation, such as aspirin or warfarin; discontinue if platelets are less than $100,000/mm^3$ or if prolonged bleeding time. Pancreatitis, hyperammonemic encephalopathy, polycystic ovary syndrome, increased testosterone, and menstrual irregularities have been reported; not recommended during first trimester of pregnancy due to risk of neural tube defects.

Data from Refs. 47 (with permission), 48, and 50–56.

predisposing to lithium toxicity include fluid and sodium loss from hot weather or exercise or drug interactions that increase serum lithium.[26]

Drug Interactions. Drug interactions involving lithium are common. Because lithium is not metabolized or protein bound, it is not associated with metabolic drug interactions that occur with other mood-stabilizing drugs. Common and significant drug interactions involve thiazide diuretics, nonsteroidal anti-inflammatory drugs, and angiotensin-converting enzyme (ACE) inhibitor drugs. If a diuretic must be used with lithium and a thiazide is not required, loop diuretics such as furosemide are less likely to increase lithium retention. The ACE inhibitors and by extension, angiotensin receptor blockers (ARB), can abruptly increase serum lithium with the potential of acute and fatal toxicity, even after months of no change in the serum lithium concentration. This combination is strongly discouraged.[27]

Divalproex Sodium and Valproic Acid Divalproex sodium is composed of sodium valproate and valproic acid (VPA). The delayed-release and extended-release formulations are converted in the small intestine into VPA, which is the systemically absorbed form. It was developed as an anticonvulsant but also has efficacy for mood stabilization and migraine headaches. It is FDA approved for the treatment of the manic phase of bipolar disorder. It is generally equal in efficacy to lithium and some other drugs for bipolar mania. It has particular utility in bipolar disorder patients with rapid cycling, mixed mood features, and substance abuse comorbidity. Although not FDA approved for relapse prevention, studies support this use, and it is widely prescribed for maintenance therapy. DVP can be used as monotherapy or in combination with lithium or an antipsychotic drug.[28]

Mechanism of Action. The mechanism of action of DVP is not well understood. It is known to affect ion transport and enhances the activity of γ-aminobutyric acid (GABA). Similar to lithium, it has possible neuroprotective effects through enhancement of BDNF.[8]

Dosing and Monitoring. DVP is usually initiated at 500 to 1,000 mg/day, but studies indicate a therapeutic serum VPA concentration can be reached more quickly through a loading dose approach of 20 to 30 mg/kg/day. Using this approach, patients may respond with a significant reduction in symptoms within the first few days of treatment. The dosage is then titrated according to response, tolerability, and serum concentration. The most often referenced desired VPA serum concentration is 50 to 125 mcg/mL (347 to 866 μmoles/L), but it is not unusual for patients to require more than 100 mcg/mL (693 μmoles/L) for optimal efficacy. Some patients require high milligram dosages in order to reach a desired serum concentration. The suggested serum concentration range is based on trough values. Serum concentration monitoring is recommended at least every 2 weeks until stabilized, then less frequently, sometimes as infrequently as twice yearly. The extended-release formulation can be taken once daily (see Table 39–4). If the extended-release formulation is administered at night, a morning blood sampling is a

peak, not a trough. The drug should be given in the morning so that blood sampling the following morning would be a trough value and more easily interpreted if the typical blood sampling time is in the morning. The systemic bioavailability of extended-release DVP is about 15% less than that of the delayed-release formulation. Patients who have difficulty swallowing large tablets can use the sprinkle formulation. The immediate-release formulation, either capsules or syrup, is generally given three or four times per day.[28]

Adverse Effects. The most common adverse effects of DVP are GI (loss of appetite, nausea, dyspepsia, diarrhea), tremor, and drowsiness. GI distress can be reduced by coadministration with food. The delayed-release and extended-release formulations are less likely to cause gastric distress than immediate-release VPA. This is an advantage for DVP, along with fewer daily doses, which can improve patient adherence to treatment. Dosage reduction can reduce all of the common DVP side effects. As with lithium, a low-dose β-blocker may alleviate the tremor. Weight gain is also common, occurring in up to 50% of patients on maintenance therapy.[28]

Other adverse effects that are less common include alopecia or a change in hair color or texture. Hair loss can be minimized by supplementation with a vitamin containing selenium and zinc. Polycystic ovarian syndrome associated with increased androgen production has been reported. Thrombocytopenia is not uncommon, and the platelet count should be monitored periodically. It is a dose-related adverse effect and usually asymptomatic, but the drug is usually stopped if the platelet count decreases to less than $100 \times 10^3/mm^3$ ($100 \times 10^9/L$). More rare are hepatic toxicity and pancreatitis, which are not always dose related. Severe GI symptoms of hepatic or pancreatic toxicity include vomiting, pain, and loss of appetite. When these occur, the patient should be evaluated for possible hepatitis or pancreatitis. DVP has a wide therapeutic index. Acute toxicity for high dosages or overdosage is not life threatening.[28]

Drug Interactions. Drug interactions involving DVP are common. It is a weak inhibitor of some of the drug metabolizing liver enzymes and can affect the metabolism of other drugs. These include other anticonvulsants and tricyclic antidepressants. The interaction between DVP and lamotrigine is particularly important. The risk of a dangerous rash caused by lamotrigine is increased when given concurrently with DVP. When lamotrigine is added to DVP, the initial lamotrigine dosage should be one-half the typical starting dosage, and lamotrigine should be titrated more slowly than usual. When DVP is added to lamotrigine, the lamotrigine dosage should be reduced by 50%. Conversely, the metabolism of DVP can be increased by enzyme-inducing drugs such as carbamazepine and phenytoin, but DVP may simultaneously slow metabolism of the other agents.[27]

Carbamazepine Although long used as a mood-stabilizing drug, only the extended-release formulation of carbamazepine has received FDA approval for treatment of bipolar disorder. Similar to DVP, it has efficacy for mood stabilization, but it is considered possibly less desirable as a first-line agent because of safety and drug interactions. It is sometimes reserved for patients who fail to respond to lithium or for patients with rapid cycling or mixed bipolar disorder. Carbamazepine can be used as monotherapy or in combination with lithium or an antipsychotic drug.[29]

Mechanism of Action. The mechanism of action of carbamazepine is not well understood. It blocks ion channels and inhibits sustained repetitive neuronal excitation, but whether this explains its efficacy as a mood-stabilizing drug is not known.[29]

Dosing and Monitoring. Carbamazepine is usually initiated at 400 to 600 mg/day. The sustained-release formulation can be given in two divided doses. In addition to a formulation that is completely sustained release, an additional extended-release formulation contains a matrix of 25% immediate-release, 40% extended-release, and 35% enteric-release beads.[29] The suggested therapeutic serum concentration is 4 to 12 mcg/mL (17 to 51 µmol/L). As with DVP, some patients require high milligram dosages to achieve a desired serum concentration and therapeutic effect. The dosage can be increased by 200 to 400 mg/day as often as every 2 to 4 days to achieve the desired effect. Serum concentration monitoring is suggested at least every 2 weeks until stabilized and then less frequently.[29]

Adverse Effects. The most common adverse effects are drowsiness, dizziness, ataxia, lethargy, and confusion. At mildly toxic serum concentrations, it also causes diplopia and dysarthria. These effects can be minimized through dosage adjustments, use of sustained-release formulations, and giving more of the drug late in the day. GI upset is also common. Carbamazepine has an antidiuretic effect similar to the syndrome of inappropriate antidiuretic hormone secretion and can cause hyponatremia. Mild elevations in liver enzymes can occur, but hepatitis is less common. Mild, dose-related leukopenia is not unusual and not usually an indication for stopping the drug. More serious blood count abnormalities such as aplastic anemia and agranulocytosis are rare but life threatening.[29] Suggested baseline and routine laboratory monitoring is reviewed in Table 39–6.

Drug Interactions. Carbamazepine induces the hepatic metabolism of many drugs, including other anticonvulsants, antipsychotics, some antidepressants, oral contraceptives, and antiretroviral agents. Carbamazepine is also an autoinducer (i.e., it induces its own metabolism). The dosage may require an increase after 1 month or so of therapy because of this effect. Conversely, the metabolism of carbamazepine can be slowed by enzyme inhibiting drugs such as some antidepressants; macrolide antibiotics, including erythromycin and clarithromycin; azole antifungal drugs, including ketoconazole and itraconazole; and grapefruit juice. Carbamazepine should not be given concurrently with clozapine because of the additive risk of agranulocytosis.[27]

Lamotrigine Lamotrigine is effective for the maintenance treatment of bipolar disorder. It is more effective for depression relapse prevention than for mania relapse prevention. Its primary limitation as an acute treatment is the time required for titration to an effective dosage. In addition to maintenance monotherapy, it is sometimes used in combination with lithium or DVP, although combination with DVP increases the risk of rash, and lamotrigine dosage adjustment is required.[30]

Mechanism of Action. The mechanism of action of lamotrigine appears to involve blockage of ion channels and effects on glutamate transmission, although the precise mechanism in bipolar disorder is not clear.[30]

Dosing and Monitoring. Lamotrigine is usually initiated at 25 mg/day for the first 1 to 2 weeks, then increasing in a dose-doubling fashion every 1 to 2 weeks to a target dosage of 200 to 400 mg/day. If lamotrigine is added to DVP, the starting dosage is 25 mg every other day with a slower titration to reduce the risk of rash. If DVP is added to lamotrigine, the lamotrigine dosage should be reduced by 50% for the same reason. If lamotrigine therapy is interrupted for more than a few days, it should be restarted at the initial dosage and retitrated. Serum concentration monitoring is not routinely recommended for patients with bipolar disorder.[30]

Adverse Effects. The lamotrigine adverse effect of greatest significance is a maculopapular rash, occurring in up to 10% of patients.[30] Although usually benign and temporary, some rashes can progress to life-threatening Stevens-Johnson syndrome. The risk of rash is greater with a rapid dosage titration and when given concurrently with DVP or other metabolic enzyme inhibitors. The risk is minimal when the dosage titration schedule is slow. Other side effects include dizziness, drowsiness, headache, blurred vision, and nausea. In contrast to other mood-stabilizing drugs such as lithium and DVP, lamotrigine does not significantly influence body weight.

Drug Interactions. The mechanisms of drug–drug interactions involving lamotrigine are unclear. Lamotrigine's primary route of metabolism is conjugative glucuronidation, although it is known to exhibit metabolic autoinduction. It is not significantly metabolized by the CYP P450 enzyme system. It does not affect drug metabolizing hepatic enzymes on its own. In particular, DVP slows the rate of elimination of lamotrigine by about half, necessitating dosage reduction. Conversely, carbamazepine increases the rate of lamotrigine metabolism, which would appear to indicate an effect on oxidative metabolism. Upward adjustment in the lamotrigine dosage may be needed as a result.[27]

Oxcarbazepine Oxcarbazepine is an analogue of carbamazepine, developed as an anticonvulsant. An advantage over carbamazepine is that routine monitoring of hematology profiles and serum concentrations are not indicated because the drug is less likely to cause hematologic abnormalities.[31] Additionally, drug interactions are less significant, although it is at least a mild inducer of certain metabolic pathways. Vigilance for drug interactions is needed, especially with oral contraceptives. Oxcarbazepine appears in the most recent treatment algorithms for bipolar disorder,[32] but clinical trial data are limited. A systematic review concluded that there are insufficient data from well-designed clinical trials to provide guidance on its use.[33]

Adverse Effects. Adverse effects from oxcarbazepine include drowsiness, dizziness, GI upset, and hyponatremia, the latter two of which may be more likely than with carbamazepine.[31]

Others High-potency benzodiazepine agents such as clonazepam and lorazepam have been used as adjunctive therapy, especially during acute mania episodes, to reduce anxiety and improve sleep.[34] As complementary or alternative medicines gain wider usage, omega-3 fatty acids have been used in mood disorders. Insufficient well-designed studies exist to support a recommendation of routine use or to establish a place in therapy relative to usual therapies.[35]

▶ Antipsychotic Drugs

First-generation antipsychotic drugs such as chlorpromazine and haloperidol have long been used in the treatment of acute mania. SGA drugs, including aripiprazole, asenapine, olanzapine, quetiapine, risperidone, and ziprasidone, are approved for the treatment of bipolar mania or mixed mood episodes as monotherapy or in combination with mood-stabilizing drugs.[15] Aripiprazole, olanzapine, and quetiapine are also approved for maintenance therapy for prevention of manic relapse. The combination of olanzapine and fluoxetine is approved for treatment of acute bipolar depression. Quetiapine is approved as monotherapy for acute bipolar depression and as adjunctive therapy with lithium or DVP for prevention of bipolar depression relapse. Approval of antipsychotic drugs in patients with bipolar disorder applies without regard to the presence of psychotic symptoms. In comparative studies, the SGAs are equivalent or better in efficacy to lithium and DVP for treatment of acute mania. Treatment guidelines include antipsychotic drugs as first-line therapy.[14,32] Of interest is evidence that the combination of mood-stabilizing drugs and antipsychotic drugs is more likely to achieve remission of acute manic episodes than monotherapy with either.[32] The quetiapine data in relapse prevention of both manic and bipolar depression episodes favored combination therapy over mood-stabilizing drug monotherapy.[36]

The mechanisms of action, usual dosages, pharmacokinetics, adverse effects, and drug interactions involving antipsychotic drugs are discussed in detail in the chapter on schizophrenia. Dosages in bipolar disorder are similar to those used in schizophrenia. Higher dosages are often required to treat an acute episode than to prevent relapse. The recommended dosage of aripiprazole for bipolar disorder is 20 to 30 mg/day, somewhat higher than the average dosage used in schizophrenia.[37] The recommended dosage for quetiapine in treatment of acute bipolar depression is 300 mg/day, less than the 600 mg/day recommended in acute mania.[38]

The SGAs are less likely than the FGAs to cause neurologic side effects, especially movement abnormalities. As a group, however, the SGAs are more likely to cause metabolic side effects, such as weight gain, glucose dysregulation, and dyslipidemia.[39] Among the SGAs approved for treatment of bipolar disorder, olanzapine is most likely to cause metabolic side effects. Asenapine, quetiapine, and risperidone cause less metabolic effects than olanzapine. Aripiprazole and ziprasidone are least associated with effects on weight, glucose, and lipids, although asenapine has not been compared directly with aripiprazole and ziprasidone. Paliperidone, iloperidone, and lurasidone are not FDA approved for bipolar disorder at

present. The chapter on schizophrenia discusses the adverse effects of antipsychotic drugs in more detail.

▶ Antidepressants

Treatment of depressive episodes in patients with bipolar disorder presents a particular challenge because of the risk of a drug-induced mood switch to mania, although there is not complete agreement about such risk. The FDA requires the product label of all antidepressant drugs to contain language about the potential risk of inducing a mood switch to mania. Most research shows no advantage for adjunctive antidepressant use compared with mood stabilizer therapy alone.[19,20] Treatment guidelines and current FDA approvals indicate lithium or quetiapine as first-line therapy.[32,38] When usual treatment fails, evidence supports use of antidepressants.[19,20]

Guidelines agree that when antidepressants must be used, they should be combined with a mood-stabilizing drug to reduce the risk of mood switch to hypomania or mania. The question of which antidepressant drugs are less likely to cause a mood switch is not resolved, but the tricyclic antidepressants are thought to carry a greater risk of treatment-emergent mania. A randomized comparison of venlafaxine, sertraline, and bupropion as adjunctive therapy to a mood stabilizer showed venlafaxine with the highest risk of a mood switch to mania or hypomania and bupropion with the least.[40]

Special Populations

Assessment and management by appropriate psychiatric specialists is important for special populations, such as pediatric, geriatric, and pregnant patients.

▶ Pediatrics

Evidence regarding treatment of bipolar disorder in children and adolescents is more limited than in adults. Children and adolescents are particularly sensitive to medication side effects, including metabolic side effects of the SGAs. With these caveats, evidence supports the use of mood-stabilizing drugs and the SGAs in children and adolescents with bipolar disorder. Lithium is FDA approved for treatment of bipolar disorder in children and adolescents as young as age 12 years. Aripiprazole, olanzapine, quetiapine, and risperidone are FDA approved in children and adolescents as young as age 10 years.[41,42]

Initial dosages of drug therapy in the pediatric population are lower than in adults. Metabolic elimination rates of many drugs are increased in children, however, so they may actually require higher dosages on a weight-adjusted basis. Dosages are titrated carefully according to response and tolerability. For lithium, DVP, and carbamazepine, serum concentration monitoring is recommended as a guide to dosage adjustment and minimizing adverse effects.

Children and adolescent patients are often more sensitive to drug side effects than adults. In particular, they are likely to experience significant weight gain from atypical antipsychotic drugs.[43] Cognitive toxicity, manifested as confusion, memory or concentration impairment, or impaired learning, is often difficult to detect and is a special consideration in the pediatric population so that intellectual and educational development is not hindered by drug therapy.

Comorbid conditions must be addressed to maximize desired outcomes. For comorbid bipolar disorder and attention-deficit hyperactivity disorder when stimulant therapy is indicated, treatment of mania is recommended before starting the stimulant o avoid exacerbation of mood symptoms by the stimulant.

▶ Geriatrics

Treatment of elderly patients with bipolar disorder requires special care because of increased risks associated with concurrent medical conditions and drug–drug interactions. General medical conditions, including endocrine, metabolic, or infectious diseases, can mimic mood disorders. Patients should be evaluated for such medical illnesses that may cause or worsen mood symptoms. As physiologic systems change with aging, elimination of drugs is often slowed. Examples are slowed renal elimination of lithium and slowed hepatic metabolism of carbamazepine and VPA. As a result, dosages of drugs required for therapeutic effect are generally lower in geriatric patients. Also, changes in membrane permeability with aging increase the risk of CNS side effects. An increased frequency of patient monitoring is often required, including serum drug concentration monitoring.

Vigilance for drug–drug interactions is required because of the greater number of medications prescribed to elderly patients and enhanced sensitivity to adverse effects. Pharmacokinetic interactions include metabolic enzyme induction or inhibition and protein binding displacement interactions (e.g., DVP and warfarin). Pharmacodynamic interactions include additive sedation and cognitive toxicity, which increase the risk of falls and other impairments.

▶ Pregnancy and Postpartum

Treatment of bipolar disorder during pregnancy is fraught with controversy and conflicting recommendations. The key issue is the relative risk of teratogenicity with drug use during pregnancy versus risk of bipolar relapse without treatment with consequent potential harm to both the pregnant patient and the fetus. Therapeutic judgments depend on the history of the patient and whether the pregnancy is planned or unplanned. Treatment is best managed when the pregnancy is planned. Clinicians should discuss the issue with every patient with bipolar disorder who is of childbearing potential. A pregnancy test should be obtained before initiating drug therapy. For a patient with severe bipolar disorder, a history of multiple mood episodes, rapid cycling, or suicide attempts, discontinuing treatment, even for a planned pregnancy, is unwise. For a patient with a remote history of a single mood episode with subsequent long stability and who is contemplating pregnancy, the answer is less clear. Patients should be provided clear and reliable information about the risks versus the benefits of stopping or continuing therapy so they can make an informed decision. Patients who decide to discontinue drug therapy before pregnancy should taper medications slowly to reduce the risk of relapse.[44,45]

Lithium administration during the first trimester is associated with Ebstein's anomaly in the infant, a downward displacement of the tricuspid valve into the right ventricle. Although more likely to occur in children of patients who took lithium during pregnancy, the absolute risk is considered small, around 0.1%. Pharmacokinetic handling of lithium changes as pregnancy progresses. Renal lithium clearance increases, which requires a dosage increase to maintain a therapeutic serum concentration. It may be advisable to decrease or discontinue lithium at term or the onset of labor to avoid toxicity postpartum when there is a large reduction in fluid volume.[45]

Lithium can cause hypotonicity and cyanosis in the neonate, termed the "floppy baby" syndrome. Most data indicate normal neurobehavioral development when these symptoms resolve. Lithium is readily transferred via breast milk. Breast-feeding is not advised for patients who are taking lithium.[26]

Valproic acid and carbamazepine are human teratogens. Neural tube defects such as spina bifida occur in up to 9% of infants exposed during the first trimester. The risk of neural tube defects is related to exposure during the third and fourth weeks after conception. As such, women with unplanned pregnancies may not know they are pregnant until after the risk of exposure has occurred. Carbamazepine can cause fetal vitamin K deficiency. Vitamin K is important for facial growth and for clotting factors. The risk of facial abnormalities is increased with carbamazepine and VPA, and neonatal bleeding is increased in infants of mothers who are treated with carbamazepine during pregnancy.[44,45]

Patient Encounter, Part 4: Outcome Evaluation

After an initial assessment, including evaluation of potential suicidality, support systems, and need for inpatient versus outpatient treatment, Roger was hospitalized briefly and then followed in the community on medication along with psychotherapy. He has cut back significantly on his intake of alcohol, is considering attending Alcoholics Anonymous meetings, and has stopped using marijuana. His job performance has returned to normal. He has responded well to treatment with sustained-release lithium carbonate 1200 mg po once daily at bedtime with a snack. Steady-state 12-hour serum lithium concentrations have stabilized at approximately 1.0 mEq/L (mmol/L). He now returns to clinic for routine follow-up. He has tolerated the lithium except for a slight weight gain of 5 lb (2.3 kg) and some facial acne, which he is willing to accept for now. However, he asks how long he must take this medication because he is now feeling well.

How would you assess therapeutic and adverse effects of treatment for this patient?

How would you educate the patient regarding the need for continued maintenance treatment?

Fewer data are available on other anticonvulsant mood-stabilizing drugs. Lamotrigine may be associated with an increased risk of oral clefts in association with first trimester exposure.[44,45]

The FGAs have been available for many years, and more data are available on their use in pregnancy compared with the SGAs, but treatment guidelines for bipolar disorder do not otherwise support the FGAs as an initial choice in treatment.

Use of antidepressant drugs during pregnancy is discussed in the chapter on depression.

OUTCOME EVALUATION

Assessment of Therapeutic Effects

Effective interviewing skills and a therapeutic relationship with the patient are essential to assessing response to treatment. Understand the particular symptom profile and needs of individual patients. These become the primary therapeutic monitoring parameters. In addition to the clinical interview, some clinicians use symptom rating scales such as the Young Mania Rating Scale (YMRS) for mania and the Hamilton Depression Rating Scale (Ham-D, discussed in the chapter on depression). The YMRS is composed of 11 items based on a patient's perception of his or her clinical condition over the preceding 48 hours. Adjunctive information is obtained from clinical observations made by the clinician during the patient interview. Items are chosen based on published descriptions of core symptoms of mania. Four items are scored on a scale of 0 to 8 (irritability, speech, thought content, and disruptive/aggressive behavior), and the other seven are graded on a 0 to 4 scale. These initial four items are given twice the weight of the remaining items to compensate for an inability to cooperate by severely ill patients. The YMRS's popularity stems from its ease of administration, widely accepted use, and brief format. The scale takes approximately 15 to 30 minutes to complete.[46]

Check serum concentrations of mood-stabilizing drugs as a guide to dosage adjustment for optimal efficacy. The frequency of follow-up visits depends on response, tolerability, adherence, and other factors.

Assessment of Adverse Effects

Adverse effects cause more nonadherence to prescribed therapy than any other factor. Monitor patients regularly for adverse effects and health status, especially because mood-stabilizing drugs and antipsychotic drugs commonly cause metabolic side effects such as weight gain. Repeat laboratory tests for renal and thyroid function for patients taking lithium and hematology and liver function for patients taking carbamazepine or DVP. Annual measurement of serum lipase may be advisable for patients taking DVP. More specific discussion of metabolic side effect monitoring of patients taking SGAs is provided in the chapter on schizophrenia.

Patient Education

8 *Patient education regarding benefits and risks of drug therapy and the importance of adherence to treatment must*

be integrated into management. This is especially important because responsiveness to treatment declines as the number of mood episodes increases. Discuss the nature and chronic course of bipolar disorder and the risks of repeated relapses. Help patients understand that treatment of bipolar disorder is not a cure but that many patients can enjoy symptom-free or nearly symptom-free function. Make it clear that long-term recovery is dependent on adherence to both pharmacologic and nonpharmacologic treatment. Explain the purpose of medication, common side effects to expect, and how to respond to side effects. Provide the patient and family with written information about medication indications, benefits, risks, and side effects. Discuss less frequent but more dangerous side effects of drugs and give written instructions on seeking medical attention immediately should they occur.

Patient Care and Monitoring

1. Assess the patient's symptoms and review the history. Review the family history, including the history of response to treatment by family members.

2. Obtain an initial medical evaluation to rule out other causes of mood episodes.

3. Obtain a thorough medication use history, including present and past drugs, prescription and nonprescription drugs, the patient's self-assessment of response and side effect problems, alcohol, tobacco, caffeine, illicit substances, herbal products, dietary supplements, allergies, and adherence.

4. Assess potential drug–disease, drug–drug, and drug–food interactions.

5. Evaluate physiologic parameters that may influence pharmacokinetics.

6. Develop a plan for monitoring therapeutic outcomes, focusing on the individual symptom profile and level of function of the patient. Include a plan for dosage adjustments or alternate therapy if the patient fails to respond adequately. Include serum drug concentration monitoring as appropriate.

7. Develop a monitoring plan for drug side effects. Include measures to prevent side effects as well as management if they occur. Include appropriate laboratory measures.

8. Determine the role of nonpharmacologic therapy and how it is to be integrated with drug therapy.

9. Educate the patient on the nature of bipolar disorder, its treatment, and what to expect with regard to response and side effects, and stress the need for adherence to treatment even when feeling well.

10. Encourage a healthy lifestyle, including eliminating or stopping substance abuse, smoking cessation, and encouraging proper nutrition and exercise.

Abbreviations Introduced in This Chapter

5-HT	5-hydroxytryptamine
Abd	Abdomen
ACE	Angiotensin-converting enzyme
ARB	Angiotensin receptor blocker
BDNF	Brain-derived neurotrophic factor
BP	Blood pressure
CBC	Complete blood count
CBT	Cognitive-behavioral therapy
CN	Cranial nerve
CNS	Central nervous system
DA	Dopamine
DSM-IV-TR	*Diagnostic and Statistical Manual of Mental Disorders,* 4th edition, text revision
DVP	Divalproex
ECG	Electrocardiogram
ECT	Electroconvulsive therapy
Exts	Extremities
FDA	Food and Drug Administration
FGA	First-generation antipsychotic
fMRI	Functional magnetic resonance imaging
FOI	Flight of ideas
GABA	γ-aminobutyric acid
GI	Gastrointestinal
Ham-D	Hamilton Depression Rating Scale
HIV	Human immunodeficiency virus
JVD	Jugular venous distention
MDD	Major depressive disorder
MRI	Magnetic resonance imaging
NE	Norepinephrine
NOS	Not otherwise specified
P	Pulse
PERRLA	Pupils equal round and reactive to light and accommodation
PET	Positron emission tomography
RR	Respiration rate
SGA	Second-generation antipsychotic
T	Temperature
THC	Tetrahydrocannabinol, psychoactive substance in marijuana
VPA	Valproic acid
YMRS	Young Mania Rating Scale

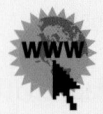 Self-assessment questions and answers are available at *http://www.mhpharmacotherapy.com/pp.html.*

REFERENCES

1. American Psychiatric Association. Diagnostic and Statistical Manual of Mental Disorders. 4th ed, text rev. Washington, DC: American Psychiatric Press; 2000.
2. Guo JJ, Keck PE, Li H, et al. Treatment costs related to bipolar disorder and comorbid conditions among Medicaid patients with bipolar disorder. Psychiatr Serv 2007;58:1073–1078.
3. Thase ME. Mood disorders: Neurobiology. In: Sadock BJ, Sadock VA, Ruiz P, eds. Kaplan and Sadock's Comprehensive Textbook of Psychiatry. 9th ed. Philadelphia, PA: Lippincott Williams & Wilkins; 2009:1664–1674.
4. Barnett JH, Smoller JW. Genetics of bipolar disorder. Neuroscience 2009;164:331–343.
5. Emsell L, McDonald C. The structural neuroimaging of bipolar disorder. Int Rev Psychiatry 2009;21:297–313.
6. Langan C, McDonald C. Neurobiological trait abnormalities in bipolar disorder. Mol Psychiatry 2009;14:833–846.
7. Serretti A, Drago A, De Ronchi D. Lithium pharmacodynamics and pharmacogenetics: Focus on inositol mono phosphatase (IMPase), inositol poliphosphatase (IPPase) and glycogen sinthase kinase 3 beta (GSK-3 beta). Curr Med Chem 2009;16:1917–1948.
8. Hashimoto K. Brain-derived neurotrophic factor as a biomarker for mood disorders: an historical overview and future directions. Psychiatry Clin Neurosci 2010;64:341–357.
9. Perugi G, Micheli C, Akiskal HS, et al. Polarity of the first episode, clinical characteristics, and course of manic depressive illness: A systematic retrospective investigation of 320 bipolar I patients. Compr Psychiatry 2000;41:13–18.
10. Judd LL, Akiskal HS, Schettler PJ, et al. The long-term natural history of the weekly symptomatic status of bipolar I disorder. Arch Gen Psychiatry 2002;59:530–537.
11. Judd LL, Akiskal HS, Schettler PJ, et al. A prospective investigation of the natural history of the long-term weekly symptomatic status of bipolar II disorder. Arch Gen Psychiatry 2003;60:261–269.
12. Hirschfeld RM, Holzer C, Calabrese JR, et al. Validity of the mood disorder questionnaire: A general population study. Am J Psychiatry 2003;160:178–180.
13. Novick DM, Swartz HA, Frank E. Suicide attempts in bipolar I and bipolar II disorder: A review and meta-analysis of the evidence. Bipolar Disord 2010;12:1–9.
14. Magalhães PV, Kapczinski F, Nierenberg AA, et al. Illness burden and medical comorbidity in the Systematic Treatment Enhancement Program for Bipolar Disorder. Acta Psychiatr Scand 2011;125(4):303–308.
15. Cipriani A, Barbui C, Salanti G, et al. Comparative efficacy and acceptability of antimanic drugs in acute mania: A multiple-treatments meta-analysis. Lancet 2011;378:1306–1315.
16. Akiskal HS. Mood disorders: Clinical features. In: Sadock BJ, Sadock VA, Ruiz P, eds. Kaplan and Sadock's Comprehensive Textbook of Psychiatry. 9th ed. Philadelphia, PA: Lippincott Williams & Wilkins; 2009:1693–1733.
17. Hollon SD, Ponniah K. A review of empirically supported psychological therapies for mood disorders in adults. Depress Anxiety 2010;27:891–932.
18. da Costa RT, Rangé BP, Malagris LE, et al. Cognitive-behavioral therapy for bipolar disorder. Expert Rev Neurother 2010;10:1089–1099.
19. Sidor MM, Macqueen GM. Antidepressants for the acute treatment of bipolar depression: A systematic review and meta-analysis. J Clin Psychiatry 2011;72:156–167.
20. Swartz HA, Thase ME. Pharmacotherapy for the treatment of acute bipolar II depression: Current evidence. J Clin Psychiatry 2011;72:356–366.
21. Nivoli AM, Murru A, Vieta E. Lithium: Still a cornerstone in the long-term treatment of bipolar disorder? Neuropsychobiology 2010;62:27–35.
22. McCarthy MJ, Leckband SG, Kelsoe JR. Pharmacogenetics of lithium response in bipolar disorder. Pharmacogenomics 2010;11:1439–1465.
23. Schneck CD. Treatment of rapid-cycling bipolar disorder. J Clin Psychiatry 2006;67(Suppl 11):22–27.
24. Cipriani A, Pretty H, Hawton K, Geddes JR. Lithium in the prevention of suicidal behavior and all-cause mortality in patients with mood disorders: A systematic review of randomized trials. Am J Psychiatry 2005;162:1805–1819.
25. Marmol F. Lithium: Bipolar disorder and neurodegenerative diseases. Possible cellular mechanisms of the therapeutic effects of lithium. Prog Neuropsychopharmacol Biol Psychiatry 2008;32:1761–1771.
26. Lithium carbonate package insert. Columbus, OH: Roxane Laboratories, 2009.

27. Sandson NB, Armstrong SC, Cozza KL. An overview of psychotropic drug-drug interactions. Psychosomatics 2005;46:464–494.

28. Depakote (divalproex sodium) package insert. North Chicago, IL: Abbott Laboratories, 2009.

29. Equetro (carbamazepine extended-release) package insert. Parsippany, NJ: Validus Pharmaceuticals, 2008.

30. Lamictal (lamotrigine) package insert. Research Triangle Park, NC: GlaxoSmithKline, 2011.

31. Trileptal (oxcarbazepine) package insert. East Hanover, NJ: Novartis Pharmaceuticals, 2011.

32. Suppes T, Dennehy DB, Hirschfeld RMA, et al. The Texas implementation of medication algorithms: Update to the algorithms for treatment of bipolar I disorder. J Clin Psychiatry 2005;66:870–886.

33. Vasudev A, Macritchie K, Watson S, et al. Oxcarbazepine in the maintenance treatment of bipolar disorder. Cochrane Database Syst Rev 2008;(1):CD005171.

34. Nardi AE, Perna G. Clonazepam in the treatment of psychiatric disorders: An update. Int Clin Psychopharmacol 2006;21:131–142.

35. Montgomery P, Richardson AJ. Omega-3 fatty acids for bipolar disorder. Cochrane Database Syst Rev 2008;(2):CD005169.

36. Vieta E, Suppes T, Eggens I, et al. Efficacy and safety of quetiapine in combination with lithium or divalproex for maintenance of patients with bipolar I disorder (international trial 126). J Affect Disord 2008;109:251–263.

37. Aripiprazole package insert. Tokyo: Otsuka Pharmaceutical. Tokyo, Otsuka Pharmaceutical, 2011.

38. Seroquel XR package insert. Wilmington, DE: AstraZeneca Pharmaceuticals, 2011.

39. American Diabetes Association, American Psychiatric Association, American Association of Clinical Endocrinologists, North American Association for the Study of Obesity. Consensus development conference on antipsychotic drugs and obesity and diabetes. Diabetes Care 2004;27:596–601.

40. Leverich GS, Altshuler LL, Frye MA, et al. Risk of switch in mood polarity to hypomania or mania in patients with bipolar depression during acute and continuation trials of venlafaxine, sertraline, and bupropion as adjuncts to mood stabilizers. Am J Psychiatry 2006;163:232–239.

41. McClellan J, Kowatch R, Findling RL, et al. Practice parameter for the assessment and treatment of children and adolescents with bipolar disorder. J Am Acad Child Adolesc Psychiatry 2007;46:107–125.

42. Thomas T, Stansifer L, Findling RL. Psychopharmacology of pediatric bipolar disorders in children and adolescents. Pediatr Clin North Am 2011;58:173–187.

43. Pringsheim T, Lam D, Ching H, et al. Metabolic and neurological complications of second-generation antipsychotic use in children: A systematic review and meta-analysis of randomized controlled trials. Drug Saf 2011;34:651–668.

44. Yonkers KA, Vigod S, Ross LE. Diagnosis, pathophysiology, and management of mood disorders in pregnant and postpartum women. Obstet Gynecol 2011;117:961–977.

45. Cohen LS. Treatment of bipolar disorder during pregnancy. J Clin Psychiatry 2007;68(Suppl 9):4–9.

46. Young RC, Biggs JT, Ziegler VE, et al. A rating scale for mania: Reliability, validity and sensitivity. Br J Psychiatry 1978;133:429–435.

47. Drayton SJ. Bipolar disorder. In: DiPiro JT, Talbert RL, Yee GC, Matzke GR, Wells BG, Posey LM, eds. Pharmacotherapy: A Pathophysiologic Approach. 8th ed. New York, NY: McGraw-Hill. 2010;1191–1208.

48. American Psychiatric Association. Practice guidelines for the treatment of patients with bipolar disorder (revision). Am J Psychiatry 2002;159:1–50.

49. Canadian Network for Mood and Anxiety Treatments (CANMAT) and International Society for Bipolar Disorders (ISBD) collaborative update of CANMAT guidelines for the management of patients with bipolar disorder: update 2009. Bipolar Disord 2009;11:225–255.

50. Goodnick PJ, ed. Mania: Clinical and Research Perspectives. Washington, DC: American Psychiatric Press; 1998.

51. McEvoy GK, Miller J, Snow EK, et al. Lithium salts. AHFS Drug Information 2007. Bethesda, MD: American Society of Health-System Pharmacists; 2007:2566–2575.

52. McEvoy GK, Miller J, Snow EK, et al. Valproate sodium, valproic acid, divalproex sodium. AHFS Drug Information 2007. Bethesda, MD: American Society of Health-System Pharmacists; 2007:2255–2262.

53. McEvoy GK, Miller J, Snow EK, et al. Carbamazepine. AHFS Drug Information 2007. Bethesda, MD: American Society of Health-System Pharmacists; 2007:2220–2225.

54. McEvoy GK, Miller J, Snow EK, et al. Oxcarbazepine. AHFS Drug Information 2007. Bethesda, MD: American Society of Health-System Pharmacists; 2007:2244–2246.

55. McEvoy GK, Miller J, Snow EK, et al. Lamotrigine. AHFS Drug Information 2007. Bethesda, MD: American Society of Health-System Pharmacists; 2007:2233–2239.

56. American Diabetes Association, American Psychiatric Association, American Association of Clinical Endocrinologists, et al. Consensus development conference on antipsychotic drugs and obesity and diabetes. Diabetes Care 2004;27:596–601.

40 Generalized Anxiety Disorder, Panic Disorder, and Social Anxiety Disorder

Sheila Botts, Sallie Charles, and Douglas Newton

LEARNING OBJECTIVES

● **Upon completion of the chapter, the reader will be able to:**

1. Describe pathophysiologic findings in patients with generalized anxiety, panic, and social anxiety disorder.

2. List common presenting symptoms of generalized anxiety, panic, and social anxiety disorders.

3. Identify the desired therapeutic outcomes for patients with generalized anxiety, panic, and social anxiety disorders.

4. Discuss appropriate lifestyle modifications and over-the-counter medication use in these patients.

5. Recommend psychotherapy and pharmacotherapy interventions for patients with generalized anxiety, panic, and social anxiety disorders.

6. Develop a monitoring plan for anxiety patients placed on specific medications.

7. Educate patients about their disease state and appropriate lifestyle modifications, as well as psychotherapy and pharmacotherapy for effective treatment.

KEY CONCEPTS

❶ The goals of therapy for generalized anxiety disorder (GAD) are to acutely reduce the severity and duration of anxiety symptoms and restore overall functioning. The long-term goal in GAD is to achieve and maintain remission.

❷ Antidepressants are considered first-line agents in the management of chronic GAD.

❸ Benzodiazepines are recommended for acute treatment of GAD when short-term relief is needed, as an adjunct during initiation of antidepressant therapy, or to improve sleep.

❹ The acute phase of panic disorder (PD) treatment lasts about 12 weeks and should result in marked reduction in panic attacks, ideally total elimination, and minimal anticipatory anxiety and phobic avoidance. Treatment should be continued to prevent relapse for an additional 12 to 18 months before attempting discontinuation.

❺ Patients with PD are more likely to experience stimulant-like side effects of antidepressants than patients with major depression. Antidepressants should be initiated at lower doses in patients with PD than in depressed patients and those with other anxiety disorders.

❻ Antidepressants should be tapered when treatment is discontinued to avoid withdrawal symptoms, including irritability, dizziness, headache, and dysphoria.

❼ The dose of benzodiazepine required for improvement in PD generally is higher than that used in other anxiety disorders.

❽ Based on their tolerability and efficacy, selective serotonin reuptake inhibitors are considered the drugs of choice for social anxiety disorder (SAD).

❾ The onset of response to antidepressants in SAD is delayed and may be as long as 8 to 12 weeks. Patients responding to medication should be continued on treatment for at least 1 year.

❿ Pharmacotherapy for patients with SAD should lead to improvement in physiologic symptoms of anxiety and fear, functionality, and overall well-being.

Anxiety is a normal response to stressful or fearful circumstances. Most people experience some degree of anxiety in reaction to stressful situations, such as final exams or giving a speech. This allows an individual to adapt to or manage the stressful or threatening situation. Anxiety symptoms generally are short lived and do not necessarily impair function. Anxiety that becomes excessive, causes irrational thinking or behavior, and impairs a person's functioning is considered an anxiety disorder.

Anxiety disorders are among the most frequent mental disorders encountered by clinicians. They often are missed or attributed incorrectly to other medical illnesses, and most patients are treated inadequately.[1] The burden of detection and diagnosis most often falls to primary care clinicians, to whom most patients present in the context of other complaints. Untreated anxiety disorders may result in increased health care utilization, morbidity and mortality, and a poorer quality of life.

EPIDEMIOLOGY AND ETIOLOGY

Epidemiology

▶ Prevalence

With a lifetime prevalence of 28.8%, anxiety disorders collectively represent the most prevalent psychiatric disorders,[2] with specific phobia (12.5%) and social anxiety disorder (SAD) (12.1%) being the most common.[3] Recent reports from the National Comorbidity Survey Revised (NCS-R) estimate the lifetime prevalence of generalized anxiety disorder (GAD) for those 18 years of age and older to be 5.7%.[3,4] Rates for panic disorder (PD) are slightly lower, with an estimated lifetime prevalence of 4.7%.

Most studies report higher rates of anxiety disorders among women (2:1 female:male ratio) and older adults.[2] Prevalence rates across the anxiety spectrum increase from the younger age group (18 to 29 years) to older age groups (30 to 44 and 45 to 59 years); however, rates are substantially lower for those older than age 59 years.[3]

▶ Course of Illness

PD and GAD have a median age of onset of 24 and 31 years, respectively, whereas specific phobia and SAD tend to develop much earlier (median age of onset, 7 and 13 years, respectively).[3] Although GAD and PD may not manifest fully until adulthood, as many as half of adult anxiety patients report subthreshold symptoms during childhood.[5]

Anxiety disorders are chronic, and symptoms tend to wax and wane, with fewer than one-third of patients experiencing spontaneous symptom remission.[6] The risk for relapse and recurrence of symptoms is also high for anxiety disorders. In a 12-year follow-up study of anxiety disorder patients, recurrence rates ranged from 58% of PD and GAD patients to 39% of SAD patients.[7]

Remission, if achieved with treatment, is most likely to occur within the first 2 years of an index episode.[6] Similarly, the highest rates of relapse are seen within the same timeframe. This suggests that many patients need ongoing maintenance treatment. Rates of remission do not appear to vary by sex.[6] Likewise, relapse rates do not appear to differ by sex; however, one study reported that women with PD without agoraphobia were three times more likely than men to experience a relapse of symptoms. Patients with anxiety disorders spend a significant portion of time "being ill" during a particular episode, ranging from 41% to 80% of the time.[7] Expectedly, anxiety disorders are associated with impaired psychosocial functioning and a compromised quality of life.[8] Appropriate treatment has been shown to improve the patient's overall quality of life and psychosocial functioning.[8]

▶ Comorbidity

More than 90% of individuals with an anxiety disorder have a lifetime history of one or more other psychiatric disorders.[9] Depression is the most common lifetime comorbid illness, followed by alcohol and substance use disorders, as well as other co-occurring anxiety disorders, especially GAD and PD.[9] Generally speaking, the onset of SAD and GAD symptoms precedes major depressive disorder (MDD), but there is an equal chance of PD onset before, during, or after MDD. Comorbid psychiatric illness is associated with lower rates of remission and higher rates of relapse. It is essential that both disorders are treated appropriately.

Etiology

Both genetic and psychosocial factors appear to play a role in the initiation and expression of anxiety disorders.[10] Documentation of moderate genetic risk has been identified for all anxiety disorders, although some conflicting data do exist. Currently, no definitive gene or set of genes has been identified as being the causative factor for a specific anxiety disorder. Additionally, it is unclear if anxiety disorders share common genetic risk factors. Genetic overlap may exist between GAD and PD and, to a lesser extent, SAD.[10]

Genetics may create a vulnerable phenotype for an anxiety disorder, and an individual's life stressors and means of coping with the stress may also play a role in precipitation and continued expression of the anxiety disorder.[11] In fact, some researchers believe that stressful life events may play a strong role in the onset of anxiety disorders, especially in GAD and PD.[10] It has been reported that those experiencing one or more negative life events have a threefold increased chance of developing GAD.[2] Similar findings have been reported with PD.[11]

PATHOPHYSIOLOGY

● The thalamus and amygdala are important in the generation of a normal fear response and play a central role in most anxiety disorders. The nervous system requires a mechanism to detect a potential threat, evaluate, and respond in a defensive or evasive manner. The thalamus provides the first real processing region to organize sensory data obtained from the environment. It passes information to higher cortical centers for finer processing and to the amygdala for rapid assessment of highly charged emotional information. The amygdala provides emotional valence or the emotional importance of the information. This helps the organism to act quickly on ambiguous but vital events. The cortex then performs a more detailed analysis and sends updates to the amygdala for comparison and any needed course corrections, thus enabling a decision on a course of action.

Anxiety becomes an anxiety disorder when the fear-response system leads to maladaptive behavior or distress. Anxiety can become independent of stimuli as in PD, be associated with benign stimuli as in phobias, or continue beyond the stimulus duration as in GAD. The precise

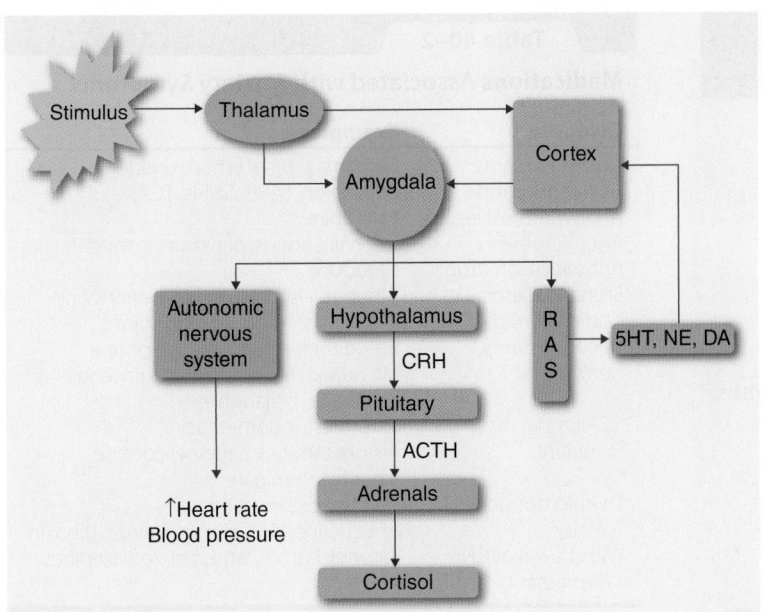

FIGURE 40–1. Neurocircuitry and key neurotransmitters involved in mediating anxiety disorders. (ACTH, adrenocorticotrophic hormone; CRH, corticotropin-releasing hormone; DA, dopamine; 5-HT, serotonin; NE, norepinephrine; RAS, reticular activating system.)

mechanism by which these changes occur is unknown, but much has been discovered regarding how this may be regulated by treatment (**Fig. 40–1**).

Direct and indirect connections to the reticular activating system (RAS), a region spanning the medulla, pons, and midbrain, help to regulate arousal, vigilance, and fear. These connections are modulated by serotonin and norepinephrine (NE), which have their primary origins in the RAS.[12] The amygdala sends projections to the hypothalamus, thus influencing the autonomic nervous system to affect heart rate, blood pressure, and stress-associated changes. It also influences the hypothalamic–pituitary–adrenal (HPA) axis, leading to a cascade of stress hormones.[13] One such hormone is cortisol, which, if elevated for prolonged periods, can damage the brain and other organs. These are important targets in our understanding of how the amygdala regulates the fear response.

Noradrenergic System

● Norepinephrine-producing cells reside primarily in a region of the brain called the locus ceruleus (LC). Increased activity in this region is associated with an increase in arousal, anxiety, and panic. Whereas drugs such as yohimbine that increase activity in the LC can be anxiogenic, drugs that decrease activity in the LC appear to improve anxiety. Furthermore, dysregulation of this region is implicated by elevated levels of NE or its metabolites in subjects with GAD, PD, and specific phobias.[13]

Serotonergic System

● The raphe nuclei and the resident cell bodies of serotonin (5-HT)-producing neurons have a complicated role related to anxiety symptoms. Activity of 5-HT cells in the raphe nuclei over time inhibits firing of noradrenergic cells in the LC. Other influences include their ability to regulate cells in

the prefrontal cortex and amygdala. Perhaps the strongest evidence for the involvement of the serotonergic system is the success of serotonin reuptake inhibitors in treatment of anxiety disorders.[13]

γ-Aminobutyric Acid

● γ-aminobutyric acid (GABA) plays an important role as an inhibitory neurotransmitter. The effects of GABA are nonspecific, and its role is complex. GABA-ergic drugs are used for acute anxiety reduction, but the lack of a specific target for their effect leads to multiple undesirable effects. Current research is focused on defining receptor subtypes that may allow for greater specificity in targeting anxiety symptoms.[14]

Hypothalamic–Pituitary–Adrenal Axis

● The HPA axis provides a critical mechanism for regulation of the stress response and its effects on the brain and other organ systems. Several important hormones, including corticotropin-releasing hormone and cortisol, are involved in this pathway. These hormones regulate the effects of anxiety on the body and provide positive feedback to the brain.[13] A cycle of anxiety and sensitization by such feedback could, if unchecked, result in escalation of symptoms. Neuropeptides may provide one mechanism to balance positive and negative feedback, helping to minimize such escalation.

Neuropeptides

● Several neuropeptides are under current investigation for their role in anxiety disorders. Important neuropeptides include neuropeptide Y (NPY), substance P, and cholecystokinin. NPY appears to have a role in reducing the effect of stress hormones and inhibiting activity of the LC. Both mechanisms may contribute to the anxiolytic properties seen experimentally. Substance P may have anxiolytic and

Clinical Presentation and Diagnosis of GAD

General

Onset is typically in early adulthood. Anxiety emerges and dissipates more gradually than in PD. Laboratory evaluation usually is reserved for later onset, atypical presentation, or poor response to treatment.

Symptoms[2]

Excessive anxiety or worry involving multiple events or activities occurring more days than not for at least 6 months and associated with at least three of the following:

- Restlessness
- Easily fatigued
- Poor concentration
- Irritability
- Muscle tension
- Insomnia or unsatisfying sleep

Differential Diagnosis

Rule out underlying medical or psychiatric disorders and medications that may cause anxiety (**Tables 40–1** and **40–2**)

Laboratory Evaluation

- Basic metabolic panel
- Thyroid-stimulating hormone
- Polysomnogram

Table 40–1

Medical Conditions That Can Cause Anxiety

Psychiatric Disorders
Mood disorders, hypochondriasis, personality disorders, alcohol or substance abuse, alcohol or substance withdrawal, other anxiety disorders

Neurologic Disorders
CVA, seizure disorders, dementia, stroke, migraine, encephalitis, vestibular dysfunction

Cardiovascular Disorders
Angina, arrhythmias, congestive heart failure, mitral valve prolapse, myocardial infarction

Endocrine and Metabolic Disorders
Hypo- or hyperthyroidism, hypoglycemia, Cushing's disease, Addison's disease, pheochromocytoma, hyperadrenocorticism, hyponatremia, hyperkalemia, vitamin B_{12} deficiency

Respiratory Disorders
Asthma, COPD, pulmonary embolism, pneumonia, hyperventilation

Other
Carcinoid syndrome, anemias, SLE

COPD, chronic obstructive pulmonary disease; CVA, cerebrovascular accident; SLE, systemic lupus erythematosus.

Data from Refs. 2 and 16.

Table 40–2

Medications Associated with Anxiety Symptoms

Category	Examples
Anticonvulsants	Carbamazepine, ethosuximide
Antidepressants	Bupropion, SSRIs, SNRIs, TCAs
Antihypertensives	Felodipine
Antimicrobials	Cephalosporins, ofloxacin, isoniazid
Antiparkinson drugs	Levodopa
Bronchodilators	Albuterol, isoproterenol, theophylline
Corticosteroids	Prednisone, methylprednisolone
Decongestants	Pseudoephedrine, phenylephrine
Herbals	Ma huang, St. John's wort, ginseng, guarana, belladonna
NSAIDs	Ibuprofen, indomethacin
Stimulants	Amphetamines, caffeine, cocaine, methylphenidate
Thyroid hormones	Levothyroxine
Toxicity	Anticholinergics, antihistamines, digoxin
Withdrawal of CNS depressants (abrupt)	Alcohol, barbiturates, benzodiazepines

CNS, central nervous system; SNRI serotonin norepinephrine reuptake inhibitor; SSRI, selective serotonin reuptake inhibitor; TCA, tricyclic antidepressant; NSAID, non-steroidal anti-inflammatory drug.

Data from Refs. 2, 16, and 17.

Patient Encounter 1, Part 1

JK is 32-year-old Hispanic woman who presents to the primary care clinic with complaints of fatigue, insomnia, and increasing irritability. She admits to "worrying" about everything, including her job; her two sons; and her father, who recently had a "heart attack." She is tearful during the interview and states that she feels "overwhelmed."

Her medical history is positive for migraine headaches and asthma.

Medications: Salmeterol inhalation, valproate 500 mg

What manifestations described above are suggestive of an anxiety disorder?

What additional information do you need to establish a diagnosis and develop a treatment plan?

What other diagnoses should be considered in your differential diagnosis?

Could her medications be contributing to her symptoms?

antidepressant properties partly because of its effects on corticotropin-releasing hormone.[15]

TREATMENT: GENERALIZED ANXIETY DISORDER

Desired Outcomes

❶ *The goals of therapy for GAD are to acutely reduce the severity and duration of anxiety symptoms and restore overall* *functioning. The long-term goal in GAD is to achieve and maintain remission.* With a positive response to treatment, patients with GAD and comorbid depression should have minimal depressive symptoms.

General Approach to Treatment

Patients with GAD may be managed with psychotherapy, pharmacotherapy, or both. The treatment plan should be individualized based on symptom severity, comorbid illnesses, medical status, age, and patient preference. Patients with severe symptoms resulting in functional impairment should receive antianxiety medication.

Nonpharmacologic Therapy

Nonpharmacologic therapy includes psychoeducation, exercise, stress management, and psychotherapy. Psycho-education should address pertinent information on GAD and its management. Patients should be instructed to avoid stimulating agents such as caffeine, decongestants, diet pills, and excessive alcohol use. Regular exercise is also recommended. Cognitive-behavioral therapy (CBT) is the most effective psychological therapy for GAD patients. It helps patients to recognize and alter patterns of distorted thinking and dysfunctional behavior. Some trials suggest that treatment gains with CBT may be maintained for up to 1 year.[18] CBT may be delivered in individual or group therapy and should often include families (children with anxiety).[19] Computerized CBT offered over the Internet is effective and may offer an alternative to face-to-face therapy for patients with access barriers.[20] The effect sizes of trials with CBT are comparable to those of pharmacologic therapies. Although there are limited data evaluating the benefit of combined CBT and medication, a recent trial in children with GAD suggests the combination was superior to either treatment alone.[21]

Patient Encounter 1, Part 2

After a medical workup, JK was diagnosed with GAD and depression NOS.

PMH: Migraine, asthma

FH: Mother treated for depression; father, alcohol dependence

SH: Drinks alcohol occasionally; lives independently with spouse and two children

Meds: Salmeterol inhalation; Valproate 500 mg/day

What are first-line treatment options for this patient?

What factors should be considered in selecting the patient's treatment?

What is the role of benzodiazepines for this patient?

How should the patient be monitored when receiving an antidepressant?

Pharmacologic Therapy

Antidepressants, benzodiazepines, pregabalin, buspirone, hydroxyzine, and the second-generation (SGA) antipsychotics have controlled clinical trial data supporting their use in GAD. Antidepressants have replaced benzodiazepines as the drugs of choice for chronic GAD owing to a tolerable side effect profile; no risk for dependency; and efficacy in common comorbid conditions, including depression, panic, obsessive-compulsive disorder (OCD), and SAD. Benzodiazepines remain the most effective and commonly used treatment for short-term management of anxiety when immediate relief of symptoms is desired. They are also recommended for intermittent or adjunctive use during GAD exacerbation or for sleep disturbance during the initiation of antidepressant treatment.[18] Buspirone and pregabalin are alternative agents for patients with GAD without depression. Hydroxyzine is usually adjunctive and is less desirable for long-term treatment owing to side effects that include sedation and anticholinergic effects.

Patients with GAD should be treated to remission of symptoms. Although data are lacking on the optimal duration of pharmacotherapy, recent guidelines recommend continuing treatment for 1 year.[18,19,22,23] Continuation of antidepressant therapy after acute response significantly decreases the risk of relapse (odds ratio, 0.2 [0.15 to 0.26]; number needed to treat [NNT], 3.23 [2.86 to 3.85]).[22] An algorithm for the pharmacologic management of GAD is shown in **Figure 40–2**.

▶ Antidepressants

❷ *Antidepressants (Table 40–3) are considered first-line agents in the management of chronic GAD.* These agents reduce the psychic symptoms (e.g., worry and apprehension) of anxiety with a modest effect on autonomic or somatic symptoms (e.g., tremor, rapid heart rate, and/or sweating). All antidepressants evaluated provide a similar degree of anxiety reduction. The onset of antianxiety effect is delayed 2 to 4 weeks. Selective serotonin reuptake inhibitors (SSRIs) or serotonin-norepinephrine reuptake inhibitors (SNRIs) are usually preferred over tricyclic antidepressants (TCAs) such as imipramine owing to improved safety and tolerability. Selection of a specific antidepressant generally is based on history of prior response, side effect profile, drug interaction profile (see Chapter 38), cost, or formulary availability.

Antidepressants modulate synaptic 5-HT, NE, and/or dopamine (DA) reuptake and receptor-activated neuronal signal transduction. These intracellular changes ultimately modify the expression of genes and proteins important in stress response (e.g., increase messenger RNA for glucocorticoid receptors and brain-derived neurotrophic factor and decrease mRNA expression for corticotropin-releasing hormone).[24] Activation of these "stress-adapting" pathways is thought to improve both somatic and psychic symptoms of anxiety.[24]

Serotonin Norepinephrine Reuptake Inhibitors Venla-faxine and duloxetine are SNRIs approved by the Food and Drug Administration (FDA) for the treatment of GAD.

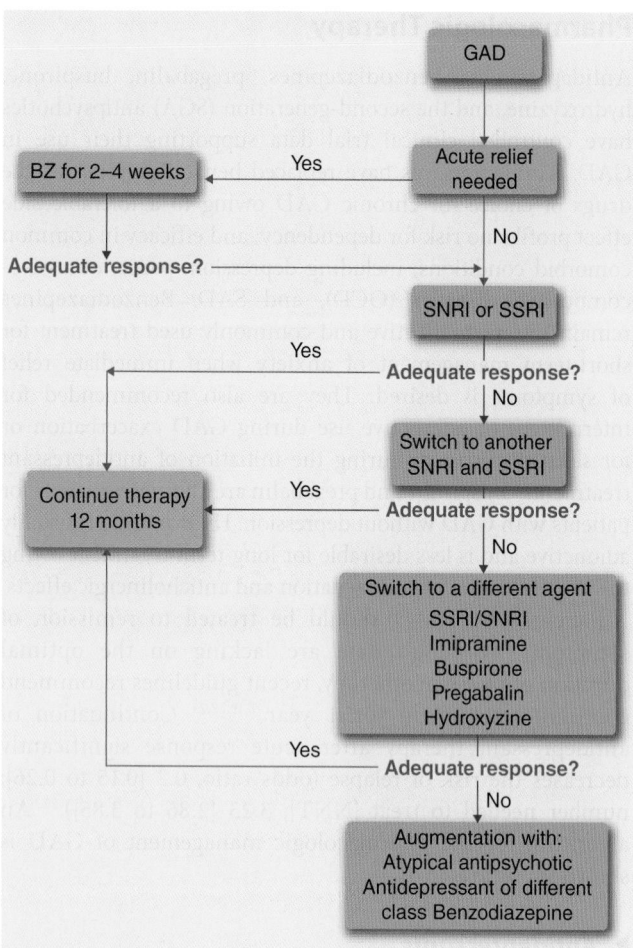

FIGURE 40–2. Treatment algorithm for generalized anxiety disorder. (BZ, benzodiazepine; SNRI, serotonin-norepinephrine reuptake inhibitor; SSRI, selective serotonin reuptake inhibitor.) (Adapted from Kirkwood CK, Melton ST. Anxiety disorders: I. Generalized anxiety, panic and social anxiety disorders. In: DiPiro JT, Talbert RL, Yee GC, et al., eds. Pharmacotherapy: A Pathophysiologic Approach. 7th ed. New York: McGraw-Hill; 2008:1166; With permission.)

They alleviate anxiety in GAD patients with and without depression. Venlafaxine is effective at doses 75 to 225 mg/day and maintains response with extended treatment.[18] Venlafaxine is also effective for the management of GAD in children and adolescents.[19] Venlafaxine has more favorable tolerability profile than TCAs. The most common side effects reported by patients with GAD are nausea, somnolence, dry mouth, dizziness, sweating, constipation, and anorexia.[18,25]

Duloxetine is effective for the treatment of GAD as well, but long-term efficacy has not yet been established. At 60 to 120 mg/day, its efficacy is noninferior to venlafaxine, and tolerability is similar.[25] For patients with concurrent pain syndromes, duloxetine has been found to improve anxiety, pain, and functional impairment more than placebo.[26]

Selective Serotonin Reuptake Inhibitors The SSRIs paroxetine, escitalopram, and sertraline have been shown to be significantly more effective than placebo in reducing anxiety symptoms in adults with GAD. Paroxetine at doses

of 20 and 40 mg/day achieved response in 62% and 68% of patients, respectively, over 8 weeks of treatment.[27] Remission occurred in 30% and 36%, respectively. In a 24-week relapse-prevention study, paroxetine was more effective than placebo at maintaining response, and patients were more likely to achieve remission with continued treatment (42.5% at 8 weeks vs. 73% at 24 weeks).[28] In GAD trials, paroxetine was associated with a high rate of somnolence, nausea, abnormal ejaculation, dry mouth, decreased libido, and asthenia compared with placebo.[27]

Escitalopram, in a dose range of 10 to 20 mg/day, was more effective than placebo in patients with GAD without depression. Fifty-eight percent of patients taking escitalopram achieved response versus 38% on placebo over the 8 weeks of treatment.[29] Side effects included headache, nausea, somnolence, upper respiratory tract infection, decreased libido, ejaculation disorder, and anorgasmia.[29]

Sertraline was more efficacious than placebo in patients with GAD being treated for 12 weeks. Sertraline treatment resulted in 56% of patients achieving response; 31% achieved remission.[30] Side effects included increased rates of nausea, insomnia, sweating, decreased libido, diarrhea, fatigue, and ejaculation disorder.[30]

Limited comparative trial data suggest comparable outcomes among these SSRIs.[31,32] SSRI therapy is better tolerated than TCAs, and tolerability is similar to that with venlafaxine. Citalopram has been shown to be efficacious in the treatment of GAD in the elderly.[33] The SSRIs, sertraline, fluoxetine, and fluvoxamine have demonstrated benefits in children and adolescents with GAD and are the preferred pharmacologic treatment in this population.[19]

Tricyclic Antidepressants Imipramine provided a higher rate of remission of anxiety symptoms than trazodone, diazepam, or placebo (e.g., 73% vs. 69% vs. 66% vs. 47%, respectively) in an 8-week controlled trial of GAD patients.[18] Antidepressants were more effective than diazepam or placebo in reducing psychic symptoms of anxiety. The use of TCAs generally is limited by bothersome adverse effects (e.g., sedation, orthostatic hypotension, anticholinergic effects, and weight gain). TCAs have a narrow therapeutic index and are lethal in overdose because of atrioventricular heart block.

Novel Antidepressants Mirtazapine, an alpha-2 adrenergic antagonist and postsynaptic serotonin (5-HT$_2$, 5-HT$_3$) receptor antagonist, is an effective antidepressant but has not been extensively evaluated in anxiety disorders. One open-label study found treatment of GAD for 12 weeks with mirtazapine 30 mg to be efficacious and well tolerated.[18] Mirtazapine is not associated with sexual dysfunction, a common antidepressant side effect, but does have a greater propensity to cause sedation and weight gain. Bupropion, a dopamine and norepinephrine reuptake-inhibitor, lacks the common antidepressant side effects of weight gain and sexual dysfunction. Bupropion has not been studied or used extensively in anxiety disorders owing to its stimulating effects that would be expected to worsen anxiety symptoms. However, a pilot controlled trial comparing bupropion XL with escitalopram found bupropion to have comparable anxiolytic efficacy and tolerability.[18]

Table 40–3

Antidepressants Used in the Treatment of Generalized Anxiety Disorder

Medication Class	Recommended Starting Dose (mg/day)	Usual Therapeutic Dosage Range (mg/day)	Hepatic Insufficiency	Renal Insufficiency
SSRIs				
Citalopram (Celexa)	20	20–40	Maximum, 40 mg/day	
Escitalopram[a] (Lexapro)	10	10–20	Maximum, 10 mg/day	
Fluoxetine (Prozac)	20	20–80	Titrate with caution	
Fluvoxamine (Luvox)	50	100–300	Titrate with caution	
Paroxetine	20	20–50	Titrate with caution	
Paroxetine CR (Paxil, Paxil CR)	25	25–62.5	Maximum, 50 mg/day	Maximum, 50 mg/day
Sertraline (Zoloft)	50–100	50–200	Reduce dose	
SNRIs				
Venlafaxine XR[a] (Effexor XR)	75	75–300	Reduce dose by 50%	Reduce dose 25%–50%
Duloxetine (Cymbalta)	30	60–120	Use not recommended	Use not recommended[b]
TCAs				
Imipramine (Tofranil)	50–75	75–200	Titrate with caution	

[a]Food and Drug Administration approved for use in generalized anxiety disorder.

[b]Duloxetine use is not recommended in severe renal impairment (creatinine clearance less than 30 mL/min [less than 0.50 mL/s])

SNRI, serotonin and norepinephrine reuptake inhibitor; SSRI, selective serotonin reuptake inhibitor; TCA, tricyclic antidepressant.

Data from Refs. 17 and 34.

▶ Benzodiazepines

③ *Benzodiazepines are recommended for acute treatment of GAD when short-term relief is needed, as an adjunct during initiation of antidepressant therapy, or to improve sleep.*[18] Benzodiazepine treatment results in a significant improvement in 65% to 75% of GAD patients, with most of the improvement occurring in the initial 2 weeks of therapy.[18] They are more effective in reducing somatic symptoms of anxiety than psychic symptoms. The major disadvantages of benzodiazepines are their lack of effectiveness in treating depression; the risk for dependency and abuse; and potential interdose rebound anxiety, especially with short-acting formulations. They should be avoided in patients with chemical dependency.

Benzodiazepines exert their effects by enhancing transmission of the inhibitory neurotransmitter GABA through interaction with the GABA$_A$-receptor complex.[17,18] Although all benzodiazepines possess anxiolytic properties, only 7 of the 13 currently marketed agents are approved by the FDA for the treatment of anxiety disorders (Table 40–4). All benzodiazepines are expected to provide equivalent benefit when given in comparable doses. Benzodiazepines differ substantially in their pharmacokinetic properties and potency for the GABA$_A$-receptor site.

Benzodiazepines are metabolized by hepatic oxidation (cytochrome P-450 3A4) and glucuronide conjugation. Because lorazepam and oxazepam bypass hepatic oxidation and are conjugated only, they are preferred agents for patients with reduced hepatic function secondary to aging or disease (e.g., cirrhosis commonly seen in patients abusing alcohol or with hepatitis B or C from intravenous drug use). Many benzodiazepines are metabolized to long-acting metabolites (see Table 40–4) that provide long-lasting anxiety relief. Drugs that either inhibit or induce CYP450 isozymes or glucuronidation are the major source of drug interactions (Table 40–5).

The most common side effects associated with benzodiazepine therapy include central nervous system (CNS) depressive effects (e.g., drowsiness, sedation, psychomotor impairment, and ataxia) and cognitive effects (e.g., poor recall and anterograde amnesia). Anterograde amnesia is more likely to occur with high-potency benzodiazepines such as lorazepam or alprazolam.[37] Some patients also may be disinhibited with benzodiazepine treatment and experience confusion, irritability, aggression, and excitement.[17,18] Discontinuation of benzodiazepines may be associated with withdrawal, rebound anxiety, and a high rate of relapse. Higher doses of benzodiazepines and a longer duration of therapy increase the severity of withdrawal and risk of seizures after abrupt or rapid discontinuation. Patients should be tapered rather than discontinued abruptly from benzodiazepine therapy to avoid withdrawal symptoms. The duration of the taper should increase with extended duration of benzodiazepine therapy.[17,18] For example, patients on benzodiazepine therapy over 2 to 6 months should be tapered over 2 to 8 weeks, but patients receiving 12 months of treatment should be tapered over 2 to 4 months. A general approach to the taper is to reduce the dose by 25% every 5 to 7 days until reaching half the original dose and then decreasing by 10% to 12% per week until discontinued. Patients should expect minor withdrawal symptoms and discomfort even when tapering. Rebound symptoms (e.g., return of original symptoms at increased intensity) are transient. The patient should be counseled so that rebound anxiety is not interpreted as a relapse. Relapse or recurrence of anxiety may occur in as many as 50% of patients discontinuing benzodiazepine treatment.[17,18] It is unclear if this relapse rate represents

Table 40–4

Comparison of the Benzodiazepines

Drug Name (Brand Name) Active Metabolites	Time to Peak Concentration (hours)	Half-Life Range (hours)	Approved Dosage Range (mg/day)	Dose Equivalent (mg)
Alprazolam[a,b] (Xanax)	1–2	12–15	1–4 (GAD) 1–10 (PD)	0.5
Chlordiazepoxide[a] (Librium)	1–4	5–30	25–100	10
Desmethylchlordiazepoxide		18		
Demoxepam		14–95		
Desmethyldiazepam		40–120		
Oxazepam		5–15		
Clonazepam[b] (Klonopin)	1–4	18–50	1–4	0.25
Clorazepate[a] (Tranzene)	1–2		7.5–60	7.5
Desmethyldiazepam		40–120		
Oxazepam		5–15		
Diazepam[a] (Valium)	0.5–2	20–80	2–40	5
Desmethyldiazepam		40–120[c]		
Temazepam		8–15		
Oxazepam		5–15		
Lorazepam[a] (Ativan)	2–4	10–20	0.5–10	0.75–1
Oxazepam[a] (Serax)	2–4	5–15	30–120	15

[a]Food and Drug Administration (FDA) approved for use in generalized anxiety disorder.

[b]FDA approved for use in panic disorder.

[c]CYP2C19 genetic polymorphisms resulting in little or no enzyme activity are present in 15% to 20% of Asians and 3% to 5% of blacks and whites, resulting in reduced clearance of desmethyldiazepam.[36]

GAD, generalized anxiety disorder; PD, panic disorder.

Data from Refs. 34 and 35.

Table 40–5

Pharmacokinetic Drug Interactions With Benzodiazepines

Drug	Effect
Alcohol (chronic)	Increased CL of BZs
Carbamazepine	Increased CL of alprazolam
Cimetidine	Decreased CL of alprazolam, diazepam, chlordiazepoxide, and clorazepate and increased $t_{1/2}$
Disulfiram	Decreased CL of alprazolam and diazepam
Erythromycin	Decreased CL of alprazolam
Fluoxetine	Decreased CL of alprazolam and diazepam
Fluvoxamine	Decreased CL of alprazolam and prolonged $t_{1/2}$
Itraconazole	Potentially decreased CL of alprazolam and diazepam
Ketoconazole	Potentially decreased CL of alprazolam
Nefazodone	Decreased CL of alprazolam, AUC doubled, and $t_{1/2}$ prolonged
Omeprazole	Decreased CL of diazepam
Oral contraceptives	Increased free concentration of chlordiazepoxide and slightly decreased CL; decreased CL and increased $t_{1/2}$ of diazepam and alprazolam
Paroxetine	Decreased CL of alprazolam
Phenobarbital	Increased CL of clonazepam and reduced $t_{1/2}$
Phenytoin	Increased CL of clonazepam and reduced $t_{1/2}$
Probenecid	Decreased CL of lorazepam and prolonged $t_{1/2}$
Propranolol	Decreased CL of diazepam and prolonged $t_{1/2}$
Ranitidine	Decreased absorption of diazepam
Rifampin	Increased metabolism of diazepam
Theophylline	Decreased alprazolam concentrations
Valproate	Decreased CL of lorazepam

AUC, area under the plasma concentration time curve; BZ, benzodiazepine; CL, clearance; $t_{1/2}$, elimination half-life.

Adapted from Kirkwood CK, Melton ST. Anxiety disorders: I. Generalized anxiety, panic and social anxiety disorders. In: DiPiro JT, Talbert RL, Yee GC, et al., eds. Pharmacotherapy: A Pathophysiologic Approach. 7th ed. New York: McGraw-Hill, 2008:1169; With permission.

an inferiority of benzodiazepines or supports the chronic nature of GAD.

▶ *Pregabalin*

Pregabalin is a calcium channel modulator, and its anxiolytic properties are attributed to its selective binding to the α_2-δ subunit of voltage-gated calcium channels. In a 4-week controlled trial versus alprazolam and placebo, pregabalin was effective for both somatic and psychic symptoms of anxiety with an onset of effect similar to that of alprazolam.[38] Compared with venlafaxine and placebo, pregabalin was found to be safe, well tolerated, and efficacious in GAD, and results were seen 1 week sooner than with venlafaxine.[39] Pregabalin reduced the risk of relapse versus placebo in a 26-week relapse prevention trial.[40] Pregabalin has short elimination half-life and must be dosed two to three times daily. It is excreted renally with a low risk of drug–drug interactions. Pregabalin is a schedule V controlled substance owing to a propensity to cause euphoria, and it has a risk of withdrawal symptoms when discontinued abruptly. It should be used cautiously in patients with a current or past history of substance abuse. It is not beneficial for depression or other anxiety disorders.

▶ *Alternative Agents*

Hydroxyzine, buspirone, and SGAs are alternative agents. Hydroxyzine may be effective for acute reduction of somatic symptoms of anxiety.[18] It does not improve psychic features of anxiety and does not treat depression or other common comorbid anxiety disorders.

Buspirone, a 5-HT$_{1A}$ partial agonist, is thought to exert its anxiolytic effects by reducing presynaptic 5-HT firing.[41] Unlike benzodiazepines, it does not have abuse potential, cause withdrawal reactions, or potentiate alcohol and sedative–hypnotic effects. It has a gradual onset of action (i.e., 2 weeks) and does not provide immediate anxiety relief. Buspirone's inconsistent data regarding its efficacy in chronic GAD or GAD with comorbid depression limit is usefulness.[18] Some research suggests that buspirone is less effective in patients who have been treated previously (4 weeks to 5 years) with benzodiazepines.[18]

Buspirone should be initiated at a dose of 7.5 mg twice daily and titrated in 5-mg/day increments (every 2 to 3 days) to a usual target dose of 20 to 30 mg/day.[18,41] The maximum daily dose is considered to be 60 mg/day.

Buspirone generally is well tolerated and does not cause sedation. The most common side effects include dizziness, nausea, and headaches. Drugs that inhibit CYP3A4 (e.g., verapamil, diltiazem, itraconazole, fluvoxamine, and erythromycin) can increase buspirone levels. Likewise, enzyme inducers such as rifampin can reduce buspirone levels significantly. Buspirone may increase blood pressure when coadministered with a monoamine oxidase inhibitor (MAOI).

The SGAs, quetiapine, olanzapine, and risperidone have demonstrated benefit in GAD. In three large placebo controlled trials, quetiapine in daily doses of 50 to 300 mg resulted in 26% greater likelihood of treatment response (effect size, ~0.3).[42] In comparative trials, quetiapine has

similar outcomes to paroxetine 20 mg/day and escitalopram 10 mg/day.[42] Risperidone and olanzapine may improve treatment outcomes in patients with inadequate response to initial pharmacotherapy.[18] SGAs are associated with an increased risk of weight gain, sedation, fatigue, and extrapyramidal symptoms in anxiety patients.

Outcome Evaluation

Assess patients for improvement of anxiety symptoms and return to baseline occupational, social, and interpersonal functioning. With effective treatment, the patient should have no or minimal symptoms of anxiety or depression. While drug therapy is being initiated, evaluate patients more frequently to ensure tolerability and response. Monitoring

Clinical Presentation and Diagnosis of PD

General

Typically presents in late adolescence or early adulthood. Onset in older adults increases suspicion of relationship to medical disorders or substance use. Laboratory evaluation must be driven by history and physical examination.

Symptoms[2]

Recurrent, discrete episodes that typically develop rapidly and peak within 10 minutes involving at least four of the following symptoms:

- Palpitations or rapid heart rate
- Sweating
- Trembling or shaking
- Sensation of shortness of breath or smothering
- Feeling of choking
- Chest pain or discomfort
- Feeling dizzy or lightheaded
- Feelings of unreality or being detached from oneself
- Fear of dying
- Numbness or tingling sensation
- Chills or hot flushes

Differential Diagnosis

Rule out underlying medical or psychiatric disorders and medications that may cause anxiety (Tables 40–1 and 40–2).

Laboratory Evaluation

- Urine drug screen
- Basic metabolic panel
- Thyroid-stimulating hormone
- Electrocardiogram
- Holter monitor
- Electroencephalogram
- Urine vanillylmandelic acid (VMA)

should include suicidal ideation and behaviors for children, adolescents, and young adults (24 years of age or younger) initiated on antidepressants.[43] Increase the dose in patients exhibiting a partial response after 2 to 4 weeks on an antidepressant or 2 weeks on a benzodiazepine. Individualize the duration of treatment because some patients require up to 1 year of treatment.[18]

TREATMENT: PANIC DISORDER

Desired Outcomes

- The main objectives of treatment are to reduce the severity and frequency of panic attacks, reduce anticipatory anxiety and agoraphobic behavior, and minimize symptoms of depression or other comorbid disorders.[44] The long-term goal is to achieve and sustain remission.

General Approach to Treatment

- Treatment options include medication, psychotherapy (e.g., CBT preferred), or a combination of both. In some cases, pharmacotherapy will follow psychotherapy treatments when full response is not realized. Patients with panic symptoms without agoraphobia may respond to pharmacotherapy alone. Agoraphobic symptoms generally take longer to respond than panic symptoms. ❹ *The acute phase of PD treatment lasts about 12 weeks and should result in marked reduction in panic attacks (ideally total elimination), minimal anticipatory anxiety, and phobic avoidance. Treatment should be continued to prevent relapse for an additional 12 to 18 months before attempting discontinuation.*[44] Patients who relapse after discontinuation of medication should have therapy resumed.[44]

Nonpharmacologic Therapy

- Patients with PD should be counseled to avoid stimulant agents (e.g., decongestants, diet pills, and caffeine) that may precipitate a panic attack. CBT generally includes psychoeducation, self-monitoring, countering anxious beliefs, exposure to fear cues, and modification of anxiety-maintaining behaviors.[18,44] Exposure therapy is useful
- for patients with phobic avoidance. CBT is considered a first-line treatment of PD, with efficacy similar to that of pharmacotherapy. Some studies suggest lower risk of relapse after CBT versus drug therapy.[44] The benefit of combination treatment is unclear; however, in a recent trial of PD with or without agoraphobia, SSRI plus CBT therapy was more effective than SSRI or CBT monotherapy after 9 months of treatment.[45] Panic-focused psychodynamic psychotherapy may be effective for some patients.[44]

Pharmacologic Therapy

- Patients with PD may be treated successfully with TCAs, SSRIs, SNRIs, or MAOIs, as well as benzodiazepines[18,44] (Table 40–6). Although all of these agents are similarly

			Table 40–6	

Antidepressants Used in the Treatment of Panic Disorder[18,23,42]

Medication Class	Recommended Starting Dose (mg/day)	Usual Therapeutic Dosage Range (mg/day)	Advantages	Disadvantages
SSRIs/SNRIs			**SSRIs (in general)**	**SSRIs (in general)**
Citalopram	10	20–60	Antidepressant activity;	Activation; delayed onset of action; may
Escitalopram	5–10	10–20	antianxiety activity; single	precipitate mania; sexual side effects;
Fluoxetine[a]	5–10	20–60	daily dosing (all but	GI side effects
Fluvoxamine	25	100–300	fluvoxamine); low toxicity;	
Paroxetine[a]	10	20–60	some available in generic	
Sertraline[a]	25	50–200		
Venlafaxine XR[a]	37.5	75–225		
TCAs			**TCAs (in general)**	**TCAs (in general)**
Clomipramine	25 mg (twice a day)	75–250	Established efficacy;	Activation; sedation; anticholinergic
			available in generic	effects; cardiovascular effects; delayed
Imipramine[a]	10–25	75–250		onset of action; may precipitate mania; sexual side effects; toxic in overdose; weight gain
MAOI				
Phenelzine	15	45–90	Antidepressant effects; available in generic	Dietary restrictions; drug interactions; weight gain; orthostasis; may precipitate mania

[a]Food and Drug Administration approved for use in panic disorder.

GI, gastrointestinal; MAOI, monoamine oxidase inhibitor; SSRI, selective serotonin reuptake inhibitor; TCA, tricyclic antidepressant.

Data from Refs. 18, 23, and 42.

effective, SSRIs have become the treatment of choice in PD. Benzodiazepines often are used concomitantly with antidepressants, especially early in treatment, or as monotherapy to acutely reduce panic symptoms. Benzodiazepines are not preferred for long-term treatment but may be used when patients fail several antidepressant trials.[18,44] PD patients with comorbid depression should be treated with an antidepressant. An algorithm for pharmacologic management of PD appears in **Figure 40–3.**

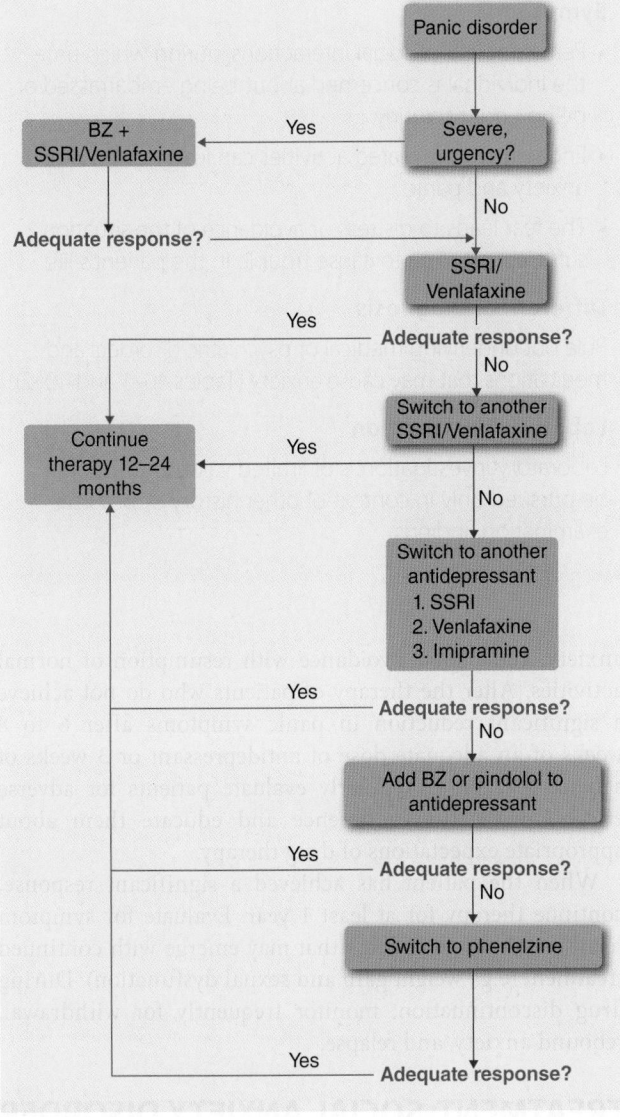

FIGURE 40–3. Algorithm for the pharmacotherapy of panic disorder. BZ, benzodiazepine; SSRI, selective serotonin reuptake inhibitor. (Adapted from Young AS, Klap R, Sherbourne CD, Wells KB. The quality of care for depressive and anxiety disorders in the United States. Arch Gen Psychiatry 2001;58:55–61 and Bruce SE, Yonkers SE, Otto MW, et al. Influence of psychiatric comorbidity on recovery and recurrence in generalized anxiety disorder, social phobia, and panic disorder: A 12-year prospective study. Am J Psychiatry 2005;162:1179–1187; With permission.)

▶ Antidepressants

● Antidepressants have a delayed onset of anti-panic effect, typically 4 weeks, with optimal response at 6 to 12 weeks. Reduction of anticipatory anxiety and phobic avoidance generally follows improvement in panic symptoms. ❺ *PD patients are more likely to experience stimulant-like side effects of antidepressants than patients with major depression. Antidepressants should be initiated at lower doses (Table 40–6) in PD patients than in depressed patients or those with other anxiety disorders. Target doses are similar to those used for depression.* ❻ *Antidepressants should be tapered when treatment is discontinued to avoid withdrawal symptoms, including irritability, dizziness, headache, and dysphoria.*

● **Tricyclic Antidepressants** Treatment with imipramine, the most studied TCA, leaves 45% to 70% of patients panic free. Both desipramine and clomipramine have demonstrated effectiveness in PD as well. Despite their efficacy, TCAs are considered second- or third-line pharmacotherapy because of poorer tolerability and toxicity on overdose.[18,44] TCAs are associated with a greater rate of treatment discontinuation than SSRIs.[44] PD patients taking TCAs may experience anticholinergic effects, orthostatic hypotension, sweating, sleep disturbances, dizziness, fatigue, sexual dysfunction, and weight gain. Stimulant-like side effects occur in up to 40% of patients.[44]

● **Selective Serotonin Reuptake Inhibitors** SSRIs are the drugs of choice for patients with PD. All SSRIs have demonstrated effectiveness in controlled trials, with 60% to 80% of patients achieving a panic-free state.[18,42] With similar efficacy reported and no trials comparing different SSRIs, drug selection generally is based on pharmacokinetics, drug interactions, side effects, and cost differences (see Chapter 38). The most common side effects of SSRIs include headaches, irritability, nausea and other gastrointestinal complaints, insomnia, sexual dysfunction, increased anxiety, drowsiness, and tremor.[44]

● **Serotonin Norepinephrine Reuptake Inhibitors** Venlafaxine, in dosages of 75 to 225 mg/day, reduced panic and anticipatory anxiety in short-term controlled trials and prevented relapse with extended treatment over 6 months.[44,46] The most common side effects include anorexia, dry mouth, constipation, somnolence, tremor, abnormal ejaculation, and sweating.

● **Monoamine Oxidase Inhibitors** MAOIs have not been evaluated systematically for treatment of PD under the current diagnostic classification and generally are reserved for patients who are refractory to other treatments.[44] They have significant side effects that limit adherence. Additionally, patients must adhere to dietary restriction of tyramine and avoid sympathomimetic drugs to avoid hypertensive crisis (see Chapter 38).

The reversible inhibitors of monoamine oxidase (RIMAs) (brofaromine and meclobemide) have been studied with mixed results.[18,44] Neither is approved for use in the United States, but they are available in Canada.

Others There is insufficient evidence to recommend the use of bupropion, trazodone, nefazodone, or mirtazapine for treatment of PD.[18,44]

► *Benzodiazepines*

Benzodiazepines are effective antipanic agents with significant effects on anticipatory anxiety and phobic behaviors. Alprazolam, the benzodiazepine most studied, is associated with significant panic reduction after 1 week of therapy (e.g., 55% to 75% panic free).[44,47] Benzodiazepines achieve outcomes similar to antidepressants over extended treatment, but benzodiazepine-treated patients are more likely to relapse when the drugs are discontinued.[44] The risk for dependence and withdrawal and lack of efficacy for depression are significant concerns for long-term treatment of patients with PD. There is no evidence that tolerance to therapeutic effect occurs. In fact, patients do not require dose escalation during extended treatment. Patients with PD do experience greater rebound anxiety and relapse when discontinuing benzodiazepines than do patients with GAD. Tapering should be done at a slower rate and over a more extended period of time than with other anxiety disorders.[18,44]

⑦ *The dose of benzodiazepine required for improvement generally is higher than that used in other anxiety disorders,* and this may explain why high-potency agents such as alprazolam and clonazepam generally are preferred. Lorazepam and diazepam, when given in equivalent doses, produce similar treatment benefits.[18,44] Doses should be titrated to response (see Table 40–4). The use of extended-release alprazolam or clonazepam may minimize breakthrough panic symptoms that are sometimes observed with immediate-release alprazolam.[47]

Side effects associated with benzodiazepines in PD patients are similar to those observed in other disorders. Sedation, fatigue, and cognitive impairment are the most commonly reported side effects.[44] Benzodiazepines should be avoided in patients with current or past substance abuse or dependence or sleep apnea. Additionally, caution should be used in older adults because they have more pronounced psychomotor and cognitive side effects.

► *β-Blockers*

Pindolol 25 mg three times a day has been shown effective as an adjunctive treatment for PD when used with an SSRI.[44] Propranolol 120 to 240 mg/day has been found equivalent to alprazolam in reduction of panic attacks.[44] β-blockers are not expected to reduce psychic anxiety or avoidance behavior. Additionally, heart rate and blood pressure reduction are dose-related adverse events that may limit use.

Outcome Evaluation

Assess patients for symptom improvement frequently (e.g., weekly) during the first 4 weeks of therapy. With effective therapy, patients should experience significant reductions in the frequency and intensity of panic attacks, anticipatory

Clinical Presentation and Diagnosis of SAD

General

Often occurs in context of other anxiety disorders. The feared social or performance situation can be limited to a specific social interaction (e.g., public speaking) or generalized to most any social interaction. Differs from specific phobia, in which the fear and anxiety are limited to a particular object or situation (e.g., insects, heights, public transportation).

Symptoms[2]

- Persistent fear of social interactions, during which time the individual is concerned about being embarrassed or being under scrutiny.
- Engaging in the feared activities can lead to extreme anxiety and panic.
- The fear leads to distress or avoidance of the situation sufficient enough to cause trouble in the patient's life.

Differential Diagnosis

Rule out underlying medical or psychiatric disorders and medications that may cause anxiety (Tables 40–1 and 40–2).

Laboratory Evaluation

Laboratory investigation is of limited value and should be pursued only in context of other history or physical examination findings.

anxiety, and phobic avoidance with resumption of normal activities. Alter the therapy of patients who do not achieve a significant reduction in panic symptoms after 6 to 8 weeks of an adequate dose of antidepressant or 3 weeks of a benzodiazepine. Regularly evaluate patients for adverse effects, medication adherence and educate them about appropriate expectations of drug therapy.

When the patient has achieved a significant response, continue therapy for at least 1 year. Evaluate for symptom relapse and adverse effects that may emerge with continued treatment (e.g., weight gain and sexual dysfunction). During drug discontinuation, monitor frequently for withdrawal, rebound anxiety, and relapse.

TREATMENT: SOCIAL ANXIETY DISORDER

Desired Outcomes

Social anxiety disorder is a chronic disorder that begins in adolescence and occurs with significant functional impairment and high rates of comorbidity. The goal of acute treatment is to reduce physiologic symptoms of anxiety, fear of social situations, and phobic behaviors. Patients with comorbid depression should have a significant reduction in depressive symptoms. The long-term goal is to restore social functioning and improve the patient's quality of life.

Patient Encounter 2

SA is an 18-year-old white woman presenting to the pediatric clinic with complaints of nausea, bloating, and stomach pain. She reports significant anxiety around school performance and social activities. She has missed 10 days of school in the past 6 weeks because of feeling ill. Her mother relates this to her avoidance of presentations and school functions. Her mother states that SA has been treated for anxiety for 15 years with Xanax 0.5 twice daily. She has considered giving her daughter a dose to get her to go to school.

Patient's medical workup is noncontributory, and she is diagnosed with generalized SAD.

What treatment options should be considered for SA?

What are the benefits of using pharmacotherapy versus psychotherapy versus both?

General Approach to Treatment

Patients with SAD may be managed with pharmacotherapy or psychotherapy. There is insufficient evidence to recommend one treatment over the other, and data are lacking on the benefits of combining treatment modalities. Pharmacotherapy often is the first choice of treatment owing to relative greater access and reduced cost compared with psychotherapy.[48] Patients with SAD generally respond slowly to treatment, and many will not achieve a full response. Relapse is common when patients are discontinued after effective short-term treatment. Patients generally are continued on treatment for at least 1 year before attempting discontinuation.

Nonpharmacologic Therapy

Patient education on disease course, treatment options, and expectations is essential, given the chronic nature and functional impairment of SAD. Support groups may be beneficial for some patients. CBT targets avoidance-learning and negative-thinking patterns associated with social anxiety by exposing the patient to a feared situation. CBT is effective for reducing anxiety and phobic avoidance and leads to a greater likelihood of maintaining response after treatment discontinuation than does pharmacotherapy.[48]

Pharmacologic Therapy

Several pharmacologic agents have demonstrated effectiveness in SAD, including the SSRIs, venlafaxine, phenelzine, RIMAs, benzodiazepines, gabapentin, and pregabalin. **8** *SSRIs are considered the drugs of choice based on their tolerability and efficacy for SAD and comorbid depression if present.* **9** *The onset of response for antidepressants may be as long as 8 to 12 weeks.*[18,49] *Patients responding to medication should be continued on treatment for at least 1 year.* Many patients relapse when medication is discontinued, and

there are no clear predictive factors for who will maintain response.[49] Some patients may elect more long-term treatment owing to fear of relapse. A suggested treatment algorithm is shown in **Figure 40–4**.

▶ Selective Serotonin Reuptake Inhibitors and Venlafaxine

The efficacy of paroxetine, sertraline, escitalopram, fluvoxamine, and venlafaxine was established in large controlled trials.[18,49] SSRIs and SNRIs improve social anxiety and phobic avoidance and reduce overall disability. Approximately 50% of patients achieve response during acute treatment. Limited data support the effectiveness of citalopram and fluoxetine in SAD.[49,50]

The initial dose of SSRI is similar to that used in depression. Patients should be titrated as tolerated to response. Many patients will require maximum recommended daily doses. Patients with comorbid PD should be started on lower doses (see Table 40–6). When discontinuing SSRIs, the dose should be tapered slowly to avoid withdrawal symptoms. Relapse rates may be as high as 50%, and patients should be monitored closely for several weeks.[48,49] Side effects of SSRIs in SAD patients are similar to those seen in depression and include nausea, sexual dysfunction, somnolence, and sweating.

Venlafaxine extended release, in doses of 75 to 225 mg/day, has similar efficacy to SSRIs.[18] As with SSRIs, doses should be tapered slowly when discontinuing therapy. Tolerability is similar to that observed in depression trials with venlafaxine extended release. Common side effects are anorexia, dry mouth, nausea, insomnia, and sexual dysfunction.

▶ Monoamine Oxidase Inhibitors and Reversible Inhibitors of Monoamine Oxidase

Phenelzine is effective in 64% to 69% of SAD patients.[49] It is generally reserved for treatment-refractory patients owing to dietary restrictions,[51] drug interactions, and side effects. The RIMAs brofaramine and meclobemide are effective in SAD.

▶ Alternative Agents

Benzodiazepines Benzodiazepines are used commonly in SAD; however, limited data support their use. Clonazepam has been effective for social anxiety, fear, and phobic avoidance, and it reduced social and work disability during acute treatment.[49] Long-term treatment is not desirable for many SAD patients owing to the risk of withdrawal and difficulty with discontinuation, cognitive side effects, and lack of effect on depressive symptoms. Benzodiazepines may be useful for acute relief of physiologic symptoms of anxiety when used concomitantly with antidepressants or psychotherapy. Benzodiazepines are contraindicated in SAD patients with alcohol or substance abuse or history of such.

Anticonvulsants Gabapentin and pregabalin, structurally similar anticonvulsant medications, have each demonstrated modest benefit in a randomized placebo controlled trial.[18,52] Gabapentin was titrated to a maximum dose of 3,600 mg/day and pregabalin to 600 mg/day. While both medications have good tolerability profiles, they should be considered for patients who have an inadequate response to SSRI/SNRIs.

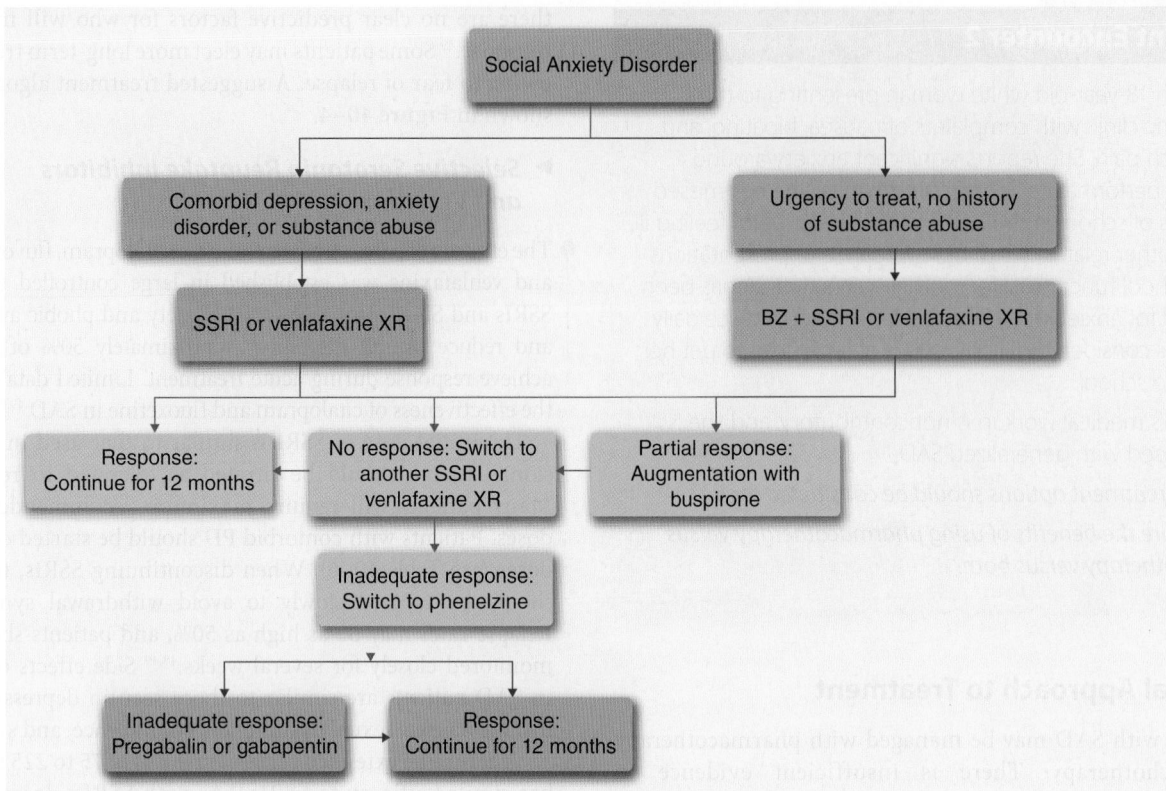

FIGURE 40–4. Algorithm for the pharmacotherapy of social anxiety disorder. BZ, benzodiazepine; SSRI, selective serotonin reuptake inhibitor. (Adapted from Melton ST, Kirkwood CK. Anxiety disorders I: Generalized anxiety, panic and social anxiety disorders. In: DiPiro JT, Talbert RL, Yee GC, et al, eds. Pharmacotherapy: A Pathophysiologic Approach. 8th ed. New York: McGraw-Hill; 2011:1209–1227; With permission.)

Patient Care and Monitoring

1. Review medical and laboratory data to rule out contributing causes of anxiety.

2. Obtain a thorough history of prescription, nonprescription, and natural product use.

3. Determine what treatments have been tried or were useful in the past. Is the patient taking medication that may cause anxiety?

4. Assess the patient's symptoms and level of functional impairment to determine if pharmacotherapy is appropriate for the anxiety disorder.

5. Provide patient education regarding disease state, lifestyle modifications, and pharmacotherapy.

   - Lifestyle changes include adequate sleep and exercise, stress management, meditation, and coping skills.

   - Potential complications of an untreated anxiety disorder

   - Potential adverse effects and risk of dependence

   - Drug interactions

   - How to record symptoms (e.g., fears, panic attacks, avoidance behaviors) for reporting back to their clinician

6. Inform patients of treatment options for anxiety disorders and the expected benefits of each (e.g., pharmacotherapy, psychotherapy, and combination treatment).

7. Develop a plan to assess the effectiveness of drug therapy during the first 12 weeks.

8. Determine an appropriate duration of treatment. Is long-term maintenance treatment needed?

9. Assess improvement in academic, social, interpersonal, and occupational functioning; quality of life; and well-being.

10. Evaluate the patient for the presence of adverse drug effects, drug–drug interactions, and drug allergies.

11. Stress the importance of adherence to medications to achieve and maintain response.

β-Blockers β-blockers decrease the physiologic symptoms of anxiety and are useful for reducing performance anxiety. Propranolol or atenolol should be administered 1 hour before a performance situation. β-blockers are not useful in generalized SAD.[49]

Outcome Evaluation

⑩ *Pharmacotherapy for patients with SAD should lead to improvement in physiologic symptoms of anxiety and fear, functionality, and overall well-being.*[18] With effective therapy, many patients will experience significant improvement in symptoms but may not achieve full remission. Monitor patients weekly during acute treatment (e.g., initiation and titration of pharmacotherapy). When patients are stabilized, monitor monthly. Inquire about adverse effects and SAD symptoms at each visit. To aid in assessing improvement, ask patients to keep a diary to record fears, anxiety levels, and behaviors in social situations.[18] Administer the Leibowitz Social Anxiety Scale (LSAS) to rate SAD severity and change, and the Social Phobia Inventory can be used as a "self-assessment" tool for patients with SAD. Last, counsel patients on appropriate expectations of pharmacotherapy in SAD, including the gradual onset of effect and the need for extended treatment of at least 1 year.

Abbreviations Introduced in This Chapter

CBT	Cognitive-behavioral therapy
CNS	Central nervous system
DA	Dopamine
FDA	Food and Drug Administration
GABA	γ-Aminobutyric acid
HPA	Hypothalamic–pituitary–adrenal
GAD	Generalized anxiety disorder
5-HT	Serotonin
LC	Locus ceruleus
LSAS	Liebowitz Social Anxiety Scale
MAOI	Monoamine oxidase inhibitor
MDD	Major depressive disorder
NCS-R	National Comorbidity Survey, Revised
NE	Norepinephrine
NPY	Neuropeptide Y
OCD	Obsessive-compulsive disorder
PD	Panic disorder
RAS	Reticular activating system
RIMA	Reversible inhibitors of monoamine oxidase A
SAD	Social anxiety disorder
SGA	Second-generation antipsychotic
SNRI	Serotonin-norepinephrine reuptake inhibitor
SSRI	Selective serotonin reuptake inhibitor
TCA	Tricyclic antidepressant
VMA	Vanillylmandelic acid

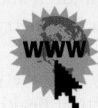 Self-assessment questions and answers are available at *http://www.mhpharmacotherapy. com/pp.html.*

REFERENCES

1. Young AS, Klap R, Sherbourne CD, Wells KB. The quality of care for depressive and anxiety disorders in the United States. Arch Gen Psychiatry 2001;58:55–61.
2. American Psychiatric Association. Diagnostic and Statistical Manual of Mental Disorders. 4th ed, text rev. Washington, DC: American Psychiatric Press; 2000:429–484.
3. Kessler RC, Berglund P, Demler O, et al. Lifetime prevalence and age-of-onset distributions of the DSM-IV disorders in the National Comorbidity Survey Replication. Arch Gen Psychiatry 2005A;62: 593–602.
4. Kessler RC, Chiu WT, Demler O, et al. Prevalence, severity, and comorbidity of 12-month DSM-IV disorders in the National Comorbidity Survey Replication. Arch Gen Psychiatry 2005;62:617–627.
5. Pollack MH. The pharmacotherapy of panic disorder. J Clin Psychiatry 2005;66(Suppl 4):23–27.
6. Yonkers KA, Bruce SE, Dyck IR, Keller MB. Chronicity, relapse, and illness-course of panic disorder, social phobia, and generalized anxiety disorder: Findings in men and women from 8 years of follow-up. Depress Anxiety 2003;17:173–179.
7. Bruce SE, Yonkers SE, Otto MW, et al. Influence of psychiatric comorbidity on recovery and recurrence in generalized anxiety disorder, social phobia, and panic disorder: A 12-year prospective study. Am J Psychiatry 2005;162:1179–1187.
8. Cramer V, Torgersen S, Kringlen E. Quality of life and anxiety disorders: A population study. J Nerv Ment Dis 2005;193:196–202.
9. Kaufman J, Charney D. Comorbidity of mood and anxiety disorders. Depress Anxiety 2000;12(Suppl 1):69–76.
10. Hettema JM, Prescott CA, Myers JM, et al. The structure of genetic and environmental risk factors for anxiety disorders in men and women. Arch Gen Psychiatry 2005;62:182–189.
11. Ninan PT, Dunlop BW. Neurobiology and etiology of panic disorder. J Clin Psychiatry 2005;66(Suppl 4):3–7.
12. Pierii JN, Lewis DA. Functional neuroanatomy. In: Sadock BJ, Sadock VA, eds. Kaplan &Sadock's Comprehensive Textbook of Psychiatry. 8th ed. Philadelphia, PA: Lippincott Williams & Wilkins; 2005:3–32.
13. Gould TD, Gray NA, Manji HK. Cellular neurobiology of severe mood and anxiety disorders: Implications for development of novel therapeutics. In: Charney DS, ed. Molecular Neurobiology for the Clinician (Review of Psychiatry Series. Vol. 22. Number 3; Oldham JM, Riba MB, series eds). Washington, DC: American Psychiatric Publishing; 2003:123–200.
14. Plata-Salaman CR, Shank RP, Smith-Swintosky VL. Amino acids as neurotransmitters. In: Sadock BJ, Sadock VA, eds. Kaplan & Sadock's Comprehensive Textbook of Psychiatry. 8th ed. Philadelphia, PA: Lippincott Williams & Wilkins, 2005:60–72.
15. Young LJ, Owens MJ, Nemeroff CB. Neuropeptides: biology, regulation, and role in neuropsychiatric disorders. In: Sadock BJ, Sadock VA, eds. Kaplan & Sadock's Comprehensive Textbook of Psychiatry. 8th ed. Philadelphia, PA: Lippincott Williams & Wilkins; 2005:3–32.
16. House A, Stark D. Anxiety in medical patients. BMJ 2002;325:207–209.
17. Melton ST, Kirkwood CK. Anxiety disorders I: Generalized anxiety, panic and social anxiety disorders. In: DiPiro JT, Talbert RL, Yee GC, et al, eds. Pharmacotherapy: A Pathophysiologic Approach. 8th ed. New York: McGraw-Hill; 2011:1209–1227.
18. Bandelow B, Zohar J, Hollander E, et al. World Federation of Societies of Biological Psychiatry (WFSBP) Guidelines for the pharmacological treatment of anxiety, obsessive-compulsive and posttraumatic stress disorders—first revision. World J Biol Psychiatry 2008;9:248–312.

19. Practice Parameter for the Assessment and treatment of children and adolescents with anxiety disorders. J Am Acad Child Adolesc Psychiatry 2007;46(2):267–283.

20. Andrews G, Cuijpers P, Craske MG, et al. Computer therapy for anxiety and depressive disorders is effective, acceptable, and practical health care: A meta-analysis. PLoS ONE 2010;5(10):e13196.

21. Walkup JT, Albano AM, Piacentini J, et al. Cognitive behavioral therapy, sertraline or a combination in childhood anxiety. N Engl J Med 2008;359(26):2753–2766.

22. Donovan MR, Glue P, Kolluri S, and Emir B. Comparative efficacy of antidepressants in preventing relapse in anxiety disorders: A meta-analysis. J Affective Disord 2010;123:9–16.

23. Davidson JR, Zhang W, Connor KM, et al. Review: A psychopharmacological treatment algorithm for generalised anxiety disorder (GAD). J Psychopharmacol 2010;24:3.

24. Shelton RC, Brown LL. Mechanisms of action in the treatment of anxiety. J Clin Psychiatry 2001;62(Suppl 12):10–15.

25. Allgulander C, Nutt D, Detke M, et al. A non-inferiority comparison of duloxetine and venlafaxine in the treatment of adult patients with generalized anxiety disorder. J Psychopharmacol 2008;22(4):417–425.

26. Hartford JT, Endicott J, Kornstein SG, et al. Implications of pain in generalized anxiety disorder: Efficacy of duloxetine. Prim Care Companion J Clin Psychiatry 2008;10(3):197–204.

27. Rickels K, Zaninelli R, McCafferty J, et al. Paroxetine treatment of generalized anxiety disorder: A double-blind, placebo-controlled study. Am J Psychiatry 2003;160:749–756.

28. Stocchi F, Nordera G, Jokinen R, et al. Efficacy and tolerability of paroxetine for the long-term treatment of generalized anxiety disorder (GAD). J Clin Psychiatry 2003;64(3):250–258.

29. Davidson JR, Bose A, Korotzer A, Zheng H. Escitalopram in the treatment of generalized anxiety disorder: Double-blind, placebo-controlled, flexible-dose study. Depress Anxiety 2004;19(4):234–240.

30. Allgulander C, Dahl AA, Austin C, et al. Efficacy of sertraline in a 12-week trial for generalized anxiety disorder. Am J Psychiatry 2004;161(9):1642–1649.

31. Ball Sg, Kuhn A, Wall D, et al. Selective serotonin reuptake inhibitor treatment for generalized anxiety disorder: A double blind, prospective comparison between paroxetine and sertraline. J Clin Psychiatry 2005;66:94–99.

32. Bielski RJ, Bose A, Chang CC. A double-blind comparison of escitalopram and paroxetine in the long-term treatment of generalized anxiety disorder. Ann Clin Psychiatry 200517(2):65–69.

33. Lenze EJ, Mulsant BH, Shear MK, et al. Efficacy and tolerability of citalopram in the treatment of late-life anxiety disorders: Results from an 8-week randomized, placebo-controlled trial. Am J Psychiatry 2005;162(1):146–150.

34. Micromedex Healthcare Series. Drugdex Evaluations. © 1974-2012 Thomson Reuters.

35. Chouinard G. Issues in the clinical use of benzodiazepines: Potency, withdrawal, and rebound. J Clin Psychiatry 2004;65(Suppl 5):7–12.

36. US Food and Drug Administration [online]. [cited 2011 Oct 10]. Available from: *http://www.fda.gov/Drugs/ScienceResearch/ResearchAreas/Pharmacogenetics/ucm083378.htm*. Accessed February 7, 2012.

37. Longo LP, Johnson B. Benzodiazepines: Side effects, abuse risk and alternatives (addiction part 1). Am Fam Physician 2000;61:2121–2128.

38. Rickels K, Pollack MH, Feltner DE, et al. Pregabalin for the treatment of generalized anxiety disorder: A 4-week, multicenter, double-blind, placebo-controlled trial of pregabalin and alprazolam. Arch Gen Psychiatry 2005;62:1022–1030.

39. Montgomery SA, Tobias K, Zornberg GL, et al. Pregabalin and venlafaxine improve symptoms of generalised anxiety disorder. Evid Based Ment Health 2007;10:23.

40. Feltner D, Wittchen HU, Kavoussi R, et al. Long-term efficacy of pregabalin in generalized anxiety disorder. Int Clin Psychopharmacol 2008;23:18–28.

41. Chessick CA, Allen MH, Thase M, et al. Azapirones for generalized anxiety disorder. Cochrane Database Syst Rev 2006;(3):CD006115.

42. Maher AR, Maglione M, Bagley S, et al. Efficacy and comparative effectiveness of atypical antipsychotic medications for off-label uses in adults: A systematic review and meta-analysis. JAMA 2011;306(12):1359–1369.

43. Bridge JA, Iyengar S, Salary CB, et al. Clinical response and risk for reported suicidal ideation and suicide attempts in pediatric antidepressant treatment: A meta-analysis of randomized controlled trials. JAMA 2007;297:1683–1696.

44. Stein MB, Goin MK, Pollack MH, et al. Practice Guideline for the Treatment of Patients with Panic Disorder. 2nd ed. Washington, DC: American Psychiatric Association; 2009. [cited 2011 Oct 10]. Available from: *http://www.psychiatryonline.com/content.aspx?aID=58560*. Accessed September 12, 2011.

45. van Apeldoorn FJ, van Hout WJ, Mersch PP, et al. Is a combined therapy more effective than either CBT or SSRI alone? Results of a multicenter trial on panic disorder with or without agoraphobia. Acta Psychiatr Scand 2008;117(4):260–270.

46. Ferguson JM, Khan A, Mangano R, et al. Relapse prevention of panic disorder in adult outpatient responders to treatment with venlafaxine extended release. J Clin Psychiatry 2007;68(1):58–68.

47. Rickels K. Alprazolam extended release in panic disorder. Expert Opin Pharmacother 2004;5(7):1599–1611.

48. Van Ameringen M, Allgulander C, Bandelow B, et al. WCA recommendations for the long-term treatment of social phobia. CNS Spectr 2003;8(Suppl 1):40–52.

49. Stein DJ, Ipser JC, Balkom AJ. Pharmacotherapy of social anxiety disorder [review]. Cochrane Database Syst Rev 2004;(4):CD001206.

50. deMenezes GB, Coutinho ESF, Fontenelle LF, et al. Second-generation antidepressants in social anxiety disorder: meta-analysis of controlled clinical trials. Psychopharmacology 2011;215:1–11.

51. Gardner DM, Shulman KI, Walker SE, Tailor SA. The making of a user friendly MAOI diet. J Clin Psychiatry 1996;57(3):99–104.

52. Schneier FR. Social anxiety disorder. N Engl J Med 2006;355:1029–1036.

41 Sleep Disorders

John M. Dopp and Bradley G. Phillips

LEARNING OBJECTIVES

● **Upon completion of the chapter, the reader will be able to:**

1. List the sequelae of undiagnosed or untreated sleep disorders and appreciate the importance of successful treatment of sleep disorders.

2. Articulate the incidence and prevalence of sleep disorders.

3. Describe the pathophysiology and characteristic features of the sleep disorders covered in this chapter, including insomnia, narcolepsy, restless legs syndrome (RLS), obstructive sleep apnea (OSA), and parasomnias.

4. Assess patient sleep complaints, conduct sleep histories, and evaluate sleep studies to recognize daytime and nighttime symptoms and characteristics of common sleep disorders.

5. Recommend and optimize appropriate sleep hygiene and nonpharmacologic therapies for the management and prevention of sleep disorders.

6. Recommend and optimize appropriate pharmacotherapy for sleep disorders.

7. Describe the components of a monitoring plan to assess safety and efficacy of pharmacotherapy for common sleep disorders.

8. Educate patients about preventive behavior, appropriate lifestyle modifications, and drug therapy required for effective treatment and control of sleep disorders.

KEY CONCEPTS

❶ Insomnia is most frequently a symptom or manifestation of an underlying disorder (comorbid or secondary insomnia) but may occur in the absence of contributing factors (primary insomnia).

❷ Patients with sleep complaints should have a careful sleep history performed to assess for possible sleep disorders and to guide diagnostic and therapeutic decisions.

❸ Although the clinical history guides diagnosis and therapy, only overnight polysomnography and multiple sleep latency tests (MSLTs) can definitively diagnose and/or guide therapy for OSA, narcolepsy, and periodic limb movements of sleep (PLMS).

❹ Treatment goals vary among different sleep disorders but generally include restoration of normal sleep patterns, elimination of daytime sequelae, improvement in quality of life, and prevention of complications and adverse effects from therapy.

❺ Early treatment of insomnia may prevent the development of persistent psychophysiologic insomnia.

❻ Benzodiazepine receptor agonists (including traditional benzodiazepines, zolpidem, zaleplon, and eszopiclone) and ramelteon are approved by the Food and Drug Administration for the treatment of insomnia and are first-line therapies.

❼ Treatment of excessive daytime sleepiness in narcolepsy and other sleep disorders may require the use of sustained- and immediate-release stimulants to effectively promote wakefulness throughout the day and at key times that require alertness.

❽ RLS treatment involves suppression of abnormal sensations and leg movements and consolidation of sleep. Dopaminergic and sedative–hypnotic medications are commonly prescribed.

❾ The primary therapy for OSA is nasal continuous positive airway pressure therapy because of its effectiveness.

❿ It is important to review patient medication profiles for drugs that may aggravate sleep disorders. Patients should be monitored for adverse drug reactions, potential drug–drug interactions, and adherence to their therapeutic regimens.

Normal humans sleep up to one-third of their lives and spend more time sleeping compared with any other single activity. Despite this, our understanding of the full purpose of sleep and the mechanisms regulating sleep homeostasis remains incomplete. Sleep is necessary to maintain wakefulness, health, and welfare. Unfortunately, disruption of normal sleep is prevalent and represents a major cause of societal morbidity, lost productivity, and reduced quality of life.[1] The link between adequate sleep and optimal health is becoming increasingly apparent, and sleep disturbances may contribute to the development and progression of comorbid medical conditions.[1]

Sleep is governed and paced by the suprachiasmic nucleus in the brain that regulates circadian rhythm. Environmental cues and amount of previous sleep also influence sleep on a daily basis. There are two main types of sleep: rapid eye movement (REM) sleep, during which eye movements and dreaming occur but the body is mostly paralyzed, and non-REM sleep, which consists of four substages (stages 1 to 4). Stage 1 serves as a transition between wake and sleep. Most of the time asleep is spent in stage 2 non-REM sleep. Stage 3 and stage 4 sleep often are grouped together and referred to as *deep sleep,* or *delta sleep,* because prominent delta waves are seen on the electroencephalogram (EEG) during these sleep stages.

EPIDEMIOLOGY AND ETIOLOGY

Sleep disorders are common. Approximately 50% of adults will report a sleep complaint over the course of their lives.[2] In general, sleep disturbances increase with age, and each disorder may have gender differences. The full extent and impact of disordered sleep on our society are not known because many patients' sleep disorders remain undiagnosed. Normal sleep, by definition, is "a reversible behavioral state of perceptual disengagement from and unresponsiveness to the environment."[3] Individuals with sleep disorders exhibit or complain about consequent symptoms (e.g., daytime sleepiness) or a bed partner will observe hallmark characteristics of the sleep disorder. Insomnia, RLS, and sleep-related breathing disorders are the most common sleep disorders.

Insomnia

The prevalence of insomnia increases with age and is nearly 1.5 times greater in women than in men. Approximately one-third of patients older than age 65 years have persistent insomnia.[4,5] In the adult population, about 10% experience chronic insomnia, and slightly more experience short-term insomnia. ❶ *Insomnia is most frequently a symptom or manifestation of an underlying disorder (comorbid or secondary insomnia) but may occur in the absence of contributing factors (primary insomnia).* Forty percent of patients with psychiatric conditions have accompanying insomnia.[6] Secondary insomnia may be triggered by acute stress and resolve when the stress resolves. Numerous coexisting medical conditions, such as pain, thyroid abnormalities, asthma, and gastroesophageal reflux, and medications, including selective serotonin reuptake

inhibitors (SSRIs), steroids, stimulants, and β-agonists, can interfere with sleep and cause insomnia. In cases of secondary insomnia, the clinician should treat the underlying cause along with insomnia symptoms.

Narcolepsy

Although difficult to estimate, the prevalence of narcolepsy is between 0.03% and 0.06%.[7] Significant differences have been reported for various ethnic groups. Narcolepsy has a higher prevalence in Japanese and a lower prevalence in Israeli populations.[8,9] Cataplexy is not required for diagnosis; however, between 50% and 80% of patients with narcolepsy have accompanying cataplexy.[10]

Restless Legs Syndrome

Restless legs syndrome occurs in 6% to 12% of the population, making it a common sleep disorder.[11,12] The prevalence of RLS increases with age and in various medical conditions such as end-stage renal disease, pregnancy, and iron deficiency.[13] RLS appears to be more common in women than in men and has a genetic link. The majority of patients (63% to 92%) report a positive family history for RLS.[14]

Obstructive Sleep Apnea

Obstructive sleep apnea is a common disorder, affecting 4% of middle-aged white men and 2% of middle-aged white women.[15] In women, the frequency of OSA increases after menopause. OSA is as common or more common in African Americans and less common in Asian populations. The risk of OSA increases with age and obesity. Individuals with OSA experience repetitive upper airway collapse during sleep, which decreases or stops airflow, with subsequent arousal from sleep to resume breathing. The severity is determined by nocturnal polysomnography (NPSG) and is graded by the number of episodes of apnea (total cessation of airflow) and hypopnea (partial airway closure with blood oxygen desaturation) experienced during sleep. The severity is expressed as the respiratory disturbance index (RDI), quantified in events per hour. People with mild sleep apnea have an RDI between 5 and 15 episodes per hour; those with moderate sleep apnea have 15 and 30; and individuals with severe OSA can exhibit more than 30 episodes per hour.

Parasomnias

Non-REM parasomnias have variable prevalence rates depending on patient age and comorbid diagnoses. Sleep talking, bruxism, sleepwalking, sleep terrors, and enuresis occur more frequently in childhood than in adulthood. Nightmares appear to occur with similar frequency in adults and children. REM behavior disorder (RBD), an REM-sleep parasomnia, has a reported prevalence of 0.5% and frequently is associated with concomitant neurologic conditions.[16] Chronic RBD is more common in elderly men and may have a familial disposition.

PATHOPHYSIOLOGY

Although the neurophysiology of sleep is complex, certain neurotransmitters promote sleep and wakefulness in different areas of the central nervous system (CNS). Whereas serotonin is thought to control non-REM sleep, cholinergic and adrenergic transmitters mediate REM sleep. Dopamine, norepinephrine, hypocretin, substance P, and histamine all play a role in wakefulness. Perturbations of various neurotransmitters are responsible for some sleep disorders and explain why various treatment modalities are beneficial.

Insomnia

Because insomnia is a complex and multifaceted disorder, there is no single pathophysiologic explanation for its various manifestations. Current hypotheses focus on a combination of possible models that incorporate physiologic, cognitive, and cortical arousal. Most insomnia models focus on hyperarousal and its interference with the initiation or maintenance of sleep.

Narcolepsy

The onset of narcolepsy–cataplexy is typically in adolescence and not at birth, suggesting that the disease may require environmental influence to develop. Currently, it is believed that narcolepsy results from autoimmune insult to the CNS because it is associated with human leukocyte antigen (major histocompatibility complex) DQB1*0602 and DQ1A1*0102.[17,18] Concentrations of hypocretin (a wake-promoting neuropeptide) in the cerebrospinal fluid of patients with narcolepsy are reduced significantly, suggesting that the autoimmune attack is against hypocretin-producing cells in the hypothalamus.[19] Intact hypocretin neurons normally stimulate arousal and wake-promoting neurons to stimulate cortical activation and behavioral arousal.

Restless Legs Syndrome and Periodic Limb Movements of Sleep

Restless legs syndrome is a neurologic medical condition characterized by an irresistible desire to move the limbs. It is thought that these abnormal sensations are a result of iron deficiency in the brain and iron-handling abnormalities in the CNS. Iron and H-ferritin concentrations, along with transferrin receptor and iron transporter numbers, are reduced in the substantia nigra of patients with RLS.[20] These iron abnormalities lead to dysfunction of dopaminergic transmission in the substantia nigra.

Obstructive Sleep Apnea

At least 20 muscles and soft tissue structures control patency of the upper airway. Patients with OSA may have differences in upper airway muscle activity during sleep and may have smaller airways, predisposing them to upper airway collapse and consequent apneic episodes during sleep. The inability of the upper airway to contend with factors that promote collapse,

including fat deposition in the neck, negative pressure in the airway during inspiration, and a smaller lower jawbone, also may play a role in the pathogenesis of OSA. Hallmarks of OSA include witnessed apneas, gasping, or both.

Poor sleep architecture and fragmented sleep secondary to OSA can cause excessive daytime sleepiness (EDS) and neurocognitive deficits. These sequelae can affect quality of life and work performance and may be linked to occupational and motor vehicle accidents. OSA is also associated with systemic disease such as hypertension, heart failure, and stroke.[21,22] OSA is likely an independent risk factor for the development of hypertension.[23] Furthermore, when hypertension is present, it is often resistant to antihypertensive therapy. Fatal and nonfatal cardiovascular events are two- to threefold higher in male patients with severe OSA.[24] OSA is associated with or aggravates biomarkers for cardiovascular disease, including C-reactive protein and leptin.[25,26] Patients with sleep apnea often are obese and may be predisposed to weight gain. Hence, obesity may further contribute to cardiovascular disease in this patient population.

Several factors suggest an association between OSA and systemic disease. Breathing against a closed upper airway during sleep causes intermittent and repetitive episodes of hypoxemia and hypercapnia, dramatic changes in intrathoracic pressure, and activation of the sympathetic nervous system. These responses can produce acute hemodynamic and humoral responses. Blood pressure can increase to 220/120 mm Hg with each apneic episode.[27] Concentrations of circulating vasoconstrictors, such as endothelin-1 and norepinephrine, are increased during OSA.[28] These acute responses to OSA may acutely impair vascular function[29] and predispose to and enhance the progression of vascular disease in the longer term.

Parasomnias

The pathogenesis of parasomnias (e.g., sleepwalking, enuresis, sleep talking) is variable and not well described and involves

---

Patient Encounter, Part 1

MC, a 53-year-old woman with a history of hypertension, depression, and anxiety, comes to your clinic complaining of difficulty initiating sleep, frequent nighttime awakenings, and sleepiness in the daytime. She reports that she falls asleep relatively easily during the day if given a chance. The sleep problems have been gradually worsening over the past weeks and occur nightly. She has been taking sertraline 150 mg/day for anxiety and depression for 4 months.

What sleep disorders do her symptoms suggest?

What additional information do you need to know in your assessment of this patient?

What are some possible contributing factors to MC's sleep complaints?

Clinical Presentation and Diagnosis

Patients with sleep disorders may complain about daytime symptoms. A bed partner may witness hallmark characteristics of the sleep disorder. ❷ *Patients with sleep complaints should have a careful sleep history performed to assess their possible sleep disorder in order to guide diagnostic and therapeutic decisions.*

Daytime symptoms and associated characteristics: EDS is the primary symptom described by patients with sleep disorders. It is usually described as not waking up refreshed in the morning or falling asleep or fighting the urge to sleep during the day despite a night of sleep. Other daytime characteristics of sleep disorders include:

- Irritability, fatigue, or depression
- Confusion or impaired performance at work or school
- Cataplexy
- Hypertension

Nighttime sleep complaints: Depending on the sleep disorder, patients may exhibit or experience various nocturnal complaints during sleep hours. Some of these complaints can be uncovered by clinical history alone (e.g., hallucinations, RLS, snoring), but others can be diagnosed during sleep studies (e.g., OSA, nighttime awakenings, somnambulism, PLMS, etc.). Frequent complaints include:

- Inability to fall asleep, nighttime awakenings
- Sleep walking (somnambulism), sleep talking (somniloquy)
- Cessation of breathing (apnea), snoring
- Sleep paralysis or hallucinations when waking or falling asleep
- Restlessness (PLMS or RLS)

state dissociation, whereby two states of being overlap simultaneously. For example, abnormal activation of the central pattern generator of the spinal cord that produces motor movements is hypothesized to underlie sleepwalking behavior. In RBD, active inhibition of motor activity in the perilocus coeruleus region is lost, resulting in loss of paralysis and dream enactment.

CLINICAL PRESENTATION AND DIAGNOSIS

❸ *Although the clinical history guides diagnosis and therapy, only overnight polysomnography and/or multiple sleep latency tests (MSLTs) can definitively diagnose and guide therapy for OSA, narcolepsy, and periodic limb movements of sleep (PLMS).* All patients presenting with sleep complaints should have a thorough inventory of their sleep habits and sleep hygiene investigated during the interview and history taking.

Insomnia (Difficulty Initiating or Maintaining Sleep)

Insomnia is often characterized by difficulty falling asleep, frequent nocturnal awakenings, early morning awakenings, and nonrestorative sleep, which may result in daytime impairments in concentration and school or work performance. In comorbid (secondary) insomnia, social factors (e.g., family difficulties, bereavement), medications (e.g., antidepressants, β-agonists, corticosteroids, decongestants), and coexisting medical or psychiatric conditions (e.g., depression, bipolar disorder) may help to explain difficulties in initiating and maintaining sleep. Insomnia may be described as transient (less than 1 week), acute (1 to 4 weeks), or chronic (more than 1 month) in duration.

Narcolepsy

The hallmark of narcolepsy is EDS and the need for unwanted episodes of sleep during the day. Patients with narcolepsy may experience repeated nighttime awakenings and terrifying dreams along with difficulty falling asleep. Patients with narcolepsy frequently experience abnormal manifestations of REM sleep, including hallucinations and sleep paralysis that occur on falling asleep and/or awakening. Cataplexy is a weakness or loss of skeletal muscle tone in the jaw, legs, or arms that is elicited by emotion (e.g., anger, surprise, laughter, or sadness).

Obstructive Sleep Apnea

Common characteristics of OSA include snoring, choking, gasping for air, nocturnal reflux symptoms, and morning headaches. A bed partner or roommate may observe these characteristics and witness episodes where the patient stops breathing during sleep. Patients with large neck sizes (more than 45 cm [~18 in] neck circumference) and a body mass index (BMI) of 30 kg/m^2 or greater are at higher risk for OSA. Hypertension, depression, and hypothyroidism are found frequently in patients with OSA.

Periodic Limb Movements of Sleep and Restless Legs Syndrome

Although RLS symptoms can vary, patients commonly report creepy-crawly, burning, tingling, or achy feelings in the legs or arms. These sensations create a desire to move the limbs and may produce motor restlessness. Symptoms are worse in the evening and are worse or exclusively present at rest, with temporary relief with movement. Symptoms also can occur during sleep and often lead to semirhythmic PLMS. PLMS are objective findings during overnight polysomnography recorded by leg electrodes. PLMS are present in most patients with RLS but can occur independently. PLMS frequently are described by a bed partner as restlessness or repeated kicking of legs or thrashing of the arms during sleep.

Parasomnias

Parasomnias are characterized by undesirable physical or behavioral phenomena that occur during sleep (e.g., sleepwalking, sleep eating, sleep talking, bruxism [grinding of teeth], enuresis, night terrors, and RBD). People with RBD act out their dreams during sleep, often in a violent manner.

Circadian Rhythm Disorders

The most common circadian rhythm disorders (CRDs) include jet lag, shift-work sleep disruption, delayed sleep-phase disorder, and advanced sleep-phase disorder. Jet lag occurs when a person travels across time zones and the external environmental time is mismatched with the internal circadian clock. Delayed and advanced sleep-phase disorders occur when bed and wake times are delayed or advanced (by 3 or more hours) compared with socially prescribed bed and wake times.

Sleep Diagnostics

Complete overnight polysomnography is the "gold standard" for diagnosing and identifying sleep-disordered breathing, PLMS, parasomnias, and nocturnal sleep irregularities related to narcolepsy. Sleep is observed and monitored in a controlled setting using an EEG, electro-oculography, electromyography, electrocardiography, air thermistors, abdominal and thoracic strain belts, and an oxygen saturation monitor. This setup assesses and records sleep onset, arousals, sleep stages, eye movements, leg and jaw movements, heart rhythm, arrhythmias, airflow during sleep, respiratory effort, and oxygen desaturations.

Evaluations of Daytime Sleepiness

The two most commonly performed objective evaluations to assess daytime sleepiness are the MSLT and the maintenance of wakefulness test (MWT). During the MSLT, the patient attempts to take a 20-minute nap every 2 hours during the day beginning 2 hours after morning awakening (after a normal night's sleep) to evaluate physiologic sleepiness. The patient is instructed not to resist the urge to fall asleep. Sleep latency of less than 5 or 6 minutes is considered pathologically sleepy. The occurrence of an REM onset period during two naps is indicative of a diagnosis of narcolepsy. The MWT is performed to assess the patient's ability to avoid succumbing to sleepiness (manifest sleepiness). Similar nap opportunities are set up for the MWT, with the exception that the patient is instructed to lie down in bed and attempt to stay awake. A subjective assessment of sleepiness can be obtained using the Epworth Sleepiness Scale (ESS). The ESS is a validated questionnaire that is easy to use and reliably predicts subjective sleepiness. The maximum score is 24, and any patient with a score greater than 10 is considered sleepy.

TREATMENT

④ *Treatment goals vary among different sleep disorders but generally include restoration of normal sleep patterns, elimination of daytime sequelae, improved quality of life, and prevention of complications and adverse effects from therapy.*

> ### Table 41–1
> ### Nonpharmacologic Therapies for Insomnia
>
> **Sleep Hygiene**
> - Keep a regular sleep schedule.
> - Exercise frequently but not immediately before bedtime.
> - Avoid alcohol and stimulants (caffeine, nicotine) in the late afternoon and evening.
> - Maintain a comfortable sleeping environment that is dark, quiet, and free of intrusions.
> - Avoid consuming large quantities of food or liquids immediately before bedtime.
>
> **Stimulus Control**
> - Go to bed only when sleepy.
> - Avoid daytime naps.
> - If you cannot sleep, get out of bed and go to another room—only return to your bed when you feel the need to sleep.
> - Bed is for sleep and intimacy only (no eating or watching TV in bed).
> - Always wake up at the same time each day.
>
> **Relaxation Training**
> - Reduce somatic arousal (muscle relaxation).
> - Reduce mental arousal (e.g., attention-focusing procedures, imagery training, meditation).
> - Use biofeedback (visual or auditory feedback to reduce tension).
>
> **Cognitive Therapy**
> - Alter beliefs, attitudes, and expectations about sleep.

Nonpharmacologic interventions for insomnia are outlined in Table 41–1. Sleep hygiene should be reinforced in all patients, and behavioral, cognitive, and stimulus-control interventions are used mainly for patients with insomnia-type complaints. Both pharmacologic and nonpharmacologic therapies are effective at improving sleep and reducing insomnia complaints. An algorithm for the initial assessment and first treatment step of EDS is provided in Figure 41–1.

Insomnia

⑤ *Early treatment of insomnia may prevent the development of persistent psychophysiologic insomnia.* The ideal hypnotic drug would be effective at reducing sleep latency and increasing total sleep time and would be free of unwanted side effects. ⑥ *Benzodiazepine receptor agonists (including traditional benzodiazepines, zolpidem, zaleplon, and eszopiclone) and ramelteon are approved by the Food and Drug Administration (FDA) for the treatment of insomnia and are first-line therapies.*[2,30,31] Not all products are available in all countries. Pharmacologic treatment of insomnia is recommended for transient and acute insomnia. Long-term use of hypnotics is not contraindicated unless the patient has another contraindication to their use. Eszopiclone is the only sedative hypnotic approved by the FDA for chronic use up to 6 months.[32] Although not first-line agents for insomnia, sedating antidepressants are also commonly prescribed.

▶ Benzodiazepine Receptor Agonists

There are currently eight benzodiazepine receptor agonists (BZDRAs) approved for insomnia, and the pharmacokinetic

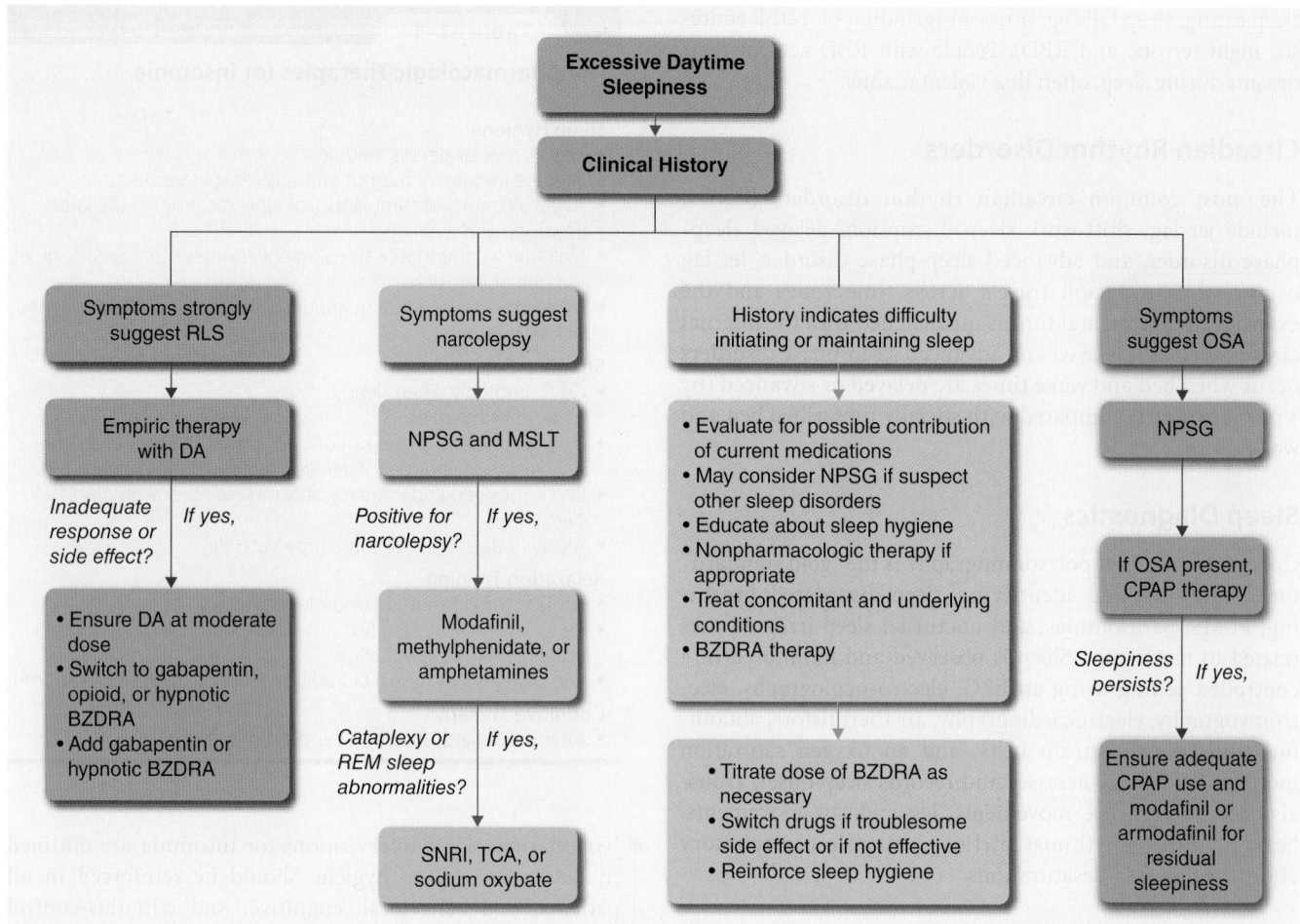

FIGURE 41–1. Primary assessment and initial treatment for complaint of excessive daytime sleepiness. BZDRA, benzodiazepine receptor agonist; CPAP, continuous positive airway pressure; DA, dopamine agonist; MSLT, multiple sleep latency test; OSA, obstructive sleep apnea; RLS, restless legs syndrome; SNRI, serotonin and norepinephrine reuptake inhibitor; NPSG, nocturnal polysomnography; TCA, tricyclic antidepressant.

differences between these agents help to guide selection depending on patient considerations and specific sleep complaints (Table 41–2). These agents occupy the benzodiazepine site on the gamma-aminobutyric acid (GABA) type A receptor complex, resulting in opening of chloride channels that facilitate GABA inhibition and promote sleepiness.[33] BZDRAs have become the first-line agents for treating insomnia and sleep-maintenance problems because they are all efficacious, have wide therapeutic indices, and in clinical use have a low incidence of abuse.[30,33]

Patients should be instructed to take BZDRAs at bedtime and to avoid engaging in activities requiring alertness after ingestion. Although BZDRAs generally are well tolerated and have good safety profiles, mild to moderate side effects can occur, and precautions are warranted, especially in high-risk populations.

Precautions and Safety The most common side effects associated with BZDRAs include residual sedation (a prolongation of the sedative effects into the waking hours after sleep), grogginess, and psychomotor impairment.[34] Careful

selection of a hypnotic agent with a duration of action matching the patient's budgeted sleep time can help minimize the risk of residual sedation. BZDRAs should be initiated at low doses, and agents with active metabolites (see Table 41–2) should be avoided in elderly patients. BZDRAs may cause anterograde amnesia, defined as memory loss of activities and interactions after ingestion of the drug. All sedatives can cause anterograde amnesia, and higher doses increase the extent of amnesia.[35,36]

On discontinuation of hypnotic BZDRAs, patients may experience rebound effects, specifically rebound insomnia that may last for one to two nights. Rebound insomnia occurs more frequently after discontinuation of shorter duration BZDRAs compared with long-duration BZDRAs. Intermittent hypnotic therapy with the lowest dose possible reduces the likelihood of tolerance, dependence, and withdrawal when therapy is stopped. Patients should be counseled that rebound insomnia is not necessarily a return of their original symptoms, and it may take a few nights for rebound symptoms to subside. In general, eszopiclone, zaleplon, and zolpidem

Table 41–2

Pharmacokinetics and Dosing of Prescription Medications[a] Approved to Treat Insomnia

Generic Name	Parent $t_{1/2}$ (hours)	Duration of Action (hours)	Daily Dose Range (mg)	Recommended Daily Dose in Elderly (mg)[b]	Dose or Action in Hepatic Impairment	Comments
Doxepin (Silenor)	15.3	Unpublished[c]	3–6	3	3 mg	Effective for sleep maintenance difficulties only
Estazolam (Prosom)	2	12–15	1–2	0.5	Dose ↓ may be needed	Moderate duration
Eszopiclone (Lunesta)	6	8	2–3	1–2	1 mg in severe impairment	Can be used up to 6 months for chronic insomnia
Flurazepam (Dalmane)	8	10–30	15–30	15	No change necessary	High risk of hangover and residual effects
Quazepam (Doral)	2	25–41	7.5–15	7.5–15	Dose ↓ may be needed	High risk of hangover and residual effects
Ramelteon (Rozerem)	1–2.6	Unpublished[c]	8	No specific recommendations	Do not use in severe hepatic impairment	Noncontrolled substance; may be useful in patients with a history of substance abuse
Temazepam (Restoril)	10–15	7	7.5–30	7.5	No change necessary	Moderate duration, well tolerated, inexpensive
Triazolam (Halcion)	2	6–7	0.125–0.25	0.125	0.125 mg	Short acting; little residual hangover
Zaleplon (Sonata)	1	6	5–10	5	5 mg	Short acting; only for difficulty falling asleep
Zolpidem (Ambien)	2–2.6	6–8	5–10	5	5 mg	Short to moderate duration; no effects on sleep architecture
Zolpidem CR (AmbienCR)	2.8	7–8	6.25–12.5	6.25	6.25 mg	Longer duration of action than regular release zolpidem
Zolpidem sublingual (Intermezzo)	2.5	Less than 4	1.75–3.5	1.75	1.75 mg	Approved for middle-of-the-night insomnia taken more than 4 hours before awakening

[a]In 2007, the Food and Drug Administration required additional information added to the safety labeling of sedative–hypnotic drugs concerning potential risks, including severe allergic reactions and complex sleep-related behaviors, which may include sleep driving. Sleep driving is defined as driving while not fully awake after ingestion of a sedative–hypnotic product with no memory of the event.

[b]If a dosing range is displayed, the first dose listed should be the starting dose.

[c]Data not available.

Adapted, with permission, from DiPiro JT, Talbert RL, Yee GC, et al (eds). Pharmacotherapy: A Pathophysiologic Approach. 8th ed. New York: McGraw-Hill; 2011:1244.

appear to be associated with lower risk of tolerance, rebound insomnia, and withdrawal than traditional benzodiazepines.

▶ Sedating Antidepressants

Sedating antidepressants, including trazodone, amitriptyline, mirtazapine, nefazodone, and doxepin are commonly used for the treatment of insomnia and may be an appealing option for insomnia in patients with concomitant depression. However, at the doses frequently used for sleep, only mirtazapine exhibits significant antidepressant activity. Furthermore, quality clinical studies demonstrating efficacy for treating insomnia are lacking. Side effects from antidepressants can be frequent and often are unpleasant, including carryover sedation, grogginess, anticholinergic effects, and weight gain. Tricyclic antidepressants (TCAs) should be used with

caution in the elderly and patients with cardiovascular and hepatic impairment. Mirtazapine can cause daytime sedation, dizziness, and weight gain, and trazodone can cause hypotension and dizziness and should be used with caution in patients with heart disease or hypertension and those taking cardiovascular agents.[37,38] Doxepin was recently approved for treatment of sleep maintenance insomnia in low doses (3 to 6 mg).

▶ Over-the-Counter and Other Miscellaneous Agents

Over-the-counter antihistamines such as diphenhydramine are frequently used (usual doses, 25 to 50 mg) for difficulty sleeping. Diphenhydramine is approved by the FDA for the treatment of insomnia and can be effective at reducing sleep latency and increasing sleep time.[39] However, diphenhydramine produces undesirable anticholinergic effects and carryover sedation that limit its use. As with TCAs and BZDRAs, diphenhydramine should be used with caution in the elderly. Valerian root is an herbal sleep remedy that has inconsistent effects on sleep but may reduce sleep latency and efficiency at commonly used doses of 400 to 900 mg valerian extract. Ramelteon, a melatonin receptor agonist, is indicated for insomnia characterized by difficulty with sleep onset. The recommended dose is 8 mg at bedtime. Ramelteon is not a controlled substance and can be a viable option for patients with a history of substance abuse, and it has documented efficacy treating sleep onset difficulties in those with mild to moderate chronic obstructive pulmonary disease and OSA.[40-42]

Patient Encounter, Part 2: Medical History, Physical Examination, and Diagnostic Test

MC undergoes further workup for her sleep complaint, and because she is also at risk for sleep apnea, it is determined she should have an overnight sleep study performed.

PMH: Hypertension × 10 years. Anxiety and depression diagnosed and treated 4 months ago but symptoms present for 1 to 2 years

FH: Father had a history of heart disease and died of a myocardial infarction at age 76 years; mother alive and well with heart disease and years of anxiety treatment

SH: Married, works as an engineer, has never smoked, drinks two or three alcoholic drinks each night

Meds: Sertraline 150 mg taken with dinner; lisinopril 20 mg/day

ROS: (+) daytime sleepiness (Epworth sleepiness score: 13 of 24); (−) symptoms of RLS

PE:

VS: BP 142/74, P 86, RR 18, T 37°C (98.6°F); BMI 29 kg/m²

Mouth: Airway crowded with large tonsils and prominent uvula

Labs: TSH 1.6 μIU/mL (mIU/L)

Overnight polysomnogram: Bedtime at 10 PM; awake at 6 AM. Frequent snoring but very infrequent hypopneas, prolonged sleep latency (75 minutes), frequent awakenings (13), 63 minutes awake after sleep onset. Awakenings occur between 11 PM and 3 AM

• RDI 3 events/h

• No significant leg movements

Given this additional information, summarize the patient's diagnosis.

Identify your treatment goals and recommendations for the patient.

What nonpharmacologic and pharmacologic alternatives are available for this patient if the prescribed therapy is not successful or not tolerated?

Narcolepsy

Therapy for narcolepsy involves two key principles: (a) treatment of EDS with scheduled naps and CNS stimulants and (b) suppression of cataplexy and REM-sleep abnormalities with aminergic signaling drugs. Modafinil (Provigil), armodafinil (Nuvigil), methylphenidate, and amphetamines are effective FDA-approved drugs for the treatment of EDS with narcolepsy.[43] Modafinil and armodafinil (the active R-isomer of modafinil) are potentially advantageous in part because they are schedule IV medications in contrast to CNS stimulants, which are schedule II. Modafinil and armodafinil prescriptions are renewable for 6 months, and these drugs may have fewer peripheral and cardiovascular effects than traditional stimulants. Selegiline, a selective monoamine oxidase B enzyme inhibitor, is metabolized to amphetamines and can be successful at reducing daytime sleepiness. In an individual patient, one wake-promoting agent may work better than another, and if the first drug selected is not successful at adequate doses, a trial with another agent should be attempted. ❼ *Treatment of EDS in narcolepsy and other sleep disorders may require the use of sustained- and immediate-release stimulants to effectively promote wakefulness throughout the day and at key times that require alertness.* One potential treatment regimen includes a sustained-release preparation first thing in the morning and again at noon followed by an immediate-release preparation as needed in the late afternoon or before driving to maintain wakefulness. One advantage of traditional CNS stimulants over modafinil is their ability to help control cataplexy and REM-sleep abnormalities.

Traditional CNS stimulants have the potential to increase blood pressure and heart rate when used long term. In addition, excessive CNS stimulation can cause tremors and tics and can carry over into evening hours, when initiation of normal nighttime sleep can be disrupted. Caution should be used in patients with underlying cardiovascular or cerebrovascular disease and in patients with a history of seizures because stimulants may lower the seizure threshold.

▶ Cataplexy

Traditionally, aminergic signaling antidepressants have been used effectively to control symptoms of cataplexy, sleep paralysis, and other REM-sleep manifestations of narcolepsy.[43] These include TCAs and certain selective serotonin and serotonin/norepinephrine reuptake inhibitors (SSRIs and SNRIs). Clomipramine, protriptyline, imipramine, venlafaxine, and fluoxetine are the agents that have been used most frequently. In addition, low-dose selegiline may be effective at reducing cataplexy. Although not approved by the FDA for treatment of cataplexy, these drugs effectively suppress REM sleep and have been the mainstay of anticataplectic therapy for years. Sodium oxybate, a potent sedative with a very short duration of action, is FDA approved for the treatment of narcolepsy with cataplexy. The mechanism whereby it reduces sleepiness and cataplexy is not entirely known. Two doses per night are taken, one at bedtime and one follow-up dose taken 2½ to

4 hours later. Sodium oxybate is tightly regulated and is only available from one central pharmacy owing to the high abuse potential of its active ingredient (γ-hydroxybutyrate).

Restless Legs Syndrome

⑧ *RLS treatment involves suppression of abnormal sensations and leg movements and consolidation of sleep. Dopaminergic and sedative–hypnotic medications are prescribed commonly.* In the past few years, dopamine agonists (DAs) have become the therapy of choice for the treatment of RLS, replacing levodopa–carbidopa as first-line agents. The DAs offer many advantages over levodopa–carbidopa, including longer half-lives to cover overnight symptoms, flexible dosing, and a reduced incidence of symptom augmentation. Up to 80% of patients who take levodopa–carbidopa eventually will experience symptom augmentation: RLS symptoms appear earlier in the day, previously unaffected body parts become involved, there is a shorter duration of relief from treatment, and higher doses of medication are required to control symptoms.[44] Ropinirole (Requip) and pramipexole (Mirapex) are FDA approved for the treatment of RLS and are available in sustained-release products.[45] Gabapentin is an effective treatment for RLS, particularly in patients with painful symptoms.[46] A new gabapentin prodrug (gabapentin enacarbil) is now FDA approved for RLS at a recommended dose of 600 mg taken with food at about 5:00 PM.[47] BZDRAs such as temazepam, clonazepam, zolpidem, and zaleplon effectively reduce arousals associated with PLMS in patients with RLS.[48] Their main benefit is derived from improving sleep continuity in patients with RLS, particularly as adjunct treatment with other pharmacologic therapies. Opioids are effective for some patients' RLS symptoms, with oxycodone, hydrocodone, and codeine being used most frequently. For both BZDRAs and opioids, caution should be used in the elderly, in patients who snore and are at risk for sleep apnea, and in patients with a history of substance abuse. Low iron levels frequently exacerbate RLS symptoms. Iron supplementation should be prescribed in patients who are iron deficient. Iron supplementation in patients with serum ferritin concentrations of less than 50 to 75 mcg/L improves RLS symptoms. Medications frequently used for RLS are shown in Table 41–3.

Obstructive Sleep Apnea

⑨ *The main therapy for OSA is nasal continuous positive airway pressure (CPAP) therapy.* CPAP alleviates sleep-disordered breathing by producing a positive pressure column in the upper airway using room air. The CPAP machine is small enough to be transportable and sits at the bedside. A flexible tube connects the CPAP machine to a mask that covers the nose. During overnight polysomnography, the pressure setting is increased until sleep-disordered breathing is eliminated. CPAP therapy has been shown to have a favorable

---

Table 41–3

Frequently Used Medications for Restless Legs Syndrome

Generic Name (Brand Name)	Half-Life (hours)	Dose Range (mg/day)[a]	Potential Side Effect or Disadvantage
Dopaminergic Agents[b]			
Levodopa–carbidopa (Sinemet)	1.5–2	100–200 of levodopa	Nausea or vomiting; high incidence of symptom augmentation
Pramipexole (Mirapex)	8–12[c]	0.125–1.5	Nausea or vomiting; risk of compulsive behaviors[d]
Ropinirole (Requip)	6[e]	0.25–3	Nausea or vomiting; risk of compulsive behaviors[d]
Anticonvulsants			
Gabapentin (Neurontin, Horizant)	5–7[c]	300–3600	Dizziness, ataxia
Hypnotic Agents			
Clonazepam (Klonopin)	30–40	0.5–2	Tolerance, carryover sedation
Temazepam (Restoril)	10–15	7.5–30	Tolerance, carryover sedation
Zolpidem (Ambien)	2–2.6[e]	5–10	Tolerance
Zaleplon (Sonata)	1[e]	5–10	Tolerance; may not last entire night
Opioids			
Hydrocodone	3.8–4.5[e]	5–10	Constipation, nausea, sedation
Codeine	2.5–3.5[e]	30–60	Constipation, nausea, sedation
Methadone	22[e]	5–20	Constipation, nausea, sedation
Oxycodone	3.2–12[c,e]	5–30	Constipation, nausea, sedation

[a]Usual range; all medications (other than dopaminergic agents) are dosed at bedtime.

[b]Dopaminergic agents are frequently given at bedtime or 2 hours before bedtime or the anticipated onset of RLS symptoms.

[c]May be longer in patients with renal dysfunction.

[d]Compulsive behaviors such as gambling, shopping, sexual behaviors, and eating have been reported in patients taking dopamine agonists.

[e]May be longer in patients with hepatic dysfunction.

Data from Earley CJ. Restless legs syndrome. N Engl J Med 2003;348:2103–2109.

impact on blood pressure and to attenuate some of the potential hemodynamic and neurohumoral responses that may link OSA to systemic disease.

Not all individuals tolerate CPAP therapy in part because it requires wearing a mask during sleep, and therapy can dry and irritate the upper airway. In some individuals, these barriers for adherence may be lessened or eliminated by properly fitting the mask, adding humidity or heat to therapy, or using bilevel positive airway pressure (BiPAP) therapy. BiPAP therapy applies a variable pressure into the airway during the inspiratory phase of respiration but, unlike CPAP, reduces the applied pressure during the expiratory phase of respiration.

There are other therapies for OSA. Obesity can worsen sleep apnea, and weight management should be implemented for all overweight patients with OSA. In obese patients with mild OSA, weight loss alone can be effective, and studies have reported improvement in the severity of OSA with gastric stapling. For patients who cannot tolerate CPAP, oral appliances can be used to advance the lower jawbone and to keep the tongue forward to enlarge the upper airway. For individuals who have OSA only during certain positions (e.g., when on their backs) during sleep, positional therapies may be effective. Surgical therapy (uvulopalatopharyngoplasty) opens the upper airway by removing the tonsils, trimming and reorienting the posterior and anterior tonsillar pillars, and removing the uvula and posterior portion of the palate. This is not a first-line option because of its invasiveness. In very severe cases, tracheostomy may be necessary. This procedure may be indicated in selected individuals who are morbidly obese, have severe facial skeletal deformity, experience severe drops in oxygen saturation (e.g., Sao$_2$ less than 70% [0.70]), or have significant cardiac arrhythmias associated with their OSA.

There is no drug therapy for OSA. Drug therapy for symptoms of OSA may be considered in selected patients. Modafinil and armodafinil are wake-promoting medications that are approved by the FDA treat residual daytime sleepiness despite CPAP therapy. Initiation of these medications should be attempted only after patients are using optimal CPAP therapy to alleviate sleep-disordered breathing. The need for treating residual sleepiness in this population is not clear because it may not be related to the OSA and is similar to sleepiness in the general population.[49] Untreated or inadequately treated sleep apnea hinders achieving blood pressure control in hypertensive patients. OSA should always be considered and evaluated in hypertensive patients who are resistant to therapy.

Parasomnias

Non-REM parasomnias usually do not require treatment. If needed, low-dose BZDRAs such as clonazepam can be prescribed for bothersome episodes. Clonazepam reduces the amount of sleep time spent in stages 3 and 4 of non-REM sleep, when most non-REM parasomnias occur. For treating RBD, clonazepam 0.5 to 2 mg at bedtime is the drug of choice, although melatonin 3 to 12 mg at bedtime also may be effective.

Patients with RBD also should have dangerous objects removed from the bedroom and cushions placed on the floor to reduce the chance of injury from breakthrough episodes.

Circadian Rhythm Disorders

Melatonin at doses of 0.5 to 5 mg taken at appropriate target bedtimes for east or west travel is becoming the drug of choice for jet lag. Melatonin significantly reduces jet lag and shortens sleep latency in travelers.[50] Hypnotic agents with relatively short durations of action (3 to 5 hours) may also be used to sustain sleep during the initial adaptation to the new time zone.

Drug–Disease and Drug–Drug Interactions

❿ *It is important to review patient medication profiles for drugs that may aggravate sleep disorders. Patients should be monitored for adverse drug reactions and potential drug–drug interactions. They should be assessed for adherence to their therapeutic regimens. Pharmacotherapy for sleep disorders should be individualized. Medications can be used commonly to treat several concomitant sleep disorders. Conversely, drug therapy may be effective for one sleep disorder and exacerbate another. For example, antidepressants may alleviate depressive symptoms but exacerbate the symptoms of RLS. Medications that block dopaminergic transmission may worsen RLS symptoms. Smoking can worsen OSA, presumably by increasing upper airway edema. Alcohol and CNS depressants, including opiate analgesics, sedatives, and muscle relaxants, can worsen OSA, even in small doses, by reducing respiratory drive and relaxing the upper airway muscles responsible for maintaining patency. CNS depressants should be avoided, and if they are necessary, they should not be administered before sleep. Drug therapy for sleep disorders should be patient specific, and careful consideration*

Patient Encounter, Part 3: Modifying the Treatment Plan

MC returns to the clinic 3 months later. The physician previously diagnosed her with sleep initiation and sleep maintenance insomnia. She received a prescription for temazepam 15 mg taken at bedtime and was instructed to take sertraline in the morning instead of evening. She reports today that the temazepam helps her sleep, but she feels groggy and hungover in the morning. Her Epworth Sleepiness Scale score today is 10 of 24.

Based on the information presented, recommend therapy suggestions for the patient.

What medications would you not want to use for MC's sleep issues?

What precautions would you want to counsel the patient on about her therapy?

Patient Care and Monitoring

Insomnia

1. Ideally limit hypnotic therapy to short-term use, and reevaluate after 2 to 3 weeks of therapy.

2. Evaluate improvement in the specific sleep complaint (e.g., how has therapy affected sleep latency or sleep maintenance?).

3. Inquire about carryover sedation and other side effects associated with the selected agent. Use a lower dose, or select a drug with a shorter duration of action if the patient experiences carryover sedation.

4. Address other psychiatric and medical conditions that frequently coexist with insomnia and medications which can worsen symptoms.

Narcolepsy

1. Administer the ESS at each visit to monitor progress with modafinil or stimulant therapy. Unfortunately, EDS in narcolepsy patients rarely is fully reversed.

2. Evaluate how sleepiness changes throughout the day to best determine how to use sustained- and immediate-release stimulants to maintain wakefulness. If the patient complains of sleep disruption from stimulant therapy, move the dosing time a few hours earlier until sleep disruption is avoided.

3. Review the patient's sleep diaries to track the number of cataplexy, sleep paralysis, and hallucinatory events and when they occur.

RLS

1. Carefully assess both the patient's and bed partner's reports of the patient's nighttime limb movements.

2. Measure sleepiness (via ESS) and RLS symptoms at each visit to track progress with therapy.

3. Evaluate potential side effects of therapy, including nausea, drowsiness, sleep attacks, compulsive behaviors, and headaches for the DA agents.

4. Review the sleep diaries and timing of RLS symptoms to screen for possible symptom augmentation.

5. If symptoms are not resolved, increase the dose of DA agent or add another agent such as gabapentin or a short- to moderate-duration sedative–hypnotic.

OSA

1. Evaluate CPAP therapy annually or at any time individuals experience symptoms (e.g., daytime sleepiness) despite CPAP therapy. For example, a change in pressure settings to alleviate OSA may be needed if weight gain occurs.

2. Monitor compliance with CPAP therapy. CPAP machines have a built-in compliance meter to measure the hours used at effective pressure. Patients should use CPAP therapy for at least 5 hours each night. In addition to alleviating sleep-disordered breathing, CPAP therapy may improve cardiovascular outcomes.

Parasomnias

1. Ask patients and family members about any bothersome or dangerous sleepwalking episodes since the last visit and if therapy has reduced the frequency of these events.

2. For RBD, review the sleep diaries and interview bed partners to determine the number and nature of episodes.

3. Inquire about carryover sedation and anterograde amnesia from therapy.

should be given to coexisting diseases, concomitant medications, and potential drug–drug and drug–disease interactions to optimize patient care and treatment.

OUTCOME EVALUATION

To determine the success of treatment, evaluate whether the treatment plan restored normal sleep patterns, reduced daytime sequelae, and improved quality of life without causing adverse effects. Schedule patients for follow-up within 3 weeks for insomnia and within 3 months for other sleep disorders. Perform a detailed clinical history to determine the patient's perception of treatment progress and symptoms along with medication effectiveness and side effects.

Instruct patients to keep sleep diaries of nightly sleep (number of hours, number of awakenings, and worsening or improved sleep) and daytime symptoms, along with documentation of episodes such as cataplexy or RBD. Increase

medication to effective doses, and if necessary, start additional therapy to control symptoms. Patients with sleep disorders should experience relief of symptoms the first night of drug therapy but may not receive maximal benefit (effect on daytime symptoms) for a few weeks. Perform a detailed history of prescription, nonprescription, and complementary or alternative medications and review the patient's sleep diary, daytime symptoms, and nonpharmacologic therapies on a regular basis.

Abbreviations Introduced in This Chapter

BiPAP	Bilevel positive airway pressure
BMI	Body mass index
BZDRA	Benzodiazepine receptor agonist
CNS	Central nervous system
CPAP	Continuous positive airway pressure

CRD   Circadian rhythm disorder
DA   Dopamine agonist
EDS   Excessive daytime sleepiness
ESS   Epworth Sleepiness Scale
GABA   γ-Aminobutyric acid
MSLT   Multiple sleep latency test
MWT   Maintenance of wakefulness test
NPSG   Nocturnal polysomnography
NREM   Non–rapid eye movement
OSA   Obstructive sleep apnea
PLMS   Periodic limb movements of sleep
RBD   REM-sleep behavior disorder
RDI   Respiratory disturbance index
RLS   Restless legs syndrome
REM   Rapid eye movement
SNRI   Serotonin/norepinephrine reuptake inhibitor
TCA   Tricyclic antidepressant

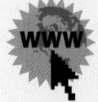 Self-assessment questions and answers are available at *http://www.mhpharmacotherapy.com/pp.html.*

REFERENCES

1. Malow B. Approach to the patient with disordered sleep. In: Kryger M, Roth T, Dement W, eds. Principles and Practice of Sleep Medicine. 5th ed. St. Louis: Elsevier Saunders; 2011:641–646.
2. NIH State-of-the-Science Conference Statement on Manifestations and Management of Chronic Insomnia in Adults [online]. 2005, [cited 2011 Oct 10]. Available from: *http://consensus.nih.gov/2005/2005InsomniaSOS026html.htm*
3. Carskadon MA, Dement WC. Normal human sleep: An overview. In: Kryger M, Roth T, Dement W, eds. Principles and Practice of Sleep Medicine. 5th ed. St. Louis: Elsevier Saunders; 2011:16–26.
4. Roth T. Insomnia: Definition, prevalence, etiology, and consequences. J Clin Sleep Med 2007;15(5 Suppl):S7–S10.
5. Kim K, Uchiyama M, Okawa M, et al. An epidemiological study of insomnia among the Japanese general population. Sleep 2000;23: 41–47.
6. McCall WV. A psychiatric perspective on insomnia. J Clin Psychiatry 2001;62(Suppl 10):27–32.
7. Silber MH, Krahn LE, Olson EJ, et al. The epidemiology of narcolepsy in Olmsted County, Minnesota: A population-based study. Sleep 2002;25:197–202.
8. Tashiro T, Kambayashi T, Hishikawa Y. An epidemiological study of narcolepsy in Japanese. Proceedings of the 4th International Symposium on Narcolepsy. Tokyo, Japan. June 16–17, 1994:13.
9. Lavie P, Peled R. Narcolepsy is a rare disease in Israel. Sleep 1987;10:608–609.
10. Mignot E, Hayduk R, Black J, et al. HLA DQB1*0602 is associated with cataplexy in 509 narcoleptic patients. Sleep 1997;20:1012–1020.
11. Berger K, Kurth T. RLS epidemiology—frequencies, risk factors and methods in population studies. Mov Disord 2007;22(Suppl):S420–S423.
12. Phillips B, Young T, Finn L, et al. Epidemiology of restless legs symptoms in adults. Arch Intern Med 2000;160:2137–2141.
13. Lee KA, Zaffke ME, Baratte-Beebe K. Restless legs syndrome and sleep disturbance during pregnancy: The role of folate and iron. J Womens Health Gend Based Med 2001;10:335–341.
14. Bonati MT, Ferini-Strambi L, Aridon P, et al. Autosomal dominant restless legs syndrome maps on chromosome 14q. Brain 2003;126:1485–1492.
15. Young T, Palta M, Dempsey J, et al. The occurrence of sleep-disordered breathing among middle-aged adults. N Engl J Med 1993;328: 1230–1235.
16. Ohayon MM, Caulet M, Priest RG. Violent behavior during sleep. J Clin Psychiatry 1997;58:369–376.
17. Mignot E, Lin X, Arrigoni J, et al. DQB1*0602 and DQA1*0102(DQ1) are better markers than DR2 for narcolepsy in Caucasian and black Americans. Sleep 1994;17:S60–S67.
18. Mignot E, Kimura A, Lattermann A, et al. Extensive HLA class II studies in 58 non-DRB1*15(DR2) narcoleptic patients with cataplexy. Tissue Antigens 1997;49:329–341.
19. Nishino S, Ripley B, Overeem S, et al. Hypocretin (orexin) deficiency in human narcolepsy. Lancet 2000;355:39–40.
20. Connor JR, Boyer PJ, Menzies SL, et al. Neuropathological examination suggests impaired brain iron acquisition in restless legs syndrome. Neurology 2003;61:304–309.
21. Somers VK, White DP, Amin R, et al. Sleep apnea and cardiovascular disease: An American Heart Association/American College of Cardiology Foundation Scientific Statement from the American Heart Association Council for High Blood Pressure Research Professional Education Committee, Council on Clinical Cardiology, Stroke Council, and Council on Cardiovascular Nursing. In collaboration with the National Heart, Lung, and Blood Institute, National Center on Sleep Disorders Research (National Institutes of Health). Circulation 2008;118:1080–1111.
22. Sahlin C, Sandberg O, Gustafson Y, et al. Obstructive sleep apnea is a risk factor for death in patients with stroke. Arch Intern Med 2008;168:297–301.
23. Peppard PE, Young T, Palta M, et al. Prospective study of the association between sleep-disordered breathing and hypertension. N Engl J Med 2000;342:1378–1384.
24. Marin JM, Carrizo SJ, Vicente E, et al. Long-term cardiovascular outcomes in men with obstructive sleep apnoea-hypopnoea with or without treatment with continuous positive airway pressure: An observational study. Lancet 2005;365:1046–1053.
25. Shamsuzzaman AS, Winnicki M, Lanfranchi P, et al. Elevated C-reactive protein in patients with obstructive sleep apnea. Circulation 2002;105:2462–2464.
26. Phillips BG, Kato M, Narkiewicz K, et al. Increases in leptin levels, sympathetic drive and weight gain in obstructive sleep apnea. Am J Physiol 2000;279:234–237.
27. Somers VK, Dyken ME, Clary MP, et al. Sympathetic neural mechanisms in obstructive sleep apnea. J Clin Invest 1995;96:1897–1904.
28. Phillips BG, Krzysztof N, Pesek CA, et al. Effects of obstructive sleep apnea on endothelin-1 and blood pressure. J Hypertens 1999;17:61–66.
29. Kato M, Roberts-Thomson P, Phillips BG, et al. Impairment of endothelium dependent vasodilation of resistance vessels in patients with obstructive sleep apnea. Circulation 2000;102:2607–2610.
30. Buscemi N, Vandermeer B, Friesen C, et al. The efficacy and safety of drug treatments for chronic insomnia in adults: A meta-analysis of RCTs. J Gen Intern Med 2007;22:1335–1350.
31. Schutte-Rodin S, Broch L, Buysse D, et al. Clinical guideline for the evaluation and management of chronic insomnia in adults. J Clin Sleep Med 2008;4:487–504.
32. Krystal AD, Walsh JK, Laska E, et al. Sustained efficacy of eszopiclone over 6 months of nightly treatment: Results of a randomized, double-blind, placebo-controlled study in adults with chronic insomnia. Sleep 2003;26:793–799.
33. Becker WC, Fiellin DA, Desai RA. Non-medical use, abuse and dependence on sedatives and tranquilizers among U.S. adults: Psychiatric and socio-demographic correlates. Drug Alcohol Depend 2007;90:280–287.
34. Roth T, Roehrs T. Issues in the use of benzodiazepine therapy. J Clin Psychiatry 1992;53(Suppl):S14–S18.
35. Roth T, Roehrs TA, Stepanski EJ, et al. Hypnotics and behavior. Am J Med 1990(Suppl);8:S43–S46.
36. Greenblatt D, Harmatz JS, Shapiro L, et al. Sensitivity to triazolam in elderly. N Engl J Med 1991;324:1691–1698.
37. Golden RN, Dawkins K, Nicholas L. Trazodone and nefazodone. In: Schatzberg A, Nemeroff, eds. The American Psychiatric Textbook of Psychopharmacology. Washington, DC: American Psychiatric Publishing; 2004:315–325.

38. Bucknall C, Brooks D, Curry PV, et al. Mianserin and trazodone for cardiac patients with depression. Eur J Clin Pharmacol 1988;33:565–569.

39. Kudo Y, Kurihara M. Clinical evaluation of diphenhydramine hydrochloride for the treatment of insomnia in psychiatric patients. J Clin Pharmacol 1990;30:1041–1048.

40. Johnson MW, Suess PE, Griffiths RR. A novel hypnotic lacking abuse liability and sedative adverse effects. Arch Gen Psychiatry 2006;63:1149–1157.

41. Kryger M, Roth T, Wang-Weigand S, et al. The effects of ramelteon on respiration during sleep in subjects with moderate to severe chronic obstructive pulmonary disease. Sleep Breath 2009;13:79–84.

42. Kryger M, Wang-Weigand S, Roth T. Safety of ramelteon in individuals with mild to moderate obstructive sleep apnea. Sleep Breath 2007;11:159–164.

43. Morganthaler TI, Kapur VK, Brown T, et al. Practice parameters for the treatment of narcolepsy and other hypersomnias of central origin an American Academy of Sleep Medicine Report. Sleep 2007;30:1705–1711.

44. Earley CJ, Allen RP. Pergolide and carbidopa/levodopa treatment of the restless legs syndrome and periodic leg movements in sleep in a consecutive series of patients. Sleep 1996;19:801–810.

45. Hening WA, Allen RP, Earley CJ, et al. Restless Legs Syndrome Task Force of the Standards of Practice Committee of the American Academy of Sleep Medicine. An update on the dopaminergic treatment of restless legs syndrome and periodic limb movement disorder. Sleep 2004;27:560–583.

46. Garcia-Borreguero D, Larrosa O, de la Llave Y, et al. Treatment of restless legs syndrome with gabapentin: A double-blind, cross-over study. Neurology 2002;59:1573–1579.

47. Product Information: Horizant, gabapentin enacarbil. Research Triangle Park, NC: GlaxoSmithKline Pharmaceuticals, 2011.

48. Earley CJ. Restless legs syndrome. N Engl J Med 2003;348:2103–2109.

49. Stradling JR, Smith D, Crosby J. Post-CPAP sleepiness—a specific syndrome? J Sleep Res 2007;16:436–438.

50. Herxheimer A, Petrie KJ. Melatonin for the prevention and treatment of jet lag. Cochrane Database Syst Rev 2005;(4):CD001520.

42 Attention-Deficit Hyperactivity Disorder

Kevin W. Cleveland and John Erramouspe

LEARNING OBJECTIVES

● **Upon completion of the chapter, the reader will be able to:**

1. Explain accepted criteria necessary for the diagnosis of attention-deficit hyperactivity disorder (ADHD).

2. Recommend a therapeutic plan, including initial doses, dosage forms, and monitoring parameters, for a patient with ADHD.

3. Differentiate among the available pharmacotherapy used for ADHD with respect to pharmacology and pharmaceutical formulation.

4. Recommend second-line and/or adjunctive agents that can be effective alternatives in the treatment of ADHD when stimulant therapy is less than adequate.

5. Address potential cost–benefit issues associated with pharmacotherapy of ADHD.

6. Recommend strategies for minimizing adverse effects of ADHD medications.

KEY CONCEPTS

❶ To meet current attention-deficit hyperactivity disorder (ADHD) diagnostic criteria, patients need to display hyperactivity, impulsivity, and/or inattentiveness before 7 years of age.

❷ The exact cause of ADHD is unknown, but dysfunction in **neurotransmitters** norepinephrine and dopamine has been implicated as a key component.

❸ ADHD is rarely encountered without comorbid conditions.

❹ Treatment goals for ADHD are to improve behavior, increase attention or **response inhibition,** and minimize side effects associated with pharmacotherapy.

❺ Pharmacotherapy is superior to behavioral therapy in the treatment of ADHD, but both should be emphasized in order to maximize outcomes.

❻ **Stimulants** are first-line agents for the treatment of ADHD. If the initial trial of a stimulant fails, then a trial of an alternative stimulant should be tried. On failure of the second stimulant, it is rational to attempt a third trial with a different stimulant formulation or select a nonstimulant agent such as bupropion, atomoxetine, guanfacine, or clonidine.

A DHD is characterized by a core triad of symptoms: hyperactivity, impulsivity, and inattention. It can have a severe impact on a patient's ability to function in both academic and social environments. Early diagnosis and appropriate treatment are essential to compensate for areas of deficit.

EPIDEMIOLOGY AND ETIOLOGY

❶ *This disorder usually begins by 3 years of age but must occur before 7 years of age to meet current diagnostic criteria.* In the United States, ADHD is the most common neurobehavioral disorder that affects children.[1–4] ADHD has been estimated to occur in 4.3% to 12% of school-aged children.[4,5] ADHD occurs more in boys than girls by a factor of approximately 3:1 in school-aged children.[6]

Although ADHD generally is considered a childhood disorder, symptoms can persist into adolescence and adulthood. The prevalence of adult ADHD is estimated to be 4%; however, 60% of adults with ADHD have symptoms that manifested in childhood.[6,7] Furthermore, problems associated with ADHD (e.g., social, marital, academic, career, anxiety, depression, smoking, and substance abuse problems) increase with the transition of patients into adulthood.

PATHOPHYSIOLOGY

❷ *The exact pathologic cause of ADHD has not been identified.* ADHD is generally thought of as a disorder of self-regulation or response inhibition. Patients who meet the criteria for ADHD have difficulty maintaining self-control, resisting distractions, and concentrating on ideas.[4,8] Furthermore, children with ADHD often alternate between inattentiveness to monotonous tasks and overexcitement. Multiple brain studies have failed to elucidate any pathophysiologic basis for ADHD.

❷ *Dysfunction of the neurotransmitters norepinephrine and dopamine is thought to be key in the pathology of ADHD.* Whereas norepinephrine is responsible for maintaining alertness and attention, dopamine is responsible for regulating learning, motivation, goal setting, and memory. Both of these neurotransmitters predominate in the frontal subcortical system, an area of the brain responsible for maintaining attention and memory. Genetics appears to play a role because a child who has a parent with ADHD has a 50% chance of developing ADHD. An association has been made between the development of ADHD and fetal alcohol syndrome, lead poisoning, maternal smoking, and hypoxia.[4,8]

CLINICAL PRESENTATION AND DIAGNOSIS

❸ *ADHD is rarely encountered without comorbid conditions and often is undiagnosed.* Between 50% and 60% of patients with ADHD will have one or more comorbidities (e.g., learning disabilities, oppositional defiant, conduct, anxiety, or depressive disorders).[2] It is important to identify coexisting conditions in patients with ADHD and to select appropriate treatment.

According to newer diagnostic and treatment guidelines, all patients 4 to 18 years of age presenting with inattention, hyperactivity, impulsivity, academic, and/or behavioral problems should be evaluated for ADHD. Additional information about behavior in various settings should be gathered from the patient, family, and teachers or supervisors. The age of onset, frequency, severity, and duration of symptoms should be documented.[9,10]

The most useful diagnostic criteria for ADHD is the *Diagnostic and Statistical Manual of Mental Disorders,* 4th edition, text revision (*DSM-IV-TR*) (Table 42–1).[10] The *DSM-IV-TR* defines three subtypes of ADHD: (a) predominately inattentive; (b) predominantly hyperactive or impulsive; and (c) combined, in which both inattentive and hyperactive or impulsive symptoms are evident.[11] Neuroimaging, electroencephalograms, and continuous performance examinations are investigational and not used clinically for diagnosis. It is recommended that parents and teachers complete a standardized rating scale based on the *DSM-IV-TR* criteria that measures various behaviors of ADHD.[12] These rating scales do not by themselves diagnose ADHD but are diagnostic aids when added to a careful history and interview.[12]

Although ADHD is considered a childhood disorder, signs and symptoms persist into adolescence in 40% to 80% of cases and into adulthood in approximately 60% of cases.[1,7] Adult ADHD is difficult to assess, and diagnosis is always suspect in patients failing to display clear symptoms before 7 years of age.[9] Untreated adults with ADHD have

Table 42–1

DSM-IV-TR Diagnostic Criteria for ADHD

I. Either A or B:
 A. *Inattention.* Must have at least six or more of the following symptoms of inattention for at least 6 months:
  1. Does not pay close attention to details in schoolwork, work, or other activities
  2. Has trouble maintaining attention to tasks or activities
  3. Has trouble actively listening when directly spoken to
  4. Has difficulty following instructions and fails to finish important daily tasks (i.e., homework, chores, and responsibilities at work)
  5. Demonstrates difficulty in organizing tasks or activities
  6. Tends to avoid or put off activities that require concentration
  7. Tends to misplace items needed to complete tasks or activities
  8. Is easily distracted from current tasks or activities
  9. Forgetful
 B. *Hyperactivity or impulsivity.* Must have at least six or more of the following symptoms of hyperactivity or impulsivity for at least 6 months:
  Hyperactivity
  1. Fidgets and is restless in a sitting position
  2. Cannot sit still for extended periods
  3. Runs around when it is not appropriate
  4. Cannot play quietly
  5. Often "on the move"
  6. Talks excessively
  Impulsivity
  1. Answers questions prematurely
  2. Has difficulty waiting one's turn
  3. Interruptive or intrudes on others
II. Above symptoms were present before 7 years of age
III. Above symptoms are present in two or more settings
IV. Impairment is clearly evident in social, school, or work functioning
V. Symptoms cannot be attributed to another mental disorder (e.g., anxiety, depression, autism, or a personality disorder)
Based on the above criteria, ADHD can be divided into three types:
  1. ADHD combined type: Both 1A and 1B
  2. ADHD inattentive type: 1A criteria are met
  3. ADHD hyperactive-impulsive type: 1B criteria are met

From American Psychiatric Association. Diagnostic and Statistical Manual of Mental Disorders. 4th ed, text rev. Washington, DC: American Psychiatric Press; 2000:39–134; With permission.

higher rates of psychopathology, substance abuse, social dysfunction, and occupational underachievement than adults without ADHD.

TREATMENT
Desired Outcomes

❹ *The primary therapeutic objectives in ADHD are to improve behavior and increase attention or response inhibition; secondary goals of treatment are to:*

• Improve relationships with family, teachers, and peers

• Decrease disruptive behavior in academic and social settings

• Improve academic performance

Clinical Presentation and Diagnosis of ADHD

General

Patients with ADHD can present with inattention, hyperactivity–impulsivity, or both. ADHD is rarely encountered without comorbid conditions.

Symptoms

- Inattention; difficulty paying attention to details in school, work, and social activities; difficulty completing tasks that require a lot of mental effort; easily distracted; forgetful

- Hyperactivity–impulsivity; difficulty sitting still, fidgets; has trouble playing quietly and waiting turns; frequently interrupts

- Combined; exhibits both inattention and hyperactivity–impulsivity

Diagnostic Criteria

- Must exhibit symptoms before 7 years of age that persist for at least 6 months

- Symptoms must be present in two or more settings and adversely affect functioning in social situations, school, or work

- Must meet the diagnostic criteria in *DSM-IV-TR* (Table 41–1)

- Symptoms cannot be better explained by another mental disorder (e.g., autism)

Patient Encounter, Part 1

The parents and their high-spirited 8-year-old boy, HA, come to your clinic. The parents are concerned because his teacher has complained about problems he is causing in her classroom. HA has difficulty finishing his classroom work, frequently disrupts his neighbor to talk, and has sudden outbursts during lessons. During recess, HA refuses to wait for his turn in games and frequently pushes others to get his way. Also, HA is not completing his homework on time. His first grade teacher also documented these problems, but the parents were told he would "grow out" of his behavior. In the after-school program, HA cannot pay attention during math tutoring. This is very distressing to HA's parents, who are barely providing for their family; the father is a full-time student, and the mother works at the local grocery store for minimum wage. They do not qualify for medical assistance. They cannot afford a more structured professional care for HA other than the free after-school program.

Which of the patient's symptoms are suggestive of ADHD?

What other comorbid conditions should the child be evaluated for before starting therapy for ADHD?

What other information do you need to assess for ADHD?

What help or suggestions could you offer to HA's parents?

- Increase independence in activities
- Minimize undesirable adverse effects of therapy

Nonpharmacologic (Behavioral) Therapy

Behavioral therapy can be used to treat patients with ADHD; however, it is generally not recommended as first-line monotherapy except in preschool-aged children (4 to 5 years of age).[6,10] ⑤ *Several studies have demonstrated that treatment with medication alone is superior to behavioral intervention alone in improving attention. However, behavioral therapy in combination with stimulant therapy is better at improving oppositional and aggressive behaviors.*[13] Behavioral modification involves training parents, teachers, and caregivers to change the physical and social environment and establish a reward or consequence system.[9,10] Success of behavioral modifications depends on the cooperation and involvement of the patient's parents and teachers.

Pharmacologic Therapy

The proposed mechanism of ADHD pharmacotherapy is to modulate neurotransmitter function in order to improve academic and social functioning. Pharmacologic therapy can be divided into two categories, stimulants and nonstimulants. Stimulant medications include methylphenidate, dexmethylphenidate, dextroamphetamine–amphetamine (amphetamine salts), dextroamphetamine and lisdexamfetamine, and nonstimulant medications include atomoxetine, bupropion, clonidine, and guanfacine.

▶ Stimulants

⑥ *Psychostimulants (e.g., methylphenidate and dextroamphetamine with or without amphetamine) are the most effective agents in treating ADHD. Once the diagnosis of ADHD has been made, a stimulant medication should be considered first-line in treating ADHD in patients 6 years of age or older* (Fig. 42–1). In preschool-aged children, methylphenidate can be added to the patient's treatment if behavioral modification monotherapy is not sufficient in managing ADHD symptoms.[10] Stimulants are safe and effective and have a response rate of 70% to 90% in patients with ADHD.[3,9,14] Generally, a trial of at least 3 months on a stimulant is appropriate, and this includes dose titration to response while balancing side effects.[7,9] ⑥ *If treatment with the first stimulant formulation fails, it is recommended to switch to a different stimulant formulation.*[9,10] For example, if the patient was started on methylphenidate but could not tolerate the side effects, switching to dextroamphetamine with or without amphetamine is appropriate. The majority of patients who fail one stimulant will respond to an alternative

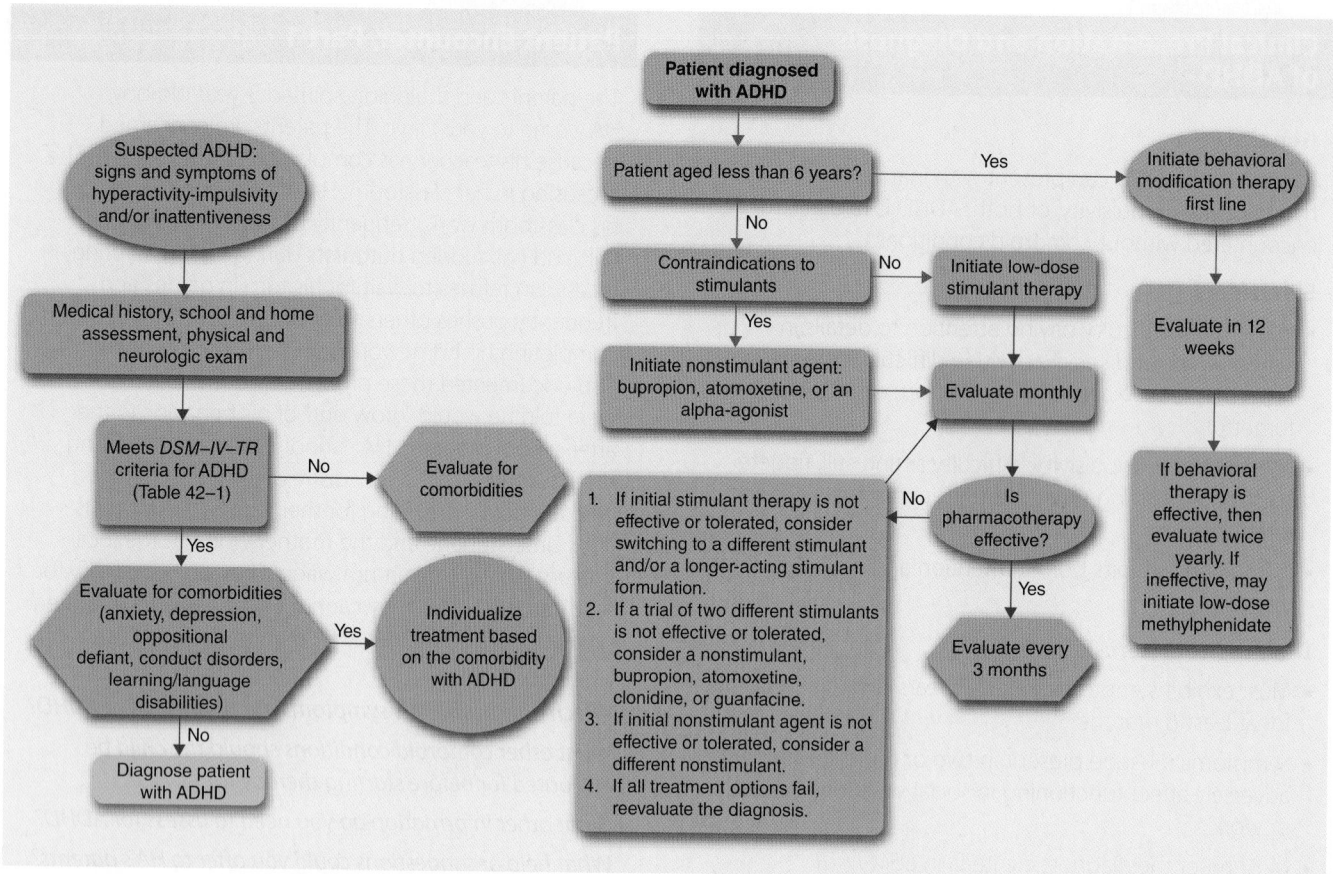

FIGURE 42-1. ADHD diagnosis and treatment algorithm. (Data from Refs. 6, 9, 10, and 16.)

stimulant.[9,10] ❻ *If the patient fails two appropriate trials of different stimulant medications, a third stimulant formulation or second-line nonstimulant such as bupropion, atomoxetine, guanfacine, or clonidine can be considered.* The diagnosis of ADHD should be revalidated as well.

Stimulants theoretically exert their primary effect by blocking the reuptake of dopamine and norepinephrine. Stimulants have been shown to decrease fidgeting and finger tapping, increase on-task classroom behavior and positive interactions at home and in social environments, and ameliorate conduct and anxiety disorders.[14]

Stimulants should be initiated at recommended starting doses and titrated up with a consistent dosing schedule to the appropriate response while minimizing side effects (Table 42–2). Generally, stimulants should not be used in patients who have glaucoma, severe hypertension or cardiovascular disease, hyperthyroidism, severe anxiety, or previous illicit or stimulant drug abuse. Furthermore, stimulants can be used, albeit cautiously, in patients with seizure disorders, Tourette's syndrome, and motor tics.[14]

Stimulant drug formulations can be divided into short-, intermediate-, and extended-acting preparations (Table 42–2). Initial response to short-acting stimulant formulations (e.g., methylphenidate and dextroamphetamine) is seen within 30 minutes and can last for 4 to 6 hours.[9,10,14] This short duration of effect frequently requires that short-acting stimulant formulations be dosed at least twice daily, thus increasing the chance of missed doses and noncompliance. Furthermore, patients using any stimulant formulation, but especially short-acting formulations, can experience a rebound effect of ADHD symptoms as the stimulant wears off.[14]

Most intermediate-acting stimulants release the medication in a slow, continuous fashion without any early release (except Dexedrine Spansules). The onset of action for this category of stimulants (typically 60 to 90 minutes) may be inadequate for some patients. Some practitioners prescribe a short-acting stimulant concurrently with an intermediate-acting stimulant to curtail the delay in onset of action of the intermediate-acting stimulant. However, this practice can increase copay costs to the patient.

To minimize rebound problems associated with short-acting formulations and still maintain early stimulant release, extended-acting formulations with rapid onsets have been developed. These formulations have an early release of medication and deliver a delayed release of stimulant in either a pulsed (Adderall XR, Focalin XR, Metadate CD, and Ritalin LA) or continuous manner (Concerta). Formulations available as capsules contain coated beads that can be opened and sprinkled on semisolid food. Concerta tablets have an immediate-release overcoat and an oral osmotic controlled-release that delivers methylphenidate in an extended manner. Furthermore, patients should be counseled that the empty tablet shell of Concerta can be detected in the stool.

Table 42–2			
Selected Medications for ADHD[a]			
Drug, Generic (Brand Name)	**Initial Dose**	**Titration Schedule Increments**	**Typical Dosing Range (Maximum Dose)**
Stimulants			
Short Acting			
Methylphenidate[b] (Methylin, Ritalin)	5 mg 2 × daily	5–10 mg/day in weekly intervals	5–20 mg 2–3 × daily (60 mg/day)
Dexmethylphenidate[b] (Focalin)	2.5 mg 2 × daily	2.5–5 mg/day in weekly intervals	5–10 mg twice daily (20 mg/day)
Dextroamphetamine[b] (Dexedrine)	2.5–5 mg every morning	2.5–5 mg/day in weekly intervals	5–20 mg twice daily (40 mg/day)
Intermediate Acting			
Methylphenidate[b] (Ritalin SR, Metadate ER, Methylin ER)	10 mg once daily	10 mg/day in weekly intervals	20–40 mg daily in the morning (60 mg/day)
Dextroamphetamine–amphetamine[b] (Adderall)	2.5–5 mg once to twice daily	2.5–5 mg/day in weekly intervals	10–30 mg every morning or 5–20 mg twice daily (40 mg/day)
Dextroamphetamine[b] (Dexedrine Spansule)	5 mg every morning	5 mg/day in weekly intervals	5–30 mg daily or 5–15 mg twice daily (40 mg/day)
Extended Acting			
Methylphenidate[b] (Concerta)	18 mg every morning	9–18 mg/day in weekly intervals	18–54 mg every morning (54 mg/day in children)
(Metadate CD)	20 mg every morning	10–20 mg/day in weekly intervals	20–40 mg daily in the morning (60 mg/day)
(Ritalin LA)	20 mg every morning	10 mg/day in weekly intervals	20–40 mg daily in the morning (60 mg/day)
Dextroamphetamine/amphetamine[b] (Adderall XR)	5–10 mg every morning (children); 20 mg once daily (adults)	5–10 mg/day in weekly intervals	10–30 mg every morning or 5–15 mg twice daily (30 mg/day, children) (60 mg/day, adult)
Dexmethylphenidate[b] (Focalin XR)	5 mg every morning (children); 10 mg every morning (adults)	5 mg/day in weekly intervals	10–20 mg daily in the morning (20 mg/day)
Lisdexamfetamine[b] (Vyvanse)	30 mg every morning (children and adults)	10–20 mg/day in weekly intervals	30–70 mg daily in the morning (70 mg/day)
Nonstimulants			
Atomoxetine[b,c] (Strattera)	Less than or equal to 70 kg: 0.5 mg/kg/day divided once to twice daily	To target dose of 1.2 mg/kg/day after 3 days	40–60 mg/day (1.4 mg/kg or 100 mg/day, whichever is less)
	Greater than 70 kg: 40 mg once daily	40 mg/day after 3 days (may ↑ to total of 100 mg/day after 2–3 weeks)	40–80 mg/day divided once to twice daily (100 mg/day)
Clonidine (Catapres)	0.05 mg once daily	0.05 mg/day every 3–7 days	0.1 mg 1 to 4 times daily (0.4 mg/day)
(Kapvay)[b]	0.1 mg at bedtime	0.1 mg/day in weekly intervals	0.1–0.2 mg twice daily (0.4 mg/day)
Guanfacine (Tenex)	0.5 mg at bedtime	0.5 mg every 3–14 days	1.5–3 mg/day divided into 2–3 × daily (4 mg/day)
(Intuniv)[b]	1 mg once daily	No more than 1 mg/week	1–4 mg daily (4 mg/day)
Bupropion (Wellbutrin, Wellbutrin SR, Wellbutrin XL)	3 mg/kg/day for 7 days (children); 150 mg once daily of SR or XL (adults)	3 mg/kg/day in weekly intervals (children); increase 150–300 mg/day in weekly intervals (adults)	6 mg/kg/day or 400 mg/day—whichever is smaller (children); 150–450 mg/day (400 mg/day SR; 450 mg/day XL—adults)

[a]Pediatric dosing except when adult dosing specified.

[b]Approved by the U.S. Food and Drug Administration for the treatment of ADHD.

[c]Dose adjustment required in patients with hepatic insufficiency.

CD, extended release (biphasic immediate release with extended release); ER, extended release; LA, long acting; SR, sustained release; XL, extended release.

Two extended-acting stimulants, Daytrana and Vyvanse, have slower onsets of action than the other extended-acting stimulants with a rapid release. Daytrana transdermal patches are to be applied for only 9 hours per day and have a delayed onset of 2 hours, and their effects persist for 3 hours after being removed. Skin sensitization and irritation have been reported in some patients. Vyvanse is a prodrug that is hydrolyzed to its active form, dextroamphetamine, after oral ingestion. Inhalation or injection abuse potential is minimized because of impeded hydrolysis by these routes.

Onset of action for Vyvanse has been reported as soon as 2 hours.[15]

● Adverse effects of stimulants can be generalized to the whole class (Table 42–3). Most of these side effects can be managed by changing the dosing routine (i.e., giving with food, dividing daily dose, or giving the dose earlier in the day). Serious side effects such as hallucinations and abnormal movements require discontinuation of medication.[9,10,14] To avoid potential drug–food interactions and absorption issues, stimulants should be given 30 to 60 minutes before eating.

● Growth suppression or delay is a major concern for parents of children taking stimulants. However, the evidence of this side effect is not clear. At present, growth delay appears to be transient and to resolve by midadolescence, but more data are needed to firmly resolve this issue. Another concern is the risk of substance abuse with stimulant use. A diagnosis of ADHD alone increases the risk of substance abuse in adolescents and adults. However, stimulant use has not been shown to further increase this risk but actually may decrease this risk, provided ADHD is treated adequately.[16]

Table 42–3

ADHD Medication Side-Effect Profiles, Management, and Monitoring

Drug	Side Effects	Management	Monitoring
Stimulants			
Methylphenidate, dextroamphetamine, dextroamphetamine–amphetamine (mixed-salts amphetamine, dexmethylphenidate, lisdexamfetamine)	GI upset, nausea, decreased appetite, potential growth delay	Administer after meals Encourage high-calorie meals Divide dose Give snacks in the evening Change to shorter acting stimulant Use drug holiday or different medication if severe growth delay	Height, weight, blood pressure, pulse ECG if warranted Eating and sleeping patterns Evaluate every 2–4 weeks until stable dose is achieved; then evaluate every 3 months
	Sleep disturbance	Move dose(s) earlier in the day and discontinue later day dose if problem persists Give clonidine or guanfacine at bedtime Change to a shorter acting stimulant	
	Rebound symptoms	Change to longer acting stimulant Overlap stimulant dosing	
	Moodiness	Decrease dose or change to longer acting stimulant Verify diagnosis and comorbidity	
	Irritability	Evaluate time of occurrence Early onset: Decrease dose or change to longer acting stimulant Late onset: Switch to longer acting stimulant Evaluate for comorbidity	
	Increased blood pressure and pulse	Decrease dose or change to longer acting stimulant	
	Tics	Discontinue or change to a different stimulant Give clonidine or guanfacine	
Nonstimulants			
Atomoxetine	Increased blood pressure and pulse, nausea, vomiting, fatigue, and insomnia	Decrease dose or change to another medication	Same as stimulants but with baseline and routine liver function tests for hepatotoxicity
	Hepatotoxicity, suicidal thoughts	Discontinue or change to a another medication	
Clonidine and guanfacine	Sedation, arrhythmia, constipation, dizziness (decreased blood pressure)	Sedation: administer later in the day Decrease dose or change medication	Same as stimulants
Bupropion	GI upset, restlessness, sleep disturbances, rash, tics, risk of seizures, tremor	Decrease dose or change medication Tics, rash, and seizures: discontinue medication	Height, weight, blood pressure, pulse every month Eating and sleeping patterns

ECG, electrocardiography; GI, gastrointestinal.

The choice of ADHD medication should be made based on the patient's condition, the prescriber's familiarity with the medications, the ease of administration, and the cost. Stimulants should be used as first-line agents in most ADHD patients, although studies in groups of patients have shown no clear advantage of using one stimulant over another.[17]

▶ Nonstimulants

Atomoxetine Atomoxetine is approved for the treatment of ADHD in both children and adults. In clinical studies, atomoxetine has demonstrated superior efficacy over placebo and either equivalent or inferior efficacy compared with a suboptimal immediate-release methylphenidate dose or Concerta (18 to 54 mg given once daily), respectively.[18–23] ⑥ *Atomoxetine may be used as a second- or third-line medication for ADHD.*

Atomoxetine selectively inhibits the reuptake of adrenergic neurotransmitters, principally norepinephrine.[18–21] Atomoxetine is metabolized through the cytochrome P450 (CYP) 2D6 pathway. Concurrent use of certain antidepressants (i.e., fluoxetine, paroxetine) may inhibit this enzyme and necessitate slower dose titration of atomoxetine. Approximately 5% to 10% of the population are CYP2D6 poor metabolizers, and atomoxetine's half-life is increased significantly in this population.[24] The recommended dosing for atomoxetine depends on the weight of the patient and is given daily in either a single or two divided doses[24] (Table 42–2). In poor metabolizers, atomoxetine should be dosed once daily at 25% to 50% of the dose typically used in normal metabolizers.[24] The maximum therapeutic effect of atomoxetine may take up to 4 weeks to be seen, which is significantly longer than what is required with stimulants. Common side effects of atomoxetine are similar to those of stimulants and include dyspepsia, nausea, vomiting, somnolence, and decreased appetite. Some studies have reported an increase in blood pressure and heart rate.[19–21] Evidence shows that atomoxetine can slow growth rate and cause weight loss; thus, height and weight should be monitored routinely in pediatric patients[19–21] (Table 42–3). Furthermore, atomoxetine's labeling includes strong warnings about severe hepatotoxicity and increased association with suicidal thinking.

Atomoxetine is similar to extended-acting stimulants in that it can be given once daily in many patients. It appears to lack any abuse potential and is not a controlled substance.[25] One big disadvantage of atomoxetine is cost compared with other ADHD medications (Table 42–4).

Because of the high cost, lack of long-term efficacy data, and few comparison studies with stimulants, atomoxetine should be advocated only if the patient has failed or is intolerant to stimulant therapy (Fig. 42–1).

Bupropion Bupropion is a monocyclic antidepressant that weakly inhibits the reuptake of norepinephrine and dopamine. Bupropion is effective for relieving symptoms of ADHD in children but is not as effective as stimulants.[26,27] Similar results have been shown in adults.[26] Specific dosing recommendations are outlined in Table 42–2. Bupropion is well tolerated with minimal side effects (e.g., insomnia,

headache, nausea, and tremor). Side effects typically disappear with continuation of therapy and are minimized with slow titration of dose. Bupropion can worsen tics and movement disorders. It is a rational choice in an ADHD patient with comorbid depression.[26] However, seizures have been associated with bupropion doses greater than 6 mg/kg/day.[28] Seizures related to high doses can be minimized by reducing the dose or switching to a longer acting formulation. Owing to the propensity of seizures with bupropion, its use is contraindicated in patients with seizure and eating disorders.

Clonidine and Guanfacine Clonidine and guanfacine are central α_2-adrenergic agonists that inhibit the release of norepinephrine presynaptically. Both of these agents are less effective than stimulants in treating symptoms of ADHD but typically are used as adjuncts to stimulants to control disruptive or aggressive behavior and alleviate insomnia.[30] The effects of immediate-release guanfacine typically will last 3 to 4 hours longer than immediate-release clonidine, and the drug requires less frequent dosing. Extended-release formulations of guanfacine (Intuniv) and clonidine (Kapvay) have been developed to minimize dosing frequency and improve treatment of oppositional conditions (anger, hostility, irritability) in patients with ADHD. Similar to other nonstimulant medications, these two dosage forms can also be used in patients who are intolerant to stimulants. However, use of these dosage forms is limited because of a lack of comparative trials to stimulants and high cost. Common side effects with clonidine and guanfacine are low blood pressure and sedation. Sedation is transient and generally subsides after 2 to 3 weeks of therapy.[29,30] Rarely, severe side effects such as bradycardia, rebound hypertension, irregular heart beats, and sudden death have been reported.

Pharmacoeconomic and Treatment Adherence Considerations

Proper ADHD treatment is a substantial financial burden.[31,32] Annual healthcare costs of patients with ADHD are more than double those of patients without ADHD ($1,343 vs. $503, respectively).[31] The financial burden of ADHD can be attributed to the direct cost of pharmacotherapy, office visits, diagnostic measurements, therapy monitoring, and indirect costs (e.g., lost work time and productivity). When selecting a treatment for an ADHD patient, the cost burden to the patient's family should be considered. Short-acting stimulants may be more cost effective in many patients compared with longer acting stimulant formulations (Table 42–4), but in certain circumstances, longer acting stimulant formulations may provide a greater benefit owing to increased adherence to the medication and prolonged control of symptoms of ADHD. All intermediate- and three extended-acting (Concerta, Ritalin LA, and Adderall XR) stimulant formulations are now available as generic products, making them potentially a more affordable current or future option for patients. In addition, some nonstimulant ADHD medications (e.g., bupropion and immediate-release α_2-adrenergic agonists) appear to be less costly than many stimulant

---

Table 42–4

Day Cost[a] of Selected ADHD Medication Regimens

Generic (Brand)	Regimen (Brand)	Cost[a]
Short-Acting Rapid-Onset Stimulants		
Methylphenidate		
Generic	5-, 10-, or 20-mg tablet twice daily	$
Methylin	5 mg/5 mL solution twice daily	$$$$
Dexmethylphenidate		
Generic	2.5-mg tablet twice daily	$
Generic	5- or 10-mg tablet twice daily	$$
Dextroamphetamine		
Generic	5- or 10-mg tablet twice daily	$
Intermediate-Acting Slower-Onset Stimulants		
Methylphenidate		
Methylin ER	10- or 20-mg ER tablet daily	$
Dextroamphetamine[b]		
Generic	5-, 10-, or 15-mg capsule daily	$$
Dextroamphetamine/amphetamine		
Generic	5-, 7.5-, 10-, 12.5-, 15-, 20-, or 30-mg tablet daily	$$
Extended-Acting Rapid-Onset Stimulants		
Methylphenidate		
Concerta (brand & generics)[b]	18-, 27-, 36-, or 54-mg tablet daily	$$$$
Metadate CD[c]	10-, 20-, or 30-mg capsule daily	$$$$
Ritalin LA[c]	10-, 20-mg capsule daily	$$$$
Dextroamphetamine/amphetamine		
Generic ER	5-, 10-, 15-, 20-, 25-, or 30-mg capsule daily	$$$$
Dexmethylphenidate		
Focalin XR[c]	5-, 10-, 15-, or 20-mg capsule daily	$$$$
Extended-Acting Slower-Onset Stimulants		
Lisdexamfetamine		
Vyvanse	20-, 30-, 40-, 50-, 60-, or 70-mg capsule daily	$$$$
Methylphenidate		
Daytrana transdermal patch	10-, 15-, 20-, or 30-mg patch daily	$$$$
Nonstimulants		
Atomoxetine		
Strattera	10-, 18-, 25-, 40-, 60-, 80-, or 100-mg capsule daily	$$$$
Clonidine		
Generic	0.1-, 0.2-, or 0.3-mg tablet twice daily	$
Kapvay	0.1- or 0.2-mg tablet twice daily	$$$$
Guanfacine		
Generic	1- or 2-mg tablet twice daily	$
Intuniv	1-, 2-, 3-, or 4-mg tablet twice daily	$$$$
Bupropion		
Generic	75- or 100-mg tablet twice daily	$
Generic	100- or 150-mg SR tablet twice daily	$
Generic	200-mg SR tablet twice daily	$$
Generic	150-mg or 300-mg XL tablet daily	$

[a]Cost based on brand regimen specified without a dispensing fee or discount for a 30-day supply. (From: Drug Topics Red Book. Montvale, NJ: Thomson Reuters Healthcare; 2010)

$, less than $40; $$, $40–$79; $$$, $80–$120; $$$$, greater than $120.

[b]Ascending release (early and then gradual or continuous).

[c]Bimodal release (early and then late; mimics twice-daily dosing of shorter acting stimulant counterpart).

CD, extended release (biphasic immediate release with extended release); ER, extended release; LA, long acting; SR, sustained release; XL, extended release.

---

formulations; however, these agents have not been proven to have superior efficacy over stimulants in treating ADHD. Decisions on selection of specific ADHD medications should not be based solely on cost but also on efficacy and safety along with adherence to the prescribed regimen.

OUTCOME EVALUATION

It is important to carefully document core ADHD symptoms at baseline to provide a reference point from which to evaluate effectiveness of treatment. Improvement in individualized patient outcomes are desired, such as (a) family and social relationships, (b) disruptive behavior, (c) completing required tasks, (d) self-motivation, (e) appearance, and (f) self-esteem. It is very important to elicit evaluations of the patient's behavior from family, school, and social environments in order to assess these outcomes. Using standardized rating scales (e.g., Conners Rating Scales—Revised, Brown Attention-Deficit Disorder Scale, and Inattentive-Overactive With Aggression [IOWA] Conners Scale) in both children and adults with ADHD helps to minimize variability in evaluation.[33] After initiation of pharmacotherapy, evaluate every 2 to 4 weeks to determine efficacy of treatment and potential effects on height, weight, pulse, and blood pressure. Use physical examinations or liver function tests as appropriate to monitor for adverse effects. In children being considered for ADHD pharmacotherapy, obtain baseline electrocardiograms (ECGs) when known or suspected cardiac disease exists or the clinician judges it necessary.[34-36] Typically, therapeutic benefits will be seen within days of initiating stimulants and within 1 or 2 months of starting bupropion and atomoxetine. When a maintenance dose has been achieved, schedule follow-up visits every 3 months. At these visits, assess height and weight, and screen for possible adverse drug effects. If a patient has failed to respond to multiple agents, reevaluate for other possible causes of behavior dysfunction. Counsel patients and their families that treatment generally is long term. Typically, appropriately treated patients learn to better control their ADHD symptoms as adults.

Patient Encounter, Part 2: Medical History, Physical Examination, and ADHD Evaluation

HA's baseline physical examination is unremarkable. The family history is positive for cardiovascular disease (father had heart attack at age 40 years), and there is no documented history of ADHD in the family.

Wt: 29.1 kg (64 lb)

Allergies: None known

Ht: 51 in (130 cm)

BP: 100/65 mm Hg

P: 91 beats/min

HA's family does not qualify for medical assistance, and they can hardly afford their monthly expenses.

What stimulants and nonstimulants are available that might control HA's symptoms? Which ADHD medications should you be concerned about using?

Which medications will maximize efficacy, facilitate adherence, minimize potential side effects, and offer an acceptable cost?

What baseline assessment do you need before starting stimulant therapy?

What are important counseling points to discuss with HA's parents before starting any ADHD medication?

Patient Care and Monitoring

1. Assess the patient's symptoms and parent–teacher evaluations to determine whether they meet the *DSM-IV-TR* diagnostic criteria for ADHD. Evaluate whether the symptoms can be explained by another disorder.

2. Interview the patient and/or caregivers to obtain a complete medical history, which should include family medical history, current and past prescription and nonprescription medications, and dietary intake. Determine whether the patient is taking medications or supplements that could interfere with the therapy.

3. Educate the patient's parents and/or caregivers that behavioral therapy is not as effective as stimulant therapy. Educate them regarding the issues of growth delay and substance abuse risks with stimulants.

4. Perform a baseline physical examination before starting stimulant therapy. Include blood pressure, pulse, and height and weight measurements. In patients taking stimulants, perform a general physical examination yearly and monitor blood pressure quarterly in adults. In children, baseline ECGs may be obtained when known or strongly suspected cardiac disease exists.

5. Start patients on a low initial dose of a stimulant, and titrate up to the desired response in order to minimize side effects and costs.

6. If the patient is not responding to therapy after an adequate trial, assess compliance with the prescribed regimen. If the patient is not compliant, counsel the patient and caregivers, and explore reasons for noncompliance. In some cases, switching to another stimulant formulation may improve compliance.

7. Important counseling points to convey to the patient and/or caregivers:
   - What is ADHD?
   - What are the complications of untreated ADHD?
   - When to take medications and what to expect with therapy.
   - What side effects to expect and what to do if these occur.
   - Controversy over substance abuse and growth delay with stimulant therapy.
   - What prescription and nonprescription medications to avoid.

Abbreviations Introduced in This Chapter

ADHD	Attention-deficit hyperactivity disorder
CYP	Cytochrome P450
DSM-IV-TR	*Diagnostic and Statistical Manual of Mental Disorders,* Fourth Edition, Text Revision
IOWA	Inattentive-Overactive With Aggression

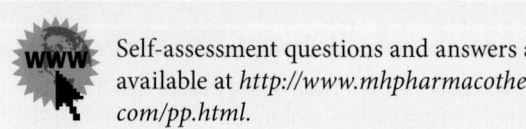

Self-assessment questions and answers are available at *http://www.mhpharmacotherapy. com/pp.html.*

REFERENCES

1. Wolraich ML, Wibbelsman CJ, Brown TE, et al. Attention-deficit/ hyperactivity disorder among adolescents: A review of the diagnosis, treatment, and clinical implications. Pediatrics 2005;115(6):1734–1746.

2. Ryan-Krause P. Attention deficit hyperactivity disorder: Part I. J Pediatr Health Care 2010;24(3):194–198.

3. Pastor PN, Reuben CA. Diagnosis of attention deficit hyperactivity disorder and learning disability: United States, 2004-2006. National Center for Health Statistics. Vital Health Stat 2008;10(237).

4. Biederman J, Faraone S. Attention-deficit hyperactivity disorder. Lancet 2005;366:237–248.

5. Centers for Disease Control and Prevention. Prevalence of diagnosis and medication treatment for attention-deficit/hyperactivity disorder—United States, 2003. MMWR Mortal Wkly Rep2005;54:842–847.

6. Rappley MD. Attention deficit-hyperactivity disorder. N Engl J Med 2005;352:165–173.

7. Elliott H. Attention deficit hyperactivity disorder in adults: A guide for the primary care physician. South Med J 2002;95:736–742.

8. Voeller KKS. Attention-deficit hyperactivity disorder (ADHD). J Child Neurol 2004;19:798–814.

9. Institute for Clinical Systems Improvement (ICSI). Health care guideline: diagnosis and management of attention deficit hyperactivity disorder in primary care for school-age children and adolescents, 8th ed. Bloominton, MN: Institute for Clinical Systems Improvement. March 2010, [cited 2011 Oct 10]. Available from: *http://www.icsi.org/ adhd/adhd_2300.html.*

10. Subcommittee on Attention-Deficit/Hyperactivity Disorder; Steering Committee on Quality Improvement and Management, Wolraich M, Brown L, Brown RT, et al. ADHD: Clinical practice guideline for the diagnosis, evaluation, and treatment of attention-deficit/hyperactivity disorder in children and adolescents. Pediatrics 2011;128(5):1007–1022.

11. American Psychiatric Association. Diagnostic and Statistical Manual of Mental Disorders. 4th ed, text rev. Washington, DC: American Psychiatric Press; 2000:39–134.

12. Pliszka S. AACAP Work Group on Quality Issues. Practice parameter for the assessment and treatment of children and adolescents with attention-deficit/hyperactivity disorder. J Am Acad Child Adolesc Psychiatry 2007;46:894–921.

13. MTA Cooperative Group. A 14-month randomized clinical trial of treatment strategies for attention-deficit/hyperactivity disorder. Arch Gen Psychiatry 1999;56(12):1073–1086.

14. Greenhill LL, Pliszka S, Dulcan MK, et al. Practice parameter for the use of stimulant medications in the treatment of children, adolescents, and adults. J Am Acad Child Adolesc Psychiatry 2002;41(Suppl 2): S26–S49.

15. Biederman J, Boellner SW, Childress A, et al. Lisdexamfetamine dimesylate and mixed amphetamine salts extended-release in children with ADHD: A double-blind, placebo-controlled, crossover analog classroom study. Biol Psychiatry 2007;62:970–976.

16. Wilens TE, Faraone SV, Biederman J, et al. Does stimulant therapy of attention-deficit/hyperactivity disorder beget later substance abuse? A meta-analytic review of the literature. Pediatrics 2003;111:179–185.

17. Brown RT, Amler RW, Freeman WS, et al. Treatment of attention-deficit/hyperactivity disorder: Overview of the evidence. Pediatrics 2005;115:749–757.

18. Michelson D, Faries D, Wernicke J, et al. Atomoxetine in the treatment of children and adolescents with attention-deficit/hyperactivity disorder: A randomized, placebo-controlled, dose-response study. Pediatrics 2001;108(5):E83.

19. Kratochvil CJ, Heiligenstein JH, Dittmann R, et al. Atomoxetine and methylphenidate treatment in children with ADHD: A prospective, randomized, open-label trial. J Am Acad Child Adolesc Psychiatry 2002;41(7):776–784.

20. Michelson D, Allen AJ, Busner J, et al. Once-daily atomoxetine treatment for children and adolescents with attention deficit hyperactivity disorder: A randomized, placebo-controlled study. Am J Psychiatry 2002;159:1896–1901.

21. Biederman J, Heiligenstein JH, Faries DE, et al. Efficacy of atomoxetine versus placebo in school-age girls with attention-deficit/hyperactivity disorder. Pediatrics 2002;110(6):E75.

22. Newcorn JH, Kratochvil CJ, Allen AJ, et al. Atomoxetine and osmotically released methylphenidate for the treatment of attention deficit hyperactivity disorder: Acute comparison and differential response. Am J Psychiatry 2008;165(6):721–730.

23. Wang Y, Zheng Y, Du Y, et al. Atomoxetine versus methylphenidate in paediatric outpatients with attention deficit hyperactivity disorder: A randomized, double-blind comparison trial. Aust N Z J Psychiatry 2007;41(3):222–230.

24. Belle DJ, Ernest S, Sauer J, et al. Effect of potent CYP2D6 inhibition by paroxetine on atomoxetine pharmacokinetics. J Clin Pharmacol 2002;42:1219–1227.

25. Heil SH, Holmes HW, Bickel WK, et al. Comparison of the subjective physiological, and psychomotor effects of atomoxetine and methylphenidate in light drug users. Drug Alcohol Depend 2002;67(2): 149–156.

26. Daviss WB, Bentivoglio P, Racusin R, et al. Bupropion sustained release in adolescents with comorbid attention-deficit/hyperactivity disorder and depression. J Am Acad Child Adolesc Psychiatry 2001;40(3): 307–314.

27. Wilens TE, Spencer TJ, Biederman J, et al. A controlled clinical trial of bupropion for attention deficit hyperactivity disorder in adults. Am J Psychiatry 2001;158:282–288.

28. Tallian K. Pharmacotherapy of ADHD. In: Schumock G, Brundage D, Chapman M, et al., eds. Pharmacotherapy Self-Assessment Program, 5th ed. Pediatrics II. Kansas City, MO: American College of Clinical Pharmacy, 2006:275–297.

29. Connor DF, Findling RL, Kollins SH, et al. Effects of guanfacine extended release on oppositional symptoms in children aged 6-12 years with attention-deficit hyperactivity disorder and oppositional symptoms: a randomized double-blind, placebo-controlled trial. CNS Drugs 2010;24(9):755–768.

30. Scrahill L. Alpha-2 adrenergic agonists in children with inattention, hyperactivity and impulsiveness. CNS Drugs 2009;23(Suppl 1):43–49.

31. Matza LS, Paramore C, Prasad M. A review of the economic burden of ADHD. Cost Eff Resour Alloc 2005;3:5.

32. Birnbaum HG, Kessler RC, Lowe SW, et al. Costs of attention deficit-hyperactivity disorder (ADHD) in the U.S.: Excess costs of persons with ADHD and their family members in 2000. Curr Med Res Opin 2005;21(2):195–205.

33. Collett BR, Ohan JL, Myers KM. Ten-year review of rating scales. V: Scales assessing attention-deficit/hyperactivity disorder. J Am Acad Child Adolesc Psychiatry 2003;42(9):1015–1037.

34. Vetter VL, Elia J, Erickson C, et al. Cardiovascular monitoring of children and adolescents with heart disease receiving medications for Attention Deficit/Hyperactivity Disorder: A scientific statement from the American Heart Association Council on Cardiovascular Disease in the Young Congenital Cardiac Defects Committee and the Council on Cardiovascular Nursing. Circulation. 2008;117:2407–2423.

35. Perrin JM, Friedman RA, KnilansTK, et al. Cardiovascular monitoring and stimulant drugs for Attention-Deficit/Hyperactivity Disorder. Pediatrics 2008; 122:451–453.

36. ECGs before stimulants in children. Med Lett Drugs Ther 2008 50(1291):60.

43   Diabetes Mellitus

Julie Sease, Susan Cornell, Kayce Shealy, and Tommy Johnson

LEARNING OBJECTIVES

● **Upon completion of the chapter, the reader will be able to:**

1. Discuss the incidence and economic impact of diabetes.

2. Distinguish clinical differences in type 1, type 2, and gestational diabetes.

3. List screening and diagnostic criteria for diabetes.

4. Discuss therapeutic goals for blood glucose, blood pressure, and lipids for a patient with diabetes.

5. Recommend nonpharmacologic therapies, including meal planning and physical activity, for patients with diabetes.

6. Compare oral agents used in treating diabetes by their mechanisms of action, time of action, side effects, contraindications, and effectiveness.

7. Select appropriate insulin therapy based on onset, peak, and duration of action.

8. Discuss the signs, symptoms, and treatment of hypoglycemia.

9. Define *diabetic ketoacidosis* and discuss treatment goals.

10. Develop a comprehensive therapeutic monitoring plan for a patient with diabetes based on patient-specific factors.

KEY CONCEPTS

❶ Diabetes mellitus (DM) describes a group of chronic metabolic disorders characterized by hyperglycemia that may result in long-term microvascular, macrovascular, and neuropathic complications.

❷ Type 1 DM (T1DM) is usually diagnosed before age 30 years but can develop at any age. Autoimmune destruction of the β cells causes insulin deficiency.

❸ Type 2 DM (T2DM) accounts for approximately 90% to 95% of all diagnosed cases of DM, is progressive in its development, and is often preceded by an increased risk for diabetes (previously known as prediabetes). A combination of insulin deficiency, insulin resistance, and other hormonal irregularities, primarily involving glucagon, are key problems with T2DM. The majority of people with T2DM are overweight, and an increasing number of cases in children have been observed.

❹ DM treatment goals include reducing, controlling, and managing long-term microvascular, macrovascular, and neuropathic complications; preserving β-cell function; preventing acute complications from high blood glucose levels; minimizing hypoglycemic episodes; and maintaining the patient's overall quality of life.

To achieve the majority of these goals, near-normal blood glucose levels are fundamental; thus, glycemic control remains a primary objective in diabetes management.

❺ Patients and clinicians can evaluate disease state control by monitoring daily blood glucose values, hemoglobin A1c or estimated average blood glucose values, blood pressure, and lipid levels.

❻ Oral and injectable agents are available to treat patients with T2DM who are unable to achieve glycemic control through meal planning and physical activity.

❼ Insulin is the primary treatment to lower blood glucose levels for patients with T1DM, and the addition of injected amylin may decrease fluctuations in blood glucose levels.

❽ Uncontrolled blood pressure plays a major role in the development of macrovascular events as well as microvascular complications, including retinopathy and nephropathy, in patients with DM. The American Diabetes Association (ADA) recommends that systolic blood pressure goals for patients with DM be individualized but generally set at less than 130 mm Hg. The diastolic blood pressure goal for patients with DM is less than 80 mm Hg.

⑨ Peripheral neuropathy is a common complication reported in T2DM. This complication generally presents as pain, tingling, or numbness in the extremities.

⑩ Lower extremity amputations are one of the most feared and disabling sequelae of long-term uncontrolled DM. A foot ulcer is an open sore that develops and penetrates to the subcutaneous tissues. Complications of the feet develop primarily as a result of peripheral vascular disease, neuropathies, and foot deformations.

INTRODUCTION

① *Diabetes mellitus (DM) describes a group of chronic metabolic disorders characterized by hyperglycemia that may result in long-term* microvascular, macrovascular, *and neuropathic complications.* These complications contribute to diabetes being the leading cause of (a) new cases of blindness among adults, (b) end-stage renal disease, and (c) nontraumatic lower limb amputations. Although prevention and treatment of DM remain challenges, several studies have shown that complications associated with DM such as retinopathy and neuropathy can be delayed or prevented through proper blood glucose management.[1,2]

The increased cardiovascular risk associated with DM contributes to its being the seventh leading cause of death in the United States.[3] In 2007, diabetes was the underlying cause of death or a contributing factor of death in approximately 284,000 decedents. The total financial impact of DM in 2007 was approximately $174 billion, with direct medical costs equaling $116 billion (2.3 times higher than what expenditures would be in the absence of diabetes) and indirect costs secondary to disability, work loss, and premature mortality equaling $58 billion.

EPIDEMIOLOGY AND ETIOLOGY

Diabetes mellitus is characterized by a complete lack of insulin, a relative lack of insulin, or insulin resistance as well as disorders of other hormones. These defects result in an inability to use glucose for energy. DM affects an estimated 25.8 million persons in the United States, or 8.3% of the population. Although an estimated 18.8 million persons have been diagnosed, another 7 million people have DM but are unaware they have the disease. The increasing prevalence of DM is partly caused by three influences: lifestyle, ethnicity, and age.

Lifestyle

A sedentary lifestyle coupled with greater consumption of high-fat, high-carbohydrate foods, and larger portion sizes have resulted in increasing rates of persons being overweight or obese. Current estimates indicate that 68% of the U.S. population is overweight, with 33.8% of this population being obese.[4] In the United States, *overweight* is defined as a body mass index (BMI) of greater than 25 kg/m², and a BMI of greater than 30 kg/m² constitutes obesity. The Centers for Disease Control and Prevention (CDC) estimates that 25.1% of Americans in 36 states engage in no leisure-time physical activity.[5]

Ethnicity

In addition to current lifestyle trends and increased body weight, certain ethnic groups are at a disproportionately high risk for developing DM. The risk of diabetes is 18% higher among Asian Americans, 66% higher among Hispanics, and 77% higher among non-Hispanic blacks compared with non-Hispanic white adults.[3] In addition, African American and Hispanic or Latino American populations are growing at a faster rate than the general U.S. population. This is a contributing factor to the rising U.S. population that has DM.

Age

The third factor contributing to the increased prevalence of type 2 DM (T2DM) is age. In 2010, 10.9 million people in the United States who were 65 years of age or older had diabetes compared with only 215,000 younger than age 20 years. As the population ages, the incidence of T2DM is expected to increase.

② *Type 1 DM (T1DM) is usually diagnosed before age 30 years but can develop at any age. Autoimmune destruction of the β cells causes insulin deficiency.* ③ *T2DM accounts for approximately 90% to 95% of all diagnosed cases of DM, is progressive in its development, and is often preceded by an increased risk for diabetes (previously known as* prediabetes*). A combination of insulin deficiency, insulin resistance, and other hormonal irregularities, primarily involving* glucagon, *are key problems with T2DM. The majority of people with T2DM are overweight, and an increasing number of cases in children have been observed.*

T1DM is an autoimmune disease in which insulin-producing β cells in the pancreas are destroyed, leaving the individual insulin deficient.[6] This is usually precipitated through genetic susceptibility and/or an environmental trigger, or both. Certain genetic markers can be measured to determine if a person is at risk of T1DM. The presence of human leukocyte antigens (HLAs), especially HLA-DR and HLA-DQ, is strongly associated with the development of T1DM. In addition, these individuals often develop islet cell antibodies, insulin autoantibodies, or glutamic acid decarboxylase autoantibodies. As more β cells are destroyed, glucose metabolism becomes compromised because of reduced insulin release after a glucose load. At the time of diagnosis of T1DM, it is commonly believed that most patients have an 80% to 95% loss of β-cell function.[7] The remaining β-cell function at diagnosis creates a "honeymoon period" during which blood glucose levels are easier to control and smaller amounts of insulin are required.[6] After this remaining β-cell function is lost, and patients become completely insulin deficient and require more exogenous insulin. Diagnosis occurs before age 16 to 18 years in 50% to 60% of those with T1DM.

Latent autoimmune diabetes in adults (LADA), slow-onset type 1, or type 1.5 DM, is a form of autoimmune T1DM that occurs in individuals older than the usual age of T1DM onset.[8] Patients often are mistakenly thought to have T2DM because the person is older and may respond initially to treatment with oral blood glucose–lowering agents. These patients do not have insulin resistance, but antibodies are present in the blood that are known to destroy pancreatic β cells.

C-peptide is the abbreviation for "connecting peptide." C-peptide is made when proinsulin is split into insulin and C-peptide. They split before proinsulin is released from endocytic vesicles within the pancreas—one C-peptide for each insulin molecule. Routine measurement of **C-peptide levels**, insulin levels, and proinsulin are not recommended in most patients.[9] However, C-peptide measurements can be used to distinguish between T1DM and T2DM. People with T1DM have C-peptide levels below 1 ng/mL (0.33 nmol/L), whereas those with T2DM will have values greater than 1 ng/mL (0.33 nmol/L).

Categories of increased risk for diabetes (commonly referred to as prediabetes) include impaired fasting glucose (IFG), impaired glucose tolerance (IGT), or hemoglobin A1c (A1c) between 5.7% and 6.4% (0.057 and 0.064; 39 and 46 mmol/mol hemoglobin [Hb]).[10] IFG is defined as having a fasting blood glucose (FBG) level between 100 and 125 mg/dL (5.6 and 6.9 mmol/L). IGT is defined by a postprandial blood glucose level between 140 and 199 mg/dL (7.8 and 11.0 mmol/L). It is currently estimated that 70 million persons in the United States have prediabetes.[3] The development of IFG, IGT, or A1c between 5.7% and 6.4% (0.057 and 0.064; 39 and 46 mmol/mol) places the individual at high risk of eventually developing diabetes. Because progression to diabetes is not predictable, early interventions are gaining popularity.

T2DM is usually slow and progressive in its development. Risk factors for T2DM include:

- First-degree family history of DM (i.e., parents or siblings)
- Overweight or obese
- Habitual physical inactivity
- Race or ethnicity (Native American, Latino or Hispanic American, Asian American, African American, and Pacific Islanders)

- Previously identified IFG, IGT, or A1c between 5.7% and 6.4% (0.057 and 0.064 or 39 and 46 mmol/mol Hb)
- Hypertension (greater than or equal to 140/90 mm Hg or on therapy for hypertension)
- High-density lipoprotein (HDL) less than 35 mg/dL (0.91 mmol/L) and/or a triglyceride level greater than 250 mg/dL (2.83 mmol/L)
- History of gestational diabetes or delivery of a baby weighing greater than 4 kg (9 lb)
- History of cardiovascular disease
- History of polycystic ovarian syndrome
- Other conditions associated with insulin resistance (e.g., **acanthosis nigricans**)[10]

Gestational diabetes mellitus (GDM) is defined as glucose intolerance in women during pregnancy. This complication develops in between 2% and 10% of all pregnancies.[3] Women who have GDM have a 35% to 60% chance of developing T2DM. Clinical detection of and therapy for GDM are important because blood sugar control produces significant reductions in perinatal morbidity and mortality. New diagnostic criteria call for all pregnant women not previously known to have diabetes to undergo screening for GDM between 24 and 28 weeks of gestation.[11] Use of these criteria resulted in an 18% GDM diagnosis rate in one multinational epidemiologic study that enrolled 25,000 pregnant women.[12]

Diabetes from other causes includes genetic defects in β-cell function, genetic defects in insulin action, diseases of the exocrine pancreas such as cystic fibrosis, and drug- or chemical-induced diabetes.[10] Table 43–1 contains a list of medications that may affect glycemic control.[13] Although the use of these medications is not contraindicated in persons with DM, caution and awareness of the effects on blood glucose should be taken into account when managing these patients.

Table 43–1

Medications That May Affect Glycemic Control[13]

Drug	Effect on Glucose	Mechanism or Comment
Angiotensin-converting enzyme inhibitors	Slight reduction	Improves insulin sensitivity
Alcohol	Reduction	Reduces hepatic glucose production
α-Interferon	Increase	Unclear
Diuretics	Increase	May increase insulin resistance
Glucocorticoids	Increase	Impair insulin action
Nicotinic acid	Increase	Impairs insulin action, increases insulin resistance
Oral contraceptives	Increase	Unclear
Pentamidine	Decrease, then increase	Toxic to β cells; initial release of stored insulin, then depletion
Phenytoin	Increase	Decreases insulin secretion
β-blockers	May increase	Decreases insulin secretion
Salicylates	Decrease	Inhibition of I-kappa-B kinase-β (IKK-β) (only high doses, e.g., 4–6 g/day)
Sympathomimetics	Slight increase	Increased glycogenolysis and gluconeogenesis
Clozapine and olanzapine	Increase	Decreases insulin sensitivity; weight gain

This list is not inclusive of all medications reported to cause glucose changes.

PATHOPHYSIOLOGY

Normal Carbohydrate Metabolism

The body's main fuel source is glucose. Cells metabolize glucose completely through glycolysis and the Krebs cycle, producing adenosine triphosphate (ATP) as energy.[14] Glucose is stored in the liver and muscles as glycogen. When energy is required, glycogenolysis converts stored glycogen back to glucose.[15] Excess glucose also may be stored in adipose tissue, which may subsequently undergo lipolysis, yielding free fatty acids.[14] In the fasting state, free fatty acids supply much of the energy needs for the body except for the central nervous system, which requires glucose to function normally.[15] Although usually reserved for other functions, proteins also can be converted to glucose through gluconeogenesis.[14] Normal homeostasis is achieved through a balance of the metabolism of glucose, free fatty acids, and amino acids to maintain a blood glucose level sufficient to provide an uninterrupted supply of glucose to the brain.[15]

Insulin and glucagon are produced in the pancreas by cells in the islets of Langerhans. β cells make up 70% to 90% of the islets and produce insulin and amylin, whereas α cells produce glucagon.[14] The main function of insulin is to decrease blood glucose levels. Glucagon, along with other counterregulatory hormones such as growth factor, cortisol, and epinephrine, increases blood glucose levels.[15] Although blood glucose levels vary, the opposing actions of insulin and glucagon, along with the counterregulatory hormones, normally maintain fasting values between 79 and 99 mg/dL (4.4 to 5.5 mmol/L).

▶ Normal Insulin Action

Fasting insulin levels in the circulation average from 43 to 186 pmol/L (6 to 26 μIU/mL).[14] After food is consumed, blood glucose levels rise, and the insulin-secretion response occurs in two phases. An initial burst, known as *first phase insulin response,* lasts approximately 5 to 10 minutes and serves to suppress hepatic glucose production and cause insulin-mediated glucose disposal in adipose tissue. This bolus of insulin minimizes hyperglycemia during meals and during the postprandial period. The *second phase of insulin response* is characterized by a gradual increase in insulin secretion, which lasts 60 to 120 minutes and stimulates glucose uptake by peripheral insulin-dependent tissues. Approximately 80% to 85% of glucose metabolism during this time occurs in muscle.[13] Slower release of insulin allows the body to respond to the new glucose entering from digestion while maintaining blood glucose levels.

Amylin is a naturally occurring hormone that is cosecreted from β cells with insulin.[14] People with diabetes have either a relative or complete lack of amylin. Amylin has three major mechanisms of action: suppression of postmeal glucagon secretion; regulation of the rate of gastric emptying from the stomach to the small intestine, which increases satiety; and regulation of plasma glucose concentrations in the bloodstream.

▶ Impaired Insulin Secretion

A pancreas with normal β-cell function is able to adjust insulin production to maintain normal blood glucose levels.[15] Hyperinsulinemia, or high blood levels of insulin, is an early finding in the development of T2DM.[16] More insulin is secreted to maintain normal blood glucose levels until eventually the pancreas can no longer produce sufficient insulin.[14] The resulting hyperglycemia is enhanced by extremely high insulin resistance, pancreatic burnout in which β cells lose functional capacity, or both. Impaired β-cell function results in a reduced ability to produce a first-phase insulin response sufficient to signal the liver to stop producing glucose after a meal.[16] As DM progresses, large numbers of patients with T2DM eventually lose all β-cell function and require exogenous insulin to maintain blood glucose control.

▶ Insulin Resistance

Insulin resistance is the primary factor that differentiates T2DM from other forms of diabetes. Insulin resistance may be present for several years prior to the diagnosis of DM and can continue to progress throughout the course of the disease.[14] Resistance to insulin occurs most significantly in skeletal muscle and the liver.[13] Insulin resistance in the liver poses a double threat because the liver becomes nonresponsive to insulin for glucose uptake, and hepatic production of glucose after a meal does not cease, which leads to elevated fasting and postmeal blood glucose levels.

▶ Impaired Glucagon Secretion

Glucagon is a counterregulatory hormone released by the α cells that raises blood glucose levels.[14] The release of insulin and the inhibition of glucagon is glucose stimulated, meaning that as glucose is consumed, the release of insulin increases and the release of glucagon decreases in people without diabetes.[17] Most patients with a 10- to 20-year history of T1DM have lost their ability to release glucagon, which increases their risk for hypoglycemic unawareness. People with T2DM have impaired phase 1 and phase 2 insulin release, and some have impaired glucagon-like peptide 1 (GLP-1) and glucose-dependent insulinotropic polypeptide (GIP) release, which further reduces the release of insulin. This leads to the liver's producing and releasing glucose even in the postprandial state.[18]

▶ Metabolic Syndrome

Insulin resistance has been associated with a number of other cardiovascular risks, including abdominal obesity, hypertension, dyslipidemia, hypercoagulation, and hyperinsulinemia. The clustering of these risk factors has been termed metabolic syndrome. It is estimated that 50% of the U.S. population older than 60 years of age has metabolic syndrome. The most widely used criteria to define metabolic syndrome were established by the National Cholesterol Education Program Adult Treatment Panel III Guidelines[19] (summarized in Table 43–2). Patients having these additional

Table 43–2

Five Components of Metabolic Syndrome[19]

Risk Factor	Defining Level
1. Abdominal obesity	
• Men	Waist circumference greater than 102 cm (40 in)
• Women	Waist circumference greater than 89 cm (35 in)
2. Triglycerides	Greater than or equal to 150 mg/dL (1.70 mmol/L)
3. HDL cholesterol	
• Men	Less than 40 mg/dL (1.03 mmol/L)
• Women	Less than 50 mg/dL (1.29 mmol/L)
4. Blood pressure	Greater than or equal to 130/85 mm Hg
5. Fasting glucose	Greater than or equal to 100 mg/dL (5.6 mmol/L)

Individuals having at least three of the five above criteria meet the diagnostic criteria for metabolic syndrome.

risk factors have been found to be at a much higher cardiovascular risk than would be expected from the individual components of the syndrome. Therefore, it is important to assume a more aggressive treatment plan for each of the individual abnormal components. As a result, a patient with prediabetes or DM having a convergence of other risk factors should be treated more aggressively than a patient having prediabetes or DM alone.

▶ Incretin Effect

A great deal of research is occurring today to develop compounds that enhance the incretin effect, either by mimicking its action or by enabling incretin hormones to remain physiologically active for longer periods of time.[18,20–22] As early as the late 1960s, Perley and others observed that insulin's response to oral glucose exceeded that of intravenous (IV) glucose administration.[22] It was concluded that factors in the gut, or incretins, affected the release of insulin after a meal is consumed.

When nutrients enter the stomach and intestines, incretin hormones are released, which stimulates insulin secretion. This was validated by measuring C-peptide and insulin response to the IV and oral glucose loads. GLP-1 and GIP are the two major incretin hormones, with GLP-1 being studied the most. GLP-1 is secreted by the L cells of the ileum and colon primarily, and GIP is secreted by the K cells.

GLP-1 was identified in the early 1980s. It is a 30/31 amino acid peptide that is a product of the glucagon gene. GLP-1 secretion is caused by endocrine and neural signals started when nutrients enter the gastrointestinal (GI) tract. Within minutes of food ingestion, GLP-1 levels rise rapidly. A glucose-dependent release of insulin occurs, and the dipeptidyl peptidase-4 (DPP-4) enzyme cleaves GLP-1 rapidly to an inactive metabolite. Much of the research on glucose-lowering products involves prolonging the action of GLP-1. Other glucose-lowering effects of GLP-1 include suppression of glucagon, slowing gastric emptying, and increasing satiety.[18,20–22]

Clinical Presentation and Diagnosis of Diabetes Mellitus

Characteristic	Type 1 Diabetes Mellitus	Type 2 Diabetes Mellitus
Usual age of onset	Childhood or adolescence	Adult
Speed of onset	Abrupt	Gradual
Family history	Negative	Positive
Body type	Thin	Obese or history of obesity
Metabolic syndrome	No	Often
Autoantibodies	Present	Rare
Symptoms	Polyuria, polydipsia, polyphagia, rapid weight loss	Asymptomatic
Ketones at diagnosis	Present	Uncommon
Acute complications	Diabetic ketoacidosis	Rare
Microvascular complications at diagnosis	Rare	Common
Macrovascular complications at or before diagnosis	Rare	Common

CLINICAL PRESENTATION AND DIAGNOSIS

Screening

Currently, the American Diabetes Association (ADA) recommends routine screening for T2DM every 3 years in all adults starting at 45 years of age.[10] Testing for T2DM should be considered in any adult, regardless of their age, who have a BMI greater than or equal to 25 kg/m². The ADA does not currently recommend widespread screening for T1DM because of the relatively low incidence in the general population, although measurement of islet autoantibodies may be appropriate for high-risk individuals, including those with transient hyperglycemia or who have relatives with T1DM. See Table 43–3[10] for complete screening guidelines.

Gestational Diabetes

All pregnant women who have risk factors for T2DM should be screened for undiagnosed T2DM at their first prenatal visit using standard diagnostic criteria. Any woman found to have diabetes at that early point in pregnancy is considered to have T2DM, not GDM. All other pregnant women, not

---

Table 43–3

American Diabetes Association Screening Recommendations for Diabetes[10]

Asymptomatic type 1
The ADA does not recommend screening for T1DM because of the low incidence in the general population and due to the acute presentation of symptoms

Asymptomatic type 2
1. The ADA recommends screening for T2DM every 3 years in all adults beginning at 45 years of age, particularly in those with a BMI greater than or equal to 25 kg/m²
2. Testing should be considered for persons younger than 45 years of age or more frequently in individuals who are overweight (BMI greater than or equal to 25 kg/m²) and have additional risk factors:
   - Habitually inactive
   - First-degree relative with diabetes
   - Member of a high-risk ethnic population (e.g., African American, Latino, Native American, Asian American, Pacific Islander)
   - Delivered a baby weighing greater than 4.1 kg (9 lb) or previous diagnosis of GDM
   - Hypertensive (greater than or equal to 140/90 mm Hg)
   - HDL cholesterol level less than 35 mg/dL (0.91 mmol/L) and/or triglyceride level greater than 250 mg/dL (2.83 mmol/L)
   - Polycystic ovary syndrome
   - Previous IGT or IFG
   - Other clinical conditions associated with insulin resistance (e.g., acanthosis nigricans)
   - History of cardiovascular disease

Type 2 in children and adolescents
Criteria:
   - Overweight (BMI greater than 85th percentile for age and sex, weight for height greater than 85th percentile, or weight greater than 120% of ideal for height)
Plus any two of the following risk factors:
   - Family history of T2DM in first- or second-degree relatives
   - Race or ethnicity (Native American, African American, Latino or Hispanic American, Asian American, Pacific Islander)
   - Signs of insulin resistance or conditions associated with insulin resistance (acanthosis nigricans, hypertension, dyslipidemia, or polycystic ovary disease)
   - Maternal history of diabetes or GDM during child's gestation

Age of initiation:
   Age 10 years or at onset of puberty, if puberty occurs at a younger age
Frequency of testing:
   Every 2 years
   Test method: FPG preferred
   Clinical judgment should be used to test for diabetes in high-risk patients who do not meet these criteria

Gestational diabetes
1. Screen for undiagnosed T2DM at first prenatal visit in those with risk factors using standard criteria
2. All women should be screened with an OGTT between weeks 24 and 28 of gestation

ADA, American Diabetes Association; BMI, body mass index; FPG, fasting plasma glucose; GDM, gestational diabetes mellitus; HDL, high-density lipoprotein; IFG, impaired fasting glucose; IGT, impaired fasting glucose; OGTT, oral glucose tolerance test; T1DM, type 1 diabetes mellitus; T2DM, type 2 diabetes mellitus.

---

currently known to have DM should be screened for GDM with a 75-g oral glucose tolerance test (OGTT) between weeks 24 and 28 of gestation. The diagnostic criteria for OGTT are listed in Table 43–4.[10]

Table 43–4

Diagnosis of Gestational Diabetes Mellitus With a 75-g Glucose Load[10]

Time	Plasma Glucose	
	mg/dL	mmol/L
75-g glucose load		
Fasting	92 or more	5.1 or more
1 hour	180 or more	10.0 or more
2 hours	153 or more	8.5 more

A positive diagnosis of diabetes is made when any of the listed glucose values are exceeded. The test should be done in the morning after an 8-hour fast.

Any woman diagnosed with GDM should be retested at 6 to 12 weeks postpartum. If screening results are normal at that point, then reassessment for DM should occur every 3 years. Family planning for subsequent pregnancies should be discussed, and monitoring for the development of symptoms of DM should be undertaken.

Diagnostic Criteria

- The diagnosis of DM includes glycemic outcomes exceeding threshold values with one of three testing options (Table 43–5).[10,23] Confirmation of abnormal values must be made on a subsequent day for diagnosis unless unequivocal symptoms of hyperglycemia exist, such as polydipsia, polyuria, and polyphagia. Either A1c, fasting plasma glucose (FPG), or OGTT are appropriate tests for detecting DM.

- The ADA categorizes patients demonstrating A1c between 5.7% and 6.4% (0.057 and 0.064 or 39 and 46 mmol/mol Hb), IFG, or IGT as having increased risk for future diabetes.

Table 43–5

ADA Criteria for the Diagnosis of Diabetes[10]

1. Symptoms of diabetes plus a casual plasma glucose concentration greater than or equal to 200 mg/dL (11.1 mmol/L). *Casual* is defined as any time of day without regard to time since the last meal. The classic symptoms of diabetes include polyuria, polydipsia, and unexplained weight loss.

or

2. FPG greater than or equal to 126 mg/dL (7 mmol/L). *Fasting* is defined as no caloric intake for at least 8 hours.

or

3. Two-hour postload glucose greater than or equal to 200 mg/dL (11.1 mmol/L) during an OGTT. The test should be performed as described by the WHO using a glucose load containing the equivalent of 75 g of anhydrous glucose dissolved in water.

or

4. A1c greater than or equal to 6.5% (0.065; 48 mmol/mol Hb). The test should be performed in a laboratory using a method that is NGSP certified to the DCCT assay.

ADA, American Diabetes Association; A1c, hemoglobin A1c; DCCT, Diabetes Control and Complications Trial; FPG, fasting plasma glucose; Hb, hemoglobin; NGSP, National Glycohemoglobin Standardization Program; OGTT, oral glucose tolerance test; WHO, World Health Organization.

In the absence of unequivocal hyperglycemia, these criteria should be confirmed by repeat testing on a different day. The OGTT is not recommended for routine clinical use.

The categorization thresholds of glucose status for FPG determination and the OGTT are listed in Table 43–6.[10,23] IFG and IGT may coexist or may be identified independently. FPG level represents hepatic glucose production during the fasting state, whereas postprandial glucose levels in the OGTT may reflect glucose uptake in peripheral tissues, insulin sensitivity, or a decreased first-phase insulin response. The OGTT identifies people with either IFG or IGT and therefore potentially more people at increased risk for DM and cardiovascular disease. The OGTT is a more cumbersome test to perform

---

Table 43–6

ADA Categorization of Glucose Status[10]

	mg/dL	mmol/L
FPG		
• Normal	Less than 100	Less than 5.6
• IFG (prediabetes)	100–125	5.6–6.9
• Diabetes	Greater than or equal to 126	7.0
2-hour postload plasma glucose (OGTT)		
• Normal	Less than 140	7.8
• IGT (prediabetes)	140–199	7.8–11.0
• Diabetes	Greater than or equal to 200	11.1

ADA, American Diabetes Association; FPG, fasting plasma glucose; IFG, impaired fasting glucose; IGT, impaired glucose tolerance; OGTT, oral glucose tolerance test.

Patient Encounter, Part 1

GH is a 56-year-old African American man who presents to his physician for a follow-up appointment for hypertension. Upon questioning, GH states that he has noticed more frequent trips to the bathroom than usual and his appetite has substantially increased. He denies much physical activity, although he has lost approximately 15 lb (6.8 kg) since his last visit 6 months ago. He is concerned about developing diabetes and heart disease like both of his parents.

PMH: Allergic rhinitis, hypercholesterolemia, hypertension

FH: Father has diabetes, hypertension, and a history of myocardial infarction at age 54 years; mother has diabetes and a history of stroke at age 70 years; brother has hypercholesterolemia

SH: Smokes ½ pack per day for 20 years; denies alcohol or illicit drug use

Allergies: sulfa and penicillin

Medications:

- Hydrochlorothiazide 25 mg by mouth once daily
- Simvastatin 20 mg by mouth once daily
- Fluticasone nasal spray, one spray each nostril daily

VS: BP 134/85 mm Hg, P 82 beats/min, RR 20, T 38°C (100°F)

Height: 6 ft, 3 in (190.5 cm)

Weight: 285 lb (129.5 kg)

Waist circumference: 46.5 in (118.1 cm)

ROS: (+) Fatigue, (−) N/V/D, HA, SOB, chest pain

What risk factors does this patient have for diabetes?

Which type of diabetes does his characteristics suggest?

What additional information is needed to diagnose this patient with diabetes?

---

than either the A1c or FPG; however, the efficacy of interventions for primary prevention of T2DM have been demonstrated among patients with IGT, not among those with IFG or specific A1c levels.

TREATMENT

Goals of Therapy

④ *DM treatment goals include reducing, controlling, and managing long-term microvascular, macrovascular, and neuropathic complications; preserving β-cell function; preventing acute complications from high blood glucose levels; minimizing hypoglycemic episodes; and maintaining the patient's overall quality of life. To achieve the majority of these goals, near-normal blood glucose levels are fundamental; thus, glycemic control remains a primary objective in diabetes management.* Two landmark trials, the Diabetes Control and Complications Trial (DCCT)[2] and the United Kingdom

Prospective Diabetes Study (UKPDS),[3] showed that lowering blood glucose levels decreased the risk of developing chronic complications. A near-normal blood glucose level can be achieved with appropriate patient education, lifestyle modification, and medications.

Proper care of DM requires goal setting and assessment for glycemic control, self-monitoring of blood glucose (SMBG), monitoring of blood pressure and lipid levels, regular monitoring for the development of complications, dietary and exercise lifestyle modifications, and proper medication use. The complexity of proper DM self-care principles has a dramatic impact on a patient's lifestyle and requires a highly disciplined and dedicated person to maintain long-term control.

▶ Setting and Assessing Glycemic Targets

⑤ *Patients and clinicians can evaluate disease state control of the patient's diabetes by monitoring daily blood glucose values, A1c or estimated average glucose (eAG) values, blood pressure, and lipid levels.* SMBG enables patients to obtain their current blood glucose level at any time easily and relatively inexpensively. The A1c test provides a weighted-mean blood glucose level from the previous 3 months.

Self-Monitoring of Blood Glucose SMBG is the standard method for routinely checking blood glucose levels. Each reading provides a point-in-time evaluation of glucose control that can vary widely depending on numerous factors, including food, exercise, stress, and time of day.

By examining multiple individual points of data, patterns of control can be established. Therapy can be evaluated from these patterns, and adjustments can be made to improve overall blood glucose control. The ADA premeal plasma glucose goals are 70 to 130 mg/dL (3.9 to 7.2 mmol/L) and peak postprandial plasma glucose goals are less than 180 mg/dL (10 mmol/L).[10] The American Association of Clinical Endocrinologists (AACE) supports tighter SMBG controls with premeal goals of less than 110 mg/dL (6.1 mmol/L) and peak postmeal goals of less than 140 mg/dL (7.8 mmol/L).[23] For patients using multiple daily insulin injections or insulin pump therapy, the ADA recommends that SMBG be performed at least three times daily.[10] The optimal frequency of testing in patients using less frequent insulin injections, non-insulin therapies, or medical nutrition therapy (MNT) is still unknown, and the cost effectiveness of routine SMBG in non–insulin-treated patients has been called into question.[10,24] Some regimen of SMBG among patients with T2DM has been associated with an A1c reduction of 0.4% (0.004; 4 mmol/mol Hb).[25] Each patient should be educated regarding how often and when to perform SMBG, and these measurements should be evaluated and used by both the patient and his or her healthcare providers to help the patient gain and maintain blood glucose control.[10]

Typically, in SMBG, a drop of blood is placed on a test strip that is then read by a blood glucose monitor. Recent technological advancements have decreased the blood sample size required to as small as 0.3 microliters, provided the capability of alternate-site testing, and allowed for the delivery of readings in as few as 5 seconds. Many SMBG devices can download or transfer information to a computer program that can summarize and produce graphs of the data. Identifying patterns in the patient's blood glucose data can aid practitioners in modifying treatment for better glucose control. Specific therapy adjustments can be made for patterns found at certain times of the day, on certain days, or with large day-to-day variances.

Although most testing occurs by lancing the fingertip to produce a blood droplet, alternate-site testing has been approved for testing the palm, arm, leg, and abdomen. Alternate-site testing was developed as a means to decrease the pain encountered with repeated fingersticks by using body locations that have a lower concentration of nerve endings.

In choosing a glucose meter for a patient, several additional factors may aid in the best selection for the patient. Larger display areas or units with audible instructions and results may be better suited for older individuals and those with visual impairment. Patients with arthritis or other conditions that decrease dexterity may prefer larger meters with little or no handling of glucose strips. Younger patients or busy professionals may prefer smaller meters with features such as faster results, larger memories, reminder alarms, and downloading capabilities. Several continuous glucose sensors are now available that work with or independently of insulin pumps. These monitors provide blood glucose readings, primarily through interstitial fluid (ISF). A small sterile disposable glucose-sensing device called a sensor is inserted into the subcutaneous tissues. This sensor measures the change in glucose in ISF and sends the information to a monitor, which stores the results. The monitor must be calibrated daily by entering several blood glucose readings obtained at different times using a standard blood glucose meter.

Hemoglobin A1c Glucose interacts spontaneously with Hb in red blood cells to form glycated derivatives. The most prevalent derivative is A1c. Greater amounts of glycation occur when blood glucose levels increase. Because Hb has a life span of approximately 3 months, levels of A1c provide a marker reflecting the average glucose levels over this timeframe.[10] The ADA goal for persons with DM is less than 7% (0.07; 53 mmol/mol Hb), whereas the AACE supports a goal of less than or equal to 6.5% (0.065; 48 mmol/mol Hb).[10,23] Testing A1c levels should occur at least twice a year for patients who are meeting treatment goals and four times per year for patients not meeting goals or those who have had recent changes in therapy.

Estimated Average Glucose The eAG is used to correlate A1c values with readings that patients obtain from their home glucose monitors.[10] The equation to convert from A1c to eAG is: eAG (mg/dL) = 28.7 × A1c − 46.7 (or eAG [mmol/L] = 1.59 × A1c − 2.59 for A1c expressed as a percentage).[26] The goal eAG is 154 mg/dL (8.5 mmol/L), which corresponds with an A1c of less than 7%, and an eAG of 240 mg/dL (13.3 mmol/L) would be equivalent to an A1c of 10%.

Ketone Monitoring Urine and blood ketone testing is important in people with T1DM, in pregnancy with preexisting diabetes, and in GDM. People with T2DM may have positive ketones and develop diabetic ketoacidosis (DKA) if they are ill.

The presence of ketones may indicate a lack of insulin or ketoacidosis, a condition that requires immediate medical attention. When there is a lack of insulin, peripheral tissues cannot take up and store glucose. This causes the body to think it is starving, and because of excessive lipolysis, ketones, primarily β-hydroxybutyric and acetoacetic acid, are produced as byproducts of free fatty acid metabolism in the liver. Glucose and ketones are osmotically active, and when an excessive amount of ketones is formed, the body gets rid of them through urine, leading to dehydration. Patients with T1DM should test for ketones during acute illness or stress or when blood glucose levels are consistently elevated above 300 mg/dL (16.7 mmol/L). This commonly occurs when insulin is omitted or when diabetes is poorly controlled due to nonadherence, illness, or other reasons. Women with preexisting diabetes before pregnancy or with GDM should check ketones using their first morning urine sample or when any symptoms of ketoacidosis such as nausea, vomiting, or abdominal pain are present. Positive ketone readings are found in normal individuals during fasting and in up to 30% of first morning urine specimens from pregnant women. Urine ketone tests using nitroprusside-containing reagents can give false-positive results in the presence of several medications, including captopril. False-negative readings have been reported when test strips have been exposed to air for an extended period of time or when urine specimens have been highly acidic, such as after large intakes of ascorbic acid. Currently, available urine ketone tests are not reliable for diagnosing or monitoring treatment of ketoacidosis. Blood ketone testing methods that quantify β-hydroxybutyric acid, the predominant ketone body, are available and are the preferred way to diagnose and monitor ketoacidosis. Home tests for β-hydroxybutyric acid are available. The specific treatment of DKA may include rehydration, correction of electrolyte imbalances, and insulin administration.

▶ Blood Pressure, Lipids, and Monitoring for Complications

The ADA standards of medical care address many of the common comorbid conditions, as well as complications that result from the progression of DM. Table 43–7 presents goals for blood pressure measurements, lipids values, and monitoring parameters for complications associated with diabetes.

General Approach to Therapy

▶ Type 1 Diabetes Mellitus

Treatment of T1DM requires providing exogenous insulin to replace the endogenous loss of insulin from the nonfunctional pancreas. Ideally, insulin therapy mimics normal insulin physiology. The basal-bolus approach attempts to reproduce

Table 43–7	
ADA Recommended Goals of Therapy	
Area	**Goals**
Glycemia	
A1c	Less than 7% (0.07; 53 mmol/mol Hb)
	Evaluate every 3 months until in goal; then every 6 months
eAG	Less than 154 mg/dL (8.5 mmol/L)
Preprandial plasma glucose	70–130 mg/dL (3.9–7.2 mmol/L)
Peak postprandial plasma glucose[a]	Less than 180 mg/dL (less than 10.0 mmol/L)
Blood Pressure	Less than 130/80 mm Hg
	Evaluate at every visit
Lipids	Evaluate at least yearly
LDL	Less than 100 mg/dL (2.59 mmol/L) or less than 70 mg/dL (1.81 mmol/L) if high risk
HDL	Greater than 40 mg/dL (1.03 mmol/L) for males; greater than 50 mg/dL (1.29 mmol/L) for females
Triglycerides	Less than 150 mg/dL (1.70 mmol/L)
Monitoring for Complications	
Eyes	Dilated eye exam yearly
Feet	Feet should be examined at every visit
Urinary microalbumin	Yearly

A1c, hemoglobin A1c; ADA, American Diabetes Association; eAG, estimated average glucose; HDL, high-density lipoprotein; LDL, low-density lipoprotein.

[a]Peak postprandial glucose measurements should be made 1 to 2 hours after the beginning of the meal.

basal insulin response using intermediate- or long-acting insulin, whereas short- or rapid-acting insulin replicates bolus release of insulin physiologically seen around a meal in nondiabetics. A number of different regimens have been used through the years to more closely follow natural insulin patterns. As a rule, basal insulin makes up approximately 50% of the total daily dose. The remaining half is provided with bolus doses around three daily meals.

Exact doses are individualized to the patient and the amount of food consumed. T1DM patients frequently are started on about 0.6 unit/kg/day, and then doses are titrated until glycemic goals are reached. Most people with T1DM use between 0.6 and 1 unit/kg/day.

Currently, the most advanced form of insulin delivery is the insulin pump, also referred to as continuous subcutaneous insulin infusion (CSII). Using rapid-acting insulin only, these pumps are programmed to provide a slow release of small amounts of insulin as the basal portion of therapy, and larger boluses of insulin are injected by the patient to account for the consumption of food. Pramlintide, a synthetic analog of the naturally occurring hormone amylin, is another injectable blood glucose–lowering medication that can be used in people with T1DM or in people with T2DM using insulin for treatment. A more in-depth description is listed in the pharmacologic treatment section.

▶ *Type 2 Diabetes Mellitus*

Treatment of patients with T2DM has changed dramatically over the past decade with the addition of a number of new drugs and recommendations to maintain tighter glycemic control. **Figures 43–1** and **43–2** summarize 2009 treatment algorithms for T2DM.[27] Algorithms from AACE for T2DM can be found at *https://www.aace.com/sites/default/files/GlycemicControlAlgorithm.pdf* and from the 2012 ADA/European Association for the Study of Diabetes joint position statement at *http://care.diabetesjournals.org/content/early/2012/04/17/dc12-0413.short*. Lifestyle modifications including education, nutrition, and exercise are paramount to managing the disease successfully. Many patients assume that once pharmacologic therapy is initiated, lifestyle modifications are no longer necessary. Practitioners should

educate patients regarding this misconception. Because T2DM generally tends to be a progressive disease, blood glucose levels will eventually increase, making insulin therapy and lifestyle modifications the eventual required therapy in many patients. It may be necessary for patients to inject insulin to lower their blood glucose levels. Figure 43–2 is an illustration of a way to start insulin therapy while keeping the patient on some oral medications. This is usually done when several oral agents have been used with inadequate glucose-lowering results.[27]

▶ *Gestational Diabetes*

An individualized meal plan consisting of three meals and three snacks per day is commonly recommended in GDM. Preventing **ketosis**, promoting adequate growth of the fetus,

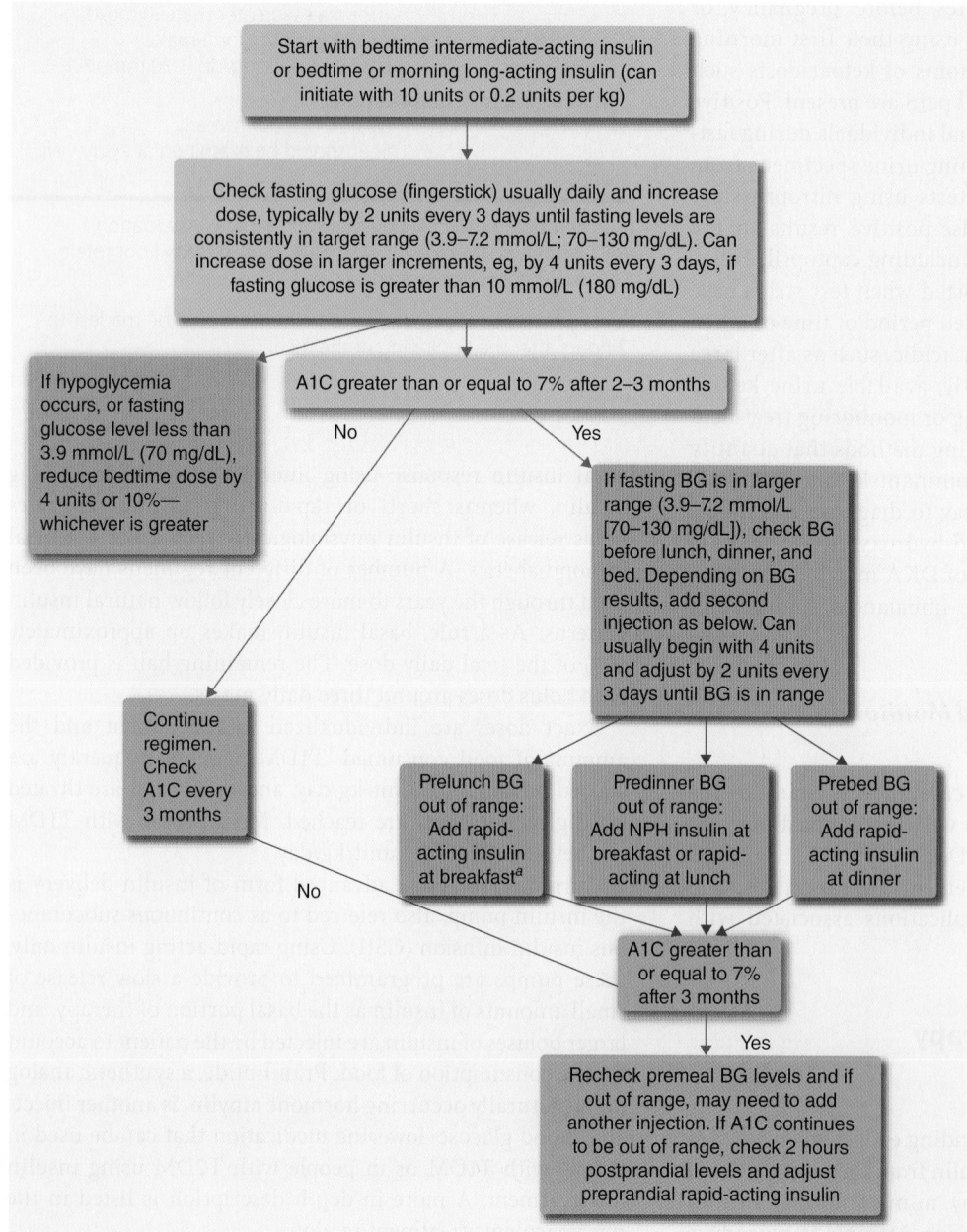

FIGURE 43–1. Initiation and adjustment of insulin regimens. Insulin regimens should be designed while taking lifestyle and meal schedule into account. The algorithm can only provide basic guidelines for initiation and adjustment of insulin. [a]Premixed insulins not recommended during adjustment of doses; however, they can be used conveniently, usually before breakfast and/or dinner, if the proportion of rapid- and intermediate-acting insulins is similar to the fixed proportions available. A1c of 7% is equivalent to 0.07 or 53 mmol/mol Hb. (A1c, hemoglobin A1c; BG, blood glucose; NPH, neutral protamine Hagedorn.) (Nathan DM, Buse JB, Davidson MB, et al. Medical management of hyperglycemia in type 2 diabetes: A consensus algorithm for the initiation and adjustment of therapy: A consensus statement from the American Diabetes Association and the European Association for the Study of Diabetes. Diabetes Care 2009;32:193–203; With permission.)

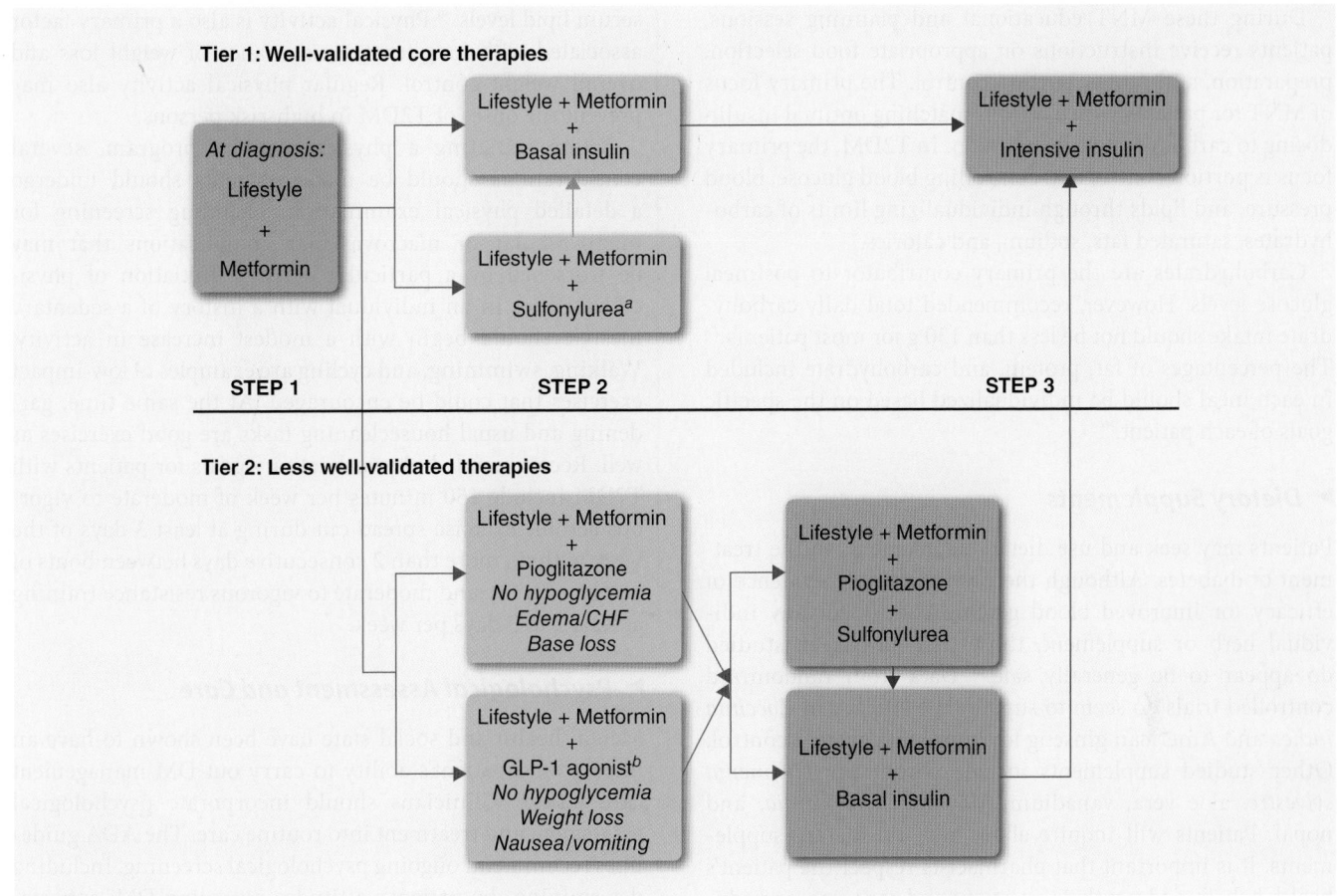

Tier 1: Well-validated core therapies

Tier 2: Less well-validated therapies

FIGURE 43–2. Algorithm for the metabolic management of type 2 diabetes mellitus; reinforce lifestyle interventions at every visit and check hemoglobin A1c every 3 months until A1c is less than 7% (0.07; 53 mmol/mol Hb) and then at least every 6 months. The interventions should be changed if A1c is greater than or equal to 7% (0.07; 53 mmol/mol Hb). [a]Sulfonylureas other than glybenclamide (glyburide) or chlorpropamide. [b]Insufficient clinical use to be confident regarding safety. See Figure 43–1 for initiation and adjustment of insulin. (CHF, congestive heart failure; GLP-1, glucagon-like peptide-1.) (Nathan DM, Buse JB, Davidson MB, et al. Medical management of hyperglycemia in type 2 diabetes: A consensus algorithm for the initiation and adjustment of therapy: A consensus statement from the American Diabetes Association and the European Association for the Study of Diabetes. Diabetes Care 2009;32:193–203; With permission.)

maintaining satisfactory blood glucose levels, and preventing nausea and other undesired GI side effects are desired goals in these patients. Controlling blood sugar levels is important to prevent harm to the baby. An abundance of glucose causes excessive insulin production by the fetus, which, if left uncontrolled, can lead to the development of an abnormally large fetus. Infant hypoglycemia at delivery, hyperbilirubinemia, and complications associated with delivery of a large baby also may occur when blood glucose levels are not controlled adequately.

Insulin should be used when blood glucose levels are not maintained adequately at target levels by diet and physical activity. Even though there have been small studies showing the safety of using glyburide, metformin, and insulin glargine during pregnancy, the use of these agents is not recommended as a general rule. In women who develop GDM and cannot control blood glucose levels with lifestyle modifications, the use of insulin detemir, insulin aspart, lispro, or regular insulin has category B safety ratings.

Nonpharmacologic Therapy

▶ *Medical Nutrition Therapy*

● Despite the popular notion, there is not a "diabetic diet," and the recommended meal plan for patients with diabetes should be low in fat, high in fiber, and low to moderate in calories and should achieve a balance of the various components and nutrients needed.[10] MNT is considered an integral component of diabetes management and diabetes self-management education. People with DM should receive individualized MNT, preferably by a registered dietitian. As part of the diabetes management plan, MNT should not be a single education session but rather an ongoing dialog. MNT should be customized to take into account cultural, lifestyle, and financial considerations. MNT plans should integrate a variety of foods that the patient enjoys and allow for flexibility to encourage patient empowerment and improve patient adherence.

During these MNT educational and planning sessions, patients receive instructions on appropriate food selection, preparation, and proper portion control. The primary focus of MNT for patients with T1DM is matching optimal insulin dosing to carbohydrate consumption. In T2DM, the primary focus is portion control and controlling blood glucose, blood pressure, and lipids through individualizing limits of carbohydrates, saturated fats, sodium, and calories.

Carbohydrates are the primary contributor to postmeal glucose levels. However, recommended total daily carbohydrate intake should not be less than 130 g for most patients.[28] The percentages of fat, protein, and carbohydrate included in each meal should be individualized based on the specific goals of each patient.[10]

▶ Dietary Supplements

Patients may seek and use dietary supplements in the treatment of diabetes. Although there is insufficient evidence of efficacy for improved blood glucose control for any individual herb or supplement, those that have been studied do appear to be generally safe.[29] Data from randomized controlled trials do seem to support the efficacy of *Coccinia indica* and American ginseng for improving glucose control. Other studied supplements include chromium, *Gymnema sylvestre*, aloe vera, vanadium, *Momordica charantia,* and nopal. Patients will inquire about and use dietary supplements. It is important that pharmacists respect the patient's health beliefs, address their questions and concerns, and educate them on the differences between dietary supplements and prescribed therapies.

▶ Weight Management

Moderate weight loss in patients with T2DM has been shown to reduce cardiovascular risk, as well as delay or prevent the onset of DM in those with prediabetes.[10,30] The recommended primary approach to weight loss is therapeutic lifestyle change (TLC), which integrates a 7% reduction in body weight and an increase in physical activity.[10] A slow but progressive weight loss of 0.45 to 0.91 kg (1 to 2 lb) per week is preferred.[31] Although individual target caloric goals should be set, a general rule for weight loss diets is that they should supply at least 1,000 to 1,200 kcal/day (about 4,200 to 5,000 kJ/day) for women and 1,200 to 1,600 kcal/day (about 5,000 to 6,700 kJ/day) for men. Because 80% of patients with T2DM are overweight, this strategy works best for these patients. Gastric reduction surgeries (gastric banding or procedures that bypass, transpose, or resect portions of the small intestine), when used as a part of a comprehensive approach to weight loss, are recommended for consideration in patients with T2DM and a BMI that exceeds 35 kg/m².[10]

▶ Physical Activity

Physical activity is also an important component of a comprehensive DM management program. Regular physical activity has been shown to improve blood glucose control and reduce cardiovascular risk factors such as hypertension and elevated serum lipid levels.[30] Physical activity is also a primary factor associated with long-term maintenance of weight loss and overall weight control. Regular physical activity also may prevent the onset of T2DM in high-risk persons.

Before initiating a physical activity program, several considerations should be made. Patients should undergo a detailed physical examination, including screening for microvascular or macrovascular complications that may be worsened by a particular activity. Initiation of physical activities in an individual with a history of a sedentary lifestyle should begin with a modest increase in activity. Walking, swimming, and cycling are examples of low-impact exercises that could be encouraged. At the same time, gardening and usual housecleaning tasks are good exercises as well. Recommended physical activity goals for patients with T2DM include 150 minutes per week of moderate to vigorous aerobic exercise spread out during at least 3 days of the week with no more than 2 consecutive days between bouts of aerobic activity and moderate to vigorous resistance training at least 2 to 3 days per week.

▶ Psychological Assessment and Care

Mental health and social state have been shown to have an impact on a patient's ability to carry out DM management care tasks.[10] Clinicians should incorporate psychological assessment and treatment into routine care. The ADA guidelines recommend ongoing psychological screening, including determining the patient's attitudes regarding DM; expectations of medical management and outcomes; mood and affect; general and diabetes-related quality of life; and financial, social, and emotional resources. Patients demonstrating poor self-management should be screened for diabetes-related distress, depression, anxiety, an eating disorder, and/or cognitive impairment.

▶ Immunizations

Influenza and pneumonia are common preventable infectious diseases that increase mortality and morbidity in persons with chronic diseases, including DM. Yearly influenza vaccinations, commonly called flu shots, are recommended for all patients with DM 6 months of age or older. Pneumococcal vaccination is also recommended for patients with DM who are 2 years of age or older as a one-time vaccination. A one-time revaccination is indicated for those older than age 64 years who were previously vaccinated when they were younger than 65 years old if the vaccine was administered more than 5 years earlier. Revaccination is also indicated in those with nephrotic syndrome or chronic renal disease and after transplantation. The hepatitis B vaccine series should also be administered as per the Center for Disease Control and Prevention's recommendations in patients with diabetes.

Pharmacotherapy

❻ *Oral and injectable agents are available to treat patients with T2DM who are unable to achieve glycemic control through meal planning and physical activity.* Currently, there are 11 classes of blood glucose–lowering agents available for the treatment of diabetes, including eight classes of oral agents and three injectable classes. Figure 43–1 shows a way to start insulin therapy for people with T2DM who are going to continue to take oral glucose-lowering medications.[27] Table 43–8[27,31,32] lists the oral agents, Figure 43–2 displays the ADA Treatment Algorithm for Patients with T2DM,[27] and Table 43–9 lists each non-insulin drug class with site of action and mechanism of action. The various classes of blood glucose–lowering agents target different organs and have different mechanisms of action. Each of these agents may be used individually or in combination with other medications that target different organs for synergistic effects.

▶ Sulfonylureas

Sulfonylureas represent the first class of oral blood glucose-lowering agents approved for use in the United States. These drugs are classified as being either first- or second-generation agents. Both classes of sulfonylureas are equally effective when given at equipotent doses. Today, the vast majority of patients receiving a sulfonylurea are prescribed a second-generation agent.

Sulfonylureas enhance insulin secretion by blocking ATP-sensitive potassium channels in the cell membranes of pancreatic β cells.[13] This action results in membrane depolarization, allowing an influx of calcium to cause the translocation of secretory granules of insulin to the cell surface, and enhances insulin secretion in a non–glucose-dependent manner. However, the extent of insulin secretion depends on the blood glucose level. Whereas more insulin is released in response to higher blood glucose levels, the additional insulin secretion from sulfonylureas is less at near-normal glucose levels. Insulin is then transported through the portal vein to the liver, suppressing hepatic glucose production.

All sulfonylureas undergo hepatic biotransformation, with most agents being metabolized by the cytochrome P450 2C9 pathway. The first-generation sulfonylureas are more likely to cause drug interactions than second-generation agents. All sulfonylureas except tolbutamide require a dosage adjustment or are not recommended in renal impairment.[32] In elderly patients or those with compromised renal or hepatic function, lower starting dosages are necessary.

Sulfonylureas' blood glucose–lowering effects can be observed in both fasting and postprandial levels. Monotherapy with these agents generally produce a 1.5% to 2% (0.015 to 0.02 or 16 to 22 mmol/mol Hg) decline in A1c concentrations and a 60- to 70-mg/dL (3.3 to 3.9 mmol/L) reduction in FBG levels.[13] Secondary failure with these drugs occurs at a rate of 5% to 7% per year as a result of continued pancreatic β-cell destruction. One limitation of sulfonylurea therapy is the inability of these products to stimulate insulin release from β cells at extremely high glucose levels, a phenomenon called glucose toxicity. Common adverse effects include hypoglycemia and weight gain. There may be some cross-sensitivity in patients with sulfa allergy.

▶ Nonsulfonylurea Secretagogues (Glinides)

Although producing the same effect as sulfonylureas, non-sulfonylurea secretagogues, also referred to as meglitinides, have a much shorter onset and duration of action. Glitinide secretagogues also produce a pharmacologic effect by interacting with ATP-sensitive potassium channels on the β cells; however, this binding is to a receptor adjacent to those to which sulfonylureas bind.

The primary benefit of nonsulfonylurea secretagogues is in reducing postmeal glucose levels. These agents have demonstrated a reduction in A1c levels between 0.8% and 1% (0.008 and 0.01; 9 to 11 mmol/mol Hb). Because they have a rapid onset and short duration of action, they are to be taken 15 to 30 minutes before a meal.

They also may be used in combination therapy with other drugs to achieve synergistic effects. Combinations with biguanides are most commonly seen.

▶ Biguanides

The only biguanide approved by the Food and Drug Administration (FDA) and currently available in the United States is metformin. Metformin was approved in the United States in 1995. This agent is thought to lower blood glucose by decreasing hepatic glucose production and increasing insulin sensitivity in both hepatic and peripheral muscle tissues; however, the exact mechanism of action remains unknown. Metformin lowers both fasting blood sugar (FBS) and post-meal blood glucose.[31] It has been shown to reduce A1c levels by 1.5 to 2% (0.015 to 0.02; 16 to 22 mmol/mol Hb) and FPG levels by 60 to 80 mg/dL (3.3 to 4.4 mmol/L) when used as monotherapy.[13] Unlike the sulfonylureas, metformin retains the ability to reduce fasting glucose levels when they are over 300 mg/dL (16.7 mmol/L). Metformin does not affect insulin release from β cells of the pancreas, so hypoglycemia is not a common side effect.[32]

Metformin significantly reduced all-cause mortality and the risk of stroke in overweight patients with T2DM compared with intensive therapy with sulfonylurea or insulin in the UKPDS.[33] It also reduced diabetes-related death and myocardial infarction compared with a conventional therapy arm. Given that metformin is the only oral antihyperglycemic medication proven to reduce mortality and is available generically, the ADA treatment algorithm (see Fig. 43–2) considers lifestyle modification and metformin as first-line therapy for T2DM.[27]

Metformin has been shown to produce beneficial effects on serum lipid levels and has become a first-line agent for T2DM patients with metabolic syndrome. On average, triglyceride and low-density lipoprotein (LDL) cholesterol levels may be reduced by as much as 18.69% and 12.09%, respectively, but HDL cholesterol may improve by as much as 1.17%.[34] Metformin is often used in combination with a sulfonylurea or a thiazolidinedione (TZD) for synergistic effects.

Metformin does not undergo significant protein binding and is eliminated from the body unchanged in the urine. Patients with a calculated creatinine clearance of

Table 43-8

Oral Agents for the Treatment of T2DM[27,31,32]

Drug Class	Target Organ	Blood Glucose Affected	Adjustment for Renal Impairment CrCl 30–50 mL/min (0.50–0.83 mL/s)	Adjustment for Renal Impairment CrCl Less Than 30 mL/min (0.50 mL/s)	Adjustment for Hepatic Impairment	Common Adverse Drug Reactions	Trade	Generic/Commercially Available	Dosing Strategy (All Agents Are Taken Orally)
α-Glucosidase Inhibitors	Brush border of small intestine	Postprandial	Serum creatinine more than 2 mg/dL (177 μmol/L): Not recommended	Serum creatinine more than 2 mg/dL (177 μmol/L): Not recommended	No specific dose adjustment recommended	GI (flatulence, diarrhea)	Precose	Acarbose/Y	25 mg 3 × daily with first bite of each main meal. Advance at 4–8 week intervals to a maximum of 100 mg 3 × daily
			Serum creatinine more than 2 mg/dL (177 μmol/L): Not recommended	Serum creatinine more than 2 mg/dL (177 μmol/L): Not recommended	No adjustment necessary	GI (flatulence, diarrhea)	Glyset	Miglitol/N	25 mg 3 × daily with first bite of each main meal. Advance at 4–8 week intervals to a maximum of 100 mg 3 × daily
Glitinides (should not be used in combination with other insulin secretagogues)	Pancreas	Postprandial	20–40 mL/min (0.33–0.67 mL/s): Initial dose: 0.5 mg with careful titration	Less than 20 mL/min (0.33 mL/s): Not studied	Use conservative initial and maintenance doses and use longer intervals between dose adjustments	Hypoglycemia (although less risk than with sulfonylureas)	Prandin	Repaglinide/N	0.5 mg 15–30 minutes before each meal. Double preprandial dose every 7 days to a maximum of 4 mg/dose or 16 mg/day (To be taken only if eating)
			No specific dose adjustment recommended	Use with caution in severe dysfunction	No dose adjustment needed in mild impairment; use with caution in moderate to severe dysfunction	Hypoglycemia (although less than with sulfonylureas)	Starlix	Nateglinide/Y	120 mg 3 × day before meals (To be taken only if eating)
Second-generation sulfonylureas	Pancreas	Fasting and postprandial	Not recommended	Not recommended	Use conservative dosing and avoid in severe disease	Hypoglycemia, weight gain	Micronase	Glyburide/Y	1.5–3 mg/day with breakfast. Increase by 1.5 mg weekly to a maximum of 12 mg/day
			Not recommended	Not recommended	Use conservative dosing and avoid in severe disease	Hypoglycemia, weight gain	DiaBeta	Glyburide/Y	2.5–5 mg/day with breakfast. Increase by 2.5 mg weekly to a maximum of 20 mg/day
			No specific dose adjustment recommended	No specific dose adjustment recommended	Initial dose: 2.5 mg/day	Hypoglycemia, weight gain	Glucotrol	Glipizide/Y	5 mg/day 30 minutes before a meal. Increase by 5 mg weekly to a maximum of 40 mg/day; divide dose if greater than 15 mg/day

(Continued)

Class	Medication (Generic)/Generic available	Brand	Site of action	Glucose effect	Adverse effects	Hepatic impairment	Renal impairment	Usual dosing
	Glipizide ER/Y	Glucatrol XL			Hypoglycemia, weight gain	No specific dose adjustment recommended	No specific dose adjustment recommended	5 mg once daily before a meal Increase by 5 mg weekly to a maximum of 20 mg/day
	Glimeperide/Y	Amaryl			Hypoglycemia, weight gain	No specific dose adjustment recommended	Less than 22 mL/min (0.37 mL/s): Initial starting dose should be 1 mg	1-2 mg with breakfast Increase by 2 mg every 1-2 weeks to a maximum of 8 mg/day
Biguanides	Metformin/Y	Glucophage Fortamet Riomet	Liver	Fasting and postprandial	GI (diarrhea, abdominal pain)	Avoid	Avoid	500 mg/day to twice daily with meals Advance weekly to a maximum of 2000-2550 mg/day
	Metformin, ER/Y	Glucophage ER, Glumetza				Avoid	Avoid	500-1000 mg/day; dose may be increased by 500 mg weekly to a maximum of 2000 mg/day
Thiazolidinediones	Pioglitazone/N	Actos	Peripheral tissue	Fasting and postprandial	Weight gain	Clearance lower in Child-Pugh grade B/C; do not start if transaminases more than 2.5 × ULN and discontinue if ALT rises to and remains at more than 3 times ULN	No adjustment necessary	15-30 mg/day Increase after 12 weeks to a maximum of 45 mg/day
Dipeptidyl peptidase-4 inhibitors	Sitagliptin/N	Januvia	GI tract (increases GLP-1)	Fasting and postprandial	Upper respiratory, diarrhea	Child-Pugh score 7-9: No dosage adjustment necessary Child Pugh score more than 9: Not studied	25 mg once daily / 50 mg once daily	100 mg/day
	Saxagliptin/N	Onglyza			UTI, headache	No dose adjustment necessary	2.5 mg once daily	2.5 or 5 mg once daily
	Linagliptin/N	Tradjenta			Headache, arthralgia, nasopharyngitis	No dose adjustment necessary	No dose adjustment necessary	5 mg/day
Dopamine receptor agonist	Bromocriptine mesylate/N	Cycloset	Hypothalamus	Postprandial	Nausea, headache	No specific dose adjustment recommended, although adjustment may be necessary because of extensive hepatic metabolism	No dose adjustment necessary	0.8 mg once daily within 2 hours of waking; may increase in weekly intervals to 4.8 mg once daily
Bile acid sequestrant	Colesevelam/N	Welchol	Intestinal lumen	Fasting	Constipation	No dose adjustment necessary	No dose adjustment necessary	1.875 g twice daily or 3.75 g once daily

ALT, alanine aminotransferase; CrCl, creatinine clearance; ER, extended release; GI, gastrointestinal; GLP-1, glucagon-like peptide-1; ULN, upper limit of normal; UTI, urinary tract infection.

> **Table 43–9**
>
> ### Site and Mechanism of Action for Non-Insulin Agents
>
> | Site of Action | Drug Class | Mechanism of Action |
> |---|---|---|
> | Pancreas | Sulfonylureas | Enhance insulin secretion |
> | | Nonsulfonylurea secretagogues | Enhance insulin secretion |
> | | GLP-1 agonists | Enhance insulin secretion and suppress glucagon secretion |
> | | Pramlintide | Suppresses glucagon secretion |
> | Liver | Biguanide | Decreases hepatic glucose production and increases insulin sensitivity |
> | | Thiazolidinedione | Increases insulin sensitivity |
> | Muscle | Biguanide | Increases insulin sensitivity |
> | | Thiazolidinedione | Increases insulin sensitivity |
> | Adipose tissue | Thiazolidinedione | Increases insulin sensitivity |
> | Intestines | GLP-1 agonists | Increase satiety and regulate gastric emptying |
> | | Pramlintide | Increases satiety and regulates gastric emptying |
> | | Dipeptidyl peptidase-4 inhibitors | Increase endogenous GLP-1 |
> | | α-Glucosidase Inhibitors | Delay the absorption of carbohydrates |

GLP-1, glucagon-like peptide-1

less than 60 mL/min (1.0 mL/s) should not receive this product.[32] It is contraindicated in patients with a serum creatinine level greater than or equal to 1.4 mg/dL (124 μmol/L) in women and 1.5 mg/dL (133 μmol/L) in men. It should not be initiated in patients 80 years of age or older unless normal renal function has been established. Additionally, therapy with metformin should be withheld in patients undergoing surgery or radiographic procedures in which a nephrotoxic dye is used. Therapy should be withheld the day of the radiographic procedure, and renal function should be assessed 48 hours after the procedure. If renal function is normal, therapy may be resumed.

Primary side effects associated with metformin therapy are GI in nature, including decreased appetite, nausea, and diarrhea. These side effects can be minimized through slow titration of the dose and often subside within 2 weeks.[27] Interference with vitamin B$_{12}$ absorption has also been reported.[13]

Biguanides such as metformin are thought to inhibit mitochondrial oxidation of lactic acid, thereby increasing the chance of lactic acidosis occurring. Fortunately, the incidence of lactic acidosis in clinical practice is rare. Patients at greatest risk for developing lactic acidosis include those with renal impairment and those who are of advanced age.[32] Metformin should be withheld promptly in cases of hypoxemia, sepsis, or dehydration. Patients should avoid consumption of excessive amounts of alcohol while taking metformin, and use of the drug should be avoided in patients with liver disease. It is common practice to evaluate liver function before initiation of metformin.

▶ Thiazolidinediones

Commonly referred to as TZDs or glitazones, thiazolidinediones have established a role in T2DM therapy. TZDs are known to increase insulin sensitivity by stimulating peroxisome proliferator-activated receptor gamma (PPAR-γ).[13] Stimulation of PPAR-γ results in a number of intracellular

and extracellular changes including increased insulin sensitivity and decreased plasma fatty acid levels. As monotherapy, TZDs reduce FPG levels by around 60 to 70 mg/dL (3.3 to 3.9 mmol/L), and the effect on A1c is an up to 1.5% (0.015; 16 mmol/mol Hb) reduction. The onset of action for TZDs is delayed for several weeks and may require up to 12 weeks before maximum effects are observed.

Additional effects of TZDs are seen in the lipid profile. Both pioglitazone and rosiglitazone increase HDL cholesterol, with rosiglitazone increasing HDL an average of 2.4 mg/dL (0.06 mmol/L) and pioglitazone increasing HDL an average of 5.2 mg/dL (0.13 mmol/L).[34] Pioglitazone has been shown to decrease serum triglycerides 51.9 mg/dL (0.59 mmol/L) on average, but an increase in triglycerides has been observed with rosiglitazone. LDL cholesterol concentrations increase by 12.3 mg/dL (0.32 mmol/L) and 21.3 mg/dL (0.55 mmol/L) on average with pioglitazone and rosiglitazone, respectively.

The TZDs may produce fluid retention and edema; the mechanism by which this occurs is not completely understood.[13] It is known that blood volume increases approximately 10% with these agents, resulting in approximately 4% to 5% of patients developing edema. Thus, these drugs are contraindicated in situations in which an increased fluid volume is detrimental such as heart failure. Fluid retention appears to be dose related and increases when combined with insulin therapy.

A few cases of hepatotoxicity have been reported with rosiglitazone and pioglitazone, but no serious complications have been reported, and symptoms typically reverse within several weeks of discontinuing therapy. Liver function tests should be performed at baseline and periodically. Patients with a baseline alanine aminotransferase (ALT) level greater than 2.5 times the upper limit of normal should not receive a TZD. If ALT levels rise to greater than three times the upper limit of normal in patients receiving a TZD and remain there, the medication should be discontinued.

Increased rates of upper and lower limb fractures are also known to occur with TZD therapy compared with other antihyperglycemic agents and, for this reason, the patient's baseline fracture risk should be considered before beginning TZD therapy. Premenopausal anovulatory women may begin to ovulate on TZD therapy, and therefore counseling should be provided to all women capable of becoming pregnant regarding this. As TZD therapy is pregnancy category C, proper precautions to avoid pregnancy should be used. In June 2011, the FDA alerted healthcare providers and patients that pioglitazone was found to be associated with an increased risk of bladder cancer after 1 year of therapy in an ongoing epidemiologic study.[32] Although this study is ongoing, risk seems highest with higher dose exposure and longer duration of therapy. For this reason, patients with active bladder cancer should not use pioglitazone, and the drug should be used with caution in those with a history of bladder cancer.

A 2007 meta-analysis conducted by Nissen and colleagues reported a significantly greater risk of myocardial infarction with rosiglitazone compared with other oral agents.[35] A subsequent prospective study found rosiglitazone use to be associated with a nonsignificant increase in myocardial infarction risk and a nonsignificant reduction in stroke, but a trend toward increased cardiovascular risk in those patients with a history of ischemic heart disease.[36] In May 2011, the FDA chose to restrict access and distribution of rosiglitazone.[32] It is currently only available through the Avandia-Rosiglitazone Medicines Access Program for patients currently clinically benefitting from the drug and in those with T2DM who cannot achieve adequate disease management with other agents or who are not willing to use pioglitazone-containing medications after counseling with their healthcare provider.

▶ α-Glucosidase Inhibitors

Acarbose and miglitol are α-glucosidase inhibitors currently approved in the United States. An enzyme that is along the brush boarder of the intestine cells called α-glucosidase breaks down complex carbohydrates into simple sugars, resulting in absorption.[13] The α-glucosidase inhibitors work by delaying the absorption of carbohydrates from the intestinal tract, which reduces the rise in postprandial blood glucose concentrations. As monotherapy, α-glucosidase inhibitors primarily reduce postprandial glucose excursions. FPG concentrations have been decreased by between 40 and 50 mg/dL (2.2 and 2.8 mmol/L); however, A1c reductions range only from 0.3% to 1% (0.003 to 0.01; 3 to 11 mmol/mol Hb). Although these agents have been popular in Europe and other parts of the world, they have failed to gain widespread use in the United States. High incidences of GI side effects, including flatulence (42% to 74%), abdominal discomfort (12% to 19%), and diarrhea (29% to 31%), have limited their use.[32] GI side effects occur as the result of intestinal bacteria in the distal gut metabolizing undigested carbohydrates and producing carbon dioxide and methane gas.[13] Low initial doses followed by gradual titration may minimize GI side effects. The α-glucosidase inhibitors are contraindicated in

patients with short bowel syndrome or inflammatory bowel disease. In addition, neither drug in this class is recommended for patients with a serum creatinine greater than 2 mg/dL (177 μmol/L).

▶ Dipeptidyl Peptidase-4 Inhibitors (Gliptins)

Sitagliptin, saxagliptin, and linagliptin are agents in a new class of diabetes drugs called dipeptidyl peptidase-4 (DPP-4) inhibitors. They are approved as adjunct to diet and exercise to improve glycemic control in adults with T2DM.[32] These agents lower blood glucose concentrations by inhibiting DPP-4, the enzyme that degrades endogenous GLP-1.[13] DPP-4 inhibitors increase the amount of endogenous GLP-1. The blood glucose–lowering effect of the gliptins is primarily on postprandial levels. Typical A1c reductions are 0.7% to 1% (0.007 to 0.01; 8 to 11 mmol/mol Hb). Common adverse effects include headache and nasopharyngitis. Hypoglycemia is not a common adverse effect with these agents because insulin secretion results from GLP-1 activation caused by meal-related glucose detection and not from direct pancreatic β-cell stimulation. Dosage adjustments for sitagliptin to 50 and 25 mg/day are recommended for patients with moderate (creatinine clearance, 30 to 49 mL/min [0.5 to 0.82 mL/s]) and severe (creatinine clearance less than 30 mL/min [0.50 mL/s]) renal impairment, respectively. Saxagliptin should be dosed at 2.5 mg/day with creatinine clearance less than 50 mL/min (0.83 mL/s) or if strong CYP3A4/5 inhibitors are being used concomitantly. Linagliptin, a substrate of CYP3A4, is dosed at 5 mg/day and requires no adjustment for renal or hepatic impairment.[32]

The FDA revised the prescribing information for sitagliptin and sitagliptin–metformin to include information on reported cases of acute pancreatitis in patients using these products after postmarketing cases of acute pancreatitis, including hemorrhagic and necrotizing pancreatitis, were reported in patients taking sitagliptin.

▶ Central-Acting Dopamine Agonist

A quick release formulation of a central-acting dopamine agonist, bromocriptine, was approved by the FDA in May 2009 for the treatment of T2DM. The mechanism of action for how bromocriptine regulates glycemic control is unknown, but data indicate that bromocriptine administered in the morning improves insulin sensitivity, and this is likely a result of its affect on dopamine oscillations.[13] When used to treat patients with T2DM, bromocriptine should be taken 2 hours after waking in the morning with food.[32] The initial dose is 0.8 mg, titrated up weekly until a maximum dosage of 4.8 mg/day is achieved. A modest A1c reduction of 0.1% to 0.4% (0.001 to 0.004; 1 to 4 mmol/mol Hb) can be expected from this drug.[13] Main side effects include rhinitis, dizziness, asthenia, headache, sinusitis, constipation, and nausea, and 24% of patients in clinical trials stopped taking bromocriptine because of untoward effects. Contraindications include syncopal migraine and women who are nursing.[32]

▶ Bile Acid Sequestrants

Colesevelam is the only bile acid sequestrant currently approved as an adjunctive therapy to improve glycemic control in conjunction with diet, exercise, and insulin or oral agents for the treatment of T2DM. It acts on the intestinal lumen to bind bile acid, but whether this is the drug's only action that results in plasma glucose lowering or if a secondary systemic effect to bile acid binding is unknown.[13] An A1c reduction of approximately 0.4% (0.004; 4 mmol/mol Hb) can be expected when added to metformin, sulfonylurea, or insulin. FPG is reduced about 5 to 10 mg/dL (0.3 to 0.6 mmol/L). LDL cholesterol is reduced 12% to 16%. Dosing for T2DM is six 625-mg tablets daily, which may be split into three tablets twice daily. Alternatively, a 3.75-g oral suspension can be used daily or a 1.875-g oral suspension packet can be used twice daily dissolved in a minimum of one-half to one cup of water. Common adverse effects include constipation and dyspepsia. Drug–drug interactions are possible because of absorption and can be particularly important in patients who are taking levothyroxine, glyburide, oral contraceptives, phenytoin, warfarin, and digoxin. These medications should not be taken together, and they should be separated by at least 4 hours before dosing colesevelam. Malabsorption of fat-soluble vitamins (A, D, E, and K) is also a concern.

▶ Insulin

Insulin is the one agent that can be used in all types of DM and has no specific maximum dose, meaning it can be titrated to suit each individual patient's needs. ❼ *Insulin is the primary treatment to lower blood glucose levels for patients with T1DM, and injected amylin can be added to decrease fluctuations in blood glucose levels.* An insulin treatment algorithm for T2DM is found in Figure 43–2.[27]

Insulin is available commercially in various formulations that vary markedly in terms of onset and duration of action. Insulin can be divided into two main classes, basal and bolus, based on their length of action to mimic endogenous insulin physiology. Most formulations are available as U-100, indicating a concentration of 100 unit/mL. Insulin is typically refrigerated, and most vials are good for 28 days at room temperature.[32] Insulin detemir can be stored at room temperature for 42 days. Specific details of insulin products are listed in Table 43–10.[32,37]

The most common route of administration for insulin is subcutaneous injection using a syringe or pen device. Patients should be educated to rotate their injection sites to minimize lipohypertrophy, a buildup of fat that decreases or prevents proper insulin absorption. Additionally, patients should understand that the absorption rate may vary among injection sites (abdomen, thigh, arm, and buttocks) because of differences in blood flow, with absorption occurring fastest in the abdomen and slowest in the buttocks. Differences in absorption of insulin based on site of injection do not appear to be significant when analog insulins such as aspart, detemir, glargine, glulisine, and lispro are administered.

Insulin syringes are distinguished according to the syringe capacity, syringe markings, and needle gauge, and length. Insulin pens are self-contained systems of insulin delivery. The primary advantage of the pen system is the patient does not have to draw up the dose from the insulin vial.

Bolus Insulins

Regular Insulin. Regular insulin is unmodified crystalline insulin commonly referred to as natural or human insulin. It is a clear solution that has a relatively short onset and duration of action and is designed to cover insulin response to meals. On subcutaneous injection, regular insulin forms small aggregates called hexamers that undergo conversion to dimers followed by monomers before systemic absorption can occur. Patients should be counseled to inject regular insulin subcutaneously 30 minutes before consuming a meal. Regular insulin is the only insulin that can be administered IV.

Rapid-Acting Insulin. Three rapid-acting insulins have been approved in the United States: aspart, glulisine, and lispro. Substitution of one or two amino acids in regular insulin results in the unique pharmacokinetic properties characteristic of these agents. The onset of action of rapid-acting insulins varies from 15 to 30 minutes, with peak effects occurring 1 to 2 hours after administration and is dosed before or with meals.

Basal Insulins

Intermediate-Duration Insulin. Neutral protamine Hagedorn, better known as NPH insulin, is prepared by a process in which protamine is conjugated with regular insulin, rendering a product with a delayed onset but extended duration of action, and is designed to cover insulin requirements in between meals and/or overnight. With the advent of the long-acting insulins, NPH insulin use has declined because of (a) an inability to predict accurately when peak effects occur and (b) a duration of action of less than 24 hours. Additionally, protamine is a foreign protein that may increase the possibility of an allergic reaction.

NPH insulin can be mixed with regular insulin and used immediately or stored for future use up to 1 month at room temperature or 3 months in refrigeration. NPH insulin can be mixed with either aspart or lispro insulins, but it must be injected immediately after mixing. Whenever mixing insulin products with NPH insulin, the shorter acting insulin should be drawn into the syringe first.

Long-Duration Insulin. Two long-duration insulin preparations are approved for use in the United States. Glargine and detemir are designed as once-daily-dosing basal insulins. Insulin glargine differs from regular insulin by three amino acids, resulting in a low solubility at physiologic pH. The clear solution is supplied at a pH of 4, which precipitates on subcutaneous administration. Detemir binds to albumin in the plasma, which gives it sustained action. Neither glargine nor detemir can be administered IV or mixed with other insulin products.

Both glargine and detemir have been shown to produce slower, more prolonged absorption and a relatively constant concentration over 24 hours as compared with NPH. Although detemir is recommended for dosing in the evening

Table 43–10

Insulin Agents for the Treatment of T1DM and T2DM[32,37]

Generic Name (Insulin)	Brand/Rx Only	Manufacturer	Strength	Onset (minutes)	Peak (hours)	Duration (hours)	Administration Options
Rapid-Acting Insulin							
Lispro	Humalog/yes	Eli Lilly	U-100	15–30	0.5–2.5	3–4	10-mL vial, 3-mL cartridge, and disposable pen
Aspart	Novolog/yes	Novo-Nordisk	U-100	15–30	1–3	3–5	10-mL vial, 3-mL cartridge, and disposable pen
Glulisine	Apidra/yes	Aventis	U-100	15–30	1–2	3–4	10-mL vial, 3-mL cartridge, and disposable pen
Short-Acting Insulin							
Regular	Humulin R/no	Eli Lilly	U-100, U-500	30–60	2–3	3–6	U-100 10-mL vial; U-500 20-mL vial
	Novolin R/no	Novo-Nordisk	U-100				10-mL vial, 3-mL cartridge, 3-mL *Innolet*
Intermediate-Acting Insulin							
Neutral protamine Hagedorn	Humulin N/no	Eli Lilly	U-100	2–4 hours	4–6	8–12	10-mL vial, 3-mL cartridge
	Novolin N/no	Novo-Nordisk	U-100				10-mL vial, 3-mL cartridge, 3-mL *InnoLet*
Long-Acting Insulin							
Glargine	Lantus/yes	Aventis	U-100	4–5 hours	Flat	22–24	10-mL vial, 3-mL cartridge for *Opticlik* (available in SoloSTAR disposable pen)
Detemir	Levemir/yes	Novo-Nordisk	U-100	3–4 hours	Flat	Up to 24	10-mL vial, 3-mL cartridge, 3-mL *Innolet*, 3-mL disposable *FlexPen*
Combination Insulin Products							
Neutral protamine Hagedorn and regular	Humulin 70/30/no	Eli Lilly	U-100	30–60	1.5–16	10–16	10-mL vial, 3-mL disposable pen
	Novolin 70/30/no	Novo Nordisk	U-100	30–60	2–12	10–16	10-mL vial, 3-mL cartridge, 3-mL *Innolet*
	Humulin 50/50/no	Eli Lilly	U-100	30–60	2–5.5	10–16	10-mL vial
Neutral protamine lispro and lispro	Humalog Mix 75/25/yes	Eli Lilly	U-100	15–30	1–6.5	15–18	10-mL vial, 3-mL disposable pen
Neutral protamine aspart and aspart	Novolog Mix 70/30/yes	Novo Nordisk	U-100	15–30	1–4	Up to 24	10-mL vial, 3-mL cartridge, 3-mL disposable *FlexPen*

if being used as a once-daily dose, it stands to reason that both glargine and detemir could be administered irrespective of meals or time of day.

Combination Insulin Products A number of combination insulin products are available commercially. NPH is available in combinations of 70/30 (70% NPH and 30% regular insulin) and 50/50 (50% NPH and 50% regular insulin). Two short-acting insulin analog mixtures are also available. Humalog mix 75/25 contains 75% insulin lispro protamine suspension and 25% insulin lispro. Novolog mix 70/30 contains 70% insulin aspart protamine suspension and 30% insulin aspart. The lispro and aspart insulin protamine suspensions were developed specifically for these mixture products and are not commercially available separately.

▶ Insulin Pump Therapy

Insulin pump therapy consists of a programmable infusion device that allows for basal infusion of insulin 24 hours daily

(Fig. 43–3), as well as bolus administration before meals and snacks. Currently, there are seven commercially available insulin pumps in the United States. Regular or rapid-acting insulin is delivered from a reservoir either by infusion set tubing or through a small canula. Most pump infusion sets are inserted in the abdomen, arm, or other infusion site by a small needle. Most patients prefer insertion in abdominal tissue because this site provides optimal insulin absorption. Infusion sets should be changed every 2 to 3 days to reduce the possibility of infection.

Patients use a carbohydrate-to-insulin ratio to determine how many units of insulin are required. More specifically, an individual's ratio is calculated to determine how many units of the specific insulin being used in the pump "covers" for a certain amount of carbohydrates to be ingested at a particular meal. The 450 rule (for regular insulin) or the 500 rule (for rapid-acting insulin) is commonly used. To calculate the ratio using the 500 rule, the patient would divide 500 by his or her total daily dose of insulin. For example, if a patient were using 25 units of insulin daily, his or her carbohydrate-to-insulin

FIGURE 43–3. Insulin pump and placement.

Skin

Catheter

Fat

Insulin

Dosage instructions are entered into the pump's small computer and the appropriate amount of insulin is then injected into the body in a calculated, controlled manner

Insulin pump

ratio would be 500:25, or 20:1. This ratio theoretically means that 1 unit of rapid-acting insulin should cover 20 g of carbohydrate. If blood sugar levels are below or above the desired blood glucose target, the amount of insulin can be adjusted. Once this ratio is determined, patients can eat more or fewer carbohydrates at a given meal and adjust the bolus dose accordingly.

In addition to mealtime boluses, correction doses based on premeal glucose readings are also used. The amount of additional insulin for the correction is based on either the 1500 rule for regular insulin or the 1800 rule for rapid-acting insulin. For example, if using rapid-acting insulin, divide 1800 by the patient's total daily insulin dose. The resulting value will represent the reduction in glucose (mg/dL) produced by one unit of insulin. If a patient is injecting 10 units of rapid-acting insulin before each of his or her 3 meals and 20 units of Lantus in the evening, his or her total daily dose would be 60 units. Using the 1800 rule, we find that 1800 divided by 60 is 30. Thus, 1 unit of rapid-acting insulin would be added for every 30 mg/dL the patient's glucose is above the premeal goal as a correction factor. The correction dose would be given in addition to the bolus dose needed based on the patient's carbohydrate-to-insulin ratio and the amount of carbohydrates present in the meal he or she is about to consume.

Insulin pump therapy may be used to lower blood glucose levels in any type of DM; however, patients with T1DM are the most likely candidates to use these devices. Use of an insulin pump may improve blood glucose control, reduce wide fluctuations in blood glucose levels, and allow individuals to have more flexibility in timing and content of meals and exercise schedules. Insulin pump therapy is not for everyone, and the complexity associated with its use, cost, increased need for blood glucose monitoring, and psychological factors may prevent individuals from using this technology optimally.

▶ Noninsulin Injectable Agents

Glucagon-Like Peptide 1 Agonists Glucagon-like peptide 1 (GLP-1) agonists enhance glucose-dependent insulin secretion while suppressing inappropriately high glucagon secretion in the presence of elevated glucose, which results in reduced hepatic glucose production.[13] These agents are also a part of the group of drugs that act as insulin agonists by producing supraphysiologic levels of GLP-1 (Table 43–11).[13,38,39] Exenatide and liraglutide are both indicated for the treatment of T2DM to improve glycemic control.[32] In a 26-week head-to-head trial in patients with T2DM with a baseline A1c between 7% and 11% (0.07 and 0.11; 53 and 97 mmol/mol Hb) who were taking metformin, sulfonylurea, or both, exenatide lowered A1c 0.8% (0.008; 9 mmol/mol Hb), but liraglutide lowered A1c a significantly greater amount at 1.1% (0.011; 12 mmol/mol Hb).[40] Both drugs produced similar weight loss, with an average reduction of 3.24 kg (7.13 lb) for liraglutide and 2.87 kg (6.31 lb) for exenatide.

GLP-1 agonists lower blood glucose levels by (a) producing glucose-dependent insulin secretion; (b) reducing postmeal glucagon secretion, which decreases postmeal glucose output; (c) increasing satiety which decreases food intake; and (d) regulating gastric emptying, which allows nutrients to be absorbed into the circulation more smoothly.[13] For exenatide, the t_{max} (defined as time after administration when the maximum plasma concentration is reached) is approximately 2 hours, and the plasma half-life is around 3.3 to 4 hours. Plasma concentrations are detected up to 10 hours after injection, although pharmacodynamic action lasts for approximately 6 hours. Hence, exenatide is recommended for twice-daily dosing in its immediate-release dosage form. A once weekly extended-release dosage form is also available.[39] Liraglutide's half-life is 13 hours, making it suitable for once-daily dosing.

Table 43–11

Noninsulin Injectable Agents for the Treatment of Diabetes[13,38,39]

Generic Name (Brand)	Type of Diabetes	Dosage Strengths[a]	Starting Dosage	Doses/Day	Titration Interval	Maximum Dose	Time to Effect (minutes)	Comments and Cautions
Pramlintide[b] (Symlin)	1	15, 30, 45, 60 mcg	15	3	3–7 days	60 mcg	20	Take just before major meals; reduce insulin by 50% Maintenance dose 30–60 mcg
	2	60, 120 mcg	60	3	3–7 days	120 mcg	20	Side effects: Hypoglycemia, nausea, vomiting Available in SymlinPen 60 and 120
Exenatide[b] (Byetta, Bydureon)	2	Immediate-release: 5 mcg, 10 mcg, extended-release: 2 mg	Immediate-release: 5 mcg, extended-release: 2 mg	Immediate-release: 2, extended-release: N/A; once-weekly	Immediate-release: 1 month, extended-release: N/A	Immediate-release: 10 mcg, extended-release: 2 mg	Immediate-release: 15–30	Inject immediate-release formulation 15–20 minutes before 2 meals of the day with 6 hours separating the meals; prefilled disposable pen; may delay absorption of oral drugs; separate doses by 1 hour Extended-release formulation can be administered regardless of meals Side effects: Nausea, vomiting, diarrhea, increased hypoglycemia with sulfonylureas
Liraglutide[b] (Victoza)	2	6 mg/3 mL pen	0.6 mg	1	1 week	1.8 mg	Not applicable	Can be dosed at any time of day regardless of meals; may delay absorption of oral drugs; separate doses by 1 hour Side effects: Nausea, vomiting, increased hypoglycemia with sulfonylureas

[a]Pramlintide supplied as 0.6 mg/mL in 5-mL vials. Exanatide immediate-release supplied as 250 mcg/mL, 1.2 mL for the 5-mcg prefilled pen, and 2.4 mL for the 10-mcg per dose prefilled pen. Exenatide extended-release supplied as 2 mg sterile powder plus 0.65 mL diluent in single use trays. Liraglutide supplied in 6 mg/3 mL prefilled pen, which can be dialed to the desired dose of 0.6, 1.2, or 1.8 mg.

[b]Generic not available in United States.

Exenatide is eliminated renally and is not recommended in patients with a creatinine clearance of less than 30 mL/min (0.50 mL/s).[32] No specific dose adjustments are recommended for liraglutide in renal impairment. An increased risk of hypoglycemia occurs when GLP-1 agonists are used in combination with a sulfonylurea.[13] Hypoglycemia is not encountered when used as monotherapy or in conjunction with metformin and/or thiazolidinedione therapy. The main side effects of GLP-1 agonist therapy include nausea, vomiting, and diarrhea. These GI adverse effects tend to lessen over time. No major drug interactions have been found with exenatide. GLP-1 agonists delay absorption of other medications, so it is best to take concomitant medications 1 hour before or 3 hours after a GLP-1 agonist if rapid absorption of the concomitant medication is required.

GLP-1 agonists have been associated with cases of acute pancreatitis. For this reason, neither drug should be used in a patient with a history of pancreatitis. Any patient presenting with symptoms of acute pancreatitis, including abdominal pain, nausea, and vomiting, should have GLP-1 agonist therapy discontinued until pancreatitis can be ruled out. Both liraglutide and exenatide extended-release packagings contain a black box warning about thyroid C-cell tumors. They are contraindicated in patients with a personal or family history of medullary thyroid cancer and in those with a history of multiple endocrine tumors.

Exenatide is currently available in 5- and 10-mcg injectable prefilled disposable pens and a 2 mg extended-release injectable suspension. Initial therapy of the immediate-release product is 5 mcg twice daily, injected zero to 60 minutes before the morning and evening meals. Patients who do not eat breakfast can take their first dose before lunch. Doses are then increased after a month to 10 mcg if the patient's blood glucose is improving and nausea is limited. Exenatide extended-release 2 mg is administered by subcutaneous injection once every 7 days immediately after the powder is suspended and can be dosed at any time of day and without regard to meals. Liraglutide is available in 6-mg/3 mL prefilled disposable pens that can be dialed to the desired dose of 0.6, 1.2, or 1.8 mg. Liraglutide should be dosed at 0.6 mg/day for at least 1 week and then increased to 1.2 mg/day for at least 1 week before being increased to the maximum dose of 1.8 mg if needed. Liraglutide can be dosed at any time of day regardless of meals.

Amylin Pramlintide acetate was approved for use in the United States in March 2005 (see Table 43–11).[38] This agent is a synthetic analog of human amylin, which is a naturally occurring neuroendocrine peptide that is cosecreted by the β cells of the pancreas in response to food. Amylin secretion is completely deficient in patients with T1DM, or relatively deficient in patients with T2DM. Pramlintide is given by subcutaneous injection before meals to lower postprandial blood glucose elevations. Pramlintide generally results in an average weight loss of 1 to 2 kg (2.2 to 4.4 lb).

Pramlintide is indicated as combination therapy with insulin in patients with types 1 or 2 DM. It has been shown to decrease A1c by an additional 0.4% to 0.5% (0.004 to 0.005; 4 to 5 mmol/mol Hb). Pramlintide slows gastric emptying without altering absorption of nutrients, suppresses glucagon secretion, and leads to a reduction in food intake by increasing satiety. By slowing gastric emptying, the normal initial postmeal spike in blood glucose is reduced.

Hypoglycemia, nausea, and vomiting are the most common side effects encountered with pramlintide therapy, although pramlintide itself does not produce hypoglycemia. To decrease the risk of hypoglycemia, doses of short-acting, rapid-acting, or premixed insulins should be reduced by 50% before pramlintide is initiated. Some practitioners will not decrease the premeal insulin dose this much because of fear of loss of glucose control. Primarily, the kidneys metabolize pramlintide, but dosage adjustments in liver or kidney impairment are not required.

Pramlintide has the potential to delay the absorption of orally administered medications. When rapid absorption is needed for the efficacy of an agent, pramlintide should be administered 2 hours before or 1 hour after this drug. Pramlintide should not be used in patients receiving medications that alter GI motility, such as anticholinergic agents, or drugs that slow the absorption of nutrients such as α-glucosidase inhibitors. A disposable pen formulation is now on the market and available as SymlinPen 60 for patients with T1DM and SymlinPen 120 for people with T2DM. The number of days the pen will last will vary depending on the daily dose. The amount of medication is 1.5 mL in the SymlinPen 60 and 2.7 mL in the SymlinPen 120.

Treatment of Concomitant Conditions

▶ *Glucose Control and Cardiovascular Health*

The results of three trials have recently been released showing the relationship between glucose control and cardiovascular health. The Action to Control Cardiovascular Risk in Diabetes (ACCORD),[41] Action in Diabetes and Vascular Disease (ADVANCE),[42] and Veterans Affairs Diabetes Trial (VADT)[43] examined if cardiovascular risks could be decreased or prevented with intensive glucose lowering. Although ACCORD was stopped early after interim analysis showed an increased risk of mortality in the intensive treatment group, both ADVANCE and VADT found that intensive therapy was no different than standard glycemic control in terms of macrovascular event rates.[41–43] The findings of these trials, when taken into context with long term follow-up information from the UKPDS[44] and DCCT[45,46] trials, seem to show the following: (1) 3 to 5 years of intensive glycemic control does not improve the risk of macrovascular complications in patients with longstanding T2DM and (2) a decrease in macrovascular risk from improved glycemic control may take more than a decade to be realized.

▶ *Coronary Heart Disease*

Cardiovascular disease is the major cause of morbidity and mortality for patients with DM.[10] Interventions targeting smoking cessation, blood pressure control, lipid management, antiplatelet therapy, and lifestyle changes (including diet and exercise) can reduce the risk of cardiovascular events and should be considered as important as glycemic control in the management of a patient with DM. All DM patients with a history of cardiovascular disease should be prescribed aspirin 75 to 162 mg/day as a secondary prevention strategy. For those with aspirin allergy, another antiplatelet option such as clopidogrel 75 mg/day should be used. Choosing if antiplatelet therapy is appropriate for a patient with DM and no history of cardiovascular disease can be more difficult because evidence is less clear regarding benefit. The ADA currently recommends that antiplatelet therapy should be considered for any patient with DM as a primary prevention strategy if that patient's risk of cardiovascular event is considered to be greater than 10% over 10 years. This includes most men older than 50 years of age and most women older than 60 years of age who have at least one additional cardiovascular risk factor. Clinical judgment is required for patients with an estimated cardiovascular risk of 5% to 10% to determine if the possible benefit of antiplatelet therapy outweighs the potential for harm from bleeding.

▶ *Dyslipidemia*

The National Cholesterol Education Program Adult Treatment Panel III guidelines classify the presence of DM to be of the same risk equivalence as coronary heart disease (CHD).[19] The primary target for lipid-lowering treatment in most patients with DM is LDL cholesterol with a goal of less than 100 mg/dL (2.59 mmol/L). For patients at high cardiovascular risk, including those with a history of cardiovascular disease, the LDL target may be set more stringently at 70 mg/dL (1.81 mmol/L). Only when triglyceride levels exceed 500 mg/dL (5.65 mmol/L) should they replace LDL as the patient's primary therapeutic goal. Because of potent LDL cholesterol-lowering ability and the known benefit in terms of improved cardiovascular morbidity and mortality, statins are considered first-line therapy for hyperlipidemia. Because statin therapy has been shown to benefit even patients with relatively low-baseline LDL cholesterol levels, it is also important to note that the ADA guidelines currently call for all patients with DM to be prescribed a statin who fall into either of the following two categories: (1) those who have overt cardiovascular disease and (2) those who do not have overt cardiovascular disease but are older than age 40 years and have one or more other cardiovascular disease risk factors.[10] Once LDL cholesterol goals are achieved with statin therapy, some patients will continue to have elevated non-HDL cholesterol produced by elevated triglyceride levels and low HDL cholesterol. Although it was common practice in the past to add niacin or fibrate therapy onto statin therapy in such patients, cardiovascular outcome benefit has not been proven with combination therapy over statin therapy alone in patients with prior cardiovascular disease or DM.[47,48]

▶ Hypertension

⑧ *Uncontrolled blood pressure plays a major role in the development of macrovascular events as well as microvascular complications, including retinopathy and nephropathy, in patients with DM. The ADA recommends that systolic blood pressure goals for patients with DM be individualized but generally set at less than 130 mm Hg.[10] The diastolic blood pressure goal for patients with DM is less than 80 mm Hg.* In addition, there are several general principles regarding the treatment of hypertension in diabetes patients. Angiotensin-converting enzyme (ACE) inhibitors or angiotensin II receptor blockers are recommended as initial therapy because of their beneficial effects on renal function. Initial combination therapy with an ACE inhibitor and dihydropyridine calcium channel blocker has been shown to reduce cardiovascular morbidity and mortality versus those receiving ACE inhibitor therapy combined with a thiazide diuretic.[49] However, thiazide diuretics work synergistically with ACE inhibitors and angiotensin II receptor blockers and can be added on for those who fail to reach blood pressure goals with a single agent alone as long as the patient's estimated glomerular filtration rate remains at 30 mL/min/1.73 m^2 (0.29 mL/s/m^2) or higher.[10] Alternatively, a loop diuretic can be used.

It can be expected that most patients will require more than one agent to reach blood pressure goal. Renal function and serum potassium levels should be monitored closely in all patients taking an ACE inhibitor, angiotensin II receptor blocker, and/or diuretic. ACE inhibitors and angiotensin II receptor blockers are contraindicated in patients who are pregnant and in those with bilateral renal artery stenosis.

Patient Encounter, Part 2: Follow-Up Visit

GH returns in 3 days with results of his fasting blood work requested by his physician. The physician also requests that his blood glucose level, A1c, and vital signs be obtained again today. The results are listed below.

VS: BP 122/76 mm Hg, P 70 beats/min, RR 19, T 38°C (100°F)

A1c (today): 7.9% (0.079; 63 mmol/mol Hb)

FPG (today): 189 mg/dL (10.5 mmol/L)

Labs (2 days ago):

- Na: 136 mEq/L (136 mmol/L)
- K: 3.6 mEq/L (3.6 mmol/L)
- Cl: 98 mEq/L (98 mmol/L)
- CO_2: 24 mEq/L (24 mmol/L)
- BUN: 15 mg/dL (5.4 mmol/L)
- SCr: 1.3 mg/dL (115 μmol/L)
- Glu: 172 mg/dL (9.5 mmol/L)

GH is diagnosed with T2DM. Identify the goals of treatment for this patient.

What nonpharmacologic and pharmacologic alternatives are available for this patient for his diabetes?

What is the most appropriate initial therapy for this patient in regards to his diabetes?

What additional interventions are recommended for this patient today?

▶ Human Immunodeficiency Virus (HIV) and Acquired Immune Deficiency Syndrome (AIDS)

Patients with risk factors for diabetes are more likely to develop diabetes when exposed to highly active antiretroviral therapy.[50] Universal screening of all HIV patients for diabetes is controversial, but most clinicians support screening for those with risk factors, especially if those risk factors include positive family history and central adiposity. Disturbances in glucose homeostasis are a known side effect of protease inhibitor therapy. Indinavir and ritonavir block insulin-mediated glucose disposal, causing insulin resistance, but amprenavir and atazanzvir have no effect on this pathway. Indinavir also increases hepatic glucose production and release and causes insulin to lose its ability to suppress hepatic glucose production. Nelfinavir, lopinavir, and saquinavir cause a 25% reduction in β-cell function, reducing first-phase insulin release. Drug selection for treating protease inhibitor–induced hyperglycemia should address the mechanism behind the adverse effect. Protease inhibitor therapy avoidance should be considered in patients with preexisting glucose abnormalities and in those with a first-degree relative with diabetes. Metformin should be used with caution in patients taking the nucleoside reverse transcriptase inhibitors stavudine, zidovudine, and didanosine because of an increased risk for lactic acidemia.

▶ *Antipsychotic Drug Therapy*

An association has been recognized between second-generation antipsychotics and the development of diabetes.[51] Risk seems to be highest with clozapine and olanzapine, but data are conflicting for risperidone and quetiapine. Aripiprazole and ziprasione have not, as of yet, shown an increased risk for diabetes with their use. Nutrition and physical activity counseling is recommended for all patients with mental illness who are overweight or obese, especially if they are beginning second-generation antipsychotic therapy. After therapy initiation, the patient's weight should be assessed at weeks 4, 8, and 12 and then every 3 months. In the event of weight gain greater than or equal to 5% of the patient's baseline weight, a therapeutic adjustment should be considered. For patients who develop worsening glycemia or dyslipidemia while on antipsychotic therapy, it is recommended that a switch to a second-generation antipsychotic with less weight gain or diabetes potential be considered.

Treatment of Acute Complications

▶ *Hypoglycemia*

Hypoglycemia, or low blood sugar, can be defined clinically as a blood glucose level of less than 50 mg/dL (2.8 mmol/L). Individuals with DM can experience symptoms of hypoglycemia at varying blood glucose levels. Patients who have regular blood glucose levels as high as 300 to 400 mg/dL (16.7 to 22.2 mmol/L) may experience symptoms of hypoglycemia when blood glucose levels are lowered to the middle to upper 100 mg/dL (5.6 mmol/L) range. Most people whose blood glucose levels are controlled adequately may experience symptoms when levels fall below 70 mg/dL (3.9 mmol/L). Symptoms of hypoglycemia include shakiness, sweating, fatigue, hunger, headaches, and confusion.

Common causes of hypoglycemia include delayed or inadequate amounts of food intake, especially carbohydrates, excessive doses of medications (e.g., sulfonylureas and insulin), exercising when insulin doses are reaching peak effect, or inadequately adjusted drug therapy in patients with impaired renal or hepatic function. Patients experiencing symptoms of hypoglycemia should check their blood glucose level, consume 15 g of carbohydrate, and wait 10 to 15 minutes for symptom resolution. Examples of acceptable treatments may include a small box of raisins, 4 oz (approximately 120 mL) of orange juice, 8 oz (approximately 240 mL) of skim milk, or three to six glucose tablets. In patients receiving an α-glucosidase inhibitor in combination with a sulfonylurea or insulin, hypoglycemia should be treated with glucose tablets or skim milk owing to the mechanism of action of the α-glucosidase inhibitors.

For patients whose blood glucose levels have dropped below 50 mg/dL (2.8 mmol/L), as much as 30 g of carbohydrate may be necessary to raise blood glucose levels adequately. For patients with hypoglycemia experiencing a loss of consciousness, a glucagon emergency kit should be administered by the intramuscular or subcutaneous route. It is important to contact emergency medical personnel in this particular situation. The patient should be rolled onto his or her side to prevent aspiration because many patients receiving the glucagon injection vomit.

▶ *Diabetic Ketoacidosis*

Diabetic ketoacidosis is a reversible but potentially life-threatening medical emergency that results from a relative or absolute deficiency in insulin.[52] Without insulin, the body

---

Patient Encounter, Part 3: Follow-Up

GH returns in 1 month for a follow-up visit. He brings his blood glucose readings from the past week for review in addition to more fasting blood work. Blood glucose readings are in units of mg/dL (mmol/L). His most recent medication list is below. There are no changes to his health record from previous visits.

Medications:

- Hydrochlorothiazide 25 mg by mouth once daily
- Simvastatin 20 mg by mouth once daily
- Fluticasone nasal spray, one spray each nostril daily as needed
- Metformin 1000 mg by mouth twice daily

VS: BP 154/96 mm Hg, P 78 beats/min, RR 18, T 38°C (100°F)

Labs:

- Total cholesterol: 240 mg/dL (6.2 mmol/L)
- HDL: 41 mg/dL (1.06 mmol/L)
- LDL: 163 mg/dL (4.22 mmol/L)
- TG: 183 mg/dL (2.07 mmol/L)
- AST: 28 U/L (0.47 µKat/L)
- ALT: 31 U/L (0.52 µKat/L)

Day	FPG	PPG
Monday	118 (6.5)	168 (9.3)
Tuesday	122 (6.8)	187 (10.4)
Wednesday	134 (7.4)	140 (7.8)
Thursday	110 (6.1)	244 (13.5)
Friday	98 (5.4)	257 (14.3)
Saturday	128 (7.1)	297 (16.5)
Sunday	116 (6.4)	240 (13.3)

Are this patient's blood glucose levels within target? What pattern seems to be established?

Based on the information available from this encounter and previous encounters, develop a care plan for this patient. The plan should include (a) identification and assessment of all drug-related needs and/or problems, (b) a detailed therapeutic plan to address each need and problem, and (c) monitoring parameters to assess safety and efficacy.

Table 43–12

Management of Diabetic Ketoacidosis[52]

1. Confirm diagnosis (increased plasma glucose, positive serum ketones, metabolic acidosis)
2. Admit to hospital; intensive care setting may be necessary for frequent monitoring or if pH less than 7 or unconscious
3. Asses serum electrolytes (K$^+$, Na$^+$, Mg^{2+}, Cl$^-$, bicarbonate, phosphate), acid–base status—pH, HCO$_3^-$, Pco$_2$, β-hydroxybutyrate, and renal function (creatinine, urine output)
4. Replace fluids: 0.9% saline 1 L/h over first 1–3 hours; subsequently, 0.45% saline at 4–14 mL/kg/h; change to 5% dextrose with 0.45% saline when plasma glucose reaches 250 mg/dL (13.9 mmol/L)
5. Administer regular insulin: IV (0.15 U/kg bolus followed by 0.1 unit/kg/h infusion), Check glucose hourly and double insulin infusion until glucose level falls at steady hourly rate of 50–70 mg/dL (2.8–3.9 mmol/h). Alternatively, could use SC or IM routes, although dosing regimen different. If initial serum potassium is less than 3.3 mmol/L (3.3 mEq/L), do not administer insulin until the potassium is corrected to greater than 3.3 mmol/L (3.3 mEq/L)
6. Assess patient: What precipitated the episode (e.g., nonadherence, infection, trauma, infarction, cocaine)? Initiate appropriate workup for precipitating event (cultures, chest x-ray, ECG)
7. Measure chemistry (especially K$^+$, bicarbonate, phosphate and anion gap) every 2–4 hours until stable
8. Replace K$^+$: If K$^+$ is less than 3.3 mEq/L (3.3 mmol/L), hold insulin and give 40 mEq (40 mmol) of K$^+$ per liter of IV fluid. If K$^+$ is greater than 5 mEq/L (5 mmol/L), do not give K$^+$ but check level every 2 hours. When K$^+$ greater than 3.3 mEq/L (3.3 mmol/L) but less than 5 mEq/L (5.5 mmol/L), ECG normal, urine flow and normal creatinine documented, administer 20–30 mEq/L (20–30 mmol/L) of IV fluid to maintain K$^+$ at 4–5 mEq/L (4–5 mmol/L)
9. Continue above until patient is stable, glucose goal is 150–250 mg/dL (8.3–13.9 mmol/L), and acidosis is resolved. Insulin infusion may be decreased to 0.05–0.1 unit/kg/h
10. Administer intermediate- or long-acting insulin as soon as patient is eating. Allow for overlap in insulin infusion and subcutaneous insulin injection

Cl, chloride; ECG, electrocardiogram; HCO$_3$, serum bicarbonate; IM, intramuscular; IV, intravenous; K, potassium; Mg, magnesium; Na, sodium; Pco$_2$, partial pressure of carbon dioxide in the arterial blood; SC, subcutaneous.

cannot use glucose as an energy source and must obtain energy via lipolysis. This process produces ketones and leads to acidosis. Although DKA occurs frequently in young patients with T1DM on initial presentation, it can occur in adults as well. Often, precipitating factors such as infection, omission, or inadequate administration of insulin can cause DKA. Signs and symptoms develop rapidly within 1 day or so and commonly include fruity or acetone breath; nausea; vomiting; dehydration; polydipsia; polyuria; and deep, rapid breathing.

Hallmark diagnostic criteria for DKA include hyperglycemia (greater than 250 mg/dL, 13.9 mmol/L), ketosis (anion gap greater than 12 mEq/L [12 mmol/L]), and acidosis (arterial pH less than or equal to 7.3). Typical fluid deficit is 5 to 7 L or more, and major deficits of serum sodium and potassium are common.

The severity of DKA depends on the magnitude of the decrease in arterial pH, serum bicarbonate levels, and the mental state rather than the magnitude of the hyperglycemia. Treatment goals of DKA consist of reversing the underlying metabolic abnormalities, rehydrating the patient, and normalizing the serum glucose. Fluid replacement with normal saline at 1 to 1.5 L/h for the first hour is recommended to rehydrate the patient and to ensure the kidneys are perfused.

Potassium and other electrolytes are supplemented as indicated by laboratory assessment. The use of sodium bicarbonate in DKA is controversial and generally only recommended when the pH is less than or equal to 7 after 1 hour of hydration. Regular insulin at 0.1 unit/kg/h by continuous IV infusion is the preferred treatment in DKA to regain metabolic control rapidly. When plasma glucose values drop below 250 mg/dL (13.9 mmol/L), dextrose 5% should be added to the IV fluids. During the recovery period, it is recommended to continue administering insulin and to allow patients to eat as soon as possible. Dietary carbohydrates combined with insulin assist in the clearance of ketones. See Table 43–12 for the management of DKA.[52]

▶ *Hyperosmolar Hyperglycemic State*

Hyperosmolar hyperglycemic state (HHS) is a life-threatening condition similar to DKA that also arises from inadequate insulin, but HHS occurs primarily in older patients with T2DM. DKA and HHS also differ in that HHS lacks the lipolysis, ketonemia, and acidosis associated with DKA. Patients with hyperglycemia and dehydration lasting several days to weeks are at the greatest risk of developing HHS. Infection; silent myocardial infarction; cerebrovascular accident; mesenteric ischemia; acute pancreatitis; and the use of medications such as steroids, thiazide diuretics, calcium channel blockers, propranolol, and phenytoin are known precipitating causes of HHS. Two main diagnostic criteria for HHS are a plasma glucose value of greater than 600 mg/dL (33.3 mmol/L) and a serum osmolality of greater than 320 mOsm/kg (320 mmol/kg). The extreme hyperglycemia and large fluid deficits resulting from osmotic diuresis are major challenges to overcome with this condition. Similar to DKA, the treatment of HHS consists of aggressive rehydration, correction of electrolyte imbalances, and continuous insulin infusion to normalize serum glucose. However, in patients with HHS, blood glucose levels should be reduced gradually to minimize the risk of cerebral edema.

Treatment of Long-Term Complications

▶ Retinopathy

Diabetic retinopathy occurs when the microvasculature that supplies blood to the retina becomes damaged. This damage permits leakage of blood components through the vessel walls. Diabetic retinopathy is the leading cause of blindness in adults 20 to 74 years of age in the United States.[10] The risk of retinopathy is increased in patients with long-standing DM, chronic hyperglycemia, hypertension, and nephropathy. Glaucoma, cataracts, and other eye disorders occur earlier and more frequently in patients with DM.

The ADA recommends that patients with DM receive a dilated eye examination annually by an ophthalmologist or optometrist. Examinations should begin within 5 years of diagnosis of T1DM and shortly after diagnosis of T2DM. Glycemic control is the best prevention for slowing the progression of retinopathy along with optimal blood pressure control. Early retinopathy may be reversed with improved glucose control.

▶ Neuropathy

⑨ *Peripheral neuropathy is a common complication reported in T2DM. This complication generally presents as pain, tingling, or numbness in the extremities.* The feet are affected more often than the hands and fingers. A number of treatment options have been tried with mixed success. Current options include pregabalin, gabapentin, low-dose tricyclic antidepressants, duloxetine, venlafaxine, topiramate, nonsteroidal anti-inflammatory drugs, and topical capsaicin.

Autonomic neuropathy is also a common complication as DM progresses. The clinical presentation of autonomic neuropathy may include gastroparesis, resting tachycardia, orthostatic hypotension, impotence, constipation, and hypoglycemic autonomic failure. Therapy for each individual autonomic complication is addressed separately.

▶ Microalbuminuria and Nephropathy

Diabetes mellitus is the leading contributor to end-stage renal disease. Early evidence of nephropathy is the presence of albumin in the urine. Therefore, as the disease progresses, larger amounts of protein spill into the urine. The ADA recommends urine protein tests annually in T2DM patients. For children with T1DM, annual urine protein testing should begin with the onset of puberty or 5 years after the diagnosis of diabetes. The most common form of screening for protein in the urine is a random collection for measurement of the urine albumin-to-creatinine ratio. The desirable value is less than 30 mcg of albumin per milligram of creatinine (3.4 mg/mmol creatinine).

Microalbuminuria is defined as between 30 and 300 mcg of albumin per milligram of creatinine (3.4 to 34 mg/mmol creatinine). The presence of microalbuminuria is a strong risk factor for future kidney disease in T1DM patients. In patients with T2DM, microalbuminuria has been found to be a strong risk factor for macrovascular disease.

Glycemic control and blood pressure control are primary measures for the prevention of progression of nephropathy. ACE inhibitors and angiotensin II receptor blockers prevent the progression of renal disease in patients with T2DM. Treatment of advanced nephropathy includes dialysis and kidney transplantation.

▶ Foot Ulcers

⑩ *Lower extremity amputations are one of the most feared and disabling sequelae of long-term uncontrolled DM. A foot ulcer is an open sore that develops and penetrates to the subcutaneous tissues. Complications of the feet develop primarily as a result of peripheral vascular disease, neuropathies, and foot deformations.*

Peripheral vascular disease causes ischemia to the lower limbs. This decreased blood flow deprives the tissues of oxygen and nutrients and impairs the ability of the immune system to function adequately. Symptoms of peripheral vascular disease include intermittent claudication, cold feet, pain at rest, and loss of hair on the feet and toes. Smoking cessation is the single most important treatment for peripheral vascular disease. In addition, exercising by walking to the point of pain and then resting and resuming can be a vital therapy to maintain or improve the symptoms of peripheral vascular disease. Pharmacologic intervention with pentoxifylline or cilostazol also may be useful to improve blood flow and reduce the symptoms of peripheral vascular disease.

Neuropathies play a large part in the development of foot ulcers. Loss of sensation in the feet allows trauma to go unnoticed. Autonomic neuropathy can cause changes in blood flow, perspiration, skin hydration, and possibly, bone composition of the foot. Motor neuropathy can lead to muscle atrophy, resulting in weakness and changes in the shape of the foot. To prevent foot complications, the ADA recommends daily visual examination of the feet and a foot check performed at every physician visit. Sensory testing with a 10-gauge monofilament can detect areas of neuropathy. Treatment consists of glycemic control, preventing infection, debriding dead tissues, applying dressings, treating edema, and limiting ambulation. Untreated foot problems may develop gangrene, necessitating surgical intervention.

Special Situations

▶ Hospitalized Care

The NICE-SUGAR (intensive versus conventional glucose in critically ill patients) trial compared intensive (81 to 108 mg/dL [4.5 to 6.0 mmol/L]) with conventional (less than 180 mg/dL [10.0 mmol/L]) glucose control using IV insulin in 6,104 intensive care unit patients.[53] At 90 days, intensively controlled patients had an increased absolute risk of death of 2.6% (829 patients in the intensively controlled and 751 patients in the conventionally controlled groups died).

Significantly more hypoglycemia was observed in the intensively controlled group.

Current recommendations call for critically ill patients to be started on IV insulin therapy at a threshold of 180 mg/dL (10.0 mmol/L).[10] A goal range of 140 to 180 mg/dL (7.8 to 10.0 mmol/L) is recommended for the majority of patients. More stringent goals may be considered for selected critically ill patients, but only if hypoglycemia can be avoided.

Scheduled subcutaneous insulin regimens with basal, nutritional, and correction components are recommended for patients who are not critically ill. Goals of less than 140 mg/dL (7.8 mmol/L) for fasting glucose and less than 180 mg/dL (10.0 mmol/L) for random glucose are recommended for noncritically ill patients.

Blood glucose levels can be measured by several methods. Arterial samples are usually 5 mg/dL (0.3 mmol/L) higher than capillary values and 10 mg/dL (0.6 mmol/L) greater than venous values. When preparing an insulin infusion for a patient, several factors must be considered. Insulin will absorb to glass and plastic, reducing the amount of insulin actually delivered by 20% to 30%. Priming the tubing decreases the variability of insulin infused. Therefore, when patients can be converted safely from infusion to needle and syringe therapy, the total daily dose should be reduced by 20% to 50% of the daily infusion amount. When transferring someone from IV insulin drip to subcutaneous insulin, basal insulin should be administered several hours before the drip is discontinued to prevent loss of glycemic control. IV drip protocols are institution specific.

▶ Sick Days

Patients should monitor their blood glucose levels more frequently during sick days because it is common for illness to increase blood glucose values.[54] Patients with T1DM should check their glucose and urine for ketones every 4 hours when sick. Patients with T2DM may also need to check for ketones when their blood glucose levels are greater than 300 mg/dL

Patient Encounter, Part 4: Insulin Therapy

GH returns to the office for his annual checkup. It has been 5 years since he was first diagnosed with diabetes. His updated information is below. His past medical and family histories are unchanged. He states that he has been adherent to his medications and lifestyle changes. He complains that he has a burning and tingling constantly in both of his feet.

SH

- Smokes ½ pack cigarettes per day for 25 years
- Drinks 6 pack of beer on the weekends
- Denies illicit drug use

Allergies

- Sulfa
- Penicillin

Medications

- Hydrochlorothiazide 25 mg by mouth once daily
- Lisinopril 20 mg by mouth once daily
- Simvastatin 40 mg by mouth once daily
- Fluticasone nasal spray, one spray each nostril daily as needed
- Metformin 1000 mg by mouth twice daily
- Pioglitazone 30 mg by mouth once daily
- Multivitamin by mouth once daily

Meal history: Has been consuming approximately 45 to 60 g of carbohydrates per meal 3 times a day; saturated fat is limited to 15 g/day, and sodium is 2,000 mg/day

Physical activity: Was walking 4 or 5 days per week for 30 minutes at moderate intensity but has not done so recently

VS: BP 145/92 mm Hg, P 85 beats/min, RR 20, T 38°C (100°F)

Height: 6 ft, 3 in (190.5 cm)

Weight: 270 lb (123 kg)

Labs:

- Na: 139 mEq/L (139 mmol/L)
- K: 5 mEq/L (5 mmol/L)
- Cl : 103 mEq/L (103 mmol/L)
- CO_2: 23 mEq/L (23 mmol/L)
- BUN: 16 mg/dL (5.7 mmol/L)
- SCr: 0.9 mg/dL (80 μmol/L)
- FPG: 190 mg/dL (10.5 mmol/L)
- A1c: 10.7% (0.107; 93 mmol/mol Hb)
- AST: 28 U/L (0.47 μKat/L)
- ALT: 31 U/L (0.52 μKat/L)
- Fasting lipid profile:
  - Total cholesterol: 202 mg/dL (5.22 mmol/L)
  - LDL: 118 mg/dL (3.05 mmol/L)
  - HDL: 43 mg/dL (1.11 mmol/L)
  - TG: 205 mg/dL (2.32 mmol/L)

What therapeutic options are available for this patient to lower his blood glucose to goal?

Which insulin and starting dose would be most appropriate for this patient?

What additional medications, screenings, labs, and/or referrals are recommended for GH at this point?

(16.7 mmol/L). Patients should continue to take their medications while sick. T1DM patients may require additional insulin coverage, and some with T2DM who are currently on oral medication regimens may require insulin during an acute illness. Patients should be advised to maintain their normal caloric and carbohydrate intake while ill as well as to drink plenty of noncaloric beverages to avoid dehydration.

When having difficulty eating a normal diet, patients may be advised to use nondiet beverages, sports drinks, broths, crackers, soups, and nondiet gelatins to provide normal caloric and carbohydrate intake and avoid hypoglycemia. With proper management, patients can decrease their chance of illness-induced hospitalization, particularly DKA and HHS.

Patient Care and Monitoring

1. Assess the patient for development or progression of DM and DM-related complications.

2. Evaluate SMBG for glycemic control, including FPG and postprandial levels.
   - Are the blood glucose values too high or low?
   - Are there specific times of day or specific days not in control?
   - Is hypoglycemia occurring?

3. Assess the patient for changes in quality-of-life measures such as physical, psychological, and social functioning and well-being.

4. Perform a thorough medication history of prescription, over-the-counter, and herbal product use.
   - Are there any medication problems, including presence of adverse drug reactions, drug allergies, and drug interactions?
   - Is the patient taking any medications that may affect blood glucose control?

5. Review all available laboratory data (some settings may have only patient-reported values) for attainment of ADA goals (Table 43–7). What therapy goals are not being met? What tests or referrals to other members of the healthcare team are needed?

6. Recommend appropriate therapy and develop a plan to assess effectiveness.

7. Stress adherence to prescribed lifestyle and medication regimen.

8. Provide patient education on diabetes, lifestyle modifications, appropriate monitoring, and drug therapy:
   - Causes of DM complications and how to prevent them.
   - How lifestyle changes including diet and exercise can affect diabetes.
   - How to perform SMBG and what to do with the results.
   - When to take medications and what to expect.
   - What adverse effects may occur?
   - What warning sign(s) should be reported to the physician?

OUTCOME EVALUATION

- The success of therapy for DM is measured by the ability of the patient to manage his or her disease appropriately between healthcare provider visits.

- Appropriate therapy necessitates adequate patient education about the disease, development of a meal plan to which patients can comply, and integration of a regular exercise program.

- Patient care plans should include a number of daily evaluations to be performed by the patient, such as examining the feet for any sores, cuts, or abrasions; checking the skin for dryness to prevent cracking and chafing; and monitoring blood glucose values as directed. Weekly appraisals of weight and blood pressure are also advised.

- Until A1c levels are at goal, quarterly visits with the patient's primary healthcare provider are recommended. Table 43–7 summarizes the specific ADA goals for therapy. The practitioner should review SMBG data and a current A1c level for progress and address any therapeutic or educational issues.

- At a minimum, yearly laboratory evaluation of serum lipids, urinary microalbumin, and serum creatinine should be performed.

Abbreviations Introduced in This Chapter

A1c	Hemoglobin A1c
AACE	American Association of Clinical Endocrinologists
ACCORD	Action to Control Cardiovascular Risk in Diabetes
ACE	Angiotensin-converting enzyme
ADA	American Diabetes Association
ADVANCE	Action in Diabetes and Vascular Disease
AIDS	Acquired immunodeficiency syndrome
ALT	Alanine aminotransferase
AST	Aspartate aminotransferase
ATP	Adenosine triphosphate
BG	Blood glucose
BMI	Body mass index
BUN	Blood urea nitrogen
CDC	Centers for Disease Control and Prevention
CHD	Coronary heart disease
CHF	Congestive heart failure
Cl	Chloride

CrCl	Creatinine clearance
CSII	Continuous subcutaneous insulin infusion
DCCT	Diabetes Control and Complications Trial
DKA	Diabetic ketoacidosis
DM	Diabetes mellitus
DPP-4	Dipeptidyl peptidase-4
eAG	Estimated average glucose
ECG	Electrocardiogram
ER	Extended release
FBG	Fasting blood glucose
FBS	Fasting blood sugar
FDA	Food and Drug Administration
FPG	Fasting plasma glucose
GDM	Gestational diabetes mellitus
GI	Gastrointestinal
GIP	Glucose-dependent insulinotropic polypeptide
GLP-1	Glucagon-like peptide-1
Hb	Hemoglobin
HCO_3	Serum bicarbonate
HDL	High-density lipoprotein cholesterol
HHS	Hyperosmolar hyperglycemic state
HIV	Human immunodeficiency virus
HLA	Human leukocyte antigen
IFG	Impaired fasting glucose
IGT	Impaired glucose tolerance
IKK-β	I-kappa-B kinase-β
IM	Intramuscular
ISF	Interstitial fluid
IV	Intravenous
K	Potassium
LADA	Latent autoimmune diabetes in adults
LDL	Low-density lipoprotein cholesterol
Mg	Magnesium
MNT	Medical nutrition therapy
Na	Sodium
NGSP	National Glycohemoglobin Standardization Program
NICE-SUGAR	Intensive versus conventional glucose control in critically ill patients
NPH	Neutral protamine Hagedorn
OGTT	Oral glucose tolerance test
Pco_2	Partial pressure of carbon dioxide in arterial blood
PPAR-γ	Proxisome proliferator activator receptor gamma
PPG	Postprandial glucose
SC	Subcutaneous
SCr	Serum creatinine
SMBG	Self-monitoring of blood glucose
T1DM	Type 1 diabetes mellitus
T2DM	Type 2 diabetes mellitus
TG	Triglycerides
TLC	Therapeutic lifestyle change
TZDs	Thiazolidinediones
UKPDS	United Kingdom Prospective Diabetes Study
ULN	Upper limit of normal
UTI	Urinary tract infection
VADT	Veterans Affairs Diabetes Trial
WHO	World Health Organization

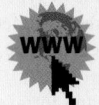 Self-assessment questions and answers are available at *http://www.mhpharmacotherapy.com/pp.html.*

REFERENCES

1. The Diabetes Control and Complications Trial Research Group. The effect of intensive treatment of diabetes on the development and progression of long-term complications in insulin-dependent diabetes mellitus. N Engl J Med 1993;329(14):977–986.
2. UK Prospective Diabetes Study (UKPDS) Group. Intensive blood-glucose control with sulfonylureas or insulin compared with conventional treatment and risk of complications in patients with type 2 diabetes (UKPDS 33). Lancet 1998;352(9131):837–853.
3. Centers for Disease Control. National Diabetes Fact Sheet, 2011 [online]. [cited 2011 Oct 10]. Available from: *http://www.cdc.gov/diabetes/pubs/pdf/ndfs_2011.pdf.* Accessed July 18, 2011.
4. Flegal KM, Carroll MD, Ogden CL, Curtin LR. Prevalence and trends in obesity among US adults, 1999–2008. JAMA 2010;303(3):235–241.
5. Centers for Disease Control. 1988–2008 No Leisure-Time Physical Activity Trend Chart [online]. [cited 2011 Oct 10]. Available from: *http://www.cdc.gov/nccdphp/dnpa/physical/stats/leisure_time.htm.* Accessed July 18, 2011.
6. Daneman D. Type 1 diabetes. Lancet 2006;367:847–858.
7. Klinke DJ. Extent of beta cell destruction is important but insufficient to predict the onset of type 1 diabetes mellitus. PLoS ONE 2008;3(1):e1374.
8. Stenström G, Gottsäter A, Bakhtadze E, et al. Latent autoimmune diabetes in adults definition, prevalence, β-cell function, and treatment. Diabetes 2005;54(Suppl):S68–S72.
9. DeFelippes M, Frank B, Chance R, et al. Insulin chemistry and pharmacokinetics. In: Porte DS, Baron A, eds. Ellenberg's and Rifkin's Diabetes Mellitus. 6th ed. New York: McGraw-Hill; 2003:481–500.
10. American Diabetes Association. Standards of medical care in diabetes—2012. Diabetes Care 2012;35(Suppl 1):S11–S63.
11. International Association of Diabetes and Pregnancy Study Groups Consensus Panel. International association of diabetes and pregnancy study groups recommendations on the diagnosis and classification of hyperglycemia in pregnancy. Diabetes Care 2010;33:676–682.
12. The HAPO Study Cooperative Research Group. Hyperglycemia and adverse pregnancy outcomes. N Engl J Med 2008;358:1991–2002.
13. Triplitt CL, Reasner CA. Diabetes mellitus. In: DiPiro JT, Talbert RL, Yee GC, et al, eds. Pharmacotherapy: A Pathophysiologic Approach. 8th ed. New York: McGraw-Hill; 2011:1255–1302.
14. Molina PE. Endocrine pancreas. In: Endocrine Physiology. 3rd ed. New York: McGraw-Hill; 2010:167–188.
15. Powers AC, D'Alessio D. Endocrine pancreas and pharmacotherapy of diabetes mellitus and hypoglycemia. In: Brunton L, Chabner B, Knollman B, eds. Goodman and Gillman's The Pharmacological Basis of Therapeutics. 12th ed. New York: McGraw Hill; 2011:1237–1274.
16. Rorsman P. Insulin secretion: function and therapy of pancreatic beta-cells in diabetes. Br J Diabetes Vasc Dis 2005;5:187–191.
17. Vinik A, Vinik E. Diabetic neuropathies. In: Mensing C, ed. The Art and Science of Diabetes Self-Management Education—A Desk Reference for Healthcare Professionals. 1st ed. Chicago, IL: American Association of Diabetes Educators; 2006:549–572.
18. Aronoff S, Berkowitz K, Shreiner B, Want L. Glucose metabolism and regulation: Beyond insulin and glucagon. Diabetes Spectr 2004;17:183–190.
19. Executive summary of the third report of the National Cholesterol Education Program (NCEP) Expert Panel on Detection, Evaluation, and Treatment of High Blood Cholesterol in Adults (Adult Treatment Panel III). JAMA 2001;285(19):2486–2497.
20. Uwaifo GI, Ratner RE. Novel pharmacologic agents for type 2 diabetes. Endocrinol Metab Clin North Am 2005;34:155–197.

21. DeFronzo RA. New concepts in pathophysiology: Incretins in type 2 diabetes. Clinical Highlights Newsletter: The Role of Incretin Mimetics and Potentiating Agents in the Prevention and Treatment of Type 2 Diabetes 2004;1:3–4.

22. Perley MJ, Kipnis DM. Plasma insulin responses to oral and intravenous glucose: Studies in normal and diabetic subjects. J Clin Invest 1967;46:1954–1962.

23. American Association of Clinical Endocrinologists. Medical guidelines for clinical practice for developing a diabetes mellitus comprehensive care plan. Endocrine Pract 2011;17(Suppl 2):1–53.

24. Diabetes Glycaemic Education and Monitoring Trial Group. Cost effectiveness of self monitoring of blood glucose in patients with non-insulin treated type 2 diabetes: Economic evaluation of data from the DiGEM trial. BMJ 2008;336:1177–1180.

25. Welschen LM, Bloemendal E, Nijpels G, et al. Self-monitoring of blood glucose in patients with type 2 diabetes who are not using insulin: a systematic review. Diabetes Care 2005;28:1510–1517.

26. Nathan D, Kuenen J, Borg R, et al. For the A1c Derived Average Glucose (ADAG) study group. Translating the A1c assay into estimated average glucose values. Diabetes Care 2008;31:1473–1478.

27. Nathan DM, Buse JB, Davidson MB, et al. Medical management of hyperglycemia in type 2 diabetes: A consensus algorithm for the initiation and adjustment of therapy: A consensus statement from the American Diabetes Association and the European Association for the Study of Diabetes. Diabetes Care 2009;32:193–203.

28. Institute of Medicine. Dietary Reference Intakes for Energy, Carbohydrate, Fiber, Fat, Fatty Acids, Cholesterol, Protein, and Amino Acids (Macronutrients). Washington, DC: National Academies Press; 2005.

29. Yeh GY, Eisenberg DM, Kaptchuk TJ, Phillips RS. Systematic review of herbs and dietary supplements for glycemic control in diabetes. Diabetes Care 2003;26:1277–1294.

30. American College of Sports Medicine and American Diabetes Association. Exercise and type 2 diabetes. Med Sci Sports Exerc 2010; 42:2282–2303.

31. Rodbard HW, Davidson JA, Garber AJ, et al. Statement by an American Association of Clinical Endocrinologists/American College of Endocrinology consensus panel on type 2 diabetes mellitus: an algorithm for glycemic control. Endocrine Pract 2009;15:540–559.

32. Lexicomp Online. Hudson, OH: Lexi-Comp. [cited 2011 Oct 10]. Available from: *http://online.lexi.com/crlsql/servlet/crlonline.* Accessed August 17, 2011.

33. UK Prospective Diabetes Study (UKPDS) Group. Effect of intensive blood-glucose control with metformin on complications in overweight patients with type 2 diabetes (UKPDS 34). Lancet 1998;352: 854–865.

34. Blake EW, Sease JM. Effect of diabetes medications on cardiovascular risk and surrogate markers in patients with type 2 diabetes. J Pharm Technol 2009;25:24–36.

35. Nissen SE, Wolski K. The effect of rosiglitazone on the risk of myocardial infarction and death from cardiovascular causes. N Eng J Med 2007;356:1–15.

36. Home PD, Pocock SJ, Beck-Nielsen H, et al. Rosiglitazone evaluated for cardiovascular outcomes in oral agent combination therapy for type 2 diabetes (RECORD): a multicentre, randomised, open-label trial. Lancet 2009;373:2125–2135.

37. Facts & Comparisons E Answers. Conshohocken, PA: Wolters Kluwer. [cited 2011 Oct 10]. Available from: *http://online.factsandcomparisons.com/login.aspx?url=/index.aspx&qs=.* Accessed August 18, 2011.

38. Amori R, Lau J, Pittas AG. Efficacy and safety of incretin therapy in type 2 diabetes: Systematic review and meta-analysis. JAMA 2007;298:194–206.

39. Bydureon [package insert]. San Diego, CA: Amylin Pharmaceuticals, Inc.; 2012 January.

40. Buse JB, Rosenstock J, Sesti G, et al. Liraglutide once a day versus exenatide twice a day for type 2 diabetes: A 26-week randomized, parallel-group, multinational, open-label trial (LEAD-6). Lancet 2009;374:39–47.

41. The Action to Control Cardiovascular Risk in Diabetes Study Group. Effects of intensive glucose lowering in type 2 diabetes. N Engl J Med 2008;358:2545–2559.

42. The ADVANCE Collaborative Group. Intensive blood glucose control and vascular outcomes in patients with type 2 diabetes. N Engl J Med 2008;358:2560–2572.

43. Duckworth W, Abraira C, Mortiz T, et al. Glucose control and vascular complications in veterans with type 2 diabetes. N Engl J Med 2009;360:1–11.

44. Holman RR, Paul SK, Bethel MA, et al. 10-year follow-up of intensive glucose control in type 2 diabetes. N Engl J Med 2008;359:1577–1589.

45. EDIC Writing Group. Sustained effect of intensive treatment of type 1 diabetes mellitus on developments and progression of diabetic neuropathy: The Epidemiology of Diabetes Interventions and Complications Study. JAMA 2003;290;2159–2167.

46. DCCT/EDIC Study Research Group. Intensive diabetes treatment and cardiovascular disease in patients with type 1 diabetes. N Engl J Med 2005;353:2643–2653.

47. Keech A, Simes RJ, Barter P, et al. Effects of long-term fenofibrate therapy on cardiovascular events in 9795 people with type 2 diabetes mellitus (the FIELD study): randomised controlled trial. Lancet 2005; 366:1849–1861.

48. AIM-HIGH Cholesterol Management Program. [cited 2011 Oct 10]. Available from: *http://www.aimhigh-heart.com.* Accessed August 19, 2011.

49. Jamerson K, Weber MA, Bakris GL, et al. Benazepril plus amlodipine or hydrochlorothiazine for hypertension in high-risk patients. N Engl J Med 2008;359:2417–2428.

50. Spollett GR. Hyperglycemia in HIV/AIDS. Diabetes Spectr 2006;19: 163–166.

51. American Diabetes Association, American Psychiatric Association, American Association of Clinical Endocrinologists, and North American Association for the Study of Obesity. Consensus development conference on antipsychotic drugs and obesity and diabetes. Diabetes Care 2004; 27:596–601.

52. Chiasson J, Aris-Jilwan N, Bélanger R, et al. Diagnosis and treatment of diabetic ketoacidosis and the hyperglycemic hyperosmolar state. CMAJ 2003;168:859–866.

53. Cook D, Dodek P, Henderson WR, et al. Intensive versus conventional glucose control in critically ill patients. N Engl J Med 2009;360: 1283–1297.

54. American Diabetes Association. When you're sick [online]. [cited 2011 Oct 10]. Available from: *http://www.diabetes.org/living-with-diabetes/treatment-and-care/who-is-on-your-healthcare-team/when-youre-sick.html.* Accessed August 21, 2011.

44 Thyroid Disorders

Michael D. Katz

LEARNING OBJECTIVES

● **Upon completion of the chapter, the reader will be able to:**

1. Explain the major components of the hypothalamic–pituitary–thyroid axis and the interaction among these components.

2. Discuss the prevalence of thyroid disorders, including subclinical (mild) and overt (typical signs and/or symptoms present) hypothyroidism and hyperthyroidism.

3. Discuss the relationship between serum thyroid-stimulating hormone (TSH) levels and primary thyroid disease and the advantages for the use of TSH levels over other tests such as serum T_4 (thyroxine) and T_3 (triiodothyronine) levels.

4. Identify the typical signs and symptoms of hypothyroidism and the consequences of inadequate treatment.

5. Describe the clinical use of levothyroxine (LT_4) in the treatment of hypothyroidism.

6. Discuss the issues regarding LT_4 product bioequivalence and the advantages of maintaining patients on the same product.

7. Describe the management of hypothyroidism and hyperthyroidism in pregnant women.

8. Identify the typical signs and symptoms of Graves' disease and the consequences of inadequate treatment.

9. Discuss the pharmacotherapy of Graves' disease, including the advantages and disadvantages of antithyroid drugs versus radioactive iodine, adverse effects, and patient monitoring.

10. Describe the potential effects of amiodarone, lithium, and interferon-α on thyroid function.

KEY CONCEPTS

❶ The thyroid gland is the largest endocrine gland in the body, residing in the neck anterior to the trachea between the cricoid cartilage and the suprasternal notch. The thyroid gland produces two biologically active hormones, thyroxine (T_4) and triiodothyronine (T_3). The parafollicular C cells of the thyroid gland produce calcitonin.

❷ In most patients with thyroid hormone disorders, the measurement of a serum thyroid-stimulating hormone (TSH) level is adequate for the initial screening and diagnosis of hypothyroidism and hyperthyroidism. Serum-free thyroxine (FT_4) and triiodothyronine (FT_3) levels may be helpful in distinguishing subclinical (mild) thyroid disease from overt disease. The target TSH for most patients being treated for thyroid disorders should be the mean normal value of 1.4 milli international units/L (mIU/L) or 1.4 micro international units/mL (μIU/mL) (target range, 0.5 to 2.5 mIU/L or 0.5 to 2.5 μIU/mL), although patients must be individually titrated based on resolution of signs and symptoms as well as biochemical tests. The target TSH may be different in patients being treated with levothyroxine (LT_4) for thyroid cancer.

❸ Hypothyroidism can affect virtually any tissue or organ in the body. The most common symptoms, such as fatigue, lethargy, sleepiness, cold intolerance, and dry skin, are nonspecific and can be seen with many other disorders. The classic overt signs, such as myxedema and delayed deep tendon reflexes, are seen uncommonly now because more patients are screened or seek medical attention earlier. Patients with mild (also known as subclinical) hypothyroidism may have subtle symptoms that progress so slowly that they are not noticed easily by the patient or family. The lack of overt or specific signs and symptoms emphasizes the importance of using the serum TSH level to identify patients with hypothyroidism. Treatment of patients with mild thyroid disease is controversial.

④ There are three major goals in the treatment of hypothyroidism: replace the missing hormones, relieve signs and symptoms, and achieve a stable biochemical euthyroid state.

⑤ Despite the availability of a wide array of thyroid hormone products, it is clear that synthetic LT_4 is the treatment of choice for almost all patients with hypothyroidism. LT_4 mimics the normal physiology of the thyroid gland, which secretes mostly T_4 as a prohormone. Peripheral tissues convert T_4 to T_3 as needed based on metabolic demands. If T_3 is used to treat hypothyroidism, the peripheral tissues lose their ability to control local metabolic rates. LT_4 also has distinct pharmacokinetic advantages over T_3. With a 7- to 10-day half-life, LT_4 provides a very smooth dose-response curve with little peak and trough effect. In a small number of patients who have impairment of conversion of T_4 to T_3, addition of T_3 may be warranted.

⑥ There is no evidence that one LT_4 product is better than another. However, given the evidence that these products do have different bioavailabilities, patients should be maintained on the same LT_4 product. Given the generic substitution regulations of most states, this is best accomplished by prescribing a brand-name product or otherwise ensuring that the product remains constant and not allowing substitution in the way allowed by state regulations or mandated by insurance companies.

⑦ The goals of treating hyperthyroidism are to relieve signs and symptoms, reduce thyroid hormone production to normal levels and achieve biochemical euthyroidism, and prevent long-term adverse sequelae.

⑧ Agranulocytosis is one of the most serious adverse effects of antithyroid drug therapy.

⑨ The growth and spread of thyroid carcinoma are stimulated by TSH. An important component of thyroid carcinoma management in many patients is the use of LT_4 to suppress TSH secretion. Early in therapy, patients receive the lowest LT_4 dose sufficient to fully suppress TSH to undetectable levels. Controlled trials show that suppressive LT_4 therapy reduces tumor growth and improves survival.

⑩ Patients receiving amiodarone must receive monitoring for thyroid abnormalities. Baseline measurements of serum TSH, FT_4, FT_3, antithyroid peroxidase antibody (anti-TPOAb), and TSH receptor-stimulating antibodies (TSHR-SAb) should be performed. TSH, FT_4, and FT_3 should be checked 3 months after initiation of amiodarone and then at least a TSH every 3 to 6 months.

Thyroid disorders are common. More than 2 billion people, or 38% of the world's population, have iodine deficiency, resulting in 74 million people with **goiters**.

Although overt iodine deficiency is not a significant problem in developed countries, a number of common thyroid conditions exist. The most common conditions are **hypothyroidism** and **hyperthyroidism**, which often require long-term pharmacotherapy. Undetected or improperly treated thyroid disease can result in long-term adverse sequelae, including increased mortality. It is important that clinicians are aware of the prevalence of thyroid disorders, the methods of identifying thyroid disorders, and the appropriate therapy. This chapter focuses on the most common pharmacologically treated thyroid disorders.

THYROID HORMONE PHYSIOLOGY AND BIOSYNTHESIS

① *The thyroid gland is the largest endocrine gland in the body, residing in the neck anterior to the trachea between the cricoid cartilage and the suprasternal notch. The thyroid gland produces two biologically active hormones, thyroxine (T_4) and triiodothyronine (T_3).* Thyroid hormones are essential for proper fetal growth and development, particularly of the central nervous system (CNS). After delivery, the primary role of thyroid hormone is in the regulation of energy metabolism. These hormones can affect the function of virtually every organ in the body. **①** *The parafollicular C cells of the thyroid gland produce calcitonin.* The function of calcitonin and its therapeutic use are discussed in other chapters in this book.

T_4 and T_3 are produced by the **organification** (binding of iodine to tyrosine residues of thyroglobulin) of iodine in the thyroid gland. Iodine is actively transported into the thyroid follicular cells. This inorganic iodine is oxidized by **thyroid peroxidase** and covalently bound to tyrosine residues of **thyroglobulin**. These iodinated tyrosine residues, monoiodotyrosine and diiodotyrosine, couple to form T_4 and T_3. Eighty percent of thyroid hormone is synthesized as T_4 and is stored in the thyroid bound to thyroglobulin. Thyroid hormones are released from the gland when needed, primarily under the influence of thyroid-stimulating hormone (TSH), which is also called thyrotropin, from the anterior pituitary. T_4 and T_3 are transported in the blood by three proteins, 70% to thyroid-binding globulin (TBG), 15% to transthyretin (thyroid-binding prealbumin), and 15% to albumin. T_4 is 99.97% protein bound, and T_3 is 99.7% protein bound, with only the unbound or free fractions physiologically active. The high degree of protein binding results in a long half-life of these hormones: approximately 7 to 10 days for T_4 and 24 hours for T_3.

Most of the physiologic activity of thyroid hormones is from the actions of T_3. T_4 can be thought of primarily as a prohormone. Eighty percent of needed T_3 is derived from the conversion of T_4 to T_3 in peripheral tissue under the influence of tissue deiodinases. These deiodinases allow end organs to produce the amount of T_3 needed to control local metabolic functions. These enzymes also catabolize T_3 and T_4 to biologically inactive metabolites.

The production and release of thyroid hormones are regulated by the hypothalamic–pituitary–thyroid axis (**Fig. 44–1**).

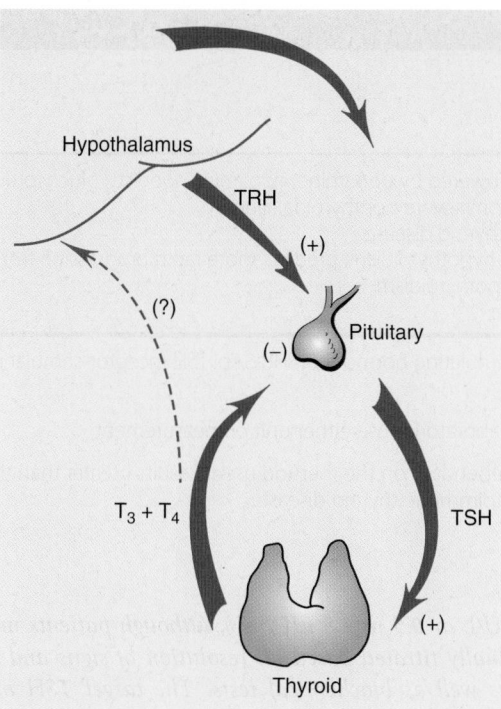

FIGURE 44–1. Hypothalamic–pituitary–thyroid axis. Thyrotropin-releasing hormone (TRH) is synthesized in the neurons within the paraventricular nucleus of the hypothalamus. TRH is released into the hypothalamic–pituitary portal circulation and carried to the pituitary, where it activates the pituitary to synthesize and release thyrotropin (TSH). TSH activates the thyroid to stimulate the synthesis and secretion of thyroxine (T_4) and triiodothyronine (T_3). T_4 and T_3 inhibit TRH and TSH secretion, closing the feedback loop.

Hypothalamic thyrotropin-releasing hormone (TRH) stimulates the release of TSH (thyrotropin) when there are physiologically inadequate levels of thyroid hormones. TSH promotes the production and release of thyroid hormones from the gland. As circulating thyroid hormone levels rise to needed levels, negative feedback results in decreased release of TSH and TRH. The release of TRH is inhibited by somatostatin and its analogs, and the release of TSH can be inhibited by dopamine, dopamine agonists, and high levels of glucocorticoids.

SPECTRUM OF THYROID DISEASE

There are two general modes of presentation for thyroid disorders: changes in the size or shape of the gland and changes in secretion of hormone from the gland. In some cases, structural changes can result in changes in hormone secretion. Thyroid nodules and goiters in euthyroid patients are common problems. Patients with a goiter who are biochemically euthyroid often require no specific pharmacotherapy unless the goiter is caused by iodine deficiency. In developing countries, iodized salt is the primary therapy in treating goiter. Thyroid nodules, seen in 4% to 7% of adults, may be

malignant or may autonomously secrete thyroid hormones. A discussion of thyroid nodules is beyond the scope of this chapter; however, thyroid cancer is discussed briefly in the context of levothyroxine (LT_4) suppressive therapy. Refer to other resources for a more extensive review of thyroid cancer management.

Changes in hormone secretion can result in hormone deficiency or excess. Although patients with overt hypothyroidism and hyperthyroidism may have dramatic signs and symptoms, most patients have subtle signs and symptoms that progress slowly over time. The availability of sensitive and specific biochemical tests for the diagnosis of thyroid hormone disorders has facilitated screening and earlier diagnosis, including in those with mild or subclinical thyroid disorders. Screening of newborns for congenital hypothyroidism has reduced the incidence of mental retardation and neonatal hypothyroidosm (**cretinism**) dramatically in the United States. However, congenital hypothyroidism owing to iodine deficiency remains a significant worldwide public health problem.

EPIDEMIOLOGY OF THYROID DISEASE

A number of studies have assessed the epidemiology of thyroid hormone abnormalities. The 1999 to 2002 National Health and Nutrition Examination Survey (NHANES) reported the prevalence of thyroid hormone disorders in 4,392 people 12 years of age and older in a sample representing the geographic and ethnic distribution of the U.S. population. Hypothyroidism was found in 3.7% (3.4% mild) and hyperthyroidism in 0.5% of the sample.[1] The prevalence of hypothyroidism was higher in older age groups and in whites and Hispanics; blacks had a lower prevalence of hypothyroidism. The prevalence of hypothyroidism correlated with age. Compared with the total population, people aged 50 to 79 years had an almost twofold higher prevalence, and those aged 80 years and older had a fivefold higher prevalence. Pregnant women also had a higher prevalence of hypothyroidism. The Colorado Thyroid Health Survey assessed thyroid function in 25,862 subjects attending a health fair.[2] The overall prevalence of an abnormal TSH level was 11.7% of the study population, with 9.4% hypothyroid (9% subclinical) and 2.2% hyperthyroid (2.1% subclinical). Of the 916 subjects taking thyroid medication, 60% were euthyroid, with an equal distribution between subclinical hypothyroidism and hyperthyroidism. The NHANES study also found that many patients receiving thyroid medications had an abnormal TSH level. These findings imply that many patients who are receiving thyroid medications are not being managed successfully.

PATIENT ASSESSMENT AND MONITORING

The assessment of patients for thyroid disorders entails a history and physical examination. In many patients with mild or subclinical thyroid disease, there may be an absence

Table 44–1

Selected Thyroid Tests for Adults

Test	Reference Range	Comments
TSH	0.5–4.5 mIU/L[a]	Gold standard; may be lowered by dopamine, dopamine agonists, glucocorticoids, octreotide, recovery from severe nonthyroidal illness
FT$_4$	0.7–1.9 ng/dL (9.0–24.5 pmol/L)	May be normal in mild thyroid disease
Anti-TPOAb	Variable[b]	Present in autoimmune hypothyroidism; predicts more rapid progression from subclinical to overt hypothyroidism
TSHR-SAb	Undetectable	Confirms Graves' disease

Anti-TPOAb, antithyroid peroxidase antibody; FT$_4$, free T$_4$ (thyroxine); TSH, thyroid-stimulating hormone; TSHR-SAb, TSH receptor-stimulating antibodies.

[a]Milli international units/L (mIU/L) = micro international units/mL (μIU/mL); clinical laboratories use either unit of measurement.

[b]Anti-TPOAb reference ranges are highly variable from one laboratory to another depending on the method used. Results greater than the upper cutoff are considered abnormal and are consistent with increased risk for autoimmune thyroid disease.

of specific signs and symptoms, and the physical examination findings may be normal. Various diagnostic tests can be used, including serum thyroid hormone(s), TSH, thyroid antibody levels, and imaging techniques to evaluate patients for thyroid disorders. Reference ranges for selected laboratory tests are given in Table 44–1. The laboratory assessment of patients with suspected thyroid disorders must be based on the continuum of disease from subclinical or mild to overt (Fig. 44–2).

TSH Levels

❷ *In most patients with thyroid hormone disorders, the measurement of a serum TSH level is adequate for the initial screening and diagnosis of hypothyroidism and hyperthyroidism. Serum free thyroxine (FT$_4$) and triiodothyronine (FT$_3$) levels may be helpful in distinguishing subclinical (mild) thyroid disease from overt disease. The target TSH for most patients being treated for thyroid disorders should be the mean normal value of 1.4 milli international units/L (mIU/L) or 1.4 micro international units/mL (μIU/mL) (target range, 0.5 to*

2.5 mIU/L or 0.5 to 2.5 μIU/mL), although patients must be individually titrated based on resolution of signs and symptoms as well as biochemical tests. The target TSH may be different in patients being treated with LT$_4$ for thyroid cancer.

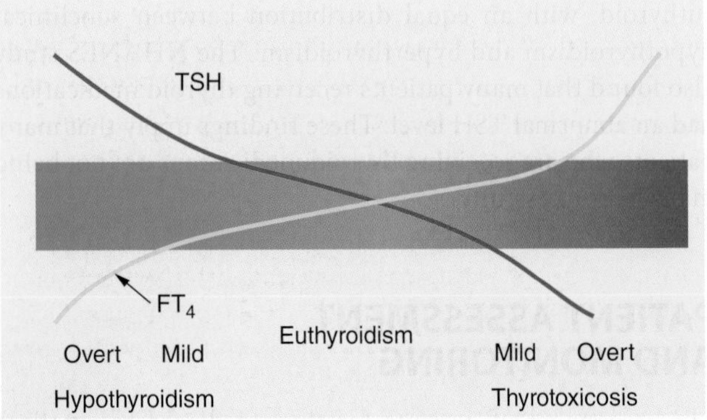

TSH is a highly sensitive bioassay of the thyroid axis. A twofold change in serum-free T$_4$ levels will result in a 100-fold change in TSH levels. This biologic magnification by TSH allows the TSH to be used in early diagnosis as well as in closely titrating therapy in hypothyroidism and hyperthyroidism. In patients with primary hypothyroidism or hyperthyroidism resulting from gland dysfunction, there is an inverse relationship between the TSH level and thyroid function. High TSH signifies hypothyroidism (or iatrogenic underreplacement), and low TSH signifies hyperthyroidism (or iatrogenic over-replacement). There is controversy regarding the normal or laboratory reference ranges for TSH. NHANES showed that the mean TSH level in a normal population was 1.46 milli international units/L (milli international units/L = micro international units/mL; clinical laboratories use either unit of measurement, usually expressed as mIU/L or μIU/mL), but the values were not normally distributed.[3] Although most laboratories quote the upper limit of normal for TSH as 4 or 5 mIU/L, 95% of subjects had a TSH level of between 0.5 and 2.5 mIU/L. The population of subjects whose TSH level was 2.5 to 4.5 mIU/L may have had mild hypothyroidism, or the non-normal distribution may reflect different normal ranges in a heterogeneous (age, sex, race) population. The mean normal TSH in the elderly appears to be higher even in people with no clinical evidence of hypothyroidism, and there is some evidence that normal TSH ranges are sex and ethnicity specific.[4] The target TSH for most patients being treated for thyroid disorders is not the same as the reference range. Ideally, the TSH should be the mean normal value of 1.4 μIU/mL or 1.4 μIU/mL (target range, 0.5 to 2.5 mIU/L or 0.5 to 2.5 μIU/mL). The upper limit of the target range may be higher in the elderly. Therapy may be titrated within the target TSH range to maximally improve patient signs and symptoms without causing adverse effects of over- or undertreatment.

FIGURE 44–2. The continuum of thyroid disorders. (FT$_4$, free T$_4$; TSH, thyroid-stimulating hormone.)

Serum T₄ and T₃ Levels

Serum T_4 and T_3 levels are used commonly to assess thyroid function. Older screening tests of thyroid function measure total serum T_4 or T_3 levels. Because of the high degree of protein binding of these hormones, the free fraction can be altered by changes in the levels of binding proteins or the degree of protein binding. Because a number of factors can alter protein binding, these older assays are very insensitive and should no longer be used even with protein-binding adjustment factors such as the free T_4 index. Free or unbound T_4 (FT_4) and T_3 (FT_3) assays are readily available and are more sensitive in identifying thyroid dysfunction than the older total assays.[6] However, patients with mild hypothyroidism or hyperthyroidism have normal FT_4 levels despite abnormal TSH levels.

Other Diagnostic Tests

Global tests of thyroid gland function can be performed to assess the rate of hormone synthesis. The radioactive iodine uptake (RAIU) is elevated in those with hyperthyroidism and can aid in identifying thyrotoxicosis owing to nonthyroid gland sources. Radionuclide thyroid scans are used in the evaluation of thyroid nodules. Because many thyroid disorders are autoimmune, measurement of various serum antithyroid antibodies can be performed. Antithyroid peroxidase antibodies (anti-TPOAb) and antithyroglobulin antibodies (anti-TGAb) are present in many patients with hypothyroidism. Most patients with Graves' disease have TSH receptor-stimulating antibodies (TSHR-SAb) as well as elevated anti-TPOAb and antimicrosomal antibodies.

HYPOTHYROIDISM

Hypothyroidism is the most common clinical disorder of thyroid function. It is the clinical syndrome that results from inadequate secretion of thyroid hormones from the thyroid gland. The vast majority of hypothyroid patients have primary gland failure, but rare patients have pituitary or hypothalamic failure. Most studies define hypothyroidism based on a serum TSH level above the upper limit of the laboratory reference range. In adults, 1.4% of women and 0.1% of men are biochemically hypothyroid. However, the incidence is highly age dependent. In the Colorado Thyroid Health Study, by age 64 years, 12% of women and 5% of men were hypothyroid, and in the over 74 years age group, the incidence in men approached that of women.[2] Most epidemiologic studies of hypothyroidism in the elderly show a prevalence of 6% to 12%. There is a strong correlation between the presence of anti-TPOAb or anti-TGAb and the risk of developing hypothyroidism. In patients with subclinical hypothyroidism and positive anti-TPOAb, 5% per year will progress to overt hypothyroidism.[7] Other risk factors for the development of hypothyroidism include the postpartum state, family history of autoimmune thyroid disorders, a previous history of head and neck or thyroid surgery, head and neck irradiation, other autoimmune endocrine disorders such as type 1 diabetes and Addison's disease, other non-endocrine autoimmune diseases

such as celiac disease and pernicious anemia, history of treatment for hyperthyroidism, treatment with amiodarone or lithium, and an iodine-deficient diet.[8]

Screening for Hypothyroidism

Because the prevalence of hypothyroidism is high in certain populations, screening may be useful. Screening for hypothyroidism in women older than age 35 years is as cost effective as screening for breast cancer and hypertension, although some organizations recommend screening of adults after the age of 50 or 60 years.[9] Others advocate a case-finding approach, defined as performing a TSH determination in patients based on risk factors or the presence of signs and symptoms.[10,11] Refer to Clinical Presentation and Diagnosis of Hypothyroidism for more information regarding screening and diagnosis.

Causes of Hypothyroidism

The most common causes of hypothyroidism are listed in Table 44–2.[8,12] Up to 90% of patients with autoimmune thyroiditis have circulating anti-TPOAbs. The autoimmune inflammatory response results in a lymphocytic infiltration of the thyroid gland and its eventual destruction.

Iatrogenic hypothyroidism can occur after thyroid irradiation or surgery and excessive doses of antithyroid drugs. Several drugs can cause hypothyroidism, including iodine-containing drugs such as amiodarone and iodinated radiocontrast media, lithium, interferon-α, multi- and tyrosine kinase inhibitors (imatinib, sunitinib, sorafenib), p-aminosalicylic acid, ethionamide, sulfonylureas, valproic acid, and aminoglutethimide.[13] Iodine deficiency is a common worldwide cause of hypothyroidism, including congenital hypothyroidism in newborns. Patients with hypothalamic or pituitary disease often have other signs of pituitary disease, such as hypogonadism, and their TSH levels are low.

Signs and Symptoms of Hypothyroidism

❸ *Hypothyroidism can affect virtually any tissue or organ in the body. The most common symptoms, such as fatigue, lethargy, sleepiness, cold intolerance, and dry skin, are nonspecific and can be seen with many other disorders. The classic overt*

Table 44–2
Common Causes of Hypothyroidism[11-13]

Primary Hypothyroidism
Autoimmune thyroiditis (Hashimoto's disease)
Iatrogenic (irradiation, surgery)
Drugs (amiodarone, radiocontrast media, lithium, interferon-α, tyrosine kinase inhibitors)
Silent thyroiditis (including postpartum)
Iodine deficiency and excess
Secondary Hypothyroidism
Pituitary disease
Hypothalamic disease

Clinical Presentation and Diagnosis of Hypothyroidism[11–13]

Symptoms

- Fatigue
- Lethargy
- Sleepiness
- Mental impairment
- Depression
- Cold intolerance
- Hoarseness
- Dry skin
- Decreased perspiration
- Weight gain
- Decreased appetite
- Constipation
- Menstrual disturbances
- Arthralgia
- Paresthesia

Signs

- Slow movements
- Slow speech

- Hoarseness
- Bradycardia
- Dry skin
- Nonpitting edema (myxedema)
- Hyporeflexia
- Delayed relaxation of reflexes

Screening/Diagnosis

A TSH level of 4.5 to 10 mIU/L may constitute mild or subclinical hypothyroidism. A TSH level greater than 10 mIU/L signifies overt hypothyroidism.[a] The free T_4 level will be normal (0.7 to 1.9 ng/dL or 9.0 to 24.5 pmol/L) in mild or subclinical hypothyroidism and low (less than 0.7 ng/dL or 9.0 pmol/L) in patients with obvious signs and/or symptoms.

---

[a]Milli international units/L (mIU/L) = micro international units/mL (µIU/mL); clinical laboratories use either unit of measurement.

---

signs, such as myxedema and delayed deep tendon reflexes, are seen uncommonly now because more patients are screened or seek medical attention earlier. Patients with mild (also known as subclinical) hypothyroidism may have subtle symptoms that progress so slowly that they are not noticed easily by the patient or family. The lack of overt or specific signs and symptoms emphasizes the importance of using the serum TSH level to identify patients with hypothyroidism. Treatment of patients with mild thyroid disease is controversial.

Mild (Subclinical) Hypothyroidism

Mild or subclinical hypothyroidism is present when a patient has an elevated TSH (usually below 10 mIU/L or 10 µIU/mL), normal FT_4, and no overt hypothyroid signs and symptoms.[12–17] Many of these patients have autoimmune thyroiditis and anti-TPO antibodies, and some will progress to overt hypothyroidism. Although patients may not express the typical symptoms of hypothyroidism, many patients do have mild, nonspecific symptoms (e.g., fatigue, cold intolerance, constipation). Recent studies have shown subclinical hypothyroidism to be a risk factor for cardiovascular mortality and to be associated with decreased myocardial contractility, decreased exercise tolerance, elevated low-density lipoprotein (LDL) cholesterol, and neuropsychiatric symptoms.[15]

Sequelae of Hypothyroidism

Hypothyroidism is a chronic disease that may result in significant long-term sequelae. Hypercholesterolemia is

associated with hypothyroidism, increasing the long-term risk of cardiovascular disease and cardiovascular mortality. Between 4% and 14% of patients with hypercholesterolemia are found to be hypothyroid. The Colorado Thyroid Health Study showed a direct correlation between the degree of TSH elevation and the rise in serum cholesterol.[2] Hypothyroidism also may result in increased systemic vascular resistance, decreased cardiac output, and increased diastolic blood pressure. Hypothyroidism can cause significant neuropsychiatric problems, including a dementia-like state in the elderly that is reversible with LT_4 therapy. Maternal hypothyroidism can have dire consequences for developing fetuses. Fetuses are almost completely dependent on maternal thyroid hormones during the first trimester, a time crucial for development of the CNS. Inadequately treated maternal hypothyroidism results in increased risk of miscarriage and developmental impairment in the child.[18]

Myxedema coma is seen in advanced hypothyroidism. These patients develop CNS depression, respiratory depression, cardiovascular instability, and fluid and electrolyte disturbances. Myxedema coma often is triggered by an underlying acute medical condition such as infection, stroke, trauma, or administration of CNS depressant drugs.

Treatment of Hypothyroidism

④ *There are three major goals in the treatment of hypothyroidism: replace the missing hormones, relieve signs and symptoms, and achieve a stable biochemical euthyroid state. Although*

Table 44–3

Thyroid Preparations

Drug (Brand Name)	Content	Relative Dose	Comments
LT$_4$ (Synthroid, Levoxyl, Unithroid), other brands, and generics	Synthetic LT$_4$; 25-, 50-, 75-, 88-, 100-, 112-, 125-, 137-, 150-, 175-, 200-, and 300-mcg tablets; 500-mcg vial for injection	60 mcg	Gold standard for treating hypothyroidism; products not therapeutically equivalent; full replacement dose, 1–1.6 mcg/kg/day; when switching from animal product, lower calculated daily dose by 25–50 mcg; IV form rarely needed
Liothyronine (Cytomel)	Synthetic T$_3$; 5-, 15-, 25-, and 50-mcg tablets	15 mcg	Rarely needed in treatment of hypothyroidism; rapid absorption and pharmacologic effect; increased toxicity versus LT$_4$; no outcome benefit to combining with LT$_4$
Thyroid (desiccated) USP (Armour, others)	Desiccated pork or beef thyroid glands; contains T$_3$ and T$_4$; 15-, 16.25-, 30-, 32.5-, 48.75-, 60-, 65-, 90-, 97.5-, 120-, 130-, 162.5-, 180-, 195-, 240-, 260-, 300-, and 325-mg tablets	65 mg	Nonphysiologic for humans; unpredictable hormone content and stability; T$_3$ content may cause toxicity; no role in modern therapy
Liotrix (Thyrolar)	Synthetic T$_4$, T$_3$ in fixed 4:1 ratio; ¼-, ½-, 1-, 2-, 3- strength tablets	12.5/50 mcg T$_3$:T$_4$ (1 strength)	Nonphysiologic T$_4$:T$_3$ ratio; T$_3$ content may cause toxicity; no role in modern therapy

IV, intravenous; LT$_4$, levothyroxine; T$_3$, triiodothyronine; T$_4$, thyroxine.

these goals should not be difficult to achieve, 20% to 40% of treated patients are not receiving optimal pharmacotherapy.

▶ Thyroid Hormone Products

A number of thyroid hormone products are marketed in the United States (Table 44–3). These products include synthetic LT$_4$ and T$_3$, combinations of synthetic LT$_4$ and T$_3$, and animal-derived products. ❺ *Despite the availability of a wide array of thyroid hormone products, it is clear that synthetic LT$_4$ is the treatment of choice for almost all patients with hypothyroidism.*[11,12] *LT$_4$ mimics the normal physiology of the thyroid gland, which secretes mostly T$_4$ as a prohormone. Peripheral tissues convert T$_4$ to T$_3$ as needed based on metabolic demands. If T$_3$ is used to treat hypothyroidism, the peripheral tissues lose their ability to control local metabolic rates. LT$_4$ also has distinct pharmacokinetic advantages over T$_3$. With a 7- to 10-day half-life, LT$_4$ provides a very smooth dose-response curve with little peak and trough effect. In a small number of patients who have impairment of conversion of T$_4$ to T$_3$, addition of T$_3$ may be warranted.* T$_3$, with a 24-hour half-life, provides a significant peak and trough effect, and many patients have symptoms of thyrotoxicosis after each dose is administered. The use of compounded T$_3$ products that have not been approved by the Food and Drug Administration (FDA) should be strongly discouraged. For patients who have difficulty adhering to a once-daily regimen, a once-weekly LT$_4$ regimen is safe and effective.[11,12]

Animal-derived products such as desiccated thyroid are obtained from cow and pig thyroid and have various degrees of purity. These products contain both LT$_4$ and T$_3$, but the amount of T$_3$ is much higher (T$_4$:T$_3$ = 4:1) than what would be found in the human thyroid gland (T$_4$:T$_3$ = 14:1). With the

desiccated thyroid products, there are concerns about standardizing the amount of hormone and lot-to-lot variability. Thyroglobulin products were removed from the U.S. market several years ago. Although some patients want to use these agents because they are "natural," they are in no way natural for humans. With the strong evidence supporting the safety and efficacy of LT$_4$ in the treatment of hypothyroidism, there is no rationale for the use of these animal-derived products. Patients who are being treated with these agents should be strongly encouraged to switch to synthetic LT$_4$. Additionally, patients should be encouraged to not purchase thyroid hormone- or iodine-containing products from health food stores or from questionable Internet sites.

Several studies have been published that evaluate the use of LT$_4$ and T$_3$ combinations in ratios that mimic human physiology. A meta-analysis of 11 randomized, controlled clinical trials comparing LT$_4$ and T$_3$ combinations with LT$_4$ monotherapy show no outcome benefit with combination therapy.[19] Except in rare circumstances (e.g., patients with impaired T$_4$-to-T$_3$ conversion), there is no rationale for using combinations of LT$_4$ and T$_3$ to treat hypothyroidism.

▶ Bioequivalence and LT$_4$ Product Selection

LT$_4$ products have a long history of bioavailability problems.[20] Over the years, LT$_4$ bioavailability has increased, so maintenance doses today are significantly lower than those seen before the early 1980s. Currently, the average bioavailability of LT$_4$ products is about 80%. Because of long-standing concerns about LT$_4$ bioequivalence and because LT$_4$ products had never undergone formal approval by the FDA under the 1938 Food, Drug, and Cosmetics Act, the FDA mandated that all manufacturers of LT$_4$ products submit an Abbreviated

New Drug Application (ANDA) to keep their products on the U.S. market after 2001.[21] Products approved under this process would have to comply with FDA manufacturing and bioequivalence standards. This FDA action has resulted in many changes in the U.S. LT_4 market, as well as renewed interest in LT_4 bioequivalence. Since 2001, a variety of brand and generic products had been approved by the FDA. Some of the generic products carry AB ratings (bioequivalence) to certain brand products.[22]

For many years, there have been concerns regarding the FDA bioequivalence methodology for LT_4 products. FDA bioequivalence standards allow a −20% to +25% variance in pharmacokinetic parameters between the test and reference products. Many people believe this degree of allowed variance is not appropriate for a narrow-therapeutic-index (NTI) drug such as LT_4.[23] Furthermore, there are unique challenges to performing bioequivalence studies with an endogenous hormone such as LT_4. Because these single-dose pharmacokinetic studies are done in healthy volunteers, the pharmacokinetic data are a combination of endogenous and exogenous LT_4. Seventy percent of the area under the curve (AUC) in these studies consists of the subjects' endogenous T_4. Thus, it is doubtful that bioavailability differences among products could be detected. Blakesley and colleagues showed the standard FDA bioequivalence methodology would rate 600-, 450-, and 400-mcg LT_4 doses as bioequivalent.[24] This study also showed that mathematically removing the subjects' endogenous T_4 level (baseline correction) improves the sensitivity of the analysis, allowing a distinction between 33% and 25% but not 12.5% dose differences. Based on these data, since 2003, the FDA has required that LT_4 bioequivalence data undergo baseline correction. Although this method has improved the ability to identify large differences in LT_4 bioequivalence, small but clinically significant differences will not be identified. In 2008, the FDA adopted stricter criteria for LT_4 tablet shelf-life potency (95% to 105% of stated potency vs. standard 90% to 110%), which may reduce the intrapatient variability seen during long-term LT_4 therapy. As of August 2011, the FDA Pharmaceutical Science and Clinical Pharmacology Advisory Committee was considering stricter guidelines for the determination of the bioequivalence of NTI drugs, including the use of TSH as a pharmacodynamic marker of LT_4 bioequivalence.

More important than bioequivalence is the therapeutic equivalence of LT_4 products. Will patients have the same outcomes if bioequivalent products are used? A study by Dong and colleagues helps to answer this question.[25] Twenty-two well-controlled hypothyroid women were randomly switched to the same dose of four different products every 6 weeks. Nonbaseline corrected bioequivalence data showed these products to be bioequivalent. However, as each product switch occurred, more of the subjects had an abnormal TSH level.[26] By the end of the third product switch, 52% had an abnormal TSH level. This is strong evidence that LT_4 products are not therapeutically equivalent even if they are rated as bioequivalent by the FDA.

Evidence does exist that small differences in the LT_4 dose can result in large changes in TSH. The impact on TSH of small changes in LT_4 dose was assessed in 21 adult therapeutically optimized hypothyroid patients.[27] When the daily dose was reduced by 25 mcg, 78% had an elevated TSH level. When the daily dose was increased by 25 mcg, 55% had a low TSH level. Clearly, differences in the LT_4 dose or bioavailability within the FDA-allowed variance for bioequivalent products can cause significant changes in TSH.

6 *There is no evidence that one LT_4 product is better than another. However, given the evidence that these products do have different bioavailabilities, patients should be maintained on the same LT_4 product. Given the generic substitution regulations of most states, this is best accomplished by prescribing a brand-name product or otherwise ensuring that the product remains constant and not allowing substitution in the way allowed by state regulations or mandated by insurance companies.* Although practitioners are pressured by insurance companies and employers to substitute LT_4 products as a cost-saving measure, such switching is not in the best interest of the patient and should not be allowed. If patients are switched to a different product, the prescriber should be notified, and a TSH determination should be done in 6 to 8 weeks to allow dose retitration. The economic impact of retitration must be considered when formularies are changed to reduce the drug acquisition cost.

▶ Therapeutic Use of LT_4

LT_4 is indicated for patients with overt hypothyroidism.[28] However, the need for treatment is controversial in patients with mild or subclinical disease. There are no large clinical trials that show an outcome benefit with treating these patients, and the therapeutic decision must be individualized. In patients without symptoms who have underlying heart disease, high cardiovascular risk, goiter, positive anti-TPOAb and/or are infertile or pregnant, LT_4 replacement should be considered.[14] Patients with mild or subclinical hypothyroidism do not need to be started on the full replacement dose because they still have some endogenous hormone production. Start these patients on 25 to 50 mcg/day and titrate every 6 to 8 weeks based on TSH levels. Over time, it is likely that the LT_4 dose will need to be increased slowly as the patient's thyroid gland loses residual function.

In patients younger than age 65 years with overt hypothyroidism, the average LT_4 replacement dose is 1.6 mcg/kg/day (use ideal body weight in obese patients[29]). However, there is wide interpatient variability in the optimal replacement dose, so individual dose titration is necessary. If there is no history of cardiac disease, these patients may be started on the full replacement dose.

The full replacement dose in patients older than age 75 years is lower, about 1 mcg/kg/day.[30] In the elderly, the starting dose should be 25 to 50 mcg/day, and the dose should then be titrated to the target TSH value. In patients with ischemic heart disease, start with 12.5 to 25 mcg/day and slowly titrate. If the patient develops angina or other forms of myocardial ischemia, lower the dose and titrate more slowly. At the start of therapy and with each change in dose, recheck the TSH in 6- to 8-week intervals. If the TSH is not in the target

Patient Encounter 1, Part 1

WM, a 49-year-old woman, comes to the clinic complaining of fatigue, lethargy, heavy periods, dry skin, and feeling cold all the time for the past 6 months. She thought it was because she was going through "the change," but the symptoms have not improved despite her primary care provider telling her she was not perimenopausal. She has noticed a 4.8-kg (10.5-lb) weight gain over the past 6 months. Her provider gave her a prescription for sertraline, but she did not get it filled because she did not think she was depressed. She takes no medications other than occasional acetaminophen for headache and milk of magnesia for constipation. Her vital signs and physical examination, including pelvic examination findings, are normal.

Labs

Serum cholesterol: 220 mg/dL (5.7 mmol/L; normal, less than 200 mg/dL, or 5.2 mmol/L); LDL cholesterol 101 mg/dL (2.6 mmol/L; normal less than 130 mg/dL or 3.36 mmol/L)

TSH: 8.6 mIU/L (reference range, 0.5 to 4.5 mIU/L)[a]

Free T$_4$: 0.9 ng/dL (11.5 pmol/L; reference range, 0.7 to 1.9 ng/dL, or 9 to 24.5 pmol/L)

PE: Wt: 74 kg (163 lb); ht: 5 ft, 5 in (165 cm); BMI: 27.2 kg/m^2

Should WM receive LT$_4$ therapy? Why or why not?

If treatment is indicated, what initial dose of LT$_4$ would you choose?

If treatment is not indicated, how would you monitor the patient?

What would you tell WM regarding the significance of her symptoms, elevated TSH level, and risk versus benefits of LT$_4$ therapy?

[a]Milli international units/L (mIU/L) = micro international units/mL (μIU/mL); clinical laboratories use either unit of measurement.

range (0.5 to 2.5 mIU/L or μIU/mL), change the dose by 10% to 20% and then recheck the TSH 6 to 8 weeks later. As the dose is titrated, assess the patient's symptoms. Many patients will improve quickly, and younger patients will feel the best if the TSH is titrated to low-normal to middle-normal levels (0.5 to 1.5 mIU/L or μIU/mL).

▶ Risks of Over- and Undertreatment

Patients receiving LT$_4$ therapy who are not maintained in a euthyroid state are at risk for long-term adverse sequelae. In general, overtreatment and a suppressed TSH are more common than undertreatment with an elevated TSH.[31] Patients with long-term overtreatment are at higher risk for atrial fibrillation and other cardiovascular morbidities, depression or mental status changes, and postmenopausal osteoporosis.

Elderly patients being treated with LT$_4$ have a dose-related risk of fractures even if their TSH is not suppressed below normal values.[32] Although studies have not defined a specific TSH target range for the elderly, these patients should receive close monitoring and dose adjustments to prevent overtreatment with LT$_4$. Patients who are undertreated are at higher risk for hypercholesterolemia and other cardiovascular problems, depression or mental status changes, and obstetric complications.

▶ Alterations in LT$_4$ Dose Requirements

A number of factors can alter LT$_4$ dose requirements (Table 44–4), including time of administration and drug–drug and drug–food interactions. LT$_4$ has the greatest and most consistent bioavailability when taken in the evening on an empty stomach.[33] The most common cause of increased dose requirement is the coadministration of LT$_4$ with calcium or iron supplements (including prenatal vitamins). Counsel patients that they should take the LT$_4$ dose at least 2 hours before or 6 hours after the calcium or iron dose. The most common cause of decreased dose requirement is aging.

Table 44–4

Factors That Alter LT$_4$ Dose Requirements

Increased Dose Requirement	Decreased Dose Requirement
Decreased LT$_4$ absorption	Aging
Malabsorption syndromes	Delivery of pregnancy
Drugs or diet	Withdrawal of interacting
Calcium	substance
Iron	
Aluminum	
Fiber	
Soy	
Cholestyramine or colestipol	
Sucralfate	
Sodium polystyrene sulfonate	
Phosphate binders	
Tube feeding	
Increased TBG	
Pregnancy	
Cirrhosis	
Estrogen therapy	
Tamoxifen, raloxifene therapy	
Hereditary	
Increased clearance	
Rifampin	
Carbamazepine	
Phenytoin	
Phenobarbital	
Impaired deiodination	
Amiodarone	
Mechanism unknown	
Sertraline, ? other serotonin-modulating drugs	
Lovastatin	
Critical illness	

LT$_4$, levothyroxine; TBG, thyroxine-binding globulin.

Table 44–5

Monitoring LT$_4$ Therapy

- Serum TSH
  - Every 6–12 months or if change in clinical status
  - 6–8 weeks after any dose or product change
  - As soon as possible in pregnancy; then monthly
- Same product prescribed and dispensed with every refill
- Watch for mg/mcg dosing errors
- Assess patient's understanding of disease, therapy, and need for adherence and tight control
- Assess for signs and symptoms of over- and undertreatment
- Identify potential interactions between LT$_4$, and foods and/or drugs

LT$_4$, levothyroxine; TSH, thyroid-stimulating hormone.

▶ Patient Monitoring

Patients on stable LT$_4$ therapy do not need frequent monitoring. In most patients, measuring a TSH every 6 to 12 months along with an assessment of clinical status is adequate (Table 44–5). If the patient's clinical status changes (e.g., pregnancy), more frequent monitoring may be necessary. LT$_4$ prescriptions should be written as microgram doses to avoid potential errors when written as milligram doses.

Patient education is an important component of care. Treatment adherence rates (at least 80% of doses taken) in hypothyroid patients are 68%, slightly less than adherence rates seen in hypertensive patients.[34] Educate patients about the benefits of proper therapy, the importance of adherence, consistency in time and method of administration, and the importance of receiving a consistent LT$_4$ product. Some patients take excessive amounts of LT$_4$ in an effort to "feel better" or as a weight loss treatment. Explain to patients that excessive amounts of LT$_4$ will not improve symptoms more than therapeutic doses will and can cause serious

Patient Encounter 1, Part 2

One year later, WM comes to you for routine follow-up stating that she has felt progressively worse since her last visit 2 months ago. Her most recent TSH determination, obtained 2 days ago, was 14.2 mIU/L (reference range, 0.5 to 4.5 mIU/L).[a]

Why is LT$_4$ therapy indicated?

What would you recommend regarding her LT$_4$ dose and monitoring?

What instructions would you give WM regarding her LT$_4$ therapy?

[a]Milli international units/L (mIU/L) = micro international units/mL (μIU/mL); clinical laboratories use either unit of measurement.

problems and that this drug is not an effective treatment for obesity.

▶ Special Populations and Conditions

Hypothyroidism and Pregnancy Hypothyroidism during pregnancy has a variety of maternal and fetal adverse effects.[18,35] During pregnancy, β-human chorionic gonadotropin (β-hCG) acts as a TSH receptor agonist, increasing the amount of thyroid hormone available for fetal growth and development. Maternal hypothyroidism results in an increased rate of miscarriage and decreased intellectual capacity of the child. Endocrinologists recommend a TSH measurement as soon as the pregnancy is confirmed. Most hypothyroid women who become pregnant will quickly need an increased dose of LT$_4$, typically 20% to 50% above the prepregnancy dose.[35] One study suggests increasing the woman's pregnancy dose by two tablets per week as soon as the pregnancy is diagnosed.[36] The increased dose should be maintained throughout the pregnancy, with monthly TSH monitoring to keep the TSH in the middle- to low-normal range. After delivery, the LT$_4$ dose usually can be reduced to prepregnancy levels, although patients with preexisting autoimmune thyroiditis may have increased postpartum dose requirements. Because prenatal vitamins contain significant amounts of calcium and iron, remind these patients to take the LT$_4$ dose at least 2 hours before or 6 hours after the vitamin.

Children Congenital hypothyroidism is still seen in the United States (fewer than 0.02% of newborns[6]), and all newborns in the United States undergo screening with a TSH level. As soon as the hypothyroid state is identified, the newborn should receive the full LT$_4$ replacement dose. The replacement dose of LT$_4$ in children is age dependent. In newborns, the usual dose is 10 to 17 mcg/kg/day. LT$_4$ tablets may be crushed and mixed with breast milk or formula, but it is best to administer LT$_4$ to infants and children on an empty stomach.[37] Serum FT$_4$ levels (target, 1.6 to 2.2 ng/dL or 20.6 to 28.3 pmol/L) are used for dose titration in infants because the TSH level may not respond to treatment as it does in older children and adults. By 6 months of age, the required dose is reduced to 5 to 7 mcg/kg/day, and from ages 1 to 10 years, the dose is 3 to 6 mcg/kg/day. After age 12 years, adult doses can be given.

Myxedema Coma This is a life-threatening condition owing to severe, long standing hypothyroidism and has a mortality rate of 60% to 70%. These patients are given 300 to 500 mcg LT$_4$ intravenously initially, using caution in patients with underlying cardiac disease. Although administration of T$_3$ would provide a more rapid onset of action, there is no evidence that T$_3$ improves outcomes in patients with myxedema coma. Historically, glucocorticoids, such as hydrocortisone 50 to 100 mg every 6 hours, are administered owing to concern about simultaneous adrenal insufficiency. Although there is no strong evidence for an outcome benefit, the use of glucocorticoids is reasonable because such treatment may be lifesaving, and the risks of a short course of corticosteroids at this dose are low. As patients improve, the LT$_4$ dose can be given orally in a typical full replacement dose.

Patient Care and Monitoring: Hypothyroidism

1. Use serum TSH to identify patients with hypothyroidism and to monitor LT_4 replacement therapy.

2. Use synthetic LT_4 as the treatment of choice for hypothyroidism.

3. Provide LT_4 replacement to patients with overt hypothyroidism.

4. Consider replacement therapy in patients with a TSH level of greater than 4.5 but less than 10 mIU/L[a] who have subtle symptoms (e.g., mild fatigue, lethargy), an elevated cholesterol level, underlying heart disease, or positive anti-TPOAbs.

5. Patients with mild hypothyroidism may be started at 25 to 50 mcg/day of LT_4.

6. Patients with overt hypothyroidism who are older than 12 and younger than 65 years of age and who do not have cardiac disease may receive the calculated full replacement LT_4 dose (1.6 mcg/kg/day based on ideal body weight if obese).

7. Elderly patients or those with cardiac disease should be started at a lower LT_4 dose (e.g., 12.5 to 25 mcg/day).

8. Measure serum TSH 6 to 8 weeks after starting or any dose change. If the TSH level is not in the target range, alter the dose by 10% to 20% increments.

9. The target TSH for patients on LT_4 replacement therapy for hypothyroidism is 0.5 to 2.5 mIU/L. Younger patients often feel best at a TSH level in the low- to middle-normal range (i.e., 0.5 to 1.5 mIU/L).

10. Provide a brand-name LT_4 product, and do not allow the patient to switch to different products. If the product is switched, check a TSH in 6 weeks and retitrate the dose.

11. Provide LT_4 prescriptions as microgram, not milligram, doses to avoid errors.

12. Check a TSH every 6 to 12 months in stable patients receiving LT_4 replacement.

13. Make sure that patients understand the importance of adherence and the risks of over- and underuse of LT_4.

14. At each visit, assess the patient for signs and symptoms of over- and undertreatment.

15. Monitor for drug interactions, such as LT_4 absorption problems caused by calcium and iron.

16. Check a TSH in pregnant women as soon as the pregnancy is diagnosed. In hypothyroid pregnant women, check the TSH monthly, and expect to increase the LT_4 dose early in the first trimester. Maintain the TSH in the low- to middle-normal range. After delivery, reduce the LT_4 dose to the prepregnancy dose.

---

[a]Milli international units/L (mIU/L) = micro international units/mL (μIU/mL); clinical laboratories use either unit of measurement.

HYPERTHYROIDISM AND THYROTOXICOSIS

Hyperthyroidism is much less common than hypothyroidism. In NHANES, 0.5% of the population was hyperthyroid, with the highest incidences in women overall and in men and women in the over 80 years of age groups.[1] The Colorado Thyroid Health Study showed a hyperthyroid incidence of 2.2% (2.1% subclinical).[2]

Causes of Thyrotoxicosis and Hyperthyroidism

Hyperthyroidism is related to excess thyroid hormone secreted by the thyroid gland. Thyrotoxicosis is any syndrome caused by excess thyroid hormone and can be related to excess hormone production (hyperthyroidism). The common causes of thyrotoxicosis are shown in Table 44–6.[38-40] Graves' disease is the most common cause of hyperthyroidism. Thyrotoxicosis in the elderly is more likely caused by toxic thyroid nodules or multinodular goiter than by Graves' disease. Excessive intake of thyroid hormone may be caused by overtreatment with prescribed therapy. Surreptitious use of thyroid hormones also may occur, especially in health professionals or as a self-remedy for obesity. Thyroid hormones can be obtained easily without a prescription from health food stores or Internet sources. Refer to Clinical Presentation and Diagnosis of Hyperthyroidism for information regarding screening and diagnosis.

Table 44–6
Causes of Thyrotoxicosis[39,40]
Primary hyperthyroidism
Graves' disease
Toxic multinodular goiter
Toxic adenoma
Thyroid cancer
Struma ovarii
Iodine excess (including radiocontrast, amiodarone)
Thyrotoxicosis without hyperthyroidism
Subacute thyroiditis
Silent (painless) thyroiditis
Excess thyroid hormone intake (thyrotoxicosis factitia)
Drug-induced (amiodarone, iodine, lithium, interferons)
Secondary hyperthyroidism
TSH-secreting pituitary tumors
Trophoblastic (hCG-secreting) tumors
Gestational thyrotoxicosis

hCG, human chorionic gonadotropin; TSH, thyroid-stimulating hormone.

Clinical Presentation and Diagnosis: Hyperthyroidism[39,40]

Symptoms

- Nervousness
- Fatigue
- Weakness
- Increased perspiration
- Heat intolerance
- Tremor
- Hyperactivity, irritability
- Palpitations
- Appetite change (usually increased)
- Weight change (usually weight loss)
- Menstrual disturbances (often oligomenorrhea)
- Diarrhea

Signs

- Hyperactivity
- Tachycardia

- Atrial fibrillation (especially in elderly adults)
- Hyperreflexia
- Warm, moist skin
- Ophthalmopathy, dermopathy (Graves' disease)
- Goiter
- Muscle weakness

Screening/Diagnosis

- Low TSH level (less than 0.5 mIU/L) signifies thyrotoxicosis.
- Free T$_4$ is elevated in overt hyperthyroidism but may be normal in mild hyperthyroidism.
- Increased radioiodine uptake in the thyroid indicates increased hormone production by the thyroid gland.
- Almost all patients with Graves' disease will have positive TSHR-SAbs and positive anti-TPOAbs.

Clinical Manifestations of Thyrotoxicosis

Many of the signs and symptoms seem to be related to autonomic hyperactivity. As with hypothyroidism, the clinical manifestations of hyperthyroidism may be subtle and slowly progressive. Screening of patients for thyroid disease may identify patients with subclinical or mild thyrotoxicosis. Patients may seek medical attention only after a long period of thyrotoxicosis or owing to an acute complication such as atrial fibrillation. The clinical manifestations of thyrotoxicosis in the elderly may be blunted or atypical. These patients may present only with atrial fibrillation, depression, or altered mental status or cognition.

Subclinical Hyperthyroidism

Subclinical or mild hyperthyroidism is defined as a low TSH level with a normal FT$_4$ level.[14] Although there may be few or no symptoms in these patients, there are several areas of concern.[17] Some patients progress to overt thyrotoxicosis. Patients with subclinical hyperthyroidism have been shown to experience long-term cardiovascular and bone sequelae. The impact of subclinical hyperthyroidism on cardiovascular mortality is not clear.[14–17] Several studies have shown that prolonged subclinical thyrotoxicosis speeds the loss of bone mineral density and increases fracture rates in postmenopausal women.[17] Treatment of patients with subclinical hyperthyroidism is controversial but should be considered in patients with TSH levels less than 0.1 mIU/L (less than 0.1 μIU/mL), postmenopausal women, and patients with underlying cardiovascular disease.[17] Patients who do not have a fully suppressed (below the lower limit of detection) TSH or

other risk factors for hyperthyroid complications (e.g., osteoporosis, cardiac arrhythmias) may just undergo observation, with TSH testing every 6 months to identify progression of the hyperthyroid state.

Graves' Disease

Graves' disease is an autoimmune syndrome that includes hyperthyroidism, diffuse thyroid enlargement, exophthalmos and other eye findings, and skin findings.[38] The prevalence of Graves' disease in the United States is approximately 0.4% in women and 0.1% in men. The peak age of incidence is 20 to 49 years, with a second peak after 80 years of age. Hyperthyroidism results from the production of TSHR-SAbs (TSH receptor-stimulating antibodies) in at least 80% of patients with clinical Graves' disease. These antibodies have TSH agonist activity, thereby stimulating hormone synthesis and release. These antibodies cross-react with orbital and fibroblastic tissue, resulting in ophthalmopathy and dermopathy. Although the underlying cause of Graves' disease is not known, heredity seems to play a role. Subclinical Graves' disease may become acutely overt in the presence of iodine excess, infection, stress, parturition, smoking, and lithium and cytokine therapy.

Several features of Graves' disease are distinct from other forms of thyrotoxicosis. Clinically apparent ophthalmopathic changes are seen in 20% to 40% of patients[38] and include exophthalmos, proptosis, chemosis, conjunctival injection, and periorbital edema. Eyelid retraction causes a typical staring or startled appearance (Fig. 44–3). Patients may complain of vague eye discomfort and excess tearing. In severe cases, the eyelids are unable to close completely, resulting in corneal damage. In very severe cases, the optic

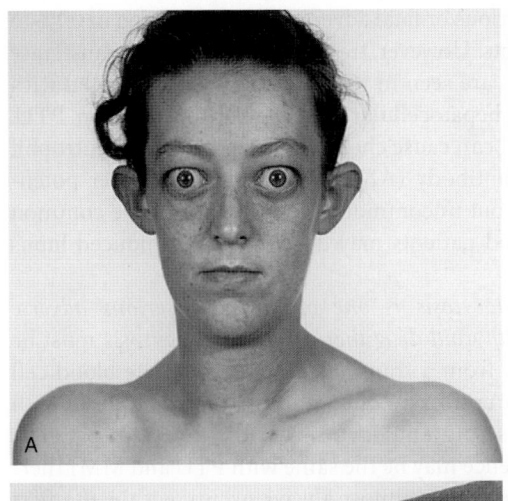

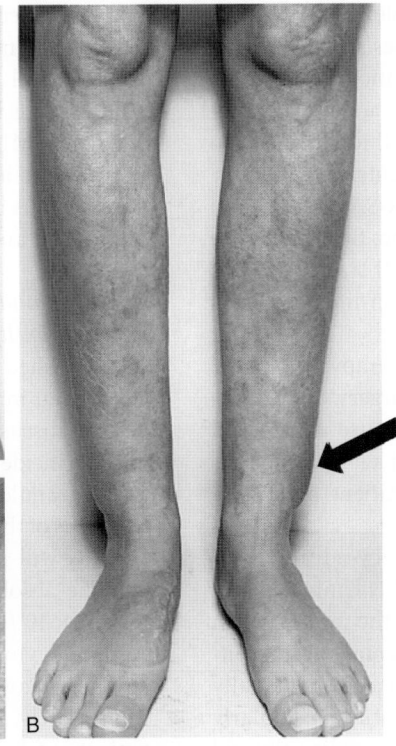

FIGURE 44–3. Features of Graves' disease. (**A**) Facial appearance: exophthalmos, eyelid retraction, periorbital edema, and proptosis. (**B**) Thyroid dermopathy over lateral aspects of the shins (*arrow*). (**C**) Thyroid clubbing, or acropachy (*arrow*). (From Jameson JL, Weetman AP. Disorders of the thyroid gland. In: Kasper DL, Braunwald E, Fauci AS, et al., eds. Harrison's Principles of Internal Medicine. 16th ed. New York: McGraw-Hill; 2004:2114.)

nerve can be compressed, resulting in permanent vision loss. All patients with suspected or known Graves' disease must be evaluated and monitored by an ophthalmologist.

Dermopathy occurs in 5% to 10% of patients with Graves' disease and usually is associated with severe ophthalmopathy. Skin findings include hyperpigmented, nonpitting induration of the skin, typically over the pretibial area (pretibial myxedema), the dorsa of the feet, and the shoulder areas. Clubbing of the digits (thyroid acropachy) is associated with long-standing thyrotoxicosis.

Treatment of Hyperthyroidism

Treatment of thyrotoxicosis caused by hyperthyroidism is similar regardless of the underlying cause.[39-44] **7** *The goals of treating hyperthyroidism are to relieve signs and symptoms, reduce thyroid hormone production to normal levels and achieve biochemical euthyroidism, and prevent long-term adverse sequelae.*

▶ *β-Blockers*

Because many of the manifestations of hyperthyroidism appear to be mediated by the β-adrenergic system, β-adrenergic blockers are used to rapidly relieve palpitations, tremor, anxiety, and heat intolerance. Because β-blockers do not reduce the synthesis of thyroid hormones, they are used only until more specific antithyroid therapy is effective. Because nonselective agents can impair the conversion of T_4 to T_3, propranolol and nadolol are used. An initial propranolol dose of 20 to 40 mg four times daily should be titrated to relieve signs (target heart rate less than 90 beats/min) and symptoms. β-Blockers should not be used in patients with decompensated heart failure or asthma. When a contraindication to β-blockers exists, clonidine or diltiazem may be used for rate control.

▶ *Methods to Reduce Thyroid Hormone Synthesis*

Excess production of thyroid hormone can be reduced in four ways: iodides, antithyroid drugs, radioactive iodine, and surgery.

Iodide Large doses of iodide inhibit the synthesis and release of thyroid hormones. Serum T_4 levels may be reduced within 24 hours, and the effects may last for 2 to 3 weeks. Iodides are used most commonly in Graves' disease patients before surgery and to quickly reduce hormone release in patients with thyroid storm. Potassium iodide is administered either as a saturated solution (SSKI) that contains 38 mg iodide per drop or as Lugol's solution, which contains 6.3 mg iodide per drop. The typical starting dose is 120 to 400 mg/day. Iodide therapy should start 7 to 14 days before surgery. Iodide should not be given before radioactive iodine treatment because the iodide will inhibit concentration of the radioactivity in the thyroid. Iodides also are used to protect the thyroid from radioactive iodine fallout after a nuclear accident or attack. Daily administration of 30 to 100 mg iodide markedly reduces thyroid gland uptake of radioactive iodine. The most frequent toxic effects with iodide therapy are hypersensitivity reactions, "iodism" (characterized by palpitations, depression, weight loss, and pustular skin eruptions), and gynecomastia.

Antithyroid Drugs The thionamide agents propylthiouracil (PTU) and methimazole (MMI) are used in the United States to treat hyperthyroidism. Carbimazole, an MMI prodrug, is used in some countries (10 mg carbimazole = 6 mg MMI). These drugs inhibit thyroid hormone synthesis by interfering with thyroid peroxidase–mediated iodination of tyrosine residues in thyroglobulin. PTU has the added effect of inhibiting the conversion of T_4 to T_3. The thionamides also have immunosuppressant effects. In patients with Graves' disease treated with thionamides, TSHR-SAb levels and other immune mediators decrease over time. Both drugs are well absorbed from the gastrointestinal (GI) tract. PTU has a half-life of 1 to 2.5 hours, whereas the half-life of MMI is 6 to 9 hours.

Antithyroid drugs are used as primary therapy for Graves' disease or as preparative therapy before surgery or radioactive iodine administration. The decision to use antithyroid drugs as primary therapy must be weighed against the risks and benefits of radioiodine or surgery. Patient preference must be considered.

In most patients, there is no clear efficacy advantage of one thionamide over the other, but in the United States, MMI use has increased dramatically since the mid-1990s in lieu of PTU.[45] Although PTU has the advantage of inhibiting T_4-to-T_3 conversion, MMI can be given as a single daily dose and may have a better overall safety profile, particularly less hepatotoxicity. MMI is preferred to normalize thyroid function before radioactive iodine therapy, although both thionamides increase the failure rate of radioactive iodine therapy.[46] The usual starting dose of MMI is 10 to 20 mg/day, and the usual starting dose of PTU is 50 to 150 mg three times daily. Thyroid hormone levels drop in 2 to 3 weeks, and after 6 weeks, 90% of patients with Graves' disease will be euthyroid. Thyroid function testing should be performed every 4 to 6 weeks until stable. After the patient becomes euthyroid, the antithyroid drug dose often can be decreased (5 to 10 mg/day MMI, 100 to 200 mg/day PTU) to maintain the euthyroid state. Excessive doses of antithyroid drugs will result in hypothyroidism.

Remission of Graves' disease occurs in 40% to 60% of patients after 1 to 2 years of therapy. Antithyroid therapy may be stopped or tapered after 12 to 24 months. Relapse usually occurs in the first 3 to 6 months after stopping antithyroid therapy. Levels of TSHR-SAb after a course of treatment may have predictive value for the risk of relapse in that antibody-positive patients almost always will relapse. However, antibody-negative patients also may relapse after therapy is stopped. About 75% of women in remission who become pregnant will have a postpartum relapse. When therapy is discontinued, a therapeutic strategy should be in place in the event of relapse. Many patients will opt for radioactive iodine as a long-term solution.

Antithyroid drugs are associated with an overall low rate of adverse effects, although serious adverse effects can occur. In 2010, the FDA released a new boxed warning on severe liver injury with PTU.[47] The warning includes a statement that PTU should only be used in patients who cannot tolerate MMI. Skin rash, arthralgias, and GI upset are seen in 5% of patients. Although the drug can be continued in the presence of a minor skin rash, the development of arthralgia warrants discontinuation. Hepatotoxicity is an uncommon but potentially serious or fatal adverse effect, occurring in 0.1% to 0.2% of patients. However, transient rises in aminotransferase enzyme levels are seen in up to 30% of patients treated with PTU. Severe hepatocellular damage can occur from PTU, whereas MMI can cause cholestatic jaundice. Antineutrophil cytoplasmic antibody (ANCA) vasculitis is another potentially serious but uncommon reaction that is more common with PTU, and patients may develop a drug-induced lupus syndrome.

❽ *Agranulocytosis is one of the most serious adverse effects of antithyroid drug therapy.* Agranulocytosis must be distinguished from a transient decrease in white blood cell count seen in up to 12% of adults and 25% of children with Graves' disease. Agranulocytosis occurs in 0.3% of patients, and the incidence may be the same with PTU and MMI therapy. Agranulocytosis almost always occurs within the first 3 months of therapy, and it occurs suddenly and unpredictably. Patients will present with fever, malaise, and a sore throat, and the absolute neutrophil count will be less than 1,000/mm^3 (1×10^9/L). Patients may develop sepsis and die rapidly. Agranulocytosis is thought to be autoimmune mediated. If agranulocytosis occurs, discontinue the antithyroid drug immediately, administer broad-spectrum antibiotics if the patient is febrile, and consider the administration of granulocyte colony-stimulating factor. The white blood cell count should recover in 1 or 2 weeks. Patients who develop agranulocytosis should not be switched to another thionamide drug. Monitoring for agranulocytosis is controversial owing to its sudden and unpredictable nature. Most practitioners do not recommend routine monitoring of the complete blood count, although early detection could improve patient outcomes. Patients initiating thionamide therapy must be informed about the signs and symptoms of agranulocytosis and other serious side effects. Patients should be counseled to report signs and symptoms suggestive of infection, such as fever and sore throat lasting more than 2 or 3 days, bruising, pruritic rash, jaundice, dark urine, arthralgias, abdominal pain, nausea or fatigue.

Radioactive Iodine Radioactive iodine, typically ¹³¹I, produces thyroid ablation without surgery. ¹³¹I is well absorbed after oral administration. The iodine is concentrated in the thyroid gland and has a half-life of 8 days. Over a period of weeks, thyroid cells that have taken up the ¹³¹I begin to develop abnormalities and necrosis. Eventually, thyroid cells are destroyed, and hormone production is reduced. After a single dose, 40% to 70% of patients will be euthyroid in 6 to 8 weeks, and 80% will be cured. In most patients, hypothyroidism will develop, and long-term LT_4 replacement will be necessary. Because ¹³¹I has a slow onset of action, most patients are treated initially with β-blockers and antithyroid drugs. MMI is the preferred agent before the administration of ¹³¹I. MMI is discontinued 3 to 5 days before the administration of ¹³¹I and is restarted 3 to 7 days later. MMI is then slowly tapered over the next 4 to 6 weeks as thyroid function normalizes. β-Blockers can be continued during ¹³¹I therapy. The dose of ¹³¹I is based on the estimated weight of the patient's thyroid gland (typical dose,

10 to 15 mCi [370 to 555 MBq]). Radioactive iodine therapy is contraindicated during pregnancy and breastfeeding. Radioactive iodine therapy may acutely worsen Graves' ophthalmopathy. Patients with prominent eye disease may be started on prednisone 40 mg/day, with the dose tapered over 2 to 3 months. Radioactive iodine also may cause a painful thyroiditis, which may necessitate anti-inflammatory therapy. No long-term carcinogenic effect of ^{131}I has been demonstrated in clinical trials.

Surgery Subtotal thyroidectomy is indicated in patients with very large goiters and thyroid malignancies and those who do not respond or cannot tolerate other therapies. Patients must be euthyroid before surgery, and they are often administered iodide preoperatively to reduce gland vascularity. The overall surgical complication rate is 2.7%. Postoperative hypothyroidism occurs in 10% of patients who undergo subtotal thyroidectomy. After thyroidectomy, serum calcium and intact parathyroid hormone levels should be monitored for early identification of postoperative hypoparathyroidism. Postoperative administration of 1,250 to 2,500 mg/day of calcium and 0.5 mcg/day of calcitriol may be given and then tapered over 1 to 2 weeks if the patient does not develop hypoparathyroidism.

▶ Special Conditions and Populations

Graves' Disease and Pregnancy[39,48] Pregnancy may worsen or precipitate thyrotoxicosis in women with underlying Graves' disease owing to the TSH agonist effect of β-hCG.

Untreated maternal thyrotoxicosis may result in increased rates of miscarriage, premature delivery, eclampsia, and low-birth-weight infants. Fetal and neonatal hyperthyroidism may occur as a result of transplacental passage of TSHR-SAbs. Because radioactive iodine is contraindicated and surgery is best avoided during pregnancy, most patients are treated with antithyroid drugs. PTU is considered the treatment of choice, particularly in the first trimester, because of a rare but well-documented teratogenic effect of MMI. Patients receiving prepregnancy MMI should be switched to PTU as soon as the pregnancy is diagnosed. The lowest possible dose of PTU to maintain maternal euthyroidism should be used. Given the potential maternal adverse effects of PTU (e.g., hepatotoxicity), it may be preferable to switch from PTU to MMI for the second and third trimesters.[47] Antithyroid therapy in excessive doses may suppress fetal thyroid function. Although PTU and MMI are found in breast milk, nursing mothers should be switched to MMI after delivery because of the risk of hepatotoxicity from PTU in the mother and infant.

Pediatric Hyperthyroidism[39] β-Blockers are administered to children who are symptomatic or have a heart rate greater than 100 beats/min. MMI is the preferred antithyroid drug therapy in children at a dose of 0.2 to 0.5 mg/kg/day. Once a euthyroid state is achieved, the MMI dose can be reduced by 50% or more to maintain euthyroidism. As in adults, antithyroid drugs are administered to children with Graves' disease for 1 to 2 years. If remission does not occur in that

---

Patient Encounter 2

TS is a 29-year-old woman who comes to the clinic stating, "I'm so jumpy and sweaty and hungry, and I'm losing weight. I think I'm losing my mind. What is wrong with me? Is it because I'm pregnant?" She first noticed these symptoms 4 months ago, and they have worsened steadily since she became pregnant 2 months ago. She feels anxious for no reason and has trouble sleeping. She has noticed that her appetite has increased, although she has lost about 1 kg (2.2 lb) over the past 2 months despite being pregnant. Sometimes she can feel her heart beating in her chest, but she denies chest pain or syncope. Her only medications are a prenatal vitamin, occasional ibuprofen for headaches, and an herbal product for boosting energy. She thinks that her mother had some kind of thyroid problem when she was pregnant.

PE:

VS: Pulse 122 beats/min, BP 106/71, RR 12, temperature 37.4°C (99.3°F)

HEENT: Diffusely enlarged thyroid; mild exophthalmos

CV: Tachycardic, RRR

Exts: Fine tremor

Skin: Warm, moist, and soft

ECG: Sinus tachycardia

Uterine ultrasound: 6-week-size fetus

Labs

Electrolytes, complete blood count normal. TSH less than 0.1 mIU/L (reference range 0.5 to 2.5 mIU/L)[a]; free T_4 (FT_4) 3.6 ng/dL (46.3 pmol/L; reference range 0.7 to 1.9 ng/dL, or 9.0 to 24.5 pmol/L); +ve TSHR-SAbs

What therapeutic options exist for TS's Graves' disease while she is pregnant?

Could the herbal product be causing any of her signs and symptoms?

What pharmacotherapy would you recommend? Would you change it after she has her baby?

How would you initiate and titrate therapy?

What would you tell TS regarding the cause of her signs and symptoms, significance of her abnormal thyroid function tests, and therapeutic options?

---

[a]Milli international units/L (mIU/L) = micro international units/mL (μIU/mL); clinical laboratories use either unit of measurement.

Patient Care and Monitoring: Hyperthyroidism

1. A low or undetectable TSH level identifies thyrotoxicosis.

2. Refer the patient for a diagnostic assessment to identify the underlying cause. Identify Graves' disease by the presence of eye and/or skin findings and the presence of TSHR-SAbs.

3. Refer patients with Graves' disease to an ophthalmologist for assessment and monitoring.

4. Treat severe or troublesome autonomic signs and symptoms with a nonselective β-blocker such as propranolol 20 to 40 mg four times daily. Titrate the β-blocker dose based on signs and symptoms.

5. In patients with excess thyroid hormone production, reduce hormone production with an antithyroid drug and/or radioactive iodine. Choose therapy based on patient-specific factors and preference.

6. Antithyroid drugs have a delayed effect. After 2 to 4 weeks of therapy, adjust the dose if the TSH is not in the target range (0.5 to 2.5 mIU/L).[a] When the patient is euthyroid, consider reducing the dose of antithyroid drug to avoid hypothyroidism.

7. MMI is the antithyroid drug of choice in most patients.

8. Treat pregnant hyperthyroid women with PTU.

9. Consider stopping antithyroid therapy in patients with Graves' disease after 12 to 18 months to see if remission has occurred.

10. Monitor patients on antithyroid drugs for signs and symptoms of adverse effects.

    a. Baseline CBC with differential and liver profile

    b. Repeat CBC when patient has a febrile illness. Routine monitoring of WBC is not recommended.

    c. Repeat liver panel if signs or symptoms of hepatotoxicity occur (some recommend routine monitoring during the first 6 months of therapy).

    d. Assess any skin rash or development of arthralgias.

11. If radioactive iodine is given, make sure that antithyroid drugs are stopped 4 to 6 days before treatment.

12. Several months after radioactive iodine, expect that the patient will require permanent LT$_4$ replacement.

---

[a]Milli international units/L (mIU/L) = micro international units/mL (μIU/mL); clinical laboratories use either unit of measurement.

---

time, long-term antithyroid drug therapy, radioactive iodine, or surgical therapy is offered. Long-term studies with ^{131}I use in children show no increased risk of thyroid cancer or leukemia.

Thyroid Storm[39,49] Thyroid storm is a life-threatening condition caused by severe thyrotoxicosis. Signs and symptoms include high fever, tachycardia, tachypnea, dehydration, delirium, coma, and GI disturbances. Thyroid storm is precipitated in a previously hyperthyroid patient by infection, trauma, surgery, radioactive iodine treatment, and sudden withdrawal from antithyroid drugs. Patients are treated with a short-acting β-blocker such as intravenous (IV) esmolol, IV or oral iodide, and large doses of PTU (500 to 1,000 mg load; then 250 mg every 4 hours) or MMI (60 to 80 mg/day). Supportive care with acetaminophen to suppress fever, fluid and electrolyte management, and antiarrhythmic agents are important components of therapy. IV hydrocortisone 300 mg initially and then 100 mg every 8 hours is used often because of the potential presence of adrenal insufficiency.

NONTHYROIDAL ILLNESS (EUTHYROID SICK SYNDROME)

A number of changes in the hypothalamic–pituitary–thyroid axis occur during acute illness.[50,51] These changes are termed *nonthyroidal illness* or *euthyroid sick syndrome*. The type and degree of abnormalities depend on the severity of

illness. Mild to moderate medical illness, surgery, or starvation causes a decrease in serum T$_3$ levels owing to decreased peripheral conversion of T$_4$ to T$_3$. The reduced T$_3$ levels do not correlate with ultimate mortality and are thought to be an adaptive response to stress. Patients with more severe illness, especially those in the intensive care unit, frequently have reduced total T$_4$ levels, although FT$_4$ levels often are normal. In critically ill patients, there is a correlation between the degree of serum T$_4$ reduction and mortality. In most acutely ill patients who are euthyroid, the TSH level is normal. However, administration of dopamine, octreotide, or high doses of glucocorticoids can reduce TSH levels. During recovery from acute illness, the TSH level may become modestly elevated to renormalize serum T$_4$ levels. During this time, thyroid function tests may be misinterpreted to indicate hypothyroidism. Despite the sometimes very low T$_4$ levels, there is no evidence that LT$_4$ administration has any benefit. Patients with possible thyroid abnormalities during acute illness should be evaluated by an endocrinologist.

THYROID CANCER AND LT$_4$ SUPPRESSION

9 *The growth and spread of thyroid carcinoma are stimulated by TSH. An important component of thyroid carcinoma management is the use of LT$_4$ to suppress TSH secretion. Early in therapy, patients receive the lowest LT$_4$ dose sufficient to* *fully suppress TSH to undetectable levels. Controlled trials show that suppressive LT$_4$ therapy reduces tumor growth and improves survival.* These patients are purposefully "over-treated" with LT$_4$, sometimes to a fully-suppressed TSH level, and rendered subclinically hyperthyroid. Postmenopausal women should receive aggressive osteoporosis therapy to prevent LT$_4$-induced bone loss. Other thyrotoxic complications, such as atrial fibrillation, should be monitored and managed appropriately.

DRUG-INDUCED THYROID ABNORMALITIES

Drugs can affect thyroid function in a number of ways.[13,52] The effects of drugs on thyroid hormone protein binding, LT$_4$ absorption, and metabolism have been discussed previously. Several commonly used medications can alter thyroid hormone secretion.

Amiodarone

Amiodarone is a commonly prescribed antiarrhythmic drug that contains two iodide atoms, constituting 38% of its mass.[53] Each 200-mg dose of amiodarone provides 75 mg of iodide. Amiodarone deiodination releases about 6 mg of free iodine daily, 20 to 40 times more than the average daily intake of iodine in the United States. Amiodarone blocks conversion of T$_4$ to T$_3$, inhibits entry of T$_3$ into cells, and decreases T$_3$ receptor binding. Amiodarone causes rapid reduction in serum T$_3$ levels, increases free and total T$_4$ levels, and increases TSH level. After 3 months of therapy, TSH levels usually return to normal, although the serum T$_3$ and T$_4$ level changes may remain. Most of these patients are euthyroid because the free T$_3$ levels are in the low-normal range. Amiodarone can frequently cause thyroid abnormalities in previously euthyroid patients. In a study of amiodarone treatment of persistent atrial fibrillation, 25.8% of patients developed subclinical hypothyroidism, and 5% developed overt hypothyroidism.[54] Hyperthyroidism occurred in 5.3%. Thyroid abnormalities, when they occurred, were seen within 6 months of initiation of amiodarone therapy in almost all patients. Amiodarone-induced hypothyroidism is more common in iodine-sufficient areas of the world. Patients with underlying autoimmune thyroiditis are much more likely to develop amiodarone-induced hypothyroidism. Amiodarone-induced hypothyroidism occurs most commonly within the first year of therapy. If amiodarone cannot be discontinued, LT$_4$ therapy will be effective in most patients. If amiodarone can be stopped, thyroid function will return to normal in 2 to 4 months.

Amiodarone is more likely to cause thyrotoxicosis in iodine-deficient areas. Type 1 amiodarone-induced thyrotoxicosis is caused by iodine excess and typically occurs in patients with preexisting multinodular goiter or subclinical Graves' disease. Type 2 amiodarone-induced thyrotoxicosis is a destructive thyroiditis that occurs in patients with no underlying thyroid disease. Amiodarone-induced thyrotoxicosis is more common in men. Because amiodarone has β-blocking activity, palpitations and tachycardia may be absent. In type 1 thyrotoxicosis, amiodarone should be discontinued. If amiodarone therapy cannot be stopped, larger doses of antithyroid drugs may be needed to control thyrotoxicosis. In type 2 thyroiditis, stopping amiodarone may not be necessary because spontaneous resolution may occur. Prednisone 40 to 60 mg/day will quickly improve thyrotoxic symptoms. Prednisone may be tapered after 1 to 2 months of therapy.

❿ *Patients receiving amiodarone must receive monitoring for thyroid abnormalities. Baseline measurements of serum TSH, FT$_4$, FT$_3$, anti-TPOAbs, and TSHR-SAbs should be performed. TSH, FT$_4$, and FT$_3$ should be checked 3 months after initiation of amiodarone and then at least a TSH every 3 to 6 months.*

Lithium

Lithium is associated with hypothyroidism in up to 34% of patients, and hypothyroidism may occur after years of therapy.[55] Lithium appears to inhibit thyroid hormone synthesis and secretion. Patients with underlying autoimmune thyroiditis are more likely to develop lithium-induced hypothyroidism. Patients may require LT$_4$ replacement even if lithium is discontinued.

Interferon-α

Interferon-α causes hypothyroidism in up to 39% of patients being treated for hepatitis C infection. Patients may develop a transient thyroiditis with hyperthyroidism before becoming hypothyroid. The hypothyroidism may be transient as well. Asians and patients with preexisting anti-TPOAbs are more likely to develop interferon-induced hypothyroidism. The mechanism of interferon-induced hypothyroidism is not known. If LT$_4$ replacement is initiated, it should be stopped after 6 months to reevaluate the need for replacement therapy.

Tyrosine Kinase Inhibitors

Tyrosine kinase inhibitors (TKIs) are an emerging class of targeted antineoplastic agents used in several types of malignancies, including thyroid cancer.[13] Several TKIs have significant effects on thyroid function, both in previously hypothyroid patients on LT$_4$ replacement and in previously euthyroid patients. Imatinib has been shown to cause a fourfold increase in TSH levels in patients being treated for thyroid cancer. Sunitinib and sorafenib have been associated with primary hypothyroidism in 20% to 40% of treated patients. Some sorafenib patients developed mild hyperthyroidism before becoming hypothyroid. Patients receiving TKI therapy should have baseline and periodic thyroid function monitoring.

OUTCOME EVALUATION

- Desired outcomes include relieving signs and symptoms and achieving a euthyroid state.

- Success of therapy for thyroid disorders must be based not only on short-term improvement of the patient's clinical status and abnormal laboratory values but also on achievement of a long-term euthyroid state. Maintaining

TSH level in the normal range improves symptoms and reduces the risk of long-term complications.

- Because pharmacotherapy often is lifelong, especially in patients with hypothyroidism, patients must undergo periodic monitoring to avoid the long-term complications of hypothyroidism and hyperthyroidism. In hypothyroid patients, such monitoring may involve simply asking the patient about signs and symptoms and a yearly measurement of the TSH level.

- Any change in the patient's clinical status, such as a new pregnancy or a major change in body weight, necessitates a reevaluation of therapy. Patients at high risk for complications, such as pregnant women, the elderly, and patients with underlying cardiac disease, must be monitored more closely.

- Patients should be educated and periodically reminded about the importance of adherence and long-term tight control, the need for periodic clinical and laboratory monitoring, and the importance of staying on one LT$_4$ product.

- In hyperthyroid patients, relieving signs and symptoms and achieving a euthyroid state are the desired outcomes. The method of achieving these outcomes may change over time with the use of antithyroid drugs versus radioactive iodine.

- Patients with hyperthyroidism also must undergo periodic clinical and laboratory monitoring, with more frequent monitoring if there is a change in the patient's clinical status.

- Patients who receive antithyroid drugs must be monitored for adverse drug events such as agranulocytosis.

- Patients who receive radioactive iodine must be monitored for the development of hypothyroidism.

- In patients with thyroid cancer, the desired outcomes with LT$_4$ therapy often are different from those in hypothyroid patients.

- LT$_4$ doses sufficient to suppress tumor growth may result in a suppressed TSH and mild hyperthyroidism. These patients must be monitored closely for complications of the mild hyperthyroid state, such as bone mineral loss and development of atrial fibrillation.

Abbreviations Introduced in This Chapter

ANCA	Antineutrophil cytoplasmic antibody
ANDA	Abbreviated New Drug Application
Anti-TGAb	Antithyroglobulin antibody
Anti-TPOAb	Antithyroid peroxidase antibody
AUC	Area under the (time-concentration) curve
β-hCG	β-Human chorionic gonadotropin
CNS	Central nervous system
FDA	Food and Drug Administration
FT$_3$	Free T$_3$
FT$_4$	Free T$_4$

GI	Gastrointestinal
hCG	Human chorionic gonadotropin
IV	Intravenous
LDL	Low density lipoprotein
LT$_4$	Levothyroxine
MMI	Methimazole
NHANES	National Health and Nutrition Examination Survey
NTI	Narrow therapeutic index
PTU	Propylthiouracil
RAIU	Radioactive iodine uptake
SSKI	Saturated solution of potassium iodide
T$_3$	Triiodothyronine
T$_4$	Thyroxine
TBG	Thyroxine-binding globulin
TKI	Tyrosine kinase inhibitor
TRH	Thyrotropin-releasing hormone
TSH	Thyroid-stimulating hormone (thyrotropin)
TSHR-SAb	Thyroid-stimulating hormone receptor-stimulating antibodies

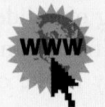 Self-assessment questions and answers are available at *http://www.mhpharmacotherapy.com/pp.html*.

REFERENCES

1. Aoki Y, Belin RM, Clickner R, et al. Serum TSH and total T$_4$ in the United States population and their association with participant characteristics: National Health and Nutrition Examination Survey (NHANES 1999–2002). Thyroid 2007;17:1211–1223.
2. Canaris GJ, Manowitz NR, Mayor G, Ridgeway EC. The Colorado thyroid disease prevalence study. Arch Intern Med 2000;160:526–534.
3. Laurberg P, Andersen S, Carle A, et al The TSH upper reference limit: Where are we at? Nature Rev Endocrinol 2011;7:232–239.
4. Surks MI, Hollowell JG. Age-specific distribution of serum thyrotropin and antithyroid antibodies in the U.S. population: Implications for the prevalence of subclinical hypothyroidism. J Clin Endocrinol Metab 2007;92:4575–4582.
5. Wartofsky L, Dickey RA. The evidence for a narrower thyrotropin reference range is compelling. J Clin Endocrinol Metab 2005;90:5483–5488.
6. Toft AD, Beckett GJ. Measuring serum thyrotropin and thyroid hormone and assessing thyroid hormone transport. In: Braverman LE, Utiger RD, eds. Werner & Ingbar's The Thyroid. A Fundamental and Clinical Text. 9th ed. Philadelphia, PA: Lippincott Williams & Wilkins; 2005:329–344.
7. Vanderpump MPJ, Tunbridge WMG, French JM, et al. The incidence of thyroid disorders in the community: A twenty year follow-up of the Whickham survey. Clin Endocrinol (Oxf) 1995;43:55–69.
8. Devdhar M, Ousman YH, Burman KD. Hypothyroidism. Endocrinol Metab Clin North Am 2007;36:595–615.
9. Danese MD, Powe NR, Sawin CT, Ladenson PW. Screening for mild thyroid failure at the periodic health examination. A decision and cost-effectiveness analysis. JAMA 1996;276:285–292.
10. Ladenson PW, Singer PA, Ain KB, Bagchi N, et al. American Thyroid Association guidelines for detection of thyroid dysfunction. Arch Intern Med 2000;160:1573–1575.

11. U.S. Preventative Services Task Force. Screening for thyroid disease: Recommendation statement. Ann Intern Med 2004;140:125–127.

12. McDermott MT. In the clinic. Hypothyroidism. Ann Intern Med 2009;151:ITC6-1–16.

13. Barbesino G. Drugs affecting thyroid function. Thyroid 2010;20:763–770.

14. Jones DD, May KE, Geraci SA. Subclinical thyroid disease. Am J Med 2010;123:502–504.

15. Singh S, Duggal J, Molnar J, et al. Impact of subclinical thyroid disorders on coronary heart disease, cardiovascular and all-cause mortality: A meta-analysis. Int J Cardiol 2008;125:41–48.

16. Ochs N, Auer R, Bauer DC, et al. Meta-analysis: Subclinical thyroid dysfunction and the risk for coronary heart disease and mortality. Ann Intern Med 2008;148:832–845.

17. Biondi B, Cooper DS. The clinical significance of subclinical thyroid dysfunction. Endocrine Rev 2008;29:76–131.

18. Glinder D. Thyroid disease during pregnancy. In: Braverman LE, Utiger RD, eds. Werner & Ingbar's The Thyroid. A Fundamental and Clinical Text. 9th ed. Philadelphia, PA: Lippincott Williams & Wilkins; 2005:1086–1108.

19. Grozinsky-Glasberg S, Fraser A, Nahshoni E, et al. Thyroxine-triiodothyronine combination therapy versus thyroxine monotherapy for clinical hypothyroidism: Meta-analysis of randomized controlled trials. J Clin Endocrinol Metab 2006;91:2592–2599.

20. Hennessey JV. Levothyroxine a new drug? Since when? How could that be? Thyroid 2003;13:279–282.

21. U.S. Department of Health and Human Services, Food and Drug Administration Center for Drug Evaluation and Research Guidance for Industry. Levothyroxine Sodium Products Enforcement of August 14, 2001 Compliance Date and Submission of New Applications [online]. [cited 2011 Oct 10]. Available from: *http://www.fda.gov/Drugs/GuidanceComplianceRegulatoryInformation/Guidances/ucm065015.htm*. Accessed September 6, 2011.

22. Food and Drug Administration Center for Drug Evaluation and Research Electronic Orange Book. Approved Drug Products with Therapeutic Equivalence Evaluations [online]. [cited 2011 Oct 10]. Available from: *http://www.accessdata.fda.gov/scripts/cder/ob/default.cfm*. Accessed September 6, 2011.

23. Benet LZ, Goyan JE. Bioequivalence and narrow therapeutic index drugs. Pharmacother 1995;15:433–440.

24. Blakesley V, Awni W, Locke C, Ludden T, et al. Are bioequivalence studies of levothyroxine sodium formulations in euthyroid volunteers reliable? Thyroid 2004;14:191–200.

25. Dong BJ, Hauck WW, Gambertoglio JG, Gee L, et al. Bioequivalence of generic and brand-name levothyroxine products in the treatment of hypothyroidism. JAMA 1997;277:1205–1213.

26. Mayor GH, Orlando T, Kurtz NM. Limitations of levothyroxine bioequivalence evaluation: An analysis of an attempted study. Am J Ther 1995;2:417–432.

27. Carr D, McLeod DT, Parry G, Thornes HM. Fine adjustment of thyroxine replacement dosage: Comparison of the thyrotrophin releasing hormone test using a sensitive thyrotrophin assay with measurement of free thyroid hormones and clinical assessment. Clin Endocrinol 1988;28:325–333.

28. Toft AD. Thyroxine therapy. New Engl J Med 1994;331:174–180.

29. Santini F, Pinchera A, Marsili A, et al. Lean body mass is a major determinant of levothyroxine dosage in the treatment of thyroid diseases. J Clin Endocrinol Metab 2005;90:124–127.

30. Laurberg P, Andersen S, Pedersen IB, Carle A. Hypothyroidism in the elderly: Pathophysiology, diagnosis and treatment. Drugs Aging 2005;22:23–38.

31. Helfand M, Crapo LM. Monitoring therapy in patients taking levothyroxine. Ann Intern Med 1990;113:450–454.

32. Turner MR, Camacho X, Fischer HD, et al. Levothyroxine dose and risk of fractures in older adults: Nested case-control study. BMJ 2011;342:d2238.

33. Bolk N, Visser TJ, Nijman J, et al. Effects of evening vs morning levothyroxine intake. A randomized double-blind crossover trial. Arch Intern Med 2010;170:1996–2003.

34. Briesacher BA, Andrade SE, Fouayzi H, Chan A. Comparison of drug adherence rates among patients with seven different medical conditions. Pharmacotherapy 2008;28:437–443.

35. Abalovich M, Amino N, Barbour LA, et al. Management of thyroid dysfunction during pregnancy and postpartum: An Endocrine Society clinical practice guideline. J Clin Endocrinol Metab 2007;92(Suppl):S1–S47.

36. Yassa L, Marqusee E, Fawcett R, Alexander EK. Thyroid hormone early adjustment in pregnancy (the THERAPY) trial. J Clin Endocrinol Metab 2010;95:3234–3241.

37. Zeitler P, Solberg P. Food and levothyroxine administration in infants and children. J Pediatr 2010;157:13–15.

38. Braverman LE, Utiger RD. Introduction to thyrotoxicosis. In: Braverman LE, Utiger RD, eds. Werner & Ingbar's The Thyroid. A Fundamental and Clinical Text. 9th ed. Philadelphia, PA: Lippincott Williams & Wilkins; 2005:453–455.

39. Bahn RS, Burch HB, Cooper DS, et al. Hyperthyroidism and other causes of thyrotoxicosis: Management guidelines of the American Thyroid Association and American Association of Clinical Endocrinologists. Thyroid 2011;21:593–646.

40. Nayak B, Hodak SP. Hyperthyroidism. Endocrinol Metab Clin North Am 2007;36:617–656.

41. Cooper DS. Approach to the patient with subclinical hyperthyroidism. J Clin Endocrinol Metab 2007;92:3–9.

42. Farwell BP, Braverman LE. Thyroid and antithyroid drugs. In: Brunton L, Lazo J, Parker K, eds. Goodman & Gilman's The Pharmacological Basis of Therapeutics. 11th ed. New York: McGraw-Hill; 2006:1511–1540.

43. Cooper DS. Treatment of thyrotoxicosis. In: Braverman LE, Utiger RD, eds. Werner & Ingbar's The Thyroid. A Fundamental and Clinical Text. 9th ed. Philadelphia, PA: Lippincott Williams & Wilkins; 2005:665–694.

44. Cooper DS. Drug therapy: Antithyroid drugs. New Engl J Med 2005;352:905–917.

45. Emiliano AB, Governale L, Parks M, Cooper DS. Shifts in propylthiouracil and methimazole prescribing practices: Antithyroid drug use in the United States from 1991 to 2008. J Clin Endocrinol Metab 2010;95:2227–2233.

46. Walker MA, Briel M, Chrit-Crain M, et al. Effects of antithyroid drugs on radioiodine treatment: Systematic review and meta-analysis of randomized controlled trials. BMJ 2007;335:1–7.

47. U.S. Food and Drug Administration FDA drug safety communication: New boxed warning on severe liver injury with propylthiouracil [online]. [cited 2011 Oct 10]. Available from: *http://www.fda.gov/Drugs/DrugSafety/PostmarketDrugSafetyInformationforPatientsandProviders/ucm209023.htm*. Accessed November 7, 2011.

48. Marx H, Amin P, Lazarus JH. Hyperthyroidism and pregnancy. BMJ 2008;336:663–667.

49. Nayak B, Burman K. Thyrotoxicosis and thyroid storm. Endocrinol Metab Clin North Am 2006;35:663–867.

50. Mebis L, Debaveye Y, Visser TJ, Van den Berghe G. Changes with the thyroid axis during the course of critical illness. Endocrinol Metab Clin North Am 2006;35:807–821.

51. Pappa TA, Apostolos G, Veganakis MA. The nonthyroidal illness syndrome in the non-critically ill patient. Eur J Clin Invest 2011;41:212–220.

52. Surks MI, Sievert R. Drugs and thyroid function. New Engl J Med 1995;333:1688–1694.

53. Padmanabhan H. Amiodarone and thyroid dysfunction. South Med J 2010;103:922–930.

54. Batcher EL, Tang C, Singh BN, et al. Thyroid function abnormalities during amiodarone therapy for persistent atrial fibrillation. Am J Med 2007;120:880–885.

55. Lazarus JH. Lithium and thyroid. Best Pract Res Clin Endocrinol Metab 2009;23:723–733.

45

Adrenal Gland Disorders

Devra K. Dang, Judy T. Chen, Frank Pucino Jr.,
and Karim Anton Calis

KEY CONCEPTS

❶ Signs and symptoms of adrenal insufficiency reflect the disturbance of normal physiologic carbohydrate, fat, and protein homeostasis caused by inadequate cortisol production and inadequate cortisol action.

❷ Lifelong glucocorticoid replacement therapy may be necessary for patients with adrenal insufficiency, and mineralocorticoid replacement therapy is usually required for those with Addison's disease.

❸ During an acute adrenal crisis, the immediate treatment goals are to correct volume depletion, manage hypoglycemia, and provide glucocorticoid replacement.

❹ Patients with known adrenal insufficiency should be educated regarding the need for additional glucocorticoid replacement and prompt medical attention during periods of excessive physiologic stress.

❺ Patients with Cushing's syndrome caused by endogenous or exogenous glucocorticoid excess typically present with similar clinical manifestations.

❻ Surgical resection is considered the treatment of choice for Cushing's syndrome from endogenous causes if the tumor can be localized and if there are no contraindications.

❼ Pharmacotherapy is generally reserved for patients (1) in whom the ectopic adrenocorticotropic hormone–secreting tumor cannot be localized, (2) who are not surgical

candidates, (3) who have failed surgery, (4) who have had a relapse after surgery, or (5) in whom adjunctive therapy is required to achieve complete remission.

❽ In drug-induced Cushing's syndrome, discontinuation of the offending agent is the best management option. However, abrupt withdrawal of the glucocorticoid can result in adrenal insufficiency or exacerbation of the underlying disease.

❾ Glucocorticoid dosages less than 7.5 mg/day of prednisone or its equivalent for less than 3 weeks generally would not be expected to lead to suppression of the hypothalamic–pituitary–adrenal axis.

INTRODUCTION

The adrenal glands are important in the synthesis and regulation of key human hormones. They play a crucial role in water and electrolyte homeostasis, as well as regulation of blood pressure, carbohydrate and fat metabolism, physiologic response to stress, and sexual development and differentiation. This chapter focuses on pharmacologic and nonpharmacologic management of the two most common conditions associated with adrenal gland dysfunction: glucocorticoid insufficiency (e.g., Addison's disease) and glucocorticoid excess (Cushing's syndrome). Other adrenal disorders such as congenital adrenal hyperplasia, pheochromocytoma, hypoaldosteronism, and hyperaldosteronism are beyond the scope of this chapter.

PHYSIOLOGY, ANATOMY, AND BIOCHEMISTRY OF THE ADRENAL GLAND

The adrenal gland is located on the upper segment of the kidney (Fig. 45–1). It consists of an outer cortex and an inner medulla. The adrenal medulla secretes the catecholamines epinephrine (also called adrenaline) and norepinephrine (also called noradrenaline), which are involved in the regulation of the sympathetic nervous system. The adrenal cortex consists of three histologically distinct zones: the outer zona glomerulosa, the zona fasciculata, and an innermost layer called the zona reticularis. Each zone is responsible for production of different hormones (Fig. 45–2).

The zona glomerulosa is responsible for the production of the mineralocorticoids **aldosterone**, 18-hydroxy-corticosterone, corticosterone, and deoxycorticosterone. Aldosterone promotes renal sodium retention and potassium excretion. Its synthesis and release are regulated by renin in response to decreased vascular volume and renal perfusion. Adrenal aldosterone production is regulated by the **renin–angiotensin–aldosterone system**.

The zona fasciculata is the middle layer and produces the glucocorticoid hormone **cortisol**. Cortisol is responsible for maintaining homeostasis of carbohydrate, protein, and fat metabolism. Its secretion follows a circadian rhythm, generally beginning to rise at approximately 4 AM and peaking around 6 to 8 AM. Thereafter, cortisol levels decrease throughout the day, approach 50% of the peak value by 4 PM, and reach their nadir around midnight.[1] The normal rate of cortisol production is approximately 8 to 15 mg/day.[2] Cortisol plays a key role in the body's response to stress. Its production increases markedly during physiologic stress, such as during acute illness, surgery, or trauma. In addition, certain conditions such as alcoholism, depression, anxiety

disorder, obsessive-compulsive disorder, poorly controlled diabetes, morbid obesity, starvation, anorexia nervosa, and chronic renal failure are associated with increased cortisol levels. High total cortisol levels are also observed in the presence of increased cortisol binding globulin (the carrier protein for 80% of circulating cortisol molecules), which is seen in pregnancy or other high-estrogen states (e.g., exogenous estrogen administration).[1] Cortisol is converted in the liver to an inactive metabolite known as cortisone.

The zona reticularis produces the androgens androstenedione, dehydroepiandrosterone (DHEA), and the sulfated form of dehydroepiandrosterone (DHEA-S). Only a small amount of testosterone and estrogen is produced in the adrenal glands. Androstenedione and DHEA are converted in the periphery, largely to testosterone and estrogen.

Adrenal hormone production is controlled by the hypothalamus and pituitary. **Corticotropin-releasing hormone** (CRH) is secreted by the hypothalamus and stimulates secretion of **adrenocorticotropic hormone** (ACTH; also known as corticotropin) from the anterior pituitary. ACTH in turn stimulates the adrenal cortex to produce cortisol. When sufficient or excessive cortisol levels are reached, a negative feedback is exerted on the secretion of CRH and ACTH, thereby decreasing overall cortisol production. The control of adrenal androgen synthesis also follows a similar negative feedback mechanism. Figure 46–1 depicts the hormonal regulation with the hypothalamic–pituitary–adrenal (HPA) axis.

ADRENAL INSUFFICIENCY

Epidemiology and Etiology

Adrenal insufficiency generally refers to the inability of the adrenal glands to produce adequate amounts of cortisol for normal physiologic functioning or in times of stress. The condition is usually classified as primary, secondary, or tertiary depending on the etiology (Table 45–1). The estimated prevalence of primary adrenal insufficiency and secondary adrenal insufficiency are approximately 60 to 143 and 150 to 280 cases per million persons, respectively. Whereas primary adrenal insufficiency is usually diagnosed in the third to fifth decades of life, secondary adrenal insufficiency is commonly detected during the sixth decade.[1,3] Adrenal insufficiency is more prevalent in women than in men, with a ratio of 2.6 to 1.[1] Chronic adrenal insufficiency is rare.

Pathophysiology

Primary adrenal insufficiency, also known as Addison's disease, occurs when the adrenal glands are unable to produce cortisol. It occurs from destruction of the adrenal cortex, usually from an autoimmune process. In general, the clinical manifestations are observed when destruction of the cortex exceeds 90%.[4] ❶ *Signs and symptoms of adrenal insufficiency reflect the disturbance of normal physiologic carbohydrate, fat, and protein homeostasis caused by inadequate cortisol production and inadequate cortisol action.* Primary adrenal

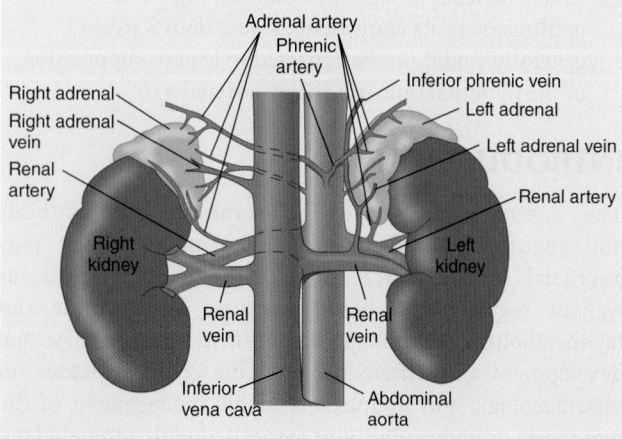

FIGURE 45–1. Anatomy of the adrenal gland. (Reprinted, with permission, from Smith SM, Gums JG. Adrenal gland disorders. In: DiPiro JT, Talbert RL, Yee GC, et al, eds. Pharmacotherapy: A Pathophysiologic Approach. 8th ed. New York: McGraw-Hill; 2011:1327.)

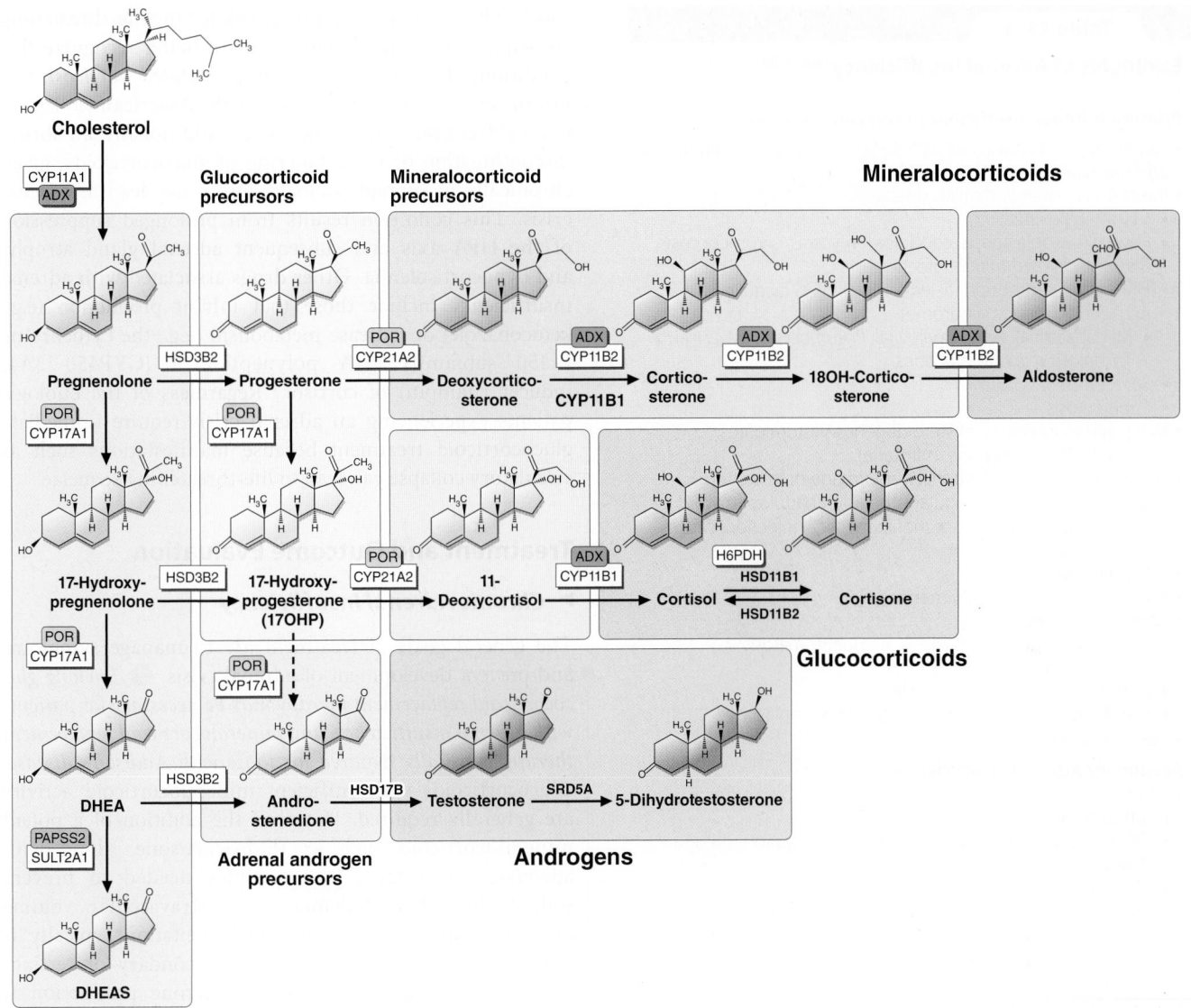

FIGURE 45–2. The adrenal cortex consists of three histologically distinct zones: the outer zona glomerulosa, the middle zona fasciculata, and an innermost layer called the zona reticularis. Each zone is responsible for production of different hormones. The zona glomerulosa is responsible for the production of mineralocorticoids such as aldosterone. The zona fasciculata produces cortisol and the zona reticularis produces androgens. (ADX, adrenodoxin; CYP11A1, side chain cleavage enzyme; CYP11B1, 11-beta-hydroxylase; CYP11B2, aldosterone synthase; CYP17A1, 17-alpha-hydroxylase/17,20 lyase; CYP21A2, 21-alpha-hydroxylase; DHEA, dehydroepiandrosterone; DHEAS, dehydroepiandrosterone sulfate; H6PDH, hexose-6-phosphate dehydrogenase; HSD3B2, 3-beta-hydroxysteroid dehydrogenase type 2; HSD11B1, 11-beta-hydroxysteroid dehydrogenase type 1; HSD11B2, 11-beta-hydroxysteroid dehydrogenase type 2; HSD17B, 17-beta-hydroxysteroid dehydrogenase; PAPSS2, PAPS synthase type 2; POR, P450 oxidoreductase; SRD5A, 5-alpha-reductase; SULT2A1, DHEA sulfotransferase.) (Adapted, with permission, from Arlt W. Disorders of the adrenal cortex. In: Longo DL, Fauci AS, Kasper DL, et al., eds. Harrison's Principles of Internal Medicine. New York: McGraw-Hill; 2012.)

insufficiency usually develops gradually. Patients may remain asymptomatic in the early stages with signs and symptoms present only during times of physiologic stress. Persistent signs and symptoms of hypocortisolism typically occur with disease progression. Additionally, primary adrenal insufficiency may be accompanied by a reduction in aldosterone and androgen production.

Secondary adrenal insufficiency occurs as a result of a pituitary gland dysfunction, whereby decreased production and secretion of ACTH leads to a decrease in cortisol synthesis. Tertiary adrenal insufficiency is a disorder of the hypothalamus that results in decreased production and release of CRH, which in turn decreases pituitary ACTH production and release. In contrast to Addison's disease (i.e., primary adrenal insufficiency), aldosterone production is unaffected in the secondary and tertiary forms of the disease. Chronic adrenal insufficiency often has a good prognosis if diagnosed early and treated appropriately.

Acute adrenal insufficiency (i.e., adrenal crisis) results from the body's inability to sufficiently increase endogenous

Table 45–1

Etiologies of Adrenal Insufficiency[1,4,6,18–20]

Primary Adrenal Insufficiency (Addison's disease)
- Autoimmune: accounts for 70% to 90% of all cases of primary adrenal insufficiency
- Infectious or granulomatous diseases
  - Cytomegalovirus
  - Fungal (histoplasmosis, coccidioidomycosis, cryptococcosis, *Blastomyces dermatitidis* infections)
  - HIV (human immunodeficiency virus), AIDS (acquired immunodeficiency syndrome)
    - Mycobacterial, cytomegaloviral, *Pneumocystis jiroveci,* and *Toxoplasma gondii* infections
  - Sarcoidosis
  - Tuberculosis
- Medications: inhibitors of steroidogenesis (etomidate, ketoconazole, metyrapone, mitotane)
- Hemorrhagic: bilateral adrenal hemorrhage or infarction usually caused by anticoagulant therapy, coagulopathy, thromboembolic disease, or meningococcal infection; causes acute adrenal insufficiency
- Adrenalectomy
- Adrenoleukodystrophy (in men)
- Adrenomyeloneuropathy
- Infiltrative disorders: amyloidosis, hemochromatosis
- Genetic causes
  - Congenital adrenal hyperplasia
  - Familial glucocorticoid deficiency and hypoplasia
- Metastatic malignancy

Secondary Adrenal Insufficiency
- Drug induced (most common cause of secondary adrenal insufficiency)
  - Chronic glucocorticoid administration at supraphysiologic doses
  - Megestrol acetate: has glucocorticoid-like activity
  - Mifepristone (RU 486): antagonizes glucocorticoid receptors
  - Possibly tyrosine kinase inhibitors: adrenal damage observed in rats and monkeys; asymptomatic decreased response to ACTH-stimulation test observed in humans
- Cushing's syndrome
- **Panhypopituitarism**
- Pituitary tumor
- Transsphenoidal pituitary microsurgery
- Pituitary irradiation
- Traumatic brain injury

Tertiary Adrenal Insufficiency
- Hypothalamic failure
- Drug-induced: chronic glucocorticoid administration at supraphysiologic doses

ACTH, adrenocorticotropic hormone.

cortisol during periods of excessive physiologic stress. Adrenal crisis can occur when patients with chronic adrenal insufficiency do not receive adequate glucocorticoid replacement during stressful conditions such as those experienced during surgery, infection, acute illness, invasive medical procedures, or trauma. Acute adrenal insufficiency can also result from bilateral adrenal infarction caused by hemorrhage, embolus, sepsis, or adrenal vein thrombosis. Patients who are critically ill may also experience impaired HPA axis function, with an overall prevalence rate of 10% to 20%, and as high as 60% in those experiencing septic

shock. These patients are also at risk for the life-threatening consequences of an adrenal crisis. To better recognize this condition, the term *critical illness–related corticosteroid insufficiency* was recently coined by the American College of Critical Care Medicine Task Force.[5] Additionally, an abrupt discontinuation or rapid tapering of glucocorticoids, given chronically in supraphysiologic doses, may lead to adrenal crisis. This condition results from prolonged suppression of the HPA axis and subsequent adrenal gland atrophy and hypocortisolemia. Other drugs associated with adrenal insufficiency include those that inhibit production (e.g., ketoconazole) or increase metabolism (e.g., the cytochrome P-450 subfamily IIIA polypeptide 4 [CYP450 3A4] inducer rifampin) of cortisol.[4] Regardless of the etiology, patients experiencing an adrenal crisis require immediate glucocorticoid treatment because manifestations such as circulatory collapse can lead to life-threatening sequelae.

Treatment and Outcome Evaluation

▶ *Chronic Adrenal Insufficiency*

The general goals of treatment are to manage symptoms and prevent development of adrenal crisis. ❷ *Lifelong glucocorticoid replacement therapy may be necessary for patients with adrenal insufficiency, and mineralocorticoid replacement therapy is usually required for those with Addison's disease.* Glucocorticoids with sufficient mineralocorticoid activity are generally required. However, the addition of a potent mineralocorticoid such as fludrocortisone, along with adequate salt intake, is sometimes needed to prevent sodium loss, hyperkalemia, and intravascular volume depletion. Mineralocorticoid supplementation typically is not indicated for the treatment of secondary or tertiary adrenal insufficiency because aldosterone production is often unaffected. Moreover, patients with secondary or tertiary adrenal insufficiency may only require replacement therapy until the HPA axis recovers. Hydrocortisone is often prescribed because it most closely resembles endogenous cortisol with its relatively high mineralocorticoid activity and short half-life and allows the design of regimens that simulate the normal circadian cycle.[6] Other glucocorticoids, however, can be used. The pharmacologic characteristics of the commonly used glucocorticoids are presented in Table 45–2. Because patients with primary adrenal insufficiency can experience DHEA deficiency, DHEA replacement also has been tried. Several small clinical studies, consisting mostly of women, suggest that treatment with DHEA can improve mood and fatigue and provide a general sense of well-being.[7-10] However, a recent meta-analysis of 10 studies found that DHEA use in women only slightly improved health-related quality of life and depression but did not affect anxiety or sexual well-being; it concluded that the totality of available data does not support routine supplementation with DHEA.[11] The use of DHEA remains controversial and requires further study. Management strategies for chronic adrenal insufficiency are outlined below:[1,3,6]

Clinical Presentation and Diagnosis of Chronic Adrenal Insufficiency[1,3,4,6]

General

- The symptoms develop gradually, especially in the early stages, may be vague, and mimic those of other medical conditions.
- The cardinal symptoms and signs are weakness and fatigue requiring rest periods, gastrointestinal symptoms, weight loss, and hypotension. These symptoms are due to cortisol deficiency.
- Patients with autoimmune adrenal insufficiency may have other autoimmune disorders such as type 1 diabetes mellitus and autoimmune thyroiditis.

Symptoms (Percent Prevalence)

- Weakness and fatigue are the most common (99%).
- Anorexia, nausea, and diarrhea (56–90%). These may range from mild to severe with vomiting and abdominal pain.
- Hypoglycemia may occur in some patients.
- Amenorrhea may occur in some women.
- Salt craving may occur in some (approximately 22%) patients with primary adrenal insufficiency due to aldosterone deficiency.

Signs

- Weight loss (97%).
- Hypotension (less than 110/70 mm Hg) and orthostasis (87%).
- Dehydration, hypovolemia, and hyperkalemia (in primary adrenal insufficiency only) due to aldosterone deficiency.
- Decreased serum sodium and chloride levels due to aldosterone deficiency. Hyponatremia can also be present in secondary adrenal insufficiency due to cortisol

deficiency and increased antidiuretic hormone secretion leading to subsequent water retention.

- Increased serum blood urea nitrogen and creatinine due to dehydration.
- Hyperpigmentation of skin and mucous membranes (92%). This is usually observed around creases, pressure areas, areolas, genitalia, and new scars. Dark freckles and patches of vitiligo may be present. Hyperpigmentation, due to increased ACTH levels, occurs in most patients with primary adrenal insufficiency but does not occur in secondary or tertiary adrenal insufficiency.
- Personality changes (irritability and restlessness) due to cortisol deficiency.
- Loss of axillary and pubic hair in women due to decreased androgen production.
- Blood count abnormalities (normocytic, normochromic anemia, relative lymphocytosis, neutrophilia, eosinophilia) due to cortisol and androgen deficiency.

Laboratory Tests (Also See Table 45–3)

- Decreased basal and stress-induced cortisol levels
- Decreased aldosterone level (in primary adrenal insufficiency only)
- Lack of increase in cortisol and aldosterone level after ACTH stimulation

Other Diagnostic Tests (Also See Table 45–3)

- Computed tomography (CT) scan or magnetic resonance imaging (MRI) of the adrenal glands, pituitary, and/or hypothalamus can aid in determining the etiology.
- The presence of anti-adrenal antibodies is suggestive of an autoimmune etiology.

Clinical Presentation and Diagnosis of Acute Adrenal Insufficiency (Adrenal Crisis)[1,3,4]

General

- Onset of symptoms is acute and precipitated by excessive physiologic stress.

Symptoms

- Severe weakness and fatigue
- Abdominal or flank pain

Signs

- Severe dehydration leading to hypotension and shock (circulatory collapse). Hypovolemia may not be responsive to intravenous hydration and may require the use of vasopressors.
- Tachycardia.
- Nausea, vomiting.
- Fever.

- Confusion.
- Hypoglycemia.
- Laboratory abnormalities are similar to those observed in chronic adrenal insufficiency.

Laboratory Tests

- The unstimulated serum cortisol and rapid ACTH stimulation tests are useful in the diagnosis of adrenal crisis (Table 45–3). The insulin tolerance test is contraindicated due to preexisting hypoglycemia. The metyrapone test is also contraindicated since metyrapone inhibits cortisol production.

Note: Due to the life-threatening nature of this condition, empiric treatment should be started before laboratory confirmation in patients who present with the clinical picture of an acute adrenal crisis.

Table 45-2

Pharmacologic Characteristics of Commonly Used Glucocorticoids

Glucocorticoid	Estimated Potency Relative to Hydrocortisone		
	Glucocorticoid (Anti-Inflammatory) Activity	Mineralocorticoid (Sodium-Retaining) Activity	Equivalent Dose (mg)
Short Acting (Half-Life Less Than 12 Hours)			
Hydrocortisone	1	1	20
Cortisone	0.8	0.8	25
Intermediate Acting (Half-Life 12–36 Hours)			
Prednisone	4	0.25	5
Prednisolone	4	0.25	5
Methylprednisolone	5	Less than 0.01	4
Triamcinolone	5	Less than 0.01	4
Long Acting (Half-Life Greater Than 48 Hours)			
Betamethasone	25	Less than 0.01	0.6-0.75
Dexamethasone	30–40	Less than 0.01	0.75

Modified from Williams GH, Dluhy RG. Disorders of the adrenal cortex. In: Kasper DL, Braunwald E, Fauci A, et al., eds. Harrison's Principles of Internal Medicine. New York: McGraw-Hill, 2005:2147.

- For the treatment of primary adrenal insufficiency (Addison's disease), 12 to 15 mg/m² of oral hydrocortisone is typically administered in two divided doses, with two-thirds of the dose given in the morning upon awakening to mimic the early morning rise in endogenous cortisol and the remaining one-third of the dose given in the late afternoon to avoid insomnia and allow for the lowest concentration in the blood at around midnight. Hydrocortisone may also be given in three doses, but this may decrease adherence. The longer acting glucocorticoids (e.g., prednisone, dexamethasone) may provide a more prolonged clinical response, thereby avoiding symptom recurrence that can occur at the end of the dosing interval with short-acting agents such as hydrocortisone. Longer acting agents also may improve adherence in some patients. Monitor the patient's weight, blood pressure, and serum electrolytes along with symptom resolution and general well-being; adjust dosages accordingly as needed. Doses of hydrocortisone, dexamethasone, prednisone, and other glucocorticoids may need to be increased or decreased in patients taking CYP450 3A4 inducers (e.g., phenytoin, rifampin, barbiturates) or inhibitors (e.g., protease inhibitors), respectively. Monitor for adverse drug reactions related to glucocorticoid administration. Glucocorticoid therapy at physiologic replacement doses should not lead to the development of Cushing's syndrome; however, careful monitoring should still be performed, and the smallest effective dose used. Educate patients regarding the need for increased glucocorticoid dosage during excessive physiologic stress. In addition, administer oral fludrocortisone at a daily dose of approximately 0.05 to 0.2 mg in the morning. Monitor for resolution of hypotension, dizziness, dehydration, hyponatremia, and hyperkalemia; and increase the dose if needed. Conversely, consider decreasing the dose if adverse reactions from mineralocorticoid administration such as hypertension, hypokalemia, fluid retention,

and other significant adverse events occur. In patients receiving hydrocortisone, it should be kept in mind that this drug also possesses mineralocorticoid activity. All patients with primary adrenal insufficiency should also maintain an adequate sodium intake (~3 to 4 g/day). Last, although controversial, consider giving 50 mg/day of DHEA (in the morning) to female patients who do not experience an improvement in mood and well-being even with adequate glucocorticoid and mineralocorticoid replacement. In these patients, monitor serum DHEA-S (aim for the middle range of normal levels in healthy young people) and free testosterone level.

- Patients with secondary and tertiary adrenal insufficiency are treated with oral hydrocortisone or a longer acting glucocorticoid in the same manner as previously described for primary adrenal insufficiency. However, patients with secondary and tertiary adrenal insufficiency may require a lower dose. Some patients (e.g., those with drug-induced adrenal insufficiency or adrenal insufficiency after treatment for Cushing's syndrome) only require glucocorticoid replacement temporarily, which can be discontinued after recovery of the HPA axis. Monitor for progression of the underlying etiology of adrenal insufficiency. Fludrocortisone therapy is generally not needed.

▶ *Acute Adrenal Insufficiency*

❸ *During an acute adrenal crisis, the immediate treatment goals are to correct volume depletion, manage hypoglycemia, and provide glucocorticoid replacement.* Volume depletion and hypoglycemia can be corrected by giving large volumes (~2 to 3 L) of intravenous (IV) normal saline and 5% dextrose solution.[1] Glucocorticoid replacement can be accomplished by administering IV hydrocortisone, starting at a dose of 100 mg every 6 hours for 24 hours, increasing to 200 to 400 mg/day if complications occur, or decreasing to 50 mg every 6 hours after achieving hemodynamic stability. The

Table 45–3

Tests for Diagnosing Adrenal Insufficiency[4,6]

Test	Procedure	Rationale	Finding in Adrenal Insufficiency	Comments
Screening and Diagnostic Tests for Adrenal Insufficiency				
Unstimulated serum cortisol measurement	Measure serum cortisol at 6–8 AM	Serum cortisol level peaks in the early morning	• Serum cortisol greater than 18 mcg/dL (497 nmol/L) is normal • Serum cortisol less than 3 mcg/dL (83 nmol/L) is indicative of adrenal insufficiency	• Used as a general initial screening test for the presence of adrenal insufficiency. Evaluate result in conjunction with those from the other tests
Rapid ACTH stimulation test (also called **cosyntropin** stimulation test)	Measure serum cortisol 30–60 minutes after administering cosyntropin 250 mcg IV	Increased cortisol secretion in normal individuals in response to ACTH stimulation but not in adrenal insufficiency	Serum cortisol concentration less than 18 mcg/dL (497 nmol/L)	• Used as the gold standard test for diagnosing primary adrenal insufficiency • False-negative results may occur if the ACTH deficiency is of recent onset (less than 1 month) • Although not widely accepted, a low-dose (1 mcg) ACTH stimulation test has been useful for the diagnosis of partial adrenal insufficiency • If measured serum cortisol concentration is low, measure plasma ACTH, aldosterone, and renin concentrations to differentiate between primary and secondary or tertiary adrenal insufficiency (see below)
Insulin tolerance test (insulin-induced hypoglycemia test)	Administer insulin IV to induce hypoglycemia; then measure serum cortisol during symptomatic hypoglycemia (confirm that blood glucose is less than 40 mg/dL [2.2 mmol/L])	Evaluates ability of entire HPA axis to respond to stress (hypoglycemia)	Serum cortisol concentration less than 18 mcg/dL (497 nmol/L) is indicative of secondary adrenal insufficiency	• If the result of the rapid ACTH stimulation test is normal, either this or the overnight metyrapone test is still needed to evaluate for secondary adrenal insufficiency. The insulin tolerance test is considered the gold standard • Contraindicated in patients with a seizure history, older than 60 years, or with cardiovascular or cerebrovascular disease • Requires close medical supervision • Contraindicated in adrenal crisis
Overnight metyrapone test	Administer metyrapone at midnight; then measure serum cortisol at 8 AM the next day	Metyrapone inhibits cortisol synthesis. Its administration leads to rise in levels of ACTH and the precursor of cortisol. Patients with adrenal insufficiency do not exhibit this	Normal response is a decrease in serum cortisol to less than 5 mcg/dL (138 nmol/L) and an increase in the cortisol precursor to more than 7 mcg/dL (193 nmol/L). Response not seen in secondary adrenal insufficiency	• Distinguishes between normal individuals and patients with secondary adrenal insufficiency • Contraindicated in adrenal crisis
Tests for Differential Diagnosis of Primary, Secondary, and Tertiary Adrenal Insufficiency				
Plasma ACTH concentration	Measure plasma ACTH	In primary adrenal insufficiency, hypocortisolism leads to elevated plasma ACTH concentration via positive HPA axis feedback	• Primary adrenal insufficiency: elevated plasma ACTH • Secondary or tertiary adrenal insufficiency: plasma ACTH low or inappropriately normal	• Evaluate result of test in combination with those from the plasma aldosterone and plasma renin tests

(Continued)

Table 45–3

Tests for Diagnosing Adrenal Insufficiency[4,6] (*Continued*)

Test	Procedure	Rationale	Finding in Adrenal Insufficiency	Comments
Plasma aldosterone concentration	Measure plasma aldosterone from same blood samples as those used in ACTH stimulation test	Patients with primary adrenal insufficiency may experience a reduction in aldosterone production	• Primary adrenal insufficiency: low plasma aldosterone • Secondary or tertiary adrenal insufficiency: aldosterone concentration is usually normal (greater than or equal to 5 ng/dL [139 pmol/L])	• Evaluate result of test in combination with those from the plasma ACTH and plasma renin tests
Plasma renin concentration or activity	Measure plasma renin concentration or activity	Mineralocorticoid deficiency occurs in primary adrenal insufficiency but is usually not present in secondary or tertiary adrenal insufficiency	• Primary adrenal insufficiency: elevated plasma renin • Secondary or tertiary adrenal insufficiency: plasma renin concentration or activity is usually normal	• Evaluate result of test in combination with those from the plasma ACTH and plasma aldosterone concentration tests

ACTH, adrenocorticotropic hormone or corticotrophin; HPA, hypothalamic–pituitary–adrenal; IV, intravenous.

Patient Encounter 1, Part 1: Presentation and Medical History

GH is a 48-year-old woman who presents to the primary care clinic with complaints of fatigue and asking for a prescription for "vitamin injections." She states that she has been feeling very tired for the past year. Upon further questioning, she also complains of dizziness, especially with positional changes, and intermittent nausea, abdominal pain, and diarrhea.

PMH:

• Tuberculosis: completed treatment course
• History of candidal vulvovaginitis
• Chronic obstructive pulmonary disease with frequent exacerbations (3 times in past 8 months) requiring prednisone taper therapy
• Depression

FH: Father with coronary artery disease, mother with diabetes

SH: Part-time factory worker, smokes 1 pack per day, denies alcohol use and illicit drug use

Current Meds:

• Fluticasone/salmeterol DPI 500/50 mcg one inhalation twice daily
• Tiotropium 18 mcg inhale contents of one capsule once daily

• Albuterol MDI two puffs q4h as needed
• Sertraline 100 mg once daily
• Loperamide 2 mg as needed for diarrhea (nonprescription)

PE

VS: Sitting BP, 106/68 mm Hg; P, 74 beats/min; standing BP, 96/68 mm Hg; RR, 14 breaths/min; weight, 130 lb (59.1 kg) with 5-lb (2.3-kg) loss in past 6 months; height, 5 ft 2 in (157.5 cm)

Skin: Hyperpigmentation increases of palms

CV: RRR, normal S_1, S_2; no murmurs, rubs, or gallops

Labs (fasting): Serum electrolytes: sodium, 133 mEq/L (133 mmol/L); potassium, 5.2 mEq/L (5.2 mmol/L); chloride, 98 mEq/L (98 mmol/L); bicarb, 30 mEq/L (30 mmol/L); blood urea nitrogen (BUN), 25 mg/dL (8.9 mmol/L); creatinine, 1.2 mg/dL (106 μmol/L); glucose, 60 mg/dL (3.3 mmol/L)

Which signs or symptoms of adrenal insufficiency does GH exhibit?

Does GH's presentation offer any clues as to the etiology or classification of adrenal insufficiency?

Which tests would be most useful for determining the etiology and confirming the diagnosis of adrenal insufficiency?

hydrocortisone dose can then be tapered to a maintenance dose by the fourth or fifth day, and fludrocortisone can be added if needed.[1] For comprehensive recommendations for the treatment of patients with critical illness–related corticosteroid insufficiency, readers are referred to the 2008 consensus statements from the American College of Critical Care Medicine Task Force.[5]

④ *Patients with known adrenal insufficiency should be educated regarding the need for additional glucocorticoid replacement and prompt medical attention during periods of excessive physiologic stress.* Although the dosage of glucocorticoid is generally individualized, a common recommendation is to double the maintenance dose of hydrocortisone if the patient experiences fever or undergoes invasive dental or diagnostic procedures.[6] Patients who experience vomiting or diarrhea may not adequately absorb oral glucocorticoids and may benefit from parenteral therapy until symptoms resolve. Before major surgery, additional glucocorticoid replacement (higher dose and parenteral route) must be given to prevent adrenal crisis. A sample protocol is as follows[1]:

- Correct electrolytes, blood pressure, and fluid status as necessary.
- Give 100 mg of hydrocortisone sodium phosphate or hydrocortisone sodium succinate intramuscularly (also,

Patient Encounter 1, Part 2: Treatment

After appropriate laboratory and diagnostic tests are performed, GH is diagnosed with Addison's disease.

How should her chronic primary adrenal insufficiency be treated?

What monitoring parameters (therapeutic and toxic) should be implemented?

make sure this is readily available to the operating room).

- Give 50 mg of hydrocortisone intramuscularly or intravenously in the recovery room and then every 6 hours for the first 24 hours.
- If patient is hemodynamically stable, reduce the dosage to 25 mg every 6 hours for 24 hours and then taper to a maintenance dosage over 3 to 5 days.
- Resume previous fludrocortisone dose when the patient is taking oral medications.
- Maintain or increase hydrocortisone dosage to 200 to 400 mg/day if fever, hypotension, or other complications occur.

Patient Care and Monitoring: Adrenal Insufficiency

1. Evaluate patients presenting with the typical clinical manifestations for chronic or acute adrenal insufficiency.
2. Perform initial screening tests to confirm the presence of adrenal insufficiency.
3. After the diagnosis is confirmed, perform further testing to differentiate between primary, secondary, and tertiary adrenal insufficiency.
4. In patients presenting with acute adrenal crisis who have not been previously diagnosed with adrenal insufficiency, immediate treatment with injectable hydrocortisone and IV saline and dextrose solutions should be initiated before confirmation of the diagnosis because of the life-threatening nature of this condition. Determine and correct the underlying cause of the acute adrenal crisis (e.g., infection).
5. Glucocorticoid replacement therapy is necessary for patients with adrenal insufficiency, and mineralocorticoid replacement therapy is required for those with Addison's disease.
6. In patients with chronic adrenal insufficiency, when excessive physiologic stress is anticipated (e.g., pending surgery), devise a strategy to give supplemental doses of glucocorticoid during this period. Monitor the patient for signs of an acute adrenal crisis and develop a plan to treat this emergency condition.
7. Monitor the patient for adequacy of treatment as well as adverse reactions from glucocorticoid and/or mineralocorticoid therapy.
8. Determine the duration of treatment for patient with secondary and tertiary adrenal insufficiency.
9. Provide patient education regarding disease state and its treatment:
   - Causes of adrenal insufficiency, including drug-induced etiologies.
   - How to recognize the clinical manifestations.
   - How to prevent an acute adrenal crisis (adhere to therapy and do not abruptly stop glucocorticoid treatment). There may be a need to increase the dose of glucocorticoid during excessive physiologic stress.
   - Administration of parenteral glucocorticoid during an acute adrenal crisis.
   - Need to notify all healthcare providers of condition.
   - Encourage wearing or carrying a medical alert (e.g., bracelet, card).
   - Counsel on dietary and pharmacologic therapy, including duration of treatment and potential adverse consequences of glucocorticoid and mineralocorticoid replacement.

HYPERCORTISOLISM (CUSHING'S SYNDROME)

Epidemiology and Etiology

Cushing's syndrome refers to the pathophysiologic changes associated with exposure to supraphysiologic cortisol concentrations (endogenous hypercortisolism) or pharmacologic doses of glucocorticoids (exogenous hypercortisolism). Cushing's syndrome from endogenous causes is a rare condition with an estimated incidence of two to five cases per million persons per year.[12] Patients receiving chronic supraphysiologic doses of glucocorticoids, such as those with rheumatologic disorders, are at high risk of developing Cushing's syndrome.

Pathophysiology

Cushing's syndrome can be classified as ACTH dependent or ACTH independent (Table 45–4). ACTH-dependent Cushing's syndrome results from ACTH-secreting (or rarely CRH-secreting) adenomas. ACTH-independent Cushing's syndrome is caused by either excessive cortisol secretion by the adrenal glands (independent of ACTH stimulation) or by exogenous glucocorticoid administration. ❺ *Patients with Cushing's syndrome caused by endogenous or exogenous glucocorticoid excess typically present with similar clinical manifestations.* The term *Cushing's disease* refers specifically to Cushing's syndrome from an ACTH-secreting pituitary adenoma. The plasma ACTH concentration is elevated in ACTH-dependent conditions but not in ACTH-independent causes because elevated cortisol concentrations suppress pituitary ACTH secretion via negative feedback. ACTH and cortisol concentrations are elevated episodically in ACTH-dependent disease caused by random hypersecretion of ACTH.[4] Other major differences among the vast etiologies of Cushing's syndrome are shown in Table 45–5.

Physiologic cortisol secretion follows a circadian pattern, with cortisol levels rising in the early morning, peaking at approximately 6 to 8 AM, and then declining steadily throughout the remainder of the day until they reach a nadir at midnight. This circadian rhythm is lost in most patients with Cushing's syndrome. As such, detection of elevated midnight cortisol concentrations can be useful in the diagnosis of Cushing's syndrome.

Cushing's disease and adrenal carcinomas cause adrenal androgen hypersecretion in high enough concentrations to result in signs of androgen excess such as acne, menstrual irregularities, and hirsutism, and cause virilization in women.[4] Drug-induced Cushing's syndrome from glucocorticoid administration occurs most commonly in patients receiving oral therapy, but other routes such as inhalation, dermal, nasal, and intraarticular have also been implicated.[13] Over-the-counter products, including dietary supplements, should also be evaluated because they may contain corticosteroids. Drug-induced Cushing's syndrome has been reported with the use of Chinese herbal products adulterated with corticosteroids.[14,15] The risk of glucocorticoid-induced Cushing's syndrome appears to increase with higher doses and/or longer treatment durations.[13]

Left untreated, patients with Cushing's syndrome may experience severe complications of hypercortisolism, resulting in up to a nearly fourfold increase in mortality.[16] Mortality in patients with Cushing's is mostly attributed to cardiovascular disease. Hypertension, hyperglycemia, and hyperlipidemia are common findings and can be associated with cardiac hypertrophy, atherosclerosis, and hypercoagulability. Osteopenia, osteoporosis, and increased fractures also have been reported.[16] Prevention and management of these conditions are discussed elsewhere in this text. Children may experience linear

---

Table 45–4

Etiologies of Cushing's Syndrome[1,13,21,22]

ACTH Dependent
- ACTH-secreting pituitary tumor (Cushing's *disease*): 70% of cases of endogenous Cushing's syndrome
- ACTH-secreting nonpituitary tumors (ectopic ACTH syndrome): 15% of cases of endogenous Cushing's syndrome; usually from small cell lung carcinoma, bronchial carcinoids, or pheochromocytoma or from thymus, pancreatic, ovarian, or thyroid tumor; the tumor is usually disseminated (difficult to localize)
- CRH-secreting nonpituitary tumors (ectopic CRH syndrome): rare

ACTH Independent: 15% of cases of endogenous Cushing's syndrome
- Unilateral adrenal adenoma
- Adrenal carcinoma
- Bilateral nodular adrenal hyperplasia: rare (less than 1%)

Drug-Induced Cushing's Syndrome (ACTH independent): most common cause of Cushing's syndrome
- Prescription glucocorticoid preparations (most routes of administration)
- Nonprescription and herbal products with glucocorticoid activity (e.g., nonprescription anti-itch products with hydrocortisone, herbal products with magnolia bark or those claiming to contain adrenal cortex extracts or other byproducts)
- Other drugs with glucocorticoid activity (e.g., megestrol acetate, medroxyprogesterone)

ACTH, adrenocorticotropic hormone or corticotropin; CRH, corticotropin-releasing hormone.

Table 45–5

Differences Among the Major Etiologies of Cushing's Syndrome[4,16,23]

	ACTH Dependent		ACTH Independent		
	Pituitary Dependent (Cushing's Disease)	**Ectopic ACTH Syndrome**	**Exogenous Glucocorticoid Administration**	**Adrenal Adenoma**	**Adrenal Carcinoma**
Onset of signs and symptoms	Gradual	Rapid	Gradual to rapid	Gradual	Rapid
Symptoms severity	Mild to moderate	Atypical	Mild to severe	Mild to moderate	Severe
Dominant sex and age	Female; 20–40 years (range, childhood to 70 years)	Male; adults	Female and male; all ages	Female	Female; children
Virilization	+	+	+	+	+++
Abdominal mass	0	0	0	0	++
Plasma ACTH concentration	Slightly elevated	Elevated	Low	Low	Low
CRH stimulation test	Response	Rare response	Decreased or no response	No response	No response
High-dose dexamethasone suppression test	Between 50% and 80% cortisol suppression	Less cortisol suppression	No cortisol suppression	No cortisol suppression	No cortisol suppression
Pituitary MRI	Tumor	Normal	Normal	Normal	Normal
Adrenal gland CT or MRI	Normal or bilateral hyperplasia	Normal or bilateral hyperplasia	No change	Mass(es)	Mass(es)

0, none; +, mild; ++, moderate; +++, pronounced; ACTH, adrenocorticotropic hormone or corticotropin; CRH, corticotropin-releasing hormone; CT, computed tomography; MRI, magnetic resonance imaging.

Adapted in part with permission from Smith SM, Gums JG. Adrenal gland disorders. In: DiPiro JT, Talbert RL, Yee GC, et al, eds. Pharmacotherapy: A Pathophysiologic Approach. 8th ed. New York: McGraw-Hill; 2011:1330.

growth retardation from reduced growth hormone secretion and inhibition of epiphysial cartilage development in long bones.[12,16]

Treatment

The goal of treatment in patients with Cushing's syndrome is reversal of hypercortisolism and management of the associated comorbidities, including the potential for long-term sequelae such as cardiac hypertrophy. ❻ *Surgical resection is considered the treatment of choice for Cushing's syndrome from endogenous causes if the tumor can be localized and if there are no contraindications.* The treatment of choice for Cushing's syndrome from exogenous causes is gradual discontinuation of the offending agent.

▶ Nonpharmacologic Therapy

Transsphenoidal pituitary microsurgery is the treatment of choice for Cushing's disease. Removal of the pituitary tumor can bring about complete remission or cure in 78% to 97% of cases. HPA axis suppression associated with chronic hypercortisolism can result in prolonged adrenal insufficiency lasting for months after surgery and requiring exogenous glucocorticoid administration. Pituitary irradiation or bilateral **adrenalectomy** is usually reserved for patients who are not surgical candidates or for those who relapse or do not achieve complete remission after pituitary surgery. Because the response to pituitary irradiation can be delayed (several months to years), concomitant treatment with cortisol-lowering medication may be necessary. Bilateral adrenalectomy is also used for the management of adrenal carcinoma and in patients with poorly controlled ectopic Cushing's disease in whom the ACTH-producing lesion cannot be localized. Bilateral laparoscopic adrenalectomy achieves an immediate and total remission (nearly 100% cure rate), but these patients require lifelong glucocorticoid and mineralocorticoid supplementation.[17,18] **Nelson syndrome** may develop in nearly 20% to 50% of patients who undergo bilateral adrenalectomy without pituitary irradiation. This condition presumably results from persistent hypersecretion of ACTH by the intact pituitary adenoma, which continues to grow because of the loss of feedback inhibition by cortisol. Treatment of Nelson syndrome may involve pituitary irradiation or surgery.[4]

The treatment of choice in patients with adrenal adenomas is unilateral laparoscopic adrenalectomy. These patients require glucocorticoid supplementation during and after surgery caused by atrophy of the contralateral adrenal gland and suppression of the HPA axis. Glucocorticoid therapy is continued until recovery of the remaining adrenal

Clinical Presentation and Diagnosis of Cushing's Syndrome[1,12,13]

General

- Patients with Cushing's syndrome caused by either endogenous or exogenous glucocorticoid excess typically present with similar clinical manifestations.

- Differential diagnoses include diabetes mellitus and the metabolic syndrome because patients with these conditions share several similar characteristics with patients who have Cushing's syndrome (e.g., obesity, hypertension, hyperlipidemia, hyperglycemia, and insulin resistance). In women, the presentations of hirsutism, menstrual abnormalities, and insulin resistance are similar to those of polycystic ovary syndrome. Cushing's syndrome can be differentiated from these conditions by identifying the classic signs and symptoms of truncal obesity, "moon facies" with facial plethora, a "buffalo hump" and supraclavicular fat pads, red-purple skin striae, and proximal muscle weakness.

- True Cushing's syndrome also must be distinguished from other conditions that share some clinical presentations (as well as elevated plasma cortisol concentrations) such as depression, alcoholism, obesity, and chronic illness—the so-called pseudo-Cushing's states.

Signs and Symptoms (Percent Prevalence)

General appearance

- Weight gain and obesity manifesting as truncal obesity (90%)
- A rounded and puffy face ("moon facies") (75%)
- Dorsocervical ("buffalo hump") and supraclavicular fat accumulation
- Hirsutism (excessive hair growth) (75%)

Skin changes from atrophy of dermis and connective tissue

- Thin skin
- Facial plethora (70%)
- Skin striae ("stretch marks" that are usually red or purple in appearance and greater than 1 cm) (50%)
- Acne (35%)
- Easy bruising (40%)
- Hyperpigmentation

Metabolic

- Hyperglycemia that can range from impaired glucose tolerance (75%) to diabetes mellitus (20% to 50%)
- Hyperlipidemia (70%)
- Polyuria (30%)
- Kidney stones (15% to 50%)
- Hypokalemic alkalosis (from mineralocorticoid effect of cortisol)

Cardiovascular

- Hypertension (from mineralocorticoid effect of cortisol) (85%)
- Patients are at risk of the cardiovascular complications of hypertension, hyperlipidemia, and hyperglycemia.
- Peripheral edema

Genitourinary

- Menstrual irregularities (the most typical presentation is amenorrhea) (70%)
- Erectile dysfunction (85%)

Other

- Psychiatric changes such as depression, emotional lability, psychosis, euphoria, anxiety, and decreased cognition (85%)
- Sleep disturbances
- Osteopenia (80%) and osteoporosis, usually affecting trabecular bone
- Linear growth impairment in children
- Proximal muscle weakness (65%)
- Avascular necrosis (more common in iatrogenic cases)
- Glaucoma and cataracts
- Impaired wound healing and susceptibility to opportunistic infections
- Hypothyroidism

Laboratory Tests

- The diagnosis of Cushing's syndrome and its etiology is often complex and generally requires the involvement of endocrinologists and specialized testing centers.

- Initial screening tests to confirm the presence of hypercortisolism and differentiate Cushing's syndrome from conditions with similar presentations include 24-hour urinary-free cortisol and overnight low-dose dexamethasone suppression test (DST) (Table 45–6).

- The midnight plasma cortisol or combined dexamethasone suppression plus CRH test are less commonly used.

- Typically, a combination of at least two screening tests is used to establish the preliminary diagnosis.

- After the diagnosis is confirmed, additional tests can be performed to determine the etiology.

Other Diagnostic Tests

Imaging studies may be used to distinguish between pituitary, ectopic, and adrenal tumors (Table 45–5).

Table 45–6

First-Line Screening Tests in Patients with Characteristics of Cushing's Syndrome[1,12,16]

Test	Test Procedure and Measurement	Rationale	Typical Finding in Cushing's Syndrome	Comments
24-hour urinary-free cortisol	Collect urine over 24 hours and measure unbound cortisol excreted by kidneys	Urinary cortisol is elevated in hypercortisolic states	Urinary-free cortisol greater than four times the upper reference limit is indicative of Cushing's syndrome. Values between one and four times the upper reference limit suggest either Cushing's syndrome or pseudo-Cushing's syndrome	• Easy to perform but should not be used alone because sensitivity and specificity depend on the assay used • To exclude periodic hypercortisolism, three or more samples should be obtained (with urinary creatinine measurement to assess completeness of the collection) • Distinguishes Cushing's syndrome from obesity (no elevation). However, false-positive results if other pseudo-Cushing's states, physiologic stress, or pregnancy • False-negative results if decreased renal function, or subclinical hypercortisolism
Overnight low-dose DST	Give 1 mg oral dexamethasone at 11 PM; then measure plasma cortisol at 8 to 9 AM the next morning	Dexamethasone administration suppresses morning plasma cortisol in normal individuals	Plasma cortisol greater than 14.3 µg/dL (395 nmol/L) is diagnostic for Cushing's syndrome. Plasma cortisol less than 1.2 µg/dL (33 nmol/L) is not suggestive of Cushing's syndrome	• Simple to perform and inexpensive • Can be used in conjunction with or instead of the urinary-free cortisol test • Can also use the 2-day 2-mg DST • False-positive result if pseudo-Cushing's states, physiologic stress, pregnancy, estrogen treatment, uremia, taking inducers of dexamethasone metabolism (e.g., phenytoin), or decreased dexamethasone absorption • False-negative result if subclinical hypercortisolism or slow metabolism of dexamethasone
Late-night salivary cortisol	Collect salivary cortisol concentration at 11 PM	Loss of circadian rhythm of cortisol secretion (no nadir at night) in Cushing's syndrome but not in pseudo-Cushing's states	Elevated late-night salivary cortisol	• Diagnostic criteria need further validation • Easiest screening test to perform (sample can be collected at home by patient) • Can be used in conjunction with or instead of the urinary-free cortisol test

DST, dexamethasone suppression test.

gland is achieved. Patients with adrenal carcinomas have a poor prognosis, with a 5-year survival rate of 20% to 58% because of the advanced nature of the condition (metastatic disease). Surgical resection to reduce tumor burden and size, pharmacologic therapy, or bilateral laparoscopic adrenalectomy are the treatment options commonly used to manage this condition.[1,18]

Pharmacologic Therapy

⑦ *Pharmacotherapy is generally reserved for patients (1) in whom the ectopic ACTH-secreting tumor cannot be localized, (2) who are not surgical candidates, (3) who have failed surgery, (4) who have had a relapse after surgery, or (5) in whom adjunctive therapy is required to achieve complete remission.*[19] The drugs used are classified according to their mechanism and site of action (Table 45–7). The most widely used therapeutic class is the adrenal steroidogenesis

inhibitors.[19] Agents in this class include ketoconazole, etomidate, and metyrapone. Steroidogenesis inhibitors can improve hypercortisolism by inhibiting enzymes involved in the biosynthesis of cortisol. Because of their potential to cause adrenal suppression, temporary glucocorticoid replacement and in some cases mineralocorticoid supplementation may be needed during and after treatment. Centrally acting neuromodulators of ACTH release such as bromocriptine, cyproheptadine, octreotide, ritanserin, and valproic acid are generally ineffective.

⑧ *In drug-induced Cushing's syndrome, discontinuation of the offending agent is the best management option. However, abrupt withdrawal of the glucocorticoid can result in adrenal insufficiency or exacerbation of the underlying disease.*[13] **⑨** *Glucocorticoid dosages less than 7.5 mg/day of prednisone or its equivalent for less than 3 weeks generally would not be expected to lead to suppression of the HPA axis.*[2,18] However, in patients receiving pharmacologic doses

Table 45-7

Pharmacologic Treatments for Cushing's Syndrome[17,24-26]

Drug	Mechanism of Action	Dosage[a]: Initial, Usual, Maximum Dosing Adjustment for Renal and/or Hepatic Failure	Common and/or Major Adverse Reactions	Comments
Inhibitors of Adrenal Steroidogenesis				
Ketoconazole[b] (oral administration)	Inhibits several cytochrome P450 enzymes, including 17,20-lyase, 17-hydroxylase, and 11β-hydroxylase; also inhibits cholesterol synthesis	*Adults:* 200 mg twice daily; 600–800 mg/day in two divided doses; NTE 1,200 mg/day in two or three divided doses *Pediatric:* safety and effectiveness have not been established Extensively metabolized by liver, and dosing adjustment should be considered in severe liver disease; dosing adjustment not needed in renal disease	Generally well tolerated Transaminase elevations, GI intolerance, and rash Gynecomastia, testicular function impairment, and adrenal insufficiency at high doses (more than 600 mg/day)	• Effective in a majority of causes; rapid clinical improvement seen • Monitor efficacy with urinary cortisol • Monitor liver transaminases for hepatotoxicity • Useful in women with hirsutism and patients with hyperlipidemia • Requires gastric acidity for dissolution and absorption, therefore not useful in patients with achlorhydria and those taking proton pump inhibitors or round-the-clock antacids or histamine-2 receptor blockers
Metyrapone[b] (oral administration)	Inhibits 11-hydroxylase. Also suppresses aldosterone synthesis	*Adults:* 750 mg/day; 500–4,000 mg/day in four divided doses; NTE 6 g/day *Pediatric:* safety and effectiveness have not been established Dosages in special populations (liver and kidney disease, elderly patients) have not been established	Generally well tolerated Hirsutism, acne, adrenal insufficiency, GI intolerance, rash, hypokalemia, edema, hypertension	• Used in Cushing's disease, ectopic ACTH syndrome, and adrenal carcinoma • Also used as a test to diagnose adrenal insufficiency
Etomidate[b] (IV administration)	Inhibits 17,20-lyase, 17-hydroxylase, and 11β-hydroxylase	*Adults:* Limited clinical experience, 1.6–4.2 mg/h intermittently *Pediatric:* safety and effectiveness have not been established Extensively metabolized in the liver to inactive metabolites; because of changes in protein binding, dosing adjustment may be needed in kidney and liver disease	Injection site pain, nausea, vomiting, myoclonus	• IV route of administration limits use
Adrenolytic Agent				
Mitotane[b] (oral administration)	Inhibits steroidogenesis at lower doses and is adrenolytic at higher doses; inhibits 11β-hydroxylase and cholesterol side-chain cleavage; reduces aldosterone synthesis	*Adults:* 2–6 g/day in three or four divided doses; 9–10 g/day in three or four divided doses; NTE 16 g/day in three or four divided doses; elderly patients may require a dose decrease *Pediatric:* safety and effectiveness have not been established Primarily metabolized by the liver and dosing adjustment may be needed in liver disease	GI intolerance (high incidence), fatigue, dizziness, somnolence, gynecomastia Hyperlipidemia requiring lipid-lowering treatment Adrenal insufficiency requiring glucocorticoid replacement therapy	• Used primarily for adrenal carcinoma but can also be used in other types of Cushing's syndrome • Efficacy takes several weeks • Lower rate of relapse when used with pituitary radiation; also enables lower doses and therefore lower rate of adverse reactions
Peripheral Glucocorticoid Antagonist				
Mifepristone (RU 486)[b] (oral administration)	Antagonizes glucocorticoid receptors	*Adults and children:* up to 20 mg/kg/day Do not exceed 600 m/d in renal impairment or mild-to-moderate hepatic impairment. Do not use in severe hepatic impairment.	Nausea, fatigue, headache, hypokalemia, arthralgia, vomiting, peripheral edema, hypertension, dizziness, decreased appetite, endometrial hypertrophy, prolonged QT interval. Has abortifacient and embryotoxic properties	• FDA-approved for the control of hyperglycemia secondary to hypercortisolism in adult patients with endogenous Cushing's syndrome who have type 2 diabetes mellitus or glucose intolerance and have failed surgery or are not candidates for surgery. Not FDA-approved in children. • Increases cortisol and ACTH levels via antagonism of negative feedback of ACTH secretion • Requires cautious use since limited clinical experiences and cannot use cortisol or ACTH levels to monitor efficacy of treatment • Quicker effectiveness compared to the other drug treatment options

[a]Dosing guidelines (including age ranges) for children have not been definitively established.

[b]These medications do not have FDA-approved indications for the treatment of Cushing's syndrome in either adults or children.

ACTH, adrenocorticotropic hormone or corticotropin; FDA, Food and Drug Administration; GI, gastrointestinal; IV, intravenous; NTE, not to exceed.

of glucocorticoids for prolonged periods, gradual tapering to near-physiologic levels (5 to 7.5 mg/day of prednisone or its equivalent) should precede drug discontinuation. Administration of a short-acting glucocorticoid in the morning and use of alternate-day dosing may reduce the risk of adrenal suppression. Testing of the HPA axis may be useful in assessing adrenal reserve. In some cases, supplemental glucocorticoid administration during excessive physiologic stress may be needed for up to 1 year after glucocorticoid discontinuation.[13] Table 45–8 lists strategies to prevent the development of hypercortisolism and hypocortisolism.

OUTCOME EVALUATION

• Monitor patients receiving surgical, medical, or radiation therapy for resolution of the clinical manifestations of hypercortisolism. Symptoms often improve immediately after surgery and soon after initiation of drug therapy. However, it may take months for symptoms to resolve after radiation therapy.

• Monitor for normalization of serum cortisol concentrations.

• Patient Care and Monitoring discusses additional evaluation strategies.

Table 45–8

Principles of Glucocorticoid Administration to Avoid Hypercortisolism or Hypocortisolism

To Prevent Hypercortisolism and Development of Cushing's Syndrome
• Give the lowest glucocorticoid dose that will manage the disease being treated and for the shortest possible duration.
• If feasible, give glucocorticoid via administration routes that minimize systemic absorption (e.g., inhalation or dermal).
• If feasible, administer glucocorticoid treatment every other day (calculate the total 48-hour dose and give as a single dose of intermediate-acting glucocorticoid in the morning).[4]
• Avoid concurrent administration of drugs that can inhibit glucocorticoid metabolism.

To Prevent Hypocortisolism and Development of Adrenal Insufficiency or Adrenal Crisis
• Assess patients at risk for adrenal insufficiency with screening tests (e.g., serum cortisol, rapid ACTH stimulation).
• If the patient requires discontinuation from chronic treatment with supraphysiologic doses of glucocorticoid, the following discontinuation protocol can be used:[4]
  • Gradually taper the dose to approximately 20 mg of prednisone or equivalent per day, given in the morning.
  • Then change glucocorticoid to every other day administration, in the morning.
  • Stop the glucocorticoid when the equivalent physiologic dose is reached (20 mg/day of hydrocortisone or 5–7.5 mg/day of prednisone or equivalent).
  • Understand that recovery of the HPA axis may take up to 1 year after glucocorticoid discontinuation during which the patient may require supplementation therapy during periods of physiologic stress.
• Evaluate patients at risk for adrenal insufficiency as a result of treatment(s) of Cushing's syndrome and initiate glucocorticoid and mineralocorticoid replacement therapy as appropriate.
• Avoid concurrent administration of drugs that can induce glucocorticoid metabolism.
• Educate patients about:
  • The need for replacement or supplemental glucocorticoid and mineralocorticoid therapy
  • How to administer parenteral glucocorticoid if unable to immediately access medical care during an emergency
  • Need to wear or carry medical identification regarding their condition (e.g., card, bracelet)

ACTH, adrenocorticotropic hormone or corticotropin; HPA, hypothalamic–pituitary–adrenal.

Patient Encounter 2

YZ is a 61-year-old man who presents to the certified diabetes educator for diabetes education and instruction in self-monitoring of blood glucose. He was recently diagnosed with type 2 diabetes based on glycosylated hemoglobin testing by his primary care physician. He also has diagnoses of hypertension, atrial fibrillation, dyslipidemia, depression, and spinal stenosis. He complains of thirst, polyuria, and fatigue. Physical examination reveals an obese (body mass index, 37 kg/m²) gentleman with truncal obesity, dorsocervical fat, reddish abdominal striae, several small bruises on abdomen and extremities, and facial plethora. The diabetes educator suggests evaluation for possible Cushing's syndrome.

Which findings are suggestive of Cushing's syndrome?

Aside from Cushing's syndrome, what are some major differential diagnoses for YZ's clinical presentation?

The primary care physician performs a 24-hour urinary-free cortisol test. The result is four times the upper reference limit. Can this result be used to establish the diagnosis of Cushing's syndrome?

Patient Care and Monitoring: Cushing's Syndrome

1. Patient evaluation should include a thorough history of all medications and herbal or dietary supplements.

2. Perform initial screening tests to confirm Cushing's syndrome and rule out those with pseudo-Cushing's conditions.

3. After the diagnosis is confirmed, perform further testing to determine etiology of Cushing's syndrome.

4. Attempt to taper glucocorticoid if Cushing's syndrome is from exogenous administration.

5. If the patient has endogenous Cushing's syndrome, determine if patient is an appropriate candidate for surgical resection of the tumor. Does the patient have any conditions that contraindicate surgical resection such as advanced disease (metastatic adrenal carcinoma)?

6. Develop a formal plan to assess the response and complications associated with surgery[17]:

   - Measure plasma cortisol post surgery to determine if the patient displays persistent hypercortisolism (surgical treatment failure) or hypocortisolism (adrenal insufficiency requiring steroid replacement therapy).

   - In patients demonstrating hypocortisolism:

      - Monitor for signs and symptoms of glucocorticoid withdrawal (headache, fatigue, malaise, myalgia).

      - Monitor for signs and symptoms of adrenal insufficiency.

      - Monitor morning cortisol or response to ACTH stimulation every 3 to 6 months to assess for HPA axis recovery. Discontinue glucocorticoid replacement therapy when cortisol concentrations are greater than 19 mcg/dL (524 nmol/L) on either test.

      - Monitor cortisol, ACTH, low-dose dexamethasone suppression, or other tests to assess for risk of relapse of hypercortisolism.

   - Monitor for development of pituitary hormone deficiency.

7. If surgical resection does not achieve satisfactory disease control or is not indicated, evaluate the patient for pituitary radiation or bilateral adrenalectomy with concomitant pituitary radiation.

   - Monitor patients treated with pituitary radiation for development of pituitary hormone deficiency.

8. Evaluate patients with adrenal adenomas for unilateral adrenalectomy.

9. Give glucocorticoid and mineralocorticoid replacement to patients who undergo adrenalectomy (permanently in the case of bilateral adrenalectomy).

10. Evaluate patient for appropriateness of pharmacologic therapy depending on the etiology of Cushing's syndrome.

11. Monitor the patient for response to therapy, need for dose adjustments, and presence of adverse drug reactions.

12. When disease control is achieved, continue to monitor biochemical markers and patient for development of complications of Cushing's syndrome, as relapse may occur.

13. Provide patient education regarding disease state and treatment:

   - Causes of Cushing's syndrome, including drug-induced etiologies
   - How to recognize the clinical manifestations of Cushing's syndrome
   - Possible sequelae of Cushing's syndrome
   - How to reduce the modifiable cardiovascular and metabolic complications
   - Advantages and disadvantages of potential treatment options
   - Possible adverse consequences of treatment
   - Need for glucocorticoid and mineralocorticoid replacement after treatment, if appropriate
   - Importance of adherence to therapy.

Abbreviations Introduced in This Chapter

ACTH	Adrenocorticotropic hormone or corticotropin
ADX	Adrenodoxin
AIDS	Acquired immunodeficiency syndrome
BUN	Blood urea nitrogen
CRH	Corticotropin-releasing hormone
CT	Computed tomography
CYP450 3A4	Cytochrome P450 subfamily IIIA, polypeptide 4
CYP11A1	Side chain cleavage enzyme
CYP17A1	17-alpha-hydroxylase/17,20 lyase
CYP21A2	21-alpha-hydroxylase
CYP11B1	11-beta-hydroxylase
CYP11B2	Aldosterone synthase
DHEA	Dehydroepiandrosterone
DHEA-S	Sulfated form of dehydroepiandrosterone
DST	Dexamethasone suppression test
GI	Gastrointestinal
H6PDH	Hexose-6-phosphate dehydrogenase
HIV	Human immunodeficiency virus
HPA	Hypothalamic–pituitary–adrenal
HSD3B2	3-beta-hydroxysteroid dehydrogenase type 2
HSD11B1	11-beta-hydroxysteroid dehydrogenase type 1
HSD11B2	11-beta-hydroxysteroid dehydrogenase type 2
HSD17B	17-beta-hydroxysteroid dehydrogenase
IV	Intravenous or intravenously
MRI	Magnetic resonance imaging
PAPSS2	PAPS synthase type 2
POR	P450 oxidoreductase
SRD5A	5-alpha-reductase
SULT2A1	DHEA sulfotransferase

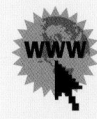 Self-assessment questions and answers are available at *http://www.mhpharmacotherapy.com/pp.html.*

REFERENCES

1. Carroll TB, Aron DC, Findling JW, Tyrrell JB. Glucocorticoids and adrenal androgens. In: Gardner DG, Shoback D, eds. Basic and Clinical Endocrinology. New York: Lange Medical Books/McGraw-Hill. 2011, [cited 2011 Oct 10]. Available from: *http://www.accessmedicine.com/content.aspx?aID=8403322.* Accessed September 27, 2011.
2. Cooper MS, Stewart PM. Corticosteroid insufficiency in acutely ill patients. N Engl J Med 2003;348:727–734.
3. Arlt W, Allolio B. Adrenal insufficiency. Lancet 2003;361:1881–1893.
4. Williams GH, Dluhy RG. Disorders of the adrenal cortex. In: Kasper DL, Braunwald E, Fauci A, Hauser S, Longo D, Jameson JL, eds. Harrison's Principles of Internal Medicine. New York: McGraw-Hill; 2005.
5. Marik PE, Pastores SM, Annane D, et al. Recommendations for the diagnosis and management of corticosteroid insufficiency in critically ill adult patients: Consensus statements from an international task force by the American College of Critical Care Medicine. Crit Care Med 2008;36:1937–1949.
6. Salvatori R. Adrenal insufficiency. JAMA 2005;294:2481–2488.
7. Arlt W, Callies F, van Vlijmen JC, et al. Dehydroepiandrosterone replacement in women with adrenal insufficiency. N Engl J Med 1999;341:1013–1020.
8. Gurnell EM, Hunt PJ, Curran SE, et al. Long-term DHEA replacement in primary adrenal insufficiency: A randomized, controlled trial. J Clin Endocrinol Metab 2008;93:400–409.
9. Hunt PJ, Gurnell EM, Huppert FA, et al. Improvement in mood and fatigue after dehydroepiandrosterone replacement in Addison's disease in a randomized, double blind trial. J Clin Endocrinol Metab 2000;85:4650–4656.
10. Johannsson G, Burman P, Wiren L, et al. Low dose dehydroepiandrosterone affects behavior in hypopituitary androgen-deficient women: A placebo-controlled trial. J Clin Endocrinol Metab 2002;87:2046–2052.
11. Alkatib AA, Cosma M, Elamin MB, et al. A systematic review and meta-analysis of randomized placebo-controlled trials of DHEA treatment effects on quality of life in women with adrenal insufficiency. J Clin Endocrinol Metab 2009;94:3676–3681.
12. Findling JW, Raff H. Screening and diagnosis of Cushing's syndrome. Endocrinol Metab Clin North Am 2005;34:385–402, ix–x.
13. Hopkins RL, Leinung MC. Exogenous Cushing's syndrome and glucocorticoid withdrawal. Endocrinol Metab Clin North Am 2005;34:371–84, ix.
14. Goldman JA, Myerson G. Chinese herbal medicine: Camouflaged prescription antiinflammatory drugs, corticosteroids, and lead. Arthritis Rheum 1991;34:1207.
15. Keane FM, Munn SE, du Vivier AW, Taylor NF, Higgins EM. Analysis of Chinese herbal creams prescribed for dermatological conditions. BMJ 1999; 318:563–564.
16. Arnaldi G, Angeli A, Atkinson AB, et al. Diagnosis and complications of Cushing's syndrome: A consensus statement. J Clin Endocrinol Metab 2003;88:5593–5602.
17. Utz AL, Swearingen B, Biller BM. Pituitary surgery and postoperative management in Cushing's disease. Endocrinol Metab Clin North Am 2005;34:459–478, xi.
18. Young WF, Jr., Thompson GB. Laparoscopic adrenalectomy for patients who have Cushing's syndrome. Endocrinol Metab Clin North Am 2005;34:489–499, xi.
19. Morris D, Grossman A. The medical management of Cushing's syndrome. Ann N Y Acad Sci 2002;970:119–133.
20. Coursin DB, Wood KE. Corticosteroid supplementation for adrenal insufficiency. JAMA 2002;287:236–240.
21. Lacroix A, Bourdeau I. Bilateral adrenal Cushing's syndrome: macronodular adrenal hyperplasia and primary pigmented nodular adrenocortical disease. Endocrinol Metab Clin North Am 2005;34:441–458, x.
22. Raff H, Findling JW. A physiologic approach to diagnosis of the Cushing syndrome. Ann Intern Med 2003;138:980–991.
23. Smith SM, Gums JG. Adrenal gland disorders. In: DiPiro JT, Talbert RL, Yee GC, Matzke GR, et al., eds. Pharmacotherapy: A Pathophysiologic Approach. New York: McGraw-Hill; 2011:1327–1344.
24. Korlym (mifepristone) package insert. California: Corcept Therapeutics Incorporated; 2012 February.
25. Chu JW, Matthias DF, Belanoff J, Schatzberg A, Hoffman AR, Feldman D. Successful long-term treatment of refractory Cushing's disease with high-dose mifepristone (RU 486). J Clin Endocrinol Metab 2001;86:3568–3573.
26. Sonino N, Boscaro M. Medical therapy for Cushing's disease. Endocrinol Metab Clin 1999;28:211–222.

46 Pituitary Gland Disorders

Judy T. Chen, Devra K. Dang, Frank Pucino Jr., and Karim Anton Calis

LEARNING OBJECTIVES

● **Upon completion of the chapter, the reader will be able to:**

1. List the mediators and primary effects of pituitary hormones.

2. Identify clinical features of patients with acromegaly.

3. Discuss the role of surgery and radiation therapy for patients with acromegaly.

4. Select appropriate pharmacotherapy for patients with acromegaly based on patient-specific factors.

5. Identify clinical features of children and adults with growth hormone (GH) deficiency and select appropriate pharmacotherapy for these patients.

6. Recommend monitoring parameters necessary to assess therapeutic outcomes and adverse effects in patients receiving GH therapy.

7. List common etiologies of hyperprolactinemia.

8. Identify clinical features of patients with hyperprolactinemia.

9. Select appropriate pharmacologic and nonpharmacologic treatments for patients with hyperprolactinemia based on patient-specific factors.

KEY CONCEPTS

❶ Surgical resection of the pituitary tumor through transsphenoidal pituitary microsurgery is the treatment of choice for most patients with growth hormone (GH)–producing pituitary adenomas.

❷ Somatostatin analogs are the mainstay of pharmacotherapy for the treatment of acromegaly when surgery is contraindicated or has failed, or as an adjuvant therapy until radiation effect is sustained.

❸ Pegvisomant, as monotherapy or adjuvant therapy to somatostatin analogs, is indicated for patients who do not tolerate or have an inadequate response to other treatment options.

❹ Dopamine agonists may be appropriate for patients with markedly elevated insulin-like growth factor-I (IGF-I) levels who have GH and prolactin cosecreting tumors, or as an additive therapy to somatostatin analog in patients with partial response to somatostatin.

❺ Prolonged exposure to elevated GH and IGF-I levels can lead to serious complications in patients with acromegaly. Comorbid conditions such as hypertension, diabetes, dysrhythmias, coronary artery disease, and heart failure should be aggressively managed to prevent vascular and neuropathic complications.

❻ Recombinant GH therapy is the main pharmacologic treatment for GH deficiency in both children and adults.

❼ Although comparative trials have not been conducted, recombinant GH products appear to have similar efficacy for treating GH deficiency as long as the regimen follows currently approved guidelines.

❽ Dopamine agonists are the first-line treatment of choice for all patients with symptomatic hyperprolactinemia; transsphenoidal surgery and radiation therapy are reserved for patients who are resistant to or severely intolerant of pharmacologic therapy.

❾ Women who become pregnant while taking a dopamine agonist should discontinue treatment immediately to minimize fetal exposure. Because cabergoline has a long half-life, women who plan to become pregnant should discontinue the drug at least 1 month before planned conception.

PHYSIOLOGY OF THE PITUITARY GLAND

The pituitary gland, located at the base of the brain in proximity to the nasal cavity, is a small endocrine gland about the size of a pea weighing approximately 600 mg. The pituitary gland is referred to as the "master gland" because it is responsible for the regulation of many other endocrine glands and body systems. Growth, development, metabolism, reproduction, and stress homeostasis are among the functions influenced by the pituitary. Functionally, the gland consists of two distinct sections: the anterior pituitary lobe (adenohypophysis) and the posterior pituitary lobe (neurohypophysis). The pituitary receives neural and hormonal input from the inferior hypothalamus via blood vessels and neurons contained in the pituitary stalk (infundibulum).

The posterior pituitary is innervated by nervous stimulation from the hypothalamus, resulting in the release of specific hormones to exert direct tissue effects. The hypothalamus synthesizes two hormones, oxytocin and vasopressin. These hormones are stored and released from the posterior pituitary lobe. Oxytocin exerts two actions, it: (a) promotes uterine contractions during labor and (b) contracts the smooth muscles in the breast to stimulate the release of milk from the mammary gland during lactation. Vasopressin, also known as antidiuretic hormone (ADH), is essential for proper fluid and electrolyte balance in the body. Specifically, vasopressin increases the permeability of the distal convoluted tubules and collecting ducts of the nephrons to water. This causes the kidneys to excrete less water in urine. Consequently, the urine becomes more concentrated as water is conserved.

In contrast to the posterior pituitary lobe, the anterior pituitary lobe is under the control of several releasing and inhibiting hormones secreted from the hypothalamus via a portal vein system. The anterior pituitary, in turn, synthesizes and secretes six major hormones. Figure 46–1 summarizes the physiologic mediators and effects of each of these hormones.

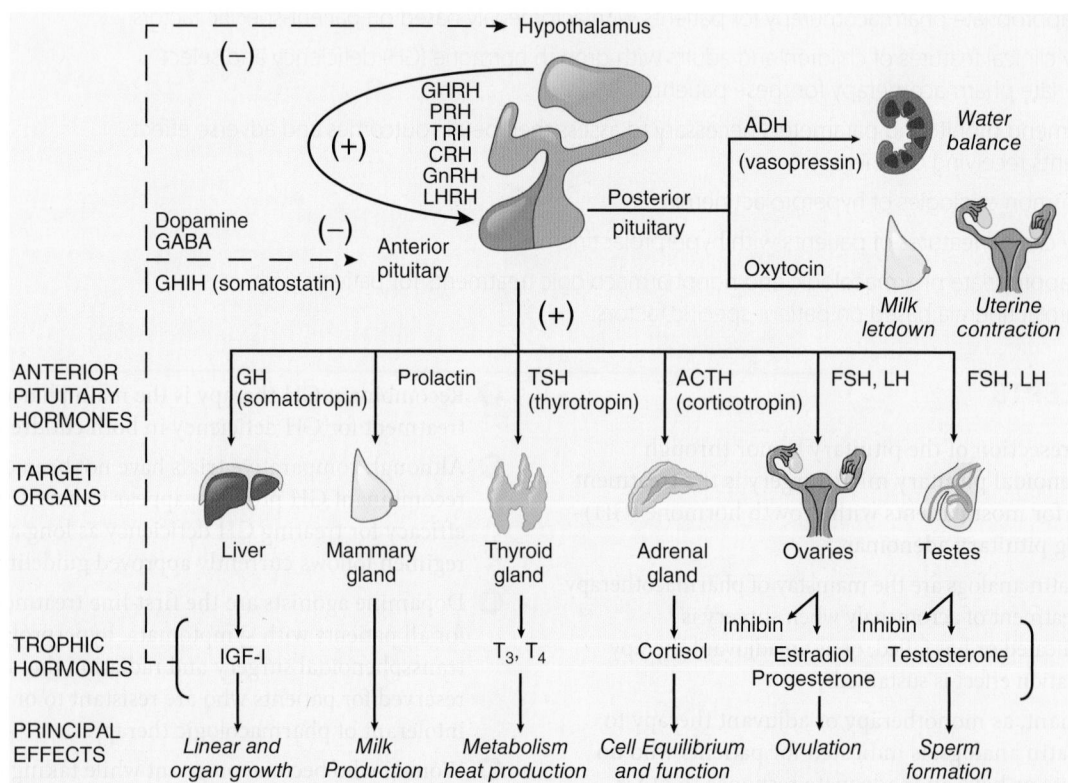

FIGURE 46–1. Hypothalamic–pituitary–target-organ axis. The hypothalamic hormones regulate the biosynthesis and release of eight pituitary hormones. Stimulation of each of these pituitary hormones produces and releases trophic hormones from their associated target organs to exert their principal effects. These trophic hormones regulate the activity of endocrine glands. Subsequently, increased serum concentration of the trophic hormones released from the target organs can inhibit both the hypothalamus and the anterior pituitary gland to maintain homeostasis (negative feedback). Inhibin is produced by the testes in men and the ovaries in women during pregnancy. Inhibin directly inhibits pituitary production of follicle-stimulating hormone (FSH) through a negative feedback mechanism. Melanocyte-stimulating hormone (MSH) produced by the anterior pituitary is not illustrated in the figure. (−), inhibit; (+), stimulate; ACTH, adrenocorticotropic hormone (corticotropin); ADH, antidiuretic hormone (vasopressin); CRH, corticotropin-releasing hormone; FSH, follicle-stimulating hormone; GABA, γ-aminobutyric acid; GH, growth hormone (somatotropin); GHIH, growth hormone–inhibiting hormone (somatostatin); GHRH, growth hormone–releasing hormone; GnRH, gonadotropin-releasing hormone; IGF-I, insulin-like growth factor-I; LH, luteinizing hormone; LHRH, luteinizing hormone–releasing hormone; PRH, prolactin-releasing hormone; T$_3$, triiodothyronine; T$_4$, thyroxine; TRH, thyrotropin-releasing hormone; TSH, thyroid-stimulating hormone (thyrotropin).

Hormonal Feedback Regulatory Systems

The hypothalamus is responsible for the synthesis and release of hormones that regulate the pituitary gland. Stimulation or inhibition of the pituitary hormones elicits a specific cascade of responses in peripheral target glands. In response, these glands secrete hormones that exert a negative feedback on other hormones in the hypothalamic–pituitary axis (see Fig. 46–1). This negative feedback serves to maintain body system homeostasis. In general, high circulating hormone levels inhibit the release of hypothalamic and anterior pituitary hormones.

Damage and destruction of the pituitary gland may result in secondary hypothyroidism, hypogonadism, adrenal insufficiency, growth hormone (GH) deficiency, hypoprolactinemia, or insufficiency or absence of all anterior pituitary hormones (i.e., panhypopituitarism). A tumor (adenoma) located in the pituitary gland may result in excess secretion of a hormone or may physically compress the gland and suppress adequate hormone release. The type, location, and size of a pituitary tumor often determine a patient's clinical presentation. This chapter discusses the pathophysiology and role of pharmacotherapy in the treatment of acromegaly, GH deficiency, and hyperprolactinemia. The following hormones are discussed elsewhere in this textbook: adreno-corticotropic hormone (ACTH or corticotropin), thyroid-stimulating hormone (TSH or thyrotropin), luteinizing hormone (LH), follicle-stimulating hormone (FSH), vasopressin (ADH), and oxytocin.

GROWTH HORMONE (SOMATOTROPIN)

Somatotropin or GH is the most abundant hormone produced by the anterior pituitary lobe. The GH-secreting somatotropes account for 50% of hormone-secreting cells in the anterior pituitary. GH is regulated primarily by the hypothalamic–pituitary axis. The hypothalamus releases growth hormone–releasing hormone (GHRH) to stimulate GH synthesis and secretion, whereas somatostatin inhibits it.[1] Upon stimulation by GHRH, somatotropes release GH into the circulation, thereby stimulating the liver and other peripheral target tissues to produce insulin-like growth factors (IGFs). These IGFs, also known as somatomedins, are the peripheral GH targets. There are two types of IGFs, IGF-I and IGF-II. IGF-I is the hormone generally responsible for growth of bone and other tissues, whereas IGF-II is primarily responsible for regulating fetal growth. High levels of IGF-I inhibit GH secretion through somatostatin, thereby inhibiting GHRH secretion at the hypothalamus.[1] The hypothalamus also may stimulate the release of somatostatin to inhibit GH secretion. The effects of IGF-I in peripheral tissues are both GH dependent and GH independent.[2] GH is an anabolic hormone with direct "anti-insulin" metabolic effects. By stimulating protein synthesis and shifting the body's energy source from carbohydrates to fats, GH promotes a diabetic state (Table 46–1).[2] GH controls somatic growth and has a critical role in the development of normal skeletal muscle, myocardial muscle, and bone.

Table 46–1		
Effects of Growth Hormone[2]		
	Mechanism of Action(s)	Effect(s)
Lipid metabolism	Increases the use of fat by stimulating triglyceride breakdown and oxidation of adipocytes	Increases breakdown of fat (lipolysis) Increases circulating fatty acid levels Increases lean body mass
Protein metabolism	Stimulates protein anabolism by increasing amino acid uptake and protein synthesis and decreasing oxidation of proteins	Increases muscle mass
Carbohydrate metabolism	Suppresses the ability of insulin to stimulate uptake of glucose in peripheral tissues	Decreases glucose utilization
	Decreases insulin receptor sensitivity	Insulin resistance
	Impairs postreceptor insulin action	Hyperglycemia
	Stimulates glucose synthesis in the liver (gluconeogenesis)	Increases hepatic glucose output

In healthy individuals, GH is secreted in a pulsatile pattern throughout a 24-hour period with several short bursts occurring mostly during the night. The most intense period of GH secretion occurs within the first 1 to 2 hours of slow-wave sleep (stage 3 or 4 deep sleep).[1] In between these bursts, basal concentration of GH falls to very low or undetectable levels because of its short half-life in the blood (~19 minutes). The amount of GH secretion fluctuates throughout a person's lifetime. Secretion of GH is lowest during infancy, increases during childhood, peaks during adolescence, and then declines gradually during the middle years.[1] These changes are parallel to an age-related decline in lean muscle mass and bone mineral density.

Growth Hormone Excess

▶ Epidemiology and Etiology

Acromegaly affects both genders equally, and the average age of presentation is 44 years. Approximately 50 to 70 people per 1 million population are affected, with an estimated annual incidence of three to four cases per 1 million people.[3,4] In more than 95% of the cases, overproduction of GH is caused by a benign pituitary tumor (adenoma), whereas malignant tumors occur in fewer than 1%.[5] Most pituitary adenomas occur spontaneously as a result of a sporadic genetic mutation acquired during life. Depending on the size of the tumor, pituitary adenomas are classified as: (a) microadenomas if they are 10 mm or less in diameter; or (b) macroadenomas

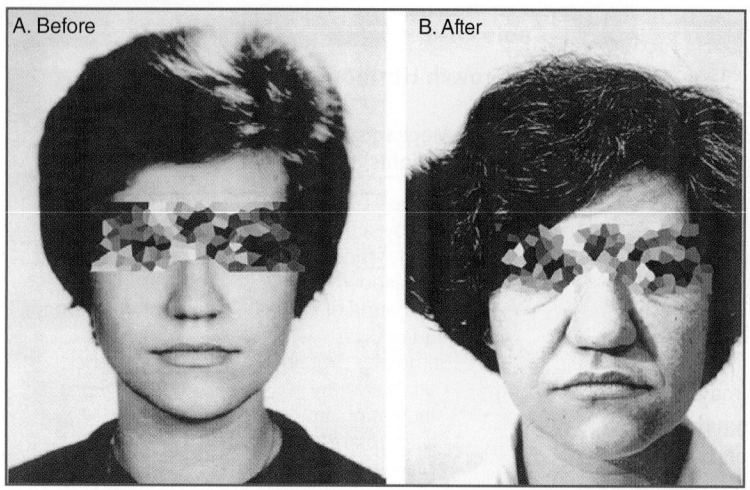

A. Before   B. After

FIGURE 46-2. Before and after photographs of a patient with acromegaly. Compare the photographs (**A**) before the onset of acromegaly and (**B**) after approximately 20 years when the diagnosis was well established. Notice the coarsening of facial features, with an enlarged nose, lips, and forehead.

if they are greater than 10 mm. Rarely, nonpituitary tumors cause acromegaly. These tumors can produce GH, but more commonly they secrete GHRH and result in excessive GH and IGF-I production.

▶ Pathophysiology

Acromegaly is a rare disorder that manifests gradually over time and typically occurs after fusion of the epiphyses (growth plates) of the long bones.[3] The facial features of an acromegalic patient are depicted in Figure 46–2. Gigantism refers to GH excess that occurs during childhood before epiphyseal closure and results in excessive linear growth (Figure 46–3).[6]

Because the signs and symptoms of acromegaly are insidious, diagnosis of this disorder is often delayed for up to 10 years after the initial presentation of symptoms. Therefore, it is important for practitioners to be vigilant in identifying

this disease in the early stages.[3] Diagnosis of acromegaly is based on both clinical and biochemical findings. Because secretion of GH fluctuates throughout the day, a single random measurement is never reliable for diagnosing GH excess.[1] However, GH-mediated IGF-I production results in relatively stable serum IGF-I concentrations during the day, which correlate positively with 24-hour mean GH levels.[1] This makes elevated IGF-I level an ideal screening test for acromegaly and a reliable monitoring biochemical marker to assess disease activity and response to therapy.[3,7] Because IGF-I levels may fluctuate with age and gender, it is important to compare IGF-I levels with age- and sex-matched population values.[7] Other conditions such as nutritional status, liver dysfunction, insulin levels, and illness also can affect IGF-I levels. The measurement of serum GH secreted by the pituitary in response to an oral glucose tolerance test (OGTT) is the primary biochemical test for diagnosing acromegaly. GH

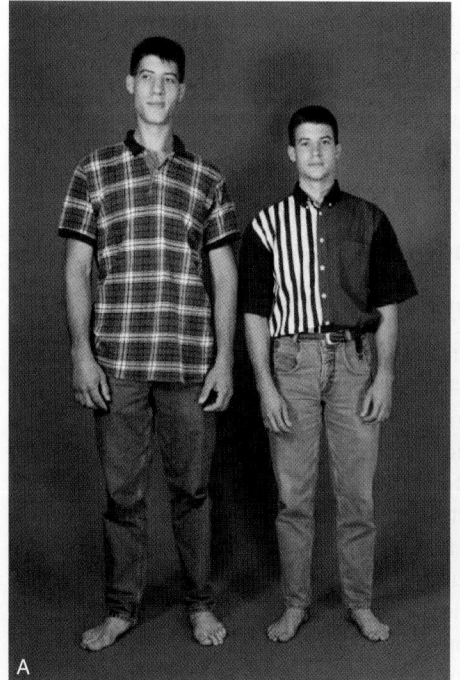

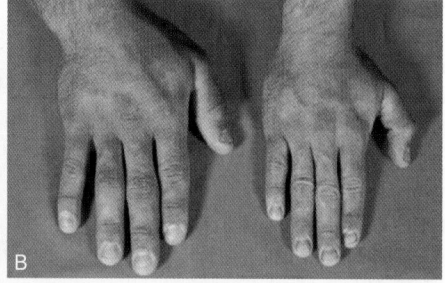

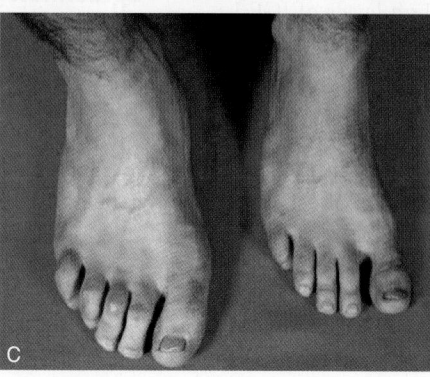

FIGURE 46-3. Example of gigantism. A 22-year-old man with gigantism caused by excess growth hormone is shown to the left of his identical twin. The increased height (**A**), enlarged hand (**B**), and enlarged foot (**C**) of the affected twin are evident. The features of the twins began to diverge at age 13 years. (Reproduced from Gagel RF, McCutcheon IE. Pituitary gigantism. New Eng J Med 1999;540:524; With permission.)

Clinical Presentation and Diagnosis of Acromegaly[3,7–9]

General

The patient will experience slow development of soft tissue overgrowth affecting many body systems. Signs and symptoms may progress gradually over 7 to 10 years.

Symptoms

- Headache and compromised visual function (loss of peripheral vision and blurred vision) caused by the actual tumor mass and its close proximity to the optic structures
- Weakness, low blood sugar, or weight loss caused by disruption of adrenal function (i.e., ACTH deficiency) by effect of tumor mass on the pituitary
- Fatigue and weight gain caused by disruption of thyroid function (i.e., TSH deficiency) by effect of tumor mass on the pituitary
- Absence of regular menstrual periods (**amenorrhea**), impotence, and decreased libido caused by disruption of the gonadotropin secretion (i.e., LH and FSH)
- Excessive sweating, joint pain, nerve pain, and abnormal neurologic sensations (paresthesias) related to elevated GH and IGF-I levels

Signs

- Coarsening of facial features
- Increased hand volume
- Increased ring and shoe size
- Increased spacing between teeth
- Increased acne or oily skin
- Enlarged tongue
- Deepening of voice
- Thick, irregular, patchy skin discoloration
- Enlarged nose, lips, and forehead (frontal bossing)
- Abnormal protrusion of the mandible (prognathia) and bite abnormalities
- Inappropriate secretion of breast milk (galactorrhea)
- Abnormal enlargement of various organs (organomegaly) such as liver, spleen, and heart
- Carpal tunnel syndrome caused by nerve compression from the swollen tissue

Laboratory Tests

- Random GH level greater than 1 ng/mL (1 mcg/L) or nadir GH level greater than 0.4 ng/mL (0.4 mcg/L) after an OGTT and elevated IGF-I level compared with age- and sex-matched control values.
- Loss of other hormonal functions caused by tumor mass compression of the anterior pituitary.
- Measure prolactin level in all patients because prolactin cosecretion is common.
- Glucose intolerance may be present in up to 50% of patients.

Additional Clinical Sequelae

- Cardiovascular diseases: hypertension, coronary heart disease, cardiomyopathy, left ventricular hypertrophy, and arrhythmia.
- Osteoarthritis and joint damage develop in up to 90% of patients.
- Respiratory disorders and **sleep apnea** occur in up to 70% of patients.
- Type 2 diabetes mellitus develops in 56% of patients.
- Increased risk for the development of esophageal, colon, and stomach cancer.

Other Diagnostic Tests

- Perform MRI examination of the pituitary to locate the tumor and validate the diagnosis.
- Obtain serum prolactin levels to assess for hyperprolactinemia and hypopituitarism.
- Without obvious pituitary tumor but proven acromegaly, measurement of GHRH may be helpful to detect ectopic tumors.

Adapted from Sheehan AH, Yanovski JA, Calis KA. Pituitary gland disorders. In: Dipiro JT, Talbert RL, Yee GC, et al, eds. Pharmacotherapy. A Pathophysiologic Approach. 8th ed. New York: McGraw-Hill; 2011:1345–1360.

---

is suppressed after administration of a 75-g oral glucose challenge because postprandial hyperglycemia inhibits secretion of GH for at least 1 hour. Measurement of GH concentrations at baseline and then every 30 minutes for a total of 2 hours after administration of OGTT is recommended.[3] If the GH level does not decline to less than 1 ng/mL (1 mcg/L) during the test, the patient is diagnosed with acromegaly.[3] With the increased sensitivity of the current GH assay, use of a lower nadir cutoff of 0.4 ng/mL (0.4 mcg/L) for GH level has been

suggested for detecting even modest elevations in GH levels.[3] In addition to clinical presentation, elevated IGF-I serum concentration helps to confirm the diagnosis.

▶ Acromegaly Treatment

Goals Patients with untreated acromegaly experience a two- to fourfold increase in mortality rate primarily because of cardiovascular and pulmonary diseases.[10] Normalization of GH and IGF-I levels lowers the mortality risk and may improve overall life expectancy. Adequate hormonal control of the disease also may alleviate associated comorbidities, especially cardiovascular, pulmonary, metabolic, and respiratory abnormalities.[11] Reduction of IGF-I levels alone does not appear to be a reliable predictor of long-term outcome.[12,13] The goals of therapy are as follows:[3]

- Normalize biochemical markers.
  - Reduce random GH to less than 1 ng/mL (1 mcg/L). When using a more sensitive GH assay, suppression of GH levels to less than 0.4 ng/mL (0.4 mcg/L) after OGTT would be indicative of disease control.
  - Normalize IGF-I levels to age- and sex-matched control values.
- Ablate or reduce tumor size to relieve tumor mass effect.
- Prevent tumor recurrence and control tumor size.
- Preserve normal pituitary function.
- Improve clinical signs and symptoms.
- Alleviate significant morbidities.
- Reduce mortality rates to those of the general population.

Surgical Treatment The American Association of Clinical Endocrinologists (AACE) published medical guidelines for the diagnosis and treatment of acromegaly (Fig. 46–4). According to these guidelines, ❶ *surgical resection of the pituitary tumor through transsphenoidal pituitary microsurgery is the treatment of choice for most patients with GH-producing pituitary adenomas.*[3] When performed by experienced surgeons, approximately 70% to 80% of patients with microadenomas and fewer than 50% of patients with macroadenomas achieve biochemical control.[10] Complete resection of a macroadenoma may be difficult if the tumor has already invaded the surrounding nerves and tissues. In such cases, debulking of the tumor along with adjunctive radiation and/or pharmacotherapy may improve treatment outcome. Infrequent surgical complications include meningitis, serious visual impairment, cerebrospinal fluid leakage, diabetes insipidus, and permanent hypopituitarism.[3] Relative contraindications to surgery include patient frailty, acromegaly-associated comorbidities, and medically unstable conditions such as airway difficulties, severe hypertension, or uncontrolled diabetes.

Pharmacologic Therapy Pharmacologic therapy is often necessary for patients in whom surgery is not an option. Somatostatin analogs, GH receptor antagonists, and dopamine agonists are the primary pharmacologic therapies used for the management of acromegaly (Table 46–2).[3,5] Pharmacologic therapy avoids hypopituitarism and other surgical risks.

Somatostatin Analog (GH-Inhibiting Hormone) ❷ *Somatostatin analogs are the mainstay of pharmacotherapy for the treatment of acromegaly when surgery is contraindicated or has failed, or as an adjuvant therapy until radiation effect is sustained.*[3] These agents mimic endogenous somatostatins and bind to somatostatin receptors in the pituitary to cause potent inhibition of GH, insulin, and glucagon secretion. Long-term treatment can sustain hormone suppression, alleviate soft tissue manifestations, and reduce tumor size. Use of the first-generation somatostatin analog octreotide is limited by its extremely short duration of action, which necessitates frequent injections of at least three times per day. The long-acting preparations of octreotide and lanreotide are considered the cornerstone of therapy because of improved patient adherence and acceptability. Typically, at least a 2-week trial of short-acting octreotide is recommended to determine efficacy and tolerance before switching to a long-acting preparation. The long-acting formulations can be administered every 14 to 28 days. Somatostatin analogs modestly reduce pituitary tumor size in 25% to 70% of patients depending in part on whether they are used as adjuvant or de novo therapy.[3] Their efficacy and safety have been demonstrated in long-term studies (up to 9 years with octreotide and 4 years with lanreotide).[14–16] Long-acting octreotide effectively suppresses GH levels and achieves normal IGF-I levels in 67% and 57% of patients, and lanreotide slow-release formulation achieved lower response rates of 48% and 47%, respectively.[17] However, the response rate of long-acting octreotide may be overestimated because of differences in subject selection.[17] The efficacy of lanreotide autogel, given by deep subcutaneous injection, is comparable to intramuscularly administered depot formulations of lanreotide and octreotide in achieving clinical and biochemical control.[3] Because somatostatin analogs can achieve substantial relief of clinical symptoms with significant reduction in tumor size, it is important to monitor patients for tumor recurrence if treatment is discontinued.[17,18] It is not yet known whether use of somatostatin analogs before surgery has additional benefits over surgery alone.[3]

Somatostatin analogs are generally well tolerated. Common adverse effects include transient gastrointestinal (GI) disturbances such as diarrhea, abdominal pain, flatulence, constipation, and nausea.[18] These adverse GI effects usually subside within the first 3 months of therapy.[4] Somatostatin analogs inhibit gallbladder contractility and decrease bile secretion; therefore, their major adverse effect is development of biliary sludge and asymptomatic gallstones (cholelithiasis). Biliary sludge is a predisposing factor for the high incidence of cholelithiasis observed in up to 20% of patients.[4] Cholelithiasis typically occurs in patients treated for 12 months or longer and is unrelated to age, gender, or dose. Somatostatin analog-induced gallstones should be managed according to standard guidelines.[4] Additionally, somatostatin analogs may alter the balance of counterregulatory hormones (i.e., glucagon, insulin, and GH), resulting in either hypoglycemia or hyperglycemia.[14] Octreotide also may suppress pituitary release of TSH, leading to decreased thyroid hormone secretion and subsequent hypothyroidism in 12% of treated patients. Close monitoring of thyroid function and glucose metabolism is recommended. Sinus bradycardia, conduction abnormalities, and arrhythmias have been reported with octreotide and lanreotide. Because of the potential adverse effects of the somatostatin analogs, concomitant use with insulin, oral hypoglycemic agents, beta-blockers, or calcium

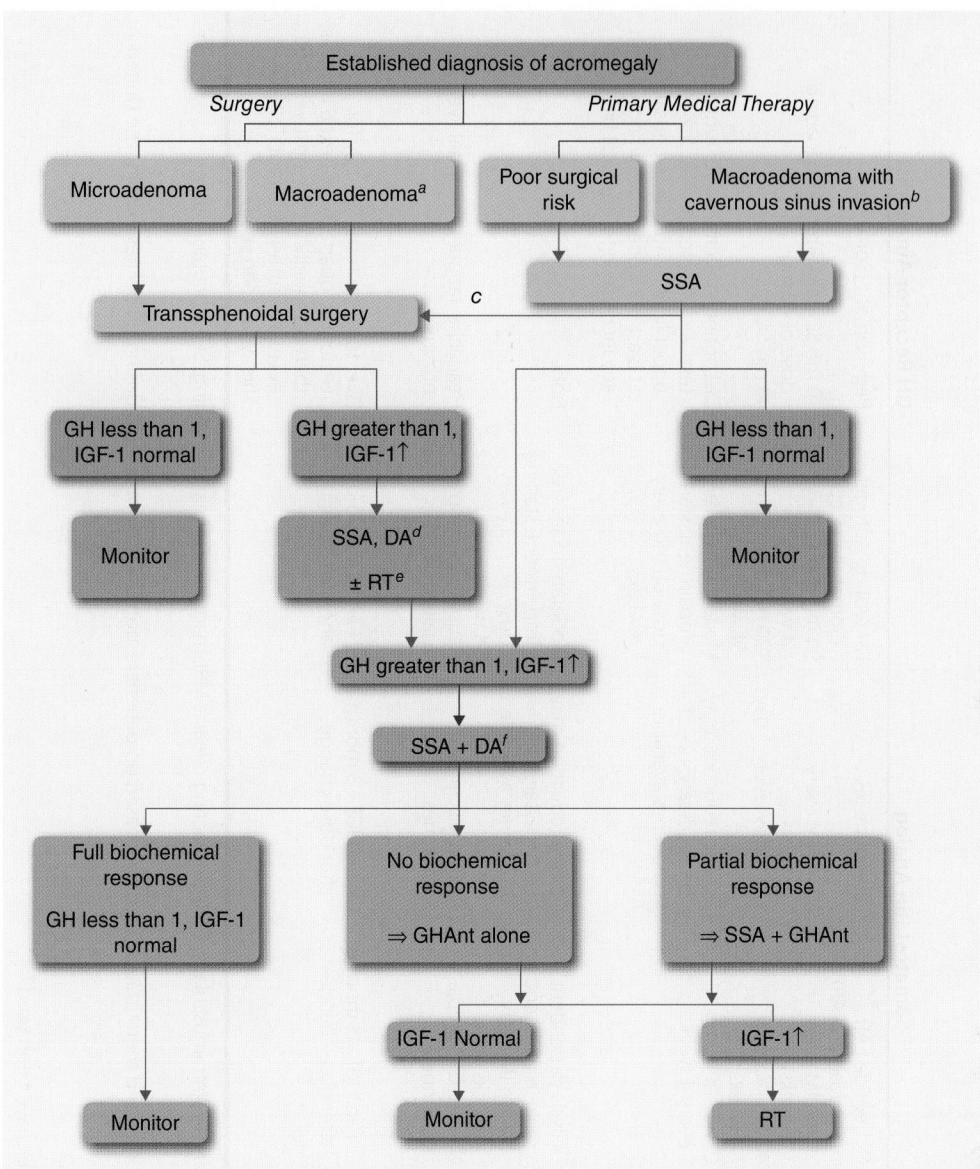

FIGURE 46–4. Treatment algorithm for acromegaly.[3] [a]Visual field compromise is absolute indication for surgery. [b]Primary medical therapy can be considered if there is no visual field deficit and there is no possibility of surgical cure because of cavernous sinus involvement. [c]Reconsider surgery to debulk tumor to improve response to medical therapy, reduce medical comorbidities, or comply with patient preference. [d]Consider a dopamine agonist (DA) in the setting of a modest disease; [e]Consider radiotherapy (RT) in patients with residual tumor after therapy. This decision is based on several factors, including age, reproductive status, pituitary function, insurance coverage, and patient preference regarding long-term medical therapy. [f]Addition of DA in the setting of modest disease. GH, growth hormone; GHAnt, growth hormone antagonist; IGF-I, insulin-like growth factor-I; SSA, somatostatin analogue. (Modified from Katznelson L, Atkinson JL, Cook DM, et al. American Association of Clinical Endocrinologists medical guidelines for clinical practice for the diagnosis and treatment of acromegaly—2011 update. Endocr Pract 2011;17(Suppl 4):1–44; With permission.

channel blockers may require careful dosage adjustment. Somatostatin analogs may also alter the bioavailability and elimination of cyclosporine, and monitoring of cyclosporine serum concentration is necessary.

GH-Receptor Antagonist The advent of a GH-receptor antagonist represents a novel approach to the treatment of acromegaly. Pegvisomant is the only genetically engineered

GH-receptor antagonist that blocks the action of GH. The effects of pegvisomant work independently of tumor characteristics, somatostatin, and dopamine receptors.[19] Up to 95% of patients with acromegaly treated with long-term pegvisomant (median dose, 15 mg/day) achieved normal age-related IGF-I levels and experienced significant improvement in clinical symptoms of GH excess.[20] In patients previously resistant to somatostatin analog therapy, normal IGF-I

Table 46–2

Comparison of Various Drugs for Treatment of Acromegaly[3,5]

Drug Class	Dopamine Agonist	Somatostatin Analog				GH Receptor Antagonist
Medication	Cabergoline	Octreotide (Sandostatin)	Octreotide LAR (Sandostatin LAR)	Lanreotide SR	Lanreotide Autogel (Somatuline Depot)	Pegvisomant (Somavert)
Starting dose	0.5–1 mg/week orally	50 mcg SC 3 × daily	20 mg IM every 4 weeks	60 mg IM every 2 weeks	90 mg deep SC every 4 weeks[a]	10 mg SC daily after initial loading dose of 40 mg
Maximal dose	4 mg/week orally	200 mcg SC 3 × daily	40 mg IM every 4 weeks[b]	120 mg IM every 7 days	120 mg deep SC every 4 weeks	40 mg SC daily[c]
Dosage in hepatic insufficiency	Dosage reduction may be recommended for patients with severe hepatic failure	—	Cirrhosis: 10 mg IM every 4 weeks	Dosage reduction may be necessary; no guidelines available	Moderate to severe impairment: starting dose 60 mg every 4 weeks	Discontinue therapy if liver function tests are elevated at least 5 × the upper limit of normal or transaminase at least 3 × upper limit of normal with any increase in serum total bilirubin
Dosage in renal failure	None	Dialysis dependent: adjustment may be necessary; no guidelines available	Dialysis-dependent renal impairment: 10 mg IM every 4 weeks	Dosage reduction may be necessary; no guidelines available	Moderate to severe impairment: starting dose, 60 mg every 4 weeks	None
Side effects	Nausea, GI cramps, headache, hypotension, nasal congestion	Nausea, GI cramps, gallstones	Nausea, GI cramps, gallstones	Nausea, GI cramps, gallstones	Nausea, GI cramps, gallstones	Headache, fatigue, abnormal liver enzymes
Monitoring suggestions	GH, IGF-I, and prolactin level 4–6 weeks after each dose change	GH and IGF-I 3 months after dose change	GH and IGF-I 3 months after dose change	GH and IGF-I 3 months after dose change	GH and IGF-I 3 months after dose change	Liver function tests monthly for 6 months, quarterly for next 6 months, then biannually for the next year; MRI every 6 months; IGF-I (not GH) after first year, then yearly

GH, growth hormone; GI, gastrointestinal; IGF-I, insulin-like growth factor-I; IM, intramuscularly; LAR, long-acting release; MRI, magnetic resonance imaging; SC, subcutaneously; SR, slow-release.

[a]In the United States, initiate lanreotide at 90 mg every 28 days for 3 months and then titrate accordingly based on patient response. Different labeled dosing guidelines exist for the United Kingdom and Canada.

[b]Product labeling recommends a maximum of 30 mg IM every 4 weeks.

[c]Alternative dose administration protocol of twice a week or once a week have been used.[3]

Adapted from AACE Medical Guidelines for Clinical Practice for the diagnosis and treatment of acromegaly. Endocr Pract 2004;10:213–225 by permission of publisher, American Association of Clinical Endocrinologists (AACE) Corp.

concentrations were achieved in 75% of patients treated with pegvisomant[21] and in 69% to 100% of patients treated with pegvisomant and somatostatin analog therapy.[22–24] Pegvisomant therapy may have favorable effects on glucose tolerance (the body's ability to metabolize glucose) and insulin sensitivity (capacity of cells to respond to insulin).[21] However, use of pegvisomant is associated with significant dose-dependent increases in GH despite declining IGF-I levels.[20] The dose-dependent increase in GH is troubling because it has been suggested that persistent elevation of GH levels may be indicative of tumor growth. Although currently available data suggest that pegvisomant does not promote tumor growth, careful monitoring with periodic imaging scans is nonetheless indicated, especially when administering pegvisomant to patients at risk for visual damage from large tumors that may impinge on the optic chiasm.[20,25]

③ *Pegvisomant, as monotherapy or adjuvant therapy to somatostatin analogs, is indicated for patients who do not tolerate or have an inadequate response to other treatment options.*[3] The long-term efficacy and safety of pegvisomant in acromegaly remain to be established. Pegvisomant appears to be well tolerated with minimal adverse effects, including self-limiting injection site reactions, elevated liver enzymes, headache, increased sweating, and abdominal complaints.[19] Although elevations of liver enzymes often are self-limiting and not associated with symptoms,[3] hepatotoxicity has been reported in clinical trials with a higher risk observed in diabetics receiving combined pegvisomant and somatostatin analogs.[20,26] Therefore, serum transaminases, total bilirubin, and alkaline phosphatase should be assessed before initiating therapy and periodically thereafter. Use caution when administering pegvisomant to patients with elevated liver function tests. Discontinue therapy if the patient presents with clinical signs and symptoms of hepatic injury.

Dopamine Agonists Dopamine is one of the neurotransmitters that can increase GH secretion in healthy adults. However, dopamine agonists administered to patients with acromegaly exert the opposite effect and suppress GH release from the tumor. The first dopamine agonist for acromegaly, bromocriptine, achieved normal IGF-I levels in fewer than 10% of patients and was associated with significant adverse effects including nausea, dizziness, and headaches.[10] The large doses of bromocriptine required to achieve the desired response are often associated with dose-limiting toxicity such as GI discomfort and orthostatic hypotension. Cabergoline, the selective long-acting agonist with improved tolerability, can effectively normalize IGF-I levels in 35% of patients and reduce GH levels in 44% of patients.[27] Acromegalic patients with coexisting hyperprolactinemia also had a more favorable response to cabergoline, with 50% of patients achieving normal IGF-I levels, 56% GH suppression, and 65% tumor shrinkage.[27] Although orally administered dopamine agonists are the least expensive medical therapy for managing acromegaly, the major disadvantage is their relative lack of efficacy compared with existing therapeutic options.

④ *Dopamine agonists may be appropriate for patients with markedly elevated IGF-I levels who have GH and prolactin*

cosecretion tumors, or as an additive therapy to somatostatin analog in patients with partial response to somatostatin.[3] Although cardiac valvular abnormalities have been observed in patients using higher doses of cabergoline for Parkinson's disease, similar findings have not been reported in patients with pituitary adenomas.[3,28] Nonetheless, patients who require prolonged therapy with higher doses of cabergoline warrant echocardiographic monitoring for potential cardiac abnormalities.[29]

● **Radiation Therapy** Radiation therapy is an important adjunctive therapy in patients with residual GH excess after surgery or pharmacologic therapy. Treatment involves the use of radiation to destroy rapidly growing tumor cells and often results in a reduction in tumor size. A major complication resulting from radiation therapy is hypopituitarism, requiring lifelong hormone replacement.[3] There is also the potential for optic nerve damage if the pituitary tumor is near the optic tracts. Radiation therapy may take 10 to 20 years before its full effects become evident.[3] Owing to delay in onset of radiation effectiveness, pharmacologic therapy with a somatostatin analog often is indicated as bridge therapy.[3] Men and women who desire to have children should be warned that pituitary irradiation therapy may impair fertility because of subsequent gonadotropin deficiency.[3]

▶ *Outcome Evaluation*

- Lifelong biochemical assessment is critical for determining therapeutic outcomes. Although some patients may experience a rapid decline in GH levels after surgery, stabilization of IGF-I levels usually occurs 3 months after surgery but rarely may be delayed for up to 12 months. Fully assess pituitary function 2 to 3 months after surgery.[3] GH and IGF-I levels should be measured 3 to 6 months postoperatively to assess treatment response.[3] Additionally, IGF-I levels should be measured annually in all postsurgical patients to monitor for potential pituitary tumor recurrence.[3]

- Assess magnetic resonance imaging (MRI) 3 to 4 months after surgery and 3 to 6 months after starting medical therapy.[7] Because up to 10% of pituitary tumors may recur within 15 years after surgery,[12] continual postoperative monitoring is recommended.

- For patients treated with somatostatin analogs, assess baseline fasting blood glucose, thyroid function tests, and heart rate. Thereafter, periodically monitor patients for adverse reactions such as GI disturbances, glucose intolerance, signs and symptoms of thyroid abnormalities, bradycardia, and arrhythmias in patients receiving long-term somatostatin analogs. Reevaluate IGF-I and GH levels at 3-month intervals to determine therapeutic response and inquire about symptoms of gallbladder disease (e.g., intermittent pain in the upper right abdomen) during follow-up appointments.[3] If normalization of GH and IGF-I levels is not fully achieved after 1 year, perform MRI 6 months later and annually thereafter to monitor tumor mass.[3]

Patient Encounter 1: Acromegaly: Medical History, Physical Examination, and Diagnostic Tests

JS is a 42-year-old man who presents to his endocrinologist with chief complaints of "not feeling like myself over the past 10 years!" He noticed dramatic physical changes and complaints of "my nose and forehead grew bigger; my face and hands became puffy!" He also noticed his shoes are too tight and "I need to be buy bigger shoes every year." He attributes the "numbness in [his] hands" to arthritis. JS reports increased fatigue, sweating, worsening headaches, and somnolence.

PMH: Hypertension for 12 years; type 2 diabetes mellitus for 5 years

FH: Mother died of diabetes at age 50. Father died of myocardial infarction at an unknown age

SH: Single, previously a successful freelance journalist, currently unemployed; graduate-level education

Meds: Enalapril/hydrochlorothiazide 10/25 mg once daily; metformin 1000 mg twice daily; glimepiride 8 mg once daily; acetaminophen 500 mg every 8 hours as needed for joint pain

ROS: (+) Deepening of voice

PE:

VS: BP 128/72 mm Hg, P 76 beats/min, RR 18 breaths/min, T 37.5°C (99.5°F)

HEENT: Ophthalmic examination reveals normal visual acuity and peripheral fields; protruding jaw and large fleshy nose

CV: RRR, normal S_1, S_2; no murmurs, rubs, gallops

Abd: Soft, nontender, nondistended; (+) bowel sounds, (–) hepatosplenomegaly

Rectal: Heme (–) stool

Labs: Electrolytes and renal function are within normal limits. Fasting blood glucose level is 180 mg/dL (10 mmol/L), HbA_{1c} is 7.9% (63 mmol/mol), and (–) microalbumin. GH level 1 hour after an OGTT is 5 ng/mL (5 mcg/L). Elevated IGF-I level at 800 ng/mL (800 mcg/L).

MRI: Reveals a pituitary tumor approximately 4 mm in diameter

Given this information, what signs and symptoms of acromegaly does JS exhibit?

What clinical complications often accompany JS's diagnosis?

Identify your treatment goals for JS.

What nonpharmacologic and pharmacologic treatment options are available for JS?

What additional considerations are needed based on patient's unemployed status?

- For patients treated with a GH receptor antagonist, GH levels are not measured because pegvisomant is a modified GH molecule that is detected in commercial GH assays, resulting in falsely elevated GH levels. Therefore, IGF-I level is the principal biochemical marker used to assess response to pegvisomant therapy. After appropriate dose titration, monitor IGF-I levels every 6 months.[3] Concern for tumor growth requires careful monitoring of tumor size; therefore, performing MRI every 6 months during the first year of therapy and annually thereafter is recommended.[3] Because of the potential for hepatotoxicity with pegvisomant therapy, it is mandatory to monitor liver enzymes prior to initiation of therapy, monthly during the first 6 months, quarterly for the next 6 months, and then biannually thereafter.[3] More frequent monitoring of liver enzymes is warranted in patients with elevated liver enzymes at baseline.[3]

- For patients receiving dopamine agonists, the maximal suppression of GH and IGF-I levels may take up to 3 months to achieve. After stable control of biochemical markers is achieved with dopamine agonists or somatostatin analogs, monitor GH and IGF-I levels annually.[3]

- With conventional multidose radiation therapy, the most rapid decline in GH serum levels occurs within the first

2 years; monitor GH levels at the second year and annually thereafter.[3,12] Patients who receive single-dose radiation therapy should be evaluated at 6-month intervals because response is observed earlier. Repeatedly assess pituitary function over the years after radiation therapy.[3]

- ⑤ *Prolonged exposure to elevated GH and IGF-I can lead to serious complications in patients with acromegaly. Aggressively manage comorbid conditions such as hypertension, diabetes, dysrhythmias, coronary artery disease, and heart failure to prevent vascular and neuropathic complications* (Table 46–3).[3,30]

Growth Hormone Deficiency

► Epidemiology and Etiology

In the United States, GH deficiency affects approximately 50,000 adults, with around 6,000 new cases diagnosed annually.[31] Approximately 10,000 to 15,000 children have growth failure owing to GH deficiency. Children may present with GH deficiency at any time during their developmental stages. The evaluation for GH deficiency in a child of short stature should be deferred until appropriate exclusion of other identifiable causes of growth failure, such as hypothyroidism, chronic illness, malnutrition, genetic syndromes, and skeletal disorders, has occurred. Also, several medications, such as somatostatin analogs, gonadotropin-releasing hormone

Table 46–3

Assessment of Acromegaly Complications at Diagnosis and Follow-up

At the Time of Diagnosis	During Long-Term Follow-Up
Glucose tolerance test (with concurrent GH sampling)	Fasting blood glucose, HbA$_{1c}$ if diabetes is present
Serum cholesterol and lipid profile	Annually
Echocardiography	Annually (in presence of cardiomyopathy)
ECG	Annually
Exercise ECG	If angina is present
Colonoscopy	Every 2–3 years
DEXA (hypogonadal only)	Every 2–3 years
Sleep assessment	Annually (if altered at diagnosis)
Blood pressure monitoring	Annually or change of treatment (if hypertensive)
Echo-Doppler of carotid artery	As indicated by clinical features

DEXA, dual-energy x-ray absorptiometry; ECG, electrocardiography; GH, growth hormone; HbA$_{1c}$, glycated hemoglobin A$_{1c}$.

From Giustina A, Casanueva FF, Cavagnini F, et al. Diagnosis and treatment of acromegaly complications. J Endocrinol Invest 2003;26:1242–1247; With permission.

(GnRH) agonists, methoxamine, phentolamine, isoproterenol, glucocorticoids, cimetidine, methylphenidate, and amphetamine derivatives, may induce GH insufficiency.[32]

▶ Pathophysiology

Growth hormone deficiency exists when GH is absent or produced in inadequate amounts. GH deficiency may be congenital, acquired, or result from disruption of the hypothalamus–pituitary axis. GH deficiency may be an isolated condition or occasionally be accompanied by other endocrine disorder (e.g., panhypopituitarism). Because GH is frequently undetectable with random sampling, a stimulation or provocative test usually is performed to confirm the diagnosis in both adults and children in whom GH deficiency is suspected. Numerous pharmacologic agents such as insulin-induced hypoglycemia, arginine plus GHRH, and glucagon have been used to stimulate the pituitary to produce GH.[33] These tests may be associated with adverse effects and therefore require close medical supervision. The gold standard for diagnosis of adults with GH deficiency is the insulin tolerance test (ITT), with glucagon as an alternative if GHRH is unavailable.[34] Adults exhibiting a peak GH level of less than 5 ng/mL (5 mcg/L) after an ITT would warrant treatment.[34] In prepubertal children, measurement of IGF-I concentrations may be useful in evaluating GH deficiency, with 100% specificity and 70% to 90% sensitivity.[35] In children, the diagnosis of GH deficiency is further supported if height is more than 2 standard deviations below the population mean (age- and sex-matched).[31] Failure of linear growth is an almost universal presenting feature of childhood GH deficiency.

Patient Care and Monitoring: Acromegaly

1. Assess the patient's clinical signs and symptoms to determine the severity of acromegaly.

2. Review the biochemical disease markers to assess the severity of acromegaly.

3. Review the available diagnostic data to determine pituitary tumor size and location. Determine if the patient has a coexisting prolactin secreting tumor. Determine if the tumor extends toward the optic chiasm or if it is continuous on the optic tracts.

4. Assess presence of acromegaly complications. Identify any significant comorbidities associated with acromegaly that require immediate treatment or early diagnosis.

5. Determine what treatment options the patient has tried in the past.

6. Evaluate patient for presence of surgical contraindications to transsphenoidal microsurgery. Determine if the patient is able or willing to undergo surgical intervention.

7. Develop a formal plan to assess patient's response and complications to surgical intervention. Measure both GH and IGF-I levels.

8. If surgical intervention does not achieve satisfactory disease control, select subsequent appropriate pharmacologic therapy based on patient-specific factors. In selecting therapy, be sure to consider if the patient has any contraindications or allergies to therapies.

9. Evaluate patient for presence of adverse drug reactions, drug allergies, and drug interactions.

10. Develop a plan to assess efficacy of pharmacologic therapy. Also consider if the patient's therapy requires any dose adjustments.

11. Assess biochemical markers annually once disease control is achieved.

12. Routinely assess acromegaly complications; include blood pressure, glucose tolerance, fasting lipid profile, cardiac evaluations (if clinically indicated), colonoscopy, dual-energy x-ray absorptiometry (DEXA) scan (hypogonadal only), evaluation of residual pituitary function and sleep apnea.

13. Provide patient education in regard to disease state, and nondrug and drug therapy. Discuss with the patient:

   • Possible complications of acromegaly

   • How to reduce the modifiable cardiovascular and metabolic risk factors

   • Potential effectiveness and disadvantages of existing treatment options

   • Importance of adherence to therapy

   • Potential adverse effects that may occur

Clinical Presentation and Diagnosis of Growth Hormone Deficiency in Children[9,31]

General

The patient will have a physical height that is greater than 2 standard deviations below the population mean for a given age and gender.

Signs

- The patient will present with reduced growth velocity and delayed skeletal maturation.
- Children with GH-deficient or GH-insufficient short stature also may present with abdominal obesity, prominence of the forehead, and immaturity of the face.

Laboratory Tests

- Patients will exhibit a peak GH level of less than 10 ng/mL (10 mcg/L) after a GH stimulation test.
- Reduced IGF-I concentration also may be present.

- Because GH deficiency may be accompanied by the loss of other pituitary hormones, hypoglycemia and hypothyroidism also may be noted.

Other Diagnostic Tests

- Perform MRI or computed tomography (CT) scan of the hypothalamic–pituitary region to detect structural or developmental anomaly.
- Perform radiography of the left wrist and hand for children older than 1 year of age to estimate bone age (knee and ankle for children younger than 1 year of age).

Adapted from Sheehan AH, Yanovski JA, Calis KA. Pituitary gland disorders. In: Dipiro JT, Talbert RL, Yee GC, et al, eds. Pharmacotherapy. A Pathophysiologic Approach. 8th ed. New York: McGraw-Hill; 2011:1345–1360.

Childhood GH deficiency may or may not continue into adulthood. The use of insulin-induced hypoglycemia as a provocative GH stimulation test is currently the gold standard for diagnosing GH deficiency in adults.[37] Most adults with GH deficiency have overt pituitary disease and present with nonspecific clinical disorders distinct from pediatric GH deficiency. Adults with more than three pituitary hormone deficiencies and a low serum IGF-I level are considered GH deficient and do not require further GH stimulation test.[36] Additionally, adult GH deficiency presumably is associated with an increased risk of death from cardiovascular diseases.[37]

▶ Treatment Goals

The goal of treatment for GH deficiency is to correct associated clinical symptoms.[31] In children, prompt diagnosis and early initiation of treatment are important to maximize final adult height. In adults, efforts should be made to achieve normal physiologic GH levels in an attempt to reverse metabolic, functional, and psychological abnormalities.[33]

▶ Pharmacologic Therapy

GH Therapy ⑥ *Recombinant GH therapy is the main pharmacologic treatment for GH deficiency in both children and adults.* It promotes skeletal, visceral, and general body growth; stimulates protein anabolism; and affects bone, fat, and mineral metabolism (see Table 46–1).[2] GH therapy requires subcutaneous or intramuscular administrations. Because two-thirds of GH secretion normally occurs during sleep, it is recommended to administer injections in the evening.[38] Many preparations of synthetic GH are available with a variety of injection devices to make administration more appealing and easier. Protropin (somatrem) and Tev-Tropin (somatropin) are approved by the Food and Drug Administration (FDA) for use in children, and other somatropin products such as

Nutropin, Nutropin AQ, Humatrope, Norditropin, Genotropin, Omnitrope, and Saizen are FDA approved in both children and adults.

⑦ *Although comparative trials have not been conducted to date, recombinant GH products appear to have similar efficacy for treating GH deficiency as long as the regimen follows currently approved guidelines.* GH secretion decreases with age. Therefore, older adults with GH deficiency often require substantially lower replacement doses than younger individuals. The optimal therapeutic approach is to initiate GH therapy at lower doses.[34] Table 46–4 lists the recommended GH replacement doses for children and adults.[34,39] Conventional weight-based regimens are not recommended in adults because of a lack of evidence supporting higher dosages in heavier individuals and greater potential for adverse effects.[33,37] Maintenance doses may be lower with chronic GH therapy.[40] For elderly patients, lower GH replacement doses often are adequate because of increased GH sensitivity.[33,34] Women with intact hypothalamic–pituitary–gonadal axis or on estrogen therapy (or oral contraceptives) generally require a higher GH dose than men.[34] Carefully monitor patients requiring replacement therapy with estrogens, thyroid hormones, or glucocorticoids because of potential interactions with GH therapy.[33] Monitor patients at 1- to 2-month intervals and titrate replacement doses in increments of 0.1 to 0.2 mg/day based on individual clinical and biochemical responses.[34] The conversion of international units (IU or mU) to milligram is a 3:1 ratio.[31] Selection of an injection device depends on patient preference because there is currently no difference in clinical outcomes among the various injection systems.[34,39]

Evidence has suggested that GH treatment in GH-deficient children can increase short-term growth and improve final adult height.[31] Beneficial effects of GH therapy in adults with GH deficiency have been demonstrated in subsequent studies to normalize body composition and metabolic process;

Clinical Presentation and Diagnosis of Growth Hormone Deficiency in Adults[33,36–38]

General

The patient likely will have a history of childhood-onset GH deficiency; hypothalamic or pituitary disorder; or the presence of three or four other pituitary hormone deficiencies caused by head trauma, tumor, infiltrative diseases, surgery, or radiation therapy.

Symptoms

- Reduced strength and exercise capacity
- Defective sweating
- Psychological problems
- Low self-esteem
- Depression
- Fatigue or listlessness
- Sleep disturbance
- Anxiety
- Social isolation
- Emotional lability and impaired self-control
- Poor marital and socioeconomic performance

Signs

- Increased fat mass (especially abdominal obesity)
- Reduced lean body mass

- Reduced muscle strength
- Reduced exercise performance
- Thin, dry skin; cool peripheries; poor venous access
- Depressed affect, labile emotions
- Impaired cardiac function as evidenced by abnormal echocardiography or stress test results

Laboratory Tests

- Patients will exhibit a peak GH level of less than 5 ng/mL (5 mcg/L) after a GH stimulation test. Insulin tolerance test (ITT) is the gold standard stimulation test. Low or low-normal IGF-I level also may be present. Presence of three or more pituitary hormone deficiencies with a low IGF-I level do not require further stimulation test.
- Increased low-density lipoprotein cholesterol, total cholesterol, triglycerides; decreased high-density lipoprotein cholesterol.
- Reduced bone mineral density associated with an increased risk of fracture.
- Increased insulin resistance and increased prevalence of impaired glucose tolerance.
- GH deficiency may be accompanied by the loss of other pituitary hormones.

Table 46–4

Dose Recommendations for Growth Hormone Deficiency in Children and Adults[34,39]

	Growth Hormone Replacement Dose	Dose Titration
Children[39]	**Dosing Range**	- Evaluate every 3–6 months based on height and height velocity.
Prepubertal children	25–50 mcg/kg/day	- Monitor IGF-I and IGFBP-3 yearly.
Adolescents	25–100 mcg/kg/day	- Monitor TSH and T$_4$ for hypothyroidism.
		- Reduce dose if serum IGF-I level is substantially above normal after 2 years of therapy.
Adults[34]	**Starting Dose**	
Age less than 30 years	0.4–0.5 mg/day[a]	- Increase dose by 0.1–0.2 mg/day based on clinical response, serum IGF-I levels, and side effects at 1- to 2-month intervals. Longer time intervals and smaller dose titration may be necessary in older adults.
Age 30–60 years	0.2–0.3 mg/day	
Age greater than 60 years	0.1–0.2 mg/day	
Diabetes or glucose intolerance (overweight, obese, or history of gestational diabetes)	0.1–0.2 mg/day	
Hepatic impairment	—	- Clearance may be reduced in patients with severe hepatic dysfunction; specific dosing suggestions are not available.
Renal impairment	—	- Patients with chronic renal failure tend to have decreased clearance; specific dosing suggestions are not available.

[a]Might require a higher dose for patients transitioning from pediatric treatment.

IGFBP-3, insulin-like growth factor-bind protein 3; IGF-I, insulin-like growth factor-I; T$_4$, thyroxine; TSH, thyroid-stimulating hormone.

improve cardiac risk profile, bone mineral density, quality of life, and psychological well-being; and increase muscle strength and exercise capacity.[37] Although long-term efficacy of GH replacement in adults has been demonstrated in a 10-year prospective study,[40] overall reduction in mortality with GH therapy remains to be established.

Practitioners should begin GH therapy as soon as possible to optimize long-term growth, especially for young children in whom GH deficiency is complicated by fasting hypoglycemia.[31] Selection of the optimal GH replacement dose will need to be individualized depending on response, financial resources, and product availability. Although the appropriate time to discontinue therapy remains controversial in childhood GH deficiency, it is reasonable to continue GH replacement until the child has reached satisfactory adult height, achieved documented epiphyseal closure, or failed to respond to therapy.[31] Management of the transition between pediatric and adult GH replacement remains a challenge because limited data are available. For patients in a transition phase who may be restarting GH therapy, the initial dose is approximately half of the pediatric and adult doses combined.[34] Starting GH therapy at a low dose and gradually titrating upward may decrease the potential for adverse effects. The optimal duration of treatment with GH therapy remains unclear, but lifelong therapy may be required. However, GH replacement should be discontinued if therapeutic benefit is not achieved after 2 years of therapy.[34]

In both children and adults, treatment with GH may mask underlying central hypothyroidism and adrenal insufficiency.[41] Treatment with GH also may induce insulin resistance and lead to the development of glucose intolerance in patients with preexisting risk factors. Adults are more susceptible to dose-related adverse effects of GH-induced symptoms, such as edema, arthralgia, myalgia, and carpal tunnel syndrome, which may necessitate dose reductions in up to 40% of adults.

Children treated with GH replacement therapy rarely experience significant adverse effects. Benign increases in intracranial pressure related to GH therapy may manifest as headaches, visual changes, or altered levels of consciousness. This condition is generally reversible upon discontinuation of treatment. Often, GH therapy can be restarted with smaller doses without symptom recurrence. In rapidly growing children, a slipped capital femoral epiphysis may occur when the femoral head shifts in a backward direction in relation to the femoral shaft.[39] There is no evidence that this problem is caused by GH therapy, but any child who experiences a change in gait during treatment should be evaluated by an orthopedic surgeon.[39] Presently, there is no compelling evidence that GH replacement therapy is associated with an increased risk of leukemia, solid tumor, or tumor recurrence.[31,33,34] GH replacement therapy is contraindicated in all patients with active malignancy.[34] However, in children with a history of malignancies, it would be prudent to wait for a 1-year tumor-free period (5 years for adults) before initiating GH therapy.[31] Any patients treated for a prior malignancy may be at risk for a second malignancy and should be monitored carefully for tumor recurrence.[31] Other rare findings associated with GH replacement therapy include

breast development, pancreatitis, juvenile osteochondritis (inflammation of a bone and its cartilage), worsening of scoliosis, and increased pigmentation.[39] Because deaths have been reported with use of GH in children with Prader-Willi syndrome who are severely obese or suffer from respiratory impairments, use of GH is contraindicated in these individuals. The ongoing multinational safety surveillance study (Safety and Appropriateness of Growth hormone treatments in Europe [SAGhE]) should provide important information on the long-term safety of GH replacement in children.[42]

Insulin-Like Growth Factor-I Therapy Mecasermin (Increlex) is the only recombinant IGF-I replacement therapy for the treatment of growth failure in children with severe primary IGF-I deficiency or with GH gene deletions who have developed neutralizing antibodies to GH. This product has not been evaluated in patients with GH deficiency aside from those with genetic abnormalities.

▶ Outcome Evaluation

- Children with GH deficiency should be evaluated by a pediatric endocrinologist every 3 to 6 months. Monitor for an increase in height and change in height velocity to assess response to GH therapy.[31,39] Every effort should be made to maximize height before the onset of puberty. After final adult height is reached and GH is discontinued for at least 1 month, retest and reevaluate the patient using the adult GH-deficiency diagnostic criteria.[34,39]

- Assess patients with scoliosis for further curvature of the spine.

- Although GH and IGF-I levels do not always correlate with growth response, measure IGF-I levels yearly to assess adherence to therapy and patient response. If the IGF-I levels are substantially above the normal range 2 years after GH replacement therapy, the dose should be reduced.[39] IGF-I level may be used as a guide to gradually reduce replacement dose after epiphyseal closure.

- Routine monitoring of fasting lipid profile, bone mineral density, and body composition in children is not typically required during GH replacement but should be done before and after discontinuation of therapy.[31,39]

- In adults, measurement of serum IGF-I, along with careful clinical evaluation, appears to be the most reliable way to assess the appropriateness of the GH dose. Measure IGF-I serum concentrations annually and 6 weeks after dosage adjustments.[37]

- Continuously monitor for dose-related adverse effects such as edema, arthralgia, myalgia, and carpal tunnel syndrome.

- Evaluate psychological well-being. Assess patients' bone mineral density every 2 to 3 years.[34]

- When maintenance therapy is achieved, assess body composition (body mass index [BMI], waist circumference, waist-to-hip ratio), metabolic status (fasting glucose level, free thyroxine serum, hemoglobin A1c), cardiac risk factors

Patient Care and Monitoring: GH Deficiency in Children

1. Assess the child's growth characteristics and compare the physical height with a population standard (e.g., Centers for Disease Control and Prevention Growth Charts).

2. Obtain a thorough history and physical examination that may indicate the possible presence of GH deficiency. Exclude other identifiable causes of growth failure, such as hypothyroidism, chronic illness, malnutrition, genetic syndromes, and skeletal disorders.

3. Perform imaging tests of the hypothalamic–pituitary region to detect structural or developmental anomalies. Perform radiography of the wrist and hand to estimate bone age.

4. Perform a provocative test to measure GH and IGF-I levels.

5. Initiate GH replacement therapy based on patient preference. Make sure that the child does not have any contraindications to GH therapy.

6. Develop a formal plan to assess response (increase in height and change in height velocity) and adverse effects of GH replacement therapy. Make dosage adjustments when appropriate.

7. May continue GH replacement therapy until child reaches satisfactory adult height, achieves documented epiphyseal closure, or fails to respond to treatment.

8. Review and retest the child using adult GH deficiency diagnostic criteria when the child reaches final adult height.

9. Provide patient education in regard to disease state and drug therapy. Discuss with the child and parents:
   - GH deficiency
   - Potential effectiveness and disadvantages of existing GH replacement therapy
   - Importance of adherence to therapy
   - Potential for adverse effects or need for lifelong replacement

Patient Care and Monitoring: GH Deficiency in Adults

1. Assess the patient's clinical signs and symptoms to determine the severity of GH deficiency.

2. Perform a provocative test to measure GH levels.

3. Evaluate the patient for the presence of metabolic abnormalities and cardiovascular and fracture risks.

4. Initiate GH replacement therapy based on patient preference. Make sure the patient does not have any contraindications to GH therapy.

5. Develop a plan to assess the efficacy and adverse effects of GH therapy and consider if the patient's therapy requires any dose adjustments based on IGF-I level, patient response, and adverse effects.

6. Provide patient education in regard to disease state and drug therapy. Discuss with the patient:
   - Possible complications of GH deficiency
   - How to reduce the modifiable cardiovascular and metabolic risk factors
   - Potential disadvantages and effectiveness of existing GH replacement therapy
   - Importance of adherence to therapy
   - Potential for adverse effects or need for lifelong replacement

(e.g., fasting lipid profile), hypothalamic–pituitary–adrenal axis function (e.g., morning serum cortisol response to ACTH stimulation), and testosterone concentrations at 6- to 12- month intervals.[33,34]

PROLACTIN

Prolactin is an essential hormone for normal production of breast milk after childbirth. It also plays a pivotal role in a variety of reproductive functions. Prolactin is regulated primarily by the hypothalamus–pituitary axis and secreted solely by the lactotroph cells of the anterior pituitary gland. Under normal conditions, secretion of prolactin is predominantly under inhibitory control by dopamine, which acts on the D_2 receptors located on the lactotroph cells. Increases of hypothalamic thyrotropin-releasing hormone in primary hypothyroidism can stimulate the release of prolactin.

Hyperprolactinemia

▶ *Epidemiology and Etiology*

Hyperprolactinemia affects women of reproductive age more than men. Although this disorder occurs in less than 1% of the general population, the estimated prevalence in

Causes of Hyperprolactinemia[9,32,43–46]

Physiologic Causes
Pregnancy
Stress (including exercise and hypoglycemia)
Breast stimulation
Breastfeeding
Coitus
Sleep
Meal

Increased Prolactin Production
Ovarian: polycystic ovarian syndrome
Oophorectomy (removal of an ovary)
Pituitary tumors
  Adenomas
  Microprolactinoma (less than 10 mm diameter)
  Macroprolactinoma (greater than or equal to 10 mm diameter)
  Hypothalamic stalk interruption (prevent dopamine from
    reaching the pituitary)
Hypophysitis (inflammation)
Ectopic tumors

Hypothalamic Prolactin Stimulation
Primary hypothyroidism
Adrenal insufficiency

Reduced Prolactin Elimination
Chronic renal failure
Hepatic cirrhosis

Neurogenic Causes
Chest wall injury (e.g., surgery, herpes zoster)
Spinal cord lesions

Abnormal Molecules
Macroprolactinemia

Medications
Dopamine antagonists: antipsychotics[a], phenothiazines,
  metoclopramide, domperidone
Dopamine-depleting agents: reserpine, α-methyldopa
Prolactin stimulators: serotonin reuptake inhibitors,
  dexfenfluramine, estrogens; progestins, antiandrogens,
  gonadotropin-releasing hormone analogs, benzodiazepines,
  tricyclic antidepressants, monoamine oxidase inhibitors,
  protease inhibitors, histamine$_2$ receptor antagonists
Other: isoniazid, cocaine, opioids, verapamil

Seizures

Idiopathic (Unknown)

[a]Atypicals (olanzapine and clozapine) other than risperidone may cause an early but transient elevation in prolactin.[32]

Adapted in part, with permission, from Sheehan AH, Yanovski JA, Calis KA. Pituitary gland disorders. In: Dipiro JT, Talbert RL, Yee GC, et al, eds. Pharmacotherapy. A Pathophysiologic Approach. 8th ed. New York: McGraw-Hill; 2011:1345–1360.

women with reproductive disorders (e.g., amenorrhea) is as high as 15% to 43%.[43] The etiologies of hyperprolactinemia are presented in Table 46–5.[9,32,43–46] Any medications that antagonize dopamine or stimulate prolactin release can induce hyperprolactinemia.[9,32,43,44] Therefore, it is important to exclude medication-induced hyperprolactinemia from other common causes such as pregnancy, primary hypothyroidism, benign prolactin-secreting pituitary adenoma (prolactinoma), and renal insufficiency. Prolactinomas are

the most common pituitary tumors. They are classified as microprolactinomas if they are less than 10 mm in diameter and as macroprolactinomas if they are 10 mm or larger in diameter.[44] In general, microprolactinomas rarely increase in size, but macroprolactinomas have the potential to enlarge and invade the surrounding tissues.[47]

▶ *Pathophysiology*

Hyperprolactinemia is a condition of elevated serum prolactin. It is the most common endocrine disorder of the hypothalamic–pituitary axis. High prolactin levels inhibit the release of gonadotropin-releasing hormone by the hypothalamus and subsequently suppress secretion of LH and FSH from the anterior pituitary. High prolactin levels result in reduced gonadal hormone levels, often leading to reproductive dysfunction and galactorrhea (inappropriate breast milk production).

In combination with clinical symptoms, one or more serum prolactin concentrations greater than 25 ng/mL (25 mcg/L) will confirm the diagnosis of hyperprolactinemia in women.[45] A number of physiologic factors such as eating, exercise, and stress can transiently elevate prolactin levels.[9] Therefore, prolactin measurements should be obtained at rest, preferably in the morning under fasting conditions.[43] If an intravenous line is present or planned, it is prudent to wait at least 2 hours after line insertion before measuring serum prolactin to decrease detecting transient physiologic increases in prolactin level (see Table 46–5).[9,32,43–46] Although medication-induced hyperprolactinemia is typically associated with prolactin concentrations of 25 to 100 ng/mL (25 to 100 mcg/L), metoclopramide, risperidone, and phenothiazines have been associated with concentrations greater than 200 ng/mL (200 mcg/L). Prolactin concentrations greater than 250 ng/mL (250 mcg/L) are almost always associated with the presence of a macroprolactinoma.[45]

▶ *Treatment Goals for Hyperprolactinemia*

Because hyperprolactinemia is often associated with hypogonadism, the goals for management of hyperprolactinemia are to correct the clinical consequences of hypogonadism and reduce its associated risk for osteoporosis, as follows[46]:

- Normalize prolactin level.
- Improve clinical symptoms.
- Restore normal fertility.
- Restore and maintain normal gonadal function.
- Protect against the development of osteoporosis.
- Prevent disease recurrence.
- If a pituitary tumor is present:
  - Ablate or reduce tumor size to relieve tumor mass effect.
  - Preserve normal pituitary function.
  - Prevent progression of pituitary tumor or hypothalamic disease.

Clinical Presentation and Diagnosis of Hyperprolactinemia[9,44,46]

General

Hyperprolactinemia most commonly affects women of reproductive age and is very rare in men.

Signs and Symptoms

Premenopausal women

- Headache and compromised or loss of vision caused by the prolactin-secreting tumor and its close proximity to the optic structures.
- Clinical presentation is associated with the degree of prolactin elevation:
  - Prolactin greater than 100 ng/mL (100 mcg/L): hypogonadism, galactorrhea, and amenorrhea
  - Prolactin 51 to 75 ng/mL (51 to 75 mcg/L): oligomenorrhea (infrequent menstruation)
  - Prolactin 31 to 50 ng/mL (31 to 50 mcg/L): decreased libido and infertility
- Increased body weight may be associated with a prolactin-secreting pituitary tumor.
- The degree of hypogonadism generally is proportionate to the degree of prolactin elevation.
- Excessive hair growth (hirsutism) and acne also may be present owing to relative androgen excess compared with low estrogen levels.

Men

- Decreased libido, decreased energy, erectile dysfunction, impotence, decreased sperm production, infertility, gynecomastia, and rarely, galactorrhea.
- Impotence is unresponsive to treatment and is associated with reduced muscle mass, loss of pubic hair, and osteoporosis.

Laboratory Tests

- Prolactin serum concentrations at rest will be greater than 20 ng/mL (20 mcg/L) in men or 25 ng/mL (25 mcg/L) in women with at least three measurements.
- Obtain β-human chorionic gonadotropin (β-hCG) level to exclude pregnancy.
- Obtain TSH level to exclude primary hypothyroidism.
- Obtain blood urea nitrogen and serum creatinine tests to exclude renal failure.

Other Diagnostic Tests

- Perform MRI to locate the tumor, exclude a pseudo-prolactinoma, and validate the diagnosis.
- Consider a bone mineral density test in patients with long-term hypogonadism.

Additional Clinical Sequelae

- The prolonged suppression of estrogen in premenopausal women with hyperprolactinemia leads to decreases in bone mineral density and significant risk for the development of osteoporosis.
- Risk for ischemic heart disease may be increased with untreated hyperprolactinemia.

Adapted, with permission, from Sheehan AH, Yanovski JA, Calis KA. Pituitary gland disorders. In: Dipiro JT, Talbert RL, Yee GC, et al, eds. Pharmacotherapy. A Pathophysiologic Approach. 8th ed. New York: McGraw-Hill; 2011:1345–1360.

▶ General Approaches to Treatment

Management of drug-induced hyperprolactinemia is to discontinue the offending agent, if clinically feasible, and replace it with an appropriate alternative that does not cause hyperprolactinemia.[45] When the offending agent cannot be discontinued, cautious use of hormone replacement, biphosphonate therapy, or dopamine agonists may be considered depending on the patient's clinical circumstances.[48] Treatment options for the management of hyperprolactinemia include (a) clinical observation, (b) pharmacologic therapy with dopamine agonists, (c) transsphenoidal pituitary adenomectomy, and (d) radiation therapy. Clinical observation and close monitoring are justifiable in patients with asymptomatic elevation of prolactin.[45] ⑧ *Dopamine agonists are the first-line treatment of choice for all patients with symptomatic hyperprolactinemia; transsphenoidal surgery and radiation therapy are reserved for patients who are resistant to or severely intolerant of pharmacologic therapy.*[47]

However, in patients with underlying psychiatric symptoms, use of dopamine agonists in addition to an antipsychotic therapy may exacerbate the underlying psychosis and should be used with caution in consultation with a mental health clinician.[32]

Pharmacologic Therapy Dopamine is the principal neurotransmitter responsible for the inhibition of prolactin secretion from the anterior pituitary. Thus, dopamine agonists are the main pharmacologic therapy used for management of hyperprolactinemia.[45] Treatment with dopamine agonists has proven to be extremely effective in normalizing serum prolactin level, restoring gonadal function, decreasing tumor size, and improving visual fields.[45] Patients with macroprolactinomas generally require a higher dose to normalize prolactin levels compared with patients with microprolactinomas.[49]

Two dopamine agonists—bromocriptine and cabergoline—are used for the management of hyperprolactinemia

Table 46–6

Comparison of Dopamine Agonists for Treatment of Hyperprolactemia[43,50]

	Bromocriptine (Parlodel)	Cabergoline
Starting dose	0.625–1.25 mg/day at bedtime	0.5 mg/week or 0.25 mg twice/week
Titrating dose	1.25 mg increments at 1-week interval	0.5 mg increment at 4-week intervals
Usually effective dose	2.5–15 mg/day	1–2 mg/week
Maximal dose	40 mg/day	4.5 mg/week
Dosing frequency	2–3 divided doses per day	Once or twice weekly
Dosage in hepatic insufficiency	May be required in acute hepatitis or cirrhosis; no guidelines are available	Dose reductions may be recommended for patients with severe hepatic failure (Child-Pugh scores of 10 or higher)
Dosage in renal failure	None	None
Adverse effects	Dizziness, headache, syncope, nausea, vomiting, GI cramps, orthostatic hypotension, nasal congestion	Similar but orthostatic hypotension less common
Cost	Moderately expensive	More expensive

GI, gastrointestinal.

(Table 46–6).[43,50] Because these two dopamine agonists are ergot derivatives, they are contraindicated in combination with potent cytochrome P-450 subfamily IIIA polypeptide 4 (CYP3A4) inhibitors, including protease inhibitors (e.g., ritonavir and indinavir), azole antifungals (e.g., ketoconazole and itraconazole), and some macrolide antibiotics (e.g., erythromycin and clarithromycin). Furthermore, ergot derivatives can cause constriction of peripheral and cranial blood vessels. These medications are also contraindicated in patients with uncontrolled hypertension, severe ischemic heart disease, or peripheral vascular disorders. Caution should be exercised with concomitant use of other ergot derivatives and in patients with impaired renal or hepatic function; dementia; concurrent antihypertensive therapy; or a history of psychosis, peptic ulcer disease, or cardiovascular disease.

Bromocriptine Bromocriptine directly binds to the D_2 receptors on the lactotroph cells to exert its effect. Bromocriptine normalizes prolactin level in more than 90% of patients, restores menstrual cycles, and reduces tumor size in 62% of patients.[43] Adverse effects such as nausea, dizziness, and orthostatic hypotension often limit 5% to 10% of patients from continuing treatment. To reduce risk of adverse effects, start bromocriptine at a low dose (e.g., 0.625 to 1.25 mg) at bedtime (taken with a snack) to decrease adverse effects.[47] Slowly titrate up to the optimal therapeutic dose (2.5 to 15 mg/day) because most adverse effects subside with continual treatment.[49] In women, if the adverse GI effects are not tolerable, bromocriptine can be administered vaginally at a reduced dose (2.5 mg/day).[51] Owing to its short half-life of only 6 hours, bromocriptine must be administered in divided doses, which may compromise patient adherence.

Cabergonline Cabergoline has a higher affinity for D_2 receptors than bromocriptine. It is a long-acting dopamine agonist capable of inhibiting pituitary prolactin secretion for at least 7 days after a single oral dose.[50] The prolonged duration of action allows for once- or twice-weekly administration. Cabergoline appears to be significantly better tolerated than bromocriptine.[43] Transient elevations of serum alkaline

phosphatase, bilirubin, and aminotransferases have been reported in a few patients treated with cabergoline. Cabergoline is more effective in normalizing prolactin levels and restoring menses than bromocriptine.[50] It also may be effective in treating hyperprolactinemia in patients who are resistant to or intolerant of bromocriptine and in men and women with micro- and macroprolactinomas.[43] Given its favorable safety and efficacy profile and ease of administration, cabergoline has replaced bromocriptine as first-line therapy for the management of hyperprolactinemia.[45] Withdrawal of pergolide from the U.S. market due to increased risk for valvular heart disease raised concerns about the safety of cabergoline. In patients with prolactinomas, tricuspid regurgitation was associated with higher cabergoline cumulative dose of more than 280 mg.[52] However, recent studies suggest the lower doses of cabergoline commonly used in the management of hyperprolactinemia do not appear to increase the risk of clinically significant valvular heart diseases.[53,54]

▶ Nonpharmacologic Therapy

In a small number of patients who have failed or are intolerant of dopamine agonists, transsphenoidal adenomectomy may be necessary.[45] Surgical treatment is also considered in patients with nonprolactin-secreting tumors or macroprolactinomas that jeopardize the optic chiasm.[44] Nonetheless, surgical intervention does not reliably lead to long-term cure and may cause permanent complications.[46] Radiation therapy is reserved for failures of both pharmacologic therapy and surgery.[44] However, normalization of prolactin levels with radiation therapy may take 20 years to show full benefit, and radiation-induced hypopituitarism may require lifelong hormone replacement.[45]

▶ Management of Hyperprolactinemia in Pregnancy

Most women with hyperprolactinemia require dopamine agonist therapy to achieve regular ovulatory cycles and pregnancy. Because restoration of the ovulatory cycle may

Patient Encounter 2: Hyperprolactinemia: Medical History, Physical Examination, and Diagnostic Tests

PR is a 23-year-old woman who presents to the primary care clinic with complaints of irregular menstruation and milky fluid discharge from both breasts for a few months. Her last menstrual period was 3 weeks ago.

PMH: Schizophrenia for 5 years, major depression for 6 years

FM: Mother has severe depression. Father, deceased, had an "unknown" mental illness and myocardial infarction at age 45.

SH: Single college student; sexually active (occasional use of condoms)

Meds: Sertraline 200 mg once daily; risperidone 8 mg once daily; ibuprofen 200 mg two tablets every 4 to 6 hours as needed for mild headaches and menstrual cramps

ROS: Negative, other than in history of present illness

PE:

HEENT: Ophthalmic examination reveals normal visual acuity and fields. (–) goiter

VS: BP 112/70 mm Hg, P 72 beats/min, RR 19 breaths/min, T 37.1°C (98.8°F)

CV: RRR, normal S$_1$, S$_2$; no murmurs, rubs, or gallops

Breasts: (+) bilateral expressible galactorrhea with no other abnormality

Abd: Soft, nontender, nondistended; (+) bowel sounds; (–) hepatosplenomegaly

Rectal: Heme (–) stool

Labs: Electrolytes, renal and thyroid function, FSH, LH, and testosterone are within normal limits. Elevated prolactin at 89 ng/mL (89 mcg/L)

Imaging: MRI did not reveal a pituitary tumor

Given this information, what signs and symptoms does PR have for hyperprolactinemia?

What other laboratory test would also be appropriate to obtain based on the patient's history and diagnosis?

What are other potential causes of hyperprolactinemia in this patient?

Identify your treatment goals for PR.

What nonpharmacologic and pharmacologic treatment options are available for PR?

occur within 1 week of initiating therapy, it is necessary to caution patients regarding their potential to become pregnant.[55]

Overall, there is reassuring worldwide evidence that bromocriptine use during pregnancy does not increase fetal malformations, spontaneous miscarriage, ectopic pregnancy, or multiple births.[43,47] Furthermore, no teratogenic effects have been reported in women who received cabergoline during pregnancy.[47,56] Despite these data, ❾ *women who become pregnant while taking a dopamine agonist should discontinue treatment immediately to minimize fetal exposure.[45] Because cabergoline has a prolonged half-life, women who plan to become pregnant should discontinue the drug at least 1 month before planned conception.[50]*

Microadenomas rarely cause complications during pregnancy. However, untreated macroprolactinomas carry about a 31% risk of tumor enlargement and potentially can jeopardize vision.[45] Therefore, monitor female patients with macroprolactinomas closely for the development of headache and visual impairments. Baseline and routine visual field examinations are essential. Evidence of abnormal visual fields may indicate tumor growth and should be followed by an MRI. If tumors enlarge, bromocriptine is the preferred choice over cabergoline because of greater experience with this drug during pregnancy.[45,47]

Outcome Evaluation

- Assess patients for tolerability to dopamine agonists.
- Monitor clinical symptoms associated with hyperprolactinemia every month for the first 3 months

to assess therapeutic efficacy and assist with dose titration.

- Evaluate the patient for symptoms, such as headache, visual disturbances, menstrual cycles in women, and sexual function in men, to assess clinical response to therapy.[45]
- When the prolactin level is normalized and clinical symptoms of hyperprolactinemia have resolved, monitor prolactin level every 6 to 12 months.[46,49]
- If the prolactin level is well controlled with dopamine agonist therapy for 2 years with significant tumor reduction, gradually taper therapy to the lowest effective dose or consider discontinuing therapy.[45] Check prolactin levels after each dose reduction.
- If the prolactin levels remain unchanged for 1 year at the reduced dose, dopamine agonist therapy may be discontinued.
- It is essential to monitor prolactin levels every 6 months or annually to detect the possibility of permanent remission of pituitary disease.[46]
- The need to continue dopamine agonists in postmenopausal women with microprolactinomas must be reassessed because these patients have a higher probability of maintaining normal prolactin levels after treatment is discontinued.[44]
- In patients with macroprolactinomas, monitor visual field at baseline and repeat the test 1 month after initiation of a dopamine agonist.

Patient Care and Monitoring: Hyperprolactinemia

1. Assess the patient's clinical signs and symptoms of hyperprolactinemia.

2. Review the available diagnostic data to determine severity and exclude other common causes of hyperprolactinemia.

3. Obtain a thorough medication history to exclude medication-induced hyperprolactinemia.

4. Determine the patient's plan regarding pregnancy because this influences treatment.

5. Educate the patient about safety and efficacy of dopamine agonists. Make sure the patient does not have any contraindications or allergies to drug therapies.

6. Develop a formal plan to assess response and adverse effects of dopamine agonists. When appropriate, be sure to make dose adjustments.

7. If the prolactin level remains normal for 2 years, reassess the need to continue treatment. Make sure the patient is taking the lowest effective dose for management of hyperprolactinemia.

8. Provide patient education in regard to disease state and nondrug and drug therapy. Discuss with the patient:

- Risk factors associated with hyperprolactinemia
- Potential disadvantages and effectiveness of existing dopamine agonist therapy
- Potential disadvantages and effectiveness of surgery and radiation treatment
- Importance of adherence to therapy
- Potential for adverse effects or long-term complications

- Repeat the MRI 6 months after initiating therapy or if an increase in symptoms or rise in prolactin levels suggests the presence of tumor growth.[49]

- Discontinuation of therapy in patients with macroprolactinomas usually leads to tumor regrowth and recurrence of hyperprolactinemia. This decision warrants careful consideration.

Abbreviations Introduced in This Chapter

AACE	American Association of Clinical Endocrinologists
ACTH	Adrenocorticotropic hormone or corticotropin
ADH	Antidiuretic hormone
β-hCG	β-Human chorionic gonadotropin
BMI	Body mass index
CRH	Corticotropin-releasing hormone
CT	Computed tomography
CYP3A4	Cytochrome P-450 subfamily IIIA polypeptide 4
DA	Dopamine agonist
DEXA	Dual-energy x-ray absorptiometry
ECG	Electrocardiography
FDA	Food and Drug Administration
FSH	Follicle-stimulating hormone
GABA	γ-Aminobutyric acid
GH	Growth hormone or somatotropin
GHIH	Growth hormone–inhibiting hormone or somatostatin
GHRH	Growth hormone–releasing hormone
GI	Gastrointestinal
GHAnt	Growth hormone antagonist
GnRH	Gonadotropin-releasing hormone
HbA$_{1c}$	Glycated hemoglobin A$_{1c}$
IGF	Insulin-like growth factor
IGF-I	Insulin-like growth factor-I
IGF-II	Insulin-like growth factor-II

IGFBP-3	Insulin-like growth factor-bind protein-3
IM	Intramuscularly
ITT	Insulin tolerance test
LAR	Long-acting release
LH	Luteinizing hormone
LHRH	Luteinizing hormone–releasing hormone
MRI	Magnetic resonance imaging
MSH	Melanocyte-stimulating hormone
OGTT	Oral glucose tolerance test
PRH	Prolactin-releasing hormone
RT	Radiation therapy
SAGhE	Safety and Appropriateness of Growth hormone treatments in Europe
SC	Subcutaneous
SR	Slow release
SSA	Somatostatin analog
SSRI	Selective serotonin reuptake inhibitor
T$_3$	Triiodothyronine
T$_4$	Thyroxine
TRH	Thyrotropin-releasing hormone
TSH	Thyroid-stimulating hormone or thyrotropin

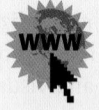 Self-assessment questions and answers are available at *http://www.mhpharmacotherapy.com/pp.html*.

REFERENCES

1. Muller EE, Locatelli V, Cocchi D. Neuroendocrine control of growth hormone secretion. Physiol Rev 1999;79:511–607.

2. Le Roith D, Bondy C, Yakar S, et al. The somatomedin hypothesis: 2001. Endocr Rev 2001;22:53–74.

3. Katznelson L, Atkinson JL, Cook DM, et al. American Association of Clinical Endocrinologists medical guidelines for clinical practice for the diagnosis and treatment of acromegaly—2011 update. Endocr Pract 2011;17(Suppl 4):1–44.

4. Melmed S. Medical progress: Acromegaly. N Engl J Med 2006;355: 2558–2573.

5. AACE Medical Guidelines for Clinical Practice for the diagnosis and treatment of acromegaly. Endocr Pract 2004;10:213–225.

6. Gagel RF, McCutcheon IE. Images in clinical medicine. Pituitary gigantism. N Engl J Med 1999;340:524.

7. Giustina A, Chanson P, Bronstein MD, et al. A consensus on criteria for cure of acromegaly. J Clin Endocrinol Metab 2010;95:3141–3148.

8. Chanson P, Salenave S. Acromegaly. Orphanet J Rare Dis 2008;3:17.

9. Sheehan AH, Yanovski JA, Calis KA. Pituitary gland disorders. In: DiPiro JT, Talbert RL, Yee GC, et al, eds. Pharmacotherapy: A Pathophysiologic Approach. 8th ed. New York: McGraw-Hill; 2010:1345–1360.

10. Katznelson L. An update on treatment strategies for acromegaly. Exp Opin Pharmacother 2008;9:2273–2280.

11. Colao A, Auriemma RS, Pivonello R, et al. Medical consequences of acromegaly: What are the effects of biochemical control? Rev Endocr Metab Disord 2008;9:21–31.

12. Biochemical assessment and long-term monitoring in patients with acromegaly: Statement from a joint consensus conference of the Growth Hormone Research Society and the Pituitary Society. J Clin Endocrinol Metab 2004;89:3099–3102.

13. Ayuk J, Clayton RN, Holder G, et al. Growth hormone and pituitary radiotherapy, but not serum insulin-like growth factor-I concentrations, predict excess mortality in patients with acromegaly. J Clin Endocrinol Metab 2004;89:1613–1617.

14. Bush ZM, Vance ML. Management of acromegaly: Is there a role for primary medical therapy? Rev Endocr Metab Disord 2008;9: 83–94.

15. Cozzi R, Montini M, Attanasio R, et al. Primary treatment of acromegaly with octreotide LAR: A long-term (up to nine years) prospective study of its efficacy in the control of disease activity and tumor shrinkage. J Clin Endocrinol Metab 2006;91:1397–1403.

16. Ronchi CL, Varca V, Beck-Peccoz P, et al. Comparison between six-year therapy with long-acting somatostatin analogs and successful surgery in acromegaly: Effects on cardiovascular risk factors. J Clin Endocrinol Metab 2006;91:121–128.

17. Freda PU, Katznelson L, van der Lely AJ, et al. Long-acting somatostatin analog therapy of acromegaly: A meta-analysis. J Clin Endocrinol Metab 2005;90:4465–4473.

18. Feelders RA, Hofland LJ, van Aken MO, et al. Medical therapy of acromegaly: Efficacy and safety of somatostatin analogues. Drugs 2009;69:2207–2226.

19. Trainer PJ. ACROSTUDY: The first 5 years. Eur J Endocrinol 2009;161(Suppl 1):S19–S24.

20. Higham CE, Chung TT, Lawrance J, et al. Long-term experience of pegvisomant therapy as a treatment for acromegaly. Clin Endocrinol 2009;71:86–91.

21. Colao A, Pivonello R, Auriemma RS, et al. Efficacy of 12-month treatment with the GH receptor antagonist pegvisomant in patients with acromegaly resistant to long-term, high-dose somatostatin analog treatment: Effect on IGF-I levels, tumor mass, hypertension and glucose tolerance. Eur J Endocrinol 2006;154:467–477.

22. Feenstra J, de Herder WW, ten Have SM, et al. Combined therapy with somatostatin analogues and weekly pegvisomant in active acromegaly. Lancet 2005;365:1644–1646.

23. Jorgensen JO, Feldt-Rasmussen U, Frystyk J, et al. Cotreatment of acromegaly with a somatostatin analog and a growth hormone receptor antagonist. J Clin Endocrinol Metab 2005;90:5627–5631.

24. Neggers SJ, van Aken MO, Janssen JA, et al. Long-term efficacy and safety of combined treatment of somatostatin analogs and pegvisomant in acromegaly. J Clin Endocrinol Metab 2007;92:4598–4601.

25. Jimenez C, Burman P, Abs R, et al. Follow-up of pituitary tumor volume in patients with acromegaly treated with pegvisomant in clinical trials. Eur J Endocrinol 2008;159:517–523.

26. Neggers SJ, van der Lely AJ. Somatostatin analog and pegvisomant combination therapy for acromegaly. Nat Rev Endocrinol 2009;5: 546–552.

27. Abs R, Verhelst J, Maiter D, et al. Cabergoline in the treatment of acromegaly: A study in 64 patients. J Clin Endocrinol Metab 1998;83:374–378.

28. Casanueva FF, Molitch ME, Schlechte JA, et al. Guidelines of the Pituitary Society for the diagnosis and management of prolactinomas. Clin Endocrinol 2006;65:265–273.

29. Melmed S, Colao A, Barkan A, et al. Guidelines for acromegaly management: An update. J Clin Endocrinol Metab 2009;94: 1509-1517.

30. Giustina A, Casanueva FF, Cavagnini F, et al. Diagnosis and treatment of acromegaly complications. J Endocrinol Invest 2003;26: 1242–1247.

31. Gharib H, Cook DM, Saenger PH, et al. American Association of Clinical Endocrinologists medical guidelines for clinical practice for growth hormone use in adults and children—2003 update. Endocr Pract 2003;9:64–76.

32. Gums JG, Anderson SD. Hypothalamic, pituitary, and adrenal disorders. In: Tisdale JE, Miller DA, eds. Drug-Induced Diseases: Prevention, Detection, and Management. 2nd ed. Bethesda, MD: American Society of Health-System Pharmacists;2010:605–628.

33. Ho KK. Consensus guidelines for the diagnosis and treatment of adults with GH deficiency II: A statement of the GH Research Society in association with the European Society for Pediatric Endocrinology, Lawson Wilkins Society, European Society of Endocrinology, Japan Endocrine Society, and Endocrine Society of Australia. Eur J Endocrinol 2007;157:695–700.

34. Cook DM, Yuen KC, Biller BM, et al. American Association of Clinical Endocrinologists medical guidelines for clinical practice for growth hormone use in growth hormone-deficient adults and transition patients—2009 update. Endocr Pract 2009;15(Suppl 2):1–29.

35. Federico G, Street ME, Maghnie M, et al. Assessment of serum IGF-I concentrations in the diagnosis of isolated childhood-onset GH deficiency: A proposal of the Italian Society for Pediatric Endocrinology and Diabetes (SIEDP/ISPED). J Endocrinol Invest 2006;29: 732–737.

36. Casanueva FF, Castro AI, Micic D, et al. New guidelines for the diagnosis of growth hormone deficiency in adults. Horm Res 2009;71(Suppl 1):112–115.

37. Nilsson AG, Svensson J, Johannsson G. Management of growth hormone deficiency in adults. Growth Horm IGF Res 2007;17: 441–462.

38. Cummings DE, Merriam GR. Growth hormone therapy in adults. Annu Rev Med 2003;54:513–533.

39. Wilson TA, Rose SR, Cohen P, et al. Update of guidelines for the use of growth hormone in children: The Lawson Wilkins Pediatric Endocrinology Society Drug and Therapeutics Committee. J Pediatr 2003;143:415–421.

40. Gotherstrom G, Bengtsson BA, Bosaeus I, et al. A 10-year, prospective study of the metabolic effects of growth hormone replacement in adults. J Clin Endocrinol Metab 2007;92:1442–1445.

41. Filipsson H, Johannsson G. GH replacement in adults: Interactions with other pituitary hormone deficiencies and replacement therapies. Eur J Endocrinol 2009;161(Suppl 1):S85–S95.

42. Safety and appropriateness of growth hormone treatments in Europe (SAGhE) [online]. [cited 2011 Oct 10]. Available from: *http://saghe.uphp.fr/site/spip.php*.

43. Crosignani PG. Current treatment issues in female hyperprolactinaemia. Eur J Obstet Gynecol Reprod Biol 2006;125:152–164.

44. Brue T, Delemer B. Diagnosis and management of hyperprolactinemia: Expert consensus—French Society of Endocrinology. Ann Endocrinol 2007;68:58–64.

45. Melmed S, Casanueva FF, Hoffman AR, et al. Diagnosis and treatment of hyperprolactinemia: An Endocrine Society clinical practice guideline. J Clin Endocrinol Metab 2011;96:273–288.

46. Serri O, Chik CL, Ur E, Ezzat S. Diagnosis and management of hyperprolactinemia. CMAJ 2003;169:575–581.

47. Gillam MP, Molitch ME, Lombardi G, Colao A. Advances in the treatment of prolactinomas. Endocr Rev 2006;27:485–534.

48. Molitch ME. Medication-induced hyperprolactinemia. Mayo Clin Proc 2005;80:1050–1057.

49. Schlechte JA. Clinical practice. Prolactinoma. N Engl J Med 2003;349:2035–2041.

50. Bankowski BJ, Zacur HA. Dopamine agonist therapy for hyperprolactinemia. Clin Obstet Gynecol 2003;46:349–362.

51. Darwish AM, Farah E, Gadallah WA, Mohammad, II. Superiority of newly developed vaginal suppositories over vaginal use of commercial bromocriptine tablets: A randomized controlled clinical trial. Reprod Sci 2007;14:280–285.

52. Colao A, Galderisi M, Di Sarno A, et al. Increased prevalence of tricuspid regurgitation in patients with prolactinomas chronically treated with cabergoline. J Clin Endocrinol Metab 2008;93:3777–3784.

53. Bogazzi F, Buralli S, Manetti L, et al. Treatment with low doses of cabergoline is not associated with increased prevalence of cardiac valve

regurgitation in patients with hyperprolactinaemia. Int J Clin Pract 2008;62:1864–1869.

54. Wakil A, Rigby AS, Clark AL, et al. Low dose cabergoline for hyperprolactinaemia is not associated with clinically significant valvular heart disease. Eur J Endocrinol 2008;159:R11–14.

55. Davis JR. Prolactin and reproductive medicine. Curr Opin Obstet Gynecol 2004;16:331–337.

56. Stalldecker G, Mallea-Gil MS, Guitelman M, et al. Effects of cabergoline on pregnancy and embryo-fetal development: Retrospective study on 103 pregnancies and a review of the literature. Pituitary 2010;13:345–350.

47 Pregnancy and Lactation: Therapeutic Considerations

Ema Ferreira, Évelyne Rey, and Caroline Morin

LEARNING OBJECTIVES

● **Upon completion of the chapter, the reader will be able to:**

1. Explain the principles of embryology and teratology.
2. Identify known teratogens and drugs of concerns during lactation.
3. Compare the main sources of drug information during pregnancy and lactation.
4. Evaluate the risks of a drug when taken during pregnancy or lactation.
5. Apply a systematic approach to counseling on the use of drugs during pregnancy and lactation.
6. Recommend the appropriate dose of folic acid to prevent congenital anomalies.
7. Describe physiologic changes during pregnancy and their impact on pharmacokinetics.
8. Choose an appropriate treatment for common conditions in a pregnant or lactating woman.

KEY CONCEPTS

❶ Although the risk of drug-induced teratogenicity is of concern, the actual risk of birth defects from most drug exposures is small.

❷ Health professionals should know which medications could be teratogenic or of concern during breast-feeding.

❸ The risk of birth defects is most often higher during organogenesis.

❹ Counsel all women of childbearing age on the use of folic acid–containing multivitamins to prevent congenital anomalies.

❺ Most drugs are safe during breast-feeding.

❻ When possible, treat conditions occurring during pregnancy with nonpharmacologic treatments instead of drug therapy.

❼ Evaluate the need for treatment, including benefits and risks. Avoid treatments that do not show evidence of benefit or that can be delayed until after pregnancy or breast-feeding.

Medication use during pregnancy and lactation is a challenge for health professionals, as pregnant and breast-feeding women are usually excluded from clinical trials. Therefore, it is important to know on which information sources to rely, how to interpret the data retrieved from these sources, and how to communicate this information to patients. This chapter reviews the available resources that help to guide therapy, general strategies to reduce risks of drug use in pregnant and lactating women, and specific recommendations for some common conditions treated during pregnancy and lactation.

EPIDEMIOLOGY AND ETIOLOGY

Use of Medications During Pregnancy and Lactation

Studies conducted in the United States have estimated that at least two-thirds of pregnant women take medications during pregnancy.[1,2] Moreover, since approximately one-half of pregnancies are unplanned, many women are exposed to medications before being aware of their pregnancy.[3]

The most popular medications are vitamins and minerals, analgesics, antacids, antibiotics, antiemetics, laxatives, asthma medication, cold and flu medications, and medications for topical administration (e.g., antifungals, antibiotics, corticosteroids).[1,2]

One study from the Netherlands indicates that 65.9% of breast-feeding women took at least one medication (53% after exclusion of vitamins and minerals) over a 6-month period.[4]

▶ Background Risks of Anomalies in Pregnancy

Table 47–1 describes the baseline risks of congenital anomalies and some obstetrical complications observed in the general

MM, a 39-year-old woman, comes to your office after a positive urine pregnancy test. You collect the following data:

Estimated gestational age: Not sure, irregular menstrual cycles

PMH: Infertility, obesity, type 2 diabetes, no previous pregnancies

FH: Diabetes, hypertension, hypothyroidism

SH: Unemployed; cigarettes, one-half pack daily; no alcohol or illicit substances

Meds: Metformin 500 mg orally twice daily, atorvastatin 20 mg daily, ramipril 2.5 mg daily; all discontinued 1 week ago

Allergy: Eggs, penicillin

ROS: Morning nausea with daily vomiting; tiredness; dizziness; abdominal bloating

VS: Weight: 198 lb (90 kg)/height: 63 inches (160 cm), BP 130/85 mm Hg, P 90 bpm, RR 12; slight enlargement of thyroid;

Last week blood glucose results between 144 to 198 mg/dL (8.0 to 11.0 mmol/L) before meals.

How will you estimate gestational age?

What prenatal screening would you perform at this time?

What is the appropriate counseling to do at this time?

What are the risks of drugs taken in the first weeks of pregnancy? What resources will you use to find the appropriate information?

What do you recommend for her pharmacologic treatment?

Table 47–1

Occurrence of Some Obstetrical Complications and Risk of Congenital Anomalies in the General Population

	Risk of Occurrence in Population (%)
Spontaneous abortion/miscarriage (pregnancy loss that occurs after the pregnancy is known and before 20 weeks of GA)	10–15
Prematurity (any birth that occur before 37 completed weeks of gestation)	12.8
Congenital anomalies (percentage of live births):	
• Minor malformations (recognized at birth or during childhood)	10–15
• Major malformations at birth	3
• Major malformations at 1 year old	6–7
Low birth weight (less than 2,500 g)	7.7

GA, gestational age.

Data from Refs. 61 and 62.

---

population. This will be important when evaluating the risks associated with drugs and in order to counsel pregnant women.

▶ Causes of Congenital Anomalies

① *Although the risk of drug-induced teratogenicity is of concern, the actual risk of birth defects from most drug exposures is small.* Medications are associated with fewer than 1% of all congenital anomalies, although they may play a more important role through interaction with genetic factors. Because it is a modifiable cause of anomalies, it is important to evaluate and manage drug use in pregnant women and women planning a pregnancy. **②** *Health professionals should know which medications could be teratogenic.* Other causes of anomalies include monogenetic conditions (8% to 18%), chromosomal disorders (7% to 10%), maternal infections (1%), maternal conditions (1% to 3%; e.g., maternal diabetes), multifactorial heredity (23% to 50%), and unknown causes (34% to 43%).[5]

PATHOPHYSIOLOGY

Age of Pregnancy

The age of pregnancy can be defined as gestational or postconceptional ages.[6] *Gestational age* (GA) is the term used in clinical practice. It is calculated from the first day of the last menstruation (or by ultrasound dating if menstrual cycles are irregular or if dates are unknown).

Postconceptional age (PCA) is calculated from the day of conception, which is 14 days shorter than gestational age if the menstrual cycle is 28 days. Some references in the field of teratology and embryology refer to PCA to describe stages of pregnancy.

Principles of Embryology

Pregnancy is usually divided into three trimesters of 13 weeks.[6] However, it can be divided more precisely into three phases: implantation and pre-differentiation, organogenesis (or embryogenesis), and fetogenesis. Table 47–2 describes these phases and the effects that drugs could have if taken during these phases, and Figure 47–1 illustrates the critical periods of human in utero development. **③** *The risk of birth defects is most often higher during organogenesis.*

▶ Teratogens

A teratogen is an exogenous agent that can modify normal embryonic or fetal development. Teratogenicity can manifest as structural anomalies, a functional deficit, cancer, growth retardation, and death (spontaneous abortion, stillbirth).

Even if we use the term *teratogen* in this chapter, we agree with some authors who have suggested to avoid this term and to use instead *teratogenic exposure*. *Teratogenic exposure* implies that we have to consider the exposure level (dose) and timing of exposure to a medication during pregnancy to

Table 47–2

Phases of Embryonic and Fetal Development

Phase of Development	Stage of Pregnancy	What Happens During This Phase of Development	Potential Teratogenic Effect
Implantation and predifferentiation	0–14 days after conception (14–28 days after last menstrual period)	*All-or-none period* Very little contact between the blastocyst and the mother's blood Cells are pluripotent, capacity to repair a damage remains Cells are fragile at this moment. If too many are killed, a miscarriage will occur before the pregnancy is detected	Spontaneous abortion or miscarriage Even if stopped during this period, prolonged half-life drugs could cause organogenesis problems
Organogenesis (embryogenesis)	From day 14 until the 9th week after conception (From day 28 until the 11th week after last menstrual period)	Organs are formed; most critical period for structural anomalies Organs are formed at different times; period of sensitivity for a potential teratogen could be different for each organ Refer to Figure 47–1 for the time frame of organ formation	Major or minor structural anomalies
Fetogenesis	After the organogenesis and until birth	The fetus grows and organs begin to function (e.g., kidneys are formed during organogenesis, but glomerular filtration begins during fetogenesis) Active cell growth, proliferation, and migration (eg., CNS)	Fetal growth retardation Functional deficit (e.g., renal insufficiency, pulmonary hypertension, neurologic impairment)

Data from Refs. 6 and 11.

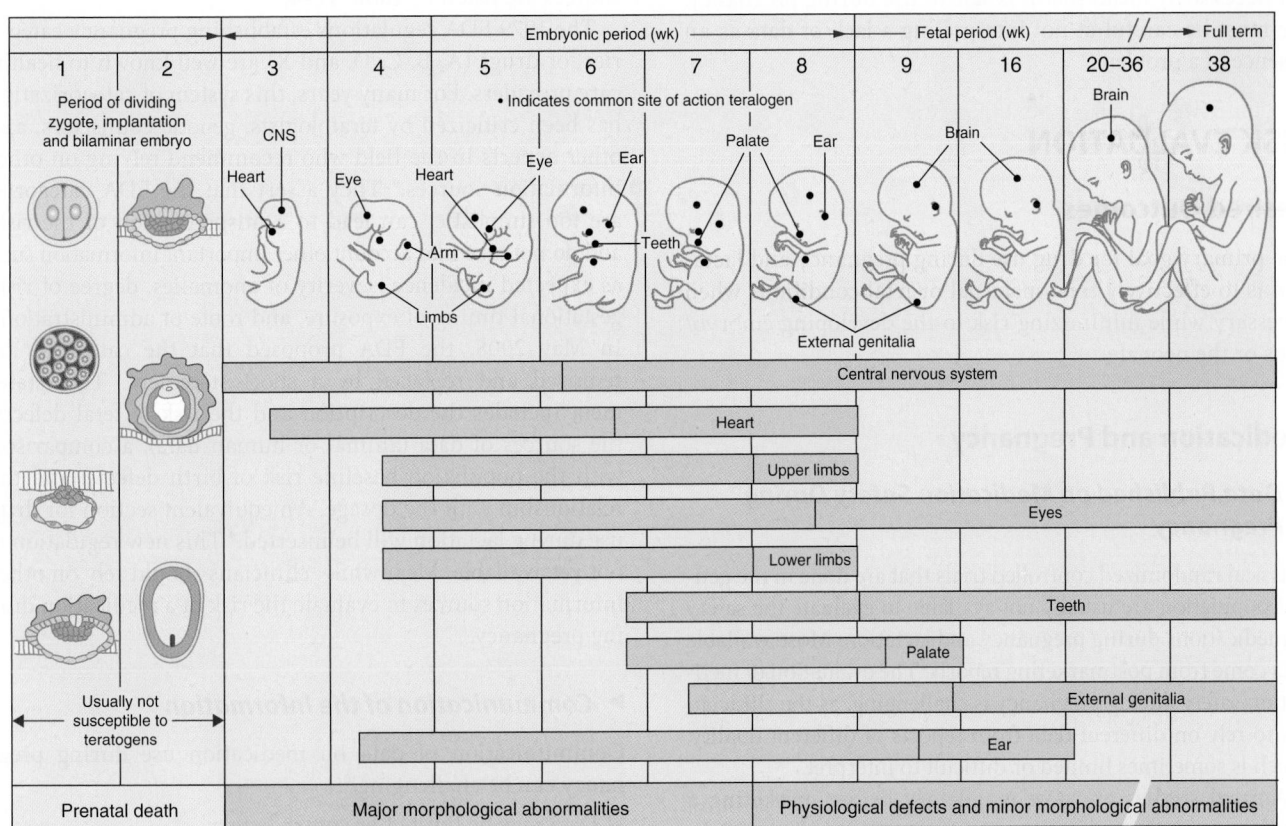

FIGURE 47–1. Embryonic and fetal development. The horizontal bars represent potential sensitivity to teratogens. The colored areas represent the more critical times. Embryonic period is in post-conceptional weeks. (Reprinted with permission from Moore KL. The Developing Human. New York: Elsevier, p 976: copyright 1974.)

determine whether it could lead to a higher risk of a specific malformation.[7]

Criteria have been proposed to determine whether a causal relationship between congenital anomalies and a medication is plausible (teratogenic effect).[3,7] Exposure to the medication must have happened during the critical period of development of the organ for which a malformation is noticed (Figure 47–1). In addition, a pattern of anomaly or a specific syndrome have to be present, and the observed effects must be reproducible in at least two studies conducted on different populations. A rare anomaly associated to a rare exposure is also indicative of a teratogenic effect (e.g., ear anomalies and isotretinoin).

Other criteria are considered (the probability of finding an association between a medication and a malformation increases with the number of criteria present):

- Strength of the association
- Same effects observed in animal studies
- Biological plausibility based on pharmacologic effect
- Higher incidence of the anomaly in the population with the use of the medication followed by a decreased incidence once the medication is no longer available (e.g., thalidomide and limb anomalies)
- Dose–response relationship

With these criteria, there are approximately 30 medications or classes of medication established to be teratogens. They are shown in Table 47–3. If a drug is not on this list, it does not necessarily mean that it is safe to use during pregnancy. We must be careful at not interpreting a lack of data as an absence of a problem.

RISK EVALUATION

Desired Outcomes

The primary goal for drug use during pregnancy and lactation is to effectively treat maternal or fetal conditions when necessary while minimizing risk to the developing embryo/fetus or the neonate.

Medication and Pregnancy

▶ Data Published on Medication Safety During Pregnancy

Classical randomized controlled trials that are done in the general population are usually not available to evaluate the safety of medications during pregnancy and lactation. Most available data come from postmarketing reports. The evaluation of medication safety during pregnancy is challenging, as the clinician has to rely on different data from reports of different quality, which is sometimes limited or difficult to interpret.

Animal studies are now mandatory before marketing a medication. Animal data are very important to identify high-risk medications and prevent congenital anomalies. However, they must be interpreted with great caution because of many limitations; the major ones are that different species do not

share the same pharmacodynamics and pharmacokinetics for a same medication, and usually much higher doses than those used in clinical settings are administered.[8]

Case reports and case series provide the first published data on the use of medications during pregnancy. A causal relationship between a single case report and an anomaly cannot usually be established unless a rare anomaly is repeatedly associated with the use of a specific medication.

Cohort studies and company registries try to compare the risks observed after exposure to a medication with the risk observed in a control group or in the general population. When studying structural anomalies, it is important to select women exposed to medication during organogenesis. Cohort studies usually evaluate the general risk of malformations and are not powerful enough to assess the risk associated with rare anomalies. When a signal of association between an anomaly and a drug exposure is observed, a case-control study can be conducted to clarify the relationship. A case-control study also has more power to detect rare anomalies. When several studies have been published using very similar methodologies, meta-analyses can be conducted to reach higher statistical power.[8]

▶ Sources of Information on the Use of Drugs During Pregnancy and Lactation

Specialized information sources provide data on the use of medications during pregnancy and lactation. Some of these sources are listed in Table 47–4.

The 1979 FDA regulations establishing pregnancy categories for drugs (A, B, C, D, and X) are well known to healthcare providers. For many years, this system of categorization has been criticized by teratologists, genetic counselors, and other experts in the field who recommend relying on other information sources.[9] They assert that the FDA categories are too simplistic, can lead to a misperception of the risk, and do not take into account other important information such as expected incidence, severity of anomalies, degree of risk, gestational timing of exposure, and route of administration.[9] In May 2008, the FDA proposed that the categories be removed and replaced by a short statement. This statement includes the description and the risk of fetal defects, the sources of data (animal or human data), a comparison with the population baseline risk of birth defects, and the relationship with the dosage. An equivalent section for drug use during lactation will be inserted.[9] This new regulation is not yet available. Meanwhile, clinicians should rely on other information sources to evaluate the risk of a medication during pregnancy.

▶ Communication of the Information

Communication of data on medication use during pregnancy can be challenging[10]:

- Data may be limited or contradictory.
- Taking medications during pregnancy is a source of anxiety for many women and for their healthcare providers.

Table 47–3

Medications with Proven Teratogenic Effects in Humans

Drug or Drug Class	Teratogenic Effects	Critical Period
Alkylating agents	Malformations of many different organs	Organogenesis
Amiodarone	Transitory hypothyroidism (17%, goiter in 18% of these cases) or hyperthyroidism (3%)	From 10th week after conception
Androgens (danazol, testosterone)	Masculinization of genital organs in female fetus	Danazol: from 6th week after conception Testosterone: not defined
Angiotensin conversion enzyme inhibitors Angiotensin II receptor antagonists	Renal failure, anuria, oligohydramnios, pulmonary hypoplasia, intrauterine growth restriction, limbs contracture, skull hypoplasia	After the first trimester
Anticonvulsants • Carbamazepine • Phenytoin • Phenobarbital • Valproic acid	NTDs (for carbamazepine and valproic acid); oral cleft, skeletal, urogenital, craniofacial, digital, and cardiac malformations; microcephalia Risk of major malformations estimated at 5–10% depending on the agent used (about 5% for carbamazepine, 10–14% for valproic acid). Valproic acid: abnormal neurologic development	7–14 weeks (gestational age); higher risk between 8 and 11 weeks. Neurologic development: not established
Systemic corticosteroids	Oral cleft (risk of 3–4/1,000 versus 1/1,000 in general population)	Organogenesis
Diethylstilbestrol	Girls: Cervical or vaginal adenocarcinoma, incidence of less than 1.4/1,000 exposures. Structural genital anomalies (e.g., of cervix, vagina) in 25% of cases Boys: Genital anomalies, spermatogenesis anomalies	First and second trimesters
Fluconazole high doses	Skeletal and craniofacial malformations, cleft palate (with chronic dose more than 400 mg/day; not reported with 150 mg single dose)	Not defined, but cases are reported where exposure was for most parts of pregnancy
Radioactive iodine (I¹³¹)	Thyroid suppression (goiter)	From 10th week after conception (consider the dosage and time to eliminate the product on a case-by-case basis)
Isotretinoin, acitretin, etretinate, and vitamin A (more than 10,000 IU/day)	CNS, skull, eyes and ears malformations, micrognathia, oral cleft, cardiac malformations, thymus anomalies, mental retardation: estimated at 25–30% (may be higher for neurologic development impairment) Contraindicated throughout pregnancy Isotretinoin: discontinue 1 month before pregnancy, prescribed under a special program called iPLEDGE Acitretin, etretinate: discontinue 2–3 years before pregnancy (alcohol consumption decreases elimination)	Organogenesis (risk of teratogenic effect after organogenesis not excluded)
Lithium	Cardiac malformations: risk of 0.9–6.8% (higher risks from small studies that included also minor cardiac anomalies) (general population risk: approximately 1%) Includes Ebstein's anomaly: risk estimated at 0.05–0.1%	Cardiac organogenesis
Methimazole/propylthiouracil	Methimazole: aplasia cutis, syndrome including choanal atresia, esophageal atresia, facial anomalies, developmental delay; risk probably low	Organogenesis
	Methimazole/propylthiouracil: fetal hypothyroidism in 2–10% of infants whose mothers were treated for Graves disease or goiter	Second and third trimesters
Methotrexate	CNS and cranial malformations, oral cleft, skeletal and limb malformations It is recommended to stop the medication 3 months before pregnancy	Organogenesis
Misoprostol	Moebius syndrome ± limb anomalies ± CNS anomalies	Organogenesis
Mycophenolate mofetil	Ear anomalies, oral cleft, other anomalies (causality to be confirmed)	Uncertain
Nonsteroidal anti-inflammatory drugs	In utero closure of ductus arteriosus (constriction is rare before 25 weeks, 50–70% at 30 weeks and 100% at 32 weeks (gestational age) and pulmonary hypertension	Third trimester
Penicillamine	Cutis laxa	Not defined
Tetracyclines	Teeth discoloration	14 weeks postconceptional
Thalidomide	Limb anomalies Cardiac, urogenital, GI, and ear malformations Prescribed under a special program called STEPS (System for Thalidomide Education and Prescribing Safety)	20–36 days after conception
Trimethoprim	Cardiac and urogenital malformations, neural tube defects, oral cleft	Organogenesis
Warfarin/acenocoumarol	Warfarin embryopathy including nasal hypoplasia, epiphysis dysplasia, vertebral malformations	Between 4th and 7th week postconception

Data from Refs. 3, 6, 7, 11, and 27.

Table 47–4

Sources of Information on Drug Use in Pregnancy and Lactation

Books
- Briggs GG, Freeman RK, Yaffe SJ. Drugs in Pregnancy and Lactation: A Reference Guide to Fetal and Neonatal Risk, 9th ed. Philadelphia: Lippincott Williams & Wilkins, 2011.
- Schaefer C, Peters PWJ, Miller RK. Drugs During Pregnancy and Lactation, Treatment Options and Risk Assessment, 2nd ed. Amsterdam: Elsevier, 2007.
- Hale TW. Medications and Mother's Milk, 14th ed. Amarillo, TX: Pharmasoft, 2010.

Databases
- Reprotox: www.reprotox.org
- Teris: http://depts.washington.edu/terisweb/teris/index.html

Websites
- www.otispregnancy.org
- www.motherisk.org
- www.marchofdimes.com
- www.cdc.gov
- www.pubmed.com
- List of pregnancy registries: http://www.fda.gov/womens/registries/registries.html
- Lactmed: http://toxnet.nlm.nih.gov/cgi-bin/sis/htmlgen?LACT

Teratology Information Service
- Organization of Teratology Information Specialists (OTIS): Go to www.otispregnancy.org to find your local Teratogen Information Service, or call at the National Toll-Free Number: (866) 626-6847

- Pregnant women tend to overestimate their risk of an anomaly associated with medication use and to lower their risk associated with the undertreatment of their disease.

- Many people, including healthcare providers, cannot properly understand numbers and probability.

The objective when transmitting information is to give precise data that will help the patient to make an informed decision for her health and the health of her baby. Unconfirmed hypotheses should not be transmitted to patients. The information should include a well-grounded assessment of risks, including baseline risks in the general population, risks associated with the medication, and those of not treating the disease during pregnancy. Women often have misconceptions and misperceptions about the use of medications during pregnancy.[3,8]

When dealing with numbers (e.g., percentages, probabilities), some authors suggest some tips to facilitate risk communication[3,10,11]:

- Absolute risks instead of relative risks should be used.

- Negatively and positively framed information should be used at the same time (e.g., 3% chance of having a malformed child; 97% chance of having a normal child).

- Visual aids should be used when appropriate.

- The same denominator should be used when discussing probabilities.

Finally, to determine a woman's risk of birth defects, it is important to obtain good medical, obstetrical, and pharmacologic histories (including nonprescribed medications) and to take into account exposure to alcohol, tobacco, and other recreational drugs.[11] All these elements can influence a woman's risk and the perception of risk.

▶ **Preconception Care**

Adverse pregnancy outcomes, which include prematurity, low birth weight, and birth defects, are major health concerns and can lead to serious health problems. One contributing factor to these adverse outcomes is the late start in prenatal care, which can delay the identification and modification of biomedical, behavioral, and social risk factors that can affect pregnancy outcomes. Strategies to improve pregnancy outcomes include taking folic acid, avoiding alcohol, smoking cessation, optimizing the treatment and management of chronic illnesses (e.g., diabetes, epilepsy, hypertension, maternal phenylketonuria), screening for infections (e.g., human immunodeficiency virus [HIV], sexually transmitted infections), appropriate vaccination, and reaching a healthy weight.[12]

▶ **Folic Acid**

Folic acid is an essential vitamin that plays an important role in the prevention of congenital anomalies, particularly neural tube defects (NTD). Approximately one in every 1000 pregnancies is affected by an NTD.[13] Recent data indicate that folic acid may also be involved in the reduction of other congenital anomalies, including cardiovascular, oral clefts, limb deformities, and urinary malformations.[14] ❹ *All women of childbearing age should be counseled on the appropriate dose of folic acid to prevent congenital anomalies.* The American College of Obstetricians and Gynecologists (ACOG) and the U.S. Services Task Force recommend that every woman of childbearing age take 0.4 to 0.8 mg of folic acid daily, beginning 1 month before pregnancy and through the first 2 to 3 months, because nutritional sources alone are not sufficient.[14,15] Women at higher risk of NTD (e.g., those who have had a previous child or a first-, second or third-degree relative with a neural tube defect, those with prepregnancy diabetes, those with epilepsy taking carbamazepine or valproic acid) are counseled to take 4 mg of folic acid per day.[15] The Society of Obstetricians and Gynecology of Canada advocates the use of higher doses of folic acid for a broader range of women including obese women and Sikh, Celtic, and Northern Chinese women, who are at higher risk of having a child with an NTD.[16]

▶ **Iron Supplements**

Anemia is a common problem during pregnancy; it is defined as a hemoglobin level less than 11 g/dL (110 g/L; 6.83 mmol/L) during the first and third trimesters and less than 10.5 g/dL (105 g/L; 6.52 mmol/L) during the second trimester.[17] Maternal symptoms of anemia include fatigue, palpitations, and decreased resistance to exercise and infections. Fetal risks are prematurity, low birth weight, and perinatal death. Recommendations are that all pregnant women be screened for anemia, and those with iron deficiency should be treated with oral iron preparations in addition to prenatal vitamins.[17] Iron supplementation decreases the prevalence of maternal anemia at delivery. It is unclear whether supplementing nonanemic pregnant women will improve perinatal outcomes.[17]

▶ Impact of Physiologic Changes During Pregnancy on Pharmacokinetics

Absorption Drug absorption is affected in several ways during pregnancy, and it is difficult to predict the final repercussion on drug efficacy. Decreased gastrointestinal transit can result in a delay in drug peak effect, prolonging the time of contact of drugs with the intestinal mucosa, and possibly enhancing absorption of certain drugs. The higher gastric pH may affect the absorption of weak bases or acids. Skin, tissue, and lung absorption might also be increased by physiologic changes during pregnancy.[18]

Distribution The volume of distribution increases for most drugs during pregnancy due to plasma volume expansion and the presence of amniotic fluid, the placenta, and the fetus. This results in a decrease in maximal concentrations of drugs and in their half-life. In addition, hypoalbuminemia and decreased protein binding of drugs increases free fraction of some medications.[18,19]

Metabolism During pregnancy the activity of some isoenzymes is increased (e.g., CYP3A4, CYP2A6, CYP2D6, CYP2C9), and the activity of others is decreased (e.g., CYP1A2, CYP2C19). It is difficult to predict the net impact on drug effect since there is a wide interindividual variability and since some drugs are metabolized by several isoenzymes.[18,19]

Renal Elimination Renal blood flow and glomerular filtration are increased significantly during pregnancy. The impact of this increase is more important for drugs that are eliminated in the urine.[19]

Table 47–5 shows clinical recommendations based on pharmacokinetic changes during pregnancy for several drugs.[6,19,20]

Table 47–5

Altered Pharmacokinetics During Pregnancy: Clinical Implications and Management

Drugs	Pharmacokinetic Changes	Recommendations and Monitoring
Aminoglycosides	$\uparrow V_d$, $\uparrow$ Cl, $\downarrow t_{1/2}$	Monitor peaks and troughs; increase doses if necessary
Antiretrovirals	Variable Cl and C_{max}	Monitor clinical response; drug levels can be useful to adjust drug dosage of some antiretrovirals
Caffeine	$\uparrow t_{1/2}$ $\downarrow$ Cl (T_1, T_2, T_3)	Risk of more frequent and prolonged side effects; decrease caffeine consumption
Carbamazepine	$\uparrow$ Cl $\downarrow t_{1/2}$	Measure free fraction (preferably); increase dose according to clinical response and levels
Digoxin	$\uparrow$ Cl $\downarrow C_{max}$	Follow plasma levels; adjust according to clinical response and plasma levels; increase doses if necessary; to treat fetal disease, higher doses might be required; digoxin-like immunoreactive substance might alter levels.
Fluoxetine and other SSRIs	$\uparrow$ Cl (T_3)	Increase dose according to clinical response; consider decreasing dose after delivery
Heparin LMWH	$\uparrow$ Cl (T_1, T_2, T_3)	Consider increasing frequency of administration If necessary, follow anti-Xa levels
Lamotrigine	$\uparrow$ Cl (T_1, T_2, T_3)	Measure drug levels at least every trimester; increase dose according to clinical response and levels; return to prepregnancy dose after delivery
Levothyroxine (T4)	$\downarrow$ ff	Increase dose at the beginning of pregnancy; follow TSH levels at least every trimester; return to prepregnancy dose after delivery
Lithium	$\uparrow$ Cl (T_1, T_2, T_3) $\downarrow t_{1/2}$	Measure drug levels at least every trimester and monthly in third trimester; increase dose according to levels if necessary; return to prepregnancy dose after delivery
Nicotine	$\downarrow t_{1/2}$ $\uparrow$ Cl (T_2, T_3)	Higher doses might be required (smoking cessation) at T2 and T3; however, increased transdermal absorption might lead to higher nicotine plasma levels
Nifedipine	$\uparrow$ Cl (T_3)	Monitor clinical effect; increase doses/frequency of administration if necessary
Phenytoin	$\downarrow C_{total}$, $\uparrow$ ff $\uparrow$ Cl (T_3) $\downarrow t_{1/2}$	Measure free fraction; increase dose according to clinical response and levels
Valproic acid	$\downarrow C_{total}$ $\uparrow$ ff	Measure free fraction if a prepregnancy reference level is available; dose will remain the same in most cases. Increase dose according to clinical response and levels.

$\uparrow$, increase; $\downarrow$, decrease; $\leftrightarrow$, unchanged; C_{max}, maximum serum concentration; Cl, clearance; ff, free fraction; T, trimester; $t_{1/2}$, elimination half-life; LMWH, low-molecular-weight heparins; C_{total}, total concentration; SSRI: selective serotonin reuptake inhibitor.

Data from Refs. 6, 19, and 20.

Medication and Lactation

According to a 2005 policy statement from the American Academy of Pediatrics (AAP), new mothers should breast-feed exclusively for 6 months. Approximately 46% of new mothers report that they breast-feed exclusively at birth. However, this figure drops to 17% at 6 months, as many new mothers supplement breast-feeding with other foods or quit entirely by this point.[21]

▶ Drug Transfer into Breast Milk

To study drug effects in a breast-fed infant, serum drug levels could be measured to help evaluate safety in the infant; however, these data are often not available. Therefore, in most instances, the approximate quantity of drug ingested by the breast-fed infant is estimated using published measured drug concentrations in breast milk. With these data, one can calculate the percentage of pediatric dose or the relative infant dose (percentage of maternal dose adjusted by weight), assuming an average of 150 mL/kg/day of milk ingested by a breast-fed infant.

- Percentage of pediatric dosage =

$$\left(\frac{\text{Quantity of medication taken from milk by the baby (mg/kg/day)}}{\text{Usual initial daily pediatric dose (mg/kg/day)}} \right) \times 100$$

- Maternal dose adjusted by weight or relative infant dose =

$$\left(\frac{\text{Quantity of medication taken from milk by the baby (mg/kg/day)}}{\text{Maternal dose adjusted by weight (mg/kg/day)}} \right) \times 100$$

In the latter equation, maternal dose refers to the dose used by patients in the published study or case report, not to the dose of your actual patient.

Usually, a percentage of less than 10% of the pediatric dose or, when a pediatric dose is not available, a percentage of less than 10% of maternal dose adjusted by weight, is acceptable in full-term healthy infants.[22]

▶ Drug Pharmacokinetics

If clinical data are not available on drug transfer into breast milk, choose drugs that are highly protein bound, have a high molecular weight, have a short half-life, have no active metabolites, and are well tolerated by children.[22]

▶ Drugs of Concern During Breast-Feeding

5 *Most drugs are safe during breast-feeding.* However, use of some drugs creates some concern and requires a more thorough assessment by the clinician (Table 47–6). **2** *Health professionals should know which medications are of concern during breast-feeding.* One should also consider the additive side effects of medication for the baby when the mother is taking a combination of medications.

Table 47–6

Drugs of Concern During Breast-Feeding

Drug or Class	Comments
Drugs that can decrease the breast milk production	
Clomiphene	Has been used to suppress lactation
Ergot derivatives (bromocriptine, cabergoline, ergotamine)	Have been used to suppress lactation
Estrogens	Hormonal contraceptives with ethinylestradiol should be delayed for 4–6 weeks following delivery.
Pseudoephedrine	Do not use in women with low milk production; a few doses will probably not have significant clinical effect
Drugs for which use during breast-feeding may expose the neonate to a significant quantity and may necessitate a strict follow-up	
β-blocking agents (acebutolol, atenolol, sotalol)	Neonatal β-blockade reported. Concern for acebutolol, atenolol and sotalol, but some other β-blocking agents are safe to use.
Amiodarone	May accumulate because of long half-life; possible neonatal thyroid and cardiovascular toxicity
Antineoplastics	Neonatal myelosuppression possible
Chloramphenicol	Severe side effects reported when used to treat babies (blood dyscrasia, grey baby syndrome)
Ergotamine	Symptoms of ergotism (vomiting and diarrhea) reported
Illicit drugs	Unknown contents and effects
Lamotrigine	A breast-fed infant could have blood concentrations between 10% and 50% of the maternal blood concentrations. One single case of apnea in a breast-fed infant, no other side effect was reported in about 100 breast-fed babies. Follow for rash and CNS side effects.
Lithium	Up to 50% of maternal serum levels have been measured in infants; cases of infant toxicity have been reported
Phenobarbital/ primidone	Drowsiness and reduced weight gain reported. Up to 25 % of a pediatric dose can be ingested via breast milk.
Radioactive iodine-131	Long radioactive half-life (21–42 days)
Tetracyclines	Chronic use may lead to dental staining or decreased epiphyseal bone growth

Data from Refs. 6 and 22.

CONDITIONS PREVALENT IN PREGNANCY AND LACTATION

6 *When possible, treat conditions occurring during pregnancy with nonpharmacologic treatments instead of drug therapy.*

7 *Evaluate the need for treatment, including benefits and risks. Avoid treatments that do not show evidence of benefit or that can be delayed until after pregnancy or breast-feeding.*

Clinical Confirmation and Associated Problems of Pregnancy and Lactation

Confirmation of Pregnancy

Positive urine human chorionic gonadotropin followed by positive ultrasound, fetal heart sounds, and/or fetal movement.

Pregnancy Dating and Gestational Age

Calculated from the first day of the last menstrual period.

Due dates typically are estimated at 40 weeks of gestation; however, infants delivered between 37 completed weeks and 42 weeks are considered full term.

Pregnancy Symptoms

First trimester: Menstrual spotting, missed menses, fatigue, breast tenderness, increased urination, mood swings, nausea/vomiting, headache, heartburn, constipation

Second trimester: Frequent urination, heartburn, constipation, dry skin, edema, **linea nigra, melasma**

Third trimester: Backache, edema, shortness of breath

Routine Pregnancy Visits

In a normal, uncomplicated pregnancy, visits should occur monthly until 28 weeks of gestation, every 2 to 3 weeks from 28 to 36 weeks of gestation, and then weekly until delivery.

Examination for each of the following is performed at each visit:

- Blood pressure
- Weight
- Urine for protein and glucose
- Uterine size
- Fetal heart rate
- Fetal movement

Routine Lab Testing for Normal Pregnancies (First Trimester Unless Otherwise Indicated)

- Human immunodeficiency virus
- Purified protein derivative (PPD) test for tuberculosis (high risk)
- Venereal Disease Research Laboratory (VDRL) slide test for syphilis
- Rubella immunity
- Cervical cytology
- Blood and Rh type
- Hepatitis B surface antigen
- Hepatitis C antibodies (if high risk)
- Bacterial vaginosis testing if symptomatic or at high risk (previous preterm labor)
- Antibody screen for Rh antibodies
- Hemoglobin and hematocrit for anemia (repeated at 26–32 weeks)
- Urinalysis with culture for asymptomatic bacteriuria

- Gonorrhea and chlamydia
- Screens for neural tube defects if indicated (at 15–20 weeks) and Down's syndrome
- Gestational diabetes screening (at 24–28 weeks)
- Group B *Streptococcus* screening (at 35–37 weeks)

Assessing Suitability of the Cervix for Labor Induction

Suitability is based on cervical dilation, length, consistency, and position. These findings are translated to a numerical rating called the Bishop score. A Bishop score of less than 6 indicates that pharmacologic therapy is needed to ripen the cervix prior to delivery.

Selected Problems Experienced During Pregnancy or Lactation

Hyperemesis gravidarum. Severe, persistent nausea and vomiting during pregnancy accompanied by dehydration, electrolyte disturbance, ketonuria, and weight loss.

Bacteriuria. Often asymptomatic in pregnancy. Diagnosed by positive urine culture.

Bacterial vaginosis. Clinically diagnosed by presence of three of the following:

- White, noninflammatory discharge
- **Clue cells** on microscopic examination
- Vaginal pH greater than 4.5
- A fishy odor before or after addition of 10% potassium hydroxide (i.e., "whiff" test)

Vulvovaginal candidiasis. Typical symptoms include vaginal itching and discharge. Clinical characteristics include:

- Vaginal pH less than 4.5
- Observation of yeast on Gram stain or wet preparation
- Thick, white, "cottage cheese–like" discharge

Chlamydia and gonorrhea. Typically asymptomatic. Diagnosed by positive culture.

Genital herpes simplex virus. Characterized by vesicular or ulcerative lesions. Diagnosis confirmed by virologic or serologic testing. Prodrome manifests as pain, burning, or itching at the site where lesions will develop.

Pelvic inflammatory disease. Difficult to diagnose in pregnancy. Symptoms may include:

- Uterine/ovarian tenderness
- Cervical motion tenderness
- Fever
- Abnormal cervical or vaginal discharge
- Presence of white blood cells in vaginal secretions
- Elevated erythrocyte sedimentation rate
- Elevated C-reactive protein

(Continued)

Clinical Confirmation and Associated Problems of Pregnancy and Lactation (*Continued*)

Syphilis. A single genital lesion may characterize early disease. Diagnosed by positive serologic testing (e.g., VDRL or rapid plasma reagin [RPR] test).

Trichomoniasis. Symptoms may include vulvar irritation and yellow-green discharge. Diagnosed after microscopic visualization of the organism.

Preterm labor. Onset of labor prior to 37 weeks of gestation.

Group B streptococcus. Diagnosed by positive culture on vaginal and rectal swab.

Mastitis. Characterized by localized redness, tenderness, and warmth on one breast accompanied by fever and flulike symptoms. Although uncommon, symptoms also may be bilateral.

Nipple candidiasis. Typical symptoms include nipple pain, itching, burning, and/or breast pain that persist after feeding.

Gestational diabetes. See Chapter 43.

Hypertension in pregnancy. Asymptomatic or presence of neurologic, hepatic, or cardiovascular symptoms. Check for proteinuria.

Nausea and Vomiting

As many as 85% of pregnant women suffer from nausea or vomiting.[23] Nonpharmacologic measures, such as lifestyle (rest, avoidance of nausea triggers) and dietary changes (small and frequent meals, fluid restriction during meals, avoiding spicy or fatty foods, consuming crackers upon rising, and elimination of pills with iron, if possible) should be used as first-line management. Acupuncture and acupressure also can be helpful.[23]

The combination of pyridoxine (vitamin B_6) and doxylamine is well studied during pregnancy and is the first-line pharmacologic treatment of nausea and vomiting during pregnancy (Table 47–7).[23] This combination is not available in the United States, and the ingredients have to be administered separately. When the combination of pyridoxine/doxylamine is insufficient, other drugs such as metoclopramide or diphenhydramine can be prescribed; ondansetron is another alternative.[23]

Constipation

Up to 40% of pregnant women will suffer from constipation.[24] Nonpharmacologic treatment is the mainstay of constipation treatment in pregnant patients. Pregnant women should be counseled to eat a high-fiber diet, drink plenty of fluids, exercise regularly, and avoid prolonged time on the toilet. Bulk-forming laxatives, such as psyllium and calcium polycarbophil, are first-line agents (Table 47–7). If these methods fail, emollients or osmotic agents can be tried. Stimulant laxatives, such as bisacodyl and senna, are acceptable second-line agents for short-term or intermittent use.[6] During lactation, bulk-forming, emollient, osmotic laxatives, and the stimulant laxatives are safe for use.[22]

Heartburn

Heartburn affects a majority of pregnant women.[25] Nonpharmacologic recommendations for the treatment of heartburn during pregnancy include small and frequent meals, remaining upright after eating, elevating the head of the bed, and avoiding factors known to decrease lower esophageal sphincter tone (e.g., smoking, chocolate, coffee, fatty foods, and peppermint).[25]

Calcium- or magnesium-containing antacids are first-line therapies. If antacids fail to improve symptoms, ranitidine can be recommended, as it is the drug with the best safety data among the H_2 blockers (Table 47–7).[25] Omeprazole, sucralfate, and metoclopramide are also safe in pregnancy (Table 47–7).[26,27]

All the drugs used for heartburn during pregnancy are acceptable during lactation.[22]

Nasal Congestion and Rhinitis

Do not underestimate the impact of nasal congestion and rhinitis, especially if it is chronic and associated with snoring and sleep disorders. Rest, fluids, humidified air, nasal saline, and acetaminophen are the mainstays of therapy for the common cold. Recommend avoiding irritants and known allergens and raising the head of the bed at 30 to 45 degrees. Nasal strips might be helpful.[28]

Treat nasal congestion as in the nonpregnant population, being mindful to do the following: (a) Avoid oral decongestants during the first trimester owing to the risk of fetal

Patient Encounter, Part 2

At 24 weeks of pregnancy, MM is admitted for acute pyelonephritis. Blood glucose levels are between 108 and 180 mg/dL (6.0 and 10.0 mmol/L). Urine culture reports the presence of *E. coli* and group B *Streptococcus*.

Medication:

Methyldopa 500 mg orally twice daily

ASA 81 mg orally at bedtime

Levothyroxine 100 mcg orally daily

Insulin NPH 46 units subcutaneously at bedtime

Insulin aspart 10 units subcutaneously before every meal

What treatment do you recommend at this time?

Table 47–7

Medication Dosing Recommendations During Pregnancy and Lactation

Drug	Dosage	Comments
Micronutrients and Vitamins		
Calcium	1,000–1,300 (elemental calcium) mg/day	To be taken with vitamin D
Folic acid	0.4–0.8 mg orally daily	RDA: 0.5 mg (breast-feeding)–0.6 mg (pregnancy)
	4 mg orally daily	Higher dose during first trimester recommended for women at higher risk of having a child with NTD, (e.g., personal or family history [FH] of NTD, medication known to cause NTD, or prepregnancy diabetes)
Iron	27 mg (elemental iron) orally daily	RDA for pregnancy RDA for breast-feeding: 9–10 mg
	60–200 mg (elemental iron) orally per day	Higher doses to treat iron-deficiency anemia
Vitamin D	600 IU orally daily	RDA during pregnancy and lactation
	400 IU orally daily (breast-fed infants)	Dose recommended for breast-fed infants
Nausea and Vomiting		
Diphenhydramine or dimenhydrinate	25–50 mg orally 4 × daily as needed	
Doxylamine	12.5 mg orally 3–4 × daily as needed	Can be taken with pyridoxine
Metoclopramide	5–15 mg orally 3–4 × daily as needed	
Meclizine	12.5–50 mg orally daily as needed	
Pyridoxine	25 mg orally 3 × daily as needed	Can be taken with doxylamine
Ondansetron	4–8 mg orally 3 times daily as needed	
Heartburn		
Antacids (calcium carbonate, magnesium hydroxide)	Product-specific dosing, refer to product monograph	
Ranitidine	150 mg orally twice daily	
Metoclopramide	5–10 mg orally 3–4 × daily	
Omeprazole	20 mg orally daily	
Sucralfate	1 g orally 4 × daily	
Constipation		
Polycarbophil	2 tablets 1–4 × daily	
Psyllium	Product specific dosing, usually 1 packet/scoopful in water up to 3 × daily	
Docusate	100–400 mg orally per day (given in 1 or 2 doses)	
Bisacodyl	5–10 mg orally (tablets) or rectally (suppositories) as needed	
Senna	17.2 mg orally (tablets or syrup) once or twice daily or rectally (suppositories) as needed	
Lactulose	15–30 mL daily or twice daily	
Nasal Congestion		
Decongestants		
Oxymetazoline	0.05% spray, 2–3 sprays in each nostril twice daily for 3–5 days	Avoid using more than 3–7 days to prevent rebound congestion
Pseudoephedrine	60 mg orally every 4–6 hours	Short term (3–5 days) second and third trimesters only.
Antihistamines		
Chlorpheniramine	4 mg every 4–6 hours	
Cetirizine	10 mg orally daily	
Loratadine	10 mg orally daily	
Sodium cromolyn	2.6 mg nasal spray, 3–4 × daily	
Nasal Corticosteroids		
Budesonide	32 mcg spray, 1–4 sprays daily	First-line agents for chronic congestion
Beclomethasone	50–100 mcg spray, twice daily	
Fluticasone	100 mcg spray daily	

(Continued)

Table 47–7

Medication Dosing Recommendations During Pregnancy and Lactation (*Continued*)

Drug	Dosage	Comments
Urinary Tract Infections		
Asymptomatic bacteriuria and uncomplicated acute cystitis		
Nitrofurantoin	100 mg orally 4 × daily	For 3 to 7 days
Cephalexin	250–500 mg orally 4 × daily	
Amoxicillin	500 mg orally 3 × daily	
Acute pyelonephritis		
Ampicillin + gentamicin	1–2 g IV every 6 hours + 1.5 mg/kg/dose IV every 8 hours	Switch to oral antibiotic after 48 hours afebrile and treat for a total of 10 to 14 days, for example: • cephalexin 500 mg orally 4 × daily • cefprozil 500 mg orally 2 × daily • amoxicillin clavulanate 875/125 mg orally 2 × daily
Cefazolin	1–2 g every IV 8 hours	
Cefuroxime	0.75–1.5 g IV every 8 hours	
Ceftriaxone	1–2 g IV or IM every 24 hours	
Prophylaxis		
Nitrofurantoin	100 mg orally at bedtime	Start after the end of the treatment for pyelonephritis and continue until 4 to 6 weeks after delivery.
Cephalexin	250 mg orally at bedtime	
Bacterial Vaginosis		
Metronidazole	250 mg orally 3 × daily for 7 days or 500 mg orally twice a day for 7 days 0.75% vaginal gel, once or twice daily for 5 days	
Clindamycin	300 mg orally twice daily for 7 days 100-mg ovules intravaginally at bedtime for 3 days	Use oral formulation during pregnancy and intravaginal formulation during breast-feeding
Vulvovaginal Candidiasis		
Butoconazole	2% cream, 5 g intravaginally for 3–6 days	Longer treatments are recommended during pregnancy
Clotrimazole	1% cream, 5 g intravaginally for 6 days 100-mg vaginal tablet daily for 7 days 2% cream, 5 g intravaginally for 3 days 200-mg vaginal tablet daily for 3 days	
Miconazole	2% cream, 5 g intravaginally for 7 days 100-mg vaginal suppository daily for 7 days 4% cream, 5 g intravaginally for 3 days 200-mg vaginal tablet daily for 3 days	
Terconazole	0.4% cream, 5 g intravaginally for 7 days 0.8% cream, 5 g intravaginally for 3 days 80-mg vaginal tablet daily for 3 days	
Nystatin	100,000-unit vaginal tablet, 1 tablet for 14 days	
Chlamydia		
Azithromycin	1 g orally (1 dose only)	Quinolones are not first choice for reasons of resistance mainly.
Amoxicillin	500 mg orally 3 × daily for 7 days	
Erythromycin base	500 mg orally 4 × daily for 7 days or 250 mg orally 4 × daily for 14 days	Avoid erythromycin estolate during pregnancy due to potential maternal hepatoxicity
Doxycycline	100 mg orally twice daily for 7 days	During lactation only. Doxycycline should be avoided in pregnant women (discoloration of teeth if used after 16 weeks of gestational age).
Gonorrhea (Uncomplicated)		
Ceftriaxone	250 mg intramuscularly once	
Cefixime	400 mg orally once	
Azithromycin	2 g orally once	For cephalosporin-allergic patients Treats chlamydia also.
Pharynx infection Ceftriaxone + azithromycin	Doses as above	

(*Continued*)

Table 47–7

Medication Dosing Recommendations During Pregnancy and Lactation (*Continued*)

Drug	Dosage	Comments
Genital Herpes Simplex Virus (Uncomplicated)		
Acyclovir	*First episode:* 400 mg orally 3 × daily for 7–10 days, or 200 mg 5 × daily for 7–10 days *Recurrent episode:* 400 mg orally 3 × daily for 5 days, or 800 mg twice daily for 5 days, or 800 mg 3 × daily for 2 days *Suppressive therapy:* 400 mg orally 3 × daily	 From 36 weeks until delivery
Syphilis		
Benzathine penicillin G	Primary, secondary, or early latent: 2.4 million units intramuscularly once Late latent or of unknown duration or tertiary: 2.4 million units intramuscularly 3 × at 1-week interval	Desensitize penicillin-allergic patients during pregnancy; first-line agent during lactation
Aqueous crystalline penicillin G	Neurosyphilis 3–4 million units 6 × daily for 10–14 days or Procaine penicillin 2.4 million units daily + probenecid 500 mg 4 × daily	Desensitize penicillin-allergic patients during pregnancy; also first-line agent during lactation
Trichomoniasis		
Metronidazole	2 g orally for 1 dose	During lactation, temporarily stop breast-feeding for 12 hours (most important for premature or very young infants).
Preterm Labor Prevention		
17-α-hydroxyprogesterone	250 mg IM each week	To prevent premature labor; start at 16–20 weeks' gestation
Progesterone (micronized)	Intravaginal suppositories 100 mg daily or 90 mg (8%) gel	To prevent premature labor; start at 16–20 weeks' gestation
Premature Rupture of Membranes		
Ampicillin	2 g IV every 6 hours for 48 hours followed by amoxicillin	Ampicillin/amoxicillin are used with erythromycin
Amoxicillin	250–500 mg orally 3 × daily for 5 days	Ampicillin/amoxicillin are used with erythromycin
Erythromycin base	250 mg IV every 6 hours × 48 hours followed by 333 mg 3 × daily for 5 days	Ampicillin/amoxicillin are used with erythromycin
Fetal Lung Maturation		
Betamethasone	12 mg IM every 24 hours for 2 doses	
Dexamethasone	6 mg IM or IV every 12 hours for 4 doses	
Preterm Labor		
Nifedipine (short acting)	30-mg oral load (divided over at least 1 hour), then 10–20 mg every 4–6 hours for 48 hours	Maternal adverse reactions include headache, flushing, dizziness, transient hypotension, and maternal pulmonary edema.
Magnesium sulfate	4–6 g IV bolus over 20 minutes, then 2–3 g/h IV drip	Contraindicated in women with myasthenia gravis, and serious complications such as maternal pulmonary edema and cardiac arrest have been reported. More benign side effects such as flushing, headache, and nausea often lead to discontinuation.
Indomethacin	50–100 mg oral load, then 25–50 mg orally every 6 hours × 48 hours	Avoid in women with a history of renal or hepatic impairment, aspirin or nonsteroidal anti-inflammatory drug (NSAID) allergy, peptic ulcer disease, other bleeding disorders, or after 32 weeks of pregnancy. Reports of increased risk of maternal postpartum hemorrhage, and neonatal complications (e.g., premature closure of the ductus arteriosus, necrotizing enterocolitis, bronchopulmonary dysplasia, renal insufficiency, and intraventricular hemorrhage) are worrisome.

(Continued)

Table 47–7

Medication Dosing Recommendations During Pregnancy and Lactation (*Continued*)

Drug	Dosage	Comments
Group B *Streptococcus*		
Penicillin G	5 million units IV initially, then 2.5–3 million units IV every 4 hours until delivery	
Ampicillin	2 g IV initially, then 1 g IV every 4 hours until delivery	
Cefazolin	2 g IV initially, then 1 g IV every 8 hours until delivery	
Clindamycin	900 mg IV every 8 hours until delivery	
Vancomycin	1 g IV every 12 hours until delivery	
Preeclampsia/Eclampsia		
Magnesium sulfate	4 g IV bolus over 20 minutes, then 1 g/h IV drip	Use same dose for fetal neuroprotection
Severe Hypertension		
First choices		
Labetalol	10–20 mg IV over 2 minutes; could be repeated every 15–30 minutes (30 mg total dose) Or 1–2 mg/minute IV drip	Not for asthmatic women. May cause fetal bradycardia
Nifedipine (short acting)	5–10 mg orally; could be repeated after 30 minutes	Maternal adverse reactions include headache, flushing, dizziness, transient hypotension, and maternal pulmonary edema.
Hydralazine	5 mg IV or IM; could be repeated IV every 30 minutes (30 mg total dose) Or 0.5–10 mg/hour IV drip	May cause tachycardia, headaches, hypotension
Second choice		
Clonidine	0.05–0.2 mg orally (maximum: 0.8 mg daily)	May cause hypotension, drowsiness
Nonsevere Hypertension		
First choices		
Methyldopa	250–500 mg orally 2–4 × daily	May cause orthostatic hypotension, drowsiness, depression, hemolytic anemia, positive antibodies antinuclear
Labetalol	100–400 mg orally 2–4 × daily	Not for asthmatic women. May cause hypotension, tiredness, headaches, hepatotoxicity
Nifedipine extended release	20–60 mg orally 1–2 × daily	May cause tachycardia, headaches, edema
Second choices		
Hydralazine	10–50 mg orally 2–4 × daily with methyldopa or labetalol	May cause tachycardia, headaches, hypotension, lupus-like syndrome
Metoprolol	25–100 mg orally 2 × daily	Not for asthmatic women; may cause fetal bradycardia
Clonidine	0.05–0.2 mg orally for a (maximum: 0.8 mg daily)	May cause hypotension, drowsiness
Hydrochlorothiazide	12.5–50 mg orally once daily	May cause hypokalemia, dehydration
Thyroid Diseases		
Hypothyroidism		
Levothyroxine	1–2 mcg/kg orally according to thyroxine-stimulating hormone (TSH) level	
Hyperthyroidism		
Propylthiouracil	50–100 mg orally 1–3 × daily according to T4 levels	Use the lowest dose to avoid fetal effects. Be aware of hepatotoxicity.
Anticoagulation		
Heparin and low-molecular-weight heparin	Same as nonpregnant and nonlactating population	

(Continued)

Table 47–7

Medication Dosing Recommendations During Pregnancy and Lactation (*Continued*)

Drug	Dosage	Comments
Mastitis		
Outpatient Treatment		
Dicloxacillin	500 mg orally 4 × daily	Treat for 10–14 days
Cephalexin	500 mg orally 4 × daily	
Amoxicillin 875 mg + 125 mg clavulanate	1 tablet orally 2 × daily	
Inpatient Treatment for More Severe Cases		
Oxacillin	2 g IV every 4 hours	Treat IV for 24–48 hours until afebrile then continue with outpatient treatment
Nafcillin	2 g IV every 4 hours	
Clindamycin	600–900 mg IV every 8 hours	
Vancomycin	1 g IV every 8–12 hours	If MRSA
Breast Candidiasis		
Mother		
Clotrimazole, miconazole, or nystatin	Topical cream	After each feeding and for 1 week after symptoms have resolved. Also treat infant even if asymptomatic
Fluconazole	200–400 mg orally for 1 dose followed by 100–200 mg orally daily	If topical treatment not efficacious, add fluconazole; use until 1 week after symptoms have resolved (minimum of 2 weeks of treatment). Also treat infant even if asymptomatic.
Infant		
Nystatin oral solution	100,000–200,000 units (1–2 mL) to be swabbed into infant's mouth 4 × daily, after feedings	
Clotrimazole or miconazole topical cream	Apply in a thin layer in infant's mouth 4 × daily, after feedings	
Other Treatments for Candidiasis		
Gentian violet 0.5–1% solution	To be swabbed into infant's mouth once daily for 5 days before a feeding	To be used if other options fail. Can stain clothes and skin. If nipples or mouth are not violet after application and the feeding, reapply the treatment

MRSA, methicillin-resistant *Staphylococcus aureus*; NTD, neural tube defect; RDA, recommended daily allowance.

Data from Refs. 6, 17, 23–25, 28–31, 33–37, 40, 41, 43, 44, 46–49, 51–54, 56, 57, 59, 60, 63–66.

gastroschisis (incidence 4 to 6 per 10,000 treated women). After the first trimester, pseudoephedrine is the preferred agent for short-term use if a topical decongestant or nasal saline solution is not effective.[6,27] (b) Stop topical decongestants after 3 to 7 days in order to minimize the incidence of rebound congestion. (c) Most first- and second-generation antihistamines are safe in pregnancy at recommended dosages. (d) Nasal corticosteroids are the best drugs for chronic rhinitis.[6,27,28]

During lactation, all the drugs previously used during pregnancy can be continued.[22,27] A lower breast milk production has been noticed in a few women following a treatment with pseudoephedrine.[22]

Urinary Tract Infections

Urinary tract infections during pregnancy, including asymptomatic disease, are associated with higher risks of hypertension, low birth weight, and preterm delivery. Asymptomatic bacteriuria and cystitis cause acute pyelonephritis more often in pregnancy than in nonpregnant women.[29] Acute pyelonephritis may lead to septic shock and adult respiratory distress syndrome and should be treated aggressively with intravenous antibiotics. Outpatient treatment with intramuscular therapy alone or followed by oral treatment is feasible for some women (e.g., stable and pregnancy less than 24 weeks).[29] Treatment reduces pregnancy complications.[30,31]

Antimicrobial therapy should target *Escherichia coli* infection.[26] Safe agents for empirical therapy include penicillins in combination with a beta-lactamase inhibitor, cephalosporins, and nitrofurantoin (Table 47-7).[29-31] Nitrofurantoin must not be used for the treatment of pyelonephritis. Sulfonamides, ampicillin, and amoxicillin are second-line choices in areas where bacterial resistance is known.[29,32] Avoid trimethoprim-sulfamethoxazole during organogenesis (congenital malformations) and near term (theoretical risk of neonatal jaundice) unless there are no other suitable choices.[27,33] Quinolones should be reserved for resistant infections due to theoretical concerns of arthropathy.[27]

Repeat urine culture 10 days after completion of therapy and monthly thereafter in case of acute pyelonephritis. After completion of the acute episode of pyelonephritis, recommend suppressive therapy prophylaxis for the remainder of the pregnancy and for 4 to 6 weeks after delivery.[29]

Bacterial Vaginosis

Bacterial vaginosis is associated with adverse pregnancy outcomes such as premature rupture of the membranes, chorioamnionitis, preterm birth, and postpartum endometritis.[34] Treatment is recommended in all symptomatic women and in asymptomatic women at high risk for preterm delivery. The Centers for Disease Control and Prevention (CDC) recommends oral metronidazole or clindamycin for the treatment of bacterial vaginosis in pregnant women (Table 47–7).[34] Metronidazole is deemed safe for use during all stages of pregnancy.[28-30] Oral antimicrobials are preferred to intravaginal antimicrobials, and clindamycin vaginal cream should be avoided due to association with low birth weight and neonatal infection.[34]

Since the cure rate is expected to be around 70%, it is important to do a culture during pregnancy 1 month after completion of therapy.[34]

During lactation, clindamycin or metronidazole vaginal formulations are the preferred therapies for bacterial vaginosis (Table 47–7).

Vulvovaginal Candidiasis

Only symptomatic vulvovaginal candidiasis should be treated in pregnant or lactating women. First-line treatment is topical azole therapy for 7 days in pregnant women; shorter courses can be used during lactation. Oral fluconazole is not a first-line treatment during pregnancy; it can be used during breast-feeding (Table 47–7).[34]

Sexually Transmitted Infections

Sexually transmitted infections (STI) have various consequences during pregnancy and require treatment. Table 47-8 presents the risks during pregnancy, the indications for treatment, and the recommended follow-up for chlamydia, gonorrhea, syphilis, herpes simplex, and trichomoniasis.

Preterm Labor

Preterm birth, especially before 32 weeks of pregnancy, is the major cause of short- and long-term neonatal mortality and morbidity. The underlying pathophysiologic conditions are diverse, and most are unknown. There is a wide variation in management, diagnosis, and treatment of preterm labor across the world.

▶ Antenatal Corticosteroids

The most beneficial intervention in preterm labor is the administration of antepartum corticosteroids. A single course of antenatal corticosteroids should be administered between 24 and 34 weeks' gestation to women at risk of preterm delivery within 7 days (Table 47–7).[35] This approach decreases the incidence and severity of neonatal respiratory distress syndrome, intraventricular hemorrhage, necrotizing enterocolitis, and death.[35] A single rescue course may be used in some women, but current guidelines do not support the use of repeated courses of corticosteroids.[36]

Table 47-8

Management of Main Sexually Transmitted Infections During Pregnancy and Lactation

	Indications of Treatment	Associated Risks During Pregnancy	When to Repeat Testing During Pregnancy	Other
Chlamydia trachomatis	All women with a positive test, even if asymptomatic	Preterm labor; neonatal infection	Third trimester: Less than 25 years of age, those at increased risk of infection or if first screening positive	Repeat testing 3–4 weeks after therapy
Gonorrhea	All women with a positive test, even if asymptomatic	Preterm labor; neonatal infection	Third trimester: (or 3–6 months after first trimester) if first screening positive or if at risk of reinfection	Repeat testing 3 weeks after therapy
Herpes Simplex	Active lesions; disseminated. Starting at 36 weeks: prevention of recurrence at term	Neonatal infection, especially if acquired near time of delivery (30–50%)		Cesarean section if active genital herpetic lesions at delivery; evaluate newborn for herpes infection
Syphilis	All women with confirmed positive serology	In utero fetal and neonatal infection; congenital malformations	At 28–32 weeks and at delivery if at risk of reinfection, if untested before, if positive serology in the first trimester, or if was previous stillborn at more than 20 weeks	Penicillin-allergic women must undergo desensitization; therapy is efficacious to treat the fetus and to prevent transmission; be aware of Jarisch-Herxheimer reaction; fetal evaluation should include ultrasounds.
Trichomoniasis	Symptomatic women	Premature rupture of membranes, preterm birth, low birth weight; neonatal infection		Therapy does not decrease perinatal mortality

Data from Workowski KA, Berman S. Sexually transmitted diseases treatment guidelines, 2010. MMWR Recomm Rep 2010;59:1–110.

▶ Tocolytic Agents

Tocolytic therapy is used to buy time to complete a course of corticosteroids and to delay delivery to allow transfer of the patient to a center with neonatal intensive care unit facilities. Agents commonly used as tocolytics in the United States include magnesium sulfate, terbutaline, indomethacin, and nifedipine (Table 47–7).[37] Few head-to-head comparisons have been made between tocolytic agents. All have limited benefits. Agent selection is based on maternal status and potential adverse drug reactions, as there is no clear first-line tocolytic drug.[37] A systematic review concludes that nifedipine offers the best benefit-to-risk ratio, but some authors opine that this conclusion is based on studies of poor quality.[38,39] Combined tocolytics and prolonged or repeated tocolytic therapy should not be used because it may lead to increased fetal risk without evidence of efficacy.[37,38]

Magnesium sulfate administered to women at risk of imminent preterm birth may prevent neonatal cerebral palsy.[40,41] The gestational age at which it should be administered is not yet established.[40,41]

The FDA has recently advised against the use of terbutaline in pregnant women due to the risk of serious side effects including increased heart rate, transient hyperglycemia, hypokalemia, cardiac arrhythmias, pulmonary edema, and myocardial ischemia.[42]

Indomethacin also prolongs pregnancy, but it has not been independently associated with decreased neonatal morbidity.[37] It may be of particular benefit in women with hydramnios.[34] Do not use after 32 weeks of pregnancy.

▶ Antibiotics

The administration of a 7-day course of parenteral (2 days) and oral therapy (5 days) with ampicillin or amoxicillin and erythromycin in the presence of premature rupture of the membranes (before 34 weeks' gestation) is associated with a delay in delivery and a reduction in maternal and neonatal morbidity.[43]

▶ Progesterone

Progesterone is recommended to prevent preterm birth in women with previous preterm delivery.[44] This medication may also be useful in women with a sonographic short cervix.[45]

Group B *Streptococcus* Infection

Maternal transmission of group B *Streptococcus* during the intrapartum period is a cause of neonatal sepsis and death. All pregnant women should be screened for group B *Streptococcus* disease using vaginal and rectal swabs between 35 and 37 weeks of gestation. Antibiotic therapy is effective in reducing the incidence of early-onset neonatal group B *Streptococcus* infection when administered to high-risk groups of women.[46] Empirical treatment should be started for group B *Streptococcus* at the time of membrane rupture and continued until delivery (Table 47–7). The antibiotic of choice for group B streptococcal disease is penicillin G, although ampicillin or clindamycin are good alternatives.[47] Resistance has developed with the use of some alternative choices for penicillin-allergic patients.

Examine the neonate for signs and symptoms of sepsis until 48 hours after birth. If present, a full diagnostic workup (including complete blood cell count and blood culture) should be initiated and empirical antibiotic therapy started.[47]

Thyroid Disorders

Care of pregestational hypothyroidism and hyperthyroidism is presented in Chapter 44.

The target thyroxine-stimulating hormone (TSH) level is below 2.5 microunits/mL (2.5 milliunits/L) in the first trimester and below 3 microunits/mL (3 milliunits/L) in the second and third trimesters.[48] Because pregnancy induces significant changes in thyroid function, transient gestational hypothyroidism or hyperthyroidism may occur and may have adverse effects on the pregnancy and the fetus/neonate, even if subclinical.[48]

Universal screening of thyroid disorders in pregnancy is debated, as well as the assessment of antibodies to thyroid peroxidase. The most appropriate management of this condition is unknown.[48]

Although there are no solid data on the impact of thyroid replacement therapy on either short-term maternal and neonatal morbidity nor on long-term infant neurologic outcomes, it is recommended to treat subclinical hypothyroidism in pregnant women.[48]

Gestational hyperthyroidism associated with hyperemesis gravidarum is self-remitting and does not require antithyroid treatment. In overt maternal hyperthyroidism, current guidelines recommend propylthiouracil in the first trimester (methimazole is associated with fetal malformations) and methimazole thereafter, because of the increased risk of hepatotoxicity with propylthiouracil (Table 47–7).[48] Check for signs of fetal hypothyroidism (induced by antithyroid drugs) or hyperthyroidism (induced by maternal thyroid-stimulating antibodies). The lowest dose necessary to keep T4 levels in the upper range of the normal should be used. I[131] should not be used in pregnancy. If required, surgery should be done in the second trimester.[48]

Evaluate TSH level 6 to 12 weeks after delivery in all women with thyroid disorders during pregnancy. All newborns must be evaluated for thyroid dysfunction. Thyroid replacement drugs and antithyroid drugs can be used during lactation.[22]

Hypertension

Hypertensive disorders in pregnancy include preexisting (chronic) hypertension and pregnancy-induced hypertension (gestational hypertension or preeclampsia). Both increase the risks of maternal and perinatal morbidity and mortality. Preeclampsia (hypertension and proteinuria) is a syndrome produced by endothelial dysfunction. Women may present with seizures (eclampsia), neurologic, hepatic, and renal and/or coagulation complications, as well as fetal death and intrauterine growth restriction. Delivery is the only treatment for preeclampsia. Intravenous magnesium sulfate may be used to prevent eclampsia (Table 47–7).[49]

Severe hypertension in pregnancy (systolic blood pressure ≥ 160 mm Hg or diastolic blood pressure ≥ 110 mm Hg) is an emergency and should be treated aggressively, under maternal and fetal monitoring (Table 47–7).[49] Treatment of nonsevere hypertension is debated. Although antihypertensive drugs do prevent severe hypertension, they do not prevent preeclampsia and could decrease fetal growth.[50] First-line drugs include methyldopa, labetalol, and nifedipine (Table 47–7). Do not use angiotensin-converting enzyme inhibitors, angiotensin receptor inhibitors, or renin inhibitors (fetopathy). Caution is advised with atenolol, as it has been associated with intrauterine growth restriction.

Low-dose aspirin (75 to 160 mg) is useful in high-risk women in preventing preeclampsia, preterm birth, and fetal/neonatal death.[51] Calcium supplements (1 g/day) are also helpful in preventing preeclampsia.[52]

See all women with hypertensive disorders 6 to 12 weeks after delivery to monitor blood pressure, proteinuria, and cardiovascular risk markers and counsel them on future pregnancy, healthy diet, and lifestyle.

Diabetes

Diabetes in pregnancy includes pregestational diabetes and gestational diabetes (Chapter 43). Women with pregestational diabetes should be counseled about the increased risk of complications such as miscarriage, fetal/neonatal death, malformations, macrosomia, and preeclampsia, as well as a need for cesarean section. Euglycemia at conception and during pregnancy is the best approach in preventing poor pregnancy outcomes. Women with type 2 diabetes may be started on insulin before pregnancy if they do not achieve optimal control with oral agents. Gestational diabetes is associated with neonatal macrosomia, preeclampsia, and cesarean section, but not with major fetal malformations.

Diet and exercise are important nonpharmacologic treatments. Weight gain during pregnancy should be adapted to prepregnancy weight.

Insulin is the first-line treatment during pregnancy. Although limited data are available on long-acting insulins (detemir, glargine), they could be continued if diabetes control is satisfactory. In women with gestational diabetes, glyburide and metformin represent interesting alternatives.[53] Metformin and glyburide do not cause fetal malformations. Limited data are available for other antidiabetic agents. Metformin may be used in women with polycystic ovary syndrome to decrease miscarriage and gestational diabetes.[54]

Intravenous drip insulin should be used during labor. After delivery, insulin doses are decreased to pregestational doses to prevent maternal hypoglycemia.

Limited data are available on use of hypoglycemic agents during lactation. Insulin should be used if glucose levels are very high. Metformin may be used during lactation based on its pharmacologic profile, but follow-up data in infants are lacking.

Evaluate for the presence of underlying diabetes in all women with gestational diabetes with a 75-g oral glucose tolerance test 6 to 12 weeks after delivery. Counsel these women on healthy diet, weight loss, and exercise.

Anticoagulation

Heparins are used for various purposes during and after pregnancy: treatment or prevention of thromboembolism, prevention of prosthetic heart valve thrombosis, and prevention of pregnancy complications. The risk of thromboembolic events is increased during pregnancy and postpartum, and anticoagulation is required in some women during these periods, even if they were not anticoagulated before pregnancy.[55]

Low-molecular-weight heparins are preferred to unfractionated heparin. Both are safe during pregnancy and lactation. Doses should be specific to the underlying condition (consult reference 55).

Women with prosthetic heart valves should be managed by a multidisciplinary specialist team. Warfarin may be used in these women in the second trimester and early third trimester since valve thrombosis has been reported with heparin therapy, but warfarin is associated with bleeding at delivery and a risk of teratogenesis during the first trimester after 6 weeks of gestational age (Table 47-3).[55]

Anticoagulation should be used after delivery in women at high risk of thromboembolism.[55]

Warfarin and heparins are safe for use during lactation.[22]

Enhancement of Lactation

Optimization of breast-feeding techniques is the first approach when decreased lactation is suspected. No drug is currently approved by the FDA for lactation enhancement, but dopamine antagonists, metoclopramide and domperidone, which increase prolactin levels are sometimes used for this purpose.[56,57] Metoclopramide's maternal side effects include fatigue, irritability, headache, and extrapyramidal symptoms. Very few side effects in the infant have been reported. However, domperidone is not available in the United States, and the FDA issued a warning against domperidone use in 2004 owing to reports of cardiac arrhythmia and sudden death associated with high IV doses prescribed for gastric disorders in cancer patients.[57]

Mastitis

Bacterial mastitis is seen typically within the first 6 weeks of breast-feeding and is characterized by localized signs of inflammation (redness, swelling, heat, or pain), and engorgement. Fever, shivering, and malaise can also occur. The most commonly encountered bacteria are *Staphylococcus aureus* (including methicillin-resistant), followed by *Streptococcus, Staphylococcus epidermidis*, and *E. coli*.[58]

Nonpharmacologic measures, such as cold or warm compresses and more frequent breast-feeding or breast pumping, should be encouraged. Several antibiotics can be used (Table 47–7). Analgesics (e.g., acetaminophen, ibuprofen, or naproxen) can be used to relieve pain.[22,58,59]

Breast Candidiasis

Diagnosis of breast candidiasis is mainly based on signs and symptoms. Candidiasis presents with severe and persistent nipple pain, which can be throbbing and radiating to the breasts and back. The pain is usually more intense during and immediately after breast-feeding. The breast-fed infant can be symptomatic or asymptomatic. *Candida albicans* is the most commonly found type of *Candida* species. It is recommended to breast-feed more frequently than usual for a shorter period of time. Milk does not have to be discarded; however, clothes and towels in contact with the breasts and the baby's mouth should be washed in hot water. Antifungal

treatment must be given to the mother and the baby simultaneously (Table 47–7). If no improvement is seen within 24 to 48 hours, the treatment should be reevaluated. Analgesics (e.g., acetaminophen, ibuprofen, or naproxen) can be used to relieve pain.[60]

Patient Care and Monitoring

1. Provide prenatal counseling regarding lifestyle modifications (healthy diet, exercise, avoidance of tobacco, alcohol, and illicit or unnecessary drugs) and medication use during pregnancy. When possible, attain good control of maternal medical conditions prior to conception. Identify patients at risk of psychosocial problems. Immunize as needed (avoid live vaccines).

2. Perform routine screening at first appointment during pregnancy
   - Hematocrit and hemoglobin levels
   - Urinalysis and urine culture
   - Determination of blood group and Rhesus type
   - Determination of immunity to rubella virus
   - Syphilis and sexually transmitted diseases
   - Cervical cytology (if needed)
   - Hepatitis B surface antigen
   - HIV antibody testing

3. Recommend appropriate folic acid and multivitamins prior to conception.

4. After pregnancy is achieved, encourage lifestyle modifications, routine pregnancy monitoring and care, and medication adherence.

5. ❻ *When possible, treat pregnancy conditions with nonpharmacologic treatments instead of using drug therapy.*

6. When considering pharmacologic treatment, evaluate the following:

   ❼ *Evaluate the need for treatment, including benefits and risks. Avoid treatments that have not shown evidence of benefit and those that can be delayed until after pregnancy and breast-feeding.*

   - Are the symptoms related to benign conditions of pregnancy (e.g., palpitations)? How bothersome are the symptoms (e.g., nausea and vomiting)? In case of chronic treatment, does it need to be continued during pregnancy (e.g., dyslipidemia)? Is the condition interfering with other pathologies (e.g., nausea and diabetes)? Could starting/continuing/stopping the treatment pose a risk for the fetus/neonate?
   - Is an effective treatment available?
   - What are the maternal side effects of the drug?
   - Which is the best drug when used alone?
   - Which is the drug with the best safety data in pregnancy/lactation?

7. Encourage breast-feeding. If maternal drug therapy is required during breast-feeding, try to choose short-acting agents with the longest history of safe use in lactation, and administer immediately after feedings.
   - Avoid treatments that have shown no evidence of benefit or that can be delayed until after breast-feeding.
   - If possible, select drugs that are used in neonates or children and that are well tolerated.
   - When possible, select drugs that yield low percentages of pediatric or relative infant doses (preferably less than 10%).
   - Consider infant age when analyzing safety of a drug during breast-feeding. Premature or very young children will be more sensitive to drug effects than older children.
   - Avoid drugs that can hinder breast milk production.

8. Monitor infants for birth defects and/or unusual reactions that may be due to maternal drug use. Report suspected drug-related reactions to the FDA or pharmaceutical companies.

Abbreviations Introduced in This Chapter

ACOG	American College of Obstetricians and Gynecologists
CDC	Centers for Disease Control and Prevention
GA	Gestational age
NSAID	Nonsteroidal anti-inflammatory drug
NTD	Neural tube defect
OTIS	Organization of Teratology Information Specialists
PCA	Postconceptional age
RPR	Rapid Plasma Reagin
STEPS	System for Thalidomide Education and Prescribing Safety
STI	Sexually Transmitted Infection
T4	Levothyroxine
TSH	Thyroxine-stimulating hormone
VDRL	Venereal Disease Research Laboratory

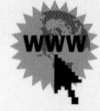 Self-assessment questions and answers are available at *http://mhpharmacotherapy.com/pp.html*.

REFERENCES

1. Refuerzo JS, Blackwell SC, Sokol RJ, et al. Use of over-the-counter medications and herbal remedies in pregnancy. Am J Perinatol 2005;22:321–324.
2. Andrade SE, Gurwitz JH, Davis RL, et al. Prescription drug use in pregnancy. Am J Obstet Gynecol 2004;191:398–407.
3. Briggs GG. Drug effects on the fetus and breast-fed infant. Clin Obstet Gynecol 2002;45:6–21.
4. Schirm E, Schwagermann MP, Tobi H, de Jong-van den Berg LT. Drug use during breastfeeding. A survey from the Netherlands. Eur J Clin Nutr 2004;58:386–390.
5. Miller R, Peters P, Schaefer C. General commentary on drug therapy and drug risks in pregnancy. In: Schaefer C, Peters P, Miller R, eds. Drugs During Pregnancy and Lactation, Treatment Options and Risk Assessment, 2nd ed. Amsterdam: Elsevier, 2007:1–26.
6. Ferreira E, ed. Grossesse et Allaitement: Guide Thérapeutique. Montreal: Editions CHU Ste-Justine, 2007.
7. Obican S, Scialli AR. Teratogenic exposures. Am J Med Genet C Semin Med Genet 2011;157:150–169.
8. Friedman JM. How do we know if an exposure is actually teratogenic in humans? Am J Med Genet C Semin Med Genet 2011;157:170–174.
9. Kweder SL. Drugs and biologics in pregnancy and breastfeeding: FDA in the 21st century. Birth Defects Res A Clin Mol Teratol 2008;82:605–609.
10. Conover EA, Polifka JE. The art and science of teratogen risk communication. Am J Med Genet C Semin Med Genet 2011;157:227–233.
11. Polifka JE, Friedman JM. Medical genetics: 1. Clinical teratology in the age of genomics. CMAJ 2002;167:265–273.
12. Centers for Disease Control and Prevention. Recommendations to improve preconception health and health care—United States. MMWR Recomm Rep 2006;55:1–23.
13. US Preventive Services Task Force [Internet]. Screening for asymptomatic bacteriuria. 2005, *http://www.ahrq.gov/clinic/3rduspstf/asymbac/asymbacrs.htm*
14. Goh YI, Koren G. Folic acid in pregnancy and fetal outcomes. J Obstet Gynaecol 2008;28:3–13.
15. Cheschier N. ACOG practice bulletin. Neural tube defects. Number 44, July 2003. (Replaces committee opinion number 252, March 2001). Int J Gynaecol Obstet 2003;83:123–133.

16. Wilson RD, Johnson JA, Wyatt P, et al. Pre-conceptional vitamin/folic acid supplementation 2007: The use of folic acid in combination with a multivitamin supplement for the prevention of neural tube defects and other congenital anomalies. J Obstet Gynaecol Can 2007;29:1003–1026.
17. ACOG Practice Bulletin No. 95: Anemia in pregnancy. Obstet Gynecol 2008;112:201–207.
18. Dawes M, Chowienczyk PJ. Drugs in pregnancy. Pharmacokinetics in pregnancy. Best Pract Res Clin Obstet Gynaecol 2001;15:819–826.
19. Anderson GD. Pregnancy-induced changes in pharmacokinetics: A mechanistic-based approach. Clin Pharmacokinet 2005;44:989–1008.
20. Hebert MF, Carr DB, Anderson GD, et al. Pharmacokinetics and pharmacodynamics of atenolol during pregnancy and postpartum. J Clin Pharmacol 2005;45:25–33.
21. Gartner LM, Morton J, Lawrence RA, et al. Breastfeeding and the use of human milk. Pediatrics 2005;115:496–506.
22. Hale T. Medications and Mother's Milk, 14th ed. Amarillo, TX: Hale Publishing, 2010.
23. ACOG Practice Bulletin: Nausea and vomiting of pregnancy. Obstet Gynecol 2004;103:803–814.
24. Cullen G, O'Donoghue D. Constipation and pregnancy. Best Pract Res Clin Gastroenterol 2007;21:807–818.
25. Dowswell T, Neilson JP. Interventions for heartburn in pregnancy. Cochrane Database Syst Rev 2008:CD007065.
26. Gill SK, O'Brien L, Einarson TR, Koren G. The safety of proton pump inhibitors (PPIs) in pregnancy: a meta-analysis. Am J Gastroenterol 2009;104:1541–1545; quiz 0, 6.
27. Briggs G, Freeman R, Yaffe S. Drugs in Pregnancy and Lactation, 9th ed. Philadephia: Lippincott Williams & Wilkins, 2011.
28. Ellegard EK. Pregnancy rhinitis. Immunol Allergy Clin North Am 2006;26:119–135, vii.
29. Jolley JA, Wing DA. Pyelonephritis in pregnancy: An update on treatment options for optimal outcomes. Drugs 2010;70:1643–1655.
30. Smaill F, Vazquez JC. Antibiotics for asymptomatic bacteriuria in pregnancy. Cochrane Database Syst Rev 2007:CD000490.
31. Vazquez JC, Abalos E. Treatments for symptomatic urinary tract infections during pregnancy. Cochrane Database Syst Rev 2011:CD002256.
32. Greer LG, Roberts SW, Sheffield JS, et al. Ampicillin resistance and outcome differences in acute antepartum pyelonephritis. Infect Dis Obstet Gynecol 2008;2008:891426.
33. ACOG Committee Opinion No. 494: Sulfonamides, nitrofurantoin, and risk of birth defects. Obstet Gynecol 2011;117:1484–1485.
34. Workowski KA, Berman S. Sexually transmitted diseases treatment guidelines, 2010. MMWR Recomm Rep 2010;59:1–110.
35. ACOG Committee Opinion No. 475: Antenatal corticosteroid therapy for fetal maturation. Obstet Gynecol 2011;117:422–424.
36. Crowther CA, McKinlay CJ, Middleton P, Harding JE. Repeat doses of prenatal corticosteroids for women at risk of preterm birth for improving neonatal health outcomes. Cochrane Database Syst Rev 2011:CD003935.
37. ACOG practice bulletin. Management of preterm labor. Number 43, May 2003. Int J Gynaecol Obstet 2003;82:127–135.
38. King JF, Flenady VJ, Papatsonis DN, et al. Calcium channel blockers for inhibiting preterm labour. Cochrane Database Syst Rev 2003: CD002255.
39. Lamont RF, Khan KS, Beattie B, et al. The quality of nifedipine studies used to assess tocolytic efficacy: A systematic review. J Perinat Med 2005;33:287–295.
40. Committee Opinion No. 455: Magnesium sulfate before anticipated preterm birth for neuroprotection. Obstet Gynecol 2010;115:669–671.
41. Doyle LW, Crowther CA, Middleton P, et al. Magnesium sulphate for women at risk of preterm birth for neuroprotection of the fetus. Cochrane Database Syst Rev 2009:CD004661.
42. FDA [Internet]. FDA Drug Safety Communication: New warnings against use of terbutaline to treat preterm labor [cited 2011 Oct 10]. Available from: *http://www.fda.gov/Drugs/DrugSafety/ucm243539.htm*
43. ACOG Committee Opinion No. 445: antibiotics for preterm labor. Obstet Gynecol 2009;114:1159–1160.
44. ACOG Committee Opinion number 419 October 2008 (replaces no. 291, November 2003). Use of progesterone to reduce preterm birth. Obstet Gynecol 2008;112:963–965.

45. Hassan SS, Romero R, Vidyadhari D, et al. Vaginal progesterone reduces the rate of preterm birth in women with a sonographic short cervix: a multicenter, randomized, double-blind, placebo-controlled trial. Ultrasound Obstet Gynecol 2011;38:18–31.

46. ACOG Committee Opinion No. 485: Prevention of early-onset group Bstreptococcal disease in newborns. Obstet Gynecol 2011;117:1019–1027.

47. Verani JR, McGee L, Schrag SJ. Prevention of perinatal group B streptococcal disease—revised guidelines from CDC, 2010. MMWR Recomm Rep 2010;59:1–36.

48. Stagnaro-Green A, Abalovich M, Alexander E, et al. Guidelines of the American Thyroid Association for the diagnosis and management of thyroid disease during pregnancy and postpartum. Thyroid 2011;21:1081–125.

49. Visintin C, Mugglestone MA, Almerie MQ, et al. Management of hypertensive disorders during pregnancy: Summary of NICE guidance. BMJ 2010;341:c2207.

50. von Dadelszen P, Ornstein MP, Bull SB, et al. Fall in mean arterial pressure and fetal growth restriction in pregnancy hypertension: A meta-analysis. Lancet 2000;355:87–92.

51. Askie LM, Duley L, Henderson-Smart DJ, Stewart LA. Antiplatelet agents for prevention of pre-eclampsia: A meta-analysis of individual patient data. Lancet 2007;369:1791–1798.

52. Imdad A, Jabeen A, Bhutta ZA. Role of calcium supplementation during pregnancy in reducing risk of developing gestational hypertensive disorders: A meta-analysis of studies from developing countries. BMC Public Health 2011;11 Suppl 3:S18.

53. Dhulkotia JS, Ola B, Fraser R, Farrell T. Oral hypoglycemic agents vs insulin in management of gestational diabetes: A systematic review and metaanalysis. Am J Obstet Gynecol 2010;203:457 e1–9.

54. Nawaz FH, Rizvi J. Continuation of metformin reduces early pregnancy loss in obese Pakistani women with polycystic ovarian syndrome. Gynecol Obstet Invest 2010;69:184–189.

55. Bates SM, Greer IA, Pabinger I, et al. Venous thromboembolism, thrombophilia, antithrombotic therapy, and pregnancy: American College of Chest Physicians Evidence-Based Clinical Practice Guidelines (8th Edition). Chest 2008;133:844S–886S.

56. ABM Clinical Protocol #9: Use of galactogogues in initiating or augmenting the rate of maternal milk secretion (First Revision January 2011). Breastfeed Med 2011;6:41–49.

57. Zuppa AA, Sindico P, Orchi C, et al. Safety and efficacy of galactogogues: substances that induce, maintain and increase breast milk production. J Pharm Pharm Sci 2010;13:162–174.

58. Dixon JM, Khan LR. Treatment of breast infection. BMJ 2011;342:d396.

59. Jahanfar S, Ng CJ, Teng CL. Antibiotics for mastitis in breastfeeding women. Cochrane Database Syst Rev 2009:CD005458.

60. Wiener S. Diagnosis and management of Candida of the nipple and breast. J Midwifery Womens Health 2006;51:125–128.

61. March of Dimes [Internet]. Peristats [cited 2011 Oct 10]. Available from: *http://www.marchofdimes.com/peristats/*

62. Schardein J, ed. Chemically induced birth defects. New York: Dekker, 2000.

63. Folic acid for the prevention of neural tube defects: U.S. Preventive Services Task Force recommendation statement. Ann Intern Med 2009;150:626–631.

64. Anotayanonth S, Subhedar NV, Garner P, et al. Betamimetics for inhibiting preterm labour. Cochrane Database Syst Rev 2004:CD004352.

65. Crowley P. Prophylactic corticosteroids for preterm birth. Cochrane Database Syst Rev 2000:CD000065.

66. Di Renzo GC, Roura LC. Guidelines for the management of spontaneous preterm labor. J Perinat Med 2006;34:359–366.

48 Contraception

Julia M. Koehler and Kathleen B. Haynes

LEARNING OBJECTIVES

● **Upon completion of the chapter, the reader will be able to:**

1. Discuss the physiology of the normal female reproductive system.

2. Compare the efficacy of oral contraceptives with that of other methods of contraception.

3. State the mechanism of action of hormonal contraceptives.

4. Discuss the risks associated with the use of contraceptives, and state absolute and relative contraindications to their use.

5. List side effects associated with the use of various contraceptives, and recommend strategies for minimizing or eliminating such side effects.

6. Describe advantages and disadvantages of various contraceptives, including both oral and nonoral formulations.

7. Cite important drug interactions that may occur with oral contraceptives.

8. Provide appropriate patient education regarding the important differences between various barrier methods of contraception.

9. Discuss how emergency contraception (EC) may be employed to prevent accidental pregnancy.

10. Provide appropriate patient education regarding the use of oral contraceptives, and recommend and discuss the use of nonoral contraceptives when appropriate.

KEY CONCEPTS

❶ Heavy smokers (greater than or equal to 15 cigarettes per day) who are 35 years of age or older as well as patients with a history of thromboembolic disease, stroke, coronary artery or ischemic heart disease, peripheral vascular disease, any estrogen-dependent neoplasm, undiagnosed abnormal uterine or vaginal bleeding, or migraine headache disorder with focal neurologic deficits should not take estrogen-containing contraceptives.

❷ Side effects associated with the use of combination oral contraceptives may be minimized by appropriately adjusting either the total estrogen or progestin content.

❸ Clinicians should be aware of the many drugs that may potentially interact with contraceptives—especially those that may reduce the effectiveness of contraceptives.

❹ Nonoral forms of contraceptives, such as the transdermal patch and the transvaginal ring, eliminate the need for daily administration and, as such, may enhance patient convenience and adherence.

❺ Oral, transdermal, and transvaginal contraceptives, as well as intrauterine devices (IUDs) and most barrier contraceptives, do not protect against sexually transmitted diseases (STDs).

❻ When a contraceptive dose is missed, the risk of accidental pregnancy may be increased. Depending on how many doses were missed, the contraceptive formulation being used, and the phase of the cycle during which doses were missed, counseling regarding the use of additional methods of contraception may be warranted.

Historically, the 1950s represented an important time in the control of human fertility. It was during that decade that the first combination oral contraceptives (COCs) were developed. Shortly after the discovery that the exogenous administration of hormones such as progesterone successfully blocked ovulation, the use of hormonal steroids quickly became the most popular method of contraception worldwide. Specifically, COCs represent the most commonly used reversible form of contraception today, and it is estimated that nearly 100 million women worldwide take oral contraceptives.[1] Of the 62 million women in the United States who are of childbearing age (15 to 44 years), it is estimated that more than 38 million are currently using a contraceptive method.[2] Although the choice of contraceptive method varies greatly according to the age of the user, oral contraceptives are the leading choice among women in the United States who are under the age of 30.[2] Since the introduction of oral contraceptives, many newer forms of contraceptives have been developed and are available for use in the United States. Today, a variety of hormone delivery systems, such as transdermal systems, transvaginal systems, and intrauterine devices (IUDs), are available and offer women effective and potentially more convenient alternatives to oral contraceptives.

EPIDEMIOLOGY

According to the National Survey of Family Growth, approximately 6.39 million pregnancies occur annually in the United States.[3] It is estimated that nearly half of all pregnancies that occur each year in the United States are unintended.[2,3] Contributing to the risk of unintended pregnancy is the fact that approximately 7% of all women who are at risk of becoming pregnant do not use any form of contraception.[2,3] In addition, many women who do use contraceptives use their chosen method of contraception imperfectly, and this also increases the risk of unintended pregnancy. For patients with certain medical conditions, such as epilepsy, hypertension, ischemic heart disease, sickle cell disease, lupus, or thromboembolic mutations, unintended pregnancy can further increase the risk for adverse health events.[4] The provision of appropriate and adequate instruction to patients regarding how to use contraceptive methods effectively is essential in order to reduce the risk of unintended pregnancy and, for some women, the associated increase in risk for adverse health-related events.

Exposure to STDs is also a concern for women who are sexually active. It is estimated that 19 million people in the United States become newly infected annually with an STD.[5] Given that not all methods of contraception protect the user against STDs, the provision of proper patient education by healthcare professionals regarding this risk is absolutely essential.

PHYSIOLOGY

The female menstrual cycle is divided into four functional phases: follicular, ovulatory, luteal, and menstrual.[6] The follicular phase begins the cycle, and ovulation generally occurs around day 14. The luteal phase then begins and continues until menstruation occurs.[6] The menstrual cycle is regulated by a negative-feedback hormone loop between the hypothalamus, anterior pituitary gland, and ovaries[6] (Fig. 48–1).

Initially, the hypothalamus releases gonadotropin-releasing hormone (GnRH), which stimulates the anterior pituitary to produce follicle-stimulating hormone (FSH) and luteinizing hormone (LH). The levels of FSH and LH released vary depending on the phase of the menstrual cycle. Just prior to ovulation, FSH and LH both are at their peak levels. The FSH helps to promote growth of the follicle in preparation for ovulation by causing granulosa cells lining the follicle to grow and produce estrogen. The LH promotes androgen production by theca cells in the follicle, promotes ovulation and oocyte maturation, and converts granulosa cells to cells that secrete progesterone after ovulation.

Conception is most likely to occur when viable sperm are present in the upper region of the reproductive tract at the time of ovulation. Fertilization occurs when a spermatozoan penetrates an ovum. Approximately 6 to 8 days after ovulation, attachment of the early embryo to the lining of the uterine cavity—implantation—occurs.

PREVENTION OF PREGNANCY: CONTRACEPTIVES AND DEVICES
Goals of Contraception/Desired Outcome

The most common goal of contraception is the prevention of pregnancy. However, some patients use contraceptive methods for other benefits, such as menstrual cycle regulation, reduction of premenstrual symptoms, or treatment of acne.

Choice of Contraceptives: Important Considerations

When helping a patient with contraceptive selection, the most important goal is finding an option the patient is comfortable with and the clinician feels is beneficial for the patient. It is imperative to explain the side effects, safety concerns, and noncontraceptive benefits of each alternative to the patient so that she may make an informed decision. Fertility goals vary for each patient. It must be determined whether the goal is to postpone conception, space out the next pregnancy, or avoid further pregnancy altogether. Also, a clinician must understand the patient's desire to have or not have a regular bleeding pattern, because many contraceptives will affect menses.

As discussed later in this chapter, contraindications exist for various forms of contraception. Patients must be evaluated by a healthcare professional to rule out medical contraindications to certain contraceptives. The physical examination also allows healthcare professionals to identify other medical concerns, such as hypertension, diabetes, or liver disease, that need to be considered when selecting an appropriate contraceptive agent. Clinicians also should review family history for potential risks with certain forms of birth control.

Sexual behavior of the female must be determined to understand the risk for STDs. Women not in a monogamous relationship must consider their risk of STDs as a factor in their contraceptive decision. Some barrier methods protect against STDs, but hormonal contraceptives do not prevent STDs if used alone.

Personal preference plays a large role when determining the best contraceptive option. For instance, if a woman is not interested in using a method that interrupts sexual activity,

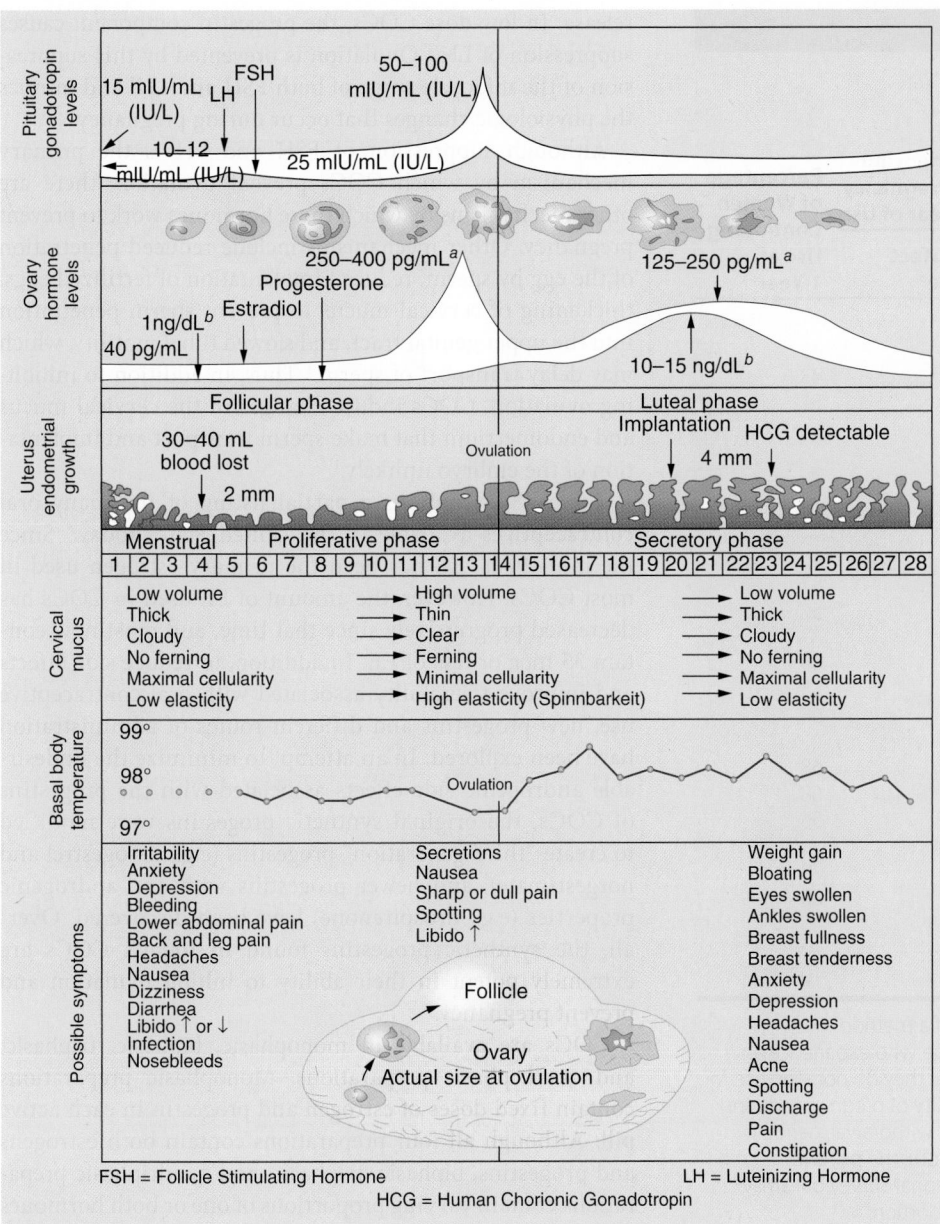

FIGURE 48-1. Menstrual cycle events. [a]Estradiol: 40 pg/mL = 147 pmol/L; 250 to 400 pg/mL = 918 to 1,468 pmol/L; 125 to 250 pg/mL = 459 to 918 pmol/L. [b]Progesterone: 1 ng/dL = 0.032 nmol/L; 10 to 15 ng/dL = 0.32 to 0.48 nmol/L. (Adapted with permission from Hatcher RA, Namnoum AB. The menstrual cycle. In: Hatcher RA, Trussel J, Nelson AL, et al. Contraceptive Technology, 19th rev. ed. New York: Ardent Media, 2007:7–18.)

then a diaphragm would be an inappropriate choice. Preference of the sexual partner may also be important. Certain agents such as male condoms require the male partner to play an active role in contraception.

Cost may also be an issue for patients. Insurance may not cover all forms of contraception, and patients may have to bear the entire cost for certain options.

Efficacy of Contraceptives

● The accidental pregnancy rate for women who do not use any form of contraception is unknown. Therefore, it is difficult to determine the true efficacy of contraceptives in preventing unwanted pregnancy. Table 48-1 shows the percentage of women who experience unintended pregnancy within 1 year of contraceptive use with ongoing sexual activity.[7]

Oral Contraceptives (Combination)

COCs contain a synthetic estrogen and one of several steroids with progestational activity. Most oral contraceptives contain one of three types of estrogen: ethinyl estradiol (EE), which is pharmacologically active; mestranol, which is converted by the liver to EE; or estradiol valerate, which is metabolized to estradiol and valeric acid. Many different progestins are found in the various oral contraceptives. These include norethindrone, norethindrone acetate, ethynodiol diacetate, norgestrel, levonorgestrel, desogestrel, norgestimate, drospirenone, and dienogest.

● The primary mechanism by which COCs prevent pregnancy is through inhibition of ovulation. FSH and LH regulate the production of estrogen and progesterone by the ovaries. Secretion of estrogen and progesterone by the

Table 48–1

Unintended Pregnancy Rates

Method	Percentage of Women Experiencing Unintended Pregnancy Within First Year of Use		Percentage of Women Continuing Use at 1 Year[c]
	Typical Use[a]	Perfect Use[b]	
No method	85	85	
Spermicides	29	18	42
Withdrawal	27	4	43
Fertility awareness–based methods	25		51
Standard days method		5	
Two-day method		4	
Sponge			
Parous women	32	20	46
Nulliparous women	16	9	57
Diaphragm	16	6	57
Condom			
Female (reality)	21	5	49
Male	15	2	53
Combination pill and mini-pill	8	0.3	68
Ortho Evra patch	8	0.3	68
NuvaRing	8	0.3	68
Depo-Provera	3	0.3	56
IUD			
ParaGard (copper T)	0.8	0.6	78
Mirena (LNG-IUS)	0.2	0.2	80
Implanon	0.05	0.05	
Female sterilization	0.5	0.5	100
Male sterilization	0.15	0.1	100

[a]Among *typical* couples who initiate use of a method (not necessarily for the first time), the percentage who experience an accidental pregnancy during the first year if they do not stop use for any other reason. Estimates of the probability of pregnancy during the first year of typical use for spermicides, withdrawal, periodic abstinence, the diaphragm, the male condom, the pill, and Depo-Provera are taken from the 1995 National Survey of Family Growth corrected for under-reporting of abortion.

[b]Among couples who initiate use of a method (not necessarily for the first time) and who use it *perfectly* (both consistently and correctly), the percentage who experience an accidental pregnancy during the first year if they do not stop use for any other reason.

[c]Among couples attempting to avoid pregnancy, the percentage who continue to use a method for 1 year.

Adapted from Trussel J. Choosing a contraceptive: Efficacy, safety, and personal considerations. In: Hatcher RA, Trussel J, Nelson AL, et al. Contraceptive Technology, 19th rev. ed. New York: Ardent Media, 2007:19–48.

ovaries occurs in a cyclic manner, which determines the regular hormonal changes that occur in the uterus, vagina, and cervix associated with the menstrual cycle. Cyclic changes in the levels of estrogen and progesterone in the blood, together with FSH and LH, modulate the development of ova and the occurrence of ovulation. The estrogen component of COCs is most active in inhibiting FSH release.[1] However, at sufficiently high doses, estrogens also may cause inhibition of LH release. In low-dose COCs, the progestin component causes suppression of LH.[1] Ovulation is prevented by this suppression of the midcycle surge of both FSH and LH[1] and mimics the physiologic changes that occur during pregnancy.

Although suppression of FSH and LH is the primary mechanism by which COCs prevent ovulation, there are other mechanisms by which these hormones work to prevent pregnancy. Other mechanisms include reduced penetration of the egg by sperm, reduced implantation of fertilized eggs, thickening of cervical mucus to prevent sperm penetration into the upper genital tract, and slowed tubal motility, which may delay transport of sperm.[1] Thus, in addition to inhibiting ovulation, COCs induce changes in the cervical mucus and endometrium that make sperm transport and implantation of the embryo unlikely.[1]

Table 48–2 contains a partial listing of the many oral contraceptives available in the United States today.[8] Since the mid-1960s, EE has been the primary estrogen used in most COCs. However, the amount of EE used in COCs has decreased progressively since that time, and most now contain 35 mcg or less of EE. In addition, to reduce side effects and improve tolerability associated with oral contraceptive use, new progestins and different routes of administration have been explored. In an attempt to minimize the undesirable androgenic side effects associated with the progestins of COCs, the original synthetic progestins were modified to create "third generation" progestins (e.g., desogestrel and norgestimate), and newer progestins with anti-androgenic properties (e.g., drospirenone) have been discovered. Overall, the synthetic progestins found in today's COCs are extremely potent in their ability to inhibit ovulation and prevent pregnancy.

COCs are available in monophasic, biphasic, triphasic, and quadriphasic preparations. Monophasic preparations contain fixed doses of estrogen and progestin in each active pill. Although all four preparations contain both estrogens and progestins, biphasic, triphasic, and quadriphasic preparations contain varying proportions of one or both hormones during the pill cycle. These preparations were introduced to reduce a patient's cumulative exposure to progestins, as well as to mimic more closely the hormonal changes of the menstrual cycle. However, there is no evidence to suggest that the multiphasic preparations offer any significant clinical advantage over monophasic pills.[8]

Most traditional COCs are packaged as 21/7 cycles (i.e., 21 days of active pills and 7 days of placebo). However, newer regimens offer either fewer hormone-free days per traditional, 28-day pill cycle or extended (or in some cases continuous) cycles, which may allow for fewer withdrawal bleeds per year and fewer menstrual-related side effects (e.g., menstrual pain, bloating, headaches) for some women.

▶ Noncontraceptive Benefits of Combination Oral Contraceptives

In addition to preventing pregnancy, there are several noncontraceptive benefits associated with the use of COCs. Some of these potential benefits are highlighted next.

Table 48–2

Some Available Oral Contraceptives

Brand Name	Estrogen (mcg/Tablet)	Progestin (mg/Tablet)
Monophasic Preparations		
Junel Fe 1/20	EE (20)	Norethindrone acetate (1)
Loestrin Fe 1/20	EE (20)	Norethindrone acetate (1)
Loestrin 24 Fe	EE (20)	Norethindrone acetate (1)
Microgestin Fe 1/20	EE (20)	Norethindrone acetate (1)
Alesse	EE (20)	Levonorgestrel (0.1)
Yaz	EE (20)	Drospirenone (3)
Beyaz[a]	EE (20)	Drospirenone (3)
Desogen	EE (30)	Desogestrel (0.15)
Ortho-Cept	EE (30)	Desogestrel (0.15)
Reclipsen	EE (30)	Desogestrel (0.15)
Levlen	EE (30)	Levonorgestrel (0.15)
Levora	EE (30)	Levonorgestrel (0.15)
Nordette	EE (30)	Levonorgestrel (0.15)
Portia	EE (30)	Levonorgestrel (0.15)
Safyral	EE (30)	Drospirenone (3)
Yasmin	EE (30)	Drospirenone (3)
Cryselle	EE (30)	Norgestrel (0.3)
Lo/Ovral	EE (30)	Norgestrel (0.3)
Low-Ogestrel	EE (30)	Norgestrel (0.3)
Junel Fe 1.5/30	EE (30)	Norethindrone acetate (1.5)
Loestrin Fe 1.5/30	EE (30)	Norethindrone acetate (1.5)
Microgestin Fe 1.5/30	EE (30)	Norethindrone acetate (1.5)
MonoNessa	EE (35)	Norgestimate (0.25)
Ortho-Cyclen	EE (35)	Norgestimate (0.25)
Balziva	EE (35)	Norethindrone (0.4)
Femcon Fe	EE (35)	Norethindrone (0.4)
Ovcon-35	EE (35)	Norethindrone (0.4)
Brevicon	EE (35)	Norethindrone (0.5)
Modicon	EE (35)	Norethindrone (0.5)
Necon 0.5/35	EE (35)	Norethindrone (0.5)
Nortrel 0.5/35	EE (35)	Norethindrone (0.5)
Necon 1/35	EE (35)	Norethindrone (1)
Norinyl 1+35	EE (35)	Norethindrone (1)
Nortrel	EE (35)	Norethindrone (1)
Ortho-Novum 1/35	EE (35)	Norethindrone (1)
Kelnor	EE (35)	Ethynodiol diacetate (1)
Zovia 1/35E	EE (35)	Ethynodiol diacetate (1)
Ogestrel 0.5/50	EE (50)	Norgestrel (0.5)
Zovia 1/50E	EE (50)	Ethynodiol diacetate (1)
Necon 1/50	Mestranol (50)	Norethindrone (1)
Norinyl 1 + 50	Mestranol (50)	Norethindrone (1)
Biphasic Preparations		
Lo Loestrin Fe	EE (10, 10)	Norethindrone acetate (1, 0)
Kariva	EE (20, 0, 10)	Desogestrel (0.15)
Mircette	EE (20, 0,10)	Desogestrel (0.15)
Triphasic Preparations		
Estrostep Fe	EE (20, 30, 35)	Norethindrone acetate (1)
Tilia Fe	EE (20, 30, 35)	Norethindrone acetate (1)
Tri-Legest Fe	EE (20, 30, 35)	Norethindrone acetate (1)
Enpresse	EE (30, 40, 30)	Levonorgestrel (0.50, 0.075, 0.125)
Triphasil	EE (30, 40, 30)	Levonorgestrel (0.05, 0.075, 0.125)
Trivora	EE (30, 40, 30)	Levonorgestrel (0.05, 0.075, 0.125)
Enpresse	EE (30, 40, 30)	Levonorgestrel (0.05, 0.075, 0.125)
Ortho Tri-Cyclen	EE (35)	Norgestimate (0.18, 0.215, 0.25)
Tri-Nessa	EE (35)	Norgestimate (0.18, 0.125, 0.25)
Tri-Previfem	EE (35)	Norgestimate (0.18, 0.125, 0.25)
Tri-Sprintec	EE (35)	Norgestimate (0.18, 0.125, 0.25)
Aranelle	EE (35)	Norethindrone (0.5, 1, 0.5)
Leena	EE (35)	Norethindrone (0.5, 1, 0.5)
Tri-Norinyl	EE (35)	Norethindrone (0.5, 1, 0.5)
Ortho-Novum 7/7/7	EE (35)	Norethindrone (0.5, 0.75, 1)
Necon 7/7/7	EE (35)	Norethindrone (0.5, 0.75, 1)
Nortrel 7/7/7	EE (35)	Norethindrone (0.5, 0.75, 1)
Ortho Tri-Cyclen Lo	EE (25)	Norgestimate (0.18, 0.215, 0.25)
TriLo Sprintec	EE (25)	Norgestimate (0.18, 0.215, 0.25)
Velivet	EE (25)	Desogestrel (0.1, 0.125, 0.15)
Cyclessa	EE (25)	Desogestrel (0.1, 0.125, 0.15)
Quadriphasic Preparations		
Natazia	Estradiol valerate (3, 2, 2, 1)	Dienogest (0, 2, 3, 0)
Extended Cycle Preparations		
Lybrel	EE (20)	Levonorgestrel (0.09)
Introvale	EE (30)	Levonorgestrel (0.15)
Quasense	EE (30)	Levonorgestrel (0.15)
Seasonale	EE (30)	Levonorgestrel (0.15)
LoSeasonique	EE (20,10)	Levonorgestrel (0.1)
Seasonique	EE (30,10)	Levonorgestrel (0.15)
Progestin-Only Preparations		
Camila		Norethindrone (0.35)
Errin		Norethindrone (0.35)
Heather		Norethindrone (0.35)
Jolivette		Norethindrone (0.35)
Micronor		Norethindrone (0.35)
Nora-BE		Norethindrone (0.35)
Nor-QD		Norethindrone (0.35)

EE, ethinyl estradiol.

[a]Each tablet also contains 451 mcg of levomefolate calcium.

Data from Anonymous. Choice of contraceptives: Treatment Guidelines from The Medical Letter. Med Lett 2010;8:89–96.

Reduction in the Risk of Endometrial Cancer The risk of endometrial cancer among women who have used oral contraceptives for at least 1 year is approximately 40% less than the risk in women who have never used oral contraceptives.[9] There is additional evidence to suggest this benefit is detectable within 1 year of use, and the reduced risk may persist for years following discontinuation of oral contraceptives.[10]

Reduction in the Risk of Ovarian Cancer When compared with women who have never used oral contraceptives, women who have used oral contraceptives for up to 4 years are 30% less likely to develop ovarian cancer. There is also additional evidence to suggest that the longer the duration of oral contraceptive use, the greater the reduction in the risk of ovarian cancer. Women who have taken oral contraceptives for 5 to 11 years are 60% less likely to develop ovarian cancer, and women who have taken oral contraceptives for more than 12 years are 80% less likely to develop ovarian cancer than those who have never used oral contraceptives. As with the reduced risk of endometrial cancer, there is evidence to suggest the reduced risk of ovarian cancer may persist for years following discontinuation of oral contraceptives.[11,12]

Improved Regulation of Menstruation Women who take oral contraceptives typically experience more regular menstrual cycles. In general, oral contraceptive use is associated with less cramping and dysmenorrhea.[1,8] Also, women who take oral contraceptives have a smaller volume of menstruum and experience fewer days of menstruation each month and consequently experience less blood loss with each menstrual period.[1,13] Some studies suggest that oral contraceptive use decreases overall monthly menstrual flow by 60% or more, which may be particularly beneficial in women who are anemic.[1]

Relief from Symptoms Associated with Premenstrual Dysphoric Disorder COCs have been widely used for the treatment of premenstrual dysphoric disorder (PMDD). Current evidence suggests that these agents are most effective at targeting the physical symptoms associated with the disorder and less effective in treating mood-related symptoms.[14] Although multiphasic COCs have been used effectively in the treatment of PMDD, monophasic preparations may yield fewer mood swings and are generally easier to manage. Yaz, which contains the progestin, drospirenone, carries an FDA-approved indication for PMDD.[8,15]

Relief of Benign Breast Disease Women who use oral contraceptives are less likely to develop benign breast cysts or fibroadenomas.[1,8]

Prevention of Ovarian Cysts Because oral contraceptives suppress ovarian stimulation, women who take them are less likely to develop ovarian cysts.[8]

Reduction in the Risk of Symptomatic Pelvic Inflammatory Disease The risk of hospitalization owing to symptomatic pelvic inflammatory disease (PID) caused by gonorrheal infection is reduced in oral contraceptive users.[4,16] Although the exact protective mechanism is unknown, it is believed that thickening of the cervical mucus and/or reduction in the ability of pathogens to enter the fallopian tubes may contribute to the lower incidence of PID experienced by oral contraceptive users.[1]

Improvement in Acne Control All COCs can improve acne by increasing the quantity of sex hormone–binding globulin and thereby decreasing free testosterone concentrations.[8] Third-generation progestins, such as desogestrel and norgestimate, are believed to have less androgenic activity compared with older progestins, and drospirenone is considered to be antiandrogenic.[8] However, it is not clear that COCs containing any of these progestins confer any advantage over other COCs with respect to their ability to improve acne control. Ortho Tri-Cyclen (EE and norgestimate), Estrostep Fe (EE and norethindrone acetate), Yaz, and Beyaz (EE and drospirenone) each carry an FDA-approved indication for the treatment of acne.[1,8]

▶ *Potential Risks of Combination Oral Contraceptives*

Although there are many noncontraceptive benefits associated with the use of COCs, their use is not without risk or potential for adverse effects.

Sexually Transmitted Diseases Because the use of COCs may decrease the use of selected barrier contraceptive methods (e.g., latex condoms) that do protect against STDs, one of the most common potential risks associated with the use of oral contraceptives is the increased risk of acquiring an STD.[4]

Cardiovascular Events and Hypertension A World Health Organization (WHO) collaborative study found that high-dose (50 mcg or more of EE) oral contraceptive users with uncontrolled hypertension have an increased risk of experiencing a myocardial infarction or stroke.[8,17] In this study, women who had the lowest risk for experiencing a myocardial infarction or stroke were those who did not smoke, took low-dose oral contraceptives, and had their blood pressure checked prior to beginning oral contraceptives.[18-20] Hypertension secondary to oral contraceptive use is thought to occur in up to 3% of women and is believed to be attributed to the effect that estrogens and progestins can have on aldosterone activity.[1] Given this and the risk for cardiovascular events, women should have their blood pressure checked prior to initiating oral contraceptives, as well as periodically throughout oral contraceptive use. If significant elevations in blood pressure are noted, oral contraceptives should be discontinued. Estrogen-containing contraceptives are not recommended for smokers who are 35 years of age or older, for women with hypertension (especially if untreated), or for women who experience migraine headaches (especially those with focal neurologic symptoms).[4,8]

Venous Thromboembolism It is believed that the estrogen component of COCs stimulates enhanced hepatic production of clotting factors. COCs have been associated with a two- to threefold increase in the risk of venous thromboembolism compared with women who do not use oral contraceptives.[8] Contraceptive users at greatest risk for the development of venous thromboembolism include those who are obese, smoke, have hypertension, have diabetes complicated by end-organ damage, are immobile, have experienced recent trauma or surgery, or have a history of prior thromboembolism. It is important to note, however, that the increase in risk of venous thromboembolism in oral contraceptive users is lower than that associated with pregnancy and the postpartum period.[8,21] Newer, less androgenic progestins, such as desogestrel and drospirenone, have been reported to be associated with a higher risk of venous thromboembolism.[22-25] Currently available studies validating this risk have produced conflicting results. A large prospective surveillance study including more than 142,000 women years of observation reported similar rates of venous thromboembolism occurrence among women taking levonorgestrel, drospirenone, and other progestins, including desogestrel.[26] However, two more recent studies published in 2011 reported a two- to threefold greater risk of venous thromboembolic events in women using oral contraceptives containing drospirenone when compared with women using levonorgestrel-containing contraceptives.[27,28] In general, progestin-only contraceptives are preferred for women who are at increased risk of cardiovascular or thromboembolic complications, including women with a prior history of thromboembolic disease.[4,8]

Glucose Intolerance Older oral contraceptive formulations containing higher doses of hormones were shown in some cases to induce hyperglycemia.[1] Because estrogens may inhibit the release of insulin from pancreatic islet cells, low-dose estrogen formulations may be preferred in patients with diabetes. Progesterone competes with insulin for binding to its receptor. Although it is thought that progestins may increase insulin resistance, the newer progestins are thought to be less androgenic and have little effect on carbohydrate and lipid metabolism. In general, the use of COCs is relatively contraindicated in patients with diabetes.

Gallbladder Disease In women with preexisting gallstones, low-dose estrogen-containing oral contraceptives may enhance the potential for the development of symptomatic gallbladder disease and may worsen existing gallbladder disease.[1,4] Although this risk has not been demonstrated with the use of higher-dose oral contraceptives, COCs containing estrogen should be used with caution in patients with a history of gallbladder disease.

Hepatic Tumors Although the use of oral contraceptives is not associated with an increased risk for the development of hepatocellular carcinoma, long-term use of high-dose oral contraceptives has been associated with the development of benign liver tumors.[1] Because even benign liver tumors may pose significant risk to the patient, oral contraceptives should be discontinued if liver enlargement is noted on physical examination. In cases of hepatoma (malignancy), the use of COCs is contraindicated.[4]

Cervical Cancer There appears to be an increased risk for the development of cervical cancer among long-term users of oral contraceptives.[1] It is uncertain whether this increase in risk is directly attributed to the use of oral contraceptives. Data suggest that oral contraceptive users tend to have more sexual partners and use condoms less frequently, and as a result, this may increase their susceptibility to infection with human papilloma virus (HPV), a known risk factor for cervical cancer.

Breast Cancer Most recent studies evaluating the relationship between oral contraceptive use and the risk for breast cancer suggest little, if any, association between the two. The baseline risk for the development of breast cancer in women with a positive family history is greater than for women without a family history. However, current data suggest that COC use (either past or current) does not further raise the risk for breast cancer in such patients.[4,29,30] Women with breast cancer susceptibility genes also have a higher baseline risk for breast cancer compared with women who do not carry such genes. Current evidence evaluating the impact of COC use on the risk for breast cancer development in women who carry the breast cancer susceptibility genes suggests that COC use does not further modify the risk in such women.[4,31] Women with a current or recent breast cancer diagnosis should not take COCs, as breast cancer tumors are sensitive to estrogen, and COC use may worsen the prognosis for such patients.[4]

❶ *Absolute and relative contraindications to the use of oral contraceptives are listed in Table 48–3.*[1,4,32]

Table 48–3

Contraindications to the Use of Combined Oral Contraceptives (COCs)

Absolute Contraindications
History of thromboembolic disease
History of stroke (or current cerebrovascular disease)
History of (or current) coronary artery disease, ischemic heart disease, or peripheral vascular disease
History of carcinoma of the breast (known or suspected)
History of any estrogen-dependent neoplasm (known or suspected)
Undiagnosed abnormal uterine or vaginal bleeding
Pregnancy (known or suspected)
Heavy smoking (defined as 15 cigarettes or more per day) by women who are 35 years of age or older
History of hepatic tumors (benign or malignant)
Active liver disease
Migraine headaches with focal neurologic symptoms
Postpartum (during the first 21 days, as well as during days 21 through 42 in women with additional risk factors for thromboembolism, including age greater than or equal to 35 years, history of previous venous thromboembolism, preeclampsia, recent cesarean delivery, obesity, and smoking)

Relative Contraindications
Smoking (less than 15 cigarettes per day) at any age
Migraine headache disorder without focal neurologic symptoms
Hypertension (NOTE: WHO considers health risk posed by COC use to be "unacceptable" when either systolic blood pressure 160 mm Hg or more, or diastolic blood pressure 90 mm Hg or more)
Fibroid tumors of the uterus
Breast-feeding
Diabetes mellitus
Family history of dyslipidemia
Sickle cell disease
Active gallbladder disease
Age greater than 50 years
Elective major surgery requiring immobilization (planned in the next 4 weeks)

Data from Refs. 1, 4, and 32.

Patient Encounter, Part 1

LM, a 24-year-old nulliparous woman, presents to your clinic requesting information on contraception. She specifically inquires about options that allow for fewer or no menstrual periods. You begin to take a history and determine that the patient is currently sexually active and is not using any method of birth control. She weighs 150 pounds (68 kg), is 66 inches (168 cm) tall, and has a blood pressure of 110/72 mm Hg. She has no history of smoking. LM does have migraines without aura, for which she takes propranolol. On further questioning, you discover that she has a positive family history of breast cancer (both her mother and maternal aunt), but no personal history. As you discuss various contraceptive options with the patient, it is clear that she has a preference for an oral contraceptive agent.

What additional information do you need to know before recommending a contraceptive for this patient?

Based on the information provided by the patient, what oral contraceptive agent would you recommend for the patient and why?

What education would you provide to this patient regarding risks associated with oral contraceptive use?

▶ *Adverse Effects of Oral Contraceptives and Their Management*

As with all medications, there are potential adverse effects with COCs. ❷ *Many side effects can be minimized or avoided by adjusting the estrogen and/or progestin content of the oral contraceptive.* It is also important to individualize the selection of oral contraceptives, because some women are at increased risk for potentially serious side effects.

Common complaints with COCs include headaches, nausea, vomiting, mastalgia, and weight gain; although studies have shown a similar percentage of patients taking placebo experience these side effects.[33] Given that oral contraceptives often are discontinued owing to side effects, proper counseling before initiation of COCs is necessary.

Between 30% and 50% of women complain of breakthrough bleeding or spotting when oral contraceptives are initiated. These side effects tend to resolve by the third or fourth cycle.[1] Before changing formulations, other more serious causes of bleeding or spotting, such as pregnancy, infection, and poor absorption of the oral contraceptive owing to drug interaction or GI problems, should be ruled out. Once these causes have been ruled out, the timing of the spotting must be determined in order to adjust the formulation appropriately.

Women who have spotting or bleeding before they finish their active pills need a higher progestin content to increase endometrial support. Either a monophasic formulation with a higher progestin or a triphasic formulation with an increasing dose of progestin would be appropriate. Women with continued bleeding after menses need more estrogen support.

Either increasing the estrogen component or having a lower early progestin component (in triphasic pills) should be sufficient. If midcycle bleeding occurs, it is more difficult to determine the cause. It may be best to increase both the estrogen and progestin component for such women.[1]

Hormonal methods of contraception usually decrease the amount of withdrawal bleeding quite significantly. Lower dose estrogen formulations may increase the risk of breakthrough bleeding. Switching to a higher estrogen formulation or to a triphasic formulation will help to minimize breakthrough bleeding and will increase the amount of withdrawal bleeding.

Acne, PMDD, and hirsutism are all side effects that may be related to progestins with higher androgenicity, such as norgestrel and levonorgestrel, although these claims have not been documented in controlled trials. Norgestimate and norethindrone have less androgenicity and claim to have greater improvement in acne. Drospirenone has both antiandrogenic and antimineralocorticoid activity and has shown improvement in PMDD, hirsutism, and acne. If patients are complaining of such side effects, switching to a product with a lower risk of androgenic effects may be appropriate.[8]

GI complaints are seen often with oral contraceptives. Estrogen can induce nausea and vomiting via the CNS, whereas progesterone slows peristalsis, causing constipation and feelings of bloating and distention.[1] Most women will adjust to the symptoms, and the symptoms often will resolve within 1 to 3 months. Taking the pill at bedtime or with food may be a potential strategy to help cope with nausea. If women are unable to tolerate the GI side effects, then either a decrease in EE to a low-dose 20-mcg formulation may minimize nausea or a decrease in progestin may minimize bloating and constipation. Progestin-only products may be considered if even low-dose EE causes nausea.

Headaches are a common occurrence for women, and they must be evaluated because they can be a major warning sign for stroke. If headaches begin or become worse after initiation of COCs, all differential diagnoses must be considered. Blood pressure should be evaluated to rule out hypertension. If any neurologic symptoms or blurred vision occur with the headache, the oral contraceptive should be stopped immediately. Migraine headaches with aura showed a significant increase in the risk for ischemic stroke in one WHO study.[17] If the headaches are not serious but still are troublesome to the patient, the following changes are suggested: (a) discontinue the oral contraceptive, (b) lower the dose of estrogen, (c) lower the dose of progestin, or (d) eliminate the pill-free interval for two to three consecutive cycles (for women with headaches during the pill-free interval only).[1]

Although rare, some women may complain of a decrease in libido. This often is found to coincide with feelings of depression. Alterations to vaginal lubrication and free testosterone levels may occur with some COCs, and both can relate to decreased libido.[34] Low levels of estrogen can decrease vaginal lubrication as well and make intercourse painful. Use of the vaginal hormonal ring (NuvaRing) may help with lubrication problems.[1]

Dyslipidemias can occur from hormone therapy. Estrogen is known to cause an increase in high-density lipoprotein cholesterol (HDL-C), triglycerides, and total cholesterol levels and to decrease low-density lipoprotein cholesterol (LDL-C). Androgenic progestins are more likely to decrease HDL-C and triglycerides and increase LDL-C. Depending on the ratio of estrogen to progestin content, the HDL-C, LDL-C, and triglyceride levels may fluctuate up or down. In women with no risk factors for dyslipidemias (e.g., women who do not smoke, have hypertension, or have a family history of heart disease), it is not necessary to obtain a baseline lipid panel. However, if the lipid panel is monitored, and if dyslipidemia occurs, then it is recommended to replace an androgenic progestin with a more estrogenic progestin. In women with triglycerides more than 350 mg/dL (3.96 mmol/L) at baseline, estrogen-containing formulations should be used only with caution, and low doses of 20 to 25 mcg EE, or a progestin-only formulation might be preferred.[1]

Mastalgia can occur in up to 30% of women taking oral contraceptives and is most likely due to the estrogen component. The average woman has a 20% increase in breast volume in the luteal phase owing to venous and lymphatic engorgement. Estrogen also causes adipose cell hypertrophy in the breast.[1] Lower dose pills (20 mcg) produce less mastalgia than those with 35 mcg of EE.[35] If tenderness occurs prior to menses, switching to a contraceptive that offers extended cycle length (see Unique Oral Contraceptives, later) may minimize problems as well.

Women often are concerned about using oral contraceptives for fear of gaining weight. It has been proven that low-dose EE oral contraceptives do not increase the risk of weight gain in women compared with placebo.[36] Estrogen can cause hypertrophy of adipose cells, and therefore, women see an increase in measurement of their breasts, hips, and thighs.[1] Weight gain associated with premenstrual fluid retention may also occur with the combination of estrogen and a higher androgenic progestin. Switching to a lower-dose estrogen and a progestin with less androgenic activity may be beneficial in this situation.[1]

Additional side effects have been noted in some women. Women wearing contact lenses may have visual changes and more disturbances with lenses. If normal saline eye drops do not help, referral to an ophthalmologist is recommended. Melasma and chloasma can occur secondary to estrogen stimulation of melanocyte production. Women with darker pigmentation are more susceptible to hyperpigmentation effects. The melasma may not be completely reversible on discontinuation. Progestin-only products may be preferable, and sunscreen use is highly recommended.[1]

As described earlier, many of the side effects of COCs may be minimized by adjusting the estrogen or progestin content of the preparation. However, although low-dose COCs may cause fewer side effects, it is important to note that in the event that doses are missed, such COCs may be more likely to result in contraceptive failure.

Progestin-Only Pills

For women unable to take estrogen-containing oral contraceptives, there is an alternative: oral contraceptives containing only the progestin, norethindrone. These agents are slightly less effective than COCs but have other advantages over COCs. Progestin-only products have not shown the same thromboembolic risk as estrogen-containing products. Therefore, women at increased risk for or with a history of thromboembolism may be good candidates for progestin-only oral contraceptives. Also, these products can minimize menses, and many women have amenorrhea after six to nine cycles. These products have also been found safe to use in women who are nursing, so they are a viable option for women who breastfeed and desire hormonal contraception. In such patients, it should not be initiated until 6 weeks postpartum. Spotting does not subside in some women, and this is a common cause for discontinuation. These products should be taken at the same time every day, and there is no pill-free or hormone-free period.

Unique Oral Contraceptives

Along with varying doses of estrogen and different progestins, there are also formulation modifications that may benefit various patient situations. In the United States, these formulations include products such as Loestrin-24 Fe and Lo-Loestrin Fe; Seasonale, Quasense, and Introvale; Seasonique and Lo Seasonique; Yasmin, Yaz, and Beyaz; Ortho Tri-Cyclen and Estrostep Fe; Mircette; Ovcon 35; and Lybrel. Each of these products may show benefit in certain women owing to their unique characteristics.

Loestrin-24 Fe and Lo-Loestrin Fe (norethindrone/EE) are extended-cycle preparations that contain a low-dose estrogen, a high amount of progestin, and medium androgenic activity. Similar to other low-dose estrogen COCs, Loestrin-24 Fe and Lo-Loestrin Fe may offer a smaller margin of error when pills are missed but provide the potential advantage of fewer estrogen-related side effects (e.g., nausea and breast tenderness). Unlike the typical 28-pill packs that contain 21 active tablets and seven placebo tablets, Loestrin-24 Fe contains 24 active tablets and four placebo (iron-only) tablets, and Lo-Loestrin Fe contains 24 combination hormone tablets, two estrogen-only tablets, and two placebo (iron-only) tablets. These products provide shorter hormone-free intervals and allow for shorter menstrual periods and fewer menstrual-related symptoms, such as menstrual-related headaches, menorrhagia, and anemia.

Seasonale, Quasense, and Introvale (levonorgestrel/EE) are each monophasic combinations that are packaged as a 91-day treatment cycles with 84 active tablets that are taken consecutively followed by seven placebo tablets. The extended cycle length of these products allows for one menstrual cycle per "season," or four per year. This type of formulation may be appealing to women with perimenstrual side effects or those at higher risk for anemia with menstrual bleeding. Seasonale, Quasense, or Introvale may improve anxiety, headache, fluid retention, dysmenorrhea, breast tenderness, bloating, and menstrual migraines. However, in the SEA 301 clinical trial comparing the efficacy of Seasonale with that of an equivalent-dosage 28-day cycle regimen, 7.7% versus 1.8% of women discontinued prematurely for unacceptable bleeding.[37] The risk of intermenstrual bleeding and/or spotting may be higher for patients taking these extended-cycle combinations than for patients taking typical 28-day-regimen COCs.

Seasonique and Lo Seasonique (levonorgestrel/EE) are also extended cycle preparations that are similar to Seasonale, Quasense, and Introvale, but instead these preparations contain seven tablets with low-dose estrogen rather than placebo. Menstruation-related problems that may improve with Seasonique or Lo Seasonique include menstrual-related headaches, menorrhagia, and anemia. In addition, endometriosis-related menstrual pain may be relieved by providing a continuous regimen without a pill-free interval.[38]

Yasmin and Yaz (drospirenone/EE) are unique oral contraceptives that contain the progestin drospirenone. This hormone not only has antiandrogenic properties, but also showed antimineralocorticoid activity in preclinical trials. It has a unique application in young women who experience problems associated with producing too much androgen. Drospirenone is a spironolactone analog, and the 3-mg dose available in COC preparations has antimineralocorticoid activity equal to 25 mg of spironolactone. It can affect the sodium and water balance in the body, although it has not shown superior efficacy for side effects such as bloating compared with other oral contraceptives. Caution should be used in women with chronic conditions or in women taking other medications that may affect serum potassium.[39] Yaz (drospirenone/EE) is an extended-cycle preparation that contains a low-dose estrogen and antimineralocorticoid and antiandrogenic activity. Like Loestrin-24 Fe, Yaz contains 24 active tablets and four placebo tablets, allowing for shorter menstrual periods and fewer menstrual-related symptoms, such as menstrual-related headaches, menorrhagia, and anemia.

In 2003, the FDA Advisory Committee for Reproductive Health Drugs recommended the development of a COC tablet containing folic acid in order to minimize the risk of neural tube defects in cases of contraceptive failure. Beyaz and Safyral, which were FDA approved in 2010, are combination tablets containing drospirenone and EE (like Yaz and Yasmin) and 451 mcg of levomefolate calcium, the primary metabolite of folic acid. Similar to Yaz, Beyaz is an extended-cycle preparation, which may allow for shorter menstrual periods and fewer menstrual-related symptoms.

In addition to the prevention of pregnancy, Yaz, Beyaz, Ortho Tri-Cyclen (norgestimate/EE), and Estrostep Fe (norethindrone acetate/EE) each carry an approved indication for treatment of moderate acne vulgaris in females 15 years of age or older desiring contraception who have not responded adequately to conventional anti-acne medication. This can help clinicians to streamline medications by serving dual purposes.

Mircette (desogestrel/EE) has a unique dosing schedule. After the usual 21 active tablets, there are only two tablets with inert ingredients. The last five tablets in the package have 10 mcg of EE. In theory, this may minimize bleeding during the menstrual cycle, although the clinical significance of this dosing schedule has not been established.[40] It is important to counsel patients to complete the entire pack and not to discard the last 7 days of medication.

Patient Encounter, Part 2: Adverse Effects

After 2 months of taking LoSeasonique, LM returns to your clinic complaining of breakthrough bleeding during her sixth week of active pills. She reports no change or increase in frequency of her migraine headaches, and her blood pressure is 112/70 mm Hg. She is frustrated with the breakthrough bleeding and wants to explore other contraceptive options.

What are some potential causes of the breakthrough bleeding that the patient has been experiencing?

What strategy would you recommend to eliminate or minimize the potential adverse effects experienced by the patient?

Another unique formulation is a chewable tablet available to women who have difficulty swallowing medications. Ovcon 35 (norethindrone/EE) has all 28 tablets in chewable form and has added spearmint flavoring.[41]

Finally, Lybrel (levonorgestrel/EE) is the first continuous-cycle COC approved by the FDA. Active pills are taken every day throughout the year with no pill-free interval. The major advantage of this product is elimination of menstrual periods, resulting in improvement in or elimination of menstrual-related symptoms. The most bothersome side effect associated with Lybrel is a high incidence of spotting and breakthrough bleeding during the initial months of use. It appears as though the incidence of breakthrough bleeding with Lybrel decreases with continued use.[42]

Drug Interactions with Oral Contraceptives

EE is metabolized in the liver primarily via cytochrome P450 (CYP450) 3A4. When reviewing drug interactions of oral contraceptives, ❸ *clinicians should be aware of the many drugs that may potentially interact with contraceptives—especially those that may reduce the effectiveness of contraceptives.* Refer to Table 48–4 for a list of some of the most common drug interactions seen with oral contraceptives.[1,43,44]

Nonoral Hormonal Contraceptives

❹ *As an alternative to oral contraceptive pills, which must be taken daily in order to reliably prevent pregnancy, nonoral contraceptives in the form of transdermal, transvaginal, and injectable preparations are available and offer patients safe and effective alternatives to the pills for prevention of pregnancy. These formulations also do not require daily administration, making them more convenient than the pill formulations.*

Ortho-Evra is a transdermal patch that contains both an estrogen (20 mcg of EE) and a progestin (150 mcg of norelgestromin). A new patch is applied to the abdomen, buttocks, upper torso, or upper (outer) arm once weekly for 3 weeks, followed by seven patch-free days.[8] Although some women

---

Table 48–4

Commonly Seen Drug Interactions With COCs

Medication	Mechanism	Clinical Effect
Anticonvulsants (carbamazepine, oxcarbazepine, phenytoin, phenobarbital, primidone, topiramate, and felbamate)	Increase metabolism of COCs via induction of various cytochrome P450 enzymes	Decrease efficacy of COCs (EE doses less than 35 mcg are not recommended in women on these medications)
Benzodiazepines (alprazolam)	COCs may inhibit oxidative metabolism	Increase side effects of benzodiazepines
Bosentan	Increase metabolism of COCs via induction of cytochrome P450 3A4 enzyme	Decrease efficacy of COCs
Colesevelam	Reduce absorption of COCs by nonspecific binding with colesevelam	Decrease efficacy of COCs
Corticosteroids (hydrocortisone, methylprednisolone, prednisone)	COCs may inhibit metabolism of corticosteroids	Increase side effects of corticosteroids
Griseofulvin	Increase metabolism of COCs	Decrease efficacy of COCs; backup method of contraception is recommended
Lamotrigine	COCs increase metabolism of lamotrigine via induction of glucuronidation	Decrease efficacy of lamotrigine; dose adjustment may be necessary
Modafinil	Increase metabolism of COCs	Decrease efficacy of COCs; alternative method of contraception is recommended
Penicillins (amoxicillin, ampicillin); tetracyclines (doxycycline, minocycline, tetracycline); Non-nucleoside reverse transcriptase inhibitors (delavirdine, efavirenz, etravirine, nevirapine)	Broad-spectrum antibiotics may alter intestinal flora, reducing enterohepatic circulation of estrogen metabolites; although the drop in estrogen levels has been shown to be only statistically significant, rather than clinically significant; Increase metabolism of COCs	Decrease efficacy of COCs; backup barrier method of contraception is controversial[a]
Rifampin, rifabutin	Increase metabolism of COCs	Decrease efficacy of COCs; backup method of contraception is recommended
Selegiline	COCs decrease metabolism of selegiline	Increase side effects of selegiline; may adjust dose of selegiline if needed
St. John's wort	Increase metabolism of COCs via induction of various cytochrome P450 enzymes	Decrease efficacy of COCs; avoid use with COCs
Theophylline	COCs decrease theophylline clearance by 34% and increase half-life by 33%	Increase side effects of theophylline

[a]Although package inserts warn of this potential interaction, no scientific literature exists to support that concomitant antibiotics and COCs is associated with contraceptive failure.[44]

Data from Refs. 1, 43, and 44.

---

have noted irregular bleeding during the first two cycles of patch use, the patch has been demonstrated to provide similar menstrual cycle control and contraceptive efficacy to that of COCs.[45] It is important to note, however, that higher contraceptive failure rates are seen when the patch is used in women weighing more than 90 kg (about 200 lb).[8,45] Further, manufacturer prescriber information indicates that women who take Ortho-Evra are exposed to approximately 60% more estrogen than women who take COCs with 35 mcg of estrogen.[46] Although the clinical significance of this is not well defined, studies have suggested a link between the use of the patch and an increased risk for venous thromboembolism. A slightly higher reported incidence of breast discomfort and local skin irritation has also been reported with the patch.[8,47]

NuvaRing is a unique transvaginal delivery system that provides 15 mcg of EE and 120 mcg of etonogestrel for the prevention of ovulation. NuvaRing is inserted into the vagina on or before day 5 of the menstrual cycle and is removed from the vagina 3 weeks later.[8] Seven days after the ring is removed, a new ring should be inserted. In clinical trials, NuvaRing demonstrated comparable efficacy and cycle control to COCs as well as a similar side effect profile.[8,48] NuvaRing should not be removed during intercourse. If the ring is dislodged or removed for more than 3 hours, efficacy could be compromised, and a backup method of contraception is recommended until a new ring has been in place for 7 days.

Depo-Provera is a progestin-only, injectable contraceptive that contains depot medroxyprogesterone acetate. Depo-Provera is administered intramuscularly as a 150-mg injection once every 3 months. An advantage of Depo-Provera is that it provides an estrogen-free method of contraception either for women in whom estrogens are contraindicated or for women who cannot tolerate estrogen-containing preparations. Depo-Provera is extremely effective in preventing pregnancy. However, the incidence of menstrual irregularities (including amenorrhea) and weight gain appears to be much greater than that seen with COCs. The use of Depo-Provera also has been demonstrated to result in significant loss of bone mineral density (BMD).[49] Although the effect is known to be reversible following product discontinuation, a black box warning within the product labeling cautions against the risk of potentially irreversible BMD loss associated with long-term use (e.g., greater than 2 years) of the injectable product. Although the extended duration of activity of this product may offer women the advantage of less frequent administration, it is important to note that on discontinuation of Depo-Provera, the return of fertility can be delayed by approximately 10 to 12 months (range 4–31 months).[8]

Depo-SubQ Provera 104 is also an injectable contraceptive product that contains only progestin (depot medroxyprogesterone acetate). This product differs from Depo-Provera in that it is given subcutaneously rather than intramuscularly, and it contains only 104 mg of medroxyprogesterone acetate (approximately 30% less hormone) administered every 3 months for the prevention of pregnancy.[50] Clinical trials have demonstrated that the subcutaneous formulation of depot medroxyprogesterone acetate is as effective as the intramuscular formulation in the prevention of pregnancy.[51] This product carries the same warning in its package labeling regarding possible effects on BMD as Depo-Provera.[50]

Long-Acting Reversible Contraception

There are currently four implantable contraceptive (three progestin-containing and one nonhormonal) devices available, also known as long-acting reversible contraception (LARC). After insertion, Mirena, a levonorgestrel-releasing intrauterine device (IUD), can provide contraceptive protection for up to 5 years.[52] ParaGard T 380A, a copper IUD, can provide contraceptive protection for up to 10 years.[53] Implanon and Nexplanon, the newest of the implantable devices, are both etonogestrel-releasing systems that can be surgically implanted under the skin of the upper arm and are effective for up to 3 years.[54,55] Surveys have shown that LARC has the highest satisfaction rate among patients using reversible contraceptives, and use within the United States is on the rise.[2]

Although the mechanism of action for IUDs is not completely understood, several theories have been suggested. The original theory is that the presence of a foreign body in the uterus causes an inflammatory response that interferes with implantation. It is believed that copper-containing IUDs may interfere with sperm transport and fertilization and prevent implantation.[53] Progestin-containing implantable contraceptives can have direct effects on the uterus, such as thickening of cervical mucus and alterations to the endometrial lining.[52] Mirena, Implanon, and Nexplanon can inhibit ovulation because they contain a progestin, but Paragard T 380A does not prevent ovulation.

It is important to evaluate a patient to determine whether she is an appropriate candidate for an implantable contraceptive. Implantable contraceptives are recommended for women with at least one child, in a monogamous relationship, who have no history of pelvic inflammatory disease (PID) and no history or risk of ectopic pregnancy. Contraindications with Implanon, the etonogestrel implant, are similar to those with COCs and include (a) known or suspected pregnancy, (b) current or past history of thrombosis or thromboembolic disorders, (c) hepatic tumors or active liver disease, (d) undiagnosed abnormal genital bleeding, (e) known or suspected carcinoma of the breast or personal history of breast cancer, and (f) hypersensitivity to any of the components of Implanon. There are also multiple contraindications to IUD use. Evaluation of the patient is essential because IUDs cannot be used in the following situations: (a) pregnancy or suspicion of pregnancy, (b) anatomically abnormal or distorted uterine cavity, (c) acute PID or current behavior suggesting a high risk for PID, (d) postpartum endometritis or infected abortion in the past 3 months, (e) known or suspected uterine or cervical malignancy, (f) genital bleeding of unknown etiology, (g) untreated acute cervicitis, (h) acute liver disease or liver tumor, (i) woman or her partner has multiple sexual partners, (j) previously inserted IUD still in place, (k) conditions associated with increased susceptibility to infections (e.g., leukemia or acquired immune deficiency syndrome), (l) hypersensitivity to any component of the IUD, (m) known or suspected carcinoma of the breast, and (n) Wilson's disease.[52,53]

There are potential side effects of IUD use. The most common adverse effects are abdominal/pelvic cramping, abnormal uterine bleeding, and expulsion of the device. Other side effects seen are ectopic pregnancy, sepsis, PID, embedment of the device, uterine or cervical perforation, and ovarian cysts.[52,53]

Nonpharmacologic Contraceptive Methods

▶ Barrier Contraceptives

As an alternative to hormonal contraceptives, several barrier contraceptive options are available for the prevention of pregnancy. Although barrier contraceptives are associated with far fewer adverse effects compared with hormonal contraceptives, their efficacy is highly user-dependent. Overall, compared with both hormonal contraceptives and IUDs, barrier contraceptives are associated with much higher accidental pregnancy rates[8] (Table 48–1).

Diaphragms and Cervical Caps Diaphragms and cervical caps are dome-shaped rubber caps that are placed over the cervix to provide barrier protection during intercourse. Both diaphragms and cervical caps require fitting by a healthcare professional, and they must be refitted in the event of weight gain or weight loss. Diaphragms or cervical caps typically can be placed over the cervix as much as 6 hours prior to intercourse. They must be left in place for at least 6 hours after intercourse before they can be removed. Diaphragms should not be left in place longer than 24 hours, and smaller cervical caps should not be left in place longer than 48 hours owing to the risk of toxic shock syndrome (TSS). Diaphragms and cervical caps are used along with spermicides to prevent pregnancy. When sexual intercourse is repeated with the diaphragm, reapplication of the spermicide is necessary.

However, when sexual intercourse is repeated with a cervical cap, reapplication of the spermicide typically is not necessary.[8] Whether or not diaphragms or cervical caps provide adequate protection against STDs remains unclear.[56]

Spermicides Nonoxynol-9, a surfactant that destroys the cell membranes of sperm, is the most commonly used spermicide in the United States.[8,57] Nonoxynol-9 is available in a variety of forms, including a cream, foam, film, gel, suppository, and tablet. Spermicides may be used alone, with a barrier method, or adjunctively with other forms of contraceptives to provide additional protection against unwanted pregnancy.[57] To be used most effectively, spermicides must be placed in the vagina not more than 1 hour prior to sexual intercourse, and they must come in contact with the cervix.[8] Although the efficacy of spermicides depends largely on how consistently and correctly they are used, their efficacy is enhanced when they are used in combination with a barrier contraceptive device.[56] Clinical trials assessing the ability of spermicides to protect against STDs have failed to produce positive results.[57] Further, there exists some evidence to suggest that frequent use of spermicides actually may increase risk for transmission of human immunodeficiency virus (HIV) secondary to vaginal mucosal tissue breakdown, which may allow a portal of entry for the virus.[8] In December 2007, the FDA issued a statement requiring manufacturers of nonoxynol-9 products to include a warning on the product label indicating that the spermicide does not provide protection against infection from HIV or other STDs.

Condoms Condoms, which are available for both male and female use, act as physical barriers to prevent sperm from coming into contact with ova.[57] Condoms are easy to use, available without a prescription, and inexpensive. Most condoms are made of latex. When used correctly, condoms can be very effective in prevention of unwanted pregnancy. Condoms should be stored in a cool, dry place, away from exposure to direct sunlight. When stored improperly or when used with oil-based lubricants, however, latex condoms can break during intercourse, increasing the risk of pregnancy.[8] For latex-sensitive individuals, condoms made from lamb intestine ("natural membrane" condoms) and synthetic polyurethane condoms are available. Unlike latex condoms, condoms made from lamb intestine contain small pores that may permit the passage of viruses and therefore do not provide adequate protection against STDs.[58] ⑤ *Both latex and synthetic condoms can provide some protection against many STDs. Data from one meta-analysis suggested that HIV transmission can be reduced by as much as 90% when condoms are consistently used.[59] This is in contrast to hormonal contraceptives (oral, transdermal, or vaginal), IUDs, and most other barrier contraceptives, which do not protect against STDs.* Relative to male condoms, female condoms may offer even better protection against STDs because they provide more extensive barrier coverage of external genitalia, including the labia and the base of the penis.[57] It is important to note that the male and female condoms are not recommended to be used together because they may adhere to one another, causing displacement of one or both condoms.[57]

Sponge The Today sponge is a small, pillow-shaped polyurethane sponge impregnated with nonoxynol-9.[56] It is an over-the-counter barrier contraceptive that has been shown to be generally less effective at preventing pregnancy than diaphragms.[60] The sponge is moistened with water and then is inserted and placed over the cervix for up to 6 hours prior to sexual intercourse. The sponge then is left in place for at least 6 hours following intercourse.[57] Although the sponge maintains efficacy for 24 hours (even if intercourse is repeated), as with diaphragms, the sponge should be removed after 24 hours owing to the risk of TSS.[8]

▶ *Fertility Awareness–Based Methods*

Fertility awareness–based methods (natural methods) represent another nonpharmacologic means of pregnancy prevention. Although failure rates of such methods can be high, some couples still prefer these types of approaches. Fertility awareness–based methods depend on the ability of the couple to identify the woman's "fertile window," or the period of time in which pregnancy is most likely to occur as a result of sexual intercourse.[61] During the fertile window, the couple practices abstinence, or avoidance of intercourse, in order to prevent pregnancy. In some cases, rather than practicing abstinence during the fertile period, some couples may prefer to employ barrier methods or spermicides as a means of preventing pregnancy rather than to avoid intercourse altogether.[8] In order to identify the fertile window, a number of different fertility awareness–based methods may be tried. The calendar (rhythm) method involves counting the days in the menstrual cycle and then using a mathematical equation to determine the fertile window.[61] The temperature method involves monitoring changes in the woman's basal body temperature using a basal thermometer.[61] The cervical mucus (or Billings ovulation) method involves observing changes in the characteristics of cervical secretions throughout the cycle.[61] Around ovulation, the mucus becomes watery. The symptothermal method, which is considered to be the most difficult to learn but potentially the most effective, is a combination of both the temperature method and the cervical mucus method.[8] In general, fertility awareness–based methods are not recommended for women who have irregular menstrual cycles or who have difficulty interpreting their fertility signs correctly.[61]

Emergency Contraception

Emergency contraception (EC) is used to prevent pregnancy after known or suspected unprotected sexual intercourse. There are three FDA-approved oral agents available for use as EC, with two being available for nonprescription sale to patients 17 years of age and older. The two over-the-counter options contain the progestin levonorgestrel and are Plan B One Step and Next Choice, both of which are available via prescription for those younger than 17 years of age. Plan B One Step allows patients to take one dose of 1.5 mg of levonorgestrel within 72 hours of unprotected intercourse. Next Choice is a two-step process of 0.75 mg of levonorgestrel

Patient Encounter, Part 3: Missed Doses

LM calls your clinic in a panic today because she forgot to take her oral contraceptive for the past 3 days, beginning the third week of active pills. Three days have elapsed since she took her last active pill, and she reports having had unprotected sexual intercourse last night. The patient is very concerned about her risk of pregnancy and is interested to learn more about emergency contraception and what her options are.

Given this patient's reported imperfect use of her oral contraceptive, what information can you provide to the patient regarding her risk of pregnancy?

What additional education should be provided to LM regarding her risk of STDs related to unprotected intercourse?

Provide appropriate patient education regarding the use of various forms of emergency contraception, in the event she decides to use EC.

taken within 72 hours of intercourse and a second equal dose taken 12 hours later. The newest EC option is ella (ulipristal acetate), a progesterone-receptor agonist/antagonist that can delay follicular rupture if taken just before ovulation and may cause endometrial changes to interfere with implantation. It is dosed as a single 30-mg tablet that can be taken up to 5 days after unprotected intercourse.[8] It is available only via prescription. It is important to note that EC is more effective the earlier it is used after unprotected intercourse. Common side effects include headache, nausea, abdominal pain, dysmenorrhea, fatigue, and dizziness. If severe abdominal pain occurs, patients should be referred to their physician for risk of an ectopic pregnancy. Patients should also contact their physician if their menstrual cycle is more than 1 week late after taking EC.

OUTCOME EVALUATION/MONITORING

Side effects of contraceptives tend to occur in the first few months of therapy. Thus schedule a follow-up visit 3 to 6 months after initiating a new contraceptive. Yearly checkups usually are sufficient for patients who are doing well on a particular product.[1] At each follow-up visit, assess blood pressure, headache frequency, and menstrual bleeding patterns, as well as compliance with the prescribed regimen. Strict adherence to the prescribed hormonal contraceptive regimen is essential for effective prevention of unintended pregnancy. ❻ *When a contraceptive dose is missed, the risk of accidental pregnancy may be increased. Depending on how many doses were missed, the contraceptive formulation being used, and the phase of the cycle during which doses were missed, counseling regarding the use of additional methods of contraception may be warranted.*

Patient Care and Monitoring

1. Obtain a thorough medical and family history and carefully evaluate each patient's risk factors prior to prescribing contraceptives.

2. Educate all women taking hormonal contraceptives to prevent pregnancy regarding self-monitoring for early warning signs that may precede adverse events. Healthcare professionals can easily recall the major warning signs by using the following two simple pneumonics:

   ACHES—for women taking hormonal contraceptives

   A = Abdominal pain. This may be an early warning sign of the presence of an abdominal thromboembolism, liver adenoma, or gallbladder disease.

   C = Chest pain. The presence of chest pain may indicate pulmonary embolism, angina, or myocardial infarction.

   H = Headaches. Headaches (particularly those associated with focal neurologic symptoms, such as blurred vision, speech impairment, and/or weakness) may represent stroke-like symptoms. Headaches also may indicate poorly controlled blood pressure.

   E = Eye problems. Blurred vision and/or ocular pain may be early warning signs for stroke and/or blood clots. In addition, visual changes may occur in patients wearing contact lenses (secondary to changes in corneal shape).

   S = Severe leg pain. Patients taking hormonal contraceptives who complain of severe leg pain should be evaluated for the presence of venous thromboembolism.

   PAINS—for women with an IUD

   P = Period late

   A = Abdominal pain, pain with intercourse

   I = Infection, abnormal or odorous vaginal discharge

   N = Not feeling well, fever, chills

   S = String (missing, shorter, longer)

3. In addition to the preceding, monitor patients taking hormonal contraceptives for missed periods, signs of pregnancy, appearance of jaundice, and/or severe mood changes. Instruct patients to consult a healthcare professional upon noticing or experiencing any of these warning signs.[1]

4. Stress the importance of adherence to the patient's chosen method of contraception in order to reliably prevent pregnancy. Educate the patient on what to do in the event of missed doses with hormonal contraception.

Abbreviations Introduced in This Chapter

BMD	Bone mineral density
COC	Combined oral contraceptive
CYP450	Cytochrome P450
EC	Emergency contraception
EE	Ethinyl estradiol
FSH	Follicle-stimulating hormone
GnRH	Gonadotropin-releasing hormone
HDL	High-density lipoprotein
HIV	Human immunodeficiency virus
HPV	Human papilloma virus
IUD	Intrauterine device
LARC	Long-acting reversible contraception
LDL	Low-density lipoprotein
LH	Luteinizing hormone
PID	Pelvic inflammatory disease
PMDD	Premenstrual dysphoric disorder
STD	Sexually transmitted disease
TSS	Toxic shock syndrome
WHO	World Health Organization

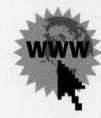 Self-assessment questions and answers are available at *http://mhpharmacotherapy. com/pp.html*.

REFERENCES

1. Nelson A. Combined oral contraceptives. In: Hatcher RA, Trussel J, Nelson AL, et al. Contraceptive Technology, 19th rev. ed. New York: Ardent Media, 2007:193–270.

2. Mosher WD, Jones J. Use of contraception in the United States: 1982–2008. Vital Health Stat 23 2010;1–44.

3. Ventura SJ, Abma JC, Mosher WD, Henshaw SK. Estimated pregnancy rates for the United States, 1990-2005: An update. Natl Vital Stat Rep 2009;58:1–14.

4. Centers for Disease Control and Prevention. U.S. Medical Eligibility Criteria for Contraceptive Use, 2010. MMWR Recomm Rep 2010; 59:1–86.

5. Centers for Disease Control and Prevention (CDC) [Internet]. Trends in sexually transmitted diseases in the United States: 2009 national data for gonorrhea, chlamydia, and syphilis. Available from: *http://www.cdc.gov/std/stats*.

6. Hatcher RA, Namnoum AB. The menstrual cycle. In: Hatcher RA, Trussel J, Nelson AL, et al. Contraceptive Technology, 19th rev. ed. New York: Ardent Media, 2007:7–18.

7. Trussel J. Choosing a contraceptive: Efficacy, safety, and personal considerations. In: Hatcher RA, Trussel J, Nelson AL, et al. Contraceptive Technology, 19th rev. ed. New York: Ardent Media, 2007:19–48.

8. Anonymous. Choice of contraceptives: Treatment Guidelines from The Medical Letter. Med Lett 2010;8:89–96.

9. Lurie G, Thompson P, McDuffie KE, Carney ME, Terada KY, Goodman MT. Association of estrogen and progestin potency of oral contraceptives with ovarian carcinoma risk. Obstet Gynecol 2007; 109:597–607.

10. Maxwell GL, Schildkraut JM, Calingaert B, et al. Progestin and estrogen: Potency of combination oral contraceptives and endometrial cancer risk. Gynecol Oncol 2006;103:535–540.

11. Ness RB, Grisso JA, Klapper J, et al. for the SHARE Study Group. Risk of ovarian cancer in relation to estrogen and progestin dose and use characteristics of oral contraceptives. Steroid hormones and reproduction. Am J Epidemiol 2000;152:233–241.

12. Schildkraut JM, Calingaert B, Marchbanks PA, et al. Impact of progestin and estrogen potency in oral contraceptives on ovarian cancer risk. J Natl Cancer Inst 2002;94:32–38.

13. Iyer V, Farquhar C, Jepson R. Oral contraceptive pills for heavy menstrual bleeding. Cochrane Database Syst Rev 2000;2:CD000154.

14. Kroll R, Rapkin AJ. Treatment of premenstrual disorders. J Reprod Med 2006;51:359–370.

15. Noncontraceptive uses of hormonal contraceptives. ACOG Practice Bulletin. No. 110. Washington, DC: The American College of Obstetricians and Gynecologists, January 2010.

16. Panser LA, Phipps WR. Type of oral contraceptive in relation to acute, initial episodes of pelvic inflammatory disease. Contraception 1991;43:91–99.

17. Tanis BC, van den Bosch MA, Kemmeren JM, et al. Oral contraceptives and the risk of myocardial infarction. Arch Intern Med 2001;161: 1065–1070.

18. Schwingl PJ, Ory HW, Visness CM. Estimates of the risk of cardiovascular death attributable to low-dose oral contraceptives in the United States. Am J Obstet Gynecol 1999;180:241–249.

19. Chang CL, Donaghy M, Poulter N. Migraine and stroke in young women: Case-control study. The World Health Organization Collaborative Study of Cardiovascular Disease and Steroid Hormone Contraception. BMJ 1999;318:13–18.

20. Curtis KM, Chrisman CE, Peterson HB, WHO Programme for Mapping Best Practices in Reproductive Health. Contraception for women in selected circumstances. Obstet Gynecol 2002;99:1100–1112.

21. Heit JA, Kobbervig CE, James AH, et al. Trends in the incidence of venous thromboembolism during pregnancy or postpartum: A 30 year population-based study. Ann Intern Med 2005;143:697–706.

22. Hennessy S, Berlin JA, Kinman JL, et al. Risk of venous thromboembolism from oral contraceptives containing gestodene and desogestrel versus levonorgestrel: A meta-analysis and formal sensitivity analysis. Contraception 2001;64:125–133.

23. Kemmeren JM, Algra A, Grobbee DE. Third generation oral contraceptives and risk of venous thrombosis: Meta-analysis. BMJ 2001;323: 131–134.

24. van Hylckama Vlieg A, Helmerhorst FM, Vandenbroucke JP, et al. The venous thrombotic risk of oral contraceptives, effects of oestrogen dose and progestin type: Results of the MEGA case-control study. BMJ 2009;339:b2921.

25. Lidegaard Ø, Løkkegaard E, Svendsen AL, Agger C. Hormonal contraception and risk of venous thromboembolism: National follow-up study. BMJ 2009;339:b2890.

26. Dinger JC, Heinemann LA, Kühl-Habich D. The safety of a drospirenone-containing oral contraceptive: Final results from the European Active Surveillance Study on oral contraceptives based on 142,475 women-years of observation. Contraception 2007;75:344–354.

27. Parkin L, Sharples K, Hernandez RK, Jick SS. Risk of venous thromboembolism in users of oral contraceptives containing drospirenone or levonorgestrel: Nested case-control study based on UK General Practice Research Database. BMJ 2011;340:d2139.

28. Jick SS, Hernandez RK. Risk of non-fatal venous thromboembolism in women using oral contraceptives containing drospirenone compared with women using oral contraceptives containing levonorgestrel: Case-control study using United States claims data. BMJ 2011;340:d2151.

29. Gaffield ME, Culwell KR, Ravi A. Oral contraceptives and family history of breast cancer. Contraception 2009;80:372–380.

30. Marchbanks PA, McDonald JA, Wilson HG, et al. Oral contraceptives and the risk of breast cancer. N Engl J Med 2002;346:2025–2032.

31. Narod SA, Dube MP, Klijn J, et al. Oral contraceptives and the risk of breast cancer in *BRCA1* and *BRCA2* mutation carriers. J Natl Cancer Inst 2002;94:1773–1779.

32. Centers for Disease Control and Prevention (CDC). Update to CDC's U.S. Medical Eligibility Criteria for Contraceptive Use, 2010: Revised

recommendations for the use of contraceptive methods during the postpartum period. MMWR Morb Mortal Wkly Rep 2011;60:878.

33. Grimes DA, Schulz KF. Nonspecific side effects of oral contraceptives: nocebo or noise? Contraception 2011;83:5–9.

34. Graham CA, Ramos R, Bancroft J, et al. The effects of steroidal contraceptives on the well-being and sexuality of women: A double-blind, placebo-controlled, two-centre study of combined and progestogen-only methods. Contraception 1995;52:363–369.

35. Rosenberg MJ, Meyers A, Roy V. Efficacy, cycle control, and side effects of low- and lower-dose oral contraceptives: A randomized trial of 20 micrograms and 35 micrograms estrogen preparations. Contraception 1999;60:321–329.

36. Burkman RT, Fisher AC, LaGuardia KD. Effects of low-dose oral contraceptives on body weight: Results of a randomized study of up to 13 cycles of use. J Rep Med 2007:52:1030–1034.

37. Duramed Pharmaceuticals. Product information for Seasonale. Pomona, NY: Duramed Pharmaceuticals, 2003.

38. Vercellini P, Frontino G, De Giorgi O, et al. Continuous use of an oral contraceptive for endometriosis-associated recurrent dysmenorrhea that does not respond to a cyclic pill regimen. Fertil Steril 2003;80:560–563.

39. Bayer HealthCare Pharmaceuticals. Product information for Yasmin. Wayne, NJ: Bayer HealthCare Pharmaceuticals, 2010.

40. Mircette Patient Information Guide [Internet]. Available from: *http://www.mircette.com/guide.html.*

41. Bristol-Myers Squibb Co. Product information for Ovcon 35. Princeton, NJ: Bristol-Myers Squibb Co, 2003.

42. Wyeth Pharmaceuticals. Product information for levonorgestrel 90 mcg and ethinyl estradiol 20 mcg (Lybrel). Philadelphia, PA: Wyeth Pharmaceuticals, 2010.

43. Tom W. Oral contraceptive drug interactions. Pharmacist's Letter/Prescriber's Letter 2005;21:210903.

44. Toh S, Mitchell AA, Anderka M. Antibiotics and oral contraceptive failure: A case-crossover study. Contraception 2011;83:418–425.

45. Anonymous. Ortho Evra—A contraceptive patch. Med Lett Drugs Ther 2002;1122:8.

46. Anonymous. An update on Ortho Evra and the risk of thromboembolism. Pharmacist's Letter/Prescribers Letter 2005;21:211202.

47. Smallwood GH, Meador ML, Lenihan JP, et al. for the Ortho Evra/Evra 002 Study Group. Efficacy and safety of a transdermal contraceptive system. Obstet Gynecol 2001;98:799–805.

48. Dieben TO, Roumen FJ, Apter D. Efficacy, cycle control, and user acceptability of a novel combined contraceptive vaginal ring. Obstet Gynecol 2002;100:585–593.

49. Westhoff C. Bone mineral density and DMPA. J Reprod Med 2002;47:795–799.

50. Pfizer. Product information for Depo-subQ Provera 104. New York: Pfizer, 2010.

51. Toh YC, Jain J, Rahnny MH, et al. Suppression of ovulation by a new subcutaneous depot medroxyprogesterone acetate (104 mg/0.65 mL) contraceptive formulation in Asian women. Clin Ther 2004;26: 1845–1854.

52. Bayer HealthCare Pharmaceuticals. Product information for Mirena. Wayne, NJ: Bayer HealthCare Pharmaceuticals, 2009.

53. Duramed Pharmaceuticals. Product information for ParaGard T 380A. N. Pomona, NY: Duramed Pharmaceuticals, 2006.

54. Shering Corporation. Product Information for Implanon. Kenilworth, NJ: Shering Corporation, 2009.

55. Merck and Co. Product Information for Nexplanon. Whitehouse Station, NJ: Merck and Co, 2011.

56. Moench TR, Chipato T, Padian NS. Preventing disease by protecting the cervix: The unexplored promise of internal vaginal barrier devices. AIDS 2001;15:1595–1602.

57. Cates W Jr, Raymond EG. Vaginal barriers and spermicides. In: Hatcher RA, Trussel J, Nelson AL, et al. Contraceptive Technology, 19th rev. ed. New York: Ardent Media, 2007:317–336.

58. Warner L, Steiner MJ. Male condoms. In: Hatcher RA, Trussel J, Nelson AL, et al. Contraceptive Technology, 19th rev. ed. New York: Ardent Media, 2007:297–316.

59. Davis KR, Weller SC. The effectiveness of condoms in reducing heterosexual transmission of HIV. Fam Plann Perspect 1999;31:272–279.

60. Kuyoh MA, Toroitich-Ruto C, Grimes DA, et al. Sponge versus diaphragm for contraception: A Cochrane review. Contraception 2003;67:15–18.

61. Jennings VH, Arevalo M. Fertility awareness-based methods. In: Hatcher RA, Trussel J, Nelson, AL, et al. Contraceptive Technology, 19th rev. ed. New York: Ardent Media, 2007:343–360.

49 Menstruation-Related Disorders

Jacqueline M. Klootwyk and Elena M. Umland

KEY CONCEPTS

❶ Nonsteroidal anti-inflammatory drugs (NSAIDs) are the treatment of choice for dysmenorrhea due to their effect on prostaglandins. In addition to their analgesic properties, NSAIDs also inhibit prostaglandin production, decreasing uterine contractions.

❷ Intrauterine devices (IUDs) are considered therapeutic options in a variety of menstrual-related disorders. Guidelines from the American College of Obstetricians and Gynecologists states that any woman (regardless of parity), including adolescents, at low risk of sexually transmitted diseases (and thus pelvic inflammatory disease) is a good candidate for IUD use.

❸ Unrecognized pregnancy remains the most common cause of amenorrhea, and a urine pregnancy test should be one of the first steps in the evaluation of this disorder.

❹ For most conditions associated with primary and secondary amenorrhea, estrogen treatment (along with a progestin to minimize the risk of endometrial hyperplasia) is utilized.

❺ Anovulatory bleeding, also referred to as dysfunctional uterine bleeding, is secondary to the effects of unopposed estrogen and does not include bleeding owing to an anatomic lesion of the uterus.

❻ The use of metformin and thiazolidinediones for anovulatory bleeding associated with polycystic ovary syndrome is beneficial for anovulatory bleeding and fertility and also improves glucose tolerance and decreases overall cardiovascular risk.

❼ Causes of menorrhagia can be divided into systemic disorders and reproductive tract abnormalities.

❽ Intrauterine pregnancy, ectopic pregnancy, and miscarriage must be at the top of the differential diagnosis list for any woman presenting with heavy menses.

❾ The reduction in menorrhagia-related blood loss with the use of NSAIDs and oral contraceptives is directly proportional to the amount of pretreatment blood loss.

Women of reproductive age commonly experience menstrual cycle-related maladies. The disorders in this chapter are most frequently encountered and include dysmenorrhea, amenorrhea, anovulatory bleeding, and menorrhagia. The need to effectively treat these disorders stems from their impact on a reduced quality of life, negative effects on reproductive health, and/or the potential for detrimental health effects over time, notably osteoporosis with amenorrhea and cardiovascular disease with polycystic ovary disease.

DYSMENORRHEA

Dysmenorrhea is pelvic pain, generally described as cramping, that occurs during or just prior to menstruation. Primary dysmenorrhea is pain in the setting of normal pelvic anatomy and physiology, whereas secondary dysmenorrhea is associated with underlying pelvic pathology.[1]

Epidemiology and Etiology

Rates of dysmenorrhea range from 20% to 90%.[2,3] Dysmenorrhea is associated with significant interference in work and school attendance for as many as 15% of women.[1,3,4] Risk factors for dysmenorrhea include young age, menarche prior to age 12, irregular or heavy menses, body mass index (BMI) less than 20 kg/m^2, smoking, and nulliparity.[1,2] Causes of secondary dysmenorrhea may include cervical stenosis, endometriosis, pelvic infections, pelvic congestion syndrome, uterine or cervical polyps, and uterine fibroids.[1,5]

Pathophysiology

① *The most significant mechanism for primary dysmenorrhea is elevated levels of arachidonic acid in the menstrual fluid leading to increased concentrations of prostaglandins and leukotrienes in the uterus.* In turn, this induces uterine contractions, stimulating pain fibers, reducing uterine blood flow, and causing uterine hypoxia.[1,3-5] This prostaglandin-mediated reaction contributes to the resulting symptoms.[1,4,5]

Clinical Presentation and Diagnosis of Dysmenorrhea

General
- Patient may or may not be in acute distress depending on the severity of menstrual pain experienced.

Symptoms
- Complaints of crampy pelvic pain beginning shortly before or at menses onset. Symptoms typically last 1 to 3 days.
- Associated symptoms may include nausea, vomiting, diarrhea, hypertension, and/or tachycardia.

Laboratory Tests
- Sexually active females should receive a pelvic examination to screen for sexually transmitted diseases.
- Gonorrhea, chlamydia cultures or PCR, wet mount.

Other Diagnostic Tests
- Pelvic ultrasound may be used to identify anatomic abnormalities such as masses/lesions or to detect ovarian cysts and endometriomas.

Patient Encounter 1, Part 1

CO is a 14 year-old white female who presents to her physician with complaints of severe pelvic pain and cramping during menses that result in 1 to 2 missed school days each menstrual cycle. She is not sexually active and does not take any routine medications. She has recently begun high school and is a member of the field hockey team.

What menstrual related disorder does this patient have?

What are the potential risk factors and etiologies for this condition?

Treatment

▶ Desired Outcomes

The medical management of dysmenorrhea should relieve the related pelvic pain and result in a reduction in lost school and work days. Table 49–1 identifies agents used to manage dysmenorrhea, their recommended doses, and their common side effects. Figure 49–1 is a treatment algorithm for dysmenorrhea management.

▶ Nonpharmacologic Therapy

Several nonpharmacologic interventions exist for the management of dysmenorrhea. Among these, topical heat therapy, exercise, and following a low-fat vegetarian diet all have been shown to reduce the intensity of dysmenorrhea.[2,4,11] Dietary changes may also shorten dysmenorrhea duration. Such interventions require little time, minimal cost, and are associated with little risk. Other nonpharmacologic options that may be considered before or after a trial of pharmacologic interventions include transcutaneous electric nerve stimulation (TENS), acupressure, and acupuncture.[2]

▶ Pharmacologic Therapy

Nonsteroidal Anti-inflammatory Drugs (NSAIDs) ①

NSAIDs are the treatment of choice for dysmenorrhea due to their effect on prostaglandins. In addition to their analgesic properties, NSAIDs also inhibit prostaglandin production, decreasing uterine contractions. Although there is not a clear difference in efficacy between the agents, switching agents may be of benefit if relief is not obtained from an initial trial (e.g., ibuprofen to mefenamic acid).[1,5] Choice of one agent over another is based on cost, convenience, and patient preference.[1-5] The most commonly used agents are naproxen and ibuprofen.

A loading dose (twice the usual single dose) of the NSAID is recommended, followed by the usually recommended dose until symptoms resolve.[11] An alternative recommendation is to begin the NSAID at menses onset or 1 to 2 days prior and continue treatment around the clock instead of

Table 49–1

Therapeutic Agents for Selected Menstrual Disorders

Specific Menstrual Disorders(s)	Agent(s)	Dose Recommended	Common Adverse Effects
Amenorrhea (primary or secondary)	CEE[a]	0.625–1.25 mg by mouth daily on days 1–25 of the cycle[6]	Thromboembolism, breast enlargement, breast tenderness, bloating, nausea, GI upset, headache, peripheral edema
	Ethinyl estradiol patch[a]	50 mcg/24 hours[6]	
	Oral CHC[a]	30–40 mcg formulations	
Amenorrhea (secondary)	Oral medroxyprogesterone acetate[a]	5–10 mg by mouth on days 14–25 of the cycle[6]	Edema, anorexia, depression, insomnia, weight gain or loss, increase in serum total and LDL cholesterol, may reduce HDL cholesterol
Amenorrhea related to hyperprolactinemia	Bromocriptine	2.5 mg by mouth 2–3 times daily[7]	Hypotension, nausea, constipation, anorexia, Raynaud's phenomenon
Anovulatory bleeding	Oral CHC[a]	Optimal dose unknown[8] For acute bleeding, product containing 35 mcg ethinyl estradiol; take one tablet by mouth 3 times daily × 1 week; then one tablet by mouth daily × 3 weeks.[9]	As noted above for CEE, ethinyl estradiol, and oral CHC (progesterone side effects with the CHC depend on agent chosen)
	Oral medroxyprogesterone acetate[a]	For acute bleeding, 20 mg by mouth 3 times daily × 1 week; then 20 mg by mouth once daily × 3 weeks.[9]	As noted above for oral medroxyprogesterone acetate
Dysmenorrhea	Oral CHC[10,a]	Less than 35 mcg formulations + norgestrel or levonorgestrel[11]; use of extended-cycle formulations are beneficial for this indication	As noted above for CEE, ethinyl estradiol, and oral CHC (progesterone side effects with the CHC depend on agent chosen)
	Depo-medroxyprogesterone acetate[a]	150 mg intramuscularly every 12 weeks	Irregular menses, amenorrhea
	Levonorgestrel IUD[12,a]	20 mcg released daily	Irregular menses, amenorrhea
	NSAIDs—any are acceptable; the most commonly studied/cited are included in this table[1,2,4,5,10]	Diclofenac 50 mg by mouth 3 times daily[b]	GI upset, stomach ulcer, nausea, vomiting, heartburn, indigestion, rash, dizziness
		Ibuprofen 800 mg by mouth 3 times daily[a]	
		Mefenamic acid 500 mg by mouth as a loading dose, then 250 mg by mouth up to 4 times daily as needed[b]	
		Naproxen 550-mg loading dose by mouth started 1–2 days prior to menses, followed by 275 mg by mouth every 6–12 hours as needed[c] Treatment should begin 1–2 days prior to the suspected onset of menses	
Menorrhagia	Oral CHC[a]	Optimal dose unknown	As noted above
	Levonorgestrel IUD[a]	20 mcg released daily	As noted above
	Medroxyprogesterone acetate (oral)[a]	5–10 mg by mouth on days 5–26 of the cycle *or* during the luteal phase[12]	As noted above
	NSAIDs	Doses as recommended for above; therapy should be initiated with the onset of menses[12]	As noted above
PCOS-related amenorrhea and/or anovulatory bleeding	Clomiphene[11]	50 mg by mouth daily × 5 days starting 3–5 days after the start of menses; doses up to 100 mg by mouth daily have been used in significantly obese patients.	Hot flashes, ovarian enlargement, thromboembolism, blurred vision, breast discomfort
	Depo-medroxyprogesterone acetate[a]	150 mg intramuscularly every 12 weeks	As noted above

(Continued)

Table 49–1			
Therapeutic Agents for Selected Menstrual Disorders (*Continued*)			
Specific Menstrual Disorders(s)	**Agent(s)**	**Dose Recommended**	**Common Adverse Effects**
PCOS-related amenorrhea and/ or anovulatory bleeding	Medroxyprogesterone acetate (oral)[a]	10 mg by mouth × 10 days[8]	As noted above
	Metformin[a]	1,500–2,000 mg by mouth daily in 2–3 divided doses[10,a,d]	Anorexia, nausea, vomiting, diarrhea, flatulence, lactic acidosis
	Thiazolidinediones[8,e]	Pioglitazone 15–45 mg by mouth daily; rosiglitazone 4–8 mg by mouth daily	Weight gain; increase in total, LDL, and HDL cholesterol; edema; headache; fatigue; hepatic injury (rare)

CEE, conjugated equine estrogen ; CHC, combination hormonal contraceptive; HDL, high-density lipoprotein; LDL, low-density lipoprotein; IUD, intrauterine device.

[a]Use is contraindicated in patients with severe hepatic impairment.

[b]Not recommended in patients with severe renal impairment.

[c]Use is contraindicated with creatinine clearance less than 30 mL/min (0.5 mL/s).

[d]Contraindicated in males with serum creatinine more than 1.5 mg/dL (133 μmol/L); females with serum creatinine more than 1.4 mg/dL (124 μmol/L); caution with creatinine clearance less than 60 mL/min (1 mL/s).

[e]Contraindicated in patients with active liver disease or if transaminases more than 2.5 times upper limit of normal at baseline, discontinue therapy if ALT is more than 3 times upper limit of normal.

Data from Refs. 1, 2, 4–14.

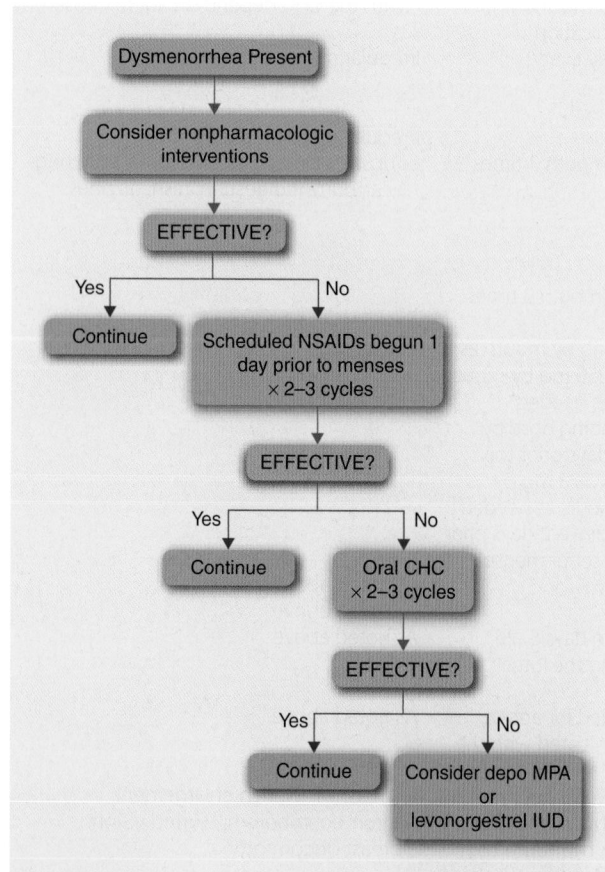

FIGURE 49–1. Treatment algorithm for dysmenorrhea. (NSAID, nonsteroidal anti-inflammatory drug; CHC, combination hormonal contraceptive; MPA, medroxyprogesterone acetate; IUD, intrauterine device.)

waiting until symptom onset. For patients in whom NSAID use is contraindicated, the agents discussed next should be considered.[1,5] The use of acetaminophen is inferior to NSAIDs for treating this disorder.[2]

● **Combination Hormonal Contraceptives (CHCs)** CHCs help to improve dysmenorrhea by inhibiting the proliferation of endometrial tissue. This reduction in tissue reduces the endometrial-derived prostaglandins that contribute to the pelvic pain.[1,3–5,11] A trial of 2 to 3 months of CHC dosing is required to establish whether the patient will be a responder or not. Significant improvements in mild, moderate, and severe dysmenorrhea have been noted with CHC use. These agents have other benefits, including pregnancy prevention, improving acne, and reducing ovarian cancer risk. Although monophasic formulations are purported to be more efficacious for this indication, the evidence supporting this is limited.[2,15] If no response occurs after 6 months of therapy, the patient should be evaluated for secondary causes.[1]

● **Progestins** The benefit of depo-medroxyprogesterone acetate in dysmenorrhea is related to its ability to render most patients amenorrheic within 1 year of use.[2] This is an expected side effect. Since the pelvic pain is related to prostaglandins released during menses, in the setting of amenorrhea, this underlying cause of dysmenorrhea is removed.

Observational data illustrate a reduction in dysmenorrhea from 60% to 29% with 3 years of levonorgestrel-releasing intrauterine device (IUD) use.[2,3] As with depo-medroxyprogesterone acetate, this reduction is likely secondary to the increasing incidence of amenorrhea observed with its use. Although data are limited, this is an option for dysmenorrhea management.[15]

Patient Encounter 1, Part 2

Additional workup of CO reveals:

PMH: seasonal allergic rhinitis

PSH: none

FH: Mother and father are alive and well. She has two younger siblings (ages 12 and 10) who are alive and well.

SH: The patient participates in high school field hockey. She denies smoking cigarettes or drinking alcohol.

Meds: Loratadine 10 mg by mouth as needed for seasonal allergies

Past Gynecologic Hx: Menarche at age 11; never pregnant and never on contraception; (–) sexual activity; (+) history of painful menses beginning at age 12; (+) heavy menstrual flow; menstrual cycle 28 to 30 days in length.

ROS: (–) fatigue; (–) headaches; (+) mild acne on shoulders; (+) moderate to severe pelvic pain with menses.

PE:

General: Thin-appearing white female, in no acute distress

VS: BP 118/62, P 74, RR 16, weight 123 lbs (55.9 kg), height 5'6" (168 cm), BMI: 19.9 kg/m2

HEENT: (–) hirsutism

Breasts: (–) galactorrhea

Pelvic exam: normal appearance of external genitalia and vagina, cervix without lesions, uterus midposition without masses, adnexa without masses

Labs:

None ordered.

Given this information, what is your assessment of this patient's condition?

Identify your treatment goals for this patient.

What therapeutic options exist for this patient? Identify those that would be most appropriate.

What monitoring parameters are necessary to employ in assessing efficacy and safety of the therapeutic options?

Dysmenorrhea in Adolescents

Dysmenorrhea is very common in adolescent females, with an incidence of 60% to 90%.[1] Any of the treatment measures discussed for dysmenorrhea would be appropriate in this population. Although NSAIDs and oral CHCs are among the top choices, levonorgestrel IUD use is also an option.[15] ❷ *The American College of Obstetricians and Gynecologists (ACOG) states that any woman, including adolescents (regardless of parity) at low risk of sexually transmitted diseases and thus pelvic inflammatory disease, is a good candidate for IUD use.*[16,17]

AMENORRHEA

Amenorrhea is either primary or secondary in nature. **Primary amenorrhea** is the absence of menses by age 15 in the presence of normal secondary sexual development or within 5 years of **thelarche** (if occurring before age 10).[18,19] **Secondary amenorrhea** is the absence of menses for three cycles or 6 months in a previously menstruating woman. The initial evaluation of amenorrhea is often the same regardless of age of onset, except in unusual clinical situations.[20]

Epidemiology and Etiology

❸ *Unrecognized pregnancy remains the most common cause of amenorrhea, and a urine pregnancy test should be one of the first steps in the evaluation of this disorder.* Amenorrhea not related to pregnancy, lactation, or menopause occurs in 3% to 4% of women.[19] After pregnancy, the five most common causes of secondary amenorrhea, in descending order of prevalence, include hypothalamic suppression (33%), chronic anovulation (28%), hyperprolactinemia (14%), ovarian failure (12%), and uterine disorders (7%).[21]

Pathophysiology

In organizing an approach to amenorrhea diagnosis and treatment, the organs involved in the menstrual cycle, including the uterus, ovaries, anterior pituitary, and hypothalamus, should be considered. Normal menstrual cycle physiology depends on a coordinated system of hormonal interactions that involve the hypothalamus, anterior pituitary gland, ovary, and endometrium. **Figures 49–2** and **49–3** summarize these points. Pulsatile gonadotropin-releasing hormone (GnRH) secretion from the hypothalamus stimulates the anterior pituitary to secrete follicle-stimulating hormone (FSH) and luteinizing hormone (LH). In the

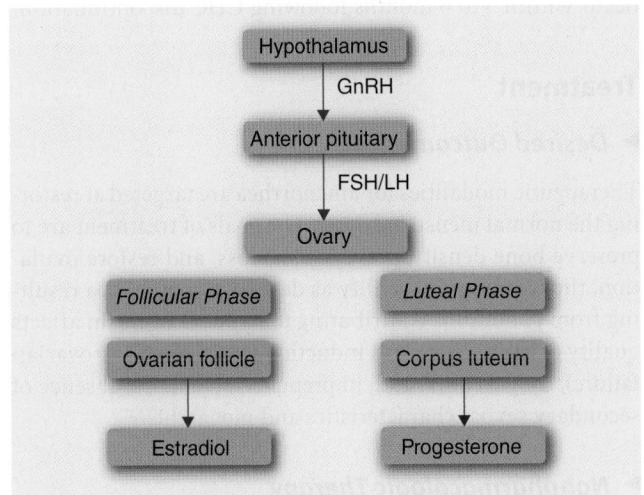

FIGURE 49–2. Summary of normal menstrual cycle. (FSH, follicle-stimulating hormone; GnRH, gonadotropin-releasing hormone; LH, luteinizing hormone.)

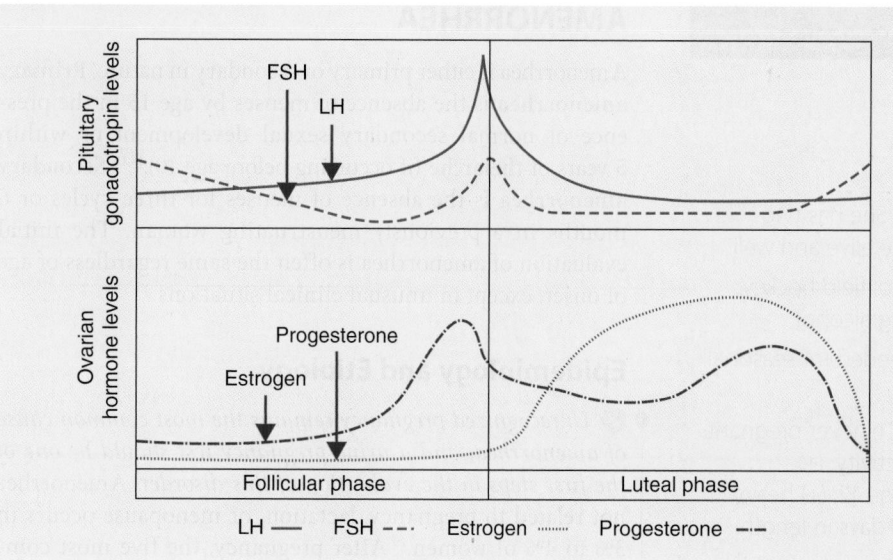

FIGURE 49–3. Hormonal fluctuations with the normal menstrual cycle. (FSH, follicle-stimulating hormone; LH, luteinizing hormone.) (Data from Umland EM, Weinstein LC, Buchanan E. Menstruation-related disorders (Chapter 89). In: Pharmacotherapy: A Pathophysiologic Approach, 8th ed. New York, NY: McGraw-Hill, 2011, with permission.)

specialized cells of the ovarian follicle, FSH and LH stimulate estradiol's release. Estradiol stimulates endometrial growth during the follicular phase of the cycle. Following the LH surge and ovulation, the follicle transforms into the corpus luteum. Progesterone secreted by the corpus luteum during the luteal phase of the cycle causes endometrial "organization." If conception does not occur, the drop in estrogen and progesterone stimulates endometrial shedding.[5,20,22] Table 49–2 illustrates amenorrhea pathophysiology relative to the organ system(s) involved, as well as the condition(s) resulting in amenorrhea. Amenorrhea is an expected, potential side effect resulting from use of low-dose oral CHCs, extended-cycle oral CHCs, or depot medroxyprogesterone acetate.[28] Many women experience delayed return of menses after CHC discontinuation. Postpill amenorrhea usually is a self-limited condition. Further evaluation for other conditions such as polycystic ovary syndrome (PCOS) should be considered if spontaneous resolution of amenorrhea does not occur within 3 to 6 months following CHC discontinuation.

Treatment

▶ Desired Outcomes

Therapeutic modalities for amenorrhea are targeted at restoring the normal menstrual cycle. The goals of treatment are to preserve bone density, prevent bone loss, and restore ovulation, thus improving fertility as desired. Amenorrhea resulting from conditions contributing to hypoestrogenism affects quality of life via hot flash induction (e.g., premature ovarian failure), dyspareunia, and, in prepubertal females, absence of secondary sexual characteristics and menarche.

▶ Nonpharmacologic Therapy

Nonpharmacologic therapy for amenorrhea varies depending on its underlying cause. Amenorrhea secondary to undernutrition or anorexia may respond to weight gain.[19]

Clinical Presentation and Diagnosis of Amenorrhea

General
- Patients may be concerned about cessation of menses and fertility implications but generally are not in acute distress.

Symptoms
- Cessation of menses
- Possible complaints of infertility, vaginal dryness, decreased libido

Signs
- Absence of menses by age 15 in the presence of normal secondary sexual development or within 5 years of thelarche (if occurs before age 10).
- Recent significant weight loss or gain
- Presence of acne, hirsutism, hair loss, or acanthosis nigricans may suggest androgen excess.

Laboratory Tests
- Pregnancy test
- TSH
- Prolactin
- If PCOS is suspected, consider free or total testosterone, 17-hydroxyprogesterone, fasting glucose, and fasting lipid panel.
- If premature ovarian failure is suspected, consider FSH and LH measurements.

Other Diagnostic Tests
- Progesterone challenge
- Pelvic ultrasound to evaluate for polycystic ovaries

Table 49–2

Pathophysiology of Selected Menstrual Bleeding Disorders

Organ System	Condition	Pathophysiology/Laboratory Findings
Amenorrhea[1,20,24]		
Uterus	Asherman's syndrome	Postcurettage/postsurgical uterine adhesions
	Congenital uterine abnormalities	Abnormal uterine development
Ovaries	Turner's syndrome	Lack of ovarian follicles
	Gonadal dysgenesis	Other genetic anomalies
	Premature ovarian failure	Early loss of follicles
	Chemotherapy/radiation	Gonadal toxins
Anterior pituitary	Pituitary prolactin-secreting adenoma	↑ Prolactin suppresses HPO axis
	Hypothyroidism	TRH causing ↑ prolactin, other abnormalities
	Medications—antipsychotics, verapamil	↑ Prolactin suppresses HPO axis
Hypothalamus	"Functional" hypothalamic amenorrhea	↓ Pulsatile GnRH secretion in the absence of other abnormalities
	Disordered eating	↓ Pulsatile GnRH secretion, ↓ FSH and LH secondary to weight loss
	Exercise	↓ Pulsatile GnRH secretion, ↓ FSH and LH secondary to low body fat
	Anovulation/PCOS	Asynchronous gonadotropin and estrogen production, abnormal endometrial growth
Anovulatory Bleeding[1,8,25,26]		
Physiologic causes	Adolescence	Immature hypothalamic-pituitary-ovarian axis: no LH surge
	Perimenopause	Declining ovarian function
Pathologic causes	Hyperandrogenic anovulation—PCOS	Hyperandrogenism: high testosterone, high LH, hyperinsulinemia, and insulin resistance
	Hypothalamic dysfunction (physical or emotional stress, exercise, weight loss)	Suppression of pulsatile GnRH secretion and estrogen deficiency: low LH, low FSH
	Hyperprolactinemia (pituitary gland tumor, psychiatric medications)	High prolactin
	Hypothyroidism	High TSH
	Premature ovarian failure	High FSH
Menorrhagia[27]		
Hematologic	von Willebrand's disease	Factor VII defect causing impaired platelet adhesion and increased bleeding time
	Idiopathic thrombocytopenic purpura	Decrease in circulating platelets—can be acute or chronic
Hepatic	Cirrhosis	Decreased estrogen metabolism, underlying coagulopathy
Endocrine	Hypothyroidism	Alterations in HPO axis
Uterine	Fibroids	Alteration of endometrium, changes in uterine contractility
	Adenomyosis	Alteration of endometrium, changes in uterine contractility
	Endometrial polyps	Alteration of endometrium
	Gynecologic cancers	Various dysplastic alterations of endometrium, uterus, cervix

↑, high; ↓, low; FSH, follicle-stimulating hormone; GnRH, gonadotropin-releasing hormone; HPO, hypothalamic-pituitary-ovarian axis; LH, luteinizing hormone; PCOS, polycystic ovary disease; TRH, thyrotropin-releasing hormone; TSH, thyroid-stimulating hormone.

Data from Refs. 1, 7, 18, 21, and 23–25.

Such patients also would benefit from psychotherapy. In young women for whom excessive exercise is an underlying cause, exercise reduction is recommended.

▶ Pharmacologic Therapy

Estrogen/Progestin Replacement Therapy ❹ *For most conditions associated with primary or secondary amenorrhea, estrogen treatment (along with a progestin to minimize the risk of endometrial hyperplasia) is utilized.* The purpose of estrogen therapy in this patient population is multifactorial: to reduce osteoporosis risk, stimulate and maintain secondary sexual characteristics, and improve quality of life.[6,13,19] Table 49–1 identifies therapeutic options for amenorrhea,

including recommended doses. **Figure 49–4** illustrates a treatment algorithm for amenorrhea management.

Bromocriptine If hyperprolactinemia is the cause of amenorrhea in women who desire conception, use of a dopamine agonist, most commonly, bromocriptine, results in a reduction in prolactin concentrations and resumption of menses.[7,19] Bromocriptine normalizes prolactin levels in 90% of women, and fertility is restored in 80% of women.[29]

Progestins Progestins have long been used to induce withdrawal bleeding in women with secondary amenorrhea. Several factors predict progesterone's efficacy for this purpose.[30] These factors include estrogen concentrations greater than or equal to 35 pg/mL (128 pmol/L) and endometrial

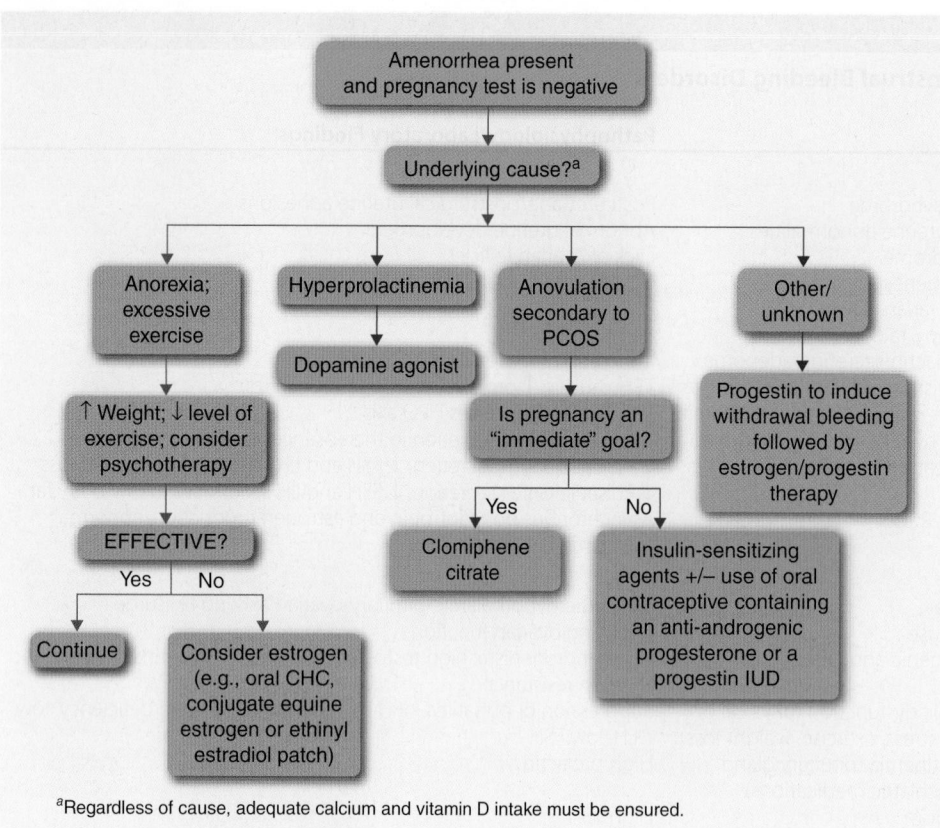

FIGURE 49–4. Treatment algorithm for amenorrhea. (CHC, combination hormonal contraceptive; IUD, intrauterine device; PCOS, polycystic ovarian syndrome.)

thickness (the greater it is, the greater the amount of withdrawal bleeding).

Progestin efficacy for secondary amenorrhea also varies depending on the formulation used. For example, progesterone in oil administered intramuscularly results in withdrawal bleeding in 70% of treated patients, whereas oral medroxyprogesterone acetate induces withdrawal bleeding in 95% of treated patients.[30] Table 49–1 identifies the types and doses of progestins used for inducing withdrawal bleeding in secondary amenorrhea. Figure 49–4 illustrates when to consider progestins for amenorrhea treatment.

Insulin-Sensitizing Agents Amenorrhea related to anovulation and PCOS may respond to the use of insulin sensitizing agents.[8] The use of metformin for this purpose will be discussed in the following anovulatory bleeding section.

For all patients experiencing amenorrhea, owing to the negative impact this has on bone health, a diet rich in calcium and vitamin D must be followed.

Amenorrhea in Adolescents

Amenorrhea in the adolescent population is very important, as this is when peak bone mass is achieved. The cause of amenorrhea and appropriate treatment must be identified promptly in this population because hypoestrogenism contributes negatively to bone development.[19] Estrogen replacement, typically via a CHC, is important. Although some recent data suggest that CHCs and depo-medroxyprogesterone acetate may reduce bone mineral density (BMD) short-term,

their long-term effects on fractures are unknown. Additionally, these negative BMD effects appear to be reversible; therefore, CHC use is still recommended in the adolescent population.[31] Ensuring adequate dietary calcium and vitamin D intake in this population is imperative.

ANOVULATORY BLEEDING

Anovulatory bleeding is irregular menstrual blood flow from the endometrium that ranges from light spotting to heavy blood flow.[32] ⑤ *Anovulatory bleeding, also referred to as dysfunctional uterine bleeding, is secondary to the effects of unopposed estrogen and does not include bleeding owing to an anatomic lesion of the uterus.* It includes noncyclic menstrual bleeding due to anovulation or oligo-ovulation.[26] Anovulatory bleeding is a diagnosis of exclusion and includes PCOS, which typically presents with irregular menstrual bleeding, hirsutism, obesity, and/or infertility.[8]

Epidemiology

Anovulatory bleeding is the most common form of noncyclic uterine bleeding.[32] Patients often seek medical care to regulate their menstrual cycle or improve fertility. All women of reproductive age should have a pregnancy test when presenting with irregular menstrual bleeding. Anovulation may be secondary to physiologic or pathologic causes. It is common at menarche and in the perimenopausal period. During adolescence, ovulatory menstrual cycles may not be regular for 12 to 18 months after menarche.[32] Ovulation frequency is related to the age at and time since menarche.[18] In the year following menarche, the feedback mechanism in the hypothalamic-pituitary-ovarian (HPO) axis may be immature, and the LH surge needed for ovulation fails to occur.[32] During perimenopause, anovulatory cycles may occur due to declining quality and quantity of ovarian follicles. As ovarian function declines, estrogen secretion continues, and progesterone secretion decreases. Chronic anovulatory cycles and unopposed estrogen secretion lead to endometrial proliferation and increased risk of polyps, endometrial hyperplasia, and endometrial carcinoma.[26]

Anovulation also may occur at any time during the reproductive years due to a pathologic cause. The most common causes of nonphysiologic ovulatory dysfunction and their prevalence rates[26] are:

- PCOS (70%)
- Hypothalamic amenorrhea (10%)
- Hyperprolactinemia (10%)
- Premature ovarian failure (10%)

PCOS, although responsible for 55% to 91% (depending on the definition) of ovulatory dysfunction cases, occurs in approximately 7% of women.[8]

Etiology

Anovulation results from dysfunction at any level of the HPO axis. In addition to physiologic life stages such as adolescence, perimenopause, pregnancy, and lactation, other causes of anovulation include the following[18,26]:

- Hyperandrogenic anovulation (PCOS, congenital adrenal hyperplasia, androgen-producing tumors)
- Hypothalamic dysfunction (anorexia nervosa, physical or emotional stress)
- Hyperprolactinemia
- Hypothyroidism
- Primary pituitary disease
- Premature ovarian failure

Pathophysiology

A normal ovulatory cycle includes follicular development, ovulation, corpus luteum development, and luteolysis. During the cycle, the endometrium proliferates and undergoes secretory changes and desquamation. This is influenced by the effects of estrogen alone, then by estrogen and progesterone, and culminates with estrogen and progesterone withdrawal. Progesterone stops endometrial growth and stimulates endometrial differentiation. In anovulatory women, a corpus luteum is not formed, and the ovary does not secrete progesterone. Without progesterone, there is no endometrial desquamation or differentiation. Chronic unopposed estrogen causes endometrial proliferation, and the endometrium becomes vascular and fragile, resulting in noncyclic menstrual bleeding. The endometrium may also become hyperplastic and progress to a precancerous state, increasing

the woman's risk of endometrial cancer.[1] See Table 49-2 for the pathophysiology of anovulatory bleeding relative to the specific conditions contributing to it.

The most common pathologic cause of anovulation is PCOS. Although PCOS does not have a universal definition, consensus criteria have been updated to include the presence of polycystic ovaries on ultrasound. The Rotterdam criteria identify PCOS as a syndrome of ovarian dysfunction diagnosed by when two of the following characteristics exist: (a) oligoanovulation or anovulation; (b) clinical signs (hirsutism, acne) or laboratory evidence of hyperandrogenism (total testosterone and sex hormone-binding globulin); and (c) polycystic ovary morphology on ultrasound.[8,33] The Androgen Excess Society (AES) recognizes hyperandrogenism as a mandatory component of diagnosis in addition to oligoanovulation or anovulation, polycystic ovaries on ultrasound, or both.[8,33] No gene or environmental substance appears to cause PCOS.[8] However, familial clustering of PCOS cases suggests that genetics play a role. Insulin resistance, hyperandrogenism, and changes in gonadotropins also influence PCOS development. The underlying cause for increased androgens is unknown.[35,36]

Recently, discussion regarding the link to cardiovascular disease has been emphasized. PCOS is associated with a two to five times increased risk of developing type 2 diabetes.[8] In women with PCOS, approximately 60% to 80% have impaired glucose tolerance (IGT). In obese women with PCOS, IGT prevalence increases to 95%,[37] and 70% have dyslipidemia.[8,37] Although rates of cardiovascular disease mortality directly related to PCOS are unknown, women with PCOS should be screened for IGT, diabetes, hypertension, and dyslipidemia.[8] If any of these are present, there is an increased risk of cardiovascular events.[37,38]

Treatment

▶ Desired Outcomes

The desired, short-term outcome of therapy is to stop acute bleeding. The long-term goals include preventing future episodes of noncyclic bleeding, decreasing long-term complications of anovulation (e.g., osteopenia and infertility), and improving overall quality of life.[26] Table 49-1 identifies the agents used in anovulatory bleeding management, their doses, and common side effects.

▶ Nonpharmacologic Therapy

Nonpharmacologic treatment options for anovulatory bleeding depend on the underlying cause. For all women with PCOS, weight loss may be beneficial. In overweight or obese women, a 5% reduction in weight has been associated with resumption of menses, improved pregnancy rates, and decreased hirsutism, glucose, and lipid levels.[8] In women who have completed childbearing or who have failed medical management, endometrial ablation or resection and hysterectomy are surgical options. It is unclear which procedure is preferred. Short term, it appears that ablation or resection

Clinical Presentation and Diagnosis of Anovulatory Bleeding

General
- May or may not be in acute distress

Symptoms
- Irregular, heavy, or prolonged vaginal bleeding, perimenopausal symptoms (hot flashes, etc.)

Signs
- Acne, hirsutism, obesity

Laboratory Tests
- If suspect PCOS, consider free or total testosterone, fasting glucose, fasting lipid panel.
- If suspect perimenopause, FSH.

Other Diagnostic Tests
- Pelvic ultrasound to evaluate for polycystic ovaries

results in less morbidity and shorter recovery periods.[39] However, a significant number of these women eventually undergo hysterectomy in the following 5 years.[26]

▶ Pharmacologic Therapy

Estrogen Estrogen is the recommended treatment for managing acute bleeding episodes because it promotes endometrial growth and stabilization.[26] Its use via CHC regimens has averted emergency surgical procedures in 95% of patients.[9] Following estrogen's initial use to control acute bleeding

Patient Encounter 2, Part 1

TP, a 32 year-old woman, presents to your office for a routine gynecologic examination. She entered menarche at the age of 12. Her last menstrual period was 3 months ago. Her periods are often irregular and occur about every 2 to 3 months. She has had all normal Pap smears in the past and no history of sexually transmitted infections. She has had a total of four sexual partners. She has never been pregnant. She is married and has noted that she is not using any form of contraception, as she and her husband have been trying, unsuccessfully, to become pregnant for the past 12 months. As you examine the patient, you note facial and chest acne, increased facial and abdominal hair, and obesity.

What anovulatory disorder is most likely present?

What signs/symptoms support this conclusion?

What diagnostic tests should be done?

episodes, it should be continued to prevent future occurrences. CHC use fulfills this role.

In addition to controlling acute bleeding, CHC use also aids in preventing recurrent anovulatory bleeding. They suppress ovarian hormones and adrenal androgen production and indirectly increase sex hormone–binding globulin (SHBG). This, in turn, binds and reduces circulating androgen.[8,26,40] For women with high androgen levels and related signs (e.g., hirsutism), low-dose CHCs (less than or equal to 35 mcg ethinyl estradiol) are the treatment of choice.[26] In theory, one may consider a CHC with a progesterone such as drospirenone that has greater impact on increasing SHBG and antiandrogenic effects.[41] However, to date there is no consensus regarding the best CHC choice for treating PCOS.[8]

Medroxyprogesterone Acetate Depot and intermittent oral medroxyprogesterone acetate suppresses pituitary gonadotropins and circulating androgens in women with PCOS.[8] Furthermore, cyclic progesterone use may benefit women over age 40 with anovulatory bleeding.[26] Similar to the use of CHCs, oral medroxyprogesterone acetate use has been observed to avert emergency surgical procedures in 100% of patients for acute uterine bleeding justifying immediate medical attention.[9]

Insulin-sensitizing Agents The use of metformin and the thiazolidinediones, pioglitazone and rosiglitazone, results in improved insulin sensitivity. In patients with PCOS, this is associated with reduced circulating androgen concentrations, increasing ovulation rates, and improving glucose tolerance.[8] These improvements can be attributed to the SHBG increase that occurs via increased insulin sensitivity. ❻ *These agents are of benefit not only for anovulatory bleeding and fertility, but also because they improve glucose tolerance and decrease overall cardiovascular risk.*[8] Metformin has an additional benefit of potentially promoting weight loss, whereas the thiazolidinediones may cause weight gain. The thiazolidinediones have fallen out of favor in recent years due to the potential negative cardiovascular effects.[42] There are no well-controlled trials lasting longer than 1 year in women with PCOS.[8] If pregnancy is a desired outcome, it is important to note that metformin is a pregnancy category B agent, whereas pioglitazone and rosiglitazone are category C.

Clomiphene Citrate Although insulin-sensitizing agent use may improve fertility, if the treatment goal is to induce ovulation, then the treatment of choice is clomiphene citrate. It is approximately three times more effective than metformin at achieving live births.[8] A recent meta-analysis has shown that combination therapy with an insulin-sensitizing agent such as metformin plus clomiphene citrate may be more effective in increasing pregnancy rates, especially in obese women with PCOS.[8,43,44] Treatment with clomiphene citrate 50 mg/day for 5 days can be initiated between days 3 and 5 of the menstrual cycle. This is often recommended following withdrawal bleeding induction with medroxyprogesterone acetate, 10 mg/day by mouth for 10 days.

Patient Encounter 2, Part 2

PMH: Obesity; acne

FH: Father is living and has hypertension. Mother is living and has diabetes mellitus and hypercholesterolemia. Both parents are obese.

SH: The patient works as a secretary. She lives with her husband. She denies any tobacco or recreational drug use. She drinks 1 to 2 alcoholic beverages per week. She denies regular exercise.

Meds: None

ROS: (+) acne, (+) hirsutism, (−) dysmenorrhea, (−) breast tenderness, (−) vaginal discharge

PE:

VS: blood pressure 128/82, pulse 80 beats per minute, respiratory rate 18, weight 170 lb (77.3 kg), height 5 ft, 3 in (160 cm), BMI 30.2 kg/m²

Abd: Obese, soft, nontender, nondistended, (+) bowel sounds, no hepatosplenomegaly

Gyn: Normal external appearance; vaginal walls normal; cervix well visualized and without lesions; midposition uterus; no cervical motion tenderness; no **adnexal** masses palpated

Labs: Urine HCG negative, free testosterone 100 ng/dL (3.47 nmol/L) (elevated), TSH 2.1 μIU/mL (2.1 milliunits/L) (within normal limits), prolactin 9 ng/mL (9 mcg/L) (within normal limits), fasting glucose 120 mg/dL (6.7 mmol/L). Fasting lipid panel: total cholesterol 181 mg/dL (4.68 mmol/L), HDL cholesterol 58 mg/dL (1.50 mmol/L), triglycerides 65 mg/dL (0.73 mmol/L), LDL cholesterol 110 mg/dL (2.84 mmol/L).

Pelvic ultrasound

15 follicles in right ovary, 14 follicles in left ovary, increased ovarian volume of 12 mL

What treatment options are available for this patient?

Anovulatory Bleeding in Adolescents

Anovulatory cycles are common in the perimenarchal reproductive years. Ovulation typically is established a year or more following menarche. When anovulatory bleeding occurs in this population, it may be excessive. In this case, the patient should be evaluated for blood dyscrasias, including von Willebrand's disease, prothrombin deficiency, and idiopathic thrombocytopenia purpura.[26,27]

In the adolescent population, specific blood dyscrasias should be treated. In addition, acute, severe bleeding is managed with high-dose estrogen. Low-dose CHCs (less than or equal to 35 mcg ethinyl estradiol) are the treatment of choice in adolescents with chronic anovulation.[26]

MENORRHAGIA

The term **menorrhagia** describes prolonged menstrual bleeding or cyclic, heavy blood loss. Menstrual cycles lasting greater than 7 days are considered prolonged, and heavy menstrual bleeding is menstrual blood loss greater than 80 mL per cycle.[25,32] The latter definition has been questioned for several reasons, including difficulty with quantifying menstrual blood loss in clinical practice. Many women with "heavy menses," but who experience less than 80 mL of blood loss, merit consideration for treatment because of containment flow problems, unpredictable heavy flow days, and other associated dysmenorrhea symptoms.[45,46]

Epidemiology and Etiology

Menorrhagia rates in healthy women range from 9% to 14%. **7** *Causes of menorrhagia can be divided into systemic disorders and reproductive tract abnormalities.* **8** *Intrauterine pregnancy, ectopic pregnancy, and miscarriage must be at the top of the differential diagnosis list for any woman presenting with heavy menses.* Additionally, genital tract malignancies and infection may present with abnormal bleeding.[25] Sys-

Clinical Presentation and Diagnosis of Menorrhagia

General
- Patient may or may not be in acute distress.

Symptoms
- Complaints of heavy/prolonged menstrual flow and fatigue and light-headedness in the case of severe blood loss. These symptoms may or may not occur with dysmenorrhea.

Signs
- Orthostasis, tachycardia, and pallor may be noted, especially with significant acute blood loss.

Laboratory Tests
- Complete blood count (CBC) and ferritin levels; hemoglobin and hematocrit results may be low.
- If the history dictates, testing may be done to identify coagulation disorder(s) as a cause.

Other Diagnostic Tests
- Pelvic ultrasound
- Pelvic magnetic resonance imaging (MRI)
- Pap smear
- Endometrial biopsy
- Hysteroscopy
- Sonohysterogram

temic disorders include coagulation dysfunction such as von Willebrand's disease and platelet function disorders.[25,27,32] Hypothyroidism is also associated with heavy menses. Specific reproductive tract causes of menorrhagia are more common in older childbearing women, and they include fibroids, adenomyosis, endometrial polyps, and gynecologic malignancies.[32]

Pathophysiology

Table 49–2 illustrates the pathophysiology of menorrhagia relative to the organ system(s) involved and the specific conditions resulting in menorrhagia.

Treatment

▶ Desired Outcomes

Menorrhagia therapy should reduce menstrual blood flow, improve the patient's quality of life, and defer the need for surgical intervention. Table 49–1 identifies agents used in managing menorrhagia. It also includes their dosing and common side effects. Figure 49–5 illustrates which treatment(s) to use and when.

▶ Nonpharmacologic Therapy

Nonpharmacologic interventions for menorrhagia include surgical interventions that are reserved for patients nonresponsive to pharmacologic treatment. These interventions vary from conservative endometrial ablation to hysterectomy.[39]

▶ Pharmacologic Therapy

Nonsteroidal Anti-inflammatory Drugs (NSAIDs) Nonsteroidal anti-inflammatory drugs (NSAIDs) are first-line treatments for menorrhagia associated with ovulatory cycles.[40] They have the advantage of being taken only during menses, and their use is associated with a significant reduction in menstrual blood loss. A 20% to 50% reduction in blood loss has been observed in 75% of treated women.[12,40] In some patients, as much as an 80% reduction has been observed. ❾ *This reduction is directly proportional to the amount of pretreatment blood loss.*[12]

Combination Hormonal Contraceptives CHC use is beneficial to women with menorrhagia who do not desire pregnancy. A 40% to 50% menstrual blood loss reduction has been observed in 68% of menorrhagia patients treated with oral CHCs containing greater than or equal to 35 mcg estradiol.[12,15]

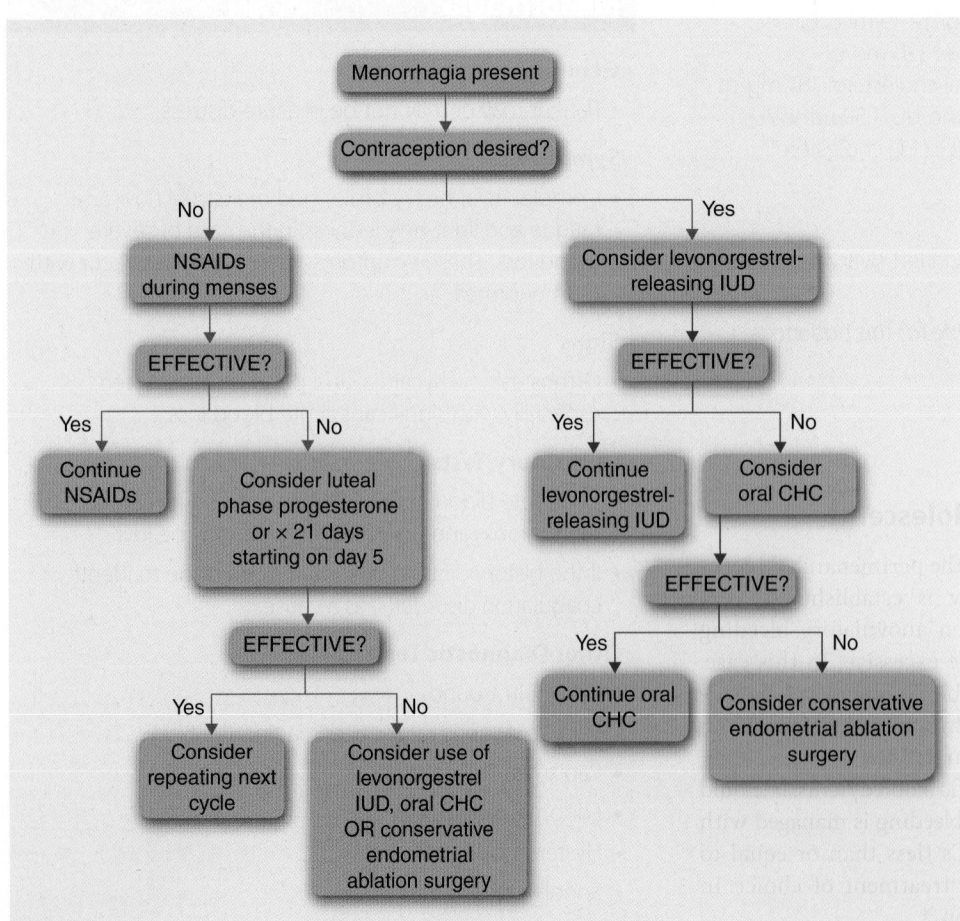

FIGURE 49–5. Treatment algorithm for menorrhagia. (CHC, combination hormonal contraceptive; IUD, intrauterine device; NSAID, nonsteroidal anti-inflammatory drug.)

Continuous and extended cycle options may also reduce the number of menstrual cycles.[15] As with NSAID use, ❾ *the reduction in blood loss is proportional to pretreatment blood loss.*

● **Progesterone** Menorrhagia also may be treated with the levonorgestrel-releasing IUD. This treatment is effective and consistently reduces menstrual flow by 75% to 95%, and after 12 months, 20% to 80% of women experience amenorrhea.[12,15,16,40,47] When compared with endometrial ablation, the progesterone IUD has similar menstrual blood loss reductions after 6, 12, and 24 months.[48] Its use has also resulted in postponing or canceling scheduled endometrial resection surgery or hysterectomy. Specifically, 60% of treated patients have avoided hysterectomy.[16,49,50]

The progesterone IUD is more effective than oral norethindrone administered cyclically.[15,51] In a small open-label study, the levonorgestrel IUD resulted in a greater menstrual blood loss reduction and number of lost days compared with oral CHCs.[52]

● Progesterone therapy either during the luteal phase of the menstrual cycle or for 21 days starting on day 5 after menses onset results in a 32% to 50% menstrual blood loss reduction.[12] Its use is not superior to other medical treatments, including NSAIDs.[12] In addition, it is not associated with contraceptive benefits.

Menorrhagia in Adolescents

● In several studies of adolescents with acute menorrhagia, underlying bleeding disorders accounted for 3% to 13%

of emergency room visits.[28] Further, 20% of adolescent females requiring hospitalization for excessive menstrual bleeding have an underlying coagulopathy.23 Although von Willebrand's disease has a 1% incidence in the general population, it is estimated that 5% to 36% of adolescents presenting with heavy menses have von Willebrand's disease.[27,28] Platelet function disorders exist in 2% to 44% of adolescents with menorrhagia.[27]

OUTCOME EVALUATION

Treatment success for menstruation-related disorders is measured by the degree to which the care plan (a) relieves or reverses the disorder's symptoms, (b) prevents or reverses the disorder's complications (e.g., osteoporosis, anemia, and infertility), and (c) results in minimal side effects. Resumption of regular menstrual cycles with minimal premenstrual or dysmenorrhea symptoms should occur. Depending on the desire for conception and related therapy, these cycles may be ovulatory or anovulatory.

Assess treatment efficacy in resuming normal menstrual cycles with minimal side effects after an appropriate treatment interval (1 to 2 months). Assess improvement in quality-of-life measures such as physical, psychological, and social functioning and well-being. Evaluate the patient for adverse drug reactions, drug allergies, and drug interactions. Table 49–1 illustrates the common side effects that require monitoring. Table 49–3 illustrates the expected outcome measures for each menstruation-related disorder discussed in this chapter.

Table 49–3	
Expected Outcome Measures for Selected Menstrual Bleeding Disorders	

Menstrual Disorder	Expected Outcome Measures
Amenorrhea	*Efficacy:* Normal breast development (especially primary amenorrhea in adolescents); BMD preservation/improvement; return of menses. *Time to relief/effect:* Menses should occur within 1–2 months of therapy.
Anovulatory bleeding	*Efficacy:* Alleviation of acute bleeding when present; ovulation and subsequent pregnancy in women desiring this; reduced risk of developing the long-term complications of PCOS (e.g., diabetes and cardiovascular disease); improved quality of life. *Time to relief/effect:* The acute treatment of heavy bleeding should reduce bleeding within 10 days of therapy onset; return of ovulation may require several months of therapy; when oral CHCs are used, abnormal bleeding control can be expected within 1–2 treatment cycles.
Dysmenorrhea	*Efficacy:* Reduction in menses-related pelvic pain; reduction in time lost from work/school; improved quality of life. *Time to relief/effect:* Improvement in pain may be observed within hours of NSAID therapy; improvement with other options such as oral CHCs may be observed after a full 1–3 cycles of use.
Menorrhagia	*Efficacy:* Decline in amount of blood loss with menses (monitor a decline in the number of times feminine hygiene products such as pads and tampons require changing during menses); increase in hemoglobin/hematocrit if anemia was present as because of menorrhagia. *Time to relief/effect:* A decline in menstrual blood loss should be realized within 1–2 cycles of therapy initiation.

BMD, bone mineral density; NSAID, nonsteroidal anti-inflammatory drug; CHCs, combination hormonal contraceptives; PCOS, polycystic ovary syndrome.

Data from Ref. 18, 25–28, 45.

Patient Care and Monitoring

1. Assess symptoms to determine whether patient-directed therapy is appropriate (e.g., NSAIDs for dysmenorrhea) or whether the patient should be evaluated by a physician (e.g., amenorrhea, menorrhagia, anovulatory bleeding, or premenstrual dysphoric disorder). Does the patient have any related complications, such as symptoms of anemia in patients presenting with menorrhagia or complaints of difficulty conceiving in women with amenorrhea or anovulatory bleeding?

2. Review any available diagnostic data, as appropriate, to determine hormonal, reproductive, and pregnancy status.

3. Obtain a thorough history of prescription, nonprescription, and natural drug product use. Determine which treatments have been helpful to the patient in the past.

4. Educate the patient on lifestyle modifications that will improve symptoms and prevent complications.

5. Is the patient taking the appropriate dose of the prescribed medication? If not, why not?

6. Develop a plan to assess effectiveness of the prescribed medication after 1 to 2 months of therapy.

7. Determine whether long-term maintenance treatment is necessary.

8. Assess improvement in quality-of-life measures such as physical, psychological, social functioning, and well-being.

9. Evaluate for adverse drug reactions, drug allergies, and drug interactions.

10. Stress the importance of adherence with the therapeutic regimen, including lifestyle modifications. Recommend a therapeutic regimen that is easy for the patient to adhere to.

11. Provide patient education regarding disease state, lifestyle modifications, and drug therapy by noting the following:

    a. What causes the menstruation-related disorder?

    b. What are the possible complications of the menstruation-related disorder?

    c. What lifestyle modifications may help to reduce the risk associated with these complications?

    d. When and how should patients take their medications?

    e. What potential adverse effects may occur?

    f. Which drugs may interact with their therapy?

 Self-assessment questions and answers are available at *http://mhpharmacotherapy.com/pp.html.*

Abbreviations Introduced in This chapter

ACOG	American College of Obstetricians and Gynecologists
BMD	bone mineral density
BMI	body mass index
CBC	complete blood count
CEE	conjugated equine estrogen
CHC	combination hormonal contraceptive
FSH	follicle-stimulating hormone
GI	Gastrointestinal
GnRH	gonadotropin-releasing hormone
HCG	human chorionic gonadotropin
HPA	hypothalamic-pituitary-adrenal
HPO	hypothalamic-pituitary-ovarian
IUD	intrauterine device
LH	luteinizing hormone
MPA	medroxyprogesterone acetate
MRI	magnetic resonance imaging
NIH	National Institutes of Health
NSAID	nonsteroidal anti-inflammatory drug
OC	oral contraceptive
PCOS	polycystic ovarian syndrome
PID	pelvic inflammatory disease
SHBG	sex hormone–binding globulin
TENS	transcutaneous electrical nerve stimulation
ULN	upper limit of normal

REFERENCES

1. Fritz MA, Speroff L. Clinical Gynecologic Endocrinology and Infertility, 8th ed. Philadelphia, PA: Lippincott Williams & Wilkins, 2010: 567–589.

2. French L. Dysmenorrhea. Am Fam Physician 2005;71:285–292.

3. Dawood MY. Primary dysmenorrhea: Advances in pathogenesis and management. Obstet Gynecol 2006;108:428–441.

4. Morrow C, Naumburg EH. Dysmenorrhea. Prim Care Clin Office Pract 2009;36:19–32.

5. Lent GM. Primary and secondary dysmenorrhea, premenstrual syndrome, and premenstrual dysphoric disorder: Etiology, diagnosis, management. In: Katz VL, ed. Comprehensive Gynecology, 5th ed. Philadelphia, PA: Mosby Elsevier, 2007:901–914.

6. Pletcher JR, Slap GB. Menstrual disorders—Amenorrhea. Pediatr Clin North Am 1999;46(3):505–518.

7. Master-Hunter T, Heiman DL. Amenorrhea: Evaluation and Treatment. Am Fam Physician 2006;73(8):1374–1382.

8. Polycystic ovary syndrome. ACOG Practice Bulletin No. 108. American College of Obstetricians and Gynecologists. Obstet Gynecol 2009; 114:936–949.

9. Munro MG, Mainor N, Basu R, et al. Oral medroxyprogesterone acetate and combination oral contraceptives for acute uterine bleeding: a randomized clinical trial. Obstet Gynecol 2006;108:924–929.

10. Wong CL, Garquhar C, Roberts H, Proctor M. Oral contraceptive pill for primary dysmenorrhoea. Cochrane Database Syst Rev 2009;4:CD002120.

11. Harel Z. Dysmenorrhea in adolescents and young adults: Etiology and management. J Pediatr Adolesc Gynecol 2006;19(6):363–371.
12. Roy SN, Bhattacharya S. Benefits and risks of pharmacological agents used for the treatment of menorrhagia. Drug Safety 2004;27(2):75–90.
13. Lobo RA. Primary and secondary amenorrhea and precocious puberty: etiology, diagnostic evaluation, management. In: Katz VL, ed. Comprehensive Gynecology, 5th ed. Philadelphia, PA: Mosby Elsevier, 2007:933–962.
14. Lexi-Comp Online. Hudson, OH: Lexi-Comp, Inc., 2012.
15. Noncontraceptive uses of hormonal contraceptives. ACOG Practice Bulletin No. 110. American College of Obstetricians and Gynecologists. Obstet Gynecol 2010;115:206–18.
16. Long-Acting Reversible Contraception: Implants and Intrauterine Devices. ACOG Practice Bulletin No. 121. American College of Obstetricians and Gynecologists. Obstet Gynecol 2011;118:184–195.
17. U.S. medical eligibility criteria for contraceptive use, 2010. Centers for Disease Control and Prevention (CDC). MMWR Recomm Rep 2010;59(RR-4):1–86.
18. Menstruation in girls and adolescents: using the menstrual cycle as a vital sign. ACOG Committee Opinion No. 349. American Academy of Pediatrics; American College of Obstetricians and Gynecologists. Obstet Gynecol 2006;108:1323–1328.
19. Current evaluation of amenorrhea. The Practice Committee of the American Society for Reproductive Medicine. Fertil Steril 2008;90:S219–S225.
20. Fritz MA, Speroff L. Clinical Gynecologic Endocrinology and Infertility, 8th ed. Philadelphia, PA: Lippincott Williams & Wilkins, 2010:435–493.
21. Reindollar RH, Novak M, Tho SP, McDonough PG. Adult-onset amenorrhea: a study of 262 patients. Am J Obstet Gynecol 1986;155(3):531–543.
22. Umland EM, Weinstein LC, Buchanan E. Menstruation-related disorders (Chapter 89). In: Pharmacotherapy: A Pathophysiologic Approach, 8th ed. New York, NY: McGraw-Hill, 2011.
23. Lobo RA. Reproductive endocrinology: Neuroendocrinology, gonadotropins, sex steroids, prostaglandins, ovulation, menstruation, hormone assay. In: Katz VL, ed. Comprehensive Gynecology, 5th ed. Philadelphia, PA: Mosby Elsevier, 2007:73–120.
24. Golden NH, Carlson JL. The pathophysiology of amenorrhea in the adolescent. Ann NY Acad Sci 2008;1135:163–178.
25. Lobo RA. Abnormal uterine bleeding: Ovulatory and anovulatory dysfunctional uterine bleeding, management of acute and chronic excessive bleeding. In: Katz VL, ed. Comprehensive Gynecology, 5th ed. Philadelphia, PA: Mosby Elsevier, 2007:915–932.
26. Management of Anovulatory Bleeding ACOG Practice Bulletin No. 14 (reaffirmed 2009). American College of Obstetricians and Gynecologists. Intl J Gynecol Obstet 2001;72:263–271.
27. Boswell HB. The adolescent with menorrhagia: Why, who, and how to evaluate for a bleeding disorder. J Pediatr Adolesc Gynecol 2011;24(4):228–230.
28. Adams Hillard PJ, Deitch HR. Menstrual disorders in the college age female. Pediatr Clin N Am 2005;52(1):179–197.
29. Lobo RA. Hyperprolactinemia, galactorrhea, and pituitary adenomas: etiology, differential diagnosis, natural history, management. In: Katz VL, ed. Comprehensive Gynecology, 5th ed. Philadelphia, PA: Mosby Elsevier, 2007:963–978.
30. Simon JA. Progestogens in the treatment of secondary amenorrhea. J Reprod Med 1999;44:185-189.
31. Tolaymat LL, Kaunitz AM. Use of hormonal contraception in adolescents: skeletal health issues. Curr Opin Obstet Gynecol 2009;21(5):396–401.
32. Fritz MA, Speroff L. Clinical Gynecologic Endocrinology and Infertility, 8th ed. Philadelphia, PA: Lippincott Williams & Wilkins; 2010:591–619.
33. Rotterdam ESHRE/ASRM-Sponsored PCOS Consensus Workshop Group. Revised 2003 consensus on diagnostic criteria and long-term health risks related to polycystic ovary syndrome. Fertil Steril 2004;81(1):19–25.
34. Azziz R, Carmina E, Dewailly D, et al. Positions statement: Criteria for defining polycystic ovary syndrome as a predominantly hyperandrogenic syndrome: An Androgen Excess Society guideline. Androgen Excess Society. J Clin Endocrinol Metab 2006;91:4237–4245.
35. Azziz R, Carmina E, Dewailly D, et al. Task Force on the Phenotype of the Polycystic Ovary Syndrome of The Androgen Excess and PCOS Society. The Androgen Excess and PCOS Society criteria for the polycystic ovary syndrome: the complete task force report. Fertil Steril 2009;91:456–488.
36. Norman RJ, Dewailly D, Legro RS, Hickey TE. Polycystic ovary syndrome. Lancet 2007;370:685–697.
37. Wild RA, Carmina E, Diamanti-Kandarakis E, et al. Assessment of cardiovascular risk and prevention of cardiovascular disease in women with the polycystic ovary syndrome: A consensus statement by the Androgen Excess and Polycystic Ovary Syndrome (AE-PCOS) Society. J Clin Endocrinol Metab 2010;95(5):2038–2049.
38. Fauser BC, Tarlatzis BC, Rebar RW, et al. Consensus on women's health aspects of polycystic ovary syndrome PCOS): the Amsterdam ESHRE/ASRM-Sponsored 3rd PCOS Consensus Workshop Group. Fertil Steril 2012;97:28–38.
39. Dickersin K, Munro MG, Clark M, et al. Hysterectomy compared with endometrial ablation for dysfunctional uterine bleeding: A randomized controlled trial. Obstet Gynecol 2007;110(6):1279–1289.
40. Casablanca Y. Management of dysfunctional uterine bleeding. Obstet Gynecol Clin N Am 2008;35:219–234.
41. Mathur R, Levin O, Azziz R. Use of ethinyl estradiol / drospirenone combination in patients with the polycystic ovary syndrome. Ther Clin Risk Manage 2008;4(2):487–492.
42. FDA. 2007 safety alerts for drugs, biologics, medical devices, and dietary supplements: Avandia (rosiglitazone maleate) tablets, Actos (pioglitazone hydrochloride) tablets, Avandaryl (rosiglitazone maleate and glimepiride) tablets, Avandamet (rosiglitazone maleate and metformin hydrochloride) tablets, Duetact (pioglitazone hydrochloride and glimepride) tablets. August 14, 2007. Available at: http://www.fda.gov/Safety/MedWatch/SafetyInformation/SafetyAlertsforHumanMedicalProducts/default.htm#rosi_pio
43. Khorram O, Helliwell JP, Katz S, et al. Two weeks of metformin improves clomiphene citrate-induced ovulation and metabolic profiles in women with polycystic ovary syndrome. Fertil Steril 2006;85(5):1448–1451.
44. Creanga AA, Bradley HM, McCormick C, et al. Use of metformin in polycystic ovary syndrome: A meta-analysis. Obstet Gynecol 2008;111(4):959–968.
45. Warner PE, Critchley HO, Lumsden MA, et al. Menorrhagia I: Measured blood loss, clinical features, and outcome in women with heavy periods: a survey with follow-up data. Am J Obstet Gynecol 2004;190(5):1216–1223.
46. Warner PE, Critchley HO, Lumsden MA, et al. Menorrhagia II: Is the 80-mL blood loss criterion useful in management of complaint of menorrhagia? Am J Obstet Gynecol 2004;190(5):1224–1229.
47. Reid PC, Virtanen-Kari S. Randomized comparative trial of levonorgestrel intrauterine system and mefenamic acid for the treatment of idiopathic menorrhagia: A multiple analysis using total menstrual fluid loss, menstrual blood loss and pictorial blood loss assessment charts. Br J Obstet Gynecol 2005;112:1121–1125.
48. Kaunitz AM, Meredith S, Inki P, et al. Levonorgestrel-releasing intrauterine system and endometrial ablation in heavy menstrual bleeding: A systematic review and meta-analysis. Obstet Gynecol 2009;113:1104–1116.
49. Hurskainen R, Paavonen J. Levonorgestrel-releasing intrauterine system in the treatment of heavy menstrual bleeding. Curr Opin Obstet Gynecol 2004;16:487–490.
50. Hurskainen R, Teperi J, Rissanen P, et al. Clinical outcomes and costs with the levonorgestrel-releasing intrauterine system or hysterectomy for treatment of menorrhagia: Randomized trial 5-year follow-up. JAMA 2004;291(12):1456–1463.
51. Lethaby A, Cooke I, Rees MC. Progesterone or progestogen-releasing intrauterine systems for heavy menstrual bleeding. Cochrane Database Syst Rev 2005;4:CD002126.
52. Shaaban MM, Zekherah MS, El-Nashar SA, Sayed GH. Levonorgestrel-releasing intrauterine system compared to low dose combined oral contraceptive pills for idiopathic menorrhagia: A randomized clinical trial. Contraception 2011;83:48–45.

50 Hormone Therapy in Menopause

Nicole S. Culhane and Kelly R. Ragucci

LEARNING OBJECTIVES

● **Upon completion of the chapter, the reader will be able to:**

1. Explain the physiologic changes associated with menopause.

2. Identify the signs and symptoms associated with menopause.

3. Determine the desired therapeutic outcomes for a patient taking hormone therapy (HT).

4. Explain how to evaluate a patient for the appropriate use of HT.

5. Recommend nonpharmacologic therapy for menopausal symptoms.

6. List the adverse effects of and contraindications to HT.

7. Differentiate between topical and systemic forms of HT.

8. Explain the risks and benefits associated with HT.

9. Educate a patient regarding the proper use and potential adverse effects of HT.

10. Describe the monitoring parameters for a patient taking HT.

11. Describe the circumstances under which nonhormonal therapies for menopausal symptoms should be considered.

KEY CONCEPTS

❶ Common symptoms of menopause include hot flashes, night sweats, vulvovaginal atrophy, vaginal dryness, and dyspareunia. Women less commonly may experience mood swings, depression, insomnia, arthralgia, myalgia, urinary frequency, and decreased libido.

❷ Hormone therapy (HT) remains the most effective treatment for vasomotor symptoms and vulvovaginal atrophy and can be considered, especially for women experiencing moderate to severe symptoms.

❸ Women should receive a thorough history and physical examination, including assessing for coronary heart disease (CHD) and breast cancer risk factors before HT is considered. If a woman does not have any contraindications to HT, including CHD or significant CHD risk factors, and also does not have a personal history of breast cancer, HT may be an appropriate therapy option.

❹ Oral or transdermal estrogen products should be prescribed at the lowest effective dose and for the shortest duration possible to provide relief of vasomotor symptoms. Topical vaginal products in the form of creams, tablets, or rings should be prescribed for women exclusively experiencing vulvovaginal atrophy.

❺ Women who have an intact uterus should be prescribed a progestogen in addition to estrogen in order to decrease the risk of endometrial hyperplasia and endometrial cancer.

❻ HT is also indicated for the prevention of osteoporosis, but is not recommended for long-term use. Traditional osteoporosis therapies such as bisphosphonates should be considered as first-line therapy for the prevention and treatment of osteoporosis, in addition to appropriate doses of calcium and vitamin D.

❼ Combined estrogen plus progestogen should not be used in the prevention of chronic diseases because it increases the risk of CHD, stroke, breast cancer, venous thromboembolism (VTE), and dementia. Estrogen alone administered to women without a uterus does not increase the risk of breast cancer. Colorectal cancer and rates of fracture are reduced with combined hormonal treatment.

❽ HT improves overall well-being and mood in women with vasomotor symptoms but has not demonstrated an improvement in quality of life (QOL) in women without vasomotor symptoms.

❾ When treating moderate to severe postmenopausal symptoms, the benefit-to-risk ratio appears to be best when HT is started close to the time of menopause. Therapy should be tapered before discontinuation in order to limit the recurrence of hot flashes.

⓾ Since the publication of the Women's Health Initiative (WHI) study, there has been an increase in the use of alternative and nonhormonal therapies for the management of menopausal symptoms, particularly for women with CHD and/or breast cancer risk factors. A wide range of therapies, both prescription and herbal, have been studied with varying degrees of success.

Menopause is the permanent cessation of menses following the loss of ovarian follicular activity. The diagnosis of menopause is primarily a clinical one and is made after a woman experiences amenorrhea for 12 consecutive months. The loss of ovarian follicular activity leads to an increase in follicle-stimulating hormone (FSH), which, on laboratory examination, may help to confirm the diagnosis.

The role of hormone therapy (HT) has changed dramatically over the years. HT has long been prescribed for relief of menopausal symptoms and, until recent years, has been purported to protect women from coronary heart disease (CHD). The reason behind recommending HT in postmenopausal women revolved around a simple theory: If the hormones lost during menopause were replaced through drug therapy, women would be protected from both menopausal symptoms and chronic diseases that often follow after a woman experiences menopause. Recent studies have disproved this theory.

In 1996, the United States Preventive Services Task Force first published its recommendations that not all postmenopausal women should be prescribed HT, but that therapy should be individualized based on risk factors. This recommendation was further supported with publication of the Heart and Estrogen/Progestin Replacement Study (HERS) in 1998, which demonstrated that women who had established CHD were at an increased risk of experiencing a myocardial infarction within the first year of HT use compared with a similar group of women without CHD risk factors. As a result, the authors concluded that HT should not be recommended for the secondary prevention of CHD.[1] Then, in 2002, the Women's Health Initiative (WHI) study was published. This trial demonstrated that HT was not protective against CHD but rather could increase the risk in women with underlying CHD risk factors. The risk of breast cancer was also increased after a woman was on combination estrogen and progestogen for approximately 3 years. It should be noted that this was not the case with estrogen alone. As a result of this study, the FDA issued a statement that HT, in general, should not be initiated or continued for the primary prevention of CHD.[2]

This series of trials led to dramatic changes in how HT is prescribed and greater understanding of the associated risks. HT, once thought of as a cure-all for menopausal symptoms, is now a therapy that should be used primarily to reduce the frequency and severity of moderate to severe **vasomotor symptoms** associated with menopause in women without risk factors for CHD or breast cancer. The changes that have occurred over the years in the use of HT further support the importance of evidence-based practice and judicious medication use.

EPIDEMIOLOGY AND ETIOLOGY

Menopause is a period of time marked by loss of ovarian follicular activity, inadequate estradiol production, and the subsequent cessation of menses. It occurs in all women usually between the ages of 40 and 58 years. The median age for a woman to experience menopause is 52 years. However, women who have undergone a total abdominal hysterectomy with bilateral salpingo-oophorectomy (surgical menopause) generally experience menopause earlier compared with women who experience natural menopause. Some other factors that may be associated with early menopause include low body weight, increased menstrual cycle length, **nulliparity,** and smoking. Smokers generally experience menopause approximately 2 years earlier than nonsmokers.[3]

The usual transitional period prior to menopause, known as **perimenopause** or the *climacteric,* is a period when hormonal and biologic changes begin to occur. These changes may begin 2 to 8 years prior to menopause and eventually lead to irregular menstrual cycles, an increase in cycle interval, and a decrease in cycle length. During this time, women also may experience physical symptoms similar to menopausal symptoms, which may require treatment depending on symptom severity.[3]

Because the perimenopausal and postmenopausal periods are marked by many biologic and endocrinologic changes, women should inform their healthcare provider when they experience any signs and symptoms in order to discuss the most appropriate therapeutic approach.

PHYSIOLOGY

Reproductive physiology is regulated primarily by the hypothalamic–pituitary–ovarian axis. The hypothalamus secretes gonadotropin-releasing hormone (GnRH), which stimulates the anterior pituitary to secrete FSH and luteinizing hormone (LH). FSH and LH regulate ovarian function and stimulate the ovary to produce sex steroids. All of these hormones are influenced by a negative-feedback system and will increase or decrease based on the levels of estradiol and progesterone.

The physiologic changes that occur during the perimenopausal and menopausal periods are caused by the decrease and eventual loss of ovarian follicular activity. As women age, the number of ovarian follicles decreases, and the remaining follicles require higher levels of FSH for maturation and ovulation. During perimenopause, anovulatory cycles are more likely, and the lack of progesterone production leads to irregular and unpredictable menses. During menopause, FSH concentrations increase 10- to 15-fold, LH concentrations increase fivefold, and levels of circulating estradiol decrease by more than 90%.[4]

Clinical Presentation and Diagnosis of HT in Menopause

❶ Menopausal Symptoms

- Vasomotor symptoms (**hot flashes**, night sweats)
- Irregular menses
- Episodic amenorrhea
- Sleep disturbances
- Mood swings
- Vaginal dryness, dyspareunia
- Depression

Less Common Symptoms

- Fatigue
- Irritability
- Migraine
- Arthralgia
- Myalgia
- Decreased libido

Diagnosis

- Amenorrhea for 1 year
- FSH greater than 40 milliunits/mL (40 units/L)
- Fivefold increase in LH

❶ *Common symptoms of menopause include vasomotor symptoms (hot flashes, night sweats), vulvovaginal atrophy, vaginal dryness, and* dyspareunia*. Women less commonly may experience mood swings, depression, insomnia, arthralgia, myalgia, urinary frequency, and decreased libido.* Menopausal symptoms tend to be more severe in women who undergo surgical menopause compared with natural menopause because of the more rapid decline in estrogen concentrations.[3] Women who seek medical treatment should undergo laboratory evaluation to rule out other conditions that may present with similar symptoms, such as abnormal thyroid function or pituitary adenoma. Once symptoms have been evaluated and other conditions have been excluded, HT may be considered.

Patient Encounter, Part 1

RJ, a 52-year-old woman with a history of hypertension, osteoarthritis, and hypothyroidism, presents to the clinic complaining of hot flashes, vaginal dryness, and insomnia. She states that she experiences approximately three hot flashes per day and is awakened from sleep at least three to four times a week in a "pool of sweat" requiring her to change her clothes and bed linens. Her symptoms began about 3 months ago, and over that time, they have worsened to the point where they have become very bothersome. On questioning, she states her last menstrual period was 1 year ago.

Which of the patient's symptoms and past medical history are consistent with menopause?

What additional information do you need to know in order to make an appropriate therapeutic plan for this patient?

TREATMENT

Desired Outcomes

❷ *HT remains the most effective treatment for vasomotor symptoms and vulvovaginal atrophy and can be considered, especially for women experiencing moderate to severe symptoms.* The goals of treatment are to alleviate or reduce menopausal symptoms and to improve the patient's quality of life (QOL) while minimizing adverse effects of therapy. The appropriate route of administration should be chosen based on individual patient symptoms, and therapy should be continued at the lowest dose for the shortest duration consistent with treatment goals for each patient.

General Approach to Treatment

There are a number of national and international guidelines and consensus statements available on the management of menopause.[5-9] The most current guidelines should always be consulted before making pharmacotherapeutic recommendations for women. Women suffering from vasomotor symptoms should attempt lifestyle or behavioral modifications before seeking medical treatment. Women who seek medical treatment usually suffer from symptoms that diminish their QOL, such as multiple hot flashes per day or week, sleep disturbances, vaginal dryness, or mood swings. HT should be considered for these women, but is not the most appropriate choice for all women. ❸ *Women should receive a thorough history and physical examination, including assessing for CHD and breast cancer risk factors and contraindications, before HT is considered. They should be informed of the risks and the benefits of HT and encouraged to be involved in the decision-making process. If a woman does not have any contraindications to HT, including CHD or significant CHD risk factors, and also does not have a personal history of breast cancer, HT could be an appropriate therapy option (*Fig. 50–1*).* Women who have undergone a hysterectomy need only be prescribed estrogen. A progestogen should be added to the estrogen only

Patient Encounter, Part 2: Medical History, Physical Exam, and Diagnostic Tests

RJ's workup reveals the following additional information:

PMH: Osteoarthritis of the lower back for 5 years controlled on acetaminophen 500 mg two tablets by mouth 3 to 4 times daily; hypertension since age 45, currently controlled; hypothyroidism since age 25, currently controlled

FH: Father: Alive with HTN and CHD (MI at age 60). Mother: Alive with hypothyroidism and GERD. Siblings: Two sisters alive and well.

SH: Occupation: nurse; nonsmoker; drinks one to two glasses of red wine with dinner on the weekends; denies illicit drug use

Meds: Acetaminophen 500 mg two tablets by mouth 3 to 4 times daily; lisinopril/HCTZ 20/12.5 mg once daily; Synthroid 0.075 mg by mouth once daily; multivitamin by mouth once daily

ROS: (+) hot flashes, night sweats, vaginal dryness and itching; (+) insomnia, myalgias, bowel changes, weight gain, constipation

PE:

VS: BP 128/78, P 78, RR 16, T 37.0°C (98.6°F), wt 74.5 kg (164 lb)

HEENT: WNL

Neck: Supple; no bruits, no adenopathy, no thyromegaly.
Breasts: Supple; no masses

CV: RRR, normal S_1 and S_2; no murmurs, rubs, or gallops

Abd: Soft, nontender, nondistended; (+) BS, no masses

Genitourinary: Pelvic examination normal except (+) mucosal atrophy

Labs:

FSH: 76 mIU/mL (76 IU/L)

TSH: 2.5 μU/mL (2.5 mIU/L)

Chem-7: Na 135 mEq/L (135 mmol/L), K 4.5 mEq/L (4.5 mmol/L), Cl 109 mEq/L (109 mmol/L), CO_2 25 mEq/L (25 mmol/L), BUN 9 mg/dL (3.21 mmol/L), SCr 0.9 mg/dL (80 μmol/L), Glucose 98 mg/dL (5.44 mmol/L)

CBC: Hgb 13 g/dL (130 g/L or 8.06 mmol/L), Hct 39% (0.39 volume fraction), WBC 5.5 × 10³/mm³ (5.5 × 10⁹/L), platelets 234 × 10³/mm³ (234 × 10⁹/L)

Fasting lipid levels: TC 232 mg/dL (6 mmol/L), low-density lipoprotein (LDL) 145 mg/dL (3.76 mmol/L), high-density lipoprotein (HDL) 45 mg/dL (1.17 mmol/L), Triglycerides (TG) 200 mg/dL (2.26 mmol/L)

Assess the patient's condition based on this additional information.

What are the goals of treatment for this patient?

Assess the patient's risk factors for heart disease and breast cancer.

Recommend nonpharmacologic and pharmacologic treatment for this patient. Justify your recommendations.

---

for women with an intact uterus. Alternative and nonhormonal treatment options are available for women who are not candidates for HT, but they are less effective than hormonal therapies. These treatments should be chosen based on the efficacy and safety profile of the treatment and the patient's past medical history and current medications.

Nonpharmacologic Therapy

Nonpharmacologic therapies for menopause-related symptoms have not been studied in large randomized trials, and evidence of benefit is not well documented. Due to the minimal adverse effects of these interventions, patients should try lifestyle or behavioral modifications before and in addition to pharmacologic therapy. The most common nonpharmacologic interventions for vasomotor symptoms include the following[3,12,13]:

- Smoking cessation
- Limit alcohol and caffeine
- Limit hot beverages (e.g., coffee/tea, soups)
- Limit spicy foods
- Keep cool, and dress in layers
- Stress reduction (e.g., meditation, relaxation exercises)
- Increase exercise
- Paced respiration

Exercise demonstrated an improvement in QOL but did not improve vasomotor symptoms. Paced respiration, a form of deep, slow breathing, improved vasomotor symptoms in a small group of patients.

Dyspareunia may result from vaginal dryness. Water-based lubricants may provide relief for several hours after application. Moisturizers may provide relief for a longer period of time and potentially can prevent infections by maintaining the acidic environment in the vagina. Both these treatments require frequent application.

A decline in estrogen concentrations also may be associated with urinary stress incontinence. **Kegel exercises** are recommended as a first-line intervention for stress incontinence, although pharmacologic therapy also may be necessary. Kegel exercises strengthen the pelvic floor muscles and help to keep the urethral sphincter from relaxing at inappropriate times, such as when lifting heavy objects, coughing, or sneezing.

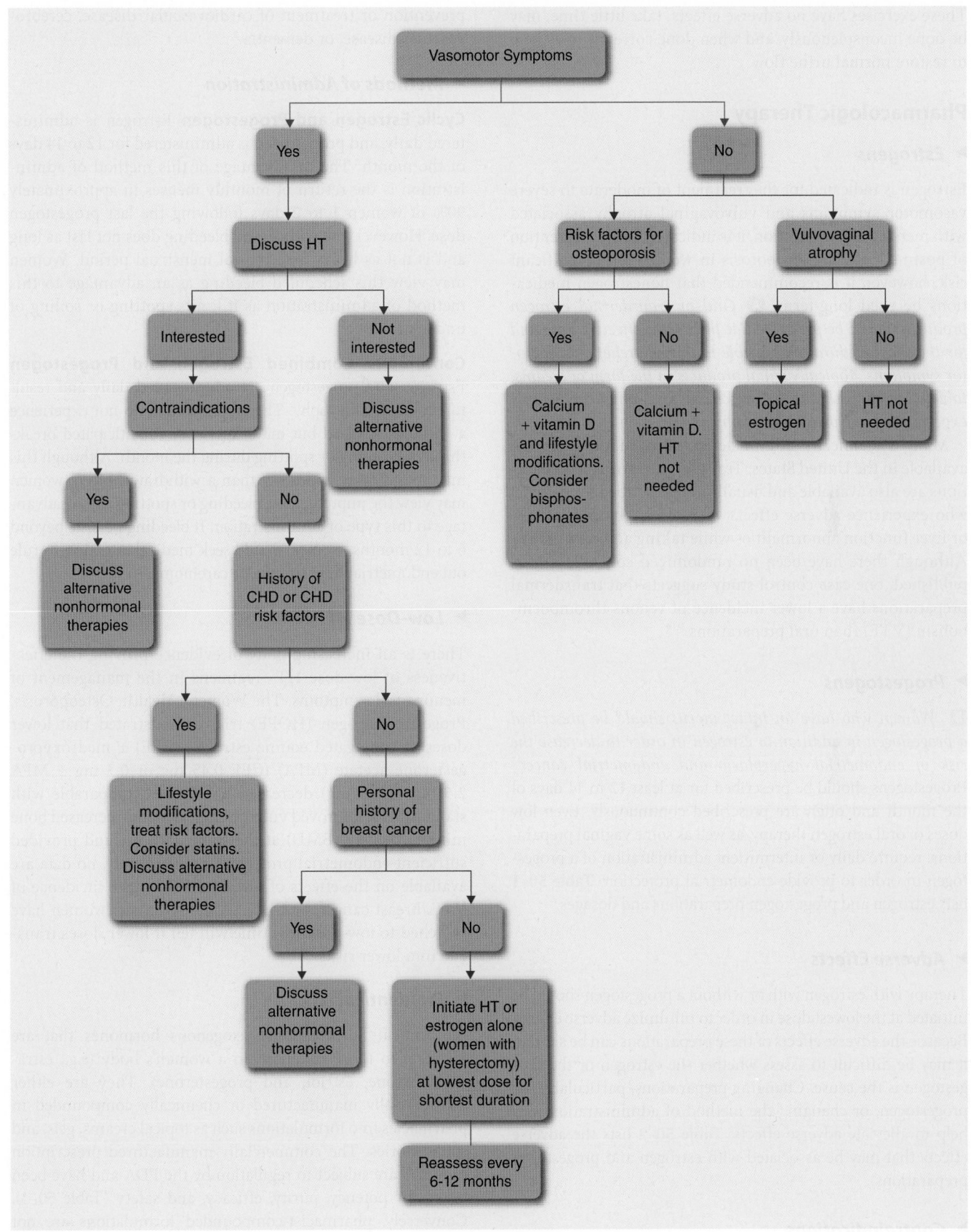

FIGURE 50–1. Treatment algorithm for postmenopausal women. (CHD, coronary heart disease; HT, hormone therapy.) (Data from Refs. 2, 10, and 11.)

These exercises have no adverse effects, take little time, may be done inconspicuously, and when done correctly, may help to restore normal urine flow.

Pharmacologic Therapy

▶ Estrogens

Estrogen is indicated for the treatment of moderate to severe vasomotor symptoms and vulvovaginal atrophy associated with menopause. In addition, it is indicated for the prevention of postmenopausal osteoporosis in women with significant risk; however, it is recommended that nonestrogen medications be used long-term. ❹ *Oral or transdermal estrogen products should be prescribed at the lowest effective dose and for the shortest duration possible to provide relief of vasomotor symptoms. Topical vaginal products in the form of creams, tablets, or rings should be prescribed for women exclusively experiencing vulvovaginal atrophy.*

Many systemically administered estrogen products are available in the United States. Transdermal estrogen preparations are also available and usually are prescribed for patients who experience adverse effects, elevated triglycerides (TG), or liver function abnormalities while taking an oral product. Although there have been no randomized controlled trials published, one case control study suggests that transdermal preparations have a lower incidence of venous thromboembolism (VTE) than oral preparations.[5,14]

▶ Progestogens

❺ *Women who have an intact uterus should be prescribed a progestogen in addition to estrogen in order to decrease the risk of endometrial hyperplasia and endometrial cancer.*[5] Progestogens should be prescribed for at least 12 to 14 days of the month and often are prescribed continuously. Even low doses of oral estrogen therapy, as well as some vaginal preparations, require daily or intermittent administration of a progestogen in order to provide endometrial protection. Table 50–1 lists estrogen and progestogen preparations and dosages.

▶ Adverse Effects

Therapy with estrogen with or without a progestogen should be initiated at the lowest dose in order to minimize adverse effects. Because the adverse effects of these preparations can be similar, it may be difficult to assess whether the estrogen or the progestogen is the cause. Changing preparations, particularly the progestogen, or changing the method of administration may help to alleviate adverse effects. Table 50–2 lists the adverse effects that may be associated with estrogen and progestogen preparations.

▶ Contraindications

HT should not be prescribed to women with a history of or active thromboembolic disease, breast cancer or estrogen-dependent neoplasm, pregnancy, liver disease, or undiagnosed vaginal bleeding. It also should not be used for the prevention or treatment of cardiovascular disease, cerebrovascular disease, or dementia.[3]

▶ Methods of Administration

Cyclic Estrogen and Progestogen Estrogen is administered daily, and progestogen is administered for 12 to 14 days of the month. The disadvantage of this method of administration is the return of monthly menses in approximately 90% of women 1 to 2 days following the last progestogen dose. However, the withdrawal bleeding does not last as long and is not as heavy as a typical menstrual period. Women may view this scheduled bleeding as an advantage to this method of administration as it limits spotting or soiling of undergarments.

Continuous Combined Estrogen and Progestogen Estrogen and progestogen are administered daily and result in endometrial atrophy. Therefore, women do not experience a withdrawal bleed but may experience unanticipated breakthrough bleeding or spotting during the month. Although this may sound more appealing than a withdrawal bleed, women may view the unpredictable bleeding or spotting as a disadvantage to this type of administration. If bleeding persists beyond 6 to 12 months, women should seek medical attention to rule out endometrial hypertrophy or carcinoma.

▶ Low-Dose HT

There is an increasing body of evidence proving the effectiveness of low-dose HT regimens in the management of menopausal symptoms. The Women's Health, Osteoporosis, Progestin/Estrogen (HOPE) trial demonstrated that lower doses of conjugated equine estrogen (CEE) ± medroxyprogesterone acetate (MPA) (CEE 0.45 mg or 0.3 mg ± MPA 2.5 mg or 1.5 mg) decreased hot flashes comparable with standard HT, improved vulvovaginal atrophy, increased bone mineral density (BMD) at the spine and hip, and provided sufficient endometrial protection.[18–21] Currently, no data are available on the effects of low-dose HT on the incidence of VTE, breast cancer, or CHD. Although many women have switched to low-dose HT, time will tell if lower doses translate into lower risks.

▶ Bioidentical HT

Bioidentical hormones are exogenous hormones that are identical to those produced in a woman's body (e.g., estradiol, estrone, estriol, and progesterone). They are either commercially manufactured or chemically compounded in pharmacies into formulations such as topical creams, gels, and suppositories. The commercially manufactured prescription products are subject to regulation by the FDA and have been tested for potency, purity, efficacy, and safety (Table 50–1). Conversely, pharmacist-compounded formulations are not subject to the same regulations and therefore, the efficacy and safety may be questionable. Often women view bioidentical hormones, particularly the pharmacist-compounded formulations, as "natural" and assume these formulations are safer than currently marketed prescription hormone products.

Table 50–1

Estrogen and Progestogen Formulations and Dosages

Product	Available Strengths	Common Dosages
Oral estrogens		
CEE (Premarin)	0.3–1.25 mg	0.3–0.625 mg/day
Synthetic conjugated estrogens (Cenestin; Enjuvia)	0.3–1.25 mg	0.3–0.625 mg/day
Esterified estrogens (Menest)	0.3–2.5 mg	0.3–0.625 mg/day
Estradiol (Estrace*a*/; Femtrace*a*)	0.5–2 mg; 0.45–1.8 mg	0.5–1 mg/day
Estropipate (Ogen*a*; Ortho-Est*a*)	0.625–5 mg; 0.625–1.25 mg	0.625 mg/day
Transdermal estrogens		
Estradiol patch (Alora, Climara, Estraderm, Vivelle, Vivelle Dot)	0.025–0.1 mg/24 hours	0.025–0.05 mg, changed weekly (Climara) or changed twice weekly
Menostar*b*	14 mcg/24 hours	14 mcg once weekly
Estradiol gel		
(Elestrin, Estrogel)	0.06%	0.87 g/day; 1.25 g/day
(Divigel)	0.1%	0.25, 0.5, 1 mg packets/day
Estradiol spray (Evamist)	1.53 mg/actuation	1–3 sprays/day
Topical estrogens		
Vaginal creams		
CEE (Premarin)	0.625 mg/g	0.5–2 g/day
Estradiol (Estrace)	0.01% estradiol	1g 1–3 times/week
Estropipate (Ogen)	1.5 mg/g	2–4 g/day
Vaginal rings		
Estradiol (Estring; Femring)	0.0075 mg/24 hours; 0.05–0.1 mg/24 hours	1 ring every 3 months
Vaginal tablet		
Estradiol (Vagifem)	10 mcg estradiol	1 tablet 2 times/week
Emulsions		
Estradiol (Estrasorb)	0.25%	3.84 g applied daily
Oral progestogens*c,d*		
MPA (Provera)	2.5–10 mg	
Micronized progesterone	100–200 mg	
Transdermal progestogens*c,d*		
Levonorgestrel	0.015 mg	
Norethindrone acetate	0.25–1 mg	
Norgestimate	0.09 mg	
Combination products		
Oral		
CEE + MPA (Prempro; Premphase)	0.3 /1.5 mg–0.625 /5 mg; 0.625/5 mg	0.3–0.625/2.5–5 mg/day
Estradiol + norethindrone (Activella)	0.5/0.1 mg–1/0.5 mg	1 tablet daily
Estradiol + drospirenone (Angeliq)	1/0.5 mg	1 tablet daily
Ethynyl estradiol + norethindrone (FemHRT)	2.5 mcg/0.5 mg; 5 mcg/1 mg	1 tablet daily
Estradiol + norgestimate (Prefest)	1/0.09 mg	1 tablet daily
Esterified estrogens + methyltestosterone (Covaryx, Covaryx HS)	1.25/2.5 mg; 0.625/1.25 mg	1 tablet daily
Transdermal		
Estradiol + norethindrone (Combipatch)	0.05/0.14–0.05/0.25 mg/24 hours	Apply one patch twice weekly
Estradiol + levonorgestrel (Climara Pro)	0.045/0.015 mg/24 hours	Apply one patch once weekly

CEE, conjugated equine estrogens; MPA, medroxyprogesterone acetate.

*a*FDA approved commercially available bioidentical product.

*b*Indicated for the prevention of postmenopausal osteoporosis only.

*c*May be administered cyclically or continuously.

*d*Dose varies based on daily or weekly administration.

Data from Refs. 10, 15, and 17.

Table 50–2
Adverse Effects of Estrogens and Progestogens

Estrogens

Common adverse effects
- Nausea
- Headache
- Bloating
- Breast tenderness
- Bleeding

Serious adverse effects
- Coronary heart disease
- Stroke
- Venous thromboembolism
- Breast cancer
- Gallbladder disease

Progestogens

Common adverse effects
- Nausea
- Headache
- Weight gain
- Bleeding
- Irritability
- Depression

Serious adverse effects
- Venous thromboembolism
- Decreased bone mineral density

Data from Refs. 4, 10, 16, and 17.

Women may feel more comfortable using compounded products that are formulated based on individual hormone levels, however, due to a lack of regulation, these products may potentially cause more harm than benefit. In addition, pharmacist-compounded formulations can result in higher costs, as they are generally not covered by third-party payers. There is little evidence comparing the safety and efficacy of conventional HT to prescription bioidentical HT, and thus the same risks and benefits should be assumed.[5,22]

▶ *Benefits of HT*

Vasomotor Symptoms HT remains the most effective treatment for vasomotor symptoms, and systemic HT should be considered only in women experiencing these symptoms. Women with mild vasomotor symptoms may benefit from nonpharmacologic therapy alone; however, many women will seek medical treatment for these symptoms. Benefits must outweigh risks, and decisions should be made only after careful consideration by the woman and her health care provider. If it is decided to use HT, it should be prescribed at the lowest dose that relieves or reduces menopausal symptoms and should be recommended only for short-term use (generally less than 5 years). Women should be reassessed every 6 to 12 months, and discontinuation of therapy should be considered.

Vulvovaginal Atrophy Approximately 50% of postmenopausal women experience vulvovaginal atrophy and seek medical attention. Vulvovaginal atrophy is associated with vaginal dryness and dyspareunia and also may be associated with recurrent urinary tract infections, urethritis, and

urinary urgency and frequency. Topical vaginal preparations generally should be prescribed as first-line therapy unless the patient is also experiencing vasomotor symptoms. Local vaginal estrogen has demonstrated increased efficacy over systemic estrogen and generally does not require supplementation with a progestogen in women with an intact uterus using low or ultralow doses.[5] Women using regular or high doses of topical estrogen products may require intermittent treatment with a progestogen. Although few data are available on the appropriate progestogen dose, some data indicate that 10 days every 12 weeks may be sufficient to prevent endometrial hyperplasia.[23] Estradiol in the form of a tablet or a ring is not significantly absorbed systemically and may be used safely in a woman with contraindications to estrogen therapy and symptoms of vulvovaginal atrophy.[5]

Osteoporosis Prevention Postmenopausal osteoporosis is a condition that affects millions of women. Fractures, particularly hip fractures, are associated with a high incidence of morbidity and mortality and a decrease in QOL. Before the WHI study, only observational data were available regarding the association of HT and the reduction of fractures. The WHI was the first randomized controlled trial (RCT) that demonstrated a reduction in total fractures, including the hip, spine, and wrist.[2,24]

❻ *Because HT should be maintained only for the short term, traditional therapies such as bisphosphonates should be considered as first-line therapy for the prevention of postmenopausal osteoporosis, in addition to appropriate doses of calcium and vitamin D.* Because of the associated risks, HT should not be prescribed solely for the prevention of osteoporosis.

Colon Cancer Retrospective observational studies suggested that HT was associated with lower rates of colorectal cancer. The mechanism was suspected to be related to reduced production of bile acids and inhibition of the growth of colon cancer cells. The WHI was the first and largest RCT to confirm that HT decreases the risk of colorectal cancer.[2] However, in the WHI estrogen alone arm, the cases of colorectal cancer were not lower in the estrogen group compared with the placebo group.[25] Data from a new analysis of the WHI suggest that there is not strong evidence for a reduction in the incidence of colorectal cancer or on mortality after 8 years with either combination HT or estrogen alone.[26] Because of these data, estrogen therapy should not be used long-term for prevention of colon cancer.

▶ *Risks of HT*

Cardiovascular Disease CHD is the leading cause of death among women in the United States. Retrospective data indicated that HT was associated with a decrease in risk of CHD by 30% to 50%.[25] However, the results of RCTs demonstrate that HT does not prevent or treat CHD in women and that it actually may cause an increase in CHD events. The HERS was the first RCT conducted in women with established CHD. This trial demonstrated an increased incidence of CHD events within the first year of treatment with HT and an increased risk of VTE and gallbladder disease. There was a trend of decreasing incidence of CHD death in years 3 to 5 that prompted a discontinuation of the study.[1] A follow-up HERS II trial also showed no difference in CHD events after 2.7 years.[27] The WHI was the first RCT conducted in women without established CHD. Women aged 50 to 79 years with an intact uterus were assigned to receive HT (CEE 0.625 mg + MPA 2.5 mg) daily for 8.5 years. The trial was stopped after only 5.2 years owing to an increased incidence of invasive breast cancer in women taking HT compared with those taking placebo. The WHI demonstrated an increased risk of CHD in the HT group compared with the placebo group (hazard ratio [HR] 1.24, 95% confidence interval [CI]) 1.00–1.54). This translates into six more cases of CHD per 10,000 women years. There also was an increased risk of stroke in the HT group compared with placebo (HR 1.31, 95% CI 1.02–1.68), which translates into seven more cases of stroke per 10,000 women years.[28,29]

The estrogen-alone arm of the WHI, which included women aged 50 to 79 years with a history of hysterectomy, continued for another 1.6 years (average follow-up 6.8 years). This arm of the study did not demonstrate an increased risk of CHD compared with placebo. However, there was an increased risk of stroke in the estrogen-alone group compared with placebo (HR 1.39, 95% CI 1.10–1.77). This translates into 12 more strokes for every 10,000 women treated per year with estrogen therapy.[25] Women who initiated hormone therapy 10 or more years after menopause tended to have an increased cardiovascular risk compared with women who initiated therapy within 10 years of menopause.[30,31]

The results of these trials demonstrate that HT should not be prescribed for the prevention of CHD or in patients with preexisting CHD. It is important to note that the average age of women included in the HERS and the WHI trials was 67 and 63 years, respectively, and they started HT a mean of 10 years after menopause. Therefore, these trials were unable to assess the true risk in younger, potentially healthier women with fewer cardiovascular risk factors.[25]

Breast Cancer Breast cancer is the most common cancer in women in the United States. Observational data indicated an association between HT and breast cancer risk. The WHI was the first RCT to demonstrate an increased risk of invasive breast cancer among women taking HT. There were eight more cases of invasive breast cancer for every 10,000 women treated per year with HT (HR 1.24, 95% CI 1.01–1.54).[2,32] The increase in risk did correlate with increased age of the women, and the risk appears to be greater in those who initiate therapy within 5 years of the start of menopause. These results are overall supported by results from a follow-up study of the WHI. During approximately 11 years of follow-up, there were 385 cases of invasive breast cancer in the combination HT group compared with 293 cases in the placebo group (95% CI 1.07–1.46, P = 0.004). There were also more deaths from breast cancer in the combination group than in the placebo group (95% CI 1.00–4.04, P = 0.049) and in deaths overall (95% CI 1.01–2.48, P = 0.045). This translates to 2.6 versus 1.3 deaths from breast cancer per 10,000 women years and 5.3 versus 3.4 deaths from all causes

after breast cancer diagnosis per 10,000 women per year.[33] It should be noted that any increase in risk for breast cancer appears to dissipate over 2 to 3 years after hormone therapy is discontinued.[5,34] Whether hormone therapy is associated with an increased risk for breast cancer recurrence is still questionable.

Breast cancer was not increased in the estrogen-alone arm of the WHI.[27] These data point to a possible link of progestogen with breast cancer risk. Whether or not the risk differs between continuous and sequential use of progestogens is questionable. Some evidence suggests that sequential use may be safer than taking progestogen each day.[5,35]

Because the WHI is the best evidence to date linking HT with breast cancer, women with a personal history of breast cancer and possibly even a strong family history of breast cancer should avoid the use of HT and consider alternative and nonhormonal therapies for the treatment of vasomotor symptoms.

Other Cancers A post-hoc analysis from the WHI suggests that combination HT therapy could be associated with an increased risk of death from lung cancer and an increased risk for certain lung tumors. However, this association was observed primarily in those who were smokers (past or present) and in women 60 years old or older.[25] The theory is that estrogen plus progestogen may promote growth of existing lung cancer in older women with a history of smoking. Data from another large observational trial suggests that the relative risk of lung cancer could be increased by approximately 50% in postmenopausal women who use combination HT for 10 years or longer.[36] Hormone therapy with estrogen alone does not appear to have this same risk.

Observational data suggested an increased risk of ovarian cancer with the use of HT in postmenopausal women. However, this increase was observed only after more than 5 years of therapy and was not seen 3 to 4 years after therapy was stopped.[5] Data from the WHI did not show an increased risk for ovarian cancer.[2]

Venous Thromboembolism The WHI demonstrated an increased risk for VTE in the HT group compared with placebo (HR 2.06, 95% CI 1.58–2.82). This translates into 18 more cases of venous thromboembolic events for every 10,000 women treated per year with HT.[2] The risk for deep vein thrombosis was also increased in the estrogen-alone arm of the WHI, but pulmonary embolism was not increased significantly.[25] The risk of thromboembolism may be dose related, and the oral route of administration is associated with a higher risk compared with the transdermal route.[14]

❼ *In summary, combined estrogen plus progestogen should not be used for the prevention of chronic diseases because it increases the risk of CHD, stroke, breast cancer, and VTE. However, colorectal cancer and rates of fracture were reduced with combined hormonal treatment.*

▶ Other Effects of HT

QOL and Cognition Although women generally consider QOL measures when deciding whether to use HT, the effects of HT on overall QOL have been inconsistent. HT did not demonstrate a clinically meaningful effect on QOL; however, women taking HT did have a small improvement in sleep disturbances, physical functioning, and bodily pain after 1 year of therapy.[37] Results from the HERS demonstrated that HT did improve emotional measures such as depressive symptoms, but only if women suffered from flushing at trial entry.[38]

Observational studies suggested a potential benefit of HT on cognitive functioning and dementia. However, the WHI Memory Study (WHIMS), conducted in postmenopausal women aged 65 years or older, failed to demonstrate an improvement in cognitive function and demonstrated a dementia rate, including Alzheimer's disease, two times greater compared with placebo.[39,40] The estrogen-alone arm of the WHIMS also demonstrated similar results.[41,42]

⑧ *HT improves overall well-being and mood in women with vasomotor symptoms, but it has not demonstrated an improvement in QOL in women without vasomotor symptoms.*

▶ Discontinuation of HT

⑨ *When treating moderate to severe postmenopausal symptoms, the benefit-to-risk ratio appears to be best when HT is started close to the time of menopause. Therapy should be tapered before discontinuation in order to limit the recurrence of hot flashes.* Although vasomotor symptoms in most women will subside within 4 years, approximately 10% of women continue to experience symptoms that interfere with their QOL. Literature suggests that one of every four women needs to be reinitiated on HT due to persistent and bothersome symptoms.[43,44]

Limited evidence is available to guide healthcare providers regarding the least disruptive way to taper HT. Slowly discontinuing HT over 3 to 6 months may be associated with less risk of symptom return. Tapering HT may be done by a dose taper or day taper. The dose taper involves decreasing the dose of estrogen over several weeks to months and

Patient Encounter, Part 4

RJ has been in good health for the past 7 years. She reports adherence with her medications, a healthy diet and exercise routine, and her medical conditions are controlled. However, 1 month ago she was diagnosed with stage 1 breast cancer following a routine mammogram. RJ is concerned that her hormone therapy may have caused the breast cancer.

Educate RJ regarding the risk of breast cancer and hormone therapy.

monitoring closely for symptom return. If symptoms recur, the next reduction in dose should not occur until symptoms resolve or stabilize on the current dose. The day taper involves decreasing the number of days of the week that a woman takes the HT dose, for example, decreasing a daily dose of 0.3 mg estrogen to 0.3 mg estrogen 5 days a week. Again, if symptoms recur, continue on the current dose until symptoms resolve or stabilize before trying a subsequent decrease. These tapering regimens have not been studied in clinical trials and may not prove to be beneficial in individual women.[44]

▶ Nonhormonal and Alternative Treatments

⑩ *Since publication of the WHI study, there has been an increase in the use of alternative and nonhormonal therapies for the management of menopausal symptoms, particularly for women with CHD and/or breast cancer risk factors. A wide range of therapies, both prescription and herbal, have been studied with varying degrees of success.* In choosing a particular therapy, it is important to match patient symptoms with a therapy that is not only effective, but also safe.

A variety of nonhormonal and alternative therapies (Table 50–3) have been studied for symptomatic management of vasomotor symptoms.[45,46] The limited and often conflicting evidence demonstrates that these agents are only modestly effective.

SSRIs and venlafaxine are theorized to reduce the frequency of hot flashes by increasing serotonin in the central nervous system and by decreasing LH. Of the SSRIs, fluoxetine, citalopram, paroxetine, and sertraline have published data demonstrating a reduction in hot flashes while treating other symptomatic complaints such as depression and anxiety.[47] These antidepressant medications offer a reasonable option for women who are unwilling or cannot take hormonal therapies, particularly those who suffer from depression or anxiety.

Phytoestrogens are plant sterols that are structurally similar to human and animal estrogen. Soy protein is a common source of phytoestrogens.[45,46] If used, at least 60 mg/day of isoflavone content is necessary for any possible benefit. Because the effect of isoflavones on breast cancer and other female related cancers is unknown, phytoestrogens should not be

Patient Encounter, Part 3: Creating a Care Plan

Based on the information presented, create a care plan for RJ's hot flashes and vaginal dryness. The plan should include:

(a) a statement identifying the patient problem and its severity

(b) goals of therapy

(c) a therapeutic plan based on individual patient-specific factors

(d) subjective and objective monitoring parameters

(e) a follow-up evaluation to assess for adverse effects and adherence and to determine whether the goals of therapy have been achieved

Table 50–3

Nonhormonal Therapies for Menopause

Agent	Demonstrated Efficacy	Dosing	Adverse Effects/Precautions
Citalopram	Nonrandomized trial demonstrated efficacy in hot flash reduction	20–60 mg daily	Nausea, dizziness, somnolence
Fluoxetine	One RCT demonstrated significant reduction in hot flashes; one RCT found drug no better than placebo	20 mg daily	Nausea, insomnia, nervousness, fatigue
Paroxetine	Two RCTs demonstrated significant reduction in and severity of hot flashes (approximately 30%)	10–20 mg daily	Headache, nausea, insomnia
Sertraline	Case series demonstrating efficacy in hot flash reduction	25–50 mg daily	Nausea, dizziness, somnolence
Venlafaxine	Two RCTs reported short-term significant reductions in and severity of hot flashes	12.5 mg twice daily	Nausea, dry mouth
Soy protein	Eighteen small RCTs demonstrated conflicting findings; modestly effective in relieving menopausal symptoms	At least 60 mg of isoflavones daily	GI upset; other adverse effects unknown; do not use in those with history of or high risk of estrogen-dependent cancer
Black cohosh	Seven small, short-term RCTs demonstrated benefit in mild-moderate hot flashes, especially when associated with sleep and mood disturbances	Varied dosing based on herbal product combination; most studied: Remifemin 40–80 mg twice daily	GI upset (take with food); potential hepatoxicity; not recommended to be taken over a 6-month period of time
Gabapentin	Four RCTs concluded that drug was significantly more effective than placebo at reducing the frequency and severity of hot flashes (approximately 50%), including those with breast cancer	900 mg daily	Dizziness and somnolence
Clonidine	Eleven studies, seven of which demonstrated significant reductions in frequency and severity of hot flashes	0.1–0.4 mg daily	Dry mouth, blood pressure lowering; monitor blood pressure
Dong quai	No demonstrated efficacy in one RCT	Not recommended	Structurally similar to coumarins—avoid with warfarin because INR can increase
Evening primrose oil, passion flowers, sage, valerian root, and wild yam	No demonstrated efficacy for any product in RCTs	Not recommended	Caution with all plant products in women with hay fever and plant allergies

INR, international normalized ratio; RCT, randomized controlled trial.

Data from Refs. 45–47.

considered in women with a history of estrogen-dependent cancers.[48] A recent trial compared the effect of dietary soy supplementation (90 mg isoflavones) with estrogen (1 mg of estradiol and 0.5 mg of norethisterone acetate) or placebo in 60 healthy, symptomatic, postmenopausal women aged 40 to 60 years.[49] The comparison between groups revealed a statistically significant improvement in hot flashes and urogenital symptoms with both soy and estrogen. There was no statistically significant difference between the groups with respect to overall menopausal symptoms. After reviewing hundreds of studies, the North American Menopause Society (NAMS) determined that soy-based isoflavones are modestly effective in relieving menopausal symptoms.[48] The efficacy of isoflavones on bone, cognitive improvement, and cardiovascular health has not been proven.

Black cohosh has been one of the most studied alternative therapies for vasomotor symptoms, but it has not demonstrated a substantial benefit over placebo. The mechanism of action, safety profile, drug–drug interactions, and adverse effects of black cohosh remain unknown. However, there have been case reports of hepatotoxicity with its use.[46,50] In non–placebo-controlled trials conducted for 6 months or less, black cohosh (40 to 80 mg/day) demonstrated small reductions in vasomotor symptoms.[45–47] Caution should be exercised when considering the use of this product, and it is not recommended for more than a 6-month period of time.

Gabapentin and clonidine have also been studied for the management of menopausal symptoms. In RCTs, gabapentin at doses of 900 mg/day demonstrated significant reductions in severity and frequency of hot flashes compared with placebo. Clonidine has been studied in several small RCTs at doses of 0.1 to 0.4 mg/day and has demonstrated statistically significant reductions in hot flashes.[47] Overall, alternative and nonhormonal therapies are less effective in treating vasomotor symptoms than HT but do offer another option for women experiencing menopausal symptoms who cannot or are unwilling to take HT. SSRIs and soy isoflavones have the best evidence for efficacy. However, healthcare providers should weigh the benefits and risks of all therapies, and women should be advised to discuss their options with their physicians and pharmacists.

OUTCOME EVALUATION

Evaluating the outcomes of any therapy for menopausal symptoms focuses primarily on the woman's report of symptom resolution. Ask women to report the resolution or reduction of hot flashes, night sweats, and vaginal dryness and any improvement or change in sleep patterns. Also ask women taking hormonal therapies to report any breakthrough bleeding or spotting. If abnormal or heavy bleeding occurs, refer the woman to her primary care provider. Monitor subjective parameters such as adverse effects and adherence to the therapy regimen, as well as monthly breast self-examinations. In addition, monitor objective parameters, including blood pressure, at every outpatient visit; encourage yearly clinical breast examinations, mammograms, lipid panel, and thyroid-stimulating hormone (TSH) determination, particularly for women with hypothyroidism on thyroid therapy, and conduct a BMD test every 2 to 5 years as indicated. Also perform endometrial studies, as necessary, in women with undiagnosed vaginal bleeding. Lastly, evaluate the patient's overall QOL. Because the management of menopause is largely symptomatic, it is important to document symptoms at the beginning of therapy and monitor symptom improvement and potential adverse effects at each visit. Frequent follow-up, proper monitoring, and education will help to ensure that the woman achieves optimal results from any therapy chosen to treat menopausal symptoms.

Patient Encounter, Part 5

It has been 6 months since RJ completed chemotherapy and radiation for breast cancer. She presents to her PCP for follow-up with a chief complaint of recurrent hot flashes. She denies recurrence of vaginal dryness or insomnia.

Recommend the most appropriate therapy for RJ's recurrent hot flashes.

Patient Care and Monitoring

1. Assess the patient for use of HT by evaluating for the presence of vasomotor symptoms. If the patient is experiencing bothersome vasomotor symptoms, consider the use of HT only after assessing for risk factors for heart disease and breast cancer. If vasomotor symptoms are tolerable and/or the patient has risk factors for heart disease and/or breast cancer, consider alternative, nonhormonal treatments for vasomotor symptoms.

2. Obtain a thorough medication history, including the use of over-the-counter and herbal products.

3. Educate the patient on lifestyle or behavioral interventions that may help to alleviate vasomotor symptoms.

4. Discuss methods of HT administration, and have the patient decide in conjunction with the healthcare provider which one she feels will work best for her.

5. Recommend the appropriate dose of HT, and use the lowest effective dose for the shortest duration of time.

6. Educate the patient regarding the proper administration, potential adverse effects, and expectations of HT.

7. Monitor the patient for a reduction in vasomotor symptoms, vaginal dryness, and improvement in sleep. Also monitor for breakthrough bleeding and spotting, adverse effects of HT, and improvement in QOL.

8. Monitor the following objective parameters:
   - Blood pressure at every outpatient visit
   - Yearly lipoprotein panels
   - Yearly fasting plasma glucose determinations
   - Yearly breast examinations and mammograms
   - Yearly TSH determinations, particularly for women with hypothyroidism on thyroid therapy
   - Endometrial studies in women with undiagnosed vaginal bleeding

9. Educate the patient regarding the importance of adhering to the medication regimen.

10. Educate the patient regarding the importance of obtaining a yearly mammogram and Papanicolaou (Pap) smear (if applicable), as well as performing a monthly breast self-examination.

11. Assess patient symptoms every 6 to 12 months, and consider tapering the HT dose and discontinuing treatment after 5 years. If vasomotor symptoms return, determine whether a longer tapering schedule is warranted or if long-term treatment is necessary. If treatment beyond 5 years is necessary, consider switching to a nonhormonal product.

Abbreviations Introduced in This Chapter

BMD	Bone mineral density
CEEs	Conjugated equine estrogen
CHD	Coronary heart disease
FSH	Follicle-stimulating hormone
GnRH	Gonadotropin-releasing hormone
HDL	High-density lipoprotein
HERS	Heart and Estrogen/Progestin Replacement Study
HOPE	Women's Health, Osteoporosis, Progestin/Estrogen trial
HT	Hormone therapy
LDL	Low-density lipoprotein
LH	Luteinizing hormone
MPA	Medroxyprogesterone acetate
NAMS	North American Menopause Society
NNTH	Number needed to treat to harm
QOL	Quality of life
PCP	Primary care provider
RCT	Randomized controlled trial
SSRI	Selective serotonin reuptake inhibitor
TG	Triglycerides
TSH	Thyroid-stimulating hormone
VTE	Venous thromboembolism
WHI	Women's Health Initiative
WHIMS	Women's Health Initiative Memory Study

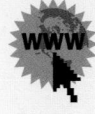 Self-assessment questions and answers are available at *http://www.mhpharmacotherapy.com/pp.html.*

REFERENCES

1. Hulley S, Grady D, Bush T, et al. for the Heart and Estrogen/progestin Replacement Study (HERS) Research Group. Randomized trial of estrogen plus progestin for secondary prevention of coronary heart disease in postmenopausal women. JAMA 1998;280(7):605–613.
2. Rossouw JE, Anderson GL, Prentice RL, et al. Risks and benefits of estrogen plus progestin in healthy postmenopausal women: Principal results from the Women's Health Initiative randomized controlled trial. JAMA 2002;288(3):321–333.
3. Nelson HD. Menopause. Lancet 2008;371:760–770.
4. Burger HG. The endocrinology of the menopause. J Steroid Biochem Mol Biol 1999;69(1–6):31–35.
5. The North American Menopause Society. Estrogen and progestogen use in postmenopausal women: 2010 position statement of The North American Menopause Society. Menopause 2010;17:242–255.
6. The North American Menopause Society. Management of postmenopausal osteoporosis: 2010 position statement of The North American Menopause Society. Menopause 2010;17:25–54.
7. The North American Menopause Society. Treatment of menopause-associated vasomotor symptoms: Position statement of The North American Menopause Society. Menopause 2004;11(1):11–33.
8. Santen RJ, Allred DC, Ardoin SP, et al. Postmenopausal hormone therapy: An endocrine society scientific statement. J Clin Endocrinol Metab 2010;95(suppl 1):S1–S66.
9. The Writing Group on behalf of the Workshop Consensus Group. Aging, menopause, cardiovascular disease and HRT. Climacteric 2009;12:368–377.
10. Kalantaridou SN, Dang DK, Davis SR, Calis KA. Hormone therapy in women. In: Dipiro, JT, Talbert RL, Yee, GC et al, eds. Pharmacotherapy: A Pathophysiologic Approach, 8th ed. New York: McGraw-Hill, 2011:1417–1436.
11. Rymer J, Wilson R, Ballard K. Making decisions about hormone replacement therapy. BMJ 2003;326(7384):322–326.
12. McKee J, Warber SL. Integrative therapies for menopause. South Med J 2005;98(3):319–326.
13. Sikon A, Thacker HL. Treatment options for menopausal hot flashes. Cleve Clin J Med 2004;71(7):578–582.
14. Canonico M, Oger E, Plu-Bureau G, et al. Hormone therapy and venous thromboembolism among postmenopausal women: impact of the route of estrogen administration and progestogens: The ESTHER Study. Circulation 2007;115:840–845.
15. Ragucci KR, Carson DS. Women's health. In: Hansen LB, Kelly W, eds. Pharmacotherapy Self-Assessment Program: Geriatrics/Special Populations, 5th ed. Kansas City: American College of Clinical Pharmacy, 2006:133–161.
16. Klasco RK. Estrogens. Accessed September 2011. Available at: DrugDex 2011. *http://www.thomsonhc.com/*
17. Klasco RK. Medroxyprogesterone. Accessed September 2011. Available at: DrugDex 2011. *http://www.thomsonhc.com/*
18. Archer DF, Dorin M, Lewis V, et al. Effects of lower doses of conjugated equine estrogens and medroxyprogesterone acetate on endometrial bleeding. Fertil Steril 2001;75(6):1080–1087.
19. Lindsay R, Gallagher JC, Kleerekoper M, et al. Effect of lower doses of conjugated equine estrogens with and without medroxyprogesterone acetate on bone in early postmenopausal women. JAMA 2002;287:2668–2676.
20. Pickar JH, Yeh I, Wheeler JE, et al. Endometrial effects of lower doses of conjugated equine estrogens and medroxyprogesterone acetate. Fertil Steril 2001;76(1):25–31.
21. Utian WH, Shoupe D, Bachmann G, et al. Relief of vasomotor symptoms and vaginal atrophy with lower doses of conjugated equine estrogens and medroxyprogesterone acetate. Fertil Steril 2001;75(6):1065–1079.
22. Bioidential hormones. The Endocrine Society position statement. 2006. Accessed January 12, 2012. Available at: *http://www.menopause.org/bioidenticalHT_Endosoc.pdf*
23. Davis S. Hormone replacement therapy. Indications, benefits and risk. Aust Fam Physician 1999;28(5):437–445.
24. Cauley JA, Robbins J, Chen Z, et al. Effects of estrogen plus progestin on risk of fracture and bone mineral density: The Women's Health Initiative randomized trial. JAMA 2003;290(13):1729–1738.
25. Anderson GL, Limacher M, Assaf AR, et al. Effects of conjugated equine estrogen in postmenopausal women with hysterectomy: The Women's Health Initiative randomized controlled trial. JAMA 2004;291(14):1701–1712.
26. Prentice RL, Pettinger M, Beresford SA, et al. Colorectal cancer in relation to postmenopausal estrogen and estrogen plus progestin in the women's health initiative clinical trial and observational study. Cancer Epidemiol Biomarkers Prev 2009;18:1531–1537.
27. Grady D, Herrington D, Bittner V, et al. Cardiovascular disease outcomes during 6.8 years of hormone therapy: Heart and Estrogen/Progestin Replacement Study followup (HERS II). JAMA 2002;288(1):49–57.
28. Manson JE, Hsia J, Johnson K, et al. Estrogen plus progestin and the risk of coronary heart disease. N Engl J Med 2003;349:523–534.
29. Wassertheil-Smoller S, Hendrix SL, Limacher M, et al. Effect of estrogen plus progestin on stroke in postmenopausal women: The women's health initiative: A randomized trial. JAMA. 2003;289:2673–2684.
30. Rossouw JE, Prentice RL, Manson JE, et al. Postmenopausal hormone therapy and risk of cardiovascular disease by age and years since menopause. JAMA 2007;297:1465–1477.
31. Toh S, Hernández-Díaz S, Logan R, et al. Coronary heart disease in postmenopausal recipients of estrogen plus progestin therapy: Does

the increased risk ever disappear? A randomized trial. Ann Intern Med 2010;152:211–217.

32. Chlebowski RT, Hendrix SL, Langer RD, et al. Influence of estrogen plus progestin on breast cancer and mammography in healthy postmenopausal women: The women's health initiative randomized trial. JAMA. 2003;289:3243–3253.

33. Chlebowski RT, Anderson GL, Gass M, et al. Estrogen plus progestin and breast cancer incidence and mortality in postmenopausal women. JAMA 2010;304:1684–1692.

34. Calle EE, Feigelson HS, Hildebrand JS, et al. Postmenopausal hormone use and breast cancer associations differ by hormone regimen and histologic subtype. Cancer 2009;115:936–945.

35. Saxena T, Lee E, Henderson KD, et al. Menopausal hormone therapy and subsequent risk of specific invasive breast cancer subtypes in the California Teachers Study. Cancer Epidemiol Biomarkers Prev 2010;19:2366–2378.

36. Slatore CG, Chien JW, Au DH, et al. Lung cancer and hormone replacement therapy: Association in the vitamins and lifestyle study. J Clin Oncol 2010;28:1540–1546.

37. Hays J, Ockene JK, Brunner RL, et al. Effects of estrogen plus progestin on health-related quality of life. N Engl J Med 2003;348(19):1839–1854.

38. Hlatky MA, Boothroyd D, Vittinghoff E, et al. Quality-of-life and depressive symptoms in postmenopausal women after receiving hormone therapy: Results from the Heart and Estrogen/Progestin Replacement Study (HERS) trial. JAMA 2002;287(5):591–597.

39. Rapp SR, Espeland MA, Shumaker SA, et al. Effect of estrogen plus progestin on global cognitive function in postmenopausal women: The Women's Health Initiative Memory Study: A randomized controlled trial. JAMA 2003;289(20):2663–2672.

40. Shumaker SA, Legault C, Rapp SR, et al. Estrogen plus progestin and the incidence of dementia and mild cognitive impairment in postmenopausal women: The Women's Health Initiative Memory Study: A randomized controlled trial. JAMA 2003;289(20):2651–2662.

41. Espeland MA, Rapp SR, Shumaker SA, et al. Conjugated equine estrogens and global cognitive function in postmenopausal women: Women's Health Initiative Memory Study. JAMA 2004;291(24):2959–2968.

42. Shumaker SA, Legault C, Kuller L, et al. Conjugated equine estrogens and incidence of probable dementia and mild cognitive impairment in postmenopausal women: Women's Health Initiative Memory Study. JAMA 2004;291(24):2947–2958.

43. Executive summary. Hormone therapy. Obstet Gynecol 2004;104 (4 suppl):1S–4S.

44. Grady D. A 60-year-old woman trying to discontinue hormone replacement therapy. JAMA 2002;287(16):2130–2137.

45. Nelson HD, Vesco KK, Haney E, et al. Nonhormonal therapies for menopausal hot flashes: Systematic review and meta-analysis. JAMA 2006;295:2057–2071.

46. Newton KM, Reed SD, LaCroix AZ, et al. Treatment of vasomotor symptoms of menopause with black cohosh, multibotanicals, soy, hormone therapy or placebo: A randomized trial. Ann Intern Med 2006;145(12):869–879.

47. Cheema D, Coomarasamy A, El-Toukhy T. Non-hormonal therapy of postmenopausal vasomotor symptoms: A structured evidence-based review. Arch Gynecol Obstet 2007;276(5):463–469.

48. NAMS 2011 Isoflavones Report. The role of soy isoflavones in menopausal health: Report of the North American Menopause Society.Menopause 2011;18:732–753.

49. Carmignani LO, Orcesi Pedro A, Costa-Paiva LH, Pinto-Neto AM. The effect of dietary soy supplementation compared to estrogen and placebo on menopausal symptoms: a randomized controlled trial. Maturitas 2010;67:262–269.

50. Lontos S, Jones RM, Angus PW, et al. Acute liver failure associated with the use of herbal preparations containing black cohosh. Med J Aust 2003;179(7):390–391.

51 Erectile Dysfunction

Cara Liday

LEARNING OBJECTIVES

● **Upon completion of the chapter, the reader will be able to:**

1. Identify the structures of the male reproductive system and describe the normal physiology of a penile erection.

2. Explain the pathophysiology of the different types of erectile dysfunction (ED).

3. Recognize risk factors and medications associated with the development of ED.

4. Identify the goals of therapy when treating ED.

5. Define the essential components of history, physical examination, and laboratory data needed to evaluate the patient presenting with ED.

6. Describe current nonpharmacologic and pharmacologic options for treating ED and determine an appropriate first-line therapy for a specific patient.

7. Compare and contrast the benefits and risks for the current phosphodiesterase (PDE) inhibitors.

8. Identify patients with significant cardiovascular risk and recommend an appropriate treatment approach for their ED.

KEY CONCEPTS

❶ Erectile dysfunction (ED) can be classified as organic, psychogenic, or mixed. Many patients may initially have organic dysfunction, but develop a psychogenic component as they cope with their inability to achieve an erection.

❷ In addition to a physical exam, a thorough medical, social, and medication history with emphasis on cardiac disease must be taken before starting any treatment for ED to assess for ability to safely perform sexual activity and to assess for possible drug interactions.

❸ Treatment options for ED include medical devices, pharmacologic treatments, lifestyle modifications, surgery, and psychotherapy. Reversible causes of ED should be identified first and treated appropriately.

❹ When determining the best treatment for an individual, the role of the clinician is to inform the patient and his partner of all available options while understanding his medical history, desires, and goals. The choice of treatment is primarily left up to the couple, but most often treatment is initiated with the least invasive option and then progresses to more invasive options if needed.

❺ Vacuum erection devices (VEDs) and intracavernosal injections are highly effective for many patients, but side effects, lack of spontaneity, and fear of needles limit their widespread use as first-line therapies.

❻ Effectiveness of the three available phosphodiesterase (PDE) inhibitors is essentially comparable, but differences exist in duration of action, absorption with a fatty meal and, to a small degree, incidence of side effects and drug interactions.

❼ Androgens are important for general sexual function and libido, but testosterone supplementation is only effective in patients with documented low serum testosterone levels.

INTRODUCTION

Erectile dysfunction (ED) is defined as the inability to achieve or maintain an erection sufficient for sexual intercourse. The definition is very subjective due to differences in desired or needed rigidity in patients of different ages and in different types of relationships. ED is the most prominent sexual problem in men, and it can lead to lower quality of life and self-esteem.[1] Patients may also develop **libido** or ejaculatory disorders, but these are not considered ED.

EPIDEMIOLOGY AND ETIOLOGY

ED becomes increasingly frequent as men age. Few men report erection problems before the age of 40, but the percentage of men experiencing ED increases to 26% in men aged 50 to 59 years and 40% in men aged 60 to 69 years.[2] The increase in incidence could be due to physiologic changes that occur with aging, the onset of chronic disease states associated with ED, increased medication use, lifestyle factors, or a combination of the above.

PATHOPHYSIOLOGY

The penis consists of three components, two dorsolateral corpora cavernosa and a ventral corpus spongiosum that surrounds the penile urethra and distally forms the glans penis. The corpora cavernosa consist of blood-filled sinusoidal or lacunar spaces, which are lined with endothelial cells, supported by trabecular smooth muscle, and surrounded by a thick fibrous sheath called the tunica albuginea. The cavernosal arteries, which are branches of the penile artery, penetrate the tunica albuginea and supply blood flow to the penis.

Sympathetic and parasympathetic nerves innervate the penis. In the flaccid state, α_2-adrenergic receptors mediate tonic contraction of the arterial and corporal smooth muscles. This maintains high penile arterial resistance, and a balance exists between blood flow into and out of the corpora. With sexual stimulation, nerve impulses from the brain travel down the spinal cord to the thoracolumbar ganglia. A decrease in sympathetic tone and an increase in parasympathetic activity then occurs, causing a net increase in blood flow into the erectile tissue. Erections may also occur as a result of a sacral nerve reflex arc while patients are sleeping (nocturnal erections). Acetylcholine-mediated parasympathetic activity leads to production of the nonadrenergic–noncholinergic transmitter nitric oxide (NO). By enhancing the activity of guanylate cyclase, NO increases the production of cyclic guanosine monophosphate (cGMP). Vasoactive peptide and prostaglandins E_1 and E_2 stimulate increased production of cyclic adenosine monophosphate (cAMP). Both cAMP and cGMP ultimately lead to a decrease in calcium concentration within smooth muscle cells of the penile arteries and the sinusoidal spaces, leading to smooth muscle relaxation and increased blood flow. As the sinusoidal spaces become engorged, intracavernosal pressure increases, subtunical venules are compressed, and the penis becomes rigid and elongated (**Fig. 51–1**).

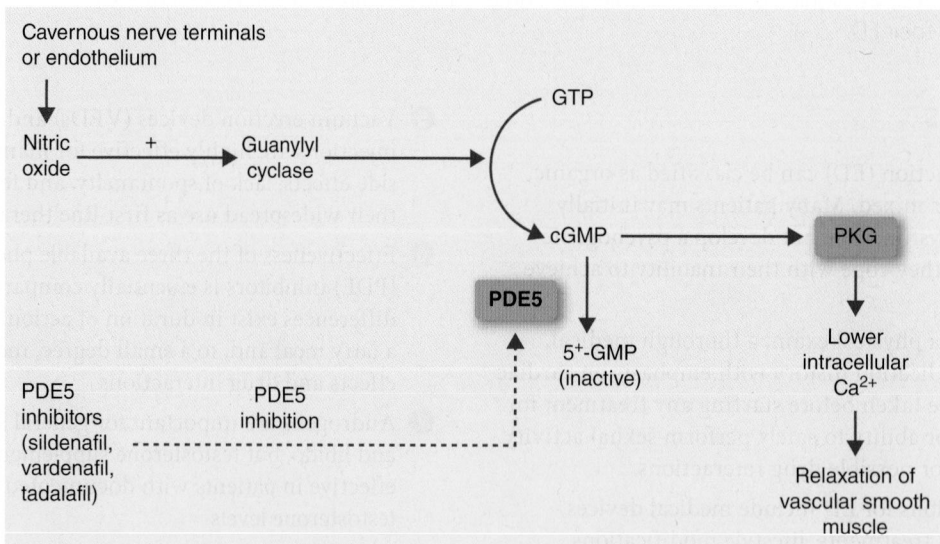

FIGURE 51–1. Mechanism of erection and sites of action of various treatment modalities for erectile dysfunction (ED). Penile erection is achieved through relaxation of smooth muscle cells lining arterial vessels and sinusoidal spaces in the corpora cavernosa, which leads to increased arterial inflow and pressure, decreased venous outflow, and increased intracavernosal pressure. Smooth muscle relaxation is mediated by intracellular generation of cyclic guanosine monophosphate (cGMP) from guanosine triphosphate (GTP) via activation of guanylate cyclase by nitric oxide. Treatment modalities for ED include oral phosphodiesterase type 5 (PDE-5) inhibitors, which inhibit the breakdown of cGMP, and local vasoactive agents. Nitric oxide–cGMP signaling in cavernous smooth muscle. (cGMP, cycle guanosine monophosphate; GTP, guanosine triphosphate; PDE5, phosphodiesterase 5; PFE, phosphodiesterase; PKG, protein kinase G.) (Reproduced, with permission, from Setter SM, Iltz JL, Fincham JE, Campbell RK, Baker DE. Phosphodiesterase 5 inhibitors for erectile dysfunction. Ann Pharmacother. 2005;39(7-8):1286-95.)

Detumescence occurs with sympathetic discharge after ejaculation. Sympathetic activity induces smooth muscle contraction of arterioles and vascular spaces leading to a reduction in blood inflow, decompression of the sinusoidal spaces, and enhanced outflow.

Testosterone also plays a significant albeit complex role in erectile function. Testosterone is responsible for much of a man's libido. With low serum concentrations, libido declines. Additionally, testosterone helps with stabilization of intracavernosal levels of NO synthase, the enzyme responsible for triggering the NO cascade. Interestingly, some patients with low or borderline-low serum concentrations of testosterone will have normal erectile function, whereas some with normal levels will have dysfunction.

Normal penile erections are complex events that require the full function of the vascular, neurologic, and hormonal systems. Anything that affects the function of these systems may lead to ED. ❶ *ED can be classified as organic, psychogenic, or a mixture of these.* Organic dysfunction includes abnormalities in the three systems responsible for a normal erection or may be medication-induced (**Tables 51–1** and **51–2**). It is estimated that 25% of ED cases are due to medications.[4] Note that many of the risk factors for ED are the same as risk factors for cardiovascular (CV) disease, including hypertension, diabetes, dyslipidemia, smoking, obesity, metabolic syndrome, and sedentary behavior.[5] In many patients, ED is the first indication of the endothelial dysfunction associated with cardiovascular disease, with two-thirds of patients with coronary artery disease having symptoms of ED before the onset of coronary symptoms.[4] The presence of ED risk factors leads to the assumption that the patient has organic dysfunction. Most commonly, medical conditions that impair arterial flow into or out of the erectile tissue or affect the innervation will be strongly associated with ED. Patients with diabetes mellitus have exceptionally high rates of ED as a result of vascular disease and neuropathy. Additionally, a relationship has been found between low testosterone levels and an increased incidence of metabolic syndrome and type 2 diabetes.[6]

Psychogenic dysfunction occurs if a patient does not respond to psychological arousal. It occurs in up to 30% of all cases of ED. Common causes include performance anxiety,

---

Table 51–1

Factors Associated with ED

Chronic medical conditions
Hypertension
Diabetes mellitus
Inflammatory conditions of the prostate
Coronary and peripheral vascular disease
Neurologic disorders (e.g., Parkinson's disease and multiple sclerosis)
Endocrine disorders (hypogonadism and pituitary, adrenal, and thyroid disorders)
Psychiatric disorders (depression, anxiety, and schizophrenia)
Dyslipidemia
Renal failure
Liver disease
Penile disease (Peyronie's disease or anatomic abnormalities)

Surgical procedures
Perineal surgery
Radical prostatectomy
Vascular surgery

Lifestyle
Age
Smoking
Excessive alcohol consumption
Obesity
Poor overall health and reduced physical activity

Trauma
Pelvic fractures
Spinal cord injuries

From Refs. 2 and 4.

Table 51–2

Medication Classes Associated with ED

Antihypertensives
β-Blockers (excluding nebivolol)
Thiazide diuretics
Centrally acting agents (clonidine, methyldopa, and reserpine)
Spironolactone
α-Blockers
Calcium-channel blockers

Lipid medications
Gemfibrozil

Antidepressants
Tricyclic antidepressants
Monoamine oxidase inhibitors
Selective serotonin reuptake inhibitors/serotonin-norepinephrine reuptake inhibitors

Antipsychotics
Phenothiazines
Risperidone
Lithium

Anticonvulsants
Carbamazepine
Phenytoin

Histamine antagonists
Cimetidine

Antiandrogens and hormones
5α-Reductase inhibitors
Progesterone and estrogen
Corticosteroids

Recreational drugs
Ethanol
Cocaine
Marijuana
Opiates

From Refs. 1, 4, and 19.

strained relationships, lack of sexual arousability, and overt psychiatric disorders such as depression and schizophrenia.[7] ❶ *Many patients may initially have organic dysfunction, but develop a psychogenic component as they try to cope with their inability to achieve an erection.*

CLINICAL PRESENTATION AND DIAGNOSIS

TREATMENT
Desired Outcomes

ED is not a life-threatening condition, but left untreated it can be associated with depression, loss of self-esteem, poor self-image, and marital discord.[9] The primary goal of therapy is achievement of erections suitable for intercourse and improvement in patient and partner quality of life. Additionally, the ideal therapy should have minimal side effects, be convenient to administer, have a quick onset of action, and have few or no drug interactions.[10]

General Approach to Treatment

After determining whether the ED is organic or psychogenic, the initial step in management is to identify associated disease states and lifestyle activities that adversely affect erectile function and treat them optimally. ❷ *In addition to*

Clinical Presentation and Diagnosis of ED

The introduction of oral medications and direct-to-consumer advertising has made patients feel more comfortable approaching practitioners for treatment advice. Despite this, some patients may only discuss their dysfunction when questioned directly by their provider or if their partner initiates the interaction. Patients may still feel that a loss in erectile function translates into a loss of masculinity.

Possible Signs and Symptoms
- Embarrassment
- Anxiousness
- Anger
- Marital difficulties
- Low self-confidence or morale, depression
- Full inability to achieve erections
- Ability to achieve partial erections, but not suitable for intercourse
- Erections sufficient for intercourse, but early **detumescence**
- The problem may have a slow or acute onset, or may wax and wane

Diagnosis

ED may be the presenting symptom of other chronic disease states.

Full medical, social, and medication histories should be taken to determine areas that can cause or exacerbate ED and to assess the patient's ability to safely perform intercourse.

- Medical history with emphasis on cardiovascular and psychiatric disorders, diabetes, trauma, and surgical procedures
- Social history including history of smoking, recreational drug use, exercise, and alcohol consumption

- Medication history including prescription, nonprescription, and dietary supplements

Physical Examination
- Review for hypogonadism (gynecomastia, testicular atrophy, reduced body hair, increase in body fat)
- Digital rectal exam to determine whether prostate is enlarged
- Vital signs
- Abnormalities of the penis or impaired vasculature and nerve function to the penis

Labs
- Fasting glucose or HbA1c
- Serum testosterone
- Fasting lipid panel
- Further cardiac testing if warranted

Determine Severity
- Use an abridged, five-item version of the International Index of Erectile Dysfunction (IIEF-5) as a diagnostic tool[12]:
  - How do you rate your confidence that you could get and keep an erection?
  - When you had erections with sexual stimulation, how often were your erections hard enough for penetration?
  - During sexual intercourse, how often were you able to maintain your erection after you had penetrated (entered) your partner?
  - During sexual intercourse, how difficult was it to maintain your erection to completion of intercourse?
  - When you attempted sexual intercourse, how often was it satisfactory for you?
  - Questions scored 1 to 5, very low to very high respectively. Score of 21 or less indicates ED likely.

a physical exam, a thorough medical, social, and medication history with emphasis on cardiac disease must be taken before starting any treatment for ED to assess for ability to safely perform sexual activity and to assess for possible drug interactions. Medications suspected to cause or worsen ED should be discontinued if possible. In patients with intermediate or high cardiovascular risk, additional testing should occur to determine whether sexual activity is safe.

③ *Treatment options for ED include medical devices, pharmacologic treatments, lifestyle modifications, surgery, and psychotherapy. Reversible causes of ED should be identified first and treated appropriately.*

④ *When determining the best treatment for an individual, the role of the clinician is to inform the patient and his partner of all available options while understanding his medical history, desires, and goals. The choice of treatment is primarily left up to the couple, but most often treatment is initiated with the least invasive option and then treatment progresses to more invasive options if needed.* Ultimately, the choice of therapy should be individualized, taking into account patient and partner preferences, concomitant disease states, response, administration route, cost, tolerability, and safety. Common drug treatment regimens for ED are listed in Table 51–3.

Table 51–3

Common Drug Treatment Regimens for ED

Route of Administration	Generic Name	Brand Name	Typical Dosing Range[a]	Maximum Dosing Frequency
Oral	Sildenafil	Viagra	25–100 mg 1 hour prior to intercourse	Once daily
	Tadalafil	Cialis	5–20 mg prior to intercourse or daily dose of 2.5–5 mg	Once daily
	Vardenafil	Levitra	5–20 mg 1 hour prior to intercourse	Once daily
	Yohimbine[b]	Aphrodyne, Yocon	5.4 mg 3 times daily	N/A
Intracavernosal	Alprostadil	Caverject, Caverject Impulse, Edex	1.25–60 mcg 5–20 minutes prior to intercourse[c]	3 times weekly, 24 hours between injections
	Papaverine[b]	N/A	Typically used in combination at variable doses[c]	3 times weekly, 24 hours between injections
	Phentolamine[b]	N/A	Typically used in combination at variable doses[c]	3 times weekly, 24 hours between injections
Intraurethral	Alprostadil	MUSE	125–1,000 mcg 5–10 minutes prior to intercourse[c]	2 times daily
Intramuscular	Testosterone cypionate	Depo-Testosterone	50–400 mg every 2–4 weeks	Once weekly
	Testosterone enanthate	Delatestryl	50–400 mg every 2–4 weeks	Once weekly
Topical	Testosterone patches	Testoderm	4–6 mg/day applied to scrotum	Once daily
		Testoderm TTS	4–6 mg/day applied to arm, back, or upper buttocks	Once daily
		Androderm	2.5–5 mg/day applied to back, abdomen, upper arms, or thighs	Once daily
	Testosterone gel	AndroGel 1%, Testim	5–10 g gel per day (50–100 mg testosterone) to shoulders, upper arms, abdomen (AndroGel 1% only)	Once daily
		AndroGel 1.62%	40.5–81 mg/day to shoulders or upper arms	Once daily
		Fortesta	10–70 mg/day to thigh	Once daily
		Axiron	30–120 mg/day to axilla	Once daily
Buccal	Testosterone	Striant	30 mg every 12 hours to gum region above incisor; rotate to alternate sides with each dose	Twice daily
Subcutaneous implantable pellet	Testosterone	Testopel	150–450 mg (150 mg for every 25 mg testosterone propionate required weekly)	Every 3–6 months

MUSE, medicated urethral system for erection.

[a]Use the lowest effective dose to limit adverse effects.

[b]Not FDA-approved for this indication.

[c]Initial dose must be titrated in physician's office.

Patient Encounter 1, Part 1

CB, a 52-year-old man with type 2 diabetes, coronary artery disease, hypertension, and dyslipidemia, returns to your clinic for follow-up on his chronic disease states. When reviewing his history, he describes problems with his erections. After further questioning, you determine that his dysfunction has progressively gotten worse over the last year. He is quite emotional and states that the problem is distressing and has caused significant marital discord. He wonders about "those ads on television" suggesting a pill.

Based on the available information, how would you classify his ED?

What additional information do you need before establishing an appropriate treatment regimen and determining his ability to safely perform intercourse?

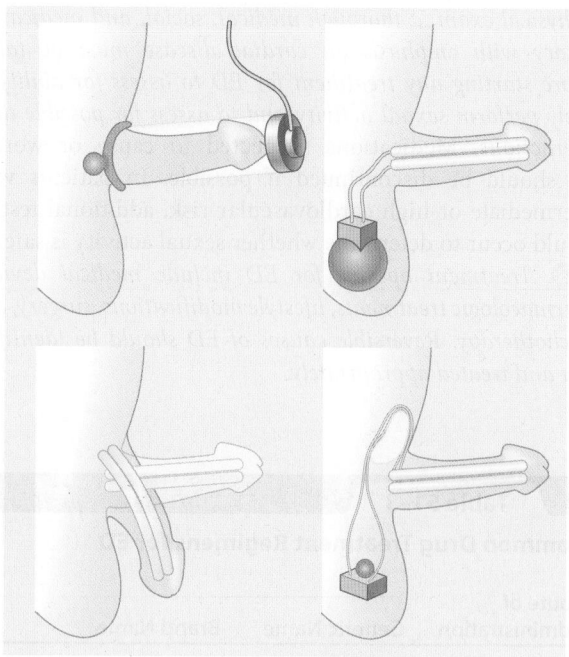

FIGURE 51–2. Available devices and prostheses used to treat ED. (From Wagner G, Saenz de Tejada I. Update on male erectile dysfunction. BMJ 1998;316:678–682.)

▶ Nonpharmacologic Therapy

Lifestyle Modifications Lifestyle modifications should always be addressed in the management of ED. A healthy diet, increase in regular physical activity, and weight loss are associated with higher International Index of Erectile Dysfunction (IIED) scores and an improvement in erectile function.[11] The clinician should also recommend smoking cessation, reduction in excessive alcohol intake, and discontinuation of illicit drug use.

Psychotherapy Psychotherapy is an appropriate treatment approach for patients with psychogenic or mixed dysfunction. It should address immediate causes of dysfunction, and if possible the partner should attend sessions as well. Effectiveness is not well documented for organic dysfunction unless combined with other therapies. Advantages include noninvasiveness and partner participation, whereas disadvantages include increased cost and time commitment.

Vacuum Erection Devices Vacuum erection devices (VEDs) induce erections by creating a vacuum around the penis; the negative pressure draws blood into the penis by passively dilating arteries and engorging the corpora cavernosa. The erection is maintained with a constriction band placed at the base of the penis to reduce venous outflow (Fig. 51–2). They may be used as often as desired, but it is recommended that the constriction band not be left in place longer than 30 minutes at a time.

⑤ *VEDs are highly effective treatment modalities for ED and are considered a second-line therapy. Efficacy rates are as high as 90% in obtaining an erection sufficient for coitus, and satisfaction rates are between 27% and 94%.*[5,13] Rigidity may be improved by using a double pump technique in which the vacuum is applied for a couple of minutes, removed, then reapplied for another few minutes. Higher efficacy rates can also be achieved by combining VEDs with other therapies.

Onset of action is slow at around 30 minutes, which limits spontaneity. In addition, patients and partners may complain of a cold, lifeless, discolored penis that has a hinge-like feel. Painful ejaculation or inability to ejaculate are additional adverse effects. VEDs are contraindicated in persons with sickle cell disease and should be used with caution in patients on oral anticoagulants or who have bleeding disorders due to the increased possibility of priapism. VEDs are generally more acceptable to older patients in stable relationships and with infrequent sexual encounters.[13]

Prostheses Penile prostheses are semirigid malleable or inflatable rods, which are inserted surgically into the corpus cavernosa to allow erections (Fig. 51–2). The malleable rods are rigid at all times, but may be bent into position by the patient when desired. The inflatable prostheses remain flaccid until the pump within the scrotum moves fluid from a reservoir to the cylinders within the penis. Detumescence is achieved when the fluid is then transferred back to the reservoir by activating a release button.

Because prostheses are the most invasive treatment available, they are only considered in patients who do not respond to medications or external devices, or those who have significant adverse effects from other therapies. Patient satisfaction rates can be as high as 95%, with partner satisfaction rates just slightly lower.[14] The primary risk of insertion is infection, although this only happens in 3% of first-time prostheses. Semirigid malleable rods may interfere with urination, are difficult to conceal, and have a higher likelihood of erosion.[14] Most devices need replacement after 10 to 15 years.

▶ Pharmacologic Therapy

Phosphodiesterase Type 5 Inhibitors Sildenafil (Viagra), tadalafil (Cialis), and vardenafil (Levitra) act by selectively inhibiting phosphodiesterase (PDE) type 5, an enzyme that breaks down cGMP. By inhibiting the breakdown of cGMP, smooth muscle relaxation is induced, leading to an erection (Fig. 51–1). However, the PDE inhibitors are only effective in the presence of sexual stimulation to drive the NO/cGMP system, making them facilitators of an erection, not initiators. Patients must be informed of the need for sexual stimulation to induce an erection, as it will not occur spontaneously.

⑥ *Effectiveness of the three available PDE inhibitors is essentially comparable, but differences exist in duration of action, absorption with a fatty meal and, to a small degree, incidence of side effects and drug interactions (Table 51–4).* Review of available data for each individual agent shows a 50% to 80% response rate depending on the dose of agent used and the etiology of dysfunction. Response rates tend to be lower in patients with radical prostatectomy as well as those with diabetes, severe nerve damage, or severe vascular disease.[15] Although efficacy rates appear to be similar between agents, there are some data to suggest that continuation rates are higher and patient preference greater with tadalafil.[16] The PDE inhibitors are considered first-line

therapies due to high efficacy rates, convenience of dosing, and minimal severe adverse effects.

The most dramatic difference among the three agents is tadalafil's extended duration of action, earning it the nickname "the weekender drug." Although sildenafil and vardenafil have average half-lives of 3 to 4 hours, tadalafil's half-life is approximately 18 hours. The extended half-life allows for more spontaneous sexual activity over a couple of days, but may increase the duration of adverse effects and likelihood of drug interactions. Tadalafil has been approved for use as a daily medication at a lower dose (2.5 to 5 mg) than the as-needed dose. The dosing efficacy appears to be similar to as-needed dosing, but cost will be prohibitive for many patients.

The most common side effects experienced with PDE inhibitors include headache, facial flushing, nasal congestion, dyspepsia, myalgia, back pain, and, rarely, priapism. Vardenafil and sildenafil may also cause difficulty in discriminating blue from green, bluish tones in vision, or difficulty seeing in dim light due to cross-reactivity with PDE 6 in the retina. Labeling for all PDE inhibitors includes a warning about nonarteritic ischemic optic neuropathy (NAION) in a small number of patients. This is a condition in which blood flow

Table 51–4
Comparison of PDE Inhibitors

	Sildenafil (Viagra)	Tadalafil (Cialis)	Vardenafil (Levitra)
Available strengths	25-, 50-, 100-mg tabs	2.5-, 5-, 10-, 20-mg tabs	2.5-, 5-, 10-, 20-mg tabs
Initial dosage in healthy adults	50 mg up to once daily taken 1 hour prior to sexual activity	10 mg up to once daily taken 1 hour prior to sexual activity or 2.5 mg daily at the same time each day	10 mg up to once daily taken 1 hour prior to sexual activity
Dosing range for healthy adults	25–100 mg	5–20 mg	5–20 mg
Dosage in the elderly	25 mg	5–10 mg	5 mg
Dosage in renal impairment	50 mg (moderate[a]) 25 mg (severe[b])	5 mg (moderate[a] and severe[b])	5–20 mg
Dosage in hepatic impairment	25 mg	10 mg[c]	5–10 mg[d]
Time to onset	30 minutes	15 minutes	Less than 1 hour
Onset delayed by high-fat meal?	Yes	No	Yes
Duration of effect	Up to 4 hours	Up to 36 hours	Up to 4 hours
Half-life	3–4 hours	18 hours	4–5 hours
Metabolism	CYP3A4 (major) CYP2C9 (minor)	CYP3A4	CYP3A4 (major) CYP3A5 (minor) CYP2C (minor)
Clinically relevant drug interactions	Nitrates, protease inhibitors, azole antifungals, erythromycin	Nitrates, a_1-blockers[e], azole antifungals, erythromycin	Nitrates, antiarrhythmic agents,[f] a_1-blockers,[e] erythromycin

CYP, cytochrome P450 isoenzyme.

[a]Moderate renal impairment = creatinine clearance (CrCl) 31 to 50 mL/min (0.51 to 0.83 mL/s).

[b]Severe renal impairment = CrCl less than 30 mL/min (0.50 mL/s).

[c]Mild to moderate only—contraindicated in severe liver disease.

[d]Mild to moderate only—not yet evaluated in severe liver disease.

[e]Selective a_1-blockers (such as alfuzosin, silodosin, and tamsulosin) are appropriate in combination.

[f]Vardenafil can cause QT-interval prolongation; this effect in combination with certain antiarrhythmic agents can lead to life-threatening arrhythmias.

is blocked to the optic nerve. If patients experience sudden or decreased vision loss, they should call a healthcare provider immediately.

Concern exists about the safety of renewing sexual activity and using PDE inhibitors in patients with cardiovascular disease. Due to the coexistence of ED and coronary artery disease, a management approach was developed to give recommendations for the use of PDE inhibitors as well as to determine the safety of intercourse in patients with cardiovascular disease[17,18] (Table 51–5). In addition to the inherent risk of renewing sexual activity, PDE inhibitors can lead to significant hypotension. Patients taking organic nitrates are at highest risk, as these drugs potentiate the drop in blood pressure. All three PDE inhibitors are absolutely contraindicated in patients taking any form of nitrate, whether scheduled or sublingual for acute situations. Caution should be used when using a PDE inhibitor in patients taking α-blockers due to an increased risk of hypotension. In addition, the labeling for vardenafil contains a precautionary statement about the possibility of QT prolongation with the use of the drug. Other drug interactions and cautions vary slightly between agents and are described in Table 51–4.

The introduction of the oral PDE inhibitors has dramatically changed the treatment of ED. Direct-to-consumer advertising has informed patients of the availability of oral drugs for treatment. However, patients must be fully informed of side effects, drug interactions, mechanism of action, and dosing before being prescribed the medication. In addition, they need to understand the need for sexual stimulation to achieve the desired result and that a single trial is not adequate. It is estimated that six to eight attempts with a medication and specific dose may be needed before successful intercourse results.[5]

Alprostadil   Alprostadil is a prostaglandin E_1 analog that induces an erection by stimulating adenyl cyclase, which leads to an increase in smooth muscle relaxation, rapid arterial inflow, and increased penile rigidity. Alprostadil is available as an intracavernosal injection (Caverject or Edex) or a transurethral suppository (MUSE, medicated urethral system for erection), but the injectable form is more effective (Fig. 51–3).[4,5] Both forms of alprostadil are considered more invasive than oral medications or VEDs and are therefore second-line therapies.

MUSE consists of a urethral pellet of alprostadil with an applicator. Onset of action is within 5 to 10 minutes and it is effective for 30 to 60 minutes. Initial dose titration should occur in a physician's office to ensure correct dose and prevent adverse events. Although effectiveness rates in clinical trials have been as high as 65%,[19] its success in practice has been lower.[20] Aching in the penis, testicles, legs, and perineum; warmth or burning sensation in the urethra, minor urethral bleeding or spotting, priapism, and lightheadedness are all possible adverse effects. In addition, partners may experience vaginal burning or itching. Disadvantages include lower effectiveness, high cost, adverse effects, complicated insertion technique, and a contraindication against use with a pregnant partner unless using a condom.

Table 51–5

Recommendations of the Second Princeton Consensus Conference for Cardiovascular Risk Stratification of Patients Being Considered for PDE Inhibitor Therapy

Risk Category	Description of Patients' Conditions	Management Approach
Low risk	Has asymptomatic CV disease with less than three risk factors for CV disease Has well-controlled hypertension Has mild, stable angina Has mild congestive heart failure (NYHA Class I) Has mild valvular heart disease Had a myocardial infarction more than 6 weeks ago	Patient can be started on PDE inhibitor
Moderate risk	Has greater than or equal to three risk factors for CV disease Has moderate, stable angina Had a recent myocardial infarction or stroke within the past 6 weeks Has moderate congestive heart failure (NYHA Class II)	Patient should undergo complete CV workup and treadmill stress test to determine tolerance to increased myocardial energy consumption associated with increased sexual activity
High risk	Has unstable or symptomatic angina, despite treatment Has uncontrolled hypertension Has severe congestive heart failure (NYHA Class III or IV) Had a recent myocardial infarction or stroke within the past 2 weeks Has moderate or severe valvular heart disease Has high-risk cardiac arrhythmias Has obstructive hypertrophic cardiomyopathy	PDE inhibitor is contraindicated; sexual intercourse should be deferred

CV, cardiovascular; NYHA, New York Heart Association; PDE, phosphodiesterase.

From Gupta BP, Murad MH, Clifton MM, et al. The effect of lifestyle modification and cardiovascular risk factor reduction on erectile dysfunction. Arch Intern Med 2011;171:1797–1803.

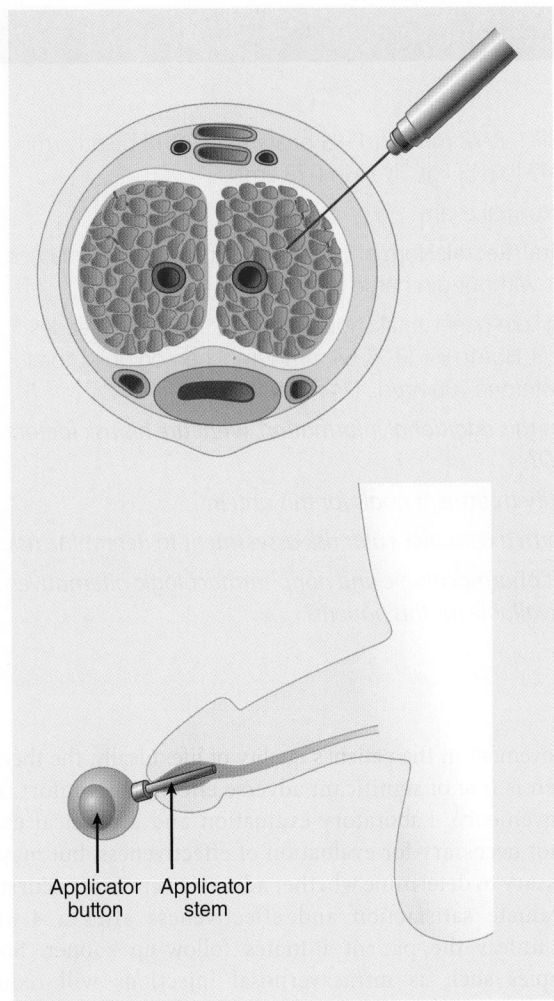

FIGURE 51–3. Intraurethral and intracavernosal administration of alprostadil. (From Wagner G, Saenz de Tejada I. Update on male erectile dysfunction. BMJ 1998;316:678–682.)

Alprostadil Alprostadil injected into the corpus cavernosum is the more effective route and is the only FDA-approved injection for ED. The onset of action is similar to transurethral alprostadil, but duration varies with dose and must be titrated in a physician's office to achieve an erection lasting no more than 1 hour. Injections should be done into one side of the penis directly into the corpus cavernosum, and then the penis should be massaged to distribute the drug. Because of cross-circulation, both corpora will become erect when massaging. Education is extremely important with intracavernosal injections. Patients must be adequately informed of technique, expectations, side effects, and when to seek help. ❺ *Intracavernosal injections are effective in up to 90% of patients, but side effects, lack of spontaneity, and fear of needles limit their widespread use as first-line therapy, and therefore this therapy is most appropriate for patients in long-term stable relationships.* Adverse effects include pain with injection, bleeding or bruising at the injection site, fibrosis, or priapism. Use with caution in patients with sickle cell disease, those on anticoagulants, or those who have

bleeding disorders, due to an increased risk of priapism and bleeding.

Papaverine and Phentolamine Papaverine and phentolamine are non–FDA-approved agents used for intracavernosal injection. Papaverine is a nonselective PDE inhibitor that induces an erection by relaxing smooth muscle and increasing blood flow. Phentolamine is a competitive α-adrenergic receptor antagonist that increases arterial inflow by opposing arterial constriction. Both drugs are rarely used alone and are most often mixed in various concentrations with alprostadil for increased effectiveness and in an effort to reduce adverse effects with smaller doses of each medication. Patients typically must see a specialist for use of these medications in mixtures, as the providers are most likely to compound them and adjust dosages.

Yohimbine Yohimbine is an indole alkaloid produced in the bark of yohimbe trees. It selectively inhibits α_2-adrenergic receptors in the brain that are associated with libido and penile erection. Because there are only limited data supporting its efficacy, yohimbine is not a recommended treatment for any form of ED.[5] Adverse effects of the drug include nausea, irritability, headaches, anxiety, tachycardia, and hypertension.

Testosterone Supplementation ❼ *Androgens are important for general sexual function and libido, but testosterone supplementation is only effective in patients with documented low serum testosterone levels.* In patients with hypogonadism, testosterone replacement is the initial treatment of choice, as it corrects decreased libido, fatigue, muscle loss, sleep disturbances, and depressed mood. Improvements in ED may occur, but they should not be expected to occur in all patients. The initial trial should be for 3 months. At that time, re-evaluation and the addition of another ED therapy is warranted. Dosage forms include oral, intramuscular, topical patches or gel, an implanted pellet, and a buccal tablet.

Injectable esters of testosterone offer the most inexpensive replacement option. Testosterone cypionate and enanthate have the longest duration of action and are therefore the preferred agents. There are several drawbacks associated with parenteral testosterone, including the need to administer deep intramuscular injections every 2 to 4 weeks. In addition, levels of hormone are well above physiologic values within the first few days. Concentrations then decline and eventually dip below physiologic levels just before the next dose. These extreme changes in concentration may lead to mood swings and a reduced sense of well-being.[21]

Treatment with topical products is attractive to patients due to convenience, but they tend to be more expensive than the injections. In a review of studies including patients with ED and primary hypogonadism, transdermal testosterone resulted in significantly higher response rates than intramuscular administration.[4] Testosterone patches and gels are administered daily and result in serum levels within the physiologic range during the 24-hour dosing period.[21] Most patients prefer the nonscrotal patch or the gel because the scrotal patch requires shaving of the area, and the patch has a tendency to fall off. Care must be taken with the use of

---

Patient Encounter 1, Part 2

PMH: Type 2 diabetes for 15 years; not controlled due to his stressful profession; he often works late, eats on the run, and has no time for exercise. Coronary artery disease; myocardial infarction with stent placement 6 months ago. Hypertension for 8 years, currently controlled. Dyslipidemia for 8 years, currently controlled.

SH: Works long hours as a business executive; drinks alcohol only occasionally; has a 20-pack-per-year smoking history, but quit 6 months ago.

Meds: Metformin 1,000 mg orally twice daily; metoprolol XL 50 mg orally once daily; lisinopril/hydrochlorothiazide 40/25 mg once daily; simvastatin 20 mg orally once daily; aspirin 81 mg once daily.

ROS: (–) Morning, nocturnal, or spontaneous erections suitable for intercourse; (–) nocturia, urgency, symptoms of prostatitis; (–) chest pain or anginal symptoms; (+) significant life stressors; (+) mild pain in feet.

PE:

VS: BP 128/78 mm Hg, P 85 beats/min, RR 18 breaths/min, Wt 249 lb (113 kg), Ht 70 in (178 cm)

CV: Normal exam

Genital/Rectal: Normal scrotum and testicles w/o masses; penis without discharge or curvature

Labs: lipid panel: total cholesterol, LDL, HDL, triglycerides at goal; HbA1c 8% (0.08; 64 mmol/mol hemoglobin), total testosterone 700 ng/dL (24 nmol/L)

Given this additional information, what are his risk factors for ED?

Identify treatment goals for this patient.

Perform a cardiovascular risk assessment to determine risk.

What pharmacologic and nonpharmacologic alternatives are available for this patient?

---

the gel to wash hands thoroughly after use and avoid baths or showers within 2 to 6 hours of application. The most common side effects of topical testosterone are dermatologic reactions caused by the absorption enhancers.

Oral testosterone products are also available for supplementation. Unfortunately, testosterone has poor oral bioavailability and undergoes extensive first-pass metabolism. Alkylated derivatives such as methyltestosterone and fluoxymesterone have been formulated to compensate for these problems, but this modification makes them considerably more hepatotoxic. This adverse effect makes oral replacement undesirable, and this route of administration should not be used.

An alternative to the oral route is the buccal mucoadhesive system. The Striant buccal system adheres to the inside of the mouth and the testosterone is absorbed through the oral mucosa and delivered to the systemic circulation. There is no first-pass effect, as the liver is bypassed by this route of administration. Patients apply a 30-mg tablet to the upper gum twice daily. The cost is similar to that of the patch or gel. Side effects unique to this dosage form include oral irritation, bitter taste, and gum edema.

General side effects of testosterone include gynecomastia, dyslipidemia, polycythemia, and acne. Weight gain, hypertension, edema, and exacerbations of heart failure also occur due to sodium retention. Before initiating testosterone, the patient should undergo evaluation for benign prostatic hypertrophy and prostate cancer. Routine follow-up includes yearly prostate-specific antigen, digital rectal exam, and hemoglobin and liver function, in addition to assessment of response.

OUTCOME EVALUATION

Successful therapy for ED results in an increase in erections suitable for intercourse and, most importantly, in an improvement in the patient's quality of life. Ideally, the therapy chosen is free of significant adverse effects, discomfort, and inconvenience. Laboratory evaluation and a physical exam are not necessary for evaluation of effectiveness, but may be necessary to determine whether adverse events are occurring.

Evaluate satisfaction and effectiveness after a 4-week trial unless the patient initiates follow-up sooner. Some therapies such as intracavernosal injections will require multiple visits over the long term to determine the correct dose and to detect adverse effects. If the initial therapy is not effective, the patient must be further evaluated to determine whether the initial assessment of comorbid disease states, type of dysfunction, and patient goals were appropriate. After providing further education, ensuring the patient is using the therapy appropriately and determining their goals are realistic, providers can then increase the dose of drug if not at maximum, switch to another therapy, or add a therapy if indicated.

Patient Encounter 1, Part 3

CB was referred to his cardiologist, and it was determined that he may safely resume sexual activity at this time. Based on the information available, create a treatment plan for this patient's ED.

Which of the available options will be your treatments of choice based on degree of invasiveness, ease of use, and side-effect profile?

What are the safety and efficacy monitoring parameters for the chosen treatment?

Patient Encounter 2, Part 1

WW is a 62-year-old man with a history of type 2 diabetes, dyslipidemia, hypertension, and ED. When in the office for a routine follow-up, he states the pill recently prescribed for his ED is not "doing the trick" so he has not been using it. He also complains that he is tired all the time, does not have much of a libido anymore, and is gaining weight.

Meds: glimepiride 4 mg orally twice daily, metformin 1,000 mg orally twice daily, losartan/hydrochlorothiazide 100/25 mg orally once daily, vardenafil 20 mg orally as needed.

ROS: (–) Morning, nocturnal, or spontaneous erections suitable for intercourse; (–) nocturia, urgency, symptoms of prostatitis.

PE:

VS: BP 132/74 mm Hg, P 82 beats/min, Wt 214 lb (97.3 kg), Ht 75 in (191 cm)

Labs: lipid panel: total cholesterol, LDL, and HDL at goal, triglycerides 191 mg/dL (2.16 mmol/L); HbA1c 8.5% (0.085; 69 mmol/mol hemoglobin)

Based on the information provided, what is your assessment of the patient's ED?

What should be recommended as the next step in treatment of his ED?

Patient Care and Monitoring

1. Assess the patient's specific symptoms to determine the type of dysfunction. Does the patient have ED or an ejaculatory or libido disorder?

2. If problems are with erectile ability, ask specific questions related to onset, frequency, and sexual relationships. Does the patient history imply psychogenic, organic, or mixed dysfunction?

3. Perform a thorough medical and social history as well as a physical exam to diagnose ED and to determine potential causes that may be treatable.

4. Perform a thorough history of prescription and nonprescription medications. Are any of the patient's medications associated with ED or are they contraindicated with possible ED therapies?

5. Generally treatment is started with the least invasive option and then progresses to more invasive options, but ultimately patient and partner preferences determine the initial therapy.

6. Discontinue medications that may cause ED if possible and optimally treat associated disease states.

7. If the patient and partner are not satisfied, provide further counseling to ensure that they are using the therapy appropriately and that they have realistic goals.

8. Provide patient education with regard to disease state, lifestyle modifications, drug therapy, and device technique:

   - The causes of ED
   - The fact that therapy will not cure ED, but may be helpful in improving erections; it is important to have realistic expectations
   - The appropriate use of medications and devices
   - Typical adverse effects
   - Drug interactions
   - Warning signs and their management (e.g., vision changes, fibrosis, pain, priapism, or hypotension)
   - The importance of frequent follow-up with the provider

Abbreviations Introduced in This Chapter

cAMP	Cyclic adenosine monophosphate
cGMP	Cyclic guanosine monophosphate
ED	Erectile dysfunction
GTP	Guanosine triphosphate
IIED	International Index of Erectile Dysfunction
MUSE	Medicated urethral system for erection
NAION	Non-arteritic ischemic optic neuropathy
PDE	Phosphodiesterase
VED	Vacuum erection device

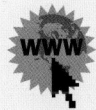 Self-assessment questions and answers are available at *http://mhpharmacotherapy.com/pp.html.*

REFERENCES

1. Heidelbaugh JJ. Management of erectile dysfunction. Am Fam Physician 2010;81:305–312.
2. Bacon CG, Mittleman MA, Kawachi I, et al. Sexual function in men older than 50 years of age: Results from the health professionals follow-up study. Ann Int Med 2003;139:161–168.

3. Morgentaler A. A 66-year-old man with sexual dysfunction. JAMA 2004;291:2994–3003.

4. McVary KT. Erectile dysfunction. N Engl J Med 2007;357:2472–2481.

5. Hatzimouratidis K, Amar E, Eardley I, et al. Guidelines on male sexual dysfunction: erectile dysfunction and premature ejaculation. Eur Urol 2010;57:804–814.

6. Shabsigh R, Arver S, Channer KS, et al. The triad of erectile dysfunction, hypogonadism and the metabolic syndrome. Int J Clin Pract 2008;62:791–798.

7. Deveci S, O'Brien K, Ahmed A, et al. Can the International Index of Erectile Function distinguish between organic and psychogenic erectile function? BJU Int 2008;102:354–356.

8. Rosen RC, Cappelleri JC, Smith MD, et al. Development and evaluation of an abridged, 5-item version of the International Index of Erectile Dysfunction (IIEF-5) as a diagnostic tool for erectile dysfunction. Int J Impot Res 1999;11:319–326.

9. DiMeo PJ. Psychosocial and relationship issues in men with erectile dysfunction. Urol Nurs 2006;26:442–446.

10. Mikhail N. Management of erectile dysfunction by the primary care physician. Clev Clin J Med 2005;293–294, 296–297, 301–305.

11. Gupta BP, Murad MH, Clifton MM, et al. The effect of lifestyle modification and cardiovascular risk factor reduction on erectile dysfunction. Arch Intern Med 2011;171:1797–1803.

12. Wagner G, Saenz de Tejada I. Update on male erectile dysfunction. BMJ 1998;316:678–682.

13. Yuan J, Hoang AN, Romero CA, et al. Vacuum therapy in erectile dysfunction: science and clinical evidence. Int J Impot Res 2010;22:211–219.

14. Brant WO, Bella AJ, Lue TF. Treatment options for erectile dysfunction. Endocrinol Metab Clin N Am 2007;36:465–479.

15. De Tejada IS. Therapeutic strategies for optimizing PDE-5 inhibitor therapy in patients with erectile dysfunction considered difficult or challenging to treat. Int J Impot Res 2004;16(Suppl 1):S40–S42.

16. Morales AM, Casillas M, Turbi C. Patients' preference in the treatment of erectile dysfunction. Int J Impot Res 2011;23:1–8.

17. Rosen RC, Jackson G, Kostis JB. Erectile dysfunction and cardiac disease: Recommendations of the Second Princeton Conference. Curr Urol Rep 2006;7:490–496.

18. Jackson G, Rosen RC, Kloner RA, Kostis JB. The second Princeton consensus on sexual dysfunction and cardiac risk: new guidelines for sexual medicine. J Sex Med 2006;3:28–36.

19. Lee M. Erectile dysfunction. In: Dipiro JT, Talbert RL, Yee GC, et al, eds. Pharmacotherapy: A Pathophysiologic Approach. 8th ed. New York: McGraw-Hill; 2011:1437–1454.

20. Padma-Nathan H, Hellstrom WJ, Kaiser FE, et al, for the Medicated Urethral System for Erection (MUSE) Study Group. Treatment of men with erectile dysfunction with transurethral alprostadil. N Engl J Med 1997;336:1–7.

21. Guay AT, Perez JB, Velasquez E, et al. Clinical experience with intra-urethral alprostadil (MUSE) in the treatment of men with erectile dysfunction. A retrospective study. Medicated urethral system for erection. Eur Urol 2000;38:671–676.

22. Traish AM, Miner MM, Morgentaler A, Zitzmann M. Testosterone deficiency. Am J Med 2011;124:578–587.

52 Benign Prostatic Hyperplasia

Mary Lee and Roohollah Sharifi

LEARNING OBJECTIVES

● **Upon completion of the chapter, the reader will be able to:**

1. Explain the pathophysiologic mechanisms underlying the symptoms and signs of benign prostatic hyperplasia (BPH).

2. Recognize the symptoms and signs of BPH in individual patients.

3. List the desired treatment outcomes for a patient with BPH.

4. Identify factors that guide selection of a particular α-adrenergic antagonist for an individual patient.

5. Compare and contrast α-adrenergic antagonists versus 5α-reductase inhibitors in terms of mechanism of action, treatment outcomes, adverse effects, and interactions when used for management of BPH.

6. Describe the indications, advantages, and disadvantages for single drug versus combination drug treatment of BPH.

7. Describe the indications for surgical intervention of BPH.

8. Formulate a monitoring plan for a patient on a given drug treatment regimen based on patient-specific information.

9. Formulate appropriate counseling information for patients receiving drug treatment for BPH.

KEY CONCEPTS

❶ The lower urinary tract symptoms (LUTS) and signs of benign prostatic hyperplasia (BPH) are due to static, dynamic, or detrusor factors. The static factor refers to anatomic obstruction of the bladder neck caused by an enlarged prostate gland. The dynamic factor refers to excessive stimulation of α-adrenergic receptors in the smooth muscle of the prostate, prostatic urethra, and bladder neck. The detrusor factor refers to irritability of hypertrophied detrusor muscle as a result of long-standing bladder outlet obstruction.

❷ Drug treatment goals for BPH include relieving obstructive and irritative voiding symptoms, preventing complications of disease, and reducing the need for surgical intervention.

❸ Watchful waiting is indicated for patients with mild symptoms that are not bothersome.

❹ Single-drug treatment with an α-adrenergic antagonist is preferred for patients with moderate or severe symptoms of BPH. Single-drug treatment with a 5α-reductase inhibitor should be reserved for patients

with moderate or severe symptoms and significantly enlarged prostates of at least 30 g (1.05 oz).

❺ Surgical intervention should be reserved for patients with severe LUTS due to BPH and those with complications of disease, such as recurrent urinary tract infections, recurrent severe gross hematuria, renal failure, and bladder calculi.

❻ α-Adrenergic antagonists reduce the dynamic factor. They competitively antagonize α-adrenergic receptors, thereby causing relaxation of the bladder neck, prostatic urethra, and prostate smooth muscle. They do not shrink an enlarged prostate. The onset of action is days to weeks, depending on the need for up-titration of the daily dose to achieve a therapeutic response. Dose-limiting adverse effects include orthostatic hypotension and syncope. In addition, delayed or retrograde ejaculation has been reported. Combined use with antihypertensives, diuretics, or phosphodiesterase inhibitors can increase the risk of hypotensive episodes, particularly with immediate release formulations of second-generation α-adrenergic antagonists.

7 Among the α-adrenergic antagonists, modified-release alfuzosin is considered functionally uroselective because usual therapeutic doses produce relaxation of the bladder neck and prostatic smooth muscle with minimal peripheral vascular relaxation. Although alfuzosin appears to produce less hypotension than immediate-release formulations of terazosin and doxazosin, it is not clear whether it has the same cardiovascular profile as tamsulosin. Although not uroselective, controlled-release doxazosin produces less hypotension than the immediate-release formulation. Tamsulosin and silodosin are pharmacologically uroselective and exert greater antagonism of $α_{1A}$-receptors, which comprise the majority of adrenergic receptors in the prostate, prostatic urethra, and bladder neck; and $α_{1D}$-receptors, which predominate in bladder detrusor muscle as compared with vascular $α_{1B}$-receptors. Therefore, tamsulosin and silodosin can be initiated with a full therapeutic dose, which achieves peak effects sooner than with immediate-release formulations of terazosin and doxazosin, which must be up-titrated. Tamsulosin appears to have the lowest potential to cause hypotension. In various clinical trials, tamsulosin is well tolerated in the elderly and in patients taking diuretics and antihypertensives. It is also commercially available in a controlled-release dosage formulation. Therefore, with chronic use, tamsulosin can be taken once daily at the patient's convenience. Fewer clinical data are available concerning silodosin than tamsulosin. Also, clinical advantages of silodosin over tamsulosin have yet to be documented. For this reason, tamsulosin is preferred over silodosin.

8 **5α-Reductase inhibitors** shrink an enlarged prostate by approximately 20% to 25%, reducing symptoms caused by the static factor. They do so by inhibiting 5α-reductase that is responsible for intraprostatic conversion of testosterone to dihydrotestosterone, the active androgen that stimulates prostate tissue growth. The onset of action is slow, with peak shrinkage of the prostate taking up to 6 months. Unlike treatment with α-adrenergic antagonists, 5α-reductase inhibitors have been shown to reduce the incidence of acute urinary retention and need for prostate surgery in patients with significantly enlarged prostate glands (more than 30 g [1.05 oz]) and those with prostate-specific antigen (PSA) serum levels of 1.5 ng/mL (1.5 mcg/L) or more. Because 5α-reductase inhibitors do not produce cardiovascular adverse effects, they are preferred for treatment of moderate to severe symptoms of BPH when the patient is at risk of hypotension, but wants to be treated medically. Adverse effects include gynecomastia, decreased libido, erectile dysfunction, and ejaculation disorders. Drug interactions are uncommon.

9 The combination of an α-adrenergic antagonist and a 5α-reductase inhibitor is a preferred drug regimen in patients with moderate to severe voiding symptoms and an enlarged prostate (more than 30 g [1.05 oz]) and who are at risk of complications of BPH as suggested by a PSA of 1.5 ng/mL (1.5 mcg/L) or more. The α-adrenergic antagonist quickly reduces the severity of obstructive voiding symptoms, and the 5α-reductase inhibitor slowly shrinks the enlarged prostate. At 2 and 4 years after the start of the combination regimen, clinical trials show that treated patients have a lower frequency of developing acute urinary retention or needing prostate surgery than patients treated with single drug therapy. Also, in patients with severe symptoms, the combination enhances the effectiveness of the α-adrenergic antagonist after the first year.

10 When monitoring efficacy of drug treatment for BPH, subjective end points include relief of obstructive and irritative voiding symptoms. Objective end points include improvements of urinary flow rates, decreased postvoid residual urinary volume, and decreased complications of disease.

INTRODUCTION

The prostate is a heart-shaped, chestnut-sized organ that encircles the portion of the proximal urethra that is located at the base of the urinary bladder. The prostate produces secretions, which are part of the ejaculate.

Benign prostatic hyperplasia (BPH) is the most common benign neoplasm in males who are at least 40 years of age. BPH can produce lower urinary tract voiding symptoms that are consistent with impaired emptying of urine from and storage of urine in the bladder. Medications are a common mode of treatment to reduce symptoms and/or delay complications of the disease. For this reason, clinicians should be knowledgeable about the medical management of this disease.

EPIDEMIOLOGY AND ETIOLOGY

BPH is present as microscopic disease in many elderly males. The prevalence increases with advancing patient age. However, only about 50% and 25% of patients with microscopic BPH disease develop an enlarged prostate on palpation and clinical voiding symptoms, respectively.[1,2] It is estimated that 25% of males 40 years of age or more have voiding symptoms consistent with BPH, and 20% to 30% of all male patients who live to the age of 80 years will require a **prostatectomy** for severe voiding symptoms of BPH.[2]

Two etiologic factors for BPH include advanced patient age and the stimulatory effect of androgens.

- Prior to 40 years of age, the prostate in the adult male stays the same size, approximately 15 to 20 g. However, in males who have reached 40 years of age, the prostate undergoes a growth spurt, which continues as the male advances in age. Enlargement of the prostate can result in clinically symptomatic BPH.

- The testes and adrenal glands produce 90% and 10%, respectively, of circulating testosterone. Testosterone enters prostate cells, where predominantly type II 5α-reductase activates testosterone to dihydrotestosterone, which combines with a cytoplasmic receptor. The complex enters the nucleus and induces changes in protein synthesis that promote glandular tissue growth of the prostate. Thus 5α-reductase inhibitors (e.g., finasteride and dutasteride) directly interfere with one of the major etiologic factors of BPH.

- The prostate is composed of two types of tissue: (a) glandular or epithelial tissue, which produces prostatic secretions, including prostate-specific antigen (PSA), and (b) muscle or stromal tissue, which can contract around the urethra when stimulated. Whereas androgens stimulate glandular tissue growth, androgens have no direct effect on stromal tissue. It has been postulated that stromal tissue growth may be stimulated by estrogen. Because testosterone is converted to estrogen in peripheral tissues in males, testosterone may be associated indirectly with stromal hyperplasia. Stromal tissue is innervated by α_{1A}-receptors. When stimulated, prostatic stroma contracts around the urethra, narrowing the urethra and causing obstructive voiding symptoms.

PATHOPHYSIOLOGY

1 *Lower urinary tract symptoms (LUTS) and signs of BPH are due to static, dynamic, and/or detrusor factors. The static factor refers to anatomic obstruction of the bladder neck caused by an enlarged prostate gland. As the gland grows around the urethra, the prostate occludes the urethral lumen. The dynamic factor refers to excessive stimulation of α_{1A}-adrenergic receptors in the smooth muscle of the prostate and urethra, which results in smooth muscle contraction. This reduces the caliber of the urethral lumen. The detrusor factor refers to bladder detrusor muscle instability, in which bladder muscle fibers have decompensated as a result of excessive hypertrophy in response to prolonged bladder outlet obstruction.* Patients with obstruction of the bladder neck or a narrowed urethral lumen due to static or dynamic factors, respectively, will develop obstructive voiding symptoms, such as decreased force of the urinary stream, urinary dribbling, an inability to completely empty the bladder. Patients with detrusor muscle instability will develop irritative voiding symptoms, such as urinary urgency and frequency.[1,3] Detrusor muscle fibers are embedded with α_{1D}-receptors. Therefore, it has been proposed that some α_{1D}-adrenergic antagonists may be particularly useful for controlling these symptoms.[4]

In an enlarged gland, the epithelial/stromal tissue ratio is 1:5.[5] Androgens stimulate epithelial, but not stromal tissue hyperplasia. Hence androgen antagonism does not induce a complete reduction in prostate size to normal. This explains one of the limitations of the clinical effect of 5α-reductase inhibitors.

Stromal tissue is the primary locus of α_1-adrenergic receptors in the prostate. An estimated 98% of the α-adrenergic receptors in the prostate are found in prostatic stromal tissue. Of the α_1-receptors found in the prostate, 70% of them are of the α_{1A}-subtype.[4] This explains why α-adrenergic antagonists are effective for managing symptoms of BPH.

Symptoms of BPH are classified as obstructive or irritative. Obstructive symptoms result from failure of the urinary bladder to empty urine when the bladder is full. The patient will complain of reduced force of the urinary stream, urinary hesitation, dribbling, and straining to empty the bladder. Irritative symptoms result from the failure of the urinary bladder to store urine until the bladder is full. With long-standing bladder outlet obstruction, detrusor muscle fibers undergo hypertrophy so that the bladder can generate higher pressure to overcome the bladder outlet obstruction and empty urine from the bladder. Once maximal bladder muscle hypertrophy occurs, the muscle decompensates. The detrusor becomes irritable, contracting abnormally in response to small amounts of urine in the bladder. As a result, the patient complains of urinary frequency and urgency.[3]

The natural history of untreated BPH is unclear in patients with mild symptoms. It is estimated that up to 38% of untreated men with mild symptoms will have symptom improvement over a 2.5- to 5-year period.[6] It may be that such patients attribute their symptoms to aging, grow tolerant of their symptoms, or adopt behavioral changes in their lifestyle that minimize their voiding symptoms. On the other hand, a significant portion of patients with mild symptoms will likely experience disease progression. Patients with moderate to severe symptoms can experience a decreased quality of life as daily activities are adjusted because of urinary incontinence. Also, such patients may develop complications of BPH, which include acute refractory urinary retention, renal failure, urinary tract infection, urinary incontinence, bladder stones, large bladder diverticuli, and recurrent gross hematuria. Predictors of disease progression include an enlarged prostate of at least 30 g (1.05 oz) or PSA of at least 1.5 ng/mL (1.5 mcg/L).[7–9]

TREATMENT

Desired Outcomes[9,10]

- **2** *Reducing or eliminating obstructive and irritative voiding symptoms. Drug treatment with an α-adrenergic antagonist or 5α-reductase inhibitor is expected to reduce the American Urological Association (AUA) Symptom Score by 30% to 50% (or a minimum decrease of 3 or more points), improve peak and mean urinary flow rate by 1 to 3 mL/s, and decrease PVR to normal (less than 50 mL total) when compared with pretreatment baseline values. The AUA Symptom Score may not correlate with response to therapy.*

- Slowing disease progression. When compared with baseline, symptoms and serum blood urea nitrogen (BUN) and creatinine should improve, stabilize, or decrease to the normal range with treatment.

- Preventing disease complications and reducing the need for surgical intervention.

- Avoiding or minimizing adverse treatment effects.

- Providing economical therapy.

- Maintaining or improving quality of life.

Clinical Presentation and Diagnosis of BPH

General

Patients may or may not be in acute distress. In early stages of disease, the patient may complain of obstructive voiding symptoms. If untreated, in late stages of disease the patient may complain of irritative voiding symptoms or acute urinary retention, which is painful due to maximal distention of the urinary bladder. Also, the patient may be symptomatic of disease complications, including urosepsis, pyelonephritis, cystitis, or overflow urinary incontinence.

Symptoms

Patients may complain of obstructive voiding symptoms (e.g., urinary hesitancy, decreased force of urinary stream, straining to void, incomplete bladder emptying, dribbling, and intermittency) and/or irritative voiding symptoms (e.g., urinary frequency, nocturia, dysuria, urgency, and urinary incontinence). Severity of symptoms should be assessed by the patient using a standardized instrument (e.g., the American Urological Association [AUA] Symptom Scoring Index; Table 52–1). However, it is important to recognize that a patient's perception of the bothersomeness of his voiding symptoms may not match with the AUA Symptom Score. In this case, after thorough evaluation of the signs and complications of BPH disease, if present, the physician and patient should discuss the bothersomeness of the patient's symptoms and decide together on the most appropriate course of treatment for the patient.[1,10] Lower urinary tract symptoms (LUTS) is a term that refers to the collection of obstructive and irritative voiding symptoms characteristic of, but not specific for, BPH. That is, other urologic diseases (e.g., urinary tract infection, prostate cancer, prostatitis, or neurogenic bladder) can also cause LUTS.

Signs

- Enlarged prostate on digital rectal exam (DRE); check for prostate nodules or induration, which would suggest prostate cancer instead of BPH as the cause of the patient's voiding symptoms
- Distended urinary bladder
- Rule out meatal stenosis or urethral stricture, which could cause voiding symptoms similar to LUTS
- Check anal sphincter tone as an indirect assessment of peripheral innervation to the detrusor muscle of the bladder

Complications of Untreated BPH

Upper and lower urinary tract infection, urosepsis, urinary incontinence refractory urinary retention, chronic renal failure, bladder diverticula, bladder stones, or recurrent gross hematuria.

Medical History

- Check the patient's general health, including previous surgery, presence of diabetes mellitus, or medications that may cause or worsen voiding symptoms.
- Have the patient provide a diary of his voiding pattern for the past week: date and time of each voiding, volume voided, and whether or not the patient had urinary leakage during the day.

Laboratory Tests

- Serum PSA: The combination of PSA and DRE of the prostate is used to screen for prostate cancer, which could also cause an enlarged prostate. Also, PSA is a surrogate marker for an enlarged prostate due to BPH. Using a PSA greater than 1.5 ng/mL (1.5 mcg/L) suggests that a patient has a prostate volume greater than 30 mm³ (30 g or 1.05 oz).[11]
- Urinalysis to rule out infection as a cause of the patient's voiding symptoms; also check urinalysis for microscopic hematuria, which typically accompanies BPH.
- Plasma blood urea nitrogen (BUN) and serum creatinine may be increased as a result of long-standing bladder outlet obstruction. These tests are not routinely performed but rather are reserved for those patients in whom renal dysfunction is suspected.

Other Diagnostic Tests (Table 52–2)

- Decreased peak and mean urinary flow rate (less than 10 to 15 mL/s) on uroflowmetry; decreased urinary flow rate is not specific for BPH; it can also be due to other urologic disorders (e.g., urethral stricture, meatal stenosis, or bladder hypotonicity)
- Increased postvoid residual urine volume (PVR) (more than 50 mL)
- DRE to check for an enlarged prostate (more than 15 to 20 g [0.5 to 0.7 oz])
- Transurethral cystoscopy reveals an enlarged prostate, which decreases urethral lumen caliber; information from this procedure helps the surgeon decide on the best surgical approach.
- Transrectal ultrasound of the prostate; a transrectal probe is inserted to evaluate prostate size and best surgical approach.
- Transrectal prostate needle biopsy to be done if the patient has areas of nodularity or induration on DRE; tissue biopsy can document the presence of prostate cancer, which can also cause enlargement of the prostate.
- IV pyelogram (IVP) will show retention of radiocontrast in the bladder if the patient has bladder outlet obstruction due to an enlarged prostate; this is only indicated in patients with recurrent hematuria, recurrent urinary tract infection, renal insufficiency, and urolithiasis.
- Filling cystometry provides information on bladder capacity, detrusor contractility, and the presence of uninhibited bladder contractions, which could also cause LUTS.

General Approach to Treatment

Until recently, the principal approach to treatment focused on reducing BPH symptoms (**Fig. 52–1**, **Tables 52–1**, **52–2**, **and 52–3**). However, treatment should also slow disease progression and decrease complications of BPH.[9]

❸ *For patients with mild symptoms that the patient does not consider to be bothersome, watchful waiting is a reasonable approach to treatment.* The patient is instructed to schedule return visits to the clinician every 3 to 6 months. At each visit, the patient's symptoms are reassessed using the AUA Symptom Scoring Index, and results are compared with baseline (Table 52–1). In addition, the patient is educated about avoiding factors that worsen obstructive and irritative voiding symptoms (**Table 52–4**). The digital rectal exam (DRE) is repeated annually. If the patient's symptoms are unchanged, then watchful waiting is continued. If the patient's symptoms worsen, then specific treatment is initiated.[10]

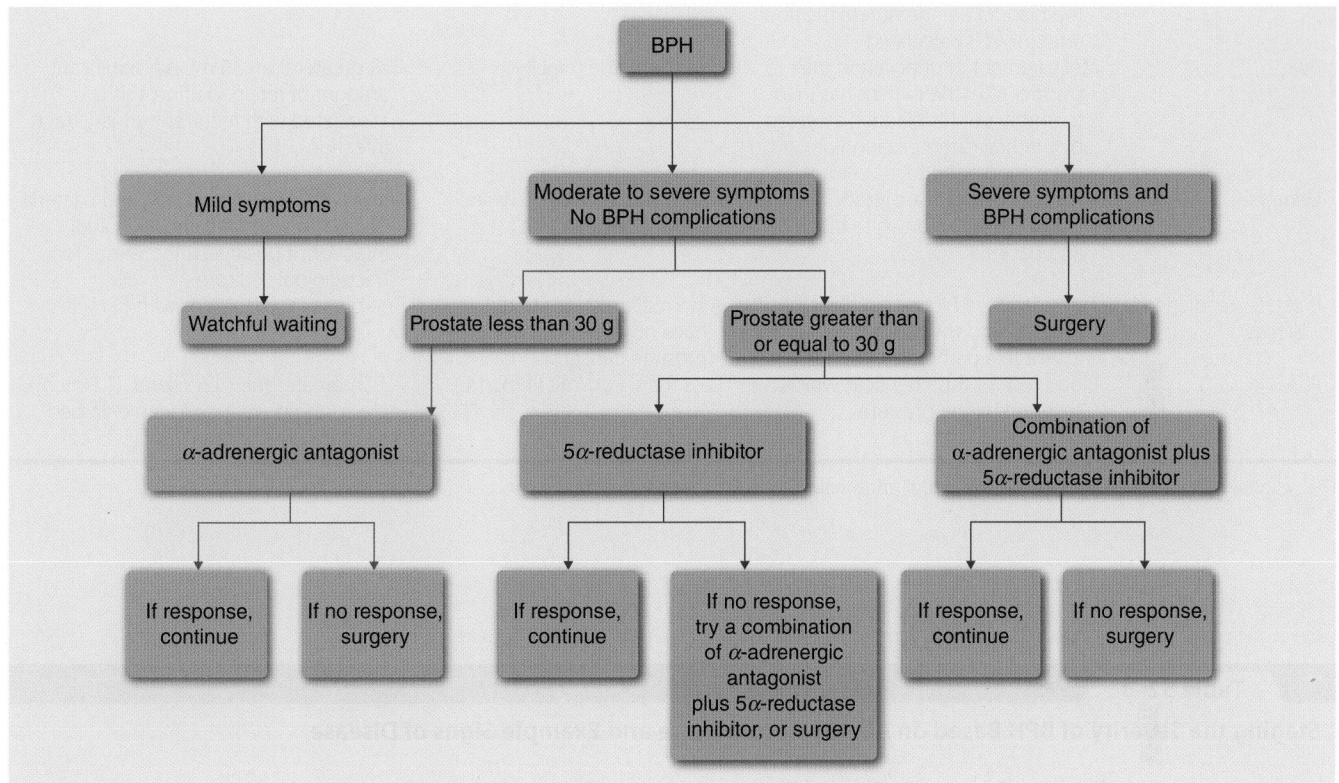

FIGURE 52–1. Algorithm for selection of treatment for BPH based on symptom severity and presence of disease complications.

Table 52–1

Questions to Determine the AUA Symptom Score

Directions for the patient: The patient should be asked to respond to each question based on the absence or presence of symptoms over the past month. For each question, the patient can respond using a 1–5 scale, where 0 = not at all or none; 1 = less than 1 time in 5; 2 = less than half of the time; 3 = about half of the time; 4 = more than half of the time; and 5 = almost always
Directions for the clinician: After the patient completes the questionnaire, the scores for individual items should be tallied for a final score. Scores of 0–7 = mild symptoms; scores of 8–19 = moderate symptoms; scores more than 20 = severe symptoms

Questions to Assess Obstructive Voiding Symptoms
1. How often have you had a sensation of not emptying your bladder completely after you finished urinating?
2. How often have you found you stopped and started again several times when you urinated?
3. How often have you had a weak urinary stream?
4. How often have you had to push or strain to begin urinating?

Questions to Assess Irritative Voiding Symptoms
5. How often have you found it difficult to postpone urination?
6. How often have you had to urinate again less than 2 hours after you finished urinating?
7. How many times did you most typically get up to urinate from the time you went to bed at night until the time you got up in the morning?

From AUA Practice Guidelines Committee. AUA guideline on the management of benign prostatic hyperplasia (2010). www.auanet.org/content/guidelines-and-quality care/clinical-guidelines.cfm?sub=bph (last accessed 8/31/2012).

Table 52–2

Objective Tests Used to Assess the Severity and Complications of BPH

Test	How the Test Is Performed	Normal Test Result	Test Result in Patients With BPH
DRE of the prostate	Prostate is palpated through the rectal mucosa; the physician inserts an index finger into the patient's rectum	Prostate is soft, symmetric, mobile; size is 15–20 g (0.5–0.7 oz)	Prostate is enlarged, more than 20 g (0.5 oz); no areas of induration or nodularity
Peak and mean urinary flow rate	Patient drinks water until bladder is full; patient empties bladder; volume of urine output and time to empty the bladder are measured; the flow rate (mL/s) is calculated	Peak and mean urinary flow rate are at least 10 mL/s	Peak and mean urinary flow rates are less than 10 mL/s
PVR	Measurement of urine left in the bladder after the patient has tried to empty out his bladder; assessed by urethral catheterization or ultrasonography	PVR should be 0 mL	PVR greater than 50 mL is a significant amount of retained urine; this is associated with recurrent urinary tract infection
Urinalysis	Midstream urine is analyzed microscopically for white blood cells and bacteria	Urine should have no white cells or bacteria in it	Urine with white blood cells and bacteria is suggestive of inflammation and infection; if positive, urine is sent for bacteriologic culture
Prostate needle biopsy	Transrectally, a biopsy needle is inserted into the prostate; tissue core is sent to a pathologist for analysis	A normal prostate should have no evidence of BPH or prostate cancer	The biopsy is consistent with BPH
PSA	Blood test for this chemical, which is secreted by the prostate	Less than 4 ng/mL (4 mcg/L)	A PSA greater than 1.5 ng/mL (1.5 mcg/L) is a surrogate marker for an enlarged prostate greater than 30 g (1.05 oz)

DRE, digital rectal exam; PVR, postvoid residual urine volume; PSA, prostate-specific antigen.

Table 52–3

Staging the Severity of BPH Based on AUA Symptom Score and Example Signs of Disease

	AUA Symptom Score	Signs of Disease
Mild	Less than or equal to 7	Enlarged prostate on DRE, peak urinary flow rate less than or equal to 10 mL/s
Moderate	8–19	All of the above, PVR greater than 50 mL, irritative symptoms
Severe	Greater than or equal to 20	All of the above plus one or more complications of BPH

AUA, American Urological Association; BPH, benign prostatic hyperplasia; DRE, digital rectal exam; PVR, postvoid residual urine volume.

The AUA Symptom Score focuses on seven items (incomplete emptying, frequency, intermittency, urgency, weak stream, straining, and nocturia) and asks that the patient quantify the severity of each complaint on a scale of 0 to 5. Thus the score can range from 0 to 35.

Table 52–4

Drugs That Can Cause Irritative or Obstructive Voiding Symptoms

Pharmacologic Class	Example Drugs	Mechanism of Effect
Androgens	Testosterone	Stimulate prostate enlargement
α-Adrenergic agonists	Phenylephrine, pseudoephedrine	Stimulate contraction of prostatic and bladder neck smooth muscle
Anticholinergic agents	Antihistamines, phenothiazines, tricyclic antidepressants, antiparkinsonian agents	Block bladder detrusor muscle contraction, thereby impairing bladder emptying
Diuretics	Thiazides diuretics, loop diuretics	Produce polyuria

Table 52–5

Comparison of α-Adrenergic Antagonists and 5α-Reductase Inhibitors for Treatment of BPH

Characteristic	α-Adrenergic Antagonists	5α-Reductase Inhibitors
Relaxes prostatic smooth muscle	Yes	No
Reduces size of enlarged prostate	No	Yes
Useful in patients with enlarged prostates	No (works independent of the size of the prostate)	Yes
Efficacy in relieving voiding symptoms and improving flow rate	++	+
Reduces the frequency of BPH-related complications	No	Yes
Reduces the frequency of BPH-related surgery	No	Yes
Frequency of daily dosing	Once or twice daily, depending on the agent and the dosage formulation	Once daily
Requirement for up-titration of dose	Yes (for terazosin and doxazosin immediate-release); no (for alfuzosin or silodosin; possibly for doxazosin extended-release and tamsulosin)	No
Peak onset of action	Days–6 weeks, depending on need for dose titration	6 months
Decreases PSA	No	Yes
Cardiovascular adverse effects	Yes	No
Drug-induced sexual dysfunction	Ejaculation disorders	Decreased libido, erectile dysfunction, ejaculation disorders

PSA, prostate-specific antigen.

❹ For patients with moderate to severe symptoms, the patient is usually offered drug treatment first. α-Adrenergic antagonists are preferred over 5α-reductase inhibitors because the former have a faster onset of action (days to a few weeks) and improve symptoms independent of prostate size. 5α-reductase inhibitors have a delayed onset of action (i.e., peak effect may be delayed for up to 6 months) and are seldom effective in patients with smaller size prostate glands (less than 30 g or 1.05 oz). Therefore, 5α-reductase inhibitors should be reserved for patients with an enlarged prostate gland, of at least 30 g, and moderate to severe symptoms. Drug treatment must be continued as long as the patient responds (Table 52–5).[10]

❺ For patients with complications of BPH disease (e.g., recurrent urinary tract infection, urosepsis, urinary incontinence, refractory urinary retention, chronic renal failure, large bladder diverticuli, recurrent severe gross hematuria, or bladder calculi secondary to prolonged urinary retention), surgery is indicated. Although it is potentially curative, surgery can result in significant morbidity, including erectile dysfunction, retrograde ejaculation, urinary incontinence, bleeding, or urinary tract infection.[12] The gold standard is a prostatectomy, which can be performed transurethrally or as an open surgical procedure, which can be performed suprapubically or retropubically. To avoid complications of prostatectomy, minimally invasive surgical procedures, such as transurethral incision of the prostate, transurethral needle ablation, or transurethral laser ablation, are options.[10,12,13] However, minimally invasive surgical procedures are associ-ated with a higher reoperation rate than a prostatectomy. Drug treatment is used in patients with severe disease when the patient refuses surgery or when the patient is not a surgical candidate because of concomitant diseases.

❻ In the Multiple Treatment of Prostate Symptoms Study (MTOPS), selected patients with moderate to severe symptoms benefited from a combination of α-adrenergic antagonist plus 5α-reductase inhibitor drug therapy.[14] Specifically, the use of doxazosin plus finasteride was more effective than doxazosin alone or finasteride alone in relieving symptoms, reducing the need for prostatectomy, and decreasing the incidence of BPH complications in patients at highest risk of developing disease complications (i.e., those with prostate size of at least 40 g [1.4 oz]). In the Combination of Avodart and Tamsulosin (CombAT) Study, which compared tamsulosin, dutasteride, and the combination of tamsulosin and dutasteride in patients with large prostates, mean volume of

Patient Encounter 1

AB is a 65-year-old man with an AUA Symptom Score of 7, urinary hesitancy, a slow urinary stream, urinary frequency, and nocturia. He wakes up three times every night to void. A DRE reveals a prostate of 40 g (1.4 oz). His PSA is 4 ng/mL (4 mcg/L). A urinary flow rate is 7 mL/s.

What stage of BPH does this patient have?

55 g (1.9 oz), and elevated PSA (mean of 4 ng/mL [4 mcg/L]), similar results were documented at 1, 2, and 4 years of follow-up.[15] Combination therapy is more expensive and also produces more adverse effects than monotherapy. Therefore, the clinician should discuss the advantages and disadvantages of combination therapy with a patient before deciding on a final treatment regimen.[16]

Nonpharmacologic Therapy

To reduce nocturia, patients should be instructed to stop drinking fluids several hours before going to bed and then void before going to sleep. During the day, patients should avoid excessive caffeine and alcohol intake, as these may cause urinary frequency. Patients should avoid taking nonprescription medications that can worsen obstructive voiding symptoms (e.g., antihistamines or decongestants) (Table 52–4). In addition, toilet mapping (knowing the location of toilets on the way to and from various destinations) may help reassure the patient that he can still continue with many of his routine daily activities. Patients are also advised to lose weight, if overweight. Because testosterone is converted to estrogen in adipose tissue, an alteration in the testosterone:estrogen ratio occurs in overweight men, similar to that which occurs in elderly males, which may contribute to the development of BPH.[17]

Although a variety of herbal agents are used for symptomatic management, including pygeum (African plum), secale cereale (rye pollen), and hypoxis rooperi (South African star grass), objective evidence of efficacy is lacking.[18,19] Also, in a randomized, double-blind, and placebo-controlled clinical trial, saw palmetto was no different than placebo in improving symptoms or increasing peak urinary flow rate.[20]

Pharmacologic Therapy

▶ α-Adrenergic Antagonist Monotherapy[21]

6 *α-Adrenergic antagonists reduce the dynamic factor causing BPH symptoms. These drugs competitively antagonize α-adrenergic receptors, thereby causing relaxation of the bladder neck, prostatic urethra, and prostate smooth muscle.*[10,21] A secondary mechanism of action may be that α-adrenergic antagonists induce prostatic apoptosis,[22] which suggests that these agents may cause some shrinkage of an enlarged prostate. However, the clinical importance of this remains to be elucidated.

All α-adrenergic antagonists are considered equally effective in relieving symptoms.[10,21] In various clinical trials, 30% to 80% of patients experience improvement in AUA Symptom Score by 30% to 45%, and 20% to 40% of patients experience urinary flow rate increases of 2 to 3 mL/s. The onset of action is days to weeks, depending on the need for titration of the dose from a subtherapeutic starting dose to a therapeutic maintenance dose. An adequate clinical trial is considered to be at least 1 to 2 weeks of continuous treatment at a full maintenance dose with any of these agents.[10] Durable

responses have been demonstrated for up to 5 years of continuous use of terazosin,[23] 10 years with doxazosin,[24] and 6 years with tamsulosin.[25] However, some patients will develop disease progression despite treatment. α-Adrenergic antagonists are hepatically metabolized. Therefore, in patients with significant hepatic dysfunction, these drugs should be used in the lowest possible dose. With the exception of silodosin, these drugs do not require dosage modification in patients with renal dysfunction.

These agents can be differentiated by their adverse effect profile. Dose-limiting adverse effects include hypotension and syncope, which are more common with immediate-release terazosin and doxazosin, less frequent with extended-release doxazosin and alfuzosin, and least frequent with pharmacologically uroselective α_{1A}-adrenergic antagonists.[26,27] Ejaculation disorders have been reported most often with tamsulosin 0.8 mg orally once a day. Combined use with antihypertensives, diuretics, or phosphodiesterase inhibitors can lead to additive blood pressure–lowering effects; however, this appears to be less of a problem with tamsulosin and silodosin.[23,26,27]

● α-Adrenergic antagonists are recommended as first-line treatment for moderate to severe voiding symptoms of BPH. The agents in this pharmacologic class can be classified by several characteristics (Table 52–6):

- *Generation of α-adrenergic antagonist.* First-generation agents (e.g., phenoxybenzamine) block presynaptic and postsynaptic α-adrenergic receptors. Whereas blockade of postsynaptic α-adrenergic receptors is desirable for BPH management, blockade of presynaptic α-adrenergic receptors is undesirable, as it results in release of catecholamines and tachycardia. Thus first-generation α-adrenergic antagonists are not used for treatment of BPH.[28] Second-generation α-adrenergic antagonists (e.g., terazosin, doxazosin, and alfuzosin) are pharmacologically not selective in blocking the subtypes of α-adrenergic receptors, which include α_{1A}-receptors in the genitourinary tract, α_{1D}- receptors in the coronary arteries and bladder, and α_{1B}-receptors in the peripheral vasculature. Hypotensive adverse effects are dose-related and common. An extended-release formulation of doxazin and a modified-release formulation of alfuzosin produce lower peak serum concentrations and less hypotension than immediate release formulations. Third-generation α-adrenergic antagonists (e.g., tamsulosin, silodosin) selectively block postsynaptic α_{1A}-receptors, which predominate in the prostate. As a result, hypotensive adverse effects are less common with third-generation agents than with second-generation agents.

- **7** *Uroselectivity.* Pharmacologic uroselectivity refers to preferential inhibition of α_{1A}-receptors, which predominate in the prostatic stroma, prostatic urethra, and bladder neck, and α_{1D}-receptors, which predominate in the bladder detrusor muscle.[21] Pharmacologically uroselective α_{1A}-adrenergic antagonists have the potential to produce less hypotension, as they have a lower

Table 52–6

Comparison of Pharmacologic Properties of α-Adrenergic Antagonists

	Terazosin	Doxazosin	Alfuzosin	Tamsulosin	Silodosin
Brand name	Hytrin	Cardura	Uroxatral	Flomax	Rapaflo
Generation	Second	Second	Second	Third	Third
Uroselective	No	No	Functionally and clinically uroselective	Pharmacologically and clinically uroselective	Pharmacologically and clinically uroselective
Need for up-titration	Yes	Yes (with immediate-release); possibly (with extended-release)	No	Minimal	No
Daily oral dose (mg)	5–20	2–8, immediate-release; 4–8, extended-release	10	0.4–0.8; (0.8 mg/day dose has not consistently produced clinical improvement over 0.4 mg/day)	8
Recommended dose reduction in patients with renal dysfunction	None needed	None needed	Manufacturer recommends caution in patients with severe renal insufficiency. No specific dosing recommendations provided.	If creatinine clearance greater than 10 mL/min (0.17 mL/s), none needed. Tamsulosin has not been studied in patients with creatinine clearance less than 10 mL/min (0.17 mL/s)	If creatinine clearance 30–50 mL/min (0.50–0.83 mL/s), use 4 mg/day. Contraindicated in patients with creatinine clearance less than 30 mL/min (0.50 mL/s)
Recommended dose reduction in patients with hepatic dysfunction	Manufacturer provides no specific recommendation. Terazosin should be used cautiously as it undergoes extensive hepatic metabolism.	Manufacturer provides no specific recommendation. Doxazosin should be used cautiously as it undergoes extensive hepatic metabolism.	Contraindicated in patients with moderate/severe hepatic impairment. Alfuzosin should be used cautiously in patients with mild hepatic impairment.	Patients with mild/moderate hepatic impairment require no dosage adjustment. Tamsulosin has not been studied in patients with severe hepatic impairment.	Patients with mild/moderate hepatic impairment require no dosage adjustment. Contraindicated in patients with severe hepatic impairment.
Best time to take doses	At bedtime	Immediate-release: anytime during the day; however, it is typically given at bedtime. Extended-release: anytime during the day	After meals for best oral absorption	On an empty stomach for best oral absorption; if taken 30 minutes after a meal, as recommended by the manufacturer, extent of absorption is reduced, thereby further reducing the potential for hypotensive adverse effects.	Take with a meal, which decreases extent of absorption. Theoretically, this would help decrease hypotensive adverse effects.
Half-life (hours)	12	22	5	10	13
Formulation	Immediate-release	Immediate-release and extended-release	Extended-release	Modified-release	Immediate-release
Cardiovascular adverse effects	++	++	+	0 to +	0 to +
Ejaculation disorders	+	+	+	++	++
Rhinitis	+	+	+	+	+
Malaise	+	+	+	+	+

+, minimal; ++ moderate

propensity to antagonize α_{1B}-adrenergic receptors in the peripheral vasculature. Tamsulosin and silodosin are the only commercially available α-adrenergic antagonists with pharmacologic uroselectivity. In contrast, despite the potential of inhibiting α-adrenergic receptors in both the prostate and peripheral vasculature, functionally uroselective α-adrenergic antagonists in usually prescribed doses produce effective relaxation of prostatic smooth muscle with minimal vascular vasodilation. *Thus blood pressure–lowering effects are mild or absent. The only functionally uroselective α-adrenergic antagonist is alfuzosin extended-release tablets. The mechanism of functional uroselectivity is unclear. It may be related to the drug formulation, which produces a higher concentration in target tissues than in nontarget tissues.*[28] Both pharmacologically and functionally uroselective agents appear to be clinically uroselective, in that they improve BPH symptoms without causing cardiovascular adverse effects in humans.[21]

Pharmacologic and functional uroselectivity are dose-related phenomena. Large daily doses of tamsulosin, silodosin, or alfuzosin may cause loss of uroselectivity, with resultant hypotension and dizziness in some patients.

- *Need for up-titration of daily dose.* Up-titration is required for immediate-release terazosin and doxazosin. It is minimally required for extended-release doxazosin and tamsulosin. It is not required for extended-release alfuzosin or silodosin. The need for up-titration with a particular α-adrenergic antagonist delays its peak onset of action and the time when the patient can experience maximal clinical benefit.

- *Plasma half-life.* α-Adrenergic receptors with short plasma half-lives (e.g., prazosin) require multiple doses during the day. This is challenging for most patients, and thus prazosin is not recommended for BPH.[10]

- *Dosage formulation.* Immediate-release formulations of terazosin and doxazosin are quickly absorbed and produce high peak plasma levels. Modified- or extended-release formulations of doxazosin, alfuzosin, and tamsulosin produce lower peak levels, but more sustained therapeutic plasma levels, than immediate-release formulations and have less potential for producing hypotensive episodes. This allows for initiation of treatment with a therapeutic dose, a shorter time to peak onset of clinical effects, and once daily dosing.[29,30]

- *Adverse effects.* Hypotensive adverse effects of α-adrenergic antagonists can range from asymptomatic blood pressure reductions to dizziness and syncope. This adverse effect is most commonly associated with immediate-release terazosin and doxazosin; is less commonly associated with extended-release alfuzosin and extended-release doxazosin, and silodosin; and least commonly associated with tamsulosin.[26,29] To minimize first-dose syncope from terazosin and

doxazosin immediate-release, a slow up-titration from a subtherapeutic dose of 1 mg/day to a therapeutic dose is essential. The first dose should be given at bedtime so that the patient can sleep through the peak serum concentration of the drug when the adverse effect is most likely to occur. A 3- to 7-day interval between each dosage increase should be allowed, and the patient should be maintained on the lowest effective dose of an α-adrenergic antagonist. If the patient is noncompliant with his regimen of terazosin or doxazosin, and he skips or interrupts treatment, the α-adrenergic antagonist should be restarted using the usual starting dose and then retitrated up. He should not be instructed to simply double up on missed doses or resume treatment with his currently prescribed daily dose, as this can lead to significant hypotension.

Ejaculation disorders, including delayed, an- and retrograde ejaculation, occur with all adrenergic antagonists. Although largely thought to be due to pharmacologic blockade of peripheral α-adrenergic receptors at the bladder neck (i.e., the bladder neck is unable to close during ejaculation in the presence of α-adrenergic blockade), a central nervous system mechanism of action cannot be discounted.[31] The incidence appears to be dose-related and highest with tamsulosin 0.8 mg daily, occurring in up to 26% of treated patients. Ejaculation disorders generally do not necessitate discontinuation of treatment. Although they may decrease the patient's satisfaction with the quality of sexual intercourse, ejaculation disorders are not harmful to the patient.

Rhinitis and malaise occur with α-adrenergic antagonists and are an extension of the pharmacologic blockade of α-adrenergic receptors in the vasculature of the nasal mucosa and in the central nervous system, respectively. Tolerance often develops to these adverse effects and they rarely require discontinuation of treatment. Avoid use of topical or oral decongestants, as these may exacerbate obstructive voiding symptoms. Cautious use of antihistamines with anticholinergic adverse effects is also recommended in patients with severe BPH and large residual urine volumes, as these drugs may cause acute urinary retention in patients with an obstructed bladder neck.

Floppy iris or small pupil syndrome has been reported with α-adrenergic antagonists, most often with tamsulosin. In response to tamsulosin, the iris dilator muscle relaxes and the pupil constricts. As a result, when the α-adrenergic antagonist–treated patient undergoes cataract surgery, the iris can become flaccid, billow out, or floppy. This plus the papillary constriction interfere with the surgical procedure and increase the risk of intraoperative and postoperative complications. A patient who plans to undergo cataract surgery is advised to inform his ophthalmologist that he is taking an α-adrenergic antagonist. Although the drug will not need to be held or discontinued, the ophthalmologist can plan to use certain surgical techniques, for example, iris hooks or iris expansion rings, to deal with the drug's effect on the iris dilator muscle.[32,33]

Patient Encounter 2

DD has essential hypertension and has been taking valsartan 160 mg and hydrochlorothiazide 12.5 mg orally every day for the past 2 years. The patient tolerates this regimen well, and his blood pressure is now 140/80 mm Hg. However, DD was recently diagnosed with moderately severe BPH, and he began taking doxazosin immediate-release tablets. Over the course of several weeks, he was slowly titrated up from an initial dose of 2 mg orally every day up to 8 mg every day. Although the patient has experienced significant improvement in his obstructive voiding symptoms, he also complains of dizziness, lightheadedness, and periodically feels like fainting.

How should this patient be managed?

Alfuzosin has been linked to two cases of hepatitis.[34,35] The cause-effect relationship remains to be elucidated.

- *Potential for drug interactions.* Hypotensive adverse effects of terazosin and doxazosin can be additive with those of diuretics, antihypertensives, and phosphodiesterase inhibitors (e.g., sildenafil). In patients at greatest risk for hypotension, or in those patients who tolerate hypotension poorly, including those with poorly controlled coronary artery disease or severe orthostatic hypotension, tamsulosin 0.4 mg appears to be the safest choice.[36,37] In patients who cannot tolerate tamsulosin, a 5α-reductase inhibitor or prostatectomy should be considered. When initiating sildenafil, tadalafil, or vardenafil, patients who are taking α-adrenergic antagonists should be stabilized first on a fixed dose of the α-adrenergic antagonist, and then patients should be started on the lowest effective dose of phosphodiesterase inhibitor to minimize the likelihood of hypotensive effects.

⑦ *Among the α-adrenergic antagonists, tamsulosin and silodosin are unique in that they are third-generation α-adrenergic antagonists. They are pharmacologically uroselective and exert greater antagonism of α_{1A}- and α_{1D}-receptors than α_{1B}-receptors. Tamsulosin exerts comparatively low antagonism of peripheral vascular α_{1B}-receptors. Therefore, tamsulosin can be started with a therapeutic dose, which achieves peak effects sooner than terazosin and doxazosin immediate-release, which must be up-titrated. Tamsulosin appears to have the lowest potential to cause hypotension.[26,36] In various clinical trials, tamsulosin had minimal hypotensive adverse effects and was well tolerated in the elderly, as well as in patients taking diuretics, antihypertensives, or phosphodiesterase inhibitors. Also, the commercially available product is a modified-release dosage formulation, which is dosed at 0.4 mg orally once a day. With chronic use, tamsulosin can be taken at any time of the day and at the patient's*

convenience. Although the package insert states that the dose can be increased to 0.8 mg daily, no consistent improvement in clinical efficacy has been observed in patients taking the higher dose. At this time, no difference in clinical efficacy or adverse effects between tamsulosin and silodosin has been documented. In addition, the amount of clinical data documenting the efficacy of silodosin is less than that with tamsulosin. For these reasons, silodosin is not considered to offer advantages over tamsulosin.[27]

In patients with BPH and hypertension, it is not recommended to use an α-adrenergic antagonist alone to treat both disorders. In the ALLHAT study,[38] where doxazosin was compared with other agents for treatment of essential hypertension, doxazosin was associated with a higher incidence of congestive heart failure. Therefore, in patients with hypertension and moderate to severe BPH, it is recommended that an appropriate antihypertensive be added to an α-adrenergic antagonist.[26]

▶ *5α-Reductase Inhibitor Monotherapy*

⑧ *5α-Reductase inhibitors reduce the static factor, which results in shrinkage of an enlarged prostate by approximately 20% to 25%. They do so by inhibiting 5α-reductase, which is responsible for intraprostatic conversion of testosterone to dihydrotestosterone, the active androgen that stimulates prostate tissue growth. In the prostate, there are two subtypes of 5α-reductase; the majority is the type II isoenzyme and the minority is the type I isoenzyme.[10,21] The onset of action is slow, with peak shrinkage of the prostate taking up to 6 months.[10] Unlike α-adrenergic antagonists, 5α-reductase inhibitors are used to prevent BPH-related complications and disease progression. Finasteride has been shown to reduce the incidence of acute urinary retention and need for prostate surgery in patients with significantly enlarged prostate glands (greater than 40 g [1.4 oz]),[14,15] and those with serum levels of PSA of at least 1.5 ng/mL (1.5 mcg/L).[11] Because 5α-reductase inhibitors do not produce cardiovascular adverse effects, they are preferred for men with moderate to severe BPH who are at risk of developing complications of BPH (i.e., the patient has an enlarged prostate of at least 30 g [1.05 oz]), and have a PSA of greater than 1.5 ng/mL (1.5 mcg/L).[8,11,39]*

With regard to their use for the symptomatic treatment of BPH, 5α-reductase inhibitors relieve BPH symptoms in 30% to 70% of patients and increase the urinary flow rate by 1 to 2 mL/s, which is less improvement than that seen with α-adrenergic antagonists.[10,14] A minimum of 6 months is required to evaluate the effectiveness of treatment. This is a disadvantage in patients with moderate to severe symptoms, as it will take that long to determine whether the drug is or is not effective. Durable responses have been demonstrated in responding patients treated up to 6 years with finasteride and 4 years with dutasteride.[40,41] These agents are hepatically metabolized. No specific recommendations for dosage modification are currently available in patients with significant hepatic dysfunction; however, due to drug specificity for its enzyme target, it is unlikely that any dosage adjustment

Table 52–7

Comparison of Pharmacologic Properties of 5α-Reductase Inhibitors

	Finasteride	Dutasteride
Brand name	Proscar	Avodart
Subtype inhibition of the 5α-reductase enzyme	Type II	Types I and II
Percentage of inhibition of serum dihydrotestosterone level	70–76	90–95
Percentage of patients with reduction in serum dihydrotestosterone	49	Greater than 85
Time to peak onset of reduction in serum dihydrotestosterone level	6 months	1 month
Percentage of inhibition of intraprostatic dihydrotestosterone	85–90	Greater than 95
Half-life	6.2 hours	3–5 hours
Daily dosage (mg)	5	0.5
Recommended dose reduction in patients with renal dysfunction	None needed	None needed
Recommended dose reduction in patients with hepatic dysfunction	Manufacturer provides no specific recommendation. Finasteride should be used cautiously as it undergoes extensive hepatic metabolism	Manufacturer provides no specific recommendation. Dutasteride should be used cautiously as it undergoes extensive hepatic metabolism

From Keam SJ, Scott LJ. Dutasteride: a review of its use in the management of prostate disorders. Drugs 2008;68:463–485.

will be required. No dosage adjustment is needed in patients with renal impairment. Adverse effects include decreased libido, erectile dysfunction, and ejaculation disorders, which generally decrease in frequency with continued use, and gynecomastia and breast tenderness. Serum testosterone levels increase by 10% to 20% in treated patients; however, the clinical significance of this is not clear at this time.[10] Drug interactions are uncommon. These drugs do produce a mean 50% decrease in serum levels of PSA. Therefore, to preserve the usefulness of this laboratory test as a diagnostic and monitoring tool, it is recommended that prescribers obtain a baseline PSA prior to the start of treatment and repeat it at least annually during treatment. A significantly elevated PSA in treated patients suggests that the patient is not compliant with his prescribed 5α-reductase inhibitor regimen or is an indicator for further diagnostic workup for prostate cancer. Exposure to 5α-reductase inhibitors is contraindicated in pregnant females, as the drugs may cause feminization of a male fetus. Pregnant females should not handle these drugs unless they are wearing gloves.

Patient Encounter 3

CC has moderately severe obstructive voiding symptoms of BPH. A DRE reveals a prostate of 20 g (0.7 oz) and a PSA of 1.2 ng/mL (1.2 mcg/L). He is started on dutasteride 0.5 mg daily by mouth. After 6 months, the patient complains that his symptoms have not significantly improved.

Explain why the patient has not responded to treatment.

Identify an alternative treatment regimen for this patient.

5α-Reductase inhibitors include finasteride and dutasteride. Finasteride is a selective type II 5α-reductase inhibitor, whereas dutasteride is a nonselective type I and II 5α-reductase inhibitor. When compared with finasteride, dutasteride produces a faster and more complete inhibition of 5α-reductase in prostate cells. However, no difference in clinical efficacy or adverse effects has been demonstrated between these two agents.[39] Thus finasteride and dutasteride are considered therapeutically interchangeable (Table 52–7).

By reducing serum levels of dihydrotestosterone, which is linked to the development of prostate cancer, it has been hypothesized that 5α-reductase inhibitors may prevent the development of prostate cancer. The Prostate Cancer Prevention Trial reported that finasteride reduced the detection of prostate cancer with prostatic needle biopsy by 25%; however, higher grade tumors were more common in treated patients.[42] This finding is likely due to the fact that the drug-induced shrinkage of the prostate increased the probability that the prostate needle biopsy procedure was able to obtain cancerous tissue.[42] The Reduce Trial compared dutasteride, tamsulosin, and the combination of dutasteride and tamsulosin. Results showed that patients treated with the combination had greater symptom improvement after 9 months and less disease progression at 4 years than patients treated with single drug therapy.[43]

▶ Combination Therapy

● *A combination of an α-adrenergic antagonist and 5α-reductase inhibitor may be considered in symptomatic patients at high risk of BPH complications, which are defined as those with an enlarged prostate of at least 30 g (1.05 oz) and a PSA of at least 1.5 ng/mL (1.5 mcg/L). In such patients, combination therapy will relieve voiding symptoms and also may reduce the risk of*

Patient Encounter 4

EE has BPH. His prostate gland is estimated to be 40 cc (1.4 oz) in size and his PSA is 3 ng/mL (3 mcg/L). The patient also suffers from recurrent urinary tract infection, renal impairment with an estimated creatinine clearance of 25 mL/min (0.42 mL/s), and gross hematuria. The patient's peak urinary flow rate is 5 mL/s, and his postvoid residual urine volume is 200 cc (200 mL). The patient's AUA Symptom Score is 25. The patient prefers medical management for his BPH.

What is the best treatment option for this patient?

developing BPH-related complications and reduce the need for prostatectomy by 67%.[14,15] Because combination therapy is more expensive and associated with the array of adverse effects associated with each drug in the combination, clinicians should discuss the advantages and disadvantages of each treatment regimen with the patient before a final decision is made.[10, 14,15]

To streamline and reduce the cost of treatment regimens, it has been suggested that the α-adrenergic antagonist may be discontinued after the first 6 to 12 months of combination therapy. However, in patients with severe symptoms and an enlarged prostate gland, the combination regimen should be continued as long as the patients are responding.[44]

Another enhancement to BPH symptom management is the addition of an anticholinergic agent to an α-adrenergic antagonist. The rationale for the anticholinergic agent is that irritative symptoms (e.g., urinary urgency and frequency) are thought to be due to hyper-reactive bladder detrusor muscle contraction, which can be ameliorated by blockade of acetylcholine receptors.[45,46] Also, α_{1D}-adrenergic receptors in the detrusor muscle, which cause muscle contraction when stimulated, can be blocked by α-adrenergic antagonists. As a result, use of an α-adrenergic antagonist may also decrease involuntary bladder muscle contraction and increase the bladder's compliance. Thus the combination may have an additive pharmacologic effect on relieving irritative voiding symptoms.[51] A recent study documenting the addition of tolterodine to tamsulosin showed significant irritative symptom improvement, more than what was observed with tamsulosin alone. No cases of urinary retention were reported. Patients at the highest risk of anticholinergic agent induced acute urinary retention include those with a high postvoid residual urine volume (250 mL or more). Thus anticholinergic agents should be used precautiously in these patients.

Finally, tadalafil is approved for treatment of LUTS. It may be prescribed alone or along with an α-adrenergic antagonist or 5 α-reductase inhibitor. It is postulated that its mechanism may be due to relaxation of smooth muscle of the urethra, prostate, and bladder neck, which is mediated by inhibiting the Rho/Rhokinase pathway or by enhancing the action of nitric oxide. Tadalafil is comparable to α-adrenergic antagonists in relieving LUTS, however, it does not increase urinary flow rate or reduce post void residual urine volume. Because tadalafil is expensive, the best candidates for treatment are those with BPH and erectile dysfunction.

OUTCOME EVALUATION

⑨ *Once the peak effects of drug treatment are expected to occur, monitor the drug for effectiveness. Assess symptom improvement using the AUA Symptom Scoring Index. A reduction in symptom score by a minimum of 3 points is anticipated with symptom improvement. However, it should be noted that the AUA Symptom Score may not match the patient's perception of the bothersomeness of his voiding symptoms. If the patient perceives his symptoms as bothersome, independent of the AUA Symptom Score, consideration should be given to modifying the patient's treatment regimen. Similarly, a patient may regard his symptoms as not bothersome even though the AUA symptom score is high. In this case, the physician should objectively assess symptoms at baseline and during treatment by performing a repeat uroflowmetry, which can detect an improvement in peak and mean urinary flow rate. If the patient shows a response to treatment, instruct the patient to continue the drug regimen and have the patient return at 6-month intervals for monitoring. If the patient shows an inadequate response to treatment, the dose of α-adrenergic antagonist can be increased (except for extended-release alfuzosin and silodosin) until the patient's symptoms improve or until the patient experiences adverse drug effects.*

For the α-adrenergic antagonists, the severity of hypotensive-related adverse effects, which may manifest as dizziness or syncope, may require a dosage reduction or a slower up-titration of immediate-release terazosin or doxazosin, or halting the up-titration of the α-adrenergic antagonist. If the patient develops adverse effects at this dose, the drug should be discontinued. Other adverse effects of α-adrenergic antagonists are nasal congestion, malaise, headache, and ejaculation disorders. None of these generally require discontinuation of treatment, and these often improve as treatment continues. For the 5α-reductase inhibitors, the most bothersome adverse effects are decreased libido, erectile dysfunction, and ejaculation disorders. In sexually active males, erectile dysfunction may be improved with erectogenic drugs; however, this adverse effect may necessitate discontinuation of treatment.

During continuing treatment of BPH, the patient should undergo an annual repeat PSA and DRE. A rising PSA level suggests that the patient has worsening BPH, new-onset prostate cancer, or that the patient is noncompliant with his regimen of 5α-reductase inhibitor. An abnormal DRE suggestive of prostate cancer would reveal a nodule or area of induration on the prostate, or a gland that is fixed in place. In such a case, a prostate biopsy is required to rule out prostate cancer.

Drug treatment failures may result from a variety of factors. Initial failure to respond to α-adrenergic antagonists occurs in 20% to 70% of treated patients. It is likely in these patients that the static factor may predominate as the cause of symptoms in these patients. In these patients, adding a 5α-reductase inhibitor may be helpful. Initial failure to respond to 5α-reductase inhibitors occurs in 30% to 70%

Table 52–8

Summary of Adverse Effects of α-Adrenergic Antagonists and 5α-Reductase Inhibitors and Management Suggestions

Drug Class	Adverse Reaction	Management Suggestion
α-Adrenergic antagonist	Hypotension	Start with lowest effective dose, give doses at bedtime, and slowly up-titrate at 0.5- to 1-week intervals to a full therapeutic dose, if using immediate-release terazosin or doxazosin Use tamsulosin, silodosin, extended-release doxazosin, or alfuzosin, as alternatives to immediate-release products, particularly in patients taking other antihypertensives
	Malaise	Educate the patient that this is a common adverse effect; tolerance may develop to malaise. Usually does not require discontinuation of treatment
	Rhinitis	Educate the patient that this is a common adverse effect; tolerance may develop to rhinitis. Usually does not require discontinuation of treatment
	Ejaculation disorders	Educate the patient that this is a common adverse effect and it is not harmful
5α-Reductase inhibitor	Gynecomastia	Educate the patient that this may be bothersome, but not harmful
	Decreased libido	If the patient is sexually active, sexual counseling may be helpful. May be reversible despite continued use of the 5α-reductase inhibitor
	Erectile dysfunction	The addition of sildenafil or another erectogenic drug may be helpful. May be reversible despite continued use of the 5α-reductase inhibitor
	Ejaculation disorders	Educate the patient that this may occur but it is not harmful. May be reversible despite continued use of the 5α-reductase inhibitor

Patient Care and Monitoring

1. Monitor the patient for the drug's effectiveness in relieving symptoms by using the AUA Symptom Scoring Index. Ensure that the score improves (by a minimum decrease of 3 points) and that the patient subjectively feels that symptoms have improved. If the patient has no improvement after several weeks of a therapeutic dose of α-adrenergic antagonist or after 6 months of a 5α-reductase inhibitor, consider surgical intervention. Alternatively, if the patient was on a 5α-reductase inhibitor alone, it may be reasonable to consider adding an α-adrenergic antagonist.

2. If the patient is started on an α-adrenergic antagonist, monitor the patient for hypotension, dizziness, or syncope. If present, assess the severity of each symptom. Reduce the drug dose, switch to a uroselective α-adrenergic antagonist, or discontinue the drug, as necessary. If the patient has malaise or rhinitis, reassure the patient that these are usual, but bothersome, adverse effects that often improve with continued therapy.

3. If the patient is started on a 5α-reductase inhibitor, monitor the patient for drug-induced decreased libido, erectile dysfunction, or ejaculation disorders. If severe, discontinue the drug.

of treated patients. It is likely that the dynamic factor may predominate as the cause of symptoms in these patients. In these patients, switching to or adding an α-adrenergic antagonist may be helpful. In contrast, drug treatment failures after an initial good response to drug therapy will likely be an indication of progressive BPH disease. In such patients, modifying the drug regimen or surgical intervention may be indicated.

Table 52–8 summarizes the adverse effects of the agents used to treat BPH and includes management suggestions for these situations.

Abbreviations Introduced in This Chapter

AUA	American Urological Association
BPH	Benign prostatic hyperplasia
BUN	Blood urea nitrogen
CombAT	Combination of Avodart and Tamsulosin Study
DRE	Digital rectal exam
IVP	Intravenous pyelogram
LUTS	Lower urinary tract symptoms
MTOPS	Multiple Treatment of Prostate Symptoms Study
PSA	Prostate specific antigen
PVR	Postvoid residual urine volume
TURP	Transurethral resection of the prostate

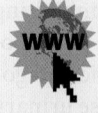

Self-assessment questions and answers are available at *http://www.mhpharmacotherapy.com/pp.html.*

REFERENCES

1. Thorner DA, Weiss JP. Benign prostatic hyperplasia: Symptoms, symptom scores, and outcome measures. Urol Clin North Am 2009;36: 417–429.

2. Berry SJ, Coffey DS, Walsh PC, et al. The development of human benign prostatic hyperplasia with age. J Urol 1984;132:474–479.

3. Wilt TJ, Dow JN. Benign prostatic hyperplasia. Part 1-diagnosis. BMJ 2008;336:146–149.

4. Pool JL, Kirby RS. Clinical significance of α_1-adrenoceptor selectivity in the management of benign prostatic hyperplasia. Int Urol Nephrol 2001;33:407–412.

5. Beckman TJ, Mynderse LA. Evaluation and medical management of benign prostatic hyperplasia. Mayo Clin Proc 2005;80:1356–1362.

6. Isaacs JT. Importance of the natural history of benign prostatic hyperplasia in the evaluation of pharmacologic intervention. Prostate 1990; 3(suppl):1–7.

7. Marks LS, Roehrborn CG, Andriole GL. Prevention of benign prostatic hyperplasia disease. J Urol 2006;176:1299–1306.

8. Patel A, Chapple C. Acute urinary retention: Who is at risk and how best to manage it. Curr Urol Rep 2006;7:252–259.

9. Wilt TJ, Down JN. Benign prostatic hyperplasia. Part 2-management. BMJ 2008;336:206–210.

10. AUA Practice Guidelines Committee. AUA guideline on the management of benign prostatic hyperplasia (2010). www.auanet.org/content/guidelines-and-quality care/clinical-guidelines.cfm?sub=bph (last accessed 8/31/2012).

11. Roehrborn CG, Boyle P, Gould AL, et al. Serum prostate-specific antigen as a predictor of prostate volume in men with benign prostatic hyperplasia. Urology 1999;53:581–589.

12. Djavan B, Eckersberger E, Johannes Handl M, et al. Durability and retreatment rates of minimally invasive-treatments of benign prostatic hyperplasia: A cross-analysis of the literature. Can J Urol 2010;17: 5249–5254.

13. Lourenco T, Pickard R, Vale L, et al. Minimally invasive treatments of benign prostatic enlargement: Systematic review of randomized controlled trials. BMJ 2008;337:a1662.

14. McConnell JD, Roehrborn CG, Bautista OM, et al. The long-term effect of doxazosin, finasteride, and combination therapy on the clinical progression of benign prostatic hyperplasia. N Engl J Med 2003;349: 2389–2398.

15. Roehrborn CG, Siami P, Barkin J, et al. The effects of combination therapy with dutasteride and tamsulosin on clinical outcomes in men with symptomatic benign prostatic hyperplasia: 4 year results from the CombAT study. Eur Urol 2010;57:123–131.

16. Hollingsworth JM, Wei JT. Does the combination of an α_1-adrenergic antagonist with a 5α-reductase inhibitor improve urinary symptoms more than either monotherapy. Curr Opin Urol 2010;20:1–6.

17. Kristal AR, Arnold KB, Schenk JM, et al. Race/ethnicity, obesity, health-related behaviors and the risk of symptomatic benign prostatic hyperplasia: Results from the prostate cancer prevention trial. J Urol 2007;177:1395–1400.

18. Avins AL, Bent S. Saw palmetto and lower urinary tract symptoms: What is the latest evidence? Curr Urol Rep 2006;7:260–265.

19. Dedhia RC, McVary KT. Phytotherapy for lower urinary tract symptoms secondary to benign prostatic hyperplasia. J Urol 2006;179: 2119–2125.

20. Bent S, Kane C, Shinohara K, et al. Saw palmetto for benign prostatic hyperplasia. N Engl J Med 2006;354:557–566.

21. Auffenberg GB, Helfand BT, McVary KT. Established medical therapy for benign prostatic hyperplasia. Urol Clin North Am 2009;36: 443–459.

22. Liao CH, Guh JH, Chueh SC. Anti-angiogenic effects and mechanism of prazosin. Prostate 2011;71:976–984.

23. Santillo VM, Lowe FC. Treatment of benign prostatic hyperplasia in patients with cardiovascular disease. Drugs Aging 2006;23:795–805.

24. Dutkiewicz S. Long term treatment with doxazosin in men with benign prostatic hyperplasia: 10 year follow up. Intern Urol Nephrol 2004;36:169–173.

25. Narayan P, Evans CP, Moon T. Long term safety and efficacy of tamsulosin for the treatment of lower urinary tract symptoms associated with benign prostatic hyperplasia. J Urol 2003;170:498–502.

26. Kaplan SA, Neutel J. Vasodilatory factors in treatment of older men with symptomatic benign prostatic hyperplasia. Urology 2006;67: 225–231.

27. Rossi M, Roumequere T. Silodosin in the treatment of benign prostatic hyperplasia. Drug Des Dev Ther 2010;4:291–297.

28. Lowe FC. Role of the newer alpha$_1$ adrenergic receptor antagonists in the treatment of benign prostatic hyperplasia-related lower urinary tract symptoms. Clin Ther 2004;26:1701–1713.

29. Goldsmith DR, Plosker GL. Doxazosin gastrointestinal therapeutic system. Drugs 2005;65(14):2037–2047.

30. Elhilali MM. Alfuzosin: An α_1-receptor blocker for the treatment of lower urinary tract symptoms associated with benign prostatic hyperplasia. Expert Opin Pharmacother 2006;7(5):583–596.

31. Hellstrom WJ, Sikka SC. Effects of acute treatment with tamsulosin versus alfuzosin on ejaculatory function in normal volunteers. J Urol 2007;177:1587–1588.

32. Friedman AH. Tamsulosin and the intraoperative floppy iris syndrome. JAMA 2009;301:2044–2045.

33. Bell CM, Hatch WV, Fischer HD, et al. Association between tamsulosin and serious ophthalmic adverse events in older men following cataract surgery. JAMA 2009;301:1991–1996.

34. Zabala S, Thomson C, Valdearcos S, et al. Alfuzosin-induced hepatotoxicity. J Clin Pharm Ther 2000;25:73–74.

35. Yolcu OF, Koklu S, Koksal AS, et al. Alfuzosin-induced acute hepatitis in a patient with chronic liver disease. Ann Pharmacother 2004;38:1443–1445.

36. Lowe FC. Coadministration of tamsulosin and three antihypertensive agents in patients with benign prostatic hyperplasia: Pharmacodynamic effect. Clin Ther 1997;19:730–742.

37. Nieminen T, Tammela TLJ, Koobi T, et al. The effects of tamsulosin and sildenafil in separate and combined regimens on detailed hemodynamics in patients with benign prostatic enlargement. J Urol 2006;176:2551–2556.

38. Davis BR, Cutler JA, Gordon DJ, et al, for the ALLHAT Research Group. Rationale and design for the antihypertensive and lipid lowering treatment to prevent heart attack trial (ALLHAT). Am J Hypertens 1996;9:342–360.

39. Keam SJ, Scott LJ. Dutasteride: A review of its use in the management of prostate disorders. Drugs 2008;68:463–485.

40. Roehrborn CG, Marks LS, Fenter T, et al. Efficacy and safety of dutasteride in the four-year treatment of men with benign prostatic hyperplasia. Urology 2004;63:709–715

41. Roehrborn CG, Bruskewitz R, Nickel JC, et al. Sustained decrease in incidence of acute urinary retention and surgery with finasteride for 6 years in men with benign prostatic hyperplasia. J Urol 2004;171: 1194–1198.

42. Thompson IM, Goodman PJ, Tangen CM, et al. The influence of finasteride on the development of prostate cancer. N Engl J Med 2003;349:215–224.

43. Roehrborn CG, Nickel JC, Andriole GL, et al. Dutasteride improves outcomes of benign prostatic hyperplasia when evaluated for prostate cancer risk reduction: Secondary analysis of the REduction of dutasteride of prostate cancer events (REDUCE) Trial. Urology 2011;78: 641–646.

44. Barkin J, Guimaraes M, Jacobi G, et al. Alpha-blocker therapy can be withdrawn in the majority of men following initial combination therapy with the dual 5-alpha reductase inhibitor dutasteride. Eur Urol 2003;44:461–466.

45. Rovner ES, Kreder K, Sussman DO, et al. Effect of tolterodine extended release with or without tamsulosin on measures of urgency and patient reported outcomes in men with lower urinary tract symptoms. J Urol 2008;180:1034–1041.

46. Roehrborn CG, Rovner ES, Kaplan SA, et al. Tolterodine and tamsulosin for treatment of men with lower urinary tract symptoms and overactive bladder. JAMA 2006;296:2319–2328.

53 Urinary Incontinence and Pediatric Enuresis

David R.P. Guay and Sum Lam

LEARNING OBJECTIVES

● **Upon completion of the chapter, the reader will be able to:**

1. Explain the pathophysiology of the major types of urinary incontinence (UI, urge, stress, overflow, and functional) and pediatric enuresis.

2. Recognize the signs and symptoms of the major types of UI and pediatric enuresis in individual patients.

3. List the treatment goals for a patient with UI or pediatric enuresis.

4. Compare and contrast anticholinergics/antispasmodics, α-adrenoceptor agonists, dual serotonin-norepinephrine reuptake inhibitors, vaginal estrogens, cholinomimetics, tricyclic antidepressants (TCAs), and vasopressin analogues in terms of mechanism of action, treatment outcomes, adverse effects, and drug–drug interaction potential when used to manage UI or pediatric enuresis.

5. Identify factors that guide drug selection for an individual patient.

6. Formulate a monitoring plan for a patient on a given treatment regimen based on patient-specific information.

7. Describe indicators for combination drug therapy of UI or pediatric enuresis.

8. Describe nonpharmacologic treatment approaches (including surgery) for UI or pediatric enuresis.

9. Formulate appropriate patient counseling information for patients undergoing drug therapy for UI or pediatric enuresis.

KEY CONCEPTS

❶ Accurate diagnosis and classification of urinary incontinence (UI) type is critical to the selection of appropriate drug therapy.

❷ Many medications can influence the lower urinary tract, including those not used for managing genitourinary disorders, and can precipitate new onset or aggravate existing voiding dysfunction and UI.

❸ Patient-specific treatment goals should be identified. This frequently requires reaching a compromise between efficacy and tolerability of drug therapy. These goals are not static and may change with time.

❹ Nonpharmacologic treatment can allow the use of lower drug doses. The combination of both therapies may have at least an additive effect on UI signs and symptoms.

❺ The anticholinergic/antispasmodic drugs are the pharmacologic first-line treatments for urge UI. They are the most effective agents in suppressing premature detrusor contractions, enhancing bladder storage, and relieving symptoms.

❻ Patient characteristics (e.g., age, comorbidities, concurrent drug therapies, and ability to adhere to the prescribed regimen) can also influence drug therapy selection.

❼ Careful dose titration is necessary to maximize efficacy and tolerability.

❽ If therapeutic goals are not achieved, a switch to an alternative agent should be made.

❾ Vaginally administered estrogen plays only a modest role in managing stress urinary incontinence (SUI, urethral underactivity), unless it is accompanied by local signs of estrogen deficiency (e.g., atrophic urethritis or vaginitis).

❿ The major impediment to using the α-adrenoceptor agonist class in SUI is the extensive list of contraindications.

⓫ The use of duloxetine in SUI is complicated by (a) the potential for multiple clinically relevant drug–drug interactions with CYP-450 2D6 and 1A2 inhibitors, (b) withdrawal reactions if abruptly discontinued,

(c) high rates of nausea and other side effects, (d) hepatotoxicity that contraindicates its use in patients with any degree of hepatic impairment, and (e) its mild hypertensive effect. Another disconcerting finding is the high discontinuation rate when duloxetine is used in a "usual use" clinic environment (66%, two-thirds due to adverse events and one-third due to lack of efficacy).

⑫ In overflow UI due to atonic bladder, a trial of bethanechol may be reasonable if contraindications do not exist.

⑬ In overflow UI due to obstruction, the goal of treatment is to relieve the obstruction.

⑭ Considering that pharmacotherapy is inferior to select nonpharmacologic treatment modalities in pediatric enuresis, pharmacotherapy will be most valuable in patients who are not candidates for nonpharmacologic therapy due to nonadherence or who do not achieve the desired outcomes on nonpharmacologic therapy alone.

⑮ Desmopressin (DDAVP) is the first-line drug choice in pediatric enuresis.

URINARY INCONTINENCE

INTRODUCTION

Urinary incontinence (UI) is defined as the complaint of involuntary leakage of urine.[1] It is often associated with other bothersome lower urinary tract symptoms such as urgency, increased daytime frequency, and nocturia. Despite its prevalence across the lifespan and in both sexes, it remains an underdetected and underreported health problem that can have significant negative consequences for the individual's quality of life. Patients with UI may be depressed due to a perceived loss of self-control, loss of independence, and lack of self-esteem, and often curtail or substantially modify their activities for fear of an "accident." Serious medical and economic consequences may also occur in untreated or undertreated patients, including perineal dermatitis and infections, worsening or lack of healing of pressure ulcers, urinary tract infections (UTIs), falls, and the need for long-term institutionalization in extended-care facilities (including skilled nursing facilities [SNFs], or nursing homes).

EPIDEMIOLOGY AND ETIOLOGY

The true prevalence of UI has been difficult to determine because of methodologic issues such as varying definitions of UI and reporting bias.[2] Although the condition occurs across the lifespan, the peak prevalence, at least in women, is around the age of menopause (approximately 50 years), which is followed by a slight decrease in the 55- to 60-year-old age group, and then a steadily increasing prevalence after age 65. In general, the median prevalences of UI are as follows[3]:

- 20% to 30% in young females
- 30% to 40% in middle-aged females

- 30% to 50% in elderly females (50% to 75% in female SNF residents)
- 10% in adult males (more than 50% in elderly male SNF residents)

UI can result from abnormalities within (intrinsic to) and outside of (extrinsic to) the urinary tract. Within the urinary tract, abnormalities may occur in the urethra (including the bladder outlet and urinary sphincters), the bladder, or a combination of both structures. Focusing on abnormalities in these two structures, a simple classification scheme emerges for all but the rarest intrinsic causes of UI. ① *Accurate diagnosis and classification of UI type is critical to the selection of appropriate drug therapy.*

PATHOPHYSIOLOGY

Stress Urinary Incontinence Related to Urethral Underactivity[4]

In stress urinary incontinence (SUI), the urethra and/or urethral sphincters cannot generate enough resistance to impede urine flow from the bladder when intra-abdominal pressures (that are transmitted to the bladder, which is an intra-abdominal organ) are elevated. Intra-abdominal pressures are suddenly elevated by exertional activities like exercise, running, lifting, coughing, and sneezing. The amount of urine lost is generally small with each episode. Nocturia and enuresis are rarely seen. The factors responsible for urethral underactivity are incompletely understood, although the loss of the trophic effects of estrogen on the uroepithelium at menopause is thought to be important. The peak of SUI prevalence in the perimenopausal years supports this hypothesis. Clearly established risk factors for SUI include[5]:

- Pregnancy (increased risk with increased parity)
- Childbirth (vaginal delivery)
- Menopause
- Cognitive impairment
- Obesity
- Increasing age

Unless the sphincter mechanism is compromised by surgery or trauma, SUI is exceedingly rare in males. The most common surgeries predisposing to SUI in males are radical prostatectomy for prostate cancer and transurethral resection of the prostate for benign prostatic hyperplasia (BPH).

Urge Urinary Incontinence Related to Bladder Overactivity[4]

In urge urinary incontinence (UUI), the detrusor (bladder) muscle is overactive and contracts inappropriately during the filling phase. Stimulation of muscarinic cholinergic receptors (especially M2 and M3 subtypes) in the bladder muscle is responsible for these contractions. The amount of urine lost per episode can be as large as the entire contents of the bladder may empty. Sleep may be disrupted by nocturia and enuresis.

In most patients, the cause of bladder overactivity is unknown (idiopathic). Clearly established risk factors for UUI include:

- Increasing age
- Neurologic disorders (e.g., stroke, Parkinson's disease, multiple sclerosis, and spinal cord injury)
- Bladder outlet obstruction (e.g., benign or malignant prostatic enlargement or hyperplasia)
- Hysterectomy
- Recurrent UTIs

Overactivity may be myogenic or neurogenic in origin or a combination of both. These etiologies appear to be interconnected and complementary.

Overflow Urinary Incontinence Related to Urethral Overactivity and/or Bladder Underactivity[4]

In overflow urinary incontinence (OUI), an important but uncommon form of UI in both sexes, the bladder is filled to capacity at all times but cannot empty, causing urine to leak out episodically. If caused by bladder underactivity, the detrusor muscle has weakened, in some cases enough to lose the ability to voluntarily contract. In this case, the bladder cannot be emptied completely, and large volumes of residual urine remain after micturition. Clinically, this is most commonly seen in the setting of long-term chronic bladder outlet obstruction due to benign or malignant prostatic enlargement. However, this may also be a manifestation of neurogenic bladder, frequently being seen in patients with diabetes, lower spinal cord injury, multiple sclerosis, or following radical pelvic surgery. If due to urethral overactivity, the resistance of the urethra and/or

sphincters cannot be overcome by detrusor contractility. This functional or anatomic obstruction results in incomplete bladder emptying. Clinically, in males this most frequently occurs in the context of long-term chronic bladder outlet obstruction, as outlined previously. In females, urethral overactivity is rare, but may result from cystocele formation or surgical overcorrection during anti-SUI surgery. In both sexes, systemic neurologic diseases such as multiple sclerosis or spinal cord injury may be the etiology.

Functional UI[4]

Functional UI is not generally caused by intrinsic urinary tract pathology. It is usually caused by factors extrinsic to the urinary tract. Examples of factors predisposing to functional incontinence include:

- Immobility (due to pain, traction, or use of nonportable medical devices)
- Lack of or slowed access to toileting facilities
- Cognitive impairment (difficulty with recognition of the urinary urge and proper response to it)
- UTIs
- Postmenopausal atrophic urethritis and/or vaginitis
- Diabetes mellitus (glucosuria leading to polyuria)
- Diabetes insipidus (polyuria due to decreased antidiuretic hormone [ADH])
- Pelvic malignancy (extrinsic pressure on urinary tract structures causing obstruction)
- Constipation or fecal impaction
- Congenital malformations
- CNS disorder resulting in a decreased level of consciousness
- Depression (apathy leading to recognition and response difficulties)

Mixed and Drug-Induced UI[4]

Frequently, two or more types of UI may coexist in a given patient, combinations termed mixed UI. This can lead to diagnostic and therapeutic difficulties due to the confusing array of presenting signs and symptoms and the opposing effects that a given treatment can have in different types of UI (i.e., a given drug may reduce the signs and symptoms of one type of UI but worsen those of other types). Another interesting type of mixed UI is coexisting bladder overactivity (UUI) and impaired bladder contractility (OUI). Most common in the elderly, this combination is called *detrusor hyperactivity with impaired contractility* (DHIC).

❷ *Many medications can influence the lower urinary tract, including those not used for managing genitourinary disorders, and can precipitate new onset or aggravate existing voiding dysfunction and UI* (Table 53–1).

CLINICAL PRESENTATION AND DIAGNOSIS

The clinical presentation of UI depends on the underlying pathophysiology. The literature evaluating the prevalences of different UI types by age and sex has produced widely varying results due to a number of factors. The clinician should thus consider a given patient as having virtually any type of UI until ruled out during diagnostic evaluation.

A complete medical history and targeted physical examination are essential to correctly classify the type(s) of UI present. It is important to assess the degree of annoyance of the patient due to UI signs and symptoms. The degree of annoyance of the patient may not correlate well with the results of quantitative tests such as symptom frequency/severity, use of absorbent products, frequency/severity of neurologic signs, and postvoid residual urine volume. This is especially the case in "hypersensitive" and "stoic" individuals. Items to address during the evaluation are illustrated in Table 53–2. Components of the physical examination include[4]:

- Abdominal examination (look for distended bladder, organomegaly, and masses)
- Neurologic evaluation of perineum and lower extremities to evaluate lumbosacral nerve function (includes digital rectal exam to check rectal tone, reflexes, ability to perform a voluntary pelvic muscle contraction in females and size and surface quality of prostate in males)
- Pelvic exam (females) (look for evidence of prolapse of bladder, small bowel, rectum, or uterus, or estrogen deficiency)
- Genital/prostate exam (men)
- Urinalysis, postvoid residual
- Direct observation of urethral meatus (opening) when patient coughs/strains (urine spurt consistent with SUI) (cough stress test)
- Perineal exam (looking for skin maceration, redness, breakdown, ulceration, and evidence of fungal skin infection)
- Optional: voiding diary, assessment of incontinence severity, quality-of-life measures

Table 53–1

Medications Influencing Lower Urinary Tract Function

Medication	Effect
Diuretics	Polyuria, frequency, urgency
α-Adrenoceptor antagonists	Urethral relaxation: may relieve obstruction in males, induces/worsens SUI in females
α-Adrenoceptor agonists	Urethral constriction: aggravates obstruction in males (may cause urinary retention), potential SUI treatment in females
Calcium channel blockers (dihydropyridines)	Urethral constriction (may cause urinary retention), especially in males
Opioid analgesics	Impaired bladder contractility (may cause urinary retention)
Sedative-hypnotics	Functional UI due to immobility, delirium, sedation
Psychotherapeutics with anticholinergic properties; anticholinergics	Urinary retention due to impaired bladder contractility or potential UUI treatment
TCAs	Combination of anticholinergic and α-adrenoceptor blocking activities can lead to unpredictable effects on UI
Ethanol	Polyuria and frequency (via effects on ADH), functional UI (delirium, sedation), urgency
ACEIs	Cough leading to SUI (ARBs do not induce cough)
Cyclophosphamide	Hemorrhagic cystitis due to acrolein metabolite (prevent with MESNA)

ACEIs, angiotensin-converting enzyme inhibitors; ADH, antidiuretic hormone (or vasopressin); ARB, angiotensin II receptor blocker; MESNA, sodium 2-mercaptoethanesulfonate; SUI, stress urinary incontinence; TCA, tricyclic antidepressant; UI, urinary incontinence; UUI, urge urinary incontinence.

Table 53–2

Items to Address During Diagnostic Evaluation of UI

Item	Comments
Urine leakage	
Use of absorbent products	Yes/no, type(s), quantity, times of day worn
	Quantity may relate more to personal preference and hygiene than to UI type and severity (e.g., use of large number of pads by a fastidiously hygienic patient with low volume loss)
Quantity lost per episode	Dribbling versus small volumes intermittently versus large volumes
	Consistent or varied quantities
Precipitants	Yes/no, physical activity, excessive fluid intake, drug(s)
Times of day	Daytime/nighttime/both
Symptoms	
Urgency	Yes/no, how often, how severe, duration from urge onset to micturition
Frequency	Yes/no, daytime/nighttime/both, how often
Nocturia	Yes/no, how often, proportion associated with UI
Obstructive symptoms	Yes/no, type(s) (hesitancy, strain to void, decreased force of stream, start and stop stream, sense of incomplete emptying), severity
Lower abdominal fullness	Yes/no, how often, how severe
Comorbidities	
Current medication use	See Table 53–1. Remember CAMs, OTCs
Evidence of preexisting or new-onset:	
Diabetes mellitus	
Metastatic or genitourinary malignancy	
Multiple sclerosis or other neurologic disease	
CNS disease above the pons	Usually UUI
Spinal cord injury	UUI or OUI, depending on level and degree of completeness of injury
Recent nongenitourinary surgery	Functional UI
Previous local surgery/radiation	Prostate surgery, lower abdominal cavity surgery (direct injury versus denervation), radiation (direct injury)
Gynecologic history	Childbirth (vaginal versus cesarean section), prior gynecologic surgery, hormonal status (pre- versus peri- versus postmenopausal)
Pelvic floor disease	Constipation, diarrhea, fecal incontinence, dyspareunia, sexual dysfunction, pelvic pain
UTI	Dysuria, CVA tenderness, frequency
Gross hematuria	Possible bladder or other genitourinary cancer

CAM, complementary and alternative medications; CVA, costovertebral angle; OTC, over-the-counter; OUI, overflow urinary incontinence; SUI, stress urinary incontinence; UTI, urinary tract infection; UUI, urge urinary incontinence.

The methods adopted for evaluating symptoms include evaluation via questioning, responses of patients to uniform questionnaires, and records in bladder diaries (recommended length of 3 days to 1 week). The Overactive Bladder Symptom Score (OABSS, see Table 53–3) has been used for the evaluation of symptoms in patients diagnosed with OAB. The recommended diagnostic criteria for OAB are "an urgency score for Question 3 of 2 or greater, and an OABSS of 3 or greater." OABSS may also be used for assessing the severity of OAB: a total score of 5 or less (mild), 6 to 11 (moderate), and 12 or more (severe). A simplified form of the OABSS can be used to screen for OAB in the general population. This three-item questionnaire has high sensitivity but low specificity for OAB.[6]

TREATMENT

❸ *Patient-specific treatment goals should be identified. This frequently requires reaching a compromise between efficacy and tolerability of drug therapy. These goals are not static and may change with time.*

Desired Outcomes

- Restoration of continence
- Reduction of the number of UI episodes (daytime and nighttime) and frequency of nocturia (must produce a minimum reduction of 50% to be clinically important)
- Prevention of disease complications (e.g., dermatologic infections and skin breakdown, delay institutionalization)
- Avoidance or minimization of adverse consequences of treatment

- Minimization of treatment costs
- Improvement in patient's quality of life

Nonpharmacologic Treatment

At the primary care level, nonpharmacologic treatment of UI constitutes the chief approach to UI management. In patients in whom pharmacologic or surgical management is inappropriate or undesirable or refused, nonsurgical nonpharmacologic treatment is the only option. Nonpharmacologic therapy has no adverse reactions, is minimally invasive, and can be utilized adjunctively with other modalities. Examples of patients fitting this scenario include:

- Those not medically fit for surgery
- Those who plan future pregnancies (as pregnancy/childbirth can compromise the long-term results of certain types of continence surgery)
- Those with OUI whose condition is not amenable to surgical or drug treatment
- Those with comorbidities that place them at high risk for significant side effects to drug therapy
- Those who wish to delay or avoid surgery
- Those with mild to moderate symptoms who do not wish to undergo surgery or take medication

Nonpharmacologic approaches include lifestyle modifications, scheduled voiding regimens, pelvic floor muscle rehabilitation (PFMR), anti-incontinence devices, and supportive interventions.[4,7] Many of these are best utilized through attendance at multidisciplinary UI clinics staffed by healthcare

---

Table 53–3

Overactive Bladder Symptom Score (OABSS)

Question	Symptom	Score	Frequency over the past
1	How many times do you typically urinate from waking in the morning until going to bed in the evening?	0	7 or less
		1	8–14
		2	15 or more
2	How many times do you typically wake up to urinate from going to sleep at night until waking in the morning?	0	0
		1	1
		2	2
		3	3 or more
3	How often do you have a sudden compelling desire to urinate, which is difficult to postpone?	0	Not at all
		1	Less than once week
		2	Once a week or more
		3	About once a day
		4	2–4 times a day
		5	5 times a day or more
4	How often do you leak urine because you cannot postpone the sudden desire to urinate?	0	Not at all
		1	Less than once week
		2	Once a week or more
		3	About once a day
		4	2–4 times a day
		5	5 times a day or more
	Sum of scores		

The sampling period is usually defined as "the past week" but, depending on the usage, it can be amended to, for example, "the past 3 days" or "the past month." Whatever the case, it is necessary to specify the sampling period.

Patient Encounter 1, Part 2: Medical History, Physical Examination, and Diagnostic Tests

PMH: Hypertension, dyslipidemia, type 2 diabetes mellitus, and osteoarthritis

FH: Mother died of breast cancer at age 70; father died of a myocardial infarction at age 65

SH: Retired certified public accountant; now volunteers as an instructor for water-color painting classes at a local senior center. Married and lives with husband. Two married daughters (ages 30 and 32 years) live in the neighborhood. Denies tobacco or alcohol use; drinks 4 cups of coffee daily

All: Erythromycin (rash)

Medications: Insulin glargine 40 units subcutaneously at bedtime; Regular insulin 10 units subcutaneously before meals; metoprolol 50 mg once daily; enalapril 5 mg once daily; atorvastatin 10 mg once daily; acetaminophen 650 mg every 6 hours as needed for knee pain

ROS: Alert, sociable, and pleasant. (–) UI, history of UTIs; (–) nocturia, enuresis, dysuria, lower abdominal fullness, decreased force of stream

PE:

Gen: Postmenopausal white woman with mild kyphosis; NAD; A & O × 3

VS: BP 120/70 mm Hg, HR 65 beats/min, RR 20 breaths/min, Temp 98.3°F (36.8°C), Wt 60 kg, Ht 5 ft 5 in (165 cm)

HEENT: PERRLA; EOMI, TMs WNL

Neck/LN: Supple w/o LAD or masses

Lungs/Thorax: CTA

CV: RRR w/o murmurs, rubs, gallops

Abd: Soft, NT/ND w/o masses; (+) BS; bladder not palpable

GU: WNL; no atrophic vaginitis or uterine prolapse

MS/Ext: WNL, no edema

Neuro: DTRs 2+, CN II – XII intact

Labs:

Na: 134 mEq/L (134 mmol/L)

K: 3.8 mEq/L (3.8 mmol/L)

Cl: 100 mEq/L (100 mmol/L)

CO_2: 22 mEq/L (22 mmol/L)

BUN: 9 mg/dL (3.2 mmol/L)

SCr: 1.0 mg/dL (88 μmol/L)

Random glucose: 180 mg/dL (10.0 mmol/L)

Hb: 12 g/dL (120 g/L; 7.45 mmol/L)

Hct: 37% (0.37)

Plts: 300,000/mm³ (300 × 10⁹/L)

WBC: 6.1 × 10³/mm³ (6.1 × 10⁹/L) with normal differential

Hemoglobin A1c 8.5% (0.085; 69 mmol/mol hemoglobin) LFTs within normal limits

UA (–)

Given this additional information, what is your assessment of the patient's condition?

What are the goals of pharmacotherapy for this patient?

What nonpharmacologic and pharmacologic alternatives are available to the patient?

---

providers. Behavioral interventions are among the first-line treatment approaches for SUI, UUI, and mixed UI. However, these lifestyle modifications, scheduling regimens, and PFMR methods require a motivated patient and/or caregiver who can play an active role in developing the treatment plan. Anything that interferes with active participation (including cognitive dysfunction) will render these approaches suboptimal. Patients/caregivers also must attend regular follow-up visits to monitor outcomes. Of interest, nonpharmacologic treatment may even be superior to pharmacologic treatment in select cases. For example, the short-term (6 months) and long-term (21 months) results of a combination of PFMR plus behavioral training produced statistically superior results compared with anticholinergic therapy in women with UUI.[8,9] Even if the results of nonpharmacologic treatment have not fully achieved the desired outcomes, if it has provided at least some improvement in UI signs and symptoms, it should be continued during pharmacologic treatment. ❹ *Nonpharmacologic treatment can allow the use of lower drug doses. The combination of both therapies may have at least an additive effect on UI signs and symptoms.*

In the recent systematic review of nonsurgical treatments for UI by Shamliyan et al., the only nonpharmacologic treatment for which true objective evidence of benefit exists is the combination of PFMR plus behavioral training (restored continence with an effect size of 0.13 [95% CI, 0.07 to 0.20], but improvement in continence was not consistent between trials). Although PFMR alone or combined with biofeedback restored and improved continence, the effect size was not consistent between trials.[10] Weight loss of 5% to 10% in overweight or obese women has an efficacy similar to that of other nonpharmacologic treatments.

Surgery is rarely a first-line treatment for UI. Surgery is generally considered only when the degree of bother or lifestyle compromise is sufficient and other nonoperative therapies are either undesired or have been ineffective. Surgery can be used to manage urethral overactivity due to benign prostatic enlargement and bladder outlet obstruction (via endoscopic incision using a cystoscope). Bladder underactivity cannot be managed surgically and rarely is surgery considered for UUI. Surgery is most effective in the management of SUI. Surgery for SUI is directed toward stabilizing the urethra and bladder neck and/or augmenting urethral resistance. This can be accomplished by injection of periurethral bulking agents, midurethral or pubovaginal sling surgeries, and lap or retropubic suspension surgeries. In males, SUI is best treated by implanting an artificial urinary sphincter.[4]

Unaddressed issues regarding nonpharmacologic therapy include uncertain long-term results, lack of standardized protocols for specific procedures in each treatment method, insurance coverage, and reimbursement concerns.[6]

Pharmacologic Treatment

▶ *Urge Urinary Incontinence*

⑤ *The anticholinergic/antispasmodic drugs are the first-line pharmacologic treatment for UUI. They are the most effective agents in suppressing premature detrusor contractions, enhancing bladder storage, and relieving symptoms.* It must be emphasized that the improvements in clinical and urodynamic parameters are modest at best, although still considered by experts in the field to be positive.[11] In the recent systematic review/meta-analysis of 50 clinical trials in UUI by Novara et al., there were no clinically important or relevant differences found among different anticholinergics.[12] Antimuscarinic agents are also the mainstay therapy for urinary symptoms, including UUI, associated with OAB. Their efficacy can be maximized by combination with nonpharmacologic therapy. These agents should be considered for patients who are bothered by OAB symptoms and have no major contraindications to therapy. They are considered equally effective based on statistical superiority over placebo or active controls, with small absolute reductions in symptom measures in most clinical trials.[13]

Currently there are few head-to-head trials that directly compare these agents, and there are no objective data suggesting the first-line drug to initiate for OAB. In the recent systematic review of Shamliyan et al., data for analysis were adequate only for oxybutynin IR (5 to 10 mg/day) and tolterodine LA (4 mg/day). Both of these agents restored continence with an effect size of 0.18 (95% CI, 0.13 to 0.22), although neither was demonstrated to be superior.[10] The ideal agent for UUI must have clinical efficacy and safety, minimal side effects, minimal drug-drug/drug-disease interactions, convenient administration, and low cost. ⑥ *Patient characteristics (e.g., age, comorbidities, concurrent drug therapies, and ability to adhere to the prescribed regimen) can also influence drug therapy selection.* Table 53–4 compares the pharmacokinetics, contraindications, precautions, and dosing of available agents (oxybutynin, tolterodine, trospium chloride, solifenacin, darifenacin, and fesoterodine) approved for OAB).[13–16]

All antimuscarinic agents have similar contraindications and precautions, including urinary retention, gastric retention, and uncontrolled narrow-angle glaucoma.[13] Older agents, such as oxybutynin IR and tolterodine IR, have been associated with higher rates of adverse effects such

as dry mouth, constipation, headache, dyspepsia, dry eyes, cognitive impairment, tachycardia, and urinary retention. Older patients are especially susceptible to adverse events associated with these agents. Significant dry mouth can be associated with dental caries, ill-fitting dentures, and swallowing difficulty. Orthostatic hypotension and sedation can be particularly troublesome to patients with cognitive impairment or at risk for falls. Issues with tolerability and multiple daily dose administration associated with IR products may jeopardize medication adherence and can prevent dose titration to achieve optimal clinical response. Thus, these products are not preferred in elderly patients with functional limitations and/or those who are already being treated with complicated drug regimens. Nevertheless, adverse events are not universal and their severity varies with individuals. Therefore, older agents (start at the lowest possible doses) are reasonable to consider in patients who cannot otherwise afford drug therapy. Extended-release agents (oxybutynin XL, tolterodine LA, trospium ER, darifenacin ER, fesoterodine ER) cause less dry mouth compared with IR products,[4,12,13] but patients are required to swallow the product whole, as these agents cannot be chewed, crushed, or divided. Oxybutynin TD patch and topical gel are alternatives for patients who cannot take or tolerate oral drugs, but they are associated with application site reactions. Similar to newer agents, they are four to five times more costly than generic oxybutynin.[13]

Most antimuscarinic agents (oxybutynin, tolterodine, fesoterodine, solifenacin, darifenacin) are tertiary amines, which can penetrate the blood–brain barrier and may lead to CNS side effects (sedation, mental status changes). Oxybutynin is also highly lipophilic, which may contribute to a greater potential for CNS side effects. Trospium chloride is a hydrophilic, positively charged quaternary amine that does not readily cross into the CNS. These characteristics have been often used to explain its lower CNS side effect potential compared with oxybutynin.[17] However, this benefit has not been confirmed in clinical studies. Patients receiving any antimuscarinic agent should be informed about sedation as a possible side effect and warned against operating heavy machinery, such as driving, especially during the initial phase of therapy. Patients with existing cognitive dysfunction or difficulty with balance should be monitored closely for mental status changes and falls, respectively. Older individuals are more likely to experience drug-induced constipation because of polypharmacy and age-related physiologic changes. A study demonstrated that solifenacin was most associated with constipation, followed by trospium chloride, oxybutynin, fesoterodine, darifenacin, and tolterodine, which was least associated with constipation.[18] Patients should be advised to contact their physician if they experience severe abdominal pain or become constipated for 3 or more days.

The appropriate dosing of drug therapy for OAB is based on drug–drug interactions and renal or hepatic function. All available OAB agents, except trospium chloride, are metabolized by CYP450 3A4 and/or 2D6

Table 53-4

Anticholinergic/Antispasmodic Drugs Recommended for UUI

Parameter	Oxybutynin	Tolterodine	Trospium Chloride	Solifenacin	Darifenacin	Fesoterodine
Dosage forms	IR tablets, solution; SR-ER tablets, SR-TD patch, topical gel	IR tablets; SR-LA capsules	IR tablets; ER tablets	IR tablets	ER tablets	ER tablets
Dosing	IR: 2.5–5 mg 2–4 times daily (pediatrics 0.3–0.5 mg/kg/day in 3 doses); SR (oral): 5–30 mg once daily (pediatrics: 0.3–0.5 mg/kg/day); SR (TD): 3.9 mg/day patch applied twice weekly; SR (gel): 1 sachet (100 mg) applied once daily	IR: 1 or 2 mg twice daily (pediatrics: 1 mg twice daily); SR: 2 or 4 mg once daily (pediatrics: 2 mg once daily)	IR: 20 mg twice daily; ER: 60 mg once daily	5–10 mg once daily	7.5–15 mg once daily	4–8 mg once daily
Kinetics	Active metabolite (N-desethyl); Not altered in renal or hepatic disease or advanced age	Active metabolite (5-hydroxymethyl); Polymorphic metabolism (CYP 2D6); Not altered in advanced age. Significantly altered in hepatic disease (decreased CL in cirrhosis) and renal disease (decreased CL)	Food: decreased BA by 70–80%; Significantly altered in renal disease (decreased CL) but not in hepatic disease or advanced age	Metabolized via CYP 3A4 but only one active metabolite (4-hydroxy); Significantly altered in severe renal impairment, moderate hepatic impairment (Child-Pugh B), and advanced age (decreased CL in all)	Complex metabolism (polymorphic CYP 2D6, CYP 3A4); Not altered in advanced age, renal impairment, mild hepatic impairment (Child-Pugh A); Significantly altered in moderate hepatic impairment (Child-Pugh B) (decreased CL)	Prodrug (for 5-hydroxmethyl tolterodine); Inactive metabolites; Not altered in advanced age; Significantly altered in renal disease (decreased CL) and moderate hepatic impairment (Child-Pugh B) (decreased CL)
Contraindications and precautions	Use with caution if CYP 3A4 inhibitors are also being taken (decreased oxybutynin CL)	Reduce dose 50% in those taking CYP 3A4 inhibitor(s) or with hepatic cirrhosis or with CrCl less than 30 mL/min (0.50 mL/s); Antacid-SR (oral) prep, interaction (dose-dumping) (not seen with PPIs)	Give on empty stomach; Decrease dose 50% when CrCl less than 30 mL/min (0.50 mL/s) and use IR formulation	Do not exceed 5 mg/day if CrCl less than 30 mL/min (0.50 mL/s), patient has moderate hepatic impairment, or patient is taking CYP 3A4 inhibitor(s); If severe hepatic impairment, do not use	Do not exceed 7.5 mg/day if patient is taking potent CYP 3A4 inhibitor(s); Use caution if patient is taking moderate CYP 3A4 inhibitor(s) or CYP 3A4 or 2D6 substrate(s); Do not chew, divide, or crush the ER tablets	Do not exceed 4 mg/day if CrCl less than 30 mL/min (0.50 mL/s) or patient is taking potent CYP 3A4 inhibitor(s); If severe hepatic impairment, do not use

BA, bioavailability; CL, total body clearance; CrCl, creatinine clearance; CYP450, cytochrome P450; TD, transdermal; ER, extended release; IR, immediate release; LA, long acting; PPIs, proton pump inhibitors; SR, sustained release.

isoenzymes. Tolterodine, solifenacin, darifenacin, and fesoterodine require dose reduction when used concurrently with CYP 3A4 inhibitor(s). In addition, darifenacin also interacts with drugs via the CYP 2D6 system. Trospium chloride, solifenacin, and fesoterodine require dose reduction in patients with CrCl less than 30 mL/min (0.50 mL/s). Tolterodine requires a 50% dose reduction in patients with hepatic cirrhosis, whereas solifenacin and fesoterodine should be avoided in patients with severe hepatic dysfunction. An important drug–drug interaction to avoid is the concurrent use of acetylcholinesterase inhibitors for dementia and anticholinergic agents of any kind due to pharmacologic antagonism.[19]

Treatment with a selected agent should be initiated at the lowest possible dose and gradually titrated upward based on clinical response; not to exceed the maximum recommended dose. A trial of at least 4 weeks is required to evaluate the efficacy of the agent. Consider switching to another agent if the patient reports intolerable side effects or inadequate relief from OAB symptoms despite optimized dose.

▶ Stress Urinary Incontinence

The goal of pharmacologic therapy of urethral underactivity is to improve the urethral closure mechanism by one or more of the following:

- Stimulating α-adrenoceptors in the smooth muscle of the proximal urethra and bladder neck
- Enhancing the supportive structures underlying the urethral mucosa
- Enhancing the positive effects of serotonin and norepinephrine in the afferent and efferent pathways of the micturition reflex

It is generally felt that there is no role for pharmacologic therapy in SUI in males resulting from surgery or trauma.[20] Initial data, however, suggest a possible role for duloxetine added to nonpharmacologic treatment (PFMR), rather than

PFMR alone, in males postradical prostatectomy, at least over the first 4 to 6 months.[21] It should be kept in mind that SUI (in contrast to UUI) is frequently curable by surgery, thus obviating years of drug therapy that may be incompletely effective in symptom relief.

Estrogens[4] ❾ *Vaginally administered estrogen plays only a modest role in managing SUI (urethral underactivity), unless it is accompanied by local signs of estrogen deficiency (e.g., atrophic urethritis or vaginitis).*

Although not supported by rigorous clinical trial evidence, local (PV) and systemic estrogens have been considered mainstays of pharmacologic management since the 1940s. They are believed to work by a trophic effect on uroepithelial cells and underlying collagenous subcutaneous tissue, enhancement of local microcirculation by increasing the number of periurethral blood vessels, and enhancement of the number and/or sensitivity of α-adrenoceptors. Open trials have supported the use of estrogens administered by the oral, TD, and local routes of administration. However, randomized controlled trials have found no significant clinical or urodynamic effects of oral estrogen compared with placebo in SUI. In fact, most trials have found that oral estrogen/hormone replacement therapy actually increases the risk of new-onset UI (SUI, UUI, mixed UI).[10] Open trials of local estrogens (estriol [not available in the United States] tablets, CEE cream, and estradiol rings) have demonstrated subjective improvement in SUI symptoms as well as positive urodynamic effects (significantly increased maximum urethral pressure, urethral closing pressure, and abdominal pressure transmission ratio to proximal urethra).[22] Systemic estrogen therapy also carries numerous short- and long-term side effect risks (mastodynia, uterine bleeding, nausea, thromboembolism, cardiac and cerebrovascular ischemic events, and enhanced breast and endometrial cancer risks). If estrogens are to be used in SUI management, only locally administered products should be used (Table 53–5). Even with locally administered products, improvement of continence has been inconsistent between trials.[10] Vaginal tablets and rings have greater acceptability than creams.

▶ α-Adrenoceptor Agonists[4]

Open and randomized controlled trials utilizing clinical and urodynamic end points have supported the use of a variety of *a*-adrenoceptor agonists, including phenylpropanolamine, ephedrine, and pseudoephedrine, in the therapy of mild and moderate SUI. In addition, several studies have demonstrated clinical and urodynamic benefits for combination estrogen–α-adrenoceptor agonist use over those of the individual agents. However, in the recent systematic review of Shamliyan et al., monotherapy with this class failed to restore continence or improve incontinence compared with placebo or PFMR.[10] Phenylpropanolamine was removed from the U.S. market in late 2000 due to the risk of ischemic stroke in women taking this drug. However, this drug is still available via the Internet, so clinicians need to monitor and discourage its

Table 53–5

Drugs Used for SUI[a]

Parameter	Estrogens	Pseudoephedrine	Duloxetine
Dosage forms	Avoid systemic (parenteral, oral, TD); use vaginal: tablet, cream, intravaginal ring	Tablets, solution	DR capsules
Dosing	Estradiol 25 mcg vaginal tablets (insert one PV daily for 14 days, then one PV twice weekly) Estradiol vaginal cream (0.1mg/gm) (2–4 g daily PV for 1–2 weeks; then 1 g PV daily or less frequently) CEE vaginal cream (0.625 mg/gm) (0.5–2 g daily PV; consider 3 weeks on, 1 week off; may be able to decrease frequency of use over time) Estradiol 2, 12.4, 24.8 mg vaginal rings (1 ring PV every 3 months)	15–60 mg 3 times daily	40–80 mg/day in one or two doses (optimal regimen from a tolerability perspective is 20 mg twice daily for 2 weeks, then titrate to 40 mg twice daily)
Kinetics	Use local route to minimize systemic BA and side effects Estradiol less likely to be absorbed; CEE 1 mg or more daily sufficiently absorbed to cause systemic side effects	Less than 1% of dose is metabolized (inactive metabolites) Primarily renal elimination of unchanged drug Would not expect hepatic impairment to have an effect (no data) Expect significant effect if renal impairment and no effect if advanced age (beyond decreased CrCl with age) (no data)	Extensive metabolism via CYP 2D6 and 1A2 (inactive metabolites) Not altered in advanced age, mild to moderate renal impairment (CrCl 31–80 mL/min [0.51–1.34 mL/s]), mild hepatic impairment (Child-Pugh A) Significantly altered in severe renal disease (CrCl less than 30 mL/min [less than 0.50 mL/s]) and moderate hepatic impairment (Child-Pugh B) Systemic exposure to duloxetine decreased by 1/3 in smokers (dose change not recommended)
Contraindications/ precautions	Contraindications include known or suspected breast or endometrial cancer Abnormal genitourinary bleeding of unknown etiology Active thromboembolism (or history of TE associated with previous estrogen use)	Contraindications include hypertension, tachyarrhythmias, coronary artery disease, MI, cor pulmonale, hyperthyroidism, renal failure, narrow-angle glaucoma	Multiple drug–drug interactions possible with CYP 2D6 and 1A2 substrates/ inhibitors Avoid if CrCl less than 30 mL/min (0.50 mL/s) and in all patients with hepatic disease Can raise BP Do not discontinue abruptly (withdrawal syndrome) Suicide risk even in patients without psychiatric disease Avoid in uncontrolled narrow-angle glaucoma (causes mydriasis) Hepatotoxic; avoid in alcoholics even if signs/symptoms of hepatic disease are absent

BA, bioavailability; BP, blood pressure; CEE, conjugated equine estrogens; CrCl, creatinine clearance; CYP, cytochrome P-450; DR, delayed-release; MI, myocardial infarction; PV, per vagina; TD, transdermal; TE, thromboembolism.

[a]None of these agents are FDA-approved for treatment of SUI.

use. Although still available by prescription, ephedrine is considerably more toxic than other α-adrenoceptor agonists and its use is not recommended. Although phenylephrine is now available in oral formulations, the lack of data regarding its use in SUI and the reported lack of efficacy in maximum recommended doses for rhinitis suggest that this agent should be avoided at present.

This leaves the clinician with only one practical agent to use: pseudoephedrine (Table 53–5). Side effects include hypertension, headache, dry mouth, nausea, insomnia, and restlessness.[23] ❿ *The major impediment to using the α-adrenoceptor agonist class is the extensive list of contraindications (Table 53–5). In the past, α-adrenoceptor agonist therapy was generally added to estrogen therapy* in those insufficiently improved with estrogen alone and in whom its use was not contraindicated. With the recent availability of duloxetine, treatment is now available for estrogen non- or hypo-responders whether they can or cannot take α-adrenoceptor agonists.

Duloxetine[24] Duloxetine is a selective serotonin-norepinephrine reuptake inhibitor similar pharmacologically to venlafaxine approved for the treatment of major depression, painful diabetic peripheral neuropathy, fibromyalgia, selected musculoskeletal pain states, and generalized anxiety disorder. Its use in SUI is off-label in the United States. Duloxetine enhances central serotonergic and adrenergic tone, which is involved in ascending and descending control of urethral smooth muscle and the internal urinary sphincter. Urethral and urinary sphincter smooth muscle tone during the filling phase are thus enhanced.[25,26] The pharmacokinetics, contraindications/precautions, and dosing of duloxetine are illustrated in Table 53–5.[24] Clearly, duloxetine has demonstrated modest efficacy in SUI, and a major question is its role in SUI compared with estrogen and α-adrenoceptor agonists as well as potentially curative surgery. In the absence of head-to-head clinical trial data, this is a difficult question to answer, at least for the comparison of duloxetine to α-adrenoceptor agonists. In the recent systematic review of Shamliyan et al., duloxetine improved incontinence with an effect size of 0.11 (95% CI, 0.07 to 0.14) but failed to restore continence.[10] Duloxetine is not the treatment of first choice in males with SUI after radical prostatectomy for prostate cancer, despite the availability of data from four clinical trials (one randomized and controlled, three case series).[27] ⓫ *The use of duloxetine in stress UI is complicated by (a) the potential for multiple clinically relevant drug–drug interactions with cytochrome P450 (CYP) 2D6 and 1A2 inhibitors, (b) withdrawal reactions if abruptly discontinued, (c) high rates of nausea and other side effects, (d) hepatotoxicity contraindicating its use in patients with any degree of hepatic impairment, and (e) its mild hypertensive effect. Another disconcerting finding is the high discontinuation rate when duloxetine is used in a "usual use" clinic environment (66% at 1 year, two-thirds due to adverse events and one-third due to lack of efficacy).[28]* Surgery (tension-free vaginal tape sling) was a more cost-effective therapy of SUI than duloxetine in women failing PFMR, due to the lower efficacy and high discontinuation rates with duloxetine.[29]

▶ Overflow Incontinence Due to Bladder Underactivity[4]

⓬ *In overflow UI due to atonic bladder, a trial of bethanechol may be reasonable if contraindications do not exist.* There is no established effective pharmacologic therapy for OUI due to poor bladder contractility (atonic bladder). The efficacy of the cholinomimetic bethanechol (25 to 50 mg three or four times daily) is uncertain, and,

in well-done clinical trials, it has had mixed results. In addition, its cholinomimetic effect is not urospecific, and its side effects are bothersome, including muscle and abdominal cramping, hypersalivation, diarrhea, and potentially life-threatening bradycardia and bronchospasm. α-Adrenoceptor antagonists such as silodosin, prazosin, terazosin, doxazosin, tamsulosin, and alfuzosin may benefit this condition by relaxing the bladder outflow tract and hence reducing outflow resistance. If pharmacologic therapy fails, intermittent urethral catheterization by the patient or caregiver three or four times per day is recommended. Less satisfactory alternatives include indwelling urethral or suprapubic catheters or urinary diversion.

▶ Overflow Incontinence Due to Obstruction

⓭ *In overflow UI due to obstruction, the goal of treatment is to relieve the obstruction.*

▶ Mixed Urinary Incontinence

Mixed urinary incontinence (MUI, usually a combination of UUI plus SUI) accounts for one-third of UI cases in women. For treatment to be considered successful, both components of the problem must be improved. Often, one component will be dominant. In such patients, a reasonable approach is a combination of lifestyle modifications and PFMR (the foundation of treatment for the individual UI types) with pharmacotherapy appropriate to the dominant type of UI (anticholinergics in UUI-predominant MUI and duloxetine or, perhaps, local estrogen and oral α-adrenoceptor agonist in SUI-predominant MUI). In some patients, the less dominant form of UI may respond, but usually not to a degree that is considered adequate by the patient. Most experts feel that SUI-predominant MUI is best treated initially using the nonpharmacologic approach just outlined plus anti-SUI surgery. Unfortunately, SUI success rates with surgery are lower in this patient subgroup compared with patients having pure SUI. In addition, the urge component may get better, stay the same, or get worse after surgery. There is no a priori way to predict the response in a given individual.[30,31]

In UUI-predominant MUI, little improvement can be expected in the SUI symptoms with anticholinergic therapy alone. Local estrogens improve the frequency and urgency symptoms of UUI but are thought to have no effect on the nocturia and incontinence symptoms. However, the latest Cochrane review suggests that local estrogens may actually improve incontinence (relative risk, 0.74; 95% CI, 0.64 to 0.86), with reductions in the numbers of micturitions, frequency episodes, and urgency episodes per day.[22] The prolongation in the interval between micturitions in pilot research in UUI patients suggests that duloxetine may help the UUI component as well. It should be emphasized that comparative trials of anticholinergic monotherapy versus anticholinergic plus local estrogen or duloxetine combination therapies have not been conducted.[30,31]

OUTCOME EVALUATION

- Monitor the patient for symptom relief. Have the desired outcomes jointly developed by the healthcare team and the patient/caregiver been achieved? If so, to what degree? Inspect the daily diary completed by the patient/caregiver since the last clinic visit and quantitate the clinical response (e.g., number of micturitions, number of incontinence episodes, and pad use). If a diary has not been used, ask the patient how many incontinence pads have been used and how they have been doing in terms of "accidents" since the last visit. If appropriate, administer a short-form instrument used to measure symptom impact and condition-specific quality of life and compare with previous result(s).

- Elicit adverse effects of drug therapy using a non-leading approach and ask the patient/caregiver to judge their severity and what measures, if any, the patient/caregiver used to ameliorate them. Assess adherence (ask patient/caregiver about missed doses or do a pill count if the prescription container was brought to the visit).

- The balance of clinical response and tolerability will dictate the approach to adjusting drug dosage. Potential approaches include dosage increase, maintenance, or decrease. If adverse effects are quite bothersome to the patient and patient safety and/or adherence are compromised, stop, or taper, the offender and initiate another drug option.

PEDIATRIC ENURESIS

INTRODUCTION

Pediatric enuresis is not a disease but a symptom, which can present alone or at the same time as other disorders, in children and adolescents. It is defined as the repeated voiding of urine into bed or clothes at least twice a week for at least 3 consecutive months in a child at least 5 years old (per the *Diagnostic and Statistical Manual of Mental Disorders*, 4th ed., Text Revision).[32,33] Enuresis can still be present even if the above frequency and duration parameters are not met, provided that associated distress or functional impairment exists. The terms "nocturnal" and "diurnal" refer to periods during sleep and while awake, respectively. Primary enuresis refers to a process wherein the patient has never been consistently dry throughout the night. Secondary enuresis refers to a process wherein the patient has resumed wetting after a period of dryness of at least 6 months in duration. Lastly, monosymptomatic and polysymptomatic enuresis should be differentiated. Monosymptomatic enuresis refers

Patient Care and Monitoring: UI

1. Identify urinary symptoms and assess their severity. Identify exacerbating factors and complications that may be related to UI. Based on patient factors, determine whether patient-directed therapy and/or triage to physician are required.

2. Review concurrent medical conditions and assess whether or not urinary symptoms could be disease-related.

3. Obtain a thorough medication history, including use of prescription, nonprescription, and complementary/alternative drug products. Determine which, if any, treatments in the past had been helpful as judged by the patient. Assess whether or not urinary symptoms could be related to drug use.

4. Educate the patient on lifestyle modifications that may improve symptoms: smoking cessation (for patients with cough-induced SUI), weight reduction (for those patients with SUI and UUI), prevention of constipation in patients at risk, caffeine reduction, and modification of diet and fluid intake (e.g., timing and quantity of fluid intake and avoidance of foods or beverages that worsen UI).

5. Evaluate whether or not the patient is taking an appropriate regimen (drug choice, dosage) for his or her type(s) of UI. If not, why?

6. Develop a plan to assess efficacy after a minimum of 4 weeks.

7. Assess changes in quality of life (physical, psychological, social functioning, and well-being).

8. Evaluate the patient for medication adherence, drug-related adverse events, allergies, and drug interactions with concomitant medications or disease states.

9. In cognitively intact elderly patients, focus communications to elicit the preferences of the patient, not those of potential proxies.

10. Stress the importance of adherence with the prescribed regimen, including lifestyle modifications. Recommend the most "patient-friendly" treatment regimen possible.

11. Provide patient education regarding the disease state, lifestyle modifications, and drug therapy:

    - Causes of UI and suggested interventions (see 2 and 4 above)

    - Possible UI complications

    - Timing of medication intake

    - Potential adverse events (limit to most frequent and/or clinically relevant)

    - Potential drug–drug or drug–disease interactions

to wetting at nighttime with no other urinary tract and no daytime symptoms. Polysymptomatic enuresis refers to wetting at nighttime associated with other urinary tract symptoms (e.g., urge or frequency without any other urinary symptoms) and daytime symptoms as well.

Enuresis is not a benign disorder that children will just "grow out of." Emotional and/or physical abuse of the child by adult caregivers lead to secondary problems such as chronic anxiety, low self-esteem, and delayed developmental milestones such as attending camp or going on "sleepovers" at the homes of friends. The emotional and developmental damage produced by enuresis may be more significant to the child than the enuresis itself.

EPIDEMIOLOGY AND ETIOLOGY

Five to seven million children and adolescents in the United States suffer from nocturnal enuresis. Primary enuresis is twice as common as secondary enuresis. Enuresis is twice as common in boys as compared with girls. The incidence of enuresis varies as a function of age[32,33]:

- 40% in 3-year-olds
- 12% to 25% in 4-year-olds
- 15% to 20% in 5-year-olds
- 10% in 6-year-olds
- 6% to 10% in 7- and 8-year-olds
- 5% in 10-year-olds
- 2% to 3% in 12-year-olds
- 1% to 3% in adolescents
- 0.5% in adults

Five to ten percent of children with enuresis will suffer from the condition as adults. It may also predispose to UUI in adults. In the enuretic population, 80% to 85% are monosymptomatic, 5% to 10% are polysymptomatic, and less than 5% have an organic cause. The spontaneous annual cure rate (i.e., restoration of continence) ranges from 14% to 16% (exception: at about 4 or 5 years of age, it may be as high as 30%).

Patient Encounter 2, Part 1

A 9-year-old female is brought into your clinic, her mother seeking advice regarding her daughter's frequent (2 to 3 nights/week) bedwetting and whether there are any nonprescription therapies that would help. After questioning both individuals separately, you determine that the child has had this problem for almost a year. It began shortly after her parent's acrimonious divorce was settled.

What should you do at this point?

The etiology of enuresis is poorly understood, but there is a clear genetic link. The incidence in children from families in whom there are no members with enuresis, where one parent had enuresis as a child, and where both parents had enuresis as children are 14%, 44%, and 77%, respectively. Loci for enuresis have been located on chromosomes 12, 13, and 22. Sleep disorders are not considered major contributors, with the exception of sleep apnea. Enuresis occurs in all sleep stages in proportion to the time spent in each stage. However, a small proportion of individuals are not aroused from sleep by bladder distention and have uninhibited bladder contractions preceding enuresis.

PATHOPHYSIOLOGY

There are potentially treatable organic causes of enuresis, as outlined in Table 53–6. However, the vast majority of children with enuresis have normal urodynamics, including nocturnal bladder capacity. Functional bladder capacity can be estimated using the formula: age in years +2 equals the ounces of capacity. In some children, there appears to be a relationship between developmental immaturity (motor and language milestones) and enuresis, but the mechanism is unknown. There is evidence that affected individuals have an attenuated vasopressin circadian rhythm (females more so than males) with lower vasopressin plasma concentrations.[34] Other contributors include detrusor overactivity at night and an increased threshold for arousal. Drugs like lithium, clozapine, risperidone, valproic acid, selective serotonin reuptake inhibitors, and theophylline can rarely cause and aggravate enuresis. However, caffeine ingestion does not correlate with enuresis (r = 0.05, p = NS).[35] Psychological factors are clearly contributory in only a minority of individuals. The most frequent example of this is secondary enuresis precipitated by a stressor such as divorce, school trauma, sexual abuse, or hospitalization. In rare cases, the family may be so dysfunctional that the child has never been properly toilet-trained.

Table 53–6

Major Potentially Treatable Organic Causes of Enuresis

Potentially Treatable by Surgery
- Ectopic ureter
- Lower UTI (correct congenital anomalies)
- Neurogenic bladder
- Bladder calculus (stone) or foreign body
- Obstructive sleep apnea

Potentially Treatable by Drugs
- UTI
- Diabetes mellitus
- Diabetes insipidus
- Fecal impaction
- Constipation

UTI, urinary tract infection.

CLINICAL PRESENTATION AND DIAGNOSIS

Clinical Presentation and Diagnosis: Pediatric Enuresis

Proper assessment of the child or adolescent with enuresis should explore every aspect of UI, especially the genitourinary and nervous systems. The minimum assessment should include[41,42,50]:

- Interview of child and parent(s), being sensitive to the emotional consequences of the enuresis.

- Direct physical examination, looking for enlarged adenoids/tonsils, bladder distention, fecal impaction, abnormal genitalia, spinal cord anomalies, and abnormal neurologic signs (look for an organic cause amenable to surgery or drugs; see **Table 53–6**).

- Obtain a urinalysis for sugar, protein, WBC, or leukocyte esterase (consider a urine culture at the same time if urinalysis is positive or has symptoms consistent with urinary tract infection).

- A 7 or more day diary of wet and dry nights prior to intervention is useful in that it can be used to monitor the response to treatment. A first-morning urine specific gravity may help to predict response to DDAVP therapy. Polysymptomatic presentation may require a more elaborate workup, including voiding cystourethrogram, renal and/or bladder ultrasound, urodynamics, and sleep studies.

Patient Encounter 2, Part 2: Medical History, Physical Examination, Diagnostic Tests, and Creating a Care Plan

PMH: Unremarkable pregnancy/delivery. All developmental milestones within normal limits. Three episodes of AOM treated with no sequelae. Current on all immunizations

FH, SH: Acrimonious divorce of parents 1 year prior, o/w noncontributory

Meds: None

ROS: (+) nocturnal incontinence 2 or 3 nights/week; (–) vaginal itching, UTIs, urgency, frequency, dysuria, lower abdominal fullness

PE:

VS: BP 90/65 mm Hg, P 72 beats/min, RR 16 breaths/min, T 37.0°C (98.6°F)

Resp: WNL

CV: WNL

Abd: Soft, nontender, nondistended; (+) bowel sounds; bladder not palpable

Neuro: WNL (gross sensory, motor, reflexes)

GU, Rectal: Deferred

Labs: Urinalysis WNL

Given this additional information, what is your assessment of this patient's condition?

Identify your treatment goals for this patient.

What nonpharmacologic and pharmacologic alternatives are available to the patient?

What initial treatment would you suggest?

TREATMENT

Desired Outcomes

- Restoration of continence, which may not initially be a realistic outcome

- Reduction in the number of enuresis episodes

- Prevention or amelioration of disease complications, including adverse psychological effects on the patient and caregivers or delay in developmental milestones

- Avoidance or prevention of adverse treatment effects

- Minimization of treatment costs

- Improvement in the patient's and caregivers' quality of life

General Approach to Treatment

Treatment is guided by the findings of the patient assessment. Daytime wetting, abnormal voiding such as unusual posturing, discomfort, straining, or poor stream, history of recurrent UTIs, and abnormalities of the genitalia suggest the need for referral to a urologist. In the rare circumstance of a true psychological cause, individual and/or family psychotherapy and crisis intervention are recommended.

In the absence of an identified cause and comorbidities, monosymptomatic nocturnal enuresis is present, which can be amenable to nonpharmacologic and pharmacologic therapies (**Fig. 53–1**). Nonpharmacologic therapy should be utilized initially, provided that the patient and family are sufficiently motivated. Use of one nonpharmacologic method at a time is reasonable, provided that each is given an adequate trial period. If response is suboptimal after 6 months, a different method should be substituted or added. There is some evidence to justify combination therapy. There is no consensus as to when pharmacologic therapy should be added to or substituted for nonpharmacologic therapy. ⑭ *Considering that pharmacotherapy is inferior to select nonpharmacologic treatment modalities in pediatric enuresis, pharmacotherapy will be most valuable in patients who are not candidates for nonpharmacologic therapy due to nonadherence or who do not achieve the desired outcomes on nonpharmacologic therapy alone.*

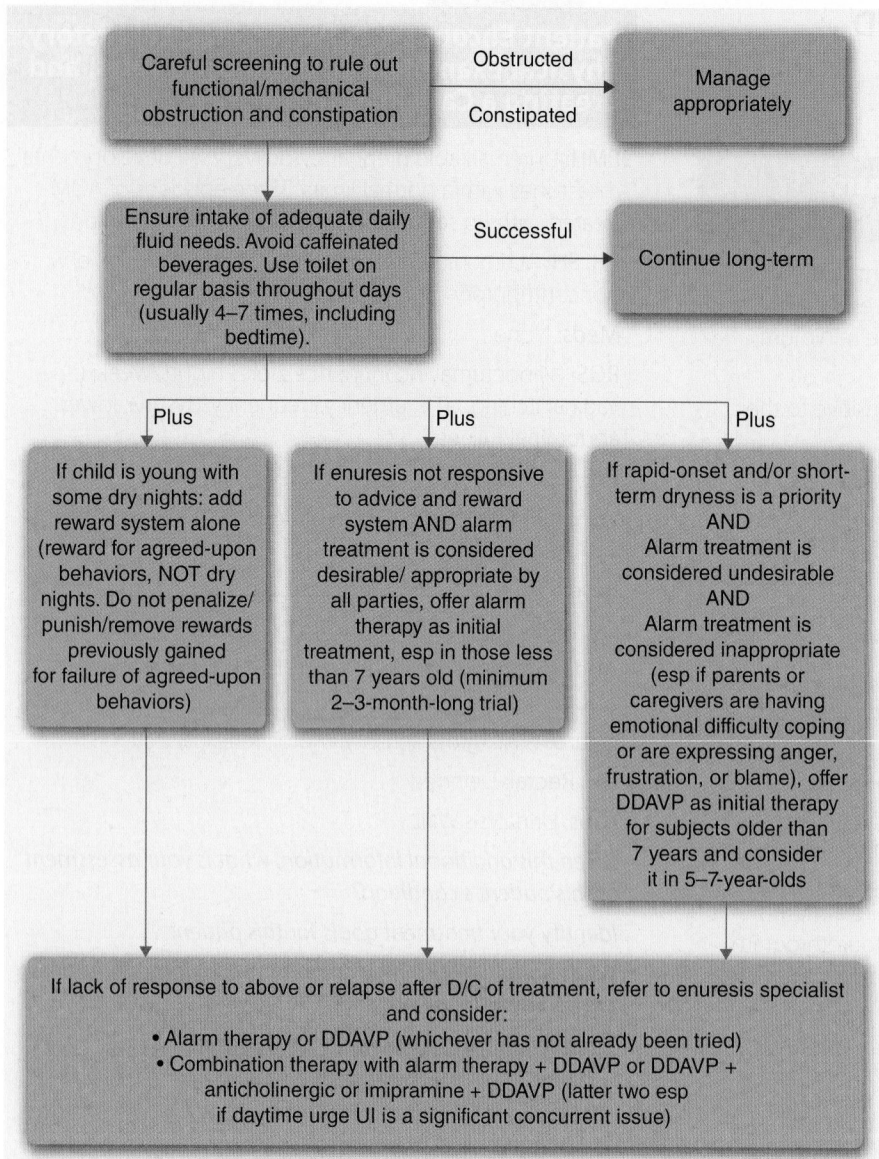

FIGURE 53–1. Enuresis treatment protocol. (DDAVP, desmopressin; HS, at bedtime; D/C, discontinuation; UI, urinary incontinence.) (Modified from Nunes VD, O'Flynn N, Evans J, Sawyer L; Guideline Development Group. Management of bedwetting in children and young people: summary of NICE guidance. BMJ 2010; 341:c5399.)

In the figure:

- Careful screening to rule out functional/mechanical obstruction and constipation → Obstructed / Constipated → Manage appropriately
- Ensure intake of adequate daily fluid needs. Avoid caffeinated beverages. Use toilet on regular basis throughout days (usually 4–7 times, including bedtime). → Successful → Continue long-term
- **Plus** — If child is young with some dry nights: add reward system alone (reward for agreed-upon behaviors, NOT dry nights. Do not penalize/punish/remove rewards previously gained for failure of agreed-upon behaviors)
- **Plus** — If enuresis not responsive to advice and reward system AND alarm treatment is considered desirable/appropriate by all parties, offer alarm therapy as initial treatment, esp in those less than 7 years old (minimum 2–3-month-long trial)
- **Plus** — If rapid-onset and/or short-term dryness is a priority AND Alarm treatment is considered undesirable AND Alarm treatment is considered inappropriate (esp if parents or caregivers are having emotional difficulty coping or are expressing anger, frustration, or blame), offer DDAVP as initial therapy for subjects older than 7 years and consider it in 5–7-year-olds
- If lack of response to above or relapse after D/C of treatment, refer to enuresis specialist and consider:
  - Alarm therapy or DDAVP (whichever has not already been tried)
  - Combination therapy with alarm therapy + DDAVP or DDAVP + anticholinergic or imipramine + DDAVP (latter two esp if daytime urge UI is a significant concurrent issue)

▶ Nonpharmacologic Treatment[36]

The standard first-line therapy is supportive in nature. This involves education about the condition, demystification, and assurance that the parents do not punish the child for enuresis. Journal keeping, fluid restriction, and nighttime awakenings of the child to preempt "accidents" make for a high level of caregiver involvement. The behavioral treatments of enuresis are explained in Table 53–7. Alarms, overlearning, and dry-bed training are the most complex and effective nonpharmacologic treatments available and compare favorably to pharmacologic therapy. A 3- to 6-month trial is recommended. Once dryness is achieved, relapse rates are low. In addition, adding alarm therapy to pharmacologic therapy can be an effective approach in partial or nonresponders to pharmacologic therapy alone. The converse applies as well.[37,38]

Measures that *do not* help or are of questionable value include:

- Bladder stretching exercises (done by delaying voiding despite the urge to do so)
- Hypnotherapy
- Dietary changes
- Desensitization to allergens
- Acupuncture[39]
- Chiropractic

▶ Pharmacologic Treatment

The two primary agents used to treat enuresis are DDAVP and imipramine (Table 53–8). ⑮ *DDAVP is the drug of choice in pediatric enuresis.* Anticholinergics have a limited role (Table 53–8). Other agents have been studied with inconclusive results.[40]

Table 53–7

Behavioral Treatments for Enuresis

Lifting	Procedure wherein the caregiver takes the child to the toilet at regular intervals during the night to urinate without fully awakening him or her
Night awakening	Procedure wherein the caregiver fully awakens the child to void shortly before he or she would usually have wet the bed; once the child is consistently dry, the frequency of awakening drops or (for single awakenings) the time of awakening is gradually moved to earlier in the night (i.e., closer to bedtime) until the child is dry when awakened 1 hour after going to bed
Alarm	An alarm device and a moisture-sensitive sensor are used in combination, with the sensor being placed under the sheets, or more commonly, attached to the child's pajamas or underwear near the urethra
Overlearning	This is commenced at a minimum of 2 weeks after the alarm has rendered the child dry; the child drinks 500 mL (about 16 oz) during the hour before going to bed; alarm use is continued until he or she is dry for 14 consecutive nights with the extra fluid intake; is used to reduce relapse rates seen with alarm use alone
Dry-bed training	This begins with an intensive first night of training that involves increased fluid consumption, hourly awakenings, praise when the bed is dry at hourly awakenings, and, when the alarm goes off, a mild reprimand and cleanliness training (child changes wet clothes and bed linens, remakes the bed, resets the alarm); before going to bed and after each wetting, the child engages in 20 practice trials of appropriate toileting (i.e., positive practice): for each practice trial, the child lies in bed, counts to 50, arises and attempts to urinate in the toilet, then returns to bed; on subsequent nights, child is woken only once, usually about 3 hours after the child has gone to bed; after a dry night, the night awakening moves up 30 minutes earlier; it is discontinued when it is scheduled to occur 1 hour after bedtime; after 7 consecutive dry nights, the alarm is discontinued, but is reinstated if two episodes of wetting occur in a 1-week period

Desmopressin[41] A synthetic analogue of ADH, DDAVP was first studied in enuresis in the 1970s. It was approved by the FDA in 1990 for the treatment of nocturnal enuresis in children at least 6 years of age. It decreases the number of wet nights per week by a mean of 1.34. The between-study variability in response to DDAVP is quite large, with a frequency of wetting ranging from 10% to 91% of patients. Only 25% to 30% become completely dry on the drug, whereas an additional 25% to 30% have a partial response. Response is dose-independent for the nasal formulation (20 = 40 = 60 mcg); however, 20 mcg is the minimum dose resulting in therapeutic benefit. Response is dose-dependent for the oral formulation (e.g., the number of wet nights fell 27%, 30%, and 40% with 0.2-, 0.4-, and 0.6-mg doses, compared with 10% with placebo in one study). Benefit exists only as long as the patient takes DDAVP, with relapse rates of up to 94% after discontinuation. Insufficient data are available to judge the relative efficacies of the two formulations. DDAVP appears to work better with monosymptomatic versus polysymptomatic enuresis and in the presence of nocturnal polyuria with a normal voided volume. The oral route is generally preferred since nasal congestion and sinusitis can reduce the bioavailability (BA) of the nasal formulation. DDAVP is an ideal agent for rapid-onset, short-term use such as attendance at camp or going on a "sleepover." If the desire is for long-term therapy and if it is sufficiently effective short term, a 3- to 6-month trial is reasonable. At the end of this period, the drug should be tapered off by 0.1 mg (oral) or 10 mcg (nasal) per month. Relapse is less likely with a tapered withdrawal compared with an abrupt discontinuation. The following factors should be considered in individuals with partial responses to DDAVP: suboptimal dosing, poor adherence, poor BA (change nasal to oral preparation), and poor fluid/dietary habits (i.e., fluid restriction and high protein intake during the day and liberal salt and fluid intake after suppertime).[42] In individuals with presumed DDAVP resistance (i.e., poor response to usual doses or deterioration after a good response has been established), oral furosemide 0.5 mg/kg in the early morning may be useful. Furosemide works by reversing the abnormal circadian rhythm of renal tubular sodium handling, which is common in such individuals.[43] In 12 patients with DDAVP-resistant enuresis, furosemide 0.5 mg/kg once daily in the morning was added to DDAVP therapy. In 9 of 12 (75%), enuresis events were reduced to less than one wet night per month. In the remaining three patients,

Table 53–8

Dosing of Pharmacologic Treatments of Enuresis

Desmopressin	Nasal: Start with 10 mcg 1 hour before bedtime and titrate upward in 10 mcg increments every week to a maximum of 40 mcg/day Oral: Start with 0.2 mg 1 hour before bedtime and titrate upward in 0.1 mg increments every week to a maximum of 0.6 mg/day
Imipramine	Start with 1 mg/kg/day (approximately 25 mg in 5- to 8-year-olds and 50 mg in older children and adolescents). Add desmopressin to augment efficacy. Only titrate in 0.5 mg/kg/day increments every 2 weeks to a maximum of 2.5 mg/kg/day if low-dose imipramine plus desmopressin combination is suboptimally effective
Anticholinergics	Refer to Table 53–4

although events were reduced from baseline (7 wet nights/week), they were still wet 2, 3, and 6 nights per week. Two of these three patients exhibited signs/symptoms of overactive bladder, and one of the two patients had to discontinue furosemide therapy due to the increased frequency of daytime symptoms.[43] With this exception, diuretics play little role in the treatment of enuresis.[43,44] Side effects to DDAVP are minor and infrequent.[45] The most serious complication, water intoxication, is extremely uncommon when DDAVP is used to treat enuresis, with only 48 reported cases, all due to the nasal formulation.[45] However, electrolyte monitoring is recommended if intercurrent illness complicates the situation. Children should also not drink more than 8 ounces (about 240 mL) of fluid at suppertime, 8 ounces (240 mL) in the evening, and none in the 2 hours prior to bed in order to reduce the risk of water intoxication.

Imipramine[46] The TCA imipramine was first used in the treatment of enuresis in the 1960s. Although trials involving other TCAs have been performed over the years, there is insufficient evidence to assess the relative performance of these agents versus imipramine, and the latter is considered the gold standard TCA in enuresis management. Its mechanism of action is unclear, although it is an anticholinergic and antispasmodic and may increase plasma ADH concentrations. About 50% of unselected patients may respond. A patient can expect approximately one less wet night per week with imipramine use. As with DDAVP, benefit only occurs as long as the drug is being taken, with relapse rates after discontinuation of therapy of up to 50%. There is no significant correlation of drug concentration with response. The usual imipramine dosage is 25 to 50 mg at bedtime, with the latter dose being used in patients greater than 9 years old. After 1 month of therapy, if some response can be discerned, DDAVP at the usual dosage should be added (but only if fluid intake can be restricted). If this combination therapy proves successful, the clinician can taper imipramine to the lowest effective dose and attempt drug holidays of 2 weeks in duration every third month to reduce the otherwise high risk of tolerance. There is a high frequency of neurologic side effects in children, including lethargy, dizziness, and headache in 5%; irritability in 11%; and anxiety in 10%; and sleep disturbances in 16%.[45] GI symptoms occur in about 25% of pediatric patients.[45] It is due to these adverse event/safety issues that imipramine has been relegated to third-line treatment status.

Anticholinergics Oxybutynin and related agents (see adult UI section of this chapter) should be used only if the patient has concurrent daytime urgency or frequency. Before adding these agents, the presence of postvoid residual urine, dysfunctional micturition, and low micturition frequency must be ruled out using frequency/volume diary, uroflowmetry, and bladder ultrasound assessments. Usual initial doses of oxybutynin and tolterodine are 5 mg and 2 mg at bedtime, respectively, and these doses can be doubled, if necessary. Maximal therapeutic effects are seen within 2 months and sometimes much sooner. Major adverse

events to be avoided include urinary retention (leads to urinary tract infections) and constipation (worsens urinary tract dysfunction). Combination therapy with DDAVP may also be worthwhile in patients refractory to combinations incorporating alarm therapy, DDAVP, and/or imipramine.

Comparison of Therapies Most of the comparisons between treatments have been made by means of meta-analyses conducted by the Cochrane Enuresis Collaborative.[40,41,46-48] Unfortunately, most enuresis treatment studies have been so poorly designed that they compromise the ability to pool studies for meta-analysis. With this in mind, the comparative efficacies of monotherapy and combination therapies using the best data available follow.

The most effective nonpharmacologic method is the use of bed alarms. Defining success as less than 1 wet night per month, the initial success rate for alarms is 66%, with long-term success after discontinuation occurring in 45% (versus 1% with no treatment). However, this method requires highly motivated families, and the development of improvement is slow (over 4 to 12 or more weeks). Data are inadequate to compare the various commercial brands of alarms available to consumers or to compare alarms to other behavioral interventions. Supplementing this method with either overlearning or dry-bed training significantly reduces the already low relapse rates seen with alarms. Alarm therapy is also significantly more effective than DDAVP, evaluated at both the end of therapy and long-term. However, a recent trial documented the equi-effectiveness of DDAVP and alarm therapy, both as primary and secondary therapies. As documented previously, relapse rates were significantly lower with alarm therapy.[49] Similar findings are noted for the alarm-versus-imipramine comparison. There are conflicting data regarding the value of supplementing the alarm method with DDAVP.

The year 2010 saw the introduction of the revised International Children's Continence Society (ICCS) and the National Institute for Health and Clinical Excellence (NICE) (UK) guidelines for the diagnosis and management of monosymptomatic nocturnal enuresis.[33,50] The algorithm (Fig. 53–1) within the NICE guideline is inclusive of the most potentially useful treatments and distinguishes approaches based on the child's age, maturity, and abilities; the frequency of enuresis; and the motivation and needs of the family.[50]

OUTCOME EVALUATION

• Monitor the patient for symptom relief. Have the desired outcomes jointly developed by the healthcare team, the patient, and his or her parents/guardians been achieved and to what degree? Evaluate the daily diary completed by the patient or parents/guardians since the last clinic visit and quantitate the clinical response (the number of dry nights versus the total number of nights, and the frequency of nights with greater than or equal to two enuresis episodes). If a diary has not been used,

Patient Care and Monitoring: Pediatric Enuresis

1. Assess the patient's symptoms to determine whether or not patient-directed therapy is appropriate or whether or not the patient should be evaluated by a physician. Assessment includes the types and severities of symptoms and the presence or absence of exacerbating factors. Does the patient have any enuresis-related complications?

2. Review any available diagnostic data to determine disease status.

3. Obtain a thorough medication history, including use of prescription, nonprescription, and complementary and alternative drug products. Determine which, if any, treatments in the past had been helpful as judged by the patient and/or caregiver(s). Could any of the patient's current medications be contributing to enuresis?

4. Educate the patient and/or caregiver(s) on lifestyle modifications that may improve symptoms or assist the clinician in monitoring the responses to therapy, including but not limited to, fluid restriction and journal keeping. The patient and/or caregiver(s) should be referred to local enuresis clinics (if available) for training in nonpharmacologic treatments such as use of bed alarms, overlearning, and dry-bed training.

5. Is the patient taking the appropriate drug(s) for his or her enuresis? Is/are the dose(s) appropriate? If no (to either question), why?

6. Develop a plan to assess efficacy after a minimum of 3 months.

7. Assess changes in quality of life (physical, psychological, and social functioning and well-being).

8. Evaluate the patient for drug-related adverse events, allergies, and interactions (drug–drug and drug–disease).

9. Stress the importance of adherence with the prescribed regimen, including lifestyle modifications and nonpharmacologic treatment. Recommend the most "patient-friendly" treatment regimen possible.

10. Provide the patient and/or caregiver(s) with education regarding the disease state, lifestyle modifications, and drug therapy:

    - The causes of enuresis and what things the patient and/or caregiver(s) can do to reduce its frequency

    - Possible enuresis complications

    - Timing of medication intake

    - Potential adverse events (limit to most frequent and/or clinically relevant)

    - Potential drug–drug interactions

elicit the clinical response, in general terms, since the last visit.

- Elicit adverse events of therapy in a nonleading manner, and ask the patient to judge their severity. Ask the patient or parents/guardians what measures if any were used to ameliorate them. Assess adherence (ask patient or parents/guardians about missed doses; do pill counts if the prescription vial is available).

- The balance of clinical response, tolerability, and burden on the family will dictate the approach to management. As most nonpharmacologic approaches are "all or none" and drug dosages after an initial titration period are fixed, the major decision process involves either changing therapy if clinical results are inadequate or beginning or continuing tapering-off and discontinuation of therapy after success. There is no consensus on which treatment approach to withdraw first, although the ICCS recommends the nonpharmacologic (alarm) therapy first, then pharmacologic (DDAVP) therapy.[33]

Abbreviations Introduced in This Chapter

ADH	Antidiuretic hormone
BA	Bioavailability
CAM	Complementary and alternative medicine
CL	Total body clearance
CrCl	Creatinine clearance
CVA	Costovertebral angle
CYP	Cytochrome P-450
DDAVP	Desmopressin
DHIC	Detrusor hyperactivity with impaired contractility
ER	Extended release
ICCS	International Children's Continence Society
IIQ	Incontinence Impact Questionnaire
IR	Immediate release
LA	Long acting
MESNA	Sodium 2-mercaptoethanesulfonate
OTC	Over the counter
OUI	Overflow urinary incontinence
PV	Per vagina
SNF	Skilled nursing facility
SR	Sustained release
SUI	Stress urinary incontinence
TCA	Tricyclic antidepressant
TD	Transdermal
UDI	Urogenital Distress Inventory
UI	Urinary incontinence
UTI	Urinary tract infection
UUI	Urge urinary incontinence

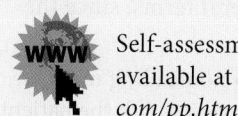 Self-assessment questions and answers are available at *http://mhpharmacotherapy.com/pp.html.*

REFERENCES

1. Abrams P, Cardozo L, Fall M, et al. The standardization of terminology of lower urinary tract function: Report from the standardization sub-committee of the International Continence Society. Neurourol Urodyn 2002;21:167–178.

2. Arnold EP, Burgio K, Diokno AC, et al. Epidemiology and natural history of urinary incontinence (UI). In: Abrams P, Khoury S, Wein AJ, eds. Incontinence. Plymouth, UK: Plymbridge Distributors; 1999:199–226.

3. Brown JS, Nyberg LM, Kusek JW, et al. Proceedings of the National Institute of Diabetes, Digestive and Kidney Diseases International Symposium on Epidemiologic Issues in Urinary Incontinence in Women. Am J Obstet Gynecol 2003;188:S77–S88.

4. Rovner ES, Wyman J, Lackner T, Guay DRP. Urinary Incontinence. In: DiPiro J, Talbert R, Hayes P, Yee G, Matzke G, Posey LM, eds. Pharmacotherapy: A Pathophysiologic Approach. 7th ed. New York: McGraw-Hill; 2008:1399–1415.

5. Groutz A, Gordon D, Keidar R, et al. Stress urinary incontinence: Prevalence among nulliparous compared with primiparous and grand multiparous premenopausal women. Neurourol Urodyn 1999;18:419–425.

6. Homma Y, Yoshida M, Seki N, et al. Symptom assessment tool for overactive bladder syndrome—overactive bladder symptom score. Urology 2006; 68:318–323.

7. Abrams P, Cardozo L, Khoury S, Wein A, eds. Incontinence. Second International Consultation on Incontinence. 2nd ed. Plymouth, UK: Health Publications Ltd; 2002.

8. Kafri R, Langer R, Dvir Z, et al. Rehabilitation vs drug therapy for urge urinary incontinence: Short-term outcome. Int Urogynecol J 2007;18:407–411.

9. Kafri R, Shames J, Raz M, et al. Rehabilitation versus drug therapy for urge urinary incontinence: Long-term outcomes. Int Urogynecol J Pelvic Floor Dyfunet 2008;19:47–52.

10. Shamliyan TA, Kane RL, Wyman J, et al. Systematic review: Randomized, controlled trials of nonsurgical treatments for urinary incontinence in women. Ann Intern Med 2008;148:459–473.

11. Chapple C, Khullar V, Gabriel Z, Dooley JA. The effects of antimuscarinic treatments in overactive bladder: A systematic review and meta-analysis. Eur Urol 2005;48:5–26.

12. Novara G, Balfano A, Secco S, et al. A systematic review and meta-analysis of randomized controlled trials with antimuscarinic drugs for overactive bladder. Eur Urol 2008;54:740–763.

13. Lam S, Hilas O. Pharmacologic management of overactive bladder. Clin Intervent Aging 2007; 2:337–345.

14. Guay DRP. Drug forecast: Solifenacin (VESIcare): An investigational anticholinergic for overactive bladder. Consult Pharm 2004;19:437–444.

15. Guay DRP. Trospium chloride: An update on a quaternary anticholinergic for treatment of urge urinary incontinence. Ther Clin Risk Manag 2005;1:157–166.

16. Guay DRP. Darifenacin: Another antimuscarinic for overactive bladder. Consult Pharm 2005;20:424–431.

17. Todorova A, Vonderheid-Guth B, Dimpfel W. Effects of tolterodine, trospium chloride, and oxybutynin on the central nervous system. J Clin Pharmacol 2001; 41:636–644.

18. Meek PD, Evang SD, Tadrous M, Roux-Lirange D. Overactive bladder drugs and constipation: A meta-analysis of randomized, placebo-controlled trials. Dig Dis Sci 2011;56:7–18.

19. Sink KM, Thomas J 3rd, Xu H, et al. Dual use of bladder anticholinergics and cholinesterase inhibitors: Long-term functional and cognitive outcomes. J Am Geriatr Soc 2008;56:847–853.

20. Peyromaure M, Ravery V, Boccon-Gibod L. The management of stress urinary incontinence after radical prostatectomy. BJU Int 2002;90:155–161.

21. Filcamo MT, LiMarzi V, DelPopolo G, et al. Pharmacologic treatment in postprostatectomy stress urinary incontinence. Eur Urol 2007;51:1559–1564.

22. Ewiles AA, Althally F. Topical vaginal estrogen therapy in managing postmenopausal urinary symptoom: A reality or a gimmick? Climacteric 2010;13:405–418.

23. Owens RG, Karram MM. Comparative tolerability of drug therapies used to treat incontinence and enuresis. Drug Saf 1998;2:123–139.

24. Guay DRP. Duloxetine. The first therapy licensed for stress urinary incontinence. Am J Geriatr Pharmacother 2005;3:25–38.

25. Fraser MO, Chancellor MB. Neural control of the urethra and development of pharmacotherapy for stress urinary incontinence. BJU Int 2003;91:743–748.

26. Burgard EC, Fraser MO, Thor KB. Serotonergic modulation of bladder afferent pathways. Urology 2003;62(Suppl 1):10–15.

27. Gajewski J, Drake MJ, Oelke M. Post-prostatectomy stress urinary incontinence: What treatment for which patient? Neurourol Urodyn 2010;29:679–683.

28. Duckett JR, Vella M, Kavalakuntla G, et al. Tolerability and efficacy of duloxetine in a nontrial situation. BJOG 2007;114:543–547.

29. Jacklin P, Duckett J, Renganathan A. Analytic model comparing the cost utility of TVT versus duloxetine in women with stress urinary incontinence. Int Urogynecol J 2010; 21:977–984.

30. Khullar V, Cardozo L, Dmochowski R. Mixed incontinence: Current evidence and future perspectives. Neurourol Urodyn 2010;29:618–622.

31. Murray S, Lemack GE. Overactive bladder and mixed incontinence. Curr Urol Rep 2010;11:385–392.

32. Fritz G, Rockney R, Bernet W, et al. Practice parameter for the assessment and treatment of children and adolescents with enuresis. J Am Acad Child Adolesc Psychiatry 2004;43:1540–1550.

33. Neveus T, Eggert P, Evans J, et al. Evaluation and treatment for monosymptomatic enuresis: A standardization document from the International Children's Continence Society. J Urol 2010;183:441–447.

34. Rittig S, Schaumberg HL, Siggaard C, et al. The circadian effect in plasma vasopressin and urine output is related to desmopressin response and enuresis status in children with nocturnal enuresis. J Urol 2008;179:2389–2395.

35. Warzak WJ, Evans S, Floress MT, Gross AC, Stoolman S. Caffeine consumption in young children. J Pediatr 2011;158:508–509.

36. Blum NJ. Nocturnal enuresis: Behavioral treatments. Urol Clin North Am 2004;31:499–507.

37. Vogt M, Lehnert T, Till H, Rolle U. Evaluation of different modes of combined therapy in children with monosymptomatic nocturnal enuresis. BJU Intern 2010;105:1456–1459.

38. Kwak KW, Park KH, Baek M. The efficacy of enuresis alarm treatment in pharmacotherapy-resistant nocturnal enuresis. Urology 2011;77:200–204.

39. Bower WF, Diao M. Acupuncture as a treatment for nocturnal enuresis. Auto Neurosci Basic Clin 2010;157:63–67.

40. Glazener CM, Evans JH, Peto RE. Drugs for nocturnal enuresis in children (other than desmopressin and tricyclics). Cochrane Database Syst Rev 2003;(4):CD002238.

41. Glazener CM, Evans JH. Desmopressin for nocturnal enuresis in children. Cochrane Database Syst Rev 2002;(3):CD002112.

42. Raes A, Dehoorne J, Van Laecke E, et al. Partial response to intranasal desmopressin in children with monosymptomatic nocturnal enuresis is related to persistent nocturnal polyuria on wet nights. J Urol 2007;178:1048–1052.

43. DeGuchtenaere A, Vande Walle C, Van Sintjan P, et al. Desmopressin resistant nocturnal polyuria may benefit from furosemide therapy administered in the morning. J Urol 2007;178:2635–2639.

44. Alawwa IA, Matani YS, Saleh AA, Al-Ghazo MA. A placebo-controlled trial of the effects of hydrochlorothiazide on nocturnal enuresis. Urol International 2010; 84:319–324.

45. Muller D, Roehr CC, Eggert P. Comparative tolerability of drug treatment for nocturnal enuresis in children. Drug Saf 2004;27:717–727.

46. Glazener CM, Evans JH, Peto RE. Tricyclic and related drugs for nocturnal enuresis in children. Cochrane Database Syst Rev 2003;(3):CD002117.

47. Glazener CM, Evans JH. Simple behavioural and physical interventions for nocturnal enuresis in children. Cochrane Database Syst Rev 2004;(2):CD003637.

48. Glazener CM, Evans JH, Peto RE. Complex behavioural and educational interventions for nocturnal enuresis in children. Cochrane Database Syst Rev 2004;(1):CD004668.

49. Kwak KW, Lee YS, Park KH, Baek M. Efficacy of desmopressin and enuresis alarm as first and second line treatment for primary mono-symptomatic nocturnal enuresis: Prospective randomized crossover study. J Urol 2010;184:2521–2526.

50. Nunes VD, O'Flynn N, Evans J, Sawyer L; Guideline Development Group. Management of bedwetting in children and young people: Summary of NICE guidance. BMJ 2010; 341:c5399.

54 Allergic and Pseudoallergic Drug Reactions

J. Russell May and Philip H. Smith

LEARNING OBJECTIVES

● **Upon completion of the chapter, the reader will be able to:**

1. Describe the potential incidence of allergic and pseudoallergic reactions and why it is difficult to obtain accurate numbers.

2. Describe the Gell and Coombs categories of reactions.

3. Identify the classes of drugs most commonly associated with allergic and pseudoallergic reactions.

4. Recommend specific treatment for a patient experiencing anaphylaxis.

5. Recommend an approach to drug selection in patients with multiple drug allergies.

6. Describe drug desensitization procedures for selected drugs.

KEY CONCEPTS

❶ Approximately 6% to 10% of adverse drug reactions are allergic or immunologic; however, allergic and pseudoallergic reactions represent 24% of reported adverse drug reactions in hospitalized patients. These reactions are costly and cause considerable morbidity and mortality.

❷ Allergy is an adverse immune response to a stimulus and has been traditionally placed in the Gell and Coombs categories: type I (immediate hypersensitivity), type II (complement-mediated antibody reactions), type III (immune complex reactions), and type IV (cellular or delayed-type hypersensitivity). Drug exposures often stimulate several or all of these types of reactions, and clinical symptoms do not always fit neatly into the categories. Only type I reactions may cause anaphylaxis.

❸ The well-known symptoms of immediate hypersensitivity include urticaria, rhinitis, bronchoconstriction, and anaphylaxis.

❹ Reactions that clinically resemble allergic reactions but lack an immune basis have been referred to as "pseudoallergic." They include almost the entire range of immediate hypersensitivity clinical patterns and range in significance from the alarming but trivial anxiety or vasovagal reactions caused by local dental anesthetics to potentially fatal reactions to ionic radiocontrast media.

❺ Penicillins and cephalosporins both have a β-lactam ring joined to an S-containing ring structure (penicillins, a thiazolidine ring; cephalosporins, a

dihydrothiazine ring). Because of this structural difference, the extent of cross-allergenicity appears to be relatively low. Cross-allergenicity is less likely with newer generation cephalosporins compared with the first-generation agents.

❻ Reactions to sulfonamide antibiotics, ranging from mild (most common) to life-threatening (rare), occur in 2% to 4% of healthy patients, with rates as high as 65% in patients with AIDS.

❼ IgE-mediated urticarial/angioedema reactions and anaphylaxis are associated with aspirin and nonsteroidal anti-inflammatory drugs (NSAIDs). Urticaria is the most common form of IgE-mediated reaction. However, most reactions are the result of metabolic idiosyncrasies, such as aspirin-induced respiratory disease, which may produce severe and even fatal bronchospasm. This class is second only to β-lactams in causing anaphylaxis.

❽ Radiocontrast media may cause serious immediate pseudoallergic reactions such as urticaria/angioedema, bronchospasm, shock, and death. These reactions have been reduced with the introduction of nonionic, lower osmolality products.

❾ Opiates (morphine, meperidine, codeine, hydrocodone, and others) stimulate mast cell release directly, resulting in pruritus and urticaria with occasional mild wheezing. Though these reactions are not allergic, many patients state that they are "allergic" to one or more of the opiates. Pretreatment with an antihistamine may reduce these reactions. These pseudoallergic reactions are rarely, if ever, life-threatening.

⑩ Drug desensitization is a potentially life-threatening procedure and requires continuous monitoring in a hospital setting, with suitable access to emergency treatment and intubation. It should only be undertaken under the direction of a physician with suitable training and experience and only when a suitable alternative is not available. In such hands, desensitization may present less risk than treatment failure with a less effective alternative medication.

INTRODUCTION

Allergic and pseudoallergic drug reactions are reported together. They are rarely confirmed by testing, making statistical analysis imprecise, with both over-reporting and under-reporting. ❶ *Approximately 6% to 10% of adverse drug reactions are allergic or immunologic; however, allergic and pseudoallergic reactions represent 24% of reported adverse drug reactions in hospitalized patients.*[1,2] *These reactions are costly and cause considerable morbidity and mortality.* Between 10% and 20% of hospitalized patients incur drug reactions (7% in the general population), with about one-third possibly due to hypersensitivity; however, most of these reactions are not reported, especially in pediatrics.[1,3,4] Patients experiencing an allergic drug reaction in the hospital result in increased costs of $275 to $600 million annually.[5] This financial burden can occur due to several reasons, including increased indirect cost of (a) time and lost labor; (b) the use of costlier alternative medications; and (c) treatment failures. Outpatient rates are not well studied and are much harder to collect. Relying on a patient's history without an attempt to verify the relationships between drugs taken and symptoms experienced results in confusion. Healthcare professionals and patients use the term "drug allergy" in such a general way that it is not medically useful and, further, perpetuates a level of fear and concern in the public and in medical practice that is inappropriate and costly. This same confusion and anxiety sometimes leads medical personnel to ignore or forget "drug allergy" with potentially catastrophic results. Clearly, an understanding of how allergic and pseudoallergic reactions occur and how they might be managed or prevented is important to healthcare professionals and their patients.

PATHOPHYSIOLOGY

Drug allergies are immune responses resulting from different mechanisms of immunologic recognition and activation, and reactions are produced by multiple physiologic pathways. This produces a confusing spectrum of clinical pictures and complex pathophysiologic mechanisms. ❷ *Allergy is an adverse immune response to a stimulus and has been traditionally placed in the Gell and Coombs categories: type I (immediate hypersensitivity), type II (complement-mediated antibody reactions), type III (immune complex reactions), and type IV (cellular or delayed-type hypersensitivity).*[6] *Drug exposures often stimulate several or all of these types of reactions, and clinical symptoms do not always fit neatly into the categories. Only type I reactions may cause anaphylaxis.*

The immune system uses many tools, such as blood vessel dilation or constriction, causing fluid to flood an infected area, or even producing special cells to kill bacteria or the infected cells in which they are harbored. The pattern of these responses is either inborn (the innate immune response) or learned from previous infections and injuries (the adaptive immune response). Most drug reactions involve the adaptive response and, in the sense that they cause more harm than good, are "mistakes."

T cells control these "learned" responses and decide which "tools" to use in each reaction. Sometimes they utilize several different tools at once, and several different reactions ensue, as when a person becomes sensitized to penicillin and may have not only anaphylaxis but hemolytic anemia and serum sickness, as well. There are different types of T cells, and they communicate either directly with other cells or by chemical messages, called "cytokines." The pattern of cytokines released is one way T cells may activate different responses. They are broadly called Th1 or Th2 responses, with Th1 mostly responding to infections and Th2 sometimes producing allergy or asthma. Here too, drug reactions often include both types of T-cell response.

Immunologic drug reactions generally represent T-cell activation. The type of T cell activated determines the type of reaction to the drug. Th1 cytokines (largely interferon-γ) produce many more chronic, and at times serious, skin reactions and destruction of cells, as in hemolytic anemia or thrombocytopenia. Sometimes these responses can damage tissues, such as the kidney (interstitial nephritis). Th2 cytokines tend to cause any antibodies produced to be switched to the immune globulin E (IgE) or allergic antibody class, which can result in hives or anaphylaxis. Other classes of antibodies are also often made, and these can produce serum sickness or indirect destruction of cells (thrombocytopenia). T-cell receptors respond to one peptide only, which makes each activation response exclusive to the original stimulus (drug) or to chemical structures with very close resemblance.

Antigens

Antigen-presenting cells recognize complex, three-dimensional protein molecules of at least 1,000 Daltons (Da) in size. Most drugs are much smaller than this and cannot be recognized on their own. Only proteins such as insulin, exogenous sera, or monoclonal antibodies are identified and their peptides presented directly to T cells.

Smaller drugs that are chemically reactive may bond covalently to body proteins, altering them and forming large enough molecules for antigen-presenting cells to recognize. This process is called haptenation, and the smaller reactive molecule, a hapten. Some other drugs are inert until they are partially metabolized (prohaptens), and it is their breakdown products that bind native proteins to serve as antigens. Metabolic variations in some patients may produce more active haptens or

		TABLE 54–1		

Reaction Classification, Clinical Symptoms, and Potential Causative Drugs[7,8]

Gell and Coombs Classification	Immune Response	Clinical Symptoms	Potential Causative Drugs[a]
Type I	IgE	Anaphylaxis, urticaria	β-Lactam antibiotics penicillins (primarily), cephalosporins, carbapenems
			Non–β-lactam antibiotics: sulfonamides, vancomycin
			Others: insulins, heparin
Type II	IgG	Hemolytic anemia thrombocytopenia	Quinidine, methyldopa penicillins, heparin
Type III	IgG, IgM	Vasculitis, serum sickness lupus	Penicillins, sulfonamides, radiocontrast agents, phenytoin
Type IV			β-Lactam antibiotics, sulfonamides, phenytoin
IVa	Th1 cytokines	Tuberculin reaction eczema	See text for examples
IVb[b]	Th2 cytokines	Maculopapular and bullous exanthema	
IVc[b]	Cytotoxic T cells (CD4 and CD8)	Same as IVb, also eczema, pustular exanthema	
IVd	T cells (IL-8)	Pustular exanthema	

[a]These drugs represent a list of causative agents. Many drugs can cause these reactions.

[b]IVb and IVc reactions may combine to produce erythema multiforme, Stevens-Johnson syndrome, and toxic epidermal necrolysis.

prevent these fragments from being detoxified, causing them to accumulate and make binding proteins and allergic sensitization more likely.

Gell and Coombs

Type I reactions occur when the drug or its bound hapten incites an IgE antibody response. IgE binds to high-affinity receptors on mast cells and basophils. ❸ *When the original antigen cross-links cell-bound IgE, the effector cell releases enormous amounts of preformed mediators, producing the well-known symptoms of immediate hypersensitivity: urticaria, rhinitis, bronchoconstriction, and anaphylaxis.*

Type II reactions are produced by IgG (or IgM) antibody. The drug or hapten that elicited the antibody response binds to target cells. When antibody attaches to a cell-bound drug, complement activation destroys the cell. **Blood dyscrasias** like thrombocytopenia or hemolytic anemia are the most common examples of type II reactions.

Type III or immune complex reactions also involve IgG antibody production. In this case, when the concentration of the sensitizing drug or hapten is in slight excess to the antibody, the two combine in the serum, producing lattices of antigen–antibody complexes. These complexes are deposited, particularly in vessel walls. Deposits of drug-antibody complexes activate complement, causing vasculitis. The classic forms of type III reaction are serum sickness (usually including arthralgias, fever, malaise, and urticaria that develop 7 to 14 days after exposure to the causative antigen) and the localized **Arthus reaction**, a local inflammatory response due to deposition of immune complexes in tissues.

Type IV reactions are mediated by T cells themselves. "Delayed-type hypersensitivity" reactions from positive tuberculin tests to allergic contact dermatitis are typical type IV reactions, but understanding T-cell function allows us to further define this category, as shown in **Table 54–1**.[7,8]

Pseudoallergic Drug Reactions

❹ *Reactions that clinically resemble allergic reactions but lack an immune basis have been referred to as "pseudoallergic." They include almost the entire range of immediate hypersensitivity clinical patterns. Pseudoallergic reactions range in significance from the alarming but trivial anxiety or vasovagal reactions caused by local dental anesthetics to sometimes fatal reactions to ionic radiocontrast media.* However, cytotoxic reactions, serum sickness, and severe dermatologic reactions (e.g., **Stevens-Johnson syndrome** and **toxic epidermal necrolysis**) are immunologic processes that are not likely to be mimicked by nonimmune processes seen with pseudoallergic reactions.

Pseudoallergic reactions are important in patient counseling and management considerations. The reactions represent common biological functions (direct histamine [H] release by vancomycin, opiates), whereas immunologic (allergic) reactions are based on the structure of the drug. Even a mild drug allergy may carry significant potential for anaphylaxis on readministration. In contrast, pseudoallergic reactions tend to remain constant whether mild or severe and are dose-related.

Pseudoallergic reactions, then, are reactions where the tools of the immune system are used in exactly the same way, but without the "learning" response by T cells and generally without the much greater danger that true immunologic sensitization implies. Pseudoallergic reactions may be thought of as a subtype of idiopathic reactions, rather than an activation of the patient's immune system. The pathophysiology of pseudoallergic reactions is generally unknown, but indicators of immune activation are not seen when they occur.

Clinical Presentation and Diagnosis of Allergic and Pseudoallergic Drug Reactions

The clinical presentation of a patient experiencing an allergic reaction varies greatly. The primary reactions are as follows:

Anaphylaxis

Anaphylaxis is an acute life-threatening allergic reaction. Signs and symptoms involve the skin (e.g., pruritus, urticaria), respiratory tract (e.g., dyspnea, wheezing), gastrointestinal tract (e.g., nausea, cramping), and cardiovascular system (e.g., hypotension, tachycardia). Onset is usually within 30 minutes, but can be as long as 2 hours. Treatment must begin immediately. Anaphylaxis may recur 6 to 8 hours after exposure, so patients experiencing anaphylaxis should be observed for at least 12 hours.

Cytotoxic Reactions

These reactions usually take the form of hemolytic anemia, thrombocytopenia, granulocytopenia, or agranulocytosis.

Immune Complex Reactions

These reactions usually involve a serum sickness-like syndrome (e.g., arthralgias, fever, malaise, and urticaria) that usually develops 7 to 14 days after exposure to the causative antigen.

Dermatologic Reactions

Rashes may range from mild to life-threatening.

- *Urticaria*: These are itchy, raised, swollen areas on the skin. Also known as hives.
- *Maculopapular rash*: A rash that contains both macules and papules. A macule is a flat, discolored area of the skin, and a papule is a small raised bump. A maculopapular rash is usually a large area that is red and has small bumps.
- *Erythema multiforme*: A rash characterized by papular (small raised bump) or vesicular lesions (blisters) and reddening or discoloration of the skin often in concentric zones about the lesion.
- *Stevens-Johnson syndrome*: A severe expression of erythema multiforme (also known as erythema multiforme major). It typically involves the skin and the mucous membranes with the potential for severe morbidity and even death.
- *Toxic epidermal necrolysis*: A life-threatening skin disorder characterized by blistering and peeling of the top layer of skin.

PROBLEMATIC DRUG CLASSES AND TREATMENT OPTIONS

The first priority is to avoid doing serious harm by administering a drug that the patient cannot tolerate. We can generally establish the likelihood of a relationship between the suspected drug and the observed reaction, and also whether it is likely to be an immune or idiopathic reaction by examining the time course and specific signs and symptoms as precisely and objectively as possible. Reevaluating the patient's physical findings and laboratory values (taking into account preexisting diseases) allows further clarification of the need to change treatments and to add therapy for the reaction itself.

Reviewing the original indications for the treatment that caused the reaction is important. For example, in many respiratory illnesses, a prescribed antibiotic may be unnecessary. If the disease persists and indications for some treatment are established, alternatives must be sought, either by adjusting dose or administration rate, finding effective and unrelated alternative medication, or desensitizing the patient to the original drug.

When adverse drug reactions occur, the healthcare provider should carefully describe all aspects of the reaction and assess the potential for it to reoccur. Many patients have frightening associations of the term "allergy" with severe and unpredictable anaphylaxis. It is difficult to undo fears created by injudiciously labeling a patient as allergic in the medical record. Labeling a person "allergic" may hamper future medical care, as patients may refuse treatment or fail to adhere to medication regimens. If the original reaction is clearly documented, healthcare providers can appropriately counsel patients about any true dangers.

Anaphylaxis is a true medical emergency and must be treated promptly. Otherwise, managing allergic reactions begins with stopping the offending agent. Understanding the allergic reaction and potential for cross-allergenicity between similar drugs will assist in selecting an alternative medication. Desensitization is a management option if the patient truly needs the medication and alternative drugs are not available. Although any drug may cause an allergic or pseudoallergic reaction, several drugs and drug classes are strongly associated with such reactions (Table 54–2). These classes will be discussed individually.

β-Lactam Antibiotics

Hypersensitivity reactions with β-lactam antibiotics, especially penicillin, may encompass any of the type I through IV Gell-Coombs classifications. The most common reactions are maculopapular and urticarial eruptions.[9] Although rare (lesser than 0.05%), anaphylactic reactions to penicillins cause the greatest concern, as they are responsible for the majority of all drug-induced anaphylaxis deaths in patients, accounting for 75% of all anaphylaxis cases in the United States.[7,10] The treatment of anaphylaxis is given in Table 54–3.[11,12]

The healthcare professional is faced with a difficult task when approaching a patient who claims a history of penicillin allergy. Although as many as 12% of hospital patients state they have an allergy to penicillin, about 90% will have negative skins tests.[13] Table 54–4 shows the traditional protocol for penicillin skin testing.[14] This test only evaluates

---

Table 54–2

Problematic Drug Classes

β-Lactam antibiotics
Sulfonamide antibiotics
Aspirin and nonsteroidal anti-inflammatory drugs
Radiocontrast media
Opiates
Cancer chemotherapy
Insulin
Anticonvulsants

IgE-mediated reactions. A patient with a history of other serious reactions such as erythema multiforme, Stevens-Johnson syndrome, or toxic epidermal necrolysis should not receive penicillins and should not be tested.

⑤ *Penicillins and cephalosporins both have a β-lactam ring joined to an S-containing ring structure (penicillins: a thiazolidine ring, cephalosporins: a dihydrothiazine ring). The extent of cross-allergenicity appears to be relatively low, with an estimate of approximately 4%.*[15] *Cross-allergenicity is less likely with newer generation cephalosporins compared with the first-generation agents. Anaphylactic reactions to cephalosporins are rare, with a predicted range of 0.0001% to 0.1%. Minor skin reactions including urticaria,* **exanthem***, and pruritus are the most common allergic reactions with cephalosporins, showing severe reactions less often than with penicillins.*[16]

For other β-lactam agents, the recommendations are fairly straightforward.[11] Carbapenems should be considered cross-reactive with penicillins. Monobactams (e.g., aztreonam) do not cross-react with any β-lactam drugs except ceftazidime because they share an identical R-group side chain.

Sulfonamide Antibiotics

Sulfonamides are compounds that contain a sulfonamide moiety (i.e., SO_2NH_2). This group includes sulfonamide antibiotics (sulfonylarylamines), and nonarylamine

---

Table 54–3

Pharmacologic Management of Anaphylactic Reactions

Immediate Intervention
Epinephrine 1:1000 (1 mg/mL)
    Adults: Give 0.2–0.5 mg intramuscularly (IM), repeat every
    5 minutes as needed
    Pediatrics: 0.01 mg/kg (maximum 0.3 mg) IM, repeat every
    5–15 minutes as needed

Subsequent Interventions
Normal saline infusion
    Adults: 1–2 L at a rate of 5–10 mL/kg in the first 5 minutes,
    followed by slow infusion
    Pediatrics: 20 mL/kg bolus repeat to a total maximum of
    60 mL/kg as needed for hypertension
Epinephrine infusion
*If patient is NOT responding to epinephrine injections and volume
    resuscitation:*
    Adults: epinephrine infusion (1 mg in 250 mL D5W):
    1–4 mcg/min, titrating based on clinical response or side effects
    Pediatrics: epinephrine 1:10,000 (0.1 mg/mL): 0.01mg/kg (up to
    0.3 mg) over several minutes

Other Considerations After Epinephrine and Fluids
Diphenhydramine
    Adults: 25–50 mg IV or IM
    Pediatrics: 1–1.25 mg/kg (maximum of 300 mg/24 hours)
Ranitidine
    Adults: 50 mg in D5W 20 mL IV over 5 minutes
    Pediatrics: 1 mg/kg (up to 50 mg) in D5W 20 mL IV over
    5 minutes
Inhaled β-agonist (bronchospasm resistant to epinephrine)
    2–5 mg in 3 mL of normal saline, nebulized, repeat as needed
Dopamine (hypotension refractory to fluids and epinephrine)
    2–20 mcg/kg/min titrated to maintain systolic blood pressure
    greater than 90 mm Hg
Hydrocortisone (severe or prolonged anaphylaxis)
    Adults: 250 mg IV (prednisone 20 mg can be given orally in
    mild cases)
    Pediatrics: 2.5–10 mg/kg/24 hours

D5W, dextrose 5% in water.

Adapted from Refs. 11 and 12.

Table 54–4

Procedure for Performing Penicillin Skin Testing

A. Percutaneous (prick) skin testing

Materials	Volume
Pre-Pen 6 x 10⁶M	1 drop
Penicillin G 10,000 Units/mL	1 drop
β-Lactam drug 3 mg/mL	1 drop
0.03% albumin-saline control	1 drop
Histamine control (1 mg/mL)	1 drop

1. Place a drop of each test material on the volar surface of the forearm.
2. Prick the skin with a sharp needle inserted through the drop at a 45° angle, gently tenting the skin in an upward motion.
3. Interpret skin responses after 15 minutes.
4. A wheal at least 2 × 2 mm with erythema is considered positive.
5. If the prick test is nonreactive, proceed to the intradermal test.
6. If the histamine control is nonreactive, the test is considered uninterruptible.

B. Intradermal skin testing

Materials	Volume
Pre-Pen 6 x 10⁶M	0.02 mL
Penicillin G 10,000 Units/mL	0.02 mL
β-Lactam drug 3 mg/mL	0.02 mL
0.03% albumin-saline control	0.02 mL
Histamine control (0.1 mg/mL)	0.02 mL

1. Inject 0.02 to 0.03 mL of each test material intradermally (amount sufficient to produce a small bleb).
2. Interpret skin responses after 15 minutes.
3. A wheal at least 6 × 6 mm with erythema and at least 3 mm greater than the negative control is considered positive.
4. If the histamine control is non-reactive, the test is considered uninterruptible.
   Antihistamines may blunt the response and cause false-negative reactions.

Adapted from Sullivan TJ. Current Therapy in Allergy. St. Louis, MO: Mosby; 1985:57–61.

Patient Encounter 1

A 10-year-old boy (38 kg [84 lb]) is admitted to the pediatric intensive care unit with an acute exacerbation of chronic bronchitis. The parents are questioned about potential allergies, but they are too upset about their child's condition to remember anything other than a mild rash with an antibiotic about 2 months ago. Ampicillin/sulbactam injection is prescribed. As the drug is infusing, the child complains of difficulty swallowing. Within seconds, he is gasping for air.

Which of the four types of allergic reactions is the child most likely having?

What treatment (dose and route) would be indicated first?

If there is no response after the first dose, how soon can a second dose be administered?

What are the subsequent interventions for this child's reaction?

Table 54–5

Multiple Antibiotic Allergies: Obtaining Background Information

For **each** antibiotic to which the patient claims to be allergic, gather the following information:
- What type of infection was being treated?
- Have you ever received the drug without experiencing a reaction?
- How many times have you received the drug and experienced a reaction?
- What was the drug dose and route of administration with the last reaction?
- How many doses did you take before the onset of the last reaction?
- How many doses did you take after the last reaction?
- Can you describe the adverse reaction?
- What was the duration of the reaction?
- What treatment was given for the reaction?
- Was there any permanent damage?

For **each** antibiotic that the patient has received and does not claim allergy, gather the following information:
- What was the last type of infection being treated?
- What was the drug dose and route of administration?
- Have you received this drug more than once without reactions?

Other information to be gathered:
- Have you had adverse reactions to any other drugs? If so, give dates and describe the reaction.
- Document any risk factors for allergic reactions such as chronic urticaria, liver or kidney disease, HIV (human immunodeficiency virus), or any other immune deficiencies.

Adapted from Macy E. Multiple antibiotic allergy syndrome. Immunol Allergy Clin North Am 2004;24:533–543.

sulfonamides such as furosemide, thiazide diuretics, sulfonylureas, and celecoxib. The sulfonamide antibiotics contain an aromatic amine at the N4 position and a substituted ring at the N1 position. Most allergists agree that most, but not all patients allergic to antimicrobial sulfonamides will tolerate nonarylamine sulfonamides.[17] Predisposition to allergic reactions is a more likely reason than cross-reactivity between these differing molecules.[18] The term "sulfa allergy" should not be used as it can be confusing to patients and healthcare providers. The sulfonamide antibiotics are significant because they account for the largest percentage of antibiotic-induced toxic epidermal necrolysis and Stevens-Johnson syndrome cases.[19]

⑥ *Reactions to sulfonamide antibiotics, ranging from mild (most common) to life-threatening (rare), occur in 2% to 4% of healthy patients, with rates as high as 65% in patients with acquired immunodeficiency syndrome (AIDS).*[20] Anaphylaxis or **anaphylactoid** reactions almost always occur within 30 minutes but may be up to 90 minutes after exposure, most commonly after parenteral administration. Isolated **angioedema** or urticaria can occur within minutes to days. Serum sickness occurs within 1 to 2 weeks. Fixed drug eruptions (lesions) occur within a half hour to 8 hours. These lesions resolve within 2 to 3 weeks after drug removal. The more severe conditions of Stevens-Johnson syndrome and toxic epidermal necrolysis tend to occur 1 to 2 weeks after initiation of therapy. Because trimethoprim-sulfamethoxazole is the drug of choice for patients with Pneumocystis jiroveci pneumonia, desensitization may be necessary. A history of Stevens-Johnson syndrome or toxic epidermal necrolysis is an absolute contraindication for the desensitization procedure.

Patients with Multiple Antibiotic Allergies

Dealing with patients who claim to have multiple antibiotic allergies can be challenging. Combining knowledge of cross-allergenicity with a careful assessment of patient history may be helpful in designing an antimicrobial regimen. Table 54–5 outlines a series of questions that can be useful in developing an effective treatment plan.[21] If available and indicated, skin testing may be useful to complete the puzzle. Often with careful assessment, an antibiotic of choice may be used when the patient's initial history would have ruled it out. Based on data gathered, the patient's record should reflect antibiotics safe to use if needed, antibiotics to be avoided, and antibiotics that can be used only after desensitization. Although Table 54–5 was designed with antibiotics in mind, it can be modified for multiple allergy situations.

Aspirin and Nonsteroidal Anti-Inflammatory Drugs

Aspirin and the nonsteroidal anti-inflammatory drugs (NSAIDs) can induce allergic and pseudoallergic reactions. Because these drugs are so widely used, with much over-the-counter use, the healthcare professional must have a basic understanding of the types of reactions that can occur and how to prevent them. Three types of reactions occur: bronchospasm with rhinoconjunctivitis, urticaria/angioedema, and anaphylaxis. Remember that patients with gastric discomfort or bruising from these agents may describe themselves as being allergic; however, these are not allergic or pseudoallergic reactions.

Patient Encounter 2

A 47-year-old woman is admitted to the hospital for treatment of community-acquired pneumonia. She is a nonsmoker, has no history of cardiopulmonary disease, and is otherwise healthy. When asked about drug allergies, she states she is allergic to penicillin, one of the "floxicin" drugs, vancomycin, and erythromycin. During your interview with the patient, the reactions are described as follows:

Penicillin: When receiving penicillin as a child, she developed "hives."

Quinolone: When receiving a drug that ended in "floxicin" for a urinary tract infection 2 years ago, she was treated in the emergency room for severe itching, shortness of breath, and nausea.

Vancomycin: When receiving vancomycin for a skin infection last year, she got a red rash on her upper body the first two times she received the drug. The nurses told her they "adjusted her dose," and she did not experience the reaction again but still believes she is allergic to it.

Erythromycin: She develops an upset stomach every time she takes a dose of erythromycin. She received it 10 years ago for bronchitis.

The physician asks you what can be used for empiric therapy pending culture results. Your hospital's treatment guidelines for community-acquired pneumonia in an otherwise healthy individual include the following choices: ceftriaxone plus azithromycin or levofloxacin (monotherapy) or ampicillin/sulbactam plus azithromycin.

Are any of the hospital's recommended regimens acceptable for this patient? If yes, which one should be recommended?

Describe your justification for your recommendation.

Two specific conditions—aspirin-exacerbated respiratory disease (AERD) and chronic idiopathic urticaria—are important because they are commonly seen. AERD may include asthma, rhinitis with nasal polyps, and aspirin sensitivity.[22] Upon exposure to aspirin or an NSAID, patients with AERD experience rhinorrhea, nasal congestion, conjunctivitis, laryngospasm, and asthma. Chronic idiopathic urticaria may also be seen with aspirin or NSAID-induced pseudoallergic reactions.[23] Patients with a history of chronic idiopathic urticaria are likely to see a flare of urticaria if aspirin or a cyclooxygenase (COX)-1 inhibiting NSAID is given. Cross-reactions between aspirin and older COX-1 inhibiting NSAIDs exist in patients with AERD and chronic idiopathic urticaria. Even though product warning labels for COX-2 inhibitors state that these agents should not be used in these two conditions, there are no reports of cross-reactivity in AERD and only rare reports in patients with chronic idiopathic urticaria.[24]

[7] *IgE-mediated urticarial/angioedema reactions and anaphylaxis are associated with aspirin and NSAIDs. Urticaria is the most common form of IgE-mediated reaction. However, most reactions are the result of metabolic idiosyncrasies, such as aspirin-induced respiratory disease which may produce severe and even fatal bronchospasm. This class is second only to β-lactams in causing anaphylaxis.* Most reactions in this class are due to a complex metabolic pattern, which causes increasingly recurrent and severe nasal polyps and often refractory asthma. The metabolic problem is constant once it emerges, accounting for the persistence and difficulty of these clinical problems. The metabolic problem is also capable of causing severe, sometimes fatal, acute reactions to aspirin or many if not all other NSAIDs. Rare reports of non–cross-reactive severe reactions suggest possible specific IgE-mediated reactions to individual NSAIDs, and there are some occurrences of urticaria related to NSAIDs as well. Because aspirin therapy is highly beneficial in primary and secondary prevention in coronary artery disease (CAD), aspirin desensitization should be considered in patients who have had reactions to aspirin. Desensitization is contraindicated in patients who have experienced aspirin-induced anaphylactoid reaction, hypotension, tachypnea, or altered consciousness. Alternate agents must be used. A comprehensive approach to aspirin-sensitive patients with CAD has been described.[25]

Radiocontrast Media

[8] *Radiocontrast media may cause serious, immediate pseudoallergic reactions such as urticaria/angioedema, bronchospasm, shock, and death. These reactions have been reduced with the introduction of nonionic, lower osmolality products.* Because a small percentage of patients who have reacted previously to radiocontrast media will react if re-exposed, several steps (listed below) should be taken to prevent reactions in these patients. These steps should also be followed in patients with high-risk factors: asthmatic patients, patients on β-blockers, and patients with cardiovascular disease.[5] The steps are as follows:

- Determine whether the study is essential.
- Be sure the patient understands the risks.
- Ensure adequate hydration.
- Use nonionic, lower osmolar agents.
- Pretreat with prednisone 50 mg orally 13, 7, and 1 hour(s) before the procedure and diphenhydramine 50 mg orally 1 hour before the procedure.

Delayed reactions with these agents occur in 1% to 3% of patients.[26] Although reactions are occasionally severe, most are mild and manifest as maculopapular rashes, fixed eruptions, erythema multiforme, and urticarial eruptions.

Opiates

[9] *Opiates (morphine, meperidine, codeine, hydrocodone, and others) stimulate mast cell release directly, resulting in*

pruritus and urticaria with occasional mild wheezing. Though these reactions are not allergic, many patients state that they are "allergic" to one or more of the opiates. Pretreatment with an antihistamine may reduce these reactions. These pseudoallergic reactions are rarely, if ever, life-threatening.[7] Avoiding other mast cell degranulating medications while patients require opiates also reduces the chances of frightening and uncomfortable reactions. Patients may state they are allergic if they have experienced gastrointestinal upset, a common side effect to opiates, with previous exposures. Obtaining a thorough history from the patient will prove useful. If a more serious reaction has occurred, a nonnarcotic analgesic should be selected.

Cancer Chemotherapy

Hypersensitivity reactions have occurred with all chemotherapy agents. Reactions are most common with the taxanes, platinum compounds, asparaginases, and epipodophyllotoxins.[9] Reactions range from mild (flushing and rashes) to severe (dyspnea, bronchospasm, urticaria, and hypotension). IgE-mediated type I reactions are the most common. To reduce the risk, patients are routinely premedicated with corticosteroids and H_1 and H_2 receptor antagonists. The platinum compounds have produced anemia, probably via a cytotoxic immunologic mechanism.

Insulin

Insulin is one of a very few medications that is itself a whole protein and can induce IgE sensitivity directly. This can result in anaphylaxis. Adverse reactions to insulin also include erythema, pruritus, and indurations, which are usually transient and may be injection site-related.[27] For the sensitivity reactions, treatment options include dexamethasone or desensitization. If the reaction is injection site-related, a change in delivery system (i.e., insulin pump or inhaled insulin) may be helpful.

Anticonvulsants

A wide range of hypersensitivity reactions, ranging from mild maculopapular skin eruptions to severe life-threatening reactions, can occur with anticonvulsants.[28] Aromatic anticonvulsants, primarily phenytoin, carbamazepine, and phenobarbital as well as some of the newer agents (lamotrigine, oxcarbazepine, felbamate, and zonisamide) can cause a life-threatening syndrome with symptoms including fever, a maculopapular rash, and evidence of systemic organ involvement. The rash may be mild at first but can progress to **exfoliative dermatitis**, erythema multiforme, Stevens-Johnson syndrome, or toxic epidermal necrolysis. This syndrome is known as anticonvulsant hypersensitivity syndrome (AHS) or drug rash with eosinophilia and systemic symptoms (DRESS). The causative agent should be withdrawn immediately. Cross-sensitivity among aromatic anticonvulsant drugs ranges between 40% and 80%.[29] If a patient is hypersensitive to an aromatic anticonvulsant, a nonaromatic agent (ethosuximide, gabapentin, levetiracetam, topiramate, and valproic acid) or the benzodiazepines may be useful.[29]

Drug Desensitization

Drug desensitization may be undertaken for some drugs in the absence of useful alternative medications. The risk of severe systemic reactions and anaphylaxis associated with desensitization must be compared with the risk of not treating the patient. Thorough evaluation should establish that the drug probably caused the reaction by an allergic mechanism. Because of the dangers involved with drug desensitization, an expert review of the patient's indication for the drug should be conducted. Consider the possibility that the patient does not really need the drug.

⑩ *Desensitization is a potentially life-threatening procedure and requires continuous monitoring in a hospital setting, with suitable access to emergency treatment and intubation if required. It should only be undertaken under the direction of a physician with suitable training and experience. In such hands, desensitization may present less risk than treatment failure with a less effective alternative medication.*

The possibility of readministering a suspected drug may be safely tested by gradual dose escalation in some cases, and there are certainly many more patients who are harmed by inappropriately withholding medications than there are those who suffer significant harm from testing and desensitization.[30]

Only type I IgE-mediated allergy may be treated by classical desensitization. Desensitization may occur within hours to several weeks, unlike specific immunotherapy injections for inhalant allergy (i.e., "allergy shots," which may take months of therapy before a patient realizes any benefit and years to complete). The mechanism of drug desensitization is poorly understood, but produces temporary drug-specific tolerance of the offending drug. Any interruption of therapy of 24 hours or more requires full repeat desensitization, and abrupt significant increases of dosage have been reported to break through the tolerance with some drugs.

The process probably involves either: (a) cross-linking small subthreshold numbers of bound IgE molecules gradually depleting mast cells of their mediators, or (b) binding of the IgE by monomers or hapten-protein entities that cannot cross-link the antibody. The low doses used at the beginning of all protocols would provide small amounts of antigen, favoring these mechanisms. Both drug-specific IgE and IgG serum concentrations increase after successful desensitization, but skin test positivity generally decreases.[31]

Oral and IV protocols are available for most drugs in this category, with the oral route producing somewhat milder reactions, but the IV route providing more precision in dosing. IV administration can also be used in unresponsive patients for whom the oral route is not feasible. Protocols generally begin at about 1% of the therapeutic dose and increase in intervals defined by the patient's reaction and the distribution and metabolism of the drug itself. Half-log$_{10}$ dose increases (about threefold) are often tolerated.

Penicillin desensitization is the most common drug desensitization protocol and is required for penicillin-allergic patients when penicillin is clearly the only treatment option, for example, when syphilis is present in pregnancy. Protocols have been adapted to most antibiotics. Tables 54–6 and 54–7 describe procedures for oral and IV penicillin desensitization, respectively.[32]

Aspirin desensitization is useful in diseases for which low-level antiplatelet action is needed and in the care of patients with aspirin sensitivity and intractable nasal polyps. Lysine aspirin availability in Europe allows desensitization by inhalation at greatly reduced risk. New procedures utilizing ketorolac as a nasal topical application may allow similar reduction of risk in the United States.[33] As with all desensitizations, constant daily administration must be maintained once the

desired dose is reached. Table 54–8 summarizes several similar aspirin desensitization protocols.[34] Table 54–9 depicts a 2-day alternative protocol.[35]

All desensitization procedures are expected to produce mild symptoms in the patient at some point, and the patient must be made to understand this before doses are started. Mild sensitivity to the drug still remains, and large dose increases as well as missing doses should be avoided. Late complications, such as urticaria, may occur with type I desensitization, and serum sickness or hemolytic anemia

Table 54–7

Parenteral Penicillin Desensitization Protocol

Injection No.	Benzylpenicillin Concentration (Units)	Volume (mL)	(Route)
1	100	0.1	ID
2	100	0.2	SC
3	100	0.4	SC
4	100	0.8	SC
5	1,000	0.1	ID
6	1,000	0.3	SC
7	1,000	0.6	SC
8	10,000	0.1	ID
9	10,000	0.2	SC
10	10,000	0.4	SC
11	10,000	0.8	SC
12	100,000	0.1	ID
13	100,000	0.3	SC
14	100,000	0.6	SC
15	1,000,000	0.1	ID
16	1,000,000	0.2	SC
17	1,000,000	0.2	IM
18	1,000,000	0.4	IM
19	Continuous IV infusion at 1,000,000 units/h		

ID, intradermal; IM, intramuscular; SC, subcutaneous.
Adapted from Weiss ME, Adkinson NF. Diagnostic testing for drug hypersensitivity. Immunol Allerg Clin North Am 1998;18:731–734.

Table 54–6

Protocol for Oral Penicillin Desensitization

Step	Phenoxymethyl Penicillin Concentration (units/mL)	Volume (mL)	Dose (units)	Cumulative Dose (units)
1	1,000	0.1	100	100
2	1,000	0.2	200	300
3	1,000	0.4	400	700
4	1,000	0.8	800	1,500
5	1,000	1.6	1,600	3,100
6	1,000	3.2	3,200	6,300
7	1,000	6.4	6,400	12,700
8	10,000	1.2	12,000	24,700
9	10,000	2.4	24,000	48,700
10	10,000	4.8	48,000	96,700
11	80,000	1.0	80,000	176,700
12	80,000	2.0	160,000	336,700
13	80,000	4.0	320,000	656,700
14	80,000	8.0	640,000	1,296,700
Observe for 30 minutes				
15	500,000	0.25	125,000	
16	500,000	0.5	250,000	
17	500,000	1.0	500,000	
18	500,000	2.25	1,125,000	

Adapted from Weiss ME, Adkinson NF. Diagnostic testing for drug hypersensitivity. Immunol Allerg Clin North Am 1998;18:731–734.

Table 54–8

Oral Aspirin Desensitization Protocols

Dose Increments (mg)	Dose Interval	Cumulative Dose (mg)
30, 60, 100, 325, 600	2 hours	1,115
1, 10, 50, 100, 300	30–40 minutes	461
1, 10, 50, 100, 300	60 minutes	661
30, 60, 120, 300, 600	2 hours	1,110
10, 20, 50, 80, 150, 300	30 minutes	610
30, 60, 125, 250, 500	60 minutes	965

Adapted from Melillo G, Balzano G, Bianco S, et al. Report of the INTERASMA Working Group on Standardization of Inhalation Provocation Tests in Aspirin-induced Asthma. Oral and inhalation provocation tests for the diagnosis of aspirin-induced asthma. Allergy 2001;56:899–911.

Table 54–9

Two-Day Oral Aspirin Desensitization Protocol

	Day 1		Day 2	
Doses (mg)[a]	Cumulative Dose (mg)	Doses (mg)	Cumulative Dose (mg)	
30	30	150	330	
60	90	325	655	
90	180	650	1,305	

[a]Doses are administered every 3 hours, with patient observed for 3 hours after final dose.

Adapted from Stevenson DD, Simon R. Sensitivity to aspirin and non-steroidal anti-inflammatory drugs. In: Middleton E, Reed CE, Ellis EF, et al., eds. Allergy Principles and Practice. St. Louis, MO: Mosby; 1998:1225.

may also occur with high-dose therapy in allergic, desensitized patients.

Some regimens are designed for outpatient administration over much longer time periods and have been used, for example, with allopurinol dermal reactions. Such late-onset morbilliform reactions, sometimes overlapping with erythema multiforme minor, are difficult to evaluate, as it is often unclear to what extent the patients were at risk for recurrent reaction.

Severe life-threatening reactions not mediated by IgE, such as Stevens-Johnson syndrome and toxic epidermal necrolysis, are absolute contraindications to testing, desensitization attempts, and readministration.

OUTCOME EVALUATION

To successfully treat a patient with a drug allergy or pseudo-allergy, several goals must be accomplished:

- If a reaction occurs, it must be identified and managed quickly.
- The patient should be educated about the reaction.
- True drug contraindications should be avoided if at all possible.
- Patients should receive the medications they need or a suitable alternative. If this is not possible due to an allergy, desensitization should be considered.
- Patients should always be monitored for adverse drug reactions.

CONCLUSION

Allergic and pseudoallergic reactions may be mild or life-threatening. Efforts to manage these reactions or change the patient's treatment due to the reactions may increase costs and prevent best therapeutic outcomes. The healthcare professional should carefully explore all available information to accurately assess potential risks from drugs after an apparent reaction to guide both avoidance and alternative treatments.

Patient Care and Monitoring

1. Before administering any medication, take a thorough drug history to establish any past allergic or adverse reactions experienced by the patient.

2. For any reaction, use questions given in Table 54–5 to establish the nature of the reaction and the likelihood it was caused by the suspected drug. For nonantibiotics, the first question regarding infection type is not needed.

3. Document the reaction, in detail, in the patient's medical record.

4. Recommend an alternative choice if the prescribed drug is contraindicated, and develop a plan to assess safety and effectiveness.

5. Consult with a physician trained in desensitization if the patient has a true allergy and no acceptable alternative medication is available.

6. Educate the patient about the allergy or pseudoallergy, so they are able to work with healthcare providers to avoid the reaction in the future.

The healthcare professional should partner with the patient to document reactions so the patient can avoid drugs that present dangers to them if possible and receive the best drug choices when needed.

Abbreviations Introduced in This Chapter

AERD	Aspirin-exacerbated respiratory disease
AHS	Anticonvulsant hypersensitivity syndrome
AIDS	Acquired immunodeficiency syndrome
CAD	Coronary artery disease
COX	Cyclooxygenase
CT	Computed tomography
Da	Dalton
D5W	Dextrose 5% in water
DRESS	Drug reaction with eosinophilia and systematic symptom
H (H1, H2)	Histamine
HIV	Human immunodeficiency virus
ID	Intradermal
Ig	Immune globulin (followed by the specific type of immune globulin: E, G, or M)
IM	Intramuscular
NSAIDs	Nonsteroidal anti-inflammatory drugs
SC	Subcutaneous

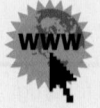 Self-assessment questions and answers are available at *http://www.mhpharmacotherapy.com/pp.html.*

REFERENCES

1. Lazarou J, Pomeranz BH, Corey PN. Incidence of adverse drug reactions in hospitalized patients. A meta-analysis of prospective studies. JAMA 1998;269:1200–1205.

2. American Academy of Allergy Asthma and Immunology [Internet]. Allergy statistics: Drug allergy [cited 2011 October 10]. Available from: *http://www.aaaai.org/about-the-aaaai/newsroom/allergy-statistics. aspx#Drug_Allergy.*

3. Gomes ER, Demoly P. Epidemiology of hypersensitivity reactions. Curr Opin Allergy Clin Immunol 2005;5(4):309–316.

4. Impicciatore P, Choonara I, Clarkson A, et al. Incidence of adverse drug reactions in paediatric in/out patients: A systematic review and meta-analysis of prospective studies. Br J Clin Pharmacol 2001;52:77–83.

5. Adkinson NF, Essayan D, Gruchalla R, et al. Task force report: Future research needs for the prevention and management of immune-mediated drug hypersensitivity reactions. J Allergy Clin Immunol 2002;109(3):S461–S478.

6. Joint Task Force on Practice Parameters, Solensky R, Kahn Da, eds. Drug allergies: an updated practice parameter. Ann Allergy Asthma Immunol 2010;105:259–373.

7. Anon, Part 1: Executive summary of disease management of drug hypersensitivity: A practice parameter. Ann Allergy Asthma Immunol 1999;83:665–700.

8. Pichler WJ. Delayed drug hypersensitivity reactions. Ann Intern Med 2003;139:683–690.

9. Gruchalla RS. Allergic disorders. J Allergy Clin Immunol 2003;111(2):S548–S559.

10. Neugut A, Ghatak A, Miller R. Anaphylaxis in the United States: An investigation into its epidemiology. Arch Intern Med 2001;161:15–21.

11. Lieberman P, Kemp SF, Oppenheimer J, et al. The diagnosis and management of anaphylaxis: An updated practice parameter. J Allergy Clin Immunol 2005;115(3):S483–S523.

12. Lane RD, Bolte RG. Pediatric anaphylaxis. Pediatr Emerg Care 2007;23(1):49–56.

13. Thethi AK, Van Dellen RG. Dilemmas and controversies in penicillin allergy. Immunol Allergy Clin North Am 2004;24:445–461.

14. Sullivan TJ. Current Therapy in Allergy. St. Louis, MO: Mosby; 1985:57–61.

15. Kelkar PS, Li JT. Cephalosporin allergy. N Engl J Med 2001;345:804–809.

16. Madaan A, Li JT. Cephalosporin allergy. Immunol Allergy Clin North Am 2004;24:463–476.

17. Dibbin DA, Montanaro A. Allergies to sulfonamide antibiotics and sulfur-containing drugs. Ann Allergy Asthma Immunol 2008;100:91–100.

18. Strom BL, Schinnar R, Apter AJ, et al. Absence of cross-reactivity between sulfonamide antibiotics and sulfonamide nonantibiotics. N Engl J Med 2003;349(17):1628–1635.

19. Slatore CG, Tilles SA. Sulfonamide hypersensitivity. Immunol Allergy Clin North Am 2004;24:477–490.

20. Greenberger PA. Drug allergy. J Allergy Clin Immunol. 2006; 117:S464–S470

21. Macy E. Multiple antibiotic allergy syndrome. Immunol Allergy Clin North Am 2004;24:533–543.

22. Fahrenholz J. Natural history and clinical features of aspirin-exacerbated respiratory disease. Clin Rev Allergy Immunol 2003;24:113–124.

23. Sanchez-Borges M, Caprilles-Hulett A, Caballero-Fonesca F. Cutaneous reactions to aspirin and NSAIDs. Clin Rev Allergy Immunol 2003;24:125–135.

24. Stevenson DD. Aspirin and NSAID sensitivity. Immunol Allergy Clin North Am 2004;24:491–505.

25. Ramanuja S, Breall JA, Kalaria VG. Approach to "Aspirin allergy" in cardiovascular patients. Circulation 2004;110:e1–e4.

26. Christiansen C. X-ray contrast media—An overview. Toxicology 2005;209:185–187.

27. Richardson T, Kerr D. Skin-related complications of insulin therapy: Epidemiology and emerging management strategies. Am J Clin Dermatol 2003;4(10):661–667.

28. Behi E, Shorvon S. Antiepileptic drugs and the immune system. Epilepsia 2011;52 (Suppl 3):40–44.

29. Bohan KH, Mansuri TF, Wilson NM. Anticonvulsant hypersensitivity syndrome: implications for pharmaceutical care. Pharmacotherapy 2007;27(10):1425–1439.

30. Adkinson NF Jr. Drug allergy. In: Middleton's Allergy: Principles & Practice. 6th ed. Philadelphia, PA: Mosby; 2003:1690.

31. Schmitz-Schumann M, Juhl E, Costabel U. Analgesic asthma-provocation challenge with acetylsalicylic acid. Atemw Lungenkrkh Jahrgang 1985;10:479–485.

32. Weiss ME, Adkinson NF. Diagnostic testing for drug hypersensitivity. Immunol Allerg Clin North Am 1998;18:731–734.

33. White A, Bigby T, Stevenson D. Intranasal ketorolac challenge for the diagnosis of aspirin exacerbated respiratory disease. Ann Allergy Asthma Immunol 2006;97:190–195.

34. Melillo G, Balzano G, Bianco S, et al. Report of the INTERASMA Working Group on Standardization of Inhalation Provocation Tests in Aspirin-induced Asthma. Oral and inhalation provocation tests for the diagnosis of aspirin-induced asthma. Allergy 2001;56(9):899–911.

35. Stevenson DD, Simon R, Sensitivity to aspirin and non-steroidal anti-inflammatory drugs. In: Middleton E, Reed CE, Ellis EF, et al., eds. Allergy Principles and Practice. St. Louis, MO: Mosby; 1998:1225.

55 Solid Organ Transplantation

Steven Gabardi, Spencer T. Martin, and Ali J. Olyaei

LEARNING OBJECTIVES

● **Upon completion of the chapter, the reader will be able to:**

1. Describe the reasons for solid organ transplantation.

2. Differentiate between the functions of cell-mediated and humoral immunity and how they relate to organ transplant.

3. Describe the roles of the antigen-presenting cells (APCs) in initiating the immune response.

4. Compare and contrast the types of rejection, including hyperacute, acute, chronic, and humoral rejection.

5. Define the terms "host–graft adaptation" and "tolerance," paying close attention to their differences.

6. Discuss the desired therapeutic outcomes and appropriate pharmacotherapy utilized to avoid allograft rejection.

7. Compare and contrast the currently available immunosuppressive agents in terms of mechanisms of action, adverse events, and drug–drug interactions (DDIs).

8. Design an appropriate therapeutic regimen for the management of immunosuppressive drug complications based on patient-specific information.

9. Develop a therapeutic drug-monitoring plan to assess effectiveness and adverse events of the immunosuppressive drugs.

10. Write appropriate patient education instructions and identify methods to improve patient adherence following transplantation.

KEY CONCEPTS

❶ T cells are the chief component initiating the immune response against the allograft. The activity of T cells is mediated by a complex system of pathways resulting from the presence of antigen and the release of multiple inflammatory markers known as cytokines.

❷ Antigen-presenting cells (APCs) are vital in initiation of the immune response and play a role in both direct and indirect allorecognition.

❸ The goal of pharmacotherapy in transplantation is to induce immunosuppression with a multidrug approach to target various points of the immune system with resultant long-term allograft and patient survival, while minimizing the complications of suppressing the immune system and drug toxicity.

❹ The goals of induction therapy are to improve short-term allograft and patient survival and to reduce the incidence of acute rejection in the immediate post-transplant period.

❺ The calcineurin inhibitors, cyclosporine and tacrolimus, block T-cell activation by inhibiting the production of interleukin 2 (IL-2). They are associated with significant adverse events, such as nephrotoxicity, cardiovascular disease, posttransplant diabetes, and neurotoxicity.

❻ The antiproliferatives, azathioprine and the mycophenolic acid derivatives, inhibit T-cell proliferation. Myelosuppression is the most significant adverse event associated with these agents.

❼ Sirolimus and everolimus, target of rapamycin (ToR) inhibitors, work by decreasing the ability of T cells to respond to IL-2. The major adverse events associated with these agents are decreased wound healing, hyperlipidemia, and myelosuppression. The promising effects of allowing calcineurin inhibitor withdrawal have been limited by the significant toxicity profile of the ToR inhibitors. However, interest in this drug class as an immunosuppressant currently surrounds its potential cardiovascular and skin malignancy protective properties.

⑧ Corticosteroids induce a nonspecific immunosuppression. Due to their overwhelming incidence of adverse events, many practitioners attempt to use low-dose maintenance therapy or, in some cases, complete steroid withdrawal. These agents are also effective in reversing acute rejection.

⑨ Belatacept is an intermittent, IV maintenance immunosuppressive agent that blocks the costimulatory pathway of T-cell activation. This agent may contribute to improved glomerular filtration rates in renal transplant recipients; however, these patients are at an increased risk of acute rejection. This medication should be avoided in patients who are Epstein-Barr virus (EBV) negative, as it is associated with an increased risk of posttransplant lymphoproliferative disorders (PTLD).

⑩ Long-term patient and allograft survival is complicated by several factors, including drug–drug interactions (DDIs) with the immunosuppressive agents, infectious disease, cardiovascular disease, new-onset diabetes after transplant, and malignancy. The goals of treating these complications are to prevent allograft damage and improve patient survival.

INTRODUCTION

The earliest recorded attempts at organ transplant date back thousands of years.[1] More than a few apocryphal descriptions exist from ancient Egypt, China, India, and Rome describing experimentation with transplantation. However, it wasn't until the early 1900s that French surgeon, Alexis Carrel, pioneered the art of surgical techniques for transplantation.[1] Together with Charles Guthrie, Carrel experimented in artery and vein transplantation. Using revolutionary methods in anastomosis operations and suturing techniques, Carrel laid the groundwork for modern transplant surgery. He was one of the first to identify the dilemma of rejection, an issue that remained insurmountable for nearly half a century.[1]

Prior to the work of Alexis Carrel, malnourishment was the prevailing theory regarding the mechanism of allograft rejection.[1] However, in 1910, Carrel noted that tissue damage in the transplanted organ was likely caused by multiple, circulating biological factors. It was not until the late 1940s with the work of Peter Medawar that transplant immunology became more understood. Medawar was able to define the immunologic nature of rejection using skin allografts. In addition, George Snell observed that grafts shared between inbred animals were accepted but were rejected when transplanted between animals of different strains.[1]

The seminal work by early transplant researchers eventually led to the concept of histocompatibility.[1,2] Histocompatibility describes the process by which polymorphic genes encode cell membrane antigens that serve as targets for

immune response, even within a species. Further research in transplant immunobiology has led to a more accurate understanding of the alloimmune response.[1,2]

Joseph Murray performed the first successful organ transplant in 1954.[1] It was a kidney transplant between identical twins. This was a success in large part because no immunosuppression was necessary due to the fact that donor and recipient were genetically identical. Murray's success laid the groundwork for modern-day transplantation.

EPIDEMIOLOGY AND ETIOLOGY
Heart

Nearly six million Americans are afflicted with heart failure.[1,3] Cardiac transplantation is the treatment of choice for patients with severe end-stage heart failure. Candidates for cardiac transplantation generally present with New York Heart Association (NYHA) class III or IV symptoms and have an ejection fraction of less than 20%. The general indications for cardiac transplantation include rapidly declining cardiac function, requirement of IV inotropes, and having a projected 1-year mortality rate of greater than 75%. Mechanical support with an implantable left ventricular assist device may be appropriate as bridge therapy while patients await the availability of a viable organ.[1,3] Most heart transplants are orthotopic; however, in certain situations, heterotopic cardiac transplants have been performed. There were 2,322 heart transplant procedures done in the United States in 2011.[3] Indications for heart transplant include:

- Cardiomyopathy (i.e., dilated myopathy, hypertrophic cardiomyopathy, restrictive myopathy)
- Congenital heart disease
- Coronary artery disease
- Valvular heart disease

Intestine

An intestine transplant may involve the use of an entire intestine or a shortened segment. Most intestine transplants completed in the United States have involved the transplant of the full organ and are often performed in conjunction with liver transplantation. Although most intestine transplants involve organs harvested from a deceased donor, recent advances in the field have made it possible for living donor intestinal segment transplants. There were 129 intestine transplants (128 deceased donors, 1 living donor) done in 2011.[3] Reasons for intestine transplant include:

- Functional bowel problems (i.e., Hirschsprung's disease, neuronal intestinal dysplasia, pseudoobstruction, protein-losing enteropathy, microvillous inclusion disease)
- Short gut syndrome (i.e., intestinal atresia, necrotizing enterocolitis, intestinal volvulus, massive resection secondary to inflammatory bowel disease, tumors, mesenteric thrombosis)

Kidneys

More than 26 million Americans have chronic kidney disease (CKD), with another 20 million more considered to be at increased risk for the development of kidney disease. End-stage renal disease (ESRD) only constitutes a small portion of those patients with CKD, with more than 450,000 patients currently diagnosed with ESRD throughout the United States. However, the ESRD population continues to increase, with projections estimating that more than 700,000 people will carry a diagnosis of ESRD by 2012. All patients with ESRD should be considered for renal transplantation if they are healthy enough to undergo the transplant surgery. A successful kidney transplant offers advantages in terms of both quality and duration of life compared with other renal replacement therapies. It is also more effective than dialysis from a medical and economic perspective.

Most kidney transplants are heterotopic, where the kidney is implanted above the pelvic bone and attached to the patient's iliac artery and vein. The ureter of the transplant kidney is attached directly to the recipient's bladder or native ureter. The native kidneys are usually not removed, and data have shown that under most circumstances, removal of the native kidneys does not influence patient and allograft survival.[1,3] There were 16,814 (11,043 deceased donors, 5,771 living donors) kidney transplants performed in 2011.[3] Reasons for kidney transplant include:

- Congenital, familial, and metabolic disorders (i.e., congenital obstructive uropathy, Fabry's disease, medullary cystic disease, nephrolithiasis)
- Diabetes mellitus (DM)
- Glomerular diseases (i.e., antiglomerular basement membrane disease, focal segmental glomerular sclerosis, IgA nephropathy, hemolytic uremic syndrome, systemic lupus erythematosus, Alport's syndrome, amyloidosis, membranous nephropathy, Goodpasture's syndrome)
- Hypertension
- Neoplasm (i.e., renal cell carcinoma, Wilms' tumor)
- Polycystic kidney disease
- Renovascular disease
- Tubular and interstitial diseases (i.e., analgesic nephropathy, drug-induced nephritis, oxalate nephropathy, radiation nephritis, acute tubular necrosis, sarcoidosis)

Liver

A liver transplant may involve the use of the entire organ or a segment. The majority of cases involve utilizing the full organ. In recent years, segmental transplants have been conducted using living donors. This procedure requires donation of the left hepatic lobe, which accounts for nearly 60% of the overall liver mass. This type of procedure is possible because the liver can regenerate; therefore, both the donor and recipient, in theory, will have normal liver function shortly after the transplant procedure.[1,3] There were 6,342 (6,095 deceased donors, 247 partial lobe-living donors) liver transplants done in 2011.[3] Reasons for liver transplant include:

- Acute hepatic necrosis (i.e., chronic or acute hepatitis B or C)
- Biliary atresia
- Cholestatic liver disease/cirrhosis (i.e., primary biliary cirrhosis)
- Metabolic disease (i.e., Wilson's disease, primary oxalosis, hyperlipidemia)
- Neoplasms (i.e., hepatoma, cholangiocarcinoma, hepatoblastoma, bile duct cancer)
- Noncholestatic cirrhosis (i.e., alcoholic cirrhosis, postnecrotic cirrhosis, drug-induced cirrhosis)

Lungs

Lung transplants may involve deceased donation of two lungs or a single lung. More recently, lobar transplants from blood group–compatible living donors have been performed for a small segment of the population. Most of the lobar transplants have been performed on cystic fibrosis patients. On rare occasions, a simultaneous heart-lung transplant occurs. This type of procedure is reserved for patients with severe pulmonary and cardiac disease. There were 1,822 (1,821 deceased donors, 1 living donor) lung transplants and 27 simultaneous heart-lung transplant procedures done in 2011.[3] Reasons for lung transplant include:

- α-1-Antitrypsin deficiency
- Congenital disease (i.e., Eisenmenger's syndrome)
- Cystic fibrosis
- Emphysema/chronic obstructive pulmonary disease
- Idiopathic pulmonary fibrosis
- Primary pulmonary hypertension

Pancreas

The exact nationwide prevalence of all diseases of the pancreas has not been fully quantified; however, DM, both types 1 and 2, affects nearly 21 million people in the United States. Some people suffering from DM may also be afflicted with ESRD. A small percentage of these patients undergo a simultaneous pancreas-kidney (SPK) transplant, which may be accomplished using organs from deceased or living donors. Transplant of a pancreas may involve either the entire organ or a pancreas segment. Currently, whole-organ transplant is the most common procedure, with a portion of the duodenum often transplanted along with the pancreas. Living donors are often the source of segmental transplants. In recent years, isolation and transplantation of β-islet cells alone have been completed. Islet transplantation is intended to treat organ dysfunction by replacing nonfunctioning islet cells with new ones. Islet transplants are still considered experimental, and long-term benefit and/or risk of this procedure needs to be studied extensively. Future success of islet cell transplantation is dependent on identifying a nontoxic immunosuppressive combination. There were 287 pancreas transplants and 795 SPK procedures done in 2011.[3] Reasons for pancreas transplants include:

- DM (i.e., type 1 and 2, DM secondary to chronic pancreatitis or cystic fibrosis)
- Pancreatic cancer

PATHOPHYSIOLOGY

Major Histocompatibility Complex

The primary target of the immune response against a transplanted organ is the major histocompatibility complex (MHC).[1,2] The MHC is a region of highly polymorphic genes located on the short arm of chromosome six. The human MHC is referred to as human leukocyte antigen (HLA). HLA is a set of glycoproteins that are expressed on the surface of most cells. These proteins are involved in immune recognition, which is the discrimination of self from nonself, but are also the principal antigenic determinants of allograft rejection.[1,2]

The protein products of the HLA have been classified into two major groups, class I and II:

- Class I: expressed on the surfaces of all nucleated cells and are recognized by CD8+ cells (i.e., cytotoxic T cells).
  - The three subclasses of MHC class I are HLA-A, HLA-B, and HLA-C.
- Class II: expressed solely on the surfaces of antigen-presenting cells (APCs). The APCs serve to stimulate CD4+ cells (i.e., helper T cells).
  - The three subclasses of MHC class II are HLA-DP, HLA-DQ, and HLA-DR.

T and B Lymphocytes

Lymphocytes are one of the five kinds of white blood cells. Mature lymphocytes are astonishingly diverse in their functions. The most abundant of the lymphocytes are T lymphocytes (i.e., T cells) and B lymphocytes (i.e., B cells).

▶ T Lymphocytes

❶ *T cells play a major role in the cell-mediated immune response.* These cells are produced in the bone marrow, but their final stage of development occurs in the thymus, hence the abbreviation "T." There are three recognized subclasses of T cells: cytotoxic T cells (CD8+), helper T cells (CD4+), and regulatory T cells (suppressor T cells):

- Cytotoxic T cells (CD8+) promote target cell destruction by activating cellular apoptosis or aggressively killing the target cell via the release of cytotoxic proteins.
- Helper T cells (CD4+) are the great communicators of the immune response. Once activated, they proliferate and secrete cytokines that regulate effector cell function. Some helper T cells secrete cytokines that recruit cytotoxic T cells, B cells, or APCs, whereas others secrete

cytokines that turn off the immune response once an antigen has been destroyed.

- Regulatory T cells, or suppressor T cells, suppress the activation of an immune response. The activity of these cells in organ transplant is not well elucidated.

▶ B Lymphocytes

B cells play a large role in the humoral immune response. In humans, B cells are produced and mature in the bone marrow. The human body produces several types of B cells. Each B cell is unique, with a distinctive cell surface receptor protein that binds to only one particular antigen. Once B cells encounter their antigen and receive a cytokine signal from helper T cells, they can further differentiate into one of two cells, plasma B cells or memory B cells. Plasma B cells secrete antibodies that induce the destruction of target antigens through complement recruitment and/or opsonization. Memory B cells play an important role in long-term immunity. Once formed to a specific antigen, memory B cells are capable of rapidly responding to subsequent exposures to their target antigen.

Antigen-Presenting Cells

❷ *APCs are vital in initiation of the immune response. An APC is a cell that displays a foreign antigen complexed with MHC on its cell surface.* Its major responsibility is to present these foreign antigens to T cells. T cells can identify this complex using their T-cell receptors (TCRs). There are three main types of APCs: dendritic cells (DCs), macrophages, and activated B cells. DCs are present in tissues that are in contact with the environment, such as the skin and the lining of the nose, lungs, stomach, and intestines. They are responsible for antigen phagocytosis. After phagocytosis, they express the foreign antigen on their cell surface and then migrate to the lymphoid tissues to interact with T and B cells to initiate the immune response. Macrophages' main role is in the removal of pathogens and necrotic debris. However, like DCs, macrophages also phagocytize antigens and express them on their cell membranes to present to T cells to initiate an immune response. The first time an antigen is encountered, the DCs and macrophages act as the primary APCs. However, if the same antigen is encountered again, memory B cells become the most important APC because they initiate the immune response quickly after antigen presentation. It appears that both the DCs and macrophages have the most activity in terms of allorecognition.

Allorecognition

❶ ❷ *Recognition of the antigens displayed by the transplanted organ (alloantigens) is the prime event that initiates the immune response against the allograft.* There are currently two accepted pathways for T-cell allorecognition:

- Direct pathway: Donor APCs migrate out of the allograft into the recipient's lymph nodes and present donor MHC molecules to the TCRs of the recipient's T cells.

Table 55–1

Organ-Specific Signs and Symptoms of an Acute Rejection Episode[1,2]

Organ	Clinical Symptoms	Laboratory Signs
Heart	Fever, lethargy, weakness, SOB, DOE, hypotension, tachycardia, atrial flutter, ventricular arrhythmias	Leukocytosis, endomyocardial biopsy positive for mononuclear infiltrates
Kidney	Fever, graft tenderness and swelling, decreased urine output, malaise, hypertension, weight gain, edema	Increased SCr, BUN, leukocytosis, renal biopsy positive for lymphocytic infiltration
Intestine	Fever and GI symptoms (i.e., bloating, cramping, diarrhea, increased stomal output)	There are no reliable biochemical markers for intestine transplant rejection, but biopsies may be helpful.
Liver	Fever, lethargy, change in color or quantity of bile in patients with biliary T-tube, graft tenderness and swelling, back pain, anorexia, ileus, tachycardia, jaundice, ascites, encephalopathy	Abnormal LFTs, increased bilirubin, alkaline phosphate, transaminases, biopsy positive for mononuclear cell infiltrate with evidence of tissue damage
Lung	Fever, impaired gas exchange, SOB, malaise, anxiety	Decreased FEV, infiltrate on CXR, biopsy positive for lymphocytic infiltration
Pancreas	Fever, graft tenderness and swelling, abdominal pain, ileus, and malaise	Increased FBS, leukocytosis, decreased human C-peptide and urinary amylase levels

BUN, blood urea nitrogen; CXR, chest x-ray; DOE, dyspnea on exertion; FBS, fasting blood sugar; FEV, forced expiratory volume; GI, gastrointestinal; LFTs, liver function tests; SCr, serum creatinine; SOB, shortness of breath.

• Indirect pathway: Recipient APCs migrate into the graft and phagocytize alloantigens. The donor MHC molecules are then expressed on the cell surface of the recipient's APCs and presented to recipient T cells in the lymph nodes.

T-Cell Activation

❶ Whether it is by the direct or indirect pathway, in order for a T cell to become activated against the allograft, two interactions or signals must take place between the APCs and the recipient's T cells[1,2]:

• Signal 1 is the interaction of the TCR with the foreign antigens presented by the APCs.

• Signal 2 is an interaction between one of several costimulatory receptors and paired ligands on the cell surfaces of the APCs and T cells, respectively. This interaction is of the utmost importance, as Signal 1, in the absence of Signal 2, induces T-cell anergy.

Once activated, T cells undergo clonal expansion under the influence of cytokines, specifically interleukin 2 (IL-2). These steps elicit an antidonor T-cell response that results in graft destruction.

Mechanisms of Acute Rejection

After activation, cytotoxic T cells emerge from lymphoid organs to infiltrate the graft and trigger the immune response. These cells induce graft destruction via two mechanisms: (a) secretion of the cytotoxic proteins perforin and granzyme B, and (b) induction of cellular apoptosis through interaction with various cell surface receptors. Besides the cytotoxic T cells, several other cell lines may play a role in allograft destruction, including B cells, granulocytes, and natural killer cells.

Types of Rejection

▶ Hyperacute Rejection

● Hyperacute rejection is an immediate recipient immune response against the allograft due to the presence of preformed recipient antibodies directed against the donor's HLA. This type of reaction generally occurs within minutes of the transplant. The organ must be removed immediately to prevent a severe systemic response. In the case of cardiac or lung transplantation in which the organ cannot be promptly removed, short-term mechanical circulatory support is required until an alternative organ becomes available. Those patients at highest risk for hyperacute rejection include any patients that have preformed HLA or ABO blood group antibodies, including patients with a history of previous organ transplant or multiple blood transfusions, as well as women who have had children. Hyperacute rejection has been largely eliminated due to routine surveillance testing completed pretransplant.

▶ Acute Rejection

● Acute rejection is a cell-mediated process that generally occurs within 5 to 90 days after transplantation; however, it can occur at any time after transplant. This reaction is mediated through alloreactive T cells, as discussed previously in the Mechanisms of Acute Rejection section. Organ-specific signs and symptoms of acute rejection can be seen in Table 55–1.[1,2]

▶ Antibody-Mediated Rejection

● Antibody-mediated rejection (AMR) is the process of creating graft-specific antibodies.[1,2,4] This type of rejection occurs less frequently than cell-mediated acute rejection. AMR is characterized by deposition of immunoglobulins and complement in allograft tissues. Treatment for this type of rejection is not well defined; however, several reports have shown that treatments such as plasmapheresis, immunoglobulin therapy, rituximab, bortezomib, or eculizumab may be effective.[6]

▶ Chronic Rejection

● Chronic rejection has traditionally been thought of as a slow, insidious form of acute rejection, resulting in worsening organ function over time. The exact immunologic processes of chronic rejection are poorly understood; however, many believe that both the cell-mediated and humoral immune systems and drug-induced toxicities play a vital role in its development. Currently, retransplantation is the only effective treatment option.[1,2,7]

▶ Host–Graft Adaptation

● The term "host–graft adaptation" describes the decreased immune response against the allograft over time.[2] This phenomenon is evident by the reduced incidence of acute rejection episodes seen months after transplantation. In theory, host–graft adaptation is thought to be secondary to a weakened T-cell response to donor antigens when patients are receiving maintenance immunosuppression.[2]

Tolerance

● Tolerance is the process that allows organ-specific antigens to be accepted as self.[2,8] This would mean the immune system would cease to respond to the allograft and immunosuppressive medications would not be required. Immune tolerance has been achieved in the lab, but has yet to be successfully accomplished in humans.[2,8] The definition of "achieved tolerance" is highly variable and subjective. Currently, a number of protocols focusing on testing clinically safe regimens to achieve chimerism or tolerance are being studied.

Immunologic Barriers to Transplantation

One of the more common barriers to successful transplantation is the presence of preformed HLA antibodies, acquired through pregnancy, blood transfusion, or previous transplant, or ABO blood group incompatibility. In cases in which these antibodies exist, if they are not adequately removed prior to transplant, they are likely to result in AMR and poor graft survival. To improve outcomes, assessment of pretransplant immune risk factors of recipients plays an important role in the prevention of immune-mediated allograft injuries. The introduction of pretransplant crossmatching and the use of ABO-compatible donors has largely eliminated hyperacute rejection episodes. However, these immunologic barriers remain intact for several transplant recipients with willing organ donors, and patients are left to wait on the deceased donor waiting list or undergo pretransplant immunomodulation in an attempt to prevent these antibodies from affecting the allograft.

▶ ABO Incompatibility

The expanding deceased donor waiting list encouraged some centers to evaluate the use of ABO desensitization protocols in order to transplant patients with ESRD that had willing but ABO-incompatible donors. The desensitization protocol most commonly used in the United States involves reducing ABO antibody titers through plasmapheresis with IV immune globulin (IVIG). Use of plasma exchange to achieve an ABO antibody titer of less than 1:8 to 1:32 has resulted in long-term renal transplant results that are comparable to those of ABO-compatible transplants, despite an incidence of acute AMR that approaches 10% to 30%.

▶ HLA Sensitization

Evaluation of the presence or absence of alloantibodies and T-cell activities to HLA antigens plays a significant role in individualization of immunosuppressive therapy. A patient's degree of sensitization is often reported as the percentage of panel-reactive antibodies (PRA), which is an estimate of the likelihood of a positive crossmatch to a pool of potential donors. Advancement in HLA antibody screening and identification through flow cytometry or solid-phase multiplex platforms has overcome many of the issues stemming from the older methods of PRA calculations. Patients are considered to be highly sensitized to HLA if they have a PRA of greater than or equal to 80%, making them less likely to receive a deceased donor organ. Patients with higher PRAs and preformed antibodies have poorer long-term allograft survival. Although PRA is a sensitive test and has predictive value, lymphocytes directly obtained from the donor is a superior method of immune monitoring before and early after transplant.[4] The assay is aimed to detect the presence of antibodies directed against the HLA antigens of the donor. In this setting, the presence of donor-specific antibodies (DSA) is identified. In one study, allograft survival was significantly lower in patients with DSA.[5] Thus detecting DSA and the presence of high PRA may indicate the need to enhance immunosuppression to improve posttransplant outcomes and allograft survival.

Like ABO incompatibilities, it is possible to desensitize patients against a willing donor despite the presence of DSA or those awaiting a deceased donor transplant with a broad array of preformed anti-HLA antibodies (PRA greater than or equal to 30%). There are two general protocols used for HLA desensitization: high-dose IVIG and low-dose IVIG with plasmapheresis. Despite the relatively high degree of AMR seen in desensitized patients, this population of patients have acceptable short-term patient and allograft survival. Unfortunately, the long-term results for graft and patient outcomes using either of these two protocols is unknown.

TREATMENT
Desired Outcome

● ❸ *The major focus of pharmacotherapy in transplantation is to achieve long-term patient and allograft survival.*[2,9] Short-term

---

Table 55–2

Currently Available Immunosuppressive Agents[2,8,9]

Generic Name (Brand Name)	Common Dosage	Common Adverse Effects
Induction Therapy Agents		
Alemtuzumab (Campath)	20–30 mg × 1–2 doses	Flu-like symptoms, chills, rigors, fever, rash, myelosuppression
Antithymocyte globulin equine (ATGAM)	15 mg/kg IV × 3–14 days	Flu-like symptoms, chills, rigors, fever, rash, myelosuppression
Antithymocyte globulin rabbit (Thymoglobulin)	1.5 mg/kg IV × 3–14 days	Flu-like symptoms, chills, rigors, fever, rash, myelosuppression
Basiliximab (Simulect)	20 mg IV × 2 doses	None reported compared to placebo
Maintenance Immunosuppressants		
Cyclosporine (Sandimmune, Neoral, Gengraf)	4–5 mg/kg by mouth twice a day	Neurotoxicity, gingival hyperplasia, hirsutism, hypertension, hyperlipidemia, glucose intolerance, nephrotoxicity, electrolyte abnormalities
Tacrolimus (Prograf)	0.05–0.075 mg/kg by mouth twice a day	Neurotoxicity, alopecia, hypertension, hyperlipidemia, glucose intolerance, nephrotoxicity, electrolyte abnormalities
Azathioprine (Imuran)	1–2.5 mg/kg by mouth once a day	Myelosuppression, GI disturbances, pancreatitis
Mycophenolate mofetil (CellCept)	0.5–1.5 gm by mouth twice a day	Myelosuppression, GI disturbances
Enteric-coated MPA (Myfortic)	720 mg by mouth twice a day	Myelosuppression, GI disturbances
Sirolimus (Rapamune)	1–10 mg by mouth once a day	Hypertriglyceridemia, myelosuppression, mouth sores, hypercholesterolemia, GI disturbances, impaired wound healing, proteinuria, lymphocele, pneumonitis
Everolimus (Zortress)	0.75 mg by mouth twice daily	Hypertriglyceridemia, myelosuppression, mouth sores, hypercholesterolemia, GI disturbances, impaired wound healing, proteinuria, lymphocele, pneumonitis
Prednisone (Deltasone)	Maintenance: 2.5–20 mg by mouth once a day	Mood disturbances, psychosis, cataracts, hypertension, fluid retention, peptic ulcers, osteoporosis, muscle weakness, impaired wound healing, glucose intolerance, weight gain, hyperlipidemia
Belatacept (Nulojix)	10 mg/kg on postop days 1 and 4	GI disturbances, electrolyte abnormalities, headache
	10 mg/kg at the end of postop weeks 2, 4, 8, and 12	
	5 mg/kg at the end of postop week 16 and every 4 weeks thereafter	

GI, gastrointestinal; MPA, mycophenolic acid.

---

outcomes (e.g., acute rejection rates, 1-year graft survival) have improved significantly since the first successful transplant due to an improved understanding of the immune system and enhancements in surgical techniques, organ procurement, immunosuppression, and posttransplant care. Despite the success in improving short-term outcomes, the overall frequency of graft loss remains higher than desired.[1,2]

It is imperative that transplant practitioners be aware of the specific advantages and disadvantages of the available immunosuppressants, as well as their adverse reactions and drug–drug interaction (DDI) profiles. There are generally considered to be three stages of medical immunosuppression: (a) induction therapy, (b) maintenance therapy, and (c) treatment of rejection. ❸ *Overall, the immunosuppressive regimens utilize multiple medications that work on different targets of the immune system.* Please refer to Table 55–2 for a list of all currently available immunosuppressive agents.[2,9,10]

Immunosuppressive Therapies—Induction Therapy

❹ *The goal of induction therapy is to provide a high level of immunosuppression in the critical early posttransplant period, when the risk of acute rejection is highest.*[2,9,11–13]

This stage of immunosuppression is initiated intraoperatively and is generally concluded within the first 1 to 10 days after transplantation. Induction therapy is not a mandatory stage of recipient immunosuppression. However, since acute rejection is a major concern in solid organ transplant recipients and its impact on chronic rejection is undeniable, induction therapy is often considered essential to optimize outcomes.[2,9,11–13]

▶ Goals of Induction Therapy

❹ *First, the induction agents are highly immunosuppressive, allowing for significant reductions in acute rejection episodes and improved 1-year graft survival. Second, due to* their unique pharmacologic effect, these agents are often considered essential for use in patients at high risk for poor short-term outcomes, such as those patients with preformed antibodies, history of previous transplants, multiple HLA mismatches, or transplantation of organs with prolonged cold ischemic time, or from expanded-criteria donors. Specifically in renal transplant recipients, induction therapy plays an important role in preventing early-onset calcineurin inhibitor–induced nephrotoxicity. With the use of induction agents, initiation of calcineurin inhibitors can be delayed until the graft regains some degree of function. [9,12,13] Transplant centers that pursue corticosteroid sparing or avoidance protocols consider induction therapy imperative due to its profound and lasting immunosuppressive effects.

The improved short-term outcomes gained from induction therapy come with a degree of risk. By using these highly immunosuppressive agents, particularly the antilymphocyte antibodies (ALA; the antithymocyte antibodies, and alemtuzumab), the body loses much of its innate ability to mount a cell-mediated immune response, which increases the risk of opportunistic infections and malignancy. [9,12,13] Cytokine release syndrome is a common complication of T-cell depleting agents and may require methylprednisolone, diphenhydramine, and/or acetaminophen 30 to 60 minutes before infusion.

▶ Currently Available Induction Therapies

Basiliximab Basiliximab is a chimeric monoclonal antibody with a high affinity for the IL-2 receptor, where it acts as a receptor antagonist.[10,13] These receptors are present on almost all activated T cells. Basiliximab inhibits IL-2–mediated activation of lymphocytes, which is an important step for the clonal expansion of T cells.

The dose of basiliximab is 20 mg IV given 2 hours prior to the transplant, followed by a second 20-mg dose on postoperative day 4.[9,10,13] This dosing schedule can be used for both children greater than or equal to 35 kg (77 lb) and adults. Two 10-mg doses with the same dosing schedule should be used for children less than 35 kg (77 lb). There is no specific dosage adjustments needed in renal or hepatic impairment.[9,10,13]

The incidence of all adverse reactions with basiliximab was similar to placebo in clinical trials.[10,13] There are no reported DDIs with basiliximab.

Antithymocyte Globulin Equine Antithymocyte globulin equine (e-ATG) is a polyclonal antibody that contains antibodies against several T-cell surface markers. After binding to these cell surface markers, e-ATG promotes T-cell depletion through opsonization and complement-mediated T-cell lysis.[9,10,12,13] The common dosing strategy for e-ATG when used for induction therapy is 10 to 30 mg/kg/day IV for 3 to 14 days.[9,10,12,13]

After T-cell lysis there is a cytokine release. Due to this phenomenon, e-ATG is associated with several adverse reactions.[9,10,12,13] The most common of these include fever (63%), chills (43.2%), headache (34.6%), back pain (43.2%), nausea (28.4%), diarrhea (32.1%), dizziness (24.7%), malaise (3.7%), and myelosuppression (leukopenia [29.6%] and thrombocytopenia

[44.4%]). The overall incidence of opportunistic infections is 27.2%, with cytomegalovirus (CMV) disease occurring in 11.1% of patients. There are currently no reported pharmacokinetic DDIs with this agent. [9,10,12,13]

Antithymocyte Globulin Rabbit Antithymocyte globulin rabbit (r-ATG) is also a polyclonal antibody that induces T-cell clearance, but more importantly, it alters T-cell activation, homing, and cytotoxic activities. Compared with e-ATG, r-ATG causes less T-cell lysis due to its secondary mechanisms of immunosuppression. It is also believed that r-ATG plays a role in inducing T-cell apoptosis. r-ATG has been dosed between 1 and 4 mg/kg/day (typically dosed at 1.5 mg/kg/day) and is usually administered for 3 to 10 days after transplantation.[9-13] Many renal transplant centers aim to initiate the first dose intraoperatively to reduce organ reperfusion injury.

Adverse reactions are common and may include fever (63.4%), chills (57.3%), headache (40.2%), nausea (36.6%), diarrhea (36.6%), malaise (13.4%), dizziness (8.5%), leukopenia (57.3%), thrombocytopenia (36.6%), and generalized pain (46.3%).[9,10,13] The incidence of infection is 36.6%, with CMV disease occurring in 13.4% of patients. There are no reported DDIs with the use of r-ATG at this time.[9-13]

Alemtuzumab Alemtuzumab is a recombinant DNA-derived monoclonal antibody that binds to CD52. CD52 is present on the surface of almost all B and T lymphocytes, many macrophages, natural killer (NK) cells, and a subpopulation of granulocytes.[10,13] This agent's mechanism of action is believed to be antibody-dependent cell lysis following its binding to CD52 cell surface markers. When used for induction therapy, alemtuzumab produces a rapid and extensive lymphocyte depletion that may take several months to return to pretransplant levels. Although it is not FDA approved for use in organ transplantation, studies have demonstrated a dose of 30 mg IV at the time of transplant to be effective in preventing acute rejection.[13] A recent retrospective analysis suggests that use of alemtuzumab as an induction therapy may be associated with an increased risk of graft loss as a result of AMR, but further study is warranted.[14]

Alemtuzumab has been associated with serious adverse reactions that include anemia (47%), neutropenia (70%), thrombocytopenia (52%), headache (24%), dysesthesias (15%), dizziness (12%), nausea (54%), vomiting (41%), diarrhea (22%), autoimmune hemolytic anemia (rare), infusion-related reactions (15% to 89%), and infection (37%; CMV viremia occurred in 15% of patients).[10,13] The FDA recommends that premedication with acetaminophen and oral antihistamines is advisable to reduce the incidence of infusion-related reactions.[10]

Comparative Efficacy—Induction Therapy Agents The improvements in short-term outcomes gained from the use of induction therapies cannot be denied. However, despite these advances, use of induction therapy has not impacted long-term allograft function or survival. There are a few studies that help to delineate the ideal induction therapy agent. Only one study has compared r-ATG to patients receiving no induction therapy and found no benefit in acute rejection, allograft loss, or death.[15] It is difficult to draw specific conclusions regarding r-ATG induction therapy from this trial due to major discrepancies in maintenance immunosuppression between the two groups. Studies comparing r-ATG and e-ATG show that r-ATG is more effective in lowering acute rejection rates and improving 1-year allograft survival.[16] Conversely, studies evaluating the use of basiliximab versus r-ATG demonstrate similar short-term efficacy between both groups.[17] However, more recent analyses of these two agents demonstrated similar results for allograft and patient survival, but a benefit for r-ATG in lowering the incidence of acute allograft rejection.[18,19] A more recent analysis showed that alemtuzumab improved transplant outcomes when compared with basiliximab in patients with a low immunologic risk, and similar outcomes in comparison with high immunologic risk patients receiving r-ATG.[20] When choosing an agent for induction therapy, one must weigh the risks versus the benefits. For the most part, the ALAs are considered to be most effective, but are associated with a higher incidence of infectious disease and malignancy.[13]

Immunosuppressive Therapies—Maintenance Therapy

The goals of maintenance immunosuppression are to prevent rejection episodes and to optimize patient and graft survival. Antirejection medications require careful selection and dosage titration to balance the risks of rejection with the risks of toxicities.

Common maintenance immunosuppressive agents can be divided into five basic medication classes:

- Calcineurin inhibitors (cyclosporine and tacrolimus)
- Antiproliferatives (azathioprine and the mycophenolic acid [MPA] derivatives)
- Target of rapamycin (ToR) inhibitors (sirolimus and everolimus)
- Corticosteroids (prednisolone derivatives and dexamethasone)
- Costimulatory pathway blocker (belatacept)

Maintenance immunosuppression is generally achieved by combining two or more medications from the different classes to maximize efficacy by specifically targeting unique components of the immune response. Please refer to **Figure 55–1** for a schematic representation of these different drug mechanisms and **Figure 55–2** for an example protocol for administration of immunosuppressive medications posttransplant. This method of medication selection also helps to minimize toxicities by choosing agents with different adverse event profiles. Immunosuppressive regimens vary between organ types and transplant centers, but most often they include a calcineurin inhibitor with an adjuvant agent, plus or minus corticosteroids. Selection of an appropriate immunosuppressive regimen should be patient-specific, and one must take into account the patient's preexisting disease states, medication regimens, and preferences.

Patient Encounter Part 1

HPI: ED is a 34-year-old man who presents to your transplant center for a living unrelated renal transplant.

PMH:
- ESRD: secondary to focal segmental glomerulosclerosis
- Anxiety
- Hypertension
- Hyperlipidemia
- Insomnia
- Gout, he has had 10 episodes of gout since the age of 21
- Secondary hyperparathyroidism

FH: Father is alive and living with a history of cardiovascular disease and mother is alive and living with a history of breast cancer.

SH: The patient works as a mechanical engineer. He admits to social alcohol use (3 or 4 drinks per week) and denies any tobacco and IV drug use.

Admission Medications:
- Bisoprolol 5 mg by mouth once a day
- Amlodipine 5 mg by mouth once a day
- Irbesartan 100 mg by mouth once a day
- Furosemide 20 mg by mouth twice a day
- Atorvastatin 20 mg by mouth once a day
- Alprazolam 0.5 mg by mouth three times a day as needed for anxiety
- Zolpidem 10 mg by mouth once a day at bedtime
- Calcitriol 0.25 mg by mouth once a day
- Epo 4000 units IV every hemodialysis session

Allergies: NKDA

Misc:
- CMV Serostatus: Donor is CMV IgG positive
- CMV Serostatus: Recipient is CMV IgG negative
- Epstein Barr Virus (EBV) Serostatus: Donor is EBV IgG positive
- EBV Serostatus: Recipient is EBV IgG negative
- Patient has documented glucose-6 phosphate dehydrogenase (G6PD) deficiency

Identify your treatment goals for this patient.

Create a plan for induction therapy (i.e., would you recommend induction therapy, if so, which agent)?

▶ Calcineurin Inhibitors

Cyclosporine and tacrolimus belong to a class of immunosuppressants called the calcineurin inhibitors. These agents are considered by many to be the cornerstone of immunosuppressive protocols. The calcineurin inhibitors work

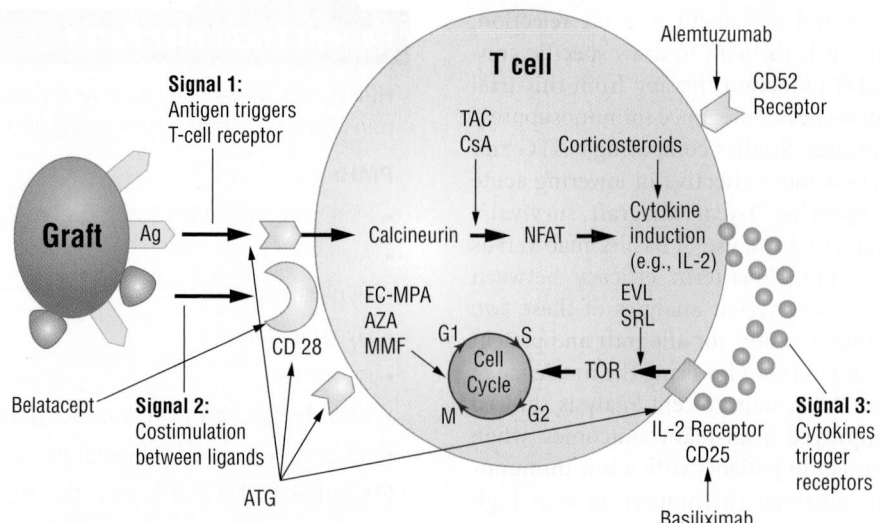

FIGURE 55–1. Identification of the sites of action of the various immunosuppressive medications. Allograft recognition through Signal 1 occurs when the antigen-major histocompatibility complex (MHC) molecule is recognized by the T-cell receptor (TCR). A costimulatory signal, Signal 2, initiates signal transduction with activation of second messengers, one of which is calcineurin. Together, Signal 1 and Signal 2 activate calcineurin phosphatase, which removes phosphates from the nuclear factors, allowing them to enter the nucleus, with a subsequent increase in IL-2 gene transcription. Signal 3 occurs with the interaction of IL-2, with the IL-2 receptor on the cell membrane surface. This culminates in a signal that passes through the mammalian target of rapamycin (ToR) and induces cell proliferation and production of cytokines specific to the T cell. (ATG, antithymocyte globulin; AZA, azathioprine; CsA, cyclosporine; EC-MPA, enteric-coated mycophenolic acid; EVL, everolimus; NFAT, nuclear factors; MMF, mycophenolate mofetil; SRL, sirolimus; TAC, tacrolimus.)

by complexing with cytoplasmic proteins (cyclosporine with cyclophilin and tacrolimus with FK binding protein-12).[9,10,21,22] These complexes then inhibit calcineurin phosphatase, which results in reduced IL-2 gene transcription. The final outcome is a decrease in IL-2 synthesis and a subsequent reduction in T-cell activation.[9,10,21,22]

Cyclosporine Cyclosporine USP was first approved in 1983, but was associated with a variable oral absorption. The development of a newer formulation, cyclosporine microemulsion USP (i.e., modified) introduced in 1994, allowed for a more consistent drug exposure due to a more reliable pharmacokinetic profile.[23] Cyclosporine modified is the formulation of choice for most transplant centers that use cyclosporine for maintenance immunosuppression due to the previously mentioned benefit. The two formulations are not interchangeable.

The usual oral adult dose of cyclosporine ranges from 3 to 7 mg/kg/day in two divided doses.[10] The appropriate selection of the starting dose usually depends on the organ type, the patient's preexisting disease states, and other concomitant immunosuppressive agents utilized. Cyclosporine modified is available as 25-mg and 100-mg individually blister-packed capsules and an oral solution. An IV formulation of conventional cyclosporine is also available. When converting a patient from oral to IV, the dosage should be reduced to approximately one-third of the total daily oral dose.[10]

Cyclosporine whole-blood trough concentrations have traditionally been obtained to help monitor for efficacy and safety.

Therapeutic trough levels (C_0) may range from 50 to 400 ng/mL (50 to 400 mcg/L or 42 to 333 nmol/L). Target levels should be individualized for each patient, usually depending on the organ transplanted, patient's condition, method of assay (high-performance liquid chromatography [HPLC], monoclonal, polyclonal), and time since transplantation. Newer studies suggest that monitoring of concentrations at 2 hours post-dose (C_2) correlates better with toxicity and efficacy when compared with C_0.[24]

Tacrolimus Tacrolimus (also known as FK506) is the second calcineurin inhibitor and was approved in 1997. Oral starting doses of tacrolimus range from 0.1 to 0.2 mg/kg/day in two divided doses. Tacrolimus is available in 0.5-, 1-, and 5-mg capsules and as an injectable.[10] Tacrolimus C_0 should be monitored (12 hours after the last administered dose) and maintained between 5 and 15 ng/mL (5 and 15 mcg/L), again depending on the transplanted organ, patient's condition, and time since transplant.[10]

The tacrolimus IV formulation is usually avoided due to the risk of anaphylaxis because of its castor oil component and nephrotoxicity. Doses for IV administration are recommended to start at 0.01 mg/kg/day. Most IV doses of tacrolimus are administered over 24 hours as a continuous infusion. To avoid drawing falsely elevated levels, it is important that trough levels are not drawn from the line that tacrolimus is being infused through. Because IV administration of tacrolimus is usually a continuous infusion, a "trough level" can be taken at any time during administration.

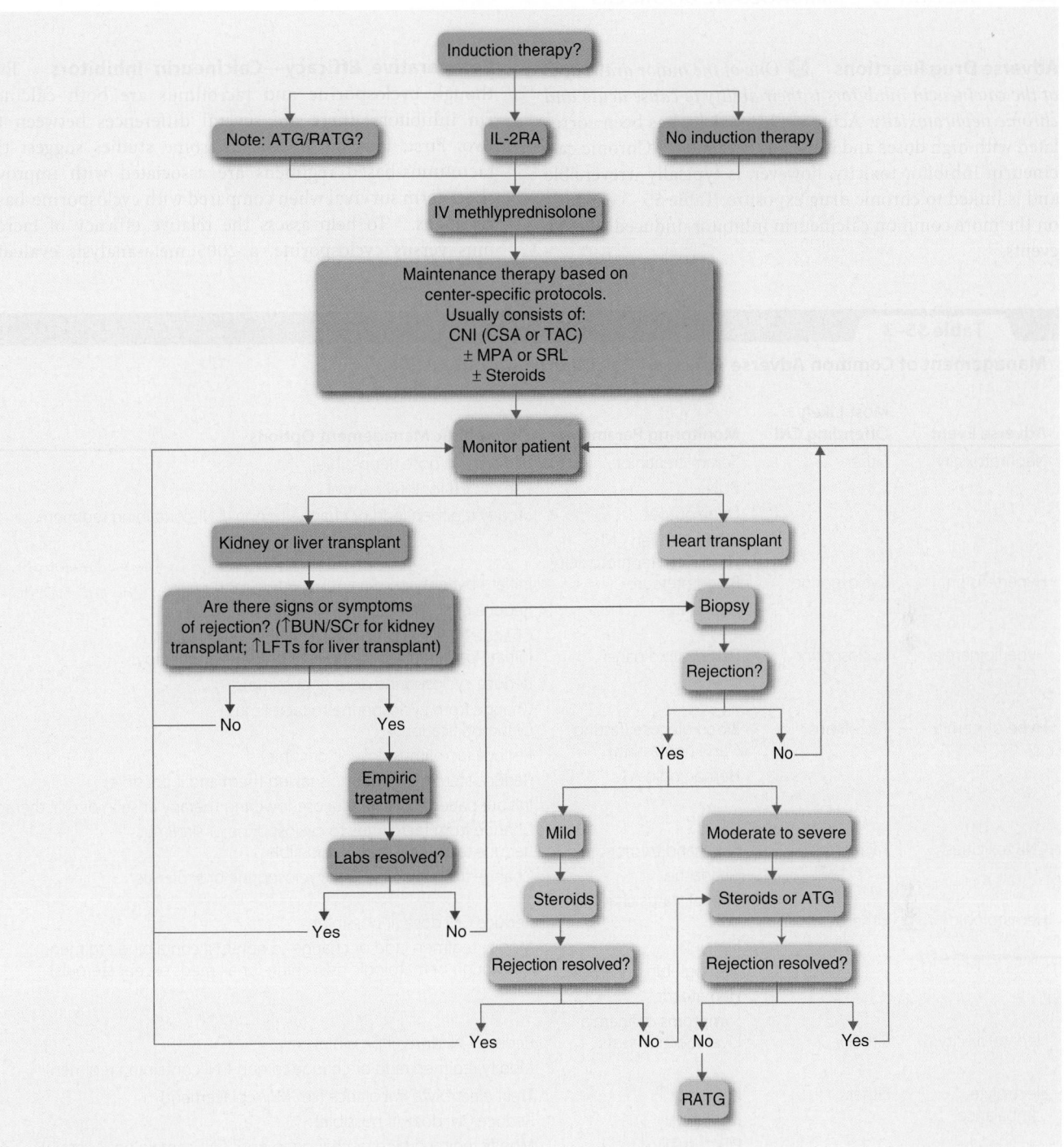

FIGURE 55–2. Example protocol of immunosuppressive medication use in organ transplantation. Center-specific protocols may use rabbit antithymocyte immunoglobulin (RATG), an interleukin-2 receptor antagonist (IL-2RA), or no induction therapy. In any situation, patients receive IV methylprednisone prior to, during, or immediately following the transplant operation. The patient then will begin the maintenance immunosuppressive regimen. The center-specific protocol will specify which calcineurin inhibitor (cyclosporine or tacrolimus) is used in combination with mycophenolate mofetil or sirolimus, with or without steroids. Patients then are monitored for signs and symptoms of rejection. If rejection is suspected, a biopsy can be done for definitive diagnosis, or the patient may be treated empirically for rejection. Empirical treatment generally involves administration of corticosteroids. If signs and symptoms of rejection are resolved with empirical therapy, the patient will continue to be monitored according to the center-specific protocol. If rejection is confirmed by biopsy, treatment may be based on the severity of rejection. High-dose corticosteroids are used most frequently for mild to moderate rejection. RATG can be used for moderate to severe rejections or steroid-resistant rejections. (ATG, antithymocyte globulin; BUN, blood urea nitrogen; CNI, calcineurin inhibitor; CSA, cyclosporine; IL-2RA, interleukin-2 receptor antagonist; LFT, liver function test; MPA, mycophenolic acid; RATG, rabbit antithymocyte immunoglobulin; SCr, serum creatinine; SRL, sirolimus; TAC, tacrolimus.) (From Schonder KS, Johnson HJ. Solid Organ Transplantation. In: DiPiro JT, Talbert RL, Yee GC, et al., eds. Pharmacotherapy: A Pathophysiologic Approach. 7th ed. New York: McGraw-Hill; 2008:1466.)

Adverse Drug Reactions ⑤ *One of the major drawbacks of the calcineurin inhibitors is their ability to cause acute and chronic nephrotoxicity.* Acute nephrotoxicity has been correlated with high doses and is usually reversible.[10] Chronic calcineurin inhibitor toxicity, however, is typically irreversible and is linked to chronic drug exposure. Table 55–3 expands on the more common calcineurin inhibitor–induced adverse events.

Comparative Efficacy—Calcineurin Inhibitors Even though cyclosporine and tacrolimus are both calcineurin inhibitors, there are several differences between the two. First, looking at efficacy, some studies suggest that tacrolimus-based regimens are associated with improved short-term survival when compared with cyclosporine-based regimens.[25] To help assess the relative efficacy of tacrolimus versus cyclosporine, a 2005 meta-analysis evaluated

Table 55–3

Management of Common Adverse Effects of Calcineurin Inhibitors[2,8,9]

Adverse Event	Most Likely Offending CNI	Monitoring Parameters	Therapeutic Management Options
Nephrotoxicity	Either	Serum creatinine BUN Urine output Biopsy-proven CNI-induced nephrotoxicity	Reduce CNI dose (if possible) Use of CCB for HTN control Modify regimen (add or change to non–CNI-containing regimen)
Hypertension[a]	Cyclosporine	Blood pressure Heart rate	Initiate patient-specific antihypertensive therapy Reduce cyclosporine dose (if possible) Change from cyclosporine to tacrolimus or sirolimus
Hyperlipidemia[a]	Cyclosporine	Fasting lipid panel	Initiate patient-specific cholesterol-lowering therapy Reduce cyclosporine dose (if possible) Change from cyclosporine to tacrolimus
Hyperglycemia[b]	Tacrolimus	Blood glucose (fasting and nonfasting) Hemoglobin A1c	Diet modifications Reduce tacrolimus dose (if possible) Reduce steroids (if patient is taking them and if possible) Initiate patient-specific glucose-lowering therapy (insulin or oral therapy) Change from tacrolimus to cyclosporine or sirolimus
CNS toxicities[b]	Tacrolimus	Fine hand tremor Headache Mental status changes	Reduce tacrolimus dose (if possible) Change from tacrolimus to cyclosporine or sirolimus
Hematologic	Either	WBC Platelets Hemoglobin Hematocrit Symptoms of anemia	Reduce CNI dose (if possible) Modify regimen (add or change to non-CNI containing regimen; although hematologic risk is high for all meds except steroids)
Hepatotoxicity	Either	Liver function tests	Reduce CNI dose (if possible) Modify regimen (add or change to non-CNI containing regimen)
Electrolyte Imbalance	Either	K (usually ↑) Mg (usually ↓) PO$_4$ (usually ↓)	Treat electrolyte imbalance (i.e., Mg replacement) Reduce CNI dose (if possible) Modify regimen (add or change to non–CNI-containing regimen)
Hirsutism	Cyclosporine	Patient complains of excessive hair growth or male-pattern hair growth	Reduce cyclosporine dose (if possible) Cosmetic hair removal Change from cyclosporine to tacrolimus or sirolimus
Alopecia	Tacrolimus	Patient complains of excessive hair loss	Reduce tacrolimus dose (if possible) Hair growth treatments (i.e., minoxidil, finasteride—males only) Change from tacrolimus to cyclosporine or sirolimus
Gingival Hyperplasia	Cyclosporine	Patient complains of excessive gum growth Recommendations for therapy from the patient's dentist	Reduce cyclosporine dose (if possible) Oral surgery (gum resection) Change from cyclosporine to tacrolimus or sirolimus

BUN, blood urea nitrogen; CCB, calcium channel blocker; CNI, calcineurin inhibitor; CNS, central nervous system; HTN, hypertension; K, potassium; Mg, magnesium; PO$_4$, phosphate; WBC, white blood cell count.

[a]Tacrolimus is also associated with hypertension and hyperlipidemia, but to a much lower extent compared with cyclosporine.

[b]Cyclosporine is also associated with hyperglycemia and CNS toxicities, but to a much lower extent compared with tacrolimus.

30 trials consisting of 4,102 patients.[26] In this meta-analysis, tacrolimus, when compared with either formulation of cyclosporine, was associated with a significantly lower risk of allograft loss at 6 months. It also appeared that late allograft loss favored tacrolimus. In addition, lower rates of acute rejection were seen at 1 year in tacrolimus-treated patients.[26] In recent years, tacrolimus has become the primary calcineurin inhibitor in many transplant centers, due in large part to a more favorable adverse reaction profile.[22]

▶ Antiproliferatives

These agents are generally considered to be adjuvant to the calcineurin inhibitors or ToR inhibitors. The medications included in this class are azathioprine and the MPA derivatives.

Azathioprine Azathioprine was originally approved in 1968 as an adjunct immunosuppressant for use in renal transplant recipients. It is available in oral and IV dosage forms.[10] Prior to the advent of cyclosporine, the combination of azathioprine and corticosteroids was the mainstay of immunosuppressive therapy. Over the past 10 years, the use of azathioprine has declined markedly, due in large part to the success of the MPA derivatives, which are more specific inhibitors of T-cell proliferation. ⑥ *Azathioprine is a prodrug for 6-mercaptopurine (6-MP), a purine analog. 6-MP acts as an antimetabolite and inhibits DNA replication with a resultant reduction in T-cell proliferation.*[10] *The typical oral dose of azathioprine for organ transplantation is 3 to 5 mg/kg once a day.*[10] *The maintenance dose is usually reduced to 1 to 2 mg/kg/day within a few weeks posttransplant.* Dose reductions due to severely impaired renal function may be necessary since 6-MP and its metabolites are renally eliminated.[10] Trough concentrations of 6-MP are not monitored; however, most clinicians often monitor for signs of myelosuppression. ⑥ *Myelosuppression (mainly leukopenia and thrombocytopenia) is a frequent, dose-dependent and dose-limiting complication (greater than 50% of patients) that often prompts dose reductions.*[10] *Other common adverse events include hepatotoxicity (2% to 10%) and adverse gastrointestinal (GI) events (10% to 15%; mostly nausea and vomiting). Importantly, pancreatitis and venoocclusive disease of the liver occur in less than 1% of patients following chronic azathioprine therapy.*[10]

Mycophenolic Acid Derivatives Mycophenolate mofetil was approved in 1995 and enteric-coated MPA in 2004. Both agents are considered to be adjunctive immunosuppressants. ⑥ *Both mycophenolate mofetil and enteric-coated MPA are prodrugs for MPA.* MPA acts by inhibiting inosine monophosphate dehydrogenase, a vital enzyme in the de novo pathway of purine synthesis. Inhibition of this enzyme prevents the proliferation of most cells that are dependent on the de novo pathway for purine synthesis, including T cells.[9,10,27-29]

Mycophenolate mofetil is available in 250-mg and 500-mg capsules, an oral suspension (100 mg/mL; in cherry syrup), and as an injectable.[10] Usual doses of mycophenolate mofetil range from 1,000 to 3,000 mg/day in two to four divided doses. The conversion between oral and IV mycophenolate

mofetil is 1:1. Enteric-coated MPA is available in 180-mg and 360-mg tablets. The appropriate equimolar conversion between mycophenolate mofetil and enteric-coated MPA is 1,000 mg of mycophenolate mofetil to 720 mg of enteric-coated MPA.[27,28,30] The recommended starting dose of enteric-coated MPA is 720 mg given twice daily.[27] Conversion of mycophenolate mofetil to enteric-coated MPA has been proven safe. MPA C_0 can be monitored; however, they are not routinely recommended.

⑥ *The most common adverse events associated with these agents are GI (18% to 54%; diarrhea, nausea, vomiting, and gastritis) and myelosuppression (20% to 40%).*[9,10,27-29] Despite being enteric-coated, enteric-coated MPA has produced the same degree of GI adverse events as mycophenolate mofetil.[27,30] However, recent data suggest that there is a benefit in converting patients with documented mycophenolate-induced GI disease from mycophenolate mofetil to enteric-coated MPA.[31]

Comparative Efficacy—Antiproliferatives Due to the results of several studies, the MPA derivatives have replaced azathioprine as the antiproliferative agent of choice in most organ transplant centers. The MPA derivatives are generally considered to provide a more specific immunosuppressive effect compared with azathioprine. Mycophenolate mofetil and enteric-coated MPA have similar safety and efficacy data in renal transplant recipients. The decision to choose one agent over another is a purely practitioner-dependent preference.

▶ Target of Rapamycin Inhibitors

Sirolimus ⑦ *Sirolimus is a macrolide antibiotic that inhibits T-cell activation and proliferation by binding to and inhibiting the activation of the mammalian ToR, which suppresses cellular response to IL-2 and other cytokines (i.e., IL-4, IL-15).*[10,32] Studies have shown that sirolimus may be used safely and effectively with either cyclosporine or tacrolimus as a replacement for either azathioprine or mycophenolate mofetil.[33] Sirolimus can also be used as an alternative agent for patients who do not tolerate calcineurin inhibitors due to nephrotoxicity or other adverse events.[34] ⑦ *At this time, the most exciting data for sirolimus point to its ability to prevent long-term allograft dysfunction when used as a substitute for the calcineurin inhibitors in renal transplant recipients.*[32,33]

Sirolimus is available in 0.5-mg, 1-mg, and 2-mg tablets and a 1-mg/mL oral solution. The current approved dosing regimen for sirolimus is a 6-mg loading dose followed by a 2-mg/day maintenance dose.[10] It was recommended that this agent does not require therapeutic drug monitoring. However, most centers do check trough concentrations and adjust doses to reach goal concentrations.[35] Most clinicians who use sirolimus utilize a loading dose of 5 to 15 mg/day for 1 to 3 days to more rapidly achieve adequate immunosuppression.[30,32] Maintenance doses of sirolimus usually range from 1 to 10 mg/day given once daily. Sirolimus blood C_0 should be maintained between 5 and 20 ng/mL, depending on the institution-specific protocols.[35] Of note, sirolimus has a half-life of approximately 62 hours, which means that it will not reach steady state after dosage changes for several days.[10]

⑦ *The most common adverse events reported with sirolimus are leukopenia (20%), thrombocytopenia (13% to 30%), and hyperlipidemia (38% to 57%).*[10,32] Other adverse effects include delayed wound healing, anemia, diarrhea, arthralgias, rash, proteinuria, pneumonitis, and mouth ulcers. ⑦ *A recent analysis suggests that use of sirolimus in kidney transplant recipients can reduce cardiovascular risk compared with calcineurin inhibitor–based regimens.*[36] Sirolimus has a black-box warning in newly transplanted liver and lung recipients.[10] In liver transplant recipients, use of sirolimus immediately after transplant is associated with an increased risk of hepatic artery thrombosis, graft loss, and death. In lung transplant recipients, bronchial anastomotic dehiscence, including some fatal cases, has been noted in patients treated with sirolimus, tacrolimus, and corticosteroids.[10]

Everolimus Everolimus is a derivative of sirolimus and has the same mechanism of action.[10,37] Everolimus is only indicated for prevention of rejection in low- to moderate-risk renal transplant recipients when given in conjunction with basiliximab induction, reduced-dose cyclosporine, and corticosteroids. This agent is available in 0.25-mg, 0.5-mg, and 0.75-mg tablets. The recommended starting dose of everolimus is 0.75 mg twice daily without the need for a loading dose. Maintenance everolimus doses should be maximized to achieve a C_0 goal of 3 to 8 ng/mL.[37,38] With a significantly shorter half-life compared with sirolimus, everolimus steady-state can be reached within 90 to 150 hours. ⑦ *The adverse event profile of everolimus is similar to that seen with sirolimus.*[10,37]

▶ Corticosteroids

Traditional triple-therapy immunosuppressive regimens have consisted of one of the following combinations:

- A calcineurin inhibitor, an antiproliferative, and a corticosteroid
- A calcineurin inhibitor, a ToR inhibitor, and a corticosteroid
- A ToR inhibitor, an antiproliferative, and a corticosteroid

In recent years, many protocols have focused on corticosteroid sparing or avoidance. Avoidance or sparing of corticosteroids has been supported in the literature, although more studies are needed to help better characterize which patients should follow these protocols.[19,39–43] A typical taper includes a bolus of IV methylprednisolone 100 to 500 mg at the time of transplant, then tapered over days to months (depending on the type of organ) to a maintenance low dose of prednisone 5 to 10 mg/day. Although most centers still use low-dose steroids for immunologically high-risk patients, a number of renal transplant programs have developed an immunosuppression protocol that completely avoids or withdraws corticosteroids at some point posttransplantation.[2,9] Therapeutic drug monitoring of corticosteroids is not employed. ⑧ *Corticosteroids are associated with a variety of acute and chronic toxicities.* The most common adverse events have been summarized in Table 55–4.

Table 55–4

Common Adverse Events Associated With Corticosteroids[9]

Body System	Adverse Event
Cardiovascular	Hyperlipidemia
	Hypertension
Central nervous system	Anxiety
	Insomnia
	Mood changes
	Psychosis
Dermatologic	Acne
	Diaphoresis
	Ecchymosis
	Hirsutism
	Impaired wound healing
	Petechiae
	Thin skin
Endocrine/metabolic	Cushing's syndrome
	Hyperglycemia
	Sodium and water retention
Gastrointestinal	Gastritis
	Increased appetite
	Nausea, vomiting, diarrhea
	Peptic ulcers
Hematologic	Leukocytosis
Neuromuscular/skeletal	Arthralgia
	Impaired growth
	Osteoporosis
	Skeletal muscle weakness
Ocular	Cataracts
	Glaucoma
Respiratory	Epistaxis

⑧ *Corticosteroids have various effects on immune and inflammatory response systems, although their exact mechanism of immunosuppression is not fully understood.* It is generally believed that at high doses, the agents are directly lymphotoxic, and at lower doses, it is believed that corticosteroids act by inhibiting the production of various cytokines that are necessary to amplify the immune response.[2,9]

The most commonly used corticosteroids are methylprednisolone (IV and oral) and prednisone (oral), although prednisolone and dexamethasone have also been shown to be effective for organ transplantation. Corticosteroid doses vary by center-specific protocols, organ type, and patient characteristics.

▶ Costimulatory Pathway Blocker

Belatacept Belatacept was approved in 2011 as the first IV biologic agent for maintenance immunosuppression in renal transplant recipients. ⑨ *Belatacept results in the blockade of the CD80 and CD86 ligands, found on APCs.*[44] The CD80 and CD86 proteins are responsible for stimulating CD28 on inactive T cells, an essential costimulatory interaction (Signal 2). As detailed in the T-Cell Activation section, Signal 1, the interaction of the TCR with a foreign antigen presented by an APC, without a complementary Signal 2 induces T-cell anergy.[45]

Studies have shown that in combination with mycophenolate mofetil and corticosteroids, belatacept may be used in place of calcineurin inhibitors. Studies demonstrated similar patient and allograft survival in patients receiving belatacept compared with those receiving a cyclosporine-based regimen.[46,47] ⑨ *Belatacept was found to improve renal function; however, the incidence of acute rejection was found to be significantly increased.* Additional benefits of belatacept when compared with calcineurin-based regimens may include improvement in blood pressure and lipid levels.[45]

Belatacept is available in a 250-mg vial that requires reconstitution prior to administration.[10] The recommended dosing regimen for belatacept is 10 mg/kg on the first day of transplantation, followed by an additional dose 4 days after transplant, and again at the end of weeks 2, 4, 8, and 12, posttransplant. Beginning at the end of week 16 posttransplant, belatacept is dosed at 5 mg/kg and every 4 weeks thereafter.[10,45] Belatacept requires access to an infusion center, a hired home infusion service, or an infusion suite to ensure appropriate IV administration.

The most common adverse effects associated with belatacept are infectious (urinary tract infection, 37%; upper respiratory infection, 15%), GI (diarrhea, 39%; constipation, 33%; nausea, 24%, vomiting, 22%), metabolic (hyperkalemia, 20%; hypokalemia 21%), and central nervous system (CNS; headache, 21%) complications.[10,45] Other adverse effects include peripheral edema, anemia, leukopenia, hypotension, arthralgia, and insomnia. ⑨ *Belatacept has a black-box warning for increased risk of developing posttransplant lymphoproliferative disorders (PTLD), especially in the CNS. Due to this risk, it is recommended that belatacept only be used in patients who present with a proven preexisting immunity to Epstein-Barr virus (EBV).* An additional black box warning states that the use of belatacept in liver transplant patients is not recommended due to an increased risk of allograft loss and patient death.[10,45]

Immunosuppressive Therapies—Future Immunosuppressive Agents

The immunosuppressant armamentarium is expanding with novel small molecules (i.e., protein kinase C and the Janus-Kinase 3 inhibitors) and other biological agents currently in clinical development. These newer agents appear promising and may represent the emergence of novel immunosuppressive agents that can deliver immunosuppression without the long-term toxicities. Some currently marketed immunosuppressants may also have beneficial effects in organ transplantation. Several agents, including alefacept, bortezomib, alemtuzumab (discussed previously), efalizumab, leflunomide and rituximab, have already been used successfully in renal transplantation.

Immunosuppressive Therapies—Treatment of Acute Rejection Episodes

Acute rejection is generally treated with a course of high-dose methylprednisolone (250 to 1,000 mg/day IV for 3 days),

which is usually sufficient to ameliorate the rejection episode. If the acute rejection episode is resistant to the initial course of steroids, a second course may be administered or the patient may begin therapy with r-ATG (1.5 mg/kg/day for 3 to 14 days).[48] Cellular acute rejection refractory to these treatments is rare and is likely due to underlying causes such as an antibody-mediated component or other diagnosis. Treatments of refractory acute rejection may include alemtuzumab, IVIG, high-dose tacrolimus, or organ irradiation. Refractory cellular acute rejections are typically related to therapeutic failures, which may require changing to an alternative protein source such as e-ATG.

Immunosuppressive Therapies—Managing Highly Sensitized Patients and Antibody-Mediated Rejection Episodes

The presence of preformed antibodies, high PRA, and donor-specific antibodies (DSA) are major barriers to successful transplantation.[49-51] This is true, mainly because traditional immunosuppressants do not significantly affect the humoral immune system and are ineffective at management of AMR, which is a leading cause of allograft loss in kidney and heart transplant recipients. Without some form of intervention, antibody formation and rejection can be a major cause of morbidity and mortality. Two major strategies are used for reduction of DSA pretransplant: (a) high-dose IV immune globulin (IVIG), and (b) plasmapheresis plus low-dose IVIG. Each approach has advantages and disadvantages.[49-51]

In plasmapheresis or plasma exchange, patients' plasma is removed and replaced with albumin or fresh-frozen plasma.[49-51] Plasmapheresis produces a rapid reduction of preformed antibodies and allows transplantation to occur. The purpose of IVIG administration is to decrease anti-HLA alloantibody synthesis. The other mechanisms of IVIG are inhibition of complement-mediated injury, reduced B-cell proliferation and NK cells, and a decrease in phagocytosis. Most patients require four to five plasmapheresis sessions and use of IVIG to remove the DSA. In patients at risk for bleeding, the use of albumin should be limited, and fresh-frozen plasma or a combination of both agents should be considered.[49-51]

In one study, Stegall compared a single dose of IVIG with two plasmapheresis sessions plus low-dose IVIG regimens. The overall success rate for desensitization was 84% to 88% in the plasmapheresis plus IVIG groups, but only 38% in the high-dose IVIG group.[51] However, they also reported that patients with high titers did not respond to either treatment.

In patients who develop AMR posttransplant, there are limited therapeutic options, none of which are FDA-approved. The potential options include plasmapheresis and IVIG, rituximab, bortezomib, and/or eculizumab.[6] All of these agents have an affect on humoral immunity, which may provide benefit to patients with AMR. The mechanisms of plasmapheresis and IVIG have been discussed earlier in this chapter. Details regarding the use of rituximab, bortezomib, and eculizumab for desensitization and treatment of AMR are provided next.[6]

Rituximab is a chimeric monoclonal anti-CD20 antibody targeting B cells.[6,10] This agent directly inhibits B-cell proliferation and induces cellular apoptosis through complement-mediated antibody-dependent cellular cytotoxicity and cell death. In an analysis of AMR treatment, the use of rituximab in conjunction with plasmapheresis/IVIG resulted in improved 3-year graft survival (92% versus 50%) and significantly reduced DSA at 3 months compared with high-dose IVIG alone.[52] Unfortunately, the majority of plasma cells lack CD20 and are unaffected by rituximab. However, rituximab may play an important role in reducing memory B-cell response. Overall, it appears that rituximab may provide beneficial effects in managing AMR when used in combination with other therapies.[6,10]

Bortezomib is a proteasome inhibitor indicated for treatment of multiple myeloma.[6,10] It works by inducing cell-cycle arrest and apoptosis of plasma cells. It also has been shown to exert numerous indirect effects on circulating B and T cells. Desensitization and treatment protocols using bortezomib have utilized doses ranging from 1 to 1.3 mg/m^2 from one to four cycles. Most commonly observed adverse effects include peripheral neuropathy, hematologic effects (thrombocytopenia, neutropenia, anemia), asthenia, paresthesia, and rash. Limited published data document bortezomib use in kidney transplantation protocols. When used in combination with other accepted modalities, it is difficult to discern whether there is any additional benefit when adding on bortezomib in patients at risk of AMR. The small case reports and case series in existence resulted in little to no added benefit in AMR treatment.[6,10] A recent analysis including less than 20 patients found treatment of AMR with bortezomib to be more efficacious compared with rituximab.[53] Future study is warranted before bortezomib can be considered as mainstay therapy of AMR.

Eculizumab is a humanized monoclonal antibody directed against complement protein C5.[6,10] It inhibits the cleavage to C5a and C5b, thus preventing the generation of the membrane attack complex (MAC) and reducing antibody-dependent cell lysis. One case report used eculizumab in combination with plasmapheresis/IVIG to salvage a kidney transplant from severe AMR.[54] In this analysis, there was a marked decrease in MAC deposition in the kidney.

Maintenance Immunosuppressive Therapies—Common Drug–Drug Interactions

⑩ *As the number of medications that a patient takes increases, so does the potential for DDIs.* Disease severity, patient age, and organ dysfunction are all risk factors for increased DDIs. In general, DDIs can be broken down into two categories: (a) pharmacokinetic, and (b) pharmacodynamic interactions.

- Pharmacokinetic interactions result when one drug alters the absorption, distribution, metabolism, or elimination of another drug.

- Pharmacodynamic interactions include additive, synergistic, or antagonistic interactions that can affect efficacy or toxicity.

▶ *Pharmacokinetic Interactions*

Pharmacokinetic DDIs pose a major dilemma with the maintenance immunosuppressants. Pharmacokinetic interactions can either result in increased concentrations of one or more agents with an increased risk for drug-induced toxicities, or lowered (i.e., subtherapeutic) drug concentrations, possibly leading to allograft rejection. As mentioned previously, pharmacokinetic DDIs can be further categorized into interactions of absorption, distribution, metabolism, and elimination.

Interactions of Absorption Most DDIs are due to altered absorption and occur within the intestines. There are a variety of potential mechanisms through which the absorption of the maintenance immunosuppressants is altered, including:

- Drug metabolism within the gut ("Interactions of Metabolism" will be discussed later)
- Alterations in the active transport process
- Changes in intestinal motility
- Chelation interactions

Active transporters (i.e., P-glycoprotein [P-gp]) play an important role in DDIs. P-gp, a plasma membrane transport protein, is present in the gut, brain, liver, and kidneys.[55,56] This protein provides a biological barrier, eliminating toxic substances and xenobiotics that may accumulate in these organ systems. P-gp plays an important role in the absorption and distribution of many medications. In the GI tract, P-gp is located in the brush borders of mature enterocytes. The colon has the largest percentage of P-gp, whereas the stomach and jejunum-ileum contain the lowest percentage. P-gp affects the absorption of cyclosporine, tacrolimus, sirolimus, and everolimus. Some medications can alter the activity of P-gp (inhibit or induce its activity). Medications that are cytochrome P450 (CYP) 3A4 substrates, inhibitors, or inducers also tend to affect P-gp; therefore, the potential exists for several DDIs with the immunosuppressants by this mechanism.[55,56] For example, medications that inhibit P-gp activity will increase concentrations of cyclosporine, tacrolimus, sirolimus, and everolimus due to a reduction in P-gp–dependent drug elimination from the hepatic circulation.

When looking at the ability of drugs that change intestinal motility and their effects on the maintenance immunosuppressants, you can see notable interactions between the prokinetic agents and the calcineurin inhibitors. Metoclopramide has been shown to increase the absorption of cyclosporine and tacrolimus by enhancing gastric mobility and emptying.[57]

Most of the interactions with mycophenolate mofetil and enteric-coated MPA are due to reductions in intestinal absorption. Proton pump inhibitor use can decrease the oral absorption of mycophenolate mofetil, but has no effect on enteric-coated MPA.[58] Aluminum, magnesium, and calcium-containing products decrease the peak level of MPA.[10] If a patient requires aluminum, magnesium, or calcium, it should be administered at least 4 hours before or after MPA. Of note, iron does not interact with the MPA preparations.[59]

Interactions of Distribution Interactions of distribution tend to occur with drugs that are highly protein bound. A drug that is extensively bound to plasma proteins can be displaced from its binding site by another agent that has greater affinity for the same binding site, thereby raising free concentrations of the displaced drug. MPA is the only highly protein bound (97% bound to albumin) maintenance immunosuppressant with a reported DDI by this mechanism. It has been shown that concomitant administration of MPA with salicylates increases the free concentrations of MPA.[10] The adverse sequelae of this drug interaction have not been assessed. DDI studies have not been completed evaluating the MPA derivatives, or the other highly protein bound maintenance immunosuppressants, when used with other highly protein bound drugs.

Interactions of Metabolism Oxidative metabolism by CYP isozymes is the primary method of drug metabolism.[60] The purpose of drug metabolism is to make drugs more water-soluble so they can be more easily eliminated. Cyclosporine, tacrolimus, sirolimus, and everolimus are all substrates of the CYP3A isozyme system. The majority of CYP-mediated metabolism takes place in the liver; however, CYP is also expressed in the intestine, lungs, kidneys, and brain. Two types of interactions usually occur with medications metabolized via the CYP enzyme system: inhibitory interactions and inducing interactions. Enzyme inhibition occurs when there is enzyme inactivation or mutual competition of substrates at a catalytic site. This usually results in a reduction of drug metabolism leading to increased medication concentrations. Enzyme induction interactions are just the opposite and occur when there is increased synthesis or decreased degradation of CYP enzymes. This type of interaction can produce decreased concentrations of medications.[60] Being CYP3A substrates, it would be anticipated that cyclosporine, tacrolimus, sirolimus, and everolimus would all experience similar pharmacokinetic DDIs. Table 55–5 details the clinically relevant DDIs that occur with the calcineurin and ToR inhibitors due to inhibition or induction of the CYP isozyme system.

One of the most often overlooked DDIs in transplant recipients is the effect corticosteroids have on drug metabolism. Dexamethasone is a CYP3A isozyme inducer, meaning that it may decrease the C_0 of cyclosporine, tacrolimus, sirolimus, and everolimus.[10,61] Conversely, methylprednisolone is a CYP3A isozyme inhibitor, and it may increase the C_0 of cyclosporine, tacrolimus, sirolimus, and everolimus.[10,61] This is usually not a noteworthy interaction, since doses of the immunosuppressants are titrated to achieve target concentrations in patients maintained on stable doses of corticosteroids. However, these DDIs may be problematic after pulse dose steroids for treatment of acute rejection or during steroid withdrawal.

Not all metabolic DDIs occur through the CYP system. Azathioprine has a considerable interaction with both allopurinol and febuxostat that is not mediated through CYP.[62] Allopurinol and febuxostat inhibit xanthine oxidase, which is the enzyme responsible for metabolizing 6-MP to inactive 6-thiouricate. Combining these agents can result in 6-MP accumulation and severe toxicities, particularly myelosuppression. It is recommended that concomitant therapy with azathioprine and allopurinol or febuxostat be avoided, but if necessary, azathioprine doses must be reduced to one-third or one-fourth of the current dose.[62]

Interactions of Elimination There are very few interactions of elimination with the maintenance immunosuppressants. However, the major interaction through this process involves MPA. MPA is metabolized to MPA-glucuronide (MPAG) via hepatic glucuronosyltransferase.[10,27] MPAG is excreted in the bile for elimination in the gut. Deconjugation of MPAG back to MPA by intestinal flora results in a secondary absorption of MPA several hours after its administration.[10,27] Several medications have been shown to interfere with the biliary excretion of MPAG, thereby eliminating its reabsorption in the intestines and lowering the overall exposure to MPA. Cyclosporine has been shown to reduce the overall exposure to the MPA derivatives through competitive inhibition of MPAG enterohepatic recirculation.[63] MPA levels are lower when administered in cyclosporine-based immunosuppression regimens compared with tacrolimus-based regimens. The bile acid sequestrants (i.e., cholestyramine, colestipol, colesevelam) have also been shown to decrease overall MPA exposure through a similar mechanism.[64,65]

▶ *Pharmacodynamic Interactions*

In addition to the numerous pharmacokinetic interactions seen with the maintenance immunosuppressants, there also exists the possibility for pharmacodynamic interactions. An in-depth review of pharmacodynamic interactions with maintenance immunosuppressive agents goes beyond the scope of this chapter. However, some common pharmacodynamic DDIs will be discussed. Pharmacodynamic interactions are the backbone of modern immunosuppressive therapies that employ multiple medications with different mechanisms of action resulting in additive immunosuppression. Unfortunately, pharmacodynamic interactions can also be problematic, such as when medications with similar adverse events are used concomitantly. For example, nephrotoxic agents, such as amphotericin B, aminoglycosides (i.e., gentamicin, tobramycin, amikacin), and nonsteroidal anti-inflammatory drugs (NSAIDs; i.e., naproxen, ibuprofen, ketorolac) may potentiate the nephrotoxic effects of the calcineurin inhibitors.[10] The use of myelosuppressive agents, such as sulfamethoxazole-trimethoprim and valganciclovir, could enhance the myelosuppressive effects of induction therapy and the maintenance immunosuppressants.[10]

The potential exists for multiple DDIs in transplant recipients due to the complexity of their medication regimens. Practitioners must be diligent in reviewing all medications for potential DDIs. In addition to reviewing prescription medications, it is essential to question patients about the use of both nonprescription and complementary and alternative medicines, as these products also have the potential for significant interactions.

Table 55–5

Potential Drug–Drug Interactions with the Calcineurin Inhibitors and Target of Rapamycin Inhibitors Mediated Through the Cytochrome P-450 System 3A (CYP3A4) Isozyme[9]

Substrates[a]		Inducers[b]	Inhibitors[c]
Alfentanil	Loratadine	Carbamazepine	Boceprevir
Alprazolam	Lovastatin	Dexamethasone	Cimetidine
Amiodarone	Nevirapine	Etravirine	Clarithromycin
Amlodipine	Nicardipine	Ethosuximide	Clotrimazole
Atorvastatin	Nifedipine	Isoniazid	Delavirdine
Boceprevir	Omeprazole	Nevirapine	Diltiazem
Cilostazol	Paclitaxel	Phenobarbital	Erythromycin
Cisapride	Propafenone	Phenytoin	Fluconazole
Chlorpromazine	Progesterone	Prednisone	Fluoxetine
Clonazepam	Quetiapine	Rifabutin	Fluvoxamine
Cocaine	Quinidine	Rifampin	Grapefruit juice
Cortisol	Rilpivirine	Rilpivirine	Indinavir
Cyclophosphamide	Rivaroxaban	St. John's wort	Itraconazole
Dantrolene	Sertraline		Ketoconazole
Dapsone	Simvastatin		Miconazole
Diazepam	Tamoxifen		Nefazodone
Disopyramide	Testosterone		Nelfinavir
Enalapril	Tolvaptan		Rilpivirine
Estradiol	Triazolam		Ritonavir
Estrogen	Vandetanib		Saquinavir
Etoposide	Venlafaxine		Telapravir
Everolimus	Vinblastine		Troleandomycin
Felodipine	Warfarin		Verapamil
Flutamide	Zolpidem		Voriconazole
Lidocaine			Zafirlukast

[a]Substrates of the CYP3A4 isozyme will compete with cyclosporine, tacrolimus, and sirolimus for metabolism; therefore, concentrations of both medications will be increased (usually by less than or equal to 20%).

[b]Inducers of the CYP3A4 isozyme will enhance the metabolism of cyclosporine, tacrolimus, and sirolimus; therefore, concentrations of these medications will be decreased.

[c]Inhibitors of the CYP3A4 isozyme will decrease the metabolism of cyclosporine, tacrolimus, and sirolimus; therefore, concentrations of these medications will be increased.

Patient Encounter Part 2

Identify your treatment goals for ED in terms of maintenance immunosuppressants.

Create a plan for maintenance therapy for ED, making sure to compare and contrast the pros and cons of the different maintenance immunosuppressants.

Identify the need to continue the patient's pretransplant medications, and identify any potential DDIs that may exist with the addition of the maintenance immunosuppressants and the medications that ED is currently taking.

Immunosuppressive Therapies—Controversies with Generic Immunosuppressants

The question of whether clinically relevant changes in drug exposure would occur with the use of generic immunosuppressants culminated with the approval of several generic formulations for cyclosporine, cyclosporine modified, mycophenolate mofetil, and tacrolimus. Generic products are considered to be therapeutically equivalent if they are both bioequivalent and pharmaceutically equivalent to the innovator product. However, bioequivalence is determined in a small group of healthy volunteers and the issue raised is would the generic products be deemed bioequivalent in a transplant population. One concern is that given the narrow therapeutic windows of both cyclosporine and tacrolimus, would generic conversion result in significant changes in drug exposure, potentially resulting in acute rejection or drug toxicities.

Generic medications are commonplace within the US healthcare system. The availability of less expensive alternatives may allow for increased access to essential drug therapy as well as defraying associated costs. Organ transplant is not immune to the financial pressures on the healthcare system. However, with few clinical studies to help guide our decision making on the use of generic immunosuppressants, appropriate clinical decisions need to balance therapeutic outcomes, patient quality of life, and the associated financial burdens. The consensus guidelines from the American Society of Transplantation advocate for use of generic immunosuppressants if they are deemed bioequivalent to the innovator product.[66] The guidelines state that use of generics offers an opportunity to reduce direct costs to the patients and potentially improve adherence.

Immunosuppressive Therapies—Management of Immunosuppressive Drug Complications

▶ *Opportunistic Infections*

🔟 *Solid organ transplant recipients are at increased risk of infectious diseases, which are a chief cause of early morbidity and mortality.*[67] The prevalence of posttransplant infection depends on many factors, including clinical risk factors, environmental exposures, and the degree of immunosuppression. Antiinfectives are universally prescribed in this population, and their use can be split into three different categories:

- Prophylaxis: antimicrobials given to prevent infection
- Empiric: preemptive therapy given based on clinical suspicion of an active infection
- Treatment: antimicrobials given to manage a documented infection

Posttransplant infections generally occur in a standard pattern; therefore, prevention is a key management strategy. The information in this section is designed to only highlight prophylaxis options routinely used in organ transplant recipients. Please refer to Table 55–6 for a list of agents used for the prevention of *Pneumocystis jiroveci* pneumonia and CMV disease.

Pneumocystis jiroveci Pneumonia 🔟 *Without prophylaxis, P. jiroveci pneumonia occurs in 5% to 15% of transplant recipients.*[68] Antipneumocystis prophylaxis is enormously helpful and is generally used in all organ transplant recipients. The duration of prophylaxis is usually 6 to 12 months after transplant, but may be prolonged in highly immunosuppressed patients (i.e., active CMV disease, treatment for rejection) or liver or lung recipients.[68] Sulfamethoxazole-trimethoprim is the preferred agent for prophylaxis. One of its major advantages is its relatively broad spectrum of activity.

Clinical Presentation of *Pneumocystis jiroveci* Pneumonia

General
- Patients may not be in acute distress or they may feel completely run down; it is very patient specific.

Symptoms
- Patients may complain of fever, cough, and progressive dyspnea.

Signs
- The most common findings are fever and tachypnea.
- Chest examination may reveal crackles and rhonchi.

Radiographic Tests
- Chest radiographs may be normal in up to 25% of patients.
- The most common radiographic abnormalities are diffuse, bilateral interstitial, or alveolar infiltrates.

Not only is it effective against *Pneumocystis* pneumonia, but it also has activity against toxoplasmosis and other common bacterial infections. Patients who have sulfa allergies, glucose-6 phosphate dehydrogenase (G6PD) deficiency, or are unable to tolerate sulfamethoxazole-trimethoprim should be given one of the second-line treatments.[10] Unfortunately, the second-line agents are antiparasitics and have no meaningful activity against common bacteria. These agents include dapsone, atovaquone, and pentamidine.[68]

Cytomegalovirus CMV is the most concerning opportunistic pathogen in transplantation due to its association with poor outcomes.[69] CMV infection is present in 30% to 97% of the general population, but CMV disease is typically restricted to immunocompromised hosts. The risk of CMV disease is highest among CMV-naive recipients who receive a CMV-positive organ (donor+/recipient−). Other factors that augment the risk of CMV disease include organ type (lung and pancreas recipients are highest risk) and immunosuppressive agents (ALA use increases risk). CMV disease characteristically occurs within the first 3 to 6 months posttransplantation, but delayed onset disease has been seen in patients receiving antiviral prophylaxis.[69] Patients with CMV infection may present with general flu-like symptoms, including fever, chills, aches, malaise, and fatigue. CMV infection may result in more profound symptoms in the immunosuppressed patient, including leukopenia, thrombocytopenia, and organ dysfunction.

🔟 *Several antivirals have proven efficacy in preventing and treating CMV.*[69] Valacyclovir and valganciclovir, prodrugs of acyclovir and ganciclovir, respectively, have improved bioavailability compared with their parent compounds and offer the advantage of less frequent dosing. CMV prophylaxis is classically continued for the first 200 days, or longer, after

---

Table 55–6

Prophylactic Options for *Pneumocystis jiroveci* Pneumonia and CMV[68,69]

Medication	Dosing	Common Adverse Events
Antipneumocystis Prophylaxis		
Sulfamethoxazole-trimethoprim (Bactrim, Septra, SMZ-TMP, cotrimoxazole)	One SS tablet by mouth once a day[a] One DS tablet by mouth once a day[a] One DS tablet by mouth every M/W/F[a]	Hyperkalemia Myelosuppression Nephrotoxicity Neutropenia Photosensitivity Rash
Pentamidine (NebuPent)	300 mg inhaled every 3–4 weeks	Bronchospasm Cough Hypo- or hyperglycemia
Dapsone (Avlosulfon)	50–100 mg tablet by mouth once a day	Hepatotoxicity Myelosuppression Nephritis
Atovaquone (Mepron)	1,500 mg suspension by mouth once a day	Elevated liver transaminases Nausea Rash
Antivirals		
Valganciclovir (Valcyte)	450–900 mg by mouth once a day[a]	Stomach upset (8–41%) Myelosuppression (2–27%) Headache (9–22%)
Ganciclovir (Cytovene)	5 mg/kg IV everyday; or 1,000 mg by mouth three times a day[a]	Stomach upset (13–40%) Myelosuppression (5–40%) Rash (10–15%)
Valacyclovir (Valtrex)	1–2 g by mouth four times a day[a]	Stomach upset (1–15%) Myelosuppression (less than 1%) Headache (14–35%)
CMV IgG (CytoGam) and polyvalent IVIG	The maximum recommended total dosage per infusion is 150 mg/kg beginning within 72 hours of transplantation. Follow-up doses and time intervals depend on the type of organ transplanted.	Stomach upset (1–6%) Fevers and chills (1–6%) Flushing (1–6%)

CMV, cytomegalovirus; DS, double-strength (800 mg SMZ, 160 mg TMP); IgG, immunoglobulin G; IVIG, intravenous immune globulin; M/W/F, Monday, Wednesday, and Friday; SS, single-strength (400 mg SMZ, 80 mg TMP); SMZ, sulfamethoxazole; TMP, trimethoprim.

[a]Dose adjustment required in renal insufficiency.

---

transplantation.[70,71] Both IV ganciclovir and oral valganciclovir may be used for preemptive therapy or for treatment of established CMV disease. Prolonged courses of low-dose ganciclovir or valganciclovir prophylaxis may be more effective in preventing CMV infection but can increase the risk of developing ganciclovir-resistant strains. The adverse events are similar among these agents and include myelosuppression and GI effects.[10]

Fungal Infections Fungal infections are an important cause of morbidity and mortality in solid organ transplant recipients.[72] Immunologic (i.e., immunosuppressants, CMV infection), anatomic (i.e., tissue ischemia and damage), and surgical (i.e., duration of surgery, transfusion requirements) factors contribute to the risk for invasive fungal infections. Mucocutaneous candidiasis (i.e., oral thrush, esophagitis) is associated with corticosteroid and ALA use. ❿ *Oral nystatin or clotrimazole troches are effective prophylactic options for the prevention of thrush.* However, clotrimazole inhibits the CYP3A system in the gut and can alter immunosuppressive levels.[10] The use of systemic antifungal prophylaxis, such as oral fluconazole, is controversial due to the potential for

DDIs and the risk of developing resistance. The American Society of Transplantation has recommended antifungal prophylaxis in liver, lung, intestine, and pancreas transplantation.[73,74] The choice of agents depends on the fungal risk in that particular population. For example, liver, intestine, and pancreas transplant recipients are at high risk for candidiasis; therefore, the use of medications that cover *Candida* spp. is crucial, such as the triazole antifungals (i.e., fluconazole, itraconazole) or the echinocandins (i.e., caspofungin, micafungin, anidulafungin). Lung transplant recipients are at high risk for aspergillosis; therefore, it is imperative to use antifungal prophylaxis that covers *Aspergillus* spp., such as the echinocandins or polyenes (i.e., amphotericin B, lipid-based amphotericin B products).[73,74]

Polyomavirus One complication of increasing significance in renal transplant recipients is polyomavirus. In humans, there are two known pathologic polyoma strains, BK and JC. These viruses are rarely associated with disease in immunocompetent individuals. During periods of immunosuppression, the virus is reactivated and can be associated with significant morbidity.[75]

In renal transplant recipients, the major diseases caused by BK virus (BKV) are tubulointerstitial nephritis and ureteral stenosis. BKV-induced nephropathy (BKVN) presents with evidence of allograft dysfunction, resulting in either an asymptomatic acute or slowly progressive rise in serum creatinine concentrations. Some studies have reported the incidence of BK viremia to be as high as 29%. It is estimated that BKVN affects up to 10% of renal transplant recipients, frequently resulting in permanent renal dysfunction or allograft loss.[75]

Currently, treatment options for BKV are limited, and management recommendations are formulated based on individual case reports and small case series. Pharmacologic options with activity against BKV are limited; therefore, a reduction in the degree of immunosuppression in patients with BK viremia is often thought to be the first-line option to prevent BKVN. Despite the lack of a directed antiviral intervention, there are several agents that have anti-BK activity, including IVIG, cidofovir, leflunomide, and the fluoroquinolone antibiotics. All of these agents have been reported to provide some benefit in managing BKV in anecdotal cases.[75]

Vaccination   Vaccination is one of the most effective means of preventing infection and related complications.[76] However, there is a valid concern that solid organ transplant recipients may mount an inadequate response to vaccination due to immunosuppression. Required vaccinations should be administered prior to transplantation so that an appropriate antibody response can develop (Table 55–7). If this strategy is pursued, the earlier a vaccine is administered, the more effective it may be, as end-stage organ failure can also contribute to a decreased immune response.[76]

In general, the weakest response to vaccine is within the first 6 months posttransplantation due to the intense level of immunosuppression during this period.[76] Vaccination within 6 months of transplant may be considered on a case-by-case basis in those patients who are at high risk of developing infection. Use of inactive vaccines is preferred in transplant recipients due to the relative risk of infection associated with live vaccines. Healthcare workers and family members who are in close contact with transplant recipients and have received a live vaccine should consider use of respiratory masks for at least 7 days after vaccination and adhere to strict oral and hand hygiene.[76]

Table 55–7

Recommended Vaccinations Pre- and Posttransplant[76]

| Vaccine | Administration | | Additional Information |
	Before SOT	After SOT	
Hepatitis A	X		Immunize as soon as possible during course of disease
Hepatitis B	X		Immunize as soon as possible during course of disease (before transplant, administer 40 mcg dose in a series of 3–4 doses)
Herpes Zoster	X		Live[a] virus, administer greater than or equal to 14 days before immunosuppressant agents are initiated (experts advise 1 month before)
Human Papilloma Virus	X		Recommended for females aged 9–26, no recommendations for SOT
Influenza	X	X	Annual vaccination with inactivated intramuscular formulation recommended before and after SOT
Measles-Rubella	X		Live[a] virus, administer to patients who are seronegative, *before* transplant, or in women of childbearing age for prevention of congenital rubella syndrome
Pneumococcal	X	X	23-valent polysaccharide vaccine should be given once before transplant and boosters at 3 and 5 years after initial dose
Tetanus/diptheria	X		TDaP booster indicated for less than 65 years old (may be given less than or equal to 2 years after last TDaP booster in SOT patients)
Varicella	X		Live[a] virus, administer to patients who are seronegative, *before* transplant

TDaP, tetanus, diphtheria, and pertussis

[a]All live vaccines are contraindicated post solid organ transplant (SOT), as they can cause serious infection.

Live vaccines:

Bacillus Calmette-Guerin

Herpes zoster

Live intranasal attenuated influenza

Live oral typhoid

Measles-rubella

Vaccinia (smallpox)

Varicella

Patient Encounter Part 3

Identify your treatment goals for ED in terms of antimicrobial prophylaxis.

Create a plan for ED's antimicrobial prophylaxis, making sure to compare and contrast the pros and cons of the different agents in this patient.

▶ Hypertension

⑩ *Cardiovascular disease has been identified as the leading causes of death in organ transplant recipients.*[77,78] Posttransplant hypertension is associated with an increase in cardiac morbidity and patient mortality in all transplant patients and is also an independent risk factor for allograft dysfunction and loss. Based on all of the available posttransplant morbidity and mortality data, it is imperative that posttransplant hypertension be identified and managed appropriately.[77,78]

There are several underlying mechanisms responsible for posttransplant hypertension. Some causes of hypertension in transplant recipients may include renal dysfunction, increased sensitivity to endothelin-1 and angiotensin, increased density of glucocorticoid receptors in the vascular smooth muscle, and decreased production of vasodilatory prostaglandins.[77,78] However, one of the most easily recognized causes of posttransplant hypertension is the use of corticosteroids and the calcineurin inhibitors. Corticosteroids usually cause sodium and water retention, thus increasing blood pressure, whereas calcineurin inhibitors are associated with a number of effects that may result in hypertension, including reduced glomerular filtration rate (GFR) and renal blood flow (RBF), increased systemic and intrarenal vascular resistance, sodium retention, reduced concentrations of systemic vasodilators (i.e., prostacyclin, nitric oxide), and increased concentrations of vasoconstrictive thromboxanes. When compared with cyclosporine in clinical trials, tacrolimus displayed significantly less severe hypertension, and patients taking tacrolimus required significantly fewer antihypertensive medications at both 24 and 60 months after transplant.[77,78]

Treatment **⑩** *Controlling hypertension after transplant is essential in preventing cardiac morbidity and mortality and prolonging graft survival.* The target blood pressure in kidney transplant recipients should be less than 130/80 mm Hg. This goal blood pressure may not be suitable for all organ transplant recipients. In such cases, the Joint National Committee Seventh Report (JNC 7) guidelines should be followed.[77,78]

Lifestyle Modifications To achieve a goal blood pressure, lifestyle modifications including diet, exercise, sodium restriction, and smoking cessation are recommended.[74] Unfortunately, lifestyle modifications alone are often inadequate to control hypertension in this high-risk population, and antihypertensive medications are usually initiated early after transplant.[77,78]

Immunosuppressive Regimen Modification Because tacrolimus has shown the propensity to cause less severe hypertension when compared with cyclosporine, conversion from cyclosporine-based immunosuppression to tacrolimus-based immunosuppression may be one way to help reduce the severity of hypertension in transplant recipients. **❼** *Conversion to a ToR inhibitor, which is not associated with increases in blood pressure, may also be an alternative to the calcineurin inhibitors in patients with difficult-to-treat hypertension.* Corticosteroid taper or withdrawal are effective strategies for lowering blood pressure, but are not warranted in all clinical situations.[77,78]

Antihypertensive Agents There is no single class of antihypertensive medications recognized as the ideal agent. Numerous factors must be considered when determining appropriate treatment for a given patient, including the safety and efficacy data of the available agents, patient-specific situations and potential comorbidities, and medication cost. A large majority of patients often require multiple medications to achieve their goal blood pressure. This conclusion is supported by the recommendations of JNC 7, where combination therapy is regarded as an appropriate first-line therapy.[77,78]

β-Blockers and thiazide diuretics have proven benefits in reducing cardiovascular disease–associated morbidity and mortality.[77,78] Tolerability permitting, these agents are to be considered first-line therapies in most transplant recipients. The angiotensin-converting enzyme (ACE) inhibitors and angiotensin receptor blockers (ARB) have definite benefits in patients with nephropathy and are believed to have renoprotective effects in most patients. However, due to their ability to cause an initial increase in serum creatinine, these agents should be used cautiously when used in combination with the calcineurin inhibitors. The dihydropyridine calcium channel blockers have demonstrated an ability to reverse the nephrotoxicity associated with cyclosporine and tacrolimus. The addition of diltiazem to patients' regimens after cardiac transplant has also been shown to retard progression of cardiac allograft vasculopathy. In general, antihypertensive therapy should focus on agents with proven benefit in reducing the progression of cardiovascular disease and should be chosen on a patient-specific basis.[77,78]

▶ Hyperlipidemia

⑩ *Hyperlipidemia is seen in up to 60% of heart, lung, and renal transplant patients and greater than 30% of liver transplant patients.*[79,80] As a result of elevated cholesterol levels, transplant recipients are not only at an increased risk of atherosclerotic events, but emerging evidence also shows an association between hyperlipidemia and allograft vasculopathy. Hyperlipidemia, along with other types of cardiovascular disease, is now one of the primary causes of morbidity and mortality in long-term transplant survivors.[79,80]

Elevated cholesterol levels in transplant patients are due to a culmination of factors such as age, genetic disposition, renal dysfunction, DM, proteinuria, body weight, and immunosuppressive therapy. Many of the immunosuppressive agents can produce elevations in serum lipid levels.[79,80]

Treatment ⑩ *Lowering cholesterol has shown to signifi-cantly decrease severe rejection and transplant vasculopathy and improve 1-year survival in heart transplant recipients.*[81] Although these results cannot be extrapolated to other transplant populations, they do demonstrate the potential benefits of aggressive cholesterol lowering in organ transplant recipients. Due to high prevalence of cardiovascular disease among organ transplant recipients, most healthcare practitioners consider these patients to fall in the highest risk category for lipid lowering as established by the National Cholesterol Education Panel (NCEP) III guidelines. These guidelines call for a calculated low-density lipoprotein cholesterol (LDL-C) target level of less than 100 mg/dL (2.59 mmol/L).[82]

Lifestyle Modifications Generally, lowering cholesterol in patients begins with therapeutic lifestyle changes. These changes are initiated either alone or in conjunction with lipid-lowering drug therapy, depending on baseline cholesterol levels and other risk factors. Therapeutic lifestyle changes entail a reduction in saturated fat and cholesterol intake and an increase in moderate physical activity.[82] As with hypertension, lifestyle modifications alone rarely are effective enough to achieve a goal LDL-C level.[79,80] Modification of the immunosuppressive regimen and use of cholesterol-lowering medications are often warranted in this patient population.

Immunosuppressive Regimen Modifications Tacrolimus has shown the propensity to cause less severe hyperlipidemia when compared with cyclosporine. Conversion from cyclosporine-based immunosuppression to tacrolimus-based immunosuppression may be one way to counteract this disease in transplant recipients.[79,80]

In past studies, steroid withdrawal in renal transplant patients did lower total cholesterol by 17% and LDL cholesterol by 16%; unfortunately, an 18% decrease in high-density lipoprotein (HDL) levels was also noted in these patients.[79,80]

Cholesterol-Lowering Agents 3-Hydroxy-3-methylglutaryl coenzyme A (HMG-CoA) reductase inhibitors, or statins, are considered to be first-line therapy for hyperlipidemia in the general population.[79,80,82] However, there is some uncertainty about the pathogenesis of cardiovascular disease in transplant recipients and whether statin therapy will have similar effectiveness in organ transplant recipients. Statins have shown definite advantages when used in heart transplantation, including a reduction in LDL-C and major adverse cardiac events (MACE), as well as an apparent cardioprotective effect. In renal transplant recipients, statins are known to lower LDL-C levels and reduce the incidence of some cardiac events; however, the ability to lower MACE may not be evident in this patient population. Despite these mixed results, statins are still considered the primary therapeutic option for hyperlipidemia in all organ transplant recipients.[79,80] Finally, when choosing a statin for management of hyperlipidemia in the transplant recipient, a focus on potential DDIs is warranted. It is recommended that doses of atorvastatin do not exceed 10 mg daily when taken with cyclosporine due to an increased risk of myopathy and

rhabdomyolysis. Use of cyclosporine in conjunction with simvastatin is considered a contraindication due to the risk of the skeletal muscle effects aforementioned.[79,80]

Fibric acid derivatives are an excellent choice for lowering triglycerides, but are not as effective as statins at lowering LDL-C.[79,80] These agents may play a role in conjunction with statins in patients with both elevated cholesterol and triglycerides. Nicotinic acid is very effective at improving the lipid panel, with excellent results in lowering LDL-C, as well as increasing HDL. However, patient tolerability issues are of concern with this agent. The bile acid sequestrants should be avoided in organ transplant recipients due to their high incidence of GI adverse events, as well as their propensity for pharmacokinetic DDIs with MPA. Ezetimibe has proven safe and effective in lowering LDL-C in renal transplant recipients. Future studies are needed to establish ideal regimens involving the antihyperlipidemic and immunosuppressive medications to decrease morbidity and mortality and ultimately prevent cardiovascular events.[79,80]

▶ *New-Onset DM After Transplantation*

⑩ *New-onset DM after transplantation (NODAT) is a serious complication that is often underestimated by transplant practitioners.*[83] Kasiske and colleagues attempted to quantify the cumulative incidence of NODAT in renal transplant recipients and found that 8.3% of patients developed NODAT at 3 months posttransplant, 12.9% at 12 months, and 22.3% at 36 months.[84] Even more alarming is that recent studies have revealed an overwhelming prevalence of impaired glucose tolerance, which is also accepted as a risk factor for long-term morbidity and mortality. NODAT is associated with increases in cardiovascular events, with an approximately 22% higher risk of mortality. Patients with NODAT are also more likely to suffer acute rejection episodes and infectious complications than patients without this complication.[83]

Prevention ⑩ *NODAT prevention mainly consists of identifying patients at risk before transplant and controlling modifiable risk factors both before and after transplantation.*[83] The major modifiable risk factors are choice of immunosuppressive therapy and body mass index (BMI). For example:

- Immunosuppressive medications: Steroid minimization and possibly withdrawal are effective strategies for the prevention of NODAT. Also, patients with worsening (increased) blood glucose after transplantation who are receiving tacrolimus may benefit from conversion to cyclosporine.[83]
- Body mass index: A reduction in body weight is always recommended in obese patients prior to the transplant procedure to help lower their NODAT risks.[83,83]

Treatment ⑩ *Lifestyle modifications are always in order in patients who have developed or those who are at increased risk of developing NODAT.*[83] Insulin therapy and oral hypoglycemic agents are often utilized in those patients in whom lifestyle modifications alone have not controlled blood glucose. Please refer to Chapter 43 for proper instruction on choosing the appropriate treatment regimens in patients with DM.[83]

▶ Neoplasia

● **Cancer Screening in Transplant Patients** Transplant recipients are at increased risk for different types of specific cancers (Table 55–8).[86] The risk of developing Kaposi's sarcoma following transplantation is over 200 times that in the general population. In addition, the risk of nonmelanocytic and melanocytic skin cancer is 10 to 20 times higher compared with the nontransplanted population. Transplant recipients are at greatest risk for the types of cancers associated with viral infections, such as PTLD, cervical, and vulvovaginal cancers. Solid organ tumors like colorectal and lung cancers are two to three times higher in transplant recipients when compared with the general population. The American Cancer Society and American Transplant Society recommend cancer screening for most adults who have undergone transplantation (Table 55–9). Although clinical research has not yet proven that the potential benefits of testing outweigh the harms of testing in transplant recipients, most believe that transplant recipients should be tested and screened very closely.[86]

● **Skin Cancer** Skin cancer remains the most common malignancy after organ transplantation. The incidence of these types of cancers increases with time posttransplant, with one study showing a prevalence rate of 35% among patients within 10 years after transplant.[85] More alarming than the high prevalence is the activity of these cancers in patients on maintenance immunosuppression. Skin cancers

in transplant recipients tend to grow more rapidly and are more likely to metastasize.[87]

The most common risk factors for skin cancer development after transplant include increased age; excessive ultraviolet (UV) light exposure; high degree of immunosuppression; Fitzpatrick skin types I, II, and III; history of skin cancers; and infection by human papillomavirus.[87] ⑦ *A recent analysis suggests that use of sirolimus in place of a calcineurin inhibitor in kidney transplant recipients can reduce the risk of nonmelanoma skin carcinomas.*[88]

It is of the utmost importance that transplant practitioners be vigilant about educating their patients about excessive exposure to the sun.[87] Patients should be warned about the risk of skin cancer and be advised on simple methods to limit their risk:

- Use of protective clothing (i.e., long-sleeved shirts and long pants, dark-colored clothing)
- Use of sunscreen daily that is applied to all sun-exposed skin
- Sun protection factor (SPF) 30 or higher is recommended

▶ Posttransplant Lymphoproliferative Disorders

⑩ *PTLDs are a major complication in patients following organ transplantation.*[89] Large series of case reports have demonstrated that the incidence of PTLD is 1% for renal patients, 1.8% for cardiac patients, 2.2% for liver patients, and 9.4% for heart-lung patients. The risk of developing non-Hodgkin's lymphoma is 28- to 49-fold higher in solid organ transplant recipients compared with the general population. Another independent risk factor is the presence of EBV.[85,89,90] Lymphomas are the most common form of PTLD in transplant recipients.[89]

The incidence of disease depends on certain factors. These factors include the type of organ transplanted, the age of the transplant recipient, the degree of immunosuppression, the type of immunosuppression, and exposure to EBV. The mortality rate in these patients is about 50%, with most patients dying shortly after diagnosis. It has also been demonstrated that the risk of developing PTLD is greater in the population of EBV seronegative patients at the time of transplant.[89]

Another risk factor for the development of PTLD is the type of immunosuppressive regimens used. Belatacept has been approved with a black box warning outlining an increased risk of PTLD, especially of the CNS. Patients who are EBV seronegative or have an unknown immunity to EBV should not be considered for therapy. ALAs have come to be widely used in the prevention and treatment of acute rejection. These agents work by causing widespread T-cell lysis. Immunosuppressive regimens utilizing the ALAs have been proven to increase the risk of PTLD.[89]

● **Treatment** ⑩ *Treatment for PTLD is still controversial; however, the most common treatment options include reduction of immunosuppression, chemotherapy, and anti–B-cell monoclonal antibodies.*[89] PTLD continues to be a long-term complication of prolonged immunosuppression. Current treatment options are all associated with certain risks.

Table 55–8

Overall Risk of Different Types of Cancer in Transplant Patients[86,87,89,90]

Cancer	Cumulative Incidence (/100,000)	Male	Female
Kaposi's sarcoma	140	17.4	62
Kidney/ureter	1,010	14.1	14.6
Lymphoma	80	6.9	29.1
Bladder	126	1.6	3.6
Esophagus	70	2.4	2.8
Cervix	180	–	5.7
Liver	220	4.2	4.5
Melanoma	320	6.9	5.2
Lung/bronchus/ trachea	690	2.3	3.6
Colorectal	510	1.6	2.8
Breast	1,050	4	1.1
Prostate	1,740	1.6	–

Table 55–9

Cancer Screening Recommendations in Transplant Patients[86,87,89,90]

Cancer Type	General Populations	Transplant Populations
Breast	Mammography every 1–2 years for all women greater than or equal to 50 years old. Clinical breast exam every 3 years in women 20–39 years old, yearly after age 40. Monthly self-exam.	Mammography every 1–2 years for all women greater than or equal to 50 years old. May undergo screening between 40 and 49 years old but no evidence for or against screening in this age group.
Cervical	Annual Pap smear & pelvic exam once sexually active; after 3 or more tests with normal results, may decrease frequency of exams.	Annual Pap smear & pelvic exam once sexually active.
Colorectal	Annual FOBT plus flexible sigmoidoscopy every 5 years for all patients greater than or equal to 50 years old or colonoscopy and DRE every 10 years.	Annual FOBT plus flexible sigmoidoscopy every 5 years for all transplant patients greater than or equal to 50 years old.
Prostate	Annual DRE & PSA for men greater than or equal to 50 years old with 10-year life expectancy or younger men at high risk.	Annual DRE & PSA measurement in all males greater than or equal to 50 years old.
Hepatocellular	Not recommended for average-risk individuals. a-Fetoprotein and ultrasound every 6 months in high-risk patients (no firm supporting data).	a-Fetoprotein and ultrasound every 6 months in high-risk patients (no firm supporting data).
Skin	Skin exam every 3 years between ages 20 and 40, annually thereafter.	Monthly self-exam. Total body skin exam every 6–12 months by dermatologists
Renal	Insufficient evidence to support routine screening.	No firm recommendations. Regular ultrasound of native kidneys.
Lung	Insufficient evidence to support routine screening.	No firm recommendations
Ovarian	Insufficient evidence to support routine screening.	No firm recommendations
Testicular	Insufficient evidence to support routine screening.	No firm recommendations
Endometrial	Insufficient evidence to support routine screening.	No firm recommendations

DRE, digital rectal exam; FOBT, fecal occult blood test; PSA, prostate-specific antigen.

Prevention is the most effective treatment for PTLD. A better understanding in the future of the disease process and the risk factors involved with the development of PTLD will aid in the prophylaxis and treatment of this disorder.[89]

▶ Pregnancy

Females of childbearing age who do not wish to become pregnant after transplantation require adequate education on preferred forms of birth control. The optimal method of birth control in this patient population is the barrier method (e.g. condom, diaphragm). Use of intrauterine devices and progestin-based oral contraceptives are controversial, and associated risks must be considered prior to initiating therapy. Intrauterine devices may be less effective in the setting of immunosuppression and predispose patients to an increased risk of infection.[91] Progestin-based oral contraceptives are considered a less effective form of birth control, but may be a safe option in those patients who have well-controlled hypertension.

Female patients considering pregnancy after transplantation should be educated extensively regarding the potential risks that transplantation and medical immunosuppression may present to a fetus. Risks to the infant include premature birth (50%) and intrauterine growth restriction (20%), which may result in death or long-term complications, including cerebral palsy, blindness, deafness, and learning deficiencies.[91] Patients hoping to become pregnant should wait at least 1 year after transplantation to ensure reconstitution of gonadal function posttransplant, as well as demonstrate a 1-year freedom from acute rejection.[91]

Understanding the associated risk of immunosuppressives while pregnant is paramount considering their ability to cross the placenta as well as enter breast milk (Table 55–10). Tacrolimus and cyclosporine, both Pregnancy Category C, are the backbone of immunosuppressive therapy and have been used safely and effectively in pregnancy posttransplant for decades.[92] Side effects associated with calcineurin inhibitors such as hypertension, diabetes, and nephrotoxicity should be monitored closely in the pregnant population. Sirolimus is also Pregnancy Category C and has not been associated with fetal malformation but has been correlated with low birth weight.[92] Corticosteroids, pregnancy category B, are recognized to be relatively safe and have been used extensively in pregnancy after transplantation. However, they carry a risk of premature membrane rupture and newborn adrenal insufficiency.[92] More common side effects associated with corticosteroids that may cause complications in pregnancy include hypertension, diabetes, weight gain, and poor wound healing. Due to teratogenic effects in animal studies, azathioprine is considered Pregnancy Category D; however, it has been used extensively as an antimetabolite in pregnant

Patient Encounter Part 4

ED continues to have his posttransplant care at your renal transplant ambulatory care clinic. He returns to your clinic 1 month after the transplant:

Labs:

Na: 141 mEq/L (141 mmol/L)

K: 4.7 mEq/L (4.7 mmol/L)

Cl: 198 mEq/L (198 mmol/L)

CO_2: 21 mEq/L (21 mmol/L)

BUN: 21 mg/dL (7.5 mmol/L)

SCr: 1.1 mg/dL (97.2 μmol/L)

Glucose: 110 mg/dL: (6.1 mmol/L)

Lipid panel: TC = 341 mg/dL (8.8 mmol/L), LDL-C = 179 mg/dL (4.6 mmol/L), HDL = 47 mg/dL (1.2 mmol/L), TG = 575 mg/dL (6.5 mmol/L)

Uric acid: 10.6 mg/dL (630.5 μmol/L)

Tacrolimus: 11.7 mg/dL

Vitals: BP 164/95 mm Hg (162/88 mm Hg repeated), HR 87 beats/min

Medications:

- Tacrolimus 6 mg by mouth twice a day
- Mycophenolate mofetil 1000 mg by mouth twice a day
- Prednisone 10 mg by mouth once a day
- Atovaquone 1500 mg by mouth once a day
- Valganciclovir 900 mg by mouth once a day
- Atorvastatin 20 mg by mouth once a day
- Metoprolol XL 100 mg by mouth once a day
- Amlodipine 5 mg by mouth once a day
- Zolpidem 10 mg by mouth once a day at bedtime
- Alprazolam 0.5 mg by mouth three times a day as needed for anxiety

Identify why ED is taking each agent listed.

What are some treatment options for ED's elevated blood pressure?

What are some treatment options for ED's elevated cholesterol?

What are some treatment options for ED's elevated uric acid?

Design a monitoring plan for ED's therapy.

transplant patients without extensive evidence of harm to the fetus. 6-Mercaptopurine has not been shown to cross the placental barrier.

Currently, the MPA derivatives, both Pregnancy Category D, are not considered optimal immunosuppressive agents for patients who become pregnant, and alternative therapies should be pursued.[92] A less teratogenic antimetabolite, aza-

thioprine, should be substituted for mycophenolate mofetil or enteric-coated MPA in patients who plan on becoming pregnant. The safety of ALAs and rituximab in transplantation has yet to be fully determined; however, IVIG has been widely used without any documented adverse events.[91] Newly available immunosuppressives, belatacept and everolimus, are pregnancy category C but are not recommended for use in pregnant patients due to inadequate human data.

▶ *Immunosuppressant Therapy Adherence*

Transplant recipients require strict adherence to their medication regimens to ensure optimal allograft and patient outcomes. Nonadherence in this population can be attributed to the complexity of the regimens coupled with the variability in drug dosing, need for therapeutic drug monitoring, avoidance of potential drug-drug interactions, infectious risks, and drug toxicities. The incidence of nonadherence to immunosuppressant therapy in the first year posttransplant has been estimated to be as high as 22.6%.[93] This is especially alarming when one considers that 35% of all graft failures can be directly attributed to nonadherence.[94] Risk factors associated with immunosuppressant therapy nonadherence include a history of substance abuse, personality disorders, and lack of social support.[95] The roll of the pharmacist in educating patients on the importance of their medication regimens and stressing the need for adherence is paramount in optimizing both patient and allograft survival after transplantation. Previous reports have suggested that intervention by a pharmacist posttransplant improves adherence.[96]

OUTCOME EVALUATION

- Successful outcomes in solid organ transplantation are generally measured in terms of several separate end points: (a) preventing acute rejection, (b) increasing 1-year graft survival, (c) preventing immunosuppressive drug complications, and (d) improving long-term allograft and patient survival.

- The short-term goals after organ transplantation revolve around reducing the incidence of acute rejection episodes and attaining a high graft survival rate. By accomplishing these goals, transplant clinicians hope to attain good allograft function to allow for an improved quality of life. These goals can be achieved through the appropriate use of medical immunosuppression and scrutinizing over the therapeutic and toxic monitoring parameters associated with each medication employed. In addition, transplant recipients should be monitored for adverse drug reactions, DDIs, and adherence with their therapeutic regimen.

- The long-term goals after organ transplant are to maximize the functionality of the allograft and prevent the complications of immunosuppression, which lead to improved patient survival. Clinicians must play multiple roles in the long-term care of transplant recipients, as not only must the patient be followed

Table 55–10

Transplant Immunosuppressants and Pregnancy[9,91,92]

Drug	Male Reproduction	Female Reproduction	Recommendations	Pregnancy Category
Prednisone	Prednisone may lead to decreased spermatogenesis.	Prednisone and prednisolone pose a small risk to the developing fetus. One of these risks appears to be orofacial clefts.	Female: No changes recommended. May need to decrease dose to improve spermatogenesis. Male: No changes recommended.	B
AZA	Treatment with azathioprine has not been associated with changes in semen quality.	Most investigators found azathioprine to be safe in pregnancy. Leukopenia and thrombocytopenia in the neonate has been seen.	Female: Continue during pregnancy. Dose adjustments may be made to maintain normal maternal leukocyte counts.	D
MPA	MPA resulted in an incidence of birth defects similar to that of the general population.	MPA in the first trimester is associated with increased risk for fetal death and structural defects. Malformations were external ear, facial anomalies, cleft lip/palate, and defects of limbs, heart, esophagus and kidney.	Male: No changes recommended. Female: Guidelines recommend against its use. Use contraception during therapy and for 6 weeks after therapy is stopped, switch to AZA.	D
ToR Inhibitors	Men on mammalian ToRs have been shown to have decreased fertility because of impaired spermatogenesis and azoospermia. This was reversible when switched to alternate agent.	Very limited data exist for human pregnancy in offspring of mothers on sirolimus; no data on everolimus.	Male: No changes recommended. Female: Guidelines recommend against its use. Use effective contraception before and during therapy and for 12 weeks after therapy is stopped.	C
CsA	No definitive evidence of malformations or major birth defects was seen in children fathered by patients on cyclosporine. Motility was affected in patients on cyclosporine only when levels exceeded normal therapeutic range.	Cyclosporine does not seem to be a human teratogen.	Male: Change to alternate agent when attempting to father a child. Female: May be used, recommend waiting to conceive until 12 months after transplant.	C
TAC	No definitive evidence of malformations or major birth defects was seen in children fathered by patients on tacrolimus. No information has been found to associate tacrolimus with oligospermia.	An abortive risk has been shown in animal models. However, human experience has shown low fetal/embryo risk.	Male: No changes recommended. Female: May be used, recommend waiting to conceive until 12 months after transplant.	C
Basiliximab	No studies have been done to assess basiliximab effects on male fertility.	No data	Male: No changes recommended. Female: Not recommended in pregnant females due to lack of evidence for safety.	C
r-ATG	No studies have been done to assess r-ATG effect on male fertility.	r-ATG use during five human pregnancies has been reported without apparent adverse fetal consequences.	Male: Avoid if attempting to have children. Female: Not recommended in pregnant females due to lack of evidence for safety.	C
Belatacept	No studies have been done to assess belatacept effect on male fertility.	No data	Male: Not recommended due to lack of evidence for safety. Female: Not recommended in pregnant females due to lack of evidence for safety.	C
Rituximab	No studies have been done to assess rituximab effect on male fertility.	Infants born to patients on rituximab were all born healthy (6 patients). Similar to research in monkey offspring. Immunosuppression was found in 1 infant and was normal at 4 months.	Males: No studies, use contraception while on rituximab therapy. Females: Appears to be safe.	C

AZA, azathioprine; CsA, cyclosporine; MPA, mycophenolic acid; r-ATG, rabbit antithymocyte immunoglobulin; TAC, tacrolimus; ToR, target of rapamycin.

from an immunologic perspective, but practitioners must be focused on identifying and treating the adverse sequelae associated with lifelong immunosuppression including cardiovascular disease, malignancy, infection, and osteoporosis among others. Again, limiting drug misadventures and ensuring adherence with the therapeutic regimen are important and should be stressed.

Abbreviations Introduced in This Chapter

6-MP	6-Mercaptopurine
ACE	Angiotensin converting enzyme
ALA	Antilymphocyte antibodies
AMR	Antibody mediated rejection
APC	Antigen-presenting cell

Patient Care and Monitoring

Early Management of Transplant Recipients

1. Review any available diagnostic and laboratory data to evaluate the function of the allograft and the health of the recipient.

2. Assess the patient's current medication regimen, including:
   - Induction therapy agent:
     - Assess for appropriate dose and duration of therapy
     - Therapeutic monitoring parameters (organ function)
     - Toxic monitoring parameters
   - Maintenance immunosuppressive agents:
     - Assess for appropriate dose and duration of therapy
     - Therapeutic monitoring parameters (organ function)
     - Toxic monitoring parameters
   - Antiinfective prophylaxis:
     - Assess suitability of chosen prophylactic agents (e.g., drug allergies, CMV donor, and recipient serostatus)
     - Therapeutic monitoring parameters
     - Toxic monitoring parameters
   - Medications used for comorbidities:
     - Assess appropriate selection of these medications for pharmacokinetic and pharmacodynamic DDIs, need (e.g., do renal transplant recipients need to continue to take erythropoietin?), and efficacy
     - Therapeutic monitoring parameters
     - Toxic monitoring parameters

3. Evaluate the patient for the presence of adverse drug reactions, drug allergies, or DDIs.

4. Develop patient-specific short-term and long-term therapeutic goals.

5. Provide patient education regarding the organ transplant, the complications associated with transplantation, the need for lifestyle modifications to reduce risk of complications (e.g., wear sunscreen, low-sodium diet), and drug therapy.

6. Stress importance of adherence with therapeutic regimen.

Outpatient Management of Transplant Recipients

1. Obtain a thorough history of prescription, nonprescription, and complimentary and alternative medication use.
   - Maintenance immunosuppressive agents:
     - Assess for appropriate dose and duration of therapy
     - Therapeutic monitoring parameters (organ function)
     - Toxic monitoring parameters

2. Antiinfective prophylaxis:
   - Assess suitability of chosen prophylactic agents (e.g., drug allergies, CMV donor, and recipient serostatus)
   - Does the patient need continued prophylaxis therapy?
   - When do you stop prophylaxis?
   - Therapeutic monitoring parameters
   - Toxic monitoring parameters

3. Medications used for comorbidities:
   - Assess appropriate selection of these medications for pharmacokinetic and pharmacodynamic DDIs, need, and efficacy
   - Therapeutic monitoring parameters (drug- and disease-specific)
   - Toxic monitoring parameters (drug-specific)

4. Evaluate the patient for the presence of adverse drug reactions, drug allergies, or DDIs.

5. Reassess your patient-specific short-term and long-term therapeutic goals.

6. Continue with patient education in regard to the complications associated with transplantation, the need for lifestyle modifications to reduce risk of the complications (e.g., wear sunscreen, low-sodium diet), and drug therapy.

7. Reemphasize the importance of adherence with therapeutic regimen.

8. Assess improvement in quality-of-life measures such as physical, psychological and social functioning, and well-being.

ARB	Angiotensin receptor blocker
ATG	Antithymocyte globulin
ATGAM	Antithymocyte globulin equine
AZA	Azathioprine
BKV	BK virus
BKVN	BK virus-induced nephropathy
BMI	Body mass index
BUN	Blood urea nitrogen
C_0	Trough concentration
C_2	Drug concentration 2 hours postdose
CCB	Calcium channel blocker
CD4+	Helper T cells
CD8+	Cytotoxic T cells
CKD	Chronic kidney disease
CMV	Cytomegalovirus
CNI	Calcineurin inhibitor
CNS	Central nervous system
CSA	Cyclosporine
CXR	Chest x-ray
CYP	Cytochrome P-450 system
CYP3A	Cytochrome P-450 system 3A isozyme
DC	Dendritic cell
DDI	Drug–drug interaction
DM	Diabetes mellitus
DOE	Dyspnea on exertion
DRE	Digital rectal exam
DSA	Donor-specific antibody
DS	Double strength
e-ATG	Antithymocyte globulin equine
EBV	Epstein-Barr virus
EC	Enteric-coated
ESRD	End-stage renal disease
EVL	Everolimus
FBS	Fasting blood sugar
FEV	Forced expiratory volume
FOBT	Fecal occult blood test
G6PD	Glucose-6-phosphate-dehydrogenase
GFR	Glomerular filtration rate
GI	Gastrointestinal
HDL	High-density lipoproteins
HLA	Human leukocyte antigen
HMG-CoA	3-Hydroxy-3-methylglutaryl coenzyme A
HPLC	High-performance liquid chromatography
HTN	Hypertension
IgG	Immunoglobulin G
IL-2	Interleukin 2
IL-2RA	Interleukin-2 receptor antagonist
IVIG	Intravenous immune globulin
JNC 7	Joint National Committee Seventh Report
K	Potassium
LDL-C	Low-density lipoprotein cholesterol
LFT	Liver function test
MAC	Membrane attack complex
MACE	Major adverse cardiac events
Mg	Magnesium
MHC	Major histocompatibility complex
MMF	Mycophenolate mofetil

MPA	Mycophenolic acid
MPAG	MPA-glucorinide
NCEP	National Cholesterol Education Program
NFAT (NFAT-P)	Nuclear factors
NK	Natural killer
NODAT	New-onset diabetes mellitus after transplantation
NSAID	Nonsteroidal anti-inflammatory drug
NYHA	New York Heart Association
P-gp	P-glycoprotein
PO_4	Phosphate
PRA	Panel of reactive antibodies
PSA	prostate-specific antigen
PTLD	Posttransplant lymphoproliferative disorders
r-ATG (RATG)	Antithymocyte globulin rabbit
RBF	Renal blood flow
SCr	Serum creatinine
SMZ-TMP	Sulfamethoxazole-trimethoprim
SOB	Shortness of breath
SOT	Solid organ transplant
SPF	Sun protection factor
SPK	Simultaneous pancreas-kidney
SRL	Sirolimus
SS	Single strength
TAC	Tacrolimus
TC	Total cholesterol
TCR	T-cell receptor
TDaP	Tetanus, diphtheria, and pertussis
TG	Triglycerides
ToR	Target of rapamycin
UV	Ultraviolet
WBC	White blood cells

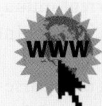 Self-assessment questions and answers are available at *http://www.mhpharmacotherapy. com/pp.html.*

REFERENCES

1. Calne RY. Transplantation: current developments and future directions. Front Biosci 2007;12:3727–3733.
2. Halloran PF. Immunosuppressive drugs for kidney transplantation. N Engl J Med 2004;351:2715–2729.
3. The Organ Procurement and Transplantation Network (OPTN) [Internet]. Data [cited 2012 August 29]. Available from: *http://optn. transplant.hrsa.gov/data/.*
4. Moll S, Pascual M. Humoral rejection of organ allografts. Am J Transplant 2005;5:2611–2618.
5. Xiaobei LI, Ishida H, Yamaguchi Y, et al. Poor graft outcome in recipients with de novo donor-specific anti-HLA antibodies after living related kidney transplantation. Transpl Int 2008;21:1145–1152.
6. Raghavaiah S, Stegall MD. New therapeutic approaches to antibody-mediated rejection in renal transplantation. Clin Pharmacol Ther 2011;90:310–315.
7. Joosten SA, Sijpkens YW, van Kooten C, Paul LC. Chronic renal allograft rejection: pathophysiologic considerations. Kidney Int 2005;68:1–13.

8. Monaco AP. The beginning of clinical tolerance in solid organ allografts. Exp Clin Transplant 2004;2:153–161.

9. Hardinger KL, Koch MJ, Brennan DC. Current and future immunosuppressive strategies in renal transplantation. Pharmacotherapy 2004;24:1159–1176.

10. Micromedex® Healthcare Series (electronic version). Greenwood Village, CO: Thomson Healthcare; 2011.

11. Mohty M, Gaugler B. Mechanisms of action of antithymocyte globulin: old dogs with new tricks! Leuk Lymphoma 2008;49:1664–1667.

12. Nashan B. Antibody induction therapy in renal transplant patients receiving calcineurin-inhibitor immunosuppressive regimens: a comparative review. BioDrugs 2005;19:39–46.

13. Gabardi S, Martin ST, Roberts KL, Grafals M. Induction immunosuppressive therapies in renal transplantation. Am J Health Syst Pharm 2011;68:211–218.

14. Willicombe M, Roufosse C, Brookes P, et al. Antibody-mediated rejection after alemtuzumab induction: incidence, risk factors, and predictors of poor outcome. Transplantation 2011;92:176-82.

15. Woodle ES, Peddi VR, Tomlanovich S, et al. A prospective, randomized, multicenter study evaluating early corticosteroid withdrawal with Thymoglobulin® in living-donor kidney transplantation. Clin Transplant 2010;24:73–83.

16. Brennan DC, Flavin K, Lowell JA, et al. A randomized, double-blinded comparison of Thymoglobulin versus Atgam for induction immunosuppressive therapy in adult renal transplant recipients. Transplantation 1999;67:1011–1018.

17. Lebranchu Y, Bridoux F, Buchler M, et al. Immunoprophylaxis with basiliximab compared with antithymocyte globulin in renal transplant patients receiving MMF-containing triple therapy. Am J Transplant 2002;2:48–56.

18. Brennan DC, Daller JA, Lake KD, Cibrik D, Del Castillo D. Rabbit antithymocyte globulin versus basiliximab in renal transplantation. N Engl J Med 2006;355:1967–1977.

19. Martin ST, Roberts KL, Malek SK, et al. Induction treatment with rabbit antithymocyte globulin versus basiliximab in renal transplant recipients with planned early steroid withdrawal. Pharmacotherapy 2011;31:566–573.

20. Hanaway MJ, Woodle ES, Mulgaonkar S, et al. Alemtuzumab induction in renal transplantation. N Engl J Med 2011;364:1909–1919.

21. Beaty CA, Cymet T. Organ transplantation for the primary care provider: what you need to know to get your patient a new liver or kidney. Compr Ther 2008;34:69–76.

22. Golshayan D, Buhler L, Lechler RI, Pascual M. From current immunosuppressive strategies to clinical tolerance of allografts. Transpl Int 2007;20:12–24.

23. Cyclosporine microemulsion (Neoral) absorption profiling and sparse-sample predictors during the first 3 months after renal transplantation. Am J Transplant 2002;2:148–156.

24. Citterio F, Scata MC, Romagnoli J, Nanni G, Castagneto M. Results of a three-year prospective study of C2 monitoring in long-term renal transplant recipients receiving cyclosporine microemulsion. Transplantation 2005;79:802–806.

25. Mayer AD, Dmitrewski J, Squifflet JP, et al. Multicenter randomized trial comparing tacrolimus (FK506) and cyclosporine in the prevention of renal allograft rejection: a report of the European Tacrolimus Multicenter Renal Study Group. Transplantation 1997;64:436–443.

26. Webster AC, Woodroffe RC, Taylor RS, Chapman JR, Craig JC. Tacrolimus versus ciclosporin as primary immunosuppression for kidney transplant recipients: meta-analysis and meta-regression of randomised trial data. BMJ 2005;331(7520):810.

27. Gabardi S, Tran JL, Clarkson MR. Enteric-coated mycophenolate sodium. Ann Pharmacother 2003;37:1685–1693.

28. Sollinger HW. Mycophenolates in transplantation. Clin Transplant 2004;18:485–492.

29. Buell C, Koo J. Long-term safety of mycophenolate mofetil and cyclosporine: a review. J Drugs Dermatol 2008;7:741–748.

30. Budde K, Durr M, Liefeldt L, Neumayer HH, Glander P. Enteric-coated mycophenolate sodium. Expert Opin Drug Saf 2010;9:981–994.

31. Reinke P, Budde K, Hugo C. Reduction of gastrointestinal complications in renal graft recipients after conversion from mycophenolate mofetil to enteric-coated mycophenolate sodium. Transplant Proc 2011;43;1641–1646.

32. Augustine JJ, Bodziak KA, Hricik DE. Use of sirolimus in solid organ transplantation. Drugs 2007;67:369–391.

33. MacDonald AS. A worldwide, phase III, randomized, controlled, safety and efficacy study of a sirolimus/cyclosporine regimen for prevention of acute rejection in recipients of primary mismatched renal allografts. Transplantation 2001;71:271–280.

34. Kreis H, Oberbauer R, Campistol JM, et al. Long-term benefits with sirolimus-based therapy after early cyclosporine withdrawal. J Am Soc Nephrol 2004;15:809–817.

35. Holt DW. Therapeutic drug monitoring of immunosuppressive drugs in kidney transplantation. Curr Opin Nephrol Hypertens 2002;11:657–663.

36. Joannidès R, Monteil C, de Ligny BH, et al. Immunosuppressant regimen based on sirolimus decreases aortic stiffness in renal transplant recipients in comparison to cyclosporine. Am J Transplant 2011;11:2414–2422.

37. Gabardi S, Baroletti SA. Everolimus: a proliferation signal inhibitor with clinical applications in organ transplantation, oncology, and cardiology. Pharmacotherapy 2010;30:1044–1056.

38. Micromedex® Healthcare Series (electronic version). Greenwood Village, CO: Thomson Healthcare, 2010.

39. Ahsan N, Hricik D, Matas A, et al. Prednisone withdrawal in kidney transplant recipients on cyclosporine and mycophenolate mofetil—a prospective randomized study. Steroid Withdrawal Study Group. Transplantation 1999;68:1865–1874.

40. Woodle ES, First MR, Pirsch J, et al. A prospective, randomized, double-blind, placebo-controlled multicenter trial comparing early (7 day) corticosteroid cessation versus long-term, low-dose corticosteroid therapy. Ann Surg 2008;248:564–577.

41. Liu CL, Fan ST, Lo CM, et al. Interleukin-2 receptor antibody (basiliximab) for immunosuppressive induction therapy after liver transplantation: a protocol with early elimination of steroids and reduction of tacrolimus dosage. Liver Transpl 2004;10:728–733.

42. Laftavi MR, Stephan R, Stefanick B, et al. Randomized prospective trial of early steroid withdrawal compared with low-dose steroids in renal transplant recipients using serial protocol biopsies to assess efficacy and safety. Surgery 2005;137:364–371.

43. Kaufman DB, Leventhal JR, Koffron AJ, et al. A prospective study of rapid corticosteroid elimination in simultaneous pancreas-kidney transplantation: comparison of two maintenance immunosuppression protocols: tacrolimus/mycophenolate mofetil versus tacrolimus/sirolimus. Transplantation 2002;73:169–177.

44. Vincenti F, Luggen M. T cell costimulation: a rational target in the therapeutic armamentarium for autoimmune diseases and transplantation. Annu Rev Med 2007;58:347–358.

45. Martin ST, Tichy EM, Gabardi S. Belatacept: a novel biologic for maintenance immunosuppression after renal transplantation. Pharmacotherapy 2011;31:394–407.

46. Vincenti F, Charpentier B, Vanrenterghem Y, et al. A phase III study of belatacept-based immunosuppression regimens versus cyclosporine in renal transplant recipients (BENEFIT study). Am J Transplant 2010;10:535–546.

47. Durrbach A, Pestana JM, Pearson T, et al. A Phase III Study of Belatacept Versus Cyclosporine in Kidney Transplants from Extended Criteria Donors (BENEFIT-EXT Study). Am J Transplant 2010;10:547–557.

48. Webster A, Pankhurst T, Rinaldi F, Chapman JR, Craig JC. Polyclonal and monoclonal antibodies for treating acute rejection episodes in kidney transplant recipients. Cochrane Database Syst Rev 2006:CD004756.

49. Jordan SC, Vo AA, Peng A, Toyoda M, Tyan D. Intravenous gammaglobulin (IVIG): a novel approach to improve transplant rates and outcomes in highly HLA-sensitized patients. Am J Transplant 2006;6:459–466.

50. Waiser J, Budde K, Schutz M, et al. Comparison between bortezomib and rituximab in the treatment of antibody-mediated renal allograft rejection. Nephrol Dial Transplant 2012;27:1246–1251.

51. Takemoto SK, Zeevi A, Feng S, et al. National conference to assess antibody-mediated rejection in solid organ transplantation. Am J Transplant 2004;4:1033–1041.

52. Stegall MD, Gloor J, Winters JL, Moore SB, Degoey S. A comparison of plasmapheresis versus high-dose IVIG desensitization in renal allograft recipients with high levels of donor specific alloantibody. Am J Transplant 2006;6:346–351.

53. Lefaucheur C, Nochy D, Andrade J, et al. Comparison of combination Plasmapheresis/IVIg/anti-CD20 versus high-dose IVIg in the treatment of antibody-mediated rejection. Am J Transplant 2009;9:1099–1107.

54. Locke JE, Magro CM, Singer AL, et al. The use of antibody to complement protein C5 for salvage treatment of severe antibody-mediated rejection. Am J Transplant 2009;9:231–235.

55. Elbarbry FA, Marfleet T, Shoker AS. Drug-drug interactions with immunosuppressive agents: review of the in vitro functional assays and role of cytochrome P450 enzymes. Transplantation 2008;85:1222–1229.

56. DuBuske LM. The role of P-glycoprotein and organic anion-transporting polypeptides in drug interactions. Drug Saf 2005;28:789–801.

57. Prescott WA Jr, Callahan BL, Park JM. Tacrolimus toxicity associated with concomitant metoclopramide therapy. Pharmacotherapy 2004;24:532–537.

58. Rupprecht K, Schmidt C, Raspe A, et al. Bioavailability of mycophenolate mofetil and enteric-coated mycophenolate sodium is differentially affected by pantoprazole in healthy volunteers. J Clin Pharmacol 2009;49:1196–1201.

59. Gelone DK, Park JM, Lake KD. Lack of an effect of oral iron administration on mycophenolic acid pharmacokinetics in stable renal transplant recipients. Pharmacotherapy 2007;27:1272–1278.

60. Lynch T, Price A. The effect of cytochrome P450 metabolism on drug response, interactions, and adverse effects. Am Fam Physician 2007;76:391–396.

61. van Duijnhoven EM, Boots JM, Christiaans MH, Stolk LM, Undre NA, van Hooff JP. Increase in tacrolimus trough levels after steroid withdrawal. Transpl Int 2003;16:721–725.

62. Baroletti S, Bencivenga GA, Gabardi S. Treating gout in kidney transplant recipients. Prog Transplant 2004;14:143–147.

63. Gregoor PJ, de Sevaux RG, Hene RJ, et al. Effect of cyclosporine on mycophenolic acid trough levels in kidney transplant recipients. Transplantation 1999;68:1603–1606.

64. Ekbal NJ, Holt DW, Macphee IA. Pharmacogenetics of immunosuppressive drugs: prospect of individual therapy for transplant patients. Pharmacogenomics 2008;9:585–596.

65. Anglicheau D, Legendre C, Beaune P, Thervet E. Cytochrome P450 3A polymorphisms and immunosuppressive drugs: an update. Pharmacogenomics 2007;8:835–849.

66. Alloway R, Isaacs R, Lake K, et al. Report of the AST conference on immunosuppressive drugs and the use of generic immunosuppressants. Am J Transplant 2003;3:1211–1215.

67. Fishman JA. Introduction: infection in solid organ transplant recipients. Am J Transplant 2009;9 Suppl 4:S3–S6.

68. Martin SI, Fishman JA. Pneumocystis pneumonia in solid organ transplant recipients. Am J Transplant 2009;9 (Suppl 4):S227–S233.

69. Humar A, Snydman D. Cytomegalovirus in solid organ transplant recipients. Am J Transplant 2009;9 (Suppl 4):S78–S86.

70. Gabardi S, Magee CC, Baroletti SA, et al. Efficacy and safety of low-dose valganciclovir for prevention of cytomegalovirus disease in renal transplant recipients: a single-center, retrospective analysis. Pharmacotherapy 2004;24:1323–1330.

71. Paya C, Humar A, Dominguez E, et al. Efficacy and safety of valganciclovir vs. oral ganciclovir for prevention of cytomegalovirus disease in solid organ transplant recipients. Am J Transplant 2004;4:611–620.

72. Gabardi S, Kubiak DW, Chandraker AK, Tullius SG. Invasive fungal infections and antifungal therapies in solid organ transplant recipients. Transpl Int 2007;20:993–1015.

73. Singh N, Husain S. Invasive aspergillosis in solid organ transplant recipients. Am J Transplant 2009;9(Suppl 4):S180–191.

74. Pappas PG, Silveira FP. Candida in solid organ transplant recipients. Am J Transplant 2009;9(Suppl 4):S173–S179.

75. Hirsch HH, Randhawa P. BK virus in solid organ transplant recipients. Am J Transplant 2009;9(Suppl 4):S136–S146.

76. Danzinger-Isakov L, Kumar D. Guidelines for vaccination of solid organ transplant candidates and recipients. Am J Transplant 2009;9 (Suppl 4):S258-S262.

77. Dunn BL, Teusink AC, Taber DJ, Hemstreet BA, Uber LA, Weimert NA. Management of hypertension in renal transplant patients: a comprehensive review of nonpharmacologic and pharmacologic treatment strategies. Ann Pharmacother 2010;44:1259–1270.

78. Gabardi S, Baroletti SA. Comment: management of hypertension in renal transplant patients: a comprehensive review of nonpharmacologic and pharmacologic treatment strategies. Ann Pharmacother 2010;44:2040–2041.

79. Olyaei A, Greer E, Delos Santos R, Rueda J. The efficacy and safety of the 3-hydroxy-3-methylglutaryl-CoA reductase inhibitors in chronic kidney disease, dialysis, and transplant patients. Clin J Am Soc Nephrol 2011;6:664–678.

80. Tannock LR, Reynolds LR. Management of dyslipidemia in patients after solid organ transplantation. Postgrad Med 2008;120:43–49.

81. Kobashigawa JA, Katznelson S, Laks H, et al. Effect of pravastatin on outcomes after cardiac transplantation. N Engl J Med 1995;333:621–627.

82. Executive Summary of The Third Report of The National Cholesterol Education Program (NCEP) Expert Panel on Detection, Evaluation, And Treatment of High Blood Cholesterol In Adults (Adult Treatment Panel III). JAMA 2001;285:2486–2497.

83. Rakel A, Karelis AD. New-onset diabetes after transplantation: risk factors and clinical impact. Diabetes Metab 2011;37:1–14.

84. Kasiske BL, Snyder JJ, Gilbertson D, Matas AJ. Diabetes mellitus after kidney transplantation in the United States. Am J Transplant 2003;3:178–185.

85. Navarro MD, Lopez-Andreu M, Rodriguez-Benot A, Aguera ML, Del Castillo D, Aljama P. Cancer incidence and survival in kidney transplant patients. Transplant Proc 2008;40:2936–2940.

86. Wong G, Chapman JR, Craig JC. Cancer screening in renal transplant recipients: what is the evidence? Clin J Am Soc Nephrol 2008;3 (Suppl 2):S87–S100.

87. Traywick C, O'Reilly FM. Management of skin cancer in solid organ transplant recipients. Dermatol Ther 2005;18:12–18.

88. Pascoe AJ, Campistol JM, Schena FP, et al. Lower malignancy rates in renal allograft recipients converted to sirolimus-based, calcineurin inhibitor-free immunotherapy: 24-month results from the CONVERT trial. Transplantation 2011;92:303–310.

89. Allen U, Preiksaitis J. Epstein-barr virus and posttransplant lymphoproliferative disorder in solid organ transplant recipients. Am J Transplant 2009;9 (Suppl 4):S87–S96.

90. Gottschalk S, Rooney CM, Heslop HE. Post-transplant lymphoproliferative disorders. Annu Rev Med 2005;56:29–44.

91. McKay DB, Josephson MA, Armenti VT, et al. Reproduction and transplantation: report on the AST Consensus Conference on Reproductive Issues and Transplantation. Am J Transplant 2005;5:1592–1599.

92. Mastrobattista JM, Gomez-Lobo V. Pregnancy after solid organ transplantation. Obstet Gynecol 2008;112:919–932.

93. Dew MA, DiMartini AF, De Vito Dabbs A, et al. Rates and risk factors for nonadherence to the medical regimen after adult solid organ transplantation. Transplantation 2007;83(7):858–873.

94. Gaston RS, Hudson SL, Ward M, et al. Late renal allograft loss: noncompliance masquerading chronic rejection. Transplant Proc 1999;31(Suppl 4A):S21–S23.

95. Shapiro PA, Williams DL, Foray AT, et al. Psychosocial evaluation and prediction of compliance problems and morbidity after heart transplantation. Transplantation 1995;60(12):1462–1466.

96. Chisholm MA, Mulloy LL, Jagadeesan M, et al. Impact of clinical pharmacy services on renal transplant patients' compliance with immunosuppressive medications. Clin Transplant 2001;15(5):330–336.

56 Osteoporosis

Beth Bryles Phillips and Maria Miller Thurston

LEARNING OBJECTIVES

● **Upon completion of the chapter, the reader will be able to:**

1. Explain the association between osteoporosis and morbidity and mortality.

2. Identify risk factors that predispose patients to osteoporosis.

3. Describe the pathogenesis of fractures.

4. List the criteria for diagnosis of osteoporosis.

5. Recommend appropriate lifestyle modifications to prevent bone loss.

6. Compare and contrast the effect of available treatment options on reduction of fracture risk.

7. Recommend an appropriate treatment regimen for a patient with osteoporosis and develop a monitoring plan for the selected regimen.

8. Educate patients on osteoporosis and drug treatment, including appropriate use, administration, and adverse effects.

KEY CONCEPTS

❶ Major risk factors for osteoporotic fracture as defined by the World Health Organization (WHO) are low bone mineral density (BMD), personal history of adult fracture, age, family history of osteoporotic fracture, current cigarette smoking, low body mass index, excessive alcohol use, and chronic glucocorticoid use.

❷ A standardized approach for diagnosing osteoporosis is recommended using central dual-energy x-ray absorptiometry (DXA) measurements.

❸ Both pharmacologic and nonpharmacologic therapies for osteoporosis are aimed at preventing fractures and their complications, maintaining or increasing BMD, preventing secondary causes of bone loss, and improving morbidity and mortality.

❹ All men and women over age 50 should be considered for pharmacologic treatment if they meet any of the following criteria: (a) history of hip or vertebral fracture, (b) *T*-score less than or equal to –2.5 at femoral neck or spine, or (c) osteopenia and at least a 3% 10-year probability of hip fracture or at least a 20% 10-year probability of major osteoporosis-related fracture as determined by FRAX.

❺ Adequate calcium and vitamin D intake is essential in prevention and treatment of osteoporosis. Calcium and vitamin D supplements to meet requirements should be added to all drug therapy regimens for osteoporosis.

❻ Bisphosphonates are first-line therapy for postmenopausal and male osteoporosis due to established efficacy in preventing hip and vertebral fractures.

❼ The American College of Rheumatology (ACR) recommends bisphosphonate therapy with alendronate or risedronate for all patients who are starting treatment with glucocorticoids (prednisone 5 mg or more daily or equivalent) that will continue for 3 months or longer.

INTRODUCTION

Osteoporosis is a common and often silent disorder causing significant morbidity and mortality and reduced quality of life. It is associated with increased risk and rate of bone fracture and is responsible for more than 1.5 million fractures in the United States annually resulting in direct healthcare costs of more than $17 billion.[1] As the population ages, these numbers are expected to increase by two- to threefold. It is estimated that postmenopausal white women have a 50% lifetime chance of developing an osteoporosis-related fracture, whereas men have a 20% lifetime chance.[1] Common sites of fracture include the spine, hip, and wrist, although almost all sites can be affected. Only a fraction of patients with osteoporosis receive optimal treatment.

The fractures associated with osteoporosis have an enormous impact on individual patients. In addition to the initial pain associated with a new fracture, several adverse long-term complications can occur, including chronic pain, loss of mobility, depression, nursing home placement, and death. Patients with vertebral fractures may experience chronic pain, height loss, kyphosis, and decreased mobility due to limitations in bending and reaching. Multiple vertebral fractures may lead to restrictive lung disease and altered abdominal anatomy. Patients with hip fractures have added risks associated with surgical intervention to repair the fracture. Some patients never fully recover or regain preinjury independence. Death is common in the year after a hip fracture.[1]

EPIDEMIOLOGY AND ETIOLOGY

Osteoporosis is the most common skeletal disorder, affecting more than 10 million Americans. Additionally, more than 34 million Americans have low bone mass. Only one in three patients with osteoporosis are diagnosed, and only one in seven receives treatment.[2] Osteoporosis can be classified as either primary (no known cause) or secondary (caused by drugs or other diseases). Primary osteoporosis is most often found in postmenopausal women and aging men, but it can occur in other age groups as well.

The prevalence of osteoporosis varies by age, gender, and race/ethnicity. The risk of fracture increases exponentially with each decade in age over 50.[3] Residents of nursing homes may be at an even higher risk of fracture. Both men and women lose bone as they age. However, women have accelerated bone loss surrounding menopause due to loss of estrogen. Men have some protection from osteoporosis due to their larger initial bone mass and size and lack of accelerated bone loss associated with menopause.[4] Fragility fractures of the hip and spine are common among men, especially as age increases. Men comprise 20% of the Americans with osteoporosis. Secondary causes of osteoporosis, such as hypogonadism, are found more commonly in men with fragility fractures.[4] Most hip fractures occur in postmenopausal white women; this group also has the highest incidence of fracture when adjusted for age. The incidence of osteoporosis and low bone mass is highest in white women, followed by Asian, Hispanic, and African American women, respectively.[5]

Many of the risk factors for osteoporosis and osteoporotic fractures are predictors of low BMD, such as age and ethnicity (Table 56–1). ❶ *Major risk factors for osteoporotic fracture as defined by the World Health Organization (WHO) are low BMD, female sex, age, race/ethnicity, personal history of fragility fracture as an adult, family history of osteoporotic fracture, low body mass index, past or present oral glucocorticoid use, current cigarette smoking, and excessive alcohol use.*[1,6] As BMD decreases, the risk of fracture increases. However, the threshold at which individual patients develop a fracture varies, and other factors may play a role in fracture susceptibility. One such factor that can influence the development of fracture is falling.

Osteoporosis can also develop from secondary causes such as concurrent disease states and drugs (Table 56–2). Approximately one-third to one-half of osteoporosis cases in men and half of all cases in perimenopausal women are due to secondary causes.[5] Common secondary causes in men

include hypogonadism and alcoholism. The most common cause of drug-induced osteoporosis is glucocorticoid use.

PATHOPHYSIOLOGY

The human skeleton is comprised of both cortical and trabecular bone. Cortical bone is dense and compact and is responsible for much of bone strength. It is the most common type of bone and accounts for approximately 80% of the skeleton. It is generally found on the surfaces of long and flat bones. Trabecular or cancellous bone has a sponge-like appearance and is generally found along the inner surfaces of long bones and throughout the vertebrae, pelvis, and ribs.

Under normal circumstances, the skeleton undergoes a dynamic process of bone remodeling. Bone tissue responds to stress and injury through continuous replacement and repair. This process is completed by the basic multicellular unit, which includes both osteoblasts and osteoclasts. Osteoclasts are involved with resorption or breakdown of bone and continuously create microscopic cavities in bone

---

Table 56–1

Risk Factors for Osteoporosis and Osteoporotic Fractures[1,2]

Risk Factors for Osteoporosis	Risk Factors for Falling and Fractures
Low bone mineral density[a]	Poor health/frailty
Female sex[a]	Impaired gait or balance
Advanced age[a]	Recent falls
Race/ethnicity[a]	Cognitive impairment
History of previous low trauma (fragility) fracture as an adult[a]	Impaired vision
Osteoporotic fracture in a first-degree relative (especially parental hip fracture[a])	Environmental factors (e.g., stairs, throw rugs, pets, poor lighting)
Low body weight or body mass index[a]	
Premature menopause (before 45 years old)[b]	
Secondary osteoporosis[b] (especially rheumatoid arthritis[a])	
Past or present systemic oral glucocorticoid therapy[a]	
Current cigarette smoking[a]	
Alcohol intake of three or more drinks per day[a]	
Low calcium intake	
Low physical activity	
Minimal sun exposure	

[a]Major risk factors used in the World Health Organization (WHO) fracture risk model.

[b]Secondary causes included in the FRAX tool question are type 1 diabetes, osteogenesis imperfecta as an adult, longstanding untreated hyperthyroidism, hypogonadism, premature menopause (before 45 years of age), chronic malnutrition, malabsorption, and chronic liver disease.

Adapted from DiPiro JT et al., eds. Pharmacotherapy: A Pathophysiologic Approach. 8th ed. New York: McGraw-Hill; 2011:1563, Table 99–1; With permission.

Table 56–2	

Medical Conditions and Drugs Associated with Osteoporosis or Low Bone Mass

Medical Conditions	Drugs
Alcoholism	Anticonvulsants (phenytoin, phenobarbital)
Chronic kidney disease	
Cushing's syndrome	Aromatase inhibitors (anastrozole, exemestane, letrozole)
Cystic fibrosis	
Diabetes mellitus	Cytotoxic drugs (e.g., methotrexate, cisplatin)
Eating disorders	
GI disorders (e.g., gastrectomy, malabsorption syndromes)	Glucocorticoids (5 mg or more of prednisone daily or equivalent for at least 3 months)
Hematologic disorders (e.g., hemophilia)	Gonadotropin-releasing hormone analogs (leuprolide acetate, nafarelin, goserelin)
Hyperparathyroidism	
Hyperthyroidism	Heparin
Hypogonadal states	Immunosuppressants (e.g., tacrolimus)
Organ transplantation	
Skeletal cancer (e.g., myeloma)	Lithium
	Medroxyprogesterone acetate
	Thyroid supplements (due to over-replacement)
	Total parenteral nutrition

tissue. Osteoblasts are involved in bone formation and continuously mineralize new bone in the cavities created by osteoclasts. Until peak bone mass is achieved between the ages of 25 and 35, bone formation exceeds bone resorption for an overall increase in bone mass. Trabecular bone is more susceptible to bone remodeling in part due to its larger surface area. **Figure 56–1** illustrates the difference between normal and osteoporotic bone.

In osteoporosis, an imbalance in bone remodeling occurs. Most commonly, osteoclastic activity is enhanced, resulting

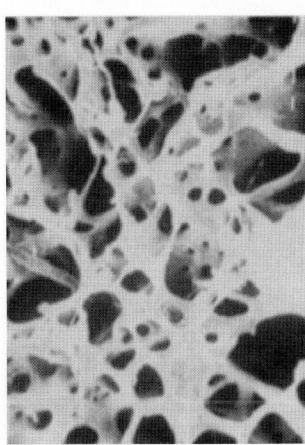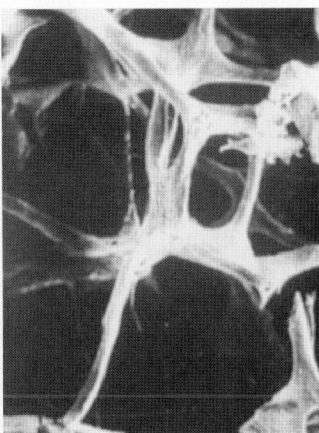

FIGURE 56–1. Normal trabecular bone (left) compared with trabecular bone from a patient with osteoporosis (right). The loss of mass in osteoporosis leaves bones more susceptible to breakage. From Barnett KE, Barman SM, Boitano S. Brooks H. Ganong's Review of Medical Physiology. 23rd ed. New York: McGraw-Hill; 2010: Figure 23–13; With permission. [cited 2011 Oct 10]. Available from: http://www.accesspharmacy.com.

General

Many patients with osteoporosis are asymptomatic unless they experience a fragility fracture.

Symptoms of Fragility Fracture

Pain at the site of the fracture or immobility.

Signs

Height loss (greater than 2 cm), spinal kyphosis ("dowager's hump"), fragility fracture especially of the hip or spine.

in overall bone loss. However, a reduction in osteoblastic activity and reduced bone formation can also occur in certain types of osteoporosis. Due to a decrease in endogenous estrogen, bone remodeling accelerates during menopause, and up to 15% of bone is lost during the first 5 years after menopause. After this initial decline, bone loss continues to occur, but at a much slower rate of up to 1% per year. The resultant bone loss and change in bone quality predispose patients to low-impact or **fragility fractures**.

CLINICAL PRESENTATION AND DIAGNOSIS

See the accompanying text box for the clinical presentation of osteoporosis.

Diagnosis

Osteoporosis has been defined by the WHO as a disease characterized by low bone density and weakening of bone tissue associated with an increase in fragility and vulnerability to fracture.[7] Because bone strength cannot be measured directly, an assessment of BMD is used, which represents 70% of bone strength. Low BMD has been associated with an increased risk of fractures. X-rays are useful only in identifying patients suspected of sustaining a fracture and are not recommended for diagnosis of osteoporosis.

▶ Measurement of Bone Mineral Density

BMD can be measured at various sites throughout the skeletal system and by various methods. The site of measurement can be either central (hip and/or spine) or peripheral (heel, forearm, or hand). Dual-energy x-ray absorptiometry (DXA) can be used to measure central and peripheral sites of BMD. Quantitative ultrasound, peripheral quantitative computed tomography, radiographic absorptiometry, and single-energy x-ray absorptiometry are used to measure peripheral sites.

❷ *The WHO recommends a standardized approach to measuring BMD for diagnosis of osteoporosis using central measurement of BMD by DXA.*[5] Central DXA is recommended for diagnosis due to inconsistencies in *T*-scores

Table 56–3	
WHO Definition of Osteoporosis	
Skeletal Disorder	**T-Score**[a]
Normal	Greater than or equal to −1
Osteopenia	Less than −1 to greater than or equal to −2.5
Osteoporosis	Less than −2.5

[a]T-score is the number of standard deviations above or below the mean bone mineral density in young adults.

measured between different sites and by different methods.[1,2] Current standards of practice consist of measuring BMD at the lumbar spine and hip, although the WHO suggests the hip is the preferred site for diagnosis.[3,7]

Some instruments used for peripheral bone densitometry are portable, which allows bone density to be measured in pharmacies and health-fair screening booths. In addition to its accessibility, peripheral measurement of BMD is generally less expensive than central DXA. These factors make it an attractive option for many patients. Peripheral BMD testing is useful in identifying patients who are candidates for central DXA and who are at increased risk of fracture.

Once the BMD report is available, T-scores and Z-scores are useful tools in interpreting the data. The T-score is the number of standard deviations from the mean BMD in healthy young white women. Osteoporosis is defined as a T-score at least −2.5 (Table 56–3). Osteopenia, or low bone mass that may eventually lead to osteoporosis, is defined as a T-score between −2.5 and −1.0. The International Society for Clinical Densitometry recommends use of the WHO definition and T-scores for diagnosis of osteoporosis in postmenopausal women and men over the age of 50.[8]

The Z-score is similar to the T-score but is corrected for both the age and sex of the patient. The Z-score is defined as the number of standard deviations from the mean BMD of age- and sex-matched controls. Z-scores may be more clinically relevant in evaluating BMD in premenopausal women, men under the age of 50, and patients who may have secondary causes for low BMD.

▶ **Screening and Risk Factor Assessment**

Screening for low bone density is an effective way to identify individuals at risk for osteoporotic fracture. A number of published osteoporosis guidelines provide recommendations for screening based on age and risk factors.[1,2,6,8] Routine BMD screening is generally recommended for all women over the age of 65 and men over the age of 70.[1] Many guidelines also recommend screening in individuals under these ages but over the age of 50 with specific risk factors such as previous fragility fracture, glucocorticoid or other high-risk medication use, or secondary cause of osteoporosis.

An additional tool, FRAX, was developed by the WHO to evaluate an individual's 10-year probability of developing hip and major osteoporotic fracture.[1] This probability is calculated based on BMD T-score, age, and other risk factors. Its intended use is for men and women over the age of 40 and may be accessed at *www.shef.ac.uk/FRAX*. Although the T-score is helpful in calculating risk of fracture with FRAX, fracture risk may be calculated without it.

▶ **Laboratory Evaluation**

Laboratory assessment has little value in diagnosing osteoporosis, but it can be beneficial in identifying or excluding secondary causes of bone loss, such as hyperparathyroidism, low 25-hydroxyvitamin D levels, hyperthyroidism (thyroid stimulating hormone levels), hypogonadism (testosterone levels), or cancer.[3] Serum creatinine, calcium, phosphorus, and complete blood count are also usually obtained. Biochemical markers of bone turnover such as pyridinoline, deoxypyridinoline, N-telopeptides, and C-telopeptides of type I collagen cross-links have been associated with an

---

Patient Encounter, Part 1: Patient History

HPI: AN is a frail 74-year-old white man who presents to the clinic for follow-up. He reports occasional forgetfulness. His erectile dysfunction, poor libido, and fatigue have improved since starting testosterone replacement therapy. He has no complaints with his current medication regimen for asthma. He also has no complaints about omeprazole but takes calcium carbonate (Tums) approximately once a week for heartburn after eating spicy meals. He usually spends his day inside his house watching television from his recliner. He states that milk upsets his stomach, so he usually drinks water or soda

PMH: Asthma, DM type 2, HTN, GERD, hypogonadism, lactose intolerance

FH: Father died at age 76 with Alzheimer's disease; mother died at age 92 with history of breast cancer and osteoporotic fractures of the hip; sister alive and well at age 69

SH: Retired construction worker; drinks 4 beers per day; nonsmoker

Meds: Albuterol inhaler two puffs as needed, metformin 500 mg twice daily; lisinopril 10 mg daily; testosterone cypionate 200 mg IM every 4 weeks; omeprazole 20 mg daily; calcium carbonate (Tums) 500 mg as needed

Do any symptoms suggest the presence of osteoporosis?

What risk factors for osteoporosis does this patient have as defined by the World Health Organization?

What secondary causes of osteoporosis does the patient have?

What are his recommended daily intakes for calcium and vitamin D?

How could he incorporate more calcium into his diet?

increased fracture risk in some trials. Variations in the normal ranges of these tests may be related to age, gender, food, and diurnal variation, making interpretation of these tests difficult.[2] For these reasons, biochemical markers of bone turnover are not recommended for diagnosis of osteoporosis.

TREATMENT

Desired Outcomes

③ *Pharmacologic and nonpharmacologic therapies are aimed at the following goals: (a) preventing fractures and their* complications; (b) maintaining or increasing BMD; (c) preventing secondary causes of bone loss; and (d) reducing morbidity and mortality associated with osteoporosis.

Nonpharmacologic Therapy

The primary goal of nonpharmacologic therapy for osteoporosis is to prevent fractures. Strategies to prevent fractures include maximizing peak bone mass, reducing bone loss, and using precautions to prevent falls leading to fragility fractures (Fig. 56–2).

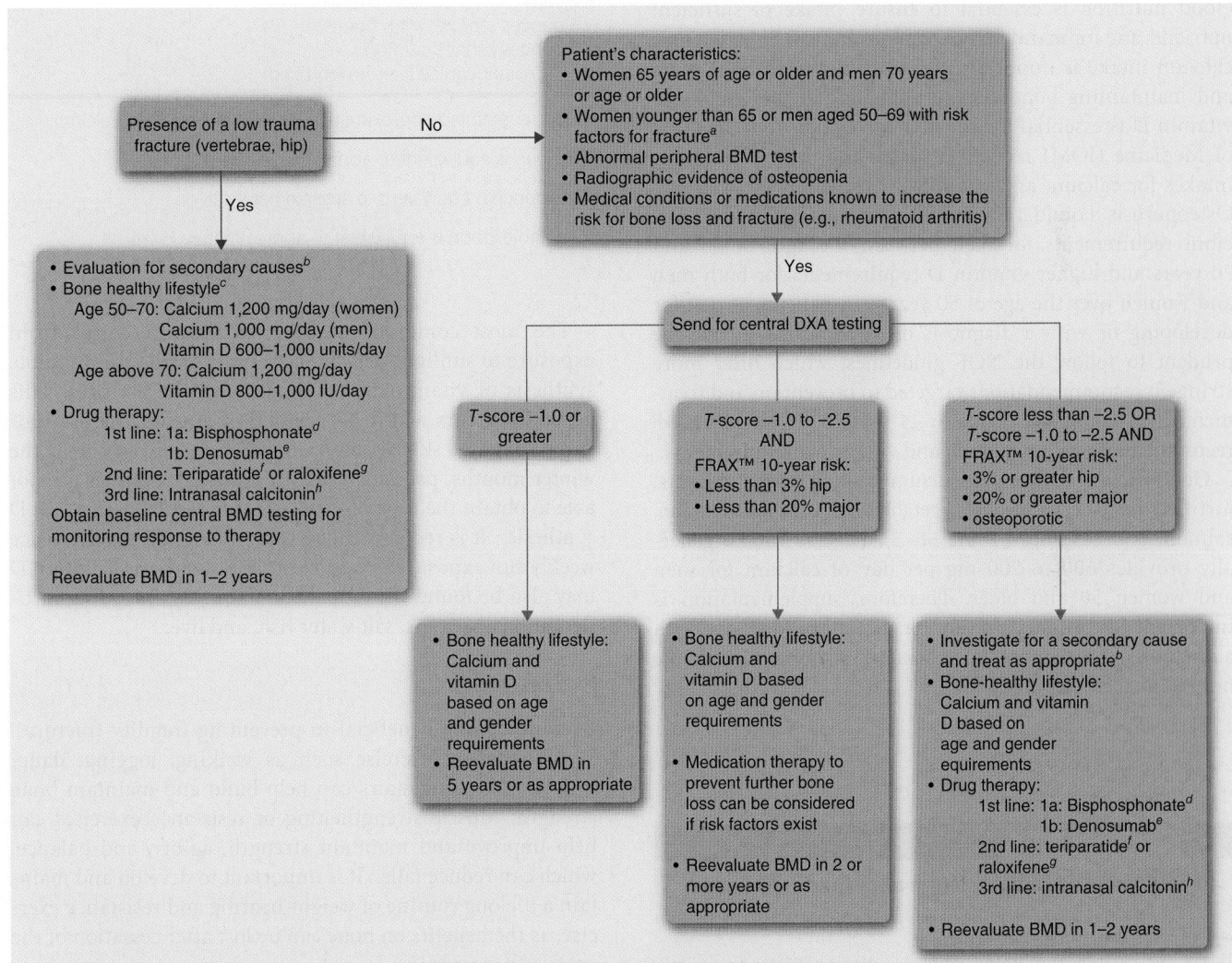

^{a}Major risk factors: Current smoker, personal history of fracture as an adult (after age 50 years), history of low-trauma fracture in a first-degree relative, low BMD, low body weight/BMI, excessive alcohol use, chronic glucocorticoid use (3 months or longer).
^{b}Secondary causes: Hypogonadism, rheumatoid arthritis, chronic obstructive pulmonary disease, systemic glucocorticoids.
^{c}Bone-healthy lifestyle: Smoking cessation, well-balanced diet, weight-bearing/resistance exercise, fall prevention for seniors, and limiting alcohol. Calcium and vitamin D values based on IOM and NOF recommendations for age and gender.
^{d}Alendronate, risedronate, and zoledronic acid are first line for men and women. Ibandronate is a second-line bisphosphonate and not FDA-approved for use in men. IV bisphosphonates are generally an option if patient cannot tolerate oral bisphosphonates or has significant adherence problems.
^{e}Denosumab may be used as a first-line agent per AACE 2010 guidelines. It is not FDA-approved for use in men.
^{f}Teriparatide is FDA-approved for use in men and can be considered a first-line option with a T-score less than –3.5 or if multiple low trauma factures.
^{g}Raloxifene may be a good option for women at high risk for breast cancer.
^{h}Calcitonin is not FDA-approved for use in men.

FIGURE 56–2. Algorithm for management of osteoporosis in women and in men aged 50 and older. Adapted from DiPiro JT et al., eds. Pharmacotherapy: A Pathophysiologic Approach. 8th ed. New York: McGraw-Hill; 2011:1567, Figure 99–3; With permission.

▶ *Modification of Risk Factors*

Some osteoporosis risk factors (see Tables 56–1 and 56–2) are nonmodifiable, including family history, age, ethnicity, gender, and concomitant disease states. However, certain risk factors for bone loss may be minimized or prevented by early intervention, including smoking, low calcium intake, poor nutrition, inactivity, heavy alcohol use, and vitamin D deficiency. To avoid certain risk factors and maximize peak bone mass, efforts must be directed toward osteoporosis prevention at an early age.

▶ *Nutrition*

Good nutrition is essential to ensure intake of sufficient nutrients and for maintenance of appropriate weight. Dietary calcium intake is important for achieving peak bone mass and maintaining bone density. Adequate dietary intake of vitamin D is essential for calcium absorption. The Institute of Medicine (IOM) recently updated the dietary reference intakes for calcium and vitamin D.[9] However, the National Osteoporosis Foundation (NOF) recommends higher calcium requirements for men between the ages of 50 and 70 years and higher vitamin D requirements for both men and women over the age of 50 years.[1] In patients at risk for developing or with a diagnosis of osteoporosis, it may be prudent to follow the NOF guidelines, which offer more stringent recommendations targeted to prevention and treatment of osteoporosis. Table 56–4 lists the IOM and NOF recommendations for calcium and vitamin D requirements.

Good dietary sources of calcium include dairy products, fortified juice, cruciferous vegetables (e.g., broccoli, kale), salmon, and sardines (Table 56–5). Dietary intake generally provides 600 to 700 mg per day of calcium for men and women 50 and older. Therefore, supplementation is important for primary prevention, as well as for those with a diagnosis of osteoporosis, to achieve recommended intake not attained by diet alone.[1]

Table 56–4
Recommended Daily Calcium and Vitamin D Intake

Age	Institute of Medicine Dietary Reference Intakes		National Osteoporosis Foundation	
	Calcium	Vitamin D	Calcium	Vitamin D
Women 50–70	1,200 mg	600 IU	1,200 mg	800–1,000 IU
Women over 70	1,200 mg	800 IU	1,200 mg	800–1,000 IU
Men 50–70	1,000 mg	600 IU	1,200 mg	800–1,000 IU
Men over 70	1,200 mg	800 IU	1,200 mg	800–1,000 IU

From references 1 and 9.

Table 56–5
Calcium-Rich Foods[a]

1 cup[b] skim milk
1 cup soy milk (calcium-fortified)
1 cup yogurt
1½ ounces[c] cheddar cheese
1½ ounces jack cheese
1½ ounces Swiss cheese
1½ ounces part-skim mozzarella
4 tablespoonfuls[d] grated Parmesan cheese
8 ounces tofu
1 cup greens (collards, kale)
2 cups broccoli
4 ounces almonds
2 cups low-fat cottage cheese
3 ounces sardines with bones
5 ounces canned salmon
1 cup orange juice (calcium-fortified)

[a]Foods containing approximately 300 mg of elemental calcium.

[b]One cup is equivalent to approximately 240 mL.

[c]One ounce is equivalent to approximately 28 g.

[d]One tablespoon is equivalent to approximately 15 mL.

The most common source of vitamin D comes from exposure to sunlight. Ultraviolet rays from the sun promote synthesis of vitamin D_3 (cholecalciferol) in the skin. This generally occurs within 15 minutes of direct sunlight exposure to exposed skin without sunscreen. However, during the winter months, patients living in northern latitudes are not able to obtain the type of exposure that results in vitamin D synthesis.[2] It is recommended that individuals receive twice weekly sun exposure to ensure optimal synthesis. Vitamin D may also be found in some dietary sources, including fortified milk, egg yolks, salt-water fish, and liver.

▶ *Exercise*

Exercise can be beneficial in preventing fragility fractures. Weight-bearing exercise such as walking, jogging, dancing, and climbing stairs can help build and maintain bone strength. Muscle-strengthening or resistance exercises can help improve and maintain strength, agility, and balance, which can reduce falls.[1] It is important to develop and maintain a lifelong routine of weight-bearing and resistance exercise, as the benefits on bone can be lost after cessation of the exercise program.[1]

▶ *Falls Prevention*

Another crucial step in avoiding fragility fractures is prevention of falls. Patients with frailty, poor vision, hearing loss, or those taking medications affecting balance are at higher risk for falling and subsequent fragility fractures.[1,2]

A number of medications have been associated with an increased risk of falling, including drugs affecting mental status such as antipsychotics, benzodiazepines, tricyclic antidepressants, sedative/hypnotics, anticholinergics, and corticosteroids. Some cardiovascular and antihypertensive drugs can also contribute to falls, especially those causing orthostatic hypotension.[1]

Efforts to decrease the risk of falling include balance training, muscle strengthening, removal of hazards in the home, installation of fall reduction measures such as handrails in the home, and discontinuation of predisposing medications.[1,2,10] Use of hip protectors also helps prevent hip fractures, although adherence to this measure may be problematic.[10]

Pharmacologic Treatment (Fig. 56–2)

4 *The NOF recommends that all men and women over age 50 be considered for pharmacologic treatment if they meet any of the following criteria: (a) history of hip or vertebral fracture, (b) T-score less than or equal to –2.5 at femoral neck or spine, or (c) osteopenia and at least a 3% 10-year probability of hip fracture or at least a 20% 10-year probability of major osteoporosis-related fracture as determined by FRAX.[1]*

▶ Calcium and Vitamin D

5 *Adequate calcium and vitamin D intake are essential for preventing and treating osteoporosis. Calcium and vitamin D supplements to meet requirements should be added to all drug therapy regimens for osteoporosis. Calcium and vitamin D supplementation increases BMD, and the combination decreases the risk of hip and vertebral fractures.[11]*

Calcium plays an important role in maximizing peak bone mass and decreasing bone turnover, thereby slowing bone loss. When the calcium supply is insufficient, calcium is taken from bone stores to maintain the serum calcium level. Adequate calcium consumption is essential to prevent this from occurring. Calcium supplementation may also correct secondary hyperparathyroidism in elderly patients.

The NOF recommends daily calcium intakes of 1,200 mg.[1] When these requirements cannot be achieved by diet alone, appropriate calcium supplementation is recommended. Intakes over 1,200 to 1,500 mg/day may increase the risk of developing kidney stones or cardiovascular disease,[1] and supplementation greater than 2,500 mg/day may lead to hypercalciuria and hypercalcemia.[6]

Calcium supplements are available in a variety of calcium salts and dosage forms. Daily calcium requirements are reported as elemental calcium. However, many product labels list calcium content in the salt form, so the percentage of elemental calcium must be known to calculate the elemental calcium content per tablet. A number of factors can limit calcium absorption, and special consideration must be given to calcium dosing to maximize absorption. Large amounts of calcium taken at once cannot be absorbed. Supplement doses should be limited to 500 to 600 mg of elemental calcium per dose. Healthcare providers can help patients find a suitable and tolerable supplement with good absorption and high elemental calcium content, necessitating fewer tablets per day. Table 56–6 lists widely available supplements with elemental calcium and vitamin D content.

Table 56–6

Calcium and Vitamin D Content of Common Supplements

Product (% Elemental Calcium)	Elemental Calcium per Tablet (mg)	Vitamin D per Tablet (IU)
Calcium Carbonate (40%)		
Tums 500 mg	200	—
Tums E-X 750 mg	300	—
Tums ULTRA 1,000 mg	400	—
Os-Cal 500	500	—
Os-Cal 500 + D	500	200
Os-Cal Ultra	600	200
Caltrate 600	600	—
Caltrate 600 + D	600	200
Caltrate 600 + Soy	600	200
One-A-Day Women's Multivitamin	450	400
Rolaids 550 mg	220	—
Viactiv	500	100
Calcium Citrate (24%)		
Citracal	200	—
Citracal 250 mg + D	250	62.5
Citracal + D	315	200
Calcium Phosphate, Tribasic (39%)		
Posture – D	600	125
Calcium Lactate (13%)	85	—
Calcium Gluconate (9%)	60	—

Calcium carbonate should be taken with food to maximize absorption. Elderly patients or patients receiving proton pump inhibitors or H_2-receptor antagonists may have added difficulty absorbing calcium supplements due to reduced stomach acidity. Better absorption may occur in this setting with calcium citrate because an acid environment is not needed for absorption; it may be taken with or without food.

Common adverse effects of calcium salts include constipation, bloating, cramps, and flatulence. Changing to a different salt form may alleviate symptoms for some patients. Calcium salts may reduce the absorption of iron and some antibiotics, such as tetracycline and fluoroquinolones.

Vitamin D is crucial for calcium absorption and maintenance of bone. The goal is to maintain a serum 25-hydroxyvitamin D level above 30 ng/mL (75 nmol/L).[1] The IOM recommends daily vitamin D intakes of 600 IU for men and women aged 51 to 70 years, and 800 IU for men and women greater than 70 years,[9] whereas the NOF recommends 800 to 1,000 IU for all men and women over 50 years of age. However, higher doses may be necessary in selected patients to meet this goal (see Table 56–4).

Vitamin D is often combined in varying amounts with calcium salts and is present in many multivitamin preparations. Vitamin D is also available as a single entity. To avoid hypercalciuria and hypercalcemia, the maximum recommended dose for most patients is 4,000 IU/day.[9] Ergocalciferol (vitamin D_2) and cholecalciferol (vitamin D_3) are available and generally reserved for patients with vitamin D deficiency. High-dose ergocalciferol is available by prescription

Patient Encounter, Part 2: Physical Exam and Diagnostic Tests

ROS: 4-cm height loss since middle age; (+) back pain

PE:

Gen: Well-developed white man in no acute distress

VS: BP 129/76, P 76, RR 18, T 36.3°C (97.3°F), wt 64.5 kg (142 lb), ht 5 ft 11 in (180 cm), BMI 19.8 kg/m²

Chest: Decreased breath sounds bilaterally, air movement decreased; no crackles or rhonchi

CV: RRR, normal S_1, S_2; no murmurs, rubs, or gallops

Abd: Soft, nontender, nondistended; normal bowel sounds, no hepatosplenomegaly

Ext: No clubbing, cyanosis, or edema

Labs:

Na 139 mEq/L (139 mmol/L)

K 4.0 mEq/L (4.0 mmol/L)

SCr 0.9 mg/dL (80 μmol/L)

A1c 6.3% (0.063; 45 mmol/mol hemoglobin)

Testosterone 308 ng/mL (10.7 nmol/L)

25(OH)D 33 ng/mL (82 nmol/L)

Bone Densitometry by DXA

- BMD of left hip: *T*-score = −2.7
- BMD of lumbar spine: *T*-score = −2.1

What additional risk factor and signs of osteoporosis are present in this patient?

What are the goals of pharmacologic and nonpharmacologic therapy?

List at least three nonpharmacologic interventions important in his treatment plan.

What factors support pharmacotherapy for osteoporosis in this patient?

What type of supplement(s) would you recommend for this patient to meet his calcium and vitamin D requirements? Why?

only, whereas cholecalciferol is available over the counter. With daily dosing, there is little difference between the potency of the two formulations, but cholecalciferol is more potent when dosed weekly or monthly.[2]

Several patient groups are at risk for vitamin D deficiency, including elderly patients with malabsorption syndromes, chronic renal insufficiency, other chronic diseases and those with limited sun exposure.[1] Elderly patients in particular are at increased risk of deficiency due to decreased exposure to sunlight and subsequent decreased vitamin D synthesis in the skin, decreased GI absorption of vitamin D, and reduction in vitamin D_3 synthesis. Individuals living in northern climates may have low vitamin D levels due to decreased sunlight exposure.

Many adults have low vitamin D levels, and vitamin D deficiency is an important secondary cause of osteoporosis.[2,12] Laboratory determination of 25-hydroxyvitamin D levels should occur prior to the start of therapy to determine whether supplementation is adequate or whether treatment of deficiency is needed. The Endocrine Society Vitamin D Deficiency Clinical Practice Guideline recommends treatment with ergocalciferol or cholecalciferol 50,000 IU once weekly (or its equivalent of 6,000 IU daily) for 8 weeks.[12] After 25-hydroxyvitamin D levels have risen above 30 ng/mL (75 nmol/L), doses of 1,500 to 2,000 IU can be used to maintain 25-hydroxyvitamin D levels between 30 and 60 ng/mL (75 and 150 nmol/L).[2,12]

▶ Bisphosphonates

⑥ *Bisphosphonates are first-line therapy for osteoporosis in both men and women due to established efficacy in preventing hip and vertebral fractures.* They are also the most commonly prescribed therapy for osteoporosis. They decrease bone resorption by binding to the bone matrix and inhibiting osteoclast activity. They remain in the bone for a prolonged period of several years and are released very slowly over time. These effects increase BMD. Although several bisphosphonates are currently available, only alendronate, ibandronate, risedronate, and zoledronic acid carry an FDA-approved indication for osteoporosis. All of these agents are approved for use in men and women, with the exception of ibandronate, which is only approved for use in postmenopausal osteoporosis. Ibandronate is generally considered a second-line bisphosphonate due to lack of documented efficacy in hip and nonvertebral fractures in prospective trials.[2] Table 56–7 contains comparative dosing and cost information for the bisphosphonates.

In placebo-controlled clinical trials, bisphosphonates increased BMD by up to 5% to 8% in the lumbar spine and up to 3% to 6% in the hip.[13–16] Additional data with oral bisphosphonates suggest that BMD continues to increase with long-term therapy of 7 to 10 years.[17,18] Although increases in BMD have been reported at other sites, most of the clinically significant fractures occur in the hip or spine, and these sites have become clinically important measures in the trials. These increases in BMD at the hip and spine are an important marker of treatment effects and are probably related to the decreases in fracture risk found in larger trials.

Large, well-designed trials have proven the benefits of bisphosphonate therapy in preventing vertebral and nonvertebral fractures. Several studies have found decreases in vertebral fracture risk by as much as 40% to 50% with oral bisphosphonates and up to 70% with zoledronic acid.[1,19] Although data suggest a similar reduction on vertebral fractures with ibandronate, only alendronate, risedronate, and zoledronic acid have been shown to decrease the incidence of hip and nonvertebral fractures as well by as much as 25% to 40%.[2,20,21] In addition to benefits in fracture reduction, the Horizon Recurrent Fracture Trial found a 28% decrease in mortality associated with hip fracture in patients treated with IV zoledronic acid.[20]

Table 56–7

Prescription Drug Therapy for Osteoporosis

Drug	Product Size	Indication/Usual Dose	Administration	Monthly Cost[a]
Bisphosphonates				
Alendronate (Fosamax)	5-, 10-, 35-, 70-mg tablets; 70-mg with cholecalciferol 2,800 IU; 70-mg with cholecalciferol 5,600 IU; 70-mg oral solution	Prevention of PM osteoporosis: 5 mg orally daily or 35 mg orally once weekly Osteoporosis (men and women): 10 mg orally once daily or 70 mg orally once weekly Glucocorticoid-induced osteoporosis: 10 mg once daily Avoid when CrCl less than 35 mL/min (0.58 mL/s)	Take after an overnight fast with 6–8 oz (180–240 mL) plain water while sitting or standing upright at least 30 minutes prior to morning meal. Do not lie down for 30 minutes after administration. Do not take with other medications or fluids. Do not chew or suck on the tablet.	As low as $9 for 70-mg weekly tablet[b]
Ibandronate (Boniva)	2.5-, 150-mg tablets; 3-mg/3 mL injection	Treatment or prevention of PM osteoporosis: 2.5 mg orally daily or 150 mg orally once monthly; 3 mg IV push over 15–30 seconds every 3 months Avoid when CrCl less than 35 mL/min (0.58 mL/s)	Same as alendronate except administer at least 1 hour prior to morning meal and refrain from lying down for 1 hour after administration.	$126 for 150-mg tablet
Risedronate (Actonel)	5-, 35-, 75-, 150-mg tablets; 35-mg with 1,250-mg calcium carbonate tablets	PM osteoporosis: 5 mg orally daily, 35 mg orally once weekly, 75 mg on 2 consecutive days each month, or 150 mg once monthly Male osteoporosis: 35 mg orally weekly or 150 mg orally monthly Glucocorticoid-induced osteoporosis: 5 mg orally daily Avoid when CrCl less than 30 mL/min (0.50 mL/s)	Same as alendronate.	$131 for 35-mg weekly tablet $144.50 for 150-mg monthly tablet
Zoledronic acid (Reclast)	5 mg/100 mL IV infusion	Prevention of PM osteoporosis: 5 mg infused IV over 15 minutes or longer every 24 months Treatment of osteoporosis (men and women), glucocorticoid-induced osteoporosis: 5 mg infused IV over 15 minutes or longer every 12 months Avoid when CrCl less than 35 mL/min (0.58 mL/s)	Infuse over at least 15 minutes. May premedicate with acetaminophen.	$1,137 for 5-mg dose
Monoclonal Antibody				
Denosumab (Prolia)	60 mg/mL SC pre-filled syringe	PM osteoporosis: 60 mg SC every 6 months	Inject in the upper arm, upper thigh, or abdomen. Keep refrigerated.	Not available
Recombinant Human Parathyroid Hormone				
Teriparatide (Forteo)	250 mcg/mL, 2.4-mL prefilled pen	Osteoporosis (men and women), glucocorticoid-induced osteoporosis: 20 mcg SC daily	Inject into thigh or abdominal wall. Keep pen refrigerated.	$1,016 per prefilled pen
Selective Estrogen Receptor Modulators				
Raloxifene (Evista)	60-mg tablets	PM osteoporosis: 60 mg daily	May be taken with or without food.	$150 for 60-mg tablet
Calcitonin				
Calcitonin salmon (Miacalcin)	200 IU/0.9 mL, 3.7-mL nasal spray	PM osteoporosis: Nasal spray: 200 IU daily	Nasal spray: Alternate nostrils on a daily basis.	$110 per 3.7-mL nasal spray

CrCl, creatinine clearance; IM, intramuscularly; PM, postmenopausal; SC, subcutaneously.

[a]Monthly cost from drugstore.com.

[b]Price available through select retail pharmacy prescription discount plans.

Several studies have evaluated the long-term efficacy and safety of bisphosphonates in postmenopausal women. One study evaluated the use of alendronate over a 10-year period and found no difference in adverse effects between women who received alendronate for 10 years compared with women who discontinued alendronate after 5 years. Women who discontinued alendronate after 5 years continued to experience sustained increases in BMD compared with baseline values and reduction in fracture rates.[17] Another study found sustained increases in BMD after discontinuation of alendronate, albeit less than in those who continued longer term alendronate therapy.[22] A 7-year follow-up study with risedronate found continued increases in BMD and no increase in adverse effects in women receiving risedronate for 7 years compared with women receiving risedronate for 2 years.[18] These findings support long-term administration of bisphosphonates in patients at high risk for fracture. However, for women who must discontinue bisphosphonate therapy due to intolerance or adverse events, improvements in BMD may be sustained.

The most notable adverse effects associated with the bisphosphonates are GI, ranging from relatively mild nausea, vomiting, and diarrhea to more severe esophageal irritation, and esophagitis. However, the most common adverse reactions reported in clinical trials include dyspepsia, abdominal pain, nausea, and esophageal reflux. Clinically significant adverse events include esophageal ulceration, erosions with bleeding, perforation, stricture, and esophagitis. Upper GI adverse effects can occur in up to 20% of patients and are often related to inappropriate administration. Advanced age, previous upper GI tract disease, and use of nonsteroidal anti-inflammatory drugs also increase the risk for GI adverse events, whereas once-weekly administration of oral bisphosphonates may decrease the risk.

The parenteral bisphosphonates (ibandronate and zoledronic acid) are associated with additional adverse effects.[2] Up to 40% of patients receiving the first dose may experience acute-phase reactions (also referred to as flu-like symptoms) that can last for days, such as headache, arthralgia, myalgia and fever.[1,2,20] Pretreatment with acetaminophen may prevent these symptoms.[2] Patients with moderate to severe renal impairment, severe dehydration, or taking concomitant diuretics or nephrotoxic drugs may be at higher risk of developing acute renal failure with zoledronic acid. Laboratory monitoring, including serum creatinine, alkaline phosphatase, phosphate, magnesium, and calcium, is recommended prior to administration of each zoledronic acid dose.

Although bisphosphonate trials have demonstrated continued efficacy over time, there may be some safety concerns associated with long-term use. Serious adverse events including osteonecrosis of the jaw (ONJ),[24,25] subtrochanteric fractures,[24] and nonvertebral atraumatic fractures[25] have been reported in the literature. These events may be related to oversuppression of bone turnover causing weakening of bone structure related to inhibition of osteoclastic activity.[23,26] Risk factors for development of ONJ include chemotherapy, radiotherapy, corticosteroids, infection, or preexisting dental disease. Most cases in the literature of ONJ occurred in patients receiving high doses of zoledronic acid for cancer-related

indications.[24] It is recommended that patients complete major dental work prior to initiation of bisphosphonate therapy. One population-based study found that older women treated with a bisphosphonate for more than 5 years had an increased risk of subtrochanteric or femoral shaft fractures.[27] The development of these fractures in patients treated with bisphosphonates are notable because they are not commonly associated with osteoporosis. The American Association of Clinical Endocrinologists (AACE) guidelines suggest that providers may consider a drug holiday of 1 to 2 years after 5 to 10 years of bisphosphonate treatment, depending on osteoporosis risk.[2] However, a recent FDA review on the risk of atypical subtrochanteric femur fractures from bisphosphonates found no clear association, and the FDA recommends to continue bisphosphonate therapy as labeled.[28] Esophageal cancer has also been reported with long-term therapy, but data are currently inconclusive.[29,30]

Oral bisphosphonates are poorly absorbed (less than 5%). Taking them in the presence of food or calcium supplementation further reduces absorption. After absorption, bisphosphonate uptake to the primary site of action is rapid and sustained. Once attached to bone tissue, bisphosphonates are released very slowly over several years. They are not recommended for use in patients with renal insufficiency because they are renally excreted and not metabolized.

Proper drug administration is important for optimal absorption and prevention of adverse effects. Oral bisphosphonates should be taken 30 to 60 minutes prior to the first meal or food in the morning after an overnight fast with 6 to 8 ounces (about 180 to 240 mL) of water (or 2 ounces [60 mL] with the oral solution). Patients should remain upright and refrain from lying down for 30 to 60 minutes after administration. The tablets should be swallowed whole without chewing or sucking. Administration should be with water only and not combined with other fluids. Bisphosphonates should not be taken with other medications or dietary supplements. Bisphosphonates are not recommended for use in patients with esophageal abnormalities that may delay transit of the tablet, such as with severe GERD, achalasia, stricture, or Barrett's esophagus. In addition, they are not recommended in patients with hypocalcemia or renal insufficiency or failure (creatinine clearance less than 30 to 35 mL/min [0.50 to 0.58 mL/s]), or in those who are pregnant. For patients unable to tolerate oral bisphosphonates, options exist for parenteral administration with ibandronate or zoledronic acid.

▶ Denosumab

Denosumab is the first human monoclonal antibody FDA approved for the treatment of postmenopausal osteoporosis. It is first-line therapy and should be considered in patients who are unable to tolerate bisphosphonates.[2] Denosumab reduces nuclear factor-kappa B ligand (RANKL) action, which leads to selective inhibition of osteoclast formation, function, and survival. In contrast to bisphosphonates, the antiresorptive effects of denosumab are reversible.

Denosumab has been shown to increase BMD in the hip and spine by up to 6% and 9%, respectively; and decrease hip, vertebral, and nonvertebral fracture risk by up to 40%, 68%, and 20%, respectively.[31] In direct head-to-head trials, patients treated with denosumab had greater increases in hip and spine BMD than patients treated with alendronate, although fracture risk was not reported.[32,33] Denosumab is a treatment alternative for patients who are unable to tolerate oral bisphosphonates due to gastrointestinal contraindications or side effects and for patients with malabsorption or adherence issues.[34]

Common adverse effects include back pain, arthralgias, fatigue, headache, dermatologic reactions, diarrhea, and nausea. Serious adverse reactions, including hypophosphatemia, hypocalcemia, dyspnea, and skin and other infections, can occur. Patients should seek medical attention if they experience any symptoms of infection. Denosumab can worsen hypocalcemia in predisposed patients, such as those with severe kidney disease. Prior to initiation of therapy, preexisting hypocalcemia should be corrected. Suppression of bone turnover has been associated with denosumab therapy, and ONJ has also been reported.[2]

Denosumab is part of a Risk Evaluation and Mitigation Strategy (REMS) program, in which the manufacturer is required by the FDA to inform patients and healthcare providers of the risks associated with its use.[35] Denosumab is administered as a subcutaneous injection once every 6 months and should be stored in the refrigerator until administration. Once at room temperature, the vial or prefilled syringe must be used within 14 days. Prescribing information recommends administration of 1,000 mg of calcium and at least 400 IU of vitamin D once daily.

▶ Teriparatide

Teriparatide, recombinant human parathyroid hormone (1–34), is the first anabolic agent approved by the FDA for treatment of postmenopausal and male osteoporosis. It is generally reserved for patients with very high fracture risk or those in whom other therapies have been ineffective.[2] This agent differs from antiresorptive therapies in that it stimulates osteoblastic activity to form new bone. It is administered as a subcutaneous injection. Teriparatide increases BMD in the spine and hip by 9% and 3%, respectively, and reduces fracture risk by 65% and 35% in vertebral and nonvertebral fractures, respectively.[36] Significant reductions in hip fracture have not been demonstrated.

Common adverse effects include nausea, headache, leg cramps, dizziness, injection site discomfort, and hypercalcemia. Orthostatic hypotension may also occur; patients should be seated after the first several doses until drug response is predictable. Observations of osteosarcoma in animal studies has led to the inclusion of a "black box warning" in the product labeling, but no cases have been reported in humans. Teriparatide should not be used in patients with preexisting hypercalcemia. Patient-related concerns regarding the use of teriparatide include cost of therapy and need for subcutaneous injections. The labeling recommends treatment for a maximum of 2 years because it has not been studied for longer periods.

▶ Raloxifene

Raloxifene is currently the only selective estrogen receptor modulator (SERM) indicated for prevention and treatment of osteoporosis. It is recommended as alternative therapy after bisphosphonates, denosumab, or teriparatide.[2] It has estrogen-like activity on bones and cholesterol metabolism and estrogen antagonist activity in breast and endometrium. It reduces bone resorption and decreases overall bone turnover.

Raloxifene has been shown to increase BMD in the vertebra (2% to 3%) and hip (1% to 2%), and reduce vertebral fracture rates by as much as 30%.[37] Significant decreases in hip and nonvertebral fractures have not been demonstrated in clinical trials.[2] In high-risk women, raloxifene has been shown to decrease the incidence of breast cancer. Although it decreases total and low-density lipoprotein (LDL) cholesterol, a large-scale trial found no benefit on cardiovascular events but did find an increased risk of fatal stroke in women treated with raloxifene.[38]

Adverse effects of raloxifene include hot flushes, leg cramps, and increased risk of venous thromboembolism. Hot flushes are very common and may be intolerable in postmenopausal women who are already predisposed to experiencing them. A more serious adverse effect is the significantly increased risk of venous thromboembolism that has been found in clinical trials.[38] A previous history of venous thromboembolism is a contraindication to therapy.

▶ Calcitonin

Calcitonin is a naturally occurring mammalian hormone that plays a major role in regulation of calcium levels. It inhibits bone resorption by binding to osteoclast receptors. Calcitonin is considered a last-line agent for the treatment of osteoporosis.[2] Calcitonin produces a modest increase in BMD at the spine of 1% to 3% and reduces vertebral fracture risk by up to 30%.[39] However, no benefit has been demonstrated in reducing hip or nonvertebral fractures.[2] Calcitonin has previously been thought advantageous for potential analgesic effects in women with back pain from vertebral fractures. However, enthusiasm for using it in this setting has waned in favor of managing fracture risk and pain separately.

Although salmon calcitonin is approved and available in injectable and intranasal formulations, only the intranasal formulation has documented benefit in clinical trials for management of osteoporosis. Adverse effects associated with the intranasal formulation include rhinitis, nasal irritation, and dryness. Hypersensitivity can develop with either formulation and should be considered before administering to patients with suspected risk of hypersensitivity.[2]

▶ Hormone Therapy

Estrogen, either alone or in combination with a progestin as hormone replacement therapy (HRT), has a long history as an effective treatment of osteoporosis. The Women's Health Initiative (WHI) trial found a 33% reduction in both vertebral and hip fractures and a 23% reduction in other fractures in postmenopausal women receiving conjugated estrogen and medroxyprogesterone.[40] However, significant risks associated with long-term HRT, including breast cancer and venous thromboembolism, have limited its use in osteoporosis.[40,41]

▶ Combination and Sequential Therapy

Interest in combination therapy with two or more osteoporosis drugs is based on the idea that using agents with differing mechanisms for inhibiting bone resorption would result in greater increases in BMD and reductions in fracture rates. Although there is some evidence to suggest modest additional increases in BMD occur with combination therapy, no significant benefits have been shown in reducing fracture rates. Combination therapy is also more expensive, and concern has been raised that significant reductions in bone turnover may promote bone that is more brittle.[42] The AACE does not recommend combination antiresorptive therapy for treating osteoporosis.[2]

Sequential therapy with teriparatide followed by bisphosphonate therapy has been studied. Its rationale is based on the limited duration (2 years) with which teriparatide can be used and the fact that increases in BMD decline rapidly after discontinuation of teriparatide.[2] Whether sequential therapy leads to reductions in fracture risk remains to be determined.

▶ Other Therapies

Investigational Agents Several anabolic and antiresorptive therapies are under investigation for treatment of osteoporosis. The most promising antiresorptive therapy may be odanacatib, a selective enzyme inhibitor of cathepsin-K.[43] This inhibition prevents enzymatic bone degradation in mature osteoclasts. It is thought that these actions lead to a more modest effect on suppression of bone turnover than other antiresorptive therapies.[43] It has been shown to progressively increase hip and spine bone BMD and reduce markers of bone resorption in postmenopausal women with low BMD. BMD levels quickly revert to baseline levels, and markers of bone remodeling rapidly increase after odanacatib discontinuation.[44]

Anabolic therapies currently under investigation include calcilytic drugs and Wnt antagonists. Calcilytic drugs increase bone formation by imitating hypocalcemia and cause parathyroid hormone secretion. The most advanced compound, MK-5442, is administered orally and could have important advantages over current therapy if efficacy and safety data are positive.[43] Wnt inhibitors bind to and block Wnt receptors and promote osteoblastic bone formation. All of these agents are currently in phase 1 and 2 trials.[43] Two other therapies with anabolic properties, strontium ranelate and PTH (1–84), are available in countries outside the United States.[43]

Complementary and Alternative Therapies Several studies have evaluated dietary supplements such as isoflavones, which are found in soy products and red clover. A well-controlled trial in more than 400 postmenopausal women evaluating a specific isoflavone, ipriflavone, found no benefits on BMD or fracture rates after 3 years.[45]

Nevertheless, because these therapies are available without prescription and are not regulated by the FDA, patients may choose to self-medicate with isoflavones. Lymphocytopenia appeared in several patients treated with ipriflavone in clinical trials. Additionally, ipriflavone should be used with caution in immunocompromised patients, those with renal disease, and patients taking drugs metabolized by CYP 1A2 and 2C9, such as warfarin.

Treatment of Special Populations

▶ Premenopausal Women

The NOF recommends measuring BMD in premenopausal women with specific risk factors for osteoporosis, such as those with a predisposing medical condition or medication, in whom treatment would be considered.[1] Premenopausal women at risk for osteoporosis should follow all nonpharmacologic recommendations for exercise and adequate calcium and vitamin D intake. Currently, no good data are available regarding pharmacologic therapy on fracture reduction in this population. Bisphosphonates should be used with caution in this population due to pregnancy risks and uncertain long-term effects.

▶ Glucocorticoid-Induced Osteoporosis

Glucocorticoids play a significant role in bone remodeling. Exogenous glucocorticoid administration results in an increase in bone resorption, inhibition of bone formation, and change in bone quality. Glucocorticoids (e.g., prednisone, hydrocortisone, methylprednisolone, and dexamethasone) promote bone resorption through reduced calcium absorption from the GI tract and increased renal calcium excretion. Bone formation is reduced through inhibition of osteoblasts. They also decrease estrogen and testosterone production.

Patients receiving long-term glucocorticoids are at increased risk of fracture. This risk is greater with higher doses and longer-term therapy. Most bone is lost during the initial 6 to 12 months of therapy, and bone mass continues to decline thereafter.[46] Due to the risk of bone loss and fractures, therapy is recommended for patients receiving long-term supraphysiologic doses of glucocorticoids.[47]

In addition to nonpharmacologic measures, the ACR has specific recommendations for preventing and treating patients receiving glucocorticoids.[47] Recommendations for optimal calcium and vitamin D intake are higher for patients receiving glucocorticoids. These recommendations include 1,200 to 1,500 mg daily of elemental calcium and 800 to 1,000 IU daily of vitamin D, or higher as needed to maintain adequate 25(OH)D levels, for all adults receiving glucocorticoids.

❼ *The ACR recommends bisphosphonate therapy with alendronate or risedronate for all patients who are starting treatment with glucocorticoids (prednisone 5 mg or more daily or equivalent) that will continue for 3 months or longer.* Therapy may also be started in other patients with lower doses or shorter duration of glucocorticoids based on risk factors for fracture. Zoledronic acid and teriparatide may also be considered for moderate- to high-risk patients. Although not FDA approved, denosumab has been studied in this population and may be considered an alternate therapy for patients nonresponsive to or intolerant of other therapies.[46]

Gastrointestinal Disease

Various GI disorders, including inflammatory bowel disease, celiac disease, and postgastrectomy states, are associated with osteoporosis due to impairment of calcium and vitamin D absorption, corticosteroid-induced bone changes, and chronic inflammatory states. Management of these patients includes stabilizing the underlying disorder, BMD measurement and screening every 1 to 2 years, and treatment in appropriate patients, including those at risk for glucocorticoid-induced osteoporosis.[48]

Transplantation Osteoporosis

Osteoporosis is an important health issue for post-transplantation patients. As survival continues to improve after transplantation, more patients are experiencing significant morbidity and mortality related to fragility fractures. These patients are at high risk for developing fractures due to pretransplantation risk factors for osteoporosis and rapid bone loss after transplantation. It is thought that significant decreases in BMD within 6 to 12 months after transplantation are due to high-dose glucocorticoids and the increase in bone resorption seen with calcineurin inhibitors such as cyclosporine.[49]

Prior to transplantation, BMD should be measured, and any secondary causes of osteoporosis should be identified and corrected. All patients should meet daily calcium and vitamin D requirements, with supplementation of vitamin D to maintain a 25(OH) D level above 30 ng/mL (75 nmol/L). Initiating therapy with a bisphosphonate before transplantation is thought to help counteract the immediate increase in bone resorption.[49]

Patient Encounter, Part 3: Development of a Treatment Plan

Considering all of the information presented, develop a treatment plan for this patient. Include the following information:

Recommendations for patient-specific drug therapy including dose and frequency.

Patient education about the chosen regimen.

Monitoring plan for efficacy and adverse effects.

Consideration of alternate therapies if the initial therapy fails or is intolerable.

OUTCOME EVALUATION

- Evaluate patients for progression of osteoporosis, including signs and symptoms of new fragility fracture (e.g., localized pain), loss of height, and physical deformity (e.g., kyphosis). Assess patients on an annual basis or more often if new symptoms present.
- Monitor for beneficial effects on bone density. The NOF recommends a follow-up DXA scan every 2 years to monitor the effects of therapy.

Patient Care and Monitoring

1. Assess patient risk factors for osteoporosis, with special attention to age, menopausal status, previous history of osteoporotic fracture, smoking status, low body weight, family history of osteoporotic fracture in first-degree relatives, and presence of secondary causes of osteoporosis.

2. Perform a thorough medication history, including prescription, over-the-counter, and alternative therapies. Pay special attention to any vitamins and calcium and vitamin D supplements the patient is taking.

3. Assess nonpharmacologic interventions for preventing osteoporotic fractures, including nutrition, weight-bearing and muscle-strengthening exercise regimens, and fall risk.

4. Determine average calcium intake from diet (Table 56–5) and supplements (Table 56–6). Compare with age-adjusted recommendations (Table 56–4). Evaluate the patient's sources of vitamin D. Recommend appropriate calcium and vitamin D supplementation.

5. Review bone densitometry (i.e., central DXA) for presence of low bone mass (i.e., T-score below −2.5 in the spine or hip). If T-score is between −1.0 and −2.5, use the FRAX risk calculator to estimate fracture risk.

6. Educate the patient about nonpharmacologic measures to prevent osteoporotic fractures.

7. If drug therapy is indicated, assess the patient for contraindications (e.g., esophageal disease or severe renal impairment for bisphosphonate therapy).

8. Educate the patient on the drug therapy selected, including drug name, dose, method of administration, common or serious adverse reactions, adherence and monitoring. Pay special attention to administration instructions and monitoring for adverse effects. Include a discussion about the therapeutic goals and expectations (e.g., changes in individual T-scores may not necessarily correlate with benefit in fracture risk reduction).

9. Develop a monitoring plan, including assessment of efficacy, adverse effects, nonpharmacologic measures to prevent fractures, and appropriate drug administration.

- Assess patients for adverse effects of therapy:
  - Oral bisphosphonates: Dyspepsia, esophageal reflux, esophageal pain, or burning
  - Injectable zoledronic acid: Influenza-type symptoms related to infusion, ONJ (rare)
  - Denosumab: Arthralgias, dermatologic reactions, and hypocalcemia
  - Teriparatide: Nausea, headache, leg cramps, hypercalcemia
  - Raloxifene: Hot flushes, signs or symptoms of thromboembolic disease (e.g., pain, redness, or swelling in one extremity, chest pain, and shortness of breath)
  - Calcitonin salmon: Nasal irritation or burning

Abbreviations Introduced in This Chapter

AACE	American Association of Clinical Endocrinologists
ACR	American College of Rheumatology
BMD	Bone mineral density
BMI	Body mass index
DXA	Dual-energy x-ray absorptiometry
HRT	Hormone replacement therapy
IOM	Institute of Medicine
NOF	National Osteoporosis Foundation
ONJ	Osteonecrosis of the jaw
PM	Postmenopausal
SERM	Selective estrogen receptor modulator
WHI	Women's Health Initiative

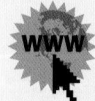 Self-assessment questions and answers are available at *http://mhpharmacotherapy.com/pp.html.*

REFERENCES

1. National Osteoporosis Foundation [Internet]. Clinician's Guide to Prevention and Treatment of Osteoporosis. Washington, DC, 2010 [cited 2011 Oct 10]. Available from: *www.nof.org.*
2. AACE Osteoporosis Task Force. American Association of Clinical Endocrinologists medical guidelines for clinical practice for the diagnosis and treatment of postmenopausal osteoporosis. Endocr Pract 2010;16(Suppl 3).
3. Raisz LG. Screening for osteoporosis. N Engl J Med 2005;353:164–171.
4. Khosla S. Update in male osteoporosis. J Clin Endocrinol Metab 2010;95:3–10.
5. NIH Consensus Development Panel on Osteoporosis Prevention, Diagnosis, and Therapy. Osteoporosis prevention, diagnosis, and therapy. JAMA 2001;285:785–795.
6. NAMS Position Statement. Management of osteoporosis in postmenopausal women: 2006 position statement of the North American Menopause Society. Menopause 2006;13:340–367.
7. Genant HK, Cooper C, Poor G, et al. Interim report and recommendations of the World Health Organization Task-Force for Osteoporosis. Osteoporosis Int 1999;10:259–264.
8. Baim S, Binkley N, Bilezikian JP, et al. Official positions of the International Society for Clinical Densitometry and Executive Summary of the 2007 ISCD Position Development Conference. J Clin Densitom 2008;11:75–91.
9. Institute of Medicine [Internet]. Dietary reference intakes for calcium and vitamin D [cited 2011 Sept 7]. Available from: *http://www.iom.edu/~/media/Files/Report%20Files/2010/Dietary-Reference-Intakes-for-Calcium-and-Vitamin-D/Vitamin%20D%20and%20Calcium%202010%20Report%20Brief.pdf.*
10. Rosen CJ. Postmenopausal osteoporosis. N Engl J Med 2005;353:595–503.
11. Trivedi DP, Doll R, Khaw KT. Effect of four monthly oral vitamin D3 (cholecalciferol) supplementation on fractures and mortality in men and women living in the community: Randomized double blind controlled trial. BMJ 2003;326:469.
12. Holick MF, Binkley NC, Bischoff-Ferrari HA, et al. Evaluation, treatment, and prevention of vitamin D deficiency: an Endocrine Society Clinical Practice Guideline. J Clin Endocrinol Metab 2011;96:1911–1930.
13. Liberman UA, Weiss SR, Broll J, et al. Effect of oral alendronate on bone mineral density and the incidence of fractures in postmenopausal osteoporosis. N Engl J Med 1995;333:1437–1443.
14. Brown JP, Kendler DL, McClung MR, et al. The efficacy and tolerability of risedronate once a week for the treatment of postmenopausal osteoporosis. Calcif Tissue Int 2002;71:103–111.
15. Chestnut CH, Skag A, Christiansen C, et al. Effects of oral ibandronate administered daily or intermittently on fracture risk in postmenopausal osteoporosis. J Bone Miner Res 2004;19:1241–1249.
16. Lyles KW, Colón-Emeric CS, Magaziner JS, et al. Zoledronic acid and clinical fractures and mortality after hip fracture. N Engl J Med 2007;357:1799–1809.
17. Boe HG, Hosking D, Devogelaer JP, et al. Ten years' experience with alendronate for osteoporosis in postmenopausal women. N Engl J Med 2004;350:1189–1199.
18. Mellström DD, Sörensen OH, Goemaere S, et al. Seven years of treatment with risedronate in women with postmenopausal osteoporosis. Calcif Tissue Int 2004;75:462–468.
19. Boe DM, Delmas PD, Eastell R, et al. Once-yearly zoledronic acid for treatment of postmenopausal osteoporosis. N Engl J Med 2007;356:1809–1822.
20. Lyes KW, Colón-Emeric CS, Magaziner JS, et al. Zoledronic acid and clinical fractures and mortality after hip fracture. N Engl J Med 2007;357:1799–1809.
21. Demas PD, Recker RR, Chesnut CH, et al. Daily and intermittent oral ibandronate normalize bone turnover and provide significant reduction in vertebral fracture risk: Results from the BONE study. Osteoporos Int 2004;14:792–798.
22. Enrud KE, Barrett-Connor EL, Schwartz A, et al. Randomized trial of effect of alendronate continuation versus discontinuation in women with low bone mineral density: Results from the Fracture Intervention Trial long-term extension. J Bone Miner Res 2004;19:1259–1269.
23. Ot SM. Long-term safety of bisphosphonates. J Clin Endocrinol Metab 2005;90:1897–1899.
24. Ruggiero SL, Mehrotra B, Rosenberg TJ, Engroff SL. Osteonecrosis of the jaws associated with the use of bisphosphonates: A review of 63 cases. J Oral Maxillofac Surg 2004;62:527–534.
25. Rizoli R, Akesson K, Bouxsein M, et al. Subtrochanteric fractures after long-term treatment with bisphosphonates: a European Society on Clinical and Economic Aspects of Osteoporosis and Osteoarthritis, and International Osteoporosis Foundation Working Group Report. Osteoporos Int 2011;22:373–390.
26. Ovina CV, Zerwekh JE, Rao DS, et al. Severely suppressed bone turnover: A potential complication of alendronate therapy. J Clin Endocrinol Metab 2005;90:1294–1301.
27. Par-Wyllie YL, Mamdani MM, Juurlink DN, et al. Bisphosphonate use and the risk of subtrochanteric or femoral shaft fractures in older women. JAMA 2011;305:783–789.
28. FDA [Internet]. FDA Drug Safety Communication: Ongoing safety review of oral bisphosphonates and atypical subtrochanteric femur

fractures [cited 2011 Sept 5]. Available from: *http://www.fda.gov/Drugs/ DrugSafety/PostmarketDrugSafetyInformationforPatientsandProviders/ ucm203891.htm.*

29. Cardwell CR, Abnet CC, Cantwell MM, Murray LJ. Exposure to oral bisphosphonates and risk of esophageal cancer. JAMA 2010;304: 657–663.

30. Green J, Czanner G, Reeves G, et al. Oral bisphosphonates and risk of cancer of oesophagus, stomach, and colorectum: case-control analysis within a UK primary care cohort. BMJ 2010;341:c4444.

31. Cummings SR, San Martin J, McClung MR, et al. Denosumab for prevention of fractures in postmenopausal women with osteoporosis. N Engl J Med 2009;361:756–765.

32. Kendler DL, Roux C, Benhamou CL, et al. Effects of denosumab on bone mineral density and bone turnover in postmenopausal women transitioning from alendronate therapy. J Bone Miner Res 2010;25: 72–81.

33. Brown JP, Prince RL, Deal C, et al. Comparison of the effect of denosumab and alendronate on BMD and biochemical markers of bone turnover in postmenopausal women with low bone mass: a randomized, blinded, phase 3 trial. J Bone Miner Res 2009;24:153–61.

34. Lewiecki EM. Treatment of osteoporosis with denosumab. Maturitas 2010;66:182–186.

35. Amgen [Internet]. Prolia (denosumab) Risk Evaluation and Mitigation Strategy [cited 2011 Sept 5]. Available from: *http://www.proliahcp.com/ risk-evaluation-mitigation-strategy/?WT.srch=1.*

36. Ner RM, Arnaud CD, Zanchetta JR, et al. Effect of parathyroid hormone (1–34) on fractures and bone mineral density in postmenopausal women with osteoporosis. N Engl J Med 2001;344:1434–1441.

37. Ettinger B, Black DM, Mitlak BH, et al. Reduction of vertebral fracture risk in postmenopausal women with osteoporosis treated with raloxifene: Results from a 3-year randomized clinical trial. JAMA 1999;282:637–645.

38. Barrett-Connor E, Mosca L, Collins P, et al., for the Raloxifene Use for the Heart (RUTH) Study Investigators. Effects of raloxifene on cardiovascular events and breast cancer in postmenopausal women. N Engl J Med 2006;355:125–137.

39. Chestnut CH, Silverman S, Andriano K, et al. A randomized trial of nasal spray salmon calcitonin in postmenopausal women with established osteoporosis: The prevent recurrence of osteoporotic fractures study. Am J Med 2000;109:267–276.

40. Rossouw JE, Anderson GL, Prentice RL, et al. Risks and benefits of estrogen plus progestin in healthy postmenopausal women: Principal results from the Women's Health Initiative randomized controlled trial. JAMA 2002;288:321–333.

41. Hulley S, Grady D, Bush T, et al. Randomized trial of estrogen plus progestin for secondary prevention of coronary heart disease in postmenopausal women. JAMA 1998;280:605–613.

42. Lecart MP, Bruyere OB, Reginster JY. Combination/sequential therapy in osteoporosis. Curr Osteoporos Rep 2004;2:123–130.

43. Rachner TD, Khosla S, Hofbauer LC. Osteoporosis: now and the future. Lancet 2011;377:1276–1287.

44. Eisman JA, Bone HG, Hosking DJ, et al. Odanacatib in the treatment of postmenopausal women with low bone mineral density: three-year continued therapy and resolution of effect. J Bone Miner Res 2011;26:242–251.

45. Alexandersen P, Toussaint A, Christiansen C, et al., for the Ipriflavone Multicenter European Fracture Study. Ipriflavone in the treatment of postmenopausal osteoporosis: A randomized controlled trial. JAMA 2001;285:1482–1488.

46. Weinstein RS. Glucocorticoid-induced bone disease. N Engl J Med 2011;365:62–70.

47. Grossman JM, Gordon R, Ranganath VK, et al. American College of Rheumatology 2010 recommendations for the prevention and treatment of glucocorticoid induced osteoporosis. Arthritis Care Res (Hoboken) 2010;62:1515–1526.

48. Katz S, Weinerman S. Osteoporosis and Gastrointestinal Disease. Gastroenterol Hepatol 2010;6:506–517.

49. Stein E, Ebeling P, Shane E. Post-transplantation osteoporosis. Endocrinol Metab Clin North Am 2007;36:937–963.

57 Rheumatoid Arthritis

Susan P. Bruce

LEARNING OBJECTIVES

● **Upon completion of the chapter, the reader will be able to:**

1. Identify risk factors for developing rheumatoid arthritis (RA).

2. Describe the pathophysiology of RA, with emphasis on the specific immunologic components.

3. Discuss the comorbidities associated with RA.

4. Recognize the typical clinical presentation of RA.

5. Create treatment goals for a patient with RA.

6. Compare the available pharmacotherapeutic options, selecting the most appropriate regimen for a given patient.

7. Propose a patient education plan that includes nonpharmacologic and pharmacologic treatment measures.

8. Formulate a monitoring plan to evaluate the safety and efficacy of a therapeutic regimen designed for an individual patient with RA.

KEY CONCEPTS

❶ Comorbidities with the greatest impact on morbidity and mortality associated with rheumatoid arthritis (RA) are: (a) cardiovascular disease, (b) infections, (c) malignancy, and (d) osteoporosis.

❷ The most clinically important features associated with poor long-term outcomes include: (a) functional limitation (defined by use of standard measurement scales such as the Health Assessment Questionnaire [HAQ] score), (b) extraarticular disease, (c) positive rheumatoid factor, (d) positive anticyclic citrullinated peptide (anti-CCP) antibodies, and/or (e) bony erosions by radiography.

❸ The goals of treatment for RA are to: (a) reduce or eliminate pain, (b) protect articular structures, (c) control systemic complications, (d) prevent loss of joint function, and (e) improve or maintain quality of life.

❹ It is imperative that the initiation of one or more disease-modifying antirheumatic drugs (DMARDs) occurs in all patients within the first 3 months of diagnosis to reduce joint erosion.

❺ Methotrexate is the nonbiologic DMARD of choice because of its documented efficacy and safety profile when monitored appropriately.

❻ The risk of infection in patients treated with biologic DMARDs must be considered when selecting and monitoring therapy.

❼ Women of childbearing potential and their partners must be counseled to: (a) use proper birth control while undergoing treatment for RA, and (b) involve healthcare providers in discussions regarding family planning to carefully consider all treatment options available.

❽ In addition to designing an individualized therapeutic regimen to control the progression of RA, the clinician must evaluate the presence of comorbidities and implement measures to control the increased risk.

INTRODUCTION

Rheumatoid arthritis (RA) is a complex systemic inflammatory condition manifesting initially as symmetric swollen and tender joints of the hands and/or feet. Some patients may experience mild **articular** (joint) disease, whereas others may present with aggressive disease and/or extraarticular manifestations. The systemic inflammation of RA leads to joint destruction, disability, and premature death. Juvenile idiopathic arthritis (JIA), formerly known as juvenile rheumatoid arthritis (JRA), is the most common form of arthritis in children.

EPIDEMIOLOGY AND ETIOLOGY

RA affects approximately 1% of the U.S. population and 1% to 2% of the world's population.[1,2] Patients with RA have a 50% increased risk of premature death and a decreased life expectancy of 3 to 10 years compared with individuals without RA.[3] The underlying causes of increased mortality in this population remain unclear. RA arises from an immunologic reaction, and there is speculation that it is in response to a genetic or infectious antigen. Risk factors associated with the development of RA include the following:

- Female gender (3:1 females to males)

- Increasing age (peak onset 35 to 50 years of age)

- Current tobacco smoking.[4] Tobacco users are more likely to have extraarticular manifestations and to experience treatment nonresponsiveness. This risk is reduced when a patient has remained tobacco-free for at least 10 years.

- Family history of RA. Genetic studies demonstrate a strong correlation between RA and the presence of major histocompatibility complex class II **human leukocyte antigens** (HLA), specifically HLA-DR1 and HLA-DR4.[5,6] HLA is a molecule associated with the presentation of antigens to T lymphocytes.

- Emerging evidence suggests that stress may influence RA onset and disease activity. It appears that individual major stressful life events do not play a significant role. Instead, chronic presence of minor stressors (daily hassles, work and relationship stress, financial pressures) may affect the immune response and RA disease activity.[9]

- The prevalence of JIA is approximately 1 in 1000 children.[10] There are no known risk factors for JIA.

PATHOPHYSIOLOGY

The characteristics of a **synovium** affected by RA are: (a) the presence of a thickened, inflamed membrane lining called **pannus**; (b) the development of new blood vessels; and (c) an influx of inflammatory cells in the synovial fluid, predominantly T lymphocytes. The pathogenesis of RA is driven by T lymphocytes, but the initial catalyst causing this response is unknown. Understanding specific components of the immune system and their involvement in the pathogenesis of RA will facilitate understanding of current and emerging treatment options for RA. The components of most significance are T lymphocytes, cytokines, and B lymphocytes.[5,11]

T Lymphocytes

The development and activation of T lymphocytes are important to maintain protection from infection without causing harm to the host.[11] Activation of mature T lymphocytes requires two signals. The first is the presentation of an antigen by antigen-presenting cells to the T-lymphocyte receptor. Second, a ligand-receptor complex (i.e., CD80/CD86) on antigen-presenting cells binds to CD28 receptors on T lymphocytes.

Once a cell successfully passes through all stages, the inflammatory cascade is activated.[12] Activation of T lymphocytes: (a) stimulates the release of macrophages or monocytes, which subsequently causes the release of inflammatory cytokines; (b) activates osteoclasts; (c) activates the release of matrix metalloproteinases or enzymes responsible for the degradation of connective tissue; and (d) stimulates B lymphocytes and the production of antibodies.[5,11]

Cytokines

Cytokines are proteins secreted by cells that serve as intercellular mediators (Table 57–1). An imbalance of proinflammatory and anti-inflammatory cytokines in the synovium leads to inflammation and joint destruction. The proinflammatory cytokines interleukin 1 (IL-1), tumor necrosis factor-α (TNF-α), IL-6, and IL-17 are found in high

---

Table 57–1

Cytokines Involved in the Pathogenesis of RA[5,7,11]

Cytokine	Source	Activity
Proinflammatory		
TNF-α	Macrophages, monocytes, B lymphocytes, T lymphocytes, fibroblasts	Induces IL-1, IL-6, IL-8, GM-CSF; stimulates fibroblasts to release adhesion molecules
IL-1	Macrophages, monocytes, endothelial cells, B lymphocytes, activated T lymphocytes	Stimulates fibroblasts and chondrocytes to release matrix metalloproteinases
IL-6	T lymphocytes, monocytes, macrophages, synovial fibroblasts	Activates T lymphocytes, induces acute-phase response, stimulates growth and differentiation of hematopoietic precursor cells; stimulates synovial fibroblasts
IL-17	T lymphocytes in synovium	Synergistic effect with IL-1 and TNF leading to increased production of proinflammatory cytokines
Anti-Inflammatory		
IL-4	CD4+ type 2 helper T lymphocytes	Inhibits activation of type 1 helper T lymphocytes, decreases production of IL-1, TNF-α, IL-6, IL-8
IL-10	Monocytes, macrophages, B lymphocytes, T lymphocytes	Inhibits production of IL-1, TNF-α, and proliferation of T lymphocytes

concentrations in synovial fluid. These proinflammatory cytokines cause the activation of other cytokines and adhesion molecules responsible for the recruitment of lymphocytes to the site of inflammation. Anti-inflammatory cytokines and mediators (IL-4, IL-10, and IL-1 receptor antagonist) are present in the synovium, although concentrations are not high enough to overcome the effects of the proinflammatory cytokines.[5,11]

B Lymphocytes

In addition to serving as antigen-presenting cells to T lymphocytes, B lymphocytes may produce proinflammatory cytokines and antibodies.[6,11] Antibodies of significance in RA are **rheumatoid factors** (antibodies reactive with the Fc region of IgG) and antibodies against **cyclic citrullinated peptide** (CCP).[6] Rheumatoid factors are not present in all patients with RA, but their presence is indicative of disease severity, likelihood of extraarticular manifestations, and increased mortality.[12] CCPs are produced early in the course of disease. High levels of anti-CCP antibodies are indicative of aggressive disease and a greater likelihood of poor outcomes. Monitoring anti-CCP antibodies may be useful to predict the severity of disease and match aggressive treatment appropriately.

Comorbidities Associated with RA

RA reduces a patient's average life expectancy, but RA alone rarely causes death. Instead, specific **comorbidities** contribute to premature death independent of safety issues surrounding the use of immunomodulating medications. ❶ *The comorbidities with the greatest impact on morbidity and mortality associated with RA are: (a) cardiovascular disease, (b) infections, (c) malignancy, and (d) osteoporosis.*

▶ *Cardiovascular Disease*

Half of all deaths in RA patients are cardiovascular related.[13] Because a patient with RA experiences inflammation and swelling in his or her joints, it is likely that there is inflammation elsewhere, such as in the blood vessels, termed **vasculitis**. C-reactive protein (CRP), a nonspecific marker of inflammation, is associated with an increased risk of cardiovascular disease; CRP is elevated in patients with RA. Traditional cardiovascular risk factors alone cannot explain the increased cardiovascular mortality in patients with RA. Increasing evidence suggests that the presence of RA is a cardiovascular risk similar to diabetes. Aggressive management of systemic inflammation and traditional cardiovascular risk factors (e.g., blood pressure, cholesterol, tobacco use) may reduce cardiovascular mortality in this population.[14]

▶ *Infections*

RA itself leads to changes in cellular immunity and causes a disproportionate increase in pulmonary infection and sepsis.[15] Because medications that alter the immune system are linked to an increased risk of infection, it is difficult to distinguish between an increased risk of infection secondary to RA and the medications used to treat RA. Patients and clinicians must pay close attention to signs and symptoms of infection because of this increased risk.[15]

▶ *Malignancy*

Patients with RA have an increased risk of developing **lymphoproliferative** malignancy (e.g., lymphoma, leukemia, and multiple myeloma) and lung cancer but a decreased risk of developing cancer of the digestive tract.[15,16] The relationship between RA and cancer is not clear. To confound the issue, medications for treating RA are undergoing review to determine whether use independently increases cancer risk. Current evidence suggests that the underlying disease process is responsible for the increased cancer risk and not the use of medications.[16] Patients presenting with new onset of symptoms (e.g., fevers, night sweats, chills, or anorexia) out of proportion with disease activity and patients not responding to conventional RA treatment should be evaluated further for lymphoproliferative malignancy.[15,17]

▶ *Osteoporosis*

Osteoporosis associated with RA follows a multifaceted pathogenesis, but the primary mechanism likely is mediated by increased **osteoclast** activity.[15] The cytokines involved in the inflammatory process directly stimulate osteoclast and inhibit **osteoblast** activity. Additionally, arthritis medications can lead to increased bone loss. Bone mineral density should be evaluated at baseline and routinely using dual-energy x-ray absorptiometry.[15]

CLINICAL PRESENTATION AND DIAGNOSIS

See the accompanying text box for the clinical presentation of RA.

Diagnosis

Both osteoarthritis and RA are prevalent in the American population, but they differ significantly in presentation (Table 57–2). Because management of the two conditions differs significantly, early evaluation and diagnosis are essential to maximize an individual patient's care.

In 2010, The American College of Rheumatology (ACR) and European League Against Rheumatism (EULAR) released new classification criteria for RA (Table 57–3).[1] The goal was to identify a subset of patients with undifferentiated synovitis who were at high risk for chronic and erosive disease. The new criteria are intended to help identify patients earlier in the course of disease. This will allow researchers to determine whether earlier introduction of medications alters

Clinical Presentation of RA

General

- About 60% of patients develop symptoms gradually over several weeks to months.
- Patients may present with systemic findings, joint findings, or both.

Symptoms

- Nonspecific systemic symptoms may include fatigue, weakness, anorexia, and diffuse musculoskeletal pain.
- Patients complain of pain in involved joints and prolonged morning joint stiffness.

Signs

- The metacarpophalangeal (MCP), proximal interphalangeal (PIP), metatarsophalangeal (MTP), and wrist joints are involved frequently.
- Joint involvement is usually symmetric.
- There is often limited joint function.
- Signs of joint inflammation are present (tenderness, warmth, swelling, and erythema).
- Low-grade fever may be present.
- Extraarticular manifestations:
  - *Skin:* Subcutaneous nodules
  - *Ocular:* Keratoconjunctivitis sicca, scleritis

- *Pulmonary:* Interstitial fibrosis, pulmonary nodules, pleuritis, pleural effusions
- *Vasculitis:* Ischemic ulcers, skin lesions, leukocytoclastic vasculitis
- *Neurologic:* Peripheral neuropathy, Felty's syndrome
- *Hematologic:* Anemia, thrombocytosis

Laboratory Tests

- Positive rheumatoid factor (the test is negative in up to 30% of patients)
- Elevated ESR (Westergren ESR: greater than 20 mm/h in men; greater than 30 mm/h in women)
- Elevated C-reactive protein (CRP) (greater than 0.7 mg/dL or 7 mg/L)
- Complete blood count: Slight elevation in WBC count with a normal differential; slight anemia; thrombocytosis
- Positive anti-CCP antibodies

Other Diagnostic Tests

- *Synovial fluid analysis:* Straw colored, slightly cloudy, WBC 5 to 25 × 10³/mm³ (5 to 25 × 10⁹/L), no bacterial growth if cultured
- *Joint x-rays:* To establish baseline and evaluate joint damage
- *MRI:* May detect erosions earlier in the course of disease than x-rays but is not required for diagnosis

---

Table 57–2

Comparison of RA and Osteoarthritis

Characteristic	RA	Osteoarthritis
Speed of onset	Rapid (weeks–months)	Slow (years)
Gender prevalence (women: men)	3:1	1:1
Usual age of onset	Juvenile or adult (35–50 years)	Greater than 50 years
Most common joints affected	Small joints of hands (MCPs, PIPs), feet	Hands (DIPs), large weight-bearing joints (hips, knees)
Joint symptoms	Pain, swelling, warmth, stiffness	Pain, bony enlargement
Presence of inflammation	Local and systemic	None or mild, local
Duration of morning joint stiffness	Usually 60 minutes or longer	Usually less than 30 minutes
Joint pattern	Symmetric	Symmetric or asymmetric
ESR	Elevated	Normal
Synovial fluid	Leukocytosis, slightly cloudy	Mild leukocytosis
Systemic manifestations	Yes	No

DIPs, distal interphalangeal joints; ESR, erythrocyte sedimentation rate; MCPs, metacarpophalangeal joints; PIPs, proximal interphalangeal joints.

---

the disease process. The criteria were developed as a tool for research purposes, but the authors acknowledge that they are also helpful to guide clinical diagnosis. Patients with at least one joint with definite clinical synovitis that is not explained by another disease should be tested for RA.

Several clinical features of RA are associated with a worse long-term prognosis. The presence of these poor prognostic features should be considered at the time initial treatment decisions are made; more aggressive treatment may be warranted if these features are present. ❷ *The most clinically important features associated with poor long-term outcomes include: (a) functional limitation (defined by use of standard measurement scales such as the Health Assessment Questionnaire [HAQ] score), (b) extraarticular disease, (c) positive rheumatoid factor, (d) positive anti-CCP antibodies, and/or (e) bony erosions by radiography.*

▶ Diagnosis of Juvenile Idiopathic Arthritis

Diagnostic criteria for JIA include: (a) age less than 16 years at disease onset, (b) arthritis in one or more joints for more than 6 weeks, (c) exclusion of other types of arthritis. JIA can be divided into three main types:

Table 57–3

ACR/EULAR 2010 Classification Criteria for Rheumatoid Arthritis[1]

Criteria	Score
Joint involvement	
1 large joint (hips, knees, ankles, elbows, shoulders)	0
2–10 large joints	1
1–3 small joints (MCPS, PIPs, MTPs, wrists)	2
4–10 small joints	3
More than 10 joints (at least 1 small joint)	5
Serology (need at least 1 result for classification)	
Negative RF and negative anti-CCP	0
Low positive RF or low-positive anti-CCP	2
High-positive RF or high-positive anti-CCP	3
Acute-phase reactants (need at least 1 result for classification)	
Normal CRP and normal ESR	0
Abnormal CRP or abnormal ESR	1
Duration of symptoms	
Less than 6 weeks	0
More than 6 weeks	1
TOTAL:	6 or greater indicates definite RA

ACR, American College of Rheumatology; anti-CCP, anti-cyclic citrullinated peptide; CRP, C-reactive protein; ESR, erythrocyte sedimentation rate; EULAR, European League Against Rheumatism; MCPs, metacarpophalangeal joints; MTPs, metatarsophalangeal joints; PIPs, proximal interphalangeal joints; RA, rheumatoid arthritis; RF, rheumatoid factor.

Patient Encounter, Part 1

RT is a 38-year-old white woman who presents to the neighborhood free medical clinic with a 4-month history of progressive stiffness and pain in her hands. She is a waitress at the local diner and has no medical or prescription insurance. She delayed seeking medical treatment for fear of the expenses she would incur. For the last 2 months, she has been taking acetaminophen for the pain but admits that it is no longer working and she needs something stronger so she can perform her job responsibilities. RT is a single mother of three children aged 6, 8, and 9. She lives in an apartment, but she is at risk of being evicted for late rent payments. She is missing work more often lately due to morning stiffness, joint pain, and general fatigue.

What risk factors does she have for RA?

What additional information do you need before creating a treatment plan for this patient?

What other variables in this scenario may inhibit optimal patient care?

1. *Systemic (approximately 10% of cases):* Occurs equally in girls and boys. There are characteristic fever spikes twice daily (greater than 38.3°C or 101°F) and the presence of a pale, pink, transient rash. The peak onset is between ages 1 and 6 years.

2. *Polyarticular (approximately 40% of cases):* More likely to affect girls than boys (3:1). Arthritis is present in five or more joints. The disorder resembles adult RA more than the other types of JIA.

3. *Pauciarticular (approximately 50% of cases):* More likely to affect girls than boys (5:1). Uveitis is more likely to be present. Arthritis is present in four or fewer joints. Categories are further divided into early onset and late onset. Early onset is more likely to occur in girls, whereas late onset is more common in boys.[18]

TREATMENT

Desired Outcomes

❸ *The goals of treatment in RA are to: (a) reduce or eliminate pain, (b) protect articular structures, (c) control systemic complications, (d) prevent loss of joint function, and (e) improve or maintain quality of life.*[8] The goals for JIA are the same, with the added goals of maintaining normal growth, development, and activity level.[19] It is a common misconception that patients with JIA grow out of the disease. Many children with JIA become adults with JIA. Knowing this, it is essential that early, aggressive treatment is initiated to achieve the goals of therapy.

General Approach to Treatment

The clinician must evaluate patient-specific factors and select appropriate treatment to maximize the care of an individual patient. Joint damage accumulates over time; therefore, early diagnosis and early aggressive treatment are necessary to reduce disease progression and prevent joint damage. Aggressive treatment is defined as one or more disease-modifying antirheumatic drugs (DMARDs) at effective doses. Delaying treatment will result in more destructive disease that is very difficult to delay or reverse to preserve joint function.

❹ *It is imperative that the initiation of one or more DMARDs occurs in all patients within the first 3 months of diagnosis to reduce joint erosion.* Depending on disease severity and whether poor prognostic features are present, combination therapy may be initiated at the time of diagnosis or after an adequate trial of a DMARD initiated as monotherapy. If a patient has more aggressive disease, a more aggressive treatment plan may be warranted. The following medication classes are prescribed commonly for the treatment of RA: (a) nonsteroidal anti-inflammatory drugs (NSAIDs), (b) glucocorticoids, (c) nonbiologic DMARDs, and (d) biologic DMARDs. Table 57–4 highlights dosing, safety, monitoring, and patient counseling information for the common nonbiologic and biologic DMARDs.

Table 57–4

FDA-Approved Nonbiologic and Biologic DMARDs for Treatment of RA

Drug	Dose^a	Route	Time to Effect (weeks)	ADRs	Dosing in Hepatic Impairment	Dosing in Renal Impairment	Monitoring	Counseling Points
Methotrexate	Adults: 7.5–20 mg once weekly Polyarticular-course JIA: Recommended starting dose: 10 mg/m² once weekly; usual max dose: 20 mg/m² once weekly	Oral or IM	4–8	N, D, hepatotoxicity, alopecia, new-onset cough or SOB, MYL	CI	CrCl (mL/min)^b: 61–80: 75% of dose 51–60: 70% of dose 10–50: 50% of dose Less than 10: Avoid use	CBC, creatinine, LFTs every 4–8 weeks; monitor for signs of infection	Use of folic acid concomitantly Avoid alcohol Use contraception if childbearing potential
Hydroxy-chloroquine	Adults: 200 mg twice daily	Oral	8–24	N, D, HA, vision changes, skin pigmentation	Use with caution	No change	Eye exam every 12 months	Sunscreen use
Sulfasalazine	Adults: 1,000 mg 2–3 × daily Polyarticular-course JIA: Initial: 10 mg/kg/day; increase weekly by 10 mg/kg/day; usual dose: 30–50 mg/kg/day in 2 divided doses; max 2 g/day	Oral	8–12	N, D, rash, yellow-orange discoloration, photosensitivity, MYL	Avoid use	CrCl (mL/min)^b: 10–30: Give twice daily; Less than 10: Give once daily	CBC every 2–4 weeks for 3 months, then every 3 months	
Leflunomide (Arava)	Adults: 100 mg daily for 3 days; then 20 mg daily	Oral	4–12	Hepatotoxicity, D, N, HTN, rash, HA, abdominal pain	Avoid use	Guidelines not available	CBC, creatinine, LFTs every months for 6 months; then every 4–8 weeks Monitor for signs of infection	Avoid alcohol Use contraception if childbearing potential
Etanercept (Enbrel)	Adults: 25 mg twice weekly or 50 mg once weekly Children ages 2–17: 0.8 mg/kg once weekly; max 50 mg/week	SC injection	1–4	ISR	No change	No change	Monitor for infection	ISR—topical corticosteroids, antipruritics, analgesics, rotate injection sites Screen for tuberculosis
Infliximab^b (Remicade)	Adults: 3–10 mg/kg at 0, 2, and 6 weeks; then every 8 weeks	IV infusion	1–4	IR (rash, urticaria, flushing, HA, fever, chills, nausea, tachycardia, dyspnea)	No change	No change	Monitor for infection	Screen for tuberculosis
Adalimumab (Humira)	Adults: 40 mg every other week Children older than 4 years and weighing 15–29 kg: 20 mg every other week Children weighing 30 kg or more: 40 mg every other week	SC injection	1–4	ISR	No change	No change	Monitor for infection	Screen for tuberculosis

Drug	Dose	Administration		Adverse effects	Hepatic	Renal	Monitoring	TB screening
Golimumab (Simponi)	Adults: 50 mg once monthly; Children: Safety and efficacy has not been established	SC injection	1–4	ISR	No change	No change	Monitor for infection	Screen for tuberculosis
Certolizumab (Cimzia)	Adults: 400 mg initially, at 2 weeks, 4 weeks, then every 4 weeks thereafter; Children: Safety and efficacy has not been established	SC injection	1–4	ISR	No change	No change	Monitor for infection	Screen for tuberculosis
Anakinra (Kineret)	Adults: 100 mg daily	SC injection	2–4	HA, N, V, D, ISR	No data available	CrCl less than 30 mL/min[b]: consider 100 mg every other day	Monitor for infection	
Abatacept (Orencia)	Adults less than 60 kg, 500 mg; 60–100 kg, 750 mg; Adults greater than 100 kg, 1,000 mg IV on days 1, 15 and every 28 days thereafter. SC Injection: Weight-based loading dose, then 125 mg SC within 1 day, 125 mg SC once weekly; or 125 mg once weekly in patients unable to receive IV. JIA (older than 6 years of age): less than 75 kg: 10 mg/kg; 75–100 kg: 750 mg; greater than 100 kg: 1,000 mg IV on days 1, 15, 28 and every 28 days thereafter	IV infusion, SC injection	2	HA, infection, IR	No change	No change	Monitor for infection	
Rituximab (Rituxan)	Adults: Two 1,000-mg infusions separated by 2 weeks	IV infusion	4	IR	No change	No change	Monitor for infection	
Tocilizumab (Actemra)	Adults: 8 mg/kg every 4 weeks; JIA (2 years and older): less than 30 kg: 12 mg/kg every 2 weeks; greater than 30 kg: 8 mg/kg every 2 weeks	IV infusion		Elevated LFTs, total cholesterol, triglycerides, and high-density lipoprotein; nasopharyngitis, infection	No data available	No data available	Monitor for infection; LFTs	

CI, contraindicated; D, diarrhea; HA, headache; HTN, hypertension; IR, infusion reactions; ISR, injection-site reactions; LFTs, liver function tests; MYL, myelosuppression (watch for fever, symptoms of infection, easy bruisability, and bleeding); N, nausea; SOB, shortness of breath.

[a]Geriatric patients should receive the usual adult dose unless renal or hepatic impairment is present. Pediatric doses are provided for drugs that have FDA-approved indications for juvenile idiopathic arthritis (JIA).

[b]To convert to SI units of mL/s, multiply by 0.0167.

From Refs. 1, 2, 8, and 20–22.

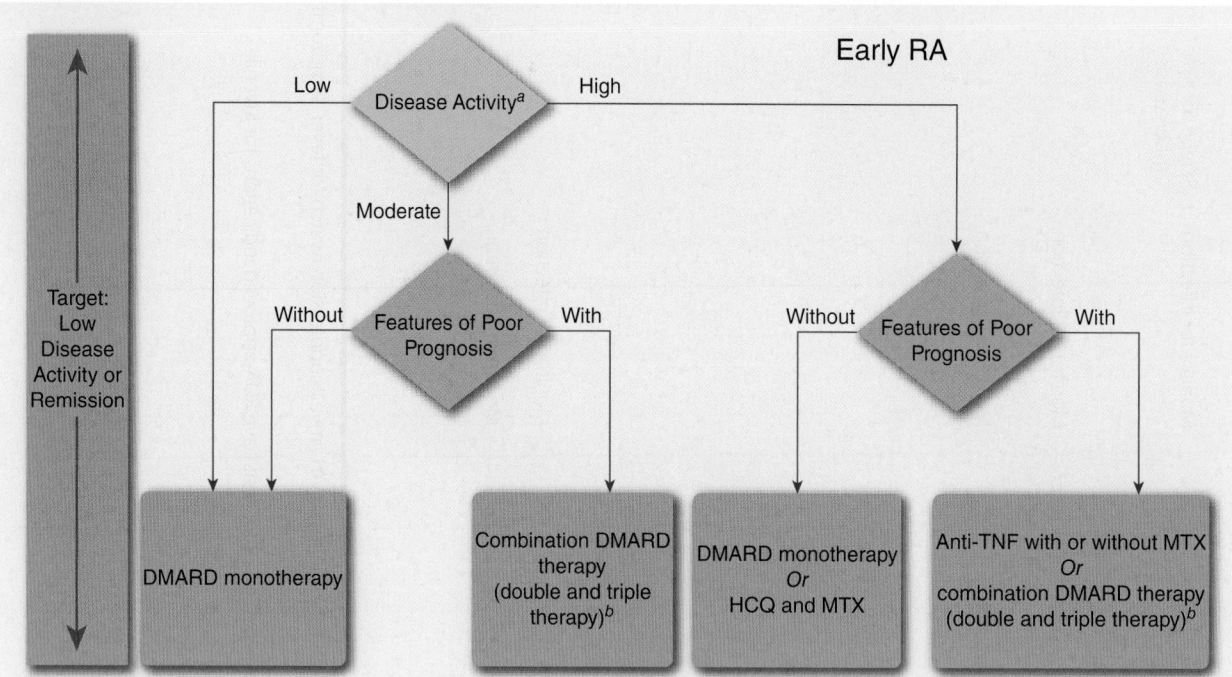

FIGURE 57–1. Recommendations for the treatment of early RA (disease duration less than 6 months). [a]See Ref. 20 for definitions of disease activity. [b]Combination DMARD therapy: methotrexate + leflunomide, methotrexate + hydroxychloroquine, methotrexate + sulfasalazine, sulfasalazine + hydroxychloroquine. Triple DMARD therapy: methotrexate + hydroxychloroquine + sulfasalazine. (Reproduced, with permission, from Singh JA, Furst DE, Bharat A, et al. 2012 Update of the 2008 American College of Rheumatology recommendations for the use of disease-modifying antirheumatic drugs and biologic agents in the treatment of rheumatoid arthritis. Arthritis Care Res 2012;64:625–639.)

Figures 57–1 and 57–2 outline the course of treatment according to the ACR 2012 Recommendations.[20] The recommendations are based on the activity level of the patient's disease, the presence or absence of poor prognostic features, and the duration of disease activity (early vs. established). Figure 57–1 applies to patients who have had RA for less than 6 months. Patients who have early RA with low disease activity may be treated with nonbiologic DMARD monotherapy (hydroxychloroquine, minocycline, leflunomide, methotrexate, or sulfasalazine). Patients with moderate or high disease activity but without poor prognostic features may receive initial treatment with DMARD monotherapy or the combination of methotrexate and hydroxychloroquine. Patients with moderate or high disease activity and evidence of poor prognostic features may receive combination therapy with methotrexate/hydroxychloroquine, methotrexate/sulfasalazine, or methotrexate/sulfasalazine/hydroxychloroquine. Alternatively, patients with high disease activity and features of poor prognosis may be started on anti-TNF therapy with or without methotrexate.

Figure 57–2 outlines the course of treatment for patients with established RA (disease duration 6 months or longer). Biologic DMARDs are usually considered in patients with established RA following inadequate response to nonbiologic or biologic DMARDs. Figure 57–2 establishes a progression of how to switch from one biologic agent to another in a patient

who experiences an inadequate response or adverse event. Because of treatment expense, biologic DMARDs should be considered only in patients who have no limitations due to cost or insurance coverage. There is no evidence that the benefits of combination therapy with biologic DMARDs outweigh the potential risks, especially the increased risk of infections.

Nonpharmacologic Therapy

All patients should receive education about the nonpharmacologic and pharmacologic measures to help manage RA and JIA. Empowered patients take an active role in care by participating in therapy-related decisions. Certain forms of nonpharmacologic therapy benefit all levels of severity, whereas others (i.e., surgery) are reserved for severe cases only.

Occupational and physical therapy may help patients preserve joint function, extend joint range of motion, and strengthen joints and muscles through strengthening exercises. Patients with joint deformities may benefit from the use of mobility or assistive devices that help to minimize disability and allow continued activities of daily living. When appropriate, patients should also be counseled about stress management (i.e., cognitive behavioral therapy, emotional disclosure, tai chi). In situations where the disease has progressed to a severe form with extensive joint erosions, surgery to replace or reconstruct the joint may be necessary.

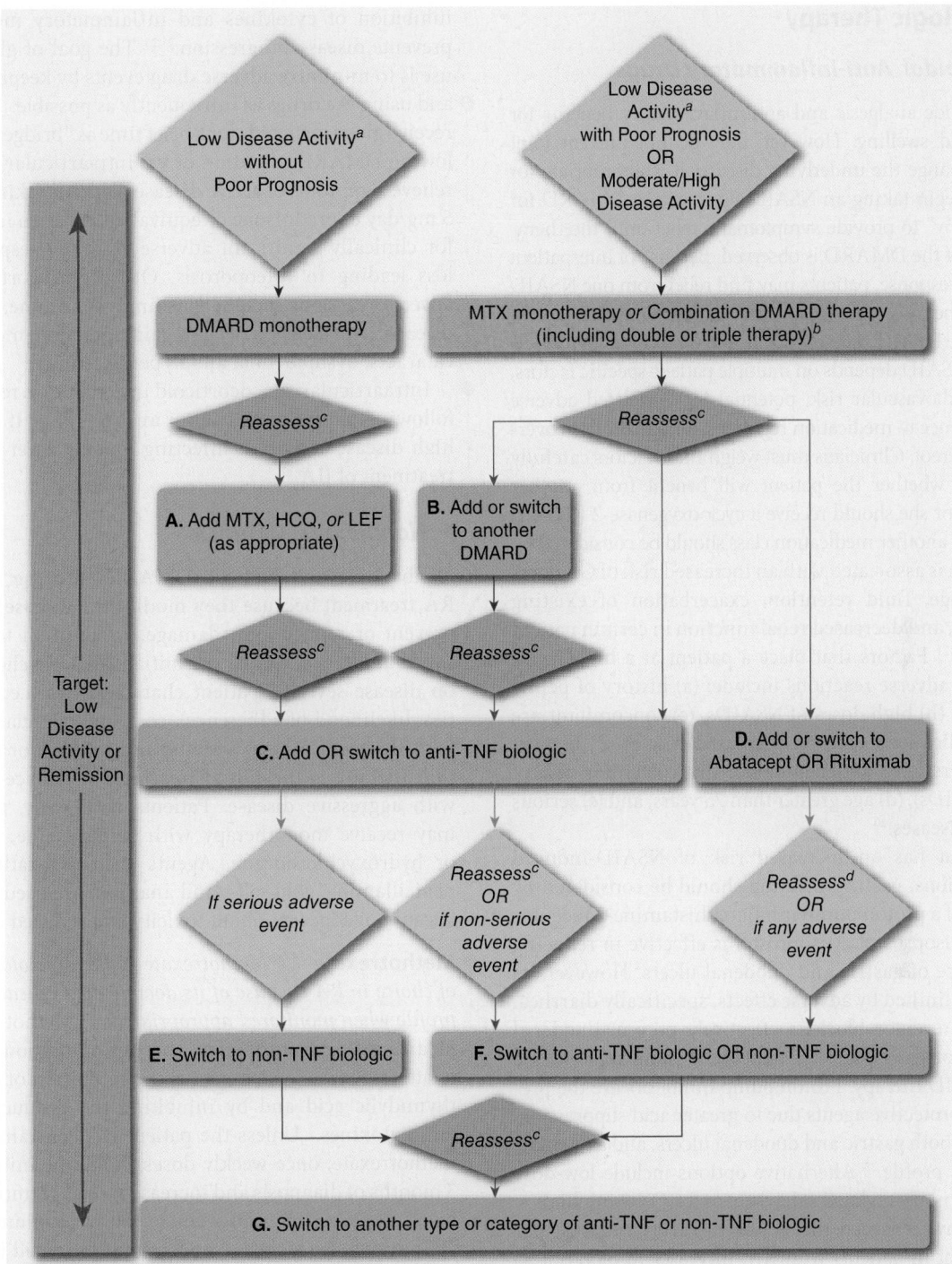

FIGURE 57–2. Recommendations for the treatment of established RA (disease duration 6 month or longer). [a]See Ref. 20 for definitions of disease activity. [b]Combination DMARD therapy: methotrexate + leflunomide, methotrexate + hydroxychloroquine, methotrexate + sulfasalazine, sulfasalazine + hydroxychloroquine. Triple DMARD therapy: methotrexate + hydroxychloroquine + sulfasalazine. [c]Reassess after 3 months of adequate therapy. [d]Reassess after 6 months of adequate therapy. (Reproduced, with permission, from Singh JA, Furst DE, Bharat A, et al. 2012 Update of the 2008 American College of Rheumatology recommendations for the use of disease-modifying antirheumatic drugs and biologic agents in the treatment of rheumatoid arthritis. Arthritis Care Res 2012;64:625–639.)

Pharmacologic Therapy

▶ *Nonsteroidal Anti-Inflammatory Drugs*

NSAIDs provide analgesic and anti-inflammatory benefits for joint pain and swelling. However, they do not prevent joint damage or change the underlying disease. It is appropriate for a patient to begin taking an NSAID along with a DMARD for "bridge therapy" to provide symptomatic relief until the therapeutic effect of the DMARD is observed. Because of interpatient variability in response, patients may find relief from one NSAID and not another. For this reason, if a patient does not receive relief from one NSAID, it is acceptable to try a second one. Selecting another NSAID depends on multiple patient-specific factors, including cardiovascular risk, potential for GI-related adverse events, adherence to medication regimens, and insurance coverage or lack thereof. Clinicians must weigh these factors carefully to determine whether the patient will benefit from another NSAID, if he or she should receive a cyclooxygenase-2 (COX-2) inhibitor, or if another medication class should be considered.

NSAID use is associated with an increased risk of GI ulcers or hemorrhage, fluid retention, exacerbation of existing hypertension, and decreased renal function in certain patient populations.[8,21] Factors that place a patient at a higher risk of GI-related adverse reactions include: (a) history of peptic ulcer disease, (b) high doses of NSAIDs, (c) concomitant use of other medications with an increased risk of GI hemorrhage or ulcers (e.g., anticoagulants, corticosteroids, use of multiple NSAIDs), (d) age greater than 75 years, and (e) serious underlying diseases.[20]

If a patient has an increased risk of NSAID-induced adverse reactions, gastroprotection should be considered by coinitiation of a proton pump inhibitor, histamine-2 receptor blocker, or misoprostol. Misoprostol is effective in reducing the occurrence of gastric and duodenal ulcers. However, its tolerability is limited by adverse effects, specifically diarrhea. Histamine-2 receptor blockers effectively prevent duodenal ulcers (but not gastric ulcers) that occur more readily as a result of NSAID therapy. Proton pump inhibitors are the preferred gastroprotective agents due to greater acid suppression, prevention of both gastric and duodenal ulcers, and a tolerable adverse-effect profile.[22] Alternative options include low-dose prednisone, a nonacetylated salicylate, or a COX-2 inhibitor.

NSAIDs may accentuate the increased risk of cardiovascular events inherent in patients with RA. Increases in blood pressure and fluid retention may exacerbate existing cardiovascular disease. With the evidence associating COX-2 inhibitors with cardiovascular disease, clinicians must carefully evaluate the potential risks of NSAID therapy against the potential benefits.[2] See Chap. 58 for additional discussion of NSAID therapy.

NSAID monotherapy is recommended as initial treatment in children with JIA with low disease activity affecting four or fewer joints. As in adults, adverse effects of NSAID therapy should be anticipated and treated accordingly in pediatrics.[10]

▶ *Glucocorticoids*

Low-dose glucocorticoid treatment (equivalent to prednisone 10 mg/day or less) effectively reduces inflammation through inhibition of cytokines and inflammatory mediators and prevents disease progression.[21,23] The goal of glucocorticoid use is to minimize adverse drug events by keeping doses low and using the drugs as infrequently as possible. Patients may receive glucocorticoids for a brief time as "bridge therapy" following DMARD initiation or via intraarticular injections to relieve symptoms of active disease. Patients taking more than 5 mg/day of prednisone or equivalent are at an increased risk for clinically significant adverse reactions, especially bone loss leading to osteoporosis. Other glucocorticoid-related adverse reactions include Cushing's syndrome, peptic ulcer disease, hypertension, weight gain, infection, mood changes, cataracts, dyslipidemia, and hyperglycemia.[2,23]

Intraarticular glucocorticoid injections are recommended following an adequate trial of an NSAID or if moderate or high disease activity is affecting four or fewer joints in the treatment of JIA.[10]

▶ *Nonbiologic DMARDs*

Nonbiologic and biologic DMARDs are the mainstay of RA treatment because they modify the disease process and prevent or reduce joint damage. In addition to relying on safety and efficacy data, the initial DMARD choice depends on disease severity, patient characteristics (i.e., comorbidities, likelihood of adherence), cost, and clinician experience with the medication.[8,20] Methotrexate alone or in combination therapy is the initial treatment of choice for patients with aggressive disease. Patients with early, mild disease may receive monotherapy with sulfasalazine, leflunomide or hydroxychloroquine. Agents such as azathioprine, D-penicillamine, gold salts, and anakinra are used rarely today because of concerns about toxicity and reduced efficacy.[1,20,21]

Methotrexate ⑤ *Methotrexate is the nonbiologic DMARD of choice in RA because of its documented efficacy and safety profile when monitored appropriately.*[1,25] Methotrexate exerts its anti-inflammatory effect through inhibition of dihydrofolate reductase, which causes the inhibition of purines and thymidylic acid and by inhibiting the production of certain cytokines.[2] Unless the patient has contraindications to methotrexate, once-weekly doses should be initiated within 3 months of diagnosis and increased steadily until the patient has symptomatic improvement or a maximum dose of 20 mg/week is reached. Concomitant folic acid is given routinely to reduce the risk of folate-depleting reactions induced by methotrexate therapy (e.g., stomatitis, diarrhea, nausea, alopecia, myelosuppression, and elevations in liver function tests).[1,25]

Serious adverse reactions include pulmonary fibrosis and hepatotoxicity. Patients should be counseled to avoid the use of alcohol, take folic acid as directed, adhere to the laboratory monitoring schedule, and immediately report symptoms of pulmonary fibrosis (e.g., cough or dyspnea) and hepatotoxicity (e.g., jaundice or abdominal pain). If monotherapy does not produce complete resolution of symptoms, methotrexate may be used in combination with other nonbiologic or biologic DMARDs. In situations in which the clinician suspects RA but a diagnosis has not yet been made, initiation of methotrexate was found to delay the diagnosis and halt joint damage without untoward adverse effects.[26]

Methotrexate is recommended as initial treatment for JIA in patients with high disease activity.[10] The usual dose is 5 to 15 mg/m² (based on body surface area) once weekly. There are insufficient published data to assess the risk of serious toxicity in children receiving doses greater than 20 mg/m²/wk. Patients will begin to notice a response in 3 to 4 weeks, with maximal response in 3 to 6 months. Methotrexate therapy in pediatric patients should be monitored the same way that is recommended in adults.[27]

Hydroxychloroquine and Sulfasalazine The exact mechanism of action of these drugs is unknown, but both agents are fairly well tolerated. Hydroxychloroquine or sulfasalazine may be initiated on diagnosis of low disease activity. Because of their slow onset of action, each drug must be given at therapeutic doses for at least 6 months before it can be deemed a treatment failure. Hydroxychloroquine and sulfasalazine are relatively inexpensive compared with the new biologic agents. If patients do not respond to methotrexate monotherapy, adding one of these agents may provide the benefit necessary to reduce symptoms satisfactorily.[2,20]

Hydroxychloroquine may cause retinal toxicity, and patients must have their eyes examined at least annually to detect this abnormality. It is not associated with renal, hepatic, or bone marrow suppression and therefore may be an acceptable treatment option for patients with contraindications to other DMARDs because of their toxicities.

Starting sulfasalazine at low doses and titrating slowly will minimize the nausea and abdominal discomfort caused by the drug. Patients receiving sulfasalazine must undergo routine blood work to monitor for leukopenia.[20] Patients with a sulfa allergy should not receive sulfasalazine.

In patients with JIA, sulfasalazine is recommended only for patients with the enthesitis-related category. Enthesitis-related arthritis is a less common form of JIA that affects boys more than girls and is characterized by lower extremity joint involvement, including heel pain and enthesitis. The dose of sulfasalazine for children older than 6 years is 30 to 50 mg/kg/day in two divided doses. Hydroxychloroquine is not recommended in patients with active arthritis associated with JIA.[10]

Leflunomide Leflunomide inhibits dihydroorotate dehydrogenase, an enzyme within the mitochondria that supplies T lymphocytes with the necessary components to respond to cytokine stimulation.[28] Thus leflunomide inhibits the T-lymphocyte response to various stimuli and halts the cell cycle. Its efficacy is similar to that of moderate doses of methotrexate or sulfasalazine.[21]Because of its extended half-life, leflunomide therapy begins with a loading dose followed by a maintenance dose. Patients with preexisting hepatic disease or a history of heavy alcohol ingestion should not receive leflunomide.[28] Leflunomide may be used in combination with methotrexate, but the added efficacy comes with a dramatic rise in the risk of hepatotoxicity. Liver function tests must be followed closely to prevent or minimize liver damage.[20] If therapy requires abrupt discontinuation (e.g.,

due to toxicity or pregnancy), administering cholestyramine will accelerate removal of leflunomide from the body.

Leflunomide is recommended as an alternative to methotrexate in patients with JIA experiencing high disease activity in five or more joints. However, leflunomide does not have an FDA-approved indication for this use.[20]

▶ *Biologic DMARDs*

Biologic DMARDs are indicated in patients who have failed an adequate trial of nonbiologic DMARD therapy or in combination with nonbiologic DMARDs in patients with early, aggressive disease. These agents may be added to nonbiologic DMARD monotherapy (e.g., methotrexate) or replace ineffective nonbiologic DMARD therapy. The decision to select a particular agent generally is based on the prescriber's comfort level with monitoring the safety and efficacy of the medications, severity of disease activity, presence of factors suggestive of poor prognosis, the frequency and route of administration, the patient's comfort level or manual dexterity to self-administer subcutaneous injections, the cost, and the availability of insurance coverage. In general, biologic DMARDs should be avoided in patients with serious infections, demyelinating disorders (e.g., multiple sclerosis or optic neuritis), or hepatitis. TNF antagonists should be avoided in patients with heart failure.[20]

Tumor Necrosis Factor Antagonists Etanercept is a recombinant form of human T receptor.[29] Etanercept provides a therapeutic effect by binding to soluble TNF and preventing its binding with TNF receptors. It is administered subcutaneously once or twice weekly; noticeable symptomatic improvement is seen in 1 to 4 weeks. Etanercept is very effective as monotherapy or in combination with other nonbiologic DMARDs. The most common adverse reactions with etanercept are injection-site reactions. If such reactions are bothersome, patients should be advised to place ice on the injection site before and after administration or apply a topical anesthetic or corticosteroid to the affected area.[30] Etanercept has an FDA-approved indication for treatment of JIA. The pediatric dose of etanercept is 0.8 mg/kg subcutaneously once weekly.

Adalimumab is a recombinant human IgG1 monoclonal antibody specific for human TNF.[31] Adalimumab binds to soluble and bound TNF-α. Patients may experience symptomatic relief in as early as 1 week. Adalimumab can be administered in combination with methotrexate or other DMARDs.[2] Adalimumab has an FDA-approved indication for JIA. Of the TNF antagonists, only etanercept and adalimumab are recommended for treating JIA with high disease activity after an adequate trial of NSAIDs, glucocorticoids, or methotrexate.[10]

Infliximab is a chimeric IgGl monoclonal antibody that binds to soluble and bound TNF-α.[32] Methotrexate typically is given with it to suppress antibody production against the mouse-derived portion of the molecule. Infliximab is delivered via IV infusion every 4 to 8 weeks; however, patients may notice benefit within 1 to 4 weeks of receiving the first infusion.

Infusion-related reactions including rash, urticaria, flushing, headache, fever, chills, nausea, tachycardia, and dyspnea may occur during treatment. Qualified healthcare personnel must be present during the infusion to respond to the infusion-related reactions, if they occur. If patients experience any of these symptoms, the reaction may be treated by: (a) temporarily discontinuing the infusion, (b) slowing the infusion rate, or (c) administering corticosteroids or antihistamines.[30] Clinicians may prescribe pretreatment regimens with corticosteroids or antihistamines if the patient continues to experience infusion reactions.[30] Infliximab was shown in clinical trials to be effective for treatment of JIA, but it has not yet received FDA approval for this indication.

Golimumab is a human monoclonal antibody that binds to membrane-bound and soluble TNF. Golimumab can be administered in combination with methotrexate in patients with moderate to severe RA. One advantage of this agent over others in the class may be the once-monthly dosing. Golimumab is not FDA-approved for use in JIA.

Certolizumab is a humanized antibody Fab fragment conjugated to polyethylene glycol, which delays the metabolism and elimination of the medication. Certolizumab can be administered as monotherapy or in combination with methotrexate in patients with moderate to severe RA. Certolizumab is not FDA-approved for use in JIA.

Interleukin-1 Receptor Antagonist Anakinra is a recombinant form of human IL-1 receptor antagonist. Anakinra inhibits the activity of IL-1 by binding to it and preventing cell signaling. It is indicated for adults with RA who have failed one or more nonbiologic DMARDs. Patients must administer a subcutaneous injection every day, which may be less desirable than other treatment options. Anakinra may be used in combination with other nonbiologic DMARDs in patients not responding to or unable to tolerate nonbiologic DMARDs or TNF antagonists. Anakinra should not be used in combination with TNF antagonists due to the increased risk of infection. Anakinra is not included in the algorithms outlined in the 2012 treatment guidelines due to its infrequent use in RA. Regarding treatment of JIA, anakinra is recommended in patients with systemic arthritis of moderate to high disease activity with active arthritis after a trial of methotrexate.[10]

Costimulation Modulators Abatacept interferes with T-cell signaling, ultimately blocking T-cell activation and leading to anergy, or lack of response to an antigen.[33] Trials conducted in patients refractory to methotrexate and anti-TNF therapy demonstrated significant clinical benefit after administration of abatacept every 28 days with a dose approximating 10 mg/kg.[33] Adverse reactions reported in clinical trials were low and similar to those of placebo, with the exception of an increased incidence of headache, infections, and infusion-related reactions in the treatment group.[33]

Abatacept is indicated as monotherapy or in combination with nonbiologic DMARDs. Its exact place in therapy is not yet clear; however, clinicians see a window of opportunity for patients who were intolerant to or did not receive therapeutic benefit from other nonbiologic or biologic DMARDs or developed antibodies to adequate trials of anti-TNF agents, specifically infliximab.[33] Abatacept is FDA approved for the treatment of moderate to severe JIA. It is recommended as a treatment option for patients who received and did not respond to an adequate trial of TNF antagonists.

Anti-CD20 Monoclonal Antibody Rituximab is a genetically engineered chimeric anti-CD20 monoclonal antibody that causes B-lymphocyte depletion in bone marrow and synovial tissue. The exact role of rituximab in RA is not clearly defined, but it is indicated for patients with moderate to severe active RA and a history of inadequate response to one or more TNF antagonist therapies. Adverse effects occurring during or up to 24 hours after the first infusion may include increases or decreases in blood pressure, cough, rash, and pruritus. The infusion-related reactions subside with subsequent infusions. Rituximab carries a black-box warning of fatal infusion reactions and severe mucocutaneous reactions, even though these events did not occur during the RA clinical trials. The benefits of rituximab must be tempered against the safety concerns reported with use of rituximab in the oncology setting. Rituximab is considered a last-line treatment option for JIA (after TNF antagonists and abatacept), although the medication is not FDA approved for this purpose.[10]

Anti–interleukin-6 Receptor Antibody Interleukin-6 (IL-6) is produced in high amounts in patients with RA. High levels are indicative of joint damage and disease activity. In addition, IL-6 plays a significant role in the pathogenesis of anemia associated with RA.[37] Tocilizumab, an anti–IL-6 receptor monoclonal antibody, inhibits the binding of IL-6 to the IL-6 receptor.[24] Studies in patients not responding to methotrexate or TNF antagonists have demonstrated decreased disease activity and improved function and quality of life in patients with RA. The tocilizumab dose is 8 mg/kg IV every 4 weeks. Adverse reactions include nasopharyngitis, infection, and elevated lab values, including liver function tests and cholesterol parameters.[38] In the 2012 recommendations, tocilizumab is considered after inadequate therapeutic response or adverse event to anti-TNF agents, abatacept, or rituximab. Tocilizumab is FDA approved for the treatment of JIA, although it was not included in the recent JIA treatment recommendations.

Kinase Inhibitors Kinases (e.g., Janus kinase 3) are intracellular molecules involved in cytokine signaling. Tofacitinib is a Janus kinase 3 inhibitor undergoing clinical trials to determine safety and efficacy in RA. Tofacitinib is an oral medication that, if approved by the FDA, may provide an alternative for patients unwilling or unable to receive injectable medications.[39]

▶ Selecting a Biologic DMARD

Developments in the treatment of RA are tempered by the lack of evidence of the long-term safety and efficacy of the biologic DMARDs. In addition, high costs can be a deterrent to use. Longer term data are emerging that suggest that patients receiving therapy with these agents early in the course of disease (within 3 years) for a defined time period have reduced disease activity and less joint destruction. If additional evidence proves this to be true, concerns regarding the cost of biologic DMARDs may be alleviated.[39] Cost analyses may indicate that the increased expenses associated with these drugs are offset by the costs avoided for treatment of advanced RA.

❻ *The risk of infection in patients treated with biologic DMARDs must be considered when selecting and monitoring therapy.*[20,40,41] Influencing the immune response to reduce symptoms of RA may influence the body's response to pathogens. Of particular concern is the use of TNF antagonists in patients with a history of tuberculosis exposure. TNF is important in the formation of granulomas that wall off tuberculosis infection. In theory, if TNF is inhibited, patients with latent tuberculosis may have a reactivated infection. Patients receiving biologic DMARD therapy should be screened for tuberculosis and other infections (hepatitis B, hepatitis, C). Antituberculosis therapy should be initiated in patients with active or latent tuberculosis.[20] Biologic therapy may be initiated after at least 1 month of antituberculosis treatment. Patients with untreated hepatitis B should not receive biologic DMARDs. Etanercept may be a potential treatment option in patients with hepatitis C.[20] Biologic DMARDs should not be initiated during an acute, serious infection and should be discontinued temporarily during times of infection.[41]

▶ *Fertility, Pregnancy, and Fetal Development*

Women of childbearing age should be counseled about the impact of antirheumatic drugs on fertility, pregnancy, fetal development, and lactation. Some women may experience a reduction in disease symptoms during pregnancy; however, many agents used to treat RA are known teratogens. In addition, some women may present with signs and symptoms of RA for the first time during the postpartum period. Women desiring motherhood must consult with their physicians to carefully plan for the pregnancy and reduce risks to the developing fetus.[42] Treatment plans selected must also consider the potential effects on breastfeeding babies. Low-dose corticosteroids generally are safe and effective. Certain NSAIDs, hydroxychloroquine, and azathioprine may be considered in severe disease.

Methotrexate use (FDA Pregnancy Category X) is associated with spontaneous abortion, fetal myelosuppression, limb defects, and CNS abnormalities; therefore, pregnancy must be avoided.[42] Methotrexate should be discontinued 3 months prior to attempting conception. Sulfasalazine, on the other hand, may be the drug of choice in women who are pregnant or planning to become pregnant due to its safety profile.[42] There is limited evidence of safety and long-term effects of the use of biologic DMARDs in pregnant women. Case reports of pregnancy during biologic DMARD therapy show no increased risk of fetal toxicity, but long-term data are needed.[29,42] Based on available data, TNF antagonists are considered safe until the time of conception, and discontinuation during pregnancy is recommended. Rituximab should be discontinued 1 year

prior to planned conception. Abatacept should be discontinued 10 weeks prior to planned conception.[42]

Male patients with RA must receive counseling about the effects of certain medications on their fertility and potential harm to the fetus. It is difficult to establish causality between use of a medication by a male and the effect on fertility or fetal development; therefore, a conservative approach must be taken. ❼ *Women of childbearing potential and their partners must be counseled to: (a) use proper birth control*

Patient Encounter, Part 2: Medical History, Physical Examination, and Laboratory Tests

PMH: Hypertension (uncontrolled), dyslipidemia (uncontrolled), depression, prediabetes (uncontrolled)

FH: Unknown, she left home at age 16

SH: She is a waitress at the local diner working 40 to 60 hours per week. She does not drink alcohol. She smokes one pack of cigarettes per day

Allergies: sulfa

Meds: She has received prescriptions for medications in the past, but she does not fill them. For the last 2 months, she has been taking acetaminophen 500 mg twice daily for joint pain. Otherwise, she takes no medications routinely

ROS: (+) fatigue, (–) N/V/D, HA, SOB, chest pain, cough

PE:

VS: BP 166/88, P 82, RR 22, T 38.0°C (100.4°F); ht 5 ft 4 in (163 cm), wt 79.5 kg (175 lb)

Skin: Warm, dry

HEENT: NC/AT, PERRLA, TMs intact

CV: RRR, normal S1 and S2, no m/r/g

Chest: CTA

Abd: Soft, NT/ND

Neuro: A & O × 3; CN II to XII intact

Ext: Bilateral tender and swollen PIPs and MCPs

Labs: ESR 82 mm/h, RF (–), HLA-DR4 (–), anti-CCP (low +)

Synovial fluid analysis: Yellow, cloudy, decreased viscosity

Hand x-rays: Soft-tissue swelling, joint space narrowing, evidence of erosions

Disease Activity Score 28 (DAS 28): 5.2

Describe whether this patient fits the classification criteria for RA.

How would you categorize this patient's disease activity—low, moderate, or high? Why? How does this affect your treatment plan?

What nonpharmacologic and pharmacologic alternatives are appropriate for this patient?

while undergoing treatment for RA, and (b) involve healthcare providers in discussions regarding family planning to carefully consider all treatment options available.[42]

OUTCOME EVALUATION

- Rheumatologists rely on standardized criteria to assess treatment interventions through measurement of disease activity. The ACR uses criteria for improvement based on percentage improvement in tender and swollen joint count and the presence of at least three or more of the following measures: (a) pain, (b) patient global assessment, (c) physician global assessment, (d) self-assessed physical disability, and (e) acute-phase reactants.[42] ACR20, ACR50, and ACR70 are common efficacy end points in clinical

---

Patient Encounter, Part 3: Creating a Care Plan

Based on the information available, create a care plan for this patient's RA. The plan should include the following:

(a) A statement of the drug-related needs and/or problems

(b) A patient-specific detailed therapeutic plan (including specific medications and associated doses)

(c) Monitoring parameters to assess safety and efficacy

Six months later, the patient returns because she just found out that she is pregnant. She has worked diligently to take care of her health and reports 80% adherence to her RA treatment regimen.

Does this change your treatment plan? If so, devise a new treatment plan for the patient.

Patient Care and Monitoring

1. Assess the patient's symptoms to determine whether they are consistent with RA. Evaluate the duration of symptoms and their impact on daily living.

2. Review available diagnostic data to determine the severity of disease and whether the patient is at risk of experiencing poor outcomes.

3. Obtain a thorough medication history, including prescription drugs, over-the-counter drugs, and dietary supplement use.

4. Educate the patient on nonpharmacologic measures that will improve symptoms.

5. Formulate a therapeutic plan, taking into consideration patient-specific factors.

6. Evaluate the patient for the presence of adverse drug reactions, drug allergies, and drug interactions.

7. Develop a plan to assess safety and efficacy of the pharmacologic treatment plan. Determine whether the appropriate doses of antirheumatic medications were used and whether all medications were given a sufficient trial to achieve therapeutic benefit.

8. Stress importance of adherence with the therapeutic regimen, including required laboratory monitoring, medication dosing, and administration. Recommend a therapeutic regimen that is convenient and consistent with the patient's lifestyle.

9. Longitudinally evaluate the patient's clinical response to therapy and the impact on quality of life and mobility.

10. Evaluate the presence of comorbidities and implement measures to control the increased risk.

   - *Cardiovascular*: Keep doses of NSAIDs and glucocorticoids low, consider initiation of folic acid to reduce homocysteine level elevations induced by methotrexate, consider initiation of low-dose aspirin and/or HMG-CoA reductase inhibitors (statins), and encourage smokers to discontinue tobacco use and assist with the development of a tobacco-cessation plan.[13,15] Screen and aggressively treat elevated blood pressure. Preferred agents in this population are angiotensin-converting enzyme inhibitors and angiotensin II blockers.

   - *Infection*: Wash hands routinely, limit contact with individuals who are ill, and report signs and symptoms of infection immediately (e.g., fever, weight loss, and night sweats).

   - *Malignancy*: Report new onset of signs and symptoms (e.g., fever, chills, anorexia, and night sweats) immediately.[17]

   - *Osteoporosis*: Encourage patients to ingest adequate amounts of calcium and vitamin D, encourage smokers to discontinue tobacco use, and consider initiation of medications for osteoporosis (e.g., bisphosphonates, calcitonin, and parathyroid hormone) if the patient is taking glucocorticoids chronically or if the patient has evidence of low bone mineral density.[21,47]

11. Provide patient education with regard to RA, lifestyle modifications, and drug therapy:

   - What causes RA?

   - What are the comorbidities associated with RA?

   - How will lifestyle modifications affect RA?

   - What are the goals of therapy in the treatment of RA?

   - When and how should the medications be administered?

   - What potential adverse drug reactions may occur?

   - Which drugs may interact with therapy?

   - What are the warning signs to report to the physician?

trials. The number corresponds with the percentage improvement. As drug development continues to evolve, the acceptable criteria for 20% improvement may be too low. For example, if a patient has 10 tender and swollen joints, reducing that by 20% to 8 tender and swollen joints is, by definition, an improvement by ACR20 criteria. However, further reduction in symptoms or disease remission may have greater clinical significance and effect on the patient's quality of life.

- A joint committee of ACR and EULAR is currently working to define criteria for disease remission in RA. At this time, different organizations define remission differently. Each criteria set has its strengths and weaknesses. A consensus definition will help to establish specific treatment targets for patients.[43]

- Physical disability from RA can be measured through the Stanford HAQ.[44,45] This patient self-assessment tool was developed to evaluate patient outcomes in five dimensions of chronic conditions: (a) disability, (b) discomfort, (c) drug adverse effects, (d) dollar costs, and (e) death. Clinicians and clinical studies in rheumatology use HAQ to assess longitudinally changes that influence the patient's quality of life.[44,45]

- Disease activity can be measured through the Disease Activity Score in 28 joints (DAS 28). Components involved in the calculation are the number of swollen and tender joints, ESR or CRP, and a subjective measure of the patient's general health. A DAS 28 score of 3.2 or less indicates low disease activity, between 3.2 and 5.1 is considered moderate activity, and 5.1 or more is considered to be high activity.[20,46] Remission, defined by DAS 28, is a score of less than 2.6.

- Before starting treatment for RA, assess the subjective and objective evidence of disease. For joint findings, this includes the number of tender and swollen joints, pain, limitations on use, duration of morning stiffness, and presence of joint erosions. Systemic findings may include fatigue and the presence of extraarticular manifestations. Obtain laboratory measurements of CRP and ESR. The impact of the disease on quality of life and functional status is also important.

- At follow-up visits, compare the patient's status to baseline or previous visits using standardized criteria for improvement of disease activity and the HAQ to assess longitudinally the influence on quality of life.

- Assess the patient's response to initiation of nonbiologic or biologic DMARD therapy after allowing adequate time for the medication to achieve its therapeutic effect.

- Determine whether any adverse reactions associated with each antirheumatic medication are present.

- Monitor laboratory parameters to ensure patient safety and reduce the risk of adverse reactions.

- ⑧ *In addition to designing an individualized therapeutic regimen to control the progression of RA, the clinician must evaluate the presence of comorbidities and implement measures to control the increased risk.*

Abbreviations Introduced in This Chapter

ACR	American College of Rheumatology
CCP	Cyclic citrullinated peptide
COX-2	Cyclooxygenase-2
CRP	C-Reactive protein
DAS	Disease Activity Score
DMARD	Disease-modifying antirheumatic drug
ESR	Erythrocyte sedimentation rate
EULAR	European League Against Rheumatism
HAQ	Health Assessment Questionnaire
HLA	Human leukocyte antigen
IL	Interleukin
JIA	Juvenile idiopathic arthritis
JRA	Juvenile rheumatoid arthritis
MCP	Metacarpophalangeal joint
MTP	Metatarsophalangeal joint
NSAID	Nonsteroidal anti-inflammatory drug
PIP	Proximal interphalangeal joint
RA	Rheumatoid arthritis
TNF	Tumor necrosis factor

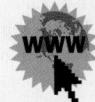 Self-assessment questions and answers are available at *http://www.mhpharmacotherapy. com/pp.html.*

REFERENCES

1. Aletaha D, Neogi T, Silman A, et al. 2010 rheumatoid arthritis classification criteria. Arthritis Rheum 2010;62:2569–2381.
2. Majithia V, Geraci SA. Rheumatoid arthritis: Diagnosis and management. Am J Med 2007;120:936–939.
3. Myasoedova E, Davis JM, Crowson CS, Gabriel SE. Epidemiology of rheumatoid arthritis: rheumatoid arthritis and mortality. Curr Rheumatol Rep 2010;12:379–385.
4. Amson Y, Shoenfeld Y, Amital H. Effects of smoking on immunity, inflammation and autoimmunity. J Autoimmun 2010;34:258–265.
5. Choy EH, Panayi GS. Cytokine pathways and joint inflammation in rheumatoid arthritis. N Engl J Med 2001;344:907–916.
6. Kotzin BL. The role of B cells in the pathogenesis of rheumatoid arthritis. J Rheumatol 2005;73(Suppl):14–18.
7. Boissier MC. Cell and cytokine imbalances in rheumatoid synovitis. Joint Bone Spine 2011;78:230–234.
8. Rindfleisch JA, Muller D. Diagnosis and management of rheumatoid arthritis. Am Fam Physician 2005;72(6):1037–1047.
9. McCray C, Agarwal SK. Stress and autoimmunity. Immunol Allergy Clin North Am 2011;31:1–18.
10. Beukelman T, Patkar NM, Saag KG. 2011 American College of Rheumatology recommendations for the treatment of juvenile idiopathic arthritis: initiation and safety monitoring of therapeutic agents for the treatment of arthritis and systemic features. Arthritis Care Res 2011;63:465–482.
11. Vital EM, Emery P. The development of targeted therapies in rheumatoid arthritis. J Autoimmun 2008;31:219–227.
12. Gonzalez A, Icen M, Kremers HM, et al. Mortality trends in rheumatoid arthritis: The role of rheumatoid factor. J Rheumatol 2008;35:1009–1014.

13. Pieringer H, Pichler M. Cardiovascular morbidity and mortality in patients with rheumatoid arthritis: vascular alterations and possible clinical implications. Q J Med 2011;104:13–26.

14. Peters MJ, Symmons DP, McCaret D, et al. EULAR evidence-based recommendations for cardiovascular risk management in patients with rheumatoid arthritis and other forms of inflammatory arthritis. Ann Rheum Dis 2010;69:325–331.

15. Magnano MD, Genovese MC. Management of co-morbidities and general medical conditions in patients with rheumatoid arthritis. Curr Rheumatol Rep 2005;7(5):407–415.

16. Szekanecz Z, Szekanecz W, Bako G, Shoenfeld Y. Malignancies in autoimmune rheumatic diseases–a mini-review. Gerontology 2011;57:3–10.

17. Chakravarty EF, Genovese MC. Associations between rheumatoid arthritis and malignancy. Rheum Dis Clin North Am 2004;30(2):271–284.

18. Hashkes PJ, Laxer RM. Medical treatment of juvenile idiopathic arthritis. JAMA 2005;294:1671–1684.

19. Wallace CA. Current management of juvenile idiopathic arthritis. Best Pract Res Clin Rheumatol 2006;20:279–300.

20. Singh JA, Furst DE, Bharat A, et al. 2012 Update of the 2008 American College of Rheumatology recommendations for the use of disease-modifying antirheumatic drugs and biologic agents in the treatment of rheumatoid arthritis. Arthritis Care Res 2012;64:625–639.

21. O'Dell JR. Therapeutic strategies for rheumatoid arthritis. N Engl J Med 2004;350:2591–2602.

22. Naesdal J, Brown K. NSAID-associated adverse effects and acid control aids to prevent them. A review of current treatment options. Drug Saf 2006;29(2):119–132.

23. Rhen T, Cidlowski JA. Antiinflammatory action of glucocorticoids—New mechanisms for old drugs. N Engl J Med 2005;353:1711–1723.

24. Ohsugi Y, Kishimoto T. The recombinant humanized anti-IL-6 receptor antibody tocilizumab, an innovative drug for the treatment of rheumatoid arthritis. Expert Opin Biol Ther 2008;8(5):669–681.

25. Cronstein BN. Low-dose methotrexate: A mainstay in the treatment of rheumatoid arthritis. Pharmacol Rev 2005;57(2):163–172.

26. vanDongen H, van Aken J, Lard LR, et al. Efficacy of methotrexate treatment in patients with probable rheumatoid arthritis: A double blind, randomized, placebo-controlled trial. Arthritis Rheum 2007;56(5):1424–1432.

27. Niehues T, Lankisch P. Recommendations for the use of methotrexate in juvenile idiopathic arthritis. Paediatr Drugs 2006;8:347–356.

28. Cannon GW, Kremer JM. Leflunomide. Rheum Dis Clin North Am 2004;30(2):295–309.

29. Genovese MC, Kremer JM. Treatment of rheumatoid arthritis with etanercept. Rheum Dis Clin North Am 2004;30(2):311–328.

30. Cush JJ. Safety overview of new disease-modifying antirheumatic drugs. Rheum Dis Clin North Am 2004;30(2):237–255.

31. Keystone E, Haraoui B. Adalimumab therapy in rheumatoid arthritis. Rheum Dis Clin North Am 2004;30(2):349–364.

32. Maini SR. Infliximab treatment of rheumatoid arthritis. Rheum Dis Clin North Am 2004;30(2):329–347.

33. Todd DJ, Costenbader KH, Weinblatt ME. Abatacept in the treatment of rheumatoid arthritis. Int J ClinPract 2007;61(3):494–500.

34. Panayi GS. B cell-directed therapy in rheumatoid arthritis—Clinical experience. J Rheumatol 2005;32(Suppl 73):19–24.

35. Buch MH, Smolen JS, Betteridge N, et al. Updated consensus statement on the use of rituximab in patients with rheumatoid arthritis. Ann Rheum Dis 2011;70:909–920.

36. Keystone E, Fleischmann R, Emery P, et al. Safety and efficacy of additional courses of rituximab in patients with active rheumatoid arthritis: an open-label extension analysis. Arthritis Rheum 2007;56(12):3896–3908.

37. Masson C. Rheumatoid anemia. Joint Bone Spine 2011;78:131–137.

38. Singh J, Beg S, Lopez-Olivo MA. Tocilizumab for rheumatoid arthritis: a Cochrane systematic review. J Rheumatol 2011;38:10–20.

39. Tak PP, Kalden JR. Advances in rheumatology: new targeted therapies. Arthritis Res Ther 2011;13(Suppl 1):S5.

40. Rychly DJ, DiPiro JT. Infections associated with tumor necrosis factor-alpha antagonists. Pharmacotherapy 2005;25:1181–1192.

41. Curtis JR, Patkar N, Xie A, et al. Risk of serious bacterial infections among rheumatoid arthritis patients exposed to tumor necrosis factor alpha antagonists. Arthritis Rheum 2007;56(4):1125–1133.

42. Parlett R, Roussou E. The treatment of rheumatoid arthritis during pregnancy. Rheumatol Int 2011;31:445–449.

43. Shammas RM, Ranganath VK, Paulus HE. Remission in rheumatoid arthritis. Curr Rheumatol Rep 2010;12:355–362.

44. Bruce B, Fries JF. The Stanford Health Assessment Questionnaire: A review of its history, issues, progress, and documentation. J Rheumatol 2003;30(1):167–178.

45. Bruce B, Fries JF. The Stanford Health Assessment Questionnaire: Dimensions and practical applications. Health Qual Life Outcomes 2003;1(1):20.

46. van der Heijde D, van 't Hof MA, van Riel PL, et al. Judging disease activity in clinical practice in rheumatoid arthritis: First step in the development of a disease activity score. Ann Rheum Dis 1990;49(11):916–920.

47. Grossman JM, Gordon R, Ranganath VK, et al. American College of Rheumatology 2010 recommendations for the prevention and treatment of glucocorticoid-induced osteoporosis. Arthritis Care Res 2010;62:1515–1526.

58 Osteoarthritis

Steven M. Smith, Eric Dietrich, and John G. Gums

KEY CONCEPTS

1 Osteoarthritis (OA) is the most common form of arthritis and is most prevalent in the middle to later years of life.

2 The most common symptoms are joint pain, reduced range of motion, and brief joint stiffness after periods of inactivity.

3 Treatment goals are to educate the patient and caregivers, relieve pain, maintain or restore mobility, minimize functional impairment, preserve joint integrity, and improve quality of life.

4 Nonpharmacologic therapy is the cornerstone of treatment; education, exercise, weight loss, and cognitive behavioral intervention are integral components.

5 Acetaminophen is the initial drug of choice; an adequate dose and duration of therapy should be used before resorting to other drug classes.

6 Nonsteroidal anti-inflammatory drugs (NSAIDs) may be initiated if acetaminophen therapy fails. At equipotent doses, all NSAIDs elicit similar analgesic and anti-inflammatory responses. Selection is based on patient preference, previous response, dosing frequency, tolerability, and cost.

7 Patients who do not respond adequately to one NSAID may respond to a different NSAID.

8 NSAIDs are associated with adverse GI, renal, hepatic, cardiovascular, and CNS effects and may increase blood pressure.

9 NSAIDs that are selective for the cyclooxygenase-2 (COX-2) enzyme are less likely to cause GI complications but may increase the risk of cardiovascular events. COX-2 inhibitors are no more effective than nonselective NSAIDs and should be reserved for patients at high risk of GI complications and low risk for cardiovascular events.

10 Glucosamine, tramadol, opioids, topical capsaicin, topical NSAIDs, intraarticular corticosteroids, hyaluronic acid, and surgery may be beneficial in certain situations.

INTRODUCTION

1 *Osteoarthritis (OA) is the most common form of arthritis.* Weight-bearing joints (e.g., hips and knees) are most susceptible, but non–weight-bearing joints, especially the hands, may also be involved. Because of its high prevalence and involvement of joints critical for daily functioning, the disease causes tremendous morbidity and financial burden.[1] OA is the leading cause of chronic mobility disability and the most common reason for total-hip and total-knee replacement.[2] ❶ *OA is strongly related to age; thus its incidence and the cost of care will increase dramatically in the coming years due to a burgeoning senior citizenry.*

EPIDEMIOLOGY AND ETIOLOGY

The National Arthritis Data Workgroup estimates that 27 million Americans have signs and symptoms of OA.[3] The true extent of the disease is much larger; nearly everyone has radiographic evidence of OA by the eighth decade of life, but individuals without symptoms often go undiagnosed. Approximately 7% of U.S. adults have daily symptomatic hand OA, whereas 6% and 3% report daily symptoms affecting the knees and hips, respectively.[3] After age 60, 10% to 17% of persons report such symptoms.[3]

The prevalence of OA is higher in women, and they have more generalized disease. Women are also more likely to have inflammation of the proximal and distal interphalangeal joints of the hands, which manifest as Bouchard's nodes and Heberden's nodes, respectively. OA of the hip occurs more frequently in men.

The prevalence of OA in whites is similar to that in African Americans, but the latter may experience more severe and disabling disease. Persons of Chinese descent rarely have hip OA; they are also less likely to develop hand OA but more likely to develop knee OA.

PATHOPHYSIOLOGY

OA is characterized by damage to diarthrodial joints and joint structures (Fig. 58–1). OA is a multifactorial disease typified by progressive destruction of joint cartilage, erratic new bone formation, thickening of subchondral bone and the joint capsule, bony remodeling, development of osteophytes, variable degrees of mild synovitis, and other changes.[4]

The earliest stages of OA are characterized by increasing water content and softening of cartilage in weight-bearing joints. As the disease progresses, proteoglycan content of cartilage declines, and eventually, cartilage becomes hypocellular.

Increasing levels of protease enzymes, such as matrix metalloproteinases (MMPs), occur before changes in cartilage, suggesting that these catabolic proteinases play an important role in the initiation and progression of OA.

Subchondral bone undergoes metabolic changes, including increased bone turnover, that appear to be precursors to tissue destruction. The normally contiguous bony surface becomes fissured. Persistent use of the joint eventually results in loss of cartilage, permitting bone-to-bone contact that ultimately promotes thickening and eburnation of exposed bone. Microfractures may appear in subchondral bone, and osteonecrosis may develop beneath the surface.

New bone is formed haphazardly, leading to the formation of osteophytes that extend into the joint capsule and ligament attachments and may encroach on the joint space. Progressive loss of joint cartilage, subchondral damage, narrowing of joint spaces, and changes in the underlying bone and soft tissues may culminate in deformed, painful joints.

Classification

OA is often divided into primary (idiopathic) and secondary disease (Table 58–1). *Primary OA* is the predominant form and occurs in the absence of a precipitating event. It may assume a localized, generalized, or erosive pattern. Localized OA is distinguished from generalized disease by the number of sites involved, whereas erosive disease is characterized by an erosive pattern of bone destruction and marked proliferation of interphalangeal joints of the hands. *Secondary OA* results from congenital or developmental disorders or inflammatory, metabolic, or endocrine diseases.

Risk Factors

OA develops when systemic factors and biomechanical vulnerabilities combine. Systemic factors include age, gender, genetic predisposition, and nutritional status. Age is the strongest predictor of OA, although advanced age alone is insufficient to cause OA.

Joints exposed to biomechanical factors are at increased risk. Occupational and recreational activities involving repetitive motion or injury can provoke OA, although most daily activities do not produce enough joint trauma to cause

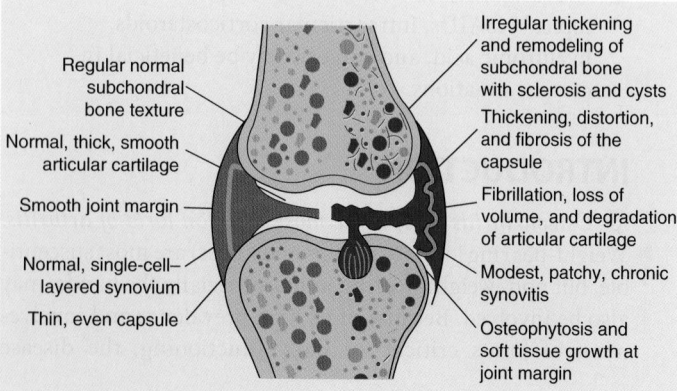

Regular normal subchondral bone texture

Normal, thick, smooth articular cartilage

Smooth joint margin

Normal, single-cell-layered synovium

Thin, even capsule

Irregular thickening and remodeling of subchondral bone with sclerosis and cysts

Thickening, distortion, and fibrosis of the capsule

Fibrillation, loss of volume, and degradation of articular cartilage

Modest, patchy, chronic synovitis

Osteophytosis and soft tissue growth at joint margin

FIGURE 58–1. Characteristics of osteoarthritis in the diarthrodial joint. (From DiPiro JT, Talbert RL, Yee GC, et al (eds.) Pharmacotherapy: A Pathophysiologic Approach. 8th ed. New York: McGraw-Hill; 2011:1601, Fig. 101–2; With permission.)

Table 58–1

Classification of Osteoarthritis

Primary Osteoarthritis
Localized (involving one or two sites)
Generalized (involving three or more sites)
Erosive

Secondary Osteoarthritis
Mechanical incongruity of joint
Congenital or developmental defect
Posttraumatic
Prior inflammatory disease (rheumatoid arthritis, chronic gouty arthritis, pseudogout, infectious arthritis)
Metabolic disorder (hemochromatosis, ochronosis, Wilson's disease, chondrocalcinosis, Paget's disease)
Endocrinopathies (diabetes mellitus, obesity, acromegaly, iatrogenic hyperadrenocorticism, sex hormone abnormalities)
Neuropathic disorders
Intraarticular corticosteroid overuse
Avascular necrosis
Bone dysplasia

OA, even after decades of repeated use. However, daily activities may lead to OA if a joint is susceptible because of previous injury, joint deformity, muscle weakness, or systemic factors. Heavy physical activity is a stronger predictor of subsequent OA than light to moderate activities.[5] This is especially true for older individuals, in whom the joint structure is less capable of coping with highly stressful activities. Obesity increases load-bearing stresses on hip and knee joints. The risk of OA increases by 10% for each kilogram of body weight above ideal body weight.[6]

CLINICAL PRESENTATION AND DIAGNOSIS

See the accompanying text box for the clinical presentation of OA. There are no laboratory tests that are specific for the diagnosis of OA. The erythrocyte sedimentation rate (ESR) and hematologic and chemistry panels are usually unremarkable. If synovial fluid is aspirated from an affected joint, it is sterile, without crystals, and has a WBC count less than $1.5 \times 10^3/\text{mm}^3$ ($1.5 \times 10^9/\text{L}$). Radiographic changes are often absent in early OA. As the disease progresses, joint-space narrowing, subchondral bone sclerosis, and osteophytes may be detected. Gross joint deformity and joint effusions may occur in late severe OA.

TREATMENT

Desired Outcomes

❸ *Goals of therapy include: (a) educating the patient and caregivers, (b) relieving pain, (c) maintaining or restoring mobility, (d) minimizing functional impairment, (e) preserving joint integrity, and (f) improving quality of life.*

Clinical Presentation of OA

General
- Patients are generally over the age of 50.
- Presentations encompass a spectrum ranging from asymptomatic to severe joint pain and stiffness with functional limitations.
- Joint involvement has an asymmetric local distribution without systemic manifestations.
- In contrast to some other arthritic conditions (e.g., rheumatoid arthritis, gout), inflammation usually is absent or mild and localized when present.

Symptoms
- ❷ *The cardinal symptoms are use-related joint pain, typically described as deep and aching in character, and stiffness. In advanced cases, pain also may be present during rest.*
- Weight-bearing joints may be unstable.
- ❷ *Joint stiffness ("gelling") abates with motion and recurs with rest.*
- ❷ *Joint stiffness generally lasts less than 30 minutes after periods of inactivity, limits the range of joint motion, impairs daily activities, and may be related to weather.*

Signs
- One or more joints may be involved, usually in an asymmetric pattern.
- The following sites are most often involved in primary OA:
  - Distal interphalangeal finger joints (Heberden's nodes)
  - Proximal interphalangeal finger joints (Bouchard's nodes)
  - First carpometacarpal joint
  - Knees, hips, and cervicolumbar spine
  - Metatarsophalangeal joint of the great toe
- The following sites are involved most often in secondary OA:
  - Metacarpophalangeal joints
  - Wrists
  - Elbows
  - Glenohumeral joints
  - Ankles
- Joint examination may reveal local tenderness, bony proliferation, soft tissue swelling, crepitus, muscle atrophy, limited motion with passive/active movement, and effusion.

Patient Encounter, Part 1

OC is a 67-year-old obese Chinese man who presents to his primary care physician with right knee pain that has significantly worsened over the past several years. He describes the pain as dull and achy, and it is most severe in the morning after awakening until he "loosens up" 10 to 15 minutes later. He believes the morning stiffness is related to a previous knee injury for which he had surgery to repair a torn ACL. OC also reports feeling "down" because he is no longer able to be on his bowling team due to his knee pain and is now forced to stay home most nights of the week. OC is retired from a factory worker position that required him to be on his feet for long hours while he assembled electronics.

What information is suggestive of osteoarthritis (OA)?

What risk factors for OA does this patient have?

What cultural or ethnic factors may contribute to his OA?

What other information will you need to differentiate OA from rheumatoid arthritis (RA)?

What potential comorbidities should be considered in this patient?

What other information will be required before formulating a treatment plan?

General Approach to Treatment

Treatment is individualized and should consider medical history, physical examination, radiographic findings, distribution and severity of joint involvement, and response to previous treatment. Comorbid diseases, concomitant medications, and allergies are integrated into a holistic treatment approach.

A comprehensive treatment algorithm for OA is given in **Figure 58–2**. Nonpharmacologic treatment is integral to achieving optimal outcomes in patients with OA. Pharmacologic therapy is used as an adjunctive measure to relieve pain; most treatments do not modify the disease course. Surgical intervention generally is reserved for patients with advanced disease complicated by unremitting pain or severely compromised function.

Nonpharmacologic Therapy

Nondrug therapy consists of a three-pronged approach of education, lifestyle modification, and physical therapy. ❹ *Educational programs include a set of systematic educational activities designed to improve health behaviors and health status, thereby slowing OA progression.* The goal is to increase patient knowledge and self-confidence in adjusting daily activities in the face of evolving symptoms. Effective programs produce positive behavioral changes, decreased pain and disability, and improved functioning. In addition to physical outcomes, psychological outcomes such as

depression, self-efficacy, and life satisfaction are positively influenced. Patients can be referred to the Arthritis Foundation (*www.arthritis.org*) for educational materials and information on support groups.

❹ *Lifestyle modification should be employed in all patients at risk for OA and in those with established disease.* In general, it is advisable to recommend low-impact exercise routinely. Aerobic exercise and strength-training programs improve functional capacity in older adults with OA. Stretching and strengthening exercises should target affected and vulnerable joints. Isometric exercises performed three to four times weekly improve physical functioning and decrease disability, pain, and analgesic use.

Obesity's association with both the onset and progression of OA make weight loss a pivotal treatment strategy in overweight and obese patients. Women who reduce body weight by 5 kg (11 lb) can cut their risk of developing OA in half. Moreover, symptomatic relief and improved quality of life occur in people with knee OA who reduce their body weight. Weight loss should be pursued through a combination of dietary modification and increased physical activity (see Chap. 102). The patient's physical capabilities should be considered when implementing an exercise program.

❹ *Application of heat or cold treatments to involved joints improves range of motion, reduces pain, and decreases muscle spasms. Practical applications of heat therapy include warm baths or warm water soaks.* Heating pads should be used with caution, especially in the elderly, and patients must be warned of the potential for burns if used inappropriately.

Referral to a physical or occupational therapist may be helpful, particularly in patients with functional disabilities. Physical therapy is tailored to the patient and may include assessment of muscle strength, joint stability, and mobility; use of heat (especially prior to episodes of increased physical activity); structured exercise regimens; and implementation of assistive devices, such as canes, crutches, and walkers. The occupational therapist ensures optimal joint protection and function, energy conservation, and use of splints and other assistive devices.

Pharmacologic Therapy

Simple analgesics such as acetaminophen and nonsteroidal anti-inflammatory drugs (NSAIDs) are first-line agents for treating OA (**Table 58–2**).

▶ Acetaminophen

Acetaminophen is a centrally acting analgesic that inhibits prostaglandin production in the brain and spinal cord. ❺ *Acetaminophen is an effective and inexpensive analgesic with a favorable risk–benefit profile. For treatment of mild-to-moderate pain, acetaminophen should be tried initially at an adequate dose and duration before considering an NSAID.*[7–10] Acetaminophen is generally considered to be as effective as NSAIDs for mild-to-moderate joint pain with a superior safety profile.[10]

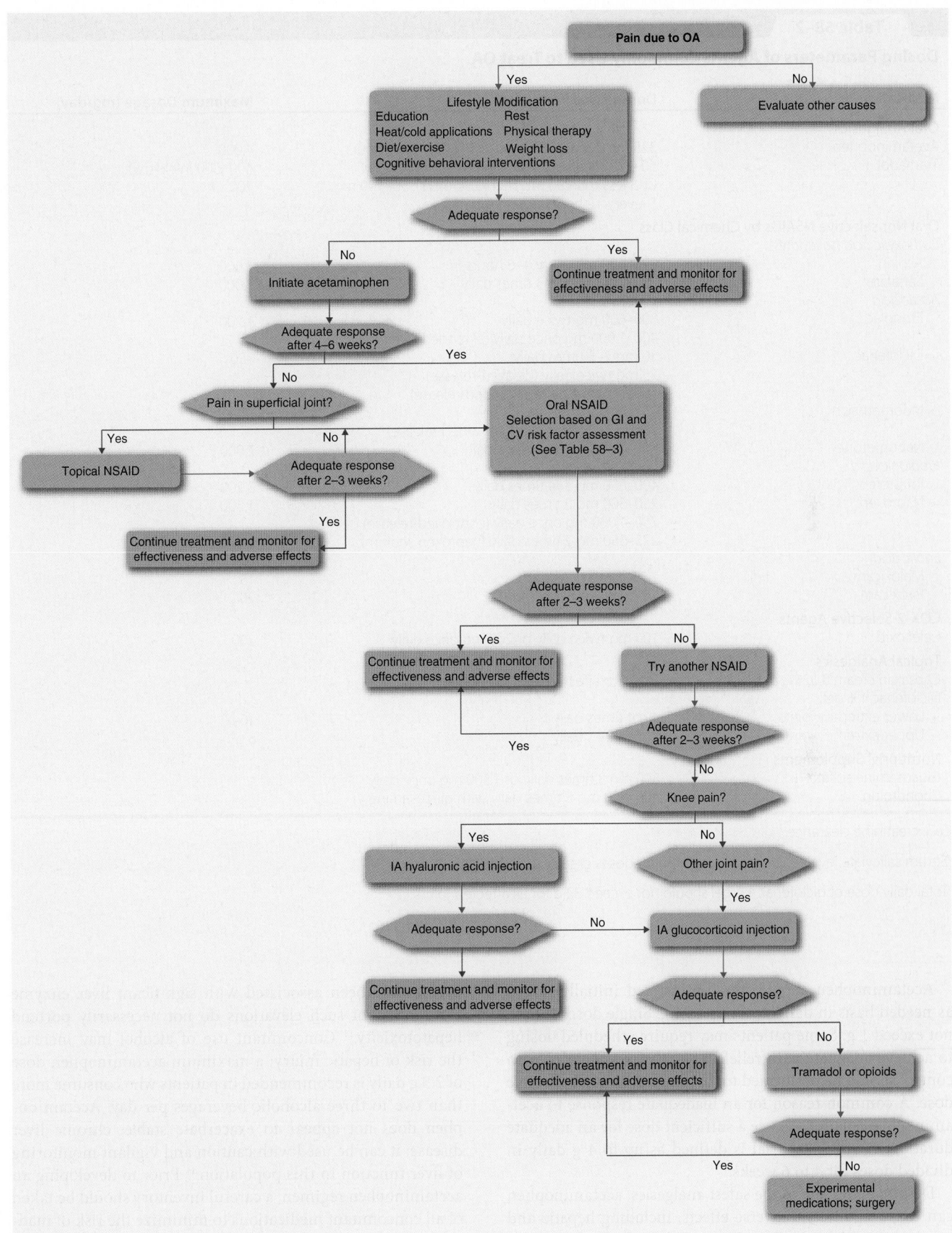

FIGURE 58-2. Treatment of osteoarthritis. (OA, osteoarthritis; COX-2, cyclooxygenase-2; CV, cardiovascular; IA, intraarticular; NSAID, nonsteroidal anti-inflammatory drug.)

Table 58–2

Dosing Parameters of Agents Commonly Used to Treat OA

Medication	Dosage and Frequency	Maximum Dosage (mg/day)
Oral Analgesics		
Acetaminophen	325 mg every 4–6 hours or 1 g every 6–8 hours	4,000
Tramadol	50–100 mg every 4–6 hours	400 (300 in elderly)
	CrCl less than 30 mL/min (0.50 mL/s): 50–100 mg every 12 hours	200
Oral Nonselective NSAIDs by Chemical Class		
Carboxylic acid (salicylates)		
Aspirin	325–650 mg every 4–6 hours	3,600[a]
Salsalate	500–1,000 mg 2–3 times daily	3,000[a]
Acetic acid		
Etodolac	300–600 mg twice daily	1,200
	400–1,000 mg once daily (extended-release)	
Diclofenac	50 mg 2–3 times daily	150
	75 mg twice daily (delayed-release)	
	100 mg once daily (extended-release)	
Indomethacin	25 mg 2–3 times daily	200
	75 mg 1–2 times daily (sustained-release)	
Nabumetone	500–1,000 mg 1–2 times daily	2,000
Propionic acid		
Ibuprofen	400–800 mg 3–4 times daily	3,200
Naproxen	250–500 mg 2 times daily	1,500
	750–1,000 mg once daily (controlled-release)	
	275–550 mg 2 times daily (naproxen sodium)	1,650
Enolic acid		
Meloxicam	7.5–15 mg once daily	15
Piroxicam	20 mg once daily	20
COX-2-Selective Agents		
Celecoxib	100 mg twice daily or 200 mg once daily	200
Topical Analgesics		
Capsaicin cream 0.025% or 0.075%	Apply to affected joint every 6–8 hours	
Diclofenac 1% gel		
Lower extremity joints	4 g 4 times daily	16 g[b]
Upper extremity joints	2 g 4 times daily	8 g[b]
Nutritional Supplements		
Glucosamine sulfate	500 mg 3 times daily or 1,500 mg once daily	
Chondroitin	400–800 mg 3 times daily with glucosamine	

CrCl, creatinine clearance.

[a]Serum salicylate levels should be monitored for doses greater than 3 g/day.

[b]Total daily dose of diclofenac 1% gel should not exceed 32 g for all affected joints.

Acetaminophen should be administered initially on an as-needed basis in daily doses up to 4 g. Single doses should not exceed 1 g. Some patients may require scheduled dosing to achieve adequate pain relief. Periodic assessment of pain control should be performed to maintain the lowest effective dose. A common reason for an inadequate response to acetaminophen is failure to use a sufficient dose for an adequate duration. A sufficient trial is defined as up to 4 g daily in divided doses for 4 to 6 weeks.

Despite being one of the safest analgesics, acetaminophen can cause significant adverse effects, including hepatic and renal toxicity.[11] Acetaminophen overdose, both intentional and unintentional, is the leading cause of acute liver injury in the United States.[12] Doses greater than 4 g are associated with an increased risk of hepatotoxicity. Total daily doses of 4 g have been associated with significant liver enzyme elevations, but such elevations do not necessarily portend hepatotoxicity.[13] Concomitant use of alcohol may increase the risk of hepatic injury; a maximum acetaminophen dose of 2.5 g daily is recommended in patients who consume more than two to three alcoholic beverages per day. Acetaminophen does not appear to exacerbate stable, chronic liver disease; it can be used with caution and vigilant monitoring of liver function in this population.[11] Prior to developing an acetaminophen regimen, a careful inventory should be taken of all concomitant medications to minimize the risk of inadvertent acetaminophen overdose from other sources.

Acetaminophen may worsen kidney function and increase blood pressure.[14,15] Nevertheless, acetaminophen remains the preferred analgesic for mild to moderate pain in patients with hypertension or kidney disease because of the greater risks associated with NSAID use.[16] Monitoring specifically for these adverse effects generally is unnecessary.

▶ *Nonsteroidal Anti-inflammatory Drugs*

Prostaglandins play an important role in the function of several organ systems. These compounds are synthesized via the interaction of two isoforms of the cyclooxygenase enzyme (COX-1 and COX-2) with their substrate, arachidonic acid (Fig. 58–3).

The COX-1 enzyme is produced normally in various body tissues (e.g., gastric mucosa, kidney, and platelets). Prostaglandins produced by the actions of the COX-1 enzyme in the GI tract preserve the integrity of the GI mucosa by increasing mucus and bicarbonate secretion, maintaining mucosal blood flow, and decreasing gastric acid secretion. COX-1–associated prostaglandins also promote normal platelet activity and function. In the kidney, COX-1–mediated prostaglandins dilate the afferent arteriole, thereby maintaining intraglomerular pressure and glomerular filtration rate when renal blood flow is reduced.

In contrast, the COX-2 enzyme is not produced normally in most tissues, but its production is increased rapidly in the presence of inflammation and local tissue injury. This change leads to the synthesis of prostaglandins involved in pain and inflammation. Consequently, blocking the COX-2 enzyme results in analgesic and anti-inflammatory effects. The beneficial effects of NSAIDs in reducing pain, decreasing joint stiffness, and improving function in patients with OA are thought to be due to inhibition of the COX-2 enzyme.

All NSAIDs inhibit both COX-1 and COX-2 isoforms to varying degrees, but most (e.g., ibuprofen, naproxen) are not particularly selective for one isoform over the other. That is, they are nonselective inhibitors of the COX enzyme system. Inhibition of COX-2 is responsible for analgesic effects, whereas inhibition of COX-1 is responsible for the most common adverse effects of NSAIDs. COX-2–selective inhibitors were developed to preserve the beneficial effects of COX-2 inhibition while avoiding the deleterious effects associated with inhibition of the COX-1 enzyme. This approach has not been entirely successful, as discussed later.

❻ *NSAIDs are a reasonable adjunctive or alternative therapy when acetaminophen fails to provide an acceptable analgesic response.* Some patients may respond well to topical NSAIDs combined with oral acetaminophen (see Topical Analgesics section later). This strategy minimizes systemic exposure to NSAIDs but is only appropriate for patients with OA of superficial joints. For patients with OA that affects other joints or those receiving no analgesic relief from acetaminophen, an oral NSAID should be considered. Some clinicians recommend NSAIDs over acetaminophen for the initial treatment of severe pain or signs and symptoms of inflammation. The rationale for this recommendation is that acetaminophen's central mechanism of action renders it ineffective against peripheral joint inflammation, and therefore less effective. Results from comparative trials of acetaminophen and NSAIDs have been equivocal, but consensus guidelines support the use of NSAIDs as an alternative to acetaminophen if clinical features of peripheral inflammation or severe pain are present.[7–9] Unfortunately, no validated

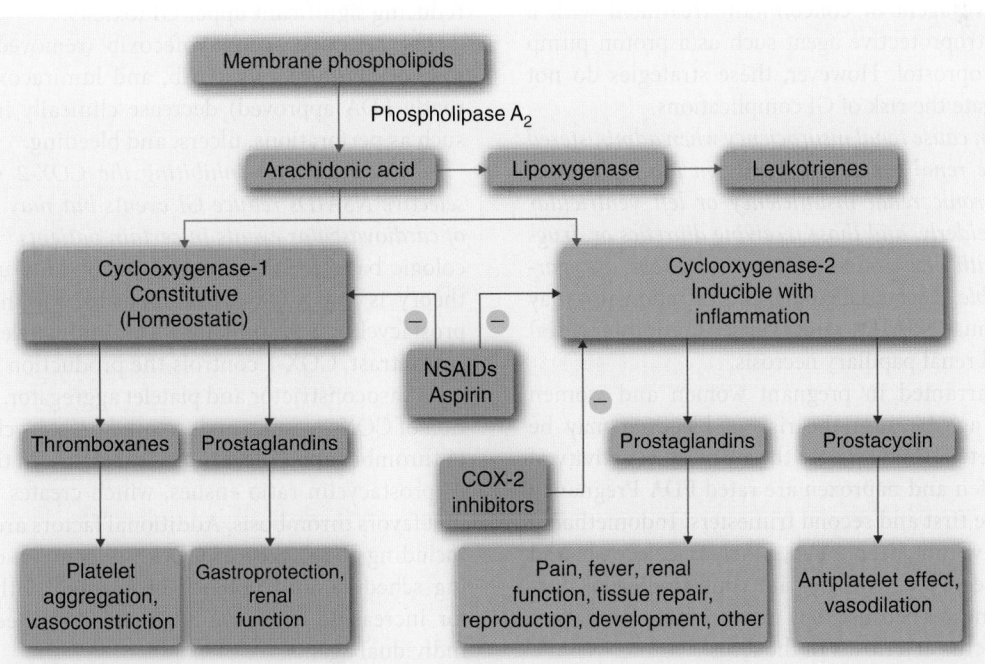

FIGURE 58–3. Synthesis pathway for prostaglandins and leukotrienes. COX-2, cyclooxygenase enzyme 2; NSAIDs, nonsteroidal anti-inflammatory drugs. (Modified from DiPiro JT, Talbert RL, Yee GC, et al (eds.) Pharmacotherapy: A Pathophysiologic Approach. 8th ed. New York: McGraw-Hill; 2011:1609, Fig. 101–5; With permission.)

mechanism exists to identify patients who are more likely to respond to NSAIDs than acetaminophen.

6 *At equipotent doses, the analgesic and anti-inflammatory activity of all oral NSAIDs are similar. The selection of a specific NSAID should be based on patient preference, previous response, tolerability, dosing frequency, and cost.* **7** *Some patients respond to one NSAID better than to another. If an insufficient response is achieved with one NSAID, another agent should be tried.* There is no convincing evidence that changing to an NSAID from a different chemical class is more likely to be effective than selecting another drug from the same chemical class. Pain relief occurs rapidly (within hours), but anti-inflammatory benefits are not realized until after 2 to 3 weeks of continuous therapy. This period is the minimal duration that should be considered an adequate NSAID trial.

Inhibition of the COX-1 enzyme is thought to be responsible primarily for the adverse effects of NSAIDs on the gastric mucosa, kidney, and platelets. Direct irritant effects also may contribute to adverse GI events. **8** *Minor GI complaints, including nausea, dyspepsia, anorexia, abdominal pain, flatulence, and diarrhea, are reported by 10% to 60% of patients treated with NSAIDs. Asymptomatic gastric and duodenal mucosal ulceration can be detected in 15% to 45% of patients.*[17] *Perforation, gastric outlet obstruction, and GI bleeding are the most severe complications and occur in 1.5% to 4% of patients annually.*[17]

Several risk factors predict a greater likelihood of GI complications in NSAID-treated patients (see Chap. 18). Detecting high-risk patients based on symptoms alone is not possible because the presence of symptoms and actual gastroduodenal damage are poorly correlated. Patients at high risk for GI complications should be evaluated for the use of a COX-2–selective agent or concomitant treatment with a prophylactic gastroprotective agent such as a proton pump inhibitor or misoprostol. However, these strategies do not completely mitigate the risk of GI complications.

8 *NSAIDs can cause renal insufficiency when administered to patients whose renal function depends on prostaglandins. Patients with chronic renal insufficiency or left ventricular dysfunction, the elderly, and those receiving diuretics or drugs that interfere with the renin–angiotensin system are particularly susceptible.* Decreased glomerular filtration also may cause hyperkalemia. NSAIDs rarely cause tubulointerstitial nephropathy and renal papillary necrosis.

Caution is warranted in pregnant women and women of childbearing age because the risk of bleeding may be increased if the fetus is subjected to the antiplatelet activity of NSAIDs. Ibuprofen and naproxen are rated FDA Pregnancy Category B in the first and second trimesters. Indomethacin and sulindac have not been rated, whereas celecoxib and etodolac are Category C. NSAIDs are contraindicated during the third trimester because they may promote premature closure of the ductus arteriosus in the fetus.

NSAIDs are prone to drug interactions due to high protein binding, detrimental renal effects, and antiplatelet activity. Interactions are encountered frequently with aspirin, warfarin, oral hypoglycemics, antihypertensives, angiotensin-converting enzyme (ACE) inhibitors, angiotensin receptor blockers (ARBs), β-blockers, diuretics, and lithium. When an interaction with an NSAID is present, vigilant monitoring is warranted for therapeutic efficacy (e.g., NSAIDs blunt the antihypertensive efficacy of diuretics) and adverse effects (e.g., NSAIDs increase the risk of bleeding in anticoagulated patients).

▶ Selective COX-2 Inhibitors

Elucidation of the activities of individual COX isoforms led to the development of drugs that selectively inhibit the inducible form of the enzyme, COX-2. Thus COX-2 inhibitors were expected to minimize NSAID GI toxicity and antiplatelet effects (see Fig. 58–3). **9** *COX-2 inhibitors are no more effective than nonselective NSAIDs in relieving pain and inflammation. In clinical trials, patients experienced similar levels of pain relief with COX-2 inhibitors and nonselective NSAIDs.* This is to be expected because both drug classes inhibit the COX-2 enzyme, which is responsible for producing prostaglandins that result in pain and inflammation.

Celecoxib is the only agent currently marketed in the United States that is classified as a true COX-2–selective inhibitor. However, meloxicam, sulindac, and diclofenac also display preferential affinity for the COX-2 enzyme. Celecoxib reduces endoscopically detected GI lesions. However, the clinical importance of this observation has been challenged because many of these lesions are asymptomatic and resolve spontaneously. Celecoxib did not reduce the incidence of significant upper GI toxicity compared with NSAIDs in a large clinical trial.[18] However, this study allowed patients to take concomitant low-dose aspirin. A post hoc analysis in patients who did not take aspirin revealed celecoxib to be effective in reducing significant upper GI toxicity.

The selective agents rofecoxib (removed from the U.S. market in 2004), etoricoxib, and lumiracoxib (neither currently FDA approved) decrease clinically important events such as perforations, ulcers, and bleeding.[19–21] **9** *By selectively inhibiting the COX-2 isoform, COX-2-selective NSAIDs reduce GI events but may increase the risk of cardiovascular events in certain patients.*[22–24] The pharmacologic basis for this finding is not fully understood. One theory is that COX-2 is responsible for the production of prostacyclin, a vasodilatory and antiplatelet prostaglandin. In contrast, COX-1 controls the production of thromboxane A_2, a vasoconstrictor and platelet aggregator. Selective inhibition of COX-2 results in decreased prostacyclin levels relative to thromboxane A_2 levels. An imbalance in the thromboxane A_2:prostacyclin ratio ensues, which creates an environment that favors thrombosis. Additional factors are likely involved, including the degree of COX-2 selectivity, dosage and dosing schedule, and potency of agents.[22] Other mechanisms for increasing cardiovascular risk have been proposed for individual agents.[25]

Concomitant use of low-dose aspirin mitigates some of the increased cardiovascular risk but also obliterates the GI safety of COX-2 selectivity.[18–20] Patients treated with a COX-2–selective agent plus aspirin experience GI complications at a rate

Table 58–3		
Treatment Options Based on Cardiovascular and Gastrointestinal Risk.		
	High CV Risk	Low CV Risk
High GI risk	NS-NSAID[a] *plus* gastroprotection[b]	COX-2[c] *or* NS-NSAID + gastroprotection[b]
Low GI risk	NS-NSAID[a]	NS-NSAID

COX-2, selective cyclooxygenase-2 inhibitor; CV, cardiovascular; NS-NSAID, non-selective nonsteroidal anti-inflammatory drug.

[a]Naproxen may be considered initially due to potentially lower CV risk compared with other NS-NSAIDs.

[b]Gastroprotection with either a proton pump inhibitor (preferred) or misoprostol.

[c]A COX-2 inhibitor + gastroprotection can be recommended for patients at very high GI risk (e.g., previous upper GI bleed attributable to NS-NSAID therapy).

commensurate with that of patients given traditional nonselective NSAIDs. Use of less selective agents (e.g., meloxicam) to avoid cardiovascular concerns with COX-2 inhibitors may not be justified because neither GI nor cardiovascular safety is optimized.

⑨ *COX-2 inhibitors should be reserved for patients at high risk for GI complications and low risk for cardiovascular events* (Table 58–3). For patients at particularly high GI risk (e.g., previous history of NSAID-induced GI bleed), a COX-2 inhibitor may be combined with a proton pump inhibitor.[26,27] In patients at risk for GI events and cardiovascular disease, a nonselective NSAID plus a proton pump inhibitor is a reasonable option. Naproxen appears to have the least cardiovascular risk of the nonselective NSAIDs and should generally be considered first in such patients.[28]

The COX-2 enzyme is also produced normally in the kidney; thus COX-2 inhibitors exert renal effects similar to those of conventional NSAIDs. Both drug classes may increase sodium reabsorption and fluid retention and can provoke renal insufficiency and hyperkalemia. COX-2 inhibitors should be used with caution in patients with heart failure or hypertension.

COX-2 inhibitors are susceptible to the same drug interactions as nonselective agents. However, the interaction with warfarin is less pronounced because platelet function is affected to a lesser degree.

▶ Glucosamine and Chondroitin

Glucosamine is believed to function as a "chondroprotective" agent, stimulating the cartilage matrix and protecting against oxidative chemical damage. Chondroitin, often administered in conjunction with glucosamine, is thought to inhibit degradative enzymes and serve as a substrate for the production of proteoglycans. Numerous clinical trials have evaluated the efficacy of these substances for the treatment

of OA. However, results vary widely, and the quality of many of these studies has been questioned.

In the landmark GAIT trial sponsored by the U.S. National Institutes of Health, glucosamine, chondroitin, and their combination were no more effective than placebo in decreasing pain symptoms in patients with knee OA after 24 weeks.[29] In the subgroup of patients with moderate to severe OA pain, the combination of glucosamine and chondroitin appeared to have a moderate effect, although this subgroup analysis must be interpreted with caution. Analysis of radiologic changes after 2 years of treatment showed no significant benefit of glucosamine, chondroitin sulfate, or the combination over placebo in preventing joint space narrowing.[30] In contrast, most industry-funded studies, many of which are limited by suboptimal study designs, have observed a significantly greater benefit with glucosamine, chondroitin, or the combination.[31] Interpretation of these results is all the more challenging given the inconsistencies in study design, differences in end points applied, quality of glucosamine preparations, and the comparator agents (celecoxib versus acetaminophen).

⑩ *In the context of study limitations, glucosamine and chondroitin appear to modestly reduce pain and improve mobility.*[31–33] *They also may slow disease progression by decreasing the rate of cartilage destruction, although the clinical impact of this effect is not clear.*[34] Glucosamine is not effective for treating acute pain since beneficial effects often mature over a period of weeks. Despite some studies suggesting the contrary, either glucosamine salt (hydrochloride or sulfate) can be recommended; both dissociate in stomach acid to the same amino sugar, glucosamine. Because these agents are loosely regulated in the United States as dietary supplements, product standards are inconsistent, and the constituents are not validated by any regulatory agency.

The use of glucosamine (derived from crab, lobster, or shrimp shells) and/or chondroitin (derived from cattle or shark cartilage) may warrant caution in patients with shellfish allergies, but preliminary evidence suggests little drug-allergy interaction.[35] Additionally, glucosamine may alter cellular glucose uptake, thus elevating blood glucose levels in diabetic patients.[36] A randomized, placebo-controlled trial of 38 diabetic participants failed to detect any significant alteration in A1C levels after 3 months of glucosamine/chondroitin therapy; however, a relatively short study period and low number of participants may account for these negative findings.[37] Blood glucose levels in diabetic patients should be monitored closely after glucosamine initiation or dosage adjustments. Given the favorable safety profile of glucosamine and chondroitin, it is reasonable to present these agents as a treatment option to patients with symptomatic knee OA in the absence of contraindicating factors.

▶ Intraarticular Therapy

⑩ *Intraarticular injection of corticosteroids or hyaluronan represents an alternative to oral agents for the treatment of joint pain.* These modalities usually are reserved for patients unresponsive to other treatments because of the relative invasiveness of intraarticular injections compared with oral drugs, the small risk of infection, and the cost of the procedure.

Hyaluronan (Hyaluronic Acid) The mechanism of action of hyaluronan is not fully understood. Healthy cartilage and synovial fluid are replete with hyaluronic acid, a viscous substance believed to facilitate lubrication and shock absorbency under varying conditions of load bearing. Patients with OA demonstrate an absolute and functional decline in hyaluronic acid; thus exogenous administration is referred to as viscosupplementation. In responders, the benefit of hyaluronan administration persists for periods that exceed its residence time in the synovium, suggesting that benefits beyond viscoelasticity are involved. Inhibition of inflammatory mediators and cartilage degradation, stimulation of the cartilage matrix, neuroprotective actions, and the ability of hyaluronan to induce its own synthesis may account in part for the benefit.

Pain and joint function have been evaluated frequently in clinical trials administering hyaluronan to patients with OA. Results are conflicting, with some suggesting dramatic improvements and others indicating no effect. A meta-analysis found that hyaluronan injections achieved a moderate reduction in pain at 7 to 10 weeks post-injection, compared with placebo.[38] This effect was generally similar to previously published effect sizes for acetaminophen, oral NSAIDs, and COX-2 inhibitors. Hyaluronan provides greater pain relief for a longer time than intraarticular corticosteroids, but corticosteroids work more rapidly.[39]

Several formulations of hyaluronan are available for the treatment of knee pain in patients with OA who are unresponsive to other measures. Administration typically consists of weekly injections for 3 to 5 weeks, depending on the specific product. Most injections are well tolerated, although some patients may report local reactions. Rarely, postinjection flares and anaphylaxis have been reported. Intraarticular injection is associated with a low risk of infection (approximately 1 joint in 50,000 injections). Patients should be counseled to minimize activity and stress on the joint for several days after each injection.

Corticosteroids Use of systemic corticosteroids is discouraged in patients with OA. ❿ *However, in a subset of patients with an inflammatory component or knee effusion, intraarticular corticosteroids can be useful as monotherapy or as an adjunct to analgesics.*[39] The affected joint can be aspirated and subsequently injected with a corticosteroid. The aspirate should be examined for the presence of crystalline formation and infection. Pain reliefs begins within days after the injection but may not persist beyond 4 weeks. A single joint should not be injected more than three to five times per year.

The crystalline nature of corticosteroid suspensions can provoke a postinjection flare in some patients. The ensuing flare mimics the flare of arthritis and inflammation that accompanies infection. Cold compresses and analgesics are recommended to treat symptoms in affected patients.

▶ *Tramadol*

Use of opioid analgesics may be warranted when pain is unresponsive to other pharmacologic agents or when such agents are contraindicated. Tramadol is an oral, centrally acting synthetic opioid analgesic that also weakly inhibits the reuptake of serotonin and norepinephrine. It is effective for treatment of moderate pain but is devoid of anti-inflammatory activity. Compared with conventional opioid analgesics, tramadol has a low abuse potential and is not scheduled as a controlled substance in the United States.

Tramadol is a reasonable option for patients with contraindications to NSAIDs or failure to respond to other oral therapies. ❿ *For the treatment of hip or knee OA, tramadol can be effective in carefully selected patients.*[40] *The addition of tramadol to NSAIDs or acetaminophen may augment the analgesic effects of a failing regimen, thereby securing sufficient pain relief in some patients.* Moreover, concomitant tramadol may permit the use of lower NSAID doses. However, the increased risk for side effects associated with tramadol may offset the benefits.[40]

Dizziness, vertigo, nausea, vomiting, constipation, and lethargy are all relatively common adverse events. These effects are more pronounced for several days after initiation and following upward dose titration. Seizures have been reported rarely; the risk is dose-related and appears to increase with concomitant use of antidepressants, such as tricyclic antidepressants or selective serotonin reuptake inhibitors. Tramadol should be avoided in patients receiving monoamine oxidase (MAO) inhibitors because tramadol inhibits the uptake of norepinephrine and serotonin.

▶ *Other Opioid Analgesics*

Opioids decrease pain, improve sleep patterns, and increase functioning in patients with OA who are unresponsive to nonpharmacologic therapy and nonopioid analgesics. Use of opioid analgesics for nonmalignant pain is increasing. Evidence suggests that patients can achieve satisfactory analgesia by using nonescalating doses of opioids with minimal risk of addiction.[41] However, clinically significant improvement in pain that is nonresponsive to NSAIDs has only been demonstrated with stronger opioids. Oxycodone is the most extensively studied of the opioids recommended for OA. However, other agents such as morphine, hydromorphone, methadone, and transdermal fentanyl are also effective.[42] The American Pain Society (APS) recommends against using codeine for OA because of the high incidence of adverse effects and limited analgesic effectiveness.[43]

❿ *Opioid analgesics should be reserved for patients who experience moderate to severe pain and do not respond to or are not candidates for other pharmacologic and nonpharmacologic strategies. Opioids also may be useful in patients with conditions that preclude the use of NSAIDs, such as renal failure, heart failure, or anticoagulation.*

These agents should be initiated at low doses in combination with acetaminophen or an NSAID when possible. Combining opioids with other analgesics reduces the opioid requirement, thereby minimizing adverse events. However, use of combination opioid products containing acetaminophen should be accompanied by clear instructions to limit additional over-the-counter acetaminophen use. Conservative initial doses of opioids are warranted, with the dose titrated to adequate response with minimal side effects. Even with these conservative strategies, adverse effects are common. In clinical trials, more than 80% of opioid-treated patients experienced at least one adverse event, compared with approximately 50% of placebo-treated patients.[42]

If opioid therapy is considered, there should be an initial comprehensive medical history and physical examination, firm documentation that nonopioid therapy has failed, clearly defined treatment goals, an understanding between the provider and the patient of the true benefits and risks of long-term opioids, use of a single provider and pharmacy whenever possible, and comprehensive follow-up.

▶ Topical Analgesics

Topical analgesics sometimes are used for mild pain or as an adjunct to systemic therapy. There are limited data to support the use of salicylate-containing rubefacients (e.g., methyl salicylate and trolamine salicylate) or other counter-irritants (e.g., menthol, camphor, and methyl nicotinate) in OA.[44] See Chap. 60 for more information on these products when used for musculoskeletal disorders.

Capsaicin achieves pain relief by depleting substance P from sensory neurons in the spine, thereby decreasing pain transmission. Capsaicin is not effective for acute pain; pain relief may take up to 2 weeks with daily administration. Capsaicin may provide the greatest benefit to painful superficial joints (e.g., hand OA). Most patients experience a local burning sensation at the site of application. The discomfort usually does not result in discontinuation and often abates within the first week. Patients should be cautioned not to allow capsaicin to come into contact with eyes or mucous membranes and to wash their hands after each application.

⑩ Topical NSAID preparations are effective for treating OA involving the superficial joints of the hands, wrists, elbows, knees, ankles, or feet. Administration via a topical vehicle targets the joints involved and decreases systemic exposure while providing pain relief comparable to that of oral NSAIDs. This may be an attractive option for patients at risk of developing adverse events from oral NSAIDs.

Diclofenac sodium gel 1% is the only commercially available topical NSAID in the United States; it decreases pain and improves joint function in patients with hand or knee OA.[45,46] Systemic absorption of topical diclofenac is approximately 17 times lower than that seen with oral diclofenac. Thus GI, cardiovascular, and renal adverse effects would not be expected with proper administration. The most common adverse effects include application site dermatitis, pruritus, and phototoxicity.

Surgery

⑩ Surgery generally is reserved for patients who fail to respond to medical therapy and have progressive limitations in activities of daily living (ADL). In joint replacement surgery (arthroplasty), the damaged joint surfaces are replaced with metal or plastic prosthetic devices. Hip and knee joints are most commonly replaced, but arthroplasty may also be performed on shoulders, elbows, fingers, and ankles. Most patients achieve significant pain relief and functional restoration after arthroplasty, and it is a reasonable option in carefully selected refractory patients.

Surgical debridement may be performed arthroscopically. With this procedure, a tiny video camera is inserted into the affected joint through a small incision, and the surgeon removes torn cartilage or other debris from the joint. The long-term benefits of arthroscopic surgery for OA are unclear, and it may be no better than optimized physical and medical therapy.[47]

Patient Encounter, Part 2: Medical History, Physical Examination, and Diagnostic Tests

PMH: Obesity (BMI 30 kg/m^2), HTN × 24 years, dyslipidemia, MI 19 years ago, COPD

PSH: Torn ACL repair on right knee 15 years ago

FH: Father had OA of the hip and knee; mother died of MI at age 68

SH: Retired factory worker. Drinks 1 to 2 beers/night; denies illicit drug use; smoked two packs of cigarettes per day for 35 years but quit 3 years ago

Allergies: NKDA; shellfish allergy

Meds: Chlorthalidone 25 mg once daily, metoprolol succinate 100 mg once daily, atorvastatin 80 mg once daily, enteric-coated aspirin 81 mg once daily, tiotropium 18 mcg once daily, albuterol 90 mcg as needed for wheezing/shortness of breath, acetaminophen 500 mg, 1 to 2 tablets 2 to 4 times/day as needed for pain.

Vital signs: BP 135/82 mm Hg, pulse 71 beats/min, RR 16 breaths/min, temperature 98.6°F (37.0°C).

Labs: Not obtained.

Radiology: Radiography of the affected knee shows joint space narrowing, minor osteophyte formation, and subchondral bone sclerosis.

What clinical parameters are consistent with a diagnosis of OA?

What are the treatment goals for this patient?

What nonpharmacologic options are available to treat this patient?

What pharmacologic options are available to treat this patient?

What factors are important to consider when selecting medications for this patient?

Patient Encounter, Part 3: Creating a Care Plan

Based on the available information, create a care plan for this patient's OA. The plan should include:

(a) A statement of the drug-related needs and/or problems

(b) An individualized, detailed therapeutic plan

(c) A plan for follow-up monitoring to document the patient's response and identify adverse reactions

Patient Care and Monitoring

1. Determine whether the patient's symptoms are consistent with OA. Review the medical history to determine whether other rheumatologic diseases may be involved.

2. Assess symptoms to determine whether pain warrants additional attention. Does the pain affect quality of life or interfere with activities of daily living?

3. Evaluate symptoms to determine what nonpharmacologic interventions can be recommended and whether pharmacologic treatment is warranted.

4. Obtain a thorough history of previous drug use, including prescription drugs, over-the-counter drugs, and dietary supplements. Determine whether and to what extent any of these treatments have been effective. Ask the patient about the dose and frequency of previous pharmacologic agents to determine whether an adequate trial was given.

5. Educate the patient about appropriate use of nonpharmacologic treatments for OA.

6. Formulate a drug therapy plan, taking into consideration the patient's medical history, concomitant medications, and previous use of medications.

7. Develop a plan to monitor the patient's response to therapy.

8. Evaluate for the presence of adverse drug reactions, drug hypersensitivity, and drug interactions.

9. Document whether the patient has had improvements in quality-of-life measures, such as improved functioning, increased ability to perform activities of daily living, and improved well-being.

10. Emphasize the value of adherence to medication regimens and lifestyle modifications. Facilitate adherence by implementing medication regimens and lifestyle plans that are simple and consistent with the patient's lifestyle.

11. Educate the patient about OA, lifestyle modifications, and medications.

OUTCOME EVALUATION

- At baseline, quantify the patient's pain using a visual analogue scale, assess range of motion of affected joints, and identify activities of daily living that are impaired.

- In patients treated with acetaminophen or oral NSAIDs, assess pain control after 2 to 3 weeks. It may take longer for the full anti-inflammatory effect of NSAIDs to ccur.

- Incorporate other measures to track disease progress. Use radiography to assess severity of joint destruction, determine 50-ft walking time and grip strength, and administer the Western Ontario and McMaster Universities Osteoarthritis Index (WOMAC) and the Stanford Health Assessment Questionnaire, where appropriate, to assess activities of daily living.

- Ask patients if they are experiencing side effects or other problems with their medications and follow-up with more specific questions.

- In patients taking oral NSAIDs, monitor for increases in blood pressure, weight gain, edema, skin rash, and CNS adverse effects such as headaches and drowsiness.

- Evaluate serum creatinine, complete blood count, and serum transaminases at baseline and at every 6 to 12 months in patients treated with oral NSAIDs or acetaminophen.

- Perform stool guaiac in patients taking oral NSAIDs when clinically indicated.

- Monitor for drug interactions, including alcohol, at every visit.

Abbreviations Introduced in This Chapter

ACR	American College of Rheumatology
APS	American Pain Society
COX	Cyclooxygenase
DJD	Degenerative joint disease
MMP	Matrix metalloproteinases
NSAID	Nonsteroidal anti-inflammatory drug
OA	Osteoarthritis
WOMAC	Western Ontario and McMaster Universities Osteoarthritis Index

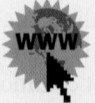 Self-assessment questions and answers are available at *http://www.mhpharmacotherapy.com/pp.html*.

REFERENCES

1. Centers for Disease Control and Prevention. National and state medical expenditures and lost earnings attributable to arthritis and other rheumatic conditions—United States, 2003. MMWR Morb Mortal Wkly Rep 2007;56(1):4–7.

2. Centers for Disease Control and Prevention. Prevalence of disabilities and associated health conditions among adults—United States, 1999. MMWR Morb Mortal Wkly Rep 2001;50:120–125.

3. The National Arthritis Data Workgroup. Estimates of the prevalence of arthritis and other rheumatic conditions in the United States: Part II. Arthritis Rheum 2008;58:26–35.

4. Bijlsma JWJ, Berenbaum F, Lafeber FPJG. Osteoarthritis: An update with relevance for clinical practice. Lancet 2011;377:2115–2126.

5. McAlindon TE, Wilson PW, Aliabadi P, et al. Level of physical activity and the risk of radiographic and symptomatic knee osteoarthritis in the elderly: The Framingham Study. Am J Med 1999;106:151–157.

6. Fife RS. Epidemiology, pathology, and pathogenesis. In: Klippel JH, ed. Primer on Rheumatic Diseases. 11th ed. Atlanta, GA: Arthritis Foundation; 1997:216–217.

7. Zhang W, Moskowitz RW, Nuki G, et al. OARSI recommendations for the management of hip and knee osteoarthritis, Part II: OARSI evidence-based, expert consensus guidelines. Osteoarthr Cartil 2008;16:137–162.

8. American College of Rheumatology Subcommittee on Osteoarthritis Guidelines. Recommendations for the medical management of osteoarthritis of the hip and knee: 2000 update. Arthritis Rheum 2000;43:1905–1915.

9. American Pain Society. Guideline for the management of pain in osteoarthritis, rheumatoid arthritis, and juvenile chronic arthritis. American Pain Society 2002;2:43–74.

10. Towheed TE, Maxwell L, Judd MG, et al. Acetaminophen for osteoarthritis. Cochrane Database Syst Rev 2006;(1): CD004257.

11. Graham GG, Scott KF, Day RO. Tolerability of paracetamol. Drug Saf 2005;28:227–240.

12. Larson AM, Polson J, Fontana RJ, et al. Acetaminophen-induced acute liver failure: results of a United States multicenter prospective study. Hepatology 2005;42:1364–1372.

13. Watkins PB, Kaplowitz N, Slattery JT, et al. Aminotransferase elevations in healthy adults receiving 4 grams of acetaminophen daily. JAMA 2006;296:87–93.

14. Fored CM, Ejerblad E, Lindblad P, et al. Acetaminophen, aspirin, and chronic renal failure. N Engl J Med 2001;345:1801–1808.

15. Curhan GC, Knight EL, Rosner B, et al. Lifetime non-narcotic analgesic use and decline in renal function in women. Arch Intern Med 2004;164:1519–1524.

16. Forman JP, Stampfer MJ, Curhan GC. Non-narcotic analgesic dose and risk of incident hypertension in U.S. women. Hypertension 2005;46:500–507.

17. Laine L. Approaches to nonsteroidal anti-inflammatory drug use in the high-risk patient. Gastroenterology 2001;120:594–606.

18. Silverstein FE, Faich G, Goldstein JL, et al. Gastrointestinal toxicity with celecoxib vs nonsteroidal anti-inflammatory drugs for osteoarthritis and rheumatoid arthritis: The CLASS study: A randomized controlled trial. Celecoxib Long-term Arthritis Safety Study. JAMA 2000;284:1247–1255.

19. Bombardier C, Laine L, Reicin A, et al. VIGOR Study Group. Comparison of upper gastrointestinal toxicity of rofecoxib and naproxen in patients with rheumatoid arthritis. N Engl J Med 2000;343:1520–1528.

20. Schnitzer TJ, Burmester GR, Mysler E, et al. Comparison of lumiracoxib with naproxen and ibuprofen in the Therapeutic Arthritis Research and Gastrointestinal Event Trial (TARGET), reduction in ulcer complications: Randomised controlled trial. Lancet 2004;364:665–674.

21. Laine L, Curtis SP, Cryer B, et al. Assessment of upper gastrointestinal safety of etoricoxib and diclofenac in patients with osteoarthritis and rheumatoid arthritis in the multinational etoricoxib and diclofenac arthritis long-term (MEDAL) programme: A randomised comparison. Lancet 2007;369:465–473.

22. Solomon SD, Wittes J, Finn PV, et al. Cardiovascular risk of celecoxib in 6 randomized placebo-controlled trials: the cross trial safety analysis. Circulation 2008;117:2104–2113.

23. McGettigan P, Henry D. Cardiovascular risk and inhibition of cyclooxygenase: a systematic review of the observational studies of selective and nonselective inhibitors of cyclooxygenase 2. JAMA 2006;296:1633–1644.

24. Bresalier RS, Sandler RS, Quan H, et al. Cardiovascular events associated with rofecoxib in a colorectal adenoma chemoprevention trial. N Engl J Med 2005;352:1092–1102.

25. Zarraga IG, Schwarz ER. Coxibs and heart disease: What we have learned and what else we need to know. J Am Coll Cardiol 2007;49:1–14.

26. Chan FKL, Wong VWS, Suen BY, et al. Combination of a cyclooxygenase-2 inhibitor and a proton-pump inhibitor for prevention of recurrent ulcer bleeding in patients at very high risk: a double-blind, randomized trial. Lancet 2007;369:1621–1626.

27. Rahme E, Barkun AN, Toubouti Y, et al. Do proton-pump inhibitors confer additional gastrointestinal protection in patients given celecoxib? Arthritis Rheum 2007;57:748–755.

28. Trelle S, Reichenbach S, Wandel W, et al. Cardiovascular safety of non-steroidal anti-inflammatory drugs: network meta-analysis. BMJ 2011;342:c7086.

29. Clegg DO, Reda DJ, Harris CL, et al. Glucosamine, chondroitin sulfate, and the two in combination for painful knee osteoarthritis. N Engl J Med 2006;354:795–808.

30. Sawitzke AD, Shi H, Finco MF, et al. The effect of glucosamine and/or chondroitin sulfate on the progression of knee osteoarthritis. Arthritis Rheum 2008;58:3183–3191.

31. Wandel S, Jüni P, Tendal B, et al. Effects of glucosamine, chondroitin, or placebo in patients with osteoarthritis of hip or knee: network meta-analysis. BMJ 2010;341:c4675.

32. Richy F, Bruyere O, Ethgen O, et al. Structural and symptomatic efficacy of glucosamine and chondroitin in knee osteoarthritis: A comprehensive meta-analysis. Arch Intern Med 2003;163:1514–1522.

33. Vlad SC, LaValley MP, McAlindon TE, Felson DT. Glucosamine for pain in osteoarthritis: Why do trial results differ? Arthritis Rheum 2007;56:2267–2277.

34. Reginster JY, Deroisy R, Rovati LC, et al. Long-term effects of glucosamine sulphate on osteoarthritis progression: A randomised, placebo-controlled clinical trial. Lancet 2001;357:251–256.

35. Gray HC, Hutcheson PS, Gray RG. Is glucosamine safe in patients with seafood allergy? J Allergy Clin Immunol 2004;114:459–460.

36. Dostrovsky NR, Towheed TE, Hudson RW, Anastassiades TP. The effect of glucosamine on glucose metabolism in humans: a systematic review of the literature. Osteoarthritis Cartilage 2011;19:375–380.

37. Scroggie DA, Albright A, Harris MD. The effect of glucosamine-chondroitin supplementation on glycosylated hemoglobin levels in patients with type 2 diabetes mellitus. Arch Intern Med 2003;163:1587–1590.

38. Bannuru RR, Natov NS, Dasi UR, et al. Therapeutic trajectory following intra-articular hyaluronic acid injection in knee osteoarthritis—meta-analysis. Osteoarthr Cartil 2011;19(6):611–619.

39. Bellamy N, Campbell J, Robinson V, et al. Intraarticular corticosteroid for treatment of osteoarthritis of the knee. Cochrane Database Syst Rev 2006;(2):CD005328.

40. Cepeda MS, Camargo F, Zea C, Valencia L. Tramadol for osteoarthritis. Cochrane Database Syst Rev 2006;3:CD005522.

41. Ballantyne JC, Mao J. Opioid therapy for chronic pain. N Engl J Med 2003;349:1943–1953.

42. Nüesch E, Rutjes AW, Husni E, et al. Oral or transdermal opioids for osteoarthritis of the knee or hip. Cochrane Database Syst Rev 2009;4:CD003115.

43. The American Academy of Pain Medicine, the American Pain Society: The use of opioids for the treatment of chronic pain: A consensus statement from the American Academy of Pain Medicine and the American Pain Society. Clin J Pain 1997;13:6–8.

44. Mason L, Moore RA, Edwards JE, et al. Systematic review of efficacy of topical rubefacients containing salicylates for the treatment of acute and chronic pain. BMJ 2004;328:995–998.

45. Baraf HS, Gloth FM, Barthel HR, et al. Safety and efficacy of topical diclofenac sodium gel for knee osteoarthritis in elderly and younger patients: pooled data from three randomized, double-blind, parallel-group, placebo-controlled, multicentre trials. Drugs Aging 2011;28:27–40.

46. Altman RD, Dreiser RL, Fisher CL. Diclofenac sodium gel in patients with primary hand osteoathritis: A randomized, double-blind, placebo-controlled trial. J Rheumatol 2009;36(9):1991–1999.

47. Kirkley A, Birmingham TB, Litchfield RB, et al. A randomized trial of arthroscopic surgery for osteoarthritis of the knee. N Engl J Med 2008;359:1097–1107.

59

Gout and Hyperuricemia

Geoffrey C. Wall

KEY CONCEPTS

❶ Gout results from deposition of uric acid crystals in joint spaces, leading to an inflammatory reaction that causes intense pain, erythema, and joint swelling.

❷ Some drugs can cause hyperuricemia and gout, such as thiazide diuretics, niacin, pyrazinamide, cyclosporine, and, occasionally, low-dose aspirin.

❸ Long-term consequences of gout and hyperuricemia include joint destruction, tophi, and nephrolithiasis.

❹ Treatment of gout involves: (a) acute relief of a gouty arthritis attack, and (b) in some patients, long-term maintenance treatment to prevent future attacks.

❺ Nonsteroidal anti-inflammatory drugs, colchicine, or corticosteroids are used for acute attacks. Selection depends on several patient factors, especially renal function.

❻ Asymptomatic hyperuricemia usually does not require treatment.

❼ Patients with recurrent attacks, evidence of tophi or joint destruction, or uric acid nephrolithiasis are candidates for maintenance therapy with allopurinol, febuxostat, probenecid, or pegloticase to lower SUA levels.

❽ Tumor lysis syndrome (TLS) is a metabolic disorder caused by rapid cell destruction (usually during chemotherapy treatment for cancer) and is associated with several electrolyte disturbances, notably hyperuricemia.

EPIDEMIOLOGY AND ETIOLOGY

Gout is the most common inflammatory arthritis in the United States and western Europe.[1] The annual incidence is approximately 62 cases per 100,000 persons in the United States.[2] The incidence increases with age and appears to be rising, probably because of a larger number of patients with risk factors for gout.[3]

PATHOPHYSIOLOGY

Gout is caused by an abnormality in uric acid metabolism. Uric acid is a waste product of the breakdown of purines contained in the DNA of degraded body cells and dietary protein. Uric acid is water soluble and excreted primarily by the kidneys, although some is broken down by colonic bacteria and excreted via the GI tract.[4,5]

The solubility of uric acid depends on concentration and temperature. At high serum concentrations, lower body temperature causes the precipitation of monosodium urate (MSU) crystals. Collections of these crystals (called microtophi) can form in joint spaces in the distal extremities.

❶ *Gout results from deposition of uric acid crystals in joint spaces, leading to an inflammatory reaction that causes intense pain, erythema, and joint swelling.* Free urate crystals can activate several proinflammatory mediators, including tumor necrosis factor α (TNF-α), interleukin 1 (IL-1), and IL-8. Activation of these mediators signals chemotactic movement of neutrophils into the joint space that "ingest" MSU crystals via phagocytosis. These neutrophils then are lysed and release proteolytic enzymes that trigger the clinical manifestations of an acute gout attack, such as pain and swelling. These inflammatory mechanisms in gout, especially in untreated disease, can lead to cartilage and joint destruction.

The increased serum uric acid (SUA) involves either the underexcretion of uric acid (80% of patients) or its overproduction. The cause of overproduction or underexcretion of uric acid in most gout patients is unknown; this is referred to as *primary gout*.[2]

The reference range for SUA is 3.6 to 8.3 mg/dL (214 to 494 μmol/L). The risk of gout increases as the SUA concentration increases. Approximately 30% of patients with levels greater than 10 mg/dL (595 μmol/L) develop symptoms of gout within 5 years.[3] However, most patients with hyperuricemia are asymptomatic. Other risk factors for gout include male gender, obesity, ethanol use (particularly beer and spirits), hypertension, and dyslipidemia.[4–7] Gout occurs frequently in patients with type 2 diabetes mellitus and coronary artery disease, but a causal relationship has not been established. Preliminary investigations have suggested a possible role of hyperuricemia in the progression of chronic kidney disease.[8]

Uric acid excretion is reduced in patients with chronic kidney disease, putting them at risk for hyperuricemia. In patients with persistently acidic urine and hyperuricemia, uric acid **nephrolithiasis** can occur in up to 25% of patients; in severe cases, uric acid stones can cause nephropathy and renal failure.[9] Extreme hyperuricemia can occur because of rapid tumor cell destruction in patients undergoing chemotherapy for certain types of cancer. This phenomenon is known as **tumor lysis syndrome** (TLS).

❷ *Some drugs can cause hyperuricemia and gout, such as thiazide diuretics, niacin, pyrazinamide, cyclosporine, and, occasionally, low-dose aspirin. In most cases, these drugs block uric acid secretion in the kidney.* ❸ *Long-term consequences of gout and hyperuricemia include joint destruction, tophi, and nephrolithiasis.*

CLINICAL PRESENTATION AND DIAGNOSIS

Aspiration of affected joint fluid is essential for a definitive diagnosis. Joint fluid containing negatively birefringent MSU crystals confirms the diagnosis. Joint fluid has an elevated white blood cell (WBC) count with neutrophils predominating (**Fig. 59–1**).[10]

Although rarely performed, a 24-hour urine collection can be obtained to determine whether the patient is an overproducer or an underexcretor of uric acid. Individuals who excrete more than 800 mg of uric acid in this collection are considered overproducers. Patients with hyperuricemia who excrete less than 600 mg/day (3.57 mmol/day) are classified as underexcretors of uric acid.

Radiographs of affected joints may have characteristic appearances of gout, including cystic changes, punched-out lytic lesions with overhanging bony edges, and soft-tissue calcified masses. These signs may appear in other arthropathies as well.[11]

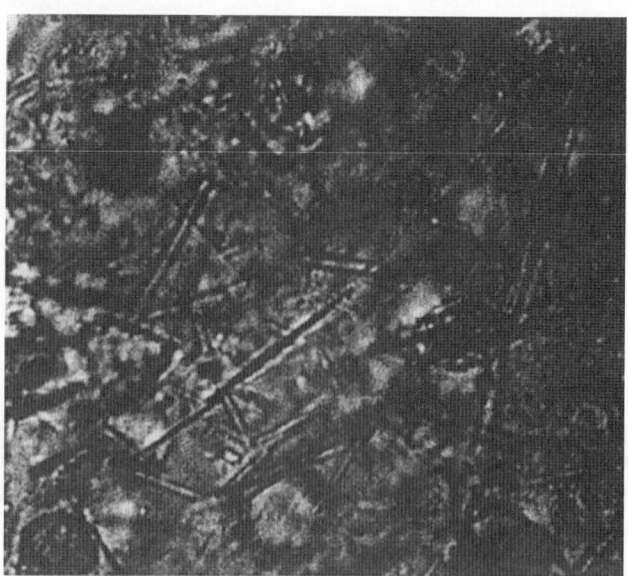

FIGURE 59–1. Synovial fluid containing extracellular and intracellular monosodium urate crystals. (From Schumacher HR, Chen LX. Gout and other crystal arthropathies. In: Fauci AS, Braunwald E, Kasper DL, et al., eds. Harrison's Principles of Internal Medicine. 17th ed. New York: McGraw-Hill; 2008:2166, Fig. 327–1. With permission.)

Clinical Presentation and Diagnosis of Acute Gouty Arthritis

General
- Patients are usually in acute distress.

Symptoms
- There is severe pain, swelling, and warmth in the affected joint(s).
- The attack is usually monoarticular; the most common sites are the metatarsophalangeal and knee joints.
- In elderly patients, gouty attacks may be atypical with insidious and polyarticular onset, often involving hand or wrist joints.

Signs
- Affected joint(s) are warm, erythematous, and swollen.
- Mild fever may be present.
- Tophi (usually on hands, wrists, elbows, or knees) may be present in chronic, severe disease.

Laboratory Tests
- The peripheral WBC count may be only mildly elevated.
- The serum uric acid level often is elevated but may be normal during an acute attack.
- Other laboratory markers of inflammation (e.g., increased erythrocyte sedimentation rate) are often present.

TREATMENT

④ *Treatment of gout involves: (a) acute relief of a gouty arthritis attack, and (b) in some patients, long-term maintenance treatment to prevent future attacks.*

Desired Outcomes

● The goals of therapy of an acute attack are: (a) achieving rapid and effective pain relief, (b) maintaining joint function, (c) preventing disease complications, (d) avoiding treatment-related adverse effects, (e) providing cost-effective therapy, and (f) improving quality of life.[12] Infrequent gouty arthritis is a self-limited disease, and treatment usually focuses on symptom relief.

Nonpharmacologic Therapy

Nondrug modalities play an adjunctive role and usually are not effective when used alone. Immobilization of the affected extremity speeds resolution of the attack. Applying ice packs to the joint also decreases pain and swelling, but heat application may be detrimental.[13]

Pharmacologic Therapy

⑤ *Nonsteroidal anti-inflammatory drugs (NSAIDs), colchicine, and corticosteroids are used for acute attacks. Selection depends on several patient factors, especially renal function* (Fig. 59–2). *Each drug class has a unique safety and efficacy profile in gout that should be considered carefully before choosing a specific agent* (Table 59–1). Generally, the earlier in the course of the arthritic attack these agents are employed, the better the outcome. Other analgesics such as opioids have little to no role in the treatment of acute gout, which results from overwhelming inflammation.[14]

▶ Nonsteroidal Anti-inflammatory Drugs

● The NSAIDs largely have supplanted colchicine as the treatment of choice, and many NSAIDs have been used successfully. These agents are most effective when given within the first 24 hours of the onset of pain. Most studies have shown similar results among agents, and all NSAIDs are considered to be effective. Doses at the higher end of the therapeutic range are often needed.[15] NSAIDs are usually continued until 24 hours after symptoms subside.

Indomethacin was used traditionally, but its relative cyclooxygenase-1 (COX-1) selectivity theoretically increases its gastropathy risk. Thus other generic NSAIDs may be preferred. Adverse effects of NSAIDs include gastropathy (primarily peptic ulcers), renal dysfunction, and fluid retention.[16] NSAIDs generally should be avoided in patients at risk for peptic ulcers, those taking warfarin, and those with renal insufficiency or uncontrolled hypertension or heart failure. Theoretically, gastroprotective agents such as proton-pump inhibitors may protect against the development of ulcers in patients receiving NSAIDs for an acute gouty flare, but no studies to date have investigated this concept.

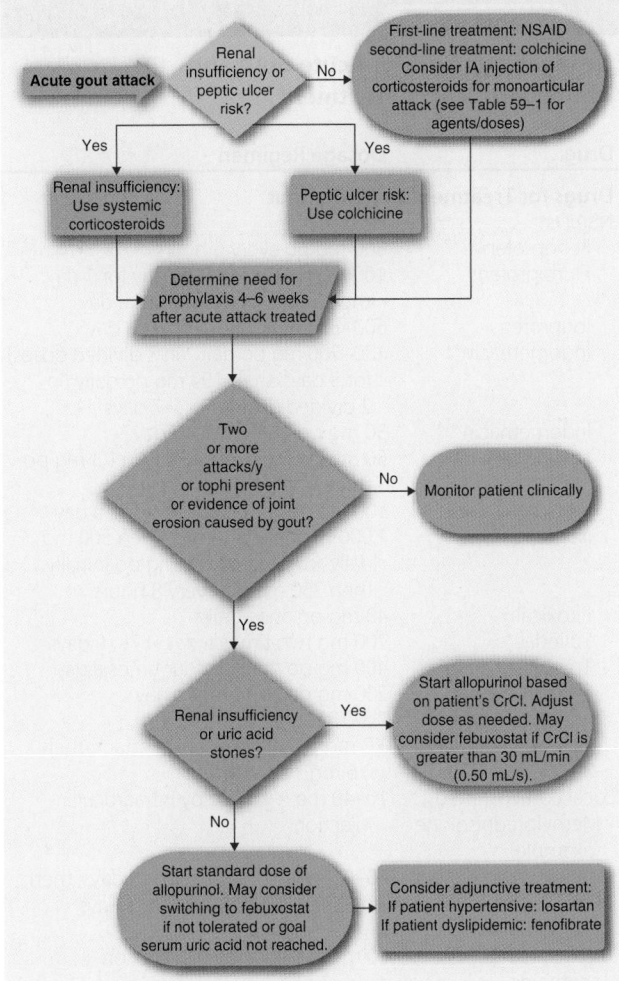

FIGURE 59–2. Treatment algorithm for gout and hyperuricemia. Renal insufficiency is defined as an estimated creatinine clearance (CrCl) of less than 30 mL/min (0.50 mL/s). (IA, intraarticular; NSAID, nonsteroidal anti-inflammatory drug.)

Cyclooxygenase-2 (COX-2)–selective inhibitors produce results comparable with those of traditional NSAIDs. However, cardiovascular safety concerns and the high cost of COX-2 inhibitors argue against their use for this disorder.

▶ Colchicine

● Colchicine has a long history of successful use and was the treatment of choice for many years. It is used infrequently today because of its low therapeutic index. Colchicine is thought to exert its anti-inflammatory effects by interfering with the function of mitotic spindles in neutrophils by binding of tubulin dimers; this inhibits phagocytic activity.[17]

About two-thirds of patients with acute gout respond favorably if it is given within the first 24 hours of symptom onset. Because NSAIDs have not been directly compared with colchicine in rigorous trials, it is unknown which modality has a faster onset. GI effects (e.g., nausea, vomiting, diarrhea, and abdominal pain) are most common and are

<table>
</table>

Table 59–1

Dosage Regimens for Acute Gout and Antihyperuricemic Treatment

Drug	Dosage Regimen
Drugs for Treatment of Acute Gout	
NSAIDs[a]	
Fenoprofen	800 mg po every 6 hours
Flurbiprofen	100 mg po four times a day for 1 day, then 50 mg po four times a day
Ibuprofen	600–800 mg po four times a day
Indomethacin*	150–200 mg po daily (in 3 divided doses) for 3 days, then 100 mg po daily (in 2 divided doses) for 4–7 days
Indomethacin*	50 mg po three times a day
Ketoprofen	50 mg po four times a day or 75 mg po three times a day
Meclofenamate	100 mg po three to four times a day
Naproxen*	1,000 mg daily × 3 days, then 500 mg daily × 7 days or 750 mg po initially, then 250 mg po every 8 hours
Piroxicam	40 mg po once daily
Sulindac*	200 mg two times a day × 7–10 days
Tolmetin	400 mg po three to four times a day
Celecoxib	200 mg po two times a day
Meloxicam	7.5–15 mg po once daily
Colchicine (Colcrys)	1.2 mg po at the onset of attack, then 0.6 mg 1 hour later
Local corticosteroids: Methylprednisolone (example)	10–40 mg × 1 dose by intraarticular injection
Systemic corticosteroids: Prednisone (example)	40–60 mg po once daily × 3 days, then decrease by 10 mg every 3 days
Triamcinolone acetonide	60 mg × 1 dose by IM injection
Antihyperuricemic Treatment	
Allopurinol	Starting dose: CrCl greater than 90 mL/min (1.50 mL/s) = 300 mg po daily; CrCl 60–90 mL/min (1.00–1.50 mL/s) = 200 mg po daily; CrCl 30–60 mL/min (0.50–1.00 mL/s) = 100 mg po daily; CrCl less than 30 mL/min (0.50 mL/s) = 50 mg po daily; Adjust dosage based on follow-up uric acid levels; maximum 800 mg po daily
Febuxostat	Starting dose 40 mg orally once daily; increase to 80 mg once daily if serum uric acid does not decline to 6.0 mg/dL (357 μmol/L) or lower after 2 weeks of treatment
Probenecid	Starting dose 250 mg po two times a day; may increase to 1,000 mg po two times a day
Pegloticase	8 mg given as an IV infusion once every 2 weeks
Rasburicase	0.2 mg/kg given as an IV infusion over 30 minutes once daily for up to 5 days

CrCl, creatinine clearance; IM, intramuscular; NSAIDs, nonsteroidal anti-inflammatory drugs; po, by mouth.

[a]NSAIDs that are FDA approved for treatment of gout are indicated with an asterisk.

Drug regimens derived from various sources.

considered a forerunner of more serious systemic toxicity, including myopathy and bone marrow suppression (usually neutropenia). However, systemic toxicity can occur with oral colchicine without prior GI effects, especially in patients with renal insufficiency.[18,19] In the presence of renal impairment, dosing should be repeated no more than once every 2 weeks. Colchicine should not be coadministered with p-glycoprotein or strong CYP3A4 inhibitors (e.g., clarithromycin). Because of these problems, oral colchicine should be reserved for patients who are at risk for NSAID-induced gastropathy or who have failed NSAID therapy.[20]

In July 2009, the FDA approved Colcrys, a single-ingredient colchicine product for treatment of acute gout attacks. As part of the approval process, a dosing study showed that one dose initially and a single additional dose after 1 hour was just as effective and less toxic than continued hourly colchicine dosing. As a result, the approved dosage regimen is 1.2 mg (two 0.6-mg tablets) at the onset of an acute flare, followed by 0.6 mg 1 hour later. This proprietary agent is much more costly than the generic compounds it replaced.

▶ Corticosteroids

When only one or two joints are affected, **intraarticular** corticosteroid injection can provide rapid relief with a relatively low incidence of side effects. Joint fluid obtained by **arthrocentesis** should be examined for evidence of joint space infection and crystal identification. If uric acid crystals are present and there is no infection, intraarticular injection can proceed.

Systemic corticosteroids are a useful option in patients with contraindications to NSAIDs or colchicine (primarily renal impairment) or polyarticular attacks, especially in elderly patients. A single intramuscular injection of a long-acting corticosteroid such as triamcinolone hexacetonide may be used. Oral agents may be needed, especially for severe attacks. Prednisone 40 to 60 mg (or an equivalent dose of another agent) is given daily, with a gradual taper over 2 weeks.[21] Oral methylprednisolone and naproxen have been shown to be equivalent in treating acute gout attacks.[22]

Short-term adverse effects from corticosteroids include fluid retention, hyperglycemia, CNS stimulation, weight gain, and increased risk of infection. Patients with diabetes should have blood glucose levels monitored carefully during the corticosteroid course.

ANTIHYPERURICEMIC GOUT PROPHYLAXIS

Gout is an episodic disease, and the number of attacks varies widely from patient to patient. Thus the benefit of long-term prophylaxis against acute gout flares must be weighed against the cost and potential toxicity of therapy that may not be necessary in all patients. ⑥ *Asymptomatic hyperuricemia usually does not require treatment.*

Nonpharmacologic Therapy

Lifestyle modifications alone usually are insufficient for lowering SUA levels in gout patients. Patients should be advised

A 58-year-old woman with a history of hypertension, gastroesophageal reflux disease, gout (with two gouty arthritis flares in the last year), and morbid obesity presents to the emergency department complaining of excruciating pain in her left big toe. This is similar to a painful episode she had with her left toe previously. On examination, her left great toe is red, swollen, and warm to the touch. She describes the pain as throbbing and rates it as a 10/10 (where 10 is the worst pain she has ever experienced). She weighs 120 kg (264 lb) and is 5 ft, 3 in (160 cm) tall. Medications include cimetidine 300 mg at bedtime, lisinopril 10 mg daily, and allopurinol 300 mg once daily. She has no prescription insurance and is currently unemployed. Serum creatinine is 1.0 mg/dL (88 μmol/L) and serum uric acid is 7.1 mg/dL (422 μmol/L). The emergency department resident would like to increase the patient's allopurinol to treat the acute gouty flare.

What information suggests gout as the cause of her symptoms?

What treatment for acute gout would you recommend for this patient?

What is the value of a serum uric acid level during an acute gout flare?

What role does allopurinol play in the treatment of acute gout?

to lose weight if obese and to discontinue ethanol consumption. Low-purine diets are not well tolerated; instead, dietary recommendations should focus on general nutrition principles. Drugs that may cause or aggravate hyperuricemia should be discontinued if possible. Few patients adhere to lifestyle modifications long term, and pharmacologic therapy usually is needed to treat hyperuricemia adequately.[23]

Pharmacologic Therapy

⑦ *Patients with recurrent attacks, evidence of tophi or joint destruction, or uric acid nephrolithiasis are candidates for maintenance therapy with allopurinol, febuxostat, probenecid, or pegloticase to lower SUA levels.* Because hyperuricemia is the strongest modifiable risk factor for acute gout, prophylactic therapy involves either decreasing uric acid production or increasing its excretion (Table 59–1). The goal of therapy is to decrease SUA levels significantly, leaving less uric acid available for conversion to MSU crystals.[12]

Ideally, the selection of long-term prophylactic therapy involves determining the cause of hyperuricemia (primarily by analyzing a 24-hour urine collection for uric acid) and tailoring therapy appropriately. If less than 600 mg of uric acid is found in the 24-hour sample, the patient is considered an underexcretor. However, this approach is not used commonly for several reasons. The urine collection is inconvenient for

patients and clinicians and does not identify patients who may be both overproducers and underexcretors of uric acid. Also, drugs used to increase uric acid excretion (**uricosurics**) generally are not as well tolerated as drugs that decrease production, and uricosurics increase the risk of uric acid nephrolithiasis.[24]

Because allopurinol (which reduces uric acid production) is effective in both overproducers and underexcretors and is generally well tolerated, many clinicians forego the 24-hour urine collection and treat patients empirically with it.

▶ *Allopurinol*

Most patients in the United States are treated with allopurinol, which usually is effective if the dosage is titrated appropriately. The drug and its primary active metabolite, oxypurinol, reduce SUA concentrations by inhibiting the enzyme xanthine oxidase, thereby blocking the oxidation of hypoxanthine and xanthine to uric acid.[12]

Allopurinol is well absorbed, with a short half-life of 2 to 3 hours. The half-life of oxypurinol approaches 24 hours, allowing allopurinol to be dosed once daily. Oxypurinol is cleared primarily renally and can accumulate in patients with reduced kidney function. Allopurinol should not be started during an acute gout attack because sudden shifts in SUA levels may precipitate or exacerbate gouty arthritis. Rapid shifts in SUA can change the concentration of MSU crystals in synovial fluid, causing more crystals to precipitate. Thus most clinicians advocate a prophylactic dose of colchicine (0.6 mg/day) during initiation of antihyperuricemic therapy. Patients receiving colchicine for this reason should be screened for drug–drug interactions (via the cytochrome p-450 system) that may increase the risk of colchicine adverse effects. NSAIDs can be used at a low dose if colchicine is contraindicated. Combined treatment is continued until uric acid levels return to normal or a maximum of 3 to 6 months. Acute episodes should be treated appropriately before maintenance treatment is started.

The initial dose of allopurinol is based on the patient's renal function. Patients with a creatinine clearance (CrCl) of 50 mL/min (0.83 mL/s) or less should receive a starting dose of less than 300 mg/day, although the product literature and other sources list alternative dosing regimens for those with renal insufficiency. The relationship between dose of allopurinol and its most severe side effects is controversial.[25] However, the dose can be adjusted upward as needed and tolerated, even in patients with mild to moderate renal insufficiency provided that patients are monitored appropriately.[26] It is reasonable to reduce the dose temporarily in patients who develop reversible acute renal failure.

SUA levels must be monitored periodically, with the first follow-up level obtained 6 months (or sooner) after starting therapy. The target SUA level is less than 6.0 mg/dL (357 μmol/L). The dose should be titrated upward (to a maximum of 800 mg/day) or downward as these levels dictate.

Allopurinol generally is well tolerated; nausea and diarrhea occur in a small percentage of patients. A generalized, maculopapular rash occurs in about 2% of patients.[27] Although usually mild, this can progress to severe skin reactions such as Stevens-Johnson syndrome. Perhaps the most feared side effect is the allopurinol hypersensitivity syndrome, which may involve severe desquamating skin lesions, high fever (usually greater than 39.0°C [102.2°F]), hepatic dysfunction, leukocytosis with predominant eosinophilia, and renal failure. Although rare, this severe reaction has a 20% mortality rate.[28] Patients with a history of the syndrome should never again receive allopurinol (including desensitization) or oxypurinol (which is available outside the United States). Patients with a mild skin rash who require allopurinol can be desensitized to it using published protocols or be switched to febuxostat.[29,30]

There are several important drug–drug interactions with allopurinol. The effects of both theophylline and warfarin may be potentiated by allopurinol. Azathioprine and 6-mercaptopurine are purines whose metabolism is inhibited by concomitant allopurinol therapy; the dose of these drugs must be reduced by 75% with allopurinol cotherapy. Patients taking allopurinol who receive ampicillin are at increased risk of skin rashes.

▶ Febuxostat

Febuxostat is a nonpurine xanthine oxidase inhibitor structurally distinct from allopurinol that is FDA approved for chronic hyperuricemia associated with gout. The initial dose is 40 mg orally once daily. The dose may be increased to 80 mg orally once daily if the SUA does not decrease to 6.0 mg/dL (357 μmol/L) or less after 2 weeks of treatment. No dosage adjustment is necessary in patients with mild or moderate renal impairment. Because of its potency and rapid reduction of SUA levels, prophylactic low-dose colchicine or an NSAID is recommended for 3 to 6 months during initiation of therapy.

Data from phase III trials suggested that febuxostat is more effective than allopurinol (at currently prescribed doses) in achieving target SUA levels of 6.0 mg/dL (357 μmol/L) or less and may be more effective in reducing the number of acute gouty flares.[31] However, fixed allopurinol doses were used rather than titrating the allopurinol dose to reach the target SUA level, which may confound these findings.

Adverse effects of febuxostat include nausea, arthralgias, rash, and transient elevation of hepatic transaminases. Periodic liver function tests are recommended (e.g., at baseline, 2 and 4 months after starting therapy, and then periodically thereafter). Due to differences in chemical structure, febuxostat would not be expected to crossreact in patients with a history of allopurinol hypersensitivity syndrome. It also appears to be safe and effective in patients with mild-to-moderate renal insufficiency.

Because of cost concerns, febuxostat should be reserved for patients who do not tolerate allopurinol or those who cannot achieve SUA levels of 6.0 mg/dL (357 μmol/L) or less despite allopurinol therapy.[2]

▶ Probenecid

Probenecid is a uricosuric agent that blocks the tubular reabsorption of uric acid, increasing its excretion. Because

Patient Encounter, Part 2

The patient is successfully treated for her symptoms and returns for a follow-up visit at your clinic 8 weeks later. She reports no pain or swelling in the joints affected previously. She is currently taking allopurinol 300 mg daily, cimetidine 300 mg at bedtime, and lisinopril 10 mg daily.

PE:

VS: BP 131/80, P 72, RR 15, T 36.1°C (96.9°F)

Ext: Trace edema in both ankles

Labs: Serum uric acid 8.1 mg/dL (482 μmol/L); serum creatinine 0.9 mg/dL (80 μmol/L).

What are the gout treatment goals for this patient?

What is your therapeutic plan to achieve these goals?

of its mechanism of action, probenecid is contraindicated in patients with a history of uric acid stones or nephropathy. Probenecid loses its effectiveness as renal function declines and should be avoided when the CrCl is 50 mL/min (0.83 mL/s) or less. Its uricosuric effect is counteracted by low aspirin doses, which many patients receive for prophylaxis of coronary heart disease.[2,12]

Although generally well tolerated, probenecid can cause GI side effects such as nausea and other adverse reactions including fever, rash, and rarely, hepatic toxicity. Patients should be instructed to maintain adequate fluid intake and urine output to decrease the risk of uric acid stone formation. Some experts advocate alkalinizing the urine to decrease this risk.

▶ Pegloticase

Gout does not occur in most nonprimate mammals because these species produce the enzyme uricase, which metabolizes uric acid into the more soluble compound allantoin, which is readily excreted. Humans lack this enzyme, which allows uric acid to accumulate, leading to gout in some individuals.

Pegloticase is a recombinant form of uricase bound to polyethylene glycol that is approved for the treatment of chronic gout refractory to other therapy. At the approved dose of 8 mg IV every 2 weeks, the drug rapidly (within 6 hours) decreased SUA in subjects in published trials.[32] However, pegloticase should be limited to patients with severe gout with tophi or nephropathy that has not responded to other agents because of significant adverse effects, including gout flares, anaphylaxis (in up to 5% of patients) that mandates pretreatment with antihistamines and corticosteroids, the inconvenience of IV therapy, and its high cost.

▶ Other Uricosuric Agents

Several other medications have mild uricosuric effects and may be appropriate adjunctive therapy in some patients.

Losartan increases both uric acid excretion and urine pH and may be an option in hypertensive patients with gout.[33] Fenofibrate is also a uricosuric and may be appropriate in selected dyslipidemic patients with gout.

TUMOR LYSIS SYNDROME

8 *Tumor lysis syndrome (TLS) is a metabolic disorder caused by rapid cell destruction (usually during chemotherapy treatment for cancer) and associated with several electrolyte disturbances, notably hyperuricemia.*

TLS is most commonly associated with the chemotherapeutic treatment of cancers, such as leukemias and lymphomas. These types of cancers have a large tumor cell burden and are highly sensitive to destruction by chemotherapy. Massive lysis of intracellular contents occurs, including the breakdown of nucleotides into hypoxanthine, xanthine and, eventually, uric acid. These large amounts of uric acid overwhelm normal urinary excretion capacities and can undergo crystalline precipitation. This can lead to acute renal failure and a host of electrolyte disturbances, including hyperkalemia and hyperphosphatemia.[34] If not prevented or treated early, TLS can lead to acute kidney damage and perhaps death; thus TLS is considered an oncologic emergency. The incidence of TLS varies according to definition, tumor type, and patient characteristics, but is thought to be approximately 5% in high-risk cancers.

Due to the potential severity of TLS, strategies to prevent this disorder are mandatory in susceptible patients. Aggressive hydration (usually with isotonic fluids such as 0.9% saline) and diuresis are the cornerstones of TLS prevention. This strategy promotes the excretion of uric acid before crystallization occurs. Alkalinization of the urine to increase uric acid solubility has not been shown to be beneficial.[35]

Allopurinol has a crucial role in the prevention of TLS. Due to its low cost and ease of administration, oral allopurinol is commonly used in doses up to 400 mg/m^2/day for the prevention of TLS. The drug is usually started several days before the initiation of chemotherapy. In patients who cannot tolerate oral allopurinol, the IV formulation can prevent hyperuricemia in up to 90% of patients treated.[36] Allopurinol does not reduce levels of uric acid formed before treatment is initiated.

Rasburicase is a recombinant form of urate oxidase indicated for the prevention and treatment of TLS. This enzyme, similar to uricase (pegloticase), also converts uric acid to allantoin. Rasburicase can dramatically reduce uric acid levels in patients with TLS and appears to be more effective than allopurinol.[37] Rasburicase is indicated for patients who have developed TLS or in patients at high risk for developing this syndrome.[38] In these patients, the drug is approved at a dose of 0.2 mg/kg as an IV infusion over 30 minutes daily for up to 5 days. Rasburicase has a much higher acquisition cost than IV allopurinol, and some investigators have studied lower doses of the drug or use it preferentially in patients with existing renal insufficiency or uric acid levels greater than 10.0 mg/dL (595 μmol/L).[38]

Rasburicase is well tolerated; mild cutaneous hypersensitivity reactions are the most common adverse effect. It can also cause hemolysis, especially in patients with glucose-6-phosphate dehydrogenase (G6PD) deficiency.

OUTCOME EVALUATION

Acute Gout

- Monitor the patient for pain relief and decreased swelling of the affected joints. Both parameters should be improved significantly within 48 hours of starting acute gout therapy.
- Assess the patient's subjective complaints and objective information for adverse effects. For NSAID therapy, be alert for new-onset epigastric pain, dark or tarry stools, blood in vomitus, dizziness or lightheadedness, development of edema, decreased urine output by more than 50% over a 24-hour period, or shortness of breath. For colchicine, monitor for nausea or vomiting, diarrhea, easy bruising, cold or flulike symptoms, lightheadedness, muscle weakness, or pain. Counsel the patient to inform you of any new medications started or stopped while taking colchicine.
- Monitor patients receiving intraarticular corticosteroid injections for increased swelling or pain at the injection site.
- Assess patients receiving systemic corticosteroids for mental status changes, fluid retention, increased blood glucose, muscle weakness, or development of new infections.

Antihyperuricemic Therapy

- Assess for new gouty arthritis attacks or the development of tophi. If neither one develops, continue antihyperuricemic therapy as prescribed.
- Obtain the first follow-up SUA level within 6 months of starting therapy. Then monitor levels at least every 6 to 12 months, and adjust the dose to achieve a target SUA level of less than 6.0 mg/dL (357 μmol/L).
- Evaluate patients taking allopurinol for development of rash, nausea, or new fever. These symptoms usually appear within the first 3 months of therapy but can occur anytime.
- Assess patients receiving probenecid for fever, nausea, or skin rash. Reevaluate therapy if a significant decrease in urine output occurs (greater than 50% in a 24-hour period).
- Reserve pegloticase for chronic gout refractory to other antihyperuricemic therapies or when other agents are not tolerated. Monitor SUA levels before each 2-week IV infusion.
- Evaluate patients on pegloticase for development of gouty flares and infusion reactions, which may include anaphylaxis. The manufacturer recommends giving an antihistamine and perhaps low-dose methylprednisolone before the infusion to minimize reactions.

Patient Care and Monitoring

1. Assess the patient's symptoms to determine the time of attack onset, which joints are affected, the level of pain, and other symptoms.

2. Review the patient history for contributing lifestyle factors and other disease states that may help guide therapy.

3. Obtain a thorough medication history for prescription drug, nonprescription drug, and dietary supplement use. Determine whether any of these products may be contributing to hyperuricemia.

4. Educate the patient on lifestyle modifications that will improve symptoms, including weight loss, if appropriate, and avoidance of ethanol.

5. If the diagnosis of gout has not been confirmed previously, consider aspiration of an affected joint to identify uric acid crystals.

6. Initiate therapy to treat the acute gout attack without delay. Develop a plan to assess this therapy after 24 and 48 hours.

7. Select therapy based on comorbidities and potential for adverse effects. In patients with no other disease states, NSAIDs are the preferred drug class.

8. Assess the need for continuous antihyperuricemic therapy. Use patient factors such as comorbidities to select an agent. Allopurinol is the standard prophylactic agent used in the United States.

9. Most patients need adjunctive therapy with low-dose colchicine or an NSAID during initiation or titration of antihyperuricemic therapy to prevent a rebound flare.

10. Do not start antihyperuricemic therapy within 4 weeks of an acute attack.

11. Evaluate the patient for the presence of adverse drug reactions, drug allergies, and drug interactions.

12. Stress the importance of adherence with the therapeutic regimen, including lifestyle modifications, to prevent future gout attacks and long-term complications.

13. Provide patient education about the disease state, lifestyle modifications, and drug therapy.

Abbreviations Introduced in This Chapter

ACTH   Adrenocorticotropic hormone
COX   Cyclooxygenase
G6PD   Glucose-6-phosphate dehydrogenase
MSU   Monosodium urate
SUA   Serum uric acid
TLS   Tumor lysis syndrome

 Self-assessment questions and answers are available at *http://www.mhpharmacotherapy.com/pp.html.*

REFERENCES

1. Mikuls TR, MacLean CH, Olivieri J, et al. Quality of care indicators for gout management. Arthritis Rheum 2004;50:937–943.
2. Neogi T. Gout. N Engl J Med. 2011;364:443–452.
3. Arromdee E, Michet CJ, Crowson CS, et al. Epidemiology of gout: Is the incidence rising? J Rheumatol 2002;29:2403–2406.
4. Cassetta M, Gorevic PD. Crystal arthritis: Gout and pseudogout in the geriatric patient. Geriatrics 2004;59:25–31.
5. Agudelo CA, Wise CM. Crystal-associated arthritis. Clin Geriatr Med 1998;14:495–513.
6. Johnson RJ, Kang DH, Feig D, et al. Is there a pathogenetic role for uric acid in hypertension and cardiovascular and renal disease? Hypertension 2003;41:1183–1190.
7. Cardona F, Tinahones FJ, Collantes E, et al. Contribution of polymorphisms in the apolipoprotein AI-CIII-AIV cluster to hyperlipidaemia in patients with gout. Ann Rheum Dis 2005;64:85–88.
8. Goicoechea M, de Vinuesa SG, Verdalles U, et al. Effect of allopurinol in chronic kidney disease progression and cardiovascular risk. Clin J Am Soc Nephrol 2010;5:1388–1393.
9. Shekarriz B, Stoller ML. Uric acid nephrolithiasis: Current concepts and controversies. J Urol 2002;168(4 Pt 1):1307–1314.
10. Terkeltaub RA. Gout. N Engl J Med 2003;349:1647–1655.
11. Schumacher Jr HR. Crystal induced arthritis: An overview. Am J Med 1996;100 (Suppl 2A):46–52.
12. Zhang W, Doherty M, Bardin T, et al. EULAR evidence based recommendations for gout. Part II: Management. Report of a task force of the EULAR Standing Committee for International Clinical Studies Including Therapeutics (ESCISIT). Ann Rheum Dis 2006;65:1312–1324.
13. Schlesinger N, Baker DK, Beutler AM, et al. Local ice therapy during bouts of acute gouty arthritis. J Rheumatol 2002;29:331–334.
14. Mandell BF, Edwards NL, Sundy JS, Simkin PA, Pile JC. Preventing and treating acute gout attacks across the clinical spectrum: a roundtable discussion. Cleve Clin J Med 2010;77(Suppl 2):S2–S25.
15. Schlesinger N. Management of acute and chronic gouty arthritis. Drugs 2004;64:2399–2416.
16. Conaghan PG, Day RO. Risks and benefits of drugs used in the management and prevention of gout. Drug Saf 1994;11:252–258.
17. Smallwood JI, Malawista SE. Colchicine, crystals, and neutrophils tyrosine phosphorylation. J Clin Invest 1993;92:1602–1603.
18. Wallace SL, Singer JZ, Duncan GJ, et al. Renal function predicts colchicine toxicity: Guidelines for the prophylactic use of colchicine in gout. J Rheumatol 1991;18:264–269.
19. Dixon AJ, Wall GC. Probable colchicine-induced neutropenia not related to intentional overdose. Ann Pharmacother 2001;35:192–195.
20. Terkeltaub R, Zelman D, Scavulli J, Perez-Ruiz F, Lioté F. Gout Study Group: update on hyperuricemia and gout. Joint Bone Spine. 2009;76:444–446.
21. Kim KY, Schumacher HR, Hunsche E, et al. A literature review of the epidemiology and treatment of acute gout. Clin Ther 2003;25:1593–1617.
22. Janssens HJ, Janssen M, van de Lisdonk EH, et al. Use of oral prednisolone or naproxen for the treatment of gout arthritis: A double-blind, randomised equivalence trial. Lancet 2008;371:1854–1860.
23. de Klerk E, van der Heijde D, Landewe R, et al. Patient compliance in rheumatoid arthritis, polymyalgia rheumatica, and gout. J Rheumatol 2003;30:44–54.
24. Pal B, Foxall M, Dysart T, et al. How is gout managed in primary care? A review of current practice and proposed guidelines. Clin Rheumatol 2000;19:21–25.

25. Vazquez-Mellado J, Morales EM, Pacheco-Tena C, Burgos-Vargas R. Relation between adverse events associated with allopurinol and renal function in patients with gout. Ann Rheum Dis 2001;60:981–983.

26. Stamp LK, O'Donnell JL, Zhang M, et al. Using allopurinol above the dose based on creatinine clearance is effective and safe in patients with chronic gout, including those with renal impairment. Arthritis Rheum 2011;63:412–421.

27. Khoo BP, Leow YH. A review of inpatients with adverse drug reactions to allopurinol. Singapore Med J 2000;41:156–160.

28. Arellano F, Sacristan JA. Allopurinol hypersensitivity syndrome: A review. Ann Pharmacother 1993;27:337–343.

29. Bardin T. Current Management of gout in patients unresponsive or allergic to allopurinol. Joint Bone Spine 2004;71:481–485.

30. Fam AG, Dunne SM, Iazzetta J, Paton TW. Efficacy and safety of desensitization to allopurinol following cutaneous reactions. Arthritis Rheum 2001;44:231–238.

31. Becker MA, Schumacher HR Jr, Wortmann RL, et al. Febuxostat compared with allopurinol in patients with hyperuricemia and gout. N Engl J Med 2005;353:2450–2461.

32. Sundy JS, Becker MA, Baraf HS, et al. Reduction of plasma urate levels following treatment with multiple doses of pegloticase (polyethylene glycol-conjugated uricase) in patients with treatment-failure gout: results of a phase II randomized study. Arthritis Rheum 2008;58:2882–2891.

33. Takahashi S, Moriwaki Y, Yamamoto T, et al. Effects of combination treatment using anti-hyperuricaemic agents with fenofibrate and/or losartan on uric acid metabolism. Ann Rheum Dis 2003;62:572–575.

34. Tiu RV, Mountantonakis SE, Dunbar AJ, Schreiber MJ Jr. Tumor lysis syndrome. Semin Thromb Hemost 2007;33:397–407.

35. Coiffier B, Altman A, Pui CH, et al. Guidelines for the management of pediatric and adult tumor lysis syndrome: An evidence-based review. J Clin Oncol 2008;26:2767–2778.

36. Holdsworth MT, Nguyen P. Role of i.v. allopurinol and rasburicase in tumor lysis syndrome. Am J Health Syst Pharm 2003;60:2213–2222.

37. Cortes J, Moore JO, Maziarz RT, et al. Control of plasma uric acid in adults at risk for tumor lysis syndrome: efficacy and safety of rasburicase alone and rasburicase followed by allopurinol compared with allopurinol alone – results of a multicenter phase III study. J Clin Oncol 2010;28:4207–4213.

38. Howard SC, Jones DP, Pui CH. The tumor lysis syndrome. N Engl J Med 2011;364:1844–1854.

60 Musculoskeletal Disorders

Jill S. Borchert

LEARNING OBJECTIVES

● **Upon completion of the chapter, the reader will be able to:**

1. Describe the pathophysiologic principles associated with tissue injury and inflammation.

2. Identify the desired therapeutic goals and outcomes for a patient with musculoskeletal injury or pain.

3. Identify the factors that guide selection of an analgesic or counterirritant for a particular patient.

4. Recommend appropriate nonpharmacologic and pharmacologic therapy for a patient with musculoskeletal injury or pain.

5. Design a patient education plan including nonpharmacologic therapy and preventative strategies.

6. Develop a monitoring plan to assess treatment of a patient with musculoskeletal disorders.

KEY CONCEPTS

❶ The two primary goals of treating musculoskeletal disorders are to: (a) relieve pain and (b) maintain functionality.

❷ The cornerstone of nonpharmacologic therapy for acute injury in the first 48 to 72 hours is known by the acronym *RICE: rest, ice, compression,* and *elevation.*

❸ Heat should not be applied during the acute injury phase (the first 48 hours) because it promotes swelling and inflammation.

❹ There are two main approaches to pharmacologic intervention for pain relief: oral (systemic) and topical agents.

❺ Localized pain may be treated effectively with local topical therapy, whereas generalized pain is best treated with systemic agents.

❻ Acetaminophen is the drug of choice for mild-to-moderate regional musculoskeletal pain without inflammation.

❼ Aspirin is not more effective than acetaminophen, and it is not recommended for treatment of acute musculoskeletal pain because its adverse effects may be more common and severe.

❽ Nonsteroidal anti-inflammatory drugs (NSAIDs) are preferred over acetaminophen in musculoskeletal disorders in which inflammation is the primary problem.

❾ Patient education on proper use of counterirritants is essential to therapeutic success.

❿ Patients using capsaicin should be advised to apply it regularly and consistently three to four times daily and that full effect may take 2 to 3 weeks or longer.

INTRODUCTION

The musculoskeletal system consists of the muscles, bones, joints, tendons, and ligaments. Disorders related to the musculoskeletal system often are classified by etiology. Acute soft-tissue injuries include strains and sprains of muscles and ligaments. Repeated movements in sports, exercise, work, or activities of daily living can lead to repetitive strain injury, where cumulative damage occurs to the muscles, ligaments, or tendons.[1,2] Although tendonitis and bursitis can arise from acute injury, more commonly these conditions occur as a result of chronic stress.[2] Other forms of chronic musculoskeletal pain, such as pain from rheumatoid arthritis (see Chap. 57) or osteoarthritis (see Chap. 58), are discussed elsewhere in this textbook.

EPIDEMIOLOGY

Musculoskeletal disorders are commonly self-treated, so true estimates of the incidence of both acute and chronic injury are difficult to obtain. Musculoskeletal disorders are among the top 10 reasons for ambulatory care visits in the United States for all age groups.[3] These disorders account for a large portion of medical care expenditures and are a leading cause of work absenteeism and disability, resulting in a substantial economic burden from lost productivity and lost wages.[4]

In addition to chronic conditions such as arthritis and low back pain, some musculoskeletal disorders are induced by trauma at the workplace either via repetition and cumulative trauma or a one-time overexertion.[5] These are more likely to occur in the setting of a rapid work pace, heavy lifting, or poor posture. For each reported incident, it is likely that there are at least 10 unreported work-related musculoskeletal events related to repetitive stress to the bones and joints.[6] In the elderly, these injuries may not be related to work but to daily life. Instability combined with activities of daily living such as stair climbing and lifting objects may lead to strains and sprains. In children and adolescents, fractures are more common than muscle and tendon injuries since growth spurts cause bones to weaken while the muscle–tendon unit tightens.[7,8]

Muscle injuries comprise the majority of sports-related injuries, and roughly half are related to overuse.[2,9] The shoulder and the knee are common sites of sports injuries.[8] Soccer, football, basketball, track and field, and other sports that require rapid acceleration or higher speeds pose a greater risk of muscle strain.[8,10] *Overuse musculoskeletal injury* is the phrase used to describe disorders arising from repetitive motion. This injury is common in activities such as running, particularly during periods of increased intensity or duration of training.[2] It also can occur in the workplace with repeated, unvaried motion.[5]

PATHOPHYSIOLOGY

Skeletal muscle consists of muscle fibers linked together by connective tissue. Tendons and ligaments are composed of collagenous fibers that have a restricted capability to stretch. Tendons connect the muscle to the bone, whereas ligaments connect bone to bone (Fig. 60–1).

Muscle Strains and Sprains

A **sprain** is an overstretching of supporting ligaments that results in a partial or complete tear of the ligament.[8,10] Although a **strain** also arises from an overstretching of the muscle–tendon unit, it is marked by damage to the muscle fibers or tendon without tearing of the ligament.[11] The key difference between a sprain and a strain is that a sprain involves damage to ligaments, whereas a strain involves damage primarily to muscle. One common example of muscle strain and sprain is low back pain.[12]

Overloading the muscle and connective tissue results in complete or partial tears of the skeletal muscle, tendons, or ligaments.[8] This usually occurs when the muscle is activated in an *eccentric contraction*, defined as a contraction in which the muscle is being lengthened.[8] Examples of this type of contraction include putting down a large, heavy laundry basket or lowering oneself from a chin-up bar. Small tears can occur in the muscle because it is lengthening while also trying to contract to support the load. This leads to

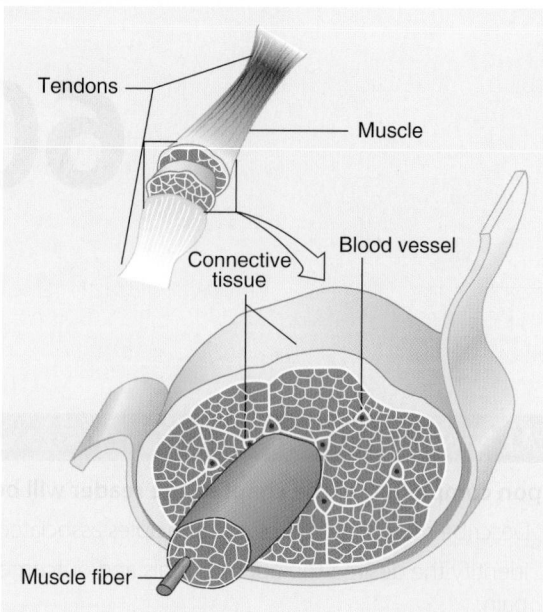

FIGURE 60–1. Skeletal muscle fiber organization. Tendons attach muscle to bone. (From Widmaier EP, Raff H, Strang KT, et al., eds. Vander, Sherman, & Luciano's *Human Physiology: The Mechanisms of Body Function.* 9th ed. New York: McGraw-Hill; 2004: Fig. 9–1.)

rupture of blood vessels at the site of the injury, resulting in the formation of a hematoma. Within 24 to 48 hours, an inflammatory response develops. In the inflammatory stage, macrophages remove necrotic fibers.[9,11,13] The activated neutrophils release growth factors that will activate myocytes for regeneration. Finally, capillaries grow into the area, and muscle fibers regenerate during the repair and remodeling phases of healing.

Bursitis and Tendonitis

Bursitis is an inflammation of the bursa, the fluid-filled sac near the joint where the tendons and muscles pass over the bone. The bursa assists with movement by reducing friction between joints. Overuse of a joint can result in an inflamed bursa. Bursitis causes stiffness and pain because the bursa serves to reduce friction within the joint space.

Tendonitis (or *tendinitis*) is an inflammation of the tendon or, more specifically, the fibrous sheath that attaches muscle to bone.[2] **Tenosynovitis** is an inflammation of the tendon sheath. Repetitive overuse of a tendon can cause cellular changes in the tissues. Specifically, collagenous tendon tissue is replaced with tissue that lacks the organized collagen arrangement of a normal tendon.[14] In fact, many patients diagnosed with chronic tendonitis may not have inflammation but instead have tendinosis, a condition marked by these collagen changes. As a result of the cellular changes, the tendon progressively loses elasticity and its ability to handle stress or weight. This makes the tendon vulnerable to rupture or inflammation (tendonitis and tenosynovitis).

Inflammation and Peripheral Pain Sensation

Inflammation is a common pathway in soft-tissue injury of musculoskeletal disorders. Inflammatory processes lead to two outcomes: swelling and pain. Inflammatory processes traditionally are considered to be a necessary part of the remodeling process because inflammatory cells remove damaged tissue.[15,16] However, inflammation also contributes to continued pain and swelling that limits range of motion.[17]

The initial injury exposes membrane phospholipids to phospholipase A_2, leading to the formation of arachidonic acid (Fig. 60-2).[15,16] Next, arachidonic acid is transformed by cyclooxygenase (COX) to thromboxanes and prostaglandins (PGs), including prostaglandin E_2 (PGE_2). PGE_2 is the most potent inflammatory mediator; it increases vascular permeability, leading to redness, warmth, and swelling of the affected area. The increased permeability also increases proteolysis, or the breakdown of proteins in the damaged tissue.

Neutrophils, lymphocytes, and monocytes are attracted to the area, and monocytes are converted to macrophages.[15] The macrophages then stimulate additional PG production. Phagocytic cells and other players in the immune system release cytokines, including interleukins, interferon, and tumor necrosis factor.

In addition to increasing vascular permeability, PGs also induce pain by sensitizing pain receptors to other substances such as bradykinin. Bradykinin, PGs, leukotrienes, and other inflammatory mediators lower the pain threshold through peripheral pain sensitization. These substances make nerve endings more excitable, and the nerve fibers are more reactive to serotonin, heat, and mechanical stimuli.[16,18] The increased sensitization in the damaged tissue causes tenderness, soreness, and hyperalgesia or an exaggerated intensity of pain sensation.[18] The process also facilitates production of additional PGs. In a cyclic fashion, the PGs then sensitize the nerves to bradykinin action.

Without interruption, the neurochemicals ultimately lead to a firing of the unmyelinated or thinly myelinated afferent neurons. This sends messages along the pain pathway in the periphery and communicates the pain message to the CNS. Interruption of this cycle occurs via anti-inflammatory agents such as aspirin and nonsteroidal anti-inflammatory drugs (NSAIDs).

Nerve receptors, or nociceptors, release substance P and other peptides when they are activated.[18] Substance P mediates the production and release of inflammatory mediators and acts as a potent vasodilator. This receptor activation also increases the sensitivity of nociceptors to painful stimuli. Capsaicin relieves pain by stimulating the release of substance P from sensory nerve fibers, which ultimately depletes stores of substance P.[19]

CLINICAL PRESENTATION AND DIAGNOSIS

See next page for information on the clinical presentation and diagnosis of musculoskeletal disorders.

TREATMENT

Desired Outcomes

❶ *The two primary goals of treating musculoskeletal disorders are to: (a) relieve pain and (b) maintain functionality.* This is accomplished by decreasing the severity and duration of pain, shortening the recovery period, and preventing acute injury pain from becoming chronic pain. If these goals are achieved, functional limitations are decreased. Ideally, a patient should be able to continue to perform activities of daily living (e.g., eating, dressing, cooking, doing laundry) and maintain normal functions in the workplace. Children ideally should be able to maintain usual play activities and sports schedules.

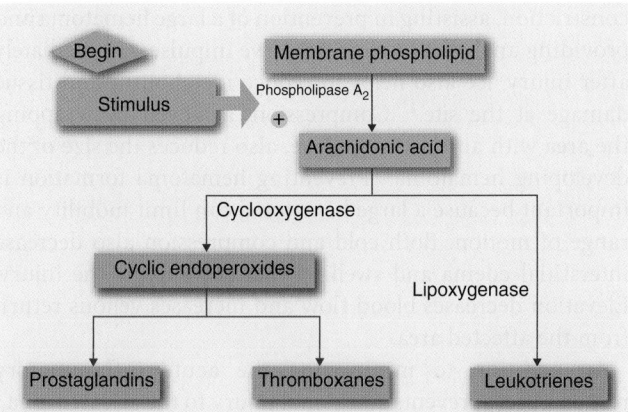

FIGURE 60-2. Eicosanoid synthesis pathway. Cyclooxygenase is inhibited by nonsteroidal anti-inflammatory drugs and aspirin. (Adapted with permission from Widmaier EP, Raff H, Strang KT. Vander's Human Physiology: The Mechanisms of Body Function. 12th ed. New York: McGraw Hill; 2011: Fig. 5–12.)

Patient Encounter 1, Part 1

A 58-year-old woman presents with left ankle pain. She was playing tennis earlier today and twisted her ankle. The pain occurs at rest and is worsened with weight-bearing on the ankle and rotation or movement. There is moderate swelling and bruising of the left ankle. She tries to avoid taking pain pills because she is on a medicine that her healthcare provider told her has lots of drug interactions. She asks for a recommendation for a topical medication.

What information is suggestive of a musculoskeletal disorder?

What is your assessment of the patient's ankle pain?

What additional information do you need to formulate a treatment plan?

Clinical Presentation and Diagnosis of Musculoskeletal Disorders

General[2,8,14,17]

- Clinical presentation varies based on the etiology of the disorder.
- Repetitive strain or overuse injuries may have a gradual onset.
- Musculoskeletal disorders due to acute injury may be associated with other signs of the injury such as abrasion.
- Low back pain is often chronic.

Signs and Symptoms of Acute Soft-Tissue Injury (Strains, Sprains)[2,8,11,17]

- Discomfort ranging from tenderness to pain; it may occur at rest or with motion
- Swelling and inflammation of the affected area
- Bruising
- Loss of motion
- Mechanical instability

Signs and Symptoms of Repetitive Strain or Overuse Injury (Tendonitis, Bursitis)[2,14]

- Pain and stiffness that occurs either at rest or with motion
- Localized tenderness on palpation

- Mild swelling of the affected area
- Decreased range of motion
- Muscle atrophy

Other Diagnostic Tests and Assessments[8]

- *Radiograph (x-ray):* Evaluate bony structures to rule out fracture, malalignment, or joint erosion as the primary cause of pain.
- *MRI:* Soft-tissue imaging to evaluate for tendon or ligament tears.
- *Ultrasound:* Superficial soft-tissue imaging to evaluate for tears in tendons or ligaments. Ultrasound does not penetrate bone, so it is of limited usefulness for assessing tendons or ligaments deep within joints.
- *Pain scale:* Patient self-rating of pain on a scale of zero (no pain) to 10 (worst possible pain). Used to assess pain both at rest and with movement. Determined at baseline and to assess response to therapy.

Further goals include a return to usual activity and prevention of future injury. It is also important to minimize the potential for adverse drug events during treatment.

General Approach to Treatment

Treatment of musculoskeletal disorders involves three phases: (a) therapy of an acute injury using the rest, ice, compression, and elevation (RICE) principle; (b) pain relief using oral or topical agents; and (c) lifestyle and behavioral modifications for rehabilitation and to prevent recurrent injury or chronic pain (Fig. 60–3).

In many cases, musculoskeletal disorders are self-treated with over-the-counter (OTC) oral or topical agents. However, further evaluation may be warranted if acute pain persists longer than 7 to 10 days, symptoms worsen or subside and then return, or there are signs of a more serious condition.[14,20,21] Warning signs of more serious conditions include joint deformity, dislocation, or lack of movement in a joint. Low back pain accompanied by burning, radiating pain, or difficulty urinating requires further evaluation.

In children and adolescents, treatment practices are similar to the approach in adults with a focus on nonpharmacologic therapy and oral analgesics. Children younger than 2 years of age, elderly persons, and pregnant women also may need special care. Elderly patients may be more prone to systemic effects because of thinning of the skin and increased absorption of topical agents and drug interactions from polypharmacy.

Nonpharmacologic Therapy: RICE

The cornerstone of nonpharmacologic therapy for acute injury in the first 48 to 72 hours is known by the acronym RICE: rest, ice, compression, and elevation[9,17] (Table 60–1). These four methods initially minimize bleeding from broken blood vessels. Rest eases pressure on the affected area and promotes pain control during the acute inflammatory phase (the first 1 to 5 days after injury). Cold causes vasoconstriction, assisting in prevention of a large hematoma and providing analgesia by slowing nerve impulses. Immediately after injury, ice also helps to reduce metabolism and tissue damage at the site.[22] Compression, achieved by wrapping the area with an elastic bandage, also reduces the size of the developing hematoma.[9] Preventing hematoma formation is important because a large hematoma can limit mobility and range of motion. Both cold and compression also decrease interstitial edema and swelling that accompany the injury. Elevation decreases blood flow and increases venous return from the affected area.

In addition to minimizing the acute inflammatory response, rest prevents additional injury to the affected area.[9] The properties of the muscle–tendon unit are altered during the acute injury, with limitations on the ability of the muscles and tendons to stretch. Movement in the injured tissue can cause further retraction of the ruptured muscle and increase the size of the gap in the muscle to be healed. Therefore, early activity predisposes a patient to further injury, but prolonged inactivity can lengthen recovery times.

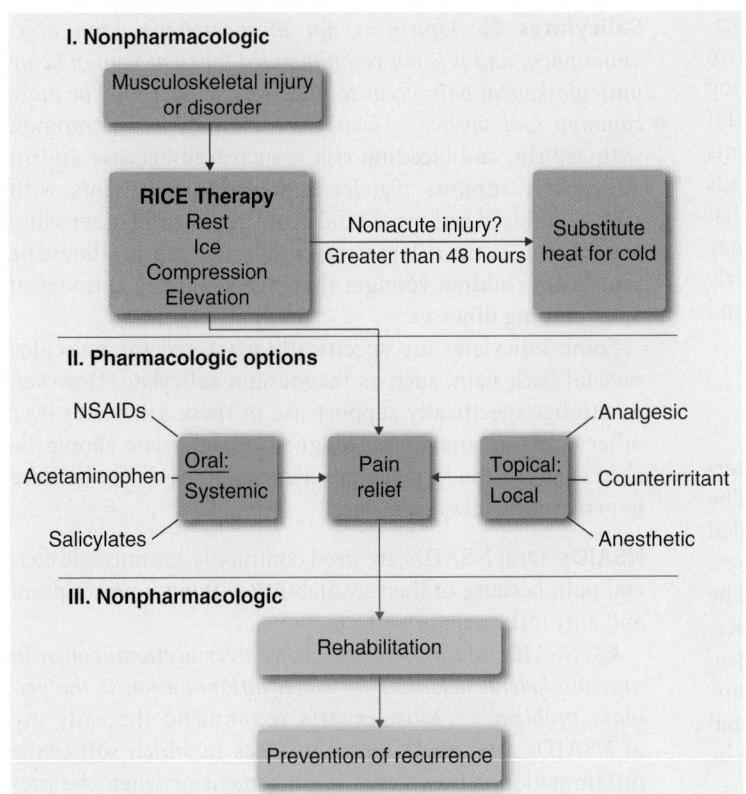

FIGURE 60-3. Treatment plan for musculoskeletal injury or disorder.

There are few studies comparing types of ice application, and recommendations vary widely.[17,22] Clinicians should instruct patients to use crushed ice or ice chips because the area will cool more evenly than with large pieces of ice. Patients should not apply ice directly to the affected area or leave it on for longer than the recommended 20 minutes, because extreme cold can cause tissue damage.[17] Similarly, patients should be instructed to wait at least 1 hour before reapplication of ice to allow the tissue to rewarm. A thin sheet or napkin will protect the skin and also allow for better cold transfer than thicker material such as a towel. Alternatively, soaking the area for 20 minutes in a cool bath (13°C [55°F]) provides effective cooling.

For small areas, an ice massage for 5 to 10 minutes can cool the area and add relief.[23] This is accomplished by freezing water in a paper cup and removing the top part of the cup to expose the ice. The exposed ice is rubbed on the affected area. Any ice application should be stopped if the area becomes white or blue.

❸ *Heat should not be applied during the acute injury phase (the first 48 hours) because it promotes swelling and inflammation.*[8] After the first 48 hours, many patients find

Table 60–1		
RICE Therapy		
Therapy	**General Guidelines**	**Therapeutic Benefit**
Rest	Rest the affected area	Analgesia
	Use supports such as slings and crutches as necessary	Anti-inflammatory
	Employ during the acute inflammatory phase, 1–5 days after injury	Prevent further injury
Ice	Cool the affected area by submersion in cool water (13°C [55°F]) or by application of crushed ice in a plastic bag covered with a thin cloth	Analgesia
	Cool the affected area for 15–20 minutes; repeat every 2 hours for the first 48 hours	Anti-inflammatory
Compression	Compress the affected area with an elastic bandage or support	Anti-inflammatory
	Begin wrapping the bandage at the point most distal to the injury (e.g., at the toes for an ankle injury); bind firmly but not tightly	Adjunctive analgesia
	If the area distal to the injury (e.g., fingers, toes) throbs or turns cold or blue, the bandage is too tight and should be loosened	
Elevation	Elevate the area (especially the extremities) above heart level	Anti-inflammatory

that heat decreases pain and eases muscle stiffness associated with immobility. A heating pad, heat wrap, or warm bath can be used on day three or later as long as no swelling develops after heat is applied. Heat should be discontinued if increased swelling occurs. Clinicians should educate patients to avoid sleeping with or sitting or lying on heating pads because this can result in burns. Low-level heat, such as that supplied by therapeutic heat wraps (e.g., ThermaCare), may provide a safer means of heat application.[24] However, elderly persons should still be cautioned about the risk of burns and be advised to wear the wrap over thin clothing.

Pharmacologic Therapy

❹ *There are two main approaches to pharmacologic intervention for pain relief: oral (systemic) and topical agents.* The choice between systemic or topical options is often guided by patient preference. For example, many topical products have a medicinal odor and require frequent applications. The extent of musculoskeletal pain also guides treatment choice. ❺ *Localized pain may be treated effectively with local topical therapy, whereas generalized pain is best treated with systemic agents.* Factors such as alcohol use, liver function, renal function, allergies, age, and comorbid conditions should be considered when choosing among therapeutic options.

▶ Oral Analgesics

Nonopioid analgesics, including acetaminophen, aspirin, and NSAIDs, are used commonly for musculoskeletal disorders. All these agents provide analgesia, but aspirin and NSAIDs also work peripherally to decrease production of the principal mediator of acute inflammation, PGE_2.[8,18] NSAIDs and aspirin inhibit the enzyme COX. Although the mechanism of action of acetaminophen is less clear, it appears that acetaminophen acts as a weak inhibitor of PG production. In contrast to aspirin and NSAIDs that inhibit PG production peripherally, acetaminophen exerts its effect centrally with little or no anti-inflammatory effect.[25]

Acetaminophen ❻ *Acetaminophen is the drug of choice for mild-to-moderate regional musculoskeletal pain without inflammation.*[26,27] Comparative trials between acetaminophen and oral NSAIDs demonstrate equivalent analgesia in some situations, but NSAIDs may be preferred in others.[27] Therefore, if adequate analgesia is not achieved with acetaminophen, switching to an NSAID is a reasonable approach. Acetaminophen offers the advantage of less GI toxicity than NSAIDs. Although tolerability of acetaminophen is high at therapeutic doses, hepatotoxicity has been reported after overdose and at therapeutic doses, especially in combination with other factors.[26] Acetaminophen should be used with caution in patients who have liver disease or consume alcohol because of the risk of hepatotoxicity. Clinicians should advise patients not to exceed 4 grams per day of acetaminophen to minimize the risk of liver injury. Due to concern over liver injury, many over-the-counter products are now labeled with a maximum of 3 grams per day; clinicians should encourage patients to follow these labeled directions.

Salicylates ❼ *Aspirin is not more effective than acetaminophen, and it is not recommended for treatment of acute musculoskeletal pain because its adverse effects may be more common and severe.*[27] Gastric irritation is more common with aspirin, and bleeding risk is increased because aspirin irreversibly inhibits platelet aggregation.[27] Patients with aspirin-induced asthma should avoid aspirin and other salicylates.[28] Due to the risk of Reye's syndrome, aspirin should be avoided in children younger than age 19 during episodes of fever-causing illnesses.

Some salicylates are specifically marketed for musculoskeletal back pain, such as magnesium salicylate. However, no studies specifically support use of these salicylates over other systemic analgesics. Magnesium salicylate should be used with caution in patients with renal impairment because hypermagnesemia can occur.[29]

NSAIDs Oral NSAIDs are used commonly for musculoskeletal pain because of their availability without a prescription and anti-inflammatory effects.[18,29]

❽ *NSAIDs are a preferred choice over acetaminophen in musculoskeletal disorders in which inflammation is the primary problem.*[26,30] Most experts recommend the early use of NSAIDs after acute injury in cases in which soft tissue inflammation causes nerve impingement or when the predominate problem is inflammation, such as in bursitis.[30]

NSAIDs are particularly beneficial for chronic overuse injury, in which inflammation is central to the pain and loss of motion. Although NSAIDs may be helpful in relieving pain and inflammation in tendonitis, many tendonopathies are not associated with inflammation. Therefore, use of a simple analgesic such as acetaminophen may relieve pain adequately.[14,29]

The analgesic effects of NSAIDs are attributed to inhibition of the COX-2 enzyme, whereas the negative GI effects are due to inhibition of COX-1.[27] Patients taking oral anticoagulants, those with a history of peptic ulcer disease, or others at high risk for GI complications may be considered candidates for a COX-2 inhibitor (e.g., celecoxib) or a combination of a nonselective NSAID with a gastroprotective agent such as a proton pump inhibitor (see Chap. 58).

COX-2 inhibitors are associated with adverse effects such as nephrotoxicity and a potential increased risk of myocardial infarction (see Chap. 58). Combination of COX-2 inhibitors with alcohol can increase GI adverse effects. All NSAIDs should be used with caution in patients with aspirin-induced asthma.[29]

Opioids Opioid analgesics can be used for patients not responding adequately to nonopioid analgesics or for moderate-to-severe pain.[27] These agents generally are given alone or in combination with simple analgesics such as acetaminophen. Tolerance and physical dependence are considerations but less of a concern when treating acute pain. When used in equivalent doses, opioids produce similar pain relief and adverse effects such as sedation, nausea, constipation, and respiratory depression (see Chap. 33).

Topical (External) Analgesics Topically (or externally) applied drugs that exert a local analgesic, anesthetic, or antipruritic effect by either suppressing cutaneous sensory receptors or by stimulating these receptors in a counterirritant fashion are termed *external analgesics*.[21] These medications are applied directly to the affected area to create high local concentrations of the drug.[19,31] Formulations include gel, cream, lotion, patch, liquid, liniment, or aerosol spray. Negligible systemic concentrations are achieved with intact skin, minimizing systemic adverse effects. Topical application should not be confused with transdermal delivery, in which drug absorption into the bloodstream produces a systemic effect. Musculoskeletal disorders often are treated with topical (but not transdermal) medications.

After application, the topical medication penetrates the skin to the soft tissue and peripheral nerves.[21] At the site, topical analgesics suppress the sensitization of pain receptors, thereby reducing pain and burning. Examples include topical NSAIDs and local anesthetics, such as lidocaine. In contrast, *counterirritant* products are external analgesics that stimulate cutaneous sensory receptors, producing a burning, warming, or cooling sensation that masks the underlying pain. In effect, the irritation or inflammation caused by the counterirritant distracts from the underlying pain. Menthol and capsaicin are examples of counterirritants.

Some patients prefer external analgesics to systemic analgesics because the rubbing during application can be comforting.[32,33] External analgesics are useful adjuvants to nonpharmacologic therapy and systemic analgesic therapy to provide additional relief. These agents also offer a therapeutic option in patients who cannot tolerate systemic analgesics. Because these agents are not in pill form and many are available without a prescription, they may be overused or misused. This prompted the FDA to caution consumers that the agents are medicines that may also cause harm.[34] Clinicians should advise patients to always read and follow directions on the labels of OTC products.

Topical NSAIDs. In acute soft-tissue injury such as strains and sprains, topical NSAIDs have efficacy that is superior to that of placebo and similar to that of oral NSAIDs.[31,37] Tissue concentrations of topical NSAIDs are high enough to produce anti-inflammatory effects, but systemic concentrations after application remain low.

Diclofenac is the only topical NSAID commercially available in the United States.[35-38] Diclofenac patch (Flector Patch) is indicated specifically for the topical treatment of acute pain from minor sprains and strains.[35] The patch is applied to the most painful area twice daily. Diclofenac gel (Voltaren Gel) is indicated for joint pain in the knees and hands secondary to osteoarthritis; it is applied up to four times daily.[36] Diclofenac solution (Pennsaid) is indicated for osteoarthritis of the knee; it is applied via a dropper to the knee four times daily.[37] Patient education for topical NSAIDs is outlined in Table 60–2.[35-37]

Theoretically, the risk of serious GI adverse events should be less than with oral NSAIDs, but long-term studies evaluating these events are lacking.[31,38] Like oral NSAIDs, topical NSAIDs should be used with caution in patients with a history of GI bleeding or ulcer.[35-37] Studies comparing topical NSAIDs with other topical products, including counterirritants, are also needed. Local cutaneous adverse reactions (e.g., erythema, rash, pruritus, and irritation) are reported and may be due in part to the vehicle used.[35-38]

Local Anesthetics. Nonprescription topical anesthetics such as lidocaine and benzocaine are available in many types of products. Local anesthetics decrease discharges in superficial somatic nerves and cause numbness on the skin surface but do not penetrate deeper structures such as muscle where the pain often lies.[19]

However, local anesthetics are helpful when abrasion accompanies the injury. Application of an OTC antibiotic ointment containing an anesthetic provides soothing relief, promotes healing of abrasions, and prevents soft-tissue infection. Minor abrasions should be cleansed thoroughly with mild soap and water before application. More severe abrasions may require removal of debris or foreign bodies by a clinician followed by irrigation with normal saline.

• ***Counterirritants.*** Counterirritants are categorized by the FDA into four groups (groups A through D) based on their

Table 60–2			
Patient Education for Topical NSAIDs			
All Topical NSAIDs	**Gel-Specific**	**Patch-Specific**	**Solution-Specific**
Do not apply to damaged or nonintact skin	Use enclosed dosing card to determine amount for application	Apply to skin at the most painful area	Recommended dose is 40 drops to the each affected knee four times daily
Wash hands after application and/or removal	Avoid bathing or showering for 1 hour after application	Do not wear during bathing or showering	Apply 10 drops at a time directly to the knee or on the hand, then the knee
Discontinue use if rash or irritation develops	Avoid sun exposure or tanning beds	Tape patch in place if it begins to peel off Discard used patches away from children and pets	Rub evenly around front, back, and sides of the knee
Do not use with oral NSAIDs	Do not use with other topical agents (e.g., sunscreens, lotions, moisturizers, and insect repellants)		Do not cover with clothing or apply other topical products onto knee until completely dry

From Refs. 35–37.

Table 60–3

Nonprescription Counterirritant External Analgesics

Group and Effect	Agents and Concentration	Example Products (If Applicable)	Comments
Group A Rubefacients: Produce redness	Allyl isothiocyanate 0.5–5%		Mustard derivative; pungent odor; avoid inhalation
	Ammonia water 1–2.5%		More concentrated solutions are highly caustic; avoid inhalation
	Methyl salicylate 10–60%	BenGay Ultra Strength[a] Flexall Plus[a] Icy Hot Stick[a]	Caution in aspirin sensitivity May produce systemic concentrations May increase INR with warfarin
Group B Produce cooling	Camphor 3–11% Menthol 1.25–16%	JointFlex BenGay Patch Icy Hot Patch Mineral Ice	Medicinal odor Sensation of heat follows cooling Mild anesthetic effects at low concentrations
Group C Produce vasodilation	Methyl nicotinate 0.25–1%		May produce systemic vasodilation
Group D Irritate without redness	Capsaicin 0.025–0.25% Capsicum oleoresin 0.025–0.25%	Capzasin-HP, Zostrix	Must use regularly Burning effect subsides with regular use

INR, International Normalized Ratio.

[a]Combination products that also contain menthol and/or camphor.

---

primary actions (Table 60–3). They produce a feeling of warmth, cooling, or irritation that diverts sensation from the primary source of pain. Because these irritant effects are central to the beneficial actions, counterirritants should not be combined with topical anesthetics or topical analgesics.

Counterirritants are indicated for the temporary relief of minor aches and pains related to muscles and joints.[21] These symptoms may be associated with simple backache, arthritis, strains, sprains, or bruises. Many are available commercially as combination products with ingredients from different counterirritant groups. Active ingredients in marketed products sometimes change; clinicians should be aware of the current ingredients before providing a product recommendation. ❾ *Patient education on proper use of counterirritants is essential to therapeutic success* (Table 60–4).[21]

Rubefacients (group A) are counterirritants that produce redness on application. Topical rubefacients containing salicylates (e.g., methyl salicylate) are used most commonly. Turpentine oil is no longer judged as either safe or effective but remains in a few products.[21] Clinical trial data evaluating the effect of rubefacients on acute pain from strains, sprains, sports injuries, and chronic musculoskeletal pain are lacking.[39] A systematic review of available evidence noted that topical salicylates are effective for pain from acute musculoskeletal conditions, but the low quality of the evidence led authors to conclude that there are no good data supporting the efficacy of rubefacients.[39]

Methyl salicylate and trolamine salicylate are topical salicylates. Methyl salicylate is considered a counterirritant, but trolamine salicylate is not considered a counterirritant because it does not produce localized irritation after application.

Table 60–4

Patient Education for Counterirritants

Apply up to 3–5 times daily to affected area.
Only for external use on the skin; do not ingest.
Do not apply to broken or damaged skin or cover large areas.
Wash hands immediately after application.
Avoid contact with the eyes and mouth.
Do not use with heating pads or other methods of heat application, because burning or blistering can occur.
Do not wrap or bandage the area tightly after application.
Consult a physician if:

- Symptoms worsen
- Symptoms persist for more than 7 days[a]
- Symptoms resolve but then recur

[a]Capsaicin may be used for chronic pain and must be applied consistently for efficacy.

From External analgesics drug products for over-the-counter human use: Tentative final monograph. Fed Regist 1983;48: 5851–5869.

Application of both topical salicylates can lead to systemic effects, especially if the product is applied liberally.[40] Repeated application and occlusion with a wrap or bandage also can increase systemic concentrations. Salicylate-containing products should be used with caution in patients in whom systemic salicylates are contraindicated, such as patients with severe asthma or aspirin allergy.[40] Topical salicylates have been reported to increase prothrombin time in patients on warfarin and should be used with caution in patients on oral anticoagulants. Methyl salicylate, including oil of wintergreen, is one of the most common sources of pediatric poisonings.[41] Clinicians should advise patients to keep products out of the reach of children.

The FDA advises that there is insufficient evidence to support the effectiveness of trolamine salicylate contained in products such as Aspercreme.[21] However, many patients choose trolamine products because of the lack of medicinal odor.

The group B counterirritants menthol and camphor exert a sensation of cooling through direct action on sensory nerve endings.[40,42] A sensation of warmth follows the cooling effect. The agents also have mild anesthetic activity at low concentrations.[42] In higher concentrations, they act as counterirritants and cause a burning sensation by stimulating cutaneous nociceptors. Menthol and camphor are used often in combination with rubefacients.

Menthol, also known as peppermint oil, is used widely in toothpastes, mouthwashes, gum, sore-throat lozenges, lip balms, and nasal decongestants. For topical analgesic use, it is available in creams, lotions, ointment, and patches. The patches can be trimmed to fit the affected area.

Menthol and camphor have caused respiratory distress in infants and should not be used in children under 2 years of age. Despite limits on the concentration of available products, camphor can be toxic to children even in small amounts.[43] Patients should be advised to keep the products out of the reach of children.

The group C counterirritants methyl nicotinate and histamine dihydrochloride produce vasodilation.[21] Methyl nicotinate is a nicotinic acid derivative that produces PG-mediated vasodilation.[44] NSAIDs and aspirin block the production of PGs and decrease methyl nicotinate–induced vasodilation. Application over a large area has been reported to cause systemic symptoms and syncope, possibly due to vasodilation and a decrease in blood pressure.[45] Patients should be educated to apply only scant amounts to the affected area to avoid this effect.

The primary counterirritant in group D is capsaicin, a natural substance found in red chili peppers and responsible for the hot, spicy characteristic when used in foods.[19,32,33] Capsaicin stimulates the release of substance P from local sensory nerve fibers, depleting substance P stores over time. A period of reduced sensitivity to painful stimuli follows, and transmission of pain impulses to the CNS is reduced.

As with other counterirritants, capsaicin and its derivatives (i.e., capsicum and capsicum oleoresin) exert a warming or burning sensation. With repeated application, desensitization occurs, and the burning sensation subsides. This typically occurs within the first 1 to 2 weeks. After discontinuation, resensitization occurs gradually and returns completely within a few weeks.[46]

Because of the lag time between initiation and effect, capsaicin is not used for treatment of acute pain from injury. Instead, topical capsaicin is used for chronic pain from musculoskeletal and neuropathic disorders. Capsaicin preparations have been studied in the treatment of pain from diabetic neuropathy, osteoarthritis, rheumatoid arthritis, postherpetic neuralgia, and other disorders.[47] It is often used as an adjuvant to systemic analgesics in these chronic pain conditions.

Although systemic adverse effects to capsaicin are rare, local adverse effects are expected and common.[19,32] Patient education regarding consistent use of capsaicin products is essential to achieving desired outcomes. Product should be applied in a thin layer and rubbed into the skin thoroughly until little remains on the surface.[40] ⑩ *Patients using capsaicin should be advised to apply it regularly and consistently three to four times daily and that full effect may take 1 to 2 weeks or longer.* Patients should be assured that the burning effects will diminish with repeated application. Adherence to therapy is essential because the burning sensation persists if applications are less frequent than recommended. Because the burning sensation is enhanced with heat, patients should avoid hot showers or baths immediately before or after application. Wearing gloves during application can decrease the potential for unintended contact with eyes or mucous membranes. Dried product residue has been reported to cause respiratory effects on inhalation,[47] and caution should be used in patients with asthma or other respiratory illnesses.

▶ *Muscle Relaxants*

Where pain is worsened by muscle spasm, oral muscle relaxants serve as a useful adjunct to therapy.[48] These agents include baclofen, metaxalone, methocarbamol, carisoprodol, and cyclobenzaprine. Muscle relaxants decrease spasm and stiffness associated with either acute or chronic musculoskeletal disorders. These agents should be used with caution because they all may cause sedation, especially in combination with alcohol or narcotic analgesics.

Lifestyle and Behavioral Modifications

After treatment of the acute injury with RICE and pharmacologic therapy, the final phase of therapy is rehabilitation and prevention of future injury. For most injuries, prolonged immobilization can lengthen the recovery time by causing wasting of the healthy muscle fibers.[14] Rehabilitation starts with the development of range of motion via stretching exercises. Patient should warm the muscle first with light activity or moderate heat.[9] Warmth produces relaxation and increases elasticity. Next, the patient should start general strengthening exercises.[49] Resistance exercises using resistance bands available at sporting goods stores are an effective method of strengthening. Strengthening and stretching exercises should be continued beyond the healing phase to prevent future injury.

After rehabilitation, the patient should be educated about behavior changes to prevent reinjury or the development of chronic pain.[14,49] The warm-up and strengthening routines learned in the rehabilitation phase should be continued. For overuse injury, correction of biomechanical abnormalities with proper footwear and changes in technique may correct misalignments and imbalances. Repetitive trauma can be decreased with proper training (e.g., by implementing a gradual increase in mileage in a running plan).

Patients with low back pain should be advised to stay active, as inactive muscles may become more sensitive to pain.[50] In the workplace, repetitive motion can be decreased through proper ergonomic design and diversification of job tasks.[51] In pain of the lower extremity, weight loss in overweight or obese patients can assist in reduction of further inflammation and help to prevent reinjury or repetitive strain injuries. Non–weight-bearing activities, such as swimming or bicycling, can be recommended for initial return to activity.[52]

OUTCOME EVALUATION

- Use a pain scale to monitor treatment interventions to ensure that pain relief is achieved. Ask the patient to rate pain on a scale of zero (no pain) to 10 (worst possible pain) both at rest and with movement. Compare the results with baseline pain assessment to monitor the response to therapy. In pediatric patients, use a visual pain scale with facial expressions depicting various degrees of pain.

- Assess range of motion at baseline and after treatment by comparing movement with the unaffected limb and functionality before the injury. Assess functionality by asking patients if they are able to perform activities of daily living or participate in exercise as desired.

- If pain from acute injury does not decrease greatly within 7 to 10 days, further diagnostic evaluation is warranted.

- For patients using capsaicin products, assess adherence to regular application for therapeutic benefit. Assess chronic pain control in 2 weeks.

- Assess medication adverse effects on a regular basis. When NSAIDs and aspirin are used, ask about GI tolerability, bruising, and bleeding. Inquire about local adverse effects, such as burning, when topical counterirritants are used for treatment.

- Evaluate adherence to preventative rehabilitation measures such as proper footwear, warm-up before activity, strength training, and proper lifting technique.

Patient Care and Monitoring

1. Assess the patient's symptoms to determine whether empirical care is appropriate or whether diagnostic evaluation is warranted. Determine the timing of injury (if applicable), duration of pain, type and degree of pain, and exacerbating factors. Determine whether the musculoskeletal disorder interferes with usual activities or range of motion.

2. Assess exacerbating or alleviating factors. Ask if the patient has tried any nonpharmacologic or pharmacologic treatments.

3. Obtain a complete medication history, including history of prescription drug, nonprescription drug, and dietary supplement use. Determine whether the patient has used any successful or unsuccessful treatments for this condition in the past.

4. Gather patient history. Assess factors involved in drug selection. Inquire about social history and alcohol use. Ask the patient about drug allergies and chronic health problems such as asthma.

5. Educate the patient on nonpharmacologic therapy, including each of the steps in RICE. If injury is the source of the pain and it occurred more than 48 hours ago, consider heat instead of ice.

6. Assess patient preference for systemic (oral) or local (topical) therapy. Would frequent application of topical medications be possible? Would the patient accept topical medications with a medicinal odor?

7. Recommend appropriate pharmacologic therapy and educate on proper use. If a counterirritant is recommended, counsel patients on the irritant effect of the product and recommend washing hands immediately after use and to avoid heating pads. For patients using a capsaicin product, emphasize that adherence to regular application is required for effectiveness.

8. Develop a plan to assess effectiveness of pharmacologic therapy. If pain is from an acute injury, assess effectiveness within 7 to 10 days. For chronic pain treated with capsaicin, begin to assess pain control in 2 weeks.

9. Evaluate for adverse effects and drug interactions. For patients on topical therapy, evaluate for local adverse effects. For patients on oral acetaminophen or NSAIDs, inquire about alcohol use.

10. Stress lifestyle modifications for rehabilitation and prevention. Recommend strength training, range-of-motion exercises, and a warm-up period before exercise. In repetitive-motion injury, recommend methods to correct biomechanical abnormalities and vary work tasks as applicable. Refer to a physical therapist or sports trainer as needed.

Abbreviations Introduced in This Chapter

COX	Cyclooxygenase
NSAIDs	Nonsteroidal anti-inflammatory drugs
PG	Prostaglandin

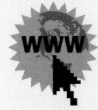 Self-assessment questions and answers are available at *http://www.mhpharmacotherapy.com/pp.html.*

REFERENCES

1. Abásolo L, Blanco M, Bachiller J, et al. A health system program to reduce work disability related to musculoskeletal disorders. Ann Intern Med 2005;143:404–414.

2. Wilder RP, Sethi S. Overuse injuries: tendinopathies, stress fractures, compartment syndrome, and shin splints. Clin Sports Med 2004;23:55–81.

3. Schappert SM, Burt CW. Ambulatory care visits to physician offices, hospital outpatient departments, and emergency departments: United States, 2001-02. Vital Health Stat 13 2006:1–66.

4. United States Bone and Joint Decade. The Burden of Musculoskeletal Diseases in the United States. Rosemont, IL: American Academy of Orthopaedic Surgeons; 2008.

5. Punnett L, Wegman DH. Work-related musculoskeletal disorders: the epidemiologic evidence and the debate. J Electromyogr Kinesiol 2004;14:13–23.

6. Morse T, Dillon C, Kenta-Bibi E, et al. Trends in work-related musculoskeletal disorder reports by year, type, and industrial sector: a capture-recapture analysis. Am J Ind Med 2005;48:40–49.

7. Caine D, Maffulli N, Caine C. Epidemiology of injury in child and adolescent sports: injury rates, risk factors, and prevention. Clin Sports Med 2008;27:19–50.

8. Audette J, Frotera W. Assessment and treatment of pain in sports injuries. In: Warfield CA, Bajwa ZH, eds. Principles and Practice of Pain Medicine. 2nd ed. New York: McGraw-Hill; 2004:35–48.

9. Järvinen TA, Järvinen TL, Kääriäinen M, et al. Muscle injuries: optimising recovery. Best Pract Res Clin Rheumatol 2007;21:317–331.

10. Ivins D. Acute ankle sprain: an update. Am Fam Physician 2006;74:1714–1720.

11. Järvinen TA, Järvinen TL, Kääriäinen M, Kalimo H, Järvinen M. Muscle injuries: biology and treatment. Am J Sports Med 2005;33:745–764.

12. Last AR, Hulbert K. Chronic low back pain: evaluation and management. Am Fam Physician 2009;79:1067–1074.

13. De Carli A, Volpi P, Pelosini I, et al. New therapeutic approaches for management of sport-induced muscle strains. Adv Ther 2009;26:1072–1083.

14. Wilson JJ, Best TM. Common overuse tendon problems: A review and recommendations for treatment. Am Fam Physician 2005;72:811–818.

15. Widmaier EP, Raff H, Strang KT. Vander's Human Physiology: The Mechanisms of Body Function. 12th ed. New York: McGraw Hill; 2011.

16. Cohen SA. Pathophysiology of pain. In: Warfield CA, Bajwa ZH, eds. Principles and Practice of Pain Medicine. 2nd ed. New York: McGraw-Hill; 2004:35–48.

17. Russell JA. Management of acute sport injury. In: Comfort P, Abrahamson E, eds. Sports Rehabilitation and Injury Prevention. Hoboken, NJ: Wiley-Blackwell; 2010:163–184.

18. Rathmell JP, Fields HL. Pain: pathophysiology and management. In: Longo D, Fauci A, Kasper D, et al., eds. Harrison's Principles of Internal Medicine. 18th ed. New York City: McGraw-Hill; 2011:93–101.

19. Stanos SP. Topical agents for the management of musculoskeletal pain. J Pain Symptom Manage 2007;33:342–355.

20. Palmer T, Toombs JD. Managing joint pain in primary care. J Am Board Fam Pract 2004;17(Suppl):S32–S42.

21. External analgesics drug products for over-the-counter human use: Tentative final monograph. Fed Regist 1983;48:5851–5869.

22. Bleakley C, McDonough S, MacAuley D. The use of ice in the treatment of acute soft-tissue injury: a systematic review of randomized controlled trials. Am J Sports Med 2004;32:251–261.

23. Mazzone MF, McCue T. Common conditions of the achilles tendon. Am Fam Physician 2002;65:1805–1810.

24. Pray WS. Treating sore muscles and tendons. US Pharm 2006;5:18–24.

25. Graham GG, Scott KF. Mechanism of action of paracetamol. Am J Ther 2005;12:46–55.

26. Hunt RH, Choquette D, Craig BN, et al. Approach to managing musculoskeletal pain: acetaminophen, cyclooxygenase-2 inhibitors, or traditional NSAIDs? Can Fam Physician 2007;53:1177–1184.

27. Sachs CJ. Oral analgesics for acute nonspecific pain. Am Fam Physician 2005;71:913–918.

28. Graham GG, Scott KF, Day RO. Tolerability of paracetamol. Drug Saf 2005;28:227–240.

29. Peterson GM. Selecting nonprescription analgesics. Am J Ther 2005;12:67–79.

30. Paoloni JA, Orchard JW. The use of therapeutic medications for soft-tissue injuries in sports medicine. Med J Aust 2005;183:384–388.

31. Haroutiunian S, Drennan DA, Lipman AG. Topical NSAID therapy for musculoskeletal pain. Pain Med 2010;11:535–549.

32. Jackson KC, Argoff CE. Skeletal muscle relaxants and analgesic balms. In: Bonica's Management of Pain. 4th ed. Baltimore, MD: Lippincott Williams & Wilkins; 2010.

33. McCleane G. Topical analgesic agents. Clin Geriatr Med 2008;24:299–312.

34. FDA Consumer Health Information [Internet]. Use Caution with Over-the-Counter Creams, Ointments[Internet]. Food & Drug Administration; 2008 [cited 2011 Sept 19]. Available from: *http://www.fda.gov/consumer/updates/otc_creams040108.html*.

35. Flector Patch (diclofenac epolamine patch 1.3%). Bristol, TN: King Pharmaceuticals; 2011.

36. Voltaren Gel (diclofenac sodium topical gel 1%) product information. Parsippany, NJ: Novartis Consumer Health; 2009.

37. Pennsaid (diclofenac sodium topical solution 1.5%) product information. Hazelwood, MO: Mallinckrodt Brand Pharmaceuticals; 2010.

38. Zacher J, Altman R, Bellamy N, et al. Topical diclofenac and its role in pain and inflammation: an evidence-based review. Curr Med Res Opin 2008;24:925–950.

39. Matthews P, Derry S, Moore RA, McQuay HJ. Topical rubefacients for acute and chronic pain in adults. Cochrane Database Syst Rev 2009;CD007403.

40. Martindale: The complete drug reference. London: Pharmaceutical Press. Electronic version, Thompson Healthcare, Greenwood Village, CO. *http://www.thomsonhc.com*.

41. Davis JE. Are one or two dangerous? Methyl salicylate exposure in toddlers. J Emerg Med 2007;32:63–69.

42. Patel T, Ishiuji Y, Yosipovitch G. Menthol: a refreshing look at this ancient compound. J Am Acad Dermatol 2007;57:873–878.

43. Dreisinger N, Zane D, Etwaru K. A poisoning of topical importance. Pediatr Emerg Care 2006;22:827–829.

44. Wilkin JK, Fortner G, Reinhardt LA, Flowers OV, Kilpatrick SJ, Streeter WC. Prostaglandins and nicotinate-provoked increase in cutaneous blood flow. Clin Pharmacol Ther 1985;38:273–277.

45. Fergusson DA. Systemic symptoms associated with a rubefacient. BMJ 1988;297:1339.

46. Mason L, Moore RA, Edwards JE, McQuay HJ, Derry S, Wiffen PJ. Systematic review of efficacy of topical rubefacients containing salicylates for the treatment of acute and chronic pain. BMJ 2004;328:995.

47. Mason L, Moore RA, Derry S, Edwards JE, McQuay HJ. Systematic review of topical capsaicin for the treatment of chronic pain. BMJ 2004;328:991.

48. Beebe FA, Barkin RL, Barkin S. A clinical and pharmacologic review of skeletal muscle relaxants for musculoskeletal conditions. Am J Ther 2005;12:151–171.

49. Windley TC, Werner S, Maffulli N, Taunton J. Lower limb muscle and tendon injuries. In: Kolt GS, Snyder-Mackler L, eds. Physical Therapies in Sport and Exercise. 2nd ed. New York: Churchill-Livingstone; 2007:440–456.

50. Duffy RL. Low back pain: an approach to diagnosis and management. Prim Care 2010;37:729–741.

51. Buckle P. Ergonomics and musculoskeletal disorders: overview. Occup Med (Lond) 2005;55:164–167.

52. Cosca DD, Navazio F. Common problems in endurance athletes. Am Fam Physician 2007;76:237–244.

61 Glaucoma

Mikael D. Jones

Mikael D. Jones

LEARNING OBJECTIVES

● **Upon completion of the chapter, the reader will be able to:**

1. Identify risk factors for the development of primary open-angle glaucoma (POAG) and acute angle-closure glaucoma.

2. Recommend a frequency for glaucoma screening based on patient-specific risk factors.

3. Compare and contrast the pathophysiologic mechanisms responsible for open-angle glaucoma and acute angle-closure glaucoma.

4. Compare and contrast the clinical presentation of chronic open-angle glaucoma and acute angle-closure glaucoma.

5. List the goals of treatment for patients with POAG suspect, POAG, and acute angle-closure glaucoma.

6. Choose the most appropriate therapy based on patient-specific data for open-angle glaucoma, glaucoma suspect, and acute angle-closure glaucoma.

7. Develop a monitoring plan for patients on specific pharmacologic regimens.

8. Counsel patients about glaucoma, drug therapy options, ophthalmic administration techniques, and the importance of adherence to the prescribed regimen.

KEY CONCEPTS

❶ Practitioners can play an important role in eye care by assessing patients for risk factors and referring to an ophthalmologist for appropriate screening and evaluation.

❷ Acute angle-closure crisis is a medical emergency and requires laser or surgical intervention.

❸ Patients with POAG typically have a slow, insidious loss of vision. This is contrasted by the course of acute angle-closure crisis, which can lead to rapid vision loss that develops over hours to days. There are exceptions in the rate of progression for both disease subtypes, and there can be mixed subtypes whereby patients exhibit features of both diseases, so-called "combined mechanism glaucoma."

❹ The goals of therapy are to prevent further loss of visual function; minimize adverse effects of therapy and impact on the patient's vision, general health, and quality of life; maintain IOP at or below a pressure at which further optic nerve damage is unlikely to occur; and educate and involve the patient in the management of their disease.

❺ Current therapy is directed at altering the flow and production of aqueous humor, which is the major determinant of IOP.

❻ Because POAG is a chronic, often asymptomatic condition, the decision of when and how to treat patients is difficult because the treatment modalities are often expensive and have potential adverse effects or complications. Therefore, the clinician should evaluate the potential effectiveness, toxicity, and the likelihood of patient adherence for each therapeutic modality.

❼ An initial target IOP should be set at least 25% lower than the patient's baseline IOP. The target IOP can be set lower (30% to 50% of baseline IOP) for patients who already have severe disease, risk factors for disease progression, or normal-tension glaucoma (NTG).

❽ Target IOP should be revised based on the course of the disease and rate of progression.

INTRODUCTION

Glaucoma refers to a spectrum of ophthalmic disorders characterized by neuropathy of the optic nerve and loss of retinal ganglion cells, which leads to permanent deterioration of the visual field and potentially total vision loss. It is often, but not always, eye pressure related. Glaucoma can be classified as primary and secondary. *Primary glaucoma* refers to glaucoma that cannot be attributed to a preexisting ocular or systemic disease, whereas *secondary glaucoma* refers to glaucoma that can be attributed to preexisting ocular or systemic disease. Examples of primary glaucoma include open-angle, closed angle, and congenital. Examples of secondary glaucoma include pigmentary glaucoma, neovascular glaucoma, traumatic glaucoma, uveitic glaucoma, steroid-responsive glaucoma, aphakic glaucoma, and pseudoexfoliative glaucoma.

Primary open-angle glaucoma (POAG) is characterized by normal anterior-chamber angles, glaucomatous changes of the optic disc, and often peripheral visual field loss (initial stages of glaucoma sometimes result in no visual field loss). Patients with ocular hypertension (elevated IOP) that have normal-appearing anterior-chamber angles anatomy and/or an eye exam suspicious of early glaucomatous damage are classified as POAG suspects. Patients with a normal eye pressure, with measurements obtained from more than one visit, and one or both optic nerves with anatomic features consistent with nerve fiber loss are also classified as glaucoma suspects. Primary angle-closure glaucoma (PACG) is characterized by the obstruction of the anterior chamber angle resulting in either intermittent or progressive (often times acutely) elevated IOP with subsequent damage to the optic nerve. PACG is associated with moderate to high elevations in IOP.[1-4] PACG can progress to acute angle-closure crisis when a large percentage of the chamber angle is obstructed, resulting in a rapid increase in IOP. POAG and PACG represent the most common types of glaucoma and therefore are the focus of this chapter.

EPIDEMIOLOGY AND ETIOLOGY

It is estimated that 60.5 million people have open-angle or angle-closure glaucoma in 2010, making it the second leading cause of blindness after cataracts. By 2020 this number may increase to almost 80 million people worldwide.[5] In the United States it is estimated that 2.22 million people are affected by POAG, and by 2020 this number will increase to 3.36 million. The prevalence varies with race and ethnicity, and it is three to five times more prevalent in African Americans than white Americans.[6] The prevalence of POAG increases with age and is rarely seen in patients younger than 40 years.[5,6] The prevalence of POAG suspects is difficult to estimate at this time, but it is estimated that 3.5% to 4.5% of white and Hispanic patients older than 40 years have ocular hypertension.[3] Other estimates indicate that 3 to 6 million of the U.S. population has ocular hypertension; however, less than 10% will have progression to POAG within 5 years, with an increase to 22% after 13 years.[7,8]

Almost 16 million people were estimated to have angle-closure glaucoma in 2010, and this is projected to increase to 21 million people by 2020.[5] The prevalence of angle-closure glaucoma is lower than POAG and varies significantly by race and ethnicity. The prevalence is lower in patients of European descent (0.09% to 0.16%) but higher in patients

Table 61–1

Recommended Frequency of Comprehensive Adult Medical Eye Evaluation

Age (Years)	With Risk Factors for Glaucoma	No Known Risk Factors for Ocular Disease
65 or above	6–12 months	1–2 years
55–65	1–2 years	1–3 years
40–54	1–3 years	2–4 years

From American Academy of Ophthalmology. Preferred Practice Pattern Guidelines Comprehensive Adult Medical Eye Evaluation. San Francisco, CA: American Academy of Ophthalmology, 2010 [cited 2011 Oct 3]. *http://www.aao.org/ppp*.

Table 61–2

Risk Factors for Glaucoma

POAG	PACG
Elevated IOP	Advancing age
African or Hispanic descent	Asian or Eskimo ethnicity
Family history of glaucoma	Female sex
Older age	Hyperopia
Thinner CCT	Shallow anterior chamber
Type 2 diabetes	Family history of
Low ocular perfusion pressures	angle-closure glaucoma
Myopia	

CCT, central corneal thickness; IOP, intraocular pressure; POAG, primary open-angle glaucoma; PACG, primary angle-closure glaucoma.

From Refs. 2, 4.

of Chinese (1.3%), Eskimo (2.9% to 5%), and Asian Indian (4.33%) descent. PACG is also more prevalent with increasing age and among females.[1,9]

POAG is a "silent disease," with patient's not experiencing vision loss until late in the disease process. ❶ *Practitioners can play an important role in eye care by assessing patients for risk factors and referring to an eye care specialist for appropriate screening and evaluation.* Risk factor evaluation is essential in determining the frequency of comprehensive eye exams for patients (Table 61–1). It is also useful in deciding when to start therapy and determining the sequence of pharmacotherapeutic or surgical treatment modalities.[1] Table 61–2 lists the major risk factors associated with POAG and PACG.

PATHOPHYSIOLOGY

The pathophysiologic alterations seen with POAG optic neuropathy are not fully understood. Elevated IOP is clearly associated with damage and eventual death of optic nerves;

Patient Encounter, Part 1

SJ, a 75-year-old Hispanic female with a history of congestive heart failure and hypertension, presents to your clinic for her yearly checkup. She states that she is concerned about losing her eyesight because her sister has started losing her vision from glaucoma. She denies any changes in her vision.

Meds: lisinopril 10 mg orally daily, carvedilol 6.25 mg orally twice daily, furosemide 20 mg PO once daily

Based on the patient's medical and family history, what risk factors does this patient have for glaucoma?

What objective assessments should be gathered in order to fully evaluate her risk factors for glaucoma?

How often would you recommend that this patient receive a comprehensive eye evaluation?

however, optic neuropathy still occurs in patients with a normal IOP. Optic nerve degeneration without elevated IOP indicates the presence of independent factors that contribute to ganglion cell death.[10,11] The key to understanding the pathophysiology and treatment of POAG relies on an understanding of aqueous humor dynamics, IOP, and optic nerve anatomy and physiology.

Aqueous Humor

The eye is separated into two segments by the lens: the anterior segment and the posterior segment (**Figs. 61–1 and 61–2**). The anterior segment of the eye is separated by the iris

into the posterior and anterior chambers. The ciliary body, a ring-like structure that surrounds and supports the lens, produces and secretes an optically neutral fluid called aqueous humor through the diffusion and ultrafiltration of plasma. The nonpigmented epithelium of the ciliary body secretes the aqueous humor into the posterior chamber. Aqueous humor formation can be modified pharmacologically

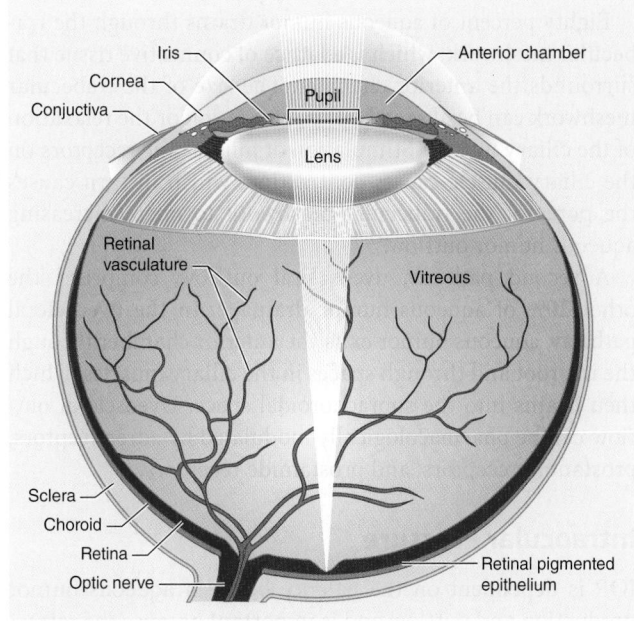

FIGURE 61–1. Anatomy of the eye. (From Lesar TS, Fiscella RG, Edward D. Glaucoma. In: DiPiro JT, Talbert RL, Yee GC, et al., eds. Pharmacotherapy: A Pathophysiologic Approach, 8th ed. New York: McGraw-Hill, 2011:1634.)

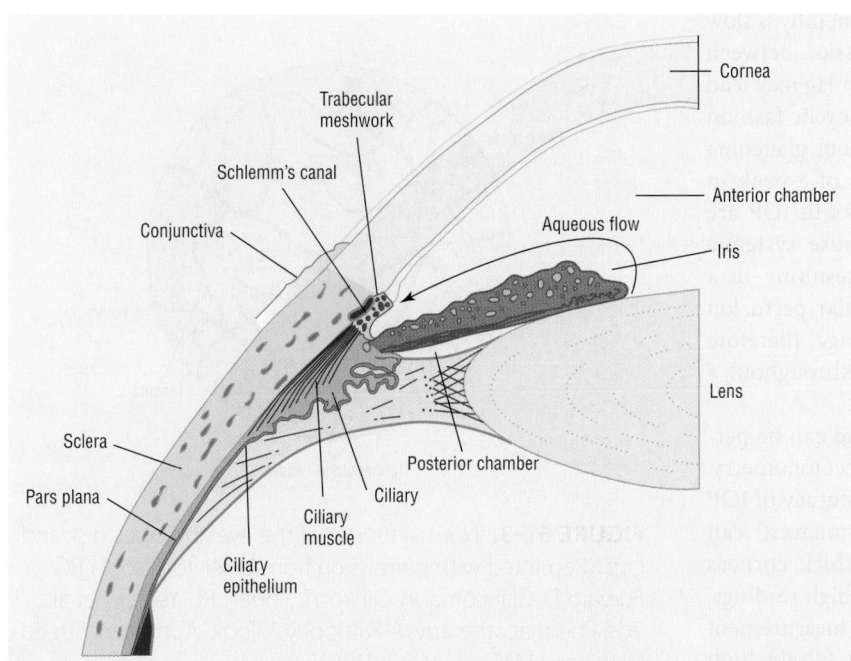

FIGURE 61–2. Anterior chamber of the eye and aqueous humor flow. (From Lesar TS, Fiscella RG, Edward D. Glaucoma. In: DiPiro JT, Talbert RL, Yee GC, et al., eds. Pharmacotherapy: A Pathophysiologic Approach, 8th ed. New York: McGraw-Hill, 2011:1634.)

through the α- and β-adrenoceptors, carbonic anhydrase, and sodium and potassium adenosine triphosphatase of the nonpigmented ciliary epithelium.[12,13]

After the transport of aqueous humor into the posterior chamber, it flows through the pupil into the anterior chamber, where it provides oxygen and nutrition to the avascular lens and cornea. Aqueous humor then exits the anterior chamber through the trabecular meshwork and drains into the Schlemm's canal, which drains aqueous humor into the episcleral venous system.[12-14]

Eighty percent of aqueous humor drains through the trabecular meshwork, which is a lattice of connective tissue that surrounds the anterior chamber. The size of the trabecular meshwork can be altered by the contraction or the relaxation of the ciliary muscle. Stimulation of muscarinic receptors on the ciliary muscle causes contraction, which in turn causes the pores of the trabecular meshwork to open, increasing aqueous humor outflow.[12,13]

A second pathway, uveoscleral outflow, comprises the other 20% of aqueous humor drainage. In the uveoscleral pathway, aqueous humor exits the anterior chamber through the iris root and through spaces in the ciliary muscles, which then drains into the suprachoroidal space. Uveoscleral outflow can be pharmacologically modulated by adrenoceptors, prostanoid receptors, and prostamide receptors.[12-14]

Intraocular Pressure

IOP is dependent on the balance between aqueous humor production and outflow and is important because the refractive properties of the eye depend on IOP to maintain the curvature of the cornea.[15] The distribution of IOP in the general population is 10 to 21 mm Hg and is slightly skewed toward higher values; however, caution should be used in assigning this range as being "normal" for IOP because optic neuropathy may be present in the normal range and may be absent at higher IOPs. Elevated IOP is generally considered greater than 21 mm Hg. Optic nerve damage generally is slow and takes several years for noticeable progression between 20 and 30 mm Hg, whereas IOP of 40 to 50 mm Hg may lead to rapid optic nerve damage.[16] IOP varies in a cyclic fashion over the 24-hour day. Patients with and without glaucoma may exhibit a circadian rhythm that consists of a peak in IOP right after falling asleep. Nighttime peaks in IOP are detrimental to patients with glaucoma, because systemic blood pressure decreases during the night, resulting in a low ocular perfusion pressure. Decreased ocular perfusion pressure can lead to further optic nerve damage, therefore highlighting the importance of IOP control throughout a 24-hour period.[17,18]

IOP is clinically measured by tonometry and can be performed via applanation, indentation, and indirect tonometry. Central corneal thickness (CCT) affects the accuracy of IOP measurements. Thin corneas (less than 540 microns) can produce falsely low IOP readings, whereas thick corneas (greater than 555 microns) may produce falsely high readings. The potential consequences of this error in measurement may lead to overtreatment of patients with falsely high IOP and undertreatment of patients with falsely low IOP. The Ocular Hypertension Treatment Study (OHTS) demonstrated that CCT is a predictive factor for the development of POAG. Patients with corneas less than 555 microns and IOP greater than 25.75 mm Hg had a 36% risk of progressing from ocular hypertension to glaucoma. The CCT of patient should be considered when evaluating a patient's IOP.[19] IOP is no longer used as a diagnostic criterion for glaucoma, because the presence of glaucomatous changes can be absent at high IOPs and can be present at lower IOPs.

Optic Nerve

The posterior segment of the eye contains vitreous humor (a clear "jellylike" substance), the retina, retinal vasculature, and the optic nerve head. The retina converts light energy into neural signals, which are transmitted out of the eye by the retinal ganglion cells. The axons of the retinal ganglion cells converge and exit the eye as a bundle through the lamina cribrosa. The converged axons forms the optic nerve (Fig. 61-3). The optic nerve contains 1 million nerve fibers and synapses at the lateral geniculate nucleus in the brain. The optic nerve head is the portion of the optic nerve that is susceptible to elevations in IOP and is visible on funduscopic examination. The optic nerve head is vertically oval and pale yellow with a depression in the center of the optic nerve, called a physiologic cup, which is formed by convergence of the axons. The area surrounding the optic nerve head is the nerve fiber layer, which consists of converging retinal ganglion cell axons. The retinal artery and vein are contained within the optic nerve head. Additionally, glial cells aid in the maintenance of homeostasis, protection, and nutrition of retinal ganglion cells.[10,11,14]

Glaucomatous changes to the optic nerve head precede visual field loss, making optic nerve head evaluation a

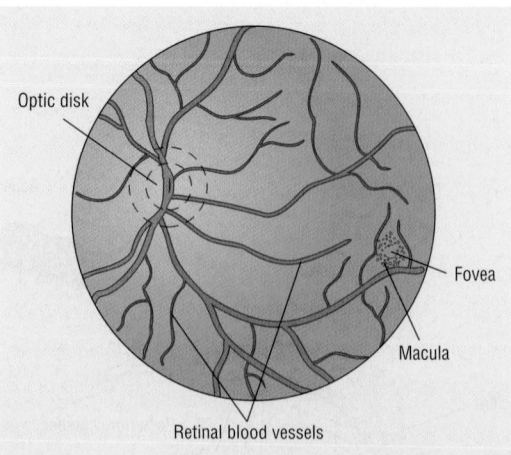

FIGURE 61-3. Normal fundus of the eye and optic disk and cup. (Reprinted with permission from Lesar TS, Fiscella RG, Edward D. Glaucoma. In: DiPiro JT, Talbert RL, Yee GC, et al., eds. Pharmacotherapy: A Pathophysiologic Approach, 8th ed. New York: McGraw-Hill, 2011:1635.)

useful screening and prognostic tool. The optic nerve head should be assessed for cupping, nerve fiber layer changes, and presence of splinter hemorrhages using a **slit-lamp biomicroscope**. Cupping refers to an increase in the size of the physiologic cup. The cup increases with the loss of retinal ganglion cell axons and the collapse of lamina cribrosa. The cup size is expressed as the ratio of the size of the cup to the size of the optic nerve head. A cup-to-disc ratio greater than 0.55 is associated with an increased risk of developing visual field loss. Other findings include atrophy and notching of the nerve fiber layer.[11,14]

Pathophysiology of Open-Angle Glaucoma

The pathophysiology of glaucomatous neurodegeneration has not been completely elucidated but appears to be caused by both IOP-dependent and IOP-independent factors. In patients with POAG, the cause of elevated IOP is not obvious, as obstruction in aqueous humor outflow is not clinically discernible. Possible causes of this increased IOP may be related to an increase in outflow resistance in the trabecular meshwork. Some forms of POAG have been associated with a mutation in the *MYOC* gene that codes a protein called myocilin. Myocilin is a protein that is produced by the ciliary body and trabecular meshwork, but its function is not known. The mutated form of myocilin may accumulate intracellularly in trabecular meshwork tissue, subsequently damaging the cells and altering aqueous humor outflow. However, this does not explain the increase in IOP in all patients with POAG.[10]

Regardless of the underlying cause, elevated IOP initiates several detrimental changes to glial cells, the lamina cribrosa, and retinal ganglion cells. The increase in IOP can lead to alterations in retinal blood flow and axonal transport of neurotrophic factors, resulting in cellular stress of the retinal ganglion cells. This stress activates the glial cells in a manner that leads to inappropriate remodeling of the extracellular matrix. Elevated IOP deforms the lamina cribrosa, which places further strain on the retinal ganglion cells. Chronic elevation of IOP ultimately causes the retinal ganglion cells to undergo apoptosis.[10,11,14,20]

Glaucomatous optic neuropathy may also occur independent of increased IOP. Pressure independent causes of optic neuropathy include abnormal blood flow, systemic hypotension, and abnormal blood coagulability.[14,16,18] Current glaucoma therapies fail to target IOP-independent glaucoma pathophysiologic factors. However, IOP reduction may still be beneficial, as the rate of visual field progression is decreased in some patients who receive IOP reduction via medical or surgical modalities.[21]

Pathophysiology of Angle-Closure Glaucoma

PACG involves a mechanical obstruction of aqueous humor outflow through the trabecular meshwork by the peripheral iris. Two major mechanisms of trabecular meshwork obstruction by the peripheral iris include pupillary block and an abnormality of the iris called *iris plateau*. Pupillary block

Clinical Presentation and Diagnosis of POAG

General
- Adult onset (usually greater than 40 years of age)
- Patients may be unaware that they have glaucoma and may be diagnosed during routine eye evaluation
- POAG is usually bilateral with asymmetric disease progression

Symptoms
- Patients with severe disease progression may report loss of peripheral vision and may describe the presence of scotomata (blind spots) in their field of vision

Signs
Ophthalmoscopic examination may reveal:
- Optic nerve head (optic disc) cupping
- Large cup-to-disc ratio
- Diffuse thinning, focal narrowing, or notching of the optic nerve head rim
- Splinter hemorrhages
- Optic nerve head/nerve fiber layer changes occur before visual field changes can be detected

Diagnostic Tests
- Gonioscopy—anterior-chamber angles are to be open
- Applanation tonometry—elevated IOP (greater than 21 mm Hg) may be present. However, patient can have signs of optic neuropathy without elevated IOP
- Pachymetry—measures central corneal thickness. Thin corneas (less than 540 μm) are considered a glaucoma risk factor.
- Automated static threshold perimetry—evaluates visual fields. Useful in diagnosis and determining whether there is progression
- Other diagnostic tests—scanning laser polarimetry, confocal scanning laser ophthalmoscopy, and optical coherence tomography

is the more common mechanism of obstruction and results from a complete or functional apposition of the central iris to the anterior lens and is associated with mid-dilation. The trapped aqueous humor in the posterior chamber increases pressure behind the iris, causing the peripheral iris to bow forward and obstruct the trabecular meshwork. Plateau iris refers to an anterior displacement of the peripheral iris caused by anteriorly positioned ciliary processes. In this configuration the peripheral iris bunches as the eye dilates. Both of these mechanisms result in the occlusion of aqueous humor outflow, causing IOP elevation at extreme levels that can lead to vision loss in hours to days.[2,11,22] The degree of iridotrabecular contact (angle closure) can be determined by **gonioscopy.**

The development of PACG is associated with several anatomical risk factors that lead to shallow anterior chambers. PACG patients may have a thick, anteriorly displaced lens that results from myopia or cataractous change. The anterior chamber depth may be shallower in some individuals with PACG, which predisposes those eyes to anatomically narrower iridocorneal inlets that are a set-up for developing critically narrow angles more susceptible to closure (from an enlarging cataractous lens or other insults).[2,22]

Medications with anticholinergic properties induce mydriasis, which can lead to angle closure in pupillary block and plateau iris. Pupillary block may also be induced by drugs that cause miosis.[23]

Patients with PACG are characterized by at least 180 degrees of iridotrabecular contact, elevated IOP, and ophthalmic exam characteristic of glaucomatous changes. Acute angle-closure crisis is the sudden obstruction of the trabecular meshwork, which leads to rapid increases in IOP resulting in pressure-induced optic neuropathy if left untreated. ❷ *Acute angle-closure crisis is a medical emergency and requires urgent laser or surgical intervention.* Recurrent attacks or a prolonged acute attack can lead to the development of peripheral anterior synechia, which partially obstructs the flow of aqueous humor through the trabecular meshwork. Patients with peripheral anterior synechia and glaucomatous changes can be classified as PACG.[2,22]

▶ Clinical Course

❸ *Patients with POAG typically have a slow, insidious loss of vision. This is contrasted by the course of acute angle-closure crisis, which can lead to rapid vision loss that develops over hours to days.* For POAG, only 4% to 8% of patients may progress to legal blindness. It may take 13 to 16 years for a patient to go blind from glaucoma. A patient's quality of life

may not be affected until significant visual field loss is present and the patient can no longer perform the activities of daily living.[24] Vision loss does not occur until there has been significant loss of the retinal ganglion cells. Peripheral vision is the most susceptible to glaucomatous damage, with central vision being preserved until advanced disease progression has occurred. Visual field abnormalities include **paracentral scotoma**, **nasal scotoma**, and **arcuate scotoma**. Patients may also have problems with depth perception and contrast sensitivity. Peripheral vision may worsen until the patient has tunnel vision and ultimately total field loss.[11,14] Visual fields can be measured by **perimetry** and can detect defects in the visual field before a patient may notice.[25]

TREATMENT
Primary Open-Angle Glaucoma

▶ Desired Outcomes and Goals

❹ *The goals of therapy are to prevent further loss of visual function; minimize adverse effects of therapy and impact on the patient's vision, general health, and quality of life; maintain IOP at or below a pressure at which further optic nerve damage is unlikely to occur; and educate and involve the patient in the management of their disease.* ❺ *Current therapy is directed at altering the flow and production of aqueous humor, which is the major determinant of IOP.*

▶ General Approach

❻ *Because POAG is a chronic, often asymptomatic condition, the decision of when and how to treat patients is difficult, as the treatment modalities are often expensive and have potential adverse effects or complications. The clinician should*

Clinical Presentation and Diagnosis of Acute Angle-Closure Crisis

General
- Medical emergency due to high risk of vision loss
- Unilateral in presentation, but fellow eye is at risk

Symptoms
- Ocular pain
- Red eye
- Blurry vision
- Halos around lights
- Systemic symptoms may develop
  - Nausea/vomiting
  - Abdominal pain
  - Headache
  - Diaphoresis

Signs
- Cloudy cornea caused by corneal edema
- Conjunctival hyperemia
- Pupil semidilated and fixed to light
- Eye will be harder on palpation through closed eye

Diagnostic Tests
- Gonioscopy—anterior-chamber angles will be closed. Peripheral anterior synechiae may be present.
- Applanation tonometry—elevated IOP (greater than 21 mm Hg, but when symptoms are present, IOP may be greater than 30 mm Hg)
- Slit-lamp biomicroscopy—reveals shallow anterior-chamber depth. Signs of previous attacks include peripheral anterior synechiae, iris atrophy, and pupillary dysfunction

evaluate the potential effectiveness, toxicity, and the likelihood of patient adherence for each therapeutic modality. The ideal therapeutic regimen should have maximal effectiveness and patient tolerance to achieve the desired therapeutic response. The American Academy of Ophthalmology (AAO) publishes Preferred Practice Patterns for POAG and POAG Suspect.[3,4]

Before the selection of a therapeutic modality, the target IOP should be determined for each patient. The target IOP ideally represents an IOP range that will slow the progression of optic neuropathy and not simply obtain an IOP in the range of 10 to 21 mm Hg. Currently, the initial target IOP is an estimate, but it should be modified based on the progression of the disease at each follow-up visit. ❼ *The AAO recommends an initial target IOP to be set at least 25% lower than the patient's baseline IOP. The target IOP can be set lower (30% to 50% of baseline IOP) for patients who already have severe disease, risk factors for disease progression, or have normal-tension glaucoma (NTG).*[4,21] Risk factors for progression include high IOP, older age, hemorrhage of the optic disc, large cup-to-disc ratio, thinner CCT, and established glaucomatous progression.

Initial IOP control can be achieved by medical, laser, surgical, or combination of these therapies. The AAO guidelines do not provide a specific recommendation on which therapeutic modality should be selected first, but patients in the early stages of glaucoma should receive treatment. In general, medical and laser trabeculoplasty are preferred as early treatment options over surgical trabeculectomy. The ophthalmologist will individualize therapy based on the risk and benefits for a specific patient. Table 61–3 describes nonpharmacologic treatment modalities for POAG.[4]

Medical treatment is the most commonly selected therapeutic modality. A well-tolerated ocular antihypertensive, at the lowest concentration, should be selected as the initial

mediation (Table 61–4). Bimatoprost, travoprost, latanoprost, and timolol are the most effective at lowering at IOP of both peak and trough measurements by at least 25% of baseline IOP.[26–29] If monotherapy alone lowers IOP but does not reach target pressure or there is evidence of progression, then combination therapy or switching to another agent is appropriate. The addition of a second agent from another class generally has an additive effect on IOP reduction. The ocular hypotensive lipids, timolol, carbonic anhydrase inhibitors, or brimonidine are reasonable choices for addition as a second agent.[30] Increasing the concentration or dose frequency can also be tried when possible. Minimizing the fluctuation of IOP between visits has also been suggested as potential target for therapy.[31]

A uniocular trial can be used to assess the safety and effectiveness of a topical medication before initiation in both eyes; however, uniocular drug trials do not always predict the IOP response of the second eye. The lack of correlation between IOP of fellow eyes may be explained by asymmetric IOP in each eye or the potential for contralateral IOP lowering of a uniocular applied medication. Uniocular trials may be more predictive of fellow eye response to a medication in POAG suspects than POAG patients. Ideally, the effect of a medication should be assessed independently using baseline IOP measurements.[32,33]

▶ *Treatment Considerations for POAG Suspects*

POAG suspects should be considered for topical medication therapy if they are at high risk for developing POAG or have a high IOP in which glaucomatous nerve damage is likely to occur. POAG suspects that develop evidence of glaucomatous damage or visual field defect have developed POAG and should be treated accordingly.[3] The Ocular Hypertension Treatment Study (OHTS) demonstrated that a 20% decrease in IOP can reduce the progression from ocular hypertension to POAG over a 5-year period. The incidence of progression to POAG in the treatment (4.4%) and control (9.5%) groups was small, which underscores the importance of selecting patients at high risk of progressing to POAG.[7] The rate of progression was similar 13 years later. POAG suspects with the highest baseline risk benefited the most from early treatment, as 40% of the observation group versus 28% of the treatment group progressed to POAG.[8] When medical therapy is indicated, a well-tolerated agent should be selected and optimized following the POAG treatment algorithm (Fig. 61–4). The benefit of therapy should be reassessed in patients who may require third- or fourth-line agents to control IOP. Surgical or laser intervention are rarely indicated in the treatment of glaucoma suspects.[3]

Primary Angle-Closure Glaucoma

▶ *Desired Outcomes and Goals*

● Therapeutic modalities for PACG are targeted at decreasing IOP. The goals of therapy are to preserve visual function by controlling the elevation in IOP, prevent damage to the optic nerve, and manage or prevent an acute attack of angle closure.[2]

Table 61–3	
Select Nonpharmacologic Treatment Options for POAG	
Treatment Option	**Description**
Laser trabeculoplasty	Laser energy aimed at trabecular meshwork Improves aqueous humor outflow
Trabeculectomy	Surgical removal of a portion of the trabecular meshwork Improves aqueous humor outflow Mitomycin C and fluorouracil are used to decrease scarring
Cyclodestructive surgery	Trans-scleral laser reduce rate of aqueous humor production Reserved for patients who have failed other options
Aqueous shunts	Drainage device that redirects the outflow of aqueous humor through a small tube into an outlet chamber placed underneath the conjunctiva

From Refs. 2, 4, 14.

Table 61–4

Topical Drugs Used in the Treatment of Glaucoma

Drug	Pharmacologic Properties	Common Brand Names	Dose Form	Strength (%)	Usual Dose[a]	Mechanism of Action
β-Adrenergic Blocking Agents						
Betaxolol	Relative β₁-selective	Generic	Solution	0.5	1 drop twice a day	All reduce aqueous production of ciliary body
		Betoptic-S	Suspension	0.25	1 drop twice a day	
Carteolol	Nonselective, intrinsic sympathomimetic activity	Generic	Solution	1	1 drop twice a day	
Levobunolol	Nonselective	Betagan	Solution	0.25, 0.5	1 drop twice a day	
Metipranolol	Nonselective	OptiPranolol	Solution	0.3	1 drop twice a day	
Timolol	Nonselective	Timoptic, Betimol, Istalol	Solution	0.25, 0.5	1 drop every day— 1–2 times a day	
		Timoptic-XE	Gelling solution	0.25, 0.5	1 drop every day[a]	
Nonspecific Adrenergic Agonists						
Dipivefrin	Prodrug	Propine	Solution	0.1	1 drop twice a day	Increased aqueous humor outflow
α₂-Adrenergic Agonists						
Apraclonidine	Specific α₂-agonists	Iopidine	Solution	0.5, 1	1 drop 2–3 times a day	Both reduce aqueous humor production; brimonidine known to also increase uveoscleral outflow
Brimonidine		Alphagan P	Solution	0.15, 0.1	1 drop 2–3 times a day	
Cholinergic Agonists Direct Acting						
Carbachol	Irreversible	Carboptic, Isopto Carbachol	Solution	1.5, 3	1 drop 2–3 times a day	All increase aqueous humor outflow through trabecular meshwork
Pilocarpine	Irreversible	Isopto Carpine Pilocar	Solution	0.25, 0.5, 1, 2, 4, 6, 8, 10	1 drop 2–3 times a day 1 drop 4 times a day	
		Pilopine HS	Gel	4	Every 24 hours at bedtime	
Cholinesterase Inhibitors						
Echothiophate		Phospholine Iodide	Solution	0.125	Once or twice a day	
Carbonic Anhydrase Inhibitors						
Topical	Carbonic anhydrase type II inhibition					All reduce aqueous humor production of ciliary body
Brinzolamide		Azopt	Suspension	1	2–3 times a day	
Dorzolamide		Trusopt	Solution	2	2–3 times a day	
Systemic						
Acetazolamide		Generic	Tablet	125 mg, 250 mg	125–250 mg 2–4 times a day	
			Injection	500 mg/vial	250–500 mg	
Methazolamide		Diamox Sequels	Capsule	500 mg	500 mg twice a day	
		Generic	Tablet	25 mg, 50 mg	25–50 mg 2–3 times a day	
Prostaglandin Analogs						
Latanoprost	Prostaglandin F₂ₐ analog	Xalatan	Solution	0.005	1 drop every night	Increases aqueous uveoscleral outflow and, to a lesser extent, trabecular outflow
Travoprost		Travatan, Travatan Z	Solution	0.004	1 drop every night	
Bimatoprost	Prostamide analog	Lumigan	Solution	0.03	1 drop every night	
Combinations						
Timolol-dorzolamide		Cosopt	Solution		Timolol 0.5% dorzolamide 2%	1 drop twice daily
Timolol-brimonidine		Combigan	Solution		Timolol 0.5% brimonide 0.2%	1 drop twice daily

[a]Use of nasolacrimal occlusion will increase the number of patients sucessfully treated with longer dosing intervals.

Adapted from DiPiro JT, Talbert RL, Yee GC, et al., (eds.) Pharmacotherapy: A Pathophysiologic Approach. 8th ed. New York: McGraw-Hill; 2011.

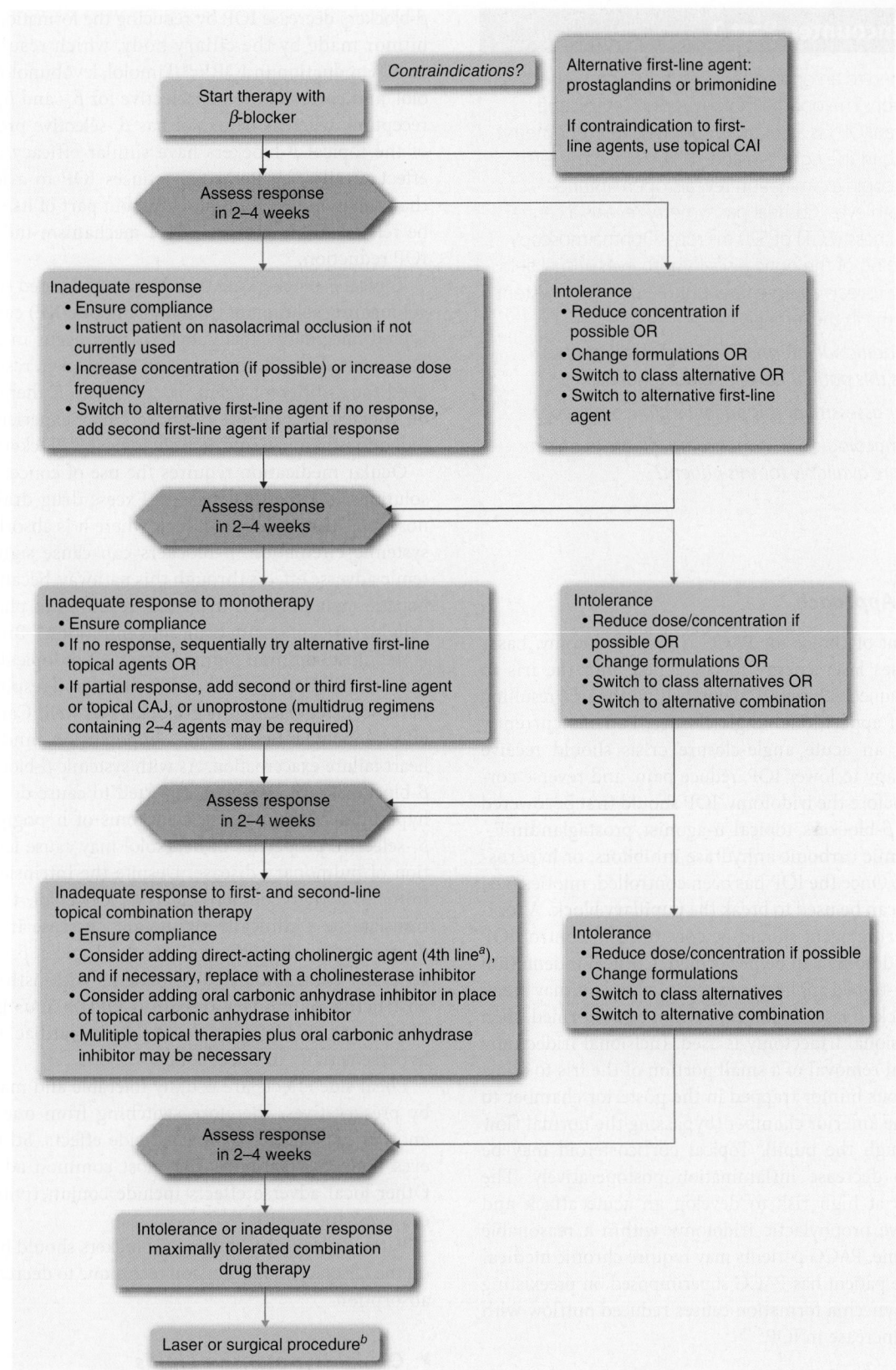

FIGURE 61–4. Algorithm for the pharmacotherapy of open-angle glaucoma. *a*Fourth-line agents not commonly used any longer. *b*Most clinicians believe laser procedures should be performed earlier (e.g., after three-drug maximum, poorly adherent patient). CAI, carbonic anhydrase inhibitor. (From Lesar TS, Fiscella RG, Edward D. Glaucoma. In: DiPiro JT, Talbert RL, Yee GC, et al., eds. Pharmacotherapy: A Pathophysiologic Approach, 8th ed. New York: McGraw-Hill, 2011:1640.)

Patient Encounter, Part 2

SJ was referred to an ophthalmologist for a comprehensive eye evaluation. The ophthalmology report reveals the patient has an IOP (as assessed by applanation tonometry) of 17 mm Hg in the right eye and 18 mm Hg in the left eye. Gonioscopic examination reveals open anterior angles in both eyes. Corneal pachymetry reveals a central corneal thickness (CCT) of 520 microns. Ophthalmoscopy reveals cupping of the optic discs in both eyes. Visual field examination reveals a nerve fiber bundle defect consistent with glaucoma in the left eye.

Given this additional information, what additional risk factors does this patient have for glaucoma?

What is your assessment this patient's glaucoma type?

What pharmacologic and nonpharmacologic treatment modalities are available for this patient?

▶ General Approach

The treatment of choice for PACG is laser iridotomy. Laser iridotomy uses laser energy to cut a hole into the iris to alleviate the aqueous humor buildup behind the iris, resulting in reversal of appositional angle closure. Patients currently experiencing an acute angle-closure crisis should receive medical therapy to lower IOP, reduce pain, and reverse corneal edema before the iridotomy. IOP should first be lowered with topical β-blockers, topical α-agonist, prostaglandin $F_{2\alpha}$ analog, systemic carbonic anhydrase inhibitors, or hyperosmotic agents. Once the IOP has been controlled, miotics (i.e., pilocarpine) can be used to break the pupillary block. A topical IOP-lowering agent should be continued to control IOP until laser iridotomy can be performed. Corneal indentation with a cotton-tipped applicator or gonioscopic lens may break pupillary block. If laser iridotomy cannot be performed, then surgical incisional iridectomy is used. Incisional iridectomy is the surgical removal of a small portion of the iris to allow flow of aqueous humor trapped in the posterior chamber to migrate to the anterior chamber (bypassing the normal flow pattern through the pupil). Topical corticosteroid may be employed to decrease inflammation postoperatively. The fellow eye is at high risk to develop an acute attack and should receive prophylactic iridotomy within a reasonable interval of time. PACG patients may require chronic medical therapy if the patient has PACG superimposed on preexisting POAG or if synechia formation causes reduced outflow with a continued increase in IOP.[2,11,34]

Pharmacologic Therapy

▶ β-Adrenergic Antagonists

Topical β-adrenergic antagonists (β-blockers) are generally considered one of the first-line agents for the treatment of POAG unless contraindications are present.[12] Topical

β-blockers decrease IOP by reducing the formation of aqueous humor made by the ciliary body, which results in a 20% to 35% reduction in IOP.[12,29] Timolol, levobunolol, metipranolol, and carteolol are nonselective for β_1- and β_2-adrenergic receptors, whereas betaxolol has β_1-selective properties. All of the topical β-blockers have similar efficacy and adverse effect profiles.[12,35] Betaxolol reduces IOP to a lesser extent than the nonselective β-blockers, but part of its efficacy may be related to a neuroprotective mechanism independent of IOP reduction.[36]

Topical β-blockers are typically administered twice daily. A gel-forming solution of timolol (Timoptic-XE) can be administered once daily. Tachyphylaxis may occur in 20% to 50% of patients on monotherapy with a β-blocker, resulting in the need for a different agent or combination therapy. Patients on concurrent systemic β-blockers may experience less IOP reduction than patients on only topical β-blockers.[12,35]

Ocular medication requires the use of concentrated drug solutions to penetrate the eye. Excess drug drains into the nose via the nasolacrimal duct, where it is absorbed into the systemic circulation. β-Blockers can cause significant systemic adverse effects through this pathway, because first-pass hepatic metabolism is bypassed, resulting in pharmacologically significant serum drug concentrations.[37] Bronchospasm is the most common pulmonary effect of topical β-blockers. Pulmonary edema, status asthmaticus, and respiratory arrest have been reported with β-blockers as well. Cardiovascular effects include bradycardia, hypotension, and congestive heart failure exacerbation. As with systemic β-blockers, topical β-blockers have also been reported to cause depression and hyperlipidemia and mask symptoms of hypoglycemia. The β_1-selective properties of betaxolol may cause less exacerbation of pulmonary disease. Despite the intrinsic sympathomimetic activity demonstrated by carteolol, this does not translate to a clinically significant decrease in pulmonary or cardiovascular adverse effects. Topical β-blockers are generally contraindicated in patients with asthma, chronic obstructive pulmonary disease (COPD), sinus bradycardia, second- or third-degree heart block, cardiac failure, and hypersensitivity to the product.[12,37]

Local side effects are usually tolerable and may be caused by preservatives, therefore switching from one product to another may alleviate the local side effects. Stinging of the eyes upon instillation is the most common adverse effect. Other local adverse effects include conjunctivitis, keratitis, dry eyes, and uveitis.[12]

Patients prescribed topical β-blockers should be counseled on the nasolacrimal occlusion technique to decrease systemic absorption.

▶ Ocular Hypotensive Lipids

The ocular hypotensive lipids in typical ophthalmology practice are considered first-line agents along with β-blockers because of their superior efficacy and safety profiles. Many clinicians may choose to use the ocular hypotensive lipids as first line, especially in patients who have an initial requirement to lower IOP by greater than 25% or in patients who have relative or absolute contraindications to topical β-blockers.[12,35] All three of the available agents currently have an FDA indication for both POAG and ocular hypertension. Latanoprost and travoprost have dosing aids that help patients administer each medication. Travoprost is available as benzalkonium chloride–free solution.

Latanoprost and travoprost are analogs of prostaglandin $F_{2\alpha}$ and are agonists of the prostanoid FP receptor, which appears to lower IOP by increasing aqueous humor outflow through the uveoscleral pathway. Bimatoprost is a prostamide analog and appears to lower IOP by activating prostamide receptors in the uveoscleral pathway and possibly through increasing outflow through the trabecular meshwork. The exact mechanism of how uveoscleral outflow is increased is still unclear, but stimulation of prostanoid FP receptors and prostamide receptors in the ciliary body cause remodeling of the extracellular matrix, making it more permeable to aqueous humor, thus increasing aqueous humor outflow through the ciliary muscles.[13,38,39]

Latanoprost, travoprost, and bimatoprost are administered once daily at bedtime and should not be increased to twice daily, as this may decrease effectiveness. The ocular hypotensive lipids can provide a consistent reduction in IOP over a 24-hour period. Peak and trough IOP reduction is approximately 28% to 30%.The prostaglandin analogs can be used as mono- or combination therapy.[28-30] For patients nonresponsive to latanoprost, switching to bimatoprost may allow some patients to reach their IOP goal, presumably because of the proposed difference in the site of action of each drug.[40,41]

The ocular hypotensive lipids are well tolerated and rarely cause systemic side effects (headache has been reported). Local effects include conjunctival hyperemia, stinging on instillation, increase in iris pigmentation, hypertrichosis, and darkening of the eyelashes. Increases in iris pigmentation occur most commonly in patients with multicolored irides on long-term prostaglandin analog therapy. The mechanism of this effect is by its action on melanocytes of the iris, in which the irides become darker because of increased production of melanin in the iris.[42] The incidence of iris pigmentation varies among the agents, with latanoprost associated with highest incidence (3% to 10%) and bimatoprost with the least (1.5%).[43-45] The increase in pigmentation may be irreversible or may reverse at a very slow rate. Increased iris pigmentation appears to be only a cosmetic effect but may affect your product selection, especially when choosing monocular therapy. Conjunctival hyperemia or engorgement of conjunctival blood vessels is a common adverse effect caused by a vasodilatory effect on scleral blood vessels. It is most prominent early in therapy and usually subsides over time. Although generally a benign adverse effect, patients may have a concern if it affects their cosmetic appearance.[43-45] The ocular hypotensive lipids should be used with caution in patients, since they may worsen anterior uveitis and herpetic keratitis. Cystoid macular edema has been reported during treatment with the ocular hypotensive lipids; therefore, use caution in patients with intraocular inflammation, aphakic patients, pseudophakic patients with a history of intraoperative

complications (e.g., torn posterior lens capsule), or in patients with risk factors for macular edema.[12,35]

Patients prescribed ocular hypotensive lipids should be counseled on potential adverse effects and appropriate administration. Patients receiving latanoprost therapy should be instructed to refrigerate the dropper bottle until opened. After the bottle has been opened it can be stored at room temperature for 6 weeks.

▶ α₂-Adrenergic Agonists

Brimonidine and apraclonidine are α_2-adrenergic agonists that decrease IOP by reducing aqueous humor production. Brimonidine has a higher selectivity to the α_2-receptor than apraclonidine and has a dual mechanism of action by increasing uveoscleral outflow.[12,13] Apraclonidine is often used for the prevention and treatment of postsurgical IOP elevations and is no longer commonly used for long-term treatment of POAG because of tachyphylaxis and high rate of blepharoconjunctivitis. Brimonidine lowers IOP by 14% to 25%. Peak IOP-lowering effect is similar to that of timolol, but the trough IOP-lowering effect is less than that of timolol.[27,29] Brimonidine may exhibit a neuroprotective effect on retinal ganglion cells and has been shown to delay visual field progression compared with timolol.[36,46]

Brimonidine is usually administered every 8 hours. A 12-hour dosing schedule may be employed when used in combination therapy. Brimonidine-purite 0.1% and 0.15% solution (Alphagan-P) has similar efficacy compared with the brimonidine 0.2% solution, because the purite solution's higher pH allows for more drug to penetrate the cornea.[12,13]

Apraclonidine and brimonidine cause both local and systemic effects. Local effects of apraclonidine include blepharoconjunctivitis, foreign body sensation, pupillary mydriasis, and eyelid retraction. Brimonidine does not cause the α_1-mediated mydriasis and eyelid retraction but does cause blepharoconjunctivitis, although at a lesser rate than apraclonidine. The brimonidine-purite solution has a lower incidence of ocular allergy. Systemic effects of both agents include headache, dry mouth, and fatigue.

Brimonidine is typically used as an adjunctive agent in combination with other agents but could be used as a first-line agent as well. The frequency of dosing and local adverse effects may lead to nonadherence in some patients. Patients prescribed brimonidine should be counseled on the nasolacrimal occlusion technique to reduce systemic adverse effects and to improve efficacy.[12] A combination product of brimonidine (0.2%) and timolol (0.5%) (Combigan) is available and can be administered twice daily.

▶ Carbonic Anhydrase Inhibitors

Carbonic anhydrase inhibitors decrease aqueous humor production by inhibition of the carbonic anhydrase isoenzyme II located in the ciliary body. In the eye, carbonic anhydrase catalyzes the conversion of H_2O and CO_2 to HCO_3^- and H^+, which is a significant step in aqueous humor production. Carbonic anhydrase inhibitors are available in systemic and topical preparations.[12,13]

Topical Carbonic Anhydrase Inhibitors Dorzolamide and brinzolamide are the only topical carbonic anhydrase inhibitors available on the market. Both medications are administered every 8 hours and are used as adjunctive therapy or as monotherapy for patients who cannot tolerate first-line therapies. Nasolacrimal occlusion may allow for an every-12-hour dosing interval. They lower peak and trough IOP by 17% to 20%.[28,29]

Local side effects include burning, stinging, itching, foreign body sensation, dry eyes, and conjunctivitis. Brinzolamide may have fewer incidences of these side effects since the drug is in a neutral pH solution. Dorzolamide has been reported to cause irreversible corneal decompensation. Taste abnormalities have been reported with each agent. Both topical carbonic anhydrase inhibitors are sulfonamides and are contraindicated in patients with history of sulfonamide hypersensitivity.[12]

A combination product of timolol (0.5%) and dorzolamide (2%) (Cosopt) is available, can be administered twice daily, and provides an additive reduction in IOP.

Systemic Carbonic Anhydrase Inhibitors There are three systemic carbonic anhydrase inhibitors: acetazolamide, dichlorphenamide, and methazolamide. These agents effectively lower IOP by 20% to 30% but are reserved as third-line to fourth-line agents because of their significant adverse effects. They are typically used as bridge therapy from maximal medical therapy to laser or surgical intervention or to control IOP in the perioperative period following a laser or surgical ocular procedure. The systemic carbonic anhydrase inhibitors can also be used to lower IOP in acute angle-closure glaucoma. Acetazolamide has an IV formulation that can be used in patients who are experiencing nausea due to the angle-closure attack. Acetazolamide and methazolamide are the best tolerated of the three agents.

The systemic carbonic anhydrase inhibitors are associated with significant adverse effects that include paresthesias of the hands and feet, nausea, vomiting, and weight loss. Patients can develop systemic acidosis, hypokalemia, hyponatremia, and nephrolithiasis due to the inhibition of renal carbonic anhydrase. Sulfonamide allergy, renal failure, hepatic insufficiency, COPD, and decreased serum potassium and sodium levels are all contraindications of systemic carbonic anhydrase inhibitor therapy. Blood dyscrasias from bone marrow suppression have been reported and include agranulocytosis, aplastic anemia, neutropenia, and thrombocytopenia.[12]

▶ Cholinergic Agents

Cholinergic agents (also called parasympathomimetics or miotics) were the first class of agents to treat glaucoma. The class can be divided into direct-acting cholinergic agents and indirect-acting cholinergic agents.

Direct-Acting Cholinergic Agents Pilocarpine directly stimulates the muscarinic (M_3) receptors of the ciliary body, which causes contraction of the ciliary muscle. This results in the widening of spaces in the trabecular meshwork, which causes an increase in aqueous humor outflow and reduces IOP by 20% to 30%.

Pilocarpine requires administration four times daily, since the IOP-lowering effect lasts only 6 hours. Pilocarpine is available in 1%, 2%, and 4% concentrations. Higher concentrations may be needed for patients with dark irides to obtain adequate IOP reduction. A pilocarpine 4% gel is available and allows for once-daily dosing at bedtime.[12] Pilocarpine is considered a third-line agent for glaucoma. In the treatment of PACG, it is important to delay use until IOP has been controlled, because pilocarpine could worsen angle closure by causing anterior displacement of the lens. Once IOP is controlled, pilocarpine can be given to break pupillary block by instilling one drop applied twice in an hour.

The adverse effects of pilocarpine are caused by the induction of miosis. The contraction of the ciliary muscle causes the lens to displace forward, which can lead to accommodation spasm and myopia, and can lead to brow ache. Pupillary constriction can also affect night vision. Pilocarpine should be avoided in patients with severe myopia as it increases the risk of developing retinal detachment. Systemic effects may occur at higher concentrations and include nausea, vomiting and diarrhea, and bradycardia.

Carbachol stimulates the same muscarinic receptor as pilocarpine and also inhibits acetylcholinesterase, the enzyme that metabolizes acetylcholine. Carbachol is more potent than pilocarpine, but it causes more accommodation spasm and brow ache and may also cause anterior uveitis. Other reported side effects include corneal clouding, persistent bullous keratopathy, and retinal detachment. Carbachol is rarely used today because of the side effect profile.

Indirect-Acting Cholinergic Agents Echothiophate iodide and demecarium bromide inhibit acetylcholinesterase. Inhibition of this enzyme increases the availability of acetylcholine at the nerve junction, thus increasing the stimulation of the muscarinic (M_3) receptors of the ciliary body. These products are given twice daily and have similar efficacy to pilocarpine in the degree of IOP reduction. The side effect profile is similar to that of pilocarpine; however, they can deplete systemic cholinesterases and pseudocholinesterases and may cause the formation of cataracts. These agents should be discontinued at least 1 week before general surgical procedures. Succinylcholine and some local anesthetics are metabolized by pseudocholinesterases; therefore, depletion of this enzyme by echothiophate or demecarium may lead to toxic effects. These agents are typically used when other topical agents have failed and are limited to patients who have had their lenses removed or who have artificial lenses.[12]

▶ Hyperosmotics

Glycerin, isosorbide, and mannitol are hyperosmotic agents that increase the osmolality of blood. These agents create an osmotic gradient that draws water from the vitreous humor, thus decreasing IOP. The resulting dehydration of the vitreous humor may cause posterior movement of the lens, which then causes the anterior chamber to deepen, thus opening the anterior angle. If the patient is not vomiting, glycerin (1 to

1.5 g/kg of a 50%) solution and isosorbide (1.5 to 2 g/kg) can be given orally. Isosorbide is preferred in patients with diabetes because it is not metabolized into glucose. If the patient has nausea or vomiting, mannitol (20%) can be given IV at a dose of 1 to 2 g/kg over 45 minutes. The hyperosmotic agents are rapid acting, reaching peak effect in 30 to 60 minutes. Headache and thirst are common complaints. Patients who are already dehydrated are at risk of developing CNS dehydration, which can lead to coma. These agents should be used with caution in patients with renal or cardiovascular disease, as extracellular water is increased.[34]

▶ *Nonselective Adrenergic Agonists*

Epinephrine and its prodrug, dipivefrin, are rarely used for the treatment of glaucoma and are considered last-line agents because of their systemic side effect profile. Dipivefrin increases the corneal penetration. Once it is absorbed through the cornea, it is enzymatically cleaved to epinephrine. Epinephrine has α- and β-agonist activity and is thought to increase the outflow of aqueous humor through the trabecular meshwork and the uveoscleral pathway. Both products are instilled twice daily and reduce IOP by 15% to 25%. Local adverse effects include mydriasis, conjunctival hyperemia, and ocular irritation. Aphakic patients should not use these medications because they cause a reversible cystoid macular edema. Epinephrine and dipivefrin should not be used in patients with narrow angles since these agents can cause acute angle closure. Systemic side effects include palpitations, increased blood pressure, and arrhythmia, and therefore, these drugs should be used with caution in patients with cardiovascular disease, cerebrovascular disease, and hyperthyroidism. Using the nasolacrimal technique may decrease systemic effects.[12]

SPECIAL CONSIDERATIONS: DRUG-INDUCED GLAUCOMAS

Medications have the potential to cause or exacerbate both POAG and PACG; however, PACG is more likely to be exacerbated by medications than POAG. The use of medications with anticholinergic or sympathomimetic properties can precipitate angle closure. Medications with anticholinergic properties include first-generation antihistamines, tricyclic antidepressants, and antipsychotics. Medications with sympathomimetic properties include phenylephrine and pseudoephedrine. PACG patients who have been treated with laser iridotomy can usually use these agents without causing an exacerbation. Sulfa-based drugs, such as topiramate, acetazolamide, and hydrochlorothiazide, cause swelling of the ciliary body, which causes an anterior displacement of the lens, resulting in a decrease in anterior-chamber depth. Patients with open or closed anterior angles can experience elevated IOP from these drugs. Controlled POAG is rarely exacerbated by anticholinergics and sympathomimetics unless the patient is concomitantly at risk for angle closure. For uncontrolled or untreated POAG, the risk–benefit ratio should be considered before employing these agents. POAG can be exacerbated by any administrated form of corticosteroids. Corticosteroids increase IOP by causing obstruction of the trabecular meshwork with extracellular material. The increase in IOP appears to increase with potency and intraocular penetration. Ophthalmic corticosteroid preparations carry the highest risk of increasing IOP. However, all administrated routes have been shown to raise IOP in some patients. The onset and extent of IOP elevation is dependent on the specific corticosteroid, dose, route, and frequency. Generally corticosteroid-induced IOP elevation typically occurs within a few weeks of beginning steroid therapy. In most cases, the IOP lowers spontaneously to the baseline within a few weeks to months upon stopping the steroid. In rare instances, the IOP remains elevated. Some patients exhibit clinically significant and dangerously high IOP as a result of steroid use.[23]

OUTCOME EVALUATION
Primary Open-Angle Glaucoma

Evaluate patients 2 to 4 weeks after the initiation or alteration of medical therapy. The clinician should elicit the status of ocular health since the last visit, systemic medical history, medication history, and presence of local and ocular adverse effects of medications. IOP measurement, visual acuity assessment, and slit-lamp biomicroscopy at every POAG follow-up visit is necessary. The frequency of visual fields and optic nerve evaluation depends on whether IOP is controlled, the length of time IOP has been controlled, and whether there is progression of the disease. Patients who are at target IOP and have no disease progression should have optic nerve head evaluation and visual field testing every 6 to 12 months. Patients with disease progression and/or who are not at target IOP should receive follow-up evaluation every 1 to 6 months. Assess the patient's ability to use topical eye drops.[4] (See Application of Ophthalmic Solutions or Suspensions textbox.) Finally, evaluate the patient's adherence to their medical regimen. Nonadherence among patients on topical medical therapy ranges from 5% to 80%. Suspect nonadherence in patients who have visual field and optic nerve progression despite a low IOP measurement, as patients may be more adherent to their medical regimen before their visit. Pharmacy refill histories may be useful in assessing adherence but do not confirm that the patient is actually taking the regimen as prescribed.[47] Specific patient factors related to the risk of nonadherence may include health literacy, medication cost, complicated medication regimens, adverse effects, and ethnicity.[48] Using adherence aids, prescribing the least complex regimen, and educating patients about their glaucoma are ways to reduce nonadherence.[49]

❽ *Target IOP should be revised based on the course of the disease and rate of progression.* Adjust therapy if the patient fails to reach his or her target IOP. Patients who have achieved target IOP yet have progressive damage of the optic nerve or who have worsening of their visual fields should have further adjustment of their therapy. Evaluate these patients further for possible reasons of continued disease progression. Consider determining the diurnal pattern of IOP and looking for signs of poor ocular perfusion pressure. Establish a lower target IOP. Adjust therapy in patients who are intolerant, are nonadherent, or develop contraindications to their drug therapy regimen. Consider increasing the target IOP and reducing drug therapy for patients who have stable disease and who have maintained a low IOP; closely follow these patients to assess their response.[4]

Patient Care and Monitoring

1. In undiagnosed patients, assess their risk factors for glaucoma and their recommended interval of glaucoma screening.

2. Obtain a thorough history of the patient's prescription, nonprescription, and natural product use. Review for potential drug–drug and drug–glaucoma interactions.

3. Evaluate diagnostic tests (IOP, visual fields, optic nerve evaluations, etc.) to determine whether the patient's current glaucoma therapy is effective.

4. Assess the patient's ability to use ophthalmic preparations.

5. Determine the patient's adherence level to prescribed medication regimen and factors contributing to poor adherence.

6. Evaluate the patient for systemic and ocular adverse drug reactions and drug allergy.

7. Provide patient education in regard to disease state, drug therapy, and surgical/laser therapy:

   - What causes glaucoma or puts people at risk for glaucoma
   - Possible complications of glaucoma
   - How to use ophthalmic preparations appropriately
   - When to take medications
   - Potential adverse drug reactions of medical therapy
   - Potential benefits and complications of laser or surgical procedures

Patient Encounter, Part 3

The practitioner and SJ agree to start medication therapy. Develop a patient-specific care plan.

Address the patient's (a) drug-related needs, (b) goals of therapy, (c) potential pharmacologic therapies, and (d) plan for follow-up of therapy.

List the monitoring parameters for effectiveness and safety for the chosen therapy.

Explain how you would counsel the patient on the chosen therapy, including the administration of an ophthalmic preparation.

Primary Angle-Closure Glaucoma

Follow-up of acute angle-closure crisis occurs in the postoperative period. Evaluate the patency of the iridotomy and IOP in the postoperative period. Perform gonioscopy and optic nerve head evaluation if not already performed. Stable patients with PACG should be evaluated at least annually, specifically for the presence of peripheral anterior synechia and optic neuropathy. Treat patients according to POAG guidelines if they have underlying POAG or areas of peripheral anterior synechia with the presence of optic neuropathy.[2]

Application of Ophthalmic Solutions or Suspension

1. Clean hands with soap and water.

2. Avoid touching the dropper tip with your fingers or against your eye to maintain sterility of product; shake dropper bottle if product is a suspension.

3. Tilt head back; pull down the lower eye lid with index finger.

4. Hold the dropper bottle with other hand as close as possible without touching the eye. The dropper should be pointing toward the eye with remaining fingers bracing against the face.

5. Gently squeeze the bottle so that one drop is placed into the pocket.

6. Close your eye for 2 to 3 minutes to allow for the maximum corneal penetration of drug.

7. Use a tissue to wipe away any excess liquid.

8. Replace and retighten the cap to the dropper bottle.

9. Wait at least 5 minutes before instilling another ophthalmic drug preparation.

10. Application of some ophthalmic preparations (suspension and gels) may cause blurring of vision.

Abbreviations Introduced in This Chapter

POAG Primary open-angle glaucoma
PACG Primary angle-closure glaucoma
IOP Intraocular pressure
CCT Central corneal thickness
NTG Normal tension glaucoma
AAO American Academy of Ophthalmology

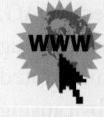 Self-assessment questions and answers are available at *http://mhpharmacotherapy.com/ pp.html.*

REFERENCES

1. Foster PJ, Buhrmann R, Quigley HA, Johnson GJ. The definition and classification of glaucoma in prevalence surveys. Br J Ophthalmol 2002;86(2):238–242.

2. American Academy of Ophthalmology Glaucoma Panel. Preferred Practice Pattern Guidelines Primary Angle Closure. San Francisco, CA: American Academy of Ophthalmology, 2010 [cited 2011 Oct 3]. Available from: *http://www.aao.org/ppp*

3. American Academy of Ophthalmology Glaucoma Panel. Preferred Practice Pattern Guidelines Primary Open-Angle Glaucoma Suspect. San Francisco, CA: American Academy of Ophthalmology; 2010 [cited 2011 Oct 3]. Available from: *www.aao.org/ppp*.

4. American Academy of Ophthalmology Glaucoma Panel. Preferred Practice Pattern Guidelines Primary Open-Angle Glaucoma. San Francisco, CA: American Academy of Ophthalmology, 2010 [cited 2011 Oct 3]. Available from: *http://www.aao.org/ppp*

5. Quigley HA, Broman AT. The number of people with glaucoma worldwide in 2010 and 2020. Br J Ophthalmol 2006;90(3):262–267.

6. Friedman DS, Wolfs RC, O'Colmain BJ, et al; Eye Diseases Prevalence Research Group. Prevalence of open-angle glaucoma among adults in the United States. Arch Ophthalmol 2004;122(4):532–538.

7. Kass MA, Heuer DK, Higginbotham EJ, et al. The Ocular Hypertension Treatment Study: A randomized trial determines that topical ocular hypotensive medication delays or prevents the onset of primary open-angle glaucoma. Arch Ophthalmol 2002;120(6):701–713; discussion 829–830.

8. Kass MA, Gordon MO, Gao F, et al; Ocular Hypertension Treatment Study Group. Delaying treatment of ocular hypertension: the ocular hypertension treatment study. Arch Ophthalmol 2010;128(3):276–287.

9. Bonomi L. Epidemiology of angle-closure glaucoma. Acta Ophthalmol Scand Suppl 2002;236:11–13.

10. Kwon YH, Fingert JH, Kuehn MH, Alward WL. Primary open-angle glaucoma. N Engl J Med 2009;360(11):1113–1124.

11. Quigley HA. Glaucoma. Lancet 2011;377(9774):1367–1377.

12. Marquis RE, Whitson JT. Management of glaucoma: Focus on pharmacological therapy. Drugs Aging 2005;22(1):1–21.

13. Woodward DF, Gil DW. The inflow and outflow of anti-glaucoma drugs. Trends Pharmacol Sci 2004;25(5):238–241.

14. Weinreb RN, Khaw PT. Primary open-angle glaucoma. Lancet 2004;363(9422):1711–1720.

15. Civan MM, Macknight AD. The ins and outs of aqueous humour secretion. Exp Eye Res 2004;78(3):625–631.

16. Shields MB. Normal-tension glaucoma: is it different from primary open-angle glaucoma? Curr Opin Ophthalmol 2008;19(2):85–88.

17. Caprioli J, Coleman AL, Blood Flow in Glaucoma D. Blood pressure, perfusion pressure, and glaucoma. Am J Ophthalmol 2010;149(5):704–712.

18. Gherghel D, Hosking SL, Orgul S. Autonomic nervous system, circadian rhythms, and primary open-angle glaucoma. Surv Ophthalmol 2004;49(5):491–508.

19. Gordon MO, Beiser JA, Brandt JD, et al. The Ocular Hypertension Treatment Study: Baseline factors that predict the onset of primary open-angle glaucoma. Arch Ophthalmol 2002;120(6):714–720; discussion 829–830.

20. Tezel G, Fourth, Arvo Pfizer Ophthalmics Research Institute Conference Working Group. The role of glia, mitochondria, and the immune system in glaucoma. Invest Ophthalmol Vis Sci 2009;50(3):1001–1012.

21. The effectiveness of intraocular pressure reduction in the treatment of normal-tension glaucoma. Collaborative Normal-Tension Glaucoma Study Group. Am J Ophthalmol 1998;126(4):498–505.

22. Quigley HA, Friedman DS, Congdon NG. Possible mechanisms of primary angle-closure and malignant glaucoma. J Glaucoma 2003;12(2):167–180.

23. Razeghinejad MR, Myers JS, Katz LJ. Iatrogenic glaucoma secondary to medications. Am J Med 2011;124(1):20–25.

24. Robin AL, Frick KD, Katz J, Budenz D, Tielsch JM. The ocular hypertension treatment study: Intraocular pressure lowering prevents the development of glaucoma, but does that mean we should treat before the onset of disease? Arch Ophthalmol 2004;122(3):376–378.

25. Sharma P, Sample PA, Zangwill LM, Schuman JS. Diagnostic tools for glaucoma detection and management. Surv Ophthalmol 2008;53Suppl1:S17–S32.

26. Cheng JW, Cai JP, Wei RL. Meta-analysis of medical intervention for normal tension glaucoma. Ophthalmology 2009;116(7):1243–1249.

27. Stewart WC, Konstas AG, Nelson LA, Kruft B. Meta-analysis of 24-hour intraocular pressure studies evaluating the efficacy of glaucoma medicines. Ophthalmology 2008;115(7):1117–1122 e1.

28. van der Valk R, Webers CA, Lumley T, Hendrikse F, Prins MH, Schouten JS. A network meta-analysis combined direct and indirect comparisons between glaucoma drugs to rank effectiveness in lowering intraocular pressure. J Clin Epidemiol 2009;62(12):1279–1283.

29. van der Valk R, Webers CA, Schouten JS, Zeegers MP, Hendrikse F, Prins MH. Intraocular pressure-lowering effects of all commonly used glaucoma drugs: A meta-analysis of randomized clinical trials. Ophthalmology 2005;112(7):1177–1185.

30. Webers CA, Beckers HJ, Nuijts RM, Schouten JS. Pharmacological management of primary open-angle glaucoma: Second-line options and beyond. Drugs Aging 2008;25(9):729–759.

31. Caprioli J, Varma R. Intraocular pressure: modulation as treatment for glaucoma. Am J Ophthalmol 2011;152(3):340–344 e2.

32. Chaudhary O, Adelman RA, Shields MB. Predicting response to glaucoma therapy in one eye based on response in the fellow eye: The monocular trial. Arch Ophthalmol 2008;126(9):1216–1220.

33. Realini T, Fechtner RD, Atreides SP, Gollance S. The uniocular drug trial and second-eye response to glaucoma medications. Ophthalmology 2004;111(3):421–426.

34. Hoh ST, Aung T, Chew PT. Medical management of angle closure glaucoma. Semin Ophthalmol 2002;17(2):79–83.

35. Cantor L. Achieving low target pressures with today's glaucoma medications. Surv Ophthalmol 2003;48Suppl 1:S8–S16.

36. Chidlow G, Wood JP, Casson RJ. Pharmacological neuroprotection for glaucoma. Drugs 2007;67(5):725–759.

37. Vander Zanden JA, Valuck RJ, Bunch CL, Perlman JI, Anderson C, Wortman GI. Systemic adverse effects of ophthalmic beta-blockers. Ann Pharmacother 2001;35(12):1633–1637.

38. Krauss AH, Woodward DF. Update on the mechanism of action of bimatoprost: A review and discussion of new evidence. Surv Ophthalmol 2004;49Suppl 1:S5–S11.

39. Eisenberg DL, Toris CB, Camras CB. Bimatoprost and travoprost: A review of recent studies of two new glaucoma drugs. Surv Ophthalmol 2002;47Suppl 1:S105–S115.

40. Bournias TE, Lee D, Gross R, Mattox C. Ocular hypotensive efficacy of bimatoprost when used as a replacement for latanoprost in the treatment of glaucoma and ocular hypertension. J Ocul Pharmacol Ther 2003;19(3):193–203.

41. Gandolfi SA, Cimino L. Effect of bimatoprost on patients with primary open-angle glaucoma or ocular hypertension who are nonresponders to latanoprost. Ophthalmology. 2003 Mar;110(3):609-14.

42. Grierson I, Jonsson M, Cracknell K. Latanoprost and pigmentation. Jpn J Ophthalmol. 2004 Nov-Dec;48(6):602-12.

43. Easthope SE, Perry CM. Topical bimatoprost: A review of its use in open-angle glaucoma and ocular hypertension. Drugs Aging 2002;19(3):231–248.

44. Netland PA, Landry T, Sullivan EK, et al. Travoprost compared with latanoprost and timolol in patients with open-angle glaucoma or ocular hypertension. Am J Ophthalmol 2001;132(4):472–484.

45. Perry CM, McGavin JK, Culy CR, Ibbotson T. Latanoprost: an update of its use in glaucoma and ocular hypertension. Drugs Aging 2003;20(8):597–630.

46. Krupin T, Liebmann JM, Greenfield DS, Ritch R, Gardiner S, Low-Pressure Glaucoma Study G. A randomized trial of brimonidine versus

timol in preserving visual function: Results from the Low-Pressure Glaucoma Treatment Study. Am J Ophthalmol 2011;151(4):671–681.

47. Olthoff CM, Schouten JS, van de Borne BW, Webers CA. Noncompliance with ocular hypotensive treatment in patients with glaucoma or ocular hypertension an evidence-based review. Ophthalmology 2005;112(6):953–961.

48. Tsai JC. A comprehensive perspective on patient adherence to topical glaucoma therapy. Ophthalmology 2009;116(11 Suppl):S30–S36.

49. Gray TA, Orton LC, Henson D, Harper R, Waterman H. Interventions for improving adherence to ocular hypotensive therapy. Cochrane Database Syst Rev 2009(2):CD006132.

50. American Academy of Ophthalmology. Preferred Practice Pattern Guidelines Comprehensive Adult Medical Eye Evaluation. San Francisco, CA: American Academy of Ophthalmology, 2010 [cited 2011 Oct 3]. Available from: *http://www.aao.org/ppp*

62 Ophthalmic Disorders

Melissa L. Hunter and Michelle L. Hilaire

LEARNING OBJECTIVES

● **Upon completion of the chapter, the reader will be able to:**

1. Differentiate between the various ophthalmic disorders based on patient-specific information.
2. Choose an appropriate treatment regimen for an ophthalmic disorder.
3. Discuss the product differences that direct the selection of ophthalmic medications.
4. Assess when further treatment is required based on patient-specific information.
5. Recommend an ophthalmic monitoring plan given patient-specific information, a diagnosis, and a treatment regimen.
6. Educate patients about ophthalmic disease states and appropriate drug and nondrug therapies.

KEY CONCEPTS

❶ The clinician must be able to distinguish ophthalmic conditions that lead to significant morbidity, including blindness.

❷ In contact lens wearers, choose an antibiotic that covers *Pseudomonas aeruginosa*.

❸ Both acute and chronic bacterial conjunctivitis are self-limiting, except if caused by *Staphylococci*.

❹ Viral conjunctivitis is usually self-limiting, resolving within 2 weeks.

❺ Nonpharmacologic measures are critical to prevent the spread of viral conjunctivitis.

❻ Use a step-care approach for treatment of allergic conjunctivitis.

❼ Untreated bacterial keratitis is associated with corneal scarring and potential loss of vision. Corneal perforation may cause the loss of the eye.

❽ There is no cure for age-related macular degeneration, and the efficacy of most treatments is low.

❾ Dry eye is a chronic condition in which symptoms can be improved with treatment, but it is not usually curable.

This chapter provides an overview of common ophthalmic disorders and their treatments. ❶ *Many ophthalmic disorders are benign or self-limited, but the clinician must be able to distinguish conditions that lead to serious morbidity, including blindness.* Preserving both visual function and cosmetic appearance should be done whenever possible.[1] The clinician must understand when referral is appropriate and the proper time frame for follow-up. These vary greatly by condition.

OCULAR EMERGENCIES

ETIOLOGY AND EPIDEMIOLOGY

Ophthalmic problems encompass 3% of all emergency department visits.[2] Falls are a frequent cause of traumatic eye injury in the elderly.[3] Corneal abrasions are the most common eye injury in children and are often due to fingernail scratches or objects swung near the eye. Even aggressive eye rubbing may damage the cornea.[4] Healthcare practitioners must know the proper treatment for ocular emergencies and the time frame for follow-up in order to prevent further morbidity (Table 62–1).

CORNEAL ABRASIONS

Treatment

▶ *Desired Outcomes*

- Complete healing of the corneal abrasion with no scarring or vision impairment
- Prevent infection and pain
- Prevent corneal loss or corneal transplant

Clinical Presentation and Diagnosis of Corneal Abrasions[4]

Symptoms

- Photophobia
- Pain with extraocular muscle movement
- Foreign body sensation
- Recent ocular trauma
- Gritty feeling
- Headache

Signs

- Excessive tearing
- Blepharospasm
- Blurred vision

Diagnostic Test

Use sterile fluorescein dye strips and visualize the cornea under a cobalt-blue filtered light; abrasions appear green; ensure that no foreign body remains in the eye.

Table 62–1

Ophthalmic Emergencies: Time to Follow-Up by Ophthalmologist

Immediate Consult Required	Within 24 Hours
Foreign body in eye	Acute angle-closure glaucoma
Acute, painless loss of vision	Orbital cellulitis
Acute chemical burn	Blood in the eye (hyphema)
Blunt trauma to eye	Macular edema
	Retinal detachment
	Sudden congestive proptosis (bulging of eye forward)
	Corneal ulcer
	Corneal abrasion

From Handler JA, Ghezzi KT. General ophthalmologic examination. Emerg Med Clin North Am 1995;13:521–538.

▶ General Approach to Treatment

The five layers of the cornea contain no blood vessels but are nourished by tears, oxygen, and aqueous humor. Minor corneal abrasions heal quickly. Moderate abrasions take 24 to 72 hours to heal. Deep scratches may scar the cornea and require corneal transplant if vision is impaired. Do not use eye patches to treat corneal abrasion, as they decrease oxygen delivery, increase pain, and increase the chance of infection.[4]

Corneal Abrasion Prevention[4]

- Wear eye protection during sports
- Wear industrial safety lenses
- Carefully fit and place contact lenses
- Clip fingernails of infants and children
- Remove low-hanging branches and objects
- Tape the eyelids closed or use gels or soft contacts during general anesthesia to prevent lagophthalmos.

Pharmacologic Therapy

▶ Topical NSAIDs

Topical nonsteroidal anti-inflammatory drugs (NSAIDs) decrease pain from corneal abrasion. Available ocular NSAIDs are bromfenac 0.09%, diclofenac 0.1%, ketorolac 0.5%, and nepafenac 0.1%. The usual dose for diclofenac and ketorolac is one drop four times daily; nepafenac is dosed three times daily, and bromfenac is dosed twice daily. Use topical NSAIDs with caution in patients with clotting disorders or those who are on systemic NSAIDs or warfarin therapy. Topical administration of NSAIDs may delay wound healing, especially with concurrent topical corticosteroid use.[4,5] Oral analgesics are not well studied for use in corneal abrasion; however, they are less expensive than topical NSAIDs and may be an option for some patients.[4]

▶ Topical Antibiotics

Because an infection slows the healing of a corneal abrasion, prophylactic antibiotics are often used. Studies on the efficacy of this are mixed. Discontinue the use of contact lenses until the abrasion is healed and the antibiotic course complete. ❷ *In contact lens wearers, choose an antibiotic that covers* Pseudomonas aeruginosa, *like gentamicin ointment or solution or a fluoroquinolone.*[4] Antibiotic resistance is an increasing problem. Resistance occurs primarily with older antibiotics, but has been reported for fluoroquinolones as well. Two newer fluoroquinolones, gatifloxacin and moxifloxacin, have low reports of resistance (2%).[6] These agents are more expensive.

Outcome Evaluation

1. Reevaluate patients in 24 hours.
2. If symptoms worsen, recheck for foreign bodies.
3. If not fully healed, evaluate again in 3 to 4 days.
4. Refer to ophthalmologist if:[4]
   - No improvement in 3 days
   - Worsening symptoms
   - Symptoms do not improve daily
   - Symptoms do not improve within a few hours of contact lens removal

OTHER OCULAR EMERGENCIES: TREATMENT

Traumatic Injuries

Attempt to remove loose foreign bodies by gentle irrigation with artificial tears or sterile saline. If removal is successful, a topical broad-spectrum antibiotic, such as erythromycin, will prevent infection. Some patients may need a short-acting cycloplegic mydriatic like cyclopentolate or tropicamide to help with pain.[2] Cycloplegic mydriatics should be used with extreme caution in children.[5] If irrigation is unsuccessful, mechanical removal of foreign objects should be completed only by ophthalmologists using a slitlamp. Protect the eye from further injury with a metal eye shield or a paper cup taped over the eye while awaiting the ophthalmologist.[2]

Splash Injuries and Chemical Exposure

● Instruct patients by phone to irrigate the eye immediately with water or saline continuously for at least 15 minutes before seeking a clinician. Irrigation dilutes and removes the chemical agent and is the best way to decrease ocular tissue
● damage. Patients should then seek immediate care from an ophthalmologist or emergency facility.[7]

Loss of Vision

A variety of disorders may lead to rapid, painless, monocular or binocular vision loss. These include central retinal artery occlusion, acute narrow-angle glaucoma, trauma, and others.[8]
● The differential diagnosis is complex and needs to be undertaken by an emergency department or ophthalmologist.

CONJUNCTIVITIS

Although no exact numbers are available, conjunctivitis, also known as red eye, is one of the most common ophthalmic complaints seen by general clinicians. An inflamed conjunctiva is the most common cause of red eye.[9] The vast majority of conjunctivitis cases are viral in nature. Use the differential diagnosis algorithm shown in Figure 62–1 to determine the proper treatment or need for referral.

BACTERIAL CONJUNCTIVITIS
Etiology and Pathophysiology

The primary cause of acute bacterial conjunctivitis is gram-positive organisms, including *Streptococcus pneumoniae and Staphylococcus aureus,* and gram-negative *Haemophilus influenzae.*[9]

Staphylococcus and *Moraxella* are common bacterial causes of chronic conjunctivitis.[10] *Moraxella* infections may cluster in groups of women who share makeup.[10] ❸ *Both acute and chronic bacterial conjunctivitis are self-limiting except if caused by* Staphylococci.[11] Because of this, the pathogens are rarely cultured unless the case is unresponsive to treatment. Although infection typically begins in one eye, it will often spread to both within 48 hours.[12]

Hyperacute bacterial conjunctivitis is associated with gonococcal infections in sexually active patients. The causative agents are *Neisseria gonorrhoeae* or *N. meningitidis.* Prompt workup and treatment is required, as corneal perforation occurs in 10% of cases within 48 hours.[12]

Treatment

▶ **Desired Outcomes**

● Complete resolution of the bacterial conjunctivitis
● Prevent adverse consequences of the infection
● Preserve functionality of the eye

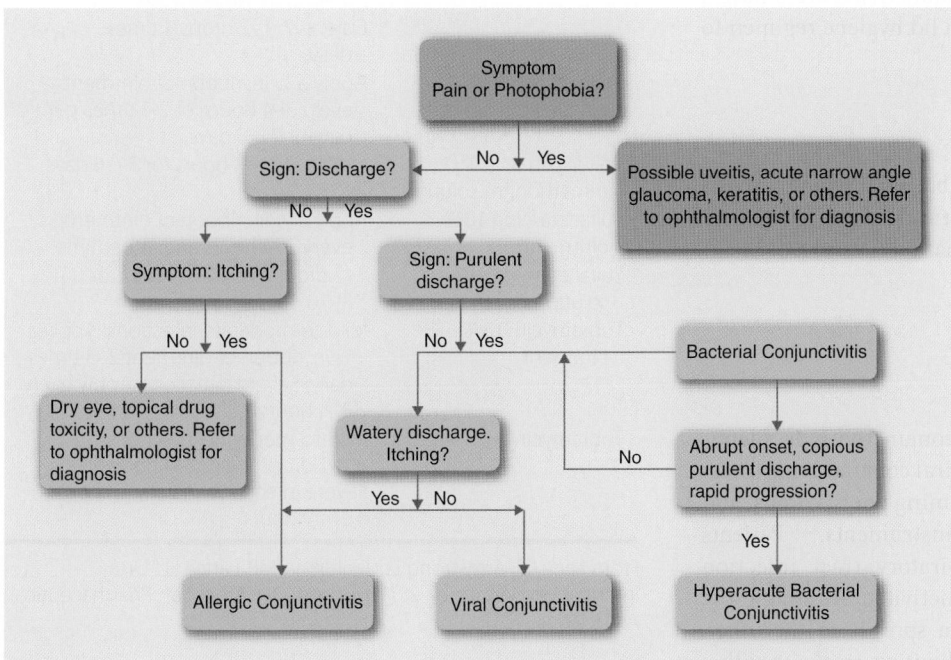

FIGURE 62–1. Differential diagnosis for red eye.

▶ General Approach to Treatment

● Treat acute bacterial conjunctivitis with broad-spectrum antibiotics. Although the condition is usually self-limiting, antibiotic treatment decreases the spread of disease to other people and prevents extraocular infection. Additionally, treatment may help decrease the risk of corneal ulceration or other complications that affect sight. Finally, treatment speeds recovery.[9]

▶ Pharmacologic Therapy

The choice of an antibiotic agent for acute bacterial con-
● junctivitis is largely empiric. The initial treatment needs to include *Staphylococcus* coverage, but also may be chosen on the basis of cost and side-effect profile.[9] In general, ointments are a good dosage form for children. Adults may prefer drops because they do not interfere with vision.[13]

● Many broad-spectrum topical antibiotics are approved to treat acute bacterial conjunctivitis (**Tables 62–2 and 62–3**). Polymyxin B/trimethoprim solution, polymyxin B with baci-tracin ointment, or erythromycin ointment are cost-effective, first-line treatments. The aminoglycosides (tobramycin, neo-mycin, and gentamicin) are alternatives but have incomplete gram-positive coverage.[13] The aminoglycosides can cause corneal epithelial toxicity. Neomycin often causes allergic reactions. Tobramycin is the best tolerated of the class, but is also the most expensive. Sulfacetamide 10% has significant resistance. If infection recurs, use a topical fluoroquinolone like ofloxacin, ciprofloxacin, gatifloxacin, moxifloxacin, or levofloxacin.[10] Fluoroquinolones are not used first-line for conjunctivitis because they have poor *Streptococcus* coverage and are expensive. Development of resistance is also a con-cern with fluoroquinolones.[13]

Treat hyperacute bacterial conjunctivitis with a single dose of 1 g of intramuscular ceftriaxone in combination with topi-cal antibiotics and refer the patient to an opthalmologist.[12]

Patients with chronic bacterial conjunctivitis often have a concurrent case of blepharitis. Add a lid hygiene regimen to topical antibiotic treatment.[9,10]

Outcome Evaluation

● Significant improvement of acute bacterial conjunctivitis should be seen within 1 week.[9,12] Terminate treatment with topical antibiotics when the inflammation is resolved.[10]

VIRAL CONJUNCTIVITIS

Etiology

The most common cause of viral conjunctivitis is adeno-virus. It is often called "pink-eye."[9] Viral conjunctivitis infec-tions are easily spread through swimming pools, camps, and contaminated fingers and medical instruments.[9,13] Patients often present with an upper respiratory tract infection or recent exposure to viral conjunctivitis. Although the infection begins in one eye, it often spreads to the other.

❹ *Viral conjunctivitis is usually self-limiting, resolving within*

Table 62–2

Adult Bacterial Conjunctivitis Dosing Guidelines for Topical Ophthalmic Antibiotics

Azithromycin 1% solution	Days 1 and 2: 1 drop twice daily, 8–12 hours apart Days 3–7: 1 drop once daily
Ciprofloxacin 3.5 mg/mL solution	Days 1 and 2: 1–2 drops every 2 hours while awake Days 3–7: 1–2 drops every 4 hours while awake
Ciprofloxacin 0.3% ointment	Apply a ½ in. ribbon of ointment 3 times daily for 2 days, then twice daily for next 5 days
Erythromycin 0.5% ointment	Apply a ½ in. ribbon of ointment up to 6 times daily
Gatifloxacin 0.3% solution	Days 1 and 2: 1 drop every 2 hours while awake up to 8 times daily Days 3–7: 1 drop every 4 hours while awake
Gatifloxacin 0.5% solution	Days 1: 1 drop every 2 hours while awake up to 8 times daily Days 2–7: 1 drop 2–4 times per day while awake
Gentamicin 0.3% solution	1–2 drops every 4 hours. In severe infections, may use up to 2 drops every hour
Gentamicin 0.3% ointment	Apply a ½ in. ribbon of ointment 2–3 times daily; up to every 3-4 hours
Levofloxacin 0.5% solution	Days 1 and 2: 1–2 drops every 2 hours while awake, up to 8 times per day Days 3–7: 1–2 drops every 4 hours while awake, up to 4 times daily
Moxifloxacin 0.5% solution	1 drop 2 times a day for 7 days (Moxeza) 1 drop 3 times a day for 7 days (Vigamox)
Ofloxacin 0.3% solution	Days 1 and 2: 1–2 drops every 2–4 hours while awake Days 3–7: 1–2 drops 4 times daily
Polymyxin B with bacitracin ointment	Apply a ½ in. ribbon of ointment every 3–4 hours, or 2-3 times per day for 7–10 days
Polymyxin B/ trimethoprim solution	1 drop every 3 hours for 7–10 days
Sulfacetamide 10% ointment	Apply a ½ in. ribbon of ointment every 3–4 hours and at bedtime
Sulfacetamide 10% solution	1–2 drops every 2–3 hours for 7–10 days
Tobramycin 0.3% ointment	Mild-to-moderate infections: Apply a ½ in. ribbon of ointment 2–3 times daily; Severe infections: Apply every 3–4 hours
Tobramycin 0.3% solution	Mild-to-moderate infections: 1–2 drops every 2–4 hours Severe infections: initially, 2 drops every hour

From Lacy CF, Armstrong LL, Goldman MP, Lance LL. Drug Information Handbook 2011. Hudson, OH: American Pharmaceutical Association, 2011.

Table 62–3

Pediatric Dosing Guidelines for Bacterial Conjunctivitis for Topical Ophthalmic Antibiotics

Azithromycin 1% solution	Children 1 year of age or older: Days 1 and 2: 1 drop twice daily, 8–12 hours apart Days 3–7: 1 drop once daily
Ciprofloxacin 3.5 mg/mL solution	Children 1 year of age or older, days 1 and 2: 1–2 drops every 2 hours while awake Days 3–7: 1–2 drops every 4 hours while awake
Ciprofloxacin 0.3% ointment	Children 2 years of age or older: Apply a ½ in. ribbon of ointment 3 times daily for 2 days, then twice daily for next 5 days
Erythromycin 0.5% ointment	Apply a ½ in. ribbon of ointment up to 6 times daily
Gatifloxacin 0.3% solution	Children 1 year of age or older, days 1 and 2: 1 drop every 2 hours while awake up to 8 times daily Days 3–7: 1 drop every 4 hours while awake
Gentamicin 0.3% solution	1–2 drops every 4 hours. In severe infections, may use up to 2 drops every hour
Gentamicin 0.3% ointment	Apply a ½ in. ribbon of ointment 2–3 times daily; up to every 3–4 hours
Levofloxacin 0.5% solution	Children 1 year of age or older, days 1 and 2: 1–2 drops every 2 hours while awake, up to 8 times daily Days 3–7: 1–2 drops every 4 hours while awake, up to 4 times daily
Moxifloxacin 0.5% solution	Children 4 months of age or older: 1 drop 2 times per day for 7 days (Moxeza) Children 1 year of age or older: 1 drop 3 times a day for 7 days
Ofloxacin 0.3% solution	Children 1 year of age or older, days 1 and 2: 1–2 drops every 2–4 hours while awake Days 3–7: 1–2 drops 4 times daily
Polymyxin B with bacitracin ointment	Apply a ½ in. ribbon of ointment every 3–4 hours for 7–10 days
Polymyxin B/trimethoprim solution	Infants and children 2 months of age or older: 1 drop every 3 hours for 7–10 days
Sulfacetamide 10% ointment	Apply a ½ in. ribbon of ointment every 3–4 hours and at bedtime
Sulfacetamide 10% solution	1–2 drops every 2–3 hours for 7–10 days
Tobramycin 0.3% ointment	Infants and children 2 months of age or older: Mild-to-moderate infections: Apply an approximately ½ in. ribbon 2–3 times daily Severe infections: Apply every 3–4 hours
Tobramycin 0.3% solution	Infants and children 2 months of age or older: Mild-to-moderate infections: 1–2 drops every 4 hours Severe infections: initially, 2 drops every hour

From Lacy CF, Armstrong LL, Goldman MP, Lance LL. Drug Information Handbook 2011. Hudson, OH: American Pharmaceutical Association, 2011.

Patient Encounter 1

This morning, a mother brings in her 7-year-old daughter who has been complaining of irritation, redness, and "goop" coming out of her left eye for the past 13 hours. She woke up terrified this morning because her left eye seemed glued shut. A warm washcloth was used to ease the eye open, and upon examination, the left eye was red and revealed a whitish discharge, whereas the right eye was just red.

What is the probable diagnosis?

Please differentiate between bacterial, hyperacute bacterial, viral, and allergic causes based on physical assessment.

What organisms should be suspected, and what are reasonable treatment regimens?

If the child would have been diagnosed with viral conjunctivitis, what nonpharmacologic measures should be employed to prevent spreading?

2 weeks.[9] Five percent of patients remain contagious 16 days after the appearance of symptoms.[12]

Treatment

▶ Desired Outcomes

- Complete resolution of the viral conjunctivitis
- Prevent adverse consequences of the infection
- Avoid spreading infection to other patients

▶ Nonpharmacologic Therapy

⑤ *Nonpharmacologic measures are critical to prevent the spread of viral conjunctivitis.* Cold compresses may relieve symptoms.[9] Patients should not share towels or other contaminated objects, should avoid close contact with other people, and avoid swimming for 2 weeks.[12] The virus remains viable on dry surfaces for more than 2 weeks.[11] Take care in the medical setting to thoroughly decontaminate instruments and wash hands.[12]

▶ Pharmacologic Therapy

Patients may obtain further symptomatic relief by using artificial tears and topical decongestants.[9] If artificial tear solutions sting, recommend a preservative-free formula.

Topical antivirals are not used to treat adenovirus conjunctivitis. Topical antibiotics are often prescribed for viral conjunctivitis, presumably to prevent bacterial superinfection. In reality, this is a case of the patient insisting on a medication to speed healing.[12] Avoid the use of antibiotics for a viral infection.[10] Eliminating superfluous antibiotic use also helps prevent the development of antibiotic resistance.

If patients have a severe subepithelial infiltration, a topical steroid may be required. However, topical steroids may cause serious ocular complications and may worsen herpetic conjunctivitis, which has similar symptoms as viral conjunctivitis. Only ophthalmologists should prescribe topical steroids.[9] Additionally, the period of virus shedding may be significantly prolonged by topical prednisolone.[14]

▶ Outcome Evaluation

● Refer patients who do not see improvement within 7 to 10 days to an ophthalmologist to rule out herpetic and other infectious processes.[12] If pain or photophobia occurs, suspect corneal involvement and refer the patient. This typically occurs 10 to 14 days after the onset of conjunctivitis.[11]

ALLERGIC CONJUNCTIVITIS

Etiology and Clinical Presentation

Ocular allergy is a broad term that includes several diseases
● with the hallmark symptom of itching, often accompanied by tearing, conjunctival swelling, photophobia, and stringy or sticky mucoid discharge.[15] Seasonal ocular allergy is the most common type of allergic conjunctivitis. This is an IgE-mediated
● hypersensitivity to pollen or other airborne allergens.[12] Often, the patient's history is positive for atopic conditions such as allergic rhinitis, asthma, or eczema.[15] Perennial allergic conjunctivitis has similar but less severe symptoms and may not be tied to a specific time of year. Finally, conjunctivitis medicamentosa is a drug-induced form of allergic conjunctivitis caused by overuse of topical vasoconstricting agents.[15]

Pathophysiology

The conjunctiva of the eye is often the initial site of contact with an environmental allergen. Mast cell degranulation occurs, resulting in the release of mediators. The earliest mediator is histamine, which causes itching, redness, and swelling. Leukotrienes and prostaglandins cause cellular infiltration and increased mucus secretion along with chemosis, resulting in conjunctival vasodilation. Mast cells release cytokines, chemokines, and growth factors, which trigger inflammatory processes.[17]

Treatment of ocular allergy is aimed at slowing or stopping these processes. Antihistamines block the histamine receptors, and some prevent histamine production and/or inhibit mediator release from the mast cells.[17] Mast cell stabilizers inhibit the degranulation of mast cells, preventing mediator release. Some topical agents have multiple mechanisms of action, combining antihistaminic, mast cell stabilization, and anti-inflammatory properties (Tables 62–4, 62–5, and 62–6).[18]

Treatment

▶ Desired Outcomes

- Relief of current allergic symptoms
- Prevention of future allergic symptoms
- No adverse effects from treatment

▶ Nonpharmacologic Therapy

● The primary treatment for ocular allergy is removal and avoidance of the allergen.[19] For conjunctivitis medicamentosa, discontinue the offending medication.[15] Apply cold compresses several times daily to reduce redness and itching and to provide symptomatic relief.

▶ Pharmacologic Therapy

❻ *Use a step-care approach for the treatment of allergic*
● *conjunctivitis.* The first step is a nonmedicated, artificial

---

Table 62–4		
Mechanisms of Action of Ocular Allergy Drugs		
Drug	**Mechanisms**	**Notes**
Azelastine	H_1-receptor antagonist, mast cell stabilizer	May inhibit cytokine release
Cromolyn sodium	Mast cell stabilizer	
Emedastine	H_1-receptor antagonist; inhibits eosinophil chemotaxis	Superior H_1-receptor binding ability
Epinastine	H_1- and H_2-receptor antagonist, mast cell stabilizer, anti-inflammatory	
Ketorolac	Prostaglandin inhibitor	
Ketotifen	H_1-receptor antagonist, mast cell stabilizer, eosinophil inhibitor, platelet-activating factor inhibitor	May inhibit eosinophil chemotaxis
Levocabastine	H_1-receptor antagonist	Downregulates intracellular adhesion molecules, decreasing the inflammatory response; may be used for up to 2 weeks
Lodoxamide	Mast cell stabilizer	May be used for up to 3 months
Loteprednol	Corticosteroid	Only 0.2% approved for seasonal allergic conjunctivitis
Nedocromil	Mast cell stabilizer, H_1-receptor antagonist	May inhibit eosinophils
Olopatadine	Antihistaminic, mast cell stabilizer	
Pemirolast	Mast cell stabilizer	
Pheniramine	H_1-receptor antagonist	Available only in combination with naphazoline

From Refs. 17–19.

Table 62–5

Adult Dosing and Common Side Effects of Ocular Allergy Drugs

Drug	Dosing[a]	Common Side Effects[b]
Azelastine 0.05%	1 drop in affected eye(s) twice daily	Ocular stinging, headache, bitter taste
Cromolyn sodium 4%	1–2 drops in each eye 4–6 times daily	Ocular stinging
Emedastine 0.05%	1 drop in affected eye up to 4 times daily	Headache
Epinastine 0.05%	1 drop in each eye twice daily	Ocular stinging, cold symptoms
Ketorolac 0.5%	1 drop 4 times a day	Ocular stinging, irritation
Ketotifen 0.025%	1 drop in affected eye(s) twice daily	Red eyes (conjunctival injection), headache
Levocabastine 0.05%	1 drop in affected eye(s) 4 times daily	Ocular stinging, headache
Lodoxamide 0.1%	1–2 drops in affected eye(s) 4 times daily	Ocular stinging, foreign body sensation
Loteprednol 0.2%	1 drop in affected eye(s) 4 times daily	Elevated intraocular pressure, cataracts, decreased wound healing, secondary ocular infections, systemic side effects possible
Nedocromil 2%	1–2 drops in each eye twice daily	Ocular stinging, bitter taste
Olopatadine 0.1%; 0.2%	0.1%:1drop in affected eye(s) 2 times daily with minimum 6- to 8-hour interval between doses 0.2%: 1 drop in affected eye(s) once daily	Headache
Pemirolast 0.1%	1–2 drops in affected eye(s) 4 times daily	Headache, cold symptoms
Pheniramine	Varies by manufacturer and product	Ocular stinging

[a]From Refs. 5, 16.

[b]From Ref. 19.

Table 62–6

Pediatric Dosing of Ocular Allergy Drugs

Drug	Dosing
Azelastine 0.05%	Children 3 years of age or older: 1 drop in affected eye(s) twice daily
Cromolyn sodium 4%	Children 4 years of age or older: 1–2 drops in each eye 4–6 times daily
Emedastine 0.05%	Children 3 years of age or older: 1 drop in affected eye up to 4 times daily
Epinastine 0.05%	Children 2 years of age or older: 1 drop in each eye twice daily
Ketorolac 0.5%	Children 3 years of age or older: 1 drop in affected eye(s) 4 times a day
Ketotifen 0.025%	Children 3 years of age or older: 1 drop in affected eye(s) twice daily
Levocabastine 0.05%	Children 12 years of age or older: 1 drop in affected eye(s) 4 times daily
Lodoxamide 0.1%	Children 2 years of age or older: 1–2 drops in affected eye(s) 4 times daily
Nedocromil 2%	Children 3 years of age or older: 1–2 drops in each eye twice daily
Olopatadine 0.1%; 0.2%	Children 3 years of age or older: 1 drop in affected eye(s) 2 times daily with minimum 6- to 8-hour interval between doses 0.2%: 1 drop in affected eye(s) once daily
Pemirolast 0.1%	Children 3 years of age or older: 1–2 drops in affected eye(s) 4 times daily
Pheniramine	Varies by manufacturer and product

From McEvoy GK, ed. AHFS Drug Information 2011. Bethesda, MD: American Society of Health-System Pharmacists, 2011.

tears solution. The solution dilutes or removes the allergen, providing relief while lubricating the eye. Solutions are applied two to four times daily as needed. Ointments may be used in the evenings to further moisturize the surface of the eye.[19] There are many products on the market. Try a preservative-free formulation if other products sting or burn. Unit-dose preservative-free products are more expensive. Some newer multidose products, such as sodium perborate (Purite), have rapidly dissociating preservatives and are more cost-effective.

If artificial tears are insufficient, the second treatment step is a topical antihistamine or antihistamine/decongestant combination. The antihistamine/decongestant combination is more effective than either agent alone. Decongestants are vasoconstrictors that reduce redness and seem to have a small synergistic effect with the antihistamine. The only topical decongestant used in combination products is naphazoline. Topical decongestants burn and sting on instillation and commonly cause mydriasis, especially in patients with lighter-colored eyes. Long-term use leads to rebound congestion. Topical decongestant use should be limited to less than 10 days.[19]

There is still debate whether oral antihistamines control ocular allergy as well as topical antihistamines. Topical antihistamines are recommended before oral agents in step therapy because of the increased risk of systemic side effects with oral drugs. Additionally, topical antihistamines provide

---

Patient Encounter 2

DJ is a 37-year-old female presenting with swollen, teary eyes, and complains of itching. Her symptoms seem to be worse in the spring and summer months. Her past medical history is positive for asthma and eczema. She has been using over-the-counter naphazoline for the past 2 weeks.

What information is suggestive of allergic conjunctivitis?

What nonpharmacologic therapies should be recommended for this patient?

What pharmacologic therapies should be recommended for this patient?

How should the patient be monitored?

---

faster relief of ocular symptoms. Consider oral antihistamines when systemic symptoms are present.[17]

If insufficient relief is obtained from these products, either a mast cell stabilizer or a multiple-action agent is appropriate.[19] Use mast cell stabilizers prophylactically throughout the allergy season. Full response may take 4 to 6 weeks.

If mast cell stabilizers or multiple-action agents are not successful, a trial of a topical NSAID is appropriate. Ketorolac is the only approved topical agent for ocular itching. NSAIDs do not mask ocular infections, affect wound healing, increase intraocular pressure, or contribute to cataract formation like the topical corticosteroids. However, in clinical trials, for allergic conjunctivitis, topical ketorolac was not as effective as olopatadine or emedastine.[17] Full efficacy of ketorolac may take up to 2 weeks.[19]

If all these avenues are ineffective, short-term topical corticosteroids and immunotherapy are the third-line treatments for ocular allergy.[15,19]

Outcome Evaluation

Monitor patients for relief of symptoms. Ensure an adequate trial of the agent. If no improvement is seen, follow a stepped-care approach to treatment. Refer severe cases that do not respond to an ophthalmologist for short-term topical corticosteroids.

BACTERIAL KERATITIS

EPIDEMIOLOGY

Thirty thousand cases of microbial keratitis occur annually in the United States.[20] Microbial keratitis encompasses bacterial, fungal, and *Acanthamoeba* keratitis.[20] Only bacterial keratitis, the most common form, is discussed here.

PATHOPHYSIOLOGY

Bacterial keratitis is a broad term for a bacterial infection of the cornea. This includes corneal ulcers and corneal abscesses.

Clinical Presentation and Diagnosis of Bacterial Keratitis[9,20]

General

The rate of progression of signs and symptoms varies depending on the infecting organism. A differential diagnosis for keratitis must include viral, fungal, and nematodal infections in addition to bacterial causes.

Symptoms

- Photophobia
- Rapid onset of ocular pain

Signs

- Red eye
- Conjunctival discharge
- Decreased vision

Laboratory Tests

Culture if keratitis is severe or sight-threatening. Otherwise, culture or smear only if the corneal infiltrate is chronic or unresponsive to broad-spectrum antimicrobial therapy.

The cornea in a healthy eye has natural resistance to infection, making bacterial keratitis rare. However, many factors may predispose a patient to bacterial infection by compromising the defense mechanisms of the eye (Table 62–7).[20]

The most common pathogens in bacterial keratitis are *Pseudomonas* (including *Pseudomonas aeruginosa*) and other gram-negative rods, *Staphylococci*, and *Streptococci*.[20] If the keratitis is related to the use of contacts, *Pseudomonas* and *Serratia marcescens* are the most common pathogens.[20] For hospitalized infants and adults on respirators, *Pseudomonas* is the most common.[20]

⑦ *Untreated bacterial keratitis is associated with corneal scarring and potential loss of vision.*[20] *Corneal perforation may occur, and the patient may lose the eye.*[20] In virulent organisms, this destruction may occur within 24 hours.[20] Central corneal scarring may result in vision loss even after successful eradication of the organism.[20]

TREATMENT

Desired Outcomes[20]

- Resolution of infection
- Resolution of corneal inflammation
- Reduced corneal pain
- Restored corneal integrity with minimal scarring
- Restored visual function

General Approach to Treatment

All cases of suspected bacterial keratitis require prompt ophthalmology consultation to prevent permanent vision loss.[9]

Table 62–7
Risk Factors for Bacterial Keratitis

Exogenous Factors
Contact lenses
Loose sutures from ocular surgeries
Previous corneal surgery
Previous ocular or eyelid surgery
Trauma, including foreign bodies, chemical and thermal injuries and local irradiation

Ocular Surface Disease
Abnormal lid anatomy or function
Misdirection of eyelashes
Ocular infection (e.g., conjunctivitis, blepharitis)
Tear film deficiencies

Systemic Conditions
Atopic dermatitis
Connective tissue disease
Debilitating illness (e.g., malnourishment or respirator dependence)
Diabetes mellitus
Factitious disease (including anesthetic abuse)
Gonococcal infection
Immunocompromised
Stevens-Johnson syndrome
Substance abuse
Vitamin A deficiency

Ocular Medications
Anesthetics
Antimicrobials
Contaminated ocular medications
Glaucoma medications
Preservatives
Steroids
Topical NSAIDs

Corneal Epithelial Abnormalities
Corneal epithelial edema
Predisposition to recurrent erosion of the cornea
Viral keratitis (e.g., herpes simplex or zoster keratitis)

From Feder RS, Dunn SP, Jones MR, et al. Bacterial keratitis, Preferred Practice Pattern – limited revision [Internet]. San Francisco: American Academy of Ophthalmology, 2011 [cited 2012 Feb 3]. Available from: http://one.aao.org/CE/PracticeGuidelines/PPP.aspx.

Table 62–8
Pharmacologic Therapies for Bacterial Keratitis

Organism	Drug
Unknown or multiple types of organisms	Cefazolin 50 mg/mL *and* tobramycin/gentamicin 9–14 mg/mL *or* Fluoroquinolones various strengths
Gram-positive cocci	Cefazolin 50 mg/mL *or* Vancomycin[a] 15–50 mg/mL *or* Bacitracin[a] 10,000 international unit *or* Moxifloxacin or gatifloxacin various strengths
Gram-negative rods	Tobramycin 9–14 mg/mL *or* Gentamicin 9–14 mg/mL *or* Ceftazidime 50 mg/mL *or* Fluoroquinolones various strengths
Gram-negative cocci	Ceftriaxone 50 mg/mL *or* Ceftazidime 50 mg/mL *or* Fluoroquinolones various strengths
Nontuberculous mycobacteria	Amikacin 20–40 mg/mL *or* Oral clarithromycin, adults: 500 mg every 12 hours Fluoroquinolones various strengths
Nocardia	Amikacin 20–40 mg/mL *or* Trimethoprim 16 mg/mL *and* sulfamethoxazole 80 mg/mL

Adult Topical Dosing
Severe keratitis: loading dose every 5–15 minutes for the first hour, then every 15 minutes to 1 hour around the clock. Less severe keratitis may use less frequent dosing

[a]Use for resistant *Enterococcus* and *Staphylococcus* species and penicillin allergy. Due to the absence of gram-negative activity, do not use vancomycin or bacitracin for single-agent empiric therapy in bacterial keratitis.

From Feder RS, Dunn SP, Jones MR, et al. Bacterial keratitis, Preferred Practice Pattern – limited revision [Internet]. San Francisco: American Academy of Ophthalmology, 2011 [cited 2012 Feb 3]. http://one.aao.org/CE/PracticeGuidelines/PPP.aspx.

Pharmacologic Therapy

▶ Dosage Considerations

- Topical antibiotic drops are preferred. Consider subconjunctival antibiotics if compliance is a concern. Systemic therapy is useful in cases of systemic infection (e.g., gonorrhea) or if the sclera is infected. Reserve ointments for minor cases or adjunctive nighttime therapy.[20]

▶ Drug Choice

- Start topical broad-spectrum antibiotics empirically. Use a loading dose for severe keratitis (Table 62–8). Single-drug therapy with a fluoroquinolone is as effective as combination therapy. Resistance is seen with some fluoroquinolones. Because of this, choose a newer fluoroquinolone such as moxifloxacin or gatifloxacin in severe keratitis cases.[6,20] Fortified antibiotic therapy is an option for severe or unresponsive infections, but may increase toxicity to the cornea and surrounding tissues. Fortified antibiotics are compounded products that are a higher concentration than the commercially available formulation.[20] All compounded formulations must comply with governmental 797 regulations concerning compounding of drug preparations.

- Topical corticosteroids are employed in some cases of bacterial keratitis. The suppression of inflammation may reduce corneal scarring. However, local immunosuppression, increased ocular pressure, and reappearance of the infection are disadvantages to their use. There is no conclusive evidence that they alter clinical outcomes. If the patient is already on topical corticosteroids when the keratitis occurs, discontinue use until the infection is eliminated.[20]

Outcome Evaluation[20]

- Monitor patient symptoms for improvement to determine therapeutic efficacy.
- Modify treatment regimen based on results of culture and sensitivity testing, if necessary.

- Modify the treatment regimen if the patient does not show improvement within 48 hours.
- Gram-negative keratitis will have increased inflammation in the first 24 to 48 hours, even on appropriate therapy.
- Taper therapy based on clinical response.
- Reculture or biopsy if negative clinical response; to improve culture results, discontinue antibiotics for 12 to 24 hours before culturing.
- Contact lenses wears should be educated about the increased risk of infection overnight and continuous wear and the importance of adherence to contact lens hygiene.

MACULAR DEGENERATION

EPIDEMIOLOGY AND ETIOLOGY

Age-related macular degeneration (AMD) is the primary cause of severe, irreversible vision impairment in developed countries (Figs. 62–2 and 62–3). The prevalence increases with age.[21] In the United States, 1.75 million people age 40 or older have advanced AMD, and another 7 million people may have intermediate AMD.[21] Because of the rapid aging of the U.S. population, it is projected that almost 3 million people will develop AMD by 2020.[22] The causes of AMD are not completely known (Table 62–9).[21]

PATHOPHYSIOLOGY

AMD is a deterioration of the macula, the central portion of the retina. The macula facilitates central vision and high-resolution visual acuity because it has the highest concentration of photoreceptors in the retina. The loss of central vision leads to irreversible loss of the ability to drive, read, and perform other

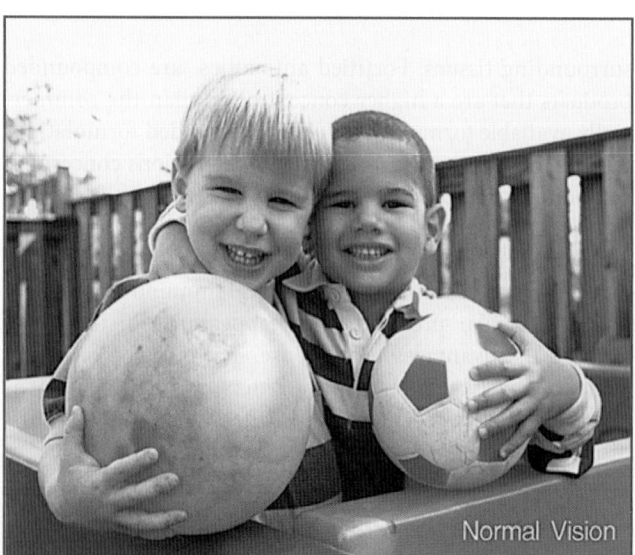

FIGURE 62–2. Normal vision. (From the National Eye Institute, National Institutes of Health Ref. No. EDS01. *http://www.nei.nih.gov/photo/*)

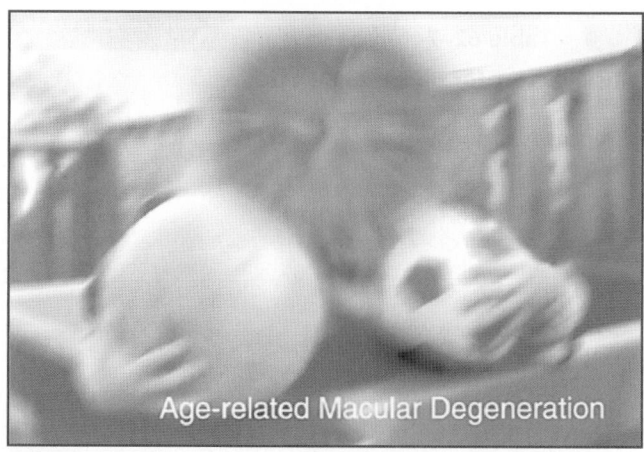

FIGURE 62–3. The scene in Figure 62–2 as it might be viewed by a person with age-related macular degeneration. (From the National Eye Institute, National Institutes of Health Ref. No. EDS05. *http://www.nei.nih.gov/photo/*)

Table 62–9	
Risk Factors for AMD	
Definite Risk Factors	**Potential Risk Factors**
Advancing age	Cardiovascular disease
Light pigmentation (white ethnicity)	Hypertension
Cigarette smoking	Low dietary intake of antioxidant vitamins or zinc
Family history	Increased body mass index
	Higher dietary fat intake

From Chew EY, Benson WE, Blodi BA, et al. Age-related macular degeneration, Preferred Practice Pattern [Internet]. San Francisco: American Academy of Ophthalmology, 2008 [cited 2011 Oct 1]. *http://one.aao.org/CE/PracticeGuidelines/PPP.aspx.*

fine visual tasks like recognize faces.[23] Peripheral vision is preserved, allowing mobility.[21] AMD is characterized by one or more of the following: drusen formation, retinal pigment abnormalities (e.g., hypo- or hyperpigmentation), geographic atrophy, and neovascular maculopathy.[21]

Based on clinical presentation, AMD is classified as early, intermediate, or advanced.[21] Early AMD is characterized by small or intermediate drusen and minimal macular pigment abnormalities.[21] These patients generally have normal central vision.[21] Intermediate AMD patients have medium or large drusen in one or both eyes.[21] Approximately 18% of these patients will progress to advanced AMD within 5 years.[21]

Advanced AMD is classified as non-neovascular (also called the atrophic, nonexudative, or dry form) or neovascular (the exudative or wet form).[21,23] In the non-neovascular form, the retina and other layers atrophy.[23] In the neovascular form, new blood vessels appear.[21,23] Generally, vision is already affected when patients progress to advanced AMD; vision loss is seen in both forms.[21] Ten to twenty percent of patients with the non-neovascular form will progress to the neovascular form.[24] Once one eye develops advanced AMD, 43% of patients will develop neovascular changes or atrophy in the other eye within 5 years.[21]

Clinical Presentation and Diagnosis of AMD[22,24]

Symptoms

- Mild blurry central vision
- Difficulty reading
- Trouble with color and contrast
- Painless, progressive, moderate to severe blurring of central vision
- Sudden loss or distortion of vision possible

Signs

- Drusen
- Retinal pigment epithelial mottling

Other Diagnostic Tests

- Amsler's grid abnormalities indicate fluid in subretinal space (Figs. 62–4 and 62–5)
- Dilated fundus examination shows drusen and pigmentary abnormalities in the macula
- Rapid sequence fluorescein angiography shows leakage in the neovascular form

TREATMENT

Desired Outcomes

The primary goal of treatment for AMD is to slow the disease progression. This includes slowing the loss of visual acuity and the progression to legal blindness, along with maintaining contrast sensitivity and slowing the rate of progression to late AMD. The secondary goals are maintaining quality of life for the patient and minimizing the adverse effects of treatment.[23]

General Approach to Treatment

❽ *There is no cure for AMD, and the efficacy of most treatments is low.* Newer drug developments show promise, but no treatment can reverse damage that has already occurred.[24] Early diagnosis is critical. High-risk patients need periodic eye examinations because some patients do not notice any changes, even when neovascularization has occurred.[21]

Nonpharmacologic Therapy

▶ *Non-neovascular AMD*

Advise patients to stop smoking, as observational data supports a causal relationship between smoking and AMD.[21]

Drusen ablation by laser has been used in non-neovascular AMD. However, it is not clear whether the treatment reduces progression to neovascular AMD.[24] There is a possibility that the treatments may induce neovascularization and retinal atrophy.[23] Other nonpharmacologic therapies are in trials,

Patient Encounter 3, Part 1

KS, a 72-year-old white female, presents with difficulty seeing license plates on cars while she is driving. She can still distinguish street signs and other cars, but notices that smaller details seem hazy. She notes that this is only occurring in her left eye, so sometimes she closes that eye and everything is fine. Her son is concerned that she shouldn't be driving.

PMH: Hypertension, osteoporosis, hyperlipidemia

SH: Denies smoking, drinking, or illicit drugs

Widowed, two adult children

FH: Mother died at 70 from "old age"

Father died at 75 from cancer

PE:

BP 136/78

P 72

R 16

Ht 5'4" (163 cm)

Wt 142 lbs (65 kg)

Medications:

Lisinopril 10 mg daily

Fosamax 70 mg q week (on Fridays)

Lipitor 20 mg daily

Aspirin 81 mg daily

Multivitamin daily

Does KS have any definitive or potential risk factors for age-related macular degeneration?

but there is insufficient evidence for experts to recommend these procedures at this time.[21]

▶ *Neovascular AMD*

Thermal laser photocoagulation reduces severe visual loss 2 to 5 years after the procedure, but leads to an immediate and permanent reduction in central vision. There is a 50% chance that leakage will recur in the next 2 years after the procedure.[23]

Use of photodynamic therapy in combination with the medication verteporfin has shown success in clinical trials.[25] Verteporfin is reconstituted to achieve the desired dose of 6 mg/m² body surface area and diluted with 5% dextrose for injection to a total infusion volume of 30 ml. The drug is given intravenously, and laser light delivery is performed on the patient 15 minutes after the start of the 10-minute infusion with verteporfin. Photodynamic therapy uses nonthermal red light to activate verteporfin, which produces reactive oxygen species that locally damage the neovascular endothelium.[25] Verteporfin treatment reduces the risk of loss of visual acuity and legal blindness over 1 to 2 years. Long-term results are not yet available. Severe photosensitivity for

3 to 5 days after the procedure is common, and some patients experience a severe loss of vision. Eventually, most patients have some visual recovery. This procedure requires multiple treatments over time.[23] Other nonpharmacologic therapies are in trials, but there is insufficient evidence for experts to recommend these procedures at this time.[21]

Pharmacologic Therapy

There are no approved pharmacologic treatments for non-neovascular AMD.[26] The Age-Related Eye Disease Study showed that a supplement containing ascorbic acid 500 mg, vitamin E 400 IU, β-carotene 15 mg, zinc oxide 80 mg, and cupric oxide 2 mg reduced the rate of clinical progression of all types of AMD by 28% in patients with at least intermediate macular degeneration.[26] No benefit was seen in patients with earlier stages of AMD; however, the duration of the study may have been insufficient to detect this benefit.[26] Currently, experts recommend antioxidant supplementation for intermediate AMD or advanced AMD in one eye.[21] Supplementation is not without risk.[24] For example, β-carotene supplementation in smokers may increase the risk of developing lung cancer.[21,24] At this time, it is not clear from the evidence whether a patient at a high risk but without symptoms of AMD would benefit from supplementation.[27]

Vascular endothelial growth factor induces angiogenesis, increases vascular permeability, and increases inflammation, all of which are thought to contribute to neovascular AMD.[28] Pegaptanib, a vascular endothelial growth factor antagonist, binds to these growth factors in an attempt to suppress neovascularization.[21,28] In clinical studies, patients treated with pegaptanib experienced a slower rate of visual decline than patients treated with a placebo injection.[29] Vision loss continued to occur in patients, and the drug was less effective in the second year of treatment.[28] Long-term efficacy studies are not available yet.[28]

Another drug, ranibizumab, binds to and inhibits the activity of vascular endothelial growth factor (VEGF) A, a critical protein in angiogenesis.[21] In one clinical study, 95% of patients treated with ranibizumab maintained visual acuity after 12 months compared with 62% of control patients.[21] Both pegaptanib and ranibizumab are administered by intravitreous injection.[21,28]

A new VEGF-A inhibitor, aflibercept, was approved in late 2011 for wet age-related macular degeneration. The dosing of 2 mg every 4 weeks for the first 3 months, followed by 2 mg every 8 weeks thereafter, results in seven injections during the first year of treatment compared with 12 injections with other products.[30] Patients treated with aflibercept or other VEGF-A inhibitors are at risk for arterial thrombotic events. Specifically, stroke, nonfatal heart attack, or vascular death were observed were observed in 1.8% of 1,824 patients in aflibercept clinical trials.[30]

Outcome Evaluation

Monitor patients for acute and chronic vision changes or loss. The Amsler's grid (Figs. 62–4 and 62–5) and frequent eye examinations may detect changes more quickly. The long-term prognosis for AMD is poor. Monitor patients for inability to drive and remove driving privileges as appropriate. Work with patients and family members to plan for lifestyle changes as vision decreases.[21]

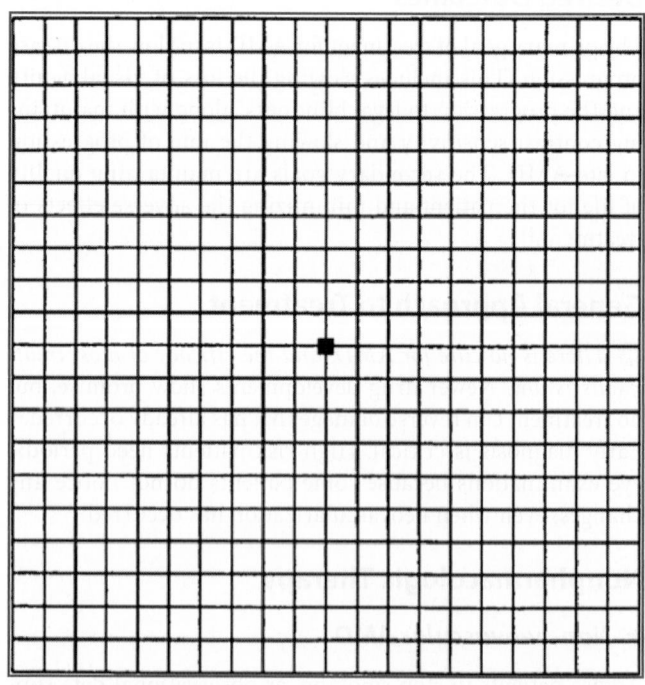

FIGURE 62–4. Amsler's grid distortions in the lines of the grid may be caused by subtle changes in central vision due to fluid in the subretinal space. This is the Amsler's grid as it appears to someone with normal vision. (From the National Eye Institute, National Institutes of Health Ref. No. EC03. *http://www.nei.nih.gov/photo/*)

Patient Encounter 3, Part 2

After meeting with a retinologist, KS has been diagnosed with early non-neovascular age-related macular degeneration. She has been advised to use a magnifying glass for her left eye instead of closing it while reading. She has been advised to not drive at night, but is still able to drive during the day.

What pharmacologic and nonpharmacologic treatment options are available for KS?

KS's daughter is very FRUSTRATED that her mother is not on a "medication," as a family friend is being treated for macular degeneration. What information is necessary to relay to KS's daughter?

What monitoring is appropriate for KS?

KS's daughter is concerned that she will develop macular degeneration because she read that it runs in families. What symptoms should KS's daughter watch for as she gets older?

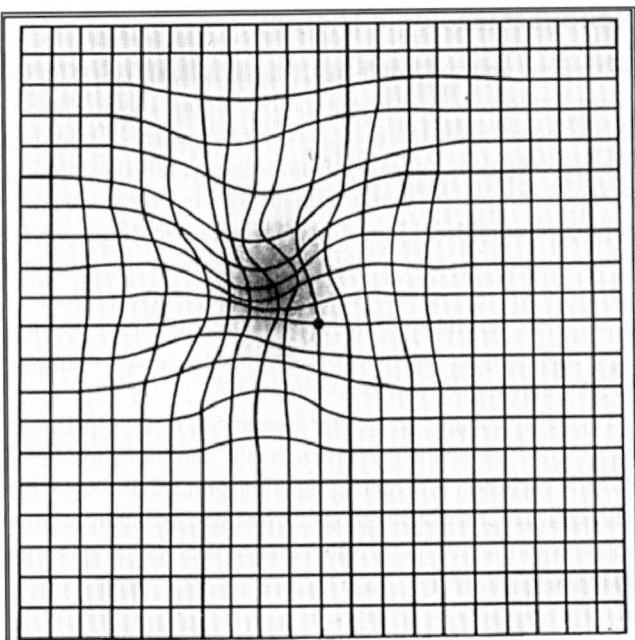

FIGURE 62–5. Amsler's grid as it might appear to someone with AMD. (From the National Eye Institute, National Institutes of Health Ref. No. EC04. *http://www. nei.nih.gov/photo/*)

DRY EYE

EPIDEMIOLOGY AND ETIOLOGY

Dry eye is a frequent cause of eye irritation. The lack of a single diagnostic test for the condition limits the available epidemiologic data. Reports of the prevalence of dry eye range from 5% to 30%, being more frequent in elderly patients.[31] The risk factors for dry eye are listed in Table 62–10. Of interest, the use of caffeine is associated with a decreased risk of dry eye. Dry eye that is left untreated can cause loss of vision, structural damage, an increased risk for infection, and compromised efficacy of ocular surgery.[32]

CLINICAL PRESENTATION

Symptoms of dry eye are similar to those of other diseases and may include blurred vision, burning, irritation, itching, soreness, and/or the sensation of a foreign body in the eye.[32]

Table 62–10

Risk Factors for Dry Eye

Older age
Female gender
Connective tissue disease
Vitamin A deficiency
Androgen deficiency
Estrogen replacement therapy

From Jackson WB. Management of dysfunctional tear syndrome: a Canadian consensus. Can J Ophthalmol 2009;44:385–394.

Clinical Presentation and Diagnosis of Dry Eye[31]

General

Many other ocular diseases have similar symptoms. Patients with suggestive symptoms without signs should be placed on a treatment trial. Repeated observations over time may be required for a clinical diagnosis.

Symptoms

- Dry or foreign body sensation
- Mild itching
- Burning
- Stinging
- Photophobia
- Ocular irritation or soreness
- Blurry vision
- Contact lens intolerance
- Diurnal fluctuation or symptoms worsening later in the day

Signs

- Redness
- Mucus discharge
- Increased blink frequency
- Tearing

Other Diagnostic Tests

- The tear break-up time test assesses the stability of precorneal tear film. Break-up times of less than 10 seconds are considered abnormal.
- Ocular surface dye staining assesses the ocular surface and will show blotchy or exposure-zone punctate areas in the dry eye.
- Schirmer's test evaluates aqueous tear production but is not diagnostic for dry eye. Results of 5 mm or less are considered abnormal.
- Assess corneal sensation if trigeminal nerve dysfunction is suspected.
- Evaluate for an autoimmune disorder if significant dry eyes or other signs and symptoms or family history are present.

PATHOPHYSIOLOGY

The surface of the eye and the tear-secreting glands work together as an integrated unit that refreshes the tear supply and clears away used tears. Dry eye may be caused by impaired tear secretion and/or increased tear evaporation.[32] It has been suggested that dry eye be called "dysfunctional tear syndrome," as all of the predisposing factors cause some disruption of the tear.[31]

Table 62-11

Associated Conditions That Cause or Worsen Dry Eye

Ocular Conditions	Environmental Factors
Blepharitis	Wind
Meibomian gland	Reduced humidity
dysfunction	Air conditioning or heating
Systemic Diseases	Exogenous irritants or allergens
Sjögren's syndrome	Prolonged use of computer or
Rosacea	reading
Lymphoma	Contact lenses
Sarcoidosis	Air travel
Hemochromatosis	Smoke exposure
Amyloidosis	**Local Trauma**
HIV	Orbital surgery
Hepatitis C	Radiation
Epstein-Barr virus	Injury
Graft-versus-host disease	Chemical exposure
Rheumatoid arthritis	**Systemic Medications**
Systemic lupus	Diuretics
erythematosus	Antihistamines
Scleroderma	Anticholinergics
Neuromuscular diseases	Antidepressants
Bell's palsy	Systemic retinoids
Parkinson's disease	Hormone antagonists
	Hormone therapy
	Cardiac antiarrhythmics
	Diphenoxylate/atropine
	β-Blockers
	Chemotherapy agents

From Refs. 31 and 32.

Dysfunction may be caused by aging, systemic inflammatory diseases, a decrease in androgen hormones, surgery, ocular surface diseases (including herpes simplex), systemic diseases, or medications that affect the efferent cholinergic nerves. Dysfunctional tear film may result in an inflammatory response on the ocular surface called **keratoconjunctivitis sicca**.[32]

Conditions that increase the evaporative loss of tears also worsen dry eye. In addition to environmental causes (Table 62-11), an abnormal blink reflex is a common cause of increased evaporative loss.[32]

TREATMENT

Desired Outcomes[32]

• Relief of the symptoms of dry eye

• Maintain or improve visual acuity

• Prevention of long-term adverse effects from dry eye

General Approach to Treatment

❾ *Dry eye is a chronic condition. Symptoms can be improved with treatment, but unless dry eye is secondary to a disease, it is not usually curable.* Because of this, patient education is critical, and a periodic reassessment of the efficacy of the treatment is appropriate. If the patient is unresponsive to treatment, refer to an ophthalmologist for additional options. If the dry eye is secondary to a systemic disease, the disease should be managed by the appropriate medical specialist.[32]

Nonpharmacologic Therapy

• Behavioral and environmental modifications may significantly improve dry eye, especially in mild cases. Patients should be counseled to increase their frequency of blinking, use eyelid hygiene and warm compresses, and stop smoking. Evaluate the patient's environment for air drafts. Consider adding a humidifier in low-humidity areas. Schedule regular breaks from computer work or reading. Lower the computer screen to below eye level to decrease lid aperture. Evaluate medication profile and therapeutically substitute medications that do not exacerbate dry eye. Spectacle side shields or goggles may reduce tear evaporation.[31,32]

If pharmacologic and other therapies are not sufficient, punctal occlusion or lateral tarsorrhaphy may be an option.[31,32] Punctal occlusion is the plugging of the punctal drainage sites with collagen or silicone plugs. Lateral tarsorrhaphy sutures portions of the lid margins together to decrease evaporative tear loss.

Pharmacologic Therapy

• Regardless of the cause, the mainstay of treatment for dry eye is artificial tears. Artificial tears augment the tear film topically and provide symptom relief. If a patient uses artificial tears more than four times daily, recommend a preservative-free formulation. Preservative-free formulations are also appropriate if the patient develops an allergy to ophthalmic preservatives. Artificial tears are available in gel, ointment, and emulsion forms that provide a longer duration of relief and may allow for less frequent instillation. Ointment use is appropriate at bedtime.[31]

Preliminary data suggest dietary or supplemental intake of omega-3 fatty acids may be beneficial.[9,31,32] Omega-3 fatty acids may block the production of inflammatory cytokines and proinflammatory mediators.[31]

Anti-inflammatory agents may be used in conjunction with artificial tears. The only approved agent is cyclosporine emulsion. Administered topically, the exact mechanism is unknown, but it is believed to act as a partial immunomodulator suppressing ocular inflammation. Cyclosporine emulsion increases tear production in some patients. Fifteen minutes should elapse after instillation of cyclosporine before artificial tears are instilled.[33] Use of topical corticosteroids for short periods (2 weeks) may suppress inflammation and ocular irritation symptoms.[32]

The oral cholinergic agonists pilocarpine and cevimeline are used for patients with Sjögren's syndrome (combined dry eye and dry mouth) or severe dry eye. By binding to muscarinic receptors, the cholinergic agonists may increase tear production. Excessive sweating is a common side effect with pilocarpine and may limit its use (Table 62-12).[32]

Outcome Evaluation[32]

• Monitor patient for relief of symptoms and ocular damage.

Table 62–12

Pharmacologic Therapies for Dry Eye

Drug (Brand Name)	Dosing
Pilocarpine 5 mg tablet (Salagen)	5 mg orally 4 times daily
Cevimeline 30 mg capsule (Evoxac)	30 mg orally 3 times daily
Cyclosporine ophthalmic emulsion 0.05% (Restasis)	One drop in each eye twice daily

From Lacy CF, Armstrong LL, Goldman MP, Lance LL. Drug Information Handbook 2011. Hudson, OH: American Pharmaceutical Association, 2011.

Patient Care and Monitoring: Patient Counseling

Wash hands before and after instilling medication(s) into the eye

Contact lenses should be removed prior to instilling eye medication, and the patient should wait 10 minutes after instilling ocular medications into the eye before inserting contact lenses

Do not touch the tip of the eye medication container with hands or surfaces, including the eye

Use of **nasolacrimal occlusion** decreases systemic absorption up to 60% and may increase ocular bioavailability of the drug. After instilling the eye drop, the patient should close the eye and press a finger gently against the nasolacrimal duct (tear duct) for 2 to 3 minutes.[34]

- Periodically reassess the patient's compliance with therapy and understanding of the disease.
- It may take 6 to 12 weeks before improvement is seen with pilocarpine therapy.[31]
- Cyclosporine therapy may take up to 3 months for full improvement.
- If a patient presents with vision loss, moderate or severe pain, corneal ulceration, or a lack of response to therapy, refer the patient to an ophthalmologist for prompt evaluation.

DRUG-INDUCED OCULAR DISORDERS

Many systemic medications can cause ocular adverse effects. Patients presenting with ocular complaints should have their medication profile evaluated for potential causative agents. Table 62–13 shows some ocular changes due to the use of certain drugs.

Table 62–13

Selected Drug-Induced Ocular Changes

Miosis
Alcohol
Narcotics
Barbiturates
Phenothiazines

Decreased Tear Volume
Anticholinergics
Diuretics
β-Blockers
Tricyclic antidepressants

Nystagmus
Phenytoin
Barbiturates

Increased Tear Volume
Cholinergic agents
Benzodiazepines
Phenothiazines

Induce Uveitis
Bisphosphonates
Sulfonamides
Cidofovir
Topical metipranolol
Topical corticosteroids
Latanoprost

Mydriasis
Anticholinergics
Corticosteroids
Tricyclic antidepressants
Sympathomimetics

Corneal Deposits
Amiodarone
Hydroxychloroquine
Tamoxifen
Gold
Indomethacin
Phenothiazines (ocular pigment deposits)

Cause or Worsen Cataracts
Corticosteroids
Phenothiazines

Decreased Blink Rate
Botulinum toxin type A
Ethanol

Lid or Corneal Edema
Chlorthalidone
Oral contraceptives
Ibuprofen
Digoxin
Phenothiazines

From Refs. 16, 35, and 36.

Abbreviations Introduced in This Chapter

AMD   Age-related macular degeneration
NSAID   Nonsteroidal anti-inflammatory drug

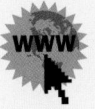 Self-assessment questions and answers are available at *http://www.mhpharmacotherapy.com/pp.html.*

REFERENCES

1. Handler JA, Ghezzi KT. General ophthalmologic examination. Emerg Med Clin North Am 1995;13:521–538.
2. Babineau MR, Sanchez LD. Ophthalmologic procedures in the emergency department. Emerg Med Clin N Am 2008:26:17–34.
3. Harlan JB Jr, Pieramici DJ. Evaluation of patients with ocular trauma. Ophthalmol Clin North Am 2002;15:153–161.
4. Wilson SA, Last A. Management of corneal abrasions. Am Fam Physician 2004;70:123–128.
5. McEvoy GK, ed. AHFS Drug Information 2011. Bethesda, MD: American Society of Health-System Pharmacists, 2011.
6. Mino de Kaspar H, Koss MJ, He L, Blumenkranz MS, Ta CN. Antibiotic susceptibility of preoperative normal conjunctival bacteria. Am J Ophthalmol 2005;139:730–733.
7. Rodrigues Z. Irrigation of the eye after alkaline and acidic burns. Emerg Nurse 2009;17(8):26–29.

8. Goold L, Durkin S, Crompton J. Sudden loss of vision—History and examination. Aust Fam Physician 2009;38:764–767.

9. Cronau H, Kankanala RR, Mauger T. Diagnosis and management of red eye in primary care. Am Fam Physician 2010;81(2):137–144; patient handout 145.

10. Thielen TL, Castle SS, Terry JE. Anterior ocular infections: An overview of pathophysiology and treatment. Ann Pharmacother 2000;34:235–246.

11. Baum J. Infections of the eye. Clin Infect Dis 1995;21:479–486; quiz 487–488.

12. Leibowitz HM. The red eye. N Engl J Med 2000;343(5):345–351.

13. Morrow GL, Abbott RL. Conjunctivitis. Am Fam Physician 1998;57:735–746.

14. Gordon YJ, Araullo-Cruz T, Romanowski EG. The effects of topical nonsteroidal anti-inflammatory drugs on adenoviral replication. Arch Ophthalmol 1998;116:900–905.

15. Bielory L. Ocular allergy. Mt Sinai J Med 2011;78:740–758.

16. Lacy CF, Armstrong LL, Goldman MP, Lance LL. Drug Information Handbook 2011. Hudson, OH: American Pharmaceutical Association, 2011.

17. Bielory L, Lien KW, Bigelsen S. Efficacy and tolerability of newer antihistamines in the treatment of allergic conjunctivitis. Drugs 2005;65:215–228.

18. Cook EB, Stahl JL, Barney NP, Graziano FM. Mechanisms of antihistamines and mast cell stabilizers in ocular allergic inflammation. Curr Drug Targets Inflamm Allergy 2002;1:167–180.

19. Bielory L. Ocular allergy guidelines: A practical treatment algorithm. Drugs 2002;62:1611–1634.

20. Feder RS, Dunn SP, Jones MR, et al. Bacterial keratitis, Preferred Practice Pattern – limited revision [Internet]. San Francisco: American Academy of Ophthalmology, 2011 [cited 2012 Feb 3]. Available from: http://one.aao.org/CE/PracticeGuidelines/PPP.aspx

21. Chew EY, Benson WE, Blodi BA, et al. Age-related macular degeneration, Preferred Practice Pattern [Internet]. San Francisco: American Academy of Ophthalmology, 2008 [cited 2011 Oct 1]. Available from: http://one.aao.org/CE/PracticeGuidelines/PPP.aspx

22. Friedman DS, O'Colmain BJ, Munoz B, et al. Prevalence of age-related macular degeneration in the United States. Arch Ophthalmol 2004;122:564–572.

23. Arnold J, Sarks S. Age related macular degeneration. Clin Evid 2004;(11):819–834.

24. Comer GM, Ciulla TA, Criswell MH, Tolentino M. Current and future treatment options for nonexudative and exudative age-related macular degeneration. Drugs Aging 2004;21:967–992.

25. Visudyne (verteporfin) for injection [package insert]. Menlo Park, CA: QLT Ophthalmics, 2010.

26. Ferris FL, Chew EY, Sperduto R, for the Age-Related Eye Disease Study Group. A randomized, placebo-controlled, clinical trial of high-dose supplementation with vitamins C and E and beta carotene for age-related cataract and vision loss: AREDS report no. 9. Arch Ophthalmol 2001;119:1439–1452.

27. Mares JA, La Rowe TL, Blodi BA. Doctor, what vitamins should I take for my eyes? Arch Ophthalmol 2004;122:628–635.

28. Macugen (pegaptanib sodium) injection [package insert]. Palm Beach Gardens, FL: Eyetech, 2011.

29. Gragoudas ES, Adamis AP, Cunningham ET Jr, et al. Pegaptanib for neovascular age-related macular degeneration. N Engl J Med 2004;351:2805–2816.

30. Eylea (aflibercept) injection [package insert]. Tarrytown, NY: Regeneron Pharmaceuticals, 2011.

31. Jackson WB. Management of dysfunctional tear syndrome: A Canadian consensus. Can J Ophthalmol 2009;44:385–394.

32. Feder RS, Dunn SP, Jones MR, et al. Dry eye syndrome, Preferred Practice Pattern – limited revision [Internet]. San Francisco: American Academy of Ophthalmology, 2011 [cited 2012 Feb 3]. Available from: http://one.aao.org/CE/PracticeGuidelines/PPP.aspx

33. Restasis (cyclosporine) emulsion [package insert]. Irvine, CA: Allergan, 2010.

34. Zimmerman TJ, Kooner KS, Kandarakis AS, Ziegler LP. Improving the therapeutic index of topically applied ocular drugs. Arch Ophthalmol 1984;102:551–553.

35. Roy FH. Ocular Differential Diagnosis [Internet]. 8th ed. Philadelphia: Lippincott Williams & Wilkins, 2007 [cited 2011 Sept 24]. Available from: http://www.eye.uthsc.edu/sections/OcularDiff.pdf

36. Li J, Tripathi RC, Tripathi BJ. Drug-induced ocular disorders. Drug Saf 2008;31:127–141.

63 Allergic Rhinitis

David A. Apgar

KEY CONCEPTS

❶ Allergic rhinitis (AR) is an allergen-induced and immunoglobulin E (IgE)-mediated inflammatory condition of the lining of the nose and upper respiratory tract.

❷ AR can be categorized in different ways.

❸ AR is a common disorder that can negatively impact quality of life to a significant degree, yet it has been trivialized in the past.

❹ The goals of treatment of AR are to reduce or minimize the frequency and severity of symptoms, prevent comorbid disorders and complications, improve the patient's quality of life, improve work attendance and productivity and/or school attendance and performance, and minimize adverse effects of therapy.

❺ The general approach for treatment of AR is fourfold: avoidance of allergen triggers, pharmacotherapy, immunotherapy, and patient/family education.

❻ Routine first-line agents for the treatment of AR are intranasal corticosteroids and oral and/or intranasal antihistamines. Adjunctive or secondary choice agents, each of which may have a first-line role in selected patients, include decongestants, cromolyn, montelukast, ipratropium, and intranasal saline irrigation.

❼ Intranasal corticosteroids are the most effective therapy for AR, especially for nasal congestion. They are first-line agents for severe manifestations and are also used for those with moderate disease not controlled with oral and/or intranasal antihistamines. Their anti-inflammatory mechanism of action probably contributes to this superiority.

❽ Second-generation antihistamines are first-line agents, especially for mild or intermittent AR. They are preferred over first-generation antihistamines because of their improved side-effect profile. Although effective for most symptoms of AR, they are less effective than intranasal corticosteroids for nasal congestion. Intranasal administration of an antihistamine is more effective than oral administration for nasal congestion.

❾ The best applications of decongestants in AR are in short-term use to overcome severe nasal congestion and to facilitate improved efficacy of intranasal agents. The intranasal administration of decongestants should usually not exceed 3 consecutive days.

❿ Generally speaking, the treatment of AR in children is the same as it is for adults, except for limitations in terms of FDA-approved products for some age groups and route of administration issues with some products.

INTRODUCTION[1-3]

Rhinitis is inflammation of the lining of the nose and other parts of the upper respiratory tract. Allergy is only one cause of rhinitis. Although there are several other types of rhinitis (see Table 63–1), and some patients can manifest a mixed form (both allergic and nonallergic rhinitis), allergic rhinitis (AR) is the focus of this chapter. Because ocular symptoms frequently occur in association with AR, another term used is allergic rhinoconjunctivitis. This acknowledges involvement of the bulbar and palpebral conjunctivae in the allergic process. ❶ *AR is an allergen-induced and immunoglobulin E (IgE)-mediated inflammatory condition of the lining of the nose and upper respiratory tract.*

❷ *AR has traditionally been categorized as either seasonal or perennial.* Seasonal allergic rhinitis (SAR) is attributed to inhaled allergens (aeroallergens) that have a seasonal variation. These allergens are usually encountered outdoors and are most often plant pollens and substances from molds and fungi. Perennial allergic rhinitis (PAR) is attributed to aeroallergens that are present in the patient's environment almost continuously throughout the year and are usually encountered indoors. Common perennial allergens are the house dust mite, indoor molds and fungi, insects (especially cockroaches), and companion animals (pets). Some patients are affected year round, but have seasonal exacerbations. These people are probably allergic to both seasonal and perennial aeroallergens. Other patients have only episodic manifestations. These people are probably allergic to aeroallergens that are only occasionally (episodically) encountered. The Joint Task Force on Practice Parameters (representing the American Academy of Allergy, Asthma and Immunology [AAAAI], the American College of Allergy, Asthma and Immunology [ACAAI], and the Joint Council of Allergy, Asthma and Immunology) published practice parameters for the diagnosis and management of AR in August 2008.[1] This document also introduces the term "episodic" AR, as a category in addition to SAR and PAR.

Recognizing that the traditional categories of seasonal and perennial AR are imperfect, another system for categorizing AR has been suggested by the international group Allergic Rhinitis and its Impact on Asthma (ARIA).[2] ❷ *This alternative system categorizes the manifestations by a combination of frequency and severity.* There are two divisions of frequency: intermittent and persistent. Intermittent frequency is defined as AR manifestations occurring less often than 4 days per week or for fewer than 4 consecutive weeks. Persistent frequency is defined as AR manifestations occurring for 4 or more days per week *and* for 4 or more consecutive weeks. Severity is categorized either as mild or as moderate–severe. Mild manifestations are those that do *not* cause interference with sleep, daily activities, or work or school performance and that are not "troublesome." Moderate–severe manifestations were combined because distinction between moderate and severe was not clinically practical. This category includes those patients with manifestations of AR that do cause interference with sleep, impairment of daily activities, problems at work or school, or are "troublesome." The ARIA document uses IAR (for intermittent) and PER (for persistent) for the two frequency categories. It is important to realize that IAR and PER are not synonymous with the classical categories of SAR and PAR, respectively. The ARIA system results in four categories: mild intermittent, mild persistent, moderate–severe intermittent, or moderate–severe persistent. The ARIA approach was updated in early 2008.[2] See Table 63–2 for a summary of these categories of AR.

Table 63–1

Types of Rhinitis

Allergic (see Table 63–2 for details)
Nonallergic
  Vasomotor (also known as perennial nonallergic rhinitis)
    (triggered by irritants, cold air, exercise/running,
    or unidentified factors)
  Food/meal related (gustatory)
  Infectious
  NARES (nonallergic rhinitis with eosinophilia syndrome)
Occupational
  Caused by protein allergens (IgE-mediated) or by irritants/
    sensitizers (probably non–IgE-mediated)
Other rhinitis syndromes
  Hormonally related (pregnancy and menstrual cycle related)
  Drug-related
    Rhinitis medicamentosa (rebound from overuse of intranasal
      decongestants)
  Drug-induced
    Angiotensin-converting enzyme inhibitors (ACEI)
    a-Antagonists (used for treatment of BPH and HT)
    Phosphodiesterase-5 inhibitors (used for treatment of ED)
    Aspirin and other NSAIDs (as an isolated side effect of AERD)
    Oral contraceptives (controversial)
  Atrophic rhinitis
  Rhinitis associated with inflammatory or immunologic
    diseases (e.g., granulomatous infections, RA, SLE, Wegener's
    granulomatosis, sarcoidosis, Churg–Strauss syndrome, and
    others)

ACEI, angiotensin-converting enzyme inhibitor; AERD, aspirin-exacerbated respiratory disease; BPH, benign prostatic hyperplasia/hypertrophy; ED, erectile dysfunction; HT, hypertension; NARES, nonallergic rhinitis with eosinophilia [on nasal smear] syndrome; NSAIDs, nonsteroidal anti-inflammatory drugs; RA, rheumatoid arthritis; SLE, systemic lupus erythematosus.

From Refs. 1–3.

EPIDEMIOLOGY

❸ *AR is one of the most common chronic disorders in the United States.*[4] One source indicates that it ranks fifth in this category.[5] It is estimated that up to 30% of adults and up to 40% of children in the United States are affected.[1,4,6–8] The total direct and indirect costs of AR in the United States for 2002 have been estimated to be in excess of 11 billion dollars.[1] AR is the most common allergic disease in children.[9] ❸ *Despite this, the disease has historically been trivialized.*

Table 63–2

Categories of Allergic Rhinitis

Based on AAAAI/ACAAI Practice Parameter
   Seasonal—symptoms present only during specific portions of the year
   Perennial—symptoms present throughout the year
   Episodic—symptoms present only during intermittent exposure to allergen trigger
Based on ARIA 2008 Update
   Mild versus moderate–severe
      Mild means no interference with sleep, daily activities, work or school function and attendance, and no troublesome symptoms
      Moderate–severe means the presence of any one of the following: abnormal sleep, impairment of daily activities, impairment of work or school function, troublesome symptoms
   Intermittent versus persistent
      Intermittent means that symptoms are present for less than 4 days/week, or for less than 4 consecutive weeks
      Persistent means that symptoms are present for more than 4 days/week and for more than 4 consecutive weeks
      Any one of the four possibilities of these variables can occur: mild intermittent, mild persistent, moderate–severe intermittent, and moderate–severe persistent

From Refs. 1–3.

The major risk factors for AR are: a family history of allergic disorder; elevated serum IgE levels, especially before the age of 6 years; higher socioeconomic class; positive skin test results; and emigration into a Western industrialized environment.[1,2]

Certain disorders occur commonly with AR. The most important example is asthma. Some sources consider AR and asthma as two manifestations on a spectrum within the same disease. As many as 78% of patients with asthma have AR, and up to 38% of patients with AR have asthma.[4,8,10] There is evidence that AR can predispose to the development of asthma.[1,4,8,10] Other conditions that can occur with AR include sinusitis, obstructive sleep apnea, otitis media with effusion, and nasal polyposis.[1]

Pathophysiology[1–3,5,10–12]

AR is an IgE-mediated disorder of people who are allergy prone. Initial contact is required to sensitize the patient to subsequent exposures. Patients with an inherited tendency to allergic disorders produce T-helper lymphocyte type 2 (Th-2)-directed responses, including production of specific IgE antibodies, to one or more allergens. The details of the process are complex and still being defined. Many types of cells, mediators, and intermediate substances (including cytokines) are involved. In response to subsequent exposures to the trigger antigen(s), there is an early-phase and often a late-phase allergic response. This distinction has therapeutic implications.

During the early phase, the trigger allergen becomes bound to IgE that is fixed to mast cells in the nasal mucosa.

This occurs within minutes of subsequent exposure to the antigen and causes the mast cells to degranulate. Degranulation results in release of preformed mediators, the most important of which is histamine. This step stimulates more mast cells, as well as macrophages, eosinophils, and basophils to produce more substances, including cysteine leukotrienes and prostaglandin D_2. These newly produced mediators bind to receptors in the nose and facilitate many of the manifestations of AR. The resultant vasodilation, mucosal edema, and hypertrophy all contribute to nasal congestion. Clear, watery, and often profuse rhinorrhea is also characteristic in this early phase, a combined result of mucous secretion and increased vascular permeability. Sneezing and nasal itch are other prominent features of the early phase. Many patients also have ocular symptoms.

The late phase occurs in up to 50% of AR sufferers. It can begin as soon as 2 hours after the early phase and usually peaks within 12 hours. The late phase involves a second release of many of the mediators of the early phase. In addition, the late phase is characterized by an inflammatory component caused by infiltration of several cell types (e.g., mast cells, eosinophils, basophils, neutrophils, and T lymphocytes) into the nasal mucosa. The most significant manifestation during the late phase is nasal congestion that is often severe and long lasting.

A phenomenon known as the priming response is also of importance. This simply means that prolonged and/or repeated allergen exposure makes it easier to stimulate the process resulting in mediator release with symptoms. The inflammatory component that characterizes the late phase probably contributes to this effect. A vicious cycle results in which smaller doses of allergen can create symptoms (i.e., the threshold is lowered). Thus, even when pollen exposure is decreased, symptoms may continue. In some patients, the threshold is lowered to the degree that even irritant substances (e.g., formaldehyde, tobacco smoke, perfumes, automobile exhaust, and other environmental pollutants) may cause symptoms, on a nonallergic basis.

TREATMENT

Desired Outcomes

4 *The goals of treatment of AR are to reduce or minimize the frequency and severity of symptoms, prevent comorbid disorders and complications, improve the patient's quality of life, improve work attendance and productivity and/or school attendance and performance, and minimize adverse effects of therapy. Until a cure is established, these are the only realistic goals.*

Nonpharmacologic Therapy

5 *The general approach for treatment of AR is fourfold: avoidance of allergen triggers, pharmacotherapy, immunotherapy, and patient/family education.* Immunotherapy will be considered nonpharmacologic, for this discussion, because it is not self-administered by the patient and its implementation requires referral to a specialist.

Clinical Presentation and Diagnosis of Allergic Rhinitis[1-4,8]

Typical Symptoms

- Rhinorrhea (usually clear and bilateral; primarily anterior but may have posterior [postnasal drip])
- Sneezing
- Itching (affecting mostly the nose, but also the palate, throat, eyes, and ears)
- Nasal congestion (usually the most troublesome symptom)

Other Symptoms

- Sleep disturbances
- Headache, mild facial or ear pain or fullness
- Cough (especially in those with concurrent asthma)
- Fatigue, asthenia, malaise, and irritability
- Ocular manifestations (itch, redness, tearing, chemosis, periorbital edema)
- Presenteeism (impaired performance at work or school)
- Absenteeism from work or school
- Quality of life impairment (including social function)
- Children (especially): rubbing the nose, snorting, sniffling, clearing the throat, learning or attention problems, poor appetite

Signs (especially common in children)

- Rubbing the nose (especially with the back of the hand or the palm; so-called allergic salute, which may create a horizontal crease just above the tip of the nose)
- Rubbing/scratching at the eyes
- Mouth breathing
- Dark circles under the eyes
- Dennie-Morgan lines or folds

Diagnosis

- Typical symptoms, especially in association with exposure to allergen triggers
- Other diagnostic testing usually optional, but may be necessary to rule out nonallergic causes of rhinitis or if immunotherapy is a consideration (physical exam, especially of the upper respiratory tract with emphasis on the nose, specific IgE antibody testing by either skin testing or in vitro serum testing, other specialized testing).

Avoidance of allergen triggers, to the extent they have been identified and to the extent such avoidance is possible, underlies the treatment for all patients with AR (see Table 63–3).[1,2]

Immunotherapy must be administered by a physician. The initial evaluation includes identification of specific allergens to determine individualized therapy. The role of a pharmacist in immunotherapy is appropriate referral of patients to an allergist or immunologist. See Clinical Presentation and Diagnosis for considerations for referral. At the time of this writing, in the United States, subcutaneous injection immunotherapy is the only option.[1-3,13,14] In other parts of the world, sublingual immunotherapy is an alternative.[9,13,15–17] The major advantage is ease of administration. Questions remain about comparative efficacy and the details of optimal dosage, frequency of administration, and duration of therapy.

Education of the patient as well as the patient's support system is essential.[1] They all need to understand the potential seriousness of AR (including complications such as asthma) and the chronic and/or recurrent nature of the disorder. The patient and significant others should be told about the various treatment options, including their relative advantages and disadvantages. Proper understanding and use of current medication in the patient's regimen should be assured. A better educated patient and support system will result in a better relationship with healthcare providers and hopefully will optimize patient outcomes.

Patient Encounter 1, Part 1

LF is a 30-year-old woman who presents to your place of work. She moved to this part of the country about 3 months ago. She complains of sneezing and runny nose, which began about 1 month ago. Her symptoms are worse when she is outdoors, especially if the weather is windy. Also, her symptoms interfere with her sleep so that often she awakens tired. This tiredness causes her to "doze off" several times a day while sitting at her computer at work. She asks your recommendation for OTC treatment.

Which of the typical symptoms consistent with AR does this patient have?

Which of the other (less typical) symptoms consistent with AR does she demonstrate?

What additional information is needed to accurately assess her current condition?

Pharmacologic Therapy

There are three guideline documents, all published in 2008, that are the basis for the summary that follows.[1-3] Although guideline documents are highly regarded by many, the patients enrolled in the randomized clinical trials that are a major basis for their conclusions and recommendations

---

Table 63–3

Allergen Avoidance Measures

Allergen avoidance underlies all other treatments of AR
There are several limitations to implementing allergen avoidance:
- Identification of allergens is necessary to successfully employ avoidance strategies.
- Literature support for a clinically significant impact on symptoms from allergen avoidance, especially any single measure, is meager.
- Quality of life may be negatively impacted by forced removal of a pet from the household.

Outdoor plant pollen and mold/fungi parts:
- Limit outdoor exposure, especially during high pollen conditions (warm sunny days with wind and low humidity) and during mold/fungi spore release (shortly after rains).
- Wear a face mask during activities that disturb the earth and decaying vegetation.
- Keep windows and doors closed.
- Use air conditioning when possible, but maintain clean equipment.

Indoor allergens (house dust mite, mold/fungi, cockroaches, and pets):
- Use air-conditioning, as above.
- Maintain humidity below 50% if possible, and maintain clean equipment.
- Clean frequently and thoroughly to prevent mold growth (dilute bleach with detergent).
- Avoid exposed food and garbage, especially in the kitchen, to deter insects.
- Clean kitchen frequently and thoroughly.
- Use roach traps that facilitate removal of allergen-containing bodies.
- Vacuum frequently, and consider use of a high-efficiency particulate air (HEPA) filter.
- Minimize carpeting, fabric covered furniture, and fabric wall/window coverings.
- Cover bedding (pillows, mattresses, box springs) with allergen-proof, zippered cases.
- Launder bedding frequently, in hot water (greater than 130°F or 54°C) if possible, to kill mite ova.
- Consider **acaricide** (e.g., benzyl benzoate) treatment of carpets to kill mites and ova.
- Put items that cannot be laundered (e.g., soft toys) in a plastic bag and freeze.
- Keep pets out of bedroom and bathe cats weekly, if possible.

Irritants:
- Avoid, to the degree possible, all exposure to smoke, chlorine fumes, formaldehyde fumes, and other substances identified as irritant triggers in the patient (e.g., perfumes, newspaper ink).

From Refs. 1 and 2.

Table 63–4

Intranasal and Oral Medications for AR

Corticosteroids
Intranasal[a] (budesonide, beclomethasone, ciclesonide, flunisolide, fluticasone [propionate and furoate], mometasone, triamcinolone)
Oral (rarely used)
Parenteral (not recommended)
Antihistamines
Intranasal[a] (azelastine, olopatadine)
Oral[b]
- First generation/sedating (cautious use in selected patients) (most OTC depending on strength: diphenhydramine, chlorpheniramine, clemastine, and others)
- Second generation/low- or nonsedating[a] (desloratadine, levocetirizine; OTC: loratadine, cetirizine, fexofenadine)
Mast cell stabilizer/cromone
Intranasal (OTC: cromolyn)
Decongestant
Intranasal (short-term use) (tetrahydrozoline; OTC: phenylephrine, naphazoline, oxymetazoline)
Oral[b] (OTC: phenylephrine; BTC[c]: pseudoephedrine)
LTRA
Oral (montelukast)
Antimuscarinic
Intranasal (ipratropium)

Note: All products are prescription unless indicated as OTC.

[a]First-line choices.

[b]Some products combine an antihistamine with a decongestant, sometimes with other ingredients.

[c]Behind the counter (OTC plus other requirements necessary; see the Decongestants section of text).

From Refs. 1–3 and 25–29.

---

the leukotriene receptor antagonist (LTRA) (montelukast), the antimuscarinic/anticholinergic (ipratropium), and intranasal saline. In all cases, therapy must be individualized, in cooperation with the patient. Considerations include frequency and severity of specific symptoms, realistic avoidance measures, patient age, patient preferences for route of administration, tolerance of side effects, adherence issues, comorbid disorders, and concurrent therapy. See Table 63–4 for intranasal and oral medications for the treatment of AR.

The guideline document on AR published in August 2008 by the Joint Task Force (for AAAAI and ACAAI) includes an action plan (similar to what is used for asthma). The entire article, with a sample Rhinitis Action Plan, is available on the AAAAI website (*http://www.aaaai.org/Aaaai/media/MediaLibrary/PDF%20Documents/Practice%20and%20Parameters/rhinitis2008-diagnosis-management.pdf*) in the public domain, for universal access.[1] The application of the differently colored zones on the Rhinitis Action Plan is explained at the bottom of the form, which is on page S25 of the document. Many patients will benefit from having an action plan.

▶ First-Line Agents

Corticosteroids Corticosteroids are usually administered by the intranasal route for the treatment of AR. Occasionally, a short course of oral therapy (burst and taper) is

are not always representative of patients in a primary practice population.[18] Other sources provide additional information for the treatment of AR.[8–10,19–29] The recommended approaches begin with allergen avoidance, emphasize patient/family education, and include immunotherapy as an option in selected patients.

The most reasonable plan may include considerations from several of these documents. ❻ *Routine first-line agents are intranasal corticosteroids and oral and/or intranasal antihistamines. Adjunctive or secondary choice agents, each of which may have a first-line role in selected patients, include decongestants, the mast cell stabilizer/cromone (cromolyn),*

Patient Encounter 1, Part 2

Further questioning of LF reveals that she had "allergies" as a child, but apparently "outgrew" them. She does not know any other details about her childhood allergies. She has not had any previous episodes as an adult. This episode started 6 weeks after her arrival to her new home. You also establish that she has had these symptoms steadily for at least the last 6 weeks and that they occur most days during the week. She also admits to almost daily nasal congestion. In fact, it is the congestion that is most bothersome to her and is the thing that interferes with her sleep. She also admits to itching of the roof of her mouth and a tickling sensation in her throat. She also has some itching and watering of both eyes. She does have some symptoms indoors, especially in the kitchen. However, the symptoms are definitely worse when she is outside, especially when doing yard work (mowing the lawn or trimming bushes and flowers). Her sleep is so disturbed that she feels tired most of the rest of the day, especially during the weekdays, while at work. The tiredness even interferes with activities during the weekend. The only things she notices that make her worse are spending a lot of time in the kitchen and especially being outdoors when the weather is windy. So far, she has tried nothing for these symptoms, because she does not know what to use. She thinks all this is due to allergies to local plants that are new to her because of her recent move.

What additional symptoms that are consistent with AR does she now demonstrate?

Presuming the patient has AR, how would you categorize her condition?

What additional information is needed to accurately assess possible causes for her symptoms other than plant allergies?

necessary. This oral use of corticosteroids is best applied to overcome severe nasal congestion, particularly that due to rhinitis medicamentosa from intranasal decongestants (see the section on Decongestants later in this chapter). Parenteral administration of corticosteroids in the management of AR is discouraged.[1]

❼ *Intranasal corticosteroids are considered the most effective therapy for AR. They are recommended as the drugs of choice for severe manifestations and for those with moderate disease not controlled with oral and/or intranasal antihistamines.* They provide very good relief for sneezing, itching, and rhinorrhea, as well as nasal congestion and even ocular symptoms. Nasal congestion is often the most bothersome symptom of AR, and the most difficult to control. This is probably because it results from inflammation that predominates in the late phase of the allergic response in AR.

❼ *Intranasal corticosteroids are the best agents for nasal congestion, probably because of their anti-inflammatory mechanism of action.*[1,19,22] Systemic corticosteroids (i.e., orally

administered) are also effective, but they are used only as a last resort due to systemic side effects.

Several meta-analyses have evaluated the relative efficacy of intranasal corticosteroids in comparison with other types of pharmacologic therapy of AR. The majority (but not all) of the literature suggests that intranasal corticosteroids are superior to intranasal antihistamines, to oral antihistamines, even when combined with a leukotriene antagonist, and to a leukotriene antagonist alone.[1,19]

There are currently eight intranasal corticosteroid products available in the United States, including two different salt forms of fluticasone. Most (e.g., budesonide, ciclesonide, fluticasone furoate, mometasone, and triamcinolone) are usually given in a single daily dose. However, fluticasone propionate may be given either once or twice daily; beclomethasone is usually given twice daily, and flunisolide is given two or three times daily. Despite some differences in formulation, potency, chemistry, and pharmacokinetic and pharmacodynamic properties among the products, there is no good evidence that any single product is superior in efficacy. Intranasal corticosteroids are best given regularly, as the onset of action usually takes up to 12 hours and the maximum effects may be delayed up to 7 to 14 days.[1,8,10] However, there is evidence that in some people the onset is within 3 to 4 hours, so these agents may even be used on an as needed basis.[1,30] When nasal congestion is severe, intranasal administration may not be effective due to limited exposure to the nasal mucosa. In that situation, short-term intranasal decongestants may facilitate better exposure. See Table 63–5 for intranasal corticosteroid products.

The correct technique for administration of intranasal medication is important for optimum efficacy. Consult the individual product labeling for specific instructions. However, also see Table 63–6 for general instructions for the optimal administration of intranasal medications. The technique described maximizes exposure of the drug to the nasal mucosa to optimize efficacy and minimizes both exposure to the nasal septum and loss of medication down the esophagus. See later for instructions about preparation and use of intranasal saline irrigations.

Most patients tolerate intranasal corticosteroids very well. Local side effects include nasal burning, irritation, and dryness, which may occur in up to 12% of patients.[1,8,10,19,23] Also, up to 10% to 12% of patients may experience mild epistaxis.[19,24] This may be partly due to the administration technique. Sore throat and headache may be noted by some patients.[24] Perforation of the nasal septum is a very rare side effect. This can be minimized by proper administration technique (see Table 63–6), specifically, directing the spray laterally and away from the (medial) nasal septum.[1,10]

The older intranasal corticosteroids (beclomethasone, flunisolide, and budesonide) have significant absorption, whereas, among the newer products, fluticasone and mometasone, have bioavailability of no more than 1% to 2%.[19] The decreased absorption minimizes systemic side effects. However, there is still some concern for growth suppression, other manifestations of hypothalamic–pituitary–adrenal (HPA) axis suppression, and bone and ocular effects.[19]

Table 63–5

Intranasal Corticosteroids

Generic (Brand) Name	mcg/spray	Usual Adult Dosage (each nostril)	Usual Pediatric Dosage (each nostril)
Beclomethasone dipropionate (Beconase AQ)	42	1–2 sprays twice daily	6 yo or more: 1–2 sprays twice daily
Budesonide (Rhinocort Aqua)	32	1–4 sprays once daily	6–11 yo or more: 1–2 sprays once daily
Ciclesonide (Omnaris)	50	2 sprays once daily	6 yo or more: 2 sprays once daily (seasonal AR) 12 yo or more: 2 sprays once daily (perennial AR)
Flunisolide	25	2 sprays two or three times daily	6–14 yo or more: 1 spray three times daily or 2 sprays twice daily
Fluticasone furoate (Veramyst)	27.5	1–2 sprays once daily	2–11 yo or more: 1–2 sprays once daily
Fluticasone propionate (Flonase)	50	1–2 sprays once daily or 1 spray twice daily	4–11 yo or more: 1–2 sprays once daily
Mometasone (Nasonex)	50	2 sprays once daily	2–11 yo or more: 1 spray once daily
Triamcinolone acetonide (Nasacort AQ)	55	2 sprays once daily	2–5 yo: 1 spray once daily 6-11 yo: 1-2 sprays once daily

mcg, micrograms; yo, years old.

Note: All products are FDA Pregnancy category C except budesonide, which is B.

From Refs. 1, 10, 25–27, and 29.

Table 63–6

Administration Instructions for Intranasal Medications

1. Clear the nose of mucus and debris to the extent possible.
2. Consult product labeling for preadministration instructions (e.g., shaking the container, priming the spray pump).
3. If seated or standing, do not just tilt head backward. This increases the amount of the dosage lost down the esophagus. This decreases efficacy and increases the potential for systemic absorption and thus systemic side effects.
4. If standing, bend the head forward (flex the chin onto the chest) so that the nose is the lowest portion of the head. This is best for nasal sprays.

    If possible, lie in the prone position with the stomach (ventral side) on a flat surface or kneel down. Then, flex chin onto neck, so that the open nostrils are pointing as far upward, toward the ceiling as possible. This position may be best for nose drops (more volume than sprays).

    An alternate position is to lie supine (on the back) on a flat surface, then bend the head backward (extend the head), again, so that the open nostrils point upward toward the ceiling.
5. Use the contralateral hand to insert the spray nozzle or dropper into one nostril (i.e., the left hand for right nostril).
6. Use the other hand to occlude the opposite nostril (the one not being medicated).
7. Aim the spray or drops toward the outer (lateral) internal surface of each nostril and away from the nasal septum (which is the inner or medial surface).
8. Breath in slowly but deeply through the medicated nostril.
9. Repeat this procedure to apply medication to the other nostril.
10. Consult the product labeling for instructions on cleaning the device.
11. See the text for information about preparation and use of saline irrigation.

From Refs. 3 and 8.

Several studies have evaluated the effects of intranasal and inhaled corticosteroids on HPA axis suppression and growth.[1,19] Most have shown little or no clinically significant effects. The product most implicated with growth suppression is beclomethasone. According to one of the guideline documents, one study demonstrated suppression in children using the drug for 1 year, but at twice the usual recommended dose.[1] There is no confirmation of a causal effect of intranasal corticosteroids on posterior subcapsular cataracts, increased intraocular pressure, or decreased bone density; however, those with risk factors for any of these conditions should be monitored carefully for their development. Ultimately, patient preference for a specific intranasal corticosteroid may be determined more by cost and by formulation differences that affect odor and aftertaste.

Antihistamines Antihistamines used for the treatment of AR are administered by either the oral or the intranasal route. These agents interact with the H_1 (histamine type 1) receptor. Histamine is involved with both the early and the late phases of AR. Activation of H_1 receptors in the nose, upper airway mucosa, and the eye produces the common manifestations of AR (sneezing, itching, rhinorrhea, nasal congestion, and ocular symptoms). The antihistamines are very effective for the sneezing, itching, and rhinorrhea of AR. There is some effect to improve nasal congestion, but less so than for the other symptoms. There is also benefit for the ocular symptoms (e.g., itch, redness, tearing). Intranasal administration is more effective than oral administration for the nasal congestion, but less effective for the ocular symptoms. The onset of action by oral administration is usually within 1 to 2 hours, and that for intranasal administration within 30 minutes.[1,8,19] All antihistamines probably provide better relief if used continuously during symptomatic periods, but they are also effective used only when needed.

Antihistamine drugs used for AR are technically inverse agonists, not competitive antagonists; however, there may be little clinical significance to the difference.[10,19,22] These drugs bind to the H_1 receptor, changing its three-dimensional conformation such that it is kept in the inactive state. This results in downregulation of H_1 receptor activity and a decrease in end organ effects. These agents do not prevent release of histamine. Research continues relative to the clinical importance of blockade of other types of histamine receptors (H_2, H_3, H_4) in the treatment of AR.[31]

The oral agents are divided into first- and second-generation drugs. The first-generation agents are distributed among six chemical classes, including the more sedating ethanolamine class (e.g., diphenhydramine) and the least sedating alkylamine class (e.g., chlorpheniramine). ❽ *Most sources now discourage the routine use of the first-generation agents for AR. This is due to their CNS and anticholinergic side effects.* The CNS effects are primarily sedation, as well as impairment of cognitive function and performance of tasks. Studies have shown that decision making and driving or work performance are impaired even when the patient is unaware of any overt effects.[1] There is also evidence of decreased performance at school and impaired learning, among pediatric patients.[1] Some controversy remains, however, about how common these problems truly are.[24] The major anticholinergic (perhaps more accurately stated as antimuscarinic) effects include blurred vision, dry mouth, urinary retention, and constipation. The only possible advantage of the antimuscarinic properties is an additional effect to decrease rhinorrhea. However, some patients complain about the increased thickness of the secretions.[22] Another disadvantage of the first-generation antihistamines is that most must be administered three to four times daily. If first-generation antihistamines are recommended by a healthcare practitioner, care must be taken to educate the patient about these CNS and anticholinergic side effects. Patients who take other sedative substances are prone to an additive effect from the antihistamine. Those taking any other medications with anticholinergic or antimuscarinic properties may experience additive effects from the antihistamine. The elderly are, in general, more sensitive to both types of adverse effects.

Currently available oral second-generation H_1 antihistamines are cetirizine, levocetirizine, loratadine, desloratadine, fexofenadine, and acrivastine. All except acrivastine are available alone, and some are marketed in combination with the decongestant pseudoephedrine. At the time of this writing, cetirizine, loratadine, and fexofenadine are available OTC. The second-generation antihistamines do not have the anticholinergic effects of the first-generation agents. Based on current literature, no single H_1 antihistamine (first or second generation) is clearly superior in efficacy; however, very few head-to-head comparative studies have been conducted. Individual variation is likely, and patients may need to try more than one product to realize optimal benefit. The oral second-generation antihistamines are effective for the sneezing, itching, and rhinorrhea of AR, but less effective for the nasal congestion. They also improve ocular symptoms. Intranasal antihistamines are better for nasal congestion.

Fexofenadine has virtually no sedative effects, even at doses higher than usually recommended. Loratadine and desloratadine are not sedative at recommended doses, but can be at higher doses. Cetirizine, levocetirizine, and acrivastine have some sedative effects, even at recommended doses.[1] All the oral second-generation agents require some dosage reduction with impaired renal function, although the specific recommendations vary with creatinine clearance.[29,32] To date, none of the currently available oral second-generation antihistamines have been reported to cause QT prolongation or torsade de pointes, as were associated with the two agents that have been removed from the U.S. market (terfenadine and astemizole).[19] Most of the oral second-generation antihistamines can be administered once daily (except for the lower dosage forms of fexofenadine). This probably improves adherence.

There are only two intranasal antihistamine products available in the U.S. market at the time of this writing. Both azelastine and olopatadine are considered second-generation agents, although they also have some mast cell stabilizing effects.[25] Both are available only by prescription. The most common side effect of these products is a bitter taste. This occurs in up to 20% of patients on azelastine and probably somewhat fewer on olopatadine.[1] Also, there is enough systemic absorption to cause sedation in some patients using azelastine (about 10%) and perhaps somewhat fewer on olopatadine.[1] There are no direct comparisons of the two agents, so definitive statements regarding their relative efficacy and side-effect incidence cannot be made. A recent manufacturer-sponsored supplement issue of an allergy journal had several articles that were favorable to the increased use of intranasal antihistamines.[33-35] However, until these changes are supported more universally, they are considered preliminary. See Table 63–7 for the single-agent second-generation antihistamine products.

❽ *Many patients with mild-to-moderate AR are adequately treated with an oral OTC first- or (preferably) second-generation antihistamine alone.* Others may prefer the intranasal administration of an antihistamine, but they require a prescription. Some patients will need or prefer combination therapy. If nasal congestion is not relieved by the above regimens, addition of a decongestant is reasonable, either alone or as a combination product (see Decongestant section that follows). Perhaps even the combination of an oral with an intranasal antihistamine is reasonable for some patients, depending on their preferences. Other pharmacologic agents can be combined with oral and/or intranasal antihistamines, as necessary for optimal control of symptoms (see later).

▶ *Adjunctive or Secondary Choice Agents*

Decongestants Decongestant drugs are useful to relieve the nasal congestion component of AR.[1-3,10,19] This is due to their α_1 adrenergic agonist activity, which results in constriction of the vasculature in the nasal mucosa. They do not prevent release of any of the mediators involved in AR. Thus they do not provide any benefit for the sneezing, itching, rhinorrhea, or the ocular manifestations. Decongestants

Table 63–7

Single-Agent Second-Generation Antihistamine Products (Oral and Intranasal)

Oral

Generic (Brand) Name	Formulation	Usual Adult Dosage	Usual Pediatric Dosage
Cetirizine[a,b] (Zyrtec, generic)	5, 10 mg tabs/chew tabs; 5 mg/mL syrup	5–10 mg once daily	6–11 mo; 2.5 mg once daily
			12–23 mo; 2.5 mg once or twice daily
			2–5 yo; 2.5–5 mg once daily or 2.5 mg twice daily
Desloratadine[b] (Clarinex)	5 mg tabs; 0.5 mg/mL syrup 2.5, 5 mg orally disintegrating tabs	5 mg once daily	6–11 mo; 1 mg once daily 1–5 yo; 1.25 mg once daily 6–11 yo; 2.5 mg once daily
Fexofenadine[a,b] (Allegra, generic)	30, 60, 180 mg tabs, 6 mg/mL suspension 30 mg orally disintegrating tabs	60 mg twice daily or 180 mg once daily	2–11 yo; 30 mg twice daily
Levocetirizine (Xyzal)	5 mg tabs 0.5 mg/mL solution	5 mg once daily	6 mo–5 yo; 1.25 mg once daily 6–11 yo; 2.5 mg once daily
Loratadine[a,b] (Claritin; Alavert, generic)	10 mg tabs; 10 mg gel cap; 1 mg/mL syrup/susp; 10 mg disintegrating tabs; 5 mg chewable tab	10 mg once daily	2–5 yo; 5 mg once daily

Intranasal Spray

Generic (Brand) Name	mcg/spray	Usual Adult Dosage (each nostril)	Usual Pediatric Dosage (each nostril)
Azelastine (Astelin, Astepro)	137	1–2 sprays twice daily	5–11 yo; 1 spray twice daily
Olopatadine (Patanase)	665	2 sprays twice daily	6–11 yo: 1 spray twice daily

Note: acrivastine is available only with pseudoephedrine and so is not included in this table.

mo, months old; yo, years old.

[a]Available OTC.

[b]Available in combination with pseudoephedrine (consult labeling for pediatric dosage).

From Refs. 1, 25–27, and 29.

Patient Encounter 1, Part 3

LF definitely denies all use of medications in an attempt to treat this episode, including OTC meds, alternative measures like herbals, and specifically any type of nose drops or spray. She notices no association of these current symptoms with fever, meals, or menstruation. She has had a diagnosis of essential hypertension for the last 6 years. Her previous PCP (where she lived before her recent move) told her that her blood pressure was "well controlled" on her current medication regimen. She does not remember the numbers of her BP readings. Her current medication is a single combination tablet that she takes regularly once daily. She says it contains a water pill and an "ace" drug. You confirm this from the prescription bottle she has in her purse, which indicates Prinzide 20/12.5 (lisinopril/hydrochlorothiazide). She admits that she is not the best housekeeper and that she has seen a few cockroaches in her kitchen.

What additional information is needed before a recommendation could be made?

can be given alone, either by the oral or by the intranasal route. Also, numerous combination products, consisting of a decongestant with an antihistamine (and sometimes other ingredients), are available as oral medications. There are some special considerations for use of decongestants in pediatric and pregnant patients (see the Special Populations section later).

Oral decongestant products are currently limited to pseudoephedrine and phenylephrine (phenylpropanolamine was removed from the market in 2000).[10] Pseudoephedrine has been changed from truly OTC to a more controlled status because it is an ingredient in the illicit manufacture of methamphetamine. The new, so-called behind-the-counter (BTC) status, established by the federal Combat Methamphetamine Act of 2005, requires: special storage; photo identification of purchasers; a log book of sales, which must be signed by purchasers; and specific limitations on daily and monthly quantities.[36,37] Subsequent to this change in status of pseudoephedrine, some manufacturers changed the ingredients of their products by replacing pseudoephedrine with phenylephrine. This was probably to maintain shelf presence in the OTC sales area. However, much controversy surrounds the efficacy of oral phenylephrine. At the time of this writing, the clinical literature suggests that the currently recommended adult dose is minimally effective as a nasal decongestant.[38-40]

The side effects of orally administered decongestants most often affect cardiovascular function or the CNS. The side effects are primarily due to sympathetic stimulation and are usually dose-related. Some elevation of blood pressure may occur, but in normotensive and well-controlled hypertensive patients, the elevation is usually small. It is not of clinical significance in most situations, especially considering that these drugs are most appropriately used only briefly or intermittently. Insomnia, nervousness, irritability, and anxiety are relatively common CNS side effects. Some patients may have decreased appetite, tremors, headache, and even hallucinations. Men with benign prostatic hyperplasia (BPH) and other patients with disorders causing bladder outlet obstruction may have increased urinary retention due to α_1 stimulation of the urethral sphincter. Theoretically, there may be some differences in the overall side effects between pseudoephedrine and phenylephrine. Pseudoephedrine stimulates both α and β receptors, whereas the effects of recommended oral doses of phenylephrine are essentially limited to stimulation of α receptors. Comparative studies are not available to confirm meaningful differences in the clinical setting.

The intranasal agents currently available include the OTC products phenylephrine, oxymetazoline, and naphazoline, and the prescription product tetrahydrozoline. Product labeling should be followed for dosage, but it is noteworthy that oxymetazoline is the longest acting of these agents and is usually given only twice daily. Intranasal application of decongestants provides rapid and effective relief of nasal congestion. This therapy may provide relief for nasal congestion, even for those patients already on intranasal corticosteroids.[41] However, the continuous use of intranasal decongestants often causes a paradoxical rebound phenomenon of persistent nasal congestion, called *rhinitis medicamentosa*.[1-3,10,42] ❾ *Although some patients do not develop rhinitis medicamentosa even after several weeks of continuous use of intranasal decongestants, the usual recommendation is to use them for no more than 3 consecutive days.*[1] Intranasal decongestants can cause local side effects, including stinging, burning, dryness, and even sneezing. These are usually mild and well tolerated. Due to very limited absorption, the intranasal route rarely causes systemic side effects.[1,8,10] Administration technique should be optimized as described in Table 63–6. Should rhinitis medicamentosa occur, the best management is first to discontinue the decongestant, possibly with a taper to minimize worsening the situation. However, the response to withdrawal is often delayed for days. Therefore, it may be necessary to start intranasal corticosteroids and/or (especially if intranasal corticosteroids are already part of the patient's regimen) begin a short course of oral corticosteroid.[42]

Despite the usual good tolerance of recommended doses of oral decongestants, caution is warranted when they are used in patients with cardiac disease (dysrhythmias, angina pectoris, heart failure), hypertension, cerebrovascular disease, bladder outlet obstruction (including BPH), glaucoma (especially closed angle), hyperthyroidism, and possibly diabetes.[1,10,19] ❾ *The best application of decongestants in AR is short-term to overcome severe nasal congestion, especially to facilitate improved efficacy of (other) intranasal agents (e.g., corticosteroids and antihistamines).* The choice between the two routes of administration is based on several considerations, including cost, convenience, patient preference, speed of onset (within 30 minutes orally, within 5 to 10 minutes intranasally), and side effects.[1,8,43]

Mast Cell Stabilizer/Cromone[1,10,22,23,43] Cromolyn is the only agent in the cromone class that is approved in the United States for treatment of AR. It is available as an OTC intranasal product. The mechanism of action in AR is mast cell stabilization. The drug binds to mast cells and prevents release of the mediators of AR that would otherwise result from allergen exposure. The drug is moderately effective, but less so than both intranasal corticosteroids and oral or intranasal antihistamines. It does have effects on both early and late phases of AR. Its effects begin within 4 to 7 days of use, but may not be maximal for up to 2 weeks.[1] However, it can be used effectively on an as needed basis for episodic exposures to allergen.[1] As with all intranasal products, if there is severe nasal congestion, contact with the nasal mucosa will be limited. Short-term use of a decongestant or an intranasal antihistamine may solve this problem. Cromolyn is very well-tolerated. The most common side effects are mild local stinging and/or burning, sneezing, unpleasant taste, and possibly nose bleed. A disadvantage is the frequency of administration. At least initially, it should be used four times daily. Some patients may need only two or three daily doses when used continuously after the first few weeks at four times daily. It is most useful for patients with mild or intermittent symptoms, especially in the pediatric population and in pregnant women.

Leukotriene Receptor Antagonist Leukotrienes are involved in the pathophysiology of AR and in particular contribute to the nasal congestion in the late phase.[1] They contribute little if anything to nasal itch and sneezing.[43] Leukotriene antagonists have been shown to be effective for some of the manifestations of AR. Montelukast is the only agent in this class with FDA approval for treatment of AR. It is marketed as oral granules and as both chewable and swallow tablets. The majority of clinical studies published to date indicate that montelukast is inferior to intranasal corticosteroids.[1,10,19,43] Montelukast is either equivalent or slightly inferior to oral H_1 antihistamines.[1,10,25,43] The combination of montelukast with an oral antihistamine shows improved efficacy over either agent alone.[19] However, even the combination is probably not better than intranasal corticosteroids.[1] The onset of action of montelukast is delayed for a day or more.[1] The drug is usually considered to be very well-tolerated with minimal side effects. However, the FDA updated their preliminary report concerning case reports of neuropsychiatric events, including suicidal ideation in association with the drug.[44] It is administered once daily, considered safe (FDA Pregnancy Category B and indicated for children as young as 6 months of age), and particularly well-suited to those patients who have concurrent asthma and AR.

Antimuscarinic (Anticholinergic) Agent[1] Ipratropium is currently the only antimuscarinic (or anticholinergic) agent indicated for treatment of AR. It is a quaternary ammonium structure, so systemic absorption is minimal. The product is available by prescription as an intranasal spray. Its use is limited to those patients whose rhinorrhea has not been controlled by other therapy (antihistamines and/or intranasal corticosteroids). There are two strengths available. The 0.03% product is approved for AR in children as young as 6 years of age. The 0.06% product is indicated for rhinorrhea associated with the common cold in children as young as 5 years old. Local side effects are essentially limited to mild epistaxis and nasal dryness.

- **Saline**[1,45,46] Nasal administration of saline is an alternative for treatment of AR. This therapy may benefit any patient with AR. Saline may be administered as drops or a spray, but the irrigation mode of administration is popularly known by several terms, including neti pot, nasal wash, nasal douche, nose bidet, and as nasal irrigation. Although less effective than intranasal corticosteroids, it has been shown to improve sneezing and nasal congestion. It can be used either alone or as add-on therapy. It is best to use canning or pickling salt, which has no iodine, preservatives, or other additives, all of which can be irritating. It appears that isotonic saline is as effective as hypertonic solutions.

An approximate isotonic concentration can be made by dissolution of one teaspoonful of noniodized salt (sodium chloride) in one pint of water. The AAAAI has another recipe.[41] Their instructions start with preparation of the dry powder component. This is done by combining three heaping teaspoonfuls of pickling salt with one rounded teaspoonful of baking soda, and mixing thoroughly. Then, one teaspoonful of the dry powder mixture is dissolved in one cup (8 oz; 237 mL) of lukewarm water. It is best if the water is distilled or has been boiled. About 4 oz (118 mL) of this solution will be used to irrigate each side of the nose. Application can be accomplished while the patient is in the shower or leaning over a sink. The head is bent forward and downward, then tilted to the side opposite the treated nostril. That is, the head is tilted to the left if the right nostril will be irrigated. Then, with a bulb syringe or similar device, slowly introduce about 4 oz (118 mL) of the warm saline solution into one side. Soon, the solution will run out of the opposite nostril. The position of the head should be adjusted as necessary to avoid the solution running into the ears or down the throat.

Nasal irrigation is one delivery method, although the optimal method (spray, drops, nebulizer, or irrigation) is not known. Optimal frequency of administration is also not known. Nasal irrigation is usually given twice daily, but use of smaller volumes as spray products may be given up to four times daily. Local side effects are usually limited to minor nasal irritation. Nausea has been reported.

Omalizumab[1,23,43] Omalizumab is a monoclonal antibody that binds to IgE. The product is approved for asthma, but not for AR. It is administered by subcutaneous injection. Dosage is determined by the patient's circulating IgE levels. The cost is high compared with that of other commonly used

---

Patient Encounter 1, Part 4

Even more questioning reveals that LF has no recent fever, facial pain, purulent nasal discharge, ear pain, or nose bleeds. She has never noticed a whistling sound to her breathing (wheezing), persistent or recurring nighttime cough, tightness in her chest, or shortness of breath. She has never been told she has polyps in her nose. She has heard about "allergy shots" but has no interest in getting them at this time. She has never been told that she has any specific allergies. She never took any medicine that caused skin rash, trouble breathing, or other bothersome symptoms. No foods have caused these types of reactions. No healthcare provider has ever told her to specifically avoid any medication. However, she does presume that she is allergic to some sort of pollen, based on her symptoms. She claims that her menstrual periods are regular and, in fact, her most recent period ended only 3 days ago.

Based on all the accumulated information, develop a comprehensive pharmaceutical care plan for this patient, including specific OTC medication recommendations.

---

modes of therapy for both asthma and AR. Investigational use has demonstrated efficacy in AR, although relative efficacy compared with other modes of therapy for AR is unknown. Its use is best limited to those with concurrent asthma and AR, pending specific approval for AR.

Complementary and Alternative Medicine Therapy Although some would consider saline in the category of complementary and alternative agents, this monograph considers it as an adjunctive mode. Complementary and alternative therapy for AR has been reviewed.[47] Consistent evidence for efficacy has not been established, and there are some safety concerns.

▶ Special Populations

- **Children** ⑩ *Generally speaking, the treatment of AR in children is the same as it is for adults. There are, however, limitations in terms of FDA-approved products for different age groups. Also, depending on the age of the patient, there may be administration issues with some products.* Most children affected by AR are more than 2 years old, although the disease may begin in children as young as 6 months of age.[1]

There has been concern about use of combination cough and cold products (many contain an antihistamine and a decongestant) in children. In October 2007, the Nonprescription Drug Advisory Committee of the FDA recommended that OTC combination cough and cold products be limited to children 6 years of age and older. This was based on reports of more than 100 deaths in association with these combination products.[1] Most of these bad outcomes seem to have resulted from inadvertent overdosage, often by giving doses of the same medication from different combination products.

In October 2008, the FDA notified consumers and healthcare providers that the Consumer Health Protection Agency (CHPA) decided to voluntarily modify the labeling of combination cough and cold products to indicate that they should not be used in children less than 4 years old. This recommendation has been published online as a reminder to consumers, including a link to a question and answer page.[48]

First-generation H_1 antihistamines are discouraged for children as they are for adults, due to the possible detrimental effects on school performance and learning. Second-generation (less sedating) H_1 antihistamines (primarily for mild or intermittent symptoms) or intranasal corticosteroids (for moderate–severe or persistent manifestations) are first-line modes of therapy. Antihistamines may need to be used even for more severe and/or persistent symptoms in those children who have difficulty with use of intranasal products. If necessary, these two classes can be combined.

See Table 63–7 for dosages of second-generation antihistamines by age groups for which they are indicated. If first-generation antihistamines are used, the healthcare practitioner should guarantee that the family members or caregivers are carefully and thoroughly educated to read and use the dosage recommendations appropriate for age or weight of the patient, as indicated on the product labeling. They should also be warned about the possibility of a paradoxical CNS stimulant side effect. Special care should be given to avoid administration of the same medication from different (especially combination) products. The most common side effects of second-generation antihistamines in children are similar to those for adults.

See Table 63–5 for dosages of intranasal corticosteroids by age groups for which they are indicated. The consensus of opinion about intranasal corticosteroids and systemic side effects, especially delay in growth, is that most products are safe. The greatest potential for problems may exist with beclomethasone.[1] Several products have been studied in children and have not been shown to delay growth. However, not every product has been studied carefully in all age groups. Some of the conclusions about safety are extrapolated from data with inhaled corticosteroids, used for asthma. The local side effects of intranasal corticosteroids are the same in children as for adults.

Other therapy options may be worth consideration for some pediatric patients. Montelukast provides an oral alternative, especially for those who are too young to cooperate with intranasal administration of corticosteroids. It may be used in combination with an oral antihistamine in hopes of providing some additional efficacy. Another advantage of montelukast is that it is indicated for children as young as 6 months. Another option for mild or intermittent symptoms is intranasal cromolyn, primarily due to its excellent safety. This OTC product is labeled for use in children 2 years of age and older. Intranasal ipratropium is indicated for patients 6 years of age or older and may benefit unresponsive rhinorrhea.

Pregnant Women[1,49] Women who have AR may suffer an exacerbation of symptoms during pregnancy. However, only minor changes in the routine approach to therapy are necessary as a result of the pregnancy. Second-generation antihistamines are generally considered safe, based on an increasing number of studies and experience.[1] The same generalization applies to intranasal corticosteroids. However, the products with the best documented safety record are beclomethasone, budesonide, and fluticasone propionate.[1] If an intranasal product is started during pregnancy, the wisest choice might be to use budesonide, based on the fact that it is FDA Pregnancy Category of B. Cromolyn is also FDA Pregnancy Category B and is considered safe. The disadvantages, however, are frequent administration and lesser efficacy than antihistamines and intranasal corticosteroids. Montelukast is also FDA Pregnancy Category B, but some recommend it be used primarily in those with concurrent asthma or in those who have demonstrated a good response prior to pregnancy.[1] Ipratropium is FDA Pregnancy Category B, despite limited data.[44] The decongestants are not considered safe, especially in the first trimester. The theoretical concern is the possibility of vasoconstriction of very small caliber fetal vasculature. If nasal congestion is severe enough to warrant consideration for a decongestant, the intranasal route of administration is preferable, due to decreased systemic exposure and the short-term duration of therapy.[1]

Elderly[1,8] Elderly patients can be treated for AR according to the approach for (younger) adults.[1,8] However, the elderly may be more sensitive to the sedative and antimuscarinic effects of antihistamines and to the cardiovascular and CNS stimulant effects of decongestants. Also, the aging process can affect the manifestations of AR. Generalized atrophy of nasal tissues can result in more nasal congestion. An increase in cholinergic activity may result in more rhinorrhea.

Athletes[1] The use of certain medications is prohibited during national and international athletic competition. The list of prohibited drugs changes each year and may not always be consistent among organizations. The most up-to-date information is available from the World Anti-Doping Agency (WADA).[50] Additional information may be obtained from the United States Anti-Doping Agency (USADA) (http://www.usantidoping.org/). This site has a link to the prohibited drugs in the form of the Global Drug Reference Online (DRO).

▶ *Ocular Symptoms*[1,25,29]

Several products are available for instillation directly into the eyes for those patients with predominant or unresponsive ocular manifestations. They may be appropriate for occasional moderate–severe flares or episodic AR when other modes of therapy are not optimally effective. The combination (antihistamine and mast cell stabilizing) agents may be the most effective, and they have the advantages of rapid onset of action and (usually) only twice daily administration. See Table 63–8 for these products.

Summary of Treatment

Once an agent appropriate for initial therapy is chosen, ongoing management requires repeated checks to ascertain

Table 63–8				
Intraocular Medications				
Category	Generic (Brand) Name	Formulation	Frequency	Age
Decongestant/vasoconstrictor	Naphazoline[a] (Naphcon, Privine, others)	0.012% + 0.025%	Four times daily	Adult
Decongestant/vasoconstrictor + antihistamine	Naphazoline + pheniramine[a] (Visine A)	0.025%/0.3%	Four times daily	6 yo or more
Antihistamine	Emedastine (Emadine)	0.05%	Four times daily	3 yo or more
	Alcaftadine (Lastacaft)	0.25%	Once daily	2 yo or more
Mast cell stabilizer	Cromolyn (generic)	4%	Every 4–6 hours	4 yo or more
	Lodoxamide (Alomide)	0.1%	Four times daily	2 yo or more
	Nedocromil (Alocril)	2%	Twice daily	3 yo or more
	Pemirolast (Alamast)	0.1%	Four times daily	3 yo or more
Antihistamine + mast cell stabilizer	Azelastine (Optivar)	0.05%	Twice daily	3 yo or more
	Epinastine (Elestat)	0.05%	Twice daily	3 yo or more
	Ketotifen[a] (Zaditor, Alaway, Claritin, Zyrtec, generic)	0.025%	Every 8–12 hours	3 yo or more
	Olopatadine (Patanol/Pataday)	0.1%/0.2%	Twice daily/once daily	3 yo or more
	Bepotastine (Bepreve)	1.5%	Twice daily	2 yo or more
NSAIDs	Ketorolac (Acular)	0.5%	Four times daily	3 yo or more
Corticosteroid	Loteprednol (Alrex)	0.2%	Four times daily	Adult

NSAID, nonsteroidal anti-inflammatory drug; yo, years old.

[a]Available OTC.

From Refs. 1, 25, 26, and 29.

Patient Encounter 2, Part 1

LW is a 60-year-old male who comes to your place of work to ask for your help. His main questions concern how to use the medications he has been given for what he calls "bad nose allergies." He says he has three different nose sprays, three different oral meds, and one bottle of eye drops. You recognize him as a regular customer. His computerized pharmacy record indicates the following information. His chronic problems are Parkinson's disease, hypertension, BPH, and moderately severe, persistent allergic rhinitis. His current medications are ropinirole (Requip) 4 mg three times a day; amantadine 100 mg three times a day; trihexyphenidyl 5 mg three times a day; Lotensin HCT 20/25 (benazepril/hydrochlorothiazide) one tablet once daily; tamsulosin 0.4 mg two tablets once daily; flunisolide nasal spray given as 2 sprays in each nostril twice daily; olopatadine nasal spray given as two sprays in each nostril twice daily; tetrahydrozoline 0.1% nasal spray given as 1 spray into each nostril, up to 3 times a day as needed for congestion, but not to exceed 3 consecutive days use; levocetirizine 5 mg once a day; diphenhydramine 25 mg tablets (OTC), pseudoephedrine 30 mg tablets (OTC), and ketotifen eye drops (OTC).

What medication-related problems does this patient's regimen present?

Explain how you would deal with his primary question about how to use his AR medications?

response and freedom from intolerable or adherence limiting side effects. Either "step-up" or "step-down" therapy may be appropriate, depending on the individual patient's response. See Table 63–9 for a summary of the approach to treatment of AR. Table 63–10 attempts to rank the relative effectiveness of the classes of agents for treatment of AR by specific symptoms.

OUTCOME EVALUATION

- Confirm the understanding of the disorder on the part of the patient and their family (see Clinical Presentation and Diagnosis).
- Confirm the understanding about allergen avoidance measures on the part of the patient and their family (see Table 63–3).
- Assess the patient's symptom response, tolerance, and adherence at each visit.
- Assess the patient's administration technique with intranasal products, especially when symptom response or tolerance is not optimal.
- Use or recommend second-generation oral antihistamine therapy for most patients with mild or intermittent (especially seasonal) symptoms (see Clinical Presentation and Diagnosis and Table 63–9).
- Recommend intranasal corticosteroid therapy for moderate–severe or persistent (especially perennial) symptoms. Advise additional adjunctive therapy for those

---

Table 63–9

Routine Approach to Therapy of AR

All patients should practice avoidance of identified allergens to the extent possible

Mild intermittent (including many patients with what some would call seasonal AR)
   First line:
      Oral antihistamine (OTC, initially; preferably second generation)
   Adjunctive/secondary (may use more than one):
      Add OTC oral decongestant for nasal congestion
      Add short-term OTC intranasal decongestant for refractory nasal congestion
      Add nasal saline (e.g., as irrigation)
      Consider intraocular medications, as needed (See Table 63–8)
      Consider prescription therapy for inadequate response (see below)
   Possibly consider referral for immunotherapy

Persistent or moderate–severe
   First line:
      Intranasal corticosteroid
      Add oral antihistamine for possible additional benefit if necessary
   Adjunctive/secondary (may use more than one):
      Add short-term intranasal decongestant for refractory nasal congestion
      Add nasal saline (e.g., as irrigation)
      Add ipratropium for inadequately controlled rhinorrhea
      Consider replacement of one first-line agent, if poorly tolerated, with montelukast
      Consider intraocular medications, as needed (See Table 63–8)
   Consider referral for immunotherapy

Episodic (no order of preference intended)
   Intranasal cromolyn (OTC)
   Intranasal antihistamine
   Intranasal corticosteroid

Special situations (children, pregnant women, elderly, athletes, ocular symptoms)
   See Special Populations section of text

From Refs. 1–3, 8, 10, 20–22, 24, 25, and 43.

Table 63–10

Relative Efficacy (Semiquantitative) by Classes of Agents for Specific Symptoms of Allergic Rhinitis

Drug Class	Nasal Congestion	Sneezing	Rhinorrhea	Nasal Itch	Ocular Symptoms
Nasal corticosteroids	3	3	3	3	2
Oral antihistamines[a]	1	2	2	3	2
Nasal antihistamines	2	2	2	3	0
Oral decongestants[a]	1½	0	0	0	0
Nasal decongestants[a,b]	3	0	0	0	0
Oral leukotriene antagonist	2	½	2	½	2
Nasal mast cell stabilizer[a]	1½	1½	1½	1½	1½
Nasal antimuscarinic	0	0	2	0	0

Note: The information in this table is a composite from numerous sources. There are different opinions about some of the rankings, partly due to inadequate study. Individual variation may create different relative efficacy in some patients. Higher number equals greater activity.

[a]Some products in these classes are available OTC.

[b]Nasal decongestants are best used for severe, unresponsive nasal congestion, or to facilitate mucosal contact of other intranasal medications, but in either case, should usually be limited to no more than 3 days.

From Refs. 1, 8, 10, and 21–23.

---

with less than optimal control (see Clinical Presentation and Diagnosis and Table 63–9).

- Consider step-up therapy for exacerbations or less than optimal response.

- Consider step-down therapy if symptoms have been minimal or stable for several months (especially if the disorder is primarily seasonal).

- Consider referral to rule out nonallergic causes of rhinitis in nonresponding patients or those with an atypical presentation (see Clinical Presentation and Diagnosis).

- Consider referral for patients who request immunotherapy.

- Consider referral for patients with comorbid conditions, especially asthma.

Patient Encounter 3, Part 1

You are at your place of work at a community pharmacy, and you receive a phone call from a medical student who is doing a rotation with a pediatrician in the neighborhood. The pediatrician advised the medical student to phone your pharmacy to ask about the use of OTC "cold medicines" in children. The student indicates that this question involves a real patient situation. The mother of a 4-year-old girl brought the child in for evaluation and advice. The child has been having sneezing, runny nose, poor appetite, and fussiness. The symptoms are present most days of every week and have been present for at least 2 months. The child is particularly fussy and "not herself" today. The student describes the child as having dark circles under her eyes and a horizontal crease about half-way up from the tip of her nose. She sniffles and rubs her nose frequently. She is a bit irritable and not always cooperative with the interview and exam. The child weighs 35 pounds (15.9 kg).

The student emphasizes that the pediatrician's evaluation has ruled out infectious causes and serious chronic disease. He thinks the child has allergic rhinitis. The mother has been giving two medications for the last week. One is called Allerfrim syrup (pseudoephedrine 30mg/5 mL and triprolidine 1.25 mg/5 mL). The other is Bromfed DM syrup (brompheniramine 2 mg/5 mL, pseudoephedrine 30 mg/5 mL, and dextromethorphan 10 mg/5 mL). She has been using ½ teaspoonful of both medicines 3–4 times daily for the last 4 days. At first, they seemed to help the girl's symptoms, but in the last day, she seems worse in some ways.

What can you tell this person about use of "cold" medicines in children?

What advice can you provide about medications that are appropriate for use to treat AR in a child of this age?

Patient Care and Monitoring

1. Determine the patient's manifestations. This is best done as a chief complaint would be evaluated: location (including referral or location of other symptoms); onset (current and past episodes); quality (the exact nature of the symptom); quantity (the severity of the symptom); setting/context (circumstances in which symptom occurs); associated symptoms (other abnormalities during primary symptom); modifying factors (what makes the symptom worse or better). This can be followed by selected questions about past medical history, allergies or intolerances (to anything, not just medicines), and current medication (OTC, prescription and herbal). Some of the most important specific questions follow.

   - What is the most troublesome symptom?
   - What is the frequency and severity of symptoms?
   - How do symptoms affect quality of life, work/school performance, and sleep?
   - What allergen or irritant triggers have been identified?

2. Attempt to rule out complications or comorbid conditions that preclude self-care (asthma, sinusitis, otitis media with effusion, and possibly nasal polyposis) and/or warrant referral to a physician, as follows:

   - Unilateral rhinitis, nasal obstruction without other typical symptoms of AR
   - Purulent rhinitis, fever, marked facial or ear pain, or recurrent nose bleeds
   - Ocular symptoms without typical symptoms of AR

   - Unilateral ocular symptoms, or photophobia, or vision changes
   - Severe symptoms
   - Failure of therapy (nonresponse or adherence limiting side effects or intolerance)
   - Desire to have specific allergen triggers identified (e.g., by skin testing)
   - Candidates for immunotherapy
   - Concurrent asthma, nasal polyposis, sinusitis, or otitis media with effusion

3. Determine past attempts at therapy. There is some overlap in this section, with 1., above (modifying factors).

   - What has the patient tried previously for these symptoms (including prescription and all nonprescription [OTC, herbal, other complementary] forms)?
   - What was the response to all previous treatments (efficacy and side effects)?

4. Determine other current disorders and treatments:

   - What conditions are present for which medications are taken regularly?
   - What medications are currently being taken regularly?

5. Assess patient's understanding of AR and its management:

   - What does the patient currently do to avoid triggers?
   - How does/did the patient administer and adhere to current or past treatments?

(Continued)

Patient Care and Monitoring (*Continued*)

6. Fill in gaps in patient's knowledge:

- Manifestations of AR and its complications

- Principles of management (allergen/trigger avoidance, pharmacologic modes, immunotherapy)

- Choices for pharmacologic therapy (OTC and prescription) and determinates (previous experience, ease of use, tolerability, cost, patient preference, and age)

- Discuss realistic goals, which may not be complete elimination of all symptoms

7. Establish a plan appropriate for and with input from the patient:

- Recommend initial OTC regimen or refer for evaluation and possible prescription therapy

- Fill in gaps in patient's knowledge about allergen avoidance and optimal adherence and administration technique (where applicable)

8. Reevaluate the patient at appropriate intervals, that will vary with the individual, but will usually be every 1 to 3 months:

- Evaluate for efficacy of therapy, including improvement in symptoms, quality of life, work/school performance and sleep pattern

- Evaluate for tolerance of side effects

- Modify the plan as needed (to increase efficacy or modify side effects), including recommendations for a change in medication and/or referral to a physician

Abbreviations

AAAAI	American Academy of Allergy, Asthma and Immunology
ACAAI	American College of Allergy, Asthma and Immunology
ACEI	Angiotensin-converting enzyme inhibitor
AERD	Aspirin-exacerbated respiratory disease
AR	Allergic rhinitis
ARIA	Allergic Rhinitis and its Impact on Asthma
BPH	Benign prostatic hyperplasia/hypertrophy
BTC	Behind-the-counter
CHPA	Consumer Health Protection Agency
H_1	Histamine type 1 (receptor)
HEPA	High-efficiency particulate air (filter)
HPA	Hypothalamic–pituitary–adrenal (axis)
HT	(essential or primary) hypertension
IAR	Intermittent allergic rhinitis (ARIA system)
IgE	Immunoglobulin E
LTRA	Leukotriene receptor antagonist
NARES	Nonallergic rhinitis with eosinophilia [on nasal smear] syndrome
NSAID	Nonsteroidal anti-inflammatory drug
OTC	Over-the-counter
PAR	Perennial allergic rhinitis (AAAAI/ACAAI system)
PDE-5	Phosphodiesterase (isoenzyme)-5
PER	Persistent allergic rhinitis (ARIA system)
QT	Interval between the Q and T waves in an ECG
SAR	Seasonal allergic rhinitis (AAAAI/ACAAI system)
USADA	United States Anti-Doping Agency
WADA	World Anti-Doping Agency

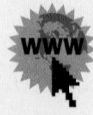 Self-assessment questions and answers are available at *http://mhpharmacotherapy.com/pp.html*.

REFERENCES

1. Wallace DV, Dykewicz MS, Bernstein DI, et al. The diagnosis and management of rhinitis: An updated practice parameter. J Allergy Clin Immunol 2008;122(2):S1–S84.

2. Bousquet J, Khaltaev N, Cruzz AA, et al. Allergic rhinitis and its impact on asthma (ARIA) 2008 update. Allergy 2008;63(Suppl 86):S8–S160.

3. Scadding GK, Durham SR, Mirakian R, et al. BSACI guidelines for the management of allergic and nonallergic rhinitis. Clin Exp Allergy 2008;38:19–42.

4. Nathan RA. The burden of allergic rhinitis. Allergy Asthma Proc 2007;28(1):3–9.

5. Broide DH. The pathophysiology of allergic rhinoconjunctivitis. Allergy Asthma Proc 2007;28(4):398–403.

6. Blaiss MS. Allergic rhinoconjunctivitis: Burden of disease. Allergy Asthma Proc 2007;28:393–397.

7. Fletcher RH. An overview of rhinitis. In: Basow DS, ed. UpToDate. Waltham, MA: UpToDate, 2011.

8. Hur SY. Allergic rhinitis. The Rx Consultant 2007;16(3):1–8.

9. Carr WW. Pediatric allergic rhinitis: Current and future state of the art. Allergy Asthma Proc 2008;29(1):14–23.

10. de Bittner MR, Sulli MM, Williams DM. The role of nonprescription antihistamines in the treatment of allergic rhinitis [continuing education monograph on the Internet]. Washington, DC: American Pharmacists Association, 2008.

11. Rosenwasser L. New insights into the pathophysiology of allergic rhinitis. Allergy Asthma Proc 2007;28(1):10–15.

12. deShazo RD, Kemp SF. Pathogenesis of allergic rhinitis (rhinosinusitis). In: Basow DS, ed. UpToDate. Waltham, MA: UpToDate, 2010.

13. Creticos PS. Oral and sublingual immunotherapy for allergic rhinitis. In: Basow DS, ed. UpToDate. Waltham, MA: UpToDate, 2011.

14. Calderon MA, Alves B, Jacobson M, et al. Allergen injection immunotherapy for seasonal allergic rhinitis [review]. 2009 [cited 2012 Feb 6]. In: The Cochrane Collaboration [Internet]. Hoboken, NJ: John Wiley & Sons. Available from: *http://onlinelibrary.wiley.com/doi/10.1002/14651858.CD001936.pub2/pdf*

15. Cox L, Nelson H, Lockey R. Allergen immunotherapy: A practice parameter third update. J Allergy Clin Immunol 2011;127(1 Suppl 1):S1–S55.

16. Radulovic S, Calderon MA, Wilson D, et al. Sublingual immunotherapy for allergic rhinitis [review]. 2011 [cited 2012 Feb 6]. In: The Cochrane Collaboration [Internet]. Hoboken, NJ: John Wiley & Sons. Available from: *http://onlinelibrary.wiley.com/doi/10.1002/14651858.CD002893.pub2/pdf*

17. Leatherman BD, Owen S, Parker M, et al. Sublingual immunotherapy: Past, present, paradigm for the future? Otolaryngol Head Neck Surg 2007;136:S1–S20.

18. Costa DJ, Amouyal M, Lambert P, et al. How representative are clinical study patients with allergic rhinitis in primary care? J Allergy Clin Immunol 2011;127(4):920–926.

19. deShazo RD, Kemp SF. Pharmacotherapy of allergic rhinitis. In: Basow DS, ed. UpToDate. Waltham, MA: UpToDate, 2011.

20. Carr WW, Nelson MR, Hadley JA. Managing rhinitis: Strategies for improved patient outcomes. Allergy Asthma Proc 2008;29(4): 349–357.

21. Lanier B. Allergic rhinitis: Selective comparisons of the pharmaceutical options for management. Allergy Asthma Proc 2007;28(1): 16–19.

22. Krouse JH. Allergic rhinitis—current pharmacotherapy. Otolaryngol Clin North Am 2008;41:347–358.

23. Marple BF, Fornadley JA, Patel AA, et al. Keys to successful management of patients with allergic rhinitis: Focus on patient confidence, compliance, and satisfaction. Otolaryngol Head Neck Surg 2007;136:S107–S124.

24. Plaut M, Valentine MD. Allergic rhinitis. N Engl J Med 2005;353(18): 1934–1944.

25. Drugs for allergic disorders. Treat Guidel Med Lett 2010;8(90):9–18.

26. U.S. Department of Health & Human Services. U.S. Food and Drug Administration. Drugs@FDA. FDA Approved Drug Products. [cited 2012 Feb 6]. Available from: *http://www.accessdata.fda.gov/scripts/cder/drugsatfda/*

27. Fluticasone furoate (Veramyst) for allergic rhinitis. Med Lett Drugs Ther 2007;49(1273):90–92.

28. Olopatadine (Patanase) nasal spray for allergic rhinitis. Med Lett Drugs Ther 2007;50(1289):51.

29. Lacy CF, Armstrong LL, Goldman MP, et al., eds. Drug Information Handbook 2010–2011. 19th ed. Hudson, OH: LexiComp, 2010.

30. Kirtsreesakul V, Chansaksung P, Ruttanaphol S. Dose-related effect of intranasal corticosteroids on treatment outcome of persistent allergic rhinitis. Otolaryngol Head Neck Surg 2008;139(4):565–569.

31. Lieberman P. The basics of histamine biology. Ann Allergy Asthma Immunol 2011;106:S2–S5.

32. Aranoff GR, Bennett WM, Berns JS, et al. Drug Prescribing in Renal Failure: Dosing Guidelines for Adults and Children, 5th ed. Philadelphia, PA: American College of Physicians, 2007.

33. Kaliner MA, Berger WE, Ratner PH, Siegel CJ. The efficacy of intranasal antihistamines in the treatment of allergic rhinitis. Ann Allergy Asthma Immunol 2011;106:S6–S11.

34. Meltzer EO, Bukstein DA. The economic impact of allergic rhinitis and current guidelines for treatment. Ann Allergy Asthma Immunol 2011;106:S12–S16.

35. Katial RK, Meltzer EO, Lieberman P, et al. Suggested updated approaches to patient management. Guest editorial. Ann Allergy Asthma Immunol 2011;106:S17–S19.

36. American Pharmacists Association (APhA). DEA interim final regulation: ephedrine, pseudoephedrine, and phenylpropanolamine requirements. 2006 September [cited 2012 Feb 6]. Available from: *http://www.pswi.org/government/Pseudoephedrine093006.pdf*

37. U.S. Department of Justice. Drug Enforcement Administration. Office of Diversion Control. Combat Methamphetamine Epidemic Act 2005 (Title VII of Public Law 109–177). [cited 2012 Feb 6]. Available from: *http://www.deadiversion.usdoj.gov/meth/index.html*

38. Kollar C, Schneider H, Waksman J, et al. Meta-analysis of the efficacy of a single dose of phenylephrine 10 mg compared with placebo in adults with acute nasal congestion due to the common cold. Clin Therap 2007;29(6):1057–1070.

39. Hendeles L, Hatton RC. Oral phenylephrine: An ineffective replacement for pseudoephedrine? J Allergy Clin Immunol 2006;118(1):279–280.

40. Hatton RC, Winterstein AG, McKelvey RP, et al. Efficacy and safety of oral phenylephrine: Systematic review and meta-analysis. Ann Pharmacother 2007;41:381–390.

41. Barnes ML, Biallosterski BT, Gray RD, et al. Decongestant effects of nasal xylometazoline and mometasone furoate in persistent allergic rhinitis. Rhinology 2005;43(4):291–295.

42. Lockey RF. Rhinitis medicamentosa and the stuffy nose. J Allergy Clin Immunol 2006;118:1017–1018.

43. Greiner AN, Meltzer EO. Pharmacologic rationale for treating allergic and nonallergic rhinitis. J Allergy Clin Immunol 2006;118:985–996.

44. U.S. Department of Health & Human Services. U.S. Food and Drug Administration. Updated information on leukotriene inhibitors: montelukast (marketed as Singulair), zafirlukast (marketed as Accolate), and zileuton (marketed as Zyflo and Zyflo CR). 2009 Aug 28. Updated Information [updated 2010 Jan 5; cited 2012 Feb 6]. Available from: *http://www.fda.gov/Drugs/DrugSafety/ PostmarketDrugSafetyInformationforPatientsandProviders/DrugSafetyInformationforHeathcareProfessionals/ucm165489.htm*

45. Rabago D, Zgierska A. Saline nasal irrigation for upper respiratory conditions. Am Fam Physician 2009;80(10)1117-9, 1121-1.

46. American Academy of Allergy Asthma & Immunology. Saline sinus rinse recipe [cited 2012 Feb 6]. Available from: *http://www.aaaai.org/conditions-and-treatments/Treatments/ Saline-Sinus-Rinse-Recipe.aspx*

47. Passalacqua G, Bousquet PJ, Kai-Hakon C, et al. ARIA update: I-systematic review of complementary and alternative medicine for rhinitis and asthma. J Allergy Clin Immunol 2006;117:1054–1062.

48. U.S. Department of Health & Human Services. U.S. Food and Drug Administration. Drugs. Resources for You. Special Features. An important FDA reminder to parents: do not give infants cough and cold products designed for older children [updated 2011 Aug 3; cited 2012 Feb 6]. Available from: *http://www.fda.gov/Drugs/ResourcesforYou/SpecialFeatures/ucm263948.htm*

49. Briggs GG, Freeman RK, Yaffe SJ. Drugs in Pregnancy and Lactation, 8th ed. Philadelphia, PA: Lippincott Williams & Wilkins, 2008.

50. World Anti-Doping Agency (WADA). Montreal, Canada. c2012 [cited 2012 Feb 6]. Available from: *http://www.wada-ama.org/*

64 Psoriasis

Rebecca M.T. Law

● **Upon completion of this chapter, the reader will be able to:**

1. Discuss the etiology of psoriasis, including genetic and immune changes.

2. Describe the pathophysiology of psoriasis, including the types of psoriasis and clinical presentations.

3. Describe the comorbidities and risks in patients with psoriasis.

4. Compare and contrast the pharmacologic treatment modalities for psoriasis, that is, topical therapies, systemic therapies including biologics, and phototherapies.

5. Recommend an appropriate treatment plan for a patient with psoriasis, including nonpharmacologic and pharmacologic therapies

6. Recommend appropriate monitoring parameters for a patient with psoriasis.

7. Provide appropriate counseling information to a patient with psoriasis.

KEY CONCEPTS

❶ Patients with psoriasis have a lifelong illness that may be very visible and emotionally distressing. There is a strong need for empathy and a caring attitude in interactions with these patients.

❷ Psoriasis is a T-lymphocyte–mediated inflammatory disease that results from a complex interplay between multiple genetic factors and environmental influences. Genetic predisposition coupled with some precipitating factor triggers an abnormal immune response, resulting in the initial psoriatic skin lesions. Keratinocyte proliferation is central to the clinical presentation of psoriasis.

❸ Diagnosis of psoriasis is usually based on recognition of the characteristic plaque lesion and is not based on lab tests.

❹ Treatment goals for patients with psoriasis are to minimize signs such as plaques and scales; alleviate symptoms such as pruritus; reduce the frequency of flare-ups; ensure appropriate management of any associated comorbidities such as psoriatic arthritis, cardiovascular disorders, Crohn's disease, or clinical depression; and minimize treatment-related morbidity.

❺ Management of patients with psoriasis generally involves both nonpharmacologic and pharmacologic therapies.

❻ Nonpharmacologic alternatives such as stress reduction and the liberal use of moisturizers may be extremely beneficial and should always be considered and initiated when appropriate.

❼ Pharmacologic alternatives for psoriasis include topical agents, phototherapy, and systemic agents, including the use of biologic response modifiers (BRMs).

❽ In initiating pharmacologic treatment, the choice of therapy is generally guided by the severity of disease: topical agents would be appropriate for mild to moderate disease, whereas a systemic agent would be a more appropriate choice for moderate to severe disease. Phototherapy or photochemotherapy is used for patients with moderate to severe psoriasis, generally when topical therapies alone are inadequate. Patient-specific concerns such as existing comorbid conditions (e.g., hypertension, hyperlipidemia, diabetes mellitus, renal impairment or hepatic disease) must also be taken into consideration in the choice of therapy. Once the disease is under control, it would be important to step down to the least potent, least toxic agent(s) that maintain control.

❾ Rotational therapy (i.e., rotating systemic drug interventions in a sequential manner) is a means to minimize drug-associated toxicities since systemic agents for psoriasis often have differing toxicities. However, continuous treatment has largely replaced rotational therapies and is now the standard of care.

❿ Some BRMs have proven efficacy for psoriasis; however, there are differences among these agents, including mechanism of action, duration of remission, and adverse-effect profile. In general, due to their immunosuppressive effects, there is an increased risk of infection with most of these agents. The use of live or live-attenuated vaccines during therapy is generally not recommended. Currently, BRMs are often considered for patients with moderate to severe psoriasis when other systemic agents are inadequate or relatively contraindicated. It has also been recommended that BRMs be considered as first-line therapy, alongside conventional systemic agents, for patients with moderate to severe psoriasis; however, in practice, drug access due to cost considerations may be a limiting factor. They may be appropriate if comorbidities exist.

INTRODUCTION

Psoriasis is a chronic illness that is never cured; however, the signs and symptoms of psoriasis may subside totally and then return. Remission may last years in some patients, whereas in others exacerbations may occur every few months. Triggers include stress, seasonal changes, and some drugs. Disease flare-ups may also occur at times of life crises. Disease severity may vary from mild to disabling. In addition, there may be associated chronic comorbid conditions that also need appropriate treatments. Thus management of patients with psoriasis is necessarily long term, and management modalities may change according to the severity of illness at the time and should be individualized to meet patient needs.

❶ *Patients with psoriasis have a lifelong illness that may be very visible and emotionally distressing. There is a strong need for empathy and a caring attitude in interactions with these patients.*

EPIDEMIOLOGY AND ETIOLOGY

Psoriasis is a common inflammatory skin disorder estimated to affect 1.5% to 3% of the white population.[1,2] Ethnic factors influence disease prevalence. In the United States, prevalence among people of African or Asian descent (0.45% to 0.7%) is lower (versus 1.4% to 4.6% in general).[1,3] It may present at any age.[4] Up to 42% of patients with psoriasis have been reported to also have psoriatic arthritis (PsA).[5] PsA generally appears much later (up to decades later) than psoriasis. However, in about 10% to 15% of psoriatic patients with arthritis, joint symptoms may appear prior to skin involvement. Furthermore, although PsA more commonly occurs in psoriatics with more extensive disease, some patients may have deforming PsA with little to no cutaneous involvement.[5]

Besides PsA, other comorbidities associated with psoriasis may have significant morbidity and mortality risks. Well-known psychiatric/psychological comorbidities include depression, anxiety, and poor self-esteem. More recently, medical comorbidities identified include cardiovascular and related conditions (hypertension, obesity, type 2 diabetes, the metabolic syndrome), inflammatory bowel disease, multiple sclerosis, and lymphoma.[6,7]

Clinical depression may present in up to 60% of patients with psoriasis[6] and may be severe enough that patients contemplate suicide. Other psychopathologies include poor self-esteem, anxiety, and sexual dysfunction. The emotional and psychological impact of psoriasis may not correlate with the severity of the skin presentation, and it is important to always evaluate the psychosocial effects of psoriasis on the patient.[6]

The incidence of inflammatory bowel diseases (e.g., Crohn's and ulcerative colitis) may be 3.8 to 7.5 times higher in psoriatic patients than in the general population.[6] This has been attributed to shared or closely linked genetic susceptibility traits, with individual susceptibility localized to a similar region of chromosome 16, among others.[6] There may also be a genetic link to multiple sclerosis.[6]

Recent research has shown that psoriatic patients have an increased risk of cardiovascular diseases.[5,7,8] There is a higher than normal incidence of myocardial infarction. The risk is increased in patients with both mild and severe psoriasis, with the highest risk in younger patients with severe disease.[8] These findings persist even when corrected for the cardiovascular risk factors.[6,8] The corrections are especially relevant since psoriatic patients also have increased incidences of type 2 diabetes, obesity, hypertension, smoking, alcohol consumption, metabolic syndrome, body mass index (BMI), and an atherogenic lipid profile.[5-8] In a recent study in hospitalized patients, the metabolic syndrome is significantly more prevalent in patients with psoriasis than those without.[6,7]

With regard to increased cancer risk, although there is controversy, some studies show an increased risk of lymphoma, with one study demonstrating a significantly increased risk of cutaneous T-cell lymphoma (relative risk of 10.75) or Hodgkin's lymphoma (relative risk of 3.18) in patients with severe disease.[6] However, the risk of melanoma and nonmelanoma skin cancer appears equal to that of the general population,[6] although risks are associated with some psoriatic treatments. Some psoriatic treatments with a known lymphoma risk may be confounding factors. Increased cancer risk may be limited to subpopulations: Caucasians with more than 250 PUVA (psoralens + UVA) treatments have a 14-fold greater risk of cutaneous squamous cell carcinoma than those with fewer treatments.[6]

❷ *Psoriasis is a T-lymphocyte–mediated inflammatory disease that results from a complex interplay between multiple genetic factors and environmental influences.*[1,5] *Genetic predisposition coupled with some precipitating factor triggers an abnormal immune response, resulting in the initial psoriatic skin lesions.* Other risk factors may exacerbate preexisting psoriasis and cause disease flare-ups. Precipitating factors include skin trauma such as a horse-fly bite (known as the Koebner phenomenon),[6] environmental changes such as cold weather, stress, a viral or streptococcal infection, or use of a β-adrenergic blocker.[2] Factors exacerbating psoriasis include drugs (e.g., lithium, NSAIDs, antimalarials, β-adrenergic blockers, and withdrawal of corticosteroids), and psoriatic patients commonly have exacerbations during times of stress.[2]

There is a clear genetic component to psoriasis. Studies conducted in twins show a risk of psoriasis that is two to three times as high in monozygotic twins versus fraternal twins.[9] As many as 71% of patients with psoriasis during childhood have some positive family history.[1,10] Similarly, psoriatic arthritis is heritable, with a prevalence 19 times higher in first-degree relatives of patients with psoriatic arthritis than in the general population.[10]

The inheritance pattern for psoriasis is complex and polygenic. Genome-wide linkage studies have identified at least nine genetic loci with statistically significant linkage to psoriasis: these are named psoriasis susceptibility 1 through 9 (PSORS1 through PSORS9).[9] PSORS1 has been considered the major gene locus for psoriasis[1,4,6,9,10]; it appears to be associated with 35% to 50% of cases of psoriasis.[9] There are three genes within this gene locus that appear to have polymorphic coding-sequence variations strongly associated with psoriasis: HLA-C with the associated HLA-Cw6 variant, CCHCRI with the associated variant WWCC, and corneodesmosin with the associated variant allele 5.[9] Current data suggest that HLA-Cw6 is the susceptibility allele within PSORS1.[9] CCHCRI and corneodesmosin encode different proteins that are overexpressed in psoriatic epidermis.[9]

Different clinical types of psoriasis appear to be associated with different genetic loci. Guttate psoriasis is strongly associated with PSORS1, but late-onset psoriasis (onset at age over 50) and palmoplantar psoriasis do not appear to be.[9] Other genetic loci of importance and under study include genes involved in IL-23 signaling (IL-23R, IL-23A, IL-12B) and susceptibility genes within the LCE gene locus on 1q21.[9] In addition, several genetic loci for psoriasis are also associated with other diseases, including Crohn's disease, rheumatoid arthritis, and diabetes.[9] There are possibly other genetic loci.

PATHOPHYSIOLOGY

❷ *Keratinocyte proliferation is central to the clinical presentation of psoriasis.* **Keratinocytes** are skin cells producing keratin, which acts as a skin barrier. Increased keratinocyte cell turnover (hyperkeratosis) with immature maturation of keratinocytes and incomplete cornification with retention of nuclei in the stratum corneum (parakeratosis)[9] result in the characteristic thick, scaly skin lesions seen in patients with psoriasis. Hyperkeratosis results from immune derangements.

The abnormal immune response seen in psoriasis is mediated primarily by T lymphocytes (T cells).[1,9] In psoriatic patients, certain types of T cells are overactive, migrating to the skin in large numbers by binding to activated endothelial cells via intracellular cell adhesion molecules (ICAM-1).[1,11] These naïve T cells then encounter antigens in the skin, presented to them by antigen-presenting cells (APCs),

and become activated T cells. There is an LFA-3–CD2 signal that plays an important part in T-cell activation: LFA-3 is the leukocyte function–associated antigen type 3 found on APCs; CD2 is a cell-surface glycoprotein expressed on T-cell subtypes.[1] When LFA-3 interacts with CD2, there is an increased proliferation of T cells.[12]

Activated T cells begin releasing cytokines including interleukin-2 (IL-2), interferon-γ (IFN-γ), tumor necrosis factor-α (TNF-α), and others.[4,12] Cytokine activity leads to a rapid proliferation and turnover of skin cells, triggering the inflammatory process and the development of psoriatic skin lesions.[4,12,13] TNF-α may have a role in disease severity; it upregulates endothelial and keratinocyte expression of ICAM-1, activates T cells, enhances T-cell infiltration, and augments keratinocyte proliferation.[11]

Dendritic cells are key sentinel cells of the immune system that bridge the gap between innate and adaptive immunity. Myeloid dermal dendritic cells are seen in increased numbers in psoriatic lesions, and they induce the auto-proliferation of T cells and production of type-1 helper T-cell cytokines. Specialized dendritic cells produce TNF-α, as well as other substances.[9]

Treatment of psoriasis is based on an understanding of the underlying pathophysiology. Agents that modulate the abnormal immune response, such as corticosteroids and biologic response modifiers (BRMs), are important treatment strategies for psoriasis. Targeted immunotherapy and phototherapy (i.e., PUVA) reduce the numbers of dendritic cells in patients with psoriasis.[9] In addition, topical therapies that affect cell turnover are effective for psoriasis. Clinically, a treatment regimen should always be individualized, taking into consideration severity of disease, patient responses, and tolerability of various interventions.

CLINICAL PRESENTATION

❸ *Diagnosis of psoriasis is usually based on recognition of the characteristic plaque lesion and is not based on lab tests.*

Patient Encounter, Part 1

A 45-year-old man with a 12-year history of plaque psoriasis presents with well-demarcated reddish-violet raised lesions on his legs, abdomen, back, elbows, and knees. The lesions are covered with loose silvery scales, which when removed show pinpoints of bleeding. When questioned, the patient says his skin was relatively clear until about a week ago; since then, the lesions have been spreading and are extremely itchy. There are signs of excoriation on the patient's legs.

What information is consistent with a flare-up of psoriasis in this patient?

Clinical Presentation and Diagnosis of Plaque Psoriasis

General

Patients have small, discrete lesions to generalized confluent lesions over a large body surface area (BSA).

Symptoms

Patients may complain of severe itching.

Signs

- Lesions are raised and are red to violet in color (commonly known as plaques).
- Lesions have sharply demarcated borders, except where confluent.
- Lesions are loosely covered with silvery-white scales, which if lifted off, show small pinpoints of bleeding (Auspitz's sign).
- Plaques appear most commonly on the elbows, knees, scalp, umbilicus, and lumbar areas, and often extend to involve the trunk, arms, legs, face, ears, palms, soles, and nails.
- Nail involvement presents as pitting, discoloration ("oil spots"), crumbling, splinter hemorrhages, growth arrest lines, or tissue buildup around the nails.

Clinical Presentation and Diagnosis of Other Types of Psoriasis

Inverse psoriasis spares the areas commonly involved in plaque psoriasis and instead appears in intertriginous areas, where scaling is minimal.

Guttate psoriasis presents as a sudden eruption of small, disseminated erythematosquamous papules and plaques, often preceded by a streptococcal infection 2 to 3 weeks prior.

Pustular psoriasis may be localized or generalized and may be an acute emergency requiring systemic therapy.

Generalized pustular psoriasis is characterized by disseminated deep-red erythematous areas and pustules, which may merge to become "lakes of pus."

Erythrodermic psoriasis is a generalized, life-threatening condition that presents with erythema, desquamation, and edema and may require life support measures as well as systemic therapy.

Psoriatic diaper rash is the most common type of psoriasis in children younger than 2 years. This usually affects inguinal folds, and greater than 90% of psoriatic diaper rash cases may have involvement outside the diaper area.

Disease severity is generally classified as mild/limited disease, moderate disease, or severe disease based on body surface area (BSA) involvement or various measurements of symptom and involvement such as the Psoriasis Area and Severity Index (PASI) and the Dermatology Life Quality Index (DLQI).[14,15]

Disease Severity Classification[14,15]

Mild or limited disease	Less than or equal to 5% BSA involvement
Moderate disease	PASI greater than or equal to 8 (higher in trials of biologics)
Severe disease	The Rule of Tens: PASI greater than or equal to 10 or DLQI greater than or equal to 10 or BSA greater than or equal to 10% (in some phototherapy trials, BSA greater than or equal to 20% is used as the lower limit)

TREATMENT

Desired Outcomes and Goals

④ *Since psoriasis is a chronic illness, goals of treatment focus on controlling the signs and symptoms, ensuring appropriate management of comorbidities, and minimizing treatment-related morbidity. Goals include the following:*

- Minimizing or eliminating the signs of psoriasis, such as plaques and scales
- Alleviating pruritus and minimizing excoriations
- Reducing flare-up frequency
- Ensuring appropriate management of associated comorbidities such as psoriatic arthritis, cardiovascular disorders, Crohn's disease, clinical depression, or itching
- Avoiding or minimizing adverse effects from treatments used
- Providing cost-effective therapy
- Providing guidance or counseling as needed (e.g., stress-reduction techniques)
- Maintaining or improving the patient's quality of life

General Approach to Treatment

⑤ *Management of patients with psoriasis generally involves both nonpharmacologic and pharmacologic therapies.* Pharmacologic alternatives for plaque psoriasis include topical treatments, phototherapy, photochemotherapy, and systemic therapies alone (orally or by injection). Systemic therapies are generally further sorted into traditional systemic therapies and biologic response modifiers (BRMs). The choice of treatment is usually dictated by the severity

Patient Encounter, Part 2

Additional relevant information was obtained from the patient, including the following history.

FH: One of his brothers has psoriasis and his sister has atopic dermatitis. His father died of a massive heart attack at age 51.

SH: He works as an assistant copywriter in a busy publishing house and is constantly struggling with multiple deadlines; he is an occasional social drinker and nonsmoker; he is a single father to an 8-year-old boy with asthma.

PE:

He appears anxious about the lesions.

VS: BP 125/70 mm Hg, P 72 beats/min, RR 16 breaths/min, T 37°C (98.6°F)

Height & Weight: Ht 5 ft 8 in (173 cm), Wt 175 lb (80 kg)

Abd: Soft, nontender; bowel sounds present; lesions on abdomen

Exts: Within normal limits; no joint pains; lesions on legs, elbows, and knees; "oil spots" on finger nails

Skin: Well-demarcated raised reddish-violet lesions on legs, abdomen, back, elbows, and knees; evidence of excoriation on legs

Labs: All within normal limits, including lipids, renal function tests, and LFTs

What risk factors does he have for psoriasis and/or its associated comorbidities?

Identify your treatment goals for the patient.

to ensure appropriate management of symptoms such as itching.

There are several recently published treatment guidelines and consensus guidelines.[5,6,14,16–23]

Efficacy Assessment

Quantitative tools to evaluate the efficacy of psoriasis treatments are generally used in clinical trials and rarely in practice. These include the Psoriasis Area and Severity Index (PASI), the Physician's Global Assessment (PGA), and the National Psoriasis Foundation—Psoriasis Score (NPF-PS). PASI is the most well known and measures overall extent and severity of psoriasis, assessing areas of coverage, erythema, induration, and scaling. Clinical efficacy is reported as a decrease in the PASI score, or an improvement (e.g., 75% improvement or PASI-75).[6]

In clinical practice, subjective qualitative assessment of disease severity is generally used to determine treatment efficacy. In addition, an assessment of the patient's quality of life (QOL) is important. The impact of psoriasis on a patient's psychological well-being may differ substantially from the severity of disease. Various QOL instruments validated for dermatologic diseases include the Dermatology Quality of Life Scales, Dermatology Life Quality Index (DLQI), Dermatology Specific Quality of Life Instrument, and Skindex-29.

Nonpharmacologic Treatment

❻ *Nonpharmacologic alternatives may be extremely beneficial in the patient with psoriasis and complement pharmacologic therapies and thus should always be considered and initiated when appropriate.* These include the following[24]:

- *Stress reduction techniques.* Psychotherapy including stress management, guided imagery, and relaxation techniques are being used more frequently as adjunctive therapies for patients with psoriasis. Stress reduction has been shown to improve both the extent and severity of psoriasis.

- *Oatmeal baths.* Regular use of oatmeal baths in tepid water may help soothe the itching associated with psoriasis and reduce the need for systemic antipruritic agents.

- *Nonmedicated moisturizers.* Maintaining adequate skin moisture helps to control the scaling associated with psoriasis. Emollients restore skin pliability, reduce skin shedding, reduce pruritus, and help prevent painful cracking and bleeding.[2] Nonmedicated moisturizers may be liberally applied several times daily to help prevent skin dryness. Fragrance-free products should be selected when available.

- *Avoid irritant chemicals on the skin.* Harsh soaps or detergents should not be used. Cleansing should be done with tepid water, preferably using lipid-free and fragrance-free cleansers.

of disease; however, the presence or absence of comorbidities, such as psoriatic arthritis, is playing a greater role in drug therapy selection. In some cases, a combination of treatment options may optimize therapy. Topical therapies can be used in patients with mild/limited to moderately severe disease. Phototherapy and photochemotherapy are generally used in moderate to severe disease. Systemic therapies are used for patients with extensive or moderate to severe disease. To minimize drug toxicities or increase efficacy, systemic therapies are sometimes used in conjunction with topical or phototherapy.[14,15] BRMs are currently recommended for consideration as first-line therapies alongside traditional systemic agents for moderate to severe disease.[14] Their safety profile in comparison with other systemic agents and relatively good acceptability by patients are all positive factors.[14] However, due to a significant cost difference, biologic agents are often reserved for cases in which traditional systemic agents provide inadequate control or for patients with comorbidities (e.g., in a patient with PsA or for whom traditional systemic agents may be inappropriate due to potential adverse effects). In addition, it is important to ensure appropriate screening and treatment of any comorbid illnesses such as depression or diabetes[7] and

- *Avoid skin trauma.* Sunburns can induce a flare-up of psoriasis. Sunscreens with a sun protection factor of at least 15 should be routinely used when outdoors; often a sun protection factor of 30 is recommended. Avoid scratching the skin, which could lead to excoriations and exacerbate psoriasis. Loose-fitting cotton garments should be worn to minimize skin irritation.

Pharmacologic Treatment

⑦ *Pharmacologic alternatives for psoriasis include topical agents, phototherapy, and systemic agents including the use of BRMs.* See **Figures 64–1** and **64–2** for treatment algorithms.

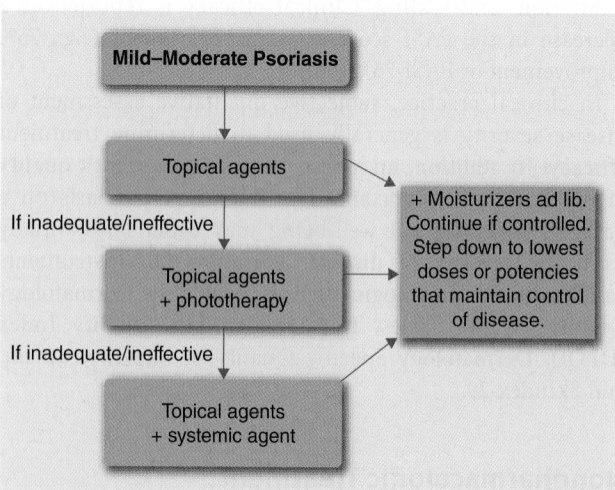

FIGURE 64–1. Treatment algorithm for mild to moderate psoriasis.

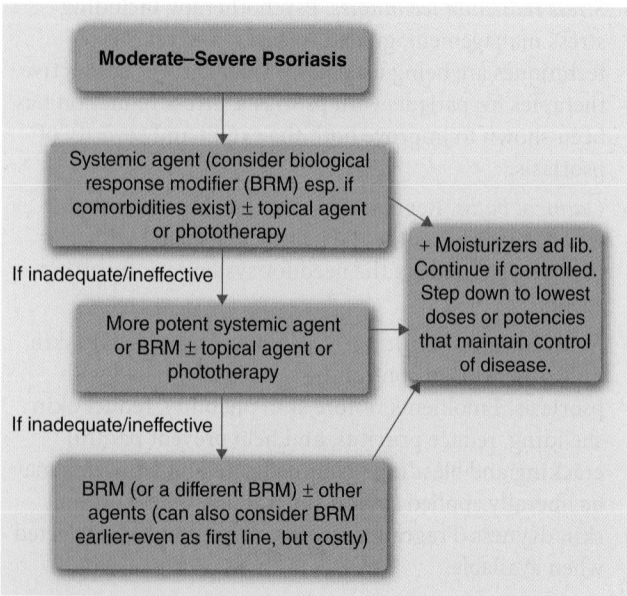

FIGURE 64–2. Treatment algorithm for moderate to severe psoriasis.

Patient Encounter, Part 3

The diagnosis is that the patient has a moderate flare-up of his plaque psoriasis.

Current meds: Nonmedicated moisturizer being applied to entire body once daily after bathing. Hydrocortisone 0.5% cream being applied to lesions twice daily (patient obtained this as an OTC product).

Identify the drug-related problems in this patient.

What nonpharmacologic alternatives are appropriate for this patient?

What pharmacologic treatments are appropriate for this patient?

▶ *Topical Therapy for Psoriasis*

⑧ *Topical therapy is the initial drug treatment strategy for patients with mild to moderate psoriasis.* Approximately 70% to 80% of psoriasis patients may be adequately managed with topical drug therapy.[1] These include corticosteroids, coal tar products, anthralin, vitamin D_3 analogues (e.g. calcipotriol), retinoids (e.g. tazarotene), and topical immunomodulators (e.g. tacrolimus, pimecrolimus).[17] Topical corticosteroids remain the mainstay of topical therapy for most psoriatic patients.[14,17] Vitamin D_3 analogues and topical retinoids all affect keratinocyte functions and the immune response and are sometimes the initial choice of therapy. Currently, these are in wider use than either anthralin or coal tar preparations.

Topical agents may be incorporated into various vehicles, including ointments, creams, gels, lotions, foams, sprays, tapes, pastes, and shampoos. Vehicle selection is an important consideration and may vary from one body part to another. Ointments and tapes provide occlusion, enhancing drug penetration to improve efficacy. Creams and lotions are easier to spread, especially in hairy areas. Gels may have drying and cooling effects in addition to easy spreadability. Foams may have enhanced drug delivery and/or efficacy versus lotions or creams and can become a cosmetically elegant liquid upon skin contact, providing good patient acceptance. Shampoos incorporating tar distillates or salicylic acid are useful for scalp psoriasis. Pastes such as Lassar's paste have an inherent stiffness, minimizing the spread of medication, and are useful for incorporating drugs such as anthralin, which, especially in higher concentrations used in short-contact methods, may cause skin irritation and burning if in contact with normal skin. It is important to remember that changing to a different vehicle may significantly alter drug potency. For example, a tape formulation (highly occlusive) is much more potent than a cream formulation. However, ultimately the optimal vehicle may be the vehicle that the patient is willing to use—occlusive ointments may be too greasy and cosmetically unappealing, resulting in poor compliance. Sometimes using a cream formulation during the day and an ointment at night may be the best option.[17]

For mild to moderate psoriasis, mid-potency corticosteroids such as betamethasone valerate (0.05% to 1%) are most frequently selected first, with escalation to higher potency corticosteroids, if needed, and stepping down to lower potency corticosteroids when the psoriasis improves. High-potency corticosteroids may be used initially in thicker plaque areas such as palms and soles, but should be considered for short-term use only. These include fluocinonide, clobetasol, halobetasol, and betamethasone dipropionate in optimized base. Low-potency corticosteroids such as hydrocortisone (0.5% to 2%) are appropriate choices if treatment of the face or flexures is necessary. Topical corticosteroids are available as ointments, creams, lotions including scalp lotions, and a few foam products and should be applied in a thin layer on the skin. Intralesional triamcinolone may be useful for specific lesions, such as nail matrix psoriasis.

Tachyphylaxis, defined as the loss of effectiveness with continued use[17] or a progressive decrease in their biological action with repeated use[14] can occur. However, this is not always seen in studies, and it remains somewhat controversial whether tachyphylaxis results from a true loss of effectiveness or reflects a loss of patient adherence.[5,17] Regardless, pulse-dosing (using a potent topical corticosteroid for only 1 to 2 days per week) has been shown to lengthen the duration of effectiveness and reduce the incidence of adverse effects.[14] Another possible concern is rebound, defined as the disease recurring worse than the pretreatment baseline after the topical corticosteroid is discontinued.[17] Rebound most typically occurs when topical corticosteroids are abruptly discontinued; however, its frequency and severity are poorly characterized.[17]

It is important to remember that adverse effects of *topical* corticosteroids may be *systemic* in nature, and hypothalamic–pituitary–adrenal axis suppression can occur, especially when high-potency corticosteroids are used. Infants and small children may be more susceptible due to their increased skin surface:body mass ratio. Much less common systemic side effects of topical corticosteroids include osteonecrosis of the femoral head, cataracts, and glaucoma.[17] Topical corticosteroids may also cause **striae**, skin atrophy, acne, **telangiectasias**, folliculitis, contact dermatitis, hypertrichosis, perioral dermatitis, traumatic purpura, and rosacea.[14,17] Atrophy can result in thin, fragile, easily lacerated skin. Striae are caused by tearing of dermal connective tissue and are irreversible. Due to their significant adverse-effect profile, it has been recommended that no topical corticosteroid be used regularly for more than 4 weeks without review and reassessment.[2] Continuous use of high-potency (class I) topical corticosteroids should normally be limited to no more than twice daily for up to 2 to 4 weeks and no more than 50 g/week[17] (based on evidence from clinical trials); however, in practice, longer durations are frequently used with judicious patient monitoring.[17] All topical corticosteroids are Pregnancy Category C and of unknown safety in nursing women.[17]

Vitamin D analogues (calcipotriol, calcitriol, tacalcitol) may also be initial pharmacotherapy for mild to moderate psoriasis.[2,5] These inhibit keratinocyte proliferation and enhance keratinocyte differentiation.[5] They are less effective than high-potency topical corticosteroids (class I)[5] and are often used in various combination regimens with topical corticosteroids to enhance efficacy and reduce steroid atrophy, as discussed later. Unlike corticosteroids, tachyphylaxis does not occur with prolonged use. Clearance of lesions should occur after 4 to 6 weeks of treatment.[2] Lack of response by 8 weeks indicates treatment failure.[2] These analogues may cause skin irritation leading to erythema, dryness, stinging, or burning. They may also cause hypercalcemia secondary to excessive absorption or use.[2,14,17] This is rare unless patients are applying more than the recommended weekly dosage or have underlying renal disease or impaired calcium metabolism.[17] Recommended dosage is 5 mg calcipotriol (i.e., 100 g of calcipotriol cream or ointment) per week.[14,17] Calcipotriol (50 mcg/g) is also available as a combination ointment product with betamethasone propionate.[17] Topical calcitriol (the active metabolite of vitamin D) has been studied for treatment of psoriasis and appears almost as effective as betamethasone dipropionate in clearance of lesions, with a longer remission period.[2] It is less irritating than calcipotriol and can be used for the face and flexures.[2,5] Calcipotriol is inactivated by UVA; thus it would be important to apply calcipotriol after and not before UVA exposure if used together.[17]

Tazarotene is a topical retinoid effective for mild to moderate psoriasis and also for acne. It normalizes keratinocyte differentiation and has antiproliferative and anti-inflammatory effects.[14,17] Tazarotene is available commercially as a 0.05% or 0.1% gel. Similar to vitamin D analogues, it is also steroid-sparing[5] and often used in combination, as discussed later. It may cause significant skin irritation, including erythema, pruritus, and burning, especially upon initial use.[14,17] Skin irritation can be minimized by using the cream formulation, the lower concentration product, moisturizers, application on alternate days, or short-contact (30 to 60 minutes) treatment.[17] Avoid use in women of child-bearing age (Pregnancy Category X), unless effective contraception is being used; there is a potential risk of systemic drug absorption, and systemic retinoids are known teratogens. Concomitant use of other topical preparations or cosmetics with a strong drying effect should be avoided.[15]

Keratolytic agents, such as salicylic acid, are often added to bath oil or shampoos (typically 3% to 4%) for scalp psoriasis.[24] Salicylic acid can also be added to topical corticosteroid preparations to enhance steroid penetration (salicylic acid breaks down keratin).[14,17] Systemic absorption of topical salicylate is rare but can occur, especially if applied to more than 20% of BSA.[17] Topical salicylate reduces the efficacy of ultraviolet B (UVB) phototherapy due to a filtering effect and should be applied after a UVB treatment if used together.[17]

Coal tar is keratolytic and may have antiproliferative and anti-inflammatory effects.[2] Coal tar products include crude coal tar and tar distillates (liquor carbonis detergens) available as ointments, creams, and shampoos in various strengths. Coal tar may cause acne, folliculitis, local irritation, and phototoxicity; it will stain clothing and has an unpleasant odor.[14,17,24] It is photosensitizing and can be combined with UVB phototherapy (Goekermann's regimen) to increase treatment response.[17]

Anthralin (dithranol) has a direct antiproliferative effect on epidermal keratinocytes[2] and is generally used only on thick plaque areas. It can be used continuously or as short-contact anthralin therapy (SCAT): exposure to anthralin for 2 hours or less.[17] SCAT is most commonly administered as 20- to 30-minute outpatient treatments, starting at 1% anthralin concentration with increasing concentration over time as tolerated.[17] Anthralin may be highly irritating, especially if SCAT treatments are misused or mistakenly applied continuously.[24] It is important to remember when compounding anthralin preparations that prescribed concentrations range from 0.1% (meant for continuous use) to 1% to 4% (meant for SCAT).[15] Normal skin surrounding the psoriasis plaques should be protected with nonmedicated paste or zinc oxide.[17,24] Persons handling the dry anthralin powder should avoid skin contact (e.g., by wearing gloves while compounding).[15]

Tacrolimus and pimecrolimus are topical calcineurin inhibitors approved for treatment of atopic dermatitis in children 2 years or older. Although currently not approved for treatment of psoriasis, they have been successfully used in treating facial and intertriginous psoriasis in several RCTs, where concerns about corticosteroid toxicity including skin atrophy is higher.[17] In fact, AAD's Work Group states that topical tacrolimus also be considered first line of therapy for intertriginous psoriasis.[5]

Combination therapy may be more efficacious and can result in reduced side effects. Topical corticosteroids used with either vitamin D analogues or retinoids are successful combinations whether used concomitantly or sequentially.[5,14] Combining tazarotene use with a topical corticosteroid (e.g., an alternate-day regimen or morning corticosteroid–evening tazarotene regimen) may minimize skin irritation and steroid-induced skin atrophy and enhance efficacy.[17] Tazarotene plus topical corticosteroid are synergistic, lengthening the duration of treatment benefit/remission.[5] Similarly, morning calcipotriol and evening halobetasol ointment resulted in reduced overall severity of psoriasis versus monotherapy.[14] Also, 2 weeks of calcipotriol followed by pulse therapy with halobetasol ointment twice daily on weekends and calcipotriol ointment twice daily on weekdays was superior to either of the two agents when pulsed with placebo.[14] Fixed-dose combination products are also more efficacious than monotherapy; however, the adverse effects of continuous corticosteroid use are not reduced. Corticosteroid/topical retinoid combination products may reduce topical irritation related to the retinoid. As mentioned earlier, salicylic acid can enhance steroid efficacy by increasing penetration, and there are combination products with corticosteroids such as betamethasone dipropionate or diflucortolone valerate.[14]

▶ *Phototherapy for Psoriasis*

8 *Phototherapy or photochemotherapy is used for patients with moderate to severe psoriasis, generally when topical therapies*

alone are inadequate. Phototherapy involves the use of either ultraviolet A (UVA) or B (UVB). Photochemotherapy is the concurrent use of phototherapy together with topical[14,17,19] or systemic agents.[14,19] UVA is a longer wavelength, and therapy with UVA is always combined with psoralens (e.g., methoxsalen or trioxsalen), which are used as photosensitizers to increase efficacy. There is an increased risk of skin cancers after prolonged use of phototherapy, and risks are greater with PUVA than UVB.[14,15,19] Narrowband UVB (NB-UVB) is generally well tolerated.

Bath PUVA, topical PUVA, and oral PUVA regimens are available.[14,19] Bath PUVA involves soaking in a bath of psoralens liquid for 15 minutes prior to UVA treatment and is commonly used in Scandinavian countries for generalized psoriasis to reduce systemic toxicities from psoralens.[19] Topical PUVA involves painting the compound on affected skin prior to UVA treatment[14] and is commonly used for psoriasis localized to palms and soles.[19] When using any form of topical PUVA, the UVA treatment should be done within 30 minutes of the psoralens skin treatment.[19] Oral PUVA involves ingesting a psoralens capsule the day prior to a UVA treatment. Oral psoralens (e.g., 5- or 8-methoxsalen) often causes nausea.[6,14] Other adverse effects of PUVA include photosensitivity (necessitating the use of eye protection and UVA-blocking sunscreen for 24 hours after a PUVA treatment), macular **melanosis** at exposed sites (PUVA **lentigines**),[19] photoaging; increased risk of cataract formation[19]; and increased risk of nonmelanoma skin cancers (especially squamous cell carcinoma; less commonly basal cell carcinomas).[14,19] One large prospective trial found an additional risk of melanoma with increasing cumulative UVA doses,[14] although other studies differ, and this is an area of controversy.[19] Regardless, it is recommended that the lifetime cumulative exposure be capped at 200 PUVA treatments.[14,19]

PUVA has been used in conjunction with other topical agents to increase treatment efficacy. Calcipotriol added to a PUVA regimen may reduce both the number of PUVA treatments and the total UVA dosage needed to clear lesions.[25,26] The rate ratio for marked improvement in patients receiving PUVA plus calcipotriol versus PUVA alone was 1.2 in a recent meta-analysis of 11 controlled studies.[27] To use calcipotriol and PUVA together, calcipotriol must be applied *after* PUVA, since UVA irradiation will inactivate calcipotriol.[28] Use with other topical agents has been limited. Tazarotene plus PUVA was studied in 12 patients with extensive plaque psoriasis, and results showed significant improvements after 3 weeks[29]; however, UVA doses should be reduced by at least one-third, since tazarotene increases the risk for immediate pigment darkening caused by UVA.[30]

PUVA can be effectively used with other systemic agents, including oral retinoids (RePUVA) and methotrexate. This will be discussed later in greater detail.

UVB treatments are often used alone.[6] Narrowband UVB (NB-UVB) is more effective than broadband UVB (BB-UVB)[19] and avoids some adverse effects of PUVA, but is slightly less effective than PUVA.[6] NB-UVB can be safely used in patients with demyelinating diseases where

TNF-α–inhibiting BRMs are contraindicated.[5] Efficacy in part depends on frequency of treatments.[14] Thrice weekly NB-UVB has been found equally effective as twice weekly PUVA, but twice weekly NB-UVB is less efficacious.[14] UVB is dosed based on either skin type or the minimal erythema dose (MED) with subsequent doses adjusted accordingly.[19] Adverse effects of BB-UVB include erythema, itching, burning, stinging, cataract formation, reactivation of herpes simplex virus infection, photoaging, and increased risk of genital tumors in men treated without genital shielding.[19] Eye goggles and genital shielding are standard practices to minimize risks, as is covering the face when there are no facial psoriasis lesions or minimizing the UVB dose to the face.[19] Lesional blistering, although uncommon, can occur with NB-UVB.[19] NB-UVB may be two to three times more carcinogenic per MED than BB-UVB; however, due to significantly greater efficacy, the total MED needed with NB-UVB is far less than BB-UVB, and a recent review found no significant association with basal cell carcinoma, squamous cell carcinoma, or melanoma in patients followed for about 5.5 years.[19]

UVB treatments have been used with topical or systemic agents to increase treatment efficacy. Topical regimens have included UVB with tazarotene, with crude coal tar (Goekermann's regimen), with anthralin (Ingram's regimen), with calcipotriol, and with topical corticosteroids.[19] UVB with tazarotene may be synergistic: The effect of each agent seems to be enhanced; efficacy is increased, whereas the number of treatment sessions and the cumulative UVB dose needed are reduced.[14,19] UVB with crude coal tar is a highly effective regimen developed early in the twentieth century; however, many patients consider it messy and time-consuming and it is less commonly used today.[14,19] UVB with SCAT has shown little additional benefit,[19] and UVB with calcipotriol has shown conflicting results.[19] UVB with topical steroids may actually shorten the remission period[31] or lead to a higher relapse rate.[19]

Several UVB and systemic therapy combinations have shown efficacy. These include UVB with acitretin (ReUVB) and UVB with methotrexate and will be discussed later.

▶ Systemic Therapy for Psoriasis

⑧ Systemic therapies are seldom used for mild to moderate psoriasis and are generally reserved for patients with moderate to severe psoriasis.[5,14,15,18] Oral agents include sulfasalazine, acitretin, methotrexate, cyclosporine, mycophenolate mofetil, azathioprine, tacrolimus, and hydroxyurea. Parenteral agents include the BRMs alefacept, etanercept, adalimumab, infliximab, ustekinumab, and many others, currently at various stages of research or approval for psoriasis.

⑧ Patient-specific concerns such as existing comorbid conditions (e.g., hypertension, hyperlipidemia, diabetes mellitus, renal impairment, or hepatic disease) must also be taken into consideration in the choice of therapy.

⑧ Once the disease is under control, it would be important to step down to the least potent, least toxic agent(s) that maintain control.

Patient Encounter, Part 4

The patient's psoriatic condition remains well controlled with topical treatments for about 11 years, then flare-ups become a frequent occurrence. Phototherapy with NB-UVB was initiated. The patient did not respond well to NB-UVB therapy used alone. He is currently presenting with fairly extensive plaque psoriasis, affecting about two-thirds of his body surface area. There are signs of excoriation as well.

Current weight: 70 kg.

Current meds: Nonmedicated moisturizer after bathing and ad lib. Betamethasone valerate 0.1% ointment bid to lesions.

Relevant social history: Patient has remarried and his son is doing well in college.

What are the drug-related problems in this patient at this time?

What pharmacologic treatments would be appropriate for this patient at this time?

Rotational therapy (i.e., rotating systemic drug interventions in a sequential manner) is a means to minimize drug-associated toxicities, since systemic agents for psoriasis often have differing toxicities. However, continuous treatment has largely replaced rotational therapies and is now the standard of care.

Sulfasalazine has variable efficacy and is of limited potency for psoriasis, although it is effective for inflammatory bowel disease. There is no FDA- or Health Canada–approved use for psoriasis.[18] However, its side-effect profile is better than that of other systemic therapies for psoriasis, and it is sometimes tried as an initial systemic agent for moderate to severe psoriasis. Usual doses are 2 to 4 g/day in divided doses,[24] starting with an initial dose of 500 mg twice daily and titrating up as tolerated.[18] Side effects include nausea/vomiting, anorexia, headache, arthralgias, and reversible oligospermia.[18]

Acitretin is an oral retinoid, likely safer than methotrexate or cyclosporine since potentially serious adverse effects can usually be minimized by appropriate patient selection, careful dosing, and monitoring.[18] It has the advantage of not being immunosuppressive.[6] The usual dose range is 10 to 50 mg once daily, with lower doses (10 to 25 mg) used more often to minimize side effects[14,18]; higher doses (70 mg/day) have been used in clinical trials.[18] Acitretin given concurrently with phototherapy (ReUVB or RePUVA) has a synergistic treatment effect: The number and duration of phototherapy sessions needed to achieve clearance is reduced.[18,19] Acitretin monotherapy is usually given for 14 days before instituting UVB or PUVA.[18] The ultraviolet light dose should be reduced by 30% to 50%.[18] ReUVB and RePUVA are well-established treatment regimens for psoriasis.[1,5,6,14,18,19]

However, acitretin is teratogenic (Pregnancy Category X) and relatively contraindicated in women of childbearing potential. It must not be used in pregnant women, those with unreliable contraception, or those who intend to become pregnant at any time during or for 3 years after discontinuation of therapy.[6,15,18] Acitretin can transform spontaneously or be converted by ethanol (transesterification) into etretinate, which may take up to 3 years for clearance.[18] Alcohol should be avoided during therapy and for at least 2 months after acitretin discontinuation—it is unknown what the minimum amount of alcohol consumption is for transesterification to occur.[15,18] Common side effects include mucocutaneous dryness and hyperlipidemia.[14,18] Long-term continuous use has caused **diffuse idiopathic skeletal hyperostosis (DISH)**[14] and periungual pyogenic granulomas.[18] Drug interactions include vitamin A (use of vitamin A should be avoided due to the increased risk of hypervitaminosis A), and caution should be used with drugs that interfere with cytochrome P450 metabolism or have significant plasma albumin binding.[18]

Methotrexate used in low doses is one of the mainstays of systemic therapy in the treatment of psoriasis.[20] Compared with cyclosporine, methotrexate has a more modest effect but can be used continuously for years, with durable benefits.[14] An initial test dose of 2.5 to 5 mg/week (single dose given once) is recommended.[15,18] If lab values are normal after 1 week, the dose can be increased to a range of 7.5 to 25 mg once weekly.[18] This can be given as a single dose or split into two or three doses given 12 hours apart to minimize GI side effects.[15,20] It may take up to 4 weeks to see a clinical response after a dose increase.[18] Always titrate to the lowest effective dosage for maintenance. Methotrexate is contraindicated in pregnancy, renal impairment, hepatitis, cirrhosis, alcoholics, unreliable patients, and patients with leukemia or thrombocytopenia.[6]

Serious side effects of methotrexate include hepatotoxicity, bone marrow suppression, and pulmonary fibrosis. Cumulative liver toxicity was shown in a Canadian study to be severe in nearly one-fourth of psoriatics receiving methotrexate over 1 to 11 years.[14] Psoriatic patients with comorbid diabetes are at particularly high risk of severe liver fibrosis and cirrhosis.[14] Psoriatic patients have a greater risk of hepatotoxicity than rheumatoid arthritis patients given similar cumulative doses of methotrexate; thus guidelines have traditionally recommended routine pretreatment liver biopsies for psoriatics[14] but not patients with rheumatoid arthritis. Currently, for psoriatics with no hepatic risk factors, a liver biopsy is suggested every time the cumulative dose of methotrexate reaches 1.5 g,[6,14] with a suggestion that 3.5 to 4 g of cumulative methotrexate may be a more appropriate time frame for the first liver biopsy.[18] However, if a history of significant liver disease exists, a liver biopsy should be considered at baseline,[20] or else delayed for 2 to 6 months (until drug efficacy and tolerability has been established),[18] with a repeated liver biopsy at a cumulative dose of 1 to 1.5 g, then repeated with every additional 1 to 1.5 g of methotrexate.[18] For lab monitoring of hepatotoxicity, patients without hepatic risk factors require liver chemistry evaluation every 1 to 3 months.[18,20] In patients with hepatic risk factors (history of or current alcohol intake greater than moderate, persistent abnormal liver chemistries, history of liver disease including chronic hepatitis B or C, family history

of inheritable liver disease, obesity, renal insufficiency, advanced age, hypoalbuminemia, on other hepatotoxic medications, etc.),[18,20] liver chemistries should be monitored more frequently.[20] Besides hepatotoxicity, methotrexate, even in low doses used in psoriasis, may cause leukopenia, megaloblastic anemia, pneumonitis, and pulmonary fibrosis. Complete blood cell counts (CBC; 7 to 14 days after starting or increasing the dose, every 2 to 4 weeks for the first few months, then every 1 to 3 months),[20] renal function tests (every 2 to 3 months),[20] and pulmonary toxicity testing should also be routinely conducted.[15,18,20,24] A pregnancy test is indicated in women of child-bearing potential, as methotrexate is an abortifacient and teratogen (Pregnancy Class X).[18] Drug interactions are numerous and include protein binding interactions (salicylates, sulfonamides, etc.), renal excretion interactions (salicylates, probenecid, acidic drugs including high-dose ascorbic acid, etc.), and concomitant hepatotoxic drug interactions (alcohol, statins, retinoids, azathioprine, etc.)[18]

Methotrexate and UVB appear synergistic; responses may occur at lower cumulative doses of both methotrexate and UVB.[31] However, stopping methotrexate may cause rebound,[31] and there is concern about photosensitivity.[14,18,20] Methotrexate and PUVA have been used in patients refractory to other treatments; however, there is increased risk of squamous cell cancer and phototoxicity.

Methotrexate has been used successfully with cyclosporine, either concurrently[32] or in rotation. Rotational therapy effectively minimizes the serious adverse effects of both agents: Hepatotoxicity from methotrexate and nephrotoxicity and hypertension from cyclosporine. However, rotational therapy is less commonly used today.

Cyclosporine is efficacious in both inducing remission and in maintenance therapy for patients with moderate to severe plaque psoriasis and is also effective in treating pustular, erythrodermic, and nail psoriasis.[14,15,21,22] Cyclosporine is used in low doses whether alone or in combination with other agents. The usual dose range is 2 to 2.5 mg/kg/day, given orally in two divided doses, for patients with stable generalized psoriasis or for moderate to severe disease.[21,22] Failing an adequate response with low-dose cyclosporine after 4 weeks of treatment, the dose can be increased in 0.5 to 1 mg/kg/day increments every 2 to 4 weeks to a maximum of 5 mg/kg/day.[18,22] For patients with severe inflammatory flares of psoriasis, or recalcitrant cases who fail to respond to numerous other therapies, or for a highly distressed patient in a crisis situation, the starting dose is higher at 4 to 5 mg/kg/day[21,22] in two divided doses. Doses can be adjusted by 0.5 to 1 mg/kg/day every 2 weeks to the lowest effective dose.[21,22] Cyclosporine should normally be used intermittently for short term (12 weeks)[14] to minimize drug toxicity. If relapse occurs, cyclosporine can be reinstituted at the previously established effective dose.[22] It has been proposed that continuous cyclosporine (for up to 2 years) may be appropriate for a subset of patients.[14,21] In the United States, cyclosporine is approved for only up to 1 year of continuous therapy at a time.[5] Cyclosporine is contraindicated in psoriatic patients with abnormal renal function, uncontrolled hypertension, malignancy (except for nonmelanoma skin cancer), prior treatment with PUVA, uncontrolled infection, and primary or secondary immunodeficiency excluding autoimmune disease.[18]

Blood pressure and serum creatinine (SCr) should be assessed prior to beginning cyclosporine therapy to obtain accurate baselines and should be reassessed biweekly once therapy is started for at least the first 12 weeks of therapy (until values stabilize), and then closely monitored during therapy (e.g., monthly). If SCr increases to greater than 25% above the patient's baseline on two occasions 2 weeks apart, the cyclosporine dosage needs to be decreased by 25% to 50% and SCr rechecked every other week for a month.[18,21] If the SCr does not return to within 10% of the patient's baseline, another dose decrease of 25% to 50% should be considered.[21] If the Scr still does not return to 10% of the patient's baseline, cyclosporine should be discontinued and only resumed when the SCr returns to within 10% of the patient's baseline.[21,23] Besides impaired renal function and hypertension, cyclosporine may cause hypertriglyceridemia, hypomagnesemia, hyperuricemia, and hypertrichosis and increase the risk of lymphomas and cutaneous malignancies after long-term treatment.[6,14,18,21] Patients should have a careful physical exam (for malignancy) and appropriate blood work prior to initiation of therapy. Testing for TB should be considered.[18] There are clinically significant drug and food interactions (e.g., grapefruit juice) since cyclosporine is metabolized by cytochrome P450 3A4.[5,18,21] Patients taking greater than 3 mg/kg/day, on drugs with potential interaction, or who have liver disease may require monitoring of cyclosporine blood levels.[18]

The combination of cyclosporine with calcipotriol, SCAT, or topical corticosteroids may all be effective.[18,21] Cyclosporine and calcipotriol may be more efficacious than either agent used alone.[33] However, cyclosporine *should not* be used concurrently with PUVA: a well-documented increased risk of squamous cell cancer exists, and the combination may have a negative effect on lesion clearance.[18] Cyclosporine alternating with methotrexate is extremely effective and minimizes toxicity from either agent. Cyclosporine has also been used successfully with mycophenolate mofetil[34] and fumaric acid esters.[22]

Mycophenolate mofetil was found useful in patients with cyclosporine-induced nephrotoxicity as a switch-over agent: although PASI increased, patients' renal function improved.[35] As adjunctive or monotherapy, there are a few studies in relatively small groups of patients with moderate to severe psoriasis that showed some benefit (at least a 50% reduction in PASI).[18,35]

Fumaric acid esters (fumarates) are commonly used in Europe for the treatment of moderate to severe psoriasis but is not approved in the United States.[18] Hydroxyurea is an older agent still used occasionally today for patients with psoriasis, although there is no FDA-approved use for psoriasis,[18] and there have been precautions about its use in the elderly and cutaneous vasculitic toxicities in patients with myeloproliferative disorders. Toxicity associated with systemic tacrolimus has limited its use in psoriasis.

Azathioprine has a slow onset and significant toxicity. Oral corticosteroids are reserved for severe or life-threatening conditions such as severe psoriatic arthritis or exfoliative psoriasis; prolonged oral steroid use should be avoided.

▶ *Biologic Response Modifiers (BRMs)*

Based on recent advances in our understanding of the pathogenesis and pathophysiology of psoriasis, there was accompanying research into the development and use of BRMs for psoriasis and psoriatic arthritis. *Some BRMs have proven efficacy for psoriasis; however, there are differences among these agents, including mechanism of action, duration of remission, and adverse-effect profile. Currently, BRMs are often considered for patients with moderate to severe psoriasis when other systemic agents are inadequate or relatively contraindicated. It has also been recommended that BRMs be considered as first-line therapy, alongside conventional systemic agents, for patients with moderate to severe psoriasis; however, in practice, drug access due to cost considerations may be a limiting factor. They may be appropriate if comorbidities exist.* ⑩ BRMs with proven efficacy for psoriasis include alefacept, etanercept, adalimumab, infliximab, and ustekinumab. These agents employ the following targeted immunosuppressive strategies: alefacept inhibits T-cell activation by targeting LFA-3–CD2 and inducing apoptosis in memory T cells[1]; etanercept, adalimumab, and infliximab are all TNF-α inhibitors[1,6,14]; ustekinumab targets IL-12 and IL-23. There are other biologic agents in clinical trials for psoriasis. ⑩ *In general, due to their immunosuppressive effects, there is an increased risk of infection (including life-threatening severe infections) with most of these agents.* In particular, efalizumab was withdrawn in the United States by the company (in consultation with the FDA) due to serious adverse CNS effects from viral causes. ⑩ *The use of live or live-attenuated vaccines during therapy is generally not recommended.*

The most promising types of BRMs are monoclonal antibodies, cytokines, and fusion proteins.[1] Monoclonal antibodies may be chimeric (fused mouse and human segments; designated "-ximab"), humanized with intermittent murine sequences (designated "-zumab"), human backbone with monkey sequences, or fully human.[35]

Alefacept is a recombinant dimeric fusion protein composed of the extracellular CD2-binding portion of lymphocyte function–associated antigen (LFA)-3 linked to the constant portion of human IgG.[6,14,35] Alefacept inhibits T-cell activation by binding to their CD2 sites and also interacts with natural killer cells to destroy already activated T cells.[1,6] It is approved for moderate to severe chronic plaque psoriasis patients who are candidates for systemic agents or phototherapy.[6] Alefacept is intended for intermittent rather than continuous use. About one-third of alefacept-treated patients enter prolonged remissions ranging from 6 to 18 months. Alefacept appears to spare helper T-cell function and does not significantly impair primary or secondary antibody responses (e.g., the ability to combat infections or respond to vaccinations). A significant risk of malignancy exists. Common side effects include lymphopenia, myalgias/chills, pharyngitis, cough, nausea, and for intramuscular (IM) injections, pain and inflammation at the injection site.[15,36] The dosage recommended is 15 mg IM once weekly for 12 weeks provided the $CD4^+$ T-cell count is normal (defined as greater than or equal to 250 cells/mm^3 [250 ×10^6 cells/L]). Biweekly monitoring of CD4 counts is required during treatment.[6] Dosing should be held for counts less than 250 cells/mm^3 (250 ×10^6 cells/L) and discontinued if the $CD4^+$ count remains below 250 cells/mm^3 (250 ×10^6 cells/L) for four consecutive weeks.[6] Maximal response generally occurs 6 to 8 weeks after the last IM injection of the 12-week course.[6,37] The regimen may be repeated when the loss of control becomes unacceptable up to twice per year[14] and if CD4 counts are normal. Although predictive markers for which patients will respond are currently unknown, those who achieve a PASI-75 or greater tend to maintain a 50% or greater reduction in PASI for a median duration of 10 months.[6] Alefacept is contraindicated in human immunodeficiency virus–positive patients due to the potential for accelerating disease progression from CD4 count reduction.[6] Alefacept in combination with NB-UVB reduces the number of UVB treatments that would otherwise be needed.[14]

The three TNF-α inhibitors etanercept, infliximab, and adalimumab discussed next share common safety concerns, including serious infections (sepsis, new-onset or reactivation tuberculosis [TB], and opportunistic infections such as histoplasmosis, cryptococcosis, aspergillosis, candidiasis, and Pneumocystis), autoimmune conditions (lupus and demyelinating disorders), and malignancies such as lymphoma.[14,15] Although the above are safety concerns common to etanercept, adalimumab, and infliximab, their safety profiles are not identical (e.g., the risk for TB is lowest with etanercept and highest with infliximab).[15]

Etanercept is a fully human dimeric fusion protein composed of human TNF-α p75 receptor fused to the Fc portion of human IgG1.[6] It acts as a TNF-α inhibitor by binding to and inactivating soluble and membrane-bound TNF-α, thus preventing interactions with its cell surface receptors.[6] Etanercept is approved for chronic moderate to severe plaque psoriasis and for psoriatic arthritis. Dosing in psoriasis is different from its other indications (rheumatoid arthritis, juvenile rheumatoid arthritis, and ankylosing spondylitis).[6] The approved psoriasis regimen is 50 mg subcutaneously twice weekly for the first 12 weeks followed by 50 mg weekly thereafter, dosing being continuous.[6] In clinical trials, 49% of patients given 50 mg subcutaneously twice weekly achieved a 75% improvement in PASI by 12 weeks.[38] Clinical responses continue to improve with longer treatment,[6,38] but some patients show a loss of response after 12 weeks when the dose is reduced to once weekly.[6] Etanercept seems well tolerated; common side effects include mild injection site reactions, headache, increased respiratory tract infections (colds and sinusitis), and GI symptoms.[6,38] There are increased risks of tuberculosis[6] and hepatitis B reactivation. Serious infections including fatalities have been reported, and there were reports of worsening congestive heart failure (CHF) and new-onset

CHF.[15] Due to rare reports of blood disorders (anemia, aplastic anemia, leukopenia, neutropenia, pancytopenia, and thrombocytopenia), patients are advised to contact their doctor if they experience persistent fever, bruising, bleeding, or paleness.[15] Baseline and yearly purified protein derivative (PPD) and periodic CBC and liver function tests (LFTs) are recommended while on treatment.[6] Etanercept is effective in children and adolescents (aged 4 to 17) with plaque psoriasis. Fifty-seven percent of patients receiving etanercept 0.8 mg/kg once weekly (to a maximum of 50 mg) achieved PASI-75.[6,39]

Infliximab is a chimeric human/murine monoclonal antibody against TNF-α that binds to both soluble and transmembrane TNF-α molecules. It is approved for both psoriasis and psoriatic arthritis. Dosing for these patients is 5 mg/kg IV over 2 to 3 hours at weeks 0, 2, and 6 and continuously every 8 weeks thereafter.[6] Approximately 80% of patients achieved PASI-75 by 10 weeks (after 3 doses of infliximab); however, by week 50, only about 60% of patients maintained PASI-75.[40,41] Significant adverse effects from postmarketing experience and clinical trials have included hematologic abnormalities (leukopenia, neutropenia, thrombocytopenia, and pancytopenia), hepatotoxicity (rarely: acute liver failure, jaundice, hepatitis, and cholestasis), hypersensitivity reactions (anaphylaxis, urticaria, and serum sickness), ocular toxicity (optic neuritis and optic neuropathy), CHF exacerbation and new-onset CHF, and increased infections (tuberculosis, hepatitis B reactivation, *Listeria monocytogenes* infections, fungal infections, and sepsis). There is an increased risk of infection by live vaccines, and vaccination with live vaccines while receiving infliximab therapy is not recommended. Recommended baseline and ongoing monitoring include yearly PPD, LFTs, and CBC.[6]

Adalimumab is a fully human TNF-α inhibitor approved for treatment of psoriasis and psoriatic arthritis. The dosage in psoriasis is 80 mg subcutaneously in the first week, followed by 40 mg the following week, and 40 mg subcutaneously every 2 weeks thereafter continuously.[6] With this regimen, 71% of patients achieved PASI-75 by 16 weeks of treatment.[42] These clinical benefits were maintained for at least 1 year with continuous therapy, although about 10% of patients who were initially considered responsive became inadequately responsive with further therapy.[14,42] Exclude patients with active or latent TB infection (tuberculin PPD skin test) prior to therapy. There is an increased risk of serious infections (especially respiratory infections including pneumonia and tuberculosis, and hepatitis B reactivation), of exacerbation in heart failure patients, and of lymphoma. Hematologic abnormalities (pancytopenia, thrombocytopenia, and leukopenia) have occurred rarely. Positive antinuclear antibody titers and a lupus syndrome have been reported. Anti-ds DNA antibody determinations are recommended in patients presenting with lupus-like symptoms during adalimumab therapy. A pruritic urticarial eruption that lessens in severity with each subsequent injection has been reported. Rebound does not usually occur.[6]

Ustekinumab is an IL-12/23 monoclonal antibody recently approved for treatment of moderate to severe psoriasis in the United States and Canada. Approximately 70% of patients achieved 75% skin clearance, and the response was maintained for 1 year with continued treatment.[43] A longer-term follow-up study indicated that clinical responses were durable, and improvements in PASI scores can be maintained through 148 weeks with continued every-12-weeks maintenance therapy.[44] Interestingly, ustekinumab was found to significantly improve symptoms of anxiety and depression, in addition to skin-related quality of life, for patients with moderate to severe psoriasis,[45] which was maintained through 3 years among responders.[46] Dosing is 45 mg for patients weighing 220 lb (100 kg) or less, and 90 mg for those over 220 lb (100 kg),[5] given subcutaneously at weeks 0, 4, then every 12 weeks thereafter. Common side effects include upper respiratory infections, headache, and tiredness. Serous side effects include those seen with other BRMs such as serious infections (e.g., tuberculosis, fungal, viral) and cancer risk; in addition, a reversible posterior leukoencephalopathy syndrome (RPLS) has been reported.[15]

▶ Natural Health Products and Treatments

Several natural health products are considered possibly effective for psoriasis. The most promising is Mahonia aquifolium (Oregon grape). This is not a grape, but a plant with blue-violet berries, native to southern British Columbia, western Oregon, and northern Idaho, and is the state flower of Oregon. An extract from the medicinal part of the plant, the rhizome and root, has been formulated into a 10% topical cream/lotion (Relieva, Apollo Pharmaceuticals) and is marketed in Canada for the treatment of psoriasis. This product was shown in several recent clinical trials to modestly decrease the severity of psoriasis and improve the quality of life for patients with mild to moderate psoriasis.[47] Preliminary research suggests similar efficacy as calcipotriene cream.[47] Adverse effects include a burning sensation, irritation, redness, itching, and possible allergic reactions. Heliotherapy is the exposure to natural ultraviolet radiation from sunlight, and there are limited randomized controlled trials of supervised heliotherapy versus no intervention that show efficacy. There are risks of photoaging and skin cancers, including basal cell and squamous cell carcinoma.

Other natural health products possibly effective include an aloe vera extract 0.5% cream and an omega-3 fatty acid–based lipid IV infusion (with docosahexaenoic acid [DHA] and eicosapentaenoic acid [EPA]). Oral supplementation with dietary fish oils containing DHA and EPA may possibly be effective. More research into these natural health products is required before they can be recommended for psoriasis.

OUTCOME EVALUATION

- Monitor for clearance of skin lesions. Depending on the agent(s) used and site of lesions, it may take 2 to 6 weeks or longer to see a response. Complete clearance may not be achieved for all patients.

Patient Encounter, Part 5

It was decided by the treating dermatologist to begin systemic therapy but not biologic therapy at this time. The choices were to treat with either methotrexate or cyclosporine to control the flare-ups. Both alternatives with their respective pros and cons were presented to the patient and discussed with the patient, with the choice being ultimately up to the patient.

What lab tests or other measurements would be important to perform prior to starting therapy with methotrexate? With cyclosporine?

What dosing regimen would be appropriate for methotrexate? For cyclosporine?

What monitoring plan would be appropriate during therapy with methotrexate? With cyclosporine?

- Monitor for specific adverse effects and drug interactions, depending on agent(s) used. Some agents are noted below, others (e.g., BRMs) were individually discussed earlier.

- Methotrexate: Monitor CBC and liver function tests at baseline and regularly, and consider liver biopsy prior to treatment and at a cumulative dose of 1.5 g for high-risk patients, as discussed earlier in the chapter. Monitor pulmonary function.

- Cyclosporine: Monitor SCr, blood urea nitrogen, serum lipids, magnesium, and blood pressure at baseline and reassess biweekly for at least 12 weeks (or longer until values stabilize), then regularly. Adjust doses when needed in response to SCr changes as discussed earlier.

- Acitretin: Monitor serum lipids and liver function tests. Pregnancy testing.

- Topical corticosteroids: Monitor for skin thinning, telangiectasias, and possible hypothalamic–pituitary–adrenal axis suppression.

SUMMARY

It is important to remember that psoriasis is a lifelong illness with no known cure and often has a significant psychosocial component. This disease may be very visible and emotionally distressing and can cause significant disability both physically and psychologically, affecting psychosocial functioning and quality of life. Empathy and a caring attitude can go a long way in the care of these patients.[48]

Acknowledgments

In the first edition, portions of this chapter had been adapted from the following article: Law RM. Psoriasis: An update. Pharm Pract 2005:21:CE 1–7. With permission from the publisher.

Patient Care and Monitoring

With respect to pharmacologic therapies, it is important to:

1. Provide patients with an approximate time frame for improvement based on the patient's areas of involvement and type of drug therapy. For example, a statement such as: "There should be less scaling and redness of your scalp lesions and a reduction in the thickly crusted areas within 1 to 2 weeks. You should notice a general improvement in your condition by 6 to 12 weeks. Your palms, soles, elbows, and knees may take longer to clear."

2. Provide appropriate advice about drug regimens, including how to apply a specific topical agent, how to use a specific systemic agent, and precautions and possible toxicities of any drug therapy, remembering that topical therapies can have significant systemic adverse effects.

3. Check the patient profile and talk with the patient to ensure that there are no significant drug interactions with other concurrent medications and therapies.

4. Reinforce the importance of adherence to therapies and specific drug regimens.

5. Reinforce the importance of regular follow-up with the patient's healthcare providers, including all appointments for follow-up care and lab work (if any).

6. Interact with the patient's other healthcare providers as needed to discuss patient concerns or issues detected, including drug interactions, nonadherence, other comorbidities, and adverse effects.

Abbreviations Introduced in This Chapter

AAD	American Academy of Dermatology
APC	Antigen-presenting cells
BB-UVB	Broadband ultraviolet B
BAD	British Academy of Dermatology
BMI	Body mass index
BRM	Biologic response modifier
BS	Bowel sounds
BSA	Body surface area
CHF	Congestive heart failure
DHA	Docosahexaenoic acid
DISH	Diffuse idiopathic skeletal hyperostosis
EPA	Eicosapentaenoic acid
ICAM-1	Intracellular cell adhesion molecules
IF-γ	Interferon-*gamma*
IL-2	Interleukin-2
IL-12/23	Interleukin-12 and interleukin-23
LFA-3	Leukocyte function–associated antigen type 3
LFT	Liver function test
MED	Minimal erythema dose
MI	Myocardial infarction
NB-UVB	Narrowband ultraviolet B
PASI	Psoriasis Area and Severity Index
PIIINP	The aminoterminal propeptide of type III procollagen
PML	Progressive multifocal leukoencephalopathy
PPD	Purified protein derivative
PsA	Psoriatic arthritis
PSORS1	Psoriasis susceptibility 1
PSORS9	Psoriasis susceptibility 9
PUVA	Psoralens + ultraviolet A
RePUVA	Oral retinoid + PUVA
ReUVB	Acitretin + ultraviolet B
RRR	Regular rate and rhythm
SCAT	Short-contact anthralin therapy
TNF	Tumor necrosis factor
UVB	Ultraviolet B

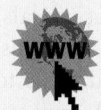 Self-assessment questions and answers are available at *http://mhpharmacotherapy.com/pp.html*.

REFERENCES

1. Schon MP, Boehncke WH. Psoriasis. N Engl J Med 2005;352: 1899–1912.
2. Clarke C. Psoriasis—First-line treatments. Pharm J 2005;274:623–626.
3. Lowes MA, Bowcock AM, Krueger JG. Pathogenesis and therapy of psoriasis. Nature 2007;445(7130):866–873.
4. Godic A. New approaches to psoriasis treatment. A review. Acta Dermatovenerol Alp Panonica Adriat 2004;13(2):50–57.
5. Menter A, Korman NJ, Elmets CA, et al. Guidelines of Care for the management of psoriasis and psoriatic arthritis. Section 6. Guidelines of care for the treatment of psoriasis and psoriatic arthritis: Case-based presentations and evidence-based conclusions. J Am Acad Dermatol 2011;65:137–174.
6. Menter A. Gottlieb A, Feldman SR, et al. Guidelines of care for the management of psoriasis and psoriatic arthritis. Section 1. Overview of psoriasis and guidelines of care for the treatment of psoriasis with biologics. J Am Acad Dermatol 2008;58:826–850.
7. Kimball AB, Gladman D, Gelfand JM, et al. National Psoriasis Foundation clinical consensus on psoriasis comorbidities and recommendations for screening. J Am Acad Dermatol 2008;58:1031–1042.
8. Kremers HM, McEvoy MT, Dann FJ, et al. Heart disease in psoriasis. J Am Acad Dermatol 2007;57:347–354.
9. Nestle FO, Kaplan DH, Barker J. Mechanisms of disease: Psoriasis. N Engl J Med 2009;361:496–509.
10. Rahman R, Elder JT. Genetic epidemiology of psoriasis and psoriatic arthritis. Ann Rheum Dis 2005;64(Suppl II):ii37–ii39.

11. Veale DJ, Ritchlin C, FitzGerald O. Immunopathology of psoriasis and psoriatic arthritis. Ann Rheum Dis 2005;64(Suppl II):ii26–ii29.

12. Ellis CN, Krueger GG. Treatment of chronic plaque psoriasis by selective targeting of memory effector T lymphocytes. N Engl J Med 2001;345:248–255.

13. Lui H, Langley R, Poulin Y, et al. Incorporating biologics into the treatment of psoriasis. J Cutan Med Surg 2004;8(Suppl):8–13.

14. Papp KA, Gulliver W, Lynde CW, Poulin Y (Steering Committee). 2009 Canadian Guidelines for the Management of Plaque Psoriasis—Canadian Guidelines for the Management of Plaque Psoriasis. Waterloo, Ontario, Canada: Canadian Dermatology Association; June 2009.

15. Law RM, Gulliver WP. Psoriasis. In: DiPiro JT, Talbert RT, Yee GCY, Matzke GR, Wells BG, Posey LM, eds. Pharmacotherapy: A Pathophysiologic Approach. 8th ed. New York: McGraw-Hill; 2011:1693–1706.

16. Gottlieb A, Korman NJ, Gordon KB, et al. Guidelines of care for the management of psoriasis and psoriatic arthritis. Section 2. Psoriatic arthritis: overview and guidelines of care for treatment with an emphasis on the biologics. J Am Acad Dermatol 2008;59:851–864.

17. Menter A, Korman NJ, Elmets CA, et al. Guidelines of care for the management of psoriasis and psoriatic arthritis. Section 3. Guidelines of care for the management and treatment of psoriasis with topical therapies. J Am Acad Dermatol 2009;60:643–659.

18. Menter A, Korman NJ, Elmets CA, et al. Guidelines of care for the management of psoriasis and psoriatic arthritis. Section 4. Guidelines of care for the management and treatment of psoriasis with traditional systemic agents. J Am Acad Dermatol 2009;61:451–485.

19. Menter A, Korman NJ, Elmets CA, et al. Guidelines of care for the management of psoriasis and psoriatic arthritis. Section 5. Guidelines of care for the treatment of psoriasis with phototherapy and photochemotherapy. J Am Acad Dermatol 2010;62:114–135.

20. Kalb RE, Strober B, Weinstein G, Lebwohl M. Methotrexate and psoriasis: 2009 National Psoriasis Foundation Consensus Conference. J Am Acad Dermatol 2009;60(5):824–837.

21. Rosmarin DM, Lebwohl M, Elewski BE, et al. Cyclosporine and psoriasis: 2008 National psoriasis Foundation Consensus Conference. J Am Acad Dermatol 2010;62:838–853.

22. Amor KT, Ryan C, Menter A. The use of cyclosporine in dermatology: Part I. J Am Acad Dermatol 2010;63:925–946.

23. Ryan C, Amor KT, Menter A. The use of cyclosporine in dermatology: Part II. J Am Acad Dermatol 2010;63:949–972.

24. Law RM, Gulliver WP. Psoriasis. In: Schwinghammer T, Koehler J, eds. Pharmacotherapy Casebook: A Patient-Focused Approach. 8th ed. New York: McGraw-Hill; 2011:289–291.

25. Speight EL, Farr PM. Calcipotriol improves the response of psoriasis to PUVA. Br J Dermatol 1994;130:79–82.

26. Frappaz A, Thivolet J. Calcipotriol in combination with PUVA: A randomized double blind placebo study in severe psoriasis. Eur J Dermatol 1993;3:351–354.

27. Ashcroft DM, Li WPA, Williams HC, Griffiths CE. Combination regimens of topical calcipotriene in chronic plaque psoriasis: Systematic review of efficacy and tolerability. Arch Dermatol 2000;136:1536–1543.

28. Lebwohl M, Hecker D, Martinez J, et al. Interactions between calcipotriene and ultraviolet light. J Am Acad Dermatol 1997;37:93–95.

29. Behrens S, Grundmann-Kollmann M, Peter RU, et al. Combination treatment of psoriasis with photochemotherapy and tazarotene gel, a receptor-selective topical retinoid. Br J Dermatol 1999;141:177.

30. Hecker D, Worsley J, Yueh G, et al. Interactions between tazarotene and ultraviolet light. J Am Acad Dermatol 1999;41:927–930.

31. Paul BS, Momtaz K, Stern RS, et al. Combined methotrexate—ultraviolet B therapy in the treatment of psoriasis. J Am Acad Dermatol 1982;7:758–762.

32. Clark CM, Kirby B, Morris AD, et al. Combination treatment with methotrexate and cyclosporin for severe recalcitrant psoriasis. Br J Dermatol 1999;141:279–282.

33. Grossman RM, Thivolet J, Claudy A, et al. A novel therapeutic approach to psoriasis with combination calcipotriol ointment and very low-dose cyclosporine: Results of a multicenter placebo-controlled study. J Am Acad Dermatol 1994;31:68–74.

34. Orvis AK, Wesson SK, Breza TS, et al. Mycophenolate mofetil in dermatology. J Am Acad Dermatol 2009;60:183–199.

35. Walsh SRA, Shear NH. Psoriasis and the new biologic agents: Interrupting a T-AP dance. Can Med Assoc J 2004;170(13):1933–1941.

36. Gottlieb G, Casale TB, Frankel E, et al. CD4+ T-cell-directed antibody responses are maintained in patients with psoriasis receiving alefacept: Results of a randomized study. J Am Acad Dermatol 2003;49:816–825.

37. Menter A, Cather JC, Baker D, et al. The efficacy of multiple courses of alefacept in patients with moderate to severe chronic plaque psoriasis. J Am Acad Dermatol 2006;54:61–63.

38. Leonardi CL, Powers JL, Matheson RT, et al. Etanercept as monotherapy in patients with psoriasis. N Engl J Med 2003;349:2014–2022.

39. Paller AS, Siegfried EC, Langley RG, et al. Etanercept treatment for children and adolescents with plaque psoriasis. N Engl J Med 2008;358:241–251.

40. Reich K, Nestle FO, Papp K, et al. Infliximab induction and maintenance therapy for moderate-to-severe psoriasis: A phase III, multicenter, double-blind trial. Lancet 2005;366:1367–1374.

41. Menter A, Feldman SR, Weinstein GD. A randomized comparison of continuous vs intermittent infliximab maintenance regimens over 1 year in the treatment of moderate-to-severe plaque psoriasis. J Am Acad Dermatol 2007;56(31):e1–e15.

42. Menter A, Tyring SK, Gordon K, et al. Adalimumab therapy for moderate to severe psoriasis: A randomized, controlled phase III trial. J Am Acad Dermatol 2008;58(1):106–115.

43. Papp KA, Langley RG, Lebwohl M, et al. Efficacy and safety of ustekinumab, a human interleukin-12/23 monoclonal antibody, in patients with psoriasis: 52-week results from a randomized, double-blind placebo-controlled trial (PHOENIX 2). The Lancet 2008;371:1675–1684.

44. Gordon K, Baker D, Guenther L, et al. P3345: Sustained efficacy of ustekinumab for the treatment of moderate to severe psoriasis in initial responders continuing with maintenance therapy through year 3. J Am Acad Dermatol 2011;64(2 Suppl 1):ABS 156.

45. Langley RG, Feldman SR, Han C, et al. Ustekinumab significantly improves symptoms of anxiety, depression, and skin-related quality of life in patients with moderate-to-severe psoriasis: Results from a randomized, double-blind, placebo-controlled phase III trial. J Am Acad Dermatol 2010;63:457–465.

46. Leonardi C, Kimball A, Schenkel B, et al. P3315: Sustained improvement in skin disease–specific quality of life in patients with moderate to severe psoriasis receiving ustekinumab maintenance therapy: Long-term results from PHOENIX 1. J Am Acad Dermatol 2011;64(2 Suppl 1):ABS 149.

47. Gulliver WP, Donsky HJ. A report on three recent clinical trials using Mahonia aquifolium 10% topical cream and a review of the worldwide clinical experience with Mahonia aquifolium for the treatment of plaque psoriasis. Am J Ther 2005;12:398–406.

48. Updike J. From the journal of a leper. Northridge, CA: Lord John Press; 1978:21.

65 Common Skin Disorders

Angie L. Goeser-Iske

KEY CONCEPTS

❶ The development of acne lesions results from four pathogenic factors, which include excess sebum production, keratinization, bacterial growth, and inflammation.

❷ Although eliminating existing lesions and preventing the development of new lesions are primary goals of acne therapy, secondary goals include relieving pain or discomfort and preventing permanent scarring.

❸ Acne is categorized as mild, moderate, or severe based on the lesion type and lesion severity. Successful treatment approaches are developed based on these categories, as well as any previous treatment information presented by the patient.

❹ Irritant contact dermatitis results from first-time exposures to irritating substances such as soaps, plants, cleaning solutions, or solvents. Allergic contact dermatitis occurs after an initial sensitivity and further exposure to allergenic substances, including poison ivy, latex, and certain types of metals.

❺ The initial treatment goal of contact dermatitis is identifying the causative substance and eliminating its exposure. The second treatment goal is symptom relief.

❻ Although many factors contribute to the etiology of diaper rash, it is most likely the result of prolonged contact of the skin with urine and feces in the diaper.

❼ The primary goal in the treatment of diaper rash is prevention and is most often accomplished through frequent diaper changes.

❽ When a diaper rash is already present, repairing the damaged skin, relieving discomfort, and preventing infection are important factors to consider when developing an effective treatment regimen.

INTRODUCTION

The skin is the largest organ of the human body. One of its most important functions is to assist the immune system by serving as a barrier that protects underlying structures from trauma, infection, and exposure to harmful environmental elements. The skin also holds in place essential organs and fluids necessary for life. Any significant injury to this outer protective layer may potentially compromise an individual's overall health.

Several thousand skin disorders are currently documented, and many patients will seek the assistance of a healthcare provider when a complication with their skin develops. Others will utilize methods of self-care to effectively treat their symptoms. Some skin problems, such as mild acne or diaper rash, may be successfully treated with over-the-counter medications and lifestyle modifications. However, if left untreated or treated inadequately, these seemingly simple disorders can worsen and require more advanced care.

As healthcare providers, it is important to be familiar with the diagnosis and treatment of skin disorders. This chapter discusses acne vulgaris, contact dermatitis (irritant and allergic), and diaper dermatitis; other common skin and soft tissue infections and superficial fungal infections are discussed in Chaps. 73 and 83, respectively. Providing patients with appropriate therapy options, as well as patient education on methods of treatment and prevention, will assist the successful resolution of many common skin disorders.

ACNE VULGARIS

Acne vulgaris, an inflammatory skin disorder of the pilosebaceous units of the skin, is the most common dermatologic reason for physician visits in the United States.[1] Although most commonly seen on the face, acne can also present on the chest, back, neck, and shoulders (Fig. 65–1).[2] Although generally a self-limiting condition, long-term physical complications of acne may include extensive scarring and psychological distress.[1,3]

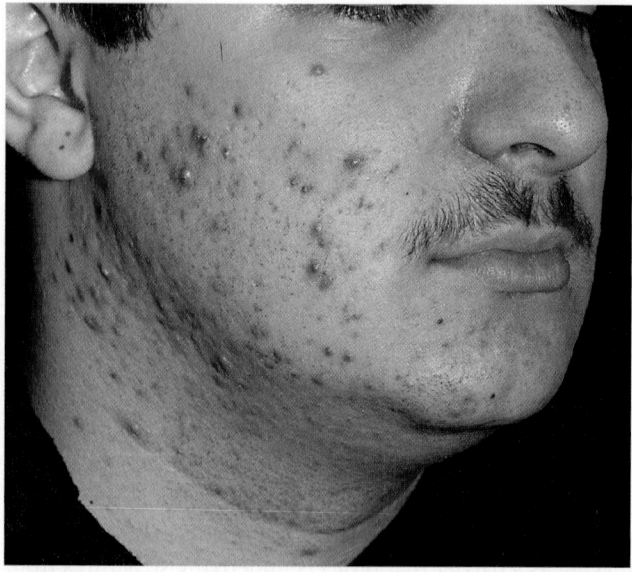

FIGURE 65–1. Twenty-year-old male. In this case of papulopustular acne, some inflammatory papules become nodular and thus represent early stages of nodulocystic acne. (From Wolff K, Johnson RA. Disorders of sebaceous and apocrine glands. Fitzpatrick's Color Atlas & Synopsis of Clinical Dermatology. 6th ed. New York: McGraw-Hill; 2009: 3.)

EPIDEMIOLOGY AND ETIOLOGY

With an estimated 40 to 50 million people affected, acne vulgaris is the number one skin disease in the United States.[3,4] Although acne affects approximately 85% of adolescents and adults aged 12 to 25 years, the disease can develop or recur

in adults aged 30 to 50 years.[5] The prevalence of acne among whites, African Americans, Hispanics, and Asians is similar, with acne occurring more often in males during adolescence and females during adulthood.[6,7]

PATHOPHYSIOLOGY

❶ *The development of acne lesions results from four pathogenic factors: excess sebum production, keratinization, bacterial growth, and inflammation.*[3,7]

The pilosebaceous unit of the skin consists of a hair follicle and the surrounding sebaceous glands. An initial acne lesion called a comedo forms when there is a blockage in the pilosebaceous unit.[8]

Sebum is released by the sebaceous glands and naturally maintains hair and skin hydration. An increase in androgen levels, especially during puberty, can cause an increase in the size of the sebaceous gland and the production of abnormally high levels of sebum within those glands. This excess sebum can result in plugged follicles and acne formation.

Keratinization, the sloughing of epithelial cells in the hair follicle, is also a natural process. In acne, however, *hyper*keratinization occurs and causes increased adhesiveness of the sloughed cells. Accumulation of these cells clogs the hair follicle, blocks the flow of sebum, and forms an acne lesion called an open comedo or "blackhead."

Propionibacterium acnes (*P. acnes*), an anaerobic organism, is also found in the normal flora of the skin. This bacteria proliferates in the mixture of sebum and keratinocytes and can result in an inflammatory response producing a closed comedo or "whitehead." More severe acne lesions such as pustules, papules, and nodules also form with inflammatory acne and result in significant scarring if treated inadequately (see Fig. 65–2 for various stages of acne development).

TREATMENT

Desired Outcomes and Goals

❷ *Although eliminating existing lesions and preventing the development of new lesions are primary goals of acne therapy, secondary goals include relieving pain or discomfort and preventing permanent scarring.*[8] In addition, acne can cause patients a significant amount of stress, anxiety, frustration, embarrassment, and even depression.[6,10] Because of these psychological symptoms, treatment compliance and patient education on both physical and psychological aspects of this skin disorder are also imperative.

General Approach to Treatment

❸ *Acne is categorized as mild, moderate, or severe based on the lesion type and lesion severity (Table 65–1). Successful treatment approaches are developed based on these categories, as well as any previous treatment information presented by the patient.* Improvement of symptoms following treatment

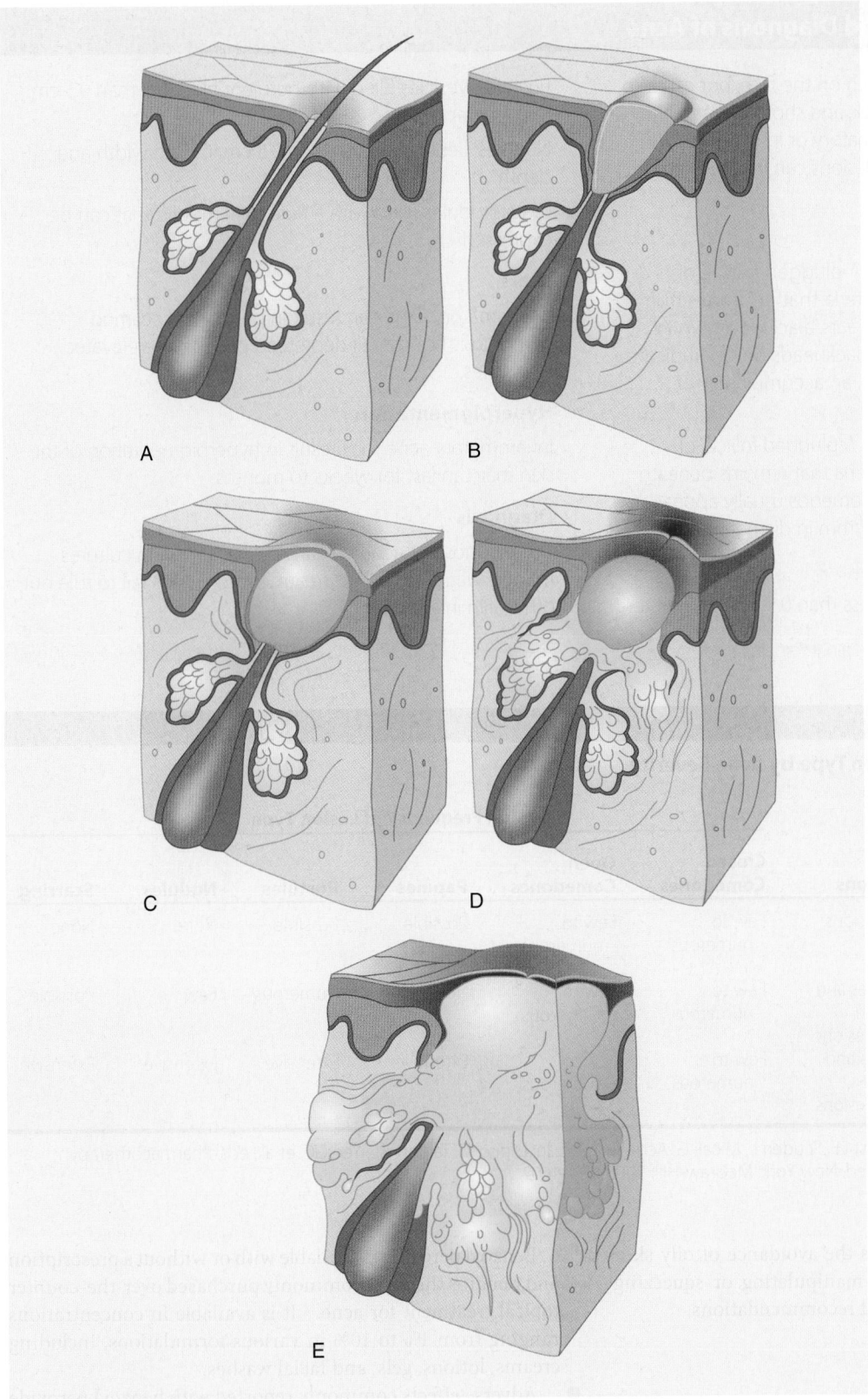

FIGURE 65–2. Stages of acne. A. Normal follicle; B. open comedo (blackhead); C. closed comedo (whitehead); D. papule; E. pustule. (From Hartsock M. Medical illustrations. Cincinnati, OH: The Medical Art Company.)

occurs gradually, sometimes taking 6 to 8 weeks for results to be physically apparent.[8] Patients need to be educated on continual treatment compliance during this time and not get discouraged if acne lesions appear to worsen before getting better during the initial 2 to 3 weeks of therapy.[11]

Nonpharmacologic Therapy

There is significant variance in the clinical benefit of many nonpharmacologic interventions for acne vulgaris. Among nondrug treatment alternatives, mild, noncomedogenic facial

Clinical Presentation and Diagnosis of Acne

Acne lesions are most often seen on the face, but can also present on the chest, back, neck, and shoulders and are described as either noninflammatory or inflammatory. In addition, severe inflammatory lesions can lead to scarring and hyperpigmentation.

Noninflammatory Lesions

Open comedo or "blackhead": A plugged follicle of sebum, keratinocytes, and bacteria that protrudes from the surface of the skin and appears black or brown in color. Although dark in color, blackheads do not indicate the presence of dirt, but rather, an accumulation of melanin.

Closed comedo or "whitehead": A plugged follicle of sebum, keratinocytes, and bacteria that remains beneath the surface of the skin. Closed comedos usually appear as small white bumps about 1 to 2 mm in diameter.

Inflammatory Lesions

Papules: Solid, elevated lesion less than 0.5 cm in diameter

Pustules: Vesicles filled with purulent fluid less than 0.5 cm in diameter

Nodules: Lesions greater than 0.5 cm in both width and depth

Cysts: Nodules filled with a fluid or semisolid that can be expressed

Scars

Inflammatory acne can result in permanent scarring that ranges from small depressed pits to large elevated blemishes.

Hyperpigmentation

Inflammatory acne may result in hyperpigmentation of the skin that can last for weeks to months.

Diagnosis

The diagnosis of acne vulgaris is clinical. Lesion cultures may be warranted when treatment regimens fail to rule out other skin infections.

Table 65–1

Predominance of Acne Lesion Type by Acne Severity

Acne Severity	Predominant Lesions	Typical Frequency of Lesion Type					
		Closed Comedones	Open Comedones	Papules	Pustules	Nodules	Scarring
Mild	Noninflammatory lesions (open and closed comedones)	Few to numerous	Few to numerous	Possible	Possible	None	None
Moderate	Inflammatory papules and pustules with some noninflammatory lesions	Few to numerous	Few to numerous	Numerous	Numerous	Few	Possible
Severe	Inflammatory lesions and scarring with some noninflammatory lesions	Few to numerous	Few to numerous	Extensive	Extensive	Extensive	Extensive

From West DP, Loyd A, Bauer KA, West LE, Scuderi L, Micali G. Acne vulgaris. In: Dipiro JT, Talbert RL, Yee GC, et al., eds. Pharmacotherapy: A Pathophysiological Approach. 7th ed. New York: McGraw-Hill; 2008:1591–1602.

---

soap used twice daily, as well as the avoidance of oily skin products and the avoidance of manipulating or squeezing lesions, are helpful self-treatment recommendations.

Pharmacologic Therapy

▶ Topical Agents

Benzoyl Peroxide Benzoyl peroxide is easy to use and is recommended as first-line therapy in the treatment of mild to moderate noninflammatory acne. Benzoyl peroxide has a comedolytic effect that increases the rate of epithelial cell turnover and helps to unclog blocked pores. It also has antibacterial activity against *P. acnes*, which appears to be the main reason for its effectiveness.[13]

Benzoyl peroxide is available with or without a prescription and remains the most commonly purchased over-the-counter topical treatment for acne.[12] It is available in concentrations ranging from 1% to 10% in various formulations, including creams, lotions, gels, and facial washes.

Adverse effects commonly reported with benzoyl peroxide are dryness, irritation, redness, and stinging of the skin. Reducing the incidence of these effects can be achieved by beginning a treatment regimen with the lowest strength and titrating up to higher effective strengths over several weeks if needed. In addition, newer formulations of benzoyl peroxide are combined with moisturizers to help decrease skin redness and irritation.[13] A disadvantage of the agent is that it can bleach and discolor hair and fabrics that come into contact.[12]

A typical regimen for benzoyl peroxide is to apply the product to clean, dry skin no more than two times a day. The strength and dosage form selected may vary from patient to patient depending on acne severity and the sensitivity of the patient's skin. Since gel preparations are the most potent dosage form, patients with dry or overly sensitive skin should be recommended a milder cream, lotion, or facial wash.[3] If severe irritation or allergic reaction develops, benzoyl peroxide use should be discontinued.

- **Retinoids** Retinoids, which are highly effective in the treatment of acne, stimulate epithelial cell turnover and aid in unclogging blocked pores. Retinoids also exhibit anti-inflammatory properties through the inhibition of neutrophil and monocyte chemotaxis.[8] Because of these comedolytic and anti-inflammatory effects, topical retinoids are recommended as first-line treatment for mild to moderate comedonal and inflammatory acne.[3] Although success is seen with monotherapy, using a retinoid in combination with benzoyl peroxide or topical antibacterials is also an appropriate and effective therapeutic treatment option.[3] Tretinoin, adapalene, and tazarotene are topical retinoids available for use in the treatment of acne. Table 65–2 describes the strengths and formulations of these agents.

- Transient erythema, irritation, dryness, and peeling at the site of application are all common adverse effects. Newer retinoids formulated in either a microsphere gel (Retin-A Micro) or an aqueous-based gel (Atralin) appear to cause less initial skin discomfort than older agents in this class.[13] Photosensitivity can also occur with retinoid use, causing increased skin irritation and redness.[14]

The topical retinoid selected should be applied once daily at bedtime, beginning with a low-potency formulation. Increased strengths are then initiated according to treatment results and tolerance. Patients should be advised that a worsening of acne symptoms generally occurs in the first few weeks of therapy, with lesion improvement occurring in 3 to 4 months.[16] The use of topical retinoids should be avoided in children younger than 12 years and in pregnant women.[14]

- **Antibacterials** Topical antibacterials directly suppress *P. acnes* and are also first-line agents used in the treatment of mild to moderate inflammatory acne.[3,16]

Clindamycin 1% and erythromycin 2% preparations, applied once or twice daily, have similar effects and are the most commonly prescribed topical antibacterial agents.[17] These agents, as well as sodium sulfacetamide, are available in various formulations for the treatment of acne.

- Adverse effects are generally mild and include dryness, erythema, and itching.[18] Although rare and seen most often with oral therapy, pseudomembranous colitis can occur with the prolonged use of topical clindamycin.[19] As with any antibacterial agent, the possibility of resistance exists with the use of topical antibiotics. However, coadministration of clindamycin or erythromycin and benzoyl peroxide has shown to decrease the incidence of resistance, as well as to improve symptoms of mild to moderate inflammatory acne.[7,20]

Azelaic Acid With antibacterial and anti-inflammatory properties, and the ability to stabilize keratinization, azelaic acid is an effective alternative in the treatment of mild to moderate acne in patients who cannot tolerate benzoyl peroxide or topical retinoids.[3,21] It can also even out skin tone and may prove effective in patients who are prone to postinflammatory hyperpigmentation resulting from acne.[22]

- Adverse effects are minimal and transient, with erythema and skin irritation most common.[21]

Azelaic acid 20% cream should be applied twice daily, with improvement of symptoms seen in 1 to 2 months.[21]

- **Dapsone** A sulfone drug, dapsone gel has antimicrobial and anti-inflammatory properties and is approved for patients with mild to moderate acne.[23,24] The development of topical dapsone marks the first new chemically based agent used in the treatment of acne vulgaris in 10 years.

Table 65–2

Topical Retinoids Available for the Treatment of Acne

Agent	Brand Name	Dosage Form	Dosage	Side Effects
Tretinoin	Retin-A	0.025%, 0.05%, and 0.1% cream 0.01%, 0.025% gel	Apply small amount once daily before bedtime	Skin irritation, dryness, photosensitivity, initially may worsen acne
	Retin-A Micro	0.04% and 0.1% gel	Apply small amount once daily before bedtime	Skin irritation, dryness, photosensitivity, initially may worsen acne
	Atralin	0.05% gel	Apply small amount once daily before bedtime	Skin irritation, dryness, peeling/flaking skin
	Ziana	0.025% with 1.2% clindamycin gel	Apply small amount once daily before bedtime	Skin irritation, erythema, scaling, itching
Adapalene	Differin	0.1% cream 0.1% and 0.3% gel 0.1% lotion	Apply small amount once daily before bedtime	Same as tretinoin but may be *less* severe
	Epiduo	0.1% with 2.5% benzoyl peroxide gel	Apply small amount once daily before bedtime	Same as tretinoin but may be *less* severe
Tazarotene	Tazorac	0.05% and 0.1% cream 0.05% and 0.1% gel	Apply small amount once daily before bedtime	Same as tretinoin but may be *more* severe

From Wickersham RM, ed. Drug Facts and Comparisons. St. Louis, MO: Drug Facts and Comparisons; 2011.

The topical gel form appears to be safer, free from the hemolysis, hemolytic anemia, and peripheral neuropathy that can result from orally administered dapsone.[23] Adverse effects are similar to what is seen with other topical acne products and include dryness, erythema, oiliness, and peeling of the skin.[24]

Dapsone 5% (Aczone) is a gritty gel that should be applied in a thin layer to the affected areas twice daily. If after 12 weeks there is no improvement, treatment with topical dapsone should be reevaluated.[24]

Keratolytics Sulfur, resorcinol, and salicylic acid are not as effective as other topical agents, but can be used as second-line therapies in the treatment of mild to moderate acne.[12]

Although these agents may cause less skin irritation than benzoyl peroxide or the topical retinoids, several disadvantages exist. Sulfur preparations produce an unpleasant odor when applied to the skin, whereas resorcinol may cause brown scaling. And although rare, the possibility of salicylism exists with continual salicylic acid use.[3,12]

▶ Oral Agents

Antibacterials Moderate to severe acne can be effectively treated with oral antibiotics, especially when treatment with topical therapy has failed. Because of their ability to decrease *P. acnes* colonization, oral antibiotics can prevent acne lesions from developing.[8] Improvement of symptoms is generally evident at 6 to 10 weeks, with maximum benefits occurring after 6 months of therapy.[25]

Tetracycline, doxycycline, and minocycline are the most commonly prescribed oral antibiotics for acne. Erythromycin and clindamycin are appropriate second-line agents for use when patients cannot tolerate or have developed resistance to tetracycline or its derivatives.[3] Other antibiotics, including trimethoprim (± sulfamethoxazole) and azithromycin, are also effective agents to use when patients fail or are unable

to tolerate conventional treatment.[7] (See Table 65–3 for antibiotic dosing guidelines.)

Adverse effects with the tetracyclines include GI upset; drug interactions with dairy products, antacids, and iron; and phototoxicity. Minocycline can also cause vestibular complications (headache, dizziness) and skin discoloration that is not typical with tetracycline and doxycycline.[16]

Although their effectiveness is similar to the tetracyclines, erythromycin and clindamycin use is often limited due to their potential adverse outcomes. Erythromycin has increased resistance to *P. acnes* and a high incidence of GI intolerance, whereas clindamycin causes diarrhea and the risk of developing pseudomembranous colitis with long-term use.[3,8]

Isotretinoin Isotretinoin is effective in up to 80% of patients with severe nodulocystic acne who are unresponsive to other topical and oral treatment regimens.[8,25,26] Isotretinoin works on the four pathogenic factors that contribute to acne development and can produce acne remission rates of up to several years.

Adverse effects with the use of isotretinoin are frequent and generally dose-related. About 90% of patients experience drying of the mucosa of the mouth, eyes, and nose.[3] Drying, peeling, and pruritus of the facial skin is also likely. Increases in cholesterol and triglyceride levels have been reported with isotretinoin use; therefore, it is recommended to monitor liver function and serum lipids at baseline and at 4 and 8 weeks of therapy to identify any complications. Other serious adverse effects from this medication include increased creatine phosphokinase, increased blood glucose, teratogenicity, photosensitivity, muscle pain, suicidality, and depression.[3] Table 65–4 lists the common adverse effects from isotretinoin therapy and management strategies for those symptoms.

Because it is teratogenic and classified as Pregnancy Category X, the FDA mandates an online registry program called iPLEDGE to ensure that females do not become pregnant while taking isotretinoin. Wholesalers, pharmacies,

---

Table 65–3				
Oral Agents Used in the Treatment of Moderate to Severe Acne				
Drug	**Dosage Form**	**Strength (mg)**	**Regimen**	**Side Effects**
Tetracycline	Tablets, capsules	250 500	500 mg twice daily before meals. Maintenance dose: 500 mg daily	GI upset, phototoxicity, tooth discoloration, drug and food interactions
Doxycycline	Tablets, capsules	50 100	100–200 mg daily before meals. Maintenance dose: 50 mg daily	GI upset, phototoxicity, drug and food interactions
Minocycline	Tablets, capsules	50 75 100	50 mg twice daily or 100 mg once daily Maintenance dose: 50 mg daily	GI upset, phototoxicity, drug and food interactions, vestibular toxicity, skin discoloration
Erythromycin	Tablets	250 500	500 mg twice daily with food Maintenance dose: 500 mg daily	GI intolerance, drug interactions
Clindamycin	Capsules	75 150 300	150–300 mg daily Maintenance dose: 150 mg daily	Diarrhea, pseudomembranous colitis
Isotretinoin	Capsules	10 20 40	0.5–1 mg/kg/day in two divided doses Maximum dose: 2 mg/kg/day Cumulative dose: 120–150 mg/day	Dry skin and mucous membranes, muscle and joint pain, elevated liver enzymes and triglycerides, depression, teratogenicity

From Wickersham RM, ed. Drug Facts and Comparisons. St. Louis, MO: Drug Facts and Comparisons; 2011

Table 65-4

Principle Adverse Effects of Oral Isotretinoin

Adverse Effect	Response
Teratogenicity	Contraindicated during pregnancy
Depression	Patient monitoring and counseling; antidepressants
Dryness	
Mouth	Hard candy
Eyes	Eyedrops; avoid contact lenses if possible during treatment course
Nose	Lubricant
Skin	Nondrying gentle skin cleansers; noncomedolytic moisturizers
Lips	Lip moisturizer with sunscreen
Muscle and joint pain	Nonsteroidal anti-inflammatory drugs
Alopecia	Reversible when drug discontinued or dose decreased
Hypertriglyceridemia	Reversible when drug discontinued or dose decreased
Acne flare at start of therapy	Continue therapy
Photosensitivity	Use sunscreens (moisturizing), protective clothing, and sun avoidance

From West DP, Loyd A, Bauer KA, West LE, Scuderi L, Micali G. Acne vulgaris. In: Dipiro JT, Talbert RL, Yee GC, et al., eds. Pharmacotherapy: A Pathophysiological Approach. 7th ed. New York: McGraw-Hill; 2008:1591–1602.

doctors, and patients must be registered in the iPLEDGE computer-based system in order to control the distribution, prescribing, and dispensing of isotretinoin. Two negative pregnancy tests prior to initiating therapy and one negative pregnancy test each month thereafter must be obtained and confirmed in the system before a prescription can be dispensed to female patients of child-bearing potential. These patients must also commit to effective measures of birth control during the course of isotretinoin therapy. Contact the program at their website: *https://www.ipledgeprogram.com/* for further details.

Initial dose ranges for treatment are 0.5 to 1 mg/kg daily in two divided doses, with beneficial results generally reported at total daily doses of 120 to 150 mg/day.[3]

Oral Contraceptives Oral contraceptives are a valuable second-line treatment option for moderate to severe acne in female patients. Although many contraceptives are effective, three agents *(Yaz, Estrostep, and Ortho Tri-Cyclen)* have been FDA approved for the treatment of acne.[27] Oral contraceptives decrease the production of androgens by the ovaries, which in turn leads to a decrease in sebum production.[3,16]

Adverse effects include nausea, weight gain, breast tenderness, and breakthrough bleeding. Oral contraceptives have also been associated with an increased incidence of thromboembolic disease, particularly in women who use tobacco products or have other risk factors for thromboembolism. The development of these complications is significantly reduced when low-dose estrogen formulations of oral contraceptives are used.[3]

Other Agents Although use is infrequent, several other agents are available as second- or third-line treatment options for acne when first-line therapies fail and include the following[3,7]:

- Corticosteroids
- Chemical peels
- Surgical extraction
- Phototherapy/photodynamic therapy
- Laser treatments

Figure 65-3 shows useful algorithms for the effective treatment of the various stages of acne.

OUTCOME EVALUATION

Depending on severity, complete resolution of acne may take weeks to months. Monitor patients after 6 weeks of pharmacologic therapy for any improvement of signs and symptoms[12]:

- Decreased number of lesions
- Decreased severity of lesions
- Relief of pain/irritation

If no improvement is reported or symptoms have worsened, patients should be reevaluated and a change in the current treatment regimen may be necessary.

Educate patients on the possibility of adverse effects. Consider a change in therapy if a patient experiences effects that are not tolerated or are considered a compromise to their health.

Patient Care and Monitoring: Acne

1. Assess patient symptoms and the presence of acne lesions. Determine severity of acne: mild, moderate, or severe.
2. Review patient history to determine treatment regimens that have been used in the past, including nonprescription, prescription, and herbal medications.
3. Obtain patient's allergy status.
4. Develop a treatment plan appropriate for improvement of acne.
5. Discuss any monitoring parameters that may be necessary throughout the course of therapy.
6. Provide patient education on acne and its treatment:
   a. What is acne and how does it develop?
   b. Physical and psychological complications that can result from acne.
   c. What drug and nondrug therapies are available for treatment?
   d. Describe the possible side effects of drug therapy.
   e. Emphasize the importance of treatment regimen compliance to ensure positive results.

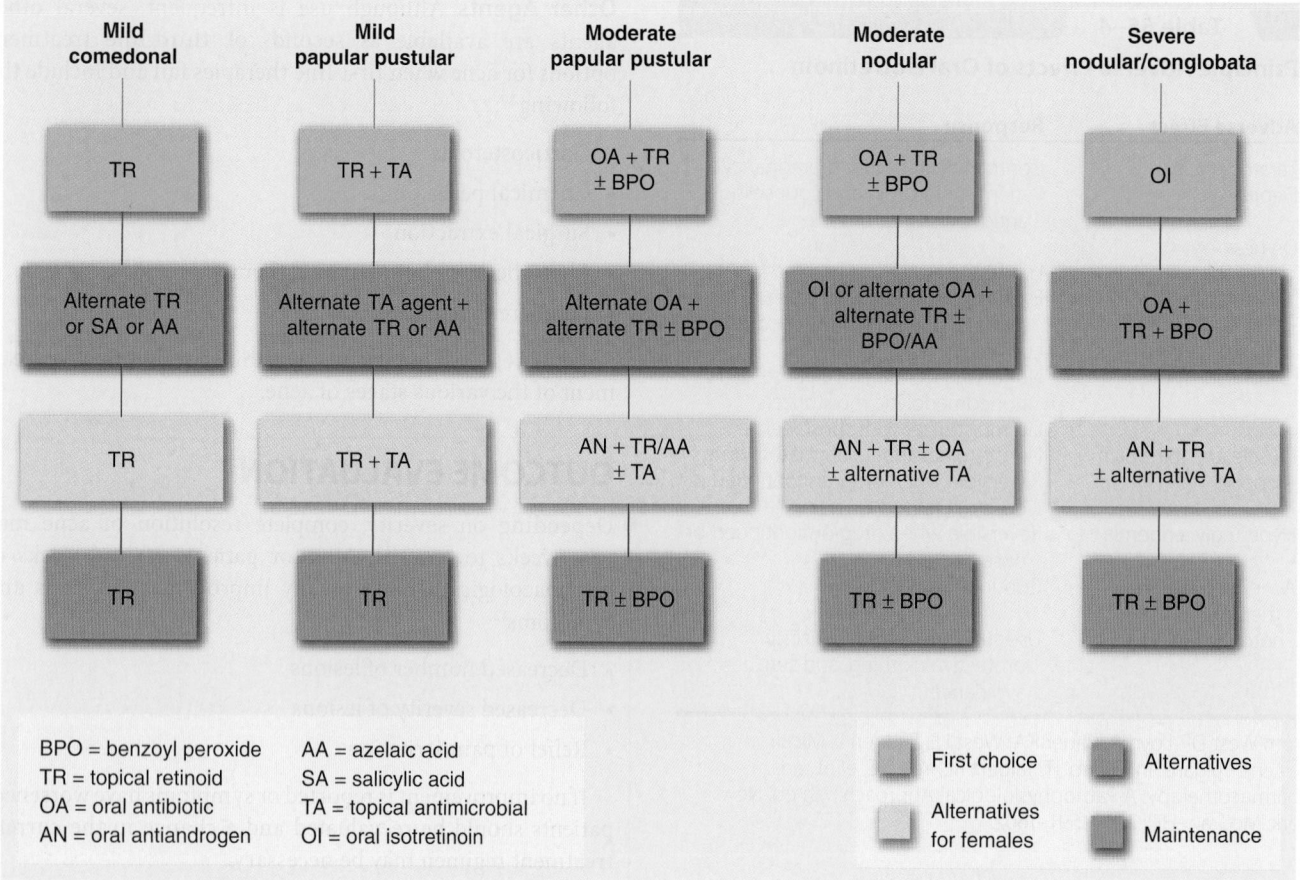

FIGURE 65–3. Algorithms for acne treatment. (From West DP, Loyd A, Bauer KA, West LE, Scuderi L, Micali G. Acne vulgaris. In: Dipiro JT, Talbert RL, Yee GC, et al., eds. Pharmacotherapy: A Pathophysiological Approach. 7th ed. New York: McGraw-Hill; 2008:1591–1602.)

Patient Encounter 1

A 16-year-old adolescent boy presents to your pharmacy with complaints of worsening acne. Upon visual examination, numerous papules, pustules, and nodules are noted on his forehead, cheeks, and chin. It is also apparent that previous breakouts have caused some scarring on his cheeks. After interviewing the patient, you conclude that his acne lesions are extremely painful. He states that he uses various over-the-counter acne washes and topical creams multiple times a day but has seen minimal improvement. He also states that he recalls being prescribed an oral antibiotic for about 3 months when he was 14 years old, but has not seen a physician since. The patient has no other medical complaints and appears to be in good physical health.

What reported symptoms support the diagnosis of acne?

What other information would you obtain from this patient before creating a treatment plan for him?

What professional recommendation would you give to this patient in regard to the current severity of his acne?

Describe your treatment goals for this patient.

What pharmacologic treatment options are available for this patient?

Given the information presented, develop a treatment regimen for this patient that includes the following:

(a) A statement of the problem

(b) A patient-specific therapeutic plan

(c) Monitoring parameters to assess efficacy and safety

CONTACT DERMATITIS

- Contact dermatitis is a condition in which exposure to an offending substance produces inflammation, erythema, and pruritus of the skin.[28] More specifically, contact dermatitis can be divided into either irritant or allergic forms.[28,29] ❹

- *Irritant contact dermatitis results from first-time exposure to irritating substances such as soaps, plants, cleaning solutions, or solvents. Allergic contact dermatitis occurs after an initial sensitivity and further exposure to allergenic substances, including poison ivy, latex, and certain types of metal.*[30] (**Figs. 65–4** and **65–5**.) **Table 65–5** lists agents commonly responsible for irritant and allergic contact dermatitis. Although generally occurring on the exposed skin, such as the hands and face, contact dermatitis can appear anywhere on the body.[28] Although most cases are easily treated, contact dermatitis remains an uncomfortable and sometimes embarrassing skin condition.

EPIDEMIOLOGY AND ETIOLOGY

Contact dermatitis is a common reason for dermatology referrals and constitutes up to 90% of all workers' compensation claims for dermatologic conditions. Although most often seen in adults, contact dermatitis can affect all age groups, with females at slightly greater risk than males.[31]

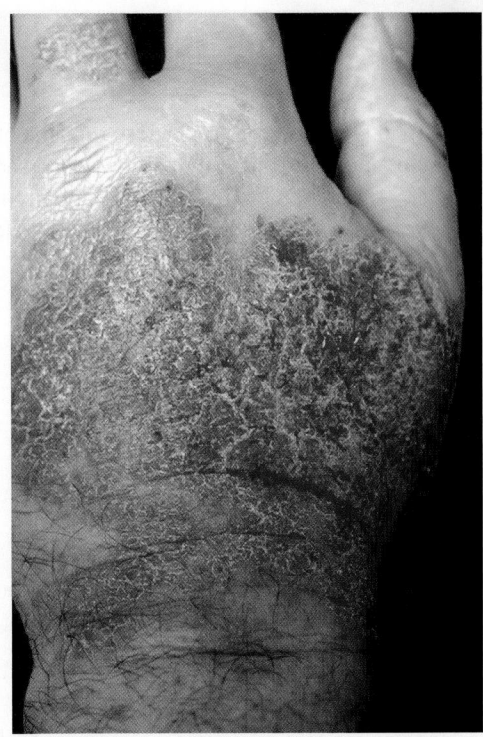

FIGURE 65–5. Allergic contact dermatitis of the hand: chromates. Confluent papules, vesicles, erosions, and crusts on the dorsum of the left hand in a construction worker who was allergic to chromates. (From Wolff K, Johnson RA. Eczema/dermatitis. Fitzpatrick's Color Atlas & Synopsis of Clinical Dermatology. 6th ed. New York: McGraw-Hill; 2009: 27.)

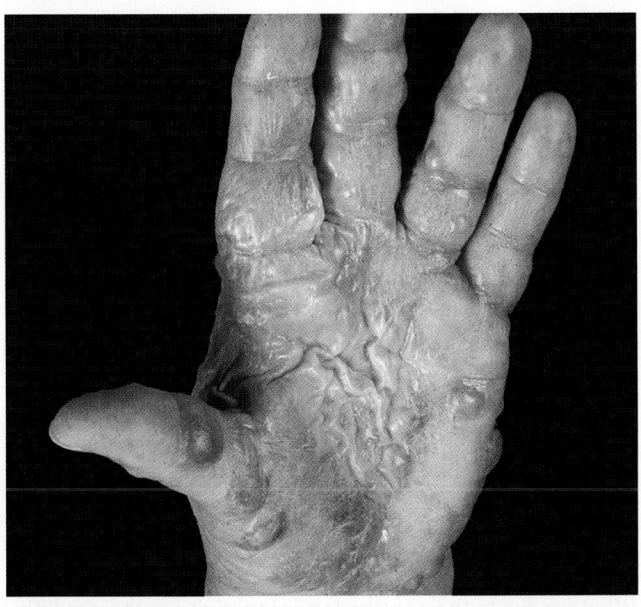

FIGURE 65–4. Acute irritant contact dermatitis on the hand due to an industrial solvent. There is massive blistering on the palm. (From Wolff K, Johnson RA. Eczema/dermatitis. Fitzpatrick's Color Atlas & Synopsis of Clinical Dermatology. 6th ed. New York: McGraw-Hill; 2009: 23.)

Table 65–5
Common Agents Causing Contact Dermatitis

Irritant Contact Dermatitis
Soaps
Detergents
Cosmetics
Solvents
Acid, mild or strong
Alkali, mild or strong

Allergic Contact Dermatitis
Plant resins, poison ivy, poison oak, sumac
Metals (nickel or gold in jewelry)
Latex and rubber
Cigarette smoke
Local anesthetics (lidocaine, benzocaine)

PATHOPHYSIOLOGY

- *Irritant* contact dermatitis is not the result of an immunologic process, but rather occurs from direct injury to the skin. An irritating agent comes into contact with the skin, damages the protective layers of the epidermis, and can cause erythema, the formation of vesicles and pruritus.[28,32,33] Symptoms occur within minutes to hours of exposure and begin to heal soon after removal of the offending substance.[30]

Clinical Presentation and Diagnosis of Contact Dermatitis

Contact dermatitis is generally confined to the area of contact, but in a highly sensitive person, a widespread or even generalized eruption may occur. Contact dermatitis is divided into two forms—irritant and allergic. Both forms may include, but are not limited to:

- Erythema
- Pruritus
- Vesicles
- Papules
- Crusts
- Burning

Irritant Form

The irritant form usually presents within hours of exposure and the rash is often localized. Irritant contact dermatitis may also result in fissuring and scaling.

Allergic Form

The allergic form can take several days to present and the condition may extend beyond the borders of the region exposed. Allergic contact dermatitis may also include oozing pustules and skin erosion.

Diagnosis

When the causative agent is known, the diagnosis of contact dermatitis is clinical. Patch testing is done if the allergens are unknown and is usually performed several weeks after the resolution of the original dermatitis.

Allergic contact dermatitis is a delayed hypersensitivity reaction.[31] Upon initial exposure, a substance penetrates the skin, binds to a protein, and develops into sensitizing antigens. Subsequent exposures to that substance will then elicit an allergic reaction.[28,32,33] Symptoms of allergic contact dermatitis are similar to those of the irritant type, but may take several hours to several days to develop following reexposure.[28,29]

TREATMENT

Desired Outcomes and Goals

⑤ *Identifying the causative substance and eliminating its exposure is the initial treatment goal for contact dermatitis.* Although physical symptoms can develop almost immediately after contact, removal of the offending agent will improve existing symptoms and prevent the occurrence of further complications. ⑤ *The second treatment goal is symptom relief.* Since inflammation and pruritus, as well as lesion formation, are likely to result from contact dermatitis, appropriate selection of nonpharmacologic and pharmacologic agents for these symptoms is necessary.

Nonpharmacologic Therapy

In many cases, contact dermatitis may not require medical treatment at all. Nondrug therapy for contact dermatitis is aimed at relieving pruritus and maintaining skin hydration.[30] Effective agents used for this include the following[28,30]:

- Colloidal oatmeal baths
- Cool or tepid soapless showers
- Cool, moist compresses applied to the area for 30 minutes three times a day
- Emollients or lubricants applied to the area after bathing (mineral oil, petrolatum)

Pharmacologic Therapy

▶ Astringents

The drying effect of **astringents** will decrease oozing from lesions and relieve itching.[28,29] Due to their ability to cause blood vessel constriction, astringents can also decrease inflammation. Aluminum acetate (Burow's solution), calamine, and witch hazel are safe and effective.[28] Patients apply solutions as a compress for 15 to 30 minutes two to four times a day.

Adverse effects reported with these agents are minimal and include drying and tightening of the skin. Because of this, their use should be limited to no more than 7 days.[28,29,31]

▶ Topical Steroids

Erythema, inflammation, pain, and itching caused by contact dermatitis can be effectively treated with topically applied corticosteroids. With such a wide range of products and potencies, an appropriate steroid selection is based on severity and location of lesions (see Table 65–6 for a list of topical steroids and potencies.) Higher potency preparations are used in areas where penetration is poor, such as the elbows and knees. Lower potency products should be reserved for areas of higher penetration, such as the face, axillae, and groin. Low-potency steroids are also recommended for the treatment of infants and children.[35,36]

Adverse effects from topical steroids are usually related to the potency of the steroid, frequency of application, duration of therapy, and the site of application. Skin atrophy, hypopigmentation, striae, and steroid-induced acne are all possible side effects associated with long-term use.[35]

Topical steroids are typically applied two to four times daily. As improvement begins, maintenance therapy should be limited to the lowest strength steroid that continues to control the condition. Once symptoms are completely resolved, use should be discontinued.

▶ Antihistamines

Whether due to their antihistaminic activity or their sedative side effects, pruritus caused by contact dermatitis can be relieved with the use of sedating oral antihistamines such as diphenhydramine or hydroxyzine. Topical antihistamines are available, but use is limited due to their high-sensitizing potential.[28,35]

Table 65–6

Topical Steroids to Treat Contact Dermatitis

Corticosteroids	Dosage Forms	Strength (%)	USP Potency Ratings[a]	Vasoconstrictive Potency Rating[b]
Alclometasone dipropionate	Cream	0.05	Low	VI
	Ointment	0.05	Low	V
Amcinonide	Lotion, ointment	0.1	High	II
	Cream	0.1	High	III
Beclomethasone dipropionate	Cream, lotion, ointment	0.025	Medium	—
Betamethasone benzoate	Cream, gel	0.025	Medium	III
	Ointment	0.025	Medium	IV
Betamethasone dipropionate	Cream AF (optimized vehicle)	0.05	Very high	I
	Cream	0.05	High	III
	Gel, lotion, ointment (optimized vehicle)	0.05	Very high	I
	Lotion	0.05	High	V
	Ointment	0.05	High	II
	Topical aerosol	0.1	High	—
Betamethasone valerate	Cream	0.01, 0.05, 0.1	Medium	V
	Lotion, ointment	0.05, 0.1	Medium	III
	Foam	0.12	Medium	IV
Clobetasol propionate	Cream, ointment, solution, foam	0.05	Very high	I
Clobetasol butyrate	Cream, ointment	0.05	Medium	—
Clocortolone pivalate	Cream	0.1	Low	—
Desonide	Cream, lotion, ointment	0.05	Low	VI
Desoximetasone	Cream	0.05	Medium	II
	Cream, ointment	0.25	High	II
	Gel	0.05	High	II
Dexamethasone	Gel	0.1	Low	VII
	Topical aerosol	0.01, 0.04	Low	VII
Dexamethasone sodium phosphate	Cream	0.1	Low	VII
Diflorasone diacetate	Cream	0.05	High	III
	Ointment	0.05	High	II
	Ointment (optimized vehicle)	0.05	Very high	II
Diflucortolone valerate	Cream, ointment	0.1	Medium	—
Flumethasone pivalate	Cream, ointment	0.03	Low	—
Fluocinolone acetonide	Cream	0.01	Medium	VI
	Cream	0.025	Medium	V
	Cream	0.2	High	—
	Ointment	0.025	Medium	IV
	Solution	0.01	Medium	VI
Fluocinonide	Gel, cream, ointment	0.05	High	II
	Solution	0.05	High	II
Flurandrenolide	Cream, ointment	0.0125	Low	—
	Ointment	0.05	Medium	IV
	Cream, lotion	0.05	Medium	V
	Tape	4 mcg/cm^2	Medium	I
Fluticasone propionate	Cream	0.05	Medium	IV
	Ointment	0.05	Medium	III
Halcinonide	Cream	0.025, 0.1	High	II
	Ointment	0.1	High	III
	Solution	0.1	High	—
Halobetasol propionate	Cream, ointment	0.05	Very high	I
Hydrocortisone	Cream, lotion, ointment	All strengths	Low	VII
Hydrocortisone acetate	Cream, lotion, ointment	All strengths	Low	VII
Hydrocortisone butyrate	Cream	0.1	Medium	V
	Ointment	0.1	Medium	—
Hydrocortisone valerate	Cream	0.2	Medium	V
	Ointment	0.2	Medium	IV
Methylprednisolone acetate	Cream, ointment	0.25	Low	VII
	Ointment	1	Low	VII
Mometasone furoate	Cream	0.1	Medium	IV
	Lotion, ointment	0.1	Medium	II

(Continued)

Table 65–6

Topical Steroids to Treat Contact Dermatitis *(Continued)*

Corticosteroids	Dosage Forms	Strength (%)	USP Potency Ratings*a*	Vasoconstrictive Potency Rating*b*
Triamcinolone acetonide	Cream, ointment	0.1	Medium	IV
	Cream, lotion, ointment	0.025	Medium	—
	Cream (Aristocort)	0.1	Medium	VI
	Cream (Kenalog)	0.1	High	IV
	Lotion	0.1	Medium	V
	Ointment (Aristocort, Kenalog)	0.1	High	III
	Cream, ointment	0.5	High	III
	Topical aerosol	0.015	Medium	—

*a*USP ratings are low, medium, high, and very high.

*b*Vasoconstriction potency scale is I (highest) to VII (lowest)—denotes unknown vasoconstrictive properties.

From West DP, Loyd A, West LE, Bauer KA, Musumeci ML, Micali G. Psoriasis. In: Dipiro JT, Talbert RL, Yee GC, et al., eds. Pharmacotherapy: A Pathophysiological Approach. 7th ed. New York: McGraw-Hill; 2008:1603–1617.

In addition to sedation, many oral antihistamines can cause hypotension, dizziness, blurred vision, and confusion.[31]

Diphenhydramine and hydroxyzine can be safely administered to children older than 2 years and adults. Table 65–7 outlines the recommended doses for these medications.

OUTCOME EVALUATION

With adequate treatment, most cases of contact dermatitis should improve within 7 days. Complete resolution of symptoms may take up to 3 weeks.[28] If a patient experiences severe symptoms associated with fever or difficulty breathing, they should be instructed to seek medical attention immediately. Furthermore, patients should return to their healthcare provider if any of the following occur:

- Rash has not improved or has worsened after several days of treatment
- Rash has increased in size or has spread to other locations
- Patient is experiencing adverse effects from the treatment regimen

Table 65–7

Oral Antihistamines Used for Pruritus

Drug	Pediatric Dosage	Adult Dosage
Diphenhydramine (Benadryl)	Not recommended for use in infants or neonates Less than 6 years old: 6.25–12.5 mg every 4–6 hours as needed 6–12 years old: 12.5–25 mg every 4–6 hours as needed	25–50 mg every 6–8 hours as needed
Hydroxyzine (Atarax)	0.6 mg/kg/dose every 6 hours as needed	25 mg every 6–8 hours as needed

From Wickersham RM, ed. Drug Facts and Comparisons. St. Louis, MO: Drug Facts and Comparisons; 2011.

Patient Care and Monitoring of Contact Dermatitis

1. Assess the patient's symptoms. Determine which form of contact dermatitis is present—irritant or allergic?

2. Obtain a thorough patient history. Has there been prior exposure to this agent? If so, what treatment regimens were used in the past to alleviate symptoms?

3. Obtain patient's allergy status.

4. Develop a treatment plan appropriate for contact dermatitis.

5. Discuss testing that may need to be performed to suggest or confirm the etiologic agent (patch testing).

6. Provide patient education on contact dermatitis and treatment:

   a. What is contact dermatitis and how does it develop?

   b. List various types of contact dermatitis.

   c. What drug therapies are available for treatment?

   d. What are the possible adverse effects of drug therapy?

   e. What are the symptoms that warrant physician referral?

   f. Explain the importance of treatment compliance.

   g. Educate on the recognition of agents that may cause contact dermatitis.

Patient Encounter 2

A 38-year-old woman presents to your clinic with complaints of a new-onset rash on the inside of both arms and wrists that is red, itching, and stinging. Upon visual examination you see that she has localized erythematous areas on the inner sides of both arms. You also note that there are small vesicles located within the affected area. After further questioning, you learn that she noticed the rash earlier that day at a medical office building where she works in the housekeeping department. She states that she uses various chemicals and cleaners at her work and thinks she may have come in to contact with bleach or "something" while she was cleaning today. The rash appeared approximately 6 hours ago, and the patient says that it has not spread since it first developed. From the information she has presented, you conclude that she came in contact with an agent at work that caused an irritant contact dermatitis to develop.

What information supports the possibility of exposure to an irritating agent?

Describe the symptoms that support this diagnosis.

Determine what the patient has tried to relieve her symptoms.

Describe the differences between allergic and irritant contact dermatitis.

What are your treatment goals for this patient?

What nonpharmacologic and pharmacologic treatment options are available for this diagnosis?

Given the information presented, develop a treatment regimen for this patient that includes the following:

(a) A statement of the problem

(b) A patient-specific therapeutic plan

(c) Monitoring parameters to assess efficacy and safety

DIAPER DERMATITIS

EPIDEMIOLOGY AND ETIOLOGY

Diaper dermatitis, more commonly known as diaper rash, is a form of irritant contact dermatitis that affects the buttocks, upper thighs, lower abdomen, and genitalia of an estimated 7% to 35% of all infants.[37,38] Onset of occurrence is usually between 3 weeks and 2 years of age, with the most cases reported between 9 and 12 months of age.[39] The rise in the number of adults who use diapers for incontinence also increases the risk of developing diaper dermatitis.[37]

PATHOPHYSIOLOGY

6 *Although many factors contribute to the etiology of diaper rash, it is most likely the result of prolonged contact of the skin with urine and feces in the diaper.* If a diaper is not changed soon after urination or defecation, the protective layer of the skin can break down and make the area more susceptible to irritation and infection from the contents of the diaper.[40] Although most mild cases of diaper rash present as erythema, moderate to severe cases can result in the formation of papules, vesicles, and even ulceration. If these cases are not effectively treated, the likelihood of secondary fungal or bacterial infections developing is greatly increased.[37]

Clinical Presentation and Diagnosis of Diaper Dermatitis

Typical Symptoms
- Erythema is the most common symptom presented with a diaper rash. The rash may begin as light to medium pink with poorly defined edges, but when further developed may become dark red and raised lesions with distinct edges.
- Rashes generally appear in the folds of the skin around the diaper area, thighs, genitals, and buttocks.
- Other typical symptoms include irritation and pruritus.

Atypical Symptoms

Patients presenting with the following symptoms may indicate the need for more aggressive antibiotic or antifungal therapy and should be referred to a primary care physician for further evaluation:
- Rashes not responding to typical creams and concurrent nonpharmacologic treatment

- Rashes extending beyond the diaper region (upper abdomen, back)
- Formation of papules, bullae, ulceration
- Excessive oozing
- Presence of genital discharge
- Concurrent fever
- Rashes appearing when diapers have not been used or rashes that fail to improve upon discontinuing diaper usage for extended periods of time (several days or more)
- Bleeding or open skin

Diagnosis

The diagnosis of diaper dermatitis is clinical. The presence of *Candida albicans* can be determined by KOH testing or culture, but is generally not necessary.

TREATMENT

Desired Outcomes and Goals

7 *The primary goal in the treatment of diaper rash is prevention and is most often accomplished through frequent diaper changes.* **8** *When a diaper rash is already present, repairing the damaged skin, relieving discomfort, and preventing secondary infections from occurring are important factors to consider when developing an effective treatment regimen.*[40]

Nonpharmacologic Therapy

Most mild cases of diaper rash can be resolved with the use of nonpharmacologic therapies. Keeping the diaper area clean and dry by changing diapers as soon as practically possible is highly effective for treatment and prevention.[37,38] Other nondrug options include[29,37]:

- Washing the area with lukewarm water and mild soap and allowing to completely dry before applying a new diaper
- Keeping diapers loose and well ventilated
- Avoiding plastic pants over diapers
- Allowing infants to take naps on an open diaper or absorbent pad to promote drying and healing

Pharmacologic Therapy

▶ Protectants

Protectants form an occlusive barrier between the skin and moisture from the diaper. Cream and ointment preparations are effective in providing a sufficient barrier in mild, irritant, and noninfected diaper rashes. For more severe cases, a paste is the topical agent of choice. Pastes are thicker and often contain additional ingredients (petrolatum, moisturizers) to help decrease discomfort and promote healing.[39] Zinc oxide is one of the most commonly used topical protectants. In addition to forming an effective barrier against moisture, it has astringent and antiseptic properties that provide added symptom relief.[37]

Protectants are generally applied to the affected area after every diaper change and can be discontinued when the rash resolves. Other available protectants that can be used alone or in combination for the safe and effective treatment of diaper rash include white petrolatum, Vitamins A and D, lanolin, and topical cornstarch. Many agents contain a combination of occlusive and protective agents such as Triple Paste and Calmoseptine.

▶ Topical Steroids

Because of the increased permeability of their skin, infants are at risk for excessive absorption and toxicity from the use of topical steroids. Although these agents are effective in decreasing inflammation and relieving pruritus, steroid use in infants for the treatment of diaper dermatitis should be limited to only the low-potency preparations.[41]

A thin layer of hydrocortisone cream (0.25% to 1%) applied twice a day for no more than 2 weeks is an appropriate treatment regimen. The use of higher potency steroids or use extending beyond 2 weeks should be at the discretion of a physician only.

▶ Antifungals

Diaper rashes lasting longer than 48 to 72 hours are at increased risk for the development of fungal infections. These complications are most frequently caused by *Candida albicans* and will require treatment with a topical antifungal.[38,39] (Fig. 65–6.)

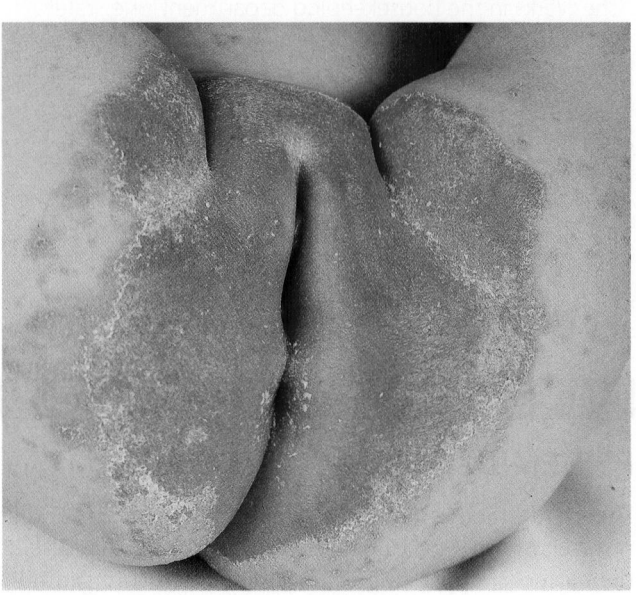

FIGURE 65–6. Candidiasis: diaper dermatitis. Confluent erosions, marginal scaling, and "satellite pustules" in the area covered by a diaper in an infant. (From Wolff K, Johnson RA. Cutaneous fungal infections. Fitzpatrick's Color Atlas & Synopsis of Clinical Dermatology. 5th ed. New York: McGraw-Hill; 2009: 723.)

Adverse events with the use of topical antifungals are generally limited to local irritation at the site of application.

Nystatin, clotrimazole, and miconazole creams or ointments applied two to four times daily with diaper changes have all shown to be effective in the treatment of candidal diaper rash. Although some of these products are available over the counter, parents and caregivers should be advised to initiate treatment with antifungal agents only after physician recommendation.

▶ Antibacterials

If conventional treatment fails, unresolved diaper rash can also lead to secondary bacterial infections. *Staphylococcus aureus* and *Streptococcus* are the most likely pathogens responsible for these infections and require treatment with systemic antibiotics.[39,40] While topical protectants may be used as an adjunct in treatment, suspected bacterial infections should always be referred to a physician for accurate diagnosis and the selection of an appropriate antibacterial regimen.[37] Figure 65–7 shows a useful algorithm for the effective treatment of diaper dermatitis.

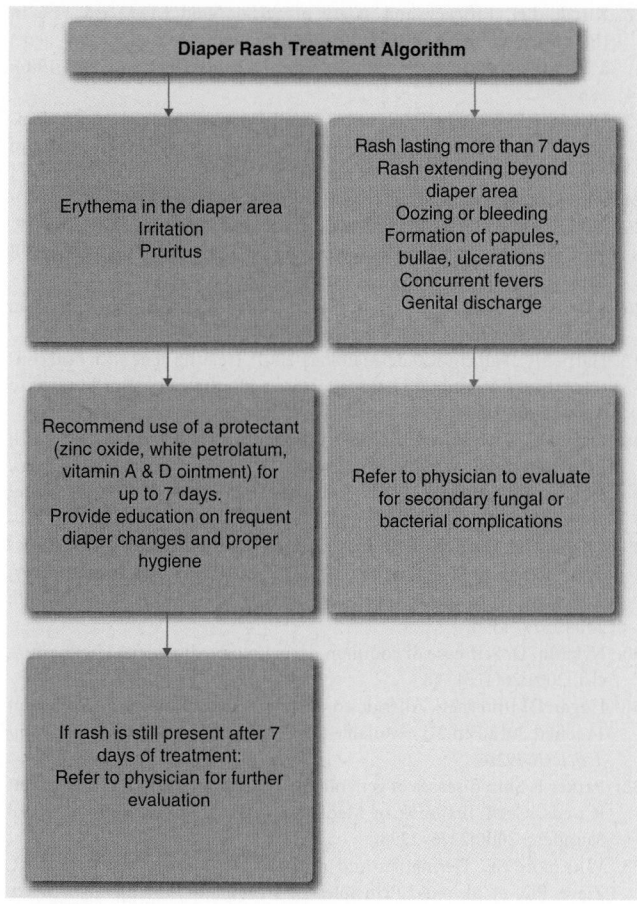

Diaper Rash Treatment Algorithm

Erythema in the diaper area
Irritation
Pruritus

Rash lasting more than 7 days
Rash extending beyond
diaper area
Oozing or bleeding
Formation of papules,
bullae, ulcerations
Concurrent fevers
Genital discharge

Recommend use of a protectant
(zinc oxide, white petrolatum,
vitamin A & D ointment) for
up to 7 days.
Provide education on frequent
diaper changes and proper
hygiene

Refer to physician to evaluate
for secondary fungal or
bacterial complications

If rash is still present after 7
days of treatment:
Refer to physician for further
evaluation

FIGURE 65–7. Diaper dermatitis treatment algorithm.

Patient Encounter 3

A woman presents to a community pharmacy inquiring about a product to purchase for her 3-month-old son who recently developed a rash in his diaper area. She says the rash is bright red and seems to fluctuate in severity from diaper change to diaper change. After further questioning, it is determined that the rash has lasted about 4 to 5 days and seems to be painful for her son when she cleans him with diaper wipes during changing. She has tried using white petrolatum a few times and is now concerned about the rash becoming infected.

What reported symptoms support the diagnosis of diaper rash?

Elicit additional information to aid in your assessment of this patient.

What are your treatment goals for this patient?

What nonpharmacologic and pharmacologic treatment options are available for this diagnosis?

Given the information presented, develop a treatment regimen for this patient that includes the following:

(a) A statement of the problem

(b) A patient-specific therapeutic plan

(c) Monitoring parameters to assess efficacy and safety

OUTCOME EVALUATION

Most diaper rashes can be effectively treated in less than 1 week. If symptoms do not resolve or begin to worsen, advise caregivers to seek medical attention to determine the presence of secondary fungal or bacterial infections. In addition, provide educational information on proper diaper hygiene techniques in order to prevent the development of future diaper rashes.

Patient Care and Monitoring: Diaper Dermatitis

1. Assess rash symptoms. Determine the level of severity—is there a possibility of a secondary fungal or bacterial infection?

2. Identify signs and symptoms that require immediate physician referral.

3. Inquire about the patient's history, including any similar rashes in the past.

4. Educate the caregiver on the importance of frequent diaper changes and proper hygiene.

5. Obtain patient allergy status.

6. Discuss labs that may be necessary if a secondary infection is suspected (cultures, biopsies).

7. Develop a treatment regimen for the patient, including a plan for assessing improvement of the condition.

8. Provide patient education about diaper rash etiology, treatment, and prevention:

   a. What is diaper rash and how does it develop? What exacerbates diaper rash?

   b. Symptoms to report to a physician (blistering, oozing, bleeding, changes in rash, or no improvement in symptoms within 2 to 3 days)

   c. Available treatment options, including proper usage instructions and potential side effects

   d. Importance of treatment compliance

   e. Prevention measures

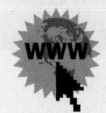

Self-assessment questions and answers are available at *http://mhpharmacotherapy. com/pp.html.*

REFERENCES

1. Bello CE. Optimizing acne vulgaris treatment. US Pharmacist. 2002;27(4):63–75.
2. Fitzpatrick TB, Johnson RA. Color Atlas and Synopsis of Clinical Dermatology: Common and Serious Diseases. 6th ed. New York: McGraw-Hill; 2009:3, 23, 27, 723.
3. West DP, Loyd A, Bauer KA, West LE, Scuderi L, Micali G. Acne vulgaris. In: Dipiro JT, Talbert RL, Yee GC, et al., eds. Pharmacotherapy: A Pathophysiological Approach. 7th ed. New York: McGraw-Hill; 2008:1591–1602.
4. Keri JE, Nijhawan RI. Diet and acne. Exp Rev Dermatol. 2008;3(4): 437–440.
5. Whitmore SE. Disorders of the pilosebaceous unit: Acne and related disorders and hair loss. In: Barker LB, Burton JR, Zieve PD, et al., eds. Principles of Ambulatory Medicine. 7th ed. Philadelphia, PA: Lippincott Williams & Wilkins; 2007:1897–1904.
6. Baxi S. OTC products for the treatment of acne. US Pharmacist. 2007;32(7):13–17.
7. Fulton J [Internet]. Acne Vulgaris. Emedicine. 2011 Aug 26 [cited 2012 Feb 21]. Available from: *http://emedicine.medscape.com/ article/1069804.*
8. Rhinard EE. Acne. In: Koda-Kimble MA, Young LY, Kradjan WA, et al., eds. Applied Therapeutics: The Clinical Use of Drugs. 9th ed. Maryland: Lippincott Williams & Wilkins; 2009:40–1–40–11.
9. Hartsock M. Medical Illustrations. Cincinnati, OH: The Medical Art Company.
10. Ayer J, Burrows N. Acne: more than skin deep. Postgrad Med J 2006;82:500–506.
11. Johnson BA, Nunley JR. Topical therapy for acne vulgaris: How do you choose the best drug for each patient? Postgrad Med 2000;107:69–80.
12. Foster KT, Coffey CW. Acne. In: Krinsky DL, Berardi RR, Ferreri SP, et al., eds. The Handbook of Nonprescription Drugs. 17th ed. Washington, DC: American Pharmaceutical Association; 2012:693–705.
13. Del Rosso JQ. Fall clinical dermatology 2007: An update on advances in acne and excerpts from what's new in the medicine cabinet. Skin Aging 2008;3(Suppl):1–11.
14. Ortho Dermalogics. Retin-A Micro Package Insert. Los Angeles, CA: Ortho-McNeil-Janssen Pharmaceuticals; 2010.
15. Wickersham RM, ed. Drug Facts and Comparisons. St. Louis, MO: Drug Facts and Comparisons; 2011.
16. Feldman S, Careccia RE, Barham KL, Hancox, J. Diagnosis and treatment of acne. Am Fam Physician 2004;69(9):2123–2130.
17. Russell JJ. Topical therapy for acne. Am Fam Physician 2000;61: 357–368.
18. Yang DJ, Hsu S, Quan LT. Topical antibacterial agents. In: Wolverton SE, ed. Comprehensive Dermatologic Drug Therapy. Philadelphia, PA: WB Saunders; 2007:525–546.
19. Stiefel Laboratories. Duac Topical Gel Package Insert. Research Triangle Park, NC: Stiefel Laboratories; 2011.
20. Zaenglein AL, Thiboutot DM. Expert committee recommendations for acne management. Pediatrics 2006;118:1188–1199.
21. Allergan Azelex package insert. Irvine, CA: Allergan; 2004 (May).
22. Kircik, LH. Efficacy and safety of azelaic acid (AzA) gel 15% in the treatment of post-inflammatory hyperpigmentation and acne: a 16-week, baseline-controlled study. J Drugs Dermatol 2011;10(6): 586–590.
23. Draelos ZD, Carter E, Maloney JM, et al. Two randomized studies demonstrate the efficacy and safety of dapsone gel, 5% for the treatment of acne vulgaris. J Am Acad Dermatol 2007;56:439.e1–e10.
24. Allergan. Aczone Package Insert. Irvine, CA: Allergan; 2010.
25. Ashourian N, Cohen PR. Systemic antibacterial agents. In: Wolverton SE, ed. Comprehensive Dermatologic Drug Therapy. Philadelphia, PA: WB Saunders; 2007:39–74.
26. Thielitz A, Gollnick, H. Topical retinoids in acne vulgaris: update on efficacy and safety. Am J Clin Derm 2008;9(6):369–381.
27. Harper JC. Fall clinical dermatology 2007: Treating acne with oral contraceptives: A guide for safe, effective and efficient prescribing. Skin Aging 2008;3(Suppl):12–14.
28. Plake KS, Darbishire PL. Contact dermatitis. In: Krinsky DL, Berardi RR, Ferreri SP, et al., eds. Handbook of Nonprescription Drugs. 17th ed. Washington, DC: American Pharmaceutical Association; 2012:645–659.
29. Cheigh NH. Dermatologic drug reactions and self-treatable skin disorders. In: Dipiro JT, Talbert RL, Yee GC, et al., eds. Pharmacotherapy: A Pathophysiological Approach. 7th ed. New York: McGraw-Hill; 2008:1577–1590.
30. Nykamp D. Self-care of common dermatologic disorders. US Pharmacist. 2001;26(4):31–48.
31. Hogan DJ [Internet]. Allergic contact dermatitis. Emedicine. 2011 Sept 14 [cited 2012 Feb 21]. Available from: *http://emedicine.medscape.com/ article/1049216.*
32. Parker F. Skin diseases of general importance. In: Goldman L, Bennett JC, eds. Cecil Textbook of Medicine. 21st ed. Philadelphia, PA: WB Saunders; 2000:2276–2298.
33. Whitmore SE. Dermatitis and psoriasis. In: Barker LB, Burton JR, Zieve PD, et al., eds. Principles of Ambulatory Medicine. 7th ed. Philadelphia, PA: Lippincott Williams & Wilkins; 2007:1905–1913.
34. West DP, Loyd A, West LE, Bauer KA, Musumeci ML, Micali G. Psoriasis. In: Dipiro JT, Talbert RL, Yee GC, et al., eds. Pharmacotherapy: A Pathophysiological Approach. 7th ed. New York: McGraw-Hill; 2008:1603–1617.
35. Cheigh NH. Atopic dermatitis. In: Dipiro JT, Talbert RL, Yee GC, et al., eds. Pharmacotherapy: A Pathophysiological Approach. 7th ed. New York: McGraw-Hill; 2008:1619–1626.
36. Burkhart C, Morrell D, Goldsmith L. Dermatological Pharmacology. In: Brunton LL, Chabner BA, Knollman BC, eds. Goodman & Gillman's: The Pharmacological Basis of Therapeutics. 12th ed. New York: McGraw-Hill; 2011:1803–1832.
37. Hagemeir NE. Diaper dermatitis and prickly heat. In: Krinsky DL, Berardi RR, Ferreri SP, et al., eds. Handbook of Nonprescription Drugs. 17th ed. Washington, DC: American Pharmaceutical Association; 2012:661–674.
38. Agrawal R, Sammeta V, Thomas I [Internet]. Diaper Dermatitis. Emedicine. 2011 Jan 4 [cited 2012 Feb 21]. Available from: *http://emedicine. medscape.com/article/911985.*
39. Borkowski S. Diaper rash care and management. Pediatr Nurs 2004;30(6):467–470.
40. Atherton JD. A review of the pathophysiology, prevention and treatment of irritant diaper dermatitis. Curr Med Res Opin 2004;20(5):645–649.
41. Raimer SS. The safe use of topical corticosteroids in children. Pediatr Ann 2001;30(4):225–229.

66 Anemia

Robert K. Sylvester

LEARNING OBJECTIVES

● **Upon completion of the chapter, the reader will be able to:**

1. Identify common causes of anemia.

2. Describe common signs and symptoms of anemia.

3. Describe diagnostic evaluation required to determine the etiology of anemia.

4. Recommend a treatment regimen for anemia considering the underlying cause and patient-specific variables.

5. Compare and contrast commonly prescribed oral and parenteral iron preparations.

6. Explain the optimal use of folic acid and vitamin B_{12} in patients with macrocytic anemia.

7. Evaluate the proper use of epoetin and darbepoetin in anemia patients with cancer chemotherapy associated or chronic kidney disease.

8. Develop a plan to monitor the outcomes of anemia pharmacotherapy.

KEY CONCEPTS

❶ Anemia is a below-normal concentration of hemoglobin (Hgb) that results in a reduction of the oxygen-carrying capacity of the blood.

❷ Common signs and symptoms of anemia include fatigue, lethargy, dizziness, shortness of breath, headache, edema, and tachycardia.

❸ A complete blood count (CBC) is the laboratory evaluation that provides objective characteristics of red blood cells (RBCs) useful in determining etiology and appropriate treatment.

❹ The goal of anemia therapy is to increase Hgb concentrations to levels that improve RBC oxygen-carrying capacity, alleviate symptoms, and prevent anemia complications.

❺ The underlying cause of anemia (e.g., iron, folic acid, or B_{12} deficiency; blood loss; or chronic disease) must be determined and used to guide therapy.

❻ In patients with iron-deficiency anemia (IDA), appropriate oral iron therapy should be attempted before giving parenteral iron.

❼ Anemia from vitamin B_{12} or folic acid deficiency is effectively treated by administration of the deficient nutrient.

❽ In patients with anemia related to cancer chemotherapy or chronic kidney disease (CKD), administration of erythropoietin-stimulating agents (ESAs) can increase Hgb and decrease transfusion requirements.

❾ ESAs have significant safety risks that require careful monitoring. Use the lowest dose of epoetin alfa and darbepoetin alfa to avoid RBC transfusions.

❿ At appropriate intervals, patients should be monitored for Hgb response, symptom resolution, and adverse effects and treatment regimens adjusted accordingly.

INTRODUCTION

❶ *Anemia is a reduction in the concentration of hemoglobin (Hgb) that results in reduced oxygen-carrying capacity of the blood.* Some patients with anemia may be asymptomatic initially, but eventually, the lack of oxygen to tissues results in fatigue, lethargy, shortness of breath, headache, edema, and tachycardia. Common causes of anemia include blood loss, decreased red blood cell (RBC) production, increased RBC destruction, or a combination of these events. Determination of the underlying cause of anemia is essential for successful management. Appropriate treatment of anemia will result in an increase in Hgb, with a corresponding increase in oxygen-carrying capacity and reduction in symptoms.

Table 66–1	
Prevalence of Anemia[1,2]	
Children (1–16 years)	6–9%
Males (16–69 years)	2%
Males (85+ years)	26%
Females (16–19 years)	16%
Females (20–49 years, nonpregnant)	12%
White, non-Hispanic	10%
Black, non-Hispanic	19%
Mexican American	22%
Females (85+ years)	20.1%

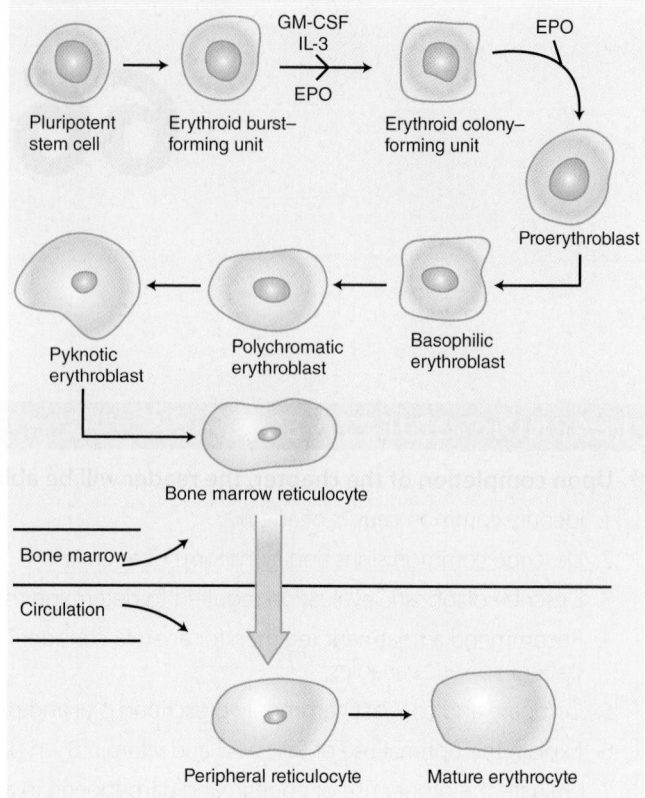

FIGURE 66–1. The process of erythropoiesis.

EPIDEMIOLOGY AND ETIOLOGY

Anemia is a common diagnosis with a prevalence that varies widely based on age, gender, and race/ethnicity (see Table 66–1).[1,2] Patients with specific comorbidities such as cancer and chronic kidney disease (CKD) have significantly higher rates of anemia. The incidence of anemia in cancer patients ranges from 30% to 90%.[3] Contributing factors include the underling malignancy and myelosuppressive antineoplastic therapy.[4] The prevalence of anemia in patients with CKD ranges from 15% to 20% in patients with CKD stages 1 through 3 and up to 70% in patients with stage 5.[5]

Causes of anemia can be divided into three main categories: decreased production, increased destruction, and blood loss. Drug therapy is the mainstay of treatment for anemias caused by reduced production of erythrocytes and is the focus of this chapter; anemia due to destruction of erythrocytes will not be discussed.

A decrease in erythrocyte production can be multifactorial. Nutritional deficiencies (iron, vitamin B_{12}, and folic acid) are common causes and often easily treatable. Patients with cancer or CKD are at risk for developing anemia caused by dysregulation of iron and erythropoietin (EPO) hemostasis. Patients with chronic immune-related diseases such as rheumatoid arthritis and systemic lupus erythematosus are also at increased risk to develop anemia as a complication of their disease. Anemia related to these chronic inflammatory conditions is termed *anemia of chronic disease* (ACD).[6]

PATHOPHYSIOLOGY

Erythropoiesis

Erythropoiesis is a process that begins with a pluripotent stem cell in the bone marrow undergoing differentiation and ends with the appearance of erythrocytes (RBCs) in peripheral blood. The production of RBCs is stimulated by EPO, a hormone that is secreted by the kidney in response to detection of decreased oxygen-carrying capacity of blood. EPO stimulates RBC production by stimulating differentiation of RBC precursors in the bone marrow to become reticulocytes (Fig. 66–1). Reticulocytes become erythrocytes after 1 to 2 days in the bloodstream.[7]

Decreased-Production Anemias

▶ Nutritional Deficiencies

Deficiencies in nutrients such as folic acid and vitamin B_{12} may hinder the process of erythrocyte maturation. Folic acid and vitamin B_{12} are required for the formation of DNA. Significant decreases in the amount of these nutrients inhibits DNA synthesis and consequently RBC production.[7,8] Poor diet can contribute to folic acid and vitamin B_{12} deficiencies. Patients with pernicious anemia are unable to absorb B_{12} due to inadequate production of intrinsic factor, a glycoprotein produced by gastric parietal cells that binds to vitamin B_{12} and facilitates its absorption in the ileum. This condition results in B_{12} deficiency despite adequate dietary B_{12} intake.[9]

Iron is another nutrient essential for production of RBCs. It is required for formation of Hgb. Lack of iron leads to a decrease in Hgb synthesis and decreased RBC production. Normal homeostasis of iron transport and metabolism is depicted in Figure 66–2.[10] Approximately 1 to 2 mg of iron is absorbed through the duodenum each day, and the same amount is lost via blood loss, desquamation of mucosal cells, or menstruation.

Iron-deficiency anemia (IDA) typically occurs because of inadequate absorption of iron or excessive blood loss. Inadequate absorption may occur in patients who have congenital or acquired intestinal conditions, such

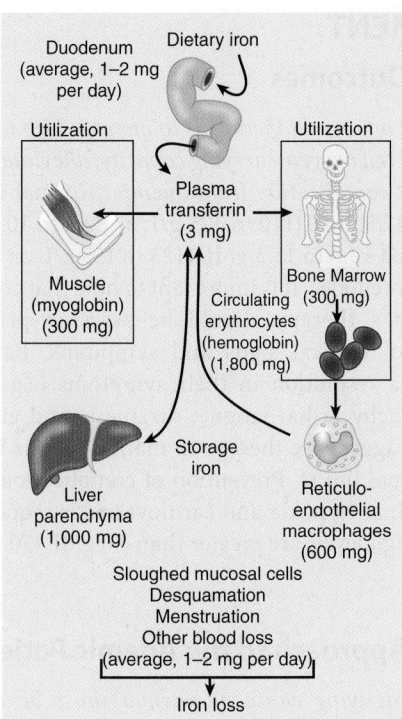

FIGURE 66–2. The distribution of iron use in adults. (From Andrews NC. Disorders of iron metabolism. N Engl J Med 1999;341:1986–1995.)

as inflammatory bowel disease, celiac disease, or bowel resection. Achlorhydria and diets poor in iron also may contribute to iron deficiency states. Iron deficiency also may occur in patients following excessive rates of iron loss from the body. Common etiologies include excessive menstruation, ulcers or neoplastic lesions in the gastrointestinal tract, and excessive bleeding following surgery or trauma.[10]

▶ *Dysregulation of Iron Homeostasis and Impaired Marrow Production*

Chronic diseases associated with ACD include infection, autoimmune disease, CKD, and cancer. A major contributing factor for development of ACD is disturbance of iron homeostasis related to activation of the immune system. Hepcidin is an acute-phase protein expressed in response to upregulation of interleukin-6 and exposure to lipopolysaccharide. Increased expression of hepcidin causes decreased iron absorption from the gastrointestinal tract and inhibition of iron release from macrophages. In addition, immune activation can cause upregulation of cytokines (interferons, interleukin-1, tumor necrosis factor-α) known to impair the proliferation and differentiation of erythroid precursors. Decreased production and blunted responsiveness to EPO can also contribute to ACD; this is best documented in patients with CKD. Finally, disruption of erythropoiesis secondary to infiltration of the bone marrow by cancer can significantly contribute to anemia in patients with cancer.[4–6]

Clinical Presentation and Diagnosis of Anemia

Signs and Symptoms

❷ Generally, the signs and symptoms of anemia are nonspecific and *may include* the following:

- Fatigue, lethargy, dizziness
- Shortness of breath
- Headache
- Edema
- Tachycardia

Other findings that may be present in some patients include:

- Dry skin, chapped lips
- Nail brittleness
- Hunger for ice, starch, or clay (termed pica)

Past Medical History

Inquire about the following conditions:

- History of blood loss, such as hemorrhoids, melena, or menorrhagia (IDA)
- Malnourished or recent weight loss (vitamin B_{12} or folate deficiency)
- Alcoholism (folate deficiency)
- Cancer or chronic kidney disease (CKD)
- Chronic autoimmune disorders or infections, such as HIV infection or rheumatoid arthritis (anemia of chronic disease)

Physical Examination

These findings aid the clinician in determining the severity of the anemia:

- Orthostatic hypotension and tachycardia secondary to volume depletion
- Cutaneous changes such as pallor, jaundice, and nail brittleness

Laboratory Evaluation

Table 66–2 describes common tests used to determine the etiology of anemia. A diagnostic and treatment algorithm for anemia is outlined in Figure 66–3.

1. ❸ A CBC is a necessary first step in evaluating a patient with anemia. If the Hgb and Hct are less than the normal range, the patient is anemic. *Subsequent evaluations of RBC indices and the peripheral smear often are necessary to determine the etiology (and ultimately, the treatment) of the* anemia.

2. Evaluating the mean corpuscular volume (MCV) is the next step in an anemia workup. It is classified as microcytic, normocytic, or macrocytic if the MCV is below, within, or above the normal range of 80 to 96 fL/cell, respectively.

(Continued)

Clinical Presentation and Diagnosis of Anemia (*Continued*)

Microcytic Anemia and Iron Evaluation

Iron studies (see Table 66–2) should be evaluated in the setting of a low MCV. These include:

- Serum iron
- **Serum ferritin**—the best indirect determinant of body iron stores. It is commonly decreased in patients with IDA
- Total iron-binding capacity (TIBC)—quantifies the iron-binding capacity of transferrin and is increased in IDA
- **Transferrin saturation** (serum iron/TIBC)—indicates the amount of transferrin that is bound with iron; it is lower in IDA

Macrocytic Anemia

- Evaluate folic acid and vitamin B_{12} levels in the setting of an elevated MCV
- Further investigation by administering radiolabeled B_{12} (i.e., Schilling test) to determine if lack of intrinsic factor
- Consider obtaining homocysteine and methylmalonic acid levels

Normocytic Anemia

- Evaluate reticulocytes and CBC
- High reticulocyte counts may indicate RBCs loss via acute blood loss, hemolysis, or splenic sequestration
- Low reticulocyte counts may indicate a diseased bone marrow (e.g., aplastic anemia, myelodysplasia, or leukemia)

Patient Encounter 1, Part 1

A 24-year-old Mexican mother returns for an appointment with her primary healthcare provider for a 1-week postpartum visit. She has two healthy children (aged 2 years and 4 years); past medical history is negative. She has experienced several episodes of dizziness and shortness of breath after walking up stairs. She states her postpartum bleeding seemed to last a few days longer than previous deliveries.

What aspects of this patient's history suggest she may be anemic?

What laboratory assessments are required to make an appropriate diagnosis and therapeutic plan?

How would the requested laboratory parameter(s) aid your decision making?

TREATMENT

Desired Outcomes

❹ *The goal of anemia therapy is to increase Hgb to levels that improve red cell oxygen-carrying capacity, alleviate symptoms, and prevent complication from anemia.* Normal Hgb values are 14.0 to 17.5 g/dL (140 to 175 g/L or 8.69 to 10.9 mmol/L) for males and 12.3 to 15.3 g/dL (123 to 153 g/L or 7.63 to 9.50 mmol/L) for females. It is important to note that continuation of a patient's therapy should be assessed primarily by resolution of clinical signs and symptoms. Patients who experience a resolution in their symptoms (e.g., shortness of breath, tachycardia, fatigue, dizziness, and edema) may not require aggressive therapy to maintain their Hgb values within normal limits. Prevention of complications owing to anemia such as hypoxia and cardiovascular sequelae can be avoided if Hgb levels are greater than 7.0 g/dL (70 g/L or 4.34 mmol/L).[11]

General Approach to the Anemic Patient

❺ *The underlying cause of anemia must be determined and used to guide therapy. The mean corpuscular volume (included in a CBC) and determination of iron, ferritin, folate, and vitamin B_{12} levels are required to correctly determine the etiology of a patient's anemia.* **Figure 66–3** and Table 66–2 illustrate how laboratory test results determine the correct diagnosis.

Nonpharmacologic Therapy

The most important nonpharmacologic treatment of anemia is transfusion of RBCs. Safety concerns, cost, and the limited availability of this therapy support efforts to establish the "optimum" threshold for administering RBC transfusions. A Cochrane review of 17 controlled studies concluded that it is appropriate to use "restrictive transfusion triggers in patients who are free of serious cardiac disease." The authors concluded a reasonable "trigger for transfusion" for patients without significant cardiovascular disease is 7.0 g/dL (70 g/L or 4.34 mmol/L).[12] The Transfusion Requirements In Critical Care trial reported no significant differences in in-hospital mortality between patients randomly assigned to maintain Hgb levels of 7.0 to 9.0 g/dL (70 g/L to 90 g/L or 4.34 mmol/L to 5.59 mmol/L) and 10.0 to 12.0 g/dL (100 g/L to 120 g/L or 6.21 mmol/L to 7.45 mmol/L).[13] Typically, only patients with acute symptoms (i.e., dyspnea, chest pain) and Hgb concentrations in the range of 7.0 to 9.0 g/dL (70 g/L to 90 g/L or 4.34 mmol/L to 5.59 mmol/L) require blood transfusions.

Certainly, anemia can be attributed to diets poor in iron, folic acid, or vitamin B_{12}. However, in the United States, nutrient-poor diets are rarely the sole cause of anemia. Therefore, ingesting a diet that is rich in iron, folic acid, or vitamin B_{12} should be encouraged, but is rarely the sole modality of treatment. Food sources of iron, folic acid, and vitamin B_{12} are listed in **Table 66–3**.[8]

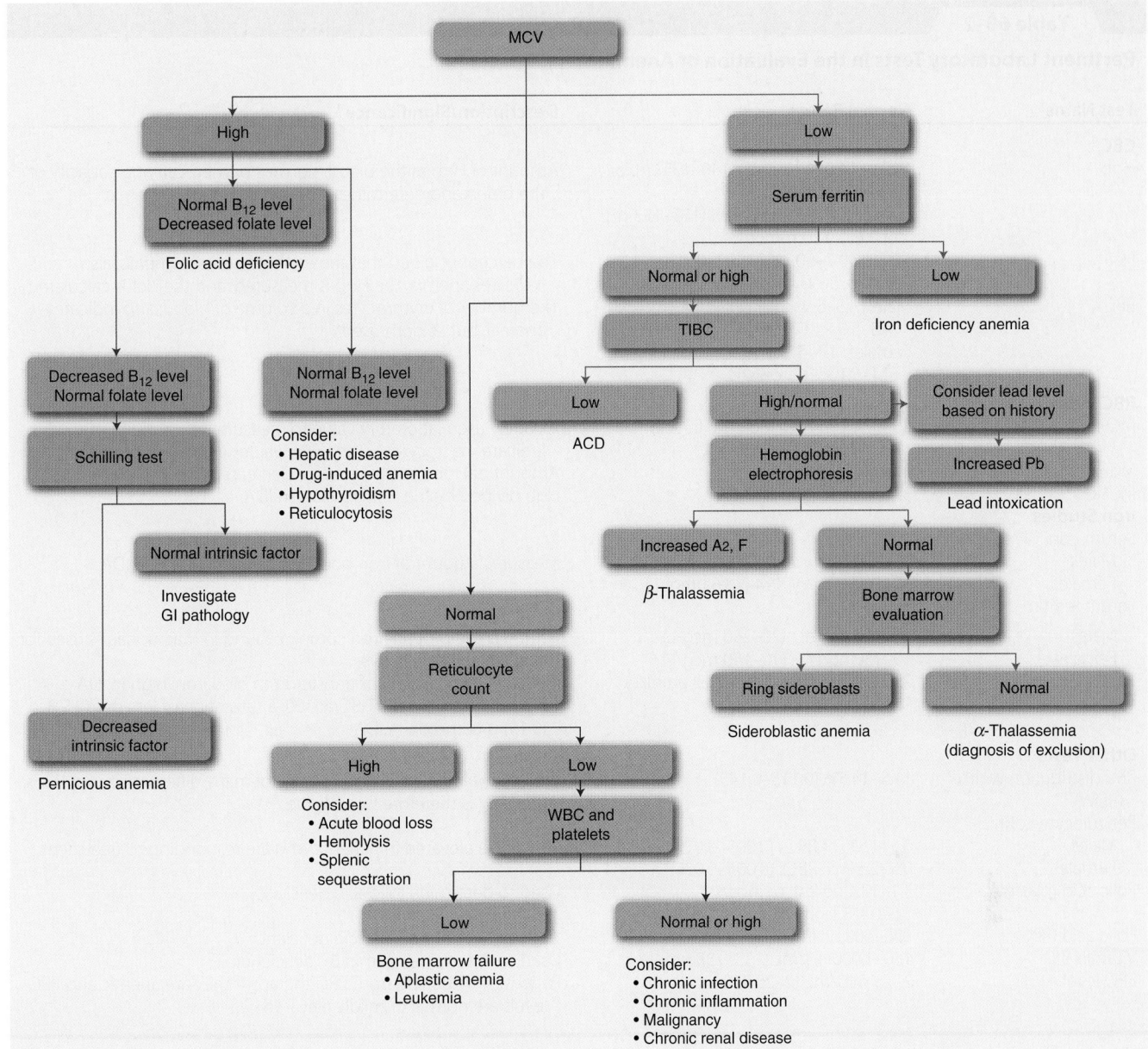

FIGURE 66–3. The anemia evaluation process. ACD, anemia of chronic disease; MCV, mean corpuscular volume; Pb, lead; TIBC, total iron-binding capacity.

Pharmacologic Therapy

▶ *Iron-Deficiency Anemia*

❻ *The initial treatment of IDA is oral iron therapy that provides 150 to 200 mg of elemental iron daily.* Many different iron products and salt forms are available. **Table 66–4** lists commonly prescribed oral iron products and the amount of elemental iron provided by each.

Iron supplementation resolves anemia by replenishing iron stores to levels necessary for RBC production and maturation. If treated properly, reticulocytosis should be seen in 7 to 10 days, and Hgb values should rise by about 1.0 g/dL (10 g/L or 0.62 mmol/L) per week. Patients should be

reassessed if Hgb does not increase by 2.0 g/dL (20 g/L or 1.24 mmol/L) in 3 weeks.[14]

The preferred dosing regimen for oral iron is to administer 50 to 65 mg of elemental iron two to three doses daily on an empty stomach. Administration on an empty stomach (1 hour before or 2 hours after a meal) is preferred for maximal absorption. However, if patients develop intolerable GI side effects (i.e., heartburn, nausea, bloating) after taking iron on an empty stomach, they should be advised to take it with meals. After absorption, iron binds to transferrin in the plasma and is transported to the muscles (for myoglobin), liver (for storage), or bone marrow (for red cell production). Common toxicities associated with oral iron products include

---

Table 66–2

Pertinent Laboratory Tests in the Evaluation of Anemia

Test Name	Normal Range	Description/Significance
CBC		
Hgb	Males: 14.0–17.5 g/dL (140–175 g/L or 8.69–10.9 mmol/L) Females: 12.35–15.3 g/dL (123–153 g/L or 7.63–9.50 mmol/L)	Amount of Hgb in the blood; signifies oxygen-carrying capacity of the blood and determines whether a patient is anemic
Hct	Males: 40.7–50.3% (0.407–0.503) Females: 36.1–44.3% (0.361–0.44.3)	The percent of blood that the erythrocytes encompass; also indicates anemia; the Hgb is measured, and the Hct is calculated
RBC	Males: 4.5–5.9 × 10⁶ cells/μL (4.5–5.9 × 10¹² cells/L) Females: 4.1–5.1 × 10⁶ cells/μL (4.1–5.1 × 10¹² cells/L)	The number of erythrocytes in a volume of blood; also indicates anemia, but seldom used
RBC Indices		
MCV	80–97.6 μm³/cell (80–97.6 fL/cell)	A widely used laboratory value to measure RBC "size"; higher values indicate macrocytosis and lower values indicate microcytosis
MCH	27–33 pg/cell	Amount of Hgb per RBC; may be decreased in IDA
MCHC	32–36 g/dL (320–360 g/L)	Hgb divided by the Hct; also low in IDA
Iron Studies		
Serum iron		
Males	45–160 mcg/dL (8.1–28.6 μmol/L)	Measures amount of iron bound to transferrin; low in IDA
Females	30–160 mcg/dL (5.4–28.6 μmol/L)	
Serum ferritin		
Males	20–250 ng/mL (20–250 mcg/L)	Ferritin is the protein–iron complex found in macrophages used for iron storage; low in IDA
Females	10–150 ng/mL (10–150 mcg/L)	
TIBC	220–420 mcg/dL (39.4–75.2 μmol/L)	Measures the capacity of transferrin to bind iron; high in IDA
TSAT	15–50% (0.15–0.50)	TSAT(%) = (serum iron/TIBC) × 100; a saturation of less than 15% (0.15) is common in IDA
Other Tests		
RBC distribution width (RDW)	11.5–14.5% (0.115–0.145)	A higher value means the presence of many different sizes of RBCs; the MCV is therefore less reliable
Reticulocyte count		
Males	0.5–1.5% of RBCs (0.005–0.015)	Should be elevated in patients who are responding to treatment
Females	0.5–2.5% of RBCs (0.005–0.025)	
Folic acid (plasma)	3.1–12.4 ng/mL or mcg/L (7.0–28.1 nmol/L)	Used to determine folic acid deficiency
Folic acid (RBC)	125–600 ng/mL (283–1,360 nmol/L)	Used to determine folic acid deficiency
Vitamin B₁₂	180–1,000 pg/mL (133–738 pmol/L)	Used to determine vitamin B₁₂ deficiency
EPO level	2–25 mIU/mL (2–25 IU/L)	Patients may benefit from EPO therapy if they are anemic and EPO levels are normal or mildly elevated

EPO, erythropoietin; Hct, hematocrit; Hgb, hemoglobin; IDA, iron-deficiency anemia; MCH, mean cell hemoglobin; MCHC, mean cell hemoglobin concentration; MCV, mean cell volume; RDW, RBC distribution width; TIBC, total iron-binding capacity; TSAT, transferrin saturation.

---

abdominal pain, nausea, heartburn, constipation, and dark stools.[14] Potentially clinically significant drug interactions involving iron products include fluoroquinolones, tetracyclines, and mycophenolate mofetil. Iron decreases the absorption of these drugs. To minimize this effect, oral iron should be administered not less than 3 hours before or 2 hours after the affected drug.[15]

Parenteral iron therapy is indicated when patients cannot tolerate oral formulations, are noncompliant, or fail to respond to oral iron because of malabsorption syndromes. Five parenteral iron formulations are available in the United States.[16–20] Use and availability of parenteral iron formulations have changed significantly since introduced over 30 years ago. The initial iron dextran formulation approved for use in the United States was a high-molecular-weight product

(HMW ID). The relatively infrequent occurrence of severe acute hypersensitivity reactions associated with this product resulted in a "black box warning" and recommendation for administration of a test dose. In 1991, this product was withdrawn from market. The same year, a low-molecular-weight iron dextran (LMW ID) was approved for use and became an established component in combination with ESAs for treating anemia in patients with CKD.[16] Although total dose infusion (TDI) is not an approved method of administration in the United States, LMW ID is approved for TDI in Europe. TDI administration has been shown to achieve similar patient outcomes (equal efficacy and safety) while lowering cost. In 1996, a new HMW ID received FDA labeling for the treatment of IDA. Sodium ferric gluconate complex, iron sucrose, and ferumoxytol received

Patient Encounter 1, Part 2

Laboratory parameters are ordered, and the following is observed:

CBC

- *WBC:* 6.50 × 10³/μL (6.50 × 10⁹/L)
- *Hgb:* 8.3 g/dL (83 g/L or 5.15 mmol/L)
- *Hct:* 24.8% (0.248)
- *Plt:* 210 × 10³/μL (210 × 10⁹/L)

Red blood Cell Indices

- *MCV:* 75 μm³/cell (75 fL/cell)
- *MCH:* 26 pg/cell
- *MCHC:* 30.3 g/dL (303 g/L)

Others

- *RBC count:* 3 × 10⁶ /μL (3 × 10¹²/L)
- *RDW:* 15% (0.15)
- *Retic%:* 3% (0.03)

Iron Studies

- *Serum iron:* 28 mcg/dL (5.3 μmol/L)
- *Serum ferritin:* 7 mcg/L (15.7 pmol/L)
- *TIBC:* 462 mcg/dL (82.7 μmol/L)
- *Transferrin saturation:* 10% (0.10)

B₁₂ and Folate

- *Serum folate:* 10 mcg/dL (22.7 nmol/L)
- *Serum B₁₂:* 496 pg/mL (366 pmol/L)

Is this a macrocytic or microcytic anemia?

Specifically, what is the etiology of the anemia?

Recommend the most appropriate drug regimen (drug, dosage form, and schedule).

FDA labeling for the treatment of patients with anemia and CKD in the last decade.[17–20] Although the occurrence of life-threatening adverse events caused by parenteral iron is extremely low, the absolute rate of life-threatening events is substantially higher for HMW ID.[21,22] **Table 66–5** provides details pertinent to the use of these products.

The dose of iron dextran can be calculated by the following equation: dose (mL) = 0.0442 (desired Hgb – observed Hgb) × body weight + (0.26 × body weight). The body weight that should be used is lean body weight for adults and children weighing more than 15 kg and actual body weight for children weighing 5 to 15 kg. The dose in milligrams can be calculated based on a standard concentration of 50 mg of elemental iron per milliliter.[16] Prescribing information recommends administering iron dextran in 100-mg aliquots daily until the total dose is achieved. However, anecdotal evidence reports that the total calculated dose can be administered safely over 4 to 6 hours in 1 day. Because of the risk of anaphylaxis, a test dose of iron dextran (0.5 mL over at least 30 seconds) must be administered to patients before their first dose of iron dextran. Patients should be monitored for signs of anaphylaxis for at least 1 hour before administering the total dose. Other adverse effects include arthralgias, arrhythmias, hypotension, flushing, and pruritus.[21]

Table 66–3

Food Sources of Iron, Folic Acid, or Vitamin B₁₂

Nutrient	Food Sources
Iron	Red meat, organ meats, wheat germ, egg yolks, oysters
Folic acid	Green vegetables, liver, yeast, fruits
Vitamin B₁₂	Animal by-products, legumes

▶ Vitamin B₁₂ and Folic Acid Anemia

❼ *Anemia from vitamin B₁₂ or folic acid deficiency is treated effectively by replacing the missing nutrient.* Both folic acid and vitamin B₁₂ are essential for erythrocyte production and maturation. Replacing these nutrients allows for normal DNA synthesis and, consequently, normal erythropoiesis.

Oral and parenteral Vitamin B₁₂ (cyanocobalamin) replacement therapies are equally effective. Vitamin B₁₂ is absorbed completely following parenteral administration, whereas oral vitamin B₁₂ is absorbed poorly via the GI tract. Furthermore, parenteral vitamin B₁₂ may circumvent the need to perform a Shilling test used to diagnose a deficiency of intrinsic factor. Consequently, cyanocobalamin is commonly administered as an intramuscular injection. A typical cyanocobalamin dosing regimen is 1,000 mcg/day for 1 week, followed by 1,000 mcg/week for a month or until the Hgb normalizes. Life-long maintenance therapy (1,000 mcg/month)

Table 66–4

Oral Iron Products and Elemental Iron Content

Salt Form	Brand Name(s)	Elemental Iron Content per Dose Form
Ferrous sulfate	Feosol	65 mg/325-mg tablet 60 mg/300-mg tablet
Ferrous sulfate, anhydrous	N/A	65 mg/200-mg tablet
Ferrous gluconate	Fergon	39 mg/325-mg tablet 37 mg/300-mg tablet
Ferrous fumarate	Feostat	33 mg/100-mg tablet
Polysaccharide–iron complex	Niferex, Ferrex	150 mg/150-mg capsule 50 mg/ 50-mg tablet

---

Table 66–5

Parenteral Iron Products

Product (Brand name)	Mol. Wt. (Da)	Max. Approved Dose (mg)	Max. Infusion Rate Undiluted	TDI Possible	Test Dose Required	Black Box Warning	Absolute Rates LT ADEs/Million
Iron dextran injection (Dexferrum)[a]	265,000	100	50 mg/min	Yes	Yes	Yes	11.3
Iron dextran injection (INFed)	165,000	100	50 mg/min	Yes	Yes	Yes	3.3
Sodium ferric gluconate complex (Ferrlecit)	289,000–444,000	125	12.5 mg/min	No	No	No	0.9
Iron sucrose injection (Venofer)	34,000–60,000	200	40 mg/min	No	No	No	0.6
Ferumoxytol injection (Feraheme)	750,000	510	30 mg/sec	No	No	No	NR

Mol. Wt. (Da), molecular weight (Daltons); Max., maximum; TDI, total dose infusion; NR, not reported.

[a]HMW DI marketed in the United States in 1996, different manufacturer than HMW DI withdrawn in 1991.

From Auerbach M, Ballard H. Clinical use of intravenous iron: Administration, efficacy and safety. Hematology Am Soc Hematol Educ Program 2010:338–347.

---

is required for patients with pernicious anemia or surgical resection of the terminal ileum. If the etiology was a dietary deficiency or reversible malabsorption syndrome, treatment can be discontinued after the underlying cause is corrected and vitamin B_{12} stores normalized. A common oral dosing regimen is from 1,000 to 2,000 mcg/day. If parenteral cyanocobalamin is used initially, oral vitamin B_{12} can be useful as maintenance therapy. Typically, resolution of neurologic symptoms, disappearance of megaloblastic RBCs, and increased Hgb levels occur within a week of therapy.

Vitamin B_{12} is well tolerated. Reported adverse effects include injection-site pain, pruritus, and rash. Clinical significance of decreases in protein-bound cyanocobalamin related to proton pump inhibitor therapy has not been established.[15]

The effective dose of folic acid is 1 mg/day by mouth. Absorption of folic acid generally is rapid and complete. However, patients with malabsorption syndromes may require doses up to 5 mg/day. Resolution of symptoms and reticulocytosis occurs within days of commencing therapy. Typically a patient's Hgb will start to rise after 2 weeks of therapy and normalize after 2 to 4 months of therapy.

Folic acid is well tolerated. Nonspecific adverse effects include allergic reactions, flushing, malaise, and rash. A small study evaluating the effect of folic acid doses of 10 mg/day on phenytoin levels reported decreased phenytoin levels in 3 of 4 subjects. However, the occurrence of this interaction at folic acid doses of 1 mg/day has not been reported.[15]

▶ Anemia of Chronic Disease

⑧ *Decreased RBC transfusion requirements is an outcome achieved in patients with ACD treated with the ESAs. However, in 2007, the FDA product labeling for epoetin and darbepoetin were revised to include new data documenting safety concerns. Subsequently, the Centers for Medicare and Medicaid Services (CMS) implemented more restrictive ESA coverage determination guidelines. In 2010, the FDA implemented a risk evaluation and mitigation strategy (REMS) for ESAs administered to treat patients with cancer who are undergoing chemotherapy.* Table 66–6 summarizes the FDA-labeled dosing regimens for patients whose anemia is related to cancer chemotherapy, CKD, or zidovudine treatment.

Anemia Due to Chemotherapy in Patients with Cancer Epoetin, a recombinant human EPO, and darbepoetin, a synthetic EPO analog, bind to the EPO receptors on RBC precursor cells in the bone marrow and result in increased RBC production. Darbepoetin differs from epoetin in that it is a glycosylated protein and exhibits a longer half-life, allowing for a longer dosing interval. Clinical practice guidelines consider epoetin and darbepoetin to be therapeutic equivalents.[4,23] ⑨ *ESAs should only be used to prevent a transfusion and should not be initiated unless the hemoglobin is less than or equal to 10.0 g/dL (100 g/L,*

Patient Encounter 1, Part 3

The patient is diagnosed with iron-deficiency anemia and is started on ferrous sulfate 325 mg orally three times daily to be taken on an empty stomach. Follow-up CBC 1 month later reveals an Hgb of 10 g/dL (100 g/L or 6.21 mmol/L), previously 8.3 g/dL (83 g/L or 5.15 mmol/L). The patient reports improvement in shortness of breath and less frequent episodes of dizziness. She also states she occasionally misses doses due to her hectic days and remembering to take it on an empty stomach.

What hemoglobin level would constitute a therapeutic response in this patient?

How can compliance be improved in this patient?

Table 66–6		
ESA Products and Usual Doses for Anemia from Cancer/Chemotherapy, CKD, and Zidovudine/HIV Infection[a]		
	Epoetin-alfa (Epogen, Procrit)	**Darbepoetin-alfa (Aranesp)**
Cancer/chemotherapy dosing regimens	150 units/kg SC or IV 3 × per week. 40,000 units SC or IV once every week	2.25 mcg/kg SC or IV once every week 500 mcg SC or IV fixed dose every 3 weeks
CKD dosing regimens	50–100 units/kg SC or IV 3 × per week	0.45 mcg/kg SC or IV once every week[b] 0.75 mcg/kg SC or IV once every 2 weeks[b] 0.45 mcg/kg SC or IV once every 4 weeks[c]
Zidovudine/HIV dosing regimen[d]	100 units/kg IV or SC 3 × per week	

[a]Indications and dosage regimens per FDA product labeling.[32-34]
[b]for patients on dialysis
[c]for patients not on dialysis
[d]FDA labeled indication for Procrit (epoetin alfa), not Epogen (epoetin alfa) or darbepoetin

6.21 mmol/L). ESA-labeled dosing regimens for treatment of patients receiving chemotherapy are summarized in Table 66–6.

A number of clinical trials and a recent meta-analysis revealed that patients administered ESAs experienced increased thrombotic events and shorter progression-free and overall survival.[23] In the meta-analysis, a total of 13,933 cancer patients from 53 trials were analyzed. ESAs increased on study mortality (combined hazard ratio [cHR] 1.17; 95% CI 1.06 to 1.30) and worsened overall survival (cHR 1.06; 95% CI 1.00 to 1.12). This corresponds to a 17% increased risk of mortality for patients treated with ESAs while on study and a 6% increase overall. Based on these data, the FDA revised ESA product labeling, restricting their administration to patients with chemotherapy-induced anemia without a curative intent. The 2010 update of the American Society of Clinical Oncology/American Society of Hematology clinical practice guideline on the use of ESAs in patients with cancer adopted FDA recommendations calling for more restrictive use of ESA in patients with cancer.[24]

CMS published more restrictive national coverage criteria for ESA treatment of anemia associated with cancer chemotherapy in 2008. Patients should be monitored every 4 weeks. If Hgb has not increased by 1.0 g/dL (10 g/L, 0.62 mmol/L) after 4 weeks and remains less than 10.0 g/dL (100 g/L, 6.21 mmol/L), a one-time dose escalation of 25% is appropriate. If Hgb increases by more than 1.0 g/dL (10 g/L, 0.62 mmol/L), or is more than 10.0 g/dL (100 g/L, 6.21 mmol/L), the ESA should be discontinued. At 8 weeks if Hgb has increased by 1 g/dL (10 g/L, 0.62 mmol/L) but remains less than 10.0 g/dL(100 g/L, 6.21 mmol/L), continued ESA administration is covered. However, if after 8 weeks Hgb fails to increase by 1 g/dL (10 g/L, 0.62 mmol/L), CMS payment of therapy is not covered. CMS covers ESA therapy for up to 8 weeks after completion of chemotherapy for patients achieving responses.[25]

"Functional" iron deficiency has been described in patients with ACD. Therefore, it is imperative that patients starting ESA therapy have laboratory studies performed to assess

Patient Encounter 2 , Part 1

A 65-year-old woman with a diagnosis of metastatic, hormone-refractory breast cancer returns to the infusion center for her fifth paclitaxel infusion. She states her level of energy seems to be dropping. Her CBC reveals the following:

CBC

- WBC: $3.50 \times 10^3/\mu L$ ($3.50 \times 10^9/L$)
- Hgb: 9.3 g/dL (93 g/L or 5.77 mmol/L)
- Hct: 24.8% (0.248)
- Plt: $210 \times 10^3/\mu L$ ($210 \times 10^9/L$)

Red Blood Cell Indices

- MCV: $85 \mu M^3$/cell (85 fL/cell)
- MCH: 30 pg/cell
- MCHC: 35.3 g/dL (303 g/L)

Others

- RBC count: $3.8 \times 10^6 /\mu L$ ($3.8 \times 10^{12}/L$)
- RDW: 12% (0.15)

Iron studies

- *Serum iron:* 38 mcg/dL (5.8 μmol/L)
- *Serum ferritin:* 100 ng/mL (100 mcg/L)
- *TIBC:* 462 mcg/dL (82.7 μmol/L)
- *Transferrin saturation:* 10% (0.10)

B$_{12}$ and folate

- *Serum folate:* 20 mcg/dL (45 nmol/L)
- *Serum B$_{12}$:* 707 pg/mL (498 pmol/L)

In addition to the order for paclitaxel, you receive the following orders:

Epoetin 40,000 units SC weekly, ferrous sulfate 325 mg tablet three times daily.

What is your assessment of the orders for epoetin and ferrous sulfate?

What discussion must be presented to the patient before ESA therapy can be initiated?

iron stores. If results document a patient has suboptimal iron stores, iron replacement therapy is indicated.

Anemia Due to CKD Patients with CKD progress through five stages of disease based on glomerular filtration rate (GFR).[27] As discussed previously, anemia is common in patients with CKD. Early treatment of anemia in patients with CKD on dialysis has been associated with slower disease progression and lower risk of death. Therefore, it is essential to evaluate and treat anemia in patients before they progress to stage 5 CKD (GFR of less than 15 mL/min/1.73 m² [0.14 mL/s/m²]).[25,26]

Patients with CKD typically develop normocytic, normochromic anemia as a result of EPO deficiency. However, a thorough workup of anemia should be performed to rule out other etiologies.[25-28] Regardless, ESA therapy is effective in treating CKD anemia. The National Kidney Foundation Clinical Practice Recommendations 2007 update recommend a Hgb target range of 11.0 to 12.0g/dL (110 g/L to 120 g/L or 6.83 mmol/L to 7.45 mmol/L) in dialysis and nondialysis patients.[29] However, in June 2011, the FDA notified healthcare providers that the target Hgb range in patients with CKD was lowered to 11.0 g/dL (110 g/L or 6.83 mmol/L) in patients on hemodialysis and to 10.0 g/dL (100 g/dL or 6.21 mmol/L) in CKD patients not on hemodialysis.[30] This revision was adopted because data documented that the use of ESAs to achieve an Hgb greater than 11.0 g/dL (110 g/L or 6.83 mmol/L) resulted in increased risk of serious adverse cardiovascular events. The product labels previously recommended administration of ESAs to reach a Hgb target range of 10.0 to 12.0 g/dL (100 g/L to 120 g/L or 6.21 mmol/L to 7.45 mmol/L) for these patients. This target range was deleted from the revised product package inserts.[31-33] ESA-labeled dosing regimens for patients with CKD are summarized in Table 66–6.

Although EPO deficiency is the primary cause of CKD anemia, iron deficiency may also exist. Iron stores in patients with CKD should be maintained so that transferrin saturation is greater than 20% (0.20) and serum ferritin is greater than 100 ng/mL (100 mcg/L or 225 pmol/L). If iron stores are not maintained appropriately, epoetin or darbepoetin will not be effective. Most CKD patients will require iron supplementation.[28]

Anemia Due to Zidovudine in HIV-Infected Patients Early clinical trials evaluating the efficacy of zidovudine in HIV-infected patients documented that nearly 50% of patients treated with zidovudine develop anemia requiring RBC transfusions. Subsequently, results from four double-blind, placebo-controlled, multicenter studies reported that epoetin resulted in statistically significant decreases in transfusion requirements for patients with serum erythropoietin levels less than 500 mUnits/mL (500 U/L). Currently, epoetin has a labeled indication for the treatment of anemia in patients with EPO levels less than 500 mUnits/mL (500 U/L) and administered zidovudine doses less than 4,200 mg/week.[35]

Other Chronic Diseases Patients with infections and autoimmune disorders such as rheumatoid arthritis and systemic lupus erythematosus can also develop ACD. The appropriate treatment of the underlying disease is the primary therapeutic intervention in these patients. However, because functional iron deficiency and blunted EPO responsiveness are frequent complications in these patients, parenteral iron and EPO are effective adjunctive therapies for correcting anemia.

OUTCOME EVALUATION

⑩ *Patients should be monitored for Hgb response, symptom resolution, and adverse effects at appropriate intervals, and treatment regimens adjusted accordingly.* The goal of anemia therapy is to correct the underlying etiology of the anemia, normalize the Hgb, and alleviate associated symptoms.

- To ensure response for patients with IDA, monitor CBC with special attention to occurrence of reticulocytosis and iron studies.

- A 1.0-g/dL (10 g/L or 0.62 mmol/L) per week increase in Hgb is desirable in patients with IDA. Reevaluate patients with increases less than 2.0 g/dL (20 g/L or 1.24 mmol/L) in 3 weeks.

- For patients with folic acid deficiency, monitor Hgb periodically and reevaluate patients who fail to normalize Hgb levels after 2 months of therapy.

- For patients with vitamin B₁₂ deficiency, monitor for resolution of neurologic symptoms (i.e., confusion and paresthesias), if applicable, and Hgb levels weekly until the levels normalize.

- For patients treated with chemotherapy, initiate ESA treatment when Hgb levels are less than 10.0 g/dL (100 g/L or 6.21 mmol/L) and monitor Hgb levels weekly. If Hgb increases exceed 1.0 g/dL (10 g/L or 0.62 mmol/L) or exceed 10.0 g/dL (100 g/L or 6.21 mmol/L), hold therapy until the level drops below 10.0 g/dL (100 g/L or 6.21 mmol/L). Restart the ESA at the lowest dose sufficient to reduce transfusions

- For patients with CKD on dialysis, initiate ESA treatment when Hgb levels are less than 10.0 g/dL (100 g/L or 6.21 mmol/L) and monitor Hgb levels weekly. If Hgb levels approach or exceed 11.0 g/dL, reduce or hold further doses until the level drops below 10.0 g/dL (100 g/L or 6.21 mmol/L). Restart the ESA at the lowest dose sufficient to reduce transfusions.

- For patients with CKD not on dialysis, initiate ESA treatment when Hgb levels are less than 10.0 g/dL (100 g/L or 6.21 mmol/L) and monitor Hgb levels weekly. If Hgb levels exceed 10.0 g/dL (100 g/L or 6.21 mmol/L), reduce or hold further doses until the level drops below 10.0 g/dL (100 g/L or 6.21 mmol/L). Restart the ESA at the lowest dose sufficient to reduce transfusions.

Patient Care and Monitoring

1. Identify and treat the underlying cause of anemia.

2. Determine whether immediate correction of anemia is required with a transfusion or if chronic therapy can be initiated.

3. Monitor symptoms such as fatigue, shortness of breath, lethargy, headache, edema, and tachycardia for resolution.

4. Monitor the CBC monthly.

5. When initiating ESAs, assess the patient's iron status.

6. Monitor side effects of therapy, such as

   • *Oral iron*: nausea, vomiting, abdominal pain, heartburn, constipation, and dark stools

   • *Parenteral iron*: anaphylaxis (test dose required for iron dextran and observe for 1 hour after), injection-site pain/irritation, arthralgias, myalgias, flushing, malaise, and fever

   • *Folic acid*: bad taste and nausea, rash, and allergic reactions

   • *Vitamin B$_{12}$*: pain and erythema at injection site

   • *ESAs*: hypertension (monitor blood pressure), thrombosis (e.g., deep vein thrombosis/pulmonary embolism, myocardial infarction, cerebrovascular accident, and transient ischemic attack), arthralgias, and headache

Abbreviations Introduced in This Chapter

CFU-E	Erythroid colony-forming unit
CKD	Chronic kidney disease
EPO	Erythropoietin
ESA	Erythropoietin stimulating agent
GFR	Glomerular filtration rate
GM-CSF	Granulocyte-monocyte colony-stimulating factor
Hct	Hematocrit
Hgb	Hemoglobin
IDA	Iron-deficiency anemia
IL-3	Interleukin 3
MCV	Mean corpuscular volume
MCH	Mean corpuscular hemoglobin
NCCN	National Comprehensive Cancer Network
NKF-K/DOQI	National Kidney Foundation Kidney Disease Outcomes Quality Initiative
TIBC	Total iron-binding capacity

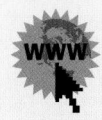

Self-assessment questions and answers are available at *http://mhpharmacotherapy. com/pp.html.*

REFERENCES

1. Centers for Disease Control and Prevention. Iron deficiency—United States, 1999-2000. MMWR Morb Mortal Wkly Rep 2002;51:897–899.

2. Guralnik JM, Eisenstaedt RS, Ferrucci L, et al. Prevalence of anemia in persons 65 years and older in the United States: Evidence for a high rate of unexplained anemia. Blood 2004;104(8):2263–2268.

3. Knight K, Wade S, Balducci L. Prevalence and outcomes of anemia in cancer: a systematic review of the literature. Am J Med 2004;116(Suppl 7A):S11–S26.

4. National Comprehensive Cancer Network [Internet]. Cancer- and chemotherapy-induced anemia. NCCN Practice Guidelines in Oncology- V.2.2012 [cited 2011 June 30]. Available from: *http://www.nccn.org/professionals/physician_gls/pdf/anemia.pdf.*

5. McFarlane SI, Chen SC, Whaley-Connell AT, et al. Prevalence and associations of anemia of CKD: Kidney Early Evaluation Program (KEEP) and National Health and Nutrition Examination Survey (NHANES) 1999-2004. Am J Kidney Dis 2008;51(Suppl 2):S46–S55.

6. Weiss G, Goodnough LT. Anemia of chronic disease. N Engl J Med 2005;352(10):1011–1023.

7. Guyton AC, Hall JE. Red blood cells, anemia, and polycythemia. In: Guyton AC, Hall JE, eds. Textbook of Medical Physiology. 11th ed. Philadelphia, PA: WB Saunders; 2006:419–428.

8. Kaushansky K, Kipps TJ. Hemapoietic Agents: growth factors, minerals, and vitamins. In: Brunton LL, Laza LS, Parker KL, eds. Goodman & Gilman's the Pharmacological Basis of Therapeutics. 11th ed. New York: McGraw-Hill; 2006:1433–1466.

9. Toh BH, van Driel IR, Gleeson PA. Pernicious anemia. N Engl J Med 1997;337(20):1441–1448.

10. Andrews NC. Disorders of iron metabolism. N Engl J Med 1999;341(26):1986–1995.

11. Aird William C. Anemia. In: Furie Bruce, Cassileth Peter A, Atkins Michael B, Mayer Robert J, eds. Clinical Hematology and Oncology. Philadelphia, PA: Churchill Livingstone; 2003:232–240.

12. Carless PA, Henry DA, Carson JL, et al. Transfusion thresholds and other strategies for guiding allogeneic red blood cell transfusion. Cochran Database Syst Rev 2010; 6:CD002042.

13. Hebert PC, Wells G, Blajchman MA, et al. A multicenter, randomized, controlled clinical trial of transfusion requirements in critical care. N Engl J Med 1999;340:409–417.

14. Alleyne M, Horne MK, Miller JL. Individualized treatment for iron-deficiency anemia in adults. Am J Med 2008;121:943–948.

15. Zucchero FJ, Hogan MJ, Sommer CD, eds. Evaluations of Drug Interactions. San Bruno, CA: First DataBank; 2007.

16. INFed (iron dextran) prescribing information. Morristown, NJ: Watson Pharma; July 2009.

17. Dexferrum (iron dextran) prescribing information. Shirley, NY: American Regent; August 2008.

18. Ferrlecit (sodium ferric gluconate complex in sucrose injection) prescribing information. Bridgewater, NJ: Sanofi-Aventis; August 2011.

19. Venofer (iron sucrose injection) prescribing information. Shirley, NY: American Regent; June 2011.

20. Feraheme (ferumoxytol injection) prescribing information. Lexington, MA: AMAG Pharmaceuticals; June 2011.

21. Auerbach M, Ballard H. Clinical use of intravenous iron: Administration, efficacy and safety. Hematology Am Soc Hematol Educ Program 2010:338–347.

22. Chertow GM, Mason PD, Vaage-Nilsen O, et al. Update on adverse drug events associated with parenteral iron. Nephrol Dial Transplant 2006;21:378–382.

23. Bohlius J, Schmidlin K, Brillant C, et al. Erythropoietin or darbepoetin for patients with cancer—meta-analysis based on individual patient data. Cochrane Database Syst Rev 2009;8:CD007303.

24. Rizzo JD, Brouwers M, Hurley P, et al. American Society of Clinical Oncology/American Society of Hematology clinical practice guideline update on the use of epoetin and darbeopetin in adult patients with cancer. J Clin Oncol 2010;28:4996–5010.

25. Centers for Medicare and Medicaid Services [Internet]. Decision memo for erythropoiesis stimulating agents (ESAs) in cancer and related

neoplastic conditions [cited 2011 Oct 27]. Available from: *https://www. cms.gov/transmittals/downloads/R80NCD.pdf.*

26. Levey AS, Coresh J, Balk E, et al. National Kidney Foundation practice guidelines for chronic kidney disease: Evaluation, classification, and stratification. Ann Intern Med 2003;139(2):137–147.

27. Jungers P, Choukroun G, Oualim Z, Robino C, Nguyen AT, Man NK. Beneficial influence of recombinant human erythropoietin therapy on the rate of progression of chronic renal failure in predialysis patients. Nephrol Dial Transplant 2001;16(2):307–312.

28. Eschbach J, DeOreo PB, Adamson J, et al [Internet]. NKF-K/DOQI Clinical Practice Guidelines. National Kidney Foundation—Kidney Disease Outcomes Quality Initiative (NKF K/DOQI) 2000 [cited 2011 Oct 12]. Available from: *http://www.kidney.org/professionals/kdoqi/ guidelines_updates/doqi_uptoc.html#an.*

29. KDOQ1; National Kidney Foundation. Am J Kid Dis 2006;47: S109–S116.

30. National Kidney Foundation Kidney Disease Outcomes Quality Initiative [Internet]. NKF-K/DOQI Clinical Practice Guideline and Clinical Practice Recommendations for Anemia in Chronic Kidney Disease: 2007 Update of Hemoglobin Target [cited 2011 Oct 14]. Available from: *http://www.kidney.org/professionals/kdoqi/guidelines_anemia/cpr21. htm.*

31. FDA [Internet]. FDA Drug Safety Communication: Modified dosing recommendations to improve the safe us of erythropoiesis-stimulating agents (ESAs) in chronic kidney disease [cited 2011 Oct 27]. Available from: *http://www.fda.gov/drugs/drugsafety/ucm259639.htm.*

32. Aranesp (darbepoetin alfa) prescribing information. Thousand Oaks, CA: Amgen; June 2011.

33. Epogen (epoetin alfa) prescribing information. Centocor Ortho Biotech Products, June 2011.

34. Procrit (epoetin alfa) prescribing information. Thousand Oaks, CA: Amgen; June 2011.

35. Henry DH, Beall GN, Benson CA, et al. Recombinant human erythro-poietin in the treatment of anemia associated with human immuno-deficiency virus (HIV) infection and zidovudine therapy. Overview of four clinical trials. Ann Intern Med 1992;117:739–748.

67

Coagulation and Platelet Disorders

Anastasia Rivkin

LEARNING OBJECTIVES

● **Upon completion of this chapter, the reader will be able to:**

1. Describe the basics of the regulation of hemostasis and thrombosis.

2. Determine which factor replacement preparation is appropriate in a given clinical situation.

3. Calculate an appropriate factor-concentrate dose for a product, given the percentage correction desired based on clinical situation.

4. List the complications from hemophilia bleeding episodes.

5. Choose appropriate treatment strategy for patients with factor VIII or IX inhibitors.

6. Devise a treatment plan for a patient with a specific variant of von Willebrand's disease (vWD).

7. Describe various recessively inherited coagulation disorders (RICDs) and role of specific factor replacement in RICD management.

8. Formulate an appropriate treatment plan based on presentation of disseminated intravascular coagulation (DIC).

9. Recommend first-line and a second-line treatment approaches for immune thrombocytopenic purpura (ITP).

10. Identify basic clinical features, causes, and management of thrombotic thrombocytopenic purpura (TTP).

KEY CONCEPTS

❶ IV replacement with recombinant or plasma-derived products to treat or prevent bleeding is the primary treatment of hemophilia.

❷ Patients with type 1 von Willebrand's disease (vWD) unresponsive to desmopressin, patients with types 2 and 3 vWD, and major surgery patients require replacement therapy with plasma-derived intermediate- and high-purity factor VIII, virus-inactivated factor VIII concentrate containing von Willebrand's factor (vWF).

❸ The primary treatment of recessively inherited coagulation disorders (RICDs) is single-donor fresh-frozen plasma (FFP) that contains all coagulation factors.

❹ The cornerstone of the management of disseminated intravascular coagulation (DIC) is aggressive treatment of the underlying primary illness. Supportive measures may be used as necessary; however, owing to the heterogeneity of the DIC etiology, treatment should be guided by predominant symptoms (bleeding or clotting).

❺ The treatment of immune thrombocytopenic purpura (ITP) is determined by the symptom severity. In some cases, no therapy is needed.

❻ The present standard of treatment for thrombotic thrombocytopenic purpura (TTP) is urgent plasma exchange (PEX). If PEX is unavailable, treatment with plasma infusion and glucocorticoids is indicated until PEX is available.

INTRODUCTION

Components of the Hemostatic System

● Following endothelial injury, vessel-wall response involves vasoconstriction, platelet plug formation, coagulation, and **fibrinolysis** regulation. In normal circumstances, platelets circulate in the blood in an inactive form. After injury, platelets undergo activation, which consists of (a) adhesion to the subendothelium, (b) secretion of granules containing chemical mediators (e.g., adenosine diphosphate, thromboxane A2, thrombin, etc.), and (c) aggregation. Chemical factors released from the injured tissue and platelets

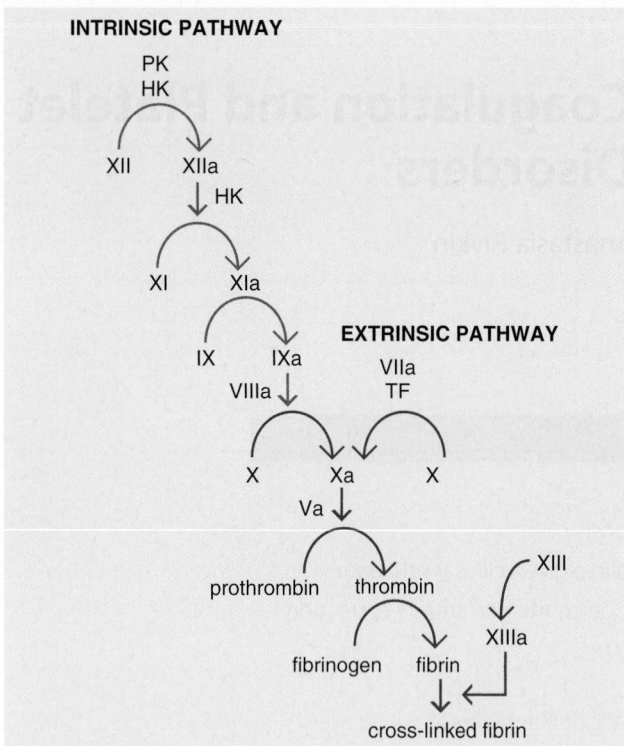

FIGURE 67–1. Cascade model of coagulation demonstrates activation via the intrinsic or extrinsic pathway. This model shows successive activation of coagulation factors proceeding from the top to the bottom where thrombin and fibrin are generated. (PK, prekallikrein; HK, high–molecular weight kininogen; TF, tissue factor.) (From Roberts HR et al. Molecular biology and biochemistry of the coagulation factors and pathways of hemostasis. In: Lichtman MA, Beutler E, Coller BS et al, eds. Williams Hematology, 7th ed. New York: McGraw-Hill, 2006:1665–1694.)

stimulate the coagulation cascade and thrombin formation. In turn, thrombin catalyzes the conversion of fibrinogen to fibrin and its subsequent incorporation into plug.

The coagulation system consists of intrinsic and extrinsic pathways. Both pathways are composed of a series of enzymatic reactions that ultimately produce thrombin, fibrin, and a stable clot. In parallel with the coagulation, the fibrinolytic system is activated locally. Plasminogen is converted to plasmin, which dissolves the fibrin mesh (Fig. 67–1).[1]

INHERITED COAGULATION DISORDERS

HEMOPHILIA

Etiology and Epidemiology

Hemophilia A and B are coagulation disorders that result from defects in the genes encoding for plasma coagulation proteins. Hemophilia A (classic hemophilia) is caused by the deficiency of factor VIII, and hemophilia B (Christmas disease) is caused

by the deficiency of factor IX. The incidences of hemophilia A and B are estimated at 1 in 5,000 and 1 in 30,000 male births, respectively. Both types of hemophilia are evenly distributed across all ethnic and racial groups.[1]

Pathophysiology

The pathophysiology of hemophilia is based on the deficiency of factor VIII or IX resulting in inadequate thrombin generation and an impaired intrinsic-pathway coagulation cascade (see Fig. 67–1). Factor VIII and IX genes are located on the X chromosome. Hemophilias are recessive X-linked diseases. Generally, affected males carrying either defective allele on their X chromosome do not transmit the gene to their sons. However, their daughters are obligate carriers. Over 2,100 mutations, deletions, and inversions have been identified throughout the factor VIII and IX genes.[2]

Consequently, hemophilia is not a result of a single genetic mutation. However, inversion at intron 22 of the factor VIII gene accounts for 45% of severe hemophilia A cases. Owing to the high incidence, this mutation is used for carrier and prenatal testing.[3]

Complications of Hemophilia

The severity of bleeding associated with hemophilia correlates with the degree of factor VIII or factor IX deficiency as measured against the normal plasma standard. Table 67–1 summarizes the age at onset and laboratory and clinical manifestations of hemophilia A and B.[4]

Treatment

▶ Desired Outcomes

Currently, there is no cure for hemophilia A or B. The life expectancy of hemophiliacs was only 8 to 11 years in the 1920s and 1930s. With the development of effective treatment strategies, life expectancy is currently about 63 to 75 years, or nearly that of the normal population.[5]

The short-term goals of hemophilia treatment are to:

- Decrease the number of bleeding episodes per year or bleeding frequency
- Normalize or improve clotting factor concentrate levels

The long-term goals of hemophilia treatment are to:

- Maintain clinical joint function
- Normalize orthopedic joint score
- Normalize radiologic joint score
- Maintain quality-of-life measurements

▶ General Approach to Treatment

❶ *IV factor replacement with recombinant or plasma-derived products to treat or prevent bleeding is the primary treatment of hemophilia.* Primary prophylaxis is defined as the regular administration of factor concentrates with the intention of preventing joint bleeds.[6] The rationale for primary

Table 67–1

Laboratory and Clinical Manifestations of Hemophilia

	Severe (Less Than 0.01 IU/mL [10 IU/L])[a]	Moderate (0.01–0.05 IU/mL [10–50 IU/L])[a]	Mild (More Than 0.05 IU/mL [50 IU/L])[a]
Age at onset	1 year or less	1–2 years	2 years–adult
Neonatal symptoms			
PCB	Usual	Usual	Rare
ICH	Occasional	Uncommon	Rare
Muscle/joint hemorrhage	Spontaneous	Minor trauma	Minor trauma
CNS hemorrhage	High risk	Moderate risk	Rare
Postsurgical hemorrhage (without prophylaxis)	Frank bleeding, severe	Wound bleeding, common	Wound bleeding
Oral hemorrhage following trauma, tooth extraction	Usual	Common	Common

CNS, central nervous system; ICH, intracranial hemorrhage; PCB, postcircumcisional bleeding.

Normal range of factor VIII/IX activity level is 0.5–1.5 IU/mL (50–150 IU/L). 1 IU/mL (1,000 IU/L) corresponds to 100% of the factor found in 1 mL of normal plasma.

[a]0.01 IU/mL = 10 IU/L; 0.05 IU/mL = 50 IU/L; 0.5 IU/mL = 500 IU/L; 1 unit/mL = 1 IU/mL = 1,000 IU/L; 1.5 IU/mL = 1,500 IU/L.

prophylaxis is that individuals with factor levels of greater than 0.02 IU/mL (20 IU/L) rarely suffer from spontaneous bleeds and arthropathy. Therefore, to maintain a trough level above this might convert "severe" hemophilia to "moderate" disease, with the abolition of joint bleeds and the associated arthropathy.[7]

Although primary prophylaxis is expensive, historical cohorts show progressively better outcomes (joint function and radiologic appearances) with its use. The Medical and Scientific Advisory Council of the National Hemophilia Foundation of the United States recommends primary prophylaxis in patients with severe hemophilia A and B (factor VIII or factor IX less than 1%). The optimal duration of prophylactic therapy is unknown.[8,9] Vaccination against hepatitis A and B is recommended in all hemophiliacs.

▶ Nonpharmacologic Therapy

Supportive Care Rest, ice, compression, elevation (RICE) can be used during the bleeding episode, following with casts, splints, and crutches after the bleeding has been controlled.

Surgery Surgical arthroscopic synovectomy reduces replacement therapy–resistant disease and repetitive hemarthrosis of a single joint. This procedure removes inflamed joint tissue. Patients may have decreased range of motion after the surgery.

Orthotics Joint prostheses do not deal with the deformities directly. Orthotics in hemophilia serve as an important supportive measure before or after surgery.

Clinical Presentation and Diagnosis of Hemophilias A and B

Hemophilias A and B are clinically indistinguishable.

Symptoms

- Ecchymoses
- **Hemarthrosis**—bleeding into joint spaces[a] (especially knee, elbow, and ankle)
  - Joint pain, swelling, and erythema
  - Cutaneous warmth
  - Decreased range of motion
- Muscle hemorrhage
  - Swelling
  - Pain with motion of affected muscle
  - Signs of nerve compression

- Potential life-threatening blood loss, especially with thigh bleeding
- Mouth bleeding with dental extractions or trauma
- Genitourinary bleeding
- GI bleeding
- Hematuria
- Intracranial hemorrhage (spontaneous or following trauma), with headache, vomiting, change in mental status, and focal neurologic signs
- Excessive bleeding with surgery

---

[a]Hallmark of hemophilia; recurrent inadequately managed hemarthrosis leads to deformity and chronic pain (hemophilic arthropathy).

► *Pharmacologic Therapy*

Hemophilia A

DDAVP. Primary therapy is based on disease severity and type of hemorrhage.[10] Most patients with mild to moderate disease and a minor bleeding episode can be treated with 1-desamino-8-D-arginine vasopressin (desmopressin acetate [DDAVP]), a synthetic analog of the antidiuretic hormone, vasopressin. DDAVP causes release of von Willebrand's factor (vWF) and factor VIII from endothelial storage sites. DDAVP increases plasma factor VIII levels by three- to five-fold within 30 minutes. The recommended dose is 0.3 mcg/kg IV (in 50 mL of normal saline infused over 15 to 30 minutes) or subcutaneously (in less than 1.5 mL) or 150 to 300 mcg intranasally via concentrated nasal spray every 12 hours. Peak effect with intranasal administration occurs 60 to 90 minutes after administration, which is somewhat later than with IV administration. Desmopressin infusion may be administered daily for up to 2 to 3 days. Facial flushing, hypertension or hypotension, GI upset, and headache are common side effects of desmopressin. Water retention and hyponatremia may occur; patients should be instructed to limit water intake while taking desmopressin. Serious side effects include seizures related to hyponatremia, most frequently seen in children younger than 2 years of age, and myocardial infarction in the elderly. Tachyphylaxis, an attenuated response with repeated administration, may occur after several doses.[11]

According to the manufacturer, use of DDAVP is contraindicated in patients with creatinine clearance less than 50 mL/min (0.83 mL/s); however, it has been used off label in patients with impaired renal function.

Antifibrinolytic Therapy. Aminocaproic acid and tranexamic acid are antifibrinolytic agents that reduce plasminogen activity leading to inhibition of clot lysis and clot stabilization. These agents are usually used as adjuncts in dental procedures or in difficult-to-control epistaxis and menorrhagia episodes.

Factor VIII Replacement. Patients with severe hemophilia may receive primary (before the first major bleed) or secondary (after the first major bleed) prophylaxis. All hemophiliacs with a major bleed require factor VIII replacement.[12] The therapy may include recombinant (produced via transfection of mammalian cells with the human factor VIII gene) or plasma-derived (concentrate from pooled plasma) factor VIII (Table 67–2). The choice of product and dose are based on the overall clinical scenario because the efficacy of various

---

Table 67–2			
Factor Concentrates			
Brand Name	**Product Type**	**Viral Inactivation or Exclusion Method**	**Other Contents**
Factor VIII Concentrates			
Alphanate	Plasma	Solvent detergent, dry heat	Albumin, heparin, vWF
Advate	Recombinant	None	Trehalose
Bioclate	Recombinant	None	Albumin
Helixate FS	Recombinant	Solvent detergent	Sucrose
Hemofil M	Plasma	Solvent detergent, monoclonal antibody	Albumin
Humate-P	Plasma	Pasteurization	Albumin, vWF
Koāte-DVI	Plasma	Solvent detergent, dry heat	Albumin, vWF
Kogenate FS	Recombinant	Solvent detergent, monoclonal antibody	Sucrose
Monoclate P	Plasma	Pasteurization, monoclonal antibody	Albumin
Recombinate	Recombinant	Monoclonal antibody	Albumin
ReFacto	Recombinant B domain deleted	None	Sucrose
XYNTHA	Recombinant B domain deleted	Solvent-detergent, nanofiltration	Sucrose
Factor IX Concentrates			
AlphaNine SD	Plasma	Solvent detergent, nanofiltration	Heparin
BeneFIX	Recombinant	None	Sucrose
Mononine	Plasma	Monoclonal antibody, nanofiltration	
APCC			
Feiba VH or NF	Plasma	Vapor heat	II, VIIa, IX, X, factor VIII coagulant antigen
PCC			
Bebulin VH	Plasma	Vapor heat	Heparin, II, IX, X
Profilnine SD	Plasma	Solvent detergent	II, VII, IX, X
Proplex T	Plasma	Dry heat	Heparin, II, VII, IX, X
Other			
NovoSeven RT	Recombinant VII	None	Sucrose
Wilate	Plasma vWF/VIII complex	Solvent detergent and dry heat	Sucrose

APCC, activated prothrombin complex concentrate; PCC, prothrombin complex concentrate; vWF, von Willebrand's factor.

Table 67–3

Guidelines for Replacement Dosing with Factor VIII and Factor IX

Type of Hemorrhage	Desired Plasma Factor VIII Level (% of Normal)	Desired Plasma Factor XI Level (% of Normal)	Duration of Therapy (days)
CNS, intracranial, retropharyngeal, retroperitoneal, surgical prophylaxis	80–100	80–100	Factor VIII: every 8–12 hours over 10–14 days Factor IX: every 12 hours over 10–14 days
Mild hemarthrosis, mucosal (e.g., epistaxis), superficial hematoma	30	20–30	Factor VIII: every 8–12 hours over 1–2 days Factor IX: every 12–24 hours over 1–2 days

preparations does not differ. Newer generation plasma-derived coagulation factor concentrates are considerably safer owing to advancements in viral testing and inactivation technology. Although original recombinant factor VIII concentrates were stabilized with human serum albumin, potentially creating a source for viral contamination, new-generation recombinant factor VIII concentrates are stabilized with sucrose, eliminating the concern for viral transmission.

The severity of hemorrhage and its location are major determinants of percentage correction to target, as well as duration of therapy (Table 67–3). The normal range of factor VIII activity level is 1 IU/mL (1000 IU/L), which corresponds to 100% of the factor found in 1 mL of normal plasma. Minor bleeding may be treated with a goal of 25% to 30% (0.25 to 0.30 IU/mL [250 to 300 IU/L]) of normal activity, whereas serious or life-threatening bleeding requires greater than 75% of normal activity. Factor VIII is a large molecule that remains in the intravascular space, and its estimated volume of distribution is approximately 50 mL/kg. Generally, factor VIII levels increase by 2% (0.02 IU/mL [20 IU/L]) for every 1 unit/kg of factor VIII concentrate infused. To calculate factor VIII replacement dose, the following equation can be used:

Dose of factor VIII (units)
= weight (kg) × (desired percentage increase) × 0.5

Thus, to increase factor VIII levels by 50% (e.g., from 0 to 50%) in a 70-kg (154-lb) patient, an IV dose of 1,750 units is required. The half-life of factor VIII ranges from 8 to 15 hours. Half the initial dose is given every half-life (every 8 to 12 hours) to maintain the desired factor VIII level.[13]Although intermittent bolus infusions of factor VIII concentrates have been used successfully, continuous-infusion protocols are being instituted successfully in patients requiring prolonged treatment of acute hemorrhage to avoid dangerously low trough levels and decrease the overall cost of therapy. Factor VIII can be administered as a continuous infusion at 2 to 4 units/kg/h with daily factor level monitoring to ensure appropriate rate of infusion.[14,15]

▶ Hemophilia B

Factor IX Replacement Hemophilia B therapy may include recombinant (produced via transfection of mammalian cells with the human factor IX gene) or plasma-derived (concentrate from pooled plasma) factor IX (see Table 67–2). Guidelines for choosing the factor-concentrate formulation

for hemophilia B are similar to the guidelines for hemophilia A. However, older generation factor IX concentrates containing other vitamin K–dependent proteins (e.g., factors II, VII, and IX), called prothrombin complex concentrates (PCCs), have been associated with thrombogenic side effects. Consequently, these products are not first-line treatment for hemophilia B. Because it is a small protein, the factor IX molecule passes into both the intravascular and the extravascular spaces. Therefore, the volume of distribution of recombinant factor IX is twice that of factor VIII. Consequently, 1 unit of factor IX administered per kilogram of body weight yields a 1% rise in the plasma factor IX level (0.01 IU/mL [10IU/L]). To calculate the factor IX replacement dose, the following equation can be used:

Dose of factor IX (units)
= weight (kg) × (desired percentage increase) × F

Where F = 1 for human plasma-derived products and 1.2 for recombinant factor IX.

Thus, to increase factor IX levels by 50% (e.g., from 0 to 50%) in a 70-kg (154-lb) patient, the required dose of factor IX is 4,200 units IV (using the recombinant factor IX product). The half-life of factor IX ranges from 18 to 22 hours; therefore, doses are given every 12 to 24 hours.

▶ Treatment of Patients with Factor VIII or IX Inhibitors

Factor VIII and IX inhibitors are antibodies that develop in 20% and 5% of hemophilia A and hemophilia B patients, respectively, in response to replacement therapy. These antibodies bind to and neutralize the activity of infused factor concentrates. Although the inhibitors do not increase hemorrhage frequency, their existence challenges the treatment of bleeding episodes. Titers of inhibitors are measured and reported in Bethesda units (BU), and this measurement is used to guide therapy (Fig. 67–2). Management options for acute bleeding in patients with factor inhibitors include the administration of factor VIII concentrates, PCCs, recombinant factor VIIa (rFVIIa), and porcine factor VIII (currently, recombinant porcine factor VIII is in phase II/III clinical trials in the United States). Immune tolerance induction can be attempted to prevent future bleeding episodes.

Factor VIII concentrates can be used in patients with low inhibitor levels to control acute bleeding episodes. The dose

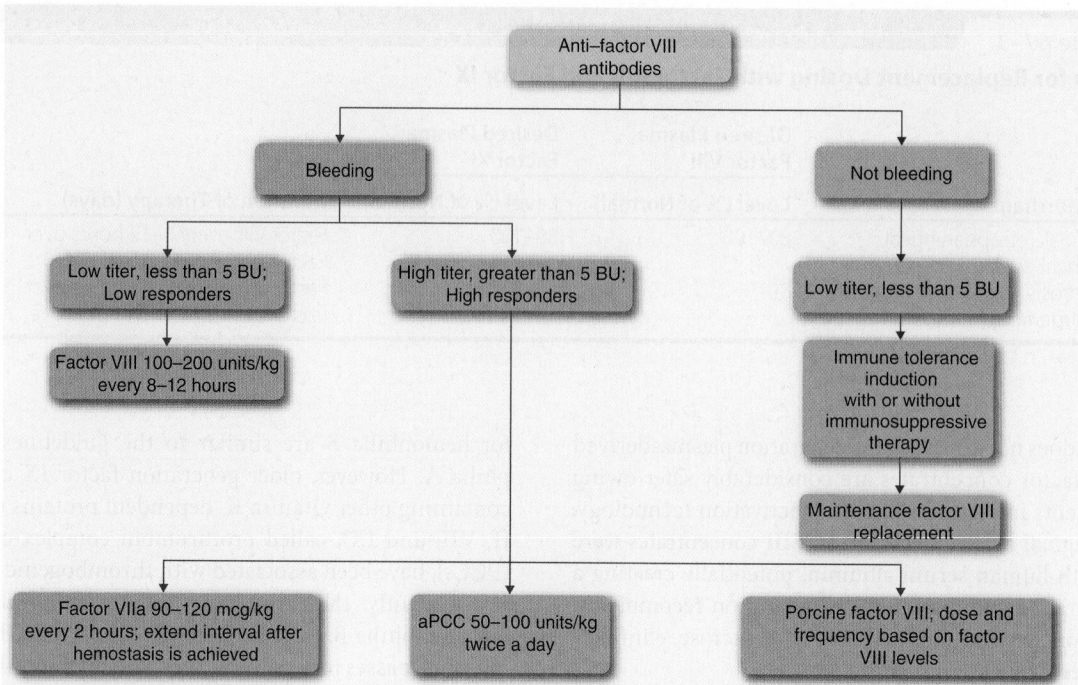

FIGURE 67–2. Treatment algorithm for the management of patients with hemophilia A and factor VIII antibodies. Porcine factor VIII is not available in the United States; recombinant porcine factor VIII is currently in phase II/III clinical trials. (BU, Bethesda unit; aPCC, activated prothrombin complex concentrate.) (Modified from DiPiro JT, Talbert RL, Yee GC, et al., eds. Pharmacotherapy: A Pathophysiologic Approach. 8th ed. New York: McGraw-Hill; 2011:1751, Figure 110–3.)

of factor VIII is determined based on clinical response (see Fig. 67–2).

PCCs contain the vitamin K–dependent factors II, VII, IX, and X. These agents bypass factor VIII at which the antibody is directed (see Fig. 67–2). However, PCCs carry the risk of serious thrombotic complications.

Factor VIIa (rFVIIa) is a bypassing agent designed to generate thrombin only at tissue injury sites, where it binds tissue factor. Due to its local action, rFVIIa is associated with fewer systemic thrombotic events than PCC. rFVIIa is used effectively in surgeries and spontaneous bleeds.[16]

Plasma-derived porcine factor VIII participates in the coagulation cascade in place of human factor VIII. However, due to contamination with parvovirus, it is no longer available. Recombinant porcine factor VIII is currently under review and could serve as a third-line agent (only after factor VIIa and a PCC have failed) owing to the relatively high incidence of cross-reactivity with factor VIII inhibitors.

Induction of immune tolerance is often performed with the goal of eliminating the inhibitor. Immune tolerance induction is accomplished by the administration of repetitive doses of factor VIII or IX with or without immunosuppressive therapy. It is effective in 70% of patients with hemophilia A and 30% of patients with hemophilia B.

Pain Associated with Hemophilia

Pain commonly occurs in patients with hemophilia. Acute bleeding episodes and long-term joint destruction

are common sources of pain. Acetaminophen and opioid analgesics are recommended to control mild to moderate and severe pain, respectively. Nonsteroidal anti-inflammatory drugs and aspirin should be avoided if possible, because these drugs bind to platelets and increase the risk of bleeding episodes. Cyclooxygenase-2 (COX-2) inhibitors can be used with caution.[17]

Outcome Evaluation

The main goal of hemophilia treatment is to prevent bleeding episodes and their long-term complications. Clinicians should evaluate patients for the following:

- Musculoskeletal status, including joint range of motion and radiologic assessment, as indicated.

- Number and type of bleeding episodes to assess adequacy of prophylactic treatment and home therapy.

- Use of clotting-factor concentrates to check for the development of inhibitors, especially in patients with severe disease and poor treatment responders.

VON WILLEBRAND'S DISEASE
Epidemiology and Etiology

von Willebrand's disease (vWD) is the most common inherited bleeding disorder caused by a deficiency or dysfunction of vWF. It is classified based on the quantitative deficiency of vWF or qualitative abnormalities of vWF.

Table 67–4

Classification of vWD

Phenotype	Mechanism of Disease	Percentage of Cases	Genetic Transmission
Type 1 vWD	Partial (mild to moderate) quantitative deficiency of vWF and factor VIII	70–80	Autosomal dominant
Type 2 vWD	Qualitative abnormalities of vWF	10–30	
2A	Decreased platelet-dependent vWF function owing to lack of larger multimers	10–15	Autosomal dominant (or recessive)
2B	Increased platelet-dependent vWF function owing to lack of larger multimers	Uncommon	Autosomal dominant
2M	Defective platelet-dependent vWF functions not associated with multimer defects	Uncommon	Autosomal dominant (or recessive)
2N	Defective vWF binding to factor VIII	Uncommon	Autosomal recessive
Type 3 vWD	Severe quantitative deficiency of vWF	Rare	Autosomal recessive

The disease prevalence is estimated at 30 to 100 cases per million. In contrast to hemophilia, the majority of vWD cases are inherited as an autosomal dominant disorder, ensuing equal frequency in males and females.[18]

Pathophysiology

vWF is a large multimeric glycoprotein with two main functions in hemostasis: to aid platelet adhesion to injured blood vessel walls and to carry and stabilize factor VIII in plasma. Table 67–4 represents three main vWD phenotypes, their frequency, and genetic transmission.[19]

Treatment

▶ Desired Outcomes

Unlike hemophilia, the bleeding tendency in vWD is less frequent and generally less severe. Consequently, chronic

prophylaxis is usually unwarranted. The goal of two mainstay therapeutic options in vWD is:

- To stop spontaneous bleeding as necessary
- To prevent surgical and postpartum bleeding

▶ Nonpharmacologic Therapy

Local measures, including pressure and ice, may be used to control superficial bleeding.

▶ Pharmacologic Therapy

Systemic therapy is used to prevent bleeding associated with surgery, childbirth, and dental extractions and to treat bleeding that cannot be controlled with local measures. The two systemic approaches involve using desmopressin, which stimulates the release of endogenous vWF, or administering products that contain vWF. The general approach to the

Clinical Presentation and Diagnosis of vWD

Clinical manifestations vary depending on the subtype. Patients with mild disease may be asymptomatic into adulthood.

Symptoms

- Bruising
- Mucocutaneous bleeding
  - Epistaxis
  - Oral cavity bleeding
  - Menorrhagia
  - GI bleeding
- Joint and deep tissue bleeding
- Postoperative bleeding

Laboratory Testing

- Low or normal von Willebrand's factor antigen concentration in plasma (vWF:Ag)
- Low or normal factor VIII coagulation assay (FVIII:C)[a]
- Low ristocetin cofactor activity (vWF:RCo)[b]

[a]Factor VIII coagulation assay measures the ability of vWF to bind and maintain adequate levels of factor VIII.

[b]Ristocetin cofactor activity (vWF:RCo) assay measures the ability of vWF to interact with intact platelets (normal 50–200 IU/dL).

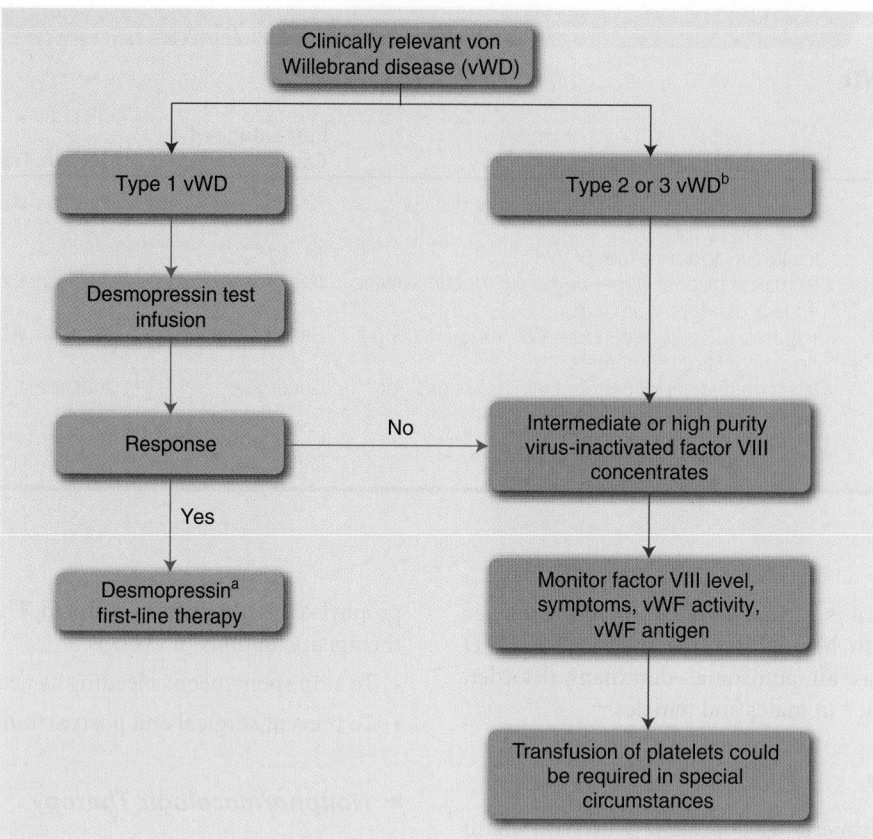

FIGURE 67–3. Guidelines for the treatment of vWD. [a]Use factor VIII concentrate for life-threatening bleeding. [b]Some patients with type 2 or 3 vWD may respond to desmopressin. (From DiPiro JT, Talbert RL, Yee GC, et al., eds. Pharmacotherapy: A Pathophysiologic Approach. 8th ed. New York: McGraw-Hill; 2011:1754, Figure 110–4.)

treatment of vWD is depicted in Figure 67–3. In 2008, The National Heart, Lung, and Blood Institute issued comprehensive evidence-based guidelines for the diagnosis and management of vWD.[20]

● **DDAVP** Most patients with type 1 vWD (functionally normal vWF) and a minor bleeding episode can be treated successfully with desmopressin, which induces release of factor VIII and vWF from endothelial cells through interaction with vasopressin V2 receptors. The recommended dose is the same as that used to treat mild factor VIII deficiency (0.3 mcg/kg IV in 50 mL of normal saline infused over 15 to 30 min or 150 to 300 mcg intranasally via concentrated nasal spray every 12 hours). This therapy is generally ineffective in type 2A patients, who secrete abnormal vWF, and is controversial in type 2B patients because it may increase the risk of postinfusion thrombocytopenia. Type 3 vWD patients who lack releasable stores of vWF do not respond to DDAVP therapy.[21]

The individual responsiveness to desmopressin is consistent, and a test dose administered at the time of diagnosis or prior to therapy is the best predictor of response. Generally, DDAVP is more effective in vWD than in hemophilia patients, with an average two- to five-fold increase in vWF and factor VIII levels over baseline. In patients with an adequate response, desmopressin is first-line therapy because

it allows for once-daily administration (elevates plasma levels for 8 to 10 hours), does not pose a threat in terms of viral transmission, and costs substantially less than that of the plasma-derived products.

● **Antifibrinolytic Therapy** Fibrinolysis inhibitors and oral contraceptives are used successfully in the management of epistaxis and menorrhagia or as adjuvant treatments. Fibrinolysis inhibitors include aminocaproic acid (25 to 60 mg/kg orally or IV (or 4 to 5 g) every 4 to 6 hours, to a maximum dose of 24 g/day) and tranexamic acid (10 mg/kg IV every 8 hours). Oral tranexamic acid recently received FDA approval for the treatment of cyclic heavy menstrual bleeding; its use is currently not approved for vWD patients. The IV form of tranexamic acid given as swish and swallow or spit every 6 to 8 hours has been used as bleeding prophylaxis in dental surgery. Both aminocaproic acid and tranexamic acid are dose adjusted for patients with renal insufficiency.

● **Replacement Therapy** ❷ *Type 1 patients unresponsive to desmopressin, patients with types 2 and 3 vWD, and major surgery patients require replacement therapy with plasma-derived, intermediate- and high-purity factor VIII virus-inactivated factor VIII concentrates containing vWF.*

Table 67–5 provides typical dosing guidelines and target levels of replacement therapy–concentrates to control various

---

Table 67–5

Replacement Therapy in vWD

Condition	Therapy	Recommended Dosage
Major surgery	Maintain vWF:RCo and factor VIII levels at least 100 IU/dL (1000 IU/L) followed by 50 IU/dL (500 IU/L) for 7–14 days To minimize risk of thrombosis: vWF:RCo levels should not exceed 200 IU/dL (2000 IU/L), and factor VIII levels should not exceed 250 IU/dL (2500 IU/L)	40–60 units/kg^a loading dose, followed by 20–40 units/kg every 8–24 hours DDAVP may be added after a few days
Minor surgery	Prophylaxis: maintain vWF:RCo and factor VIII levels at least 30 IU/dL (300 IU/L) (preferably greater than 50 IU/dL [greater than 500 IU/L]) Minor surgery: maintain vWF:RCo and factor VIII levels at least 30 IU/dL (300 IU/L) (preferably greater than 50 IU/dL [greater than 500 IU/L]) for 3–5 days	30–60 units/kg loading dose, followed by 20–40 units/kg every 12–48 hours DDAVP may be added after a few days

^{a}vWF concentrates are dosed based on vWF:RCo units concentration in the preparation to achieve the desired vWF:RCo levels.

types of hemorrhage. Ultra-high-purity (monoclonal) plasma-derived and recombinant factor VIII concentrates do not contain vWF and should not be used in the treatment of vWD.

Outcome Evaluation

The main goal of vWF treatment is to prevent bleeding with surgery or dental procedures. Clinicians should evaluate patients every 6 to 12 months for the following:

- Number and type of bleeding episodes to assess the need for prophylactic treatment.
- Ensure adequate levels of vWF and factor VIII prior to minor and major surgical procedures and for the treatment of bleeding.

- Vaccination against hepatitis A and B is recommended in all patients with vWF deficiency.

OTHER CLOTTING FACTOR DEFICIENCIES

Etiology and Epidemiology

Recessively inherited coagulation disorders (RICDs) refer to relatively rare deficiencies in factor II, V, VII, and X to XIII resulting in either decreased clotting factor production or production of a dysfunctional molecule with reduced activity.[22] The clinical severity of bleeding varies and generally is poorly correlated with the factor blood levels. Table 67–6 illustrates these clotting factor deficiencies and some of their characteristics.

Table 67–6

Clotting Factor Deficiency Characteristics

Factor Deficient	Inheritance Pattern	Estimated Incidence	Laboratory Abnormalities	Severity and Site of Bleeding
II	Autosomal dominant or recessive	Extremely rare	Prolonged PT and aPTT	Mild to moderate umbilical cord, joint, and mucosal tract
V	Autosomal recessive	1:1,000,000	Prolonged PT and aPTT	Mild to moderate mucosal tract
VII	Autosomal recessive	1:500,000	Prolonged PT	Mild to severe mucosal tract and joint
X	Autosomal recessive	1:1,000,000	Prolonged PT and aPTT	Mild to severe umbilical cord, joint, and muscle
XI	Autosomal recessive	4% of Ashkenazi Jews: otherwise rare	Prolonged aPTT	Mild to moderate posttraumatic bleeding
XII	Unknown	Unknown	Prolonged aPTT	No bleeding
XIII	Autosomal recessive	Less than 1:2,000,000	Normal PT and aPTT	Moderate to severe umbilical cord, intracranial, and joint bleeding; recurrent miscarriages, impaired wound healing

aPTT, activated partial thromboplastin time; PT, prothrombin time.

Pathophysiology

The RICDs are rare genetic disorders. Mutations in the genes responsible for the respective clotting factors result in impaired functionality or production of the factor.

Treatment

▶ Desired Outcomes

Therapeutic options for RICDs improve hemostasis via replacement of deficient blood coagulation factors while minimizing the development of immune tolerance.[23]

Hemostatic levels should be maintained for the following conditions:

- Spontaneous bleeding—until bleeding stops
- Minor surgery—for 2 to 3 days
- Major surgery—until incision site has healed

▶ Nonpharmacologic Therapy

Transfusional Therapies ❸ *The primary treatment of RICDs is single-donor fresh-frozen plasma (FFP) that contains all coagulation factors.* Disadvantages of FFP treatment include the risk of the patient becoming volume overloaded, especially when repeated infusions are administered to improve and maintain hemostasis; risk of infections; and risk of inhibitor development. PCCs licensed for the treatment of hemophilia B also contain significant levels of vitamin K–dependent factors and may be used off label for treatment of RICD. Table 67–7 lists the recommended RICD treatment schedules in different clinical scenarios.

▶ Pharmacologic Therapy

Less severe hemorrhages may be treated successfully with antifibrinolytic amino acids alone or in combination with factor replacement therapy. Tranexamic acid and aminocaproic acid may be administered IV or orally (for doses, see von Willebrand's Disease, Pharmacologic Therapy above).

ACQUIRED COAGULATION DISORDERS

DISSEMINATED INTRAVASCULAR COAGULATION

Etiology and Epidemiology

Disseminated intravascular coagulation (DIC) is a systemic thrombohemorrhagic disorder characterized by an increased propensity for clot formation secondary to a wide variety of clinical conditions (Table 67–8). Central to the etiology of DIC is excessive and unregulated generation of thrombin, leading to an aggressive compensatory **fibrinolysis**. Therefore, clinical manifestations of DIC result from a loss of balance between the clot-promoting (leading to thrombosis) and the clot-lysing (leading to hemorrhage) systems. Although this balance may tip in either direction, presenting as bleeding or clotting, bleeding is most common. Incidence of bleeding, end-organ dysfunction, and other manifestations depend on the etiology of DIC.[24]

Pathophysiology

Once injured or activated by a toxic substance (e.g., bacterial toxins, placenta chemicals, snake venom, etc.), endothelial cells and monocytes respond by generating tissue factor on the cell surface. Generation of tissue factor–factor VIIa complexes leads to extrinsic pathway activation, excessive generation of thrombin and fibrin, generation of systemic microthrombi, and consumption of coagulation factors and platelets. In addition, inhibition of naturally occurring endothelium-linked anticoagulant pathways (e.g., antithrombin, protein C, and tissue factor pathway inhibitor) and fibrinolytic system (due to a rise in plasminogen activator inhibitor, PAI-1 concentrations) leads to a vast procoagulant state. Although bleeding into the subcutaneous tissues, skin, and mucous membranes takes place, microvascular thrombosis exacerbates tissue ischemia and organ damage.[25]

Table 67–7

Treatment of Factor Deficiencies

Factor Deficient	Major Surgery	Spontaneous Bleeding
II	1. PCC: 20–30 units/kg 2. FFP: 15–20 mL/kg	1. FFP: 15–20 mL/kg
V	1. FFP: 15–20 mL/kg	1. FFP: 15–20 mL/kg
VII	1. rFVIIa: 15–30 mcg/kg every 4–6 hours	1. rFVIIa: 15–30 mcg/kg every 4–6 hours
X	1. PCC: 20–30 units/kg 2. FFP: 15–20 mL/kg	1. PCC: 20–30 units/kg 2. FFP: 15–20 mL/kg
XI	1. FFP: 15–20 mL/kg	1. FFP: 15–20 mL/kg
XIII	1. Pasteurized plasma concentrate: 10–20 units/kg 2. FFP: 15–20 mL/kg 3. Cryoprecipitate (1 bag per 10 kg)	1. FFP: 3–5 mL/kg

Numbers indicate lines of therapy. FFP, fresh-frozen plasma; PCC, prothrombin complex concentrates.

Table 67–8

Conditions Associated with DIC

Cardiovascular
Acute myocardial infarction
Angiopathy
Aortic aneurysm
Aortic balloon assist devices
Giant hemangiomas
Peripheral vascular disease
Postcardiac arrest
Prosthetic devices
Raynaud's syndrome

Infectious
Arbovirus
Aspergillus
Candida albicans
Cytomegalovirus
Ebola virus
Gram-negative bacteria
Gram-positive bacteria
Herpesvirus
Histoplasma
Human immunodeficiency virus
Influenza
Kala-azar
Malaria
Mycobacteria
Mycoplasma
Paramyxoviruses
Rocky Mountain spotted fever
Rubella
Typhoid
Varicella
Variola

Intravascular Hemolysis
Hemolytic transfusion reaction
Hemolytic uremic syndrome
Minor hemolysis
Massive transfusion

Newborn
Birth asphyxia
Hypothermia
Meconium or amniotic fluid aspiration
Necrotizing enterocolitis
Respiratory distress syndrome
Shock

Obstetrics
Abortion
Amniotic fluid embolism
Fatty liver of pregnancy
Placental abruption
Preeclampsia/eclampsia
Retained fetus syndrome

Pulmonary
Empyema
Hyaline membrane disease
Pulmonary embolism
Pulmonary infarction

Tissue injury
Burns
Crush injuries
Extensive surgery
Head trauma
Multiple trauma

Miscellaneous
Acid–base imbalance
Acute liver failure
Amphetamines
Anaphylaxis
Autoimmune diseases
Cholestasis
Chronic inflammatory diseases
Collagen vascular disease
Craniotomy
Extracorporeal circulation
Extracorporeal membrane oxygenation
Fat embolism
Heat stroke
Hemorrhagic telangiectasia
Hepatitis
Leukemia
Lightning strikes
Near drowning
Organic solvent poisoning
Paroxysmal nocturnal hemoglobinuria
Peritoneovenous or pleurovenous shunts
Polycythemia rubra vera
Renal vascular disorders
Severe anoxia
Snake bite
Solid tumors
Transplant rejection

Treatment

▶ Desired Outcomes

❹ The cornerstone of the management of DIC is aggressive treatment of the underlying primary illness. Supportive measures may be used as necessary, but owing to the heterogeneity of DIC etiology, treatment should be guided by predominant symptoms (bleeding or clotting).[26]

Goals of DIC treatment include:

- Replace missing blood components
- Interrupt coagulation
- Treat underlying disease

Clinical Presentation of DIC

Clinical manifestations generally are associated with underlying primary illness, as described in Table 67–8.

Signs and Symptoms

- Thrombosis, hemorrhage, or both
- Hemorrhagic bullae
- Peripheral cyanosis
- Petechiae and purpura

Thrombus and End-Organ Dysfunction

- Skin
- Lungs
- Kidneys
- Liver
- Adrenal glands
- Heart
- Evidence of end-organ dysfunction or failure

Laboratory Testing

- Increased D-dimer
- Thrombocytopenia
- Decreased fibrinogen
- Increased fibrin degradation products (FDP)
- Increased prothrombin time (PT)

Patient Encounter 1, Part 1: DIC

A 74-year-old man with a history of chronic obstructive pulmonary disease (COPD) and coronary artery disease (CAD) was admitted to the intensive care unit with severe COPD exacerbation that required mechanical ventilation. Upon admission, his arterial blood gas analysis showed acute on chronic respiratory acidosis. His other laboratory parameters were within normal limits. After 4 days of invasive mechanical ventilation, he started having episodes of fever and hypotension and had to be started on vasopressor support. Peripheral blood cultures show gram-positive cocci in clusters.

What are this patient's risk factors for disseminated intravascular coagulation (DIC)?

What additional information do you need to create a treatment plan for this patient?

What is the most important intervention at this time?

Antithrombin concentrate has been evaluated in clinical trials and has not been associated with reduced mortality in septic patients. rFVIIa can be used in DIC after all other options fail; however, its efficacy and toxicity is not supported by sufficient clinical data.

Platelets and FFP Treatment with platelet concentrates and plasma is indicated in patients who are bleeding or who require an invasive procedure. In a bleeding patient, the platelet count should be maintained above $50 \times 10^3/mm^3$ ($50 \times 10^9/L$), and platelet concentrates should be given at a dose of 1 unit/10 kg of body weight. For patients who are not bleeding, a lower threshold of less than 10 to $20 \times 10^3/mm^3$ or less than 10 to $20 \times 10^9/L$ is used. FFP contains all the coagulant factors as well as fibrinogen. Adding fibrinogen to the blood system in a situation where the level of antithrombin is already low may predispose patients to widespread microvascular thrombosis and may aggravate end-organ damage. Therefore, FFP use is reserved for actively bleeding patients who have significantly elevated prothrombin time and a fibrinogen concentration less than 50 mg/dL (0.5 g/L). The recommended FFP dose is 10 to 15 mL/kg.

▶ *Pharmacologic Therapy*

Anticoagulants Although bleeding is the most frequently observed symptom of DIC, thrombotic events cause most of the mortality. Heparin is an effective anticoagulant that activates the antithrombin system and inhibits factors II (thrombin), IXa, and Xa; however, its use is limited by the potential for bleeding. Clinical trials of heparin in DIC have not shown a consistent improvement in organ function or mortality benefit; thus treatment-dose heparin is used infrequently in DIC management. DIC patients most likely to benefit from heparin are those with chronic symptomatic thromboemboli, extensive fibrin deposition, and solid tumors. Heparin is contraindicated in DIC patients with serious or life-threatening bleeding, such as intracranial bleeding.[27]

Heparin may be given IV or subcutaneously; there is no universally accepted dose. Heparin administered subcutaneously for venous thromboembolism prophylaxis (5,000 units every 8 to 12 hours) can be beneficial in DIC patients without serious or life-threatening bleeding. Full-dose heparin therapy in adults is a bolus of 5,000 units, followed by a continuous infusion of 1,000 units/h. In general, full-dose heparin should be avoided in patients with DIC due to increased risk of bleeding, and a lower dose of 500 units/h can be used. Since the activated partial thromboplastin time (aPTT) is already elevated in many patients with DIC, monitoring heparin therapy may be difficult. Low-molecular-weight heparins can also be used in place of heparin. Venous thromboembolism prophylaxis is recommended in nonbleeding critically ill patients with DIC.[28]

Patient Encounter 1, Part 2: DIC

Medications

- Albuterol/ipratropium via nebulizer
- Methylprednisolone 40 mg IV every 6 hours
- Levofloxacin 750 mg IV every 24 hours
- Insulin via sliding scale SC
- Fentanyl 50 mcg/h continuous infusion
- Norepinephrine 10 mcg/min continuous infusion
- Heparin 5,000 U SQ every 8 hours
- Aspirin 325 mg po daily
- Clopidogrel 75 mg po daily
- Pantoprazole 40 mg IV every 24 hours

Laboratory findings

- Platelet count: $45 \times 10^3/mm^3$ ($45 \times 10^9/L$) (normal 140–$440 \times 10^3/mm^3$ [140–$440 \times 10^9/L$])
- aPTT: 50 seconds (normal 25–40 seconds)
- INR 4 (normal 0.8–1.2)
- D-dimer: 1 mcg/mL (1 mg/L; 5.5 nmol/L) (normal 0.250 mcg/mL [0.25 mg/L; 1.4 nmol/L])
- Fibrinogen: 0.7 g/L (normal 2–4 g/L)

Given this additional information, is this patient's presentation consistent with DIC?

Identify your treatment goals for this patient.

● **Cryoprecipitate** If FFP cannot maintain fibrinogen concentration above 100 mg/dL (1 g/L) in a symptomatic patient, cryoprecipitate may be administered. One bag of cryoprecipitate contains 200 mg of fibrinogen and will raise plasma fibrinogen level by about 0.07 g/L.[28]

Outcome Evaluation

- With each therapeutic option, postinfusion monitoring parameters (platelets, prothrombin time [PT], aPTT, and fibrinogen) should be checked within 30 to 60 minutes and every 6 hours thereafter, and the dose should be adjusted accordingly.
- Monitor the patient for relief of symptoms and signs of hemorrhage.

PLATELET DISORDERS

IMMUNE THROMBOCYTOPENIC PURPURA

Etiology and Epidemiology

Immune (or idiopathic) thrombocytopenic purpura (ITP) is one of the most common causes of acquired thrombocytopenia. The estimated incidence is 100 cases per 1 million persons per year, about half of whom are children. ITP is an autoimmune disorder caused by the binding of antibodies (usually immunoglobulin G [IgG]) to platelet surface antigens, resulting in shortened platelet life span. ITP can occur as an isolated condition or secondary to an underlying disorder. Childhood-onset and adult-onset ITP present very differently. Adult-onset ITP is generally chronic (greater than 6 months) and affects women two to three times more often than men. By contrast, childhood-onset ITP is acute in onset and usually follows an infectious illness, and both sexes are equally affected. Childhood ITP typically resolves on its own within 4 to 6 weeks without major sequelae. In adults presenting with ITP, testing for human immunodeficiency virus (HIV) and hepatitis C virus (HCV) is recommended, because treating these infections may improve ITP course. ITP occurs in 1 to 2 of every 1,000 pregnancies. In pregnant women with preexisting ITP, both maternal and fetal complications may occur, requiring separate management.[29]

Pathophysiology

In ITP, IgG autoantibodies bind to platelet-antigen complex and are cleared from the blood via binding to mononuclear

phagocytes by macrophage Fcγ receptor, leading to thrombocytopenia. Platelet survival time is significantly shorter in patients with ITP (from minutes to 2 to 3 days compared with normal 7 to 10 days). Sequestration in spleen, liver, and bone marrow is partially responsible for decreased platelet survival. Megakaryopoiesis may be reduced due to antibody binding to megakaryocyte precursors in the bone marrow.

Treatment

▶ Desired Outcomes

In children, the main goal of ITP treatment is to maintain the platelet count associated with sufficient hemostasis, while awaiting spontaneous or treatment-induced remission. In adults, the main goal is to maintain platelet count greater than $30 \times 10^3/mm^3$ ($30 \times 10^9/L$), because below this count, the incidence of bleeding in increased.[30]

▶ General Approach to Treatment

⑤ *The treatment of ITP is determined by the symptom severity. In some cases, no therapy is needed* (Table 67–9). The initial treatment of children with ITP is controversial because greater than 75% to 80% of cases resolve spontaneously irrespective of pharmacologic intervention. Therapy may be given in children with severe hemorrhage or platelet counts less than $10 \times 10^3/mm^3$ ($10 \times 10^9/L$) and mucocutaneous bleeding. In adults, treatment is indicated when platelet counts are less than $30 \times 10^3/mm^3$ ($30 \times 10^9/L$).[30]

▶ Nonpharmacologic Therapy

● In adults, splenectomy is generally considered after 3 to 6 months if the patient continues to require 10 to 20 mg/day of prednisone to maintain the platelet count greater than $30 \times 10^3/mm^3$ ($30 \times 10^9/L$). Splenectomy may also be considered for urgent treatment of neurologic symptoms or for managing relapse despite an adequate trial of corticosteroids, IV immunoglobulin (IVIg), or anti-Rh(D). Even though individual patient response cannot be predicted, approximately two-thirds of refractory adult patients have a favorable response to splenectomy within several days; however, 30% to 40% will have no response or will experience a relapse some time after splenectomy. In children, splenectomy is usually reserved due to the self-limited nature of ITP and

● fear of infectious complications of splenectomy. Splenectomy is recommended in children with ITP duration greater than 1 year with significant bleeding symptoms and unresponsive or intolerant of pharmacological therapies. Between 70% and 80% of children attain complete remission following splenectomy. Laparoscopic splenectomy is preferable to open splenectomy because it speeds the recovery and shortens the duration of hospitalization. The major drawback of splenectomy is bacterial sepsis, occurring at incidence rates of approximately 1%. Immunization with *Haemophilus influenzae* type b, pneumococcal, and meningococcal vaccines is indicated in all patients 2 weeks prior to splenectomy.[31]

▶ Pharmacologic Therapy

● The general approach to management of ITP in adults is summarized in Table 67–9.

Glucocorticoids Glucocorticoids may decrease splenic sequestration of antibody-coated platelets, diminish antibody

Table 67–9	
Guidelines for the Management of Adult ITP	
Greater than 30×10^3 platelets/mm^3 ($30 \times 10^9/L$), no bleeding	No treatment
First line Less than 30×10^3 platelets/mm^3 ($30 \times 10^9/L$), bleeding symptoms	Prednisone (1–1.5 mg/kg/day) Anti-D immune globulin (75 mcg/kg/day, × 1 dose) if corticosteroids contraindicated IVIg (1 g/kg/day × 1 dose, repeat as necessary) if corticosteroids contraindicated
Second line Reserved for patients with bleeding symptoms and platelets less than 30×10^3 platelets/mm^3 ($30 \times 10^9/L$) after an adequate trial of first-line agents	Splenectomy Rituximab (375 mg/m^2 once weekly for 4 doses) Eltrombopag (25–75 mg daily) Romiplostim (1–10 mcg/kg) Immunosuppressants
Hemorrhage	Platelet transfusion IVIg (1 g/kg/day × 1 dose, repeat as necessary) Methylprednisolone (1 g/day for 3 days)

generation by the spleen and the bone marrow, and increase platelet output by the bone marrow. In adults, the response rate to oral prednisone (1 to 1.5 mg/kg/day) is 50% to 75%, with patients usually responding within the first 2 to 3 weeks. In children, oral or parenteral corticosteroids (prednisone, dexamethasone, methylprednisolone) can be used; various dosage regimens have been studied with no specific dose or dosage regimen showing superiority.[32]

IV Immunoglobulin (IVIg) IVIg impairs the clearance of platelets coated with IgG by activating inhibitory receptor FcRγIIb. Roughly 80% of adults will respond to IVIg, but remission usually is not sustained. In adults, use of IVIg (1 g/kg/day) is reserved for situations in which rapid increase in platelet count is necessary, for example, for severe life-threatening bleeding and platelet counts less than $5 \times 10^3/mm^3$ ($5 \times 10^9/L$), with extensive purpura. If treatment is indicated in children, a single dose of IVIg (0.8 to 1 g/kg) is usually effective. IVIg use is complicated by many serious adverse effects and high cost.

Anti-Rh(D) Anti-Rh(D) can be used only in Rh(D)-positive patients who have not had splenectomy. It is as efficacious as IVIg and is generally less expensive. The indications for use of anti-Rh(D) are identical to those for IVIg. Anti-Rh(D) is a desirable form of treatment in chronic ITP when the goal is to circumvent long-term exposure to corticosteroids. At doses of 50 to 75 mcg/kg/day, anti-Rh(D) may increase the platelet count in about 70% to 80% of children with ITP. Dosage adjustment is recommended based on hemoglobin levels. Response to anti-Rh(D) lasts about 3 to 5 weeks, and substantial numbers of patients treated repetitively with Rh(D) can postpone or avoid splenectomy. Rare fatal intravascular hemolysis has been reported with use of anti-Rh(D); special monitoring for this side effect is recommended.

Immunosuppressants Immunosuppressant therapy is generally utilized for patients who are refractory to or intolerant of all other ITP treatments. Rituximab (375 mg/m² once weekly for 4 doses) can induce long-term response in 18% to 35% of patients.[33] Progressive multifocal leukoencephalopathy has been rarely reported with rituximab use. Rituximab can be considered as a second- or third-line therapy in patients who have experienced treatment failure with corticosteroids, IVIg, or splenectomy. Azathioprine and cyclophosphamide produce response rates of 20% to 40% in adult patients who are treated for 2 to 6 months. Other medications used in ITP include vincristine, vinblastine, cyclosporine, danazol, and mycophenolate mofetil; due to major toxicities and lack of adequate evidence-based recommendations, their use is reserved for refractory ITP.

Thrombopoietic Growth Factors New treatment options for ITP include a thrombopoiesis-stimulating protein and a small-molecule thrombopoietin (TPO) receptor agonist. These agents stimulate the bone marrow to make enough platelets to overcome the body's premature destruction of platelets. Romiplostim and eltrombopag are two TPO mimetics that have been approved by the FDA for the treatment of thrombocytopenia in patients with chronic ITP who

have had an insufficient response to corticosteroids, immunoglobulins, or splenectomy. Use of TPO-mimetic agents is reserved for refractory ITP due to cost considerations, lack of durability of response after discontinuation, and limited knowledge of long-term side effects. Currently, these agents are not FDA approved for use in children.

Romiplostim is a TPO peptide mimetic that binds to and activates the human TPO receptor. As a once weekly subcutaneous injection, romiplostim stimulates megakaryopoiesis, resulting in enhanced platelet production. Initial dose of romiplostim is based on the actual body weight, adjusted weekly by increments of 1 mcg/kg until a maximum of 10 mcg/kg and the patient achieves a platelet count greater than or equal to $50 \times 10^3/mm^3$ ($50 \times 10^9/L$) as necessary to reduce the risk for bleeding. In clinical studies, most patients who responded to romiplostim achieved and maintained platelet counts greater than or equal to $50 \times 10^3/mm^3$ ($50 \times 10^9/L$), with a median dose of 2 mcg/kg. Both agents need to be discontinued if platelet counts do not increase after 4 weeks at a maximum dose.

Eltrombopag is a once-daily oral nonpeptide thrombopoietin receptor agonist with a low immunogenic potential that stimulates megakaryocyte proliferation and differentiation.

For most patients, the initial dose of eltrombopag is 50 mg once daily. The daily dose is subsequently adjusted to a maximum dose of 75 mg daily in order to achieve and maintain a platelet count greater than or equal to $50 \times 10^3/mm^3$ ($50 \times 10^9/L$) in order to reduce the risk for bleeding.

Romiplostim and eltrombopag are effective in increasing platelet counts in patients with ITP and can be used in combination with therapies that inhibit platelet destruction. Although usually well tolerated, a number of rare but serious risks have been reported, including changes in the bone marrow, worsened thrombocytopenia and the risk of bleeding after cessation of the medication, thrombotic/thromboembolic complications (including portal vein thrombosis with eltrombopag), and worsening of blood cancers. Eltrombopag carries a "black box warning" regarding hepatic toxicity. It is also associated with development of cataracts and has drug–drug interactions with antacids and several minerals (calcium, iron, aluminium, magnesium, selenium, zinc).

To enhance patient safety, both romiplostim and eltrombopag are available only through restricted access programs. For both programs, each institution must enroll in the program to receive drug and training kits, and only prescribers, pharmacists, and patients registered with the

---

Patient Encounter 2, Part 3: ITP: Creating a Care Plan

Based on the information presented, create a care plan for this patient. Please include whether pharmacologic therapy is indicated, and if so, please list first-line and alternative therapies.

program are able to prescribe, dispense, and receive the product, respectively.

Outcome Evaluation

- Monitor platelet counts as indicated clinically.
- In adults, the goal of therapy is to maintain platelet count greater than or equal to $30 \times 10^3/mm^3$ ($30 \times 10^9/L$).
- Monitor for signs and symptoms of bleeding.

THROMBOTIC THROMBOCYTOPENIC PUPURA

Etiology and Epidemiology

Thrombotic thrombocytopenic purpura (TTP) is a severe systemic disorder characterized by thrombi formation within the circulation that results in the platelet consumption and subsequent thrombocytopenia. Acute idiopathic TTP is more common in women and African Americans and most frequently occurs in people between 30 and 40 years of age. The estimated annual incidence of TTP is 3.8 cases per million.[34] Common conditions associated with TTP are summarized in Table 67–10.

Pathophysiology

Endothelial cells normally synthesize vWF in the form of a high-molecular-weight multimer composed of smaller identical monomers. Each monomer is able to bind platelets, and the number of monomers on the vWF multimer is directly proportional to its platelet-binding capacity. Consequently, particularly adherent ultra-large molecules of the vWF (ULvWF) are broken down to smaller size by vWF-cleaving proteases such as ADAMTS13 (a disintegrin and metalloprotease with thrombospondin type 1 repeats) to avoid undesired clot formation. TTP results from genetic or acquired deficiency in the vWF-cleaving protease ADAMTS13 activity. This, in turn, elevates circulating levels of ULvWF, leading to inappropriate platelet agglutination. Thrombocytopenia develops because the rate of aggregated platelet consumption is faster than megakaryocyte bone marrow production. Microangiopathic hemolytic anemia

---

Table 67–10

Conditions Associated with TTP

- Infections
  Bacterial, fungal, viral, atypical
- Transplantation
  Solid organ or bone marrow
- Malignancy
- Pregnancy
- Collagen vascular diseases
- Medications
  Antineoplastic agents, ticlopidine, clopidogrel, antibiotics, immunosuppressants, others

---

Clinical Presentation and Diagnosis of TTP

Typical Pentad of Symptoms (Rare That All Five Are Present)[a]

1. Thrombocytopenia
   - Thrombocytopenic purpura
   - Bleeding
2. Fever
3. Microangiopathic hemolytic anemia
4. Neurologic symptoms
   - Headache, confusion, difficulty speaking, transient paralysis, numbness
5. Renal abnormalities
   - Proteinuria, hematuria, mild renal insufficiency

Laboratory Testing

- Decreased hemoglobin, hematocrit, and platelets
- Peripheral blood smear showing schistocytes
- Decreased serum haptoglobin
- Elevated lactate dehydrogenase (LDH)
- Elevated indirect bilirubin level
- Elevated reticulocyte count
- Normal PT and aPTT
- Elevated urine protein, red blood cells, and/or serum creatinine

---

[a]TTP diagnosis can be based on the presence of thrombocytopenia and microangiopathic hemolytic anemia in the absence of other possible causes.

---

generally follows as a consequence of red blood cell damage by platelet clumps occluding the microcirculation. Occlusive ischemia of the brain or GI tract is common, and renal dysfunction may occur.

Patient Encounter 3, Part 1: TTP

A 35-year-old Hispanic woman is brought by her husband to the emergency department. He states that she had been complaining of headache, weakness, fever, and bloody nasal discharge over the past few days. He also noticed increased confusion and slurred speech today. She had undergone a liver transplantation 2 years ago, and her medication regimen had recently been adjusted to include tacrolimus.

What information could be suggestive of thrombotic thrombocytopenic purpura (TTP)?

What additional information do you need to create a treatment plan for this patient?

Patient Encounter 3, Part 2: TTP

Meds at Home: Tacrolimus 5 mg po twice daily; mycophenolate mofetil 1,500 mg po twice daily; dapsone 100 mg po daily; fluconazole 100 mg po daily.

PE: Wt 55 kg

Labs

- Platelet count: $11 \times 10^3/mm^3$ (11×10^9/L) (normal $140–440 \times 10^3/mm^3$ [$140–440 \times 10^9$/L])
- aPTT: 30 seconds (normal 25–40 seconds)
- PT: 10 seconds (normal 10–12 seconds)
- Haptoglobin 10 mg/dL (100 mg/L) (normal 30–200 mg/dL or 300–2,000 mg/L)
- LDH 2,550 U/L (42.5 μkat/L) (normal 100–250 U/L, or 1.67–4.17 μkat/L)
- Hemoglobin 10.5 g/dL (105 g/L or 6.52 mmol/L) (normal 12.1–15.1 g/dL or 121–151 g/L or 7.51–9.37 mmol/L)
- Blood peripheral smear: numerous schistocytes (11–12 per high power field)
- Serum creatinine 2mg/dL (177 μmol/L) (increased from 0.8 mg/dL [71 μmol/L] on record 2 month prior) (normal 0.6–1.2 mg/dL [53–106 μmol/L])

Given this additional information, is this patient's presentation consistent with TTP?

What is the likely etiology of this patient's TTP?

Identify your treatment goals for this patient.

Patient Encounter 3, Part 3: TTP: Creating a Care Plan

Based on the information presented, create a care plan for this patient's TTP.

Treatment

▶ Desired Outcomes

The main goal of TTP treatment is to prevent end-organ damage.

▶ Nonpharmacologic Therapy

❻ *The present standard of treatment for TTP is urgent plasma exchange (PEX). If PEX is unavailable, treatment with plasma infusion and glucocorticoids is indicated until PEX is available.*[30]

Plasma Exchange The procedure involves removal of the patient's plasma and its substitution with donor plasma. In this manner, circulating antibody inhibitor of ADAMTS13 is removed and enzyme is replenished. PEX involves placement of two IV lines (cannulae) into two separate veins. Blood removed through one cannula is centrifuged to separate the blood cells from the plasma. The blood cells are mixed subsequently with donor plasma and returned to the patient via the second cannula. The goal is to exchange 1 to 1.5 plasma volumes (40 to 60 mL/kg). The procedure generally

Patient Care and Monitoring

1. Obtain a complete history.

2. In a patient presenting with a bleeding or clotting disorder, an initial evaluation should include bleeding time, prothrombin time (PT), activated partial thromboplastin time (aPTT), thrombin time, and platelet count.

   - Activated partial thromboplastin time: aPTT is performed by adding calcium phospholipids and kaolin to citrated blood and measuring the time required for a fibrin clot to form. In this manner, aPTT measures the activity of intrinsic and common pathways. Prolongation of aPTT may be due to a deficiency or inhibitor for factors II, V, VIII, IX, X, XI, and XII. It also may be due to heparin, direct thrombin inhibitors, vitamin K deficiency, liver disease, or lupus anticoagulant.

   - Prothrombin time: PT is performed by adding thromboplastin (tissue) factor and calcium to citrate-anticoagulated plasma, recalcifying the plasma, and measuring the clotting time. The major utility of PT is

   to measure the activity of the vitamin K–dependent factors II, VII, and X. The PT is used in evaluation of liver disease, to monitor warfarin anticoagulant effect, and to assess vitamin K deficiency.

   - Thrombin time is an assessment of the time required for the appearance of the fibrin clot after thrombin is added to plasma. It may be affected by thrombin inhibitors or fibrinogen abnormalities. Most commonly, thrombin time is used to monitor fibrinolytic therapy.

   - Bleeding time indicates how well platelets interact with blood vessel walls to form blood clots by assessing the length of time to arrest the bleeding after a standardized skin cut. The bleeding time is prolonged in thrombocytopenia, fibrinogen disorders, and collagen defects.

3. After a diagnosis is made, institute specific therapy.

4. Monitor resolution of laboratory and clinical symptoms with treatment.

is repeated daily until neurologic symptoms resolve and normal lactate dehydrogenase (LDH) and platelet counts are maintained for several days. After complete remission is achieved, PEX frequency can be reduced to every other day for an additional few days, with subsequent PEX discontinuation and close patient follow-up. When PEX is started immediately upon diagnosis, remission and survival rates at 6 months are approximately 80%. Although generally considered safe, complications from catheter insertion or catheter infection may occur and include hemorrhage, pneumothorax, sepsis, and thrombosis. Allergic reactions to plasma can cause severe hypotension and hypoxia.[35]

● **Splenectomy** Splenectomy is reserved for patients with frequently relapsing disease who are refractory to PEX or immunosuppressive therapy.

▶ *Pharmacologic Therapy*

● **Corticosteroids** Corticosteroids can be used for their immunosuppressive effect in combination with PEX; however, they are not as efficacious as monotherapy in TTP. The most commonly used agents are methylprednisolone 250 mg/day to 1 g/day IV for 3 days or prednisone 1 to 2 mg/kg/day orally for the duration of PEX therapy.

● **Immunosuppressants** TTP that fails to respond adequately to PEX can be treated with immunosuppressive agents. Cytotoxic immunosuppressive therapies with the most potential benefit in refractory TTP include cyclosporine and rituximab. Other agents that had been used include vincristine, cyclophosphamide, azathioprine, and IVIg.[30]

Outcome Evaluation

Monitor platelet counts, hemoglobin, and LDH.

Abbreviations Introduced in This Chapter

ADAMTS13	A disintegrin and metalloprotease with thrombospondin type 1 repeats (vWF-cleaving metalloprotease)
BU	Bethesda units
DDAVP	1-Desamino-8-D-arginine vasopressin (desmopressin acetate)
DIC	Disseminated intravascular coagulation
FFP	Fresh-frozen plasma
HCV	Hepatitis C virus
ICH	Intracranial hemorrhage
ITP	Immune thrombocytopenic purpura
IVIg	IV immunoglobulin
PCC	Prothrombin complex concentrate
PEX	Plasma exchange
rFVIIa	Recombinant factor VIIa
RICD	Recessively inherited coagulation disorder
TTP	Thrombotic thrombocytopenic purpura
ULvWF	Ultra-large molecules of vWF
vWD	von Willebrand's disease
vWF	von Willebrand's factor

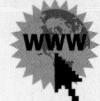 Self-assessment questions and answers are available at *http://mhpharmacotherapy.com/pp.html.*

REFERENCES

1. Soucie JM, Evatt B, Jackson D. Occurrence of hemophilia in the United States. The Hemophilia Surveillance System Project Investigators. Am J Hematol 1998;59:288–294.
2. Bolton-Maggs PH, Pasi KJ. Haemophilias A and B. Lancet 2003;361:1801–1809.
3. Stobart K, Iorio A, Wu JK. Clotting factor concentrates given to prevent bleeding and bleeding-related complications in people with hemophilia A or B. Cochrane Database Syst Rev 2006;CD003429.
4. Astermark J, Petrini P, Tengborn L, et al. Primary prophylaxis in severe haemophilia should be started at an early age but can be individualized. Br J Haematol 1999;105:1109–1113.
5. Darby SC, Kan SW, Spooner RJ, et al. Mortality rates, life expectancy, and causes of death in people with hemophilia A or B in the United Kingdom who were not infected with HIV. Blood 2007;110:815–825.
6. Berntorp E. Prophylactic therapy for haemophilia: early experience. Haemophilia 2003;9(Suppl 1):5–9; discussion.
7. Blanchette VS, Manco-Johnson M, Santagostino E, Ljung R. Optimizing factor prophylaxis for the haemophilia population: where do we stand? Haemophilia 2004;10(Suppl 4):97–104.
8. Manco-Johnson MJ, Abshire TC, Shapiro AD, et al. Prophylaxis versus episodic treatment to prevent joint disease in boys with severe hemophilia. N Engl J Med 2007;357:535–544.
9. MASAC Recommendation Concerning Prophylaxis (Regular Administration of Clotting factor Concentrate to Prevent Bleeding). MASAC Document #179. New York: National Hemophilia Foundation; 2007.
10. Fiebig EW, Busch MP. Emerging infections in transfusion medicine. Clin Lab Med 2004;24:797–823.
11. Srivastava A. Optimizing clotting factor replacement therapy in hemophilia: a global need. Hematology 2005;10(Suppl 1):229–230.
12. MASAC Recommendations Concerning the Treatement of Hemophilia and Other Bleeding Disorders. MASAC Document #182. New York: National Hemophilia Foundation, 2008.
13. Mannucci PM, Tuddenham EG. The hemophilias—from royal genes to gene therapy. N Engl J Med 2001;344:1773–1779.
14. Batorova A, Martinowitz U. Continuous infusion of coagulation factors: current opinion. Current OpinHematol 2006;13:308–315.
15. Schulman S. Continuous infusion. Haemophilia 2003;9:368–375.
16. Shord SS, Lindley CM. Coagulation products and their uses. Am J Health Syst Pharm 2000;57:1403–1417; quiz 1418–1420.
17. MASAC Recommendations on Use of COX-2 Inhibitors in Patients with Bleeding Disorders. MASAC Document #162. New York: National Hemophilia Foundation; 2005.
18. Rodeghiero F, Castaman G, Dini E. Epidemiological investigation of the prevalence of von Willebrand's disease. Blood 1987;69:454–459.
19. Werner EJ, Broxson EH, Tucker EL, etal. Prevalence of von Willebrand disease in children: a multiethnic study. J Pediatr 1993;123:893–898.
20. Nichols WL, Hultin MB, James AH, et al. von Willebrand disease (VWD): evidence-based diagnosis and management guidelines, the National Heart, Lung, and Blood Institute (NHLBI) Expert Panel report (USA). Haemophilia 2008;14:171–232.
21. Mannucci PM. Treatment of von Willebrand's Disease. N Engl J Med 2004;351:683–694.
22. Mannucci PM, Duga S, Peyvandi F. Recessively inherited coagulation disorders. Blood 2004;104:1243–1252.
23. Roberts HR, Escobar MA. Other clotting factor deficiencies. In: Hoffman R, Benz EJJ, Shattil SJ, eds. Hematology: Basic Principles and Practice. 4th ed. Philadelphia, PA: Elsevier; 2005:2047–2069.
24. Okajima K, Sakamoto Y, Uchiba M. Heterogeneity in the incidence and clinical manifestations of disseminated intravascular coagulation: a study of 204 cases. Am J Hematol 2000;65:215–222.

25. Levi M. Disseminated intravascular coagulation. Crit Care Med 2007;35:2191–2195.

26. Rodgers GM. Acquired coagulation disorders. In: Greer JP, Foerster J, Lukens JN, Rogers GM, Parasvekas F, Glader B, eds. Wintrobe's Clinical Hematology. 11th ed. Philadelphia, PA: Lippincot Williams and Wilkins; 2004:1669.

27. Levi M. Disseminated intravascular coagulation: What's new? Crit Care Clin 2005;21:449–467.

28. Levi M, Toh CH, Thachil J, Watson HG. Guidelines for the diagnosis and management of disseminated intravascular coagulation. British Committee for Standards in Haematology. Br J Haematol 2009;145:24–33.

29. Frederiksen H, Schmidt K. The incidence of idiopathic thrombocytopenic purpura in adults increases with age. Blood 1999;94:909–913.

30. Neunert C, Lim W, Crowther M, et al. The American Society of Hematology 2011 evidence-based practice guideline for immune thrombocytopenia. Blood 2011;117:4190–4207.

31. George JN, Woolf SH, Raskob GE, et al. Idiopathic thrombocytopenic purpura: a practice guideline developed by explicit methods for the American Society of Hematology. Blood 1996;88:3–40.

32. Blanchette V, Carcao M. Approach to the investigation and management of immune thrombocytopenic purpura in children. Semin Hematol 2000;37:299–314.

33. Medeot M, Zaja F, Vianelli N, et al. Rituximab therapy in adult patients with relapsed or refractory immune thrombocytopenic purpura: long-term follow-up results. Eur J Haematol 2008;81:165–169.

34. Furlan M, Robles R, Galbusera M, et al. von Willebrand factor-cleaving protease in thrombotic thrombocytopenic purpura and the hemolytic-uremic syndrome. N Engl J Med 1998;339:1578–1584.

35. Sadler J, Poncz M. Antibody-mediated thrombotic disorders: idiopathic thrombotic thrombocytopenic purpura and heparin-induced thrombocytopenia. In: Lichtman M, ed. Williams Hematology. 7th ed. New York: McGraw-Hill; 2006:2031–2054.

68

Sickle Cell Anemia

Tracy M. Hagemann and Teresa V. Lewis

- **Upon completion of the chapter, the reader will be able to:**

1. Explain the underlying causes of sickle cell disease (SCD) and their relationship to patient signs and symptoms.

2. Identify the typical characteristics of SCD as well as symptoms that indicate complicated disease.

3. Identify the desired therapeutic outcomes for patients with SCD.

4. Recommend appropriate pharmacotherapy and nonpharmacotherapy interventions for patients with SCD.

5. Recognize when chronic maintenance therapy is indicated for a patient with SCD.

6. Describe the components of a monitoring plan to assess effectiveness and adverse effects of pharmacotherapy for SCD.

7. Educate patients about the disease state, appropriate therapy, and drug therapy required for effective treatment and prevention of complications.

KEY CONCEPTS

❶ Sickle cell disease (SCD) is an inherited disorder caused by a defect in the gene for hemoglobin. Patients may have one defective gene (sickle cell trait [SCT]) or two defective genes (SCD).

❷ Although most often seen in persons of African ancestry, other ethnic groups can be affected.

❸ SCD involves multiple organ systems.

❹ Prophylaxis against pneumococcal infection reduces death during childhood.

❺ Hydroxyurea has been shown to decrease the incidence of painful crises. However, the patient population that receives hydroxyurea should be carefully monitored.

❻ Chronic transfusion therapy programs have been shown to be beneficial in decreasing the occurrence of stroke in children with SCD.

❼ Patients with fever greater than 38.5°C (101.3°F) should be evaluated, and appropriate antibiotics should include coverage for encapsulated organisms, especially pneumococcal.

❽ Pain episodes can usually be managed at home. Hospitalized patients usually require parenteral analgesics. Analgesic options include opioids, nonsteroidal anti-inflammatory agents, and acetaminophen. The patient characteristics and the severity of the crisis should determine the choice of agent and regimen.

INTRODUCTION

❶ *"Sickle cell syndrome" refers to a collection of autosomal recessive genetic disorders that are characterized by the presence of at least one sickle hemoglobin gene (HbS).*[1,2]

Sickle cell disease (SCD) is a chronic illness that is associated with frequent crisis episodes. Acute complications are unpredictable and potentially fatal. Common symptoms include excruciating musculoskeletal pain, life-threatening pneumonia-like illness, cerebrovascular accidents, and splenic and renal dysfunction.[2] As the disease progresses, patients may develop organ damage from the combination of hemolysis and infarction. Because of the complexity and severity of SCD, it is imperative that patients have access to comprehensive care with providers who have a good understanding of the countless clinical presentations and the management options of this disorder.

EPIDEMIOLOGY AND ETIOLOGY

Sickle cell trait (SCT) is the heterozygous form (HbAS) of SCD in which a person inherits one normal adult hemoglobin (HbA) gene and one sickle hemoglobin (HbS) gene. These individuals are carriers of the SCT and are usually asymptomatic.[2] Symptomatic disease is seen in homozygous and compound heterozygous genotypes of SCD. Sickle cell anemia (SCA) is the homozygous (HbSS) state of SCD.[2] It is the most common and severe form of SCD. Compound heterozygosity is seen when individuals inherit one copy of the mutation that causes HbS and one copy of another abnormal hemoglobin gene. Compound heterozygosity may also include the coinheritance of HbS and one of the many different mutations of β-thalassemia (HbSβ^0-thalassemia and HbSβ^+-thalassemia).[1-3] SCA affects both males and females equally because it is not a sex-linked disease.

❷ *Nine percent of African Americans possess the SCT and 1 in 600 has HbSS.*[4] Two thousand infants are identified with SCD annually in the United States.[5] For every infant diagnosed with SCD, 50 are identified as carriers.[5] HbSS (approximately 45%) is the most common genotype, followed by HbSC (approximately 25%), HbSβ^+-thalassemia (approximately 8%), and HbSβ^0-thalassemia (approximately 2%). Other variants account for fewer than 1% of patients.[2,5]

Having the sickle hemoglobin gene protects heterozygous carriers from succumbing to *Plasmodium falciparum* (malaria) infection.[1] The microorganism cannot parasitize abnormal red blood cells (RBCs) as easily as normal RBCs. Consequently, persons with heterozygous sickle gene (SCT) have a selective advantage in tropical regions where malaria is endemic.

The highest incidence of SCD is seen in those with African heritage, but SCD also affects persons of Indian, Saudi Arabian, Mediterranean, South and Central American, and Caribbean ancestry.[5,6]

Normal adult hemoglobin (HbA) is composed of two α-chains and two β-chains ($\alpha2\beta2$).[3] A single substitution of the amino acid valine for glutamic acid at position 6 of the β-polypeptide chain is responsible for the production of a defective form of hemoglobin called sickle hemoglobin (HbS).[1] Different genetic mutations encode for other hemoglobin variants such as hemoglobin C (HbC). HbC is produced by the substitution of lysine for glutamic acid at the sixth amino acid position in the β-globulin chain.[3] The α-chains of HbS, HbA, and HbC are structurally identical. The chemical differences in the β-chain are responsible for RBC sickling and its associated sequelae.

SCA is the homozygous (HbSS) state of SCD in which individuals inherit the mutant hemoglobin gene (HbS) from both parents. The progeny of two carriers will have a 25% probability of having SCD and a 50% risk of being a carrier (Fig. 68–1). β-Thalassemia can be found in conjunction with HbS. Patients with HbSS and HbSβ^0-thalassemia do not have normal β-globulin production and usually have a more severe course than those with HbSC and HbSβ^+-thalassemia.

Impaired circulation, destruction of RBCs, and vascular stasis are three known problems that are primarily responsible for the clinical manifestations of SCD (Fig. 68–2).

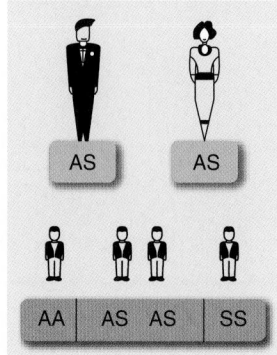

FIGURE 68–1. Sickle gene inheritance scheme for both parents with sickle cell trait (SCT). Possibilities with each pregnancy: 25% normal (AA); 50% SCT (AS); 25% sickle cell anemia (SS). (A, normal hemoglobin; S, sickle hemoglobin.) (From Chan CYJ, Moore R. Sickle cell disease. In: DiPiro JT, Talbert RL, Yee GC, et al., eds. Pharmacotherapy: A Pathophysiologic Approach. 8th ed. New York: McGraw-Hill; 2011.)

PATHOPHYSIOLOGY

Erythrocyte Physiology

A review of RBC physiology is important to understand the pathophysiology of SCD. Pediatric RBCs possess normal hemoglobin concentrations between 9.0 and 18.5 g/dL (90 and 185 g/L or 5.59 and 11.5 mmol/L), depending on the age of the child.[7] Adult RBCs contain 12.0 to 15.5 g/dL (120 to 155 g/L or 7.45 to 9.62 mmol/L) hemoglobin.[7] The predominant form of hemoglobin is adult hemoglobin or HbA (96%). Other forms of hemoglobin include HbA2 and fetal hemoglobin (HbF). HbA2 makes up less than 1% of hemoglobin in newborns. In adults, HbA2 constitutes approximately 1.6% to 3.5%.[7] Fetal hemoglobin (HbF) is present primarily in fetal RBCs (60% to 90%), whereas adult RBCs contain less than 1% HbF.[7] HbF is the primary oxygen transport protein in the fetus. After birth, only a small proportion of red cell clones remain to produce HbF. The elasticity of young erythroid cells enables them to deform and squeeze through capillaries. As RBCs age, mean corpuscular hemoglobin concentration (MCHC) increases, deformability decreases, and the cells are removed by the reticuloendothelial system.

❸ *SCD involves multiple organ systems, and its clinical manifestations vary greatly between and among genotypes.*

Sickle Hemoglobin Polymerization

The primary event in the molecular pathogenesis of SCD involves polymerization of deoxygenated HbS. Since RBCs are packaged with such a high concentration of hemoglobin (32.0 to 34.0 g/dL, 320 to 340 g/L, or 19.9 to 21.1 mmol/L), it is important that the proteins be extremely soluble.[1] HbS carries oxygen normally, and when oxygenated, the solubility of HbS and HbA are the same. Once the oxygen

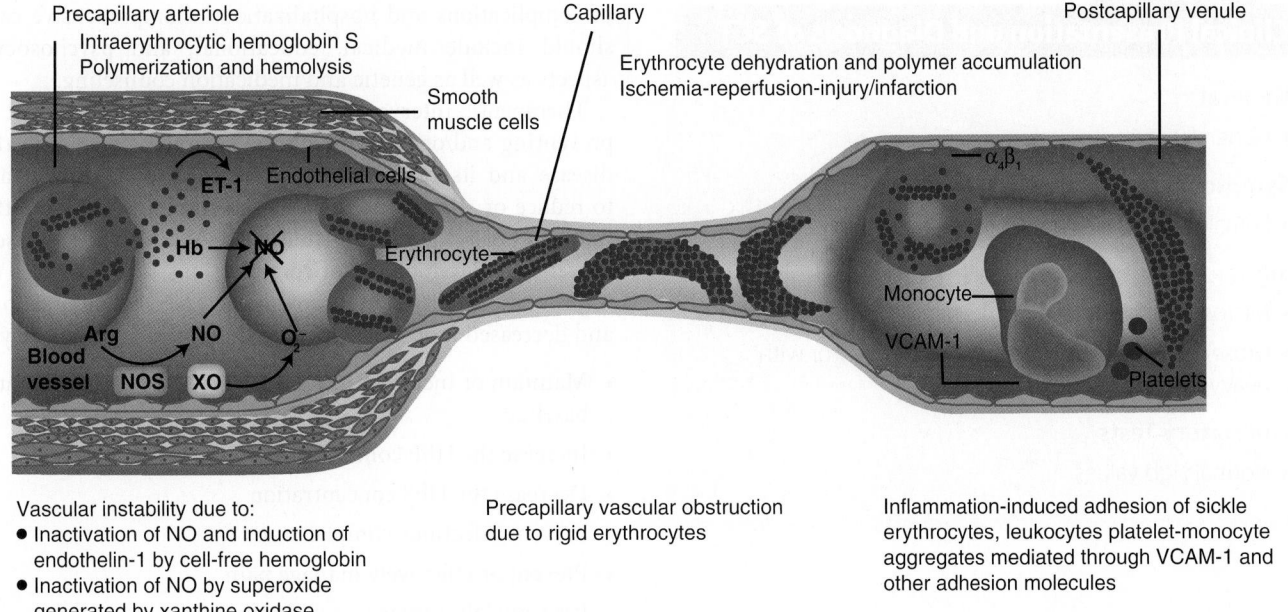

FIGURE 68–2. Pathophysiology of SCD. (Arg, arginine; ET-1, endothelin-1; Hb, hemoglobin; NO, nitric oxide; NOS, nitrous oxide synthase; VCAM-1, vascular cell adhesion molecule 1; XO, xanthine oxidase.) (From Kato GJ, Gladwin MT. Sickle cell disease. In: Hall JB, Schmidt GA, Wood LDH, eds. Principles of Critical Care. 3rd ed. New York: McGraw-Hill; 2005:1658.)

is unloaded to the tissues, HbS solubility decreases. This promotes hydrophobic interactions between the hemoglobin molecules and polymerization, which leads to the distortion of the RBC into the characteristic crescent or sickle shape.[1] Polymerization of deoxy-HbS is influenced by the degree of red cell deoxygenation, MCHC, temperature, intracellular pH, intraerythrocytic HbS concentration, and intracellular HbF concentration.[1]

Viscosity of Erythrocytes and Sickle Cell Adhesion

When HbS becomes reoxygenated, the polymers within the RBCs disappear, and the cells eventually return to normal shape. Vasoocclussion is caused by a combination of factors. Repeated assaults on RBCs from sickling and unsickling can lead to cell membrane damage, loss of membrane flexibility, and rearrangement of surface phospholipids. Damage to cell membranes can interfere with ion transport, leading to loss of potassium and water. This creates dehydrated, dense sickle cells and irreversible sickle cells (ISCs). ISCs are the densest cells, and they tend to remain sickled even when oxygenated. Rigid ISCs can become trapped in microvasculature, leading to cell fragmentation and chronic hemolysis, thus contributing to short survival of RBCs. The life span of sickled RBCs is markedly shorter (10 to 20 days) than that of normal RBCs (100 to 120 days). As intracellular membrane viscosity of HbS-containing RBCs increases, blood viscosity increases, which further contributes to vasoocclussion.[8] There is also increasing evidence that suggest sickle cells adhere to vascular endothelium.[1,8] The combined effects

of decreased RBC deformability, slow transit through microcirculation, and adhesion to vascular endothelium contribute to obstruction of small and sometimes large blood vessels. The resulting local tissue hypoxia can accentuate the pathologic process of SCD.

Protective Hemoglobin Types

Fetal hemoglobin binds oxygen more tightly than HbA, and it has a decreased propensity to sickling. HbA2 also possesses this characteristic but to a lesser extent. RBCs that contain HbF sickle less readily than cells without. ISCs are found to have low HbF concentrations. In some patients, higher HbF may ameliorate the disease.

Other Pathophysiologic Effects

Other factors may be responsible for the pathogenesis of some of the clinical features of SCD. Sickle cells can obstruct blood flow to the spleen leading to functional asplenia. Impaired splenic function can increase the propensity to infection by encapsulated organisms, particularly *Streptococcus pneumoniae*.[1] Additionally, coagulation abnormalities are not uncommon since almost every component of hemostasis is altered in SCD.

TREATMENT
Desired Outcomes

Multidisciplinary, regularly scheduled care is required over the lifetime of the SCD patient, with the goal of reduction

Clinical Presentation and Diagnosis of SCT

General
- Generally asymptomatic

Symptoms
- Females may have frequent urinary tract infections

Signs
- Microscopic hematuria occurs rarely
- Gross hematuria may occur spontaneously or with heavy-intensity exercise

Laboratory Tests
- Normal Hgb values

Clinical Presentation and Diagnosis of SCD

General
- Indentified by neonatal screening before 2 months of age

Symptoms
- Painful vasoocclusive crises are the hallmark of SCD
- Dactylitis (hand–foot syndrome) before age 1 year
- May develop infarction of the spleen, liver, bone marrow, kidney, brain, and lungs
- Gallstones
- Priapism in males
- Slow-healing lower extremity ulcers after trauma or infection
- Weakness, fatigue

Signs
- Chronic hemolytic anemia is common
- Enlargement of spleen and heart
- Scleral icterus

Laboratory Tests
- Hgb 7.0 to 10.0 g/dL (70 to 100 g/L or 4.34 to 6.21 mmol/L)
- Low HgF and increased reticulocytes, platelets, and WBCs
- Presence of sickled cells on blood smear (see Fig. 68–2)
- Neonatal screening: hemoglobin electrophoresis, isoelectric focusing, or DNA analysis

of complications and hospitalizations. Comprehensive care should include medical, educational, and psychosocial aspects as well as genetic and medication counseling.

Therapeutic interventions for SCD should be targeted at preventing and/or minimizing the symptoms related to the disease and its complications. The goals of treatment are to reduce or eliminate the patient's symptoms; decrease the frequency of sickle crises, including vasoocclusive pain crises; prevent the development of complications; and maintain or improve the quality of life through decreased hospitalizations and decreased morbidity. Specific therapeutic options may:

- Maintain or increase the hemoglobin level to the patient's baseline
- Increase the HbF concentration
- Decrease the HbS concentration
- Prevent infectious complications
- Prevent or effectively manage pain
- Prevent CNS damage, including stroke

General Approach to Treatment

Patients should be educated to recognize the signs and symptoms of complications that would require urgent evaluation. Patients and parents of children with SCD should be educated to read a thermometer properly and to seek immediate medical care when a fever develops or signs of infection occur. With acute illnesses, prompt evaluation is important, as deterioration may occur rapidly. Fluid status should be monitored to avoid dehydration or overhydration, both of which may worsen complications of SCD. Patients in acute distress should maintain oxygen saturation at 92% (0.92) or at their baseline. Any supplemental oxygen requirements should be evaluated.[5]

Nonpharmacologic Therapy

Patients should avoid smoking and excessive alcohol intake. Patients with SCD should maintain adequate hydration in order to help decrease blood viscosity and should be educated to avoid extreme temperature changes and to dress properly in hot and cold weather. Physical exertion that leads to complications should be avoided.[5] Regular exams, including ophthalmic, renal, pulmonary, and cardiac function, are required to monitor for organ damage. A treatment overview is shown in Table 68–1.

Pharmacologic Therapy

► *Health Maintenance*

Immunizations Children with SCD should receive the required immunizations as recommended by the American Academy of Pediatrics and the Advisory Committee on Immunization Practices.[9] Additionally, influenza vaccine should be administered yearly to SCD patients 6 months of age and older, including adult patients. Any SCD patient who

Table 68–1

Management of SCD

	Options and Comments
Health maintenance	
Infection prophylaxis	• Pneumococcal vaccines (PCV 13 and PPV 23) • Penicillin prophylaxis for children less than 5 years of age • Annual influenza vaccine
Induction of fetal hemoglobin	• Hydroxyurea is the primary agent • Other agents are butyrates (arginine butyrate and sodium phenylbutyrate), decitabine, clotrimazole, and erythropoietin • Combination HbF inducers have been proposed
Chronic transfusion therapy	• Primary indication: stroke prevention in pediatric patients • May also reduce pain crisis and acute chest syndrome • Goal: maintain HbS less than 30% (0.30)
Future prospects	
Transplantation	• May potentially cure the disease • Most experience is with HLA-matched donors; umbilical cord blood transplantation is being evaluated
Crises and complications	
Fever and infection	• Broad-spectrum antibiotic: cefotaxime or ceftriaxone (clindamycin for cephalosporin allergy); vancomycin for staphylococcal and resistant pneumococcal organisms
Stroke	• Fluids • Acetaminophen or ibuprofen for fever • Exchange transfusion • Initiate chronic transfusion therapy to prevent recurrent strokes
Acute chest syndrome	• Broad-spectrum antibiotics (include Mycoplasma coverage) • Bronchodilator if wheezing or history of reactive airway disease • Fluids • Pain management • Transfusion
Pain crisis	• Hydration • Analgesics

is scheduled for splenectomy should receive the vaccine for meningococcal disease if over 2 years of age.[9]

Because patients with SCD have impaired splenic function, they are less adequately protected against encapsulated organisms such as *Streptococcus pneumoniae, Haemophilus influenzae,* and *Salmonella.* ❹ *The use of pneumococcal vaccine in SCD patients has dramatically decreased the rates of morbidity and mortality; however, there are still groups of SCD children who continue to have high rates of invasive pneumococcal infections.*[10–12] Infection is the leading cause of death in children younger than 3 years of age.[4,12,13] Two pneumococcal vaccines are available. The 13-valent conjugate vaccine (PCV 13: Prevnar) is indicated for infants and children and provides good protection against the 13 most common isolates seen in this age range. Administer the first dose of PCV 13 between 6 weeks and 6 months of age, followed by two additional doses at 2-month intervals and a fourth dose at 12 to 15 months of age. The 23-valent polysaccharide vaccine (PPV 23: Pneumovax 23) is indicated for children over 2 years of age and adults. Because PPV 23 is a polysaccharide vaccine, children less than 2 years of age do not respond well. PPV 23 contains the 23 most common isolates of *S. pneumoniae* seen in older children and adults. Because of the different serotypes seen in the two vaccines, it is recommended that SCD children receive both vaccines, with a dose of PPV 23 administered after the child turns 2 years of age. The dose of PPV 23 should be separated from

the last dose of PCV 13 by at least 2 months. An additional dose of PPV 23 should be considered in children 3 to 5 years of age to ensure antibody response. All adults with SCD should be vaccinated once with PPV 23 also. Because some children fall behind on their childhood vaccinations, a catch-up schedule is presented in Table 68-2.[9]

Patient Encounter 1

A 3-year-old boy with SCD is currently taking penicillin V potassium 125 mg orally twice daily, folic acid 0.4 mg orally daily, and acetaminophen/codeine 120/12 mg per 5 mL orally every 6 hours as needed for pain. He fully completed all his routine childhood vaccinations at age 2 years. He was hospitalized 1 month ago for aplastic crisis.

What are the general pneumococcal prophylaxis recommendations for children with SCD?

What interventions do you want to make today to his medication/immunization regimens?

Design an infection prevention plan for this patient.

Table 68-2

Pneumococcal Immunization for Children with SCD[10]

	Recommended Schedule
Previously unvaccinated	
Age 2–6 months	PCV 13 (Prevnar): three doses 8 weeks apart; then 1 dose at 12–15 months
Age 7–11 months	PCV 13 (Prevnar): two doses 8 weeks apart; then 1 dose at 12–15 months
Age 12–23 months	PCV 13 (Prevnar): two doses 8 weeks apart
Age 24–71 months	PCV 13 (Prevnar): two doses 8 weeks apart
	PPV 23 (Pneumovax): two doses; first dose at least 8 weeks after last PCV 13 dose; second dose 5 years after the first PPV 23 dose
Age 5 years or older	PCV 13 (Prevnar): one dose
	PPV 23 (Pneumovax): one dose at least 8 weeks after last PCV 13 dose; second dose 5 years after the first PPV 23 dose
Previously vaccinated	
Age 12–23 months, incomplete PCV 13 series	PCV 13 (Prevnar): two doses 8 weeks apart
Age 24–71 months, any incomplete schedule or completed less than 3 doses with PCV 13	PCV 13 (Prevnar): two doses 8 weeks apart
	PPV 23 (Pneumovax): two doses; first dose at least 6–8 weeks after last PCV 13 dose; second dose 5 years after the first PPV 23
Age 24–71 months, any incomplete schedule of 3 doses or 4 doses of PCV 13	PCV 13 (Prevnar): one dose at least 8 weeks after the most recent dose
	PPV 23 (Pneumovax): two doses; first dose at least 6–8 weeks after last PCV 13 dose; second dose 5 years after the first PPV23
Age 24–71 months, 1 dose PPV 23 given	PCV 13 (Prevnar): one dose at least 8 weeks after PPV 23 dose
	PPV 23 (Pneumovax): second dose 5 years after first PPV 23
Age 5 to 18 years, received 1 dose PPV 23	PCV 13 (Prevnar): one dose at least 8 weeks after PPV 23
	If only received one dose of PPV 23 (Pneumovax): second dose 5 years after the first PPV 23 dose

Penicillin ④ *Children with SCD should receive prophylactic penicillin until at least the age of 5 years, even if they have been appropriately immunized with PCV 13 against pneumococcal infections.* Penicillin V potassium is typically initiated at age 2 months, with a dose of 125 mg orally twice daily until age 3 years, then 250 mg orally twice daily until 5 years of age. The intramuscular use of benzathine penicillin 600,000 units every 4 weeks from age 6 months to 6 years is also an option for noncompliant patients. Penicillin-allergic patients may receive erythromycin 10 mg/kg twice daily. Penicillin prophylaxis usually is not continued in children over the age of 6 years, but may be considered in patients with a history of invasive pneumococcal infection or surgical splenectomy.[5,14,15]

Folic Acid Folic acid supplementation with 1 mg daily is generally recommended in adult SCD patients, women considering pregnancy, and any SCD patient with chronic hemolysis.[5] Because of accelerated erythropoiesis, these patients have an increased need for folic acid. There are conflicting studies in the SCD population, especially among infants and children, but if the child has chronic hemolysis, supplementation is recommended.[16]

Fetal Hemoglobin Inducers Fetal hemoglobin (HbF) induction in patients with SCD, especially those with frequent crises, has been shown to decrease RBC sickling and RBC adhesion. A direct relationship between HbF concentrations and the severity of disease has been demonstrated in studies.[2]

Hydroxyurea Hydroxyurea is a ribonucleotide reductase inhibitor that prevents DNA synthesis and traditionally has been used in chemotherapy regimens. Studies in the 1990s also found that hydroxyurea increases HbF levels as well as increasing the number of HbF-containing reticulocytes and intracellular HbF. Other beneficial effects of hydroxyurea include antioxidant properties, reduction of neutrophils and monocytes, increased intracellular water content leading to increased red cell deformability, decreased red cell adhesion to endothelium, and increased levels of nitric oxide, which is a regulator involved in physiologic disturbances.[17]

⑤ *Hydroxyurea reduced the frequency of hospitalizations and the incidences of pain, acute chest syndrome, and blood transfusions by almost 50% in a landmark trial in adult SCD patients with moderate to severe disease.* Hemoglobin and HbF concentrations increased and hemolysis decreased.[17] A follow-up study demonstrated a 40% reduction in mortality over a 9-year period in patients continuing to receive hydroxyurea.[18] Not all patients responded equally; therefore, hydroxyurea may not be the best option for all patients.

The use of hydroxyurea in children and adolescents with SCD has been investigated, and similar results were reported as in adult trials, with no adverse effects on growth and development.[5,19,20] Hydroxyurea is recommended as an option for children with moderate to severe SCD.[21]

The most common adverse effect of hydroxyurea in reported studies is myelosuppression. Long-term adverse effects are unknown, but myelodysplasia, acute leukemia, and chronic opportunistic infections have been reported.[17] Hydroxyurea is teratogenic in high doses in animal studies and this is a concern, which should be addressed with patients. Normal pregnancies with no birth defects have been reported in some women receiving hydroxyurea, but close monitoring and weighing risk versus benefit to the patient are vitally important. Hydroxyurea is excreted in breast milk and should be avoided in lactating mothers.[17]

Hydroxyurea should be considered in SCD with frequent vasoocclusive crises, severe symptomatic anemia, repeated history of acute chest syndrome (ACS), or other history of severe vasoocclusive crisis (VOC) complications.[5] The prevention of organ damage or reversal of previous damage has not been shown to occur with chronic use of hydroxyurea.[18] The goals of therapy with hydroxyurea are to decrease the acute complications of SCD, improve quality of life, and reduce the number and severity of pain crises.

Hydroxyurea is available in 200-, 300-, 400-, and 500-mg capsules. Extemporaneous liquid preparations can be prepared for children who cannot swallow capsules. Doses should start at 10 to 15 mg/kg daily in a single oral dose, which can be increased after 8 to 12 weeks if blood counts are stable and there are no side effects. Individualize the dosage based on the patient's response and the toxicity seen. With close monitoring, doses can be increased 5 mg/kg/day up to 35 mg/kg daily.[17] In patients with renal failure, dosing of hydroxyurea will need to be adjusted according to the creatinine clearance, as shown in Table 68–3.

Closely monitor patients for efficacy and toxicity while they are receiving hydroxyurea. Monitor mean corpuscular volume (MCV), since it increases as the level of HbF increases. If the MCV does not increase with hydroxyurea use, the marrow may be unable to respond, the dose may not be adequate, or the patient may be noncompliant.[17] HbF levels can also be monitored to assess response with a goal of increasing HbF to 15% to 20% (0.15 to 0.20). Assess blood counts every 2 weeks during dose titration and then every 4 to 6 weeks once the dose is stabilized. Temporary discontinuation of therapy is warranted if hemoglobin level is less than 5.0 g/dL (50 g/L or 3.10 mmol/L), absolute neutrophil count is less than $2 \times 10^3/mm^3$ (2×10^9/L), platelets are less than $80 \times 10^3/mm^3$ (80×10^9/L), or the reticulocytes are less than $80 \times 10^3/mm^3$ (80×10^9/L). Monitor for increases in serum creatinine and transaminases. Once the patient's blood counts have returned to baseline, hydroxyurea may be restarted with a dose that is 2.5 to 5 mg/kg less than the dose associated with the patient's toxicity. Doses may then be increased by 2.5 to 5 mg/kg daily after 12 weeks with no toxicity.

Administer prophylactic folic acid supplementation to SCD patients receiving hydroxyurea, because folate deficiency may be masked by the use of hydroxyurea.

5-Aza-2′-Deoxycytine (Decitabine) For patients who do not respond to hydroxyurea, 5-azacytidine and 5-aza-2′-deoxycytidine (decitabine) may be useful. Both induce HbF by inhibiting methylation of DNA, preventing the switch from γ- to β-globin production. Decitabine appears to be safer and more potent than 5-azacytadine. In a small study in adults refractory to hydroxyurea, decitabine 0.2 mg/kg subcutaneously one to three times weekly was associated

Table 68–3

Dosage Adjustments for Renal and Hepatic Dysfunction

Medication	Renal Adjustment	Hepatic Adjustment
Decitabine (Decagon)	For Scr greater than or equal to 2 mg/dL (177 μmol/L): hold therapy until values return to baseline	For serum alanine transaminase (ALT), serum glutamic pyruvic transaminase (SGPT), or total bilirubin values greater than 2 times the upper limit of normal: hold therapy until values return to baseline
Deferoxamine (Desferal)	Cl$_{cr}$ less than 10 mL/min (0.17 mL/s): decrease the dose by 50%	
Deferasirox (Exjade) children	Greater than 33% increase in Scr (on two consecutive readings) and above the age-appropriate upper limits of normal: decrease daily dose by 10 mg/kg	Severe or persistent elevations in liver function tests: decrease the daily dose or discontinue therapy
Adults	Greater than 33% increase in Scr above pretreatment values on two consecutive readings: decrease daily dose by 10 mg/kg	Severe or persistent elevations in liver function tests: decrease the daily dose or discontinue therapy
Folic acid	No adjustment necessary	No adjustment necessary
Hydroxyurea	Cl$_{cr}$ less than 60 mL/min (1.00 mL/s): Initial dose of 7.5 mg/kg/day Cl$_{cr}$ 10–50 mL/min (0.17-0.83 mL/s): reduce the daily dose by 50% Cl$_{cr}$ less than 10 mL/min (0.17 mL/s): administer 20% of the usual dose Hemodialysis: 7.5 mg/kg/day given after dialysis	Monitor patient for bone marrow toxicity

From Refs. 22–27.

Patient Encounter 2

SC is a 22-year-old African American woman with SCD. She was admitted to the hospital for progressive neck, shoulder, back, and chest pain that began 2 days ago. The patient denies injury. She also has productive cough and subjective fever but denies chills.

PMH

- Sickle cell anemia (*HbSS*)
- Admitted for vasoocclusive crises 5 times over the past year
- Acute chest syndrome at age 14, 16, and 20
- Multiple blood transfusions

PSH

- Cholecystectomy
- Splenectomy
- Port placement × 3

FH: Father with SC trait. Mother with SCD.

Allergies: NKDA

SH: Occasional alcohol use. Is sexually active.

Home Meds

- Hydrocodone/acetaminophen 7.5/500 mg, one tablet every 6 hours prn for pain
- Folic acid 1 mg daily by mouth

PE

VS: T 39° C (102.2° F), BP 113/66, P 78, RR 22, O$_2$ Sat 99% on 2 L nasal cannula, Ht 162.56 cm, Wt 62.7 kg

Gen: awake, alert × 3, in no acute distress, but obviously in pain

HEENT: Normocephalic, atraumatic. PERRLA. No lymphadenopathy

Chest: Normal to inspection and palpation. No rhonchi, rales, or wheezes. Lower lobe crackles with left greater than right

CV: RRR, no m/g/r

Abd: Soft, NT/ND

Ext: No clubbing, cyanosis, or edema. Shoulder pain with palpation

Neuro: Cranial nerves II through XII are grossly intact. Nonfocal

Labs: Hgb 7.3 g/dL (73 g/L or 4.53 mmol/L), Hct 23.1% (0.231 fraction), WBC 19 × 10³/microliter (19 × 10⁶/L), BMP WNL

Chest x-ray showed a left lower lobe atelectasis and right hemidiaphragm consistent with possible left lower lobe pneumonia.

What is your assessment of this patient's condition?

List treatment goals for this patient.

Devise a detailed therapeutic plan for this patient's hospital management.

Is the patient a candidate for hydroxyurea? Why or why not?

---

with an increase in HbF in all patients. Additionally, RBC adhesion was reduced. Neutropenia was the only significant toxicity reported.[28]

Combinations of HbF Inducers Very limited information is available on the use of combination therapy for potentiation of HbF production. Erythropoietin has shown inconsistent results in small numbers of patients. When used with hydroxyurea, erythropoietin has been shown to increase HbF to a greater extent than hydroxyurea alone, and although more studies are needed, this may provide an option for patients who do not respond to hydroxyurea alone.

Patient Encounter 3

Four months later, SC is seen on follow-up in the outpatient clinic for management of her SCD. She reports that she is 3 months pregnant.

Is the patient a candidate for hydroxyurea? Why or why not?

Chronic Transfusion Therapy Chronic transfusion therapy is warranted to prevent serious complications from SCD, including stroke prevention and recurrence. ❻ *Especially in children, chronic transfusions have been shown to decrease stroke recurrence from approximately 50% to 10% over 3 years.* Without chronic transfusions, approximately 70% of ischemic stroke patients will have another stroke. Chronic transfusion therapy also may be used to prevent vasoocclusive pain and ACS, as well as prevent progression of organ damage. Patients receiving chronic transfusion therapy report increased energy levels, improved quality of life, and better exercise tolerance. Patients in whom chronic transfusion therapy should be considered include those with severe or recurrent ACS, debilitating pain, splenic sequestration, recurrent priapism, chronic organ failure, transient ischemic attacks, abnormal transcranial Doppler studies, intractable leg ulcers, severe chronic anemia in the presence of cardiac failure, and complicated pregnancies.[5]

Several methods of transfusion may be used, including simple transfusion, exchange transfusion, or erythrocytapheresis. The goal of chronic transfusion therapy is to maintain the HbS level at less than 30%

(0.30) of total hemoglobin concentration. Transfusions are usually administered every 3 to 4 weeks depending on the HbS concentration. For secondary stroke prevention, current studies have indicated that lifelong transfusion may be required, with increased incidence of recurrence once transfusions are stopped.[5]

The benefits of transfusion should be weighed with the risks. Risks associated with transfusions include alloimmunization (sensitization to the blood received), hyperviscosity, viral transmission, volume overload, iron overload, and transfusion reactions. Approximately 18% to 30% of SCD patients who receive transfusions will experience alloimmunization, which can be minimized by the use of leukocyte-reduced RBCs or HLA-matched units. Viral transmission is still a concern, despite increased screening of blood donors and units. Although the risk of contraction of AIDS has decreased dramatically, hepatitis C remains a concern. All SCD patients should be vaccinated for hepatitis A and B and should be serially monitored for hepatitis C and other infections. Parvovirus occurs in 1 of every 40,000 units of RBCs and can be associated with acute anemia and multiple sickle cell complications.[5] Iron overload remains a concern among those patients maintained on chronic transfusions for greater than 1 year. Counsel patients to avoid excessive dietary iron, and monitor serum ferritin regularly. Chelation therapy with deferoxamine or deferasirox should be considered when the serum ferritin level is greater than 1,500 to 2,000 ng/mL (1,500 to 2,000 mcg/L). Deferoxamine should be initiated at 20 to 40 mg/kg daily (to a maximum of 1 to 2 g/day) over 8 to 12 hours subcutaneously and has been associated with growth failure.[5] Monitor children receiving deferoxamine for adequate growth and development on a regular basis. Deferasirox should be initiated at 20 mg/kg daily and is available in a tablet that should be dispersed in water, orange juice, or apple juice and taken orally 30 minutes before food.[29,30] Monitor all chelation patients for auditory and ocular changes on a yearly basis. Exchange transfusions may also be helpful in cases of iron overload.

Sickle cell hemolytic transfusion reaction syndrome is a unique problem in SCD patients. Due to alloimmunization, an acute or delayed transfusion reaction may occur. Delayed reactions typically occur 5 to 20 days posttransfusion. Alloantibodies and autoantibodies resulting from previous transfusions can trigger the reaction, in which patients develop symptoms suggestive of a pain crisis or worsening symptoms if they are already in crisis. A severe anemia after transfusion also may occur due to a rapid decrease in hemoglobin and hematocrit, along with a suppression of erythropoiesis. Further transfusions may worsen the clinical picture due to autoimmune antibodies. Recovery may occur only after ceasing all transfusions and is evidenced by a gradual increase in hemoglobin with reticulocytosis, which indicates the patient is now making their own RBCs.[5]

Allogeneic Hematopoietic Stem Cell Transplant
Allogeneic hematopoietic stem-cell transplantation (HSCT) is the only potential cure for SCD. The best candidates are children with SCD who are younger than 16 years of age with severe complications, who have an identical HLA-matched donor, usually a sibling. The transplant-related mortality rate is between 5% and 10%, and graft rejection is approximately 10%. Other risks include secondary malignancies, development of seizures or intracranial bleeding, and infection in the immediate posttransplant period.[5,31,32]

Experience with HSCT in adult patients with SCD is very limited. Umbilical cord blood and hematopoietic cells from nonmatched donors are potential alternatives in some patients, but use is limited.[5,32]

▶ Acute Complications

Transfusions for Acute Complications Red cell transfusion is indicated in patients with acute exacerbations of baseline anemia; in cases of severe vasoocclusive episodes, including ACS, stroke, and acute multiorgan failure; and in preparation for procedures that will require the use of general anesthesia or ionic contrast products. Transfusions also may be useful in patients with complicated obstetric problems, refractory leg ulcers, refractory and prolonged pain crises, or severe priapism. Hyperviscosity may occur if the hemoglobin level is increased to greater than 10.0 to 11.0 g/dL (100 to 110 g/L or 6.21 to 6.83 mmol/L). Volume overload leading to congestive heart failure is more likely to occur if the anemia is corrected too rapidly in patients with severe anemia and should be avoided.[5]

Infection and Fever ❼ *Any fever greater than 38.5°C (101.3°F) in a SCD patient should be immediately evaluated, and the patient should have a blood culture drawn and be started on antibiotics that provide empirical coverage for encapsulated organisms.*[5]

Patients who should be hospitalized include the following:

- Infants younger than 1 year of age
- Patients with a previous sepsis or bacteremia episode
- Patients with temperatures in excess of 40°C (104°F)
- Patients with WBC counts greater than $30 \times 10^3/mm^3$ ($30 \times 10^9/L$) or less than $0.5 \times 10^3/mm^3$ ($0.5 \times 10^9/L$) and/or platelets less than $100 \times 10^3/mm^3$ ($100 \times 10^9/L$) with evidence of other acute complications
- Acutely ill-appearing individuals

Broad IV antibiotic coverage for the encapsulated organisms can include ceftriaxone or cefotaxime. For patients with true cephalosporin allergy, clindamycin may be used. If staphylococcal infection is suspected due to previous history or the patient appears acutely ill, vancomycin should be initiated. Macrolide antibiotics, such as erythromycin or azithromycin, may be initiated if mycoplasma pneumonia is suspected. While the patient is receiving broad-spectrum antibiotics, their regular use of penicillin for prophylaxis can be suspended. Fever should be controlled with acetaminophen or ibuprofen. Because of the risk of dehydration during infection with fever, increased fluid may be needed.[1,5]

Clinical Presentation and Diagnosis of Infection in SCD

General

- Patients may become acutely distressed very rapidly
- A low threshold to begin empiric therapy is recommended

Symptoms

- Patients may complain of lethargy, nausea, cough, or a general "unwell" feeling

Signs

- Temperature greater than 38.5°C (101.3°F)

Laboratory Tests

- CBC with reticulocyte count
- Cultures (urine, blood, and throat)
- Lumbar puncture if toxic-looking or signs of meningitis
- Urinalysis
- Chest x-ray

Potential Pathogens

- *Streptococcus pneumoniae* (most common), *Haemophilus influenzae*, *Salmonella*, *Mycoplasma pneumoniae*, *Chlamydia*, and viruses (parvovirus B19)

Clinical Presentation and Diagnosis of Stroke in SCD

General

- Most common cause is cerebrovascular occlusion
- Initial episode most often occurs during first 10 years of life
- Silent infarcts seen on MRI have been reported in 22% of patients and may be associated with increased risk of stroke and decreased neurocognitive function

Symptoms

- Patients may present with headache, vomiting, stupor, hemiparesis, aphasia, visual disturbances, and seizure

Evaluation

- CT scan and MRI for acute event
- Magnetic resonance angiography for asymptomatic infarction
- Transcranial Doppler to detect abnormal velocity and identify high-risk patients
- Electroencephalography if there is history of seizure
- Chest x-ray

Bone infarcts or sickling in the periosteum usually is indicated by pain and swelling over an extremity. Osteomyelitis also should also be considered. *Salmonella* species are the most common cause of osteomyelitis in SCD children, followed by *Staphylococcus aureus*.[1] Select an appropriate antibiotic to cover the suspected organisms empirically.

Cerebrovascular Accidents Acute neurologic events, such as stroke, will require hospitalization and close monitoring. Patients should have physical and neurologic examinations every 2 hours.[5] Acute treatment may include exchange transfusion or simple transfusion to maintain hemoglobin at approximately 10.0 g/dL (100 g/L or 6.21 mmol/L) and HbS concentration at less than 30% (0.30). Patients with a history of seizure may need anticonvulsants, and interventions for increased intracranial pressure should be initiated if necessary. Children with history of stroke should be initiated on chronic transfusion therapy. Adults presenting with ischemic stroke should be considered for thrombolytic therapy if it has been less than 3 hours since the onset of symptoms.[5]

Early detection of ischemic stroke can be done with the use of transcranial Doppler ultrasonography. In the Stroke Prevention Trial in Sickle Cell Anemia (STOP) study, screening with this method followed by chronic transfusion therapy significantly reduced the incidence of stroke.[33–35] Screening is recommended in all patients over the age of 2 years.

Acute Chest Syndrome ACS will require hospitalization for appropriate management of symptoms and to avoid complications. Patients should be encouraged to use incentive spirometry at least every 2 hours. Incentive spirometry helps the patient take long, slow breaths to increase lung expansion. Appropriate management of pain is important, but analgesic-induced hypoventilation should be avoided. Patients should maintain appropriate fluid balance because overhydration can lead to pulmonary edema and respiratory distress. Infection with gram-negative, gram-positive, or atypical bacteria is common in ACS, and early use of broad-spectrum antibiotics, including a macrolide, quinolone, or cephalosporin is recommended. Fat emboli, from infarction of the long bones, may lead to ACS. Oxygen therapy should be utilized in any patient presenting with respiratory distress or hypoxia. Oxygen saturations, measured by pulse oximeter, should be maintained at 92% (0.92) or above. Transfusions are often indicated, and patients who present with wheezing may require inhaled bronchodilators.[5,36,37]

The use of corticosteroids is controversial. Although they may decrease the inflammation and endothelial cell adhesion seen with ACS, their use has also been associated with higher readmission rates for other complications. Tapered corticosteroids, nitric oxide therapy, and L-arginine are being evaluated for use in ACS in studies.[36,37]

Priapism By age 18, approximately 90% of SCD males will have had at least one episode of priapism. Stuttering priapism, where erection episodes last anywhere from a few minutes to

Clinical Presentation and Diagnosis of ACS in SCD

General
- Occurs in 15% to 43% of patients and is responsible for 25% of deaths
- Risk factors include young age, low HbF level, high Hgb and WBCs, winter seasons, reactive airway disease
- Recurrences are up to 80% and can lead to chronic lung disease

Symptoms
- Patients may complain of cough, fever, dyspnea, chest pain

Signs
- Temperature greater than 38.5°C (101.3°F)
- Hypoxia
- New infiltrate on chest x-ray

Laboratory Tests
- CBC with reticulocyte count
- Blood gases
- Oxygen saturation
- Cultures (blood and sputum)

Other
- Closely monitor pulmonary status

Clinical Presentation and Diagnosis of Priapism in SCD

General
- Mean age of initial episode is 12 years of age
- Most males with SCD will have one episode by age 20
- Repeated episodes can lead to fibrosis and impotence

Symptoms
- Patients may complain of painful and unwanted erection lasting anywhere from less than 2 hours (stuttering type) to more than 2 hours (prolonged type)

Signs
- Urinary obstruction

Laboratory Tests
- CBC with reticulocyte count

Other
- Monitor for duration of episode
- Prolonged episodes should be considered medical emergencies

Clinical Presentation and Diagnosis of Acute Aplastic Crisis in SCD

General
- Transient suppression of RBC production in response to bacterial or viral infection
- Most commonly due to infection with parvovirus B19

Symptoms
- Patients may complain of headache, fatigue, dyspnea, pallor, or fever
- Patients may also complain of upper respiratory or GI infection symptoms

Signs
- Temperature greater than 38.5°C (101.3°F) may occur
- Hypoxia
- Tachycardia
- Acute decrease in Hgb with decreased reticulocyte count

Laboratory Tests
- CBC with reticulocyte count
- Chest x-ray
- Parvovirus titers
- Cultures (blood, urine, and throat)

less than 2 hours, resolves spontaneously. Erections lasting more than 2 hours should be evaluated promptly. Goals of therapy are to provide pain relief, reduce anxiety, provide detumescense, and preserve testicular function and fertility. Initial treatment should include aggressive hydration and analgesia. Transfusion may or may not be helpful, but should be considered in anemic patients. Avoid the use of ice packs due to the risk of tissue damage.[5]

Both vasoconstrictors and vasodilators have been used in the treatment of priapism. Vasoconstrictors are thought to work by forcing blood out of the cavernosum and into the venous return. Aspiration of the penile blood followed by intracavenous irrigation with epinephrine (1:1,000,000 solution) has been effective with minimal complications.[38] In severe cases, surgical intervention to place penile shunts has been used, but there is a high failure rate, and the risk of complications, from skin sloughing to fistulas, limits its use.

Pseudoephedrine dosed at 30 to 60 mg/day taken at bedtime has been used to prevent or decrease the number of episodes of priapism.[5] Terbutaline 5 mg has been used orally to prevent priapism, with mixed results.[38,39] Leuprolide, a gonadotropin-releasing hormone, also has been used for this indication. Hydroxyurea may be helpful in some patients.[38,40] The use of antiandrogens is under investigation.[5]

Clinical Presentation and Diagnosis of Sequestration Crisis in SCD

General

- Acute exacerbation of anemia due to sequestration of large blood volume by the spleen
- More common in patients with functioning spleens
- Onset often associated with viral or bacterial infections
- Recurrence is common and can be fatal

Symptoms

- Sudden onset of fatigue, dyspnea, and distended abdomen
- Patients may present with vomiting and abdominal pain

Signs

- Rapid decrease in Hgb and Hct with elevated reticulocyte count
- Splenomegaly
- May exhibit hypotension and shock

Evaluation

- Vital signs
- Spleen size changes
- Oxygen saturations
- CBC with reticulocyte count
- Cultures (blood, urine, throat)

Clinical Presentation and Diagnosis of Vasoocclusive Crisis in SCD

General

- Most often involves the bones, liver, spleen, brain, lungs, and penis
- Precipitating factors include infection, extreme weather conditions, dehydration, and stresses
- Recurrent acute crises result in bone, joint, and organ damage and chronic pain

Symptoms

- Patients may complain of deep throbbing pain, local tenderness

Signs

- Erythema and swelling of painful area
- Dactylitis in young infants
- Temperature greater than 38.5°C (101.3°F)
- Leukocytosis

Laboratory tests

- CBC with reticulocyte count
- Urinalysis
- Abdominal studies (if symptoms exist)
- Cultures (blood and urine)
- Liver function tests and bilirubin
- Chest x-ray

▶ *Treatment of Acute Complications*

Aplastic Crisis Most patients in aplastic crisis will recover spontaneously and therefore treatment is supportive. If anemia is severe or symptomatic, transfusion may be indicated. Infection with human parvovirus B19 is the most common cause of aplastic crisis. Isolate infected patients because parvovirus is highly contagious. Pregnant individuals should avoid contact with infected patients because midtrimester infection with parvovirus may cause hydrops fetalis and still birth.[1,5]

Sequestration Crisis RBC sequestration in the spleen in young children may lead to a rapid drop in hematocrit, resulting in hypovolemia, shock, and death. Treatment is RBC transfusion to correct the hypovolemia, as well as broad-spectrum antibiotics, because infections may precipitate the crisis.[1,5]

Recurrent episodes are common and can be managed with chronic transfusion and splenectomy. Observation is used commonly in adults because their episodes are milder. Splenectomy is usually delayed until after 2 years of age to lessen the risk of postsplenectomy septicemia. Patients with chronic hypersplenism should be considered for splenectomy.[5,41]

Vasoocclusive Pain Crisis The mainstay of treatment for vasoocclusive crisis includes hydration and analgesia (Table 68–4). Pain may involve the extremities, back, chest, and abdomen. ❽ *Patients with mild pain crisis may be treated as outpatients with rest, warm compresses to the affected (painful) area, increased fluid intake, and oral analgesia.* Patients with moderate to severe crises should be hospitalized. Infection should be ruled out because it may trigger a pain crisis, and any patient presenting with fever or critical illness should be started on empirical broad-spectrum antibiotics. Patients who are anemic should be transfused to their baseline. IV or oral fluids at 1.5 times maintenance is recommended. Close monitoring of the patient's fluid status is important to avoid overhydration, which can lead to ACS, volume overload, or heart failure.[5]

Aggressive pain management is required in patients presenting in pain crisis. Assess pain on a regular basis (every 2 to 4 hours), and individualize management to the patient. The use of pain scales may help with quantifying the pain rating. Obtain a good medication history of what has worked well for the patient in the past. Use acetaminophen or a nonsteroidal anti-inflammatory drug (NSAID) for treatment of mild to moderate pain. Patients with bone or joint pain

Table 68–4

Management of Acute Pain of SCD

Principles

- Treat underlying precipitating factors.
- Avoid delays in analgesia administration.
- Use pain scale to assess severity.
- Choice of initial analgesic should be based on previous pain crisis pattern, history of response, current status, and other medical conditions.
- Schedule pain medication; avoid as-needed dosing.
- Provide rescue dose for breakthrough pain.
- If adequate pain relief can be achieved with one or two doses of morphine, consider outpatient management with a weak opioid; otherwise hospitalization is needed for parenteral analgesics.
- Frequently assess to evaluate pain severity and side effects; titrate dose as needed.
- Treating adverse effects of opioids is part of pain management.
- Consider nonpharmacologic intervention.
- Transition to oral analgesics as the patient improves; choose an oral agent based on previous history, anticipated duration, and ability to swallow tablets; if sustained-release products are used, a fast-release product is also needed for breakthrough pain.

Analgesic Regimens

Mild to moderate pain:
Acetaminophen with codeine
- Dose based on codeine—children: 1 mg/kg per dose every 6 hours; adults: 30–60 mg/dose

Hydrocodone + acetaminophen:
- Dose based on hydrocodone—children: 0.2 mg/kg per dose every 6 hours; adults: 5–10 mg/dose

Anti-inflammatory agents
- Use with caution in patients with renal failure (dehydration) and bleeding
- Ibuprofen (oral): children: 10 mg/kg every 6–8 hours; adults: 200–400 mg/dose
- Naproxen: 5 mg/kg every 12 hours; adults: 250–500 mg/dose
- Ibuprofen + hydrocodone: Each tablet contains 200 mg ibuprofen and 7.5 mg hydrocodone per tablet; only for older children who can swallow tablets

Moderate to severe pain:
Morphine—children: 0.1–0.15 mg/kg per dose every 3–4 hours; adults: 5–10 mg/dose
- Continuous infusion: 0.04–0.05 mg/kg/h; titrate to effect

Hydromorphone—children: 0.015 mg/kg per dose every 3–4 hours; adults: 1.5–2 mg/dose
- Continuous infusion: 0.004 mg/kg/h; titrate to effect

IV anti-inflammatory agents:
- Ketorolac: 0.5 mg/kg up to 30 mg/dose every 6 hours

Patient-controlled analgesics:
- Morphine: 0.01–0.03 mg/kg/h basal; demand 0.01–0.03 mg/kg every 6–10 minutes; 4 hours lockout 0.04–0.06 mg/kg
- Hydromorphone: 0.003–0.005 mg/kg/h basal; demand 0.003–0.05 mg/kg every 6–10 minutes; 4 hours lock out 0.4–0.6 mg/kg

who require IV medications may be helped by the use of ketorolac, an injectable NSAID. Because of the concern for side effects, including GI bleeding, ketorolac should be used only for a maximum of 5 consecutive days. Monitor for the total amount of acetaminophen given daily, because many products contain acetaminophen. Maximum daily dose of acetaminophen for adults is 4 g/day, and for children, five doses over a 24-hour period.[42] Add an opioid if pain persists or if pain is moderate to severe in nature. Combining an opioid with an NSAID can enhance the analgesic effects without increasing adverse effects.[43-46]

Severe pain should be treated with an opioid such as morphine, hydromorphone, methadone, or fentanyl. Moderate pain can be effectively treated in most cases with a weak opioid such as codeine or hydrocodone, usually in combination with acetaminophen. Meperidine should be avoided because of its relatively short analgesic effect and its toxic metabolite, normeperidine. Normeperidine may

accumulate with repeated dosing and can lead to CNS side effects including seizures.

IV opioids are recommended for use in treatment of severe pain because of their rapid onset of action and ease in titration. Intramuscular injection should be avoided. Analgesia should be individualized and titrated to effect, either by scheduled doses or continuous infusion. The use of continuous infusion will avoid the fluctuations in blood levels between doses that is seen with bolus dosing. As-needed dosing of analgesia is only appropriate for breakthrough pain or uncontrolled pain. Patient-controlled analgesia (PCA) is commonly used and allows the patient to have control over his or her analgesic breakthrough dosing. As the pain crisis resolves, the pain medications can be tapered. Physical therapy and relaxation therapy can be helpful adjuvants to analgesia.[43-46]

Tolerance to opioids is seen when patients have had continuous long-term use of the medications and can be managed during acute crises by using a different potent opioid or using a larger dose of the same medication. Adverse effects associated with the use of opioids include respiratory depression, itching, nausea and vomiting, constipation, and drowsiness. Patients on continuous infusions of opioids should be on continuous pulse oximeter to assess oxygen saturations. Monitor the patient for oxygen saturations less than 92% (0.92). Oxygen should be administered as needed to keep the saturations above 92% (0.92). Itching can be managed with an antihistamine such as diphenhydramine. Nausea and vomiting can be treated and managed with the administration of antiemetics such as promethazine or the 5HT3 antagonists, but the use of promethazine is contraindicated in children younger than 2 years of age. Assess stool frequency in all patients on a continuous opioid, and start stool softeners or laxatives as needed. Excessive sedation is difficult to control, and the concurrent use of an opioid with diphenhydramine or other sedative medications can exacerbate the drowsiness, leading to hypoxemia. A continuous very low dose of naloxone, an opioid antagonist, has been used successfully when the adverse effects such as itching are unbearable.[47]

OUTCOME EVALUATION

SCD treatment and prevention are considered successful when complications are minimized. The major outcome parameters are a decrease in morbidity and mortality,

measured by the number of hospitalizations, and the extent of end-organ damage seen over time. Today, with longer survival for SCD, chronic manifestations of the disease contribute to the morbidity later in life (Table 68–5). Thirty years ago, complications from SCD contributed to high mortality. It was estimated that approximately 50% of patients with SCD did not survive to reach adulthood.[4] Since that time, data suggest improvement in mortality rates for patients with SCD. The survival age for individuals with HbSS has increased to at least the fifth decade of life. Recent reports suggest 85% survival by 18 years of age.[4] SCD is a chronic disease and cannot be cured, except in some patients with transplant.

Starting with birth, SCD patients should have regularly scheduled health assessments and interventions when necessary. Obtain a urine analysis, complete blood count, liver function tests, ferritin or serum iron level and total iron-binding capacity, blood urea nitrogen (BUN), and creatinine on at least a yearly basis and more often for children younger than 5 years of age to monitor for complications. All SCD patients should have regular screening of their hearing and vision.

All patients and parents of children with SCD should have a plan for what to do in the event of symptoms of infection or pain. Obtain a medication history when patients are admitted to the hospital. Assess compliance with prophylactic penicillin and childhood immunization schedules in all pediatric SCD patients.

Table 68–5

Chronic Complications of SCD

System	Complications
Auditory	Sensorineural hearing loss due to sickling in cochlear vasculature with hair cell damage
Cardiovascular	Cardiomegaly, myocardial ischemia, murmurs, and abnormal ECG; patients with SCD have lower BP than the normal population; normal BP values for SCD should be used for diagnosis of hypertension ("relative" hypertension); heart failure usually is related to fluid overload
Dermatologic	Painful leg ulcers; failure to heal occurs in 50% of patients; recurrences are common
Genitourinary	Renal papillary necrosis, hematuria, hyposthenuria, proteinuria, nephrotic syndrome, tubular dysfunction, chronic renal failure, impotence
Growth and development	Delay in growth (weight and height) and sexual development; decreased fertility; increased complications during pregnancy; depression may be more prevalent than in general population, especially in patients with unstable disease
Hepatic and biliary	Cholelithiasis, biliary sludge, acute and chronic cholecystitis, and cholestasis (can be progressive and life-threatening)
Neurologic	"Silent" brain lesions on MRI are associated with poor cognitive and fine motor functions; pseudotumor cerebri (rare)
Ocular	Retinal or vitreous hemorrhage, retinal detachment, transient or permanent visual loss; central retinal vein occlusion
Pulmonary	Pulmonary fibrosis, pulmonary hypertension, cor pulmonale
Renal	Hematuria, hyposthenuria (inability to concentrate urine maximally), tubular dysfunction, enuresis during early childhood, acute renal failure can also occur
Skeletal	Aseptic necrosis of ball-and-socket joints (shoulder and hip); prostheses may be needed due to permanent damage; bone marrow hyperplasia resulting in growth disturbances of maxilla and vertebrae
Spleen	Asplenia (autosplenectomy or surgical splenectomy)

Patient Care and Monitoring

1. Assess the patient's symptoms to determine whether the patient should be evaluated by a physician and/or receive immediate care. Determine the type of symptoms, onset of symptoms, frequency and exacerbating factors. Does the patient have evidence of SCD-related complications?

2. Review any available diagnostic data to determine the severity and status of the patient's SCD. When was the patient last hospitalized for SCD complications?

3. Obtain a thorough history of prescription, nonprescription, and natural drug product use. For pain control, determine which treatments have been helpful to the patient in the past. Is the patient currently taking any medications on a chronic basis?

4. Educate the patient on lifestyle modifications that may lessen complications. These include maintaining adequate hydration status, avoiding extreme temperature changes, dressing appropriately for hot or cold weather, and avoiding physical exertion, smoking, and excessive alcohol intake.

5. Is the patient up-to-date on immunizations? Have they received their annual influenza vaccine? If not, why?

6. Is the patient taking appropriate doses of their pain medication to achieve effect? If not, why?

7. Develop a plan to assess the effectiveness of pain medications.

8. Determine whether the patient is a candidate for hydroxyurea therapy.

9. Assess improvement in quality-of-life measures, such as physical, psychological, and social functioning and well-being.

10. Evaluate the patient for the presence of adverse drug reactions, drug allergies, and drug interactions.

11. Stress the importance of adherence with the therapeutic regimen, including lifestyle modifications. Recommend a therapeutic regimen that is easy for the patient/parent to accomplish.

12. Provide patient education on disease state, lifestyle modifications, and drug therapy:

    - Possible complications of SCD, both long and short term
    - When to take their medications
    - Adverse effects and how to mange them
    - Which drugs may interact with their medication therapy
    - Warning signs to report to the physician (increased or new pain, sudden headache, bleeding or bruising, fever, loss of energy, loss of appetite)

Abbreviations Introduced in This Chapter

ACS	Acute chest syndrome
HbA	Normal adult hemoglobin
HbAS	One normal and one sickle hemoglobin gene
HbC	Hemoglobin C
HbF	Fetal hemoglobin
HbS	Sickle hemoglobin
HbSβ^0-thalassemia	One sickle hemoglobin and one β^0-thalassemia gene
HbSβ^+-thalassemia	One sickle hemoglobin and one β^+-thalassemia gene
HbSC	One sickle hemoglobin and one hemoglobin C gene
HbSS	Homozygous sickle hemoglobin
Hgb	Hemoglobin
HSCT	Hematopoietic stem cell transplantation
ISC	Irreversibly sickled cell
MCHC	Mean corpuscular hemoglobin concentration
MCV	Mean corpuscular volume
NSAID	Nonsteroidal anti-inflammatory drug
PCA	Patient-controlled analgesia
PCV 13	13-Valent pneumococcal conjugate vaccine
PPV 23	23-Valent pneumococcal polysaccharide vaccine
SCA	Sickle cell anemia
SCD	Sickle cell disease
SCT	Sickle cell trait
STOP	Stroke Prevention Trial in Sickle Cell Anemia
VOC	Vasoocclusive crisis

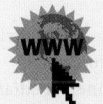 Self-assessment questions and answers are available at *http://mhpharmacotherapy.com/pp.html.*

REFERENCES

1. Stuart MJ, Nagel RL. Sickle-cell disease. Lancet 2004;364(9442):1343–1360. Review.
2. Ashley-Koch A, Yang Q, Olney RS. Sickle hemoglobin (HbS) allele and sickle cell disease: A huge review. Am J Epidemiol 2000;151:839–844.

3. Steinberg MH. Pathophysiologically based drug treatment of sickle cell disease. Trends Pharmacol Sci 2006;27(4):204–210.

4. Quinn CT, Rogers ZR, Buchanan GR. Survival of children with sickle cell disease. Blood 2004;103(11):4023–4027.

5. National Institutes of Health. The Management of Sickle Cell Disease. NIH Pub. No. 02–2117. Bethesda, MD: Division of Blood Diseases and Resources, Public Health Service, U.S. Department of Health and Human Services; June 2002:1–88.

6. World Health Organization [Internet]. Fifty-Ninth World Health Assembly 2006 [cited 2011 Oct 10]. Available from: *http://www.who.int/gb/ebwha/pdf_files/WHA59/A59_9-en.pdf*.

7. Lanzkowsky P. Manual of Pediatric Hematology and Oncology. 4th ed. New York: Churchill Livingstone; 2005:160.

8. Rees DC, Williams TN, Gladwin MT. Sickle-cell disease. Lancet 2010;376:2018–2031.

9. American Academy of Pediatrics Policy Statement. Recommended Childhood and Adolescent Immunization Schedule—United States, 2011. Pediatrics 2011;127;387–388.

10. Nuorti JP, Whitney CG. Prevention of pneumococcal disease among infants and children—use of 13-valent pneumococcal conjugate vaccine and 23-valent pneumococcal polysaccharide vaccine—recommendations of the Advisory Committee on Immunization Practices (ACIP). MMWR Recomm Rep 2010;59:1–18.

11. Adamkiewicz TV, Silk BJ, Howgate J, et al. Effectiveness of the 7-valent pneumococcal conjugate vaccine in children with sickle cell disease in the first decade of life. Pediatrics 2008;121:562–569.

12. Battersby AJ, Knox-Macaulay HHM, Carrol ED. Susceptibility to invasive bacterial infections in children with sickle cell disease. Pediatr Blood Cancer 2010;55:401–406.

13. Quinn CT, Lee NJ, Shull EP, Ahmad N, Rogers ZR, Buchanan GR. Prediction of adverse outcomes in children with sickle cell anemia: a study of the Dallas Newborn Cohort. Blood 2008;111:544–548.

14. Falletta JM, Woods RM, Verter JI, et al. Discontinuing penicillin prophylaxis in children with sickle cell anemia. J Pediatr 1995;127:685–690.

15. Hirst C, Owusu-Ofori S. Cochrane Review: Prophylactic antibiotics for preventing pneumococcal infections in children with sickle cell disease. Evidence-Based Child Health 2007;2:993–1009.

16. Kennedy TS, Fung EB, Kawchak DA, et al. Red blood cell folate and serum B12 status in children with sickle cell disease. J Pediatr Hematol Oncol 2001;23:165–169.

17. Brawley OW, Cornelius LJ, Edwards LR, et al. National Institutes of Health consensus development conference statement: hydroxyurea treatment for sickle cell disease. Ann Intern Med 2008;148:932–938.

18. Steinberg MH, Bartin F, Castro O, et al. Effect of hydroxyurea on mortality and morbidity in adult sickle cell anemia. Risks and benefits up to 9 years of treatment. JAMA 2003;289:1645–1651.

19. Kinney TR, Helms RW, O'Branski EE, Ohene-Frempong K, et al. Safety of hydroxyurea in children with sickle cell anemia: Results of the HUG-KIDS study, a phase I/II trial. Pediatric Hydroxyurea Group Blood 1999;94(5):1550–1554.

20. Strouse JJ, Lanzkron S, Beach MC, et al. Hydroxyurea for sickle cell disease: a systematic review for efficacy and toxicity in children. Pediatrics 2008;122:1332–1342.

21. Hankins JS Ware RE, Rogers ZR, et al. Long-term hydroxyurea therapy for infants with sickle cell anemia: The HUSOFT extension study. Blood 2005;106:2269–2275.

22. Lexi-Comp. Hydroxyurea monograph. Lexi-Comp Online,™ Pediatric Lexi-Drugs Online.™ Hudson, OH: Lexi-Comp; October 10, 2011.

23. Lexi-Comp. Deferoxamine monograph. Lexi-Comp Online,™ Pediatric Lexi-Drugs Online.™ Hudson, OH: Lexi-Comp; October 10, 2011.

24. Lexi-Comp. Deferasirox monograph. Lexi-Comp Online,™ Pediatric Lexi-Drugs Online.™ Hudson, OH: Lexi-Comp; October 10, 2011.

25. Lexi-Comp. Decitabine monograph. Lexi-Comp Online,™ Lexi-Drugs Online,™ Hudson, OH: Lexi-Comp, October 10; 2011.

26. Lexi-Comp. Folic acid monograph. Lexi-Comp Online,™ Lexi-Drugs Online,™ Hudson, OH: Lexi-Comp; October 10, 2011.

27. Aronoff GR, Bennett WM, Berns JS, et al., eds. Drug Prescribing in Renal Failure. 15th ed. Philadelphia, PA: American College of Physicians; 2007.

28. Hankins J, Aygun B. Pharmacotherapy in sickle-cell disease—state of the art and future prospects. Br J Haematol 2009;145:296–308.

29. Porter J, Vinchinsky E, Rose C, et al. A phase II study with ICL670 (Exjade), a once-daily oral iron chelator, in patients with various transfusion dependent anemias and iron overload (abstract). Blood 2004;104:3193.

30. Brittenham GM. Iron-chelating therapy for transfusional iron overload. N Engl J Med 2011;364:146–156.

31. Bolanos-Meade J, Brodsky RA. Blood and marrow transplantation for sickle cell disease: overcoming barriers to success Curr Opin Oncol 2009;21:158–161.

32. Bhatia M, Walters MC. Hematopoietic cell transplantation for thalassemia and sickle cell disease: past, present and future. Bone Marrow Transplant 2008;41:109–117.

33. Adams RJ, Brambilla DJ, Granger S, et al. Stroke and conversion to high risk in children screened with transcranial Doppler ultrasound during the STOP study. Blood 2004;103:3689–3694.

34. Lee MT, Piomelli S, Granger S, et al. Stroke Prevention Trial in Sickle Cell Anemia (STOP): extended follow-up and final results. Blood 2006;108:847–852.

35. Kwiatkowski JL, Granger S, Brambilla DJ, Brown RC, Miller ST, Adams RJ. Elevated blood flow velocity in the anterior cerebral artery and stroke risk in sickle cell disease; extended analysis from the STOP trial. B J Haematol 2006;134:333–339.

36. Caboot JB, Allen JL. Pulmonary complications of sickle cell disease in children. Curr Opin Pediatr 2008;20:279–287.

37. Johnson CS. The acute chest syndrome. Hematol Oncol Clin North Am 2005;198:857–879.

38. Maples BL, Hagemann TM. Treatment of priapism in pediatric patients with sickle cell disease. Am J Health Syst Pharm 2004;61:355–363.

39. Fuh BR, Perkin RM. Sickle cell disease emergencies in children. Ped Emer Med Report 2009;14:145–155.

40. Saad STO, Lajolo C, Gilli S, et al. Follow-up of sickle cell disease patients with priapism treated by hydroxyurea. Am J Hematol 2004;77:45–49.

41. Owusu-Ofori S, Riddington C. Splenectomy versus conservative management for acute sequestration crises in people with sickle cell disease. Cochrane Database Syst Rev 2002;(4):CD003425.

42. Changes for acetaminophen-containing prescription products. Pharm Lett Prescribe Lett 2011;27(2):270203.

43. Field JJ, Knight-Perry JE, Debaun MR. Acute pain in children and adults with sickle cell disease: management in the absence of evidence-based guidelines. Curr Opin Hematol 2009;16:173–178.

44. Jerrell JM, Tripathi A, Stallworth JR. Pain management in children and adolescents with sickle cell disease. Am J Hematol 2011;86:82–84.

45. Frei-Jones MJ, Baxter AL, Rogers ZR, Buchanan GR. Vaso-occlusive episodes in older children with sickle cell disease: emergency department management and pain assessment. J Pediatr 2008;152:281–285.

46. Mousa SA, Al Momen A, Al Sayegh F, et al. Management of painful vaso-occlusive crisis of sickle-cell anemia: consensus opinion. Clin Appl Thromb Hemost 2010;16:365–376.

47. Miller JM, Hagemann TM. Use of pure opioid antagonists for management of opioid-induced pruritus. Am J Health-Syst Pharm 2011;68:1419–1425.

69 Antimicrobial Regimen Selection

Catherine M. Oliphant and Karl Madaras-Kelly

LEARNING OBJECTIVES

● **Upon completion of the chapter, the reader will be able to:**

1. Recognize that antimicrobial resistance is an inevitable consequence of antimicrobial therapy.

2. Describe how antimicrobials differ from other drug classes in terms of their effects on individual patients as well as on society as a whole.

3. Identify two guiding principles to consider when treating patients with antimicrobials, and apply these principles in patient care.

4. Differentiate between microbial colonization and infection based on patient history, physical examination, and laboratory and culture results.

5. Evaluate and apply at least six major drug-specific considerations when selecting antimicrobial therapy.

6. Evaluate and apply at least seven major patient-specific considerations when selecting antimicrobial therapy.

7. Select empirical antimicrobial therapy based on spectrum-of-activity considerations that provide a measured response proportional to the severity of illness. Provide a rationale for why a measured response in antimicrobial selection is appropriate.

8. Identify and apply five major principles of patient education and monitoring response to antimicrobial therapy.

9. Identify two common causes of patients failing to improve while on antimicrobials, and recognize other less common but potential reasons for antimicrobial failure.

KEY CONCEPTS

❶ An inevitable consequence of exposing microbes to antimicrobials is that some organisms will develop resistance to the antimicrobial.

❷ Antimicrobials are different from other classes of pharmaceuticals because they exert their action on bacteria infecting the host as opposed to acting directly on the host.

❸ Two guiding principles to consider when treating patients with antimicrobials are (a) make the diagnosis and (b) do no harm!

❹ Only bacteria that cause disease should be targeted with antimicrobial therapy, and colonizing flora should be left intact whenever possible.

❺ Bacterial cultures should be obtained prior to antimicrobial therapy in patients with a systemic inflammatory response, risk factors for antimicrobial resistance, or infections where diagnosis or antimicrobial susceptibility is uncertain.

❻ Drug-specific considerations in antimicrobial selection include the spectrum of activity, effects on nontargeted microbial flora, appropriate dose, pharmacokinetic and pharmacodynamic properties, adverse-effect and drug-interaction profile, and cost.

❼ Empirical therapy should be based on patient- and antimicrobial-specific factors such as the anatomic location of the infection, the likely pathogens associated with the presentation, the potential for adverse effects, and the antimicrobial spectrum of activity.

❽ Key patient-specific considerations in antimicrobial selection include recent previous antimicrobial exposures, identification of the anatomic location of infection through physical examination and diagnostic imaging, history of drug allergies, organ dysfunction that may affect drug clearance, immunosuppression, pregnancy, and adherence.

❾ Patient education, de-escalation of antimicrobial therapy based on culture results, monitoring for clinical response and adverse effects, and appropriate duration of therapy are important treatment components.

⑩ Inadequate diagnosis resulting in poor initial antimicrobial selection, poor source control, or the development of a new infection with a resistant organism are relatively common causes of antimicrobial failure.

The discovery of antimicrobials is among the greatest medical achievements of the 20th century. Prior to the antimicrobial era, patients who contracted common infectious diseases developed significant morbidity or perished. The discovery of penicillin in 1927, followed by the subsequent discovery of other antimicrobials, contributed to a significant decline in infectious disease–related mortality during the next five decades. However, since 1980, infectious disease–related mortality in the United States has increased, in part owing to increases in antimicrobial resistance. The discovery of virtually every new class of antimicrobials has occurred in response to the development of bacterial resistance and loss of clinical effectiveness of existing antimicrobials. ❶ *An inevitable consequence of exposing microbes to antimicrobials is that some organisms will develop resistance to the antimicrobial.* Today, there are dozens of antimicrobial classes and hundreds of antimicrobials available for clinical use. However, in many cases, differences in mechanisms of action between antimicrobials are minor, and the microbiologic properties of the agents are similar. ❷ *Antimicrobials are different from other classes of pharmaceuticals because they exert their action on bacteria infecting the host as opposed to acting directly on the host.* Because use of an antimicrobial in one patient affects not only that patient but also other patients if they become infected with resistant bacteria, correct selection, use, and monitoring of clinical response are paramount.

❸ *There are two guiding principles to consider when treating patients with antimicrobials: (a) make the correct diagnosis and (b) do no harm!* Patients with infections frequently present with signs and symptoms that are nonspecific for infection and may be confused with other noninfectious disease. Not only is it important to determine whether a disease process is of infectious origin, but it is also important to determine the specific causative pathogen of the infection. Antimicrobials vary in their spectrum of activity, the ability to inhibit or kill different species of bacteria. Antimicrobials that kill many different species of bacteria are called *broad-spectrum antimicrobials,* whereas antimicrobials that kill only a few species of bacteria are called *narrow-spectrum antimicrobials.* One might argue that treating everybody with broad antimicrobial antimicrobials will increase the likelihood that a patient will get better even without knowing the bacteria causing infection. However, counter to this argument is the principle of "Do no harm!" Broad antimicrobial coverage does increase the likelihood of empirically killing a causative pathogen; unfortunately, the development of

secondary infections can be caused by selection of antimicrobial-resistant nontargeted pathogens. In addition, adverse events are thought to complicate up to 10% of all antimicrobial therapy, and for select agents, the adverse-event rates are similar to high-risk medications such as warfarin, digoxin, or insulin.[1] Therefore, the overall goal of antimicrobial therapy should be to cure the patient's infection; limit harm by minimizing patient risk for adverse effects, including secondary infections; and limit societal risk from antimicrobial-resistant bacteria.

EPIDEMIOLOGY AND ETIOLOGY

Infectious disease–related illnesses, particularly respiratory tract infections, are among the most common reasons patients seek medical care.[2] Antimicrobial prescribing in the past has been associated with inappropriate use of antimicrobial agents. During the late 1990s/early 2000s, many organizations initiated campaigns to promote appropriate antimicrobial use. Recent trends in prescribing suggest a modest reduction in antimicrobial use for these infections, suggesting an increased recognition of the negative consequences of antimicrobial use.[4] Prescribing of antimicrobials in hospitalized patients is also common, as up to one-half of all patients receive at least one antimicrobial during hospitalization. In 2002, the estimated number of nosocomial infections was 1.8 million, with an estimated 99,000 deaths.[5] In 2009, the CDC reported 25,000 fewer central line–associated bloodstream infections than in 2001, a 58% reduction.[6] Nosocomial infections tend be associated with antimicrobial-resistant strains of bacteria. However, there has been a shift in the etiology of some community-acquired infections. Increasingly, infections caused by antimicrobial-resistant pathogens, traditionally nosocomial in origin, are being identified in ambulatory care settings. Reasons for this change include an aging populace, improvement in the management of chronic comorbid conditions including immunosuppressive conditions, and increases in outpatient management of more debilitated patients. The majority of infections caused by antimicrobial-resistant pathogens in the ambulatory care setting occur in patients who have had recent exposure to some aspect of the healthcare system and are therefore defined as healthcare–associated infections. The converging bacterial etiologies and increasing resistance in all healthcare environments emphasize the need to "make the diagnosis."

PATHOPHYSIOLOGY
Normal Flora and Endogenous Infection

Many areas of the human body are colonized with bacteria—this is known as *normal flora.* Infections often arise from one's own normal flora (also called an *endogenous infection*). Endogenous infection may occur when there are alterations in the normal flora (e.g., recent antimicrobial use may allow for overgrowth of other normal flora) or disruption of host defenses (e.g., a break or entry in the skin). Knowing what organisms reside where can help to guide empirical

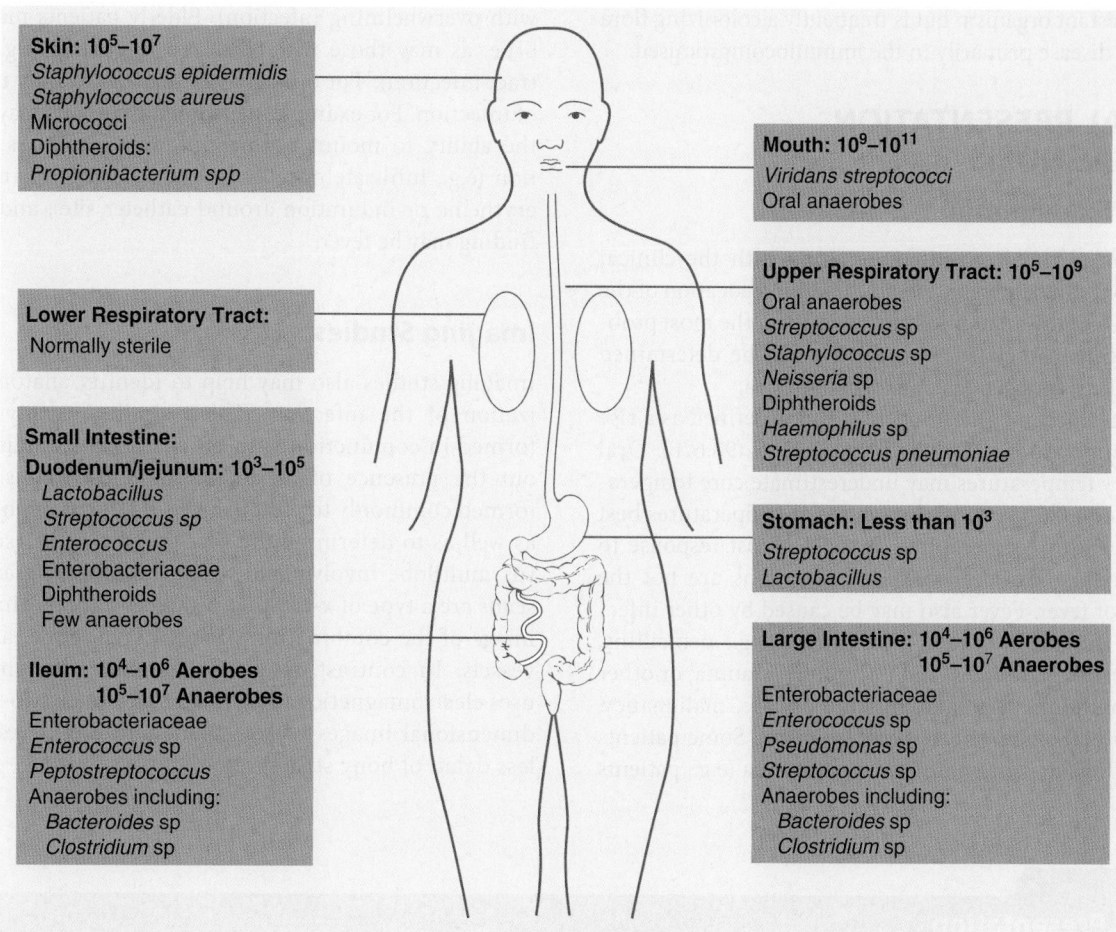

Skin: 10^5–10^7
Staphylococcus epidermidis
Staphylococcus aureus
Micrococci
Diphtheroids:
Propionibacterium spp

Mouth: 10^9–10^{11}
Viridans streptococci
Oral anaerobes

Upper Respiratory Tract: 10^5–10^9
Oral anaerobes
Streptococcus sp
Staphylococcus sp
Neisseria sp
Diphtheroids
Haemophilus sp
Streptococcus pneumoniae

Lower Respiratory Tract:
Normally sterile

Small Intestine:
Duodenum/jejunum: 10^3–10^5
Lactobacillus
Streptococcus sp
Enterococcus
Enterobacteriaceae
Diphtheroids
Few anaerobes

Stomach: Less than 10^3
Streptococcus sp
Lactobacillus

Ileum: 10^4–10^6 Aerobes
          10^5–10^7 Anaerobes
Enterobacteriaceae
Enterococcus sp
Peptostreptococcus
Anaerobes including:
  Bacteroides sp
  Clostridium sp

Large Intestine: 10^4–10^6 Aerobes
                   10^5–10^7 Anaerobes
Enterobacteriaceae
Enterococcus sp
Pseudomonas sp
Streptococcus sp
Anaerobes including:
  Bacteroides sp
  Clostridium sp

FIGURE 69–1. Normal flora and concentrations of bacteria (organisms per milliliter).

antimicrobial therapy (Fig. 69–1). In addition, it is beneficial to know what anatomic sites are normally sterile. These include the cerebrospinal fluid, blood, and urine.

Determining Colonization Versus Infection

Infection refers to the presence of bacteria that are causing disease (e.g., the organisms are found in normally sterile anatomic sites or in nonsterile sites with signs/symptoms of infection). *Colonization* refers to the presence of bacteria that are not causing disease. ❹ *Only bacteria that cause disease should be targeted with antimicrobial therapy, and non-disease-producing colonizing flora should be left intact.* It is important to differentiate infection from colonization because antimicrobial therapy targeting bacterial colonization is inappropriate and may lead to the development of resistant bacteria.

Exogenously Acquired Bacterial Infections

Infections acquired from an external source are referred to as *exogenous infections.* These infections may occur as a result of human-to-human transmission, contact with exogenous

bacterial populations in the environment, and animal contact. Resistant pathogens such as methicillin-resistant *Staphylococcus aureus* (MRSA) and vancomycin-resistant *Enterococcus* spp. (VRE) may colonize hospitalized patients or patients who access the healthcare system frequently. It is key to know which patients have acquired these organisms because patients generally become colonized prior to developing infection, and colonized patients should be placed in isolation (per infection-control policies) to minimize transmission to other patients.

Contrasting Bacterial Virulence and Resistance

Virulence refers to the pathogenicity or disease severity produced by an organism. Many bacteria may produce toxins or possess growth characteristics that contribute to their pathogenicity. Some virulence factors allow the organism to avoid the immune response of the host and cause significant disease. Virulence and resistance are different microbial characteristics. For example, *Streptococcus pyogenes,* a common cause of skin infections, produces toxins that can cause severe disease, yet it is very susceptible to penicillin. *Enterococcus faecium* is a highly resistant organism but is frequently a colonizing flora that causes disease primarily in the immunocompromised.

CLINICAL PRESENTATION AND DIAGNOSIS

Physical Examination

Findings on physical examination, along with the clinical presentation, can help to provide the anatomic location of the infection. Once the anatomic site is identified, the most probable pathogens associated with disease can be determined based on likely endogenous or exogenous flora.

Fever often accompanies infection and is defined as a rise in body temperature above the normal 37°C (98.6°F). Oral and axillary temperatures may underestimate core temperature by at least 0.6°C (1°F), whereas rectal temperatures best approximate core temperatures. Fever is a host response to bacterial toxins. However, bacterial infections are not the sole cause of fever. Fever also may be caused by other infections (e.g., fungal or viral), medications (e.g., penicillins, cephalosporins, salicylates, and phenytoin), trauma, or other medical conditions (e.g., autoimmune disease, malignancy, pulmonary embolism, and hyperthyroidism). Some patients with infections may present with hypothermia (e.g., patients with overwhelming infection). Elderly patients may be afebrile, as may those with localized infections (e.g., urinary tract infection).[7] For others, fever may be the only indication of infection. For example, neutropenic patients may not have the ability to mount normal immune responses to infection (e.g., infiltrate on chest x-ray, pyuria on urinalysis, or erythema or induration around catheter site), and the only finding may be fever.

Imaging Studies

Imaging studies also may help to identify anatomic localization of the infection. These studies usually are performed in conjunction with other tests to establish or rule out the presence of an infection. Radiographs are performed commonly to establish the diagnosis of pneumonia, as well as to determine the severity of disease (single versus multilobe involvement). Computed tomography (CT) scans are a type of x-ray that produces a three-dimensional image of the combination of soft tissue, bone, and blood vessels. In contrast, magnetic resonance imaging (MRI) uses electromagnetic radio waves to produce two- or three-dimensional images of soft tissue and blood vessels with less detail of bony structures.

Clinical Presentation

- Review of symptoms consistent with an infectious etiology?
- Signs and symptoms may be nonspecific (e.g., fever) or specific.
- Specific signs and symptoms are beyond the scope of this chapter (see disease state–specific chapters for these findings).

Patient History
- History of present illness
- Comorbidities
- Current medications
- Allergies
- Previous antibiotic exposure (may provide clues regarding colonization or infection with new specific pathogens or pathogens that may be resistant to certain antimicrobials)
- Previous hospitalization or healthcare utilization (also a key determinant in selecting therapy because the patient may be at risk for specific pathogens and/or resistant pathogens)
- Travel history
- Social history
- Pet/animal exposure

- Occupational exposure
- Environmental exposure

Physical Findings
- Findings consistent with an infectious etiology?
- Vital signs
- Body system abnormalities (e.g., rales, altered mental status, localized inflammation, erythema, warmth, edema, pain, and pus)

Diagnostic Imaging
- Radiographs (x-rays)
- CT scans
- MRI
- Labeled leukocyte scans

Nonmicrobiologic Laboratory Studies
- White blood cell count (WBC) with differential
- Erythrocyte sedimentation rate (ESR)
- C-reactive protein
- Procalcitonin

Microbiologic Studies
- Gram stain
- Culture and susceptibility testing

Nonmicrobiologic Laboratory Studies

Common nonmicrobiological laboratory tests include the white blood cell count (WBC) and differential, erythrocyte sedimentation rate (ESR), and determination of biomarkers C-reactive protein (CRP) or procalcitonin levels. In most cases, the WBC count is elevated in response to infection, but it may be decreased owing to overwhelming or long-standing infection. The differential is the percentage of each type of WBC (Table 69–1). In response to physiologic stress, neutrophils leave the bloodstream and enter the tissue to "fight" against the offending pathogens (i.e., leukocytosis). It is important to recognize that leukocytosis is nonspecific for infection and may temporarily occur in response to non-infectious conditions such as acute myocardial infarction. During an infection, immature neutrophils (e.g., bands) are released at an increased rate to help fight infection, leading to what is known as a bandemia or left shift. Therefore, a WBC count differential is key to determining whether an infection is present. Some patients may present with a normal total WBC with a left shift (e.g., the elderly). ESR and CRP are

Table 69–1

WBC and Differential

Type of Cell	Normal Value (% or Fraction)	Function	Abnormalities
Neutrophil	Segs 40–60 (0.40–0.60) Bands 3–5 (0.03–0.05)	Phagocytic	Leukocytosis • Bacterial infections • Fungal infections • Physiologic stress • Tissue injury (e.g., myocardial Infarction) • Medications (e.g., corticosteroids) Leukopenia • Long-standing infection • Cancer • Medications (e.g., chemotherapy)
Lymphocyte	20–40 (0.20–0.40)	T cells (cell-mediated immunity) B cells (humoral antibody response)	Lymphocytosis • Viral infections (e.g., mononucleosis) • Tuberculosis • Fungal infections Lymphopenia • HIV
Monocyte	2–8 (0.02–0.08)	Phagocytic Precursor to macrophage	Monocytosis • Tuberculosis • Protozoal infections • Leukemia
Eosinophil	1–4 (0.01–0.04)	Antigen-antibody reactions	Eosinophilia • Hypersensitivity reactions, including medications • Parasitic infections
Basophil	Less than 1 (0.01)		Hypersensitivity reactions

Patient Encounter 1

HPI: An 87-year-old woman with a history of hypertension, hyperlipidemia, atrial fibrillation, and recent cerebrovascular accident is transported from a nursing home facility to the emergency room. Nursing staff report a several day history of fatigue, anorexia, nausea, and increasing confusion. She awoke this morning with a fever of 38.1°C and shortness of breath. She received cephalexin 14 days ago for a lower extremity cellulitis.

PMH: Hypertension, hyperlipidemia, atrial fibrillation, cerebrovascular accident 2 months ago for which she was hospitalized for 10 days.

FH: Father died of pneumonia at age 68. Mother died of lung cancer at age 81.

SH: Lives in a nursing home. Has 3 daughters and 2 sons.

Allergies: Sulfa (rash).

Meds:

Lisinopril 10 mg daily

Simvastatin 20 mg daily

Metoprolol XL 50 mg daily

Warfarin 2.5 mg daily

Alendronate 70 mg weekly

Calcium carbonate 500 mg BID

Multivitamin 1 daily

What information in the history supports an infectious etiology?

Is this patient at risk for resistant pathogens? Why?

nonspecific markers of inflammation that increase as a result of the acute-phase reactant response, which is a response to inflammatory stimuli such as infection or tissue injury. These tests may be used as markers of infectious disease response because they are elevated when the disease is acutely active and usually fall in response to successful treatment. Clinicians may use these tests to monitor a patient's response to therapy in osteomyelitis and infective endocarditis. These tests should not be used to diagnose infection because they may be elevated in noninfectious inflammatory conditions (e.g., rheumatoid arthritis, polymyalgia rheumatica, and temporal arteritis). In contrast, procalcitonin, a prohormone of calcitonin, is rapidly produced in response to bacterial infection. Procalcitonin serum levels in conjunction with clinical findings are increasingly being utilized to assess both the need to initiate antibiotic therapy as well as determine when antibiotic therapy may be safely discontinued.

A full discussion of the role of procalcitonin in diagnosing and treating disease is beyond the scope of this chapter.[8,9]

Microbiologic Studies

Microbiologic studies that allow for direct examination of a specimen (e.g., sputum, blood, or urine) also may aid in a presumptive diagnosis and give an indication of the characteristics of the infecting organism. Generally, microbial cultures are obtained with a Gram stain of the cultured material.

A Gram stain of collected specimens can give rapid information that can be applied immediately to patient care. A Gram stain is performed to identify whether bacteria are present and to determine morphologic characteristics of bacteria (e.g., gram-positive or gram-negative or shape—cocci, bacilli). Certain specimens do not stain well or at all and must be identified by alternative staining techniques (*Mycoplasma* spp., *Legionella* spp., *Mycobacterium* spp.). Figure 69–2 identifies bacterial pathogens as classified by

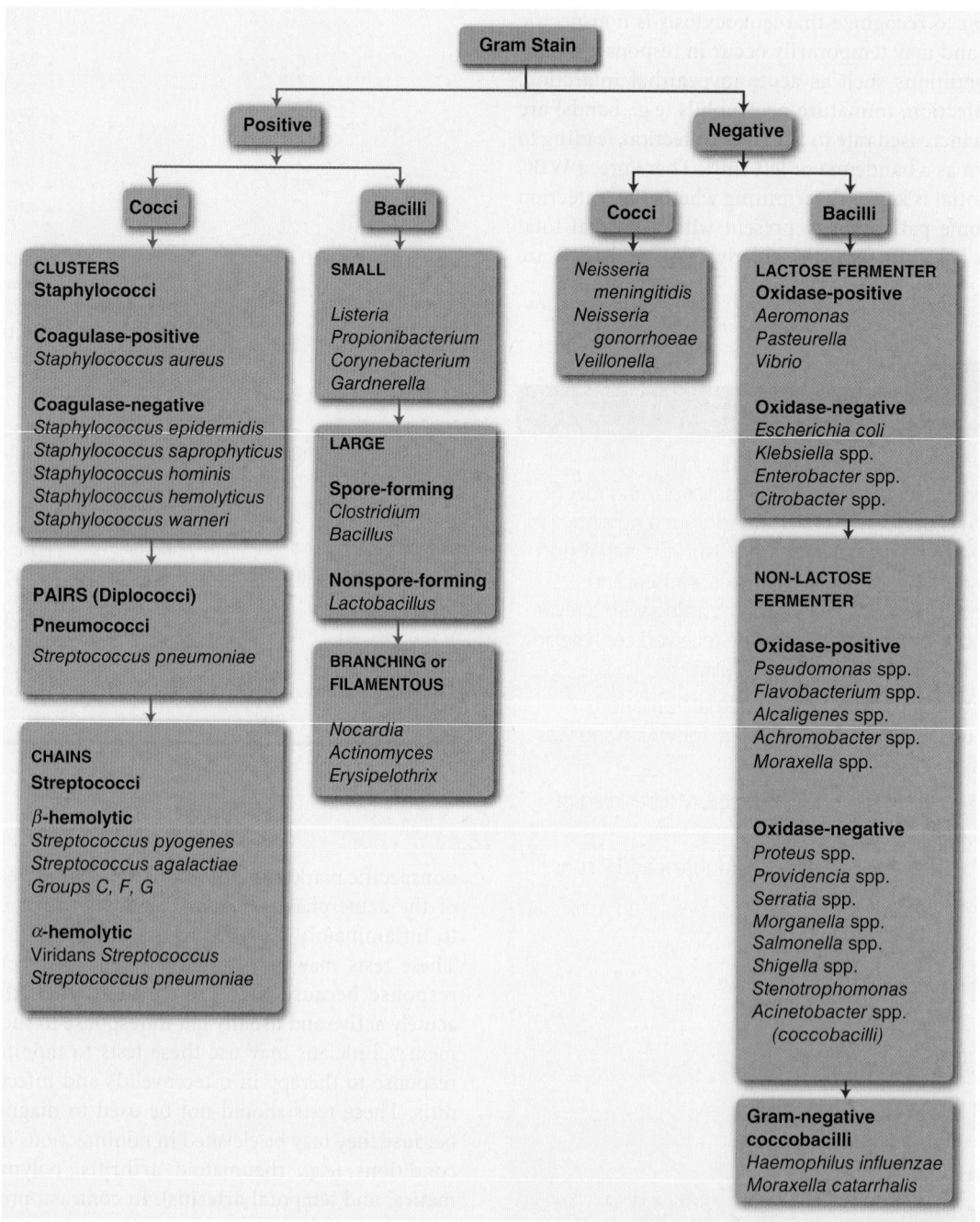

FIGURE 69–2. Important bacterial pathogens classified according to Gram stain and morphologic characteristics. (From Rybak MJ, Aeschlimann JR. Laboratory tests to direct antimicrobial pharmacotherapy. In: In DiPiro JT, Talbert RL, Yee GC, et al., eds. Pharmacotherapy: A Pathophysiologic Approach. 8th ed. New York: McGraw-Hill; 2011.)

Gram stain and morphologic characteristics. The presence of WBCs on a Gram stain indicates inflammation and suggests that the identified bacteria are pathogenic. The Gram stain may be useful in judging a sputum specimen's adequacy. For example, the presence of epithelial cells on sputum Gram stain suggests that the specimen is either poorly collected or contaminated. A poor specimen can give misleading information regarding the underlying pathogen and is a waste of laboratory personnel time and patient cost.

Culture and susceptibility testing provides additional information to the clinician to select appropriate therapy. Specimens are placed in or on culture media that provide the proper growth conditions. Once the bacteria grow on culture media, they can be identified through a variety of biochemical tests. Once a pathogen is identified, susceptibility tests can be performed to various antimicrobial agents. The *minimum inhibitory concentration* (MIC) is a standard susceptibility test. The MIC is the lowest concentration of antimicrobial that inhibits visible bacterial growth after approximately 24 hours (Fig. 69–3). Breakpoint and MIC values determine whether the organism is susceptible (S), intermediate (I), or resistant (R) to an antimicrobial. The *breakpoint* is the concentration of the antimicrobial that can be achieved in the serum after a normal or standard dose of that antimicrobial. If the MIC is below the breakpoint, the organism is considered to be susceptible to that agent. If the MIC is above the breakpoint, the organism is said to be resistant. Reported culture and susceptibility results may not provide MIC values but generally report the S, I, and R results.

5 *In general, bacterial cultures should be obtained prior to initiating antimicrobial therapy in patients with a systemic inflammatory response, risk factors for antimicrobial resistance, or infections where diagnosis or antimicrobial susceptibility is uncertain.* The decision to collect a specimen for culture depends on the sensitivity and specificity of the physical findings, diagnostic examination findings, and whether or not the pathogens are readily predictable. Culture and susceptibility testing usually is not warranted in a young, otherwise healthy woman who presents with signs and symptoms consistent with a urinary tract infection (UTI) because the primary pathogen, *Escherichia coli*, is readily predictable. Cultures and susceptibility testing are routine for sterile-site specimens (e.g., blood and spinal fluid), as well as for material presumed to be infected (e.g., material obtained from joints and abscesses). Cultures need to be interpreted with caution. Poor specimen collection technique and processing speed can result in misleading information and inappropriate use of antimicrobials.

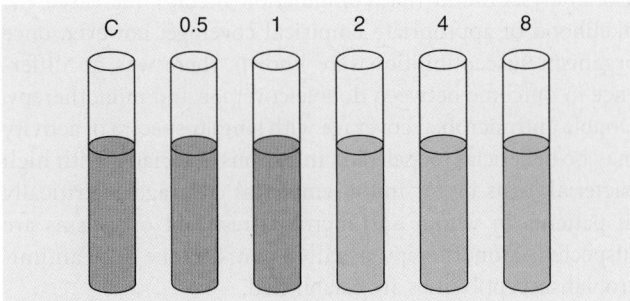

FIGURE 69–3. Macrotube minimal inhibitory concentration (MIC) determination. The growth control (C), 0.5 mg/L, and 1 mg/L tubes are visibly turgid, indicating bacterial growth. The MIC is read as the first clear test tube (2 mg/L). (From Rybak MJ, Aeschlimann JR. Laboratory tests to direct antimicrobial pharmacotherapy. In: In DiPiro JT, Talbert RL, Yee GC, et al., eds. Pharmacotherapy: A Pathophysiologic Approach. 8th ed. New York: McGraw-Hill; 2011.)

Patient Encounter 2: Review of Symptoms, Physical Examination, and Laboratory Data

ROS: Elderly woman who is confused and unable to answer questions. No reports of emesis or diarrhea but with decreased appetite per nursing staff.

PE:

- **VS:** BP 100/58 P 84, RR 30, T 38.5°C, O$_2$ sat 84% (0.84) on room air, Ht 5 ft 1 in (155 cm), Wt 50 kg
- **HEENT:** Dry mucous membranes
- **Chest:** Diminished breath sounds, rales, and rhonchi LLL
- **CV:** Tachycardic with irregularly irregular rhythm

Labs:

- WBC 17.6 × 10^3/mm^3 (17.6 × 10^9/L), segs 75% (0.75), bands 15% (0.15), lymphs 10% (0.10)
- SCr 2.1 mg/dL (186 μmol/L)
- Glucose 142 mg/dL (7.9 mmol/L)
- INR 3.5
- Procalcitonin 0.5 μg/L
- Sputum Gram stain: less than 10 epithelial cells/lpf, greater than 25 WBCs/lpf; gram-negative bacilli

Blood Cultures: Pending

What findings on physical examination are suggestive of an infectious process?

What laboratory findings and/or diagnostic studies have been performed to help establish the presence of an infection?

Are the findings of these laboratory and diagnostic studies suggestive of an infection?

What is your working diagnosis based on this patient encounter?

TREATMENT

General Approach to Treatment, Including Nonantimicrobial Treatment

While selection of antimicrobial therapy may be a major consideration in treating infectious diseases, it may not be the only therapeutic intervention. Other important therapies may include adequate hydration, ventilatory support, and other supportive medications. In addition, antimicrobials are unlikely to be effective if the process or source that leads to the infection is not controlled. *Source control* refers to this process and may involve removal of prosthetic materials such as catheters and infected tissue or drainage of an abscess. Source control considerations should be a fundamental component of any infectious diseases treatment. It is also important to recognize that there may be many different antimicrobial regimens that may cure the patient. While the following therapy sections provide factors to consider when selecting antimicrobial regimens, an excellent and more in-depth resource for selecting antimicrobial regimens for a variety of infectious diseases are the *Infectious Diseases Society of America Guidelines*.[10]

Antimicrobial Considerations in Selecting Therapy

⑥ *Drug-specific considerations in antimicrobial selection include spectrum of activity, effects on nontargeted microbial flora, appropriate dose, pharmacokinetic and pharmacodynamic properties, adverse-effect and drug-interaction profile, and cost* (**Table 69–2**).

▶ Spectrum of Activity and Effects on Nontargeted Flora

Most initial antimicrobial therapy is empirical because cultures usually have not had sufficient time to allow identification of a pathogen. ⑦ *Empirical therapy should be based on patient- and antimicrobial-specific factors such as the anatomic location of the infection, the likely pathogens associated with the presentation, the potential for adverse effects in a given patient, and the antimicrobial spectrum of activity.* Prompt initiation of appropriate therapy is paramount in hospitalized patients who are critically ill. Patients who receive initial antimicrobial therapy that provides coverage against the causative pathogen

---

Table 69–2

Considerations for Selecting Antimicrobial Regimens

Drug Specific	Patient Specific
Spectrum of activity and effects on nontargeted flora	Anatomic location of infection
	Antimicrobial history
Dosing	Drug allergy history
Pharmacokinetic properties	Renal and hepatic function
Pharmacodynamic properties	Concomitant medications
Adverse-effect potential	Pregnancy or lactation
Drug-interaction potential	Compliance potential
Cost	

---

survive at twice the rate of patients who do not receive adequate therapy initially.[11] Empirical selection of antimicrobial spectrum of activity should be related to the severity of the illness. Generally, acutely ill patients may require broader-spectrum antimicrobial coverage, whereas less ill patients may be managed initially with narrow-spectrum therapy. While a detailed description of antimicrobial pathogen-specific spectrum of activity is beyond the scope of this chapter, this information can be obtained readily from a number of sources.[12,13]

Collateral damage is defined as the development of resistance occurring in a patient's nontargeted antimicrobial flora that can cause secondary infections. Clostridium difficile infection (CDI) is an example of a disease that occurs secondary to collateral damage from antimicrobial therapy. Antibiotics can increase the risk of CDI by suppressing normal intestinal flora, resulting in overgrowth of the non-susceptible *C. difficile* bacteria. In addition, CDI is associated with the prior use of broad-spectrum antibiotics, particularly fluoroquinolones.[14] If several different antimicrobials possess activity against a targeted pathogen, the antimicrobial that is least likely to be associated with collateral damage may be preferred.

▶ Single Versus Combination Therapy

A common subject of debate involves the need to provide similar bacterial coverage with two antimicrobials for serious infections. Proponents state that double coverage may be synergistic, prevent the emergence of resistance, and improve outcome. However, there are few clinical examples in the literature to support these assertions. Examples where double coverage is considered superior are limited to infections associated with large bacterial inocula and in species that are known to readily develop resistance such as active tuberculosis or enterococcal endocarditis.[15,16] A study of patients with *Pseudomonas aeruginosa* infections, an intrinsically resistant organism, demonstrated that empirical double coverage with two antipseudomonal antimicrobials improved survival.[17] The analysis found that combination therapy increased the likelihood of appropriate empirical coverage; however, once organism susceptibilities were known, there was no difference in outcome between double coverage and monotherapy. Double antimicrobial coverage with similar spectra of activity may be beneficial for selected infections associated with high bacterial loads or for initial empirical coverage of critically ill patients in whom antimicrobial-resistant organisms are suspected. Monotherapy usually is satisfactory once antimicrobial susceptibilities are established.

▶ Antimicrobial Dose

Clinicians should be aware that dosage regimens with the same drug may be different depending on the infectious process. For example, ciprofloxacin, a fluoroquinolone, has various dosage regimens based on site of infection. The dosing for uncomplicated UTIs is 250 mg twice daily for 3 days. For complicated UTIs, the dose is 500 mg twice daily for 7 to 14 days. Severe complicated pneumonia requires a dosage regimen of

750 mg twice daily for 7 to 14 days. Clinicians are encouraged to use dosing regimens designed for treatment of the specific diagnosed infection because they have demonstrated proven efficacy and are most likely to minimize harm.

▶ Pharmacokinetic Properties

Pharmacokinetic properties of an antimicrobial may be important in antimicrobial regimens. *Pharmacokinetics* refers to a mathematical method of describing a patient's drug exposure in vivo in terms of absorption, distribution, metabolism, and elimination. *Bioavailability* refers to the amount of antimicrobial that is absorbed orally relative to an equivalent dose administered IV. Drug-related factors that may affect oral bioavailability include the salt formulation of the antimicrobial, the dosage form, and the stability of the drug in the gastrointestinal tract. Frequently, absorption may be affected by gastrointestinal tract blood flow. All patients that manifest systemic signs of infection such as hypotension or hypoperfusion should receive intravenous antimicrobials to ensure drug delivery. In almost all cases where patients have a functioning gastrointestinal tract and are not hypotensive, antimicrobials with almost complete bioavailability (greater than 80%) such as the fluoroquinolones, fluconazole, and linezolid may be given orally. With antimicrobials with modest bioavailability (e.g., many β-lactams), the decision to choose an oral product will depend more on the severity of the illness and the anatomic location of the infection. In sequestered infections, where higher systemic concentrations of antimicrobial may be necessary to reach the infected source (e.g., meningitis) or for antimicrobials with poor bioavailability, IV formulations should be used.

Several points regarding how the antimicrobial distributes into tissue are worth mentioning. First, only antimicrobials not bound to albumin are biologically active. Protein binding is likely clinically irrelevant in antimicrobials with low or intermediate protein binding. However, highly protein-bound antimicrobials (greater than 50%) also may not be able to penetrate sequestered compartments, such as cerebral spinal fluid, resulting in insufficient concentration to inhibit bacteria. Second, some drugs may not achieve sufficient concentrations in specific compartments based on distribution characteristics. For example, *Legionella pneumophila* is a nonenteric gram-negative organism that causes severe pneumonia. The organism is known to survive and reside inside pulmonary macrophages. Treatment with an antibiotic that works by inhibiting bacterial cell wall synthesis, such as a cephalosporin, will be ineffective because it only distributes into extracellular host tissues. However, macrolide or fluoroquinolone antimicrobials, which concentrate in human pulmonary macrophages, are highly effective against pneumonia caused by this organism.

Many antimicrobials undergo some degree of metabolism once ingested. Metabolism may occur via hepatic, renal, or non–organ-specific enzymatic processes. The route of elimination of the metabolic pathway may be exploited for infections associated with tissues related to the metabolic pathways. For example, many fluoroquinolone antimicrobials are metabolized only in part and undergo renal elimination.

Urinary concentrations of active drug are many times those achieved in the systemic circulation, making several of these agents good choices for complicated urinary tract infections.

▶ Pharmacodynamic Properties

Pharmacodynamics describes the relationship between drug exposure and pharmacologic effect of antibacterial activity or human toxicology. Antimicrobials generally are categorized based on their concentration-related effects on bacteria. Concentration-dependent pharmacodynamic activity occurs where higher drug concentrations are associated with greater rates and extents of bacterial killing. Concentration-dependent antimicrobial activity is maximized when peak antimicrobial concentrations are high. In contrast, *concentration-independent (or time-dependent) activity* refers to a minimal increase in the rate or extent of bacterial killing with an increase in antimicrobial dose. Concentration-independent antimicrobial activity is maximized when these antimicrobials are dosed to maintain blood and/or tissue concentrations above the MIC in a time-dependent manner. Fluoroquinolones, aminoglycosides, and metronidazole are examples of antimicrobials that exhibit concentration-dependent activity, whereas β-lactam and glycopeptide antimicrobials exhibit concentration-independent activity. Pharmacodynamic properties have been optimized to develop new dosing strategies for older antimicrobials. Examples include single-daily-dose aminoglycoside or β-lactam therapy administered by continuous or extended infusion. The product labeling for many new antimicrobials takes pharmacodynamic properties into account.

Antimicrobials also can be classified as possessing bactericidal or bacteriostatic activity in vitro. Bactericidal antibiotics generally kill at least 99.9% (3 log reduction) of a bacterial population, whereas bacteriostatic antibiotics possess antimicrobial activity but reduce bacterial load by less than 3 logs. Clinically, bactericidal antibiotics may be necessary to achieve success in infections such as endocarditis or meningitis. A full discussion of the application of antimicrobial pharmacodynamics is beyond the scope of this chapter, but excellent sources of information are available.[18]

▶ Adverse-Effect and Drug-Interaction Properties

A major concern when selecting antimicrobial regimens should be the propensity for the regimen to cause adverse effects and the potential for interaction with other drugs. Patients may possess characteristics or risk factors that increase their likelihood of developing an adverse event, emphasizing the need to obtain a good patient medical history. In general, if several different antimicrobial options are available, antimicrobials with a low propensity to cause specific adverse events should be selected, particularly for patients with risk factors for a particular complication. Risk factors for adverse events may include the coadministration of other drugs that are associated with a similar type of adverse event. For example, coadministration of the known nephrotoxin gentamicin with vancomycin increases the risk for nephrotoxicity compared with administration of either drug alone.[19] Other drug interactions may predispose the patient to dose-related toxicity through inhibition of drug metabolism. For example, erythromycin has the potential to prolong cardiac QT intervals in a dose-dependent manner, potentially increasing the risk for sudden cardiac death. A cohort study of patients taking oral erythromycin found that patients with concomitantly prescribed medications that inhibited the metabolism of erythromycin exhibited a fivefold increase in cardiac death versus controls.[20]

▶ Antimicrobial Cost

A final consideration in selecting antimicrobial therapy relates to cost. It is important to remember that the most inexpensive antimicrobial is not necessarily the most cost-effective antimicrobial. Antimicrobial costs constitute a relatively small portion of the overall cost of care. Frequently, regulatory studies are not designed to identify differences in hospital length of stay, less common adverse events, monitoring costs, collateral damage, or antimicrobial-specific resistance issues, all of which may contribute to medical costs. Careful consideration of antimicrobial microbiologic, pharmacologic, and patient-related factors such as compliance and a variety of clinical outcomes is necessary to establish the cost versus benefit of an antimicrobial in a given patient. If there is no difference or a small difference in these factors, the least costly antimicrobial may be the best choice.

Patient Considerations in Antimicrobial Selection

⑧ *Key patient-specific considerations in antimicrobial selection include recent previous antimicrobial exposures, identification of the anatomic location of infection through physical examination and diagnostic imaging, history of drug allergies, pregnancy or breast-feeding status, organ dysfunction that may affect drug clearance, immunosuppression, compliance, and the severity of illness (see Table 69–2).*

▶ Host Factors

Host factors can help to ensure selection of the most appropriate antimicrobial agent. Age is an important factor in antimicrobial selection. With regard to dose and interval, renal and hepatic function varies with age. Populations with diminished renal function include neonates and the elderly. Hepatic function in the neonate is not fully developed, and drugs that are metabolized or eliminated by this route may produce adverse effects. For example, sulfonamides and ceftriaxone may compete with bilirubin for binding sites and may result in hyperbilirubinemia and kernicterus. Gastric acidity also depends on age; the elderly and children younger than 3 years of age tend to be achlorhydric. Drugs that need an acidic environment (e.g., ketoconazole) are not well absorbed, and those whose absorption is enhanced in an alkaline environment will have increased concentrations (e.g., penicillin G).

Disruption of host defenses due to IV or indwelling Foley catheters, burns, trauma, surgery, and increased gastric pH

(secondary to antacids, H_2 blockers, and proton pump inhibitors) may place patients at higher risk for infection. Breaks in skin integrity provide a route for infection because the natural barrier of the skin is disrupted. Increased gastric pH can allow for bacterial overgrowth and has been associated with an increased risk of pneumonia.[21]

Recognizing the presumed site of infection and most common pathogens associated with the infectious source should guide antimicrobial choice, dose, and route of administration. For example, community-acquired pneumonia is caused most commonly by *S. pneumoniae*, *E. coli* is the primary cause of uncomplicated UTIs, and staphylococci and streptococci are implicated most frequently in skin and skin-structure infections (e.g., cellulitis).

Patients with a history of recent antimicrobial use may have altered normal flora or harbor resistant organisms. If a patient develops a new infection while on therapy, fails therapy, or has received antimicrobials recently, it is prudent to prescribe a different class of antimicrobial because resistance to the current treatment is likely. Previous hospitalization or healthcare utilization (e.g., residing in a nursing home, hemodialysis, and outpatient antimicrobial therapy) are risk factors for the acquisition of nosocomial pathogens, which are often resistant organisms.

Antimicrobial allergies are some of the most common drug-related allergies reported and have significant potential to cause adverse events. In particular, penicillin-related allergy is common and can be problematic because there is an approximately 4% cross-reactivity with cephalosporins as well as carbapenems.[22,23] In general, a patient's medical history should be reviewed to determine the offending β-lactam and nature of the allergic reaction. In some cases, patients with mild or nonimmunologic reactions may receive a β-lactam antimicrobial with low cross-reactive potential. However, patients with a history of physical findings consistent with IgE-mediated reactions such as anaphylaxis, urticaria, or bronchospasm should not be administered any type of β-lactam antimicrobial, including cephalosporins, unless there are no other alternatives, and even then they should be administered with caution. Administration of potentially cross-reactive agents in this situation should occur only under controlled conditions, and some patients may need to undergo desensitization. If the specific medical history relating to a reported allergy cannot be obtained, the patient should be assumed to have had an IgE-mediated reaction and should be managed in a similar manner. Monobactams (i.e., aztreonam) may be administered to patients with IgE-mediated allergic reactions to penicillin and are therefore an appropriate choice in these patients.

Renal and/or hepatic function should be considered in every patient prior to initiation of antimicrobial therapy. In general, most antimicrobials undergo renal elimination and exhibit decreased clearance with diminished renal function, and dosing adjustments are frequently necessary and recommendations for adjustment are available in the literature.[24] In contrast, dosing adjustments for antimicrobials that undergo nonrenal elimination are less well documented. Failure to adjust the antimicrobial dose or interval may result in drug accumulation and an increase in adverse effects.

Concomitant administration of other medications may influence the selection of the antimicrobial, dose, and monitoring. Medications that commonly interact with antibiotics include, but are not limited to, warfarin, rifampin, phenytoin, digoxin, theophylline, multivalent cations (e.g., calcium, magnesium, and zinc), and sucralfate. Drug interactions between antimicrobials and other medications may occur via the cytochrome P-450 system, protein-binding displacement, and alteration of vitamin K–producing bacteria. Interactions may result in increased concentrations of one or both agents, increasing the risk of adverse effects or additive toxicity. A key consideration in selecting antimicrobial regimens starts with obtaining a good patient medical and drug history, recognizing drug-specific adverse-event characteristics, and anticipating potential problems proactively. If it is necessary to use an antimicrobial with a relatively high frequency of adverse effects, informing patients of the risks and benefits of therapy, as well as what to do if an adverse effect occurs, may improve patient compliance and may facilitate patient safety.

Antimicrobial agents must be used with caution in pregnant and nursing women. Some agents pose potential threats to the fetus or infant (e.g., quinolones, tetracyclines, and sulfonamides). For some agents, avoidance during a specific trimester of pregnancy is warranted (e.g., the first trimester with trimethoprim/sulfamethoxazole). Pharmacokinetic variables also are altered during pregnancy. Both the clearance and volume of distribution are increased during pregnancy. As a result, increased dosages and/or more frequent administration of certain drugs may be required to achieve adequate concentrations. This information can be obtained from a number of sources.[25,26]

Adherence is essential to ensure efficacy of a particular agent. Patients may stop taking their antibiotics once the symptoms subside and save them for a "future" infection. If the patient does not complete the course of therapy, the infection may not be eradicated, and resistance may emerge. Self-medication of saved antibiotics may be harmful, leading to overtreatment, which may further contribute to antibiotic resistant. Poor patient adherence may be due to adverse effects, tolerability, cost, and lack of patient education.

OUTCOME EVALUATION

Figure 69–4 provides an overview of patient- and antimicrobial agent–specific factors to consider when selecting an antimicrobial regimen. It further delineates monitoring of therapy and actions to take depending on the patient's response to therapy. The duration of therapy depends on patient response and type of infection being treated.

Modifying Empirical Therapy Based on Cultures and Clinical Response

If a successful clinical response occurs and culture results are available, therapy should be de-escalated. Antibiotic *de-escalation* generally refers to the discontinuation of antibiotics that are providing a spectrum of activity greater than necessary to treat the infection, discontinuation of duplicative spectrum antibiotics, or switching to a narrower spectrum antibiotic once a patient is clinically stable. De-escalation of empirical therapy may also include discontinuing antibiotics based on clinical criteria and negative culture results, such as the absence of antibiotic-resistant pathogens.[27] The purpose of de-escalation therapy is to minimize the likelihood of secondary infections owing to antimicrobial-resistant organisms. In cases in which a specific organism is recovered that has a known preferred agent of choice, therapy might be changed to that specific agent. For example, antistaphylococcal penicillins are considered to be the agents of choice for methicillin-susceptible *S. aureus* owing to their bactericidal activity and narrow-spectrum activity and may be preferable to other antibiotic regimens. In other cases, empirical coverage might be discontinued if a specific suspected pathogen is excluded by culture or an alternative, noninfectious diagnosis is established. In addition, IV antimicrobials frequently are more expensive than oral therapy. Therefore, it is usually desirable to convert therapy to oral antimicrobials with a comparable antimicrobial spectrum or specific pathogen sensitivity as soon as the patient improves clinically.[28]

Failure of Antimicrobial Therapy

While many infections respond readily to antimicrobials, some infections do not. A relatively common question when a patient's condition fails to improve relates to whether the antimicrobial therapy has failed. Changing antimicrobials generally is one of the easiest interventions relative to other options. However, it is important to remember that antimicrobial therapy comprises only a portion of the overall disease treatment, and there may be many factors that contribute to a lack of improvement. ❿ *In general, inadequate diagnosis resulting in poor initial antimicrobial or other nonantibiotic drug selection, poor source control, or the development of a new infection with a resistant organism are relatively common causes of antimicrobial failure.* An infection-related diagnosis may be difficult to establish and generally has two components: (a) differentiating infection from noninfection-related disease and (b) providing adequate empirical spectrum of activity if

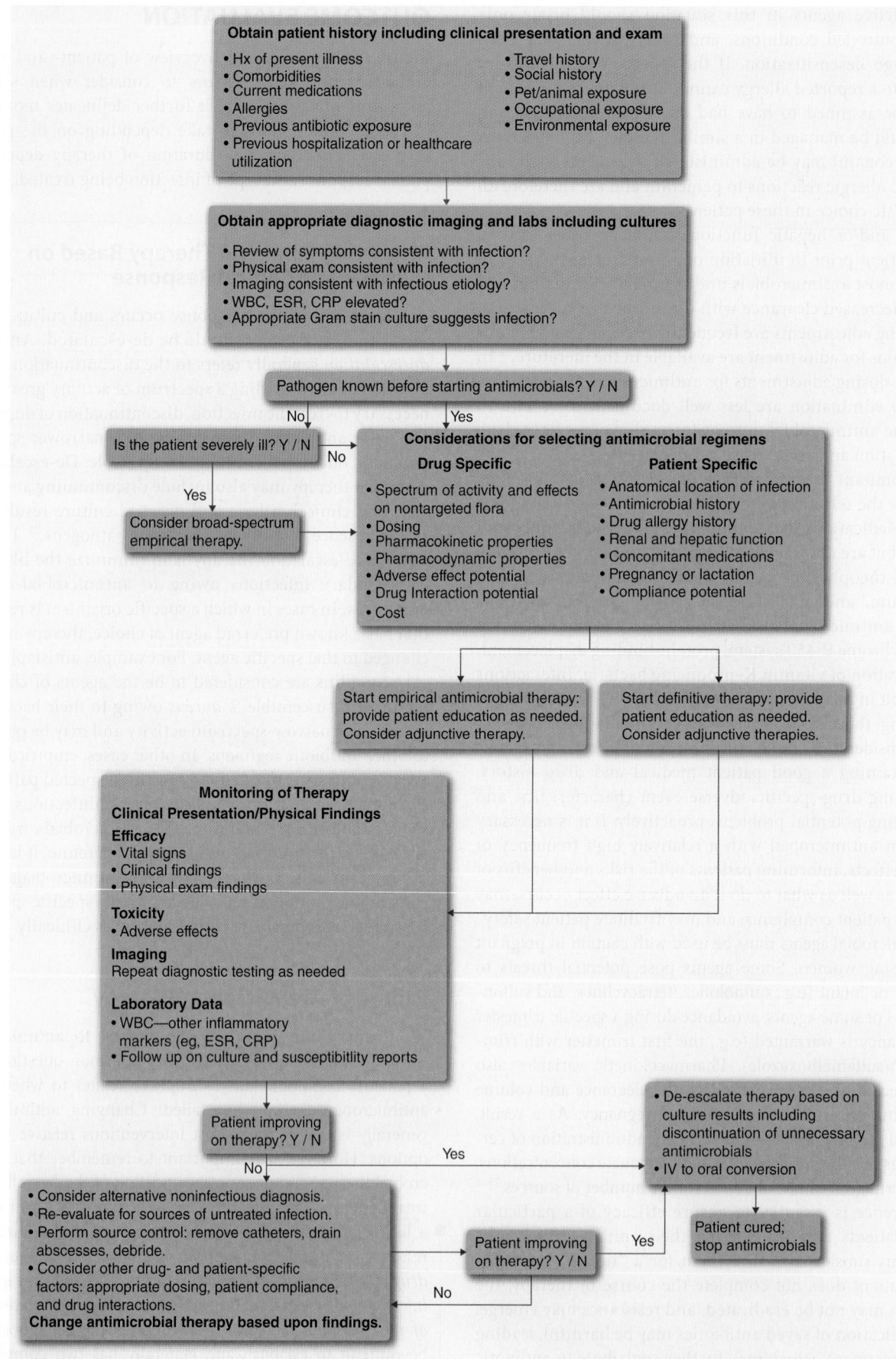

FIGURE 69-4. Approach to selection of antimicrobial therapy.

Patient Encounter 4: Patient Care and Monitoring

Update: The patient was admitted to the hospital with a presumptive diagnosis of healthcare-associated pneumonia. She received IV hydration with normal saline, 4 L oxygen, and empirical antibiotic therapy with cefepime, levofloxacin, and vancomycin.

After 48 hours of therapy, the following parameters are obtained:

PE:

- VS: BP 120/72, P 70, RR 22, T 37.9°C (100.2°F), O_2 sat 92% (0.92) on 2 L
- Repeat CXR: Infiltrate unchanged

Labs:

- WBC $11.2 \times 10^3/mm^3$ ($11.2 \times 10^9/L$)
- SCr 1.5 mg/dL (133 μmol/L)
- Glucose 116 mg/dL (6.4 mmol/L)
- Blood cultures × 2: Negative
- Sputum culture: *Klebsiella pneumoniae*

Sensitivity Report:

Cefepime sensitive (MIC = 1 mg/L)

Ceftazidime sensitive (MIC = 2 mg/L)

Ceftriaxone sensitive (MIC = 1 mg/L)

Piperacillin/taz sensitive (MIC = 8 mg/L)

Meropenem resistant (MIC greater than 64 mg/L)

Gentamicin sensitive (MIC = 0.5 mg/L)

Amikacin sensitive (MIC = 0.5 mg/L)

Ciprofloxacin resistant (MIC greater than 4 mg/L)

What information suggests improvement in the patient's condition?

Do any of the antimicrobial doses need to be adjusted for changes in organ function?

Should antimicrobial therapy be modified based on the culture results?

Can the antimicrobial therapy be converted from IV to oral therapy?

---

of secondary infections. In this case, the patient generally improves, but then develops a new infection caused by an antimicrobial-resistant pathogen and relapses. The emergence of resistance to a targeted pathogen while on antimicrobial therapy can be associated with clinical failure but usually is limited to tuberculosis, pseudomonads, or other gram-negative enterics. Drug- and patient-specific factors such as appropriate dosing, patient compliance, and drug interactions can be associated with therapeutic failure and also should be

Patient Care and Monitoring

After selection and initiation of antimicrobial regimen, there are a number of additional patient care and monitoring considerations that should be addressed to improve the likelihood of a successful outcome. ❾ *Patient education, de-escalation of antimicrobial therapy based on culture results, monitoring for clinical response and adverse effects, and appropriate duration of therapy are important.*

Patient Education

Provide patient education with regard to appropriate use of antimicrobials (e.g., dose, interval), adverse effects, and drug interactions (which may play a role in therapy failure and increased toxicity).

Therapeutic Monitoring

Monitor for therapeutic response by assessing efficacy and toxicity of the antimicrobial regimen.

- Clinical presentation/physical findings
- *Efficacy:* Assess vital signs (monitor for return to normal or lack of altered findings; e.g., fever), physical examination findings, patient's subjective impression
- *Toxicity:* Monitor and assess for adverse effects and evaluate antimicrobial serum concentrations when appropriate to minimize toxicity and improve outcomes
- *Diagnostic imaging:* Diagnostic testing is disease state–dependent
- Laboratory data
- Monitor and assess laboratory data: WBC with differential (goal is a reduction in WBC if elevated initially and resolution of left shift), renal and/or hepatic function (consider need for dosage adjustments), other labs as indicated (e.g., ESR, CRP)
- Follow up on culture and susceptibility reports with subsequent de-escalation of therapy, if possible
- Reculture of specimens is not performed routinely except in few cases (e.g., endocarditis) or where a secondary infection is suspected because data may be misleading and lead to the addition of broader or more powerful antimicrobials

---

the cause is infectious. Failure of improvement in a patient's condition should warrant broadening the differential diagnosis to include noninfection-related causes, as well as considering other potential infectious sources and/or pathogenic organisms. Another common cause of failure is poor source control. A diagnostic search for unknown sources of infection and removal of indwelling devices in the infected environment or surgical drainage of abscesses should be undertaken if the patient's condition is not improving. Less common but still frequent causes of therapeutic failure include the development

considered. A common assumption is that the correct diagnosis was made, but the patient was not treated long enough with antimicrobials. There are certain types of infections (e.g., endocarditis or osteomyelitis) where the standard of care is to treat for prolonged periods of time (i.e., weeks or months). However, the optimal duration of therapy for many infectious diseases is somewhat subjective. Recently, studies of several infectious processes have suggested that shorter durations of therapy can result in similar clinical outcomes as longer durations of therapy, frequently with fewer complications or secondary infections.[29-31] The general trend has been to treat these disease processes with shortened courses of antibiotic therapy. In this period of extensive antimicrobial resistance, clinicians should keep abreast of changing recommendations emphasizing shorter durations of therapy.

CONCLUSION

Antimicrobial regimen selection is a complex process involving the integration of a multitude of factors. The guiding principles to make the diagnosis and do no harm must be considered when choosing an antimicrobial for a given patient. In summary, when infection is suspected, rapid and accurate diagnosis should be followed by early intervention that includes administration of appropriately dosed antibiotics with appropriate empirical spectra. De-escalation to suitable narrow-spectrum antibiotics if susceptibilities are known should occur as soon as possible, and therapy should be stopped as soon as the patient is cured. These fundamental actions improve infectious disease outcomes and minimize collateral damage and adverse effects.

Abbreviations Introduced in This Chapter

CDC	Centers for Disease Control and Prevention
CRP	C-reactive protein
ESR	Erythrocyte sedimentation rate
HPI	History of present illness
MIC	Minimum inhibitory concentration
MRSA	Methicillin-resistant *Staphylococcus aureus*
PMH	Past medical history
UTI	Urinary tract infection
VRE	Vancomycin-resistant *Enterococcus*
WBC	White blood cell count

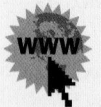 Self-assessment questions and answers are available at http://mhpharmacotherapy. com/pp.html.

REFERENCES

1. Shehab N, Patel PR, Srinivasan A, Budnitz DS. Emergency department visits for antibiotic-associated adverse events. Clin Infect Dis 2008;47:735–743.

2. Chow AC, Benninger MS, Brook I, et al. IDSA clinical practice guideline for acute bacterial rhinosinusitis in children and adults. Clin Infect Dis 2012;54(8):e72–e112.

3. Centers for Disease Control and Prevention. Get Smart Campaign. www.cdc.gov/getsmart.

4. Vanderweil SG, Pelletier AJ, Hamedani AG, Gonzales R, Metlay JP, Camargo CA Jr. Declining antibiotic prescriptions for upper respiratory infections, 1993–2004. Acad Emerg Med 2007;14:366–369.

5. Klevens RM, Edwards JR, Richards CL, et al. Estimating healthcare-associated infections and deaths in U.S. hospitals, 2002. Public Health Rep 2007;122:160–166.

6. Centers for Disease Control. Vital Signs: Central line associated blood stream infections—United States 2001, 2008, and 2009. MMWR March 4, 2011;60(8):243–248. www.cdc.gov/mmwr/preview/mmwrhtml/mm6008a4.htm.

7. Mackowiak PA. Temperature regulation and the pathogenesis of fever. In: Mandell GL, Bennett JE, Dolin R. Mandell, Douglas, Bennett's, eds. Principles and Practice of Infectious Diseases. 5th ed. Philadelphia, PA: Churchill Livingstone; 2000:604–620.

8. Simon L, Gauvin F, Amre DK, Saint-Louis P, Lacroix J. Serum calcitonin and C-reactive protein levels as markers of bacterial infection: a systematic review and meta-analysis. Clin Infect Dis 2004;39:206-217.

9. Agarwal R, Schwartz DN. Procalcitonin to guide duration of antimicrobial therapy in intensive care units: a systematic review. Clin Infect Dis 2011;53(4):379-387.

10. Infectious Diseases Society of America. Practice Guidelines from the Infectious Diseases Society of America [online]. [cited 2011 Oct 10]. Available from: www.idsociety.org/IDSA-Practice_Guidelines.

11. Kollef MH, Sherman G, Ward S, Fraser VJ. Inadequate antimicrobial treatment of infections: A risk factor for hospital mortality among critically ill patients. Chest 1999;115:462-474.

12. Antimicrobial spectra. In: Gilbert DN, Moellering RC, Eliopoulos GM, Sande MA, eds. The Sanford Guide to Antimicrobial Therapy. 41st ed. Sperryville, VA: Antimicrobial Inc; 2011.

13. John Hopkins University Division of Infectious Diseases. Antibiotic Guide [online]. [cited 2011 Oct 10]. Available from: *http://www.hopkins-abxguide.org.*

14. Cohen SH, Gerding DN, Johnson S, et al. Clinical Practice Guidelines for Clostridium difficile Infection in Adults: 2010n Update by the Society for Healthcare Epidemiology of America (SHEA) and the Infectious Diseases Society of America (IDSA). Infect Control Hosp Epidemiol 2010;31(5):431–455.

15. Peloquin CA. Tuberculosis. In: DiPiro JT, Talbert RL, Yee GC, et al., eds. Pharmacotherapy: A Pathophysiological Approach. 6th ed. New York: McGraw-Hill; 2005:2015–2334.

16. Baddour LM, Wilson WR, Bayer AS, et al. Infective endocarditis: diagnosis, antimicrobial therapy, and management of complications: a statement for healthcare professionals from the Committee on Rheumatic Fever, Endocarditis, and Kawasaki Disease, Council on Cardiovascular Disease in the Young, and the Councils on Clinical Cardiology, Stroke, and Cardiovascular Surgery and Anesthesia, American Heart Association: endorsed by the Infectious Diseases Society of America. Circulation 2005;111:394–434.

17. Chamot E, Boffi E, Amari E, et al. Effectiveness of combination antimicrobial therapy for Pseudomonas aeruginosa bacteremia. Antimicrob Agents Chemother 2003;47:2756–2764.

18. Craig WA. Pharmacodynamics of antimicrobials. In: Nightingale CH, Murakawa T, Ambrose PG, eds. Antimicrobial Pharmacodynamics in Theory and Clinical Practice. 1st ed. New York: Marcel Dekker; 2002:1–22.

19. Rybak MJ. The pharmacokinetic and pharmacodynamic properties of vancomycin. Clin Infect Dis 2006;42(Suppl 1):S35–S39.

20. Ray WA, Murray KT, Meredith S, et al. Oral erythromycin and the risk of sudden death from cardiac causes. N Engl J Med 2004;351:1089–1096.

21. Laheij RJ, Sturkenboom MC, Hassing R, et al. Risk of community-acquired pneumonia and use of gastric acid-suppressing drugs. JAMA 2004;292:1955–1960.

22. Gruchalla RS, Pirmohamed M. Clinical practice. Antibiotic allergy. N Engl J Med 2006;354:601–609.

23. Weiss ME, AdkinsonNF. β-lactam allergy. In: Mandell GL, Bennett JE, Dolin R, eds. Principles and Practice of Infectious Diseases. 7th ed. Philadelphia, PA: Churchill Livingstone; 2009:347–354.

24. Frye RF, Matzke GR. Drug therapy individualization for patients with renal insufficiency. In: DiPiro JT, Talbert RL, Yee GC, et al., eds. Pharmacotherapy: A Pathophysiological Approach. 6th ed. New York: McGraw-Hill; 2005:919–933.

25. Briggs GG, Freeman RK, Yaffe SJ. Drugs in Pregnancy and Lactation. 7th ed. Philadelphia, PA: Lippincott Williams & Wilkins; 2005.

26. Hale TW. Medications and Mothers' Milk. 11th ed. Amarillo, TX: Pharmasoft; 2004.

27. Dellit TH, Owens RC, McGowan JE, et al. Infectious Diseases Society of America and the Society for Healthcare Epidemiology of America Guidelines for Developing an Institutional Program to Enhance Antimicrobial Stewardship. Clin Infect Dis 2007;44(2):159–177.

28. Press RA. The use of fluoroquinolones as antiinfective transition-therapy agents in community-acquired pneumonia. Pharmacotherapy 2001;21(7 pt 2):S100–S104.

29. Goff DA. Short-duration therapy for respiratory tract infections. Ann Pharmacother 2004;38(Suppl 9):S19–S23.

30. Chastre J, Wolff M, Fagon JY, et al. For the PneumA Trial Group. Comparison of 8 vs 15 days of antibiotic therapy for ventilator-associated pneumonia in adults: A randomized trial. JAMA 2003;290:2588–2598.

31. Kollef MH, Napolitano LM, Solomkin JS, et al. Healthcare-associated infection (HAI): A critical appraisal of the emerging threat-proceedings of the HAI Summit. Clin Infect Dis 2008;2(Suppl 47):S55–S99.

70 Central Nervous System Infections

P. Brandon Bookstaver and April D. Miller

LEARNING OBJECTIVES

● **Upon completion of the chapter, the reader will be able to:**

1. Discuss the pathophysiology of CNS infections and the impact on antimicrobial treatment regimens (e.g., antimicrobial dosing and CNS penetration).

2. Describe the signs, symptoms, and clinical presentation of CNS infections.

3. List the most common pathogens causing CNS infections and identify risk factors for infection with each pathogen.

4. State the goals of therapy for CNS infections.

5. Design appropriate empirical antimicrobial regimens for patients suspected of having CNS infections caused by each of the following pathogens (taking age, vaccine history, and other patient-specific information into account), and analyze the impact of antimicrobial resistance on both empirical and definitive therapy: *Neisseria meningitidis* meningitis, meningitis, *Haemophilus influenzae* meningitis, *Listeria monocytogenes* meningitis, group B *Streptococcus* meningitis, gram-negative bacillary meningitis, postneurosurgical infection, CNS shunt infection, herpes simplex encephalitis.

6. Modify empirical antimicrobial regimens based on laboratory data and other diagnostic criteria.

7. Discuss the management of close contacts of patients diagnosed with CNS infections.

8. Identify candidates for vaccines and other prophylactic therapies to prevent CNS infections.

9. Describe the role of adjunctive agents (e.g., dexamethasone) in the management of CNS infections.

10. Formulate a monitoring plan to assess efficacy and adverse effects of therapy for CNS infections.

KEY CONCEPTS

❶ Meningitis is a neurologic emergency that requires prompt recognition, diagnosis, and management to prevent death and residual neurologic defects. Patients with fever, headache, and neck stiffness should be evaluated for meningitis.

❷ Ideally, lumbar puncture (LP) to obtain cerebrospinal fluid (CSF) for direct examination and laboratory analysis, as well as blood cultures and other relevant cultures, should be obtained before initiation of antimicrobial therapy. However, initiation of antimicrobial therapy should not be delayed if a pretreatment LP cannot be performed.

❸ The treatment goals for CNS infections are to prevent death and residual neurologic deficits, eradicate or control causative microorganisms, ameliorate clinical signs and symptoms, and identify measures (e.g., vaccination and suppressive therapy) to prevent future infections.

❹ Prompt initiation of IV high-dose bactericidal antimicrobial therapy directed at the most likely pathogen(s) is essential due to the high morbidity and mortality associated with CNS infections.

❺ IV antimicrobial therapy is administered for the full course of therapy for CNS infections to ensure adequate CSF penetration throughout the course of treatment.

❻ Empirical antimicrobial therapy should be directed at the most likely pathogen(s) for a specific patient, taking into account age, risk factors for infection (including underlying disease and immune dysfunction, vaccine history, and recent exposures), CSF Gram stain results, CSF antibiotic penetration, and local antimicrobial resistance patterns.

❼ Empirical antimicrobial therapy should be modified on the basis of laboratory data and clinical response.

❽ Close contacts of patients with CNS infections should be evaluated for possible antimicrobial prophylaxis.

❾ Components of a monitoring plan to assess the efficacy and safety of antimicrobial therapy of CNS infections include clinical signs and symptoms and laboratory data (e.g., CSF findings, culture, and sensitivity data).

The term *CNS infections* describes a variety of infections involving the brain and spinal cord and associated tissues, fluids, and membranes, including meningitis, encephalitis, brain abscess, shunt infections, and postoperative infections (see Glossary). ❶ *CNS infections, such as meningitis, are considered neurologic emergencies that require prompt recognition, diagnosis, and management to prevent death and residual neurologic deficits.* Improperly treated, CNS infections are associated with high rates of morbidity and mortality. Despite advances in care, the overall mortality of bacterial meningitis in the United States remains at approximately 15%, and at least 10% to 30% of survivors are afflicted with neurologic impairment, including hearing loss, hemiparesis, and learning disabilities.[1-4] Antimicrobial therapy and preventive vaccines have revolutionized management and improved outcomes of bacterial meningitis and other CNS infections dramatically.

EPIDEMIOLOGY AND ETIOLOGY

CNS infections are uncommon, and rates of bacterial meningitis are declining, with an incidence of two cases per 100,000 in 1998 and 1999 down to 1.38 cases per 100,000 in 2006 and 2007.[3] Increased rates of vaccination appear to prevent four to six cases of meningitis reported per 100,000 adults annually.[5] However, the severity of these infections demands prompt medical intervention and treatment. CNS infections can be caused by bacteria, fungi, mycobacteria, viruses, parasites, and spirochetes.

Bacterial meningitis is the most common cause of CNS infections. *Streptococcus pneumoniae* (pneumococcus) was the most common pathogen for bacterial meningitis (0.8 to 1.09 cases/100,000), followed by *Neisseria meningitidis* (meningococcus, 0.19 to 0.44 cases/100,000), group B *Streptococcus* (0.21 to 0.3 cases/100,000), *Haemophilus influenzae* (0.08 to 0.12 cases/100,000), and *Listeria monocytogenes* (0.03 to 0.1 cases/100,000).[3,5] Vaccines directed against bacteria causing meningitis and related infections (e.g., pneumonia and ear infections) have reduced the risk of infections due to *S. pneumoniae*, *N. meningitidis*, and *H. influenzae* type b (Hib) dramatically. Prior to the availability of Hib conjugate vaccines, Hib meningitis or other invasive disease was documented in one in 200 children by the age of 5 years.[6] Widespread use of the Hib vaccine has reduced the incidence of invasive Hib disease by 99% and has reduced the incidence of Hib meningitis in children by 35%.[1,3,7] The routine use of the 7-valent conjugate pneumococcal vaccine (PCV7) in children has reduced the incidence of pneumococcal meningitis from PCV7 serotypes from 3.37 cases per 100,000 in 1998 and 1999 to 0.07 cases per 100,000 in 2006 and 2007 in children under the age of 5 years. In addition, cases of PCV7 serotype

pneumococcal meningitis in adults aged 65 years or more declined between the same time periods from 0.77 to 0.11 cases per 100,000.[3] Despite use of the PCV7, *S. pneumoniae* remains the most common pathogen for pediatric bacterial meningitis, with nearly 50% of cases due to nonvaccine serotypes.[3,9] From 2003 to 2007, PCV13 serotypes, reflecting a new 13-valent vaccine licensed for use in 2010, accounted for 57.2% and 41.6% of meningitis cases in children and adults, compared with only 15.5% and 16.0% accounted for by PCV7 serotypes, respectively.[3] Introduction of the PCV13 vaccine may have a significant impact on the epidemiology of pneumococcal meningitis in the future.

● Encephalitis may result from viral, bacterial, parasitic, and other noninfectious causes. Herpes simplex virus (HSV) is the most common cause of encephalitis in the United States, accounting for 10% of all cases.[10] The annual incidence of viral encephalitis is 3.5 to 7.4 infections per 100,000 persons.[10] Other pathogens include common bacterial meningitis causes, *Ricksettsia* species, enteroviruses, arboviruses, varicella-zoster virus, rotavirus, coronavirus, influenza viruses A and B, West Nile virus, and Epstein-Barr virus may be associated with a meningo-encephalopathic presentation.[11] Approximately 20,000 hospitalizations each year are secondary to encephalitis, accounting for $650 million in healthcare costs.[12] Over the past 10 to 20 years, mortality secondary to encephalitis has remained constant, correlating well with the increased number of people living with human immunodeficiency virus (HIV) and acquired immune deficiency syndrome (AIDS). HIV infection is concurrent in nearly 20% of patients dying from encephalitis.[13]

Neurosurgical procedures may place patients at risk for meningitis due to bacteria (e.g., *Staphylococcus aureus*, coagulase-negative staphylococci, and gram-negative bacilli) acquired at the time of surgery or in the postoperative period. In addition to bacteria, other pathogens may cause meningitis in at-risk patients. Immunocompromised patients, such as solid-organ transplant patients and patients living with HIV infection, are at risk for fungal meningitis with *Cryptococcus neoformans* and encephalitis secondary to *Toxoplasma gondii* and JC virus (see Chap. 84). Tuberculosis can spread from pulmonary sites to cause clinical disease in the CNS. Life-threatening viral encephalitis and meningitis can occur in otherwise healthy, young individuals, as well as in patients immunocompromised by age or other factors. Because the treatments for different types of CNS infections are often different, it is important to pay close attention to patients' risk factors when choosing empirical antimicrobial therapy. Patients at extremes of age, those living in close contact with others, and those with immune defects are most susceptible to meningitis. Risk factors for CNS infections can be classified as follows:

- *Environmental*—recent exposures (e.g., close contact with meningitis or respiratory tract infection, contaminated foods), active or passive exposure to cigarette smoke, close living conditions

- *Recent infection in the patient*—respiratory infection, otitis media, sinusitis, mastoiditis

Table 70–1

Most Likely Pathogens and Recommended Empirical Therapy, by Risk Factor, for Bacterial Meningitis

Predisposing Factor	Most Likely Pathogens	Recommended Empirical Antibiotic Therapy
Age		
Less than 3 months	Group B *Streptococcus* *Escherichia coli* *Klebsiella pneumoniae* *Listeria monocytogenes*	Ampicillin *plus* cefotaxime *or* aminoglycoside
3 months to less than 18 years	*Streptococcus pneumoniae* *Neisseria meningitidis* *Haemophilus influenzae*	Cefotaxime *or* ceftriaxone *plus* vancomycin
18 years to less than 60 years	*S. pneumoniae* *N. meningitidis*	Cefotaxime *or* ceftriaxone *plus* vancomycin
60 years *or* older	*S. pneumoniae* Gram-negative bacilli *L. monocytogenes*	Cefotaxime *or* ceftriaxone *plus* vancomycin *plus* ampicillin
Immunocompromised	*S. pneumoniae* *N. meningitidis* *L. monocytogenes* Gram-negative bacilli (including *Pseudomonas aeruginosa*)	Cefotaxime *or* ceftriaxone *plus* vancomycin *plus* ampicillin (consider double antibiotic coverage against *Pseudomonas* spp. if suspected)
Surgery, Trauma		
Postneurosurgical infection	*S. aureus* (including MRSA) Coagulase-negative *Staphylococcus* (including MRSE) Gram-negative bacilli (including *P. aeruginosa*)	Vancomycin *or* linezolid *plus* ceftazidime *or* cefepime *or* meropenem (consider double antibiotic coverage against *Pseudomonas* spp. if suspected)
Penetrating head trauma	*S. aureus* (including MRSA) coagulase-negative *Staphylococcus* Gram-negative bacilli (including *P. aeruginosa*)	Vancomycin *or* linezolid *plus* ceftazidime *or* cefepime *or* meropenem (consider double antibiotic coverage against *Pseudomonas* spp. if suspected)
CSF shunt	Coagulase-negative *Staphylococcus* (including MRSE) *S. aureus* (including MRSA) Gram-negative bacilli (including *P. aeruginosa*)	Vancomycin *or* linezolid *plus* ceftazidime *or* cefepime *or* meropenem (consider double antibiotic coverage against *Pseudomonas* spp. if suspected)

MRSA, methicillin-resistant *Staphylococcus aureus*; MRSE, methicillin-resistant *Staphylococcus epidermidis*.

From Refs. 15 and 25.

Patient Encounter 1, Part 1

NB is a 67-year-old woman resident of an elderly singles assisted living facility. She maintains her activities of daily living on her own. NB participates in group activities with co-residents on a weekly basis, with the most recent being a wine and cheese party about 1 week ago. She now presents to the emergency department with a 2-day history of headache, fever, and photophobia. Physical findings and laboratory values include temperature of 38.3°C (101°F) and WBC of $13.4 \times 10^3/mm^3$ ($13.4 \times 10^9/L$), with 70% (0.70) polymorphonuclear cells. Examination reveals nuchal rigidity; remainder is benign for additional findings. NB also reports occasional nausea. She has a significant history for osteoporosis for which she takes alendronate and calcium with vitamin D. She receives the influenza vaccine yearly.

What signs and symptoms consistent with meningitis are present in NB?

What causative pathogens should be suspected in NB?

What empiric antimicrobials should be started?

- *Immunosuppression*—anatomic or functional asplenia, sickle cell disease, alcoholism, cirrhosis, immunoglobulin or complement deficiency, cancer, HIV/AIDS, uncontrolled diabetes mellitus, debilitated state of health
- *Surgery, trauma*—neurosurgery, head trauma, CSF shunt, cochlear implant
- Noninfectious causes of meningitis include malignancy, medications (e.g., sulfonamides, nonsteroidal anti-inflammatory drugs [NSAIDs], IV immunoglobulin), autoimmune disease (e.g., lupus), and trauma.[9,10]
- The most common pathogens causing bacterial meningitis, by age group and other risk factors, are found in Table 70–1.

PATHOPHYSIOLOGY

Meningitis is an inflammation of the membranes of the brain and spinal cord (meninges) and the CSF in contact with these membranes, whereas encephalitis is an inflammation of the brain tissue. CSF flows through the subarachnoid space, insulating and protecting delicate CNS tissue. CSF is produced within the ventricles of the brain and flows downward through the spinal cord, serving as a continuous flushing mechanism for the CNS.

The blood–brain barrier and blood–CSF barrier are made of specialized tissue capillaries that isolate the brain from substances circulating in the bloodstream or colonizing nearby tissues. To initiate a CNS infection, pathogens must gain entry into the CNS by **contiguous** spread, **hematogenous** seeding, direct inoculation, or reactivation of latent infection. **Contiguous** spread occurs when infections in adjacent structures (e.g., sinus cavities or the middle ear) invade directly through the blood–brain barrier (e.g., Hib). **Hematogenous** seeding occurs when a more remote infection causes bacteremia that seeds the CSF (e.g., pneumococcal pneumonia). Reactivation of latent infection results from dormant viral, fungal, or mycobacterial pathogens in the spine, brain, or nerve tracts. Direct inoculation of bacteria into the CNS is the result of trauma, congenital malformations, or complications of neurosurgery.

Once through the blood–brain barrier, pathogens thrive and replicate due to limited host defenses in the CNS. **Figure 70–1** depicts the pathophysiologic changes associated with meningitis. Neurologic tissue damage is the result of the host's immune reaction to bacterial cellular components (e.g., lipopolysaccharide, teichoic acid, and peptidoglycan), which triggers **cytokine** production, particularly tumor necrosis factor alpha (TNF-α) and interleukin 1 (IL-1), as well as other mediators of inflammation.[15] Bacteriolysis resulting from antibiotic therapy further contributes to the inflammatory process. **Cytokines** increase permeability of the blood–brain barrier,

allowing influx of neutrophils and other host defense cells that contribute to the development of cerebral edema and increased intracranial pressure characteristic of meningitis.[16] The increase in intracranial pressure is responsible for the hallmark clinical signs and symptoms of meningitis: headache, neck stiffness, altered mental status, photophobia, and seizures. Unaltered, these pathophysiologic changes may result in cerebral ischemia and death.

The CNS response to infection is evident by demonstrable changes in the CSF. ❷ *Ideally, LP to obtain CSF for direct examination and laboratory analysis, as well as blood cultures and other relevant cultures, should be obtained before initiation of antimicrobial therapy. However, initiation of antimicrobial therapy should not be delayed if a pretreatment LP cannot be performed.*

Normal CSF has a characteristic composition in terms of protein and glucose content, as well as cell count. **Table 70–2** lists CSF findings observed in the absence of infection, as well as in patients with bacterial, viral, fungal, and tuberculous meningitis.

CLINICAL PRESENTATION AND DIAGNOSIS

A high index of suspicion should be maintained for patients at risk for CNS infections. Prompt recognition and diagnosis are essential so that antimicrobial therapy can be initiated as quickly as possible. A medical history (including risk factors for infection and history of possible recent exposures) and

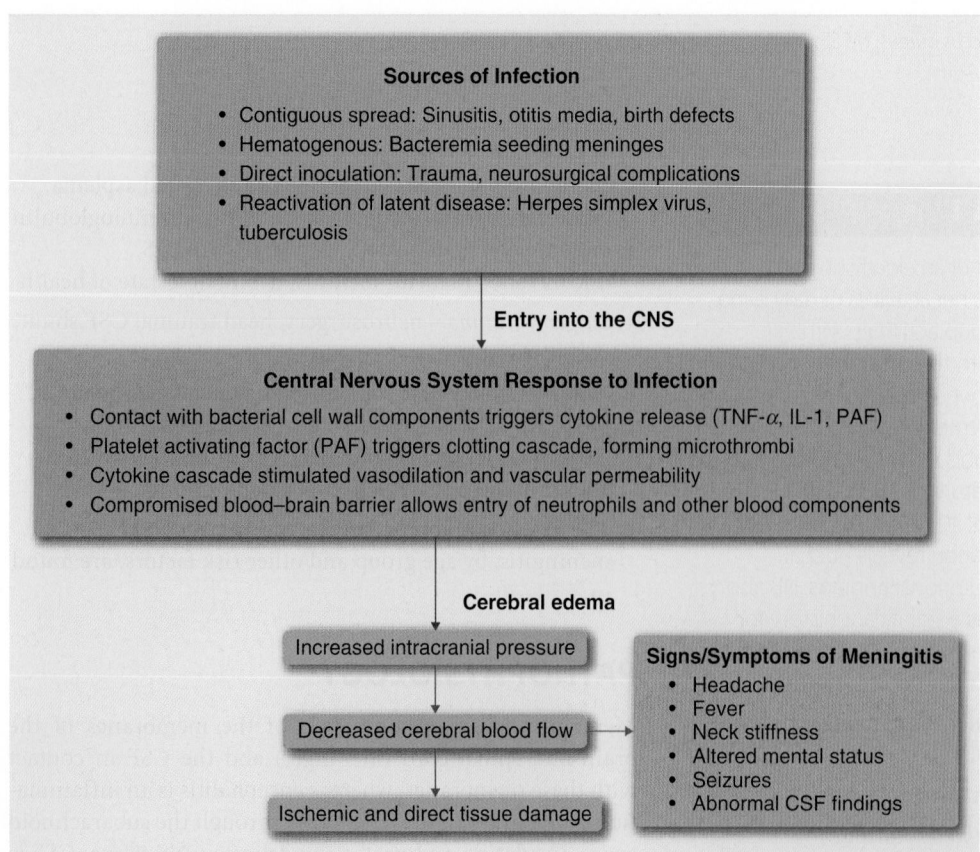

FIGURE 70–1.

Pathophysiology of bacterial meningitis.

Table 70–2

CNS Response to Infection (CSF Findings)

	Normal CSF	Bacterial Infection	Viral Infection	Fungal Infection	Tuberculosis
WBC ($\times 10^3$/mm³ *or* $\times 10^9$/L)	Less than 0.005	1.0–greater than 5.0	0.1–1	0.1–0.4	50–500
WBC differential (% or fraction in brackets, predominant cell type)	Greater than 85% (0.85) monocytes	At least 80% (0.80) PMNs	50% (0.50) lymphocytes (PMN early)	Greater than 50% (0.50) lymphocytes	Greater than 80% (0.80) lymphocytes (PMNs early)
Protein (mg/dL, mg/L)	20–45 (200–450)	Greater than 100 (greater than 1,000)	50–100 (500–1,000)	100–200 (1,000–2,000)	40–150 (400–1,500)
Glucose (mg/dL, mmol/L)	45–80 (2.5–4.4)	5–40 (0.3–2.2)	30–70 (1.7–3.9)	Less than 30–70 (less than 1.7–3.9)	Less than 30–70 (less than 1.7–3.9)
CSF: serum glucose ratio	At least 0.6 serum glucose	Less than 0.4 serum glucose	At least 0.6 serum glucose	Less than 0.4 serum glucose	Less than 0.4 serum glucose
CSF stain	Negative	Positive Gram stain (60–90%)	Negative	Positive India ink stain (Cryptococcus)	Positive acid-fast bacilli stain
Opening pressure	Less than 20 mm Hg	Greater than 20 mm Hg	Less than 20 mm Hg	Greater than 20 mm Hg	Greater than 20 mm Hg

CSF, cerebrospinal fluid; PMNs, polymorphonuclear neutrophils.

From Refs. 5, 11, 20, and 33.

Clinical Presentation and Diagnosis of CNS Infections

General
- Evaluate patient risk factors and recent exposures
- Evaluate other possible causes: space-occupying lesion (which may *or* may not be malignant), drug-induced CNS pathology autoimmune disease, and trauma[12,13]

Signs and Symptoms[2]
- 95% of patients with bacterial meningitis have two of the following: headache, fever, neck stiffness, and altered mental status
- Headache (87%)
- Nuchal rigidity (stiff neck) (83%)
- Fever (77%)
- Nausea (74%)
- Altered mental status (i.e., confusion, lethargy, and obtundation) (69%)
- Focal neurologic defects (including positive Brudzinski's sign and Kernig's sign) (33%)
- Seizures
- Malaise, restlessness
- Photophobia
- Skin lesions (diffuse petechial rash observed in 50% of patients with meningococcal meningitis)
- Signs and symptoms in neonates, infants, and young children: nonspecific findings, such as altered feeding and sleep patterns, vomiting, irritability, lethargy, bulging fontanel, seizures, respiratory distress, and petechial/purpuric rash[17]
- Predictors of an unfavorable outcome: seizures, focal neurologic findings, altered mental status, papilledema, hypotension, septic shock, and pneumococcal meningitis[4]

Laboratory Tests[5,18,19]
- CSF examination via lumbar puncture (LP, spinal tap); contraindicated in patients with cardiorespiratory compromise, increased intracranial pressure and papilledema, focal neurologic signs, seizures, bleeding disorders, abnormal level of consciousness, and possible brain herniation (a CT scan should be performed before LP if there is a question of a CNS mass to avoid potential for brain herniation) (see Table 70–2 for specific CSF findings)
- Elevated opening pressure (may be decreased in neonates, infants, and children)
- Cloudy CSF
- Decreased glucose
- Elevated protein
- Elevated WBC (differential provides clues to offending pathogen)
- Gram stain (adequate for diagnosis in 60% to 90% of patients with bacterial meningitis)
- Culture and sensitivity (positive in 70% to 85% without prior antibiotic therapy, positive in less than 20% who have had prior therapy)
- If CSF Gram stain and/or culture is negative, rapid diagnostic tests (such as latex agglutination) may be useful; these tests are positive even if bacteria are dead
- Polymerase chain reaction (PCR; DNA amplification of the most common bacterial meningitis pathogens) may be useful to help exclude bacterial meningitis
- Elevated CSF lactate and C-reactive protein
- Blood cultures (at least two cultures, one "set"; positive in 66%)
- Scraping of skin lesions (e.g., rash) for direct microscopic examination and culture
- Other cultures should be obtained as clinically indicated (e.g., sputum)
- WBC with differential
- Fungal meningitis: CSF culture, CSF and serum cryptococcal antigen titers, microscopic examination of CSF specimens
- Tuberculous meningitis: CSF culture, PCR evaluation (preferred), and acid-fast stain

physical examination yield important information to help guide the diagnosis and treatment of meningitis. Common signs and symptoms include fever, headache, nuchal rigidity (stiff neck), and photophobia. As common meningeal signs are not typically present in infants, nonspecific signs and symptoms including excessive irritability or crying, vomiting or diarrhea, tachypnea, altered sleep pattern, and poor eating should be noted. Depending on involved pathogens and disease severity, patients may also present with altered mental status, stupor, and seizures.

TREATMENT

Goals of Therapy

The introduction of antibiotic therapy and vaccines has reduced dramatically the mortality associated with bacterial meningitis.[20] Prior to these advances, bacterial meningitis was almost universally fatal, and those few patients who survived often suffered from debilitating residual neurologic deficits, such as permanent hearing loss. Although significant improvements have been made, the fatality rate of meningitis remains above 15% in adults, likely due to its occurrence in debilitated patient populations.

❸ *The treatment goals for CNS infections are to prevent death and residual neurologic deficits, eradicate or control causative micro-organisms, ameliorate clinical signs and symptoms, and identify measures to prevent future infections (e.g., vaccination and suppressive therapy).* These goals should be accomplished with minimal adverse drug reactions and interactions. Surgical debridement should be employed, if appropriate (as in postneurosurgical infections and brain abscess). Supportive care, consisting of hydration, electrolyte replacement, antipyretics, antiemetics, analgesics, antiepileptic drugs,

and wound care (for surgical wounds), is an important adjunct to antimicrobial therapy, particularly early in the treatment course.

Treatment Principles

❹ *Prompt initiation of IV high-dose bactericidal antimicrobial therapy directed at the most likely pathogen(s) is essential due to the high morbidity and mortality associated with CNS infections.* Although there are no prospective studies that relate timing of antibiotic administration to clinical outcome in bacterial meningitis, a longer duration of symptoms and more advanced disease before treatment initiation increase the risk of a poor outcome.[4,18,21] Initiation of antibiotic therapy as soon as possible after bacterial meningitis is suspected or proven (even before hospitalization) reduces mortality and neurologic sequelae, as long as antibiotics were started before patients deteriorate to a score of 10 on the Glasgow Coma Scale.[22,23] Rapid sterilization of CSF is important; delayed CSF sterilization after approximately 24 hours of antibiotic therapy increases the risk of neurologic sequelae, including moderate to profound hearing loss.[24,25]

Meningitis occurs in a tissue with limited host defenses. Bacterial replication occurs rapidly in the absence of complement and specific antibodies directed toward common bacterial pathogens.[26] High-dose parenteral bactericidal antibiotic therapy is required to treat meningitis effectively. Data from animal studies and patients demonstrate better outcomes when bactericidal antibiotic therapy (versus bacteriostatic therapy) is used to sterilize the CSF.[27] However, successful treatment of meningitis has been reported with bacteriostatic agents. High doses of parenteral therapy are required to achieve CSF antibiotic concentrations adequate to rapidly sterilize the CSF and reduce the risk of complications. The presence of infection in the CSF reduces the activity of some classes of antibiotics. For example, the decreased pH of CSF associated with meningitis significantly reduces the activity of aminoglycoside antibiotics.[28]

Antimicrobial pharmacokinetics and pharmacodynamics must be considered when designing treatment regimens for CNS infections. Ability of antibiotics to reach and achieve effective concentrations at the infection site is the key to treatment success. In experimental models of meningitis, maximum bactericidal activity is achieved when CSF concentrations exceed the minimum bactericidal concentration (MBC) of the infecting pathogen by 10- to 30-fold.[17] In general, low-molecular-weight lipophilic antibiotics that are unionized at physiologic pH and not highly protein bound penetrate best into CSF and other body tissues and fluids.[26,28] In addition to drug characteristics, integrity of the blood–brain barrier determines antibiotic penetration into CSF. The CSF penetration of most, but not all, antibiotics is enhanced by the presence of infection and inflammation. Sulfonamides, trimethoprim, chloramphenicol, rifampin, and most antitubercular drugs achieve therapeutic CSF levels even without meningeal inflammation.[10] Most β-lactams and related antibiotics (i.e., carbapenems and monobactams), vancomycin, quinolones, acyclovir, linezolid, daptomycin, and colistin achieve therapeutic CSF levels in the presence of meningeal inflammation.[11] Aminoglycosides, first-generation cephalosporins, second-generation cephalosporins (except cefuroxime), clindamycin, and amphotericin do not achieve therapeutic CSF levels, even with inflammation, but clindamycin does achieve therapeutic brain tissue levels.[11]

An adequate duration of therapy is required to treat meningitis successfully (Table 70–3). ⑤ *Parenteral (IV) therapy is administered for the full course of therapy for CNS infections to ensure adequate CSF penetration throughout the course of treatment.* Antibiotic treatment (and dexamethasone, if used as a treatment adjunct) reduces the inflammation associated with meningitis, which, in turn, reduces the penetration of some antibiotics into the CSF. To ensure adequate antibiotic concentrations throughout the treatment course, parenteral administration is continued for the full treatment course. Carefully selected patients who have close medical monitoring and follow-up may be able to receive a portion of their parenteral meningitis treatment on an outpatient basis.[18,29] A management algorithm for adults with suspected bacterial meningitis, as recommended by the Infectious Diseases Society of America (IDSA), is summarized in Figure 70–2.

Empirical Antimicrobial Therapy

After expeditious workup (i.e., evaluation of risk factors, clinical signs and symptoms, and laboratory data) and diagnosis, prompt and aggressive antimicrobial therapy is initiated. Appropriate empirical treatment is of the utmost importance in patients with suspected CNS infections. In most patients, a diagnostic LP will be performed before beginning antibiotics, but this never should delay initiation of antimicrobials. Antibiotic pretreatment may alter the CSF profile and complicate interpretation. ⑥ *Empirical therapy should be directed at the most likely pathogen(s) for a specific patient, taking into account age, risk factors for infection (including underlying disease and immune dysfunction, vaccine history, and recent exposures), CSF Gram stain results, CSF antibiotic penetration, and local antimicrobial resistance patterns.* Results of the CSF Gram stain may be used to help narrow empirical therapy for bacterial meningitis. In the absence of a positive Gram stain, empirical therapy should be continued for at least 48 to 72 hours, when meningitis may, in most cases, be ruled out by CSF findings inconsistent with bacterial meningitis, negative CSF culture, and negative polymerase chain reaction (PCR) evaluations. A repeat LP may be useful in the absence of other findings. Table 70–1 outlines recommendations for empirical antibiotic therapy for bacterial meningitis by most likely pathogen(s) and patient risk factors.

Impact of Antimicrobial Resistance on Treatment Regimens for Meningitis

Development of resistance to β-lactam antibiotics, including penicillins and cephalosporins, has significantly impacted the management of bacterial meningitis. Approximately 17% of U.S. pneumococcal CSF isolates are resistant to penicillin, and 3.5% of CSF isolates are resistant to cephalosporins.[30] The Clinical and Laboratory Standards Institute (CLSI) has set a lower ceftriaxone susceptibility breakpoint for pneumococcal CSF isolates (1 mg/L) than for isolates from non-CNS sites (2 mg/L). Increasing pneumococcal resistance to penicillin G has changed empirical treatment regimens to the combination of a third-generation cephalosporin plus vancomycin. Recognition of relative and high-level resistance to *N. meningitidis* in the laboratory, as well as in clinical treatment failures, has led to greater use of third-generation cephalosporins for empirical therapy of meningococcal meningitis.[21] Traditionally, ampicillin was the cornerstone of treatment for *H. influenzae* meningitis. Now, treatment of suspected or proven β-lactamase-mediated Hib meningitis requires a third-generation cephalosporin. Increasing rates of methicillin-resistant *S. aureus* (about one-third of staphylococcal CSF isolates) and coagulase-negative staphylococci require the use of vancomycin for empirical therapy when these pathogens are suspected.[29] As previously mentioned, hospitalized patients, especially those residing in an intensive care unit, are at risk for developing meningitis secondary to gram-negative pathogens. The emergence and continued rise of multidrug resistant strains of gram-negative organisms such as *Pseudomonas aeruginosa*, *Acinetobacter* species, AmpC, and extended spectrum β-lactamase (ESBL) producing strains of Enterobacteriaceae have become a recognized threat nationally. Global and local resistance patterns should be taken into account and combined with optimized pharmacodynamic dosing strategies when designing empirical treatment regimens for bacterial meningitis.

Pathogen-Directed Antimicrobial Therapy

⑦ *Empirical antimicrobial therapy should be modified on the basis of laboratory data and clinical response.* If cultures or other diagnostics, such as CSF Gram stain or bacterial antigen or antibody tests, indicate a specific pathogen, therapy should be adjusted quickly as needed to ensure adequate

---

Table 70–3

Pathogen-Based Definitive Treatment for CNS Infections

Pathogen	Recommended and Alternative Antimicrobial Therapy (Adult Doses)	Adverse Effects/Safety Monitoring	Renal and Hepatic Dose Adjustment	Duration (Days)
Neisseria meningitidis Penicillin MIC 0.1 mg/L	*Standard Therapy* Penicillin G 4 million units IV every 4 hours or	Hypersensitivity (rash, anaphylaxis), diarrhea	*Renal*: CrCl less than 50 mL/min (0.83 mL/s): 3 million units IV every 4 hours; CrCl less than 10 mL/min (0.17 mL/s): 2 million units IV every 4 hours *Hepatic*: No dose adjustment	7
	Ampicillin 2 g IV every 4 hours	Hypersensitivity (rash, anaphylaxis), diarrhea	*Renal*: CrCl less than 50 mL/min (0.83 mL/s): 2 g IV every 8 hours; CrCl less than 30 mL/min (0.50 mL/s): 2 g IV every 12 hours; CrCl less than 10 mL/min (0.17 mL/s): 2 g IV every 24 hours *Hepatic*: No dose adjustment	
	Alternative Therapies Ceftriaxone 2 g IV every 12 hours or	LFT elevation, cholecystitis	*Renal*: No dose adjustment *Hepatic:* Caution in severe hepatic impairment	
	Cefotaxime 2 g IV every 4 hours	Pseudocholelithiasis	*Renal*: CrCl less than 80 mL/min (1.34 mL/s): 2 g IV every 6–8 hours; CrCl less than 50 mL/min (0.83 mL/s): 2 g IV every 8–12 hours; CrCl less than 30 mL/min (0.50 mL/s): 2 g IV every 12 hours; CrCl less than 10 mL/min (0.17 mL/s): 2 g IV every 24 hours *Hepatic:* No dose adjustment	
Penicillin MIC 0.1–1 mg/L	*Standard Therapy* Ceftriaxone or cefotaxime			
	Alternative Therapies Moxifloxacin 400 mg IV every 24 hours or	Nausea/vomiting/diarrhea, dizziness, headache, QT prolongation	*Renal*: No dose adjustment *Hepatic*: Caution in severe hepatic impairment	
	Meropenem 2 g IV every 8 hours or	Rash, hypersensitivity, diarrhea, decreased seizure threshold	*Renal*: CrCl less than 50 mL/min (0.87 mL/s): 2 g IV every 12 hours; CrCl less than 30 mL/min (0.50 mL/s): 500 mg to 1 g IV every 12 hours; CrCl less than 10 mL/min (0.17 mL/s): 500 mg to 1 g IV every 24 hours *Hepatic*: No dose adjustment	
	Chloramphenicol 1–1.5 g IV every 6 hours	Rash, diarrhea, seizures, anemia, gray baby syndrome, hypersensitivity, neurotoxicity (last choice due to toxicities)	*Renal*: No dose adjustment *Hepatic*: Reduce dose in moderate to severe impairment; consider serum drug monitoring	
Streptococcus pneumoniae Penicillin MIC 0.1 mg/L	*Standard Therapy* Penicillin G or ampicillin *Alternative Therapies* Ceftriaxone or cefotaxime or chloramphenicol			10–14

(Continued)

Table 70–3

Pathogen-Based Definitive Treatment for CNS Infections (*Continued*)

Pathogen	Recommended and Alternative Antimicrobial Therapy (Adult Doses)	Adverse Effects/Safety Monitoring	Renal and Hepatic Dose Adjustment	Duration (Days)
Penicillin MIC 0.1–1 mg/L (ceftriaxone/cefotaxime-sensitive strains)	*Standard Therapy* Ceftriaxone *or* cefotaxime *Alternative Therapies* Cefepime 2 g IV every 8 hours *or* meropenem	Hypersensitivity (rash, anaphylaxis), decreased seizure threshold	*Renal:* CrCl less than 50 mL/min (0.83 mL/s): 2 g IV every 12–24 hours; CrCl less than 30 mL/min (0.50 mL/s): 1–2 g IV every 24 hours *Hepatic:* No dose adjustment	
Penicillin MIC 2 mg/L *or* greater	*Standard Therapy* Vancomycin 15 mg/kg IV every 8–12 hours (with dosing based on serum levels) plus ceftriaxone *or* cefotaxime *Alternative Therapies* Moxifloxacin	Vancomycin: rash, red man's syndrome (if infused too quickly) nephrotoxicity, thrombocytopenia	*Renal:* CrCl less than 50 mL/min (0.83 mL/s): dosing every 24 hours; CrCl less than 20 mL/min (0.33 mL/s): dosing based on serum concentrations; all dose adjustments should be made based on serum concentrations *Hepatic:* No dose adjustment	
Cefotaxime/ceftriaxone MIC at least 1 mg/L	*Standard Therapy* Vancomycin *plus* ceftriaxone *or* cefotaxime *Alternative Therapies* Moxifloxacin			
H. influenzae β-Lactamase-negative	*Standard Therapy* Ampicillin *Alternative Therapies* Ceftriaxone *or* cefotaxime *or* cefepime *or* moxifloxacin *or* chloramphenicol			7
β-Lactamase-positive	*Standard Therapy* Ceftriaxone *or* cefotaxime *Alternative Therapies* Cefepime *or* moxifloxacin *or* chloramphenicol			
Listeria monocytogenes	*Standard Therapy* Ampicillin *or* penicillin G *plus* gentamicin (5 mg/kg/day, dosing based on serum levels) *Alternative Therapies* Trimethoprim-sulfamethoxazole (10–20 mg/kg trimethoprim) IV per day in divided doses every 6–8 hours *or* meropenem	Gentamicin: nephrotoxicity, ototoxicity Trimethoprim-sulfamethoxazole: rash, SJS, bone marrow suppression, hepatotoxicity, elevated serum creatinine, hyperkalemia	*Renal:* CrCl less than 60 mL/min (1.00 mL/s): Use of traditional pharmacokinetic dosing; dose adjustments per serum levels *Hepatic:* No dose adjustment *Renal:* CrCl less than 50 mL/min (0.83 mL/s): 10–15 mg/kg trimethoprim IV per day divided every 8 hours; CrCl less than 10 mL/min (0.17 mL/s): 7–10 mg/kg trimethoprim IV per day divided every 8–12 hours *Hepatic:* No dose adjustment	21

(Continued)

Table 70–3

Pathogen-Based Definitive Treatment for CNS Infections (*Continued*)

Pathogen	Recommended and Alternative Antimicrobial Therapy (Adult Doses)	Adverse Effects/Safety Monitoring	Renal and Hepatic Dose Adjustment	Duration (Days)
Streptococcus agalactiae (group B. *Streptococcus*)	*Standard Therapy* Ampicillin *or* penicillin G			14–21
	Alternative Therapies Ceftriaxone *or* cefotaxime			
Enterobacteriaceae	*Standard Therapy* Ceftriaxone *or* cefotaxime			
	Alternative Therapies Aztreonam 2 g IV every 6–8 hours	Phlebitis, fever, rash, headache, confusion, seizures	*Renal*: CrCl less than 50 mL/min (0.83 mL/s): 2 g IV every 8 hours; CrCl less than 30 mL/min (0.50 mL/s): 2 g IV every 12 hours; CrCl less than 10 mL/min (0.17 mL/s): 1 g IV every 12 hours *Hepatic*: No dose adjustment	
	Moxifloxacin *or* meropenem *or* trimethoprim-sulfamethoxazole *or* ampicillin			
Pseudomonas aeruginosa	*Standard Therapy* cefepime *or* ceftazidime 2 g IV every 8 hours *or* meropenem (addition of aminoglycoside should be considered)	Hypersensitivity, rash, anemia, neutropenia, eosinophilia, LFT elevation	*Renal*: CrCl less than 50 mL/min (0.83 mL/s): 1–2 g IV every 12 hours; CrCl less than 30 mL/min (0.50 mL/s): 1–2 g IV every 24 hours; CrCl less than 10 mL/min (0.17 mL/s): 1 g IV every 24 hours *Hepatic*: No dose adjustment	
	Alternative Therapies Aztreonam *or* ciprofloxacin 400 mg IV every 8–12 hours (addition of aminoglycoside should be considered)	Nausea/vomiting/diarrhea, dizziness, headache, rash, confusion, seizures	Ciprofloxacin: *Renal*: CrCl less than 30 mL/min (0.50 mL/s): 400 mg IV every 24 hours *or* 200 mg IV every 12 hours *Hepatic*: No dose adjustment	
Staphylococcus aureus Methicillin-susceptible	*Standard Therapy* Nafcillin *or* oxacillin 1.5–3 g every 4 hours	Rash, nausea/vomiting/diarrhea, acute interstitial nephritis	*Renal*: No dose adjustment *Hepatic*: No dose adjustment (combined renal and hepatic impairment may require dose adjustment)	
Methicillin-resistant	*Alternative Therapies* Vancomycin *or* meropenem *Standard Therapy* Vancomycin *plus* Rifampin 600 mg orally *or* IV daily if shunt involved	Rifampin: Hepatotoxicity, red-orange discoloration of body fluids, skin rash, hepatic enzyme induction	*Renal*: No dose adjustment *Hepatic*: Caution in moderate/ severe hepatic impairment	
	Alternative Therapies Linezolid 600 mg IV every 12 hours *or* trimethoprim-sulfamethoxazole	Linezolid: blood dyscrasias, myalgias, arthralgias, neuropathy	*Renal*: No dose adjustment *Hepatic*: No dose adjustment	

(Continued)

Table 70–3

Pathogen-Based Definitive Treatment for CNS Infections (*Continued*)

Pathogen	Recommended and Alternative Antimicrobial Therapy (Adult Doses)	Adverse Effects/Safety Monitoring	Renal and Hepatic Dose Adjustment	Duration (Days)
Staphylococcus epidermidis	*Standard Therapy* Vancomycin *plus* rifampin 600 mg orally *or* IV daily if shunt involved *Alternative Therapies* Linezolid			
Herpes simplex virus	*Standard Therapy* Acyclovir 10 mg/kg IV every 8 hours (adults); 20 mg/kg IV every 8 hours (neonates)	Nephrotoxicity, crystalluria, nausea/vomiting, neurotoxicity, phlebitis	*Renal*: CrCl less than 50 mL/min (0.83 mL/s): 10 mg/kg IV every 12 hours; CrCl less than 30 mL/min (0.50 mL/s): 10 mg/kg IV every 24 hours; CrCl less than 10 mL/min (0.17 mL/s): 5 mg/kg IV every 24 hours *Hepatic*: No dose adjustment	
	Alternative Therapy Foscarnet 120–200 mg/kg IV per day in divided doses every 8–12 hours	Nephrotoxicity, electrolyte imbalances, nausea/vomiting, headache, penile ulceration, thrombophlebitis, seizures	*Renal*: CrCl: 1.0–1.4 mL/min/kg (0.017-0.023 mL/s/kg): 70 mg/kg IV every 12 hours; CrCl: 0.8–1.0 mL/min/kg (0.013-0.017 mL/s/kg): 50 mg/kg IV every 12 hours; CrCl: 0.6–0.8 mL/min/kg (0.010-0.013 mL/s/kg): 80 mg/kg IV every 24 hours; CrCl: 0.5–0.6 mL/min/kg (0.008-0.010 mL/s/kg): 60 mg/kg IV every 24 hours; CrCl: 0.4–0.5 mL/min/kg (0.007–0.008 mL/s/kg): 50 mg/kg IV every 24 hours; CrCl less than 0.4 mL/min/kg (0.007 mL/s/kg) *or* less than 20 mL/min (0.33 mL/s) not recommended. *Hepatic*: No dose adjustment	
Cryptococcus neoformans	Amphotericin B 0.7mg/kg IV daily *plus* flucytosine 100–150 mg/kg/day in divided doses every 6 hours (induction) Fluconazole 400–800 mg (maintenance) Fluconazole 200 mg (secondary prophylaxis)	Amphotericin: nephrotoxicity, electrolyte imbalances Flucytosine: bone marrow suppression, rash Fluconazole: transaminitis; QTc prolongation	*Renal*: Caution in severe renal dysfunction; consider alternative dosing strategy or change to lipid formulation *Hepatic*: No dose adjustment *Flucytosine* *Renal*: CrCl 25–50 mL/min (0.42–0.83 mL/s): every 12 hours; CrCl 10–25 mL/min (0.17–0.42 mL/s) every 24 hours; CrCl less than 10 mL/min (0.17 mL/s) 12.5mg/kg every 24 hours *Hepatic*: No dose adjustment Fluconazole *Renal*: CrCl less than 50 mL/min (0.83 mL/s) decrease dose by 50% *Hepatic*: Consider 50% reduction in mild-moderate hepatic insufficiency; risk-benefit in severe hepatic dysfunction	

(Continued)

Table 70–3

Pathogen-Based Definitive Treatment for CNS Infections (*Continued*)

Pathogen	Recommended and Alternative Antimicrobial Therapy (Adult Doses)	Adverse Effects/Safety Monitoring	Renal and Hepatic Dose Adjustment	Duration (Days)
Toxoplasmosis gondii	Pyrimethamine 200 mg orally x 1, then 50 mg (less than 60 kg) to 75 mg (more than or equal to 60 kg) daily *plus* sulfadiazine 1,000 mg (less than 60 kg) to 1,500 mg (more than or equal to 60 kg) orally every 6 hours plus leucovorin 10–25 mg orally daily	Pyrimethamine: bone marrow suppression, high-risk for anemia Sulfadiazine: nephrotoxicity, bone marrow suppression, rash, SJS	*Renal*: No dose adjustment *Hepatic*: No dose adjustment *Renal*: CrCL 25–50 mL/min (0.42–0.83 mL/s): every 12 hours; CrCl 10–25 mL/min (0.17–0.42 mL/s) every 24 hours; CrCl less than 10ml/min (less than 0.17 mL/s) caution use due to high risk of crystalluria *Hepatic*: No dose adjustment	

LFTs, liver function tests; MIC, minimum inhibitory concentration; SJS, Stevens-Johnson Syndrome.

Adapted, with permission, from Refs. 14 and 55.

coverage for the offending pathogen(s). Table 70–3 outlines recommended definitive pathogen-directed treatment regimens, recommended treatment duration, and key adverse effects that should be monitored during antibiotic therapy for meningitis. Treatment considerations for selected pathogens causing CNS infections are summarized next. Table 70–4 provides pediatric doses of selected agents used in bacterial meningitis treatment.

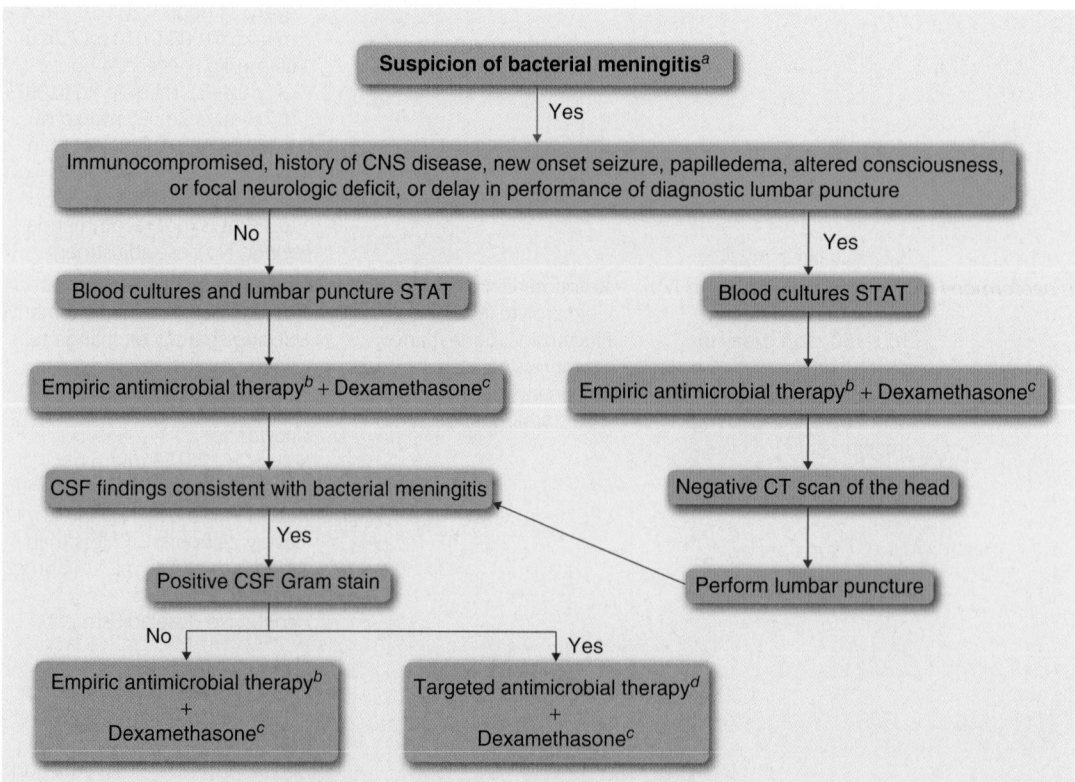

FIGURE 70–2. Management algorithm for adults with suspected bacterial meningitis. [a]Management algorithm is similar for infants and children with suspected bacterial meningitis. [b]See Table 70–1 for empirical treatment recommendations. [c]See text for specific recommendations for use of adjunctive dexamethasone in adults with bacterial meningitis. [d]See Table 70–3 for pathogen-based definitive treatment recommendations. (Adapted, with permission, from Moris G, Garcia-Monco JC. The challenge of drug-induced aseptic meningitis. Arch Intern Med 1999;159:1185–1194.)

Table 70–4			
Pediatric Doses of Selected Agents Used in Bacterial Meningitis Treatment			
	Neonates, 0–7 Days	**Neonates, 8–28 Days**	**Infants and Children**
Ampicillin	150 mg/kg IV per day in divided doses every 8 hours	200 mg/kg IV per day in divided doses every 6–8 hours	300 mg/kg IV per day in divided doses every 8 hours
Cefepime	—	—	150 mg/kg per day in divided doses every 8 hours
Cefotaxime	100–150 mg/kg IV per day in divided doses every 8–12 hours	150–200 mg/kg IV per day in divided doses every 6–8 hours	225–300 mg/kg per day in divided doses every 6–8 hours
Ceftriaxone	—	—	80–100 mg/kg IV per day in divided doses every 12 hours
Gentamicin	5 mg/kg IV per day in divided doses every 12 hours (with dosing based on serum levels)	7.5 mg/kg IV per day in divided doses every 8 hours (with dosing based on serum levels	7.5 mg/kg IV per day in divided doses every 8 hours based on serum levels)
Meropenem	—	—	120 mg/kg IV per day in divided doses every 8 hours
Nafcillin/oxacillin	75 mg/kg IV per day in divided doses every 8–12 hours	Nafcillin: 100–150 mg/kg IV per day in divided doses every 6–8 hours; Oxacillin: 150–200 mg/kg IV per day in divided doses every 6–8 hours	200 mg/kg IV per day in divided doses every 6 hours max, 2 g pediatrics greater than 3 months of age
Penicillin G	0.15 million units/kg IV per day in divided doses 8–12 hours	0.2 million units/kg IV per day in divided doses every 6–8 hours	0.3 million units/kg IV per day in divided doses every 4–6 hours
Vancomycin	20–30 mg/kg IV per day in divided doses every 8–12 hours	30–45 mg/kg IV per day in divided doses every 6–8 hours	60 mg/kg IV per day in divided doses every 6 hours

LFTs, liver function tests; MIC, minimum inhibitory concentration.

Adapted, with permission, from Scheld WM, Koedel U, Nathan B, Pfister HW. Pathophysiology of bacterial meningitis: mechanism(s) of neuronal injury. J Infect Dis 2002;186(Suppl 2):S225–S233.

▶ Neisseria meningitidis *Meningitis*

N. meningitidis CNS infections most commonly occur in children and young adults. *N. meningitidis* accounts for 13.9% of all cases of bacterial meningitis annually. Its overall incidence has declined by 58% between 1998 and 2007, largely due to the use of vaccines. In 2006 and 2007, there were 0.19 cases per 100,000 of meningococcal meningitis.[3] From 11% to 19% of survivors of meningococcal meningitis experience long-term sequelae, including hearing loss, limb loss, and neurologic deficits.[31] Nearly all meningococcal disease is caused by five serogroups: A, B, C, Y, and W-135. In the United States, serotypes B, C, and Y each are responsible for approximately 30% of cases.

Meningococcal meningitis is observed most commonly in individuals living in close quarters (e.g., college students, military personnel). Infants younger than 1 year of age are at highest risk, possibly because pneumococcal vaccination reduces bactericidal antibodies.[33] However, nearly 60% of cases occur in patients over 11 years of age.[31,34] *N. meningitidis* colonizes the nasopharynx and usually is transmitted via inhaled respiratory droplets from patients or asymptomatic carriers. A subclinical bacteremia typically ensues, seeding the meninges. Meningococcal disease is often (approximately 50%) associated with a diffuse petechial rash, and patients may experience behavioral changes. Patients may develop fulminant meningococcal sepsis, characterized by shock, disseminated intravascular coagulation, and multiorgan failure.[31,32] Meningococcal sepsis has a poor prognosis and carries a mortality rate of up to 80%, whereas the mortality rate with meningococcal meningitis alone is 13%.[21,35] Patients with suspected meningococcal infection should be kept on respiratory isolation for the first 24 hours of treatment.[5]

Traditionally, high-dose penicillin G was the treatment standard for meningococcal disease. However, increasing penicillin resistance requires that third-generation cephalosporins now be used for empirical treatment until in vitro susceptibilities are known.[28] Patients with a history of type I penicillin allergy or cephalosporin allergy may be treated with vancomycin. Treatment should be continued for 7 days, after which no further treatment is necessary.

Prevention of meningococcal disease by vaccination is a key to reducing the incidence of meningococcal meningitis. Adolescents should be routinely immunized with a 2-conjugate vaccine series beginning at age 11 or 12 years. In addition, individuals aged 2 through 54 years who are immunocompromised (including those with complement deficiencies, who have HIV, or who have asplenia) should receive a 2-polysaccharide vaccine series.[36] The quadrivalent conjugate meningococcal vaccine protects against four of the five serotypes causing invasive disease (A, C, Y, and W-135). Meningococcal vaccines do not protect against serotype B, which causes more than 50% of the cases of meningococcal meningitis in children younger than 2 years of age.[37] Meningococcal vaccines can be used in outbreak situations, with protective antibodies measurable within 7 to 10 days. **⑧** *Close contacts of patients with meningococcal infections should be evaluated for antimicrobial prophylaxis.* Close contacts include members of the same household, individuals who share sleeping quarters, daycare contacts, and individuals exposed to oral secretions of meningitis patients. After consultation with the local health department, close contacts should receive prophylactic antibiotics to eradicate nasopharyngeal carriage of the organism. Household contacts of patients with meningococcal meningitis have a 400- to 800-fold increased risk of developing meningitis.[32] Prophylactic antibiotics should be started as soon as possible, preferably within 24 hours of exposure (and within 14 days, after which the benefit is significantly reduced). Recommended regimens, all of which are 90% to 95% effective, for adults include rifampin 600 mg orally every 12 hours for 2 days, ciprofloxacin 500 mg orally for one dose, or ceftriaxone 250 mg intramuscularly for one dose. Regimens for children include rifampin 5 mg/kg orally every 12 hours for 2 days (less than 1 month of age), rifampin 10 mg/kg orally every 12 hours for 2 days (greater than 1 month of age), or ceftriaxone 125 mg intramuscularly for one dose (less than 12 years of age).[31,32] It is not known whether close contacts who have been vaccinated will benefit from prophylaxis. Patients with meningococcal meningitis who are treated with antibiotics other than third-generation cephalosporins also should be considered for prophylaxis to eradicate the nasopharyngeal carrier state.[34]

▶ Streptococcus pneumoniae *Meningitis*

S. pneumoniae is the most common cause of meningitis in adults and in children younger than 2 years of age. Pneumococcus is associated with the highest mortality observed with bacterial meningitis in adults (14–18%), and coma and seizures are more common in pneumococcal meningitis.[1–4] Patients at high risk for pneumococcal meningitis include

the elderly, alcoholics, splenectomized patients, patients with sickle cell disease, and patients with cochlear implants. At least 50% of pneumococcal meningitis cases are due to a primary infection of the ears, sinuses, or lungs.

High-dose penicillin G traditionally has been the drug of choice for the treatment of pneumococcal meningitis. However, due to increases in pneumococcal resistance, the preferred empirical treatment now includes a third-generation cephalosporin in combination with vancomycin.[18] All CSF isolates should be tested for penicillin and cephalosporin resistance by methods endorsed by the CLSI. Once in vitro sensitivity results are known, therapy may be tailored (Table 70–3). Patients with a history of type I penicillin allergy or cephalosporin allergy may be treated with vancomycin. Treatment should be continued for 10 to 14 days, after which no further maintenance therapy is required. Antimicrobial prophylaxis is not indicated for close contacts.

Administration of vaccines to high-risk individuals is a key strategy to reduce the risk of invasive pneumococcal disease. The 23-valent pneumococcal vaccine targets serotypes that account for more than 90% of invasive disease in high-risk patients. However, the 23-valent vaccine does not produce a reliable immunologic response in children younger than 2 years of age, nor does it reduce pneumococcal carriage. The 7-valent pneumococcal protein-polysaccharide conjugate vaccine used between 2000 and 2010 targeted the seven most common serotypes in children and provided protection (94% reduction) against invasive pneumococcal disease (such as sepsis and meningitis) in children younger than 5 years of age.[37] Widespread administration of the 7-valent conjugate vaccine to children has also contributed to a 28% reduction in invasive pneumococcal disease in adults.[8] There are some concerns about an apparent increase in cases caused by nonvaccine serotypes including 19A, 22F, and 35B, including strains with increased antimicrobial resistance.[35] In 2010, a 13-valent vaccine, PCV13, was introduced that confers protection against 1,3,4, 5, 6A, 6B, 7F, 9V, 14, 18C, 19A, 19F, and 23F. It is intended for use in children younger than 18 years in the same schedule as the 7-valent conjugate vaccine.[38] Immunization schedules provided by the U.S. Centers for Disease Control and Prevention (CDC) are updated at least annually and should be consulted for additional details. The impact of PCV13 on the incidence of pneumococcal disease is unknown at this time, but should be anticipated to further reduce disease burden in both children and adults.

▶ Haemophilus influenzae *Meningitis*

Prior to the introduction of the Hib conjugate vaccine, *H. influenzae* type b was the most common cause of bacterial meningitis in the United States.[5] Routine inoculation of pediatric patients against Hib has reduced the incidence of Hib meningitis by 38% between 1998 and 2007.[3] The Hib vaccine is also recommended for patients undergoing splenectomy. Hib meningeal disease is often associated with a parameningeal focus such as a sinus or middle ear infection. Increases in β-lactamase–mediated resistance have changed the empirical treatment of choice from ampicillin to

---

Patient Encounter 2, Part 1

BB is a 4-year-old boy who is brought to the ED with a 3-day history of fever and irritability. In the past 24 hours, he has become more lethargic, sleeping for 18 hours, and is difficult to arouse. Vital signs and laboratory values include a rectal temperature of 39.4°C (103°F), respirations 40 per minute, heart rate 145 beats per minute, and peripheral WBC of $15.9 \times 10^3/\text{mm}^3$ ($15.9 \times 10^9/\text{L}$), with 68% (0.68) PMNs. Physical examination reveals that the patient is more comfortable when lying flat and has some nuchal rigidity. BB also has a 9-year-old brother with autism and therefore he has not received any routine vaccinations.

What signs and symptoms consistent with meningitis are present in BB?

What clues to causative pathogen are present in BB?

What empiric antimicrobial regimen should be started?

Patient Encounter 2, Part 2

BB underwent lumbar puncture. Initial results from CSF studies are WBC $1.76 \times 10^3/mm^3$ ($1.76 \times 10^9/L$) with 79% (0.79) PMNs, protein 265 mg/dL (2,650 mg/L), glucose 30 mg/dL (1. 7 mmol/L), with a concurrent serum glucose of 110 mg/dL (6.1 mmol/L). Gram stain shows gram-negative rods and culture results identify *H. influenzae* infection. The patient is admitted to an acute care unit and remains clinically stable.

What complications is BB at risk for acutely? What potential long-term complications may result?

How can his antibiotic regimen be streamlined at this time?

How long should the antibiotics be continued?

third-generation cephalosporins (e.g., ceftriaxone and cefotaxime). Treatment should be continued for 7 days, after which no further maintenance therapy is required.

⑧ *Close contacts of patients with H. influenzae type B meningitis should be evaluated for antimicrobial prophylaxis.* The risk of Hib meningitis in close contacts may be up to 200- to 1,000-fold higher than in the general population.[11] Invasive Hib disease, including meningitis, should be reported to the local health department and the CDC. Prophylaxis to eliminate nasal and oropharyngeal carriage of Hib in exposed individuals should be initiated after consultation with local health officials. Rifampin (600 mg/day for adults; 20 mg/kg/day for children, maximum of 600 mg/day) is administered for 4 days.[17] Rifampin prophylaxis is not necessary for individuals who have received the full Hib vaccine series. Exposed, unvaccinated children between 12 and 48 months of age should receive one dose of vaccine, and unvaccinated children 2 to 11 months of age should receive three doses of vaccine, as well as rifampin prophylaxis.[17] Because of prior vaccine shortages, it cannot be assumed that all children have been vaccinated. Further, some children have not received all childhood vaccines because of parental fears regarding vaccine safety.

▶ Listeria monocytogenes *Meningitis*

L. monocytogenes is an intracellular gram-positive bacillus that has been reported to contaminate certain foods, such as soft cheese, unpasteurized milk, raw meats and fish, processed meats, and raw vegetables. Bacteria from contaminated foods colonize the GI tract, pass into the bloodstream, and overcome natural cellular immune responses to cause infection. *L. monocytogenes* meningitis, usually observed in patients at extremes of age and in immunocompromised patients with depressed cellular immunity (including patients with leukemia, solid-organ transplants, and HIV/AIDS) has an overall mortality rate of up to 30%.[39,40]

Only a limited number of antibiotics show bactericidal activity against *Listeria*. The combination of high-dose ampicillin or penicillin G and an aminoglycoside is synergistic and bactericidal against *Listeria*. A total treatment course of at least 3 weeks is required. Because of concerns about the risk of nephrotoxicity with an extended treatment course of aminoglycosides, patients are treated with combination therapy for 10 days and may finish out the remainder of their treatment with ampicillin or penicillin alone.[40] In penicillin-allergic patients, trimethoprim-sulfamethoxazole is the agent of choice due to documented in vitro bactericidal activity against *Listeria*, as well as good CNS penetration. Vancomycin and cephalosporins are not effective treatments for *Listeria* meningitis. Prophylaxis is not needed for close contacts, nor is suppressive therapy indicated. Patients with severe depression of cell-mediated immunity should be advised to avoid foods that may be contaminated with *Listeria*.

▶ Group B Streptococcus *Meningitis*

Infection with group B *Streptococcus* (e.g., *S. agalactiae*) is the most common cause of neonatal sepsis and meningitis. Fifteen to 35% of pregnant women are a carrier of group B *Streptococcus* in the vagina or rectum. Group B streptococci can be acquired during childbirth after exposure to infected secretions from the mother's birth canal or rectum. Neonates born to women who are carriers are at very high risk (1 of every 100–200 babies) of developing invasive group B streptococcal disease, including sepsis and meningitis.[41] Neonatal meningitis is associated with significant morbidity and mortality. Synergistic treatment with penicillin or ampicillin, plus gentamicin, for 14 to 21 days is recommended for the treatment of group B streptococcal meningitis.[18]

To reduce the risk of clinical group B streptococcal disease in neonates, pregnant women should be screened at 35 to 37 weeks' gestation to determine whether they are carriers of group B streptococci.[41] Intrapartum antibiotics (e.g., penicillin or ampicillin) are recommended for pregnant women with the following characteristics: group B streptococcal carrier state detected at screening, history of group B streptococcal bacteriuria at any time during pregnancy, and history of delivery of infant with invasive group B streptococcal disease.[41]

▶ Gram-Negative Bacillary Meningitis

Meningitis caused by enteric gram-negative bacilli is an important cause of morbidity and mortality in populations at risk, including those with diabetes, malignancy, cirrhosis, immunosuppression, advanced age, parameningeal infection, and/or a defect allowing communication from skin to CNS (e.g., neurosurgery, congenital defects, cranial trauma).[11]

The optimal treatment for gram-negative bacillary meningitis is not well defined. The introduction of extended-spectrum cephalosporins has improved patient outcomes significantly. Although the third-generation cephalosporins ceftriaxone and cefotaxime provide good coverage for most Enterobacteriaceae, these antibiotics are not active against *P. aeruginosa*. Ceftazidime, cefepime, and carbapenems are effective in pseudomonal meningitis.[26,28] Addition of an aminoglycoside may improve treatment results; however, CNS penetration of aminoglycosides is extremely poor, even in the setting of inflamed meninges. Intrathecal or intraventricular administration of aminoglycosides may be useful, but intra-ventricular antibiotics have been associated with increased mortality in neonates.[26,42] Intrathecal therapy is accomplished by administering the antibiotic into the CSF via LP, whereas intraventricular therapy is usually administered into a reservoir implanted in the ventricles of the brain.

Initial therapy of suspected or documented pseudomonal meningitis should include an extended-spectrum β-lactam (e.g., ceftazidime, cefepime, meropenem) plus an aminoglycoside (preferably tobramycin or amikacin). Although the carbapenem imipenem-cilastatin has similar activity to these β-lactams, its use is not recommended in meningitis because of the risk of seizures. Aztreonam, high-dose ciprofloxacin, and colistin are alternative treatments for pseudomonal meningitis. Local therapy (i.e., intrathecal or intraventricular therapy) may be indicated in patients with gram-negative bacillary meningitis (especially infections caused by multidrug-resistant *P. aeruginosa*) or in patients who fail to improve on IV antibiotics alone. In cases of multidrug-resistant pathogens, alternative pharmacodynamic dosing strategies such as continuous or extended infusion of β-lactam antimicrobials may be considered to optimize target attainment (time greater than minimum inhibitory concentration). Given the differences in local hospital resistance patterns, administration of pathogen-directed treatment is very important after microbiology results become available. Therapy for gram-negative bacillary meningitis should be continued for at least 21 days.

▶ Postoperative Infections in the Neurosurgical Patient and Shunt Infections

Patients who undergo neurosurgical procedures or have invasive or implanted foreign devices (e.g., CSF shunts, intraspinal pumps or catheters, epidural catheters) are at risk for CNS infections. Key pathogens in postneurosurgical infections include coagulase-negative staphylococci, *S. aureus*, streptococci, propionibacteria, and gram-negative bacilli, including *P. aeruginosa*. Clinical signs and symptoms may be similar to those of other CNS infections, and there also may be evidence of malfunction of implanted hardware or visible signs of a postoperative wound infection.

Empirical therapy for postoperative infections in neurosurgical patients (including patients with CSF shunts) should include vancomycin in combination with either cefepime, ceftazidime, or meropenem. Linezolid reaches adequate CSF concentrations and resolves cases of meningitis refractory to vancomycin.[40,43] However, data with linezolid are limited. The addition of rifampin should be considered for treatment of shunt infections. When culture and sensitivity data are available, pathogen-directed antibiotic therapy should be administered. Removal of infected devices is desirable; aggressive antibiotic therapy (including high-dose IV antibiotic therapy plus intraventricular vancomycin and/or tobramycin) may be effective for patients in whom hardware removal is not possible.[44] If methicillin-resistant *S. aureus* is identified as the causative organism, daptomycin may be considered an alternative therapy.[45]

The use of prophylactic antibiotics against meningitis postcraniotomy remains controversial. A meta-analysis suggests that prophylaxis reduces rates of postoperative meningitis by nearly one-half.[47] Other studies have demonstrated no benefit, and there are limited data on organism-specific reductions in infection rate.[48,49] Additionally, breakthrough meningitis that does occur may be a result of drug-resistant pathogens.[48]

Brain abscesses are localized collections of pus within the cranium. These infections are difficult to treat due to the presence of walled-off infections in the brain tissue that are hard for some antibiotics to reach. In addition to appropriate antimicrobial therapy (a discussion of which is beyond the scope of this chapter), surgical debridement is often required as an adjunctive measure. Surgical debridement may also be required in the management of neurosurgical postoperative infections.

▶ Viral Encephalitis and Meningitis

Viral encephalitis and meningitis may mimic bacterial meningitis on clinical presentation but often can be differentiated by CSF findings (Table 70–2). The most common viral pathogens are enteroviruses, which cause approximately 85% of cases of viral CNS infections.[11] Other viruses that may cause CNS infections include arboviruses, HSV, cytomegalovirus, varicella-zoster virus, rotavirus, coronavirus, influenza viruses A and B, West Nile virus, and Epstein-Barr virus. Viral CNS infections are acquired through hematogenous or neuronal spread.[11] Most cases of enteroviral meningitis or encephalitis are self-limiting with supportive treatment.[46] However, arbovirus, West Nile virus, and Eastern equine virus infections are associated with a less favorable prognosis.

In contrast to other viral encephalitides, HSV type 1 and 2 encephalitis are treatable. Although rare (one case per 250,000 population per year in the United States), HSV encephalitis is a serious, life-threatening infection.[50] More than 90% of HSV encephalitis in adults is due to HSV type 1, whereas HSV type 2 predominates in neonatal HSV encephalitis (greater than 70%).[51] HSV encephalitis is the result of reactivation of a latent infection (two-thirds of cases) or a severe case of primary infection (one-third). Without effective treatment, the mortality rate may be as high as 85%, and survivors often have significant residual neurologic deficits. In accordance with 2008 IDSA guidelines, high-dose IV acyclovir is the drug of choice, given for 2 to 3 weeks at a dose of 10 mg/kg IV every 8 hours in adults, based on ideal body weight, and for 3 weeks at a dose of 20 mg/kg IV every 8 hours in neonates.[52,53] Patients receiving acyclovir should maintain adequate hydration (consider continuous IV hydration in those receiving high-dose acyclovir) to help prevent acute kidney injury secondary to crystal nephropathy.[52,53] Foscarnet 120 to 200 mg/kg/day divided every 8 to 12 hours for 2 to 3 weeks is the treatment of choice for acyclovir-resistant HSV isolates.[52,53]

▶ Opportunistic CNS Infections

Cerebral Toxoplasmosis Across the globe, cerebral toxoplasmosis represents the most common focal brain infection in HIV-infected patients. Infection rates in the United

States vary but are reported to be approximately 15% among patients with AIDS.[54] Nearly all cases occur in patients with CD4+ cell counts less than 200 cells/mm³ (less than 200 × 10⁶/L), and the greatest risk is in severely immunocompromised hosts with CD4+ cell counts less than 50 cells/mm³ (less than 50 × 10⁶/L). Potent antiretroviral therapy and primary prophylaxis in IgG-positive patients has greatly reduced the disease burden. First-line therapy in toxoplasmosis encephalitis is pyrimethamine plus sulfadiazine, given concomitantly with leucovorin to prevent severe hematologic adverse effects secondary to pyrimethamine (see tables for dosing). Clindamycin may be substituted for sulfadiazine in cases of contraindications to sulfa-based therapy. Sulfamethoxazole-trimethoprim may also be an option, specifically in patients unable to take oral therapy. Adjunctive corticosteroids and anticonvulsant therapy should be considered to reduce sequelae from the inflammatory process and control active seizures, respectively.[55]

Cryptococcal Meningitis CNS disease secondary to *Cryptococcus neoformans* is primarily observed in severely immunocompromised hosts, such as those with HIV infection. Potent antiretroviral therapy has significantly reduced the disease burden from pre–antiretroviral therapy rates of 5% to 8% in developed countries. The majority of disease occurs in patients with CD4+ cell counts less than 50 cells/mm³ (less than 50 × 10⁶/L). First-line therapy is considered amphotericin B deoxycholate 0.7 mg/kg IV daily plus flucytosine 100mg/kg/day orally in four divided doses for a minimum of 2 weeks. Therapeutic drug monitoring may be considered for flucytosine to help reduce the risk of adverse effects. Development of renal dysfunction as a result of disease and/or drug toxicity should be closely monitored and may prompt dose reduction or possible switch to alternative lipid formulations of amphotericin, which may be less nephrotoxic. High-dose fluconazole is considered an alternative first-line therapy, especially in resource-limited areas. Secondary prophylaxis with fluconazole for an indefinite period is recommended following the completion of at least 2 weeks of induction therapy and 8 weeks of maintenance therapy with fluconazole.[55]

▶ Adjunctive Dexamethasone Therapy

The adjunctive agent dexamethasone improves outcomes in selected patient populations with meningitis. Dexamethasone inhibits the release of proinflammatory cytokines and limits the CNS inflammatory response stimulated by infection and antibiotic therapy.

Clinical benefit in reducing neurologic deficits (primarily by reducing hearing loss) has been observed in infants and children with *H. influenzae* meningitis, as well as other pathogens causing meningitis, if dexamethasone is initiated prior to antibiotic therapy.[1,14] The American Academy of Pediatrics recommends dexamethasone (0.15 mg/kg IV every 6 hours for 2 to 4 days) for infants and children at least 6 weeks of age with Hib meningitis and consideration of dexamethasone in pneumococcal meningitis.[18,56] In contrast to this recommendation, a large multicenter cohort study failed to show any mortality benefit of adjunctive dexamethasone therapy

regardless of age or responsible pathogen (*S. pneumoniae* or *N. meningitidis*).[57] Dexamethasone should be initiated 10 to 20 minutes before or no later than the time of initiation of antibiotic therapy; it is not recommended for infants and children who have already received antibiotic therapy because it is unlikely to improve treatment outcome in these patients. There are insufficient data to make a recommendation regarding the use of adjunctive dexamethasone therapy in neonatal meningitis.

In adults, a significant benefit was observed with dexamethasone over placebo in reducing meningitis complications, including death, particularly in patients with pneumococcal meningitis.[58] The IDSA recommends dexamethasone 0.15 mg/kg IV every 6 hours for 2 to 4 days (with the first dose administered 10 to 20 minutes before or with the first dose of antibiotics) in adults with suspected or proven pneumococcal meningitis.[18] Dexamethasone is not recommended for adults who have already received antibiotic therapy. Some clinicians would administer dexamethasone to all adults with meningitis pending results of laboratory tests. Benefit of dexamethasone in bacterial meningitis in a HIV-positive population has not been clearly established.[59]

There is some controversy regarding the administration of dexamethasone to patients with pneumococcal meningitis caused by penicillin- or cephalosporin-resistant strains, for which vancomycin would be required. Animal models indicate that concurrent steroid use reduces vancomycin penetration into the CSF by 42% to 77% and delays CSF sterilization due to reduction in the inflammatory response.[28] A prospective evaluation in patients with pneumococcal meningitis receiving vancomycin and adjunctive dexamethasone demonstrated that adequate concentrations of vancomycin, nearly 30% of serum concentrations, were achievable in the CSF, provided appropriate vancomycin dosage was utilized.[60] Treatment failures have been reported in adults with resistant pneumococcal meningitis who were treated with dexamethasone, but the risk–benefit of using dexamethasone in these patients cannot be defined at this time. Animal models indicate a benefit of adding rifampin in patients with resistant pneumococcal meningitis whenever dexamethasone is used.[26,28]

OUTCOME EVALUATION

Monitor patients with CNS infections continuously throughout their treatment course to evaluate their progress toward achieving treatment goals, including relief of symptoms, eradication of infection, and reduction of inflammation to prevent death and the development of neurologic deficits. These treatment goals are best achieved by appropriate parenteral antimicrobial therapy, including empirical therapy to cover the most likely pathogens, followed by directed therapy after culture and sensitivity results are known. ❾ *Components of a monitoring plan to assess efficacy and safety of antimicrobial therapy of CNS infections include clinical signs and symptoms and laboratory data (e.g., CSF findings, culture, sensitivity data).*

Patient Encounter 2, Part 3

As noted, BB had not received any vaccinations since birth. The parents are concerned and inquire about the need for antibiotic prophylaxis for the family and now are considering vaccination for BB.

Who should receive antimicrobial prophylaxis for H. influenzae?

Who should receive vaccination against Hib disease?

How is vaccination important in the prevention of Hib disease, especially for BB?

During the patient's treatment course, monitor clinical signs and symptoms at least three times daily. Trends are more important than one-time assessments. Expect fever, headache, nausea and vomiting, and malaise to begin to improve within 24 to 48 hours of initiation of antimicrobial therapy and supportive care. Evaluate the patient for resolution of neurologic signs and symptoms, such as altered mental status and nuchal rigidity, as the infection is eradicated and inflammation is reduced within the CNS. Expect improvement and subsequent resolution of signs and symptoms as the treatment course continues. At the time of hospital discharge, arrange outpatient follow-up for several weeks to months depending on the causative pathogen, clinical treatment course, and patient's underlying comorbidities. Specifically evaluate patients for the presence of residual neurologic deficits.

Monitoring of laboratory tests is important in patients receiving treatment for CNS infections. Monitor CSF and blood cultures so that antimicrobial therapy can be tailored to the etiologic organisms. Follow-up cultures may be obtained to prove eradication of the organism(s) or treatment failure. Although repeat LP generally is not performed, consider repeat LP for patients who do not respond clinically after 48 hours of appropriate antimicrobial therapy, especially those with resistant pneumococcus who receive dexamethasone.[14] Other candidates for repeat LP include those with infection

Patient Care and Monitoring

1. Assess the patient's signs, symptoms, and risk factors for meningitis. Do these offer any clues to the offending pathogen?

2. Determine whether the patient can undergo an immediate LP or if the LP should be delayed until a CNS mass lesion can be ruled out. If the LP is delayed, blood cultures should be drawn and appropriate empirical antimicrobial therapy initiated immediately.

3. Based on patient-specific data, local resistance patterns, and other relevant data, design an appropriate empirical antimicrobial regimen directed at the most likely pathogens; empirical regimens should consist of high-dose IV bactericidal therapy.

4. Determine whether adjunctive dexamethasone therapy is indicated; if so, start steroid therapy 15 to 20 minutes before the first dose of antimicrobial therapy.

5. Provide supportive care for patients with CNS infections, including hydration, electrolyte replacement, antipyretics, analgesics, and antiepileptic drugs.

6. Monitor culture and sensitivity data from the microbiology laboratory to determine whether any refinements are needed in the patient's treatment regimen. Design a therapeutic plan to finish out the patient's course of therapy for acute meningitis.

7. Monitor the patient's response to therapy (i.e., clinical signs/symptoms and laboratory data), as well as the development of complications, including seizures and hearing loss. Dexamethasone therapy may reduce antibiotic penetration, so antimicrobial drug dosing may have to be increased (especially vancomycin) to achieve adequate CSF levels. Serum levels of vancomycin should be measured and doses titrated to ensure adequate CNS concentrations. Evaluate whether intraventricular or intrathecal antibiotics are indicated.

8. Perform ongoing surveillance for adverse drug reactions, drug allergies, and drug interactions.

9. Determine whether prophylaxis is indicated for close contacts of patients with CNS infections. Close contacts should be located for patients with suspected meningococcal or Hib meningitis. After consultation with the local health department, antibiotic prophylaxis should be provided promptly to these individuals to avoid secondary disease.

10. Evaluate whether the patient is a candidate for finishing out his or her course of parenteral treatment on an outpatient basis. If so, the importance of close medical follow-up and medication compliance should be stressed to the patient and his or her family.

11. Consider how to minimize the patient's risk of contracting the current (and other) CNS infections in the future; administer appropriate vaccines after recovery from the acute infection.

12. Arrange for patient follow-up after discharge from the hospital. Continue to monitor for neurologic sequelae for several months after completion of treatment, and educate the patient and family in this regard. Serious complications that may occur include, among others, hearing loss, hemiparesis, quadriparesis, muscular hypertonia, ataxia, seizure disorders, mental retardation, learning disabilities, and obstructive hydrocephalus.

with gram-negative bacilli, prolonged fever, and recurrent meningitis. Repeat the LP in neonates to determine the duration of therapy. Repeat LP also may be performed to relieve elevated intracranial pressure. Expect repeat blood cultures to become negative quickly during therapy and the serum WBC count to improve and normalize with appropriate antimicrobial therapy.

Evaluate antimicrobial dosing regimens to ensure efficacy of the treatment regimen. Trough vancomycin concentrations of 15 to 20 mg/L (10 to 14 µmol/L) are recommended for the treatment of CNS infections.[18] Monitor patients for drug adverse effects, drug allergies, and drug interactions. The specific safety monitoring plan will depend on the antibiotic(s) used (Table 70–3). Pay close attention to concomitant medications in patients on rifampin for treatment or prophylaxis. Rifampin is a potent inducer of hepatic metabolism and may reduce the efficacy of other drugs metabolized by the cytochrome P-450 3A enzyme pathway.

Abbreviations Introduced in This Chapter

CDC	Centers for Disease Control and Prevention
CLSI	Clinical and Laboratory Standards Institute
CNS	Central nervous system
CSF	Cerebrospinal fluid
DIC	Disseminated intravascular coagulation
ESBL	Extended spectrum beta-lactamase
GBS	Group B *Streptococcus*
Hib	*Haemophilus influenzae* type B
HSV	Herpes simplex virus
IDSA	Infectious Diseases Society of America
IL-1	Interleukin 1
LP	Lumbar puncture
MBC	Minimum bactericidal concentration
MIC	Minimum inhibitory concentration
MRSA	Methicillin-resistant *Staphylococcus aureus*
MRSE	Methicillin-resistant *Staphylococcus epidermidis*
NSAIDS	Nonsteroidal anti-inflammatory drugs
PCR	Polymerase chain reaction
PMN	Polymorphonuclear cell
SJS	Stevens-Johnson Syndrome
TNF-α	Tumor necrosis factor-alpha

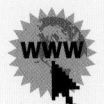 Self-assessment questions and answers are available at *http://mhpharmacotherapy.com/pp.html*.

REFERENCES

1. van de Beek D, de Gans J, McIntyre P, Prasad K. Corticosteroids for acute bacterial meningitis. Cochrane Database Syst Rev 2003;3:CD004405.
2. van de Beek D, de Gans J, Spanjaard L, et al. Clinical features and prognostic factors in adults with bac terial meningitis. N Engl J Med 2004;351(18):1849–1859.
3. Thigpen MC, Whitney CG, Messonnier NE, et al. Bacterial meningitis in the United States, 1998-2007. N Engl J Med 2011;364(21):2016–2025.
4. Aronin SI, Peduzzi P, Quagliarello VJ. Common-acquired bacterial meningitis: Risk stratification for adverse clinical outcome and effect of antibiotic timing. Ann Intern Med 1998;129(11):862–869.
5. van de Beek D, de Gans J, Tunkel AR, Wijdicks EFM. Community-acquired bacterial meningitis in adults. N Engl J Med 2006;354:44–53.
6. Schuchat A, Robinson K, Wenger JD, et al. Bacterial meningitis in the United States in 1995. N Engl J Med 1997;337(14):970–976.
7. Centers for Disease Control and Prevention. Progress toward elimination of Haemophilus influenzae type b invasive disease among infants and children—United States, 1998–2000. MMWR Recomm Rep 2002;51(RR11):234–237.
8. Lexau CA, Lynfield R, Danila R, et al. Changing epidemiology of invasive pneumococcal disease among older adults in the era of pediatric pneumococcal conjugate vaccine. JAMA 2005;294(16):2043–2051.
9. Nigrovic LE, Kuppermann N, Malley R, et al. Children with bacterial meningitis presenting to the emergency department during the pneumococcal conjugate vaccine era. Acad Emerg Med 2008;15:522–528.
10. Sejvar JJ. The evolving epidemiology of viral encephalitis. Curr Opin Neurol 2006;19:350–357.
11. Mitropoulous IF, Hermsen ED, Schafer JA, Rotschafer JC. Central nervous system infections. In: DiPiro JT, Talbert RL, Yee GC, et al., eds. Pharmacotherapy: A Pathophysiologic Approach. 7th ed. New York City: McGraw-Hill; 2008:1743–1760.
12. Khetsuriani N, Holman RC, Anderson LJ. Burden of encephalitis-associated hospitalizations in the United States, 1988–1997. Clin Infect Dis 2002;35:175–182.
13. Chamberlain MC. Neoplastic meningitis. J Clin Oncol 2005;23(15):3605–3613.
14. Moris G, Garcia-Monco JC. The challenge of drug-induced aseptic meningitis. Arch Intern Med 1999;159(11):1185–1194.
15. Scheld WM, Koedel U, Nathan B, Pfister HW. Pathophysiology of bacterial meningitis: mechanism(s) of neuronal injury. J Infect Dis 2002;186(Suppl 2):S225–S233.
16. Kim KS. Pathogenesis of bacterial meningitis: From bacteraemia to neuronal injury. Nat Rev Neurosci 2003;4:376–385.
17. Bashir HE, Laundy M, Booy R. Diagnosis and treatment of bacterial meningitis. Arch Dis Child 2003;88:615–620.
18. Tunkel AR, Hartman BJ, Kaplan SL, et al. Practice guidelines for the management of bacterial meningitis. Clin Infect Dis 2004;39:1267–1284.
19. Choi C. Bacterial meningitis in aging adults. Clin Infect Dis 2001;33:1380–1385.
20. Swartz MN. Bacterial meningitis—A view of the past 90 years. N Engl J Med 2004;351(18):1826–1828.
21. van Deuren M, Brandtzaeg P, van der Meer JWM. Update on meningococcal disease with emphasis on pathogenesis and clinical management. Clin Microbiol Rev 2000;13(1):144–166.
22. Lu CH, Huang CR, Chang, WN, et al. Community-acquired bacterial meningitis in adults: The epidemiology, timing of appropriate antimicrobial therapy, and prognostic factors. Clin Neurol Neurosurg 2002;104:352–358.
23. Miner JR, Heegaard W, Mapes A, Biros M. Presentation, time to antibiotics, and mortality of patients with bacterial meningitis at an urban county medical center. J Emerg Med 2001;21:387–392.
24. Radetsky M. Duration of symptoms and outcome in bacterial meningitis: An analysis of causation and the implications of a delay in diagnosis. Pediatr Infect Dis J 1992;11:694–698.
25. Schaad UB, Suter S, Gianella-Borradori A, et al. A comparison of ceftriaxone and cefuroxime for the treatment of bacterial meningitis in children. N Engl J Med 1990;322(3):141–147.
26. Quagliarello VJ, Scheld WM. Treatment of bacterial meningitis. N Engl J Med 1997;336(10):708–716.
27. Pankey GA, Sabath LR. Clinical relevance of bacterio-static versus bactericidal mechanisms of action in the treatment of gram-positive bacterial infections. Clin Infect Dis 2004;38:864–870.
28. Sinner SW, Tunkel AR. Antimicrobial agents in the treatment of bacterial meningitis. Infect Dis Clin N Am 2004;18:581–602.
29. Tice AD, Strait K, Ramey R, et al. Outpatient parenteral antimicrobial therapy for central nervous system infections. Clin Infect Dis 1999;29:1394–1399.
30. Jones ME, Draghi DC, Karlowsky JA, Sahm DF, Bradley JS. Prevalence of antimicrobial resistance in bacteria isolated from central nervous system specimens as reported by U.S. hospital laboratories from

2000 to 2002 (Online. Updated March 25, 2004). Ann Clin Microb 2004;3:3 (online journal published March 25, 2004).

31. Centers for Disease Control and Prevention. Prevention and control of meningococcal disease. MMWR Recomm Rep 2005;54(RR07): 1–21.

32. Rosenstein NE, Perkins BA, Stephens DS, Popovic T, Hughes JM. Meningococcal disease. N Engl J Med 2001;344(18):1378–1388.

33. Kim KS. Acute Bacterial Meningitis in Infants and Children. Lancet Infect Dis 2010;10(1):32–42.

34. Campos-Outcalt D. Meningococcal vaccine: New product, new recommendations. J Fam Pract 2005;54(4):324–326.

35. Nudelman Y, Tunkel AR. Bacterial Meningitis Epidemiology, Pathogenesis, and Management Update. Drugs 2009;69(18):2577–2596.

36. Updated recommendations for use of meningococcal conjugate vaccines—Advisory Committee on Immunization Practices, 2010. Morb Mortal Wkly Rep 2011;60(3):72–76.

37. Centers for Disease Control and Prevention. Direct and indirect effects of routine vaccination of children with 7-valent pneumococcal conjugate vaccine on incidence of invasive pneumococcal disease—United States, 1998–2003. Morb Mortal Wkly Rep 2005;54(36):893–897.

38. Advisory Committee on Immunization Practices (ACIP). Prevention of pneumococcal disease among infacts and children—use of 13-valent pneumococcal conjugate vaccine and 23-valent pneumococcal polysaccharide vaccine. Morb Mortal Wkly Rep 2011;59:RR-11.

39. Mylonakis D, Hohmann EL, Calderwood SB. Central nervous system infection with Listeria monocytogenes: 33 years' experience at a general hospital and review of 776 episodes from the literature. Medicine 1998;77(5):313–336.

40. Hof H. An update on the medical management of Listeriosis. Expert Opin Pharmacother 2004;5(8):1727–1735.

41. Department of Health and Human Services/CDC. Prevention of Perinatal Group B Streptococcal Disease. Morb Mortal Wkly Rep 2010;59:RR-10.

42. Shah S, Ohlsson A, Shah V. Intraventricular antibiotics for bacterial meningitis in neonates. Cochrane Database Syst Rev 2004;4:CD004496.

43. Villani P, Regazzi MB, Marubbi F, et al. Cerebrospinal fluid linezolid concentrations in postneurosurgical central nervous system infections. Antimicrob Agents Chemother 2002;46(3):936–937.

44. Anderson EJ, Yogev R. A rational approach to the management of ventricular shunt infections. Pediatr Infect Dis J 2005;24:557–558.

45. Lee DH, Palermo B, Chowdhury M. Successful treatment of methicillin-resistant Staphylococcus aureus meningitis with daptomycin. Clin Infect Dis 2008;47:588–589.

46. Sawyer MH. Enterovirus infections: Diagnosis and treatment. Pediatr Infect Dis J 1999;18(12):1033–1040.

47. Barker FG. Efficacy of prophylactic antibiotics against meningitis after craniotomy: A meta-analysis. Neurosurgery 2007;60:887–894.

48. Korinek AM, Golmard JL, Elcheick A, et al. Risk factors for neurosurgical site infections after craniotomy: A critical reappraisal of antibiotic prophylaxis on 4,578 patients. Br J Neurosurg 2005;19: 155–162.

49. Reichert MC, Medeiros EA, Ferraz FA. Hospital-acquired meningitis in patients undergoing craniotomy: Incidence, evolution, and risk factors. Am J Infect Control 2002;30:158–164.

50. Tyler KL. Herpes simplex virus infections of the central nervous system: Encephalitis and meningitis, including Mollaret's. Herpes 2004;11(Suppl 2):57A–64A.

51. Kimberlin D. Herpes simplex virus, meningitis and encephalitis in neonates. Herpes 2004;11(Suppl 2):65A–76A.

52. Tunkel AR, Glaser CA, Bloch KC, et al. The management of encephalitis: Clinical practice guidelines by the Infectious Diseases Society of America. Clin Infect Dis 2008;47:303–327.

53. Roos KL. Encephalitis. Neurol Clin 1999;17:813–833.

54. Pereira-Chioccola VL, Vidal JE, Su C. Toxoplasma gondii infection and cerebral toxoplasmosis in HIV-infected patients. Future Microbiol 2009;4(10):1363-1379

55. Centers for Disease Control and Prevention Guidelines for Prevention and Treatment of Opportunistic Infections in HIV-infected Adults and Adolescents. Morb Mortal Wkly Rep 2009;58:RR-4.

56. American Academy of Pediatrics. Pneumococcal infections. In: Pickering, LK, ed. Red Book: 2003 Report of the Committee on Infectious Diseases. 26th ed. Elk Grove Village, IL: American Academy of Pediatrics; 2003:490–500.

57. Mongelluzzo J, Mohamad Z, Ten Have TR, Shah SS. Corticosteroids and mortality in children with bacterial meningitis. JAMA 2008;299(17):2048–2055.

58. de Gans J, van de Beek D, for the European Dexamethasone in Adulthood Bacterial Meningitis Study Investigators. N Engl J Med 2002;347(20):1549–1556.

59. Scarborough M, Gordon SB, Whitty CJM, et al. Corticosteroids for bacterial meningitis in adults in Sub-Saharan Africa. N Engl J Med 2007;357:2441–2450.

60. Ricard JD, Wolff M, Lacherade JC, et al. Levels of vancomycin in cerebrospinal fluid of adult patients receiving adjunctive corticosteroids to treat pneumo-coccal meningitis: A prospective multicenter observational study. Clin Infect Dis 2007;44:250–255.

71

Lower Respiratory Tract Infections

Diane M. Cappelletty

LEARNING OBJECTIVES

● **Upon completion of the chapter, the reader will be able to:**

1. List the common pathogens that cause community-acquired pneumonia (CAP), aspiration pneumonia, ventilator-associated pneumonia (VAP; early versus late onset), and healthcare-associated pneumonia.

2. Explain the host defenses that protect against infection.

3. Explain the pathophysiology of pneumonia.

4. List the signs and symptoms associated with CAP and VAP.

5. Identify patient and organism factors required to guide the selection of a specific antimicrobial regimen for an individual patient.

6. Design an appropriate empirical antimicrobial regimen based on patient-specific data for an individual with CAP, aspiration pneumonia, and VAP or healthcare-associated pneumonia (early versus late onset).

7. Design an appropriate antimicrobial regimen based on both patient- and organism-specific data.

8. Develop a monitoring plan based on patient-specific information for a patient with CAP and healthcare-associated pneumonia or VAP.

9. Formulate appropriate educational information to be provided to a patient with pneumonia.

KEY CONCEPTS

❶ There are five classifications of pneumonia: community-acquired, aspiration, hospital-acquired, ventilator-associated, and healthcare-associated.

❷ The etiology of bacterial pneumonia varies in accordance with the type of pneumonia.

❸ *Streptococcus pneumoniae* is the most common bacterial pathogen associated with community-acquired pneumonia (CAP).

❹ The signs and symptoms and severity of pneumonia are needed not only to diagnose the infection but also to determine and assess response to therapy.

❺ The goal of therapy is to eliminate the patient's symptoms, minimize or prevent complications, and decrease mortality.

❻ Antimicrobial treatment of CAP is predominantly empirical.

❼ Selection of antimicrobial therapy for ventilator-associated, health-care associated, and hospital-associated pneumonia is empirical and broad spectrum; however, once culture and susceptibility information are

available, the antimicrobial therapy should be narrowed (de-escalation) to cover the identified pathogen(s).

❽ Duration of antimicrobial therapy should be kept to the shortest length possible.

❾ Monitoring response to therapy is essential for determining efficacy, identifying adverse reactions, and determining the duration of therapy.

❿ Prevention of both pneumococcal and influenza pneumonia by use of vaccination is a national goal.

Pneumonia is inflammation of the lung with consolidation. The cause of the inflammation is infection, which can be caused by a wide range of organisms. ❶ *There are five classifications of pneumonia: community-acquired, aspiration, hospital-acquired, ventilator-associated, and healthcare-associated.* Patients who develop pneumonia in the outpatient setting and have not been in any healthcare facilities, which include wound care and hemodialysis clinics, have community-acquired pneumonia (CAP). Pneumonia can be caused by aspiration of either oropharyngeal or gastrointestinal contents. Hospital-acquired pneumonia (HAP) is defined as pneumonia that occurs 48 hours or more after admission.[1,2] Ventilator-associated pneumonia (VAP) requires endotracheal intubation for at least 48 to 72 hours before the onset of pneumonia.[2,3] The newest category is healthcare-associated pneumonia (HCAP), which is defined as pneumonia occurring in any patient hospitalized for at least 2 days within 90 days of the onset of the infection; residing in a nursing home or long-term care facility; received IV antibiotic therapy, wound care, or chemotherapy within the last 30 days prior to the onset of the infection; or having attended a hemodialysis clinic.[2,4]

EPIDEMIOLOGY AND ETIOLOGY

Etiology and Mortality Rates

❷ *The etiology of bacterial pneumonia varies in accordance with the type of pneumonia.* Table 71–1 lists the more common pathogens associated with the various types or classifications of pneumonia. *Streptococcus pneumoniae* colonizes the nasopharyngeal flora in up to 50% of healthy adults and may colonize the lower airways in individuals with chronic bronchitis.[5,6] It possesses many virulence factors, enhancing its ability to cause infection in the respiratory tract. ❸ Therefore, *it is not surprising that S. pneumoniae is the predominant bacterial pathogen associated with CAP.* The second most common pathogen is one of the atypical organisms, *Mycoplasma pneumoniae.* Nontypeable *Haemophilus influenzae* intermittently colonizes about 80% of the population, and the incidence of permanent colonization increases in chronic obstructive pulmonary disease (COPD) patients and those with cystic fibrosis. Therefore, the likelihood of nontypeable *H. influenzae* causing pneumonia increases in COPD patients. *Moraxella catarrhalis* is a more common

cause of pneumonia in the very young and the very old. *Chlamydia pneumoniae* and *Legionella pneumophila* are less frequent causes than the other bacterial and atypical organisms. Community-acquired methicillin-resistant *Staphylococcus aureus* (CA-MRSA) is associated with necrotizing and severe pneumonia in healthy children and young adults. Less than 2% of all CA-MRSA infections are pneumonia (most are skin and soft tissue); however, the number of reports of pneumonia are increasing.[7]

Viruses are a common cause of CAP in children (about 65%) and much less common in adults (about 15%).[8] Viruses often associated with pneumonia in adults include influenza A and B and adenoviruses, whereas less common causes include rhinoviruses, enteroviruses, cytomegalovirus, varicella-zoster virus, herpes simplex virus, and others. In children, viral pneumonia is more commonly caused by respiratory syncytial virus, influenza A, and parainfluenza, and less commonly the viruses are similar to those listed previously for adults. Influenza is associated with seasonal local outbreaks (epidemics) and global outbreaks (pandemics). Influenza viruses are characterized and named for the hemagglutinin (H) and neuraminidase (N) proteins on the surface of the viruses. There are 16 hemagglutinin and nine neuraminidase subtypes of influenza A, and H1–3 and N1 and 2 are the principal antigenic types found in humans.[9]

Mortality associated with CAP is dependent on the severity of the illness and the age of the patient. In elderly patients admitted to the hospital with severe pneumonia, the mortality rate is up to 40%.[10–13] In the outpatient setting (mild to moderate disease), the mortality rate is less than 5%.[14] Mortality among case reports of CA-MRSA necrotizing pneumonia is 42%.[7] Pneumonia owing to aspiration of oral contents is caused by a variety of anaerobes (*Bacteroides spp., Fusobacterium spp., Prevotella spp.,* and anaerobic gram-positive cocci) as well as *Streptococcus spp. Moraxella catarrhalis* and *Eikenella corrodens* may be involved but much less frequently.[15,16] When gastric contents are aspirated, enteric gram-negative bacilli and *Staphylococcus aureus* are more commonly the pathogens.[16]

HAP, VAP, and HCAP may be caused by a wide spectrum of organisms. HCAP, early onset HAP and VAP are commonly caused by enteric gram-negative bacilli in addition to the bacteria listed previously for CAP. Late-onset HAP and VAP are more likely to be caused by more resistant enteric gram-negative bacilli, *Pseudomonas aeruginosa, Acinetobacter spp.,* or *S. aureus.* Rarely are viruses or fungi a cause of HAP, VAP, or HCAP. The number of infections caused by multidrug-resistant (MDR) bacteria is increasing significantly in hospitalized patients.[4,13,17–19]

PATHOPHYSIOLOGY

Local Host Defenses

Local host defenses of both the upper and lower respiratory tract along with the anatomy of the airways are important in preventing infection. Upper respiratory defenses include the mucociliary apparatus of the nasopharynx, nasal hair,

---

Table 71–1	
Common Pathogens by Type of Pneumonia	
Type of Pneumonia	**Common Pathogens**
Community	Aerobic bacteria: *S. pneumoniae, H. influenzae, M. catarrhalis*
	Atypical: *M. pneumoniae, C. pneumoniae, L. pneumophila,* respiratory viruses
Aspiration	Oral contents: Anaerobes, *Viridans* streptococci
	GI contents with pH increase
	Enteric gram-negative bacilli
Hospital	(Early onset, no risk factors for resistant pathogens)
Ventilator health care	*S. pneumoniae,* MSSA, *E. coli, K. pneumoniae,* (*M. pneumoniae, C. pneumoniae* are rare)
Hospital	(Late onset and/or risk factors for resistant pathogens)
Ventilator health care	MRSA, extended-spectrum β-lactamase-producing *K. pneumoniae, P. aeruginosa, Acinetobacter* spp.

MRSA, methicillin-resistant *Staphylococcus aureus;* MSSA, methicillin-susceptible *S. aureus.*

normal bacterial flora, IgA, and complement. Local host defenses of the lower respiratory tract include cough, mucociliary apparatus of the trachea and bronchi, antibodies (IgA, IgM, and IgG), complement, and alveolar macrophages. Mucous lines the cells of the respiratory tract, forming a protective barrier for the cells. This minimizes the ability of organisms to attach to the cells and initiate the infectious process. The squamous epithelial cells of the upper respiratory tract are not ciliated, but those of the columnar epithelial cells of the lower tract are. The cilia beat in a uniform fashion upward, moving particles up and out of the lower respiratory tract.

Particles greater than 10 microns (μm) are efficiently trapped by mechanisms of the upper airway and are removed from the nasopharynx either by swallowing or by expulsion. The mucociliary apparatus of the trachea and bronchi along with the sharp angles of the bronchi often are effective at trapping and eliminating particles that are 2 to 10 μm in size. Particles in the range of 0.5 to 1 μm may consistently reach the alveolar sacs of the lung. Microorganisms fall within this size range, and if they reach the alveolar sacs, then infection may result if alveolar macrophages and other defenses cannot contain the organisms.

Aspiration

Aspiration of the oropharyngeal or gastric contents may lead to aspiration pneumonia or chemical (acid) pneumonitis. Risk factors for aspiration include dysphagia, change in oropharyngeal colonization, gastroesophageal reflux (GER), and decreased host defenses.

Dysphagia can be caused by stroke or other neurologic disorders, seizures, alcoholism, and aging.[15] Oropharyngeal colonization may be altered by oral/dental disease, poor oral hygiene, tube feedings, or medications. This could result in a higher number of anaerobic organisms in the oral cavity or colonization with enteric gram-negative bacilli.[15] GER occurs in all individuals to a degree; however, those with

GER disease (GERD) have it more frequently. Acid suppression is an important factor in the treatment of GERD, which may allow enteric gram-negative bacilli to colonize the gastric contents. Finally, impaired mucous production or cilia function, decreased immunoglobulin in secretions, and altered cough reflex may increase the likelihood of infection following an aspiration. The infection can result in a necrotizing pneumonia or lung abscess.

HAP, VAP, HCAP

Risk factors for the development of HAP fall into four general categories: intubation and mechanical ventilation, aspiration, oropharyngeal colonization, and hyperglycemia.

Intubation and mechanical ventilation increase the risk of HAP/VAP 6- to 21-fold.[2,20] VAP may also be related to colonization of the ventilator circuit.[21] Risk of aspiration is increased in these patients due to the supine positioning of the patient, the presence of the endotracheal tube preventing the closure of the epiglottis over the glottis, enteral feedings, GER, and medications.[21] Oropharyngeal colonization is affected by the use of antibiotics, oral antiseptics, and poor infection control measures, which may decrease normal commensal flora and allow pathogenic organisms to colonize the oral cavity. Hyperglycemia may directly or indirectly promote infection; two proposed mechanisms are inhibiting phagocytosis and providing additional nutrients for bacteria.

Once breakdown of the local host defenses occurs and organisms invade the lung tissue, an inflammatory response is generated either by the organisms causing tissue damage or by the immune response to the presence of the organisms. This inflammatory response either can remain localized in the infected tissue or can become systemic. The role of the alveolar macrophages is two-fold. First, to engulf the organisms and to contain the infection, and second, to process the antigens for presentation in order to generate a specific immune response by either the cell-mediated or humoral system,

---

Patient Encounter 1, Part 1

A 36-year-old woman presents to your ED complaining of difficulty breathing and shortness of breath. Her physical examination reveals that she is alert and oriented ×3, has decreased breath sounds on the right side compared with the left, and has rales and crackles in the right lower lobe. Her temperature is 38.6°C (101.5°F), respiratory rate is 18 breaths/min, and blood pressure is 120/80 mm Hg.

What are her signs and symptoms of pneumonia?

What are the top two organisms that could be causing the pneumonia?

What additional information do you need to know before creating a treatment plan for this patient?

Patient Encounter 2, Part 1

A 63-year-old man was admitted to the hospital secondary to a motor vehicle accident. Five days after admission he developed respiratory failure and was intubated. The chest x-ray revealed bilateral lower lobe infiltrates. He is sedated but does respond to commands. His temperature is 38.2°C (100.8°F), his blood pressure is 110/70 mm Hg, and his WBC is $16.8 \times 10^3/mm^3$ ($16.8 \times 10^9/L$) with a cell differential of 74% (0.74) neutrophils, 6% (0.06) bands, 17% (0.17) lymphocytes, and 3% (0.03) monocytes.

What are his signs and symptoms of pneumonia?

What are the top three organisms that could be causing the pneumonia?

What additional information do you need to know before creating a treatment plan for this patient?

or both. The macrophages release cytokines in the area of the infection, which result in increased mucous production, constricting the local vasculature and lymphatic vessels and attraction of other immune cells to the site. The increase in mucous is associated with symptoms such as cough and sputum production. If tumor necrosis factor alpha (TNF-α) and interleukins-1 and -6 are released systemically, then the symptoms become more severe and include hypotension, organ dysfunction, and/or a septic or septic-shock clinical presentation.

CLINICAL PRESENTATION AND DIAGNOSIS

Several scoring systems are available for assessing the severity of the pneumonia: the Pneumonia Severity Index (PSI); Confusion, Uremia, Respiratory Rate, Blood pressure (CURB); CURB-65 (for those 65 years of age and older), and Systolic BP, Oxygenation, Age, and Respiratory rate (SOAR).[10,13,22] Some of the characteristics evaluated with these models include but are not limited to age, comorbidities, blood pressure, mental status, respiratory rate, oxygenation, and organ function. PSI or CURB-65 scores less than or equal to 70 and less than 2 respectively, correlate with mild disease that should be treated in the outpatient setting. These models are used by physicians to help determine the severity of illness, prognosis (mortality risk), and the need for hospitalization and then to help guide in the selection of antimicrobial therapy, along with the use of published guidelines.[10,13,14]

Clinical Presentation of CAP or Aspiration Pneumonia

General

Patients may experience nonrespiratory symptoms in addition to respiratory symptoms. With increasing age, both respiratory and nonrespiratory symptoms decrease in frequency.

④ Symptoms

- Respiratory—cough (productive or nonproductive), shortness of breath, and difficulty breathing
- Nonrespiratory—fever, fatigue, sweats, headache, myalgias, mental status changes

Signs

- Temperature may increase or decrease from baseline, but most often it is elevated. The temperature may be sustained or intermittent.
- Respiratory rate is often increased. Cyanosis, increased respiratory rate, and use of accessory muscles of respiration are suggestive of severe respiratory compromise.
- Breath sounds may be diminished. Rales or rhonchi may be heard.
- Confusion, lethargy, and disorientation are relatively common in elderly patients.

Diagnostic Tests

- Chest x-ray should reveal single or multiple infiltrates.
- Oxygen saturation should be over 90% (0.90), as determined by pulse oximetry.
- Arterial blood gases are beneficial primarily in patients with severe pneumonia.

Laboratory Tests

- The WBC may or may not be elevated. In elderly patients, a drop in WBCs also can be a sign of infection. The differential should show a predominance of neutrophils if a bacterial infection is present. The presence of bands also could be an indicator of bacterial infection. Elevated lymphocytes are an indication of viral infection.
- Blood urea nitrogen (BUN) and serum creatinine are needed to dose antibiotics appropriately and to minimize or prevent drug toxicity (especially in the elderly patient).

Microbiology Tests

- Sputum Gram stain should demonstrate the presence of WBCs and the absence of squamous epithelial cells. It may or may not show a predominance of one type of organism.
- Sputum culture and susceptibility are not obtained in the outpatient setting. The value of culturing is debated owing to the rapidity in which *S. pneumoniae* dies in transport media and the inability to reliably or routinely culture atypical organisms.
- Bronchoscopy may be performed to improve the ability to diagnose pneumonia. Tracheal secretions often are better specimens than sputum owing to the lack of oral contamination.
- Serology (IgM and IgG) is useful in determining the presence of atypical organisms such as *Mycoplasma* and *Chlamydia*.
- Urinary Legionella antigen is used to diagnose *L. pneumophila*.
- Polymerase chain reaction (PCR) is being used more frequently to detect the DNA of respiratory pathogens.
- Blood cultures must be obtained in all patients hospitalized with pneumonia to comply with Joint Commission on Accreditation of Healthcare Organizations (JCAHO) pneumonia guidelines. Positive blood cultures are present in about 1% to 20% of patients with CAP.

Clinical Presentation of Severe CAP or Aspiration Pneumonia

General

In approximately 10% of patients, CAP will be severe enough to require intensive care or mechanical ventilation.

Symptoms ❹

- Respiratory—cough (productive or nonproductive), shortness of breath, difficulty breathing
- Nonrespiratory—fever, fatigue, sweats, headache, myalgias, mental status changes

Signs

- Temperature may increase or decrease from baseline, but most often it is elevated. The temperature may be sustained or intermittent.
- Respiratory rate greater than 30 breaths per minute. Cyanosis and use of accessory muscles of respiration along with the increased respiratory rate are suggestive of severe respiratory compromise.
- Hypotension (systolic blood pressure less than 90 mm Hg or diastolic blood pressure less than 60 mm Hg).

- Requirement for vasopressors.
- Breath sounds may be diminished. Rales or rhonchi may be heard.
- Urine output less than 20 mL/h or less than 80 mL over 4 hours.
- Confusion, lethargy, and disorientation are relatively common in elderly patients.

Diagnostic Tests

As stated in the clinical presentation of community-acquired or aspiration pneumonia

Laboratory Tests

As stated in the clinical presentation of community-acquired or aspiration pneumonia

Microbiology Tests

As stated in the clinical presentation of community-acquired or aspiration pneumonia

Diagnosis of VAP

Clinical Strategy

- Chest x-ray should reveal a new infiltrate *plus* two of the following:
  - Temperature greater than 38.0°C (100.4°F)
  - Leukocytosis or leukopenia
  - Purulent secretions
  - Semiquantitative cultures are obtained to identify the pathogen(s)
- Tracheal aspirates grow more organisms than invasive quantitative cultures and often result in overuse of antibiotics
- The major limitation of the clinical strategy is the consistent overprescribing of antibiotics

Bacteriologic Strategy

- Uses quantitative culture of endotracheal aspirates, bronchoalveolar lavage (BAL), or protected specimen brush (PSB)
- Greater than or equal to 10^6 cfu/mL (10^9 cfu/L) for endotracheal aspirates
- Greater than or equal to 10^4 to 10^5 cfu/mL (10^7 to 10^8 cfu/L) for BAL
- Greater than or equal to 10^3 cfu/mL (10^6 cfu/L) for PSB
- The advantage of this method is that it separates colonization from infection better than culturing tracheal aspirates.

- The limitation is the potential misinterpretation of negative culture results. These samples should be obtained prior to antibiotics being started.

Recommended Diagnostic Strategy

- Combination of the preceding two methods
- Obtain either a quantitative or semiquantitative culture of a lower respiratory sample. Initiate empirical broad-spectrum antibiotic therapy
- Days 2 and 3: Check culture results, and assess clinical response to therapy: temperature, WBCs, chest x-ray, oxygenation, purulent sputum, hemodynamic changes, and organ function
- Assess clinical improvement at 48 to 72 hours:
  - Improvement and culture negative—stop antibiotics
  - Improvement and culture positive—narrow antibiotic therapy
  - No improvement and culture negative—consider other pathogens, complications, or other diagnosis
  - No improvement and culture positive—change antibiotic therapy and consider other pathogens, complications, or other diagnosis

TREATMENT

Desired Outcomes

⑤ *The goal of antibiotic therapy is to eliminate the patient's symptoms, minimize or prevent complications, and decrease mortality.* Potential complications secondary to pneumonia include further decline in pulmonary function in patients with underlying pulmonary disease, prolonged mechanical ventilation, bacteremia/sepsis/septic shock, and death. Use of an antimicrobial agent with the narrowest spectrum of activity that covers the suspected pathogen(s) without having activity against organisms not involved in the infection is preferred to minimize the development of resistance.

General Approach to Treatment

● Designing a therapeutic regimen for any patient with any type of pneumonia begins with three general categories of consideration:

1. Patient specific factors that will impact therapy.

2. The top one to three organisms likely causing the infection and resistance issues associated with each organism.

3. The antimicrobials that will cover these organisms. The spectrum should not be too broad or narrow; they should penetrate into the site of infection and be the most cost effective.

Patient factors that need to be considered include age, renal function, drug allergies and/or drug intolerances, immune status (diabetes, neutropenia, or immunocompromised host), cardiopulmonary disease, pregnancy, medical insurance and prescription coverage, exposure to resistant organisms, and prior antibiotic exposure(s) (what agents and when).

- The most common pathogens vary with the type of pneumonia, and they are listed in Table 71–1. *M. pneumoniae* lack a cell wall; therefore, β-lactam drugs have no activity against this organism. The atypical organisms have not changed in recent years with respect to antibiotic resistance. β-Lactamase production in *H. influenzae* has remained relatively steady over the last 5 to 10 years, and the rate is approximately 25%.[23] *S. pneumoniae* has developed resistance mechanisms against many classes of antimicrobials, and the mechanisms include:

- Alteration of the penicillin-binding proteins (PBPs), inactivating β-lactams

- Efflux or methylation of the ribosome-inactivating macrolides

- Ribosome protection (tetM gene) inactivating tetracyclines

- Alteration of DNA gyrase or topoisomerase IV inactivating fluoroquinolones

Resistance to commonly prescribed antimicrobials such as the penicillins and macrolides/azalides dramatically increased in the late 1980s through the mid- to late 1990s and has remained relatively flat in the 2000s. Resistance information

---

Patient Encounter 1, Part 2: Medical History, Physical Examination, and Diagnostic Tests

A 36-year-old woman presents to your ED complaining of difficulty breathing and shortness of breath.

PMH: IDDM for 15 years; hypertension for 1 year, currently controlled

FH: Father died of lung cancer at the age of 68 years; mother died of natural causes

SH: Denies tobacco and alcohol use. Lives with her husband and 2 children aged 4 and 7 years. The past 3 days she has been caring for her 4-year-old daughter who has been home from daycare with acute otitis media and possible URI. She is 5 ft 3 in (160 cm) and weighs 180 lb (81.8 kg).

Allergies: NKDA

Meds: Humalog 75/2540 units once daily; Lisinopril 10 mg orally once daily

ROS: (+) difficulty breathing and shortness of breath; (−) chest pain, N/V/D, change in appetite

PE:

VS: BP 120/80, P 82, RR 28, T 38.6°C (101.5°F)

CV: RRR, normal S_1, S_2; no murmurs, rubs, or gallops

Lungs: Decreased breath sounds on the right side compared with the left with rales and crackles in the right lower lobe

Abd: Soft, nontender, nondistended; (+) bowel sounds, no hepatosplenomegaly, heme (−) stool

Neuro: Oriented ×2, somewhat confused and disoriented to place

Diagnostic Tests: Chest x-ray: right lower lobe infiltrates; oxygen saturation 86% (0.86) on room air

Labs: WBCs $19.2 \times 10^3/\text{mm}^3$ ($19.2 \times 10^9/\text{L}$) with a cell differential of 70% (0.70) neutrophils, 8% (0.08) bands, 16% (0.16) lymphocytes, and 6% (0.06) monocytes; BUN 9 mg/dL (3.2mmol/L), SCr 0.9 mg/dL (80 μmol/L), glucose 360 mg/dL (20.0mmol/L); sputum Gram stain: moderate gram-positive diplococci, many WBCs; sputum culture is pending

Given this additional information, what is your assessment of the patient's condition?

Identify your treatment goals for the patient.

---

collected nationally using the Tracking Resistance in the US Today (TRUST) surveillance database, along with susceptibility testing for a new antimicrobials, demonstrates that average national rates of resistance to penicillin and macrolides were approximately 13% and 38%, respectively.[24,25] Resistance to trimethoprim/sulfamethoxazole is approximately 25%, and fluoroquinolone resistance remains less than 0.5%.[25] Susceptibility results alone do not account for clinical success or failures when treating pneumonia. Therefore, despite the 13% and 32% resistance to penicillin and macrolides, the clinical failure rate is less than this. Because CAP in the outpatient setting is treated empirically, establishing a meaningful clinical failure rate with any therapy is difficult to do. No studies have been performed establishing a correlation between clinical failure rates with a particular antimicrobial agent and the percentage of resistance.

For HCAP, HAP, and VAP, the risk of infection from an MDR pathogen is relatively high. The number and type of organisms that are MDR vary from hospital to hospital, making it more difficult to generate guidelines for treatment. Therefore, the treatment recommendations may be too broad or too narrow for any given institution. Treating patients with HCAP, HAP, or VAP is more complex than treating patients with CAP. There are many factors to consider, and one of those relates to the timing of infection to the most likely pathogens. Early-onset infection is less likely to be caused by MDR pathogens than late-onset infection. In early-onset infection, community pathogens such as pneumococcus, *Legionella*, and *Mycoplasma* need to be considered as well as some of the hospital pathogens. Patients developing late-onset pneumonia are at increased risk of have a resistant pathogen or MDR pathogen such as MRSA, enteric gram-negative bacilli, *Pseudomonas*, and *Acinetobacter*. Another issue is how HCAP and HAP are studied compared with VAP. The majority of studies were performed using patients that were intubated. Therefore, the body of literature supporting the treatment recommendations is greatest for VAP and not for HCAP or HAP. The evidence-based guidelines generated by the American Thoracic Society and Infectious Diseases Society of America were derived from VAP and applied to HCAP and HAP.

Risk factors for developing infection caused by a resistant pathogen are generally related to the prior use of antibiotics, insertion of catheters or other invasive devices, and hospitalization in a unit contaminated/colonized with resistant organisms. The following is a more complete list of factors influencing infection from a resistant organism.

- Antimicrobial therapy in preceding 90 days
- Current hospitalization of at least 5 days
- High occurrence of antibiotic resistance in the community or in the specific hospital unit
- Immunosuppressive disease and/or therapy
- Presence of risk factors for HCAP:
  - Hospitalization for 2 days or more in the preceding 90 days
  - Residence in a nursing home or extended-care facility
  - Home infusion therapy (including antibiotics)
  - Peritoneal or hemodialysis within 30 days
  - Home wound care
  - Close contact family member with MDR pathogen

Once these issues are addressed, antimicrobial therapy can be selected and initiated. The patient- and drug-related categories are common to all types of pneumonia, but the organisms vary with the type of pneumonia. Guidelines have been

Patient Encounter 2, Part 2: Medical History, Physical Examination, and Diagnostic Tests

A 63-year-old man was admitted to the hospital secondary to a motor vehicle accident. Five days after admission he developed respiratory failure and was intubated. The chest x-ray revealed bilateral lower lobe infiltrates. He is sedated but does respond to commands.

PMH: Two surgeries in the last 5 days for fractures of the femur, tibia and humerus; hypertension for 15 years, currently controlled

FH: Father and mother deceased from natural causes. Both had hypertension.

SH: Smoked 1 pack per week ×40 years, quit 3 years ago; drinks 2–3 beers per week. He lives with his wife; occupation—carpenter. He is 5 ft 10 in (178 cm) and weighs 80 kg (176 lb).

Allergies: Penicillin—hives

Meds: Losartan 50 mg orally once daily

PE:

VS: BP 110/70, P 78, T 38.2°C (100.8°F)

CV: RRR, normal S_1, S_2; no murmurs, rubs, or gallops

Abd: Soft, nontender, nondistended; (+) bowel sounds, no hepatosplenomegaly, incision looks good and is healing

Diagnostic Tests: Chest x-ray: bilateral lower lobe infiltrates; oxygen saturation 98% (0.98) on ventilator

Labs: WBC is 16.8×10^3/mm³ (16.8×10^9/L) with a cell differential of 74% (0.74) neutrophils, 6% (0.06) bands, 17% (0.17) lymphocytes, and 3% (0.03) monocytes; BUN 10 mg/dL (3.6 mmol/L), SCr 0.9 mg/dL (80 µmol/L); sputum gram stain: many gram-negative bacilli, moderate Gram-positive cocci in clusters, many WBCs; sputum culture is pending

Given this additional information, what is your assessment of the patient's condition?

Identify your treatment goals for the patient.

generated by experts in the field for all types of pneumonia. These guidelines were generated to provide practitioners with evidence-based therapeutic options for the management of patients with pneumonia.

Pharmacologic Therapy for CAP

6 *Treatment of CAP is predominantly empiric, that is, treatment is started without knowing the causative pathogen.* As a way of incorporating an evidence-based approach to antibiotic selection, several different organizations have generated guidelines for the treatment of bacterial or atypical CAP in adults. The most recent guidelines are the result of a collaboration between the Infectious Diseases Society of America and the American Thoracic Society.[26] The approach to patient

Table 71–2

Summary of CAP Treatment

Adult outpatient otherwise healthy Empirical coverage against *S. pneumoniae*, *M. pneumoniae*, *C. pneumoniae*, and *H. influenzae*	*Monotherapy* Azithromycin, clarithromycin, erythromycin, doxycycline
Adult outpatient comorbidities Empirical coverage against *S. pneumoniae*, *M. pneumoniae*, *C. pneumoniae*, and *H. influenzae*	*Combination therapy* High-dose amoxicillin, high-dose amoxicillin-clavulanate (alternatives are cefpodoxime, or cefuroxime, or ceftriaxone) *plus* azithromycin, or clarithromycin or, doxycycline *Monotherapy* Gemifloxacin, levofloxacin, moxifloxacin
Adult inpatient (non-ICU) Empirical coverage against *S. pneumoniae*, *H. influenzae*, *M. pneumoniae*, and *C. pneumoniae*	*Combination therapy* Cefotaxime, or ceftriaxone, or ampicillin-sulbactam, or ertapenem *plus* azithromycin, or clarithromycin, or doxycycline *Monotherapy* Gemifloxacin, levofloxacin, moxifloxacin
Adult inpatient ICU (no Pseudomonas) Empirical coverage against *S. pneumoniae*, *L. pneumophila*, *H. influenzae*, enteric GNB, and *S. aureus*	*Combination therapy* Cefotaxime or ceftriaxone *plus* azithromycin, or levofloxacin, or moxifloxacin
Adult inpatient ICU (Pseudomonas is a concern) Empirical coverage against *P. aeruginosa*, *S. pneumoniae*, *L. pneumophila*, *H. influenzae*, enteric GNB, and *S. aureus*	*Combination therapy* Cefepime, or ceftazidime, or piperacillin-tazobactam, or imipenem, or meropenem *plus* or ciprofloxacin or levofloxacin or an aminoglycoside If an aminoglycoside is chosen, then add azithromycin or levofloxacin or moxifloxacin
Adult inpatient non-ICU or ICU (CA-MRSA is a concern) Empirical coverage against *S. pneumoniae*, *L. pneumophila*, *H. influenzae*, enteric GNB, and *S. aureus* (*Pseudomonas* if ICU)	Add vancomycin or linezolid to the regimens listed above
Pediatric outpatient Empirical coverage against *S. pneumoniae*, *M. pneumoniae*, and *C. pneumoniae*	*Monotherapy* High-dose amoxicillin, or high-dose amoxicillin-clavulanate, or intramuscular ceftriaxone, or azithromycin, or clarithromycin
Pediatric inpatient (non-ICU) Empirical coverage against *S. pneumoniae*, *H. influenzae*, *M. pneumoniae*, and *C. pneumoniae*	*Combination therapy* IV cefuroxime, or cefotaxime, or ceftriaxone, or ampicillin-sulbactam plus azithromycin, or clarithromycin
Pediatric inpatient ICU Empirical coverage against *S. pneumoniae*, *L. pneumophila*, *H. influenzae*, enteric GNB, and *S. aureus*	*Combination therapy* Cefotaxime, or ceftriaxone plus azithromycin, or clarithromycin

CA-MRSA, community-acquired methicillin-resistant *Staphylococcus aureus*; GNB, gram-negative bacteria; ICU, intensive care unit.

care is based on the classification of patients into two broad categories, outpatient and inpatient, and then further dividing the groups by comorbid conditions and location in the hospital, respectively. These guidelines use patient-specific data along with predominant pathogen information to design appropriate empirical antimicrobial regimens. Table 71–2 summarizes these therapeutic options. If influenza virus is the cause, supportive care is the best medical intervention available; antiviral agents against influenza are not effective.

▶ Adult Outpatient Previously Healthy

First-line therapeutic options for treating previously healthy adults include use of a macrolide (erythromycin, clarithromycin) or an azalide (azithromycin) or doxycycline.[26] If a patient has failed therapy with a macrolide, azalide, or doxycycline, one has to consider why the patient failed. The most common reasons are either medication adherence issues or the presence of resistant organisms. If a resistant organism is suspected, then use of one of the respiratory fluoroquinolones active against *S. pneumoniae* (gemifloxacin, levofloxacin, or moxifloxacin) is warranted.

▶ Adult Outpatient With Comorbid Conditions

The comorbid conditions that can impact therapy and outcomes in patients with CAP include diabetes mellitus; COPD; chronic heart, liver, or renal disease; alcoholism; malignancy; asplenia; and immunosuppressive condition or use of immunosuppressive drugs.[26] If the patient did not receive antibiotics in the last 3 months, then either a respiratory fluoroquinolone alone or a combination of an oral β-lactam agent plus a macrolide or azalide is recommended. If the patient received an antibiotic in the last 3 months, the recommendation is to use an agent from a different class. Doxycycline is an acceptable alternative to a macrolide or azalide.

Patient Encounter 1, Part 3: Creating a Care Plan

Based on the information presented, create a care plan for this patient's pneumonia. Your plan should include:

(a) The goals of therapy

(b) A patient-specific detailed therapeutic plan

(c) A plan for follow-up to determine whether the goals have been achieved and adverse effects avoided

The preferred β-lactam agents are high-dose (3 g daily) amoxicillin or high-dose (4 g daily) amoxicillin-clavulanate. Alternative β-lactams are second- and third-generation cephalosporins such as cefuroxime, cefpodoxime, or ceftriaxone.

Telithromycin, a ketolide antibiotic approved for the treatment of mild to moderate CAP, is not included in the recommendations because of safety issues related to hepatotoxicity, loss of consciousness, and visual disturbances. Telithromycin is similar in spectrum of activity to clarithromycin and azithromycin in that it covers primarily the respiratory pathogens and not gram-negative bacilli.

▶ Adult Inpatient Not in the ICU

For patients admitted to the hospital with CAP, the severity of illness is generally increased (caused either by the organism itself or underlying comorbidities in the patient), and the pathogens are essentially the same as in the outpatient setting. Recommendations are to use either a respiratory fluoroquinolone alone or a combination of an IV β-lactam agent plus an advanced macrolide/azalide (clarithromycin/azithromycin) or doxycycline. The recommended β-lactams include cefotaxime, ceftriaxone, ampicillin-sulbactam, or ertapenem.[26] Therapy should be initiated in the emergency room; however, due to the controversy with a first antibiotic dose time of less than 4 or 8 hours, no recommendations have been made regarding time to the first antibiotic dose. Conversion to oral therapy should occur when the patient is hemodynamically stable, improving clinically, and able to take oral medications, which often is within 48 to 72 hours for most patients. Discharge from the hospital should be as soon as the patient is stable and without other medical complications. The need to observe the patient in the hospital on their oral antibiotic is not necessary.[26]

▶ Adult Inpatient in the ICU

Patients admitted to the ICU have severe pneumoniae, and the likely etiology includes S. pneumoniae and H. influenzae as in the other categories; however, the incidence of L. pneumophila increases in this setting and should be considered a potential pathogen. In addition, enteric gram-negative bacilli and S. aureus are more frequently the cause of the pneumonia in these patients. The recommendations are to treat with an IV β-lactam plus either azithromycin or a respiratory fluoroquinolone. This combination therapy minimizes the risk of treatment failure due to a resistant pathogen as well as provides coverage against all of the potential pathogens.[26] The preferred β-lactams are ceftriaxone, cefotaxime, or ampicillin-sulbactam. If the patient is allergic to β-lactams, then aztreonam plus a respiratory fluoroquinolone are preferred.

If P. aeruginosa is suspected, then the antimicrobial treatment must be broadened to cover Pseudomonas as well as the organisms listed previously. Owing to the high resistance rates observed in Pseudomonas, the recommended regimens empirically double cover the Pseudomonas to ensure at least one of the antibiotics is active against Pseudomonas. The regimens include the use of an antipneumococcal, antipseudomonal β-lactam (cefepime, ceftazidime, piperacillin/tazobactam, imipenem, or meropenem), plus either ciprofloxacin or levofloxacin or an aminoglycoside. If the aminoglycoside is chosen, then either IV azithromycin or a respiratory fluoroquinolone should be added to cover S. pneumoniae and the atypical bacterial organisms.[26]

If CA-MRSA is suspected in the patient, then the addition of vancomycin or linezolid to the preceding regimen should be considered. Daptomycin cannot be used because surfactant in the lung inactivates the drug, thus rendering it ineffective for pneumonia. CA-MRSA can cause a necrotizing pneumonia, and the cause is believed to be due to its many virulence factors, including the Panton-Valentine leukocidin toxin.[7] In these patients the use of an agent that decreases toxin production may be beneficial. Linezolid decreases toxin production; the other recommended agents to decrease toxin production and added to vancomycin therapy are clindamycin or a respiratory fluoroquinolone.[26]

▶ Influenza

Influenza viruses A and B can cause pneumonia in pediatric and adult patients. Amantadine and rimantadine are available oral agents with activity against influenza virus type A. If started within 48 hours of the onset of the first symptoms, they reduce the duration of the illness by about 1.3 days. Oseltamivir and zanamivir also are oral agents active against both type A and B influenza that reduce the duration of the illness by about 1.3 days if initiated within 40 to 48 hours of the first symptoms.[27] For active infection beyond the first 48 hours, none of these agents are effective in treating infection, and supportive care is the best treatment for these patients.

▶ Aspiration

Anaerobes and Streptococcus spp. are the primary pathogens if a patient aspirates his or her oral contents and develops pneumonia. Antibiotics active against these organisms include penicillin G, ampicillin/sulbactam, and clindamycin. If the patient aspirates oral and gastric contents, then anaerobes and gram-negative bacilli are the primary pathogens. The preferred treatment regimen is a β-lactam/β-lactamase inhibitor combination (ampicillin/sulbactam, amoxicillin/clavulanate, piperacillin/tazobactam, or ticarcillin/clavulanate).[26]

Patient Encounter 2, Part 3: Creating a Care Plan

Based on the information presented, create a care plan for this patient's pneumonia. Your plan should include:

(a) The goals of therapy
(b) A patient-specific detailed therapeutic plan
(c) A plan for follow-up to determine whether goals have been achieved and adverse effects avoided

▶ Pediatric Outpatient

Guidelines have been published for treating CAP in children. The most predominant pathogens in preschool children in the outpatient setting are viruses, and often supportive therapy (maintaining hydration, antipyretics) is all that is needed.[28] For appropriately immunized infants, children, and adolescents with mild-to-moderate pneumonia in an area lacking high-level penicillin-resistant pneumococcus, high-dose amoxicillin is the recommended first-line therapy. If atypical organisms are considered likely, then a macrolide is recommended. If moderate to severe CAP is diagnosed and it is during influenza season, then treatment with oseltamivir, zanamivir (Relenza), amantadine, or rimantadine is recommended.[28] Fluoroquinolones and tetracyclines should not be used in children younger than 5 years of age. Dosing of antibiotics for pediatric patients is presented in Table 71–3.

▶ Pediatric Inpatient

If the infant or child is fully immunized, then the guidelines recommend the use of IV penicillin G or ampicillin. If an atypical organism is highly suspected, then azithromycin in combination with a β-lactam is recommended. Alternative β-lactams include IV cefotaxime or ceftriaxone. If the infant or child is not fully immunized, then the third-generation cephalosporins (cefotaxime or ceftriaxone) should be administered.[28] Again, if atypical organisms are suspected, add azithromycin to the β-lactam. If community-acquired MRSA is suspected, then vancomycin or clindamycin should be added to the regimen.[28]

Pharmacologic Therapy for HCAP/HAP/VAP

Nosocomial pneumonia was the term used to describe pneumonia that developed in patients in an institutional setting. This has since been replaced by the terms *healthcare-associated pneumonia, hospital-associated pneumonia,* and *ventilator-associated pneumonia.* ❼ *Empirical selection of antimicrobial therapy for ventilator-, healthcare-, and hospital-associated pneumonia is broad spectrum; however, once culture and susceptibility information are available, the therapy should be narrowed (de-escalation) to cover the identified pathogen(s).* Two factors important to the empirical selection of antibiotics for these types of pneumonia are onset time after admission and risk factors for MDR organisms. If it is early onset (less than or equal to 5 days since admission), and there are no risk factors for MDR organisms, then the most frequent pathogens include *S. pneumoniae, H. influenzae,* methicillin-susceptible *Staphylococcus aureus* (MSSA), and enteric gram-negative bacilli. Recommendations for therapy include third-generation cephalosporins such as ceftriaxone or cefotaxime; a respiratory fluoroquinolone such as gemifloxacin, levofloxacin, or moxifloxacin; ampicillin/sulbactam; or ertapenem.[29] If it is late-onset pneumonia and/or there are risk factors for MDR organisms, then the pathogen list includes *P. aeruginosa,* extended-spectrum β-lactamase–producing *K. pneumoniae, Acinetobacter spp.,* and MRSA. Empirical antibiotic selection must cover *P. aeruginosa,* which often then covers the other gram-negative pathogens. Available antibiotics

---

Table 71–3

CAP Antimicrobial Dosing in Pediatric Patients

Drug (Route)	Body Weight Less Than 2,000 g		Body Weight Greater Than 2,000 g		Greater Than 28 Days Old
	0–7 Days Old	7–28 Days Old	0–7 Days Old	7–28 Days Old	
Amoxicillin (orally)				15 mg/kg every 12 hours	17 mg/kg every 8 hours
Amoxicillin-clavulanate (orally)			15 mg/kg every 12 hours	15 mg/kg every 12 hours	45 mg/kg every 12 hours
Cefotaxime (IV)	50 mg/kg every 12 hours	50 mg/kg every 8 hours	50 mg/kg every 12 hours	50 mg/kg every 8 hours	50 mg/kg every 8 hours
Ceftriaxone (IM/IV)	25 mg/kg every 24 hours	50 mg/kg every 24 hours	25 mg/kg every 24 hours	50 mg/kg every 24 hours	50 mg/kg every 24 hours
Cefuroxime (orally)					15 mg/kg every 12 hours
Azithromycin (orally/IV)	5 mg/kg every 24 hours	10 mg/kg every 24 hours	5 mg/kg every 24 hours	10 mg/kg every 24 hours	10 mg/kg every 24 hours
Clarithromycin (orally)					7.5 mg/kg every 12 hours

Table 71–4				
Empirical Therapy for Late-Onset HAP, HCAP, or VAP in Adults				
Antibiotic (Route)	**CrCl[a] Greater Than 50 mL/min (0.83 mL/s)**	**CrCl 30–50 mL/min (0.50-0.83 mL/s)**	**CrCl 10–30 mL/min (0.17-0.50 mL/s)**	**CrCl Less Than 10 mL/min (0.17 mL/s)**
Cefepime (IV)	1–2 g every 12 hours	1–2 g every 24 hours	1 g every 24 hours	0.5–1 g every 24 hours
Ceftazidime (IV)	1–2 g every 8 hours	1–2 g every 12 hours	1–2 g every 12–24 hours	1–2 g every 24 hours
Imipenem (IV)	500 mg every 6 hours or 1 g every 8 hours	500 mg every 6–8 hours	500 mg every 8–12 hours	250 mg every 12 hours
Meropenem (IV)	1 g every 8 hours	1 g every 12 hours	500 mg every 12 hours	500 mg every 24 hours
Piperacillin-tazobactam (IV)	4.5 g every 6 hours or 3.375 g every 4 hours	4.5 g every 8 hours or 3.375 g every 6 hours	4.5 g every 8–12 hours or 3.375 g every 6–8 hours	4.5 g every 12 hours or 3.375 g every 8 hours or 2.25 g every 6 hours
Ticarcillin-clavulanate (IV)	3.1 g every 4–6 hours	2 g every 4–6 hours	2 g every 8 hours	2 g every 12 hours
Levofloxacin (IV/orally)	750 mg every 24 hours	750 mg every 48 hours	750 mg × 1 then 500 mg every 48 hours	750 mg × 1 then 500 mg every 48 hours
Ciprofloxacin (IV)	400 mg every 8 hours	400 mg every 8 hours	400 mg every 12 hours	400 mg every 24 hours
Ciprofloxacin (orally)	750 mg every 8 hours	750 mg every 8 hours	750 mg every 12 hours	750 mg every 24 hours
Gentamicin or Tobramcyin[b] (IV)	5–7 mg/kg every 24 hours	1.7–2 mg/kg every 12–24 hours	1.7–2 mg/kg every 36 hours	1.7–2 mg/kg every 48 hours
Amikacin[b] (IV)	20 mg/kg every 24 hours	7.5 mg/kg every 12–24 hours	7.5 mg/kg every 36 hours	7.5 mg/kg every 48 hours
Vancomycin[c] (IV)	15–20 mg/kg every 12 hours	15–20 mg/kg every 24 hours	15–20 mg/kg every 48 hours	15–20 mg/kg every 72 hours
Linezolid (IV/orally)	600 mg every 12 hours	600 mg every 12 hours	600 mg every 12 hours	600 mg every 12 hours

[a]CrCl, creatinine clearance.

[b]Trough concentrations ideally should be nondetectable; less than 1 mcg/mL for gentamicin (1 mg/L; 2 μmol/L) and tobramycin (1 mg/L; 2 μmol/L) and less than 4 to 5 mcg/mL (4–5 mg/L; 7–9 μmol/L) for amikacin are potentially acceptable.

[c]Trough concentrations should be between 15 and 20 mcg/mL (15 and 20 mg/L; 10 and 14 μmol/L).

include cefepime, ceftazidime, imipenem, meropenem, piperacillin/tazobactam, ticarcillin/clavulanate, levofloxacin, ciprofloxacin, gentamicin, tobramycin, and amikacin. Empirical therapy for late-onset pneumonia (listed in Table 71–4) could include any of the β-lactams, carbapenems, or fluoroquinolones alone or in combination with one of the aminoglycosides. If MRSA is suspected, then either vancomycin or linezolid should be added to the regimen. Recommendations for vancomycin trough concentrations of 15 to 20 mcg/mL (15 to 20 mg/L; 10 to 14 μmol/L) were based on expert opinion, not evidence from clinical trials.[29]

Currently there is debate over whether or not double coverage for *Pseudomonas* is required. In vitro studies have shown that aminoglycosides exhibit synergistic killing against gram-negative bacilli when combined with β-lactams. Dosing of the aminoglycosides is dependent on the patient's renal function. A high-dose once-daily regimen (e.g., 4 to 7 mg/kg gentamicin or tobramycin or 15 to 20 mg/kg amikacin) can be utilized in patients with good renal function. Most of the studies enrolled patients with estimated creatinine clearances of at least 70 mL/min (1.17 mL/s). Meta-analyses have shown high-dose once-daily regimens to be as efficacious as and less toxic than divided daily dosing.[30–34] Divided daily dosing (e.g., 1 to 2 mg/kg gentamicin or tobramycin or 7.5 mg/kg amikacin) has been utilized since the 1970s,

and the dosing interval is based on the patient's renal function to achieve a trough concentration of less than 2 mcg/mL (2 mg/L; 4 μmol/L) for gentamicin and tobramycin and less than 5 mcg/mL (5 mg/L; 9 μmol/L) for amikacin.

In addition to obtaining a synergistic effect, another reason for double coverage when treating VAP, HAP, or HCAP is to broaden the coverage empirically to increase the likelihood of covering the majority of resistant pathogens. VAP is the most studied of these types of pneumonias and is often the most severe. There is an increase in mortality when inadequate therapy is initiated for VAP. Crude mortality ranges are quite large (35% to 92%) compared with estimates of attributable mortality (approximately 9%); however, attributable mortality studies are limited by the large sample size needed to accurately measure this outcome.[35–37]

❼ *Once a pathogen or pathogens have been identified, therapy should be narrowed to cover only those pathogens.* Use of broad-spectrum antibiotics for prolonged durations increases the risk of colonization with MDR pathogens.

Duration of Antimicrobial Therapy

❽ *The duration of therapy for pneumonia should be kept as short as possible* and depends on several factors: type of pneumonia, inpatient or outpatient status, patient comorbidities, bacteremia/sepsis, and the antibiotic chosen. If the duration of therapy is too prolonged, then it can have a negative impact on the patient's normal flora in the respiratory and gastrointestinal tracts, vaginal tract of women, and on the skin. This can result in colonization with resistant pathogens, *Clostridium difficile* colitis, or overgrowth of yeast. In addition, the longer antibiotics are administered, the greater the chance for toxicity from the agent, as well as an increase in cost.

For treating adult outpatient CAP, two antibiotics are approved for a 5-day duration of therapy, levofloxacin (the 750-mg dose) and azithromycin. The recommended duration of therapy for all other therapies is 7 to 10 days. For treatment of CAP in adult patients admitted to the hospital, the duration is dependent on whether or not blood cultures were positive. In the absence of positive blood cultures, the duration of therapy is 7 to 10 days. If blood cultures were positive, the duration of therapy should be 2 weeks from the day blood cultures first became negative. The duration of therapy in pediatric patients is 10 days for uncomplicated CAP, with the exception of azithromycin, which is approved for 5 days.[28]

The duration of therapy cited in the literature for HCAP, HAP, or VAP ranges from 10 to 21 days. Efforts should be made to shorten the duration of therapy from the traditional 14 to 21 days to periods as short as 7 days, provided that the etiologic pathogen is not P. aeruginosa and that the patient has a good clinical response with resolution of clinical features of infection. Shortening the duration of therapy is acknowledged as beneficial because of the colonization, toxicity, and cost issues. Several studies evaluated mortality, clinical success, recurrence, or the development of resistance with shorter courses of therapy for VAP and found no differences when compared with longer courses of therapy.[36,38] The Clinical Pulmonary Infection Score (CPIS) has been used to determine when to end therapy for VAP. Luna and colleagues[39] used the CPIS and found that patients who survived VAP and were treated with adequate therapy clinically improved within 3 to 5 days. This study was instrumental in recommending a shortened duration of therapy of 6 days.

OUTCOME EVALUATION

For CAP, outcomes include preventing hospitalization, shortening the duration of hospitalization, and minimizing mortality. For patients admitted to the hospital, if antibiotics are initiated within 4 hours of presentation, the duration of hospitalization is decreased compared with when antibiotics are started after 4 hours.[40]

Improvement of symptoms should occur within 48 to 72 hours after initiation of therapy for most patients with CAP. Response to therapy could be slowed in patients with underlying pulmonary disease such as moderate to severe asthma, COPD, or emphysema. In patients not responding to therapy and when there are no underlying factors that would suggest a slowed response to therapy, then other infectious and noninfectious reasons must be considered. The infection could be caused by a pathogen not covered by the initial therapy, a drug-resistant isolate could be present, or more

---

Patient Care and Monitoring

⑨ *Monitoring response to therapy is essential for determining efficacy, identifying adverse reactions, and determining the duration of therapy.*

1. Assess the patient's symptoms and status (i.e., inpatient, outpatient, or intubated) to determine the type of pneumonia and comorbid conditions. Does the patient have moderate to severe asthma, COPD, or emphysema or is a current smoker?

2. Review any available diagnostic data to determine severity of the disease.

3. Obtain a history of prescription and nonprescription medication use, as well as allergies and drug intolerances, noting the severity of the reaction.

4. What are the top two to three organisms associated with the type of pneumonia the patient has?

5. Select an appropriate empirical antibiotic regimen for the patient, ensuring that the doses are correct for renal function.

6. Develop a plan to assess the effectiveness of the antibiotic therapy after 24 to 72 hours. If the patient is not improving, then reevaluate the diagnosis and pathogen list, and make appropriate changes to therapy. Develop a plan to assess the effectiveness of the antibiotic therapy again at the end of therapy. When can conversion from IV to oral therapy occur?

7. Evaluate the patient for the presence of adverse drug reactions, drug allergies, and drug interactions.

8. For patients who meet the qualifications, discuss the value of vaccination against *S. pneumoniae* and/or influenza.

---

severe infection could be present (nonpulmonary), and the patient should be reevaluated. Noninfectious reasons to consider include pulmonary embolus, congestive heart failure, carcinoma, lymphoma, intrapulmonary hemorrhage, and certain inflammatory lung diseases.

Outcome parameters for VAP, HAP, and HCAP are similar to those with CAP. Clinical improvement should occur within 48 to 72 hours of the start of therapy. If a patient is not responding to therapy, then, again, consider infectious and noninfectious reasons. Infectious explanations are the same as for CAP, but noninfectious are not. They include atelectasis, acute respiratory distress syndrome (ARDS), pulmonary embolism or hemorrhage, cancer, empyema, or lung abscess.

PREVENTION

⑩ *Prevention of both pneumococcal and influenza pneumonia by use of vaccination is a national goal.* Vaccination is used to prevent or minimize the severity of pneumonia caused by *S. pneumoniae* or the influenza virus.

The influenza vaccine is available in two forms, injectable and nasal inhalation. There are two forms of the injectable inactivated vaccine (containing killed virus). The regular influenza vaccine is approved for use in people older than 6 months of age, including healthy people and people with chronic medical conditions. Fluzone® intradermal vaccine is indicated for adults 18 through 64 years of age against influenza disease caused by virus subtypes A and type B. This vaccine utilizes a microinjection delivery system with a needle significantly smaller than other intradermal needles, which may decrease the fear associated with injections and increase immunization rates. The high-dose influenza vaccine is recommended for those 65 years of age and older. The nasal-spray influenza vaccine is made with live, weakened influenza viruses that do not cause the influenza (live attenuated influenza vaccine). This formulation is approved for use in healthy people 2 to 49 years of age who are not pregnant. The ability of influenza vaccine to protect a person depends on two key factors: the age and health status of the person getting the vaccine, and the similarity or "match" between the virus strains in the vaccine and those in circulation. Given these factors, the vaccine is effective and protective antibodies are detected approximately 2 weeks after vaccination. In February 2010, the Centers for Disease Control and Prevention (CDC) adopted a universal influenza vaccination policy, thus recommending all persons 6 months of age and older to be vaccinated annually. The CDC indentifies high risk groups in whom vaccination is especially important[41]:

1. Pregnant women
2. Children younger than 5, but especially children younger than 2 years old
3. People 50 years of age and older
4. People of any age with certain chronic medical conditions
5. People who live in nursing homes and other long-term care facilities
6. People who live with or care for those at high risk for complications from flu, including:
   - Healthcare workers
   - Household contacts of persons at high risk for complications from the flu
   - Household contacts and out-of-home caregivers of children less than 6 months of age (these children are too young to be vaccinated)

There are three pneumococcal vaccines, 7- and 13-valent conjugated vaccines for children younger than 5 years of age (6 years if chronic health conditions are present) and a 23-purified-capsular polysaccharide antigen vaccine for children 5 years of age and older and adults. The 7-valent conjugated vaccine has been replaced with the 13-valent conjugated vaccine. The serotypes in the 13-valent conjugated vaccine include those in the 7-valent, along with six serotypes that emerged as disease-causing strains after the implementation of the 7-valent vaccine.[42,43] The minimum age to receive the conjugated vaccine is 6 weeks, and the recommended age range is between 12 and 15 months. A reliable immunologic response

to the 13-valent conjugated vaccine has been demonstrated, along with a favorable safety profile.[43,44] The 23 capsular types in the vaccine represent at least 85% to 90% of the serotypes that cause invasive pneumococcal infections among children and adults in the United States. Ten years after vaccination, a sample of elderly individuals demonstrated significant quantity of protective antibodies.[45] Those who should receive the polysaccharide vaccine include the following[41]:

1. *All adults 65 years of age or older should receive one dose.*
2. *Anyone over 6 years of age who has a long-term health problem* such as heart disease, lung disease, sickle cell disease, diabetes, alcoholism, cirrhosis, and leakage of cerebrospinal fluid.
3. *Anyone over 6 years of age who has a disease or condition or is taking any drug that lowers the body's resistance to infection,* such as Hodgkin's disease, lymphoma, leukemia, kidney failure, multiple myeloma, nephrotic syndrome, HIV infection or AIDS, damaged spleen or no spleen, organ transplant, long-term steroids, certain cancer drugs, or radiation therapy.

Abbreviations Introduced in This Chapter

ARDS	Acute respiratory distress syndrome
ATS	American Thoracic Society
BUN	Blood urea nitrogen
CA-MRSA	Community-acquired methicillin-resistant *Staphylococcus aureus*
CAP	Community-acquired pneumonia
CDC	Center for Disease Control and Prevention
COPD	Chronic obstructive pulmonary disease
CPIS	Clinical Pulmonary Infection Score
DFA	Direct fluorescence antigen
GER(D)	Gastroesophageal reflux (disease)
H	Hemagglutinin
HCAP	Health care–associated pneumonia
HAP	Hospital-acquired pneumonia
IDDM	Insulin-dependent diabetes mellitus
IDSA	Infectious Diseases Society of America
MDR	Multidrug resistant
MRSA	Methicillin-resistant *Staphylococcus aureus*
MSSA	Methicillin-susceptible *S. aureus*
N	Neuraminidase
Pao_2/Fio_2	Arterial oxygen pressure/fraction of inspired oxygen
PBP	Penicillin-binding protein
PCR	Polymerase chain reaction
TNF-α	Tumor necrosis factor alpha
TRUST	Tracking Resistance in the United States Today
VAP	Ventilator-associated pneumonia

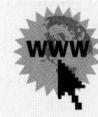

Self-assessment questions and answers are available at *http://www.mhpharmacotherapy. com/pp.html.*

REFERENCES

1. Masterton R. The place of guidelines in hospital-acquired pneumonia. J Hosp Infect 2007;66(2):116–122.

2. Tablan OC, Anderson LJ, Besser R, Bridges C, Hajjeh R. Guidelines for preventing health-care--associated pneumonia, 2003: recommendations of CDC and the Healthcare Infection Control Practices Advisory Committee. MMWR Recom Rep 2004;53(RR-3):1–36.

3. Hugonnet S, Eggimann P, Borst F, Maricot P, Chevrolet J-C, Pittet D. Impact of ventilator-associated pneumonia on resource utilization and patient outcome. Infect Control Hosp Epidemiol 2004;25(12):1090–1096.

4. Polverino E, Dambrava P, Cill, et al. Nursing home-acquired pneumonia: a 10 year single-centre experience. Thorax 2010;65(4):354.

5. Lees AW, McNaught W. Bacteriology of lower-respiratory-tract secretions, sputum, and upper-respiratory-tract secretions in "normals" and chronic bronchitics. Lancet 1959;2:1112–1115.

6. Hendley JO, Sande MA, Stewart PM, Gwaltney JMJ. Spread of *Streptococcus pneumoniae* in families. I. Carriage rates and distribution of types. J Inect Dis 1975;132(1):55–61.

7. Wallin TR, Hern HG, Frazee BW. Community-associated methicillin-resistant *Staphylococcus aureus*. Emerg Med Clin North Am 2008;26(2):431–455, ix.

8. Howard LS, Sillis M, Pasteur MC, Kamath AV, Harrison BDW. Microbiological profile of community-acquired pneumonia in adults over the last 20 years. J Infect 2005;50(2):107–113.

9. Petric M, Comanor L, Petti C. Role of the laboratory in diagnosis of influenza during seasonal epidemics and potential pandemics. J Infect Dis. 2006;194(Suppl)2:S98.

10. Barlow GD, Lamping DL, Davey PG, Nathwani D. Evaluation of outcomes in community-acquired pneumonia: a guide for patients, physicians, and policy-makers. Lancet Infect Dis 2003;3(8):476–488.

11. Lim WS, van der Eerden MM, Laing R, et al. Defining community acquired pneumonia severity on presentation to hospital: an international derivation and validation study. Thorax 2003;58(5):377–382.

12. Ewig S, de Roux A, Bauer T, et al. Validation of predictive rules and indices of severity for community acquired pneumonia. Thorax 2004;59(5):421–427.

13. Myint PK, Kamath AV, Vowler SL, Maisey DN, Harrison BDW. Severity assessment criteria recommended by the British Thoracic Society (BTS) for community-acquired pneumonia (CAP) and older patients. Should SOAR (systolic blood pressure, oxygenation, age and respiratory rate) criteria be used in older people? A compilation study of two prospective cohorts. Age Ageing 2006;35(3):286–291.

14. Aujesky D, Auble TE, Yealy DM, et al. Prospective comparison of three validated prediction rules for prognosis in community-acquired pneumonia. Am J Med 2005;118(4):384–392.

15. Kikawada M, Iwamoto T, Takasaki M. Aspiration and infection in the elderly: epidemiology, diagnosis and management. Drugs Aging 2005;22(2):115–130.

16. Allewelt M, Schuler P, Bolcskei PL, Mauch H, Lode H. Ampicillin + sulbactam vs clindamycin +/- cephalosporin for the treatment of aspiration pneumonia and primary lung abscess. Clin Microbiol Infect. 2004;10(2):163–170.

17. Wunderink RG. Nosocomial pneumonia, including ventilator-associated pneumonia. Proc Am Thorac Soc 2005;2(5):440–444.

18. Edwards JR, Peterson KD, Andrus ML, et al. National Healthcare Safety Network (NHSN) Report, data summary for 2006, issued June 2007. Am J Infect Control 2007;35(5):290–301.

19. Hidron A, Edwards J, Patel J, et al. NHSN annual update: antimicrobial-resistant pathogens associated with healthcare-associated infections: annual summary of data reported to the National Healthcare Safety Network at the Centers for Disease Control and Prevention, 2006-2007. Infect Control Hosp Epidemiol 2008;29(11):996.

20. Kollef MH. Prevention of hospital-associated pneumonia and ventilator-associated pneumonia. Crit Care Med 2004;32(6):1396–1405.

21. Bonten MJ, Kollef MH, Hall JB. Risk factors for ventilator-associated pneumonia: from epidemiology to patient management. Clin Infect Dis 2004;38(8):1141–1149.

22. Levy ML, Le Jeune I, Woodhead MA, Macfarlaned JT, Lim WS, on behalf of the British Thoracic Society Community Acquired Pneumonia in Adults Guideline G. Primary care summary of the British Thoracic Society Guidelines for the management of community acquired pneumonia in adults: 2009 update. Primary Care Resp J 2010;19(1):21–27.

23. Darabi A, Hocquet D, Dowzicky MJ. Antimicrobial activity against Streptococcus pneumoniae and Haemophilus influenzae collected globally between 2004 and 2008 as part of the Tigecycline Evaluation and Surveillance Trial. Diagnost Microbiol Infect Dis 2010;67(1):78–86.

24. Ortho-McNeil Pharmaceutical. TRUST Surveillance Database, 1999-2007. Raritan, NJ: Ortho-McNeil Pharmaceutical.

25. Jones R, Farrell D, Mendes R, Sader H. Comparative ceftaroline activity tested against pathogens associated with community-acquired pneumonia: results from an international surveillance study. J Antimicrobiol Chemother 2011;66(Suppl 3):iii69.

26. Mandell LA, Wunderink RG, Anzueto A, et al. Infectious Diseases Society of America/American Thoracic Society consensus guidelines on the management of community-acquired pneumonia in adults. Clin Infect Dis 2007;44(Suppl 2):S27–S72.

27. Clark N, Lynch J. Influenza: epidemiology, clinical features, therapy, and prevention. Semin Resp Crit Care Med 2011;32(4):373.

28. Bradley J, Byington C, Shah S, et al. The management of community-acquired pneumonia in infants and children older than 3 months of age: clinical practice guidelines by the pediatric infectious diseases society and the infectious diseases society of america. Clin Infect Dis 2011;53(7):e25.

29. Niederman MS, Craven DE. Guidelines for the management of adults with hospital-acquired, ventilator-associated, and healthcare-associated pneumonia. Am J Resp Crit Care Med 2005;171(4):388–416.

30. Contopoulos-Ioannidis DG, Giotis ND, Baliatsa DV, Ioannidis JPA. Extended-interval aminoglycoside administration for children: a meta-analysis. Pediatrics 2004;114(1):e111–118.

31. Ferriols-Lisart R, Alos-Alminana M. Effectiveness and safety of once-daily aminoglycosides: a meta-analysis. Am J Health-Sys Pharm 1996;53(10):1141–1150.

32. Hatala R, Dinh T, Cook DJ. Once-daily aminoglycoside dosing in immunocompetent adults: a meta-analysis. Ann Intern Med 1996;124(8):717–725.

33. Munckhof WJ, Grayson ML, Turnidge JD. A meta-analysis of studies on the safety and efficacy of aminoglycosides given either once daily or as divided doses. J Antimicrob Chemother 1996;37(4):645–663.

34. Nestaas E, Bangstad HJ, Sandvik L, Wathne KO. Aminoglycoside extended interval dosing in neonates is safe and effective: a meta-analysis. Arch Dis Child 2005;90(4):F294–300.

35. Melsen WG, Rovers MM, Koeman M, Bonten MJM. Estimating the attributable mortality of ventilator-associated pneumonia from randomized prevention studies. Crit Care Med 2011;39:2736–2742.

36. Chastre J, Wolff M, Fagon J, et al. Comparison of 8 vs 15 days of antibiotic therapy for ventilator-associated pneumonia in adults: a randomized trial. JAMA 2003;290(19):2588.

37. Klompas M, Khan Y, Kleinman K, et al. Multicenter evaluation of a novel surveillance paradigm for complications of mechanical ventilation. PLoS ONE 2011;6(3):e18062.

38. Pugh RJ, Cooke RPD, Dempsey G. Short course antibiotic therapy for Gram-negative hospital-acquired pneumonia in the critically ill. J Hosp Infect 2010;74(4):337–343.

39. Luna CM, Blanzaco D, Niederman MS, et al. Resolution of ventilator-associated pneumonia: prospective evaluation of the clinical pulmonary infection score as an early clinical predictor of outcome. Crit Care Med 2003;31(3):676–682.

40. Ziss DR, Stowers A, Feild C. Community-acquired pneumonia: compliance with centers for Medicare and Medicaid services, national guidelines, and factors associated with outcome. Southern Med J 2003;96(10):949–959.

41. Center for Disease Control and Prevention. Seasonal Influenza [cited 2011 Oct 10]. Available from: *www.cdc.gov/flu*.

42. Greenberg D. The shifting dynamics of pneumococcal invasive disease after the introduction of the pneumococcal 7-valent conjugated vaccine: toward the new pneumococcal conjugated vaccines. Clin Infect Dis 2009;49(2):213.

43. Paradiso PR. Advances in pneumococcal disease prevention: 13-valent pneumococcal conjugate vaccine for infants and children. Clin Infect Dis 2011;52(10):1241–1247.

44. Nunes M, Madhi S. Review on the immunogenicity and safety of PCV-13 in infants and toddlers. Exp Rev Vac 2011;10(7):951.

45. Musher D, Manoff S, McFetridge R, et al. Antibody persistence 10 years after 1st and 2nd doses of 23-valent pneumococcal polysaccharide vaccine, and immunogenicity and safety of 2nd and 3rd doses in older adults. Hum Vac 2011;7(9).

72 Upper Respiratory Tract Infections

Heather L. VandenBussche

LEARNING OBJECTIVES

● **Upon completion of the chapter, the reader will be able to:**

1. List the most common bacterial pathogens that cause acute otitis media (AOM), acute bacterial rhinosinusitis (ABRS), and acute pharyngitis.

2. Explain the pathophysiologic causes of and risk factors for AOM, bacterial rhinosinusitis, and acute pharyngitis.

3. Identify clinical signs and symptoms associated with AOM, bacterial rhinosinusitis, streptococcal pharyngitis, and the common cold.

4. List treatment goals for AOM, bacterial rhinosinusitis, streptococcal pharyngitis, and the common cold.

5. Develop an appropriate antibiotic regimen for each infection based on patient-specific data.

6. Recommend appropriate adjunctive therapy for a patient with AOM or ABRS.

7. Recommend an appropriate treatment plan for a patient with the common cold.

8. Create a monitoring plan for a patient being treated for an upper respiratory tract infection (URI) using patient-specific information and prescribed therapy.

9. Educate patients about URIs and proper use of antibiotic therapy.

KEY CONCEPTS

❶ Most upper respiratory tract infections (URIs) are caused by viruses, have nonspecific symptoms, and resolve spontaneously.

❷ Antibiotic resistance greatly influences the treatment options for bacterial URIs.

❸ Proper diagnosis of bacterial URIs is essential to identify when antibiotic use is appropriate.

❹ Antibiotic therapy for acute otitis media (AOM) should be reserved for children who are most likely to benefit from therapy and is dependent on patient age, illness severity, and diagnostic certainty.

❺ For AOM, high-dose amoxicillin (80 to 90 mg/kg/day) is the drug of choice, but high-dose amoxicillin-clavulanate is an alternative agent for children with severe illness or when a broader spectrum agent is desired.

❻ Antibiotic therapy for sinusitis should be reserved for patients with moderate persistent symptoms, clinical decompensation, or severe symptoms.

❼ Amoxicillin and amoxicillin-clavulanate are first-line antibiotics for acute bacterial rhinosinusitis (ABRS).

❽ The goals of therapy for streptococcal pharyngitis are to eradicate infection, reduce symptoms and infectivity, and prevent complications.

❾ Penicillin is the drug of choice for streptococcal pharyngitis.

❿ Treatment for the common cold focuses on symptom relief and is influenced by patient age, comorbid conditions, and balance of medication effectiveness and safety.

INTRODUCTION

Upper respiratory tract infection (URI) is a term that encompasses many upper airway infections, including otitis media, sinusitis, pharyngitis, laryngitis, and the common cold. More than 1 billion URIs occur annually in the United States, triggering millions of ambulatory care visits each year.[1] ❶ *Most URIs are caused by viruses, have nonspecific symptoms, and resolve spontaneously.*[2] Antibiotics do not impact the resolution of viral URIs, and their excessive use for these infections has contributed to antibiotic resistance. Guidelines have been established to reduce inappropriate antibiotic therapy for viral URIs.[2] This chapter focuses on **acute otitis media** (AOM), sinusitis, and pharyngitis because these infections are frequently caused by bacteria, and their complications can be minimized with appropriate antibiotic therapy. Proper management of the common cold is also reviewed.

OTITIS MEDIA

Otitis media, or inflammation of the middle ear, is the most common illness treated with antibiotics in children. It usually results from a nasopharyngeal viral infection and can be subclassified as AOM or otitis media with effusion (OME). AOM is a rapid, symptomatic infection with effusion, or presence of fluid, in the middle ear. OME does not have signs of acute illness but is characterized by the presence of middle ear fluid. It is important to distinguish between AOM and OME because antibiotics are only useful for the treatment of AOM.

EPIDEMIOLOGY AND ETIOLOGY

Otitis media occurs in all age groups but is most common in children between 6 months and 2 years of age. By 3 years of age, up to 85% of children have had at least one episode of otitis media, and up to 20% have recurrent infections by 12 months of age.[3] In 2000, approximately 13 million antibiotic prescriptions were written in the United States for otitis media, resulting in $2 billion in direct costs.[4,5] From 1995 to 2006, rates of antibiotic prescriptions for otitis media declined by 36%, but the proportion of healthcare visits for otitis media that resulted in antibiotic prescriptions remained stable at 80%.[6] Many factors (Table 72–1) predispose children to otitis media, and some are associated with antibiotic resistance, such as daycare attendance, prior antibiotic exposure, and age younger than 2 years.[3,7,8]

Bacteria are isolated from middle ear fluid in up to 70% of children with AOM, but viruses can also cause AOM.[7] Historically, *Streptococcus pneumoniae* was the most common organism, responsible for up to half of bacterial cases.[4,9] *Haemophilus influenzae* and *Moraxella catarrhalis* caused 15% to 30% and 3% to 20% of cases, respectively. After the introduction of routine childhood pneumococcal vaccination, the prevalence of *H. influenzae* increased, and it now causes more than half of all bacterial cases.[9–11] Bacteria that are less frequently associated with AOM include *Staphylococcus aureus*, *Streptococcus pyogenes*, and *Pseudomonas aeruginosa*. Viruses such as respiratory syncytial virus, influenza, parainfluenza, enteroviruses, rhinovirus, and adenoviruses are isolated from middle ear fluid with or without concomitant bacteria in about half of AOM cases.[7,12] Lack of improvement with antibiotic treatment is often a result of viral infection and subsequent inflammation rather than antibiotic resistance.

❷ *Antibiotic resistance has great influence on the treatment options for AOM.* Penicillin-resistant *S. pneumoniae* (PRSP) exhibit either intermediate resistance (minimum inhibitory concentrations between 0.1 and 1.0 mcg/mL [0.1 and 1.0 mg/L]) or high-level resistance (minimum inhibitory concentration of 2.0 mcg/mL [2.0 mg/L] and higher). Altered penicillin-binding proteins cause penicillin resistance in approximately 40% of pneumococcal isolates, almost half of which are highly penicillin-resistant.[13] Amoxicillin-clavulanate resistance is less common, occurring in approximately 17% of pneumococci.[13] PRSP are commonly resistant to other drug classes, including sulfonamides, macrolides, and clindamycin, but are usually susceptible to levofloxacin. Treatment should be aimed at *S. pneumoniae* because pneumococcal AOM is unlikely to resolve spontaneously and commonly results in recurrent infections.[7] β-Lactamase production occurs in 30% and nearly 100% of *H. influenzae* and *M. catarrhalis*, respectively.[14] Although infections caused by these organisms are more likely to resolve without treatment, they should be considered in cases of treatment failure.

PATHOPHYSIOLOGY

AOM is caused by an interplay of multiple factors. Nasopharyngeal viral infections impair eustachian tube function and cause mucosal inflammation, which impairs mucociliary clearance and promotes bacterial proliferation and infection. Children are predisposed to AOM because their eustachian tubes are shorter, more flaccid, and more horizontal than those of adults, which make them less functional for drainage and protection of the middle ear from bacterial entry.[7] Clinical manifestations of AOM are the result of host immune response and cellular damage from inflammatory mediators such as tumor necrosis factor and interleukins that are released from bacteria.[3]

Viscous middle ear effusions caused by allergy or irritant exposure may contribute to impaired mucociliary clearance and AOM in susceptible individuals.[3] Middle ear effusions can persist for up to 6 months after an episode of AOM. OME occurs chronically in atopic children and may require tympanostomy tube placement to reduce complications such as hearing and speech impairment and recurrent otitis media.

Table 72–1	
Risk Factors for Otitis Media	
Allergies	Native American or Inuit ethnicity
Anatomic defects such as cleft palate	Pacifier use
Daycare attendance[a]	Positive family history/genetic predisposition
Gastroesophageal reflux	Siblings
Immunodeficiency	Tobacco smoke exposure
Lack of breast-feeding	Viral respiratory tract infection/winter season
Low socioeconomic status	Young age at first diagnosis[a]
Male sex	

[a]Risk factors for infection with a resistant pathogen (daycare attendee, age under 2 years, recent antibiotic use in previous 3 months).

From Refs. 3, 7, and 8.

Patient Encounter 1, Part 1

A 22-month-old boy presents to the evening pediatric clinic with 2 days of fever (38.6°C [101.5°F]), nasal congestion, and fussiness. His mother reports that he was rubbing his left ear throughout the day. She states that he is more irritable than usual and was crying intermittently throughout the night last night. He is not eating as much as usual today. He attends daycare 5 days a week and has a 4-year-old sister who recently had a cold.

What information is suggestive of acute otitis media (AOM)?

What risk factors does this child have for AOM?

Is there any additional information you need to know before recommending a treatment plan?

TREATMENT

Desired Outcomes

Treatment for AOM focuses on symptom relief and prevention of complications. The goals of treatment are to alleviate ear pain and fever, if present; eradicate infection; prevent complications; and minimize unnecessary antibiotic use.

General Approach to Treatment

❶ *The majority of uncomplicated AOM cases resolve spontaneously without significant morbidity.* Untreated AOM improves in almost 80% of all children between days 2 and 7 of illness without increasing the risk of complications.[15] Antibiotics improve ear pain in only 6% of all children between days 2 and 7 of therapy while *increasing* the risk of adverse events by 5%.[15] Antibiotics significantly improve recovery in children younger than 2 years of age with bilateral AOM and in those with AOM and otorrhea.[15] Children younger than 2 years of age have a higher incidence of PRSP infections, and children between 6 months and 3 years of age have higher clinical and bacteriologic failure rates and complications when not treated initially with antibiotics as compared with older children.[4,16] Patients with severe illness, defined by degree of fever and pain severity, have lower spontaneous recovery rates than those with less severe disease, particularly in children less than 2 years of age.[13,17] ❸ ❹ *Therefore, antibiotics should be reserved for children most likely to benefit from therapy, which is dependent on patient age, illness severity, and diagnostic certainty.* Current guidelines recommend stratifying patients based on these criteria in order to identify those most likely to benefit from antibiotic therapy.[4]

Nonpharmacologic Therapy

Watchful waiting and "safety-net" antibiotic prescriptions (to be filled only if symptoms do not resolve after 48 to 72 hours

Clinical Presentation and Diagnosis of Acute Otitis Media

It is important to differentiate AOM from OME because they are treated differently. Patients with AOM usually have cold symptoms, including rhinorrhea, cough, or nasal congestion, before or at diagnosis.

Symptoms

- Young children: ear tugging, irritable, poor sleeping and eating habits
- Older patients: ear pain (mild, moderate, or severe), ear fullness, hearing impairment

Signs[4,7]

- Fever: present in fewer than 25% of patients; often in younger children
- Middle ear effusion
- Otorrhea (middle ear perforation with fluid drainage): uncommon
- Bulging tympanic membrane
- Limited or absent mobility of tympanic membrane
- Distinct erythema of tympanic membrane
- Opaque or cloudy tympanic membrane obscuring or reducing visibility of middle ear

Laboratory Tests

Gram stain, culture, and sensitivities of ear fluid if draining spontaneously or obtained via tympanocentesis (not performed routinely in practice)

Complications

- Infectious: mastoiditis, meningitis, osteomyelitis, intracranial abscess
- Structural: perforated eardrum, **cholesteatoma**
- Hearing and/or speech impairment

Diagnosis[4]

Certain AOM: Requires *all* the following:

- Rapid onset of signs and symptoms
- Middle ear effusion findings with **pneumatic otoscopy**
- Inflammation indicated by either otoscopic evidence (distinct erythema) or otalgia

Uncertain AOM: not all three criteria are present

Severe AOM: moderate to severe ear pain or fever of 39°C (102.2°F) or greater

Nonsevere AOM: mild ear pain and fever of less than 39°C (102.2°F) in past 24 hours

of observation) are approaches being used more frequently to attenuate microbial resistance and avoid unnecessary adverse events and costs of antibiotics. Delayed antibiotic therapy in older children and those with less severe disease does not result in more infectious complications, such as mastoiditis or meningitis, when compared with routine initial antibiotic treatment.[15,18] Use of an observation approach or use of a safety-net antibiotic prescription can reduce antibiotic use by 67% without increasing complications.[18] Observation or delayed antibiotic therapy should be considered only in otherwise healthy children without recurrent disease (Fig. 72–1) and only if proper follow-up and good communication exist between clinicians and the parent/caregiver.[3,4,18]

Other nondrug approaches include the use of external heat or cold to reduce postauricular pain and surgery. Tympanostomy tubes are most useful for patients with recurrent disease or chronic OME with impaired hearing or speech. Adenoidectomy may be necessary for children with chronic nasal obstruction, but tonsillectomy is rarely indicated.[3]

Pharmacologic Therapy

▶ Antibiotic Therapy

When antibiotic therapy is needed, many factors influence initial drug selection. Clinicians must consider drug factors such as antimicrobial spectrum, likelihood of clinical response, middle ear fluid penetration, incidence of side effects, drug interactions, and cost, as well as patient factors, including risk factors for bacterial resistance, allergies, ease of dosing regimen, medication palatability, and presence of other medical conditions. Studies in uncomplicated AOM have not revealed significant differences between antibiotics in clinical response rates, but most were confounded by spontaneous resolution in children likely to have had viral illnesses. Bacteriologic response varies among antibiotics and does not always correlate well with clinical response but is considered important when selecting an agent.[4,7]

Guidelines from the American Academy of Pediatrics and the American Academy of Family Physicians are available for children between 2 months and 12 years of age with uncomplicated AOM (Fig. 72–2) and are based on published trials and expert opinion.[4] ⑤ *Amoxicillin is the drug of choice in most patients because of its proven effectiveness in AOM, high middle ear concentrations, excellent safety profile, low cost, good-tasting suspension, and relatively narrow spectrum of activity* (Table 72–2). High-dose amoxicillin (80 to 90 mg/kg/day) is preferred over conventional doses (40 to 45 mg/kg/day) because higher middle ear fluid concentrations can overcome pneumococcal penicillin resistance without substantially increasing adverse effects.[19] ⑤ *In cases of severe illness or when coverage for β-lactamase-producing organisms is desired, high-dose amoxicillin-clavulanate is the preferred agent.* Pneumococcal resistance to trimethoprim-sulfamethoxazole and macrolides is problematic and strikingly common in PRSP, making these agents less desirable

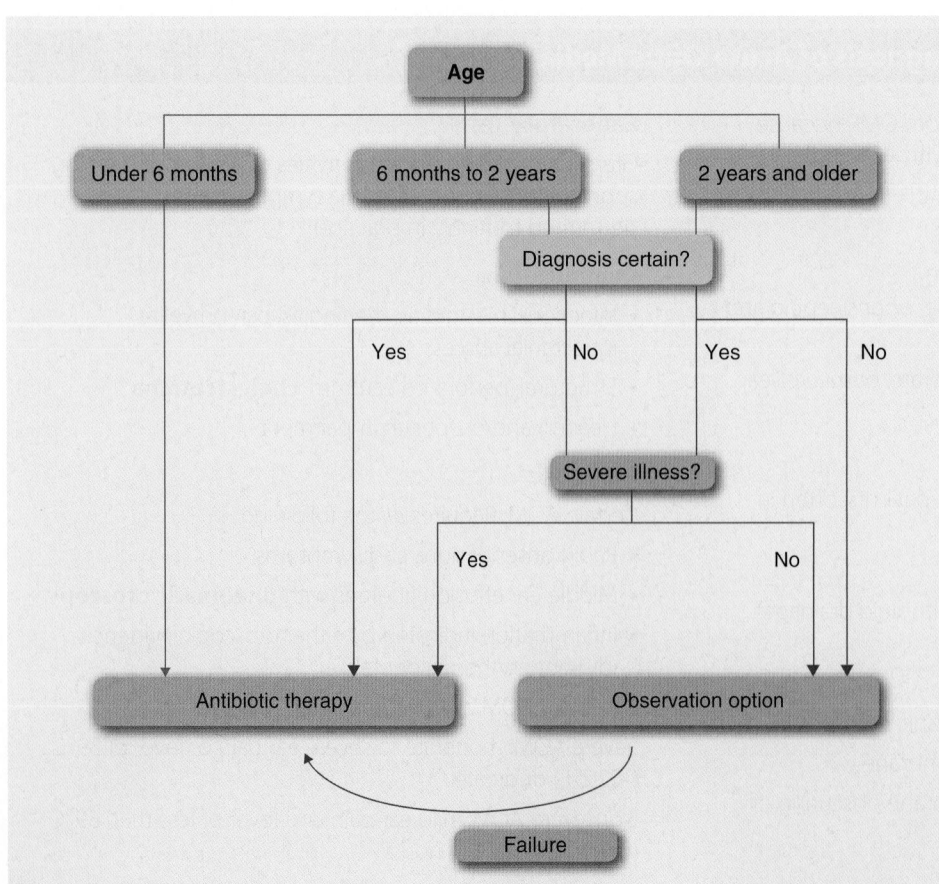

FIGURE 72–1. Treatment algorithm for initial antibiotics or observation in children with suspected or certain uncomplicated AOM. (From American Academy of Pediatrics and American Academy of Family Physicians. Diagnosis and management of acute otitis media. Pediatrics 2004;113:1451–1465.)

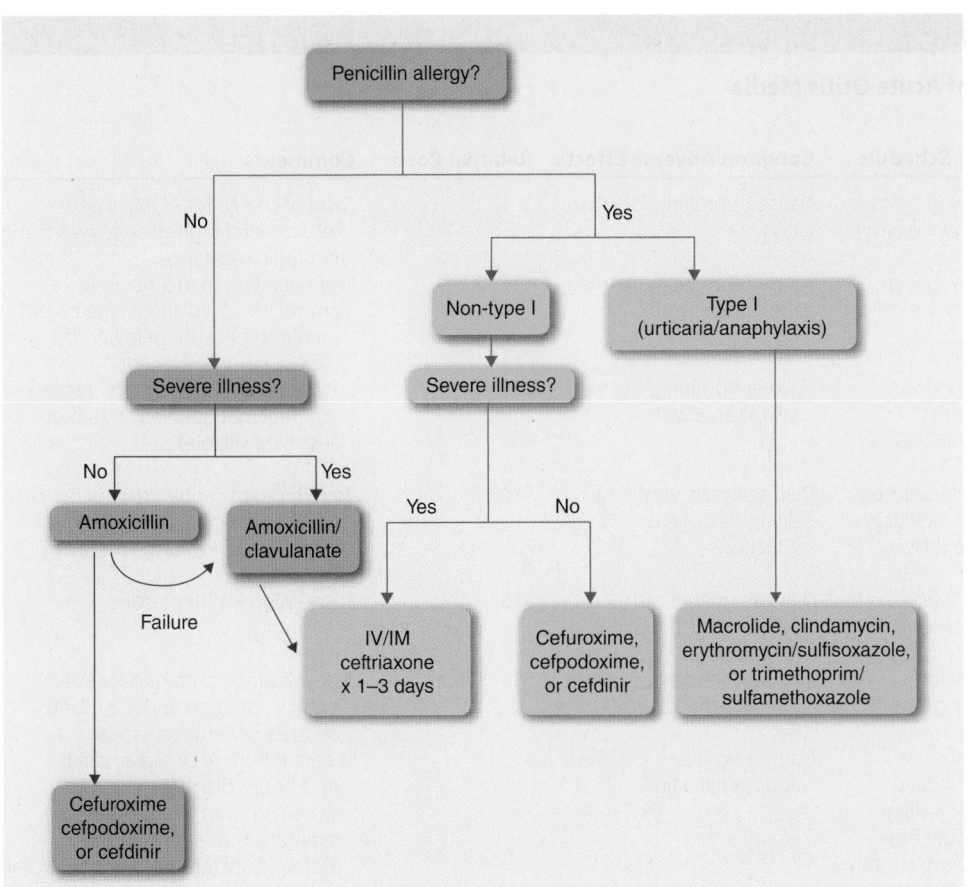

FIGURE 72–2. Treatment algorithm for uncomplicated AOM in children 2 months to 12 years of age. (From Refs. 4 and 8.)

for most patients.[8,13] Patients with penicillin allergies require alternative first-line therapy (Fig. 72–2). Children who have received an antimicrobial in the previous month are more likely to harbor resistant organisms and should also receive alternative therapy (Table 72–2).[8] A single dose of intramuscular ceftriaxone is effective for children who cannot tolerate oral medications, but a 3-day course may be preferred because of increasing pneumococcal resistance and reports of treatment failure with single doses.[20] Ototopical antibiotics are an alternative to systemic agents for AOM in patients with otorrhea or tympanostomy tubes.[21]

If there is a lack of improvement or worsening with initial therapy during the first 48 to 72 hours, antibiotic selection must be reassessed and other contributing diseases must be excluded.[4,8] **Tympanocentesis** can assist with guiding therapy in difficult cases.

The duration of antibiotic therapy depends on antibiotic selection, patient characteristics, and acceptability of clinical failure if a short treatment course is used. Standard 10-day oral therapy is more effective than shorter courses when comparing clinical outcomes between 8 and 19 days after initiating antibiotics, but failure rates are equivalent at 30 days following antibiotic initiation.[22] Failure rates of short-course therapy are significantly higher in children with perforated eardrums and in children less than 2 years of age treated with azithromycin.[22] Short-course antibiotics may result in fewer gastrointestinal adverse events but only when compared with 10-day treatment courses of amoxicillin-clavulanate.[22]

Short-course ceftriaxone is no more effective than standard 10-day oral regimens and is associated with significantly more gastrointestinal adverse effects.[22] Clinicians must balance the increased risk of failure with short-course therapies against the inconvenience of longer courses when selecting a duration of treatment.

▶ Adjunctive Therapy

Pain is a central feature of AOM but its management is often overlooked. Acetaminophen and ibuprofen are commonly used nonprescription agents for mild to moderate pain. Ibuprofen has a longer duration of effect than acetaminophen but is not used routinely in children younger than 6 months of age because of increased toxicity concerns. Alternating ibuprofen with acetaminophen is not recommended because of the potential for dosing confusion and error in an ambulatory setting and a lack of safety and efficacy data with combination therapy exceeding 24 to 48 hours. Topical anesthetic drops such as benzocaine (in Auralgan) provide pain relief within 30 minutes of administration and may be preferred over systemic analgesics when fever is absent. **Myringotomy** provides immediate relief but is performed rarely. Other medications such as decongestants, antihistamines, and corticosteroids have no role in the treatment of AOM and can, in some cases, prolong effusion duration.[4,23] Data are lacking on the safety and efficacy of complementary and alternative treatments.

Table 72-2

Antibiotics^a for the Treatment of Acute Otitis Media

Drug	Usual Dose and Schedule	Common Adverse Effects	Relative Cost^b	Comments
Amoxicillin	80–90 mg/kg/day in 2 doses (adult: 875 mg twice daily)	Nausea, vomiting, diarrhea, rash	$	Drug of choice for AOM; experts recommend high-dose to overcome penicillin resistance
Amoxicillin-clavulanate	80–90 mg/kg/day in 2 doses (adult: 875 mg twice daily)	Nausea, vomiting, diarrhea, rash, diaper rash	$$$–$$$$	More diarrhea than amoxicillin, amoxicillin:clavulanate ratio of 14:1 preferred because of lower daily clavulanate component
Cefuroxime axetil	30 mg/kg/day in 2 doses (max 1 g/day with suspension; adult: 250 mg twice daily)	Nausea, vomiting, diarrhea, rash, diaper rash	$$$	Suspension gritty and bitter tasting, not interchangeable with tablets (less bioavailable)
Cefdinir	14 mg/kg/day in 1–2 doses (adult: 300 mg twice daily or 600 mg once daily)	Diarrhea, rash, vomiting, diaper rash, yeast infections	$$$	Preferred oral cephalosporin (good taste); separate from Al or Mg antacids and Fe supplements by 2 hours
Cefpodoxime proxetil	10 mg/kg/day in 2 doses (adult: 200 mg twice daily)	Diarrhea, diaper rash, vomiting, rash, yeast infections	$$$	Suspension is bitter tasting
Ceftriaxone	50 mg/kg IM or IV for 1–3 days (max 1 g/dose)	Injection site pain, swelling, or erythema, diarrhea, rash	$$$–$$$$	3-day regimen preferred for PRSP; avoid in children under 2 months because of kernicterus risk
Azithromycin	10 mg/kg × 1 day, 5 mg/kg/day × 4 days; 10 mg/kg/day × 3 days; or 30 mg/kg single dose (adult dose 500 mg × 1 day, 250 mg × 4 days)	Nausea, vomiting, diarrhea, abdominal pain	$$	Separate from Al or Mg antacids by 2 hours; diarrhea/vomiting more common with single-dose regimen; 3- or 5-day courses preferred; increasing pneumococcal resistance; many failures with *H. influenzae* infection
Clarithromycin	15 mg/kg/day in 2 doses (adult: 250 mg twice daily)	Diarrhea, vomiting, rash, abnormal taste, abdominal pain	$$	Many drug interactions (inhibits cytochrome P-450 3A4); suspension cannot be refrigerated and has metallic taste; same microbiologic issues as azithromycin
Erythromycin-sulfisoxazole	50 mg/kg/day of erythromycin component in 3–4 doses	Nausea, vomiting, abdominal pain, diarrhea, rash	$$	Many drug interactions (like clarithromycin), contraindicated in children under 2 months because of kernicterus risk; increasing pneumococcal resistance
Trimethoprim-sulfamethoxazole	8–10 mg/kg/day of trimethoprim component in 2 doses	Nausea, vomiting, anorexia, rash, urticaria	$	Increasing pneumococcal resistance; contraindicated in children under 2 months because of kernicterus risk
Clindamycin	20–30 mg/kg/day in 3–4 doses (adult: 300 mg 4 times daily or 450 mg 3 times daily)	Nausea, diarrhea, C. difficile colitis, anorexia	$	Oral liquid poor tasting; only for pneumococcal infection

^{a}Other FDA-approved antibiotics for AOM not included in AAP/AAFP guidelines: cefaclor, cephalexin, cefprozil, cefixime, loracarbef, and ceftibuten.

^{b}Approximate cost per course: $ (under $25), $$ ($25–$50), $$$ ($50–$100), $$$$ (over $100).

AOM, acute otitis media. Al, aluminum; Mg, magnesium; Fe, iron; IM, intramuscular; PRSP, penicillin-resistant *S. pneumoniae*.

From American Academy of Pediatrics and American Academy of Family Physicians. Diagnosis and management of acute otitis media. Pediatrics 2004;113:1451–1465.

▶ *Prevention*

Vaccinations may prevent AOM in certain patients, such as older children and those with recurrent infections. Influenza vaccine is more effective in preventing AOM in children older than 2 years of age than in younger patients, possibly from impaired immune responses and immature host defenses in infants and toddlers.[24] The live attenuated influenza vaccine is more effective than the injectable inactivated influenza vaccine in protecting children older than 2 years against influenza-associated AOM.[25] Pneumococcal conjugate vaccine is protective against infection by vaccine serotypes only with a limited overall benefit for AOM.[26] Antibiotic prophylaxis is not recommended for otitis-prone children because of antibiotic resistance trends. Avoidance or minimization

Patient Encounter 1, Part 2

On further questioning, you discover that the child is allergic to amoxicillin. He developed a nonurticarial rash last year during treatment for a urinary tract infection. He has not received antibiotics since that time, and this is his first ear infection.

Immunizations: up-to-date

Medications: acetaminophen drops 120 mg orally every 4 to 6 hours as needed for fever

ROS: (+) nasal congestion and rhinorrhea, (–) vomiting, diarrhea, or cough

PE:

- **Gen:** irritable child but consolable
- **VS:** BP 100/60 mm Hg, P 124 beats/min, RR 20 breaths/min, T 38.4°C (101.1°F)
- **HEENT:** erythema and bulging of the left tympanic membrane with the presence of middle ear fluid; the right tympanic membrane is obscured with cerumen.

Identify your treatment goals for this child.

Given this information, what nonpharmacologic and pharmacologic therapy do you recommend?

Patient Care and Monitoring of Acute Otitis Media (AOM)

1. Assess the patient's signs and symptoms. Are they consistent with AOM?

2. Review diagnostic information to determine whether acute infection is present. Are all three diagnostic criteria present? Was the proper method used for diagnosis (pneumatic otoscopy)?

3. Does the patient require antibiotic therapy, or is observation an appropriate option?

4. Obtain a complete medication history, including prescription drugs, nonprescription drugs, and natural product use, as well as allergies and adverse effects.

5. Determine what medication should be used for pain, if present.

6. If applicable, determine which antibiotic to use and the duration of therapy.

7. Develop a plan to assess effectiveness of the chosen therapy and course of action to take if the patient does not improve or worsens.

8. Provide patient education on:

   - What to expect from prescribed medication, including potential adverse effects

   - Avoidance of antihistamines and decongestants

   - Signs of treatment failure

9. Stress the importance of adherence to therapy, including antibiotic resistance concerns.

10. Determine the need for influenza and pneumococcal vaccinations.

11. Educate the family regarding risk factors for otitis media.

of risk factors associated with otitis media, such as tobacco smoke and bottle feeding, is advised, but the effects of these interventions remain unproven.

OUTCOME EVALUATION

Improvement of signs and symptoms (i.e., pain, fever, and tympanic membrane inflammation) should be evident by 72 hours of therapy. Children can appear clinically worse during the first 24 hours of treatment but often stabilize during the second day with defervescence and improved eating and sleeping patterns. If symptoms persist or worsen, reevaluation must occur to determine the proper diagnosis and treatment. Counsel patients and caregivers regarding common antibiotic adverse events such as rash, diarrhea, and vomiting that may prompt additional medical attention.

Presence of middle ear effusion in the absence of symptoms is not an indicator of treatment failure. Persistent effusion greater than 3 months in duration requires a hearing evaluation in children who are otherwise healthy.[27] Preschool-aged and younger children or those at risk for developmental difficulties may need reexamination earlier because speech and hearing impairment is more difficult to assess in these populations.

SINUSITIS

Sinusitis, or inflammation of the paranasal sinuses, is often described as **rhinosinusitis** because it involves inflammation of contiguous nasal mucosa, which occurs in nearly all cases of viral respiratory infections. Acute rhinosinusitis is characterized by symptoms that persist for up to 4 weeks, whereas chronic rhinosinusitis manifests as cough, rhinorrhea, and/or nasal obstruction for more than 12 weeks. Acute bacterial rhinosinusitis (ABRS) refers to an acute bacterial infection of the sinuses that occurs independently of or is superimposed on chronic sinusitis. This section will focus on ABRS and its appropriate treatment.

EPIDEMIOLOGY AND ETIOLOGY

Rhinosinusitis is one of the most common medical conditions in the United States, affecting about 1 billion people annually.[1] It is caused mainly by respiratory viruses but can also be triggered by allergies or environmental irritants. Viral rhinosinusitis is complicated by secondary bacterial infection in 0.2% to 2% of adults and 5% to 13% of children.[1,28] Upper respiratory infections of less than 7 days' duration are usually viral, whereas more prolonged disease or severe symptoms are often caused by bacteria. Risk factors

Table 72–3
Risk Factors for Acute Bacterial Rhinosinusitis

Allergic or nonallergic rhinitis	Intranasal medications or illicit drugs
Anatomic defects (e.g., septal deviation)	Mechanical ventilation
Aspirin allergy, nasal polyps, and asthma	Nasogastric tubes
Cystic fibrosis or ciliary dyskinesia	Swimming or diving
Dental infections or procedures	Tobacco smoke exposure
Female sex	Traumatic head injury
Immunodeficiency	Viral respiratory tract infection or winter season

From Refs. 29 and 30.

for ABRS include prior viral respiratory infection, allergic rhinitis, anatomic defects, and certain medical conditions (Table 72–3).[29,30]

Bacteria that cause sinusitis are similar to those that cause AOM. *S. pneumoniae* and *H. influenzae* are responsible for more than half of the cases in all patients, with an additional 20% of cases caused by *M. catarrhalis* in children.[29,30] Similar to AOM, an increased prevalence of *H. influenzae* has been reported in ABRS, and certain factors predict the presence of drug-resistant pathogens.[1,31] Other bacteria that cause sinusitis include *S. pyogenes* (up to 5%), anaerobic organisms such as *Bacteroides* and *Peptostreptococcus* species (up to 9% of adults), and *S. aureus* (up to 10% of adults).[29,32] Chronic sinusitis is often polymicrobial with a higher incidence of anaerobes, gram-negative bacilli, and fungi.

PATHOPHYSIOLOGY

Rhinosinusitis is caused by mucosal inflammation and local damage to mucociliary clearance mechanisms from viral infection or allergy. Increased mucus production and reduced clearance of secretions can lead to blockage of the sinus ostia, or the opening of the sinuses to the upper airway. This environment is ideal for bacterial growth and promotes a cycle of local inflammatory response and mucosal injury characterized by increased concentrations of interleukins, histamine, and tumor necrosis factor.[29,30] Factors that contribute to sinus invasion include nose blowing, reduced local immunity, viral virulence, and nasopharyngeal colonization with bacteria.[29,33] Damage to the host defense system perpetuates bacterial overgrowth and persistence of infection.

TREATMENT
Desired Outcomes

The goals of treatment for ABRS are to eradicate bacteria and prevent serious sequelae. Specific aims are to relieve symptoms, normalize the nasal environment, use antibiotics when appropriate and select effective antibiotics that minimize resistance, and prevent development of chronic disease or complications.

General Approach to Treatment

Initial management of rhinosinusitis focuses on symptom relief for patients with mild disease of less than 7 to 10 days in duration. Clinicians often inappropriately prescribe antibiotics for rhinosinusitis, which usually is viral and self-limited.

Clinical Presentation and Diagnosis of Acute Bacterial Rhinosinusitis

Sinusitis symptoms typically last 7 to 10 days after a viral infection and are caused by activation of the immune system and parasympathetic nervous system.

Acute Signs and Symptoms[28,29,33]

- *Adults*: nasal congestion or obstruction, purulent nasal or postnasal discharge, facial pain or pressure or fullness (especially unilateral in a sinus area), diminished sense of smell, fever, cough, maxillary tooth pain, fatigue, ear fullness or pain

- *Children*: purulent nasal or postnasal drainage, nasal congestion and mouth breathing, persistent cough (particularly at night) or throat clearing, fever, pharyngitis, ear discomfort, halitosis, morning periorbital edema or facial swelling, fatigue, facial or tooth pain

Complications

Orbital cellulitis or abscess, periorbital cellulitis, meningitis, cavernous sinus thrombosis, ethmoid or frontal sinus erosion, chronic sinusitis, and exacerbation of asthma or bronchitis

③ **Diagnosis**[28,29,33]

- *Clinical diagnosis*: most common method; acute rhinosinusitis signs and symptoms (as noted previously) that have not resolved after 10 days or that worsen within 10 days after initial improvement. Respiratory secretion color is unreliable for diagnosis of bacterial infection because neutrophil presence causes color and can be found in viral sinusitis.

- *Radiographic studies*: useful for assessing presence of abscess or intracranial complication

- *Paranasal sinus puncture*: "gold standard"; not performed routinely but can be useful in complicated or chronic cases

- *Laboratory studies/nasopharyngeal cultures*: not recommended for routine diagnosis

Studies comparing antibiotics to placebo in ABRS report a high spontaneous improvement rate of more than 70% after 7 to 12 days of nonsevere symptoms and only modest symptom improvements but more adverse events in patients treated with antibiotics.[33,34] Withholding antibiotics is an option in nonsevere ABRS for up to 7 to 10 days duration if adequate follow-up can be assured.[1,33] ❻ *Antibiotic therapy should be reserved for persistent, worsening, or severe ABRS, such as patients with moderately severe symptoms that have persisted for greater than 10 days or worsened within 10 days after initial improvement and patients with severe symptoms regardless of duration.*[28,29,33] Empiric antibiotic selection is usually employed and should target commonly infecting bacteria because sinus cultures are rarely obtained.

Nonpharmacologic Therapy

Ancillary treatments such as humidifiers, vaporizers, and saline nasal sprays or drops are used to moisturize the nasal canal and impair crusting of secretions along with promoting ciliary function. Although many patients report benefit from such therapies, there are no controlled studies that support their use. Nasal irrigation with isotonic or hypertonic saline may improve quality of life, reduce medication usage, and improve symptoms, especially in patients with recurrent or chronic sinusitis.[33]

Pharmacologic Therapy

▶ Adjunctive Therapy

Medications that target URI symptoms are used widely in patients with rhinosinusitis, particularly in the early stage of infection. There is a lack of evidence supporting their use in ABRS, but they may provide temporary relief in certain patients.[28,33] Analgesics are used to treat fever and pain from sinus pressure. Oral decongestants relieve congested nasal passages but should be avoided in children younger than 4 years and patients with ischemic heart disease or uncontrolled hypertension. Intranasal decongestants can be used for severe congestion in most patients 6 years of age or older, but use should be limited to 3 days or less to avoid rebound nasal congestion. Guaifenesin, a mucolytic, has no evidence to support its use in rhinosinusitis. Antihistamines should be avoided because they thicken mucus and impair its clearance, but they may be useful in patients with predisposing allergic rhinitis or chronic sinusitis. Similarly, intranasal corticosteroids usually are reserved for patients with allergies or chronic sinusitis, but they may be beneficial as monotherapy or with antibiotics in ABRS.[35]

▶ Antibiotic Therapy

Although many antibiotics have been studied for ABRS, no randomized, double-blind, placebo-controlled studies have used pre- and posttreatment sinus aspirate cultures as an outcome measure. In some studies, antibiotics result in faster symptom resolution and lower failure rates and complications compared with no treatment, particularly in more severe disease.[28,33] Because diagnosis is based on clinical presentation and not sinus aspirate cultures, clinicians must attempt to differentiate ABRS from viral rhinosinusitis in order to minimize inappropriate antibiotic use. ❸ ❻ *Antibiotic use should be limited to cases where infection is unlikely to resolve without causing prolonged disease: patients with moderately severe symptoms that persist for greater than 10 days or worsen after initial improvement and patients with severe symptoms.*[28,29,33]

Treatment guidelines outline antibiotic choices that are likely to result in favorable clinical and bacteriologic outcomes based on causative pathogens, spontaneous resolution rates, and nationwide resistance patterns.[28,29,33] ❷ *These guidelines (**Figs. 72–3** and **72–4**) stratify therapy based on disease severity and risk of infection with resistant bacteria, defined as antibiotic use within the previous 4 to 6 weeks. Other risk factors for resistance include daycare attendance, frequent*

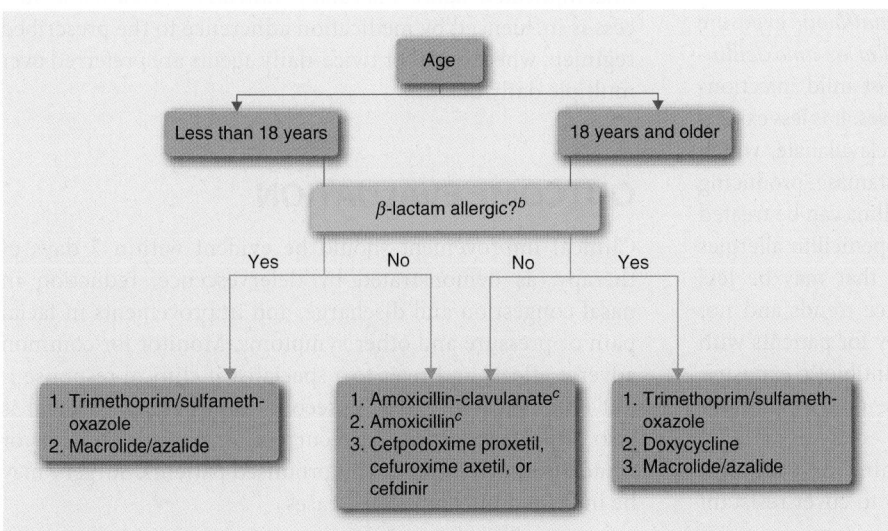

FIGURE 72–3. Treatment algorithm[a] for ABRS in patients with mild disease without recent antibiotic exposure. [a]Antibiotics are listed in order of predicted efficacy based on predicted clinical and bacteriologic efficacy rates, clinical studies, safety, and tolerability. Doses can be found in Table 72–4. [b]Cephalosporins should be considered for patients with non–type I hypersensitivity to penicillins; they are more likely to be effective than the alternative agents. [c]High doses are recommended for adults with daycare contacts or frequent infections and most children. (From Refs. 28 and 29.)

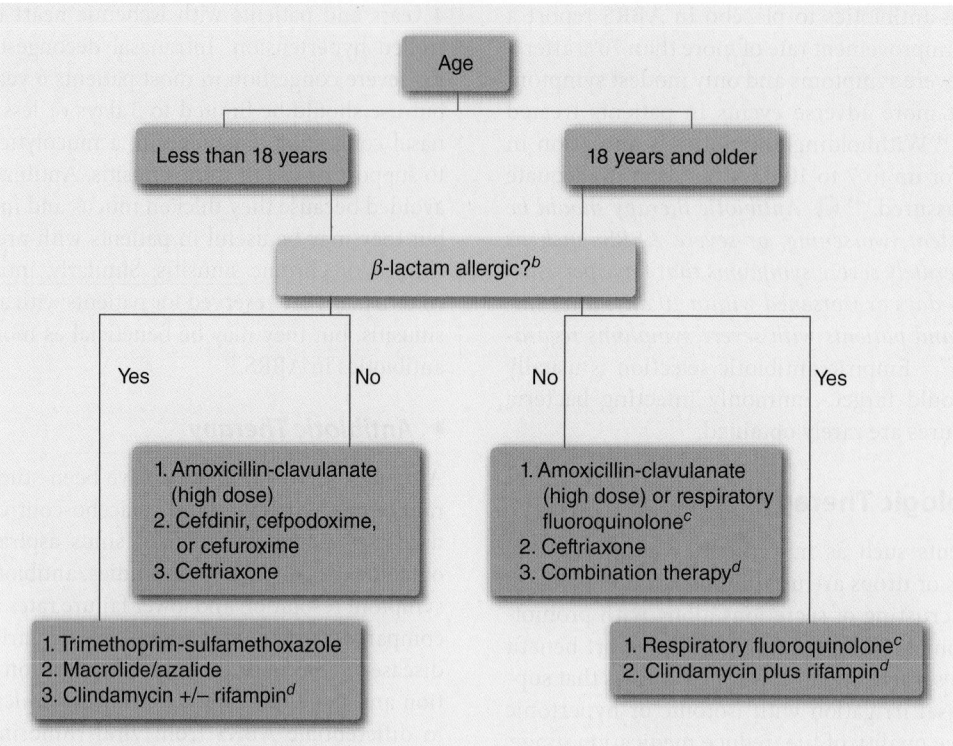

FIGURE 72–4. Treatment algorithm[a] for ABRS in patients with mild disease and recent antibiotic exposure or moderate disease. [a]Antibiotics are listed in order of predicted efficacy based on predicted clinical and bacteriologic efficacy rates, clinical studies, safety, and tolerability. Doses can be found in Table 72–4. [b]Cephalosporins should be considered for patients with non–type I hypersensitivity to penicillins; they are more likely to be effective than the alternative agents. [c]Respiratory fluoroquinolone = levofloxacin, moxifloxacin. [d]Combination therapy should provide gram-positive and gram-negative coverage. Examples are high-dose amoxicillin or clindamycin plus rifampin or cefixime. There are no published clinical studies to support such combinations. (From Refs. 28 and 29.)

exposure to children in daycare, and recurrent disease. Severe disease requires evaluation and treatment in conjunction with specialized physicians such as otolaryngologists.

Antibiotic therapy (Table 72–4) should target *S. pneumoniae*, but consideration must be given to other bacteria, including *H. influenzae, M. catarrhalis, S. aureus,* and PRSP. ❼ *Patients with mild disease and no prior antibiotic exposure should receive initial therapy with amoxicillin or amoxicillin-clavulanate.* Amoxicillin is effective for most mild infections and covers most PRSP when used in high doses. It is less expensive and better tolerated than amoxicillin-clavulanate, which provides expanded coverage against β-lactamase–producing bacteria. Patients who are allergic to penicillins can be treated with an appropriate cephalosporin; severe penicillin allergies require treatment with alternative agents that may be less effective based solely on bacterial resistance trends and not clinical data[13,28,29] (Fig. 72–3). Initial therapy for patients with moderate symptoms or those with recent antibiotic exposure includes high-dose amoxicillin-clavulanate or a respiratory fluoroquinolone[23,24] (Fig. 72–4).

Failure to respond to initial therapy within 7 days requires reevaluation to consider changing therapy to cover resistant organisms and to examine for complications.[33] Antibiotics traditionally have been given for at least 10 to 14 days, with up to 21 days needed for resolution in some patients.[29] Five-day treatment courses of some fluoroquinolones or β-lactams are as effective as longer courses in adults with uncomplicated acute maxillary sinusitis.[36] Treatment success is influenced by medication adherence to the prescribed regimen, where once- or twice-daily agents are preferred over multiple daily doses.

OUTCOME EVALUATION

Clinical improvement should be evident within 7 days of therapy, as demonstrated by defervescence, reduction in nasal congestion and discharge, and improvements in facial pain or pressure and other symptoms. Monitor for common adverse effects and refer to a specialist if clinical response is not obtained with first- or second-line therapy. Referral is also important for severe, recurrent, or chronic sinusitis or acute disease in immunocompromised patients. Surgery may be indicated in complicated cases.

Table 72–4

Antibiotics^a for the Treatment of Acute Bacterial Rhinosinusitis

Drug	Adult Dose	Pediatric Dose^b	Comments
Amoxicillin	1.5–4 g/day in 2–3 doses	90 mg/kg/day in 2 doses	Lacks coverage against β-lactamase producers
Amoxicillin-clavulanate	1.75–4 g/day in 2–3 doses	90 mg/kg/day in 2 doses	Broad coverage particularly with high doses; Augmentin XR (2 g every 12 hour) targeted toward PRSP
Cefdinir	600 mg/day in 1–2 doses	14 mg/kg/day in 1–2 doses	Preferred oral liquid cephalosporin owing to good palatability
Cefpodoxime proxetil	200 mg twice daily	10 mg/kg/day in 2 doses	
Cefuroxime axetil	250–500 mg twice daily	15–30 mg/kg/day in 2 doses	
Ceftriaxone	1 g IM/IV every 24 hour	50 mg/kg IM/IV every 24 hour	Experts recommend a 5-day treatment course
Trimethoprim-sulfamethoxazole	160/800 mg (1 DS tablet) twice daily	8–10 mg/kg/day of trimethoprim component in 2 doses	Considerable pneumococcal resistance limits use of this agent
Azithromycin	500 mg × 1 day, 250 mg/day × 4 days; 500 mg/day × 3 days; 2 g × 1 dose	10 mg/kg × 1 day, 5 mg/kg/day × 4 days; 10 mg/kg/day × 3 days	Increasing pneumococcal resistance and limited *H. influenzae* activity; single-dose regimen has high incidence of nausea, vomiting, and diarrhea
Clarithromycin	500 mg twice daily or 1 g once daily (XL only)	15 mg/kg/day in 2 doses	XL tablets reported to have fewer GI problems and taste disturbances than twice-daily preparation
Doxycycline	100 mg twice daily	Avoid in children under 8 years	Can cause photosensitivity, GI problems, tooth staining in young children; many drug–drug interactions (antacids, iron, calcium)
Levofloxacin	500–750 mg once daily (750 mg × 5 days)	Not available	Common fluoroquinolone side effects are nausea, vaginitis, diarrhea, dizziness; many drug–drug interactions (antacids, iron, calcium); tendon rupture, photosensitivity, QT prolongation possible; cost similar to amoxicillin/clavulanate
Moxifloxacin	400 mg once daily	Not available	
Clindamycin	150–450 mg 3–4 times daily	20–40 mg/kg/day in 3–4 doses	No gram-negative coverage; use in combination

^{a}Refer to Table 72–2 for more information on antibiotics. Other FDA-approved antibiotics for ABRS not included in the Sinus and Allergy Health Partnership or American Academy of Pediatrics guidelines: cefaclor, cefprozil, cefixime, ciprofloxacin, erythromycin, loracarbef.

^{b}Maximum dose not to exceed adult dose.

ABRS, acute bacterial rhinosinusitis; PRSP, penicillin-resistant *S. pneumoniae*; IM, intramuscular.

From Refs. 28 and 29.

PHARYNGITIS

Pharyngitis is an acute and often painful inflammation of the throat typically caused by viral or bacterial infection. Other conditions, such as gastroesophageal reflux, postnasal drip, or allergies, also can cause pharyngitis and must be distinguished from infectious causes. Acute pharyngitis is responsible for 1% to 2% of physician visits in adults and 6% to 8% of pediatric visits, but it is generally self-limited without serious sequelae.[37,38] Antibiotics are frequently prescribed because of the inability to easily distinguish between viral and bacterial infections and the fear of untreated streptococcal illness.

EPIDEMIOLOGY AND ETIOLOGY

Pharyngitis is a common manifestation of upper respiratory infections caused by rhinovirus, coronavirus, adenovirus, influenza virus, parainfluenza virus, or Epstein-Barr virus. Group A *Streptococcus*, or *S. pyogenes*, is the most common bacterial cause of acute pharyngitis, responsible for 20% to 30% of cases in children and 5% to 15% of adult infections.[39] Infection is most common in late winter and early spring and is spread easily through direct contact with contaminated secretions. Clusters of infection are common within families, classrooms, and other crowded areas. Less common causes of bacterial pharyngitis are *Corynebacterium diphtheriae*, groups C and G streptococci, *Chlamydia pneumoniae*, *Mycoplasma pneumoniae*, and *Neisseria gonorrhoeae*. This section will focus on group A streptococcal disease in which antimicrobial therapy is indicated.

PATHOPHYSIOLOGY

Pharyngeal colonization with group A streptococci occurs in up to 20% of children and is a risk factor for developing streptococcal pharyngitis after a break in upper respiratory mucosal integrity.[40] Clinicians should recognize that the symptoms of streptococcal pharyngitis usually are self-limited and resolve within 7 days of onset without antibiotic treatment.[39] Historically, untreated or inappropriately treated disease caused acute **rheumatic fever**, potential permanent heart valve damage, and infectious complications such as peritonsillar and retropharyngeal abscesses. Delayed antibiotic therapy given up to 9 days after symptom onset can prevent these particular sequelae, so ❸ *proper diagnosis is important to minimize unnecessary antibiotic use for viral pharyngitis and prevent complications of untreated streptococcal infection.*[37,39–41]

TREATMENT

Desired Outcomes

❽ *The goals of therapy for streptococcal pharyngitis are to eradicate infection in order to shorten the disease course, reduce infectivity and spread to close contacts, and prevent complications.* Antibiotic use only prevents peritonsillar or retropharyngeal abscesses, cervical lymphadenitis, and rheumatic fever. Immune-mediated, nonsuppurative complications

Patient Care and Monitoring of Streptococcal Pharyngitis

1. Assess the patient's signs and symptoms. Are they consistent with streptococcal pharyngitis? Are symptoms of viral infection present?

2. Perform laboratory testing to confirm the presence of group A streptococci.

3. Does the patient require antibiotic therapy? Avoid antibiotic use in viral illness.

4. Obtain a complete medication history, including prescription drugs, nonprescription drugs, and natural product use, as well as allergies and adverse effects.

5. Recommend antipyretic or analgesic therapy, if needed.

6. If applicable, determine which antibiotic to use and the duration of therapy.

7. Develop a plan to assess effectiveness of chosen therapy and course of action to take if the patient does not improve or worsens.

8. Provide patient education on:
   • What to expect from the antibiotic, including potential adverse effects
   • Avoidance of close contacts for 24 hours
   • Signs of treatment failure

9. Stress the importance of medication adherence and the need to complete therapy, including antibiotic resistance concerns.

of streptococcal infection are not impacted by antibiotic treatment. These conditions include acute **glomerulonephritis** and reactive arthritis.[37]

Pharmacologic Therapy

Pain is often a central feature of pharyngitis, regardless of its cause. Oral analgesics such as acetaminophen or ibuprofen provide pain relief and can allow patients to maintain normal eating and drinking habits. ❸ *Antibiotics should be used only in cases of laboratory-documented streptococcal pharyngitis that is associated with clinical symptoms in order to avoid unnecessary treatment* (Fig. 72–5).[37,39–41] Effective therapy (Table 72–5) reduces the infectious period from approximately 10 days to 24 hours and shortens symptom duration by 1 to 2 days.[37] ❾ *Treatment guidelines recommend penicillin*

as the drug of choice because of its narrow antimicrobial spectrum, documented safety and history of nasopharyngeal streptococcal eradication, and low cost.[37,40,41] Amoxicillin is an alternative first-line agent, particularly for children requiring a liquid formulation because of its improved taste as compared with penicillin and its enhanced adherence with once-daily dosing.[41] Studies proving that antibiotics prevent rheumatic fever used intramuscular procaine penicillin, but other antibiotics can also eradicate nasopharyngeal streptococci and presumably are effective for preventing rheumatic heart disease.[37,41] Cephalosporins may be more effective than penicillin for relapse prevention and nasopharyngeal eradication of streptococci, particularly in asymptomatic carriers.[39,41,42] Usual duration of antibiotic therapy is 10 days, but 5-day courses of certain cephalosporins are just as effective for streptococcal eradication as 10 days of penicillin.[43]

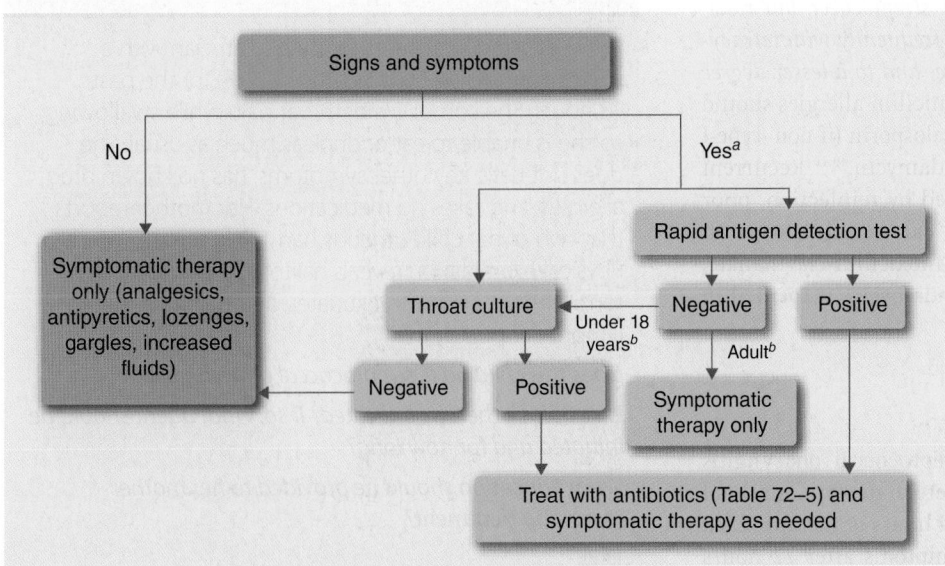

FIGURE 72–5. Treatment algorithm for management of pharyngitis in children and adults. [a]Rapid antigen detection tests (RADTs) are preferred if the test sensitivity exceeds 80%. [b]Parents, teachers, or other adults with significant pediatric contact should also be cultured if RADT is negative. (From Bisno AL, Gerber MA, Gwaltney JM, et al. Practice guidelines for the diagnosis and management of group A streptococcal pharyngitis. Clin Infect Dis 2002;35:113–125.)

Table 72–5

Antibiotics[a] for the Treatment of Streptococcal Pharyngitis

Drug	Adult Dose	Pediatric Dose	Duration	Comments
Penicillin V	500 mg 2–3 times daily	250 mg 2–3 times daily (if less than or equal to 27 kg), 500 mg 2-3 times daily (if more than 27 kg)	10 days	Drug of choice but increasing reports of treatment failures
Penicillin G benzathine	1.2 million units	600,000 units (if less than or equal to 27 kg); 1.2 million units (if more than 27 kg)	1 IM dose	Useful for patients with poor adherence or emesis; painful injection but pain can be reduced if warmed to room temperature prior to administration
Amoxicillin	775 mg–1 g once daily (Moxatag 775 mg is a time-released formulation given once daily for patients 12 years of age and older)	50 mg/kg once daily; max 1 g	10 days	Preferred drug for young children because of improved palatability and once daily dosing
Cephalexin	250–500 mg 4 times daily	25–50 mg/kg/day in 4 doses	10 days	Recommended in non–type I penicillin allergy
Cefadroxil	500 mg twice daily	30 mg/kg/day in 2 doses	10 days	Recommended in non–type I penicillin allergy
Cefuroxime axetil	250 mg twice daily	20 mg/kg/day in 2 doses	10 days	
Cefdinir	300 mg twice daily or 600 mg once daily	14 mg/kg/day in 1–2 doses	5–10 days	Broad spectrum; expensive
Azithromycin	500 mg once daily	12 mg/kg once daily	5 days	Recommended in immediate-type penicillin hypersensitivity; increasing resistance
Clindamycin	300 mg 3 times daily	20 mg/kg/day in 3 doses	10 days	Recommended in immediate-type penicillin hypersensitivity; useful for recurrent infections

[a]Other FDA-approved agents include amoxicillin-clavulanate, cefixime, cefaclor, cefprozil, cefpodoxime, erythromycin, clarithromycin, and others.

IM, intramuscular.

From Refs. 40 and 41.

Antibiotic resistance plays a smaller role in pharyngitis therapy compared with other URIs. ❷ *Penicillin resistance has not been documented in group A streptococci, but resistance and clinical failures occur more frequently with tetracyclines, trimethoprim-sulfamethoxazole, and to a lesser degree macrolides.* As such, patients with penicillin allergies should be treated with a first-generation cephalosporin (if non–type I allergy), a macrolide/azalide, or clindamycin.[40,41] Recurrent infections or treatment failures caused by reinfection, poor adherence, or true antibiotic failure can be retreated with the same antibiotic or treated with amoxicillin-clavulanate, a first-generation cephalosporin, clindamycin, or penicillin G benzathine.[40,41]

OUTCOME EVALUATION

Antibiotics relieve symptoms of streptococcal pharyngitis within 3 to 5 days, and patients can return to work or school if improved clinically after the first 24 hours of therapy. Lack of improvement or worsening of symptoms after 72 hours

Patient Encounter 3

A 9-year-old girl presents to the pediatrician with a sore throat and fever of 39.0°C (102.2°F) for the past 18 hours. She complains of throat pain while swallowing, so she is unable to eat or drink as much as usual. She does not have any other symptoms, has no known drug allergies, and takes no medications. Her mother reports that two of her child's friends had "strep throat" recently. Physical examination reveals halitosis, pharyngeal and tonsillar erythema with exudates, and painful cervical lymphadenopathy.

Does this child have streptococcal pharyngitis?

Is antibiotic therapy indicated? If so, what agent should be initiated and for how long?

What education should be provided to her mother regarding treatment?

Clinical Presentation and Diagnosis of Streptococcal Pharyngitis

Children between 5 and 15 years of age have the highest incidence of streptococcal pharyngitis. Parents and adults with significant pediatric contact are also at increased risk.

Signs and Symptoms of Streptococcal Pharyngitis[39–41]

- Sudden onset of sore throat with severe pain on swallowing
- Fever
- Headache, abdominal pain, nausea, or vomiting (especially in children)
- Pharyngeal and tonsillar erythema with possible patchy exudates
- Tender, enlarged anterior cervical lymph nodes
- Swollen and red uvula
- Halitosis
- Soft palate petechiae

- **Scarlatiniform rash**
- General absence of conjunctivitis, hoarseness, cough, rhinorrhea, discrete ulcerations, and diarrhea (suggestive of viral etiology)

Diagnosis[37,40,41]

- Rapid antigen detection test (RADT): 80% to 90% sensitivity; results available within minutes.
- Throat swab and culture: "gold standard"; results available within 24 to 48 hours. Should be performed in all negative RADTs in children and adolescents, and adults with significant pediatric contact. Also recommended in outbreaks and to monitor for antibiotic resistance.
- These tests should be performed *only* if there is a clinical suspicion of streptococcal pharyngitis. Pharyngeal carriage of group A streptococci is 5% to 20% in children.

of therapy requires reevaluation. Follow-up throat cultures are not recommended to test for bacterial eradication unless symptoms persist or recur. Recurrent symptoms following an appropriate treatment course should prompt reevaluation for possible retreatment.

COMMON COLD

The common cold is a self-limited viral URI that occurs frequently throughout life. It is responsible for millions of missed school and work days and is associated with significant healthcare resource utilization, including physician office and emergency department visits and nearly universal use of cough and cold medication for treatment or prevention.[44,45] Clinicians

must be aware of evidence regarding the use of cough and cold products in order to make appropriate treatment recommendations for this commonly encountered condition.

EPIDEMIOLOGY AND ETIOLOGY

Hundreds of different viruses cause the common cold, including rhinoviruses (most common), coronaviruses, parainfluenza viruses, respiratory syncytial virus, and adenoviruses. Infection rates increase during the fall through spring seasons and are highest in the winter months. Adults experience 2 to 4 colds each year, whereas children have 6 to 10 colds per year.[44,46] Colds can last for 10 to 14 days and can be complicated by bacterial superinfections, including AOM and ABRS. Factors associated with an increased incidence

Clinical Presentation and Diagnosis of the Common Cold

Symptoms begin 24 to 72 hours after infectious contact. They usually peak around day 3 to 4 and begin to wane by day 7; colds typically last 10 to 14 days.

Signs and Symptoms[44,45]

- *Onset*: malaise, fatigue, headache, pharyngitis, low-grade fever (can be higher in infants and children); these symptoms usually resolve over a few days.
- *Secondary*: nasal and/or postnasal drainage (often clear at onset, but can become thick and purulent); nasal congestion; cough and/or throat clearing; sneezing; conjunctivitis; irritability; loss of smell or taste

Complications

AOM, bacterial sinusitis, chronic bronchitis, bronchiolitis (in infants and children under 2 years of age), pneumonia, asthma exacerbation

Diagnosis

- *Clinical diagnosis*: most common method; based on history, presence of symptoms, and physical examination
- *Radiographic studies*: not recommended routinely; useful for assessing complications such as pneumonia
- *Laboratory studies*: not recommended routinely; rapid viral antigen tests and nasopharyngeal cultures helpful for epidemiology and diagnosis in acutely ill young infants

of colds are young age, contact with school-age children, crowded conditions and poorly ventilated areas, and cigarette smoking. Children are more likely than adults to transmit viruses because of poorer hand hygiene, closer casual contacts, and sharing of toys.[45] Viral antigenic drifts and host immune system evasion contribute to the persistence of URIs in the community.

PATHOPHYSIOLOGY

Viruses enter the upper respiratory tract mucosa via inhalation of aerosols or infected droplets or direct contact with contaminated secretions. After cell entry, viral replication and shedding occur for several days to weeks. Clinical symptoms arise from epithelial cell damage, inflammation, vasodilation, edema from increased vascular permeability, increased mucus production, and impaired mucociliary clearance. Tracheobronchial inflammation and irritation induce cough via afferent nerve impulse transmission to the medulla.[45] Antibody production halts viral replication and inflammation as symptoms diminish.

TREATMENT

Desired Outcomes

● The treatment goal for the common cold is to minimize discomfort from symptoms to allow patients to function as normally as possible. Preventative measures are also a focus to limit the spread of infection to others.

General Approach to Treatment

Antibiotics have no role in the treatment of the common cold. They are often prescribed inappropriately to patients with viral URIs and purulent secretions, which has contributed to increased antibiotic resistance.[2] Antimicrobials do not shorten symptom severity or duration and do not prevent bacterial complications from occurring in patients with the common cold.[2,44] Treatment measures should focus on symptom relief.

Nonpharmacologic Therapy

Patient discomfort can be managed with supportive measures that include cool mist air humidification, use of intranasal saline drops or sprays with or without bulb suctioning, increased fluid intake, throat lozenges or saline gargles, and rest. Nasal strips have been advocated to relieve congestion by lifting the nares and opening the anterior nasal passages. These nondrug measures are particularly important for infants, children under 6 years of age, and pregnant women, for whom medication safety is a significant concern. Although studies proving their benefits are lacking, these nondrug treatments are safe.

Pharmacologic Therapy

Nonprescription cough and cold preparations are used frequently to manage cold symptoms despite the lack of evidence to support their safety and efficacy. Reports of serious adverse events and deaths have led to efforts to eliminate use of nonprescription cough and cold medications in young children.[47] Manufacturers have removed product labeling for all children under 4 years of age.

Hundreds of nonprescription cough and cold products are available to manage cold symptoms. ❿ *Choice of therapy is influenced by patient age, presence of comorbid conditions, and balance of effectiveness and safety.* Single-ingredient agents are preferred over multi-ingredient products in order to target only symptoms that are present and to minimize the toxicity and overdose risk that can result from confusion and lack of knowledge on active ingredients in marketed formulations. Cautious use of nonprescription preparations is warranted in certain patient populations: pregnant and/or lactating women, elderly, those with cardiovascular disease including hypertension, patients with diabetes, and patients with glaucoma. Table 72–6 summarizes some of the available nonprescription agents used for cold symptoms. Antipyretics and analgesics can be used for fever, pain, and discomfort from cold symptoms. Local anesthetics (e.g., benzocaine, dyclonine) relieve throat pain and are available in lozenges and sprays. Decongestants cause vasoconstriction that can modestly improve nasal airway resistance and congestion, but use of intranasal products should be limited to 3 days to avoid rebound congestion.[44,49]

Antihistamines should be avoided when treating cold symptoms: first-generation antihistamines may help dry watery secretions through their anticholinergic effects, but they impair mucociliary clearance of thick mucus, which can worsen congestion, and studies have not shown clear benefits for cough or cold symptoms.[44,49] Cough suppressant use is not supported by strong evidence showing benefit. They can cause significant neurologic adverse effects and have been linked to abuse by teens for their euphoric effects in high doses.[44-46,49] Guaifenesin, an expectorant, may reduce cough frequency and sputum thickness in adults, but it has been poorly studied in children.[49] Routine high-dose vitamin C (more than 200 mg/day) supplementation does not significantly impact cold severity or duration, but it may be useful for prevention in certain populations exposed to severe physical exercise or cold stress.[49] Use of Echinacea purpurea extracted from aerial parts may have benefit in adults when started early for treatment, but its use is discouraged for prevention and in all children.[50] Other forms of echinacea have not shown consistent benefit for treatment of cold symptoms. Zinc lozenges are not effective for treating cold symptoms, and concerns exist regarding the loss of smell with intranasal zinc preparations, so they should be avoided.

PREVENTION

Prevention of the common cold is best achieved by minimizing contact with infected people and secretions.

Table 72–6

Select Nonprescription Medications for the Common Cold for Patients 6 Years of Age and Above

Class/Drug	Adult Dose[a]	Pediatric Dose[b]	Comments
Analgesics/Antipyretics			
Acetaminophen[c][d]	325–1,000 mg every 4–6 hours (max 4 g/day)	10–15 mg/kg/dose every 4–6 hours (max 5 doses/day)	Use with caution in preexisting liver disease
Ibuprofen[e]	200–400 mg every 6–8 hours (max 1,200 mg/day)	5–10 mg/kg/dose every 6–8 hours (max 4 doses/day)	Use with caution in cardiovascular disease; avoid use in elderly, renal impairment, and heart failure; avoid in third trimester of pregnancy
Decongestants			
Intranasal:			
Oxymetazoline 0.05%[d]	2–3 sprays every 12 hours (max 2 doses/24 hours)	1–2 sprays every 12 hours (max 2 doses/24 hours)	Limit use of intranasal decongestants to 3 to 5 days to minimize risk of rebound congestion; use with caution in patients with cardiovascular disease
Phenylephrine 0.25%, 0.5%, 1%	2–3 sprays no more than every 4 hours	2–3 sprays no more than every 4 hours (0.25% only)	
Systemic:			
Pseudoephedrine	60 mg every 4–6 hours (max 240 mg/day)	30 mg every 4–6 hours (max 120 mg/day)	Avoid use in patients with cardiovascular disease; children and elderly have increased risk of adverse effects (cardiovascular or CNS stimulation); use with caution in patients with diabetes, hyperthyroidism, prostatic hypertrophy; avoid in first trimester of pregnancy
Phenylephrine	10 mg every 4 hours (max 60 mg/day)	5 mg every 4 hours (max 30 mg/day)	
Cough Suppressants			
Dextromethorphan[d]	10–20 mg every 4 hours or 30 mg every 6–8 hours or 60 mg every 12 hours (max 120 mg/day)	5–10 mg every 4 hours or 15 mg every 6–8 hours or 30 mg every 12 hours (max 60 mg/day)	Increased adverse effects in children and poor metabolizers (5–10% of white patients); can cause dysphoria and serotonin syndrome; use caution in those taking psychotropic medications
Expectorants			
Guaifenesin	200–400 mg every 4 hours or 600–1,200 mg every 12 hours (max 2.4 g/day)	100–200 mg every 4 hours (max 1.2 g/day)	May cause nausea and abdominal pain, particularly in higher doses
Anticholinergics			
Intranasal ipratropium 0.06%[d]	2 sprays 3–4 times/day	2 sprays 3 times/day	Used for rhinorrhea only; does not improve congestion, postnasal drip, or sneezing

[a]Also for children greater than 12 years of age.

[b]For children 6 to 12 years of age.

[c]Preferred antipyretic/analgesic for children; can be used in newborns.

[d]Safe to use in pregnancy.

[e]Can be used in children older than 6 months of age.

From Refs. 44 and 48.

Frequent handwashing with soap and water or use of alcohol-based products is the cornerstone of prevention. Coughing and sneezing into the arm sleeve should be taught rather than using tissues or covering the mouth and nose with hands. Other methods that are often advocated for preventing the spread of colds include smoking cessation, maintenance of a healthy lifestyle through diet and exercise, and minimizing stress.

OUTCOME EVALUATION

Most colds will resolve within 7 to 10 days. Monitor patients for symptoms that persist for longer than 10 to 14 days, worsening symptoms, and complications such as wheezing, difficulty breathing, moderate to severe facial or ear pain, and high fevers. If complications are suspected, referral to a physician is warranted.

Patient Encounter 4

A 20-year-old female presents to the university health center clinic with a "sinus infection." Three days ago, she developed a sore throat and a "runny nose." Today, the nasal discharge is a thicker and yellow-green color, and she has a mild headache. She also has nasal congestion and a dry, nonproductive cough that started yesterday. She took acetaminophen 650 mg this morning, which provided some headache relief. She has no medical conditions, but she does experience colds three to four times per year. She attends college and lives in an apartment with three friends. Two of her roommates also have similar symptoms.

Immunizations: up-to-date; needs influenza vaccine this season

Meds: vitamin C 1,000 mg orally daily, Ortho Tri-Cyclen orally daily

Allergies: sulfa drugs (rash)

PE:

Gen: no apparent distress; pleasant

VS: BP 126/78 mm Hg, P 72 beats/min, RR 18 breaths/min, T 37.5°C (99.5°F), wt 61.4 kg (135 lb)

HEENT: conjunctiva clear; no photophobia; green-yellow nasal discharge with mucosal hypertrophy and narrowed passages; erythematous pharynx with no exudates; no facial pain upon palpation; tympanic membranes normal appearing

Lungs: clear to auscultation; occasional wheeze with cough; no crackles

What signs and symptoms are suggestive of the common cold? Which are suggestive of ABRS?

What other diagnostic studies, if any, should be performed?

Create a care plan that includes nonpharmacologic and pharmacologic therapies and a monitoring plan. Include preventative measures in your plan.

Patient Care and Monitoring of Common Cold

1. Assess the patient's signs and symptoms. Are they consistent with the common cold?

2. How long have the patient's symptoms been present? If symptoms have been present for fewer than 7 to 10 days, the common cold is likely. Persistent moderate or acute severe symptoms are more indicative of bacterial infections.

3. Has the patient tried any medications or nonpharmacologic methods to treat the symptoms? If yes, do they provide any relief?

4. Obtain a medication and medical history, including prescription and nonprescription drugs, natural product use, allergies, and current medical conditions.

5. Determine whether nonprescription medications should be used to alleviate symptoms, such as pain and congestion.

6. Develop a treatment plan (including use of nonpharmacologic measures) to assess effectiveness of the chosen therapy and course of action to take if the patient does not improve or worsens.

7. Provide patient education on:

   - Role of viruses in colds, symptom resolution expectations, and how to prevent transmission to others

   - What to expect from the chosen therapy, including proper dosing and potential adverse effects

   - Avoidance of antibiotics to treat colds

   - When to seek additional medical care

8. Stress the importance of handwashing and limiting spread to others.

Abbreviations Introduced in This Chapter

ABRS	Acute bacterial rhinosinusitis
AOM	Acute otitis media
OME	Otitis media with effusion
PRSP	Penicillin-resistant *S. pneumoniae*
RADT	Rapid antigen detection test
URI	Upper respiratory tract infection

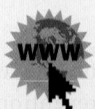

Self-assessment questions and answers are available at *http://www.mhpharmacotherapy.com/pp.html.*

REFERENCES

1. Anon JB. Upper respiratory infections. Am J Med 2010;123:S16–S25.
2. Gonzales R, Bartlett JG, Besser RE, et al. Principles of appropriate antibiotic use for treatment of nonspecific upper respiratory tract

infections in adults: Background. Ann Intern Med 2001;134:490–494.

3. Rovers MM, Schilder AGM, Zielhuis GA, Rosenfeld RM. Otitis media. Lancet 2004;363:465–473.

4. American Academy of Pediatrics and American Academy of Family Physicians. Diagnosis and management of acute otitis media. Pediatrics 2004;113(5):1451–1465.

5. McCaig LF, Besser RE, Hughes JM. Trends in antimicrobial prescribing rates for children and adolescents. JAMA 2002;287:3096–3102.

6. Grijalva CG, Nuorti JP, Griffin MR. Antibiotic prescription rates for acute respiratory tract infections in US ambulatory settings. JAMA 2009;302:758–766.

7. Corbeel L. What is new in otitis media? Eur J Pediatr 2007;166:511–519.

8. Dowell SF, Butler JC, Giebink GS, et al. Acute otitis media: Management and surveillance in an era of pneumococcal resistance—a report from the Drug-Resistant *Streptococcus pneumoniae* Therapeutic Working Group. Pediatr Infect Dis J 1999;18:1–9.

9. Coker TR, Chan LS, Newberry SJ, et al. Diagnosis, microbial epidemiology, and antibiotic treatment of acute otitis media in children: a systematic review. JAMA 2010;304:2161–2169.

10. Casey JR, Pichichero ME. Changes in frequency and pathogens causing acute otitis media in 1995–2003. Pediatr Infect Dis J 2004;23:839–841.

11. Pichichero ME, Casey JR. Evolving microbiology and molecular epidemiology of acute otitis media in the pneumococcal conjugate vaccine era. Pediatr Infect Dis J 2007;26:S12–S16.

12. Nokso-Koivisto J, Räty R, Blomqvist S, et al. Presence of specific viruses in the middle ear fluids and respiratory secretions of young children with acute otitis media. J Med Virol 2004;72:241–248.

13. Jones RN, Sader HS, Moet GJ, Farrell DJ. Declining antimicrobial susceptibility of *Streptococcus pneumoniae* in the United States: report from the SENTRY Antimicrobial Surveillance Program (1998-2009). Diagn Microbiol Infect Dis 2010;68:334–336.

14. Johnson DM, Stilwell MG, Fritsche TR, Jones RN. Emergence of multidrug resistant *Streptococcus pneumoniae*: Report from the SENTRY Antimicrobial Surveillance Program (1999–2003). Diagn Microbiol Infect Dis 2006;56:69–74.

15. Sanders S, Glasziou PP, Del Mar CB, Rovers MM. Antibiotics for acute otitis media in children. Cochrane Database Syst Rev 2004;CD000219.

16. Tähtinen PA, Laine MK, Huovinen P, et al. A placebo-controlled trial of antimicrobial treatment for acute otitis media. N Engl J Med 2011;364:116–126.

17. Hoberman A, Paradise JL, Rockette HE, et al. Treatment of acute otitis media in children under 2 years of age. N Engl J Med 2011;364:105–115.

18. Spiro DM, Arnold DH. The concept and practice of a wait-and-see approach to acute otitis media. Curr Opin Pediatr 2008;20:72–78.

19. Piglansky L, Leibovitz E, Raiz S, et al. Bacteriologic and clinical efficacy of high dose amoxicillin for therapy of acute otitis media in children. Pediatr Infect Dis J 2003;22:405–413.

20. Leibovitz E, Piglansky L, Raiz S, et al. Bacteriologic and clinical efficacy of one day vs. three day intramuscular ceftriaxone for treatment of nonresponsive acute otitis media in children. Pediatr Infect Dis J 2000;19:1040–1045.

21. Schmelzle J, Birtwhistle RV, Tan AK. Acute otitis media in children with tympanostomy tubes. Can Fam Physician 2008;54:1123–1127.

22. Kozyrskyj AL, Klassen TP, Moffatt M, Harvey K. Short-course antibiotics for acute otitis media. Cochrane Database Syst Rev 2010;CD001095.

23. Coleman C, Moore M. Decongestants and antihistamines for acute otitis media in children. Cochrane Database Syst Rev 2008;CD001727.

24. Jenson HB, Baltimore RS. Impact of influenza and pneumococcal vaccines on otitis media. Curr Opin Pediatr 2004;16:58–60.

25. Block SL, Heikkinen T, Toback SL, Zheng W, Ambrose CS. The efficacy of live attenuated influenza vaccine against influenza-associated acute otitis media in children. Pediatr Infect Dis J 2011;30:203–207.

26. Jansen AG, Hak E, Veenhoven RH, et al. Pneumococcal conjugate vaccines for preventing otitis media. Cochrane Database Syst Rev 2009;CD001480.

27. American Academy of Family Physicians; American Academy of Otolaryngology—Head and Neck Surgery; American Academy of Pediatrics Subcommittee on Otitis Media With Effusion. Otitis media with effusion. Pediatrics 2004;113:1412–1429.

28. American Academy of Pediatrics. Clinical practice guideline: Management of sinusitis. Pediatrics 2001;108:798–808.

29. Sinus and Allergy Health Partnership. Antimicrobial treatment guidelines for acute bacterial rhinosinusitis. Otolaryngol Head Neck Surg 2004;130:S1–S45.

30. Sande MA, Gwaltney JM. Acute community-acquired bacterial sinusitis: Continuing challenges and current management. Clin Infect Dis 2004;39:S151–S158.

31. Benninger MS. Acute bacterial rhinosinusitis and otitis media: changes in pathogenicity following widespread use of pneumococcal conjugate vaccine. Otolaryngol Head Neck Surg 2008;138:274–278.

32. Payne SC, Benninger MS. *Staphylococcus aureus* is a major pathogen in acute bacterial rhinosinusitis: a meta-analysis. Clin Infect Dis 2007;45:e121–e127.

33. Rosenfeld RM, Andes D, Bhattacharyya N, et al. Clinical practice guideline: Adult sinusitis. Otolaryngol Head Neck Surg 2007;137:S1–S31.

34. Rosenfeld RM, Singer M, Jones S. Systematic review of antimicrobial therapy in patients with acute rhinosinusitis. Otolaryngol Head Neck Surg 2007;137:S32–S45.

35. Zalmanovici A, Yaphe J. Intranasal steroids for acute sinusitis. Cochrane Database Syst Rev 2009;CD005149.

36. Falagas ME, Karageorgopoulos DE, Grammatikos AP, Matthaiou DK. Effectiveness and safety of short vs. long duration of antibiotic therapy for acute bacterial sinusitis: a meta-analysis of randomized trials. Br J Clin Pharmacol 2009;67:161–171.

37. Cooper RJ, Hoffman JR, Bartlett JG, et al. Principles of appropriate antibiotic use for acute pharyngitis in adults: background. Ann Intern Med 2001;134:509–517.

38. Linder JA, Bates DW, Lee GM, Finkelstein JA. Antibiotic treatment of children with sore throat. JAMA 2005;294:2315–2322.

39. Wessels MR. Streptococcal pharyngitis. N Engl J Med 2011;364:648–655.

40. Bisno AL, Gerber MA, Gwaltney JM, et al. Practice guidelines for the diagnosis and management of group A streptococcal pharyngitis. Clin Infect Dis 2002;35:113–125.

41. Gerber MA, Baltimore RS, Eaton CB, et al. Prevention of rheumatic fever and diagnosis and treatment of acute streptococcal pharyngitis. A scientific statement from the American Heart Association Rheumatic Fever, Endocarditis, and Kawasaki Disease Committee of the Council on Cardiovascular Disease in the Young, the Interdisciplinary Council on Functional Genomics and Translational Biology, and the Interdisciplinary Council on Quality of Care and Outcomes Research: endorsed by the American Academy of Pediatrics. Circulation 2009;119:1541–1551.

42. van Driel ML, De Sutter AI, Keber N, et al. Different antibiotic treatments for group A streptococcal pharyngitis. Cochrane Database Syst Rev 2010;CD004406.

43. Casey JR, Pichichero ME. Metaanalysis of short course antibiotic treatment for group a streptococcal tonsillopharyngitis. Pediatr Infect Dis J 2005;24:909–917.

44. Simasek M, Blandino DA. Treatment of the common cold. Am Fam Physician 2007;75:515–520.

45. Kelley LK, Allen PJ. Managing acute cough in children: evidence-based guidelines. Pediatr Nurs 2007;33:515–524.

46. Pratter MR. Cough and the common cold. ACCP evidence-based clinical practice guidelines. Chest 2006;129:S72– S74.

47. Ryan T, Brewer M, Small L. Over-the-counter cough and cold medication use in young children. Pediatr Nurs 2008;34:174–180.

48. Erebara A, Bozzo P, Einarson A, Koren G. Treating the common cold during pregnancy. Can Fam Physician 2008;54:687–689.

49. Arroll B. Non-antibiotic treatments for upper-respiratory tract infections (common cold). Respir Med 2005;99:1477–1484.

50. Linde K, Barrett B, Bauer R, et al. Echinacea for preventing and treating the common cold. Cochrane Database Syst Rev 2006;CD000530.

73 Skin and Soft Tissue Infections

Jaime R. Hornecker

LEARNING OBJECTIVES

● **Upon completion of the chapter, the reader will be able to:**

1. Discuss characteristics of the skin that render it resistant to infection.

2. Describe the epidemiology, etiology, pathogenesis, clinical manifestations, diagnostic criteria, and complications associated with skin and soft tissue infections (SSTIs).

3. Identify the desired therapeutic outcomes for patients with SSTIs.

4. Recommend appropriate empirical and definitive antimicrobial regimens when given a diagnosis, patient history, physical examination, and laboratory findings.

5. Monitor chosen antimicrobial therapy for safety and efficacy.

KEY CONCEPTS

❶ Impetigo commonly afflicts young children, is usually caused by group A streptococci or *Staphylococcus aureus*, and is characterized by numerous blisters that rupture and form crusts. Dicloxacillin, cephalexin, and topical mupirocin are considered the antibiotics of choice for treatment of impetigo.

❷ Folliculitis, furuncles, and carbuncles refer to the inflammation of one or more hair follicles, often attributed to infection with *S. aureus*. Treatment depends on severity and may involve local heat, incision and drainage, and/or oral or topical antibiotic therapy.

❸ Erysipelas is a superficial infection of the upper dermis and superficial lymphatics distinguished from cellulitis by its well-defined borders and slightly raised lesions. It is usually caused by β-hemolytic streptococci and treated with penicillin.

❹ Cellulitis, a bacterial infection of the dermis and subcutaneous tissue, is most commonly caused by *S. aureus* and β-hemolytic streptococci. Although β-lactams active against penicillinase-producing strains of *S. aureus* have historically been the drugs of choice, in areas with high rates of community-acquired methicillin-resistant *S. aureus* (CA-MRSA), or in patients with risk factors for CA-MRSA infection, treatment with antibiotics active against this organism should be initiated due to its increasing prevalence.

❺ Persons who are immunocompromised, have diabetes or vascular insufficiency, or use injection drugs are at risk for polymicrobial cellulitis, often requiring broad-spectrum antibiotic coverage.

❻ Necrotizing fasciitis (NF) is an uncommon, rapidly progressive, life-threatening infection that causes necrosis of the subcutaneous tissue and fascia. Immediate surgical débridement is key to reducing its associated mortality.

❼ The pathogenesis of diabetic foot infection stems from three key factors: neuropathy, angiopathy, and immunopathy. Aerobic gram-positive cocci, such as *S. aureus* and β-hemolytic streptococci, are the predominant pathogens in acutely infected diabetic foot ulcers. However, chronically infected wounds are subject to polymicrobial infection and require treatment with broad-spectrum antibiotics.

❽ Prevention is key in the management of pressure sores. Mild superficial pressure sore infections may be treated with topical antimicrobial agents. Systemic antibiotics are indicated for serious pressure ulcer infections, including those associated with spreading cellulitis, osteomyelitis, or bacteremia.

❾ Bite wound infections generally are polymicrobial. Amoxicillin-clavulanate is the drug of choice for treating infected bite wounds and is also used as infection prophylaxis for human bites, deep punctures, and bites to the hand, or those requiring surgical repair.

❿ Every patient receiving treatment for skin and soft tissue infections (SSTIs) must be educated on prevention measures and monitored for efficacy and safety. Efficacy typically is manifested by reductions in temperature, white blood cell count, erythema, edema, and pain that begin within 48 to 72 hours after treatment initiation. To ensure safety, adjust antibiotic dosages for renal and hepatic dysfunction as appropriate, and monitor for and minimize adverse drug reactions, allergic reactions, and drug interactions.

Skin and soft tissue infections (SSTIs) are frequently encountered in both acute and ambulatory care settings. They can range in severity from mild, superficial, and self-limiting, to life-threatening deep tissue infections that require intensive care, surgical intervention, and IV broad-spectrum antibiotics. *S. aureus* and β-hemolytic streptococci (*Streptococcus pyogenes* and *Streptococcus agalactiae*) are the most common causative bacteria.[1-3] Complicated infections that may involve deeper layers of the skin, fascia, or muscle in persons with immune suppression, diabetes, vascular insufficiency, burns, decubitus ulcers, or traumatic wounds are often polymicrobial.[3]

The role of methicillin-resistant *S. aureus* (MRSA), particularly community-acquired methicillin-resistant *S. aureus* (CA-MRSA), is of increasing importance. In many U.S. cities, MRSA has become the most frequently isolated pathogen from patients presenting to emergency departments with SSTI.[4] From 2000 to 2004, hospital admissions for SSTIs increased by 29%, presumably due to the emergence of CA-MRSA.[5] MRSA infections were historically associated with exposures to healthcare settings (including hospitals or long-term care facilities), but have recently become problematic in previously healthy persons. Although risk factors for acquisition of CA-MRSA are not well established, outbreaks of CA-MRSA infection have occurred in prison inmates, homosexual males, injection drug users, athletes, military recruits, Native Americans, individuals with lower socioeconomic status, and children, especially those with daycare exposure. In both adults and children, recent antibiotic exposure is also associated with a dose-dependent increase in the risk of CA-MRSA infection.[6,7] In these high-risk groups, in those with recurrent infections or infections that persist despite appropriate antimicrobial therapy, or in areas with high rates of CA-MRSA, empiric therapy including antibiotics active against this pathogen must be considered.[3] This chapter covers the epidemiology, pathogenesis, clinical manifestations, and pharmacologic management of the more common and severe bacterial SSTIs.

Intact skin generally is resistant to infection. In addition to providing a mechanical barrier, its relative dryness, slightly acidic pH, colonizing bacteria, frequent desquamation, and production of various antimicrobial defense chemicals, including sweat (which contains IgG and IgA), prevent invasion by various microorganisms.[8] Conditions that predispose a patient to SSTIs include: (a) high bacterial load (greater than 10^5 microorganisms); (b) excessive skin moisture; (c) decreased skin perfusion; (d) availability of bacterial nutrients; and (e) damage to the corneal layer of the skin.[9]

IMPETIGO

EPIDEMIOLOGY AND ETIOLOGY

Impetigo, which stems from the Latin word for "attack," is a common skin infection worldwide.[10] ❶ *It predominately afflicts children between 2 and 5 years of age but may occur in any age group.*[2] β-Hemolytic streptococci and *S. aureus* are the most common causative pathogens.[2,10] Impetigo is a superficial infection and is spread easily, especially in settings of poor hygiene and crowding, and particularly during the summer months. The offending microorganisms colonize the skin surface and invade through abrasions, insect bites, or other small traumas. The scabby, crusty eruption of impetigo ensues. These lesions may occur anywhere on the body, but are most common on the face and extremities.[2]

CLINICAL PRESENTATION AND DIAGNOSIS

Impetigo lesions are numerous, well-localized, and erythematous. ❶ *They develop either as small, thin-walled blisters (impetigo contagiosum), or as larger blisters (bullous impetigo), which may be associated with mild systemic symptoms.*[2,10,11] *S. aureus* is most often implicated in bullous impetigo. The blisters rupture easily, leaving behind a friable crust reminiscent of cornflakes. The lesions of impetigo are rarely painful, but are pruritic. Scratching the lesions can spread the infection to other areas of the body.[10]

In order to avoid further spread and complications, antibiotic therapy is usually indicated. If left untreated, mild, localized cases of impetigo typically resolve within 2 to 3 weeks.[10,11] Sequelae of impetigo are uncommon, and when complications do occur, they seem to be more frequent in adults. Rarely, glomerulonephritis secondary to group A *Streptococcus* (GAS) may occur in nonbullous impetigo. Development of impetigo into more serious infections such as cellulitis or sepsis is another rare, but serious consequence.

TREATMENT
Desired Outcomes

The primary goals of therapy for impetigo include preventing the spread of infection within the patient and to others, resolution of infection, and preventing recurrence. Secondarily, relief of symptoms associated with impetigo, such as itching, and improving cosmetic appearance are also important. Prevention of the rare, but serious complications of impetigo is an alternative goal.[12]

Nonpharmacologic Treatment

Because impetigo is rarely painful, there is often a delay in seeking medical attention. However, the lesions will often resolve with time and increased hygiene. Soaking and cleansing the lesions with mild soap and water and the use of skin emollients to dry skin areas may reduce spread.[10]

Pharmacologic Treatment

Antibiotic therapy is recommended to achieve the desired outcomes of preventing the spread of infection and complications. Because GAS historically has been the primary causative organism, penicillin has been the mainstay of therapy. ❶ *However, the incidence of* S. aureus *impetigo is increasing significantly, so oral penicillinase-stable penicillins or first-generation cephalosporins are now preferred.* Clindamycin or a macrolide are alternative choices when penicillin allergy is a concern; however, erythromycin-resistant strains of staphylococci and streptococci are increasing in prevalence. ❶ *Topical mupirocin or retapamulin may be used alone in mild cases with few lesions.*[2,11]

FOLLICULITIS, FURUNCLES, AND CARBUNCLES

See **Table 73–1.**

CELLULITIS AND ERYSIPELAS

EPIDEMIOLOGY AND ETIOLOGY

● Cellulitis and erysipelas are bacterial infections involving the skin. ❸ and ❹ *Cellulitis is an infection of the dermis and subcutaneous tissue, whereas erysipelas is a more superficial infection of the upper dermis and superficial lymphatics. Although both can occur on any part of the body, about 90% of infections involve the leg.*[14] These infections develop after a break in skin integrity, resulting from trauma, surgery, ulceration, burns, tinea infection, or other skin disorder.

Table 73–1

Folliculitis, Furuncles, and Carbuncles

	Folliculitis	Furuncles	Carbuncles
Epidemiology/etiology	❷ *Folliculitis is a superficial inflammatory reaction involving the hair follicle. The most familiar form of folliculitis is acne.* It can be infectious, caused by microorganisms such as *S. aureus, Pseudomonas, and Candida.* Folliculitis can also be chemically induced.	Also known as boils, furuncles might be described as a deep form of folliculitis. A furuncle is a bacterial infection that has spread into the subcutaneous skin layers but still only involves individual follicles. Furuncles occur primarily in young men. Diabetes and obesity are other predisposing factors. Staphylococci are the most common cause.	Carbuncles share all the characteristics of furuncles. However, a carbuncle is larger and involves several adjacent follicles and may extend into the subcutaneous fat. Carbuncles are more likely to occur in patients with diabetes and tend to form on the back of the neck.
Presentation and diagnosis	Folliculitis presents as small, pruritic, erythematous papules. Location of the lesions and a good patient history are often all that are required in the diagnosis of folliculitis. Although Gram stain and culture of the papules may be considered to help determine the causative agent, they are not generally required as folliculitis typically resolves spontaneously.	Furuncles most commonly develop on the face, neck, axilla, and buttock. A furuncle typically starts as a small, red, tender nodule. Within a few days, the nodule becomes painful and pustular. Typically, a furuncle will spontaneously discharge pus, heal, and leave a small scar.	Carbuncles are similar to furuncles; only they are larger and exquisitely painful.
Desired outcomes	The goals of therapy for folliculitis, furuncles, and carbuncles are resolution of infection with no or minimal scarring. A secondary goal of therapy for larger furuncles and all carbuncles is to minimize the risk of endocarditis or osteomyelitis by reducing bloodstream invasion.		
Nonpharmacologic treatment	❷ *Warm compresses are generally sufficient.*	*Moist heat is indicated to facilitate drainage. Large furuncles require incision and drainage.*	*Incision and drainage are indicated.*
Pharmacologic treatment	❷ *Often resolves spontaneously. A topical antibiotic or antifungal may be used to control the spread of infection but generally is unnecessary.* For staphylococcal or streptococcal folliculitis, antibiotic ointments such as mupirocin might be administered three times daily. Antifungal shampoo can be used for dermatophytes.	*Carbuncles and furuncles that have surrounding cellulitis and fever or are located midline on the face must be treated systemically with an antibiotic that will cover S. aureus, such as dicloxacillin or cephalexin. Trimethoprim-sulfamethoxazole DS, doxycycline, or clindamycin are preferred if CA-MRSA is suspected or if the patient has a severe allergy to penicillin.* Treatment should continue until acute inflammation has resolved, usually a 5- to 10-day course. Prevention for recurrent episodes may be warranted, including adequate skin hygiene with the use of antimicrobial soap and water, and handwashing after contact with lesions. Proper care of clothing and dressings is also recommended to prevent autoinoculation.	

From Refs. 2, 11, and 13.

Patient Encounter 1, Part 1: Cellulitis

A 49-year-old woman presents to the ambulatory care clinic with a 3-day history of progressively worsening pain and swelling of her right lower extremity. Upon examination, you notice that in addition to the patient's complaints, the area is visibly erythematous. Poorly defined areas of redness and streaking extend from just below the knee up toward her hip. A small, nonpurulent scabbed area is present over the kneecap. She reports running a low-grade fever and some feelings of fatigue, but otherwise feels fine. When questioned, she indicates that she recently fell on the sidewalk and "skinned" her knee after tripping while walking her dog. Her vitals at the clinic reveal a temperature of 38.2°C, pulse 92 beats/min, blood pressure 122/82 mm Hg, and respiratory rate 18 breaths/min. The physician diagnoses the patient with cellulitis.

What subjective and objective clinical manifestations are suggestive of cellulitis?

What additional information do you need before developing a therapeutic plan for this patient?

However, they may occur after an inapparent break in the skin, and the skin may appear previously intact. In rare cases, cellulitis develops from bloodborne or contiguous spread of pathogens.[2,15]

Etiologic microorganisms vary according to the area involved, host factors, and exposures. ❸ *Erysipelas is generally caused by β-hemolytic streptococci, mainly GAS, and rarely by S. aureus.* ❹ *The predominant pathogens associated with cellulitis are S. aureus, including methicillin-resistant strains, and β-hemolytic streptococci.* ❺ *Persons who are immunocompromised, have diabetes or vascular insufficiency, or use injection drugs are at risk for polymicrobial cellulitis.*[2,3]

CLINICAL PRESENTATION AND DIAGNOSIS

● The manifestations of and diagnostic criteria for erysipelas and cellulitis are presented in Table 73–2. Once diagnosed, cellulitis may be characterized as complicated or uncomplicated. Complicated infections are those that involve abnormal skin or wounds, occur in immunocompromised hosts, require substantial surgical intervention, or are polymicrobial in origin.[16]

With early diagnosis and appropriate therapy, the prognoses for cellulitis and erysipelas are excellent. Severe or repeated episodes can cause lymphedema. Rare complications include the spread of infection to deeper skin and soft tissue layers, bacteremia, and sepsis.[2] Although rates of bacteremia were traditionally low, prevalence may be increasing and associated with increased length of hospitalization and costs, and higher readmission rates.[17] If the circumference of an extremity is cellulitic, compartment syndrome becomes a concern, and a surgical consult may be required. Recurrent cellulitis can be problematic. About 30% of patients hospitalized with cellulitis will develop a recurrent episode within 3 years. Vascular and lymphatic insufficiencies increase the risk of recurrences.[15]

Table 73–2

Presentation of Erysipelas and Cellulitis

Symptoms

- The infected area is described as painful or tender. In the case of erysipelas, the patient may complain of "burning pain" at the lesion site. CA-MRSA infections often start as a localized skin lesion and may be described by the patient as looking like a "spider bite."

Signs

- Both erysipelas and cellulitis are manifested by rapidly spreading areas of redness, edema, and heat. **Lymphangitis** and regional lymphadenopathy may be observed.
- Important clinical differences between erysipelas and cellulitis exist:
  - In erysipelas, low-grade fever and flu-like illness are common prior to development of the lesion. The lesion is fiery red, raised above the level of surrounding skin, and has well-defined borders. The affected area may have an "orange peel" appearance.
  - In cellulitis, the lesion is not raised and has poorly defined margins.

Laboratory Tests

- Leukocytosis may be present.
- Cultures and sensitivities:
  - Blood cultures should be obtained for complicated or severe cases, although their yield is often low as bacteremia is an infrequent, but growing, occurrence; facial cellulitis may increase risk. Cultures aspirated from the lesion have an organism isolation rate of less than 20%, but also may be considered.
  - Abscess drainage and débrided tissue, if obtainable, should be cultured and will yield the causative organism(s) up to 90% of the time.

Imaging Studies

- Imaging studies may identify abscess formation, gas in the soft tissues, or osteomyelitis.

From Refs. 2, 14, and 15.

TREATMENT

Desired Outcomes

The goals of therapy for cellulitis and erysipelas are rapid and successful eradication of the infection and prevention of related complications.

Nonpharmacologic Treatment

Nonpharmacologic treatment includes elevating and immobilizing the involved limb to decrease swelling. Sterile saline dressings should be placed on any open lesions to cleanse them of **purulent** materials. Surgical débridement is indicated occasionally for severe infection. Drainage of abscesses is imperative to achieving clinical cure and may be the only treatment necessary if the abscess is small (less than 5 cm) with limited cellulitis.[15,18]

Pharmacologic Treatment

Most patients with erysipelas or cellulitis are not hospitalized. Hospitalization and treatment with IV antibiotics should be considered if there are systemic signs and symptoms of infection (e.g., fever, chills, or hypotension), the patient has significant comorbid conditions (e.g., immunocompromise, diabetes, cirrhosis, cardiac failure, or renal insufficiency), or the cellulitis is spreading rapidly, involves a large area of the body, or is chronic.[15]

③ *Penicillin is the treatment of choice for erysipelas.* In uncomplicated cases, a 5-day course is as effective as a 10-day course.[2] Other agents that are acceptable for treatment include clindamycin, cephalexin, and dicloxacillin.

④ Although β-lactams, such as dicloxacillin, active against penicillinase-producing strains of *S. aureus* (commonly known as methicillin-sensitive *S. aureus*, or MSSA), have historically been the drugs of choice for acute bacterial cellulitis in otherwise healthy individuals, the increasing prevalence of infection with CA-MRSA is concerning, particularly in patients presenting with abscess.[2,19,20] Even in settings in which a drainable abscess is absent but the cellulitis is purulent or exudative, empiric therapy for CA-MRSA should be initiated.[21] Treatment active against CA-MRSA should also be initiated in areas with a high prevalence (e.g., greater than 15% of community *S. aureus* isolates show methicillin resistance) and in patients with risk factors for CA-MRSA infection.[3,19] Vancomycin continues to be the drug of choice for severe cellulitis due to MRSA because of its efficacy, safety, and low cost. Daptomycin, linezolid, telavancin, or ceftaroline are also acceptable and should be considered over vancomycin when the isolated organism has a minimum inhibitory concentration (MIC) of greater than 2 mcg/mL (greater than 2 mg/L) (e.g., vancomycin-intermediate *S. aureus* [VISA] or vancomycin-resistant *S. aureus* [VRSA]).[21] Tigecycline is an alternative; however, due to its broad spectrum of activity, it is best reserved for patients with intolerances to the aforementioned drugs or in those with polymicrobial infections. For less severe, uncomplicated infections, many CA-MRSA strains can be treated with clindamycin (isolates resistant to erythromycin should be evaluated with a D-test), doxycycline, minocycline, or trimethoprim-sulfamethoxazole.[2,3,19-22] However, it should be mentioned that although these agents are widely used for uncomplicated SSTI, this is an off-label use supported predominantly by data from observational and small interventional trials.[23] Also, trimethoprim-sulfamethoxazole

---

Patient Encounter 1, Part 2: Cellulitis: Medical History, Physical Examination, and Diagnostic Tests

PMH: GERD. C-section × 2.

FH: Father (age 70) and mother (age 68) are both alive. Father has type 2 diabetes; mother is otherwise healthy. One sister, age 43, is healthy.

SH: Denies alcohol or illicit drug use. Married, with two sons who attend the local community college. Works part-time in retail sales.

Meds: Omeprazole 20 mg daily prn, multivitamin daily.

Allergies: No known drug allergies.

ROS: (+) pain, edema, and erythema in the right lower extremity; (−) headache, chest pain, shortness of breath, cough, nausea, vomiting, diarrhea, and weight loss.

PE:

Gen: Patient is in no acute distress. Wt 68.0 kg (149.6 lb); ht 5 ft 5 in (165 cm).

Chest: Lungs bilaterally clear to auscultation.

CV: Regular rate, rhythm. No murmurs/rubs/gallops.

Ext: Right lower extremity with erythema and edema from the knee to just below the hip. Warm to the touch. LLE within normal limits.

Labs: WBC 15.8 × 10³/mm³ (15.8 × 10⁹/L), serum creatinine 0.8 mg/dL (71 μmol/L).

What are the most likely causative organisms in this case of cellulitis?

What are the goals of therapy for this patient?

What nonpharmacologic interventions would you recommend for her?

What antimicrobial therapy would you recommend? Include drug, dosage, route, interval, and duration of therapy.

How would you monitor your selected regimen for safety and efficacy?

How would your initial choice of an antimicrobial agent change if this patient was at high risk for CA-MRSA?

and doxycycline have less than optimal activity against GAS and should be empirically combined with an agent with such activity (e.g., cephalexin) if GAS is also a suspected causative organism.[19,20]

⑤ In addition to being at risk for staphylococcal and streptococcal cellulitis, patients with immune suppression, diabetes, vascular insufficiency, or wounds are also at risk for disease caused by gram-negative bacilli such as *Escherichia coli* and *Pseudomonas aeruginosa*, with or without anaerobes.[3] Empirical broad-spectrum antimicrobial coverage, including coverage for resistant organisms such as healthcare-associated MRSA (HA-MRSA) and *P. aeruginosa*, is appropriate for severe cellulitis and/or severe systemic illness. The clinician should be diligent in attempting to isolate a causative pathogen in these individuals.[2]

Injection drug use also predisposes individuals to polymicrobial cellulitis. The antecubital region of the arm is usually the site of infection. *S. aureus,* the most common isolate, is frequently associated with abscess formation. Because some injection drug users lick their needles to "clean" them, antibiotics that cover oropharyngeal anaerobes should be included. Occasionally, *Candida* spp. are isolated, and the patient may require antifungal therapy.[24]

Table 73–3 lists some recommended antibiotic regimens for the treatment of cellulitis. Because antimicrobial susceptibilities vary considerably between geographic locations, clinicians should select empirical treatment based on the antibiograms at their respective institutions. To decrease the spread of resistance, antibiotic therapy should be narrowed based on culture and sensitivity results whenever possible. The duration of therapy for uncomplicated cellulitis typically ranges from 7 to 10 days. For complicated cellulitis, therapy with IV antibiotics is generally initiated, and a switch to oral therapy can be made once the patient is afebrile and skin findings begin to resolve. Typically, this is done after 3 to 5 days. The complete duration of therapy can range from 10 to 14 days and longer in cases in which abscess, tissue necrosis, underlying skin wounds, or delayed response to therapy are involved.[2,15]

Patient Encounter 1, Part 3: Cellulitis: Clinical Course

Three days later, the patient returns to the clinic with moderate improvement of her cellulitis, but with a new presentation of a maculopapular skin rash. It is presumed that she has developed an allergy to penicillin.

What would you suggest for modification of her antimicrobial regimen?

How would you monitor her new regimen for safety and efficacy?

How would your choice of an agent change if this patient's cellulitis was severe enough to warrant hospitalization?

NECROTIZING FASCIITIS
EPIDEMIOLOGY AND ETIOLOGY

Necrotizing fasciitis (NF) is an uncommon, rapidly progressive, life-threatening infection that causes necrosis of the subcutaneous tissue and fascia. When due to GAS infection, its associated mortality rate approaches 25%.[25] NF can affect any age group. Although the risk of NF is higher in injection drug users and in patients with diabetes, immune suppression, or obesity, healthy hosts can become infected as well.[26]

NF typically erupts after an initial trauma, which can range from a small abrasion to a deep penetrating wound. The infection begins in the fascia, where bacteria replicate and release toxins that facilitate their spread.[27]

In approximately 70% of cases, NF is polymicrobial and typically involves anaerobes (i.e., *Bacteroides* or *Peptostreptococcus*), facultative anaerobes (i.e., β-hemolytic streptococci), and Enterobacteriaceae (e.g., *Escherichia coli, Enterobacter, Klebsiella*). *P. aeruginosa* is occasionally implicated as well.[26] Polymicrobial NF develops in the following clinical settings: after surgery or deep penetrating wounds involving the bowel; from decubitous ulcer, perianal, or vulvovaginal infection; or from the injection site in an IV drug user.[2,11]

The remaining 30% are monomicrobial, caused by invasive GAS, or less frequently, *Clostridium perfringens.* CA-MRSA is being implicated in these infections as well.[26] Monomicrobial NF is generally more severe than polymicrobial NF. GAS NF often occurs after minor trauma, such as an insect bite or abrasion, whereas infection with *C. perfringens* typically develops from surgical or traumatic wounds.[2,28] Once introduced, these organisms produce toxins that induce systemic toxicity, multiorgan failure, and shock.[28,29] Clostridial myonecrosis is more commonly known as gas gangrene.[2,28]

CLINICAL PRESENTATION AND DIAGNOSIS

Patient outcomes rely on the clinician's ability to recognize NF early in the course of disease. This is often difficult because early disease tends to be indistinguishable from cellulitis. The clinical presentation of NF is presented in Table 73–4.

NF is perhaps the most devastating SSTI. Left untreated, it can invade the muscles and circulation, resulting in myonecrosis and septic shock, respectively. Half of the cases caused by GAS are accompanied by GAS toxic shock–like syndrome. The syndrome is endotoxin-mediated, manifested by hypotension and multiorgan dysfunction, and highly lethal.[9,26] Amputation is required in up to 50% of patients with extremity infections.[30] Once the patient recovers from acute NF, he or she often requires skin and/or muscle grafting and consequent physical rehabilitation depending on the amount and types of tissues removed during surgical intervention and the duration of hospital stay.[31]

Table 73–3

Empirical Antimicrobial Therapy for Cellulitis

Host Factors	Probable Etiologic Bacteria	Mild Infection or Step-Down Therapy[a] (Oral Antibiotic Therapy)	Moderate–Severe Infection[a] (IV Antibiotic Therapy)
Previously healthy	MSSA GAS CA-MRSA	Dicloxacillin 500 mg every 6 hours Cephalexin 500 mg every 6 hours Clindamycin 300–600 mg every 6–8 hours CA-MRSA suspected or allergy to PCNs: Clindamycin[b] 300–600 mg every 6–8 hours Trimethoprim-sulfamethoxazole DS[c] 1–2 tabs every 12 hours Doxycycline[c] 100 mg every 12 hours Minocycline[c] 100 mg every 12 hours	Nafcillin 1–2 g every 4 hours Cefazolin 1–2 g every 8 hours Clindamycin 600–900 mg every 8 hours CA-MRSA suspected or allergy to PCNs: Vancomycin 15–20 mg/kg every 8–12 hours (individualize dose to achieve a trough of 15–20 mcg/mL [15–20 mg/L; 10.4–13.8 μmol/L]) Linezolid 600 mg every 12 hours Daptomycin 4 mg/kg every 24 hours Telavancin 10 mg/kg every 24 hours Ceftaroline[f] 600 mg every 12 hours
Immunocompromise, diabetes mellitus, vascular insufficiency, pressure ulcer infection, or other polymicrobial infection suspected	MSSA HA-MRSA CA-MRSA Enterobacteriaceae *P. aeruginosa* Anaerobes	Amoxicillin-clavulanate[d] 875 mg every 12 hours Levofloxacin[e] 750 mg every 24 hours + clindamycin 300–600 mg every 6 hours Moxifloxacin[d] 400 mg every 24 hours	Vancomycin, daptomycin, linezolid or telavancin[g] In combination with one of the following choices: Piperacillin-tazobactam[e] 3.375 g every 6 hours Ampicillin-sulbactam 3 g every 6 hours Imipenem-cilastatin[e] 500 mg every 6 hours Ertapenem 1 g every 24 hours Meropenem 500 mg every 8 hours Cefepime[e] 2 g every 12 hours ± metronidazole 500 mg every 8 hours Ceftazidime[e] 2 g every 8 hours + clindamycin 600–900 mg every 8 hours Levofloxacin[e] 750 mg every 24 hours ± clindamycin 600 mg every 8 hours OR Ceftaroline 600 mg every 12 hours + clindamycin 600–900 mg every 8 hours or metronidazole 500 mg every 8 hours OR Tigecycline 100 mg load, then 50 mg every 12 hours

[a]Doses given are for adults with normal renal function. IV therapy can be switched to oral therapy (as for mild infection) when the patient is afebrile and signs of infection are resolving.

[b]CA-MRSA isolates resistant to erythromycin should be evaluated for inducible clindamycin resistance via a D-test.

[c]Limited clinical data exist for the treatment of MRSA infections. Poor activity against GAS; consider using in combination with clindamycin or cephalexin if empirical coverage for GAS is desired.

[d]If CA-MRSA suspected, clindamycin, trimethoprim-sulfamethoxazole, or doxycycline must be added to this regimen.

[e]*P. aeruginosa* generally is susceptible to this agent.

[f]Use caution in patients with known hypersensitivity to beta-lactam antibiotics.

[g]MRSA coverage indicated for patients with severe cellulitis or systemic illness, who have risk factors for HA-MRSA or CA-MRSA infection, or reside in areas with high CA-MRSA prevalence. Otherwise, the broad-spectrum regimens listed below, without MRSA coverage, are appropriate.

From Refs. 2, 3, 11, 15, and 18–23.

Table 73-4

Presentation of Necrotizing Fasciitis

Symptoms

- Early: Severe pain that is disproportionate to clinical signs and extends beyond the margins of the infected area.
- Late: Area may become numb secondary to muscle and nerve involvement.

Signs

- Early: Skin is erythematous, edematous, and warm; the clinical presentation is similar to that of cellulitis.
- Intermediate (within 24–48 hours): Blisters and bullae indicate severe skin and tissue ischemia.
- Late: The skin becomes violaceous and progressively gangrenous; hemorrhagic bullae may be present. Systemic signs may include fever, tachycardia, hypotension, and shock.

Laboratory Tests

- White blood count, serum creatinine, and C-reactive protein may be elevated.
- Deep tissue specimens obtained during surgical irrigation and débridement should be sent for Gram stain, culture, and sensitivity.

Imaging Studies

- MRI and CT scans may reveal fluid and gas along fascial planes.
- Typically, imaging studies are avoided when making a diagnosis because they may delay surgical intervention and increase mortality.

NF, Necrotizing fasciitis.

From Refs. 2, 26, and 27.

TREATMENT

Desired Outcomes

The goals of therapy for NF include eradication of infection and reduction of related morbidity and mortality.

Nonpharmacologic Treatment

6 After resuscitation and hemodynamic stabilization, *prompt surgical intervention is key in the treatment of NF. Delayed operative débridement increases mortality.*[2,27] Some clinicians recommend hyperbaric oxygen (HBO) as an adjunct treatment for NF, although its use is controversial. Clinical data supporting the use of HBO in NF are inconsistent, with some trials showing reduced mortality rates and others showing no benefit.[32]

Pharmacologic Treatment

As an adjunct to surgery, high-dose, broad-spectrum IV antibiotic therapy should be initiated immediately in patients with NF. Piperacillin-tazobactam or a carbapenem is appropriate for empiric therapy. These agents should be used in combination with vancomycin, daptomycin, or linezolid until MRSA infection is ruled out. The protein synthesis

inhibitors clindamycin or linezolid are often utilized to decrease bacterial toxin production, thereby limiting tissue damage. This is particularly beneficial in streptococcal or clostridial infection.[26]

If GAS or *C. perfringens* is identified as the sole causative organism from deep tissue culture, antimicrobial therapy can be narrowed to high-dose IV penicillin G plus clindamycin. Antibiotic therapy should be continued until further operative débridements are unnecessary, the patient displays substantial clinical improvement, and fevers have abated for at least 48 to 72 hours.[2]

IV immune globulin (IVIG) dosed at 2 g/kg may also be a useful adjunctive treatment in patients with GAS NF who present with shock. Anecdotal evidence and data from small studies strongly support its use in improving 30-day survival and reducing mortality.[33,34]

DIABETIC FOOT INFECTIONS

EPIDEMIOLOGY AND ETIOLOGY

Foot ulcers and related infections are among the most common, severe, and costly complications of diabetes mellitus. Fifteen percent of all patients with diabetes develop at least one foot ulcer, resulting in direct healthcare expenditures of approximately $9 billion annually in the United States.[35]

Infected diabetic foot ulcers typically contain a multitude of microorganisms. **7** *Aerobic gram-positive cocci, such as S. aureus and β-hemolytic streptococci, are the predominant pathogens in acutely infected diabetic foot ulcers. However, chronically infected wounds are subject to polymicrobial infection.* The clinician should suspect the involvement of gram-negative (Enterobacteriaceae and *P. aeruginosa*) and possibly low-virulence pathogens (including enterococci and *S. epidermidis*) in chronic or necrotic wounds. Foul-smelling, necrotic, or gangrenous wounds are also commonly infected with anaerobic bacteria. Patients recently hospitalized or treated with broad-spectrum antibiotics are at risk for infection with antibiotic-resistant organisms, including MRSA and vancomycin-resistant enterococci (VRE).[36]

PATHOPHYSIOLOGY

7 *The pathogenesis of diabetic foot infection stems from three key factors: neuropathy, angiopathy, and immunopathy.*[37,38] Neuropathy, the most prominent risk factor for diabetic foot ulcers, develops when continuously high blood glucose levels damage motor, autonomic, and sensory nerves. Damage to motor neurons that supply the small intrinsic muscles of the foot causes deformation, resulting in altered muscular balance, abnormal areas of pressure on tissues and bone, and repetitive injuries. Damage to autonomic neurons results in the shunting of blood through direct arteriole-venous communications, thereby decreasing capillary flow. The secretion of sweat and oil is also diminished, producing dry, cracked skin that is more prone to infection. Finally, damage to sensory neurons produces a loss of protective sensation so that the patient becomes unaware of injury or ulceration.[37,38]

Angiopathy of large (macroangiopathy) and small (microangiopathy) vessels is also the result of high blood glucose concentrations. Angiopathy results in ischemia and skin breakdown.[37,38]

Finally, persons with diabetes have altered immune function that predisposes them to infection. Although their humoral immune responses remain intact, leukocyte function and cell-mediated immunity are compromised in poorly controlled disease. Achieving and maintaining tightly controlled blood glucose levels can wholly or partially reverse diabetic immunopathy.[37,38]

CLINICAL PRESENTATION AND DIAGNOSIS

Not all diabetic foot ulcers are infected. However, infection is often difficult to detect when perfusion and the inflammatory response are limited in the patient with diabetes. The common signs and symptoms (i.e., pain, erythema, and edema) of infection may be absent.[39] Still, the diagnosis of diabetic foot infection depends mostly on clinical evaluation.

Purulent drainage from the ulcer is indicative of infection. When pus and inflammatory symptoms are not present, the clinician must be astute to more subtle findings. These include delayed healing, increase in lesion size, prolonged exudate production, malodor, and tissue friability. Abnormal granulation tissue also may be present, as evidenced by color change (from bright red to dark red, brown, or gray) and increased bleeding. The ability to probe the ulcer to the underlying bone is highly indicative of osteomyelitis.[39]

Diabetic foot infections are classified into four categories based on clinical presentation using the PEDIS scale (perfusion, extent/size, depth/tissue loss, infection, sensation). Grade 1 signifies no infection; grade 2, involvement of skin and subcutaneous tissue only; grade 3, extensive cellulitis or deeper infection; and grade 4, systemic inflammatory response syndrome.[36] Grade 2 infections are classified as non–limb-threatening infections, whereas grade 3 and 4 infections are limb-threatening.[36,38] Table 73–5 provides detailed information regarding these grades.

Imaging studies, such as x-ray and magnetic resonance imaging (MRI), can identify osteomyelitis. Blood cultures should be obtained from all patients with signs and symptoms of systemic illness. Deep tissue cultures may help to direct therapy. Bone also may be sent for culture in cases of osteomyelitis. Superficial cultures of ulcers are unreliable and should be avoided.[36]

Spreading soft tissue infection and osteomyelitis are often the first complications that develop from diabetic foot infection. Some patients develop bacteremia and sepsis.

The most feared complication of infected diabetic foot ulcers is lower extremity amputation. More than 60% of all nontraumatic lower extremity amputations performed each year in Western nations are linked to diabetic foot infection; nearly 71,000 were performed in the United States in 2004.[40]

TREATMENT
Desired Outcomes

● The goals of therapy for diabetic foot infection are eradication of the infection and avoidance of soft tissue loss and amputation.

Prevention

● Comprehensive foot care programs can reduce the rate of diabetic foot ulcers and associated amputations by 45% to 85%.[37] Periodic foot examinations with monofilament testing and patient education regarding proper foot care, optimal glycemic control, and smoking cessation are key preventative strategies. Custom orthotic footwear and prophylactic reconstructive foot surgeries also may be effective in reducing the incidence of foot ulcers.[35]

Patient Encounter 2, Part 3: Diabetic Foot Infection: Clinical Course

The patient received the empiric therapy you recommended for his diabetic foot infection. Two days later, deep wound cultures were reported positive for *P. aeruginosa*. Blood cultures revealed no growth. The patient remained hospitalized for an additional week, during which time his cellulitis improved on directed antimicrobial therapy. He was discharged to complete his antibiotic therapy and to follow up as an outpatient in 1 week.

What modifications would you make to this patient's antimicrobial regimen knowing that the causative agent is P. aeruginosa?

What individualized foot care strategies can you suggest to this patient to prevent further infections?

Table 73–5

Clinical Classification of a Diabetic Foot Infection

Infection Severity	PEDIS Grade	Clinical Manifestations of Infection
Uninfected	1	Wound lacking purulence or any manifestations of inflammation
Mild	2	Presence of at least two manifestations of inflammation (purulence or erythema, pain, tenderness, warmth, or induration), but any cellulitis/erythema extends no more than 2 cm around the ulcer, and infection is limited to the skin or superficial subcutaneous tissues; no other local complications or systemic illness
Moderate	3	Infection (as above) in a patient who is systemically well and metabolically stable but who has at least one of the following characteristics: cellulitis extending greater than 2 cm, lymphangitic streaking, spread beneath the superficial fascia, deep tissue abscess, gangrene, and involvement of muscle, tendon, joint, or bone
Severe	4	Infection in a patient with systemic toxicity or metabolic instability (e.g., fever, chills, tachycardia, hypotension, confusion, vomiting, leukocytosis, acidosis, severe hyperglycemia, or azotemia)

From Lipsky BA, Berendt AR, Deery G, et al. Diagnosis and treatment of diabetic foot infections. Clin Infect Dis 2004;39:885–910.

Nonpharmacologic Treatment

The nonpharmacologic treatment of diabetic foot ulcers may include off-loading, chemical or surgical débridement of necrotic tissue, wound dressings, HBO, vascular or orthopedic surgery, and the use of human skin equivalents.[38]

Pharmacologic Treatment

● The severity of a patient's infection, based on the PEDIS scale, guides the selection of empirical antimicrobial therapy. Although most patients with grade 2 diabetic foot infections can be treated as outpatients with oral antimicrobial agents, all grade 4 and many grade 3 infections require hospitalization, stabilization of the patient, and broad-spectrum IV antibiotic therapy.[36]

Multiple antibiotic options exist for the treatment of diabetic wound infections. Table 73–6 provides both general treatment strategies and specific, although not all-inclusive, antibiotic recommendations. The duration of therapy correlates with infection severity. Antibiotics should be continued until the infection has resolved, but not necessarily until the ulcer has healed. Grade 2 infections generally require 7 to 14 days of therapy, whereas grade 3 to 4 necessitate treatment durations of 14 to 28 days.

Table 73–6			
Empirical Pharmacologic Treatment of Diabetic Foot Infection			
Infection Severity	**PEDIS Grade**	**General Approach to Empirical Pharmacologic Treatment**	**Examples of Appropriate Empirical Antibiotics**[a]
Uninfected	1	None. Avoid treating uninfected diabetic foot ulcers.	Not applicable
Mild	2	Oral, narrow-spectrum antibiotic therapy with activity against *S. aureus* and streptococcal species. Include coverage for MRSA (HA- or CA-MRSA) according to patient history and resistance patterns in the area.	MRSA not suspected: cephalexin, dicloxacillin, or clindamycin HA-MRSA suspected: vancomycin (IV), daptomycin (IV), linezolid, telavancin (IV), or ceftaroline (IV) CA-MRSA suspected: clindamycin[b], trimethoprim-sulfamethoxazole[c], doxycycline[c], or minocycline[c]
Moderate	3	Difficult to define a general approach. In many patients, highly bioavailable oral therapy is appropriate. IV therapy should be initiated in patients with more extensive or chronic infections, or those with abscess, deep tissue or bone involvement or gangrene.	Oral options for grade 3 infections: Amoxicillin-clavulanate, levofloxacin[d] + clindamycin, or moxifloxacin CA-MRSA suspected: Include clindamycin[b], trimethoprim-sulfamethoxazole[c], doxycycline[c], or minocycline[c]
Severe	4	Parenteral, broad-spectrum antibiotic therapy should be initiated. Ideally, drugs with activity against gram-positive, gram-negative, and anaerobic bacteria (especially if wound is malodorous) should be selected. Include coverage for MRSA.	IV options for grade 3–4 infection: Vancomycin, daptomycin, linezolid, or telavancin[e] In combination with one of the following choices: Piperacillin-tazobactam[d], ampicillin-sulbactam, imipenem-cilastatin[d], ertapenem, moxifloxacin, levofloxacin[d] + clindamycin, cefepime[d] + metronidazole, ceftazidime[d] + clindamycin *OR* Ceftaroline[f] + clindamycin or metronidazole *OR* Tigecycline[f] monotherapy

[a]Please refer to Table 73–3 for dosing in adults with normal renal function.

[b]CA-MRSA isolates resistant to erythromycin should be evaluated for inducible clindamycin resistance via a D-test.

[c]Limited clinical data exist for the treatment of MRSA infections. Poor activity against GAS; consider using in combination with clindamycin or cephalexin if empirical coverage for GAS is desired.

[d]*P. aeruginosa* generally is susceptible to this agent.

[e]MRSA coverage indicated for patients with severe cellulitis or systemic illness who have risk factors for HA-MRSA or CA-MRSA infection, or reside in areas with high CA-MRSA prevalence. Otherwise, the broad-spectrum regimens listed below, without MRSA coverage, are appropriate.

[f]Not currently approved for the treatment of diabetic foot infections.

From Refs. 36 and 40–42.

If osteomyelitis is present, treatment duration depends on whether infected and necrotic bone is surgically debrided. In the case of amputation, where all infected bone and tissue is removed, 2 to 5 days of therapy is sufficient. Residual infection, status-postsurgical debridement, requires 2 to 6 weeks of antibiotic therapy. Without surgery, antibiotic therapy should continue for at least 12 weeks.[36]

INFECTED PRESSURE SORES

EPIDEMIOLOGY AND ETIOLOGY

Pressures sores, also known as *decubitus ulcers* or *bedsores,* affect approximately 7% to 24% of long-term care and 10% to 18% of hospitalized patients. Patients of advanced age and those with spinal cord or orthopedic injuries are at highest risk.[43]

A pressure sore is a chronic wound that results from continuous pressure on the tissue overlying a bony prominence. This pressure impedes blood flow to the dermis and subcutaneous fat, resulting in tissue damage and necrosis.[44,45]

Pressure sore infections develop from breaks in skin integrity and contamination from dirty areas of close proximity. Pressure sore infections generally are polymicrobial.[46]

CLINICAL PRESENTATION AND DIAGNOSIS

Approximately two-thirds of all pressure sores occur on the sacrum and heels. The remaining one-third occur predominately on the elbows, ankles, trochanters, ischia, knees, scapulas, shoulders, or occiput.[47] Pressure sores are classified according to the extent of tissue destruction.[48] The most commonly used system for staging of pressure sores is presented in Table 73–7.

Bacterial colonization of pressure sores is common. Because infection impairs wound healing and may require systemic antimicrobial therapy, the clinician must be able to distinguish it from colonization. Table 73–8 describes the clinical presentation of infected pressure sores.

Most complications are infectious. The most common is osteomyelitis, which is present in approximately 38% of infected pressure sores.[44] Less frequently, NF, clostridial myonecrosis, and sepsis can occur.

TREATMENT

Desired Outcomes

The goals of therapy for infected pressure sores include resolution of infection, promotion of wound healing, and establishment of effective infection control.[45]

Prevention

❽ *Prevention is the most humane and cost-effective component in the management of pressure sores.* Key prevention strategies include monitoring of high-risk patients, reducing skin

Table 73–7
Staging of Pressure Ulcers

Suspected Deep Tissue Injury
- Intact skin with localized area of purple or maroon discoloration or presence of a blood-filled blister
- The area may be preceded by tissue that is painful, firm, mushy, boggy, and warmer or cooler as compared with adjacent tissue

Stage I
- Intact skin with localized area of nonblanchable redness, usually over a bony prominence
- May be difficult to detect in darkly pigmented skin; its color may differ from the surrounding area

Stage II
- Partial-thickness loss of dermis presenting as a shallow open ulcer with a red pink wound bed or an intact or ruptured serum-filled blister
- This stage should not be used to describe skin tears, tape burns, perineal dermatitis, maceration, or excoriation

Stage III
- Full-thickness tissue loss. Subcutaneous fat may be visible, but bone, tendon, or muscle are not exposed. Slough may be present but does not obscure the depth of tissue loss. May include undermining and tunneling.

Stage IV
- Full-thickness tissue loss with exposed bone, tendon, or muscle. Slough or eschar may be present on some parts of the wound bed. Often include undermining and tunneling.

Unstageable
- Full-thickness tissue loss in which the base of the ulcer is covered by slough (yellow, tan, gray, green, or brown) and/or eschar (tan, brown, or black) in the wound bed
- Until enough slough and/or eschar is removed to expose the base of the wound, the true depth, and therefore stage, cannot be determined. Stable (dry, adherent, intact without erythema or fluctuance) eschar on the heels serves as "the body's natural (biological) cover" and should not be removed.

From National Pressure Ulcer Advisory Panel. Updated staging system [online]. 2007. [cited 2011 Oct 10]. Available from: *http://www.npuap.org/pr2.htm.*

exposure to pressure and moisture, and promoting good nutritional status.

Careful monitoring and preventative care of high-risk patients can begin once these patients are identified. Intrinsic or host-related risk factors for the development of pressure sores include age greater than 75 years, limited mobility, loss of sensation, unconsciousness or altered sense of awareness, and malnutrition. Extrinsic or environmental risk factors include pressure, friction, shear stress, and moisture.[44]

Turning and repositioning the patient at least every 2 hours can reduce skin pressure and prevent pressure sores. However, because this level of care is difficult to achieve in most hospital and nursing home environments, multitudes of pressure-reducing mattresses have been manufactured. Although these can help to decrease

Table 73–8

Presentation of Infected Pressure Sores

Symptoms
- Because many high-risk patients lack sensation, pain may not be a primary symptom.

Signs
- Infection generally is diagnosed when erythema and edema of the surrounding skin, purulent drainage, malodor, or delayed wound healing are present.
- Patients with bacteremia often develop fever, chills, confusion, and/or hypotension.

Laboratory Tests
- Deep tissue cultures may help to direct therapy. Bone also may be sent for culture in cases of osteomyelitis. Superficial cultures are unreliable and should be avoided.

Imaging Studies
- Imaging studies, such as CT, MRI, or bone scan, can be used to detect osteomyelitis and to determine the depth and extent of tissue destruction.

From Refs. 45 and 47.

pressure on susceptible areas, they do not negate the need for position changes.[44]

Maintaining a clean, dry environment can prevent skin maceration and subsequent tissue damage. This can be accomplished with frequent changes of bed sheets and clothing, thorough drying of skin after bathing, and prompt disposal of incontinent stool or urine.

Malnutrition is a significant but reversible risk factor. High-protein diets have been shown in multiple studies to improve wound healing in patients with pressure sores.[44]

Nonpharmacologic Treatment

Pressure relief, adequate nutrition (high-protein diet), and surgical débridement or abscess drainage are the mainstays of nonpharmacologic treatment.[45]

Pharmacologic Treatment

8 *Systemic antibiotics are indicated for serious pressure ulcer infections, including those associated with spreading cellulitis, osteomyelitis, or bacteremia.*[45] Pressure ulcer infections are generally polymicrobial. Thus antimicrobial agents with a broad spectrum of activity should be initiated and narrowed according to the results of cultures obtained surgically. The duration of treatment is generally 10 to 14 days, unless osteomyelitis is present.[45]

Mild superficial infections, such as those that present clinically with delayed wound healing or minimal cellulitis, may be treated with topical antimicrobial agents such as silver sulfadiazine 1% cream or combination antibiotic ointments.[44] Systemic options for more extensive cellulitis are available in Table 73–3.

INFECTED BITE WOUNDS

EPIDEMIOLOGY AND ETIOLOGY

Fifty percent of Americans will be bitten by an animal at least once during their lifetimes. Although most of these injuries are minor, approximately 20% will require medical treatment.[2]

Dogs cause approximately 80% of all bites, of which approximately 15% to 25% become infected. These bites most commonly involve the extremities, and young children are particularly at risk.[49]

Cat bites are the second most common animal bite, most often occurring in women and elderly individuals. Most involve the hand. Because cats have long, thin teeth that cause puncture wounds, their bites are more likely to become infected than a dog bite. Approximately 50% of cat bites become infected.[49]

Human bites are third most common and the most serious. Before the availability of antibiotics, up to 20% resulted in amputation. Currently, human bite–associated amputation rates remain at 5%, secondary to vascular compromise and infectious complications.[49]

There are two types of human bite injuries. Occlusal injuries are inflicted by actual biting, whereas clenched-fist injuries are sustained when a person's closed fist hits another's teeth. Of the two, clenched-fist injuries typically are more prone to infectious complications.[49]

9 *Bite wound infections generally are polymicrobial.* On average, five different bacterial species can be isolated from an infected animal bite wound.[2] Both the normal flora of the biter's mouth and that of the bite recipient's skin can be implicated. The bacteriology of the cat and dog mouth is quite similar. *Pasteurella multocida*, a gram-negative aerobe, is one of the predominant pathogens, isolated in up to 50% of dog and 75% of cat bites. Viridans streptococci are the most frequently cultured bacteria from human bite wounds, although empiric treatment should also provide coverage for *Eikenella corrodens*.[2,49] Table 73–9 provides a comprehensive list of cat-, dog-, and human bite-wound pathogens.

CLINICAL PRESENTATION AND DIAGNOSIS

The clinical presentation of infected bite wounds is presented in Table 73–9.

Complications of infected bite wounds include lymphangitis, abscess, septic arthritis, tenosynovitis, and osteomyelitis. Bites to the hand are particularly complication-prone.[49]

TREATMENT
Desired Outcomes

The goals of therapy for an infected bite wound are rapid and successful eradication of infection and prevention of related complications.

Table 73–9

Etiology and Presentation of Infected Bite Wounds

Bacterial Pathogens

- *Dog and cat: Pasteurella multocida*, staphylococci, streptococci *Moraxella* spp., *Eikenella corrodens*, *Capnocytophaga canimorsus*, *Actinomyces*, *Fusobacterium*, *Prevotella*, and *Porphyromonas* spp.
- *Human:* Viridans streptococci, *S. aureus*, *E. corrodens*, *Haemophilus influenzae*, and β-lactamase–producing anaerobic bacteria

Signs and Symptoms

- The onset of infectious symptomatology is typically 12–24 hours after the bite.
- Pain at the wound site is common.
- Erythema, edema, and purulent or malodorous drainage at the wound site are manifestations of infected wounds. The patient may be febrile.
- Limited range of motion may be present, especially if the hand is bitten.

Laboratory Tests

- Leukocytosis may be present.
- The clinician should obtain anaerobic and aerobic wound cultures only if the wound appears clinically infected.

Imaging Studies

- X-rays should be obtained if the bite is on the hand, could have damaged bone or joints, or if an embedded object or tooth fragment is suspected.

From Bower MG. Managing dog, cat, and human bite wounds. Nurs Pract 2001;26:36–38, 41, 42, 45.

Nonpharmacologic Treatment

Thorough irrigation with normal saline is the first step in the care of an infected bite wound. The wound should be elevated and immobilized. Surgical closure may be advocated, especially for facial wounds. Wounds that are infected, at higher risk for infection, or older than 24 hours should be left open because premature closure can lead to disastrous infectious complications. ❾ *Wounds at higher risk for infection include human bites, deep punctures, and bites to the hand.*[49]

Pharmacologic Treatment

Most bite wounds require antibiotic therapy only when clinical infection is present. *However, prophylactic therapy is recommended for wounds at higher risk for infection and bites requiring surgical repair.*[49]

The most effective agent for the treatment (and prophylaxis) of human and animal bite-wound infections is amoxicillin-clavulanate. Alternatives for patients with significant penicillin allergies include either a fluoroquinolone (e.g., ciprofloxacin) or trimethoprim-sulfamethoxazole in combination with clindamycin. The durations of prophylaxis and treatment generally are 3 to 5 and 10 to 14 days, respectively.[2]

If the wound is associated with significant cellulitis and edema, systemic signs of infection, or possible joint or bone involvement, hospitalization and IV antibiotics (typically

ampicillin-sulbactam 3 g IV every 6 hours) should be initiated. Bone and joint infections will require longer durations of therapy of up to 6 weeks.[2,49]

OUTCOME EVALUATION

Education of the patient, caregivers, and household members is important to limit further spread of infection and is a key component in SSTI case management. Table 73-10 lists several key prevention messages for patients with SSTIs.

❿ *Patients receiving antibiotic therapy for SSTIs require monitoring for efficacy and safety. Efficacy typically is manifested by reductions in temperature, white blood cell count, erythema, edema, and pain.* Initially, signs and symptoms of infection may worsen owing to toxin release from certain organisms (i.e., GAS); however, they should begin to resolve within 48 to 72 hours of treatment initiation. If no response or worsening infection is noted after the first 3 days of antibiotics, reevaluate the patient.[2] Lack of response may be due to a noninfectious or nonbacterial diagnosis, a pathogen not covered by or resistant to current antibiotic therapy, poor patient adherence, drug or disease interactions causing decreased antibiotic absorption or increased clearance, immunodeficiency, or the need for surgical intervention. *To ensure the safety of the regimen, dose antibiotics according to renal and hepatic function as appropriate, and monitor for or minimize adverse drug reactions, allergic reactions, and drug interactions.*

Table 73–10

Prevention Education for Patients with SSTIs

1. Draining wounds should be covered with clean, dry bandages.
2. Hands should be cleaned regularly with soap and water (or with alcohol-based hand gel if not visibly soiled) and immediately after touching infected skin or any item directly contacting a draining wound.
3. General hygiene should be maintained with regular bathing.
4. Items that may become contaminated with wound drainage or that directly touch the skin should not be shared.
5. Wash and dry thoroughly any clothing that has come in contact with wound drainage after each use.
6. If the wound is unable to be covered with a clean, dry bandage at all times, avoid activities with skin-to-skin contact until the wound is healed.
7. Equipment and environmental surfaces with bare skin contact should be cleaned with *S. aureus*–active detergents or disinfectants.

From Gorwitz RF, Jernigan DB, Powers JH, et al. Strategies for clinical management of MRSA in the community: summary of an experts' meeting convened by the Centers for Disease Control and Prevention [online]. 2006. [cited 2011 Oct 10]. Available from: *http://www.cdc.gov/ncidod/dhqp/ar_mrsa_ca.html.*[50]

Patient Care and Monitoring

Choosing antibiotic therapy for SSTIs:

1. To select the most effective *empirical* antibiotic agent(s) for SSTIs, review the following:
   - The diagnosis
   - Clinical manifestations and severity of illness (to assess the need for IV versus oral therapy)
   - Past medical history, chronic disease states (to determine suspected pathogens)
   - Patient's ability to adhere to the regimen (if outpatient treatment indicated)

In pediatric patients especially, consider duration of therapy, frequency of dosing, method and ease of administration, and palatability and tolerability of oral formulations.

2. To ensure the safety of your selected antibiotic agent(s), review the following:
   - Current medications (over-the-counter, prescription, and alternative) for potential drug interactions
   - History of medication allergies and adverse effects
   - Current laboratory analyses to determine renal and hepatic function
   - Chronic disease states or acute conditions that could be worsened by certain antimicrobial agents (e.g., QT prolongation or acute renal failure)
   - Other disease modifiers that may preclude use (e.g., pregnancy, age)

Monitoring antibiotic therapy for SSTIs:

1. Ensure that antimicrobial therapy is effective by monitoring for:
   - Resolution of local and systemic signs and symptoms of infection
   - Resolution of laboratory evidence of infection

2. Narrow antibiotic coverage when possible with the use of culture and sensitivity data.

3. Assess patient adherence.

4. Ensure that antimicrobial therapy is safe by monitoring for and treating (as appropriate):
   - Common and severe adverse effects
   - Drug interactions

Patient education regarding antibiotic therapy for SSTIs:

1. It is imperative to take the antibiotic as prescribed and to finish the therapy.

2. If no symptomatic improvement is noted within 3 days, contact your healthcare provider.

3. Many antibiotics cause diarrhea. If it is severe, contact your healthcare provider.

4. Consider health initiatives to improve wound healing, such as smoking cessation and glycemic control.

Abbreviations Introduced in This Chapter

CA-MRSA	Community-acquired methicillin-resistant *S. aureus*
GAS	Group A *Streptococcus* (also known as *Streptococcus pyogenes*, one of the β-hemolytic streptococci)
HA-MRSA	Health care-associated methicillin-resistant *S. aureus*
HBO	Hyperbaric oxygen
MIC	Minimum inhibitory concentration
MRI	Magnetic resonance imaging
MRSA	Methicillin-resistant *S. aureus*
MSSA	Methicillin-sensitive *S. aureus*
NF	Necrotizing fasciitis
SSTI	Skin and soft tissue infection
VISA	Vancomycin-intermediate *S. aureus*
VRE	Vancomycin-resistant enterococci
VRSA	Vancomycin-resistant *S. aureus*

 Self-assessment questions and answers are available at *http://www.mhpharmacotherapy.com/pp.html.*

REFERENCES

1. Pallin DJ, Espinola JA, Leung DY, et al. Epidemiology of dermatitis and skin infections in United States physicians offices, 1993-2005. Clin Infect Dis 2009;49:901–907.
2. Stevens DL, Bisno AL, Chambers HF, et al. Practice guidelines for the diagnosis and management of skin and soft tissue infections. Clin Infect Dis 2005;41:1373–1406.
3. Choice of antibacterial drugs. Treatment Guidelines. Med Lett 2007;5(57):33–50.
4. Moran GJ, Krishnadasan A, Gorwitz RJ, et al. Methicillin-resistant *S. aureus* infection among patients in the emergency department. N Engl J Med 2006;355(7):666–674.
5. Edelsberg J, Taneja C, Zervos M, et al. Trends in US hospital admissions for skin and soft tissue infections. Emerg Infect Dis 2009;15(9):1516–1518.
6. Boucher HW, Corey GR. Epidemiology of methicillin-resistant *Staphylococcus aureus*. Clin Infect Dis 2008;46(Suppl 5):S344–S349.
7. Schneider-Lindner V, Quach C, Hanley JA, Sulssa S. Antibacterial drugs and the risk of community-acquired methicillin-resistant *Staphylococcus aureus* in children. Arch Pediatr Adolesc Med 2011;165(12):1107–1114.
8. Dieffenbach CW, Tramont EC, Plaeger SF. Innate (general or nonspecific) host defense mechanisms. In: Mandell GL, Bennett JE, Dolin R, eds. Principles and Practice of Infectious Diseases. 7th ed. Philadelphia, PA: Elsevier; 2010:37–47.
9. Yagupski P. Bacteriologic aspects of skin and soft tissue infections. Pediatr Ann 1993;22:217–224.
10. Watkins P. Impetigo: Aetiology, complications, and treatment options. Nurs Stand 2005;19(36):50–54.
11. Pasternack MS, Swartz MN. Cellulitis, necrotizing fasciitis, and subcutaneous tissue infections. In: Mandell GL, Bennett JE, Dolin R, eds. Principles and Practice of Infectious Diseases. 7th ed. Philadelphia, PA: Elsevier; 2010:1289–1312.

12. Cole C, Gazewood J. Diagnosis and treatment of impetigo. Am Fam Physician 2007;75:859–864, 868.

13. Luelmo-Aguilar J, Santandreu MS. Folliculitis: Recognition and management. Am J Clin Dermatol 2004;5(5):301–310.

14. Bonnetlanc JM, Bedane C. Erysipelas: Recognition and management. Am J Clin Dermatol 2003;4(3):157–163.

15. Swartz MN. Clinical practice. Cellulitis. N Engl J Med 2004;350(9):904–912.

16. DiNubile MJ, Lipsky BA. Complicated infections of skin and skin structures: When the infection is more than skin deep. J Antimicrob Chemother 2004;53(Suppl S2):ii37–ii50.

17. Micek ST, Hoban AP, Pham V, Doherty JA, Kollef MH. Institutional perspective on the impact of positive blood cultures on the economic and clinical outcomes of patients with complicated skin and skin structure infections: focus on gram-positive infections. Clin Ther 2011;33:1759–1768.

18. Segarra-Newnham M. Revision of a treatment algorithm for community-associated methicillin-resistant *Staphylococcus aureus* skin infections. Hosp Pharm 2009;44:392–396.

19. Stryjewski ME, Chambers HF. Skin and soft-tissue infections caused by community-acquired methicillin-resistant *Staphylococcus aureus*. Clin Infect Dis 2008;46(Suppl 5):S368–S377.

20. Cohen P. Community-acquired methicillin-resistant *Staphylococcus aureus* skin infections: Implications for patients and practitioners. J Clin Dermatol 2007;8(5):259–270.

21. Liu C, Bayer A, Cosgrove SE, et al. Clinical practice guidelines by the Infectious Diseases Society of America for the treatment of methicillin-resistant *Staphylococcus aureus* infections in adults and children. Clin Infect Dis 2011;52:1–38.

22. Ruhe JJ, Monson T, Bradsher RW, et al. Use of long-acting tetracyclines for methicillin-resistant *Staphylococcus aureus* infections: Case series and review of the literature. Clin Infect Dis 2005;40(10):1429–1434.

23. Cenizal MJ, Skiest D, Luber S, et al. Prospective randomized trial of empiric therapy with trimethoprim-sulfamethoxazole or doxycycline for outpatient skin and soft tissue infections in an area of high prevalence of methicillin-resistant *Staphylococcus aureus*. Antimicrob Agents Chemother 2007;51(7):2628–2630.

24. Bisbe J, Miro J, Latorre, et al. Disseminated candidiasis in addicts who use brown heroin: Report of 83 cases and review. Clin Infect Dis 1992;15:910–923.

25. Group A Streptococcal (GAS) Disease [online]. Department of Health and Human Services. Centers for Disease Control and Prevention. April 3, 2008. [cited 2011 Oct 10]. Available from: *http://www.cdc.gov/ncidod/dbmd/diseaseinfo/groupastreptococcal_t.htm*.

26. Anaya DA, Dellinger EP. Necrotizing soft-tissue infection: Diagnosis and management. Clin Infect Dis 2007;44:705–710.

27. Wong C, Wang Y. The diagnosis of necrotizing fasciitis. Curr Opin Infect Dis 2005;18:101–106.

28. Finsterer J, Hess B. Neuromuscular and CNS manifestations of *Clostridium perfringens* infections. Infection 2007;35(6):396–405.

29. Wolf JE, Rabinowitz LG. Streptococcal toxic shock-like syndrome. Arch Dermatol 1995;131:73–77.

30. Jallali N. Necrotising fasciitis: Its aetiology, diagnosis and management. J Wound Care 2003;12(8):297–300.

31. Cunningham JD, Silver L, Rudikoff D. Necrotizing fasciitis: A plea for early diagnosis and treatment. Mt Sinai J Med 2001;68(4–5):253–261.

32. Jallali N, Withey S Butler PE. Hyperbaric oxygen as adjuvant therapy in the management of necrotizing fasciitis. Am J Surg 2005;189:462–466.

33. Kaul R, McGeer A, Norrby-Teglund A, et al. Intravenous immunoglobulin therapy for streptococcal toxic shock syndrome—a comparative observational study. Clin Infect Dis 1999;28:800–807.

34. Darenberg J, Ihendyane N, Sjolin J, et al. IV immunoglobulin G therapy in streptococcal toxic shock syndrome: A European randomized, double-blind, placebo-controlled trial. Clin Infect Dis 2003;37(3):333–340.

35. Singh N, Armstrong DG, Lipsky BA. Preventing foot ulcers in patients with diabetes. JAMA 2005;293(2):217–228.

36. Lipsky BA, Berendt AR, Deery G, et al. Diagnosis and treatment of diabetic foot infections. Clin Infect Dis 2004;39:885–910.

37. National Diabetes Fact Sheet, United States [online]. Department of Health and Human Services. Centers for Disease Control and Prevention, 2007. [cited 2011 Oct 10]. Available from: *http://www.cdc.gov/diabetes/pubs/pdf/ndfs_2007.pdf*.

38. Calhoun JH, Overgaard KA, Stevens CM, et al. Diabetic foot ulcers and infections: Current concepts. Adv Skin Wound Care 2002;15:31–45.

39. Williams DT, Hilton JR, Harding KG. Diagnosing foot infection in diabetes. Clin Infect Dis 2004;39(2):S83–S86.

40. Bader MS. Diabetic foot infection. Am Fam Physician 2008;78(1):71–79,81–82.

41. Matthews PC, Berendt AR, Lipsky BA. Clinical management of diabetic foot infection: Diagnostics, therapeutics and the future. Expert Rev Anti Infect Ther 2007;5(1):117–127.

42. Lipsky BA, Giordano P, Shurjeel C, et al. Treating diabetic foot infections with sequential IV moxifloxacin compared with piperacillin-tazobactam/amoxicillin-clavulanate. J Antimicrob Chemother 2007;60:370–376.

43. National Pressure Ulcer Advisory Panel Board of Directors. Pressure ulcers in America: Prevalence, incidence, and implications for the future. Adv Skin Wound Care 2001;14:208–215.

44. Thomas DR. Prevention and treatment of pressure ulcers: What works? What doesn't? Cleve Clin J Med 2001;68(8):704–707.

45. Livesley NJ, Chow AW. Pressure ulcers in elderly individuals. Clin Infect Dis 2002;35:1390–1396.

46. Darouiche R. Infections in patients with spinal cord injury. In: Mandell GL, Bennett JE, Dolin R, eds. Principles and Practice of Infectious Diseases. 6th ed. Philadelphia, PA: Elsevier; 2005; 3512–3517.

47. Cannon BC, Cannon JP. Management of pressure ulcers. Am J Health Syst Pharm 2004;61:1895–1907.

48. National Pressure Ulcer Advisory Panel. Updated staging system [online]. 2007. [cited 2011 Oct 10]. Available from: *http://www.npuap.org/pr2.htm*.

49. Bower MG. Managing dog, cat, and human bite wounds. Nurs Pract 2001;26(4):36–38, 41, 42, 45.

50. Gorwitz RF, Jernigan DB, Powers JH, et al. Strategies for clinical management of MRSA in the community: summary of an experts' meeting convened by the Centers for Disease Control and Prevention [online]. 2006. [cited 2011 Oct 10]. Available from: *http://www.cdc.gov/ncidod/dhqp/ar_mrsa_ca.html*.

74

Infective Endocarditis

Ronda L. Akins and Katie E. Barber

KEY CONCEPTS

❶ For infective endocarditis (IE) to develop, several factors are required, including alterations to the endocardial surface that allow bacterial adherence and eventual infection.

❷ Persistent fever is the most common symptom present in patients with IE.

❸ Blood cultures are the essential laboratory test for the diagnosis and treatment of IE. Typically, patients with IE have a low-grade consistent bacteremia. Blood culture results are critical for determining the most appropriate therapy.

❹ Echocardiograms are used for detecting the presence of a vegetation. Either a transthoracic echocardiogram (TTE) or a transesophageal echocardiogram (TEE) may be used depending on certain patient characteristics.

❺ Choosing the appropriate antimicrobial therapy is crucial to achieve adequate organism kill.

❻ An extended treatment course of 4 to 6 weeks (in most cases) is required to achieve an adequate cure.

❼ The overall goal of therapy is to eradicate the infection and minimize/prevent any complications.

❽ In an effort to prevent the development of IE, prophylactic treatment generally is considered appropriate for patients with high-risk factors.

❾ Monitoring the patient's clinical course is necessary to assess the effectiveness of therapy, detect the potential development of bacterial resistance, and determine outcome.

Infective endocarditis (IE) is a serious infection affecting the lining and valves of the heart. Although this disease is mostly associated with infection of the heart valves, the septal defects may become involved in some cases. Infections also occur in patients with prosthetic or mechanical devices or who are intravenous drug users (IVDUs). Bacteria are the primary cause of IE; however, fungi and atypical organisms may also be responsible pathogens.

Typically IE is classified into two categories: acute or subacute. The difference between the two categories is based on the progression and severity of the disease. Acute disease is more aggressive, characterized by high fevers, leukocytosis, and systemic toxicity, with death occurring within a few days to weeks. This type of IE is often caused by more virulent organisms, particularly *Staphylococcus aureus*. Subacute disease is typically caused by less virulent organisms, such as viridans group streptococci, producing a slower and more subtle presentation. It is characterized by weakness, fatigue, low-grade fever, night sweats, weight loss, and other nonspecific symptoms, with death occurring in several months.

Successful management of patients with IE is based on proper diagnosis, treatment with adequate therapy, and monitoring for complications, adverse events, or development of resistance. The treatment and management of IE are best determined through identification of the causative organism. IE has varied clinical presentations; therefore, patients with this infection may be found in any medical subspecialty (i.e., medicine, surgery, critical care, etc.).

EPIDEMIOLOGY AND ETIOLOGY

Despite IE being a fairly uncommon infection, in the United States, there are about 10,000 to 20,000 new cases annually, and IE accounts for an incidence of approximately five to seven cases per 100,000 persons-years.[1] Although the exact number of cases is often difficult to determine owing to the diagnostic criteria and reporting methods for this disease, it continues to rise. IE is now considered the fourth leading cause of serious infectious disease syndromes following urosepsis, pneumonia, and intra-abdominal sepsis.[2] Men are affected more commonly than women at a ratio of 1.7:1. Although IE occurs at any age, more than 50% of cases occur in patients older than 50 years.[1] IE in children continues to be uncommon and is mainly associated with underlying structural defects, surgical repair of the defects, or nosocomial catheter-related bacteremia.[1] With the increased use of mechanical valves, prosthetic-valve endocarditis (PVE) now accounts for approximately 10% to 30%.[3] Patients who are IVDUs are also at an increased risk for IE, with 150 to 2,000 cases per 100,000 persons per year, most being younger adults.[4] Additionally, other patients at high risk for IE include patients with any congenital or structural cardiac defects, including valvular disease; long-term hemodialysis; diabetes mellitus; poor oral hygiene; major dental treatment; previous endocarditis; hypertrophic cardiomyopathy; and mitral valve prolapse with regurgitation.[5–8]

Although almost any type of microorganism is capable of causing IE, the majority of cases are caused by gram-positive organisms. These consist primarily of streptococci, staphylococci, and enterococci. Consideration of gram-negative, fungal, and other atypical organisms must be taken into account, particularly in certain patient populations. In Table 74–1,

---

Patient Encounter, Part 1

A 72-year-old man with a history of hypertension, benign prostate hyperplasia (BPH), and coronary artery diseases (CAD) s/p tricuspid valve replacement 2 years ago presents to the emergency department with complaints of weakness, fever, and chills. His current weight is 50 kg (110 lb). On interviewing the patient, you determine that he had a transurethral resection (TUR) of the prostate to treat his BPH 21 days ago. He denies any use of alcohol, illicit drugs, or smoking.

What information would make you suspect IE?

Does he have any risk factors for IE?

What additional information would you like to know before deciding on an empirical treatment for this patient?

Table 74–1

Etiologic Organisms of Infective Endocarditis

	Native-Valve IE		PVE (Indicated in Months After Valve Surgery)			IVDU (Right- and Left-Sided)
Organism	**Community-Acquired**	**Healthcare-Associated**	**Less Than 2**	**2–12**	**Greater Than 12**	**Total**
Streptococci[a]	40	9	1	9	31	12
Pneumococci	2	—	—	—	—	—
Enterococci	9	13	8	12	11	9
Staphylococcus aureus	28	53[b]	22	12	18	57
CNS	5	12	33	32	11	—
HACEK group	3	—	—	—	6	—
Gram-negative bacilli	1	2	13	3	6	7
Fungi (*Candida* spp.)	Less than 1	2	8	12	1	4
Polymicrobial/miscellaneous	3	4	3	6	5	7
Diphtheroids	—	Less than 1	6	—	3	0.1
Culture-negative	9	5	5	6	8	3

CNS, coagulase-negative staphylococci; HACEK, *Haemophilus* spp. (primarily *H. paraphrophilus*, *H. parainfluenzae*, and *H. aphrophilus*), *Actinobacillus actinomycetemcomitans*, *Cardiobacterium hominis*, *Eikenella corrodens*, and *Kingella kingae*.

[a]Includes viridans group streptococci; *S. bovis*; other nongroup A, groupable streptococci; and nutritionally variant streptococci.

[b]Methicillin resistance is common among these *S. aureus* strains.

Modified from Karchmer AW. Infective endocarditis. In: Fauci AS, Braunwald E, Kasper DL, Hauser SL, Longo DL, Jameson JL, Loscalzo J, eds. Harrison's Principles of Internal Medicine. 18th ed. New York: McGraw Hill; 2012: Chap. 124.

approximate percentages are given for each organism based on the type of IE, including native valve (community-acquired versus health care–associated), prosthetic valve (grouped by months postsurgery), and IVDUs.

PATHOGENESIS AND PATHOPHYSIOLOGY

❶ *For IE to develop, the occurrence of several factors is required. Typically, there must be an alteration of the endothelial surfaces of the heart valves to allow for organism attachment and colonization.* These alterations may be produced by an inflammatory process such as rheumatic heart disease or by injury from turbulent blood flow. Platelets and fibrin now deposit on the damaged valves, forming a **nonbacterial thrombotic endocarditis** (NBTE). At this point, bacteria through hematogenous spread (i.e., bacteremia) adhere to and colonize the **nidus**, forming a vegetation. Further deposits of platelets and fibrin cover the bacteria, providing a protective coating that allows for the development of a suitable environment for continued organism and vegetation progression, often producing an organism density of 10^9 to 10^{10} **colony-forming units** (CFU) per gram. This sequence of events is summarized in **Figure 74–1**.

Acquisition of PVE differs in early stages, where direct inoculation may occur during surgery instead of through hematogenous seeding. In addition, causative organisms in early PVE are typically nosocomial, with more likelihood of being drug resistant.[8,9] The prosthetic valve also has a greater propensity for organism colonization than native valves.[9] However, in late PVE, the process of colonization and vegetation formation is similar to that of native-valve IE, as described earlier.[8,9]

Typically, vegetations are located on the line along valve closure on the atrial surface of the atrioventricular valves (tricuspid and mitral) or on the ventricular surface of the semilunar valves (pulmonary and aortic) (**Fig. 74–2**). The vegetations can vary significantly in size, ranging from millimeters to several centimeters and may be single or multiple masses. Often, destruction of underlying tissue occurs and may cause perforation of the valve leaflet or rupture of the chordae tendinae, interventricular septum, or papillary muscle. Valve ring abscesses may occur, resulting in fistulas penetrating into the myocardium or pericardial sac, particularly with staphylococcal endocarditis.

Embolic events are also common. Embolization occurs as portions of the friable vegetation break lose and enter the bloodstream. These infected pieces are called *septic emboli*. Pulmonary abscesses are commonly formed as a result of septic emboli from right-sided IE (tricuspid and pulmonary valves). However, left-sided IE (mitral and aortic valves) is more likely to have an embolus travel to any organ system, especially the kidneys, spleen, and brain. Along with emboli, immune complex deposition may occur in organ

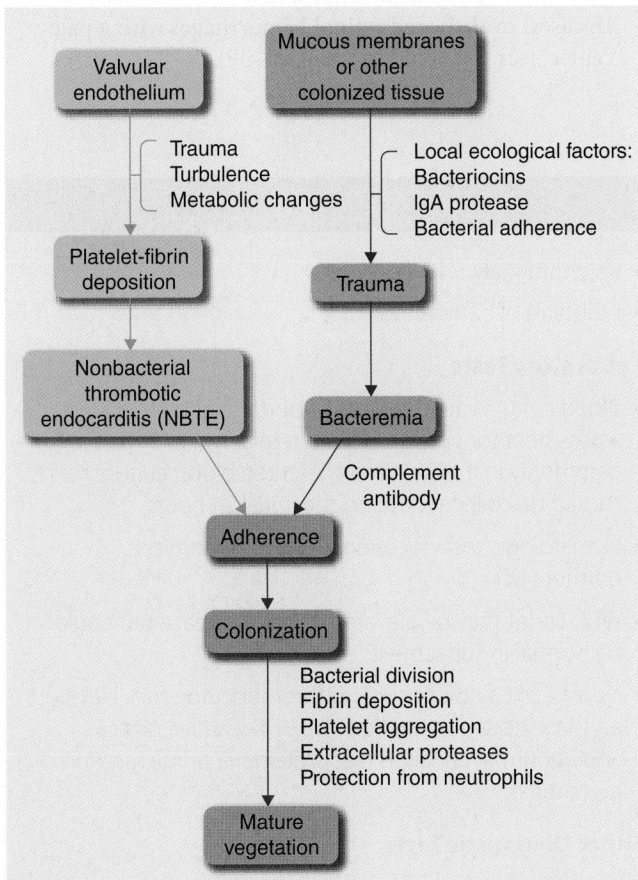

FIGURE 74–1. Pathogenesis of infective endocarditis. (From Fowler VG Jr, Scheld WM, Bayer AS. Endocarditis and intravascular infections. In: Mandell GL, Bennett JE, Dolin R, eds. Principles and Practice of Infectious Diseases, 6th ed. Philadelphia, PA: Elsevier; 2005:975-1022; With permission from Elsevier.)

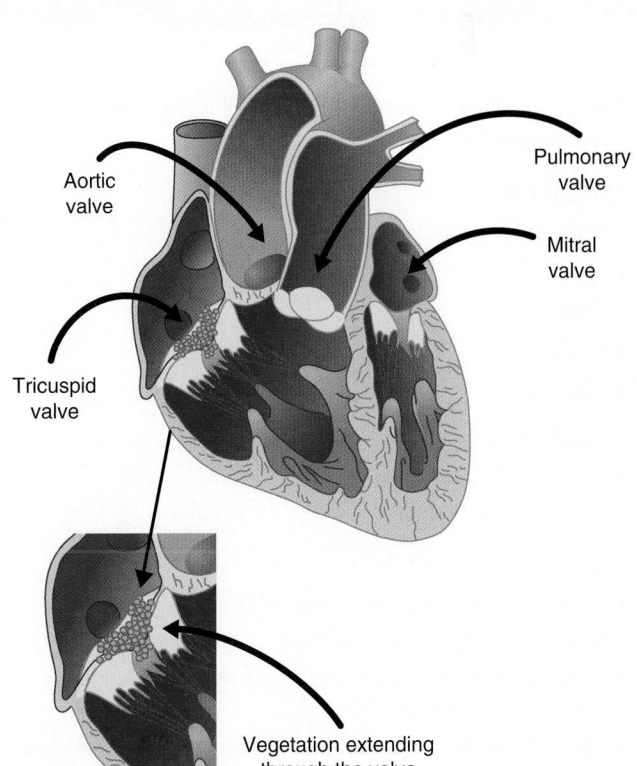

FIGURE 74–2. Diagram of the heart indicating common sites of infection.

systems, causing extracardiac manifestations of the disease. This commonly occurs in the kidneys, producing abscesses, infarction, or glomerulonephritis. Immune complexes or emboli also may produce skin manifestations of the disease, as seen with petechiae, Osler's nodes, and Janeway's lesions, or within the eye (e.g., Roth's spots).

CLINICAL PRESENTATION AND DIAGNOSIS

The clinical presentation for IE is quite variable and often nonspecific. ❷ *A fever is the most frequent and persistent symptom in patients but may be blunted with previous antibiotic use, congestive heart failure, chronic liver or renal failure, or infection caused by a less virulent organism (i.e., subacute disease).*[1,3,4] Other signs and symptoms that also may occur are listed in the Clinical Presentation box, with some discussed further in detail next.

Heart murmurs are heard frequently on auscultation (more than 85% of cases), but a new murmur or change in murmurs is only found in 3% to 5% or 5% to 10%, respectively.[1] Additionally, more than 90% of patients who have a new murmur will develop congestive heart failure, which is a major cause of morbidity and mortality. Splenomegaly and mycotic aneurysms are also noted in many cases of IE.

This disease is also characterized by the following peripheral manifestations. Some of these clinical findings are found in up to one-half of adult patients with IE, although recently the prevalence has been decreasing and are rarely seen in children.[1,3,10]

- **Skin:** *Petechiae* are very small (usually less than 3 mm), pinpoint, flat red spots beneath the skin surface caused by microhemorrhaging. They occur in 20% to 40% of patients with chronic IE and are often found on the buccal mucosa, conjunctivae (Fig. 74–3A), and extremities.[1] *Splinter hemorrhages* appear as small dark streaks beneath the finger- or toenails and occur most commonly proximally with IE, typically occurring as a result of local vasculitis or microemboli occurring in about 20% of patients (Fig. 74–3B). *Osler's nodes* are small (usually 2 to 15 mm), painful, tender subcutaneous nodules located on the pads of the fingers and toes (Fig. 74–3D) caused primarily by either septic emboli or vasculitis. These nodes are rare in acute disease but are also nonspecific for IE despite occurring in 10% to 25% of all patients.[1] *Janeway's lesions* are small, painless, hemorrhagic macular plaques on the palms of the hands or soles of the feet due to septic emboli (in approximately 5% of patients) and more commonly associated with acute *S. aureus* IE (Fig. 74–3E).

- **Extremities:** *Clubbing* of the finger tips typically occurs in long-standing illness and is present in approximately 10% to 20% of patients (Fig. 74–3C).[1]

- **Eye:** *Roth's spots* occur rarely and are (in less than 5% of IE cases) oval-shaped retinal hemorrhages with a pale center near the optic disc (Fig. 74–3F).

Clinical Presentation of IE ❷ ❸ ❹

General

Patients typically present with nonspecific and variable signs or symptoms.

Symptoms

Complaints from patients may include:

- Fever
- Chills
- Night sweats
- Weakness
- Dyspnea
- Weight loss
- Myalgia or arthralgias

Signs

- Fever is the most common sign of IE
- New or changing heart murmur
- Embolic phenomena (emboli affect the heart, lungs, abdomen, or extremities)
- Skin manifestations (e.g., petechiae, splinter hemorrhages, Osler's nodes, Janeway's lesions)
- Splenomegaly
- Clubbing of extremities

Laboratory Tests

- Blood cultures are the most important laboratory assessment for persistent bacteremia, which occurs commonly in IE. A minimum of three blood culture sets should be collected during the initial 24 hours
- Hematologic tests for anemia (normochromic, normocytic)
- WBC count may be elevated in acute disease but could be normal in subacute IE
- Nonspecific findings such as thrombocytopenia, elevated erythrocyte sedimentation rate or C-reactive protein, and abnormal urinalysis (i.e., proteinuria or microscopic hematuria)

Other Diagnostic Tests

An echocardiogram (TTE or TEE) should be performed on any patient with suspected IE to detect the presence of vegetations.

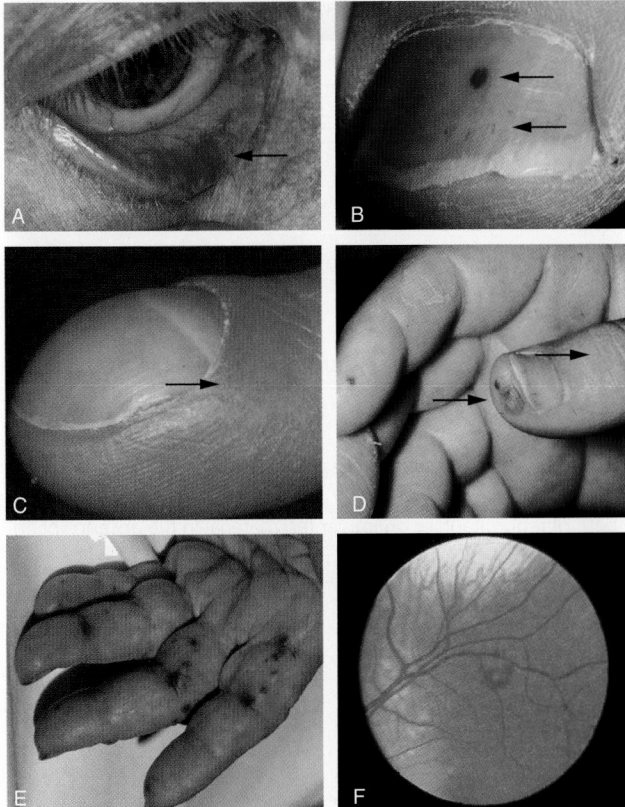

FIGURE 74–3. A. Conjunctival petechiae. (From Wolff K, Johnson RA, Suurmond D. In: Fitzpatrick's Color Atlas & Synopsis of Clinical Dermatology. 5th ed. New York: McGraw Hill. Copyright 2005.) **B.** Splinter hemorrhage. (From Collins SP. In: Atlas of Emergency Medicine. 2nd ed. New York: McGraw Hill. Copyright 2002.) **C.** Clubbing of finger. (From Tosti A, Piraccini BM. In: Fitzpatrick's Dermatology in General Medicine. 7th ed. New York: McGraw Hill. Copyright 2007.) **D.** Osler's nodes. (From Collins SP. In: Atlas of Emergency Medicine. 2nd ed. New York: McGraw Hill. Copyright 2002.) **E.** Janeway's lesions. (From Wolff K, Johnson RA, Suurmond D. In: Fitzpatrick's Color Atlas & Synopsis of Clinical Dermatology. 5th ed. New York: McGraw Hill. Copyright 2005.) **F.** Roth's spots (From Effron D, Forcier BC, Wyszynski RE. In: Atlas of Emergency Medicine. 2nd ed. New York: McGraw Hill. Copyright 2002.)

Laboratory Studies

❸ *Blood cultures are the essential laboratory test for the diagnosis and treatment of IE. Typically, patients with IE have a low-grade consistent bacteremia, with approximately 80% of cases having less than 100 CFU/mL (100,000 CFU/L) in the bloodstream.[1] Blood culture results are critical for determining the most appropriate therapy.* Three blood culture sets should be drawn within the initial 24 hours to determine the etiologic agent. Approximately 90% of the first two cultures will yield a positive result. If a positive blood culture is not obtained from a patient with suspected IE, the microbiology laboratory should be notified and cultures requested to be monitored for growth of fastidious organisms for up to 1 month.

❹ *Another important tool aiding in the diagnosis of IE is the echocardiogram. This imaging tool is used to visualize*

vegetations. Two methods of the echocardiogram are used: the transthoracic echocardiogram (TTE) and the transesophageal echocardiogram (TEE). The TTE has been used since the 1970s; however, it is less sensitive (45% to 65%) than the TEE (85% to 95%).[3] Despite the TEE being more sensitive, use of the TTE for patients with suspected native-valve IE is usually sufficient.[11,12] The TEE may be used as a secondary test for patients whose TTE was negative and in whom a high clinical suspicion of IE exists. Additionally, a TEE is often preferred in patients who have complicated disease, including left-sided IE, prosthetic valves, or perivalvular extension of the vegetation.[2,12,13] Echocardiograms also may be employed to assess the need for surgical intervention or to determine the possible source of emboli.[10,12]

Additional nonspecific tests for IE may be performed. These include hematologic parameters to determine whether the patient is anemic, which occurs in a majority of patients. The WBCs may be elevated, particularly in acute disease. However, in a subacute infection, the WBCs may be normal. An erythrocyte sedimentation rate (ESR) may also be obtained to determine the presence of inflammation, although this test is highly nonspecific and almost always elevated in IE.

Diagnostic Criteria

A definitive diagnosis of IE would consist of a biopsy or culture directly from pathologic specimens from the endocardium. However, this would be a highly invasive test. Therefore, diagnosis of IE relies on clinical presentation as well as laboratory and echocardiogram results. To guide this clinical diagnosis, criteria have been established to assess major and minor criteria for IE[14,15] (Table 74–2A). Depending on the number of major or minor criteria a patient demonstrates, he or she will be classified as having a definite, possible, or rejected diagnosis of IE (Table 74–2B).

Causative Organisms

Gram-positive bacteria are the most common organisms that produce IE. Streptococci and staphylococci species account for the majority of cases at more than 80%.[1,8] Viridans group streptococci have been considered the primary pathogens in IE. However, staphylococci have been increasing in prevalence as causative organisms and are the dominant causative organisms in some reports (Table 74–1).[5,15,16] Other gram-positive, gram-negative, atypical, and fungal organisms are less common but still must be considered in certain patient populations.

▶ *Streptococci*

Streptococci causing IE are most commonly a group of species called viridans group streptococci. The most common of this group are *Streptococcus salivarius, Streptococcus mutans, Streptococcus mitis*, and *Streptococcus sanguis*. This group of bacteria, considered normal flora in the human mouth, is α-hemolytic, and typically, most clinical microbiology laboratories do not differentiate the exact species. These organisms

Table 74–2

Modified Duke's Criteria for IE

2A. Definitions of Modified Duke's Criteria

Major Criteria

Blood culture positive for IE:

Typical microorganisms consistent with IE from two separate blood cultures:

Viridans streptococci, *S. bovis*, HACEK group, *S. aureus*, or community-acquired enterococci in the absence of a primary focus, or

Microorganisms consistent with IE from persistently positive blood cultures, defined as follows:

At least two positive cultures of blood samples drawn greater than 12 hours apart, or

All of three or a majority of four separate cultures of blood (with first and last sample drawn at least 1 hour apart)

Single positive blood culture for *C. burnetii* or antiphase I IgG antibody titer greater than 1:800

Evidence of endocardial involvement:

Echocardiogram positive for IE (TEE recommended in patients with prosthetic valves, rated at least "possible IE" by clinical criteria, or complicated IE [paravalvular abscess] TTE as first test in other patients), defined as follows:

Oscillating intracardiac mass on valve or supporting structures, in the path of regurgitant, or on implanted material in the absence of an alternative anatomic explanation, or

Abscess, or

New partial dehiscence of prosthetic valve

New valvular regurgitation (worsening or changing of preexisting murmur not sufficient)

Minor Criteria

Predisposition: predisposing heart condition or injection drug use

Fever: temperature greater than 38°C (100.4°F)

Vascular phenomena: major arterial emboli, septic pulmonary infarcts, mycotic aneurysm, intracranial hemorrhage, conjunctival hemorrhages, and Janeway's lesions

Immunologic phenomena: glomerulonephritis, Osler's nodes, Roth's spots, and rheumatoid factor

Microbiologic evidence: positive blood culture but does not meet a major criterion as noted above[a] or serologic evidence of active infection with organism consistent with IE

2B. Modified Duke's Criteria for the Diagnosis of IE

Definite IE

Pathologic criteria:

(1) Microorganisms demonstrated by culture or histologic examination of a vegetation that has embolized, or an intracardiac abscess specimen, or

(2) Pathologic lesions; vegetation or intracardiac abscess confirmed by histologic examination showing active endocarditis

Clinical criteria[b]:

(1) Two major criteria, or

(2) One major criterion and three minor criteria, or

(3) Five minor criteria

Possible IE

(1) One major criterion and one minor criterion, or

(2) Three minor criteria

Rejected

(1) Firm alternate diagnosis explaining evidence of IE, or

(2) Resolution of IE syndrome with antibiotic therapy for less than or equal to 4 days, or

(3) No pathologic evidence of IE at surgery or autopsy, with antibiotic therapy for less than or equal to 4 days, or

(4) Does not meet criteria for possible IE, as above

CNS, coagulase-negative staphylococci; TEE, transesophageal echocardiography; TTE, transthoracic echocardiography.

[a]Excludes single positive cultures for CNS and organisms that do not cause endocarditis.

[b]See above for definitions of major and minor criteria.

From Li JS, Sexton DJ, Mick N, et al. Proposed modifications to the Duke criteria for the diagnosis of infective endocarditis. Clin Infect Dis 2000;30:633–638; With permission. University of Chicago Press, 2000 by the Infectious Diseases Society of America. All rights reserved.

may cause bacteremia after dental procedures, which can lead to the development of IE in at-risk patients. Viridans group streptococci are also the predominant pathogen of IE associated with mitral valve prolapse and native valves and in children.[18] Another streptococci species that is commonly associated with IE is *Streptococcus bovis*, classified as group D streptococci, found in the GI tract. However, owing to the similarities of these streptococci, including microbiologic susceptibility, treatment is similar regardless of the species.

IE caused by these streptococci typically has a subacute clinical course. The current cure rate is often greater than 90% unless complications occur, and they do occur in more than 30% of patients.[18,19] The majority of viridans group streptococci remain very susceptible to penicillin, with most strains having a minimum inhibitory concentration (MIC) of less than 0.125 mcg/mL (0.125 mg/L).[20] Isolation of organisms with decreased susceptibilities is increasing. Therefore, antibiotic susceptibilities need to be assessed in order to determine the most appropriate treatment regimen.

▶ Staphylococci

Staphylococcal endocarditis is increasing in prevalence, causing 30% or more of all cases of IE, with the majority (80% to 90%) being due to *S. aureus* (a coagulase-positive staphylococci).[17,21] This increase in staphylococci has been primarily attributed to expanded use of venous catheters, more frequent valve replacement, and increased IVDU.[21] Coagulase-negative staphylococci (CNS) also cause IE; however, these organisms typically infect prosthetic valves or indwelling catheters.[22]

Historically, *S. aureus* was considered community acquired[21]; however, now almost half the cases are nosocomial in origin.[17] Any patient who is bacteremic with *S. aureus* is at an increased risk of developing IE. *S. aureus* also may infect "normal" heart valves (no prior detected valvular disease) in a third of cases.[1,21] Therefore, it is imperative to assess these patients adequately for the presence of vegetations. Any heart valve may be affected; however, when the mitral or aortic valve is involved, it often results in extensive systemic infection with a mortality rate of approximately 20% to 65%.[1,21] When treating *S. aureus* IE, one must consider whether the isolate displays methicillin resistance, the location of the infection (right or left side), presence of prosthetic valves, and history of IVDU. Despite significant resistance to penicillinase-resistant penicillins (e.g., methicillin and nafcillin), most isolates remain susceptible to vancomycin. However, there is an increasing incidence of *S. aureus* intermediately resistant or fully resistant to vancomycin.[23-25] Fortunately, they are not widespread enough to affect empirical antibiotic selection. Susceptibility reports should be assessed to ensure antibiotic activity.

Over the past decade there has been an increasing emergence of community-acquired methicillin-resistant *S. aureus* (CA-MRSA) that differs from healthcare-associated MRSA. This organism tends to be less resistant to many antibiotics, with sensitivity to clindamycin, trimethoprim-sulfamethoxazole, and minocycline, as well as vancomycin, linezolid, and daptomycin. However, this organism has a virulence gene (Panton-Valentine leukocidin), which produces a toxin that causes necrosis. To date this organism primarily causes skin/skin-structure infections or pneumonias (see Chap. 73, Skin and Soft Tissue Infections). There have been a limited number of cases of IE caused by CA-MRSA.[26] If CA-MRSA is suspected, treatment with vancomycin with or without gentamicin and/or rifampin remains the standard of care.

The predominant coagulase-negative organism causing IE has been *S. epidermidis*. However, in the past few years, an increase in isolation of another coagulase-negative species (*S. lugdunensis*) has been noted.[27-29] Typically, coagulase-negative staphylococcal IE has a subacute course with numerous complications. Treatment (with or without surgical intervention) is usually successful. On the other hand, *S. lugdunensis* produces a more virulent infection and, despite similar antibiotic susceptibilities, has a much higher mortality rate.[28,29]

▶ Enterococci

Enterococci are normal flora of the human GI tract and sometimes found in the anterior urethra. Historically, enterococci were considered part of the streptococci genus but now are separated despite similarities, such as group D classification and causing subacute disease. Frequently affected patients are older males who have undergone genitourinary manipulations or younger females who have had obstetric procedures. Although enterococci are a less common cause of IE, there are two predominant species: *Enterococcus faecium* and *Enterococcus faecalis*. *E. faecalis* is the most common and the more susceptible of the strains. However, enterococci overall are more intrinsically resistant, with enterococcal IE representing one of the most problematic gram-positive infections to treat and cure. Frequently, enterococci display resistance to multiple antibiotics, including penicillins, vancomycin, aminoglycosides, and has been described in some of the newer agents (e.g., linezolid or quinupristin/dalfopristin, daptomycin).[30]

▶ Gram-Negative Organisms

Gram-negative IE is much less common (approximately 2%) but is typically much more difficult to treat than gram-positive infections.[1,31] Fastidious organisms, such as the HACEK group, tend to be seen most commonly, causing approximately 3% of all IE.[4,32,33] This group consists of *Haemophilus* spp. (primarily *H. paraphrophilus*, *H. parainfluenzae*, and *H. aphrophilus*), *Actinobacillus actinomycetemcomitans*, *Cardiobacterium hominis*, *Eikenella corrodens*, and *Kingella kingae*. The clinical presentation of IE by these organisms is subacute, with approximately 50% of patients developing complications. These complications are primarily due to the presence of large, friable vegetations and numerous emboli along with the development of acute congestive heart failure often requiring valve replacement.[33,34] It is important to allow cultures sufficient incubation time (often 2 to 3 weeks) in order to isolate these organisms. Often these organisms may not be isolated on culture and thus present as culture-negative IE.

Other gram-negative organisms, such as *Pseudomonas* spp., cause IE, especially in IVDUs and patients with prosthetic valves. Additionally, IE may be caused by *Salmonella* spp.,

Escherichia coli, Citrobacter spp., *Klebsiella* spp., *Enterobacter* spp., *Serratia marcescens, Proteus* spp., and *Providencia* spp.[1,31]

Historically, gram-negative IE typically had a poor prognosis with high mortality rates. However, as nondrug therapy advances to include cardiac surgery in more than half of patients, the in-hospital mortality has improved to 24%.[1,31] Treatment usually consists of high-dose combination therapy, with valve replacement often a necessity in many patients.

▶ Culture Negative

Negative blood cultures are reported in approximately 5% of confirmed IE cases, often delaying diagnosis and treatment.[1,4,35] Sterile cultures may be the result of previous antibiotic use, subacute right-sided disease, slow growth of fastidious organisms, nonbacterial endocarditis (e.g., fungal or intracellular parasitic infections), noninfective endocarditis, or improper collection of blood cultures. If nonbacterial or fastidious organisms are suspected, additional testing is essential. The choice of treatment regimen depends on patient history and risk factors.

▶ Other Organisms

Numerous bacteria, including gram-positive bacilli, unusual gram-negative bacteria, atypical bacteria, and anaerobes, as well as spirochetes, may cause IE, but these infections are rare.[32] Some of the more common organisms include *Legionella, Coxiella burnetii* (Q fever), and *Brucella*. These rare organisms occur primarily in at-risk patients such as those who have a prosthetic valve or are IVDUs. A comprehensive discussion of these organisms is not feasible for this chapter; for further information, other references sources (particularly references 1 to 5) should be examined. Treatment of these organisms is difficult, and cure rates are low. Therefore, consulting an infectious diseases specialist is warranted.

▶ Fungi

Fungal endocarditis is quite uncommon but has significant mortality, typically affecting patients who have had cardiovascular surgery, received a prolonged course of broad-spectrum antibiotics, have long-term catheter placement, are immunocompromised, or are IVDUs.[3,36,37] Survival rates have remained poor, at approximately 15%, but improvements (survival rates approximately 30%) have been reported owing to advances in diagnosis and treatment.[36] The poor prognosis has been attributed to large vegetations, propensity for organism invasion into the myocardium, extensive septic emboli, poor antifungal penetration into the vegetation, and low toxic-to-therapeutic ratio and lack of cidal activity of certain antifungals.[33,36] The two most commonly associated organisms are *Candida* spp. and *Aspergillus* spp. Lack of clinical studies makes treatment decisions difficult. Typically, combination and/or high-dose therapy in conjunction with surgery is required.

TREATMENT
Therapeutic Considerations

Treatment of IE often is complicated and difficult. Numerous factors involving the vegetation influence the effectiveness of the antimicrobial agents. The vegetation consists of a fibrin matrix (as discussed earlier) that provides an environment where organisms are relatively free to replicate unimpeded, allowing the microbial density to reach very high concentrations (10^9 to 10^{10} CFU/g). Once the organism density has reached this level, the organisms are virtually in a static growth phase. These factors hinder host defenses, as well as the ability of antimicrobials to produce sufficient kill. This is seen often with β-lactams and glycopeptides because their effectiveness can be significantly affected by the bacterial inoculum.

5 *Selection of an appropriate antimicrobial agent must combine characteristics such as the ability to penetrate into the vegetation, the ability to achieve adequate drug concentrations, and the ability to be minimally affected by high bacterial inoculum in order to achieve adequate kill rates.*

6 *To accomplish this, antimicrobials typically have to be given parenterally at high doses, with an extended treatment course of 4 to 6 weeks (in most cases).* Other desirable drug characteristics include bactericidal and synergistic activity.

Empirical Therapy

7 *The overall goal of therapy is to eradicate the infection and minimize/prevent any complications.* Patients with suspected IE should be evaluated for risk factors that may provide some indication of the most likely organism causing the infection. If no risk factors can be determined, empirical therapy should primarily cover gram-positive organisms. Generally, if streptococci are suspected, empirical treatment should consist of penicillin plus gentamicin. However, if staphylococci or enterococci are suspected, empirical treatment should consist of vancomycin plus gentamicin. It is important to monitor the patient's response to therapy closely until cultures and susceptibilities are determined to ensure adequate treatment.

Specific Therapy

The American Heart Association (AHA) has published guidelines for the management of IE, including specific treatment recommendations.[5] A summary of these treatments for the most common organisms (streptococci, staphylococci, and enterococci) is provided in Tables 74–3 through 74–6. However, for more detailed information (including dosing, length of treatment, etc.) for these organisms or less common organisms, refer to the complete guidelines.[5] These guidelines include primary and alternative regimens, as indicated in the treatment tables under strength of recommendation.

▶ Streptococci

Most isolates are highly susceptible to penicillin; therefore, penicillin G remains the regimen of choice. However, ceftriaxone may be used as an alternative agent if the patient is

Patient Encounter, Part 2: Medical History, Physical Examination, and Diagnostic Tests

PMH

- CAD s/p tricuspid valve replacement 2 years ago
- BPH s/p TUR of the prostate 21 days ago

FH

Mother had a history of CAD and died at the age of 70 from a heart attack; father died at 81 from prostate cancer

SH

Denies alcohol, illicit drugs, and smoking

Meds

- Simvastatin 80 mg daily
- Lisinopril 20 mg daily
- Warfarin 5 mg Monday through Friday, 7.5 mg Saturday and Sunday

Allergies: penicillin (patient reports hives)

ROS

Fatigue, decreased appetite

PE

- Vital signs: BP 174/90 mm Hg, P 105 beats/minute, RR 22 breaths/minute, T 39.0°C
- Cardiovascular: Tachycardia, positive new murmur
- Abdomen: Underweight, soft, nontender, nondistended; (+) bowel sounds

Labs

Within normal limits, except WBC = 18.6 × 10³/µL (18.6 × 10⁹/L)

Given this additional information, what is your assessment of the patient's condition?

Identify your empirical treatment recommendations for this patient.

What other information would be beneficial to obtain?

Patient Encounter, Part 3: Additional Laboratory and Diagnostic Tests

Blood cultures

All cultures are positive for gram-positive cocci in pairs and chains. *Enterococcus faecalis*.

Labs

Within normal limits.

Echo

0.7 × 1.2 cm vegetation on the tricuspid valve.

Given this additional information, are there any changes in your assessment of the patient?

How would you tailor your treatment based on these new data?

What would be your treatment goals, including length of treatment?

What other information would be beneficial to have?

or equal to 0.5 mcg/mL [0.5 mg/L]), treatment doses are increased, and 4 weeks of treatment is suggested. In addition, combination therapy with gentamicin is recommended during the first 2 weeks. In patients who are allergic or intolerant to either of the β-lactams, vancomycin is an alternative treatment option. Additionally, in patients with resistant strains of viridans group streptococci (MIC greater than 0.5 mcg/mL [0.5 mg/L]), treatment should employ antimicrobial agents for enterococcal IE (precise agents determined by the susceptibility report).

Patients with PVE caused by penicillin-susceptible strains of viridans streptococci require treatment for 6 weeks with penicillin G or ceftriaxone with or without gentamicin during the initial 2 weeks of therapy. However, if the organism demonstrates less susceptibility to penicillin (MIC greater than 0.12 mcg/mL [0.12 mg/L]), a combination therapy with penicillin G or ceftriaxone plus gentamicin should be given for the entire 6 weeks. Vancomycin remains the primary alternative if the patient is allergic to β-lactams (e.g., penicillins, cephalosporins).

▶ Staphylococci

It is important to determine (a) whether the isolate is methicillin-susceptible versus methicillin-resistant and (b) whether the patient has a native valve versus prosthetic valve. For patients with no prosthetic material, methicillin-susceptible staphylococci treatment should consist of a penicillinase-resistant penicillin (e.g., nafcillin or oxacillin) with or without gentamicin, and for methicillin-resistant strains, therapy should consist of vancomycin (see Table 74–4). Combination therapy with aminoglycosides, when used in these patients, typically is given only during the first 3 to 5 days of therapy to decrease the bacterial burden. In the absence of prosthetic material, some treatment guidelines do not recommend combination therapy against MRSA.

allergic or resistance is suspected to penicillin. Typically, the length of treatment is 4 weeks and remains the most common regimen. However, a shorter course (i.e., 2 weeks) may be employed for a patient with uncomplicated IE due to highly penicillin-susceptible strains with no extracardiac infection or whose creatinine clearance is greater than 20 mL/min (0.33 mL/s). If the shorter length of therapy is chosen, gentamicin should be added to the previous regimens for the entire course (i.e., 2 weeks). Recommended therapies for highly penicillin-susceptible viridans streptococci are summarized in Table 74–3.

When penicillin MICs for viridans group streptococci increase (greater than 0.12 mcg/mL [0.12 mg/L] but less than

Table 74–3

Therapy of Native-Valve Endocarditis Caused by Highly Penicillin-Susceptible Viridans Group Streptococci and *S. bovis*

Regimen	Dosage[a] and Route	Duration (weeks)	Strength of Recommendation[b]	Comments
Aqueous crystalline penicillin G sodium *OR*	12–18 million units/24 hours (IV either continuously or in 4 or 6 equally divided doses	4	IA	Preferred in most patients 65 years of age or older or patients with impairment of eighth cranial nerve function or renal function
Ceftriaxone sodium	2 g/24 hours IV/IM in 1 dose *Pediatric dose[c]*: penicillin 200,000 units/kg per 24 hours IV in 4–6 equally divided doses; ceftriaxone 100 mg/kg per 24 hours IV/IM in 1 dose	4	IA	
Aqueous crystalline penicillin G sodium *OR*	12–18 million units/24 hours IV either continuously or in 6 equally divided doses	2	IB	2-week regimen not intended for patients with cardiac or extracardiac abscess or for those with creatinine clearance of less than 20 mL/min (0.33 mL/s), impaired eighth cranial nerve function, or *Abiotrophia, Granulicatella,* or *Gemella* spp. infection; gentamicin dosage should be adjusted to achieve peak serum concentration of 3–4 mcg/mL (3-4 mg/L; 6.3–8.4 μmol/L) and trough serum concentration of less than 1 mcg/mL (1 mg/L; 2.1 μmol/L) when 3 divided doses are used; nomogram used for single daily dosing[e]
Ceftriaxone plus gentamicin sulfate[d]	2 g/24 hours IV/IM in 1 dose 3 mg/kg per 24 hours IV/IM in 1 dose *Pediatric dose*: penicillin 200,000 units/kg per 24 hours IV in 4–6 equally divided doses; ceftriaxone 100 mg/kg per 24 hours IV/IM in 1 dose; gentamicin 3 mg/kg per 24 hours IV/IM in 1 dose or 3 equally divided doses[f]			
Vancomycin hydrochloride[g]	30 mg/kg per 24 hours IV in 2 equally divided doses not to exceed 2 g/24 hours unless concentrations in serum are inappropriately low *Pediatric dose*: 40 mg/kg per 24 hours IV in 2–3 equally divided doses MIC less than or equal to 0.12 mcg/mL (0.12 mg/L)	4	IB	Vancomycin therapy recommended only for patients unable to tolerate penicillin or ceftriaxone; vancomycin dosage should be adjusted to obtain peak (1 hour after infusion completed) serum concentration of 30–35 mcg/mL (30–35 mg/L; 21–24 μmol/L) and a trough concentration range of 10–15 mcg/mL (10–15 mg/L; 6.9–10.4 μmol/L)

IM, intramuscularly; MIC, minimum inhibitory concentration.

[a]Dosage recommended are for patients with normal renal function.

[b]IA, condition with evidence and/or general agreement that a procedure or treatment is useful and effective, based on data from multiple randomized clinical trials; IB, condition with evidence and/or general agreement that a procedure or treatment is useful and effective based on data from a single randomized trial or nonrandomized studies.

[c]Pediatric dose should not exceed that of a normal adult.

[d]Other potentially nephrotoxic drugs (e.g., nonsteroidal anti-inflammatory drugs) should be used with caution in patients receiving gentamicin therapy.

[e]See Nicolau DP, Freeman CD, Belliveau PB, et al. Experience with a once-daily aminoglycoside program administered to 2184 adult patients. Antimicrob Agents Chemother 1995;39:650–655.

[f]Data for once-daily dosing of aminoglycosides for children exist, but no data for treatment of IE exist.

[g]Vancomycin dosages should be infused during course of at least 1 hour to reduce risk of histamine-release "red man" syndrome.

Reprinted with permission. Baddour LM, Wilson WR, Bayer AS, et al. American Heart Association Scientific Statement. Infective endocarditis: Diagnosis, antimicrobial therapy, and management of complications. Circulation 2005;111:e394–e433. ©2005, American Heart Association, Inc.

Table 74–4

Therapy for Endocarditis Caused by Staphylococci in the Absence of Prosthetic Materials

Regimen	Dosage[a] and Route	Duration (weeks)	Strength of Recommendation[b]	Comments
Oxacillin-Resistant Strains				
Nafcillin or oxacillin[c]	12 g/24 hours IV in 4–6 equally divided doses	6	IA	For complicated right-sided IE and for left-sided IE, 6-week treatment; for uncomplicated right-sided IE, 2-week treatment
with optional addition of gentamicin sulfate[d]	3 mg/kg per 24 hours IV/IM in 2 or 3 equally divided doses *Pediatric dose[e]*: nafcillin or oxacillin 200 mg/kg per 24 hours IV in 4–6 equally divided doses; gentamicin 3 mg/kg per 24 hours IV/IM in 3 equally divided doses	3–5 days		Clinical benefit of aminoglycosides has not been established
For penicillin-allergic (nonanaphylactoid type) patients: cefazolin	6 g/24 hours IV in 3 equally divided doses	6	IB	Consider skin testing for oxacillin-susceptible staphylococci and questionable history of immediate-type hypersensitivity to penicillin; cephalosporins should be avoided in patients with anaphylactoid-type hypersensitivity to β-lactams; vancomycin should be used in these cases[e]
with optional addition of gentamicin sulfate	3 mg/kg per 24 hours IV/IM in 2 or 3 equally divided doses *Pediatric dose*: cefazolin 100 mg/kg per 24 hours IV in 3 equally divided doses; gentamicin 3 mg/kg per 24 hours IV/IM in 3 equally divided doses	3–5 days		Clinical benefit of aminoglycosides has not been established
Oxacillin-Resistant Strains				
Vancomycin hydrochloride[f]	30 mg/kg per 24 hours IV in 2 equally divided doses *Pediatric dose*: 40 mg/kg per 24 hours IV in 2–3 equally divided doses	6	IB	Adjust vancomycin dosage to achieve 1 hour (peak) serum concentration of 30–45 mcg/mL (30-45 mg/L; 21–31 μmol/L) and trough concentration of 10–15 mcg/mL (10-15 mg/L; 6.9–10.4 μmol/L) (see text for vancomycin alternatives)

MIC, minimum inhibitory concentration; IM, intramuscular.

[a]Dosages recommended are for patients with normal renal function.

[b]IA, condition with evidence and/or general agreement that a procedure or treatment is useful and effective, based on data from multiple randomized clinical trails; IB, condition with evidence and/or general agreement that a procedure or treatment is useful and effective based on data from a single randomized trial or nonrandomized studies.

[c]Penicillin G 24 million units/24 hours IV in 4 to 6 equally divided doses may be used in place of nafcillin or oxacillin if strain is penicillin-susceptible (MIC less than or equal to 0.1 mcg/mL [0.1 mg/L]) and does not produce β-lactamase.

[d]Gentamicin should be administered in close temporal proximity to vancomycin, nafcillin, or oxacillin dosing.

[e]Pediatric dose should not exceed that of a normal adult.

[f]For specific dosing adjustment and issues concerning vancomycin, see Table 74–3 footnotes.

Reprinted with permission. Baddour LM, Wilson WR, Bayer AS, et al. American Heart Association Scientific Statement. Infective endocarditis: diagnosis, antimicrobial therapy, and management of complications. Circulation 2005;111:e394–e433. ©2005, American Heart Association, Inc.

Table 74–5

Therapy for PVE Caused by Staphylococci

Regimen	Dosage[a] and Route	Duration (weeks)	Strength of Recommendation[b]	Comments
Oxacillin-Susceptible Strains				
Nafcillin or oxacillin	12 g/24 hours IV in 4–6 equally divided doses	6 weeks or longer	IB	Penicillin G 24 million units/24 hours IV in 4 to 6 equally divided doses may be used in place of nafcillin or oxacillin if strain is penicillin-susceptible (MIC less than or equal to 0.1 mcg/mL [0.1 mg/L]) and does not produce β-lactamase; vancomycin should be used in patients with immediate-type hypersensitivity reactions to β-lactam antibiotics (see Table 74–3 for dosing guidelines); cefazolin may be substituted for nafcillin or oxacillin in patients with nonimmediate-type hypersensitivity reactions to penicillins
plus Rifampin	900 mg per 24 hours IV/orally in 3 equally divided doses	6 weeks or longer		
plus Gentamicin sulfate[c]	3 mg/kg per 24 hours IV/IM in 2 or 3 equally divided doses	2		
	Pediatric dose[d]: nafcillin or oxacillin 200 mg/kg per 24 hours IV in 4–6 equally divided doses; rifampin 20 mg/kg per 24 hours IV/oral doses; in 3 equally divided doses; gentamicin 3 mg/kg per 24 hours in 3 equally divided doses			
Oxacillin-Resistant Strains				
Vancomycin hydrochloride	30 mg/kg per 24 hours IV in 2 equally divided doses	6 weeks or longer	IB	Adjust vancomycin to achieve 1 hour (peak) serum concentration of 30–45 mcg/mL (30–45 mg/L; 21–31 μmol/L) and trough concentration of 10–15 mcg/mL (10–15 mg/L; 6.9–10.4 μmol/L)
plus Rifampin	900 mg/24 hours IV/oral in 3 equally divided doses	6 weeks or longer		
plus Gentamicin sulfate	3 mg/kg per 24 hours IV/IM in 2 or 3 equally divided doses	2		
	Pediatric dose: vancomycin 40 mg/kg per 24 hours IV in 2 or 3 equally divided doses; rifampin 20 mg/kg per 24 hours IV/oral in 3 equally divided doses (up to adult dose); gentamicin 3 mg/kg per 24 hours IV/IM in 3 equally divided doses			

[a]Dosages recommended are for patients with normal renal function.

[b]IB, condition with evidence and/or general agreement that a procedure or treatment is useful and effective, based on data from a single randomized trial or nonrandomized studies.

[c]Gentamicin should be administered in close proximity to vancomycin, nafcillin, or oxacillin dosing.

[d]Pediatric dose should not exceed that of a normal adult.

Reprinted with permission from Baddour LM, Wilson WR, Bayer AS, et al. American Heart Association Scientific Statement. Infective endocarditis: Diagnosis, antimicrobial therapy, and management of complications. Circulation 2005;111:e394–e433. ©2005, American Heart Association, Inc.

However, many clinicians may combine either gentamicin or rifampin with vancomycin if the patient is unresponsive to monotherapy.

Increasing resistance of staphylococci necessitates the expanded use of alternative therapies. A clinical study demonstrated similar activity for daptomycin compared with standard therapy (i.e., penicillinase-resistant penicillin for methicillin-sensitive *S. aureus* [MSSA] or vancomycin for MRSA) in staphylococcal IE.[38] Based on this study, the FDA has approved an indication of daptomycin for the treatment of right-sided IE or bacteremia caused by *S. aureus*. Recommended dosing for these indications are 6 mg/kg/day

Table 74–6

Therapy for Native-Valve or Prosthetic-Valve Enterococcal Endocarditis Caused by Strains Susceptible to Penicillin, Gentamicin, and Vancomycin

Regimen	Dosage[a] and Route	Duration (weeks)	Strength of Recommendation[b]	Comments
Ampicillin sodium OR	12 g/24 hours IV in 6 divided doses	4–6	IA	Native valve: 4-week therapy recommended for patients with symptoms of illness less than or equal to 3 months; 6-week therapy recommended for patients with symptoms greater than 3 months
Aqueous crystalline penicillin G sodium	18–30 million units/24 hours IV either continuously or in 6 equally divided doses	4–6	IA	Prosthetic valve or other prosthetic cardiac material: minimum of 6 weeks of therapy recommended
plus gentamicin sulfate[c]	3 mg/kg per 24 hours IV/IM in 3 equally divided doses *Pediatric dose[d]*: ampicillin 300 mg/kg per 24 hours IV in 4–6 equally divided doses; penicillin 300,000 units/kg per 24 hours IV in 4–6 equally divided doses; gentamicin 3 mg/kg per 24 hours IV/IM in 3 equally divided doses	4–6		
Vancomycin hydrochloride[e]	30 mg/kg per 24 hours IV in 2 equally divided doses	6	IB	Vancomycin therapy recommended only for patients unable to tolerate penicillin or ampicillin
plus gentamicin sulfate	3 mg/kg per 24 hours IV/IM in 3 equally divided doses *Pediatric dose*: vancomycin 40 mg/kg per 24 hours IV in 2 or 3 equally divided doses; gentamicin 3 mg/kg per 24 hours IV/IM in 3 equally divided doses	6		6 weeks of vancomycin therapy recommended because of decreased activity against enterococci

[a]Dosages recommended are for patients with normal renal function.

[b]IA, condition with evidence and/or general agreement that a procedure or treatment is useful and effective, based on data from multiple randomized clinical trials; IB, condition with evidence and/or general agreement that a procedure or treatment is useful and effective, based on data from a single randomized trial or nonrandomized studies.

[c]Dosage of gentamicin should be adjusted to achieve peak serum concentration of 3 to 4 mcg/mL (3–4 mg/L; 6.3–8.4 µmol/L) and a trough concentration of less than 1 mcg/mL (1 mg/L; 2.1 µmol/L). Patients with a creatinine clearance of less than 50 mL/min (0.83 mL/s) should be treated in consultation with an infectious diseases specialist.

[d]Pediatric dose should not exceed that of a normal adult.

[e]See Table 74–3 for appropriate dosage of vancomycin.

Reprinted with permission from Baddour LM, Wilson WR, Bayer AS, et al. American Heart Association Scientific Statement. Infective endocarditis: Diagnosis, antimicrobial therapy, and management of complications. Circulation 2005;111:e394–e433. ©2005, American Heart Association, Inc.

(unless renal adjustments are necessary); although dosages of 8 to 10 mg/kg/day have been suggested in IE.[38,39] This study, along with another retrospective study, reported daptomycin to be safe and well tolerated.[38,40] Additionally, other antibiotics, such as ceftaroline, linezolid, quinupristin/dalfopristin and telavancin, or tigecycline alone or in combination, have been used in patients who were unresponsive to standard therapy, although they have had variable response rates.[41–44] These therapies often are reserved for patients who have been unresponsive to traditional therapy (e.g., β-lactams or vancomycin) or for organisms that remain susceptible to these agents when resistant to traditional therapy.

For staphylococcal PVE, treatment length increases significantly, typically requiring a minimum of 6 weeks (see Table 74–5). For MSSA, a penicillinase-resistant penicillin is still employed, as well as vancomycin for MRSA. However, with either regimen, the addition of both gentamicin for first 2 weeks and rifampin for the entire length of treatment is recommended.

▶ Enterococci

For enterococci, it is imperative to determine species and antibiotic susceptibilities. If the organism is susceptible to penicillin and vancomycin, treatment may consist of high-dose penicillin G, ampicillin, or vancomycin plus an aminoglycoside (gentamicin [see Table 74–6] or streptomycin for gentamicin-resistant strains). Treatment length is usually 4 to 6 weeks, with the aminoglycoside used over the entire course. As resistance develops to penicillin, ampicillin and vancomycin remain treatment options. Once the isolate becomes resistant to ampicillin, vancomycin is considered the treatment of choice.

If the isolate is determined to be vancomycin-resistant, it is most important to know the exact species because some of the treatment options, such as quinupristin/dalfopristin, are not active against *E. faecalis*. Currently, the treatment options for vancomycin-resistant enterococci (VRE) are not well established by clinical studies or patient experience. The treatment recommendations for vancomycin-resistant *E. faecium* include linezolid or quinupristin/dalfopristin for a minimum of 8 weeks. However, newer agents, such as daptomycin, may provide another option for treatment for either enterococci species (*E. faecium* and *E. faecalis*). Additionally, guidelines suggest the use of imipenem/cilastatin plus ampicillin or ceftriaxone plus ampicillin for the treatment of *E. faecalis*, with a minimum of 8 weeks of therapy. Consultation with an infectious diseases specialist is recommended.

▶ Gram-Negative Organisms

Identification of the exact isolate is crucial in gram-negative IE because treatment decisions depend on which organism is isolated. Therapy is usually targeted to the most susceptible antibiotics. Combination therapy (usually the addition of an aminoglycoside) is commonly used. For example, *Pseudomonas* spp. are treated with an antipseudomonal (e.g., piperacillin/tazobactam, cefepime, imipenem/cilastatin) plus high-dose aminoglycoside (typically tobramycin 8 mg/kg/day). However, exact dosing of antibiotics depends on the organism isolated. Length of treatment is usually a minimum of 6 weeks.

▶ HACEK Group

The HACEK group is difficult to isolate, often taking weeks for identification. If one of these organisms is suspected (e.g., subacute disease, embolism, large vegetations), it is important to initiate appropriate empirical treatment. The preferred regimen is ceftriaxone (or another third- or fourth-generation cephalosporin), followed by ampicillin-sulbactam. However, for patients who are intolerant of these treatments, ciprofloxacin may be used. The length of treatment typically is 4 weeks for these organisms.

▶ Culture-Negative

Treatment for culture-negative IE presents a significant dilemma. Therapeutic regimens are guided by specific isolated organisms. When cultures fail to identify a specific organism, decisions regarding treatment should cover the most common causative organisms. If the patient is unresponsive to this initial treatment, then additional coverage for less common organisms is warranted. An infectious diseases specialist should be consulted for managing a patient with this type of infection.

▶ Fungi

Treatment of fungal IE is exceptionally difficult. There is a significant lack of studies to identify and recommend the most appropriate therapy. Currently, amphotericin B is the most common treatment. However, valve replacement surgery is often considered an adjunct therapy. IV antifungal therapy requires high doses for a minimum of 8 weeks of treatment. Oral azoles (e.g., fluconazole) are used as long-term suppressive therapy to prevent relapse. The exact role of some of the newer antifungals (e.g., voriconazole and caspofungin) is unknown, but they should provide a viable option.[45,46]

Surgery

Surgical intervention has become an integral therapy in combination with pharmacologic management of IE. Valve replacement is the predominant intervention, and it is used in almost one-half of all cases of IE.[1] Surgery may be indicated if the patient has unresolved infection, ineffective antimicrobial therapy (often associated with fungal IE), more than one episode of serious emboli, refractory congestive heart failure, significant valvular dysfunction, a mycotic aneurysm requiring resection, local complications (perivalvular or myocardial abscesses), or a prosthetic-valve infection associated with a pathogen that demonstrates higher antimicrobial resistance (e.g., staphylococci, gram-negative organisms, and fungi).[47,48] Often a patient's hemodynamic status (i.e., blood pressure, heart rate, pulmonary artery pressure, etc.) is used to determine when surgical intervention is warranted.[1] Despite appropriate medical management and cure, a significant number of people who develop native-valve endocarditis require valve replacement surgery. Involvement of the aorta or development of IE complications is considered an indication for surgery in the majority of patients with PVE.[49,50]

Dosing Considerations

The majority of antibiotic and antifungal agents used for the treatment of IE require dosing modifications based on renal or hepatic function. However, the most closely monitored are vancomycin and aminoglycosides. This is due in part because (a) therapeutic levels are normally monitored, and (b) the increased likelihood of developing toxicities (i.e., nephrotoxicity) if the level is too high or adverse outcomes (i.e., clinical failure or resistance development) if level is too low.

Table 74–7

Dosage Considerations for Standard Antibiotics for Treatment of IE[a]

Drug	Renal Adjustments	Hepatic Adjustments	Comments
Penicillin G	Required	None	Extension of dosing interval primarily used for adjustment
Ampicillin	Required	None	Seizures most common AE if dosing not adjusted
Nafcillin	None	Severe (see comment)	Adjustments necessary ONLY in patients with severe hepatic AND renal impairment
Oxacillin	Severe (see comment)	None	Adjustments for CrCl less than 10 mL/min (0.17 mL/s) to lower range of normal dose
Cefazolin	Required	None	Dose and/or dosing interval require adjustment. Based on patient's CrCl
Ceftriaxone	Severe (see comment)	None	Do not exceed 2 g/day if patient has BOTH severe renal AND hepatic impairment
Vancomycin	Required	None	Monitor therapeutic levels to guide dosage adjustments (see treatment guidelines for target ranges)
Gentamicin	Required	None	Used for synergy only with gram-positives. Therapeutic levels vary for gram-negative organisms Monitor therapeutic levels to guide dosage adjustments Synergy target levels: peak 3–4 mcg/mL (3–4 mg/L; 6.3–8.4 μmol/L) and trough less than 1 mcg/mL (1 mg/L; 2.1 μmol/L)
Rifampin	None	Required	Adjustment based on hepatic dysfunction
Newer and Salvage Drugs			
Ceftaroline	Required	None	Adjustments in dose (33–67% reduction) are based on patient's CrCl. Suggested dosages in off-label use for IE are higher than standard dosing (i.e., 600 mg every 8 hours).
Daptomycin	Required	None	Adjustment in dosing interval CrCl less than 30 mL/min (0.50 mL/s) CPK should be monitored prior to and during therapy
Linezolid	None	None	Metabolites may accumulate in severe renal impairment Monitor for hematologic AE Use in severe hepatic impairment not established
Quinupristin/dalfopristin	None	Possibly	Adjustments suggested based on pharmacokinetic data. However, no specific recommendations are described
Telavancin	Required	None	Decrease daily dose by 25% if CrCl 30–50 mL/min (0.50–0.83 mL/s) or if CrCl less than 30 mL/min (0.50 mL/s)—extend interval to every 48 hours
Tigecycline	None	Severe (see comment)	In severe hepatic impairment (Child-Pugh class C)—decrease maintenance dose 50%
Streptomycin	Required	None	Used for synergy only with gram-positives. Therapeutic levels vary for gram-negative organisms Monitor therapeutic levels to guide dosage adjustments Synergy target levels: peak 20–35 mcg/mL (20–35 mg/L; 34–60 μmol/L) and trough less than 10 mcg/mL (10 mg/L; 17 μmol/L)

AE, adverse event; CPK, creatinine phosphokinase; CrCl, creatinine clearance.

[a]Gram-negative bacteria, fungal, or atypical treatments are not listed. It is suggested that an Infectious Diseases Consult be obtained if a patient has IE caused by one of these organisms due to the complexity and difficulty in managing these patients.

General dosing considerations are included in Table 74–7 for the most commonly used drugs for treating IE. However, specific dosing adjustments for individual patients should be determined by referring to an appropriate drug dosing reference.

Prophylaxis

⑧ *Certain conditions have been associated more commonly with IE due to preexisting cardiac disease in the presence of a* *transient bacteremia. In an effort to prevent the development of IE, prophylactic treatment generally is considered appropriate for these at-risk patients.* Although there are no well-controlled clinical studies of these recommendations, it is thought that if antibiotics are given just prior to a procedure, the number of bacteria may be decreased in the bloodstream and prevent the bacteria from adhering to the valves.

Cardiac conditions in which prophylaxis is reasonable include presence of prosthetic valves or material, prior IE,

---

Patient Encounter, Part 4: Additional Laboratory

Susceptibility Report: *Enterococcus faecalis*

Drug	Ampicillin	Vancomycin	Gentamicin Synergy	Streptomycin Synergy
MIC (mg/L)	2	4	More than 500	Less than 1,000

Given this additional information, are there any changes in your assessment of the patient?

Do you need to adjust your treatment regimen based on these data?

Would your treatment goals, particularly length of treatment, change?

Patient Encounter, Part 5: Create a Care Plan

Based on this patient's information, create a care plan for the management of his IE. Be sure to include:

(a) A statement regarding treatment requirements and/or possible problems

(b) Goals of therapy

(c) A patient-specific plan, including preventive plans

(d) A follow-up plan to assess whether the goals have been met and to determine whether the patient experienced any adverse effects

---

congenital cardiac disease (specific forms only), and cardiac transplant patients with cardiac valvulopathy (Table 74–8).[7] Although many patients have other cardiac dysfunction, only patients with these conditions are considered to be at a high risk of developing IE. No prophylaxis is advised in other patients.

Transient bacteria may occur due to many types of dental and surgical procedures. However, the AHA has recently published new guidelines significantly limiting the types of procedures where prophylaxis is appropriate. Only dental procedures involving manipulation of gingival tissue or the periapical region of teeth or perforation of the oral mucosa are considered to increase the likelihood that high-risk patients will develop IE.[7] Viridans group streptococci are the primary bacteria targeted for prophylaxis in this circumstance. On the other hand, prophylaxis for GI or genitourinary surgeries primarily targets enterococci.

The AHA guidelines include suggested antibiotic regimens for dental procedures for which prophylaxis is warranted.[7] Recommended regimens for dental procedures are listed in Table 74–9. These guidelines recommend a single oral or intramuscular/IV dose initiated shortly before the procedure. The regimen for dental procedures consists primarily of a penicillin as first choice, with a cephalosporin for nonanaphylactic penicillin-allergic patients and clindamycin or a macrolide for penicillin-allergic patients. A second prophylactic dose is not recommended. However, if an infection develops at the procedure site, additional antibiotics (i.e., a therapeutic course) may be required.

Table 74–8

Cardiac Conditions Associated With the Highest Risk of Adverse Outcome From Endocarditis for Which Prophylaxis With Dental Procedures Is Reasonable[a]

Prosthetic cardiac valve or prosthetic material used for cardiac-valve repair

Previous IE

Congenital heart disease[b]

Unrepaired cyanotic congenital heart disease, including palliative shunts and conduits

Completely repaired congenital heart defect with prosthetic material or device, whether placed by surgery or by catheter intervention, during the first 6 months after the procedure[c]

Repaired congenital heart disease with residual defects at the site or adjacent to the site of a prosthetic patch or prosthetic device (which inhibit endothelialization)

Cardiac transplantation recipients who develop cardiac valvulopathy

[a]All dental procedures that involve manipulation of gingival tissue or the periapical region of teeth or perforation of the oral mucosa is reasonable to give prophylaxis in the patient conditions listed above.

[b]Except for the conditions listed above, antibiotic prophylaxis is no longer recommended for any other form of CHD.

[c]Prophylaxis is reasonable because endothelialization of prosthetic material occurs within 6 months after the procedure.

Reprinted with permission from Wilson W, Taubert KA, Gewitz M, et al. Prevention of infective endocarditis: Guidelines from the American Heart Association. Circulation 2007;116:1736–1754. ©2007, American Heart Association, Inc.

OUTCOME EVALUATION

Monitoring for successful therapy is critical in this serious infection to prevent complications, prevent resistance development, and decrease mortality. Routine assessment of clinical signs and symptoms, as well as laboratory tests (i.e., repeat blood cultures), microbiologic testing, and serum drug concentrations (if appropriate), must be performed.

Resolution of signs and symptoms typically occurs within a few days to a week in most cases. Monitor the patient daily for febrile episodes, as well as other vital signs, with expected normal values within 2 to 3 days of initiating antimicrobial

Table 74–9

Prophylactic Regimens for Dental Procedure

Situation	Agent	Regimen: Single Dose 30–60 Minutes Before Procedure	
		Adults	Children
Oral	Amoxicillin	2 g	50 mg/kg
Unable to take oral medications	Ampicillin or Cefazolin or Ceftriaxone	2 g IM or IV	50 mg/kg IM or IV
Allergic to penicillins or ampicillin—oral	Cephalexin[a,b] or Clindamycin or Azithromycin or Clarithromycin	2 g 600 mg 500 mg	50 mg/kg 20 mg/kg 15 mg/kg
Allergic to penicillins or ampicillin and unable to take oral medications	Cefazolin or Ceftriaxone[b] or Clindamycin	1g IM or IV 600 mg IM or IV	50 mg/kg IM or IV 20 mg/kg IM or IV

IM, intramuscular.

[a]Or other first- or second-generation oral cephalosporin in equivalent adult or pediatric dosage.

[b]Cephalosporins should not be used in an individual with a history of anaphylaxis, angioedema, or urticaria with penicillins or ampicillin.

Reprinted with permission from Wilson W, Taubert KA, Gewitz M, et al. Prevention of infective endocarditis: Guidelines from the American Heart Association. Circulation 2007;116:1736–1754. ©2007, American Heart Association, Inc.

therapy.[4] Persistent signs or symptoms could be indicative of inadequate treatment or development of resistance.

Blood cultures are the primary laboratory evaluation to assess response to therapy. Typically, with appropriate treatment, they should become negative within 3 to 7 days. Use subsequent blood cultures if the patient appears not to be responding to therapy or on completing treatment to confirm eradication of infection. Evaluate all susceptibility reports to assess antimicrobial therapy.

Additionally, the patient needs to be counseled on the necessity of prophylactic antibiotics prior to major dental treatments (in appropriate patients) in order to prevent recurrent infections. This is critical in patients with risk factors that predispose them to developing IE, such as prosthetic heart valves, other valvular defects, or previous IE.

Develop a follow-up plan to determine whether the patient has achieved a cure, which includes a clinical evaluation of signs/symptoms, repeat blood cultures, and possibly a repeat echocardiogram. The patient should also be assessed for any adverse events. This should be performed usually within a few weeks after the completion of therapy.

❾ Patient Care and Monitoring

1. Assess the patient's symptoms and/or laboratory results to determine whether the empirical therapy is effective. Is the patient's fever resolving? Is the patient's WBC decreasing?

2. Review available microbiologic cultures and sensitivity to assess whether the initial antimicrobial regimen needs to be tailored?

3. Review any additional diagnostic tests to determine if treatment may be needed to prevent/minimize complications (e.g., emboli, congestive heart failure).

4. Evaluate therapeutic serum drug concentrations as appropriate (e.g., vancomycin and gentamicin).

5. Monitor serum creatinine in order to make appropriate renal adjustments of the antimicrobials as necessary.

6. Assess any repeat blood cultures and vital signs to determine continued treatment effectiveness.

7. Evaluate the patient for occurrence of any adverse drug reactions and possible drug allergies and/or drug interactions.

8. Develop a plan if the patient is going to continue therapy at home. Once defervescence has occurred, the patient may complete therapy outside the hospital by receiving the antimicrobials from an outpatient infusion center or through a home health agency.

9. Develop a follow-up plan to assess the resolution of infection once the patient has completed therapy. Assessment of any adverse events also should be conducted at this time.

10. Educate high-risk patients on the importance of taking prophylactic antibiotics prior to having certain dental procedures in an effort to prevent the future development of another infection. Stress the potential complications as well as the morbidity and mortality that are associated with IE and that taking precautions can minimize or prevent them.

Abbreviations Introduced in This Chapter

AHA	American Heart Association
CFU	Colony-forming units
CNS	Coagulase-negative staphylococci
ESR	Erythrocyte sedimentation rate
HACEK	Group of bacteria consisting of *Haemophilus* spp., *Actinobacillus actinomycetemcomitans, Cardiobacterium hominis, Eikenella corrodens,* and *Kingella kingae*
IE	Infective endocarditis

IVDUs   Intravenous drug users
MIC   Minimum inhibitory concentration
MRSA   Methicillin-resistant *S. aureus*
MSSA   Methicillin-sensitive *S. aureus*
NBTE   Nonbacterial thrombotic endocarditis
PVE   Prosthetic-valve endocarditis
TEE   Transesophageal echocardiogram
TTE   Transthoracic echocardiogram
VRE   Vancomycin-resistant enterococci

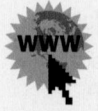 Self-assessment questions and answers are available at *http://mhpharmacotherapy .com/pp.html.*

REFERENCES

1. Fowler VG Jr, Scheld WM, Bayer AS. Endocarditis and intravascular infections. In: Mandell GL, Bennett JE, Dolin R, eds. Principles and Practice of Infectious Diseases. 7th ed. Philadelphia, PA: Elsevier; 2009:1067–1111.
2. Bayer AS, Bolger AF, Taubert KA, et al. Diagnosis and management of infective endocarditis and its complications. Circulation 1998;98:2936–2948.
3. Karchmer AW. Infective endocarditis. In: Bonow: Braunwald E, ed. Heart Disease: A Textbook of Cardiovascular Medicine. 9th ed. Philadelphia, PA: Saunders; 2012:1540–1560.
4. Mylonakis E, Calderwood SB. Infective endocarditis in adults. N Engl J Med 2001;345:1318–1320.
5. Habib B. Management of infective endocarditis. Heart 2006;92: 124–130.
6. Baddour LM, Wilson WR, Bayer AS, et al. American Heart Association Scientific Statement. Infective endocarditis: Diagnosis, antimicrobial therapy, and management of complications. Circulation 2005;111:e394–e433.
7. Wilson W, Taubert KA, Gewitz M, et al. Prevention of infective endocarditis: Guidelines from the American Heart Association. Circulation 2007;116:1736–1754.
8. Que Y, Moreillon P. Infective endocarditis. Nat Rev Cardiol 2011;8: 322–336.
9. Knoll BM, Baddour LM, Wilson WR. Prosthetic valve endocarditis. In: Mandell GL, Bennett JE, Dolin R, eds. Principles and Practice of Infectious Diseases. 7th ed. Philadelphia, PA: Elsevier; 2009:1113–1126.
10. Hoyer A, Silberbach M. Infective Endocarditis. Pediatr Rev 2005;26: 394–400.
11. Cecchi E, Imazio M, Trinchero R. Infective endocarditis: Diagnostic issues and practical clinical approach based on echocardiography. J Cardiovasc Med 2008;9:414–418.
12. Mestres CA, Fita G, Azqueta M, Miro JM. Role of echocardiogram in decision making for surgery in endocarditis. Curr Infect Dis Rep 2010;12:321–328.
13. Habib G, Badano L, Tribouilloy C, Vilacosta I, Zamorano JL. Recommendations for the practice of echocardiography in infective endocarditis. Eur J Echocardiogr 2010;11:202–219.
14. Durack DT, Lukes AS, Bright DK, Duke Endocarditis Service. New criteria for diagnosis of infective endocarditis: Utilization of specific echocardiographic findings. Am J Med 1994;96:200–209.
15. Li JS, Sexton DJ, Mick N, et al. Proposed modifications to the Duke criteria for the diagnosis of infective endocarditis. Clin Infect Dis 2000;30:633–638.
16. Murdoch DR, Corey GR, Hoen B, et al. Clinical presentation, etiology, and outcome of infective endocarditis in the 21st century. Arch Intern Med 2009;169:463–473.
17. Fowler VG Jr., Miro JM, Hoen B, et al. Staphylococcus aureus endocarditis: A consequence of medical progress. JAMA 2005;293: 3012–3021.
18. Ferrieri P, Gewitz MH, Gerber MA, et al. Unique features of infective endocarditis in childhood. Circulation 2002;105:2115–2127.
19. Knoll B, Tleyjeh IM, Steckelberg JM, et al. Infective endocarditis due to penicillin-resistant viridans group streptococci. Clin Infect Dis 2007;44:1585–1592.
20. Upton A, Drinkovic D, Pottumarthy S, et al. Culture results of heart valves resected because of streptococcal endocarditis: Insights into duration of treatment to achieve valve sterilization. J Antimicrob Chemother 2005;55:234–239.
21. Murray RJ. Staphylococcus aureus infective endocarditis: Diagnosis and management guidelines. Intern Med J 2005;35:S25–S44.
22. Lopez J, Revilla A, Vilacosta I, et al. Definition, clinical profile, microbiological spectrum, and prognostic factors of early-onset prosthetic valve endocarditis. Eur Heart J 2007;28:760–765.
23. Huang YT, Hsiao CH, Liao CH, Lee CW, Hsueh PR. Bacteremia and infective endocarditis caused by a non-daptomycin-susceptible, vancomycin-intermediate, and methicillin-resistant Staphylococcus aureus strain in Taiwan. J Clin Microbiol 2008;46:1132–1136.
24. Bae IG, Federspiel JJ, Miro JM, et al. Heterogeneous vancomycin-intermediate susceptibility phenotype in bloodstream methicillin-resistant Staphylococcus aureus isolates from an international cohort of patients with infective endocarditis: prevalence, genotype, and clinical significance. J Infect Dis 2009;200:1355–1366.
25. Woods CW, Cheng AC, Fowler VG Jr, et al. Endocarditis caused by Staphylococcus aureus with reduced susceptibility to vancomycin. Clin Infect Dis 2004;38:1188–1191.
26. Millar BC, Prendergast BD, Moore JE. Community-associated MRSA (CA-MRSA): An emerging pathogen in infective endocarditis. J Antimicrob Chemother 2008;61:1–7.
27. Anguera I, Del Rio A, Miro JM, et al. Staphylococcus lugdunensis infective endocarditis: Description of 10 cases and analysis of native valve, prosthetic valve, and pacemaker lead endocarditis clinical profiles. Heart 2005;91:e10.
28. Van Hoovels L, De Munter P, Colaert J, et al. Three cases of destructive native valve endocarditis caused by Staphylococcus lugdunensis. Eur J Clin Microbiol Infect Dis 2005;24:149–152.
29. Frank KL, Luiz del Pozo J, Patel R. From clinical microbiology to infection pathogenesis: How daring to be different works for Staphylococcus lugdunensis. Clin Microbiol Rev 2008;21:111–133.
30. Linden PK. Optimizing therapy for vancomycin-resistant enterococci (VRE). Semin Respir Crit Care Med 2007;28:632–645.
31. Morpeth S, Murdoch D, Cabell CH, et al. Non-HACEK gram-negative bacillus endocarditis. Ann Intern Med 2007;147:829–835.
32. Brouqui P, Raoult D. Endocarditis due to rare and fastidious bacteria. Clin Microbiol Rev 2001;14:177–207.
33. Durante-Mangoni E, Tripodi MF, Albisinni R, Utili R. Management of Gram-negative and fungal endocarditis. Int J Antimicrob Agents 2010;36S:s40–s45.
34. Raza SS, Sultan OW, Sohail MR. Gram-negative bacterial endocarditis in adults: state-of-the-heart. Expert Rev Anti Infect Ther 2010;8: 879–885.
35. Houpikian P, Raoult D. Blood culture-negative endocarditis in a reference center: Etiologic diagnosis of 348 cases. Medicine 2005;84: 162–173.
36. Ellis ME, Al-Abdely H, Sandridge A, et al. Fungal endocarditis: Evidence in the world literature, 1965–1995. Clin Infect Dis 2001;32: 50–62.
37. Millar BC, Jugo J, Moore JE. Fungal endocarditis in neonates and children. Pediatr Cardiol 2005;26:517–536.
38. Fowler V, Boucher HW, Corey GR, et al. Daptomycin versus standard therapy for bacteremia and infective endocarditis caused by Staphylococcus aureus. N Engl J Med 2006;355:653–665.
39. Liu C, Bayer A, Cosgrove SE, et. al. Clinical practice guidelines by the Infectious Diseases Society of America for the treatment of methicillin-resistant Staphylococcus aureus infections in adults and children: executive summary. Clin Infect Dis 2011;52:285–292.

40. Segreti JA, Crank CW, Finney MS. Daptomycin for the treatment of gram-positive bacteremia and infective endocarditis: A retrospective case series of 31 patients. Pharmacotherapy 2006;26:347–352.

41. Tascini C, Bongiorni MG, Doria R, et al. Linezolid for endocarditis: a case series of 14 patients. J Antimicrob Chemother 2011;66:679–682.

42. Ho TT, Cadena J, Childs LM, et al. Methicillin-resistant *Staphylococcus aureus* bacteraemia and endocarditis treated with ceftaroline salvage therapy. J Antimicrob Chemother 2012; 67:1267–1270.

43. Drees M, Boucher H. New agents for *Staphylococcus aureus* endocarditis. Curr Opin Infect Dis 2006;19:544–550.

44. Marcos LA, Camins BC. Successful treatment of vancomycin-intermediate *Staphylococcus aureus* pacemaker lead infective endocarditis with telavancin. Antimicrob Agents Chemother 2010;54:5376–5378.

45. Rajendram R, Alp NJ, Mitchell AR, et al. Candida prosthetic valve endocarditis cured by caspofungin therapy without valve replacement. Clin Infect Dis 2005;40:e72–e74.

46. Reis LJ, Barton TD, Pochettino A, et al. Successful treatment of Aspergillus prosthetic valve endocarditis with oral voriconazole. Clin Infect Dis 2005;41:752–753.

47. Sohail MR, Martin KR, Wilson WR, et al. Medical versus surgical management of Staphylococcus aureus prosthetic valve endocarditis. Am J Med 2006;119:147–154.

48. Rivas P, Alonso J, Moya J, et al. The impact of hospital-acquired infections on the microbial etiology and prognosis of late-onset prosthetic valve endocarditis. Chest 2005;128:764–771.

49. Head SJ, Mokhles MM, Osnabrugge RLJ, et al. Surgery in current therapy for infective endocarditis. Vascular Health and Risk Management 2011;7:255–263.

50. Leontyev S, Borger MA, Modi P, et al. Surgical management of aortic root abscess: a 13 year experience in 172 patients with 100% follow-up. J Thorac Cardiovasc Surg 2012;143:332–337.

75 Tuberculosis

Charles Peloquin and Rocsanna Namdar

LEARNING OBJECTIVES

Upon completion of the chapter, the reader will be able to:

1. Compare the risk for active tuberculosis (TB) disease among patients based on their age, immune status, place of birth, and time since exposure to an active case.

2. Design an appropriate therapeutic plan for an immunocompetent, immunocompromised, pregnant, and pediatric patient with pulmonary TB.

3. Distinguish between the diagnostic tests used for patients potentially infected with tuberculosis.

4. Assess the effectiveness of therapy in TB patients.

5. Describe the common and important adverse drug effects caused by TB drugs.

6. Select patients for whom therapeutic drug monitoring (TDM) may be valuable and identify the necessary laboratory monitoring parameters for patients on antituberculosis medications.

7. Design appropriate antimicrobial regimens for the treatment of latent TB infection (LTBI) in all patient populations.

KEY CONCEPTS

1. Tuberculosis (TB) is the most prevalent communicable infectious disease on earth and remains out of control in many developing nations. These nations require medical and financial assistance from developed nations in order to control the spread of TB globally.

2. In the United States, TB disproportionately affects ethnic minorities as compared with whites, reflecting greater ongoing transmission in ethnic minority communities. Additional TB surveillance and preventive treatment are required within these communities.

3. Coinfection with HIV and TB accelerates the progression of both diseases, thus requiring rapid diagnosis and treatment of both diseases.

4. Mycobacteria are slow-growing organisms; in the laboratory, they require special stains, special growth media, and long periods of incubation to isolate and identify.

5. TB can produce atypical signs and symptoms in infants, the elderly, and immunocompromised hosts, and it can progress rapidly in these patients.

6. Latent tuberculosis infection (LTBI) can lead to reactivation disease years after the primary infection occurred.

7. The patient suspected of having active TB disease must be isolated until the diagnosis is confirmed and he or she is no longer contagious. Often, isolation takes place in specialized "negative pressure" hospital rooms to prevent the spread of TB.

8. Isoniazid and rifampin are the two most important drugs to treat TB; organisms resistant to both these drugs (multidrug-resistant tuberculosis [MDR-TB]) are much more difficult to treat.

9. Never add only a single antituberculosis drug to a failing regimen for active TB!

10. Directly observed therapy (DOT) should be used whenever possible to reduce treatment failures and the selection of drug-resistant isolates.

INTRODUCTION

Worldwide, tuberculosis (TB) kills about 1.5 million people each year, more than any other infectious organism. TB is caused by *Mycobacterium tuberculosis*, and it presents either as latent TB infection (LTBI) or as progressive active disease.[1] The latter typically causes progressive destruction of the lungs, leading to death in most patients who do not receive treatment. Currently, one-third of the world's population is infected, and drug resistance is increasing in many areas.[1]

EPIDEMIOLOGY

❶ *Roughly one of every three people on earth is infected by* Mycobacterium tuberculosis.[1-3] *The distribution is uneven, with the highest incidences found in southern Asia and sub-Saharan Africa. In the United States, about 13 million people have LTBI, evidenced by a positive skin test (purified protein derivative ([PPD]) but no signs or symptoms of disease.* Such patients have roughly a one in 10 chance of active disease during their lives, with the greatest risk in the first 2 years after infection. In 2010, about 11,182 TB cases were reported in the United States; a 3.1% decline from 2009.

The most recent data from the Centers for Disease Control and Prevention (CDC) indicate that TB deaths in the United States have decreased by 7%, from 590 deaths in 2008 to 547 deaths in 2009.[4] (For details, visit the CDC website at *www.cdc.gov/nchstp/tb.*)

Risk Factors for Infection

▶ Location and Place of Birth

California, New York, Florida, and Texas accounted for 50% of all TB cases in 2011, reflecting the high immigration rates into these states.[4] Mexico, the Philippines, Vietnam, India, and China account for the largest numbers of these immigrants.[4] TB is most prevalent in large urban areas and is exacerbated by crowding in poor immigrant neighborhoods.[3,4] Those in close contact with patients with active pulmonary TB are most likely to become infected.[2,3] These include family members, coworkers, or co-residents in places such as prisons, shelters, and nursing homes.

▶ Race, Ethnicity, Age, and Gender

❷ *In the United States, the incidence of TB is more concentrated in nonwhite individuals. In 2010, Hispanics accounted for 29% of new TB cases, followed by Asians (28%) and non-Hispanic blacks (24%), whereas non-Hispanic whites accounted for only 16% of new TB cases.*[5] TB is most common among people 25 to 44 years of age (33% of all cases), followed by those 45 to 64 years of age (31%) and 65 or more years of age (20%).[5]

▶ Coinfection with HIV

❸ *HIV is the most important risk factor for active TB because the immune deficit prevents patients from containing the initial infection.*[2,3,5,6] In 2010, data on HIV status was available in approximately 70% of reported TB cases. Based on this information, *roughly 9% of TB patients ages 25 to 44 years are coinfected with HIV.*[4,5] Consistent with HIV in general, HIV-associated TB is most common among 25- to 44-year-olds. Substance abuse and other risk factors are shared among some TB and HIV-infected individuals, promoting the spread of both diseases.[2,7]

Risk Factors for Disease

Once infected with *M. tuberculosis*, a person's lifetime risk of active TB is about 10%, with about half this risk evident during the first 2 years after infection.[2,3,6] Young children, the elderly, and immunocompromised patients have greater risks. HIV-infected patients with *M. tuberculosis* infection

are roughly 100 times more likely to develop active TB than normal hosts due to the lack of normal cellular immunity.[3,8,9]

ETIOLOGY

❹ *Microscopic examination of infected material ("smear") detects about 8 to 10 × 10³ organisms/mm³/(8 to 10 × 10⁹/L) of specimen using the older AFB (acid-fast bacillus) stain. The newer auramine-rhodamine fluorescent technique is one-third more sensitive. A smear-negative patient still can grow* M. tuberculosis *on culture, which is more sensitive than either staining technique. Unfortunately, culture is much slower than staining due to the roughly 20-hour doubling time of the bacilli.* Further, microscopic examination cannot determine which of over 90 mycobacterial species is present. The usual practice is to assume the worst (TB) until confirmed by genetic probe or positive culture.

Culture and Susceptibility Testing

Susceptibility testing is essential for directing proper treatment. The most common agar method, known as the *proportion method*, takes many weeks to produce results. The recently discontinued BACTEC and newer mycobacterial growth indicator tube (MGIT) systems use liquid media and detect live

---

Patient Encounter, Part 1

HPI: AF is a 56-year-old HIV-positive man who presents to the medical clinic complaining of a 1-month history of a persistent cough that has become productive over the past 2 weeks. He also complains of malaise and a 6-kg (13-lb) weight loss over the past 2 months.

PMH: HIV positive; last CD4⁺ 28% (0.28); type 2 diabetes mellitus (NIDDM)—well controlled; hypertension (HTN) × 5 years—well controlled

FH: Mother and father died in an MVA 10 years ago; one brother, age 54, lives with the patient; one sister, age 50, is alive and has had breast cancer

SH: Single, one daughter. He reports IV drug use but last use was 20 years ago. He had a 20-year history of alcohol abuse but has been sober for 10 years. He owns his own import/export business and travels internationally.

Meds: Atripla (emtricitabine, efavirenz, tenofovir) 1 tablet daily; lisinopril 20 mg daily; amlodipine 5 mg daily; metformin 500 mg twice daily. Patient reports that he tries to be compliant with his therapies and takes them regularly except when he is unable to get his refills; over the past 2 months, he has only gone 3 to 4 days without medication.

What information is suggestive of TB?

What factors place this patient at increased risk for acquiring TB?

mycobacteria in about 2 weeks.[1,10,11] Rapid-identification tests include nucleic acid probes and DNA fingerprinting using restriction fragment length polymorphism (RFLP) analysis, and polymerase chain reaction (PCR).[1,6,10,12–15] The Hain (pronounced "Hine") GenoType® MTBDR plus test, a new and improved molecular test for multidrug-resistant tuberculosis (MDR-TB), has been approved in Europe.[14] The Cepheid MTB/RIF Assay performed on the GeneXpert® System is a qualitative test designed for rapid detection of *M. tuberculosis* and rifampicin resistance.[15] New tests looking for specific mutations such as the katG gene associated with isoniazid resistance may facilitate rapid drug therapy decisions in the future. Nitrate reductase assays and porous ceramic support systems are among other rapid drug susceptibility testing techniques currently being investigated.[16]

PATHOPHYSIOLOGY

Primary Infection

M. tuberculosis is transmitted from person to person by coughing or sneezing.[2,6,17,18] This produces small particles known as *droplet nuclei* that float in the air for long periods of time. Primary infection usually results from inhaling droplet nuclei that contain *M. tuberculosis*.[2,6,17] The progression to clinical disease depends on three factors: (1) the number of *M. tuberculosis* organisms inhaled (infecting dose), (2) the virulence of these organisms, and (3) the host's cell-mediated immune response.[2,4,6,12,18,19] If pulmonary macrophages inhibit or kill the bacilli, the infection is aborted.[18] If not, *M. tuberculosis* eventually spreads throughout the body through the bloodstream.[2,6,18] *M. tuberculosis* most commonly infects the posterior apical region of the lungs, where conditions are most favorable for its survival.

T lymphocytes become activated over the course of 3 to 4 weeks, producing interferon-γ (IFN-γ) and other cytokines. These stimulate microbicidal macrophages to surround the tuberculous foci and form granulomas to prevent further extension.[18] At this point, the infection is largely under control, and bacillary replication falls off dramatically. Any remaining mycobacteria are believed to reside primarily within granulomas or within macrophages that have avoided detection and lysis. Over 1 to 3 months, tissue hypersensitivity occurs, resulting in a positive tuberculin skin test.[2,6,17]

⑤ *Progressive primary disease occurs in roughly 5% of patients, especially children, the elderly, and immunocompromised patients.*[20,21] *This presents as a progressive pneumonia and frequently spreads, leading to meningitis and other severe forms of TB, even before patient skin tests become positive.*[20]

Reactivation Disease

⑥ *About 10% of infected patients develop reactivation TB, with half occurring in the first 2 years after infection.*[2,6,12] Upper lobe pulmonary disease is the most common (85% of cases).[2] **Caseating granulomas** result from the vigorous immune response, and liquefaction leads to local spread. Eventually, a pulmonary cavity results, and this provides a portal to the outside that allows for person-to-person spread. Bacterial counts in the cavities can be as high as 10^8/mL (10^{11}/L) of cavitary fluid.[2,18] Prior to the chemotherapy era, pulmonary TB usually was associated with hypoxia, respiratory acidosis, and eventually death.

Extrapulmonary and Miliary Tuberculosis

Caseating granulomas, regardless of location, can undergo liquefaction, spread tubercle bacilli, and cause symptoms.[2,6] Because of muted or altered symptoms, the diagnosis of TB is difficult and often delayed in immunocompromised hosts.[2,3,6] HIV-infected patients may present with only extrapulmonary TB, which is uncommon in HIV-negative persons. A widely disseminated form of the disease called *miliary TB* can occur, particularly in children and immunocompromised hosts, and it can be rapidly fatal.[17] Immediate treatment is required.

Influence of HIV Infection on Pathogenesis

HIV infection is the most important risk factor for active TB.[2,6,17] As CD4+ lymphocytes multiply in response to the mycobacterial infection, HIV multiplies within these cells and selectively destroys them, gradually eliminating the TB-fighting lymphocytes.[17] Patients coinfected with HIV and TB have a substantially higher risk of early mortality compared with HIV-negative patients with TB. Approximately 5% of HIV-infected patients with pulmonary TB will have positive results on acid-fast staining yet have a normal chest radiograph.

CLINICAL PRESENTATION AND DIAGNOSIS

Fever, night sweats, weight loss, fatigue, and a productive cough are the classic symptoms of TB.[1,2,6,19] Onset may be gradual, and the diagnosis is easily missed if the symptoms are muted, such as in the elderly.[2,6,19] Progressive pulmonary disease leads to cavitation visible on x-ray. Physical examination is nonspecific but may be consistent with pneumonia. Dullness to chest percussion, rales, and increased vocal **fremitus** may be observed on examination. Laboratory data often are uninformative, but a modest increase in the white blood cell (WBC) count with a lymphocyte predominance can be seen.

Atypical presentations are common in patients coinfected with HIV.[1,2,6,19,24,25] HIV-positive patients often have negative skin tests and fail to produce **cavitary lesions**, and fever may be absent.[22,23] Symptoms for these patients range from classic pulmonary to muted and nonspecific. Extrapulmonary TB typically presents as a slowly progressive decline in organ function, and lymphadenopathy is relatively common.[26,18,19] Abnormal behavior, headaches, or convulsions suggest tuberculous meningitis, although other acute CNS infections must be excluded.[6,19]

The Elderly

⑤ *Many clinical findings are muted in the elderly or absent altogether, so there can be considerable diagnostic uncertainty.*

Positive skin tests, fevers, night sweats, sputum production, or hemoptysis may be absent, making TB hard to distinguish from other bacterial or viral infections or chronic lung diseases.[2,19,26,27] In contrast, mental status changes are twice as common in the elderly, and CNS disease must be considered when TB is entertained. Mortality is six times higher in the elderly in part owing to delays in diagnosis.[2,19,26] Ethnic distributions of disease are different in the elderly and include more white patients because these patients often were infected decades ago, when TB was more prevalent in the United States.

Children

⑤ *Because children less than 5 years old have immature cellular immunity, TB can be particularly dangerous in this population. TB in children may present as atypical bacterial pneumonia, called progressive primary TB, and often involves the lower and middle lobes.*[17,19–21] Extrapulmonary TB is more common in children; dissemination is fairly common to the lymph nodes, GI and genitourinary tracts, bone marrow, and meninges. For these reasons, Bacille Calmette-Guérin (BCG) vaccinations are administered in countries where TB remains common. BCG appears to stimulate children's immune systems just enough to ward off the most serious forms of the disease. However, BCG does not block infection, and these same children often experience reactivation TB as young adults. Because cavitary lung lesions are uncommon, children do not spread TB readily. From the public health perspective, pediatric TB is the clearest indication of recent spread of TB.

Skin Testing

TB skin testing with the 5-TU strength of Tubersol PPD, also known as the *Mantoux test*, is a method for skin testing.[2,19,22] The product is injected into the skin (not subcutaneously) with a fine (27-gauge) needle and produces a small, raised, blanched wheal to be read by an experienced professional in 48 to 72 hours. Criteria for interpretation are listed in Table 75–1.[1,2,6,19,22] The chance of a false-negative result is increased when the patient is immunosuppressed.

The CDC does not recommend the routine use of anergy panels.[22,28] The "booster effect" occurs in patients who do not respond to an initial skin test but show a positive reaction if retested 1 to 3 weeks later.[19,28] In order to reduce the likelihood that a boosted reaction is misinterpreted as a new infection, the two-step method is recommended at the time of initial testing for individuals such as healthcare workers or nursing home residents who may be tested periodically. If the first PPD skin test is negative, repeat the test in 1 to 3 weeks. If the second test is positive, it is most likely a boosted reaction, and the person should be classified as previously infected.

Newer Diagnostic Tests

The sensitivity and specificity of the PPD tests are estimated to be 71% and 66%, respectively. Newer technology has lead to the development of blood tests or interferon-γ release assays (IGRAs) that may replace the PPD test.[28–33] These methods measure the release of interferon-γ in blood in response to TB antigens. The sensitivity of IGRAs ranges from 76% to 90%, and specificity ranges from 92% to 97%. The IGRAs do not cause the booster phenomenon and are unaffected by BCG, or infection by most nontuberculosis mycobacteria. Results of the IGRAs are available in less than 24 hours, versus the 3 days required for the traditional PPD skin test. Data are limited for use of IGRAs in children younger than 5 years of age, persons recently exposed to TB, healthcare workers, and immunodeficient patients.[28] The CDC has concurred with the use of these tests in all circumstances in which the PPD is currently used. IGRAs are approved for the diagnosis of LTBI in HIV-infected patients, but they are not recommended for the diagnosis of active TB in HIV-infected persons.[28] As seen with the PPD test, there is a theoretical concern that the sensitivity of the IGRA test may be lower in patients with advanced immunodeficiency.

Table 75–1		
Criteria for Tuberculin Positivity, by Risk Group		
Reaction Greater Than or Equal to 5 mm of Induration	**Reaction Greater Than or Equal to 10 mm of Induration**	**Reaction Greater Than or Equal to 15 mm of Induration**
HIV-positive persons	Recent immigrants (i.e., within the last 5 years) from high-prevalence countries	Persons with no risk factors for TB
Patients with TB	Injection drug users	
Fibrotic changes on chest radiograph consistent with prior TB	Residents and employees[a] of the following high-risk congregate settings: prisons and jails, nursing homes and other long-term facilities for the elderly, hospitals and other healthcare facilities, residential facilities for patients with AIDS, and homeless shelters	
Patients with organ transplants and other immunosuppressed patients (receiving the equivalent of 15 mg/d or more of prednisone for 1 month or more)[b]	Mycobacteriology laboratory personnel, persons with the following clinical conditions that place them at high risk: silicosis, diabetes mellitus, chronic renal failure, some hematologic disorders, other specific malignancies, gastrectomy, and jejunoileal bypass	
	Children younger than 4 years of age or infants, children, and adolescents exposed to adults at high risk	

[a]For persons who are otherwise at low risk and are tested at the start of employment, a reaction of 15 mm or more of induration is considered positive.

[b]Risk of TB in patients treated with corticosteroids increases with higher dose and longer duration.

IGRAs are preferred for testing patients who have received BCG and in patients who have poor rates of return for PPD skin test reading. Testing with both PPD and IGRA generally is not recommended, but may be useful in certain situations (e.g., if the initial PPD test is negative and the risk for infection, clinical suspicion, or the risk for poor outcome is high; or if the initial PPD test is positive and additional evidence of infection is required; or the patient has a low risk of infection or progression).[31-33]

Additional Tests

Morning sputum collections have the highest yield of organisms.[2,10,19] Daily sputum collections over 3 consecutive

---

Patient Encounter, Part 2

VS: BP 126/78, P 90 beats/min, RR 18, T 37.2°C (99°F), O_2 sat 82% (0.82) on room air, wt 51 kg (112 lb)

HEENT: PERRLA; EOMI

Neck: Supple; no lymphadenopathy, bruits, or JVD; no thyromegaly

Chest: Diffuse rhonchi, decreased breath sounds on left

CV: RRR; no murmurs, rubs, gallops

Abd: (+) BS; nontender, nondistended

Neuro: A&O ×3

Laboratory Values (U.S. Units)

Lab	Normal	Lab	Normal
Na 139 mEq/L	135–145 mEq/L	Hgb 13.5 g/dL	13.5–17.5 g/dL
K 3.9 mEq/L	3.5–5 mEq/L	Hct 40%	40%–54%
Cl 98 mEq/L	95–105 mEq/L	RBC 4.6×10^6 mm³	$4.6–6.0 \times 10^6$ mm³
CO_2 38 mEq/L	22–30 mEq/L	WBC 3.5×10^3 mm³	$4.0–10 \times 10^3$ mm³
BUN 20 mg/dL	5–25 mg/dL	PMN 42%	50–65%
SCr 1.0 mg/dL	0.8–1.3 mg/dL	Lymph 24%	25–35%
Gluc 123 mg/dL	Less than 140 mg/dL	Mono 2%	2–6%
AST 36 IU/L	5–40 IU/L	Other: HIV positive	
ALT 28 IU/L	5–35 IU/L	CD4$^+$ 28%	31–61% total lymphocytes
Tbili 1 mg/dL	0.1–1.2 mg/dL		
PT 10 seconds	10–12 seconds		

Laboratory Values (SI Units)

Lab	Normal	Lab	Normal
Na 139 mmol/L	135–145 mmol/L	Hgb 135 g/L or 8.38 mmol/L	135–175 g/L or 8.38–10.86 mmol/L
K 3.9 mmol/L	3.5–5 mmol/L	Hct 0.40 vol fraction	0.40–0.54 vol fraction
Cl 98 mmol/L	95–105 mmol/L	RBC 4.6×10^{12}/L	$4.6–6.0 \times 10^{12}$/L
CO_2 38 mmol/L	22–30 mmol/L	WBC 3.5×10^9/L	$4.0–10.0 \times 10^9$/L
BUN 7.1 mmol/L	1.8–8.9 mmol/L	PMN 0.42	0.50–0.65
SCr 88 µmol/L	71–115 µmol/L	Lymph 0.25	09.25–0.35
Gluc 6.8 mmol/L	Less than 7.8 mmol/L	Mono 0.02	0.02–0.06
AST 0.60 µkat/L	0.08–0.67 µkat/L	CD4$^+$ 0.28	0.31–0.61 total lymphocytes
ALT 0.47 µkat/L	0.08–0.58 µkat/L	Other: HIV positive	
Tbili 17.1 µmol/L	1.7–20.5 µmol/L		
PT 10 second	10–12 second		

CXR: Bilateral upper lobe infiltrates with cavitation on left; small left pneumothorax

Clinical Course: The patient was admitted and placed on respiratory isolation. Three separate sputum AFB stain specimens were reported to contain 3+ AFB. IFGA was sent and a PPD tuberculin skin test was placed. Sputum samples were sent for AFB, fungi, and bacterial cultures and sensitivities. After 48 hours, the PPD skin test was read as a 5-mm area of induration

Assessment: Active pulmonary TB in an HIV-positive patient; pneumothorax; HTN; type 2 diabetes mellitus

Which signs, symptoms, and other findings are consistent with active TB infection?

days improve the yield of positive results. Sputum induction with aerosolized hypertonic saline may produce a diagnostic sample in patients unable to produce sputum. Bronchoscopy or aspiration of gastric fluid via a nasogastric tube may be attempted in selected patients, the latter being used more often in children.[19] For patients with suspected extrapulmonary TB, samples of draining fluid, biopsies of the infected site, or both may be attempted. Blood cultures are positive occasionally, especially in AIDS patients who have low CD4+ counts.[19,25,29]

Advances in TB diagnosis include methods for rapid identification of patients with suspected TB. Improved smear microscopy, automated liquid cultures, nucleic acid amplification tests, antibody detection tests, and antigen detection tests are under development.[30] The Hain and the Cepheid tests, described earlier, are for the rapid identification of certain types of drug resistance.[14,15]

TREATMENT

General Approaches to Treatment

Monotherapy can be used only for infected patients who do not have active TB (LTBI, as shown by a positive skin test or IGRA in the absence of signs or symptoms of disease). Once active disease is present, a minimum of two drugs and typically *three or four drugs* must be used simultaneously from the outset of treatment.[2,6,12,34] For most patients, the shortest duration of treatment is 6 months, and 2 to 3 years of treatment may be necessary for advanced cases of MDR-TB.[2,6,12,34] Directly observed treatment (DOT) is a method used to ensure compliance in which patients are directly observed by a healthcare worker while taking their antituberculosis medication.[35] This is also a cost-effective way to ensure completion of treatment.[2,6,12,34–36]

Nonpharmacologic Therapy

7 *Steps should be taken to (a) prevent the spread of TB (respiratory isolation); (b) find where TB has already spread (contact investigation); and (c) return the patient to a state of normal weight and well-being.* The older term for TB is *consumption* because wasting was a primary symptom of disease progression in the prechemotherapy era and remains descriptive today. Items (a) and (b) are performed by public health departments. Clinicians involved in the treatment of TB should verify that the local health department has been notified of all new cases of TB. Surgery may be needed to remove destroyed lung tissue, space-occupying infected lesions (tuberculomas), and certain extrapulmonary lesions.[2,12,34]

Pharmacologic Therapy

▶ *Treating LTBI*

Isoniazid is used for treating LTBI.[2,6,12,34] Typically, isoniazid 300 mg daily (5–10 mg/kg of body weight) is given alone for 9 months. Lower doses usually are less effective.[2,37] The treatment of LTBI reduces a person's lifetime risk of active TB from about 10% to about 1%.[22] Rifampin 600 mg daily for 4 months can be used when isoniazid resistance is suspected or when

the patient cannot tolerate isoniazid.[2,21,37,38] Rifabutin 300 mg daily might be substituted for rifampin in patients at high risk of drug interactions. The combination of pyrazinamide and rifampin is no longer recommended because of unacceptable rates of hepatotoxicity.[39] Recently, 12 directly observed, once-weekly doses of isoniazid 900 mg and rifapentine 900 mg were shown to be as effective as 9 months of self-administered isoniazid 300 mg daily.[40] When resistance to isoniazid and rifampin is suspected in the isolate causing infection, there is no regimen proven to be effective[34] (Table 75–2). Note that patients with LTBI are not expelling organisms, so there is no isolate on which to perform susceptibility testing. Susceptibility patterns must be inferred based on the most likely source of infection. This is in contrast to active disease, described next.

▶ *Treating Active Disease*

In the United States, all patients diagnosed with TB can receive treatment free of charge through the local health department, and this is encouraged because local health departments generally have the greatest expertise. Treating active TB disease requires combination chemotherapy. Generally, *four drugs are given at the onset of treatment.* **8** *Isoniazid and rifampin should be used together for most cases because they are the best drugs for preventing drug resistance.*[2,6,34,40,41] Drug susceptibility testing should be done on the initial isolate for all patients with active TB and should be used to guide the selection of drugs over the course of treatment.[2,6,12,34] Susceptibility testing may be repeated in cases where the patient remains culture-positive 8 weeks or more into therapy.

8 *The standard TB treatment regimen is isoniazid, rifampin, pyrazinamide, and ethambutol for 2 months, followed by isoniazid and rifampin for 4 months, for a total of 6 months of treatment.*[2,12,34] *Extending treatment to 9 months of isoniazid and rifampin treatment is recommended for patients at greater risk of failure and relapse, including those with cavitation on initial chest radiograph or positive cultures at the completion of the initial 2-month phase of treatment, as well as for patients treated initially without pyrazinamide. Treatment should be continued for at least 6 months from the time that patients convert to a negative smear and culture.*[2,6,12,34] Some authors recommend therapeutic drug monitoring (TDM) for such patients because one of the proven reasons for treatment failure is malabsorption of orally administered drugs.[2,34,41,42] Table 75–3 shows the recommended treatment regimens for TB. When intermittent therapy is used, DOT is essential. Doses missed during an intermittent TB regimen decrease the efficacy of the regimen and increase the relapse rate. Further, outcomes appear to be worse for immunocompromised patients when intermittent treatment, especially twice-weekly treatment, is used. Therefore, HIV-positive TB patients should receive TB drugs daily during the first 2 months of treatment, and at least three times weekly thereafter.[43] When the patients' sputum smears convert to negative, the risk of them infecting others is greatly reduced, but it is not zero.[2,15,34] Such patients can be removed from respiratory isolation, but they must be careful not to cough on others and should meet only in well-ventilated places.

Table 75–2

Recommended Drug Regimens for Treatment of LTBI in Adults

Drug	Interval and Duration	Comments	Rating[a] HIV–	Evidence HIV+
Isoniazid	Daily for 9 months[c,d]	In HIV-infected patients, isoniazid may be administered concurrently with nucleoside reverse transcriptase inhibitors (NRTIs), protease inhibitors, or non-NRTIs (NNRTIs)	A (II)	A (II)
	Twice weekly for 9 months[c,d]	Directly observed treatment (DOT) must be used with twice-weekly dosing	B (II)	B (II)
Isoniazid	Daily for 6 months[d]	Not indicated for HIV-infected persons, those with fibrotic lesions on chest radiographs, or children	B (I)	C (I)
	Twice weekly for 6 months[d]	DOT must be used with twice-weekly dosing	B (II)	C (I)
Rifampin	Daily for 4 months	For persons who are contacts of patients with isoniazid-resistant rifampin-susceptible TB	B (II)	B (III)
		In HIV-infected patients, protease inhibitors or NNRTIs generally should not be administered concurrently with rifampin; rifabutin can be used as an alternative for patients treated with indinavir, nelfinavir, amprenavir, ritonavir, or efavirenz, and possibly with nevirapine or soft-gel saquinavir[e]		

[a]Strength of recommendation: A = preferred; B = acceptable alternative; C = offer when A and B cannot be given.

[b]Quality of evidence: I = randomized clinical trial data; II = data from clinical trials that are not randomized or were conducted in other populations; III = expert opinion.

[c]Recommended regimen for children younger than 18 years.

[d]Recommended regimens for pregnant women. Some experts would use rifampin and pyrazinamide for 2 months as an alternative regimen in HIV-infected pregnant women, although pyrazinamide should be avoided during the first trimester.

[e]Rifabutin should not be used with hard-gel saquinavir or delavirdine. When used with other protease inhibitors or NNRTIs, dose adjustment of rifabutin may be required.

Table 75–3

Drug Regimens for Culture-Positive Pulmonary Tuberculosis Caused by Drug-Susceptible Organisms

| | | Initial Phase | | Continuation Phase | |
Regimen	Drugs	Interval and Doses[a] (Minimal Duration)	Drugs	Interval and Doses[a,b] (Minimal Duration)	Range of Minimal Doses (mg)
1	Isoniazid Rifampin Pyrazinamide Ethambutol	7 days/wk for 56 doses (8 weeks) or 5 days/wk for 40 doses (8 weeks)[c]	Isoniazid/Rifampin	7 days/wk for 126 doses (18 weeks) or 5 days/wk for 90 doses (18 weeks)[c]	182–130 (26 weeks)
			Isoniazid/Rifampin	Twice weekly for 36 doses (18 weeks)	92–76 (26 weeks)[d]
			Isoniazid/Rifapentine	Once weekly for 18 doses (18 weeks)	74–58 (26 weeks)
2	Isoniazid Rifampin Pyrazinamide Ethambutol	7 days/wk for 14 doses (2 weeks)[c], then twice weekly for 12 doses (6 weeks) or 5 days/wk for 10 doses (2 weeks), then twice weekly for 12 doses (6 weeks)	Isoniazid/Rifampin	Twice weekly for 36 doses (18 weeks)	62–58 (26 weeks)[d]
			Isoniazid/Rifapentine	Once weekly for 18 doses (18 weeks)	44–40 (26 weeks)
3	Isoniazid Rifampin Pyrazinamide Ethambutol	3 × weekly for 24 doses (8 weeks)	Isoniazid/Rifampin	3 × weekly for 54 doses (18 weeks)	78 (26 weeks)
4	Isoniazid Rifampin Ethambutol	7 days/wk for 56 doses (8 weeks) or 5 days/wk for 40 doses (8 weeks)[c]	Isoniazid/Rifampin	7 days/wk for 217 doses (31 weeks) or 5 days/wk for 155 doses (31 weeks)[c]	273–195 (39 weeks)
			Isoniazid/Rifampin	Twice weekly for 62 doses (31 weeks)	118–102 (39 weeks)

Adjustments to the regimen should be made once the susceptibility data are available.[2,12,34] Drug resistance should be expected in patients who have been treated previously for TB. Two or more drugs with in vitro activity against the patient's isolate and that were not used previously should be added to the regimen as needed.[2,12,34] When isoniazid and rifampin cannot be used, treatment durations typically become 2 years or more, regardless of immune status.[2,12,34,41] TB specialists should be consulted regarding cases of drug-resistant TB or in any setting where there is uncertainty regarding appropriate treatment.[2,12,34] ⑨ *It is critical to avoid adding only a single drug to a failing regimen.*[2,12,34]

Special Populations

Patients with CNS TB usually are treated for longer periods (up to12 months instead of 6 months) because the consequences of undertreatment are severe.[2,12,34] Isoniazid and pyrazinamide cross the blood–brain barrier well, but rifampin, ethambutol, and streptomycin can penetrate inflamed meninges. TB of the bone typically is treated for up to 9 months, occasionally with surgical débridement.[2,12,34] Drug selection is the same as for pulmonary disease. Extrapulmonary TB of the soft tissues can be treated with conventional regimens.[2,12,34] TB in children may be treated with regimens similar to those used in adults, although some physicians extend treatment to 9 months.[2,12,19,20,34,38,43] Pediatric doses of isoniazid and rifampin on a milligram per kilogram basis are higher than those used in adults[34] (Table 75–4).

Pregnant women receive the usual treatment of isoniazid, rifampin, and ethambutol for 9 months.[2,34,38,41] Pyrazinamide has not been studied in large numbers of pregnant women, but anecdotal data suggest that it may be safe.[34] B vitamins should be provided. Streptomycin, other aminoglycosides, capreomycin, and ethionamide generally are avoided because they have been associated with toxic effects on the fetus.[34,44] *Para*-aminosalicylic acid and cycloserine are used sparingly.[44] Quinolones generally are avoided in pregnancy because of concern about adverse effects on cartilage development.[34,44] Although most antituberculosis drugs are excreted in breast milk, the amount of drug received by the infant through nursing appears to be insufficient to cause toxicity. Quinolones should be avoided in nursing mothers, if possible, for the same reason as mentioned previously.

▶ Human Immunodeficiency Virus

The recommended regimen for susceptible TB in HIV-infected adults is a 6-month regimen consisting of an initial phase of isoniazid, a rifamycin, pyrazinamide, and ethambutol for the first 2 months followed by a continuation phase of isoniazid and a rifamycin for 4 months.[2,12,34] Some clinicians extend treatment for 9 months for such patients. Rifabutin is the rifamycin of choice in this population due to drug interactions with some protease inhibitors and non-nucleoside reverse transcriptase inhibitors. Because of the large pill burden, overlapping toxicities, and the risk of immune reconstitution

inflammatory syndrome when TB and HIV treatments are initiated simultaneously, most clinicians elect to begin TB treatment first. Recent data support the early introduction of antiretroviral therapy (within 2 weeks of starting TB drugs) in patients with low CD4+ counts (less than or equal to 50/mm³ [less than or equal to 50×10^6/L]).[45–47] Treatment for HIV has been recommended to start after 2 months of TB treatment, although individual circumstances often dictate the exact timing. Highly intermittent regimens (twice or once weekly) are not recommended for HIV-positive TB patients.[34] It is advisable that such patients are managed by TB-HIV experts because the challenges are many. Prognosis has been particularly poor for HIV-infected patients infected with MDR-TB. Some patients with AIDS malabsorb their oral medications, and drug interactions are common so therapeutic drug monitoring can be useful.[2,34,41,42] Recommendations for regimens for the concomitant treatment of tuberculosis and HIV infection are provided in Table 75–5.

▶ Multidrug-Resistant TB

Drug-resistant TB may be suspected based on a patient's history or epidemiologic information. If drug-resistant TB is suspected, the empiric regimen should be modified based on patterns of suspected resistance. Once susceptibilities are confirmed, regimens can be modified appropriately. Patients with MDR-TB are at high risk of failure and should be treated by specialists.

▶ Renal Failure

Because they are primarily hepatically cleared, isoniazid and rifampin usually do not require dose modification in renal failure.[41,44,48] Pyrazinamide and ethambutol typically are reduced to three times weekly to avoid accumulation of the parent drug (ethambutol) or metabolites (pyrazinamide).[34,48] Renally cleared TB drugs include the aminoglycosides (e.g., amikacin, kanamycin, streptomycin), capreomycin, ethambutol, cycloserine, and levofloxacin.[34,41,44] Dosing intervals need to be extended for these drugs. Serum concentration monitoring should be performed for cycloserine and ethambutol to avoid dose-related toxicities in renal failure patients.[37,41,42]

▶ Hepatic Failure

Elevations of serum transaminase concentrations generally are not correlated with the residual capacity of the liver to metabolize drugs, so these markers cannot be used directly as guides for residual metabolic capacity. Hepatically cleared TB drugs include isoniazid, rifampin, pyrazinamide, ethionamide, and *p*-aminosalicylic acid.[44] Ciprofloxacin and moxifloxacin are about 50% cleared by the liver. Further, isoniazid, rifampin, pyrazinamide, and to a lesser degree ethambutol, *p*-aminosalicylic acid, and rarely ethambutol may cause hepatotoxicity.[34,41,44] These patients require close monitoring, and serum concentration monitoring may be the most accurate way to dose them.

Table 75–4

Antituberculosis Drugs for Adults and Children[a]

Drug	Daily Doses[b]	Adverse Effects	Monitoring
Isoniazid	*Adults*: 5 mg/kg (300 mg) *Children*: 10–15 mg/kg (300 mg)	Asymptomatic elevation of aminotransferases, clinical hepatitis, fatal hepatitis, peripheral neurotoxicity, CNS system effects, lupus-like syndrome, hypersensitivity, monoamine poisoning, diarrhea	LFT monthly in patients who have preexisting liver disease or who develop abnormal liver function that does not require discontinuation of drug Dosage adjustments may be necessary in patients receiving anticonvulsants or warfarin
Rifampin	*Adults*[c]: 10 mg/kg (600 mg) *Children*: 10–20 mg/kg (600 mg)	Cutaneous reactions, GI reactions (nausea, anorexia, abdominal pain), flu-like syndrome, hepatotoxicity, severe immunologic reactions, orange discoloration of bodily fluids (sputum, urine, sweat, tears), drug interactions owing to induction of hepatic microsomal enzymes	Rifampin causes many drug interactions. For a complete list of drug interactions and effects, refer to CDC website: *www.cdc.gov/nchstp/tb/tb*
Rifabutin	*Adults*[c]: 5 mg/kg (300 mg) *Children*: Appropriate dosing unknown	Hematologic toxicity, uveitis, GI symptoms, polyarthralgias, hepatotoxicity, pseudojaundice (skin discoloration with normal bilirubin), rash, flu-like syndrome, orange discoloration of bodily fluids (sputum, urine, sweat, tears)	Drug interactions are less problematic than rifampin
Rifapentine	*Adults*: 10 mg/kg (continuation phase) (600 mg) dosed weekly. *Children*: The drug is not approved for use in children	Similar to those associated with rifampin	Drug interactions are being investigated and are likely similar to rifampin
Pyrazinamide	*Adults*: Based on IBW: 40–55 kg: 1,000 mg; 56–75 kg: 1,500 mg; 76–90 kg: 2,000 mg *Children*: 15–30 mg/kg	Hepatotoxicity, GI symptoms (nausea, vomiting), nongouty polyarthralgia, asymptomatic hyperuricemia, acute gouty arthritis, transient morbilliform rash, dermatitis	Serum uric acid can serve as a surrogate marker for compliance LFTs in patients with underlying liver disease
Ethambutol[d]	*Adults*: Based on IBW: 40–55 kg: 800 mg; 56–75 kg: 1,200 mg; 76–90 kg: 1,600 mg *Children*[c]: 15–20 mg/kg daily	Retrobulbar neuritis, peripheral neuritis, cutaneous reactions	Baseline visual acuity testing and testing of color discrimination Monthly testing of visual acuity and color discrimination in patients taking greater than 15–20 mg/kg, renal insufficiency, or receiving the drug for greater than 2 months
Cycloserine	*Adults*[e]: 10–15 mg/kg/day, usually 500–750 mg/day in 2 doses *Children*: 10–15 mg/kg/day	CNS effects	Monthly assessments of neuropsychiatric status Serum concentration may be necessary until appropriate dose is established
Ethionamide	*Adults*[f]: 15–20 mg/kg/day, usually 500–750 mg/day in a single daily dose or 2 divided doses *Children*: 15–20 mg/kg/day	GI effects, hepatotoxicity, neurotoxicity, endocrine effects	Baseline LFTs Monthly LFTs if underlying liver disease is present TSH at baseline and monthly intervals
Streptomycin	*Adults*[g] *Children*: 20–40 mg/kg/day	Ototoxicity, neurotoxicity, nephrotoxicity	Baseline audiogram, vestibular testing, Romberg testing and SCr Monthly assessments of renal function and auditory or vestibular symptoms
Amikacin/kanamycin	*Adults*[g] *Children*: 15–30 mg/kg/day IV or intramuscular as a single daily dose	Ototoxicity, nephrotoxicity	Baseline audiogram, vestibular testing, Romberg testing and SCr Monthly assessments of renal function and auditory or vestibular symptoms

(Continued)

| Table 75–4 | | | |

Antituberculosis Drugs for Adults and Children[a] (Continued)

Drug	Daily Doses[b]	Adverse Effects	Monitoring
Capreomycin	Adults[g] Children: 15–30 mg/kg/day as a single daily dose	Nephrotoxicity, ototoxicity	Baseline audiogram, vestibular testing, Romberg testing and SCr Monthly assessments of renal function and auditory or vestibular symptoms Baseline and monthly serum K+ and Mg2+
p-Aminosalicylic acid (PAS)	Adults: 8–12 g/day in 2 or 3 doses Children: 200–300 mg/kg/day in 2–4 divided doses	Hepatotoxicity, GI distress, malabsorption syndrome, hypothyroidism, coagulopathy	Baseline LFTs and TSH TSH every 3 months
Levofloxacin	Adults: 500–1,000 mg daily Children[h]: Not recommended	GI disturbance, neurologic effects, cutaneous reactions	No specific monitoring recommended
Moxifloxacin	Adults: 400 mg daily Children[i]: Not recommended		

IBW, ideal body weight; LFT, liver function test; SCr, serum creatinine; TSH, thyroid-stimulating hormone.

[a]For purposes of this document, adult dosing begins at age 15 years.

[b]Dose per weight is based on ideal body weight. Children weighing more than 40 kg should be dosed as adults.

[c]Dose may need to be adjusted when there is concomitant use of protease inhibitors or nonnucleoside reverse transcriptase inhibitors.

[d]The drug likely can be used safely in older children but should be used with caution in children younger than 5 years, in whom visual acuity cannot be monitored. In younger children, ethambutol at the dose of 15 mg/kg/day can be used if there is suspected or proven resistance to isoniazid or rifampin.

[e]It should be noted that although this is the dose recommended generally, most clinicians with experience using cycloserine indicate that it is unusual for patients to be able to tolerate this amount. Serum concentration measurements are often useful in determining the optimal dose for a given patient.

[f]The single daily dose can be given at bedtime or with the main meal.

[g]Dose: 15 mg/kg/day (1 g) and 10 mg/kg in persons older than 50 years of age (750 mg). Usual dose: 750–1,000 mg administered intramuscularly or IV, given as a single dose 5–7 days/wk, and reduced to 2–3× per week after the first 2–4 months or after culture conversion, depending on the efficacy of the other drugs in the regimen.

[h]The long-term (more than several weeks) use of levofloxacin in children and adolescents has not be approved because of concerns about effects on bone and cartilage growth. However, most experts agree that the drug should be considered for children with TB caused by organisms resistant to both isoniazid and rifampin. The optimal dose is not known.

[i]The long-term (more than several weeks) use of moxifloxacin in children and adolescents has not been approved because of concerns about effects on bone and cartilage growth. The optimal dose is not known.

Patient Encounter, Part 3

Based on the information provided, what are the goals of therapy for this patient?

Select and recommend a therapeutic plan for treatment of this patient's TB infection. What drugs, dose, schedule, and duration of therapy are best for this patient?

How should any contacts infected by this patient be evaluated and treated?

Who else should be tested and how should they be treated?

The TB Drugs

The interested reader is referred to several other publications for more detailed information regarding these drugs.[2,11,34,41–42,44] A summary of daily doses, adverse effects, and monitoring parameters of first- and common second-line antituberculosis drugs is provided in Table 75–4.[34] Isoniazid and rifampin are considered the two key drugs for the treatment of active TB, followed by pyrazinamide, which has a special role in the first 2 months of treatment. Other drugs are used to suppress the emergence of drug resistance in conjunction with the first-line drugs or for preexisting drug-resistant TB. In general, the most important toxicity with first-line drugs is hepatotoxicity, whereas various organs may be affected by each of the second-line drugs. Pyridoxine can reduce the risk of peripheral neuropathy associated with isoniazid. Quinolones such as moxifloxacin are gaining interest in the treatment of TB. The role of these agents in the first 2-month intensive phase of therapy is currently being evaluated. In the future these agents may be considered drugs of first choice.[49–50] Other new therapies include investigational vaccines, and investigational drugs such as PA-824, OPC-67683 (Delamanid), TMC 207 (Bedaquiline), and SQ109, which are in clinical trials.[51]

Table 75–5

Recommendations for Regimens for the Concomitant Treatment of Tuberculosis and HIV Infection

Combined Regimen for Treatment of HIV and Tuberculosis	PK Effect of the Rifamycin	Tolerability/Toxicity	Antiviral Activity When Used With Rifampin	Recommendation (Comments)
Efavirenz-based antiretroviral therapy[a] with rifampin-based TB treatment	Well-characterized, modest effect	Low rates of discontinuation	Excellent	Preferred (efavirenz should not be used during the first trimester of pregnancy)
PI-based antiretroviral therapy[a] with rifabutin-based TB treatment	Little effect of rifabutin on PI concentrations, but marked increases in rifabutin concentrations	Low rates of discontinuation (if rifabutin is appropriately dose-reduced)	Favorable, though published clinical experience is not extensive	Preferred for patients unable to take efavirenz[b]
Nevirapine-based antiretroviral therapy with rifampin-based TB treatment	Moderate effect	Concern about hepatotoxicity when used with isoniazid, rifampin, and pyrazinamide	Favorable	Alternative for patients who cannot take efavirenz and if rifabutin not available
Zidovudine/lamivudine/abacavir/tenofovir with rifampin-based TB treatment	50% decrease in zidovudine, possible effect on abacavir not evaluated	Anemia	No published clinical experience	Alternative for patients who cannot take efavirenz and if rifabutin not available
Zidovudine/lamivudine/tenofovir with rifampin-based TB treatment	50% decrease in zidovudine, no other effects predicted	Anemia	Favorable, but not evaluated in a randomized trial	Alternative for patients who cannot take efavirenz and if rifabutin not available
Zidovudine/lamivudine/abacavir with rifampin-based TB treatment	50% decrease in zidovudine, possible effect on abacavir not evaluated	Anemia	Early favorable experience, but this combination is less effective than efavirenz-based regimens in persons not taking rifampin	Alternative for patients who cannot take efavirenz and if rifabutin not available
Super-boosted lopinavir-based ART with rifampin-based TB treatment	Little effect	Hepatitis among healthy adults, but favorable experience, among young children (younger than 3 years)	Good, among young children (younger than 3 years)	Alternative if rifabutin not available; preferred for young children when rifabutin not available

ART, antiretroviral therapy; PK, pharmacokinetic; TB, tuberculosis.

[a]With two nucleoside analogues.

[b]Includes patients with NNRTI-resistant HIV, those unable to tolerate efavirenz, and women during the first 1–2 trimesters of pregnancy.

OUTCOME EVALUATION

Effectiveness of TB therapy is determined by AFB smears and cultures. Sputum samples should be sent for AFB staining and microscopic examination (smears) every 1 to 2 weeks until two consecutive smears are negative. This provides early evidence of a response to treatment.[34] Once on maintenance therapy, **sputum cultures** can be performed monthly until two consecutive cultures are negative, which generally occurs over 2 to 3 months. If sputum cultures continue to be positive after 2 months, drug susceptibility testing should be repeated, and serum concentrations of the drugs should be checked.

⑩ *The most serious problem with TB therapy is patient nonadherence to the prescribed regimens.*[35,52] *Unfortunately, there is no reliable way to identify such patients a priori. The most effective way to achieve this end is with DOT.*[2,11,34] The use of DOT in noncompliant patients will be of benefit.[53] DOT also provides increased opportunities to observe the patient for any apparent toxicities, thus improving overall care.[53]

Serum chemistries, including blood urea nitrogen (BUN), creatinine, aspartate transaminase (AST), and alanine transaminase (ALT) and a complete blood count with platelets should be performed at baseline and periodically thereafter depending on the presence of other factors that may increase the likelihood of toxicity (e.g., advanced age, alcohol abuse, pregnancy).[2,34] Hepatotoxicity should be suspected in patients whose transaminases exceed five times the upper limit of normal (ULN) or whose total bilirubin exceeds 3 mg/dL (51 μmol/L) and in patients with symptoms such as nausea, vomiting, and jaundice with liver enzyme elevations of more than three times ULN. At this point, the offending agent(s) should be discontinued. Typically, all TB drugs are stopped, followed by the sequential reintroduction of the drugs, along with frequent testing of liver enzymes. This usually is successful in identifying the offending agent; other agents may be continued[34] (Table 75–4).

Patient Care and Monitoring

1. Rapidly identify a new TB case.

2. Assess the patient's risk factors and signs and symptoms to determine whether the patient might be infected with TB.

3. Isolate the patient with active disease to prevent the spread of the disease.

4. Collect appropriate samples for smears and cultures.

5. Obtain a thorough medication history.

6. Select and recommend appropriate antituberculosis treatment. Consider HIV status, pregnancy, type of TB infection, renal function, liver function, etc.

7. Ensure adherence to the treatment regimen by the patient.

8. Obtain AFB stains to evaluate the effectiveness of treatment.

9. Consider TDM if no clinical improvement.

10. Secondary goals are identification of the index case that infected the patient, identification of all persons infected by both the index case and the new case of TB, and the completion of appropriate treatments for those individuals.

Patient Encounter, Part 4

Based on the information provided, which clinical and laboratory parameters should be monitored in this patient to determine efficacy and avoid toxicity?

Is this patient a candidate for therapeutic drug monitoring? Why or why not?

Therapeutic Drug Monitoring

TDM or applied pharmacokinetics is the use of serum drug concentrations to optimize therapy.[34,41,42] Non-AIDS patients with drug-susceptible TB generally do well. TDM may be used if patients are failing appropriate DOT (no clinical improvement after 2 to 4 weeks or smear-positive after 4 to 6 weeks). On the other hand, patients with AIDS, diabetes, and various GI disorders often fail to absorb these drugs properly and are candidates for TDM. Also, patients with hepatic or renal disease should be monitored, given their potential for overdoses. In the treatment of MDR-TB, TDM may be particularly useful.[44,48] Finally, TDM of the TB and HIV drugs is perhaps the most logical way to untangle the complex drug interactions that take place. For a complete list of drug interactions, visit the CDC website at *www.cdc.gov/nchstp/tb/tb_hiv_drugs/toc. htm*.[54,55] In particular, interactions between the rifamycins (e.g., rifampin, rifapentine, rifabutin) and the HIV protease

inhibitors and non-nucleoside reverse transcriptase inhibitors are common and require dose and frequency modifications in many cases. Because these are constantly being updated, the preceding link is an excellent way to keep current.

Abbreviations Introduced in This Chapter

AIDS	Acquired immunodeficiency syndrome
ALT	Alanine transaminase
AST	Aspartate transaminase
BCG	Bacille Calmette-Guérin
CDC	Centers for Disease Control and Prevention
CNS	Central nervous system
DOT	Directly observed therapy
HIV	Human immunodeficiency virus
HTN	Hypertension
IGRA	Interferon gamma release assay
INF	Interferon
LTBI	Latent tuberculosis infection
MDR-TB	Multidrug-resistant tuberculosis
MGIT	Mycobacterial growth indicator tube
NIDDM	Non–insulin-dependent diabetes mellitus
PCR	Polymerase chain reaction
PPD	Purifies protein derivative
RFLP	Restriction fragment length polymorphism
TB	Tuberculosis
TDM	Therapeutic drug monitoring
ULN	Upper limit of normal
WBC	White blood cell

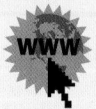 Self-assessment questions and answers are available at http://mhpharmacotherapy. com/pp.html.

REFERENCES

1. World Health Organization Report on the Global Tuberculosis Control 2011 [online]. [cited 2011 Oct 10]. Available from: *http://www.who.int/tb/publications/global_report/en/*.

2. Iseman MD. A Clinician's Guide to Tuberculosis. Philadelphia, PA: Lippincott Williams & Wilkins; 2000.

3. Schneider E, Moore M, Castro KG. Epidemiology of tuberculosis in the United States. Clin Chest Med 2005;26:183–195.

4. Centers for Disease Control and Prevention. Trends in Tuberculosis Morbidity–United States, 2011. MMWR 2012;61:181–185.

5. Centers for Disease Control and Prevention. Reported tuberculosis in the United States, 2010. Atlanta, GA: U.S. Department of Health and Human Services; October 2011.

6. Fitzgerald DW, Sterling TR, Haas DW. Mycobacterium tuberculosis. In: Mandell GL, Bennett JE, Dolin R, eds. Principles and Practice of Infectious Diseases. 7th ed. New York: Churchill Livingstone; 2009:3129–3165.

7. Centers for Disease Control and Prevention. Plan to combat extensively drug resistant tuberculosis. Recommendations of the Federal Tuberculosis Task Force. MMWR 2009;41(RR-03):1–43.

8. Heifets L. Mycobacteriology laboratory. Clin Chest Med 1997;18:35–53.

9. Heifets LB. Drug susceptibility tests in the management of chemotherapy of tuberculosis. In: Heifets LB, ed. Drug Susceptibility in the Chemotherapy of Mycobacterial Infections. Boca Raton, FL: CRC Press; 1991:89–122.

10. Daley CL, Chambers HF. Mycobacterium tuberculosis complex. In: Yu VL, Weber R, Raoult D, eds. Antimicrobial therapy and vaccines, Volume I: Microbes. 2nd ed. New York: Apple Trees Productions; 2006:841–865.

11. Issa R, Mohd Hassan NA, Abdul H, Hashim SH, Seradja VH, Abdul Sani A. Detection and discrimination of Mycobacterium tuberculosis complex. Diagn Microbiol Infect Dis 2012;72:62–67.

12. Kiraz N, Sglik I, Kiremitci A, Kasifoglu N, Akgun Y. Evaluation of the genotype mycobacteria direct assay for direct detection of the Mycobacterium tuberculosis complex obtained from sputum samples. J Med Microbiol 2010;59:930–934.

13. Drobniewski FA, Caws M, Gibson A, Young D. Modern laboratory diagnosis of tuberculosis. Lancet Infect Dis 2003;3:141–147.

14. Hillemann D, Weizenegger M, Kubica T, Richter E, Niemann S. Use of the genotype MTBDR assay for rapid detection of rifampin and isoniazid resistance in Mycobacterium tuberculosis complex isolates. J Clin Microbiol 2005;43:3699–3703.

15. Marlowe EM, Novack-Weekley SM, Cumpio J, et al. Evaluation of the Cepheid Xpert MTB/RIF assay for direct detection of Mycobacterium tuberculosis complex in respiratory specimens. J Clin Microbiol 2011;49:1621–1623.

16. Martin A, Panaiotov S, Portaels F, Hoffner S, Palomino JC, Angeby K. The nitrate reductase assay for the rapid detection of isoniazid and rifampicin resistance in Mycobacterium tuberculosis: A systematic review and meta-analysis. J Antimicrob Chemother 2008;62(1):56–64.

17. Daniel TM, Boom WH, Ellner JJ. Immunology of Tuberculosis. In: Reichman LB, Hershfield ES. Tuberculosis. A Comprehensive International Approach. 4th ed. New York: Marcel Dekker; 2006:60–81.

18. Woolwine SC, Bishai WR. Pathogenesis of tuberculosis from a cellular and molecular perspective. In: Reichman LB, Hershfield ES. Tuberculosis. A Comprehensive International Approach. 3rd ed. New York: Marcel Dekker; 2006:101–17.

19. American Thoracic Society/Centers for Disease Control and Prevention. Diagnostic standards and classification of tuberculosis in adults and children. Am J Respir Crit Care Med 2000;161:1376–1395.

20. Cruz AT, Starke JR. Clinical manifestations of tuberculosis in children. Paediatr Respir Rev 2007; 8:107–117.

21. Schaaf HS, Shean K, Donald PR. Culture-confirmed multidrug-resistant tuberculosis in children: diagnostic delay, clinical features, response to treatment and outcome. Arch Dis Child 2003;88:1106–11.

22. American Thoracic Society/Centers for Disease Control and Prevention. Targeted tuberculin skin testing and treatment of latent tuberculosis infection. Am J Respir Crit Care Med 2000;161: S221–S247.

23. Zumla A. Malon P, Henderson J, Grange JM. Impact of HIV infection on tuberculosis. Postgrad Med J 2000;76:259–268.

24. Wendel KA, Alwood KS, Gachuhi R, Chaisson RE, Bishai WR, Sterling RT. Paradoxical worsening of tuberculosis in HIV-infected persons. Chest 2001;120:193–197.

25. Kwan CK, Ernst JD. HIV and tuberculosis: a deadly human syndemic. Clin Microbiol Rev 2011;24:351–376.

26. Zevallos M, Justman JE. Tuberculosis in elderly. Clin Geriatr Med 2003;19:121–138.

27. Umeki S. Comparison of younger and elderly patients with pulmonary tuberculosis. Respiration 1989;55:75–83.

28. Centers for Disease Control and Prevention. Guidelines for using interferon gamma release assays to detect Mycobacterium tuberculosis infection–United States, 2010. MMWR 2010;59(RR-5):1–25.

29. Barnes PF, Lakey DL, Burman WJ. Tuberculosis in patients with HIV infection. Infect Dis Clin North Am 2002;16:107–126.

30. Pai M, O'Brien R. New Diagnostics for latent and active tuberculosis: State of the art and future prospects. Semin Respir Crit Care Med 2008;29:560–568.

31. Nienhaus A, Schablon A, Diel R. Interferon-gamma release assay for the diagnosis of latent TB infection—Analysis of discordant results, when compared to the tuberculin skin test. PLoS ONE 2008;3(7):e2665.

32. Pai M, Zwerling A, Menzies D. Systematic review: T-cell based assays for the diagnosis for latent tuberculosis infection. Ann Intern Med 2008;149:177–184.

33. Pai M, Dheda K, Cunningham J, Scano F, O'Brien R. T-cell assays for the diagnosis of latent tuberculosis infection: moving the research agenda forward. Lancet Infect Dis 2007;7:428–438.

34. American Thoracic Society/Centers for Disease Control/Infectious Disease Society of America. Treatment of tuberculosis. Am J Respir Crit Care Med 2003;167:603–662.

35. Fujiwara PI, Larkin C, Frieden TR. Directly observed therapy in New York City. Clin Chest Med 1997;18:135–148.

36. Volmink J, Garner P. Directly observed therapy for treating tuberculosis. Cochrane Database Syst Rev 2007;17:CD003343.

37. Malone RS, Fish DN, Spiegel DM, Childs JM, Peloquin CA. The effect of hemodialysis on cycloserine, ethionamide, para-aminosalicylate, and clofazimine. Chest 1999;116:984–990.

38. Mnyani CN , McIntyre JA. Tuberculosis and pregnancy. BJOG: An International J Obstet Gynaecol 2010;118:226–231.

39. Centers for Disease Control and Prevention. Update: Fatal and severe liver injuries associated with rifampin and pyrazinamide for latent tuberculosis infection, and revisions in the American Thoracic Society/CDC recommendations. MMWR 2001;50(34):733–735.

40. Sterling T. PREVENT TB: Results of a 12-dose, once-weekly treatment of latent tuberculosis infection (LTBI). Press release, CDC May 16, 2011. [cited 2011 Oct 10]. Available from: *http://www.cdc.gov/nchhstp/ newsroom/PREVENTTBPressRelease.html.*

41. Peloquin CA. Pharmacological issues in the treatment of tuberculosis. Ann NY Acad Sci 2001;953:157–164.

42. Peloquin CA. Therapeutic drug monitoring in the treatment of tuberculosis. Drugs 2002;62:2169–2183.

43. Centers for Disease Control and Prevention. Guidelines for prevention and treatment of opportunistic infections in HIV-infected adults and adolescents: recommendations from CDC, the National Institutes of Health, and the HIV Medicine Association of the Infectious Diseases Society of America. MMWR 2009;58:1–207.

44. Peloquin CA. Antituberculosis drugs: Pharmacokinetics. In: Heifets LB, ed. Drug Susceptibility in the Chemotherapy of Mycobacterial Infections. Boca Raton, FL: CRC Press; 1991:59–88.

45. Onyebujoh PC, Ribeiro I, Whalen CC. Treatment options for HIV-associated tuberculosis. J Infect Dis 2007;196:S35–S45.

46. Karim SSA, Naidoo K, Grobler A, et al. Integration of antiretroviral therapy with tuberculosis treatment. N Engl J Med 2011;365:1492–1501.

47. Blanc FX, Sok T, Laureillard D, Borand L, Rekacew C, Nerrienet E. Earlier versus later start of antiretroviral therapy in HIV-infected adults with tuberculosis. N Engl J Med 2011;365:1471–1481.

48. Malone RS, Fish DN, Spiegel DM, Childs JM, Peloquin CA. The effect of hemodialysis on isoniazid, rifampin, pyrazinamide, and ethambutol. Am J Respir Crit Care Med 1999;159:1580–1584.

49. Burman WJ. Moxifloxacin versus ethambutol in the first 2 months of treatment for pulmonary tuberculosis. Am J Respir Crit Care Med 2006;174:331–338.

50. Conde MB, Efron A, Loredo C, et al. Moxifloxacin versus ethambutol in the initial treatment of tuberculosis: a double-blind, randomized, controlled phase II trial. Lancet 2009;373:1183–1189.

51. Zhang Y. Advances in the treatment of tuberculosis. Clin Pharmacol Ther 2007;82:595–600.

52. Mahmoudi A, Iseman MD. Pitfalls in the care of patients with tuberculosis: Common errors and their association with the acquisition of drug resistance. JAMA 1993;270:65–68.

53. Volmink J, Garner P. Directly observed therapy for treating tuberculosis. Cochrane Database Syst Rev 2009;4:CD0003343.

54. Namdar R, Ebert S, Peloquin CA. Drugs for Tuberculosis. In: Piscitelli SC, Rodvold KA, Pai M, eds. Drug Interactions in Infectious Diseases. 3rd ed. Totowa, NJ: Humana Press; 2011:191–214.

55. Centers for Disease Control and Prevention. Drug Interactions in the Treatment of HIV-Related Tuberculosis [online]. [cited 2011 Oct 10]. Available from: *www.cdc.gov/tb/publications/guidelines/TB_HIV_Drugs/ default.htm.* Accessed Nov 2011.

76 Gastrointestinal Infections

Bradley W. Shinn, Elizabeth D. Hermsen, and Ziba Jalali

LEARNING OBJECTIVES

● **Upon completion of the chapter, the reader will be able to:**

1. Describe the epidemiology and clinical presentation of commonly encountered GI infections.

2. Summarize common risk factors associated with the development of a GI infection.

3. Given a patient with a GI infection, develop an individualized treatment plan.

4. Outline the impact of widespread antimicrobial resistance on current treatment recommendations for GI infections.

5. Discuss the effect of host immunosuppression on the risk of disease complications and treatment strategies associated with GI infections.

6. Educate patients on appropriate prevention measures of GI infections.

7. Describe the role of antimicrobial prophylaxis and/or vaccination for GI infections.

KEY CONCEPTS

❶ Rehydration is the foundation of therapy for GI infections.

❷ The indiscriminate use of proton-pump inhibitor (PPI) therapy leads to GI-tract bacterial colonization and increased susceptibility to enteric bacterial infections.

❸ Blood in the stool indicates the possibility of inflammatory mucosal disease of the colon such as enterohemorrhagic *Escherichia coli* (EHEC), which is an important cause of bloody diarrhea in the United States.

❹ Traveler's diarrhea is most commonly caused by bacteria such as *Shigella, Salmonella, Campylobacter,* and enterotoxigenic *E. coli* (ETEC), although viruses are increasingly recognized as a significant cause of traveler's diarrhea as well.

❺ The education of travelers about high-risk food and beverages is an important component in the prevention of traveler's diarrhea.

❻ Nosocomial *Clostridium difficile*–associated diarrhea (CDAD) is almost always associated with antimicrobial use; therefore, unnecessary and inappropriate antibiotic therapy should be avoided. Almost all antibiotics except aminoglycosides have been associated with CDAD.

❼ Viruses are the most common cause of diarrheal illness in the world. A live, oral vaccine is licensed and recommended for use in infants for the prevention of rotavirus infection.

INTRODUCTION

One of the primary concerns related to GI infection, regardless of the cause, is dehydration, which is the second leading cause of worldwide morbidity and mortality.[1] Worldwide, dehydration is especially problematic for children younger than age 5. However, the highest rate of death in the United States occurs among the elderly.[1] ❶ *Rehydration is the foundation of therapy for GI infections, and oral rehydration therapy (ORT) is usually preferred* (Table 76–1).

In the United States, each year 31 major pathogens cause about 9 million episodes of foodborne illness, almost 56,000 hospitalizations, and 1,350 deaths. Most illnesses are caused by norovirus, nontyphoidal *Salmonella* (NTS), *C. perfringens,* and *Campylobacter.*[2] ❷ *The indiscriminate use of proton-pump inhibitor (PPI) therapy leads to GI-tract bacterial colonization and increased susceptibility to enteric bacterial infections.*[3]

BACTERIAL INFECTIONS

SHIGELLOSIS

Epidemiology

● *Shigella* causes bacillary dysentery, which refers to diarrheal stool containing pus and blood. Worldwide, there are an estimated 165 million annual cases of shigellosis, with 1 million associated deaths,[4] and approximately 450,000 infections each year in the United States, which results in more than

Table 76–1

Clinical Assessment of Degree of Dehydration in Children Based on Percentage of Body Weight Loss

Variable	Mild (3–5%)	Moderate (6–9%)	Severe (10% or More)
Blood pressure	Normal	Normal	Normal to reduced
Quality of pulses	Normal	Normal to slightly decreased	Moderately decreased
Heart rate	Normal	Increased	Increased (bradycardia in severe cases)
Skin turgor	Normal	Decreased	Decreased
Fontanelle	Normal	Sunken	Sunken
Mucous membranes	Slightly dry	Dry	Dry
Eyes	Normal	Sunken orbits/decreased tears	Deeply sunken orbits/decreased tears
Extremities	Warm, normal capillary refill	Delayed capillary refill	Cool, mottled
Mental status	Normal	Normal to listless	Normal to lethargic to comatose
Urine output	Slightly decreased	Less than 1 mL/kg/hr	Less than 1 mL/kg/h
Thirst	Slightly increased	Moderately increased	Very thirsty
Fluid replacement	ORT 50 mL/kg over 2–4 hours	ORT 100 mL/kg over 2–4 hours	Lactated Ringer's 40 mL/kg in 15–30 minutes, then 20–40 mL/kg if skin turgor, alertness, and pulse have not returned to normal or Lactated Ringer's or normal saline 20 mL/kg, repeat if necessary, and then replace water and electrolyte deficits over 1–2 days, followed by ORT 100 mL/kg over 4 hours

From Martin S, Jung R. Gastrointestinal infections and enterotoxigenic poisonings. In: DiPiro JT, Talbert RL, Yee GC, et al, eds. Pharmacotherapy: A Pathophysiologic Approach. 8th ed. New York: McGraw-Hill; 2011:1951–1967.

6,000 hospitalizations.[4,5] Shigellosis usually affects children 6 months to 10 years of age. In the United States, shigellosis is a serious problem in daycare centers and in areas with crowded living conditions or poor sanitation. Most cases of shigellosis are transmitted through the fecal–oral route. Activities that may lead to shigellosis include handling toddlers' diapers, ingesting pool water, or consuming vegetables from a sewage-contaminated field. *Shigella* transmission from contaminated food (e.g., salads, raw vegetables, dairy products, and meat) and water, although less common, is associated with large outbreaks. Several large *Shigella* outbreaks have been reported on cruise ships associated with poor sanitation.

Pathogenesis

Shigella organisms are nonmotile, nonlactose-fermenting, gram-negative rods and are members of the Enterobacteriaceae family. There are four species of *Shigella*: *S. dysenteriae* (serogroup A), *S. flexneri* (serogroup B), *S. boydii* (serogroup C), and *S. sonnei* (serogroup D), which is responsible for most shigellosis cases in the United States. Infection with *Shigella* occurs after ingestion of as few as 10 to 100 organisms, which may explain the ease of person-to-person spread and the high secondary attack rate when an index case is introduced into a family. On average, symptoms develop about 3 days (range, 1 to 7) after contracting the bacteria.[6]

Shigella strains invade intestinal epithelial cells, with subsequent multiplication, inflammation, and destruction. The organism infects the superficial layer of the gut, rarely penetrates beyond the mucosa, and seldom invades the bloodstream. However, bacteremia can occur in malnourished

children and immunocompromised patients and is associated with a mortality rate as high as 20%.[7]

Treatment and Monitoring

Although infection with *Shigella* is generally self-limited and responds to supportive care, antibiotic therapy is indicated because it shortens the duration of illness and shedding and consequently reduces the risk of transmission. Antibiotic resistance is a growing worldwide problem for enteric bacterial pathogens. Antibiotic susceptibility testing is recommended for the management of patients with suspected *Shigella* infection. When antimicrobial susceptibility of the organism is unknown, the recommended treatment of choice is a fluoroquinolone such as levofloxacin or ciprofloxacin. Alternative agents include azithromycin and ceftriaxone.[8] These antibiotics should be administered for 3 days at the following doses: levofloxacin 500 mg orally once daily, ciprofloxacin 500 mg twice daily, or azithromycin 500 mg once daily. Azithromycin may also be given to children at a dose of 10 mg/kg daily for 3 days. Antimotility agents are not recommended because they can worsen dysentery and may be related to the development of toxic megacolon. No vaccines are licensed currently for the prevention of shigellosis.

SALMONELLOSIS

Epidemiology

Salmonella typhi and *Salmonella paratyphi*, which cause typhoid fever, have high host specificity for humans. In the

Clinical Presentation and Diagnosis of Shigellosis

- Biphasic illness
  - Early—high fever, watery **diarrhea** without blood
  - Later—after approximately 48 hours, colitis develops with urgency, **tenesmus,** and dysentery.
  - Low-grade fever
  - More frequent small-volume stools ("fractional stools")
  - Abdominal cramping
  - Vomiting (35%)
- Complications of shigellosis
  - Proctitis or rectal prolapse—more common in infants and young children
  - Toxic megacolon—more commonly associated with *S. dysenteriae* 1 infection
  - Intestinal obstruction
  - Colonic perforation
  - Bacteremia—more common in children
  - Metabolic disturbances
  - Leukemoid reaction—WBC count more than 50,000/mm³ (more than 50×10^9/L)
  - Neurologic disease—most commonly seizures (approximately 10% of patients)
  - Reactive arthritis or Reiter's syndrome—most common in men aged 20 to 40 years
  - Hemolytic-uremic syndrome (HUS)—mortality rate greater than 50%
- Microscopic examination of stool is extremely useful and reveals multiple polymorphonuclear leukocytes and red blood cells (RBCs). Diagnosis is usually confirmed by stool culture

Patient Encounter 1

A 55-year-old man presents with headache, fever, abdominal pain, and bloody diarrhea for 48 hours. He states that his wife had similar symptoms several days ago. His stool Gram stain reveals the presence of leukocytes, and his WBC is 52×10^3/mm³ (52×10^9/L).

What test should you send?

Stool culture showed many Shigella sonnei.

What treatment do you recommend?

United States, typhoid fever is now a rare disease with approximately 300 clinical cases reported per year. However, infections secondary to these organisms cause an estimated 20 million cases and 200,000 deaths annually worldwide.[9]

Nontyphoidal *Salmonella* (NTS) are important causes of reportable food-borne infection. There are an estimated 1.4 million cases of NTS illness annually in the United States, and almost 94 million worldwide.[10] The highest incidence is in those younger than 1 year of age and older than 65 years of age or in those with HIV/AIDS. Outbreaks of intestinal salmonellosis have been associated with undercooked poultry and eggs, unpasteurized orange juice, tomatoes, cantaloupe, alfalfa sprouts, and cilantro. Exotic pets, especially reptiles (e.g., snakes, turtles, and iguanas), are an increasing source of human salmonellosis, accounting for 3% to 5% of all cases. NTS strains may also result in bacteremia and focal disease, such as endovascular infections, osteomyelitis, meningitis, and septic arthritis. Antimicrobial-resistant strains are associated with excess bloodstream infections and hospitalizations.[11] Recurrent *Salmonella* bacteremia is an AIDS-defining illness.

Risk factors for salmonellosis include extremes of age; alteration of endogenous GI flora due to antimicrobial therapy, surgery, or acid-suppressive therapy[3]; diabetes; malignancy; rheumatologic disorders; HIV infection; and therapeutic immunosuppression. Proper food handling and storage can help prevent *Salmonella* gastroenteritis. Effective handwashing is important, especially when handling eggs and poultry.

Pathogenesis

Salmonella are motile, nonlactose-fermenting, gram-negative rods. In salmonellosis, the organisms penetrate the epithelial lining to the lamina propria with production of diffuse inflammation. The distal ileum and colon are sites of infection.

Treatment and Monitoring

▶ *Gastroenteritis*

Salmonella gastroenteritis is usually self-limited, and antibiotics have no proven value. Patients respond well to ORT. Symptoms typically diminish in 3 to 7 days without sequelae. Antibiotic use may result in a higher rate of chronic carriage and relapse. Antimicrobial use should be limited to preemptive therapy among patients at higher risk for extraintestinal spread or invasive disease (Table 76–2). Antimotility agents should not be used. Avoiding milk products and following a BRAT diet (bananas, rice, applesauce, toast) may help reduce diarrhea associated with gastroenteritis.

▶ *Enteric Fever*

The current drug of choice for typhoid fever is a fluoroquinolone, such as ciprofloxacin. The recommended adult dose of ciprofloxacin for uncomplicated typhoid fever is 500 mg orally twice daily for 5 to 7 days; however, decreased susceptibility to ciprofloxacin is a significant problem in the Indian subcontinent, Southeast Asia, Mexico, the Arabian Gulf, and Africa. All *S. typhi* isolates should be tested for fluoroquinolone resistance. In the United States, *S. typhi* with decreased ciprofloxacin susceptibility is associated with

Clinical Presentation and Diagnosis of Salmonellosis

Gastroenteritis

- Onset 8 to 48 hours after ingestion of contaminated food.
- Fever, diarrhea, and cramping.
- Stools are loose, of moderate volume, and without blood.
- Headache, myalgias, and other systemic symptoms can occur.
- Diagnosis relies on isolation of the organism from stool or ingested food.
- Certain underlying conditions (e.g., AIDS, inflammatory bowel disease, and prior gastric surgery) predispose the patient to more severe disease.

Enteric Fever

- Febrile illness 5 to 21 days after ingestion of contaminated food or water. The fever may progress in stepwise manner to become persistent and high grade. Relative bradycardia may be noted at the fever peak.
- Chills, diaphoresis, headache, anorexia, cough, weakness, sore throat, dizziness, and muscle pains may be present before onset of fever.
- Diarrhea is an early symptom and occurs in approximately 50% of cases.
- Intestinal hemorrhage or perforation, leukopenia, anemia, and subclinical disseminated intravascular coagulopathy may be seen.
- Rose spots, a coated tongue, and/or hepatosplenomegaly may be noted.
- Culture of stool, blood, or bone marrow for *Salmonella* species is helpful.

Table 76–2

Antimicrobial Indications for Nontyphoidal Salmonellosis (NTS)

Age 3 months or less or 65 years or more
Fever and systemic toxicity
HIV/AIDS
Other immunodeficiency (e.g., steroid use, organ transplantation)
Uremia or hemodialysis or renal transplant
Malignancy
Sickle cell anemia or hemoglobinopathy
Inflammatory bowel disease
Aortic aneurysm, prosthetic heart valve, vascular or orthopedic prosthesis

travel to the Indian subcontinent.[9] If ciprofloxacin resistance is present, ceftriaxone may be used; however, this agent may be less suitable in some low- and middle-income countries due to cost and route of administration. Azithromycin

(500 mg once daily for 7 days for adults or 20 mg/kg/day up to a maximum of 1000 mg/day for 7 days for children) is an effective alternative for uncomplicated typhoid fever.[12]

- Two typhoid vaccines are available currently for use in the United States: an oral live-attenuated vaccine (Vivotif Berna-TM vaccine, Swiss Serum and Vaccine Institute) and a parenteral capsular polysaccharide vaccine (Typhim Vi, Pasteur Merieux). Immunization is recommended only for travelers going to endemic areas such as Latin America, Asia, and Africa; household contacts of a chronic carrier; and laboratory personnel who frequently work with *S. typhi*.

▶ Bacteremia and Focal Infections

- Treatment of *Salmonella* bacteremia should be initiated with either a fluoroquinolone) (e.g., levofloxacin, ciprofloxacin) or a third-generation cephalosporin (e.g., ceftriaxone).[8] Given increasing antimicrobial resistance, life-threatening infections should be treated with both agents until susceptibilities are available.[10] If there is no evidence of an endovascular infection, therapy for bacteremia should continue for 10 to 14 days. For patients with suspected meningitis, high-dose ceftriaxone is preferred because of its optimal penetration of the blood–brain barrier. Osteomyelitis and joint infections, often associated with sickle-cell anemia, are difficult to eradicate and require longer durations of antimicrobial therapy (at least 4 to 6 weeks).[10] In persons with HIV infection and an initial episode of *Salmonella* bacteremia, a longer-duration of antibiotic therapy (1 to 2 weeks of parenteral therapy followed by 4 weeks with an oral fluoroquinolone) is recommended to prevent relapse of bacteremia.

▶ Chronic Carrier State

A chronic carrier state, defined as positive stool or urine cultures for more than 12 months, develops in 1% to 4% of adults with typhoid fever. Persistence of the organism is often due to biliary tract carriage, which is higher in persons with biliary tract abnormalities. In patients with normal gallbladder function, effective agents for eradication of chronic carriage include amoxicillin (3 g orally divided three times a day in adults for 3 months), trimethoprim-sulfamethoxazole (one double-strength tablet orally twice a day for 3 months), or ciprofloxacin (750 mg orally twice daily for 4 weeks). Surgery in combination with antibiotic therapy is indicated in patients with biliary tract abnormalities.

CAMPYLOBACTERIOSIS

Epidemiology

- *Campylobacter jejuni* is the most commonly identified cause of bacterial diarrhea worldwide. In the United States, this organism accounts for an estimated 1.4 million infections, 13,000 hospitalizations, and 100 deaths annually.[13] Risk factors for *Campylobacter* infection include consumption of contaminated foods of animal origin, especially undercooked poultry or other foods that are cross-contaminated by raw poultry meat during food preparation; unpasteurized milk;

Patient Encounter 2

A 45-year-old Hispanic man with AIDS presents to the emergency department (ED) with fever, nausea, two episodes of vomiting, abdominal pain, and nonbloody diarrhea for 2 days. He reports that his diarrhea is improving, but he developed fever and chills a few hours before he came to the ED. Other history is noncontributory. His physical examination is positive for fever and diffuse abdominal pain. An abdominal ultrasound did not show any abnormal findings. Two sets of blood cultures were sent to the laboratory, and he is admitted to the hospital.

What primary risk factor does this patient have for a disseminated Salmonella infection?

Do any further tests need to be performed before you can decide on a treatment recommendation?

What treatment do you recommend? Are there any special considerations due to this patient's HIV infection?

Clinical Presentation and Diagnosis of Campylobacteriosis

- Incubation period of 1 to 7 days.
- A brief prodrome of fever, headache, and myalgias is followed by crampy abdominal pain, a high fever, and several bowel movements per day, which may be watery or bloody.
- The abdominal pain and tenderness may be localized, and pain in the right lower quadrant may mimic acute appendicitis. Abdominal pain is more prevalent in *Campylobacter* infection than in either *Shigella* or *Salmonella* infections.
- Tenesmus occurs in approximately 25% of patients.
- Fecal leukocytes and red blood cells (RBCs) are detected in the stools of 75% of infected individuals. Diagnosis of *Campylobacter* is established by stool culture.

contaminated water; foreign travel; contact with farm animals and pets; and the use of antimicrobial therapy.[14] Between 25% and 50% of *C. jejuni* infections in the United States appear to be related to chicken exposure or consumption. People should be instructed to wash their hands after contact with raw meats and animals.

The age and sex distributions of *Campylobacter* infections are unique among bacterial enteric pathogens. In developed countries, there are two age peaks: younger than 1 year of age and 15 to 44 years of age. There is a mild male predominance among infected persons. The reason for this distinct age and sex distribution remains unknown. The epidemiology of *Campylobacter* infections is quite different in developing countries; *Campylobacter* diarrhea is primarily a pediatric disease in developing countries.

Pathogenesis

Campylobacter spp. are gram-negative bacilli that have a curved or spiral shape. *Campylobacter* are sensitive to stomach acidity; as a result, diseases or medications that buffer gastric acidity may increase the risk of infection. The infectious dose for *C. jejuni* is low, similar to that for *Salmonella* spp. After an incubation period, infection is established in the jejunum, ileum, colon, and rectum.

Treatment and Monitoring

Effective fluid and electrolyte replacement is the cornerstone of therapy for patients with *Campylobacter* infection. In most cases, this can be accomplished with the use of oral glucose–electrolyte solutions; however, severe cases may require IV fluids. Antibiotic therapy should be considered in patients with high fevers, bloody stools, symptoms lasting longer than 1 week, pregnancy, infection with HIV, and other immunocompromising conditions.

Macrolides are the recommended first-line drug class for the treatment of *Campylobacter* infections.[8] The recommended dosage of azithromycin for adults is 500 mg orally daily for 3 days and it is 500 mg orally four times daily for 5 days for erythromycin. The recommended regimen for children is azithromycin 20 mg/kg (up to 1 g) orally daily. A fluoroquinolone or a tetracycline are alternatives; however, the widespread use of these agents in food animals has resulted in fluoroquinolone-resistant *Campylobacter* strains worldwide.[13,14] In 1999, 18% of human *Campylobacter* isolates in the United States were fluoroquinolone resistant, and this rate is much higher in many developing countries.[15]

Campylobacter fetus is the most commonly identified species in patients with bacteremia, which primarily occurs in patients who are elderly or immunocompromised. In addition, focal infections such as cellulitis, vascular infections, meningitis, and abscesses may be present. *C. fetus* has a predilection for the vascular endothelium and implanted medical devices.[16] For these serious infections, treatment with a third-generation cephalosporin, gentamicin, ampicillin, or a carbapenem is recommended.[8] Antimotility agents should be avoided because they may prolong the duration of symptoms and have been associated with worse outcomes. Postinfectious complications associated with *Campylobacter* infection include reactive arthritis (1%) and Guillain-Barré syndrome (0.1%).[17]

ENTEROHEMORRHAGIC *ESCHERICHIA COLI*

Epidemiology

Blood in the stool indicates the possibility of inflammatory mucosal disease of the colon such as enterohemorrhagic Escherichia coli (EHEC), a pathogenic subgroup of shiga toxin–producing organisms and an important cause of bloody diarrhea in the United States. Acute hemorrhagic colitis has been primarily

Patient Encounter 3

A 55-year-old woman presents with a 3-day history of high fevers, headaches, and diarrhea. She reports having 7 to 10 loose watery stools per day. She had chicken for lunch in a local restaurant last week, which she really liked. Otherwise, she denies any unusual foods, any recent travel, or any sick contacts. She doesn't have any pets at home. She is able to keep food down. The only positive physical findings are diffuse abdominal tenderness, fever, and high blood pressure. Fecal leukocytes were negative. A stool culture was sent, which showed moderate *Campylobacter jejuni*.

How would you treat this patient?

Clinical Presentation and Diagnosis of EHEC

- Incubation period of 3 to 5 days
- Bloody stools
- Fever usually absent
- Leukocytosis
- Abdominal tenderness
- HUS in 2% to 10% of patients (especially children 1 to 5 years of age and the elderly in nursing homes); develops on average 1 week after the onset of diarrhea.
- EHEC belonging to serotype O157:H7 characteristically do not ferment sorbitol, whereas more than 70% of intestinal floral *E. coli* do. To properly screen EHEC strains in cases of diarrhea, stool should be placed on special sorbitol-MacConkey agar. Colonies of *E. coli* O157:H7, which do not ferment the sorbitol, can be identified readily and confirmed by serotyping with specific antisera. In addition, stool should be tested directly for the presence of Stx I and II by enzyme immunoassay (EIA).

associated with the O157:H7 serotype. This serotype has been responsible for large outbreaks of infection, has higher rates of complications, and appears to be more pathogenic than non-EHEC STEC strains. The spectrum of disease associated with *E. coli* O157:H7 includes bloody diarrhea, which is seen in as many as 95% of patients; nonbloody diarrhea; hemolytic-uremic syndrome (HUS); and thrombotic thrombocytopenic purpura (TTP). HUS is the most common cause of acute kidney injury in children in the United States and frequently leads to prolonged hospitalization, dialysis, and extended follow-up medical care.[18]

Approximately 70,000 cases of EHEC illness occur every year in the United States and lead to more than 2,000 hospitalizations. The highest incidence is in patients aged 5 to 9 years and 50 to 59 years. This organism is also associated with significant morbidity and mortality in elderly, institutionalized patients. Both young and old patients are at particular risk to develop postinfectious complications, TTP, and HUS.[19] Outbreaks of diarrhea due to *E. coli* O157:H7 and other STECs have occurred following ingestion of contaminated beef, hamburgers from fast-food chains, unpasteurized milk and other dairy products, vegetables (e.g., alfalfa sprouts, coleslaw, and lettuce), and apple juice. The most important reservoir for *E. coli* O157:H7 is the GI tract of cattle. Person-to-person transmission also occurs, and swimming in infant pools or contaminated lakes or drinking municipal water are additional risk factors. The incidence of diagnosed *E. coli* O157:H7 infections in the United States are greater among rural than urban populations; *E. coli* O157:H7 infections occur in summer and autumn.

Pathogenesis

The infectious dose of EHEC is very low, between 1 and 100 colony-forming units (CFUs). The two major virulence factors for EHEC are the production of two Shiga-like cytotoxins (Shiga toxin [Stx] I and II) and adhesion-causing attachment–effacement lesions. These cytotoxins are responsible for vascular damage and systemic effects such as HUS. Adhesion mediates initial attachment of EHEC to intestinal epithelial cells. Following attachment, these organisms produce lesions on individual intestinal epithelial cells in the small or large intestine and cause diarrhea.

Treatment and Monitoring

The only recommended treatment of EHEC infection is supportive, including fluid and electrolyte replacement, often in the form of ORT. Most illnesses resolve in 5 to 7 days. Patients should be monitored for the development of HUS. Antibiotics are currently contraindicated because they can induce the expression and release of toxin. Antimotility agents should be avoided because they delay clearance of the pathogen and toxin, which increases the risk of systemic complications. The use of narcotics and nonsteroidal anti-inflammatory drugs (NSAIDs) should also be avoided in acutely infected patients.[20]

Prevention of EHEC infection is especially important because once an infection is established, no therapeutic interventions are available to lessen the risk of the development of HUS.[18] Hamburgers should be cooked thoroughly until the temperature of the thickest part of the patty is 72°C. All surfaces and utensils that contact raw meat should be washed thoroughly before reuse. Fruits and vegetables should be washed thoroughly, especially those that will not be cooked. Handwashing is also very important and should include the supervision of handwashing by children in daycare centers.

CHOLERA

Epidemiology

Cholera is an intestinal infection that is caused by the bacterium *Vibrio cholerae* that leads to a massive loss of fluid through the GI tract and often results in life-threatening

Patient Encounter 4

A very pleasant 73-year-old white woman with a 48-hour history of hematochezia and hemoptysis presents to the ED. She denies any recent travel, exotic foods, raw foods, or sick contacts. She does note that she ate cold-cut sandwiches at a fundraiser approximately 3 days before her symptoms started. She also noticed that she has three friends who developed bloody diarrhea who also ate at this same fundraiser. She denies any fevers, shakes, chills, cough, sore throat, shortness of breath, chest pain, nausea or vomiting, dysuria, hematuria, edema, or night sweats. On her initial presentation, she had a CT that showed pancolitis and terminal ileitis. She was started on antibiotic therapy including ciprofloxacin and metronidazole. Fecal leukocytes were negative. A stool culture was sent and was positive for Stx. The final culture result was positive for *Escherichia coli* O157:H7.

What would be your recommendation for this patient?

Two days later, she develops acute kidney injury and thrombocytopenia.

What is the most likely diagnosis?

Clinical Presentation and Diagnosis of Cholera

- Incubation period of 18 hours to 5 days.
- Abrupt, painless onset of watery diarrhea and vomiting. The diarrheal fluid is usually clear and may be as much as 10 to 20 liters per day.
- Large volumes of rice-water stools, which may have fishy odor.
- Dehydration, which may be severe. Patients suffering from severe dehydration owing to rapid fluid loss are at risk for death within several hours of disease onset. Typical symptoms of severe dehydration include low blood pressure, poor skin turgor, sunken eyes, and rapid pulse.
- Severe muscle cramps in extremities owing to the electrolyte imbalances are caused by fluid loss. These cramps should resolve with treatment.
- Metabolic acidosis.

dehydration and shock.[21] The biotypes of *V. cholerae* responsible for pandemics are serogroup O1 (El Tor) and serogroup O139.[22] Worldwide this infection affects 3 to 5 million people and causes more than 100,000 deaths per year. Although not associated with pandemics, serogroups O75 and O141 have caused small outbreaks of severe diarrhea in the United States. Cholera can be transmitted by water or by food tainted with contaminated water, particularly undercooked seafood. Research on cholera has led to the refinement of general rehydration therapy, including the proper use of IV and oral rehydration solutions.[21]

Pathogenesis

V. cholerae is a gram-negative bacillus. Vibrios pass through the stomach to colonize the upper small intestine. They possess filamentous protein extensions that attach to receptors on the intestinal mucosa, and their motility assists with penetration of the mucus layer.[21] The cholera enterotoxin consists of two subunits, one of which (subunit A) is transported into the cells and causes an increase in cyclic adenosine monophosphate (cAMP), which leads to the secretion of fluid into the small intestine. This large volume of GI fluid results in the watery diarrhea that is characteristic of cholera. The stools consist of an electrolyte-rich isotonic fluid that is highly infectious.[21]

Treatment and Monitoring

The cornerstone of cholera treatment is fluid replacement. Without treatment, the case-fatality rate for severe cholera is approximately 50%. For cholera, rice-based ORT is better than glucose-based ORT because it reduces the number of stools.[23] Antibiotic prophylaxis is not warranted. A short course of antibiotic therapy shortens the course of the disease and decreases the severity of symptoms. The current WHO treatment protocol recommends antibiotics for only "severe" symptoms; however, the International Center for Diarrheal Disease Research, Bangladesh (ICDDR,B) recommends antibiotics for both severe and moderate cases.[24] The WHO recommendation is usually interpreted to provide antibiotics only to patients with severe dehydration (i.e. greater than 10% body weight loss). With effective antibiotic therapy, the illness is shortened by about 50%, and the duration of excretion of *V. cholerae* in the stool is shortened to 1 or 2 days.[24] Several experts argue that antibiotics should be used more liberally in significant outbreaks.[24,25] A tetracycline (e.g., doxycycline) is recommended as first-line therapy; however, some strains are resistant. Other therapeutic options include a fluoroquinolone, trimethoprim-sulfamethoxazole, and azithromycin.[8] Fluoroquinolones are not recommended for children. Single-dose azithromycin demonstrated a dramatic resolution of diarrhea at 24 hours in one study.[26] This agent is increasingly utilized in areas where multidrug-resistant strains are prevalent.[25]

Primary preventive strategies include ensuring a safe water supply and safe food preparation, improving sanitation, and patient education. A number of safe and effective oral vaccines for cholera are available, which can prevent 50% to 60% of cholera episodes during the first 2 years after vaccination.[27] However, cholera vaccination is not recommended by the Centers for Disease Control and Prevention (CDC) for most people traveling from the United States to endemic areas. The WHO recommends immunization of high-risk groups, such as children and patients infected with HIV, in countries where the disease is endemic.[25]

TRAVELER'S DIARRHEA
Epidemiology

Traveler's diarrhea (TD) commonly occurs when visitors from developed countries travel to developing countries. More than 50 million people are at risk for TD each year.[28] These infections arise following the consumption of food or water contaminated with bacteria, viruses, or parasites. ❹ *Bacteria such as* Shigella, Salmonella, Campylobacter, *and enterotoxigenic* E. coli *(ETEC) are responsible for 60% to 85% of TD cases.*[28] *Noroviruses are increasingly recognized as a significant cause of TD as well.*[29] *Most of these illnesses occur during the first 2 weeks of travel and last about 4 days without therapy.*[30] Protozoans are an uncommon cause but should be suspected if diarrhea lasts for more than 2 weeks.

Food and water contaminated with fecal matter are the main sources of pathogens that lead to TD. Particularly problematic foods and beverages include salads, unpeeled fruits, raw or poorly cooked meats and seafood, unpasteurized dairy products, and tap water (including ice).[30] Bottled water is generally safe if the cap and seal are intact. Food from street vendors and buffet-style meals are particularly risky.[31] The consumption of more than five alcoholic drinks per day has been demonstrated to be a risk factor for TD, especially in males.[32] Providing effective education about the types of foods and activities to avoid during travel may decrease the number of cases of TD.

Pathogenesis

Enterotoxigenic *E. coli*, one of the most common causes of TD and responsible for up to 70% of cases in Mexico, produces both heat-labile enterotoxins (LT) and heat-stable enterotoxins (ST). Both toxins demonstrate cellular mechanisms similar to those of cholera toxins and lead to a great increase in both fluid and electrolyte secretion. These *E. coli* strains are not invasive, as are the Shiga-toxin–producing EHEC strains. These organisms do not cause inflammation and lead to a profuse, watery diarrhea without blood, leukocytes, or abdominal cramping.

Clinical Presentation and Diagnosis of Traveler's Diarrhea

- Frequent, loose stools
- Associated with nausea and vomiting
- Abdominal pain
- Fecal urgency
- Dysentery
- Signs and symptoms related to specific causative pathogen

Treatment and Monitoring

The goal of treatment is to maintain hydration and functional status and to prevent disruption of travel plans. For travelers with mild cases of diarrhea, oral rehydration salts can prevent and treat dehydration and may be particularly important for children and the elderly.[33] Loperamide (4-mg loading dose, then 2 mg orally after each loose stool to a maximum of 16 mg/day) may be used for milder diarrhea; however, this agent is not recommended if bloody diarrhea or fever is present. Antibiotics are effective at reducing the duration of illness to 1 or 2 days. Providing the traveler with a means for empiric self-treatment is an effective method of treating this illness without promoting the inappropriate use of antibiotics. Therapy should be initiated after the first episode of diarrhea that is uncomfortable or interferes with activities.[34]

Trimethoprim-sulfamethoxazole and doxycycline are no longer recommended because of widespread resistance. In general, levofloxacin (500 mg orally once daily for 1 to 3 days) or ciprofloxacin (500 mg orally twice daily for 1 to 3 days) are recommended as first-line agents for travel to most parts of the world.[30,33] Azithromycin (1,000 mg as a single oral dose or 500 mg daily for 1 to 3 days) is an alternative and is preferred in areas where quinolone-resistant *Campylobacter* is prevalent (e.g., Thailand, India).[30] Azithromycin can also be used in pregnant women and children (10 mg/kg/day orally for 3 days).[33] Rifaximin (200 mg orally three times daily for 3 days), a nonabsorbed oral antibiotic, is approved for treatment of TD caused by ETEC in persons at least 12 years old. This agent may be a good choice for persons traveling to destinations where ETEC is the predominant pathogen, such as Mexico.[30] One meta-analysis found that use of an antimicrobial agent plus loperamide was more effective than use of an antimicrobial alone in decreasing the duration of illness.[35] Thus many clinicians will recommend the use of loperamide in dysentery if it is combined with an antibiotic.[30]

❺ *The education of travelers about high-risk food and beverages is an important component in the prevention of TD.* Slogans such as "peel it, boil it, cook it, or forget it" can help to remind travelers of the foods that may be contaminated. However, many travelers find it difficult to follow dietary recommendations. In a study of American travelers, almost 50% developed diarrhea despite receiving advice on preventive dietary measures.[36] Antibiotic prophylaxis is not recommended by the CDC because it can lead to drug-resistant organisms and may give travelers a false sense of security.[30] However, some healthcare professionals do prescribe prophylactic antibiotics for those who are at high risk of developing TD (e.g., immunocompromised persons, patients with impaired gastric acid production) or for those who cannot risk temporary incapacitation (e.g., athletes, diplomats, business people). A fluoroquinolone antibiotic, such as levofloxacin or ciprofloxacin, is usually used first line for this purpose at a dose of one tablet daily during travel and for 2 days following return.[33] Although not approved for prophylaxis, rifaximin may be an excellent option for travelers to Mexico because it is not absorbed and should be less likely to select out resistant organisms than are the fluoroquinolones.[37] Bismuth subsalicylate (Pepto-Bismol; 525 mg orally four times daily for up to 3 weeks) provides a rate of protection of about 60% against TD.[30] However, this agent should not be used in persons taking anticoagulants or other salicylates. Probiotics colonize the GI tract and may prevent pathogenic organisms from causing infections. These agents may provide protection rates as high as 50%,[38] but additional studies are needed, and these products suffer from lack of standardization. No effective vaccines are available for TD.

CLOSTRIDIUM DIFFICILE INFECTION

Epidemiology

C. difficile is the primary cause of nosocomial infectious diarrhea in hospitalized patients. Both the incidence and severity of C. difficile infection (CDI) have been increasing in the United States.[39] The number of C. difficile cases that were reported in 2005 (84 per 100,000) was nearly three times higher than the 1996 rate.[40] There has also been a significant increase in severe cases, colectomies, and death related to CDI.[41] A more virulent, epidemic strain (NAP1/B1/027) was initially identified in the 1980s and is now commonly associated with outbreaks. These strains are associated with an increased production of toxins A and B, which are the primary virulence determinants for C. difficile.[40] In addition, an increasing proportion of CDI patients have a community-acquired infection. These patients are often younger, lack traditional risk factors, and generally have less severe disease compared with those with hospital-acquired infections.[39] A primary risk factor for these community-acquired infections appears to be therapeutic gastric acid suppression.[42] Common risk factors for hospital-acquired CDI include increasing age, severe underlying illness, intensive care unit admission, gastric acid suppression,[43] and exposure to antimicrobials, especially broad-spectrum, multiple-drug regimens.[44] ⑥ *Nosocomial Clostridium difficile-associated diarrhea (CDAD) is almost always associated with antimicrobial use; therefore, unnecessary and inappropriate antibiotic therapy should be avoided. Clindamycin, cephalosporins, and penicillins are the antibiotics most commonly associated with CDAD, but almost all antibiotics except aminoglycosides have been implicated.*[45] Fluoroquinolones are also strongly associated with CDAD.[46]

Pathogenesis

C. difficile, a gram-positive, spore-forming anaerobe, is spread by the fecal–oral route, and patient-to-patient spread is an important mode of transmission within the hospital. The organism is ingested either as the vegetative form or spores, which can survive for long periods in the environment and can traverse the acidic stomach. In the small intestine, spores germinate into the vegetative form. Once the GI tract is colonized with spores, disruption of the gut flora, which occurs with antibiotic therapy, allows C. difficile to proliferate.

Toxin production is essential for the disease to occur and is responsible for the inflammation, fluid and mucus secretion, and mucosal damage that lead to diarrhea or colitis.

Treatment and Monitoring

Patients who develop CDI while receiving an antibiotic should have the antibiotic discontinued, if possible. If antimicrobial therapy must continue, an attempt should be made to switch the patient to an agent with a lower risk of CDI.[47] The use of concurrent antibiotics during CDI therapy, or soon thereafter, lowers the chances of both a clinical and global cure (i.e., clinical cure with no recurrence after 4 weeks).[48] Although a systematic review has concluded that no antimicrobial agent is clearly superior for the initial cure of CDI,[49] clinical practice guidelines recommend that initial antimicrobial therapy should be based on the degree of illness.[50] If severe or complicated disease is present, empiric antimicrobial therapy should begin as soon as the diagnosis is suspected. If relatively mild symptoms are present, antimicrobial therapy may be delayed until stool toxin assay results are available.[50]

Metronidazole (500 mg orally three times daily for 10 to 14 days) is the recommended first-line drug for initial treatment of mild-to-moderate CDI. Oral vancomycin (125 mg four times daily for 10 to 14 days) is the recommended first-line drug therapy for initial treatment of severe CDI,[50] which is usually defined as a serum creatinine increase to more than 1.5 times baseline or a white blood cell count greater than 15,000 cells/mm³(15×10^9/L). Other risk factors for severe disease include age greater than 65 years, hypoalbuminemia, immunosuppression, and severe underlying disease.[44] For the treatment of severe, complicated CDI (refractory hypotension, ileus, and/or toxic megacolon), a higher dose of vancomycin (500 mg orally four times daily) may be combined with IV metronidazole (500 mg every 8 hours). Vancomycin may be given as a retention enema (500 mg in 100 mL of normal saline every 6 hours) if a complete ileus is present.[50] The use of antimotility agents should be avoided because they may precipitate toxic megacolon. Surgical intervention may be lifesaving, particularly in cases complicated by toxic megacolon or colonic perforation.

A study from a single, tertiary care hospital suggests that Infectious Diseases Society of America guidelines regarding the initial use of oral vancomycin may not be consistently followed in practice. Although not statistically significant, these data support the guidelines by noting a trend toward lower mortality and hospital length of stay in patients with severe CDI who were given oral vancomycin. These authors conclude that antimicrobial stewardship teams could play an important role in better assuring that initial CDI therapy is based on severity.[51] The cost of oral vancomycin capsules (approximately $1,000 for a 10-day course) is much higher than metronidazole; however, vancomycin for IV use can be prepared for oral use at a much lower cost.[44] The FDA has also approved fidaxomicin, an oral macrolide antibiotic, for the treatment of CDI in patients who are at least 18 years old. This drug is minimally absorbed and has no activity against organisms other than

Clinical Presentation and Diagnosis of CDAD

- Symptoms can start as early as the first day of antimicrobial therapy or several weeks after antibiotic therapy is completed.
- Asymptomatic carriage.
- Diarrhea:
  - Acute watery diarrhea with lower abdominal pain, low-grade fever, and mild or absent leukocytosis.
  - Mild, with only three or four loose watery stools per day.
  - *C. difficile* toxins are present in stool, but sigmoidoscopic examination is normal.
- Colitis:
  - Profuse, watery diarrhea with 5 to 15 bowel movements per day, abdominal pain, abdominal distention, nausea, and anorexia
  - Left or right lower quadrant abdominal pain and cramps that are relieved by passage of diarrhea
  - Dehydration and low-grade fever
  - Sigmoidoscopic examination may reveal a nonspecific diffuse or patchy erythematous colitis without pseudomembranes
- Pseudomembranous colitis: Same symptoms as colitis, but sigmoidoscopic examination reveals a characteristic membrane with adherent yellow or off-white plaques, usually in distal colon.
- Toxic megacolon: Suggested by acute dilation of the colon to a diameter greater than 6 cm, associated systemic toxicity, and the absence of mechanical obstruction. It carries a high mortality rate.

- Fulminant colitis: Acute abdomen and systemic symptoms such as fever, tachycardia, dehydration, and hypotension. Some patients have marked leukocytosis (up to 40×10^3 white blood cells/mm^3 [40×10^9/L]). Diarrhea is usually prominent but may not occur in patients with paralytic ileus and toxic megacolon.
- Recurrent disease:
  - Risk factors include increased age, recent abdominal surgery, increased number of *C. difficile* diarrheal episodes, and leukocytosis.
  - 20% to 25% of patients develop a second episode of CDAD within 2 months of the initial diagnosis.
- In most cases, *C. difficile* toxin testing of a single unformed stool specimen effectively establishes the diagnosis. Stool culture is the most sensitive test, but it is not clinically practical due to slow turnaround time. Enzyme immunoassay (EIA) testing for toxin A and B is used in most labs. This test is rapid, but less sensitive, and repeat testing may be necessary if the initial test is negative. Newer tests, such as EIA detection of glutamate dehydrogenase (GDH) or use of polymerase chain reaction (PCR) technology, may ultimately improve diagnostic testing for CDI.
- Leukocytosis, hypoalbuminemia, and fecal leukocytes are nonspecific but suggestive of *C. difficile* infection.
- In selected patients, sigmoidoscopy, colonoscopy, or abdominal CT scan can provide useful diagnostic information.

clostridia, which allows for preservation of normal gut flora.[52] The recommended dose of fidaxomicin is 200 mg orally twice daily for 10 days. In clinical trials, fidaxomicin resulted in clinical cure rates that were similar to those achieved with oral vancomycin, but there were significantly fewer recurrences in those treated with fidaxomicin.[53] However, recurrence rates were similar among patients infected with the more virulent NAP1/B1/027 strain. One study did suggest that fidaxomicin might provide improved cure rates versus vancomycin if a patient must continue antibiotics while receiving therapy for CDI.[48] However, fidaxomicin is very costly (approximately $3,000 for a 10-day course).

The recurrence rate after an initial episode of CDI is approximately 20% to 25%, with the highest risk within the first 2 weeks.[44] This rate is independent of which first-line agent is used. Treatment of the first recurrence of CDI is usually treated with the same regimen used for the initial episode; however, this choice should also depend on the clinical condition of the patient, as recommended for the initial therapy choice.[50] Metronidazole should not be used beyond the first recurrence or for long-term

chronic treatment due to the risk of neurotoxicity. The treatment of second or later recurrences of CDI should be undertaken with vancomycin using a tapered and/or pulse regimen.[40,50] Fidaxomicin may be superior to vancomycin at preventing CDAD recurrences secondary to non-NAP1/B1/027 strains. Rifaximin, approved for the treatment of TD, and nitazoxanide, approved for the treatment of *Giardia* or *Cryptosporidium*, may be useful for the prevention of recurrent CDI episodes.[44] Rifaximin, administered directly following a course of metronidazole or vancomycin, may be an option for the prevention of recurrent episodes of CDI in some patients. Fecal microbiota transplantation has a reported efficacy of about 90% in preventing recurrent CDI, and one report suggests that this therapy might emerge as a first-line therapy for severe infection.[54]

Strict infection control measures, including contact precautions, should be instituted for all patients with CDAD. Environmental cleaning with chlorine-containing agents should be used to eliminate *C. difficile* spores. Because alcohol is ineffective in killing spores, it is essential that healthcare workers wash their hands with soap and water rather than

Patient Encounter 5

A 70-year-old man presents to the ED because of diffuse abdominal pain and nonbloody diarrhea. One day earlier he had been discharged from the hospital, where he had received ceftriaxone and levofloxacin for 7 days for an upper respiratory infection. Soon after going home, he passed numerous liquid brown stools. A few hours later, the patient became disoriented, and an ambulance was called. His medical history is unremarkable. Laboratory values: WBC count $50 \times 10^3/mm^3$ ($50 \times 10^9/L$), hematocrit 43% (0.43), sodium 125 mEq/L (125 mmol/L), potassium 5.6 mEq/L (5.6 mmol/L), CO_2 14 mEq/L (14 mmol/L), and metabolic acidosis. An abdominal radiograph series show no evidence of obstruction. The patient was admitted to the hospital.

What GI disease do you suspect based on this information?

From your suspicion, what diagnostic tests and treatment would you recommend for this patient?

In the hospital, he receives fluids and vancomycin 125 mg orally four times daily. Stool was sent for *C. difficile* toxin assay, which came back positive. The patient continues to have abdominal pain but no bowel movement. On day 3 of hospitalization, his abdomen is distended with diffuse pain. His WBC count remains elevated. A CT scan of the abdomen showed colonic dilation to greater than 6 cm. The patient became febrile and hypotensive, requiring multiple pharmacologic support for hypotension.

What are this patient's risk factors for Clostridium difficile–*associated diarrhea (CDAD)?*

What do these new findings suggest?

How does this progression change your treatment recommendations?

---

using alcohol-based hand sanitizers. Meticulous handwashing is the single most important strategy to decrease the patient-to-patient transmission of *C. difficile*. The administration of currently available probiotic agents is not recommended to prevent primary CDI or to treat recurrences.[44,50]

CRYPTOSPORIDIOSIS

Epidemiology

Cryptosporidiosis has been recognized as a human disease since the 1970s, with increasing importance in the 1980s and 1990s because of its relationship with HIV/AIDS. *Cryptosporidium* accounts for 2.2% and 6.1% of diarrhea cases in immunocompetent people in developed and developing countries, respectively.[55] In the United States, the number of reported cases of cryptosporidiosis increased from 6,479 in 2006 to 10,500 in 2008. This increase was partially attributed to multiple large recreational water outbreaks and likely reflects increased use of communal swimming venues (e.g., lakes, swimming pools, and water parks) by young children.[56]

Cryptosporidiosis is spread person-to-person, usually via the fecal–oral route; by animals, particularly cattle and sheep; and through the environment, especially water. People at increased risk of contracting cryptosporidiosis include household and family contacts and sexual partners of someone with the disease, healthcare workers, daycare workers, users of public swimming areas, and people traveling to regions of high endemicity.[55]

Pathogenesis

Cryptosporidium is an intracellular protozoan parasite that is capable of completing its entire life cycle within one host. Humans become infected on ingestion of the oocysts, and

Clinical Presentation and Diagnosis of Cryptosporidiosis

General

- 7- to 10-day incubation period.
- Profuse, watery diarrhea with mucus but not blood or leukocytes that lasts for approximately 2 weeks.
- Nausea, vomiting, and abdominal cramps often accompany the diarrhea.
- Fever may be present.
- Simplest method of diagnosis is detection of oocysts by modified acid-fast staining of a stool specimen. Standard ova and parasite test does not include *Cryptosporidium*.

Immunocompetent

- May manifest as asymptomatic disease, acute diarrhea, or persistent diarrhea lasting for several weeks
- Usually self-limiting

Immunocompromised

- May manifest as asymptomatic disease; transient infection for less than 2 months; chronic diarrhea lasting at least 2 months, or fulminant infection, with at least 2 L of watery stool per day
- Asymptomatic disease more common in those with a CD4+ cell count greater than 200 cells/mm³ ($200 \times 10^6/L$), and fulminant infection more common in those with a CD4+ cell count of less than 50 cells/mm³ ($50 \times 10^6/L$)

autoinfection and persistent infections are possible owing to repeated life cycles within the GI tract. As few as 10 to 100 oocysts can cause infection.[55]

Treatment and Monitoring

● In general, immunocompetent persons and those with asymptomatic infection do not require antimicrobial therapy. In patients with HIV/AIDS, the optimal therapy is restoration of immune function through the use of antiretroviral therapy (ART). In persons in whom antimicrobial therapy is deemed necessary or in HIV/AIDS patients in whom ART is ineffective, a combination of an antimicrobial and an antidiarrheal agent is recommended.[55]

Nitazoxanide is the only FDA-approved agent for the treatment of cryptosporidiosis in adults and children. This agent has demonstrated efficacy in cryptosporidiosis in immunocompetent persons, malnourished children, and HIV/AIDS patients.[57] Patients who are infected with both HIV and *Cryptosporidium* usually require longer therapy durations and higher doses than immunocompetent patients.[57] Alternative agents include paromomycin, azithromycin, and clarithromycin.[58]

Patient Encounter 6

A 35-year-old man with a past medical history significant for recent kidney transplant presents with diarrhea for 1 month. He reports four to five watery stools per day. He also complains of abdominal pain and weight loss. He denies any fever, nausea, and vomiting. Stool studies including fecal leukocytes, culture, and ova and parasites were all negative.

What additional diagnostic test should you order and why?

An acid-fast staining of stool was positive for Cryptosporidium parvum. What treatment would you recommend for this patient?

Prevention of cryptosporidiosis can prove difficult because the oocysts are resilient to many disinfectants and antiseptics, including ammonia, alcohol, and chlorine.[55] Most traditional water-treatment methods, including filtration, do not eradicate all oocysts, which is problematic in the face of the small dose of *Cryptosporidium* that is necessary for infection.

● Routine screening of drinking water should be considered for water-treatment plants, and severely immunocompromised individuals should be advised to avoid water in lakes and streams and contact with young animals.[55]

VIRAL GASTROENTERITIS

⑦ *Viruses are the most common cause of diarrheal illness in the world and, in the United States, account for 450,000 illnesses and 160,000 hospitalizations for adults and children, respectively, and more than 4,000 deaths.*[59] Many viruses may cause gastroenteritis, including rotaviruses, noroviruses, astroviruses, enteric adenoviruses, and coronaviruses (Table 76–3). This chapter focuses on rotaviruses.

ROTAVIRUS

● Rotavirus causes between 600,000 and 875,000 deaths each year, with the highest rates in the very young and in developing countries. Rotavirus is the leading cause of childhood gastroenteritis and death worldwide. Most infections occur in children between 6 months and 2 years of age, typically during the winter season, but adults may be infected as well. Rotavirus causes more than 2 million hospitalizations and 600,000 deaths per year in children younger than 5 years of age.[60] Person-to-person transmission occurs through the fecal–oral route.

The mechanism of diarrhea has not been clearly elucidated, but theories include a reduction in the absorptive surface along with impaired absorption owing to cellular damage, enterotoxigenic effects of a rotavirus protein, and stimulation of the enteric nervous system.

| Table 76–3 |

Agents Responsible for Acute Viral Gastroenteritis and Diarrhea

Virus	Peak Age	Peak Time	Duration	Transmission	Symptoms
Rotavirus	6 months–2 years	Winter	3–8 days	Fecal–oral, water, food	Diarrhea, vomiting, fever, abdominal pain
Enteric adenovirus	Less than 2 years	Year-round	7–9 days	Fecal–oral	Diarrhea, respiratory symptoms, vomiting, fever
Astrovirus	Less than 7 years	Winter	1–4 days	Fecal–oral, water, shellfish	Vomiting, diarrhea, fever, abdominal pain
Noroviruses	More than 5 years	Variable	12–24 hours	Fecal–oral, food, aerosol	Nausea, vomiting, diarrhea, abdominal cramps, headache, fever, chills, myalgia

Modified from Martin S, Jung R. Gastrointestinal infections and enterotoxigenic poisonings. In: DiPiro JT, Talbert RL, Yee GC, et al, eds. Pharmacotherapy: A Pathophysiologic Approach. 8th ed. New York: McGraw-Hill; 2011:1951–1967.

Clinical Presentation and Diagnosis of Rotavirus Infection

- Incubation period of 2 days
- 2- to 3-day **prodrome** of fever and vomiting
- Profuse diarrhea without blood or leukocytes (up to 10 to 20 stools per day)
- Severe dehydration
- Anorexia
- Fever may be present
- Presentation in adults may vary from asymptomatic to nonspecific symptoms of headache, malaise, and chills to severe diarrhea, nausea, and vomiting
- Diagnosis can be made by polymerase chain reaction (PCR) of the stool

Patient Encounter 7

A 12-month-old infant was brought to the ED for 10 watery stools in the last 36 hours. She attends a home daycare center. Her mom reports that three other kids at the same daycare center developed the same symptoms. She also vomited four times today. Positive physical findings include low-grade fever plus hyperactive bowel sounds.

What diagnostic test would you recommend?

What treatment would you recommend for this patient?

How can you prevent this infection?

The cornerstone of rotavirus treatment is supportive care and rehydration with ORT or IV fluids if necessary. Antimotility and antisecretory agents should not be used owing to their potential side effects in children and the self-limited nature of the disease. ❼ *A live, oral rotavirus vaccine is approved by the FDA for use in infants aged 6 weeks to 32 weeks and provides protection against rotavirus infection for at least 24 months.* The CDC Advisory Committee on Immunization Practices recommends vaccination at 2, 4, and 6 months.

FOOD POISONING

Each year in the United States, approximately 76 million foodborne illnesses occur, leading to 325,000 hospitalizations and more than 5,000 deaths. Many bacterial and viral pathogens that have been discussed previously in this chapter (e.g., *Salmonella, Shigella, Campylobacter, E. coli,* and noroviruses) can cause food poisoning. Other bacteria that can cause foodborne illness include *Staphylococcus aureus, C. perfringens, C. botulinum,* and *Bacillus cereus* (Table 76–4). Food poisoning should be suspected if at least two individuals present with similar symptoms after the ingestion of a common food in the prior 72 hours.

OUTCOME EVALUATION

Patients with GI infections should be evaluated for resolution of GI symptoms, as well as any related systemic signs and symptoms. If antimicrobial therapy was used, completion of the course of therapy should be assessed. Documented clearance of the offending microorganism is not necessary.

Table 76–4

Food Poisonings

Organism	Onset (Hours)	Associated Foods	Duration	Symptoms	Treatment
Staphylococcus aureus	1–6	Salad, pastries, ham, poultry	12 hours	Nausea, vomiting	Supportive
Bacillus cereus—emetic	0.5–6	Rice, noodles, pasta, pastries	24 hours	Vomiting	Supportive
Bacillus cereus—diarrheal	8–16	Meats, vegetables, soups, sauces, milk products	24 hours	Diarrhea, abdominal pain	Supportive
Clostridium perfringens (type A)	8–12	Meats, poultry	24 hours	Nausea; abdominal cramps; profuse, watery diarrhea	Supportive
Clostridium botulinum	18–24	Canned fruits, vegetables, meats, honey, salsa, relish	Weeks	Acute GI symptoms followed by symmetric, descending, flaccid paralysis; death is possible	Supportive (including mechanical ventilation); trivalent antitoxin

Patient Care and Monitoring

1. Observe the patient for signs and symptoms of dehydration, and rehydrate as necessary (see Tables 76–1 and 76–2).

2. Monitor for increase in stool consistency and decrease in stool frequency.

3. If pharmacologic agents are used, monitor for any adverse effects.

4. Evaluate the patient for any complications or effects specific to the afflicting pathogen.

Abbreviations Introduced in This Chapter

AAD	Antibiotic-associated diarrhea
ART	Antiretroviral therapy
cAMP	Cyclic adenosine monophosphate
BRAT	Bananas, rice, applesauce, toast
CDAD	*Clostridium difficile*–associated diarrhea
CDC	Centers for Disease Control and Prevention
CDI	*Clostridium difficile* infection
CFUs	Colony-forming units
EHEC	Enterohemorrhagic *Escherichia coli*
ETEC	Enterotoxigenic *Escherichia coli*
EIA	Enzyme immunoassay
ELISA	Enzyme-linked immunosorbent assay
GBS	Guillain-Barré syndrome
HUS	Hemolytic-uremic syndrome
ICDDR, B	International Center for Diarrheal Disease Research, Bangladesh
ORT	Oral rehydration therapy
LT	Heat-labile enterotoxin
NSAID	Nonsteroidal anti-inflammatory drug
MIC	Minimum inhibitory concentration
NTS	Nontyphoidal *Salmonella*
PCR	Polymerase chain reaction
STEC	Shiga toxin-producing *E. coli*
ST	Heat-stable enterotoxin
Stx	Shiga toxin
TD	Traveler's diarrhea
TTP	Thrombotic thrombocytopenic purpura
VRE	Vancomycin-resistant *Enterococcus*
WHO	World Health Organization

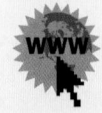

Self-assessment questions and answers are available at *http://www.mhpharmacotherapy. com/pp.html.*

REFERENCES

1. Martin S, Jung R. Gastrointestinal infections and enterotoxigenic poisonings. In: DiPiro JT, Talbert RL, Yee GC, et al, eds. Pharmacotherapy: A Pathophysiologic Approach. 8th ed. New York: McGraw-Hill; 2011:1951–1967.

2. Scallan E, Hoekstra RM, Angulo FJ, et al. Foodborne illness acquired in the United States—major pathogens. Emerg Infect Dis 2011;17:7–15.

3. Bavishi C, Dupont HL. Systematic review: The use of proton pump inhibitors and increased susceptibility to enteric infection. Aliment Pharmacol Ther 2011;34:1269–1281.

4. Kotloff KL, Winickoff JP, Ivanoff B, et al. Global burden of *Shigella* infections: Implications for vaccine development and implementation of control strategies. Bull World Health Organ 1999;77:651–666.

5. Sivapalasingam S, Nelson JM, Joyce K, et al. High prevalence of antimicrobial resistance among *Shigella* isolates in the United States tested by the National Antimicrobial Resistance Monitoring System from 1999 to 2002. Antimicrob Agents Chemother 2006;50:49–54.

6. Dupont HL. *Shigella* species (bacillary dysentery). In: Mandell GL, Bennett JE, Dolin R, eds. Principles and Practice of Infectious Diseases. 7th ed. Philadelphia, PA: Elsevier Churchill Livingstone; 2009: Chap 224.

7. Moralez EI, Lofland D. Shigellosis with resultant septic shock and renal failure. Clin Lab Sci Summer 2011;24(3):147–152.

8. The choice of antibacterial drugs. Treat Guidel Med Lett 2010;8:e1–e6.

9. Lynch MF, Blanton EM, Bulens S, et al. Typhoid fever in the United States, 1999-2006. JAMA 2009;302:859–865.

10. Hohmann EL. Nontyphoidal salmonellosis. Clin Infect Dis 2001;32:263–269.

11. Crump JA, Medalla FM, Joyce KW, et al. Antimicrobial resistance among invasive nontyphoidal *Salmonella enterica* isolates in the United States: National Antimicrobial Resistance Monitoring System, 1996 to 2007. Antimicrob Agents Chemother 2011;55:1148–1154.

12. Crump JA, Mintz ED. Global trends in typhoid and paratyphoid fever. Clin Infect Dis 2010;50:241–246.

13. Nelson JM, Chiller TM, Powers JH, Angulo FJ. Fluoroquinolone-resistant *Campylobacter* species and the withdrawal of fluoroquinolones from use in poultry: A public health success story. Clin Infect Dis 2007;44:977–980.

14. Luangtongkum T, Jeon B, Han J, et al. Antibiotic resistance in *Campylobacter*: Emergence, transmission, and persistence. Future Microbiol 2009;4:189–200.

15. Gupta A, Nelson JM, Barrett TJ, et al. Antimicrobial resistance among *Campylobacter* strains, United States, 1997-2001. Emerg Infect Dis 2004;10:1102–1109.

16. Pacanowski J, Lalande V, Lacombe K, et al. *Campylobacter* bacteremia: Clinical features and factors associated with fatal outcome. Clin Infect Dis 2008;47:790–796.

17. Vucic S, Kiernan MC, Cornblath DR. Guillain-Barre syndrome: An update. J Clin Neurosci 2009;16:733–741.

18. Pennington H. *Escherichia coli* O157. Lancet 2010;376:1428–1435.

19. Reiss G, Kunz P, Koin D, Keeffe EB. *Escherichia coli* O157:H7 infection in nursing homes: Review of literature and report of recent outbreak. J Am Geriatr Soc 2006;54:680–684.

20. Tarr PI, Gordon CA, Chandler WL. Shiga-toxin-producing *Escherichia coli* and hemolytic uremic syndrome. Lancet 2005;365:1073–1086.

21. Sack DA, Sack RB, Nair GB, Siddique AK. Cholera. Lancet 2004;363:223–233.

22. Faruque SM, Chowdhury N, Kamruzzaman M, et al. Reemergence of epidemic Vibrio cholerae O139, Bangladesh. Emerg Infect Dis 2003;9:1116–1122.

23. Zaman K, Yunus M, Rahman A, et al. Efficacy of a packaged rice oral rehydration solution among children with cholera and cholera-like illness. ActaPaediatr 2001;90:505–510.

24. Nelson EJ, Nelson DS, Salam MA, Sack DA. Antibiotics for both moderate and severe cholera. N Engl J Med 2011;364:5–7.

25. Sack DA, Sack RB, Chaignat CL. Getting serious about cholera. N Engl J Med 2006;355:649–651.

26. Saha D, Karim MM, Khan WA, et al. Single-dose azithromycin for the treatment of cholera in adults. N Engl J Med 2006;354:2452–2462.

27. Sinclair D, Abba K, Zaman K, et al. Oral vaccines for preventing cholera. Cochrane Database Syst Rev 2011;16:CD008603.

28. Okhuysen PC. Current concepts in travelers' diarrhea: Epidemiology, antimicrobial resistance and treatment. CurrOpin Infect Dis 2005;18:522–526.

29. Chapin AR, Carpenter CM, Dudley WC, et al. Prevalence of norovirus among visitors from the United States to Mexico and Guatemala who experience traveler's diarrhea. J Clin Microbiol 2005;43:1112–1117.

30. Yates J. Traveler's diarrhea. Am Fam Physician 2005;71:2095–2100.

31. Ansdell VE, Ericsson CD. Prevention and empiric treatment of traveler's diarrhea. Med Clin North Am 1999;83:745–773, vi.

32. Huang DB, Sanchez AP, Triana E, et al. United States male students who heavily consume alcohol in Mexico are at greater risk of travelers' diarrhea than their female counterparts. J Travel Med 2004;11:143–145.

33. Advice for travelers. Treat Guidel Med Lett 2009;7:83–94.

34. Ericsson CD. Travelers' diarrhea: Epidemiology, prevention, and self-treatment. Infect Dis Clin North Am 1998;12:285–303.

35. Riddle MS, Arnold S, Tribble DR. Effect of adjunctive loperamide in combination with antibiotics on treatment outcomes in traveler's diarrhea: A systematic review and meta-analysis. Clin Infect Dis 2008;47:1007–1014.

36. Hill DR. Occurrence and self-treatment of diarrhea in a large cohort of Americans traveling to developing countries. Am J Trop Med Hyg 2000;62:585–589.

37. DuPont HL, Jiang ZD, Okhuysen PC, et al. A randomized, double-blind, placebo-controlled trial of rifaximin to prevent travelers' diarrhea. Ann Intern Med 2005;142:805–812.

38. Hilton E, Kolakowski P, Singer C, Smith M. Efficacy of Lactobacillus GG as a diarrheal preventive in travelers. J Travel Med 1997;4:41–43.

39. Khanna S, Pardi DS, Aronson SL. The epidemiology of community-acquired *Clostridium difficile* infection: A population-based study. Am J Gastroenterol 2012;107:89–95.

40. Kelly CP, LaMont JT. *Clostridium difficile*—more difficult than ever. N Engl J Med 2008;359:1932–1940.

41. Oake N, Taljaard M, van Walraven C, et al. The effect of hospital-acquired *Clostridium difficile* infection on in-hospital mortality. Arch Intern Med 2010;170:1804–1810.

42. Dial S, Delaney JA, Barkun AN, Suissa S. Use of gastric acid-suppressive agents and the risk of community-acquired *Clostridium difficile*-associated disease. JAMA 2005;294:2989–2995.

43. King RN, Lager SL. Incidence of *Clostridium difficile* infections in patients receiving antimicrobial and acid-suppression therapy. Pharmacotherapy 2011;31:642–648.

44. Treatment of *Clostridium difficile* infection. Med Lett Drugs Ther 2011;53:14–16.

45. Wistrom J, Norrby SR, Myhre EB, et al. Frequency of antibiotic-associated diarrhoea in 2462 antibiotic-treated hospitalized patients: A prospective study. J Antimicrob Chemother 2001;47:43–50.

46. Pepin J, Saheb N, Coulombe MA, et al. Emergence of fluoroquinolones as the predominant risk factor for *Clostridium difficile*-associated diarrhea: A cohort study during an epidemic in Quebec. Clin Infect Dis 2005;41:1254–1260.

47. Gerding DN, Muto CA, Owens RC Jr. Treatment of *Clostridium difficile* infection. Clin Infect Dis 2008;46(Suppl 1):S32–S42.

48. Mullane KM, Miller MA, Weiss K, et al. Efficacy of fidaxomicin versus vancomycin as therapy for *Clostridium difficile* infection in individuals taking concomitant antibiotics for other concurrent infections. Clin Infect Dis 2011;53:440–447.

49. Drekonja DM, Butler M, MacDonald R, et al. Comparative effectiveness of *Clostridium difficile* treatments: a systematic review. Ann Intern Med 2011;155:839–847.

50. Cohen SH, Gerding DN, Johnson S, et al. Clinical practice guidelines for *Clostridium difficile* infection in adults: 2010 update by the Society for Healthcare Epidemiology of America (SHEA) and the Infectious Diseases Society of America (IDSA). Infect Control Hosp Epidemiol 2010;31:431–455.

51. Le F, Arora V, Shah DN, et al. A real-world evaluation of oral vancomycin for severe *Clostridium difficile* infection: Implications for antibiotic stewardship programs. Pharmacotherapy 2012;32:129–134.

52. Fidaxomicin (Dificid) for *Clostridium difficile* infection. Med Lett Drugs Ther 2011;53:7374.

53. Louie TJ, Miller MA, Mullane KM, et al. Fidaxomicin versus vancomycin for *Clostridium difficile* infection. N Engl J Med 2011;364:422–431.

54. Brandt LJ, Reddy SS. Fecal microbiota transplantation for recurrent *Clostridium difficile* infection. J Clin Gastroenterol 2011;45(Suppl): S159–S167.

55. Chen XM, Keithly JS, Paya CV, LaRusso NF. Cryptosporidiosis. N Engl J Med 2002;346:1723–1731.

56. Yoder JS, Harral C, Beach MJ. Cryptosporidiosis surveillance—United States, 2006-2008. MMWR Surveill Summ 2010;59:1–14.

57. Rossignol JF. Nitaazoxanide in the treatment of acquired immune deficiency syndrome-related cryptosporidiosis: Results of the United States compassionate use program in 365 patients. Aliment Pharmacol Ther 2006;24:887–894.

58. Smith HV, Corcoran GD. New drugs and treatment for cryptosporidiosis. Curr Opin Infect Dis 2004;17:557–564.

59. Mead PS, Slutsker L, Dietz V, et al. Food-related illness and death in the United States. Emerg Infect Dis 1999;5:607–625.

60. Parashar UD, Hummelman EG, Bresee JS, et al. Global illness and deaths caused by rotavirus disease in children. Emerg Infect Dis 2003;9:565–572.

77 Intra-Abdominal Infections

Joseph E. Mazur and Joseph T. DiPiro

LEARNING OBJECTIVES

● **Upon completion of the chapter, the reader will be able to:**

1. Define and differentiate between primary and secondary intra-abdominal infections (IAIs).

2. Describe the microbiology typically seen with primary and secondary IAIs.

3. Describe the clinical presentation typically seen with primary and secondary IAIs.

4. Describe the role of culture and susceptibility information for diagnosis and treatment of IAIs.

5. Recommend the most appropriate drug and nondrug measures to treat IAIs.

6. Recommend an appropriate antimicrobial regimen for treatment of a primary and a secondary IAIs.

7. Describe the patient-assessment process during the treatment of IAIs.

KEY CONCEPTS

❶ Most intra-abdominal infections (IAIs) are "secondary" infections that are caused by a defect in the GI tract that must be treated by surgical drainage, resection, and/or repair.

❷ Primary peritonitis generally is caused by a single organism (*Staphylococcus aureus* in patients undergoing continuous ambulatory peritoneal dialysis [CAPD] and *Escherichia coli* in patients with cirrhosis).

❸ Secondary IAIs usually are caused by a mixture of enteric gram-negative bacilli and anaerobes. This mix of organisms enhances the pathogenic potential of the bacteria.

❹ For peritonitis, early and aggressive IV fluid resuscitation and electrolyte replacement therapy are essential. A common cause of early death is hypovolemic shock caused by inadequate intravascular volume expansion and tissue perfusion.

❺ Cultures of secondary (IAI) sites generally are not useful for directing antimicrobial therapy. Treatment generally is initiated on a "presumptive" or empirical basis.

❻ Antimicrobial regimens for secondary IAIs should include coverage for enteric gram-negative bacilli and anaerobes. Antimicrobial agents that may be used for treatment of secondary IAIs include the following: (a) a carbapenem, (b) piperacillin-tazobactam, or (c) ceftazidime or cefepime plus metronidazole. An aminoglycoside or colistin may be another treatment option.

❼ Treatment of primary peritonitis for CAPD patients should include an antistaphylococcal antimicrobial such as a first-generation cephalosporin (cefazolin) or vancomycin, usually given by the intraperitoneal (IP) route.

❽ The duration of antimicrobial treatment should be for a total of 4 to 7 days for most secondary IAIs.

❾ Healthcare-associated infections are becoming more common for IAIs secondary to acute care hospital admissions or admissions from chronic care settings. The major pathogens include more resistant gram-negative flora, *Candida* infections causing peritonitis, and Enterococcal species.

Intra-abdominal infections (IAIs) are those contained within the peritoneal cavity or retroperitoneal space. The peritoneal cavity extends from the undersurface of the diaphragm to the floor of the pelvis and contains the stomach, small bowel, large bowel, liver, gallbladder, and spleen. The duodenum, pancreas, kidneys, adrenal glands, great vessels (aorta and vena cava), and most mesenteric vascular structures reside in the retroperitoneum. IAIs may be generalized or localized. They may be contained within visceral structures, such as the liver, gallbladder, spleen, pancreas, kidney, or female reproductive organs. Two general types of IAI are discussed throughout this chapter: peritonitis and abscess.

Peritonitis is defined as the acute inflammatory response of the peritoneal lining to microorganisms, chemicals, irradiation, or foreign-body injury. This chapter deals only with peritonitis of infectious origin.

An *abscess* is a purulent collection of fluid separated from surrounding tissue by a wall consisting of inflammatory cells and adjacent organs. It usually contains necrotic debris, bacteria, and inflammatory cells. Peritonitis and abscess differ considerably in presentation and approach to treatment.

EPIDEMIOLOGY AND ETIOLOGY

Peritonitis may be classified as primary, secondary, or tertiary. Primary peritonitis, also called *spontaneous bacterial peritonitis*, is an infection of the peritoneal cavity without an evident source of bacteria from the abdomen.[1,2] In secondary peritonitis, a focal disease process is evident within the abdomen. Secondary peritonitis may involve perforation of the GI tract (possibly because of ulceration, ischemia, or obstruction), postoperative peritonitis, or posttraumatic peritonitis (e.g., blunt or penetrating trauma). Tertiary peritonitis occurs in critically ill patients, and it is an infection that persists or

recurs at least 48 hours after apparently adequate management of primary or secondary peritonitis.

❶ *Primary peritonitis develops in 10% to 30% of hospitalized patients with alcoholic cirrhosis.*[3] Patients undergoing continuous ambulatory peritoneal dialysis (CAPD) average one episode of peritonitis every 2 years.[4] Secondary peritonitis may be caused by perforation of a peptic ulcer; traumatic perforation of the stomach, small or large bowel, uterus, or urinary bladder; appendicitis; pancreatitis; diverticulitis; bowel infarction; inflammatory bowel disease; cholecystitis; operative contamination of the peritoneum; or diseases of the female genital tract such as septic abortion, postoperative uterine infection, endometritis, or salpingitis. Appendicitis is one of the most common causes of IAI. In 2007, 326,000 appendectomies were performed in the United States for suspected appendicitis.[5]

Primary peritonitis in adults occurs most commonly in association with alcoholic cirrhosis, especially in its end stage, or with ascites caused by postnecrotic cirrhosis, chronic active hepatitis, acute viral hepatitis, congestive heart failure, malignancy, systemic lupus erythematosus, and nephrotic syndrome. It also may result from the use of a peritoneal catheter for dialysis with renal failure or CNS ventriculoperitoneal shunting for hydrocephalus. Abscesses are the result of chronic inflammation and may occur without preceding generalized peritonitis. They may be located within the peritoneal cavity or in a visceral organ and may vary in size, taking a few weeks to years to form. The causes of intra-abdominal abscess overlap those of peritonitis and, in fact, may occur sequentially or simultaneously. Appendicitis is the most frequent cause of abscess.

PATHOPHYSIOLOGY

IAI results from bacterial entry into the peritoneal or retroperitoneal spaces or from bacterial collections within intra-abdominal organs. In primary peritonitis, bacteria may enter the abdomen via the bloodstream or the lymphatic system by transmigration through the bowel wall, through an indwelling peritoneal dialysis (PD) catheter, or via the fallopian tubes in females. Hematogenous bacterial spread (through the bloodstream) occurs more frequently with tuberculosis peritonitis or peritonitis associated with cirrhotic ascites. When peritonitis results from PD, skin-surface flora are introduced via the peritoneal catheter. In secondary peritonitis, bacteria most often enter the peritoneum or retroperitoneum as a result of perforation of the GI or female genital tracts caused by diseases or traumatic injuries.

If bacteria that enter the abdomen are not contained by cellular and humoral defense mechanisms, bacterial dissemination occurs throughout the peritoneal cavity, resulting in peritonitis. This is more likely to occur in the presence of a foreign body, hematoma, necrotic tissue, large bacterial inoculum, continuing bacterial contamination, and contamination involving a mixture of synergistic organisms.

The fluid and protein shift into the abdomen (called *third spacing*) may be so dramatic that circulating blood volume is decreased, which causes decreased cardiac output and hypovolemic shock. Accompanying fever, vomiting, or diarrhea may worsen the fluid imbalance. A reflex sympathetic response, manifested by sweating, tachycardia, and vasoconstriction, may be evident. With an inflamed peritoneum, bacteria and endotoxins are absorbed easily into the bloodstream (translocation), and this may result in septic shock.[1] Other foreign substances present in the peritoneal cavity potentiate peritonitis, notably feces, dead tissues, barium, mucus, bile, and blood.

Many of the manifestations of IAIs, particularly peritonitis, result from cytokine activity. Inflammatory cytokines are produced by macrophages and neutrophils in response to bacteria and bacterial products or to tissue injury, resulting from the surgical incision.[1] The outer membrane components of gram-negative and gram-positive organisms contribute to the cascade of proinflammatory cytokines, ultimately leading to end-organ dysfunction (lungs, heart, kidneys) and septic shock.[6] Peritonitis may result in death because of the effects on major organ systems.

An abscess occurs if peritoneal contamination is localized but bacterial elimination is incomplete. The location of the abscess often is related to the site of primary disease. For example, abscesses resulting from appendicitis tend to appear in the right lower quadrant or the pelvis; those resulting from diverticulitis tend to appear in the left lower quadrant or pelvis. A mature abscess may have a fibrinous capsule that isolates bacteria and the liquid core from antimicrobials and immunologic defenses.

Microbiology of Intra-Abdominal Infection

❷ *Primary bacterial peritonitis is often caused by a single organism.* In children, the pathogen is usually *Streptococcus pneumoniae* or a group A *Streptococcus*, *E. coli*, *S. pneumoniae*, or *Bacteroides* species.[4,7] When peritonitis occurs in association with cirrhotic ascites, *E. coli* and *Klebsiella* are isolated most frequently.[8] Other potential pathogens are *Haemophilus pneumoniae*, *Klebsiella*, *Pseudomonas*, anaerobes, and *S. pneumoniae*.[9] Occasionally, primary peritonitis may be caused by *Mycobacterium tuberculosis*. Peritonitis in patients undergoing PD is caused most often by common skin organisms ranging from *S. aureus* to *S. epidermidis*, to *Pseudomonas aeruginosa*.[10] Occasionally, aerobic gram-negative bacilli may cause infections, particularly in patients undergoing dialysis during hospitalization.

❸ *Because of the diverse bacteria present in the GI tract, secondary intra-abdominal infections are often polymicrobial.*[2,11] The mean number of different bacterial species isolated from infected intra-abdominal sites ranged from three when infection involves the small intestine to 26 with the colon.[11]

Bacterial Synergism and Other Factors

A combination of aerobic and anaerobic organisms appears to increase the severity of infection. Facultative bacteria (e.g., *E. coli*) may provide an environment conducive to the growth of anaerobic bacteria.[2] Although many bacteria isolated in mixed infections are nonpathogenic by themselves, their presence may be essential for the pathogenicity of the bacterial mixture.[3] Facultative bacteria in mixed infections have the ability to:

- Promote an appropriate environment for anaerobic growth through oxygen consumption
- Produce nutrients necessary for anaerobes
- Produce extracellular enzymes that promote tissue invasion by anaerobes

Complicating the clinical picture for treatment are polymicrobial IAIs with certain bacterial species being isolated such as Enterococci or *P. aeruginosa*. Depending on the patients' immune system (immunocompromised host), targeting these organisms may be necessary to avoid treatment failure or mortality.[12]

Clinical Presentation of Primary Peritonitis

General

Patients may not be in acute distress, particularly with peritoneal dialysis.

Symptoms

Patient may complain of nausea, vomiting (sometimes with diarrhea), and abdominal tenderness.

Signs

- Temperature may be only mildly elevated or not elevated in patients undergoing peritoneal dialysis.
- Bowel sounds are hypoactive.
- Cirrhotic patients may have worsening encephalopathy.
- There may be cloudy dialysate fluid with peritoneal dialysis.

Laboratory Tests

- The WBC may be only mildly elevated.
- Ascitic fluid usually contains more than $0.3 \times 10^3/mm^3$ $(0.3 \times 10^9/L)$ leukocytes, and bacteria may be evident on Gram stain of a centrifuged specimen.

Other Diagnostic Tests

Culture of peritoneal dialysate or ascitic fluid should be positive.

Clinical Presentation of Secondary Peritonitis

General

Patients may be in acute distress.

Symptoms

- Patients may complain of nausea, vomiting, and generalized abdominal pain.
- Patients may demonstrate abdominal guarding and a "boardlike abdomen."

Signs

- Tachypnea and tachycardia are present.
- Temperature is normal initially, then may increase to 100°F to 102°F (37.8–38.9°C) within the first few hours, and may continue to rise for the next several hours.
- Hypotension and shock may develop if intravascular volume is not restored.
- Decreased urine output may develop owing to dehydration.
- Bowel sounds are faint initially and eventually cease.

Laboratory Tests

- The WBC is high (WBCs $15–20 \times 10^3/mm^3$ [$15–20 \times 10^9/L$]), with neutrophils predominating and an elevated percentage of immature neutrophils (bands).
- The hematocrit and blood urea nitrogen increase because of dehydration.
- Hyperventilation and vomiting result in early alkalosis, which changes to acidosis and lactic academia to reduced intravascular volume and diminished tissue perfusion.

Other Diagnostic Tests

Abdominal radiographs may be useful because free air in the abdomen (indicating intestinal perforation) or distension of the small or large bowel is often evident.

CLINICAL PRESENTATION AND DIAGNOSIS

IAIs have a wide spectrum of clinical features. Peritonitis usually is easily recognized, but intra-abdominal abscess often may continue unrecognized for long periods of time. Patients with primary and secondary peritonitis present quite differently.

TREATMENT

Desired Outcomes

The primary goals of treatment are correction of the intra-abdominal disease processes or injuries that have caused infection and drainage of collections of purulent material (abscess). A secondary objective is to resolve the infection without major organ system complications (e.g., pulmonary, hepatic, cardiovascular, or renal failure) or adverse drug effects. Ideally, the patient should be discharged from the hospital with full function for self-care and routine daily activities.

General Approach to Treatment

The treatment of IAI most often requires the coordinated use of three major modalities: (a) prompt drainage; (b) support of vital functions; and (c) appropriate antimicrobial therapy to treat infection not eradicated by surgery.[13] Antimicrobials are an important adjunct to drainage procedures in the treatment of secondary IAIs; however, the use of antimicrobial agents without surgical intervention usually is inadequate. For most cases of primary peritonitis, drainage procedures may not be required, and antimicrobial agents become the mainstay of therapy.

④ *In the early phase of serious IAIs, attention should be given to preserving major organ system function.* With generalized peritonitis, large volumes of IV fluids are required to maintain intravascular volume, to improve cardiovascular function, and to ensure adequate tissue perfusion and oxygenation. Adequate urine output should be maintained to ensure appropriate fluid resuscitation and to preserve renal function. A common cause of early death is hypovolemic

Patient Encounter 1, Part 2: Physical Examination and Diagnostic Tests

PE: The patient is still encephalopathic and somnolent.

The patient is placed on ECG monitoring revealing atrial fibrillation. Ascitic fluid analysis is reported as following: hazy yellow color with 2,446 cu/mm³ (2.446×10^9/L) WBC, (31% [0.31] neutrophils, 3% [0.03] lymphocytes, 66% [0.66] macrophages). Urinalysis is not significant because the patient is anuric. Other physical exam findings are nonsignificant.

VS: As noted previously

Labs: As noted previously

Serum: As noted previously

KUB: Negative findings

DPL (diagnostic peritoneal lavage): 2,446 cu/mm³ (2.446×10^9/L)

Microbiological cultures: 4/4 bottles from the blood positive for gram-negative rods resembling *Pseudomonas aeruginosa*, and *E coli*. cultured in the dialysate fluid.

Discuss the most appropriate pharmacologic course of treatment, outlining medications, dosing, and monitoring parameters.

List the goals of treatment and follow-up plan that should be developed by the clinician to ensure positive patient outcomes.

Patient Encounter 2, Part 2

The patient's clinical status grows worse over the next couple of hours despite the efforts of the team. She is now placed on vasopressor therapy combined with fluid, antibiotics are begun emergently, and steroids are also begun. Urine output is less than 10 mL/h and the patient is still mechanically ventilated.

What are your next steps in terms of a care plan as well as monitoring parameters for this patient?

Detail the limitations to certain pharmacologic versus surgical treatments for this patient, and comment on the overall prognosis based on the clinical findings.

shock caused by inadequate intravascular volume expansion and tissue perfusion.

An additional important component of therapy is nutrition. IAIs often involve the GI tract directly or disrupt its function (paralytic ileus). The return of GI motility may take days, weeks, and occasionally, months. In the interim, enteral or parenteral nutrition as indicated facilitates improved immune function and wound healing to ensure recovery.

Nonpharmacologic Therapy

▶ Drainage Procedures

Primary peritonitis is treated with antimicrobials and rarely requires drainage. Secondary peritonitis requires surgical removal of the inflamed or gangrenous tissue to prevent further bacterial contamination. If the surgical procedure is suboptimal, attempts are made to provide drainage of the infected or gangrenous structures.

The drainage of purulent material is the critical component of management of an intra-abdominal abscess. This may be performed surgically or with percutaneous image-guided techniques.[14] Without adequate drainage of the abscess, antimicrobial therapy and fluid resuscitation can be expected to fail. The most valuable microbiologic information may be obtained at the time of percutaneous or operative abscess drainage.

▶ Fluid Therapy

In patients with peritonitis, hypovolemia is often accompanied by acidosis, and large volumes of a solution such as lactated Ringer's may be required initially to restore intravascular volume. Maintenance fluids should be instituted (after intravascular volume is restored) with 0.9% sodium chloride and potassium chloride (20 mEq/L [20 mmol/L]) or 5% dextrose and 0.45% sodium chloride with potassium chloride (20 mEq/L [20 mmol/L]). The administration rate should be based on estimated daily fluid loss through urine and nasogastric suction, including 0.5 to 1.0 L for insensible fluid loss. Potassium would not be included routinely if the patient is hyperkalemic or has renal insufficiency. Aggressive fluid therapy often must be continued in the postoperative period because fluid will continue to sequester in the peritoneal cavity, bowel wall, and lumen.

Pharmacologic Therapy

▶ Antimicrobial Therapy

The goals of antimicrobial therapy are as follows:

- To control bacteremia and prevent the establishment of metastatic foci of infection
- To reduce suppurative complications after bacterial contamination
- To prevent local spread of existing infection

After suppuration has occurred (e.g., an abscess has formed), a cure by antibiotic therapy alone is difficult to achieve; antimicrobials may serve to improve the results with surgery.

⑤ *An empirical antimicrobial regimen should be started as soon as the presence of IAI is suspected and before identification of the infecting organisms is complete.* Therapy must be initiated based on the likely pathogens, which vary depending on the site of IAI and the underlying disease process. Cultures of secondary IAI sites generally are not useful for directing antimicrobial therapy. Table 77–1 lists the likely pathogens against which antimicrobial agents should be directed.

Table 77–1		
Likely Intra-Abdominal Pathogens		
Type of Infection	Aerobes	Anaerobes
Primary Bacterial Peritonitis		
Children (spontaneous)	Group A *Streptococcus, Escherichia coli, pneumococci*	
Cirrhosis	*E. coli, Klebsiella, pneumococci* (many others)	—
Peritoneal dialysis	*Staphylococcus, Streptococcus*	—
Secondary Bacterial Peritonitis		
Gastroduodenal	*Streptococcus, E. coli*	—
Biliary tract	*E. coli, Klebsiella,* enterococci	*Clostridium* or *Bacteroides* (infrequent)
Small or large bowel	*E. coli, Klebsiella* spp., *Proteus* spp.	*Bacteroides fragilis* and other *Bacteroides; Clostridium*
Appendicitis	*E. coli, Pseudomonas*	*Bacteroides* spp.
Abscesses	*E. coli, Klebsiella,* enterococci	*B. fragilis* and other *Bacteroides, Clostridium,* anaerobic cocci
Liver	*E. coli, Klebsiella,* enterococci, staphylococci, amoeba	*Bacteroides* (infrequent)
Spleen	*Staphylococcus, Streptococcus*	

From DiPiro JT, Talbert RL, Yee GC, et al, eds. Pharmacotherapy: A Pathophysiologic Approach. 8th ed. New York: McGraw-Hill; 2011.

▶ *Antimicrobial Experience*

Many studies have been conducted evaluating or comparing the effectiveness of antimicrobials for treatment of IAIs. Substantial differences in patient outcomes from treatment with a variety of agents generally have not been demonstrated.[15]

Important findings from the last 20 years of clinical trials regarding selection of antimicrobials for IAIs are as follows:

- Antimicrobial regimens for secondary IAIs should cover a broad spectrum of aerobic and anaerobic bacteria from the GI tract. Worrisome is the development of hospital-acquired IAIs such as *P. aeruginosa, Acinetobacter spp., Proteus* spp., B-lactamase producing bacteria, methicillin-resistant *S. aureus* (MRSA), *Enterobacteriaceae, Candida* spp., and Enterococci that make the clinical management of these patients challenging.

- Single-agent regimens (such as antianaerobic cephalosporins, extended-spectrum penicillins with β-lactamase inhibitors, or carbapenems) are as effective as combinations of aminoglycosides or fluoroquinolones with antianaerobic agents. This is also true for antimicrobial treatment of acute bacterial contamination from penetrating abdominal trauma.

- Newer agents such as tigecycline and ertapenem may offer some theoretical advantages in the treatment of IAIs, but have some limitations. Tigecycline has a broad spectrum of activity against both aerobic and anaerobic gram negative rods, but lacks sufficient anti-*Pseudomonal* activity. Ertapenem is an example of a carbapenem that has a favorable pharmacokinetic profile (once daily dosing) and, like the other agents, lacks MRSA activity.

- Clindamycin and metronidazole appear to be equivalent in efficacy when combined with agents effective against aerobic gram-negative bacilli (e.g., gentamicin or aztreonam).

- For most patients, antimicrobial treatment can be completed orally with moxifloxacin, ciprofloxacin and metronidazole, levofloxacin plus metronidazole, or amoxicillin–clavulanate or the combination of ciprofloxacin and metronidazole.

- Four to 7 days of antimicrobial treatment are sufficient for most IAIs of mild to moderate severity.

IAI presents in many different ways and with a wide spectrum of severity. The antibiotic regimen employed and duration of treatment depend on the specific clinical circumstances (i.e., the nature of the underlying disease process and the condition of the patient).

Recommendations

6 *For most IAIs, the antimicrobial regimen should be effective against both aerobic and anaerobic bacteria.*[16] Although it is impossible to provide antimicrobial activity against every possible pathogen, agents with activity against enteric gram-negative bacilli, such as *E. coli* and *Klebsiella,* and anaerobes, such as *B. fragilis* and *Clostridia* spp., should be administered. Table 77–2 presents the recommended agents for treatment of community-acquired and complicated IAIs from the Infectious Diseases Society of America and the Surgical Infection Society.[16] These recommendations were formulated using an evidence-based approach. Most community-acquired infections are "mild to moderate," whereas healthcare-associated infections tend to be more severe and difficult to treat. Table 77–3 presents guidelines for treatment and alternative regimens for specific situations. These are general guidelines; there are many factors that cannot be incorporated into such a table.

When used for IAI, aminoglycosides should be combined with agents that are effective against the majority of *B. fragilis*; however, their side-effect profile may prohibit use secondary to nephrotoxicity. Clindamycin or metronidazole is the agent of first choice, but others, such as antianaerobic cephalosporins (e.g., cefoxitin, cefotetan, or ceftizoxime), piperacillin, mezlocillin, and combinations of extended-spectrum penicillins

---

Table 77–2

Recommended Agents for the Treatment of Community-Acquired Complicated Intra-Abdominal Infections in Adults

Agents Recommended for Mild to Moderate Infections	Agents Recommended for High-Severity Infections
β-Lactam/β-Lactamase Inhibitor Combinations	
Ticarcillin-clavulanate	Piperacillin-tazobactam
Carbapenems	
Ertapenem	Imipenem/cilastatin
Others	
Tigecycline	Meropenem, Doripenem
Combination Regimens	
Cefazolin, cefuroxime, cefotaxime, or ceftriaxone plus metronidazole	Third- or fourth-generation cephalosporins (ceftazidime, cefepime) plus metronidazole
Ciprofloxacin or levofloxacin in combination with metronidazole	Ciprofloxacin or levofloxacin, in combination with metronidazole
	Aztreonam plus metronidazole
	Tigecycline plus ciprofloxacin
	Piperacillin-tazobactam + aminoglycoside
	Imipenem or meropenem + aminoglycoside[a]

[a]From Ball CG, Hansen G, Harding G, et al. Canadian practice guidelines for surgical intra-abdominal infections. Can J Infect Dis Med Microbiol 2010; 21:11–37.

From Solomkin JS, Mazuski JE, Bradley JS, et al. Diagnosis and management of complicated intra-abdominal infection in adults and children: guidelines by the Surgical Infection Society and the Infectious Diseases Society of America. Clin Infect Dis 2010;50:133–164.

Table 77–3

Guidelines for Initial Antimicrobial Agents for Intra-Abdominal Infections

Primary Agents		Alternatives
Primary Bacterial Peritonitis		
Cirrhosis	Cefotaxime	1. Add clindamycin or metronidazole if anaerobes are suspected.
		2. Other third-generation cephalosporins, extended-spectrum penicillins, aztreonam, and imipenem as alternatives.
		3. Piperacillin-tazobactam.
Peritoneal dialysis	Initial empiric regimens: Cefazolin or cephalothin plus ceftazidime or cefepime	1. An aminoglycoside may be used in place of ceftazidime or cefepime.
		2. Imipenem/cilastin or cefepime may be used alone.
		3. Quinolones may be used in place of ceftazidime or cefepime if local susceptibilities allow.
	Staphylococcus: penicillinase-resistant penicillin or first-generation cephalosporin	1. Alternative for methicillin-resistant staphylococci is vancomycin.
		2. For vancomycin-resistant *Staphylococcus aureus*, linezolid, daptomycin, or quinupristin-dalfopristin must be used.
	Streptococcus or *Enterococcus:* ampicillin	1. An aminoglycoside may be added for enterococcal peritonitis.
		2. Linezolid or quinupristin-dalfopristin should be used to treat vancomycin-resistant enterococcus not susceptible to ampicillin.
	Aerobic gram-negative bacillic ceftazidime or cefepime	1. The regimen should be based on in vitro sensitivity tests.
	Pseudomonas aeruginosa: two agents with differing mechanisms of actions, such as an oral quinolone plus ceftazidime, cefepime, tobramycin, or piperacillin	

(Continued)

Table 77–3

Guidelines for Initial Antimicrobial Agents for Intra-Abdominal Infections (*Continued*)

Primary Agents		Alternatives
Secondary Bacterial Peritonitis		
Perforated peptic ulcer	First-generation cephalosporins	1. Antianaerobic cephalosporins[a] 2. Possibly add aminoglycoside if patient condition is poor 3. Aminoglycoside with clindamycin or metronidazole; add ampicillin if patient is immunocompromised or if biliary tract origin of infection
Other	Imipenem-cilastatin, meropenem, ertapenem, or extended-spectrum penicillins with β-lactamase inhibitor	1. Ciprofloxacin with metronidazole 2. Aztreonam with clindamycin or metronidazole 3. Antianaerobic cephalosporins[a]
Abscess		
General	Imipenem-cilastatin, meropenem, ertapenem, or extended-spectrum penicillins with β-lactamase inhibitor	1. Aztreonam with clindamycin or metronidazole 2. Ciprofloxacin with metronidazole 3. Aminoglycoside with clindamycin or metronidazole
Liver	As above but add a first-generation cephalosporin	1. Use metronidazole if amoebic liver abscess is suspected
Spleen	Aminoglycoside plus penicillinase-resistant penicillin	1. Alternatives for penicillinase-resistant penicillin are first-generation cephalosporins or vancomycin
Appendicitis		
Normal or inflamed	Antianaerobic cephalosporins[a] (discontinued immediately postoperation)	1. Ampicillin-sulbactam
Gangrenous or perforated	Imipenem-cilastatin, meropenem, ertapenem, antianaerobic cephalosporins or extended-spectrum penicillins with β-lactamase inhibitor	1. Aztreonam with clindamycin or metronidazole 2. Ciprofloxacin with metronidazole 3. Aminoglycoside with clindamycin or metronidazole
Acute cholecystitis	First-generation cephalosporin	1. Aminoglycoside plus ampicillin if severe infection
Cholangitis	Aminoglycoside with ampicillin with or without clindamycin or metronidazole	1. Use vancomycin instead of ampicillin if patient is allergic to penicillin
Acute contamination from abdominal trauma	Antianaerobic cephalosporins[a] or ampicillin-sulbactam	1. A carbapenem 2. Ciprofloxacin plus metronidazole
Pelvic inflammatory disease	Cefotetan or cefoxitin with doxycycline	1. Clindamycin with gentamicin 2. Ampicillin-sulbactam with doxycycline 3. Ciprofloxacin with doxycycline and metronidazole

[a]Cefoxitin, cefotetan, and ceftizoxime.

From DiPiro JT, Talbert RL, Yee GC, et al, eds. Pharmacotherapy: A Pathophysiologic Approach. 8th ed. New York: McGraw-Hill; 2011.

with β-lactamase inhibitors would be suitable alternative. Pre-emptive antifungal therapy should maybe be indicated with either an azole antifungal (fluconazole) or an echinocandin (caspofungin) in patients who are immunocompromised or postsurgical with recurrent infection.

In immunocompromised patients or patients with valvular heart disease or a prosthetic heart valve, there is justification to provide specific antimicrobial activity against enterococci. Ampicillin or other penicillins that are active against enterococci (e.g., penicillin, piperacillin, and mezlocillin) should be used in patients at high-risk, patients with persistent or recurrent intra-abdominal infection, or patients who are immunosuppressed, such as after organ transplantation. Ampicillin remains the drug of choice for this indication because it is most active in vitro against enterococci and is relatively inexpensive. Vancomycin is active against most enterococci; however, resistance is increasing, and this agent should be reserved for established infections when first-line therapies cannot be used.

Intraperitoneal (IP) administration of antibiotics is preferred over IV therapy in the treatment of peritonitis that occurs in patients undergoing CAPD.[17] The International Society of Peritoneal Dialysis revised its guidelines for the diagnosis and pharmacotherapy of PD-associated infections.[10] The guidelines provide dosing recommendations for intermittent and continuous therapy based on the modality of dialysis (CAPD or automated peritoneal dialysis [APD]) and the extent of the patient's residual renal function.

7 *Antimicrobial agents effective against both gram-positive and gram-negative organisms should be used for initial IP empirical therapy for peritonitis in PD patients.* The most important factors to take into consideration for initial antimicrobial selection are the dialysis center's and the patient's history of infecting organisms and their sensitivities. The use of cefazolin (loading dose [LD] 500 mg/L, maintenance dose [MD] 125 mg/L) plus ceftazidime (LD 500 mg/L, MD 125 mg/L) or cefepime (LD 500 mg/L, MD 125 mg/L) or an aminoglycoside (gentamicin-tobramycin LD 8 mg/L, MD 4 mg/L) is suitable for initial empirical therapy; if patients are allergic to cephalosporin antibiotics, vancomycin (LD 1,000 mg/L, MD 25 mg/L) or an aminoglycoside should be substituted. Aztreonam is an alternative to ceftazidime or cefepime in this patient population. Another option is monotherapy with imipenem-cilastin (LD 750 mg/L, MD 50 mg/L) or cefepime. Antimicrobial doses should be increased empirically by 25% in patients with residual renal function (more than 100 mL/day urine output).[10] Antimicrobial therapy should be continued for at least 1 week after the dialysate fluid is clear and for a total of at least 14 days. The reader is referred to these guidelines for additional information.[10]

After acute bacterial contamination, such as with abdominal trauma where GI contents spill into the peritoneum, combination antimicrobial regimens are not required. If the patient is seen soon after injury (within 2 hours) and surgical measures are instituted promptly, antianaerobic cephalosporins (e.g., cefoxitin or cefotetan) or extended-spectrum penicillins are effective in preventing most infectious complications. Antimicrobials should be administered as soon as possible after injury.[18]

For appendicitis, the antimicrobial regimen used should depend on the appearance of the appendix at the time of operation, which may be normal, inflamed, gangrenous, or perforated. Because the condition of the appendix is unknown preoperatively, it is advisable to begin antimicrobial agents before the appendectomy is performed. Reasonable regimens would be antianaerobic cephalosporins or, if the patient is seriously ill, a carbapenem or β-lactam–β-lactamase-inhibitor combination. If, at operation, the appendix were normal or inflamed, postoperative antimicrobials would not be required. If the appendix is gangrenous or perforated, a treatment course of 5 to 7 days with the agents listed in Table 77–2 is appropriate.

⑧ *Acute intra-abdominal contamination, such as after a traumatic injury, may be treated with a short course (24 hours) of antimicrobials.*[18] *For established infections (i.e., peritonitis or intra-abdominal abscess), an antimicrobial course limited to 4 to 7 days is justified.* Under certain conditions, therapy for longer than 7 days would be justified, for example, if the patient remains febrile or is in poor general condition, when relatively resistant bacteria are isolated, or when a focus of infection in the abdomen still may be present. For some abscesses, such as pyogenic liver abscess, antimicrobials may be required for a month or longer.

OUTCOME EVALUATION

Whether diagnosed with primary or secondary peritonitis, monitor the patient for relief of symptoms. Once antimicrobials are initiated and the other important therapies described earlier are used, most patients should show improvement within 2 to 3 days. Successful antimicrobial therapy with resolution of infection will result in decreased pain, manifested as resolution of abdominal guarding and decreased use of pain medications over time. The patient should not appear in distress, with the exception of recognized discomfort and pain from incisions, drains, and a nasogastric tube.

Monitor vital signs and WBC count with differential; each should normalize as the infection resolves. At 24 to 48 hours, aerobic bacterial culture results should be available.

If a suspected pathogen is not sensitive to the antimicrobial agents being given, the regimen should be changed if the patient has not shown sufficient improvement. If the isolated pathogen is extremely sensitive to one antimicrobial and the patient is progressing well, concurrent antimicrobial therapy often may be discontinued.

With anaerobic culturing techniques and the slow growth of these organisms, anaerobes often are not identified until 4 to 7 days after culture, and sensitivity information is difficult to obtain. For this reason, anaerobic culture information generally is not helpful for selection of the antianaerobic component of the antimicrobial regimen. A report indicating that anaerobes were not isolated should not be the sole justification for discontinuing antianaerobic drugs because anaerobic bacteria that were present in the infectious process may not have been transported properly to the microbiology laboratory, or other problems may have led to bacterial death in vitro.

Once the patient's temperature is normal for 48 to 72 hours and the patient is eating, consider changing the IV antibiotic to an oral regimen for the duration of antibiotic treatment. Monitor the serum creatinine level to evaluate for renal complications as well as potential drug toxicity, especially if an aminoglycoside is a component of the antibiotic regimen. Bowel sounds should return to normal. Evaluate the patient daily for development of rash or other drug-related adverse effects.

For patients with primary peritonitis, if peritoneal dialysate cultures were positive initially, repeat cultures should be negative. For patients with secondary peritonitis, monitor the amount of fluid draining if a drain was placed. The volume of drainage should lessen as the infection resolves. Repeat abdominal radiographs should return to normal.

If symptoms do not improve, the patient should be evaluated for persistent infection. There are many reasons for poor patient outcome with IAI; improper antimicrobial selection is only one. The patient may be immunocompromised, which decreases the likelihood of successful outcome with any regimen. It is impossible for antimicrobials to compensate for a nonfunctioning immune system. There may be surgical reasons for poor patient outcome. Failure to identify all intra-abdominal foci of infection or leaks from a GI anastomosis may cause continued IAI. Even when IAI is controlled, accompanying organ system failure, most often renal or respiratory, may lead to patient demise. ⑨ *Healthcare-associated infections are becoming more common for IAIs secondary to acute care hospital admissions or admissions from chronic care settings. The major pathogens include more resistant gram-negative flora,* Candida *infections causing peritonitis, and Enterococcal species.*

The outcome from IAI is not determined solely by what transpires in the abdomen. Unsatisfactory outcomes in patients with IAIs may result from complications that arise in other organ systems. Infectious complications commonly associated with mortality after IAI are urinary tract infections and pneumonia.[19] Reasons for antimicrobial failure may not always be apparent. Even when antimicrobial susceptibility tests indicate that an organism is susceptible

Patient Care and Monitoring

1. A thorough patient medication history should be taken at the time of admission to document all recent medication use, including nonprescription medications and use of complementary or alternative medicines. Any drug allergies or intolerances also should be documented.

2. The initial antimicrobial regimen should conform to standard guidelines unless an appropriate justification for an alternative regimen is evident. With the first few doses of antimicrobial, assess the patient for hypersensitivity reactions or other acute intolerances.

3. Review the dosages of all medications to be sure that they are appropriate for age, weight, and major organ function. Verify that the drugs selected are not contraindicated in the patient with allergies or other intolerances.

4. Confirm that all necessary acute and chronic medications are continued postoperatively.

5. Monitor vital signs (i.e., temperature and heart rate) and laboratory assessments (i.e., WBC count) daily to assess resolution of infection and efficacy of pain medications. When possible, interview the patient to obtain additional information about pain control.

6. Evaluate fluid status to ensure that the patient is not hypovolemic. In a seriously ill patient, assess intravascular volume by monitoring blood pressure and heart rate, but do so more accurately by measuring central venous pressure or urinary output via a urinary bladder catheter. Urine output should equal or exceed 0.5 mL/kg of body weight per hour.

7. Review results of cultures obtained preoperatively or during the surgical procedure. Evaluate the appropriateness of antibiotic therapy based on susceptibility information. Although some investigators suggest that routine culturing of patients with community-acquired intra-abdominal infections contributes little to their management, other investigators suggest that antimicrobial therapy should be based on susceptibility of the bacteria collected from the operative site because this has been shown to correlate with clinical outcome.[20]

8. Assess serum creatinine and aminoglycoside serum concentrations if the patient is being treated with an aminoglycoside. Adjust aminoglycoside dose based on serum concentrations; target peak concentration with multiple doses per day = 6 mcg/mL (6 mg/L; 12.5 μmol/L gentamicin or 12.8 μmol/L tobramycin).

9. On the fifth day of antimicrobial treatment or when GI function returns, determine whether parenteral antimicrobial agents can be switched to oral agents to complete therapy.

10. Assess nutritional needs and recommend appropriate supplementation. When the patient is tolerating an oral diet, determine whether any parenteral medications can be switched to the oral route.

11. Monitor the patient for the development of potential complications of treatment such as delayed hypersensitivity reactions, antibiotic-induced diarrhea, pseudomembranous colitis, or fungal superinfections (manifested as oral thrush).

12. Provide information to the patient concerning the medications administered in the hospital as well as any new medications prescribed for use at home. Advise the patient to contact his or her doctor or pharmacist if he or she experience any adverse effects from medications.

---

in vitro to the antimicrobial agent, therapeutic failures may occur. Possibly there is poor penetration of the antimicrobial agent into the focus of infection, or bacterial resistance may develop after initiation of antimicrobial therapy. Also, it is possible that an antimicrobial regimen may encourage the development of infection by organisms not susceptible to the regimen being used. Superinfection in patients being treated for IAI can be caused by *Candida*; however, Enterococci or opportunistic gram-negative bacilli such as *Pseudomonas* and *Serratia* may be involved.

Treatment regimens for IAI can be judged as successful if the patient recovers from the infection without recurrent peritonitis or intra-abdominal abscess and without the need for additional antimicrobials. A regimen can be considered unsuccessful if a significant adverse drug reaction occurs, reoperation or percutaneous drainage is necessary, or patient improvement is delayed beyond 1 or 2 weeks.

Abbreviations Introduced in This Chapter

APD   Automated peritoneal dialysis
CAPD   Continuous ambulatory peritoneal dialysis
DPL   Diagnostic peritoneal lavage
IAIs   Intra-abdominal infections
IP   Intraperitoneal
LD   Loading dose
MD   Maintenance dose
MRSA   Methicillin-resistant *S. aureus*
PD   Peritoneal dialysis

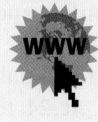 Self-assessment questions and answers are available at *http://mhpharmacotherapy.com/pp.html.*

REFERENCES

1. Ordonez CA, Puyana JC. Management of peritonitis in the critically ill patient. Surg Clin North Am 2006;86:1323–1349.
2. Marshall JC. Intra-abdominal infections. Microbes Infect 2004;6:1015–1025.
3. Mowat C, Stanley AJ. Spontaneous bacterial peritonitis—Diagnosis, treatment, and prevention. Aliment Pharmacol Therap 2001;15:1851–1859.
4. Vas S, Oreopoulos DG. Infections in patients undergoing peritoneal dialysis. Infect Dis Clin North Am 2001;15:743–774.
5. Hall MJ, DeFrances CJ, Williams SN, et al. National Hospital Discharge Survey: 2007 Summary. Natl Health Stat Report 2010;29:1–20,24.
6. Sartelli M, Viale P, Koike K, et al. WSES consensus conference: Guidelines for first-line management of intra-abdominal infections. World J Emerg Surg 2011;6:1–29.
7. Thompson AE, Marshall JC, Opal SM. Intraabdominal infections in infants and children: Descriptions and definitions. Pediatr Crit Care Med 2005;6:S30–S35.
8. Căruntu FA, Benea L. Spontaneous bacterial peritonitis: Pathogenesis, diagnosis, treatment. J Gastroint Liver Dis 2006;15:51–56.
9. Johnson DH, Cuhna BA. Infections in cirrhosis. Infect Dis Clin North Am 2001;15:363–371.
10. Li PK, Szeto CC, Piraino B, et al. Peritoneal dialysis-related infections: 2010 update. Perit Dial Int 2010;30:393–423.
11. Brook I. Microbiology and management of abdominal infections. Dig Dis Sci 2008;53:2585–2591.
12. Ball CG, Hansen G, Harding G, et al. Canadian practice guidelines for surgical intra-abdominal infections. Can J Infect Dis Med Microbiol 2010; 21:11–37.
13. Gauzit R, Pean Y, Barth X, etal. Epidemiology, management, and prognosis of secondary non-postoperative peritonitis: A French prospective observational multicenter study. Surg Infect 2009;10(2):119–127.
14. Jaffe TA, Nelson RC, Delong DM, Paulson EK. Practice patterns in percutaneous image-guided intraabdominal abscess drainage: Survey of academic and private practice centers. Radiology 2004;233:750–756.
15. Wong PF, Gilliam AD, Kumar S, Shenfine J, O'Dair GN, Leaper DJ. Antibiotic regimens for secondary peritonitis of gastrointestinal origin in adults. Cochrane Database Syst Rev 2005;(2):CD004539.
16. Solomkin JS, Mazuski JE, Bradley JS, et al. Diagnosis and management of complicated intra-abdominal infection in adults and children: guidelines by the Surgical Infection Society and the Infectious Diseases Society of America. Clin Infect Dis 2010;50:133–164.
17. Wiggins KJ, Craig JC, Johnson DW, Strippoli GF. Treatment for peritoneal dialysis-associated peritonitis. Cochrane Database Syst Rev 2008;(1):CD005284.
18. Bozorgzadeh A, Pizzi WF, Barie PS, et al. The duration of antibiotic administration in penetrating abdominal trauma. Am J Surg 1999;172:125–135.
19. Merlino JI, Yowler CJ, Malangoni MA. Nosocomial infections adversely affect the outcomes of patients with serious intraabdominal infections. Surg Infect (Larchmt) 2004;5:21–27.
20. Nathens AB. Relevance and utility of peritoneal cultures in patients with peritonitis. Surg Infect (Larchmt) 2001;2:153–160.

78 Parasitic Diseases

J. V. Anandan

LEARNING OBJECTIVES

● **Upon completion of the chapter, the reader will be able to:**

1. Identify the primary reasons why some parasitic diseases may be more prevalent in the U.S. population.

2. Describe the treatment algorithm for giardiasis and amebiasis.

3. List one effective therapy for nematodes and select the drugs of choice for strongyloidiasis and tapeworms.

4. List three major reasons why travelers are infected with malaria.

5. Describe the presenting signs and symptoms of malaria.

6. List some specific toxicities of mefloquine.

7. Identify the monitoring parameters for quinidine gluconate in severe malaria.

8. Define the major complications of falciparum malaria.

9. Discuss the cardiovascular complications of chronic South American trypanosomiasis.

10. Describe the steps to take to eradicate lice infestation and scabies.

KEY CONCEPTS

❶ For treatment of giardiasis (or as empirical treatment), metronidazole 250 mg three times daily for 7 days or tinidazole 2 g as a single dose is recommended.

❷ Diagnostic tests for amebiasis include stool for ova, antigen detection, or polymerase chain reaction (PCR) testing.

❸ The drug of choice for nematode infestations (hookworm, enterobiasis, and ascariasis) is mebendazole, whereas ivermectin is indicated for strongyloidiasis and praziquantel is indicated for tapeworms.

❹ The primary reasons why travelers are infected with malaria are failure to take chemotherapy, inappropriate chemotherapy, and delay in seeking medical care.

❺ Falciparum malaria must be considered a life-threatening medical emergency.

❻ Treatment of serious malarial infection requires admission to an acute care service, IV administration of quinidine gluconate, and symptomatic support.

❼ Complications of falciparum malaria include hypoglycemia, acute renal failure, pulmonary edema, seizure, and coma.

❽ The chronic presentation of American trypanosomiasis includes cardiovascular, GI, and CNS manifestations.

❾ Lice infestation should be treated with 1% permethrin followed by treatment of immediate family members and sexual partners. Bedding and clothes should be sterilized by washing in the hot cycle of the washing machine.

❿ The diagnosis of scabies is made by obtaining skin scrapings and detecting the mite in a wet mount. Topical therapy is 5% permethrin.

Parasitic medicine is an ever-changing field. The increased desire of large segments of the U.S. population to travel to Asia, Africa, and other parts of the world can expose them to parasitic infections that are endemic in those areas. The influx of refugees and new immigrant populations from Asia and other parts of the world have brought new parasitic infections to our shores. Migrant farm workers who work and live in substandard hygienic conditions, the large and growing Central and South American immigrant population, and the presence of immunosuppressed populations (e.g., those with the AIDS and transplant patients) represent other significant sources of parasitic infections in the United States.[1–10] Clearly, there is a need for health professionals in the United States to be familiar with the pathophysiology and treatment of parasitic diseases.

Defined next are some terms that are frequently used when discussing parasitic diseases.[9] *Symbiosis* is defined as "living together," when two species are dependent on each other for food and protection. The term *commensalism*, from the Latin translation of "eating at the same table," implies a mutual association in which both organisms may benefit, or at least one benefits but does no harm to the other. In contrast, *parasitism*, although resembling symbiosis in one aspect (i.e., it is also an intimate relationship between two species), does not represent a mutually beneficial association. One species (the host) does not benefit from the relationship, and in fact the relationship may be detrimental to its very survival. Parasites have made morphologic, biochemical, reproductive, and defensive adaptations over time. These adaptations have increased the ability of parasites to survive host defenses and have allowed them to utilize the host's biochemical systems to synthesize necessary cellular components. Beef and pork tapeworms (cestodes) possess highly developed reproductive systems that allow them to transfer easily to new hosts. Because of the lack of digestive systems, cestodes are completely host-dependent for all nutrients. Cestodes (tapeworms) (*Taenia saginata* and *Taenia solium*) use specialized suckers that enable them to obtain blood and vital nutrients from their host. *Entamoeba histolytica*, the causative agent for amebiasis, once it has gained access to the human colon or large intestine is able to invade and utilize its specialized proteolytic enzyme to penetrate and erode the GI mucosa. *E. histolytica* is also able to survive in adverse conditions when it leaves the host by walling itself off and forming **cysts**; this protects the parasite from environmental conditions until it is ready to infect the next host.

Although acquired immunity to some parasitic diseases may lower the level of infection, absolute immunity as seen in bacterial and viral infections is seldom seen in parasitic diseases. Since parasitic infections produce a wide variety of antigens because of the many life cycle phases, it is more difficult to identify a constant antigenic protein against which specific antibodies are protective. However, malaria remains a likely candidate for a vaccine and there are ongoing studies to develop one.

Space constraints do not allow detailed discussions of the world of parasites, and clinicians and students are directed to some excellent resources for further details on parasites and parasitic diseases.[9,11] Discussion in this chapter includes those parasitic diseases that are more likely to be seen in the United States and includes GI parasites (primarily giardiasis and amebiasis), protozoan infections (malaria and South American trypanosomiasis), some common helminthic diseases (specifically those caused by nematodes and cestodes), and ectoparasites (lice and scabies).

GIARDIASIS

Epidemiology and Etiology

Giardia lamblia (also known as *G. intestinalis* or *G. duodenalis*), an enteric protozoan, is the most common intestinal parasite responsible for diarrheal syndromes throughout the world.

Giardia is the most frequently identified intestinal parasites in the United States, with a prevalence rate of 5% to 15% in some areas. G. lamblia has been identified as the first enteric pathogen seen in children in developing countries, with prevalence rates between 15% and 30%.[11]

There are two stages in the life cycle of *G. lamblia*: the trophozoite and the cyst. *G. lamblia* is found in the small intestine, the gallbladder, and in biliary drainage.[9] The distribution of giardiasis is worldwide, with children being more susceptible than adults.

Pathophysiology

Giardiasis is caused by ingestion of *G. lamblia* cysts in fecally contaminated water or food.[9-15] The protozoan excysts in the low gastric pH to release the trophozoite. Colonization and multiplication of the trophozoite lead to mucosal invasion, localized edema, and flattening of the villi, resulting in malabsorption states in the host. Achlorhydria, hypogammaglobulinemia, or deficiency in secretory immunoglobulin A (IgA) predispose to giardiasis.[11] Individuals with HIV infection and AIDS may have higher carriage rates than the general population. Some patients may develop lactose intolerance after chronic giardiasis.

Clinical Presentation and Diagnosis of Giardiasis

Acute Onset

- Diarrhea, cramp-like abdominal pain, bloating, and flatulence
- Malaise, anorexia, nausea, and belching

Chronic Symptoms

- Diarrhea: Foul-smelling, copious, light-colored, and greasy stools
- Weight loss, steatorrhea, and vitamin B_{12} and fat-soluble vitamin deficiencies
- Constipation alternating with diarrhea

Diagnosis

- Diagnosis is made by examination of fresh stool or a preserved specimen during acute diarrheal phase
- Fresh stool may show trophozoites, whereas preserved specimens yield cysts. (*Note:* stool for ova may show the presence of other parasites [e.g., *Cryptosporidium parvum*, *E. histolytica*, or *E. hartmanni*]; multiple stool samples may be needed.)
- Even though stool examination for ova and parasites has remained the major means of diagnosis, other diagnostic tests include enzyme-linked immunosorbent assay (ELISA), which is considered to be between 85% and 98% sensitive and almost 100% specific (ProSpec T, Giardia Microplate Assay, Remel, Lenexa, KS).

Patient Encounter 1: Giardiasis

AD is a 33-year-old artist from San Francisco who had traveled to Playa Melague in Mexico to complete a painting assignment for a permanent Canadian resident. While there he rented a small house out of town and occasionally ate at local restaurants. Three weeks after his return from Mexico he developed diarrhea, alternating with constipation. When he is seen at the travel clinic at University of California, he reports nausea and crampy diarrhea with foul-smelling stools in the last 2 weeks.

Are his symptoms characteristic of giardiasis?

How would you differentiate giardiasis from possible Escherichia coli–induced diarrhea?

Clinical Presentation and Diagnosis

▶ *Pharmacologic Therapy*

1 *All symptomatic adults and children over the age of 8 years with giardiasis should be treated with metronidazole 250 mg three times daily for 7 days, or tinidazole 2 g as a single dose, or nitazoxanide (Alina) 500 mg twice daily for 3 days.*[12,13,16] The pediatric dose of metronidazole is 15 mg/kg/day three times daily for 7 days. Alternative drugs include furazolidone 100 mg four times daily or paromomycin 25 to 35 mg/kg/day in divided doses daily for 7 days. Paromomycin may be used in pregnancy instead of metronidazole. Pediatric patients can also be treated with suspensions of furazolidone 6 mg/kg/day in four divided doses for 7 days.

Quinacrine 100 mg three times in adults or 5 mg/kg/day in pediatric patients for 5 to 7 days, is available from a specialized pharmacy (e.g., Panorama Compounding Pharmacy).[12]

Outcome Evaluation

Patients with symptomatic giardiasis and positive stool samples or positive enzyme-linked immunosorbent assay

Patient Care and Monitoring: Giardiasis

1. Metronidazole produces cure rates between 85% and 95%.

2. Diarrhea will cease within a few days, although in some patients it may take 1 to 2 weeks.

3. Cyst excretion will cease within days.

4. Intestinal dysfunction (manifested as increased transit time) and radiologic changes primarily due to chronic infection may take months to resolve.

5. Patients who fail therapy with metronidazole should receive a second course with either metronidazole or an alternative agent; nitazoxanide has been shown to be effective in resistant giardiasis.

(ELISA) tests should be treated with metronidazole for 7 days. Patients who fail initial therapy with metronidazole should receive a second course of therapy. Pregnant patients can receive paromomycin 25 to 35 mg/kg/day in divided doses for 7 days. Giardiasis can be prevented by good hygiene and by using caution in food and drink consumption.

AMEBIASIS

Epidemiology and Etiology

Amebiasis remains one of the most important parasitic diseases because of its worldwide distribution and serious GI manifestations. The major causative agent in amebiasis is *E. histolytica*, which invades the colon and must be differentiated from *Entamoeba dispar*, which is associated with an asymptomatic carrier state and is considered nonpathogenic.[17–20] Invasive amebiasis is almost exclusively the result of ingesting *E. histolytica* cysts found in fecally contaminated food or water. Approximately 50 million cases of invasive disease result each year worldwide, leading to an excess of 100,000 deaths. In the general population, the highest incidence is found in institutionalized mentally retarded patients, sexually active homosexuals, AIDS patients, the Native American population, and new immigrants from endemic areas (e.g., Mexico, South and Southeast Asia, West and South Africa, and portions of Central and South America).[18,20]

Pathophysiology

E. histolytica invades mucosal cells of colonic epithelium, producing the classic flask-shaped ulcer in the submucosa. The trophozoite toxin has a cytocidal effect on cells. If the trophozoite gets into the portal circulation, it will be carried to the liver, where it produces abscess and periportal fibrosis. Liver abscesses are more common in men than women and are rarely seen in children.[18,20] Amebic ulcerations can affect the perineum and genitalia, and abscesses may occur in the lung and brain.

Erosion of liver abscesses can result in peritonitis. Liver abscesses that are located in the right lobe can spread to the lungs and pleura. Pericardial infection, although rare, may be associated with extension of the amebic abscesses from the liver.[21–23]

Pharmacologic Therapy

Metronidazole (Flagyl), dehydroemetine, and chloroquine (Aralen) are tissue-acting agents, and iodoquinol (Yodoxin), diloxanide furoate (Furamide), and paromomycin (Humatin) are luminal amebicides. A systemic or tissue-acting agent may be so well absorbed that the amounts of the drug remaining in the bowel may be insufficient to have luminal or local effects. A luminally active agent, on the other hand, may not attain effective enough levels in the tissue to be efficacious. Asymptomatic cyst passers (identified by stool examinations, and who may develop invasive disease)

Clinical Presentation and Diagnosis of Amebiasis

Review of the patient's history should include the following: recent travel, type of foods ingested (e.g., salads or unpeeled fruit), the nature of water and fluid consumed, and description of any symptoms of friends or relatives who ate the same food.

Intestinal Disease

- Vague abdominal discomfort
- Symptoms may range from malaise to severe abdominal cramps, flatulence, and nonbloody or bloody diarrhea (heme-positive in 100% of cases) with mucus
- May have low-grade fever, but this may be absent in many patients
- Eosinophilia is usually absent, although mild leukocytosis is not unusual

Note: Fecal screening may show other intestinal parasites, including *Cryptosporidium* spp., *Balantidium coli, Dientamoeba fragilis, Isospora belli, G. lamblia,* or *Blastocystis hominis.*

Amebic Liver Abscess

- May present with high fever with significant leukocytosis with left shift, anemia, elevated alanine aminotransferase, and dull abdominal pain on palpation

- *Physical findings:* Right upper quadrant pain, hepatomegaly, and liver tenderness, with referred pain to the left or right shoulder (*Note:* Erosion of liver abscesses may present as peritonitis.)

❷ Diagnosis

- *Intestinal amebiasis is diagnosed by demonstrating* E. histolytica *cysts or trophozoites (may contain ingested erythrocytes) in fresh stool or from a specimen obtained by sigmoidoscopy.*
- *Microscopy may not differentiate between the pathogenic* E. histolytica *and the nonpathogenic (commensal)* E. dispar *or* E. moshkovskii *in stools.*
- *Sensitive techniques are available to detect* E. histolytica *in stool: antigen detection, antibody test (ELISA) and PCR.*
- Endoscopy with scrapings or biopsy and stained slides (iron hematoxylin or trichrome) may provide more definitive diagnosis of amebiasis.
- Diagnosis for liver abscess includes serology and liver scans (using isotopes by ultrasound or CT) or MRI; however, none of these are specific for liver abscess. In rare instances, needle aspiration of hepatic abscess may be attempted using ultrasound guidance.

---

and patients with mild intestinal amebiasis should receive a luminal agent: paromomycin 25 to 35 mg/kg/day three times daily for 7 days, or iodoquinol 650 mg three times daily for 20 days. These regimens have cure rates of between 84% and 96%. The pediatric dose of paromomycin is the same as

---

Patient Encounter 2: Amebiasis

PL is a 23-year-old college student who has recently returned from a holiday trip to Malaysia and Thailand. While there he had consumed the local food and traveled extensively in Thailand. PL now presents in the emergency department with complaints of a 3-week history of sharp, crampy, and postprandial abdominal pain. The pain is more intense over the right lower quadrant and associated with watery nonbloody diarrhea and tenesmus. PL indicates that he had some diarrhea while he was in Thailand and received some medications from a local physician.

What specific findings in this patient suggest that he may have giardiasis or amebiasis?

What other information do you need to confirm a diagnosis of amebiasis?

What is the major complication of amebiasis?

---

that used in adults, whereas the pediatric dose of iodoquinol is 30 to 40 mg/kg (maximum: 2 g) per day in three doses for 20 days, and the pediatric dose of diloxanide furoate is 20 mg/kg/day in three doses for 10 days. Paromomycin is the preferred agent in pregnant patients.[12]

Patients with severe intestinal disease or liver abscess should receive metronidazole 750 mg three times daily for 10 days, followed by the luminal agents indicated previously. The pediatric dose of metronidazole is 50 mg/kg/day in divided doses, which should be followed by a luminal agent. An alternative regimen of metronidazole is 2.4 g/day for 2 days in combination with the luminal agent.[20,21] Tinidazole administered in a dose of 2 g daily for 3 days (pediatric dose: 50 mg/kg for 3 days; can be crushed and added to cherry syrup) is an alternative to metronidazole.[12] If there is no prompt response to metronidazole or aspiration of the abscess, an antibiotic regimen should be added. Patients who cannot tolerate oral doses of metronidazole should receive an IV dose of metronidazole.[19]

Outcome Evaluation

Follow-up in patients with amebiasis should include repeat stool examinations, serology, colonoscopy (in colitis), or computed tomography (CT) a month after the end of therapy. Serial liver scans have demonstrated healing of liver abscesses over 4 to 8 months after adequate therapy.[18]

Patient Care and Monitoring: Amebiasis

1. Follow-up in patients with amebiasis should include repeat stools (1 to 3), colonoscopy (in colitis) or CT (in liver abscess) between days 5 and 7, at the end of the course of therapy, and a month after the end of therapy.

2. Most patients with either intestinal amebiasis or colitis will respond in 3 to 5 days with amelioration of symptoms.

3. Those with liver abscess may take up to 7 days before there will be decreases in pain and fever. In liver abscess, patients not responding by the fifth day may require aspiration of the abscesses or exploratory laparotomy.

4. Serial liver scans have demonstrated that healing of liver abscesses take from 4 to 8 months following adequate therapy.

Preventive Measures

- Travelers and tourists visiting endemic areas should avoid local tap water, ice, salads, and unpeeled fruits. Boiled water is safe.

- Water can be disinfected by the use of iodine 2% (5 drops/L) or chlorine 6% (laundry bleach: 4 drops/L) or use of a commercial water purifier, such as Portable Aqua tablets (Wisconsin Pharmaceutical).

HELMINTHIC DISEASES

Helminthic infections include three groups of organisms: roundworms or nematodes, flukes (trematodes), and tapeworms (cestodes). Because of space constraints, only brief descriptions of some of the helminthic infections most commonly seen in North America and their treatments are provided here. Although helminthic infections may not produce clinical manifestations, they can cause significant pathology. One factor that determines the pathogenicity of helminthic infections is their population density; a high-density population ("worm burden") results in predictable disease presentation. In the United States, these infections are reported most frequently in recent immigrants from Southeast Asia, the Caribbean, Mexico, and Central America.[1,24–28] Populations at risk include institutionalized patients (both young and elderly), preschool children in daycare centers, residents of Native American reservations, and homosexuals.[24,25] Certain conditions and drugs (anesthesia and corticosteroids) can cause atypical localization of worms. Immunocompromised hosts can be overwhelmed by some helminthic infections, such as *Strongyloides stercoralis*.

Nematodes

▶ Hookworm Disease

Hookworm infection is caused by *Ancylostoma duodenale* or *Necator americanus*. *N. americanus* is found in the southeastern United States.[24–25] Infective larvae enter the host in contaminated food or water or penetrate the skin and migrate to the small intestine. The adult worm attaches to GI mucosa and causes injury by lytic destruction of the tissue. Over a period of time, the adult worm can cause anemia and hypoproteinemia in the host.[26–28]

▶ Treatment

❸ *The drug of choice is mebendazole (Vermox), which is also active against ascariasis, enterobiasis, trichuriasis, and hookworm.*[12] The adult and pediatric (age more than 2 years) oral dose of mebendazole for hookworm is 100 mg twice daily for 3 days. An alternative agent that can be used in both pediatric and adult patients is albendazole (Zentel), 400 mg as a single oral dose. Diagnosis is by detection of eggs or larvae in stool. Stool examination for eggs and the larvae should be repeated in 2 weeks and the patient retreated if necessary.

Ascariasis

The causative agent in ascariasis is the giant roundworm *Ascaris lumbricoides*, which is found worldwide and is responsible for about 4 million infections in the United States (it primarily affects residents of the Appalachian mountain range and the Gulf Coast states).[29–31] Migration of the worm into the lungs usually produces pneumonitis, fever, cough, eosinophilia, and pulmonary infiltrates. *Ascaris* infection can also cause abdominal discomfort, intestinal obstruction, and appendicitis. Diagnosis is made by detection of the characteristic eggs in the stool or passed worms.

▶ Treatment

In both adults and pediatric patients older than 2 years of age, mebendazole 100 mg orally twice daily for 3 days is the treatment to use. An alternative agent is pyrantel pamoate (Antiminth).[12] The stool should be checked within 2 weeks and the patient retreated when warranted.

Enterobiasis

Enterobiasis, or pinworm infection, is caused by *Enterobius vermicularis*. It is the most widely distributed helminthic infection in the world.[24,32] There are approximately 42 million cases in the United States, primarily affecting children. The most common manifestation of the infection is cutaneous irritation in the perianal region, resulting from the migrating female or the presence of eggs. The intense pruritus may lead to dermatitis and secondary bacterial infections. Diagnosis is made by the use of a perianal swab and cellophane tape sampling, which will aid in egg identification.

▶ Treatment

The three agents that are administered for enterobiasis include pyrantel pamoate, mebendazole, and albendazole.[12] The oral dose of pyrantel pamoate is 11 mg/kg (maximum: 1 g) as a single dose that can be repeated in 2 weeks. The oral dose of mebendazole for both adults and children older than 2 years of age is 100 mg as a single dose. This may be repeated in 2 weeks.[12] Following treatment, to eradicate the eggs, all bedding and underclothing should be sterilized by steaming or washing in the hot cycle of the washing machine.

Strongyloidiasis

Strongyloidiasis is caused by *Strongyloides stercoralis,* which has a worldwide distribution and is predominantly prevalent in South America (Brazil and Columbia) and in Southeast Asia.[33-38] Strongyloidiasis is primarily seen among institutionalized populations (those in mental hospitals and children's hospitals) and immunocompromised individuals (those with HIV infection, AIDS, and patients with hematologic malignancies).[33,36,37] The worm is usually found in the upper intestine, where the eggs are deposited and hatch to form the rhabditiform larvae. The rhabditiform larva (male and female) migrate to the bowel where they may be excreted in the feces. If excreted in the feces, the larva can evolve into either one of two forms after copulation: a free-living non-infectious rhabditiform larvae, or an infectious filariform larvae. The filariform larva can penetrate host skin and migrate to the lungs and produce progeny, a process called autoinfection. This can result in hyperinfection (i.e., an increased number of larva in the intestine, lungs, and other internal organs), especially in an immunocompromised host.

Patients with acute infection may develop a localized pruritic rash, but heavy infestations can produce eosinophilia (10% to 15% [0.10 to 0.15]), diarrhea, abdominal pain, and intestinal obstruction. Administration of corticosteroids or other immunosuppressive drugs to an infected individual can result in hyperinfections and disseminated strongyloidiasis.[33-35] Diagnosis of strongyloidiasis is made by identification of the rhabditiform larva in stool, sputum, or duodenal fluid, or from small bowel biopsy specimens. Even though antigen testing (ELISA essay) remains the most sensitive method, stool examinations and other body fluids should also be utilized in the diagnosis.[36,38]

▶ Treatment

③ *The drug of choice for strongyloidiasis is oral ivermectin 200 mcg/kg/day for 2 days, whereas albendazole 400 mg twice daily is given for 7 days as an alternative.*[12,38] With hyperinfection or disseminated strongyloidiasis, immunosuppressive drugs should be discontinued and treatment should be initiated with ivermectin 200 mcg/kg/day until all symptoms are resolved. Failure with ivermectin therapy has been reported.[39] Patients should be tested periodically to ensure the elimination of the larva. Individuals from an endemic area who are candidates for organ transplantation must be screened for *S. stercoralis.*[38]

Cestodiasis

Cestodiasis (tapeworm infection) is caused by species of the phylum Platyhelminthes (flatworms) and include, among others, the pork tapeworm (*Taenia solium*) and the beef tapeworm (*T. saginata*).[9,40] The tapeworm attaches itself to the mucosal wall of the upper jejunum by the scolex (mouth parts) and by two to four cup-shaped suckers and a structure called a rostellum, which may have hooks in some species. Since the parasite lacks a digestive system, it obtains all nutrients directly from the host. The scolex, proglottids (segments), and eggs are specific for each species and used for identification of tapeworms. Tapeworm infections are caused by ingestion of poorly cooked meat that contains the larva or cysticerci. Cysticerci, when released from the contaminated meat by host digestive juices, mature in the host jejunum. Cystericercosis is a systemic disease caused by the larva of *T. solium* (oncosphere or hexacanth) and is usually acquired by ingestion of eggs in contaminated food or by autoinfection.[41-45] The larvae can penetrate the bowel and migrate through the bloodstream to infect different organs, including the CNS (neurocysticercosis). Diagnosis of both *T. saginata* and *T. solium* is accomplished by recovery of the gravid proglottids and the scolex in the stool. Newer diagnostic tools for neurocysticercosis include serum and cerebrospinal antigen and antibody testing.[45]

▶ Treatment

③ *Tapeworm infections (*T. saginata *and* T. solium*) are treated with praziquantel 5 to 10 mg/kg as a single dose (use the same dose for adults and pediatric patients).*[12] The treatment for cysticercosis and neurocysticercosis may include surgery, anticonvulsants (neurocysticercosis can cause seizures), and anthelmintic therapy. The anthelmintic therapy of choice is albendazole 400 mg twice daily for 8 to 30 days.[45,46] The pediatric dose of albendazole is 15 mg/kg (maximum: 800 mg) in two divided doses for 8 to 30 days. The doses for both adults and pediatric subjects can be repeated if necessary. Praziquantel is an alternative therapy.[12]

Outcome Evaluation

Morbidity and disease due to helminthic infections is related to the intensity of infection. The major adverse effects of helminthic infections are malnutrition, fatigue, and diminished work capacity. Unlike other helminthic infections, strongyloidiasis can cause autoinfection, and in the presence of immunosuppression, it can cause CNS and disseminated infections, which have high mortality.[42]

The most serious complication of cysticercosis is neurocysticercosis that can cause strokes and seizures.[44,45] Treatment of neurocysticercosis with anthelmintic treatment remains controversial.

MALARIA

Malaria is one of the most devastating parasitic diseases, affecting a population in excess of 500 million and causing between 700,000 and 2.7 million deaths a year worldwide.[3,5,7] In the year 2000, approximately 27 million U.S. travelers visited countries where malaria is endemic.

Patient Encounter 3, Part 1: Malaria

CP is a 43-year-old Vietnamese man who had returned recently from a visit to Vietnam and Cambodia. He indicates that he had also visited a refugee camp on the border between Thailand and Cambodia. He was well since returning from Asia until 2 days ago, when he developed a temperature as high as 39°C (102.2°F), with anorexia, headache, chills, sweats, myalgias, and abdominal pain. He took a few doses of acetaminophen, which relieved his headache, but his fever only subsided transiently and came back after a few hours. CP is brought in by his daughter to the emergency department with high fever (greater than 39.8°C [greater than 103.6°F]), headache, abdominal pain, nausea, stiffness of the neck, and back pain. The patient's daughter indicates that CP did not take any antimalarial drugs on his trip.

Are the symptoms in this patient consistent with malaria?

What places this patient at risk for malaria?

What additional information do you need to develop a therapeutic plan for this patient?

In 2009, the Centers for Disease Control and Prevention indicated that there were 1,484 cases of malaria, of which 661 were in U.S. civilians, 18 cases in U.S. military personnel, 201 cases among foreign residents, and 604 among patients of unknown status.[5] There were four fatalities, three due to *Plasmodium falciparum* (the malaria species in the fourth case was not reported). ❹ *The primary reasons for morbidity and death in malaria are failure to take recommended chemoprophylaxis, inappropriate chemoprophylaxis, delay in seeking medical care or in initiating therapy promptly, and misdiagnosis.* Evaluation of a patient should include specific travel history, details of chemoprophylaxis, and physical findings (e.g., splenomegaly).

Malaria is transmitted by the bites of the *Anopheles* mosquitoes, which introduce into the bloodstream one of four species of sporozoites of the plasmodia (*Plasmodium falciparum, P. ovale, P. vivax,* or *P. malariae*).[47–56] Initial symptoms of malaria are nonspecific and may resemble influenza and include chills, headache, fatigue, muscle pain, rigors, and nausea. The onset of the symptoms is between 1 and 3 weeks following exposure. Fever may appear 2 to 3 days after initial symptoms and may follow a pattern and occur every 2 or 3 days (*P. vivax, P. ovale,* and *P. malariae*). Fever with *P. falciparum* can be erratic and may not follow specific patterns. It is not unusual for patients to have concomitant infections with *P. vivax* and *P. falciparum*. Falciparum malaria must always be regarded as a life-threatening medical emergency.

Epidemiology and Etiology

The distribution of the various species of malaria is not well defined, but *P. vivax* is reported to be prevalent in the Indian subcontinent, Central America, North Africa, and the Middle East, whereas *P. falciparum* is predominantly in Africa (including sub-Saharan Africa), both East and West Africa, Haiti, the Dominican Republic, the Amazon region of South America, Southeast Asia, and New Guinea.[5,48,51] Most *P. ovale* infections occur in Africa, whereas the distribution of *P. malariae* is worldwide.[7] Most infections in the United States are reported in American travelers, recent immigrants, or immigrants who have visited friends and family in an endemic area.[4,7] Placental transmission and blood transfusions are also sources of malaria.

Within minutes after the bite of the *Anopheles* mosquito, the sporozoites invade hepatocytes in the liver and begin an asexual phase called schizonts (exoerythrocytic stage or schizogony). The patient may be asymptomatic during this period. After a lapse of between 5 and 15 days (depending on the species), schizonts rupture to release daughter cells (merozoites) into the blood, which then invade erythrocytes. In erythrocytes, the merozoites undergo a number of sequential forms: a ring form, trophozoite, schizont, and merozoite, which then invade new erythrocytes. This asexual phase is about 48 hours for *P. falciparum, P. vivax,* and *P. ovale,* and 72 hours for *P. malariae*. Subsequently, the merozoites develop into gametocytes and undergo a sexual phase (sporogony) in the *Anopheles* mosquito. In the mosquito, the gametocytes undergo a number of stages: zygote, ookinete, and oocyst, and finally transform into sporozoites in the salivary glands, where it is again able to infect the next host. Unlike *P. falciparum* and *P. malariae,* which only remain in the liver for about 3 weeks before invading erythrocytes, *P. ovale* and *P. vivax* can remain in the liver for extended periods in a latent stage (as hypnozoites); this can result in the recurrence of the infection after weeks or months. Primaquine therapy is necessary to eradicate this stage of the infection.

Pathophysiology

The clinical presentation of malaria can be quite variable. Normally, the appearance of a prodrome with headache, abdominal pain, fatigue, fever, and chills, which coincides with the erythrocytic phase of malaria, occurs frequently between 10 and 21 days after being exposed.[48,51] This phase causes extensive hemolysis, which results in anemia and splenomegaly. The most serious complications are caused by *P. falciparum* infections. Infants and children under the age of 5 years and nonimmune pregnant women are at high risk for severe complications with falciparum infections.[52–58] The complications associated with falciparum malaria are related to two unique features of *P. falciparum*: (a) its ability to produce high parasitism (up to 80%) of red cells of all ages; and (b) the propensity to be sequestered in postcapillary venules of critical organs such as brain, liver, heart, lungs, and kidneys.[51,53,54] It has been postulated that tissue hypoxia from anemia, together with *P. falciparum*–parasitized red blood cell adherence to endothelial cells in capillaries, contributes to severe ischemia and metabolic derangements. *P. malariae* is implicated in immune-mediated glomerulonephritis and nephrotic syndrome.[51]

Patient Encounter 3, Part 2: Falciparum Malaria

CP presents with fever, nausea, headache, myalgias, chills, and body aches including back pain.

PMH: Otherwise healthy 43-year-old male

FH: Father died of stroke at age 87 years; mother, who is 82-year-old, has rheumatoid arthritis and lives with an unmarried daughter

SH: Owns a dry-cleaning business; infrequently drinks a beer

Meds: Acetaminophen 325 mg

ROS: In addition to the complaints noted previously, he complains of severe nausea and fatigue

PE

Gen: Patient is slightly agitated and febrile

VS: BP 125/70 mm Hg; P 120 beats/min, RR 36 breaths/min, T 40.1°C (104.2°F)

Skin: Warm and dry to touch

HEENT: Slightly dry oral mucosa

ABD: Splenomegaly

Rest of the systems were WNL

Labs: Sodium 131 mEq/L (131 mmol/L); hemoglobin 10.2 g/dL (102 g/L or 6.33 mmol/L); potassium 4.9 mEq/L (4.9 mmol/L); hematocrit 31% (0.31); chloride 96 mEq/L (96 mmol/L); WBC 14.8 × 10³/mm³ (14.8 × 10⁹/L); BUN 28 mg/dL (10 mmol/L); total bilirubin 1.8 mg/dL (30.8 μmol/L); Scr 1.4 mg/dL (124 μmol/L); platelets 110 × 10³/mm³ (110 × 10⁹/L); glucose 77 mg/dL (4.3 mmol/L); aspartate aminotransferase 87 U/L (1.45 μkat/L); albumin 3.2 g/dL (32 g/L); alanine aminotransferase 94 U/L (1.57 μkat/L); blood smear (Giemsa stain): *P. falciparum*

In view of the above information, what is your assessment of this patient?

Identify your treatment goals and monitoring parameters.

Clinical Presentation and Diagnosis of Malaria

Initial Presentation

Include a careful travel history of patient and physical findings (e.g., splenomegaly) and details of antimalarial chemoprophylaxis, when obtainable.

Erythrocytic Phase

1. Prodrome: Headache, anorexia, malaise, fatigue, and myalgia
2. Nonspecific complaints include abdominal pain, diarrhea, chest pain, and arthralgia
3. Paroxysm: High fever, chills, and rigor
4. Cold phase: Severe pallor, cyanosis of the lips and nail beds
5. Hot phase: Fever between 40.5°C (104.9°F) and 41°C (105.8°F) (seen more frequently with *P. falciparum*)
6. Sweating phase: Follows the hot phase by 2 to 6 hours
7. When fever resolves, it is followed by marked fatigue and drowsiness, warm dry skin, tachycardia, cough, headache, nausea, vomiting, abdominal pain, diarrhea and delirium, anemia, and splenomegaly

⑤ *P. falciparum malaria is a life-threatening emergency. Complications include hypoglycemia, acute renal failure, pulmonary edema, severe anemia (high parasitism), thrombocytopenia, heart failure, cerebral congestion, seizures, coma, and adult respiratory distress syndrome.*

Diagnostic Procedures for Malaria

1. To ensure a positive diagnosis, blood smears (both thick and thin films) should be obtained every 12 to 24 hours for 3 consecutive days.
2. The presence of parasites in the blood 3 to 5 days after initiation of therapy suggests resistance to the drug regimen.

Clinical Presentation and Diagnosis

Innovations for detecting malaria include DNA or RNA probes by polymerase chain reaction (PCR) and monoclonal antibody testing.[59] These, however, are not widely available for clinical use. A *P. falciparum*–specific monoclonal antibody test, histidine-rich protein 2 (HRP-2), has been evaluated and considered to be fairly sensitive for *P. falciparum* and is recommended by the World Health Organization as an alternative for microscopic test (the "gold standard"). However, the rapid malaria diagnostic tests (MRDTs) are restricted from wide use by cost, regulatory standards, operative expertise, and availability.[59]

Treatment

The primary goal in the management of malaria is the rapid identification of the *Plasmodium* species by blood smears (both thick and thin smears repeated every 12 hours for 3 days). Antimalarial therapy should be initiated promptly to eradicate the infection within 48 to 72 hours and avoid complications such as hypoglycemia, pulmonary edema, and renal failure.[48,54]

Pharmacologic Therapy

The chemoprophylaxis regimen for malaria is outlined in **Table 78–1**.[12]

▶ Chemotherapy for Malarial Infection

In an uncomplicated attack of malaria (for all plasmodia except chloroquine-resistant *P. falciparum and P. vivax*),

Table 78–1

Chemoprophylaxis for Malaria

Plasmodia-Sensitive	Drug	Dose	Pediatric Dose	Comments
Chloroquine-sensitive	Chloroquine phosphate (oral)[a]	300 mg (base) once weekly beginning 1 week prior to departure and continued for 4 weeks after leaving endemic area	5 mg (base) per kg of body weight once weekly (maximum 300 mg)	Hydroxychloroquine sulfate 310 (base) or 400 mg salt once a week may be used instead of chloroquine; regimen will be similar to chloroquine
When leaving an area endemic for *P. vivax* or *P. ovale*	Primaquine (oral)	30 mg base (52.6 mg salt) daily for 14 days after departure, in addition to the above	0.6 mg/kg base (1 mg/kg salt) daily for 14 days after departure	*Contraindicated* in those with G6PD deficiency and in pregnancy and lactation
Chloroquine-resistant *P. falciparum*	Atovaquone-proguanil (oral)	250 mg atovaquone and 100 mg proguanil (1 tablet) once daily	62.5 mg atovaquone and 25 mg proguanil once daily 11–20 kg: 1 tablet 21–30 kg: 2 tablets 31–40 kg: 3 tablets Greater than or equal to 40 kg: 1 adult tablet daily	Begin 1–2 days before departure and continue for 1 week after leaving high-risk area Recommended also for primary prophylaxis in mefloquine-resistant *P. falciparum*
	Alternatives			
	Doxycycline (oral)	100 mg daily	Greater than or equal to 8 years of age 2 mg/kg (maximum 100 mg)	Effective for mefloquine-resistant *P. falciparum*. Start 1–2 days before departure, continue through stay in endemic area, and continue regimen for 4 weeks after returning
	Mefloquine (oral)	228 mg (base) (250 mg salt) weekly	Less than or equal to 5–10 kg: 4.6 mg/kg base (5 mg/kg salt) once weekly 11–20 kg: 1/4 tablet 21–30 kg: 1/2 tablet 31–45 kg: 3/4 tablet Greater than or equal to 45 kg: 1 tablet	Start 1–2 week before departure and continue for 4 week after leaving endemic area; may start 3–4 week earlier to assess tolerance *Contraindications:* History of seizure, psychiatric disorders (including depression and anxiety), or arrhythmias
	Primaquine (oral)	30 mg base (1 mg/kg salt for adult) daily	0.6 mg/kg base (1 mg/kg salt up to adult dose)	Alternative or second-line regimen; see above for contraindications

G6PD, glucose-6-phosphate dehydrogenase deficiency.

[a]Pediatric dose can be calculated and tablet pulverized and placed in gelatin capsules. Parents can be instructed to suspend dose in food, simple syrup, or drink.

For further information, see Ref 21: Rao S, Solaymani-Mohammadi S, Petri WA Jr, Parker SK. Hepatic amebiasis: A reminder of the complications. Curr Opin Pediat 2009;21:145–149 (Table 73.19 on p. 1276).

the recommended oral regimen is chloroquine 600 mg (base) initially, followed by 300 mg (base) 6 hours later, and then 300 mg (base) daily for 2 days.[12] ❻ *In severe illness or falciparum malaria, patients should be admitted to an acute care unit, and quinidine gluconate 10 mg salt/kg as a loading dose (maximum 600 mg) in 250 mL normal saline should be administered IV slowly over 1 to 2 hours. This should be followed by continuous infusion of 0.02 mg/kg/min of quinidine for at least 24 hours until oral therapy can be started. In patients who have received either quinine or mefloquine, the loading dose of quinidine should be omitted. Oral quinine salt (650 mg every 8 hours) plus doxycycline 100 mg twice daily should follow the IV dose of quinidine to complete 7 days of therapy.*[12,52,54] The pediatric dose of IV quinidine

gluconate is the same as the dose for adults. The pediatric dose of oral quinine is 25 mg/kg/day in three divided doses, whereas the dose of doxycycline (children older than 8 years) is 4 mg/kg in two divided doses for 7 days. An alternative to doxycycline is clindamycin 900 mg (20 mg/kg/day) three times daily for 3 days. The pediatric dose of clindamycin is the same as in adults. *(In patients who cannot tolerate quinidine or if quinidine is not readily available, IV artesunate 2.4 mg/kg/dose × 3 days, at 0, 12, 24, 48, and 72 hours may be used, followed by oral therapy. Artesunate is available from the Centers for Disease Control and Prevention (CDC) under an investigational new drug application. The pediatric dose of artesunate is same as in adults. Oral therapy may include atovaquone/proguanil, doxycycline, mefloquine or clindamycin.)*[12]

Patient Encounter 3, Part 3: Malaria

Following treatment of falciparum malaria, CP has remained well for 3 weeks. However, 2 days ago, he started developing fever and chills, nausea, and abdominal pain. When seen in the emergency department he has a fever of 38.4°C (101.1°F) and complains of severe headache. Examinations of a thick and thin blood smear of the patient's blood identified *P. falciparum* infection. When CP is questioned about his compliance with his medication, he is not very cooperative. He is admitted to the hospital and received a course of IV quinidine and oral quinine for 7 days. In a follow-up exam 4 weeks later, a repeat blood smear was negative for parasites and the patient was asymptomatic.

In *P. falciparum, P. vivax, P. ovale,* or *P. malariae* (chloroquine-resistant) infections, a dose of 750 mg of mefloquine followed by 500 mg 12 hours later is recommended.[12] The pediatric dose of mefloquine is 15 mg/kg (less than 45 kg) followed by 10 mg/kg 8 to 12 hours later. Mefloquine is associated with sinus bradycardia, confusion, hallucinations, and psychosis and should be avoided in patients with a history of cardiovascular problems or depression. IV quinidine gluconate followed by quinine plus doxycycline or clindamycin should be administered for severe illness as indicated previously. The IV quinidine regimen requires close monitoring of the ECG (QT-segment) and other vital signs (hypotension and hypoglycemia). An alternative oral treatment for *P. falciparum* infections in adults, especially those with history of seizures, psychiatric disorders, or cardiovascular problems, is the combination of atovaquone 250 mg and proguanil 100 mg (Malarone) (two tablets twice daily for 3 days).[12] The pediatric dose of Malarone is as follows: it is not indicted for children less than 5 kg; 9 to 10 kg: 3 pediatric tablets/day × 3 days; 11 to 20 kg: one adult tablet/day × 3 days; 21 to 30 kg: 2 adult tablets/day 3 days; 31 to 40 kg: 3 adult tablets/day 3 days; greater than 40 kg: 2 adults tablets twice daily × 3 days. ❼ *Since falciparum malaria is associated with serious complications, including pulmonary edema, hypoglycemia, jaundice, renal failure, confusion, delirium, seizures, coma, and death, careful monitoring of fluid status and hemodynamic parameters is mandatory.* Exchange transfusion that may be required in patients with *P. falciparum* malaria in whom parasitemia may be between 5% and 15% remains a controversial modality.[12,57] Either peritoneal or hemodialysis may be indicated in renal failure.[48,51]

Outcome Evaluation

When advising potential travelers on prophylaxis for malaria, be aware of the incidence of chloroquine-resistant *P. falciparum* malaria and the countries where it is prevalent.[60–74] In patients who have *P. vivax* or *P. ovale* malaria (note that some patients can have *P. falciparum* and one of these species), following the treatment of the acute phase of malaria and screening for glucose-6-phosphate dehydrogenase

---

Patient Care and Monitoring: Malaria

1. Acute *P. falciparum* malaria resistant to chloroquine should be treated with IV quinidine via central venous catheter and fluid status and the electrocardiogram (ECG) should be monitored closely.

2. The loading dose of quinidine should be omitted in those patients who have received quinine or mefloquine.

3. Hypoglycemia that is associated with both *P. falciparum* and quinidine administration should be checked every 4 to 6 hours and corrected with dextrose infusions (5% to 10%).

4. Quinidine infusions should be slowed temporarily or stopped if the QT interval is greater than 0.6 second, the increase in the QRS complex is greater than 25%, or hypotension unresponsive to fluid challenge results.

5. The suggested quinidine levels should be maintained at 3 to 7 mg/dL (9.2 to 21.6 μmol/L). If quinidine is not readily available, artesunate obtained from the Centers for Disease Control and Prevention on an investigational protocol should be utilized (contact:www.cdc.gov/malaria/features/artesunate_ now available.htm).[12]

6. Blood smears should be checked every 12 hours until parasitemia is less than 1%.

7. Resolution of fever should take place between 36 and 48 hours after initiation of the IV quinidine therapy, and the blood should be clear of parasites in 5 days.

8. When parenteral therapy is required for more than 48 hours or the patient's renal function deteriorates, the dose of quinidine should be lowered by half.

Advice to Travelers

All travelers to endemic areas should be advised to remain in well-screened areas, to wear clothes that cover most of the body, and sleep in mosquito nets. Travelers should adhere to malaria chemoprophylaxis regimens and carry the insect repellant DEET (*N, N-diethylmetatoluamide*) or other insect sprays containing DEET for use in mosquito-infested areas. Relapse of *P. falciparum* between 2 and 4 weeks may take place if the initial therapeutic regimen is not completed.

---

deficiency, patients should receive a regimen of primaquine for 14 days to ensure eradication of the hypnozoite stage of *P. vivax* or *P. ovale*.[61,62] For detailed recommendations for prevention of malaria, go to *www.cdc.gov/travel/*.

AMERICAN TRYPANOSOMIASIS
Etiology

Two distinct forms of the genus *Trypanosoma* occur in humans. One is associated with African trypanosomiasis (sleeping sickness) and the other with American trypanosomiasis (Chagas' disease). *Trypanosoma brucei gambiense* and *Trypanosoma brucei rhodesiense* are the causative organisms for the East African and West African trypanosomiasis, respectively. *T. brucei rhodesiense* causes the acute disease and is the more virulent of the two species. Both East and West African trypanosomiasis are transmitted by various species of tsetse fly belonging to the genus *Glossina*. Further discussion of this subject will focus on American trypanosomiasis.

Trypanosoma cruzi is the agent that causes American trypanosomiasis. American trypanosomiasis is transmitted by a number of species of reduviid bugs *(Triatoma infestans and Rhodium prolixus)* that live in wall cracks of houses in rural areas of North, Central, and South America.[75-79] The reduviid bug is infected by sucking blood from animals (e.g., opossums, dogs, and cats) or humans infected with circulating trypomastigotes. American trypanosomiasis is endemic in all Latin American countries and can be transmitted congenitally, by blood transfusion, and by organ transplantation.

Clinical Presentation and Diagnosis

▶ *Pharmacologic Therapy*

The drugs used for *T. cruzi* include nifurtimox (Lampit) and benznidazole (Rochagan). Oral nifurtimox is available from the CDC, whereas benznidazole is only available in Brazil.[12,80-83] The adult dose of nifurtimox is 8 to 10 mg/kg/day in divided doses for 120 days. Since children seem to tolerate

Clinical Presentation and Diagnosis of Trypanosomiasis

Acute

- Unilateral orbital edema (Romana's sign)
- Granuloma (chagoma)
- Fever, hepatosplenomegaly, and lymphadenopathy

Chronic ❽

- *Cardiac: cardiomyopathy and heart failure*
- *ECG: first-degree heart block, right bundle-branch block, and arrhythmias*
- *GI: enlargement of the esophagus and colon ("mega" syndrome)*
- *CNS: meningoencephalitis, strokes, seizures, and focal paralysis*

Diagnosis

Positive history of exposure and use of serology: indirect hemagglutination test, ELISA (Chagas EIA, Abbott Labs, Abbott Park, IL), and complement fixation (CF) test. (*Note*: CF may produce false-positive reactions in those exposed to leishmaniasis, syphilis, and malaria. PCR may be more definitive for diagnosis.)

Patient Care and Monitoring of Trypanosomiasis

1. It is essential to identify *T. cruzi*–infected patients by serology and to monitor the cardiovascular status of these patients by ECG periodically.
2. Some patients will benefit from implantation of pacemakers.
3. All transplant candidates from areas endemic for Chagas' disease need to be screened for *T. cruzi*. Immunosuppression in these patients can lead to overwhelming infections.

the dose better than adults, the pediatric dose of nifurtimox for 1- to 10-year-old children is 15 to 20 mg/kg/day, and for 11- to 16-year-old children is 12.5 to 15 mg/kg/day in divided doses.[12] Symptomatic treatment for heart failure associated with Chagas' disease should be initiated. The GI complications may require surgical revisions and reconstruction.

Outcome Evaluation

Treatment of the acute phase of the disease (i.e., fever, malaise, edema of the face, and hepatosplenomegaly) is nifurtimox. The congestive heart failure associated with cardiomyopathy of Chagas' disease is treated the same way as cardiomyopathy from other causes.[76,79]

ECTOPARASITES

A parasite that lives outside the body of the host is called an ectoparasite. Approximately 6 to 12 million subjects become infested with pediculosis (lice infestation) yearly in the United States. Pediculosis is usually associated with poor hygiene, and infections are passed from person to person through social and sexual contact.

Lice

The two species that belong to this group include *Pediculus humanus capitis* (head louse) and *Pediculus humanus corporis* (body louse).[84-88] The eggs (or nits) remain firmly attached to the hair, and in about 10 days the lice hatch to form nymphs, which mature in 2 weeks. The lice become attached to the base of the hair follicle and feed on the blood of the host.[10] Pubic or crab lice is found on the hairs around the genitals but may occur in other parts of the body (e.g., eyelashes or axillae). Hypersensitivity to the secretions from lice can produce macular swellings and lead to secondary bacterial infections.

▶ *Treatment*

❾ *The agent of choice for all three infections (body, head, and crab lice) is 1% permethrin (Nix).[12]* Permethrin has both pediculicidal and ovicidal activity against *P. humanus capitis*. The cure rate is reported to be between 90% and 97%. A cream rinse of permethrin 1% (Nix-Crème Rinse) is also available. Individuals with a history of hypersensitivity to ragweed or chrysanthemum may react to permethrin and should avoid this preparation. An alternative agent is oral ivermectin 100 mcg/kg for 3 days (days 1, 2, and 10). Permethrin can cause itching, burning, stinging, and tingling with application. Permethrin 1% should be applied to the dry scalp after shampooing and be left on the scalp for 10 minutes. The application may need to be repeated. Because of the reports of resistance to permethrin, an alternative agent is 0.5% malathion (Ovide), which has to be left on the scalp for 90 minutes and has also been found to be effective. Two applications of malathion, 7 days apart, may be necessary to eradicate the infection.[12] An alternative for head lice is Spinosad 0.9% Creme which became available for patients who may not tolerate permethrin.[91] For the relief of pruritus, calamine lotion with 0.1% menthol or an equivalent agent may be used. *All individuals, including immediate family members and sexual partners of the primary host, should be treated. All bedding and clothes should be sterilized as previously indicated for enterobiasis.*

SCABIES

⑩ *Scabies is caused by the itch mite* Sarcoptes scabiei hominis, *which affects both humans and animals. Infection usually affects the interdigital and popliteal folds, axillary folds, the umbilicus, and the scrotum.* The infection causes severe itching and excoriations in the interdigital web spaces, buttocks, groin, and scalp.[89,90] *Diagnosis is made by identifying the mite from skin scrapings on a wet mount.*

Treatment

⑩ *The agent of choice for scabies is permethrin 5% (Elimite) cream.*[12] Alternative agents in subjects who cannot use permethrin are crotamiton 10% (Eurax) and oral ivermectin (Stromectol) 200 mcg/kg as a single dose. To initiate the treatment with permethrin, the skin should be scrubbed in a warm soapy bath to remove the scabs. The permethrin lotion should then be applied to the whole body, avoiding the face, mucous membranes, and eyes, and left on for 8 to 14 hours. A single application eradicates 97% of scabies. However, in subjects with poor response, permethrin application can be combined with oral ivermectin therapy.[90] All close contacts should be treated appropriately. The pruritus associated with scabies may persist for 2 to 4 weeks because of the remnants of mite parts in the skin.

Outcome Evaluation

Infections due to arthropods can be controlled by preventing their access to the host. Improving living conditions and avoiding sharing common personal items like hats and hair brushes may minimize these infections due to arthropods. Permethrin (1% to 5%) is an effective agent for all these infections.

Abbreviations Introduced in This Chapter

CDC   Centers for Disease Control and Prevention
CF   Complement fixation
DEET   *N,N*-Diethylmetatoluamide
ELISA Enzyme-linked immunosorbent assay
IgA   Immunoglobulin A
PCR   Polymerase chain reaction

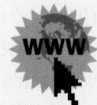 Self-assessment questions and answers are available at *http://www.mhpharmacotherapy.com/pp.html.*

REFERENCES

1. Goswami ND, Shah JS, Corey GR, Stout JE. Short report: Persistent eosinophilia and *Strongyloides* infection in Montagnard refugees after presumptive albendazole therapy. Am J Trop Med Hyg 2009;81:302–304.
2. Freedman DO, Weld LH, Kozarsky PE, et al. Spectrum of disease and relation to place of exposure among ill returned travelers. N Engl J Med 2006;354:119–130.
3. Garcia LS. Malaria. Clin Lab Med 2010;30:93–129.
4. Chen LH, Wilson ME, Schlagenhauf P. Controversies and misconceptions in malaria chemoprophylaxis for travelers. JAMA 2007;297: 2251–2263.
5. Mali S, Tan KR, Arguin PM. Malaria Surveillance—United States, 2009. MMWR SurveillSumm 2011;60:1–15.
6. Munoz P, Valerio M, Puga D, Bouza E. Parasitic infections in solid organ transplant recipients. Infect Dis Clin N Amer 2010;24:461–495.
7. Franco-Paredes C, Santos-Preciado JI. Problem pathogens: Prevention of malaria in travelers. Lancet Infect Dis 2006;6:139–149.
8. Biggs B-A, Caruana S, Mihrshahi S, et al. Short report: Management of chronic strongyloidiasis in Immigrants and Refugees: Is serologic testing useful? Am J Trop Med Hyg 2009;80:788–791.
9. John DT, Petri WA Jr. Markell and Voge's Medical Parasitology. 9th ed. Philadelphia, PA: Saunders; 2006.
10. Escobedo AA, Cimerman S. Giardiasis: A Pharmacotherapy Review. Expert Opin Pharmacother 2007;8(12):1885–1902.
11. Hill DR, Nash TE. Giardia lamblia. In: Mandell GL, Bennett JE, Dolin R, eds. Principles and Practice of Infectious Diseases. 7th ed. New York: Elsevier Churchill-Livingstone; 2010:3527–3534.
12. Drugs for parasitic infections. In: Handbook of Antimicrobial Therapy. 18th ed. New Rochelle, NY: Medical Letter; 2008:225–280.
13. Escobedo AA, Cimerman S. Giardiasis: A pharmacotherapy review. Expert Opin Pharmacother 2007;8:1885–1902.
14. Eisenstein L, Bodager D, Ginzl D. Outbreak of Giardiasis and Cryptosporidiosis associated with a neighborhood interactive water fountain–Florida, 2006. J Environ Health 2008;71:18–22.
15. Grazioli B, Matera G, Laratta C, et al. *Giardia lamblia* infection in patients with irritable bowel syndrome and dyspepsia: A prospective study. World J Gastroenterol 2006;12:1941–1944.
16. Escobedo AA, Alvarez G, Gonzalez ME, et al. The treatment of giardiasis in children: a single-dose tinidazole comparing with 3 days of Nitazoxanide. Ann Trop Med Parasitol 2008;102:199–207.
17. Solaymani-Mohammadi S, Petri WA Jr. Intestinal invasion by *Entamoeba histolytica*. Subcell Biochem 2008;47:221–232.
18. Farthing MJG. Intestinal protozoa. *Entamoeba histolytica*. In: Manson's Tropical Diseases. 22nd ed. London: WB Saunders; 2009:1375–1386.
19. Kimura M, Nakamura T, Nawa Y. Experience with intravenous metronidazole to treat moderate-to-severe amebiasis in Japan. Am J Trop Med Hyg 2007;77:381–385.

20. Petri WA Jr, Haque R. Entamoeba species, including amebiasis. In: Mandell GL, Bennett JA, Dolin R, eds. Principles and Practice of Infectious Diseases. 7th ed. New York: Elsevier Churchill-Livingstone; 2010:3411–3425.

21. Rao S, Solaymani-Mohammadi S, Petri WA Jr, Parker SK. Hepatic amebiasis: A reminder of the complications. Curr Opin Pediat 2009;21:145–149.

22. Bercu TE, Petri WA Jr, Behm BW. Amebic colitis: New insights into pathogenesis and treatment. Curr Gastroenterol Rep 2007;9:429–433.

23. Athie-Gutierrez C, Rodea-Rosas H, Guizar-Bermudez C, Alcantara A, MontalvoJave E. Evolution of surgical treatment of amebiasis-associated colon perforation. J Gastrointest Surg 2010;14:82–87.

24. Maguire JH. Intestinal nematodes (roundworms). In: Mandell GL, Bennett JE, Dolin R, eds. Principles and Practice of Infectious Diseases. 7th ed. New York: Elsevier Churchill-Livingstone; 2010:3577–3586.

25. Bethony J, Brooker S, Albonico M, et al. Soil-transmitted helminth infection: Ascariasis, trichuriasis, and hookworm. Lancet 2006;367:1521–1532.

26. Pasricha S-R, Caruana SR, Phu TQ, et al. Anemia, iron deficiency, meat consumption, and hookworm infection in women of reproductive age in Northwest Vietnam. Am J Trop Med Hyg 2008;78:375–381.

27. Jardin-Botelho A, Raff S, Hoffman HJ, et al. Hookworm, *Ascaris lumbricoides* infection and polyparasitism associated with poor cognitive performance in Brazilian schoolchildren. Trop Med Int Health 2008;13:994–1004.

28. Shah JJ, Maloney SA, Liu Y, et al. Evaluation of the impact of overseas pre-departure treatment for infection with intestinal parasites among Montagnard refugees migrating from Cambodia to North Carolina. Am J Trop Med Hyg 2008;78:754–759.

29. Shah OJ, Zargar SA, Robbani I. Biliary ascariasis: A Review. World J Surg 2006;30:1500–1506.

30. Keiser J, Utzinger J. Efficacy of current drugs against soil-transmitted helminth infections. Systematic review and meta-analysis. JAMA 2008;299:1937–1948.

31. Huratado RM, Sahani DV, Kradin RL. Case records of the Massachusetts General Hospital. Case 9-2006. A 35-year-old woman with recurrent-upper-quadrant pain. N Engl J Med 2006;354:1295–1303.

32. Sodergren MH, Jethwa P, Wilkinson S, Kerwat R. Presenting features of *Enterobius vermicularis* in the vermiform appendix. Scand J Gastroenterol 2009;44:457–461.

33. Balagopal A, Mills L, Shah A, Subramaniam A. Detection and treatment of Strongyloides hyperinfection syndrome following lung transplantation. Transpl Infect Dis 2009;11:149–154.

34. Basile A, Simzar S, Benton J, et al. Disseminated *Strongyloides* stercoralis. Hyperinfection during medical immunosuppression. J Am AcadDermatol 2010;63:896–902.

35. Rodriguez-Hernandez MJ, Ruiz-Perez-Pipaon M, Canas E, Bernal C, Gavilan F. Strongyloides stercoralis hyperinfection transmitted by liver allograft in a transplant recipient. Am J Transplant 2009;9:2637–2640.

36. Bush LM, de Almeida KNF, Perez MT. Severe strongyloidiasis associated with subclinical Human T-Cell Leukemia/Lymphoma Virus-1 infection. Infect Dis Clin Pract 2009;17:84–89.

37. Aregawi D, Lopez D, Wick M, Scheld WM, Schiff D. Disseminated strongyloidiasis complicating glioblastoma therapy: a case report. J Neurooncolog 2009;94:439–443.

38. Marty FM. Editorial. Strongyloides hyperinfection syndrome and transplantation: a preventable, frequently fatal infection. Transpl Infect Dis 2009;11:97–99.

39. Leung V, Al-Rawahi GN, Grant J, Fleckenstein L, Bowie W. Case report: Failure of subcutaneous ivermectin in treating Strongyloides hyperinfection. Am J Trop Med Hyg 2008;79:853–855.

40. King CH, Fairley JK. Cestodes (tapeworms). In: Mandell GL, Dolin R, Bennett JE, eds. Principles and Practice of Infectious Diseases. 7th ed. New York: Elsevier Churchill-Livingstone; 2010:3607–3616.

41. Cardenas G, Jung H, Rios C, Fleury A, Sato-Hernandez JL. Severe cysticercal meningitis: clinical and imaging characteristics. Am J Trop Med Hyg 2010;82:121–125.

42. Serpa JA, Graviss EA, Kass JS, White AC Jr. Neurocysticercosis in Houston, Texas. An Update. Medicine 2011;90:81–86.

43. Sorrillo F, Wilkins P, Shafir S, Eberhard M. Public health implications of cysticercosis acquired in the United States. Emerging Infect Dis 2011;17:1–6.

44. Hajek J, Keystone J. Intraventricular neurocysticercosis managed with albendazole and dexamethasone. Can J Neurol Sci 2009;36:102–104.

45. White AC Jr. New developments in the management of neurocysticercosis. Clin Infect Dis 2009;199:1261–1262.

46. Gongora-Rivera F, Soto-Hernandez JL, Esquivel DG, et al. Albendazole trial at 15 or 30 mg/kg/day for subarachnoid and intraventricular cysticercosis. Neurology 2006;66:436–438.

47. Fairhurst RM, Wellems TE. Plasmodium species (malaria). In: Mandell GL, Dolin R, Bennett JE, eds. Principles and Practice of Infectious Diseases. 7th ed. New York: Elsevier Churchill-Livingstone; 2010:3437–3462.

48. White NJ, Breman JG. Malaria and babesiosis: Diseases caused by red blood cell parasites. In: Harrison's Principles of Internal Medicine. 18th ed. New York: McGraw-Hill; 2008:1280–1294.

49. Newman RD, Parise ME, Barber AM, Steketee RW. Malaria-related deaths among travelers, 1963-2001. Ann Intern Med 2004;141:547–555.

50. Scuracchio P, VieraSD, Dourado DA, et al. Transfusion-transmitted malaria: a case report of asymptomatic donor harboring *Plasmodium malariae*. Rev Inst Med Trop Sao Paulo 2011;53:55–59.

51. White NJ. Malaria. In: Cook GC, Zumla A, eds. Manson's Tropical Diseases. 22st ed. London: WB Saunders; 2009:1201–1300.

52. Crawley J, Chu C, Mtove G, Nosten F. Malaria in children. Lancet 2010;375:1468–1481.

53. John CC, Bangirana P, Byarugaba J et al. Cerebral malaria in children is associated with long-term cognitive impairment. Pediatr 2008;122:e92–e99.

54. Day N, Dondorp AM. The management of patients with severe malaria. Am J Trop Med Hyg 2007;77(Suppl): 29–35.

55. Ehrich JHH, Eke FU. Malaria-induced renal damage: facts and myths. Pediatr Nephrol 2007;22:626–637.

56. Mishra SK, Wiese L. Advances in the management of cerebral malaria in adults. Curr Opin Neurol 2009;22:302–307.

57. Szczepiorkowsi Z, Winters JL, Bandarenko N, et al. Guidelines on the use of therapeutic apheresis in clinical practice—evidence-based approach from the Apheresis Applications Committee of the American Society of Apheresis. J Clin Apheresis 2010;25:83–177.

58. Schantz-Dunn J, Nour NM. Malaria and Pregnancy: A Global Health Perspective. Rev Obstet Gynecol 2009;2:186–192.

59. Murray CK, Gasser RA Jr, Magill AJ, Miller RS. Update on rapid diagnostic testing of malaria. Clin Microbiol Rev 2008;21:97–110.

60. Freedman DO. Malaria prevention in short-term travelers. N Engl J Med 2008;359:603–612.

61. Schlagenhauf P, Petersen E. Malaria chemoprophylaxis: strategies for risk groups. Clin Microbiol Rev 2008;21:466–472.

62. Chen LH, Wilson ME, Schlagenhauf P. Controversies and misconceptions in malaria chemoprophylaxis for travelers. JAMA 2007;297:2257–2263.

63. Taylor WRJ, White NJ. Antimalarial drug toxicity. Drug Saf 2004;27:25–61.

64. Ward SA, Sevene EJP, Hastings IM, Nosten F, McGreasly R. Antimalarial drugs and pregnancy: safety, pharmacokinetics, and pharmacovigilance. Lancet Infect Dis 2007;7:136–144.

65. Goodman AL, Draper SJ. Blood-stage malaria vaccines—recent progress and future challenges. Ann Trop Med Parasitol 2010;104:189–211.

66. Winzeler EA. Malaria research in the post-genomic era. Nature 2008;455:751–756.

67. Roestenberg M, McCall M, Hopman J, et al. Protection against a malaria challenge by sporozoite inoculation. N Engl J Med 2009;361:468–477.

68. Griffith KS, Lewis LS, Mali S, et al. Treatment of malaria in the United States: A systematic review. JAMA 2007;297:2185–2186.

69. Rathore D, McCutchan TF, Sullivan M, Kumar S. Antimalarial drugs: Current status and new developments. Expert Opin Investig Drugs 2006;14:871–883.

70. Feachem R, Sabot O. A new global malaria eradication strategy. Lancet 2008;371:1633–1635.

71. Rosenthal PJ. Artesunate for the treatment of severe Falciparum malaria. N Engl J Med 2008;358:1829–1836.

72. Noedl H, Socheat D, Satimai W. Artemisinin-resistant malaria in Asia. N Engl J Med 2009;361:540–541.

73. Douglas NM, Anstey NM, Angus BJ, Nosten F, Price RN. Artemisinin combination therapy for vivax malaria. Lancet Infect Dis 2010;10: 405–416.

74. Rosenthal PJ. Antiprotozoal drugs. In: Katzung BG, ed. Basic and Clinical Pharmacology. 11th ed. New York: Lange Medical Books/ McGraw-Hill; 2009:899–921.

75. Rassi A Jr, Rassi A, Marin-Neto AM. Chagas disease. Lancet 2010;375:1388–1402.

76. Marin-Neto JA, Cunha-Neto E, Maciel BC, Simoes MV. Pathogenesis of chronic Chagas heart disease. Circulation 2007;115:1109–1123.

77. Kirchhoff LV. Trypanosoma species (American trypanosomiasis, Chagas' disease): Biology of trypanosomes. In: Mandell GL, Bennett JE, Dolin R, eds. Principles and Practice of Infectious Diseases. 7th ed. New York: Elsevier Churchill-Livingstone; 2010:3481–3488.

78. Milei J, Guerri-Guttenberg A, Grana DR, Storino R. Prognostic impact of Chagas Disease in the United States Am Heart J 2009;157:22–29.

79. Nunes MCP, Barbosa MM, Ribeiro AL, Barbosa FBL, Rocha MOC. Ischemic cerebrovascular events in patients with Chagas cardiomyopathy: A prospective followup study. J Neurol Sci 2009;278:96–101.

80. Bern C, Montgomery SP, Katz L, Caglioti S, Stramer SL. Chagas disease and the US blood supply. Curr Opin Infect Dis 2008;21:476–482.

81. Kun H, Moore A, Mascola L, et al. Transmission of *Trypanosoma cruzi* by heart transplantation. Clin Infect Dis 2009;48:1534–1540.

82. Viotti R, Vigliano C, Lococo B, et al. Long-term cardiac outcomes of treating chronic Chagas disease with benznidazole versus no treatment. A nonrandomized trial. Ann Intern Med 2006;144: 724–734.

83. Rosenthal PJ. Clinical pharmacology of the anthelmintic drugs. In: Katzung BG, ed. Basic and Clinical Pharmacology. 11th ed. New York: Lange Medical Books/McGraw-Hill; 2009:923–934.

84. Diaz SH. Lice (pediculosis). In: Mandell GL, Bennett JR, Dolin R, eds. Principles and Practice of Infectious Diseases. 7th ed. New York: Elsevier Churchill-Livingstone; 2010:3629–3632.

85. Diamantis S, Morrell DS, Burkhart CN. Treatment of head lice. Dermatologic Therapy 2009;22:273–278.

86. Idriss S, Levitt J. Malathion for head lice and scabies: treatment and safety considerations. J Drugs Dermatology 2009;8:715–720.

87. Chosidow O, Giraudeau B, Cottrell J, et al. Oral ivermectin versus malathion lotion for difficult-to-treat head lice. N Engl J Med 2010;362: 896–905.

88. Lebwohl M, Clark L, Levitt J. Therapy for head lice based on life cycle, resistance, and safety. Pediatr 2007;119:965–974.

89. Hicks MI, Elston DM. Scabies. Derm Ther 2009;22:279–292.

90. Currie BJ, McCarthy JS. Permethrin and ivermectin for scabies. N Engl J Med 2010;362:717–725.

91. Stough D, Shellabager S, Quiring J, Gabrielsen Jr AA. Efficacy and safety of Spinosad and Permethrin Creme for Pediculosis Capitis (Head Lice). Pediatr 2009;124:e389.

79 Urinary Tract Infections

Warren E. Rose and Kathryn R. Matthias

● **Upon completion of the chapter, the reader will be able to:**

1. Determine the diagnostic criteria for significant bacteriuria.

2. Interpret the signs and symptoms of urinary tract infections (UTIs) and differentiate those of upper versus lower urinary tract disease.

3. Identify the organism responsible for the majority of uncomplicated UTIs.

4. Assess the laboratory tests that help in diagnosing patients with UTI.

5. Recommend appropriate drug, dose, and duration for uncomplicated and complicated UTI prophylaxis and empiric treatment.

6. Evaluate and select therapy for uncomplicated and complicated UTIs based on specific urine culture results and patient characteristics.

7. Formulate appropriate monitoring and education information for patients with UTIs.

KEY CONCEPTS

❶ Urinary tract infections (UTIs) are thought of as either uncomplicated or complicated. Generally this refers to absence or presence, respectively, of functional or structural abnormalities within the urinary tract.

❷ The majority of uncomplicated UTIs are the result of a single causative organism, which is primarily *Escherichia coli* in up to 85% of cases. The remaining 15% are caused by *Staphylococcus saprophyticus* along with *Klebsiella* species (spp.), *Proteus* spp., *Pseudomonas* spp., *Enterobacter* spp., and *Enterococcus* spp.

❸ Symptoms of lower UTIs include **dysuria,** gross hematuria, suprapubic heaviness, **nocturia,** increased urinary frequency, and urgency.

❹ Symptoms of upper UTIs include fever, nausea, vomiting, malaise, and often severe flank pain.

❺ The goals of treatment are to eradicate the causative pathogen, to prevent or treat consequences of infection, and to prevent, if possible, recurrence of infection.

❻ Uncomplicated UTIs may be managed with a short course antimicrobial therapy with one-dose, 3-day, or 5-day regimens, depending on the clinical factors.

❼ Complicated UTIs including acute pyelonephritis should be treated for at least 7 days and sometimes 2 weeks or longer.

❽ Treatment of catheterized patients with bacteriuria should follow one of two treatment algorithms: (a) for

asymptomatic patients, hold antibiotics and remove the catheter if possible; or (b) for symptomatic patients, initiate antibiotic therapy and remove the catheter if possible.

❾ Any urinary tract infection in a male is considered complicated and should be treated with at least 2 weeks of targeted antimicrobial therapy. Male patients with prostatic sources or prior treatment failure should be treated for up to 6 weeks.

Urinary tract infections (UTIs) are comprised of a diverse array of syndromes depending on the location of the infection within the urinary tract.[1-3] UTIs occur frequently and are responsible for approximately 5.3 million annual visits to primary care and surgical specialty offices along with approximately 2.6 million annual visits to hospital outpatient and emergency departments.[4,5] In simplest of terms, a UTI is defined by microorganism(s) in the urinary tract, which does not represent contamination.

Bacteriuria, or bacteria in the urine, does not always represent infection. For this reason a number of quantitative diagnostic criteria have been created (Table 79–1) to identify the amount of bacteria in the urine that most likely represents true infection (hence the term "significant bacteriuria").[6] Furthermore, UTIs are classified as lower tract or upper tract disease. Patients can present differently with upper versus lower tract disease, and upper tract disease is thought of as a

---

Table 79–1

Diagnostic Criteria for Significant Bacteriuria

- Greater than or equal to 10^2 CFU coliforms/mL (10^5 CFU/L) or greater than or equal to 10^5 CFU noncoliforms/mL (10^8 CFU/L) in a symptomatic female
- Greater than or equal to 10^3 CFU organisms/mL (10^6 CFU/L) in a symptomatic male
- Greater than or equal to 10^5 CFU same organisms/mL (10^8 CFU/L) in asymptomatic individuals on two consecutive specimens
- Any growth of bacteria on suprapubic catheterization in a symptomatic patient
- Greater than or equal to 10^2 CFU organisms/mL in a catheterized patient

---

Patient Encounter, Part 1

BM is a 25-year-old female who presents to a local primary care physician with complaints of painful urination, blood in her urine with last menstrual cycle 3 weeks ago, and frequent need to urinate especially at night, which began 5 days ago. She denies vomiting, fever, nausea, or flank pain. Upon questioning she does admit that she is sexually active with only one partner and uses oral contraceptives. She also uses spermicidal jellies occasionally when she is noncompliant with the daily oral contraceptive regimen. She states that she had a similar episode approximately 3 months earlier.

What symptoms are suggestive of a lower urinary tract infection (UTI)?

What risk factors does she have for a UTI?

What additional patient information is required before creating an appropriate treatment plan for this patient?

---

much more severe infection since patients are more likely to be admitted to the hospital. An example of lower tract syndrome is cystitis, which involves inflammation of the bladder and commonly causes symptoms such as dysuria, nocturia, gross hematuria, and occasional suprapubic tenderness. An example of upper urinary tract disease is pyelonephritis. Pyelonephritis is an inflammation of the kidney that is usually due to infection. Patients with uncomplicated UTI are more frequently treated as outpatients as compared with those patients with complicated UTIs.

EPIDEMIOLOGY AND ETIOLOGY

The prevalence and type of UTIs generally vary by age and gender.[7-9] UTIs may occur at any age, even in infants. Premature infants, for example, have a higher rate than full-term infants, and neonatal boys are five to eight times more likely to have UTIs than neonatal girls. In young children 1 to 5 years of age, significant bacteriuria occurs more in girls than boys, 4.5% compared with 0.5%, respectively.[10] Once adulthood is reached, bacteriuria increases in young, nonpregnant women (range, 1% to 3%), yet remains low in men (up to 0.1%).[11] Symptomatic UTI affects 30% of women between 20 and 40 years of age, which represents a prevalence that is 30 times greater than that of men in the same age group. Upwards of 40% to 50% of the female population will experience a symptomatic UTI at some time during their life.[4]

The etiology of UTIs has remained relatively unchanged over the past several decades. ❶ *UTIs are either uncomplicated or complicated.* There is a lack of consensus regarding the definition of what makes a UTI complicated (specifically in postmenopausal women or patients with diabetes mellitus), but in general, a complicated UTI refers to a structural or functional abnormality of the urinary tract.[1] Patients with complicated UTIs are typically given longer treatment durations than those patients with uncomplicated infections. Those with complicated UTIs by definition are also prone to more frequent infections. It is important to note that an upper UTI does not necessarily imply complicated UTI, nor does lower UTI imply uncomplicated UTI.

The frequency of causative organisms changes depending on the location of infection and patient characteristics. ❷ Almost all uncomplicated UTIs are the result of a single causative organism, which is primarily *Escherichia coli* in up to 85% of cases.[12] A variety of other organisms may cause uncomplicated UTIs, but represent the minority of pathogens. Other organisms include gram-positives such as *Staphylococcus saprophyticus* and *Enterococcus* spp. and gram-negative bacteria such as *Pseudomonas aeruginosa*, *Klebsiella pneumoniae*, *Proteus* spp., and *Enterobacter* spp.[13-15] The chances of isolating an organism other than *E. coli* are higher in patients who have recurrent UTIs, particularly those patients whose UTIs are considered complicated. It is also more common for organisms other than *E. coli* to cause UTIs in the hospitalized population than in the general population.[16,17]

PATHOPHYSIOLOGY

There are three potential ways for bacteria to enter into the urinary tract and cause infection: the ascending, hematogenous, and lymphatic pathways.

Ascending Pathway

The ascending pathway occurs when bacteria colonizing the urethra subsequently travel upwards, or ascend, the urethra to the bladder and cause cystitis (Fig. 79–1). The ascending route may help to explain why UTIs occur more commonly in women than in men. Women have a shorter urethra than men, and colonization of the female urethra is likely due to its proximity to the perirectal area. The use of spermicidal agents increases the colonization of the vagina with uropathogens.[18] Additionally, massage of the urethra in women as well as sexual intercourse may

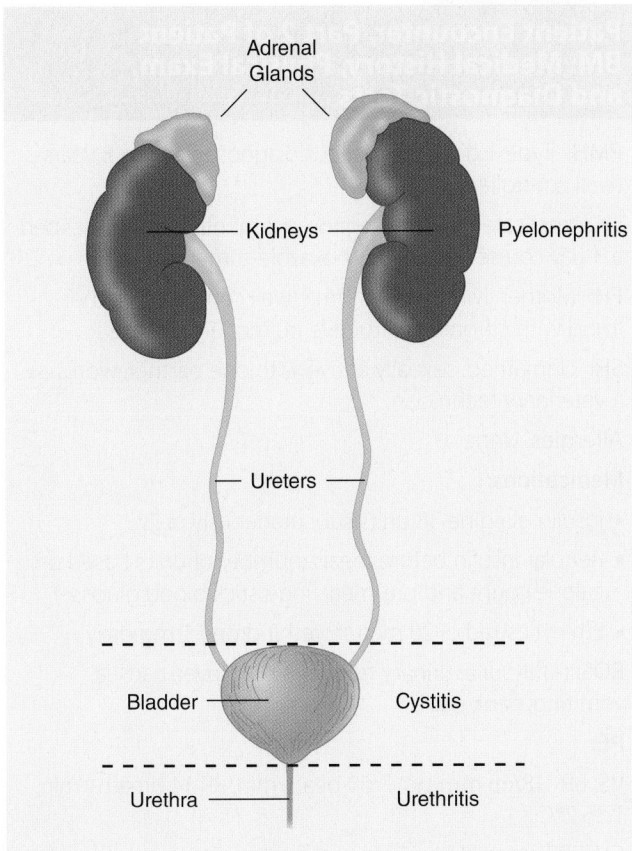

FIGURE 79–1. Anatomy and associated infections of the urinary tract. (From Sprandel KA, Lesch CA, Rodvold KA. Lower urinary tract infection. In: Schwinghammer TL (ed). Pharmacotherapy Casebook: A Patient-Focused Approach. 6th ed. New York City: McGraw-Hill; 2005:315; With permission).

lead to bacteria gaining entrance into the bladder.[19,20] Once in the bladder, bacteria are not limited to causing cystitis. These bacteria may continue to ascend the urinary tract via the ureters and cause more complicated infections, such as pyelonephritis.

Hematogenous Pathway

The hematogenous route occurs through the seeding of the urinary tract with pathogens carried by the blood supply. These pathogens represent an infection at some other primary site in the body. *Staphylococcus aureus* bacteremia, for example, can cause renal abscesses via the hematogenous route, and pyelonephritis can be experimentally produced in rabbits by IV injection of *Salmonella* spp., *Mycobacterium tuberculosis*, or even yeast (*Candida* spp.).[21] However, experimentally creating this pathway has not been successful with all organisms. Experimental hematogenous seeding of the kidneys could not be created with the IV injection of large inocula of *E. coli* or *P. aeruginosa* in a mouse model.[22]

Lymphatic Pathway

The lymphatic system, also known as the secondary circulatory system, connects the bladder to the kidney and may represent a way for bacteria to be transported and subsequently cause infection. Although this pathway is classically included as a route of infection, there is a lack of data showing the lymphatic pathway as a significant mechanism for development of infection. As a result this pathway is not believed to be a significant host mechanism.

Host Defense Mechanisms

Urine possesses characteristics that are less than ideal for bacterial metabolism and growth. Some of these characteristics include low pH, significant urea concentration, and high osmolality. Also, bacteria in the bladder can stimulate an urge to urinate. Additionally, prostatic fluid secretions in men can inhibit bacterial growth, whereas normal vaginal flora in women such as *Lactobacillus* spp. can secrete lactic acid, which can decrease the pH of the enviroment.[23-25]

There are several other host factors that inhibit bacterial virulence factors. These virulence factors are mechanisms that bacteria utilize to cause infection and/or ensure their survival. The first is glycosaminoglycan, a compound produced by the body that coats the epithelial cells of the bladder. This compound essentially separates the bladder from the urine by forming a protective layer against bacterial adhesion.[26] A second compound known as Tamm-Horsfall protein is secreted into the urine and prevents *E. coli* from binding to receptors present on the surface of the bladder. Other factors implicated in contributing to host defense mechanisms against UTIs include immunoglobulins, specifically IgA.

Risk Factors

There are several risk factors for development of UTIs.[11] Common risk factors for UTIs in women include sexual intercourse, use of a cervical diaphragm, use of spermicidal jellies, diabetes, and pregnancy.[27-29] In men, the risks are increased in uncircumcised males and older age men with **prostatic hyperplasia**. Common risk factors for both men and women include urologic instrumentation, urethral catheterization, renal transplantation, neurogenic bladder, and urinary tract obstruction.[30,31]

TREATMENT
Desired Outcomes

⑤ *The goals of treatment are to eradicate the causative pathogen, prevent or treat consequences of infection, administer targeted antimicrobial therapy for the identified or most likely pathogen, and prevent, if possible, recurrence of infection.* Therapy is directed at microbiologic eradication of the offending organism through antibiotics with a defined duration of treatment based on the UTI classification.

Clinical Presentation and Diagnosis of UTIs

General

- Most women present with hematuria; however, this is not a presentation restricted only to UTIs.
- Elderly patients frequently will not present with common signs and symptoms of UTI, but may present with altered mental status.
- More than 95% of uncomplicated UTIs are caused by a single organism.
- Patients may present with urosepsis.

③ *Signs and Symptoms of Lower UTI*

- *Dysuria, gross hematuria, suprapubic heaviness, nocturia, increased urinary frequency and urgency*

④ *Signs and Symptoms of Upper UTI*

- *Fever, nausea, vomiting, malaise, and often severe flank pain*

Laboratory Tests

Urinalysis should show:

- **Pyuria** typically greater than 10 white blood cells/mm³ urine (10×10^6/L)
- Bacteriuria, usually greater than 10^5 CFU organisms/mL (10^8 CFU/L)
- Nitrites present
- Leukocyte esterase present

Other Diagnostic Tests

- Bacterial urine culture
- Presence of costovertebral tenderness (upper UTI only)

Patient Encounter, Part 2 of Patient BM: Medical History, Physical Exam, and Diagnostic Tests

PMH: Type 1 diabetes mellitus diagnosed at age 8 years (well controlled)

Uncomplicated cystitis diagnosed 3 months ago (prescribed a 3-day course of sulfamethoxazole-trimethoprim)

FH: Mother living with asthma (well controlled); father living with chronic obstructive pulmonary disease

SH: Unmarried, sexually active with one partner, works as a veterinary technician

Allergies: None

Medications:

- Insulin glargine 38 units subcutaneously daily
- Regular insulin before meals (number of units based on calorie count and pre-meal fingerstick blood glucose)
- Ethinyl estradiol 20 mcg/norethindrone 1 mg daily

ROS: (+) dysuria, urinary frequency; (–) fever, nausea, vomiting, flank pain

PE:

VS: BP 118/68 mm Hg, P 60 beats/min, RR 14 breaths/min, T 36.2°C

CV: RRR, normal S1, S2; normal findings

Abd: Soft, nontender, nondistended; (+) bowel sounds, no hepatosplenomegaly, heme (–) stool

Lab: Within normal limits including blood glucose; (–) pregnancy test

Urinalysis: Greater than 200 white blood cells/mm³; urine nitrates negative

Urine Gram stain: Gram-negative rods, more than 10^5 CFU/mL

Given this additional information, what is your assessment of the patient's condition?

Identify your treatment goals for the patient.

What nonpharmacologic and pharmacologic alternatives are available for the patient?

General Approach to Treatment

Antimicrobial therapy is the cornerstone of treatment in UTIs. The selected antimicrobial should ideally be well tolerated, lend itself to patient compliance (low total number of doses), have adequate concentrations at the site of the infection in the urinary tract, have good oral bioavailability, and be narrow in antimicrobial spectrum to limit collateral damage and resistance development in human flora not affiliated with the infection.[1] Table 79–2 reviews oral and IV antibiotics frequently used to treat UTIs with comments on their use, and Table 79–3 reviews frequency, duration, and doses of oral antibiotics used commonly for outpatient treatment of UTIs.

Nonpharmacologic Therapy

Although there are limited data in the literature and sometimes conflicting results, several nonpharmacologic therapies have been proposed for prevention of UTIs. The intake of large volumes of cranberry juice has been associated with a decrease in the number of UTIs over a year period in patients with recurrent UTIs in small randomized controlled trials. The efficacy is uncertain in the general population and with smaller intake volumes.[32–34] Probiotics such as *Lactobacillus* spp. have been used to decrease vaginal pH in women and potentially reduce the growth of pathogenic bacteria.[24,25] Topical estrogen replacement therapy significantly decreases the incidence of UTIs in postmenopausal women as compared with placebo.[35] Methenamine hippurate and methenamine mandelate have no antimicrobial properties but decrease the incidence of UTIs when used for prophylaxis. Patient education of common risk factors is important.

Table 79–2

Commonly Used Antimicrobial Agents for the Treatment of UTIs

Agent	Comments
Oral Therapy	

Penicillins
  Amoxicillin
  Amoxicillin-
    clavulanic acid
  Pivmecillinam
	Increasing *E. coli* resistance has limited amoxicillin use in acute cystitis despite broad-spectrum activity. Amoxicillin-clavulanic acid is empirically preferred due to resistance. Ampicillin is the drug of choice for enterococci-sensitive to penicillin, but oral bioavailability is approximately 50%.
	Pivmecillinam is a prodrug of mecillinam and is recommended for treatment of acute cystitis. It should be avoided in patients with suspected pyelonephritis. Neither pivmecillinam nor mecillinam are currently approved for use by the U.S. FDA.

Cephalosporins
  Cefaclor
  Cefadroxil
  Cefixime
  Cefpodoxime
  Cefuroxime
  Cephalexin
  Cephradine
	There are no major advantages of these agents over other oral agents in the treatment of UTIs, and they may have inferior efficacy as compared with other oral agents such as fluoroquinolones. They may be useful in cases of resistance to amoxicillin and trimethoprim-sulfamethoxazole, but concern exists for use as a first-line agent for uncomplicated cystitis therapy due to potential selection of cephalosporin resistant organisms (collateral damage). These agents are not active against enterococci. Susceptibility of cephalexin cannot be accurately predicted based on cefazolin susceptibility testing.

Tetracyclines
  Doxycycline
  Minocycline
  Tetracycline
	These agents have been effective for initial episodes of UTI; however, resistance can develop rapidly. Avoid during pregnancy.

Fluoroquinolones
  Ciprofloxacin
  Levofloxacin
  Norfloxacin
  Ofloxacin
	The newer quinolones have a greater spectrum of activity; rates of resistance are increasing. Concern for use as a first-line agent for uncomplicated UTI therapy exists due to potential selection of multidrug resistant organisms (collateral damage). These agents are often effective for pyelonephritis. Avoid in pregnancy and children. Moxifloxacin is not listed due to limited urinary excretion.

Miscellaneous
  Trimethoprim-
    sulfamethoxazole
	This combination is highly effective against most aerobic enteric bacteria except *P. aeruginosa*. High urinary tract tissue levels and urine levels are achieved, which may be important in complicated UTI treatment. Also effective as prophylaxis for recurrent infections. Generally well tolerated and low cost but increasing resistance rates above 20% in certain regions has limited empiric use. Its use may be precluded in patients with sulfa allergies.

Nitrofurantoin	This agent is effective in treatment and prophylaxis in patients with uncomplicated or recurrent lower tract UTIs. Should not be used in patients with low estimated CrCl (less than 40 to 60 mL/min [0.67 to 1.00 mL/s]) due to limited urine concentrations and potential increased risk of neuropathy.
Azithromycin	Commonly used for sexually transmitted diseases (i.e., chlamydia infections) rather than for UTIs.
Fosfomycin	Single-dose therapy for uncomplicated cystitis. Has been recommended for empiric therapy since resistance rates are low but may have inferior efficacy when compared with short courses of other oral antibiotic agents.
Parenteral Therapy	

Aminoglycosides
  Amikacin
  Gentamicin
  Tobramycin
	Gentamicin and tobramycin are generally equally effective, whereas tobramycin has slightly better coverage of certain *Pseudomonas* spp. Amikacin generally is reserved for multidrug-resistant bacteria. Typically used as a short course of therapy followed by a switch to an oral agent. Concern for neurotoxicity and ototoxicity generally limit use, especially in patients with impaired renal function.

Penicillins
  Ampicillin
  Ampicillin-sulbactam
  Ticarcillin-clavulanate
  Piperacillin
  Piperacillin-tazobactam
	These agents are generally effective for susceptible bacteria. The extended-spectrum penicillins are active against certain strains of *Pseudomonas* spp. They are very useful in renally impaired patients since urine concentration can remain adequate or when an aminoglycoside is avoided. Empiric use of ampicillin with an aminoglycoside is recommended only in patients with suspected infection due to *Enterococcus* spp.

Cephalosporins
  First-, second-, third-, and
    fourth-generation
	Second- and third-generation cephalosporins have a broad spectrum of activity against gram-negative bacteria, but are not active against enterococci. Only ceftazidime and cefepime have activity against certain strains of *Pseudomonas* spp. They are useful for nosocomial infections and urosepsis due to susceptible pathogens. A single ceftriaxone dose could be used in lieu of an IV fluoroquinolone for acute uncomplicated pyelonephritis.

Carbapenems
  Doripenem
  Ertapenem
  Imipenem-cilastatin
  Meropenem
	These agents have broad-spectrum activity, including gram-positive, gram-negative, and anaerobic bacteria. Ertapenem is not active against *Pseudomonas* spp. All may be associated with *Candida* spp. superinfections. Rarely used for UTIs.

(Continued)

Table 79–2

Commonly Used Antimicrobial Agents for the Treatment of UTIs (*Continued*)

Agent	Comments
Fluoroquinolones Ciprofloxacin Levofloxacin	These agents have broad-spectrum activity against both gram-negative and gram-positive bacteria. They provide high urine and tissue concentrations and are actively secreted in reduced renal function. Switch to oral therapy when possible due to excellent bioavailability.
Monobactam Aztreonam	Only active against gram-negative bacteria, including some strains of *P. aeruginosa*. Generally useful for nosocomial infections when aminoglycosides are to be avoided and in patients with type 1/immediate hypersensitivity to penicillins.
Glycopeptide Vancomycin	May be considered in combination for empiric therapy based on patient risk factors for multidrug-resistant organisms and gram-positive cocci shown in urinalysis.

Table 79–3

Overview of Outpatient, Oral Antimicrobial Therapy for Lower and Upper Tract UTIs

Indications	Antibiotic	Adult Dose[a]	Frequency	Duration
Lower Tract UTIs				
Uncomplicated	Nitrofurantoin macrocrystals	100 mg	Every 12 hours	5–7 days
	Nitrofurantoin monohydrate	100 mg	Every 12 hours	5–7 days
	Trimethoprim-sulfamethoxazole	1 DS[b] tablet	Every 12 hours	3 days
	Trimethoprim	100 mg	Every 12 hours	3 days
	Fosfomycin	3,000 mg	Single dose	1 day
	Pivmecillinam[c]	400 mg	Every 12 hours	3–7 days
Alternative options:	Ciprofloxacin	250 mg	Every 12 hours	3 days
	Levofloxacin	250 mg	Every 24 hours	3 days
	Ofloxacin	200 mg	Every 12 hours	3 days
	Amoxicillin-clavulanic acid	500 mg	Every 8 hours	3 days
	Cefdinir	100 mg	Every 12 hours	7 days
	Cefaclor	250–500 mg	Every 8 hours	7 days
	Cefpodoxime-proxetil	100 mg	Every 12 hours	7 days
Complicated	Trimethoprim-sulfamethoxazole	1 DS[b] tablet	Every 12 hours	7–10 days
	Trimethoprim	100 mg	Every 12 hours	7–10 days
	Ciprofloxacin	500 mg	Every 12 hours	7–10 days
	Norfloxacin	400 mg	Every 12 hours	7–10 days
	Levofloxacin	250 mg	Every 24 hours	7–10 days
	Amoxicillin-clavulanic acid	500 mg	Every 8 hours	7–10 days
Recurrent infections—continuous prophylaxis	Trimethoprim-sulfamethoxazole	½ SS[d] tablet	Every 24 hours	6 months
	Trimethoprim	100 mg	Every 24 hours	6 months
	Ciprofloxacin	125 mg	Every 24 hours	6 months
	Nitrofurantoin	50 *or* 100 mg	Every 24 hours	6 months
	Cefaclor	250 mg	Every 24 hours	6 months
	Cephalexin	125 mg	Every 24 hours	6 months
Upper Tract UTIs				
Uncomplicated Acute pyelonephritis[e]	Ciprofloxacin	500 mg	Every 12 hours	7 days
	Ciprofloxacin (extended release)	1,000 mg	Every 24 hours	7 days
	Levofloxacin (extended release)	750 mg	Every 24 hours	5 days
	Trimethoprim-sulfamethoxazole	1 DS[b] tablet	Every 12 hours	14 days

[a]Majority of listed antimicrobial agents require dosage adjustment in patients with significant renal dysfunction.

[b]DS, double strength (160 mg trimethoprim/800 mg sulfamethoxazole).

[c]Not approved for use by the U.S. FDA as of November 2011.

[d]SS, single strength (80 mg trimethoprim/400 mg sulfamethoxazole).

[e]Doses listed for acute pyelonephritis are for oral regimens.

Pharmacologic Therapy

▶ Uncomplicated UTIs

Cystitis Uncomplicated cystitis in patients with absence of fever or flank pain represents the most common type of UTIs. It is frequently managed in the outpatient setting and occurs mostly in women of childbearing age.[1] *E. coli* represent the vast majority of causal organisms in this setting, but a minority of cases may be caused by *S. saprophyticus*, *K. pneumoniae*, *Proteus mirabilis*, *Enterococcus* spp., and a small percentage of other organsims.[12–15] As such, treatment in the outpatient setting is frequently relegated to a urinalysis and empiric therapy without a urine culture.[1,36,37] Patients are subsequently monitored for resolution of signs and symptoms. ❻ *Uncomplicated UTIs may be managed with a short course antimicrobial therapy with one-dose, 3-day, or 5-day regimens depending on the clinical factors involved.*

For acute uncomplicated UTIs, it is reasonable to pursue oral empiric therapy with one dose (3,000 mg) of fosfomycin, a 3-day course of trimethoprim-sulfamethoxazole (one double-strength tablet twice daily), or a 5-day course of nitrofurantoin (100 mg twice daily) depending on the patient's characteristics and risk factors.[1] The antibiotic selection for empiric therapy partly depends on known resistance rates in the geographic region, particularly *E. coli* resistance to trimethoprim-sulfamethoxazole.[12,38,39] Empiric therapy with trimethoprim-sulfamethoxazole should be considered only if the local resistance rates in *E. coli* is less than 20%, due to poor UTI treatment responses with trimethoprim-sulfamethoxazole when resistance rates are above this threshold.[1,40] Although fluoroquinolone antibiotics and certain β-lactam agents can be highly active and efficacious against *E. coli*, these agents should be considered alternative agents in uncomplicated UTIs due to their broad-spectrum activity and risk of resistance development in bacteria unaffiliated with the infection.[1]

▶ Complicated UTIs

❼ Complicated UTIs including acute pyelonephritis should be treated for at least 7 days and sometimes 2 weeks or longer.

▶ Acute Pyelonephritis

In contrast to patients who present with lower UTIs, those who present with pyelonephritis usually have high-grade fever (greater than 38.3°C [100.9°F]) and severe flank pain. Select patients with pyelonephritis may be treated in the outpatient setting; however, patients whose infection is severe enough to cause vomiting, decreased food intake, and dehydration may need to be treated in an inpatient hospitalized setting. These patients will often receive IV antibiotics initially before being switched to oral therapy depending on susceptibility testing.

Patients with pyelonephritis are traditionally given 14 days of therapy; however, there are limited data showing success in treating acute uncomplicated pyelonephritis for 7 to 10 days. More studies need to be conducted to determine the efficacy for shorter duration regimens.[1] Gram stain and culture are important in ensuring that appropriate antimicrobial coverage is selected. Stratification is used to manage patients with acute pyelonephritis. Women who present with mild cases of pyelonephritis (defined as low-grade fever and a normal to slightly elevated peripheral white blood count, without nausea or vomiting) may be treated as outpatients.[1] Those patients who exhibit more severe signs and symptoms will need to be admitted to an acute care setting for appropriate treatment. The same holds true for antibiotic selection in these patients. Those who are treated in an outpatient setting can be treated with trimethoprim-sulfamethoxazole, fluoroquinolones, or even β-lactam/β-lactamase inhibitors, such as amoxicillin-clavulanic acid. In cases where an initial, one-time IV antibiotic is used as supplemental therapy, a single ceftriaxone dose or single high-dose aminoglycoside therapy could be used in lieu of an IV fluoroquinolone. This practice is a recommended addition to therapy if local prevalence of fluoroquinolone resistance exceeds 10%.[1] In those patients who are admitted to the hospital, antibiotic therapy is usually broader in nature, especially in patients suspected of having bacteremia or **urosepsis**. These patients will typically receive IV therapy such as a fluoroquinolone or a β-lactam plus an aminoglycoside.[1,41,42] When selecting fluoroquinolone antibiotics for treatment of gram-negative pyelonephritis, ciprofloxacin may be ideal due to its relatively narrow spectrum of activity against these organisms.[1]

⚲ Special Populations

▶ Pregnant Women

Changes to the urinary tract in pregnant women predispose them to an increased incidence of bacteriuria and subsequent UTIs that may follow. These changes include alterations in amino acid and other nutrient concentrations in the urine along with physiologic changes such as reduced bladder tone and dilation of the renal pelvis and ureters.[43,44]

An association exists between maternal UTI during pregnancy and fetal death, mental retardation, and developmental delay.[45] Due to this known association and because up to 7% of pregnant women will develop an asymptomatic bacteriuria that may progress to pyelonephritis, screening for UTI is necessary.[2,27] In pregnant patients with significant bacteriuria, whether symptomatic or asymptomatic, treatment is recommended to avoid these complications. In the majority of patients, a sulfonamide (with the exception of use during the third trimester due to concerns for hyperbilirubinemia), amoxicillin-clavulanic acid, cephalexin, or nitrofurantoin are effective treatment options. Tetracyclines and fluoroquinolones should be avoided due to risk of teratogenicity and ability to inhibit cartilage and bone development, respectively. Follow-up usually consists of a urine culture 1 to 2 weeks after completion of therapy and then subsequent monthly urine cultures until birth.

▶ *Catheterized Patients*

An indwelling catheter is commonly used in various healthcare settings and is associated with UTIs.[30,46] Bacteria may be introduced into the bladder via the catheter in several ways, including direct infection introduction during catheterization (via colonization and subsequently traveling the length of the catheter through bacterial motility or capillary action). UTIs as a result of an indwelling catheter are common and occur at a rate of 5% per day of catheter presence.[47]

The approach to management of a patient with bacteriuria and an indwelling urinary catheter follows two paths.[46] ⑧ *The first, in asymptomatic patients with catheterization, is to hold antibiotics and remove the catheter if possible. The second, in symptomatic patients with catheterization, is to initiate antibiotic therapy and remove the catheter if possible.* In both of the above situations, if discontinuation of the catheter is not possible, the patient should be recatheterized with a new urinary catheter if the previous catheter is greater than 2 weeks old.[46]

▶ *UTIs in Men*

⑨ *Although UTIs in men are not always complicated by definition, due to the relative infrequency of UTIs in men compared with women, an abnormality (structural or functional) should be suspected and therefore treated as a probable complicated infection until proven otherwise.*[48] For this reason, men should not be treated with a single dose or short course of therapy if diagnosed with a UTI. Typically these patients will receive 2 weeks of therapy and in situations of failure may be treated up to 6 weeks, particularly if a prostatic source of infection is suspected. Prostatic enlargement, as previously mentioned, is a risk

---

Patient Encounter, Part 3: Creating a Care Plan

Based on the information presented, create a care plan for this patient's UTI. Your plan should include:

(a) A statement of the drug-related needs and/or problems

(b) A patient-specific detailed therapeutic plan

(c) Monitoring parameters to assess efficacy and safety

---

factor in men, and the prevalence of benign prostatic hyperplasia in the elderly population may predispose this population to UTIs.

OUTCOME EVALUATION

- Monitor the patient for resolution of symptoms, with a goal of 48 to 72 hours to resolution after start of antimicrobial therapy.

- If possible, follow up on susceptibilities of the infecting organism (urine culture).

- Repeat culture is necessary only if symptoms do not acutely abate or reinfection or recurrence occurs. Resistance rates to *E. coli* are increasing to several of the agents commonly prescribed for UTI, and certain isolates are multidrug resistant.[49]

- Depending on chosen antibiotic therapy, evaluate the patient based on drug therapy monitoring parameters including those presented in Table 79–4 to optimize therapy and decrease incidence of adverse drug events.

Table 79–4			
Monitoring Parameters for Select Antibiotics Used in the Treatment of UTIs			
Drug Class or Drug	**What to Monitor**	**Frequency**	**Endpoint**
Aminoglycosides	SCr, urine output	Every 24 hours	Prevention of nephrotoxicity manifested by a rise in SCr
	Aminoglycoside serum concentrations	Depends on duration of therapy. At least once weekly; more frequently if evidence of changing renal function	Trough serum concentrations less than 2 mg/L (less than 4.2 μmol/L for gentamicin and less than 4.3 μmol/L for tobramycin) or less than 8 mg/L (13.7 μmol/L) for amikacin,[a] to decrease risk of nephrotoxicity and ototoxicity
Nitrofurantoin	SCr	Only if renal function changing or unstable	Nitrofurantoin metabolites may accumulate in renal insufficiency and lead to neuropathy; avoid if CrCl less than 40 mL/min (0.67 mL/s)
	Liver profile	Periodic monitoring	Prevention of cholestasis
Aminoglycosides Nitrofurantoin Tetracyclines Sulfonamides	SCr	Only if renal function changing or unstable	Decreases in glomerular filtrate rate can significantly decrease the urine concentration of these agents

[a]Streptomycin concentrations are different than those listed here; because streptomycin is not used to treat UTIs, monitoring for this agent is not included.

Patient Care and Monitoring

1. Assess the patient's symptoms to determine response to the antimicrobial regimen you have chosen.

2. Review any microbiologic data:
   - Based on urinalysis and Gram stain (if available), is your empiric selection reasonable?
   - Based on culture and susceptibility data (if available), are there any changes that need to be made from your initial empiric antimicrobial selection (i.e., resistance to the regimen initially selected)?

3. Determine whether the patient may benefit from prophylactic therapy (i.e., recurrent UTIs secondary to chronic urinary catheterization due to paraplegia).

4. Evaluate the patient for the presence of adverse drug reactions, drug allergies, and potential drug interactions.

5. Stress the importance of complying with the prescribed antimicrobial regimen and to follow up with the healthcare provider if signs and symptoms recur.

Abbreviations Introduced in This Chapter

CFU   Colony-forming units
CrCl   Creatinine clearance
SCr   Serum creatinine
UTI   Urinary tract infection

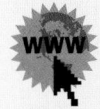 Self-assessment questions and answers are available at *http://mhpharmacotherapy.com/pp.html*.

REFERENCES

1. Gupta K, Hooton TM, Naber KG, et al. International clinical practice guidelines for the treatment of acute uncomplicated cystitis and pyelonephritis in women: a 2010 update by the Infectious Diseases Society of America and the European Society of Microbiology and Infectious Diseases. Clin Infect Dis 2011;52(5):e103–e120.
2. Nicolle LE, Bradley S, Colgan R, et al. Infectious Diseases Society of America guidelines for the diagnosis and treatment of asymptomatic bacteriuria in adults. Clin Infect Dis 2005;40:643–654.
3. Fihn SD. Clinical practice. Acute uncomplicated urinary tract infection in women. N Engl J Med 2003;349:259–266.
4. Foxman B. Epidemiology of urinary tract infections: Incidence, morbidity, and economic costs. Am J Med 2002;113(Suppl 1A):5S–13S.
5. Schappert SM, Rechtsteiner EA. Ambulatory medical care utilization estimated for 2007. National Center for Health Statistics. Vital Health Stat 2011;13:29.
6. Bent S, Nallamothu BK, Simel DL, et al. Does this woman have an acute, uncomplicated urinary tract infection? JAMA 2002;287:2701–2710.
7. American Academy of Pediatrics, Subcommittee on Urinary Tract Infection, Steering Committee on Quality Improvement Management. Urinary tract infection: clinical practice guideline for the diagnosis
8. and management of the initial UTI in febrile infants and children 2 to 24 months. Pediatrics 2011;128:595–610.
8. Alper BS, Curry SH. Urinary tract infection in children. Am Fam Physician 2005;72:2483–2488.
9. Shortliffe LM, McCue JD. Urinary tract infections at the age extremes: Pediatrics and geriatrics. Am J Med 2002;113(Suppl 1A):S55–S66.
10. Smellie JM, Prescod NP, Shaw PJ, et al. Childhood reflux and urinary infection: A follow-up of 10–41 years in 225 adults. Pediatr Nephrol 1998;12:727–736.
11. Ronald AR, Pattullo AL. The natural history of urinary tract infection in adults. Med Clin North Am 1991;75:299–312.
12. Zhanel GG, Hisanaga TL, Laing NM, et al. Antibiotic resistance in Escherichia coli outpatient urinary isolates: Final results from the North American Urinary Tract Infection Collaborative Alliance (NAUTICA). Int J Antimicrob Agents 2006;27:468–475.
13. Stamm WE, Hooton TM. Management of urinary tract infections in adults. N Engl J Med 1993;329:1328–1334.
14. Ronald A. The etiology of urinary tract infection: Traditional and emerging pathogens. Am J Med 2002;113(Suppl 1A):S14–S19.
15. Raz R, Colodner R, Kunin CM. Who are you—Staphylococcus saprophyticus? Clin Infect Dis 2005;40:896–898.
16. Wagenlehner FM, Naber KG. Hospital-acquired urinary tract infections. J Hosp Infect 2000;46:171–181.
17. Lundstrom T, Sobel J. Nosocomial candiduria: A review. Clin Infect Dis 2001;32:1602–1607.
18. Hooten TM, Hillier S, Johnson C, et al. Escherichia coli bacteriuria and contraceptive method. JAMA 1991;265:64–69.
19. Stamatiou C, Bovis C, Panaguopoulos P, et al. Sex-induced cystitis—patient burden and other epidemiological features. Clin Exp Obstet Gynecol 2005;32:180–182.
20. Bran JL, Levison ME, Kaye D. Entrance of bacteria into the female urinary bladder. N Engl J Med 1972;286:626–629.
21. Freedman LR. Experimental pyelonephritis. VI. Observation on susceptibility of the rabbit kidney to infection by a virulent strain of Staphylococcus aureus. Yale J Biol Med 1960;32:272–279.
22. Gorrill RH, DeNavasquez SJ. Experimental pyelonephritis in the mouse produced by Escherichia coli, Pseudomonas aeruginosa, and Proteus mirabilis. J Pathol Bacteriol 1964;87:79–87.
23. Stamey TA, Fair WR, Timothy MM, et al. Antibacterial nature of prostatic fluid. Nature 1968;218:444–447.
24. Kwok L, Staphleton AE, Stamm WE, et al. Adherence of Lactobacillus crispatus to vaginal epithelial cells from women with or without a history of recurrent urinary tract infection. J Urol 2006;176:2050–2054.
25. Gupta K, Stapleton AE, Hooton TM, et al. Inverse association of H_2O_2-producing lactobacilli and vaginal Escherichia coli colonization in women with recurrent urinary tract infections. J Infect Dis 1998;178:446–450.
26. Parsons CL, Schrom SH, Hanno P, et al. Bladder surface mucin: Examination of possible mechanisms for its antibacterial effect. Invest Urol 1978;6:196–200.
27. U.S. Preventive Services Task Force. Screening for asymptomatic bacteriuria in adults: U.S. Preventive Services Task Force reaffirmation recommendation statement. Ann Intern Med 2008;149:43–47.
28. Nicolle LE. Urinary tract infection in diabetes. Curr Opin Infect Dis 2005;18:49–53.
29. Harding GK, Zhanel GG, Nicolle LE, et al. Antimicrobial treatment in diabetic women with asymptomatic bacteriuria. N Engl J Med 2002;347:1576–1583.
30. Niël-Weise BS, van den Broek PJ. Urinary catheter policies for long-term bladder drainage. Cochrane Database Syst Rev 2005;1:CD004201.
31. Sobel JD, Kaye D. Urinary tract infection. In: Mandell GL, Bennett JE, Dolin R, eds. Principles and Practice of Infectious Diseases. 7th ed. Philadelphia, PA: Elsevier; 2009:966.
32. Jepson RG, Craig JC. Cranberries for preventing urinary tract infection. Cochrane Database Syst Rev 2008;1:CD001321.
33. Salo J, Uhari M, Helminen M, et al. Cranberry juice for the prevention of recurrences of urinary tract infections in children: a randomized placebo-controlled trail. Clin Infect Dis 2012;54:340–346.

34. Barbosa-Cesnik C, Brown MB, Buxton M, et al. Cranberry juice fails to prevent recurrent urinary tract infection: results from a randomized placebo-controlled trail. Clin Infect Dis 2011;52:23–30.

35. Raz R, Stamm WE. A controlled trial of intravaginal estriol in post-menopausal women with recurrent urinary tract infections. N Engl J Med 1993;329:753–756.

36. Carson C, Naber KG. Role of fluoroquinolones in the treatment of serious bacterial urinary tract infections. Drugs 2004;64:1359–1373.

37. Miller LG, Tang AW. Treatment of uncomplicated urinary tract infections in an era of increasing antimicrobial resistance. Mayo Clin Proc 2004;79:1048–1054.

38. Wagenlehner FME, Naber KG. Treatment of bacterial urinary tract infections: Presence and future. Eur Urol 2006;49:235–244.

39. Gupta K, Sahm DF, Mayfield D, et al. Antimicrobial resistance among uropathogens that cause community-acquired urinary tract infections in women: A nationwide analysis. Clin Infect Dis 2001;33:89–94.

40. Perfetto EM, Gondek EK. *Escherichia coli* resistance in uncomplicated urinary tract infection: A model for determining when to change first-line empirical antibiotic choice. Manag Care Interface 2002;6:35–42.

41. Wagenlehner FM, Pilatz A, Naber KG, et al. Anti-infective treatment of bacterial urinary tract infections. Curr Med Chem 2008;15:1412–1427.

42. Rubenstein JN, Schaeffer AJ. Managing complicated urinary tract infections: The urologic view. Infect Dis Clin North Am 2003;17:333–351.

43. Ovalle A, Levancini M. Urinary tract infections in pregnancy. Curr Opin Urol 2001;11:55–59.

44. Christensen B. Which antibiotics are appropriate for treating bacteriuria in pregnancy? J Antimicrob Chemother 2000;46(suppl S1):29–34.

45. McDermott S, Daguise V, Mann H, et al. Perinatal risk for mortality and mental retardation associated with maternal urinary tract infections. J Fam Pract 2001;50:433–437.

46. Hooton TM, Bradley SF, Cardenas DD, et al. Diagnosis, prevention, and treatment of catheter-associated urinary tract infection in adults: 2009 international clinical practice guidelines from the Infectious Diseases Society of America. Clin Infect Dis 2010;50:625-663.

47. Warren JW. The catheter and urinary tract infection. Med Clin North Am 1991;75:481–493.

48. Naber KG, Bergman B, Bishop MC, et al. EAU guidelines for management of urinary and male genital tract infections. Urinary Tract Infection Working Group of the Health Care Office of the European Associated of Urology. Eur Urol 2001;40:576–588.

49. Johnson JR, Johnston B, Clabots C, et al. *Escherichia coli* sequence Type ST131 as the major cause of serious multidrug-resistant *E. coli* in the United States. Clin Infect Dis 2010;51:286–294.

80 Sexually Transmitted Infections

Marlon S. Honeywell and Evans Branch III

LEARNING OBJECTIVES

● **Upon completion of the chapter, the reader will be able to:**

1. Analyze the behavioral considerations and assess the importance of contraception with regard to the contributing factors of sexually transmitted infections (STIs).

2. Apply the "expedited partner treatment" method when recommending treatment for STIs.

3. Identify the patient populations that are typically affected by specific STIs.

4. Identify causative organisms for STIs.

5. Devise a list of the clinical signs and symptoms corresponding to each type of STI and classify patients based on recommended criteria.

6. Select appropriate diagnostic procedures for STIs.

7. Identify STI treatment regimens and recommend therapy when appropriate.

8. Design a patient care plan based on the monitoring parameters.

KEY CONCEPTS

❶ Optimal detection and treatment of sexually transmitted infections (STIs) depends on counseling by a patient-friendly and knowledgeable clinician who can establish open communication with the patient. Patients, especially adolescents, should be counseled on the importance of using condoms, spermicides, and diaphragms properly.

❷ Generally, when treating an STI, the patient being treated should be provided with a sufficient quantity of medication for his/her partner, increasing the probability that the initial infection will be cured in both individuals. Counseling regarding the appropriate use of condoms, cervical diaphragms, spermicides, and emergency contraception is also important to mitigate the occurrence of reinfection.

❸ Patients treated for gonorrhea should be assumed to be coinfected with *Chlamydia trachomatis*; treatment recommendations should cover both organisms. Treatment of *Neisseria gonorrhoeae* with fluoroquinolones is inadvisable in those with a history of recent foreign travel, infections acquired in California or Hawaii, infections in other areas with increased gonococcal resistance, or in men who have sex with men (MSM). Additionally, treatment on gonorrhea over time has resulted in drug resistance to some cephalosporins.

❹ Parenterally administered penicillin G is recommended for all stages of syphilis.

❺ Metronidazole and tinidazole are the standard agents for trichomoniasis; advise patients to avoid the consumption of alcohol during treatment.

❻ Due to the variable appearance of genital warts, treatment may be based on the size, site, and morphology of the lesions. Treatment options include podofilox, imiquimod, sinecatechins, podophyllin resin, and bichloro- and trichloroacetic acid. The Gardasil® vaccine was FDA approved for the prevention of vulvar, vaginal, and cervical cancer and genital warts.

❼ Acyclovir, valacyclovir, and famciclovir may be prescribed to treat first and intermittent episodes of genital herpes and to suppress active herpetic infections.

❽ Bacterial vaginosis (BV) is a clinical syndrome categorized by an overgrowth of polymicrobial anaerobic organisms, such as *Gardenella vaginalis*, *Prevotella* species, *Mycoplasma hominis*, and *Mobiluncus* species. BV infection leads to the replacement of the normal hydrogen peroxide–producing lactobacillus and an increase in vaginal pH from 4.5 to 7.

❾ In patients with pelvic inflammatory disease (PID), resolution of infection (i.e., *N. gonorrhoeae*, *C. trachomatis*, *Streptococcus* spp., and gram-negative facultative bacteria) and mitigation of sequelae should be the main goal of pharmacologic therapy.

Though we have made progress in medicine, age-old problems of infectious disease continue to plague us.[1] Even with the discovery of newly improved antibiotics, sexually transmitted infections (STIs) have not been eradicated. Many have reemerged secondary to modern social trends of sexual activity, and some as a result of the HIV epidemic, socioeconomic concerns, and the global lack of preventive education. Educating the public decreases the probability of infection in some individuals; however, this tactic alone may not be sufficient. ❶ *Optimal detection and treatment of STIs depends on counseling by a patient-friendly and knowledgeable clinician who can establish open communication with the patient.*

BEHAVIORAL CONSIDERATIONS

The correlation between risky sexual behavior and STIs is well documented.[2] Inconsistent and incorrect condom use increases the incidence of new STIs. ❶ *Assuming that patients, especially adolescents, consistently use and understand how to use condoms, spermicides, or diaphragms can be detrimental and may contribute to nonpharmacologic mismanagement.*[3] Healthcare providers who manage persons at risk for STIs should counsel women concerning the option for emergency contraception, if indicated, and provide it in a timely fashion if desired by the woman or the couple. Plan B (two 750 mcg of levonorgestrol) is approved in the United States for the prevention of unintended pregnancy.[4]

In addition to the increasing number of adolescents engaging in unsafe sexual practices is a high incidence of men who have sex with men (MSM) and women who have sex with women (WSW). Many MSM do not disclose their HIV status. This "don't ask, don't tell" practice has been linked to an upsurge in newly diagnosed HIV infections and STIs among previously noninfected people.[5] Although limited data are available with regard to STIs in WSW, risk of transmission probably varies by the specific STI and sexual techniques. Sharing penetrative items or employing practices involving digital vaginal or digital anal contact most likely represent common modes of transmission. This possibility is supported by reports of metronidazole-resistant trichomoniasis and genotype-specific HIV transmitted sexually between women who reported such behaviors and an increased prevalence of bacterial vaginosis (BV) among monogamous WSW.[6]

Sexual abuse in adolescents and children is being reported more often in the United States. Any child or adolescent with an STI should be evaluated for sexual abuse.[7] In cases of abusive contact, commonly found infections include *Neisseria gonorrhoeae* or *Chlamydia trachomatis*. Abusive cases should be reported to the police.

The emergence of "swingers" (a person who engages in the exchanging of spouses for sexual activities) as a new category of at-risk patients has been seen in STI clinics throughout the world. In fact, one clinic in South Limburg reports that swingers comprise approximately 12% of total consultations since 2007, most of which involved a predominantly older group of people (median age 43 years).[8] To this end, swingers now represent a group with risky behaviors that must be identified and treated when necessary.

❷ *Optimally, both sex partners should be treated simultaneously for an STI; however, this is difficult to accomplish. Clinics and health departments often proactively attempt dual treatment by providing a prescription for the partner to the* index patient *(the patient who is evaluated by a clinician), a practice commonly known as expedited partner treatment.* Counseling regarding the appropriate use of condoms, cervical diaphragms, spermicides, and emergency contraception is also important to mitigate the occurrence of reinfection.

Accurate reporting of STIs is imperative to the evaluation of trends in sexual behaviors; reporting may be provider- or laboratory-based. State and local health departments may assist with the mechanism by which STIs are reported, and cases must be conveyed in accordance with statutory requirements. Confidentiality should always be exercised in such cases.[9,10]

GONORRHEA

Gonorrhea is a curable STI caused by the gram-negative diplococcus *Neisseria gonorrhoeae*. Proper therapeutic management with antimicrobial agents is essential to eradicate this infection and prevent the development of associated sequelae such as a urethritis, cervicitis, or dysuria.

In the United States, the highest rate of gonococcal infection is seen within the 15- to 24-year-old age groups for both sexes; although more cases are reported in men. Approximately 700,000 new cases occur annually in the United States.[9,10] Factors associated with an increased risk of infection include ethnicity, low socioeconomic status, and illicit drug use. The risk of a cervical infection after a single episode of vaginal intercourse is approximately 50% and increases with multiple exposures. Furthermore, rates of reinfection are significantly higher among ethnic minorities.

Patient Encounter 1, Part 1

KL is a 27-year-old African American female who visits a clinic complaining of profuse urethral discharge for the past several days. She also informs the nurse that she did not have a menstrual cycle last month and that a home pregnancy test taken this morning revealed that she was indeed pregnant. The patient admits to having sexual intercourse without barrier contraception (condoms) with her boyfriend within the past week or two and is not sure of other sexual encounter(s) in which he may have been involved.

What information is suggestive of gonorrhea?

What potential risk factors for STIs are present?

What impact will pregnancy have on diagnostic and treatment plans for STI management?

PATHOPHYSIOLOGY

Attachment to mucosal epithelium, mediated in part by pili and opa (outer membrane opacity proteins), is followed by penetration of *N. gonorrhoeae* through epithelial cells to the submucosal tissue within 24 to 48 hours. A vigorous response by neutrophils begins with sloughing of the epithelium, development of submucosal microabscesses, and exudation of pus. Stained smears usually reveal large numbers of gonococci within a few neutrophils, whereas most cells contain no organisms.[11]

DIAGNOSIS

Several laboratory tests are available to aid in the diagnosis of gonorrhea and include Gram-stained smears, endocervical or vaginal specimens, culture, or the DNA hybridization probe. A Gram stain of a male urethral specimen that demonstrates polymorphonuclear leukocytes with intracellular gram-negative diplococci may be considered diagnostic in symptomatic men. A negative Gram stain should not be considered sufficient for ruling out infection in asymptomatic men.[9] Additionally, Gram stain of endocervical, pharyngeal, or rectal specimens are also insufficient to detect infections. All patients who test positive for gonorrhea should be tested for other STIs, including chlamydia, syphilis, and HIV.

Patient Encounter 1, Part 2

PMH: Currently receiving no medications; no prior history of STIs; no drug allergies noted

FH: Noncontributory

SH: Admits to having unprotected sex with boyfriend. Does not smoke or drink alcohol

ROS: C/o vaginal discharge, recent nonpruritic rash development across abdominal area noted over past 3 to 5 days

PE:

VS: BP 130/80 mm Hg, P 70 beats/min, T 37°C (98.6°F)

Lab: Urethral discharge swab revealed *N. gonorrhoeae*; rapid plasma reagin (RPR) test was positive.

Given this additional information, what is your assessment of the patient's condition?

What consideration should be given to other STIs?

Identify your treatment goals for this patient.

What pharmacologic alternatives are available for this patient?

TREATMENT

Desired Outcome

The desired outcome is complete eradication of *N. gonorrhoeae* and avoidance of sequelae.

Pharmacologic Therapy[4,9,12,13]

❸ *Patients infected with gonorrhea often are coinfected with* Chlamydia trachomatis *and should receive therapy to eradicate both organisms concurrently.* Although fluoroquinolones and broad-spectrum cephalosporins have been effective in the treatment of gonorrhea, resistant strains of *N. gonorrhoeae* have emerged. In Far-Eastern countries, as many as 50% of gonococcal strains exhibit decreased susceptibility to fluoroquinolones. Although ciprofloxacin is still an option for treatment, gonococcal resistance to ciprofloxacin is usually indicative of its resistance to other fluoroquinolones. As a result, monitoring for fluoroquinolone resistance is now essential to ensure proper treatment and to ascertain the maximum time that this class may be employed as a treatment option.

Fluoroquinolones should not be prescribed for infections in MSM, in those with a history of recent foreign travel or partners' travel, or for infections acquired in California or Hawaii or infections in other areas with increased gonococcal resistance.[14]

Gonoccocal resistance to some cephalosporins has emerged.[15] Presently, the recommended first-line treatment for gonorrhea in most countries is third-generation cephalosporins, and in some cases, spectinomycin and azithromycin.[16] However, resistance to oral third-generation

---

Clinical Presentation of Gonorrhea[9,10]

General

- Purulent discharge

Signs

- Painful or swollen testicles
- Tubal scarring

Symptoms

Men:

- May be asymptomatic, although acute urethritis is the predominant manifestation
- Urethral discharge and dysuria, usually without urinary frequency or urgency
- When compared with nongonococcal urethritis, the discharge in gonococcal urethritis is generally more profuse and purulent
- Dysuria

Women:

- Cervicitis, urethritis, increased vaginal discharge, dysuria and intermenstrual bleeding
- Abdominal pain

Unprotected sex is a major risk factor for contracting STIs. Although the purulent discharge is consistent with gonorrhea infection, a positive urethral swab coupled with an incubation period consistent with gonorrhea confirms the diagnosis. A serologic test for syphilis should be performed on all pregnant women at the first prenatal visit, and a RPR should be performed at the time pregnancy is confirmed and treatment provided. Although the patient has confirmed gonorrhea, infection with *Chlamydia trachomatis* occurs commonly in this setting. Additionally, pregnant patients should be tested for this infection during the first prenatal visit and treated appropriately. Further, the presence of a rash could possibly suggest that the patient may have contracted syphilis previously, potentially indicative of secondary syphilis.

If this patient had an allergy to penicillin, how would the therapeutic management of the identified problems change?

cephalosporins has developed in Asia and Australia and in other parts of the world. The mechanism of resistance appears to be associated with a mosaic penicillin-binding protein in addition to other chromosomal mutations previously found to confer resistance to β-lactam antimicrobials. To mitigate the prevalence of cephalosporin resistance, strong antimicrobial management programs, expanding surveillance networks and procedures, and STI control and prevention are warranted.

Combined hormonal contraception has been evaluated to determine whether it deters the acquisition of gonnococal infections in women. Although the transmission of *N. gonorrhea* is poorly understood, data from an original study suggested that combined hormonal therapy may lessen the probability of infection.[17] More studies are required to support this theory as a viable option for prevention.

Treatment of gonorrhea may vary according to clinical presentation and are indicated as follows[9]:

Uncomplicated Gonococcal Infection of the Cervix, Urethra, and Rectum* Ceftriaxone 250 mg intramuscularly *or* cefixime 400 mg orally *or* single-dose injectable cephalosporin regimens *plus* azithromycin 1 g orally *or* doxycycline 100 mg orally twice daily for 7 days. Several alternative agents possess notable activity; however, they should not be used if pharyngeal infection is suspected. Alternatives include cefpodoxime 400 mg orally or cefuroxime axetil 1 g orally or azithromycin 2 g. Although unavailable in the United States, spectinomycin has also been prescribed.

MSM or Heterosexuals with a History of Recent Travel* Ceftriaxone 250 mg intramuscularly *or* cefixime 400 mg

orally *plus* treatment for chlamydial infection if it has not been ruled out.

Uncomplicated Gonococcal Infection of the Pharynx* Ceftriaxone 250 mg intramuscularly plus azithromycin 1 g orally or doxycycline 100 mg orally twice daily for 7 days.

Coverage for Coinfection with *Chlamydia Trachomatis* Azithromycin 1 g orally as a single dose *or* doxycycline 100 mg orally twice daily for 7 days.

▶ **Treatment of Gonorrhea in Special Situations**

Uncomplicated infections of the cervix, urethra, and rectum can be treated with one of the following regimens in adults:

Recommendations During Pregnancy

- Pregnant women should be treated with a recommended or alternative cephalosporin. For women who cannot tolerate a cephalosporin, azithromycin 2 g orally may be prescribed. For treatment of presumptive or diagnosed *C. trachomatis*, azithromycin or amoxicillin is recommended.

- Doxycycline and fluoroquinolones are contraindicated.

Recommendations for Disseminated Gonococcal Infection (Regimens Should Be Continued for 24 to 48 Hours) Ceftriaxone 1 g intramuscularly or IV every 24 hours *or* cefotaxime 1 g IV every 8 hours *or* ceftizoxime 1 g IV every 8 hours. Continue regimens for 24 to 48 hours after improvement is noted. Once improvement begins, therapy should be converted to Cefixime 400 mg orally twice daily for at least 1 week.

Uncomplicated Infections of the Cervix, Urethra, and Rectum in Children Weighing Less Than 45 kg Ceftriaxone 250 mg intramuscularly as a single dose *or* spectinomycin 40 mg/kg intramuscularly as a single dose (not to exceed 2 g).

Gonococcal Conjunctivitis Ceftriaxone 1 g intramuscularly once for adults has demonstrated excellent response rates. Lavage of the infected eye(s) once with saline solution should also be considered. Patients treated for gonococcal conjunctivitis should also be treated empirically for *C. trachomatis* infection.

Ophthalmic Neonatorum or Prophylactic Treatment for Infants Whose Mothers Have Gonococcal Infection Ceftriaxone 25 to 50 mg/kg IV *or* intramuscularly in a single dose, not to exceed 125 mg.

Ophthalmic Neonatorum Prophylaxis Erythromycin (0.5%) ophthalmic ointment in a single application to the eyes *or* tetracycline (1%) ophthalmic ointment in a single application to the eyes.

PATIENT CARE AND MONITORING

Monitoring is generally not required.

---

*Regimens are given for one dose only.

CHLAMYDIA

EPIDEMIOLOGY

Infection with *C. trachomatis* has increased dramatically in recent years. This bacterium is the most common cause of nongonococcal urethritis, accounting for as many as 50% of cases. Worldwide, this intracellular, gram-negative bacterium produces approximately 92 million new genital infections. The prevalence is highest in individuals less than 25 years of age. Associated sequelae include pelvic inflammatory disease (PID), ectopic pregnancy, and infertility.

PATHOPHYSIOLOGY

C. trachomatis possesses characteristics resembling both bacteria and viruses. Its major membrane is comparable to that of gram-negative bacteria, although it lacks a peptidoglycan cell wall and requires cellular components from the host for replication. Chlamydia transmission risk is thought to be less than that of gonorrhea.

DIAGNOSIS

Common tests used to diagnose *C. trachomatis* include culture, the enzyme immunoassay, the DNA hybridization probe, or the direct fluorescent monoclonal antibody test. Diagnosis has been confirmed in women through urine or swab specimen collected from the endocervix and in men using a urethral swab or urine specimen. Most women are asymptomatic; therefore, an annual screening or physical is necessary, as early detection may reduce rates of transmission.

Clinical Presentation of Chlamydia[9,10,13]

General
- Asymptomatic

Signs
- Beefy red cervix that bleeds easily (women)

Symptoms
- When present, the urethral discharge is watery and less purulent than that seen with acute gonococcal urethritis. Complications resulting from lack of treatment or inadequate treatment include epididymitis (in males) and PID including associated complications in women.

Other Diagnostic Tests
- Culture is usually positive for both chlamydia and gonorrhea.

TREATMENT[9,18]

Uncomplicated Urethral, Endocervical, or Rectal Infection in Adults

The recommended adult regimen is azithromycin 1 g orally in a single dose *or* doxycycline 100 mg orally twice daily for 7 days. An alternate regimen is erythromycin ethylsuccinate 800 mg orally four times daily for 7 days *or* erythromycin base 500 mg orally four times daily for 7 days *or* levofloxacin 500 mg orally once daily for 7 days.

The recommended regimen for pregnancy is azithromycin 1 g orally in a single dose *or* amoxicillin 1 g orally in a single dose *or* amoxicillin 500 mg orally three times daily for 7 days.

Alternate regimens include erythromycin base 500 mg orally four times daily for 7 days *or* 250 mg orally four times daily for 14 days *or* erythromycin ethylsuccinate 800 mg orally four times daily for 7 days *or* 400 mg orally four times daily for 14 days.

C. trachomatis Infection in Infants

Treatment of ophthalmia neonatorum or infant pneumonia should be with erythromycin base or ethylsuccinate 50 mg/kg/day orally divided into four doses daily for 14 days.

PATIENT CARE AND MONITORING

Monitoring is generally not required.

SYPHILIS

Syphilis, attributed to the spirochete *Treponema pallidum*, can have numerous and complex manifestations. Clinician familiarity, stage-specific diagnosis, and effective treatment are vital. Missed or inappropriately treated syphilis may result in cardiovascular complications, neurologic disease, or congenital syphilis.

EPIDEMIOLOGY

After the 1940s, the incidence of syphilis declined drastically following the introduction of penicillin, but rose when HIV arrived from obscurity in the 1980s. In 2009, rates of primary and secondary syphilis increased for the tenth consecutive year, reaching the highest rate reported since 1995. Although increases have occurred mostly among men, in 2009, 62% of cases from 44 states and the District of Columbia occurred in MSM. Increases also were observed among women during 2004 through 2008; cases were mostly noted in the south. The primary and secondary syphilis rate among blacks was nine times the rate among whites, emphasizing the need for enhanced preventive measures among blacks and MSM. The disparity among men and women has been observed across racial and ethnic groups and is highest in the South and among non-Hispanic blacks.[19]

PATHOPHYSIOLOGY

T. pallidum rapidly penetrates intact mucous membranes or microscopic dermal abrasions, and within a few hours, enters the lymphatics and blood to produce systemic illness. During the secondary stage, examinations commonly demonstrate abnormal findings in the cerebrospinal fluid (CSF). As the infection progresses, the parenchyma of the brain and spinal cord may subsequently be damaged.

Stages of Syphilis

▶ Primary Syphilis

Usually manifests as a solitary, painless chancre. Primary syphilis develops at the site of infection approximately 3 weeks after exposure to *T. pallidum*; the chancre is highly infectious.[9,20]

▶ Secondary Syphilis

Without appropriate treatment, primary syphilis will advance to secondary syphilis, a stage usually apparent from its clinical symptomatology. Symptoms include fatigue, diffuse rash, fever, lymphadenopathy, and genital or perineal condyloma latum. Additionally, the skin is most often affected and a rash may present as macular, macropapular, or pustular lesions or may involve skin surfaces including the palms of the hands and soles of the feet.

▶ Latent Syphilis

Early Latent Usually occurs during the first year after infection and may be established in patients who have seroconverted, who have had symptoms of primary or secondary syphilis, or who have had sex with a partner with primary, secondary, or latent syphilis.

Late Latent Patients should be considered to have late latent syphilis if the aforementioned criteria (early latent) are not met. In both stages, patients are usually asymptomatic and the lesions noted in the primary and secondary phase usually resolve; however, individuals are still seropositive for *T. pallidum*.

Tertiary Syphilis Develops years after the initial infection and may involve any organ in the body.

Congenital Syphilis

Congenital syphilis is a condition in which the fetus is infected with *T. pallidum* as a result of the hematogenous spread from an infected mother, although transmission may also occur from direct contact with the infectious genitalia of the mother. Since the primary stage of syphilis is characterized by spirochetemia, infectious rates of the fetus are nearly 100% if the mother has primary syphilis.[20,21]

DIAGNOSIS

Diagnostic procedures include dark-field microscopy, nontreponemal exams[9,20] (i.e., the Venereal Disease Research Laboratory [VDRL] and the rapid plasma reagin [RPR]

Patient Encounter 2

KG is an HIV-positive male who complains of the appearance of a "sore" on his penis. He reports having unprotected sexual intercourse with another male approximately 5 to 7 days prior to the appearance of the lesion. He denies pain or itching at the site of the lesion, dysuria, or frequent urination. Additionally, there appears to be no vesicles in the genital area.

What information is suggestive of syphilis?

What potential risk factors for STIs are present?

How should the diagnosis of syphilis be confirmed in this patient?

If the diagnosis of syphilis is confirmed, what therapeutic options exist for this patient?

---

test), and treponemal exams (i.e., enzyme immunoassay, the *T. pallidum* hemagglutination test, the fluorescent treponemal antibody test, and the enzyme-linked immunosorbent assay).

TREATMENT

Desired Outcome

After confirming the diagnosis of syphilis, the desired outcome is a fourfold decrease in quantitative nontreponemal titers over a 6-month period and within 12 to 24 months after treatment of latent or late syphilis. An algorithm for the treatment of syphilis is shown in **Figure 80–1**.

With regard to neurosyphilis, a reduction in neurologic manifestations is desired, which may include seizures, paresis, meningitis, stroke, hyperreflexia, visual disturbances, hearing loss, neuropathy, or loss of bowel and bladder function. In late neurosyphilis, vascular lesions (meningovascular neurosyphilis) may also be observed; thus a reduction in the number of observed lesions is warranted. A diminution in CSF white blood cell count (WBC) (less than $10 \times 10^3/\text{mm}^3$ [$10 \times 10^9/\text{L}$]) or protein levels (0.05 g/dL [0.5 g/L]) is also preferred.

Pharmacologic Therapy

❹ *Parenterally administered penicillin G is recommended for all stages of syphilis* (*Table 80–1*). Although penicillin G is the drug of choice, combinations of benzathine penicillin with procaine penicillin or oral penicillin preparations are not considered appropriate treatment regimens. Several reports have demonstrated the misuse of the benzathine–procaine combination (Bicillin C-R) instead of the standard benzathine penicillin (Bicillin L-A).[20,22] Clinicians and purchasing agents should be aware of the similarities in product names to avoid errors in the prescribing and administration of these agents. Pertinent information germane to benzathine penicillin G is found in Table 80–1.

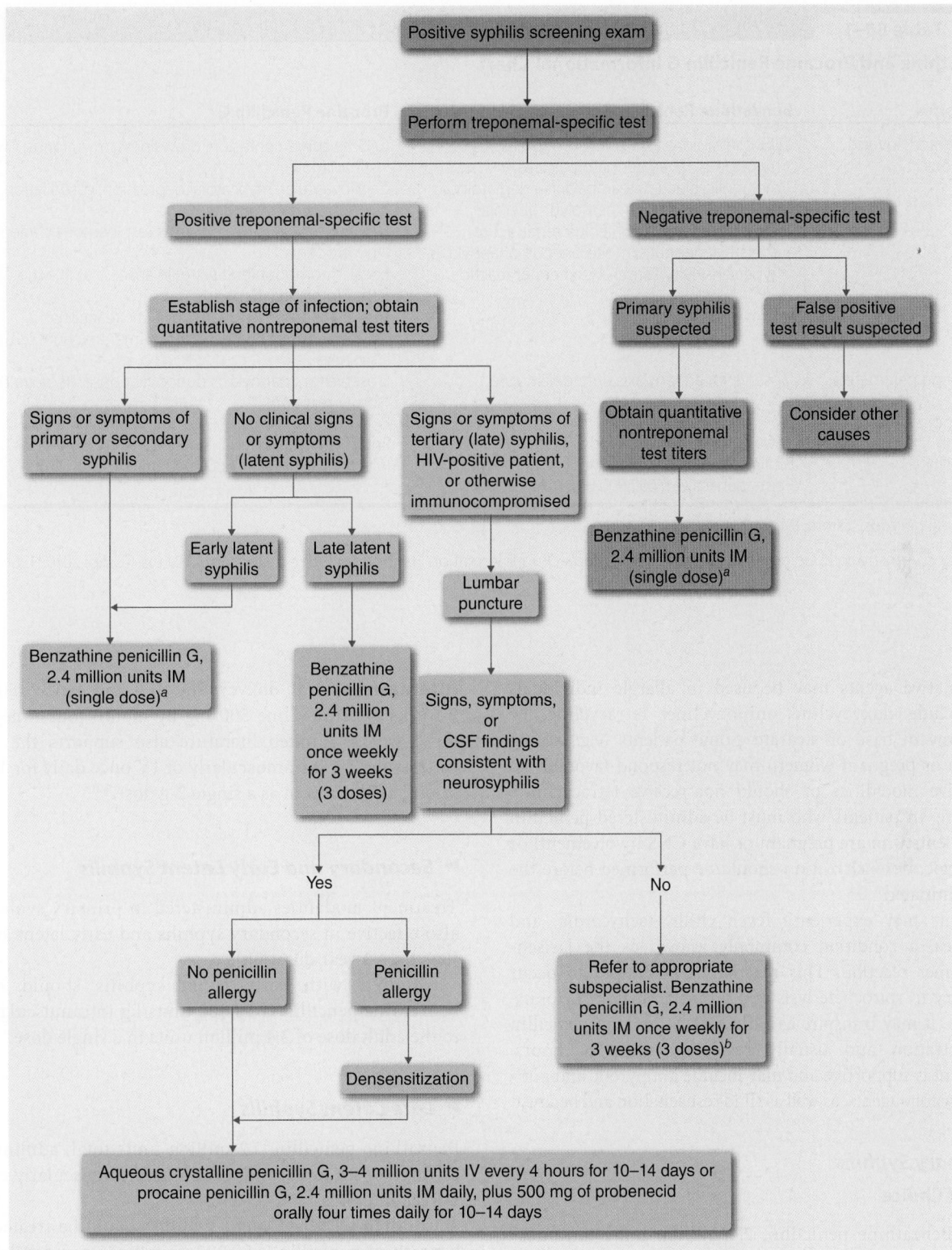

FIGURE 80–1. Treatment of syphilis. (CSF, cerebrospinal fluid; IM, intramuscularly.) (From Brown D, Frank J. Diagnosis and management of syphilis. Am Fam Physician 2003;68(2):283–290.) [a]Alternative treatments for nonpregnant penicillin-allergic patients: doxycycline 100 mg orally twice daily for 2 weeks or tetracycline 500 mg four times daily for 2 weeks; limited data support ceftriaxone 1 g once daily IM or IV for 8 to 10 days; or azithromycin 2 g orally (single dose). [b]Alternative treatments for nonpregnant penicillin-allergic patients: doxycycline 100 mg orally twice daily for 4 weeks, or tetracycline 500 mg orally four times daily for 4 weeks.

Table 80–1		
Benzathine and Procaine Penicillin G Informational Chart		
Categories	**Benzathine Penicillin G**	**Procaine Penicillin G**
Drug-related adverse reactions	CNS: convulsions, confusion, drowsiness, myoclonus, fever; dermatologic: rash; metabolic: electrolyte imbalance; hematologic: positive Coombs test, hemolytic anemia; local: pain, thrombophlebitis; renal: acute interstitial nephritis; miscellaneous: anaphylaxis, hypersensitivity, Jarisch-Herxheimer reaction	CNS: seizures, confusion, drowsiness, myoclonus, CNS stimulation Cardiovascular: myocardial depression, vasodilation, conduction disturbances Hematologic: positive Coombs test, hemolytic anemia, neutropenia Local: thrombophlebitis, sterile abscess at injection site Renal: interstitial nephritis Miscellaneous: pseudoanaphylactic reactions, hypersensitivity, Jarisch-Herxheimer reaction, serum sickness
Monitoring parameters	Observe for anaphylaxis during first dose	Observe for anaphylaxis during first dose. Remove the other reactions
Pregnancy category	B	B
Lactation	Enters breast milk	Enters breast milk
Availability	Bicillin L-A: 600,000 units/mL (1, 2, and 4 mL); Permapen Isoject: 600,000 units/mL (2 mL)	Injection, suspension: 600,000 units/mL (1, 2 mL)

CNS, central nervous system; IM, intramuscular.

From Lacy C, Armstrong L, Goldman M, Lance L. Lexi-Comp's Drug Information Handbook. 19th ed. Hudson, OH: Lexi-Comp; 2010:1128–1132.

Alternative agents may be used in allergic individuals and include doxycycline, minocycline, tetracycline, or erythromycin base or stearate. Some patients (e.g., young children or pregnant women) may not respond favorably to alternative modalities or should not receive tetracyclines. Therefore, in patients who must be administered penicillin (i.e., patients who are pregnant or have CNS involvement) or are allergic, desensitization should be performed before the drug is initiated.

Patients may experience fever, chills, tachycardia, and tachypnea, a condition commonly known as the Jarisch-Herxheimer reaction. This reaction is postulated to occur secondary to spirochete lysis and proinflammatory cytokine cascades. It may transpire as early as 2 hours after penicillin administration and usually resolves within 24 hours. Treatment is supportive and may include antipyretic and anti-inflammatory agents, as well as fluid resuscitation and bed rest.

▶ Primary Syphilis

Drug of Choice

Adults. Benzathine penicillin, 2.4 million units intramuscularly as a single dose. Additional doses of benzathine penicillin or other antibiotics do not enhance efficacy, regardless of HIV status.[9]

Children. Benzathine penicillin 50,000 units/kg intramuscularly, up to the adult dose of 2.4 million units in a single dose. Infants less than 1 month of age diagnosed with syphilis should have a CSF test to determine whether asymptomatic neurosyphilis is present. Patient records should be reviewed to decipher whether syphilis is congenital or acquired.

Alternatives Oral doxycycline 100 mg twice daily for 2 weeks *or* tetracycline 500 mg by mouth four times daily for 2 weeks. Limited literature also supports the use of ceftriaxone 1 g intramuscularly or IV once daily for 10 days *or* oral azithromycin as a single 2-g dose.[9,21]

▶ Secondary and Early Latent Syphilis

Treatment modalities administered in primary syphilis are also effective in secondary syphilis and early latent syphilis (less than 1 year duration).

Children with early latent syphilis should receive benzathine pencillin G 50,000 units/kg intramuscularly, up to the adult dose of 2.4 million units in a single dose.

▶ Late Latent Syphilis

Benzathine penicillin, 7.2 million units total, administered as three doses of 2.4 million units intramuscularly each at 1-week intervals.

Children with late latent syphilis should be treated with benzathine penicillin G 50,000 units/kg intramuscularly, up to the adult dose of 2.4 million units, administered as three doses at 1-week intervals (total 150,000 units/kg up to the adult dose of 7.2 million units).

▶ Tertiary Syphilis

Drug of Choice Benzathine penicillin 2.4 million units administered intramuscularly once weekly for 3 weeks. A total of 7.2 million units should be administered.

Alternatives In nonpregnant patients with a penicillin allergy, alternative regimens include doxycycline 100 mg orally two times daily for 4 weeks *or* tetracycline 500 mg orally four times daily for 4 weeks.

▶ Gummatous and Cardiovascular Syphilis

As long as no evidence of CNS involvement exists, antibiotic therapy for gummatous and cardiovascular syphilis is identical to that for tertiary syphilis.

▶ Neurosyphilis

As an effective treatment for neurosyphilis, the Centers for Disease Control and Prevention (CDC) endorses two regimens of penicillin. Alternatively, ceftriaxone may also be prescribed.[25]

The regimens of choice are aqueous penicillin G 3 to 4 million units administered IV every 4 hours or continuous infusion for 10 to 14 days *or* procaine penicillin G 2.4 million units administered intramuscularly once daily, plus probenecid 500 mg orally four times daily, both for 10 to 14 days. Limited data suggest that ceftriaxone 2 g daily either IM or IV for 10 to 14 days can be used as an alternative treatment for patients with neurosyphilis.

Congenital Syphilis[23-25]

The decision to treat an infant should be based on a diagnosis of syphilis in the mother and confirmation of adequacy of maternal treatment. Clinical, laboratory, or radiographic evidence of syphilis in the infant should be documented. Maternal nontreponemal titers (at delivery) should be compared with the infant's nontreponemal titers. Because diagnosis based on neonatal serologic testing is complicated by the transplacental transfer of maternal IgG antibodies, which can cause a positive test in the absence of infection, neonatal titers are assessed. A titer greater than four times the maternal titer would not generally result from passive transfer, and diagnosis is considered confirmed or highly probable.

The following regimens are recommended for treatment of maternal syphilis: benzathine penicillin G 2.4 million units weekly or 7.2 million units intramuscularly over 3 weeks if the duration of syphilis has been at least a year. An alternative regimen is procaine penicillin 0.6 to 0.9 million units daily intramuscularly for 10 to 14 days, or ceftriaxone 1 g daily intramuscularly or IV for 8 to 10 days.

In women who experience uterine cramping, pelvic pain, or fever, administer acetaminophen to combat these symptoms. Additionally, the patient should be well hydrated and rested.

Treatment of asymptomatic neonates is with 50,000 units/kg of benzathine penicillin G in a single intramuscular dose. Symptomatic neonates should receive 50,000 units/kg of aqueous crystalline penicillin G every 12 hours intramuscularly for the first 7 days of life, then every 8 hours for 3 days *or* procaine penicillin G 50,000 IU/kg intramuscularly as a single dose daily for 10 days.

PATIENT CARE AND MONITORING

The CDC has provided patient care monitoring guidelines for syphilis (**Fig. 80–2**).[9,11,20]

Primary and Secondary Syphilis

- After 6, 12, and 24 months of treatment, reexamine the patient and recommend a follow-up quantitative nontreponemal titer. More frequent assessment might be sensible if follow-up is uncertain. If the patient is asymptomatic, yet has a fourfold increase in nontreponemal titer or persistent or recurrent symptoms are observed, order an HIV test and a lumbar puncture; if the patient is HIV positive, suggest an infectious disease consult.

- In patients who are both negative for HIV and the lumbar puncture, administer benzathine penicillin G 2.4 million units intramuscularly once weekly for 3 weeks. Perform a patient follow-up in 6 months, including a clinical examination and another nontreponemal titer. In HIV-negative patients with lumbar puncture findings compatible with neurosyphilis, treat the patient accordingly for neurosyphilis.

- Six months after the original diagnosis, institute a standard clinical follow-up exam in patients who show no symptomatology and a fourfold decrease in nontreponemal titers. By testing and observing the patient for signs of remission, you may be able to initiate proper treatment or recommend a consult in a timely fashion, thereby decreasing the propensity of the patient's condition to advance to a higher stage.

  - If serologic titers do not decline despite a negative CSF examination and a repeated course of therapy, it is unclear whether additional therapy or CSF examinations are needed; additional testing or repeated therapy is not generally recommended.

Early and Late Latent Syphilis

- Order nontreponemal titers 6, 12, and 24 months after instituting treatment for early or late latent syphilis. Neurosyphilis should be strongly considered in patients who show a fourfold increase in titers, patients who have an initially high titer (1:32 or greater) that fails to decline at least fourfold within 12 to 24 months of therapy, HIV-infected patients, and patients who develop signs or symptoms associated with neurosyphilis.

Neurosyphilis

- Follow-up is dependent on the CSF findings. If pleocytosis is present, reexamine the CSF every 6 months until the WBC count normalizes. Consider recommending a second course of treatment if the CSF white count does not decline after 6 months or completely normalize after 2 years.[4,9,20] Failure to normalize may require retreatment; most treatment failures occur in immunocompromised patients.

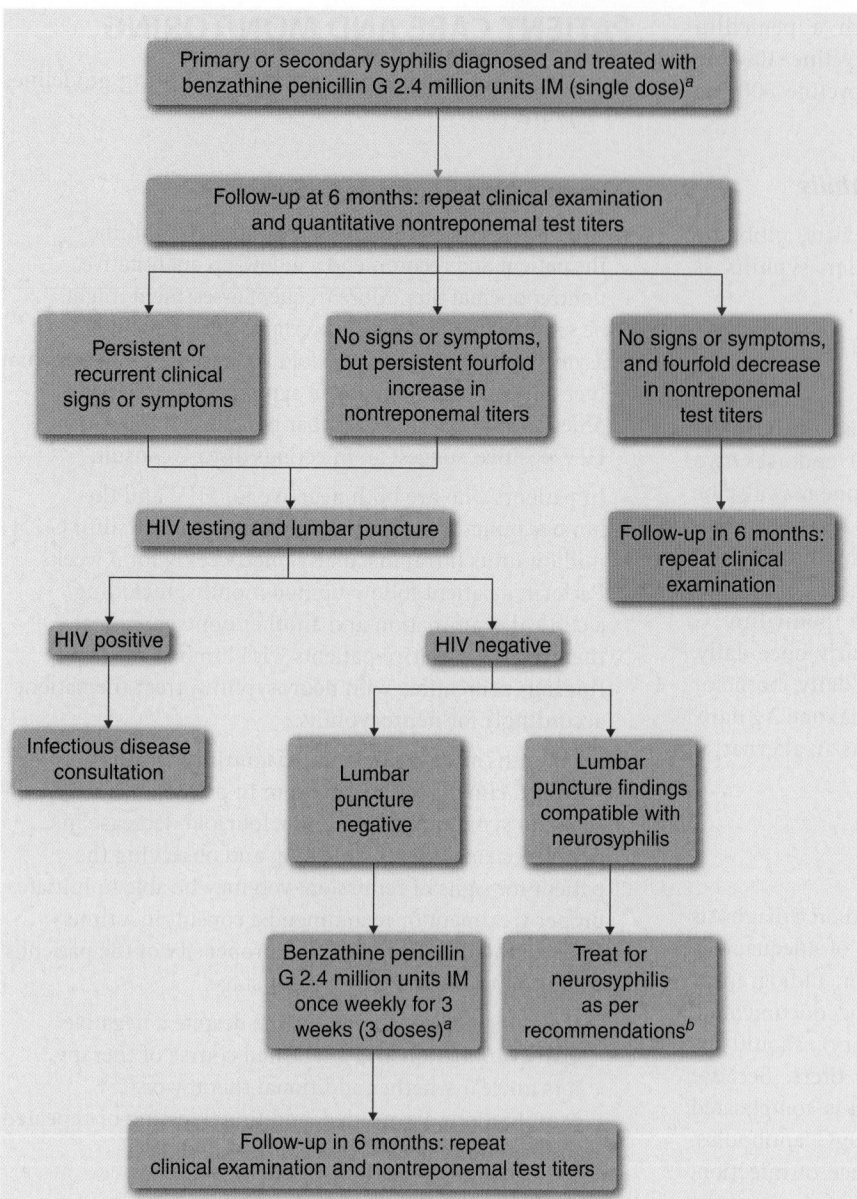

FIGURE 80–2. Patient care monitoring for syphilis. (From Brown D, Frank J. Diagnosis and management of syphilis. Am Fam Physician 2003;68(2):283–290.) (^aSee text for alternative treatment recommendations for nonpregnant penicillin-allergic patients. ^bSee text for treatment recommendations for neurosyphilis.)

Congenital Syphilis

- Observe the patient for changes in clinical features; hepatomegaly, jaundice, and bone changes will usually resolve in 3 months.
- Monitor elevated serologic markers (nontreponemal tests) for reduction in titer levels. Given effective treatment, clinical features will usually disappear after 6 months. On this basis, evaluate seropositive infants periodically for at least 6 months.[24]

TRICHOMONIASIS

Trichomoniasis is caused by the protozoan *Trichomonas vaginalis* and is far more prevalent than *C. trachomatis* or *N. gonorrhoeae*. In the United States, approximately 5 million new cases appear annually, compared with 3 million chlamydial and 650,000 gonococcal cases annually.[26]

PATHOPHYSIOLOGY

T. vaginalis, a protozoa, may be isolated from the vagina, urethra, and Bartholin's or Skene's glands. After attachment to the host cells, it ignites an inflammatory response exhibited as a discharge containing elevated levels of polymorphonuclear leukocytes. The protozoal pathogen causes direct damage to the epithelium, leading to microulcerations.

DIAGNOSIS

Diagnosis is usually performed with a wet mount or Papanicolaou smear. In women, symptoms are characterized

Clinical Presentation of Trichomoniasis[9,26]

General
- Asymptomatic

Signs
- Strawberry cervix (women)
- Colpitis macularis (women)
- Prostatitis or epididymitis (men)

Symptoms
- Vaginal/vulvar erythema
- Excessive yellow-green discharge
- Vulvar itching
- Vaginal odor
- Urethral discharge or irritation
- Dysuria
- Vaginal pH greater than 4.5

by diffuse, malodorous, yellow-green vaginal discharge with vulvar irritation. Some women may be asymptomatic.

TREATMENT

Desired Outcome

The desired outcome is the complete eradication of *T. vaginalis* in the patient and sexual partner(s) and elimination of the signs and symptoms observed.

Pharmacologic Therapy

⑤ *The 5-nitroimidazoles have been the standard therapy for trichomoniasis for over 45 years.* Drugs included in this class are metronidazole, tinidazole, ornidazole, and secnidazole; metronidazole and tinidazole are the only drugs in this class available in the United States. When recommending the 5-nitroimidazoles, advise patients to avoid the consumption of alcohol.

▶ *Metronidazole*

Metronidazole may be administered orally as a single 2-g dose or 500 mg twice daily for 7 days.[9,26] Pregnant women should be prescribed the single dose of metronidazole. Cure rates are greater than 90% when metronidazole is administered as either a single 2-g dose or a 7-day regimen. Possible adverse effects include an unpleasant metallic taste, reversible neutropenia, urticaria, rash, flushing, dry mouth, darkened urine, and a disulfiram-like reaction.

▶ *Tinidazole*

Tinidazole, a second-generation nitroimidazole with protozoal and anaerobic activity, has been available outside the United States for over 35 years.[27] As a single 2-g dose,

tinidazole has an efficacy equivalent to a 2-g dose of metronidazole. Tindazole also has a longer half-life than metronidazole, 14 and 7 hours respectively, and penetrates into male reproductive tissue better than metronidazole.

Tinidazole is effective for metronidazole-resistant trichomoniasis.[26,27] Possible side effects include an unpleasant metallic taste, dizziness, loss of coordination, seizures, severe diarrhea, darkened urine, nausea, vomiting, and a swollen or discolored tongue.

PATIENT CARE AND MONITORING

Monitoring for *T. vaginalis* is generally not required unless symptoms persist or recur.

GENITAL WARTS

● Genital warts, caused by the human papillomavirus (HPV), usually appear in the genital area as very contagious, small bumps. Responsible for various visible, keratotic, and nonkeratotic manifestations, HPV has more than 120 noted strains, some of which have been linked to squamous cell carcinoma.[28] More than 40 strains have been linked to the genital area.[9]

EPIDEMIOLOGY

Affecting more than 20 million Americans, HPV is the most common newly diagnosed STI in the United States, with prevalence just about 15.2%. Approximately 6.2 million new HPV infections occur every year in the United States.[29] The frequency of cervicovaginal HPV infection among sexually active women has been observed at 43%, with the greatest incidence noticed in men with three or more sex partners and women whose most recent regular sexual partner had two or more lifetime partners. Most people with HPV do not develop symptoms. At least half of sexually active persons will become infected at least once in their lifetime. In 90% of the cases, the body's immune system clears HPV naturally within 2 years. HPV types 16 and 18 cause over 70% of all cervical cancer, whereas HPV types 6 and 11 are responsible for about 90% of genital warts.[30]

PATHOPHYSIOLOGY

HPV replicates in terminally differentiated squamous cells in the intermediate layers of the genital mucosa. Hence these effects of the viral early region genes on DNA synthesis are critical for viral survival. Genital warts are the clinical manifestation of active viral replication and virion production at the infection site.

DIAGNOSIS

- A definitive diagnosis of HPV is based on DNA or RNA or capsid protein detection.
- Diagnosis is generally made from the clinical presentation and may be classified into several categories: classic

Clinical Presentation of Genital Warts[9,30,31]

General
- Appear as rough, thick, cauliflower-like lesions

Signs
- Black dots within warts
- Disrupted surface

Symptoms
- Anogenital pruritus
- Burning
- Vaginal discharge or bleeding
- Although rare, dyspareunia may occur with vulvovaginal condyloma

Table 80–2

Comparison of Adverse Effects Seen with Treatments for Genital Warts

Treatment	Adverse Effects
Podofilox	Burning at site of application, pain, inflammation
Imiquimod	Erythema, irritation, ulceration, pain, burning, edema, pigmentary changes
Sinecatechins	Burning at site of application, erythema, pruritus, edema
Podophyllin resin	Local irritation, erythema, burning, soreness at application site; possibly oncogenic
Bichloroacetic and trichloroacetic acid	Local irritation and pain, minimal systemic effects
Cryotherapy	Pain or blisters at application site
Surgical excision	Pain, bleeding, scarring; possible burning or allergic reaction to local anesthetic
Vaporization	Pain, bleeding, scarring; risk of HPV spreading via smoke plumes
Intralesional interferon	Burning, itching, irritation at injection site, systemic myalgia, headache, fever, chills, leukopenia, elevated liver enzymes, and thrombocytopenia

HPV, human papillomavirus.

From Refs. 9, 28, and 31.

condyloma acuminata, which are pointed or cauliform; keratotic warts with a thick, horny surface resembling common skin warts; and flat warts, frequently observed on the *outer layer of skin.*
- Tissue biopsy or viral typing is only indicated if the diagnosis is uncertain and is not recommended for patients with routine or typical lesions.
- Since HPV is highly associated with cervical cancer and has more than 20 different cancer-associated HPV types, patients who are diagnosed with HPV should be tested for cervical cancer.

TREATMENT

Desired Outcome

Removal of visible warts and reduction of infectivity are the goals of treatment.

Pharmacologic Therapy[9,31]

⑥ *Currently, the choice of therapy is based on the size, site, and morphology of lesions, as well as patient preference, treatment costs, convenience, adverse effects, and clinician experience. Factors that might affect response include the presence of immunosuppression and patient compliance.* Assuming that the diagnosis is correct, switching to alternate therapy is appropriate if there has been no response observed after three treatment cycles. A comparison of adverse effects related to treatment options may be found in Table 80–2.

▶ *Patient-Applied Treatment*

Podofilox Available as a 0.5% gel or solution containing purified extract of the most active compound of podophyllin, podofilox arrests the formation of the mitotic spindle, prevents cell division, and may also induce damage in blood vessels within the warts. The surface area treated must not exceed 10 cm², and a maximum of 0.5 mL should be used on a daily basis.

Apply twice daily for 3 consecutive days followed by 4 consecutive days without treatment. This cycle may be repeated until there are no visible warts or for a maximum of 4 weeks. Side effects are generally local and may include erythema, swelling, and erosions. Podofilox is not recommended for use in the vagina, anus, or during pregnancy.

Imiquimod Imiquimod is a cell-mediated immune-response modifier, available as a topical 5% cream in single-dose application packets. Imiquimod is applied at bedtime, three times a week for up to 16 weeks.

The treatment area should be washed with soap and water 6 to 10 hours after application. Mild to moderate erythema has been noted with imiquimod use; however, this generally suggests that the drug is reaching a therapeutic range and may be clearing the lesion.[32,33]

Sinecatechins A green tea extract with an active product (catechins) is available as a 15% ointment. Apply a thin layer (0.5 cm) using a finger to each wart three times a day until complete clearance of warts. Do not wash off after use, and all sexual contact should be avoided while ointment is on the skin. This product should not be continued for longer than 16 weeks.[9]

▶ *Physician-Applied Treatments*

Podophyllin Resin A 10% to 25% solution of podophyllin resin has been the standard in-office treatment for genital warts. Because podophyllin is neurotoxic and easily systemically absorbed, only a small amount (no more than 0.5 mL) should be applied, avoiding normal tissue. Application should be limited to less than 0.5 mL of podophyllin on an area of less than 10 cm² of warts per session, and no open lesions or wounds should exist in the area to which treatment is administered. The affected area will likely become erythematous and painful within 48 hours of application.[34]

Topical podophyllin is applied once weekly and the area should be allowed to dry. Immediately following treatment, the dried drug should be removed using alcohol or soap and water. It is contraindicated in pregnant patients.

Bichloracetic and Trichloroacetic Acids These products are available in 80% to 90% concentrations and are not systemically absorbed. The products are effective when used to treat a few, small, moist lesions. They may be applied to both keratinized epithelial and mucosal surfaces and may be used in pregnancy.

A noted reaction to these medications is transient burning; contact with surrounding epithelium may prove to be painful, producing significant local erythema and swelling. To avoid these effects, place petroleum jelly around the external lesion, including unaffected skin, and carefully apply the agent with a small applicator. If an excess amount of acid is used, talc or sodium bicarbonate (baking soda) may be used to neutralize unreacted acid.

Other Treatments Additional treatments may include fluorouracil/epinephrine/bovine collagen gel, an intralesional injection that has been proven effective in clinical trials for refractory patients or an intralesional injection of interferon.[31]

▶ Ablative Therapy

Several ablative options have been employed in the treatment of genital warts and include cryotherapy, surgical removal, and vaporization.

▶ Special Therapeutic Issues[31,34]

Large Warts Treat warts greater than 10 mm in diameter with surgical excision. Use imiquimod for three to four treatment cycles to reduce the number of warts and improve surgical outcomes. Fifty percent reduction in wart size after four treatment cycles warrants continued use of imiquimod until warts clear or eight cycles have been completed; less than 50% reduction warrants surgical excision or other ablative therapy.

Subclinical Warts Subclinical warts may be identified through colonoscopy, biopsy, acetic acid application, or laboratory serology. However, early treatment has not been linked to a favorable effect during the course of therapy in the index patient or the partner with regard to reduction of the transmission rate.

Pregnancy Agents contraindicated in pregnancy include podofilox, sinecatechins, fluorouracil, and podophyllin. Imiquimod is not approved for use in pregnancy, although it has been considered after signed consent has been obtained.

Bichloroacetic and trichloroacetic acids have been used without problems. Ablative therapy is also a viable option.

PATIENT CARE AND MONITORING

Monitor patients every 3 to 6 months for a reduction in lesions or disease remission. Monitoring parameters include patient compliance, disease remission, and benign or cancerous tumors. Sexually active people can lower their chances of getting HPV by limiting their number of partners.

Vaccinations

Several HPV genotypes have been linked to the development of cervical cancer. Gardasil®, developed to protect against HPV genotypes 6, 11, 16, and 18, was the first vaccine employed to prevent cervical cancer, precancerous genital lesions, and genital warts due to HPV. Cervarix® vaccine helps prevent cervical cancer and precancers caused by HPV types 16 and 18. The CDC recommends the HPV vaccine for all 11- and 12-year-old males and females. Vaccination is also recommended for all teens, girls, and women through 26 years who have not been previously vaccinated or who have not completed the full series of shots.[40]

Both vaccines are given in a series of three injections over a 6-month period. The second and third doses should be given at 2 and 6 months (respectively) after the first dose. HPV vaccine may be given at the same time as other vaccines.

GENITAL HERPES

Genital herpes (GH) is caused by herpes simplex virus (HSV) types 1 and 2. HSV is a chronic, life-long viral infection for which there is no cure. Once latency is established, neither competent host immunity nor therapeutic agents can eradicate the virus.[9] Currently, there is no vaccine available for HSV, and it seems that the development of one is unlikely in the near future.

EPIDEMIOLOGY

Approximately 50 million Americans have GH. HSV-2 is the most common cause of recurrent genital herpes. Roughly one in six people in the United States (16.2%) aged 14 to 49 is infected with HSV-2. Prevalence of HSV-2 infection has grown slightly since the late 1970s (16.4% to 17.2%), and currently more than 500,000 new cases of HSV-2 occur annually.

PATHOPHYSIOLOGY

Nearly all HSV-2 infections are sexually acquired. Since HSV is only found in humans, infection may only be transmitted from infectious secretions onto mucosal surfaces (i.e., cervix or urethra) or direct contact with an active lesion (abraded skin). The virus may survive for a limited amount of time on environmental surfaces.

DIAGNOSIS

Ulcerative or multiple vesicular lesions are absent in many infected persons. Laboratory confirmation is vital to effective treatment of HSV, especially in individuals in whom a clinical diagnosis cannot be obtained. There are several methods by which a definitive diagnosis may be acquired, and these include virologic typing, serologic diagnosis, rapid point-of-care antigen detection, enzyme-linked immunosorbent assay (ELISA), immunoblot, and DNA polymerase chain reaction.[35] Additionally, the FDA recently approved glycoprotein G-based assays to aid in the diagnosis of HSV.

TREATMENT

Desired Outcome

The desired outcome is to curtail the number of episodic prodromes and to minimize any side effects experienced due to the antivirals. Counseling of infected persons and their partners is vital to the management of HSV.

Pharmacologic Therapy[9]

⓻ *Treatment is based on several factors, including likelihood of patient compliance, whether it is the first or a recurrent episode, host immunity, and pregnancy.* However, patient response has been linked to the time it takes to initiate treatment with acyclovir, or its analogues, after symptom onset.

▶ *First Episode*

The first episode is a systemic illness associated with the vesicular lesions, may last up to 21 days, usually has an uncomplicated course of infection, and in severe cases may require hospitalization. Several agents are effective during this period (Table 80–3).[36–38] At the cited dosages, these agents have had excellent outcomes with regard to lesion healing time, viral shedding, and resolution of pain. Common adverse effects are nausea, headache, and diarrhea.

▶ *Episodic Therapy*

In a patient with a previous diagnosis of genital herpes, the appearance of new vesicular lesions is synonymous with HSV reactivation. For most patients, genital herpes recurrence is self-limiting and short-lived, lasting approximately 6 to 7 days.

▶ *Suppressive Therapy*

Suppressive therapy is effective for controlling all symptoms related to the disease and may impact troublesome complications of infection. Daily suppressive therapy is used in patients who have six or more episodes per year. Before beginning suppressive therapy, discuss patient expectations. Encourage patients to record any breakthrough episodes, as this may require treatment reevaluation and adjustment.

▶ *Preventive Therapy*

Valacyclovir 500 mg orally once daily has been implicated to prevent the sexual transmission of HSV to an uninfected partner. In addition to pharmacologic therapy, counsel patients regarding safe sex practices.

▶ *Drug Resistance*

All acyclovir-resistant strains are resistant to valacyclovir, and the majority are resistant to famciclovir. Foscarnet, cidofovir, and trifuridine have been administered in acyclovir-resistant patients.[39] These agents are usually reserved for use after other medications have failed because of their associated toxicities.

▶ *Pregnancy*

Women who are pregnant may transmit the virus to the neonate during delivery. There are two management strategies: cesarean section and antiviral therapy. A few

Table 80–3

Comparison of Antivirals Used for Herpes Simplex Infection

Agent	Dose	Side Effects
First Episode		
Acyclovir	*200 mg orally 5 times a day × 7–10 days* 400 mg orally 3 times daily × 7–10 days	Headache, confusion, nausea, vomiting, thrombocytopenia, renal insufficiency, rash, pruritus, fever, arthralgias, myalgia, thrombotic thrombocytopenic purpura, hallucinations, somnolence, depression
Valacyclovir	*1 g orally 2 times daily × 7–10 days*	Refer to acyclovir
Famciclovir	250 mg orally 3 times daily × 7–10 days	Refer to acyclovir
Episodic		
Acyclovir	*200 mg orally 5 times daily × 5 days* *Or* 400 mg orally every 8 hours × 5 days *Or* 800 mg orally 2 times daily × 5 days *Or* 800 mg orally 3 times daily × 2 days	Refer to acyclovir
Valacyclovir	*500 mg orally 2 times daily × 3 days* *Or* 1 g orally once daily × 5 days	Refer to acyclovir
Famciclovir	125 mg orally 2 times daily × 5 days 1000 mg orally twice daily × 1 day	Refer to acyclovir *Or*
Suppressive		
Acyclovir	400 mg orally 2 times daily continuously *Or*	Refer to acyclovir
Valacyclovir	500 mg orally once daily continuously *Or*	Refer to acyclovir
Valacyclovir	1000 mg orally once daily continuously *Or*	Refer to acyclovir
Famciclovir	250 mg orally 2 times daily continuously	Refer to acyclovir
Reserved Agents		
Foscarnet	40 mg/kg IV every 8 hours until clinical resolution is attained	Renal insufficiency, metabolic disturbances, hypophosphatemia
Cidofovir	1% topical agent (gel) used daily on a compassionate basis for acyclovir-resistant herpes lesions × 5 days	Application site reactions, lesion recrudescence
Imiquimod	Topical alternative used daily on a compassionate basis for acyclovir-resistant herpes lesions × 5 days	Application site reactions, lesion recrudescence

Italicized data indicate recommended dosages.

From Refs. 9 and 33.

studies indicate that acyclovir 200 to 400 mg every 8 hours has been administered from 38 weeks gestation until delivery. Suppressive treatment includes the use of acyclovir or valacyclovir from week 36 until delivery. The goal of therapy is to reduce the number of lesions and asymptomatic shedding at delivery.

▶ Neonates

The risk for transmission from an infected mother to a neonate is high among women who acquired GH near time of delivery. HSV infections should be considered in all neonates who present with nonspecific symptoms such as fever, poor feeding, lethargy, or seizures in the first month of life. Infants suspected to have or who are diagnosed with an HSV infection should be treated parenterally. Acyclovir can be administered 20 mg/kg/day in three divided doses IV for 21 days for disseminated and CNS disease or 14 days for disease limited to skin, eyes, and mucous membranes.

PATIENT CARE AND MONITORING

Reevaluation of the patient's condition and therapy adjustment are key elements in effective monitoring. Parameters may include:

- The patient's psychosocial and psychosexual status
- Frequent reassessment of recurrent episodes and therapy adjustment

- Ordering tests for malignancy
- Yearly testing of HIV status
- Side effects of drugs

BACTERIAL VAGINOSIS

8 *Bacterial vaginosis (BV) is a clinical syndrome categorized by an overgrowth of polymicrobial anaerobic organisms, such as* Gardenella vaginalis, Prevotella *species,* Mycoplasma hominis, *and* Mobiluncus *species. BV infection leads to the replacement of the normal hydrogen peroxide-producing lactobacillus and an increase in vaginal pH from 4.5 to 7.*[41] BV is the most prevalent cause of vaginal discharge and malodor.

EPIDEMIOLOGY

BV is associated with having multiple male or female partners, a new sex partner, douching, lack of condom use, and lack of vaginal lactobacilli. It is estimated that one in three women will develop BV at some point in their lives. BV has been found in 12% to 25% of women in routine clinic populations, 10% to 26% of women in obstetrics clinics, and 32% to 64% of women in clinics for STIs. BV infection usually results from sexual activity, although some cases have been reported in women who are not sexually active.

PATHOPHYSIOLOGY

A complex and intricate balance of microorganisms maintains the normal vaginal flora (i.e., lactobacilli, corynebacteria, and yeast). The normal postmenarchal and premenopausal vaginal pH is 3.8 to 4.2. At this pH, growth of pathogenic organisms is usually inhibited; however, disturbance of the normal vaginal pH can alter the vaginal flora, leading to overgrowth of pathogens.

DIAGNOSIS

BV is diagnosed according to the Amsel criteria. In order for diagnosis to be confirmed, three of the four criteria must be present:

1. Thin, white, homogenous discharge
2. Clue cells on microscopy (clue cells are epithelial cells of the vagina that get their distinctive stippled appearance by being covered with bacteria)
3. pH of vaginal fluid greater than 4.5
4. Release of a fishy odor upon the addition of an alkali (10% potassium hydroxide) to a vaginal sample

Alternatively, a gram-stain vaginal smear may be used to diagnose BV using the Nugent criteria. This relies on estimating the proportions of bacteria morphotypes to

Clinical Presentation of Bacterial Vaginosis[9,42,43]

General
- Offensive fishy-smelling vaginal discharge

Signs
- Thin, white, homogenous discharge, coating the walls of the vagina

Symptoms
- Many women are asymptomatic; usually not associated with soreness, itching, or irritation

provide a score between 0 and 10. A score of less than 4 is normal, 4 to 6 is intermediate, and greater than 6 is consistent with BV. Isolation of G. *vaginalis* may not be diagnostic because it can be cultured from the vagina in some normal women, although a high concentration may be indicative of infection.[42]

TREATMENT
Desired Outcome

Reduction in the number of causative bacteria, cessation of vaginal discharge, and decrease in vaginal pH are the desired outcomes.

Pharmacologic Therapy[9,43]

▶ *Adults*

Recommended adult regimens include metronidazole 500 mg orally twice daily for 7 days *or* metronidazole gel (0.75%), one full applicator (5 g) intravaginally once daily for 5 days *or* clindamycin cream (2%), one full applicator (5 g) intravaginally at bedtime for 7 days.

Alternative regimens include clindamycin ovules 100 mg intravaginally once at bedtime for 3 days, clindamycin 300 mg orally twice daily for 7 days, tinidazole 2 g orally once daily for 2 days, or Tinidazole 1 g orally daily for 5 days.

▶ *Pregnancy*

Pregnant symptomatic women should receive treatment. Treatment of BV in asymptomatic women at high-risk for preterm delivery with a recommended oral regimen mitigates preterm delivery. Screening should be performed during the first prenatal visit. Recommended regimens for pregnant women include metronidazole 500 mg orally twice daily for 7 days *or* metronidazole 250 mg orally three times daily for 7 days *or* clindamycin 300 mg orally twice daily for 7 days. Metronidazole is not recommended for use in the first trimester of pregnancy.

PATIENT CARE AND MONITORING

A test to determine whether the patient has been cured is generally not recommended, thus follow-up visits are unnecessary if symptoms resolve. However, in patients with recurrent symptomatic BV, a follow-up after the course of therapy may be warranted. If treatment has been prescribed during pregnancy to reduce preterm birth, perform a repeat exam in 1 month and advise further treatment for recurrent BV. Patients taking metronidazole should be cautioned not to consume alcohol while taking this medication for up to 24 hours after taking the last dose.

PELVIC INFLAMMATORY DISEASE

Pelvic inflammatory disease (PID) usually affects young, sexually active, reproductive-age women. PID includes a spectrum of inflammatory disorders of the upper female genital tract. In the majority of cases, the pathogens responsible are *C. trachomatis* and *N. gonorrhoeae,* although anaerobes, enteric gram-negative rods, and cytomegalovirus have also been implicated in the pathogenesis.[44] PID has been correlated with ectopic pregnancy, infertility, tubo-ovarian abscess, and chronic pelvic pain.[46]

EPIDEMIOLOGY

More than 750,000 women are affected by PID each year in the United States. The highest rates of PID occur in teenagers and first-time mothers. Up to 10% to 15% of these women may become infertile as a result of PID. The CDC estimates that more than 1 million women experience an episode of PID every year. The disease leads to approximately 2.5 million office visits annually. Because many cases of PID go unrecognized and some episodes are asymptomatic, the potential for damage to the reproductive health of women is substantial.

PATHOPHYSIOLOGY

PID occurs when bacteria move upward from a woman's vagina into her reproductive organs. *Chlamydia* may produce a heat-shock protein that causes tissue damage through a delayed hypersensitivity reaction. *C. trachomatis* may also possess DNA evidence of toxin-like genes that code for high-molecular-weight proteins with structures similar to *Clostridium difficile* cytotoxins, enabling inhibition of immune activation. This may explain the observation of a chronic *C. trachomatis* infection in subclinical PID.

DIAGNOSIS[44,45]

To be diagnosed with PID, patients must have uterine tenderness, cervical motion tenderness, lower abdominal pain, painful intercourse, and adnexal tenderness with no other cause of these signs. Additional criteria include:

- Oral temperature greater than 38.3°C (101°F)
- Abnormal cervical or vaginal discharge
- WBC presence on saline microscopy of vaginal secretions
- Elevated erythrocyte sedimentation rate
- Elevated C-reactive protein
- Laboratory documentation of cervical infection with *N. gonorrhoeae* or *C. trachomatis*

TREATMENT
Desired Outcome

The eradication of causative bacteria and reduction of any related sequelae are the desired goals of treatment.

Table 80–4

Treatment Regimens for Pelvic Inflammatory Disease

Parenteral Option A
Cefotetan 2 g IV every 12 hours plus doxycycline 100 mg orally or IV every 12 hours
or
Cefoxitin 2 g IV every 6 hours plus doxycycline 100 mg orally or IV every 12 hours

Parenteral Option B
Clindamycin 900 mg IV every 8 hours plus gentamicin, loading dose IV or IM (2 mg/kg) followed by maintenance dose (1.5 mg/kg) every 8 hours. A single daily dose of gentamicin (3–5 mg/kg) may be used.

Alternative Parenteral treatment
Ampicillin-sulbactam 3 g IV every 6 hours plus doxycycline 100 mg orally or IV every 12 hours

Oral
Ceftriaxone 250 mg IM single dose plus doxycycline 100 mg orally twice daily for 14 days with or without metronidazole 500 mg orally twice daily for 14 days
Or
Cefoxitin 2 g IM single dose and probenecid 1 g single dose, plus doxycycline 100 mg orally twice daily for 14 days with or without metronidazole 500 mg orally twice daily for 14 days
Or
Third-generation cephalosporin (ceftizoxime or cefotaxime) plus doxycycline 100 mg orally twice daily for 14 days with or without metronidazole 500 mg orally twice daily for 14 days

From Refs. 9, 45, and 46.

Pharmacologic Treatment[9]

[9] *Resolution of infection (i.e., N. gonorrhoeae, C. trachomatis, Streptococcus spp., and gram-negative facultative bacteria) and mitigation of sequelae should be the main goal of pharmacologic therapy.* CDC-approved treatment regimens are shown in Table 80–4.[9,44] Optimal management of PID should be individualized based on clinical setting and patient characteristics. For some patients, hospitalizations, IV antibiotics, and surgical treatment of complications may be needed. Although outpatient management remains contentious, many feel that outpatient management should be limited to individuals who remain afebrile, have a WBC count less than $11 \times 10^3/\text{mm}^3$ ($11 \times 10^9/\text{L}$), have minimal evidence of peritonitis, have active bowel sounds, and can tolerate oral nourishment. Nonetheless, outpatient therapy with a parenteral cephalosporin followed by doxycycline and metronidazole is recommended.

PATIENT CARE AND MONITORING

If no clinical improvement has occurred within 3 days after parenteral or outpatient oral therapy, further assessment should be performed. The goals of monitoring patients with PID are related to reducing long-term complications. To this end, the primary approach should be prevention and education of at-risk women. Secondary prevention may include screening by conducting a pelvic exam during a routine checkup. The male sex partners of women with PID should be examined if the patient's onset of symptoms occurred within the previous 60 days. It is imperative that women understand that the more sex partners she encounters, the greater her risk of developing PID.

PREVENTION STRATEGIES

A combination of prevention efforts is advised. Alteration in sexual behavior should undoubtedly be the first counseling concern, as promiscuous sexual activity has been shown to augment the probability of infection.

Abstinence is the best course of action, especially in patients with herpes during lesional episodes. However, compliance in some may be minimal, in which case, appropriate condom use should always be recommended. To alleviate any possible misconceptions about condom application, either demonstrate how to apply a condom or

Patient Encounter 4, Part 2

PMH: History of bacterial vaginosis 2 years ago. Allergy to clindamycin.

FH: Noncontributory.

SH: Has two children from two different fathers. Admits to having six sexual partners in the last 3 years. Smokes ½ pack of Newport cigarettes per day to remain calm.

ROS: Painful vesicles, frequent urination, and urticaria in the genital area. Recently developed a fishy smelling vaginal (white) discharge.

PE:

VS: BP = 135/85 mm Hg, Height = 5 ft 2 in (157 cm), Weight = 217 lb (98.6 kg), Temp = 97.8°F (36.6°C)

Lab: Vaginal pH = 4.7

What information is suggestive of bacterial vaginosis?

If the diagnosis of bacterial vaginosis is confirmed, what therapeutic options exist for this patient?

Patient Encounter 4, Part 3

SM is young and uneducated about the ramifications of her sexual actions. She continues to have unprotected sex with multiple men. Although taking birth control pills may protect her from pregnancy, they will not protect her from STIs. The incidence of STIs has increased dramatically over the last 25 years.

What impact will pregnancy have on the treatment plan for the two STIs?

What consideration should be given to other STIs?

ask the patient to demonstrate. During the demonstration, explicitly educate the patient with regard to application, storage, and the use of lubricants.[47]

Abbreviations Introduced in This Chapter

BV	Bacterial vaginosis
CSF	Cerebrospinal fluid
ELISA	Enzyme-linked immunosorbent assay
GH	Genital herpes
HPV	Human papillomavirus
HSV	Herpes simplex virus
MSM	Men who have sex with men
PID	Pelvic inflammatory disease
RPR	Rapid plasma reagin
STI	Sexually transmitted infection
WSW	Women who have sex with women

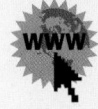 Self-assessment questions and answers are available at *http://mhpharmacotherapy.com/pp.html*.

REFERENCES

1. Birley H, Duerden B, Hart C. Sexually transmitted diseases: Microbiology and management. J Med Microbiol 2002;51:793–807.
2. Aral S. Sexually risky behaviour and infection: Epidemiological considerations. Sex Transm Infect 2004;80(Suppl II):ii8–ii12.
3. Biddlecom A. Trends in sexual behaviours and infections among young people in the United States. Sex Transm Infect 2004;80(Suppl II):ii74–ii79.
4. Sexually Transmitted Diseases. MMWR Recommendations and Reports 2006;55 RR-11:1–92.
5. Gorbach P, Galea J, Amani A, et al. Don't ask, don't tell: Patterns of HIV disclosure among HIV positive men who have sex with men with recent STI practicing high risk behaviour in Los Angeles and Seattle. Sex Transm Infect 2004;80:512–517.
6. Fethers K, Marks C, Mindel A, et al. Sexually Transmitted Infections and risk behaviors in women who have sex with women. Sex Transm Infect 2000;76:345–349.
7. Bechtel K. Sexual abuse and sexually transmitted infections in children and adolescents. Curr Opin Ped 2010;22:94–99.
8. Dukers-Muijrers N, Niekamp A, Brouwers E, et al. Older and swinging; need to identify hidden and emerging risk groups at STI clinics. Sex Transm Infect 2010;86: 315–317.
9. Sexually Transmitted Diseases. MMWR Treatment Guidelines, 2010 [online]. [cited 2011 Oct 10]. Available from: *www.cdc.gov/mmwr.* Accessed May 14, 2011.
10. Kodner C. Sexually transmitted infections in men: Primary care. Clin Office Pract 2003;30:173–191.
11. Mandell GL, Bennet JE, Dolin R. Mandell, Douglas, and Bennet's Principles and Practice of Infectious Diseases. 7th ed. Philadelphia, PA: Church Livingstone; 2010.
12. Moran J. Gonorrhea. Clin Evid 2004;(11):2104–2112.
13. Lyss S, Kamb M, Peterman T, et al. Chlamydia trachomatis among patients infected with and treated for Neisseria gonorrhea in sexually transmitted disease clinics in the United States. Ann Intern Med 2003;139:178–185.
14. Tapsall JW. What management is there for gonorrhea in the postquinolone era? Sex Transm Dis 2006;33:8–10.
15. Barry P, Klausner J. The use of cephalosporins for gonorrhea: the impending problem of resistance. Expert Opin Pharmacother 2009;10 (4):555–577.
16. Manju B, Semma S. Cephalosporin resistance in *Neisseria gonorrhoeae.* J Global Infect Dis 2010;23:284–296.
17. Gursahaney P, Meyn L, Hiller S, et. al. Combined hormonal contraception may be protective against *Neisseria gonorrhoeae* infection. Sex Transm Dis 2010;37(6):356–360.
18. Young F. Sexually transmitted infections. Genital chlamydia: Practical management in primary care. J Fam Health Care 2005;15:19–21.
19. Summary of Notifiable Diseases in the United States, 2009 [online]. Morbidity and Mortality Weekly Report. [cited 2011 Oct 10]. Available from: *http://www.cdc.gov/mmwr/preview/mmwrhtml/mm5853a1.htm.* Accessed September 14, 2011.
20. Brown D, Frank J. Diagnosis and management of syphilis. Am Fam Physician 2003;68:283–290.
21. Saloojee H, Sithembiso V, Goga Y, et al. The prevention and management of congenital syphilis: An overview and recommendations. Bull World Health Organ 2004;82(6):424–430.
23. Berman S. Maternal syphilis: Pathophysiology and treatment. Bull World Health Organ 2004;82(6):433–438.
24. Peeling R, Ye H. Diagnostic tools for preventing and managing maternal and congenital syphilis: An overview. Bull World Health Organ 2004;82(6):439–446.
25. Berman S. Maternal syphilis: Pathophysiology and treatment. Bull World Health Organ 2004;82(6):433–438.
26. Soper D. Trichomoniasis: Under control or undercontrolled? Am J Obstet Gynecol 2004;190:281–290.
27. Tindamax [online]. [cited 2011 Oct 10]. Available from: *www.tindamax.com.*
28. Kodner C, Nasraty S. Management of genital warts. Am Fam Physician 2004;70:2335–2342, 2345–2346.
29. Ault K. Epidemiology and natural history of human papillomavirus infections in the female genital tract. Infect Dis Obstet Gynecol 2006:1–5.
30. Smith G, Travis L. Getting to know human papillomavirus (HPV) and the HPV vaccine. J Am Osteopath2001;111 (3 suppl 2):S29–S34.
31. Gunter J. Genital and perianal warts: New treatment opportunities for human papillomavirus infection. Am J Obstet Gynecol 2003;189:S3–S11.
32. Bowden F, Tabrizi S, Garland S, et al. Sexually transmitted infections: New diagnostic approaches and treatments. MJA 2002;176:551–557.
33. World Health Organization. Guidelines for the management of sexually transmitted infections, 2003 [online]. [cited 2011 Oct 10]. Available from: *http://www.who.int/HIV/pub/sti/en/STIGuidelines2003.pdf.*
34. Woodward C, Fisher M. Drug treatment of common STDs: Part II. Vaginal infections, pelvic inflammatory disease and genital warts. Am Fam Physician 1999;60:1716–1722.
35. Patel R. Progress in meeting today's demands in genital herpes: An overview of current management. J Infect Dis 2002;186(Suppl I):S47–S56.
36. Alexander L, Naisbett B. Patient and physician partnerships in managing genital herpes. J Infect Dis 2002;186(Suppl I):S57–S65.
37. Lacy C, Armstrong L, Goldman M, Lance L. Lexi-Comp's Drug Information Handbook. 19th ed. Hudson, OH: Lexi-Comp; 2010:1128–1132.
38. Kimberlin D, Rouse D. Genital Herpes. N Engl J Med 2004;350:1970–1977.
39. Wald A. New therapies and prevention strategies for genital herpes. Clin Infect Dis 1999;28(Suppl 1):S4–S13.
40. Gardasil [online]. [cited 2011 Oct 10]. Available from: *http://www.cdc.gov/vaccines/vpd-vac/hpv/vac-faqs.html.*
41. Klebanoff M, Hauth J, MacPherson C, et al. Time course of the regression of asymptomatic bacterial vaginosis in pregnancy with and without treatment. Am J Obstet Gynecol 2004;190:363–370.
42. Sobel J. What's new in bacterial vaginosis and trichomoniasis? Infect Dis Clin North Am 2005;19:387–406.
43. Clinical Effectiveness Group. National guidelines for the management of bacterial vaginosis. Sex Transm Infect 1999;75(Suppl I):S16–S18.
44. Miller K, Ruiz D, Graves J. Update on the prevention and treatment of sexually transmitted diseases. Am Fam Physician 2003;67(9):1915–1922.
45. Beigi R, Wiesenfeld H. Pelvic inflammatory disease: New diagnostic criteria and treatment. Obstet Gynecol Clin North Am 2003;30(4):777–793.
46. Epperly AT, Viera AJ. Pelvic inflammatory disease. Clin Fam Pract 2005;7:67–78.
47. FDA. Condoms and Sexually Transmitted diseases [online]. [cited 2011 Oct 10]. Available from: *http://www.fda.gov/oashi/aids/condom.html.* Accessed August 24, 2011.

81 Osteomyelitis

Melinda M. Neuhauser and Susan L. Pendland

KEY CONCEPTS

❶ Osteomyelitis, an infection of the bone, can be an acute or chronic process.

❷ Osteomyelitis is most often classified by duration of disease and route of infection.

❸ *Staphylococcus aureus* is the predominant pathogen seen in all types of osteomyelitis, with methicillin-resistant *S. aureus* (MRSA) being increasingly reported. However, the spectrum of potential causative pathogens varies with patient-specific risk factors and route of infection.

❹ The gold standard for diagnosis of osteomyelitis is a bone biopsy with isolation of microorganism(s) from culture and the presence of inflammatory cells and osteonecrosis on histologic exam. Due to the invasive nature of the bone biopsy, the diagnosis of osteomyelitis is often based on clinical findings, laboratory tests, and imaging studies rather than bone biopsy.

❺ Typical signs and symptoms of osteomyelitis include local pain and tenderness over the affected bone, as well as inflammation, erythema, edema, and decreased range of motion. Patients with acute hematogenous osteomyelitis may also present with fever, chills, and malaise.

❻ The treatment goals for acute and chronic osteomyelitis are to eradicate the infection and prevent recurrence. Higher cure rates are seen with acute compared with chronic osteomyelitis. Therefore, in chronic osteomyelitis, a common treatment goal for many patients is to prevent complications such as amputation.

❼ Treatment of osteomyelitis is dependent on the extent of bone necrosis. For acute osteomyelitis with minimal bone destruction, an extended course of antimicrobial therapy should effectively treat the infection; however, in chronic osteomyelitis, surgical intervention is also typically required.

❽ Empiric antimicrobial therapy should target likely causative pathogen(s) based on patient-specific risk factors and route of infection. *With the increased incidence of MRSA, the use of anti-MRSA antimicrobials should be considered as first-line therapy for empiric coverage of suspected staphylococcal osteomyelitis.* However, therapy should be modified based on culture and sensitivity data.

❾ The duration of antimicrobial therapy is usually 4 to 8 weeks.

❿ Patients should be monitored for clinical and laboratory response, development of adverse drug reactions, and potential drug–drug interactions. Patients should also be closely monitored for adherence in the outpatient setting.

INTRODUCTION

❶ *Osteomyelitis is an infection of the bone that is associated with high morbidity and increased healthcare costs. The inflammatory response associated with acute osteomyelitis*

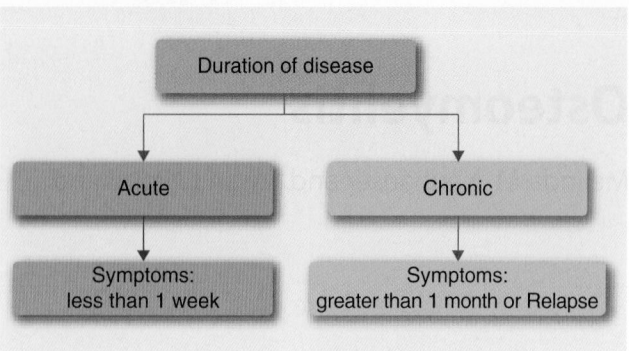

FIGURE 81–1. Classification by duration of disease.

can lead to bone necrosis and subsequently chronic infections. Bacterial pathogens, particularly *Staphylococcus aureus*, are the most common microorganisms implicated in these infections. Diagnosis and treatment are often difficult due to the heterogeneous nature of osteomyelitis. Medical management is the mainstay of treatment for acute infections; however, surgical intervention is necessary for chronic cases that involve bone necrosis. Outcomes may vary based on patient-specific risk factors, duration of disease, and site of infection.

❷ *There are multiple classification schemes for osteomyelitis.[1-5] Due to the heterogeneity of bone infections, no single classification system has been universally accepted.[1,6] Two of the most common classification schemes are based on* duration of disease *and* route of infection.[1,3,4,6,7]

Historically, osteomyelitis has been classified as acute or chronic based on duration of disease (**Fig. 81–1**).[1,2,6] However, there are no established definitions for acute and chronic infections.[1,6] Acute infection has been defined as first episode or recent onset of symptoms (within 2 weeks).[2,3,8] Chronic osteomyelitis is generally defined as relapse of the disease or symptoms persisting beyond 2 months.[2,3] Because there is no abrupt demarcation, but rather a gradual shift from acute to chronic infection, others describe chronic osteomyelitis as the presence of necrotic bone.[1,5,6,9]

Waldvogel classified osteomyelitis based on the route of infection and the presence of vascular insufficiency.[7] In this classification scheme, the route of infection is categorized as either hematogenous or contiguous (**Fig. 81–2**). Osteomyelitis

secondary to a contiguous focus is further subdivided into infections with or without vascular insufficiency. This classification, based on etiology of the infections, does not provide therapeutic guidance.[1,3]

An alternative classification, the Cierny-Mader staging system, is based on anatomic site and physiologic status of the patient.[4] This classification scheme was developed for chronic osteomyelitis involving long bones, but has limited application for small bones and digits. The detailed stratification has the greatest utility in clinical trials since it permits comparison of treatment regimens in patients with diverse comorbidities and infection sites.

EPIDEMIOLOGY AND ETIOLOGY

Osteomyelitis due to contiguous spread accounts for approximately 80% of all cases and is the most common type in adults.[3] Hematogenous spread accounts for the remaining 20% of bone infections and is the most common type of osteomyelitis in children.[1-3,6,7,10] Hematogenous osteomyelitis is reported in older adults and IV drug users, with the spine (vertebral osteomyelitis) being the most common site of infection.[1-3,11,12]

❸ The etiology of osteomyelitis has remained relatively unchanged, with *S. aureus being the predominant pathogen seen in all types of osteomyelitis.*[1-3,5,6,8,13-15] However, the susceptibility of *S. aureus* has been shifting from methicillin-sensitive to methicillin-resistant in both the healthcare and community settings.[1,2,5,8,10,12-14,16-21] Although it is more common in skin and soft tissue infections,[22] MRSA has been increasingly reported in osteomyelitis.[1,2,5,8,10,12-14,16-21] Risk factors for healthcare-associated MRSA include previous antimicrobial therapy, prolonged hospitalization, hemodialysis, or presence of an indwelling catheter.[23] In contrast, community-associated MRSA has emerged in patients with no prior healthcare exposure or apparent risk factors.[23]

Host factors such as age, comorbidities, medication, and presence of foreign devices can influence the spectrum of infection (i.e., bone and pathogen involvement).[1,2,6,11,14,24]

• Patients with uncontrolled diabetes and/or peripheral vascular disease (PVD) have poor wound healing and often present with nonhealing skin ulcers.

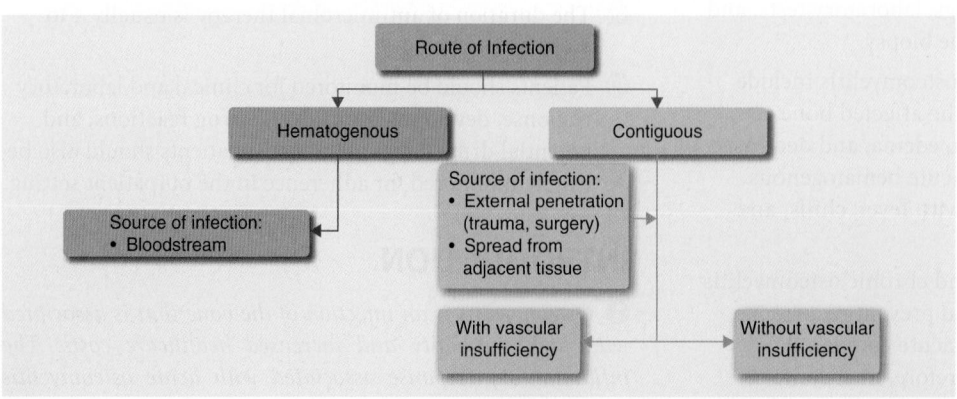

FIGURE 81–2. Classification by route of infection.

These wounds are typically colonized with a mixture of aerobic and anaerobic microorganisms, which can lead to polymicrobial osteomyelitis.[1,2,6,14,25] Common aerobic pathogens in this setting may include MRSA, *Enterococcus* spp, Enterobacteriaceae, and *Pseudomonas aeruginosa*.[25] Therefore, if a wound is deep or extensive, these patients should be evaluated for underlying osteomyelitis.[2,14,24]

- Other special populations with a varied pathogen spectrum include:
  - IV drug users (MRSA)[1,2,6,11,14]
  - Elderly (*Eschericia coli* secondary to urinary tract infections)[1,11,14]
  - Sickle cell patients (*Salmonella* spp)[1,2,5,6,13,14]
  - Individuals with prosthetic implants (coagulase-negative staphylococci)[1,5,14]
  - Neonates (*E. coli* or group B streptococci)[2,5,13]
  - Patients with pressure sores (polymicrobial—aerobes and anaerobes)[1,2,14]
- Typical bone involvement in osteomyelitis depends on the route of infection.
  - Hematogenous: long bones (femur, tibia) in neonates and prepubertal children and vertebra in the elderly[1–3,5,10,11,13]
  - Contiguous with vascular insufficiency: lower extremities[25]
  - Contiguous without vascular insufficiency: bones affected by trauma, surgery, or adjacent to soft-tissue infection[6]
  - Osteomyelitis of the jaw has been reported in patients receiving bisphosphonate therapy.[26] Risk factors include cancer, chemotherapy, corticosteroids, tooth extraction and poor oral hygiene. Bisphosphates may induce osteoclast apoptosis and slow wound healing, leaving oral lesions susceptible to infection from oral microflora.[26]

PATHOPHYSIOLOGY

Both microbial and host factors are important determinants in the development of osteomyelitis.[1,6,25] Healthy bone tissue is normally resistant to infection but may become susceptible under certain conditions.[1,2,6,25] Bone can become infected: (a) via the presence of bacteria in the bloodstream, (b) by direct inoculation from trauma or surgery, and (c) by spread from an adjacent site (e.g., soft-tissue infection).[1,6,25] The latter is particularly problematic in patients with foreign body implants (e.g., hip replacement) and chronic skin ulcers.[1] *Staphylococcus* species possess bacterial adhesins, which promote their attachment to tissues and foreign devices.[1,13,25] Microbial adherence to bone elicits an inflammatory response.[1] The subsequent release of leukocytes and cytokines leads to edema and ischemia. In some cases, these processes can lead to bone necrosis.[1,25] Pieces of dead bone may become separated, forming sequestra (**Fig. 81–3**).[1,25] These

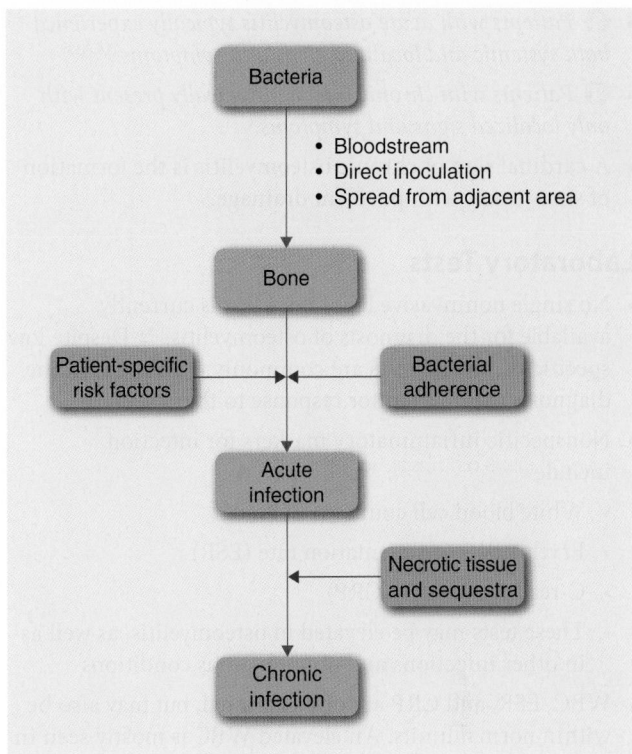

FIGURE 81–3. Pathogenesis of osteomyelitis.

areas typically cannot be penetrated by antimicrobials and phagocytic cells and thus require surgical intervention to eradicate the bacterial nidus.[1]

CLINICAL PRESENTATION AND DIAGNOSIS

General

- The clinical presentations of osteomyelitis may vary depending on route and duration of infection, as well as patient-specific factors such as infection site, age, and comorbidities.[1,5,6,10,13]
- ❹ *The gold standard for diagnosis of osteomyelitis is a bone biopsy with isolation of microorganism(s) from culture and the presence of inflammatory cells and osteonecrosis on histologic exam.*[1–3,6,13,24,25,27] Due to the invasive nature of the bone biopsy, the diagnosis of osteomyelitis is often based on clinical findings, laboratory tests, and imaging studies rather than bone biopsy.[1,27] A thorough history and physical examination are especially important for diagnosis in patients with limited or atypical symptoms.[1,24]

Symptoms and Signs

- *Systemic:* Fever, chills, malaise[1,5,6,10,13]
- *Localized:* Pain or tenderness, edema, erythema, inflammation, decreased range of motion of infected area[1,5,6,10,14]

- ⑤ *Patients with acute osteomyelitis typically experience both systemic and localized signs and symptoms.*[5,6,8,13]
- ⑤ *Patients with chronic infection typically present with only localized signs and symptoms.*[6]
- A cardinal sign of chronic osteomyelitis is the formation of sinus tracts with purulent drainage.[1]

Laboratory Tests

- No single noninvasive laboratory test is currently available for the diagnosis of osteomyelitis.[1,3,6] Despite low specificity, several tests are commonly used to aid in the diagnosis and to monitor response to therapy.
- Nonspecific inflammatory markers for infection include[1,3,5,6,9,11,12,21,25,28]:
  - White blood cell count (WBC)
  - Erythrocyte sedimentation rate (ESR)
  - C-reactive protein (CRP)
  - These tests may be elevated in osteomyelitis, as well as in other infections and noninfectious conditions
- WBC, ESR, and CRP are often elevated, but may also be within normal limits. An elevated WBC is mostly seen in patients with acute osteomyelitis.[1,3,6]
- CRP rises faster than ESR during early stages of infection and also returns to normal levels more quickly than ESR. This makes CRP a more useful tool for both diagnosis and monitoring of therapeutic response.[2,5,6,11,21]

Microbiologic evaluation

- Isolation of causative pathogen is essential for targeted antimicrobial therapy.[1–3,6,24,25]
- Positive culture and histology from bone biopsy samples provide definitive diagnosis of osteomyelitis.[1,5,14,25] However, bone biopsies are rarely performed due to the invasive nature of the procedure.[1,3,6,25]
- If bone biopsy is not done, quality specimens (e.g., two consecutive samples with bone contact [deep samples] in patients with contiguous osteomyelitis[3,24,29] or blood cultures in patients with acute hematogenous osteomyelitis[1,5,11,13]) should be obtained to provide pathogen identification. Superficial swabs often represent colonization rather than infecting organism(s).[1,3,14]
- *S. aureus* is the predominant pathogen in all types of bone infection.[1–3,5,6,13–15]
- A single pathogen is most often isolated in hematogenous osteomyelitis, whereas multiple organisms are often isolated in contiguous osteomyelitis.[2,3,6]

Imaging Studies

- A number of different imaging tests are used to assist in the diagnosis of osteomyelitis.[2,6,25,28,30]
- Plain film radiographs (x- rays) are the initial imaging study of choice for skeletal infections.[1,2,11,13,24,28] Although changes in soft tissue may appear within 3 days of infection, bone lesions may not be visible for 10 to 21 days.[1–3,6,28]
  - Advantages: accessibility, cost, low radiation exposure, readily repeatable[28]
  - Disadvantages: inability to detect early bone infections[1–3,5,13,28]
- Magnetic resonance imaging (MRI) is generally considered the best overall imaging modality for the diagnosis of osteomyelitis.[1–3,5,8,13,21,27,28,30]
  - Advantages: early detection (i.e., 3 to 5 days after onset of infection), no radiation exposure, high resolution[1–3,13,28,30]
  - Disadvantages: expense, inconvenience to patients (long examination time), movement artifacts, limitations to scanning patients with pacemakers and other implantable metal devices[2,3,5,8,30]
- Computed tomography (CT) scans have high resolution and reproducibility.[3,30] CT scans have reduced sensitivity compared with MRI and should not be routinely used to diagnose osteomyelitis.[28]
  - Advantages: useful for the identification of sequestra, less expensive than MRI[3,5,28,30]
  - Disadvantages: exposure of the patient to radiation, inability to use contrast medium to enhance images in patients with impaired renal function or previous allergic reactions[5,28,30]
- Radionuclide imaging is also used for the early diagnosis of bone infections. The most widely used nuclear medicine test is the three-phase bone scan.[28,30]
  - Advantages: early detection within 24 to 48 hours after onset of symptoms[3,13,28]
  - Disadvantages: low specificity (increased risk of false positives) in patients with recent trauma, surgery, orthopedic prosthesis, diabetes, and ischemia[1,3,13,28]

TREATMENT

Desired Outcomes

⑥ *The treatment goals for osteomyelitis are to eradicate the infection and prevent recurrence.*[13,24] *Cure rates of greater than*

Patient Encounter, Part 1

A 38-year-old male with history of diabetes comes to the emergency department complaining of a painful ulcer on his right bottom foot. After questioning him, you determine that the wound has been present for several months and has not responded to multiple debridements and oral antibiotic therapy. On physical examination, a large wound with purulent drainage is seen.

What information is suggestive of osteomyelitis?

What risk factors, if any, does he have for osteomyelitis?

85% have been reported for acute hematogenous osteomyelitis.[8] In contrast, chronic osteomyelitis is associated with higher failure rates, largely due to the presence of necrotic bone.[6] These patients typically require surgical intervention to remove the necrotic bone and tissue, and if applicable, to replace infected hardware.[14] Comorbidities such as vascular insufficiency can further contribute to the poor outcomes seen with chronic osteomyelitis.[14] Due to the high failure rates, treatment in this patient population may require prolonged therapy, with the primary goal of preventing amputation of infected areas.[1,6]

General Approach to Treatment

❼ *Antimicrobial therapy alone is the mainstay of treatment for acute osteomyelitis.*[5,11,14] *In comparison, treatment for chronic osteomyelitis typically requires a combination of antimicrobial therapy and surgical intervention.*[3,14] If the patient is not a candidate for surgical intervention, prolonged antimicrobial therapy is generally necessary.[25]

▶ Nonpharmacologic Therapy

In addition to medical and surgical management, nonpharmacologic interventions that reduce risk factors for developing osteomyelitis should be communicated to the patient. Examples include smoking cessation, weight-control, exercise, and good nutrition.[1,6] Additionally, a diabetic patient should be counseled regarding the necessity of controlled blood glucose, routine care and self-examination of lower extremities, and aggressive wound care.[2] Patients with chronic immobility should be counseled on skin care and techniques to prevent the development of pressure ulcers.

▶ Pharmacologic Therapy

❽ *Empiric antimicrobial therapy should target likely causative pathogen(s) based on patient-specific risk factors and route of infection.*[13] *Empiric antimicrobial coverage against* S. aureus *should be considered for all classifications of osteomyelitis.*[2] *With MRSA increasingly being reported in both the hospital and community setting, the use of anti-MRSA antimicrobials (e.g., vancomycin) should be considered as first-line therapy for empiric coverage of suspected staphylococcal osteomyelitis.*[1,2,5,13–16,18,19] In addition to anti-MRSA coverage, patients with contiguous osteomyelitis with vascular insufficiency (e.g., diabetic) should also receive

empiric antimicrobial therapy to cover P. aeruginosa *and anaerobes.*[2,24] *Specific recommendations may vary based on factors such as patient allergies, potential for harboring a resistant organism, institution formulary, and cost considerations.*[10,14] *Antimicrobial therapy should be modified based on culture and sensitivity data of appropriately collected specimens* (Table 81–1).[6,25]

Once culture and sensitivity results are available, therapy can be targeted against specific pathogens based on susceptibility data.[5,13] If MRSA is isolated, vancomycin is considered first-line therapy unless the minimum inhibitory concentration is greater than 2 mcg/mL (2 mg/L).[5,21,31] Alternate agents include daptomycin, linezolid, clindamycin, and trimethoprim-sulfamethoxazole in combination with oral rifampin.[1,3,6,10,14,21,32–36] Clindamycin is commonly used in pediatric patients.[5,8,10,15,21] However, microbiology laboratories must screen with a disk diffusion test (D-test) for inducible resistance via the macrolide-lincosamide-streptogramin (MLS) gene, as clindamycin failures have been associated with infections caused by these isolates.[5,8,10,15,17,21,37] In addition, many experts recommend the use of oral rifampin in combination with an anti-MRSA antibiotic in patients with MRSA osteomyelitis.[1–3,14,21] If methicillin-sensitive S. aureus is isolated and the patient has no β-lactam allergy, therapy should be changed to nafcillin/oxacillin or cefazolin (Table 81–1).[1–3,11,13–15] Changes or addition of other antimicrobial agents should be based on the identification and susceptibility of other aerobic or anaerobic gram-positive and gram-negative bacteria isolated in appropriately collected cultures (Table 81–1).[1,5,11,13–15]

Treatment is initiated with IV antimicrobials to optimize drug concentrations in bone.[1,6] *IV therapy can be administered in the inpatient or outpatient setting.*[6,14] *Following 1 to 2 weeks of IV therapy, a switch to oral antibiotics may be considered in patients with good clinical response, strict adherence, and outpatient follow-up.*[5,6,13,21] Oral agents should possess such characteristics as high bio-availability, good bone penetration, and long half-life (i.e., extended dosing interval).[1,6,13,14,21] Antimicrobials commonly used as oral therapy for osteomyelitis include fluoroquinolones, clindamycin, linezolid, and trimethoprim-sulfamethoxazole.[1,3,6,8,13–15,21,37] Additionally, oral rifampin may be used in combination with another antibiotic in patients with foreign devices or MRSA osteomyelitis.[1,14,21]

For chronic osteomyelitis, some clinicians recommend placement of antibiotic impregnated beads or cement.[5,6,14] This enables antibiotics such as aminoglycosides and vancomycin to be delivered in high concentrations at the site of infection.[5,6,14]

❾ *The duration of treatment had typically been 4 to 6 weeks for acute and chronic osteomyelitis.*[1,2,5,6,9,11,13] *Recent guidelines recommend a minimum of 8 weeks for treatment of MRSA osteomyelitis.*[21] *In patients who have undergone surgery, the total length of therapy should be counted after the last major surgical intervention.*[6] *Therapy should be continued until the infection has resolved.* Prolonged therapy (greater than 3 months) may be necessary for certain populations such as patients with vascular insufficiency or patients with

---

Table 81–1

Pathogen-Targeted Antimicrobial Therapy and Dosing Recommendations in Adults and Pediatrics

Microorganism	Antimicrobial Agent	Adult Dose	Pediatric Dose[a]
S. aureus			
MRSA	Vancomycin[b]	15–20 mg/kg IV every 8–12 hours	15 mg/kg IV every 6 hours
	Daptomycin[b]	6 mg/kg IV every 24 hours	6–10 mg/kg IV every 24 hours
	Linezolid	600 mg IV/oral every 12 hours	10 mg/kg IV/oral every 8 hours (less than 12 years old)
	Clindamycin[c]	600 mg IV/oral every 8 hours	10–13 mg/kg/dose IV/oral every 6–8 hours
	trimethoprim-sulfamethoxazole[b] (+ rifampin[c] 600 mg oral daily)	3.5–4.0 mg/kg of trimethoprim component IV/oral every 8–12 hours (trimethoprim-sulfamethoxazole single strength tablet is 80 mg/400 mg; double strength tablet is 160 mg/800 mg)	——
MSSA	Nafcillin[d]/oxacillin[b]	1–2 g IV every 4–6 hours	100–200 mg/kg/day IV in divided doses every 4–6 hours
	Cefazolin[b]	1–2 g IV every 6–8 hours	50–100 mg/kg/day IV in divided doses every 6–8 hours
Enterococcus spp.			
Ampicillin-sensitive	Ampicillin[b]	2 g IV every 4–6 hours	100–400 mg/kg/day IV in divided doses every 6 hours
Ampicillin-resistant	Vancomycin[b]	15 – 20 mg/kg IV every 8–12 hours	15 mg/kg IV every 6 hours
Vancomycin-resistant	Daptomycin[b]	4–6 mg/kg IV every 24 hours	—
	Linezolid	600 mg IV/oral every 12 hours	10 mg/kg IV/oral every 8 hours (less than 12 years old)
Streptococcus spp.	Penicillin G[b]	2–4 million units IV every 4–6 hours	250,000-400,000 units/kg/day IV in divided doses every 4–6 hours
P. aeruginosa			
	Doripenem[b]	500 mg IV every 8 hours	—
	Imipenem/cilastatin[b]	500 mg IV every 6 hours	25 mg/kg IV every 6 hours
	Meropenem[b]	1 g IV every 8 hours	10–20 mg/kg IV every 8 hours
	Ceftazidime[b]	2 g IV every 8 hours	50 mg/kg IV every 8 hours
	Cefepime[b]	2 g IV every 12 hours	50 mg/kg IV every 8–12 hours
	Piperacillin/tazobactam[b]	4.5 g IV every 6 hours	100 mg/kg IV piperacillin component every 8 hours
	Ciprofloxacin[b,e]	400 mg IV every 8–12 hours; 750 mg oral every 12 hours	—
	Levofloxacin[b,e]	750 mg IV/oral every 24 hours	—
Enterobacteriaceae (in addition to antipseudomonal agents listed above)	Ceftriaxone[d]	1–2 g IV every 24 hours	50–100 mg/kg/day IV in divided doses every 12–24 hours
	Cefotaxime[b,d]	1–2 g IV every 8 hours	50–200 mg/kg/day IV in divided doses every 6–8 hours
	Ertapenem[b]	1 g IV every 24 hours	—
	Moxifloxacin[c,e]	400 mg IV/oral every 24 hours	—
Anaerobes[f]	Clindamycin[e]	600–900 mg IV every 8 hours; 300–450 mg oral every 6–8 hours	25–40 mg/kg/day IV in divided doses every 6–8 hours
	Metronidazole[b,c]	500 mg IV/oral every 6–8 hours	30 mg/kg/day IV/oral in divided doses every 6–8 hours

[a]Refer to specialized pediatric reference for maximum neonatal and pediatric dosing recommendations.

[b]Dosage adjustment necessary in renal dysfunction.

[c]Dosage adjustment necessary in severe hepatic dysfunction.

[d]Dosage adjustment necessary in patients with concomitant renal and hepatic dysfunction.

[e]Fluoroquinolones: Not approved by the U.S. FDA for use in children except for anthrax (ciprofloxacin, levofloxacin) and complicated UTI and pyelonephritis (ciprofloxacin).

[f]May consider β-lactam/β-lactamase inhibitor or carbapenem for broad-spectrum activity including anaerobes.

From Refs. 1, 6, 10, 11, 14, 17, 18, 21, 31, and 36–38.

recalcitrant infections that do not respond to 4 to 6 weeks of therapy.[1,5,6,9,21,25]

OUTCOME EVALUATION

● Therapeutic success is measured by the extent to which the care plan (a) resolves signs and symptoms, (b) eradicates the microorganism(s), (c) prevents relapses, and (d) prevents complications such as amputation.[13] Patients should be evaluated for resolution of clinical signs and symptoms and normalization of laboratory tests (WBC, CRP, ESR, and cultures).[13] Hospitalized patients should be examined daily. Improvement in clinical manifestations should be seen within 48 to 72 hours of initiation of IV antimicrobial therapy. In the outpatient setting, patients should be evaluated weekly during the initial 4 to 8 weeks of therapy.[5,11] A reduction in CRP should be seen within 1 week of therapy and should be monitored weekly throughout therapy for a continued downward trend.[5,8] ESR can also be monitored weekly, although normalization will be slower than for CRP.[8] Patients should also be monitored for antimicrobial tolerability and toxicity (Table 81–2).

If poor response is noted, the following should be evaluated: (a) patient adherence, (b) significant drug–drug or drug–food interactions, (c) appropriate dosage to achieve therapeutic concentrations, (d) development of antimicrobial resistance necessitating a change in the treatment regimen, (e) need for additional imaging studies, and (f) diagnostic reevaluation. Treatment is considered successful if all clinical signs and symptoms are resolved and all laboratory tests have returned to normal following 4 to 8 weeks of appropriate treatment. Due to high rates of relapse, patients should have medical follow-up for at least 1 year following resolution of symptoms. Patients should be evaluated at 3- to 6-month intervals for any clinical manifestations of recurring infection and continued normalization of laboratory tests. Follow-up imaging studies at 1 to 2 years may be useful in some patients to confirm therapeutic success.

Table 81–2

Monitoring Considerations for Select Antistaphylococcal Agents

Antimicrobial	Monitoring Considerations
Daptomycin	Muscle pain or weakness particularly of the distal extremities; monitor CPK weekly with more frequent monitoring in patients with renal insufficiency or receiving (or recent discontinuation) of HMG-CoA reductase inhibitors Consider temporarily discontinuing HMG-CoA reductase inhibitors while patient receiving daptomycin
Linezolid	Myelosuppression: monitor CBC once weekly if more than 2 weeks of therapy Mild MAO inhibitor; evaluate for potential drug–drug or drug–food interactions Peripheral and/or optic neuropathy has been reported with long-term therapy; perform routine neurologic and ophthalmic evaluations in these patients
Vancomycin	Targeted steady state trough is 15–20 mcg/mL (15–20 mg/L; 10–14 μmol/L) for serious infections such as osteomyelitis Renal dysfunction: monitor weekly renal function (BUN/SCr) and troughs in stable patients Potential for additive renal toxicity if being coadministered with a nephrotoxic agent (e.g., aminoglycoside)

BUN, blood urea nitrogen; CBC, complete blood count; CPK, creatine phosphokinase; MAO, monoamine oxidase; SCr, serum creatinine.

From Refs. 1, 3, 5, 6, 10, 14, 18, 21, 31, 34, 35, and 38.

Patient Encounter, Part 3: The Medical History, Physical Exam, and Diagnostic Tests

PMH: Type 1 diabetes mellitus

SH: Tobacco smoker (2 packs per day for the past 20 years), denies alcohol and illicit drug use. Self-employed

Allergies: NKDA

Meds: Novolin 70/30: 40 units every morning and at bedtime

PE:

Gen: No apparent distress with tenderness and pain in the region of the nonhealing skin ulcer

Skin: 4 cm ulcer on the 5th metatarsal with purulent drainage

VS: BP 130/85 mm Hg, P 72 beats/min, RR 15 breaths/min, T 36.9°C (98.4°F), ht 5 ft 9 in (175 cm), wt 77.3 kg (170 lb)

Labs: WBC $7 \times 10^3/mm^3$ ($7 \times 10^9/L$), BUN 19 mg/dL (6.8 mmol/L), serum creatinine (Scr) 0.9 mg/dL (80 μmol/L), fasting blood glucose 290 mg/dL (16.1 mmol/L), ESR 70 mm/h, CRP 74 mg/dL (740 mg/L)

Microbiology: Culture from bone biopsy during debridement grew *S. aureus* (sensitive to linezolid, vancomycin, TMP/SMX but resistant to oxacillin, erythromycin, and clindamycin) and *P. aeruginosa* (sensitive to all antibiotics tested including amikacin, cefepime, levofloxacin, meropenem, piperacillin, tobramycin)

Based on the information presented, create a care plan for this patient's osteomyelitis. Your plan should include:

(a) Goals of therapy

(b) Patient-specific detailed therapeutic plan

(c) Nonpharmacologic interventions

(d) Follow-up plan to determine whether outcomes have been achieved

Patient Encounter, Part 4

The patient received 4 weeks of IV antimicrobial therapy following debridement. The patient has shown clinical and laboratory improvement. The multidisciplinary medical team plans to complete therapy with an oral antibiotic.

What oral antimicrobial therapy would you recommend for this patient?

Evaluate the patient's medication profile for drug–drug interactions.

Counsel the patient regarding this drug therapy.

Patient Care and Monitoring

1. ⑩ *Assess the patient's symptoms and laboratory test results to determine whether patient-directed therapy is appropriate.*

2. Obtain a thorough history of prescription, nonprescription, and natural drug product use.

3. Educate the patient on lifestyle modifications that will reduce the risk of recurrent infections.

4. Develop a plan to assess the effectiveness of antimicrobial therapy.

5. Evaluate the patient for the presence of adverse drug reactions, drug allergies, and drug interactions.

6. Stress the importance of adherence to the therapeutic regimen.

7. Provide patient education with regard to disease state and drug therapy. Explain the following:

   - Causes of osteomyelitis

   - Complications associated with osteomyelitis

   - The drug, dose, duration, and route of administration of the patient's antimicrobial regimen

   - Optimal medication administration time for the patient's lifestyle and other concurrent medications

   - Available options for missed dose(s)

   - Adverse effects that may occur

   - Provide patient education monographs for antibiotic(s)

Disclaimer

The views expressed in this chapter are those of the authors and do not necessarily reflect the position or policy of the Department of Veterans Affairs or the United States government.

Abbreviations Introduced in This Chapter

BUN	Blood urea nitrogen
CBC	Complete blood count
CRP	C-reactive protein
CPK	Creatine phosphokinase
CT	Computed tomography
CYP	Cytochrome P-450 isoenzyme
ESR	Erythrocyte sedimentation rate
IV	Intravenous
LFT	Liver function test
MAO	Monoamine oxidase
MRI	Magnetic resonance imaging
MRSA	Methicillin-resistant *Staphylococcus aureus*
MSSA	Methicillin-sensitive *Staphylococcus aureus*
Scr	Serum creatinine
TMP-SMX	Trimethoprim-sulfamethoxazole
UTI	Urinary tract infection
WBC	White blood cell

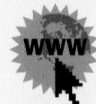 Self-assessment questions and answers are available at *http://mhpharmacotherapy.com/pp.html.*

REFERENCES

1. Chihara S, Segreti J. Osteomyelitis. Dis Mon 2010;56:6–31.
2. Howell WR, Goulston C. Osteomyelitis: an update for hospitalists. Hosp Pract (Minneap) 2011;39(1):153–160.
3. Esposito S, Leone S, Bassetti M, et al. Italian guidelines for the diagnosis and infectious disease management of osteomyelitis and prosthetic joint infections in adults. Infect 2009;37:478–496.
4. Mader JT, Shirtliff M, Calhoun JH. Staging and staging application in osteomyelitis. Clin Infect Dis 1997;25:1303–1309.
5. Harik NS, Smeltzer MS. Management of acute hematogenous osteomyelitis in children. Exp Rev Anti-Infect Ther 2010;8:2:175.
6. Calhoun JH, Manring MM. Adult osteomyelitis. Infect Dis Clin N Am 2005;19:765–786.
7. Waldvogel FA, Medoff G, Swartz MN. Osteomyelitis: A review of clinical features, therapeutic considerations and unusual aspects. N Engl J Med 1970;282:198–206.
8. Gutierrez K. Bone and joint infections in children. Pediatr Clin North Am 2005;52:779–794.
9. Conterno LO, da Silva Filho CR. Antibiotics for treating chronic osteomyelitis in adults. Cochrane Database Syst Rev 2009;CD004439.
10. Geist A, Kuhn R. Pharmacological approaches for pediatric patients with osteomyelitis: current issues and answers. Orthopedics 2009;32:573–577.
11. Zimmerli W. Vertebral osteomyelitis. N Engl J Med 2010;362:1022–1029.
12. Livorski DJ, Daver NG, Atmar RL, Shelburne SA, White AC, Musher DM. Outcomes of treatment for hematogenous *Staphylococcus aureus* vertebral osteomyelitis in the MRSA era. J Infect 2008;57:128–131.
13. Conrad DA. Acute hematogenous osteomyelitis. Pediatr Rev 2010;31:464–471.
14. Rao N, Ziran BH, Lipsky BA. Treating osteomyelitis: antibiotics and surgery. Plast Reconstr Surg 2011;127(Suppl 1):S177–S187.
15. Kaplan SL. Osteomyelitis in children. Infect Dis Clin North Am 2005;19:787–797.

16. Allison DC, Holtom PD, Patzakis MJ, Zalavras CG. Microbiology of bone and joint infections in injecting drug abusers. Clin Orthop Relat Res 2010;468(8):2107–2112.

17. Eleftheriadou I, Tentolouris N, Argiana V, Jude E, Boulton AJ. Methicillin-resistant *Staphylococcus aureus* in diabetic foot infections. Drugs 2010;70(14):1785–1797.

18. Boucher H, Miller LG, Razonable RR. Serious infections caused by methicillin-resistant *Staphylococcus aureus*. Clin Infect Dis 2010;51(Suppl 2):S183–S197.

19. Bhavan KP, Marschall J, Olsen MA, Fraser VJ, Wright NM, Warren DK. The epidemiology of hematogenous vertebral osteomyelitis: a cohort study in a tertiary care hospital. BMC Infect Dis 2010;10:158.

20. Ascione T, Rosario P, Pempinello R, et al. Impact of therapeutic choices on outcome of osteomyelitis caused by MRSA. J Infect 2011;63:102–104.

21. Liu C, Bayer A, Cosgrove SE, et al. Clinical practice guidelines by the Infectious Diseases Society of America for the treatment of methicillin-resistant Staphylococcus aureus infections in adults and children. Clin Infect Dis 2011;52:1–38.

22. Talan DA, Krishnadasan A, Gorwitz RJ, et al. Comparison of *Staphylococcus aureus* from skin and soft tissue infections in US emergency department patients, 2004 and 2008. Clin Infect Dis 2011;53:144–149.

23. David MZ, Daum RS. Community-associated methicillin-resistant *Staphylococcus aureus*: epidemiology and clinical consequences of an emerging epidemic. Clin Microbiol Rev 2010;23:616–687.

24. Byren I, Peters EJG, Hoey C, Berendt A, Lipsky BA. Pharmacotherapy of diabetic foot osteomyelitis. 2009;10(18):3033–3047.

25. Hartemann-Heurtier A, Senneville E. Diabetic foot osteomyelitis. Diabetes Metab 2008;34:87–95.

26. Wimalawansa SJ. Insight into bisphosphonate-associated osteomyelitis of the jaw: pathophysiology, mechanisms and clinical management. Expert Opin Drug Saf 2008;7(4):491–512.

27. Game F. Management of osteomyelitis of the foot in diabetes mellitus; Nat Rev Endocrinol 2010;6:43–47.

28. Hankin D, Bowling FL, Metcalfe SA, Whitehouse RA, Boulton AJ. Critically evaluating the role of diagnostic imaging in osteomyelitis. Foot Ankle Spec 2011;4(2):100–105.

29. Bernard L, Assal M, Garzoni C, Uckay. Predicting the pathogen of diabetic toe osteomyelitis by two consecutive ulcer cultures with bone contact. Eur J Clin Microbiol Infect Dis 2011;30:279–281.

30. Gotthardt M, Bleeker-Rovers CP, Boerman OC, Oyen WJG. Imaging of inflammation by PET, conventional scintigraphy, and other imaging techniques. J Nucl Med 2010;51:1937–1949.

31. Rybak M, Lomaestro B, Rotschafer JC, et al. Therapeutic monitoring of vancomycin in adult patients: A consensus review of the American Society of Health-System Pharmacists, the Infectious Diseases Society of America, and the Society of Infectious Diseases Pharmacists. Am J Health-Syst Pharm 2009;66:82–98.

32. Lamp KC, Friedrich LV, Mendez-Vigo L, Russo R. Clinical experience with daptomycin for the treatment of osteomyelitis. Am J Med 2007;120:S13–S20.

33. Falagas ME, Giannopoulou KP, Ntziora F, Papagelopoulous PJ. Daptomycin for treatment of patients with bone and joint infections: A systemic review of the clinical evidence. Int J Antimicrob Agents 2007;30:202–209.

34. Rice DAK, Medendez L. Daptomycin in bone and joint infections: a review of the literature. Arch Orthop Trauma Surg 2009;129:1495–1504.

35. Falagas ME, Siempos II, Papagelopoulos P, Vardakas KZ. Linezolid for the treatment of adults with bone and joint infections. Int J Antimicrob Agents 2007;29:233–239.

36. Toma MB, Smith KM, Martin CA, Rapp RP. Pharmacokinetic considerations in the treatment of methicillin-resistant *Staphylococcus aureus* osteomyelitis. Orthopedics 2006;29(6):497–501.

37. Moellering RC Jr. Current treatment options for community-acquired methicillin-resistant *Staphylococcus aureus* infection. Clin Infect Dis 2008;46:1032–1037.

38. Lexi-Drugs Online. [cited 2011 Oct 10]. Available from: *www.crlonline.com*.

82

Sepsis and Septic Shock

S. Scott Sutton, Christopher M. Bland, and
Gowtham A. Rao

LEARNING OBJECTIVES

● **Upon completion of the chapter, the reader will be able to:**

1. Compare and contrast the definitions of syndromes related to sepsis.

2. Identify the pathogens associated with sepsis.

3. Discuss the pathophysiology of sepsis as it relates to pro- and anti-inflammatory mediators.

4. Identify patient symptoms as early or late sepsis and evaluate diagnostic and laboratory tests for patient treatment and monitoring.

5. Assess complications of sepsis and discuss their impact on patient outcomes.

6. Design desired treatment outcomes for septic patients.

7. Formulate a treatment and monitoring plan (pharmacologic and nonpharmacologic) for septic patients.

8. Evaluate patient response and devise alternative treatment regimens for nonresponding septic patients.

KEY CONCEPTS

❶ Sepsis is a continuum of stages defined by physiologic measures and signs and symptoms of a sepsis process.

❷ Gram-positive and gram-negative bacteria, fungal species, and viruses may cause sepsis.

❸ Inflammation is the key factor in the development of sepsis. Patients with severe infections, trauma, debilitating conditions, or an immunocompromised status may experience an imbalance among inflammatory mediators that progresses to sepsis.

❹ The cumulative burden of sepsis complications is the leading factor of mortality. The risk of death increases 20% with failure of each additional organ. Severe sepsis averages two failed organs, with a mortality rate of 40%.

❺ Treatment is aimed at early goal-directed resuscitation; reducing or eliminating organ failures; treating and eliminating the source of infection; avoiding adverse reactions of treatment; and providing cost-effective therapy.

❻ Appropriate empiric anti-infective therapy administered within 1 hour of the recognition of sepsis decreases complications and 28-day mortality.

Sepsis is a continuum of physiologic stages characterized by infection, systemic inflammation, and hypoperfusion with widespread tissue injury.[1] ❶ The American College of Chest Physicians and the Society of Critical Care Medicine developed definitions to utilize for sepsis (Table 82–1).[2] *Physiologic parameters categorize patients as having bacteremia, infection, systemic inflammatory response syndrome (SIRS), sepsis, severe sepsis, septic shock, or multiple-organ dysfunction syndrome (MODS).*[2] Standardized definitions have been developed for infections in critically ill patients.[3]

EPIDEMIOLOGY AND ETIOLOGY

Sepsis is the leading cause of morbidity and mortality for critically ill patients and the tenth leading cause of death overall.[1,4] Additionally, care of septic patients has a significant economic impact in the United States.[1,4–6]

Risk factors for sepsis include age, cancer, immunodeficiency, chronic organ failure, genetic factors (male sex and nonwhite ethnic origin in North America), and bacteremic patients.[4,7–10] Pulmonary, GI, genitourinary, and bloodstream infections account for the majority of sepsis cases.[4,7,8]

Table 82–1

Definitions Related to Sepsis

Bacteremia (fungemia): Presence of viable bacteria or fungi in the bloodstream.

Infection: Inflammatory response to invasion of normally sterile host tissue by microorganisms.

SIRS: A systemic inflammatory response to a variety of clinical insults that can be infectious, but can have a noninfectious etiology. The response is manifested by two or more of the following conditions: temperature greater than 38.0°C (100.4°F) or less than 36.0°C (96.8°F); pulse greater than 90 beats/min; respiratory rate greater than 20 breaths/min or $Paco_2$ less than 32 torr or mm Hg (4.26 kPa); WBC count greater than $12 \times 10^3/mm^3$ ($12 \times 10^9/L$), less than $4 \times 10^3/mm^3$ ($4 \times 10^9/L$), or greater than 10% (0.10) immature (band) forms.

Sepsis: The SIRS and documented infection (culture or Gram stain of blood, sputum, urine, or normally sterile body fluid positive for pathogenic microorganisms).

Severe sepsis: Sepsis associated with organ dysfunction due to hypoperfusion or hypotension (systolic blood pressure less than 90 mm Hg). Hypoperfusion and perfusion abnormalities may include, but are not limited to, lactic acidosis, oliguria, or acute alteration in mental status.

Septic shock: Sepsis with hypotension, despite fluid resuscitation, along with the presence of perfusion abnormalities. Patients who are on inotropic or vasopressor agents may not be hypotensive at the time perfusion abnormalities are measured.

MODS: Presence of altered organ function requiring intervention to maintain homeostasis.

MODS, multiple-organ dysfunction syndrome; $Paco_2$, partial pressure of carbon dioxide; SIRS, systemic inflammatory response syndrome.

From American College of Chest Physicians, Society of Critical Care Medicine Consensus Conference. Definitions for sepsis and organ failure and guidelines for the use of innovative therapies in sepsis. Crit Care Med 1992;20:864–874.

---

❷ *Gram-positive and gram-negative bacteria, fungal species, and viruses cause sepsis (Table 82–2).* Gram-positive infections account for 30% to 50% of sepsis and septic shock cases.[4,7,8] The percentages of gram-negative, polymicrobial, and viral sepsis cases are 25%, 25%, and 4%, respectively.[4,7,8,11] Multidrug-resistant (MDR) bacteria are responsible for approximately 25% of sepsis cases, are difficult to treat, and increase mortality.[7,8] The rate of fungal infections has significantly increased.[4] *Candida albicans* is the most common fungal species; however, non-albicans species (*C. glabrata, C. krusei,* and *C. tropicalis*) have increased from 24% to 46%.[4,11,12] Other fungi identified as causes of sepsis include species of *Cryptococcus, Coccidioides, Fusarium,* and *Aspergillus.*

PATHOPHYSIOLOGY

The development of sepsis is complex and multifactorial. The normal host response to infection is designed to localize and control bacterial invasion and initiate repair of injured tissue through **phagocytic** cells and inflammatory mediators.[1] Sepsis results when the inflammatory response becomes

---

Table 82–2

Pathogens in Sepsis

Organism	Frequency (%)
Gram-positive bacteria	30–50
Methicillin-susceptible *Staphylococcus aureus*	14–24
Methicillin-resistant *Staphylococcus aureus*	5–11
Other *Staphylococcus species*	1–3
Streptococcus pneumoniae	9–12
Other *Streptococcus* species	6–11
Enterococcus species	3–13
Anaerobes	1–2
Other gram-positive bacteria	1–5
Gram-negative bacteria	25–30
Escherichia coli	9–27
Pseudomonas aeruginosa	8–15
Klebsiella pneumoniae	2–7
Enterobacter species	6–16
Haemophilus influenzae	2–10
Anaerobes	3–7
Other gram-negative bacteria	3–12
Fungi	
Candida albicans	1–3
Other *Candida* species	1–2
Parasites	1–3
Viruses	2–4

From Refs. 4–7.

---

exaggerated and extends to normal tissue distant from the initial tissue site.

Pro- and Anti-inflammatory Mediators

❸ *The key factor in the development of sepsis is inflammation, which is intended to be a local and contained response to infection or injury. Infection or injury is controlled through pro- and anti-inflammatory mediators.* Proinflammatory mediators facilitate clearance of the injuring stimulus, promote resolution of injury, and are involved in processing of damaged tissue.[1,13–16] To control the intensity and duration of the inflammatory response, anti-inflammatory mediators are released that act to regulate proinflammatory mediators.[15,16] The balance between pro- and anti-inflammatory mediators localizes infection/injury of host tissue.[13–16] However, systemic responses ensue when equilibrium in the inflammatory process is lost.

The inflammatory process in sepsis is linked to the coagulation system. Proinflammatory mediators may be procoagulant and antifibrinolytic, whereas anti-inflammatory mediators may be fibrinolytic. A key factor in the inflammation of sepsis is activated protein C, which enhances fibrinolysis and inhibits inflammation. Protein C levels are decreased in many septic patients.

CLINICAL PRESENTATION AND DIAGNOSIS

The clinical presentation of sepsis varies, and the rate of development of clinical manifestations may differ from patient to patient. Immunosuppressed patients and patients

Physical Examination Results in Sepsis

HEENT: Scleral icterus, dry mucous membranes, pinpoint pupils, dilated and fixed pupils, nystagmus

Neck: Jugular venous distention, carotid bruits

Lungs: Crackles (rales), consolidation, egophony, absent breath sounds

CV: Irregular rhythm, S_3 gallop, murmurs

Abd: Tense, distended, tender, rebound, guarding, hepatosplenomegaly

Rectal: Decreased tone, bright red blood

Exts: Swollen calf, disparity of blood pressure between upper extremities

Neurologic: Agitation, confusion, delirium, obtundation, coma

Skin: Cold, clammy, or warm; hyperemic skin; rashes

with meningococcemia or *Pseudomonas aeruginosa* infections may progress to late sepsis more rapidly.

A physical examination should be performed rapidly and efficiently, with efforts directed toward uncovering the most likely cause of sepsis. The patient may not provide any

medical history; therefore, historical data may be obtained from medical records and/or family. The patient's medical condition, recent illnesses, infections, or activities may provide valuable information about the cause of sepsis.

Diagnostic and Laboratory Tests

Microbiologic cultures should be obtained before anti-infective therapy is initiated. However, cultures take 6 to 48 hours for results to be completed and often are negative (no growth of bacterial organisms). Negative cultures do not rule out infection. Administering anti-infectives before obtaining cultures may lead to a false-negative culture.

Two sets of blood cultures should be obtained to rule out contamination. At least one set should be drawn percutaneously and one drawn through each vascular access device, unless the device was recently (less than 48 hours) inserted.

Cultures of urine (with urinalysis), respiratory secretions, cerebrospinal fluid, and wounds should be obtained if the clinical situation suggests infection of these specific fluids, tissues, or organs. Laboratory tests should be performed to evaluate infection or complications of sepsis, including complete blood count (CBC) with differential, coagulation parameters, basic metabolic panel, serum lactate concentration, and arterial blood gas.

The use of biomarkers of sepsis has been controversial. Measurement of endotoxin, procalcitonin, or other markers in blood or serum is not routinely recommended. Concentrations

Clinical Presentation and Diagnosis of Sepsis

The signs and symptoms of septic patients are referred to as early and late sepsis.

Signs and Symptoms

The initial clinical signs and symptoms represent early sepsis, and they include fever, chills, and change in mental status. Other signs and symptoms include:

- Tachycardia
- Tachypnea
- Nausea and vomiting
- Hyperglycemia
- Myalgias
- Lethargy and malaise
- Proteinuria
- Leukocytosis
- Hypoxia
- Hyperbilirubinemia

Septic patients may have an elevated, low, or normal temperature. The absence of fever is common in neonates and elderly patients. Hypothermia is associated with a poor prognosis. Hyperventilation may occur before fever and

chills and may lead to respiratory alkalosis. Disorientation and confusion may develop early in septic patients, particularly in the elderly and patients with preexisting neurologic impairment. Disorientation and confusion may be related to the infection or due to sepsis signs and symptoms (e.g., hypoxia).

Late sepsis represents a slow process that develops over several hours of hemodynamic instability. Signs and symptoms of late sepsis include:

- Lactic acidosis
- Oliguria
- Leukopenia
- Thrombocytopenia
- Myocardial depression
- Pulmonary edema
- Hypotension
- Hypoglycemia
- GI hemorrhage

Oliguria often follows hypotension because of decreased perfusion. Metabolic acidosis ensues because of diminished clearance by the kidneys and liver of lactic acid.

of procalcitonin in serum are usually increased in sepsis, but fail to differentiate between infection and inflammation. However, procalcitonin has a high negative predictive value and could allow for the discontinuation of antibiotics.

Complications of Sepsis

4 *Recognition and treatment of sepsis complications, particularly organ failure, is essential to improve outcomes. The cumulative burden of sepsis complications is the leading factor of mortality. The risk of death increases 20% with failure of each additional organ. Severe sepsis averages two failed organs, with a mortality rate of 40%.* The most common complications are disseminated intravascular coagulation, acute respiratory distress syndrome (ARDS), acute kidney injury (AKI), and hemodynamic compromise.

▶ Disseminated Intravascular Coagulation

Disseminated intravascular coagulation (DIC) complicates 25% to 50% of septic patients and is an independent predictor of mortality.[17] DIC is a syndrome characterized by coagulation and activation and production of proinflammatory cytokines, culminating in intravascular fibrin formation and deposition in the microvasculature. Bleeding results from consumption and exhaustion of coagulation proteins and platelets, because of continued activation of the coagulation system.[17] DIC may produce AKI, hemorrhagic necrosis of the GI mucosa, liver failure, acute pancreatitis, ARDS, and pulmonary failure.[17]

▶ Acute Respiratory Distress Syndrome

ARDS is an acute and persistent lung inflammatory process with increased vascular permeability leading to severe hypoxia that can affect 20% of septic shock patients.[18,19] Lung deterioration is a multiphase process that begins after infection, injury, or exacerbation of the medical condition. The patient appears stable; however, the chest radiograph reveals parenchymal infiltrates. At this time the patient has pulmonary edema and may be hyperventilating.[18,19] During the next phase, the patient develops respiratory insufficiency and pulmonary edema can be seen on chest radiographs. Severe hypoxia may ensue, leading to mechanical ventilation.

▶ Acute Kidney Injury

AKI occurs in 19% of septic patients, 25% of severe septic patients, and 51% of septic shock patients.[20] Sepsis and AKI together have a 70% mortality, compared with 45% among patients with AKI alone.[20] AKI leads to fluid in the extravascular space, including the lungs, followed by impairment in gas exchange and severe hypoxemia. Hypoxemia will exacerbate ischemia and organ damage. Renal replacement therapy with the use of continuous venovenous hemofiltration, continuous venovenous hemofiltration, and dialysis or intermittent hemodialysis can be used to manage volume and electrolytes.[20]

▶ Hemodynamic Compromise

Arterial vasodilatation is the hallmark of hemodynamic effects related to sepsis. High cardiac output and low systemic vascular resistance characterize sepsis. Inflammatory cytokines (i.e., tumor necrosis factor-α [TNF-α]) and endotoxin directly depress cardiovascular function. Persistent hypotension offsets the delivery of oxygen to tissues (Do_2) and oxygen consumption by tissues (Vo_2).[21] Certain tissues may receive adequate oxygen during sepsis; however, in other tissues, oxygen demands may not be met because of decreased perfusion. This perfusion defect is accentuated by increased precapillary atrioventricular shunt. If perfusion decreases, oxygen extraction increases, and the atrioventricular oxygen gradient widens. Cellular Do_2 is decreased, but Vo_2 remains unchanged. If perfusion decreases significantly, reserve Do_2 will be exceeded, and tissue ischemia results. Tissue ischemia leads to organ failure. Therefore, increasing oxygen delivery or decreasing oxygen consumption in a hypermetabolic patient should optimize systemic Do_2 relative to Vo_2.[21]

TREATMENT AND OUTCOME EVALUATION

Desired Outcomes

5 *The primary treatment goal of sepsis is to prevent morbidity and mortality.* Treatment is aimed at early goal-directed resuscitation, reducing or eliminating organ failures, treating and eliminating the source of infection, avoiding adverse reactions of treatment, and providing cost-effective therapy.[22-28]

General Approach to Treatment

The speed and appropriateness of therapy administered in the initial hours after sepsis develops influences outcome, as is the case for acute myocardial infarction and cerebrovascular accidents.[22]

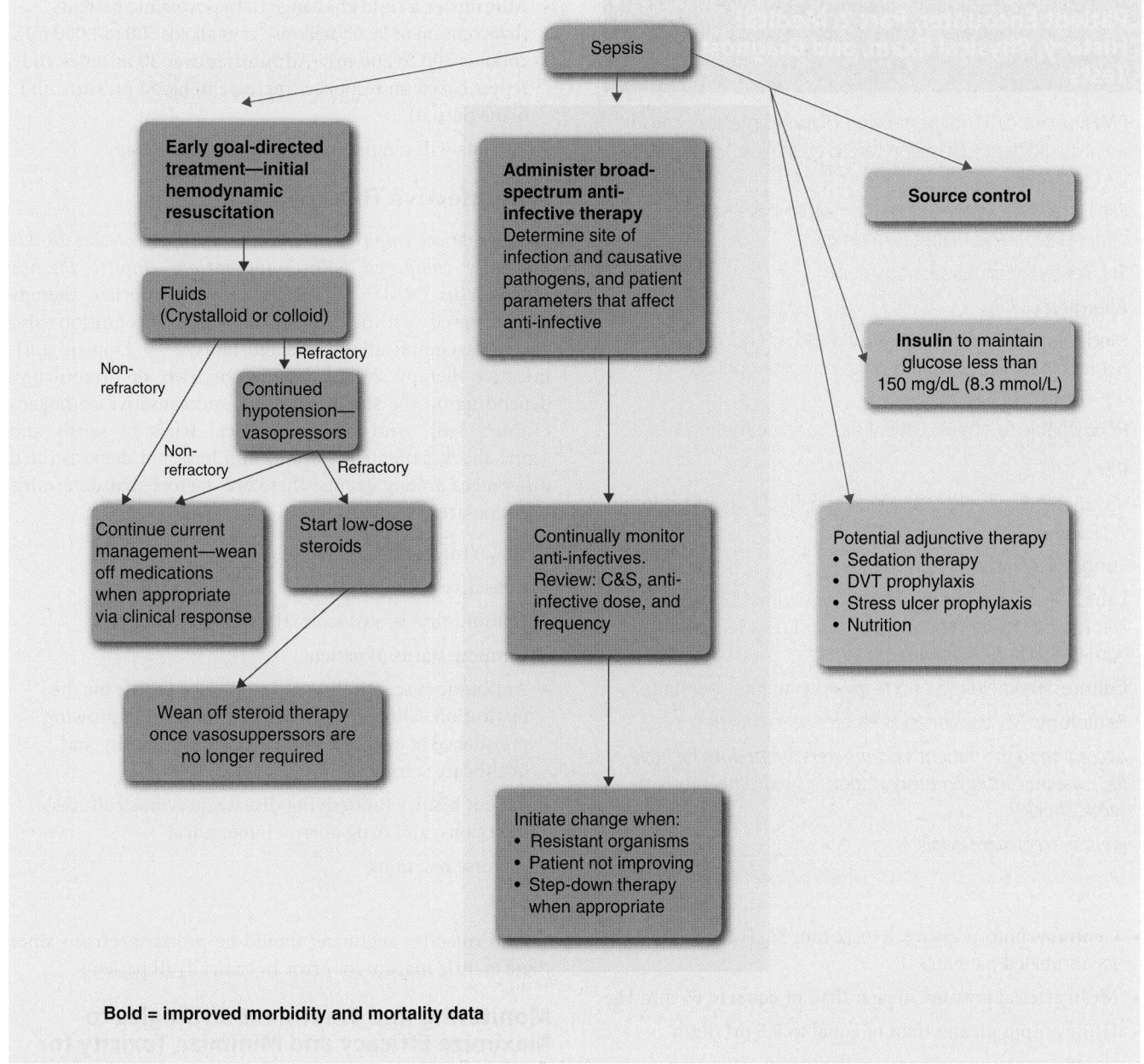

FIGURE 82–1. Therapeutic approach to sepsis. (C&S, culture and sensitivity.)

Pertinent issues in the management of septic patients are as follows (Fig. 82–1):[24]

1. Early goal-directed resuscitation of septic patients during the first 6 hours after recognition.

2. Early administration of broad-spectrum anti-infective therapy.

3. Hydrocortisone for septic shock patients refractory to resuscitation and vasopressors.

4. Glycemic control via infusion of insulin and glucose, to maintain a glucose level less than 150 mg/dL (8.3 mmol/L).

5. Adjunctive therapies: nutrition, deep vein thrombosis (DVT) prophylaxis, stress ulcer prophylaxis, and sedation for mechanically ventilated patients.

Pharmacologic Therapy

Treatment for sepsis focuses on infection, inflammation, hypoperfusion, and widespread tissue injury. Septic patients may require multiple simultaneous treatment regimens to achieve desired outcomes of decreased morbidity and mortality.

Initial Resuscitation

❺ *Early goal-directed resuscitation decreases 28-day mortality in septic patients.* The treatment goals of sepsis-induced hypoperfusion (hypotension or lactic acidosis) during the first 6 hours include[24,27–29]:

- Central venous pressure: 8 to 12 mm Hg (12 to 15 mm Hg for intubated patients)
- Mean arterial pressure greater than or equal to 65 mm Hg
- Urine output greater than or equal to 0.5 mL/kg/h
- Central venous or mixed venous oxygen saturation greater than or equal to 70% (0.70) or 65% (0.65), respectively.

Crystalloid (such as 0.9% sodium chloride or lactated Ringer's solutions) or colloid fluids (5% albumin or 6% hetastarch) are used for resuscitation, and clinical studies comparing the fluids have found them to be equivalent.[29] Crystalloids require more fluids, which may lead to more edema (utilize caution in patients at risk for fluid overload, e.g., congestive heart failure and ARDS); however, colloids are significantly more expensive. Most patients require aggressive fluid resuscitation during the first 24 hours because of persistent venodilation and capillary leak.[24]

Monitoring Parameters and Alternative Treatment for Resuscitation[24,27–29]

- An elevated serum lactate concentration may be an early marker for tissue hypoperfusion.

- Administer a fluid challenge to hypovolemic patients (hypotension or lactic acidosis): crystalloids 500 to 1,000 mL; colloids 300 to 500 mL. Administer over 30 minutes and repeat based on response (increase in blood pressure and urine output).
- Patients will require maintenance fluid therapy.

Anti-infective Therapy

❻ *Appropriate empiric anti-infective therapy decreases 28-day mortality compared with inappropriate empiric therapy (24% versus 39%).*[22,23,30] Additionally, appropriate therapy administered within 1 hour of sepsis recognition also decreases complications and mortality.[22,23,30] Empiric anti-infective therapy should include one, two, or three drugs, depending on the site of infection and causative pathogens (Table 82–3). Anti-infective clinical trials in sepsis and septic shock patients are scarce and have not demonstrated differences among agents; therefore, factors that determine selection are:

- Site of infection
- Causative pathogens
- Community- or nosocomial-acquired infection
- Immune status of patient
- Antibiotic susceptibility and resistance profile for the institution. Clinicians should be cognizant of growing prevalence of bacterial resistance in community and healthcare setting
- Patient history (underlying disease, previous cultures or infections, and drug allergy/intolerance)
- Adverse reactions
- Cost

Anti-infective regimens should be broad-spectrum since there is little margin for error in critically ill patients.

Monitoring and Treatment Strategies to Maximize Efficacy and Minimize Toxicity for Anti-infectives

- Administer broad-spectrum anti-infectives for initial therapy, as early as possible and within first hour of recognition of sepsis.
- Appropriate cultures should be obtained before initiating antibiotic therapy, but should not prevent prompt administration of treatment.
- Administer antibiotics that concentrate at the site of infection.
- Monitor patient parameters to ensure adequate dosing.
- Abnormal renal and hepatic function will increase drug concentration and predispose the patient to toxicity.
  - Ensure antibiotic dosing is changed to normal doses once renal dysfunction has resolved to limit the development of antimicrobial resistance.
- Septic patients may have altered volume of distribution due to initial resuscitation.

Table 82–3

Empirical IV Antimicrobial Regimens in Sepsis

Infection (Site or Type)	Community Acquired	Hospital Acquired
Urinary tract	Third-generation cephalosporin (ceftriaxone) or fluoroquinolone (levofloxacin or ciprofloxacin)	Antipseudomonal penicillin or antipseudomonal cephalosporin or antipseudomonal carbapenem plus aminoglycoside
Community-acquired pneumonia	Third-generation cephalosporin or ampicillin-sulbactam plus a macrolide or fluoroquinolone (levofloxacin or moxifloxacin)	
Healthcare-associated, ventilator-associated, or nosocomial pneumonia (early onset; no risk factors for MDR pathogens)		Third-generation cephalosporin or fluoroquinolone or ampicillin-sulbactam or ertapenem
Healthcare-associated, ventilator-associated, or nosocomial pneumonia (late onset and/or MDR pathogen risk factors)		Antipseudomonal penicillin or antipseudomonal cephalosporin or antipseudomonal carbapenem plus aminoglycoside or antipseudomonal fluoroquinolone plus vancomycin or linezolid
Intra-abdominal	Ertapenem or ciprofloxacin or levofloxacin + metronidazole or moxifloxacin	Piperacillin-tazobactam or imipenem or meropenem or cefepime plus metronidazole or ciprofloxacin or levofloxacin plus metronidazole
Skin and soft-tissue	Nafcillin or cefazolin	Ceftriaxone ± vancomycin
Catheter-related		Vancomycin
Unknown source of infection		Antipseudomonal penicillin ± antipseudomonal cephalosporin or antipseudomonal carbapenem plus aminoglycoside plus vancomycin

MDR, multidrug resistant.

From Refs. 31–37.

Clinical Parameters for Aminoglycosides

Tobramycin is more active against *Pseudomonas aeruginosa* than gentamicin, whereas gentamicin is more active against *Serratia* species. Amikacin is the most potent aminoglycoside against the Enterobacteriaceae; however, it should be reserved for bacterial organisms resistant to gentamicin and tobramycin. Select an aminoglycoside based on:

- Local susceptibility patterns
- Patient parameters (infection and microbiologic culture history)
- Cost

Aminoglycosides may be administered by traditional methods (1.5 to 2 mg/kg every 8 hours) or by an extended-dosing interval method (7 mg/kg every 24 hours) in patients with normal renal function. The extended-dosing method maximizes the pharmacodynamic properties of aminoglycosides (concentration-dependent killing and postantibiotic effect) and reduces the incidence of nephrotoxicity. Extended-dosing interval aminoglycosides have prolonged drug-free periods, during which the saturable uptake of aminoglycosides into the proximal renal tubular cells can be completed. Extended-dosing interval aminoglycosides should not be used in pediatric patients, burn victims, pregnant patients, or patients with preexisting or progressive renal insufficiency.[38]

- Reevaluate the initial regimen daily to optimize activity, prevent development of resistance, reduce toxicity, and decrease costs.
- Initiate step-down therapy based on microbiologic cultures to: prevent resistance, reduce toxicity, and cost.
- Monotherapy is equivalent to combination therapy once a causative pathogen has been identified. Empiric therapy should include combination regimens to ensure coverage of causative organisms.

Selection of Antimicrobial Agents

▶ Urinary Tract Infections

Septic patients with a community-acquired urinary tract infection should be treated with a third-generation cephalosporin (ceftriaxone or cefotaxime) or a fluoroquinolone (ciprofloxacin or levofloxacin). ❷ The causative pathogen is commonly an enteric gram-negative bacilli (i.e., *Escherichia coli*). Nosocomially acquired urinary tract infections are often related to catheters and are caused by fermenting and nonfermenting (*Pseudomonas*) gram-negatives and *enterococci* (see Table 82–3). β-Lactam/β-lactamase inhibitor combinations (i.e., piperacillin-tazobactam), an antipseudomonal cephalosporin (i.e., cefepime or ceftazidime), or an antipseudomonal carbapenem (imipenem, meropenem, or doripenem), plus an aminoglycoside are recommended treatment options until susceptibilities are known (see Table 82–3).[31]

▶ *Community-Acquired Pneumonia*

Septic patients with community-acquired pneumonia (CAP) are treated with a third-generation cephalosporin (ceftriaxone or cefotaxime) plus a macrolide (azithromycin or clarithromycin) or doxycycline, or a respiratory fluoroquinolone (levofloxacin, moxifloxacin, gemifloxacin) (see Table 82–3).[32] ❷ *The causative organisms for CAP are* Streptococcus pneumoniae, Haemophilus influenzae, Moraxella catarrhalis, *and atypical organisms* (Mycoplasma pneumoniae, Chlamydia pneumoniae, *and* Legionella pneumophila). *S. pneumoniae* accounts for 60% of the deaths associated with CAP and is resistant to penicillin and macrolides (multidrug resistant *S. pneumoniae*; MDRSP) 30% to 40% of the time.[32,33] Controversy exists relating to the clinical significance of this resistance for nonmeningitis infections. Respiratory fluoroquinolones (levofloxacin, moxifloxacin, and gemifloxacin) may be utilized for MDRSP; however, clinical data have not shown them to be superior to cephalosporins plus a macrolide or doxycycline. The Centers for Disease Control and Prevention recommends reserving fluoroquinolones as last-line options in order to maintain their broad-spectrum antibacterial activity.[33] Treatment of methicillin-resistant *Staphylococcus aureus* (MRSA) or *P. aeruginosa* is a potential reason to modify the standard empirical regimen for CAP. Risk factors for the development of these pathogens are listed in Table 82–4.

▶ *Hospital-, Ventilator-, and Healthcare–Associated Pneumonia*

Treatment for septic patients with hospital-acquired, ventilator-acquired, and healthcare-associated pneumonia is dependent on risk factors for MDR organisms (Fig. 82–2). Recommended treatment for patients with no MDR risk factors are third-generation cephalosporins (ceftriaxone or cefotaxime), fluoroquinolones (levofloxacin and moxifloxacin),

Table 82–4

Risk Factors for MRSA, *Pseudomonas*, and Gram-Negatives in Community-Acquired Pneumonia

Methicillin-Resistant *Staphylococcus aureus*
End-stage renal disease
Injection drug abuse
Prior influenza
Prior antibiotic therapy (especially fluoroquinolones)
Pseudomonas aeruginosa
Structural lung disease
Exacerbations of severe chronic obstructive pulmonary diseases leading to frequent steroid and/or antibiotic use, as well as prior antibiotic therapy
Other Gram-negatives (*Klebsiella pneumoniae* or *Acinetobacter* species)
Chronic alcoholism

From Heffelfinger JD, Dowell SF, Jorgensen JH, et al. Management of community-acquired pneumonia in the era of pneumococcal resistance: A report from the Drug-Resistant Streptococcus pneumoniae Therapeutic Working Group. Arch Intern Med 2000;160:1399–1408.

Clinical Dilemma About Antibiotic-Resistant Bacteria

- MRSA is a common hospital-acquired pathogen and is also increasing in the community. MRSA presented a problem in the past because it required treatment with vancomycin. Community-acquired MRSA presents a major therapeutic challenge. MRSA can cause pneumonia, cellulitis, and other infections. Clinicians should be aware of the rate of hospital and community MRSA in their geographic area. New treatment options are available for MRSA. They include linezolid, tigecycline, daptomycin, telavancin, and ceftaroline. Prospective clinical trials have not demonstrated improved efficacy of these agents over vancomycin.[39,40]

- Extended-spectrum β-lactamase (ESBL) gram-negative bacteria are increasing in frequency. ESBLs most often occur in fermenting (lactose positive) Enterobacteriaceae and may be difficult to treat. ESBLs most commonly occur in urinary tract infections in patients with chronic Foley catheters, but they can occur in any infection. Carbapenem antibiotics are the most utilized agents for the treatment of ESBL infections.

ampicillin-sulbactam, or ertapenem (see Table 82–3).[34] Recommended treatment for patients with MDR risk factors are: β-lactam/β-lactamase inhibitor combinations (piperacillin/tazobactam), antipseudomonal cephalosporin (cefepime or ceftazidime), or an antipseudomonal carbapenem (imipenem, meropenem, or doripenem), plus an aminoglycoside, plus vancomycin or linezolid (see Table 82–3).[34] If an aminoglycoside is undesirable, an antipseudomonal fluoroquinolone (ciprofloxacin or levofloxacin) may be utilized with a antipseudomonal β-lactam (piperacillin/tazobactam, cefepime, ceftazidime, imipenem, meropenem, or doripenem).

▶ *Skin and Soft-Tissue Infections*

❷ *Community-acquired skin and soft-tissue infections are caused by* Streptococcus pyogenes *and* S. aureus. Treatment with nafcillin or cefazolin is recommended (see Table 82–3).[35] Local susceptibility rates may warrant empiric coverage for MRSA with anti-MRSA agents, especially in geographical areas with MRSA rates greater than 50%. Soft-tissue infections caused by *S. pyogenes* can lead to streptococcal toxic shock syndrome. Although penicillins and cephalosporins are efficacious, experimental models show clindamycin to be more effective than penicillin.[31] Hospital-acquired skin and soft-tissue infections are caused by *S. pyogenes*, *S. aureus*, and enteric gram-negatives. Recommended treatment is a third-generation cephalosporin (cefotaxime or ceftriaxone), ampicillin-sulbactam, or ertapenem, plus vancomycin (see Table 82–3).[35]

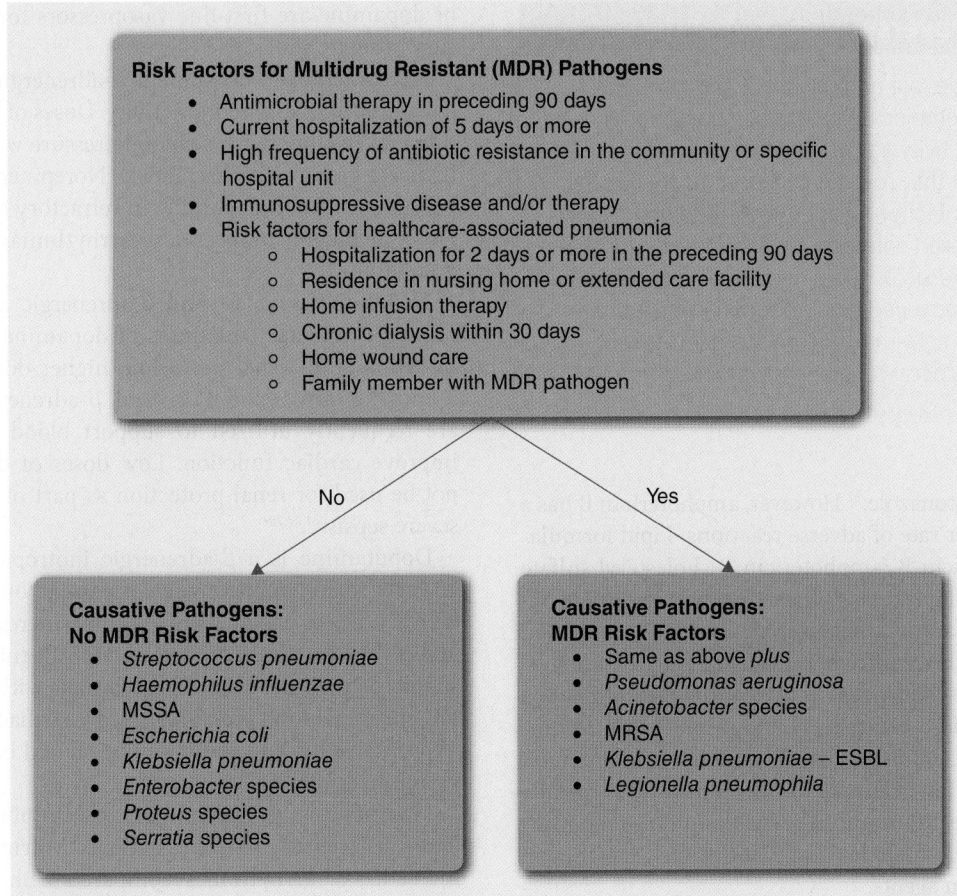

FIGURE 82–2. Risk factors for multidrug-resistant pathogens and causative pathogens for hospital-, ventilator-, and healthcare-associated pneumonia.[34] (ESBL, extended-spectrum β-lactamase; MDR, multidrug resistant; MRSA, methicillin-resistant *Staphylococcus aureus*; MSSA, methicillin-sensitive *Staphylococcus aureus*.)

▶ Intra-Abdominal Infections

❷ *Intra-abdominal infections are polymicrobial, including enteric aerobes and anaerobes.* Patients with community-acquired intra-abdominal infections of mild to moderate severity should be administered antibiotics with activity against enteric gram-negative bacilli, gram-negative anaerobes, and gram-positive cocci. Recommended treatment agents for mild to moderate community-acquired intra-abdominal infections include cefoxitin, cephalosporins (ceftriaxone or cefotaxime) plus metronidazole, fluoroquinolones (levofloxacin, ciprofloxacin) plus metronidazole or moxifloxacin monotherapy, ticarcillin-clavulanic acid, and ertapenem (see Table 82–3).[36] Patients with nosocomial-acquired, high-severity intra-abdominal infections or immunosuppression should receive empiric treatment with broad-spectrum antibiotics. Broad-spectrum antibiotics such as antipseudomonal β-lactam/β-lactamase inhibitor combinations (piperacillin/tazobactam), carbapenems (imipenem, meropenem, or doripenem), antipseudomonal cephalosporins (cefepime or ceftazidime) plus metronidazole, or antipseudomonal fluoroquinolones (ciprofloxacin or levofloxacin) plus metronidazole are recommended (see Table 82–3).[36]

Antifungal Therapy

❷ *Septic patients not responding to conventional antibiotics should be evaluated for fungal infections. Candida albicans is the most common fungal species; however, the prevalence of nonalbicans species is increasing.* Amphotericin B is utilized in septic patients with fungal or suspected fungal infections because of greater activity against nonalbicans *Candida*

Patient Encounter, Part 3

Treatment and Outcome Evaluation

The patient has continued hypotension despite previous intervention. Continued hypoxia has led to mechanical ventilation. The patient's serum creatinine has risen to 6.8 mg/dL (601 μmol/L). Blood and urine cultures reveal lactose-positive gram-negative rods.

Design a therapeutic regimen for this patient. Include all necessary medications.

compared with fluconazole.[37] However, amphotericin B has a significantly higher rate of adverse reactions. Lipid formulations of amphotericin B (amphotericin B cholesteryl sulfate complex, lipid complex, and liposomal amphotericin B) are available that are less nephrotoxic and have decreased infusion-associated side effects. Efficacy among the amphotericin products is equivalent, but the lipid formulations are significantly more expensive. Lipid products are recommended for patients intolerant of conventional amphotericin. Other alternatives for treatment of fungal infections include voriconazole and echinocandins (anidulafungin, caspofungin, micafungin). Data are lacking that demonstrate clinical superiority between agents.

Duration of Anti-Infective Therapy

● Average duration of anti-infective therapy for septic patients is 7 to 10 days. However, the durations vary depending on the site of infection and response to therapy. Step-down therapy from IV to oral anti-infectives is recommended for hemodynamically stable patients, patients afebrile for 48 to 72 hours, patients with normalized WBC, and patients able to take oral medications.

Vasopressors and Inotropic Therapy

● When fluid resuscitation does not provide adequate arterial pressure and organ perfusion, vasopressors and/or inotropic agents should be initiated. Vasopressors are recommended in patients with a systolic blood pressure less than 90 mm Hg or mean arterial pressure (MAP) lower than 60 to 65 mm Hg, after failed treatment with crystalloids.[24,27,28] Vasopressors and inotropes are effective in treating life-threatening hypotension and improving cardiac index, but complications such as tachycardia and myocardial ischemia require slow titration of the adrenergic agents to restore MAP without impairing stroke volume. Vasopressor therapy may also be required transiently to sustain life and maintain perfusion in the face of life-threatening hypotension, even when fluid resuscitation is in progress and hypovolemia has not yet been corrected. Agents commonly considered for vasopressor or inotropic support include dopamine, dobutamine, norepinephrine, phenylephrine, and epinephrine. Norepinephrine

or dopamine are first-line vasopressors to correct hypotension in septic shock.[24,27,28]

Norepinephrine is a potent α-adrenergic agent with less pronounced β-adrenergic activity. Doses of 0.01 to 3 mcg/kg/min can reliably increase blood pressure with small changes in heart rate or cardiac index. Norepinephrine is a more potent agent than dopamine in refractory septic shock.[24,27,28] Norepinephrine induces less arrhythmias compared with dopamine.[41]

Dopamine is an α- and β-adrenergic agent with dopaminergic activity. Low doses of dopamine (1 to 5 mcg/kg/min) maintain renal perfusion; higher doses (greater than 5 mcg/kg/min) exhibit α- and β-adrenergic activity and are frequently utilized to support blood pressure and to improve cardiac function. Low doses of dopamine should not be used for renal protection as part of the treatment of severe sepsis.[24,27,28]

Dobutamine is a β-adrenergic inotropic agent that can be utilized for improvement of cardiac output and oxygen delivery. Doses of 2 to 20 mcg/kg/min increase cardiac index; however, heart rate increases significantly. Dobutamine should be considered in septic patients with adequate filling pressure and blood pressure, but low cardiac index. If used in hypotensive patients, dobutamine should be combined with vasopressor therapy.[24,27,28]

Milrinone is a phosphodiesterase inhibitor with vasodilatory as well as inotropic actions. Milrinone has a lower incidence of arrhythmias compared with dobutamine. Its vasodilatory properties limit its use in the setting of hypotension due to sepsis.

Phenylephrine is a fast-acting, short-duration α_1 agonist. Phenylephrine has primarily vascular effects and does not impair cardiac or renal function. Phenylephrine is useful when tachycardia limits the use of other vasopressors.[24,27,28]

Epinephrine is a nonspecific α- and β-adrenergic agonist that can increase cardiac index and produce significant peripheral vasoconstriction. However, it can also increase lactate levels and impair blood flow to the splanchnic system. Because of these undesirable effects, epinephrine should be reserved for patients who fail to respond to traditional therapies.[24,27,28]

Vasopressin levels are increased during hypotension to maintain blood pressure by vasoconstriction. However, there is a vasopressin deficiency in septic shock. Low, fixed doses of vasopressin increase MAP, leading to the discontinuation of vasopressors. However, routine use of vasopressin with norepinephrine is not recommended because of no difference in mortality compared with norepinephrine monotherapy.[42] Vasopressin is a direct vasoconstrictor without inotropic or chronotropic effects and may result in decreased cardiac output and hepatosplanchnic flow. Vasopressin use may be considered in patients with refractory shock despite adequate fluid resuscitation and high-dose vasopressors.[24,27,28]

Steroids

● Stress-induced adrenal insufficiency complicates 9% to 24% of septic patients and is associated with increased mortality.

Patient Encounter, Part 4

During medical rounds, you are asked to discuss clinical trials and resistant bacteria.

What antibiotics are found to be superior in septic patients?

What are examples of resistant bacteria?

Is this patient a candidate for antipseudomonal therapy?

Corticosteroid therapy's effect on mortality in the treatment of septic shock is conflicting. Septic shock patients refractory to resuscitation and vasopressors may be administered IV hydrocortisone 200 to 300 mg/day in three divided doses.[24,43,44] Patients should be weaned from steroid therapy when vasopressors are no longer required.

Sedation and Neuromuscular Blockade

Patients with ARDS and progressive hypoxia require mechanical ventilation. Critically ill patients may require sedation when high ventilator settings are used or when patients fight the ventilator. Mechanically ventilated patients should receive sedation by a protocol that includes a daily interruption or lightening of a sedative infusion until the patient is awake.[24] The utilization of sedation protocols decreases the duration of mechanical ventilation, length of hospitalization, and tracheostomy rates.

Paralysis usually is reserved for patients in whom sedation alone does not improve the effectiveness of mechanical ventilation. Neuromuscular blockers may lead to prolonged skeletal muscle weakness and should be avoided if possible. Patients requiring neuromuscular blockade should be monitored, and intermittent boluses or continuous infusion should be utilized. Monitor depth of neuromuscular blockade with train-of-four stimulation when using continuous infusion.

Glucose Control

Glycemic control improves survival in postoperative surgical patients and is recommended in septic patients. Following initial stabilization of septic patients, current guidelines recommend maintaining blood glucose concentrations less than 150 mg/dL (8.3 mmol/L).[24,45,46] There is an increase in mortality in tightly controlled patients (81 to 108 mg/dL [4.5 to 6.0 mmol/L]) versus moderately controlled patients (less than 180 mg/dL [10.0 mmol/L]). Septic patients with high glucose concentrations should receive insulin and glucose with frequent blood glucose monitoring (every 1 to 2 hours until glucose values and insulin infusion rates are stable, then every 4 hours).

Adjunctive Therapies

Enteral nutrition is recommended in septic patients to meet the increased energy and protein requirements. Protein requirements are increased to 1.5 to 2.5 g/kg/day. Nonprotein caloric requirements range from 25 to 40 kcal/kg/day (105 to 167 kJ/kg/day).[24]

DVT prophylaxis is recommended for septic patients. Low-dose unfractionated heparin, low-molecular-weight heparin (e.g., enoxaparin or dalteparin), or pentasaccharide therapy (e.g., fondaparinux) may be utilized. Graduated compression stockings or an intermittent compression device is recommended for patients with a contraindication to heparin products (thrombocytopenia, severe coagulopathy, active bleeding, or recent intracerebral hemorrhage).[24] Patients with severe sepsis and history of DVT, trauma, or orthopedic surgery should receive a combination of pharmacologic and mechanical therapy unless contraindicated or not practical.

Stress ulcer prophylaxis is recommended in septic patients. Patients at greatest risk for stress ulcers include those who are coagulopathic, mechanically ventilated (more than 48 hours), and hypotensive. Histamine-receptor antagonists (e.g., ranitidine) are more efficacious than sucralfate, and proton pump inhibitors (e.g., omeprazole) have shown no added benefit over histamine-receptor antagonists. However, they do demonstrate equivalence in the ability to increase gastric pH.[24] The benefit of prophylaxis must be weighed against the potential effect of an increased stomach pH and development of hospital-acquired pneumonia.

Nonpharmacologic Therapy

Evaluate septic patients for the presence of a localized infection amenable to source control measures. Common source control measures include drainage and debridement, device removal, and prevention.[24-26] Implementation of source control methods should be instituted as soon as possible following initial fluid resuscitation. The selection of optimal source control methods must weigh benefits and risks of the intervention. Source control measures may cause complications (bleeding, fistulas, and organ injury); therefore, the method with the least risk should be employed.[24]

Prognosis

There are various factors that influence outcome. Gram-negative bacteria are more likely to produce septic shock than gram-positive bacteria (50% versus 25%) and have a higher mortality rate than other pathogens. This may be related to the severity of the underlying condition. Patients with rapidly fatal conditions, such as leukemia, aplastic anemia, and burns, have a worse prognosis than patients with nonfatal underlying conditions, such as diabetes mellitus or chronic renal insufficiency. Other factors that worsen the prognosis of septic patients include advanced age, malnutrition, resistant bacteria, utilization of medical devices, and immunosuppression. Data for long-term mortality are lacking (it is estimated that the mortality for sepsis survivors within the first year is 20%).[5] Patients may have prolonged physical disability related to muscle weakness and posttraumatic stress.

Patient Care and Monitoring

1. Evaluate patient parameters and classify as infection, SIRS, sepsis, severe sepsis, septic shock, or MODS.

2. Review available diagnostic and laboratory data.

3. Evaluate early goal-directed resuscitation therapy. Understand what parameters define efficacy and failure of initial therapy. Recommend alternative resuscitation therapy if the patient does not respond to initial fluid challenge.

4. Evaluate the source of infection and make recommendations to remove potential source(s).

5. Analyze anti-infective therapy (dose, frequency, and duration) and revise as necessary based on clinical response, culture and sensitivity reports, and renal/hepatic function. Prepare an appropriate step-down therapy for the patient.

6. Determine the risk of sepsis complications and construct recommendations for treatment and monitoring.

7. Formulate appropriate doses of medications involved in patient therapy and revise as needed. Patient parameters may change frequently, thus requiring different doses and/or medications. Examples include antibiotic therapy, analgesics, sedatives, insulin, fluids, or vasopressors.

8. Continually monitor patient parameters to ensure optimal therapy to maximize outcomes.

Abbreviations Introduced in This Chapter

ARDS	Acute respiratory distress syndrome
AKI	Acute kidney injury
CAP	Community-acquired pneumonia
CBC	Complete blood count
DIC	Disseminated intravascular coagulation
Do_2	Delivery of oxygen to tissues
DVT	Deep vein thrombosis
ESBL	Extended-spectrum β-lactamase
MAP	Mean arterial pressure
MDR	Multidrug resistant
MDRSP	Multidrug-resistant *Streptococcus pneumonia*
MODS	Multiple-organ dysfunction syndrome
MRSA	Methicillin-resistant *Staphylococcus aureus*
MSSA	Methicillin-sensitive *S. aureus*
$Paco_2$	Partial pressure of carbon dioxide
SIRS	Systemic inflammatory response syndrome
TNF-α	Tumor necrosis factor-α
Vo_2	Oxygen consumption by tissues

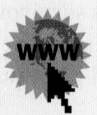 Self-assessment questions and answers are available at *http://www.mhpharmacotherapy.com/pp.html.*

REFERENCES

1. Hotchkiss RS, Karl IE. The pathophysiology and treatment of sepsis. N Engl J Med 2003;348:138–150.
2. American College of Chest Physicians, Society of Critical Care Medicine Consensus Conference. Definitions for sepsis and organ failure and guidelines for the use of innovative therapies in sepsis. Crit Care Med 1992;20:864–874.
3. Calandra T, Cohen J. The international sepsis forum consensus conference on definitions of infection in the intensive care unit. Crit Care Med 2005;33:1538–1548.
4. Martin GS, Mannino DM, Eaton S, Moss M. The epidemiology of sepsis in the United States from 1979 through 2000. N Engl J Med 2003;348:1546–1554.
5. Cartin-Ceba R, Kojicic M, Li G, et al. Epidemiology of critical care syndromes, organ failures, and life-support interventions in a suburban US community. Chest 2011;140(6):1447–1455.
6. Angus DC, Linde-Zwirble WT, Lidicker J, et al. Epidemiology of severe sepsis in the United States: Analysis of incidence, outcome, and associated costs of care. Crit Care Med 2001;29:1303–1310.
7. Hoste E, Lameire NH, Vanholder RC, et al. Acute renal failure in patients with sepsis in a surgical ICU: predictive factors, incidence, comorbidity, and outcome. J Am Soc Nephrol 2003;14:1022–1030.
8. Poutsiaka DD, Davidson LE, Kahn KL, et al. Risk factors for death after sepsis in patients immunosuppressed before the onset of sepsis. Scand J Infect Dis 2009;41(6-7):469–479.
9. Wafaisade A, Lefering R, Bouillon B, et al. Epidemiology and risk factors of sepsis after multiple trauma: An analysis of 29,829 patients from the trauma registry of the German society for trauma surgery. Crit Care Med 2011;39(4):621–628.
10. Lin MT, Albertson TE. Genomic polymorphisms in sepsis. Crit Care Med 2004;32:569–579.
11. Bodey GP, Mardani M, Hanna HA, et al. The epidemiology of Candida glabrata and Candida albicans fungemia in immunocompromised patients with cancer. Am J Med 2002;112:380–385.
12. Costa SF, Marino I, Araujo EA, et al. Nosocomial fungemia: A 2-year prospective study. J Hosp Infect 2000:45:69–72.
13. Marie C, Muret J, Fitting C, et al. Interleukin-1 receptor antagonist production during infectious and noninfectious systemic inflammatory response syndrome. Crit Care Med 2000;28:2277–2282.
14. Opal SM, Girard TD, Ely EW. The immunopathogenesis of sepsis in elderly patients. Clin Infect Dis 2005;41:S504–S512.
15. Kim PK, Deutschman CS. Inflammatory responses and mediators. Surg Clin North Am 2000;80:885–894.
16. van der Poll T, van Deventer SJH. Cytokines and anticytokines in the pathogenesis of sepsis. Infect Dis Clin North Am 1999;13:413–426.
17. Zeerleder S, Hack CE, Wuillemin WA. Disseminated intravascular coagulation in sepsis. Chest 2005;128:2864–2875.
18. Wheeler AP, Bernard GR. Treating patients with severe sepsis. N Engl J Med 1999;340:207–214.
19. Hirrela E. Advances in the management of acute respiratory distress syndrome. Arch Surg 2000;135:126–134.
20. Schrier RW, Wang W. Acute renal failure and sepsis. N Engl J Med 2004;351:159–169.
21. Awad SS. State-of-the-art therapy for sepsis and multisystem organ failure. Am J Surg 2003;186:S23–S30.
22. Harbarth S, Garbino J, Pugin J, et al. Inappropriate initial antimicrobial therapy and its effects on survival in a clinical trial of immunomodulating therapy for severe sepsis. Am J Med 2003;115:529–535.
23. Garnacho-Montero J, Garcia-Garmendia JL, Barrero-Almodovar A, et al. Impact of adequate empirical antibiotic therapy on the outcome of patients admitted to the intensive care unit with sepsis. Crit Care Med 2003;31:2742–2751.
24. Dellinger RP, Levy MM, Carlet JM, et al. Surviving Sepsis Campaign: International guidelines for the management of severe sepsis and septic shock:2008. Crit Care Med 2008;36:296–327.
25. Jimenez MF, Marshall JC. Source control in the management of sepsis. Intensive Care Med 2001;27:S49–S62.
26. Centers for Disease Control and Prevention. Guidelines for the prevention of catheter-related infections. MMWR 2002;51:1–29.

27. Rivers E, Nguyen B, Havstad S, et al., for the Early Goal-directed Therapy Collaborative Group. Early goal-directed therapy in the treatment of severe sepsis and septic shock. N Engl J Med 2001;345:1368–1377.

28. Hollenberg SM, Ahrens TS, Annane D, et al. Practice parameters for hemodynamic support of sepsis in adult patients: 2004 update. Crit Care Med 2004;32:1928–1948.

29. Finfer S, Bellomo R, Boyce N, et al. A comparison of albumin and saline for fluid resuscitation in the intensive care unit. N Engl J Med 2004;350:2247–2256.

30. MacArthur RD, Miller M, Albertson T, et al. Adequacy of early empiric antibiotic treatment and survival in severe sepsis: Experience from the MONARCS trial. Clin Infect Dis 2004;38:284–288.

31. Simon D, Trenholme G. Antibiotic selection for patients with septic shock. Crit Care Clin 2000;16:215–231.

32. Mandell LA, Wunderink RG, Anzueto A, et al. Infectious Diseases Society of America/American Thoracic Society Consensus Guidelines on the Management of Community-Acquired Pneumonia in Adults. Clin Infect Dis 2007;44:S27–S72.

33. Heffelfinger JD, Dowell SF, Jorgensen JH, et al. Management of community-acquired pneumonia in the era of pneumococcal resistance: A report from the Drug-Resistant Streptococcus pneumoniae Therapeutic Working Group. Arch Intern Med 2000;160:1399–1408.

34. American Thoracic Society and the Infectious Diseases Society of America. Guidelines for the management of adults with hospital-acquired, ventilator-associated, and healthcare-associated pneumonia. Am J Respir Crit Care Med 2005;171:388–416.

35. Stevens DL, Bisno AL, Chambers HF, et al. Practice guidelines for the diagnosis and management of skin and soft-tissue infections. Clin Infect Dis 2005;41:1373–1406.

36. Solomkin JS, Mazuski JE, Bradley JS, et al. Diagnosis and management of complicated intra-abdominal infection in adults and children: Guidelines by the Surgical Infection Society and the Infectious Diseases Society of America. Clin Infect Dis 2010;50:133–164.

37. Pappas PG, Kauffman CA, Andes D, et al. Clinical practice guidelines for the management of candidiasis: 2009 Update by the Infectious Diseases Society of America. Clin Infect Dis 2009;48:503–535.

38. Wallace AW, Jones M, Bertino JS. Evaluation of four once-daily aminoglycoside dosing nomograms. Pharmacotherapy 2002;22:1077–1083.

39. Zetola N, Francis JS, Nuermberger EL, Bishai WR. Community-acquired methicillin-resistant Staphylococcus aureus: An emerging threat. Lancet Infect Dis 2005;5:275–286.

40. Crum NF. The emergence of severe, community-acquired methicillin-resistant Staphylococcus aureus infections. Scand J Infect Dis 2005;39:651–656.

41. De Backer D, Biston P, Devriendt J, et al. Comparison of dopamine and norepinephrine in the treatment of shock. N Engl J Med 2010;362:779–789.

42. Russell JA, Walley KR, Singer J, et al. Vasopressin versus norepinephrine infusion in patients with septic shock. N Engl J Med 2008;358:877–887.

43. Annane D, Sebille V, Charpentier C, et al. Effect of treatment with low doses of hydrocortisone and fludrocortisone on mortality in patients with septic shock. JAMA 2002;288:862–871.

44. Sprung CL, Annane D, Keh D, et al. Hydrocortisone therapy for patients with septic shock. N Engl J Med 2008;358:111–124.

45. Van den Berghe G, Wilmer A, Hermans G, et al. Intensive insulin therapy in the medical ICU. N Engl J Med 2006;354:449–461.

46. van den Berghe G, Wouters P, Weekers F, et al. Intensive insulin therapy in the critically ill patient. N Engl J Med 2001;345:1359–1367.

83 Superficial Fungal Infections

Lauren S. Schlesselman

LEARNING OBJECTIVES

● **Upon completion of the chapter, the reader will be able to:**

1. Explain the underlying pathophysiology of vulvovaginal candidiasis, oropharyngeal candidiasis, esophageal candidiasis, and fungal skin infections.

2. Identify symptoms of vulvovaginal candidiasis, oropharyngeal candidiasis, esophageal candidiasis, and fungal skin infections.

3. Identify the desired therapeutic outcomes for patients with uncomplicated and complicated vulvovaginal candidiasis, oropharyngeal candidiasis, esophageal candidiasis, and fungal skin infections.

4. Recommend appropriate lifestyle modifications and pharmacotherapy interventions for patients with vulvovaginal candidiasis, oropharyngeal candidiasis, esophageal candidiasis, and fungal skin infections.

5. Recognize when long-term suppressive therapy is indicated for a patient with vulvovaginal candidiasis.

6. Recognize when topical versus oral treatment is indicated for a patient with oropharyngeal candidiasis, esophageal candidiasis, vulvovaginal candidiasis, and fungal skin infections.

7. Educate patients about the disease state, appropriate lifestyle modifications, and medication therapy required for effective treatment of vulvovaginal candidiasis, oropharyngeal candidiasis, esophageal candidiasis, and fungal skin infections.

KEY CONCEPTS

❶ The predominant pathogen associated with vulvovaginal candidiasis is *Candida albicans*, although a small percentage of cases are caused by *Candida glabrata, Candida tropicalis, Candida krusei,* and *Candida parapsilosis.*

❷ A variety of factors may increase the risk of developing symptomatic vulvovaginal candidiasis, including antibiotic use, diabetes, and immunosuppression. No risk factors are consistently associated with all cases of vulvovaginal candidiasis.

❸ Asymptomatic vaginal colonization of *Candida albicans* is not diagnostic of vulvovaginal candidiasis since 10% to 20% of women are asymptomatic carriers of *Candida* species. Asymptomatic vaginal colonization does not require treatment.

❹ Selection of antifungal agents to treat uncomplicated vulvovaginal candidiasis is influenced by patient preference, including route of administration, duration of therapy, cost, risk of adverse effects, and potential for medication interactions.

❺ Recurrent vulvovaginal candidiasis, defined as four or more infections per year, requires long-term suppressive therapy for 6 months.

❻ The occurrence of oropharyngeal and esophageal candidiasis is an indicator of immune suppression, often developing in infants, the elderly, and the immunocompromised.

❼ Topical antifungal agents are first-line therapy for oropharyngeal candidiasis, although oral agents may be used for severe or unresponsive cases.

❽ Esophageal candidiasis is a severe form of extension of oropharyngeal candidiasis that requires oral antifungal therapy.

❾ Because dermatophyte hyphae seldom penetrate into the living layers of the skin, instead remaining in the stratum corneum, most mycotic infections of the skin can be treated with topical antifungals. Infections covering large areas of the body or infections involving nails or hair may require oral therapy.

❿ Onychomycosis, fungal infections involving the nails, requires oral antifungal therapy. Topical agents do not adequately penetrate the nail.

VULVOVAGINAL CANDIDIASIS

Vulvovaginal candidiasis (VVC), whether symptomatic or asymptomatic, refers to infections in women whose vaginal cultures are positive for *Candida* species.

EPIDEMIOLOGY AND ETIOLOGY

Vulvovaginal candidiasis, also known as moniliasis, is a common form of vaginitis, accounting for 20% to 25% of vaginitis cases. Although VVC is uncommon prior to **menarche**, nearly 50% of women will experience one or more episodes by the age of 25 years.[1] A survey of women in the United States found that 6.5% of women over the age of 18 years reported experiencing at least one episode of vaginitis during the previous 2 months.[2]

According to the treatment guidelines of the Centers for Disease Control and Prevention (CDC),[3] VVC can be classified as uncomplicated or complicated. Uncomplicated infections occur sporadically, cause mild to moderate symptoms, and occur in nonimmunocompromised women. Uncomplicated infections, most often caused by *Candida albicans*, often have no identifiable precipitating cause. Complicated infections, including recurrent, severe infections, and those in women with uncontrolled diabetes, debilitation, or immunosuppression, may be caused by nonalbicans or azole-resistant fungal organisms. Immunocompromise, including immunosuppression, uncontrolled diabetes, pregnancy, or debilitation, is also a risk factor for developing recurrent infection. Recurrent VVC, defined as four or more infections per year, occurs in less than 5% of women.[3] Recurrent infection is distinguishable from a persistent infection by the presence of a symptom-free interval between infections.

❶ *Candida albicans* is the primary pathogen responsible for VVC, accounting for approximately 70% of cases.[4] Other cases are caused by nonalbicans species including *Candida glabrata*, *Candida tropicalis*, *Candida krusei*, and *Candida parapsilosis*. In patients with recurrent vaginitis, the causative *Candida* is twice as likely to be nonalbicans.[5] The incidence of nonalbicans VVC is increasing, possibly due to overuse of nonprescription vaginal antifungal products, short-course antifungal treatments, and long-term suppressive therapy with antifungals.

PATHOPHYSIOLOGY

The normal vaginal environment protects women against vaginal infections. Under the influence of estrogen, vaginal epithelium cornifies to reduce the risk of infection. Vaginal discharge, comprised of exfoliated cells, cervical mucus, and colonized bacteria, cleans the vagina. The volume of discharge varies during pregnancy, during oral contraceptive use, with age, and at midmenstrual cycle near ovulation. The normal pH of vaginal secretions, near 4.0, is maintained by *Lactobacillus acidophilus*, diphtheroids, and *Staphylococcus epidermidis*. The low pH is toxic to many pathogens.

Any alteration in the vaginal environment allows for overgrowth of organisms that are normally suppressed. Increases in the vaginal pH are associated with increased vulvovaginitis.

Clinical Presentation and Diagnosis of VVC

Patients with VVC may present with vulvar and/or vaginal symptoms. Symptoms often develop the week before menses and resolve with the onset of menses.

Symptoms include:
- Vaginal itching
- Vaginal soreness
- Vaginal burning
- Irritation
- External dysuria
- Dyspareunia

Signs include:
- Nonodorous vaginal discharge (may vary from watery to curd-like)
- Yellow or yellowish-green discharge
- Erythema and edema of the labia and vulva
- Fissures
- Pustulopapular lesions
- Normal cervix

Diagnostic Testing

- Microscopic investigation for the presence of blastospores or pseudohyphae; saline wet mount has a sensitivity of 40% to 50%, whereas a potassium hydroxide (KOH) preparation has a sensitivity of 50% to 70%.[7] *Asymptomatic vaginal colonization of* Candida albicans *is not diagnostic of VVC since 10% to 20% of women are asymptomatic carriers of* Candida *species. Asymptomatic vaginal colonization does not require treatment; therefore the presence alone of* Candida *should not determine care.*

- Vaginal pH less than or equal to 4.5; pH should remain normal in cases of fungal infection, whereas an elevated pH suggests bacterial infection.

- *Candida* cultures should be obtained only if signs and microscopy are inconclusive or in cases of recurrent VVC.

---

pH changes are caused by stress, changes in hormone level, sexual activity, pregnancy, phases of the menstrual cycle, contraceptive use, presence of foreign bodies or necrotic tissue, use of douches, or the use of antibiotics. An increase in glycogen production, associated with altered estrogen and progesterone levels, can also increase the risk of infection through increased adherence of *Candida albicans* to epithelial cells.

RISK FACTORS

❷ *Although no risk factors are consistently associated with conversion to symptomatic infection, a variety of factors may increase the risk of developing symptomatic VVC in certain women* (Table 83–1).

Table 83–1

Possible Risk Factors Associated with VVC

Risk Factor	Proposed Mechanism
Broad-spectrum antibiotic use	Altered vaginal flora allowing overgrowth of *Candida* organisms; risk increases with duration of antibiotic use
Systemic corticosteroid or immunosuppressant use	Reduced vaginal protection by immunoglobulins
Sexual activity	VVC is often associated with the onset of sexual activity; partners may have penile or oral colonization; use of vaginal irritants or devices, including diaphragms and intrauterine systems, can irritate vaginal mucosa
Tight-fitting and nonabsorbent clothing	Promotes warm, moist environment for fungus growth
Elevated estrogen levels, hormonal contraceptives, and pregnancy	Estrogen enhances *Candida* adherence to vaginal epithelial cells and yeast-mycelial transformation; this is supported by the fact that infection rates are lower before menarche and after menopause (except in women taking hormone replacement therapy), whereas rates are higher during pregnancy
Vaginal pH	Changes in glycogen and lactic acid levels
Gastrointestinal reservoir of *Candida* organisms	Transfer of organism from rectum to vagina; irritation of the vulvovaginal area during sexual intercourse may enhance invasion of organisms
Diabetes	Enhanced binding of *Candida* to epithelial cells due to hyperglycemia; asymptomatic colonization is more common in patients with diabetes; elevated sugar levels may cause conversion to symptomatic infection

Patient Encounter 1

A 19-year-old woman presents to your clinic complaining of what she calls "itching and burning in my private areas." After questioning her, you determine that she has vaginal burning, soreness, and itching, accompanied by a curd-like discharge. Although she has had vaginal infections before, she admits to recently becoming sexually active and is very concerned that she may have contracted a sexually transmitted disease. On examination, she has erythema of the labia and a nonodorous discharge.

What information is suggestive of VVC?

What additional information do you need to know before creating a treatment plan for this patient?

TREATMENT

The goals of treatment of VVC are as follows:

- Relief of symptoms
- Eradication of infection
- Reestablishment of normal vaginal flora
- Prevention of recurrent infections in complicated infections

Nonpharmacologic Treatments

● In combination with pharmacologic treatment, the practitioner should recommend basic nonpharmacologic approaches to treatment and prevention of VVC:

- Keep the genital area clean and dry
- Avoid prolonged use of hot tubs
- Avoid constrictive clothing
- Avoid vaginal douching
- Wear underwear made of breathable materials, such as cotton
- To reduce vulvar irritation, avoid soaps and perfumes in the genital area
- Although study results are conflicting, the daily consumption of active *Lactobacillus acidophilus* may reduce recurrence. One study found that the daily ingestion of oral *Lactobacillus* reduced fungal concentrations and produced a normal balance of colonized organisms,[6] whereas other studies found no difference in infection rates in women who ingested yogurt[7,8]

Pharmacologic Treatment of Uncomplicated VVC

Most cases of uncomplicated VVC will resolve with a single course of antifungal therapy. Treatment with an oral or vaginal antifungal agent, either prescription or nonprescription, is appropriate for most uncomplicated cases. Nonprescription azole antifungal products are available as 1-night, 3-night, and 7-night regimens in a variety of formulations, including cream, suppository, and vaginal tablets (Table 83–2). Oral fluconazole offers the option of treatment with one dose administered without regard to time of day. Some practitioners opt to re-treat with a second dose of fluconazole 3 days later. Due to the risk of severe hepatotoxicity, the use of oral ketoconazole should be reserved for severe fungal infections resistant to other antifungal options.

To avoid inappropriate use of nonprescription products, the practitioner should only recommend them to women who have previously been diagnosed with VVC. Estimates of how accurately women self-diagnose VVC are difficult to assess. One study found that only one-third of women accurately diagnosed an episode of vaginitis.[9] Women with a previous clinically based diagnosis of VVC are no more accurate at self-diagnosing than women without prior clinical diagnosis.[9]

Table 83–2
Treatment Options for Uncomplicated VVC

1-Day Therapies

Butoconazole 2% sustained-release cream, 5 g intravaginally as a single application
Fluconazole 150 mg, one tablet orally as a single dose
Tioconazole 6.5% ointment, 5 g intravaginally as a single application

3-Day Therapies

Butoconazole 2% cream, 5 g intravaginally for 3 nights
Clotrimazole 100-mg vaginal tablet, two tablets for 3 nights
Miconazole 200-mg vaginal suppository, one suppository for 3 nights
Terconazole 0.8% cream, 5 g intravaginally for 3 nights
Terconazole 80-mg vaginal suppository, one suppository for 3 nights

7- to 14-Day Therapies

Boric acid 600-mg vaginal suppository, one suppository intravaginally twice daily for 14 days
Clotrimazole 1% cream, 5 g intravaginally for 7–14 nights
Clotrimazole 100-mg vaginal tablet, one tablet for 7 nights
Miconazole 2% cream, 5 g intravaginally for 7 nights
Miconazole 100-mg vaginal suppository, one suppository for 7 nights
Nystatin 100,000-unit vaginal tablet, one tablet for 14 nights
Terconazole 0.4% cream, 5 g intravaginally for 7 nights

Inability to resolve an infection may indicate a mixed infection, infection owing to a nonalbicans strain, or an infection that is not fungal. Difficulty treating VVC can also be indicative of serious underlying conditions, such as diabetes or human immunodeficiency virus (HIV) infection. For these reasons, if infection does not resolve easily with a single course of antifungal therapy or if symptoms return within 2 months, practitioners should check cultures and further evaluate the patient's health status or refer the patient to a physician.

④ *Due to the numerous treatment options available, a variety of factors can influence product selection, with patient preference playing a significant role.* To improve adherence with therapy, the practitioner should discuss with the patient what options are available and what her preferences are.

Adherence rates are greater with oral treatment than with vaginal therapy. This may be due to the ease of administration, short duration, and flexibility on time of administration. Vaginal creams provide rapid relief of itching and burning. The practitioner may wish to advise a patient to apply a vaginal cream externally to reduce itching and burning if using an oral agent. The need to clean the vaginal applicator for reuse is unappealing for some women. Many nonprescription vaginal products are now packaged with sufficient disposable applicators to prevent the need for reuse with subsequent doses. Available regimens range from 1 to 7 days for topical preparations and fluconazole. Cure rates are similar among different durations of therapy.[10] Most OTC products cost $10 to $20 per course of therapy. The cost of prescription products can vary based on if and what type of insurance coverage the patient has. If the patient does not have prescription coverage, nonprescription products may prove less expensive than even one or two fluconazole tablets.

▶ Risk of Adverse Effects and Interactions

Systemic adverse effects associated with vaginal azoles are less frequent than with oral products. With topical products, local discomfort such as burning, itching, stinging, and redness may occur, particularly with the first application. In contrast, common adverse effects associated with fluconazole include headache, diarrhea, nausea, dizziness, abdominal pain, and taste alterations. Fifteen percent of patients experience gastrointestinal side effects with orally administered antifungal agents.[11] Oral ketoconazole is associated with hepatic toxicity at a rate of 1 in 15,000.[12]

Oral azoles are associated with significant interactions, particularly due to cytochrome P-450 isoenzymes. Medications that interact with azoles include warfarin, phenytoin, theophylline, rifampin, cyclosporine, and zidovudine. For patients receiving only a few doses, these interactions do not pose a significant risk. These interactions may pose a risk for patients receiving long-term suppressive therapy for recurrent infections.

TREATMENT OF RECURRENT VVC

The goal of treating recurrent VVC is control of the infection, rather than cure. First, any acute episodes are treated, followed by maintenance therapy. For the treatment of acute episodes, intravaginal or oral azoles can be utilized. Although acute episodes of recurrent VVC will respond to azole therapy, some patients may require prolonged therapy to achieve remission. To achieve remission, a second dose of oral fluconazole 150 mg repeated 3 days after the first dose or 14 days of topical azole therapy can be used. The practitioner should consider that nonalbicans infections are more common in recurrent VVC; therefore, fluconazole and itraconazole resistance may make these agents less effective.

⑤ *After achieving remission, recurrent VVC requires long-term suppressive therapy for 6 months* (Table 83–3). To improve adherence to long-term suppressive therapy, oral therapy, typically with fluconazole, is preferred. Fluconazole 150 mg weekly for 6 months will prevent recurrence of

Table 83–3
Treatment Options for Maintenance Therapy

Daily

Boric acid 600 mg in gelatin capsule vaginally daily during menses (5 days)
Itraconazole 100 mg orally once daily
Ketoconazole 100 mg orally once daily

Weekly

Clotrimazole 500 mg vaginal suppository once weekly
Fluconazole 100 or 150 mg orally once weekly
Terconazole 0.8% cream 5 g vaginally once weekly

Monthly

Fluconazole 150 mg orally once monthly
Itraconazole 400 mg orally once monthly

infection in 90% of women.[13] Cessation of suppressive therapy is associated with resurgence of symptomatic infection in 50% of women.[14]

TREATMENT OF NONALBICANS INFECTIONS

Treatment response rates are lower for nonalbicans infections. Although an optimal regimen is unknown, use of intravaginal azole therapy for 7 to 14 days is recommended. Terconazole may prove more effective than other azoles in the treatment of nonalbicans infections since *C. glabrata* and *C. tropicalis* are more susceptible to terconazole.[15] For second-line therapy, boric acid 600 mg in a gelatin capsule administered vaginally twice daily for 2 weeks followed by once daily during menstruation is effective.[16] Local irritation often limits the use of boric acid. Topical 4% flucytosine is also effective, but use should be limited due to the potential for resistance.

VVC DURING PREGNANCY

During pregnancy, VVC may prove difficult to treat due to elevated estrogen levels, accompanied by concern about harm to the fetus. Response rates are lower and recurrences are frequent during pregnancy. Vaginal antifungals remain the preferred treatment during pregnancy, although therapy should continue for 1 to 2 weeks to ensure effectiveness.[14] Most topical antifungals are classified as risk category C, whereas clotrimazole is classified as risk category B. Fluconazole's risk category classification was recently changed to category D for all indications other than vaginal candidiasis, for which it remains a risk category C. Despite oral fluconazole's classification, studies have not demonstrated an increased risk to the fetus when the pregnant mother was exposed to low-dose fluconazole,[17,18] although case studies have reported congenital limb deformities with doses of 400 to 800 mg daily during the first trimester.[19]

Cultural Awareness During Treatment of VVC

As with all gynecologic issues, the practitioner is faced with cultural perceptions of female genitalia. In particular, practitioners are treating an increased number of patients who have undergone female genital mutilation. More than 100 million women and girls worldwide have undergone such procedures for cultural and religious reasons.[20] Female genital mutilation, formerly known as female circumcision, describes the intentional alteration or injury of female genitalia. Some authorities suggest using the term "genital cutting" when dealing with patients to avoid appearing judgmental.[21] Regardless of the terminology used, many immigrants are aware of common cultural views in the United States pertaining to female genital mutilation. Women who have undergone this procedure suffer acute and chronic complications. Within the scope of this chapter, the practitioner may find that patients with female genital mutilation suffer from recurrent VVC due to

inadequate drainage of vaginal fluids. Regardless of what the practitioner's opinion is about female genital mutilation, the practitioner must be sensitive to the patient's feeling and cultural values.

Patient Care and Monitoring of VVC

1. Assess the patient's symptoms to determine whether self-treatment with OTC antifungal therapy is appropriate or whether the patient should be evaluated by a practitioner or physician. OTC preparations should only be recommended for patients who have previously been diagnosed with VVC. Patients who experience more than four episodes per year should be referred to a physician for culturing and initiation of maintenance therapy.

2. Review any available diagnostic data, including cultures and KOH preps.

3. Obtain a thorough history of prescription, nonprescription, and natural drug product use. Is the patient taking any medications, such as steroids, antibiotics, or immunosuppressants, that may contribute to VVC? Is the patient taking any medications that may interfere with treatment?

4. If the patient has had VVC previously, determine what treatments were helpful to the patient in the past.

5. Educate the patient on lifestyle modifications that may prevent recurrence, including decreased consumption of sucrose and refined carbohydrates, increased consumption of yogurt containing live cultures, and wearing cotton underwear.

6. Develop a plan to assess effectiveness of antifungal therapy.

7. Determine whether long-term suppressive therapy is necessary.

8. Evaluate the patient for the presence of adverse drug reactions, drug allergies, and drug interactions.

9. Stress the importance of adherence with the antifungal regimen, including lifestyle modifications.

10. Provide patient education pertaining to vulvovaginal candidiasis and antifungal therapy.
    - Causes of vulvovaginal candidiasis
    - How to administer vaginal antifungal creams
    - Vaginal antifungal creams' and suppositories' adverse effects on latex condoms and diaphragms
    - Potential adverse effects that may occur with antifungal therapy
    - Medications that may interact with antifungal therapy
    - Preventing the spread of infection
    - Warning signs to report to a physician (recurrent or difficult-to-cure infections, infections with malodorous discharge)

OUTCOME EVALUATION

● Whether using a topical or an oral agent, patients should notice relief of itching and discomfort within 1 to 2 days. The volume of discharge should also begin to decrease within a few days. The entire course of therapy should be continued even if symptoms have resolved. If the condition does not resolve or worsens, the patient should be referred to a physician for aggressive therapy. If the condition recurs within 4 weeks or more than four times per year, the patient should be further evaluated or referred to a physician for evaluation of possible non-*Candida* infections, resistant organism, or other complicating factors, along with assessment of need for long-term suppressive therapy.

OROPHARYNGEAL AND ESOPHAGEAL CANDIDIASIS

Oropharyngeal candidiasis (OPC) is a common fungal infection, usually associated with immune suppression. If left untreated, it will progress to more serious oral disease. Esophageal candidiasis, representing a serious progression of oropharyngeal candidiasis, is associated with increased morbidity.

EPIDEMIOLOGY AND ETIOLOGY

❻ *The occurrence of oropharyngeal and esophageal candidiasis is an indicator of immune suppression, often developing in infants, the elderly, and the immunocompromised.* One-third to one-half of geriatric inpatients develop oropharyngeal candidiasis. Denture stomatitis is present in approximately 40% of denture wearers,[22] more commonly in women than men. Oral candidiasis is the most commonly reported adverse drug event reported by patients receiving inhaled corticosteroids.[23] The prevalence of esophageal candidiasis is 37% among patients treated with inhaled corticosteroids.[24] The incidence is highest among patients receiving high doses of corticosteroids or those with diabetes.

The prevalence of HIV infection plays a significant role in the incidence of oropharyngeal and esophageal candidiasis. In the 1980s, the incidence of oropharyngeal candidiasis increased fivefold, in association with the spread of HIV infections.[25] Although HIV infection remains a risk factor for candidiasis, the introduction of highly active antiretroviral therapy precipitated a decline in the incidence of both infections by 50% to 60%.[26]

Oropharyngeal candidiasis remains the most common opportunistic infection in patients with HIV. Ninety percent of HIV-positive patients develop oropharyngeal candidiasis.[27] For 70% of these patients, it is the first manifestation of HIV infection.[28] The incidence of oropharyngeal infection increases with decreasing CD4+ lymphocyte counts, with an incidence of 60% in patients with a CD4+ count less than 200 cells/mm³ (200×10^6/L).

Although esophageal candidiasis represents the first manifestation of HIV infection in less than 10% of cases, it is the most common acquired immunodeficiency syndrome (AIDS)–defining disease.[29] As with oropharyngeal candidiasis, the incidence of esophageal candidiasis increases with decreasing CD4+ counts.

Candida albicans accounts for 80% of cases of OPC and esophageal candidiasis. Over the last 20 years, an increasing incidence of *C. albicans* resistance has been accompanied by an increased incidence of nonalbicans species infections, including *Candida glabrata, Candida tropicalis, Candida krusei,* and *Candida parapsilosis.* In patients with cancer, nonalbicans *Candida* species account for almost half of all cases.[27]

PATHOPHYSIOLOGY

● Similar to VVC, the development of OPC occurs when the normal environment is altered. *Candida* organisms frequently colonize the oropharynx and mucous membranes. These organisms do not become pathogenic until the environmental balance is disturbed. This occurs in the setting of broad-spectrum antibiotic use, tissue damage (due to chemotherapy, catheter tubing, trauma), or immune deficiency.

RISK FACTORS

Risk factors for OPC can be found in Table 83–4.

Table 83–4	
Risk Factors for Oropharyngeal and Esophageal Candidiasis	
Factor	**Proposed Mechanism**
Extremes of age	Immature immunity in infants and reduced immunity in the elderly
Impaired mucosal integrity	Breaks in the protective barrier allows fungal invasion; often due to radiation, surgery, or mucositis
Dentures	Adherence of fungus to dentures, along with reduced salivary flow under dentures; ill-fitting dentures may impair mucosal integrity
Xerostomia	Reduced cleansing and defense factors of saliva
Use of antibiotics	Altered flora of mucosa allowing fungal overgrowth
Use of steroids	Suppression of immunity
Use of immunosuppressants	Suppression of immunity
HIV infection	Decreased CD4 T lymphocytes
Diabetes mellitus	Elevated glucose levels and defense factors in saliva
Nutritional deficiencies	Altered defense mechanisms, impaired mucosal integrity, or enhanced pathogenic potential of fungus

CLINICAL PRESENTATION AND DIAGNOSIS

● See text boxes for clinical presentation and diagnosis of OPC and esophageal candidiasis.

TREATMENT

● Along with selecting an effective treatment, selection of an appropriate antifungal agent requires consideration of

---

Clinical Presentation and Diagnosis of OPC

OPC is often a presumptive diagnosis based on signs and symptoms, along with the resolution of them after treatment with antifungal agents.

Symptoms

- Sore, painful mouth and tongue
- Burning tongue
- Dysphagia
- Metallic taste

Signs

Signs vary depending on the type of oropharyngeal candidiasis.

- Diffuse erythema on the surface of buccal mucosa, throat, tongue, and gums
- White patches on tongue, gums, or buccal mucosa; removal of patches reveals erythematous and bloody tissue; ability to remove patches distinguishes OPC from oral hairy leukoplakia
- Angular cheilitis presents with small cracking lesions, erythema, and soreness at the corners of the mouth; associated with vitamin and iron deficiency
- Denture stomatitis presents with flat, red lesions on mucosa beneath dentures; signs of chronic erythema and edema on mucosa
- Hyperplastic OPC presents with discrete, transparent raised lesions on the inner mucosa of the cheek; typically found in men who smoke
- Pseudomembranous OPC presents with yellow-white plaques that may be small and discrete or confluent; most common form found in HIV patients

Diagnostic Testing

Diagnosis is primarily based on identification of characteristic lesions. Although rarely necessary, diagnostic testing is possible if a definitive diagnosis is required.

- Cytology, although presence of *Candida* is not diagnostic since colonization is common
- Culture to identify species of yeast or presence of resistance
- Biopsy

Clinical Presentation and Diagnosis of Esophageal Candidiasis

Symptoms

- Fever
- Odynophagia
- Dysphagia
- Retrosternal pain

Signs

- Fever
- Hyperemic or edematous white plaques
- Ulceration of esophagus
- Increased mucosal friability
- Narrowing of lumen

Diagnostic Testing

Unlike OPC, diagnosis of esophageal candidiasis is not based solely on clinical presentation, instead requiring endoscopic visualization of lesions and culture confirmation. Due to the invasive nature of these procedures, most practitioners opt to treat the infection presumptively, reserving endoscopic evaluation for patients who fail therapy.

- Cytology and culture to identify species of yeast or presence of resistance
- Barium esophagogram
- Endoscopy revealing whitish plaques with progression to superficial ulceration of the esophageal mucosa
- Mucosal biopsy

---

location and severity of infection, medication adherence, potential drug interactions, concomitant medical conditions, and presence of sucrose or dextrose. Topical agents require frequent dosing and prolonged contact time with oral mucosa. Rough surfaces of tablets and troches may irritate sensitive mucosa. Patients with xerostomia may have inadequate saliva to dissolve troches. Topical agents containing sucrose or dextrose may increase the risk of caries or cause elevated blood sugar in patients with diabetes. Along with being expensive, oral azoles exhibit an increased risk of toxicity and drug interactions due to cytochrome P-450.

Because oropharyngeal and esophageal candidiasis are signs of immunocompromise, the immune status of the patient should be considered in the therapeutic care plan. For HIV-infected patients, this should also include an evaluation of the patient's antiretroviral therapy since fungal infections may represent deterioration in immune status.

❼ *For low-risk patients, topical agents are first-line therapy for oropharyngeal candidiasis, although systemic agents may be used for severe or unresponsive cases.* For patients with mild infections, nystatin suspension provides an inexpensive option for treatment of oropharyngeal candidiasis, although it must be dosed 4 times per day. In small children, 0.5 to 1 mL of the suspension can be squirted into the cheeks using an oral syringe, whereas older children and adults can receive 5 mL per dose. Despite the convenience of once-daily dosing, fluconazole is typically reserved for more severe or unresponsive cases. For patients with severe OPC, oral fluconazole remains the agent of choice. Oral fluconazole administered for 2 weeks exhibits a mycological cure rate of 48% and a clinical cure rate of 84% in HIV patients.[30] Response occurs within 5 days in patients receiving 100 to 200 mg daily.[14] Doses as low as 50 mg are effective, but clinical response is slow and potentially leads to resistance. Two weeks of oral itraconazole solution is as effective as fluconazole but is less well tolerated. Due to variable absorption, risk of toxicity, and potential for drug interactions, ketoconazole and itraconazole capsules are considered second-line alternatives to fluconazole.

For non–HIV-infected patients who have suppressed immune systems, the practitioner must consider the patient's risk of dissemination. Patients with cell-mediated immune deficiency but near-normal granulocyte function, such as patients with diabetes, solid organ transplant, or solid tumors, are at low risk for dissemination. The risk of dissemination is higher for patients who develop neutropenia, including patients with leukemia or bone marrow transplant. These patients should be treated aggressively to prevent invasive fungal infection.

For the treatment of OPC in HIV-infected individuals, initial episodes can be adequately controlled with topical agents, such as clotrimazole troches, so long as symptoms are not severe and no esophageal involvement is suspected.[26] Topical nystatin is the least effective agent, especially in severely immunocompromised patients.[31] Topical clotrimazole appears to be the most effective topical antifungal, exhibiting clinical responses equivalent to oral fluconazole and itraconazole solution, but mycological cure rates are lower and relapse rates higher with clotrimazole.[29]

⑧ *Representing a severe extension of oropharyngeal candidiasis, esophageal candidiasis requires systemic antifungal therapy.* The significant morbidity associated with esophageal candidiasis warrants aggressive treatment. The diagnosis of esophageal candidiasis requires endoscopic evaluation, but rather than employing invasive procedures, patients can be treated with an appropriate course of antifungal based on clinical presentation. If patients do not respond, endoscopy should be considered.

Two to 3 weeks of fluconazole or itraconazole solution are highly effective and demonstrate similar clinical response rates.[32] Oral doses of 100 to 200 mg are effective in immunocompetent patients, but doses up to 400 mg are recommended for immunocompromised patients. Due to variable absorption, ketoconazole and itraconazole capsules should be considered second-line therapy. In severe cases, oral azoles may prove ineffective, warranting the use of IV amphotericin B for 10 days. Although echinocandins, voriconazole, and posaconazole are effective in treatment of esophageal candidiasis, experience remains limited and

Patient Encounter 2

An 89-year-old woman presents to the dental clinic complaining that her dentures must not be fitting correctly because "my mouth is very sore." She comments that she noticed "these white spots" on her gums that "make everything taste funny." On initial examination, she has white patches on her tongue, gums, and buccal mucosa. These patches are easily removed, revealing erythematous tissue underneath.

Her medical record shows that she recently completed a course of azithromycin and steroids for bronchitis.

What additional information do you need to know before creating a treatment plan for this patient?

What underlying medical conditions might make her susceptible to fungal infections?

How is the treatment care plan altered if the patient has a history of frequent and severe OPC? If the patient is HIV-positive? If the patient is neutropenic?

their role has yet to be established, particularly in light of less expensive alternatives

Fluconazole-Resistant Infections

Twenty percent of HIV-infected patients develop fluconazole-resistant *Candida albicans* isolates after repeated exposure to fluconazole.[33] To treat fluconazole-resistant oropharyngeal candidiasis, daily itraconazole for 2 to 4 weeks may be used. Oral itraconazole solution exhibits a mycological cure rate of 88% and a clinical cure rate of 97% in immunocompromised patients.[34] Fluconazole-resistant esophageal candidiasis should be treated with IV amphotericin B or caspofungin.

Recurrent Infections

If immunocompromised patients experience frequent or severe recurrences, particularly of esophageal candidiasis, chronic maintenance therapy with fluconazole 100 to 200 mg daily should be considered. In patients with infrequent or mild cases, secondary prophylaxis is not recommended. The rationale for not giving prophylaxis includes availability of effective treatments for acute episodes, risk of developing resistant organisms, potential for drug interactions, and the cost of therapy.

OUTCOME EVALUATION

- Patients should notice symptomatic relief within 2 to 3 days of initiating therapy. Complete resolution typically occurs within 7 to 10 days. The entire course of therapy should be continued even if symptoms have resolved. If the condition does not resolve or worsens, the patient should be referred to a specialist for aggressive therapy.

Patient Care and Monitoring of OPC

1. Assess the patient's symptoms to determine whether symptoms are consistent with oropharyngeal or esophageal candidiasis. All patients with suspected oropharyngeal or esophageal candidiasis should be referred to a practitioner or physician since no antifungal products appropriate for oral use are available without a prescription.

2. Review any available diagnostic data, including cultures.

3. Obtain a thorough history of prescription, nonprescription, and natural drug product use. Is the patient taking any medications that may contribute to candidiasis? Is the patient taking any medications that may interfere with treatment?

4. If the patient has had oropharyngeal or esophageal candidiasis previously, determine what treatments were helpful to the patient in the past.

5. If the patient has had oropharyngeal or esophageal candidiasis previously, determine whether the patient has risk factors for recurrent infection.

6. Develop a plan to assess effectiveness of antifungal therapy.

7. Determine whether long-term suppressive therapy is necessary.

8. Evaluate the patient for the presence of adverse drug reactions, drug allergies, or drug interactions.

9. Stress the importance of adherence with the antifungal regimen.

10. Provide patient education pertaining to oropharyngeal or esophageal candidiasis and antifungal therapy.

    - Causes of oropharyngeal or esophageal candidiasis
    - Risk factors for developing candidiasis
    - How to administer topical antifungal agents, including cleaning the oral cavity prior to administration, shaking suspensions prior to use, administering after meals, how to dissolve troches, and how to swish suspensions
    - Importance of completing the course of therapy
    - Potential adverse effects that may occur with antifungal therapy
    - Medications that may interact with antifungal therapy
    - Warning signs to report to a physician (recurrent or difficult-to-cure infections, or worsening symptoms)

- Short courses of oral azoles are associated with gastrointestinal upset, whereas courses lasting longer than 7 to 10 days are associated with increased risk of hepatotoxicity. In patients receiving prolonged therapy lasting more than 3 weeks, periodic monitoring of liver function tests should be considered.

- Immunocompetent patients generally do not require reassessment after treatment. Patients with neutropenia exhibit an increased risk of dissemination of infection and therefore should be monitored for signs of systemic fungal infection. Due to an increased risk of recurrence, HIV-positive patients should routinely be evaluated for recurrence at each visit.

MYCOTIC INFECTIONS OF THE SKIN, HAIR, AND NAILS

Tinea infections are superficial fungal infections in which the pathogen remains within the keratinous layers of the skin or nails (Table 83–5). Typically these infections are named for the affected body part, such as tinea pedis (feet), tinea cruris (groin), and tinea corporis (body). Tinea infections are commonly referred to as ringworm due to the characteristic circular lesions. In actuality, tinea lesions can vary from rings to scales and single or multiple lesions.

EPIDEMIOLOGY AND ETIOLOGY

Tinea infections are second only to acne in frequency of reported skin disease.[35] The common tinea infections are tinea pedis, tinea corporis, and tinea cruris. Tinea pedis, the most prevalent cutaneous fungal infection, afflicts more than 25 million people annually in the United States.

Fungal skin infections are primarily caused by dermatophytes such as *Trichophyton*, *Microsporum*, and *Epidermophyton*. *Trichophyton rubrum* accounts for more than 75% of all cases in the United States.[36] To a lesser extent, *Candida* and other fungal species cause skin infections. With tinea infections, the causative dermatophyte typically

Clinical Presentation and Diagnosis of Mycotic Infections

Symptoms and Signs (see Table 83–5)

Diagnostic Testing

- KOH prep
- Wood's ultraviolet lamp
- Microscopic examination
- Fungal cultures
- Periodic acid-Schiff (PAS) staining of nail

Treatment of Skin and Hair Infections

The goals of treatment include:

- Providing symptomatic relief
- Resolution of infection
- Preventing spread of infection

Table 83–5

Signs, Symptoms, and Risk Factors of Superficial Fungal Infections

Infection	Symptoms, Signs, and Risk Factors
Tinea pedis	• Involves plantar surface and interdigital spaces of foot • Interdigital infections produce itching; presents as fissures, scaling, or macerated skin; can occur between any toes but most often between fourth and fifth toes; may cause foul smell due to superinfection with *Pseudomonas* or diphtheroids • Hyperkeratotic infections present with slivery white scales on a thickened, red base; usually covers entire foot; occasionally may also affect hand • Vesiculobullous tinea pedis presents as pustules or vesicles on soles of feet; associated with maceration, itching, and thickening of sole; may cause lymphangitis and cellulitis; most common during summer months • Ulcerative tinea pedis presents as macerated, denuded, and weeping ulcers on soles; may produce extreme pain and erosion of interdigital spaces; typically complicated by opportunistic gram-negative infections • Risk factors include occlusive footwear, foot trauma, and use of public showers
Tinea manuum	• Infection of the interdigital and palmar surfaces • Presents as white scales in palmar folds; may also develop scales on remainder of palm; may present as singular plaque • More commonly affecting only one hand • Presents with hyperkeratotic skin
Tinea cruris	• Presents with follicular papules and pustules on the medial thigh and inguinal folds • Ringed lesions may extend from inguinal fold over adjacent inner thigh • Lesions usually spare the penis and scrotum, in contrast to candidiasis • Frequency increases during summer • Primarily develops in young men • Risk factors include tight-fitting clothing, excessive sweating, poor hygiene, increased humidity and temperatures • Commonly referred to as "jock itch"
Tinea corporis	• Presents with circular, scaly patch with enlarged border • Lesions may have red papules or plaque in center that clears, leaving hypopigmentation or hyperpigmentation • Itching may be present • Commonly referred to as ringworm of the body • Risk factors include animal to human contact
Tinea versicolor	• Characterized by skin depigmentation but can present as hyperpigmentation, particularly in dark-skinned patients • Typically occurs in areas with sebaceous glands, including neck, trunk, and arms • Depigmentation may persist for years • Primarily develops in young and middle-aged adults • Risk factors include application of oil, greasy skin, high ambient temperature, high relative humidity, tight-fitting clothing, immunodeficiency, malnutrition, hereditary predisposition
Tinea barbae	• Infection of beard area
Tinea capitis	• Infection of the head and scalp • May be asymptomatic initially, then progresses to inflammatory alopecia • "Black dot" alopecia may develop due to breakage of hair at the root • May form kerions (nodular swellings) • Scaling or favus may develop on scalp • Cervical lymphadenopathy is common • Primarily found in infants, children, and young adolescents, often in African-American and Hispanic populations • Can be spread from person to person or animal to person
Onychomycosis (tinea unguium)	• Infection of nail plate and bed • Nail becomes opaque, thick, rough, yellow or brownish, and friable; nail may separate from bed • Toenails affected more frequently than fingernails • Prevalence increases with advanced age

invades the stratum corneum without penetration into the living tissues, leading to a localized infection.

PATHOPHYSIOLOGY

The primary mode of transmission of tinea infections is direct contact with other persons or surface reservoirs. Upon contact, the dermatophytes attach to the keratinized cells, leading to thickening of the cells. Although infection remains localized, bacterial superinfections may develop.

The pathophysiology of onychomycosis depends on the clinical type. With the most common form of onychomycosis, distal lateral subungual, the fungus spreads from the plantar skin. The fungus invades the underside of the nail through the distal lateral nail bed, leading to inflammation of the area. In cases of white superficial onychomycosis, the fungus invades the surface of the nail plate directly. With white superficial onychomycosis, the nail bed and hyponychium are infected secondarily. Proximal subungual onychomycosis infections begin in the cuticle and the proximal nail fold, then penetrate the dorsum of the nail plate.

RISK FACTORS

- Prolonged exposure to sweaty clothing
- Excessive skin folds
- Sedentary lifestyle
- Warm, humid climate
- Use of public pools
- Walking barefoot in public areas
- Skin trauma
- Poor nutrition
- Diabetes mellitus
- Immunocompromise
- Impaired circulation

TREATMENT

Nonpharmacologic Therapy

- Because fungi thrive in warm, moist environments, the practitioner should encourage patients to wear loose-fitting clothing and socks, preferably garments made of cotton or other fabrics that wick moisture away from the body. Avoid clothing made with synthetic fibers or wool.
- Clean the infected area daily with soap and water.
- The infected area should be dried completely prior to dressing, paying particular attention to skin folds.
- To allow circulation of air, the infected area should not be bandaged.
- For foot infections, cotton socks are recommended, although these should be changed two to three times a day to reduce moisture.

Patient Encounter 3

A mother presents to the clinic with her 15-year-old daughter. The mother explains that her daughter's feet "look awful—they are red and raw looking with cracks between her toes." The daughter adds that "it is starting to get embarrassing to take off my running shoes in the locker room after track practice."

What information is suggestive of tinea pedis?

What risk factors are present for tinea pedis?

What nonpharmacologic approaches can be recommended to prevent recurrence?

- To prevent spread, towels, clothing, and footwear should not be shared with other persons.
- Wear protective footwear in public showers and pool areas.

Pharmacologic Therapy of Tinea Infections

⑨ *Since dermatophyte hyphae seldom penetrate into the living layers of the skin, instead remaining in the stratum corneum, most infections can be treated with topical antifungals. Infections covering large areas of the body or infections involving nails or hair may require systemic therapy.* Treatment is typically initiated based on symptoms, rather than on microscopic evaluation. For infections accompanied by inflammation, combination therapy with a topical steroid can be considered (Tables 83–6 and 83–7). Patients with chronic infections or infections that do not respond to topical therapy are also candidates for systemic therapy (Table 83–8).

For the treatment of tinea pedia, corporis, and cruris, topical agents can be utilized unless the infection is refractory. Typically, tinea pedis requires treatment one to two times daily for 4 weeks, whereas tinea corporis and tinea cruris require treatment one to two times daily for 2 weeks. When applying treatment, the medication should be applied at least 1 in beyond the affected area. Treatment of any infection should continue at least 1 week after resolution of symptoms. Many practitioners opt to initiate therapy with nonprescription clotrimazole, tolnaftate, miconazole, or terbinafine, reserving prescription topical agents, such as naftifine, ciclopirox, and butenafine, for second-line therapy or refractory cases. For refractory cases or widespread lesions, systemic therapy can be prescribed.

When recommending topical therapy, the selection of vehicle is based on the type of lesion and location of the infection. Solutions and lotions are recommended for hairy areas and oozing lesions, whereas creams and ointments should be avoided in these area. Creams are better for moderately scaling and nonoozing lesions. For hyperkeratotic lesions, ointments can be considered. The selected formulation should be applied to the affected area

Table 83–6

Available Topical Antifungal Agents

Medication	Rx/OTC	Cream/Ointment	Gel	Lotion	Spray/Solution	Powder
Butenafine	OTC	X				
Ciclopirox	Rx	X		X	Lacquer & shampoo	
Clotrimazole	OTC	X		X	X	X
Econazole	Rx	X				
Haloprogin	Rx	X			X	
Ketoconazole	Rx/OTC	X			Shampoo	
Miconazole	OTC	X		X	X	X
Naftifine	Rx	X	X			
Nystatin	Rx	X		X		X
Oxiconazole	Rx	X		X		
Sertaconazole	Rx	X				
Sulconazole	Rx	X				
Terbinafine	OTC	X	X		X	
Tolnaftate	OTC	X			X	

Table 83–7

Dosing of Topical Agents for Tinea Infections

Agents	Topical Dosing Frequency
Butenafine	Once daily
Ciclopirox	Twice daily; at bedtime (lacquer)
Clotrimazole	Twice daily
Econazole	Once daily
Haloprogin	Twice daily
Ketoconazole	Once daily
Miconazole	Twice daily
Naftifine	Once daily (cream); twice daily (gel)
Oxiconazole	Twice daily
Sertaconazole	Twice daily
Sulconazole	Twice daily
Terbinafine	Twice daily
Tolnaftate	2–3 times daily

Table 83–8

Dosing of Systemic Therapy for Tinea Infections

Medication	Adult Dosing	Pediatric Dosing
Fluconazole	150 mg/week	6 mg/kg/week
Griseofulvin	0.5–1 g/day	10–20 mg/kg/day
Itraconazole	200 mg twice daily	Not studied
Ketoconazole	200–400 mg/day	3.3–6.6 mg/kg/day
Terbinafine	250 mg/day	Less than 25 kg: 125 mg/day; 25–35 kg: 187.5 mg/day; more than 35 mg: 250 mg/day

after it is cleaned and dried. The medication should be rubbed into the infected area for improved penetration. Because most patients do not rub in sprays and powders, penetration of the epidermis is minimal, making them less effective than other formulations. Sprays and powders should be considered as adjuvant therapy with a cream or lotion or as prophylactic therapy to prevent recurrence (Table 83–7).

Due to the severity of infection and inflammation, tinea capitis does not adequately respond to topical agents. Oral agents for 6 to 8 weeks are recommended for eradication of tinea capitis. Griseofulvin has long been considered the treatment of choice due to its ability to achieve high levels within the stratum corneum. Itraconazole has also demonstrated effectiveness. Due to its lipophilicity, itraconazole achieves high levels in the skin. These levels are maintained for 4 weeks after medication is discontinued. Some practitioners recommend adjunct therapy with the oral agent to decrease dissemination, including ketoconazole or selenium sulfide shampoos.

Treatment of Onychomycosis

Onychomycosis is a chronic infection that rarely remits spontaneously. Adequate treatment is essential to prevent spread to other sites, secondary bacterial infections, cellulitis, or gangrene. ❿ *Due to the chronic nature and impenetrability of nails, topical agents have low efficacy rates for treating onychomycosis.* Oral agents that can penetrate the nail matrix and nail base, such as itraconazole and terbinafine, are more effective than ciclopirox lacquer. Itraconazole and terbinafine demonstrate mycological cure rates of 62%[37] and 76%,[38] respectively, whereas ciclopirox has a cure rate of 29% to 36%.[39]

Itraconazole can be administered continuously (200 mg orally daily) or as pulse therapy (200 mg orally twice daily for 1 week per month). Terbinafine is administered orally 250 mg per day as continuous therapy. Whether administered continuously or as pulse therapy, oral treatment for toenail infections should continue for at least 3 months, whereas treatment for fingernail infections should continue for at least 2 months. Terbinafine is an inhibitor of CYP450 2D6 isozyme. When administered with other medications metabolized via this isozyme, the other medication should be started at a low dose if it has a narrow therapeutic range. Griseofulvin is also effective for the treatment of onychomycosis, but therapy must be continued for 4 months for fingernail infections or 6 months for toenail infections. For patients with liver disease or who are unable to use oral agents, ciclopirox nail lacquer remains a reasonable alternative, although it requires 48 weeks of therapy.

The FDA has released warnings pertaining to itraconazole and terbinafine as there is a small but real risk of developing congestive heart failure with itraconazole therapy due to its negative inotropic effects. Itraconazole should not be administered to patients with ventricular dysfunction such as congestive heart failure. The FDA also released warnings that itraconazole and terbinafine are associated with serious hepatic toxicity, including liver failure and death. Liver failure associated with these medications has occurred in patients with no preexisting living disease or serious underlying medical conditions. Treatment with itraconazole or terbinafine for prolonged periods requires laboratory monitoring of liver function tests before initiation of therapy and at monthly intervals.

Cultural Awareness When Treating Mycotic Infections

Awareness of cultural beliefs related to feet and hands is essential when treating patients with fungal infections. In Arab countries, showing the bottom of the foot is a grave insult. The foot is considered the dirtiest part of the body. As such, patients from these countries may be hesitant to show their feet to the practitioner. In other countries, the open palm "high five" gesture is considered insulting. When treating patients with infections on the hand, the practitioner should refrain from making this gesture while discussing the patient's hand infection.

OUTCOME EVALUATION

● For infections of the skin, patients should notice relief of symptoms, including pruritus, scales, and inflammation, within 1 to 2 weeks. Therapy should be continued at least 1 week after complete resolution of symptoms. If the

Patient Care and Monitoring of Mycotic Infections

1. Assess the patient's symptoms to determine whether self-treatment with OTC antifungal therapy is appropriate or whether the patient should be evaluated by a practitioner. Exclusions for self-treatment include infection of nails or hair, unsuccessful initial treatment, worsening condition, signs of secondary bacterial or systemic infection, large infected areas, or chronic medical conditions such as diabetes, immunosuppression, or impaired circulation.

2. Review any available diagnostic data, including cultures and KOH preps.

3. Obtain a thorough history of prescription, nonprescription, and natural drug product use.

4. If the patient has had a mycotic infection previously, determine what treatments were helpful to the patient in the past.

5. Educate the patient on lifestyle modifications that will prevent recurrence, including keeping the area dry, wearing shower shoes, washing clothing in hot water, using drying powders, avoiding sharing towels or clothing, and wearing loose-fitting clothing.

6. Develop a plan to assess effectiveness of antifungal therapy.

7. Determine whether long-term prophylactic therapy is necessary to prevent recurrence.

8. Evaluate the patient for the presence of adverse drug reactions, drug allergies, and drug interactions.

9. Stress the importance of adherence with the antifungal regimen.

10. Provide the patient education pertaining to mycotic infections and antifungal therapy.
    - Causes of mycotic infections of the skin, hair, or nails
    - Different types of OTC antifungal products, such as creams, sprays, shampoos, ointments, gel, lotions, solutions, and powders
    - How to apply various OTC antifungal products
    - How long therapy should be continued
    - How to avoid spread of infection
    - How to avoid recurrent infection
    - Potential adverse effects that may occur with antifungal therapy
    - Dietary modifications that are necessary with oral agents
    - Medications that may interact with antifungal therapy, particularly with oral agents used for nail infections
    - Warning signs to report to a physician (recurrent or difficult-to-cure infections, infections with malodorous discharge or bleeding)

condition worsens or does not resolve within 4 weeks, the patient should be treated with oral therapy.

For onychomycosis, relief of symptoms is slow. The infected nail will need months to grow out. The practitioner should advise the patient not to become frustrated by the slow resolution. Despite the slow progress, the antifungal agent is curing the infection. The practitioner should also advise the patient that even after the infection is cured, the nail may not look "normal."

Abbreviations Introduced in This Chapter

AIDS   Acquired immunodeficiency syndrome
CDC   Centers for Disease Control and Prevention
HIV   Human immunodeficiency virus
KOH   Potassium hydroxide
OPC   Oropharyngeal candidiasis
OTC   Over the counter
PAS   Periodic acid-Schiff test
VVC   Vulvovaginal candidiasis

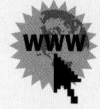
Self-assessment questions and answers are available at *http://mhpharmacotherapy.com/ pp.html.*

REFERENCES

1. Cleveland A. Vaginitis: finding the cause prevents treatment failure. Cleve Clin J Med 2000;67:634–646.
2. Foxman B, Barlow R, D'Arcy H, et al. Candida vaginitis: self-reported incidence and associated costs. Sex Transm Dis 2000;27:230–235.
3. Center for Disease Control and Prevention. Sexually transmitted diseases treatment guidelines, 2010 [online]. [cited 2011 Oct 10]. Available from: *http://www.cdc.gov/mmwr/preview/mmwrhtml/rr5912a1.htm.*
4. Ozcan SK, Budak F, Yucesoy G, Susever S, Willke A. Prevalence, susceptibility profile and proteinase production of yeasts causing vulvovaginitis in Turkish women. APMIS 2006;114:139–145.
5. Richter SS, Galask RP, Messer SA, et al. Antifungal susceptibilities of Candida species causing vulvovaginitis and epidemiology of recurrent cases. J Clin Microbiol 2005;43:2155–2162.
6. Reid G, Charbonneau D, Erb J, et al. Oral use *of Lactobacillus rhamnosus* GR-1 and *L. fermentum* RC-14 significantly alters vaginal flora: randomized, placebo-controlled trial in 64 healthy women. FEMS Immun Med Microbiol 2003;35:131–134.
7. Shalev E, Battino S. Weiner E, et al. Ingestion of yogurt containing Lactobacillus acidophilus compared with pasteurized yogurt as prophylaxis for recurrent candidal vaginitis and bacterial vaginosis. Arch Fam Med 1996;5:593–596.
8. Pirotta M, Chondros, P, Grover S, et al. Effect of lactobacillus in preventing post-antibiotic vulvovaginal candidiasis: a randomized controlled trial. BMJ 2004;329:548.
9. Ferris DG, Nyirjesy P, Sobel JD, et al. Over-the-counter antifungal drug misuse associated with patient-diagnosed vulvovaginal candidiasis. Obstet Gynecol 2002;99:419–425.
10. Edelman DA, Grant S. One-day therapy for vaginal candidiasis a review. J Reprod Med 1999;44:543–547.
11. American Society of Health-System Pharmacists. AHFS drug information, 2006.
12. Janssen Pharmaceutical. Nizoral® package insert. Titusville, NJ: Janssen Pharmaceutical; 1997.
13. Sobel JD, Wiesenfeld HC, Martens M, et al. Maintenance fluconazole therapy for recurrent vulvovaginal candidiasis. N Engl J Med 2004;351:876–883.
14. Vazquez JA, Sobel JD. Mucosal candidiasis. Infect Dis Clin N Am 2002;16:793–820.
15. Ringdahl EN. Treatment of recurrent vulvovaginal candidiasis. Am Fam Physician 2000;61:3306–3312, 3317.
16. Ray D, Goswami R, Dadhwal V, et al. Prolonged (3-month) mycological cure rate after boric acid suppositories in diabetic women with vulvovaginal candidiasis. J Infection 2007;55:374–377.
17. Mastroiacovo P, Mazzone T, Botto L, et al. Prospective assessment of pregnancy outcomes after first-trimester exposure to fluconazole. Am J Obstet Gynecol 1996;175:1645–1650.
18. Jick SS. Pregnancy outcomes after maternal exposure to fluconazole. Pharmacotherapy 1999;19:221–222.
19. Pursley TJ, Blomquist IK, Abraham J, et al. Fluconazole-induced congenital anomalies in three infants. Clin Infect Dis 1996;22:336–340.
20. World Health Organization Website. Female genital mutilation [online]. [cited 2011 Oct 10]. Available from: *http://www.who/int/ mediacentre/factsheets/fs241/en/print.html.*
21. Braddy CM, Files JA. Female genital mutilation: cultural awareness and clinical considerations. J Midwifery Womens Health 2007;52:159–163.
22. Kossioni A. The prevalence of denture stomatitis and its predisposing conditions in an older Greek population. Gerodontology 2011;28:85–90.
23. Kaliner M, Amin A, Gehling R, et al. Impact of inhaled corticosteroid-induced oropharyngeal adverse effects on treatment patterns and costs in asthmatic patients: results from a Delphi panel. P&T 2005;30:573–589.
24. Kanda N, Yasuba H, Takahashi T, et al. Prevalence of esophageal candidiasis among patients treated with inhaled fluticasone propionate. Am J Gastroenterol 2003;98:2146–2148.
25. Fotos PG, Lilly JP. Clinical management of oral and perioral candidosis. Dermatol Clin 1996;14:273–280.
26. Powderly WG, Mayer KH, Perfect JR. Diagnosis and treatment of oropharyngeal candidiasis in patients infected with HIV: a critical reassessment. AIDS Res Hum Retroviruses 1999;15:1405–1412.
27. Leigh JE, Shetty K, Fidel P. Oral opportunistic infections in HIV-positive individuals: review and role of mucosal immunity. AIDS Patient Care STDs 2004;18:443–456.
28. Minamoto GY, Rosenberg AS. Fungal infection in patients with acquired immunodeficiency syndrome. Med Clin North Am 1997;81:381-409.
29. Buchacz K, Baker RK, Palella FJ, et al. AIDS-defining opportunistic illnesses in US patients, 1994-2007: a cohort study. AIDS 2010;24:1549–1559.
30. Hay RJ. Overview of studies of fluconazole in oropharyngeal candidiasis. Rev Infect Dis 1990;12:S334–S337.
31. Epstein JB, Polsky B. Oropharyngeal candidiasis: a review of its clinical spectrum and clinical therapies. Clin Ther 1998;20:40–57.
32. Dewit S, Urbain D, Rahir F, et al. Efficacy of oral fluconazole in the treatment of AIDS-associated esophageal candidiasis. Eur J Clin Microbiol Infect Dis 1991;10:503–505.
33. Ruhnke M, Eigler A, Tennagen I, et al. Emergence of fluconazole-resistant strains of candida albicans in patients with recurrent oropharyngeal candidosis and human immunodeficiency virus infection. J Clin Microbiol 1994;32:2092–2098.
34. Saag MS, Fessel WJ, Kaufman CA, et al. Treatment of fluconazole-refractory oropharyngeal candidiasis with itraconazole oral solution in HIV-positive patients. AIDS Res Hum Retroviruses 1999;15:1413–1417.
35. Stern RS. The epidemiology of dermatophyte infections. In: Freedberg IM, Fitzpatrick TB, eds. Fitzpatrick's Dermatology in General Medicine. 5th ed. New York: McGraw-Hill; 1999:7–12.
36. Kemna ME, Elewski BE. A U.S. epidemiologic survey of superficial fungal diseases. J Am Acad Dermatol 1996;35:539–542.
37. Gupta AK, Maddin S, Arlette J, et al. Itraconazole pulse therapy is effective in dermatophyte onychomycosis of the toenail: a double-blind placebo-controlled study. J Dermatolog Treat 2000;11:33–37.
38. Evans EG, Sigurgeirsson B. Double-blind, randomized study of continuous terbinafine compared with intermittent itraconazole in treatment of toenail onychomycosis. The LION study group. BMJ 1999;318:1031–1035.
39. Dermik Laboratories. Penlac nail lacquer topical solution prescribing information. Berwyn, PA: Dermik Laboratories; 2000.

84 Invasive Fungal Infections

Russell E. Lewis

LEARNING OBJECTIVES

● **Upon completion of the chapter, the reader will be able to:**

1. Differentiate epidemiologic differences and host risk factors for acquisition of primary and opportunistic invasive fungal pathogens.

2. Recommend appropriate empiric or targeted antifungal therapy for the treatment of invasive fungal infections.

3. Describe the components of a monitoring plan to assess effectiveness and adverse effects of pharmacotherapy for invasive fungal infections.

4. Evaluate the role of antifungal prophylaxis in the prevention of opportunistic fungal pathogens.

KEY CONCEPTS

① The diagnosis of endemic fungal infections is often prompted by a patient history of prolonged infectious symptoms, travel or residence in an endemic area, and/or participation in activities that result in exposures to soil contaminated by endemic fungi.

② The approach to antifungal therapy in patients with endemic fungal infections is determined by the severity of clinical presentation, the patient's underlying immunosuppression, and potential toxicities and drug interactions associated with antifungal treatment.

③ Commensal or environmental fungi that are typically harmless can become invasive mycoses when the host immune defenses are impaired. Host immune suppression and risk for opportunistic mycoses can be broadly classified into three categories: (a) quantitative or qualitative deficits in neutrophil function, (b) deficits in cell-mediated immunity, and (c) disruption of integument and/or microbiologic barriers.

④ It is important to be familiar with the relative epidemiology and frequency of non-*albicans Candida* species in the institution or intensive care unit (ICU) before selecting empiric antifungal therapy for invasive candidiasis, as fluconazole is not recommended for the treatment of *C. glabrata* and *C. krusei* infections

⑤ If a patient is nonneutropenic, clinically stable (i.e., normotensive with relatively normal organ function), and has never received prior azole therapy, fluconazole 12 mg/kg/day loading dose followed by 6 mg/kg/day is still considered an appropriate first-line therapy for

invasive candidiasis in many centers until speciation of the *Candida* isolate is confirmed.

⑥ Clinical trials performed by the National Institute of Allergy and Infectious Diseases (NIAID) Mycoses Study Group demonstrated that 2 weeks of induction antifungal therapy with combination amphotericin B (0.7 mg/kg/day) plus flucytosine (100 mg/kg/day) achieved the highest clinical cure rates with reduced toxicity for cryptococcal meningitis.

⑦ Immunocompromised patients on fluconazole with progressive sinus or pulmonary disease by radiography should be considered to have a possible mold infection and receive empiric antifungal therapy directed (at minimum) against *Aspergillus species*.

Invasive fungal infection or invasive mycoses are general terms for diseases caused by invasion of living tissue by fungi. Unlike superficial mycoses (see Chap. 83), invasive mycoses invade internal organs, can disseminate throughout the body, and are associated with high rates of morbidity and mortality, particularly in the immunocompromised host. Invasive fungal infections are broadly categorized as either primary or opportunistic invasive mycoses. Primary invasive fungal infections are caused by fungal spores or conidia in the soil that, when disturbed, can become aerosolized and inhaled leading to infection, even in an immunocompetent patient. Because these fungi are often endemic to certain soil types and hence geographically restricted, primary invasive fungal pathogens are also known as endemic fungi. In the United States, three species (*Histoplasma capsulatum*, *Blastomyces dermatitidis*, and *Coccidioides immitis*) account

Table 84–1

Invasive Mycoses

Primary (Endemic) Invasive Fungi
Histoplasma capsulatum[a]
Coccidioides immitis[a]
Blastomyces dermatitidis[a]

Opportunistic Invasive Fungi
Yeast
  Candida species (*C. albicans, C. glabrata, C. parapsilosis,
    C. tropicalis, C. krusei,* and others)[a]
  Cryptococcus neoformans[a]
  Trichosporon spp. and others

Mold
Hyalohyphomycoses (nondematiaceous)
  Aspergillus fumigatus and other species[a]
  Fusarium solani and *Fusarium oxysporum*
  Mucorales (formally zygomycosis) (*Mucor, Absidia, Rhizopus,
    Cunninghamella,* and *Rhizomucor*)
  Penicillium
Phaeohyphomycoses (dematiaceous)
  Pseudallescheria boydii (*Scedosporium* spp.)
  Bipolaris
  Alternaria

Other
  Pneumocystis jiroveci (formerly *P. carinii*)[a]

[a]Most common.

for most of these infections (Table 84–1). In contrast, opportunistic fungal infections occur only in the setting of compromised host immune defenses and are caused by a wider spectrum of less virulent fungal species that are generally

incapable of causing infection in healthy patients (see Table 84–1). Hence, the spectrum, severity, and outcome of opportunistic fungal infections are heavily influenced by the degree, type, and severity of host immunosuppression. As a general rule, opportunistic fungal infections are difficult to diagnose, uniformly fatal if not treated early and aggressively, and associated with high rates of morbidity and mortality.

ENDEMIC MYCOSES

EPIDEMIOLOGY

Endemic mycoses are capable of infecting otherwise healthy individuals. In immunocompromised patients, endemic fungal infections often present with a more fulminant course (in the case of primary infections) or reactivate to cause life-threatening infection. Because initial symptoms of an endemic fungal infection are nonspecific and produce symptoms indistinguishable from other slowly progressing infections (e.g., tuberculosis), a careful patient history concerning travel and activities associated with potential exposure to soil contaminated with endemic fungi is essential for the diagnosis.

Two of the most common endemic fungal infections (histoplasmosis and North American blastomycosis) are found in overlapping regions in the eastern and central river basins of the United States (Fig. 84–1).[1] *Histoplasma capsulatum* var. *capsulatum*, the causative fungus of histoplasmosis, grows heavily in soil contaminated with bird or bat excreta, which serve to enhance sporulation of the fungus.[2] Activities

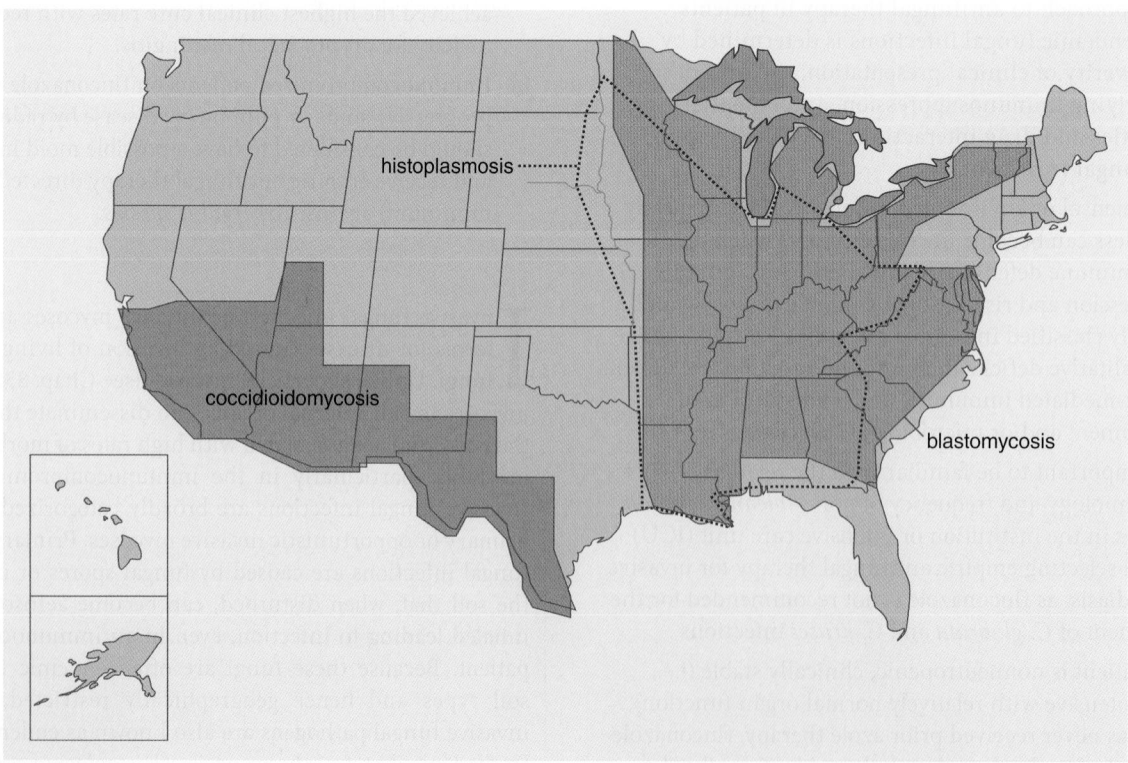

FIGURE 84–1. Geographic localization of primary (endemic) fungi in the United States.

in endemic regions that are classically associated with high exposures to *Histoplasma capsulatum* include cave exploration (spelunking), working in or demolishing chicken coops, or demolition of older buildings, woodcutting in forests with large bird roosts, or spreading avian excreta as fertilizer. For blastomycosis, decaying organic matter, warm humid conditions, and proximity to water or frequent rainfall seem to support growth of this fungus.[3] Occupational or recreational activities that disturb soil heavily contaminated with *Blastomyces dermatitidis* are a common feature in the social history of patients who develop blastomycosis. Coccidioidomycosis differs from histoplasmosis and blastomycosis, as the fungus is associated with arid to semiarid climates, hot summers, low altitude, alkaline soil, and sparse flora. Hence the fungus is found in the southwestern regions of the United States stretching from western Texas to southern California (see Fig. 84–1).[4] Epidemics of coccidioidomycosis have been reported in California following dust storms and earthquakes, including cycles of intense drought and rain, which favor the growth cycle of the fungus and enhance dispersion of its specialized spore forms, called arthroconidia.

PATHOPHYSIOLOGY

Endemic fungi share several key biologic and ecologic characteristics that contribute to their pathogenicity in humans. All endemic fungi exhibit temperature-dependent dimorphism, meaning they can propagate as either yeast (single cells that reproduce by budding into daughter cells) or molds (multicellular filamentous fungi that reproduce through production of conidia or spores). At environmental temperatures (25–30°C [77–86°F]), *H. capsulatum*, *B. dermatitidis*, and *C. immitis* grow in the mold form, producing 2- to 10-µm round- to oval-shaped (*Histoplasma* and *Blastomyces*) or barrel-shaped conidia (*Coccidioides*) that are dispersed throughout the environment and in air currents. At physiologic temperatures, the conidia germinate into yeast (*Histoplasma* and *Blastomyces*) or in specialized cell forms called spherules (*Coccidioides*) that are resistant to killing by resident alveolar macrophages and neutrophils in the host lung. Control of infection is mediated by the development of antigen-specific T-lymphocyte response that enhances macrophage fungicidal activity and formation of a granuloma to contain the fungus.[5] Not surprisingly, patients with T-cell–mediated immune deficiency (e.g., AIDS patients and transplant recipients) or suppressed cellular immunity due to drug therapy (e.g., chemotherapy, high-dose corticosteroids, or tumor necrosis-α blockers such as infliximab) are especially prone to severe reactivation of fungal disease.

The most common route of infection for endemic fungi is the respiratory tract, where conidia aerosolized from contaminated soil are inhaled into the lung. Once in the lung, conidia are phagocytosed but not destroyed by resident macrophages and neutrophils in the alveoli and bronchioles. Within 2 to 3 days, conidia germinate into facultative yeast resistant to phagocytosis and killing by macrophages and neutrophils

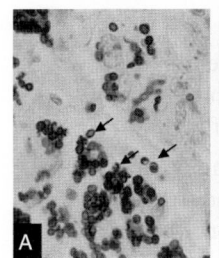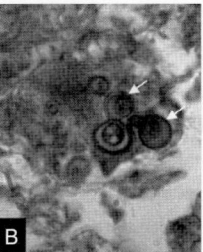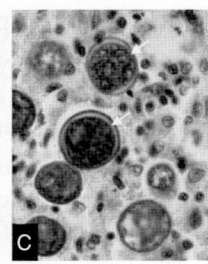

FIGURE 84–2. Histopathology of endemic mycoses in tissue. *A.* Histoplasmosis (yeast). *B.* Blastomycoses (broad-based budding yeast). *C.* Coccidioidomycoses (spherules with endospores).

(Fig. 84–2A and B). For *C. immitis*, germination of the arthroconidia results in the formation of a sac-like structure called a spherule filled with endospores (Fig. 84–2C). Spherules then rupture to release large numbers of endospores, which are the propagating form of the infection. Control of infection in the lungs is typically accomplished through formation of **granulomas**. However, in patients exposed to an overwhelming inoculum, or lower inocula in the setting of suppressed T-cell–mediated immunity, dissemination outside the lung to the skin and oral mucosa (especially blastomycoses), adrenal glands, bone, spleen, thyroid, GI tract, heart, and CNS is possible and uniformly fatal if left untreated.

CLINICAL PRESENTATION AND DIAGNOSIS

Histoplasmosis and coccidioidomycosis are frequently asymptomatic infections in immunocompetent patients or present as a self-limiting, influenza-like illness 1 to 3 weeks after inhalation of conidia. The clinical presentation of blastomycosis can range from asymptomatic infection, to acute or chronic pneumonia that develops 30 to 40 days after exposure, to full-blown disseminated disease.

Symptomatic endemic fungal infections often present as persistent pneumonia despite antibiotic therapy that is accompanied by fever, chills, cough, arthralgia, night sweats, and weight loss that is indistinguishable from other chronic infections such as pulmonary tuberculosis. ❶ *The diagnosis of endemic fungal infection is often prompted by a patient history of prolonged infectious symptoms, travel or residence in an endemic area, and/or participation in activities that result in exposures to soil contaminated by endemic fungi.*

Radiographs

- Chest radiographs often reveal either diffuse or nodular infiltrates in the lung, accompanied by enlargement of the hilar and/or mediastinal lymph nodes.

- Fulminant pneumonia may be seen with high inoculum exposures, resulting in diffuse lung infiltrates that precede to acute respiratory distress syndrome (ARDS) and respiratory failure.

Signs and Symptoms

- Rheumatologic symptoms such as severe arthritis, pericarditis, and erythema nodosum may be seen in 10% to 30% of patients with endemic fungi.[1,2,6]

- Dissemination outside the lung is common in patients with suppressed cellular immunity and frequently produces signs of progressing infection.

- Ulcerative oral and cutaneous lesions may also arise with any endemic fungal infections.

- Verrucose skin lesions on sun-exposed areas on the face are particularly suggestive of progressing blastomycosis and are frequently mistaken for cutaneous malignancy.[6]

- Dissemination of the fungi to bone marrow may result in anemia or thrombocytopenia.

- Hepatomegaly, splenomegaly, and adrenal insufficiency can also occur with dissemination of the endemic fungi to these internal organs.

- Seizures, meningeal signs, and hydrocephalus are common findings with dissemination of the infection to the CNS and portend an especially poor prognosis in the setting of disseminated coccidioidomycosis.

Definitive diagnosis of an endemic fungal infection requires growth of the fungus from body fluids or tissue, or evidence of cellular or tissue invasion in clinical samples by histopathology. However, cultures may only be positive in the setting of high inoculum exposures, pneumonia, or disseminated disease.[7] Serologic testing is helpful in the diagnosis and management of patients with histoplasmosis or coccidioidomycosis but lacks sufficient specificity for diagnoses of *B. dermatitidis*.[6] In general, a fourfold rise in antibody or complement fixation titers of *Histoplasma* or *Coccidioides* or any titer greater than 1:16 suggests active infection. However, many clinicians still consider titers as low as 1:8 as evidence

of active disease because undetectable titers may be present in one-third of all active infections.[4] Enzyme-linked immunosorbent assays (ELISAs) have been developed for detection of *Histoplasma* antigen in serum and urine, and a new radioimmunoassay directed against surface proteins of *B. dermatitidis* has shown promising sensitivity and specificity. Serial antigen testing can also provide a means for assessing response to antifungal therapy and early detection of relapse in patients with histoplasmosis or coccidioidomycosis.

The clinical presentation of blastomycosis covers a wide spectrum ranging from asymptomatic infections to flu-like illness resembling other upper respiratory tract illnesses; to infections resembling bacterial pneumonia with acute onset, high fever, lobar infiltrates, and cough; to subacute or chronic respiratory illness with complex symptoms resembling tuberculosis or lung cancer. At the other end of the spectrum, blastomycosis can also present with fulminant lung infections with high fever, diffuse infiltrates, and an ARDS-like presentation.[6] As mentioned previously, the skin is the most common site of dissemination, typically involving sunlight exposed body areas (i.e., nose, face, and arms) and mucous membranes.

TREATMENT

General Approach

❷ *The approach to antifungal therapy in patients with endemic fungal infections is determined by the severity of clinical presentation, the patient's underlying immunosuppression, and potential toxicities and drug interactions associated with antifungal treatment.* Immunocompetent patients with mild disease following exposure to *H. capsulatum* or *C. immitis* often experience a benign course of infection and rarely require antifungal therapy. Persons of Filipino or African descent have a higher risk for dissemination with *C. immitis*, and this may also be taken into consideration for more aggressive treatment.[4] Typically, patients are followed in the outpatient setting with serial antigen testing to confirm resolving infection. Patients without clinical improvement within the first month are typically treated with oral itraconazole for 6 to 12 weeks (Table 84–2).[1,4,6] Broader spectrum triazoles such as voriconazole and posaconazole appear to have good activity against endemic fungi; however, there are currently insufficient data to recommend their routine first-line use. Fluconazole (400 to 800 mg/day) is somewhat less effective than itraconazole (higher relapse rates) but has fewer GI adverse effects and drug interactions versus itraconazole.[1,4,6] Patients with progressive symptoms for longer than 2 weeks or titers greater than 1:8 of histoplasmosis or coccidioidomycosis antigen are candidates for immediate antifungal therapy.[1,4] Any patient with underlying immunosuppression should also receive immediate antifungal therapy. The following signs and symptoms are considered to be indicators of severe disease that require hospitalization and initial treatment with systemic amphotericin B (see Table 84–2).[1,4,6]

- Hypoxia indicated by a partial pressure of oxygen less than 80 mm Hg (10.6 kPa)

- Hypotension (systolic blood pressure less than 90 mm Hg)

Patient Encounter 1, Endemic Fungal Infection, Part 1

A 64-year-old woman from Indianapolis, Indiana, with a history of rheumatoid arthritis chronically treated with prednisone and methotrexate presents with a 4-week history of cough, fever, and night sweats and 9-kg weight loss. Approximately 6 weeks before this presentation, she was treated with infliximab for an arthritis flare. The patient complained of fatigue but was afebrile (37°C), with a normal resting respiratory rate. Laboratory studies revealed anemia (hemoglobin less than 8.7 g/dL [87 g/L or 5.4 mmol/L]). Computer tomography (CT) of the chest revealed several pulmonary nodules.

What are this patient's risk factors for developing an endemic fungal infection?

What is the most likely endemic fungal pathogen based on this patient's area of residence?

Table 84–2

Common Treatment Regimens for Endemic Fungal Infections

Mycosis	Recommended Treatment Regimens	Comments
Histoplasmosis		
Mild to moderate	Observation or itraconazole 200 mg 3 × daily for three days, then 1 to 2 × daily for 6–12 weeks	Fluconazole has a higher rate of relapse than itraconazole, but is better tolerated by many patients than itraconazole. Echinocandins are not clinically effective against endemic mycoses.
	Fluconazole 12 mg/kg/day PO for 6–12 weeks adjusted for renal function[a]	Lipid formulation may be more effective than conventional formulations, especially for CNS disease. Patients initially treated with amphotericin B–based regimens are transitioned to itraconazole or fluconazole once they are clinically stable. Corticosteroid therapy should be considered in hypoxic patients with acute pulmonary infection. Itraconazole is less effective for CNS infections.
Severe including CNS disease or immunocompromised host	Amphotericin B 0.7 mg/kg per day IV or liposomal AMB 3–5 mg/kg per day for 12 weeks or until clinically stable	
Blastomycosis		
Mild to moderate	itraconazole 200 mg 3 × daily for 3 days, then 1 to 2 × daily for 6–12 weeks OR Fluconazole 6–12 mg/kg/day PO adjusted for renal function[a]	Relapses are common in immunocompromised host Suppressive therapy with itraconazole 200 mg/day PO or fluconazole 800 mg PO daily for 6 months is common in immunocompromised patients.
Severe including CNS disease or immunocompromised host	Amphotericin B 0.7 mg/kg per day IV until patient is clinically stable, then Itraconazole (non-CNS) or fluconazole 12 mg/kg/day PO adjusted for renal function[a]	
Coccidioidomycosis		
Mild to moderate	Observation or itraconazole 200 mg 3 × daily for three days, then 1 to 2 × daily for 6–12 weeks OR Fluconazole 6–12 mg/kg/day PO daily adjusted for renal function[a]	Itraconazole demonstrated trend toward superiority over fluconazole in a randomized controlled trial for progressive, nonmeningeal coccidioidomycosis; however, fluconazole is better tolerated than itraconazole.
Diffuse pneumonia or disseminated infection	Amphotericin B 1–1.5 mg/kg per day with dose and frequency decreased as improvement occurs OR Lipid Amphotericin B formulations 3–5 mg/kg per day	Fluconazole 800–1,000 mg/day adjusted for renal function[a] is often recommended after initial AMB therapy for meningitis.

CNS, central nervous system; IV, intravenous; PO, oral.

[a]CrCl more than 50–90 mL/min (more than 0.83–1.50 mL/s), 100% of dose; CrCl 10–50 mL/min (0.17–0.83 mL/s), 50% of dose; CrCl less than 10 mL/min (less than 0.17 mL/s) 50%.

- Impaired mental status
- Anemia (hemoglobin less than 10 g/dL [100 g/L or 6.2 mmol/L])
- Leukopenia (less than $1 \times 10^3/mm^3$ [1×10^9/L])
- Elevated hepatic transaminases (greater than five times upper limit of normal) or bilirubin (greater than 2.5 times upper limit of normal)
- Coagulopathy
- More than 10% loss in body weight with onset of illness
- Evidence of dissemination, including cutaneous manifestations
- Meningitis

The treatment of blastomycosis is heavily dependent on the severity of clinical manifestations. Generally, patients with mild disease can be managed as outpatients with oral itraconazole.[6] Patients with evidence of severe pulmonary disease or dissemination require initial treatment in the hospital with amphotericin B–based regimens until they are clinically stable, whereupon they can complete a 6- to 12-month treatment course as outpatients with oral triazoles.[6] Methylprednisolone (0.5 to 1 mg/kg daily IV) during the first 1 to 2 weeks of antifungal therapy is recommended for patients who develop respiratory complications during initial treatment, including hypoxemia or significant respiratory distress.

PATIENT MONITORING

Response to antifungal therapy may be slow in patients with a prolonged history of infection or severe manifestations. However, gradual improvements in symptoms and reduction in fever are indicators of response to antifungal therapy. For histoplasmosis and coccidioidomycosis, decreasing antigen titers are also indicative of response to antifungal therapy.[1,4]

Antifungals used for the treatment of endemic mycoses can be associated with clinically significant drug interactions and toxicities, especially with the prolonged treatment courses that are often required in the management of endemic mycoses. Itraconazole is available as a capsule formulation and as a cyclodextrin-solubilized solution. The liquid formulation of itraconazole has several advantages over the capsule: It has a better oral bioavailability and does not require the low gastric pH that is required for dissolution and absorption of the capsule. However, the oral solution is somewhat dilute, has an unpalatable aftertaste (an issue when taking months of therapy), and has a much higher rate of GI intolerance. Therefore, the capsule formulation is often preferred provided patients are not on acid-suppression therapy (i.e., proton pump inhibitors, histamine antagonists, or antacids). Posaconazole is formulated as a micronized suspension that is best absorbed when taken with high-fat meals in divided doses up to 800 mg per day. Similar to the capsule formulation of itraconazole, the coadministration of posaconazole with acid-suppression therapy significantly reduces drug absorption, especially if the patient has poor appetite, nausea, or diarrhea. Absorption of voriconazole is not affected by gastric pH, but is generally administered 1 hour prior to or 2 hours after eating.

Drug interactions are an important concern in patients taking long-term triazole therapy. Itraconazole and voriconazole are substrates of the cytochrome P450 (CYP) 3A4 enzyme. Coadministration of itraconazole, voriconazole, and to lesser extent fluconazole and posaconazole, with inducers of this CYP 3A4 (e.g., rifampin, phenytoin, and phenobarbital) increases drug clearance resulting in ineffective plasma and tissue concentrations of the drug.[8–11] In general, coadministration of the broader spectrum triazoles (itraconazole, voriconazole, posaconazole) with these inducers should be avoided. Itraconazole, voriconazole, and posaconazole are also potent inhibitors of CYP 3A4, which predisposes these agents to a large number of clinically significant pharmacokinetic drug–drug interactions. Posaconazole is also a substrate and inhibitor of P-glycoprotein, although the impact of this pathway on drug absorption is unknown. Even in the absence of drug interactions, serum drug levels of the broader spectrum triazoles (itraconazole, voriconazole, posaconazole) are often variable.[12] For voriconazole, pharmacokinetic variability results primarily from pharmacogenetic differences in CYP2C19 metabolism, with some patients classified as homozygous rapid metabolizers, heterozygous metabolizers, or homozygous poor metabolizers. Consequently, serum drug exposures are often difficult to predict from one patient to the next administered fixed drug doses. Impaired absorption is a primary factor influencing the variability of itraconazole and posaconazole serum concentrations. Serum drug concentration monitoring has been recommended in patients receiving triazole antifungals for documented infections, or when inadequate serum concentrations are suspected (Table 84–3).

As potent inhibitors of CYP3A4, itraconazole, voriconazole, and posaconazole can dramatically decrease the clearance of many medications with narrow therapeutic indices, leading to potentially dangerous drug interactions. Patients receiving anticoagulation therapy with warfarin, immunosuppressive therapy with cyclosporine or tacrolimus, those taking midazolam, HMG-CoA reductase inhibitors (statins), rifabutin, chemotherapy agents (e.g., vinca alkaloids, busulfan, and cyclophosphamide), and digoxin will require dosage adjustment and careful monitoring while receiving therapy with triazole antifungals[12] Although fluconazole is not as potent an inhibitor of CYP3A4 as other triazoles, clinically significant drug interactions may still be observed at higher fluconazole dosages (i.e., 800 mg/day).[12]

All azole antifungals carry the potential for rash, photosensitivity, and hepatotoxicity. In general, hepatotoxicity is mild and reversible, presenting as asymptomatic increases in liver transaminases or with cholestatic toxicity with increases in total bilirubin. Fulminant hepatic failure is less common and typically mediated by immunologic mechanisms. Therefore, serial monitoring of liver function is recommended in all patients receiving triazole antifungals. Long-term therapy with itraconazole has also been associated with reversible adrenal suppression and cardiomyopathy associated with the drug's negative inotropic effects. These adverse effects can be prevented or managed with close monitoring and follow-up of patients on long-term therapy. Voriconazole has also been

Table 84–3

Recommendations for Antifungal Therapeutic Drug Monitoring

Drug	Indication for Monitoring	Time of First Measurement	Target Conc. for Efficacy (mcg/mL or mg/L)	Target Conc. for Safety (mcg/mL or mg/L)
Flucytosine	Routine during first week of therapy, renal insufficiency, or poor clinical response	3–5 days	Peak greater than 20 (greater than 155 μmol/L)	Peak less than 50 (less than 388 μmol/L) to reduce risk of marrow toxicity
Itraconazole	Routine during first week of therapy, GI dysfunction, suspected drug interactions	4–7 days	Prophylaxis greater than 0.5 (greater than 0.7 μmol/L); therapy trough greater than 1–2 (greater than 1.4–2.8 μmol/L)	Some evidence to suggest trough greater than 4 mcg/mL (greater than 5.7 μmol/L) increased cardiac toxicity
Voriconazole	Lacking response, GI dysfunction, suspected drug interactions, pediatrics,[a] IV to oral switch, unexplained neurological changes	4–7 days	Prophylaxis trough greater than 0.5 (greater than 1.4 μmol/L); therapy trough 1–2 (2.9–5.7 μmol/L)	Trough less than 6 (17.2 μmol/L) to reduce risk of CNS toxicities
Posaconazole	Lacking response, GI dysfunction, potent acid suppression therapy (i.e, proton pump inhibitor) therapy, suspected drug interactions	4–7 days	Prophylaxis trough greater than 0.5 (greater than 0.7 μmol/L); therapy trough 0.5–1.5 (0.7–2.1 μmol/L)	Not established

[a]Pediatric patients display accelerated linear clearance of voriconazole. Therefore, higher daily voriconazole dosing (7 mg/kg every 12 hours) without a loading dose are recommended to achieve similar exposures to adults. Some children may require doses as high as 12 mg/kg every 12 hours to achieve similar serum drug exposures to adults. Therefore, therapeutic drug monitoring is recommended.

associated with severe phototoxic reactions and cutaneous erythema in sun-exposed skin, which may not be preventable with sunscreen alone. These reactions have been recently linked to development of squamous cell carcinoma or melanoma. Therefore, patients should be instructed to avoid sun exposure while on voriconazole therapy and have frequent skin examinations by a dermatologist.

Amphotericin B is the mainstay of treatment of patients with severe endemic fungal infections. The conventional deoxycholate formulation of the drug can be associated with substantial infusion-related adverse effects (e.g., chills, fever, nausea, rigors, and in rare cases hypotension, flushing, respiratory difficulty, and arrhythmias). As-needed premedication with low doses of hydrocortisone, acetaminophen, nonsteroidal anti-inflammatory agents, and meperidine can be used to reduce acute infusion-related reactions. Venous irritation associated with the drug can also lead to thrombophlebitis; hence central venous catheters are the preferred route of administration in patients receiving more than a week of therapy.

The most severe adverse effect associated with amphotericin B therapy is nephrotoxicity, which occurs through the renal vascular effects of the drug (constriction of the afferent arterioles in the kidney tubule), and direct toxicity to the kidney tubular membrane.[12] Generally, nephrotoxicity with amphotericin B is reversible provided the drug is stopped. However, treatment interruptions can be problematic in patients with severe infections. Precipitous decreases in glomerular filtration may occur in patients with marked dehydration or during aggressive diuresis. Infusion of normal saline before and after amphotericin B, a practice known as "sodium loading," can blunt precipitous decreases in renal

perfusion pressure and slow the rate of decline in the glomerular filtration rate. Administration of amphotericin B by continuous infusion has also been reported to reduce the nephrotoxicity of the drug, but is generally not advocated because of unproven efficacy when the drug is administered by this approach. Tubular toxicity can be delayed by avoiding the use of other drugs with known tubular toxicity such as aminoglycosides, cyclosporine, cisplatin, or foscarnet. Generally, tubular toxicity manifests in patients with severe wasting of potassium and magnesium in the urine. Therefore, patient electrolytes must be carefully monitored and potassium and magnesium supplementation is always necessary. Hypokalemia and hypomagnesaemia frequently precede decreases in glomerular filtration (increased serum creatinine), especially in patients who are adequately hydrated.[12] Continued tubular damage eventually results in decreases in renal blood flow and glomerular filtration through tubuloglomerular feedback mechanisms that further constrict the afferent arteriole.

During the 1990s, amphotericin B was reformulated into three different lipid-based formulations (Abelcet, AmBisome, and Amphotec) that have reduced rates of nephrotoxicity compared with the conventional deoxycholate formulation (Fungizone). Two of the formulations (Abelcet and AmBisome) have also shown reductions in the rates of infusion-related reactions. Although these lipid formulations are generally considered to be as effective as conventional amphotericin B deoxycholate, they are not dosed equivalently to the standard formulation (Table 84–2).

Unlike conventional amphotericin B, which is administered at dosages ranging from 0.6 to 1.5 mg/kg/day, lipid formulation doses are threefold to fivefold higher on a milligram-per-milligram basis, ranging from 3 to 6 mg/kg/day.[12] Only one prospective study has directly compared the efficacy of a lipid amphotericin formulation with that of the conventional formulation in AIDS patients with disseminated histoplasmosis.[13] Liposomal amphotericin B (AmBisome) was found to be more effective than amphotericin B, with response rates of 84% and 64%, respectively. AmBisome may also be the preferred agent in patients with CNS infections over other lipid formulations, due to its improved CNS penetration.[14]

PROPHYLAXIS

Primary prophylaxis, before development of infection, is generally not recommended for endemic fungi but may be considered in specific situations, including the following:

1. Patients with HIV infection with CD4+ cell counts less than 150 cells/mm³ (150 × 10⁶/L) (histoplasmosis) or less than 250 cells/mm³ (250 × 10⁶/L)(coccidioidomycosis) living in regions with high endemic case rates (greater than 10 cases per 100 patient-years), or in any patient with positive IgM or IgG antibodies. The recommended regimen is itraconazole 200 mg daily.[1,4,6]

2. *Secondary prophylaxis or suppressive therapy with itraconazole 200 mg daily is recommended to prevent recurrence of blastomycosis in immunosuppressed patients if immunosuppression cannot be reversed.*[6]

3. In patients with prior CNS disease, fluconazole or voriconazole are preferred over itraconazole due to the limited penetration of itraconazole into the CNS.

OPPORTUNISTIC MYCOSES

❸ *Commensal or environmental fungi that are typically harmless can become invasive mycoses when the host immune defenses are impaired. Host immune suppression and risk for opportunistic mycoses can be broadly classified into three categories:*

1. *Quantitative or qualitative deficits in neutrophil function*

2. *Deficits in cell-mediated immunity*

3. *Disruption of the integument and/or microbiologic barriers*

Quantitative defects in neutrophils (neutropenia) resulting from neoplastic diseases, cytotoxic chemotherapy, marrow transplantation, or aplastic anemia are among the most common risk factors for opportunistic mycoses. Qualitative defects may be seen in certain disease states (e.g., advanced diabetes mellitus and chronic granulomatous disease) or with high-dose corticosteroid therapy. Deficits in T-cell–mediated immunity secondary to AIDS, high-dose corticosteroid therapy, cyclosporine or other immunosuppressive drugs, chemotherapy, transplantation, bone marrow failure, and various other disorders have become increasingly common with the prolonged survival of transplant patients on chronic immunosuppressive therapy.

Immune deficits arising from disruption of the integument or GI/genitourinary barriers can also predispose patients to fungal infections. The most common types of barrier disruptions include surgery or infections/perforation of the abdominal viscus, use of central venous and urinary catheters, hyperalimentation, and mucositis associated with cytotoxic chemotherapy. Broad-spectrum antibacterial therapy can also predispose patients to fungal infections through disruption of the microbiologic flora in the gut, which allows overgrowth of *Candida* species. Successful management of opportunistic fungal pathogens, therefore, requires the reversal or reduction of underlying deficits in the host immune system.

All of the opportunistic mycoses are difficult to diagnose and often must be treated empirically before diagnosis is proven. Deciding when to initiate antifungal therapy and what opportunistic pathogens to cover is a decision governed largely by the *cumulative* immune deficits and clinical status of the host.

INVASIVE CANDIDIASIS

EPIDEMIOLOGY

Candida species are the most common opportunistic fungal pathogens encountered in hospitals, ranking as the third to fourth most common cause of nosocomial bloodstream infections in United States.[15] The incidence of nosocomial candidiasis has increased steadily since the early 1980s, with the widespread use of central venous catheters, broad-spectrum antimicrobials, and other advancements in the supportive care of critically ill patients. In the 1980s, *C. albicans* accounted for more than 80% of all bloodstream yeast isolates cultured from patients. By the late 1990s, this relative frequency of *C. albicans* had decreased to 50% in national surveys of bloodstream infections without a corresponding decrease in infections caused by non-*albicans* species. Because of the inherent resistance (e.g., *C. krusei*) or diminished susceptibility (e.g., *C. glabrata*) of many of the non-*albicans* species, the introduction of fluconazole in the early 1990s is often cited as the key element driving the shift in the microbiology of invasive candidiasis.[16] However, it is likely that other institution-specific factors (e.g., increasing use of central venous catheters and increasing intensity of cytotoxic/mucotoxic chemotherapy) and use of broad-spectrum antibiotic therapy have contributed equally to this trend. ❹ *It is important to be familiar with the relative epidemiology and frequency of nonalbicans* Candida *species in the institution or intensive care unit (ICU) before selecting empiric antifungal therapy for invasive candidiasis, as fluconazole is not recommended for the treatment of* C. glabrata *and* C. krusei *infections.*

CLINICAL PRESENTATION AND DIAGNOSIS

Invasive candidiasis is not a single syndrome, rather a spectrum of infections that differ in terms of clinical presentation and course depending on the type of host immune immunosuppression. However, disseminated infection is associated with crude mortality rates approaching 30% to 40%, underscoring the potential severity of infection.[17] The most common form of invasive candidiasis is seen in nonneutropenic patients with disruption of the GI, skin, or microbiologic barriers giving rise to a bloodstream infection (fungemia) from, or seeding to, a central venous catheter. Catheter-related candidemia carries a good prognosis if appropriate antifungal therapy is instituted early with catheter removal.[17] Fungemia can be of high density, however, leading to metastatic sites of infection and invasion of deep organs with increased morbidity. Therefore, the infection must be taken seriously, especially in patients with poor performance status (i.e., a high Acute Physiology, Age, and Chronic Health Evaluation [APACHE] II score) in the ICU.

Patients with acute disseminated candidiasis share many similar features as patients with catheter-related candidemia, except infection generally arises from the gut following mucotoxic chemotherapy, and the patients are often profoundly ill. Hematogenous spread to noncontiguous organs is common in patients with acute disseminated candidiasis, and outcome is heavily dependent upon recovery from neutropenia.[17] Fluconazole prophylaxis has markedly decreased the incidence of acute disseminated candidiasis among high-risk patient groups such as bone marrow transplant and acute leukemia patients.[17] However, breakthrough infections with fluconazole-resistant *C. glabrata* and *C. krusei* are still a concern.

Some forms of invasive candidiasis are dominated by deep-organ infection and may never be detected by blood cultures. Chronic disseminated candidiasis or hepatosplenic candidiasis is a unique presentation of candidemia seen after recovery from neutropenia. Candidemia during the period of neutropenia may be initially localized to the portal circulation with dissemination to contiguous organs. After recovery of neutrophils, an inflammatory response is seen against areas of focal infection in the liver and spleen. This inflammatory response produces abdominal pain that is associated with increases in alkaline phosphatase levels and hepatocellular enzymes.[17] Diagnosis is typically confirmed by patient history (recent neutropenia), and multiple areas of lucency in the liver and spleen on CT.

Focal invasive candidiasis has been reported for virtually every organ, even following apparently uncomplicated catheter-related fungemia. The most common sites of infection are the kidney, eye, and bone. *Candida* in the urine can be an indication of renal candidiasis or an obstructing fungus ball; however, it must be distinguished from more benign colonization of the urinary tract, especially in patients with chronic indwelling urinary catheters.[17] All patients with candidemia should undergo an eye exam to rule out *Candida* endophthalmitis, which can be sight-threatening if not recognized early.[17]

Laboratory diagnosis of invasive candidiasis is established by detection of the yeast in blood cultures or another sterile site (Fig. 84–3A).[17] Growth of *Candida* from urine, sputum, or respiratory secretions (including bronchoalveolar lavage) is not considered to be evidence of invasive infection, as these areas frequently become colonized with *Candida*

species in patients receiving broad-spectrum antibiotics.[17] Colonization at multiple body sites or with high density of *Candida* species, however, may precede invasive infection. Therefore, preemptive antifungal therapy may be indicated in colonized high-risk populations such as those with neutropenic fever, transplant recipients, or following major abdominal surgery.[17] Although *Candida* are not particularly fastidious organisms, the sensitivity of blood cultures is relatively poor (less than 60%), and a negative culture does not rule out infection.[17] The poor sensitivity of blood cultures for detecting invasive disease has led to the study of novel serodiagnostic tests to detect antibodies, fungal metabolites, fungal cell wall antigens, or nucleic acids of *Candida* species. Of the four approaches, testing of patient serum for fungal cell wall β-glucan polymers (i.e., Fungitell®(1→3)-β-D-glucan test, Associates of Cape Cod Inc.) appear most promising; however, these tests may not be routinely performed in many hospitals.

Laboratory identification of *Candida* in clinical samples must be performed to the species level whenever possible, as *Candida* species differ considerably in their susceptibility to antifungal agents.[17-20] Rapid discrimination of *C. albicans* from common nonalbicans *Candida* species can be accomplished by the germ-tube test, which presumptively identifies *C. albicans* by the early formation (less than 4 hours) of a hyphae-like structure when the yeast is incubated in serum at 37°C (98.6°F). Definitive species identification, however, may require an additional 48 to 72 hours after the organism is isolated on agar. Fluorescent in situ hybridization (FISH) of *Candida* species-specific DNA sequences can reduce the time needed for definitive species identification, but may not be offered in many clinical microbiology laboratories.

C. albicans remains the most common cause of invasive candidiasis and is the most virulent of *Candida* species, but is the most susceptible to commonly used antifungals including fluconazole.[17,19,20] Like *C. albicans*, *C. tropicalis* is a relatively virulent species that has a tropism for causing deep tissue invasion. *C. tropicalis* is generally sensitive to antifungals, including fluconazole.[17,19,20] *C. parapsilosis* is a less virulent species seen frequently in neonates and in adults with central venous catheters. Although *C. parapsilosis* is less virulent, many isolates form thick biofilms on prosthetic materials and catheters that make the organism difficult to eradicate.[17] *C. parapsilosis* is generally susceptible to most antifungals, including fluconazole. However, this species is inherently less susceptible to echinocandin antifungals, although many patients still respond to treatment, perhaps due to the lower virulence of this species. *C. krusei* is a less common species associated with breakthrough infections in heavily immunocompromised patients and should always be considered resistant to fluconazole.[17,19,20] Most fluconazole-resistant isolates of *C. krusei* retain susceptibility to itraconazole, voriconazole, and posaconazole based on laboratory testing.

C. glabrata has become a common cause of both de novo and breakthrough candidemia in heavily immunocompromised hosts and breakthrough infection in patients on fluconazole prophylaxis. Although *C. glabrata* is generally

Patient Encounter 2, Opportunistic Fungal Infection, Part 1

A 45-year-old man in the surgical ICU with necrotizing pancreatitis develops fever while receiving broad-spectrum antibacterial therapy (meropenem 1 g every 8 hours, gentamicin 120 mg every 8 hours, and linezolid 600 mg every 12 hours). The patient has a central venous catheter and a Foley catheter. Blood cultures are negative at the time, but the patient has yeast growing in the sputum and urine. A serum $(1\rightarrow3)$-β-D-glucan test is positive at 90 pg/mL (90 ng/L). Laboratory studies reveal a white blood cell count of 12,500 cells/mm³ (12.5 × 10⁹/L).

What are this patient's risk factors for developing an invasive fungal infection?

What current evidence suggests that this patient has an invasive fungal infection?

If antifungal therapy is started in this patient, which species need to be treated?

less virulent than other *C. albicans*, infections with this organism are typically seen in patients with poor performance status, and therefore mortality remains high. The marginal susceptibility of *C. glabrata* to fluconazole dictates that other agents such as echinocandins and possibly amphotericin B be considered as first-line therapy until susceptibility to fluconazole can be documented.[19,20] The effectiveness of voriconazole or posaconazole for fully fluconazole-resistant *C. glabrata* fungemia is not well established, and cross-resistance among these triazole antifungals has been documented in laboratory studies.[19,20]

TREATMENT

Six antifungals (amphotericin B, fluconazole, voriconazole, caspofungin, micafungin, and anidulafungin) have been studied as monotherapy in prospective, randomized comparative clinical trials for the treatment of invasive candidiasis.[16,21–25] Although these treatment options are considered to have relatively equivalent efficacy, they differ somewhat in toxicity and associated drug–drug interaction profiles. Lipid amphotericin B formulations are probably as effective as the aforementioned agents; however, evidence supporting their use is derived principally from open-label observational studies and empiric therapy trials of febrile neutropenia.[17] Moreover, the acquisition cost of lipid amphotericin B formulations may be relatively higher in many institutions compared with fluconazole and the echinocandins. As a result, their first-line use is not prominently recommended in evidence-based guidelines for proven infection.[17] No prospective randomized, controlled clinical trials have been published comparing antifungal therapies for proven acute disseminated candidiasis in neutropenic patients, chronic

disseminated candidiasis, or other forms of deep-organ candidiasis.[17]

A majority of patients are treated empirically for invasive candidiasis before conclusive evidence of infection is available to direct therapy. Empiric therapy for invasive candidiasis should be considered in any patient with persistent, unexplained fever and host deficits that predispose patients to candidemia, including broad-spectrum antibacterial therapy, presence of a central venous catheter, patients with severe organ dysfunction or on dialysis, recent history of surgery that damages or opens the GI viscera, patients with neutropenia or qualitative deficiencies in host immunity (e.g., due to high-dose corticosteroid therapy), or colonization with *Candida* at one or more body sites.

⑤ If a patient is nonneutropenic, clinically stable (i.e., normotensive with relatively normal organ function), and has never received prior azole therapy, fluconazole 12 mg/kg/day loading dose followed by 6 mg/kg/day is still considered an appropriate first-line therapy for invasive candidiasis in many centers until speciation of the *Candida* isolate is confirmed.[17] However, echinocandins (caspofungin, micafungin, anidulafungin) are preferred as first-line agents in more critically ill patients with compromised renal function, hypotension/sepsis, or in institutions/ICUs with higher rates (greater than 10%) of *C. glabrata* or *C. krusei* (Table 84–4).[19] Treatment is continued for at least 2 weeks for uncomplicated catheter infections that respond quickly to antifungals and catheter removal or at least 4 to 6 weeks for complicated infections arising from an endovascular source or infections associated with a high risk of metastatic seeding.

One caveat is that cryptococcosis, endemic fungi, or other rare yeast (e.g., *Trichosporon* species) occasionally produce fungemia in lymphopenic patients that may initially be mistakenly assumed to be *Candida*. Therefore, initial treatment with a lipid amphotericin B formulation may be judicious in profoundly lymphopenic patients (i.e., CD4⁺ less than 250/mm³ [250 × 10⁶/L]) with yeast in blood cultures until fungal identification is confirmed, as echinocandins have poor activity against non-*Candida* yeast. Timely initiation of appropriate antifungal therapy is critical, as any delay in the initiation of antifungal therapy once a patient has a positive blood culture significantly increases mortality and the potential for metastatic infections.[26]

Amphotericin B deoxycholate 0.7 mg/kg/day or an echinocandin (i.e., caspofungin, micafungin, or anidulafungin); voriconazole; or a lipid amphotericin B formulation are recommended as empiric therapy in patients with neutropenic (i.e., absolute neutrophil count less than 500 PMN/mm³ [500 × 10⁶/L]) fever.[17,21] If the neutropenia is of shorter duration and the patient is at lower risk for mold infections (e.g., solid tumor patients with 2 weeks or less of neutropenia), higher dose fluconazole (i.e., 800 mg/day or 12 mg/kg) could be considered.[17,21] Lipid amphotericin B formulations, an echinocandin, or voriconazole are often the preferred agents in febrile patients with 3 weeks or more of neutropenia to expand coverage against molds.[17,27] If the yeast is identified as *C. glabrata*, treatment guidelines recommend the use of an echinocandin or possibly amphotericin B formulations.[17,27]

Table 84–4

Therapeutic Approach to Opportunistic Invasive Fungal Infections

Mycoses	Recommended Treatment Regimens	Comments
Candidiasis Catheter-related and acute hematogenous	Fluconazole 12 mg/kg loading dose, then 6–12 mg/kg/day IV every 24 hours adjusted for renal function[a] OR Echinocandin[b] OR Voriconazole 6 mg/kg every 12 hours IV for 1 day, then 3 mg/kg every 12 hours IV *Second line:* Lipid amphotericin B formulation 3–5 mg/kg per day[c] OR Amphotericin B 0.7 mg/kg per day IV OR Amphotericin B + fluconazole	Treat for 14 days after the last positive blood culture and resolution of signs and symptoms; catheter should be removed whenever possible Patients can be switched to oral fluconazole when clinically stable if isolate is susceptible The IV cyclodextrin formulation of voriconazole is not recommended in patients with estimated creatinine clearance less than 50mL/min (less than 0.83 mL/s) due to concerns of accumulation of the cyclodextrin vehicle Echinocandins and amphotericin B are preferred agents for fluconazole-resistant species. Voriconazole appears to be effective against fluconazole-resistant *C. krusei*
Empirical therapy in neutropenic patient	Fluconazole 6–12 mg/kg/day (low risk) adjusted for renal function[a] OR Liposomal amphotericin B 3 mg/kg every 24 hours OR Echinocandin OR Amphotericin B 0.7 mg/kg every 24 hours	Antifungals with coverage of *Aspergillus* should be used in higher risk patients or prolonged neutropenia (i.e., longer than 3 weeks)
Urinary candidiasis	Fluconazole 200 mg IV or PO for 7–14 days OR Amphotericin B 0.3 mg/kg per day IV for 1–7 days	Asymptomatic candiduria does not require therapy
Cryptococcosis Pulmonary-isolated	Fluconazole 6 mg/kg/day IV or PO for 6–12 mo adjusted for renal function[a]	
Severe pulmonary infection and meningitis	*Induction:* Amphotericin B 0.7–1 mg/kg per day + flucytosine 100 mg/kg per day PO divided every 6 hours for 2 weeks adjusted for renal function[c] *Consolidation:* Fluconazole 6–12 mg/kg/day for 10 weeks adjusted for renal function[a] *Second line:* Fluconazole + flucytosine for 2 weeks, then fluconazole for 10 weeks adjusted for renal function[a,c] OR Amphotericin + fluconazole for 2 weeks, then fluconazole for 10 weeks adjusted for renal function[a] OR Liposomal amphotericin B 5 mg/kg per day × 2 weeks, then fluconazole for 10 weeks adjusted for renal function[a]	Therapeutic drug monitoring is required for safe use of flucytosine, see Table 84–3. Amphotericin B +5-flucytosine, Amphotericin B + fluconazole, liposomal amphotericin B (4–6 mg/kg/day) Echinocandins have no activity against cryptococci

(Continued)

Table 84–4

Therapeutic Approach to Opportunistic Invasive Fungal Infections (*Continued*)

Mycoses	Recommended Treatment Regimens	Comments
Aspergillosis	Voriconazole 6 mg/kg IV every 12 hours × 2 doses, then 4 mg/kg IV every 12 hours OR Lipid formulations of amphotericin B OR Echinocandin[b] OR Posaconazole 200 mg PO 4 times daily × 14 days, then 400 mg PO twice daily OR Combination therapy	Voriconazole can be administered as oral therapy in patients taking oral medications Therapeutic drug monitoring should be considered in patients receiving voriconazole or posaconazole, see Table 84–3. Preclinical studies suggest mold-active azoles (i.e., voriconazole) plus echinocandins[c] have enhanced activity vs. triazole monotherapy. *A. terreus* should be considered resistant to amphotericin B

[a]Fluconazole renal dosing adjustments: CrCl greater than 50–90 mL/min (0.83–1.50 mL/s), 100% of dose; CrCl 10–50 mL/min (0.17–0.83 mL/s), 50% of dose; CrCl less than 10 mL/min (less than 0.17 mL/s) 50%.

[b]Anidulafungin 200 mg loading dose day 1, then 100 mg daily, caspofungin 70 mg loading dose day 1, then 50 mg daily; or micafungin 100 mg daily.

[c]Flucytosine renal dosing adjustments: CrCl greater than 50–90 mL/min (0.83–1.50 mL/s), 25 mg/kg every 12 hours; CrCl 10–50 mL/min (0.17–0.83 mL/s), 25 mg/kg every 12–24 hours; CrCl less than 10 mL/min (less than 0.17 mL/s) 25 mg/kg every 24 hours. Therapeutic drug monitoring is required for safe use of flucytosine (see Table 84–3).

Voriconazole or posaconazole are generally avoided because of concerns of cross-resistance.[19,20] *C. krusei* infections can be treated with an echinocandin, amphotericin B, or newer triazoles such as voriconazole and posaconazole, as cross-resistance among triazoles is less problematic than with *C. glabrata*.[19,20] Patients who respond to therapy are medically stable, are not neutropenic, and are taking oral medications can be transitioned to oral fluconazole or voriconazole preferably after documentation of susceptibility to fluconazole with minimum inhibitory concentration testing.

Treatment recommendations for other forms of invasive candidiasis are based primarily on anecdotal evidence and expert opinion. Deep-organ candidiasis requires prolonged therapy to achieve a cure; therefore, importance is placed on the use of convenient and nontoxic long-term treatment regimens. Fluconazole (400 mg/day or 6 mg/kg/day) is the preferred regimen in clinically stable patients. Echinocandins, amphotericin B, or lipid amphotericin B formulations can be considered for refractory cases or clinically unstable patients. Infections of the eye, bone, pancreas, or gallbladder are typically treated with either amphotericin B, fluconazole, or possibly voriconazole. Although echinocandins are effective for intra-abdominal infections, their limited penetration into the eye makes them unsuitable agents for *Candida* endophthalmitis.

Urinary candidiasis is a term for an ill-defined group of syndromes that can range from benign colonization (candiduria) in the bladder to invasive disease of the renal parenchyma. Asymptomatic nonneutropenic patients with candiduria do not require antifungal therapy, as no study has demonstrated the value of transiently clearing *Candida* from the urine. Patients should receive 7 to 14 days of antifungal therapy for urinary candidiasis if they are (a) symptomatic, (b) have clinical or laboratory evidence of infection, (c) are neutropenic, (d) are low-birth-weight infants; (e) will undergo urologic manipulations, or (f) have renal allografts. Removal of urinary tract instruments, including Foley catheters and stents, is essential to prevent relapse. The preferred therapy is fluconazole 200 mg daily, although IV amphotericin B deoxycholate 0.3 to 1 mg/kg/day is also effective. Other antifungal agents (with the exception of flucytosine) do not achieve appreciable concentrations in the urine and therefore should not be considered for urinary candidiasis. Irrigation with amphotericin B is not effective for infections above the bladder and should not be used in higher risk patients with the exception of its use as a diagnostic tool for confirming a localized infection of the bladder. *Candida* infections of the renal parenchyma secondary to metastatic seeding from the bloodstream are treated in a similar fashion to candidemia.

Mucocutaneous candidiasis is not invasive and can be treated with topical azoles (clotrimazole troches), oral azoles (fluconazole, ketoconazole, or itraconazole), or oral polyenes (such as nystatin or oral amphotericin B). Orally administered and absorbed azoles (ketoconazole, fluconazole, or itraconazole solution), amphotericin B suspension, IV echinocandins, or IV amphotericin B are recommended for refractory or recurrent infections.[17]

Although more severe than mucocutaneous candidiasis, esophageal candidiasis typically does not evolve into a life-threatening infection unless the esophagus is ruptured. However, topical therapy is ineffective. Triazole antifungals (fluconazole, itraconazole solution, or voriconazole), echinocandins, or IV amphotericin B (in cases of unresponsive infections) are effective treatment options. Parenteral therapy should be used in patients who are unable to take oral medications.[17]

Patient Encounter 2, Opportunistic Fungal Infection, Part 2

Selecting Antifungal Therapy

The patient is started on fluconazole 400 mg/day, but 3 days later has persistent fever and develops hypotension and decreased urine output. Blood cultures are now growing a germ tube–negative yeast. Laboratory studies revealed a white blood cell count of 14,200/mm³ (14.2 × 10⁹/L), aspartate aminotransferase 68 IU/L (1.13 µkat/L), alanine aminotransferase 75 IU/L (1.25 µkat/L), alkaline phosphatase 168 IU/L (2.80µkat/L), and normal bilirubin. Serum creatinine has increased from 1.2 to 1.8 mg/dL (106 to 159 µmol/L) over the last 3 days.

What factors suggest empiric antifungal therapy should be changed in this patient?

What other procedures should be recommended in this patient to improve response to antifungal therapy?

PATIENT MONITORING

Response to antifungal therapy in invasive candidiasis is often more rapid than for endemic fungal infections. Resolution of fever and sterilization of blood cultures are indications of response to antifungal therapy with the caveat that the growth of *Candida* from blood cultures is often delayed by 48 to 72 hours. Adverse effects associated with antifungal therapy are similar in these patients as described earlier, except some toxicities may be more pronounced in critically ill patients with invasive candidiasis. Nephrotoxicity and electrolyte disturbances with amphotericin B can be especially problematic and may not be avoidable even with lipid amphotericin B formulations. Therefore, current treatment guidelines emphasize less toxic treatment options, such as the first-line use of fluconazole in lower-risk patients and echinocandins in higher risk patients. Decisions to use one class of antifungal agents over the other are principally driven by concerns of nonalbicans species, patient tolerability, or history of prior fluconazole exposure (risk factor for nonalbicans species.).

PROPHYLAXIS

Fluconazole (400 mg/day) has been extensively studied as a prophylactic regimen to prevent invasive candidiasis in patients with prolonged (greater than 2 weeks) neutropenia.[28-32] Placebo-controlled, prospective randomized trials performed in the 1990s demonstrated that fluconazole was effective in reducing the frequency, morbidity, and, in some trials, mortality due to invasive candidiasis if administered until marrow recovery. However, the major limitation with fluconazole is its lack of mold coverage

needed for high-risk patients with persistent neutropenia. Studies have examined the use of itraconazole, voriconazole, posaconazole, or the echinocandin micafungin as prophylaxis in hematopoietic cell transplant recipients until engraftment to provide protection against both *Candida* and *Aspergillus* species.[32-35]Although each of these studied antifungals has demonstrated a benefit in reducing fungal infections, all of the drugs have limitations with respect to prolonged administration in high-risk patients. Therefore, the approach toward antifungal prophylaxis is highly institution-specific depending on the patient population, epidemiology of invasive fungal infections, and options for outpatient IV drug therapy.

Use of antifungal prophylaxis for invasive candidiasis in nonneutropenic patients remains an area of controversy. Prophylaxis should be targeted toward clearly defined high-risk transplant populations (e.g., liver, pancreatic, or small-bowel transplantation) or ICU patients (i.e., neonatal intensive care) with rates of invasive candidiasis exceeding 10%, despite aggressive infection-control procedures.[36,37] Fluconazole prophylaxis (400 mg/day) reduces the rate of *Candida* peritonitis in patients with refractory GI perforation and trended toward decreased rates of invasive candidiasis in select adult patients admitted to a surgical ICU for more than 3 days.[36,37] Fluconazole is also effective in reducing the rate of invasive candidiasis in neonates.[37] However, prophylaxis can result in excessive antifungal use in lower-risk patients; therefore, many experts have advocated preemptive (i.e., starting therapy based on biomarkers of infection such as serum beta glucan) or empirical (symptoms of infection) treatment approaches in this population in lieu of prophylaxis. A multi-institutional prospective randomized trial of administering empirical fluconazole (800 mg/day versus placebo) in ICU patients with persistent fever, however, did not demonstrate a benefit for the nonneutropenic population.[38] It is hoped that ongoing studies will better define the risks versus benefits of routine antifungal prophylaxis or preemptive treatment approaches in the ICU setting.

CRYPTOCOCCOSIS

EPIDEMIOLOGY

Cryptococcus neoformans is an encapsulated yeast that can infect apparently normal hosts but is more frequently associated with severe infections in immunocompromised patients. *C. neoformans* is divided into two varieties based on serotype: *C. neoformans* var. *neoformans* (serotypes a and d) that is associated with infections in immunocompromised patients, and *C. neoformans* var. *gattii* (serotypes b and c) that is associated with infections in healthy hosts. *C. neoformans* var. *gattii* is found predominantly in tropical and subtropical climates with eucalyptus trees, and more recently has been linked to infectious outbreaks around Vancouver Island and the U.S. Pacific Northwest. *C. neoformans* var. *neoformans* is found worldwide and is associated with pigeon droppings and other avian excreta. Before the AIDS pandemic, cryptococcosis was a relatively uncommon disease, but became a leading cause of meningitis among HIV-infected patients. Although the incidence of this infection has declined somewhat with the widespread use of highly active antiretroviral therapy (HAART), *C. neoformans* remains an important pathogen in the developing regions with high rates of AIDS and also in immunocompromised patients, including transplant and cancer patients who may present with the pulmonary form of the infection.

CLINICAL PRESENTATION AND DIAGNOSIS

C. neoformans is acquired primarily through inhalation of the desiccated yeast particles found in the environment. Inhaled cells reach distal alveolar spaces where they gradually rehydrate and form their characteristic polysaccharide capsules that enable resistance to phagocytosis. Defects in cellular immunity allow reconstitution of the protective capsule and multiplication of yeast in the lungs. Although alveolar macrophages phagocytose the yeast, containment and killing require a coordinated response between innate and adaptive humoral (complement and anticryptococcal antibodies) and T-cell–mediated host responses.[5] Deficiencies in cell-mediated immunity allow the yeast to survive as a facultative intracellular pathogen in macrophages as they migrate from the lung to draining lymph nodes, leading to dissemination via the bloodstream to the meninges.

Unlike most opportunistic fungi, true virulence factors have been identified for *C. neoformans*. The capsules, including the soluble polysaccharides released from the yeast cells during infection, impair phagocytosis and binding of anticryptococcal antibodies. Primary cryptococcal infection begins in the lung, presenting as a mildly symptomatic or asymptomatic infection that resolves spontaneously or undergoes encapsulation in noncalcified lung nodules. It is common for these isolated nodules to be detected on chest x-rays during routine workup. Diagnosis of primary cryptococcosis is only made if the nodule is aspirated or removed because of concerns of primary lung cancer.

In the immunocompromised host, infection of the lung may present with more diffuse, bilateral, and interstitial disease that mimics the presentation of *Pneumocystis jiroveci (carinii)* pneumonia (PCP). Dissemination to other organs, particularly the CNS, eye, and possibly the skin, is more likely to occur in patients with severe deficits in cell-mediated immunity. Fever, cough, dyspnea, and pleural pain are common at presentation, with accompanying hypoxemia that can rapidly evolve to acute respiratory failure. Because the features of diffuse pulmonary cryptococcosis overlap with other opportunistic pathogens, early diagnosis requires bronchoalveolar lavage or transbronchial biopsy, which can effectively diagnose 80% to 100% of cases.[39] The clinical course of diffuse cryptococcal pneumonia can be as severe as PCP, with mortality rates approaching 100% in untreated patients by 48 hours.

C. neoformans is strongly neurotropic and readily disseminates from the lung to the CNS, specifically the leptomeninges, and occasionally the parenchyma of the brain. The clinical characteristics of cryptococcal meningitis differ somewhat, however, between patients with and without underlying AIDS. In patients without AIDS, disease presentation is more insidious, and symptoms such as dizziness, irritability, decreased comprehension, and unstable gait may present many weeks to months before the diagnosis is established.[39] Patients with AIDS generally present much later in the course of disease with severe meningoencephalitis.[39] The most common signs and symptoms on presentation are fever, headache, meningismus, photophobia, mental status changes, and seizures. CT or more sensitive MRI may reveal cerebral edema, multiple areas of enhanced nodules, or a single mass lesion (cryptococcoma). Examination of the cerebrospinal fluid (CSF) often reveals increased opening pressure upon lumbar puncture, but glucose, protein, and leukocyte levels can be normal.[39]

LABORATORY DIAGNOSIS

Clinical diagnosis is confirmed by cultures from the blood, CSF, or other clinically relevant fluids or tissue. However, early diagnosis is suggested by either direct observation of *C. neoformans* in the CSF by India ink staining (Fig. 84–3B).[39] Similarly, detection of cryptococcal antigen in either serum or CSF can provide a rapid diagnosis with greater than 95% sensitivity and specificity and appears to correlate with fungal burden.[39] A positive serum antigen test of greater than 1:4 strongly suggests cryptococcal infection, and greater than or equal to 1:8 is indicative of active disease. Antigen titers in serum are positive in 99% of patients with cryptococcal meningitis and typically exceed titers of 1:2,048 in patients with

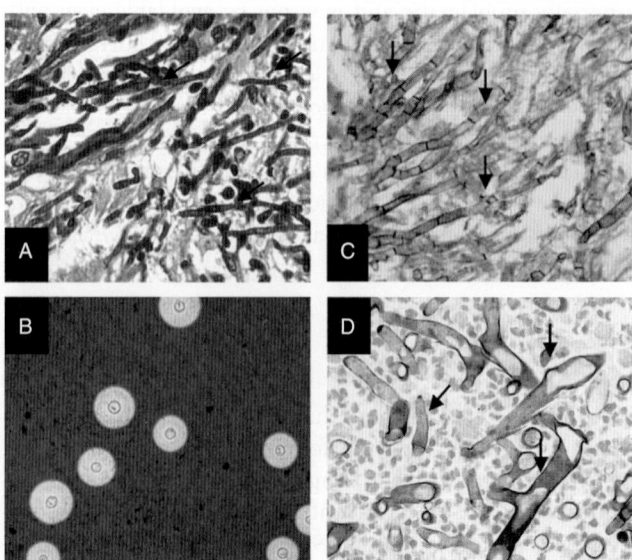

FIGURE 84–3. Opportunistic mycoses in clinical samples. *A.* Candidiasis (tissue). *B.* Cryptococcosis (India ink stain of CSF). *C.* Aspergillosis (tissue). *D.* Mucormycosis (tissue).

AIDS.[39] However, the time course of cryptococcal antigen elimination is unknown, and a positive test result can persist for many years. Changes in the CSF cryptococcal antigen titers have limited value in the monitoring of drug therapy for cryptococcal meningitis, although it is expected that a decrease should be seen after 2 or more weeks of antifungal therapy.[39]

TREATMENT

Cryptococcal meningitis is fatal if left untreated. Because pneumonia frequently precedes dissemination of disease and subsequent meningitis, all patients with culture-, histopathology-, or serology-proven disease should receive antifungal therapy. In patients with isolated pulmonary cryptococcosis, fluconazole is generally considered to be the therapy of choice (see Table 84–2).[39] Alternatively, itraconazole, voriconazole, or combination therapy (fluconazole plus flucytosine) has also been used with some success, but these regimens are generally considered inferior to amphotericin B and are recommended only for persons unable to tolerate or unresponsive to standard treatment. Echinocandins do not have activity against *C. neoformans*.

Disseminated or CNS cryptococcosis requires a more aggressive treatment approach. Pretreatment predictors of poor outcome with antifungal therapy include the following:

- Progressive underlying disease or immune dysfunction
- Abnormal mental status at the time of presentation
- Increased opening pressure on lumbar puncture (greater than 260 mm H₂O [2.55 kPa])
- High fungal burden as reflected by a CSF antigen titer (in AIDS patients) of greater than 1:2,048

Prospective randomized trials completed prior to the recognition of AIDS demonstrated high response rates (approximately 80%) with the combined use of amphotericin B and flucytosine for 4 to 6 weeks. Although sterilization of the CSF could be achieved in most patients within 2 weeks with this regimen, a substantial number of patients (30% to 40%) developed dose-limiting toxicities, and relapse was seen in roughly 50% of patients. Therefore, a treatment approach was devised that consists of distinct treatment phases to minimize toxicity and reduce the risk of relapse. ❻ *Clinical trials performed by the National Institute of Allergy and Infectious Diseases (NIAID) Mycoses Study Group after the recognition of AIDS showed that 2 weeks of induction antifungal therapy with combination amphotericin B (0.7 mg/kg/day) plus flucytosine (100 mg/kg/day) for cryptococcal meningitis, followed by consolidation therapy with fluconazole (400 mg daily) for 8 weeks, was as effective as 4 weeks of combination therapy, with fewer toxicities* (see Table 84–2).[12,41] Lipid formulations of amphotericin B can be substituted in patients at higher risk for nephrotoxicity. Other studies have suggested that fluconazole plus amphotericin or high-dose fluconazole alone (more than 800 mg/day) may be an acceptable alternatives in patients who cannot tolerate therapy with flucytosine (see Table 84–2).[36]

PROPHYLAXIS

Fluconazole (200 mg/day) is recommended as maintenance therapy for life in patients with persistent underlying immune dysfunction to prevent recurrent cryptococcal meningitis.[36] Available data have demonstrated that it is safe to discontinue maintenance therapy in AIDS patients who have had a sustained immunologic response on effective antiretroviral therapy (i.e., CD4⁺ count greater than 100 cells/microliter (greater than 100 × 10⁶/L) with undetectable or very low viral RNA) if they have received at least 12 months of antifungal therapy.[36] Occasionally, initiation of HAART can result in the reactivation of a subclinical, immunologic manifestation of cryptococcal infection (or other opportunistic infections). Manifestations of this *immune reconstitution inflammatory syndrome* (IRIS) may include exacerbations of meningitis or necrotizing pneumonia. Antifungal therapy plus a nonsteroidal anti-inflammatory agent or prednisone have been used successfully in patients with cryptococcal-associated immune reconstitution syndrome.[39] However, the optimal management of this recently defined clinical entity remains unknown.

INVASIVE ASPERGILLOSIS

EPIDEMIOLOGY

Invasive molds, particularly *Aspergillus*, are a common complication of intensive cancer chemotherapy required for hematologic malignancies as well as hematopoietic and solid organ transplant recipients. More than 180 species within the genus *Aspergillus* have been described, but only four species are commonly associated with invasive infection: *Aspergillus fumigatus*, *Aspergillus flavus*, *Aspergillus terreus*, and *Aspergillus niger*. Of these four species, *A. fumigatus* accounts for most of human infections. However, identification of *Aspergillus* mold in culture to the species level is still essential because the incidence of amphotericin B–resistant *Aspergillus terreus* and *Aspergillus flavus* have increased over the last 10 years in many centers. Additionally, less common mold infections such as fusariosis and mucormycosis often present with similar clinical features aspergillosis, but require different treatment approaches due to their inherent resistance to many antifungal agents. Early and accurate diagnosis of invasive aspergillosis (IA) improves the outcome of infection, reducing mortality rates by 30% to 50% with the timely administration of effective antifungal therapy.[40]

CLINICAL PRESENTATION AND DIAGNOSIS

The pathogenesis of IA is defined largely by the underlying immune dysfunction of the host. The most common route of acquisition for *Aspergillus* is through the respiratory tract. Conidia dispersed in air currents are continuously

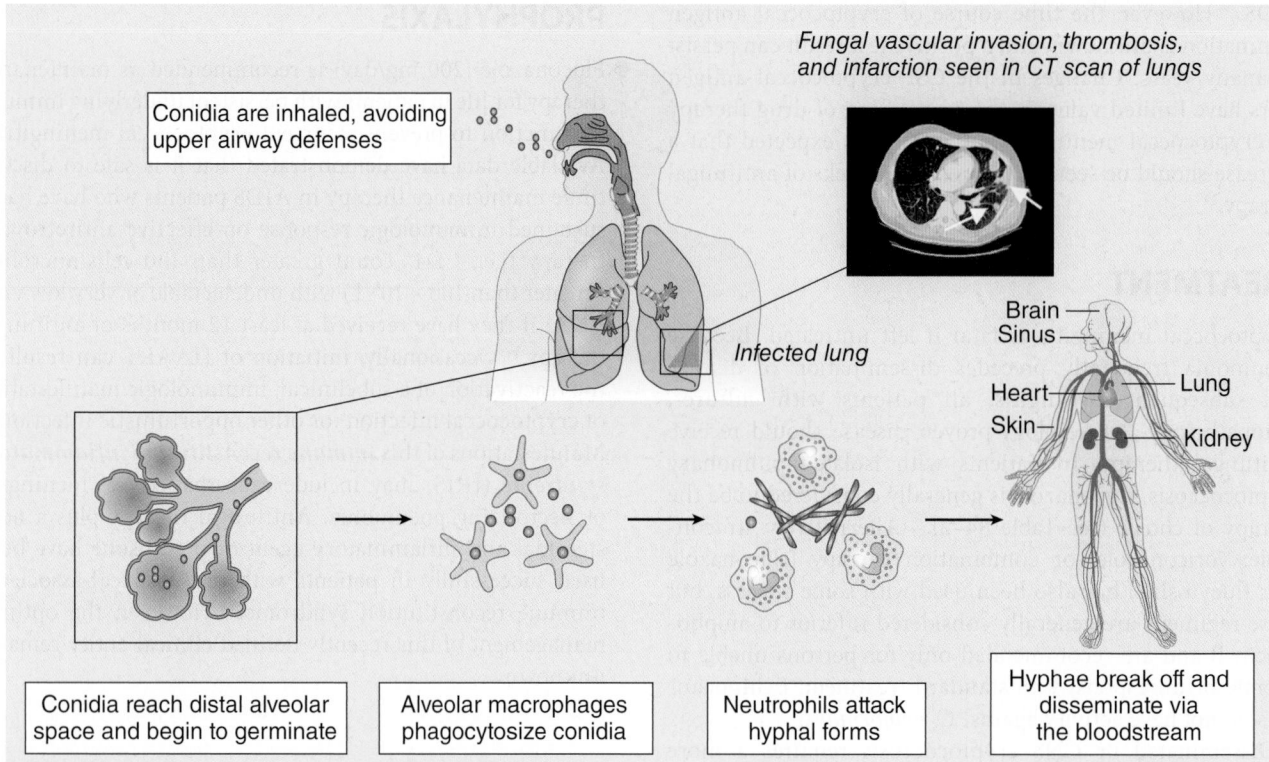

FIGURE 84–4. Pathogenesis of invasive aspergillosis (IA).

inhaled through the sinuses and mouth and penetrate down to distal alveolar spaces (see Fig. 84–4). Most conidia are rapidly phagocytosed and removed by resident macrophages and neutrophils in the upper and lower respiratory tract.[5] However, macrophage function may be suppressed following transplantation, cytotoxic chemotherapy, or in patients who have received high-dose corticosteroid therapy. Conidia that escaped phagocytosis begin to germinate into hyphal forms that invade blood vessels or contiguous tissues or bone (in sinuses), resulting in hemorrhage and/or infarction and coagulative necrosis. Once in the bloodstream, viable hyphal fragments can break off and disseminate to distal organs including the brain. Control of the infection at this stage requires development of an adaptive Th1 or TH17 response to enhance the fungicidal activity of professional effector cells (i.e., neutrophils) against hyphal elements.[5] Patients with dysregulated, suppressed T-cell–mediated immunity or prolonged neutropenia are unable to control fungal growth and are at high risk for dissemination of the infection. Without early diagnosis and antifungal therapy, IA in persistently immunosuppressed patients is uniformly fatal.

Signs and symptoms of IA are predictably muted in the immunocompromised host. Fever is common but nonspecific for infection and may be accompanied by pleuritic chest pain, cough, hemoptysis, and/or friction rub.[40] Neurologic signs, including seizures, hemiparesis, and stupor, may be present in patients with dissemination to the brain. Cutaneous plaques or papules characterized by a central

necrotic ulcer or eschar occur in up to 10% of patients with disseminated disease; however, concomitant blood cultures are often negative. Chest radiographs cannot detect early forms of disease and may remain negative in up to 10% of patients within 1 week of death.[41,42] Nodular lesions detected by high-resolution computed tomography (HRCT) scans, along with fever, are often the first indication of invasive pulmonary aspergillosis in severely immunocompromised patients. Typically these radiographs reveal wedge-shaped or nodular lesions, surrounded by intermediate attenuation called the "halo sign" (Fig 84–5).[40,43] These early lesions on CT scans represent hemorrhage and edema surrounding

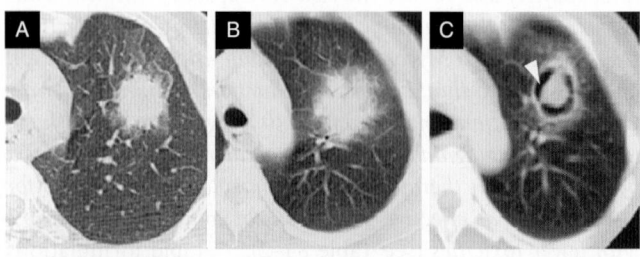

FIGURE 84–5. Radiographic evolution of invasive pulmonary aspergillosis in a neutropenic patient. A. Early halo sign of ground glass opacity surrounding nodular lesions. B. Nonspecific infiltrate of increased diameter. C. Air crescent sign observed with neutrophil recovery, cavitation of infected lung in walled off cavity with air (arrow).

Patient Encounter 3

Invasive Mold Infection

A 53-year-old man with acute myelogenous leukemia at day 80 after matched-allogeneic donor hematopoietic stem-cell transplantation presents to the clinic with increasing complaints of nausea, stomach cramping, and rash on the back and chest. He also complains of sharp pain in the left side of his chest during deep inspiration. By laboratory examination, he is noted to have an alanine aminotransferase of 119 IU/L (1.98 μkat/L), aspartate aminotransferase 107 IU/L (1.78μkat/L), and total bilirubin of 1.8mg/dL (31 μmol/L). The patient has an absolute neutrophil count of 950 cells/mm³ (950 × 10⁶/L). His current medications include tacrolimus 5 mg twice daily (most recent level: 9 ng/mL [9 mcg/L; 11 nmol/L]), prednisone 20 mg daily, levofloxacin 500 mg daily, fluconazole 200 mg/day, valacyclovir 500 mg twice daily. He is admitted to the hospital for suspected graft-versus-host disease exacerbation. However, computed tomography scan of the chest reveals a single dense pleural-based lung nodule in the left lung. A serum galactomannan test is reported to be negative (index 0.4; positive when more than 0.5). The primary service wishes to start voriconazole.

What are the patient's risk factors for developing an invasive mold infection?

Is voriconazole an acceptable option in this patient? Are there any drug interaction concerns?

What mold infections need to be considered if the patient had presented to the hospital with these findings while already receiving voriconazole prophylaxis?

an infarcted blood vessel. Despite "effective" antifungal therapy, lesions on CT scan may continue to increase in size in neutropenic patients until neutrophil counts recover, at which time they begin to cavitate, forming the "air-crescent sign" on chest radiographs, indicative of resolving infection. ⑦ *Immunocompromised patients on fluconazole with progressive sinus or pulmonary disease by radiography should be considered to have a possible mold infection and receive empiric antifungal therapy directed (at minimum) against* Aspergillus *species.*[40]

LABORATORY DIAGNOSIS

Like other invasive mycoses, definitive diagnosis of aspergillosis requires histopathologic evidence of hyphal invasion in tissue (Fig. 84–3). However, procedures needed to establish a definitive diagnosis by sampling of suspicious lesions (e.g., fine-needle aspiration or thoracoscopic lung biopsy) are not feasible in many patients with underlying thrombocytopenia secondary to hematologic malignancies or chemotherapy. Even if hyphae are observed in tissue, histopathology alone cannot distinguish Aspergillus from other angioinvasive

septate molds, such as *Fusarium*, which have different patterns of antifungal susceptibility (see Table 84–1).[40] Therefore, respiratory and/or wound cultures (if cutaneous or sinus/hard palate lesions are present) are important factors in the modification of empiric antifungal therapy.

Respiratory cultures including sputum, bronchial washings, or bronchoalveolar lavage have a low sensitivity for diagnosis of IA but a high positive predictive value in immunocompromised patients.[40] Therefore, a negative bronchoalveolar lavage culture does not rule out invasive pulmonary aspergillosis, but a positive culture in a high-risk patient (e.g., allogeneic hematopoietic cell transplant patients) indicates pulmonary aspergillosis in at least 60% of such patients. Blood cultures have little diagnostic value for IA but may reflect true disease with *A. terreus*. Patients with limited lung involvement or on prophylactic or empiric antifungal therapy may continue to be culture-negative for *Aspergillus* species, despite the appearance of progressing disease.[40] Therefore, negative cultures are never the sole indication for stopping antifungal therapy in patients with suspected or proven aspergillosis.

Considerable effort has been focused in the last decade to develop non–culture-based laboratory methods (antigen detection, polymerase chain reaction [PCR], and antigen detection) for the diagnosis of IA. The hope is that these surrogate tests could detect early evidence of *Aspergillus* infection before significant target organ damage eventually detected by CT scans occurs. The FDA has approved an enzyme-linked immunosorbent assay (ELISA)–based assay for the detection of a polysaccharide component of the *Aspergillus* cell wall called galactomannan. Although several large prospective studies have found that the sensitivity and specificity of the assay exceeded 90% in neutropenic patients with hematologic malignancies, the median time span between galactomannan detection and clinical signs and symptoms of IA averages less than 6 days.[40] The sensitivity of the galactomannan may be enhanced if the test is performed on bronchial lavage fluid. Other factors such as patient immune status (neutropenia versus graft-versus-host disease), antibacterial therapy, and diet may affect the interpretation of the galactomannan test.[40] For example, false-positive results have been reported to be higher in the pediatric population, patients receiving piperacillin-tazobactam for neutropenic fever, and following the ingestion of certain cereals, pastas, nutritional supplements, or soy sauce.[40] Accumulating clinical data suggest that rising galactomannan levels are a harbinger of breakthrough infection, and declining galactomannan concentrations are an early indicator of response to treatment. However, antifungal therapy is rarely stopped in patients once the serum galactomannan becomes negative, especially in persistently immunosuppressed patients. Hence, the galactomannan test and other non–culture-based strategies, such as serum β-glucan, which can also be detected during *Aspergillus* infection, serve as complementary methods to confirm results from microbiologic, histopathologic, and radiographic investigations directed toward diagnosing IA.

TREATMENT

To date, only two comparative randomized controlled clinical trials have evaluated antifungal therapies for the treatment of diagnosis-proven IA, and only one study was sufficiently powered to measure differences in response to antifungal therapy.[43] In that study, unblinded investigators compared patients initially randomized to the newer triazole, voriconazole, with patients initially treated with amphotericin B deoxycholate.[43] The study design was unique in that it allowed a change from the randomized drug to any other licensed antifungal therapy, without requiring that the patient be classified as a treatment failure on randomized therapy. Nearly 80% of patients randomized to receive amphotericin B deoxycholate were switched to other licensed antifungal therapies (mean duration 10 days) versus 36% of patients in the voriconazole arm (mean duration 77 days). The poor tolerability of amphotericin B deoxycholate was not surprising given the relatively higher dosages (1 mg/kg/day IV) and prolonged treatment courses required in the treatment of IA. At the end of the study (12 weeks), a higher proportion of patients in the voriconazole arm remained alive (70.8%) compared with amphotericin B deoxycholate–treated patients (57.9%). On the basis of these results, many experts now consider voriconazole as the initial drug of choice for IA in patients without significant contraindications (e.g., drug interactions or preexisting liver dysfunction) to azole therapy (see Table 84–2).[40] Voriconazole also appears to have some efficacy in CNS aspergillosis, a form of IA with historical mortality rates approaching 100%. Itraconazole has activity against *Aspergillus* and is sometimes used as prophylaxis, but is not considered a particularly effective treatment option for invasive disease.[40]

Lipid formulations of amphotericin B, echinocandins, or posaconazole can be considered as possible alternatives to voriconazole therapy and may be preferred agents in patients with breakthrough infection on azole antifungals (including itraconazole or fluconazole). Several recent open-label case series have suggested that combination therapy, with an echinocandin and mold-active triazole such as voriconazole, may be more effective than voriconazole alone for patients with IA who have failed amphotericin B–based therapy.[40] An ongoing multicenter prospective trial comparing voriconazole monotherapy versus voriconazole plus anidulafungin should provide insights (if any) into the benefits of starting with combination regimens during the initial treatment of IA. Once antifungal therapy has begun, the duration and intensity of antifungal therapy is directed by host-specific factors, including clinical response, underlying immunosuppression, tolerability, and plans for future chemotherapy/immunosuppression. In the heavily immunocompromised patient, complete eradication of the fungus is unlikely, and suppressive therapy may be required until well after recovery of cellular immune function. Reactivation from residual infarcts or devitalized tissue in the sinus or lung harboring aspergillosis is a concern if the patient will receive further immunosuppressive therapy. Therefore, surgical debridement of the sinus or excision of large lung lesions is often pursued if the patient is not profoundly thrombocytopenic. Relapsing or breakthrough *Aspergillus* infections respond less favorably to antifungal therapy than de novo IA and may require more aggressive measures (combination therapy, immunotherapy, or surgery) to stabilize the infection.

PROPHYLAXIS

Although recently published guidelines for preventing opportunistic infections in hematopoietic cell transplant recipients do not provide concrete recommendations for antifungal prophylaxis against *Aspergillus*, prophylaxis should be considered in certain high-risk subgroups with rates of IA exceeding 10%. These groups include (a) patients with prolonged pre-engraftment periods (e.g., cord-blood transplant recipients), (b) patients with a history of IA prior to transplantation, (c) patients receiving transplants with a high risk of graft-versus-host disease (e.g., haploidentical allogeneic transplant) or infection (e.g., T-cell–depleted transplant), any patient with graft-versus-host disease on high-dose corticosteroid therapy (greater than 1 mg/kg prednisone equivalent) with or without antithymocyte globulin or tumor necrosis factor blockade (i.e., infliximab), and (d) any transplant recipient with active cytomegalovirus disease, which is associated with an increased risk of subsequent mold infections due to the immunosuppressive effects of the virus. Posaconazole was shown in two prospective randomized trials to reduce *Aspergillus*-associated death in patients with acute high-risk leukemia and reduce mold infections in patients with graft-versus-host disease following hematopoietic stem cell transplantation.[33,34] Similar data are available for voriconazole,[35] but less benefit was observed versus standard fluconazole prophylaxis plus intensive galactomannan monitoring in the hematopoietic stem cell transplant patients. Prophylactic approaches, however, are often institution and patient specific.

PATIENT MONITORING

Response to antifungal therapy in invasive molds is slow and difficult to judge by clinical signs alone. Resolution of fever and eventual clearing of CT scans (in the case of lung infections) are indications of response to antifungal therapy. Toxicity associated with antifungal therapy is similar in these patients as in those described earlier. In addition to the adverse effects mentioned earlier, voriconazole may cause transient visual changes (photopsia) in approximately one-third of patients with the first few doses of therapy. Occasionally, these visual disturbances are accompanied by hallucinations and may require discontinuation of therapy. The risk of phototoxic reactions and cutaneous malignancies with voriconazole is of special concern in transplant patients, who are often receiving calcineurin inhibitors that increase the risk for secondary malignancies. Voriconazole and posaconazole exhibit wide intrapatient and interpatient pharmacokinetic variability due to variable absorption and metabolism, respectively.[44,45] Therefore, many experts advocate therapeutic drug monitoring in patients with documented disease receiving the drugs as monotherapy, or in patients with suspected breakthrough infection (voriconazole, posaconazole) or toxicities (voriconazole) while on therapy (see Table 84–3).[40,44–46] Patients who develop breakthrough infections on voriconazole should also undergo a careful clinical workup for other invasive mold pathogens such as mucormycosis (see Table 84–1), which are not susceptible to voriconazole. In most cases, antifungal therapy may be continued until immunosuppression has resolved.

Abbreviations Introduced in This Chapter

AIDS	Acquired immunodeficiency syndrome
ARDS	Acute respiratory distress syndrome
CNS	Central nervous system
CSF	Cerebrospinal fluid
CrCl	Estimated creatinine clearance
CT	Computed tomography
CYP	Cytochrome P-450 isoenzyme
ELISA	Enzyme-linked immunosorbent assay
FISH	Fluorescent in situ hybridization
HAART	Highly active antiretroviral therapy
HRCT	High-resolution computed tomography
IA	Invasive aspergillosis
ICU	Intensive care unit
IRIS	Immune Reconstitution Inflammatory Syndrome
IV	Intravenous
NIAID	National Institute of Allergy and Infectious Diseases
PCP	*Pneumocystis jiroveci (carinii)* pneumonia
PCR	Polymerase chain reaction
PO	Oral

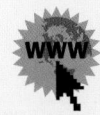 Self-assessment questions and answers are available at *http://mhpharmacotherapy.com/pp.html*.

REFERENCES

1. Wheat LJ, Freifeld AG, Kleiman MB, et al. Clinical practice guidelines for the management of patients with histoplasmosis: 2007 update by the Infectious Diseases Society of America. Clin Infect Dis 2007;45:807–825.
2. Wheat LJ, Kauffman CA. Histoplasmosis. Infect Dis Clin North Am 2003;17:1–19.
3. Pappas PG. Blastomycosis. Semin Respir Crit Care Med 2004;25:113–121.
4. Galgiani JN, Ampel NM, Blair JE, et al. Coccidioidomycosis. Clin Infect Dis 2005;41:1217–1223.
5. Romani L. Immunity to fungal infections. Nat Rev Immunol 2004;4:11–23.
6. Chapman SW, Dismukes WE, Proia LA, et al. Clinical practice guidelines for the management of blastomycosis: 2008 update by the Infectious Diseases Society of America. Clin Infect Dis 2008;46:1801–1812.
7. Lortholary O, Denning DW, Dupont B. Endemic mycoses: A treatment update. J Antimicrob Chemother 1999;43:321–331.
8. Brüggemann RJM, Alffenaar JC, Blijlevens NMA, et al. Clinical relevance of the pharmacokinetic interactions of azole antifungal drugs with other coadministered agents. Clin Infect Dis 2009;48:1441–1458.

9. Todd JR, Arigala MR, Penn RL, King JW. Possible clinically significant interaction of itraconazole plus rifampin. AIDS Patient Care STDS 2001;15:505–510.
10. Nicolau DP, Crowe HM, Nightingale CH, Quintiliani R. Rifampin-fluconazole interaction in critically ill patients. Ann Pharmacother 1995;29:994–996.
11. Gubbins PO, McConnell SA, Penzak SR. Antifungal agents. In: Piscitelli SC, Rodvold KA, eds. Drug Interactions in Infectious Diseases. Totowa, NJ: Humana Press; 2001.
12. Dodds-Ashley E, Lewis RE, Lewis JS II, et al. Pharmacology of systemic antifungal agents. Clin Infect Dis 2006;43(Suppl 1):S28–S39.
13. Johnson PC, Wheat LJ, Cloud GA, et al. Safety and efficacy of liposomal amphotericin B compared with conventional amphotericin B for induction therapy of histoplasmosis in patients with AIDS. Ann Intern Med 2002;137:105–109.
14. Groll AH, Giri N, Petraitis V, et al. Comparative efficacy and distribution of lipid formulations of amphotericin B in experimental Candida albicans infection of the central nervous system. J Infect Dis 2000;182:274–282.
15. Wisplinghoff H, Seifert H, Wenzel RP, Edmond MB. Current trends in the epidemiology of nosocomial bloodstream infections in patients with hematological malignancies and solid neoplasms in hospitals in the United States. Clin Infect Dis 2003;36:1103–1110.
16. Rex JH, Bennett JE, Sugar AM, et al. A randomized trial comparing fluconazole with amphotericin B for the treatment of candidemia in patients without neutropenia. N Engl J Med 1994;331:1325–1330.
17. Pappas PG, Rex JH, Sobel JD, et al. Guidelines for treatment of candidiasis. Clin Infect Dis 2004;38:161–189.
18. Rex JH, Pfaller MA, Walsh TJ, et al. Antifungal susceptibility testing: Practical aspects and current challenges. Clin Microbiol Rev 2001;14:643–658.
19. Pfaller MA, Moet GJ, Messer SA, et al. *Candida* bloodstream infections: Comparison of species distribution and antifungal resistance patterns in community-onset and nosocomial infections in the SENTRY Antimicrobial Surveillance Program 2008–2009. Antimicrob Agent Chemother 2011;55:561–566.
20. Pfaller MA, Castanheira M, Messer SA, et al. Variation in the *Candida* spp. distribution and antifungal resistance rates among bloodstream infections isolates by patient age: report from the SENTRY Antimicrobial Surveillance Program 2008–2009. Diagn Microbiol Infect Dis 2010;68:278–283.
21. Mora-Duarte J, Betts R, Rotstein R, et al. Comparison of caspofungin and amphotericin B for invasive candidiasis. N Engl J Med 2002;347:2020–2029.
22. Kullberg BJ, Sobel JD, Ruhnke M, et al. Voriconazole versus a regimen of amphotericin B followed by fluconazole for candidaemia in non-neutropenic patients: A randomised non-inferiority trial. Lancet 2005;366:1435–1442.
23. Kuse E, Chetchotisakd P, da Cunha C, et al. Micafungin versus liposomal amphotericin B for candidemia and invasive candidiasis: A phase III randomized double-blind trial. Lancet 2007;369:1519–1527.
24. Pappas P, Kauffman CA, Andes DA, et al. Clinical Practice Guidelines for the Management of Candidiasis: 2009 Update by the Infectious Diseases Society of America. Clin Infect Dis 2009;48:503–535.
25. Morrell M, Fraser V, Kollef M. Delaying the empiric treatment of Candida bloodstream infection until positive blood culture results are obtained: A potential risk factor for hospital mortality. Antimicrob Agent Chemother 2005;49:3640–3645.
26. Freifeld AG, Bow EJ, Sepkowitz KA, et al. Clinical practice guidelines for the use of antimicrobial agents in neutropenic patients with cancer. Clin Infect Dis 2011;52:e56–e93.
27. Goodman JL, Winston DJ, Greenfield RA, et al. A controlled trial of fluconazole to prevent fungal infections in patients undergoing bone marrow transplantation. N Engl J Med 1992;326:845–851.
28. Winston DJ, Chandrasekar PH, Lazarus HM, et al. Fluconazole prophylaxis of fungal infections in patients with acute leukemia. Results of a randomized placebo-controlled, double-blind, multicenter trial. Ann Intern Med 1993;118:495–503.
29. Slavin MA, Osborne B, Adams R, et al. Efficacy and safety of fluconazole prophylaxis for fungal infections after bone marrow transplantation—a prospective, randomized, double-blind study. J Infect Dis 1995;171:1545–1552.

30. Winston DJ, Maziarz RT, Chandrasekar PH, et al. Intravenous and oral itraconazole versus intravenous and oral fluconazole for long-term antifungal prophylaxis in allogeneic hematopoietic stem-cell transplant recipients—a multicenter, randomized trial. Ann Intern Med 2003;138:705–713.

31. Van Burik J, Ratanatharathorn V, Lipton J, et al. Randomized, double-blind trial of micafungin versus fluconazole for prophylaxis of invasive fungal infections in patients undergoing hematopoietic stem cell transplant. Clin Infect Dis 2004;39:1407–1416.

32. Cornely O, Maertens J, Winston D, et al. Posaconazole versus fluconazole or itraconazole prophylaxis in patients with neutropenia. N Engl J Med 1007;356:348–359.

33. Ullman A, Lipton J, Vesole D, et al. Posaconazole or fluconazole for prophylaxis in severe graft versus host disease. N Engl J Med 2007;356:335–347.

34. Wingard J, Carter S, Walsh T, et al. Randomized, double-blind trial of fluconazole versus voriconazole for prevention of invasive fungal infection after allogeneic hematopoietic cell transplantation. Blood 2010;116:5111–5118.

35. Pelz RK, Hendrix CW, Swoboda SM, et al. Double-blind placebo-controlled trial of fluconazole to prevent candidal infections in critically ill surgical patients. Ann Surg 2001;233:542–548.

36. Rex JH, Sobel JD. Prophylactic antifungal therapy in the intensive care unit. Clin Infect Dis 2001;32:1191–1200.

37. Shuster M, Edward J, Sobel J, et al. Empirical fluconazole versus placebo for intensive care unit patients: A randomized trial. Ann Intern Med 2008;149:83–90.

38. Perfect JR, Dismukes WE, Dromer F, et al. Clinical practice guidelines for the management of cryptococcal disease. Clin Infect Dis 2010;50:291–322.

39. Walsh TJ, Anaissie EJ, Denning DW, et al. Treatment of aspergillosis: Clinical Practice Guidelines of the Infectious Diseases Society of America. Clin Infect Dis 2008;46:327–360.

40. Caillot D, Mannone L, Cuisenier B, Couaillier JF. Role of early diagnosis and aggressive surgery in the management of invasive pulmonary aspergillosis in neutropenic patients. Clin Microbiol Infect 2001;7:54–61.

41. Caillot D, Casasnovas O, Bernard A, et al. Improved management of invasive pulmonary aspergillosis in neutropenic patients using early thoracic computed tomographic scan and surgery. J Clin Oncol 1997;15:139–147.

42. Herbrecht R, Denning DW, Patterson TF, et al. Voriconazole versus amphotericin B for the primary treatment of aspergillosis. N Engl J Med 2002;347:408–415.

43. Walsh T, Raad I, Patterson T, et al. Treatment of invasive aspergillosis with posaconazole in patients who are refractory to or intolerant of conventional therapy: An externally controlled trial. Clin Infect Dis 2007;44:2–12.

44. Pascual A, Calandra T, Bolay S. Voriconazole therapeutic drug monitoring in patients with invasive mycoses improves safety and efficacy outcomes. Clin Infect Dis 2007;46:201–211.

45. Andes DA, Pascual A, Marchetti O. Antifungal therapeutic drug monitoring: established and emerging indications. Antimicrob Agent Chemother 2009;53:24–34.

85 Antimicrobial Prophylaxis in Surgery

Mary A. Ullman and John C. Rotschafer

LEARNING OBJECTIVES

● **Upon completion of the chapter, the reader will be able to:**

1. Discuss the epidemiology and impact of surgical site infections (SSIs) on patient outcomes and healthcare costs.

2. Name and differentiate the four different types of wound classifications.

3. Recognize at least three risk factors for postoperative SSIs.

4. Identify likely pathogens associated with different surgical operations.

5. Compare and contrast antimicrobials used for surgical prophylaxis and identify potential advantage and disadvantages for each antibiotic.

6. Discuss the importance of β-lactam allergy screening and how this could impact resistance and healthcare costs.

7. Identify nonantimicrobial methods that can reduce the risk of postoperative infection.

8. Discuss the possible impact of antimicrobial-impregnated bone cement and how this affects the use of antimicrobial prophylaxis in surgery.

9. Discuss the importance of timing, duration, and redosing in relation to antimicrobial prophylaxis in surgery.

10. Recommend appropriate prophylactic antimicrobial(s) given a surgical operation.

KEY CONCEPTS

❶ Surgical site infections (SSIs) are a significant cause of morbidity and mortality.

❷ The distinction between prophylaxis and treatment influences the choice of antimicrobial and duration of therapy.

❸ Surgical operations are classified as clean, clean-contaminated, contaminated, or dirty.

❹ Choosing the appropriate prophylactic antimicrobial relies on anticipating which organisms are likely to be encountered during the operation.

❺ A thorough drug allergy history should be taken to discern true drug allergy (anaphylaxis) from other adverse events (stomach upset).

❻ For prevention of SSIs, correct timing of antimicrobial administration is imperative so as to allow the persistence of therapeutic concentrations in the blood and wound tissues during the entire course of the operation.

❼ The goal of antimicrobial dosing for surgical prophylaxis is to optimize the pharmacodynamic

parameter of the selected agent against the suspected organism for the duration of the operation.

❽ The duration of antimicrobial prophylaxis should not exceed 24 hours (48 hours for cardiac surgery); additional doses of antimicrobial past this time point do not demonstrate added benefits.

❾ According to Centers for Disease Control and Prevention criteria, SSIs may appear up to 30 days after an operation and up to 1 year if a prosthesis is implanted.

❶ *Surgical site infections (SSIs) are a significant cause of morbidity and mortality.* Approximately 2% to 5% of patients undergoing clean **extra-abdominal** operations and 20% undergoing **intra-abdominal** operations will develop an SSI.[1] SSIs have become the second most common cause of nosocomial infection, and these data are likely underestimated.[1] More than 70% of surgical procedures are now performed on an outpatient basis, creating a significant potential for under-reporting.[2]

SSIs negatively affect patient outcomes and increase health-care costs. Patients who develop SSIs are five times more likely to be readmitted to the hospital and have twice the mortality of patients who do not develop an SSI.[1] A patient with an SSI is also 60% more likely to be admitted to an ICU.[1] SSIs increase lengths of hospital stay and costs.[1,3,4] The type of SSI can also affect the severity of a patient's negative outcome due to surgery. Deep SSIs, involving organs or spaces, result in longer durations of hospital stay and higher costs compared with SSIs that are limited to the incision.[5] Additionally, since 2008, Medicare and Medicaid Services no longer reimburses the hospitals for any cost incurred from treating certain hospital-acquired infections, including SSIs.[6] Thus, even greater importance is placed on preventing infection, and, if infection should occur, treatment of the infection should be for the shortest duration possible and in the most cost-effective manner.

SSIs are defined and reported according to Centers for Disease Control and Prevention (CDC) criteria.[5] SSIs are classified as either incisional or organ/space. Incisional SSIs are further divided into superficial incisional SSI (skin or subcutaneous tissue) and deep incisional SSI (deeper soft tissues of the incision). Organ/space SSIs involve any anatomic site other than the incised areas. For example, a patient who develops meningitis after removal of a brain tumor could be classified as having an organ/space SSI. An infection is considered as SSI if any of the above criteria is met and the infection occurs within 30 days of the operation. If a prosthetic is implanted, the timeline extends out to 1 year.

EPIDEMIOLOGY AND ETIOLOGY

Numerous **risk factors** for SSIs have been identified in the literature.[5,7,8] These factors can be divided into two categories: patient and operative characteristics. Patient risk factors for SSI include age, comorbid disease states (especially chronic lung disease and diabetes), malnutrition, immunosuppression, nicotine or steroid use, and colonization of the nares with *Staphylococcus aureus*. Many patients developing postoperative wound infections bring the organism with them into the hospital. Modifying risk factors may decrease the threat of SSI. Malnutrition can be corrected using enteral or parenteral feedings. Additional nonantimicrobial strategies to reduce SSIs will be discussed later.

Operative characteristics are based on the actions of both the patient and the operating staff. Shaving of the surgical site prior to operating can produce microscopic lacerations and increase the chance of SSI and is, therefore, not accepted as a method of hair removal.[5] Maintaining aseptic technique and proper sterilization of medical equipment is effective in preventing SSI. Surgical staff should wash their hands thoroughly. In clean surgeries, most bacterial inoculums introduced postoperatively are generally small. However, subsequent patient contact between contaminated areas (nares or rectum) and the surgical site can lead to SSI. Finally, the appropriate use of **antimicrobial prophylaxis** can have a significant impact on decreasing SSIs.

PATHOPHYSIOLOGY

Prophylaxis Versus Treatment

Properly identifying the state of an infection is important when using antimicrobial prophylaxis in surgery. Antibiotic prophylaxis begins with the premise that no infection exists but that during surgery there can be a low-level inoculum of bacteria introduced into the body. However, if sufficient antimicrobial concentrations are present, the situation can be controlled without infection developing. This is the case when surgery is done under controlled conditions, there are no major breaks in sterile technique or spillage of GI contents, and perforation or damage to the surgical site is absent. An example would be an elective hysterectomy done with optimal surgical technique.

If an infection is already present, or presumed to be present, then antimicrobial use is for treatment, not prophylaxis, and the goal is to eliminate the infection. This is the case when there is spillage of GI contents, gross damage or perforation is already present, or the tissue being operated on is actively infected (pus is present and cultures are positive). An example would be a patient undergoing surgery for a ruptured appendix with diffuse peritonitis.

❷ *The distinction between prophylaxis and treatment influences the choice of antimicrobial and duration of therapy.* Appropriate antimicrobial selection, dosing, and duration of therapy differ significantly between these two situations. A regimen for antimicrobial prophylaxis ideally involves one agent and lasts less than 24 hours. Treatment regimens can involve multiple antimicrobials with durations lasting weeks to months depending on desired antimicrobial coverage and the surgical site.

Types of Surgical Operations

❸ *Surgical operations are classified at the time of operation as clean, clean-contaminated, contaminated, or dirty.* Antimicrobial prophylaxis is appropriate for clean, clean-contaminated, and contaminated operations. Dirty operations take place in situations of existing infection and antimicrobials are used for treatment, not prophylaxis (Table 85–1).

Microbiology

❹ *Choosing the appropriate prophylactic antimicrobial relies on anticipating which organisms will be encountered during the operation.* SSIs associated with extra-abdominal operations are the result of skin flora organisms in nearly all cases. These organisms include gram-positive cocci, with *S. aureus* and *Staphylococcus epidermidis* being among the most frequently isolated SSI pathogens according to the National Nosocomial Infections Surveillance System (NNIS)[5] (Table 85–2). *Streptococcus* spp. and other gram-positive aerobes may also be implicated.

Intra-abdominal operations involve a diverse flora with the potential for polymicrobial SSIs. *Escherichia coli* make up a large portion of bowel flora and are frequently isolated as pathogens according to the NNIS.[5] Other enteric

---

Table 85–1

National Red Cross Wound Classification, Risk of SSI, and Antibiotic Indication

Classification	Description	SSI Risk	Antibiotic Prophylaxis
Clean	No acute inflammation or transection of GI, oropharyngeal, GU, biliary, or respiratory tracts; elective case, no technique break	Low	Indicated
Clean-contaminated	Controlled opening of aforementioned tracts with minimal spillage or minor technique break; clean procedures performed emergently or with major technique breaks	Medium	Indicated
Contaminated	Acute, nonpurulent inflammation present; major spillage or technique break during clean-contaminated procedures	High	Indicated
Dirty	Obvious preexisting infection present (abscess, pus, or necrotic tissue present)	—	Not indicated; antibiotics used for treatment

GU, genitourinary.

From Refs. 7 and 9.

---

gram-negative bacteria, as well as anaerobes (especially *Bacteroides* spp.), may be encountered during intra-abdominal operations.

Candida albicans is being implicated as the cause of a growing number of SSIs. According to the NNIS, from 1991 to 1995, the incidence of fungal SSIs rose from 0.1 to 0.3 per 1,000 discharges.[5] Increased use of broad-spectrum antimicrobials and rising prevalence of immunocompromised and human immunodeficiency virus-infected individuals are factors in fungal SSIs. Despite this increase, antifungal prophylaxis for surgery is not currently recommended.

Table 85–2

Major Pathogens in Surgical Wound Infections

Pathogen	Percentage of Infections[a]
Staphylococcus aureus	20
Coagulase-negative staphylococci	14
Enterococci	12
Escherichia coli	8
Pseudomonas aeruginosa	8
Enterobacter spp.	7
Proteus mirabilis	3
Klebsiella pneumoniae	3
Other *Streptococcus* spp.	3
Candida albicans	3
Group D streptococci	2
Other gram-positive aerobes	2
Bacteroides fragilis	2

[a]Data reported by the NNIS from 1990 to 1996, adapted from National Academy of the Sciences National Research Council. Postoperative wound infections: The influence of ultraviolet irradiation of the operating room and of various other factors. Ann Surg 1984;160:32–135.

From Kanji S, Devlin JW. Antimicrobial prophylaxis in surgery. In: DiPiro JT, Talbert RL, Yee GC, et al. (eds.) Pharmacotherapy: A Pathophysiologic Approach. 6th ed. New York: McGraw-Hill; 2005: 2219; With permission.

Choosing an Antibiotic

An antimicrobial used in surgical prophylaxis should meet certain criteria. Selecting an antimicrobial with a spectrum that covers expected pathogens is crucial. The antimicrobial should be inexpensive, available in a parenteral formulation, and easy to use. Adverse-event potential should be minimal. Choosing an agent with a longer half-life reduces the likely need to redose unless the surgical procedure is prolonged.

Operations can be separated into two basic categories: extra-abdominal and intra-abdominal. SSIs resulting from extra-abdominal operations are frequently caused by gram-positive aerobes. Thus an antimicrobial with strong gram-positive coverage is useful. Cefazolin provides a benign adverse-event profile, simple dosing, and low cost, making cefazolin the mainstay for surgical prophylaxis of extra-abdominal procedures. For patients with a β-lactam allergy, clindamycin or vancomycin can be used as an alternative.

Intra-abdominal operations necessitate broad-spectrum coverage of gram-negative organisms and anaerobes. Anti-anaerobic cephalosporins, cefoxitin and cefotetan, are widely used. Fluoroquinolones or aminoglycosides, paired with clindamycin or metronidazole, should provide adequate coverage for intra-abdominal operations; these regimens are recommended as appropriate regimens for use in patients with β-lactam allergies.

The Hospital Infection Control Practices Advisory Committee allows for the use of vancomycin for surgical prophylaxis when methicillin-resistant *S. aureus* (MRSA) rates at an institution are "high."[1] Unfortunately, a "high" rate of MRSA has not been standardized. Additionally, vancomycin use in institutions where MRSA rates are "high" may not translate into a lower incidence of SSI. Finkelstein and associates found that the incidence of SSI for patients on cefazolin or vancomycin did not differ despite a high MRSA rate at the study institution. However, patients who received cefazolin were more likely to develop an SSI due to MRSA.[10] The increasing prevalence of community-associated methicillin-resistant *S. aureus* (CA-MRSA) in patients admitted to the hospital creates an added concern, although this pathogen is often sensitive to clindamycin. Vancomycin should be considered appropriate surgical prophylaxis for those patients identified as being colonized with MRSA (prior to or at admission).[1]

Due to antimicrobial shortages of the recommended antimicrobials and development of newer antimicrobials (e.g., carbapenems, third- and fourth-generation cephalosporins, and antipseudomonal penicillins), some interest has been generated in the use of these newer antimicrobials for surgical prophylaxis. Ertapenem was superior to standard cefotetan in the prevention of SSIs after elective colorectal surgery.[11] However, the ertapenem treatment group had a larger proportion of *Clostridium difficile* infections than those in the cefotetan treatment group. Ertapenem has been included as an approved antibiotic for colon surgery.[12] At this time, it is not considered appropriate to use these newer antimicrobials for surgical prophylaxis; overuse of these antimicrobials may contribute to collateral damage and the development of bacterial resistance. Further research is needed before any of these newer agents are routinely used for surgical prophylaxis. New guidelines are likely to be published soon and may offer guidance on the use of newer antimicrobials.

β-Lactam Allergy

Allergy to β-lactams such as penicillin is one of the most common reported drug allergies. Concerns over cross-reactivity may limit the use of β-lactams for surgical prophylaxis. ❺ *A thorough drug allergy history should be taken to discern true allergy (e.g., anaphylaxis) from adverse event (e.g., stomach upset).* Allergy testing may be helpful in confirming a patient's penicillin allergy and could spare vancomycin. However, practitioners should be aware allergy testing may be difficult to perform due to the removal of a major component (penicilloyl-polylysine) of the testing from the commercial market.[13] If a practitioner desires to perform allergy testing, the individual reagents required for penicillin allergy testing must be prepared at the healthcare facility, on a case-by-case basis. Cross-allergenicity between penicillin and cephalosporins is low. The increased risk of cephalosporin allergy in patients with a history of penicillin allergy may be as low as 0.4% for first-generation cephalosporins and nearly zero for second- and third-generation agents.[14] Other studies also found the risk of cross-reactivity to be very low.[15] However, in the case of severe penicillin allergy (anaphylaxis), cephalosporins should be avoided.

Alternative Methods to Decrease SSI

Several nonantimicrobial methods have been studied for reducing the risk of SSI.[16] Providing supplemental warming to patients (36.7°C [98°F]) during the intraoperative period reduced infection rates compared with control patients (34.7°C [94.5°F]).[17] Intensive glucose control (maintaining blood glucose to 80 to 110 mg/dL [4.4 to 6.1 mmol/L]) versus conventional control (blood glucose less than 220 mg/dL [less than 12.2 mmol/L]) reduced infections and improved outcomes in cardiac patients who received intensive insulin

control in the ICU after surgery.[18] Also, patients randomized to 80% (0.80) inspired oxygen had lower SSI rates compared with patients on 30% (0.30) oxygen after colorectal resection.[19] Despite these findings, there are insufficient data to make definitive recommendations on the use of these therapies.

Antimicrobial-impregnated bone cement is being used as an adjunct or alternative to traditional antimicrobial prophylaxis for orthopedic operations. Cefuroxime-impregnated cement lowered the risk of deep infection after primary total knee arthoplasty.[20] Other studies have been inconclusive regarding superiority of antimicrobial-impregnated bone cement versus conventional therapies.[21] Confounding this issue is the lack of standards regarding antimicrobial-impregnated cements. An array of drugs, from aminoglycosides to macrolides, is used in these preparations. Some cements are produced commercially, whereas others are made in the operating room. The long-term durability of impregnated cements is also unknown, as the addition of antimicrobials may reduce the tensile strength of bone cement. Further study is needed before antimicrobial-impregnated bone cements can be recommended as an alternative to preoperative prophylaxis with traditional antimicrobials.

Antimicrobial irrigation may also be encountered in the surgical arena as an adjunct or alternative to traditional parenteral antimicrobial prophylaxis. Irrigation of wounds allows debris removal as well as an additional way to lessen bacterial contamination simply by dislodging, diluting, or evacuating possible microbes. However, as with the antimicrobial bone cement, evidence is mixed on the advantages of using this approach. Irrigation with detergent solutions, rather than antimicrobials, appears to provide the same results but with less wound-healing problems encountered with antimicrobial irrigation.[22] Additionally, because antimicrobial irrigation solutions are not commercially available, irrigants are often made in the operation rooms, allowing for the possibility of higher than or lower than desired concentrations. If concentrations are higher than desired, local chemical irritation may occur as well as systemic absorption and toxicity. If concentrations fall below desired targets, development of resistant organisms may occur. Further study is required before antimicrobial irrigation is recommended for use in surgical prophylaxis.

With the increase of CA-MRSA, increased importance has been placed on screening for *S. aureus,* especially MRSA and decolonization. Surgical patients with nasal colonization of *S. aureus* have a higher risk of an SSI due to *S. aureus,* and decolonization leads to a lower incidence of SSIs.[23–25] However, although this evidence may imply the opportunity for some real benefits in the surgical population, a clear consensus on how the nasal colonization should be approached has not been reached. British guidelines recommend an attempt at decolonization for patients undergoing planned surgical procedures to minimize the risk of infection.[26] Harbarth and colleagues suggest that MRSA screening should be targeted to patients undergoing elective surgical procedures that have a high risk of MRSA infection. In addition, each hospital's infection control team, along with the surgical team, should analyze their patient population and MRSA epidemiology to appropriately select screening guidelines,[27] keeping in mind state and federal statutes regarding the use of active surveillance cultures. Screening methods that utilize rapid, polymerase chain reaction (PCR)–based testing may provide an advantage in quickly identifying colonized patients and allowing decolonization to occur prior to surgery.

The most studied approach to eradication of methicillin-sensitive *S. aureus* (MSSA) and/or MRSA has been mupirocin applied to the anterior nares for 5 days prior to surgery.[28] Additionally, skin decolonization with 4% chlorhexidine for 5 days prior to surgery has also been recommended. Although decolonization of the anterior nares is the most common and most studied, some controversy exists because patients may be colonized elsewhere (rectum, throat, vagina, etc.) and often do not receive complete decolonization.[28] Furthermore, decolonization usually does not lead to life-long eradication. Other drugs, both topical and systemic, have been studied for decolonization/eradication of MRSA, but a review of randomized controlled trials for the eradication of MRSA found insufficient evidence for the use of any agent for eradication of MRSA.[29] In one study, surgical patients were assessed for nasal colonization by *S. aureus*. A significantly lower incidence of infections was demonstrated in patients who were colonized with *S. aureus* and completed a 5-day treatment of intranasal mupirocin twice daily and chlorhexidine wash daily. Although no MRSA infections were noted in the patients included in this study, the authors suggest that this treatment strategy would be beneficial in MRSA-colonized patients as long as those strains were susceptible to mupirocin. Although MRSA screening has gained more acceptance, less than 10% of centers screen for mupirocin and/or chlorhexidine resistance.[31] Mupirocin resistance rates have varied from 1.9 to 5.6% of *S. aureus* isolates.[32] Further studies are needed to elucidate this area of surgical prophylaxis, including cost-effectiveness.

Principles of Antimicrobial Prophylaxis

▶ Route of Administration

IV antimicrobial administration is the most common delivery method for surgical prophylaxis. IV administration ensures complete bioavailability while minimizing the impact of patient-specific variables. Oral administration is also used in some bowel operations. Nonabsorbable compounds such as erythromycin base and neomycin are given up to 24 hours prior to surgery to cleanse the bowel. Note that oral agents are used adjunctively and do not replace IV agents.

▶ Timing of First Dose

6 *For prevention of SSIs, correct timing of antimicrobial administration is imperative so as to allow the persistence of therapeutic concentrations in the blood and wound tissues during the entire course of the operation.* The National Surgical Infection Prevention Project recommends infusing antimicrobials for surgical prophylaxis within 60 minutes of the first incision. Exceptions to this rule are fluoroquinolones and vancomycin, which can be infused 120 minutes prior to avoid

infusion-related reactions.[1] No consensus has been reached on whether the infusion should be complete prior to the first incision. However, if a proximal tourniquet is used, antimicrobial administration should be complete prior to inflation.

Administration of the antimicrobial should begin as close to the first incision as possible. This is important for antimicrobials with short half-lives so that therapeutic concentrations are maintained during the operation and reduce the need for redosing. Beginning the antimicrobial infusion after the first incision is of little value in preventing SSI. Administration of the antimicrobial after the first incision had SSI rates similar to patients who did not receive prophylaxis.[33]

▶ Dosing and Redosing

7 *The goal of antimicrobial dosing for surgical prophylaxis is to optimize the pharmacodynamic parameter of the selected agent against the suspected organism for the duration of the operation.* Dosing recommendations can vary between institutions and guidelines. Clinical judgment should be exercised regarding dose modifications for renal function, age, and especially weight. Obese patients often require higher doses than do nonobese patients.[1] Morbidly obese patients (body mass index greater than 40 kg/m²) who received 2 g of cefazolin had a lower incidence of SSI compared with patients receiving 1 g.[34] An advisory statement from the National Surgical Infection Prevention Project suggested that for patients weighing less than 80 kg, cefazolin should be dosed at 1 g; patients who weigh 80 kg or more should receive 2 g of cefazolin for adequate prophylaxis.[1]

If an operation exceeds two half-lives of the selected antimicrobial, then another dose should be administered.[1] Repeat dosing reduces rates of SSI. For example, cefazolin has a half-life of about 2 hours, thus another dose should be given if the operation exceeds 4 hours. The clinician should have extra doses of antimicrobial ready in case an operation lasts longer than planned.

▶ Duration

The National Surgical Infection Prevention Project and published evidence suggest that the continuation of antimicrobial prophylaxis beyond wound closure is unnecessary.[1] **8** *The duration of antimicrobial prophylaxis should not exceed 24 hours (48 hours for cardiac surgery); additional doses of antimicrobial past this time point do not demonstrate added benefits. Longer durations of antimicrobial prophylaxis are advocated by some guidelines and will be discussed later.*

TREATMENT

Antimicrobial Prophylaxis in Specific Surgical Procedures

▶ Gynecologic and Obstetric

Enteric gram-negative bacilli, anaerobes, group B streptococci, and enterococci are all possible pathogens that may be encountered in gynecologic or obstetric surgeries. For

Table 85–3

Recommended Regimens for Antimicrobial Prophylaxis of Specific Surgical Procedures[a]

Type of Operation	Recommended Prophylaxis Regimen	Alternative Regimen
Vascular	Cefazolin 1–2 g IV every 8 hours for a total of 24 hours *or* cefuroxime 1.5 g IV × 1, then 750 mg every 8 hours for a total of 24 hours	Clindamycin 600–900 mg IV every 6 hours for a total of 24 hours *or* vancomycin 1 g IV every 8–12 hours for a total of 24 hours
Neurosurgery	Cefazolin 1–2 g IV every 8 hours for a total of 24 hours	Vancomycin 1 g IV every 8–12 hours for a total of 24 hours
Head and neck	Cefazolin 1–2 g IV every 8 hours for a total of 24 hours	Clindamycin 600–900 mg IV every 6 hours for a total of 24 hours
Urologic	Cefazolin 1–2 g IV × 1	Ciprofloxacin 400 mg IV × 1
Cesarean section	Cefazolin 1–2 g IV × 1	See hysterectomy
Hysterectomy	Cefotetan 1 g IV × 1, cefazolin 1–2 g IV × 1, cefoxitin 1–2 g IV × 1	Antianaerobic agent (metronidazole 0.5–1 g IV × 1 *or* clindamycin 600–900 mg IV × 1 combined with gentamicin 1.5 mg/kg IV × 1, aztreonam 1–2 g IV × 1, *or* ciprofloxacin 400 mg IV × 1) Ampicillin/sulbactam 3 g IV × 1
Gastroduodenal (high-risk only: obstruction, acid suppression, morbid obesity, hemorrhage, malignancy)	Cefazolin 1–2 g IV × 1	Ciprofloxacin 400 mg IV × 1
Biliary tract (high-risk only: age greater than 70 years, acute cholecystitis, obstructive jaundice, duct stones, nonfunctioning gallbladder)	Cefazolin 1–2 g IV × 1 *or* cefoxitin 1–2 g IV × 1	Ciprofloxacin 400 mg IV × 1
Colorectal	[b]Oral: neomycin 1 g plus erythromycin base 1 g (give 19, 18, and 9 hours prior to procedure) IV: cefoxitin 1–2 g × 1	Cefazolin 1–2 g IV plus metronidazole 0.5–1 g IV × 1 *or* hysterectomy regimens Ertapenem 1 g × 1
Appendectomy	Cefoxitin 1–2 g IV × 1; cefotetan 1 g IV × 1	Metronidazole 0.5–1 g IV *plus* gentamicin 1.5 mg/kg IV × 1
Orthopedic	Cefazolin 1–2 g IV every 8 hours for a total of 24 hours	Vancomycin 1 g IV every 12 hours *or* clindamycin 600–900 mg IV q 6 h
Cardiothoracic	Cefazolin 1–2 g IV every 8 hours for a total of 48 hours *or* cefuroxime 1.5 g IV every 12 hours for a total of 48 hours	Vancomycin 1 g IV every 12 hours for a total of 48 hours *or* clindamycin 600–900 mg IV every 6 hours

[a]Dosing recommendations are based on common clinical doses for adult patients with normal renal function; dosing for individual patients and institutions may vary.

[b]Oral regimens should be used in conjunction with IV prophylaxis.

From Refs. 1, 9, and 15.

patients undergoing hysterectomy, cefoxitin or cefotetan are appropriate therapies (Table 85–3). Cefazolin or ampicillin/sulbactam may be used. In the case of β-lactam allergy, the following regimens are appropriate: clindamycin combined with gentamicin, aztreonam, or ciprofloxacin; metronidazole combined with gentamicin or ciprofloxacin, or clindamycin monotherapy. Metronidazole monotherapy is also indicated but is less effective than other regimens.[1]

Cesarean sections are stratified into low- and high-risk groups. Patients who undergo emergency operations or have cesarean sections after the rupture of membranes and/or onset of labor are considered high risk. Prophylactic antimicrobials are most beneficial for high-risk patients but are used in both groups. Antimicrobial regimens similar to those for hysterectomy are appropriate. Antimicrobials should not be administered until after the first incision and the umbilical cord has been clamped. This practice prevents potentially harmful antimicrobial concentrations from reaching the newborn.

▶ Orthopedic Surgery

Orthopedic operations are generally clean and are done under controlled conditions. Likely pathogens include gram-positive cocci, mostly staphylococci. In the case of total joint (knee and hip) arthroplasty, cefazolin is the antimicrobial of choice. Patients with a β-lactam allergy should receive either clindamycin or vancomycin. Antimicrobial prophylaxis should not exceed 24 hours and does not need to be continued until all drains and catheters have been removed. Antimicrobial-impregnated bone cement can be useful in lowering infection rates in orthopedic surgery but has not been approved for prophylaxis.

▶ Cardiothoracic and Vascular Surgery

Cefazolin or cefuroxime are appropriate for prophylaxis in cardiothoracic and vascular surgeries. In the case of β-lactam allergy, vancomycin or clindamycin are advised. Debate exists on the duration of antimicrobial prophylaxis. SSIs are rare after cardiothoracic operations, but the potentially devastating consequences lead some clinicians to support longer periods of prophylaxis. The National Surgical Infection Prevention Project cites data that extending prophylaxis beyond 24 hours does not decrease SSI rates and may increase bacterial resistance.[1] However, the Society of Thoracic Surgeons issued practice guidelines in 2006 to extend the duration of antibiotics to 48 hours following cardiac surgeries.[35] Duration of therapy should be based on patient factors and risk of development of an SSI.

▶ Colorectal Surgery

Antimicrobial prophylaxis for colorectal operations must cover a broad range of gram-positive, gram-negative, and anaerobic organisms. Strategies include oral antimicrobial bowel preparations, parenteral antimicrobials, or both. Oral prophylaxis combinations of neomycin and erythromycin or neomycin and metronidazole are common. Oral antimicrobials should be administered at 19, 18, and 9 hours prior to surgery. A delay in surgery may require a redose, depending on the length of postponement. For parenteral prophylaxis, cefoxitin, cefotetan, or ertapenem is appropriate. Cefazolin combined with metronidazole or ampicillin/sulbactam is an effective alternative

---

Patient Encounter Part 1

RP is a 50-year-old man with a history of rectal bleeding and recent diagnosis of sigmoid colon cancer. He presents today for a colon resection (colorectal surgery). He has a history of nausea with cephalexin. You have been asked for recommendation for surgical prophylaxis.

Height: 68 in (173 cm)

Weight: 214 lb (97.3 kg)

VS: BP 127/83 mm Hg, HR 63 beats/min, RR 21 breaths/min, T 98.6°F (37°C)

Labs: WBC 3×10^3 mm^3 (3×10^9/L), serum creatinine 0.9 mg/dL (80 μmol/L), glucose 95 mg/dL (5.3 mmol/L)

What organisms are likely to be encountered for this operation and why?

What agents need to be avoided considering this patient's previous reaction with cephalosporins?

What drug would you choose for this operation and why?

The surgeon agrees with your decision and wants to begin infusing the antibiotic 3 hours prior to the first incision. Comment on this.

What other interventions besides antibiotic use could prove useful in lowering RP's risk of SSI?

Patient Encounter Part 2

RP is transferred to the oncology ward after completion of his surgery. In the procedure notes, the surgeon notes that part of the small bowel was nicked and possible intra-abdominal contamination may have occurred.

Does this patient still require surgical site prophylaxis?

The surgeon asks for your opinion for which antibiotic the patient should receive. Which antibiotic do you recommend?

How long should this patient remain on antibiotics?

---

if antianaerobic cephalosporins are not available. For patients with β-lactam allergies, use clindamycin combined with gentamicin, aztreonam, or ciprofloxacin; metronidazole combined with gentamicin or ciprofloxacin is also appropriate.

Appendectomy is one of the most common intra-abdominal operations. Antimicrobial prophylaxis used for appendectomy is similar to that used for colorectal regimens. In the case of ruptured appendix, antimicrobials are used for treatment, not prophylaxis.

OUTCOME EVALUATION

The clinician should consistently follow up postoperative patients and screen for any sign of SSI. ❾ *According to CDC criteria, SSIs may appear up to 30 days after an operation and up to 1 year if a prosthesis is implanted.*[5] This period often extends beyond hospitalization, so patients should be educated on warning signs of SSI and be encouraged to contact a clinician immediately if necessary. The presence of fever or leukocytosis in the immediate postoperative period does not constitute SSI and should resolve with proper patient care. Distal infections, such as pneumonia, are not considered

---

Patient Encounter Part 3

RP was treated appropriately for his surgical complications based on your recommendations following his surgery. He presents to a 3-week follow-up appointment to the surgical clinic. He notes that his wound site has been increasing in redness over the past 1 to 2 days, accompanied by a slight discharge that started this morning prior to the clinic visit.

VS: BP 104/78 mm Hg, P 82 beats/min, RR 21 breaths/min, T 100.7°F (38.2°C)

Labs: WBC 13×10^3/mm^3 (13×10^9/L) serum creatinine 1 mg/dL (88 μmol/L)

Based on the available data, does RP have an SSI?

What further steps should be taken in regard to this possible SSI?

Patient Care and Monitoring

1. Conduct a thorough medication history, including prescription and nonprescription medications, as well as herbals and vitamins.

2. Verify the patient's allergy history and the type of reaction experienced. Attempt to discern between true allergy and adverse event. β-Lactam–allergic patients may receive clindamycin, vancomycin, or other antimicrobials. Cross-reactivity between penicillin allergy and cephalosporins is low, but cephalosporins should be avoided in patients with a history of anaphylaxis to penicillins.

3. Document the type of operation the patient is undergoing. Verify the surgical procedure with the patient.

4. Prophylactic antimicrobials should be started within an hour of the first incision to optimize patient outcomes. Exceptions to this include vancomycin and fluoroquinolones.

5. The patient should be monitored for signs of an allergic reaction during the operation. These include rash, hives, difficulty breathing, or substantial drops in blood pressure.

6. Major breaks in surgical technique may cause the classification of the operation to change and require adjustments in antimicrobial prophylaxis.

7. The patient should be monitored for signs and symptoms of infection postoperatively. These could include pus, erythema, and fever. If signs consistent with SSI appear, cultures should be taken and additional antimicrobial therapy should be considered.

8. Patients being discharged should be counseled on recognizing signs and symptoms of SSI. An SSI can appear up to 30 days after an operation is completed.

SSIs even if these infections occur in the 30-day period. The appearance of the surgical site should be checked regularly and changes should be documented (e.g., erythema, drainage, or pus). The presence of pus or other signs suggestive of SSI must be treated accordingly. Any wound requiring incision and drainage is considered an SSI regardless of appearance. Prompt cultures should be collected and appropriate antimicrobial therapy initiated to reduce any chance of morbidity and mortality.

Abbreviations Introduced in This Chapter

ASHP	American Society of Health-System Pharmacists
CA-MRSA	Community-associated methicillin-resistant *Staphylococcus aureus*
MIC	Minimum inhibitory concentration
MRSA	Methicillin-resistant *Staphylococcus aureus*
MSSA	Methicillin-sensitive *S. aureus*
NNIS	National Nosocomial Infections Surveillance System
SSI	Surgical site infection

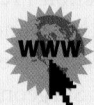 Self-assessment questions and answers are available at *http://www.mhpharmacotherapy.com/pp.html.*

REFERENCES

1. Bratzler DW, Houck PM, for the Surgical Infection Prevention Guideline Writers Workgroup. Antimicrobial prophylaxis for surgery: An advisory statement from the National Surgical Infection Prevention Project. Am J Surg 2005;189:395–404.

2. Barie PS, Eachempati SR. Surgical site infections. Surg Clin North Am 2005;85:1115–1135.

3. Kirkland KB, Briggs JP, Trivette SL, et al. The impact of surgical site infections in the 1990s: Attributable mortality, excess length of hospitalization, and extra costs. Infect Control Hosp Epidemiol 1999;20:725–730.

4. Hollenbeak CS, Murphy D, Dunagan WC, et al. Nonrandom selection and the attributable cost of surgical-site infections. Infect Control Hosp Epidemiol 2002;23:174–176.

5. Mangram AJ, Horan TC, Pearson ML, et al. Guideline for prevention of surgical site infection, 1999. Infect Control Hosp Epidemiol 1999;20:247–266.

6. Department of Health and Human Services: Centers for Medicare & Medicaid Services. Medicare Program; Changes to the Hospital Inpatient Prospective Payment Systems and Fiscal Year 2008; Final Rule. Federal Register 2007;72:47200–47206.

7. Dionigi R, Rovera F, Dionigi G, et al. Risk factors in surgery. J Chemother 2001;13:6–11.

8. Pessaux P, Atallah D, Lermite E, et al. Risk factors for prediction of surgical site infections in "clean surgery." Am J Infect Control 2005;33:292–298.

9. Devlin JW, Kanji S, Janning SW, et al. Antimicrobial prophylaxis in surgery. In: Dipiro JT, Talbert RL, Yee GC, et al. Pharmacotherapy: A Pathophysiologic Approach. 5th ed. New York: McGraw-Hill; 2002:2111–2122.

10. Finkelstein R, Rabino G, Mashiah T, et al. Vancomycin versus cefazolin prophylaxis for cardiac surgery in the setting of a high prevalence of methicillin-resistant staphylococcal infections. J Thorac Cardiovasc Surg 2002;123:326–332.

11. Itanu KMF, Wilson SE, Awad SS, et al. Ertapenem versus cefotetan prophylaxis in elective colorectal surgery. N Engl J Med 2006;355:2640–2651.

12. Centers for Medicare & Medicaid Services and The Joint Commission. *The Specifications Manual for National Hospital Inpatient Quality Measures (Specifications Manual)* Version 3.0b [online]. [cited 2011 Oct 10]. Available from: *http://www.qualitynet.org/dcs/contentserver?cid=11 41662756099&pagename=Qnetpublic%2Fpage%2FQnetTier2&c=page.* Last accessed September 25, 2011.

13. Schafer JA, Mateo N, Parlier GL, Rotschater JC. Penicillin allergy skin testing: What do we do know? Pharmacotherapy 2007;27:542–545.

14. Pichichero ME. A review of evidence supporting the American Academy of Pediatrics recommendation for prescribing cephalosporin antibiotics for penicillin-allergic patients. Pediatrics 2005;115:1048–1057.

15. Apter AJ, Kinman JL, Bilker WB, et al. Is there cross-reactivity between penicillins and cephalosporins? Am J Med 2006;119:354.e11–e20.

16. Weed HG. Antimicrobial prophylaxis in the surgical patient. Med Clin North Am 2003;87:59–75.

17. Kurz A, Sessler D, Lenhardt R. Perioperative normothermia to reduce the incidence of surgical-wound infection and shorten hospitalization. Study of Wound Infection and Temperature Group. N Engl J Med 1996;334:1209–1215.

18. Ingels C, Debaveye Y, Milants I, et al. Strict blood glucose control with insulin during intensive care after cardiac surgery: Impact on 4-years survival, dependency on medical care, and quality of life. Eur Heart J 2006;27(22):2716–2724.

19. Greif R, Akca O, Horn E, et al., for the Outcomes Research Group. Supplemental perioperative oxygen to reduce the incidence of surgical-wound infection. N Engl J Med 2000;342:161–167.

20. Chiu FY, Chen CM, Lin CF, et al. Cefuroxime-impregnated cement in primary total knee arthroplasty. J Bone Joint Surg 2002; 84:759–762.

21. Joseph TN, Chen AL, Di Cesare PE. Use of antibiotic-impregnated cement in total joint arthroplasty. J Am Acad Orthop Surg 2003;11:38–47.

22. Fletcher N, Sofianos D, Berkes MB, Obremskey WT. Prevention of perioperative infection. J Bone Joint Surg Am 2007;89:1605–1618.

23. Wilcox MH, Hall J, Pike H, et al. Use of perioperative mupirocin to prevent methicillin-resistant staphylococcus aureus (MRSA) orthopaedic surgical site infections. J Hosp Infect 2003;54:196–201.

24. Perl TM, Cullen JJ, Wenzel RP, et al. Intranasal mupirocin to prevent postoperative *Staphylococcus aureus* infections. N Engl J Med 2002;346:1871–1877.

25. Munoz P, Hortal J, Giannella M, et al. Nasal carriage of *S. aureus* increases the risk of surgical site infection after major heart surgery. J Hosp Infect 2008;68:25–31.

26. Coia JE, Duckworth GJ, Edwards DI, et al. Guidelines for the control and prevention of meticillin-resistant *Staphylococcus aureus* (MRSA) in healthcare facilities. J Hosp Infect 2006;63:S1–S44

27. Harbath S, Fankhauser C, Schrenzel J, et al. Universal screening for methicillin-resistant Staphylococcus aureus at hospital admission and noscomial infection in surgical patients. JAMA 2008;299:1149–1157.

28. Loveday HP, Pellowe CM, Jones SRLJ, Pratt RJ. A systematic review of the evidence for interventions for the prevention and control of meticillin-resistant *Staphylococcus aureus* (1996 – 2004): Report to the Joint MRSA Working Party (Subgroup A). J Hosp Infect. 2006;63: S45–S70.

29. Loeb M, Main C, Walker-Dilks C, Eady A. Antimicrobial drugs for treating methicillin-resistant Staphylococcus aureus colonization. Cochrane Database Syst Rev 2003;CD003340.

30. Bode LGM, Kluytmans JAJW, Wertheim HFL, et al. Preventing surgical-site infections in nasal carriers of *Staphylococcus aureus*. N Engl J Med 2010;362:9–17.

31. Diekema D, Johannsson B, Herwaldt, et al. Current practice in *Staphylococcus aureus* screening and decolonization. Infect Control Hosp Epidemiol 2011;32:1042–1044.

32. Deshpande LM, Fix AM, Pfaller MA, et al. Emerging elevated mupirocin resistance rates among staphylococcal isolates in the SENTRY Antimicrobial Surveillance Program (2000): correlations of results from disk diffusion, Etest, and reference dilution methods. Diagn Microbiol Infect Dis 2002;42:283–290.

33. Stone HH, Hooper CA, Kolb LD, et al. Antibiotic prophylaxis in gastric, biliary and colonic surgery. Ann Surg 1976;184:443–452.

34. Forse RA, Karam B, MacLean LD, et al. Antibiotic prophylaxis for surgery in morbidly obese patients. Surgery 1989;106:750–756.

35. Edwards FH, Engelman RM, Houck P, et al. The Soceity of Thoracic Surgeons practice guideline series: antibiotic prophylaxis in cardiac surgery, part I: duration. Ann Thorac Surg 2006;81:397–404.

86 Vaccines and Toxoids

Marianne Billeter

KEY CONCEPTS

❶ Vaccines provide active immunity against viral and bacterial pathogens.

❷ Polysaccharide vaccines are poorly immunogenic in children younger than 2 years of age.

❸ Combination vaccines decrease the number of injections and increase the likelihood of completing the immunization schedule.

❹ Healthcare professionals should report vaccine-adverse events.

❺ Live virus vaccines should not be given to an immunocompromised host.

❻ Vaccines are cost effective in preventing disease.

The development and widespread use of vaccines is one of the greatest public health achievements of the 20th century. Other than safe drinking water, no other modality has had a greater impact on reducing mortality from infectious diseases. The first accounts of deliberate inoculation to prevent disease date back as far as the 10th century. However it wasn't until 1798 that Edward Jenner published his work on inoculation of natural cowpox as a means to prevent infection with smallpox. This was the first scientific attempt to prevent infection by inoculation. Since 1900, vaccines have been developed against more than 20 diseases, with half of these recommended for routine use. The widespread use of vaccines has resulted in the eradication of smallpox worldwide and wild-type poliovirus from

the Western hemisphere. There have also been dramatic declines in the incidence of diphtheria, pertussis, tetanus, measles, mumps, rubella, and *Haemophilus influenzae* type b.

❶ *Vaccines have traditionally been preparations of killed or attenuated microorganisms that provide active immunity against a variety of viral and bacterial infections.* Most vaccines are designed to prevent acute infections that can be rapidly controlled and cleared by the immune system. Successful immunization involves activation of antigen-presenting cells with processing of the antigen by lysosomal or cytoplasmic pathways. T and B lymphocytes will be activated to replicate and differentiate to form large pools of memory cells for protection against subsequent exposure to the antigen.[1]

Vaccines against viral infections may be **attenuated** live viruses or inactivated viral particles. Attenuation may be accomplished by several methods to decrease the viruses' virulence while retaining their **immunogenicity**. Bacterial vaccines utilize antigenic particles of the outer membrane to elicit an immune response. ❷ *Outer membrane polysaccharides are poorly immunogenic in children younger than 2 years of age* unless conjugated with a carrier protein. Also, bacterial toxins may undergo chemical treatment to render them nontoxic to form **toxoids** against infectious agents.

Often the terms *vaccination* and *immunization* are used interchangeably even though they are distinct concepts. Vaccination refers to the act of administering a vaccine, whereas immunization refers to the development of immunity to a pathogen. The delivery of a vaccine does not imply that the individual mounted an adequate immune response to the vaccine to elicit protection. However, immunization implies that the act of vaccination resulted in the development of protective immunity.

Patient Encounter 1

A mother is taking her 11-year-old girl to the pediatrician for a routine sports physical. The pediatrician notices that the girl is due for several vaccines.

Which vaccines should the girl receive?

Will any booster doses be required for the administered vaccines?

The mother voices concerns about vaccinating her daughter against a sexually transmitted disease. What is an appropriate response?

Herd immunity refers to high levels of immunization in one population, resulting in protection of another unvaccinated population. For example, concentrated vaccination of children with the 7-valent pneumococcal conjugate vaccine resulted in decreased invasive *Streptococcus pneumoniae* infection not only in the vaccinated children, but also in elderly persons within the same community.

Cocoon immunization is a strategy used to immunize all persons surrounding another high-risk individual, such as vaccinating parents, siblings, and grandparents of a new infant who is too young to be vaccinated. This strategy is used to protect individuals who are not able to be vaccinated themselves.

THE ROUTINE VACCINES

Diphtheria, Tetanus, and Pertussis Vaccines

▶ *Diphtheria Toxoid*

Diphtheria is a bacterial respiratory infection characterized by membranous pharyngitis. The membrane may cover the pharynx, tonsillar areas, soft palate, and uvula. Diphtheria may also cause anal, cutaneous, vaginal, and conjunctival infections. The impact of diphtheria is not from the causative bacteria, *Corynebacterium diphtheriae*, but rather from complications attributed to its exotoxin, such as myocarditis and peripheral neuritis. In the late 1800s, the annual death rate from diphtheria ranged from 46 to 196 cases per 100,000. Mortality from diphtheria dropped in the 1900s mostly due to the availability of diphtheria antitoxin, which elicited passive immunity. Diphtheria is rarely reported in the United States since the introduction of vaccination with diphtheria toxoid; however, diphtheria continues to be a major problem in developing countries.

In the early 1900s, a balanced mixture of diphtheria toxin and antitoxin was found to produce active immunity in both animals and humans. This preparation gained widespread acceptance and protected approximately 85% of recipients. Several years later, diphtheria toxoid was developed by treating the toxin with small amounts of formalin. This process caused the toxin to lose its toxic properties while maintaining its immunogenic properties. In the mid-1920s, the addition of an alum precipitate enhanced the immunogenic properties of the toxoid.

In the 1940s, diphtheria toxoid was combined with tetanus toxoid and whole-cell pertussis vaccines and later with the acellular pertussis vaccine. The diphtheria toxoid, tetanus toxoid, and acellular pertussis vaccine are part of the routine childhood immunization schedule. Diphtheria toxoid is also combined with tetanus toxoid and is commonly used as a booster vaccine. The pediatric product (DT) has a higher amount of diphtheria toxoid than does the adult product (Td). Diphtheria toxoid is not available as an individual vaccine.

Recent outbreaks of diphtheria have demonstrated that immunity wanes in adulthood. Approximately 50% of all adults no longer have immunity to diphtheria. Regular boosters with tetanus and diphtheria toxoids every 10 years will provide adequate recall immunity to diphtheria provided the adult was previously immunized.[2]

▶ *Tetanus Toxoid*

The tetanus vaccine differs from others in that it does not protect against a contagious disease such as diphtheria, but rather against an environmental pathogen. *Clostridium tetani* is widely found in the environment, especially in dirt and soils. Additionally, animals and humans may harbor and excrete the organism. *C. tetani* produces two neurotoxins, tetanospasmin and tetanolysin, which are responsible for producing the painful muscular contractions associated with tetanus. Tetanus continues to be a major problem in the developing world, causing approximately 1 million deaths each year.[3] Approximately 40% of the cases are neonatal tetanus and most likely associated with the use of nonsterile instruments or poultices on the umbilical cord. Tetanus is rarely seen in developed countries.

Immunity to tetanus decreases with increasing age; therefore, a regular booster every 10 years with tetanus toxoid is recommended. The preferred agent to use in adults is tetanus and diphtheria toxoid (Td) in order to give a booster for diphtheria. Tetanus immunization status should be assessed in the management of wounds in individuals seeking medical care. A tetanus booster should be administered if a tetanus-containing vaccine has not been given in the preceding 5 years for moderate and severe wounds or contaminated wounds. If the wound is minor and uncontaminated, then a tetanus booster is needed if the previous tetanus vaccination was more than 10 years ago.

▶ *Pertussis*

Pertussis is a highly contagious respiratory tract infection caused by the bacteria *Bordetella pertussis*. Pertussis is characterized by a protracted severe cough with or without posttussive vomiting, whoop, difficulty breathing, difficulty sleeping, and rib fractures. It is often referred to as "whooping cough" or the 100-day cough. In the prevaccine era, pertussis accounted for more than 250,000 cases of severe illness and 10,000 deaths per year in the United States. Pertussis has always been thought of as a pediatric disease since most cases occurred in preschool-aged children with relatively no cases seen in adolescents and adults. The first pertussis vaccine was introduced in the 1940s and within 30 years resulted in a 99% reduction in disease. However, during the past two decades, there has been a steady increase in reported cases of pertussis among adolescents and adults, indicating a waning immunity after primary immunization.[4]

The first pertussis whole-cell vaccine was a mixture of killed organisms that was associated with frequent local and systemic reactions. In the late 1980s, an acellular pertussis (aP) vaccine was introduced that contains purified pertussis components that are immunogenic but associated with fewer adverse reactions. Acellular pertussis vaccine is available in combination with tetanus and diphtheria toxoids. Pertussis is not available as a separate vaccine component. In the spring of 2005, the FDA-approved tetanus toxoid, reduced diphtheria toxoid, and acellular pertussis vaccines for use in adolescents and adults.

▶ Use of Diphtheria, Tetanus, and Acellular Pertussis Vaccine

Diphtheria and tetanus toxoids and acellular pertussis (DTaP) vaccine should be administered in a five-shot series to all children beginning at 2 months of age (Table 86–1). The shots are given at 2, 4, 6, and 15 to 18 months, and 4 to 6 years. Complete immunity to diphtheria and tetanus is achieved after the third vaccination.

Tetanus toxoid, reduced diphtheria toxoid, and acellular pertussis vaccine (Tdap) is recommended as a single booster for the following groups in place of a tetanus booster.[5]

- *Adolescents 11 to 18 years of age*: regardless of the interval from the last tetanus-containing vaccine.
- *Adults 19 to 64 years of age*: Tdap should replace the next routine tetanus booster regardless of the interval from the last tetanus-containing vaccine.
- *Tetanus prophylaxis in wound management*: Adolescents and adults 11 to 64 years of age who have completed a primary series and require a tetanus-containing product should receive Tdap instead of Td if they have not already received Tdap.
- *Prevention of pertussis among infants younger than 12 months of age*: Adults who have close contact with infants younger than 12 months of age, especially parents, grandparents, and child care providers, should receive a single dose of Tdap. Ideally, Tdap should be given 2 weeks prior to contact with the infant.
- *Postpartum women*: Women should receive a single dose of Tdap in the immediate postpartum period if Tdap has not been previously received. Ideally this should be administered prior to discharge from the hospital or birthing center.
- *Healthcare workers with direct patient contact*: Such workers should receive a single dose of Tdap.

Haemophilus Influenzae Type b Vaccine

Haemophilus influenzae is a bacterial respiratory pathogen that causes a wide spectrum of disease ranging from colonization of the airways to bacterial meningitis. It causes considerable morbidity and mortality, especially in children younger than 5 years of age. *H. influenzae* is either encapsulated or unencapsulated. The encapsulated strains can be further differentiated into six antigenically distinct serotypes, designated by the letters a through f. *H. influenzae* type b was primarily found in cerebrospinal fluid and blood of children with meningitis, whereas the unencapsulated strains were found in the upper respiratory tract of adults. Before the introduction of the vaccine, *H. influenzae* was responsible for 20,000 to 25,000 cases of invasive disease annually and was the most common cause of bacterial meningitis. Since the introduction of the vaccine, invasive disease due to *H. influenzae* type b has been nearly eliminated.

The *H. influenzae* type b vaccine is a protein conjugate that utilizes a carrier-hapten for antigen presentation. The polysaccharide is conjugated to an immunogenic protein carrier, which is recognized by T cells and macrophages, which stimulates T-dependent immunity. The conjugated vaccine elicits an immune response characterized by T-helper cell activation. The T-dependent antigens induce an enhanced immune response in younger children. Within 10 years of its introduction, the *H. influenzae* type b vaccine use has resulted in widespread herd immunity.

H. influenzae type b conjugate vaccine is a recommended routine childhood vaccine given at 2, 4, 6, and 12 to 15 months of age. Adolescents and adults with functional or anatomic asplenia should also receive a booster dose of *H. influenzae* type b vaccine. The currently available vaccines are labeled for pediatric use, but can be used in adults when vaccination is indicated. There are several *H. influenzae* type b vaccines on the market that differ in the size of the polysaccharide and type of carrier protein; however, the immune response to *H. influenzae* type b is similar among the different vaccines. The different brands are interchangeable without affecting the primary immune response or booster response.

H. influenzae type b and influenza vaccines have the potential for confusion and medication errors because of the similarity of the names. Care should be taken when ordering, dispensing, and administering these vaccines.

Hepatitis A Vaccine

Hepatitis A virus continues to be a frequent cause of illness despite the availability of a highly effective vaccine. Hepatitis A typically has an abrupt onset of symptoms including fever, malaise, nausea, abdominal discomfort, and jaundice. Frequently, children younger than 6 years of age are asymptomatic, whereas adults typically have symptomatic disease. Symptoms may persist for 2 months or longer. There is wide geographic variation in the incidence of hepatitis A infection, with the number of cases ranging from 50 to more than 700 cases per 100,000 persons annually. The economic burden of hepatitis A is greater than $300 million annually in combined direct and indirect costs. Widespread use of the vaccine offers the opportunity to substantially decrease the disease burden caused by hepatitis A infection.[6]

Table 86–1

Vaccine Dosing

Vaccine	Common Abbreviation	Dose	Route	Cautions and Adverse Effects
Diphtheria and tetanus toxoid	DT	0.5 mL	Intramuscular	
Diphtheria, tetanus, acellular pertussis	DTaP	0.5 mL	Intramuscular	Systemic neurologic reaction from previous vaccine Brachial neuritis Cries for 3 hours nonstop after previous dose Temperature greater than 40.6°C (105°F)
Haemophilus influenzae type b	HIB	0.5 mL	Intramuscular	
Hepatitis A	HAV	C: 0.5 mL A: 1 mL	Intramuscular	
Hepatitis B	HBV	C: 0.5 mL A: 1 mL	Intramuscular	Allergic reaction to yeast (baking yeast)
Human papillomavirus	HPV	0.5 mL	Intramuscular	Pregnant women
Inactivated influenza	TIV	0.5 mL	Intramuscular	Severe egg allergy History of Guillain-Barré syndrome
Live attenuated influenza	LAIV	0.5 mL	Intranasal	Severe egg allergy Asthma Chronic health problems Immunocompromised host Pregnant women History of Guillain-Barré syndrome
Measles, mumps, rubella	MMR	0.5 mL	Subcutaneous	Allergic reaction to gelatin or neomycin Pregnant women Immunocompromised host Recently received a blood transfusion Severe egg allergy
Meningococcal polysaccharide	MPSV4	0.5 mL	Subcutaneous	History of Guillain-Barré syndrome
Meningococcal conjugate	MCV4	0.5 mL	Intramuscular	History of Guillain-Barré syndrome
Pneumococcal 13-valent conjugate	PCV13	0.5 mL	Intramuscular	
Pneumococcal polysaccharide	PPV23	0.5 mL	Intramuscular route preferred; subcutaneous	Children younger than 2 years of age
Poliovirus, inactivated	IPV	0.5 mL	Intramuscular, subcutaneous	Allergic reaction to neomycin, streptomycin, polymyxin B
Rotavirus vaccine	RV	2 mL	Oral	Immunocompromised host
Tetanus and diphtheria toxoid	Td	0.5 mL	Intramuscular	
Tetanus, reduced diphtheria, acellular pertussis	Tdap	0.5 mL	Intramuscular	History of Guillain-Barré syndrome Systemic neurologic reaction from previous vaccine
Varicella	VAR	0.5 mL	Subcutaneous	Allergic reaction to gelatin or neomycin Pregnant women Immunocompromised host Recently received a blood transfusion Hematopoietic stem-cell transplant
Zoster	ZOS	0.65 mL	Subcutaneous	Allergic reaction to gelatin or neomycin Immunocompromised host Recently received a blood transfusion Hematopoietic stem-cell transplant

C, children; A, adult.

Hepatitis A vaccine was licensed in the United States in 1995. It is an inactivated whole virus vaccine that is administered in a two-dose series. More than 94% of children, adolescents, and adults will have protective antibodies 1 month after receiving the first dose and 100% following the second dose.[6] Recommended use of the hepatitis A vaccine utilizes an incremental implementation schedule beginning with high-risk populations or those at increased risk for serious complications from the disease. Currently, hepatitis A vaccine is recommended for all children following the first birthday, with the second dose administered 6 months later. Adults who are at high risk for hepatitis A should receive two doses at least 6 months apart. High-risk adults include persons with clotting disorders or chronic liver disease, men who have sex with men, illicit drug users, international travelers going to areas with high to intermediate endemicity of hepatitis A, persons with anticipated close contact with an international adoptee, or any other person who wishes to become immune.

Hepatitis B Vaccine

Hepatitis B virus is a blood-borne or sexually transmitted virus. Most acute infections occur in adults, whereas chronic infections usually occur in individuals infected as infants or children. However, about 10% of adults who contract hepatitis B virus will fail to clear their infection and develop chronic hepatitis B infection. Individuals with chronic hepatitis B infection are at risk for cirrhosis or hepatocellular carcinoma. Vaccination with hepatitis B vaccine is the most effective way to prevent hepatitis B infection.[7]

Hepatitis B vaccine is manufactured using recombinant DNA technology to express hepatitis B surface antigen (HBsAg) in yeast. This is further purified with biochemical separation techniques to produce the vaccine. The vaccines are formulated to contain 10 to 40 mcg of HBsAg protein/mL. Hepatitis B vaccine is available as a single component or in combination vaccines.

Hepatitis B vaccine is recommended for routine use in children. The first dose should be given within 12 hours of birth. The second and third doses are given at 2 months and 6 months, respectively, after the first dose if using the single-component vaccine or at 2, 4, and 6 months if using a hepatitis B–containing combination vaccine. If the infant weighs less than 2,000 g at birth, the birth dose is not counted in the three-dose series. Infants less than 2,000 g do not produce an adequate immune response to the birth dose of hepatitis B vaccine. Adolescents should receive the three-dose series if not previously vaccinated.[7]

Adults at high risk for hepatitis B because of occupation or lifestyle should receive the hepatitis B vaccine series. The typical series has the second and third doses given 1 month and 6 months after the first dose. Accelerated schedules may also be used. Frequently, individuals do not follow through with the complete three-dose series and questions arise about restarting the series. Hepatitis B vaccine produces an amnesic response; therefore, the series may be continued at any time in order to complete the three doses.

Following vaccination with hepatitis B vaccine, hepatitis B virus serologic markers will remain negative, with the exception of anti-HBs (antibody to hepatitis B surface antigen), which will be positive indicating immunity. Persons with anti-HBs concentration greater than 10 mIU/mL (10 IU/L) after vaccination will have complete protection against acute and chronic infection.[7] There is no need for booster doses in immunocompetent individuals when anti-HBs concentrations fall below 10 mIU/mL (10 IU/L), since a good memory response will occur following exposure to hepatitis B virus. However, a booster dose is warranted in immunocompromised individuals.

Human Papillomavirus Vaccine

Human papillomavirus (HPV) is the most common sexually transmitted virus and is associated with a wide range of diseases, including genital warts and cervical cancer. More than 100 HPVs have been sequenced and classified as low-risk nononcogenic or high-risk oncogenic types based on their ability to cause malignant disease. The predominant low-risk types HPV 6 and 11 are associated with 90% of genital warts. High-risk types HPV 16 and 18 are associated with 70% of cervical cancer cases and cervical intra-epithelial neoplasia.[8] HPV is also associated with other gynecologic cancers, such as vaginal and vulvovaginal tumors.

Two HPV L-1 virus-like particle vaccines have been developed. The quadrivalent vaccine contains HPV types 6, 11, 16, and 18. The bivalent vaccine contains HPV types 16 and 18. Both vaccines have shown greater than 95% efficacy in preventing precancerous lesions of the cervix, vulva, and vagina. Additionally, the quadrivalent vaccine is also effective against genital warts. Both HPV vaccines are safe and adverse events are similar to other vaccines administered to adolescents.

These vaccines are unique in that preventing infection by HPV will translate into prevention of cancer, making these the first cancer prevention vaccines. Clinical trials are utilizing surrogate markers, prevention of precancerous lesions, to determine efficacy of the vaccines. However, the true impact on preventing cancerous tumors will not be known for years. The HPV vaccine is recommended for use in girls and women 9 through 26 years of age.[9] Ideally it should be administered to girls before they become sexually active. However, sexually active girls and women should still receive the vaccine. Additionally, girls and women who have been infected with HPV should still receive the vaccine since the vaccine provides protection against more than one type of HPV. The quadrivalent HPV vaccine is also recommended for use in boys and men aged 9 through 26 years to prevent genital warts.

Influenza Vaccine

Influenza is a contagious viral respiratory infection that usually occurs during the winter months in the Northern Hemisphere and all year round in the Southern Hemisphere. All age groups are affected by influenza; however, children have the highest rate of infection. Serious illness and death due to influenza usually occurs in extremes of age, those over 65 years or under 2 years. Influenza is responsible for approximately 36,000 deaths annually in the United States.[10]

Influenza A and B viruses are responsible for causing human disease. Influenza A is further categorized into subgroups by its surface antigens, hemagglutinin and neuraminidase (e.g., influenza A H1N1 virus). Influenza B virus is not subtyped. Both influenza A and B undergo frequent antigenic drift, creating new influenza variants. Immunity to the surface antigens decreases the likelihood of infection. Unfortunately, antibody to one influenza subgroup does not give complete protection against other influenza subtypes. Therefore, annual influenza vaccination is recommended from September through November, and continuing until the vaccine supply is exhausted.

The best way to protect against influenza is through vaccination. The influenza vaccine is composed of two influenza

A subtypes and one influenza B subtype. The viral subtypes contained in the vaccine usually changes each year. The exact composition is selected by a panel of experts and announced by the Centers for Disease Control and Prevention (CDC) in March or April each year. The vaccine becomes available for use in August. Two types of influenza vaccine are licensed for use in the United States; both vaccines contain the same viral subunits. The influenza viruses for both vaccine preparations are grown in eggs. Therefore, the vaccines are contraindicated in individuals with severe allergy to eggs.

The influenza vaccine should be administered to all persons aged 6 months and older. The trivalent inactivated influenza vaccine can be administered to all age groups and risk populations; high-dose influenza vaccine should be administered to persons 65 years and older. The live attenuated influenza vaccine may be administered to healthy individuals between the age of 2 and 49 years. If the child is less than 8 years old and is receiving influenza vaccine for the first time, two doses separated by 4 to 6 weeks should be given.[10]

Measles, Mumps, and Rubella Vaccine

▶ Measles

Measles, also known as rubeola, is characterized by a rash that is often complicated by diarrhea, middle ear infection, or pneumonia. Encephalitis occurs in 1 of every 1,000 reported cases. Individuals who recover from encephalitis usually have permanent brain damage. Death occurs in 1 to 2 of every 1,000 reported measles cases.[11]

Prior to measles vaccine availability, the number of cases of measles approached the birth rate of approximately 3 to 4 million annually. The first measles vaccine was licensed in 1963. Since that time there has been a 99% reduction in reported measles cases. Currently, there is a goal to eliminate measles transmission in the United States through aggressive immunization programs.

There have been several types of measles vaccines used since its introduction. The current vaccine uses a live attenuated preparation of the Enders-Edmonston virus strain. Following vaccination with measles-containing vaccine, a mild noncommunicable infection develops. Approximately 95% of individuals will develop antibodies following a single dose if administered after 12 months of age. More than 99% of individuals who receive two inoculations will develop long-term, probably lifelong, immunity to measles.[11]

▶ Mumps

Mumps is usually thought of as a disease of children, but it has also gained notoriety as a prominent illness affecting military units. Mumps produces a typical acute parotitis, but may also cause nonspecific respiratory symptoms. In postpubertal males, mumps may also cause orchitis in 38% of those infected, which may result in infertility.[11]

Since the introduction of the mumps vaccine in 1967, there has been a 99% reduction in reported cases. The mumps vaccine is a live virus preparation of the Jeryl-Lynn strain. It produces a subclinical, noncommunicable infection following vaccination. Single doses of mumps vaccine will elicit immunity in 75% to 95% of individuals. Vaccine-induced immunity lasts for more than 30 years.

▶ Rubella

German measles, also known as rubella, is a mild exanthematous illness in children and young adults; however, rubella infection in pregnant women can cause a variety of congenital malformations in the infant. Congenital rubella syndrome occurs in approximately 25% of infants whose mother acquires rubella during the first trimester. Congenital rubella syndrome is characterized by congenital cataracts, heart disease, deafness, thrombocytopenia, mental retardation, and numerous other abnormalities.[11]

The first rubella vaccine was licensed in 1969. Initial vaccination campaigns were targeting young children, as this age group had the highest rate of rubella infection. This strategy significantly decreased rubella cases in children, but did not have the desired effect on infection in adolescents and adults or on congenital rubella syndrome. Adolescents, especially young girls, were then targeted for vaccination. This has resulted in a significant reduction in the number of cases of congenital rubella syndrome.

The live rubella vaccine available in the United States contains the RA 27/3 strain of the virus. Following a single dose of rubella vaccine after the first birthday, more than 90% of individuals will develop long-term immunity. Rarely has congenital rubella syndrome been reported in infants born to mothers with adequate rubella immunization.

▶ Use of Measles, Mumps, and Rubella Vaccine

Measles, mumps, and rubella vaccines are no longer available as single-component vaccines because authorities recommend use of the measles, mumps, and rubella combination. Two doses of the measles, mumps, and rubella vaccine are recommended for all individuals born after 1957. The first dose should be administered soon after the first birthday and the second prior to entering school. For high-risk adolescents and adults who do not have adequate immunity, two doses of the vaccine should be separated by a minimum of 28 days.[11]

Measles, mumps, and rubella vaccine is a live virus vaccine that should be used with caution in immunosuppressed children, such as those with cancer receiving chemotherapy, undergoing solid organ or bone marrow transplantation, or receiving other immunosuppressive drugs, such as steroids in a dose equivalent to prednisone 1 mg/kg/day or higher or 20 mg/day for 2 weeks or longer. If possible, vaccines should be given prior to becoming immunosuppressed. Otherwise, it may be prudent to defer the vaccine until after the immunosuppression resolves.

Meningococcal Vaccines

Neisseria meningitidis is a significant cause of meningitis and severe sepsis. Meningococcus causes an estimated 2,500 cases of invasive disease each year in the United States. Invasive meningococcal disease is associated with

Patient Encounter 2

A mother brings her 4-year-old child to the pediatrician for a routine exam. The child is due for some vaccines.

Which vaccines should the child receive?

The mother is concerned about the number of shots. How can the number of shots be minimized?

The mother is concerned about her child developing autism from one of the vaccines. What is an appropriate response?

an estimated 15% mortality rate. Morbidity in survivors is substantial, with approximately 20% having loss of limb or neurologic sequelae. The highest rates of meningococcal disease are among young children; however, rates have been increasing in adolescents and young adults aged 16 to 21 years. Thirteen meningococcal serogroups have been identified; however, five serogroups, A, B, C, Y, and W-135, are responsible for epidemic and endemic disease worldwide. Despite the availability of highly active antibacterial agents against *N. meningitidis*, there has been little impact on decreasing the morbidity and mortality due to invasive meningococcal disease.[12]

A meningococcal polysaccharide diphtheria toxoid conjugate vaccine was approved by the FDA in 2005, and contains meningococcal serogroups A, C, Y, and W-135. Use of the conjugate meningococcal vaccine in adolescents has shown a significant decrease in meningococcal disease among person aged 11 to 14, but not among persons aged 15 to 18. This indicates waning immunity as adolescents become older.

The meningococcal conjugate vaccine is recommended for routine vaccination at age 11 to 12 years, with a booster dose at age 16 to 18 years. Persons aged 2 through 54 years with complement component deficiencies or asplenia should receive a two-dose primary series administered 2 months apart and a booster dose every 5 years.

Pneumococcal Vaccines

Streptococcus pneumoniae is the most common bacterial cause of community-acquired respiratory tract infections. *S. pneumoniae* causes approximately 3,000 cases of meningitis, 50,000 cases of bacteremia, 500,000 cases of pneumonia, and more than 1 million cases of otitis media each year. The increasing prevalence of drug-resistant *S. pneumoniae* has highlighted the need to prevent infection through vaccination. Both licensed pneumococcal vaccines are highly effective in preventing disease from the common *S. pneumoniae* serotypes that cause human disease.

The 23-valent pneumococcal polysaccharide vaccine contains 23 serotypes that are responsible for causing more than 80% of invasive *S. pneumoniae* infections in adults. The vaccine includes those serotypes that are associated with drug resistance. Use of the vaccine will not prevent the development of antibiotic-resistant *S. pneumoniae*, but is likely to prevent infection from drug-resistant strains. The 23-valent

pneumococcal polysaccharide vaccine has demonstrated good immunogenicity in adults, but an individual will not develop immunity to all 23 serotypes following vaccination.[13]

The 23-valent pneumococcal polysaccharide vaccine is recommended for use in all adults 65 years of age or older and adults less than 65 years who have medical comorbidities that increase the risk for serious complications from *S. pneumoniae* infection, such as chronic pulmonary disorders, cardiovascular disease, diabetes mellitus, chronic liver disease, chronic renal failure, functional or anatomic asplenia, immunosuppressive disorders, and cigarette smokers. Children over the age of 2 years may be vaccinated with the 23-valent pneumococcal polysaccharide vaccine if they are at increased risk for invasive *S. pneumoniae* infections, such as children with sickle cell anemia or those receiving cochlear implants.

Revaccination with the 23-valent pneumococcal polysaccharide vaccine is recommended for adults over the age of 65 years if the first dose was administered when they were less than 65 years of age and at least 5 years have passed. Revaccination results in a blunted immune response and increased local adverse reactions; therefore, routine revaccination is not recommended.[13] Adults vaccinated at age 65 or greater do not require revaccination.

The 7-valent pneumococcal conjugate vaccine was licensed in February 2000 for use in children. Widespread use of the 7-valent pneumococcal conjugate vaccine has resulted in herd immunity and decreased the incidence of invasive *S. pneumoniae* disease among unvaccinated adults over 20 years of age.[13] A 13-valent pneumococcal vaccine was introduced in 2010 and is part of the routine childhood immunization schedule beginning at 2 months of age. It is given at 2, 4, 6, and 12 to 18 months of age.

Poliovirus Vaccine

Poliomyelitis is a highly contagious disease that is often asymptomatic; however, approximately 1 in every 100 to 1,000 cases will develop a rapidly progressive paralytic disease. Polio is caused by poliovirus, which has three serotypes; type 1 is most frequently associated with paralytic disease. Poliovirus replicates in the oropharynx and intestinal tract and is excreted in oral secretions and feces, which can infect others. As a result, more than 90% of unvaccinated individuals will become infected with poliovirus following household exposure to wild-type poliovirus. Since the introduction of the first poliovirus vaccine, there has been a significant reduction in the number of polio cases. Today, polio caused by wild-type poliovirus has been eradicated from the Western hemisphere with the goal of eradicating it from the world.[14]

The first inactivated poliovirus vaccine was introduced in the 1950s in an injectable formulation, and replaced in the 1960s by a live oral poliovirus vaccine. The oral poliovirus vaccine not only elicits systemic immunogenicity but also a localized immune response in the intestinal tract. Unfortunately, the oral poliovirus vaccine has the risk of vaccine-associated paralytic poliomyelitis occurring in approximately 1 case of every 2.4 million doses distributed. The risk with the first dose of oral poliovirus vaccine is 1 case in 750,000 doses.[14]

The last reported case of indigenous wild-type poliovirus in the United States was in 1979; subsequent cases were all vaccine-associated. In 1997, a transition period to the inactivated poliovirus vaccine was begun to reduce the risk of vaccine-associated paralytic poliomyelitis. By January 2000, the oral vaccine was no longer recommended for routine use. Currently, the inactivated poliovirus vaccine is recommended for routine use in the United States. The oral poliovirus vaccine is still widely used in some countries where poliovirus eradication has been more difficult.

The enhanced potency inactivated poliovirus vaccine contains all three serotypes. After two doses, more than 90% of those vaccinated will have immunity to the three serotypes, and 99% will have immunity after three doses. Inactivated poliovirus vaccine is recommended to be given at 2, 4, 6 to 18 months, and 4 to 6 years of age.

Rotavirus Vaccine

Rotavirus is the most common cause of diarrhea worldwide. Most children will become infected by the age of 5 years. In the United States, rotavirus is responsible for approximately 50,000 hospitalizations for severe diarrhea and dehydration, and 20 to 40 deaths annually. Most hospitalizations occur in children younger than 3 years. Rotavirus infections follow a winter–spring seasonal pattern. Rotavirus G1 is the most prevalent strain found in the United States. However, in any given year, other strains (G2, G3, G4, and G9) may predominate.

The first rotavirus vaccine was a tetravalent rhesus-based rotavirus strain. It was licensed in the United States in 1998 and subsequently withdrawn from the market within the first year due to an association with intussusception. A pentavalent human-bovine reassortant rotavirus vaccine was approved by the FDA in February 2006. This vaccine contains outer capsid proteins for G1, G2, G3, G4 and P1. A monovalent, G1 vaccine has been approved for use in the United States.[15] The exact mechanism by which these vaccines produce an immune response is unknown; however, these live virus vaccines replicate in the small intestine and induce immunity.

The rotavirus vaccine is administered in either a two-dose or three-dose series that is orally administered. The first dose is given to infants between 6 and 12 weeks of age.[15] One year after the introduction of the rotavirus vaccine, the CDC reported a 50% reduction in reported cases of rotavirus in the United States.

Varicella Vaccine

Varicella zoster virus is a herpes virus that infects nearly all humans. Primary infection with Varicella zoster causes chickenpox (varicella), which is one of the most common childhood diseases. Chickenpox has always been thought to be a benign disease causing few serious complications in children. The rate of chickenpox prior to the vaccine becoming available was thought to approximate the birth rate, with 3 to 4 million cases annually resulting in 11,000 hospitalizations and 100 deaths. Adults who develop chickenpox have a 25% greater risk for developing serious complications from varicella compared with children. Chickenpox is highly contagious and has a secondary household transmission rate of 87%. Following resolution of the primary infection, varicella becomes latent in cranial nerve, dorsal routs, and autonomic ganglia.

The varicella vaccine is made up of an attenuated Oka strain of varicella zoster virus. This is a live attenuated vaccine. Attenuation was achieved by performing serial passages through human embryonic lung cells, embryonic guinea pig cells, and human diploid cells.

Children younger than 12 years will have a 97% seroconversion rate following a single vaccination. Adolescents and adults more than 13 years old will only have 78% seroconversion after a single inoculation, but will have 99% conversion after the second vaccination administered 4 to 8 weeks after the first. Antibody titers appear to persist for at least 20 years following immunization. Despite excellent seroconversion rates, breakthrough chickenpox is reported at a rate of 1 case per 10,000 doses distributed. Most cases occurred within the first year following vaccination, and were due to wild-type varicella zoster virus. The majority of breakthrough cases were mild and of short duration.[16]

Secondary transmission to household contacts is always a concern with administration of a live vaccine. There are a few cases of possible secondary transmission of varicella following vaccination. Of the cases that varicella typing was done, 62% were wild-type virus, indicating exposure to an unvaccinated person. There are fewer than 10 confirmed cases of secondary transmission of the Oka vaccine strain following vaccination. A mild rash occurring in less than 5% of persons has been reported following vaccination. The varicella virus may be shed from the rash. Rashes due to the Oka vaccine strain typically occur more than 20 days following vaccination.[16]

Varicella vaccine should be administered after 12 months of age and a second dose at 4 years of age. Adolescents and adults without evidence of immunity to varicella zoster should receive two doses of varicella vaccine given 4 to 8 weeks apart. Varicella vaccine is available as a single-component vaccine or in combination with measles, mumps, and rubella vaccine.

Zoster Vaccine

Later in life, approximately 15% of the population will develop herpes zoster (shingles). Zoster is the reactivation of latent varicella zoster virus in the sensory ganglia. It produces a classic rash along a single nerve track. Approximately 20% of persons with herpes zoster will develop postherpetic neuralgia, which is a painful debilitating condition that can persist for months after resolution of the herpes zoster rash. Adults get a boost in immunity with repeated exposure to children with the chickenpox. Zoster most frequently occurs in the elderly and immunocompromised individuals who have decreased circulating antibodies to varicella zoster virus.[17]

Zoster vaccine is a more concentrated form of the varicella vaccine. It is recommended for use in individuals 60 years of age and older even if they have had a previous episode of shingles. Use of the zoster vaccine has shown a 60% reduction in the incidence of zoster and postherpetic neuralgia. There is decreased effectiveness of the vaccine with increasing age.

The varicella vaccine is relatively new and has only been recommended for use since 1996; therefore, its true impact on chickenpox and zoster is not yet known. Continued use of the varicella vaccine will undoubtedly change the epidemiology of both of these diseases. As the prevalence of chickenpox declines, the rate of zoster will likely increase in the elderly, making vaccination with the zoster vaccine more prudent.[17]

COMBINATION VACCINES

The childhood immunization schedule is complex and requires a large number of injections. In small infants, the large number of injections can be intolerable to the infant, parent, and healthcare provider. Limiting the number of injections at each visit can lead to missed vaccinations and increased expense for return visits. ❸ *Use of combination vaccines decreases the number of injections and increases the likelihood that the immunization schedule will be completed.*

Many factors have to be considered when developing combination vaccines. First, the selected components need to be given on a similar schedule, and all components should already be licensed in the United States. The excipients contained in the individual vaccines may interfere with another component when combined, altering a component's immunogenicity. Finally, the immunogenicity of the combination must be similar (within 10%) to the immune response when the components are administered separately.[18]

There are several combination vaccines available in the United States. Two of the most popular pediatric combinations are Pediarix and Pentacel, which are used in the primary infant vaccination series. The only combination available for adults is Twinrix, which has hepatitis A and hepatitis B vaccines.

VACCINE ADMINISTRATION SCHEDULES

Most vaccines are administered in two- to four-shot series in order to elicit the best protection. Childhood and adult immunization schedules are revised frequently and published annually by the CDC Advisory Committee on Immunization Practices. Current immunization schedules can be found at *www.cdc.gov*. Recommendations will be published throughout the year in the *Morbidity and Mortality Weekly Report* (*MMWR*) as new vaccines are licensed or new information necessitates a change in previous recommendations.

VACCINE SAFETY

Vaccination is one of the most powerful tools used to prevent disease. As with all drugs, most vaccines have been reported to cause adverse reactions. The reactions are either acute, such as local reactions, or are related to the risk of developing another disease. Healthcare professionals are to give vaccine information sheets (VIS) to individuals or caregivers prior to vaccination; these provide information about the risks and benefits of each vaccine.

Vaccine safety is monitored by the FDA and CDC through a passive reporting system that allows anyone, health professionals or lay public, to report any event. ❹ *Healthcare professionals are bound by federal regulation to report certain adverse events* (*Table 86-2*). Additionally, any serious, life-threatening or unusual reactions should also be reported. The Vaccine Adverse Event Reporting System (VAERS) can be found at *http://vaers.hhs.gov*.

The VAERS database is continually monitored to determine whether the prevalence of reactions is changing and to identify previously unreported reactions to a particular vaccine. One of the limitations of the VAERS data is that it does not contain denominator data. Therefore, it is not possible to calculate a true rate of reaction occurrence: the number of cases of reaction per dose of vaccine administered. Rates are usually calculated using the number of doses distributed from the manufacture as the denominator. This makes the assumption that each dose distributed is administered.

Local Reactions

Pain at the injection site is one of the most commonly reported adverse effects of vaccination. The reaction is usually mild, with complaints of pain and tenderness at the injection site that may or may not be accompanied by erythema. Local reactions tend to be more frequent with repeated doses or booster doses of vaccine. The frequency and degree of the reactions appear to be related to the amount of preformed antibodies and rapid immunologic responses reflective of priming from previous doses. More serious Arthus reactions are infrequently reported. Arthus reactions are classified as type III hypersensitivity reactions and are characterized by a massive local response involving the entire thigh or deltoid. Arthus reactions are also related to preformed antibody complexes that induce an inflammatory lesion.[19]

Tetanus-containing vaccines are well known for causing localized reactions; however, all vaccines can cause local reactions.

Fever

Fever is the most frequently reported adverse effect in children and adolescents. Fever associated with vaccination is defined as a temperature of greater than or equal to 38°C (100.4°F) measured at any site using a validated device. Fever is caused by a complex reaction induced by the production of cytokines that affect the hypothalamic neurons. This

Table 86–2		
Vaccine Reportable Events		
Vaccine/Toxoid	**Event**	**Interval From Vaccination**
Tetanus in any combination (DTaP, DTP, DTP-Hib, DT, Tdap, Td, or TT)	Anaphylaxis or anaphylactic shock	7 days
	Brachial neuritis	28 days
	Systemic allergic reaction	7 days
	Systemic neurologic reaction	
Pertussis in any combination (DTaP, DTP, DTP-Hib, or Tdap)	Anaphylaxis or anaphylactic shock	7 days
	Encephalopathy or encephalitis	7 days
	Progressive neurologic disorders, such as infantile spasms or uncontrolled epilepsy	7 days
Measles, mumps, and rubella in any combination (MMR, MR, M, or R)	Anaphylaxis or anaphylactic shock	7 days
	Encephalopathy or encephalitis	15 days
Rubella in any combination (MMR, MR, or R)	Chronic arthritis	42 days
Measles in any combination (MMR, MR, or M)	Thrombocytopenic purpura	7–30 days
	Vaccine strain measles in immunodeficient recipient	6 months
Oral polio (OPV)	Paralytic polio	30 days to 6 months
	Vaccine strain polio infection	30 days to 6 months
Inactivated polio (IPV)	Anaphylaxis or anaphylactic shock	7 days
	Systemic allergic reaction	7 days
Hepatitis B	Anaphylaxis or anaphylactic shock	7 days
	Systemic allergic reaction	7 days
Haemophilus influenzae type b (conjugate)	Anaphylaxis or anaphylactic shock	7 days
	Systemic allergic reaction	7 days
Varicella (chickenpox)	Anaphylaxis or anaphylactic shock	7 days
	Systemic allergic reaction	7 days
Rotavirus	Intussusception	30 days
Pneumococcal conjugate	Anaphylaxis or anaphylactic shock	7 days
	Systemic allergic reaction	7 days

results in raising the hypothalamic set point. Temperature elevations above 40°C (104°F) can result in cellular and multiorgan dysfunction. Excessive temperature elevations rarely result from fever alone, but are usually coupled with other thermoregulatory dysfunction.[20]

The whole-cell pertussis vaccine has been highly associated with temperature elevations; however, the prevalence has significantly decreased since the introduction of the acellular pertussis vaccine. Live virus vaccines are also associated with fever.

Guillain-Barré Syndrome

Guillain-Barré syndrome is a transient neurologic disorder involving inflammatory demyelination of the peripheral nerves. The syndrome is characterized by progressive symmetric weakness of the legs and arms with loss of reflexes. Occasionally, sensory abnormalities and paralysis of respiratory muscles will occur.[21]

The etiology of Guillain-Barré syndrome is unknown, but increasing evidence suggests it is probably a humoral and cellular autoimmune disease induced by infection with a variety of microorganisms. The background rate of Guillain-Barré syndrome is 1 to 2 cases per 100,000 persons annually. Guillain-Barré syndrome has been associated with several vaccines. An influenza vaccine used in the mid-1970s (swine flu vaccine) increased the incidence of Guillain-Barré syndrome by a factor of eight.[21] Warnings about Guillain-Barré

syndrome continue to be given with annual influenza vaccinations. The hepatitis B vaccine derived from pooled plasma was also associated with Guillain-Barré syndrome; however, Guillain-Barré has not been reported with use of the currently available hepatitis B vaccines produced through recombinant DNA technology. Most recently, Guillain-Barré syndrome has been reported to occur with the meningococcal conjugate vaccine.

Other Safety Concerns

A clear cause-and-effect relationship between vaccine administration and chronic diseases, such as diabetes mellitus, multiple sclerosis, and chronic arthritis, has never been scientifically proven.

Thimerosal is a preservative used in vaccines that has been purported to cause autism in children. The assumption is that thimerosal, also known as ethyl mercury, causes similar effects as methyl mercury, which has neurotoxic and nephrotoxic effects at high doses. Several epidemiologic studies have not shown a higher rate of autism among children receiving thimerosal-containing vaccines when compared with the normal background rate of autism. Additionally, the mercury exposure with vaccination is much lower than through many other environmental exposures. Despite the lack of evidence of thimerosal causing neurologic disorders, vaccine manufacturers are producing vaccines that are thimerosal-free or only contain trace amounts of thimerosal.[19]

SPECIAL POPULATIONS

Immunocompromised Host

The number of immunocompromised persons is continually increasing as advances are made in medicine. The life expectancy for persons with cancer, HIV infection, and solid organ or bone marrow transplantation is increasing. Vaccination provides one tool to prevent infection in the immunocompromised host; however, the individual's immunosuppressed state will alter the response to the vaccine. In general, all vaccinations should be updated prior to the person becoming immunosuppressed, if possible. ⑤ *Once a person becomes significantly immunosuppressed, live virus vaccines should be avoided.*

Adults with HIV infection should be vaccinated with the 23-valent pneumococcal polysaccharide and hepatitis B vaccines as early in the course of the disease as possible. Inactivated influenza vaccine should be given yearly. Children should continue to receive vaccinations on the standard childhood immunization schedule. The individual may experience a transient elevation in HIV viral load following vaccination.[22]

Following hematopoietic stem-cell transplantation, the patient will need virtually all routine vaccines to be administered again; however, the patient will not be able to mount an adequate response for 6 to 12 months posttransplant. Diphtheria, tetanus, acellular pertussis, *H. influenzae* type b, hepatitis B, pneumococcal, and inactivated poliovirus should be given at 12, 14, and 24 months posthematopoietic stem cell transplantation. Inactivated influenza vaccine should be given yearly, starting 6 months after transplant. Measles, mumps, and rubella can be given 2 years after transplant and varicella and zoster vaccines are contraindicated.[22]

Solid organ transplant recipients have a blunted immune response to vaccines because the immunosuppressive regimens used to prevent organ rejection inhibit both T- and B-cell proliferation. Many of these patients will also have secondary hypogammaglobulinemia posttransplantation. Prior to transplant, children should complete primary immunization schedules if possible; accelerated schedules may be used. Adults should have all vaccinations updated prior to transplantation.[22]

Household contacts of immunocompromised persons should have all routine vaccines as scheduled, including yearly influenza vaccination. Children in the household may receive live virus vaccines without special precautions; however, if a rash develops following varicella vaccination, contact should be avoided with the immunocompromised host until the rash resolves.

Patient Encounter 3

A 70-year-old patient goes to the physician for a routine physical. The patient reports not seeing a doctor for more than 5 years. The last time he was at the doctor he had shingles.

Which vaccines should the patient be screened for?

Should this patient receive the zoster vaccine?

Pregnancy

Immunization during pregnancy is done to ensure that the infant has sufficient antibodies during the period the infant is most vulnerable to disease. Maternal antibodies are actively transported to the fetus throughout the pregnancy. However, in the last 4 to 6 weeks of gestation, the active transport of immunoglobulins substantially increases. Vaccines administered during pregnancy should produce high antibody concentrations following a single vaccination and are administered in the second and third trimester, but no later than 2 weeks prior to delivery. Maternal vaccination has not shown any harmful effects to the developing fetus. However, live virus vaccines are avoided due to theoretical concerns of the virus being transported across the placenta and infecting the fetus. It is recommended that pregnant women be up-to-date on tetanus vaccine and receive the influenza vaccine if the second and third trimester will occur during the winter months.[23]

Healthcare Workers

Most healthcare workers are at risk for exposure to many diseases in the normal course of their work. Additionally, healthcare workers may transmit vaccine-preventable diseases to their patients. At the time of employment and on a regular basis, healthcare workers should be screened for immunity to measles, mumps, rubella, and varicella; if found to be nonimmune, the measles, mumps, and rubella, and varicella vaccines should be administered. The hepatitis B series should be given if not already completed. Tetanus should be updated and given every 10 years. Healthcare personnel in hospitals and ambulatory settings with direct patient contact should receive Tdap if not already received.

All healthcare personnel should receive the influenza vaccine yearly in order to prevent transmission of influenza within the healthcare facility and to decrease employee absenteeism for influenza-related reasons. The vaccine should be made available to employees at the workplace free of charge. Employees should be asked to sign a declination if refusing to receive the influenza vaccine. Additionally, healthcare facilities should report the number of healthcare personnel receiving influenza vaccine as a patient safety measure.[24]

OUTCOME MEASURES

⑥ *Vaccines are a cost-effective means for disease prevention.* For every dollar spent on routine childhood vaccines, there will be a savings of $0.90 to $24.00 in direct medical expense. The rates of vaccination for children are well over 90%. This has been attributed to the requirements for proof of vaccination by states for enrollment into day care centers and school. Additionally, children (18 years of age or younger) may receive routine vaccinations free of charge through state health departments or other assistance programs, such as the national Vaccines for Children program. Many states have developed universal immunization databases to document pediatric and adult vaccination status. This eliminates the problems of lost immunization records if a child changes healthcare providers.

The vaccination rate in adults is much lower than that in children. Only 50% to 60% of adults who meet criteria have received pneumococcal or influenza vaccination. Comprehensive initiatives need to be implemented to increase the adult vaccination rate. Some proven concepts are providing reminders to patients that vaccines are due and implementation of standing orders for vaccines. This latter concept allows nurses and pharmacists to screen patients to determine whether pneumococcal, influenza, or other vaccines are needed and to vaccinate without a physician's order.

The Centers for Medicare and Medicaid Services has incorporated pneumococcal and influenza immunization rates into some of their quality standards. Patients admitted to a hospital for community-acquired pneumonia should be screened for, offered, and vaccinated with pneumococcal and influenza vaccines prior to discharge if not previously administered. In physicians' office practice, all persons older than 65 years who have been hospitalized in the past year should be screened for, offered, and vaccinated with pneumococcal and influenza vaccines if not previously administered. Both of these standards will affect payment if the standard is not met. The Joint Commission has also incorporated these standards into their accreditation reviews of healthcare facilities.

Abbreviations Introduced in This Chapter

anti-HBs	Antibody to hepatitis B surface antigen
CDC	Centers for Disease Control and Prevention
HBsAg	Hepatitis B surface antigen
TT	Tetanus toxoid
VAERS	Vaccine Adverse Event Reporting System
VIS	Vaccine information sheets

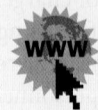 Self-assessment questions and answers are available at *http://mhpharmacotherapy.com/pp.html*.

REFERENCES

1. MacKay IR, Rosen FS. Vaccines and vaccination. N Engl J Med 2001;345:1042–1053.
2. Mattos-Guaraldi AL, Moreira LO, Damasco PV, Junior RH. Diphtheria remains a threat to health in the developing world—An overview. Mern Inst Oswaldo Cruz 2003;98:987–993.
3. Rhee P, Nunley MK, Demetriades D, Velmahos G, Doucet JJ. Tetanus and trauma: A review and recommendations. J Trauma 2005;58:1082–1088.
4. Hewlett El, Edwards KM. Pertussis—Not just for kids. N Engl J Med 2005;352:1215–1222.
5. Centers for Disease Control and Prevention. Preventing tetanus, diphtheria, and pertussis among adults: Use of the tetanus toxoid, reduced diphtheria toxoid and acellular pertussis vaccine. MMWR 2006;55 (No. RR-17):1–34.
6. Centers for Disease Control and Prevention. Prevention of hepatitis A through active and passive immunization: Recommendations of the Advisory Committee on Immunization Practices (ACIP). MMWR 1999; 48(No. RR-12):1–37.
7. Centers for Disease Control and Prevention. A comprehensive immunization strategy to eliminate transmission of hepatitis B virus infection in the United States: recommendations of the Advisory Committee on Immunization Practices (ACIP); Part 1 immunization of infants, children, and adolescents. MMWR 2005; 55(No. RR-16):1–32.
8. Govan VA. A novel vaccine for cervical cancer: Quadrivalent human papillomavirus (types 6, 11, 16 and 18) recombinant vaccine (Gardasil®). Ther Clin Risk Manag 2008;4:65–70.
9. Centers for Disease Control and Prevention. Quadrivalent human papillomavirus vaccine: Recommendations of the Advisory Committee on Immunization Practices (ACIP). MMWR 2007;57 (No. RR-2):1–23.
10. Centers for Disease Control and Prevention. Prevention and control of influenza: Recommendations of the Advisory Committee on Immunization Practices (ACIP), 2008. MMWR 2008;57(No. RR-7): 1–59.
11. Centers for Disease Control and Prevention. Measles, mumps, and rubella—Vaccine use and strategies for elimination of measles, rubella, and congenital rubella syndrome and control of mumps: recommendations of the Advisory Committee on Immunization Practices (ACIP). MMWR 1998;47(No. RR-8):1–57.
12. Centers for Disease Control and Prevention. Prevention and control of meningococcal disease recommendations of the Advisory Committee on Immunization Practices (ACIP). MMWR 2005;54(No. RR-7): 1–21.
13. American Society of Health-Systems Pharmacists. ASHP therapeutic position statement on strategies for identifying and preventing pneumococcal resistance. Am J Health-Syst Pharm 2004;61: 2430–2435.
14. Centers for Disease Control and Prevention. Poliomyelitis in the United States: Updated recommendations of the Advisory Committee on Immunization Practices (ACIP). MMWR 2000;49(No. RR-5): 1–22.
15. Centers for Disease Control and Prevention. Prevention of rotavirus gastroenteritis among infants and children: Recommendations of the Advisory Committee on Immunization Practices (ACIP). MMWR 2006;55 (No. RR-12):1–13.
16. Sharrar RG, LaRussa P, Galea SA, et al. The postmarketing safety profile of varicella vaccine. Vaccine 2001;19:916–923.
17. Quan D, Cohrs RJ, Mahalingam R, Gilden DH. Prevention of shingles: Safety and efficacy of live zoster vaccine. Ther Clin Risk Manag 2007;3:633–639.
18. Edwards KM, Decker MD. Combination vaccines. Infect Dis Clin N Am 2001;15:209–230.
19. Moylett EH, Hanson IC. Mechanistic actions of the risks and adverse events associated with vaccine administration. J Allerg Clin Immunol 2004;114:1010–1020.
20. Kohl KS, Marcy SM, Blum M, et al. Fever after immunization: Current concepts and improved future scientific understanding. Clin Infect Dis 2004;39:389–394.
21. Shoenfeld Y, Aron-Maor A. Vaccination and autoimmunity –'vaccinosis': A dangerous liaison? J Autoimmune 2000;14:1–10.
22. Weber DJ, rutala WA. Immunization of immunocompromised persons. Immunol Allergy Clin North Am 2003;23:605–634.
23. Munoz FM, Englund JA. Vaccines in pregnancy. Infect Dis Clin North Am 2001;15:253–271.
24. Centers for Disease Control and Prevention. Influenza vaccination of health-care personnel: Recommendations of the Healthcare Infection Control Practices Advisory Committee (HICPAC) and the Advisory Committee on Immunization Practices (ACIP). MMWR Recomm Rep 2006;55 (RR-2):1–16.

87

Human Immunodeficiency Virus Infection

Jessica L. Adams, Julie B. Dumond,
Angela D.M. Kashuba, and Amanda Corbett

LEARNING OBJECTIVES

● **Upon completion of the chapter, the reader will be able to:**

1. Explain the routes of transmission for HIV and its natural disease progression.

2. Identify typical and atypical signs and symptoms of acute and chronic HIV infection.

3. Identify the desired therapeutic outcomes for patients with HIV infection.

4. Recommend appropriate first-line pharmacotherapy interventions for patients with HIV infection.

5. Recommend appropriate second-line pharmacotherapy interventions for patients with HIV infection.

6. Describe the components of a monitoring plan to assess effectiveness and adverse effects of pharmacotherapy for HIV infection.

7. Educate patients about the disease state, appropriate lifestyle modifications, and drug therapy required for effective treatment.

KEY CONCEPTS

❶ The treatment goals for HIV infection are to maximally and durably suppress HIV replication, avoid the development of drug resistance, restore and preserve immune function, prevent opportunistic infections, and minimize adverse effects.

❷ HIV RNA plasma concentrations and CD4+ T-cell counts are used to assess risk of progression to AIDS (or risk for opportunistic infection) and to monitor efficacy and durability of treatment.

❸ Effective and complete treatment of HIV infection involves a multidisciplinary approach, which includes pharmacists, other clinicians, and social workers.

❹ Treatment with two nucleoside reverse transcriptase inhibitors (NRTIs) *and* a nonnucleoside reverse transcriptase inhibitor (NNRTI) *or* a ritonavir-boosted protease inhibitor (PI) *or* an integrase stand transfer inhibitor (INSTI) is the mainstay of initial treatment for HIV infection.

❺ All patients with HIV infection relapse if medication is withdrawn. Therefore, long-term maintenance treatment is required.

❻ HIV mutates easily, and strict adherence to the drug regimen and avoidance of deleterious drug interactions is critical to preventing the development of drug resistance and treatment failure.

❼ The majority of antiretroviral medications are metabolized by the cytochrome P-450 enzyme system (CYP). Therefore, it is important to review patient medication profiles for drugs that may interact with antiretroviral drugs.

❽ Most antiretroviral medications cause acute and chronic adverse effects. Patients should be closely monitored for these toxicities so that interventions can occur quickly.

The acquired immune deficiency syndrome (AIDS) was first recognized in 1981 and was described in a cohort of young homosexual men with significant immune deficiency. Since then, human immunodeficiency virus type 1 (HIV-1) has been clearly identified as the major cause of AIDS. HIV-2 is much less prevalent than HIV-1, but also causes AIDS. HIV primarily targets CD4+ lymphocytes, which are critical to proper immune system function. If left untreated, patients experience a prolonged asymptomatic period followed by rapid, progressive immunodeficiency. Therefore, most complications experienced by patients with AIDS involve opportunistic infections and cancers.

HIV is primarily transmitted by sexual contact, by contact with blood or blood products, and from mother to child during gestation, delivery, or breast-feeding. The prevalence and incidence of HIV is rising globally, and to date there are no treatments that eradicate HIV from the body. Combinations of potent antiretroviral agents (called highly active antiretroviral therapy, or HAART) can suppress HIV replication to undetectable levels, delay the onset of AIDS, and prolong survival. However, there are a number of drug-induced, long-term toxicities that challenge effective patient management. This chapter addresses HIV treatment options and challenges and gives practical suggestions for patient management.

EPIDEMIOLOGY

Since the first cases of AIDS were identified in 1981, close to 30 million people have died as a result of HIV infection. This makes AIDS one of the most destructive epidemics in recorded history. The epidemic remains extremely dynamic, and no country in the world is unaffected. In 2009, HIV infected approximately 33 million people worldwide. Approximately 68% of these cases are in sub-Saharan Africa, with a prevalence of approximately 5%. East Asia, Central Asia, and Eastern Europe are also seeing rapidly rising infection rates.[1]

In 2009 alone, approximately 1.8 million people died from AIDS and 2.6 million people were newly infected with HIV. Most of these infections were acquired through heterosexual transmission. As of December 2009, women accounted for 52% of all people living with HIV worldwide. Persons aged 15 to 24 years accounted for approximately 40% of new HIV infections worldwide.[1]

In the United States, at the end of 2008, an estimated 1,000,000 persons were living with HIV/AIDS. Approximately 20% of these are undiagnosed and unaware of their HIV infection and could be unknowingly transmitting the virus to others. In 2008, of the total number of HIV-infected patients, approximately one-half were living with AIDS, whereas approximately 18,000 died with AIDS. The cumulative estimated number of diagnoses of AIDS through 2006 was 1,014,797, one-half of whom (565,927) had died. Approximately 56,300 people are newly infected with HIV each year.[2]

Compared with their distribution in the U.S. population, African American and Hispanic populations are disproportionately affected by HIV/AIDS, representing 46% and 17% of cases, respectively. HIV/AIDS is among the top four causes of death for African American men aged 25 to 44 years and is among the top three causes of death for African American women of the same age. In 2008, HIV/AIDS rates for African American males were six times those for white males and three times those for Hispanic males. HIV/AIDS rates for African American females were 15 times the rates for white females and four times the rates for Hispanic females.[2]

ETIOLOGY AND PATHOGENESIS

HIV-1 is a retrovirus and member of the genus *Lentivirus*. These viruses have a characteristically prolonged latency period. There are two molecularly and serologically distinct but related types of HIV: HIV-1 and HIV-2. HIV-2 is a less common cause of the epidemic and is found primarily in West Africa. HIV-1 is categorized by phylogenetic lineages into three groups (M [main], N [new], and O [outlier]). HIV-1 group M can be further categorized into nine subtypes: A through D, F through H, and J and K. HIV-1 subtype B is primarily responsible for the North American and Western European epidemic.

HIV in humans is believed to result from cross-species transmission from primates infected with simian immunodeficiency virus (SIV). HIV-2 is closely related to the SIV found in sooty mangabeys in West Africa, and HIV-1 is similar to the SIV found in chimpanzees. The earliest known human HIV infection was in central Africa in 1959. Cultural practices such as the preparation and eating of bush-meat, or keeping primates as pets, may have allowed the virus to transmit from animal to human. The rapid spread of the virus throughout the world can be primarily attributed to sexual promiscuity, drug abuse, and high mobility due to modern transportation.

HIV infection occurs through three primary modes of transmission: sexual, parenteral, and perinatal. The most common method for transmission is receptive anal and vaginal intercourse, with the probability of transmission up to 30% per sexual contact. The probability of transmission increases when the index partner has a high level of viral replication (which occurs at the beginning of infection or late in disease) or when the uninfected partner has ulcerative disease or compromised mucosal surfaces or (in the case of men) has not been circumcised.

Parenteral transmission of HIV primarily occurs through injection drug use by sharing contaminated needles or injection-related supplies. As a result of a comprehensive North American screening program, less than 1% of all cases of HIV infection occur as a result of transfusions of contaminated blood or blood products, or infected transplant organs. Healthcare workers have a 0.3% estimated risk of acquiring HIV infection through percutaneous needle-stick injury.

Perinatal infection (also known as vertical transmission or mother-to-child transmission [MTCT]) can occur during gestation, at or near delivery, and during breast-feeding. The risk of MTCT up to and including delivery is approximately 25%, whereas the risk of transmission during breast-feeding is approximately 15% to 20% within the first 6 months of life. Because a high rate of HIV replication in the blood is a significant risk factor for transmission of HIV, it is important to treat women for their HIV infection during pregnancy. After delivery, mothers are strongly recommended not to breast-feed if safe alternatives are available.

Understanding the life cycle of the virus is important to know how antiretroviral drugs are combined for optimal therapy (Fig. 87–1). Once HIV enters the body, an outer glycoprotein called gp120 binds to CD4 receptors found on the surface of dendritic cells, T lymphocytes, monocytes, and macrophages. This allows further binding to other chemokine receptors on the cell surface called CCR5 and CXCR4. Greater than 95% of newly infected patients have viruses that preferentially use CCR5 to enter the cell, and most patients with advanced disease have viruses that preferentially use

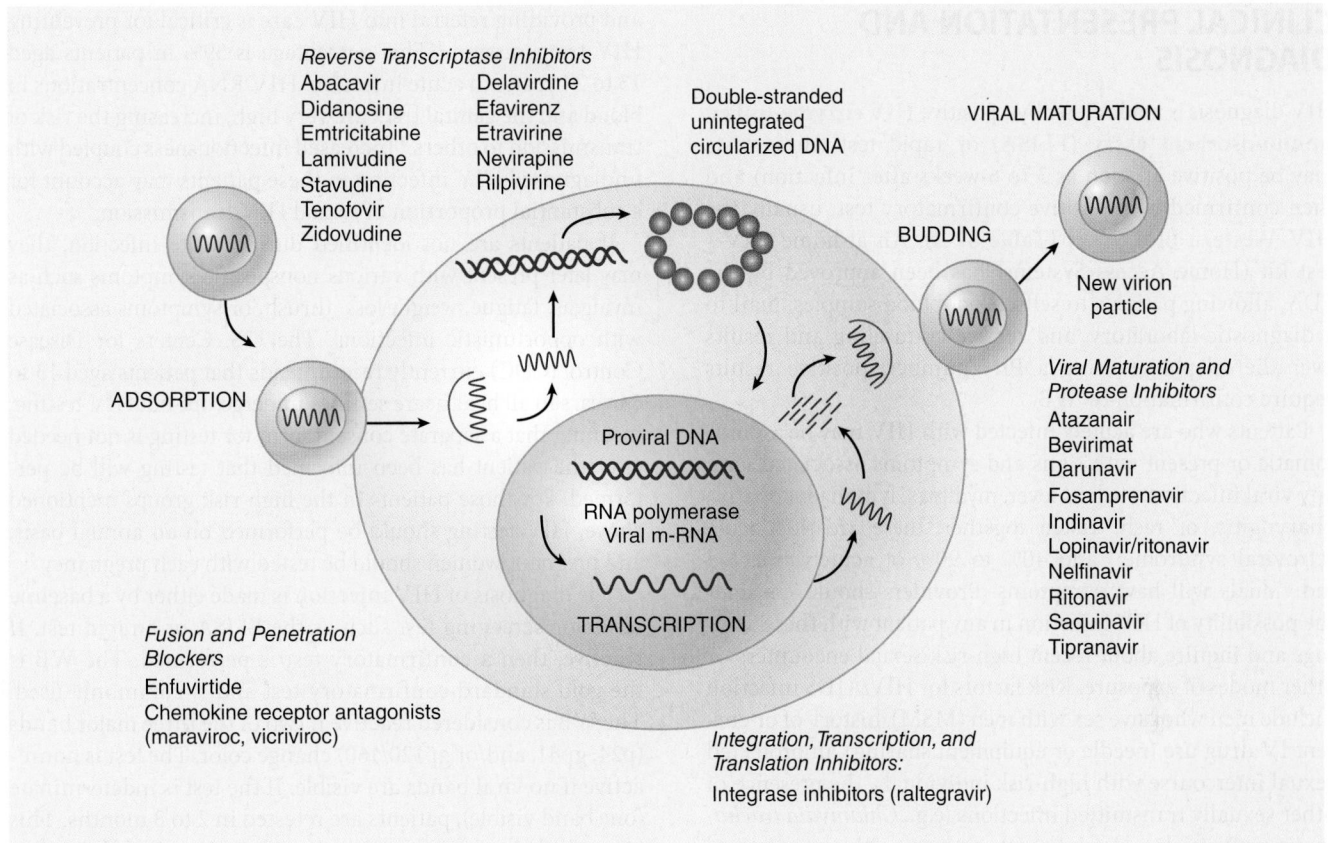

FIGURE 87–1. Life cycle of HIV and targets for antiretroviral drugs. (From Fletcher CV, Kakuda TN. Human immunodeficiency virus infection. In: DiPiro JT, Talbert RL, Yee GC, et al., eds. Pharmacotherapy: A Pathophysiologic Approach. 8th ed. New York: McGraw-Hill; 2005: 2258; With permission.)

CXCR4 to enter the cell. This becomes important in understanding the place in therapy for some of the new drugs in development.

After the virus has attached to CD4 and chemokine receptors, another viral glycoprotein (gp41) assists with viral fusion to the cell and internalization of the viral contents. The viral contents include single-stranded RNA, an RNA-dependent DNA polymerase (also known as reverse transcriptase), and other enzymes. Using the single-stranded viral RNA as a template, reverse transcriptase synthesizes a complementary strand of DNA. The single-stranded viral RNA is removed from the newly formed DNA strand by ribonuclease H, and reverse transcriptase completes the synthesis of double-stranded DNA. The viral reverse transcriptase enzyme is highly error-prone, and many mutations occur in the conversion of RNA to DNA. This inefficient reverse transcription activity is responsible for HIV's ability to rapidly mutate and develop drug resistance.

A chronic infection is established when the double-stranded DNA migrates to the host cell nucleus and is integrated into the host cell chromosome by an HIV enzyme called integrase. Once the cell becomes activated by antigens or cytokines, HIV replication starts: Host DNA polymerase transcribes viral DNA into messenger RNA, and messenger RNA is translated into viral proteins. These proteins assemble beneath the bilayer of the host cell, a nucleocapsid

forms containing these proteins, and the virus buds from the cell. After budding, the virus matures when an HIV protease enzyme cleaves large polypeptides into smaller functional proteins. Without this process, the virus is unable to infect other cells.

During the early stages of infection, approximately 10 billion virions can be produced each day. Most of the cells containing these viruses will be lysed as a result of budding virions, killed by cytotoxic T-lymphocytes, or undergo apoptosis. However, virus will be protected within some cells (macrophages, T cells in lymph nodes), which can stay dormant for years. The initial immune response against HIV is relatively effective, but it is unable to completely clear the infection, and the patient enters a latent, asymptomatic, or mildly symptomatic stage lasting 5 to 15 years. During this time, a high rate of viral replication can be seen in the lymph nodes. Eventually immune deficiency occurs when the body is no longer able to replenish helper T cells at a rate equal to that at which HIV is destroying them.

❶ *The goal of therapy is to maximally and durably suppress HIV replication to restore and preserve immune system function and minimize morbidity and mortality.* Because HIV replication has been found in all areas of the body, it is important to use potent drug therapy that can achieve adequate concentrations in all tissues, including protected sites such as the brain and genital tract.

CLINICAL PRESENTATION AND DIAGNOSIS

HIV diagnosis is made either by a positive **HIV enzyme-linked immunosorbent assay (ELISA)** or rapid test (these tests may be positive as soon as 3 to 6 weeks after infection) and then confirmed by a positive confirmatory test, usually the HIV **Western blot (WB)** (Table 87–1). An at-home HIV-1 test kit (Home Access Systems) has been approved by the FDA, allowing patients to self-collect blood samples, mail to a diagnostic laboratory, and receive counseling and results over the telephone using a PIN number; positive results require confirmation by WB.

Patients who are acutely infected with HIV may be asymptomatic or present with signs and symptoms associated with any viral infection, such as fever, myalgias, lymphadenopathy, pharyngitis, or rash. Taken together, these are the "acute retroviral syndrome," and 40% to 90% of acutely infected individuals will have symptoms. Providers should consider the possibility of HIV infection in any patient with these findings and inquire about recent high-risk sexual encounters or other modes of exposure. Risk factors for HIV/AIDS infection include men who have sex with men (MSM), history of or current IV drug use (needle or equipment sharing), unprotected sexual intercourse with high-risk individuals, the presence of other sexually transmitted infections (e.g., *Chlamydia trachomatis or Neisseria gonorrhoeae*), persons with coagulation/hemophilia disorders, and previous blood product recipients. In the United States, 20% of HIV-infected individuals are not aware of their status, thus identifying acutely infected patients and providing referral into HIV care is critical for preventing HIV transmission.[2] This percentage is 59% in patients aged 13 to 24 years. In acute infection, HIV RNA concentrations in blood and the genital tract are very high, increasing the risk of transmission to others.[3] Increased infectiousness coupled with undiagnosed HIV infection in these patients may account for a substantial proportion of sexual HIV transmission.

If patients are not identified during acute infection, they may later present with various nonspecific symptoms such as myalgias, fatigue, weight loss, thrush, or symptoms associated with opportunistic infections. The U.S. Centers for Disease Control (CDC) currently recommends that patients aged 13 to 64 years in all healthcare settings undergo opt-out HIV testing, meaning that a separate consent form for testing is not needed after the patient has been informed that testing will be performed. For those patients in the high-risk groups mentioned above, HIV testing should be performed on an annual basis, and pregnant women should be tested with each pregnancy.[4]

The diagnosis of HIV infection is made either by a baseline serologic screening test such as the ELISA or a rapid test. If reactive, then a confirmatory test is performed. The WB is the gold standard confirmatory test and is commonly used. The WB is considered reactive if two of the three major bands (p24, gp41, and/or gp120/160) change color. The test is nonreactive if no viral bands are visible. If the test is indeterminate (one band visible), patients are retested in 2 to 3 months. This is most likely if a recent (i.e., less than 3 to 6 weeks) infection has occurred, and HIV antibodies have not yet been fully formed. In this case, a plasma HIV RNA concentration (reverse transcriptase polymerase chain reaction [RT-PCR])

Table 87–1

HIV Diagnostic Tests

Test	Minimum Time to Detection After Exposure	Sample(s) Tested	Comments
Initial Screening Tests			
ELISA	3–6 weeks	Plasma	If nonreactive, no further testing is required, unless acute infection suspected
HIV RNA assay	Up to 14 days	Plasma	Obtain if recent high-risk exposure; if initially negative, repeat at months 1, 3, and 6
Rapid tests (currently FDA-approved products):	Detects HIV antibodies within minutes of sample application		
OraQuick ADVANCE	3–6 weeks	Whole blood, plasma, or oral fluid	Detects HIV-1 and HIV-2
HIV 1/2 STAT-PAK	3–6 weeks	Whole blood, plasma, or serum	Detects HIV-1 and HIV-2
SURE CHECK HIV 1/2	3–6 weeks	Whole blood, plasma, or serum	Detects HIV-1 and HIV-2
Multispot HIV-1/HIV-2 Rapid Test	3–6 weeks	Plasma or serum	Detects HIV-1 and HIV-2
Reveal Rapid HIV-1 Antibody Test	3–6 weeks	Plasma or serum	Detects HIV-1
Uni-Gold Recombigen HIV Test	3–6 weeks	Whole blood, plasma, or serum	Detects HIV-1
INSTI™ HIV-1 Antibody Kit	3–6 weeks	Plasma or whole blood	Detects HIV-1
Confirmatory Tests			
Western blot (WB)	3–6 weeks	Plasma	Gold standard confirmatory test
Indirect immunofluorescence assay (IFA)	3–6 weeks	Plasma	Simple to perform, but requires expertise to interpret results

ELISA, enzyme-linked immunosorbent assay.

Clinical Presentation and Diagnosis of HIV

Patients with acute HIV infection may display symptoms described as "acute retroviral syndrome." Patients with chronic HIV infection may present with these same nonspecific symptoms and/or opportunistic infections.

Acute Retroviral Syndrome

The majority of patients may present with fever, lymphadenopathy, pharyngitis, and/or rash. Other symptoms include:

- Myalgia or arthralgia
- Diarrhea
- Headache
- Nausea and vomiting
- Hepatosplenomegaly
- Weight loss
- Thrush
- Neurologic symptoms (meningoencephalitis, aseptic meningitis, peripheral neuropathy, facial palsy, or cognitive impairment or psychosis)

Opportunistic Infections

Depending on the severity of immunosuppression (the CD4+ T lymphocyte count), patients may present with the following opportunistic infections (grouped by CD4+ count):

Any CD4+ count

- *Mycobacterium tuberculosis* disease

- Bacterial pneumonia (commonly *Streptococcus pneumoniae, Haemophilus influenzae, Pseudomonas aeruginosa,* and *Staphylococcus aureus*)
- Herpes simplex virus disease
- Varicella zoster virus disease
- Bacterial enteric disease (most commonly *Salmonella, Campylobacter,* and *Shigella*)
- Syphilis
- Bartonellosis

Less than 250 cells/mm³ (250 × 10⁶/L)

- Coccidioidomycosis
- *Pneumocystis jiroveci* (formerly *carinii*) pneumonia (PCP)
- Oropharyngeal and esophageal candidiasis
- Kaposi's sarcoma or human herpesvirus-8 disease

Less than 150 cells/mm³ (150 × 10⁶/L)

- Disseminated histoplasmosis

Less than 100 cells/mm³ (100 × 10⁶/L)

- Cryptosporidiosis
- Microsporidiosis

Less than 50 cells/mm³ (50 × 10⁶/L)

- Disseminated *Mycobacterium avium* complex disease
- Cytomegalovirus disease
- Cryptococcosis, aspergillosis, and *Toxoplasma gondii* encephalitis

---

should be evaluated. Patients with acute infection will generally have HIV RNA concentrations greater than 10⁶ copies/mL (10⁹ copies/L). ❷ *HIV severity is determined by following: (a) the CD4+ lymphocyte count (CD4 count) and percentage and (b) HIV RNA (viral load).* The CD4 percentage is followed because the absolute count may fluctuate and does not necessarily indicate a change in the patient's condition.

TREATMENT

❶ *The goals of treatment are to maximally and durably suppress viral replication, avoid the development of drug resistance, restore and preserve immune function, prevent opportunistic infections, and minimize drug adverse effects.* Elimination of HIV is not possible with currently available therapies. Instead, maximal suppression of viral replication (defined as HIV RNA concentrations undetectable by the most sensitive assay available) is desired. After the initiation of antiretroviral therapy, a rapid decline to undetectable HIV RNA in 16 to 24 weeks is a predictor of improved clinical outcomes.[5]

❷ *Degree of immune function preservation is also correlated with decreased viral replication, and is measured by CD4+ T-cell counts. CD4 measures are the best predictor of*

progression to AIDS and help clinicians determine when to initiate treatment. At CD4+ T-cell counts of 200 cells/mm³ (200 × 10⁶/L) and lower, patients require drug prophylaxis for opportunistic infections. Table 87–2 details the monitoring end points of HIV treatment for HIV RNA and CD4+ T-cell counts. In addition to these parameters, basic blood chemistry tests, liver function tests, complete blood counts, and lipid profiles should be monitored every 3 to 6 months in patients receiving antiretroviral therapy.[5]

Six classes of drugs are available to treat HIV infection: **nucleoside (NRTI)/nucleotide (NtRTI) reverse transcriptase inhibitor, protease inhibitor (PI), nonnucleoside reverse transcriptase inhibitor (NNRTI), fusion inhibitors, CCR5 inhibitors, and integrase strand transfer inhibitors (INSTI).** ❸ *Currently, combination antiretroviral drug therapy with three or more active drugs is the standard of care,* which increases the durability of viral suppression and decreases the potential for the development of resistance. ❹ *Two nucleoside (nucleotide) reverse transcriptase inhibitors AND a NNRTI OR a ritonavir-boosted PI OR an INSTI are the mainstay regimens of combination therapy in initial treatment.* Use of two NRTIs/NtRTIs with a CCR5 inhibitor may also be considered as an initial regimen. In the late

Patient Encounter 1, Part 1

A 22-year-old African American man presents to the emergency department of your hospital complaining of a fever, malaise, and pharyngitis that has been present for about a week.

PMH: No significant past medical history

FH: Noncontributory

SH: College student; reports multiple sexual partners in the past few months with condom use about 50% of the time. He denies illicit drugs, but drinks 5 to 10 alcoholic drinks weekly.

Meds: None

ROS: (–) weight loss, decreased appetite, shortness of breath, and cough, chest pain, nausea, vomiting, diarrhea

PE: Within normal limits

VS: BP 124/84 mm Hg, P 73 beats/min, RR 18 breaths/min, T 39.3°C

HEENT: Within normal limits

CV: RRR, normal S1, S2; no murmurs, rubs, gallops

Abd: Soft, nontender, nondistended; (+) bowel sounds, no hepatosplenomegaly

Rectal: Deferred

Labs: Sodium 135 mEq/L (135 mmol/L), potassium 3.6 mEq/L (3.6 mmol/L), chloride 100 mEq/L (100 mmol/L), bicarbonate 24 mEq/L (24 mmol/L), blood urea nitrogen 14 mg/dL (5 mmol/L), creatinine 1.0 mg/dL (88 μmol/L), WBC 5.2×10^3/mm^3 (5.2×10^9/L), hemoglobin 11.5 g/dL (115 g/L or 7.14 mmol/L), hematocrit 34.1% (0.341), platelets 151×10^3/mm^3 (151×10^9/L), neutrophils 58% (0.58), bands 9% (0.09), lymphocytes 32% (0.32), monocytes 1% (0.01), eosinophils 0% (0.00), basophils 0% (0.00)

What information is suggestive of HIV?

What is the likely time frame of this patient's HIV infection?

What are the risk factors present for having HIV?

How can the diagnosis of HIV be made in this patient?

What additional laboratory measurements would be useful?

Table 87–2

Monitoring End Points for CD4⁺ T-Cell Counts and HIV RNA

CD4⁺ T Cell Counts			HIV RNA Concentration		
When to Monitor?	**Why?**	**Goal**	**When to Monitor?**	**Why?**	**Goal**
Initial diagnosis	Assess need for ART	Start therapy in appropriate patients	Initial diagnosis/ evaluation	Establish baseline and assess need for ART	Start ART in appropriate patients
	Assess need for OI chemoprophylaxis	Start therapy when counts less than 200 cells/mm³ (less than 200 × 10⁶/L)	2–8 weeks after starting or changing ART^a	Early assessment of regimen efficacy	Undetectable concentrations
Every 3–6 months	Receiving ART: monitor success of treatment^b	Average increase of 100–150 cells/mm³/year (100 × 10⁶-150 × 10⁶/L/ year)	Every 3–6 months	Receiving ART: assess success and durability of virologic suppression with current regimen	Steadily decreasing and/or consistently undetectable concentrations
	Not receiving ART: assess need to begin therapy	Start ART in appropriate patients	Every 3–4 months	Not receiving ART: monitor changes in viral load	Start therapy in appropriate patients
	Assess need for OI chemoprophylaxis	Start therapy when counts less than 200 cells/mm³ (less than 200 × 10⁶/L)		Not receiving ART: monitor changes in viral load	Start therapy in appropriate patients

ART, antiretroviral therapy; OI, opportunistic infection.

^{a}If viral load is detectable, repeat every 4 to 8 weeks until less than 200 copies/mL (less than 200 × 10³/L), then resume every 3- to 6-months schedule.

^{b}In clinically stable patients with viral loads less than 50 copies/mL (less than 50 × 10³/L) for more than 2 years, monitoring can be extended to every 6 to 12 months.

Adapted from Panel on Antiretroviral Guidelines for Adults and Adolescents. Guidelines for the use of antiretroviral agents in HIV-1-infected adults and adolescents [online]. Department of Health and Human Services. October 14, 2011;1–166. [cited 2011 Oct 10]. Available from: *http://www.aidsinfo.nih.gov/ContentFiles/AdultandAdolescentGL.pdf.*

1980s, when only zidovudine was available, achieving and maintaining viral suppression for more than 4 months was rarely possible. As more agents became available in the mid-1990s (most notably the PIs), HIV RNA was suppressed to undetectable concentrations and maintained there for long periods of time. Currently recommended combination regimens decrease HIV RNA to less than 50 copies/mL (50×10^3 copies/L) in 80% to 90% of patients in clinical trials. Therefore, monotherapy with any agent or the use of NRTIs without another drug class are not routine treatment options. Fusion inhibitors are only FDA-approved for use in treatment experienced patients with drug resistance to NRTIs, NNRTIs, and/or PIs. Figure 87–1 details the mechanisms of action of the drug classes within the life cycle of HIV.

Nonpharmacologic Interventions

6 *Patient adherence is a key component in treatment success.* Drug therapy is required for a lifetime, as the virus begins to replicate at high levels when medications are stopped. Early HIV combination therapy was exceedingly complicated for patients, with multiple daily doses, varying food restrictions, and large pill burdens. Advances in delivery and formulations now make possible once- or twice-daily dosing with fewer pills per day. Currently, two combination tablets providing one pill, once daily NNRTI-containing regimens are available: tenofovir + emtricitabine + efavirenz (Atripla) and tenofovir + emtricitabine + rilpivirine (Complera). The use of low-dose ritonavir to enhance the concentrations of other PIs (known as pharmacokinetic enhancement, or "boosting") allows for significantly fewer doses and lower pill burdens. Atazanavir or darunavir with ritonavir boosting are potent, once-daily PI options; once-daily lopinavir/ritonavir or fosamprenavir/ritonavir may be used in selected treatment-naïve patients. These advances, however, do not replace the need for patient counseling by a trained pharmacist and a multidisciplinary approach to promoting adherence.

Counsel all patients initially and repeatedly on ways to prevent viral transmission. Preventing the spread of resistant virus is particularly important. Patients receiving antiretroviral therapy can still transmit virus to sexual partners and to those with whom they share needles or other drug equipment. Where both partners are HIV-positive, safe sex and needle practices reduce the risk of superinfection with differing strains of HIV and the transmission of other sexually transmitted diseases. General guidelines for preventing viral transmission include using condoms with a water-based lubricant for vaginal or anal intercourse, using condoms without lubricant or dental dams for oral sex, and not sharing equipment used to prepare, inject, or inhale drugs. Treating other sexually transmitted infections (STIs), particularly genital herpes, in HIV-infected patients may help to prevent HIV transmission. The presence of STIs increases genital tract HIV viral load and, correspondingly, the risk of HIV transmission to sexual partners.

3 *Nutrition and dietary counseling should also be included in the care of the HIV patient, as poor nutrition leads to poorer outcomes and complicates treatment.* Antiretroviral therapy itself introduces a host of nutritional issues, including drug–food interactions, GI adverse effects that may affect appetite and limit dietary intake, lipid abnormalities, and fat redistribution. The American Dietetics Association currently recommends assessing HIV-infected patients for their level of nutritional risk and involving a registered dietician as part of the clinical team for optimal nutrition care.[6]

Pharmacologic Therapy for Antiretroviral-Naïve Patients

Two major panels of experts publish guidelines for the treatment of HIV-infected individuals. Although the recommendations are quite similar, slight differences do exist between the Department of Health and Human Services (DHHS) Guidelines[5] and the International AIDS Society–USA (IAS-USA) Panel Recommendations.[7] The DHHS Guidelines are updated frequently, and current and archived versions are available online at *www.aidsinfo.nih.gov*. The IAS-USA Guidelines were last updated in 2010, and in 2008 prior to that revision. Due to the intense research and constant modifications to therapeutic approaches in the treatment of HIV, the majority of the treatment algorithms and recommendations presented herein follow the most up-to-date information found in the October 2011 DHHS recommendations.

2 *The decision of when to begin antiretroviral therapy is complex. Recommendations are based on the CD4+ T-cell count, which predicts disease-free survival, and other comorbid conditions (Table 87–3).* Other factors to consider include the patient's viral load, decline in CD4+ counts over time, hepatitis C status, risk for cardiovascular disease, risk of

---

Table 87–3

Summary of Recommendations for Initiating Antiretroviral Therapy

Clinical Indicator/CD4+ Count	Recommended Action
Symptomatic HIV disease or opportunistic infection Asymptomatic infection with CD4+ count less than 350 cells/mm³ (less than 350×10^6/L) CD4 count 200–350 cells/mm ($200 \times 10^6 - 350 \times 10^6$/L) Pregnant women HIV-associated nephropathy HBV coinfection, where HBV treatment is indicated	Start ART
CD4+ count greater than 350 mm³	Currently panels of experts are divided; depends on the patient characteristics and individual risk-benefit assessment

ART: antiretroviral therapy; HBV, hepatitis B virus.

Adapted from Panel on Antiretroviral Guidelines for Adults and Adolescents. Guidelines for the use of antiretroviral agents in HIV-1-infected adults and adolescents [online]. Department of Health and Human Services. October 14, 2011;1–166. [cited 2011 Oct 10]. Available from: *http://www.aidsinfo.nih.gov/ContentFiles/AdultandAdolescentGL.pdf*.

transmission to sex partners, willingness to begin therapy and maintain medication adherence, and the risk versus benefit of treating an asymptomatic patient. The clinical evidence is strongest for beginning treatment at CD4$^+$ counts less than 200 cells/mm³ (200 × 10⁶/L), but more recent evidence from long-term studies and the availability of potent drugs with improved tolerability support earlier treatment at higher CD4$^+$ counts. Many experts recommend starting treatment at CD4$^+$ counts greater than 500 cells/mm³ (greater than 500 × 10⁶/L), including the IAS-USA Panel. Once the decision is made to initiate treatment, the regimen is selected based on patient-specific factors. ④ *All recommended regimens for initial treatment contain an NNRTI, a ritonavir-boosted PI, or an INSTI in combination with tenofovir (NtRTI) and emtricitabine (NRTI).* The preferred agents are as follows:

1. NRTI/NtRTI combination:
   a. Tenofovir *and* emtricitabine (dosed once daily)
2. PIs:
   a. Atazanavir/ritonavir (dosed once daily)
   b. Darunavir/ritonavir (dosed once daily)
3. NNRTI:
   a. Efavirenz (dosed once daily)
4. INSTI:
   a. Raltegravir (dosed twice daily)

The decision to choose an NNRTI- or PI-based regimen as initial therapy is based on many patient- and clinician-specific factors. Drug resistance testing should be performed at diagnosis and again prior to initiating treatment if time has elapsed between diagnosis and treatment (see Pharmacologic Therapy for Antiretroviral-Experienced Patients for further discussion of drug resistance testing). The results of resistance testing may dictate which drug class is preferred; a minimum of 6% to 16% of newly diagnosed patients will have drug-resistant virus. This initial resistance pattern often involves the NNRTIs, but may involve other drug classes. NNRTI-based regimens have low pill burdens and may have decreased incidences of long-term adverse effects (e.g., dyslipidemia) in comparison with some PI-based regimens. However, this class also has a low threshold for drug resistance (the K103N mutation causes high level cross-class resistance), and patient adherence is a critical consideration. In pregnant women, or women with the potential to become pregnant, a PI-based regimen is preferred due to the potential teratogenicity of efavirenz in early pregnancy (Pregnancy Category D). INSTI-based regimens have the advantage of avoiding many complex drug–drug interactions and toxicities seen with NNRTIs and PIs; however, raltegravir must be dosed twice daily and also has a low threshold for drug resistance. Transmitted INSTI resistance is not yet a major clinical concern, but may develop as raltegravir comes into wider use. If transmitted INSTI resistance is a concern, integrase resistance testing must be ordered separately from standard HIV genotyping, which only includes the protease and reverse transcriptase genes.

In patients who cannot tolerate the above preferred first-line therapies, or have a compelling reason to choose a different agent, the following alternative regimens are recommended.

1. PI-based:
   a. Atazanavir/ritonavir + abacavirlamivudine
   b. Darunavir/ritonavir + abacavir/lamivudine
   c. Fosamprenavir/ritonavir (dosed once or twice daily) + either tenofovir/emtricitabine OR abacavir/lamivudine
   d. Lopinavir/ritonavir (dosed once or twice daily) + either tenofovir/emtricitabine OR abacavir/lamivudine
2. NNRTI:
   a. Efavirenz + abacavir/ lamivudine
   b. Rilpivirine/tenofovir/emtricitabine in patients with viral load less than 100,000 copies/mL (less than 100 × 10⁶ copies/L) (due to a more frequent incidence of virologic failure with development of broad NNRTI resistance in patients with high viral loads)
   c. Rilpivirine + abacavir/lamivudine in patients with viral load less than 100,000 copies/mL (less than 100 × 10⁶ copies/L)
3. INSTI:
   a. Raltegravir + abacavir/lamivudine

If abacavir is included in a regimen, patients should undergo HLA-B*5701 testing prior to initiation to reduce the risk of abacavir hypersensitivity. Patients who test positive for the allele are at high risk (approximately 61%) of developing this reaction and should not be given abacavir. An abacavir allergy should also be documented in the patient's medical record to prevent future administration. Those patients with a negative test may receive abacavir, but should still be monitored for the development of hypersensitivity.

A number of acceptable regimens that have demonstrated efficacy but are less desirable than the preferred and alternative regimens are listed in the DHHS Guidelines. These regimens include CCR5-based regimens (maraviroc with lamivudine/zidovudine, tenofovir/emtricitabine, or abacavir/lamivudine), nevirapine-based regimens (with lamivudine/zidovudine, tenofovir/emtricitabine, or abacavir/lamivudine), and other first-line or preferred agents with zidovudine/lamivudine-based regimens (efavirenz, rilpivirine, raltegravir, darunavir/ritonavir, fosamprenavir/ritonavir, atazanavir/ritonavir, lopinavir/ritonavir) and unboosted atazanavir with non-tenofovir-based NRTI regimens. Boosted saquinavir with two NRTIs is acceptable, but should be used with caution. One of these regimens should only be selected if a first-line regimen is intolerable or the patient has a compelling reason to avoid drugs in a first-line regimen. If maraviroc is under consideration, viral tropism testing should be performed to ensure CCR5-tropic virus for optimal efficacy.

Therapies *not recommended* for initial treatment due to poor potency or significant toxicity include triple-NRTI regimens, delavirdine, nevirapine in patients with moderate to high CD4$^+$ T-cell counts, indinavir ± ritonavir, saquinavir or fosamprenavir used without ritonavir ("unboosted"), ritonavir used without another PI, nelfinavir, tipranavir/ritonavir, and tenofovir, lamivudine, or emtricitabine with didanosine. Because of limited data in antiretroviral naïve patients, etravirine is not recommended in the DHHS Guidelines at this time.

Drugs that should *not be combined* due to overlapping toxicities include atazanavir plus indinavir (due to enhanced hyperbilirubinemia), two NNRTIs, and didanosine plus stavudine. Emtricitabine and lamivudine should not be combined because of their similar chemical structures, and antagonism can result when stavudine is combined with zidovudine.

Pharmacologic Therapy for Antiretroviral-Experienced Patients

⑥ *Ongoing viral replication, whether at low levels in the face of adequate drug concentrations or at higher levels due to inconsistent systemic concentrations (or low concentrations in sanctuary sites, e.g., male and female genital fluids, cerebrospinal fluid, or lymph nodes), will eventually lead to resistance to the prescribed medications.* There is no consensus on the optimal time to change therapy based on virologic or immunologic failure **②** *Virologic failure is defined as the inability to obtain or maintain an HIV RNA less than 200 copies/mL (less than 200 × 10³ copies/L), whereas incomplete virologic suppression is defined as two consecutives HIV RNA greater than 200 copies/mL (greater than 200 × 10³ copies/L) after 24 weeks of therapy.*[5] Immunologic failure is defined as the failure to achieve and/or maintain an adequate CD4+ count in the setting of virologic suppression. A typical CD4+ count should increase at least 150 cells/mm³ (150 × 10⁶/L) over the first year of therapy. The goal of therapy for patients with antiretroviral resistance is to reestablish virologic suppression or HIV RNA less than 48 copies/mL (less than 48 × 10³ copies/L).

Treatment considerations for antiretroviral-experienced patients are much more complex than for patients who are naïve to therapy. Prior to changing therapy, the reasons for treatment failure should be identified. A comprehensive review of the patient's severity of disease, antiretroviral treatment history, adherence to therapy, intolerance or toxicity, concomitant drug therapies, comorbidities, and results of current and past HIV resistance testing should be performed. If patients fail therapy due to poor adherence, the underlying reasons must be determined and addressed prior to initiation of new therapy. Reasons for poor adherence include problems with medication access, active substance abuse, depression and/or denial of the disease, and a lack of education on the importance of 100% adherence to therapy. Medication intolerance or toxicity can be remedied with therapy for the adverse event, exchanging the drug causing the toxicity with another in the same class, or changing the entire regimen. Pharmacokinetics or systemic drug exposure can be optimized by ensuring maximal drug absorption (taking the drug with or without food can alter exposure by up to 30%) and avoiding interactions with concomitant prescription or nonprescription medications and dietary supplements or natural products. When causes for treatment failure are identified, appropriate strategies for therapy can be determined.

An additional consideration when stopping or changing therapy is a staggered discontinuation of antiretrovirals with different half-lives. For example, in patients taking Atripla (tenofovir, emtricitabine, and efavirenz), tenofovir, and emtricitabine should be continued for at least 4 to 7 days after discontinuation of efavirenz due to the much prolonged half-life of efavirenz as compared with tenofovir and emtricitabine. Otherwise, the potential for monotherapy with efavirenz exists. If new antiretroviral therapy is to be initiated immediately, no overlap is necessary; however, it should be noted that efavirenz concentrations will persist for some period of time.

Drug interactions between antiretrovirals and between antiretrovirals and concomitant medications should be evaluated for each patient to avoid under- and/or overexposure of either therapy. **⑦** *NNRTIs and PIs are metabolized by CYP450 enzymes and are inducers and/or inhibitors of this enzyme system.* In addition, some of the antiretrovirals are substrates, inhibitors, and/or inducers of transporters such as P-glycoprotein and therefore may lead to drug interactions. Information provided in Table 87–4 describes the drug interaction potential of each antiretroviral. Due to the ever-changing drug interactions with this class of medications, the regularly updated DHHS Guidelines for the Use of Antiretroviral Agents in HIV-1–Infected Adults and Adolescents are a recommended source of specific drug interactions.[5]

The goals of therapy differ for antiretroviral-experienced patients who have limited drug exposure (i.e., developing resistance to their first antiretroviral regimen) versus those with extensive exposure (i.e., developing resistance to their third or fourth antiretroviral regimen). It is reasonable to expect maximal viral suppression in those with limited drug exposure. However, this may not be feasible for patients with prior exposure to multiple medications. **①** *In antiretroviral-experienced patients, a reasonable goal is to simply preserve immune function and prevent clinical progression.*

Several issues need to be considered in choosing a salvage regimen for HIV infection. Knowing prior medication exposure can assist in identifying which drugs to avoid. However, direct HIV resistance testing can better identify the resistance and susceptibility patterns of the major viral strains. Because HIV may be susceptible to certain components of the failing antiretroviral regimen, these drugs can be recycled into future regimens. Resistance testing should be used when all patients enter into care, in patients with virologic failure on a current antiretroviral regimen, or with suboptimal suppression after initiation of antiretroviral therapy. Testing is generally preferred for antiretroviral naïve patients. For resistance testing to be useful, the patient should have a plasma HIV RNA of at least 1,000 copies/mL (1 × 10⁶ copies/L) and should be currently taking their antiretroviral medications (or be within 4 weeks of discontinuing antiretroviral therapy). This viral concentration is necessary to yield reliable amplification of the virus, and the antiretroviral medications are needed because the dominant viral species reverts to wild-type within 4 to 6 weeks after medications are stopped.

Two types of HIV resistance testing are available, an HIV genotype and an HIV phenotype. Genotyping involves detecting mutations by genetically sequencing the virus, whereas phenotyping determines the ability of the virus to

Table 87–4

Summary of Currently Available Antiretroviral Agents

Generic Name [Abbreviation] (Trade Name)	Dosage Forms	Commonly Prescribed Doses	Dose Adjustments	Food Restrictions	Significant Adverse Events	Drug Interaction Potential
Nucleoside (tide) Reverse Transcriptase Inhibitors						
Abacavir (Ziagen)	300-mg tablet; 20 mg/mL oral solution	300 mg twice daily or 600 mg once daily	None	None (alcohol increases abacavir conc. by 41%)	Potentially fatal hypersensitivity reaction (rash, fever, malaise, nausea, vomiting, shortness of breath, sore throat, loss of appetite)	Alcohol dehydrogenase and glucuronyl transferase, 82% renal excretion of metabolites
Didanosine (Videx EC) Generic didanosine EC	125-, 200-, 250-, 400-mg capsules 125-, 200-, 250-, 400-mg capsules	Greater than 60 kg: 400 mg daily Less than 60 kg: 250 mg daily	CrCl (mL/min [mL/s]): Greater than 60 kg: / Less than 60 kg: 30–59 [0.50–0.99]: 200 mg / 125 mg 10–29 [0.17–0.49]: 125 mg / 100 mg less than 10 [0.17]: 125 mg / 75 mg	Take 30 minutes prior or 2 hours after meal (conc. decrease 55% with food)	Pancreatitis; peripheral neuropathy; nausea; diarrhea	Renal excretion
Emtricitabine (Emtriva)	200-mg capsule; 10 mg/mL oral solution	200 mg daily; 240 mg (24 mL) oral solution daily	Capsule: CrCl (mL/min[mL/s]): Solution: 30–49 [0.50–0.82]: 200 mg every 48 hours / 120 mg every 24 hours 15–29 [0.25–0.49]: 200 mg every 72 hours / 80 mg every 24 hours Less than 15/HD [0.25/HD]: 200 mg every 96 hours / 60 mg every 24 hours (Dose after dialysis on dialysis days)	None	Minimal	Renal excretion
Lamivudine (Epivir)	150-mg and 300-mg tabs or 10 mg/mL oral solution	150 mg twice daily or 300 mg once daily	CrCl (mL/min): Dose: 30–49 [0.50–0.82]: 150 mg qday 15–29 [0.25–0.49]: 150 mg, then 100 mg every day 5–14 [0.08–0.24]: 150 mg, then 50 mg every day Less than 5/HD [0.08/HD]: 50 mg, then 25 mg every day (Dose after dialysis on dialysis days)	None	Minimal	Renal excretion
Stavudine (Zerit)	15, 20, 30, 40-mg capsules or 1 mg/mL for oral solution	Greater than 60 kg: 40 mg twice daily Less than 60 kg: 30 mg twice daily	CrCl (mL/min): Greater than 60 kg: / Less than 60 kg: 26–50 [0.43–0.83]: 20 mg every 12 hours / 15 mg every 12 hours 10–25/HD [0.17–0.42/HD]: 20 mg every 24 hours / 15 mg every 24 hours	None	Peripheral neuropathy; lipodystrophy; rapidly progressive ascending neuromuscular weakness (rare); pancreatitis; lactic acidosis with hepatic steatosis (higher incidence with stavudine than with other NRTIs); hyperlipidemia	Renal excretion

Drug	Formulation	Usual dose	Dosage adjustment (renal)	Dosage adjustment (hepatic)	Adverse events	Elimination
Tenofovir disoproxil fumarate (Viread)	300-mg tablet	300 mg daily	**CrCl (mL/min): Dose:** 30–49 [0.50–0.82]: 300 mg every 48 hours; 10–29 [0.17–0.49]: 300 mg twice weekly; ESRD/HD: 300 mg every 7 days (Dose after dialysis on dialysis days)	None	Asthenia, headache, diarrhea, nausea, vomiting, and flatulence; renal insufficiency	Renal excretion
Zidovudine (Retrovir)	100-mg capsule, 300-mg tablet, 10 mg/mL IV solution, 10 mg/mL oral solution	300 mg twice daily	100 mg 3 times daily or 300 mg once daily in severe renal impairment or HD	None	Bone marrow suppression: macrocytic anemia or neutropenia; GI intolerance, headache, insomnia, asthenia	Glucuronyl transferase and renal
Zidovudine + lamivudine (Combivir)	Zidovudine 300 mg + Lamivudine 150-mg tablet	1 tablet twice daily	Do not use with CrCl less than 50 mL/min (0.83 mL/s)	None	See adverse events for zidovudine and lamivudine	See zidovudine and lamivudine
Abacavir + lamivudine + zidovudine [abacavir/lamivudine/zidovudine] (Trizivir)	Abacavir 300 mg + lamivudine 150 mg + zidovudine 300-mg tablet	1 tablet twice daily	Do not use with CrCl less than 50 mL/min (0.83 mL/s)	None	See adverse events for zidovudine, lamivudine, and abacavir	See zidovudine, lamivudine, and abacavir
Abacavir + lamivudine [abacavir/lamivudine] (Epzicom)	Abacavir 600 mg + lamivudine 300-mg tablet	1 tablet daily	Do not use with CrCl less than 50 mL/min (0.83 mL/s)	None	See adverse events for abacavir and lamivudine	See abacavir and lamivudine
Tenofovir + emtricitabine [Tenofovir/emtricitabine] (Truvada)	Tenofovir 300 mg + emtricitabine 200-mg tablet	1 tablet daily	**CrCl (mL/min [mL/s]): Dose:** 30–49 [0.50–0.82]: 1 tablet every 48 hours; less than 30 [less than 0.50]: Not recommended	None	See adverse events for tenofovir and emtricitabine	See tenofovir and emtricitabine
Nonnucleoside Reverse Transcriptase Inhibitors						
Delavirdine (Rescriptor)	100-, 200-mg tablets	400 mg 3 times daily (100-mg tablet can be dispersed in 3 oz or more of water to produce slurry); 200-mg tablet should be administered whole; separate dosing from buffered didanosine or antacids by 1 hour	Use with caution in patients with hepatic impairment	None	Rash; increased LFTs, headaches	Metabolized by cytochrome P-450 (CYP); CYP3A inhibitor; 51% excreted in urine (less than 5% unchanged); 44% in feces

(Continued)

Table 87–4

Summary of Currently Available Antiretroviral Agents (Continued)

Generic Name [Abbreviation] (Trade Name)	Dosage Forms	Commonly Prescribed Doses	Dose Adjustments	Food Restrictions	Significant Adverse Events	Drug Interaction Potential
Efavirenz (Sustiva)	50-, 100-, 200-mg capsules or 600-mg tablet	600 mg daily at or before bedtime	Use with caution in patients with hepatic impairment	Take on an empty stomach (high-fat/calorie meals increases C_{max} of capsule 39% and C_{max} of tablet 79%	Rash; CNS symptoms (insomnia, irritability, lethargy, dizziness, vivid dreams) usually resolve in 2 weeks; increased LFTs; false-positive cannabinoid test; teratogenic in monkeys	Metabolized by CYP2B6 and CYP3A (3A mixed inducer/inhibitor); 14–34% excreted in urine (glucuronidated metabolites, less than 1% unchanged); 16–61% in feces
Etravirine (Intelence)	100-, 200-mg tablets	200 mg twice daily following a meal	No dosage adjustment for Child Pugh Class A or B. Has not been evaluated for Class C	Take following a meal. Fasting decreases by 50%	Rash, nausea	Metabolized by CYP3A, 2C9, and 2C19; Induces 3A4 and inhibits 2C9 and 2C19
Nevirapine (Viramune)	200-mg tablet or 50 mg/5 mL oral suspension	200 mg once daily for 14 days; then 200 mg twice daily	Use with caution in patients with hepatic impairment; avoid use with moderate to severe hepatic impairment	No food restrictions	Rash including Stevens-Johnson syndrome; symptomatic hepatitis, including fatal hepatic necrosis	Metabolized by CYP2B6 and CYP3A (3A inducer); 80% excreted in urine (glucuronidated metabolites; less than 5% unchanged); 10% in feces
Rilpivirine (Edurant)	25-mg tablet	25 mg daily	No dosage adjustment for Child Pugh Class A or B. Has not been evaluated for Class C; Use with caution in severe or end-stage renal impairment	Take with a normal- to high-calorie meal Absorption dependent on gastric pH–special considerations needed when coadministered with antacids	Rash; depressive disorders;	Metabolized by CYP3A4

Drug	Formulations	Usual Dose	Dose in Hepatic Impairment	Dose in Renal Impairment	Administration	Adverse Effects	Metabolism/Interactions
Tenofovir + emtricitabine + efavirenz [tenofovir/emtricitabine/efavirenz] (Atripla)	Tenofovir 300 mg Emtricitabine 200 mg Efavirenz 600 mg	1 tablet daily		Do not use in patients with CrCl less than 50 mL/min (0.83 mL/s)	High-fat/high-caloric meals increase peak plasma concentrations of efavirenz capsules by 39% and efavirenz tablets by 79%; take on empty stomach	See adverse events of tenofovir, emtricitabine, and efavirenz	See tenofovir, emtricitabine, and efavirenz
Tenofovir + emtricitabine + rilpivirine [tenofovir/emtricitabine/rilpivirine] (Complera)	Tenofovir 300 mg Emtricitabine 200 mg Rilpivirine 25mg	1 tablet daily		Do not use in patients with CrCl less than 50 mL/min (0.83 mL/s)	Take with a meal (preferrably high fat)	See adverse events of tenofovir, emtricitabine, and rilpivirine	See tenofovir, emtricitabine, and rilpivirine
Protease Inhibitors							
Atazanavir (Reyataz)	100-, 150-, 200-, 300-mg capsules	400 mg daily If taken with tenofovir use the following: atazanavir 300 mg daily + ritonavir 100 mg daily If taken with efavirenz in treatment of naïve patients only: atazanavir 400 mg daily + ritonavir 100 mg daily (do not use efavirenz in treatment of experienced patients)	Child-Pugh Class 7–9 Greater than 9	Dose 300 mg daily Not recommended; Treatment-naïve patients on hemodialysis: atazanavir 300 mg + ritonavir 100 mg daily; treatment-experienced patients on hemodialysis: Not recommended	Take with food (AUC increases 30%); pH-sensitive dissolution—special considerations needed when coadministered with antacids	Indirect hyperbilirubinemia; prolonged PR interval (asymptomatic first-degree AV block); use with caution in patients with underlying conduction defects or on concomitant medications that can cause PR prolongation; hyperglycemia; fat maldistribution; increased bleeding episodes in patients with hemophilia	CYP3A4 inhibitor and substrate; UGT1A1 inhibitor
Darunavir (Prezista)	400-, 600-mg tablets	Darunavir 600 mg + ritonavir 100 mg twice daily	Use with caution in patients with hepatic impairment		Should be given with food	Skin rash (has a sulfonamide moiety, Stevens Johnson and erythema multiforme have been reported); diarrhea, nausea; headache; hyperlipidemia; transaminase elevation; hyperglycemia; fat maldistribution; possible increased bleeding episodes in patients with hemophilia	CYP3A4 inhibitor and substrate

(Continued)

Table 87–4

Summary of Currently Available Antiretroviral Agents (*Continued*)

Generic Name [Abbreviation] (Trade Name)	Dosage Forms	Commonly Prescribed Doses	Dose Adjustments	Food Restrictions	Significant Adverse Events	Drug Interaction Potential
Fosamprenavir (Lexiva)	700-mg tablet; 50 mg/mL oral suspension	ARV-naïve patients: fosamprenavir 1,400 mg twice daily, Fosamprenavir 700 mg + ritonavir 100 mg twice daily, or fosamprenavir 1,400 mg + ritonavir 200 mg once daily; PI-experienced *patients:* fosamprenavir 700 mg + ritonavir 100 mg twice daily Coadministration with efavirenz: fosamprenavir 700 mg + ritonavir 100 mg twice daily or fosamprenavir 1,400 mg + ritonavir 300 mg once daily	Child-Pugh Class / Dose: 5–8 / 700 mg twice daily; 9–12 / Not recommended. Ritonavir should not be used in patients with hepatic impairment	None	Skin rash; diarrhea, nausea and vomiting; headache; hyperlipidemia; LFT elevation; hyperglycemia; fat maldistribution; increased bleeding episodes in patients with hemophilia	CYP3A4 inhibitor, inducer, and substrate
Indinavir (Crixivan)	200-, 333-, 400-mg capsules	800 mg every 8 hours; indinavir 800 mg + ritonavir 100 twice daily; indinavir 800 mg + ritonavir 200 mg twice daily	Mild to moderate hepatic insufficiency due to cirrhosis: 600 mg every 8 hours	*For unboosted indinavir:* Take 1 hour before or 2 hours after heavy meals, or concomitantly with low-fat meal. No restrictions when used with ritonavir	Nephrolithiasis; GI intolerance, nausea; indirect hyperbilirubinemia; hyperlipidemia; headache, asthenia, blurred vision, dizziness, rash, metallic taste, thrombocytopenia, alopecia, hemolytic anemia; hyperglycemia; fat maldistribution; increased bleeding episodes in patients with hemophilia	CYP3A4 inhibitor (less than ritonavir)

Drug	Formulation	Dose	Hepatic impairment	Administration	Adverse effects	Metabolism
Lopinavir + ritonavir (Kaletra)	Lopinavir 200 mg + ritonavir 50-mg tablet, lopinavir 400 mg + ritonavir 100 mg/5 mL oral solution (contains 42% alcohol)	2 tablets or 5 mL twice daily 4 tablets once daily; tablets once daily with efavirenz or nevirapine: 3 tablets or 6.7 mL twice daily	Use with caution in patients with hepatic impairment	Take with food (AUC increases 48–80%)	Nausea, vomiting, diarrhea; asthenia; hyperlipidemia; LFT elevation; hyperglycemia; fat maldistribution; increased bleeding episodes in hemophiliacs	CYP3A4 inhibitor and susbstrate CYP2C9, 2C19, 1A2 inducer
Nelfinavir (Viracept)	250–625-mg tablets, 50 mg/g oral powder	1,250 mg twice daily or 750 mg 3 times daily	Use with caution in patients with hepatic impairment	Take with meal or snack	Diarrhea; hyperlipidemia; hyperglycemia; fat maldistribution; increased bleeding in hemophiliacs; LFT elevation	CYP3A4 inhibitor and substrate
Ritonavir (Norvir)	100-mg tablet, 600 mg/7.5-mL solution	600 mg twice daily (when ritonavir is used as sole PI); 100–200 mg/dose when used as pharmacokinetic enhancer	No dosage adjustment in mild hepatic impairment. No data for moderate to severe impairment; use with caution	Take with food to improve tolerability	GI intolerance, nausea, diarrhea; paresthesias; hyperlipidemia; hepatitis; asthenia; taste perversion; hyperglycemia; fat maldistribution; increased bleeding in hemophiliacs	CYP3A4 inhibitor (potent) and substrate; CYP2D6 substrate; mixed dose-dependent induction and inhibition of other phase I and II enzymes
Saquinavir tablets and hard gel capsules (Invirase)	200-mg capsule, 500-mg tablet	Unboosted saquinavir not recommended *With ritonavir:* (ritonavir 100 mg + saquinavir 1,000 mg) twice daily	Use with caution in patients with hepatic impairment	Take within 2 hours of a meal when taken with ritonavir	Nausea, diarrhea; headache; LFT elevation; hyperlipidemia; hyperglycemia; fat maldistribution; increased bleeding in hemophiliacs	CYP3A4 inhibitor and substrate

(Continued)

Table 87-4

Summary of Currently Available Antiretroviral Agents (*Continued*)

Generic Name [Abbreviation] (Trade Name)	Dosage Forms	Commonly Prescribed Doses	Dose Adjustments	Food Restrictions	Significant Adverse Events	Drug Interaction Potential
Tipranavir (Aptivus)	250-mg capsules	500 mg twice daily with ritonavir 200 mg twice daily	Contraindicated in patients with moderate to severe hepatic insufficiency	Take with food	Hepatotoxicity; skin rash; hyperlipidemia; hyperglycemia; fat maldistribution; possible increased bleeding in hemophiliacs	Tipranavir/ritonavir mixed CYP inhibitor/inducer; Tipranavir is CYP3A4 substrate
Fusion Inhibitors						
Enfuvirtide (Fuzeon)	Injectable, in lyophilized powder Each single-use vial contains 108 mg of enfuvirtide to be reconstituted with 1.1 mL of sterile water for injection for delivery of approximately 90 mg/1 mL	90 mg (1 mL) subcutaneously 2 times per day	No dosage recommendation	N/A	Local injection site reaction (pain, erythema, induration, nodules and cysts, pruritus, eachymosis) in most patients; increased rate of bacterial pneumonia; less than 1% hypersensitivity reaction (rash, fever, nausea, vomiting, chills, rigors, hypotension, or elevated serum transaminases); do not rechallenge	Catabolism to amino acids, with subsequent recycling in the body pool

Chemokine Receptor Antagonists (CCR5 Antagonists)

Drug	Formulation	Dose	Special Considerations	Food	Adverse Effects	Metabolism
Maraviroc (Selzentry)	150-mg and 300-mg tablets	150 mg twice daily when given with strong CYP3A inhibitors (with or without CYP3A inducers) including PIs (except tipranavir/ritonavir) 300 mg twice daily when given with NRTIs, enfuvirtide, tipranavir/ritonavir, nevirapine and other drugs that are not potent P450 inhibitors 600 mg twice daily when given with CYP3A inducers, including efavirenz, rifampin, etc. (without a CYP3A inhibitor)	Patients with CrCl less than 50 mL/min (0.83 mL/s) should receive maraviroc with a CYP3A inhibitor only if benefit outweighs the risk	No food restrictions	Abdominal pain; cough; dizziness; musculoskeletal symptoms; pyrexia; rash; upper RTI; hepatotoxicity; orthostatic hypotension	CYP3A substrate

Integrase Inhibitors

Drug	Formulation	Dose	Special Considerations	Food	Adverse Effects	Metabolism
Raltegravir (Isentress)	400-mg tablet	400 mg twice daily	No dosage adjustment	No food restrictions	Nausea; headache; diarrhea; pyrexia; CPK elevation	UGT1A1 substrate (glucuronidation)

AUC, area under the time-concentration curve; ARV, antiretroviral; AV, atrioventricular; C_{max}, maximum concentration; CrCl, creatinine clearance; ESRD, end-stage renal disease; HD, hemodialysis; LFT, liver function test; NRTI, nucleoside reverse transcriptase inhibitor; UGT, uridine diphosphate-glucuronosyltransferase.

Adapted from the DHHS Guidelines for the Use of Antiretroviral Agents in HIV-1-Infected Adults and Adolescents, January 29, 2008.

replicate in the presence of varying ARV concentrations. Genotyping is more rapid and less costly than phenotyping, but results in a list of mutations that may be more difficult to interpret than phenotyping. An **HIV virtual phenotype** report may also be obtained when genotypes are ordered.[5] This compares the patient's viral sequence to a database of matched genotypes and drug susceptibilities. Because the predictability of virtual phenotypes are dependent on the robustness of the database from which they are derived, some clinicians believe their utility is limited. Web-based tools are available to assist with interpretation of resistance mutations (e.g., Stanford University's HIV Drug Resistance Database; *http://hivdb. stanford.edu/index.html*). However, expert interpretation of genotype and phenotype reports is recommended.

Certain guiding principles should be considered when treating antiretroviral-experienced patients, and expert opinion is advised before selecting therapy. ❹ *As with antiretroviral-naïve patients, three or more active drugs should be prescribed.*[5] Because considerable cross-resistance can occur between medications within an antiretroviral class, simply using drugs to which the patient has not been exposed may be insufficient. Complete cross-resistance occurs within the first generation of NNRTIs, whereas the NRTIs and PIs have variable overlapping resistance patterns. For this reason, HIV resistance assays are important tools for choosing subsequent effective therapies. The following factors are associated with superior virologic response: lower viral load at the time therapy is changed, using a new class of antiretroviral agent, and using ritonavir-enhanced PIs in patients previously exposed to PIs.[5]

If patients fail therapy with resistance to only one drug, one or two active agents may be substituted for this drug while retaining the remaining drugs in the regimen. If patients fail therapy with resistance to more than one drug, changing classes of antiretrovirals and/or adding new active drugs is warranted. New NRTIs should be selected from resistance testing. If this is not available, the assumption should be made that resistance has developed to all NRTIs used in the failing regimen. In general, HIV that is resistant solely to lamivudine and/or emtricitabine will be susceptible to other NRTIs. If HIV develops resistance solely to tenofovir, then it may have reduced susceptibility to didanosine and likely abacavir but should remain susceptible to zidovudine, stavudine, lamivudine, and emtricitabine. Cross-resistance occurs between zidovudine and stavudine.

If a patient appears to fail an antiretroviral regimen without detectable HIV resistance, adherence should be investigated, and the adequacy of the plasma HIV RNA concentration in the resistance sample confirmed. Options include continuing the current regimen or starting a new regimen and repeating the resistance test 2 to 4 weeks after adherence is verified. An increasing number of patients have extensive HIV resistance, such that antiretroviral regimens cannot be designed to which the virus is fully susceptible. For these patients, continuing the current regimen may be beneficial because drug-resistant virus may have a compromised **replication capacity.** Other strategies may be considered for this type of patient, including pharmacokinetic enhancement with ritonavir, retreatment with prior antiretroviral agents, treatment with multidrug regimens (four or more antiretroviral drugs), and the use of new agents through expanded access programs or clinical trials.

Treatment Considerations in Special Populations

▶ *Acute HIV Infection*

Diagnosis of acute HIV infection is difficult, since many patients are asymptomatic or have nonspecific clinical symptoms similar to other common respiratory infections. If acute HIV infection is suspected, HIV antibody tests and a plasma HIV RNA concentration should be obtained. A clear diagnosis is made when an HIV antibody test is negative and the plasma HIV RNA concentration is high. Some centers are utilizing pooled testing methods on HIV antibody–negative patients to test for HIV RNA in order to more readily diagnosis acute infection. This method involves combining 50 to 100 patient samples that are negative for HIV antibody and testing the pooled sample for HIV RNA. This is a more complex and expensive test, and combining samples for initial screening limits the need to test all patient samples separately. If this pooled sample is negative for HIV RNA, no further testing is required. If the pooled sample is positive, individual patient samples will then be tested to determine which one is acutely infected with HIV (ie, HIV antibody negative, HIV RNA positive).

There are limited outcome data for treating acutely infected patients. Treatment of acute infection can decrease the severity of acute disease and decrease the viral set point; this may decrease progression rates and reduce the rate of viral transmission.[5] Limitations include an increased risk of chronic drug-induced toxicities and the development of viral resistance. Resistance testing should be performed prior to initiation of therapy due to an increase in resistance of antiretroviral naïve patients.[5]

▶ *Adolescent and Young Adult Patients*

As a result of similar modes of HIV transmission, adolescents infected after puberty are treated as adults. In this population, dosing of antiretroviral drugs should not be based on age, but on the Tanner stage (which considers external primary and secondary sexual characteristics). Adolescents in early puberty should be dosed according to pediatric guidelines, whereas those in late puberty should be dosed as adults. During growth spurts, adolescents should be monitored closely for drug efficacy and toxicity, since rapid changes in weight can lead to altered drug concentrations. Adherence is of concern in this population due to denial of the disease, misinformation, distrust of healthcare professionals, low self-esteem, and lack of family and/or social support. Additionally, asymptomatic patients this age find it more difficult to adhere to therapy while feeling well.

▶ *Pediatric Patients*

There are unique considerations in the treatment of HIV-infected children. Specific treatment guidelines exist,[8] but a thorough review is outside the scope of this chapter.

Most children acquire HIV infection through perinatal transmission either in utero, intrapartum, or postpartum through breast-feeding, although antiretroviral interventions have dramatically reduced transmission rates.[5] Antiretroviral therapy is limited in pediatric patients, as some drugs have no dosing recommendations for this population or are not available in a formulation that can be easily administered to children. Additionally, drug exposures can change dramatically during early childhood development due to altered drug-metabolizing enzyme and drug transporter activities.

▶ Illicit Drug Users

Treatment challenges in illicit drug users include comorbidities (such as hepatitis infection), limited access to care, inadequate adherence to therapy, side effects and toxicities, and the need for treatment of substance abuse, which can lead to drug interactions. *Many drugs of abuse have the potential to interact with antiretroviral medications, and a number of case reports have documented drug overdose when combined with PI therapy.*[9] In these populations, without addiction control, adherence is suboptimal and treatment failure is common. Most PIs and NNRTIs decrease methadone concentrations up to 50%. As this can result in the development of withdrawal symptoms, patients should be closely monitored for 4 to 8 weeks after initiation of antiretroviral therapy. Withdrawal symptoms can be alleviated with a methadone dose increase of 5 to 10 mg. Although there are fewer data, buprenorphine concentrations may be similarly affected, and therefore this drug requires close monitoring.

▶ Pregnancy and Women of Reproductive Potential

The goals of antiretroviral therapy for women of reproductive age and pregnant women are the same as for other adult patients. Specific guidelines for HIV-infected pregnant women are available.[10] If a women is already virally suppressed on an antiretroviral regimen at the time she becomes pregnant, it is recommended that she remain on that regimen unless it contains efavirenz, which is Pregnancy Category D. If not already on antiretroviral therapy, recommended therapies in pregnancy include zidovudine, lamivudine, lopinavir/ritonavir, and, if the CD4+ count is less than 250 cells/mm^3 (250 × 10^6/L), nevirapine. A dual nucleoside reverse transcriptase inhibitor (NRTI) backbone that includes one or more NRTIs with high levels of transplacental passage, if possible, is recommended. Drugs to be avoided include efavirenz (due to potential teratogenicity), the combination of didanosine and stavudine (due to a high incidence of lactic acidosis), and nevirapine in patients with a CD4+ count greater than 250 cells/mm^3 (250 × 10^6/L) (due to an increased risk of hepatotoxicity). The goal of therapy is to reduce plasma HIV RNA below 1,000 copies/mL (1 × 10^6 copies/L) and prevent MTCT of HIV. Limited data are available on antiretroviral pharmacokinetics in pregnancy, and standard doses of antiretroviral drugs are currently recommended, with close HIV RNA and CD4+ monitoring in the third trimester of pregnancy.

Women of reproductive potential prescribed efavirenz should be counseled on its potentially teratogenic effects

---

Patient Encounter 1, Part 2

After receiving the diagnosis of HIV and assessing his laboratory values, the patient from Part 1 and his medical team decide to start antiretrovirals.

What is the guidance for when to start therapy in a treatment-naïve patient?

What are the recommended regimens according to the October 2011 DHHS Guidelines?

What is the drug interaction potential with each of the recommended regimens?

What adverse effects does the patient need to be counseled on with each of the recommended regimens?

---

and the importance of birth control. ❼ *Additionally, efavirenz, nevirapine, ritonavir, lopinavir/ritonavir, and tipranavir/ritonavir, darunavir/ritonavir, fosamprenavir/ritonavir, and saquinavir/ritonavir decrease the concentrations of different estrogens and/or progestins in oral contraceptives, which could lead to failure.*[5] For patients prescribed these drugs, barrier forms of contraception are preferred to prevent pregnancy. Atazanavir may be taken with oral contraceptives with caution, as it can increase or decrease the exposure to estrogen and progesterone, depending on whether it is used in combination with ritonavir. DepoProvera may be a safe alternative, as it does not affect nelfinavir, efavirenz, or nevirapine concentrations; although the effect of antiretrovirals on medroxyprogesterone concentrations has not been examined, no evidence of ovulation has been seen in women on these combinations.[11] Maraviroc and raltegravir have not shown clinically significant effects when used with oral contraceptive and are safe to use in combination.

▶ Hepatitis B Coinfection

HIV-infected patients coinfected with hepatitis B virus (HBV) have higher concentrations of DNA and hepatitis B early antigen (HBeAg) and higher rates of HBV-associated liver disease. Therapy for HBV should be offered to patients who are HBeAg-positive or have HBV DNA greater than 10^5 copies/mL (10^8 copies/L) and have either liver serologies (serum alanine aminotransferase) greater than two times the upper limit of normal or histologic evidence of moderate disease or fibrosis. Options include interferon-α 2a or 2b and nucleoside/tide analogs. Nucleoside/tide analogs that treat HBV but not HIV are adefovir and entecavir. Nucleoside/tide analogs that treat HBV and HIV are lamivudine, emtricitabine, and tenofovir. These latter agents should be considered when treating HIV infection in HBV-coinfected patients.[12] When changing HIV therapy in a patient with HBV viral suppression, the lamivudine, emtricitabine, or tenofovir should be continued for treatment of HBV in addition to the new HIV regimen.[5]

▶ *Hepatitis C Coinfection*

Patients coinfected with hepatitis C virus (HCV) and HIV have a threefold increase in rate of progression to cirrhosis compared with those with HCV alone. Therapy for HCV is considered in patients with detectable plasma HCV RNA and results of liver biopsy and or liver imaging. Patients with HCV genotype 2 and 3 (and a CD4$^+$ count greater than 200 cells/mm^3 [200 × 10^6/L]) treated with pegylated interferon plus ribavirin have a better sustained viral response at 48 weeks (60% to 70%) compared with those with HCV genotype 1 (15% to 28%). Comprehensive treatment guidelines for HIV/HCV-coinfected patients are available.[12–14] Important considerations addressed in these guidelines include avoiding the combination of ribavirin with didanosine, and stavudine (due to increased risk of pancreatitis and/or lactic acidosis) and ribavirin with zidovudine (due to increased risk of anemia). Growth factors and erythropoietin may be needed to treat neutropenia from interferon and anemia from ribavirin. Two new protease inhibitors, telaprevir and boceprevir, that inhibit HCV protease have been approved for use in combination with peg interferon-α and ribavirin to treat HCV genotype 1. These agents have potentially significant drug–drug interactions with antiretrovirals for which there are limited data available at this time.[15,16] Careful consideration should be taken when deciding on HIV and HCV regimens in coinfected patients. Antiretrovirals such as nevirapine, efavirenz, and tipranavir are hepatotoxic and in most cases should be avoided in HCV/HIV-infected patients.

OUTCOME EVALUATION

① *The success of antiretroviral therapy is measured by the degree to which the therapy(a) restores and preserves immunologic function, (b) maximally and durably suppresses HIV RNA, (c) improves quality of life, (d) reduces HIV-related morbidity and mortality, and (e) prevents opportunistic infections.* **②** *The major outcome parameters are CD4$^+$ lymphocyte absolute count and percentage and plasma HIV RNA.* Adequate immunologic response in antiretroviral-naïve patients consists of an increase in CD4$^+$ cell count that

averages 50 to 150 cells/mm^3 (50 × 106 to 150 × 10^6/L) (with a faster response in the first 3 months), and a 1-log decrease in HIV RNA by 2 to 8 weeks after starting medications, followed by concentrations less than 50 copies/mL (50 × 103 copies/L) by 12 to 16 weeks (if HIV RNA less than 100,000/mL [100 × 10^6/L]or by 16 to 24 weeks if HIV RNA greater than 100,000/mL [100 × 10^6/L]). Upon initiating or changing antiretroviral therapy, HIV RNA should be measured after 2 to 8 weeks and every 4 to 8 weeks until undetectable. Once stable, HIV RNA and CD4$^+$ count are monitored generally every 3 to 6 months. In highly treatment-experienced patients, adequate immunologic response may be only a stable, or slightly increased, CD4$^+$ T-cell count and a stable HIV RNA. This may be enough to prevent clinical progression. However, with the new agents and new therapeutic classes of antiretrovirals available for treatment-experienced patients, the goal of treatment should be to reestablish maximal viral suppression to less than 50 HIV RNA copies/mL (50 × 10^3 copies/L).[5]

Each patient should have a plan to assess the effectiveness of antiretroviral therapy after initiation. At each clinic visit, patients should be evaluated for the presence of adverse drug reactions, drug allergies, medication adherence, and potential drug interactions. **⑧** *Antiretrovirals have both class-associated and drug-specific adverse effects* (see Table 87–4). If the patient experiences any of the serious, life-threatening effects (Table 87–5), the offending agent should be discontinued promptly, and in most cases the patient cannot be rechallenged. Potential long-term complications that may reduce the quality of life are listed in Table 87–6. For drugs with a high likelihood of intolerability (such as nelfinavir-associated diarrhea), patients should be counseled to anticipate these effects and have concomitant prescriptions available for pre-emptive management (such as an antidiarrheal agent). Patients should have follow-up within the first week after initiating a new drug regimen. If the patient does not tolerate a medication despite all efforts to the contrary, consider changing the drug.[5]

⑤ *Currently, treatment of HIV infection is lifelong.* Unplanned short-term treatment interruptions may be necessary due to drug toxicity or illness that precludes administration of oral therapy. If a patient must interrupt therapy due to toxicity, all drugs of the regimen should be stopped at the same time, regardless of half-life. The strategy of scheduling elective treatment interruptions (where patients stop and start antiretroviral therapy based on CD4$^+$ T-cell count criteria) has been evaluated in several clinical trials. Viral rebound occurs quickly after stopping therapy and worsens immune function, causes clinical progression, and may even result in death. If either short-term (less than 7 days) or long-term treatment interruption is needed, drug half-life must be taken into consideration. For regimens in which all components have similar half-lives, all drugs can be stopped simultaneously. If the regimen contains components with significantly different half-lives (e.g., Atripla), stopping all drugs at the same time could result in the drug with the longest half-life (usually NNRTIs) lingering in the body and functioning as monotherapy. The ideal time to stop the NNRTIs (efavirenz, etravirine, or nevirapine) is unknown, as these drugs can continue to be detectable 1 to 3+ weeks in patients. Options

---

Patient Encounter 2

A 43-year-old white woman presents to your clinic with significant psychiatric effects after starting a regimen consisting of emtricitabine, tenofovir, and efavirenz 2 weeks prior. Because the side effects have been interfering with her job, she has had intermittent adherence and would like to switch therapy.

What laboratory tests do you recommend?

What additional information do you need to know before creating a treatment plan for this patient?

What monitoring assessments and follow-up would you recommend?

Table 87-5

Serious Adverse Effects and Management

Adverse Effects	Drug	Signs and Symptoms	Risk Factors	Prevention/Monitoring	Management
Hepatotoxicity	Nevirapine	**Onset:** Up to 18 weeks postinitiation **Symptoms:** Abrupt onset of flu-like symptoms, abdominal pain, jaundice, fever ± rash	Increased CD4+ count at initiation Female Elevated baseline AST/ALT Any liver disease High nevirapine concentration	2-week dose escalation Avoid starting nevirapine in women with CD4+ greater than 250 cells/mm³ (250 × 10⁶/L), men with CD4+ greater than 400 cells/mm³ (400 × 10⁶/L) AST/ALT every 2 weeks for 1st month, monthly for 3 months, then every 3 months	D/C antiretrovirals; D/C all hepatotoxic agents; rule out other causes; do not rechallenge with nevirapine
	Other NNRTIs, PIs, most NRTIs, and MVC	**Onset:** NNRTI—60% within first 12 weeks PI—weeks to months NRTI—months to years **Symptoms:** NNRTI—asymptomatic to nonspecific symptoms, such as anorexia, weight loss, or fatigue PI—generally asymptomatic, some with anorexia, weight loss, jaundice Didanosine NRTI—zidovudine, didanosine, stavudine may cause hepatotoxicity associated with lactic acidosis; lamivudine, emtricitabine, or tenofovir may cause HBV flare when these drugs are withdrawn	HBV or HCV coinfection Alcoholism Concomitant hepatotoxic drugs	Monitor LFTs at least every 3–4 months	Rule out other causes. For symptomatic patients: D/C all antiretrovirals and other potential hepatotoxic agents; after symptoms and LFTs normalize, begin new antiretroviral regimen (without the potential offending agents). For asymptomatic patients: If ALT greater than 5–10 × ULN, may consider D/C antiretrovirals or continue with close monitoring; after symptoms and LFTs normalize, begin new antiretroviral regimen (without the potential offending agents)
Lactic acidosis/hepatic steatosis ± pancreatitis	NRTIs (esp. stavudine, didanosine, zidovudine)	**Onset:** Months after initiation **Symptoms:** Nonspecific GI (nausea, anorexia, abdominal pain, vomiting, weight loss, fatigue) Laboratory values: ↑ lactate, ↓ arterial pH, ↓ serum bicarbonate, ↑ AST/ALT, ↑ PT, ↑ T.bili, ↓ serum albumin, ↑ amylase/lipase (with pancreatitis)	Stavudine + didanosine Female sex Obesity Pregnancy Didanosine + hydroxyurea or ribavirin ↑ Duration of NRTI use	None unless symptoms present Consider lactate concentrations in patients with ↓ serum bicarbonate or ↑ anion gap	D/C all antiretrovirals; symptomatic support with fluids; some patients require IV bicarbonate, hemodialysis, parenteral nutrition, or mechanical ventilation; once syndrome resolves, consider using NRTIs with ↓ mitochondrial toxicity (abacavir, tenofovir, lamivudine, or emtricitabine); monitor lactate after restarting NRTIs; some clinicians use NRTI-sparing regimens

(Continued)

Table 87–5

Serious Adverse Effects and Management (Continued)

Adverse Effects	Drug	Signs and Symptoms	Risk Factors	Prevention/Monitoring	Management
Stevens-Johnson syndrome/toxic epidermal necrosis	Nevirapine greater than efavirenz, delavirdine, etravirine; also, amprenavir, abacavir, zidovudine, didanosine, indinavir lopinavir/r, atazanavir	**Onset:** 1st day–weeks after therapy start **Symptoms:** Skin eruption with mucosal ulcerations; fever, tachycardia, malaise, myalgia, arthralgia; for nevirapine may also have hepatic toxicity	Nevirapine—female, black, Asian, Hispanic	Nevirapine: use 2-week lead in 200 mg daily, then 200 mg twice a day Avoid corticosteroid use during dose escalation— may increase rash incidence Educate patients to report symptoms as soon as they appear	D/C all antiretrovirals as well as any other possible cause; aggressive symptom support; do not rechallenge patient with offending agent; if caused by nevirapine, avoid NNRTI class, if possible
Hypersensitivity reaction (HSR)	Abacavir	**Onset:** Median = 9 days; 90% within first 6 weeks **Symptoms:** Acute onset of symptoms (most frequent to least): high fever, diffuse skin rash, malaise, nausea, headache, myalgia, chills, diarrhea, vomiting, abdominal pain, dyspnea, arthralgia, respiratory symptoms	HLA-B*5701, HLA-DR7, HLA-DQ3 Antiretroviral-naive patients Higher incidence with 600 mg every day compared with twice a day dosing	HLA-B*5701 screening prior to abacavir if (+), label as abacavir allergic in medical chart Educate patients about signs and symptoms of HSR and the need of prompt report	D/C abacavir and other antiretrovirals; rule out other causes of symptoms, most signs and symptoms resolve 48 hours after abacavir/DC; do not rechallenge with abacavir after suspected HSR
Lactic acidosis/rapidly progressive ascending neuromuscular weakness	Stavudine	**Onset:** Months, then striking motor weakness within days–weeks **Symptoms:** Rapidly progressive ascending demyelinating polyneuropathy (similar to Guillain-Barré); respiratory paralysis	Prolonged stavudine use	Early recognition and D/C of offending agent to avoid progression	D/C antiretrovirals; supportive care; recovery may take months, sometimes irreversible; do not rechallenge with offending agent
Bleeding events	Tipranavir/ ritonavir: intracranial hemorrhage (ICH); other PIs: ↑ bleeding in hemophiliacs	**Onset:** ICH: median = 525 days on tipranavir/ ritonavir Hemophiliacs: Few weeks **Symptoms:** ↑ Spontaneous bleeding tendency (in joints, muscles, soft tissues, and hematuria)	ICH: CNS lesions, head trauma, recent neurosurgery, coagulopathy, alcohol abuse, or on anticoagulant or antiplatelet agents Hemophiliac patients: PI use	ICH: Avoid tipranavir/ritonavir use in high risk patients Hemophiliacs: Consider using an NNRTI-based regimen; monitor for spontaneous bleeding	ICH: D/C tipranavir/ritonavir; supportive care Hemophiliacs: May require increased use of factor VIII products
Bone marrow suppression	Zidovudine	**Onset:** Few weeks–months **Symptoms:** Fatigue, risk of ↑ bacterial infections due to neutropenia; anemia, neutropenia	Advanced HIV High-dose zidovudine Preexisting anemia or neutropenia Concomitant use of bone marrow suppressants	Avoid in patients at high risk for bone marrow suppression; avoid other suppressing agents; monitor CBC with differential at least every 3 months	Switch to another NRTI; D/C concomitant bone marrow suppressant, if possible; for anemia: Identify and treat other causes; consider erythropoietin treatment or blood transfusion, if indicated; for neutropenia: Identify and treat other causes; consider filgrastim treatment, if indicated

		Onset/Symptoms	Risk factors	Management
Nephrolithiasis/ urolithiasis/crystalluria	Indinavir	**Onset:** Any time after initiation of therapy, especially if ↓ fluid intake **Symptoms:** Flank pain and/or abdominal pain, dysuria, frequency; pyuria, hematuria, crystalluria; rarely, ↑ serum creatinine and acute renal failure	History of nephrolithiasis Patients unable to maintain adequate fluid intake High peak indinavir concentration ↑ duration of exposure	Drink at least 1.5–2 L of noncaffeinated fluid per day; ↑ fluid intake at first sign of darkened urine; monitor urinalysis and serum creatinine every 3–6 months	Increased hydration; pain control; may consider switching to alternative agent; stent placement may be required
Nephrotoxicity	Indinavir, tenofovir	**Onset:** Indinavir—months after therapy Tenofovir—weeks to months after therapy **Symptoms:** Indinavir—asymptomatic; rarely develop end-stage renal disease; ↑ serum creatinine, pyuria; hydronephrosis, renal atrophy Tenofovir—asymptomatic to symptoms of nephrogenic diabetes insipidus, Fanconi syndrome; ↑ serum creatinine, proteinuria, hypophosphatemia, glycosuria, hypokalemia, non–anion gap metabolic acidosis	History of renal disease Concomitant use of nephrotoxic drugs	Avoid use of other nephrotoxic drugs; adequate hydration if on indinavir; monitor creatinine, urinalysis, serum potassium and phosphorus in patients at risk	D/C offending agent, generally reversible; supportive care; electrolyte replacement as indicated
Pancreatitis	Didanosine; didanosine + stavudine; didanosine + hydroxyurea or ribavirin; tenofovir	**Onset:** Usually weeks to months **Symptoms:** Postprandial abdominal pain, nausea, vomiting; ↑ serum amylase and lipase	High intracellular and/ or serum Didanosine concentrations History of pancreatitis Alcoholism Hypertriglyceridemia Concomitant use of didanosine with stavudine, hydroxyurea, or ribavirin Use of didanosine + tenofovir without Didanosine dose reduction	Didanosine should not be used in patients with history of pancreatitis; avoid concomitant use of didanosine with stavudine, hydroxyurea, or ribavirin; ↓ didanosine dose when used with tenofovir	D/C offending agents; symptomatic management of pancreatitis—bowel rest, IV hydration, pain control, gradual resumption of oral intake

AST, aspartate aminotransferase; ALT, alanine aminotransferase; CBC, complete blood cell count; CPK, creatine phosphokinase; D/C, discontinue; HBV, hepatitis B virus; HCV, hepatitis C virus; LFT, liver function tests; NNRTI, nonnucleoside reverse transcriptase inhibitor; NRTI, nucleoside reverse transcriptase inhibitor; PI, protease inhibitor; PT, prothrombin time; T.bili, total bilirubin; ULN, upper limit of normal.

Table 87-6

Other Adverse Effects and Management

Adverse Effects	Drug	Signs and Symptoms	Risk Factors	Prevention/Monitoring	Management
Potential Long-Term Complications					
Cardiovascular	Potentially all PIs and other antiretrovirals (efavirenz, stavudine—unfavorable lipid effect; abacavir, didanosine—unknown)	Onset: months to years after therapy initiation; symptoms: premature CVD	Other risk factors for CVD	Consider non-PI-based regimen; lifestyle modification, counseling	Early diagnosis, prevention, and pharmacologic therapy for hyperlipidemia, HTN, insulin-resistance/diabetes mellitus; assess cardiac risk factors; switch to NNRTI- or atazanavir-based regimen; avoid stavudine
Hyperlipidemia	All PIs (except atazanavir); stavudine; efavirenz (to a lesser extent)	Onset: weeks to months after therapy initiation; symptoms: all PIs except atazanavir—↑ LDL and total cholesterol (TC), ↓↑ HDL; lopinavir/r and ritonavir—disproportionate ↑ TG; stavudine—↑ TG; may also ↑ LDL and TC; efavirenz or nevirapine—↑ HDL, slight ↑ TG	Underlying hyperlipidemia PI: Tipranavir/r greater than lopinavir/r and ritonavir greater than nelfinavir and amprenavir greater than indinavir and saquinavir greater than atazanavir NNRTI: less than PIs; efavirenz greater than nevirapine, etravirine, or rilpivirine NRTI: stavudine greater than zidovudine and tenofovir most common	Use non-PI, non–stavudine-based regimens; use atazanavir-based regimen; monitor fasting lipid profile at baseline, 3–6 months after new regimen, then at least annually	Assess cardiac risk factor; lifestyle modification; switch to antiretrovirals with fewer lipid effects; total cholesterol greater than 200 mg/dL (5.17 mmol/L), LDL, TG 200–500 mg/dL (2.26–5.65 mmol/L) ⇒ pravastatin or atorvastatin; TG greater than 500 mg/dL (5.65 mmol/L) gemfibrozil or micronized fenofibrate
Insulin resistance/diabetes mellitus	All PIs	Onset: weeks to months after therapy initiation; symptoms: polyuria, polydipsia, polyphagia, fatigue, weakness; exacerbation of hyperglycemia in patients with underlying diabetes	Underlying hyperglycemia, family history of diabetes mellitus	Use PI-sparing regimens; monitor fasting blood glucose 1–3 months after starting new regimen, then at least every 3–6 months	Diet and exercise; consider switching to an NNRTI-based regimen; if need for pharmacologic therapy, consider metformin, sulfonylurea, "glitazones," or insulin, where indicated
Osteonecrosis	All PIs	Onset: insidious; symptoms: mild to moderate periarticular pain; 85% of cases involve one or both femoral heads	Diabetes Prior steroid use Advanced age Alcohol use Hyperlipidemia	Risk reduction (limit steroid and alcohol use); for asymptomatic cases with less than 15% bony head involvement, monitor with MRI every 3–6 months × 1 year, then every 6 months × 1 year, then annually	Conservative: reduce weight-bearing activity on affected joint; reduce risk factors; analgesics as needed; surgical: core decompression ± bone grafting (early disease); total joint arthroplasty (severe disease)
Quality-of-Life Complications					
CNS effects	Efavirenz	Onset: first few doses; symptoms: one or more of the following: drowsiness, insomnia, abnormal dreams, dizziness, impaired concentration, depression, hallucination; exacerbation of psychiatric disorders; psychosis; suicidal ideation	Preexisting or unstable psychiatric illness Use of other drugs with CNS effects May be more common in African Americans due to genetic predisposition of ↓ clearance	Take no earlier than 2–3 hours before bedtime; take on an empty stomach; counsel patients to avoid operating machinery during first 2–4 weeks of therapy	Symptoms usually diminish or resolve after 2–4 weeks; may consider discontinuing therapy if symptoms persist and significantly impair daily function or exacerbate psychiatric illness

Adverse Effect	Associated Agents	Onset and Symptoms	Risk Factors	Monitoring	Management/Comments
Fat maldistribution	PIs, thymidine analogs (stavudine more common than zidovudine)	Onset: gradually, months after therapy initiation; symptoms: lipoatrophy—peripheral fat loss (facial thinning, thinning of extremities and buttocks); lipohypertrophy—increase in abdominal girth, breast size, and dorsocervical fat pad (buffalo hump)	Lipoatrophy—low baseline body mass index	DEXA scan; lipoatrophy: avoid thymidine analogs or switch from zidovudine or stavudine to abacavir or tenofovir	Switching to other agents may slow or stop progression, but may not reverse effects; injectable poly-L-lactic acid for facial lipoatrophy
GI intolerance	All PIs, zidovudine, didanosine	Onset: first few doses; symptoms: nausea, vomiting, abdominal pain; diarrhea commonly seen with nelfinavir, lopinavir/ritonavir, and didanosine-buffered formulations	All patients		Taking with food may reduce symptoms (not for didanosine or unboosted indinavir); may preemptively need antiemetics or antidiarrheals
Injection site reactions	Enfuvirtide	Onset: first new doses; symptoms: pain, pruritus, erythema, ecchymosis, warmth, nodules, rarely injection site infection	All patients		Educate regarding use of sterile technique, solution at room temperature, rotation of injection sites, avoidance of sites with little subcutaneous fat or existing reactions
Peripheral neuropathy	Didanosine, stavudine	Onset: weeks to months after therapy initiation; symptoms: begins with numbness and paresthesias of toes and feet; may progress to painful neuropathy; upper extremities less frequently involved; may be irreversible despite drug discontinuation	Preexisting peripheral neuropathy; Combined use of these NRTIs or other drugs which may cause neuropathy; Advanced HIV; High dose of offending drugs or drugs that may increase didanosine intracellular activities (hydroxyurea, ribavirin)		Consider D/C offending agent prior to onset of disabling pain; pharmacologic treatment (variable effectiveness): gabapentin, tricyclic antidepressants, lamotrigine, oxcarbamazepine, topiramate, tramadol, narcotic analgesics, capsaicin cream, topical lidocaine

CVD, cardiovascular disease; D/C, discontinue; DEXA, dual-energy x-ray absorptiometry; HDL, high-density lipoprotein; HTN, hypertension; LDL, low-density lipoprotein; NNRTI, nonnucleoside reverse transcriptase inhibitor; NRTI, nucleoside reverse transcriptase inhibitor; PI, protease inhibitor; TG, triglyceride.

include either (a) stopping the NNRTI first and continuing the other drugs in the regimen for up to 4 weeks or (b) substituting the NNRTI with a PI and continuing the PI with dual NRTIs for up to 4 weeks. In this situation, therapeutic drug monitoring of the long half-life drug can be useful in determining when to stop the NRTI ± PI coverage.[5]

Patient Care and Monitoring

Patient Assessment

1. Medication history

- Get a thorough history of prescription, nonprescription, and natural drug product use. Determine what prior antiretroviral regimens, if any, were used in the past.

- *Is the patient taking the appropriate dose of each medication? Are the doses adjusted for renal or hepatic failure? Are the doses adjusted for drug interactions with concomitant medications?*

- Evaluate the patient for the presence of adverse drug reactions, drug allergies, and drug interactions.

- Assess improvement in quality-of-life measures such as physical, psychological, and social functioning and well-being. *Is the patient experiencing any drug-induced adverse effects? What can you do to help manage these adverse effects?*

2. Review any available diagnostic data to determine status of his HIV/AIDS.

3. Determine whether initiation of antiretroviral therapy is indicated. Evaluate the patient's ability to adhere to medications, daily routine, social support, and financial stability. *Is the patient taking any medications that may interfere with the individual components of potential regimens? Does the patient have medical insurance and prescription coverage?*

4. Develop a plan to assess the effectiveness and tolerability of antiretroviral therapy.

Patient Education

1. Educate the patient on HIV/AIDS disease and the importance of strict adherence to medication (the patient must ideally take his or her medications at the same time every day). Recommend a therapeutic regimen that is as easy as possible for the patient to take. Talk to the patient specifically about when and how the patient will be taking the medications. *What time do they eat meals? When do they wake up? What other medications are they taking at the same time?* Educate patients whether to take their medications with or without food.

2. Educate the patient on common adverse drug effects and a few of the key signs and symptoms of severe toxicity (i.e., jaundice and abacavir hypersensitivity reaction). Tell them to call their provider immediately if any of those symptoms occur. Make sure they have the correct telephone number for the clinic.

Abbreviations Introduced in This Chapter

AIDS	Acquired immunodeficiency syndrome
ALT	Alanine aminotransferase
ART	Antiretroviral therapy
AST	Aspartate aminotransferase
CPK	Creatine phosphokinase
CVD	Cardiovascular disease
CYP	Cytochrome P-450 isoenzyme
D/C	Discontinue
DEXA	Dual-energy x-ray absorptiometry
DHHS	Department of Health and Human Services
ELISA	Enzyme-linked immunosorbent assay
GERD	Gastroesophageal reflux disease
gp	Glycoprotein
HAART	Highly active antiretroviral therapy
HBeAg	Hepatitis B early antigen
HBV	Hepatitis B virus
HCV	Hepatitis C virus
HDL	High-density lipoprotein
HIV	Human immunodeficiency virus
HLA	Human leukocyte antigen
HSR	Hypersensitivity reaction
HTN	Hypertension
IAS-USA	International AIDS Society–USA
ICH	Intracranial hemorrhage
IFA	Indirect immunofluorescence assay
LDL	Low-density lipoprotein
LFT	Liver function tests
MSM	Men who have sex with men
MTCT	Mother-to-child transmission
NNRTI	Nonnucleoside reverse transcriptase inhibitor
NRTI	Nucleoside reverse transcriptase inhibitor
NtRTI	Nucleotide reverse transcriptase inhibitor
PCP	*Pneumocystis jiroveci* (formerly *carinii*) pneumonia
PI	Protease inhibitor
PT	Prothrombin time
RT-PCR	Reverse transcriptase polymerase chain reaction
SIV	Simian immunodeficiency virus
STI	Sexually transmitted infection
T.bili	Total bilirubin
TDF	Tenofovir disoproxil fumarate
TG	Triglyceride
ULN	Upper limit of normal
WB	Western blot

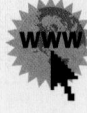 Self-assessment questions and answers are available at *http://mhpharmacotherapy.com/pp.html.*

REFERENCES

1. World Heath Organization. UNAIDS Report on the Global AIDS Epidemic 2010 [online]. [cited 2011 Oct 10]. Available from: *http://www. unaids.org/globalreport/.*

2. Centers for Disease Control and Prevention. HIV Surveillance in the United States, 1981-2008. MMWR 2011;61(21):689–728.

3. Wawer MJ, Gray RH, Sewankambo NK, et al. Rates of HIV-1 transmission per coital act, by stage of HIV-1 infection, in Rakai, Uganda. J Infect Dis 2005;191:1403–1409.

4. Branson BM, Handsfield HH, Lampe MA, et al. Revised recommendations for HIV testing of adults, adolescents, and pregnant women in health-care settings. MMWR Recomm Rep 2006;55:1–17.

5. Panel on Antiretroviral Guidelines for Adults and Adolescents. Guidelines for the use of antiretroviral agents in HIV-1-infected adults and adolescents [online]. Department of Health and Human Services. October 14, 2011;1–166. [cited 2011 Oct 10]. Available from: *http://www.aidsinfo.nih.gov/ContentFiles/AdultandAdolescentGL.pdf.* Accessed October 14, 2011.

6. Fields-Gardner C, Campa A for the America Dietetics Assocation. Position of the American Dietetic Association: Nutrition Intervention and Human Immunodeficiency Virus Infection. J Am Diet Assoc 2010:110(7):1105–1119.

7. Thompson MA, Aberg JA, Cahn P, et al. Antiretroviral treatment of adult HIV infection: 2010 Recommendations of the International AIDS Society-USA panel. JAMA 2010;304(3):321–333.

8. Panel on Antiretroviral Therapy and Medical Management in HIV-infected Children. Working Guidelines for the Use of Antiretroviral Agents in Pediatric HIV Infection [online]. August 11, 2011. [cited 2011 Oct 10]. Available from: *http://aidsinfo.nih.gov/contentfiles/ PediatricGuidelines.pdf.*

9. Institute NYSDoHA. Drug Interactions Between ARVs and Recreational Drugs [online]. February 2009. In HIV and Substance Use. [cited 2011 Oct 10]. Available from: *http://www.hivguidelines.org.*

10. Public Health Service Task Force. Recommendations for Use of Antiretroviral Drugs in Pregnant HIV-Infected Women for Maternal Health and Interventions to Reduce Perinatal HIV-1 Transmission in the United States [online]. September 14, 2011. [cited 2011 Oct 10]. Available from: *http://aidsinfo.nih.gov/contentfiles/PerinatalGL.pdf.*

11. Cohn SE, Watts D, Lertora J, Park JG, Yu S. Depo-medroxyprogesterone in women on antiretroviral thearpy: Effective contraception and lack of clinically significant interactions. Clin Pharmacol Ther 2007;81:222–227.

12. Koziel MJ, Peters MG. Viral hepatitis in HIV infection. N Engl J Med 2007;356:1445–1454.

13. Tien PC. Management and treatment of hepatitis C virus infection in HIV-infected adults: Recommendations from the Veterans Affairs Hepatitis C Resource Center Program and National Hepatitis C Program Office. Am J Gastroenterol 2005;100:2338–2354.

14. European AIDS Clinical Society (EACS) Guidelines Part IV: Clinical management and treatment of chronic hepatitis B and C coinfection in HIV-infected adults. Version 6.0, October 2011. [cited 2011 Oct 10]. Available from: *www.europeanaidsclinicalsociety. org.*

15. Dore GJ, Matthews GV, Rockstroh J. Future of Hepatitis C Therapy: development of direct acting antivirals. Curr Opin HIV AIDS 2011;6:508–513.

16. R van Heeswijk, A Vandevoorde, G Boogaerts, et al. Pharmacokinetic Interactions between ARV Agents and the Investigational HCV Protease Inhibitor TVR in Healthy Volunteers. 18th Conference on Retroviruses and Opportunistic Infections (CROI 2011), Boston, MA, February 27–March 2, 2011. Abstract 119.

88   Cancer Chemotherapy and Treatment

Amy Robbins Williams

KEY CONCEPTS

❶ The word *cancer* covers a diverse array of tumor types that affect a significant number of Americans and individuals worldwide and are a significant cause of mortality.

❷ Numerous cellular changes occur in the genetic material of the cancer cell so that programmed cell death, or **apoptosis**, does not occur. Proliferation of cancer cells goes unregulated.

❸ Most solid tumors are staged according to the tumor, nodes, metastases (TNM) classification system. The size of the primary tumor, extent of nodal involvement, and presence of metastases are used to determine the stage. Metastases are cancer cells that have spread to sites distant from the primary tumor site and have started to grow. The most frequently occurring sites of metastases of solid tumors are the brain, bone, liver, and lungs. After TNM staging, most cancers types are then classified by a more simplified staging (i.e., stages I to IV), which indicates disease severity.

❹ Traditional chemotherapy agents have some similar side effects, usually manifested on the most rapidly proliferating cells of the body. However, various pharmacological categories of antineoplastic agents do possess unique toxicities. Anthracyclines (e.g., doxorubicin) have the potential to cause cardiac toxicity, which is related to the cumulative dose. Microtubule-targeting agents (e.g., vincristine) are associated with various forms of neurotoxicity. Alkylating agents (e.g., melphalan) are associated with secondary malignancies.

❺ Because of the risk of severe toxicities associated with many of the chemotherapy agents, safety and handling precautions must be in place to prevent chemotherapy errors and/or accidental chemotherapy exposures to health care professionals or patients.

❻ Clinicians should play a role in ensuring chemotherapy safety, patient education, and monitoring patient response to therapy. For example, cumulative doses of anthracyclines should be monitored along with signs and symptoms of heart failure. Clinicians should also monitor for drug interactions between other current medications and chemotherapy agents.

EPIDEMIOLOGY

❶ *The word cancer covers a diverse array of tumor types that affect a significant number of Americans and individuals worldwide and are a significant cause of mortality.* The term cancer actually refers to more than 100 different diseases. What is common to all cancers is that the cancerous cell is uncontrollably growing and has the potential for invading local tissue and spreading to other parts of the body, a process called **metastases**. Cancer is now the leading cause of death in Americans younger than the age of 85 years of age.[1] In 2011, it was projected that almost 1.6 million Americans will be diagnosed with cancer, and more than 570,000 Americans will die from the cancer.[2] **Figure 88–1** describes cancers by gender, new cases, and deaths.

Once diagnosed, a cancer patient may encounter many different health care professionals. All health care professionals need to collaborate to ensure safe and appropriate

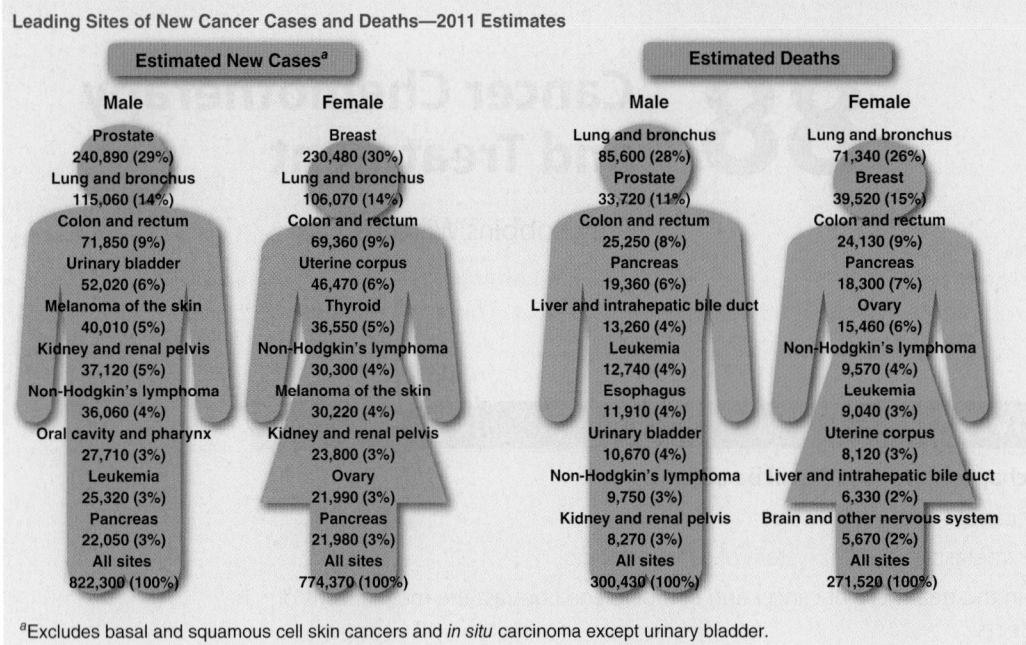

FIGURE 88–1. Cancer incidences (*left*) and deaths (*right*) in the United States for males and females—2011 estimates. (Reproduced from American Cancer Society. Cancer facts and figures–2011. Atlanta: American Cancer Society; 2011.)

Leading Sites of New Cancer Cases and Deaths—2011 Estimates

Estimated New Cases[a]

Male	Female
Prostate 240,890 (29%)	Breast 230,480 (30%)
Lung and bronchus 115,060 (14%)	Lung and bronchus 106,070 (14%)
Colon and rectum 71,850 (9%)	Colon and rectum 69,360 (9%)
Urinary bladder 52,020 (6%)	Uterine corpus 46,470 (6%)
Melanoma of the skin 40,010 (5%)	Thyroid 36,550 (5%)
Kidney and renal pelvis 37,120 (5%)	Non-Hodgkin's lymphoma 30,300 (4%)
Non-Hodgkin's lymphoma 36,060 (4%)	Melanoma of the skin 30,220 (4%)
Oral cavity and pharynx 27,710 (3%)	Kidney and renal pelvis 23,800 (3%)
Leukemia 25,320 (3%)	Ovary 21,990 (3%)
Pancreas 22,050 (3%)	Pancreas 21,980 (3%)
All sites 822,300 (100%)	All sites 774,370 (100%)

Estimated Deaths

Male	Female
Lung and bronchus 85,600 (28%)	Lung and bronchus 71,340 (26%)
Prostate 33,720 (11%)	Breast 39,520 (15%)
Colon and rectum 25,250 (8%)	Colon and rectum 24,130 (9%)
Pancreas 19,360 (6%)	Pancreas 18,300 (7%)
Liver and intrahepatic bile duct 13,260 (4%)	Ovary 15,460 (6%)
Leukemia 12,740 (4%)	Non-Hodgkin's lymphoma 9,570 (4%)
Esophagus 11,910 (4%)	Leukemia 9,040 (3%)
Urinary bladder 10,670 (4%)	Uterine corpus 8,120 (3%)
Non-Hodgkin's lymphoma 9,750 (3%)	Liver and intrahepatic bile duct 6,330 (2%)
Kidney and renal pelvis 8,270 (3%)	Brain and other nervous system 5,670 (2%)
All sites 300,430 (100%)	All sites 271,520 (100%)

[a]Excludes basal and squamous cell skin cancers and *in situ* carcinoma except urinary bladder.

prescribing, preparation, administration, and monitoring of anticancer agents; management of toxicities; resolution of reimbursement issues; and participation in clinical trials.[3]

As a result of advances in research and technology, available cancer treatments have increased dramatically in the last couple of decades. The fields of radiation therapy, surgery, and drug development have made enormous progress over the years; therefore, patients may not only be receiving less toxic treatments but also treatments that have better outcomes than in the past. Supportive care therapies have improved, and patients now may be at less risk for toxicity and have a better quality of life than patients in the past. In the early 1990s, most patients received chemotherapy in the hospital because of side effects. Today, most patients are able to receive chemotherapy in the outpatient clinics and/or take oral anticancer agents at home.

Cancer Prevention

Because most cancers are not curable in advanced stages, cancer prevention is an important and active area of research. Both lifestyle modifications and chemoprevention agents may significantly reduce the risk of developing cancer. Although still an active area of investigation, the Food and Drug Administration (FDA) has approved two vaccines that can help prevent cancer. One of these vaccines prevents infection with human papillomavirus, which can cause cervical cancer and anal cancer. The other vaccine prevents infection with hepatitis B virus, which can cause liver cancer. In addition, both tamoxifen and raloxifene are approved for the prevention of breast cancer, and celecoxib is approved for the prevention of familial adenomatous polyposis (FAP) variant of colon cancer.

Tobacco

Tobacco smoking increases the risk of developing not only lung cancer but also many other types of cancer, including cancer of the bladder, mouth, pharynx, larynx, and esophagus as well as renal cell cancer. Smoking cessation is associated with a gradual decrease in the risk of cancer, but more than 5 years is needed before a major decline in risk is detected. In addition, most studies have found that passive smoking (i.e., secondhand smoke) also increases a person's risk of developing lung cancer.[4]

Sun Exposure

Ultraviolet light and increased skin exposure may increase the risk of melanoma and other skin cancers, especially in individuals who have a positive family history and who are fair skinned, and have light-colored eyes, high degrees of freckling, and a tendency to burn instead of tan. Practitioners can counsel patients on proper sun protection, including minimizing sun exposure, using sunscreens with a sun protection factor (SPF) of 15 or greater on exposed areas, wearing protective clothing, avoiding tanning beds, and the importance of early detection.

CARCINOGENESIS

●The exact cause of cancer remains unknown and is probably very diverse given the vast array of diseases called cancer. It is thought that cancer develops from a single cell in which the normal mechanisms for control of growth and proliferation are altered. Current evidence indicates that there are four stages in the cancer development process.

The first step, **initiation**, occurs when a carcinogenic substance encounters a normal cell to produce genetic damage and results in a mutated cell. The environment is altered by carcinogens or other factors to favor the growth of the mutated cell over the normal cell during **promotion**, the second step. The main difference between initiation and promotion is that promotion is a reversible process. Third, **transformation** (or **conversion**) occurs when the mutated cell becomes malignant. Depending on the type of cancer, up to 20 years may elapse between the carcinogenic phases and the development of a clinically detectable tumor. Finally, **progression** occurs when cell proliferation takes over and the tumor spreads or develops metastases.

There are substances known to have carcinogenic risks, including chemicals, environmental factors, and viruses. Chemicals in the environment, such as aniline and benzene, are associated with the development of bladder cancer and leukemia, respectively. Environmental factors, such as excessive sun exposure, can result in skin cancer, and smoking is widely known as a cause of lung cancer. Viruses, including human papilloma virus (HPV), Epstein-Barr virus, and hepatitis B virus, have been linked to cervical cancers, lymphomas, and liver cancers, respectively. Anticancer agents such as the alkylating agents (e.g., melphalan), anthracyclines (e.g., doxorubicin), and epipodophyllotoxins (e.g., etoposide) can cause secondary malignancies (e.g., leukemias) years after therapy has been completed. Additionally, factors such as the patient's age, gender, family history, diet, and chronic irritation or inflammation may be considered to be promoters of carcinogenesis.

Cancer Genetics

Because the human genome has been sequenced and with the great improvements in genetic technology, there is growing knowledge regarding the genetic changes of cancer. There are two major classes of genes involved in carcinogenesis, **oncogenes** and **tumor suppressor genes**. **Protooncogenes** are normal genes that, through some genetic alteration caused by carcinogens, change into oncogenes. Protooncogenes are present in all normal cells and regulate cell function and replication. Genetic damage of the protooncogene may occur through point mutation, chromosomal rearrangement, or an increase in gene function, resulting in the oncogene. The genetic damage may either be inherited from an individual's parents (germline mutations) or by way of carcinogenic agents (e.g., smoking). The oncogene produces abnormal or excessive gene product that disrupts normal cell growth and proliferation.[5] As a result, this may cause the cell to have a distinct growth advantage, increasing its likelihood of becoming cancerous. Table 88-1 provides examples of oncogenes by their cellular function and associated cancer.

Tumor suppressor genes inhibit inappropriate cellular growth and proliferation by gene loss or mutation. This results in loss of control over normal cell growth. The *p53* gene is one of the most common tumor suppressor genes, and mutations of *p53* may occur in up to 50% of all malignancies. This gene stops the cell cycle to enable "repairs" of the cell.

If *p53* is inactivated, then the cell allows the mutations to occur. Although mutations of the *p53* gene are found in many tumors, such as breast, colon, and lung cancer, it is also associated with drug resistance of cancer cells. DNA repair genes fix errors in DNA that occur because of environmental factors or errors in replication and can be classified as *tumor suppressor genes*. Mutations in DNA repair genes have been reported in hereditary nonpolyposis colon cancer and in some breast cancer syndromes.

❷ *Numerous cellular changes occur in the genetic material of the cancer cell so that programmed cell death, or apoptosis, does not occur. Proliferation of cancer cells goes unregulated.* If mutations persist and cells are not repaired or suppressed, cancer may develop. **Apoptosis**, or programmed cell death, may prevent the mutated cell from becoming cancerous. Loss of *p53* and overexpression of *bcl-2* are two examples of changes within the cell that occur to result in enhanced cell survival. Cellular senescence refers to cell death that occurs after a preset number of cell doublings. Telomeres are DNA segments at the ends of chromosomes that shorten with each replication to the point where senescence is triggered.

Identification of genes involved in cancer may be conducted for various reasons, including cancer screening to determine if an individual is at an increased risk of cancer, to develop new anticancer agents, to aid in diagnosis, and to predict response and/or the toxicity of the agents used in individual patients.

Principles of Tumor Growth

It takes about 10^9 cancer cells to be clinically detectable by palpation or radiography. Figure 88-2 demonstrates the classic Gompertzian kinetics tumor growth cycle. From the diagram, one can see that malignant cell growth occurs many times before a mass may be detected. The number of malignant cells may decrease drastically because of surgery or in decreasing steps by each administration of chemotherapy. One dosing round, or cycle, of chemotherapy does not eliminate all malignant cells; therefore, repeated cycles of chemotherapy are administered to eliminate tumor cell burden. The cell kill hypothesis states that a fixed percentage of tumor cells will be killed with each cycle of chemotherapy. According to this hypothesis, the number of tumor cells will never reach zero. This theory assumes that all cancers are equally responsive and that anticancer drug resistance and metastases do not occur, which is not the case.[6]

Metastases

A **metastasis** is a growth of the same cancer cell found at some distance from the primary tumor site.[7] The metastasis may be large, or it may be just a few cells that may be detected through polymerase chain reaction (PCR); however, the presence of metastasis at staging usually is associated with a poorer prognosis than the patient with no known metastatic disease. As the technology to detect malignant cells evolves, the dilemma exists on how to treat patients based on current guidelines that were not based on cellular detection technology.

Table 88–1

Examples of Oncogenes and Tumor Suppressor Genes

Gene	Function	Associated Human Cancer
Oncogenes		
Genes for growth factors or their receptors		
EGFR or Erb-B1	Codes for epidermal growth factor (EGFR) receptor	Glioblastoma, breast, head and neck, and colon cancers
HER-2/neu or Erb-B2	Codes for a growth factor receptor	Breast, salivary gland, prostate, bladder, and ovarian cancers
RET	Codes for a growth factor receptor	Thyroid cancer
Genes for cytoplasmic relays in stimulatory signaling pathways		
K-RAS and N-RAS	Code for guanine nucleotide-proteins with GTPase activity	Lung, ovarian, colon, pancreatic binding cancers
		Neuroblastoma, acute leukemia
Genes for transcription factors that activate growth-promoting genes		
c-MYC		Leukemia and breast, colon, gastric, and lung cancers
N-MYC		Neuroblastoma, small cell lung cancer, and glioblastoma
Genes for cytoplasmic kinases		
BCR-ABL	Codes for a nonreceptor tyrosine kinase	Chronic myelogenous leukemia
Genes for other molecules		
BCL-2	Codes for a protein that blocks apoptosis	Indolent B-cell lymphomas
BCL-1 or PRAD1	Codes for cyclin D_1, a cell-cycle clock stimulator	Breast, head, and neck cancers
MDM2	Protein antagonist of p53 tumor suppressor protein	Sarcomas
Tumor-suppressor genes		
Genes for proteins in the cytoplasm		
APC	Step in a signaling pathway	Colon and gastric cancer
NF-1	Codes for a protein that inhibits the stimulatory Ras protein	Neurofibroma, leukemia, and pheochromocytoma
NF-2	Codes for a protein that inhibits the stimulatory Ras protein	Meningioma, ependymoma, and schwannoma
Genes for proteins in the nucleus		
MTS1	Codes for p16 protein, a cyclin-dependent kinase inhibitor	Involved in a wide range of cancers
RB1	Codes for the pRB protein, a master brake of the cell cycle	Retinoblastoma, osteosarcoma, and bladder, small cell lung, prostate, and breast cancers
p53	Codes for the p53 protein, which can halt cell division and induce apoptosis	Involved in a wide range of cancers
Genes for protein whose cellular location is unclear		
BRCA1	DNA repair, transcriptional regulation	Breast and ovarian cancers
BRCA2	DNA repair	Breast cancer
VHL	Regulator of protein stability	Renal cell cancer
MSH2, MLH1, PMS1, PMS2, MSH6	DNA mismatch repair enzymes	Hereditary nonpolyposis colorectal cancer

From DiPiro JT, Talbert RL, Yee GC, et al. (eds.) Pharmacotherapy: A Pathophysiologic Approach. 8th ed. New York: McGraw-Hill; 2011: Table 135-2.

Cancers spread usually by two pathways: hematogenous (through the bloodstream) or through the lymphatics (drainage through adjacent lymph nodes). The malignant cells that split from the primary tumor find a suitable environment for growth. It is believed that malignant cells secrete mediators that stimulate the formation of blood vessels for growth and oxygen, the process of angiogenesis. The usual metastatic sites for solid tumors are the brain, bone, lung, and liver.

PATHOPHYSIOLOGY

Tumor Origin

Tumors may arise from the four basic tissue types: epithelial, connective (i.e., muscle, bone, and cartilage), lymphoid, or nerve tissue. The suffix -oma is added to the name of the cell type if the tumor cells are benign. A *lipoma* is a benign growth that resembles fat tissue.

Precancerous cells have cellular changes that are abnormal but not yet malignant and may be described as *hyperplastic* or *dysplastic*. Hyperplasia occurs when a stimulus is introduced and reverses when the stimulus is removed. Dysplasia is an abnormal change in the size, shape, or organization of cells or tissues.

Malignant cells are divided into categories based on the cells of origin. Carcinomas arise from epithelial cells, whereas sarcomas arise from muscle or connective tissue. Adenocarcinomas arise from glandular tissue. *Carcinoma in situ* refers to cells limited to epithelial origin that have not yet invaded the basement membrane. Malignancies of

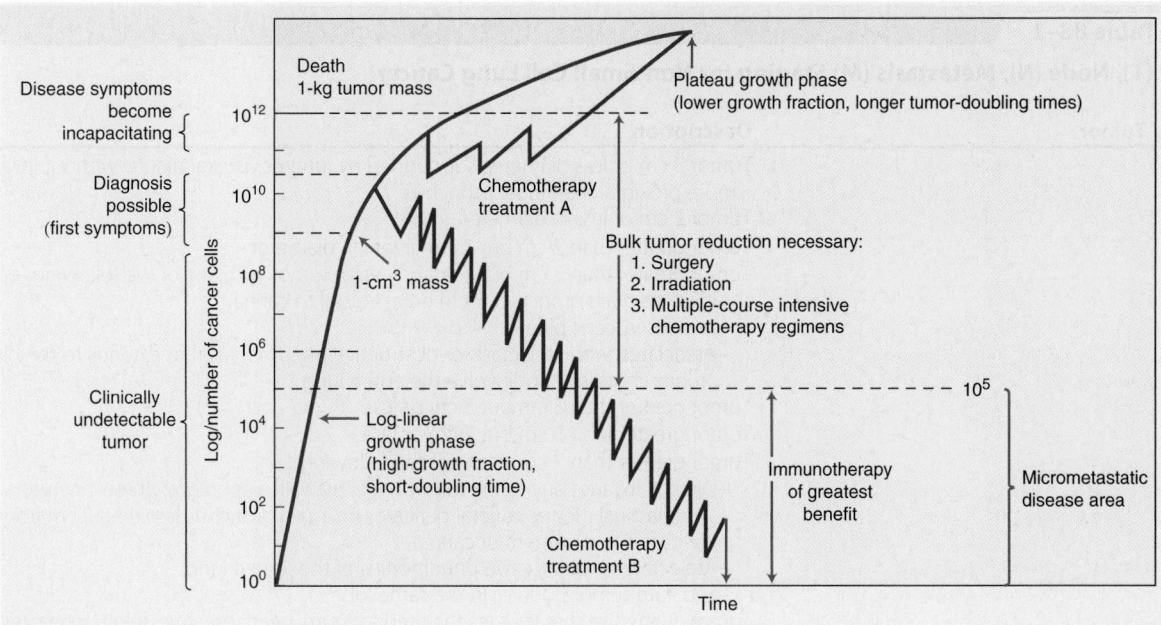

FIGURE 88–2. The Gompertzian growth curve demonstrating symptoms and treatments versus tumor volume. (From Buick RN. Cellular basis of chemotherapy. In: Dorr RT, Von Hoff DD, eds. Cancer Chemotherapy Handbook. 2nd ed. New York: Elsevier; 1994: 3–14.)

the bone marrow or lymphoid tissue, such as leukemias or lymphomas, are named differently.

Tumor Characteristics

Tumors are either benign or malignant.[8] Benign tumors often are encapsulated, localized, and indolent; they seldom metastasize; and they rarely recur once removed. Histologically, the cells resemble the cells from which they developed. Malignant tumors are invasive and spread to other locations even if the primary tumor is removed. The cells no longer perform their usual functions, and their cellular architecture changes. This loss of structure and function is called *anaplasia*. Despite improvements in screening procedures, many patients have metastatic disease at the time of diagnosis. Usually, once distant metastases have occurred, the cancer is deemed to be incurable.

DIAGNOSIS OF CANCER

Cancer can present as a number of different signs and symptoms as well as pain and loss of appetite. Unfortunately, many people fear a diagnosis of cancer and may not seek medical attention at the first warning signs when the disease is at its most treatable stage. After the initial visit with the physician, a variety of tests will be performed, which are somewhat dependent on the initial differential diagnosis. Appropriate laboratory tests, radiologic scans, and tissue samples are necessary. The sample of tissue may be obtained by a biopsy, fine-needle aspiration, or exfoliative cytology. No treatment of cancer should be initiated without

a pathologic diagnosis of cancer. During the pathologic workup, cytogenetics may be done. Depending on the type of cancer, the cytogenetics can provide the additional information on prognosis of the malignancy and whether certain therapies may be appropriate.

❸ Once the pathology of cancer is established, then the staging of the disease is done before treatment is initiated. Each chapter describing a cancerous disease state will discuss the specifics of staging of the disease. Cancer staging is usually done according to the primary tumor size, extent of lymph node involvement, and the presence or absence of metastases, also referred to as the tumor, nodes, metastases (TNM) system (Table 88–2). The stage of the disease is a compilation of the primary tumor size, the nodal involvement, and metastases and is usually referred to as stages I, II, III, or IV. Not all cancers can be staged according to this system, but many of the solid tumors are classified this way.

Why are tumors staged? First, the stage of the disease is an important part of determining the prognosis of the cancer. Second, staging of the cancers allows comparison of patient groups when examining data from clinical trials; staging reflects the extent of disease. Finally, the clinician uses it as a guide to treatment and may use restaging after treatment to guide further treatment.

Some cancers produce substances (e.g., proteins) that are detected by a blood test, that may be useful in following response to therapy or detecting a recurrence; these are referred to as tumor markers. An example of a clinically used tumor marker is the prostate-specific antigen (PSA). The PSA serum level can be used as a screening test for prostate cancer. Unfortunately, some tumor markers are nonspecific

Table 88–2

Tumor (T), Node (N), Metastasis (M) Staging for Non-Small Cell Lung Cancer

Primary Tumor		Description
T_1		Tumor 3 cm or less diameter, surrounded by lung or visceral pleura, without invasion more proximal than lobar bronchus
	T_{1a}	Tumor 2 cm or less in diameter
	T_{1b}	Tumor greater than 2 cm but 3 cm or less in diameter
T_2		Tumor greater than 3 cm but 7 cm or less, or tumor with any of the following features: –Involves main bronchus, 2 cm or less distal to carina –Invades visceral pleura –Associated with atelectasis or obstructive pneumonitis that extends to the hilar region but does not involve the entire lung
	T_{2a}	Tumor greater than 3 cm but 5 cm or less
	T_{2b}	Tumor greater than 5 cm but 7 cm or less
T_3		Tumor greater than 7 cm or any of the following: –Directly invades any of the following: chestwall, diaphragm, phrenic nerve, mediastinal pleura, parietal pericardium, main bronchus less than 2 cm from carina (without involvement of carina) –Atelectasis or obstructive pneumonitis of the entire lung –Separate tumor nodules in the same lobe
T_4		Tumor of any size that invades the mediastinum, heart, great vessels, trachea, recurrent laryngeal nerve, esophagus, vertebral body, carina, or with separate tumor noçdules in a different ipsilateral lobe

Regional lymph nodes (N)

N_0		No regional lymph node metastases
N_1		Metastasis in ipsilateral peribronchial and/or ipsilateral hilar lymph nodes and intrapulmonary nodes, including involvement by direct extension
N_2		Metastasis in ipsilateral mediastinal and/or subcarinal lymph node(s)
N_3		Metastasis in contralateral mediastinal, contralateral hilar, ipsilateral or contralateral scalene, or supraclavicular lymph node(s).

Distant metastasis (M)

M_0		No distant metastasis
M_1		Distant metastasis
	M_{1a}	Separate tumor nodule(s) in a contralateral lobe; tumor with pleural nodules or malignant pleural or pericardial effusion
	M_{1b}	Distant metastasis

Stage	T	N	M	5 Yr Survival
Stage IA:	T_{1a}–T_{1b}	N_0	M_0	73%
Stage IB:	T_{2a}	N_0	M_0	58%
Stage IIA:	$T_{1a}, T_{1b}, T_{2a} T_{2b}$	$N_1 N_0$	$M_0 M_0$	46%
Stage IIB:	$T_{2b} T_3$	$N_1 N_0$	$M_0 M_0$	36%
	$T_{1a}, T_{1b}, T_{2a}, T_{2b}$	N_2	M_0	
Stage IIIA:	T_3	N_1, N_2	M_0	24%
	T_4	N_0, N_1	M_0	
Stage IIIB:	T_4	N_2	M_0	9%
	Any T	N_3	M_0	
Stage IV:	Any T	Any N	M_{1a} or M_{1b}	13%

From DiPiro JT, Talbert RL, Yee GC, et al. (eds.) Pharmacotherapy: A Pathophysiologic Approach. 8th ed. New York: McGraw-Hill; 2011: Table 137-2.

and may be elevated from nonmalignant causes. In the case of PSA, nonmalignant causes such as prostatitis, trauma, surgery, ejaculation, some medications, benign prostatic hypertrophy, or riding on an exercise bicycle can all cause increased PSA levels.[9] Some tumors may express a marker in some patients and not in others. The full role of tumor markers has not been fully elucidated.

TREATMENT

Desired Outcome

Surgery may be able to remove all macroscopic disease; however, microscopic cells may still be present near the surgical site or may have traveled to other parts of the body. When malignant cells have traveled to other parts of the body and become established there and are able to grow in this new environment, they are called *metastatic cancer cells*. Thus, for chemotherapy-sensitive diseases, systemic therapies may be administered after surgery to destroy these microscopic malignant cells; this is called *adjuvant chemotherapy*. The goals of adjuvant chemotherapy are to decrease the recurrence of the cancer and to prolong survival. Chemotherapy may also be given before surgical resection of the tumor; this is referred to as neoadjuvant chemotherapy. Chemotherapy given before surgery should decrease the tumor burden to be removed (which may result in a shorter surgical procedure or less physical disfigurement to the patient) and make the surgery easier to perform because the tumor has shrunk away from vital organs or vessels. Neoadjuvant chemotherapy also gives the clinician an idea of the responsiveness of the tumor to that particular chemotherapy.

Chemotherapy may be given to cure cancers that are curable, or it may be given to help control the symptoms of an incurable cancer, which is referred to as palliative therapy.

Response

The responses to chemotherapy may be referred to as complete response (CR), partial response (PR), stable disease (SD), or disease progression. A cure in oncology implies that the cancer is completely gone, and the patient will have the same life expectancy as a patient without cancer. The Response Evaluation Criteria in Solid Tumors (RECIST)

was developed in 2000 and revised in 2009 and is considered to be the standard criteria to evaluate a response to therapy (Table 88–3). A CR refers to complete disappearance of all cancer for 1 month after treatment. PR is defined as a 30% or greater decrease in tumor diameter along with no new disease for 1 month. The term overall objective response rate refers to the combination of PR and CR. SD occurs in a patient whose tumor size neither grows nor shrinks by the

Table 88–3

RECIST 1.1 Criteria

Term	Description
Complete response (CR)	Disappearance of all targeted lesions
Partial response (PR)	At least a 30% decrease in the sum of the longest diameter of target lesions from baseline
Progressive disease (PD)	At least a 20% increase in the sum of the longest diameter of target lesions from baseline, including new lesions discovered during treatment
Stable disease (SD)	Neither sufficient shrinkage to qualify for PR nor sufficient increase to qualify for PD

Adapted from Eisenhauer E, Therasse P, Bogaerts J, et al. New response evaluation criteria in solid tumours: Revised RECIST guideline (version 1.1). Eur J Cancer 2009;45:228–247.

Clinical Presentation and Diagnosis: Cancer Chemotherapy and Treatment

Signs and Symptoms

- The seven warning signs of cancer are:
  - Change in bowel or bladder habits
  - A sore that does not heal
  - Unusual bleeding or discharge
  - Thickening or lump in breast or elsewhere
  - Indigestion or difficulty in swallowing
  - Obvious change in a wart or mole
  - Nagging cough or hoarseness
- The eight warning signs of cancer in children are:
  - Continued, unexplained weight loss
  - Headaches with vomiting in the morning
  - Increased swelling or persistent pain in bones or joints
  - Lump or mass in abdomen, neck, or elsewhere
  - Development of a whitish appearance in the pupil of the eye
  - Recurrent fevers not caused by infections
  - Excessive bruising or bleeding
  - Noticeable paleness or prolonged tiredness

Diagnostic Procedures

- Laboratory tests: CBC, lactate dehydrogenase (LDH), renal function, and liver function tests
- Radiologic scans: x-rays, CT scans, MRI, position emission tomography (PET)
- Biopsy of tissue or bone marrow with pathologic evaluation
- Cytogenetics
- Tumor markers
- Staging determination of the primary tumor size, extent of lymph node involvement, and the presence or absence of metastases, referred to as the TNM system (see Table 88–2). ❸ *Most solid tumors are staged according to the tumor, nodes, metastases (TNM) classification system. The size of the primary tumor, extent of nodal involvement, and presence of metastases are used to determine the stage. Metastases are cancer cells that have spread to sites distant from the primary tumor site and have started to grow. The most frequently occurring sites of metastases of solid tumors are the brain, bone, liver, and lungs.*

above criteria. Disease progression refers to tumor that has spread or the primary tumor that has increased in size by 20% while the patient is receiving treatment. Some cancers, such as leukemia, cannot be measured by size, so biopsy of the bone marrow provides a cellular indication of the absence or presence of disease.[10]

Cancer chemotherapy and the treatment of cancers are analogous to antiinfectives and the treatment of infections. Cancer cells may be sensitive to certain chemotherapy agents, but then with repeated exposure, the cells may become resistant to treatment. The resistant cells then may grow and multiply. A number of genetic mutations, including *EGFR*, *KRAS*, and *BRAF*, predict sensitivity to chemotherapy agents that target these mutations. These mutations will be discussed in the oncology disease-specific chapters where the agents are used.

Nonpharmacologic Therapy

The four primary treatment modalities of cancer are surgery, radiation, biotherapy, and pharmacologic therapy. Surgery is useful to gain tissue for diagnosis of cancer and for treatment, especially those cancers with limited disease. Radiation plays a key role not only in the treatment and possible cure of cancer but also in palliative therapy. Together, surgery and radiation therapy may provide local control of symptoms of the disease. However, when cancer is widespread, surgery may play little or no role, but radiation therapy localized to specific areas may palliate symptoms.

Pharmacologic Therapy

Chemotherapy of cancer started in the early 1940s when nitrogen mustard was first administered to patients with lymphoma. Since then, numerous agents have been developed for the treatment of different cancers.

Dosing of Chemotherapy

Chemotherapeutic agents typically have a very narrow therapeutic index. If too much is administered, the patient may suffer from fatal toxicities. If too little is given, the desired effect on cancer cells may not be achieved. Many chemotherapy agents have significant organ toxicities that preclude using steadily increasing doses to treat the cancer. The doses of chemotherapy must be given at a frequency that allows the patient to recover from the toxicity of the chemotherapy; each period of chemotherapy dosing is referred to as a *cycle*. Each cycle of chemotherapy may have the same dosages; the dosages may be modified based on toxicity; or a chemotherapy regimen may alternate from one set of drugs given during the first, third, and fifth cycles to another set of different drugs given during the second, fourth, and sixth cycles. The dose density of chemotherapy refers to shortening of the period between cycles of chemotherapy. This can accomplish two things: First, the tumor has less time between cycles of chemotherapy to grow, and second, patients receive

the total number of required cycles in a shorter time period. Administration of dose-dense chemotherapy regimens often requires the use of colony-stimulating factors (e.g., filgrastim also known as granulocyte colony-stimulating factor [G-CSF]) to be administered. These agents shorten the duration and severity of neutropenia. The chemotherapy regimens that are dose dense tend to be adjuvant regimens, and the goal of therapy is cure.

When a chemotherapy regimen is used as palliative therapy (to control symptoms), the dosages of chemotherapy may be decreased based on toxicity or the interval between cycles may be lengthened to maintain quality of life.

Patient and tumor biology also affect how cancer therapy is dosed. Patients with a uridine diphosphate–glucuronosyltransferase 1A1 enzyme deficiency can have life-threatening diarrhea and complications from irinotecan related to a decreased ability to metabolize the parent drug. The patient may have a blood test before irinotecan therapy to determine if this genetic mutation is present (Table 88–4). In the case of some monoclonal antibodies, flow cytometry results reveal whether the tumor has the receptor where the drug will bind and exert the pharmacologic effect.

Another consideration of chemotherapy administration is the patient. Factors that affect chemotherapy selection and dosing are age, concurrent disease states, and performance status. Performance status can be assessed through either the Eastern Cooperative Oncology Group (ECOG) Scale or the Karnofsky Scale (Table 88–5). Performance status is a very important prognostic factor for many types of cancer. If a patient has renal dysfunction and the chemotherapy is eliminated primarily by the kidney, dosing adjustments will need to be made. If a patient has had a myocardial infarction recently or preexisting heart disease, the clinician will weigh the risks of anthracycline therapy against the benefit of the treatment of the cancer.

Another important consideration for treatment of cancers is reimbursement by third-party payors for off-label use of chemotherapy agents because of the high expense. The American Association of Cancer Centers (*www.accc-cancer.org*) provides a drug compendium quarterly to which clinicians may refer to verify coverage by Medicare based on ICD-9 codes. Drugs used according to FDA-approved indications are usually reimbursed. If sufficient supportive literature exists, an insurer may pay for an off-label use.

During the time of chemotherapy administration, patients will likely experience various toxicities. The National Cancer Institute (NCI) has provided a standardized system for evaluating and grading the toxicity from chemotherapy to provide uniform grading of toxicity and evaluation of new agents and new regimens (Table 88–6).

Combination Chemotherapy

The underlying principles of using combination therapy are to use (1) agents with different pharmacologic actions, (2) agents with different organ toxicities, (3) agents that are

Table 88–4

Oncology Drugs With Valid Genomic Biomarkers

Biomarker	Drug	Approved Label Content
Biomarkers for Selection of Therapy		
ALK	Crizotinib	Crizotinib is specifically approved for the treatment of locally advanced or metastatic non–small cell lung cancer that is ALK positive as detected by an FDA-approved test.
BRAF	Vemurafenib	Vemurafenib is indicated for the treatment of unresectable or metastatic melanoma with BRAF^{V600E} mutation (found in approximately 70% of malignant melanomas), as detected by an FDA-approved test. It is not recommended for treatment of wild-type BRAF.
CD20	Rituximab, tositumomab	Rituximab and tositumomab are indicated for the treatment of patients with CD20-positive lymphomas
CD30	Brentuximab	Brentuximab binds to CD-30–expressing cells and is indicated for the treatment of Hodgkin's lymphoma patients after failure of ASCT or after failure of at two prior multidrug regimens and not eligible for ASCT and for patients with anaplastic large cell lymphoma who have failed at least one chemotherapy regimen.
c-kit	Imatinib	Imatinib is indicated for the treatment of patients with kit (CD117)-positive unresectable and/or metastatic malignant GIST.
Chromosome 5 deletion	Lenalidomide	Lenalidomide is indicated for the treatment of patients with transfusion-dependent anemia caused by low- or intermediate-1-risk myelodysplastic syndromes associated with a deletion 5q cytogenetic abnormality with or without additional cytogenetic abnormalities.
EGFR expression	Erlotinib[b], panitumumab[a] Cetuximab[a]	Erlotinib is indicated for advanced NSCLC and advanced pancreatic cancer. EGFR expression was determined using the EGFR pharmDx kit. In contrast to the 1% cutoff specified in the pharmDx kit instructions, a positive EGFR expression status was defined as having at least 10% of cells staining for EGFR. Cetuximab is indicated for EFFR-expressing colorectal cancer and for cancers of the head and neck. Panitumomab is indicated for metastatic colorectal cancer after disease progression on other therapies. Patients enrolled in the clinical studies were required to have immunohistochemical evidence of positive EGFR expression using the DakoCytomation EGFR pharmDx test kit.
Flp1L1-PDGFRa	Imatinib	Imatinib is indicated in adult patients with HES and /or CEL who have this fusion kinase and for patients with HES and/or CEL who are negative or unknown.
HER-2/neu	Trastuzumab, lapatinib	Detection of HER-2 protein overexpression is necessary for selection of patients appropriate for trastuzumab and lapatinib therapy.
PDGFR	Imatinib	Imatinib is indicated in adult patients with MDS/MPD associated with PDGFR gene rearrangements.
Philadelphia chromosome	Busulfan, imatinib, dasatinib, nilotinib	Busulfan is clearly less effective in patients with CML who lack the Philadelphia (Ph1) chromosome. Imatinib is indicated for patients with newly diagnosed adult and pediatric patients with Ph⁺ chronic CML in chronic phase, and in Ph⁺ CML patients in blast crisis, accelerated phase, or chronic phase after failure of interferon-a therapy. It is also indicated in relapsed or refractory Ph⁺ acute lymphoblastic leukemia. Dasatinib is indicated for the treatment of adults with Ph⁺ ALL. Nilotinib is indicated for the treatment of adult patients with newly diagnosed Philadelphia Ph+ CML in chronic phase. It is also indicated for the treatment of chronic phase and accelerated phase Ph⁺ CML in adult patients resistant or intolerant to prior therapy that included imatinib.
PML/RAR fusion gene	Tretinoin, arsenic trioxide	Initiation of therapy with tretinoin may be based on the morphologic diagnosis of APL. Confirmation of the diagnosis of APL should be sought by detection of the t (15; 17) genetic marker by cytogenetic studies. If these are negative, PML/RAR (a) fusion should be sought using molecular diagnostic techniques. The response rate of other AML subtypes to tretinoin has not been demonstrated; therefore, patients who lack the genetic marker should be considered for alternative treatment. Arsenic trioxide is indicated for induction of remission and consolidation in patients with APL who are refractory to or have relapsed from retinoid and anthracycline therapy and APL that has demonstrated the presence of the t(15;17) translocation or PML/RAR-a gene expression.
Biomarkers for Preventing Toxicity		
TPMT	Azathioprine, Mercaptopurine	Thiopurine methyltransferase deficiency or lower activity caused by mutation at increased risk of myelotoxicity. TPMT testing is recommended and consideration be given to either genotype or phenotype patients for TPMT.
UGT1A1	Irinotecan, nilotinib	Individuals who are homozygous for the UGT1A*28 allele are at increased risk for neutropenia following initiation of irinotecan treatment. A reduced initial dose should be considered for patients known to be homozygous for the UGT1A*28 allele. Heterozygous patients may be at increased risk of neutropenia; however, clinical results have been variable that patients have been shown to tolerate normal starting doses.

(Continued)

Table 88–4

Oncology Drugs With Valid Genomic Biomarkers (*Continued*)

Biomarker	Drug	Approved Label Content
DPD deficiency	5-FU, Capecitabine	Nilotinib is a competitive inhibitor of UGT1A1 in vitro, which could increase the concentrations of nilotinib. In a pharmacogenetic analysis, patients with (TA)7/(TA)7 genotype (UGT1A1*28) had a statistically significant increase in bilirubin over other genotypes. Rarely, unexpected, severe toxicity (e.g., stomatitis, diarrhea, neutropenia, neurotoxicity) associated with 5-FU has been attributed to a deficiency of DPD activity. A link between decreased levels of DPD and increased, potentially fatal toxic effects of 5-FU therefore cannot be excluded.

ALK, anaplastic lymphoma kinase; ALL, acute lymphoblastic leukemia; APL, acute promyelocytic leukemia; ASCT, autologous stem cell transplant; CEL, chronic eosinophilic leukemia; CML, chronic myeloid leukemia; DPD, dihydropyrimidine dehydrogenase; EGFR, epidermal growth factor receptor; FDA, Food and Drug Administration; 5-FU, 5-fluorouracil; GIST, gastrointestinal stromal tumor; HES, hypereosinophilic syndrome; MDS, myelodysplastic disease; MPD, myeloproliferative disease; NSCLC, non–small cell lung cancer; PDGFR, platelet-derived growth factor receptor; TPMT, thiopurine *S*-methyltransferase.

*a*Panitumumab and cetuximab are not recommended for the treatment of colorectal cancer with *KRAS* mutations in codon 12 or 13. Retrospective subset analyses have not shown a treatment benefit for these mutations.

*b*Erlotinib is recommended as first-line therapy in patients with activating EGFR mutations.

---

active against the tumor and ideally synergistic when used together, and (4) agents that do not result in significant drug interactions (although these can be studied carefully and the interactions addressed). When two or more agents are used together, the risk of development of resistance may be lessened, but toxicity may be increased.

❹ *Traditional chemotherapy agents have some similar side effects, usually manifested on the most rapidly proliferating cells of the body. However, there are unique toxicities of various* pharmacologic categories of antineoplastic agents. Anthracyclines (e.g., doxorubicin) have the potential to cause cardiac toxicity, which is related to the cumulative dose. Microtubule-targeting agents (e.g., vincristine) are associated with various forms of neurotoxicity. Alkylating agents (e.g., melphalan) are associated with secondary malignancies.

● Currently, anticancer agents are categorized by the mechanism of action. As depicted in **Figure 88–3**, different agents work in different parts of the cell.

Table 88–5

Performance Status Scales

Description: Karnofsky Scale	Karnofsky Scale (%)	Zubrod Scale (ECOG)	Description: ECOG Scale
No complaints; no evidence of disease	100	0	Fully active; able to carry on all predisease activity
Able to carry on normal activity; minor signs or symptoms of disease	90		
Normal activity with effort; some signs or symptoms of disease	80	1	Restricted in strenuous activity but ambulatory and able to carry out work of a light or sedentary nature
Cares for self; unable to carry on normal activity or to do active work	70		
Requires occasional assistance but is able to care for most personal needs	60	2	Out of bed more than 50% of time; ambulatory and capable of self-care but unable to carry out any work activities
Requires considerable assistance and frequent medical care	50		
Disabled; requires special care and assistance	40	3	In bed more than 50% of time; capable of only limited self-care
Severely disabled; hospitalization indicated, although death not imminent	30		
Very sick; hospitalization necessary; requires active supportive treatment	20	4	Bedridden; cannot carry out any self-care; completely disabled
Moribund; fatal processes progressing rapidly	10		
Dead	0		

ECOG, Eastern Cooperative Oncology Group.

Table 88–6

Selected National Cancer Institute Common Toxicity Criteria

Toxicity	Grade 1	Grade 2	Grade 3	Grade 4	Grade 5
General Neutropenia	Mild Lowest baseline: 1,500/mm³ (1.5 × 10⁹/L)	Moderate Less than 1,500–1,000/ mm³ (1.5–1 × 10⁹/L)	Severe Less than 1,000–500/mm³ (1–0.5 × 10⁹/L)	Life threatening Less than 500/mm³ (5 × 10⁹/L)	Death
Thrombocytopenia	Lowest baseline: 75,000/mm³ (75 × 10⁹/L)	Less than 75,000–50,000/ mm³ (75–50 × 10⁹/L)	Less than 50,000–25,000/mm³ (50–25 × 10⁹/L)	Less than 25,000 mm³ (25 × 10⁹/L)	Death
Diarrhea	Increase of less than 4 stools per day over baseline or mild increase in ostomy output	Increase of 4–6 stools per day over baseline; IV fluids indicated less than 24 hours of moderate increase in ostomy output compared with baseline; not interfering with ADLs	Increase of greater than or equal to 7 stools per day over baseline; incontinence; IV fluids greater than or equal to 24 hours; hospitalization; severe increase in ostomy output compared with baseline; interfering with ADLs	Life-threatening consequences (e.g., hemodynamic collapse)	Death
Esophagitis	Asymptomatic pathologic, radiographic, or endoscopic findings only	Symptomatic altered eating or swallowing; IV fluids indicated less than 24 hours	Symptomatic and severely altered eating or swallowing; IV fluids, tube feedings, or TPN indicated 24 hours or more	Life-threatening consequences	Death
Nausea	Loss of appetite without alteration in eating habits	Oral intake decreased without significant weight loss, dehydration, or malnutrition; IV fluids indicated less than 24 hours	Inadequate oral caloric or fluid intake; IV fluids, tube feedings, or TPN indicated greater than 24 hours	Life-threatening consequences	Death
Vomiting	1 episode in 24 hours	2–5 episodes in 24 hours; IV fluids indicated less than 24 hours	6 episodes or more in 24 hours; IV fluids or TPN indicated greater than or equal to 24 hours	Life-threatening consequences	Death

ADL, activity of daily living; IV, intravenous; TPN, total parenteral nutrition.

Antimetabolites: Pyrimidine analogs

▶ Fluorouracil

5-Fluorouracil, commonly referred to as 5-FU, is a fluorinated analog of the pyrimidine uracil. Once administered, this prodrug is metabolized by dihydropyrimidine dehydrogenase. 5-FU ultimately is metabolized to fluorodeoxyuridine monophosphate (FdUMP), which interferes with the function of thymidylate synthase, which is required for synthesis of thymidine. The triphosphate metabolite of 5-FU is incorporated into RNA to produce the second cytotoxic effect of 5-FU. Inhibition of thymidylate synthesis occurs with the continuous infusion regimens, whereas the triphosphate form is associated with bolus administration. Patients with a low activity of dihydropyrimidine dehydrogenase appear to be at risk for life-threatening toxicities.[11] Folates appear to increase the stability of FdUMP–thymidylate synthase inhibition, which enhances the activity of the drug in certain cancers. 5-FU is metabolized extensively by the liver, but up to 15% of a dose may be found unchanged in the urine.

Age does not appear to alter the pharmacokinetics. 5-FU has shown clinical activity in the treatment of colorectal, breast, esophageal, pancreas, stomach, anal, and head and neck cancers. Adverse effects may include stomatitis, diarrhea, cardiac abnormalities, and rarely reported cerebellar toxicities. Esophagitis and gastric ulcerations also may occur. Some alopecia may occur, but hair regrowth may occur with subsequent doses. Cryotherapy (using ice chips in the mouth) for 30 minutes while receiving bolus 5-FU may decrease the severity of mucositis.[12] Neurotoxicity may consist of headaches, visual disturbances, and cerebellar ataxia. Cardiac toxicity may consist of ST-segment elevation, which appears to be more common in patients with a history of coronary artery disease.

▶ Capecitabine

Capecitabine is an orally active prodrug of 5-FU and has shown to be active in tumors of the colon, rectum, and breast. It not only shares the same mechanism but the toxicity profile is also similar to that of 5-FU. Toxicities include diarrhea,

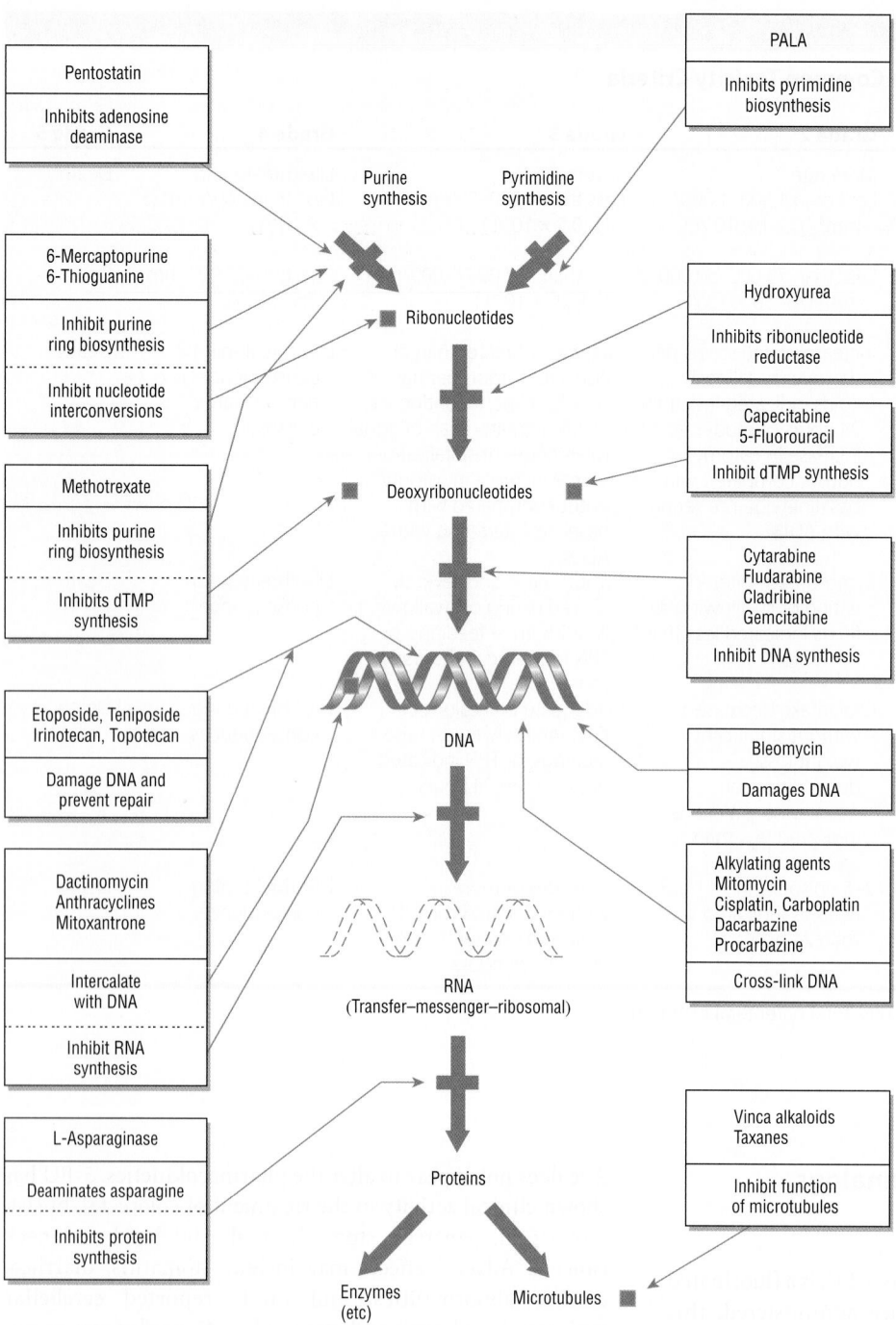

FIGURE 88–3. The mechanisms of action of commonly used antineoplastic agents. (dTMP, deoxythymidylic acid; PALA, N-phosphonacetyl-l-aspartate.) (From Chabner BA, Amrein PC, Druker BJ, et al. Antineoplastic agents. In: Brunton LL, Lazo JS, Parker KL, eds. Goodman & Gilman's The Pharmacologic Basis of Therapeutics, 11th ed. New York: McGraw-Hill; 2006: 1319.)

mucositis, palmar-plantar erythrodysesthesia, nausea, and **myelosuppression**. Palmar-plantar erythrodysesthesia, also referred to as hand–foot syndrome, refers to redness, itching, and blistering of the palms of the hands and soles of the feet. Patients should be counseled to notify the prescriber when this adverse effect occurs. Significant increases in international normalization ratio (INR) and prothrombin time may occur within several days when capecitabine is initiated in patients concomitantly receiving warfarin. The INR should be monitored closely or the patient may be switched to a low-molecular-weight heparin. Phenytoin levels

may become elevated related to possible CYP2C9 inhibition by capecitabine; therefore, plasma levels of phenytoin should be monitored. Patients should be instructed to take capecitabine within 30 minutes of a meal to increase absorption of the drug.

▶ *Cytarabine*

Cytarabine, also known as Ara-C, is a structural analog of cytosine and is phosphorylated intracellularly to the active triphosphate form, which inhibits DNA polymerase.

Patient Encounter 1, Part 1

BM is a 58-year-old previously healthy woman who has had symptoms of an upper respiratory tract infection for about 4 weeks. She has been treated with two courses of antibiotics without improvement of symptoms. She has also noticed an increase in bruising and bleeding gums after brushing her teeth. She reports feeling extraordinarily tired recently. Today, she presents to an urgent care center with worsening cough. Her complete blood count (CBC) reveals a high white blood cell (WBC) count (39 x 10³/mm³ [39 x 10⁹/L]) and peripheral blasts (60% [0.60]). She is emergently admitted to the hospital for further evaluation.

After a bone marrow biopsy and further cytogenetic testing, a diagnosis of acute myeloid leukemia (AML) is made and treatment is planned to start as soon as possible.

What signs and symptoms does BM have that are consistent with a cancer presentation?

What is your desired outcome when treating this patient?

The triphosphate form also may be incorporated into DNA to result in chain termination to prevent DNA elongation. The drug may be administered as a low-dose continuous infusion, high-dose intermittent infusion, and into the subdural space via intrathecal or intraventricular administration. There is also a liposomal formulation available for less frequent administration into the central nervous system (CNS). Cytarabine is eliminated by the kidneys with a renal clearance of 90 mL/min (1.5 mL/s). Cytarabine has shown efficacy in the treatment of acute leukemias and some lymphomas. The toxicities of cytarabine in high doses include myelosuppression; cerebellar syndrome (i.e., nystagmus, dysarthria, and ataxia); and chemical conjunctivitis, an eye irritation that requires prophylaxis with steroid eye drops. The risk of neurotoxicity is increased with high doses (greater than 1 g/m²), advanced age, and renal dysfunction. If cerebellar toxicity does occur, the drug needs to be discontinued immediately, and decisions regarding further therapy need to be carefully considered.[13]

▶ Gemcitabine

Gemcitabine is a deoxycytidine analog that is structurally related to cytarabine. Gemcitabine inhibits DNA polymerase activity and ribonucleotide reductase to result in DNA chain elongation. Gemcitabine has shown activity in cancers of the pancreas, breast, lung, ovary, and some lymphomas. The toxicities include myelosuppression; flu-like syndrome with fevers during the first 24 hours after administration; rash that appears 48 to 72 hours after administration; and hemolytic uremic syndrome, a rare but life-threatening adverse effect. Patients should be counseled to use acetaminophen to treat the fevers during the first 24 hours; however, fevers occurring 7 to 10 days after gemcitabine are likely to be febrile neutropenias and need prompt treatment with broad-spectrum antibiotics.

▶ Azacitidine and Decitabine

Azacitidine and decitabine, both nucleoside analogs, were recently approved for the treatment of patients with myelodysplastic syndrome, a hematopoietic disorder that can transform into acute myeloid leukemia. Both of these agents cause cytotoxicity by directly incorporating in the DNA and inhibiting DNA methyltransferase, which causes hypomethylation of DNA. Hypomethylation of DNA appears to normalize the function of the genes that control cell differentiation and proliferation to promote normal cell maturation. The major side effects reported are myelosuppression and infections.

▶ Nelarabine

Nelarabine is indicated for the treatment of patients with T-cell acute lymphoblastic leukemia and T-cell lymphoblastic lymphoma, whose disease has been already treated with at least two other chemotherapy regimens. Nelarabine is a prodrug that accumulates as the active 5′-triphosphate form in leukemic blasts to result in inhibition of DNA synthesis and cell death. The most common adverse effects are hematologic toxicities, neutropenic fever, headaches, and gastrointestinal toxicities. Severe neurologic toxicities, including mental status change, convulsions, peripheral neuropathies, and effects similar to Guillain–Barré syndrome, have been reported.

Antimetabolites: Purine Analogs

▶ Mercaptopurine and Thioguanine

6-Mercaptopurine (6-MP) and thioguanine are oral purine analogues that are converted to ribonucleotides that inhibit purine synthesis. Mercaptopurine is converted into thiopurine nucleotides, which are catabolized by thiopurine *S*-methyltransferase (TPMT), which is subject to genetic polymorphisms and may cause severe myelosuppression. TPMT status may be assessed before therapy to reduce drug-induced morbidity and the costs of hospitalizations for neutropenic events. Both of these agents are used in the treatment of acute lymphocytic leukemia (ALL) and chronic myeloid leukemia (CML). Because the agents are similar structurally, cross-resistance is observed. Significant side effects include myelosuppression; mild nausea; skin rash; cholestasis; and rarely, veno-occlusive disease. Mercaptopurine is metabolized by xanthine oxidase, an enzyme that is inhibited by allopurinol. This represents a major drug–drug interaction. To avoid toxicities of mercaptopurine when these drugs are used concomitantly, the dose of mercaptopurine must be reduced by 66% to 75%.

▶ Fludarabine

Fludarabine is an analog of the purine adenine. It interferes with DNA polymerase to cause chain termination and inhibits transcription by its incorporation into RNA. Fludarabine is dephosphorylated rapidly and converted to 2-fluoro-Ara-AMP (2-FLAA), which enters the cells and is phosphorylated to 2-fluoro-Ara-ATP, which is cytotoxic. Fludarabine is used in the treatment of chronic lymphocytic leukemia (CLL), some lymphomas, and refractory acute myeloid leukemia (AML). This drug is given intravenously (IV) usually daily for 5 days every 4 weeks. Significant myelosuppression may occur, along with immunosuppression, so patients are susceptible to opportunistic infections. Prophylactic antibiotics and antivirals are recommended until CD4 counts return to normal. Mild nausea and vomiting and diarrhea have been observed. Rarely, interstitial pneumonitis has occurred.

▶ **Cladribine**

Cladribine (2-chlorodeoxyadenosine, or 2-CDA) is a purine nucleoside that is a prodrug, activated via phosphorylation to a 5′-triphosphate derivative, which is incorporated into DNA, resulting in inhibition of DNA synthesis and chain termination. It may be administered as a continuous 7-day IV infusion or as a 2-hour infusion daily for 5 days; both regimens deliver the same total dose of drug. The primary indication for cladribine is hairy cell leukemia, although it has been used in the management of other hematologic conditions, including pediatric leukemias, and non-Hodgkin's lymphoma. Although fairly well tolerated, patients may experience myelosuppression and opportunistic infections. Fever, which is thought to be as a result of cell lysis and endogenous pyrogens being released into the bloodstream, can prompt the clinician to consider initiation of antibiotics. Even though it is likely drug induced, it may be difficult to rule out an infectious cause. Rash occurs in approximately 50% of patients.

▶ **Clofarabine**

Clofarabine was developed based on the structures of fludarabine and cladribine with the hope it would be resistant to deamination by adenosine deaminase. Clofarabine has shown activity in myeloid leukemia and myelodysplastic syndrome.[14] Side effects include bone marrow suppression, severe but transient liver dysfunction in 15% to 25% of patients, skin rashes, and hand–foot syndrome.

▶ **Pentostatin**

Pentostatin is an inhibitor of adenosine deaminase, an enzyme important in purine base metabolism. Pentostatin irreversibly inhibits adenosine deaminase, which blocks DNA synthesis through inhibition of RNA ribonucleotide reductase. Side effects include bone marrow suppression, myalgias, conjunctivitis, and rash.

Antimetabolites: Folate antagonists

Folates carry one-carbon groups in transfer reactions required for purine and thymidylic acid synthesis. Dihydrofolate reductase is the enzyme responsible for supplying reduced folates intracellularly for thymidylate and purine synthesis.

▶ **Methotrexate**

Methotrexate inhibits dihydrofolate reductase of both malignant and nonmalignant cells. When high doses of methotrexate are given, the "rescue drug" leucovorin, a reduced folate, is administered to bypass the methotrexate inhibition of dihydrofolate reductase of normal cells and is usually initiated 24 hours after methotrexate administration. This is done to prevent potentially fatal myelosuppression and mucositis. For safety purposes, the term *folinic acid*, another term used for leucovorin, should not be used because of the potential for a medication error in which folic acid might be given instead. Methotrexate concentrations should be monitored to determine when to stop leucovorin administration. Generally, leucovorin administration may be stopped when methotrexate concentrations decrease to 5×10^{-8} M, although this may vary by the chemotherapy regimen. High dosages of methotrexate may cause methotrexate to crystallize out in the kidney, which may result in acute renal failure and decreased methotrexate clearance. Administration of IV hydration with sodium bicarbonate to maintain urinary pH greater than or equal to 7 is necessary to prevent methotrexate-induced renal dysfunction. Methotrexate is eliminated by tubular secretion; therefore, concomitant drugs (e.g., probenecid, salicylates, penicillin G, and ketoprofen) that may inhibit or compete for tubular secretion should be avoided. Methotrexate doses must be adjusted for renal dysfunction. A recommended dosing adjustment is to divide the creatinine clearance of the patient by 70 mL/minute (1.17 mL/s), which is the average creatinine clearance of patients who received methotrexate during clinical trials, and then to multiply this fraction by the dosage recommended for that disease state. Again, close monitoring of methotrexate concentrations in patients with renal impairment is advised. Methotrexate has shown activity in lymphoma, gastric, esophageal, bladder, and breast cancer and ALL. Side effects of methotrexate include myelosuppression, nausea and vomiting, and mucositis. Methotrexate also may be administered via the intrathecal route or via an Ommaya reservoir in very low doses as small as 12 mg to doses of 20 g IV, so it is crucial for the clinician to know the correct dose by the correct route in order to avoid substantial toxicity. The methotrexate used for intrathecal and intraventricular injection must be preservative-free to prevent CNS toxicity.

▶ **Pemetrexed**

Pemetrexed inhibits four pathways in thymidine and purine synthesis. Pemetrexed has shown activity in the treatment of mesothelioma and non–small cell lung cancer (NSCLC). Side effects include myelosuppression, rash, diarrhea, and nausea and vomiting. Patients should receive folic acid and cyanocobalamin to reduce bone marrow toxicity and diarrhea. Doses of folic acid of at least 400 mcg/day starting 5 days before treatment and continuing throughout therapy, as well as for 21 days after the last pemetrexed dose, have been used. Cyanocobalamin 1,000 mcg is given intramuscularly the week before pemetrexed and then every 3 cycles thereafter. Dexamethasone 4 mg twice daily the day before, the day of, and the day after pemetrexed administration helps to decrease the incidence and severity of rash.[15]

▶ Pralatrexate

Pralatrexate is a folate analogue metabolic inhibitor that is transported into tumor cells via the reduced folate carrier (RFC-1) and competitively inhibits dihydrofolate reductase. It also competitively inhibits for polyglutamylation by the enzyme folylpolyglutamyl synthetase, resulting in the depletion of thymidine and other molecules. It is an intravenously administered agent indicated for the treatment of patients with refractory or relapsed peripheral T-cell lymphoma. Pralatrexate was approved based on overall response rates, not survival benefits. Common adverse reactions include mucositis, thrombocytopenia, nausea, and fatigue. In an effort to reduce the treatment-related mucositis and hematologic toxicity associated with pralatrexate, patients should be counseled to take low-dose oral folic acid on a daily basis and vitamin B_{12} intramuscular injections every 8 to 10 weeks.

Microtubule-Targeting Agents

▶ Vinca Alkaloids (Vincristine, Vinblastine, and Vinorelbine)

The vinca alkaloids (vincristine, vinblastine, and vinorelbine) are derived from the periwinkle (vinca) plant and cause cytotoxicity by binding to tubulin, disrupting the normal balance between polymerization and depolymerization of microtubules, and inhibiting the assembly of microtubules, which interferes with the formation of the mitotic spindle. As a result, cells are arrested during the metaphase of mitosis. The vinca alkaloids are used primarily to treat hematologic malignancies (including Hodgkin's disease and ALL); lung, breast, and testicular cancers; Wilm's tumor; and sarcomas. Even though these agents have similar structures, the incidence and severity of toxicities vary among the agents. The dose-limiting toxicity of vincristine is neurotoxicity, which can consist of depressed tendon reflexes, paresthesias of the fingers and toes, toxicity to the cranial nerves, or autonomic neuropathy (constipation or ileus, abdominal pain, and/or orthostatic hypotension.) In contrast, the dose-limiting toxicity associated with vinorelbine and vinblastine is myelosuppression. All of the vinca alkaloids are vesicants and can cause tissue damage; therefore, the clinician must take precautions to avoid extravasation injury. Biliary excretion accounts for a significant portion of elimination of vincristine and its metabolites, so doses need to be adjusted for obstructive liver disease.

Vincristine, vinblastine, and vinorelbine have similar sounding names, which is a potential cause of medication errors. As with all chemotherapy prescribing, dispensing, and administration, the clinician must be very careful with sound-alike, look-alike medications. Unfortunately, vincristine has been involved in numerous cases of fatal chemotherapy errors, including inadvertent intrathecal administration. Because the drug is a vesicant, intrathecal administration of the drug can cause widespread tissue damage in the brain and death. An example of a strategy that health systems can use to decrease the likelihood of an error such as this is for the pharmacy to only dispense vincristine in a mini-bag for IV administration. Many clinicians cap IV vincristine doses at 2 mg to prevent severe neuropathic side effects; however, if the intent of chemotherapy is curative, the vincristine dose may be dosed above the 2-mg cap.[16]

▶ Taxanes (Paclitaxel, Docetaxel, and Cabazitaxel)

Paclitaxel and docetaxel are taxane plant alkaloids that, similar to the vinca alkaloids, exhibit cytotoxicity during the M phase of the cell cycle by binding to tubulin. Unlike the vinca alkaloids, however, the taxanes do not interfere with tubulin assembly. Rather, the taxanes promote microtubule assembly and inhibit microtubule disassembly. Once the microtubules are polymerized, the taxanes stabilize against depolymerization.

Hepatic metabolism and biliary excretion account for the majority of paclitaxel's elimination. Paclitaxel has demonstrated activity in ovarian, breast, non–small cell lung, prostate, esophageal, gastric, and head and neck cancers. Considerable variability exists in paclitaxel dosing, from weekly 1-hour infusions to 24-hour infusions administered every 3 weeks. The diluent for paclitaxel, Cremophor EL, is composed of ethanol and castor oil. Infusions must be prepared and administered in non–polyvinyl chloride–containing bags and tubings, and solutions must be filtered. Patients receive dexamethasone, diphenhydramine, and an H_2 blocker to prevent hypersensitivity reactions caused by Cremophor EL. Patients also may have asymptomatic bradycardia during the infusion. Approximately 3 to 5 days after administration, patients may complain of myalgias and arthralgias that may last several days. Myelosuppression, flushing, neuropathy, ileus, and total-body alopecia are other common side effects. Because paclitaxel is a substrate for CYP 3A4, steady-state concentrations of paclitaxel were 30% lower in patients receiving phenytoin than in patients not receiving phenytoin. Paclitaxel clearance was decreased by 33% when it was administered after cisplatin, so paclitaxel is administered before cisplatin.

A nanoparticle albumin-bound paclitaxel product is also available for the treatment of metastatic breast cancer. This product does not have the serious hypersensitivity reactions encountered with paclitaxel solubilized in Cremophor EL, so premedication with H_1 and H_2 blockers and steroids is not necessary. The dose is infused over 30 minutes and does not require a special IV bag, tubing, or filter. The dosing of this product is different from that of the original paclitaxel, so practitioners need to be aware of which product is being prescribed. The pharmacokinetics of the albumin-bound paclitaxel display a higher clearance and larger volume of distribution than paclitaxel. The drug is eliminated primarily via fecal excretion.[17] Bone marrow suppression, neuropathy, ileus, arthralgias, and myalgias still occur.

Docetaxel has activity in the treatment of breast, non–small cell lung, prostate, bladder, esophageal, stomach, ovarian, and head and neck cancers. Dexamethasone, 8 mg twice daily for 3 days starting the day before treatment, is used to prevent the fluid-retention syndrome associated with docetaxel and possible hypersensitivity reactions. The fluid-retention syndrome is characterized by edema and weight gain that is unresponsive to diuretic therapy and is associated with cumulative doses greater than 800 mg/m^2. Myelosuppression, alopecia, and neuropathy are other side effects associated with docetaxel treatment.

Cabazitaxel is a newer taxane used in combination with prednisone for the treatment of metastatic hormone-refractory prostate cancer in patients previously treated with a docetaxel-containing treatment regimen. Cabazitaxel has shown to have similar adverse effects as paclitaxel and docetaxel. Premedication with an antihistamine, corticosteroid, and H$_2$ antagonist to prevent hypersensitivity reactions is required.

▶ Eribulin Mesylate

Eribulin mesylate is classified as a nontaxane microtubule dynamics inhibitor. It is a synthetic analog of halichondrin B, which is a product isolated from the sea sponge *Halichondria okadai*. While taxanes inhibit cell division by stabilizing microtubules, eribulin arrests the cell cycle through inhibition of the growth phase of microtubules without interfering with microtubule shortening. The cytotoxicity results from its effects via a tubulin-based antimitotic mechanism, resulting in G$_2$/M cell-cycle arrest and mitotic blockage. Apoptotic cell death results from prolonged mitotic blockage. Eribulin mesylate is an IV medication that is specifically indicated for the treatment of patients with metastatic breast cancer who have received at least two previous chemotherapy regimens (containing an anthracycline and taxane) for metastatic disease. The most common adverse effects reported are neutropenic fever, anemia, asthenia or fatigue, alopecia, peripheral neuropathy, nausea, and constipation. Eribulin has been reported to cause significant neutropenia and QT interval prolongation. It has vesicant properties. Dosages should be adjusted in renal and hepatic impairment.[18]

▶ Estramustine

Estramustine, an oral drug, also inhibits microtubule assembly and has weak estrogenic activity at the estradiol hormone receptors of the cell. This drug is used primarily for the treatment of prostate cancer, but its use is limited by the side effects, which include nausea and vomiting, diarrhea, thromboembolic events, and gynecomastia.

▶ Ixabepilone

Ixabepilone, an epothilone analog, binds to β-tubulin subunits on microtubules, which results in suppression of microtubule dynamics. Ixabepilone is primarily eliminated by the liver by oxidation through the CYP3A4 system.

Ixabepilone is indicated for the treatment of metastatic or locally advanced breast cancer after failures of anthracyclines and a taxane. Side effects include hypersensitivity reactions, myelosuppression, and peripheral neuropathy. To minimize the occurrence of hypersensitivity reactions, patients must receive both H1 and H2 antagonists before therapy. If a reaction still occurs, corticosteroids should be added to the premedications.

Topoisomerase Inhibitors

Topoisomerase is responsible for relieving the pressure on the DNA structure during unwinding by producing strand breaks. Topoisomerase I produces single-strand breaks, whereas topoisomerase II produces double-strand breaks.

▶ Epipodophyllotoxins (Etoposide and Teniposide)

Etoposide and teniposide are semisynthetic podophyllotoxin derivatives that inhibit topoisomerase II, causing multiple DNA double-strand breaks. Etoposide has shown activity in the treatment of several types of lymphoma, testicular and lung cancer, retinoblastoma, and carcinoma of unknown primary. The IV preparation has limited stability. Stability is concentration dependent, with a concentration of 0.4 mg/dL having 24 hours' stability. Oral bioavailability is approximately 50%, so oral dosages are approximate two times those of IV doses. Teniposide has shown activity in the treatment of ALL, neuroblastoma, and non-Hodgkin's lymphoma. Both of these agents should be slowly administered to prevent hypotension. Side effects of these agents include mucositis, myelosuppression, alopecia, phlebitis, hypersensitivity reactions, and secondary leukemias. Hypersensitivity reactions may be life threatening.

▶ Camptothecin Derivatives (Irinotecan and Topotecan)

Irinotecan and topotecan, both camptothecins, inhibit the topoisomerase I enzyme to interfere with DNA synthesis through the active metabolite SN38. Topoisomerase I enzymes stabilize DNA single-strand breaks and inhibit strand resealing. Irinotecan has shown activity in the treatment of cancers of the colon, rectum, cervix, and lung. Irinotecan-induced diarrhea is a serious complication and may be life threatening. One form of diarrhea (acute) can occur during or immediately after the infusion. This is a result of a cholinergic process in which the patient may experience facial flushing, diaphoresis, and abdominal cramping. IV atropine should be administered to treat diarrhea that occurs any time during the first 24 hours of administration. Another form of diarrhea (chronic) can occur several days after administration and can result in severe dehydration. This adverse effect should be treated immediately with loperamide at a dosage of 2 mg every 2 hours or 4 mg every 4 hours until diarrhea has stopped for 12 hours. Other side effects include myelosuppression, fatigue, and alopecia. Individuals homozygous for *UGT1A1* 28* have an increased risk of febrile neutropenia and diarrhea and should be considered for an upfront dose reduction of one level; heterozygotes should receive closer monitoring, including more frequent complete blood counts (CBCs) to detect myelosuppression.

Topotecan has shown clinical activity in the treatment of ovarian and lung cancer, myelodysplastic syndromes, and AML. The IV infusion may be scheduled daily for 5 days or once weekly. Side effects include myelosuppression, mucositis, and diarrhea. Diarrhea is less common than with irinotecan.

Anthracene Derivatives

▶ *Daunorubicin, Doxorubicin, Idarubicin, and Epirubicin*

Anthracyclines (daunorubicin, doxorubicin, idarubicin, and epirubicin) are also referred to as antitumor antibiotics or topoisomerase inhibitors when considering their mechanism of action. All of the anthracyclines contain a four-membered anthracene ring, a chromophore, with an attached sugar portion. Free radicals formed from the anthracyclines combine with oxygen to form superoxide, which can make hydrogen peroxide. These agents are able to insert between base pairs of DNA to cause structural changes in DNA. However, the primary mechanism of cytotoxicity appears to be the inhibition of topoisomerase II. These drugs are widely used in a variety of cancers.

Oxygen-free-radical formation is a cause of cardiac damage and extravasation injury, which is common with these drugs. Daunorubicin, doxorubicin, epirubicin, and idarubicin can cause cardiac toxicity as manifested by a congestive heart failure or cardiomyopathy symptomatology, alopecia, nausea or vomiting, mucositis, myelosuppression, and urinary discoloration. These drugs are vesicants; significant tissue damage may occur with extravasation. Dosage alterations should be made in the presence of biliary dysfunction.[20]

To reduce the risk of cardiotoxicity associated with doxorubicin, the maximum lifetime cumulative dose is 550 mg/m². Ventricular ejection fractions should be measured before therapy and periodically if therapy is continued. Therapy should be halted if there is a 10% to 20% decrease from baseline in ejection fraction. Patients at increased risk of cardiotoxicity include patients reaching the upper limit of cumulative lifetime dose; those taking concomitant or previous cardiotoxic drugs, concurrent paclitaxel, or bolus administration; patients with preexisting cardiac disease or mediastinal radiation; and the very young and elderly. Cardioprotectants (e.g., dexrazoxane) have been used to decrease risk in some cases. Clinical guidelines exist recommending when cardioprotective agents are warranted.[19]

Liposomal doxorubicin is an irritant, not a vesicant, and is dosed differently from doxorubicin, so clinicians need to be very careful when prescribing these two drugs. Liposomal doxorubicin has shown significant activity in the treatment of breast and ovarian cancer along with multiple myeloma and Kaposi's sarcoma. Side effects include mucositis, myelosuppression, alopecia, and palmar-plantar erythrodysesthesia. The liposomal doxorubicin may be less cardiotoxic than doxorubicin.

▶ *Mitoxantrone*

This royal blue–colored drug is an anthracenedione that inhibits DNA topoisomerase II. Mitoxantrone has shown clinical activity in the treatment of acute leukemias, breast and prostate cancer, and non-Hodgkin's lymphomas. Myelosuppression, mucositis, nausea and vomiting, and cardiac toxicity are side effects of this drug. The total cumulative dose limit is 160 mg/m² for patients who have not received prior anthracycline or mediastinal radiation. Patients who have received prior doxorubicin or daunorubicin therapy should not receive a cumulative dose greater than 120 mg/m² of mitoxantrone. Patients should be counseled that their urine will turn a blue-green color.[21]

Alkylating Agents

Although still widely used for many malignancies, the alkylating agents are the oldest class of anticancer drugs. The agents cause cytotoxicity via transfer of their alkyl groups to nucleophilic groups of proteins and nucleic acids. The major site of alkylation within DNA is the N7 position of guanine, although alkylation does occur to a lesser degree at other bases. These interactions can either occur on a single strand of DNA (monofunctional agents) or on both strands of DNA through a cross-link (bifunctional agents), which leads to

---

Patient Encounter 1, Part 2

The decision to treat BM with a systemic chemotherapy regimen is made. She will be receiving the standard induction regimen of 7 + 3 (idarubicin 12 mg/m²/day IV every day for 3 days + cytarabine 100 mg/m²/day continuous IV infusion for 7 days).

Before initiating this chemotherapy regimen in the patient, what patient specific issues need to be addressed?

What adverse effects will BM likely experience with these two chemotherapy drugs?

Patient Encounter 1, Part 3

BM goes into complete remission (or a complete response), and now consolidation therapy with high-dose cytarabine (2 gm/m²/dose IV every 12 hr for 6 doses) will be initiated.

What is the mechanism of action of cytarabine?

How do the toxicities of high-dose cytarabine differ from those of conventional (low-dose) cytarabine? What are the risk factors, prophylaxis, and treatment for these toxicities?

strand breaks. The major toxicities of the alkylating agents are myelosuppression, alopecia, nausea or vomiting, sterility or infertility, and secondary malignancies.

▶ Nitrogen Mustards (Cyclophosphamide and Ifosfamide)

Cyclophosphamide and ifosfamide are commonly used bifunctional alkylating agents, therefore causing cross-linking of DNA. They each share similar adverse effects and spectrum of activity, being used in a variety of solid and hematologic cancers. Cyclophosphamide and ifosfamide are both prodrugs, requiring activation by mixed hepatic oxidase enzymes to get to their active forms, phosphoramide and ifosfamide mustard, respectively. During the activation process, additional byproducts (acrolein and chloroacetaldehyde) are formed. Acrolein has no cytotoxic activity but is responsible for the hemorrhagic cystitis associated with ifosfamide and high-dose cyclophosphamide. Acrolein produces cystitis by directly binding to the bladder wall. Prophylaxis is necessary with aggressive hydration, administration of 2-mercaptoethane sulfonate sodium (MESNA, which binds to and inactivates acrolein in the bladder), frequent voiding, and patient monitoring in patients receiving ifosfamide and high-dose cyclophosphamide. Patients should be counseled to drink plenty of fluids; void frequently; and report any hematuria, irritation, or flank pain. Dosing regimens of MESNA range from an equal milligram dose to the ifosfamide mixed in the same IV bag to 20% of the dose before ifosfamide and 20% of the dose repeated at 4 and 8 hours after the dose.

Chloroacetaldehyde, a metabolite of ifosfamide, can result in encephalopathy, especially in patients receiving ifosfamide that exhibit risk factors such as renal dysfunction or advanced age. This adverse effect can occur within 48 to 72 hours of administration and is usually reversible.

▶ Busulfan

Busulfan is an alkylating agent that forms DNA–DNA and DNA–protein cross-links to inhibit DNA replication. Oral busulfan is well absorbed, has a terminal half-life of 2 to 2.5 hours, and is eliminated primarily by metabolism. It is also available in an IV formulation, which is useful when using the high doses required in blood and marrow transplantation. Busulfan has shown significant clinical activity in the treatment of AML and chronic myelocytic leukemia. Side effects include bone marrow suppression; hyperpigmentation of skin creases; and rarely, pulmonary fibrosis. High doses used for bone marrow transplant preparatory regimens result in severe nausea and vomiting, tonic–clonic seizures, and sinusoidal obstruction syndrome (formerly known as *veno-occlusive disease*). Patients receiving high-dose busulfan should receive anticonvulsant prophylaxis.

▶ Nitrosureas (Carmustine and Lomustine)

Carmustine (BCNU) and lomustine (CCNU) are nitrosureas that are lipophilic in nature and therefore able to cross the blood–brain barrier. Carmustine, which is reconstituted with ethanol, crosses the blood–brain barrier when given IV. It also comes as a biodegradable wafer formulation that may be implanted to treat residual tumor tissue after surgical resection of brain tumors. Lomustine is available in an oral formulation. Carmustine has shown clinical activity in the treatment of lymphoma, melanoma, and brain tumors. Lomustine has shown clinical activity in the treatment of non-Hodgkin's lymphoma and melanoma. Patients should receive only enough lomustine for one cycle at a time to prevent confusion with their drug regimens and the prolonged neutropenia that can occur. Side effects include myelosuppression, severe nausea and vomiting, and pulmonary fibrosis with long-term therapy.

▶ Nonclassic Alkylating Agents (Procarbazine and Temozolomide)

Although the exact mechanism of action remains unclear, dacarbazine and temozolomide appear to inhibit DNA, RNA, and protein synthesis. Dacarbazine has shown clinical benefit in the treatment of patients with melanoma, Hodgkin's lymphoma, and soft tissue sarcomas. Side effects include myelosuppression, severe nausea and vomiting, and a flu-like syndrome that starts about 7 days after treatment and lasts 1 to 3 weeks.

Temozolomide is an orally active agent that is well absorbed and crosses the blood–brain barrier. Temozolomide is converted via pH-dependent hydrolysis to the active metabolite 5-(3-methyltriazeno)-imidazole-4-carboxamide. Temozolomide may be used in the treatment of melanoma, refractory anaplastic astrocytoma, and glioblastoma multiforme. Nausea may be minimized by administering the drug at bedtime. Because patients receiving temozolomide may have confusion secondary to their brain tumors and because dosing can consist of multiple capsule sizes, care must be taken by all providers to simplify regimens to prevent chemotherapy overdose.[22]

▶ Procarbazine

Although the exact mechanism of action of procarbazine is unknown, it does inhibit DNA, RNA, and protein synthesis. Procarbazine is used most often in the treatment of lymphoma. Myelosuppression is the major side effect. Nausea, vomiting, and a flu-like syndrome occur initially with therapy. Patients must be counseled to avoid tyramine-rich foods because procarbazine is a monoamine oxidase inhibitor. Patients should be provided a list of foods and beverages to avoid a hypertensive crisis. A disulfiram-like reaction can occur with the ingestion of alcohol.

▶ Bendamustine

Bendamustine has three chemically active groups: a 2-chlorethyl group, a butyric acid side chain, and a benzimidazole ring. The 2-chloroethyl group, which confers alkylating properties, is shared with chlorambucil and other agents from the nitrogen mustard class. The butyric acid side chain, also common to chlorambucil, confers water solubility. The benzimidazole ring, structurally similar to a purine ring, occupies the position of the benzene ring in chlorambucil. Bendamustine has shown activity in chronic lymphocytic leukemia and non-Hodgkin's lymphoma. The recommended dose of bendamustine is 100 mg/m² given IV over 30 minutes on days 1 and 2 of a 28-day cycle. Side effects include nausea, vomiting, bone marrow suppression, headache and dyspnea.

▶ *Thiotepa*

Thiotepa is an alkylating agent that reacts with DNA phosphate groups to produce chromosomal cross-linkage. Thiotepa has shown clinical activity in the treatment of breast, bladder, and ovarian cancer, along with carcinomatous meningitis and malignant effusions, and usually is administered IV or as an intravesicular infusion. It also may be used intrathecally. Side effects include myelosuppression, nausea and vomiting, and venous irritation.

Heavy Metal Compounds

Platinum drugs form reactive platinum complexes that bind to cells, so the pharmacokinetics of the individual drug may be of the platinum, both free and bound, rather than of the parent drug.

▶ *Cisplatin*

Cisplatin forms inter- and intrastrand DNA cross-links to inhibit DNA synthesis. Cisplatin has shown clinical activity in the treatment of numerous tumor types, from head and neck cancers to anal cancer, including many types of lymphoma and carcinoma of unknown primary. Cisplatin is highly emetogenic, even when low doses are given daily for 5 days, and causes delayed nausea and vomiting as well; patients require aggressive antiemetic regimens for both delayed and acute emesis. Significant nephrotoxicity and electrolyte abnormalities can occur if inadequate hydration occurs. Ototoxicity, which manifests as a high-frequency hearing loss, and a glove-and-stocking neuropathy may limit therapy.

▶ *Carboplatin*

Although carboplatin has the same mechanism of action as cisplatin, its side effects are similar but less intense than those of cisplatin. Many chemotherapy regimens dose carboplatin based on an area under the curve (AUC), which is also called the *Calvert equation*. According to the Calvert equation, the dose in milligrams = (CrCl + 25) × AUC desired.[23] Carboplatin has shown clinical activity in the treatment of ovarian, lung, breast, testicular, esophageal, and head and neck cancers, as well as lymphomas. Thrombocytopenia, nausea and vomiting, and hypersensitivity reactions are side effects.

▶ *Oxaliplatin*

Oxaliplatin has shown clinical activity in the treatment of colorectal cancer. Oxaliplatin, although similar in action to cisplatin and carboplatin, causes a cold-induced neuropathy. Patients should be counseled to avoid cold beverages, to use gloves to remove items from the freezer, and to wear protective clothing in cold climates for the first week after treatment. A glove-and-stocking neuropathy also occurs with long-term dosing. Hypersensitivity reactions and moderate nausea and vomiting are also side effects.[24]

mTOR Inhibitors

▶ *Temsirolimus and Everolimus*

The mammalian target of rapamycin (mTOR) is a downstream mediator in the phosphatidylinositol 3-kinase/Akt signaling pathway that controls translation of proteins that regulate cell growth and proliferation but also angiogenesis and cell survival. The mTOR is an intracellular component that stimulates protein synthesis by phosphorylating translation regulators, and contributes to protein degradation and angiogenesis.

Temsirolimus is approved for the treatment advanced renal cell carcinoma. Temsirolimus and its metabolite sirolimus are substrates of the cytochrome P4503A4/5 isoenzyme system. The primary side effects of temsirolimus include mucositis, diarrhea, maculopapular rash, nausea, leucopenia, thrombocytopenia, and hyperglycemia.

Everolimus is an oral inhibitor of mTOR that is approved for the treatment of patients with advanced renal cell cancer after failure of treatment with sunitinib or sorafenib and most recently for the treatment of advanced pancreatic neuroendocrine tumors. Drug interactions and adverse reactions are similar to those of temsirolimus.

Miscellaneous Agents

▶ *Altretamine*

Altretamine, formerly known as hexamethylmelamine, is similar in structure to alkylating agents but is known to have anticancer activity in cancer cells resistant to alkylating agents. Altretamine has shown activity in the treatment of ovarian and lung cancer. This orally administered drug has the dose-limiting side effects of anorexia, nausea, vomiting, diarrhea, and abdominal cramping. Other side effects include neuropathy, agitation, confusion, and depression.

▶ *Bleomycin*

Bleomycin is a mixture of peptides with drug activity expressed in units, where 1 unit equals 1 mg. Bleomycin causes DNA strand breakage. Bleomycin has shown clinical activity in the treatment of patients with testicular cancer and malignant effusions, squamous cell carcinomas of the skin, and Kaposi's sarcoma. Hypersensitivity reactions and fever may occur, so premedication with acetaminophen may be required. The most serious side effect is the pulmonary toxicity that presents as a pneumonitis with a dry cough, dyspnea, rales, and infiltrates. Pulmonary function studies show decreased carbon monoxide diffusing capacity and restrictive ventilatory changes. "Bleomycin lung" is associated with cumulative dosing greater than 400 units and occurs rarely with a total dose of 150 units. The pulmonary toxicity is potentiated by thoracic radiation and by hyperoxia. Additional side effects include fever with or without chills, mild to moderate alopecia, and nausea and vomiting. Bleomycin has been used to manage malignant effusions at doses of 15 to 60 units through installation into the affected area. The drainage tube of the effusion is clamped off for some period of time after administration of bleomycin (time varies based on the location of the effusion), and then the amount of drainage is monitored to determine efficacy of the bleomycin treatment.[25]

▶ Hydroxyurea

Hydroxyurea is an oral drug that inhibits ribonucleotide reductase, which converts ribonucleotides into the deoxyribonucleotides used in DNA synthesis and repair. Hydroxyurea has shown clinical activity in the treatment of chronic myelocytic leukemia, polycythemia vera, and thrombocytosis. The major side effects are myelosuppression, nausea and vomiting, diarrhea, and constipation. Rash, mucositis, and renal tubular dysfunction occur rarely.

▶ L-Asparaginase

L-Asparaginase is an enzyme that may be produced by *Escherichia coli*. Asparaginase hydrolyzes the reaction of asparagine to aspartic acid and ammonia to deplete lymphoid cells of asparagine, which inhibits protein synthesis. L-Asparaginase has shown clinical activity in the treatment of ALL and childhood AML. Severe allergic reactions may occur when the interval between doses is 7 days or greater, so while a skin test result may be negative, patients should be observed closely after asparaginase administration. Pancreatitis and fibrinogen depletion may also occur during therapy. Repletion of fibrinogen should be done to prevent disseminated intravascular coagulation and fatal bleeding. If the patient suffers an allergic reaction to L-asparaginase, pegaspargase, which is L-asparaginase modified through a linkage with polyethylene glycol, which extends the half-life and allows for lower doses and less frequent administration, may be given. Cost and limited availability are some reasons pegaspargase may not be used first.

▶ Arsenic Trioxide

Arsenic trioxide, which is approved for the treatment of acute promyelocytic leukemia (APL), induces the growth of cancer cells into mature, more normal cells and induces programmed cell death, or apoptosis. Arsenic trioxide causes QT-interval prolongation, so frequent electrocardiograms need to be done before each dose, and other drugs that may prolong the QT interval need to be avoided during therapy. Monitoring of potassium and magnesium should be performed and active replacement undertaken to prevent QT prolongation. Other side effects include dry skin with itching, nausea and vomiting, loss of appetite, and elevations of serum

hepatic enzymes. A serious side effect is APL differentiation syndrome, which appears similar to pneumonia but is related to the arsenic therapy.[26]

▶ Mitomycin C

Mitomycin C forms cross-links with DNA to inhibit DNA and RNA synthesis. Mitomycin C has shown clinical activity in the treatment of anal, bladder, cervix, gallbladder, esophageal, and stomach cancer. Side effects consist of myelosuppression and mucositis, and it is a vesicant.

▶ Tretinoin

Tretinoin, also referred to *ATRA*, which stands for all-trans-retinoic acid, is a retinoic acid that is not cytotoxic but promotes the maturation of early promyelocytic cells and is specific to the t(15;17) cytogenetic marker. The most significant side effect is the APL differentiation syndrome, which may occur anywhere from the first couple of days of therapy until the end of therapy and consists of symptoms of fever, respiratory distress, and hypotension. Chest radiographs are consistent with a pneumonia-like process. The syndrome can be confused easily with pneumonia in a patient with possible neutropenia. The treatment for retinoic acid syndrome is dexamethasone 10 mg IV every 12 hours; the syndrome may resolve within 24 hours of the start of dexamethasone therapy. However, the use of steroids in a febrile neutropenic patient may further compromise the treatment of infection.[27]

▶ Thalidomide

Thalidomide was introduced into the market on October 1, 1957, as a sedative–hypnotic, and when it was taken by pregnant women, it resulted in severe limb deformities (phocomelia). Thalidomide is indicated for the treatment of leprosy and multiple myeloma. Thalidomide is an angiogenesis inhibitor, but the full the mechanism of action is still unknown. Possible mechanisms of action include free radical oxidative damage to DNA, inhibiting tumor necrosis factor α production, altering the adhesion of cancer cells, and altering cytokines that affect the growth of cancer cells.[28,29] Thalidomide has shown clinical activity in the treatment of multiple myeloma and is still being studied for the treatment of several other cancers. Because of thalidomide's potential to cause phocomelia, each patient must be counseled on the risks of thalidomide not only for the patient but also the patient's reproductive partner. Physicians must be registered to prescribe thalidomide. Pharmacists can fill prescriptions only when both the patient and the physician have completed surveys on a monthly basis.

▶ Lenalidomide

Lenalidomide is approved for the treatment of myelodysplastic syndrome when the 5q deletion is present and multiple myeloma. Because lenalidomide is an analog of thalidomide, all of the same precautions must be taken to prevent phocomelia. Dosing adjustments are necessary for renal dysfunction. Lenalidomide is used in the treatment of myelodysplastic syndrome and multiple myeloma. Other side effects are neutropenia, thrombocytopenia, deep vein thrombosis (DVT), and pulmonary embolus.

▶ Bexarotene

Bexarotene is a retinoid that selectively activates retinoid X receptors, which affects cellular differentiation and proliferation. Bexarotene is eliminated primarily by the hepatobiliary system. Bexarotene is indicated for the treatment of cutaneous manifestations of cutaneous T-cell lymphoma in patients who are refractory to other therapy. Side effects include hypercholesterolemia, elevations in triglycerides, pancreatitis, hypothyroidism, and leukopenia, headache, and dry skin.

▶ Bortezomib

The proteasome is an enzyme complex that exists in all cells and plays an important role in degrading proteins the control the cell cycle. When the proteasome is inhibited, the numerous pathways that are necessary for the growth and survival of cancer cells is disrupted. Bortezomib specifically inhibits the 26S proteasome, which is a large protein complex that degrades ubiquitinated proteins. This pathway plays an essential role in regulating the intracellular concentration of specific proteins, causing the cells to maintain homeostasis. Inhibition of the 26S proteasome prevents this to occur, ultimately causing a disruption in the homeostasis and cell death.

Bortezomib is approved for the treatment of multiple myeloma and mantle cell lymphoma. It is administered as an IV injection. The most commonly reported adverse effects are asthenia, gastrointestinal disturbances (nausea, diarrhea, decreased appetite, constipation, vomiting), thrombocytopenia, peripheral neuropathy, anemia, headache, insomnia, and edema. Reactivation of varicella zoster infection is also common with bortezomib, and antiviral prophylaxis with acyclovir should be considered.

▶ HDAC Inhibitors (Vorinostat and Romidepsin)

Vorinostat is indicated for the treatment of cutaneous T-cell lymphoma in patients with progressive, persistent, or recurrent disease after treatment with two systemic therapies. Romidepsin was approved in 2009 for the treatment of cutaneous or peripheral T-cell lymphoma in patients who have received at least one systemic therapy. These agents catalyze the removal of acetyl groups from acetylated lysine residues in histones, resulting in the modulation of gene expression. Vorinostat is an orally available agent, and romidepsin is only available in an IV formulation. These drugs are metabolized by CYP3A4, so caution should be exercised with monitoring for drug–drug interactions. Side effects include diarrhea, fatigue, nausea and anorexia, hypercholesterolemia, hypertriglyceridemia, and hyperglycemia. Despite anemia, thrombocytopenia, and neutropenia, patients have developed pulmonary embolism and DVT while on therapy.[30]

Patient Encounter 2

RA is a 43-year-old man receiving doxorubicin and ifosfamide for a newly diagnosed osteosarcoma. While receiving chemotherapy, he begins to complain of flank pain and hematuria. His serum creatinine has risen from 0.9 mg/dL to 1.8 mg/dL (80 to 159 μmol/L) in the last 3 days.

What is the likely diagnosis?

What drug should always be included as part of this regimen?

What should patients be counseled to do while receiving ifosfamide therapy?

Immune Therapies

▶ Interferons

The categories of α, β, and γ interferons exist; the α-interferons are used in the treatment of cancer. Interferon enhances the immune system's attack on cancer cells, can decrease new blood vessel formation, and can augment expression of antigen on tumor cell surfaces. Interferon has shown clinical activity in the treatment of melanoma, kidney cancer, Kaposi's sarcoma, and chronic myelocytic and lymphocytic leukemia. Unfortunately, interferon is not well tolerated by patients because it causes a flu-like syndrome that consists of fevers and chills; depression, malaise, and fatigue are other side effects. Premedication with acetaminophen helps alleviate the flu-like symptoms, which decrease with chronic administration.

▶ Aldesleukin

Aldesleukin, which is a human recombinant *interleukin-2 (IL-2)*, is a lymphokine that promotes B- and T-cell proliferation and triggers a cytokine cascade to attack the tumor. Aldesleukin has shown clinical activity in the treatment of kidney cancer and melanoma. Side effects of IL-2 vary by dose and route. IV high-dose IL-2 causes a drug-induced shocklike picture. Patients may develop hypotension despite aggressive IV hydration. Patients develop a red, itching skin; liver and kidney function tests change; via immune complex formation in the kidneys, fluid and electrolyte imbalances occur; and high fevers occur while receiving scheduled acetaminophen and nonsteroidal anti-inflammatory agents. Severe rigors and chills may require IV meperidine for symptom control. All the side effects reverse within 24 hours of stopping the drug. The toxicity profile is much less with subcutaneous administration. However, with subcutaneous administration, nodules form at the injection site and may take months to resolve. Corticosteroids should not be administered to patients while they are receiving aldesleukin unless a life-threatening emergency occurs. Steroids reverse all the symptoms and the antitumor effect even with topical administration. The itching, red skin may be treated with topical creams and antihistamines.

▶ *Denileukin Diftitox*

Denileukin diftitox is a combination of the active moieties of IL-2 and diphtheria toxin. It binds to high-affinity IL-2 receptors on the cancer cell (and other cells), and the toxin portion of the molecule inhibits protein synthesis to result in cell death. Denileukin diftitox is used for the treatment of persistent or recurrent cutaneous T-cell lymphoma whose cells express the CD25 receptor. Side effects include vascular leak syndrome, fevers or chills, hypersensitivity reactions, hypotension, anorexia, diarrhea, and nausea and vomiting.

▶ *Peginterferon Alfa-2b*

Sylatron, approved in April 2011, is a covalent conjugate of recombinant alfa-2b interferon with monomethoxy polyethylene glycol (PEG). The mechanism of cytotoxicity in patients with melanoma is unknown. This agent is specifically indicated for the adjuvant treatment of melanoma with microscopic or gross nodal involvement up to 84 days after definitive surgical resection (including complete lymphadenectomy). Adverse effects include fatigue, increased liver enzymes, pyrexia, headache, anorexia, myalgia, nausea, chills, and pain at the injection site.[31]

▶ *Sipuleucel-T*

Sipuleucel-T is a novel autologous cellular immunotherapy, approved in 2010, for the treatment of asymptomatic or minimally symptomatic metastatic hormone refractory prostate cancer. Sipuleucel-T is designed to induce an immune response targeted at prostatic acid phosphatase (PAP), which is an antigen expressed in greater than 95% of prostate cancers. Patients receiving sipuleucel-T undergo leukapheresis to collect their own antigen-presenting cells. These cells are then sent to a manufacturing facility and cultured with a recombinant antigen (PAP-GM-CSF, composed of PAP and GM-CSF, an immune cell activator). The cellular product, which is made specifically for each patient, is then delivered to the patient's clinic and infused intravenously into the patient on day 3 or 4. Each course consists of three infusions of activated cells given at 2-week intervals. Adverse effects include chills, fatigue, fever, back pain, nausea, joint pain, and headache.[32]

Monoclonal Antibodies

The cell surface contains molecules, which are referred to as *CD*, which stands for "cluster of differentiation." The antibodies are produced against a specific antigen. When administered, usually by an IV injection, the antibody binds to the antigen, which may trigger the immune system to result in cell death through complement-mediated cellular toxicity, or the antigen–antibody cell complex may be internalized to the cancer cell, which results in cell death. Monoclonal antibodies also may carry radioactivity, sometimes referred to as *hot antibodies*, and are referred to as *radioimmunotherapy*, so the radioactivity is delivered to

Table 88–7	
Syllable Source Indicators for Monoclonal Antibodies[a]	
U	Human
O	Mouse
A	Rat
E	Hamster
I	Primate
Xi	A cross between humanized and animal source

[a]These letters appear before mab, which stands for monoclonal antibody.

From Programme on International Nonproprietary Names (INN) Division of Drug Management and Policies, World Health Organization, Geneva. 1997.

the cancer cell. Antibodies that contain no radioactivity are referred to as *cold antibodies*.

All monoclonal antibodies end in the suffix -*mab*. The syllable before -*mab* indicates the source of the monoclonal antibody (Table 88–7). When administering an antibody for the first time, one should consider the source. The less humanized an antibody, the greater the chance for the patient to have an allergic-type reaction to the antibody. The more humanized the antibody, the lower the risk of a reaction. The severity of the reactions may range from fever and chills to life-threatening allergic reactions (which have resulted in death). Premedication with acetaminophen and diphenhydramine is common before the first dose of any antibody. If a severe reaction occurs, the infusion should be stopped and the patient treated with antihistamines, corticosteroids, or other supportive measures.

▶ *Alemtuzumab*

Alemtuzumab is an antibody to the CD52 receptor present on B and T lymphocytes. Alemtuzumab has shown clinical activity in the treatment of chronic lymphocytic leukemia. Severe and prolonged (6 months) immunosuppression may result, which necessitates pneumocystis carinii pneumonia (PCP) prophylaxis and antifungal and antiviral prophylaxis to prevent opportunistic infections.

▶ *Bevacizumab*

Bevacizumab is a humanized monoclonal antibody that binds to vascular endothelial growth factor (VEGF), which prevents it from binding to its receptors, ultimately resulting in inhibition of angiogenesis. Bevacizumab has shown clinical activity in the treatment of colorectal, kidney, lung, breast, and head and neck cancer. Patients may develop hypertension requiring chronic medication during therapy. Impaired wound healing, thromboembolic events, proteinuria, bleeding, and bowel perforation are serious side effects that occur with this drug.

▶ *Brentuximab*

Brentuximab vedotin is a CD30-directed antibody–drug conjugate (ADC) that consists of the antibody specific for

CD30, a microtubule disrupting agent called monomethyl auristatin E (MMAE), and a protease-cleavable linker that covalently attaches MMAE to the antibody. It is reported that the cytotoxic activity is a result of the binding of the ADC to CD30-expressing cells followed by internalization of the ADC–CD30 complex, and then proteolytic cleavage and release of MMAE into the cell. Binding of MMAE to tubulin disrupts the microtubule network, resulting in cell cycle arrest and apoptosis. This IV agent, which was granted accelerated approval in 2011, is indicated for Hodgkin's lymphoma patients after failure of autologous stem cell transplant (ASCT) or after failure of at least two multidrug regimens in patients who are not eligible for ASCT and for patients with systemic anaplastic large cell lymphoma who have failed at least one systemic chemotherapy regimen. In vitro data suggests that MMAE is a substrate and an inhibitor of CYP3A4/5; therefore, patients need to be monitored for drug–drug interactions. The most common adverse effects are neutropenia, peripheral neuropathy, fatigue, nausea and vomiting, diarrhea, anemia, thrombocytopenia, and upper respiratory infection. Dosing modifications guidelines for peripheral neuropathy can be found in the prescribing information.[33]

▶ Cetuximab

Cetuximab is a chimeric antibody that binds to the epidermal growth factor receptor (EGFR) to block its stimulation. Tumors that have *KRAS* mutations do not respond to treatment with cetuximab; therefore, tumors should be tested for *KRAS* mutations before initiating therapy. Cetuximab has shown clinical activity in the treatment of colorectal and head and neck cancers. An acne-like rash may appear on the face and upper torso 1 to 3 weeks after the start of therapy. Other side effects include hypersensitivity reactions, interstitial lung disease, fever, malaise, diarrhea, abdominal pain, and nausea and vomiting.

▶ Gemtuzumab Ozogamicin

Gemtuzumab ozogamicin is a humanized antibody to the CD33+ receptor present on about 80% of AML cells. The antibody is linked to calicheamicin, a cellular toxin that is released intracellularly after the antigen–antibody complex is internalized. Inside the cell, calicheamicin binds to DNA in the minor groove, resulting in DNA double-strand breaks and cell death. Shortly after receiving accelerated approval in 2000 for elderly patients with relapsed CD33+ AML, hepatotoxicity (specifically veno-occlusive disease) and hypersensitivity reactions, including anaphylaxis, infusion reactions, and pulmonary events, were observed, which led to the addition of black box warnings. Unfortunately, the confirmatory postapproval clinical trial did not confirm the clinical benefit of gemtuzumab ozogamicin. Based on these safety and efficacy concerns, in 2010, gemtuzumab ozogamicin was voluntarily withdrawn from the market in the United States.

▶ Ibritumomab Tiuxetan

This "hot antibody" is linked to yttrium and binds to the CD20 receptor of B lymphocytes (see Rituximab later). Hematologic toxicity may occur several weeks after administration and may take weeks to resolve.

▶ Ipilimumab

Ipilimumab is a recombinant, human monoclonal antibody that binds to the cytotoxic T lymphocytic–associated antigen 4 (CTLA-4), which is a molecule on T cells that causes a suppression of the immune response. CTLA-4 is a negative regulator of T-cell activation. Ipilimumab binds to CTLA-4 and blocks the interaction of CTLA-4 with its ligands. This blockage has been reported to enhance T-cell activation and proliferation. Ipilimumab is approved for patients with unresectable or metastatic melanoma. The antitumor effects appear to be T-cell–mediated immune responses. This medication is given through IV administration and is dosed at 3 mg/kg over 90 minutes every 3 weeks for a total of four doses. Ipilimumab administration can result in severe and fatal immune-mediated adverse reactions, including enterocolitis, hepatitis, toxic epidermal necrolysis, neuropathy, and endocrine abnormalities. These symptoms can occur during treatment or weeks to months after discontinuation of the drug. Liver and thyroid function tests should be performed at baseline and before each dose. If this occurs, treatment should be initiated with systemic corticosteroids and the drug should be discontinued permanently. Progressive multifocal leukoencephalopathy has been reported. Additional less serious adverse effects include fatigue, diarrhea, pruritus, rash, and colitis.

▶ Ofatumumab

Ofatumumab is a fully human monoclonal antibody to CD20 that received accelerated approval as single-agent therapy in 2009 for patients with chronic lymphocytic leukemia that is refractory to fludarabine and alemtuzumab therapy. Data suggest that possible mechanisms of anticancer activity are through complement-dependent and antibody-dependent cell-mediated cytotoxicity. The most common adverse effects include infusion-related reactions, neutropenia, infections, pyrexia, anemia, diarrhea, and nausea. Serious adverse events, including fatal infections, progressive multifocal leukoencephalopathy, and reactivation of hepatitis B, have been reported.

▶ Panitumumab

Panitumumab binds to the EGFR to prevent receptor autophosphorylation and activation of receptor-associated kinases, which results in inhibition of cell growth and induction of apoptosis. Panitumumab has demonstrated activity against tumors of the colon and rectum. However, panitumumab is not recommended for the treatment of colorectal cancer with *KRAS* mutations in codon 12 or 13. Retrospective subset analyses have not shown a treatment benefit for these mutations. Side effects include dermatitis, pruritus, exfoliative rash, infusion reactions, pulmonary fibrosis, diarrhea, hypomagnesemia, hypocalcemia, and photosensitivity.

▶ *Rituximab*

Rituximab is a monoclonal antibody to the CD20 receptor expressed on the surface of B lymphocytes; the presence of the antibody is determined during flow cytometry of the tumor cells. Cell death results from antibody-dependent cellular cytotoxicity. Rituximab has shown clinical activity in the treatment of B-cell lymphomas that are CD20 positive. Side effects include hypersensitivity reactions, hypotension, fevers, chills, rash, headache, and mild nausea and vomiting.

▶ *Tositumomab*

This "hot antibody" is linked to radioactive iodine and binds to the CD20 receptor present on B lymphocytes (see Rituximab earlier). Tositumomab has shown activity in non-Hodgkin's lymphoma. Hematologic toxicity occurs several weeks after administration and may persist for months. Because radioactive iodine may have adverse effects on the thyroid, all patients must receive thyroid-blocking agents.

▶ *Trastuzumab*

Trastuzumab is the antibody directed against human epidermal receptor 2 (*HER-2*), which is overexpressed by 25% to 30% of breast cancers and is associated with aggressive disease and decreased survival. Breast cancer tissue must be tested for the presence of *HER-2* because patients who do not express *HER-2* do not respond to trastuzumab. Trastuzumab is also indicated for the treatment of gastric cancer. Severe congestive heart failure may occur with concurrent anthracycline administration. Cardiac toxicity may be seen when the drug is administered months after anthracycline administration, so patients must be counseled on the signs and symptoms of heart failure. Other side effects include hypersensitivity reactions, fever, diarrhea, infections, chills, cough, headache, rash, and insomnia.[34]

Tyrosine Kinase Inhibitors

There are more than 100 different types of tyrosine kinases present in the body. Tyrosine kinase inhibitors (TKIs) are also referred to as small-molecule inhibitors. Each of the following drugs was developed to block either several or a specific tyrosine kinase.

▶ *Imatinib*

Imatinib was the first FDA-approved TKI. The drug was designed to block the breakpoint cluster region tyrosine kinase (BCR-ABL) produced by the Philadelphia chromosome associated with CML and ALL. Imatinib also has shown activity against gastrointestinal stromal tumors (GIST) that are positive for c-kit (CD117). Numerous drug interactions have been reported for imatinib. CYP450 3A4 inducers, such as rifampicin and St. John's wort, increase the clearance of

imatinib.[35,36] Ketoconazole, a CYP450 3A4 inhibitor, has been shown to decrease imatinib clearance by almost 30%.[37] Imatinib also may increase the exposure of simvastatin, a CYP450 3A4 substrate.[38]

▶ *Dasatinib*

Dasatinib is a second-generation TKI that shares the same binding site on the BCR-ABL cluster region as imatinib but maintains activity despite imatinib resistance, with higher potency than imatinib. Dasatinib also inhibits SRC kinases, which are tyrosine kinases that mediate cellular differentiation, proliferation, and survival. Dasatinib is used front line in the treatment of CML and in CML with resistance or intolerance to imatinib, as well as for the treatment of Philadelphia-chromosome-positive acute lymphoblastic leukemia. Side effects of dasatinib include myelosuppression, nausea and vomiting, headache, fluid retention, hypocalcemia, and pleural effusions.

▶ *Nilotinib*

Nilotinib also blocks the breakpoint cluster region tyrosine kinase (BCR-ABL) produced by the Philadelphia chromosome associated with CML and ALL. Nilotinib is also indicated for the treatment of Philadelphia-chromosome-positive CML. Nilotinib is a competitive inhibitor of UGT1A1 in vitro, which could increase the concentrations of nilotinib. In a pharmacogenetic analysis, patients with (TA)7/(TA)7 genotype (UGT1A1*28) had a statistically significant increase in bilirubin over other genotypes.[39] Nilotinib should be administered on an empty stomach or 2 hours after a meal. Side effects include QT prolongation, bone marrow suppression, elevations in lipase, and hepatotoxicity.

▶ *Erlotinib*

Erlotinib, whose pharmacology is not entirely understood, is believed to inhibit the intracellular phosphorylation of the EGFR. Erlotinib is about 60% absorbed after oral administration. Food increases bioavailability to almost 100%, but this is variable, and experts recommend administering erlotinib on an empty stomach. Erlotinib is eliminated predominately by CYP450 3A4. Smoking increases the clearance of erlotinib by 24%, which may result in treatment failure.[40] Erlotinib is used in the treatment of NSCLC and cancer of the pancreas. Side effects include interstitial lung disease, rash, diarrhea, anorexia, pruritus, conjunctivitis, and dry skin. Again, significant drug interactions have been documented with CYP450 3A4 inducers and inhibitors.

▶ *Lapatinib*

Lapatinib inhibits the intracellular kinase domains of both EGFR and *HER-2* and has been shown to retain activity against breast cancer cells that have become resistant to trastuzumab. The drug is dosed at 1000 mg/day in combination with trastuzumab, 1250 mg/day in combination with capecitabine, and 1500 mg/day in combination with letrozole. Patients with Child-Pugh class C liver disease should have a dosage reduction to 750 mg/day to adjust the AUC to the normal range. Lapatinib is indicated for the treatment of patients with breast cancer whose tumors overexpress *HER-2*. Side effects of lapatinib include decreased left ventricular ejection fraction, diarrhea, hepatotoxicity, rash, and QT prolongation.

▶ *Sorafenib*

Sorafenib is a multikinase inhibitor that inhibits both intracellular and extracellular kinases to decrease renal cell cancer proliferation. Sorafenib is metabolized primarily by the liver by CYP450 3A4. Sorafenib is used for the treatment of renal cell cancer. The primary side effects of sorafenib include rash, hand–foot skin reaction, diarrhea, pruritus, and elevations in serum lipase.

▶ *Sunitinib*

Sunitinib blocks several tyrosine kinases, including platelet-derived growth factor, VEGF receptor, stem cell factor receptor, fms-like receptor growth factor, colony-stimulating growth factor receptor type 1, and glial cell line–derived neurotrophic factor receptor. The active metabolite of sunitinib blocks these same enzymes with similar potency. It is indicated for the treatment of GISTs after disease progression or intolerance to imatinib. It is also indicated for the treatment of advanced renal cell cancer and pancreatic neuroendocrine tumors. Significant side effects include left ventricular dysfunction, hemorrhage, asthenia, hypertension, nausea and vomiting, and diarrhea. Approximately one-third of patients may develop a yellow color of the skin along with dryness and cracking of the skin. Also, hair may become depigmented with doses of 50 mg/day or more; the depigmentation is reversible when therapy is stopped. Clinically significant drug interactions exist with drugs metabolized via the CYP450 3A4 system; ketoconazole has been shown to increase concentrations of sunitinib, whereas rifampin has been shown to decrease concentrations of sunitinib.

▶ *Pazopanib*

Pazopanib is a vascular epidermal growth factor receptor (VEGFR) TKI that acts at VEGFR-1, VEGFR-2, and VEGFR-3. It is specifically indicated for the treatment of patients with advanced renal cell carcinoma. Pazopanib is metabolized through CYP3A4; therefore, drug–drug interactions should be monitored. Pazopanib is an orally administered agent that should be taken on an empty stomach. Common adverse effects include diarrhea, hypertension, hair color change, nausea and vomiting, fatigue, and anorexia. Serious toxicities that have been observed are increases in liver enzymes and bilirubin, including fatal hepatotoxicity, prolonged QT intervals and torsades de pointes, hemorrhagic events, arterial thrombotic events, gastrointestinal perforation, and proteinuria.

▶ *Vemurafenib*

Vemurafenib, formerly known as PLX4032, is a potent inhibitor of mutated *BRAF*. In August 2011, the agent received FDA approval for the treatment of unresectable or metastatic melanoma in patients with documented *BRAFV600E* mutation as determined by an FDA-approved test. Vemurafenib produced improved rates of overall and progression-free survival in a phase III trial when compared with dacabarazine. Vemurafenib is not indicated for patients with wild-type BRAF. The orally administered vemurafenib is dosed at 960 mg twice daily without regards to meals. Common adverse effects include arthralgia, rash, fatigue, alopecia, keratoacanthoma or squamous cell cancer, photosensitivity, nausea, and diarrhea. Approximately 40% of patients require dosage modifications because of adverse effects.[41]

▶ *Crizotinib*

Crizotinib is a small-molecule inhibitor of the anaplastic lymphoma kinase gene (ALK) and mesenchymal epithelial transition growth factor (c-MET). This orally available agent was approved in August 2011 for the treatment of locally advanced or metastatic NSCLC that is ALK positive (about 2% to 7% of NSCLC patients) as detected by an FDA-approved test. Crizotinib is dosed at 250 mg orally twice daily without regards to meals. Adverse effects reported include mild gastrointestinal symptoms, edema, and visual disturbances, which have been described as trails of light following objects as they move.[42]

▶ *Vandetanib*

Vandetanib is an orally available receptor TKI that blocks both the VEGF and EGF receptor kinase. This agent is indicated for the treatment of symptomatic or progressive medullary thyroid cancer in patients with unresectable locally advanced or metastatic disease. It is an orally administered agent dosed at 300 mg/day without regards to meals. Common adverse effects include diarrhea, rash, acne, nausea, hypertension, headache, fatigue, decreased appetite, and abdominal pain.

Hormonal Therapies

Hormonal therapies have shown activity in the treatment of cancers whose growth is affected by gonadal hormonal control. Hormonal treatments either block or decrease the production of endogenous hormones.

▶ *Antiandrogens: Bicalutamide, Flutamide, and Nilutamide*

The antiandrogens block androgen receptors to inhibit the action of testosterone and dihydrotestosterone in prostate cancer cells. Unfortunately, prostate cancer cells may become hormone refractory.

Side effects common to these agents are hot flashes, gynecomastia, and decreased libido. Flutamide tends to be associated with more diarrhea and requires three times daily administration, whereas bicalutamide is dosed once daily. Nilutamide may cause interstitial pneumonia and is associated with the visual disturbance of delayed adaptation to darkness.

▶ Luteinizing Hormone–Releasing Hormone Agonists: Goserelin and Leuprolide

Initially, luteinizing hormone–releasing hormone (LHRH) agonists increase levels of luteinizing hormone and follicle-stimulating hormone, but testosterone and estrogen levels are decreased because of continuous negative-feedback inhibition. Major side effects are testicular atrophy, decreased libido, gynecomastia, and hot flashes. Goserelin is injected as a pellet under the skin, therefore, subcutaneous injection of lidocaine around the injection site before administration helps to decrease the pain associated with goserelin administration. Numerous dosage forms are available for leuprolide with varying strengths and dosing intervals. Antiandrogens may be administered during initial therapy to decrease symptoms of tumor flare (e.g., bone pain and urinary tract obstruction).

▶ Ketoconazole

Although ketoconazole is an antifungal agent, it has been used for treatment of prostate cancer. In high doses of 400 mg three times daily, ketoconazole blocks the production of testosterone.

▶ Luteinizing Hormone–Releasing Hormone Antagonist: Degarelix

Degarelix is a gonadotropin-releasing hormone (GnRH) receptor antagonist that works by binding reversibly to the pituitary GnRH receptors, thereby reducing the release of gonadotropins and consequently testosterone. Degarelix was approved in 2008 and is indicated for the treatment of advanced prostate cancer. Adverse events include hot flashes, injection site reactions, and an increase in liver enzymes. An advantage of degralix over LHRH agonists is the lack of the tumor flare. [43]

▶ Abiraterone

Abiraterone, approved in 2011, is an orally available androgen biosynthesis inhibitor that inhibits 17α-hydroxylase/C17,20-lyase (CYP17), which is expressed in testicular, adrenal, and prostatic tumor tissues. Abiraterone is indicated in combination with prednisone for the treatment of metastatic castration–resistant prostate cancer who have received prior chemotherapy containing docetaxel. Adverse effects include joint swelling, hypokalemia, edema, muscle discomfort, hot flashes, diarrhea, urinary tract infections, nocturia, urinary frequency, dyspepsia, cough, hypertension, and arrhythmia. The patient must be counseled to take the oral medication on an empty stomach because food increases absorption and results in adverse reactions. [44]

▶ Anastrozole

Anastrozole is a selective nonsteroidal aromatase inhibitor that lowers estrogen levels. Anastrozole is used for the adjuvant treatment of postmenopausal women with hormone-positive breast cancer and in breast cancer patients who have had disease progression following tamoxifen. Side effects include hot flashes, arthralgias, osteoporosis or bone fractures, and thrombophlebitis.

▶ Exemestane

Exemestane is an irreversible aromatase inactivator that binds to the aromatase enzyme to block the production of estrogen from androgens. Exemestane is indicated for the treatment of advanced breast cancer in postmenopausal women who have had disease progression following tamoxifen therapy. Side effects include hot flashes, fatigue, osteoporosis or bone fractures, and flu-like symptoms.

▶ Letrozole

Letrozole is another selective aromatase that inhibits the conversion of androgens to estrogen. Letrozole is used in the treatment of postmenopausal women with hormone receptor–positive or unknown advanced breast cancer. Side effects include bone pain, hot flashes, back pain, nausea, arthralgia, osteoporosis or bone fractures, and dyspnea.

▶ Fulvestrant

Fulvestrant is an estrogen receptor antagonist that binds to the estrogen receptor and is given as a monthly intramuscular injection. Fulvestrant is used for the treatment of hormone receptor–positive metastatic breast cancer in postmenopausal women with disease progression following antiestrogen therapy. Side effects are hot flashes, abdominal pain, depression, and myalgias.

▶ Megestrol Acetate

Megestrol is a synthetic progestin with antiestrogen properties that is used for breast cancer and in higher doses for weight gain. Side effects include fluid retention, hot flashes, vaginal bleeding and spotting, breast tenderness, and thrombosis.

▶ Tamoxifen

Tamoxifen is a selective estrogen receptor modulator (SERM). Tamoxifen is used for the treatment of metastatic hormone receptor–positive breast cancer, adjuvant and primary treatment of breast cancer, and prevention of breast cancer in high-risk women. Side effects include hot flashes, fluid retention, mood swings, thrombosis, endometrial and uterine cancer, and corneal changes and cataracts. Because tamoxifen is a substrate of CYP450 3A4, decreased tamoxifen levels have occurred with use of St. John's wort, and decreased tamoxifen levels have been observed with the use of rifampin. Tamoxifen is also a substrate for CYP450 2D6, and evidence suggests that those who are CYP2D6*4/*4 may have a poorer response and more toxicity with tamoxifen.[45] Significant drug interactions exist with antidepressants that may be used to treat depression or help relieve hot flashes.

▶ *Raloxifene*

Raloxifene is an SERM usually used for the treatment of osteoporosis in postmenopausal women, although it is also indicated for the prevention of breast cancer in high-risk women at a dose of 60 mg/day. When compared head to head with tamoxifen for breast cancer prevention, it was demonstrated to have equal efficacy with less toxicity. The only advantage of tamoxifen for the prevention of breast cancer is that it can be used in premenopausal women. Hot flashes, arthralgias, and peripheral edema occur frequently with raloxifene, but thrombosis is a rare but serious adverse effect.

▶ *Toremifene*

Toremifene is an SERM. Toremifene is used for the treatment of metastatic breast cancer in postmenopausal women with estrogen receptor–positive or unknown tumors. Toremifene causes hot flashes, vaginal bleeding, thromboembolism, and visual acuity changes.

ADMINISTRATION ISSUES

Extravasation

One issue of chemotherapy safety is extravasation. Antineoplastic agents that cause severe tissue damage when they escape from the vasculature are called vesicants. Some examples of vesicants are the anthracyclines and the vinca alkaloids. The tissue damage may be severe, with tissue sloughing and loss of mobility, depending on the area of extravasation. Patients need to be educated to notify the nurse immediately if there is any pain on administration. If extravasation of a vesicant occurs, the injection should be stopped and any fluid aspirated out of the injection site. If an antidote should be administered, such as with nitrogen mustard extravasation, the pharmacy should be notified immediately so that the sodium thiosulfate can be prepared and delivered quickly. Cold compresses should be applied (heat should be used for vincas) to the affected area. The area of extravasation should be recorded and inked and followed closely to detect early signs of infection and to treat pain. Obviously, prevention of extravasation is very important. Good IV access is key, which may include the placement of a central venous catheter along with free-flowing IV fluids. During administration of a vesicant, blood return should be checked to be sure that the drug is going into the vein. Central venous catheters can be placed for patients needing infusions of vesicants or for patients with small, friable veins to prevent extravasation.

Hypersensitivity Reactions

Hypersensitivity reactions of cancer treatments is problematic because of cross-reactivity between agents and the desire to continue active therapies against the cancer.[46] For documented immediate hypersensitivity reactions to a particular agent, further administration of the agent may be achieved through extensive premedication with H1 and H2 antihistamines and corticosteroids and through use of escalating doses of the offending agent given at doses of one-hundredth, one-tenth, and the balance of the dose (so the total dose administered is equivalent to the normally prescribed dose) administered over a much longer period of time. These treatments must be given in an environment where resuscitation is readily available in case of medical emergency.

Secondary Malignancies

Chemotherapy and radiation therapy treatments may cause cancers later in life; these are referred to as secondary cancers. The most common type of secondary cancer is myelodysplastic syndrome, or AML. The antineoplastic agents most commonly associated with secondary malignancies are alkylating agents, etoposide, teniposide, topoisomerase inhibitors, and anthracyclines. Although the risk for secondary cancers is extremely low, it must outweigh the risk of survival produced by treatment of the primary malignancy. Because secondary malignancies may not occur for several years after treatment, patients with relatively short-term survival owing to the primary malignancy should consider the more immediate benefits of chemotherapy. Radiation therapy rarely may cause solid tumors as secondary cancers decades after treatment. The most common example of radiation therapy–induced secondary malignancy is breast cancer, which rarely occurs after mantle field radiation therapy for Hodgkin's disease.

CHEMOTHERAPY SAFETY

One of the first Institute of Medicine reports, the health arm of the National Academy of Sciences, starts out with a patient who died from an overdose of chemotherapy; the patient did not have an immediately life-threatening cancer, so her death was hastened by a medication error. Chemotherapy agents may cause harm to patients, health care workers, and the environment if not handled correctly. ⑤ *Because of the risk of severe toxicities associated with many of the chemotherapy agents, safety precautions must be in place to prevent chemotherapy errors or accidental chemotherapy exposures of health care professionals or patients.* The Oncology Nursing Society and the American Society of Health-System Pharmacists have information to assist in the safe handling of chemotherapy agents.[16] National, state, and local regulations regarding the safe disposal of chemotherapy agents and the equipment used to administer them need to be followed to protect the environment.

Each organization should have chemotherapy safety checks built into the prescribing, preparation and administration of chemotherapy.[16] Dosing based on patient-specific information should be included on every order for chemotherapy, whether it is oral or parenteral. Many chemotherapy regimens are referred to by acronyms (e.g., AC, which is doxorubicin cyclophosphamide); these should not be allowed as the only reference to drugs in the prescribing of chemotherapy. Also, abbreviations for the names of chemotherapy agents should be avoided because one abbreviation may stand for two different drug entities. For drugs such as doxorubicin and liposomal doxorubicin, the names should be written out fully, and in this case, the addition of the brand name may help to prevent a mistake.

The measured height and weight, along with the body surface area (BSA), if applicable, should be readily available, along with the dosage in milligrams per meter squared or kilogram, so that the dosage may be checked. If a chemotherapy regimen is a continuous infusion of 800 mg/m²/day for 4 days, an added safety feature would be to include the total dosage of 3200 mg in order to prevent any ambiguity. In cases where the clinician wants to decrease the dosage based on a laboratory value or side effect, it is recommended that the clinician include that information with the order so that everyone understands what the correct dosage is for that patient. Chemotherapy dosages should be checked for route and dose to determine that the dosages prescribed are correct according to the regimen and do not exceed dosing guidelines. Appropriate laboratory values should be checked to verify that dosages are correct for any organ dysfunction present, and drug interactions should be scrutinized closely (Tables 88–8 and 88–9). Health care practitioners administering chemotherapy should check the dosage calculation for the patient's weight or BSA along with the five Rs of administering medication (i.e., right patient, right medication, right dose, right route, at the right time). If there is any question about the safe dosage or safe administration of a chemotherapy agent, the chemotherapy should not be administered until the question is resolved.

An area of controversy with chemotherapy dosing: What weight should be used for patients who are morbidly obese? Currently, there is no consensus. Some clinicians cap BSA at some value; some clinicians will use an adjusted weight for the BSA calculation even though there is no recommendation on what adjusted weight to use. This is an area for future research.

Many of the newer agents used to treat cancer are orally administered agents. Clinicians need to be aware of drug–herbal interactions, timing of agents with respect to meals, patient education on correct dosing when multiple dosage forms are used, and reimbursement issues. Table 88–10 presents a summary of timing of oral chemotherapy with respect to food. Information should be provided to the patient both in writing and verbally, as well as to patient

Table 88–8

Empiric Dose Modifications in Patients with Renal Dysfunction

Agent	Organ Dysfunction	Dose Modification
Bleomycin	CrCl = 30–60 mL/min (0.50–1.0 mL/s)	25%–50% decrease
	CrCl = 10–30 mL/min (0.17–0.50 mL/s)	25%–50% decrease
	CrCl less than 10 mL/min (less than 0.17 mL/s)	50% decrease
Capecitabine	CrCl = 30–50 mL/min (0.50–0.84 mL/s)	25% decrease
	CrCl less than 30 mL/min (less than 0.50 mL/s)	Do not use
Carboplatin	Renal insufficiency	Total Dose = AUC × (CrCl [in mL/min] + 25)
Cisplatin	Use with caution in patients with CrCl less than 50 mL/min (less than 0.84 mL/s)	
Cyclophosphamide	Renal failure	Decrease dose 25%
Etoposide	Decrease in proportion to CrCl: 15–50 mL/min (0.25–0.84 mL/s)	Decrease dose 25%
Fludarabine, hydroxyurea	Use in caution in patients with CrCl less than 60 mL/min (less than 1.0 mL/s)	Decrease dose in proportion to CrCl
Ifosfamide	CrCl = 10–50 mL/min (0.17–0.84 mL/s)	Decrease dose 25%
	CrCl = less than 10 mL/min (less than 0.17 mL/s)	Decrease dose 50%
Methotrexate	Decrease in proportion to CrCl	80 mL/min (1.34 mL/s)–full dose
	Monitor levels closely in all patients receiving high-dose therapy (e.g., 150 mg/m² or greater)	80 mL/min (1.34 mL/s)–75%
		60 mL/min (1.00 mL/s)–63%
		50 mL/min (0.84 mL/s)–56%
		Less than 50 mL/min (less than 0.84 mL/s)–use alternative chemotherapy
Pentostatin	Dose in proportion to CrCl	
Streptozocin	Renal Failure	Decrease dose 50%–75%
Topotecan	CrCl 20–39 mL/min (0.33–0.65 mL/s)	Decrease dose 50%
	CrCl less than 20 ml/min (less than 0.33 mL/s)	Do not use

Adapted from DiPiro JT, Talbert RL, Yee GC, et al. (eds.) Pharmacotherapy: A Pathophysiologic Approach. 8th ed. New York: McGraw-Hill; 2011: Table 135-8.

Table 88–9

Empiric Dose Modifications for Patients with Hepatic Dysfunction

Anthracyclines	Bilirubin 1.2–3.0 mg/dL (20.5– 51.3 μmol/L)	Decrease dose 50%
	Bilirubin 3.1–5.0 mg/dL (53.0– 85.5 μmol/L)	Decrease dose 75%
	Bilirubin greater than 5.0 mg/dL (greater than 85.5 μmol/L)	Omit
Docetaxel	Bilirubin greater than ULN	Do not give
	AST or ALT greater than 1.5 ULN and	Do not give
	Alk Phos greater than 2.5 ULN	
Etoposide	Bilirubin 1.5–3.0 mg/dL (25.7– 51.3 μmol/L)	Decrease dose 50%
	Bilirubin 3.1–5.0 mg/dL (53.0– 85.5 μmol/L)	Omit
Imatinib	Bilirubin greater than 3 × ULN	Withhold until less than 1.5 ULN
Ixabepilone	As a monotherapy agent if AST or ALT greater than 10 × ULN or bilirubin greater than 3 × ULN	Contraindicated
	In combination with capecitabine AST or ALT greater than 2.5 × ULN or bilirubin greater than 1 × ULN	
Lapatinib	Child–Pugh class C hepatic dysfunction	Dose reduction to 750 mg/day
Paclitaxel	Use with caution in hepatic failure	
Thiotepa	Use with caution in hepatic failure	
Vinblastine, vincristine	Bilirubin 1.5–3.0 mg/dL (25.7–51.3 μmol/L)	Decrease dose 50%
	Bilirubin 3.1–5.0 mg/dL (53.0–85.5 μmol/L)	Omit
Vinorelbine	Bilirubin 2.1–3.0 mg/dL (35.9–51.3 μmol/L)	Decrease dose 50%
	Bilirubin greater than 3 mg/dL (51.3 μmol/L)	Decrease dose 75%

Adapted from DiPiro JT, Talbert RL, Yee GC, et al. (eds.) Pharmacotherapy: A Pathophysiologic Approach. 8th ed. New York: McGraw-Hill; 2011: Table 135-8.

Table 88–10

Oral Chemotherapy Administration with Respect to Food

	With Food	Empty Stomach	With or Without Food
Abiraterone		X	
Anastrozole			X
Bexarotene	X		
Bicalutamide			X
Capecitabine	X		
Crizotinib			X
Dasatinib			X
Erlotinib		X	
Estramustine			X
Etoposide			X
Everolimus			X
Exemestane	X		
Imatinib	X		
Lapatinib		X	
Lenalidomide			X
Letrozole			X
Nilotinib		X	
Nilutamide			X
Pazopanib		X	
Sorafenib		X	
Sunitinib			X
Tamoxifen			X
Temozolomide		X	
Thalidomide			X
Toremifene			X
Vandetanib			X
Vemurafenib			X
Vorinostat	X		

caregivers. Particular attention should be paid to educating patients on regimens given Monday through Friday only, daily times 4 weeks and then off 2 weeks. Patients should be encouraged to bring in oral medications with visits so adherence can be checked.

OUTCOME EVALUATION

Once a pathologic diagnosis of cancer is made, the patient may be evaluated by a radiation oncologist, a surgical oncologist, and a medical oncologist. Options for treatment are presented that may include surgery, radiation, chemotherapy biotherapy, or some combination of these modalities. The goals of treatment vary by the cancer and the stage of disease. For example, the patient who has metastatic kidney cancer could be presented with several options. They may have a possible cure with high-dose aldesleukin or receive palliative therapy with sorafenib or sunitinib, or the patient may decline any therapy because of fears of significant toxicity that would decrease quality of life. In this case, if the patient's performance status is poor, such as an ECOG performance status 3, then the patient would not be a candidate for aldesleukin therapy because of significant toxicity or even death from treatment. The patient with the poor performance status will receive palliative therapy to control symptoms of the disease to improve the quality of life at the end of life. For the patient with a poor performance status and extensive metastatic disease, no treatment of the cancer may be appropriate, and the patient may be enrolled in a hospice program or provided comfort care.

Patient Care and Monitoring

6 *Clinicians should play a role in chemotherapy safety, patient education, and monitoring patient response to therapy.*

Chemotherapy Administration

1. Evaluate the chemotherapy regimen to ensure the correct dose and route of administration.

2. Check patient laboratory values to ensure that the CBC and organ function studies are normal or within acceptable limits before administering chemotherapy.

3. If a patient has renal or hepatic impairment or a poor metabolizer genotype, adjust chemotherapy doses if necessary.

4. Ensure appropriate antiemetic therapy for the degree of emetogenicity.

5. Assess the regimen to determine if primary prophylaxis with colony-stimulating factors is needed.

6. Assess the patient's concurrent medications for the possibility of drug interactions and discontinue potentially interacting medications, if possible.

7. Use safe handling and disposal methods.

Monitoring

1. Efficacy:

   - Monitor CT scans or other imaging studies, and categorize patient with a complete response (CR), partial response (PR), stable disease (SD), or progressive disease.

2. Toxicity:

   - Monitor CBC and other laboratory tests

   - Monitor patient for other known toxicities of the chemotherapy regimen and decrease the dose or discontinue the regimen if necessary

Abbreviations Introduced in This Chapter

2-CDA	2-Chlorodeoxyadenosine
2-FLAA	2-Fluoro-Ara-AMP
5-FU	Fluorouracil
6-MP	6-Mercaptopurine
6-TG	6-Thioguanine
ADC	Antibody–drug conjugate
ALK	Anaplastic lymphoma kinase gene
ALL	Acute lymphocytic leukemia
AML	Acute myeloid leukemia
Ara-C	Cytarabine
ASCT	Autologous stem cell transplant
ATRA	All-trans-retinoic acid
AUC	Area under the-curve
CD	Cluster of differentiation
c-MET	Mesenchymal epithelial transition
CML	Chronic myeloid leukemia
CTC	Common toxicity criteria
CTLA-4	Cytotoxic T-lymphocytic-associated antigen 4
ECOG	Eastern Cooperative Oncology Group
EGFR	Epidermal growth factor receptor
FdUMP	Fluorodeoxyuridine monophosphate
GIST	Gastrointestinal stromal tumor
HER-2	Human epidermal receptor-2
HPV	Human papillomavirus
IL	Interleukin
LHRH	Luteinizing hormone releasing hormone
MMAE	Monomethyl auristatin E
NCI	National Cancer Institute
NSCLC	Non–small cell lung cancer
PCR	Polymerase chain reaction
PSA	Prostate Specific Antigen
TNM	Tumor, nodes, metastases
TPMT	Thiopurine S-methyltransferase
VEGFR	Vascular Epidermal Growth Factor Receptor

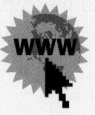 Self-assessment questions and answers are available at *http://www.mhpharmacotherapy. com/pp.html.*

REFERENCES

1. Jemal A, Murray T, Ward E, et al. Cancer Statistics, 2005. CA Cancer J Clin 2005;55(1):10-30.

2. American Cancer Society. Cancer Facts & Figures 2011. [Internet]. Atlanta: American Cancer Society; 2011 [cited 2011 Aug September 24]. Available from: http://www.cancer.org/research/cancerfactsfigures/index.

3. Sessions J, Valgus J, Barbour S, Iacovelli I. Role of Oncology clinical pharmacists in light of the oncology workforce study. J Oncol Pract 2010;6(5):270-272.

4. Schottenfeld D, Searle JG. The etiology and epidemiology of lung cancer. In: Pass HI, Carbone DP, Johnson DH, Minna JD, Turrisi AT, eds. Lung Cancer: Principles and Practice, 3rd ed. Philadelphia: Lippincott, Williams & Wilkins; 2005:3–24.

5. Blagosklonny MV. Molecular theory of cancer. Cancer Biol Ther 2005;4(6):621–627.

6. Buick RN. Cellular basis of chemotherapy. In: Dorr RT, Von Hoff DD, eds. Cancer Chemotherapy Handbook, 2nd ed. New York: Elsevier, 1994:3–14.

7. Folkman J. Angiogenesis. Annu Rev Med 2006;57:1–18.

8. Mountford CE, Doran S, Lean CL, Russell P. Cancer pathology in the year 2000. Biophys Chem 1997;68(1–3):127.

9. Chang S, Harshman L, Presti J. Impact of common medications on serum total prostate-specific antigen levels: Analysis of the National Health and Nutrition Examination Survey. J Clin Oncol 2010;28(5):3951–3957.

10. Eisenhauer E, Therasse P, Bogaerts J, et al. New response evaluation criteria in solid tumours: Revised RECIST guideline (version 1.1). Eur J Cancer 2009;45:228–247.

11. Paolo A, Danesi R, Vannozzi F, et al. Limited sampling model for the analysis of 5-fluorouracil pharmacokinetics in adjuvant chemotherapy for colorectal cancer. Clin Pharmacol Ther 2002;72:627–637.

12. Baydar M, Dikilitas M, Sevinc A, Aydogdu I. Prevention of oral mucositis due to 5-Fluorouracil treatment with oral cryotherapy. J Natl Med Assoc 2005;97(5):1161–1164.

13. Baker J, Royer G, Weiss R. Cytarabine and neurological toxicity. J Clin Oncol 1991;9(4):679–693.

14. Kantarjian H, Gandhi V, Cortes J, et al. Phase 2 clinical and pharmacologic study of clofarabine in patients with refractory or relapsed acute leukemia. Blood 2003;1202:2379–2386.

15. Villela LR, Stanford BL, Shah SR. Pemetrexed, a novel antifolate therapeutic alternative for cancer chemotherapy. Pharmacotherapy 2006;26(5):641–654.

16. American Society of Health-System Pharmacists. ASHP guidelines on preventing medication errors with antineoplastic agents. Am J Health Syst Pharm 2002;59:1648–1668.

17. Sparreboom A, Scripture CD, Trieu V, et al. Comparative preclinical and clinical pharmacokinetics of a Cremophor-free, nanoparticle albumin-bound paclitaxel (ABI-007) and paclitaxel formulated in Cremophor (Taxol). Clin Cancer Res 2005;11(11):4136–4143.

18. Cortes J, O'Shaughnessy J, Loesch D, et al. Eribulin monotherapy versus treatment of physician's choice in patients with metastatic breast cancer (EMBRACE): A phase 3 open-label randomised study. Lancet 2011;377(9769):914–923.

19. Hensley M, Hagerty K, Kewalramani T, et al. American Society of Clinical Oncology clinical practice guideline update: Use of chemotherapy and radiation therapy protectants. J Clin Oncol 2009;27(1):127–145.

20. Ormrod D, Holm K, Goa K, Spencer C. Epirubicin: A review of its efficacy as adjuvant therapy and in the treatment of metastatic disease in breast cancer. Drugs Aging 1999;5:389–416.

21. Faulds D, Balfour JA, Chrisp P, Langtry HD. Mitoxantrone: A review of its pharmacodynamic and pharmacokinetic properties, and therapeutic potential in the chemotherapy of cancer. Drugs 1991;41(3):400–449.

22. Rudek MA, Donehower RC, Statkevich P, et al. Temozolomide in patients with advanced cancer: Phase I and pharmacokinetic study. Pharmacotherapy 2004;24(1):16–25.

23. Calvert AH, Newell DR, Gumbrell LA, et al. Carboplatin dosage: Prospective evaluation of a simple formula based on renal function. J Clin Oncol 1989;7(11):1748–1756.

24. Graham MA, Lockwood GF, Greenshade D, et al. Clinical pharmacokinetics of oxaliplatin: A critical review. Clin Cancer Res 2000;6:1205–1218.

25. Dorr RT. Bleomycin pharmacology: Mechanism of action and resistance, and clinical pharmacokinetics. Semin Oncol 1992;19(2 suppl 5):3–8.

26. Zhi-Xiang S, Chen, G, Ni J, et al. Use of arsenic trioxide in the treatment of acute promyelocytic leukemia: II. Clinical efficacy and pharmacokinetics in relapsed patients. Blood 1997;89(9):3354–3360.

27. Avvisati G, Tallman MS. All-trans retinoic acid in acute promyelocytic leukaemia. Best Pract Res Clin Haematol 2003;16(3):419–432.

28. Wohl DA, Aweeka FT, Schmitz J, et al. Safety, tolerability, and pharmacokinetic effects of thalidomide in patients infected with human immunodeficiency virus: AIDS clinical trials group 267. J Infect Dis 2002;185:1359–1363.

29. Chen N, Lau H, Kong L, et al. Pharmacokinetics of lenalidomide in subjects with various degrees of renal impairment and in subjects on hemodialysis. J Clin Pharmacol 2007;47:1466–1475.

30. Dokmanovic M, Clarke C, Marks P. Histone deacetylase inhibitors: Overview and perspectives. Mol Cancer Res 2007;5:981–989.

31. Bouwhuis MG, Suciu S, Testori A, et al. Phase III trial comparing adjuvant treatment with pegylated interferon alfa-2b versus observation: prognostic significance of autoantibodies—EORTC 18991. J Clin Oncol 2010;28(14):2460–2466.

32. Kantoff P, Higano C, Shore N, et al. Sipuleucel-T immunotherapy for castration-resistant prostate cancer. N Eng J Med 2010;363(5):411–422.

33. Adcetris (Brentuximab) package insert. Bothell, WA: Seattle Genetics, 2011

34. Leyland-Jones B, Gelman K, Ayoub J, et al. Pharmacokinetics, safety, and efficacy of trastuzumab administered every three weeks in combination with paclitaxel. J Clin Oncol 2003;21:3965–3971.

35. Bolton AE, Peng B, Hubert M, et al. Effect of rifampicin on the pharmacokinetics of imatinib mesylate in healthy subjects. Cancer Chemother Pharmacol 2004;53(2):102–106.

36. Frye RF, Fitzgerald SM, Lagattuta TF, et al. Effect of St. John's Wort on imatinib mesylate pharmacokinetics. Clin Pharmacol Ther 2004;76(4):323–329.

37. Dutreix C, Peng B, Mehring G, et al. Pharmacokinetic interaction between ketoconazole and imatinib mesylate in healthy subjects. Cancer Chemother Pharmacol 2004;54(4):290–294.

38. O'Brien SG, Meinhardt P, Bond E, et al. Effects of imatinib mesylate on the pharmacokinetics of simvastatin, a cytochrome p450 3A4 substrate, in patients with chronic myeloid leukaemia. Br J Cancer 2003;89(3):1855–1859.

39. Singer JB, Shou Y, Giles F, et al. UGT1A1 promoter polymorphism increases risk of nilotinib-induced hyperbilirubinemia. Leukemia 2007;21(11):2311–2315.

40. Hamilton M, Wolf JL, Rusk J, et al. Effects of smoking on the pharmacokinetics of erlotinib. Clin Cancer Res 2006;12:2166–2171.

41. Chapman PB, Hauschild A, Robert C, et al. Improved survival with vemurafenib in melanoma with BRAF V600e mutation. N Eng J Med 2011;264(26):2507–2516.

42. Kwak EL, Bang YJ, Carnidge DR, et al. Anaplastic lymphoma kinase inhibition in non-small cell lung cancer. N Eng J Med 2010;363(18):1693–1703.

43. Firmagon (Degarelix) package insert. Parsippany, NJ: Ferring Pharmaceuticals, 2009.

44. Bono JS, Logothetis CJ, Molina A, et al. Abiraterone and increased survival in metastatic prostate cancer. N Eng J Med 2011;364(21):1995–2005.

45. Goetz MP, Knox SK, Suman VJ, et al. The impact of cytochrome P450 2D6 metabolism in women receiving adjuvant tamoxifen. Breast Cancer Res Treat 2007;101:113–121.

46. Gonzalez ID, Saez RS, Rodilla EM, Yges EL, Toledano FL. Hypersensitivity reactions to chemotherapy drugs. Allerg Immunol Clin 2000;15:151–181.

89

Breast Cancer

Gerald Higa

LEARNING OBJECTIVES

● **Upon completion of the chapter, the reader will be able to:**

1. List factors associated with an increased risk of breast cancer in the United States.

2. Assess patients for signs and symptoms related to breast cancer in early and late stages of the disease.

3. List all modalities that are appropriate screening tools for breast cancer and determine how they should best be used in the public domain.

4. Discuss available options for breast cancer prevention.

5. Critique available prognostic variables for clinical utility.

6. Determine which patient populations may benefit from systemic adjuvant therapy for breast cancer.

7. Determine the treatment goals for early stage, locally advanced, and metastatic breast cancer.

8. Determine appropriate indications for endocrine therapy, chemotherapy, and biologic therapy for patients with metastatic breast cancer.

9. Evaluate available chemotherapy options for patients with metastatic breast cancer based on pertinent patient and disease state characteristics.

10. Discuss the role of trastuzumab in the management of early and advanced stage breast cancer.

KEY CONCEPTS

❶ Breast cancer is the most common neoplasm diagnosed in American women, although the disease risk varies by ethnicity.

❷ Classic breast cancer risk factors, initially derived from epidemiologic studies, now include genetic and nongenetic components.

❸ Most patients diagnosed with breast cancer have early stage, and potentially curable, disease.

❹ Early breast cancer is now treated with less aggressive surgical procedures that involve the primary tumor and regional lymph nodes.

❺ The presence of two receptors, estrogen and HER2/neu, guides the application of systemic therapy for both early and advanced breast cancers.

❻ Appropriate application of adjuvant endocrine therapy with or without chemotherapy plus trastuzumab (if indicated) reduces the rates of relapse and death.

❼ Goals of therapy differ between early and metastatic breast cancer—cure in the former and preserving or improving quality of life in the latter.

❽ In the absence of acute life-threatening complications, initial therapy of estrogen receptor (ER)–positive advanced breast cancer is endocrine therapy.

❾ Approximately 50% to 60% of women who have not received prior chemotherapy for metastatic disease will respond to chemotherapy regimens; anthracycline- and taxane-containing regimens are the most active.

❿ Chemotherapy plus trastuzumab (if indicated) is the strategy of choice for ER-negative metastatic disease.

After a sharp increase in new breast cancer diagnoses during the early 1980s and a more modest rise during the latter half of the 1990s, the incidence of invasive disease has decreased slightly over the past 10 years.[1] Moreover, the 5-year survival rates has also improved significantly from 75% to 89% during the mid-1970s and 1996 to 2004, respectively. The latter finding is likely attributable to early detection and the development of effective treatment regimens. Treatment strategies for most breast cancer patients include surgical, radiologic, and pharmacologic therapies.

EPIDEMIOLOGY AND ETIOLOGY

Breast cancer is the most common type of cancer and is second only to lung cancer as a cause of cancer death in American women. In 2012 alone, an estimated 229,000 new cases of invasive breast cancer were diagnosed; and nearly 40,000 women died of complications of the disease.[1] The median age for the diagnosis of breast cancer is 63 years.[2] Notably, the annual incidence does not include approximately 40,000 patients diagnosed with DCIS or LCIS. ❶ *Although the disease occurs more frequently in white women than any other ethnic group, the mortality rate is highest among African Americans.*

Most breast cancers diagnosed are small (2 cm or less), with disease localized in all racial and ethnic groups. However, African American and other minority women have proportionally more cases of advanced disease compared with white women. The reason for the latter finding is believed to be related to barriers in access to care, reduced screening mammography and biological factors.

Although the etiology of breast cancer is largely unknown, a number of factors that increase the risk of developing the disease have been identified. ❷ *Additionally, information regarding breast cancer biology suggests that a complex interplay exists among one's sex hormones, genetic factors, environment, and lifestyle. These external and internal factors contribute to the pathogenesis of disease.*

The two variables most strongly associated with the development of breast cancer are gender and age. Although breast cancer is a disease primarily of women, about 1% of the total incidence occur in men.[1] When the stage and other known prognostic factors are controlled for, men have similar treatments and prognoses as women.

The incidence of breast cancer increases with advancing age. Perhaps the most frequently quoted breast cancer statistic is that one in seven women will develop the disease sometime during her lifetime. It should be emphasized that this is a cumulative lifetime risk from birth to 110 years of age and that the estimates are weighted by the probability of surviving through each decade of life.[3] Feuer and colleagues developed a more useful method of presenting the risk data based on age intervals.[3] As Table 89–1 demonstrates, the risk of a woman developing breast cancer before the age of 40 years is about one in 250. It is apparent from this table that although the cumulative probability of developing breast cancer increases with age, more than half the risk occurs after the age of 60 years. It is also important to note that the cysts found it fibrocystic breast disease do not develop into breast cancer. As many as 85% of American women have "lumpy breasts," which are typically benign cysts and may have a clinical diagnosis of fibrocystic or benign breast disease. Data suggest that this condition is not typically associated with an increased risk for developing breast cancer.[4] However, it must be noted that "lumpy breasts" may delay a diagnosis of breast cancer because of an inability of the patient or physician to detect a true malignant lesion.

Table 89–1	
Risk of Developing Breast Cancer: SEER Areas, Women, All Races, 1998 to 2000	
Age Interval (years)	**Probability (%) of Developing Invasive Breast Cancer During the Interval**
30–40	0.40 or 1 in 250
40–50	1.45 or 1 in 69
50–60	2.78 or 1 in 36
60–70	3.81 or 1 in 26
From birth to death	13.51 or 1 in 7

SEER, Surveillance, Epidemiology and End Results.

From Ries LAG, Eisner MP, Kosary CL, et al. SEER Cancer Statistics Review, 1975–2001. Bethesda, MD, National Cancer Institute. 2004, *http://seer.cancer.gov/csr/1975-2001.*

Endocrine Factors

❷ *A number of endocrine factors have been linked to an increased risk for breast cancer.*[5,6] Many of the risks relate to the total duration of estrogen exposure. Hence, early menarche (before age 12 years) and late menopause (after age 55 years) are associated with an increased risk of the disease. Support for this belief is the finding that bilateral oophorectomy before age 35 years decreases the relative risk of developing breast cancer.[5,6] Nulliparity and a late age at first birth (30 years or older) have been reported to increase the lifetime risk of developing breast cancer twofold.[5,6]

Long-term use of hormone replacement therapy and concurrent use of progestins appear to contribute to breast cancer risk.[7] Use of postmenopausal estrogen replacement therapy in women with a history of breast cancer is generally contraindicated. However, most experts believe that the safety and benefits of low-dose oral contraceptives currently outweigh the potential risks and that changes in the prescribing practice for the use of oral contraceptives are not warranted. Oral contraceptives are known to reduce the risk of ovarian cancer by about 40% and the risk of endometrial cancer by about 60%.

Genetic Factors

❷ *Both personal and family histories influence a woman's risk of developing breast cancer.* A medical history of breast cancer is associated with about a fivefold increased risk of contralateral breast cancer. Cancer of the uterus and ovary also has been associated with an increased risk of developing breast cancer.

For some time, it has been recognized that a family history of breast cancer is strongly associated with a woman's risk for developing the disease. The percentage of all breast cancers in the population that are attributed to family history ranges between 6% and 12%.[8] Empirical estimates of the risks associated with particular patterns of family history of breast cancer indicate the following:

1. Having any first-degree relative (i.e., mother or sister) with breast cancer increases the risk up to threefold, depending on age.

2. The relative risk is even higher if the first-degree relative was diagnosed with breast cancer at an age younger than 45 years.

3. Having multiple first-degree relatives affected has been inconsistently associated with elevated risks.

4. Having a second-degree relative with breast cancer increases the risk of developing breast cancer by approximately 50% (relative risk, 1.5).

5. Affected family members on the maternal side and the paternal side contribute similarly to the risk.

② *In the early 1990s, the* BRCA1 *gene on the long arm of chromosome 17 (17q21) was identified as abnormal in a large percentage of hereditary breast and ovarian cancer patients.*[9,10] A second breast cancer gene, called BRCA2, has been mapped to chromosome 13. Both *BRCA1* and *BRCA2* are tumor suppressors. A woman with a strong family history of breast or ovarian cancer, or both, who carries a germ-line mutation of *BRCA1* faces roughly an 85% lifetime risk of breast cancer and a 60% risk of ovarian cancer.[11] Carriers of the *BRCA2* mutation have similar risks for breast cancer but much lower risks for ovarian cancer. Jewish people of Eastern European descent (Ashkenazi Jews) have an unusually high (2.5%) carrier rate of germ-line mutations in *BRCA1* and *BRCA2* compared with the rest of the U.S. population.

Women with a strong family history of breast cancer are candidates for genetic testing. A genetic test that evaluates for *BRCA1* and *BRCA2* mutations is commercially available and should be done under the guidance of a genetic counselor. It is recommended for high-risk carriers of *BRCA1* and *BRCA2* mutations to undergo an oophorectomy at completion of childbearing. Bilateral total mastectomy does reduce the risk of breast cancer occurrence; however, both breast and ovarian cancer have been reported in patients who have had prophylactic removal of these organs. It is recommended for *BRCA* carriers who do not opt for surgical prophylaxis to have mammography every 6 months. Carriers may also consider tamoxifen therapy.

Environmental and Lifestyle Factors

② *Experimental and epidemiologic evidence suggests an association between breast cancer and the Western diet (high in calories, fat, and cooked meats). Obesity in postmenopausal women and distribution of body fat around the abdominal region also appear to increase the risk of breast cancer.* A recent meta-analysis[12] indicates both a modest positive association between alcohol ingestion and breast cancer in a dose–response relationship. Cigarette smoking and augmentation mammoplasty do not appear to increase the risk of breast cancer. Exercise may provide modest protection against breast cancer[12].

Radiation, an environmental risk factor, is associated with an increased risk of breast cancer in survivors of the atomic bomb, patients given radiation for postpartum mastitis, women receiving multiple fluoroscopic examinations during therapy for tuberculosis, and patients who receive mediastinal radiation for malignancies. Interestingly, this risk appears to be confined to radiation exposure before age 40 years, which suggests that a "window of initiation" for breast cancer occurs at a relatively early age. Exposure to diagnostic x-rays, including annual screening mammography, does not impart a sufficient dose of radiation for clinical concern.

It should be emphasized that more than 60% of women with breast cancer have no identifiable major risk factor, indicating that the search for the etiology of this disease is largely incomplete.

A number of calculators are available on the Internet to estimate a patient's risk of developing breast cancer. The National Cancer Institute (NCI) has an online version of the Breast Cancer Risk Assessment Tool that is considered to be the most authoritative and accurate standard (*www.cancer.gov/bcrisk-tool*). The Breast Cancer Risk Assessment Tool was designed for health professionals to project a women's individualized risk for invasive breast cancer over a 5-year period and over her lifetime.

PATHOPHYSIOLOGY

The pathologic evaluation of breast lesions serves to establish histologic diagnosis and confirm the presence or absence of other factors believed to influence prognosis. These **prognostic factors** include the presence of necrosis, lymphatic or vascular invasion, nuclear grade, hormone receptor status, proliferative index, amount of aneuploidy, and *HER-2/neu* gene amplification or protein expression.

Invasive Carcinoma

Invasive breast cancers are a histologically heterogeneous group of lesions. Most breast carcinomas are adenocarcinomas and are classified on the basis of their microscopic appearance as ductal or lobular, corresponding to the ducts and lobules of the normal breast. The various histologic types of breast cancer have different prognoses, but it is unknown whether their response to therapy differs because patients in therapeutic trials typically are not stratified according to histologic type. Infiltrating lobular carcinoma commonly metastasizes to meningeal and serosal surfaces, whereas ductal carcinomas usually metastasize to the bone, brain, or liver.

Noninvasive Carcinoma

As with invasive carcinoma, the noninvasive lesions may be divided broadly into ductal and lobular categories. During the past decade, the widespread use of screening mammography and subsequent biopsy, coupled with recognition of noninvasive breast carcinoma by pathologists, has resulted in a significant increase in diagnosis of in situ breast cancer. A detailed discussion of the biology and appropriate management of noninvasive breast cancer is beyond the scope of this chapter, but some of the more salient characteristics of ductal carcinoma in situ (DCIS) and lobular carcinoma in situ (LCIS) are described below, and readers are referred to a number of excellent reviews for a more comprehensive discussion.[13,14]

DCIS is diagnosed more frequently than LCIS. Simple or total mastectomy (without lymph node dissection) has been the standard treatment of DCIS for several decades. Breast conservation (i.e., wide local excision followed by irradiation of breast tissue) may be an effective alternative to mastectomy. Although radiation following lumpectomy does not appear to change the survival rate of patients with DCIS, it significantly reduces the incidence of local recurrences and enhances the breast preservation rate in these women. Axillary dissection generally is not indicated because there is only a 1% incidence of axillary node involvement. There is currently no proven benefit for the use of cytotoxic chemotherapy in patients who receive local therapy for DCIS. However, subgroups of patients with DCIS, such as hormone receptor-positive patients, may benefit from the addition of tamoxifen to lumpectomy plus radiation.[15]

CLINICAL PRESENTATION AND DIAGNOSIS

Prevention and Early Detection

Current efforts at breast cancer prevention are directed toward the identification and removal of risk factors. Unfortunately, a number of risk factors associated with the development of breast cancer, such as family history of breast cancer or personal history of breast or other gynecologic malignancies, cannot be modified. Isolation and cloning of breast cancer susceptibility genes allow screening of women with histories suggestive of "breast cancer families" and identification of appropriate candidates for prophylactic bilateral mastectomy. Currently, no absolute indications for prophylactic bilateral mastectomy exist. This surgery is

considered for high risk, particularly if the woman's breasts are difficult to evaluate by both physical examination and mammography and if she presents with persistent, disabling fears of breast cancer diagnosis.

The idea that prevention can be achieved pharmacologically is based on clinical trials of tamoxifen, an antiestrogen used as adjuvant therapy for early breast cancer. These trials demonstrate reduced development of contralateral breast cancer and a survival advantage in women who received tamoxifen for 2 to 5 years following mastectomy.[16–18] Several clinical trials were conducted with tamoxifen, which provided proof of principle that breast cancer risk reduction could be achieved through chemoprevention.[19–21] A recent meta-analysis of these trials indicates a consistent (and significant) benefit in reducing the risk of developing estrogen receptor (ER)–positive breast cancers in premenopausal and postmenopausal women.[22]

Patient Encounter, Part 1

In September 2005, AD, a 41-year-old business executive mother of two girls, ages 11 and 9 years, had a routine screening mammography. Upon radiographic review, an amorphous abnormality is seen in the upper outer quadrant of the right breast. Fine-needle aspirate of the abnormal area was performed the following day. Frozen section of the specimen indicated hyperplastic changes of ductal epithelial cells. Diagnosis was confirmed on complete pathologic review.

Plan: Repeat the mammogram in 6 months.

What factors are relevant when screening for any disease?

Why is close surveillance necessary in this patient?

Clinical Presentation and Diagnosis of Breast Cancer

Common early signs and symptoms include:

- Painless lump (90% of cases) that is:
  - Solitary
  - Unilateral
  - Solid
  - Hard
  - Irregular
  - Nontender
- Stabbing or aching pain (10% of cases) as the first symptom

Uncommon early signs and symptoms include:

- Nipple discharge (3% of women and 20% of men), retraction, or dimpling

- Eczema appearance of the nipple (Paget's carcinoma)
- Prominent skin edema, redness, warmth, and induration of the underlying tissue (inflammatory carcinoma)

Metastatic signs and symptoms—tissues most commonly involved with metastases are lymph nodes (other than axillary or internal mammary), skin, bone, liver, lungs, and brain. The following symptoms of metastases will be present in about 10% of patients when they first seek treatment:

- Bone pain
- Difficulty breathing
- Abdominal enlargement
- Jaundice
- Mental status changes

Table 89–2

Guidelines for Early Detection of Breast Cancer

	American Cancer Society[18]	U.S. Preventive Services Task Force[19]	National Cancer Institute[20]
BSE	Age 20 years and older: Risk-to-benefit discussion	All ages: NR	NR
CBE	Age 20 to 30 years: Every 3 years Age 40 years and older: Every year	All ages: ± (recommended with mammography)	All ages: Every year
Mammography	Age 40 years and older: Interval not designated	Age 50 years or older: Every 1–2 years (with or without CBE)	Age 40–49: Every 1–2 years Age 50 years and older: Every 1–2 years

±, insufficient data to recommend for or against; BSE, breast self-examination; CBE, clinical breast examination; NR, not recommended.

However, results of the prevention trials also confirmed the increased incidence of tamoxifen-induced endometrial cancer. Because this outcome could have a direct impact on patient acceptance of chemoprevention, a search began for an agent with a better safety profile. A compound related to tamoxifen known as raloxifene was found to reduce the incidence of spinal fractures in postmenopausal women at high risk for osteoporosis.[23] Raloxifene is also an antiestrogen, so its effects on breast and endometrial tissue were closely monitored. After 3 years of raloxifene therapy, investigators found a significant decrease in the incidence of breast cancer without the carcinogenic effect on the endometrium.[24]

The Study of Tamoxifen and Raloxifene (STAR) trial compared the two agents in postmenopausal women who were considered to be at increased risk (as determined by the Gail model)[25] for developing invasive breast cancer.[26] Although there was a similar reduction in the incidence of breast cancer, raloxifene had a superior safety profile with regards to uterine cancer and thromboembolic events. Thus, raloxifene is the chemopreventive agent of choice for high-risk postmenopausal women. Because premenopausal women were not included in the STAR trial, tamoxifen is the only agent approved for reducing the risk of breast cancer in younger patients.

The impressive data of the aromatase inhibitors (AIs) in the adjuvant setting provided the rationale and impetus for studying their potential as breast cancer chemoprevention agents. Exemestane is more effective than placebo in reducing the risk of breast cancer in high risk postmenopausal women, although it has not been compared with either tamoxifen or raloxifene. Based on indirect comparisons with tamoxifen and raloxifene, cardiovascular and endometrial toxicity with exemestane may be less, with hot flashes and arthralgias reported most frequently.[27]

The rationale for early detection of breast cancer is based on the clear relationship between stage of breast cancer at diagnosis and probability of cure. Thus, if breast cancer is detected at a very early stage (i.e., small primary tumor and negative lymph nodes), then conceivably more patients with the disease could be cured. Screening guidelines for early detection of breast cancer have been put forward by the American Cancer Society, the United States Preventive

Services Task Force (USPSTF), and the NCI[28-30] (Table 89–2). All include recommendations for women at average risk, with some general statements regarding screening for high-risk women as well. Nearly 75% of all breast cancer occurs in women 50 years of age or older, and regular use of screening mammography can reduce mortality from breast cancer by 20% to 40% in this age group. Controversy regarding the use of screening mammography is largely confined to women younger than 50 years of age. After many years of debate, three organizations recommended mammograms in this age group of women every 1 to 2 years except for the USPSTF, which modified its recommendation in 2009.[28-31]

Patient Encounter, Part 2

HPI: In August of 2006, AD returns for her biannual mammogram. The abnormal area previously visualized appears to be calcified with the lesion measuring 1.2 cm. An ultrasound-guided core biopsy of the lesion was performed the following day. Frozen section of the specimen indicated dysplastic changes with focal nests of neoplastic cells invading the ducts. Pathological review of the tissue sample confirmed a diagnosis of invasive intraductal breast cancer.

PMH: No comorbid medical problems; oral contraceptives between 19 and 24 years of age and for the past 5 years.

FH: Mother with breast cancer at age 45 years (succumbed to disease 2 years after initial diagnosis). Father is alive.

Plan: Discuss management of the cancer with the multidisciplinary breast cancer team.

Is hyperplasia one of the steps in the tumorigenic process?

What are the patient's risk factors for developing breast cancer?

What issues should be considered regarding testing for BRCA1 and BRCA2 mutations in this patient? In her two daughters?

Diagnosis

The initial workup for a woman presenting with signs or symptoms suggestive of breast cancer should include a careful history, physical examination of the breast, three-dimensional mammography, and possibly other imaging techniques such as magnetic resonance imaging. Most (80% to 85%) breast cancers are visualized on a mammogram as a mass, a cluster of calcifications, or a combination of both. A breast biopsy is indicated for a mammographic abnormality that suggests malignancy or for a palpable mass on physical examination.

Clinical Staging

Stage (anatomic extent of disease) is defined on the basis of the primary tumor size (T_{1-4}), presence and extent of lymph node involvement (N_{1-3} or pN_{1-3} if pathologic examination of lymph nodes is conducted), and presence or absence of distant metastases (M_{0-1}) (Table 89–3). For a more complete description of the **staging** system, readers are referred to the guidelines.[32] Although many possible combinations of T and N are possible within a given stage, simplistically, stage 0

Table 89–3

Tumor, Nodes, Metastasis Stage Grouping for Breast Cancer

Stage Grouping

0	T_{is}	N_0	M_0
I	$T_1{}^a$	N_0	M_0
IIA	$T_0{}^a$	N_1	M_0
	$T_1{}^a$	N_1	M_0
	T_2	N_0	M_0
IIB	T_2	N_1	M_0
	T_3	N_0	M_0
IIIA	$T_0{}^a$	N_2	M_0
	$T_1{}^a$	N_2	M_0
	T_2	N_2	M_0
	T_3	N_1	M_0
	T_3	N_2	M_0
IIIB	T_4	N_0	M_0
	T_4	N_1	M_0
	T_4	N_2	M_0
IIIC	Any T	N_3	M_0
IV	Any T	Any N	M_1

T_0, no evidence of tumor; T_{is}, carcinoma in situ or Paget's disease of the nipple with no tumor; T_1, less than or equal to 2 cm; T_2, greater than 2 to 5 cm; T_3, greater than 5 cm; T_4, any size; direct extension to chest wall (excluding pectoral muscle) or skin infiltration; regional lymph nodes (N); N_x, regional lymph nodes cannot be assessed (e.g., previously removed); N_0, no regional lymph node metastasis; pN, metastasis in one to three lymph nodes; N_2, metastasis in four to nine lymph nodes; N_3, metastasis in 10 or more lymph nodes; metastasis (M); M_0, no distant metastases; M_1, distant metastasis.

^{a}T_1 includes T_1mic tumor (T).

Adapted with permission of the American Joint Committee on Cancer (AJCC), Chicago, IL. The original source for this material is the AJCC Cancer Staging Manual, 6th ed. Published by Springer-Verlag New York, 2002.

Table 89–4

Estimated Stage at Presentation and 5-Year Disease-Free Survival (DFS): Breast Cancer

	Percentage of Total Cases	5-Year DFS^a (%)
Stage I	40	70–90
Stage II	40	50–70
Stage III	15	20–30
Stage IV	5	0–10^b

^{a}With current conventional local and systemic therapy.

^{b}Patients in stage IV are rarely free of disease; however, 10% to 20% of these patients may survive with minimal disease for 5 to 10 years.

---

represents carcinoma in situ (T_{is}) or disease that has not invaded the basement membrane. Stage I represents small primary tumor without lymph node involvement, and the majority of stage II disease involves regional lymph nodes. Stages I and II are often referred to as early breast cancer. It is in these early stages that the disease is curable. Stage III, also referred to as locally advanced disease, usually represents a large tumor with extensive nodal involvement in which either node or tumor is fixed to the chest wall. Stage IV disease is characterized by the presence of metastases to organs distant from the primary tumor and is often referred to as advanced or metastatic disease, as described earlier. Most cancer today presents in early stages, when prognosis is favorable (Table 89–4).

Prognostic Factors

A number of potential prognostic factors have been identified for breast cancer. *Prognostic factors* are biological or clinical indicators associated with survival independent of therapy. Poor prognostic factors include:

- *Age* younger than 35 years
- *Larger tumor size*
- *High nuclear grade* signifies that a tumor is growing quickly
- *Lymph node involvement*
- *Negative tumor receptor status (i.e., ER-, PR-, and HER2-)*
- *Over-expression of HER-2/neu*

EARLY BREAST CANCER

TREATMENT

Desired Outcome

❸ *Most patients presenting with breast cancer today have an in situ tumor, a small tumor with negative lymph nodes (stage I), or a stage II cancer. The goal of therapy in early breast cancer is cure.* Surgery alone can cure most, if not all, patients with in situ cancers and approximately half of all patients with stage II cancers.

Nonpharmacologic Local-Regional Therapy

Surgical procedures have changed drastically over the past 50 years. ❹ *Less aggressive surgical options for early invasive breast cancer include the modified radical mastectomy (also termed total mastectomy with ipsilateral axillary lymph node dissection) and breast conservation.* In the modified radical mastectomy, the pectoralis minor muscle may be excised, divided, or left intact; more important, there may be variation in the extent of axillary lymph node dissection, ranging from sampling to full dissection. It is important to note that in the elderly patients with comorbid conditions, patients with particularly favorable tumors, or patients whose adjuvant therapy would not be affected by node status, axillary dissection is an optional. Breast conservation consists of lumpectomy, also referred to as segmental or partial mastectomy, and is defined as excision of the primary tumor and adjacent breast tissue followed by radiation therapy to reduce the risk of local recurrence. Removal of level I/II axillary lymph nodes is recommended for completeness of staging and prognostic information. The National Institutes of Health (NIH) Consensus Conference on the Treatment of Early-Stage Breast Cancer addressed the roles of modified radical mastectomy versus breast conservation and concluded that primary therapy for breast cancer stages I and II should be breast conservation.[33] The reason for favoring breast conservation therapy is that it achieves similar results to more extensive surgical procedures and cosmetically superior. Additionally, breast conservation helps to preserve a woman's emotional and psychological well-being.

In most instances, external-beam radiation therapy used in conjunction with breast-conserving procedures involves 4 to 6 weeks of therapy directed to eradicate residual disease. Complications associated with radiation therapy are minor and include erythema of the breast tissue and subsequent shrinkage of total breast mass beyond that predicted on the basis of breast tissue removal alone. Some clinical situations also require postmastectomy radiation therapy as well (see section on locally advanced breast cancer).

Several contraindications to breast conservation must be considered when selecting patients:

- Multiple sites of cancer within the breast
- Pregnancy (patient cannot receive radiation)
- Inability to attain negative pathologic margins on the excised breast specimen
- Preexisting collagen vascular diseases (e.g., scleroderma, systemic lupus erythematosus)
- Diffuse malignant-appearing microcalcifications on mammography
- Prior radiation treatment to the breast or chest wall
- Large tumor volume in a woman with small breasts (better cosmetic results often can be obtained with mastectomy and reconstruction).

The importance of stage I/II axillary dissection is being challenged. Although highly accurate, its morbidity rate is significant, with rates of acute complication and chronic lymphedema of 20% to 30%.[34,35] Across the United States, a new procedure involving lymphatic mapping and sentinel lymph node biopsy is becoming more acceptable at many academic centers.[36] The sentinel lymph node is the first lymph node that drains a cancer. Injection of a dye around the primary breast tumor results in identification of the sentinel lymph node in the majority of patients, and the status of this lymph node may predict the status of the remaining nodes in the nodal basin. A sentinel lymph node can be identified in 90% of patients and can accurately predict the status of the remaining axillary nodes in 95% of patients.[37]

Pharmacologic Systemic Adjuvant Therapy

Unfortunately, breast cancer cells often spread by contiguity, lymph channels, and through the blood to distant sites. This often occurs early in cancer growth, and deposits of tumor cells form in distant sites (micrometastases) that cannot be detected with current diagnostic methods and equipment. *Systemic adjuvant therapy* is defined as the administration of systemic therapy following definitive local therapy (i.e., surgery, radiation, or a combination of these) when there is no evidence of metastatic disease but a high likelihood of disease recurrence. ❺❻ *Most published results confirm that chemotherapy (in all patients) and hormonal therapy (in patients with hormone receptor–positive disease) or chemotherapy plus trastuzumab (if tumor is HER2 positive) result in improved disease-free survival (DFS) and/or overall survival (OS) for patients with early-stage breast cancer.*

A standard approach was formalized at the NIH's 2000 Consensus Development Conference on adjuvant therapy for breast cancer.[33] The panel recommended the consideration of adjuvant hormonal therapy for women whose tumors contain hormone receptor protein regardless of age, menopausal status, involvement of axillary lymph nodes, or tumor size. They also recommended that adjuvant chemotherapy be given for essentially all patients with lymph node metastases or breast tumors 1 cm or larger in size.[33]

Another group, the St. Gallen expert panel, is convened every 2 years to review new information and establish evidence-based recommendations regarding the treatment of patients with early breast cancer.[38] In 2007, the panel

---

Table 89–5

St. Gallen Risk Classification and Therapy Recommendations

Risk Classification	Low Risk	Intermediate Risk	High Risk
Tumor and patient criteria	Node negative (and all of the following):	1–3 nodes involved with tumor and HER-2 negative	Greater than 4 nodes involved with tumor
	ER/PR positive; *HER-2* negative; 2 cm or smaller in size; grade 1; no vascular invasion; 35 years of age or older	*or* Node negative (and at least one of the following): *HER-2* overexpressed greater than 2 cm in size; grade greater than 1; presence of vascular invasion; younger than 35 years of age	*or* 1–3 nodes involved with tumor and *HER-2* positive
Adjuvant therapy	Endocrine or no therapy	Endocrine responsive: Endocrine therapy or chemotherapy followed by endocrine therapy; add trastuzumab if *HER-2* positive	Endocrine responsive or uncertain: Chemotherapy followed by endocrine therapy; add trastuzumab if *HER-2* positive
		Endocrine uncertain: Chemotherapy followed by endocrine therapy; add trastuzumab if *HER-2* positive	Endocrine nonresponsive: Chemotherapy; add trastuzumab if *HER-2* positive
		Endocrine nonresponsive: Chemotherapy; add trastuzumab if *HER-2* positive	

From Morrow M, Harris JR. Local management of invasive breast cancer. In: Diseases of the Breast, 2nd ed. Lippincott Philadelphia, Williams & Wilkins, 2000:515–560.

endorsed the concept and definition of "endocrine-responsive" tumors, as well as the classification of patients into three risk groups. Tumors are categorized as endocrine responsive (10% or greater number of ER-positive tumor cells), endocrine nonresponsive (0% ER-positive tumor cells), and endocrine responsive uncertain (1% to 9% ER-positive tumor cells). Risk classification is based on a number of tumor and patient characteristics with the regional lymph node status being the major criterion. The most prominent recommendation in 2007 was the addition of adjuvant trastuzumab for all patients with HER-2/neu overexpressing tumors. A summary of risk classification and therapy recommendations is provided in Table 89–5.

The National Comprehensive Cancer Network (NCCN) also has developed practice guidelines for the treatment of early breast cancer.[39] These guidelines recommend, though the prognosis of patients with tumors 1 cm or smaller and negative or micro tumor–involved nodes is generally good, the decision to use trastuzumab must consider the relative clinical benefits and drug-associated toxicities. Additionally, adjuvant trastuzumab should be given for at least 1 year in the absence of treatment-limiting toxicity. Finally, the use of preoperative (*neoadjuvant*) systemic therapy is gaining favor in both early stage and locally advanced breast cancers. When used before surgery, treatments incorporating trastuzumab should be given for at least 9 weeks before the operation is performed.

Although neoadjuvant therapy most often consists of cytotoxic chemotherapy, hormonal agents may be preferable in patients with significant comorbidities. Nonetheless, this strategy can be used to determine tumor response in vivo (an important prognostic indicator) as well as

minimize the amount of breast tissue resected. Although this approach to therapy generally is reserved for patients with inoperable tumors (locally advanced), early-stage breast cancer patients who meet the criteria for breast-conserving therapy, excluding tumor size, may be considered for preoperative systemic therapy.

▶ Adjuvant Chemotherapy

⑥ *Cytotoxic drugs that have been used most frequently in combination as adjuvant therapy of breast cancer include doxorubicin, epirubicin, cyclophosphamide, paclitaxel, docetaxel, methotrexate, and fluorouracil.* The most common chemotherapy regimens used in the adjuvant and metastatic settings are listed in Table 89–6. The dose-limiting toxicities and other significant toxicities are listed for each chemotherapeutic agent in Table 89–7.

The basic principle of adjuvant therapy for any cancer type is that the regimen with the highest response rate in advanced disease should be the optimal regimen for use in the adjuvant setting. Theoretically, early administration of effective combination chemotherapy at a time when the tumor burden is low should increase the likelihood of cure and minimize the emergence of drug-resistant tumor cell clones. Anthracyclines (e.g., doxorubicin and epirubicin) historically have been referred to as the most active class of chemotherapy agents in the treatment of metastatic breast cancer. This has led to the assumption that anthracycline-containing regimens are associated with a higher cure rate than non–anthracycline-containing regimens.

The taxanes (e.g., paclitaxel and docetaxel) are a relatively newer class of agents that rival the anthracyclines in their

Patient Encounter, Part 4

HPI: Staging workup for the patient AD thus far included bone and CT scans, which were negative for objective evidence of distant disease. Liver function tests were normal. After presenting all of the information to the patient, it was decided (with the patient's concurrence) that management of the cancer would include surgery followed by external beam radiation, then systemic adjuvant therapy. Ten days after the diagnosis, a lumpectomy was performed with surgical margins free of tumor. The tumor measured 1.7 cm at its greatest dimension. Sentinel node biopsy was positive for tumor. Tumor ER and PR were both positive; HER2 gene amplification was negative by FISH. *BRCA1* and *BRACA2* mutations were present.

Plan: Complete staging and plans for managing the patient.

What is the stage of the breast cancer in this patient?

What would be the rationale for giving systemic adjuvant therapy?

If systemic therapy is used, what agents should this patient receive?

When should endocrine therapy begin?

Is there a role for oophorectomy in this patient?

Should the patient receive zoledronic acid?

activity in metastatic breast cancer, becoming the most active class of chemotherapy for this disease.

Although the optimal duration of adjuvant chemotherapy administration is unknown, it appears to be 12 to 24 weeks depending on the adjuvant regimen. Chemotherapy is usually initiated within 3 weeks of surgical removal of the primary tumor. Dose intensity and dose density appear to be critical factors in achieving optimal outcomes in adjuvant breast cancer therapy. *Dose intensity* is defined as the amount of drug administered per unit of time and typically is reported in milligrams per square meter of body surface area per week (mg/m²/wk). Increasing dose, decreasing time, or both can increase the dose intensity. *Dose density* is equivalent to the concept of increasing dose intensity by decreasing the time between treatment cycles. Reducing the dose for standard treatment regimens should be avoided unless necessitated by severe toxicity. On the other hand, increasing doses beyond those contained in standard treatment regimens does not appear to add benefit because there is a threshold for dosing adjuvant chemotherapy above which only additional toxicity is seen without any improvement in patient outcomes. The short-term toxic effects of chemotherapy used in the adjuvant setting generally are well tolerated. Although a number of investigators have demonstrated a reduction in quality of life, most patients are able to maintain a reasonable level of functional, emotional, and social well-being during treatment.[40] In general, supportive therapy of the patient receiving systemic adjuvant chemotherapy has improved in the past decade. Increased attention to the impact of symptoms on quality of life may account for some of this improvement. In addition, antiemetics that block serotonin and substance P have become available to assist in managing chemotherapy-induced nausea and vomiting, and colony-stimulating factors often are helpful in preventing febrile neutropenia, particularly in elderly patients or patients receiving dose-dense chemotherapy regimens. A number of side effects are common with the regimens used, and patients should be counseled appropriately regarding the likelihood of alopecia, weight gain, and fatigue. Patients who are menstruating usually experience a cessation of menses that may or may not return. Along with cessation of menses are accompanying signs and symptoms of menopause. Deep vein thrombosis has been reported in women receiving combination chemotherapy regimens.[41] A recent study estimated that 1–10 of 10,000 patients treated for 6 months with cyclophosphamide-based regimens are expected to have leukemia within 10 years of diagnosis of breast cancer.[42] Cardiomyopathy induced by doxorubicin occurs less than 1% of the time in women whose total dose of doxorubicin is less than 320 mg/m².[43] It should be noted that epirubicin in the adjuvant setting is given at a dose of 100 to 120 mg/m².[44] At this dose, epirubicin has an equal chance of causing cardiomyopathy as standard doxorubicin doses when both agents are given as bolus or short infusions. Taxanes often are associated with hypersensitivity reactions, peripheral neuropathy, and/or myalgias and arthralgias for a few days following the infusion.

It is important to note that the magnitude of survival benefit for chemotherapy appears to be small, with an absolute reduction in the mortality rate of only 5% at 10 years for patients with negative axillary lymph nodes and 10% for patients with positive axillary lymph nodes. Regardless, it has been reported that most patients with early breast cancer would accept drug-related toxicities to achieve the modest overall benefits.[45,46] Because the risks are not insignificant, investigators have been searching for ways to identify patients who could avoid chemotherapy without altering the disease prognosis. Recently, three potential gene expression assays (e.g., Oncotype DX, MammaPrint, and H/I) have become commercially available. Of the three, Oncotype DX provides the strongest evidence that a subset of patients, especially those with ER-positive, lymph node–negative tumors, derive little or no benefit from adjuvant chemotherapy when compared with the use of hormonal therapy alone.[47] Newer data suggest this is also true for patients with lymph node–positive disease.[48] In essence, genomic analyses may play an important role in improving risk stratification and determining chemotherapy benefit.[49]

▶ Adjuvant Biologic Therapy

Trastuzumab is a monoclonal antibody directed against the HER-2/neu receptor. HER-2/neu is a member of the erbB (or HER) growth factor receptor family and is expressed

Table 89–6

Common Chemotherapy Regimens for Breast Cancer

Adjuvant Chemotherapy Regimens

AC

Doxorubicin 60 mg/m^2 IV, day 1

Cyclophosphamide 600 mg/m^2 IV, day 1

Repeat cycles every 21 days for 4 cycles[a]

FAC[w]

Fluorouracil 500 mg/m^2 IV, days 1 and 4

Doxorubicin 50 mg/m^2 IV continuous infusion over 72 hours[w]

Cyclophosphamide 500 mg/m^2 IV, day 1

Repeat cycles every 21–28 days for 6 cycles[c]

CAF

Cyclophosphamide 600 mg/m^2 IV, day 1

Doxorubicin 60 mg/m^2 IV bolus, day 1

Fluorouracil 600 mg/m^2 IV, day 1

Repeat cycles every 21–28 days for 6 cycles[e]

FEC

Fluorouracil 500 mg/m^2 IV, day 1

Epirubicin 100 mg/m^2 IV bolus, day 1

Cyclophosphamide 500 mg/m^2 IV, day 1

Repeat cycle every 21 days for 6 cycles[g]

CEF

Cyclophosphamide 75 mg/m^2 orally on days 1–14

Epirubicin 60 mg/m^2 IV, days 1 and 8

Fluorouracil 500 mg/m^2 IV, days 1 and 8

Repeat cycles every 28 days for 6 cycles (requires prophylactic antibiotics or growth factor support)[i and j]

AC → Paclitaxel (CALGB 9344)

Doxorubicin 60 mg/m^2 IV, day 1

Cyclophosphamide 600 mg/m^2 IV, day 1

Repeat cycles every 21 days for 4 cycles

Paclitaxel 175 mg/m^2 on day 1

TAC (BCIRG 001)

Docetaxel 75 mg/m^2 IV, day 1

Doxorubicin 50 mg/m^2 IV bolus, day 1

Cyclophosphamide 500 mg/m^2 IV, day 1

(doxorubicin should be given first)

Repeat cycles every 21–28 days for 6 cycles[d]

Paclitaxel → FAC[f,w]

Paclitaxel 80 mg/m^2/wk IV over 1 hour every week for 12 weeks

Followed by:

Fluorouracil 500 mg/m^2 IV, days 1 and 4

Doxorubicin 50 mg/m^2 IV continuous infusion over 72 hours

Cyclophosphamide 500 mg/m^2 IV, day 1

Repeat cycles every 21–28 days for 4 cycles[n]

CMF

Cyclophosphamide 100 mg/m^2/day orally, days 1–14

Methotrexate 40 mg/m^2 IV, days 1 and 8

Fluorouracil 600 mg/m^2 IV, days 1 and 8

Repeat cycles every 28 days for 6 cycles[h,j]

or

Cyclophosphamide 600 mg/m^2 IV, day 1

Methotrexate 40 mg/m^2 IV, day 1

Fluorouracil 600 mg/m^2 IV, days 1 and 8

Repeat cycles every 28 days for 6 cycles[i]

Dose-Dense AC → Paclitaxel

Doxorubicin 60 mg/m^2 IV bolus, day 1

Cyclophosphamide 600 mg/m^2 IV, day 1

Repeat cycles every 14 days for 4 cycles (must be given with growth factor support)

Followed by:

Paclitaxel 175 mg/m^2 IV over 3 hours

Repeat cycles every 14 days for 4 cycles (must be given with growth factor support)[k]

Followed by:

Paclitaxel 175 mg/m^2 IV over 3 hours

Repeat cycles every 21 days for 4 cycles[b]

Metastatic Single-Agent Chemotherapy

Paclitaxel

Paclitaxel 175 mg/m^2 IV over 3 hours

Repeat cycles every 21 days[l]

or

Paclitaxel 80 mg/m^2/wk IV over 1 hour

Repeat dose every 7 days[m]

Vinorelbine

Vinorelbine 30 mg/m^2 IV, days 1 and 8

Repeat cycles every 21 days

or

Vinorelbine 25–30 mg/m^2/wk IV

Repeat cycles every 7 days (adjust dose based on absolute neutrophil count; see product information)[n]

(Continued)

Table 89–6

Common Chemotherapy Regimens for Breast Cancer (*Continued*)

Metastatic Single-Agent Chemotherapy

Docetaxel

Docetaxel 60–100 mg/m^2 IV over 1 hour
Repeat cycles every 21 days[o]
or
Docetaxel 30–35 mg/m^2/wk IV over 30 minutes
Repeat dose every 7 days[p]

Capecitabine

Capecitabine 2,000–2,500 mg/m^2/day orally, divided twice daily
for 14 days
Repeat cycles every 21 days[q,r]

Docetaxel + Capecitabine

Docetaxel 75 mg/m^2 IV over 1 hour, day 1
Capecitabine 2,000–2,500 mg/m^2/day orally divided twice
daily for 14 days
Repeat cycles every 21 days[t]

Epirubicin + Docetaxel[x]

Epirubicin 70–90 mg/m^2 IV bolus
Followed by:
Docetaxel 70–90 mg/m^2 IV over 1 hour
Repeat cycles every 21 days[v]

Gemcitabine

Gemcitabine 600–1,000 mg/m^2/wk IV, days 1, 8, and 15
Repeat cycles every 28 days (may need to hold day-15 dose based on
blood counts)[q]

Liposomal Doxorubicin

Liposomal doxorubicin 30–50 mg/m^2 IV over 90 minutes
Repeat cycles every 21–28 days[s]

Doxorubicin + Docetaxel[x]

Doxorubicin 50 mg/m^2 IV bolus, day 1
Followed by:
Docetaxel 75 mg/m^2 IV over 1 hour, day 1
Repeat cycles every 21 days[u]

[a]From Fisher B, et al. J Clin Oncol 1990;8:1483. [b]From Henderson CI, et al. J Clin Oncol 2003;21:976. [c]From Buzdar AU, et al. In: Salmon S, ed. Adjuvant Therapy of Cancer, VIII. Philadelphia, Lippincott-Raven, 1997:93–100. [d]From Martin et al. San Antonio Breast Cancer Symposium 2003; A43. [e]From Wood WC, et al. N Engl J Med 1994;330:1253. [f]From Green, et al. Proc Am Soc Clin Oncol 2002; A135. [g]French Adjuvant Study Group. J Clin Oncol 2001;19:602. [h]From Bonadonna G, et al. N Engl J Med 1976;294:405. [i]From Fisher B, et al. N Engl J Med 1989;32:473. [j]From Levine MN, et al. J Clin Oncol 1998;16:2651. [k]From Citron et al. J Clin Oncol 2003;21;1431. [l]From Taxol (paclitaxel) product information. Bristol-Myers Squibb, April 2003. [m]From Perez EA, et al. Clin Oncol 2001;19:4216. [n]From Zelek L. Cancer 2001;92:2267. [o]From Taxotere (docetaxel) product information. Aventis Pharmaceuticals Inc., April 2003. [p]From Hainsworth JD, et al. J Clin Oncol 1998;16:2164. [q]From Carmichael J, et al. J Clin Oncol 1995;13:2731. [r]From Michaud et al. Proc Am Soc Clin Oncol 2000; A402, and Xeloda product information. [s]From Ranson MR, et al. J Clin Oncol 1997;15:3185. [t]From O'Shaughnessy et al. J Clin Oncol 2002;20:2812. [u]From Nabholtz JM, et al. J Clin Oncol 2003;21:968. [v]From Levin MN, et al. J Clin Oncol 1998;16:2651. [w]FAC may also be given with bolus doxorubicin administration, and the fluorouracil dose is then given on days 1 and 8. [x]Paclitaxel may also be given concurrently with doxorubicin or epirubicin as a combination regimen. Pharmacokinetic interactions make these regimens more difficult to give.

IV, intravenous.

at low levels in the epithelial cells of normal breast tissue. Overexpression of HER-2/neu is associated with increased signaling in pathways that mediate cellular growth and division. Most experts agree that women whose tumors overexpress HER-2/neu appear to be relatively resistant to alkylating agent–based adjuvant therapy and may derive greater benefit from an anthracycline-based adjuvant therapy regimen.[50-52]

Although HER-2/neu positively, though not absolutely, predicts response to trastuzumab therapy, receptor overexpression is also considered a poor prognostic factor. ⑥ *Currently, the use of trastuzumab is indicated for treatment of adjuvant and metastatic breast cancer in patients who have tumors that overexpress HER-2/neu.*[39] It is important to note that trastuzumab therapy should not be given concurrently with the anthracyclines because of increased risk of cardiotoxicity (see section on metastatic breast cancer).

▶ *Adjuvant Endocrine Therapy*

⑥ *Hormonal therapies that have been studied in the treatment of primary or early breast cancer include selective estrogen receptor modulators (SERMs), oophorectomy, ovarian irradiation, luteinizing hormone–releasing hormone (LHRH) agonists, and AIs.*

⑤ *Hormone receptors are used clinically as indicators of prognosis and to* predict response *to hormone therapy.* Hormone receptors are cytoplasmic proteins that transmit signals to the nucleus of the cell for growth and proliferation. The hormone receptors clinically useful in discussions of breast cancer include the ER and the progesterone receptor (PR). The presence of these proteins in the primary tumor is measured routinely by enzyme-linked immunochemical assays and radio assays (enzyme-linked immunosorbent assay). About 50% to 70% of patients with primary or

---

Table 89–7

Toxicities of Common Chemotherapies Used for Breast Cancer

Class	Drug	Dose-Limiting Toxicities	Other Toxicities
Anthracyclines	Doxorubicin, epirubicin	Myelosuppression, cardiomyopathy	Alopecia, nausea, vomiting, stomatitis, ulceration, and necrosis with extravasation, red-colored urine, radiation-recall effect
	Liposomal doxorubicin	Myelosuppression, palmar-plantar erythrodysesthesia (hand–foot syndrome)	Alopecia, infusion reactions, stomatitis, fatigue, nausea, vomiting
Taxanes	Paclitaxel	Neutropenia, peripheral neuropathy, hypersensitivity reactions	Alopecia, fluid retention, myalgia, skin reactions, ulceration, and necrosis with extravasation, bradycardia, stomatitis
	Docetaxel	Myelosuppression, severe fluid retention	Alopecia, fatigue, stomatitis, nausea, vomiting, diarrhea, peripheral neuropathy, nail disorder, skin reactions, hypersensitivity reactions
Antimetabolites	Capecitabine	Diarrhea, palmar-plantar erythrodysesthesia (hand–foot syndrome)	Myelosuppression, stomatitis, nausea, vomiting
	Gemcitabine	Myelosuppression (especially thrombocytopenia)	Flulike syndrome (fever, chills, myalgias, and arthralgias), nausea
	Fluorouracil	Myelosuppression	Stomatitis, diarrhea, alopecia
	Methotrexate	Myelosuppression, stomatitis	Diarrhea, nausea, vomiting, renal toxicity
Vinca alkaloids	Vinorelbine	Neutropenia	Fatigue, nausea, vomiting, ulceration, and necrosis with extravasation
Alkylating agents	Cyclophosphamide	Myelosuppression, hemorrhagic cystitis	Alopecia, stomatitis, amenorrhea, aspermia

---

metastatic breast cancer have hormone receptor–positive tumors. Tumors that are hormone receptor positive are associated with superior response to hormone therapy, a longer disease-free interval between primary and subsequent metastatic disease, and a favorable prognosis. Hormone receptor–positive tumors are more common in postmenopausal patients than in premenopausal patients. Many experts believe that breast cancer in postmenopausal women is substantially different from that occurring in premenopausal women.

Tamoxifen traditionally was the "gold standard" adjuvant hormonal therapy and has been used in the adjuvant setting for 3 decades. Tamoxifen is antiestrogenic in breast cancer cells, but it appears to have estrogenic properties in other tissues and organs.[53,54] Newer information confirms that tamoxifen and other similar drugs have many estrogenic and antiestrogenic effects that depend on the tissue and the gene in question. Women receiving adjuvant tamoxifen therapy have a reduction in recurrence and mortality compared with women not receiving tamoxifen therapy.[55] This observation, coupled with evidence of tamoxifen's tolerability, including beneficial estrogenic effects on the lipid profile and bone density, led to tamoxifen being the hormonal agent of choice.

Tamoxifen therapy is initiated shortly after surgery or as soon as pathology results are known. Because many patients receive chemotherapy, administration of tamoxifen should begin after completion of chemotherapy. This practice is supported by a study which showed after a median follow-up of 8.5 years, the administration of sequential tamoxifen resulted in an estimated DFS advantage of 18% (hazard ratio [HR], 1.18) compared with the *concurrent* use of tamoxifen with chemotherapy.[56] Data suggest the growth-inhibitory effect of tamoxifen diminished the cytotoxic effect of chemotherapy, resulting in a shorter DFS in women who received these two agents concurrently.

Patient Encounter, Part 5

HPI: Five years have passed since the original diagnosis. AD returns for her annual checkup. She continues tamoxifen, and except for occasional hot flashes, she is doing very well. Laboratory tests are all within normal limits. There is no abnormal bleeding. Psychosocial evaluation reports a well-adjusted woman, devoted mother, and consummate professional.

Plan: Complete 5 years of tamoxifen. Monitor bone density. Judicious surveillance for disease recurrence.

Should the patient be continued on endocrine therapy for an additional 5 years?

If zoledronic acid was not used initially, should the agent be implemented if the patient chooses to continue endocrine therapy?

How much longer does the patient need to be followed for her breast cancer?

Table 89–8

Breast Cancer Pharmacogenomics

Gene or Gene Product	Drug	Effect on Drug	Comment
CYP2D6	Tamoxifen	Enzyme responsible for metabolic activation of tamoxifen	Genetic variants of *CYP2D6* with low metabolizing activity or co-prescribed drugs that inhibit CYP2D6 (e.g., fluoxetine and paroxetine) are inconsistently associated with increased risk of disease recurrence and shorter DFS
HER2/neu	Anthracycline-containing chemotherapy regimens	Precise mechanistic effect on drug therapy not known	Clinical trial data indicate a differential benefit of the anthracyclines; these data also support the belief that the anthracyclines are one of the most active class of drugs for breast cancer
	Trastuzumab	Gene amplification and protein overexpression have predictive value	Predictive value relates to the likelihood of response to trastuzumab (conversely, the agent is of no benefit in patients with *HER-2*–negative disease)
	Lapatinib	Gene amplification and protein overexpression has predictive value	Beneficial in patients with trastuzumab resistant disease; may be beneficial in brain metastasis
Dihydropyrimidine dehydrogenase	5-FU	Inactivates 5-FU	Low DPD activity associated with increased normal tissue toxicity
Thymidine phosphorylase	Capecitabine	Converts drug to 5-FU	Oral TP/DPD ratio appears to determine tumor 5-FU levels

DFS, disease-free survival; 5-FU, 5-fluorouracil.

From Refs. 50, 51, 57–61, 83, and 89.

Adjuvant tamoxifen (20 mg/day) is currently given for 5 years,[57] but two ongoing clinical trials are evaluating whether tamoxifen treatment for 10 years results in improved patient outcome.. Because of the significant side effects of tamoxifen, all patients must be counseled properly about warning signs of endometrial cancer (i.e., vaginal bleeding or groin pain or pressure) and thromboembolism (i.e., chest pain, trouble breathing, changes in vision, one-sided weakness, or pain or swelling in the legs).

An intriguing observation associated with the adjuvant tamoxifen trials is related to the role of pharmacogenomics in tailoring therapy to individual patients (Table 89–8). For example, evidence indicates that germline variants of CYP2D6 are associated with substantially lower concentrations endoxifen, the metabolite of tamoxifen, significant disease recurrence, and shorter DFS.[58,59] Consistent with these findings, additional data demonstrate that concomitant administration CYP2D6 inhibitors result in reduced plasma levels of endoxifen and is an independent predictor of breast cancer outcome.[60-62] However, discordant results of a more recent study have been presented.[63]

In premenopausal women, the use of LHRH agonists or other means of ovarian ablation have been shown beneficial in the adjuvant setting.[64] The use of goserelin, an LHRH agonist, alone or with tamoxifen, has been compared with standard chemotherapy regimens (see Table 89–6). As a single agent, goserelin appears to provide similar benefit to CMF for node-positive, ER-positive tumors in premenopausal breast cancer patients.[65] In another trial, a

significant advantage of endocrine therapy in terms of DFS over chemotherapy alone was demonstrated after a median follow-up of 6 years.[66] Retrospective reviews have found that premenopausal women who cease to menstruate with chemotherapy may have a better survival than women who continue to menstruate.[67] Therefore, the role of an LHRH agonist after chemotherapy in women who continue to menstruate is being investigated.

In postmenopausal women, the use of adjuvant AIs has been studied in three different ways: (a) direct comparison with tamoxifen for adjuvant hormonal therapy, (b) sequential use after 5 years of adjuvant tamoxifen therapy, and (c) sequential use after 2 to 3 years of adjuvant tamoxifen. Based on the positive results of several studies, oncology groups recommend AIs as the endocrine therapy of choice for postmenopausal women with ER-positive breast cancer.[38,68] However, it is still unclear if AIs should be used instead of or sequentially when tamoxifen has been given for 2 to 5 years.[38] Nonetheless, a survival benefit appears to be emerging with sequential administration of anastrozole after 2 to 5 years of initial tamoxifen therapy.[69]

The NCCN Practice Guidelines recommend "bone mineral density determination at initiation of AI therapy and periodically thereafter."[39] Other concerns related to changes in blood lipids and cardiovascular disease requires further study. Successful coadministration of bisphosphonates with the AIs has been accomplished in many patients in the metastatic setting. The three available AIs are exemestane, anastrozole, and letrozole (Table 89–9).

Table 89–9

Endocrine Therapies Used for Metastatic Breast Cancer

Class	Drug	Dose	Side Effects
Aromatase inhibitors			
Nonsteroidal	Anastrozole	1 mg/day PO	Hot flashes, arthralgias, myalgias, headaches, diarrhea, mild nausea
	Letrozole	2.5 mg/day PO	
Steroidal	Exemestane	25 mg/day PO	
Antiestrogens			
SERMs	Tamoxifen	20 mg/day PO	Hot flashes, vaginal discharge, mild nausea, thromboembolism, endometrial cancer
	Toremifene	60 mg/day PO	
SERDs	Fulvestrant	250 mg IM every 28 days	Hot flashes, injection-site reactions, possibly thromboembolism
LHRH analogs	Goserelin	3.6 mg SC every 28 days	Hot flashes, amenorrhea, menopausal symptoms, injection-site reactions
	Leuprolide	7.5 mg IM every 28 days	
	Triptorelin	3.75 mg IM every 28 days	
Progestins	Megestrol acetate	40 mg PO 4 for a day	Weight gain, hot flashes, vaginal bleeding, edema, thromboembolism
	Medroxyprogesterone	400–1,000 mg IM every week	
Androgens	Fluoxymesterone	10 mg PO twice a day	Deepening voice, alopecia, hirsutism, facial or truncal acne, fluid retention, menstrual irregularities, cholestatic jaundice
Estrogens	Diethylstilbestrol	5 mg PO 3 for a day	Nausea or vomiting, fluid retention, anorexia, thromboembolism, hepatic dysfunction
	Ethinyl estradiol	1 mg PO 3 for a day	
	Conjugated estrogens	2.5 mg PO 3 for a day	

IM, intramuscular; LHRH, luteinizing hormone–releasing hormone; PO, oral; SC, subcutaneous; SERD, selective estrogen-receptor downregulator; SERM, selective estrogen-receptor modulator.

LOCALLY ADVANCED BREAST CANCER (STAGE III)

TREATMENT

Desired Outcome

Locally advanced breast cancer generally refers to breast carcinomas with significant primary tumor and nodal disease but in which distant metastases cannot be documented. A wide variety of clinical scenarios can be seen within this group of patients, including neglected tumors that have spread locally and inflammatory breast cancers that are a unique clinical entity. Patients with inflammatory breast cancer are often treated inappropriately for cellulitis for several weeks to months.

Treatment of stage III breast cancer generally consists of a combination of surgery, radiation, and chemotherapy (i.e., **combined modality**) administered in an aggressive approach with the treatment goal of a cure. In patients with locally advanced breast cancer, systemic relapse and death are common even when local-regional control is accomplished.[70] These observations led to the use of neoadjuvant or primary chemotherapy as an approach to render inoperable tumors resectable even with the possibility of breast-conserving surgery. Theoretical advantages to this method include potential benefits related to early initiation of systemic therapy, delivery of drugs through an intact vasculature, in vivo assessment of treatment response, and an opportunity to evaluate the biologic effects of the systemic therapy. However, the use of this approach does not use well-validated pathologic prognostic markers, such as initial tumor size and involvement of axillary lymph nodes.

Pharmacologic Therapy

For patients with inoperable breast cancer, including inflammatory breast cancer, the treatment objective is to obtain tumor resectablity using neoadjuvant chemotherapy. After neoadjuvant chemotherapy, most tumors respond with more than a 50% decrease in tumor size, and about 70% of patients experience tumor downstaging. Chemotherapy regimens used in stage III breast cancer are similar to those used in the adjuvant setting. Supporting evidence for each individual regimen differs, but available data support the use of anthracycline-containing regimens, incorporation of the taxanes, and approaches to improve dose density or dose intensity.[70] Neoadjuvant endocrine therapy may be an option for patients who have unresectable, hormone receptor–positive tumors and unable to receive chemotherapy (e.g., multiple comorbid conditions). Even though not an approved indication, several preliminary clinical studies have demonstrated the efficacy of neo-adjuvant trastuzumab in patients with HER-2-overexpressing tumors. In terms of local therapy, the extent of surgery will be determined by a patient's response to chemo- or endocrine therapy, the wishes of the patient, and the cosmetic results likely to be achieved. Adjuvant radiation therapy should be administered to all patients with locally advanced breast cancer to minimize local recurrences regardless of the type of surgery used for that individual patient (e.g., mastectomy or segmental mastectomy). Inoperable tumors that are unresponsive to systemic chemotherapy may require radiation for local management; however, these tumors may be ineligible for subsequent surgical resection. Such patients have a very poor prognosis and are not commonly seen. For most patients in this category, cure is still the primary goal of therapy.

METASTATIC BREAST CANCER (STAGE IV)

TREATMENT

Desired Outcome

❼ *The goal of therapy with early and locally advanced breast cancer is to cure the disease. Currently, breast cancer is incurable after it has advanced beyond local-regional disease.* Goals for treatment of metastatic breast cancer are to improve symptoms; maintain quality of life; and if possible, prolong survival. Thus, it is important to choose therapy with good activity while minimizing toxicities. Treatment of metastatic breast cancer with either cytotoxic or endocrine therapy often results in regression of disease and improvement in quality of life.

General Approach to Treatment

❺ *The choice of therapy for metastatic disease is based on the site of disease involvement and presence or absence of certain characteristics (i.e., hormone and HER-2 receptor status of the primary tumor).* For example, patients with ER-positive tumors who experience a long DFS following local-regional therapy or have disease located primarily in bone or soft tissue often respond to endocrine therapy. Patients with asymptomatic visceral involvement (e.g., liver or lung) may be candidates for hormonal therapy. **❽** *Patients who are hormone receptor positive generally receive initial endocrine therapy followed by combination chemotherapy when endocrine therapy fails.* Patients who respond to initial endocrine therapy often respond to a second (or even third) hormonal manipulation, although the response rate is lower and duration of response is shorter with second- and third-line hormonal therapies. About 50% to 60% of ER-positive patients and 75% to 80% of ER- and PR-positive patients respond to hormonal therapy; however, the response rate of ER- and PR-negative tumors is less than 10%. Thus, the primary factor determining the choice of endocrine versus cytotoxic chemotherapy is the presence of hormone receptors in the primary breast tumor.

Patients who are hormone receptor negative with rapidly progressive or symptomatic disease involving the liver, lung, or central nervous system and those having progressed on initial endocrine therapy usually are treated with cytotoxic chemotherapy. **❾** *Chemotherapy results in an objective response in about 50% to 60% of patients previously unexposed to chemotherapy.* Most patients have partial responses, but complete disappearance (i.e., **complete response**) of disease occurs in fewer than 20% of patients. The median duration of response is 5 to 12 months, although some patients have an excellent response to an initial course of chemotherapy and may live 5 to 10 years without evidence of disease. In general, survival of patients after treatment with commonly used drug combinations for metastatic breast cancer is a median of 14 to 33 months. The response rate to second- and third-line combination chemotherapy varies from 20% to 40% depending on the previous chemotherapy regimens the patients have received. Combinations of different hormonal therapies or chemotherapy plus hormones are not used in the setting of metastatic breast cancer owing to the lack of increased efficacy and evidence of increased toxicity. **❿** *Patients with tumors that overexpress HER-2/neu should be considered for treatment with trastuzumab, usually in combination with chemotherapy.*

Pharmacologic Systemic Therapy

▶ *Endocrine Therapy*

The pharmacologic goals of endocrine therapy for breast cancer are to decrease circulating levels of estrogen and/or to prevent the effects of estrogen on the breast cancer cell (targeted therapy) through blocking the hormone receptors or downregulating the presence of those receptors. Achievement of these goals is independent of menopausal status. Many endocrine therapies are available to target these goals. Combination studies also have been conducted in an attempt to improve patient outcomes. Unfortunately, many combinations do not improve efficacy but they do increase toxicity. Therefore, therapy involving combinations of endocrine agents is not recommended outside the context of a clinical trial. Thus, patients are often treated with a series of endocrine agents over several years before chemotherapy is considered.

Until recently, there was little evidence supporting improved response or survival benefit from one endocrine therapy superior to that achieved with other therapies. Given this equality in efficacy, the choice of a particular endocrine therapy was primarily based on toxicity (Table 89–9), resulting in the use of tamoxifen as the preferred initial agent when metastasis is present. An exception to this occurs if a patient is receiving adjuvant tamoxifen at the time or within 1 year of occurrence of metastatic disease.

Over the past decade, new information has been published regarding the use of a new generation of AIs. These data have changed the way patients with metastatic breast cancer and early stage breast cancer are treated. In postmenopausal and women without functioning ovaries, the main source of estrogen is derived from peripheral conversion of androstenedione and testosterone produced by the adrenal gland to estrone and estradiol. This conversion process requires aromatase. This enzyme also catalyzes the conversion of androgens to estrogens in the ovary in premenopausal women and in extraglandular tissue, including the breast itself, in postmenopausal women. Therefore, AIs effectively reduce the level of circulating estrogens, as well as estrogens in the target organ. Their toxicity profile consists mainly of skeletal complications such as fractures, nausea, hot flashes, arthralgias or myalgias, and mild fatigue. Anastrozole and letrozole are nonsteroidal compounds that exhibit reversible, competitive inhibition of aromatase. Exemestane is a steroidal compound that binds irreversibly to aromatase, forming a covalent bond. However, clinical evidence does not demonstrate superior results with exemestane over the other agents in this class.

The AIs are used as first-line therapy for ER-positive advanced breast cancer in postmenopausal women. Large trials have compared these agents with tamoxifen and have found similar response rates and a longer median time to progression for patients receiving the selective AIs.[50] A consistent finding in these trials was a lower incidence of thromboembolic events and vaginal bleeding in patients treated with an AI. This led to the conclusion that the new AIs were superior to tamoxifen as first-line therapy for advanced breast cancer in postmenopausal women. Use of exemestane after treatment with a nonsteroidal inhibitor may provide some benefit. This is a common practice based on small clinical trials investigating this sequential approach to therapy.[71] The opposite sequence also has shown some benefit. Therefore, patients may receive two AIs (first and second line sequentially), especially patients who progress while on adjuvant tamoxifen therapy.

The AIs are only used in postmenopausal women. Premenopausal or perimenopausal women with functioning ovaries are not appropriate candidates for these therapies, at least based on the available evidence. Use of the AIs in addition to ovarian ablation (e.g., oophorectomy or LHRH agonists) is currently being investigated. The use of AIs in men with advanced breast cancer should be avoided. Available data suggest the use of these agents in men increases circulating levels of testosterone, which may negate the therapeutic effects of the drug.[72]

Antiestrogens bind to ERs, preventing receptor-mediated gene transcription, and therefore are used to block the effect of estrogen on the end target. This class of agents now is subdivided into two pharmacologic categories, SERMs and pure antiestrogens. SERMs include tamoxifen and toremifene and demonstrate tissue-specific activity, both estrogenic and antiestrogenic, as described previously. The agonistic activity is thought to be responsible for many of the adverse reactions seen with these agents, including the increased risk of endometrial cancer. In an effort to minimize this agonistic activity, research has led to the development of pure estrogen receptor antagonists that lack estrogen agonist activity. Pure antiestrogens are a new class of agents that are also referred to as *selective estrogen-receptor downregulators* (SERDs). These molecules bind to ER and degrade the drug–ER complex. Fulvestrant is the only pure antiestrogen available commercially in the United States.

Tamoxifen can be used in both premenopausal and postmenopausal women with metastatic breast cancer who have tumors that are hormone receptor positive. The toxicities of tamoxifen are described in the section on adjuvant endocrine therapy. The only additional toxicity that one might expect to find in the setting of metastatic breast cancer (specifically bone metastases) is a tumor flare or hypercalcemia, which occurs in approximately 5% of patients following the initiation of any SERM therapy and is not an indication to discontinue SERM therapy. It is generally accepted that this is a positive indication that the patient will respond to endocrine therapy.

Fulvestrant is approved as second-line therapy of postmenopausal metastatic breast cancer patients who have tumors that are hormone receptor positive. Studies examining the role of fulvestrant in the treatment of metastatic breast cancer have compared this agent with anastrozole. Given anastrozole's mechanism of action, only postmenopausal women were eligible for these trials. In the comparative trials with fulvestrant and anastrozole, similar efficacy and safety were demonstrated with both agents when given after patients progressed on tamoxifen therapy.[73,74] Adverse events related to fulvestrant include injection-site reactions, hot flashes, asthenia, and headaches. This agent is a good option for patients who are unable to take an oral medication because it is given as an intramuscular injection every 28 days. There is no biological reason why fulvestrant should not produce similar outcomes in premenopausal women; however, data supporting this hypothesis have not been published confirming the safety or efficacy in this group. Another goal of antitumor treatment is to reduce estrogen production in premenopausal women using surgery, irradiation, or medication. Statistical significance was not found in two randomized trials evaluating the overall response rate between tamoxifen and oophorectomy in premenopausal women. However, the secondary response rate to oophorectomy after tamoxifen treatment was somewhat higher than the response to tamoxifen after primary oophorectomy (33% versus 11%).[75] Some experts interpret this as suggesting that tamoxifen does not completely antagonize available estrogen, particularly in premenopausal women. Ovarian ablation (surgically or chemically) is still used commonly in some parts of the United States and is considered by many specialists to be the endocrine therapy of choice in premenopausal women. The mortality rate with surgical oophorectomy is low (less than 2% to 3% in appropriately selected patients). Medical inhibition of estrogen production castration with LHRH analogs is used increasingly in lieu of oophorectomy in premenopausal women.

Medical inhibition of estrogen production castration with LHRH analogs has been used in premenopausal metastatic breast cancer patients and induces remission in about one-third of unselected patients. The mechanism of action of LHRH analogs in breast cancer is thought to result from downregulation of LHRH receptors in the pituitary. Decreased levels of luteinizing hormone (LH) subsequently results in a significant decrease in estrogen to castrate levels. The three agents available in the United States for medical inhibition of estrogen production are leuprolide, goserelin, and triptorelin, but only goserelin is approved for the treatment of metastatic breast cancer. These agents are administered as an injection and are associated with primarily nuisance side effects such as amenorrhea; hot flashes; and occasionally, nausea. A recent meta-analysis of premenopausal women reported on the combined use of tamoxifen and LHRH agonists versus LHRH agonists alone in patients with metastatic breast cancer.[76] With a median follow-up of 6.8 years, combined treatment demonstrated a significant survival benefit and progression-free survival (PFS) benefit. The overall response rate was also significantly higher on combined endocrine treatment. However, this analysis did not compare tamoxifen alone against the combination of an LHRH agonist with tamoxifen. LHRH agonists also may produce a flare response owing to an initial surge in LH and estrogen production for the first 2 to 4 weeks. This flare response is similar to that seen with tamoxifen, and patients should be monitored for increasing pain and/or hypercalcemia during the initiation period.

In randomized trials, progestins such as megestrol acetate and medroxy-progesterone acetate have been compared with tamoxifen and have been found to yield equal response rates. Medroxyprogesterone acetate is used more frequently in Europe, and megestrol acetate is used more frequently in the United States. Based on efficacy and tolerability, these agents generally are reserved as third-line therapy after patients have received an AI and an SERM (i.e., tamoxifen or toremifene). The most common side effect is weight gain, occurring in 20% to 50% of patients. Patients experiencing weight gain may have fluid retention, but fluid retention is not totally responsible for the weight gain. In cachectic cancer patients, the weight gain may be desirable, but this is not uniformly true of all patients with metastatic breast cancer. Additional side effects associated with progestins include vaginal bleeding in 5% to 10% of patients, either while patients are taking the progestational agent or when it is discontinued, and somewhat less than a 10% incidence of hot flashes. Thromboembolic complications are also significant with these agents. High-dose estrogens and androgens are rarely used because they are more toxic than other hormonal agents. About one-third of patients placed on high-dose estrogens will discontinue the use of these agents because side effects, the most important of which are thromboembolic events, vomiting, and fluid retention. Given the recent availability of the AIs, use of androgens and estrogens has become rare.

▶ Cytotoxic Chemotherapy

Cytotoxic chemotherapy is eventually required in most patients with metastatic breast cancer. Patients with hormone receptor–negative tumors require chemotherapy as initial treatment of symptomatic metastases. In general, the median survival time of patients after treatment with commonly used drug combinations for metastatic breast cancer is 14 to 33 months. In most studies, the median time to response has ranged from 2 to 3 months, but this period depends in large part on the site of measurable disease. The median time to appearance of response is between 3 and 6 weeks in patients whose disease is primarily in the skin and lymph nodes, 6 to 9 weeks in patients with metastatic lung involvement, 15 weeks in patients with hepatic involvement, and nearly 18 weeks in patients with bone involvement. Thus, an immediate response to therapy is often not apparent, and in general, once a chemotherapy regimen has been initiated, it is continued until there is unequivocal evidence of disease progression.

Currently well-defined clinical characteristics or established tests to identify patients likely to benefit from chemotherapy are not available. Factors associated with an increased probability of response include good performance status, limited number (one or two) of disease sites, and previous response to chemotherapy with a long disease-free interval. Patients who have progressive disease during chemotherapy have a lower probability of response to a different type of chemotherapy. Patients who do not respond to endocrine therapy are as likely to respond to chemotherapy as patients who are treated with chemotherapy as their initial treatment modality. Age; menopausal status; and, in some instances, receptor status have not been associated with a favorable or unfavorable response to chemotherapy.

Although many chemotherapeutic agents have demonstrated activity in the treatment of breast cancer, the most frequently used agents include doxorubicin, epirubicin, paclitaxel, nab-paclitaxel, docetaxel, capecitabine, fluorouracil, cyclophosphamide, methotrexate, vinorelbine, ixabepilone, and gemcitabine. ❿ *The most active classes of chemotherapy in metastatic breast cancer are the anthracyclines and the taxanes, producing response rates as high as 50% to 60% in patients who have not received prior chemotherapy for metastatic disease.*[77] In the metastatic setting the most effective weekly dose of paclitaxel appears to be 80 mg/m^2/wk with no breaks in therapy. With this approach, the toxicity profile of paclitaxel changes with less myelosuppression and delayed onset of peripheral neuropathy but slightly more fluid retention and skin and nail changes. Patients should be premedicated with a steroid (dexamethasone), H$_1$ antagonist (diphenhydramine), and H$_2$ antagonist (ranitidine or famotidine) before treatment to minimize hypersensitivity reactions. A randomized study comparing doses of 60, 75, and 100 mg/m^2 docetaxel was published recently and demonstrates a dose–response relationship with regard to response rates only.[78] Time to progression and OS were similar among all dose levels. Therefore, dose remains important for symptomatic patients who require a rapid response to therapy. In asymptomatic patients requiring docetaxel chemotherapy, lower doses may be appropriate. Results from a single randomized trial indicate that docetaxel is associated with less neuropathy, myalgia, and hypersensitivity than paclitaxel given every 3 weeks, but febrile neutropenia, fluid retention, and skin reactions appear to occur more frequently with the newer taxane.[79] The median cumulative docetaxel dose to the onset of fluid retention is 400 mg/m^2 in nonpremedicated patients. Premedication with a steroid (dexamethasone) before beginning docetaxel and continued for 3 days helps to prevent hypersensitivity reactions and fluid retention.

Regardless of the minor controversy regarding whether a new formulation of an old drug can be considered a "new" drug, nanoparticle albumin-bound paclitaxel or nab-paclitaxel exhibits some advantages over conventional paclitaxel. In a clinical study designed to compare the efficacy and safety of nab-paclitaxel with the older formulation, patients with metastatic breast cancer were enrolled into a randomized trial.[80] Patients received either 260 mg/m^2 nab-paclitaxel or 175 mg/m^2 conventional paclitaxel. Because the albumin-bound drug does not require solvents, standard premedications to prevent acute drug reactions were not given to those randomized to the newly formulated product. Results of the trial indicated significantly better outcomes in patients treated with nab-paclitaxel than those receiving standard paclitaxel. The overall response rates of 33% and 19% favored patients in the nab-paclitaxel arm ($P = .001$); the median time to progression for the nab-paclitaxel group and conventional paclitaxel group was 23 weeks versus 16.9 weeks, respectively ($P = .006$). However, no survival advantage was noted. Despite the higher dosage, the incidence of severe neutropenia was significantly lower with nab-paclitaxel than paclitaxel (9% versus 22%, respectively; $P < .001$). In addition, even in the absence of premedication, no acute hypersensitivity reactions were observed with nab-paclitaxel administration. Nab-paclitaxel is currently indicated for patients with metastatic breast cancer resistant to conventional chemotherapy or progressing within 6 months of receiving an adjuvant anthracycline-containing chemotherapy regimen.

Ixabepilone is a member of a distinct class of microtubule-targeted agents known as the epothilones. In vitro studies show that the antitumor activity of ixabepilone, similar to the taxanes, occurs primarily by blocking disassembly, thus kinetically "stabilizing" the microtubule structure. The results of an international phase III clinical trial demonstrated that the combination of ixabepilone plus capecitabine significantly prolonged PFS by approximately 1.6 months compared with capecitabine alone (median, 5.8 months versus 4.2 months, respectively; $P = 0.0003$).[81] This relatively modest improvement represented a 38% overall increase in PFS. The objective response rate (ORR) was more than twice as high with the combination compared with capecitabine alone (35% versus 14%, respectively). Notably, the response rates were nearly identical to the ORRs (33% versus 14%) in patients who had disease that was intrinsically resistant to previous taxane therapy. The findings from this study support preclinical data that the antitumor activity between ixabepilone and capecitabine are at least additive and may in fact, be synergistic.[82]

However, a much higher incidence of adverse effects involving the bone marrow and peripheral nervous system was apparent in those receiving ixabepilone plus capecitabine. Five infection-related deaths were associated with abnormal liver function at the time of enrollment. In addition, two-thirds of the patients developed variable grades of sensory neuropathy; 21% of the all patients discontinued treatment because of this adverse effect. Ixabepilone is approved for use in combination with capecitabine for patients with advanced breast cancer resistant to or progressing on previous anthracycline and taxane therapy or for patients in whom anthracyclines are contraindicated. The use of single-agent ixabepilone is approved for use in patients with disease resistant capecitabine as well as any drugs in the two classes mentioned earlier.

Capecitabine is a novel oral agent approved in the mid-1990s with significant activity in metastatic breast cancer patients who have progressed on an anthracycline-containing regimen as well as a taxane regimen. This agent is a prodrug for fluorouracil with somewhat targeted activity toward malignant cells. The parent compound undergoes a three-step enzymatic conversion to become fluorouracil (see Table 89–8).[83] The third and final step in this conversion is more likely to occur in malignant cells than normal cells owing to the presence of higher levels of the responsible enzyme in malignant tissues. Approximately 85% of fluorouracil is degraded by dihydropyrimidine dehydrogenase (see Table 89–8). In patients who have been exposed to an anthracycline and a taxane, capecitabine produces response rates of about 25%, which is impressive compared with other tested chemotherapy agents.[84]

Vinorelbine, a microtubule interactive agent, also has shown impressive response rates in metastatic breast cancer.[85] Vinorelbine was approved by the Food and Drug Administration (FDA) in 1994 for the treatment of non–small cell lung cancer. It is not approved for breast cancer, but response rates to vinorelbine range from 30% to 50%, with an overall 5% complete response rate in phase I and phase II studies in patients with advanced breast cancer. Importantly, paclitaxel, docetaxel, and vinorelbine do not appear to be cross-resistant with anthracyclines, which are arguably considered first-line treatment of metastatic breast cancer.

Gemcitabine is another agent that is used quite frequently in patients who have received the aforementioned chemotherapy regimens, who still have a good performance status and who may benefit from additional chemotherapy. This is a nucleotide analog that inhibits DNA synthesis. Response rates ranging from 13% to 42% have been reported in a number of phase II trials.[85] In patients who have been exposed to an anthracycline and a taxane, gemcitabine appears to provide similar benefit to capecitabine. This agent appears to affect platelets more frequently than other chemotherapy previously mentioned, and close monitoring is required for patients receiving this agent.

Combination chemotherapy regimens are associated with higher response rates than are single-agent therapies in the treatment of metastatic breast cancer, but the higher response rates usually have not translated into significant differences in time to progression and OS. The use of sequential single-agent chemotherapies versus the combination regimens has been debated widely for metastatic breast cancer. Current consensus is that first-line chemotherapy includes sequential single agents or combination chemotherapy.[39] In the palliative metastatic setting, using the least toxic approach is preferred when efficacy is considered equal. In clinical practice, patients who require a rapid response to chemotherapy (e.g., those with symptomatic bulky metastases) often receive combination therapy despite the added toxicity. This decision is complex and should be made on an individual patient basis.

Because most patients are given adjuvant chemotherapy, regimens chosen for first-line use in the metastatic setting often are different from those used in the adjuvant setting. If a patient's cancer recurs within 1 year of finishing adjuvant chemotherapy, those chemotherapy agents are not considered effective for treatment of the metastatic disease. However, if the patient recurs more than 1 year after the end of her adjuvant chemotherapy, the same agents also may be helpful in the metastatic setting.

▶ Biologic Therapy

Trastuzumab is a humanized monoclonal antibody that binds with a specific epitope of the HER-2/neu protein. Single-agent treatment with trastuzumab has a response rate of 15% to 20% and a clinical benefit rate of nearly 40% in patients with HER-2/neu-overexpressing cancers.[86] Trastuzumab has additive and perhaps synergistic activity with other chemotherapeutic agents.[87] In the pivotal trial, patients who received the doxorubicin-trastuzumab combination had a very high incidence of cardiotoxicity (27%), leading to a black-box warning regarding this combination in the product information for trastuzumab. Cardiotoxicity is reduced when trastuzumab is given after all cycles of the anthracyclines have been completed. An alternative regimen that may be considered is concurrent administration of docetaxel, carboplatin, and trastuzumab.[88]

Other chemotherapy agents that are being evaluated in combination with trastuzumab include vinorelbine, gemcitabine, capecitabine, and the platinum agents (e.g., cisplatin and carboplatin).[89]

Trastuzumab is reasonably well tolerated. The most common adverse effects (e.g., chills) are infusion related and occur in about 40% of patients during the initial infusion. To alleviate the symptoms, acetaminophen and diphenhydramine may be given and/or the infusion rate may be reduced. The rare adverse effects of severe hypersensitivity and/or pulmonary reactions have been reported. It is important to educate patients regarding the pulmonary reactions because they may occur up to 24 hours after the infusion and if not treated promptly can be fatal. Trastuzumab may increase the incidence of infection, diarrhea, and/or other adverse events when given with chemotherapy. When trastuzumb is given with an anthracycline, the rates of heart failure are unacceptably high, but even as a single agent, there is a 5% incidence of heart failure. Fortunately, the heart failure seen with trastuzumab is somewhat reversible with pharmacologic management. Some patients have continued therapy with trastuzumab after their left ventricular ejection fraction has returned to normal. Close monitoring for clinical signs and symptoms of heart failure is important in order to intervene with appropriate cardiac treatments. It should be noted that only 20% to 25% of patients with metastatic breast cancer overexpress HER-2/neu, and commercially available immunohistochemistry (IHC) tests that score 2+ for HER-2/neu are often negative by the more sensitive and specific fluorescence in situ hybridization (FISH) technique. To date, little benefit is associated with the administration of trastuzumab to the subset of patients who are HER-2/neu-negative and a very questionable benefit associated with administration of trastuzumab to women who are 2+ for HER-2/neu by IHC staining alone. The patients who benefit most from trastuzumab therapy include those whose tumors overexpress HER-2 protein at the 3+ level and/or demonstrate gene amplification by FISH testing.[90]

Lapatinib is a dual inhibitor of HER-2/neu and the epidermal growth factor receptor (EGFR). In contrast to the extracellular recognition site of trastuzumab, the specific targets of lapatinib are the receptors' intracellular kinase domain. A critical phase III trial was conducted to assess the efficacy and safety of lapatinib plus capecitabine versus capecitabine alone in patients with trastuzumab-refractory advanced breast cancer.[91] Of note, the trial was terminated early when a preplanned interim analysis indicated a significant reduction in risk of disease progression (time to progression [TTP], $P < 0.001$) that favored the group receiving the combination to capecitabine alone. Efficacy data were reanalyzed 4 months later. Based on an independent review, the median TTP was 27.1 weeks and 18.6 weeks ($P = 0.00013$; HR, 0.57), and response rates were 23.7% and 13.9% for the lapatinib combination arm and capecitabine monotherapy arm, respectively. Interestingly,

tumor cell expression of EGFR was not an eligibility criterion. This is especially notable because results from an earlier study of lapatinib suggested that clinical response may be higher in breast tumors that coexpressed EGFR and HER2.[92] Another relevant outcome was the significantly lower incidence of brain metastasis in the lapatinib-treated group compared with capecitabine alone (2% versus 11%, respectively; $P = 0.0445$).[93]

Clinical trials of lapatinib have revealed a remarkably similar side effect profile that included non–treatment-limiting diarrhea, rash, nausea, and fatigue among the most frequently reported side effects. The incidence of diarrhea, dyspepsia, and rash was higher when lapatinib was combined with capecitabine.[81] Cardiac events were also monitored because severe toxicity related to blockade of the HER-2/neu signaling pathway has been previously reported.[94,95] Although addition of lapatinib was not associated with any cardiac event resulting in subject withdrawal, the answer related to this issue is not final as the possibility of selection bias and the relatively short observation period.

Based on these data, lapatinib in combination with capecitabine was approved in March 2007 for patients with HER-2/neu-overexpressing metastatic breast cancer progressing on prior anthracycline, taxane, and trastuzumab therapy.

Bevacizumab is a humanized monoclonal antibody that targets vascular endothelial growth factor (VEGF), thereby preventing angiogenesis, which is a necessary process to support tumor growth and metastasis. Based on results from a phase III clinical trial,[39] the antibody received FDA approval in February 2008 as first-line therapy in combination with paclitaxel for metastatic HER-2–negative breast cancer. However, in late 2010, the FDA rescinded its prior approval after two clinical trials failed to reproduce the clinically meaningful benefit observed in the earlier study. Additional studies are being conducted to elucidate bevacizumab's role in the treatment of breast cancer and its efficacy in combination with trastuzumab.

A novel HER-2 targeted agent called pertuzumab was recently approved by the FDA for use as first-line therapy (in combination with docetaxel) for HER-2-positive metastatic breast cancer. Unlike the monoclonal antibody trastuzumab, pertuzumab binds to a specific epitope on the ectodomain of the receptor and sterically hinders the dimerization process.

▶ Bisphosphonates

For women whose breast cancer has metastasized to bone, bisphosphonates are recommended, in addition to chemotherapy or endocrine therapy, to reduce bone pain and fractures.[39,96] Pamidronate (90 mg) and zoledronate (4 mg) can be given IV once each month. These bisphosphonates are given in combination with calcium and vitamin D.

Local-Regional Control

▶ Radiation Therapy

Radiation is an important modality in the treatment of symptomatic metastatic disease. The most common indication for treatment with radiation therapy is painful bone metastases or other localized sites of disease refractory to systemic therapy. Approximately 90% of patients who are treated for painful bone metastases experience significant pain relief with radiation therapy. Additionally, radiation is an important modality in the palliative treatment of metastatic brain lesions and spinal cord lesions, which respond poorly to systemic therapy, as well as eye or orbit lesions and other sites where significant accumulation of tumor cells occurs. Skin and/or lymph node metastases confined to the chest wall area also may be treated with radiation therapy for palliation (e.g., open wounds or painful lesions).

OUTCOME EVALUATION

Early breast cancer is resected completely with curative intent and adjuvant chemotherapy and/or hormonal therapy with trastuzumab in selected patients are initiated to prevent recurrence. During adjuvant chemotherapy, laboratory values to monitor chemotherapy toxicity are obtained before each cycle of chemotherapy. After completion of adjuvant therapy, patients are monitored every 3 months for the first few years after diagnosis, with intervals between examinations extended as time from diagnosis lengthens.

- Physical examination to detect breast cancer recurrence
- Annual mammography
- Symptom-directed workup

Patients with locally advanced breast cancer are often treated with neoadjuvant therapy to make the tumor surgically resectable. During neoadjuvant chemotherapy, laboratory values to monitor chemotherapy toxicity are obtained before each cycle of chemotherapy, and a physical and ultrasound examinations to detect size of tumor are performed after the cycles of neoadjuvant therapy are completed. After complete surgical resection, monitoring proceeds as described for early breast cancer.

Metastatic breast cancer is not curable, and therapy is intended to palliate symptoms. In most cases, hormonal therapy is the mainstay for tumors that are ER positive. While on therapy, patients are monitored monthly for signs of disease progression or metastasis to common sites, such as the bones, brain, or liver. Evaluations include:

- Pain
- Mental status or other neurologic findings
- Laboratory tests
- Liver function tests
- Complete blood count
- Calcium, electrolytes

Patient Care and Monitoring

1. Review the patient's diagnostic information to determine the stage of disease, overall prognosis, and goals of therapy.

2. Obtain a thorough history of prescription, nonprescription, and natural drug product use. Is the patient taking any medications that may contribute to breast cancer and require discontinuation?

3. Review the patient's medical history to determine the risks associated with any potential therapies and/or surgery and/or radiation therapy.

4. Educate the patient on the chemotherapy or endocrine therapy regimen chosen for the patient, focusing on what adverse events to expect, when to expect them, and how to manage them if they do occur. Also include in the initial education an overall plan of care, including the duration of therapy, other treatment modalities that will follow (e.g., radiation therapy, surgery, endocrine therapy), and when the patient will receive them.

5. Develop a premedication and postmedication plan for the chemotherapy or endocrine therapy regimen chosen based on the patient's risk factors for adverse events; chemotherapy or endocrine therapy drugs chosen; and dose, route, and timing of administration chosen.

6. Develop a plan to assess effectiveness of the overall treatment plan, focusing on educating the patient on ways to monitor and track adverse events and/or disease-related symptoms throughout therapy.

7. Determine success of the overall treatment plan by obtaining a thorough history of adverse events experienced with the previous chemotherapy or endocrine therapy treatment and objective measures of response to therapy. Assess effects on quality of life measures such as physical, psychological, and social function and well-being.

8. Address any adverse events the patient experienced and alter the premedication and postmedication plan for the next treatment accordingly.

9. Provide follow-up patient education regarding the new plan for side effect management.

10. Stress importance of reporting adverse events and adherence with the prescribed medication regimen. Attempt to develop a therapeutic regimen that is easy for the patient to accomplish.

Abbreviations Introduced in This Chapter

AI	Aromatase inhibitor
DCIS	Ductal carcinoma in situ
DFS	Disease-free survival
ER	Estrogen receptor
HER2/neu	Human epidermal growth factor receptor 2
LCIS	Lobular carcinoma in situ
LHRH	Luteinizing hormone-releasing hormone
MRI	Magnetic resonance imaging
OS	Overall survival
PFS	Progression-free survival
PR	Progesterone receptor
SERM	Selective estrogen receptor modulator
TNM	Tumor, node, metastasis (staging system)

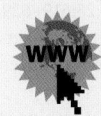 Self-assessment questions and answers are available at *http://mhpharmacotherapy. com/pp.html.*

REFERENCES

1. Jemal A, Siegel R, Xu J, Ward E. Cancer statistics, 2010. CA Cancer J Clin 2010;60:277–300.
2. Ries LAG, Eisner MP, Kosary CL, et al. SEER Cancer Statistics Review, 1975–2001. Bethesda, MD, National Cancer Institute. 2004, *http://seer. cancer.gov/csr/1975-2001.*
3. Feuer EJ, Wun LM, Boring CC, et al. The lifetime risk of developing breast cancer. J Natl Cancer Inst 1993;85:892–897.
4. Dupont WD. Risk factors for breast cancer in women with proliferative breast disease. N Engl J Med 1985;312:146–151.
5. Clemons M, Goss P. Estrogen and the risk of breast cancer. N Engl J Med 2001;344:276–285.
6. Kelsey JL, Gammon MD, John EM. Reproductive factors and breast cancer. Epidemiol Rev 1993;15:36.
7. Risks and benefits of estrogen and progestin in healthy postmenopausal women: Principal results from the Women's Health Initiative randomized controlled trial. JAMA 2002;288:321.
8. Familial breast cancer: Collaborative reanalysis of individual data from 52 epidemiological studies including 58,209 women with breast cancer and 101,986 women without the disease. Lancet 2001;358:1389.
9. Weber BL, Abel JK, Brody LC, et al. Familial breast cancer. Cancer 1994;74:1013–1020.
10. Wooster R, Weber BL. Genomic medicine: Breast and ovarian cancer. N Engl J Med 2003;348:2339–2347.
11. King MC, Marks JH, Mandell JB. Breast and ovarian cancer risks due to inherited mutations in BRCA1 and BRCA2. Science 2003;302: 643–646.
12. Longnecker MP. Alcohol consumption in relation to risk of breast cancer. Cancer Causes Control 1994;5:73–82.
13. Frykberg ER, Bland KI. Overview of the biology and management of ductal carcinoma in situ of the breast. Cancer 1994;74:350–361.
14. Frykberg ER, Ames FC, Bland KI. Current concepts for management of early (in situ and occult invasive) breast carcinoma. In: Bland KI, Copeland EM, eds. The Breast: Comprehensive Management of Benign and Malignant Diseases. Philadelphia: WB Saunders, 1991:731–751.
15. Goldhirsch A, Wood WC, Gelber RD, et al. Meeting highlights: Updated international expert consensus on the primary therapy of early breast cancer. J Clin Oncol 2003;21:3357–3365.
16. Cuzick J, Baum M. Tamoxifen and contralateral breast cancer. Lancet 1985;2:282.
17. Baum M, Brinkley DM, Dossett JA, et al. Improved survival among patients treated with adjuvant tamoxifen after mastectomy for early breast cancer. Lancet 1983;2:450.
18. Edinburgh SCTO. Adjuvant tamoxifen in the management of operable breast cancer: The Scottish Trial: Report from the Breast Cancer Trials Committee. Lancet 1987;2:171–175.
19. Fisher B, Costantino JP, Wickerham DL, et al. Tamoxifen for prevention of breast cancer: Report of the National Surgical Adjuvant Breast and Bowel Project P-1 Study. J Natl Cancer Inst 1998;90:1371–1388.
20. Powles TJ, Ashley S, Tidy A, et al. Twenty-year follow-up of the Royal Marsden randomized double-blinded tamoxifen breast cancer prevention trial. J Natl Cancer Inst 2007;99:283–290.
21. Cuzick J, Forbes FJ, Sestak I, et al. Long-term results of tamoxifen prophylaxis for breast cancer-96-month follow-up of the randomized IBIS-1 trial. J Natl Cancer Inst 2007;99:272–282.
22. Cuzick J, Powles T, Veronesi U, et al. Overview of the main outcomes in breast cancer prevention trials. Lancet 2003;361:296–300.
23. Ettinger B, Black DM, Mitlak BH, et al. Reduction of vertebral fracture risk in postmenopausal women with osteoporosis treated with raloxifene: Results from a 3-year randomized clinical trial: Multiple Outcomes of Raloxifene Evaluation (MORE). JAMA 1999;282:637–645.
24. Cummings SR, Eckert S, Krueger KA, et al. The effect of raloxifene on risk of breast cancer in postmenopausal women: Results from the MORE randomized trial. JAMA 1999;281:2189–2197.
25. Gail MH, Brinton LA, Byar DP, et al. Projecting individualized probabilities of developing breast cancer for white females who are being examined annually. J Natl Cancer Inst 1989;81:1879–1886.
26. Vogel VG, Costantino JP, Wickerham DL, et al. The study of tamoxifen and raloxifene (STAR): Report of the National Surgical Adjuvant Breast and Bowel Project P-2 trial. JAMA 2006;295:2727–2741.
27. Barton MK Exemestane is effective for the chemoprevention of breast cancer. CA Cancer J Clin 2011;61(6):363–364.
28. Smith RA, Cokkinides V, Eyre HJ. American Cancer Society guidelines for the early detection of cancer, 2006. CA Cancer J Clin 2006;56:11–25.
29. U.S. Preventive Services Task Force. Breast cancer screening. February 2002, *www.ahcpr.gov/clinic/uspstf/uspsbrca.htm.*
30. National Cancer Institute. NCI statement on mammography screening. *http://www.cancer.gov/newscenter/mammstatement31jan02.*
31. U.S. Preventive Services Task Force. Screening for breast cancer: U.S. Preventive Services Task Force recommendation statement. Ann Intern Med 2009;151:716–726.
32. Singletary SE, Allred C, Ashley P, et al. Revision of the American Joint Committee on cancer staging system for breast cancer. J Clin Oncol 2002;20:3628–3636.
33. NIH Consensus Development Conference Statement. Adjuvant Therapy for Breast Cancer. November 1–3;17:1–23, 2000, *http://www.nih.gov website.*
34. Ivens D, Hoe AL, Podd TJ, et al. Assessment of morbidity from complete axillary dissection. Br J Cancer 1992;66:136–138.
35. Keramopoulos A, Tsionou C, Minaretzis D, et al. Arm morbidity following treatment of breast cancer with total axillary dissection: A multivariated approach. Oncology 1993;50:445–449.
36. Hsueh EC, Hansen N, Giuliano A. Intraoperative lymphatic mapping and sentinel lymph node dissection in breast cancer. CA Cancer J Clin 2000;50:279–291.
37. Morrow M, Harris JR. Local management of invasive breast cancer. In: Diseases of the Breast, 2nd ed. Lippincott Philadelphia, Williams & Wilkins, 2000:515–560.
38. Persing M, Große R. Current St. Gallen recommendations on primary therapy of early breast cancer. Breast Care 2007;2:137–140.
39. NCCN Practice Guidelines in Oncology—v.1. 2009, *http://www.nccn. org.*
40. Winer EP. Quality-of-life research in patients with breast cancer. Cancer 1994;74:410–415.
41. Levine MN, Gent M, Hirsh J, et al. The thrombogenic effect of anticancer drug therapy in women with stage II breast cancer. N Engl J Med 1988;318:404–407.
42. Smith RE, Bryant J, DeCillis A, et al. Acute myeloid leukemia and myelodysplastic syndrome after doxorubicin-cyclophosphamide

adjuvant therapy for operable breast cancer: The National Surgical Adjuvant Breast and Bowel Project experience. J Clin Oncol 2003;21:1195–1204.

43. Henderson IC, Sloss JL, Jaffe N, et al. Serial studies of cardiac function in patients receiving Adriamycin. Cancer Treat Rep 1978;62:923–929.

44. Ellence (epirubicin) product information. Pfizer, New York, NY, August 2012.

45. Ravdin PM, Siminoff IA, Harvey JA. Survey of breast cancer patients concerning their knowledge and expectations of adjuvant therapy. J Clin Oncol 1998;16:515–521.

46. Lindley C, Vasa S, Sawyer WT, Winer EP. Quality of life and preferences for treatment following systemic adjuvant therapy for early stage breast cancer. J Clin Oncol 1998;16:380–387.

47. Paik S, Tang G, Shak S, et al. Gene expression and benefit of chemotherapy in women with node-negative, estrogen receptor-positive breast cancer. J Clin Oncol 2006;24:3726–3734.

48. Albain K, Barlow W, Shak S, et al. Prognostic and predictive value of the 21–gene recurrence score assay in postmenopausal, node–positive, ER–positive breast cancer (S8814, INT0100) [abstract 10]. Program and abstracts of the 30th Annual San Antonio Breast Cancer Symposium, December 13–16, 2007.

49. Marchionni L, Wilson RF, Wolff AC, et al. Systematic review: Gene expression profiling assays in early-stage breast cancer. Ann Intern Med 2008;148:358–369.

50. Hayes DF, Thor AD. c-erbB-2 in breast cancer: Development of a clinically useful marker. Semin Oncol 2002;29:231–245.

51. Pritchard KI, Shepherd LE, O'Malley FP, et al. HER2 and responsiveness of breast cancer to adjuvant chemotherapy. N Engl J Med 2006;354:2177–2179.

52. Paik S, Bryant J, Tan-Chiu, et al. HER2 and choice of adjuvant chemotherapy for invasive breast cancer. J Natl Cancer Inst 2000;92:1991–1998.

53. Love RR, Mazess RB, Barden HS, et al. Effects of tamoxifen on bone mineral density in postmenopausal women with breast cancer. N Engl J Med 1992;326:852–856.

54. Love RR, Wiebe DA, Newcomb PA, et al. Effects of tamoxifen on cardiovascular risk factors in postmenopausal women. Ann Intern Med 1992;115:860–864.

55. Early Breast Cancer Trialists' Collaborative Group. Tamoxifen for early breast cancer: An overview of the randomized trials. Lancet 1998;351:1451–1467.

56. Albain KS, Green SJ, Ravdin PM, et al. Adjuvant chemohormonal therapy for primary breast cancer should be sequential instead of concurrent: Initial results from intergroup trial 0100 (SWOG-8814) [meeting abstract]. Proc Am Soc Clin Oncol 2002;A143.

57. Fisher B, Dignam J, Bryant J, et al. Five versus more than five years of tamoxifen for lymph node-negative breast cancer: Updated findings from the National Surgical Adjuvant Breast and Bowel Project B-14 randomized trial. J Natl Cancer Inst 2001;93:684–690.

58. Jin Y, Desta Z, Stearns V, et al. CYP2D6 genotype, antidepressant use, and tamoxifen metabolism during adjuvant breast cancer treatment. J Natl Cancer Inst 2005;97:30–39.

59. Schroth W, Antoniadou L, Fritz P, et al. Breast cancer treatment outcome with adjuvant tamoxifen in relation to patient CYP2D6 and CYP2C19 genotypes. J Clin Oncol 2007;25:5187–5193.

60. Goetz MP, Rae JM, Suman VJ, et al. Pharmacogenetics of tamoxifen biotransformation is associated with clinical outcomes of efficacy and hot flashes. J Clin Oncol 2005;23:9312–9318.

61. Goetz MP, Knox SK, Suman VJ, et al. The impact of cytochrome P4502D6 metabolism in women receiving adjuvant tamoxifen. Breast Cancer Res Treat 2007;101:113–121.

62. Gonzalez-Santiago S, Zarate R, Haba-Rodriguez JA, et al. CYP2D6*4 polymorphism as blood predictive biomarker of breast cancer relapse in patients receiving adjuvant tamoxifen [meeting abstract]. J Clin Oncol 2007;A590.

63. Dezentje VO, Van Schaik RH, Vletter-Bogaartz JM, et al. Pharmacogenetics of tamoxifen in relation to disease-free survival in a Dutch cohort of the tamoxifen exemestane adjuvant multinational (TEAM) trial [abstract 508]. J Clin Oncol 2010;28(15 Suppl):70S.

64. Early Breast Cancer Trialists' Collaborative Group. Ovarian ablation for early breast cancer: An overview of the randomized trials. Cochrane Database Syst Rev 2000;CD000485.

65. Jonat W, Kaufmann M, Sauerbrei W, et al. Goserelin versus cyclophosphamide, methotrexate and fluorouracil as adjuvant therapy is premenopausal patients with node-positive breast cancer: The Zoladex Early Breast Cancer Research Association Study. J Clin Oncol 2002;20:4628–4635.

66. Jakesz R, Hausmaninger H, Kubista E, et al. Randomized adjuvant trial of tamoxifen and goserelin versus cyclophosphamide, methotrexate, and fluorouracil: Evidence for the superiority of treatment with endocrine blockade in premenopausal patients with hormone-responsive breast cancer—Austrian Breast and Colorectal Cancer Study Group Trial 5. J Clin Oncol 2002;20:4621–4627.

67. Laurentiis MD, Martignetti A, Isernia G, et al. Amenorrhea induced by adjuvant chemotherapy in breast cancer patients strongly correlates with a better survival: A long follow-up study [meeting abstract]. Proc Am Soc Clin Oncol 1998;A519.

68. Winer EP, Hudis C, Burstein HJ, et al. American Society of Clinical Oncology technology assessment on the use of aromatase inhibitors as adjuvant therapy for postmenopausal women with hormone receptor-positive breast cancer: Status report 2004. J Clin Oncol 2005;23:619–629.

69. Mouridsen H, Giobbie-Hurder A, Goldhirsch A, et al. Letrozole therapy alone or in sequence with tamoxifen in women with breast cancer. N Engl J Med 2009;361:766–776.

70. Giordano SH. Update on locally advanced breast cancer. Oncologist 2003;8:521–530.

71. Assikis VJ, Buzdar AU. Recent advances in aromatase inhibitor therapy for breast cancer. Semin Oncol 2002;29(3 Suppl 11):120–128.

72. Mauras N, O'Brien KO, Klein KO. Estrogen suppression in males: Metabolic effects. J Clin Endocrinol Metab 2000;85:2370–2377.

73. Osborne CK, Pippen J, Jones SE, et al. Double-blind, randomized trial comparing the efficacy and tolerability of fulvestrant versus anastrozole in postmenopausal women with advanced breast cancer progressing on prior endocrine therapy: Results of a North American Trial. J Clin Oncol 2002;20:3386–3395.

74. Howell A, Robertson JFR, Albano JQ, et al. Fulvestrant, formerly ICI 182,780, is as effective as anastrozole in postmenopausal women with advanced breast cancer progressing after prior endocrine treatment. J Clin Oncol 2002;20:3396–3403.

75. Ingle JN, Krook JE, Green SJ, et al. Randomized trial of bilateral oophorectomy versus tamoxifen in premenopausal women with metastatic breast cancer. J Clin Oncol 1986;4:178–185.

76. Klijn JGM, Blamey RW, Boccardo F, et al. Combined tamoxifen and luteinizing hormone-releasing hormone (LHRH) agonist versus LHRH agonist alone in premenopausal advanced breast cancer: A meta-analysis of four randomized trials. J Clin Oncol 2001;19:343–353.

77. Michaud LB, Valero V, Hortobagyi G. Risks and benefits of taxanes in breast and ovarian cancer. Drug Saf 2000;23:401–428.

78. Mouridsen H, Harvey V, Semiglazov V, et al. Phase III trial of docetaxel 100 versus 75 versus 60 mg/m² as second-line chemotherapy in advanced breast cancer [meeting abstract]. San Antonio Breast Cancer Symposium 2002;A327.

79. Jones S, Erban J, Overmoyer B, et al. Randomized trial comparing docetaxel and paclitaxel in patients with metastatic breast cancer [meeting abstract]. San Antonio Breast Cancer Symposium 2003;A10.

80. Gradishar WJ, Tjulandin S, Davidson N, et al. Phase III trial of nanoparticle albumin-bound paclitaxel compared with polyethylated castor oil-based paclitaxel in women with breast cancer. J Clin Oncol 2005;23:7794–7803.

81. Thomas ES, Gomez HL, Li RK, et al. Ixabepilone plus capecitabine for metastatic breast cancer progressing after anthracycline and taxane treatment. J Clin Oncol 2007;25:5210–5217.

82. Lee FY, Camuso A, Castenada C, et al. Preclinical efficacy evaluation of ixabepilone (BMS-247550) in combination with cetuximab or capecitabine in human colon and lung carcinoma xenografts [meeting abstract]. J Clin Oncol 2006;A12017.

83. Innocenti F, Ratain MJ. Update on pharmacogenetics in cancer chemotherapy. Eur J Cancer 2002;38:639–644.

84. Xeloda (capecitabine) product information. Hoffman–LaRoche Pharmaceuticals, Florence, SC, April 2003.

85. Esteva FJ, Valero V, Pusztai L, et al. Chemotherapy of metastatic breast cancer: What to expect in 2001 and beyond. Oncologist 2001;6: 133–146.

86. Cobleigh MA, Vogel CL, Tripathy D, et al. Multinational study of the efficacy and safety of humanized anti-HER2 monoclonal antibody in women who have HER2-overexpressing metastatic breast cancer that progressed after chemotherapy for metastatic disease. J Clin Oncol 1999;17:2639–2648.

87. Slamon DJ, Leyland-Jones B, Shak S, et al. Use of chemotherapy plus a monoclonal antibody against HER2 for metastatic breast cancer that overexpresses HER2. N Engl J Med 2001;344:783–792.

88. Slamon D, Eiermann W, Robert N, et al. Phase III randomized trial comparing doxorubicin and cyclophosphamide followed by docetaxel (AC->T) with doxorubicin and cyclophosphamide followed by docetaxel and trastuzumab (AC->TH) with docetaxel, carboplatin and trastuzumab (TCH) in Her2neu positive early breast cancer patients: BCIRG 006 Study. *Cancer Res* 2010;69:62.

89. Yeon CH, Pegram MD. Anti-erbB-2 antibody trastuzumab in the treatment of HER2-amplified breast cancer. Invest New Drugs 2005;23: 391–409.

90. Vogel CL, Cobleigh MA, Tripathy D, et al. Efficacy and safety of trastuzumab as a single agent in first-line treatment of HER2-overexpressing metastatic breast cancer. J Clin Oncol 2002;20:719–726.

91. Geyer CE, Forster J, Lindquist D, et al. Lapatinib plus capecitabine for HER2-positive advanced breast cancer. N Engl J Med 2006;355: 2733–2743.

92. Burris HA III, Hurwitz HI, Dees EC, et al. Phase I study, pharmacokinetics, and clinical activity study of lapatinib (GW572016), a reversible dual inhibitor of epidermal growth factor receptor tyrosine kinases, in heavily pretreated patients with metastatic carcinomas. J Clin Oncol 2005;23:5305–5313.

93. Geyer CE, Martin A, Newstat B, et al. Lapatinib (L) plus capecitabine (C) in HER2+ advanced breast cancer (ABC): Genomic and updated efficacy data [meeting abstract]. Proc Am Soc Clin Oncol 2007;A1035.

94. Campone M, Bourbouloux E, Fumoleau P. Cardiac dysfunction induced by trastuzumab. Bull Cancer 2004;91(Suppl 3):166–173.

95. Grazette LP, Boecker W, Matsui T, et al. Inhibition of erbB2 causes mitochondrial dysfunction in cardiomyocytes: Implications for herceptin-induced cardiomyopathy. J Am Coll Cardiol 2004;44:2231–2238.

96. Hillner BE, Ingle JN, Chlebowski RT, et al. American Society of Clinical Oncology 2003 update on the role of bisphosphonates and bone health issues in women with breast cancer. J Clin Oncol 2003;21:4042–4057.

90 Lung Cancer

Val Adams and Justin Balko

LEARNING OBJECTIVES

● **Upon completion of the chapter, the reader will be able to:**

1. Identify major risk factors for the development of lung cancer.

2. Explain the pathologic progression of lung cancer and its relationship with signs and symptoms of the disease.

3. Make appropriate recommendations for screening or preventive measures in high-risk patients.

4. Understand staging of lung cancer patients and how it influences treatment decisions.

5. List the rationale, advantages, disadvantages, and place in therapy for adjuvant and neoadjuvant chemotherapy.

6. Identify the chemotherapeutic regimens of choice for limited and extensive small cell lung carcinoma, as well as local, locally advanced, and advanced non–small cell lung carcinoma.

7. Monitor patients for chemotherapy-associated toxicity and recommend appropriate management.

8. Distinguish the treatment goals of palliative care versus those of first-line treatment.

KEY CONCEPTS

❶ The most important risk factor for the development of lung cancer is smoking, and the most effective way for high-risk patients to reduce their risk is to stop smoking. Additional recommendations should include an increase in dietary intake of fruits and vegetables.

❷ The signs and symptoms of lung cancer can be classified as pulmonary, extrapulmonary, and paraneoplastic. These classifications relate to disease progression.

❸ The treatment goals in lung cancer are cure (early-stage disease), prolongation of survival, and maintenance or improvement of quality of life through alleviation of symptoms.

❹ The performance status (PS) of the patient represents an important aspect of chemotherapy treatment decisions. Patients with a PS of 0 to 1 may be treated with chemotherapy. Patients with a PS of 2 may be treated with less aggressive regimens that have a decreased risk of major toxicities.

❺ Surgical resection of the tumor is the mainstay of treatment in early-stage non–small cell lung cancer and produces the longest survival rates.

❻ Doublet chemotherapy regimens offer superior response rates compared to single-agent regimens and should be used when the patient can tolerate the associated toxicity. Platinum-containing doublets are first-line treatment in most cases.

❼ Knowing when and how to treat adverse events from chemotherapy is an important aspect of patient care. Unmanaged events may cause delays in chemotherapy administration and reduced chemotherapy doses and may contribute to treatment failure.

❽ Although some evidence suggest that the use of a colony-stimulating factor reduces the number of neutropenic fever episodes, hospital stay, and antibiotic administration in certain subsets of lung cancer patients, routine front-line (prophylactic) use of a colony-stimulating factor is not recommended owing to lack of a survival benefit.

Lung cancer has a major health impact both in the United States and worldwide. Before 1930, lung cancer was a relatively rare disease, but a sharp incline in industrialization and smoking in the early 1900s has bred an epidemic. Lung cancer has a high mortality rate, and although treatment can cure selected patients, most therapies only prolong survival for months. Recent advances in lung cancer research provide good reason for optimism. However, despite the emergence of new therapies, antismoking campaigns still appear to offer the best opportunity to reduce lung cancer incidence and mortality.

EPIDEMIOLOGY AND ETIOLOGY

Incidence and Mortality

Cancer is the second leading cause of death in the United States. Cancers of the lung and bronchus rank first in cancer-related mortality, comprising more than 28% of cancer-related deaths.[1] In 2011, more than 220,000 new cases of lung cancer are expected. A close correlation exists between incidence and mortality of lung cancer, reflecting the reality that approximately 70% of lung cancer patients ultimately die of the disease.

Gender

Lung cancer incidence and mortality are slightly higher in men, but the rate in women is expected to match that of men in future years owing to changes in smoking patterns.[2] Typically, women with lung cancer are diagnosed at an earlier age, which has raised the question that there may be inherent genetic differences between men and women in their susceptibility to lung cancer. Furthermore, there are differences in the prevalence of histologic subtypes of tumors. Interestingly, historical studies have shown improved prognosis and survival times for women diagnosed with lung cancer.[3]

Race

Although no significant difference is noted in incidence or mortality between black and white women, black mens have a markedly higher incidence and mortality rate than white men. Proposed contributions to this gap include differences in smoking habits, such as increased menthol cigarette use.[2] Black Americans also have a significantly lower 5-year survival rate than white Americans regardless of gender. They present with more advanced disease and are less likely to be treated, suggesting that genetic, psychosocial, and socioeconomic components contribute to this disparity. Although it remains a significant health care issue, Asians, Hispanics, and Native Americans have lower rates of lung cancer than both whites and African Americans.[2,4,5]

Clinical Risk Factors

▶ Smoking

❶ *The most important risk factor for the development of lung cancer is smoking.* One of the most predictive factors on lung cancer epidemiology is trends in population cigarette smoking. Because lung cancer is a fatal disease in most cases, both incidence and mortality strongly reflect the smoking trends of the population on a 20- to 30-year lag. In other words, decreases in tobacco use now would be expected to affect lung cancer incidence in 2030. With this knowledge, the current expectation is that lung cancer incidence and mortality will decrease steadily until 2020, reflecting decreases in cigarette smoking between 1970 and 1990. Because smoking has

continued at a steady rate since 1990, lung cancer incidence is expected to plateau.[2] Correlation between smoking and lung cancer continues to drive antismoking campaigns and should be considered an investment in the future health care of the nation. Furthermore, smoking cessation plays an important role in reducing lung cancer risk on a patient-to-patient basis, and appropriately guiding such therapy is a crucial part of treating at-risk patients.[6] Both total smoke exposure and current use correlate with the individual's risk of developing malignancy. The risk of lung cancer decreases to near-normal levels 10 to 15 years following successful smoking cessation. Total smoke exposure is reported as pack-years. One pack-year is the equivalent of smoking 1 pack per day for 1 year. A patient who smokes 40 cigarettes per day (2 packs) for 5 years would have a 10 pack-year history (2 packs/day × 5 years).

▶ Other Air-Related Risks

In addition to direct inhalation of cigarette smoke, other environmental factors have been identified as risks for the development of primary lung tumors. Environmental tobacco smoke (ETS) presents a significant occupational hazard for nonsmokers working in environments that have a high smoking population, such as bars or restaurants. Most states have instituted laws banning public smoking in order to protect individuals working in these locations. Each year approximately 3000 cases of lung cancer in nonsmokers are caused by ETS. Other environmental factors linked to lung cancer include radon, arsenic, nickel, and chloromethyl ethers. Those who live in an urban environment are also at an increased risk for lung cancer owing to exposure to high concentrations of combustion fumes.[4] Asbestos exposure increases the risk of developing a distinct type of lung cancer called mesothelioma, which is rare and beyond the scope of this chapter.

▶ Nutrition

Diet and nutrition have long been suspected to play a role in cancer susceptibility, and many studies have sought to define specific foods or nutrients that influence cancer risk. Because not all heavy smokers develop lung cancer, it is thought that nutritional factors may explain part of this variation. Epidemiologic studies focusing on diet and nutrition in lung cancer have shown reduced rates of lung cancer in individuals who report higher fruit and vegetable consumption. However, studies attempting to identify specific chemical components of fruits and vegetables that are responsible for this effect have not been successful. ❶ *Recommendations to patients who are at risk owing to smoking or other factors or those who are simply interested in reducing their risk of cancer should include an increase in dietary intake of fruits and vegetables.*

Hereditary or Genetic Risk Factors

Although smoking is a key risk factor for lung cancer, the majority of people who smoke never develop lung cancer. Genetic risk factors may predispose certain smokers to lung cancer. After adjustments for age, smoke exposure, occupation, and gender, relatives of a lung cancer patient have approximately a twofold risk of developing lung cancer. The degree of inherited risk inversely correlates with the age of the relative at the time of diagnosis. First-degree relatives of a lung cancer patient diagnosed between the ages of 40 and 59 years have a sixfold relative risk for lung cancer. Familial lung cancer that develops at an early age in nonsmokers fits a Mendelian codominant inheritance model. However, a lung cancer gene has not been identified.

Other genetic links to lung cancer involve metabolic enzymes that process carcinogens. The damaging effects of tobacco smoke are thought be a result of bulky aromatic hydrocarbons that damage DNA. These chemicals are activated by certain phase I metabolic enzymes and are deactivated by phase II conjugating enzymes such as the glutathione-S-transferases. People with elevated cytochrome CYP 2D6, 1A1, or 1A2 have greater risk of DNA damage and subsequent cancer owing to higher formation rates of active carcinogens. Those with deficient phase II metabolism (*GSTM1* or *GSTT1*) similarly may have increased risk owing to lower clearance of carcinogens.

Chemoprevention

Chemoprevention refers to the use of prophylactic medications to prevent the development of cancer. Many studies of potential chemopreventatives, including nonsteroidal anti-inflammatory drugs (NSAIDs), retinoids, inhaled glucocorticoids, vitamin E, selenium, and green tea extracts, have been conducted, but none have been successful. Large randomized clinical trials have evaluated β-carotene and vitamin E as lung cancer chemopreventative agents in high-risk patients (older smokers). Although vitamin E has no influence on lung cancer, the trials show that older people who smoke have a higher risk of developing and dying of lung cancer if they take a β-carotene supplement. Nonsmokers do not appear to have an altered risk of lung cancer with β-carotene consumption. Interestingly, data from a placebo-controlled double blind study demonstrated that selective cyclooxygenase-2 (COX-2) inhibition with celecoxib reduces the proliferation of bronchial epithelial cells, lowers inflammatory markers, and may resolve benign or premalignant lung nodules in former smokers.[7] Existing data suggest that bronchial epithelial cell proliferation may be a surrogate endpoint for chemopreventative lung cancer trials. Thus, COX-2 inhibition may be a viable strategy for lung cancer chemoprevention, but requires additional validation. In the absence of this validation, and given the long-term cardiovascular effects of selective COX-2 inhibitors, routine use of celecoxib as a chemopreventative agent is not warranted.

Screening and Early Detection

Overall 5-year survival in lung cancer is only 15%, but those who are diagnosed at a localized stage exhibit a 5-year survival rate of 50%. Currently, more than three-quarters of newly diagnosed lung cancers present with locally advanced or metastatic disease, and therefore, very few patients are able to undergo surgical resection.[1] In an attempt to identify tumors when they are localized and have higher cure rates, many investigators are evaluating different screening modalities. Effective screening methods have the potential to save thousands of lives. The use of spiral computed tomography (CT) has been shown to be more sensitive in detecting small nodules compared with chest radiography. However, spiral CT scanning alone has limited benefit owing to the high rate of false-positive results (i.e., lack of specificity) leading to excessive patient anxiety and workup, which can have a negative effect on morbidity and mortality. Nonetheless, a landmark trial, the National Lung Screening Trial, which randomized more than 53,000 patients at high risk for lung cancer to triannual CT or chest radiography demonstrated a significant impact (20% reduction) on lung cancer mortality using CT as a screening tool.[8] However, the number of false-positive results in the CT arm was greater than triple that of the chest radiography arm. Thus, screening using CT can significantly reduce mortality but at the cost of higher false-positive results. Future trials will likely be aimed at reducing false-positive results associated with spiral CT using additional screening tools for follow-up of suspicious lesions.

Because lung cancer tumors are hypermetabolic, they can typically be visualized with 5-FDG (5-fluorodeoxyglucose) positron emission tomography (PET). The combination of spiral CT scanning and follow-up PET scanning for positive lesions is a promising method for the identification of false-positive results. In a recent study, this combination resulted in 90% specificity and 100% sensitivity for detection of cancer when a 3-month follow-up CT was used after a negative PET scan result. Furthermore, 92% of non–small cell tumors were diagnosed at stage IA or IB.[9] Additional studies evaluating the benefits on mortality of this approach are underway. Spiral CT and PET scanning are currently the most promising screening tools for patients at a high risk for lung cancer. High-risk individuals should be encouraged to enter randomized controlled trials aimed at demonstrating a survival benefit from screening.

PATHOPHYSIOLOGY

Most lung cancers arise from the epithelium of the airways and are classified as carcinomas. There are four major and several rare histologic types of lung cancer. They appear to form through different mutagenic pathways; however, they all appear to transition through a premalignant state. The presence of a transitional state from normal tissue to cancerous tissue is important because the premalignant cells contain damage that is generally thought to be reversible. Researchers are currently trying to develop methods to identify people with premalignant lesions as well as drugs that can reverse the damage.

Continued damage to premalignant cells can lead to cancer. The first appearance of cancer cells that have not yet become invasive is referred to as *carcinoma in situ*. Patients are rarely diagnosed with this early stage of cancer owing to a lack of symptoms and relatively rapid progression from

Table 90–1

Lung Tumor Histopathology[43]

Tumor Type	Percent of Tumors	Approximate Cell Doubling Time (days)	Sensitivity to Chemotherapy and Radiotherapy	Relative Risk of Metastasis
Small cell	15–20	30	High	High
Non–small cell				
Adenocarcinoma	30–35	180	Low	Medium
Large cell (giant)	9	100	Low	Low
Squamous (epidermoid)	30–35	180	Low	Low

this state to larger invasive tumors. As the tumor grows, cells may become dislodged from the tumor bulk and enter the hematologic or lymphatic circulatory systems, where they can travel to either local or distant parts of the body. Hematologic spread usually results in metastatic sites in the bones, liver, and central nervous system (CNS). Lymphatic spread is more orderly in nature, with the hilar and mediastinal lymph nodes in the pleural cavity commonly being involved. Once the tumor has spread to multiple locations, curative treatment is rare because surgical excision and radiotherapy cannot remove all or nearly all of the cancer cells.

Histologic Classification

Histologic classification of lung cancer involves determining the cellular origin of the tumor. Knowing the histology of the tumor influences treatment decisions as well as prognosis. For histologic classification to be carried out, the pathologist must obtain a tissue sample. Methods of tissue sampling are discussed in the section on diagnostic principles.

There are four major histologic types of lung cancer that are divided into two classes based on response to treatment and prognosis: small cell lung cancer (SCLC) and non–small cell lung cancer (NSCLC). However, it is important to note that certain other rare malignancies can be seen and many lung cancers may consist of multiple histologic subtypes. Furthermore, a recent phenomenon has been observed where pharmacologic treatments may selectively kill different components of the

tumor, resulting in a conversion of the remaining tumor to a different subtype (i.e., NSCLC becomes SCLC after treatment). Therefore, repeat biopsies of lung tumors before each line of treatment may become a standard of care, although it is not routinely performed at this time. The four major types of lung cancer are outlined by class in Table 90–1.

CLINICAL PRESENTATION AND DIAGNOSIS

Clinical symptoms are not commonly seen until lung cancer tumors become large and/or have metastasized. This is a key factor in the poor prognosis associated with lung cancer. Patients who are diagnosed at an earlier clinical stage have improved prognosis compared with those diagnosed at later stages. Therefore, diagnosing lung cancer earlier through screening and identification of initial signs and symptoms is important. Patients with multiple risk factors for lung cancer; including smoking, may be screened for suspicious lesions using spiral CT triannually because this method has been shown to beneficially impact lung cancer mortality in a high-risk population. However, it should be noted that screening using CT predisposes patients to a greater number of false-positive test results, which may lead to unnecessary evaluation procedures and patient anxiety and stress.

Diagnosis

The diagnosis of lung cancer requires both visualization of the cancerous lesion and tissue sampling for pathologic assessment. Visualization of the suspected tumor provides the clinician with the information necessary to choose the most appropriate sampling technique. Although some lung tumors may be apparent using relatively simple techniques such as a chest x-ray (CXR), many can be either too small to detect or located in an anatomically difficult area to visualize. Therefore, multiple methods of visualization are often used. Once the tumor has been located, sampling provides tissue to confirm malignancy and to determine the histology (e.g., squamous cell, adenocarcinoma, large cell, or small cell). The advantages and disadvantages of various sampling methods must be weighed carefully so that the procedure performed is the least invasive with a high likelihood of providing an accurate diagnosis. Tools used in the diagnosis of lung cancer are outlined in Table 90–2.

Patient Encounter, Part 1

A 57-year-old Asian woman, LT, presents at your clinic complaining of new-onset cough. She has had several upper respiratory infections in the past 2 months with occasional hemoptysis. She smoked about a half a pack of cigarettes per day beginning in her early 30s but quit about 10 years later and has not smoked since. She lives downtown in the city and has worked at her own restaurant and bar since she bought the establishment 10 years ago.

What risk factors for lung cancer are present?

Calculate this patient's pack-year history.

Clinical Presentation and Diagnosis of Lung Cancer

❷ *Signs and symptoms of lung cancer can be classified into three subdivisions: pulmonary, extrapulmonary, and paraneoplastic syndromes. Distinguishing among these classes of symptoms is important because it can aid in determining the severity of the disease, guide treatment options, and affect prognosis.*

Pulmonary Symptoms

Symptoms owing to the direct effects of the primary tumor are often the first to appear and are the most common. These include:

- Cough
- Chest pain
- Superior vena cava obstruction
- Shortness of breath
- Dysphagia
- Hemoptysis
- Pleural effusion

Extrapulmonary Symptoms

Once the tumor invades tissues outside the pleural cavity, it can produce a wide array of symptoms, including:

- General bone pain
- Adrenal insufficiency
- Nausea
- Focal neurologic symptoms
- Confusion
- Personality changes
- Enlarged lymph nodes
- Weight loss
- Seizures
- Horner's syndrome
- Fatigue
- Headache
- Vomiting
- Subcutaneous skin nodules

Paraneoplastic Syndromes

Symptoms that are not a result of the direct effects of the tumor are termed *paraneoplastic syndromes*. They may be caused by substances secreted by the tumor or in response to the tumor and often occur in tissues far from the site of malignancy. Paraneoplastic syndromes are numerous and affect a wide variety of systems, including the endocrine, neurologic, skeletal, renal, metabolic, vascular, and hematologic systems.

Diagnosis

Diagnosis requires visualization of one or more lesions as well as biopsy of the lesion to confirm malignancy. Both visualization and sampling can be performed by invasive or noninvasive methods. These methods are summarized in Table 90–2.

Table 90–2

Diagnostic Tools

	Technique	Description
Visualization	Chest x-ray	The least expensive visualization method in the diagnosis of lung cancer. Readily accessible and does not require systemic administration of contrast dye. However, it often detects lesions that are not cancerous and is not capable of assessing lymph node status.
	CT	More accurate when providing information on size, location, and invasion than chest radiography. It is recommended as part of the standard workup in most cases.
	PET scanning	Uses a substance called 5-FDG to produce a functional image of the lungs. Cells that are actively growing and dividing use greater amounts of glucose and therefore take up more 5-FDG. Focal regions of fluorescence can be visualized in cancerous lesions. PET scanning combined with a CT scan is more accurate than CT scan alone; however, the exact role of PET scanning in staging and monitoring is unclear. The apparent benefit and common role in staging is to evaluate mediastinal disease when it can influence the tumor resectability.
Tumor sampling	Fine-needle aspiration	A method of aspirating cells from the tumor via insertion of a small-bore needle into the lesion and aspirating. Commonly used to evaluate lymph nodes or other poorly accessible sites, it has the advantage of being faster and less invasive than other biopsy methods; however, it does not preserve the architecture of the tumor and may return cells that are undergoing cell death, which negates histologic analysis.
	Bronchoscopy	A fiberoptic camera is inserted through the airways to examine the site of the suspected lesion. Once the lesion is visualized, a tool attached to the camera allows for a tissue biopsy. Newer technologies incorporate fluorescence to differentiate malignant tissue from premalignant lesions.
	Core needle biopsy	A method of obtaining tissue and preserving the tumor architecture. A large-bore needle is inserted into a lesion, where it cuts a core of tissue out that then can be evaluated.
	Thoracentesis	Involves removal of fluid in the pleural cavity via a needle. The fluid then is assayed for presence cancerous cells. This procedure has low sensitivity and depends on the presence of a pleural effusion.
	Sputum cytology	Detects cancerous cells that become dislodged from the airways into the sputum. Sputum cytology is useful because it is not invasive, but it has much lower sensitivity for detecting cancer.

CT, computed tomography; 5-FDG, 5-fluorodeoxyglucose; PET, positron emission tomography.

Clinical Staging

Once the diagnosis of lung cancer is confirmed through visualization and biopsy, the extent of disease must be determined. NSCLC is staged using the American Joint Committee on Cancer (AJCC) tumor, node, and metastasis (TNM) staging system. SCLC is typically staged using the Veterans Administration Lung Cancer Study Group method. Clinical staging serves two primary purposes: predicting prognosis and guiding therapy.

► Non–Small Cell Lung Cancer

Clinical staging of NSCLC with the TNM system evaluates the size of the tumor (T), extent of nodal involvement (N), and presence of metastatic sites (M). The combination of these three evaluations determines the stage. Clinical stages and associated survival rates are outlined in Table 90–3. Local disease includes tumors that are confined to a single hemithorax and those cancers which have spread to the ipsilateral hilar lymph nodes. Once malignancy invades the mediastinal lymph nodes or contralateral hilar nodes, the disease becomes locally advanced. When signs of cancer are detected outside the pleural cavity, it is classified as advanced disease. Local disease is associated with the highest cure and survival rates, whereas those with advanced disease have a 5-year survival rate of less than 5%.

► Small Cell Lung Cancer

The most common system for staging SCLC was developed originally by the Veterans Administration Lung Cancer Study Group. This system categorizes SCLC into two classifications, limited and extensive disease.[10]

- Limited disease: evidence of the tumor is confined to a single hemithorax and can be encompassed by a single radiation port

- Extensive disease: any progression beyond limited disease

TABLE 90–3

Clinical Stage and Prognosis[10]

Clinical Stage	TNM Staging			Survival Rate (%)	
	Tumor	Node	Metastasis	1 Year	5 Year
Local					
IA	1	0	0	94	67
IB	2	0	0	87	53
IIA	1	1	0	89	40
Locally Advanced					
IIB	2	1	0	73	30
	3	0	0		
IIIA	1	2	0	58	15
	2	2	0		
	3	1	0		
	3	2	0		
IIIB	Any	3	0	37	10
Advanced					
IIIB	4	Any	0	37	10
IV	Any	Any	1	18	Less than 5

Patient Encounter, Part 2: Medical History, Physical Examination, and Diagnosis

PMH: GERD (controlled with PPIs) and moderate hypertension (controlled)

FH: Father recently diagnosed with colorectal cancer, but alive, mother living and healthy.

Meds:

- Lisinopril 20 mg/day
- Lansoprazole 30 mg/day

ROS: (+)chest pain, shortness of breath, hemoptysis; (–) recent weight loss

PE

VS: BP 125/69, RR 26, P 80, T 99°F (37.2°C)

CV: RRR

Labs:

Slightly elevated ionized calcium and LFTs; all others WNL.

Chest radiograph reveals a solitary nodule in right lower lobe.

Fine-needle aspiration confirms adenocarcinoma of the lung.

Further evaluation with CT and PET scans reveal a 3-cm mass with possible ipsilateral lymph node involvement.

What clinical stage is this patient's disease?

What is the estimated survival time for this stage of NSCLC?

Does this patient have any factors that may negatively or positively influence survival?

TREATMENT

Desired Outcome and General Approach to Patient

The treatment of lung cancer depends on tumor histology; stage of disease; and patient characteristics such as age, gender, history, and performance status (PS). All of these aspects must be assessed before appropriate treatment can be recommended. The general approach to treatment of lung cancer is outlined in Figure 90–1. In the development of a patient care plan, keep in mind the ultimate goals of therapy. ❸ *In patients with early stage disease, a definitive cure is the primary goal of treatment, although this end point is not always met. Additional goals of treating lung cancer patients include prolongation of survival and improvement of quality of life through alleviation of symptoms.* The goals of treatment must be considered when selecting a therapeutic plan. Some treatments may prolong survival by a few months but at the expense of significant decreases in patient quality of life. Treatment decisions must include both the health care team and an informed and well-counseled patient.

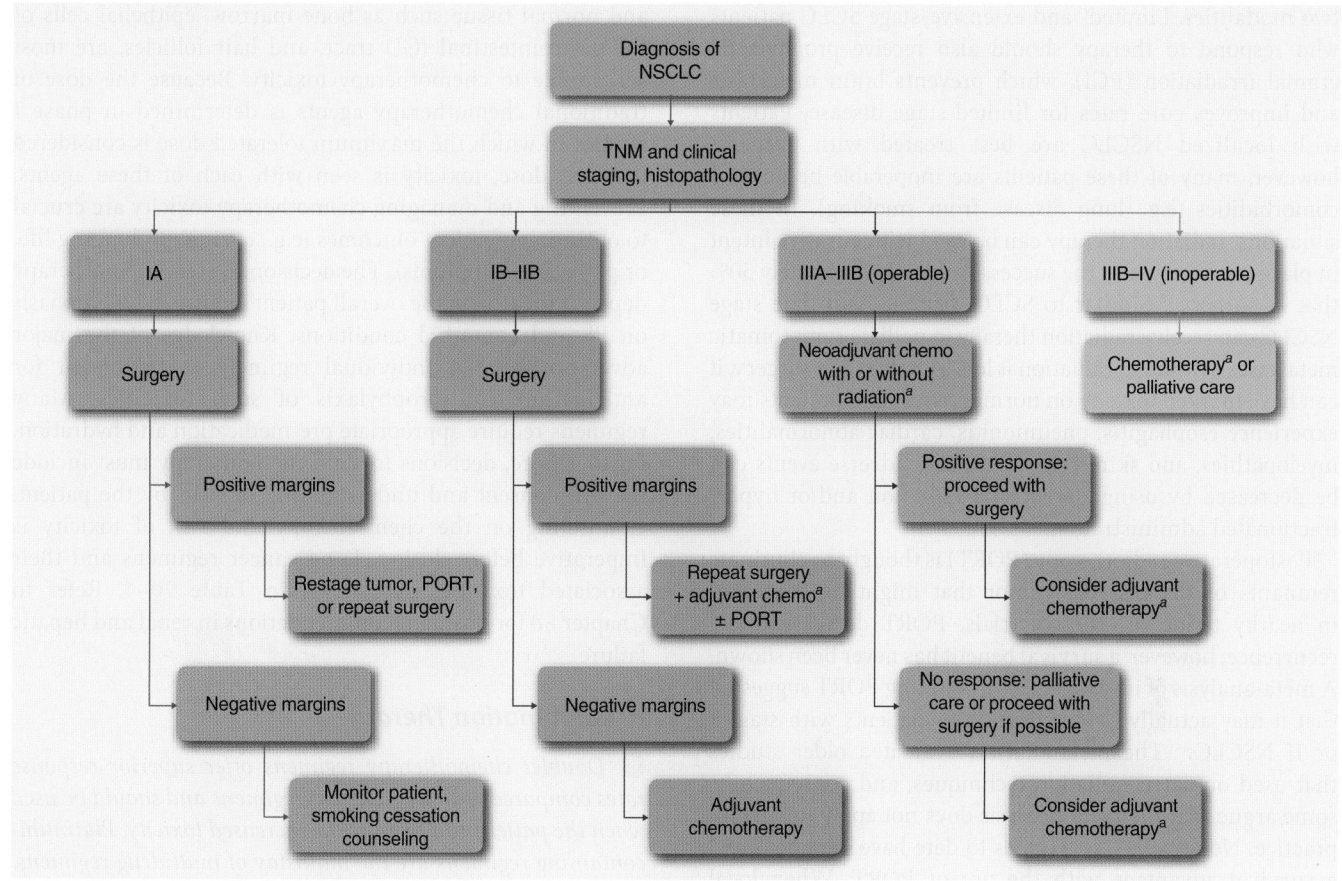

FIGURE 90–1. Clinical pathway for non–small cell lung cancer. *See text for specific treatment recommendations. (chemo, chemotherapy; NSCLC, non–small cell lung cancer; PORT, postoperative radiotherapy; TNM, tumor, node, metastasis.)

▶ *Performance Status*

The PS of an individual patient predicts response and likelihood of toxicity to chemotherapy as well as overall survival. The PS scaling system used most frequently was developed by the Eastern Cooperative Oncology Group (ECOG) (see Chap. 88). ❹ *Categorizing patients by their ECOG PS allows for an objective measure of capability to tolerate systemic therapies that may severely compromise the patient's health. patients with a good PS (0 to 1) are more likely to tolerate intense therapy. PS 2 may receive chemotherapy, and PS 3–4 may receive supportive therapy or treatment with targeted therapies if they have activating mutations.* Patients with less advanced disease may be treated more aggressively in this scenario because the intent of treatment is curative.

Nonpharmacologic Therapy

▶ *Surgery*

❺ *Of all treatment modalities, surgical resection of the affected lobe or lung leads to the greatest improvement in survival for patients with early stage and locally advanced NSCLC tumors (clinical stage IA, IB, or IIA).* The candidacy of the tumor for resection should only be determined by an experienced

thoracic surgeon who routinely works with cancer patients. During surgery, peripheral lymph nodes may be removed if they are thought to be involved, and mediastinal nodes are often dissected for biopsy to determine their involvement. In patients with advanced disease NSCLC, surgery is not curative and as a general approach does not prolong survival. However, surgery for advanced disease is an important palliative treatment that can improve quality of life in some patients. In this respect, surgery is limited to local sites where the tumor is causing significant morbidity (e.g., spinal cord compression). Patients with small cell carcinomas are rarely treated with surgery because the results of a randomized trial published in 1969 showed that surgery did not result in any 5- or 10-year survivors, but radiation produced a 4% survival rate at 5 and 10 years.[11] With improved imaging and surgical techniques as well as the use of effective adjuvant therapy, some clinicians believe that surgery does have a role in early stage SCLC. However, this has yet to be proven in a clinical trial.

▶ *Radiotherapy*

As mentioned earlier, radiotherapy is the treatment of choice for limited-stage SCLC. Optimal patient outcomes are achieved when radiation is administered concurrently with chemotherapy because of synergy between the two modalities. Limited- and extensive-stage SCLC patients who respond to therapy should also receive prophylactic cranial irradiation (PCI), which prevents brain metastasis and improves cure rates for limited-stage disease. Patients with localized NSCLC are best treated with surgery; however, many of these patients are inoperable because of comorbidities (e.g., lung disease from smoking). In these situations, radiation therapy can be used with curative intent in place of surgery, and the success rate is approximately 50% that of surgery.[12] Similar to SCLC, patients with late stage NSCLC can receive radiation therapy to palliate symptomatic metastases. Although radiation is less invasive than surgery, it can have marked toxicity on normal tissue, and patients may experience esophagitis, pneumonitis, cardiac abnormalities, myelopathies, and skin irritation. These adverse events can be decreased by using stereotactic radiation and/or hyper-fractionated administration.[13]

Postoperative radiotherapy (PORT) is thought to eliminate remnants of the resected tumor that might be deposited in nearby tissue. In clinical trials, PORT decreases local recurrence; however, a survival benefit has never been shown. A meta-analysis of investigations evaluating PORT suggested that it may actually be detrimental to patients with stage I or II NSCLC.[14] The meta-analysis evaluated older studies that used outdated radiation techniques, and consequently, some argue that the meta-analysis does not apply to current practice. Nonetheless, no studies to date have demonstrated a survival advantage with the use of PORT. When local recurrence is a significant risk, PORT still may be a viable option. In fact, current guidelines recommend that patients with positive surgical margins (i.e., cancerous cells are detected on the surface of the excised tissue) undergo re-resection or systemic chemotherapy or PORT.[15] Outside of this recommendation, adjuvant radiotherapy without concurrent chemotherapy is not considered beneficial, especially in early-stage disease.

Pharmacologic Therapy

▶ Chemotherapy

Traditional chemotherapeutic agents interfere with processes during cell division or affect DNA replication in nondividing cells, resulting in cell death. Unfortunately, these agents are not specific for cancer cells, and other tissues in the body often are affected. Rapidly cycling cells, both tumor

and normal tissue such as bone marrow, epithelial cells of the gastrointestinal (GI) tract, and hair follicles, are most susceptible to chemotherapy toxicity. Because the dose of traditional chemotherapy agents is determined in phase I studies in which the maximum tolerated dose is considered the best dose, toxicity is seen with each of these agents. Preventing and managing chemotherapy toxicity are crucial to optimizing patient outcomes (e.g., curing, prolonging life, or palliating symptoms). The decision to start chemotherapy depends greatly on the overall patient picture, with emphasis on PS and comorbid conditions. Knowledge of the major adverse effects of individual regimens is important for anticipation and prophylaxis of such toxicities. Many regimens require appropriate pre-medication and hydration. Furthermore, decisions to start chemotherapy must include the full consent and understanding of risks by the patient. Counseling on the chemotherapy and risk of toxicity is imperative before dosing. Lung cancer regimens and their associated toxicities are shown in Table 90-4. Refer to Chapter 88 for dosing recommendations in renal and hepatic failure.

▶ Combination Therapy

6 *Doublet chemotherapy regimens offer superior response rates compared with single-agent regimens and should be used when the patient can tolerate the increased toxicity. Platinum-containing regimens are the mainstay of multidrug regimens.* Several regimens contain either cisplatin or carboplatin combined with another chemotherapy agent; these are known as platinum doublets. Cisplatin and carboplatin are structurally related but have distinct toxicity profiles, and it is unclear if they are equally efficacious.

Non–Small Cell Lung Cancer Both carboplatin and cisplatin show the most pronounced improvements in survival in patients with advanced stage NSCLC when combined with newer agents such as gemcitabine, vinorelbine, docetaxel, or paclitaxel. Because of reduced neurotoxicity, nephrotoxicity, and GI toxicity, many clinicians favor carboplatin over cisplatin.[16] There is also interest in developing non–platinum-containing doublets. Recent studies suggest that gemcitabine combined with paclitaxel or docetaxel is just as effective in advanced stage NSCLC as a platinum doublet; however, guidelines maintain that a platinum-containing doublet should be used when feasible.[15]

Small Cell Lung Cancer In SCLC, a platinum agent combined with an older agent (e.g., etoposide) is the treatment of choice. There are also a number of non–platinum-containing three-drug anthracycline-containing regimens that are as effective as a platinum doublet in extensive-stage disease. However, the three-drug regimens are more toxic and are rarely used in the United States. In limited-stage disease, cisplatin and etoposide are superior to the three-drug anthracycline-containing regimens and provide optimal outcomes when combined with concurrent radiation.[17]

A direct comparison of etoposide combined with either cisplatin or carboplatin in SCLC found similar results.

Table 90–4

Chemotherapy Regimens in Lung Cancer and Associated Toxicities[19,23,31,44–50]

	Dose	Cycle Length (days)	Neutropenia Grade III (%)	Neutropenia Grade IV (%)
Non–Small Cell				
Paclitaxel–carboplatin–bevacizumab	Carboplatin, dose targeted to AUC of 6 IV (day 1), paclitaxel 200 mg/m² IV over 3 hours (day 1), bevacizumab 15 mg/kg IV (day 1)	21		24
Cisplatin–paclitaxel	Paclitaxel 135 mg/m² IV over 24 hours (day 1) and cisplatin 75 mg/m² IV (day 2)	21	18	57
Cisplatin–docetaxel	Cisplatin 75 mg/m² IV (day 1) and docetaxel 75 mg/m² IV (day 1)	21	21	48
Cisplatin–gemcitabine	Cisplatin 100 mg/m² IV (day 1) and gemcitabine 1000 mg/m² IV (days 1, 8, and 15)	28	24	39
Cisplatin–vinorelbine–cetuximab	Cisplatin 80 mg/m² (day 1) and vinorelbine 25 mg/m² (days 1 and 8) +/- cetuximab 400 mg/m² initial dose; then 250 mg/m²/wk)	21	14	38
Cisplatin–vinorelbine	Cisplatin 80 mg/m² (day 1) and vinorelbine 25 mg/m² weekly (days 1 and 8)	21	14	38
Carboplatin–paclitaxel	Carboplatin, dose targeted to AUC of 6 IV (day 1), and paclitaxel 225 mg/m² IV over 3 hours (day 1)	21	20	43
Gemcitabine–paclitaxel	Paclitaxel 200 mg/m² IV (day 1) and gemcitabine 1000 mg/m² (days 1 and 8)	21	10	5
Gemcitabine–docetaxel	Gemcitabine 1100 mg/m² IV (days 1 and 8) and docetaxel 100 mg/m² IV (day 8)	21	11	11
Gemcitabine	Gemcitabine 1125 mg/m² (days 1 and 8)	21		19
Pemetrexed	Pemetrexed 500 mg/m² (day 1), vitamin B₁₂ 1 mg IM 1–2 weeks before treatment initiation and every 9 weeks thereafter; folic acid 1 mg/day beginning 3 weeks before treatment initiation	21		5–6
Paclitaxel	Paclitaxel 200 mg/m² IV over 3 hours (day 1)	21	34	3
Docetaxel	Docetaxel 35 mg/m² IV over 1 hour (days 1, 8, 15)	28		5
Small Cell				
EP	Etoposide 100 mg/m² IV (days 1–3) and cisplatin 100 mg/m² IV (day 2)	28	85	18
CAV	Cyclophosphamide 800 mg/m² IV (day 1), doxorubicin 50 mg/m² (day 1), and vincristine 1.4 mg/m² (maximum, 2 mg) IV (day 1)	21–28	15	72
EC	Etoposide 100 mg/m² IV (days 1–3) and carboplatin AUC 5–6 IV (day 1)	21	10–20	5–15
IC	Irinotecan 60 mg/m² (days 1, 8, 15) and cisplatin 60 mg/m² (day 1)	28	40	25
Topotecan	Topotecan 1.5 mg/m² IV over 30 minutes (days 1–5)	21	18	70

	Other Significant Toxicities	Nausea/Vomiting Potential
Non–Small Cell		
Paclitaxel–carboplatin–bevacizumab	Diarrhea, fever, headache, hypertension, hemoptysis, infection, leukopenia, nausea, neuropathy, peripheral neuritis, vomiting, thrombocytopenia, thrombotic events, bleeding, proteinuria	High (day 1 only)
Cisplatin–paclitaxel	Febrile neutropenia or infection, thrombocytopenia, nausea, vomiting, diarrhea, cardiac toxicity, renal toxicity, neuropathy, weakness, hypersensitivity reactions, anemia	High (day 2 only)
Cisplatin–docetaxel	Infection, thrombocytopenia, nausea, vomiting, diarrhea, cardiac, renal, neuropathy, weakness, hypersensitivity, anemia	High (day 1 only)
Cisplatin–gemcitabine	Febrile neutropenia or infection, thrombocytopenia, nausea, vomiting, diarrhea, cardiac, renal, neuropathy, weakness, anemia	High (day 1) mild (days 8/15)
Cisplatin–vinorelbine–cetuximab	Data not available	High (day 1 only)
Cisplatin–vinorelbine	Neutropenia, infection, anorexia, thrombocytopenia, nausea, vomiting, dyspnea, constipation, neuropathy, anemia	High (days 1 and 8)
Carboplatin–paclitaxel	Infection, thrombocytopenia, nausea, vomiting, diarrhea, cardiac, renal, neuropathy, weakness, hypersensitivity, anemia	High (day 1 only)
Gemcitabine–paclitaxel	Alopecia, nausea and vomiting, neurotoxicity, thrombocytopenia	Moderate
Gemcitabine–docetaxel	Nausea and vomiting, diarrhea, thrombocytopenia, asthenia, neurotoxicity	Moderate
Gemcitabine	Thrombocytopenia	Mild
Pemetrexed	Anemia	Mild
Paclitaxel	Infection, nausea, vomiting, diarrhea, mucositis, arthralgia, asthenia, peripheral neuropathy, alopecia, cardiovascular	Mild (day 1 only)
Docetaxel	Fatigue, nausea, vomiting, skin toxicity, neuropathy, anemia, hypersensitivity, alopecia	Mild

(Continued)

Table 90–4

Chemotherapy Regimens in Lung Cancer and Associated Toxicities[19,23,31,44–50] (*Continued*)

	Other Significant Toxicities	Nausea/Vomiting Potential
Small Cell		
EP	Infection, nausea, vomiting, thrombocytopenia, anemia	High (day 2 only)
CAV	Nausea, vomiting, thrombocytopenia, neuropathy, hepatic, renal, alopecia	High
EC	Infection, thrombocytopenia, alopecia	High (day 1 only)
IC	Fever, infection, thrombocytopenia, anemia, diarrhea, nausea and vomiting, elevated liver enzymes	High (day 1), moderate (days 8/15)
Topotecan	Neutropenic fever, neutropenic sepsis, anemia, thrombocytopenia, nausea, fatigue, vomiting, stomatitis, anorexia, diarrhea, fever	Mild (days 1–5)

AUC, area under the curve; CAV, cyclophosphamide–doxorubicin–vincristine; EC, etoposide–carboplatin; EP, etoposide–cisplatin; IM, intramuscular; IC, irinotecan–cisplatin; IV, intravenous.

See Chapter 88 for dose reductions for hepatic and renal dysfunction.

This leads some clinicians to consider the agents interchangeable; however, this trial primarily enrolled patients with extensive-stage disease. A direct comparison in patients with limited-stage disease has not been performed, and most clinicians consider cisplatin and etoposide to be the treatment of choice because this combination has been used in nearly all the large comparative trials.

Single-Agent Chemotherapy First-line therapy for advanced-stage NSCLC and SCLC is best done with a two-drug regimen. However, patients who have a recurrence after the initial regimen are best treated with a single chemotherapy agent. Single-agent therapy is also acceptable for patients with poor health and advanced disease because toxicities tend to be lower with one-drug regimens. Chemotherapeutic agents used in monotherapy in lung cancer include pemetrexed, docetaxel, gemcitabine, paclitaxel, topotecan, and vinorelbine (see Table 90–4).

● **Adjuvant Chemotherapy** Surgery has a limited role in the treatment of SCLC, making adjuvant chemotherapy primarily applicable to NSCLC. The rationale behind adjuvant chemotherapy is to eradicate micrometastases or other tumor cells that may have been missed during removal of the primary tumor. The recent results of five relatively large prospective trials ($n = 344$ to 1867) suggest that there is benefit from adjuvant chemotherapy. The largest study, the International Adjuvant Lung Trial (IALT),[18] led to the conclusion that adjuvant chemotherapy following surgical resection of non–small cell tumors results in a 4% improvement in survival. However, the majority of patients in IALT were treated with a cisplatin and etoposide, which has been proven inferior to newer combinations of cisplatin in the advanced disease setting. In support of this criticism, the intergroup JBR-10 study evaluated adjuvant cisplatin–vinorelbine (a current standard regimen for advanced stage disease) and found a survival advantage of 15%.[19] Consequently, adjuvant therapy has become the standard of care in resectable NSCLC and should be offered to patients after resection, particularly those with stage II to III disease. Although the regimen of choice is unclear, cisplatin–vinorelbine appears to be the regimen with the most evidence.

● **Neoadjuvant Therapy** *Neoadjuvant* or *induction therapy* refers to the use of chemotherapy regimens or radiotherapy before surgery. Again, because surgery has a limited role in SCLC, this section applies primarily to NSCLC. The rationale behind neoadjuvant therapy is to decrease the size of the tumor so that it can be extracted more easily with clean margins, as well as to eliminate distant micrometastases before invasive local treatment. Furthermore, patients with marginally resectable or nonresectable tumors may respond sufficiently to induction therapy that surgery becomes an option. Neoadjuvant chemotherapy has been shown to yield benefits in NSCLC (i.e., increase in median survival and disease-free survival and decreased risk of metastasis) for both local and locally advanced disease. One concern is that the toxicity of induction regimens may delay surgery, and if the tumor does not respond to the treatment, there is a risk of disease progression. Nonetheless, current data suggest that more than 90% of patients who are treated with neoadjuvant therapy maintain their scheduled surgery.[20] This approach is most common in patients with locally advanced tumors (stage III).[21] Current studies are aimed at comparing neoadjuvant with adjuvant therapy in earlier stage NSCLC patients. The benefit of combining adjuvant therapy with induction therapy and surgery is also being investigated but is of unknown value at this time.

▶ *Monoclonal Antibodies*

Bevacizumab and cetuximab are IgG monoclonal antibodies that have activity in NSCLC. Bevacizumab targets vascular endothelial-derived growth factor (VEGF), which facilitates angiogenesis, a process contributing to growth and maintenance of the tumor environment. Bevacizumab has been shown to improve survival of advanced stage non–squamous cell NSCLC patients in a large phase III trial[22] and has been incorporated into current guidelines.[15] Squamous cell carcinoma of the lung should not be treated with bevacizumab due to the increased risk of bleeding events (an adverse event associated with bevacizumab administration) in this histologic subtype.

Cetuximab targets epidermal growth factor receptor (EGFR), a cytokine receptor on tumor cells that is frequently involved with tumor survival and proliferation. This monoclonal antibody has a different and less extensive toxicity profile than traditional chemotherapy agents and appears to be synergistic when combined with chemotherapy. Cetuximab has recently been shown to be beneficial in NSCLC when added to cisplatin and vinorelbine in recurrent or metastatic NSCLC (stages IIIB–IV).[23]

▶ Tyrosine Kinase Inhibitors

The tyrosine kinase inhibitors (TKIs) work by targeting specific intracellular messenger proteins that transmit growth and survival signals. The three TKIs are currently available for treatment of lung cancer are erlotinib, gefitinib, and crizotinib. Erlotinib and gefitinib, similar to cetuximab, target the EGFR, which has been shown to be mutated or overexpressed in some lung tumors. Both gefitinib and erlotinib are structurally related and presumably have the same mechanism of action; however, data show that erlotinib prolongs survival, but gefitinib does not in unselected patient populations. Consequently, gefitinib availability is currently restricted in the United States.

Crizotinib targets the *EML4–ALK* fusion gene, which results from a chromosomal translocation that fuses *EML4* gene to the ALK kinase, resulting in a constitutively active oncogenic protein product which is not present in normal cells. *EML4–ALK* fusions occur in about 5% of lung cancer patients and are also more common in never smokers. *EML4–ALK* fusion-positive lung cancer patients benefit significantly from crizotinib, which selectively targets the ALK kinase.[24]

Pharmacogenomics and pharmacogenetics now play a major role in the selection of NSCLC patients who should receive oral EGFR inhibitors such as gefitinib or erlotinib. Large bodies of preclinical and clinical data demonstrate that certain mutations in the kinase domain of EGFR (L858R and del746-750) are associated with significant responses to such agents.[25] The presence of other mutations in EGFR (T790M) are associated with resistance to such inhibitors through decreased drug binding to the receptor. EGFR mutations are more frequent in women, Asians, patients with adenocarcinoma histology, and nonsmokers. Additionally, the presence of activating mutations in KRAS, another oncogene known to play a role in lung cancer, is also associated with clinical resistance to EGFR inhibitors. These findings have prompted clinical guidelines to suggest that assessment of the mutation status of EGFR and/or KRAS is critical in selecting patients for EGFR kinase inhibitor therapy.[15] Patients with mutations in exons 19 or 21 of EGFR demonstrate the greatest likelihood of benefit, while those with mutations in exon 20 of EGFR or those with mutations in exons 1 or 2 of KRAS demonstrate the lowest likelihood of benefit. Furthermore, advanced stage NSCLC patients with EGFR mutations in exons 19 or 21 demonstrate improved survival and tolerability of therapy when treated with gefitinib or erlotinib versus chemotherapy. Therefore, use of genotyping KRAS and EGFR should now be routinely used in selecting lung cancer

patients who will benefit from EGFR TKIs. In addition to erlotinib and gefitinib, several "multitargeted" TKIs that target the EGFR and other cell-signaling cascades are in clinical trials and show promise for the treatment of patients with lung cancer. Likewise, fluorescence in situ hybridization techniques to detect the EML4–ALK fusion event are also now approved and required for selection of patients to receive crizotinib.

Small Cell Lung Cancer

Small cell lung cancer typically presents as extensive disease (approximately 60% to 70% of new cases) and progresses very quickly. Small cell carcinomas are very responsive to chemotherapy and radiation but have a short duration of response. Radiotherapy became the standard in 1969, when a randomized trial showed that it offered the potential for cure, whereas surgery did not.[26] In the vast majority of patients, chemotherapy with or without radiotherapy is the treatment of choice. Even after a complete response to therapy, the cancer usually recurs within 6 to 8 months, and the survival time following recurrence is typically short (approximately 4 months). This yields a typical survival rate of 14 to 20 months for limited disease and 8 to 13 months for extensive disease.[27] Figure 90–2 illustrates the general treatment path of SCLC.

▶ Limited Disease

- The regimen of choice for limited-disease SCLC is etoposide–cisplatin (EP). In patients who are able to tolerate combined modality therapy, concomitant chemoradiotherapy offers the greatest survival benefit. Carboplatin may be substituted for cisplatin in patients who cannot tolerate cisplatin toxicity. Cisplatin is preferred over carboplatin because of a small study that randomized patients to cisplatin or carboplatin plus etoposide. There was a numerically higher complete response rate with cisplatin, which is believed to be requisite for cure. In European countries, a three-drug combination containing an anthracycline has been the mainstay of therapy; however, mounting clinical evidence shows that these regimens are inferior to EP plus concurrent radiation and have more toxicity. Consequently, the guidelines recommend that the EP regimen be used with concurrent radiotherapy.[27]

Because patients with SCLC commonly have a recurrence in the CNS, trials have been performed to evaluate the benefit of PCI. A pivotal study showed that PCI reduces the incidence of brain metastasis and increases the 3-year survival rate from 15% to 21%.[28] Patients with limited stage SCLC who achieve a complete response with treatment should be offered PCI.

▶ Extensive Disease

- Platinum regimens, particularly EP, are the treatment of choice in extensive disease. In one Japanese study, a combination of irinotecan and cisplatin demonstrated an increased median survival time by approximately 3 months over the EP regimen. This irinotecan–cisplatin regimen also had a lower incidence of severe neutropenic side effects but exhibited higher rates of middle- to high-grade diarrhea.

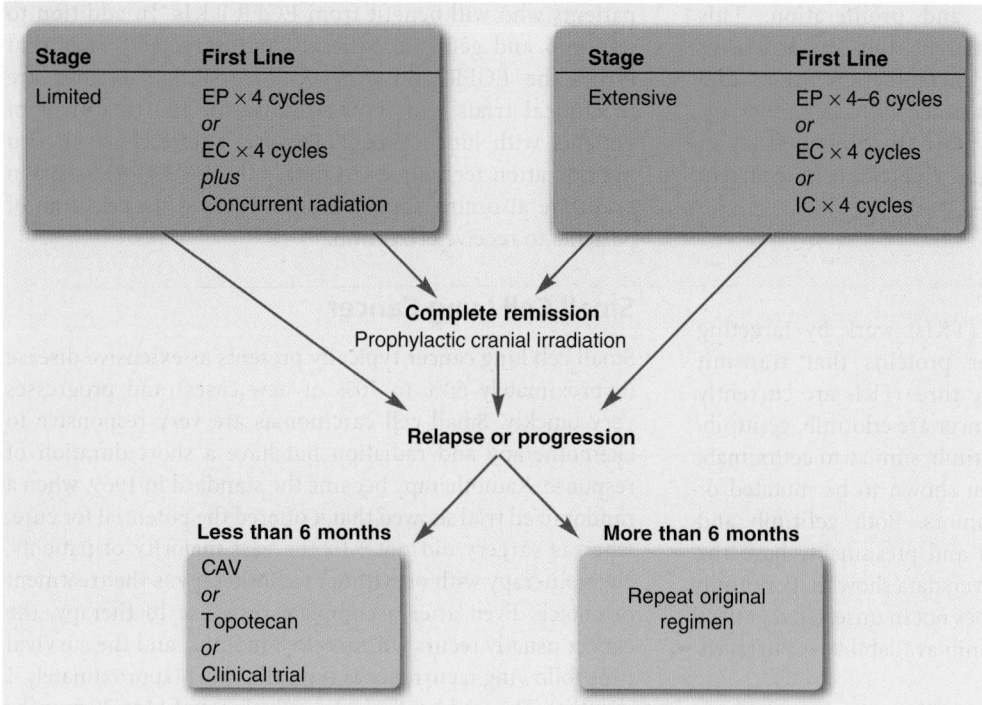

FIGURE 90–2. Small cell lung cancer treatment overview.[27] (CAV, cyclophosphamide, doxorubicin [Adriamycin], and vincristine; EC, etoposide–carboplatin; EP, etoposide–cisplatin; IC, irinotecan–cisplatin.)

However, this study was repeated in the United States and did not show a similar improvement over the EP regimen.[29] Therefore, EP remains the regimen of choice for treating extensive SCLC in the United States. Because of the high sensitivity of treatment-naïve SCLC to chemotherapy, it is imperative that these patients be monitored for signs of tumor lysis syndrome and possibly treated with prophylactic therapy.

Concurrent radiotherapy is not used routinely in extensive disease; however, PCI provides significant benefit in patients responding to chemotherapy. A pivotal study demonstrated that median survival from the time of randomization increased from 5.4 to 6.7 months and 1-year survival rates increased from 13.3% to 27.1% with PCI. An additional benefit was a lower rate of brain metastasis (14.6% versus 40.4%).[30]

▶ Recurrent Disease

● The treatment of recurrent SCLC depends on the time to recurrence. If the time to recurrence is less than 6 months, second-line therapy should be considered if the patient has an acceptable PS (see Patient Care and Monitoring). The most widely accepted second-line therapies in SCLC are topotecan alone or CAV (cyclophosphamide, doxorubicin [Adriamycin], and vincristine). Relapses occurring more than 6 months after treatment warrant a repeat of the initial regimen. Patients with a poor PS (3 to 4) are typically managed with best supportive care, including palliative care therapies.

Non–Small Cell Lung Cancer

The first step in treatment of NSCLC involves confirmation of the clinical stage and determination of resectability

of the tumor. This decision should always be made by a thoracic surgeon who routinely performs lung cancer surgery. Treatment options depend on the advancement of disease (i.e., local, locally advanced, or metastatic), PS, and eligibility for resection.

▶ Local Disease (Stages 1A, 1B, and IIA)

● Local disease encompasses stages IA through IIA and is associated with a favorable prognosis because approximately 40% to 60% of patients are expected to live more than 5 years from diagnosis. Goals of therapy are curative in local disease, and surgery is the mainstay of treatment. Stage IA tumors are rarely seen clinically and may be treated with surgery alone. In this case, neoadjuvant or adjuvant therapy has not been adequately studied to know if it conveys a benefit. If surgical margins are positive, radiotherapy or re-resection is recommended.[15] Stage IB, IIA, and locally advanced IIB NSCLC are treated with adjuvant chemotherapy. Patients who have positive or questionable margins may receive radiation therapy, which typically is administered with the adjuvant chemotherapy. The regimen of choice in this setting is not clear; however, clinical trials demonstrating the most benefit used cisplatin–vinorelbine.

▶ Locally Advanced Disease (Stages IIB and IIIA)

● Patients with locally advanced disease should also be considered for surgery. Neoadjuvant chemotherapy with or without concurrent radiotherapy can be used before surgery, although this practice varies from institution to institution. Progression of disease during induction therapy may preclude surgery, and the regimen should be altered. If there is a response, surgical resection can be attempted, with or without additional adjuvant chemotherapy. Nonresectable locally advanced disease may be treated with both an active platinum-containing regimen and radiotherapy.

▶ *Advanced or Metastatic Disease (Stages IIIB and IV)*

● Advanced disease is treated with chemotherapy if the patient has an acceptable ECOG PS score (0–1). Historically, platinum-containing doublets have produced the highest overall response rates (25% to 35%) and survival times (30% to 40% 1-year survival) in well-performing patients with advanced disease. A number of different platinum doublet treatment regimens have been used in this setting. In some patients with stage IIIB disease, cisplatin and etoposide may be given concurrently with radiotherapy. However, treating unresectable stage III patients with a platinum-containing doublet regimen and omitting the radiation is common. The optimal regimen has yet to be determined. NSCLC chemotherapy doublets that are considered generally equivalent include:

- Paclitaxel–cisplatin
- Paclitaxel–carboplatin
- Cisplatin–gemcitabine
- Cisplatin–docetaxel
- Carboplatin–docetaxel
- Cisplatin–vinorelbine
- Gemcitabine–paclitaxel
- Gemcitabine–docetaxel
- Cisplatin–pemetrexed

A large randomized trial comparing the first four regimens reported similar response rates and survival with all treatments, although there were less life-threatening toxicity and treatment-related deaths associated with paclitaxel–carboplatin.[31] Consequently, one may argue that paclitaxel–carboplatin is the treatment of choice. However, the carboplatin–paclitaxel regimen used in the trial infused paclitaxel over 24 hours, which is uncommon in clinical practice. The most common carboplatin–paclitaxel regimen infuses a higher dose of paclitaxel over 3 hours in the clinic rather than admit patients to the hospital for a 24-hour infusion. It is unfair to extrapolate the toxicity advantage from this trial to the commonly used 3-hour paclitaxel infusion, and consequently, there is not a single best regimen. A subset analysis of the cisplatin–pemetrexed data shows that only patients with a nonsquamous histology benefit from pemetrexed. Additionally, two non–platinum-containing regimens have been shown to have similar survival benefits. Both gemcitabine–paclitaxel and gemcitabine–docetaxel produce response durations and survival times similar to the platinum-containing doublet regimens. These regimens may be substituted when patients are unlikely to tolerate the toxicity of platinum regimens owing to comorbidities or other factors.[32]

● **Targeted agents** Although it is unclear which chemotherapy combination is the best, research aimed at integrating targeted agents into therapy have proven successful but only in defined subgroups. Adding bevacizumab to the carboplatin–paclitaxel

(3-hour infusion) regimen increases response rates and prolongs progression-free survival by 1.7 months and overall survival by 2.3 months.[22] Consequently, carboplatin–paclitaxel and bevacizumab are arguably the new standard of care. However, bevacizumab is only appropriate for patients with non–squamous cell histology because of a high risk of fatal hemoptysis seen in patients with squamous histology.[32]

Interestingly, bevacizumab does not show the same level of synergy with all regimens; when combined with cisplatin and gemcitabine, better progression-free survival and response were seen, but there was no difference was in overall survival. Early data suggest a large benefit from combining bevacizumab with a platinum and pemetrexed, but it is not currently the standard of care. Based on the current peer review data, bevacizumab should only be used with carboplatin and paclitaxel as the initial treatment.[32]

The anti-EGFR monoclonal antibody cetuximab has been shown to improve survival when combined with cisplatin and vinorelbine. The FLEX trial demonstrated a 1.2-month survival advantage of cetuximab when added to cisplatin and vinorelbine in recurrent or metastatic NSCLC (stages IIIB–IV).[23] The study population consisted of chemotherapy-naïve patients with PSs of 0 to 2 that demonstrated positive tumor staining for EGFR by immunohistochemistry. It is unclear how this regimen compares with bevacizumab plus carboplatin and paclitaxel. Because bevacizumab was proven effective first and the survival advantage appears superior, cisplatin, vinorelbine, and cetuximab will likely only be used in patients with a contraindication to bevacizumab (e.g., squamous cell histology).

Individualized therapy has blossomed with the use of EGFR TKIs. Demographic, pathology, and genetic markers can help identify patients most likely to respond to these treatments. Early studies showed that nonsmokers with adenocarcinoma were most likely to benefit from therapy; correlative studies demonstrated that patients with mutations in exon 19 and/or 21 also defined a population likely to respond to treatment. This knowledge has now been tested prospectively. Gefitinib, an EGFR TKI, was compared with carboplatin–paclitaxel as first-line therapy in patients with adenocarcinoma who were never smokers or light former smokers. They reported that gefitinib was noninferior and improved quality of life. A subset analysis showed that those with a mutation in exon 19 or 21 had the highest objective response rates and appeared to have the most benefit.[33] A similar trial comparing erlotinib to a platinum-based doublet in patients with an exon 19 or 21 mutation found that erlotinib improved progression free survival.[34] Based on this data, erlotinib is recommended as first-line therapy in patients with an activating EGFR mutation.

Crizotinib is a new targeted therapy that appears to be very effective for a subset of patients with an ALK rearrangement (approximately 5% of patients). It recently received accelerated approval based on a single arm trial in the salvage setting that resulted in a 55% survival rate at 2 years.[24] Despite the lack of data in the first-line setting, the NCCN guidelines recommend that patients with a known ALK rearrangement can be treated with crizotinib in the first-line setting, which is based on its activity as salvage treatment.

In summary, targeted therapy as monotherapy or in combination with chemotherapy has become a mainstay in first-line treatment of advanced NSCLC.

● **Poorly Performing Patients** Treating patients with a PS of 2 is a subject of debate. Although patients with a PS of 2 typically have inferior survival rates and higher toxicity to platinum chemotherapy than higher performing patients, low-toxicity single-agent regimens may offer a survival advantage in this subset. Use of these regimens also presents a method of providing symptomatic care for advanced stage patients. Agents such as pemetrexed, gemcitabine, and docetaxel may be used in this scenario. In patients with a PS of 3 or 4, chemotherapy typically results in high rates of toxicity and fails to convey a survival benefit. Consequently, treatment should be aimed at relief of symptoms instead of a definitive cure. Because targeted agents typically have less severe toxicity, they also have been used in appropriate subsets of patients with a poor PS (ECOG PS of 2 or 3). Unfortunately, we do not have peer review clinical trial data regarding the efficacy and toxicity of targeted agents in these patients. In summary, debilitated patients should not be treated with combination chemotherapy with or without targeted agents because of historically high rates of toxicity without benefit. Single-agent therapy with less toxicity can be used to help palliate symptoms.

Duration of Therapy Because advanced stage NSCLC is not curable, an argument can be made that the goal is to extend the number of quality days, rather than just overall survival. With this goal in mind and an assumption that quality of life is lower during chemotherapy treatment, it is important to consider the duration of therapy. Over the last decade, treatment has moved toward fewer chemotherapy cycles. Typical therapy regimens have decreased from planning eight cycles to six cycles, to four cycles, which was the standard until several years ago. It was at this time that positive data were reported from two studies using pemetrexed, erlotinib, and bevacizumab as maintenance therapy. Both key studies included patients who had a response or stable disease after 4 cycles of a platinum-based doublet who were then randomized to placebo or treatment.[35] The pemetrexed study reported a 3-month survival advantage with maintenance therapy. A subgroup analysis of this study demonstrated that patients with squamous histology did not benefit from therapy leaving an overall survival benefit of 5 months for the non–squamous cell group. Similarly, the erlotinib maintenance study reported a 1-month overall survival advantage, which does not appear as robust; however, the subset analysis showed benefit was much more likely in nonsmokers and those with adenocarcinoma histology and particularly in patients who had an activating mutation (exon 19 or 21). Similar to the pemetrexed study, patients whose tumor was of squamous cell histology did not appear to benefit from maintenance. In summary, the duration of therapy depends highly on histology; patients with squamous

cell histology will likely be treated for four cycles, but patients with non–squamous cell histology will be treated until progression.[35]

▶ *Recurrent and Progressive Disease*

● Although patients frequently experience a response to initial therapy, disease recurs in most cases. If the recurrence is localized, surgery options may be assessed. If the patient's PS remains acceptable (0 to 1), second-line systemic chemotherapy has been shown to improve survival. Although platinum doublets may be used at this point in care, a single-agent therapy with docetaxel, pemetrexed, erlotinib, or crizotinib is recommended.[24,36] Recurrences in poorly performing patients (3–4) usually are not treated with chemotherapy and are instead treated with supportive care. Additional recurrences (e.g., third-line therapy) may be treated with single-agent therapy not previously used or best supportive care.

PATIENT CARE AND MONITORING
Management of Toxicity

⑦ *Knowing when and how to treat adverse events from chemotherapy is an important aspect of patient care. Unmanaged events may cause delays in chemotherapy administration and reduced chemotherapy doses and may contribute to treatment failure.* Given the fatal nature of untreated lung cancer, patients and health care professionals are willing to tolerate high risks of severe and life-threatening side effects provided that the therapy has been shown to benefit the patient. There are multiple methods of preventing or reducing toxicity from chemotherapeutic agents. These methods usually are agent specific but commonly include maintenance of adequate hydration, use of appropriate premedications, dose reduction of the causative agent, and use of growth factors to combat toxicities associated with cytopenias.

▶ *Grading Toxicity*

● In order to standardize grading of adverse events, the National Cancer Institute (NCI) has developed the Common Toxicity Criteria for Adverse Events (CTC, V4.0) (see Chap. 88). In most cases, patients who experience grade 3 or 4 toxicity require a change in therapy with the next cycle of treatment. Common changes include a chemotherapy dose reduction or pharmacologic intervention to prevent or treat the toxicity. The CTC is an invaluable tool to determine what serious toxicity is most likely with a particular regimen and improves the pharmacist's ability to counsel the patient as well as determine appropriate toxicity-prevention measures.

▶ *Dose Intensity and Growth Factors*

● The term *dose intensity* refers to the percent of drug delivered compared with the planned amount as measured by milligrams per meter squared per week. Maintaining dose intensity (i.e., delivering the planned dose according to the scheduled time course) has been shown to influence survival in some cancers, such as breast cancer; however, the importance of dose intensity in lung cancer is not well established. In order to maintain dose intensity, pharmacologic agents are sometimes used to combat serious toxicities that may prohibit or delay administration of subsequent doses.

With most lung cancer chemotherapy regimens, the most common grade 3 or 4 toxicity is neutropenia. Patients who experience grade 3 or 4 neutropenia are at a high risk of developing a severe or life-threatening bacterial infection. Consequently, patients with neutropenia who develop a fever are empirically given broad-spectrum antibiotics. If a patient experiences neutropenic fever, dose reduction, or intervention with growth factors (e.g., pegfilgrastim, filgrastim, or sargramostim) to maintain dose intensity should occur before the next cycle of chemotherapy. In lung cancer patients, no survival benefit has been demonstrated by using a colony-stimulating factor to maintain dose intensity. ❽ *Although some evidence suggest that the use of a colony-stimulating factor reduces the number of neutropenic fever episodes, hospital stay, and antibiotic administration in certain subsets of lung cancer patients, routine front-line (prophylactic) use of a colony-stimulating factor is not recommended owing to a lack of a survival benefit.*[37,38]

▶ Nausea and Vomiting

● Platinum agents are the most active lung cancer agents and historically have very high rates of nausea and vomiting. This is particularly true of high-dose cisplatin, which is used in many regimens. Understanding how to prevent and treat chemotherapy-induced nausea and vomiting (CINV) in lung cancer patients is crucial because nearly all the regimens are highly emetogenic. Although the pathology of CINV is not fully understood, there are three classifications of CINV based on the time of occurrence in relationship to chemotherapy administration: acute CINV (1–24 hours after the dose), delayed (24 hours to 5 days after the dose), and anticipatory (before the dose following one or more previous cycles).

Acute CINV appears to be influenced predominantly by serotonin binding to 5-HT$_3$ receptors on the vagal nerve, where it innervates the GI tract. Delayed CINV has been attributed to a variety of mechanisms but appears to be influenced by substance P stimulation of neurokinin-1 (NK-1) receptors in the CNS, as well as a corticosteroid-responsive element. Anticipatory CINV is thought to be a learned or conditioned behavior. The major influencing factors appear to be prior acute or delayed CINV and anxiety. Anticipatory CINV may be prevented or treated with benzodiazepines such as lorazepam or alprazolam not because they possess antiemetic properties but rather because they contain amnesic and antianxiety properties.

The three main drug targets that are antagonized to prevent or treat acute and delayed CINV are 5-HT$_3$ receptors, dopamine type 2 receptors (D$_2$), and NK-1 receptors. 5-HT$_3$ receptor antagonists are the most effective agents for preventing acute CINV. However, they are only recommended for moderate to high emetogenic potential regimens, primarily owing to cost (see Table 90–5 for a comparison of agents). Because ondansetron's patent has expired, several generics are available, and the cost for this class of agents has dropped significantly. Aprepitant is the only available NK-1 receptor

---

Table 90–5

Pharmacotherapy for Chemotherapy-Induced Nausea and Vomiting

Class	Indication	Drug	Dose	Half-life
NK-1 inhibitors	Acute or delayed NV	Aprepitant	125 mg PO on day 1 80 mg PO daily on days 2–3	9–13 hours
		Fosaprepitant	115 mg IV on day 1 80 mg PO aprepitant daily on days 2–3	9–13 hours
5-HT$_3$ inhibitors	Acute NV	Ondansetron	16–24 mg PO or 8–12 mg IV on day 1 16 mg PO daily or 8 mg IV daily on days 2–4	3–6 hours
		Palonosetron	0.25 mg IV on day 1	40 hours
		Granisetron	1–2 mg PO or 0.01 mg/kg IV on days 1–4	4–12 hours
		Dolasetron	100 mg PO or 100 mg IV daily on days 1–4	8 hours (active metabolite)
D$_2$ antagonists	Acute or delayed NV, PRN breakthrough treatment	Haloperidol	1–2 mg PO q4–6 hours or 1–3 mg IV q4–6 hours	20 hours
		Olanzapine	Olanzapine 2.5–5 mg PO twice a day PRN	20–50 hours
Corticosteroids	Adjunctive treatment for acute or delayed NV	Dexamethasone	12 mg IV or PO on day 1 8 mg IV or PO daily on days 2–4	2–4 hours biologic half-life of 36–54 hours
Benzodiazepines	Anticipatory NV	Lorazepam	0.5–2 mg PO once on night before and once on morning of treatment	12–16 hours
	Anticipatory NV	Alprazolam	0.5–2 mg PO three times a day starting the night before treatment	12–16 hours

5-HT$_3$, 5-hydroxytryptamine receptor; IV, intravenous; NK-1, neurokinin-1; NV, nausea and vomiting; PO, oral; PRN, as needed.

antagonist that is approved to prevent CINV. It has modest but additive activity in acute CINV and appears to be highly active in preventing delayed CINV. It was approved for use in highly emetogenic regimens but also works in patients receiving moderately emetogenic chemotherapy. The use of aprepitant is somewhat limited by the cost. Dopamine type 2 receptor antagonists, which are approved for schizophrenia, also have antiemetic activity in both acute and delayed CINV. As a group, these agents do not appear to be as effective as 5-HT$_3$ receptor antagonists in acute CINV or as effective as aprepitant in delayed CINV. Consequently, their use is frequently limited to patients receiving mild emetogenic chemotherapy as prevention or as treatment following full-dose 5-HT$_3$ receptor antagonist and/or aprepitant. They are attractive owing to their relatively low cost but cause a significant number of side effects. Interestingly, corticosteroids, most commonly dexamethasone, is an active antiemetic agent that can be used as monotherapy to prevent acute CINV in patients receiving mild to moderate emetogenic chemotherapy. They are also synergistic with 5-HT$_3$ receptor antagonists, aprepitant, and D$_2$-receptor antagonists in acute and delayed CINV. Although antiemetic choices typically are guided by chemotherapy, patient-specific risk factors that may play a role include the following high-risk features: very young age, very old age, female gender, emesis associated with pregnancy or motion sickness, and those with low alcohol intake.[39]

▶ Diarrhea

Chemotherapy-induced diarrhea can be a significant toxicity in cancer patients and should be managed pharmacologically when necessary. The most common offending agent in the treatment of lung cancer is irinotecan. Treatment may include loperamide (4 mg at the onset followed by 2 mg every 2 hours until resolution; may use 4 mg every 4 hours during sleep) or octreotide (starting at 100 mcg subcutaneously every 8 hours and titrated to effect). The goals of therapy are resolution of diarrhea and improvement in quality of life.

Surveillance

Following response to surgery or pharmacologic treatment, the patient should be monitored regularly to detect recurrence. NCCN guidelines suggest a physical examination and chest x-ray every 3 to 4 months for 2 years. If no disease is detected during this time, follow-up frequency can be prolonged to every 6 months for 3 years and then annually. Low-dose spiral CT scanning is also recommended annually. Additionally, smoking cessation counseling with or without pharmacologic treatment should be a priority. Although studies have shown that patients who continue to smoke through treatment in NSCLC do not perform more poorly compared with those that quit before treatment, those who respond to treatment and continue to smoke probably have an increased risk of developing secondary malignancies.[40] In contrast to NSCLC, some data suggest that SCLC patients with limited stage disease have poorer outcomes if they continue to smoke during treatment.[41]

Complications

▶ Cachexia and Anorexia

Cachexia is a severe wasting syndrome that is seen in many cancer patients. Although it is more common in advanced disease, it is often seen in localized disease as well. Cachexia is characterized by a catabolic state that leads to significant loss of body mass, both lean muscle and fat. The causes of cachexia are poorly understood, but it is thought that they involve inflammatory cytokines such as tumor necrosis factor alpha (TNF-α, originally described as cachexin). Anorexia is a patient's loss of appetite or willingness to eat. The presence of anorexia can aggravate cachexia and contribute to morbidity. When anorexia contributes to cachexia, it is important to assess the patient for the underlying cause of the anorexia.

Causes for anorexia in lung cancer patients can be widespread and include CINV, esophagitis and mucosal irritation from combined radiotherapy and chemotherapy, GI obstruction owing to tumors, constipation from opioid analgesics, and psychological factors such as anxiety or depression. Many of these issues may be improved with pharmacologic treatment of the underlying cause (i.e., antidepressant therapy for psychological factors) or with palliative treatment of the offending tumor.[42] Additionally, appetite stimulants such as the cannabinoid, dronabinol (2.5 mg twice daily with meals, titrated to a maximum of 20 mg/day) and megestrol acetate (400–800 mg/day orally) can aid in increasing caloric intake.

Cachexia is more difficult to treat, although it may resolve following treatment of the underlying malignancy. Nutritional consultation may be of aid, although cachexia is thought to be more attributable to internal pathophysiologic processes than malnutrition.

▶ Paraneoplastic Syndromes

Paraneoplastic syndromes are clinical syndromes caused by nonmetastatic systemic effects of cancer. Tumors make and secrete biologically active products that can stimulate or inhibit hormone production, autoimmunity, immune complex production, or cause immune suppression. Lung cancer, particularly SCLC, is associated with a high rate of paraneoplastic syndromes. Pharmacologic therapy is necessary when the abnormality causes the patient acute physical or psychological stress or adversely affects his or her health. When possible, therapy should be directed at the primary tumor, and a response often leads to resolution of symptoms.

▶ Palliative Care

Ultimately, most lung cancer patients succumb to their disease. Palliative care involves management of symptoms and improvement of quality of life when curative treatment options are no longer available. Often, problematic metastases can be removed by surgery (depending on location) or can be treated with radiotherapy to reduce tumor size. In selecting options at this point in treatment, it is important to keep the goals of therapy (i.e., maximizing the duration and quality of life)

Patient Encounter, Part 4

LT undergoes surgery for her disease, which is successful, with negative margins. After 1 year, however, the patient returns for routine follow-up and is found to have recurrent disease, with metastases present in both the brain and in the liver. Molecular diagnostics reveals a mutation in exon 19 of the *EGFR* gene.

What is the patient's new clinical stage?

Discuss the significance of the mutation identified in the tumor.

Based on the information provided, develop a care plan for this patient. Include (a) treatment goals, (b) monitoring parameters for anticipated toxicities, and (c) a follow-up plan to determine response to treatment and surveillance.

Patient Care and Monitoring

1. Review the patient's medical and social history. Was the patient exposed to clinical risk factors for lung cancer?

2. Verify the histology and clinical stage of disease. Evaluate the patient's performance status. Is the patient a surgical candidate? How does this influence your treatment recommendations?

3. Develop a care plan based on treatment goals. If the goal is palliative care, how does treatment-related toxicity influence therapy?

4. If chemotherapy is the treatment of choice, counsel the patient on the risks and benefits of undergoing such therapy. Be sure that the patient understands the issues fully before moving forward.

5. Verify dosing of all agents in the chemotherapy regimen. What are the major expected toxicities?

6. Evaluate toxicity as treatment progresses. Is the toxicity severe enough to warrant dose reduction or pharmacologic treatment? Record graded toxicities according to the NCI CTC V4.0 criteria.

7. Evaluate the response to treatment. Did the patient experience a complete response, partial response, stable disease, or disease progression? How does this change future treatment?

8. If the patient is in remission, develop a monitoring plan. What signs or symptoms denote disease progression?

9. Recommend a smoking cessation program or other risk reduction plan for the patient.

in mind. Low-toxicity single-agent chemotherapy, targeted therapy, and best supportive care (including fatigue and pain management) are commonly the mainstays of palliative care.

OUTCOME EVALUATION

Following treatment, evaluate the goals of therapy versus the response that was achieved. Was there response to treatment or progression of disease? If the patient is being treated with supportive care, then alleviation of symptoms and improvement in quality of life should be of primary importance. Be sure to document objective evaluations of the outcome in the care plan.

Abbreviations Introduced in This Chapter

5-FDG	5-Fluorodeoxyglucose
CAV	Cyclophosphamide, doxorubicin, vincristine
CT	Computed tomography
ECOG	Eastern Cooperative Oncology Group
EGF	Epidermal growth factor
EGFR	Epidermal growth factor receptor
EP	Etoposide, cisplatin
ETS	Environmental tobacco smoke
NSCLC	Non–small cell lung cancer
PCI	Prophylactic cranial irradiation
PET	Positron-emission tomography
PS	Performance status
SCLC	Small cell lung cancer
TNM	Tumor, node, and metastasis staging
VEGF	Vascular endothelial-derived growth factor

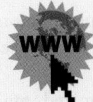 Self-assessment questions and answers are available at *http://www.mhpharmacotherapy.com/pp.html.*

REFERENCES

1. Siegel R, Ward E, Brawley O, Jemal A. Cancer statistics, 2011: The impact of eliminating socioeconomic and racial disparities on premature cancer deaths. CA Cancer J Clin 2011;61(4):212–236.
2. Alberg AJ, Brock MV, Samet JM. Epidemiology of lung cancer: Looking to the future. J Clin Oncol 2005;23(14):3175–3185.
3. Fu JB, Kau TY, Severson RK, Kalemkerian GP. Lung cancer in women: Analysis of the national Surveillance, Epidemiology, and End Results database. Chest 2005;127(3):768–77.
4. Ginsberg MS. Epidemiology of lung cancer. Semin Roentgenol 2005;40(2):83–89.
5. Tammemagi CM, Neslund-Dudas C, Simoff M, Kvale P. In lung cancer patients, age, race-ethnicity, gender and smoking predict adverse comorbidity, which in turn predicts treatment and survival. J Clin Epidemiol 2004;57(6):597–609.
6. Westmaas JL, Brandon TH. Reducing risk in smokers. Curr Opin Pulm Med 2004;10(4):284–288.

7. Mao JT, Roth MD, Fishbein MC, et al. Lung cancer chemoprevention with celecoxib in former smokers. Cancer Prev Res (Phila) 2011;4(7):984–993.

8. Aberle DR, Adams AM, Berg CD, et al. Reduced lung-cancer mortality with low-dose computed tomographic screening. N Engl J Med 2011 Aug 4;365(5):395–409.

9. Bastarrika G, Garcia-Velloso MJ, Lozano MD, et al. Early lung cancer detection using spiral computed tomography and positron emission tomography. Am J Respir Crit Care Med 2005;171(12):1378–1383.

10. Micke P, Faldum A, Metz T, et al. Staging small cell lung cancer: Veterans Administration Lung Study Group versus International Association for the Study of Lung Cancer—what limits limited disease? Lung Cancer 2002;37(3):271–276.

11. Fox W, Scadding JG. Medical Research Council comparative trial of surgery and radiotherapy for primary treatment of small-celled or oat-celled carcinoma of bronchus. Ten-year follow-up. Lancet 1973;2(7820):63–65.

12. Jeremic B, Shibamoto Y, Acimovic L, Milisavljevic S. Hyperfractionated radiotherapy for clinical stage II non-small cell lung cancer. Radiother Oncol 1999;51(2):141–145.

13. Spira A, Ettinger DS. Multidisciplinary management of lung cancer. N Engl J Med 2004;350(4):379–392.

14. Postoperative radiotherapy for non-small cell lung cancer. Cochrane Database Syst Rev 2005;(2):CD002142.

15. NCCN Practice Guidelines in Oncology: Non-small Cell Lung Cancer. National Comprehensive Cancer Network. 2012, http://www.nccn.org.

16. Milton DT, Miller VA. Advances in cytotoxic chemotherapy for the treatment of metastatic or recurrent non-small cell lung cancer. Semin Oncol 2005;32(3):299–314.

17. Johnson DH. "The guard dies, it does not surrender!": Progress in the management of small-cell lung cancer? J Clin Oncol 2002;20(24): 4618–4620.

18. Arriagada R, Bergman B, Dunant A, et al. Cisplatin-based adjuvant chemotherapy in patients with completely resected non-small-cell lung cancer. N Engl J Med 2004;350(4):351–360.

19. Winton T, Livingston R, Johnson D, et al. Vinorelbine plus cisplatin vs. observation in resected non-small-cell lung cancer. N Engl J Med 2005;352(25):2589–2597.

20. Belani CP. Adjuvant and neoadjuvant therapy in non-small cell lung cancer. Semin Oncol 2005;32(2 Suppl 2):S9–S15.

21. De Marinis F, Gebbia V, De Petris L. Neoadjuvant chemotherapy for stage IIIA-N2 non-small cell lung cancer. Ann Oncol 2005;16(Suppl 4): iv116–iv22.

22. Sandler A, Gray R, Perry MC, et al. Paclitaxel-carboplatin alone or with bevacizumab for non-small-cell lung cancer. N Engl J Med 2006;355(24):2542–2550.

23. Pirker R, Szczesna A, Von Pawel J, et al. FLEX: A randomized, multicenter, phase III study of cetuximab in combination with cisplatin/vinorelbine (CV) versus CV alone in the first-line treatment of patients with advanced non-small cell lung cancer (NSCLC). J Clin Oncol 2008;26(Suppl).

24. Shaw AT, Yeap BY, Solomon BJ, et al. Effect of crizotinib on overall survival in patients with advanced non-small-cell lung cancer harbouring ALK gene rearrangement: A retrospective analysis. Lancet Oncol 2011;12(11):1004–1012.

25. Sequist LV, Joshi VA, Janne PA, et al. Epidermal growth factor receptor mutation testing in the care of lung cancer patients. Clin Cancer Res 2006;12(14 Pt 2):4403S–4408S.

26. Miller AB, Fox W, Tall R. Five-year follow-up of the Medical Research Council comparative trial of surgery and radiotherapy for the primary treatment of small-celled or oat-celled carcinoma of the bronchus. Lancet 1969;2(7619):501–505.

27. NCCN Practice Guidelines in Oncology: Small Cell Lung Cancer. National Comprehensive Cancer Network. 2012, http://www.nccn.org.

28. Auperin A, Arriagada R, Pignon JP, et al. Prophylactic cranial irradiation for patients with small-cell lung cancer in complete remission. Prophylactic Cranial Irradiation Overview Collaborative Group. N Engl J Med 1999;341(7):476–484.

29. Hanna N, Bunn PA, Jr., Langer C, et al. Randomized phase III trial comparing irinotecan/cisplatin with etoposide/cisplatin in patients with previously untreated extensive-stage disease small-cell lung cancer. J Clin Oncol 2006;24(13):2038–2043.

30. Slotman B, Faivre-Finn C, Kramer G, et al. Prophylactic cranial irradiation in extensive small-cell lung cancer. N Engl J Med 2007;357(7): 664–672.

31. Schiller JH, Harrington D, Belani CP, et al. Comparison of four chemotherapy regimens for advanced non-small-cell lung cancer. N Engl J Med 2002;346(2):92–98.

32. Azzoli CG, Baker S Jr, Temin S, et al. American Society of Clinical Oncology Clinical Practice Guideline update on chemotherapy for stage IV non-small-cell lung cancer. J Clin Oncol 2009;27(36):6251–6266.

33. Mok TS, Wu YL, Thongprasert S, et al. Gefitinib or carboplatin-paclitaxel in pulmonary adenocarcinoma. N Engl J Med 2009;361(10):947–957.

34. Rosell R, Gervais R. Erlotinib versus chemotherapy (CT) in advanced non-small cell lung cancer (NSCLC) patients (p) with epidermal growth factor receptor (EGFR) mutations: Interim results of the European Erlotinib Versus Chemotherapy (EURTAC) phase III randomized trial. J Clin Oncol 2011;29(Suppl).

35. Stinchcombe TE, Socinski MA. Maintenance therapy in advanced non-small-cell lung cancer: Current status and future implications. J Thorac Oncol 2011;6(1):174–182.

36. Pfister DG, Johnson DH, Azzoli CG, et al. American Society of Clinical Oncology Treatment of Unresectable Non-Small-Cell Lung Cancer Guideline: Update 2003. J Clin Oncol 2004;22(2):330–353.

37. Berghmans T, Paesmans M, Lafitte JJ, et al. Role of granulocyte and granulocyte-macrophage colony-stimulating factors in the treatment of small-cell lung cancer: A systematic review of the literature with methodological assessment and meta-analysis. Lung Cancer 2002;37(2):115–123.

38. Kasymjanova G, Kreisman H, Correa JA, et al. Does granulocyte colony-stimulating factor affect survival in patients with advanced non-small-cell lung cancer? J Thorac Oncol 2006;1(6):564–570.

39. Jordan K, Kasper C, Schmoll HJ. Chemotherapy-induced nausea and vomiting: Current and new standards in the antiemetic prophylaxis and treatment. Eur J Cancer 2005;41(2):199–205.

40. Tsao AS, Liu D, Lee JJ, et al. Smoking affects treatment outcome in patients with advanced nonsmall cell lung cancer. Cancer 2006;106(11):2428–2436.

41. Videtic GM, Stitt LW, Dar AR, et al. Continued cigarette smoking by patients receiving concurrent chemoradiotherapy for limited-stage small-cell lung cancer is associated with decreased survival. J Clin Oncol 2003;21(8):1544–1549.

42. MacDonald N, Easson AM, Mazurak VC, et al. Understanding and managing cancer cachexia. J Am Coll Surg 2003;197(1):143–161.

43. Ruckdeschel JC, Schwartz AG, Bepler G, et al. Cancer of the Lung: NSCLC and SCLC. In: Abeloff MD, Armitage JO, Niederhuber JE, Kastan MB, McKenna WG, eds. Clinical Oncology, 3rd ed. Orlando: Churchill Livingston, 2004.

44. NCCN Practice Guidelines in Oncology: Small Cell Lung Cancer. National Comprehensive Cancer Network. 2008, http://www.nccn.org.

45. NCCN Practice Guidelines in Oncology: Non-small Cell Lung Cancer. National Comprehensive Cancer Network. 2008, http://www.nccn.org.

46. Hanna N, Shepherd FA, Fossella FV, et al. Randomized phase III trial of pemetrexed versus docetaxel in patients with non-small-cell lung cancer previously treated with chemotherapy. J Clin Oncol 2004;22(9):1589–1597.

47. Kosmidis P, Mylonakis N, Nicolaides C, et al. Paclitaxel plus carboplatin versus gemcitabine plus paclitaxel in advanced non-small-cell lung cancer: A phase III randomized trial. J Clin Oncol 2002;20(17):3578–3585.

48. Noda K, Nishiwaki Y, Kawahara M, et al. Irinotecan plus cisplatin compared with etoposide plus cisplatin for extensive small-cell lung cancer. N Engl J Med 2002;346(2):85–91.

49. Scagliotti GV, Kortsik C, Dark GG, et al. Pemetrexed combined with oxaliplatin or carboplatin as first-line treatment in advanced non-small cell lung cancer: A multicenter, randomized, phase II trial. Clin Cancer Res 2005;11(2 Pt 1):690–696.

50. Shepherd FA, Dancey J, Ramlau R, et al. Prospective randomized trial of docetaxel versus best supportive care in patients with non-small-cell lung cancer previously treated with platinum-based chemotherapy. J Clin Oncol 2000;18(10):2095–2103.

91

Colorectal Cancer

Emily B. Borders and Patrick J. Medina

LEARNING OBJECTIVES

● **Upon completion of the chapter, the reader will be able to:**

1. Identify the risk factors for colorectal cancer.

2. Recognize the signs and symptoms of colorectal cancer.

3. Describe the treatment options for colorectal cancer based on patient-specific factors, such as stage of disease, age of patient, genetic mutations, and previous treatment received.

4. Outline the pharmacologic principles for agents used to treat colorectal cancer.

5. Develop a monitoring plan to assess the efficacy and toxicity of agents used in colorectal cancer.

6. Educate patients about the adverse effects of chemotherapy that require specific patient counseling.

7. Outline preventive and screening strategies for individuals at average and high risk for colorectal cancer.

KEY CONCEPTS

❶ Although there are numerous risk factors for developing colorectal cancer, age is the biggest risk factor for sporadic colorectal cancer.

❷ Diets high in fat and low in fiber are associated with increased colorectal cancer risk, whereas the regular use of aspirin (and nonsteroidal anti-inflammatory drugs [NSAIDs]) and calcium supplementation may decrease the risk of colorectal cancer.

❸ Effective colorectal cancer screening programs incorporate annual fecal occult blood testing in combination with regular examination of the entire colon starting at age 50 years for average-risk individuals and should be recommended by all health care providers.

❹ Most patients with colorectal cancer are asymptomatic early but may develop changes in bowel or eating habits, fatigue, abdominal pain, and blood in stool.

❺ The stage of colorectal cancer is determined by the tumor-node-metastasis (TNM) staging system and is the most important prognostic factor for patient survival. Disease stages I to III are curable, but patients with stage IV disease are treated with the goal of palliation.

❻ Adjuvant chemotherapy is not needed in patients with stage I colon cancer, may be beneficial in selective high-risk patients with stage II colon cancer, and is

standard of care in patients with stage III colon cancer. 5-Fluorouracil (5-FU), leucovorin and oxaliplatin chemotherapy (FOLFOX) is the standard regimen used in adjuvant colon cancer. It is usually given for 6 months.

❼ Triple-drug therapy consisting of 5-FU and leucovorin with oxaliplatin or irinotecan improves survival compared with 5-FU plus leucovorin alone and is considered standard first-line therapy for metastatic disease. The addition of bevacizumab is recommended to be added to 5-FU–based regimens based on improvements in overall survival.

❽ Pharmacogenetic testing for KRAS mutation status should occur in all patients before starting an epidermal growth factor receptor (EGFR) targeted agent. EGFR inhibitors should be considered for addition to standard chemotherapy regimens only in patients with metastatic disease and a wild-type KRAS mutation status.

❾ Treatment of relapsed or refractory metastatic disease uses agents not given in the first-line setting; patients who receive all effective chemotherapy options have improved outcomes compared with those who do not.

❿ Adjuvant therapy consisting of 5-FU–based chemotherapy in combination with radiation therapy should be offered to patients with stage II or III cancer of the rectum. Metastatic rectal cancer is treated similar to metastatic colon cancer.

INTRODUCTION

Colorectal cancer is one of the three most common cancers diagnosed in the United States and includes cancers of the colon and rectum. It was projected that, in 2011, an estimated 141,210 new cases would be diagnosed and an estimated 49,380 deaths would occur, making colorectal cancer the second leading cause of cancer-related deaths in the United States.[1] The prognosis is primarily determined by the stage of disease with the majority of patients with early stage (I or II) disease cured. Treatment options for colorectal cancer include surgery, radiation, chemotherapy, and new targeted molecular therapies.

EPIDEMIOLOGY AND ETIOLOGY

Colorectal cancer occurs at a much higher rate in industrialized parts of the world such as North America and Europe, while the lowest rates are seen in less-developed areas, suggesting that environmental and dietary factors influence the development of colorectal cancer. In addition to these environmental factors, colorectal cancers are known to develop more frequently in certain families, and genetic predisposition to this cancer is well known.

The incidence of colorectal cancer is greatest among men, who have an approximately 1.5 times greater risk for developing colorectal cancer than women. Overall, colon and rectal cancers make up approximately 10% of all cancer diagnoses in men and women in the United States.[1] The median age at diagnosis is 72 years with very few cases occurring in individuals younger than 45 years of age.[2] ❶ *Age appears to be the biggest risk factor for the development of colorectal cancer with 70% of cases diagnosed in adults older than 65 years of age.*

Although still the third leading cause of cancer death, mortality rates for colorectal cancer have declined over the past 30 years as a result of better and increasingly used screening modalities and more effective treatments.

RISK FACTORS

Besides age, the development of colorectal cancer appears to be caused by variety of dietary or environmental factors, inflammatory bowel disease, and genetic susceptibility to the disease. Table 91–1 lists well-known risk factors for developing colorectal cancer. Epidemiologic studies of the worldwide incidence of colorectal cancer suggest that dietary habits strongly influence its development.

❷ *High-fat, low-fiber diets, which usually occur in tandem, have been associated with an increased risk of colorectal cancer.* The association between red meat consumption and colorectal cancer is strongest, possibly a result of the heterocyclic amines formed during cooking or the presence of specific fatty acids in red meat such as arachidonic acid. Although data indicate that animal meat and saturated fat intake are associated with an increased risk of colorectal cancer, the exact increase in risk is unknown. The evidence

Table 91–1
Risk Factors for Colorectal Cancer
General
Age is the primary risk factor
Dietary
High-fat, low-fiber diets
Lifestyle
Alcohol
Smoking
Obesity or physical inactivity
Comorbid Conditions
Inflammatory bowel disease (ulcerative colitis and Crohn's disease)
Hereditary or Genetic
FAP and HNPCC
Family history

FAP, familial adenomatous polyposis; HNPCC, hereditary nonpolyposis colorectal cancer.

for low-fiber diets as a risk factor is based on the ingestion of large amounts of dietary fiber being associated with a small, inconsistent, reduced colorectal cancer risk. Foods that are high in fiber include vegetables, fruit, grains, and cereals. The protective effects of fiber may be a result of reduced absorption of carcinogens in the bowel, reduced bowel transit time, or a reduction in dietary fat intake associated with high-fiber diets.[3]

The degree of colorectal cancer risk reduction associated with increased consumption of vegetables and fruit is variable but generally modest and has ranged from no difference to a 25% decrease in cancer risk in prospective studies.[3] A large pooled analysis of 13 prospective cohort studies found dietary fiber intake to be inversely associated with the risk of colorectal cancer; however, upon multivariate analysis for other dietary risk factors, the benefit was no longer observed.[3] This analysis does not consider for the known benefits of a fiber-rich diet for noncancerous conditions such as diabetes and coronary artery disease.

❷ *The risk of colorectal cancer appears to be inversely related to calcium and folate intake.* Higher intake of calcium and vitamin D has been associated with a reduced risk of colorectal cancer in epidemiologic studies and polyp recurrence in polyp-prevention trials. However, daily supplementation of calcium (1,000 mg) with vitamin D3 (400 IU) for 7 years had no effect on the incidence of colorectal cancer among postmenopausal women compared with a placebo group in the randomized trial involving 18,106 women The benefit of calcium and vitamin D for preventing colon cancer may require longer follow-up.[4]

Calcium's protective effect may be related to a reduction in mucosal cell proliferation rates or through its binding to bile salts in the intestine, and dietary folate helps maintain normal bowel mucosa. Based on its role in DNA methylation, folate intake has been associated with modifying the risk of colorectal cancer. Epidemiologic evidence suggests that higher intake of folate decreases the risk for the development of colorectal cancer. However, studies are inconsistent, and whether benefit is limited to certain patient populations requires further study. In addition, the timing of folate intake may be important with early intake preventing colorectal cancer and later intake promoting the progression of disease.[5] Micronutrient deficiencies, including selenium, vitamin C, vitamin D, vitamin E, and β-carotene, appear to increase colorectal cancer risk; however, the benefit of dietary supplementation of these micronutrients does not appear to be substantial.[6]

Chronic use of several medications has been shown to influence the risk of developing colorectal cancer. ❷ *Studies have consistently demonstrated that regular (at least two doses per week) nonsteroidal anti-inflammatory drug (NSAID) and aspirin use is associated with a reduced risk of colorectal cancer.*[7,8] Additional studies support these findings that regular aspirin or NSAID use may decrease the risk of colorectal cancer by as much as 50%.[7,8] The potential mechanisms by which these agents exert their protective effects appear to be linked primarily to their inhibition of cyclooxygenase-2 (COX-2), and protective effects may be limited to those precancerous lesions that overexpress COX-2.[9] Colorectal cancers with weak or absent expression of COX-2 may not derive the same benefit from long-term COX-2 inhibition.[9] Exogenous hormone use, particularly postmenopausal hormone replacement therapy, is associated with a significant reduction in colorectal cancer risk in most studies with the greatest benefit in women who are on current hormone replacement therapy.[10] Unfortunately, the known risks of hormone replacement therapy outweigh this benefit, and routine use of hormone replacement therapy to prevent colorectal cancer is not recommended.

Physical inactivity and elevated body mass index (BMI) are associated with up to a twofold increase in the risk of colorectal cancer. Decreased bowel transit time and exercise-induced alterations in body glucose, insulin levels, and perhaps other hormones may reduce tumor cell growth.[6,11] Type 2 diabetes mellitus, independent of body mass size and physical activity level, is also associated with an increased risk of colorectal cancer in women and supports a role for hyperinsulinemia as a possible link between obesity, sedentary lifestyle, diabetes mellitus, and colorectal cancer.[11] Additional lifestyle choices that increase the risk of colorectal cancer include alcohol consumption and smoking that may increase the risk of colorectal cancer by generating carcinogens or their direct toxic effects on bowel tissue.[6]

Inflammatory bowel diseases, such as chronic ulcerative colitis, particularly when it involves the entire large intestine, and to lesser extent Crohn's disease, confer increased risk for colorectal cancer. Overall, persons diagnosed with either disease constitute about 1% to 2% of all new cases of colorectal cancer each year.

Finally, as many as 10% of cases are thought to be hereditary, resulting from genetic mutations. The two most common forms of hereditary colorectal cancer are familial adenomatous polyposis (FAP) and hereditary nonpolyposis colorectal cancer (HNPCC). FAP is a rare autosomal dominant trait that is caused by mutations of the adenomatous polyposis coli (APC) gene and accounts for 1% of all colorectal cancers. The disease is manifested by hundreds to thousands of polyps arising during adolescence.[12] The risk of developing colorectal cancer for individuals with untreated FAP is virtually 100%, and patients require early screening for the disease and likely prophylactic total colectomy. HNPCC, also an autosomal dominant syndrome, accounts for up to 5% of colorectal cancer cases.[12] In contrast to FAP, juvenile polyps occur rarely, and the average age of colorectal cancer in these patients is closer to that of average risk patients, with most patients diagnosed in their forties. Testing for HNPCC mutations is available but reserved for individuals who meet strict diagnostic criteria.

Up to 25% of patients who develop colorectal cancer have a family history of colorectal cancer unrelated to a mutation described earlier.[8] First-degree relatives of patients diagnosed with colorectal cancer have an increased risk of the disease that is at least two to four times that of persons in the general population without a family history.

Summary of Risk Factors

In summary, the true association between most dietary factors and the risk of colorectal cancer is unclear. The protective effects of fiber, calcium, and a diet low in fat are not completely known at this time. NSAID use and hormonal use appear to decrease the risk of colorectal cancer while physical inactivity, alcohol use, and smoking appear to increase the risk of colorectal cancer. Clinical risk factors and genetic mutations are well-known risks for colorectal cancer.

SCREENING

❸ *Health care professionals must be aware of and promote appropriate screening recommendations for colorectal cancer in their patients.* Effective screening programs incorporate fecal occult blood tests (FOBTs) and regular examinations. Appropriate screening of patients at normal and high risk for colorectal cancer leads to the detection of smaller, localized lesions and higher cure rates.[13] Screening techniques include FOBTs and imaging of the colon. The use of FOBTs annually in combination with digital rectal examinations has led to earlier diagnosis of early stages of disease and may reduce colorectal cancer mortality by up to one-third.[13] However, FOBT using a single stool sample collected during a digital rectal examination is not a recommended option for screening because this method has a decreased sensitivity for detecting advanced disease.[8] Recommendations for adequate FOBT require the patient to collect two stool samples from three consecutive specimens using at-home testing procedures.[13] Two main methods are available to detect occult blood in the feces: guaiac dye and immunochemical methods. The Hemoccult II is the most commonly used FOBT in the United States and is a guaiac-based test. Proper counseling by health care providers is required to receive accurate test results. Table 91–2 lists common reasons for inaccurate results with the guaiac tests and requires appropriate counseling on the

Table 91–2

Common Reasons for Inaccurate Results from Guaiac Stool Tests

False-Positive Results	False-Negative Results
Red meat, blood soup, blood sausage[a]	Vitamin C[a]
Vegetables with peroxidase activity[a]	Dehydrated samples
Iron[a]	
Gastric irritation (NSAIDs)[a]	

NSAID, nonsteroidal anti-inflammatory drug.

[a]Avoid these foods and medications for 3 days before the test.

use of these tests. Fecal immunochemical tests (FITs) (InSure and others), which use antibodies to detect hemoglobin, are also available for use. One advantage of FITs is that they do not react with dietary factors or medications. Both FOBTs can be recommended in screening protocols for patients.

In addition, imaging of the colon with a sigmoidoscopy, colonoscopy, or double-contrast barium enema is required every 5 to 10 years in most individuals. Colonoscopy is the preferred procedure as it allows for greater visualization of the entire colon and simultaneous removal of lesions found during screening.[13] A sigmoidoscopy only examines the lower half of the colon, and a double-contrast barium enema requires a supplemental colonoscopy to remove any lesions found during the screening process. Several revisions to the colorectal cancer screening guidelines have been made in an attempt to increase the compliance to screening guidelines. These include the use of computed tomographic colonography (CTC) and stool DNA testing as acceptable screening methods. CTC, also known as "virtual colonoscopy," uses integrated two- and three-dimensional images to detect and characterize polyps. Although noninvasive compared with colonoscopy, adequate

Patient Encounter, Part 1

HB is a 68-year-old man who presents to your clinic with a chief complaint of abdominal discomfort and blood in his stool for the past 3 months. He also states he has felt tired and has had diarrhea and a reduced appetite over the past month. HB has a medical history positive for hypercholesterolemia, gastroesophageal reflux disease (GERD), and obesity. He states that he consumes a moderate amount of alcohol (3 or 4 beers most days of the week after work), quit smoking a few weeks ago (previously smoked ½ pack per day for 40 years), and does not follow any particular diet (mostly red meat and fried foods).

What risk factors does HB have for colon cancer?

Does he have clinical symptoms suggestive of colon cancer?

What additional tests need to be ordered to diagnosis colon cancer?

Table 91–3

Colon Cancer Screening Guidelines

Average risk	Annual FOBT or FIT after age 50 years
	Stool DNA testing may be used as an alternative *and*
	One of the following after age 50 years:
	Sigmoidoscopy every 5 years
	Colonoscopy every 10 years
	Barium enema every 5 years
	CTC every 5 years
Family history	Screening at ages 35–40 years
HNPCC	Screening at age 30 years
FAP	Screening at ages 10–12 years

CTC, computed tomographic colonography; DRE, digital rectal examination; FAP, familial adenomatous polyposis; FIT, fecal immunochemical tests; FOBT, fecal occult blood tests; HNPCC, hereditary nonpolyposis colorectal cancer.

bowel preparation, which is often cited as the reason for noncompliance, is still required. In addition, any lesions found on examination require a follow-up colonoscopy.

Stool DNA testing detects molecular markers associated with advanced colorectal cancer. Because this test is not dependent on the detection of bleeding, which can be sporadic, it requires only a single stool collection. How often and what molecular markers to test for are undergoing further evaluation. ❸ Table 91–3 *is a summary of the current American Cancer Society guidelines for screening and surveillance for early detection of colorectal polyps and cancer.*[13]

COLORECTAL CANCER PREVENTION

Strategies to prevent colorectal cancer can be done with pharmacologic or surgical interventions and involve either preventing the initial development of colorectal cancer (primary prevention) or preventing cancer in patients who demonstrate early signs of colorectal cancer (secondary prevention).

The most widely studied agents for the chemoprevention of colorectal cancer are agents that inhibit COX-2 (aspirin, NSAIDs, and selective COX-2 inhibitors) and calcium supplementation.[14] COX-2 appears to play a role in polyp formation, and COX-2 inhibition suppresses polyp growth. In 1999, the Food and Drug Administration (FDA) approved the use of celecoxib to reduce the number of colorectal polyps in patients with FAP as an adjunct to usual care. This may delay the need for surgical intervention in these patients, but the results cannot be extrapolated to the general population. The dose of celecoxib for this indication is 400 mg orally twice daily, and the risk of cardiovascular damage from COX-2 inhibition needs to be assessed carefully in these patients. The use of aspirin as both a primary and secondary chemoprevention agent has also been studied. In a prospective, randomized trial, low-dose (81 mg/day) aspirin was shown to decrease the incidence of additional polyps by 19% in patients with a previous history of at least one polyp.[15]

Calcium supplementation appears to be associated with a moderate reduction in risk of recurrent colorectal adenomas with prospective studies demonstrating a nonstatistical decrease in adenoma recurrence, and its role as a chemoprevention agent remains under investigation.[14]

Additional agents, including selenium and folic acid, show promise as chemopreventive agents in colorectal cancer and preliminary, and confirmatory studies evaluating their effectiveness have been completed or are ongoing.[14]

Surgical resection remains an option to prevent colorectal cancer in individuals at extremely high risk for its development such as patients diagnosed with FAP. Individuals with FAP who are found to have polyps on screening examinations require total abdominal colectomy. In addition, removal of noncancerous polyps detected during screening colonoscopy is considered the standard of care to prevent the progression of premalignant polyps to cancer.

PATHOPHYSIOLOGY

Anatomy and Bowel Function

The large intestine consists of the cecum; ascending, transverse, descending, and sigmoid colon; and rectum (Fig. 91–1). The function of the large intestine is to receive contents from the ileum, absorb water, and package solid waste for excretion. Absorption of materials occurs in segments of the colon proximal to the middle of the transverse colon, with movement and storage of fecal material in the left colon and distal segments of the colon.

Four major tissue layers, from the lumen outward, form the large intestine: the mucosa, submucosa, muscularis externa, and serosa (Fig. 91–2). Complete replacement of surface epithelial cells occurs every 7 to 10 days with the

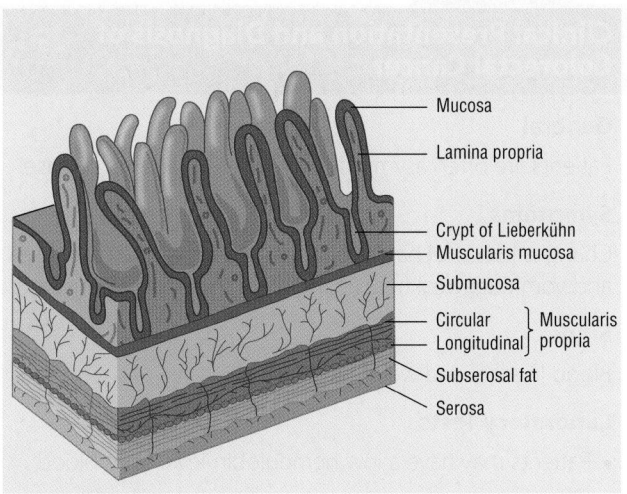

FIGURE 91–2. Cross-section of bowel wall. (From DiPiro JT, Talbert RL, Yee GC, et al., eds. Pharmacotherapy: A Pathophysiologic Approach, 6th ed. New York: McGraw-Hill, 2005; Fig. 127–3.)

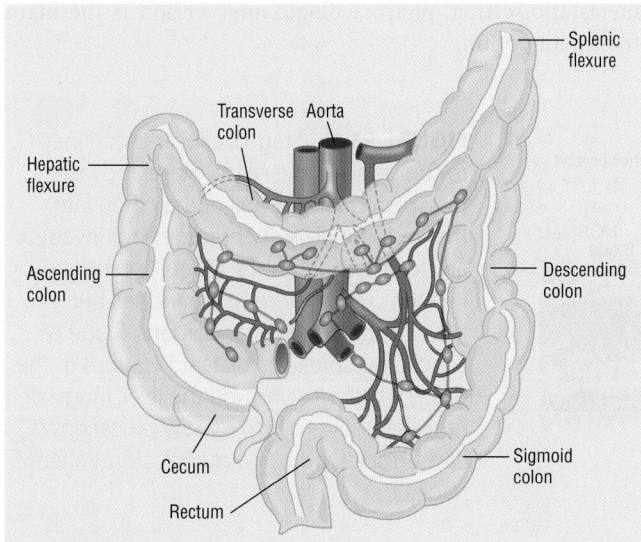

FIGURE 91–1. Colon and rectum anatomy. (From DiPiro JT, Talbert RL, Yee GC, et al., eds. Pharmacotherapy: A Pathophysiologic Approach, 6th ed. New York: McGraw-Hill, 2005; Fig. 127–2.)

total number of epithelial cells remaining constant in normal colonic tissue. As patients age, abnormal cells accumulate on the surface epithelium and protrude into the stream of fecal matter; their contact with fecal mutagens can lead to further cell mutations and eventual adenoma formation.[12]

Colorectal Tumorigenesis

The development of a colorectal neoplasm is a multistep process of several genetic and phenotypic alterations of normal bowel epithelium leading to unregulated cell growth, proliferation, and tumor development. A genetic model has been proposed for colorectal tumorigenesis that describes a process of transformation from adenoma to carcinoma. This model of tumor development reflects an accumulation of mutations within colonic epithelium that give a selective growth advantage to the cancer cells.[12] Genetic changes include activating mutations of oncogenes, mutations of tumor suppressor genes, and defects in DNA mismatch repair genes.

Additional genes and protein receptors are believed important in colorectal tumorigenesis. COX-2, which is induced in colorectal cancer cells, influences apoptosis and other cellular functions in colon cells, and overexpression of the EGFR, a transmembrane glycoprotein involved in signaling pathways that affect cell growth, differentiation, proliferation, and angiogenesis, occurs in the majority of colon cancers.[16] These mechanisms are potentially important because of the availability of pharmacologic agents targeted to inhibit these processes.

More than 90% of colorectal cancers that develop are adenocarcinomas and are assigned a grade of I to III based on how similar they are compared with normal colorectal cells. Grade I tumors most closely resemble normal cellular structure, but grade III tumors have frequently lost the characteristics of mature normal cells. Grade III tumors are associated with a worse prognosis than grade I turmors.[17]

Clinical Presentation and Diagnosis of Colorectal Cancer

General

Patients are often asymptomatic in early stages of disease

Symptoms

Changes in bowel habits, abdominal pain, anorexia, nausea and vomiting, weakness (if anemia is severe), and tenesmus

Signs

Blood in stool and weight loss

Laboratory Tests

- Patients may have a low hemoglobin level from blood loss
- Positive FOBT
- Liver function tests (INR, activated partial thromboplastin time, and bilirubin) may be abnormal if disease has metastasized to the liver
- CEA level may be high; normal level is less than 2.5 ng/mL (2.5 mcg/L) in nonsmokers and less than 5 ng/mL (5 mcg/L) in smokers

Imaging Tests

Chest x-ray, CT scan, or PET scan results may be positive if cancer has spread to the lungs, liver, or peritoneal cavity

CLINICAL PRESENTATION AND DIAGNOSIS

④ *The signs and symptoms associated with colorectal cancer can be extremely varied, subtle, and nonspecific. Most patients are asymptomatic but may develop changes in bowel or eating habits, fatigue, abdominal pain, and blood in the stool.*

TREATMENT

Desired Outcome

Staging is required to determine the extent of disease and is necessary in developing patient treatment options and determining patient prognosis. The tumor, node, metastasis (TNM) classification system that takes into account T (tumor size and depth of tumor invasion), N (lymph node involvement), M (presence or absence of metastases) is used to stage patients from stage I to stage IV. Computed tomography (CT) and appropriate assessment of lymph node involvement during surgical resection are essential in determining the stage of disease and subsequent treatment options. At this time, routine magnetic resonance imaging and positron emission tomography (PET) scans for initial staging are not recommended. **Figure 91–3** depicts how the three categories are used in combination to determine the stage of disease. **⑤** *The stage of colorectal cancer upon diagnosis is the most important prognostic factor for survival and disease recurrence. Stages I, II, and III disease are considered potentially curable and are aggressively treated in an attempt to cure these patients. Patients who develop stage IV disease are treated to reduce symptoms, avoid disease-related complications, and prolong survival.*

General Approach to Treatment

The treatment approaches for colorectal cancer reflect two primary treatment goals: curative therapy for localized disease (stages I to III) and palliative therapy for metastatic cancer (stage IV). Surgical resection of the primary tumor is the most important part of therapy for patients in whom cure is possible.[18] Depending on the stage of disease and whether the tumor originated in the colon or rectum, further adjuvant chemotherapy or chemotherapy plus radiation may be needed after surgery to cure these patients. In the metastatic setting, pharmacologic intervention is the main treatment option.

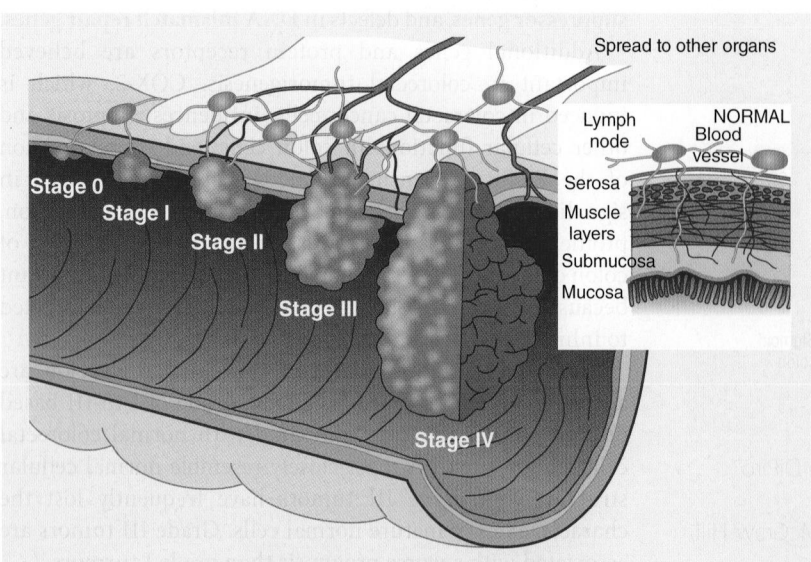

FIGURE 91–3. Stage I: cancer is confined to the lining of the colon. Stage II: cancer may penetrate the wall of the colon into the abdominal cavity but does not invade any local lymph nodes. Stage III: cancer invades one or more lymph nodes but has not spread to distant organs. Stage IV: cancer has spread to distant locations in the body, which may include the liver, lungs, or other sites. (From http://www.cancer.gov/cancertopics/pdq/treatment/colon/Patient/page2.)

Pharmacogenetic and pharmacogenomic testing has become an integral component to designing the optimal pharmacologic intervention for patients with colorectal cancer. The choice of treatment agents is largely dictated by individualized patient and tumor specific factors. For example, recent data have demonstrated specific tumor characteristics that may assist clinicians in predicting who will respond to EGFR inhibitors. Early immunohistochemical staining for EGFR status is not useful in predicting response because both EGFR-positive and -negative patients respond at the same rate. Fluorescence in situ hybridization (FISH) of EGFR copy number and *KRAS* gene mutation status have demonstrated predictive value. Patients with high EGFR gene copy number and wild-type (WT) (nonmutated) *KRAS* are more likely to benefit from cetuximab or panitumumab therapy.[17] In particular, testing for *KRAS* mutational status is now part of the disease workup to define patients who may derive benefit from cetuximab or panitumumab. Characteristics of the tumor are also vital in making treatment decisions for patients with stages II and III disease. The degree of microsatellite instability (MSI) within a tumor tells clinicians information about both prognosis and treatment options. More detail on specific pharmacogenetic and pharmacogenomic information is provided the pertinent pharmacologic therapy sections.

Nonpharmacologic Therapy

▶ Operable Disease (Stages I–III)

Surgery Individuals with stage I to III colorectal cancer should undergo a complete surgical resection of the tumor mass with removal of regional lymph nodes as a curative approach for their disease.[18] Surgery for rectal cancer depends on the region of tumor involvement with attempts to retain rectal function as a goal of the surgical procedure. Overall, surgery for colorectal cancer is associated with low morbidity and mortality rates. Common complications associated with colorectal surgery include infection, anastomotic leakage, obstruction, adhesion formation, and malabsorption syndromes.

Radiation Therapy There is currently no role for adjuvant radiation in colon cancer. However, patients who receive surgery for rectal cancer receive radiation therapy to reduce local tumor recurrence. Adjuvant radiation plus chemotherapy is considered standard treatment for patients with stage II or III rectal cancer after the surgical procedure is complete.[19] Preoperative radiation may be used to reduce the initial size of rectal cancers to make the surgical procedure easier.

▶ Metastatic Disease (Stage IV)

Surgery Unlike stages I to III disease, the benefit of surgical resection in most patients with metastatic disease is limited to symptomatic improvement. Select patients who have from one to three small nodules isolated to the liver, lungs, or abdomen may have a prolongation of survival, although cure is rare. Five-year survival for patients who undergo surgical resection of metastases isolated to the liver is approximately double that of patients who are not surgical candidates with approximately 33% of patients alive at 5 years.[20] Alternatives to surgery include destroying the tumor through freezing and thawing (cryoablation), heat (radiofrequency), or alcohol injection, although these appear to be less successful than surgical resection.[18,20] Because the majority of these patients will relapse, many practitioners offer adjuvant chemotherapy

---

Patient Encounter, Part 2

PMH: Hypercholesterolemia and GERD since age 40 years; obesity; the patient is 60% over his ideal body weight

FH: Father died at age 60 years following a stroke. Mother died at age 75 years with breast cancer; older sister with breast cancer; maternal aunt died at age 47 years from rectal cancer.

SH: Works on a farm. Widowed with three children.

Meds: Simvastatin 20 mg daily, omeprazole 20 mg daily, aspirin 81 mg daily

ROS: (+) Abdominal cramping, loss of appetite, blood in stool, and fatigue

PE:

VS: 164/88 mm Hg, P 80, RR 17, T 37.1°C (98.8°F), ht 190 cm (75 in), wt 125 kg (275 lb)

Abd: Distended and tender to touch, (+) bowel sounds, and heme (+) stools

Labs: Positive hemoglobin 11.6 g/dL (116 g/L or 7.20 mmol/L) decreased from 14.6 g/dL (146 g/L or 9.06 mmol/L) last year.

Imaging and Diagnostic Studies

- Colonoscopy revealed multiple polyps in his transverse colon.
- Biopsy revealed three polyps positive for adenocarcinoma of the colon
- Staging CT scan negative for disease outside of his colon.
- Four lymph nodes positive for disease.

Because HB has stage III colon cancer, how does this affect the goal of your treatment plan compared with stage IV disease?

What nonpharmacologic and pharmacologic options are available to HB?

to select patients following potentially curative resection, but further studies are needed to determine an optimal treatment regimen.[20] Additionally, neoadjuvant approaches to patients with isolated hepatic lesions are discussed later in the chapter.

Radiation Symptom reduction is the primary goal of radiation for patients with advanced or metastatic colorectal cancer.

Pharmacologic Therapy

Table 91–4 lists common chemotherapy regimens used in colorectal cancer and the abbreviations used in the literature to describe them.

▶ Operable Disease (Stages I–III)

⑥ *Adjuvant chemotherapy is administered after tumor resection to decrease relapse rates and improve survival in patients with colon cancer by eliminating micrometastatic disease that is undetected on imaging studies. Patients diagnosed with stage I colon or rectal cancer are usually cured by surgical resection, and adjuvant chemotherapy is not indicated in these patients.*[18] The role of adjuvant chemotherapy for stage II colon cancer is controversial but may benefit certain high-risk groups. Table 91–5 lists adjuvant treatment regimens based on stage and performance status (PS). Adjuvant chemotherapy for patients with stage II disease has not been shown to be superior to surgery alone with the exception of high-risk patients. High-risk patients who may benefit include those with inadequate nodes sampled for staging, bowel perforation upon diagnosis, T4 lesions, and those with unfavorable histology.[17] The risks and benefits of adjuvant chemotherapy should be discussed with medically fit patients who have stage II disease with high-risk features. However, the American Society of Clinical Oncology does not recommend the routine use of adjuvant chemotherapy in the general patient population unless part of a clinical trial.[21]

The use of tumor gene profiling may predict patients with stage II disease that would benefit from adjuvant chemotherapy but requires further validation in prospective trials.[17]

Table 91–4	

Dosing Schedules of Chemotherapy Regimens for Colon Cancer[a]

Regimen	Dosing
5-FU + leucovorin (bolus)	Leucovorin 500 mg/m² IV 5-FU 500 mg/m² IV Every week × 6 weeks followed by 2-week rest
5-FU + leucovorin (continuous infusion)	Leucovorin 200 mg/m² IV 5-FU 400 mg/m² IV bolus and then 600 mg/m² of 5-FU as a 22-hour continuous infusion On days 1 and 2; repeat every 2 weeks
FOLFIRI	Irinotecan 180 mg/m² IV day 1 Folinic acid (leucovorin) 400 mg/m² IV day 1 5-FU 400–500 mg/m² IV bolus after folinic acid; then 2,400–3,000 mg/m² of 5-FU IV over 46 hours Repeat every 14 days
FOLFOX4	Oxaliplatin 85 mg/m² IV + leucovorin 200 mg/m² IV followed by 5-FU 400 mg/m² IV bolus and then 5-FU 600 mg/m² IV over 22 hours day 1 Leucovorin 200 mg/m², followed by 5-FU 400 mg/m² IV bolus and then 5-FU 600 mg/m² IV over 22 hours day 2 Repeat every 2 weeks
mFOLFOX6	Oxaliplatin 85 mg/m² IV day 1 Leucovorin 400 mg/m² IV over 2 hrs, followed by 5-FU 400 mg/m² IV bolus day 1 followed by 2400 mg/m² IV over 46 hours Repeat every 2 weeks
Bevacizumab + 5-FU regimen	Bevacizumab 5 mg/kg every 2 weeks + a 5-FU–containing regimen (FOLFOX, FOLFIRI, or 5-FU + leucovorin) Bevacizumab 7.5 mg/kg every 3 weeks with CapeOX
Cetuximab ± irinotecan	Cetuximab 400 mg/m² first infusion, then 250 mg/m² weekly ± irinotecan 125 mg/m² every week for 4 weeks Repeat irinotecan every 6 weeks (after a 2-week break)
Panitumumab	6 mg/kg every 2 weeks
Capecitabine	1,250 mg/m² twice a day orally for 14 days Repeat every 3 weeks
CapeOX	Capecitabine 1,000 mg/m² twice a day orally for 14 days Oxaliplatin 130 mg/m² IV on day 1 Repeat every 3 weeks
CAPIRI	Capecitabine 1,000 mg/m² twice a day for 14 days Irinotecan 100 mg/m² IV days 1 and 8 Repeat every 22 days

CAPIRI–capecitabine and irinotecan; CapeOX, capecitabine–oxaliplatin; 5-FU, 5-fluorouracil; IV, intravenous.

[a]Note that many variations exist, and current literature should be checked before administering any chemotherapy regimen.

Table 91–5

Treatment Regimens for Adjuvant Colon Cancer

Stage II[a]	Stage III
High Risk	**Good Performance Status**
• Capecitabine or 5-FU plus leucovorin	• FOLFOX
• FOLFOX	• Capecitabine or 5-FU plus leucovorin
Low Risk[b]	**Poor Performance Status**
• Observation or clinical trial	• Capecitabine
• Capecitabine or 5-FU plus leucovorin	

5-FU, 5-fluorouracil.

[a]Individualized assessment of patient risk is necessary to determine if treatment is required. Clinical trials or observation may be an appropriate option.

[b]T3 lesions may be considered high risk by some clinicians.

An additional consideration for deciding on adjuvant therapy is the status of MSI within the tumor. MSI results from defective DNA mismatch repair (dMMR) genes leading to damaged DNA. Tumors that display high-levels of MSI appear to be associated with better prognosis for patients than those with microsatellite-stable (MSS) tumors. Despite being associated with a better prognosis, tumors that display high-levels of MSI do not respond as well to certain chemotherapy, including 5-fluorouracil (5-FU).[22] It is recommended that stage II patients should be tested for the status of MSI if 5-FU alone is being considered for therapy, and an alternative therapy should be considered if high levels of MSI are displayed.[17] In general, patients with stage II colon cancer should be enrolled into carefully controlled clinical trials to assess the impact of new agents and prognostic models. ⑥ *Adjuvant chemotherapy is standard therapy for patients with stage III colon cancer.* The presence of lymph node involvement in the resected specimen places patients with stage III colon cancer at high risk for relapse; the risk of death within 5 years of surgical resection alone is as high as 70%.[18] In this population of patients, adjuvant chemotherapy significantly decreases the risk of cancer recurrence and death and is considered the standard of care.

⑥ *5-FU, leucovorin, and oxaliplatin (FOLFOX)–based chemotherapy is the standard regimen used in adjuvant colon cancer. It is usually given for 6 months.* 5-FU alone results in a small improvement in survival that can vary based on the method of 5-FU administration and the status of MSI. Studies suggest that continuous IV 5-FU infusion treatment schedules are more effective as adjuvant therapy and tumors with high levels of MSI display increased resistance to the single agent.[22]

More often, 5-FU is administered as part of a combination regimen. The most frequently used combination is that of 5-FU, oxaliplatin, and leucovorin. The combination of 5-FU plus leucovorin has undergone extensive study in the adjuvant setting with decreased rates of recurrence and improved survival seen in patients receiving 5-FU plus leucovorin compared with surgery alone. A pooled analysis demonstrated that 5-year disease-free survival (DFS) and overall survival were increased by 12% and 7% with adjuvant 5-FU–based chemotherapy, respectively.[23] 5-Fluorouracil and leucovorin can be administered in a variety of treatment schedules, but none has proven superior with regard to overall patient survival. In the past, the United States has favored bolus regimens based on patient convenience. However, improved availability and comfort in use of portable infusion pumps has led to an increase in use of the continuous IV schedule of 5-FU commonly advocated in Europe. Patients are treated with 6 months of adjuvant therapy. Longer regimens do not improve patient outcomes. No standard exists for the best schedule of 5-FU and leucovorin administration, although continuous infusions may be less toxic and have improved response rates (although no survival advantage) compared with bolus regimens.

Oxaliplatin added to the combination of 5-FU and leucovorin has further improved response rates in the adjuvant setting. The MOSAIC trial, conducted in more than 2,200 patients, demonstrated that the addition of oxaliplatin to 5-FU and leucovorin decreases disease recurrence and improves DFS and overall survival in patients with stage III disease.[24] These results led to the approval of the FOLFOX4 regimen, given for 6 months, for the adjuvant treatment of colon cancer. FOLFOX is considered standard of care for patients with stage III disease unless their PS is so poor that clinicians do not believe the patients could tolerate intensive combination therapy. Age alone should not determine whether patients receive combination adjuvant therapy or not because elderly patients have been found to equally benefit from this approach with minimal addition of adverse effects. Every effort should be made to minimize adverse treatment effects and use this regimen in patients with stage III colon cancer because this is the only regimen demonstrated to improve overall survival in these patients.[18,24] Several variations on the original FOLFOX regimen have been studied with mFOLFOX6 being the most routinely used in clinical practice. Table 91-4 displays selected variations of the FOLFOX regimen.

Capecitabine is an oral prodrug of 5-FU that is also effective in the adjuvant setting and is being evaluated as a replacement in certain regimens for 5-FU for patient convenience and possible economic and safety reasons. Data suggest that capecitabine is at least equivalent to bolus 5-FU and leucovorin in efficacy and is better tolerated by patients.[25] An increase in hand–foot syndrome and decreased mucositis and neutropenia are seen with capecitabine compared with bolus 5-FU. Consequently, most practitioners feel that capecitabine is an acceptable alternative to IV 5-FU plus leucovorin. The role of capecitabine in combination with additional chemotherapy agents such as oxaliplatin has been investigated. The addition of oxaliplatin to capecitabine resulted in improved DFS compared with bolus 5-FU–leucovorin in stage III patients and is considered an acceptable adjuvant regimen in this patient population.[17,26] Use of capecitabine as part of additional chemotherapy regimens should not be done outside of clinical trials.

Targeted therapies are being evaluated for their role in their adjuvant treatment of colon cancer. In particular, cetuximab and bevacizumab are in or have recently completed phase III trials. Trials comparing mFOLFOX6 with and without bevacizumab have failed to show a benefit of bevacizumab in the adjuvant setting.[27] At this time, no targeted agents are approved for use as adjuvant therapy in stage II or III colorectal cancer patients. Additionally, irinotecan should not be used in the adjuvant setting because its addition to 5-FU–based regimens has increased toxicity without therapeutic benefit.[17]

▶ Metastatic Disease (Stage IV)

Traditional chemotherapy and targeted biological therapies are the mainstay of treatment for metastatic colon or rectal cancer and have improved the median survival time of these patients to more than 20 months.[18] Most often, a combination of chemotherapy agents with biological therapies is administered to these patients. Currently, metastatic colorectal cancer is incurable, and treatment goals are to reduce patients' symptoms, improve quality of life, and extend survival. Combination chemotherapy regimens have been demonstrated to result in prolongation of survival with tolerable adverse effects. Similar to the adjuvant setting, 5-FU plus leucovorin continues to be in most first-line chemotherapy regimens used for metastatic colorectal cancer. A variety of continuous intravenous (IV) infusion 5-FU and bolus regimens can be used; however, compared with IV bolus 5-FU, response rates with continuous infusion 5-FU are approximately doubled. In a meta-analysis of six randomized trials evaluating more than 1,200 patients with advanced colorectal cancer, continuous infusions of 5-FU had a significantly higher tumor response rate, a small increase in survival, and lower incidence of myelosuppression, diarrhea, and mucositis when compared with bolus regimens.[28]

Additional agents have been added to the 5-FU and leucovorin regimen with superior response and survival rates compared to the two drugs used alone. The addition of irinotecan to 5-FU plus leucovorin (IFL) significantly improves response rates and survival without adversely affecting quality of life. This regimen was superior to 5-FU plus leucovorin with regard to tumor response, survival, and quality of life.[29] As a result, irinotecan received approval from the FDA in 2000 as first-line therapy for metastatic colorectal cancer in combination with 5-FU and leucovorin. Soon thereafter, oxaliplatin in combination with 5-FU and leucovorin (FOLFOX4) demonstrated improvement in median survival compared with the IFL regimen described earlier. A comparison of oxaliplatin plus 5-FU and leucovorin (FOLFOX4) with weekly IFL showed superior efficacy with FOLFOX4 compared with IFL with regard to response rates and survival.[30] Several study design questions including the crossover design and differing methods of 5-FU administration led several practitioners to debate the significance of these results. Patients in the IFL arm received weekly IV bolus 5-FU, and FOLFOX4 patients received 5-FU as IV bolus followed by continuous infusion IV, which is

thought to increase response rates. A larger European study validated these concerns when it compared a combined bolus and infusional 5-FU regimen plus irinotecan (FOLFIRI) with the FOLFOX regimen (using a slightly different schedule) with crossover to the opposite arm upon relapse.[31] No difference in patient survival was seen with either regimen, and toxicity was as expected. Neuropathy and neutropenia were more common with FOLFOX, and diarrhea, nausea, vomiting, dehydration, and febrile neutropenia were more common with FOLFIRI. Based on improved survival data with the FOLFOX and FOLFIRI regimens, irinotecan administered in a bolus fashion, as described in the IFL regimens, is no longer recommended for routine use. When irinotecan-based combination chemotherapy is to be given for the metastatic treatment of colon cancer, it should be as FOLFIRI described in Table 91–4.

Capecitabine also has activity in the metastatic setting. When combined with oxaliplatin in regimens known as CapeOx or XELOX, capecitabine appears to be as safe as 5-FU–based regimens.[17] Additionally, progression-free survival (PFS) with capecitabine and oxaliplatin is similar to that of FOLFOX and is considered noninferior to the FOLFOX regimen as first-line therapy in advanced disease.[32] This noninferiority with capecitabine may be specific to its use with oxaliplatin because capecitabine in combination with irintoecan (CAPIRI) demonstrated decreased PFS compared with FOLFIRI and the routine substitution of 5-FU with capecitabine in irinotecan-based regimens is not recommended.[17,33]

5-Fluorouracil plus leucovorin or capecitabine alone is appropriate first-line treatment only for individuals for whom three-drug combination regimens are believed to toxic. The site(s) of tumor involvement, history of prior chemotherapy, and patient-specific factors help define the appropriate management strategy. ❾ *The most important factor in patient survival is not the initial regimen but whether or not patients receive all three active chemotherapy drugs (5-FU, irinotecan, and oxaliplatin) at some point in their treatment course.*[34]

Targeted or biologic agents have been approved for use in metastatic colorectal cancer. Bevacizumab in combination with IV 5-FU–based chemotherapy is approved by the FDA for initial treatment of patients with metastatic colorectal cancer. Results from randomized trials show increased benefit compared with chemotherapy alone. One phase III trial of bevacizumab in combination with IFL as first-line therapy in patients with metastatic colorectal cancer has also been completed with a 5-month increase in median survival seen with the addition of bevacizumab with manageable adverse effects.[35] The results of this study show the relevance of angiogenesis as an important target for the treatment of metastatic colorectal cancer. Similar to when used without bevacizumab, FOLFIRI is superior to IFL in combination with bevacizumab. Survival time was improved by approximately 9 months with FOLFIRI plus bevacizumab compared with IFL plus bevacizumab.[33]

The addition of bevacizumab when added to first-line oxaliplatin-based chemotherapy has also been demonstrated to improve PFS but did not positively impact response rates or overall survival.[36] Similar results were demonstrated with bevacizumab in combination with capecitabine and oxaliplatin.[47]

Based on these results, bevacizumab is recommended as part of all 5-FU–based chemotherapy regimens used for the first-line treatment of metastatic colorectal cancer unless contraindicated. Bevacizumab should not be used in patients who present with or develop the following conditions until they are stabilized or treated, including patients with gastrointestinal (GI) perforation or fistulas involving a major organ, recent (within 28 days) major surgeries or open wounds, wound dehiscence requiring medical intervention, hypertensive crisis or uncontrolled severe hypertension, hypertensive encephalopathy—serious bleeding, a severe arterial thromboembolic event, moderate or severe proteinuria (2 g or higher of proteinuria/24 hours); nephrotic syndrome, and reversible posterior leukoencephalopathy syndrome.

The EGFR inhibitors, cetuximab and panitumumab, demonstrate improved PFS as first-line therapy in the metastatic setting when individually combined with either the FOLFOX or FOLFIRI regimens.[37-40] ❽ *Before using these agents, testing for KRAS mutation status should occur. Extensive literature exists documenting evidence demonstrating failure of EGFR inhibitors in patients whose tumors have a mutation in codon 12 or codon 13 of the KRAS gene.*[17] To illustrate the importance of *KRAS* mutation status, in a retrospective analysis of data from a large phase III trial investigating panitumumab versus best supportive care in the metastatic setting, patients with WT *KRAS* had a 17% response rate, but those with mutant *KRAS* had a 0% response rate to panitumumab.[41] Similar findings have been replicated with cetuximab as well. Consequently, cetuximab or panitumumab may be used in the first-line setting in combination with traditional chemotherapy agents in *KRAS* WT patients only.[17]

Attempts to combine the vascular endothelial growth factor (VEGF) inhibitor bevacizumab with cetuximab and panitumumab as part of traditional chemotherapy regimens have resulted in inferior outcomes to regimens with bevacizumab alone.[42] Based on these results, the use of bevacizumab with either EGFR inhibitor is not recommended.[17]

❼ *In summary, most practitioners select first-line treatment for metastatic colorectal cancer from among these currently approved treatments: oxaliplatin plus 5-FU plus leucovorin (FOLFOX); irinotecan plus 5-FU plus leucovorin (FOLFIRI); capecitabine plus oxaliplatin (CapeOx or XELOX); bevacizumab plus 5-FU– or capecitabine-based chemotherapy (FOLFIRI or FOLFOX or CapeOx); or cetuximab or panitumumab plus 5-FU based chemotherapy (FOLFOX or FOLFIRI) in* KRAS *WT patients.*[17]

▶ Second-Line Therapy

❾ *Treatment of relapsed or refractory metastatic disease uses agents not given in the first-line setting.* Because most patients will have received a combination of 5-FU or capecitabine with either irinotecan or oxaliplatin, second-line therapy with the alternate regimen should be considered.[17] For example, a patient who received FOLFOX plus bevacizumab as first-line therapy for metastatic disease should be offered FOLFIRI as part of their second-line regimen. EGFR inhibitors are an additional option for use in the second-line setting in patients with WT *KRAS only*. Patients who did not have an EGFR inhibitor in their first-line regimens are candidates for single-agent cetuximab or panitumumab or either agent in combination with 5-FU and irinotecan (FOLFIRI + EGFR inhibitor). Additionally cetuximab plus irinotecan can be used without the inclusion of 5-FU. The use of EGFR inhibitors may be beneficial as monotherapy, but response rates and PFS appear to be increased in combination with irinotecan-based chemotherapy.[43-47] The results appear to be best when irinotecan is continued because of synergy demonstrated between the two classes of agents.[17,43]

If targeted agents such as bevacizumab were not part of the initial regimen, addition to the second-line regimen should be strongly considered. In the phase III randomized Eastern Cooperative Oncology Group trial, patients with metastatic colorectal who had failed first-line therapies were randomized into three treatment arms: FOLFOX4, FOLFOX4 plus bevacizumab, and single-agent bevacizumab. The addition of bevacizumab to FOLFOX increased the overall survival time from 10.8 to 12.9 months.[48] Bevacizumab as monotherapy was shown to be inferior to FOLFOX4 in efficacy and should not be considered as a treatment option in the second-line setting.

▶ Salvage Therapy

Third-line options for patients with metastatic colorectal cancer are limited. Panitumumab is approved for patients who have progressed after 5-FU, oxaliplatin, and irinotecan. Compared with best supportive care, it was demonstrated to improve disease progression.[17] Patients who fail standard treatment for metastatic colorectal cancer should be encouraged to participate in a clinical trial evaluating new treatment approaches for this incurable disease. Table 91–6 lists treatment options for first- and second-line treatment of metastatic colorectal cancer. Patients with good PS are treated more aggressively than those with poor PS because of their ability to better tolerate chemotherapy.

▶ Metastatic Patients With Isolated Hepatic Metastasis

Patients with metastatic lesions in the liver that remain unresectable have a poor outcome with limited chance for long-term survival. One approach to treating these patients is to resect the lesion and then give adjuvant chemotherapy. Unfortunately, the majority of patients with hepatic lesions have unresectable lesions at diagnosis. For these patients, neoadjuvant chemotherapy should be considered in attempt to convert their tumors unresectable to resectable.[17]

FOLFOX and FOLFIRI have both been demonstrated to allow for an increase in surgical resection and increase the potential for long-term survival.[17] A systematic review

Table 91–6

Treatment Options for Metastatic Colon Cancer[a]

First-Line Therapy	Second-Line Therapy
Good Performance Status • FOLFOX with or without bevacizumab • FOLFIRI with or without bevacizumab • 5-FU + leucovorin with bevacizumab	**If First-Line Irinotecan** • FOLFOX with or without bevacizumab[b] • Irinotecan with or without cetuximab[c] • Capecitabine or 5-FU plus leucovorin
Poor Performance Status • Capecitabine or 5-FU plus leucovorin with or without bevacizumab	**If First-Line Oxaliplatin** • FOLFIRI with or without bevacizumab[b] • Irinotecan with or without cetuximab[c]

5-FU, 5-fluorouracil.

[a]CapeOX may replace FOLFOX in selected patients.

[b]Bevacizumab may be given if not part of the first-line therapy.

[c]If *KRAS* wild type.

published on the outcomes of surgical resection in patients with colorectal liver metastasis found that a subgroup of patients with hepatic metastases receive a large benefit from surgical resection.[20] Five year-survival rates in the reviewed studies ranged from 15% to 67% (median, 30%). Recent studies have added bevacizumab to combination chemotherapy regimens with success. No more than 8 to 10 weeks of chemotherapy should be given to avoid liver complications associated with it, and health care practitioners should take precautions to ensure that bevacizumab is not given within 6 weeks of surgery in this setting.[17] Additionally, EGFR inhibitors can be considered for part of the neoadjuvant regimen in patients with WT status.

Hepatic arterial infusion pumps have been used in the setting of isolated liver metastases, but this practice has fallen

Patient Encounter, Part 3

Based on the information presented, create a care plan for this patient's colon cancer.

Your plan should include:

(a) The patient's drug- and nondrug-related needs and problems

(b) The goals of therapy

(c) A treatment plan specific to HB that includes strategies to prevent adverse effects of chemotherapy

(d) A follow-up plan to determine whether the goals have been achieved and the adverse effects of chemotherapy have been minimized

(e) A plan for treatment options when the initial therapy is no longer achieving the goals of therapy.

out of favor given improvements in local therapy such as radiofrequency ablation, cryoablation, and chemoembolization.

SPECIFIC AGENTS USED IN COLORECTAL CANCER

Table 91–7 lists all FDA-approved drugs used in colorectal cancer along with their mechanisms of action, common toxicities, and recommended dose adjustments for hepatic and renal dysfunction.

5-Fluorouracil

5-Fluorouracil acts as a "false" pyrimidine inhibiting the formation of the DNA base thymidine.[18] The main mechanism by which it accomplishes this is by inhibiting the enzyme thymidylate synthase, the rate-limiting step in thymidine formation. 5-Fluorouracil must first be metabolized to its active metabolite, fluoro-deoxy-uridine monophosphate (F-dUMP). Additionally, metabolites of 5-FU may incorporate into RNA inhibiting its synthesis.

5-Fluorouracil is commonly used in the adjuvant and metastatic treatment of colon and rectal cancers. Various dosing administration techniques and schedules have been developed with 5-FU, including IV bolus every 3 to 4 weeks, IV continuous infusion, weekly IV boluses, and IV boluses followed by continuous infusions of 5-FU. Clinical studies comparing efficacy of bolus and continuous infusion schedules generally favor continuous infusion of 5-FU. This is consistent with evidence that suggests that the duration of infusion may be an important determinant of the biologic activity of 5-FU, particularly because of its short plasma half-life, S-phase specificity, and relatively slow growth of colon tumors.[18,49]

Clinically significant differences in toxicity also differ based on the dose, route, and schedule of 5-FU administration. Leukopenia and mucositis are the primary dose-limiting toxicities of bolus 5-FU, whereas palmar-plantar erythrodysesthesia ("hand–foot syndrome") and diarrhea occur most frequently with continuous infusions of 5-FU.[18,49] Health care practitioners can offer valuable patient advice to decrease the impact of these adverse effects. Patients can be informed to suck on ice chips before and for up to 30 minutes after 5-FU boluses to decrease the incidence of mucositis. Hand–foot syndrome, characterized by painful swelling and redness of the soles of the feet and palms of the hand, can be minimized with loose-fitting clothing and keeping skin moist. Additional toxicities include moderate nausea and vomiting, skin discoloration, nail changes, photosensitivity, and neurologic toxicity.

An additional determinate of 5-FU toxicity, regardless of the method of administration, is related to its catabolism and pharmacogenomic factors. Dihydropyrimidine dehydrogenase (DPD) is the main enzyme responsible for the catabolism of 5-FU to inactive metabolites.[50] A number of polymorphisms in DPD have been identified in which patients have a complete or near-complete deficiency of this enzyme. This results in unusually severe toxicity, including

Table 91–7

FDA-Approved Drugs Used in Colon Cancer

Generic Name (Trade Name)	Mechanism of Action	Common Toxicities	Dosing Adjustments for Renal or Hepatic Dysfunction or Pharmacogenetic Considerations
5-FU	Inhibition of the enzyme thymidylate synthase, the rate-limiting step in thymidine formation	*Dose limiting:* Myelosuppression and mucositis with bolus administration Diarrhea and hand–foot syndrome with continuous infusion *Additional toxicities:* Skin discoloration, nail changes, photosensitivity, and neurologic toxicity	Do not give if bilirubin greater than 5 mg/dL (86 μmol/L) DPD deficiency may result in increased toxicity. Testing not routine, but may be considered in those with excessive toxicity.
Capecitabine (Xeloda)	Orally active prodrug of 5-FU. Once activated, the mechanism of action is the same	Similar to continuous infusion 5-FU	CrCl 30–50 mL/min (0.50–83 mL/s) decrease starting dose to 75% of the original dose Do not give if CrCl less than 30 mL/min (0.50 mL/s)
Irinotecan (Camptosar)	Topoisomerase inhibitor that forms a complex with the covalently bound DNA topoisomerase enzyme and interferes with the DNA breakage-resealing process	*Dose limiting:* Early and late diarrhea *Additional toxicities:* Neutropenia, nausea, and vomiting	Decrease dose one level in patients with a homozygous UGT1A1*28 allele. Having this allele decreases the hepatic metabolism of irinotecan and increases the toxicity
Oxaliplatin (Eloxatin)	Similar to other platinum analogs (cisplatin) in that it binds to the N-7 position of guanine, which results in cross-linking of DNA and double-stranded DNA breaks	*Dose limiting:* Acute (within first 2 days) and persistent (greater than 14 days) neuropathies *Additional toxicities:* Anaphylactic-like reactions, dyspnea, nausea, vomiting	No formal dose adjustment, though use with caution in patients with mild to moderate renal dysfunction
Bevacizumab (Avastin)	Monoclonal antibody that binds to VEGF and inhibits angiogenesis	*Dose limiting:* Hypertension, bleeding episodes, thrombotic events *Additional toxicities:* Rare perforation of the bowel, proteinuria	None
Cetuximab (Erbitux)	Binds to the cell surface EGFR, preventing EGF and TGF-α binding. This decreased cell proliferation of cancer cells	*Dose limiting:* Infusion-related reactions, acneiform skin rash *Additional toxicities:* Diarrhea, hypomagnesemia, hypocalcemia, interstitial lung disease	*KRAS* WT only
Panitumumab (Vectibix)	Similar to cetuximab	*Dose limiting:* Acneiform skin rash *Additional toxicities:* Infusion-related reactions, diarrhea, hypomagnesemia, hypocalcemia, interstitial lung disease	*KRAS* WT only

CrCl, creatinine clearance; EGF, epidermal growth factor; EGFR, epidermal growth factor receptor; 5-FU, 5-fluorouracil; TGF, transforming growth factor; VEGF, vascular endothelial growth factor; WT, wild type.

death, after the administration of 5-FU. Approximately 3% of patients have a complete lack of DPD activity with other patients demonstrating a partial deficiency in enzyme activity. Although patients may be tested for level of DPD activity, it is not routinely done but may be considered in patients who develop severe toxicity after 5-FU administration. The response to 5-FU is also influenced by the status of MSI within the tumor. Tumors with high levels of MSI are generally more resistant to 5-FU despite being associated with better prognosis.

Leucovorin is commonly given with 5-FU. Leucovorin acts to increase the affinity of 5-FU to thymidine synthase, thus increasing the pharmacologic activity of 5-FU.[18] Leucovorin is most effective when administered before 5-FU and can be given by IV bolus or as a continuous infusion. Health care practitioners can also expect an increase in 5-FU toxicities (leukopenia, mucositis, and diarrhea) when leucovorin is given in combination with 5-FU.

Capecitabine

Capecitabine (Xeloda) is an oral prodrug of 5-FU that is designed to be selectively activated by tumor cells. Capecitabine undergoes a three-step conversion to 5-FU, the last step being phosphorylation by thymidine phosphorylase (TP). TP levels are reported to be higher in tumor cells than normal tissues; therefore, the systemic exposure of active drug is minimized, and tumor concentrations of the active drugs are optimized.[18,25] After the drug is converted to 5-FU, it has the same mechanism of action. The current FDA-approved indication for capecitabine is for use in metastatic and adjuvant colorectal cancer when monotherapy is desired, although it is actively being investigated as a replacement for 5-FU in most combinations of colon and rectal cancer regimens. Capecitabine has been demonstrated to be at least equivalent to bolus IV 5-FU in the metastatic and adjuvant setting with improved patient tolerability.[25,51] Hand–foot syndrome and diarrhea are common with capecitabine because its toxicities (and pharmacologic activity) appear to mimic those of continuous infusions of 5-FU. Both irinotecan and oxaliplatin have been combined with capecitabine. Capecitabine in combination with oxaliplatin appears to be as safe and effective as IV-based 5-FU in the treatment of patients with colorectal cancer.[17,49] Combinations with irinotecan have had mixed results and are not routinely recommended.[17,33]

The dose of capecitabine ranges from 1,000 to 1,250 mg/m^2 twice a day when used by itself; lower doses are often used when it is given in combination with irinotecan or oxaliplatin or in patients with renal insufficiency. The dose should be taken on a full stomach with breakfast and dinner. Capecitabine administered with warfarin can result in significant increases in patients' international normalized ratio (INR) and requires close monitoring. The convenience of oral administration, potentially requiring fewer clinic visits, and an improvement in toxicity make capecitabine a useful alternative to IV 5-FU both by itself and incorporated into other regimens used in colorectal cancer.

Irinotecan

Irinotecan (Camptosar) is a **topoisomerase-I** inhibitor that forms a complex with the covalently bound DNA topoisomerase I enzyme and interferes with the DNA breakage–resealing process.[49] Binding permits uncoiling of the double-stranded DNA, but it prevents subsequent resealing of the DNA, resulting in double-stranded DNA breaks. Irinotecan is a prodrug that is converted by carboxylesterases to its active form, SN-38. Irinotecan is indicated for the first-line treatment of metastatic colorectal cancer in combination with 5-FU and leucovorin or as a single agent in patients who fail first-line therapies. Irinotecan is not recommended as part of the adjuvant treatment of colorectal cancer at this time.

The major toxicity of irinotecan is diarrhea, which can occur both early and late in therapy.[17,49] The early diarrhea is a cholinergic reaction that occurs in the first 24 hours (often during the infusion) in up to 10% of patients and responds to atropine 0.25 to 1 mg IV. The late diarrhea seen in a larger percent of patients occurs 7 to 14 days after the irinotecan infusion. Health care practitioners have to be diligent in counseling patients on this adverse reaction and counseling them on the proper use of antidiarrheals. At the first change

in bowel habits, an intensive loperamide regimen should be started by patients (4 mg initially followed by 2 mg every 2 hours until diarrhea free for 12 hours). If diarrhea does not stop or if it worsens, patients should be instructed to call their health care provider immediately. Late-onset diarrhea may require hospitalization or discontinuation of therapy, and fatalities have been reported. Additional toxicities with irinotecan include leukopenia (including neutropenic fever) and moderate nausea and vomiting. Toxicities of irinotecan appear to be greater when the drug is given weekly compared with other administration schedules.

Similar to 5-FU, a pharmacogenomic abnormality is associated with irinotecan toxicity. UDP-glucuronosyltransferase (UGT1A1) is an enzyme that is responsible for the glucuronidation of SN-38 to inactive metabolites, and reduced or deficient levels of this enzyme correlate with irinotecan-induced diarrhea and neutropenia.[17,49] Recently, the FDA approved a blood test that detects variations in this gene. This test may assist health care providers in predicting which patients may develop severe toxicities from "normal" doses of irinotecan and can be ordered before patients receive irinotecan.[17] The package insert recommends dose reductions of one levels in patients who are UGT1A1 homozygous variants. Irinotecan is administered as an IV bolus over 60 to 90 minutes in a variety of dosing schedules.

Oxaliplatin

Oxaliplatin (Eloxatin) is similar to other platinum analogs (cisplatin) in that it binds to the N-7 position of guanine that results in cross-linking of DNA and double-stranded DNA breaks.[49] Oxaliplatin differs from cisplatin in that the DNA damage induced by oxaliplatin may not be as easily recognized by DNA repair genes often seen in colorectal cancer. Oxaliplatin, in combination with 5-FU-based regimens, is indicated for the first- and second-line treatment of metastatic colorectal cancer as well as the adjuvant treatment of colorectal cancer.

The dose-limiting toxicity of oxaliplatin is acute and chronic neuropathy.[18] Acute neuropathies occur within 1 to 2 days of dosing, resolve within 2 weeks, and usually occur peripherally. These acute neuropathies occur in almost all patients to some degree and are exacerbated by exposure to cold temperature or cold objects. Health care providers should instruct patients to avoid cold drinks, avoid use of ice, and cover skin before exposure to cold or cold objects. In addition, carbamazepine, gabapentin, amifostine, and calcium and magnesium infusions have been used to both prevent and treat oxaliplatin-induced neuropathies, although use of these agents is not widely accepted.[18] Persistent neuropathies generally occur after eight cycles of oxaliplatin and are characterized by defects that can interfere with daily activities (e.g., writing, buttoning, swallowing, and walking). Patients may receive predefined breaks from oxaliplatin to decrease the onset of these toxicities with reinitiation of therapy.[30] This strategy varies among protocols but involves administering a certain number of predefined oxaliplatin cycles and then stopping. Maintenance therapy with another agent is usually administered and then the oxaliplatin-based regimen is restarted based on the protocol. These neuropathies occur in up to half of patients receiving oxaliplatin but usually resolve with dosage reductions or after oxaliplatin is stopped.[18] A recent phase III trial in the adjuvant setting demonstrated a decrease in greater than grade 2 chronic sensory neuropathies in patients receiving IV calcium and magnesium infusions before and after oxaliplatin infusion.[52] Oxaliplatin has minimal renal, myelosuppressive effects, and nausea and vomiting when compared with other platinum drugs. Oxaliplatin is given IV in a variety of dosing schedules with a typical dose of 85 mg/m^2 IV every 2 weeks.

Bevacizumab

Bevacizumab (Avastin) is a recombinant, humanized monoclonal antibody that inhibits VEGF. VEGF is a proangiogenic growth factor found in many cancers, including colorectal, and is thought to promote blood vessel formation and metastasis of the tumor by binding to VEGF receptors on tumors. Bevacizumab inhibits circulating VEGF, preventing it from binding to receptors and decreasing the formation of new blood vessels.[17,18] Additionally, bevacizumab may allow for increased concentrations of traditional chemotherapy such as irinotecan to reach the tumor to exert its pharmacologic effect. Bevacizumab is not effective alone and must be used in combination with other agents effective in colorectal cancer. It is indicated for first-line treatment of patients with metastatic colorectal cancer in combination with IV 5-FU–based regimens. Bevacizumab has also been shown to increase survival in the second-line setting when used in combination with the FOLFOX regimen in patients who have not yet received bevacizumab.[17]

Adverse effects associated with bevacizumab include hypertension, which is common but easily managed with oral antihypertensive agents.[35,53] Thrombotic events (including myocardial infarctions, pulmonary embolisms, and deep vein thrombosis) occur more frequently in the elderly patients with cardiovascular risk factors and need to be monitored routinely. Because bevacizumab interferes with normal wound healing, it should not be given shortly before or after surgical procedures.[53] Initiation within 28 days of surgery is not recommended to allow for proper wound healing and decrease the risk of bleeding. The amount of time needed after bevacizumab discontinuation to perform elective surgical procedures is less clear, but health care providers should take into consideration bevacizumab's half-life of approximately 20 days when making clinical decisions.[38] Patients should have their urine checked for protein before each dose of bevacizumab to check for potential kidney damage. Patients who have developed 2+ protein on the urinalysis require additional testing before receiving therapy. These patients will have their 24-hour urine collected and assessed for protein. Therapy is interrupted for 2 g or more of proteinuria/24 hours and resumed when proteinuria was less than 2 g/24 hours.

Finally, there is a risk of GI perforation that is rare but potentially fatal. Patients complaining of abdominal pain associated with vomiting or constipation should be counseled to call their physician immediately. Bevacizumab is commonly given at a dose of 5 mg/kg IV every 14 days until disease progression. Once disease progresses and salvage chemotherapy is initiated, the benefit of continuing bevacizumab is unclear.

Cetuximab and Panitumumab

Cetuximab (Erbitux) and panitumumab (Vectibix) are monoclonal antibodies directed against the EGFR. Cetuximab is a chimeric antibody, whereas panitumumab is a fully human monoclonal antibody. EGFR is overexpressed in colorectal cancers and leads to an increase in tumor proliferation and growth.[49] Cetuximab received FDA approval for use in EGFR-expressing metastatic colorectal cancer in irinotecan-relapsed or -refractory patients. Cetuximab should be administered in combination with irinotecan but can be used as a single agent in patients who cannot tolerate irinotecan-based chemotherapy. Panitumumab is approved as monotherapy agent and should not be used in combination with other agents outside of clinical trials.

Both agents are well tolerated with infusion-related reactions being cetuximab's dose-limiting toxicity and rash most commonly seen with panitumumab. Patients receiving cetuximab require premedication with acetaminophen and diphenhydramine and may require modifications to their administration schedule or permanent discontinuation if they develop severe allergic toxicity. A skin rash and diarrhea are also commonly seen with both agents, and health care practitioners should provide counseling to patients about these adverse effects. Treatment options include common medications used to treat acne (doxycycline), topical and systemic steroids, and general skin care. Development of rash may be a surrogate marker of response, and clinicians should attempt to minimize the complications of the rash before discontinuing therapy.[17] Other toxicities common to both agents include low magnesium, calcium, and potassium levels that require checking levels and replacement therapy as clinically indicated. A rare (less than 1%) interstitial lung disease is seen with all agents that inhibit EGFR, and patients should be instructed to report any new-onset shortness of breath. Cetuximab has an initial loading dose of 400 mg/m^2 IV infusion. Weekly doses of 250 mg/m^2 are then administered starting the following week. Panitumumab is given 6 mg/kg every 2 weeks.

Patient Encounter, Part 4

Despite completing 6 cycles of adjuvant chemotherapy, HB's disease progresses, and a CT scan reveals metastases to his bone and liver. The tumor is sent for pharmacogenomic profiling and is found to have a mutation in the *KRAS* gene.

What pharmacologic treatment options are available for the treatment of his metastatic disease?

RECTAL CANCER

Although often treated similarly to colon cancer, there are some important differences in the treatment of rectal cancer, especially in the adjuvant setting. Rectal cancer involves tumors found in the distal 15 cm of the large bowel and, as such, is very distinct from colon cancer in that it has a propensity for both local and distant recurrence. The higher incidence of local failure and poorer overall prognosis associated with rectal cancer are attributable to limitations in surgical techniques. Therefore, multimodality therapies with a combination of chemotherapy, radiation, and surgery are at the forefront in the treatment of rectal cancer with the main goal of survival and quality of life by preserving the function of the anal sphincter. In addition, because treatment with surgery, radiation, or systemic chemotherapy at the time of the recurrence is often suboptimal, adjuvant therapy after tumor resection is an important aspect of treatment of the primary tumor. Similar to adjuvant therapy for colon cancer, 5-FU provides the basis for chemotherapy regimens for rectal cancer. ❿ *Adjuvant therapy consisting of 5-FU–based chemotherapy in combination with radiation therapy should be offered to patients with stage II or III cancer of the rectum.*[54] Radiation therapy decreases the rate of local recurrences, but the 5-FU decreases the risk of distant tumor recurrence as well as acting as a radiosensitizer. Toxicities from combined modality therapy include severe hematologic toxicity, enteritis, and diarrhea. Additional trials have sought to determine optimal combinations of concurrent radiation and 5-FU. Similar to tumors in the colon, continuous infusions of 5-FU appear to be superior to bolus doses. However, leucovorin does not appear to improve efficacy of adjuvant treatment for rectal cancer. Use of oral alternatives to 5-FU that are also known to enhance radiation effects, such as capecitabine, are under investigation with preliminary data suggesting the combination of capecitabine and radiation will be safe and effective. In addition, based on the efficacy in colon cancer, FOLFOX regimens have moved into clinical trials in the adjuvant setting.

Another unique aspect of rectal cancer is the use of neoadjuvant therapy. Preoperative radiation (with or without chemotherapy) is given to downstage the tumor before surgical resection to improve sphincter preservation.[54] The issue of pre- versus postoperative radiation is a subject of debate and investigation in the United States and requires further data to determine the superiority of a specific neoadjuvant protocol.

❿ *Finally, once rectal cancer is metastatic, similar regimens as outlined in the colon cancer section are used for palliation of symptoms.*[54]

OUTCOME EVALUATION

• The goals of monitoring are to evaluate whether the patient is receiving any benefit from the management of the disease, detect recurrence, and minimize the adverse effects of treatment. During treatment for active disease, patients should undergo monitoring for measurable tumor response, progression, or new metastases; these tests may include chest CT scans or x-rays, abdominal or pelvic CT scans or x-rays, depending on the site of disease being evaluated for response; and carcinoembryonic antigen (CEA) measurements every 3 months if the CEA level is or was previously elevated.[17] A PET scan can be considered to identify localized sites of metastatic disease when a rising CEA level suggests metastatic disease but results of CT scans and other imaging studies are negative. Symptoms of recurrence such as pain, changes in bowel habits, rectal bleeding, pelvic masses, anorexia, and weight loss develop in fewer than 50% of patients. Patients who undergo curative surgical resection, with or without adjuvant therapy, require close follow-up because early detection and treatment of recurrence could still result in patient cures. In addition, early treatment for asymptomatic metastatic colorectal cancer appears superior to delayed therapy. Colorectal cancer surveillance guidelines published by the American Society of Clinical Oncology recommend against routinely monitoring liver function tests, complete blood count (CBC), FOBT, CT scans, annual chest x-rays, or pelvic imaging in asymptomatic patients.[55]

In addition, a CBC should be obtained before each course of chemotherapy administration to ensure that hematologic values are adequate. In particular, white blood cell counts and absolute neutrophil counts can be decreased in patients receiving chemotherapy such as irinotecan and 5-FU. Baseline liver function tests and an assessment of renal function should be evaluated before and periodically during therapy. Other selected laboratory tests include checking for the presence of protein in the urine in patients receiving bevacizumab and monitoring of magnesium, calcium, and potassium in patients receiving cetuximab or panitumumab.

Patients should be evaluated during every treatment visit for the presence of anticipated side effects from their treatment, and health care practitioners should anticipate these adverse reactions and aggressively treat and prevent them from occurring. These generally include loose stools or diarrhea from irinotecan, 5-FU, and capecitabine; hand–foot syndrome from 5-FU and capecitabine; nausea or vomiting from irinotecan, 5-FU, and oxaliplatin; mouth sores from 5-FU; neuropathies from oxaliplatin; bleeding and hypertension from bevacizumab; and skin rash associated with cetuximab and panitumumab.

SUMMARY

Recent advances in the treatment of cancer of the colon and rectum now offer the potential to improve patient survival, but for many patients, improved DFS and PFS represent equally important therapeutic outcomes. In the absence of the ability of a specific treatment to demonstrate improved survival, important outcome measures should include the effects of the treatment on patient symptoms, daily activities, PS, and other quality-of-life indicators. Individualized patient care to balance the risks associated with treatment and benefits of a specific treatment regimen is necessary to optimize patient outcomes.

Patient Care and Monitoring

1. Review any available diagnostic data to determine the status of the colon cancer.

2. Obtain a thorough history of prescription, nonprescription, and natural drug product use.

3. Evaluate patient-specific factors that may dictate treatment regimen. Does the patient have a known pharmacogenomic deficiency? What lifestyle issues are important to the patient?

4. Determine if any dose modifications are required in the chemotherapy regimen prescribed. Does the patient have adequate blood counts to receive chemotherapy?

5. Educate the patient on drug therapy and possible treatment-related adverse effects and counsel the patient on appropriate recommendations to prevent or minimize these adverse effects. What medications are for the treatment of cancer, and what medications are to prevent the adverse effects of chemotherapy?

6. Develop a plan to prevent treatment-related adverse effects. Are the antiemetics appropriate? Does the patient understand the possible adverse effects and when to call the physician versus when patient-directed care is appropriate?

7. Warning signs to report to the physician (depends on regimen used) include fever, diarrhea, mucositis, and hand–foot syndrome.

8. Evaluate the patient for the presence of adverse drug reactions, drug allergies, and drug interactions.

Abbreviations Introduced in This Chapter

APC	Adenomatous polyposis coli
CapeOX	Capecitabine and oxaliplatin
CBC	Complete blood count
CEA	Carcinoembryonic antigen
COX-2	Cyclooxygenase-2
CTC	Computed tomographic colonoscopy
DFS	Disease-free survival
DPD	Dihydropyrimidine dehydrogenase
EGFR	Epidermal growth factor receptor
FAP	Familial adenomatous polyposis
F-dUMP	Fluoro-deoxy-uridine monophosphate
FISH	Fluorescence in situ hybridization
FIT	Fecal immunochemical test
FOBT	Fecal occult blood test
FOLFIRI	Folinic acid, fluorouracil, and infusional irinotecan
FOLFOX	Folinic acid, fluorouracil, and oxaliplatin
HNPCC	Hereditary nonpolyposis colorectal cancer
IFL	Irinotecan, fluorouracil, and leucovorin

INR	International normalized ratio
MSI	Mircrosatellite instability
NSAID	Nonsteroidal anti-inflammatory drug
PET	Positron emission tomography
PFS	Progression-free survival
TNM	Tumor, node, metastasis
TP	Thymidine phosphorylase
UGT	UDP-glucuronosyltransferase
VEGF	Vascular endothelial growth factor

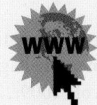 Self-assessment questions and answers are available at *http://www.mhpharmacotherapy.com/pp.html.*

REFERENCES

1. Siegel R, Ward E, Brawley O, Jemal A. Cancer statistics, 2011. CA Cancer J Clin 2011;61:212–236.
2. Ries LAG, Eisner MP, Kosary CL, et al, eds. SEER Cancer Statistics Review, 1975–2000. Bethesda, MD: National Cancer Institute. *http://seer.cancer.gov/csr/1975_2000.*
3. Park Y, Hunter DJ, Spiegelman D, et al. Dietary fiber intake and risk of colorectal cancer: A pooled analysis of prospective cohort studies. JAMA 2005;294:2849–2857.
4. Wactawski-Wende J, Kotchen JM, Anderson GL. Calcium plus vitamin D supplementation and the risk of colorectal cancer. N Engl J Med 2006;354:684–696.
5. Kim YI. Folate and colorectal cancer: An evidence-based critical review. Mol Nutr Food Res 2007;51:267–292.
6. Giovannucci E. Modifiable risk factors for colon cancer. Gastroenterol Clin North Am 2002;31:925–943.
7. Chan AT, Giovannucci EL, Meyerhardt JA, et al. Long-term use of aspirin and nonsteroidal anti-inflammatory drugs and risk of colorectal cancer. JAMA 2005;294:914–923.
8. NCCN Guidelines—Colorectal Cancer Screening v.2. 2011, *http://www.nccn.org.*
9. Chan AT, Ogino S, Fuchs CS. Aspirin and the risk of colorectal cancer in relation to the expression of COX-2. N Engl J Med 2007;356:2131–2142.
10. Nelson HD, Humphrey LL, Nygren P, et al. Postmenopausal hormone replacement therapy: Scientific review. JAMA 2002;288:872–881.
11. Giovannucci E. Metabolic syndrome, hyperinsulinemia, and colon cancer: A review. Am J Clin Nutr 2007;86(Suppl):S836–S842.
12. Calvert PM, Frucht H. The genetics of colorectal cancer. Ann Intern Med 2003;137:603–612.
13. Levin B, Lieberman DA, McFarland B, et al. Screening and surveillance for the early detection of colorectal cancer and adenomatous polyps, 2008: A joint guideline from the American Cancer Society, the US Multi-Society Task Force on Colorectal Cancer, and the American College of Radiology. American Cancer Society guidelines for the early detection of cancer. CA Cancer J Clin 2008;58:130–160.
14. Hawk ET, Levin B. Colorectal cancer prevention. J Clin Oncol 2005;23:378–391.
15. Baron JA, Cole BF, Sandler RS, et al. A randomized trial of aspirin to prevent colorectal adenomas. N Engl J Med 2003;348:891–899.
16. Grunwald V, Hidalgo M. Developing inhibitors of the epidermal growth factor receptor for cancer treatment. J Natl Cancer Inst 2003;95:851–867.
17. NCCN Guidelines—Colon Cancer v.1. 2012, *http://www.nccn.org.*
18. Libutti SK, Saltz LB, Tepper JE. Colon cancer. In: DeVita VT, Lawrence TS, Rosenberg SA, eds. Cancer: Principles and Practice of Oncology, 9th ed. Philadelphia: Lippincott Williams & Wilkins, 2011:1084–1126.

19. Libutti SK, Tepper JE, Saltz LB. Rectal cancer. In: DeVita VT, Lawrence TS, Rosenberg SA, eds. Cancer: Principles and Practice of Oncology, 9th ed. Philadelphia: Lippincott Williams & Wilkins, 2011:1127–1141.

20. Simmonds PC, Primrose JN, Colquitt JL, et al. Surgical resection of hepatic metastases from colorectal cancer: A systematic review of published studies. Br J Cancer 2006;94:982–999.

21. Benson AB, Schrag D, Somerfield MR, et al. American Society of Clinical Oncology recommendations of adjuvant chemotherapy for stage II colon cancer. J Clin Oncol 2004;22:3408–3419.

22. Sargent DJ, Marsoni S, Monges G, et al. Defective mismatch repair as a predictive marker for lack of efficacy of fluorouracil-based adjuvant therapy in colon cancer. J Clin Oncol 2010;28:3219–3226.

23. Gill S, Loprinzi CL, Sargent DJ, et al. Pooled analysis of fluorouracil-based adjuvant therapy for stage II and III colon cancer: Who benefits and by how much? J Clin Oncol 2004;22:1797–1806.

24. Andre T, Boni C, Navarro M, et al. Improved overall survival with oxaliplatin, fluorouracil, and leucovorin as adjuvant treatment in stage II or III colon cancer in the MOSAIC trial. J Clin Oncol. 2009;27:3109–3116

25. Twelves C, Wong A, Nowacki MP, et al. Capecitabine as adjuvant treatment for stage III colon cancer. N Engl J Med 2005;352:2696–2704.

26. Haller DG, Tabernero J, Maroun J, et al. Capecitabine plus oxaliplatin compared with fluorouracil and folinic acid as adjuvant therapy for stage III colon cancer. J Clin Oncol 2011;29:1465–1471.

27. Allegra CJ, Yothers G, O'Connell MJ, et al. Phase III trial assessing bevacizumab in stages II and III carcinoma of the colon: Results of NSABP protocol C-08. J Clin Oncol 2011;29:11–16.

28. Saltz LB, Cox JV, Blanke C, et al. Efficacy of intravenous continuous infusion of fluorouracil compared with bolus administration in advanced colorectal cancer. Meta-analysis Group in Cancer. J Clin Oncol 1998;16:301–308.

29. Saltz LB, Cox JV, Blanke C, et al. Irinotecan plus fluorouracil and leucovorin for metastatic colorectal cancer. N Engl J Med 2000;343:905–914.

30. Goldberg RM, Sargent DJ, Morton RF, et al. A randomized controlled trial of fluorouracil plus leucovorin, irinotecan, and oxaliplatin combinations in patients with previously untreated metastatic colorectal cancer. J Clin Oncol 2004;22:23–30.

31. Tournigand C, André T, Achille E, et al. FOLFIRI followed by FOLFOX6 or the reverse sequence in advanced colorectal cancer: A randomized GERCOR study. J Clin Oncol 2004;22:229–237.

32. Cassidy J, Clarke S, Diaz-Rubio E, et al. Randomized phase III study of capecitabine plus oxaliplatin compared with fluorouracil/folinic acid plus oxaliplatin as first-line therapy for metastatic colorectal cancer. J Clin Oncol. 2008;26:2006–2012.

33. Fuchs CS, Marshall J, Barrueco J. Randomized, controlled trial of irinotecan plus infusional, bolus, or oral fluoropyrimidines in first-line treatment of metastatic colorectal cancer: Updated results from the BICC-C study. J Clin Oncol 2008;26:689–690.

34. Grothey A, Sargent D, Goldberg RM, Schmoll H. Survival of patients with advanced colorectal cancer improves with the availability of fluorouracil-leucovorin, irinotecan, and oxaliplatin in the course of treatment. J Clin Oncol 2004;22:1204–1214.

35. Hurwitz H, Fehrenbacher L, Novotny W, et al. Bevacizumab plus irinotecan, fluorouracil, and leucovorin for metastatic colorectal cancer. N Engl J Med 2004;350:2335–2342

36. Saltz LB, Clarke S, Díaz-Rubio E, et al. Bevacizumab in combination with oxaliplatin-based chemotherapy as first-line therapy in metastatic colorectal cancer: A randomized phase III study. J Clin Oncol 2008;20:2013–2019.

37. Bokemeyer C, Bondarenko I, Makhson A, et al. Fluorouracil, leucovorin, and oxaliplatin with and without cetuximab in the first-line treatment of metastatic colorectal cancer. J Clin Oncol. 2009;27:663–671.

38. Van Cutsem E, Kohne CH, Hitre E, et al. Cetuximab and chemotherapy as initial treatment for metastatic colorectal cancer. N Engl J Med. 2009;360:1408–1417.

39. Douillard JY, Siena S, Cassidy J, et al. Randomized, phase III trial of panitumumab with infusional fluorouracil, leucovorin, and oxaliplatin (FOLFOX4) versus FOLFOX4 alone as first-line treatment in patients with previously untreated metastatic colorectal cancer: The PRIME study. J Clin Oncol. 2010;28:4697–4705.

40. Tol J, Koopman M, Cats A, et al. Chemotherapy, bevacizumab, and cetuximab in metastatic colorectal cancer. N Engl J Med 2009;360:563–572.

41. Amado RG, Wolf M, Peters m, et al. Wild-type KRAS is required for panitumumab efficacy in patients with metastatic colotrectal cancer. J Clin Onc 2008;26:1626–1634.

42. Hecht JR, Mitchell E, Chidiac T, et al. A randomized phase IIIB trial of chemotherapy, bevacizumab, and panitumumab compared with chemotherapy and bevacizumab alone for metastatic colorectal cancer. J Clin Oncol 2009;27:672–680.

43. Cunningham D, Humblet Y, Siena S, et al. Cetuximab monotherapy and cetuximab plus irinotecan in irinotecan-refractory metastatic colorectal cancer. N Engl J Med 2004;351:337–345.

44. Jonker DJ, O'Callaghan CJ, Karapetis CS, et al. Cetuximab for the treatment of colorectal cancer. N Engl J Med. 2007;357:2040–2048.

45. Karapetis CS, Khambata-Ford S, Jonker DJ, et al. *KRAS* mutations and benefit from cetuximab in advanced colorectal cancer. N Engl J Med. 2008;359:1757–1765.

46. Peeters M, Price TJ, Cervantes A, et al. Randomized phase III study of panitumumab with fluorouracil, leucovorin, and irinotecan (FOLFIRI) compared with FOLFIRI alone as second-line treatment in patients with metastatic colorectal cancer. J Clin Oncol 2010;28:4706–4713.

47. Sobrero AF, Maurel J, Febrenbacher L, et al. EPIC: phase III trial of cetuximab plus irinotecan after fluoropyrimidine and oxaliplatin failure in patients with metastatic colorectal cancer. J Clin Onc 2008;26(14):2311–2319.

48. Giantonio BJ, Catalano PJ, Meropol NJ, et al. Bevacizumab in combination with oxaliplatin, fluorouracil, and leucovorin (FOLFOX4) for previously treated metastatic colorectal cancer: Results from the Eastern Cooperative Oncology Group Study E3200. J Clin Onc 2007;25:1539–44.

49. Wolpin BM, Mayer RJ. Systemic treatment of colorectal. Gastroenterology 2008;134:1296–1310.

50. Mercier C, Ciccolini J. Profiling dihydropyrimidine dehydrogenase deficiency in patients with cancer undergoing 5-fluorouracil/capecitabine therapy. Clin Colorectal Cancer 2006;6:288–296.

51. Twelves C. Capecitabine as first-line treatment in colorectal cancer: Pooled data from two large, phase III trials. Eur J Cancer 2002;38(Suppl):15–20.

52. Grothey A, Nikcevich DA, Sloan JA, et al. Intravenous calcium and magnesium for oxaliplatin-induced sensory neurotoxicity in adjuvant colon cancer: NCCTG N04C7. J Clin Onc 2011;29:421–427.

53. Motl S. Bevacizumab in combination chemotherapy for colorectal and other cancers. Am J Health Syst Pharm 2005;62:1021–1032.

54. NCCN Guidelines—Rectal Cancer v.1. 2012, *http://www.nccn.org.*

55. Desch CE, Benson AB, Smith TJ, et al. Recommended colorectal cancer surveillance guidelines by the American Society of Clinical Oncology. J Clin Oncol 1999;17:1312–1321.

92 Prostate Cancer

Trevor McKibbin

KEY CONCEPTS

❶ Prostate cancer is the most frequent cancer in U.S. men. Increasing age and family history are the primary risk factors for prostate cancer.

❷ Prostate-specific antigen (PSA) is a useful marker for predicting outcome for localized disease and monitoring response to androgen-deprivation therapy or chemotherapy for advanced-stage disease. An elevated PSA may detect asymptomatic prostate cancer at an early stage.

❸ The prognosis for prostate cancer patients depends on the histologic grade, tumor size, and disease stage. More than 85% of patients with stage 1 disease but fewer than 1% of those with stage D can be cured.

❹ Androgen ablation with a luteinizing hormone–releasing hormone (LHRH) agonist plus an antiandrogen should be used before radiation therapy for patients with locally advanced prostate cancer to improve outcomes over radiation therapy alone.

❺ Androgen ablation therapy with orchiectomy, an LHRH agonist alone or an LHRH agonist plus an antiandrogen (combined hormonal blockade) can be used to provide palliation for patients with advanced (stage D) prostate cancer. The effects of androgen deprivation are most pronounced in patients with minimal disease at diagnosis.

❻ For patients having progressive disease while receiving combined hormonal blockade with an LHRH agonist plus an antiandrogen, antiandrogen withdrawal can provide additional symptomatic relief. Mutations in the androgen receptor have been documented that cause antiandrogen compounds to behave like receptor agonists.

❼ Chemotherapy with docetaxel and prednisone improves survival in patients with castrate-resistant prostate cancer (CRPC).

❽ Chemotherapy with cabazitaxel and prednisone improves survival in patients with CRPC who have either progressed or are intolerant to docetaxel

❾ Hormonal manipulation with abiraterone and prednisone improves survival in patients previously treated with docetaxel and prednisone.

❿ Immunotherapy with sipuleucel-T improves survival in patients with minimally symptomatic CRPC.

INTRODUCTION

Prostate cancer is the most commonly diagnosed cancer in U.S. men.[1] The disease course varies from a slow growing, asymptomatic tumor that may not require treatment to a rapidly progressing, aggressive tumor resulting in mortality. Prostate cancers are hormonally sensitive, and their growth is increased by androgen signaling. In most men, prostate cancer has a prolonged course. The treatment of clinically localized prostate cancer is based on risk features that may predict a more aggressive cancer. Treatment options for clinically localized disease include active surveillance (also referred to as observation, or watchful waiting) for low-risk patients to surgery, and/or radiation for higher risk patients.

With active surveillance, patients are monitored for disease progression or development of symptoms. In patients with certain high-risk features, a course of adjuvant androgen deprivation therapy may be used after surgery or radiation. Although clinically localized prostate cancer can be cured by surgery or radiation therapy, advanced prostate cancer is not yet curable. Treatment for advanced prostate cancer can provide significant disease palliation for many patients for several years after diagnosis. Advances in the understanding of the biology of the disease resulted in the availability of multiple treatment options and improved survival for patients with advanced prostate cancer.

EPIDEMIOLOGY AND RISK FACTORS

❶ *Prostate cancer is the most frequently diagnosed cancer among U.S. men and represents the second leading cause of cancer-related deaths in all men.*[1] In the United States alone, it was predicted that more than 240,000 new cases of prostatic carcinoma will be diagnosed and more than 33,000 men would die from this disease in 2011.[1] Although prostate cancer incidence increased during the late 1980s and early 1990s owing to widespread prostate-specific antigen (PSA) screening, deaths from prostate cancer have been declining since 1995.

Table 92–1 summarizes the possible factors associated with risk for prostate cancer.[2,3] The widely accepted risk factors for prostate cancer are age, race or ethnicity, and family history of prostate cancer. The disease is rare under the age of 40, but the incidence sharply increases with each subsequent decade of life, most likely because with older age an individual has had a greater lifetime exposure to testosterone, a known growth signal for the prostate. In an evaluation of autopsies from men in Michigan dying of unrelated causes, prostate cancer was identified in 2%, 29%, 32% 55%, and 64% of men in their third, fourth, fifth, sixth and eighth decades of life, respectively.

Race and Ethnicity

The incidence of clinical prostate cancer varies across geographic regions. Scandinavian countries and the United States report the highest incidence of prostate cancer, but the disease is relatively rare in Japan and other Asian countries.[5] African American men have the highest rate of prostate cancer in the world, and in the United States, prostate cancer mortality in African Americans is approximately twice that seen in the white population.[1] Hormonal, dietary, and genetic differences, as well as differences in access to health care, may contribute to the altered susceptibility to prostate cancer in these populations.[2,3] Testosterone, commonly implicated in the pathogenesis of prostate cancer, is 15% higher in African American men compared with white men. Activity of 5-α-reductase, the enzyme that converts testosterone to its more active form, dihydrotestosterone (DHT), in the prostate, is decreased in Japanese men compared with African Americans and whites.[2,3] In addition, genetic variations in

Table 92–1	
Risk Factors Associated With Prostate Cancer	
Factor	**Possible Relationship**
Probable Risk Factors	
Age	More than 70% of cases are diagnosed in men older than 65 years
Race	African Americans have a higher incidence and death rate
Genetic	Familial prostate cancer inherited in an autosomal dominant manner
	Mutations in *p53*, *Rb*, E-cadherin, α-catenin, androgen receptor, *KAI1*, and microsatellite instability; loss of heterozygosity at 1, 2q, 12p, 15q, 16p, and 16q; *BRCA1* and *BRCA2* mutations
	Candidate prostate cancer gene locus identified on chromosome 1
Possible Risk Factors	
Environmental	Clinical carcinoma incidence varies worldwide
	Latent carcinoma similar between regions' nationalized men adopt intermediate incidence rates between that of the United States and their native country
Occupational	Increased risk associated with cadmium exposure
Dietary	Increased risk associated with high-meat and high-fat diets
	Decreased intake of 1,25-dihydroxyvitamin D, lycopene, and β-carotene increases risk
Hormonal	Does not occur in castrated men
	Low incidence in cirrhotic patients
	Up to 80% are hormonally dependent
	African Americans have 15% increased testosterone
	Japanese have decreased 5-α-reductase activities
	Polymorphic expression of the androgen receptor

the androgen receptor exist. Activation of the androgen receptor is inversely correlated with trinucleotide (CAG) repeat length. Shorter CAG repeat sequences have been found in African Americans. Therefore, the combination of increased testosterone and increased androgen receptor activation may account for the increased risk of prostate cancer in African American men.[2,3] The Asian diet generally is considered to be low in fat and high in fiber with a high concentration of phytoestrogens, potentially explaining their decreased risk.[5,6]

Family History

Men with a brother or father with prostate cancer have twice the risk for prostate cancer compared to the rest of the population.[6] Genome-wide scans have identified potential prostate cancer susceptibility candidate genes, and there appears to be a familial clustering of a prostate cancer syndrome. Male carriers of germline mutations of *BRCA1* and *BRCA2* are known to have an increased risk for developing prostate cancer.[7] Common exposure to environmental and other risk factors may also contribute to increased risk among patients with first-degree relatives with prostate cancer.[6]

An alternative explanation for the familial clustering may be polymorphisms in genes important for prostate cancer function and development.[8] Candidate **polymorphisms** include a polymorphism in the androgen receptor, which has two different nucleotide repeat variants, the CAG or the GCC. The CAG repeat varies in repeat number from 11 to 31 repeats in healthy individuals, and the number of repeats is inversely proportional to the activity of the androgen receptor. Some studies have demonstrated that shorter CAG repeats are associated with increased prostate cancer risk. Another candidate polymorphism is *SRD5A2*, which is the gene that codes for 5-α-reductase, the enzyme that converts testosterone to the more active DHT. A variant in *SRD5A2*, the Ala49Thr, increases the activity and may increase prostate cancer risk.[8]

Diet

A number of epidemiologic studies support an association between high fat intake and risk of prostate cancer. A strong correlation between national per capita fat consumption and national prostate cancer mortality has been reported, and prospective case-control studies suggest that a high-fat diet doubles the risk of prostate cancer.[6] This relationship between high fat intake and prostate cancer may be explained by differences in insulin-like growth factor-1 (IGF-1). High-calorie and high-fat diets stimulate production of IGF-1 by the liver. This factor is involved in the regulation of proliferation of cancer cells and may also prevent them from undergoing apoptosis. High levels of IGF-1 are associated with an increased risk of prostate cancer.[8]

Other dietary factors implicated in prostate cancer include retinol, carotenoids, lycopene, and vitamin D consumption.[5] Retinol, or vitamin A, intake, especially in men older than 70 years, is correlated with an increased risk of prostate cancer, but intake of its precursor, β-carotene, has a protective or neutral effect. Lycopene, obtained primarily from tomatoes, decreased the risk of prostate cancer in small cohort studies. Men who developed prostate cancer in one cohort study had lower levels of $1,25(OH)_2$-vitamin D than matched control participants, although a prospective study did not support this. Clearly, dietary risk factors require further evaluation, but because fat and vitamins are modifiable risk factors, dietary intervention may be promising in prostate cancer prevention. Investigations of selenium and vitamin E supplementation are discussed further in the chemoprevention section.

Other Factors

Benign prostatic hyperplasia (BPH) is a common problem among elderly men, affecting more than 40% of men older than the age of 70 years. BPH results in the urinary symptoms of hesitancy and frequency. Because prostate cancer affects a similar age group and often has similar presenting symptoms, the presence of BPH often complicates the diagnosis of prostate cancer, although it does not appear to increase the risk of developing prostate cancer.[2,9]

Smoking has been associated with an increased risk of aggressive prostate cancer and smokers with prostate cancer have an increased mortality resulting from the disease compared with nonsmokers with prostate cancer (relative risk [RR], 1.5 to 2).[10]

PATHOPHYSIOLOGY

The prostate gland is a solid, rounded, heart-shaped organ positioned between the neck of the bladder and the urogenital diaphragm (Fig. 92–1). The normal prostate is composed of acinar secretory cells arranged in a radial shape and surrounded by a foundation of supporting tissue. The size, shape, or presence of acini is almost always altered in a gland that has been invaded by prostatic carcinoma. Adenocarcinoma, the major pathologic cell type, accounts for more than 95% of prostate cancer cases.[11,12] Much rarer tumor types include small cell neuroendocrine cancers, sarcomas, and transitional cell carcinomas.

Prostate cancer can be graded systematically according to the histologic appearance of the malignant cell and then grouped into well, moderately, or poorly differentiated grades.[11,12] Gland architecture is examined and then rated on a scale of 1 (well differentiated) to 5 (poorly differentiated). Two different specimens are examined, and the score for each specimen is added. Groupings for total Gleason score are 2 to 4 for well differentiated, 5 or 6 for moderately differentiated, and 7 to 10 for poorly differentiated tumors. Poorly differentiated tumors grow rapidly (poor prognosis), while well-differentiated tumors grow slowly (better prognosis).

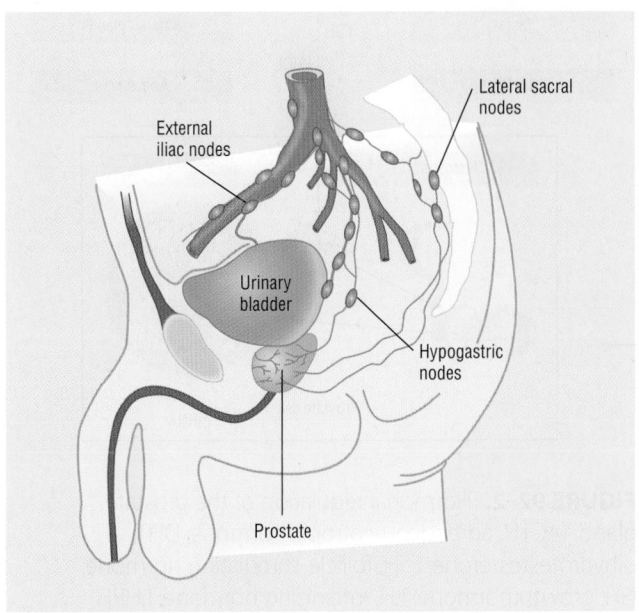

FIGURE 92–1. The prostate gland. (From DiPiro JT, Talbert RL, Yee GC, et al, eds. Pharmacotherapy: A Pathophysiologic Approach, 6th ed. New York: McGraw-Hill, 2005:1856.)

Metastatic spread can occur by local extension, lymphatic drainage, or hematogenous dissemination.[11,12] Lymph node metastases are more common in patients with large, undifferentiated tumors that invade the seminal vesicles. The pelvic and abdominal lymph node groups are the most common sites of lymph node involvement (Fig. 92–1). Skeletal metastases from hematogenous spread are the most common sites of distant spread. Typically, the bone lesions are osteoblastic or a combination of osteoblastic and osteolytic. The most common site of bone involvement is the lumbar spine. Other sites of bone involvement include the proximal femurs, pelvis, thoracic spine, ribs, sternum, skull, and humerus. The lung, liver, brain, and adrenal glands are the most common sites of visceral involvement, although these organs usually are not involved initially. About 25% to 35% of patients have evidence of lymphangitic or nodular pulmonary infiltrates at autopsy. The prostate is rarely a site for metastatic involvement from other solid tumors.

Normal growth and differentiation of the prostate depends on the presence of androgens, specifically DHT.[13,14] The testes and the adrenal glands are the major sources of circulating androgens. Hormonal regulation of androgen synthesis is mediated through a series of biochemical interactions among the hypothalamus, pituitary, adrenal glands, and testes (Fig. 92–2). Luteinizing hormone–releasing hormone (LHRH) released from the hypothalamus stimulates the release of luteinizing hormone (LH) and follicle-stimulating hormone (FSH) from the anterior pituitary gland. LH complexes with receptors on the Leydig cell testicular membrane and stimulates the production of testosterone and small amounts of estrogen. FSH acts on the Sertoli cells within the testes to promote the maturation of LH receptors and to produce an androgen-binding protein. Circulating testosterone and estradiol influence the synthesis of LHRH, LH, and FSH by a negative feedback loop operating at the hypothalamic and pituitary level.[15,16] Prolactin, growth hormone, and estradiol appear to be important accessory regulators for prostatic tissue permeability, receptor binding, and testosterone synthesis.

Testosterone, the major androgenic hormone, accounts for 95% of the androgen concentration. The primary source of testosterone is the testes; however, 3% to 5% of the testosterone concentration is derived from direct adrenal cortical secretion of testosterone or C19 steroids such as androstenedione.[13,17]

In early stage prostate cancers, aberrant tumor cell proliferation is promoted by the presence of androgens. For these tumors, blockade of androgens induces tumor regression in most patients. Hormonal manipulations to ablate or reduce circulating androgens can occur through several mechanisms (Table 92–2).[15,16] The organs responsible for androgen production can be removed surgically (orchiectomy, hypophysectomy, or adrenalectomy). Hormonal pathways that modulate prostatic growth can be interrupted at several steps (see Fig. 92–2). Interference with LHRH or LH (by estrogens, LHRH agonists, progesterones, and cyproterone acetate) can reduce testosterone secretion by the testes. Estrogen administration reduces androgens by directly inhibiting LH release, acting directly on the prostate cell, or decreasing free androgens by increasing steroid-binding globulin levels.[15,16]

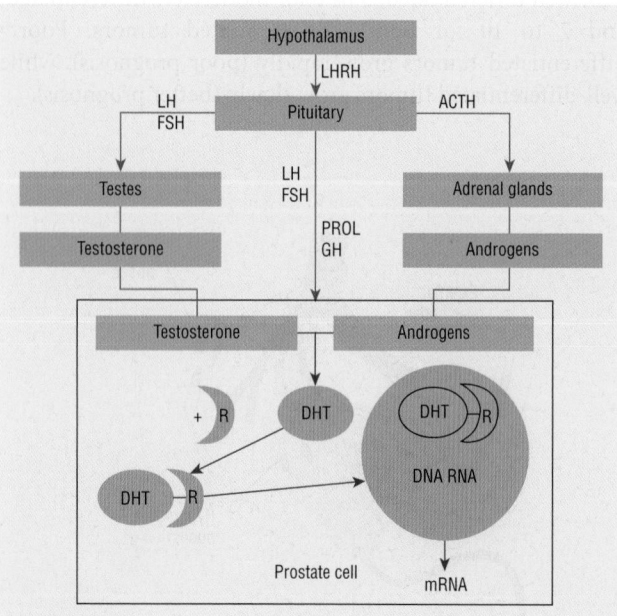

FIGURE 92–2. Hormonal regulation of the prostate gland. (ACTH, adrenocorticotropic hormone; DHT, dihydrotestosterone; FSH, follicle-stimulating hormone; GH, growth hormone; LH, luteinizing hormone; LHRH, luteinizing hormone–releasing hormone; PROL, prolactin; R, receptor.) (From DiPiro JT, Talbert RL, Yee GC, et al, eds. Pharmacotherapy: A Pathophysiologic Approach, 6th ed. New York: McGraw-Hill, 2005:1856.)

Table 92–2
Hormonal Manipulations in Prostate Cancer

Androgen source ablation	Antiandrogens
Orchiectomy	Flutamide
Adrenalectomy	Bicalutamide
Hypophysectomy	Nilutamide
LHRH or LH inhibition	Cyproteroneacetate[b]
Estrogens	Progesterones
LHRH agonists	5-α-Reductase inhibition
Progesterones[a]	Finasteride[b]
Cyproteroneacetate[b]	Dutasteride[b]
Gonadotropin receptor antagonists	
Abarelix	
Degarelix	
Androgen synthesis inhibition	
Abiraterone	
Aminoglutethimide	
Ketoconazole	
Progesterones[a]	

LH, luteinizing hormone; LHRH, luteinizing hormone–releasing hormone.

[a]Minor mechanisms of action.

[b]Investigational compounds or use.

Isolation of the naturally occurring hypothalamic decapeptide hormone LHRH has provided another group of effective agents for advanced prostate cancer treatment. The physiologic response to LHRH depends on both the dose and the mode of administration. Intermittent pulsed LHRH administration, which mimics the endogenous release pattern, causes sustained release of both LH and FSH, but high dose or continuous intravenous administration of LHRH inhibits gonadotropin release caused by receptor downregulation.[14-16] Structural modification of the naturally occurring LHRH and innovative delivery have produced a series of LHRH agonists that cause a similar downregulation of pituitary receptors and a decrease in testosterone production.[16]

Androgen synthesis can also be inhibited in the testes or adrenal gland. Aminoglutethimide inhibits the desmolase–enzyme complex in the adrenal gland, thereby preventing the conversion of cholesterol to pregnenolone. Pregnenolone is the precursor substrate for all adrenal-derived steroids, including androgens, glucocorticoids, and mineralocorticoids. Ketoconazole, an imidazole antifungal agent, causes a dose-related reversible reduction in serum cortisol and testosterone concentration by inhibiting both adrenal and testicular steroidogenesis.[15] Megestrol is a synthetic derivative of progesterone that exhibits a secondary mechanism of action by inhibiting the synthesis of androgens. This inhibition appears to occur at the adrenal level, but circulating levels of testosterone also are reduced, suggesting that inhibition at the testicular level also may occur.[15]

Antiandrogens inhibit the formation of the DHT–receptor complex and thereby interfere with androgen-mediated action at the cellular level. Megestrol acetate, a progestational agent, also is available and has antiandrogen actions.[18] Finally, the conversion of testosterone to DHT may be inhibited by 5-α-reductase inhibitors.[9]

In advanced stages of the disease, prostate cancer cells may be able to survive and proliferate without the signals normally provided by circulating androgens.[18] When this occurs, the tumors are no less sensitive to therapies that are dependent on androgen blockade. These tumors are referred to as *castrate resistant* and were formally known as *hormone refractory* or *androgen independent*.

PREVENTION AND EARLY DETECTION
Chemoprevention

Significant decreases in the risk of prostate cancer have been demonstrated by the 5-α-reductase inhibitors finasteride and dutasteride.[9,19] These medications work by inhibiting 5-a-reductase, an enzyme that converts testosterone to its more active form, DHT, which is involved in prostate epithelial proliferation. There are two types of 5-α-reductase, types I and II; both are implicated in the development of prostate cancer. Finasteride selectively inhibits the 5-α-reductase type-II isoenzyme, whereas dutasteride inhibits both isoenzymes. Both finasteride and dutasteride lower the PSA by approximately 50% within 1 year.[9,19] However this lowering may vary across individuals or within the same individual

over time. Although no prospective studies have validated a specific threshold for PSA monitoring in patients receiving a 5-α-reductase inhibitor, common clinical practice is to lower the PSA threshold by one-half.

The Prostate Cancer Prevention Trial compared 5 mg/day of finasteride for 7 years with placebo for the prevention of prostate cancer in men 55 years of age or older with normal digital rectal examination findings and a PSA of 3.0 ng/mL (3.0 mcg/L) or less.[9,20] When compared with placebo, the prevalence of prostate cancer was reduced for those on finasteride by 24.8% (95% confidence interval [CI], 18.6% to 30.6%) (hazard ratio, 0.75). However, in those who did develop prostate cancer, there was an increase in the number of high-grade (Gleason grade, 7 to 10) tumors detected at biopsy in the finasteride group. Overall, finasteride did reduce the frequency of prostate cancer; however, the prostate cancers that were diagnosed in the finasteride group were more aggressive. There were no differences in overall survival. Common adverse events included decreased libido, erectile dysfunction, and gynecomastia.

Dutasteride was evaluated in a different population of men.[19] They randomized men that were 50 to 75 years of age with PSA levels of 2.5 to 10 ng/mL (2.5 to 10 mcg/L) and a recent negative prostate biopsy result to dutasteride 0.5 mg/day or placebo. Treatment with dutasteride resulted in a significant reduction in the risk for prostate cancer (RR reduction of 22.8%) as well as a reduction in acute urinary retention. There were no significant differences in overall survival.[20]

The use of finasteride to prevent prostate cancer is the subject of a joint consensus statement. The American Society of Clinical Oncology (ASCO) and the American Urological Association (AUA) used the results from a systematic review of the literature to develop evidence-based recommendations for the use of 5-α-reductase inhibitors for prostate cancer chemoprevention.[21] 5-α-Reductase inhibitors decrease the period prevalence of for-cause prostate cancer by approximately 26% (RR, 0.74; 95% CI, 0.67 to 0.83). The absolute risk reduction is about 1.4% (4.9% in controls versus 3.5% in the treatment arms), although this may vary with the age of the treated population. On the basis of these outcomes, the ASCO and AUA recommend that asymptomatic men with a PSA less than or equal to 3 ng/mL (3 mcg/L) who are regularly screened with PSA may benefit from a discussion of both the benefits of 5-α-reductase inhibitors for 7 years for the prevention of prostate cancer and the potential risks (including the possibility of high-grade prostate cancer). Men who are taking 5-α-reductase inhibitors for benign conditions such as lower urinary tract symptoms may benefit from a similar discussion, understanding that the improvement of symptoms should be weighed with the potential risks of high-grade prostate cancer.

Selenium and vitamin E alone or in combination were evaluated in the *Sele*nium and Vitamin *E* Cancer Prevention *Trial* (SELECT), a clinical trial investigating their effects on the incidence of prostate cancer. The data and safety monitoring committee found that after 5 years, selenium and vitamin E taken alone or together did not prevent prostate cancer.

On the basis of these data and safety concerns, the trial was halted.[22] Other agents, including vitamin D, lycopene, green tea, nonsteroidal anti-inflammatory agents, isoflavones, and statins, are under investigation for prostate cancer and show promise; however, none are currently recommended for routine use outside of a clinical trial.[23]

Screening

Early detection of potentially curable prostate cancers is the goal of prostate cancer screening. For cancer screening to be beneficial, it must reliably detect cancer at an early stage, and identify those cancers that would benefit from an early intervention and decrease mortality. Whether prostate cancer screening fits these criteria has generated considerable controversy.[24,25] Digital rectal examination (DRE) has been recommended since the early 1900s for the detection of prostate cancer. The primary advantage of DRE is its specificity, reported at greater than 85%, for prostate cancer. Other advantages of DRE include low cost, safety, and ease of performance. However, DRE is relatively insensitive and is subject to interobserver variability. DRE as a single screening method has poor compliance and had little effect on preventing metastatic prostate cancer in one large case-control study.[26]

❷ *Prostate-specific antigen is a useful marker for detecting prostate cancer at early stages, predicting outcome for localized disease, monitoring disease-free status, and monitoring response to androgen-deprivation therapy or chemotherapy for advanced-stage disease.* PSA is used widely for prostate cancer screening in the United States, with simplicity as its major advantage and low specificity as its primary limitation.[24,27] Although PSA is often elevated in men with prostate cancer, the PSA may also be elevated in men with acute urinary retention, acute prostatitis, and prostatic ischemia or infarction, as well as BPH, a nearly universal condition in men at risk for prostate cancer. PSA elevations between 4.1 ng/mL (4.1 mcg/L) and 10 ng/mL (10 mcg/L) cannot distinguish between BPH and prostate cancer, limiting the utility of PSA alone for the early detection of prostate cancer. Additionally, only 38% to 48% of men with clinically significant prostate cancer have a serum PSA outside the reference range.[28]

Neither DRE nor PSA is sensitive or specific enough to be used alone as a screening test. Although the relative predictability of DRE and PSA is similar, the tumors identified by each method are different. Catalona and associates[29] confirmed that the combination of a DRE plus PSA determination is a better method of detecting prostate cancer than DRE alone.

The common approach to prostate cancer screening today involves offering a baseline PSA and DRE between the age of 40 and 50 years with annual evaluations beginning at the age of 50 years to all men of normal risk with a 10-year or greater life expectancy. Men with an increased risk of prostate cancer, including men of African American ancestry and men with a family history of prostate cancer, may begin screening earlier, at age 40 to 45 years.

Patient Encounter 1: Prevention and Screening

OC is a 56-year-old white man who comes into the pharmacy for a refill of his finasteride, which he is taking for BPH. He wants to know what he can do to reduce his risk of prostate cancer.

OC does not have a family history of prostate cancer. He has never been screened for prostate cancer.

What do you recommend for prostate cancer screening?

What do you recommend for prostate cancer chemoprevention?

Despite this common practice, the benefits of prostate cancer screening are unproven.[24,30] PSA measurements can identify small, subclinical prostate cancers, in which no intervention may be required. Detecting prostate cancer in those not needing therapy not only increases the cost of care through unnecessary screening and workups but also increases the toxicity of therapy, by subjecting some patients to unnecessary therapy.[31,32] Currently, the American College of Physicians recommends that rather than screening all men for prostate cancer as a matter of routine, physicians should describe the potential benefits and known risks of screening, diagnosis, and treatment; listen to the patient's concerns; and then decide on an individual's screening method. The United States Preventative Task Force recently downgraded PSA screening for prostate cancer to a grade D, intended to "discourage the use of the service."[24]

CLINICAL PRESENTATION AND DIAGNOSIS

Before the implementation of routine screening, prostate cancers were frequently identified on the investigation of symptoms that included urinary hesitancy, retention, painful urination, hematuria, and erectile dysfunction. With the introduction of screening techniques, most prostate cancers are now identified before the development of symptoms.[33]

There are two commonly recognized staging classification systems (Table 92–3). The formal international classification system (tumor, node, metastases [TNM]), adopted by the International Union Against Cancer in 1974, was last updated in 2002. The AUA classification is also commonly used in the United States (Table 92–4). Patients are assigned to stages A through D and corresponding subcategories based on the size of the tumor (T), local or regional extension, presence of involved lymph node groups (N), and presence of metastases (M). Some studies classify patients who have progressed after hormonal therapy as stage D_3. On the basis of men diagnosed with prostate cancer at Walter Reed Army Medical Center from 1988 to 1998, including

Clinical Presentation of Prostate Cancer

Localized Disease

Asymptomatic

Locally Invasive Disease

Ureteral dysfunction, frequency, hesitancy, and dribbling

Impotence

Advanced Disease

Back pain

Cord compression

Lower extremity edema

Pathologic fractures

Anemia

Weight loss

more than 2,042 prostate cancer diagnoses, localized prostate cancer (stage T_1 and T_2) was diagnosed more frequently (89% versus 68%), and advanced disease (stages T_3, T_4, and D) was diagnosed less frequently (11% versus 32%) when comparing the incidence rates in 1998 with the 1988 rates, respectively. This largely reflects the impact of widespread PSA screening. Prostate cancer is usually initially diagnosed by PSA and DRE and confirmed by a biopsy when the Gleason score is assigned.

Table 92–3

Diagnostic and Staging and Classification Systems Workup for Prostate Cancer

Initial tests	DRE
	PSA
	TRUS if either DRE is positive or PSA is elevated
	Biopsy
Staging tests	Gleason score on biopsy specimen
	Bone scan
	CBC
	Liver function tests
	Serum phosphatases (acid/alkaline)
	Excretory urography
	Chest radiography
Additional staging tests (depends on tumor classification, PSA, and Gleason score)	Skeletal films
	Lymph node evaluation
	Pelvic CT
	^{111}In-labeled capromab pendetide scan
	Bipedal lymphangiogram
	Transrectal MRI

CBC, complete blood count; CT, computed tomography; DRE, digital rectal examination; MRI, magnetic resonance imaging; PSA, prostate-specific antigen; TRUS, transrectal ultrasongraphy.

❸ *The prognosis for patients with prostate cancer depends on the histologic grade, tumor size, and local extent of the primary tumor and PSA.*[11,34] One of the most important prognostic criteria appears to be the histologic grade, assessed by Gleason score. Poorly differentiated tumors are highly associated with both regional lymph node involvement and distant metastases. Once the tumor has spread into locoregional lymph nodes, there is a significantly increased risk of recurrence of disease after curative intent therapy.[11] The 10-year cancer-specific survival is estimated as 95% for stage A_1, 80% for stages A_2 to B_2, 60% for stage C, 40% for stage D_1, and 10% for stage D_2.[32] It is estimated that more than 85% of patients with stage A_1 can be cured, but fewer than 1% of patients with stage D_2 will be cured.

TREATMENT

Desired Outcome

The desired outcome in early stage prostate cancer is to minimize morbidity and mortality from prostate cancer with special consideration that some degree of morbidity may be caused by the toxicity of treatment.[34] The most appropriate therapy of early stage prostate cancer is a matter of debate. Early stage disease may be treated with surgery, radiation, or watchful waiting. Although surgery and radiation are curative, they are associated with significant morbidity and mortality. Because the overall goal is to minimize morbidity and mortality associated with the disease, watchful waiting is appropriate in selected individuals with a low risk of rapid disease progression.[34] Advanced prostate cancer (metastatic spread) is not currently curable, and treatment should focus on providing symptom relief and maintaining quality of life.[35]

General Approach to Treatment

The initial treatment for prostate cancer depends on the disease stage, Gleason score, presence of symptoms, and life expectancy of the patient.[33] For asymptomatic patients determining risk for disease progression and recurrence are critical for determining treatment options. Asymptomatic patients with a low risk of recurrence, those with a T_1 or T_{2a} tumor, with a Gleason score of 2 through 6, and a PSA of less than 10 ng/mL (10 mcg/L) may be managed by active surveillance, radiation, or radical prostatectomy (Table 92–5). Because patients with asymptomatic, early stage disease generally have an excellent 10-year survival rate, immediate morbidities of treatment must be balanced with the lower likelihood of dying from prostate cancer. In general, more aggressive treatments of early stage prostate cancer are reserved for younger men, although patient preference is a major consideration in all treatment decisions. In a patient with a life expectancy of less than 10 years, expectant management or radiation therapy may be offered. In those with a life expectancy of equal to or greater than 10 years, expectant management, radiation (**external beam** or **brachytherapy**), or radical **prostatectomy** with a pelvic

Table 92–4

Staging and Classification Systems for Prostate Cancer

AUA[a] Stage (A–D)	AJCC-UICC[b] Classification (TNM)
A (occult, nonpalpable)	$T_x N_x M_x$ (cannot be assessed)
A$_1$: Focal	$T_0 N_0 M_0$ (nonpalpable)
A$_2$: Diffuse	T_0: Focal or diffuse
B (confined to prostate)	$T_1 N_0 M_0$, $T_2 N_0 M_0$
B$_1$: Single nodule in 1 lobe, less than 1.5 cm	T_1 (Clinically inapparent tumor not palpable or visible by imaging)
	T_{1a}: Tumor incidental histologic finding in 5% or less of tissue resected
	T_{1b}: Tumor incidental histologic finding in 5% or more of tissue resected
	T_{1c}: Tumor identified by needle biopsy (e.g., because of elevated PSA)
B$_2$: Diffuse involvement of whole gland, greater than 1.5 cm	T_2: (Tumor confined within the prostate[c])
	T_{2a}: Tumor involves half of a lobe or less
	T_{2b}: Tumor involves more than half a lobe, but not both lobes
	T_{2c}: Tumor involves both lobes
C (localized to periprostatic area)	$T_3 N_0 M_0$, $T_4 N_0 M_0$
C$_1$: No seminal vesicle involvement, less than 70 g	T_3: (Tumor extends through the prostatic capsule[d])
	T_{3a}: Unilateral extracapsular extension
	T_{3b}: Bilateral extracapsular extension
	T_{3c}: Tumor invades the seminal vesicle(s)
C$_2$: Seminal vesicle involvement, greater than 70 g	T_4: Tumor is fixed or invades adjacent structures other than the seminal vesicles
	T_{4a}: Tumor invades any of bladder neck, external sphincter, or rectum
	T_{4b}: Tumor invades levator muscles and/or is fixed to the pelvic wall
D (metastatic disease)	Any T, $N_{1–4}$, M_0 or $N_{0–4}$, M_1
D$_1$: Pelvic lymph nodes or ureteral obstruction	N_1: Metastasis in a single lymph node, 2 cm or less in greatest dimension
	N_2: Metastasis in single lymph node more than 2 cm but not more than 5 cm in greatest dimension; or multiple lymph node metastases, none more than 5 cm in greatest dimension
	N_3: Metastasis in lymph node more than 5 cm in greatest dimension
D$_2$: Bone, distant lymph node, organ, or soft tissue metastases	M_{1a}: Nonregional lymph node(s)
	M_{1b}: Bone(s)
	M_{1c}: Other site(s)

[a]American Urologic Association.

[b]American Joint Committee on Cancer–International Union Against Cancer.

[c]Tumor found in one or both lobes by needle biopsy, but not palpable or visible by imaging, is classified as T_{1c}.

[d]Invasion into the prostatic apex or into (but not beyond) the prostatic capsule is not classified as T_3 but as T_2.

Table 92–5

Management of Prostate Cancer With Low and Intermediate Recurrence Risk

Recurrence Risk	Expected Survival (years)	Initial Therapy
Low	Less than 10	Expectant management or radiation therapy
T$_1$-T$_{2a}$ and Gleason 2–6 and PSA less than 10 ng/mL (10 mcg/L) and less than 5% tumor in specimen	10 or more	Expectant management or radical prostatectomy with or without pelvic lymph node dissection or radiation therapy
Intermediate		
T$_{2b}$ or Gleason 7 or PSA 10–20 ng/mL (10–20 mcg/L)	Less than 10	Expectant management or radical prostatectomy with or without pelvic lymph node dissection or radiation therapy with or without 4–6 months of androgen deprivation therapy
	10 or more	Radical prostatectomy with or without pelvic lymph node dissection or radiation therapy with or without 4–6 months of androgen deprivation therapy

PSA, prostate-specific antigen.

lymph node dissection may be offered. Radical prostatectomy and radiation therapy generally are considered therapeutically equivalent for localized prostate cancer, although neither has been proven to be better than observation alone.[35,36] Complications from radical prostatectomy include blood loss, stricture formation, incontinence, lymphocele, fistula formation, anesthetic risk, and impotence. Nerve-sparing radical prostatectomy can be performed in many patients; 50% to 80% regain sexual potency within the first year. Acute complications from radiation therapy include cystitis, proctitis, hematuria, urinary retention, penoscrotal edema, and impotence (30% incidence).[11] Chronic complications include proctitis, diarrhea, cystitis, enteritis, impotence, urethral stricture, and incontinence.[11] Because radiation and prostatectomy have significant and immediate morbidity compared with expectant management alone, many patients may elect to postpone therapy until symptoms develop.

Individuals with T_{2b} disease or a Gleason score of 7 or a PSA ranging from 10 to 20 ng/mL (10 to 20 mcg/L) are considered at intermediate risk for prostate cancer recurrence.[34] Individuals with less than a 10-year expected survival may be offered expectant management, radiation therapy, or radical prostatectomy with or without a pelvic lymph node dissection, and those with a greater than or equal to 10-year life expectancy may be offered either radical prostatectomy with or without a pelvic lymph node dissection or radiation therapy (see Table 92–5).

The patients at high risk of recurrence (stages T_{2c}, a Gleason score ranging from 8 to 10, or a PSA value greater than 20 ng/mL [20 mcg/L]) should be treated with androgen ablation for 2 to 3 years combined with radiation therapy (Table 92–6).[34] Selected individuals with a low tumor volume may receive a radical prostatectomy with or without a pelvic lymph node dissection.

Table 92–6

Management of Prostate Cancer With High and Very High Recurrence Risk

Recurrence Risk	Initial Therapy[a]
High T_{2c} or T_{3a}, Gleason 8–10, PSA greater than 20 ng/mL (20 mcg/L)	Androgen ablation[b] (2–3 years) and radiation therapy, or radiation therapy or radical prostatectomy with or without pelvic lymph node dissection
Locally Advanced, Very High $T_{3b–T4}$	Androgen ablation[b] (2–3 years) or radiation therapy + androgen ablation (2–3 years)
Very High Any T, N_1	Androgen ablation[b] or radiation therapy + androgen ablation
Any T, Any N, M_1	Androgen ablation[b]

[a]Androgen ablation = serum testosterone levels less than 50 ng/mL (1.74 nmol/L).

[b]Luteinizing hormone–releasing hormone agonist (medical castrations or surgical are equivalent).

Patients with T_{3b} and T_4 disease have a very high risk of recurrence and are not candidates for radical prostatectomy because of extensive local spread of the disease.[33]

④ *Androgen ablation with an LHRH agonist plus an antiandrogen should be used before radiation therapy for patients with locally advanced prostate cancer to improve outcomes over radiation therapy alone.* Recent evidence suggests that a course of androgen ablation therapy should be instituted at diagnosis rather than waiting disease recurrence. In a clinical trial enrolling 500 men with locally advanced prostate cancer who were randomized to either immediate initiation of androgen ablation with either orchiectomy or androgen ablation or deferred hormonal therapy, individuals with immediate therapy had a median actuarial cause-specific survival duration of 7.5 years for immediate treatment and 5.8 years for deferred treatment.[37]

⑤ *Androgen ablation therapy, with either orchiectomy, an LHRH agonist alone or an LHRH agonist plus an antiandrogen (combined androgen blockade), can be used to provide palliation for patients with advanced (stage D2) prostate cancer.* Secondary hormonal manipulations, cytotoxic chemotherapy, or supportive care is used for patients who progress after initial therapy.[37] Estrogens were once widely used; however, the primary estrogen, diethylstilbestrol (DES), was withdrawn from the U.S. market in 1997 because of an increased cardiovascular risk.

Nonpharmacologic Therapy

▶ Expectant Management

Active surveillance, also known as observation or watchful waiting, involves monitoring the course of disease and initiating treatment if the cancer progresses or the patient becomes symptomatic. A PSA and DRE are performed every 6 months with a repeat biopsy at any sign of disease progression. The advantages of expectant management are avoiding the adverse effects associated with definitive therapies such as radiation and radical prostatectomy and minimizing the risk of unnecessary therapies. The major disadvantage of expectant management is the risk that the cancer progresses and requires a more intensive therapy or metastasizes, making the disease incurable.[33]

▶ Orchiectomy

Bilateral orchiectomy, or removal of the testes, rapidly reduces circulating androgens to castrate levels (i.e., serum testosterone levels less than 50 ng/dL [1.74 nmol/L]).[12] However, many patients find this procedure psychologically unacceptable, and others are not surgical candidates owing to their advanced age.[12] Orchiectomy is the preferred initial treatment in patients with impending spinal cord compression or ureteral obstruction.

▶ Radiation

The two commonly used methods for radiation therapy are external-beam radiotherapy and brachytherapy.[33] In external-beam radiotherapy, doses of 70 to 75 Gy are delivered in 35 to 41 fractions in patients with low-grade prostate cancer and 75 to 80 Gy for those with intermediate- or high-grade prostate cancer. Brachytherapy involves the permanent implantation of radioactive beads of 145 Gy 125-iodine or 124 Gy of 103-palladium and is generally reserved for individuals with low-risk cancers.

▶ Radical Prostatectomy

Radical prostatectomy is performed in patients who are surgical candidates and in disease that requires definitive therapy based on risk factors and patient preference; additionally, the disease must be amenable to complete surgical resection. Complications from radical prostatectomy include blood loss, stricture formation, incontinence, lymphocele, fistula formation, anesthetic risk, and impotence. Nerve-sparing radical prostatectomy can be performed in many patients; 50% to 80% regain sexual potency within the first year. Acute complications from radical prostatectomy and radiation therapy include cystitis, proctitis, hematuria, urinary retention, penoscrotal edema, and impotence (30% incidence).[12,26] Chronic complications include proctitis, diarrhea, cystitis, enteritis, impotence, urethral stricture, and incontinence.[12] Because radiation and prostatectomy have significant and immediate mortality when compared with observation alone, many patients may elect to postpone therapy until symptoms develop.

Pharmacologic Therapy

▶ LHRH Agonists

LHRH agonists are a reversible method of androgen ablation and are as effective as orchiectomy in treating prostate cancer (Table 92–7).[38] Currently available LHRH agonists

Table 92–7

Luteinizing Hormone–Releasing Hormone Agonists

LHRH Agonist	Usual Dose	Adverse Effects (Similar for All Agents)
Leuprolide depot	7.5 mg every 28 days 22.5 mg every 12 weeks 30 mg every 16 weeks	Gynecomastia Hot flashes Decreased libido, impotence, Fatigue
Goserelin implant	3.6 mg every 28 days 10.8 mg every 12 weeks	Tumor flare in first 2 weeks and increased risk of cardiovascular disease Osteopenia with long-term use
Triptorelin depot	3.75 mg every 28 days 11.25 mg every 84 days	

LHRH, luteinizing hormone–releasing hormone.

include leuprolide, leuprolide depot, leuprolide implant, triptorelin depot, triptorelin implant, and goserelin acetate implant. Leuprolide acetate is administered once daily, whereas leuprolide depot and goserelin acetate implant can be administered once monthly, once every 12 weeks, or once every 16 weeks (leuprolide depot, every 4 months). The leuprolide depot formulation contains leuprolide acetate in coated pellets. The dose is administered intramuscularly, and the coating dissolves at different rates to allow sustained leuprolide levels throughout the dosing interval. Goserelin acetate implant contains goserelin acetate dispersed in a plastic matrix of D,L-lactic and glycolic acid copolymer and is administered subcutaneously. Hydrolysis of the copolymer material provides continuous release of goserelin over the dosing period. Another formulation of leuprolide is a mini-osmotic pump implanted intramuscularly that delivers 120 mcg of leuprolide daily for 12 months. After 12 months, the implant is removed, and a different implant can be placed. Triptorelin LA is administered as an intramuscular injection of 11.25 mg every 84 days. Triptorelin depot is administered once every 28 days as a 3.75-mg dose.

Several randomized trials have demonstrated that leuprolide, goserelin, and triptorelin are effective agents when used alone in patients with advanced prostate cancer.[14] Response rates around 80% have been reported, with a lower incidence of adverse effects compared with estrogens.[14] There are no direct comparative trials of the currently available LHRH agonists or the dosage formulations, but a recent meta-analysis reported that there is no difference in efficacy or toxicity between leuprolide and goserelin. Triptorelin is a more recent addition but is generally considered equally effective. Therefore, the choice between the three agents is usually made on the basis of cost and patient and physician preference for a dosing schedule.

The most common adverse effects reported with LHRH agonist therapy include a disease flare-up during the first week of therapy, hot flashes, erectile impotence, decreased libido, and injection-site reactions.[14] The disease flare-up is caused by an initial induction of LH and FSH by the LHRH agonist, leading to an initial phase of increased testosterone production. It manifests clinically as an exacerbation of disease-related symptoms, usually increased bone pain or urinary symptoms.[14] This flare reaction usually resolves after 2 weeks and has a similar onset and duration pattern for the depot LHRH products.[39,40] Initiating an antiandrogen before the administration of the LHRH agonist and continuing for 2 to 4 weeks is a frequently used strategy to minimize this initial tumor flare.[16]

LHRH agonist monotherapy can be used as initial therapy, with response rates similar to orchiectomy. There is a lower incidence of cardiovascular-related adverse effects associated with LHRH therapy than with estrogen administration. Patients should be counseled to expect worsening symptoms during the first week of therapy; appropriate pain and symptom management is required during this period, and a short course of concomitant antiandrogen therapy may need to be considered before initiating the LHRH agonist. Caution should be exercised if initiating LHRH agonist therapy in patients with widely metastatic disease involving the spinal cord or having the potential for ureteral obstruction because irreversible complications may occur.

Another potentially serious complication of androgen deprivation therapy is a resultant decrease in bone-mineral density, leading to an increased risk for osteoporosis, osteopenia, and an increased risk for skeletal fractures. Most clinicians recommend that men starting long-term androgen deprivation therapy should have a baseline bone mineral density test and be initiated on a calcium and vitamin D supplement.[16]

▶ Gonadotropin-Releasing Hormone Antagonists

An alternative to LHRH agonists is the recently approved GnRH antagonist degarelix. Degarelix works by binding reversibly to gonadotropin-releasing hormone (GnRH) receptors on cells in the pituitary gland, reducing the production of testosterone to castrate levels. The major advantage of degarelix over LHRH agonists is the speed at which it can achieve the drop in testosterone levels; castrate levels are achieved in 7 days or less with degarelix, compared with 28 days with leuprolide, eliminating the tumor flare seen and need for antiandrogens with LHRH agonists.

In a trial of 610 men with advanced prostate cancer, degarelix was shown to be equivalent to leuprolide in lowering testosterone levels for up to 1 year and is approved by the Food and Drug Administration for the treatment of advanced prostate cancer. Degarelix is available as 40-mg/mL and 20-mg/mL vials for subcutaneous injection, and the starting dose is 240 mg followed by 80 mg every 28 days. The starting dose should be split into two injections of 120 mg.

The most frequently reported adverse reactions were injection-site reactions, including pain (28%), erythema (17%), swelling (6%), induration (4%), and nodule (3%). Most were transient and mild to moderate, leading to discontinuation in fewer than 1% of study subjects. Other adverse effects included elevations in lever function tests, which occurred in approximately 10% of study subjects.

Similar to other methods of androgen deprivation therapy, osteoporosis may develop, and calcium and vitamin D supplementation should be considered.

Degarelix is not approved in combination with antiandrogens, and routine use of the combination cannot be recommended.

Antiandrogens

Three antiandrogens—flutamide, bicalutamide, and nilutamide—are currently available (Table 92-8). Cyproterone is another agent with antiandrogen activity but is not available in the United States. Antiandrogens have been used as monotherapy in previously untreated patients, but a recent meta-analysis determined that monotherapy with antiandrogens is less effective than LHRH agonist therapy.[40] Therefore, for advanced prostate cancer, all currently available antiandrogens are indicated only in combination with androgen-ablation therapy, flutamide and bicalutamide are indicated in combination with an LHRH agonist, and nilutamide is indicated in combination with orchiectomy.[41]

The most common antiandrogen-related adverse effects are listed in Table 92-7. In the only randomized comparison of bicalutamide plus an LHRH agonist versus flutamide plus an LHRH agonist, diarrhea was more common in

Table 92–8

Antiandrogens

Antiandrogen	Usual Dose	Adverse Effects
Flutamide	750 mg/day	Gynecomastia Hot flushes GI disturbances (diarrhea) Liver function test abnormalities Breast tenderness Methemoglobinemia
Bicalutamide	50 mg/day	Gynecomastia Hot flushes GI disturbances (diarrhea) Liver function test abnormalities Breast tenderness
Nilutamide	300 mg/day for first month; then 150 mg/day	Gynecomastia Hot flushes GI disturbances (nausea or constipation) Liver function test abnormalities Breast tenderness Visual disturbances (impaired dark adaptation) Alcohol intolerance Interstitial pneumonitis

GI, gastrointestinal.

flutamide-treated patients. Antiandrogens can reduce the symptoms from the flare phenomenon associated with LHRH agonist therapy.[16]

Combined Androgen Blockade

Although up to 80% of patients with advanced prostate cancer respond to initial hormonal manipulation, almost all patients progress within 2 to 4 years after initiating therapy.[12] Two mechanisms have been proposed to explain this tumor resistance. The tumor could be heterogeneously composed of cells that are hormone dependent and hormone independent, or the tumor could be stimulated by extratesticular androgens that are converted intracellularly to DHT. The rationale for combination hormonal therapy is to interfere with multiple hormonal pathways to more completely eliminate androgen action. In clinical trials, combination hormonal therapy, sometimes also referred to as maximal androgen deprivation or total androgen blockade, or combined androgen blockade (CAB), has been used. The combination of LHRH agonists or orchiectomy with antiandrogens is the most extensively studied CAB approach.

Many studies comparing CAB with conventional medical or surgical castration have been performed.[42-44] In studies with LHRH agonists, the results have varied, with no consistent benefit demonstrated for CAB. A National Cancer Institute (NCI) intergroup trial involving 1,387 evaluable stage D_2 prostate cancer patients failed to show any significant survival benefits for the combination of orchiectomy plus flutamide over orchiectomy alone.[45] Similar to other studies of CAB, overall survival was longest in patients with minimal disease. Diarrhea, elevated liver function test results, and anemia were more common in those patients who received flutamide.

A meta-analysis of 27 randomized trials in 8,275 patients (4,803 treated with flutamide, 1,683 treated with nilutamide, and 1,784 treated with cyproterone) comparing CAB with conventional medical or surgical castration showed a small survival benefit at 5 years for those treated with flutamide or nilutamide (27.6%) compared with those with castration alone (24.7%; $P = 0.0005$).

In one of the few combination androgen-deprivation studies comparing two different antiandrogens (bicalutamide versus flutamide), the time to treatment failure (the main study end point), time to progression (as defined by appearance of new or worsening bone or extraskeletal lesions), and time to death were equivalent, suggesting that the two treatments are equally effective.

Although some investigators now consider CAB to be the initial hormonal therapy of choice for newly diagnosed advanced prostate cancer patients, clinicians are left to weigh the costs of combined therapy against potential benefits in light of conflicting results in the randomized trials[41] and the modest benefit seen in the meta-analysis.[43] For trials that did show an advantage for CAB, whether these effects are specific to the testosterone-deprivation method (orchiectomy vs. leuprolide vs. goserelin), the antiandrogen, the duration of therapy, or patient selection is not clear. Until further carefully designed studies that use survival, time

to progression, quality of life, patient preference, and cost as end points are conducted, it is appropriate to use either LHRH agonist monotherapy or CAB as initial therapy for metastatic prostate cancer. CAB may be most beneficial for improving survival in patients with minimal disease and for preventing tumor flare, particularly in those with advanced metastatic disease. All other patients may be started on LHRH monotherapy, and an antiandrogen may be added after several months if androgen ablation is incomplete.

There is considerable debate concerning when to start hormonal-deprivation therapy in patients with advanced prostate cancer.[14] The original recommendation to start therapy when symptoms appeared was based on the Veterans Administration Cooperative Urologic Research Group (VACURG) trials in which no overall survival difference was demonstrated in patients who either started DES initially or crossed over to active treatment when symptoms appeared; the excess mortality rate was attributed to estrogen administration. Because LHRH agonists and antiandrogens are viable therapies with less cardiovascular toxicity, it is not clear whether delaying therapy is justified with these agents. Reanalysis of the original VACURG data and recent combined androgen-deprivation trials demonstrate a survival advantage for young, good-performance status, minimal-disease patients treated initially with hormonal therapy, suggesting that early intervention before symptoms appear may be appropriate. The issue of when best to start hormonal therapy is the subject of several ongoing clinical trials.[46]

Secondary Therapies

Secondary or salvage therapies for patients who progress after their initial therapy depend on what was used for initial management. For patients initially diagnosed with localized prostate cancer, radiotherapy can be used in the case of failed radical prostatectomy. Alternatively, androgen ablation can be used in patients who progress after either radiation therapy or radical prostatectomy.

In patients treated initially with one hormonal modality, secondary hormonal manipulations may be attempted. This may include adding an antiandrogen to a patient who incompletely suppresses testosterone secretion with an LHRH agonist. In patients who have progression while receiving CAB, withdrawing antiandrogens, or using agents that inhibit androgen synthesis may be attempted.

For patients who initially received an LHRH agonist alone, castration testosterone levels should be documented. Patients with inadequate testosterone suppression (greater than 20 ng/dL [0.7 nmol/L]) can be treated by adding an antiandrogen or performing an orchiectomy. If castration testosterone levels have been achieved, the patient is considered to have castrate-resistant disease, and palliative salvage therapy can be used. Supportive care, chemotherapy, immunotherapy, and local radiotherapy can be used in patients who have failed all forms of androgen-ablation manipulations because these patients are considered to have castrate-resistant prostate cancer

6 *Antiandrogen withdrawal for patients having progressive disease while receiving combined hormonal blockade with an*

LHRH agonist plus an antiandrogen can provide additional symptomatic relief. Mutations in the androgen receptor have been documented that cause antiandrogen compounds to act like receptor agonists.

If the patient initially received CAB with an LHRH agonist with an antiandrogen, then androgen withdrawal is the first salvage manipulation.[33] Objective and subjective responses have been noted following the discontinuation of flutamide, bicalutamide, or nilutamide in patients receiving these agents as part of combined androgen ablation with an LHRH agonist. Mutations in the androgen receptor have been demonstrated that allow antiandrogens such as flutamide, bicalutamide, and nilutamide (or their metabolites) to become agonists and activate the androgen receptor. Patient responses to androgen withdrawal manifest as significant PSA reductions and improved clinical symptoms. Androgen withdrawal responses lasting 3 to 14 months have been noted in up to 35% of patients, and predicting response seems to be most closely related to longer androgen exposure times.[44] Incomplete cross-resistance has been noted in some patients who received bicalutamide after they had progressed while receiving flutamide, suggesting that patients who fail one antiandrogen may still respond to another agent. Adding an agent that blocks adrenal androgen synthesis, such as aminoglutethimide, at the time that androgens are withdrawn may produce a better response than androgen withdrawal alone. Because of the potential for response immediately after antiandrogen withdrawal, a sufficient observation and assessment period (usually 4 to 6 weeks) is usually required before a patient can be enrolled on a clinical trial evaluating a new agent or therapy for advanced prostate cancer.

Androgen synthesis inhibitors, such as aminoglutethimide 250 mg orally every 6 hours or ketoconazole 400 mg orally three times a day, can provide symptomatic relief for a short time in approximately 50% of patients with progressive disease despite previous androgen-ablation therapy.[37] Adverse effects during aminoglutethimide therapy occur in approximately 50% of patients.[37] Central nervous system effects that include lethargy, ataxia, and dizziness are the major adverse reactions. A generalized morbilliform, pruritic rash has been reported in up to 30% of patients treated. The rash is usually self-limiting and resolves within 5 to 8 days with continued therapy. Adverse effects from ketoconazole include gastrointestinal intolerance, transient rises in liver and renal function tests, and hypoadrenalism. Additionally, ketoconazole is a strong inhibitor of CYP1A2 and CYP3A4 and is contraindicated in combination with a number of medications that are commonly used in men with prostate cancer, including cisapride, lovastatin, midazolam, and triazolam because ketoconazole inhibits their metabolism and leads to increased toxicity. Arrhythmias often fatal have been reported with the combination of cisapride and ketoconazole. Absorption of ketoconazole requires gastric acidity; therefore, ketoconazole should not be administered with H2-blockers, proton pump inhibitors, or antacids. Additionally, ketoconazole should not be administered with strong CYP3A4 inducers, such as rifampin, because this

may reduce the effectiveness of ketoconazole because it is also a substrate for CYP3A4. Ketoconazole is combined with replacement doses of hydrocortisone to prevent symptomatic hypoadrenalism.[37]

After all hormonal manipulations are exhausted, the patient is considered to have androgen-independent disease, also known as hormone-refractory prostate cancer. At this point, either chemotherapy or palliative supportive therapy is appropriate. Palliation can be achieved by pain management, using radioisotopes such as strontium-89 or samarium-153 lexidronam for bone-related pain, analgesics, corticosteroids, bisphosphonates, or local radiotherapy.[47,48]

Skeletal metastases from hematogenous spread are the most common sites of distant spread of prostate cancer. Typically, the bone lesions are osteoblastic or a combination of osteoblastic and osteolytic. Bisphosphonates may prevent skeletal related events and improve bone mineral density. A randomized, controlled trial of zoledronic acid at a dose of 4 mg every 3 weeks reduced the incidence of skeletal-related events by 25% ($P = 0.021$) compared with placebo.[49] The usual dose of pamidronate is 90 mg every month, and the usual dose of zoledronic acid is 4 mg every 3 to 4 weeks. A trial of pamidronate or zoledronic acid can be initiated in prostate cancer patients with bone pain; if no benefit is observed, the drug may be discontinued.[50]

Patient Encounter 3: Progressive Disease

JM is a 66-year-old man who was initially diagnosed with metastatic prostate cancer 5 years ago. He was initially started on leuprolide and has progressed through treatment as described in the treatment summary below.

Treatment Summary

Date	PSA	Intervention
9/2/10	25 ng/mL (25 mcg/L)	Started leuprolide 7.5 mg IM every month
12/2/10	2 ng/mL (2 mcg/L)	Continued leuprolide
6/2/11	22 ng/mL (22 mcg/L)	Added bicalutamide 50 mg PO daily
9/2/11	5 ng/mL (5 mcg/L)	Continued leuprolide and bicalutamide
10/2/12	32 ng/mL (32 mcg/L)	Continued leuprolide; stopped bicalutamide
11/1/12	7 ng/mL (7 mcg/mL)	Continued leuprolide

Today he presents to the clinic with bone pain and a serum PSA of 67 ng/mL (67 mcg/L).

Why was bicalutamide discontinued on 10/2/12?

How would you characterize the patient's disease?

What treatments are options for him?

Table 92–9

First-Line Chemotherapy for Metastatic Castrate-Resistant Prostate Cancer

Chemotherapy	Usual Dose	Adverse Effects	Dose Adjustments
Docetaxel	75 mg/m² every 3 weeks	Fluid retention, alopecia, mucositis, myelosuppression, hypersensitivity	*Hepatic* If AST/ALT is greater than 1.5 × the upper limit of normal and ALP is greater than 2.5 upper limit of normal, do not administer *Hematologic* Ensure CBC recovered
Estramustine	280 mg three times a day on days 1–5	Edema, gynecomastia, leukopenia, increased risk of thromboembolic events	*Hematologic* Ensure CBC recovered

ALP, alkaline phosphatase; ALT, alanine aminotransferase; AST, aspartate aminotransferase; CBC, complete blood count.

❼ *Chemotherapy with docetaxel and prednisone improves survival in patients with castrate-resistant prostate cancer.*

Docetaxel 75 mg/m² every 3 weeks combined with prednisone 5 mg twice a day improves survival in hormone-refractory metastatic prostate cancer.[51] The most common adverse events reported with this regimen are nausea, alopecia, and bone marrow suppression. In addition, fluid retention and peripheral neuropathy, known effects of docetaxel, are observed. Docetaxel is hepatically eliminated; patients with hepatic impairment may not be eligible for treatment with docetaxel because of an increased risk for toxicity.[51]

The combination of estramustine (280 mg three times a day, days 1 to 5) and docetaxel 60 mg/m² on day 2 every 3 weeks also improves survival in hormone-refractory metastatic prostate cancer.[52] Estramustine causes a decrease in testosterone and a corresponding increase in estrogen; therefore, the adverse effects of estramustine include an increase in thromboembolic events, gynecomastia, and decreased libido (Table 92–9). Estramustine is an oral capsule and should be refrigerated. Calcium inhibits the absorption of estramustine. Although both the docetaxel–prednisone and the docetaxel–estramustine regimens are effective in hormone-refractory prostate cancer, most clinicians prefer the docetaxel/prednisone regimen because of the cardiovascular adverse effects associated with estramustine and the improved survival seen with docetaxel–prednisone. In addition, androgen ablation is usually continued when chemotherapy is initiated.

The regimen of mitoxantrone plus prednisone has been shown to be effective in reducing pain from bone metastasis and was a standard therapy before the development of docetaxel and prednisone. The effectiveness of mitoxantrone after failure of docetaxel-based therapy has not been scientifically evaluated. Treatment options now include continued chemotherapy with cabazitaxel, additional hormonal manipulation with abiraterone, immunotherapy with sipuleucel-T, or radiation for palliation of local symptoms.

❽ *Chemotherapy with cabazitaxel and prednisone improves survival in patients with castrate-resistant prostate cancer who have either progressed or are intolerant to docetaxel.*

Cabazitaxel is a taxane with demonstrated activity in docetaxel resistant cell lines and animal models of human cancer. A partial explanation is that docetaxel is a substrate for P-glycoprotein multidrug resistance transporter while cabazitaxel has low affinity.[53] In patients previously treated with docetaxel and prednisone, treatment with cabazitaxel 25 mg/m² every 3 weeks with prednisone 10 mg/day significantly improved progression-free survival and overall survival compared with mitoxantrone and prednisone. Neutropenia, febrile neutropenia, neuropathy and diarrhea are the most significant toxicities. Hypersensitivity reactions may occur, and premedication with an antihistamine, a corticosteroid, and an H₂ antagonist is recommended. Cabazitaxel is extensively hepatically metabolized and should be avoided in patients with hepatic dysfunction (Table 92–10).

❾ *Hormonal manipulation with abiraterone and prednisone improves survival in patients previously treated with docetaxel and prednisone.*

An upregulation of androgen synthesis has been noted in castration-resistant prostate cancer, and further inhibition of androgen synthesis after failure of androgen deprivation therapy and antiandrogens can provide benefit for patients. Abiraterone is an inhibitor of CYPC17, an enzyme critical for testosterone synthesis. In patients previously treated with docetaxel, compared with prednisone alone, treatment with abiraterone 1000 mg orally once daily and prednisone 5 mg orally twice daily lead to increases in overall survival and progression-free survival of 3.9 months and 2 months, respectively. Abiraterone should be administered on an empty stomach either 2 hours after or 1 hour before a meal. The most significant adverse effects with abiraterone were fluid retention, hypokalemia, and hypertension (Table 92–10).[55]

❿ *Immunotherapy with sipuleucel-T improves survival in patients with castrate-resistant prostate cancer with minimally symptomatic disease.*

Table 92–10

Second-Line Therapy for Metastatic Castrate Resistant Prostate Cancer

Chemotherapy	Usual Dose	Adverse Effects	Dose Adjustments
Cabazitaxel	25 mg/m² every 3 weeks	Myelosuppression, neuropathy, diarrhea	*Hepatic* Extensively hepatically metabolized, usage should be avoided in hepatic dysfunction (ALT/AST greater than 1.5 × ULN or bilirubin > ULN) *Hematologic* Ensure CBC recovered
Abiraterone	1000 mg once daily	Edema, hypokalemia, hypertension, hepatotoxicity	*Hepatic* Moderate hepatic impairment (Child-Pugh class B), reduce the starting dose to 250 mg once daily; for developmen t of hepatotoxicity during treatment, hold until recovery; retreatment may be initiated at a reduced dose

ALT, alanine aminotransferase; AST, aspartate aminotransferase; CBC, complete blood count.

The approval of sipuleucel-T ushered in a new era of cancer treatment. Sipuleucel is a patient-specific anticancer vaccine.[56] Patients eligible for treatment first undergo a leukapheresis procedure to collect dendritic cells. These are then cultured at a central manufacturing facility and stimulated with a fusion protein of prostatic phosphatase and granulocyte macrophage colony-stimulating factor. These are then injected into the patient. This procedure is performed three times, at 0, 2, and 4 weeks. Treatment is well tolerated with the most common adverse effects reported being moderate and transient chills, fever, and influenza-like symptoms. In the pivotal clinical trial, the patient population was limited to minimally symptomatic men and, although most men in the trial had not received chemotherapy, approximately 15% had been previously treated with docetaxel. Patients with long-bone fractures, spinal cord compression, or visceral metastases were excluded. Although disease progression was not improved by sipuleucel-T, overall survival was significantly improved from 21.7 months with placebo to 25.8 months with sipuleucel-T.[56] High cost and limited production capacity limit the availability of this therapy. In patients who are minimally symptomatic and are able to receive treatment, sipuleucel-T is a valid treatment option. However, because disease progression was not slowed, it may not offer significant relief from disease-related symptoms. In highly symptomatic patients, a treatment that delays tumor progression may be more appropriate.

OUTCOME EVALUATION

Monitoring of prostate cancer depends on the stage of the cancer. When definitive, curative therapy is attempted, objective parameters to assess tumor response include assessment of the tumor size, evaluation of involved lymph nodes, and the response of tumor markers such as PSA to the treatment. Following definitive therapy, the PSA level is checked every 6 months for the first 5 years and then annually. Local recurrence in the absence of a rising PSA may occur, so the DRE is also performed. In the metastatic setting, clinical benefit responses can be documented by evaluating performance status changes, weight changes, quality of life, and analgesic requirements, in addition to the PSA or DRE at 3-month intervals and radiologic studies to objectively measure tumor response.

Patient Care and Monitoring

1. Obtain complete past medical history, family history, and social history.

2. Obtain complete list of any concomitant prescription and over-the-counter medications; be sure to include herbal, vitamin, and mineral supplements.

3. Verify completion of prostate cancer workup and staging.

4. Using information obtained, identify appropriate treatment options.

5. Discuss the benefits and risks of appropriate treatment options with the health care team and patient.

6. If drug therapy is selected, review patient medical history for drug–drug and drug–herbal interactions.

7. Initiate therapy. If patient is asymptomatic, monitor PSA and circulating androgens for castration level of testosterone. If patient is symptomatic, monitor symptoms for improvement or worsening.

8. Monitor for any new symptoms and adverse events from therapy.

Abbreviations Introduced in This Chapter

ASCO	American Society of Clinical Oncology
AUA	American Urological Association
BPH	Benign prostatic hyperplasia
CAB	Combined androgen blockade
CI	Confidence interval
DES	Diethylstilbestrol
DHT	Dihydrotestosterone
DRE	Digital rectal examination
FSH	Follicle-stimulating hormone
GnRH	Gonadotropin-releasing hormone
IGF-1	Insulin-like growth factor-1
IM	Intramuscular
LH	Luteinizing hormone
LHRH	Luteinizing hormone–releasing hormone
NCI	National Cancer Institute
PSA	Prostate-specific antigen
SELECT	Selenium and Vitamin E Cancer Prevention Trial
TRUS	Transrectal ultrasonography

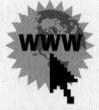

Self-assessment questions and answers are available at *http://www.mhpharmacotherapy.com/pp.html.*

REFERENCES

1. Siegel R, Ward E, Brawley O, Jemal A. Cancer statistics, 2011: The impact of eliminating socioeconomic and racial disparities on premature cancer deaths. CA Cancer J Clin 2011;61:212--236.
2. Hsieh K, Albertsen PC. Populations at high risk for prostate cancer. Urol Clin North Am 2003;30:669–676.
3. Odedina FT, Ogunbiyi JO, Ukoli FA. Roots of prostate cancer in African-American men. J Natl Med Assoc 2006;98:539–543.
4. Sakr WA, Grignon DJ, Crissman JD, et al. High grade prostatic intraepithelial neoplasia (HGPIN) and prostatic adenocarcinoma between the ages of 20-69: An autopsy study of 249 cases. In Vivo 1994;8:439–443.
5. Denis L, Morton MS, Griffiths K. Diet and its preventive role in prostatic disease. Eur Urol 1999;35:377–387.
6. Crawford ED. Epidemiology of prostate cancer. Urology 2003;62:3–12.
7. Liede A, Karlan BY, Narod SA. Cancer risks for male carriers of germline mutations in BRCA1 or BRCA2: A review of the literature. J Clin Oncol 2004;22:735–742.
8. Gurel B, Iwata T, Koh CM, Yegnasubramanian S, Nelson WG, De Marzo AM. Molecular alterations in prostate cancer as diagnostic, prognostic, and therapeutic targets. Adv Anat Pathol 2008;15:319–331.
9. Thompson IM, Goodman PJ, Tangen CM, et al. The influence of finasteride on the development of prostate cancer. N Engl J Med 2003;349:215–224.
10. Kenfield SA, Stampfer MJ, Chan JM, Giovannucci E. Smoking and prostate cancer survival and recurrence. JAMA 2011;305:2548–2555.
11. Iczkowski KA. Current prostate biopsy interpretation: Criteria for cancer, atypical small acinar proliferation, high-grade prostatic intraepithelial neoplasia, and use of immunostains. Arch Pathol Lab Med 2006;130:835–843.
12. Khauli RB. Prostate cancer: Diagnostic and therapeutic strategies with emphasis on the role of PSA. J Med Liban 2005;53:95–102.
13. Culig Z. Role of the androgen receptor axis in prostate cancer. Urology 2003;62:21–26.
14. Marks LS. Luteinizing hormone-releasing hormone agonists in the treatment of men with prostate cancer: Timing, alternatives, and the 1-year implant. Urology 2003;62:36–42.
15. Anderson J. The role of antiandrogen monotherapy in the treatment of prostate cancer. BJU Int 2003;91:455–461.
16. Sharifi N, Gulley JL, Dahut WL. Androgen deprivation therapy for prostate cancer. Jama 2005;294:238–244.
17. De Marzo AM, Meeker AK, Zha S, et al. Human prostate cancer precursors and pathobiology. Urology 2003;62:55–62.
18. Nieto M, Finn S, Loda M, Hahn WC. Prostate cancer: Re-focusing on androgen receptor signaling. Int J Biochem Cell Biol 2007;39:1562–1568.
19. Musquera M, Fleshner NE, Finelli A, Zlotta AR. The REDUCE trial: Chemoprevention in prostate cancer using a dual 5alpha-reductase inhibitor, dutasteride. Expert Rev Anticancer Ther 2008;8:1073–1079.
20. Andriole GL, Bostwick DG, Brawley OW, et al. Effect of dutasteride on the risk of prostate cancer. N Engl J Med 2010;362:1192–1202.
21. Kramer BS, Hagerty KL, Justman S, et al. Use of 5-alpha-reductase inhibitors for prostate cancer chemoprevention: American Society of Clinical Oncology/American Urological Association 2008 Clinical Practice Guideline. J Clin Oncol 2009;27:1502–1516.
22. Lippman SM, Klein EA, Goodman PJ, et al. Effect of selenium and vitamin E on risk of prostate cancer and other cancers: The Selenium and Vitamin E Cancer Prevention Trial (SELECT). JAMA 2009;301:39–51.
23. Neill MG, Fleshner NE. An update on chemoprevention strategies in prostate cancer for 2006. Curr Opin Urol 2006;16:132–137.
24. McNaughton-Collins MF, Barry MJ. One man at a time: Resolving the PSA controversy. N Engl J Med 2011;365(21):1951–1953.
25. Schmid HP, Prikler L, Semjonow A. Problems with prostate-specific antigen screening: A critical review. Recent results in cancer research. Fortschritte der Krebsforschung 2003;163:226–231; discussion 64–66.
26. Galic J, Karner I, Cenan L, et al. Role of screening in detection of clinically localized prostate cancer. Coll Antropol 2003;27(Suppl 1):49–54.
27. Wilson SS, Crawford ED. Screening for prostate cancer: Current recommendations. Urol Clin North Am 2004;31:219–226.
28. Gohagan JK, Prorok PC, Kramer BS, Hayes RB, Cornett JE. The Prostate, Lung, Colorectal, and Ovarian-Cancer Screening Trial of the National-Cancer-Institute. Cancer 1995;75:1869–1873.
29. Catalona WJ, Smith DS, Ratliff TL, et al. Measurement of prostate-specific antigen in serum as a screening test for prostate cancer. N Engl J Med 1991;324:1156–1161.
30. Screening for prostate cancer: U.S. Preventive Services Task Force recommendation statement. Ann Intern Med 2008;149:185–191.
31. Harris R, Lohr KN. Screening for prostate cancer: An update of the evidence for the U.S. Preventive Services Task Force. Ann Intern Med 2002;137:917–929.
32. Ross KS, Carter HB, Pearson JD, Guess HA. Comparative efficiency of prostate-specific antigen screening strategies for prostate cancer detection. JAMA 2000;284:1399–1405.
33. Cooperberg MR, Moul JW, Carroll PR. The changing face of prostate cancer. J Clin Oncol 2005;23:8146–8151.
34. Simmons MN, Berglund RK, Jones JS. A practical guide to prostate cancer diagnosis and management. Cleve Clin J Med 2011;78:321–331.
35. Schroder FH, de Vries SH, Bangma CH. Watchful waiting in prostate cancer: Review and policy proposals. BJU Int 2003;92:851–859.
36. Scher HI. Prostate carcinoma: Defining therapeutic objectives and improving overall outcomes. Cancer 2003;97:758–771.
37. Immediate versus deferred treatment for advanced prostatic cancer: initial results of the Medical Research Council Trial. The Medical Research Council Prostate Cancer Working Party Investigators Group. British journal of urology 1997;79:235–246.
38. Maximum androgen blockade in advanced prostate cancer: An overview of the randomised trials. Prostate Cancer Trialists' Collaborative Group. Lancet 2000;355:1491–1498.
39. Hedlund PO, Henriksson P. Parenteral estrogen versus total androgen ablation in the treatment of advanced prostate carcinoma: Effects on overall survival and cardiovascular mortality. The Scandinavian Prostatic Cancer Group (SPCG)-5 Trial Study. Urology 2000;55:328–333.

40. Seidenfeld J, Samson DJ, Hasselblad V, et al. Single-therapy androgen suppression in men with advanced prostate cancer: A systematic review and meta-analysis. Ann Intern Med 2000;132:566–577.

41. Oh WK. Secondary hormonal therapies in the treatment of prostate cancer. Urology 2002;60:87–92; discussion 3.

42. Labrie F, Dupont A, Cusan L, Gomez J, Emond J, Monfette G. Combination therapy with flutamide and medical (LHRH agonist) or surgical castration in advanced prostate cancer: 7-year clinical experience. J Steroid Biochem Mol Biol 1990;37:943–950.

43. Moul JW, Fowler JE, Jr. Evolution of therapeutic approaches with luteinizing hormone-releasing hormone agonists in 2003. Urology 2003;62:20–28.

44. Tyrrell CJ, Altwein JE, Klippel F, et al. Comparison of an LH-RH analogue (Goeserelin acetate, 'Zoladex') with combined androgen blockade in advanced prostate cancer: Final survival results of an international multicentre randomized-trial. International Prostate Cancer Study Group. Eur Urol 2000;37:205–211.

45. Eisenberger MA, Blumenstein BA, Crawford ED, et al. Bilateral orchiectomy with or without flutamide for metastatic prostate cancer. N Engl J Med 1998;339:1036–1042.

46. Weckermann D, Harzmann R. Hormone therapy in prostate cancer: LHRH antagonists versus LHRH analogues. Eur Urol 2004;46: 279–283; discussion 83–84.

47. Crawford ED, Kozlowski JM, Debruyne FM, et al. The use of strontium 89 for palliation of pain from bone metastases associated with hormone-refractory prostate cancer. Urology 1994;44:481–485.

48. Resche I, Chatal JF, Pecking A, et al. A dose-controlled study of 153Sm-ethylenediaminetetramethylenephosphonate (EDTMP) in the treatment of patients with painful bone metastases. Eur J Cancer 1997;33:1583–1591.

49. Saad F, Gleason DM, Murray R, et al. Long-term efficacy of zoledronic acid for the prevention of skeletal complications in patients with metastatic hormone-refractory prostate cancer. J Natl Cancer Inst 2004;96:879–882.

50. Posadas EM, Dahut WL, Gulley J. The emerging role of bisphosphonates in prostate cancer. Am J Ther 2004;11:60–73.

51. Tannock IF, de Wit R, Berry WR, et al. Docetaxel plus prednisone or mitoxantrone plus prednisone for advanced prostate cancer. N Engl J Med 2004;351:1502–1512.

52. Petrylak DP, Tangen CM, Hussain MH, et al. Docetaxel and estramustine compared with mitoxantrone and prednisone for advanced refractory prostate cancer. N Engl J Med 2004;351:1513–1520.

53. Beltran H, Beer TM, Carducci MA, et al. New therapies for castration-resistant prostate cancer: efficacy and safety. Eur Urol 2011;60:279–290.

54. de Bono JS, Oudard S, Ozguroglu M, et al. Prednisone plus cabazitaxel or mitoxantrone for metastatic castration-resistant prostate cancer progressing after docetaxel treatment: A randomised open-label trial. Lancet 2010;376:1147–1154.

55. de Bono JS, Logothetis CJ, Molina A, et al. Abiraterone and increased survival in metastatic prostate cancer. N Engl J Med 2011;364:1995–2005.

56. Kantoff PW, Higano CS, Shore ND, et al. Sipuleucel-T immunotherapy for castration-resistant prostate cancer. N Engl J Med 2010;363:411–422.

93 Skin Cancer

Trinh Pham

LEARNING OBJECTIVES

● **Upon completion of this chapter, the reader will be able to:**

1. Identify the risk factors associated with skin cancer.

2. Devise a plan of lifestyle modifications for the prevention of skin cancer.

3. Explain the goals of therapy for the treatment of the different stages of nonmelanoma and melanoma skin cancer.

4. Discuss the role of mutation testing in patients with newly diagnosed metastatic melanoma and the impact of the test on choosing drug therapy.

5. Compare and contrast the pharmacologic treatment options that are available for patients diagnosed with nonmelanoma and melanoma skin cancer.

6. Suggest management options for patients experiencing adverse effects of pharmacologic therapy.

KEY CONCEPTS

❶ Exposure to ultraviolet radiation from the sun is recognized as one of the primary triggers for skin cancer development.

❷ Staging of malignant melanoma is important to determine prognosis, categorize patients with regard to metastatic potential and survival probability, and aid in clinical decision making.

❸ Determination of lymph node status is important in melanoma staging because it is an independent prognostic factor, and it provides the oncologist with guidance for therapy decisions.

❹ Stages IIB, IIC, and III melanoma are considered to be high risk because of their potential for recurrence and distant metastasis. The primary treatment modality is surgical excision of the tumor and a lymphadenectomy for patients with positive lymph nodes.

❺ Stage IV melanoma is not curable, and the primary goal of therapy is local control of the disease and relief of identifiable symptoms.

❻ Melanoma is an immunogenic tumor and strategies to enhance the patient's immune response to treat the cancer are an area of active research. Ipilimumab is an immunotherapy agent that has a major role in the treatment of unresectable or metastatic melanoma.

❼ Interferon alfa 2b is indicated as adjuvant therapy for patients with bulky stages IIB, IIC, and stage III melanoma because they are at high risk for recurrence after curative surgical resection of the cancer.

❽ Advances in molecular profiling and genome sequencing have lead to the identification of the *BRAF V600E* gene mutation in patients with melanoma. Genetic testing for this mutation should be performed in patients with unresectable or metastatic melanoma to determine the patient's eligibility to start targeted therapy with vemurafenib.

❾ In patients diagnosed with basal cell carcinoma and squamous cell carcinoma, the primary goal of therapy is to cure the patient and to prevent recurrence.

Skin cancer is the most prevalent of all malignancies occurring in humans, and in the United States, it accounts for more than 50% of all cancers.[1] The most common cutaneous malignancies are basal cell carcinoma (BCC), squamous cell carcinoma (SCC), and malignant melanoma (MM). BCC and SCC are categorized as nonmelanoma skin cancer (NMSC). It is estimated that more than 3.5 million cases (in more than 2 million people) of BCC and SCC and more than 100,000 cases of melanomas are diagnosed in the United States each year.[1] Ultraviolet radiation (UVR) exposure is the leading environmental factor causing skin cancer.[2] This is a modifiable risk factor, and prevention of skin cancer development is possible through a sun protection regimen that includes wearing protective clothing; avoidance of prolonged, intense sun exposure and sunburns; and regular application of sunscreen. If skin cancer is detected in its early stage, survival is improved, and the disease is curable. Therefore, campaigns for primary and secondary prevention of skin cancer are important in combating this tumor. NMSC and MM differ with regard to prognosis, metastatic potential, mortality, curability, and treatment options. This chapter reviews the pathogenesis and risk factors for the development of skin cancer and provides current data on the recommendations for the prevention and treatment of both NMSC and MM.

MELANOMA

EPIDEMIOLOGY AND ETIOLOGY

Malignant melanoma is the most common serious form of skin cancer, and the lifetime risk of developing it is 1 in 37 for men and 1 in 56 for women.[1] Approximately 70,230 new cases of invasive melanoma were predicted to occur in 2011.[1] Melanoma represents about 2% of all skin cancers in the United States, but it accounts for 75% of all skin cancer deaths.[1] It was estimated that in 2011, 8,790 deaths would be attributable to melanoma.[1] The incidence of melanoma is not evenly distributed among all populations; race, gender, and age confer different rates. The rate of MM is 10 times higher in whites than in African Americans or Hispanics, and it is 50% higher in white men than white women.[3] In patients older than 65 years, the incidence is 10 times higher than in patients younger than 40 years.[4] The median age of diagnosis for cutaneous melanoma is 59 years, and the median age of death is 68 years.[5] The trend in 5-year survival rates for melanoma has improved from 82% to 93% in the past 4 decades; however, MM is still a major public health problem in the United States because of its dramatic rise in incidence in the past 3 decades.[3] Data from the National Cancer Institute Surveillance Epidemiology and End Results (SEER) show that the incidence of melanoma nearly tripled from 1975 to 2005.[5]

RISK FACTORS

Environmental

The risk factors for developing MM can be categorized as environmental factors and host factors. ❶ *Exposure to UVR from the sun is recognized as one of the primary triggers for skin carcinogenesis.* UV radiation (specifically UVB) is absorbed by DNA in the cells in the epidermal layer and may induce DNA damage. Gene mutations, such as UVR-induced mutation to the p53 tumor suppressor gene, may transpire, resulting in dysregulation of apoptosis, expansion of mutated keratinocytes, and initiation of skin cancer.[2] Other mechanisms of UV radiation–induced DNA damage include the generation of reactive oxygen species, which

create breaks in DNA, leading to genetic mutations and skin cancer.[2] It is estimated that 65% to 90% of MMs are attributable to UV exposure, particularly when a person has a history of intense and blistering sunburns in childhood. If a person experienced more than one severe sunburn in childhood, the risk of developing melanoma is increased twofold.[2] Since the mid 1980s, depletion of the ozone layer has been of concern because this allows more UVR to penetrate the atmosphere. Melanoma mortality may increase by 1% to 2% when there is an approximate 1% decrease in ozone levels.[2] Exposure to sources of artificial UV radiation such as tanning beds has also been linked to increased risk of skin cancer.[2]

Host Factors

Host risk factors for developing MM include individuals with phenotypic characteristics of red hair, light skin, blue eyes, sun sensitivity, and freckling. Family history of MM in a first-degree relative is another risk factor for developing MM, with a twofold likelihood compared with patients with no family history.[2] In individuals without a family history of MM (sporadic MM), the presence of benign melanocytic nevi (benign moles) is consistently identified as the strongest risk factor for the future development of MM. It has been found that the greater the number of benign nevi a person possess, the greater the susceptibility to MM growth. A personal history of MM or NMSC also increases the risk of developing subsequent MM.[5] The dysplastic nevus syndrome is another

---

Patient Encounter, Part 1

DM is a 55-year-old woman who presented to her dermatologist with a pigmented skin lesion on her left shoulder that she noticed had enlarged and changed color recently in the past few months.

History: She has the lesion since youth, and it was measured at 3 mm. She noticed the change in color and size in the past few months.

DM reports being a "sun worshiper" all her life; she spends her weekends outdoors or at the pool and vacations at the beach. DM notes that she burns initially and then eventually tans with excessive freckling. She reports using an indoor tanning bed 3 to 5 days a week for the past 20 years. She does not use sunscreen or practice sun protection measures.

What are DM's risk factors for developing malignant melanoma?

What primary prevention measures are recommended to prevent skin cancer?

What is the recommendation to detect melanoma early in a patient?

risk factor. A person with five or more dysplastic nevi has six times the risk of developing MM than a person with no dysplastic nevi.[5] Larger nevi, as in the case of congenital melanocytic nevi (greater than 20 cm), is also associated with a greater risk of developing MM.[5]

Compared with other cancers, MM occur at a younger age with a median of 62 years in men and 54 years in women, and as a person ages, the risk increases further, especially in men.[6] The risk of MM is also increased in patients with immunosuppression due to cancer, AIDS, a history of chronic lymphocytic leukemia, non Hodgkin's lymphoma, and after organ transplants.[2] Rare genetic syndromes such as xeroderma pigmentosum (XP) increases the risk of developing MM and NMSC 100-fold compared with the general population.[6] MM has been reported in breast-ovarian cancer families with a 2.6-fold risk in carriers of *BRCA2* mutations.[6] An association has been found between pancreatic cancer and MM with mutation in *CDKN2A*.[6]

PRIMARY PREVENTION OF SKIN CANCER

Ultraviolet radiation exposure from the sun is the major cause of NMSC and MM. **Primary prevention** strategies for skin cancer aim at educating people against excessive exposure to the sun and are spearheaded by the American Academy of Dermatology, American Cancer Society, Environmental Protection Agency, and Centers for Disease Control and Prevention. The aims of these programs are to increase public awareness about the harmful effects of sun exposure and the risk of skin cancer, change attitudes about the social norms related to sun protection and tanned skin, and decrease the incidence of skin cancer and deaths related to this malignancy. Recommendations for prevention of skin cancer are universal and include a variety of simple strategies to minimize exposure to UV rays:

- Avoid direct exposure to the sun between the hours of 10 AM and 4 PM, when UV rays are most intense.
- Wear hats with a broad enough brim to shade the face, ears, and neck.
- Wear protective clothing (especially tightly woven apparel) that covers as much as possible the arms, legs, and torso.
- Cover skin with a sunscreen lotion with a skin protection factor (SPF) of at least 15, protecting against UV radiation (both UVA and UVB).
- Reapply sunscreens every 2 hours (especially if sweating or swimming).
- Avoid sun lamps and tanning beds, which provide an additional source of UV radiation.
- Seek shade when outdoors.

The use of chemical sunscreen is only one of many strategies, and it should not be the sole agent used for cancer prevention. The lay public should be warned not to use sunscreen with a higher SPF with the intent to extend the duration of exposure because it is observed that DNA damage can occur long before sunburn appears, and the long-term effects of increased sun exposure are not known. Sunscreen protective agents have been proven only to reduce the risk of actinic keratosis (AK) and SCC. There is no convincing evidence that sunscreen application has protective effect against BCC or MM.[7]

SECONDARY PREVENTION OF SKIN CANCER

Secondary prevention of skin cancer involves early detection of premalignant cancers for early intervention with the hope that it will reduce mortality and increase cure. Regular screening for melanoma either by skin self examination or total skin examination performed by health care providers consistently identify smaller and thinner lesions in high-risk patients.[8] However, recommendations for melanoma screening are conflicting because there are no randomized, controlled, prospective melanoma trials demonstrating that routine screening reduces mortality. For this reason, the US Preventive Services Task Force (USPSTF) recommends neither for nor against routine screening for the general population. On the other hand, the American Cancer Society and the National Institutes of Health promote skin self-examination and recommend routine clinic-based screening for skin cancer for all individuals beginning at age 20 years. The American Academy of Dermatology, Skin Cancer Foundation, and 1992 National Institutes of Health Consensus Conference on Early Melanoma recommend annual screening for all patients.[8] The American Academy of Family Physicians and American College of Preventive Medicine recommend screening for high-risk populations with family or personal history of skin cancer, clinical evidence of precursor lesions, or increased occupational or recreational exposure to sunlight.[8] Pamphlets and online information describing the method of skin self-examination are available from agencies such as the American Cancer Society (*www.cancer.org*), American Academy of Dermatology (*www.aad.org*), and Skin Cancer Foundation (*www.skincancer.org*).

PATHOPHYSIOLOGY

Malignant melanoma is a cancer that arises from melanocytes, which are cells that synthesize melanin and contribute to hair and skin pigmentation. The overwhelming majority of MMs originate from the skin, although they may also arise less commonly from mucosal epithelial tissues such as the conjunctiva, oral cavity, esophagus, vagina, female urethra, penis, and anus. The pathway that leads to the development of melanoma is complex, and the processes by which melanocytes transform to malignant melanoma cells are thought to occur through germline predisposition, multistep accumulation of genetic and molecular alterations, and environmental factors such as UV exposure. Exposure to UVR is an important factor in MM development; however, the relationship between risk and exposure is not clear. MM may occur in individuals with either inherent genetic susceptibility or low genetic susceptibility for melanocyte proliferation. The distinguishing characteristic is that MM may develop with less solar damage and on intermittent sun exposed body sites such as the trunk for individuals with high genetic susceptibility. Conversely, in individuals with low genetic susceptibility, melanoma occurs with chronic UV exposure on commonly exposed areas such as the face and neck.[10]

Genetic Pathway to the Development of Melanoma

Recent advances in molecular profiling and genome sequencing have enabled the identification of oncogenic mutations that drive MM progression. Much attention has been focused on the BRAF melanoma oncogene and its role in MM. BRAF is a serine/threonine protein kinase that is a member of the RAF kinase family, which is a part of the RAF/MEK/ERK serine threonine cascade (also known as ERK/MAP kinase pathway or "classical" MAPK pathway).[11] Mutations in BRAF activates the ERK/MAP pathway and thus trigger melanocyte proliferation and clonal expansion. BRAF mutation is found in approximately one half of all MM, and BRAF mutant melanomas tend to occur on intermittent sun-exposed skin areas, skin phenotypes that have poor UV protection (e.g., pale skin, poor tanning response, red hair, and freckling), and younger individuals (younger than 55 years) with lower cumulative UV exposure.[12] There are more than 50 mutations in BRAF described, but the valine to glutamic acid (*BRAF V600E*) substitution accounts for 80% of all *BRAF* mutations. Furthermore, this *V600E* mutation is the most common BRAF mutation in MM.[13] The development of potent and selective BRAF kinase inhibitors has demonstrated early evidence of tumor regression and disease control in metastatic MM.

CLINICAL PRESENTATION, DIAGNOSIS, AND STAGING

There are four major subtypes of cutaneous MM: superficial spreading, nodular, lentigo maligna melanoma, and acral lentiginous (Table 93–1). They each vary in clinical and growth characteristics.[14,15]

Data from SEER show that 84% of diagnosed MM are locally confined, 8% are diagnosed after the cancer has spread regionally, 4% are diagnosed with distant metastasis, and the remaining 4% are not staged.[16] ❷ *Once skin cancer is diagnosed, it is important to determine the stage of the cancer to find out if the cancer is confined to the original tumor site or has spread to other sites, such as the lymph nodes, liver, brain, lungs, or bone. The purpose of staging is to determine prognosis, categorize patients with regard to metastatic potential and survival probability, and aid in clinical decision making.* As with most solid tumors, the tumor, node, metastasis (TNM) classification is used to stage MM,

and the latest guidelines for staging MM proposed by the American Joint Committee on Cancer were implemented in 2010 (Table 93–2).[17]

❸ *Determination of lymph node status is important in melanoma staging because it is an independent prognostic factor, and it provides the oncologist with guidance for therapy decisions.* For patients with MM that are at risk of spreading to the lymph nodes, a sentinel lymph node (SLN) biopsy is performed. The SLN, the first lymph node to receive lymph draining from the tumor, is identified by injecting a radioactive material, technetium-99m-labeled radiocolloids, and vital blue dye into the skin next to the tumor and tracing the flow of lymph from the tumor site to the nearest lymph node chain. Once the SLN is located, it is removed and analyzed for the presence of MM cells. If it is positive for the presence of MM, then the whole lymph node basin in that area is dissected; this is also known as lymphadenectomy. An SLN biopsy is the initial procedure to assess the status of lymph node involvement to prevent the morbidity associated with a total lymphadenectomy.

In addition to the stage of the disease and the status of disease involvement in the lymph nodes, other prognostic factors for outcome in MM include primary tumor thickness (Fig. 93–1), the presence of ulceration in the primary melanoma, mitotic activity, the presence of tumor infiltrating lymphocytes (TIL), and gender. Tumor thickness is defined as thin (less than 1 mm), intermediate (1 to 4 mm), and thick (greater than 4 mm). The 10-year survival rate is 92% for thin tumors and 63% to 80% for intermediate tumors and decreases further to 50% in patients with thick tumors.[17] *Ulceration* is defined as the lack of an intact dermis overlying the primary tumor on histologic evaluation. Survival rates for patients with an ulcerated melanoma are proportionately lower than those with a nonulcerated melanoma of equivalent thickness, but the survival rate is similar for a nonulcerated melanoma of the next highest level of thickness. The male sex is associated with poor prognosis and adverse outcome in MM.[18]

Skin Examination

The *ABCDE* acronym is a helpful mnemonic for recognizing the signs and symptoms of early MM (Fig. 93–2). It was devised in 1985 by clinicians working in the Melanoma Clinical Cooperative Group at New York University School of Medicine and is used to educate health care professionals who are not dermatologists in differentiating common moles from cancer.[8] It is also a useful tool to educate the lay public to assess pigmented lesions and screen for suspicious moles to help identify the MM in its early stage when it is curable. Not all MMs, including nodular melanoma, have all ABCDE characteristics, and it is not meant to provide a comprehensive list of all MM features. The characteristics for each of the letters are described in the Clinical Presentation and Diagnosis box. It should be noted that evolution of a lesion is one of the most important warning signs of danger in the assessment of moles for MM.

Table 93–1

Characteristics of Different Types of Skin Cancer

	Malignant Melanoma				Nonmelanoma Skin Cancer	
	Superficial Spreading	Nodular	Lentigo Maligna Melanoma	Acral Lentiginous	Basal Cell Carcinoma	Squamous Cell Carcinoma
Frequency	70%	10–15%	10%	Less than 10%	75%	20%
Location	Head, neck Legs in women Trunk in men	Trunk, head, neck	Sun-exposed areas, face, head, neck	Palms of the hands, soles of feet, nailbeds	Head and neck	Face, hands, forearms
Age	Fifth decade	Seventh decade	Eighth decade	Sixth decade	Incidence increases after age 40	Incidence increases after age 40
Ethnicity	White	White	White	Most frequent in ethnic groups of color	Similar between whites and African Americans	Most common in African descendants
Clinical features	Long horizontal growth phase (5–7 years); better prognosis	Very aggressive without identifiable horizontal growth phase; deeply invasive at the time of diagnosis; associated with poor prognosis	Long horizontal growth phase (10 years); lentigo maligna is the in situ form of lentigo maligna melanoma (only 5% transform to malignant melanoma)	Aggressive, rapid progression from horizontal to vertical growth; poorer prognosis	Rarely metastasize **Circumscribed types:** A: Nodular BCC, most common subtype B: Adenoid BCC C: Fibroepithelioma D: Basosquamous (metatypical) **Diffuse types:** plaque-like with horizontal spread and poorly defined margins A: Superficial BCC, second most common type of BCC, least aggressive B: Morpheaform, most aggressive C: Micronodular	Metastasize to lymph nodes and blood Have premalignant precursors and in situ variant; usually presents as raised pink papule or plaque, often scaly and sometimes ulcerated

From Refs. 14 and 15.

Table 93–2

2009 AJCC Melanoma Staging System and Classification (7th Edition)

Stage	Histologic Features	Overall Survival	
		5 Years (%)	10 Years (%)
0	Melanoma in situ (involves only the epidermis layer)	100	100
IA	Less than or 1 mm thickness, no ulceration, and mitosis less than $1/mm^2$	95	88
IB	Less than or 1 mm with ulceration or mitosis greater than or $1/mm^2$ or between 1.01 and 2 mm with no ulceration	89–91	79–83
IIA	Between 1.01 and 2 mm with ulceration or between 2.01 and 4 mm with no ulceration	77–79	64
IIB	Between 2.01 and 4 mm with ulceration or greater than 4 mm with no ulceration	63–67	51–54
IIC	Greater than 4 mm with ulceration	45	32
IIIA	Any tumor thickness with no ulceration with one lymph node involved and micrometastases or any tumor thickness with no ulceration with two to three lymph nodes involved and micrometastases	63–70	57–63
IIIB	Any tumor thickness with ulceration and one to three lymph nodes involved and micrometastases or any tumor thickness without ulceration and one to three lymph nodes involved and macrometastases or any tumor thickness with ulceration with in-transit metastases or satellite lesions without metastatic lymph nodes	46–59	36–48
IIIC	Any tumor thickness with ulceration with one lymph node involved and macrometastases	24–29	15–24
	Any tumor thickness with ulceration with two to three lymph nodes involved and macrometastases		
	Any tumor thickness with four or more metastatic lymph nodes or in-transit metastases or satellite lesions with metastatic lymph nodes		
IV	M_{1a}: Skin, subcutaneous tissue, or distant lymph nodes with normal LDH	7–19	3–16
	M_{1b}: Lung with normal LDH		
	M_{1c}: To all other visceral sites (liver) or distant metastasis at any site with elevated serum LDH		

From Refs. 5 and 17.

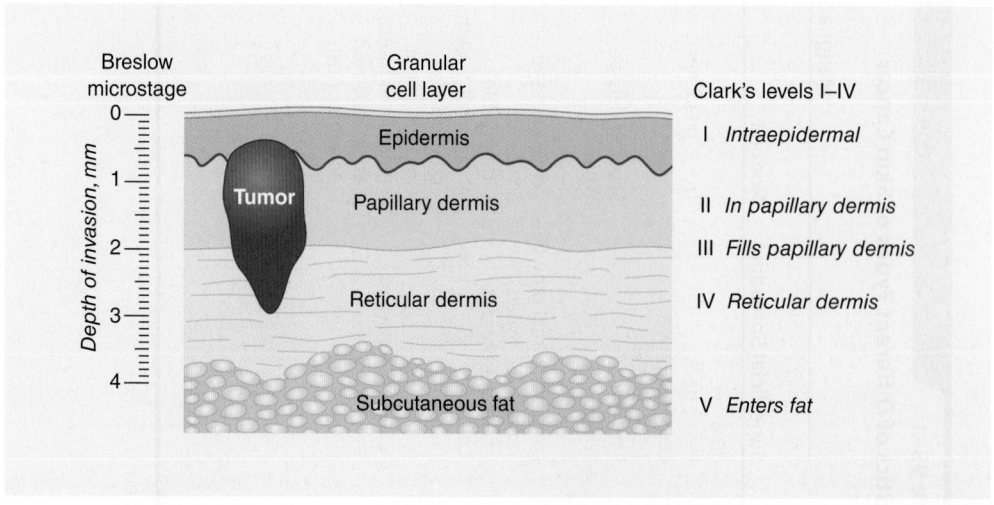

FIGURE 93–1. Skin anatomy: Breslow microstaging and Clark's levels. Clark's level refers to the level of penetration into the dermis. Breslow classification measures tumor thickness in millimeters from the epidermis to the deepest depth of penetration into the dermis. (From Langley RGB, Barnhill RL, Mihm Jr MC, et al. Neoplasms: Cutaneous melanoma. In: Freedberg IM, Eisen AZ, Wolff K, et al., eds. Fitzpatrick's Dermatologyin General Medicine, 6th ed. New York: McGraw-Hill; 2003:938.)

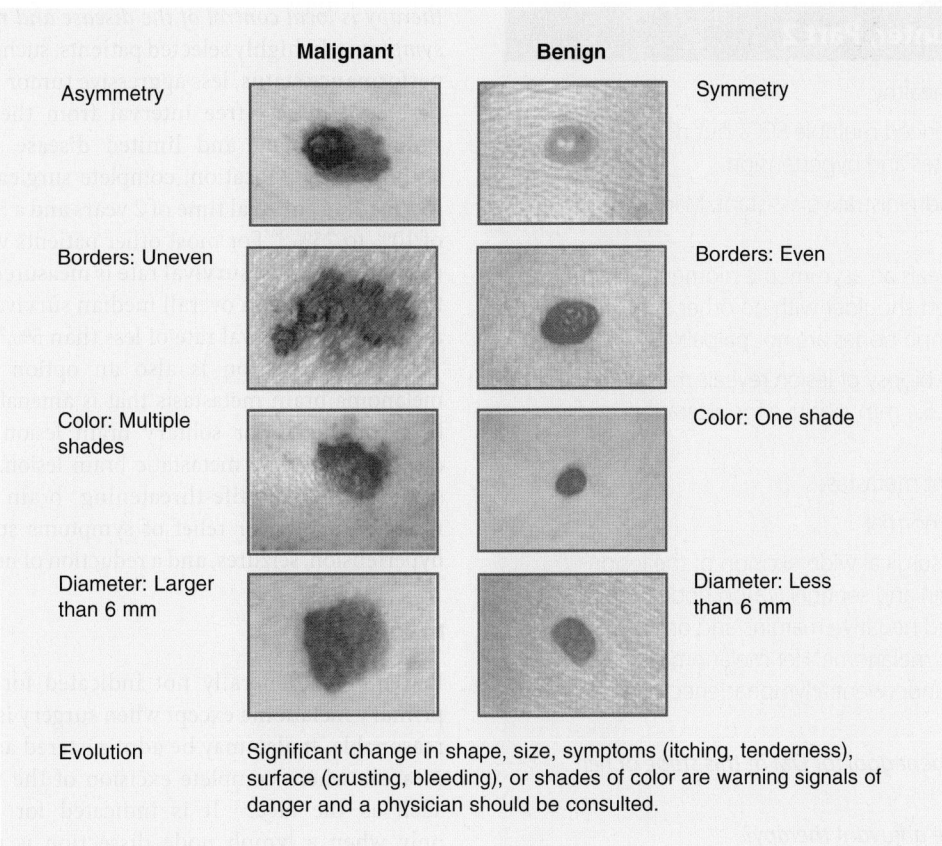

FIGURE 93–2. ABCDE features of early melanoma. (Images courtesy of the Skin Cancer Foundation, New York, *www.skincancer.org.*)

TREATMENT

Early diagnosis of skin cancer is the key to improved prognosis. On presentation to a clinician's office, patients may offer a history of a new growth or an area of irritation. Conversely, the skin cancer may have been present for years undetected by the patient. The definitive diagnosis of any suspected cutaneous malignancy should be confirmed by a biopsy before treatment.

The modality of treatment for skin cancer depends on the size, location, and stage of the tumor; the age of the patient; and the type of skin cancer. Treatment options for skin cancer include surgery, radiation, chemotherapy, immunotherapy, and targeted therapy.

Desired Outcome

The primary goals of therapy for MM are to completely eradicate the tumor and minimize the risk of tumor recurrence and metastasis. Secondary goals of therapy include preserving normal tissue, maintaining function, and providing optimal cosmetic outcomes. Patients with local disease MM (stages I and IIA) are curable with surgical resection of the tumor. Thus, the aim is to diagnose patients at the earliest stage to increase the probability of cure.

Patients with regional disease (stages IIB, IIC, and III) have a high recurrence risk, and the goal of therapy is to prevent relapse of the disease. Disseminated, metastatic MM is not curable, and the goal of therapy is local control of the disease and palliation of symptoms.

The outcome of patients diagnosed with MM depends on the stage of the disease at diagnosis. The overall 5-year survival rate for patients with localized disease (stages I and IB) is the best at 89% to 95%.[17] For patients with stage IIA to IIIA disease, the 5-year survival rate is greater than 50%, ranging from 63% to 79%.[17] In patients with more advanced regional metastatic disease (stage IIIB to IIIC), the 5-year survival rate ranges from 24% to 59%. Patients with stage IV distant metastatic disease have the worst 5-year survival rate at only 7% to 19%.[17]

Treatment Options for Malignant Melanoma

▶ *Surgery*

❹ *The primary treatment modality for local/regional (stage I to III) MM is surgical excision of the tumor and a lymphadenectomy for patients with positive lymph nodes.* The goals of therapy are to optimize local control, achieve potential cure, and minimize morbidity. Achieving adequate

Patient Encounter, Part 2

PMH: Otherwise healthy

FH: Father experienced multiple SCCs but no melanoma. Mother has diabetes and hypertension.

SH: Patient is an administrative assistant. Married with two children.

Examination: Reveals an asymmetric pigmented lesion of 6 mm on the left shoulder with no other suspicious lesions noted. Lymph nodes are not palpable.

Biopsy: Excisional biopsy of lesion reveals melanoma, Breslow thickness 5.4 mm, positive for ulceration, and mitosis 3/mm^2

CT scan: no distant metastases

Laboratory data: normal

DM underwent a surgical wide excision of the lesion with a 2-cm margin and sentinel lymph node biopsy. Pathology revealed negative margins and one of three nodes positive for melanoma. Her melanoma is diagnosed as stage IIIB. She underwent a lymphadenectomy of the left axilla.

What is the treatment goal for DM at this stage of her disease?

Should DM receive adjuvant therapy?

If it is decided that DM should receive adjuvant treatment, which is the preferred option, high-dose interferon or pegylated interferon?

surgical margins for the primary tumor is important in preventing local recurrence and improving overall survival. The thickness of the tumor dictates the extent of the surgical margin (Table 93–3).[19] The most common first site of recurrence in primary melanoma after excision of the tumor is in the lymph nodes. ⑤ *For patients with metastatic MM, surgical excision is not curative. The primary goal of*

Table 93–3

Excision Margin Based on Tumor Thickness

Tumor Thickness (mm)	Excision Margin (cm)
In situ	0.5–1
0–1	1
1–2	1 or 2[a]
2–4	2
Greater than 4	2

[a]A 2-cm margin is preferred, but a 1-cm margin is acceptable in anatomic locations where a 2-cm margin may compromise function or significantly affect cosmesis.

From Ross M, Gershenwald J. Evidence-based treatment of early-stage melanoma. J Surg Oncol 2011;104:341–353.

therapy is local control of the disease and relief of identifiable symptoms. In highly selected patients, such as those with good performance status, less aggressive tumor biology, prolonged period of disease-free interval from the time of primary tumor treatment, and limited disease that is contained within a single location, complete surgical resection results in a median survival time of 2 years and a 5-year survival rate of 10% to 25%.[20] For most other patients with stage IV MM, unfortunately, the survival rate is measured in months rather than years, with an overall median survival of 5 to 8 months and a 5-year survival rate of less than 5%.[20]

Surgical resection is also an option for patients with melanoma brain metastasis that is amenable to surgery. It is best considered for solitary brain lesion without systemic disease or a single metastatic brain lesion. For patients with symptomatic or life-threatening brain lesions, surgical resection allows for relief of symptoms such as intracranial hypertension, seizures, and a reduction of neurologic deficits.[21]

▶ *Radiation*

Radiation is generally not indicated for the treatment of primary melanoma except when surgery is impossible or not reasonable. It also may be administered as adjuvant therapy in areas where complete excision of the tumor is difficult, such as the face.[22] It is indicated for the lymph nodes only when a lymph node dissection is not complete. For patients with bone metastasis, radiation may be indicated as palliative therapy for pain, fracture risks, or spinal cord compression.[22]

Melanoma is the third cancer most commonly associated with central nervous system (CNS) metastasis after lung and breast cancer, and 10% to 40% of melanoma patients present with cerebral metastasis.[22] Patients with brain metastasis have a life expectancy of 3 to 5 months, and 1-year survival is less than 10% to 15%.[22] Headaches and seizures are the most common presenting symptoms. Radiation therapy is indicated for palliation of CNS symptoms and as adjuvant therapy after resection of the CNS metastasis.[22]

Whole-brain radiation therapy (WBRT) is indicated for patients with multiple (more than three) CNS metastases, surgically inaccessible lesions, and extensive systemic disease.[23] WBRT for metastatic CNS MM does not improve survival or provide a cure; however, it is effective in relieving neurologic symptoms,[23] preventing new metastasis, reducing symptomatic recurrence, and decreasing the need for salvage therapy.[22] It improves neurologic deficits in 50% to 75% of cases and relieves headaches in 80% of patients.[24] There are some data to suggest that surgical resection followed by WBRT in patients with a single CNS metastasis decreases the risk of local recurrence compared with resection alone.[22]

Stereotactic radiosurgery (SRS) delivers high doses of focused ionizing external-beam radiation to a well-defined target area in one session of radiation therapy.[23] This technique maximizes the dose of radiation to the tumor with a rapid dose falloff outside the target area, resulting in sparing of the surrounding nontarget normal tissue. SRS may be considered over surgery for patients with fewer than three

Clinical Presentation of MM

Patients with skin cancer generally present with a lesion that may be located anywhere on the body. The most common sites are the head, neck, trunk, and extremities. Changes in any characteristics of a lesion are important danger warning signals. Abnormal presentations of a mole or lesion indicate the need for further assessment.

- *Asymmetry*: Half the lesion does not mirror the other half
- *Border*: Sharp, ragged, uneven, and irregular borders
- *Color*: Multiple colors of various hues of light brown, dark brown, black, red, blue, or gray
- *Diameter*: Larger than 6 mm or the size of a pencil head eraser
- *Evolving*: Significant change in shape, size, symptoms, surface, or shades of color

Other signs and symptoms to monitor for in a lesion, in addition to ABCDE, include:

- Sudden or continuous enlargement of a lesion or elevation of a lesion
- Changes in the skin surrounding the nevus
- Redness, swelling, itching, tenderness, or pain
- Ulceration: friability of the lesion with bleeding or oozing. This is a danger signal.

Less Common Sites and Manifestations of MM

It is important to examine these sites for "hidden" MM:

- Nailbed
- Mucosal tissue
- Scalp
- Eye

In the nailbed, a black streak or wide variegated brown streak, elevation of nailbed, skin next to nail becomes darker, nail looks deformed or is being destroyed; size of nail streak increases over time.

Diagnostic Tests

- Dermoscopy
- Biopsy

Staging Tests (Depending on Patient's Presentation)

- Baseline chest radiography
- LDH level
- CT of chest, abdomen, pelvis
- SLN biopsy: ❸ The status of the SLN is one of the most powerful independent prognostic factors predicting survival. It also provides the oncologist with guidance for therapy decisions and accurate staging.
- PET
- MRI

From Rigel D, Russak J, Friedman R. The evolution of melanoma diagnosis: 25 years and beyond the ABCDs. CA Cancer J Clin 2010;60(5):301–316.

---

metastatic CNS lesions that are deep, nonsymptomatic, and smaller than 3 cm in size.[23]

► Chemotherapy

In general, cytotoxic chemotherapy is not considered a standard of care for metastatic melanoma even though this is an area of active research to identify the optimal chemotherapy regimen. The following review highlights the current status of the most promising chemotherapy agents in the treatment of melanoma.

The major indication for systemic chemotherapy is in patients with metastatic or inoperable MM who are not candidate for vemurafenib. The goal of chemotherapy is to reduce tumor size, and it is an accepted palliative therapy for stage IV melanoma. Dacarbazine, an alkylating agent, is the most active single-agent chemotherapy against MM, achieving response rates of 15% to 25% in older clinical trials.[25] More recent large-scale clinical trials have shown response rates of 5% to 12%.[26] It is the only chemotherapy agent approved by the Food and Drug Administration (FDA) for the treatment of metastatic MM. Temozolomide (TMZ) is an oral chemotherapy agent that is structurally and functionally similar to dacarbazine that yields the same active intermediate. TMZ possesses activity against MM cells and the ability to cross the blood–brain barrier because of its lipophilicity, thus making it an appropriate chemotherapy agent to be investigated for the treatment of MM with CNS metastases. A phase III clinical trial comparing single-agent TMZ versus dacarbazine demonstrated that TMZ is at least as effective as dacarbazine against advanced metastatic MM without CNS involvement.[25] Combining other chemotherapy agents with dacarbazine has been investigated in phase III clinical trials and has not shown improvement in median or long-term survival over single-agent dacarbazine at the risk of greater toxicity.[27] Therefore, combination chemotherapy is not a standard of care for stage IV MM. The role of TMZ, either alone or as combination therapy in the prevention and treatment of MM CNS metastasis is an area of active research (Table 93–4).

Paclitaxel with or without cisplatin or carboplatin demonstrate response rates below 20% as first- or second-line treatment for stage III or IV MM.[28,29] The combination of cisplatin, paclitaxel, and dacarbazine (CTD regimen)

Table 93–4

Dosing[a] Recommendations

Interferon[a] Regimens Used in Clinical Trials

High dose (HDI)	20 million units/m² IV daily × 5 days/week for 4 weeks followed by 10 million units/m² SC 3 times/week for 48 weeks
Intermediate dose (IDI)	10 million units × 5 days/week for 4 weeks followed by 10 million units SC 3 times/week for varying durations
Low dose (LDI)	3 million units SC 3 times/week for varying durations
	1 million units SC every other day for 1 year
Peginterferon	6 mcg/kg/week SC for 8 weeks followed by 3 mcg/kg/week for up to 5 years

Interleukin-2[a] Dosing Regimens

IL-2 600,000 or 720,000 IU/kg by 15-minute infusion every 8 hours for 14 consecutive doses over 5 days as tolerated

IL-2 720,000 IU/kg IV over 15 minutes beginning at 6 PM on day 1 and subsequently at 8 AM and 6 PM up to a maximum of eight total doses on days 1 to 5 (first treatment course) and repeated on days 15 to 19 (second treatment course)

Ipilimumab[a]

Ipilimumab 3 mg/kg every 3 weeks for four doses

Vemurafenib[a]

Vemurafenib 960 mg PO twice daily with the first dose in the morning and the second dose in the evening approximately 12 hours later. Continue treatment until disease progression or unacceptable toxicity occurs

Caution should be used in patients with severe renal or hepatic impairment; no specific guidelines exist

Vemurafenib is only indicated in patients with a BRAF mutation

Chemotherapy[a] Dosing

Dacarbazine 250 mg/m²/day IV, days 1 to 5, every 21 days

No guidelines exist for dose adjustment in patients with renal or hepatic impairment

Temozolomide 150 to 200 mg/m²/day by mouth × 5 days, every 28 days

Caution should be used in patients with severe renal or hepatic impairment; no specific guidelines exist

Measure ANC and platelets on days 22 and 29

If ANC is less than 1,000/mm³ (1.0×10^9/L) or platelet is less than 50,000/ mm³ (50×10^9/L), postpone therapy until ANC is greater than 1,500/mm³ (1.5×10^9/L) and platelet is greater than 100,000/mm³ (100×10^9/L); reduce dose by 50 mg/m² for subsequent cycle

If ANC is 1,000 to 1,500/ mm³ (1.0×10^9–1.5×10^9/L) or platelet is less than 50,000–100,000/ mm³ (50×10^9–100×10^9/L) , postpone therapy until ANC is greater than 1,500/ mm³ (1.5×10^9/L) and platelet is greater than 100,000/mm³ (100×10^9/L) ; maintain initial dose

If ANC is greater than 1,500/mm³ (1.5×10^9/L) and platelet is greater than 100,000/mm³ (100×10^9/L), increase dose to or maintain dose at 200 mg/m²/day for 4 subsequent cycles

[a]The doses presented here are general. Clinicians should refer to clinical trials to determine the specific dose based on the regimen the patient is receiving.

ANC, absolute neutrophil count; IV, intravenous; PO, oral; SC, subcutaneous.

From Refs. 26, 28, 37, 41, and 43.

demonstrated overall response rates of 41% as first-line therapy in patients with stage III or IV disease. Sensory neuropathy and myelosuppression occur with cumulative dosing of CTD and may require dose reduction.[30] A nanoparticle albumin bound paclitaxel (nab-paclitaxel) formulated in a solvent free vehicle to avoid the toxicities associated with Cremophor has been studied in combination with carboplatin for patients with stage IV MM. This regimen has shown promising activity as first line therapy in chemotherapy naïve patients and may have role in the treatment of MM[31] (see Table 93–4).

Enrollment in clinical trials is encouraged in patients with MM because there is little consensus regarding standard chemotherapy for patients with metastatic melanoma.

▶ Immunotherapy

6 *Melanoma is an immunogenic tumor and strategies to enhance the patient's immune response to treat the cancer are an area of active research.* The relationship between melanoma and the immune system was also established

after spontaneous regression of melanoma was observed, and spontaneous serologic and cellular immunity can be documented in a high proportion of patients with advanced melanoma.[32] Strategies to enhance patients' immune response for the treatment of MM have focused on cytokine therapy, immune-modulating therapy, adoptive T-cell therapy, and vaccines.

Interferon-α2b Interferon-α2b (IFN-α2b) has diverse mechanisms of action, including antiviral activity, impact on cellular metabolism and differentiation, and antitumor activity. The antitumor activity is attributable to a combination of direct antiproliferative effect on tumor cells and indirect immune-mediated effects.[33] **7** *IFN and pegylated IFN (peginterferon alfa-2b) are both approved by the FDA as adjuvant therapy for patients who are free of disease after curative surgical resection but are at high risk of MM recurrence.* This includes patients with bulky disease or regional lymph node involvement such as stage IIB, IIC, or III disease. The doses of IFN used in clinical trials can be classified into three groups: high-dose (HDI), intermediate-dose (IDI), and low-dose (LDI) interferon (see Table 93–4).

The optimum dose, schedule, and duration of IFN alfa-2b in high-risk melanoma remain to be defined. A recent meta-analysis of clinical trials of IFN in patients at high risk of recurrence after surgical resection showed improvements in relapse-free survival and overall survival.[34] However, IFN is associated with substantial toxicities, and the National Comprehensive Cancer Network (NCCN) Melanoma Guidelines recommend that the decision for IFN therapy should be made on an individual basis after explaining to the patient the potential benefits and side effects of the therapy. The NCCN Melanoma Guidelines recommend high-dose IFN for 1 year or peginterferon alfa-2b for up to 5 years if the decision is made to initiate IFN (see Table 93–4). Encouragement to participate in clinical trials is also reasonable for eligible patients.[35]

HDI has substantial side effects (Table 93–5) that can be divided into acute and chronic manifestations and categorized into four major side effect groups: constitutional, neuropsychiatric, hematologic, and hepatic.[36] Patients should be educated on the side effects to expect and counseled of the interventions available to minimize the toxicities. Peginterferon alfa-2b has a longer duration of action than IFN alfa-2b and may be administered once a week. The side effects are similar to IFN alfa-2b, although the incidence may be less. The monitoring recommendations for peginterferon alfa-2b are the same as for IFN.

Interleukin 2 Interleukin-2 (IL-2) therapy is approved by the FDA for the treatment of metastatic MM. IL-2 indirectly causes tumor cell lysis by proliferating and activating cytotoxic T lymphocytes (CTLs). The overall objective response rate for patients with metastatic MM receiving high-dose IL-2 is 16%, with a complete response in 6% of patients and a partial response in 10% of patients. The median duration of response is 8.9 months for all responding patients and 5.9 months for patients with a partial response.[37] The median duration of complete response has not been reached but is at least 59 months. Disease progression is not observed in any patient responding for longer than 30 months. The data are encouraging because for the small number of patients who responded to therapy, the effect is of a long duration, and some patients may be considered to be cured of the disease. (Refer to Table 93–4 for dosing.)

High-dose IL-2 therapy is associated with significant severe toxicities and morbidity.[38,39] This treatment option is generally only considered in patients with good performance status who will have a better chance of tolerating and completing the therapy. With the availability of new therapies such as ipilimumab and vemurafenib, IL-2 is no longer the primary option for patients with metastatic melanoma. Table 93–6 lists the most common side effects experienced by patients receiving IL-2 therapy and recommendations for management. All clinicians involved with the care of patients receiving IL-2 should be well educated on the monitoring and management of IL-2–specific side effects.

Table 93–5
IFN Toxicities

Common Acute Toxicity	Management
Flu-Like Symptoms	
Fever, rigors, chills, headaches, myalgia, nausea, emesis	Last 1–12 hours after dose and tolerance develops with continued therapy; Bedtime administration helps with tolerating side effects; Premedicate with acetaminophen or NSAID and administer meperidine for severe chills and rigors; 5-HT$_3$ antagonist, prochlorperazine, metoclopramide, fluids helps with nausea and vomiting
Neutropenia	Weekly CBC; reduce dose by 30–50%
Hepatic enzyme elevation	LFTs at baseline, weekly during induction, monthly during first 3 months of maintenance, then every 3 months; withhold treatment until LFTs normalize; restart at 30–50% dose reduction; reversible on dose reduction or cessation
Cutaneous: alopecia; transient, mild rashlike reaction	INF is contraindicated in patients with psoriasis because exacerbation of psoriasis has been noted during IFN therapy
Common Chronic Toxicity	**Management**
Fatigue, weight loss, anorexia	Reported in 70–100% of patients and increase in intensity as therapy continues; Increase aerobic activity, light exercise, improve nutrition, increase noncaffeinated fluid intake, stress management technique; pharmacologic intervention—megesterol acetate, methylphenidate, to help with either fatigue or anorexia
Depression, cognitive dysfunction. Rare—mania, mood instability	Psychiatric history before therapy and reassess every 4 to 6 weeks; antidepressants: SSRIs, mood stabilizer, bupropion, psychostimulants
Thyroid dysfunction	Initial thyroid function test (TSH), then monthly; if three sequential values are stable or normal, bimonthly or quarterly TSH

CBC, complete blood count; 5-HT$_3$, serotonin; INF, interferon; LFT, liver function test; NSAID nonsteroidal anti-inflammatory drug; SSRI, selective serotonin reuptake inhibitor; TSH, thyroid-stimulating hormone.

From Hauschild A, Gogas H, Tarhini A, et al. Practical guidelines for the management of interferon-a-2b side effects in patients receiving adjuvant treatment for melanoma. Expert opinion. Cancer 2008;112:982–994.

Table 93–6

IL-2 Toxicities

Toxicity (% of Patients)	Management
Cardiovascular	
Hypotension (64%), supraventricular tachycardia (17%)	Discontinue antihypertensive medications; IV fluids to maintain systolic blood pressure greater than 80–90 mm Hg or vasopressor support with an α-agonist such as phenylephrine as indicated; be judicious in use of IV fluids for hypotension
GI	
Vomiting and diarrhea (55%), nausea (24%), stomatitis (14%)	5-HT₃ antagonist, prochlorperazine for emesis (avoid corticosteroids), H₂ blocker for gastritis, antidiarrheal as needed (loperamide, diphenoxylate/atropine, codeine)
Neurologic	
Confusion (30%), somnolence	Haldol for agitation, lorazepam for anxiety, zolpidem for insomnia
Pulmonary	
Dyspnea (31%), pulmonary edema, and ARDS	Advise smokers to quit 2 weeks before therapy; discontinue therapy if requiring greater than 4 L O₂ or 40% O₂ mask for saturation greater than 95%
Hepatic	
Elevated bilirubin (51%), transaminase (39%), ALP	Consider discontinuing therapy if severe
Renal	
Oliguria (49%), elevated serum creatinine (35%), anuria (8%)	Normal saline or dopamine at renal perfusion dose of 2 mcg/kg/min for oliguria; monitor for electrolyte abnormalities and replace as indicated
Hematologic	
Thrombocytopenia (43%), anemia (29%), leukopenia (21%)	Transfuse with packed red blood cells and platelets as needed
Skin	
Rash (27%), exfoliative dermatitis (15%), pruritus	Hydroxyzine, diphenhydramine, oatmeal powder baths, Lubriderm lotion
General	
Fever and or chills (47%), malaise (34%), infection (15%)	Acetaminophen and NSAIDs around the clock for fever and chills; add meperidine if chills are severe; clindamycin or cefazolin to prevent infection
Hypothyroidism	May occur in one-third of patients; thyroid function tests

ALP, alkaline phosphatase; ARDS, adult respiratory distress syndrome; 5-HT₃, serotonin; IV, intravenous; NSAID, nonsteroidal anti-inflammatory drug.

From Refs. 38 and 39.

Antibody Blockade of CTLA-4 with Ipilimumab

▶ *T-Cell Activation and Inhibition*

T-cell activation involves two different signals: (a) the binding of the T-cell receptor to a peptide presented by the major histocompatibility complex (MHC) on the antigen presenting cell (APC) and (b) the interaction of a costimulatory receptor (CD28) on the T-cell surface with a costimulatory ligand (B7) on the APC. The costimulatory molecules enhance the immune response by promoting T-cell activation and proliferation.[40]

CTLA-4 is expressed in CD4+ and CD8+ T cells and regulatory T cells. It is a member of the immunoglobulin super family. After T-cell activation occurs, CTLA-4 migrates to the surface of the T cell, where it has higher affinity for the B7 ligand than CD28 and preferentially binds to B7. This results in an inhibitory signal to the T-cell and causes a downregulation on the immune response; in other words, CTLA-4 acts as a "brake" on the activation of the immune system.[40]

Ipilimumab is a fully human monoclonal immunoglobulin (IgG1 κ) specific for CTLA-4. It has a high affinity for CTLA-4 and impedes binding of CTLA-4 to B7, preventing downregulation of the immune response. This results in increased proliferation of activated T cells and increases the interactions of T cells and cancer cells.[40] Ipilimumab is approved by the FDA for the treatment of unresectable or metastatic melanoma based on a phase III study demonstrating improved survival.[41] The onset of response and regression of tumor size are slow after ipilimumab administration and may take at least 12 weeks of therapy for the response to be measurable. Furthermore, in the initial weeks of therapy, there may be apparent growth of the tumor probably because of drug-related inflammatory infiltrate from activation of T lymphocytes.[42]

The most common adverse effects observed with ipilimumab are immune related, and they follow a characteristic pattern of onset.[42] The skin side effects are seen after an average of 3 to 4 weeks with improvement in 6 weeks, the gastrointestinal tract and liver side effects occur after 6 to 7 weeks with improvement after a median of 2 weeks for

Table 93-7
Ipilimumab Toxicities[a]

Toxicity (% of patients)	Management
Dermatologic (47–68%)	
Maculopapular rash	Do not need to stop or dose reduce ipilimumab
Pruritus	Topical corticosteroid
Vitiligo	Urea-containing cream
	Antipruritic agent such as hydroxyzine
	For grade 3 or 4: oral corticosteroid with prednisone 1 mg/kg or dexamethasone 4 mg every 4 hours with a 4-week taper
GI (31–46%)	
Mild diarrhea, severe diarrhea, or colitis	Loperamide, hydration, electrolyte replacement
	Budesonide 9 mg/day or prednisone 1 mg/kg
	or high-dose IV steroids: methylprednisolone 2 mg/kg once or twice daily or dexamethasone 4 mg every 4 hours; then taper over 4 weeks after symptom resolution; some patients may require 6 to 8 weeks; taper; too rapid taper may result in recrudescence or worsening of symptoms
	If no response to steroids in 48 to 72 hours:
	Infliximab 5 mg/kg every 2 weeks. NOTE: infliximab is contraindicated in patients with bowel perforation or sepsis
	Discontinue ipilimumab for severe symptoms such as colitis
Inflammatory hepatoxicity (3–9%)	Methylprednisolone 2 mg/kg/day 1–2 times daily for LFT greater 8 × ULN or total bilirubin greater 5 × ULN
	Mycophenolate 1 g IV or 1.5 g orally two times daily if symptoms persist
Endocrine (4–6%)	
Hypophysitis	Obtain thyroid function tests, serum cortisol levels, ACTH, testosterone, FSH, LH, prolactin
	Dexamethasone 4 mg every 4 hours for 7 days and taper over at least 4 weeks
	Hormone substitution as needed
	Endocrinologist consult
Neurologic (1%)	
Guillain–Barré syndrome	If symptoms persist for more than 5 days, evaluate for neurologic disorders
Sensory or motor neuropathy	Corticosteroids
Myasthenia gravis	May need to interrupt or discontinue therapy if symptoms are severe

[a]In general, for severe grade 3 or 4 ipilimumab toxicities, therapy should be discontinued permanently.
ACTH, adrenocorticotropic hormone; FSH, follicle-stimulating hormone; LH, luteinizing hormone; ULN, upper limit of normal
From Kähler C, Hauschild A. Treatment and side effect management of CTLA-4 antibody therapy in metastatic melanoma. J Dtsch Dermatol Ges 2011;9:277–285.

GI and 4 weeks for liver toxicity, and the endocrine effects are apparent after an average of 9 weeks with improvement occurring 20 weeks later. The skin side effect is manifested as a maculopapular rash with associated pruritus. The most common GI side effect is diarrhea, which is usually mild but in some cases may be prolonged or severe and may worsen to colitis and the risk of bowel perforation. The hepatoxicity presents as an asymptomatic increase in transaminases or as immune-related hepatitis with fever and malaise. Hypophysitis (inflammation of the pituitary gland) is the presenting endocrine disorder, and it is a rare side effect of ipilimumab. Clinical symptoms of hypophysitis include headache, nausea, dizziness, vision disturbances, and weakness. Severe ophthalmologic (episcleritis and uveitis) side effects have also been reported with ipilimumab. It appears on average 2 months after beginning therapy and resolved within 1 week regardless of therapy. Fewer than 1% of patients experience neurologic side effects such as Guillain–Barré syndrome, sensory or motor neuropathy, or myasthenia gravis.[42]

Corticosteroids are the treatment of choice for ipilimumab-induced irAE. The administration of steroids to treat the side effects did not appear to result in decreased effectiveness of ipilimumab. Interestingly, there may be a correlation between immune-related adverse events and treatment success[42] (see Table 93–7 for side effects management).

Targeted Therapy with Vemurafenib

BRAF is an intermediary in signal transduction through the MAPK pathway. Activation of BRAF is associated with downstream activation of ERK, elevation of cyclin D1, and an increase in cellular proliferation.[43] BRAF is mutated in approximately 50% of melanomas, and 80% of these mutations are the *BRAF V600E* mutation.[12] Vemurafenib is an oral competitive small molecule serine threonine kinase inhibitor that functions by binding to the adenosine triphosphate binding domain of mutant BRAF.[43] **8** *Vemurafenib selectively targets the mutated BRAF V600E isoform and it is approved by the FDA as first-line therapy for unresectable stage IIIC or* *metastatic melanoma that is* BRAF V600 *mutation positive.* The Cobas 4800 BRAF V600 Mutation Test is the companion FDA-approved diagnostic tool used to test for the BRAF V600 mutation (see Table 93–4 for dosing).

A phase III clinical trial compared vemurafenib with dacarbazine in patients with previously untreated, unresectable stage IIIC or metastatic melanoma possessing the BRAFV600 E mutation.[44] Data analysis at 6 months showed that overall survival was 84% and median progression-free survival was 5.3 months for patients receiving vemurafenib compared with 64% overall survival and 1.6 months progression-free survival for patients receiving dacarbazine. The most common side effects associated with vemurafenib were arthralgia, photosensitivity, rash, diarrhea, nausea, fatigue, and alopecia. Some patients may require dose reduction for severe side effects, but doses lower than 480 mg twice daily are not recommended. Eighteen percent of patients in the phase III clinical trial reported at least one squamous cell carcinoma or keratoacanthoma. These lesions were excised, and no patients required dose modification of vemurafenib.[44] Rare side effects that led to discontinuation of the drug in some patients include liver function abnormalities, prolonged QTc, and retinal vein thrombosis.

OUTCOME EVALUATION

After diagnosis and treatment of skin cancer, the next phase of management is appropriate follow-up with the purpose of detecting recurrent disease or new malignant melanomas. Patients need to understand the importance of scheduling regular follow-up visits with the oncologist or dermatologist after the diagnosis and treatment of skin cancer. The NCCN Melanoma Guidelines recommend that patients with stage IA to IIA disease to be seen every 3 to 12 months for 5 years and then annually for life. Patients with stage IIB to IV

disease should be followed up every 3 to 6 months for 2 years, then every 3 to 12 months for 3 years, and then annually for life. Chest x-ray, computed tomography, or positron emission tomography scans every 6 to 12 months and annual brain magnetic resonance imaging may be considered for patients with stage IIB to IV disease. Routine radiologic screening for asymptomatic recurrence is not recommended after 5 years.[35]

Recurrence of MM occurs after complete resection in 30% of patients diagnosed with stage I to III disease, and 80% of the patients develop recurrence within 3 years of their diagnosis of primary MM.[45] Among patients whose melanoma recurred, the site of recurrence is local in 20% to 28% of patients; in 26% to 60%, recurrence is in regional lymph nodes; and 15 to 50% experience distant recurrence. The rate of recurrence detection by patients is reported to be 33% to 99%; thus, patients should be educated on how to perform self-examination of the skin and lymph nodes and the importance of ongoing sun protection measures.[45]

Patients who received immunotherapy for stage III or IV MM may experience fatigue and other chronic side effects. Develop a plan to order laboratory tests such as liver function tests, thyroid-stimulating hormone, and white blood cell count at baseline and on a weekly or monthly basis as indicated. Monitor and evaluate patients for side effects of IL-2, IFN, ipilimumab, and vemurafenib and educate patients on what to expect and how the side effects will be managed. Assess patients' psychological, physical, and social functioning. Counsel patients to contact the hospital's social service department or the American Cancer Society for assistance in dealing with the disease emotionally and recommend that patients consider attending support group meetings or talking to a counselor if or before they become overwhelmed with the diagnosis.

Patient Encounter, Part 5

Create a care plan for DM while she is receiving ipilimumab. The plan should include (a) the goal of therapy and (b) a plan related to dealing with the side effects of ipilimumab.

For how long should DM be monitored for side effects if they should occur?

What laboratory parameters need to be monitored?

What are the indications to discontinue ipilimumab?

What does it mean if DM develops new lesion in the first few weeks of therapy?

NONMELANOMA SKIN CANCER

EPIDEMIOLOGY AND ETIOLOGY

NMSC accounts for more than half of all newly diagnosed cancers in the United States each year, and it was estimated that more than 3.5 million new cases of BCC and SCC (in more than 2 million people) would be diagnosed in 2011.[1] The true prevalence of NMSC may be underestimated because it is treated in outpatient settings, and no formal reporting to cancer registries is required. The incidence rate of NMSC is increasing worldwide with a yearly rise of 3% to 8% since 1960.[46] BCC is the most common form of NMSC and comprises 75% of NMSC with SCC accounting for 20%.[15] The majority of NMSCs are curable, and the mortality rate is low; cure rates approach 98%, and the overall 5-year survival rate is greater than 95%.[47] Metastasis occurs in fewer than 0.1% of BCCs compared with an average of 3.6% of SCCs. Seventy-five percent of all NMSC deaths are attributed to SCC.[47] NMSC is associated with considerable morbidity related to functional and cosmetic deformity. In addition, it is an economic burden to the health care system because costs associated with NMSC treatment are estimated at approximately $426 million per year.[15]

RISK FACTORS

The risk of developing NMSC is multifactorial (Table 93–8). The most important risk factor for NMSC is UV radiation exposure, and data from epidemiologic studies indicate that greater cumulative lifetime sun exposure is associated with a higher risk of developing SCC, but intermittent and childhood sun-exposure correlates more with BCC.[46] Most cases of BCC are sporadic; however, it occurs frequently in the rare individuals with hereditary disorders such as basal cell nevus syndrome (also known as Gorlin's syndrome). It is also common in patients with genetic syndromes such as XP. The *patched* gene (*PTCH*), a tumor-suppressor gene, has been shown to be mutated in 68% of sporadic BCCs.[46] There is clear evidence linking defects of the immune system to the development of NMSC. For example, it is observed that

Table 93–8
Risk Factors for Developing Non-Melanoma Skin Cancer

	Basal Cell Carcinoma	Squamous Cell Carcinoma
Host Factors		
Phenotype	X	X
Fair skin		
Blonde or red hair		
Blue or green eyes		
Immunosuppression	X	X
Solid organ transplant		
HIV		
Chronic lymphocytic leukemia		
Lymphoma		
Increasing age	X	X
Environmental		
UV Radiation		
Sun	X	X
Ionizing	X	X
Tanning bed	X	X
Psoralen + UVA (PUVA)	X	
Arsenic	X	X
Photosensitizing drugs	X	X
Human papillomavirus	X	X
Smoking		X

UVA, ultraviolet A.

From Refs. 46 and 48.

patients receiving chronic immunosuppressant therapy for organ transplantation have a 65-fold increase in developing SCC and 10-fold increase in developing BCC.[48]

PATHOPHYSIOLOGY

NMSCs arise from epidermal keratinocytes and involve primarily squamous cells and basal cells of the epidermis and dermis skin layers. BCCs arise from interfollicular basal cells or keratinocytes in hair follicles or sebaceous glands.[48]

CLINICAL PRESENTATION, PROGNOSIS

BCC is characterized as circumscribed or diffuse, and within these two groups, it is further classified according to type, degree of differentiation, and depth of invasion (see Table 93–1).[14] The nodular BCC is the most common type of BCC followed by superficial BCC. The morpheaform BCC is the most aggressive subtype.[14] BCC has indolent growth characteristics with a very low metastatic and mortality rate.[46] Paradoxically, BCCs can cause extensive local destruction and significant disfigurement. Approximately 80% of BCCs occur on the head and neck. Superficial BCC occurs predominantly on the trunk. Early stage BCC is usually small, translucent or pearly with raised telangiectatic edges.[46] BCC may also appear as raised, yellowish-reddish lesions with a border resembling a string of pearls and telangiectasia. Dermatoscopy may distinguish between a benign and malignant lesion; however, clinical examination is usually sufficient for diagnosis of BCC. Depending on the size of the tumor, subtype, and treatment planned, a biopsy may be needed.

SCC usually presents on sun-exposed sites because of UVR damage to the skin. Unlike BCC, SCCs are preceded by premalignant lesions such as leukoplakia, actinic keratosis (AK) (a small papule that appears on areas of sun damage on the skin), or SCC in situ (Bowen's disease).[46] The rate of AK progression to SCC is 1% to 10% in 10 years and may be higher if a patient has more than five AKs.[46] Patients with Bowen's lesion present with slowly enlarging erythematous scaly or crusted plaques and have a 3% to 5% risk of progressing to SCC. A typical SCC lesion has an adherent crust and ill-defined edges; the first sign of malignant SCC is induration of the lesion. The rate of metastasis for SCC is 2% to 6% and may be as high as 10% to 14% in high-risk sites such as the ear and lip and 30% in the genital area.[47] Metastasis most commonly presents 1 to 2 years after diagnosis of the primary SCC with 80% of metastasis involving the regional lymph nodes.[49] The Skin Cancer Foundation (www.skincancer.org) provides images and descriptions of the various presentations of BCC and SCC.

High-risk factors for NMSC are outlined in Table 93–7. If a patient possesses these factors, he or she is at high risk for disease recurrence and subsequent metastasis. Patients with NMSC have a 10-fold increased risk of developing subsequent NMSC compared with the general population.[46]

Staging for NMSC uses the TNM staging system recommended by the American Joint Committee on Cancer. It is seldom done for patients with BCC because nodal and visceral metastasis is rare for this diagnosis.[46]

TREATMENT

⑨ *In patients diagnosed with BCC and SCC, the primary goal of therapy is to cure the patient and to prevent recurrence.* Although NMSC has a low mortality rate, morbidity related to tissue destruction, functional impairment, and disfigurement is a significant issue. Therefore, secondary goals of therapy for NMSC are preservation of function and restoration of cosmesis. The treatment options for NMSC involve surgery, pharmacologic therapy, or a combination of both. The choice of treatment depends on factors such as tumor size, the site of the lesion, patient comorbidities, and the histologic and clinical nature of the cancer.

Nonpharmacologic Therapy

▶ *Surgery*

Surgery is the primary treatment modality for all patients diagnosed with either BCC or SCC. Full-thickness ablative procedure in the form of surgical excision of the tumor along with a margin of normal tissue surrounding the tumor is the preferred method for high-risk tumors. Obtaining negative surgical margins is critical for cure and decreasing the risk of tumor recurrence. A margin of 4 to 5 mm in well-defined BCC and SCC ensures peripheral clearance in 95% of cases. Depending on the tumor size, degree of differentiation, and invasion of surrounding structures, larger margins of resection may be necessary.[46] The two most common surgical techniques used are electrodessication and curettage (ED&C) and Mohs' micrographic surgery (MMS). The indications of each of these procedures are described below.

Low-risk tumors defined as small, well-differentiated, and slow growing can be treated with superficial ablative techniques, including ED&C and cryotherapy.[46] ED&C is a simple, cost-effective technique that uses repeated cycles of using a curette to cut through malignant tissue followed by electrodesiccation, which involves the application of high voltage, low current to the skin, causing drying or desiccation of the tissue. ED&C is most appropriate for well-defined superficial lesions that are not located in areas with increased risk for metastasis. The disadvantage of this technique is that histologic confirmation of complete tumor removal is not possible.[48] This procedure is not recommended for treatment of recurrent disease, tumors of the face, and high-risk tumors.[48]

For high-risk NMSC or for tumors located in cosmetically or anatomically sensitive areas, MMS is the procedure of choice. The goal of this therapy is complete removal of the cancer with preservation of as much surrounding normal tissue as possible. MMS involves careful dissection, staining of frozen sections, and anatomic mapping of the tumor specimen. Sections are assessed immediately under the microscope by the surgeon, and the process is repeated until a tumor-free margin is attained. MMS cures 93% of primary NMSC and 90% to 94% of recurrent disease compared with 92% and 77% cure rate with standard excision for primary and recurrent disease, respectively.[49] Cure rates for all modalities decrease with the presence of high-risk features but are still superior with MMS.[49]

Cryotherapy is a procedure used primarily for smaller, low-risk NMSCs with clearly defined margins. It involves delivering liquid nitrogen at subzero temperatures as a spray or with a supercooled metal probe to destroy the malignant tissue in a single cycle or multiple cycles.[48] This technique can achieve comparable results to conventional surgery for well-differentiated, not too large, superficial tumors in older patients with BCC.[48] The procedure is contraindicated in the hair-bearing scalp, upper lip, and distal portion of lower leg because of delayed healing and high rates of recurrence.[48]

▶ *Radiation*

Radiation is not standard therapy for the treatment of skin cancer; however, there are circumstances in which radiation may be preferred. It may be offered to patients in whom surgery is not possible because the tumor is inoperable or surgery would lead to unacceptable cosmetic or functional impairment.[49] Radiation to the lip, ear, and nasal entrance for SCC may provide the best cosmetic and functional result. On the other hand, some patients may develop dyspigmentation, radiodystrophy, or telangiectasia at the site of radiation, resulting in poorer cosmetic outcomes. Radiation is contraindicated in treating BCC that recurred after radiotherapy. It should be used with caution in patients younger than 65 years because latent NMSC can develop after 15 to 20 years of radiation exposure.[46]

▶ *Photodynamic Therapy*

Photodynamic therapy (PDT) involves the topical application of a photosensitizing agent that is activated after exposure to a light source and causes tumor cell damage and death. The photosensitizer is converted to protoporphyrin IX after it is preferentially taken up by active tumor cells. Damage to cell membranes, organelles, and surrounding vasculature occurs when protoporphyrin IX is activated after exposure to a light source. Protoporphyrin IX has absorption bands at 408, 510, 543, 583, and 633 nm; therefore, blue light (corresponding to 408-nm band) and red light (corresponding to 633-nm band) are the most commonly used light source.[48] Blue light is used for superficial lesions because of its shorter wavelength and because it does not penetrate the skin as well as red light.[48]

δ-Aminolevulinic acid (ALA) and methyl aminolevulinate (MAL) are two photosensitizing agents that have FDA approval for the treatment of AK[50] (see **Table 93–9** for dosing). PDT has also been shown to be effective in the treatment of SCC in situ, but it is not indicated for SCC because of its extensive invasiveness and metastatic potential.[50] In patients with superficial BCC, MAL-PDT may be considered when surgery may result in suboptimal cosmetic outcomes or complications.[50] For patients with nodular BCC, MAL-PDT may be considered but not ALA-PDT.[48,50]

Pharmacologic Therapy

▶ *Fluorouracil*

Nonsurgical treatment is used frequently for superficial NMSCs. Topical 5-fluorouracil has been used for the treatment of dermatologic disorders for approximately 45 years, and it has FDA approval for the treatment of AK and superficial BCC[50,] (Table 93–4). Fluorouracil is available as solution and cream with strengths ranging from 1% to 5%. There is also a microsphere-encapsulated 0.5% cream that has reduced systemic absorption with enhanced skin retention to reduce systemic side effects. The microsphere formulation is applied only once a day, providing patient preference and convenience over the twice-daily application with the other formulations.[50] The optimal strength of fluorouracil is still under investigation, but the FDA has approved 2% to 5% cream or solution and 0.5% microsphere formulation for AK. For superficial BCC, only the 5% strength is FDA approved for this indication.[50] The most common side effects with topical fluorouracil are expected to occur within the initial 5 to 10 days of treatment, and it presents as erythema, irritation, burning sensation, pruritus, and pain along with hypo- or hyperpigmentation.[50] Patients also experience inflammatory

---

> **Table 93–9**
>
> **Topical Therapy for Nonmelanoma Skin Cancer**
>
> **Methyl Aminolevulinate Hydrochloride**
>
> **Actinic keratosis:** apply up to 1 g (half tube) of cream *topically* on lesion(s) during PDT session (2 sessions 1 week apart) followed by occlusive dressing for 3 hr (at least 2.5 hr and no more than 4 hr in duration) and then red light illumination for 7 to 10 min; maximum, 1 g (half tube) per treatment session
>
> **Aminolevulinic Acid**
>
> **Actinic keratosis:** apply *topically* to target lesion(s) on face or scalp and let dry and then repeat once; 14 to 18 hr later, gently rinse area with water and pat dry; follow by illumination from the BLU-U(R) Blue Light Photodynamic Therapy Illuminator; may retreat a second time after 8 wk
>
> Protect treated lesions from sunlight or prolonged or intense light for at least 40 hr by covering with light-opaque material; sunscreen will not protect against photosensitivity reactions caused by visible light.
>
> **Topical Fluorouracil**
>
> **Actinic keratosis:** cover lesions *topically* with 2% or 5% solution or cream twice daily for 2 to 6 weeks or with 0.5% microsphere formulation once daily for up to 4 weeks.
> **Superficial basal cell carcinoma:** cover lesions *topically* with 5% cream or solution twice daily for 3 to 6 weeks up to 10 to 12 weeks.
>
> **Imiquimod**
>
> **Superficial basal cell carcinoma on trunk, neck, or extremities when surgical methods are less appropriate and follow-up is assured: Aldara 5%** apply *topically* formulation once daily five times per week for 6 weeks; apply at bedtime and leave on skin for 8 hr

The doses presented here are general. Clinicians should refer to clinical trials to determine the specific dose based on the regimen the patient is receiving.

PDT, photodynamic therapy.

From National Comprehensive Cancer Network. Basal Cell and Squamous Cell Skin Cancer. Version 1. 2012, *http://www.nccn.org*.

---

reactions that include crusting, edema, and oozing. If the reactions are severe, the fluorouracil strength or frequency of application may be reduced. To reduce inflammation, topical steroids may be used concurrent with fluorouracil application and for 1 to 2 weeks after treatment.[50] Caution should be used in administering fluorouracil to patients with dihydropyrimidine dehydrogenase deficiency, an enzyme critical in the metabolism of fluorouracil, because increased toxicity may be observed.

▶ *Imiquimod*

Imiquimod is an immune-modulating agent that works by stimulating innate and cell-mediated immune responses. It has FDA approval for the treatment of AK and for when surgical procedure is not appropriate for superficial BCC located on the trunk, neck, or extremities and when follow up is assured. Imiquimod has been shown to have complete clearing of AK in 50% of patients and partial clearing in 75% of patients with AK compared with 5% for those treated with placebo. Cure rates for imiquimod 5% in patients with superficial BCC are greater than 90%. The response rate is much lower for nodular BCC at 75%; therefore, it should be used in these patients only if they are not able to undergo surgery, radiation, or cryotherapy and the tumor is small and in a low-risk area. Imiquimod is not recommended for the treatment of invasive SCC, but data for SCC in situ showed a 93% cure rate; thus, it may be considered for this patient population.

Imiquimod is available in 3.75% strength, which may be applied daily on larger areas of skin, the balding scalp, or the full face, and 5% strength, which may be used on areas of skin that are 25 cm^2 or smaller[50] (see Table 93–4). Imiquimod should be applied before bedtime and left on the skin for 6 to 10 hours. The most common side effects with imiquimod involve the area of application and present as erythema, pruritus, a burning or stinging sensation, and tenderness. Less commonly, hypopigmentation, fever, diarrhea, and fatigue may also occur. Temporary discontinuation of imiquimod and application of topical steroids may be necessary to alleviate the irritation symptoms. Imiquimod may be resumed at a decreased frequency after the symptoms have resolved.[50]

▶ *Vismodegib*

Genetic alterations in hedgehog signaling pathway cause loss of function of patch homolog 1 (PTCH1), which normally acts to inhibit signaling activity of Smoothened, a transmembrane protein involved in Hedgehog signal transduction. Vismodegib is a first-in-class, oral small molecule inhibitor of the Hedgehog signaling pathway; it binds to and inhibits Smoothened (SMO). Vismodegib is approved by the FDA for the treatment of adults with metastatic BCC or locally advanced BCC that has recurred following surgery or who are not candidates for surgery or radiation.

OUTCOME EVALUATION

BCC and SCC have excellent outcomes, with cure rates approaching 98%.[47] Recurrence of NMSC is around 30% to 50% during a 5-year follow-up, and 70% to 80% of recurrence develops within the first 2 years after initial therapy.[47] Therefore, it is crucial to advise patients to schedule routine follow-up visits with their dermatologist and to educate them about the value of sun protection and total-body skin self-examination. Patients with SCC at high risk for recurrence should be monitored every 1 to 3 months for the first year, every 2 to 4 months in the second year, every 4 to 6 months for years 3 to 5, and then every 6 to 12 months annually for life.[50] The follow-up recommendation for low-risk SCC patients is every 3 to 6 months for 2 years, every 6 to 12 months for year 3, and then annually for life. For patients with BCC, the recommendation is for physician follow-up with complete skin examination every 6 to 12 months for life.[50] Patients may be directed to the following websites that discuss skin cancer prevention: http://www.aafp.org/afp/2000/0715/p375.html, http://www.skincancer.org/Guidelines/, and http://www.aad.org/skin-care-and-safety/skin-cancer-prevention/skin-cancer-prevention.

Patients receiving topical agents such as fluorouracil or imiquimod should be educated to wash the treatment area with mild soap and water before applying the cream, use gloves to apply enough to cover the area with a 1-cm margin, and wash their hands thoroughly after each application. They should avoid sun exposure and be counseled to monitor for side effects such as pain, itching, and inflammation. They should consult their dermatologist if the side effects are intolerable.

Patient Care and Monitoring

1. Obtain a thorough patient medication history, both prescription and nonprescription, to prevent drug interactions with the current therapy the patient is receiving.

2. Obtain the appropriate baseline laboratory tests and determine a time interval for reevaluation of specific laboratory tests to determine toxicity.

3. Provide education on the side effects of therapy:
   - What to administer or take to prevent side effects
   - When to administer or take the medication to decrease side effects
   - Nonpharmacologic recommendations to minimize side effects
   - Drugs that may interact with therapy
   - Lab tests that need to be monitored on a regular basis
   - The parameters for discontinuing or holding therapy
   - If therapy is to be reinitiated, the new dose of therapy

4. Assess the patient for adverse drug reactions and drug–drug interactions.

5. Educate the patient on the signs and symptoms of infection.

6. Assess for changes in the patient's quality of life owing to side effects of drug therapy.

7. Educate the patient on measures that should be undertaken to limit sun exposure and prevent skin cancer.

8. Educate the patient on how to do skin self-examination for suspicious moles.

9. Educate the patient on follow-up recommendations after treatment for skin cancer is completed.

Abbreviations Introduced in This Chapter

AK	Actinic keratosis
BCC	Basal cell carcinoma
CNS	Central nervous system
CTL	Cytotoxic T lymphocyte
CTLA-4	Cytotoxic T-lymphocyte antigen-4
ED&C	Electrodessication and curettage
HDI	High-dose interferon-*a*2b
IDI	Intermediate-dose interferon-*a*2b
IFN	Interferon-*a*2b
IL-2	Interleukin 2
LDI	Low-dose interferon-*a*2b
LFT	Liver function test
MM	Malignant melanoma
MMS	Mohs' micrographic surgery
NMSC	Nonmelanoma skin cancer
SCC	Squamous cell carcinoma
SEER	Surveillance, Epidemiology, and End Results
SLN	Sentinel lymph node
SPF	Skin protection factor
SRS	Stereotactic radiosurgery
TMZ	Temozolamide
TNM	Tumor, node, metastasis
UVR	Ultraviolet radiation
WBRT	Whole-brain radiation therapy
XP	Xeroderma pigmentosum

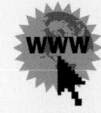

Self-assessment questions and answers are available at *http://www.mhpharmacotherapy.com/pp.html.*

REFERENCES

1. Siegel R, Ward E, Brawley O, Jemal A. Cancer statistics, 2011: The impact of eliminating socioeconomic and racial disparities on premature cancer deaths. CA Cancer J Clin 2011;61:212–236.
2. Narayanan D, Saladi R, Fox J. Ultraviolet radiation and skin cancer. Int J Dermatol 201049(9):978–886.
3. American Cancer Society. Cancer Facts and Figures. 2010, *http://www.cancer.org/acs/groups/content/@epidemiologysurveilance/documents/document/acspc-026238.pdf.*
4. Lasithiotakisa K, Petrakisa I, Garbeb C. Cutaneous melanoma in the elderly: Epidemiology, prognosis and treatment. Melanoma Res 2010;20:163–170.
5. Cho Y, Chiang M. Epidemiology, staging (new system), and prognosis of cutaneous melanoma. Clin Plastic Surg 2010;37:47–53.
6. Psaty E, Scope A, Halpern A, Marghoob A. Defining the patient at high risk for melanoma. Int J Dermatol 2010;49:362–376.
7. Gallagher R. Sunscreens in melanoma and skin cancer prevention. CMAJ 2005;173(3):244–245.
8. Rigel D, Russak J, Friedman R. The evolution of melanoma diagnosis: 25 years and beyond the ABCDs. CA Cancer J Clin 2010;60(5):301–316.
9. Palmieri G, Capone M, Ascierto M, et al. Main roads to melanoma. J Transl Med 2009;7:86.
10. Ko J, Velez N, Tsao H. Pathways to melanoma. Semin Cutan Med Surg 2010;29:210–217.
11. Wellbrock C, Hurlstone A. BRAF as therapeutic target in melanoma. Biochem Pharmacol 2010;80:561–567.
12. Ko J, Fisher D. A new era: Melanoma genetics and therapeutics. J Pathol 2011;223:241–250.
13. Fedorenko I, Paraiso K, Smalley K. Acquired and intrinsic BRAF inhibitor resistance in BRAF V600E mutant melanoma. Biochem Pharmacol 2011;82:201–209.
14. Netscher D, Leong M, Orengo I, et al. Cutaneous malignancies: Melanoma and nonmelanoma types. Plast Reconstr Surg 2011; 127:37e.
15. Neville J, Welch E, Leff D. Management of nonmelanoma skin cancer in 2007. Nat Clin Pract Oncol 2007;4(8):462–469.
16. Surveillance Epidemiology and End Results (SEER), National Cancer Institute. Surveillance Research Program [Internet]. Cited October 8, 2011. Available from: *http://seer.cancer.gov/statfacts/html/melan.html#survival.*
17. Balch C, Gershenwald J, Soong S, Thompson J, Atkins M, Byrd D, et al. Final version of 2009 AJCC melanoma staging and classification. J Clin Oncol 2009;27:6199–6206.
18. Spatz A, Batista G, Eggermontb A. The biology behind prognostic factors of cutaneous melanoma. Curr Opin Oncol 2010;22:163–168.
19. Ross M, Gershenwald J. Evidence-based treatment of early-stage melanoma. J Surg Oncol 2011;104:341–353.
20. Spanknebel K, Kaufman H. Surgical treatment of stage IV melanoma. Clin Dermatol 2004;22:240–250.
21. Tarhini A, Agarwala S. Management of brain metastases in patients with melanoma. Curr Opin Oncol 2004;16:161–166.
22. Rao N, Yu H, Trotti III A, Sondak V. The role of radiation therapy in the management of cutaneous melanoma. Surg Oncol Clin North Am 2011;20:115–131.
23. Bafaloukosa D, Gogas H. The treatment of brain metastases in melanoma patients. Cancer Treat Rev 2004;30:515–520.
24. Garbe C, Peris K, Hauschild A, et al. Diagnosis and treatment of melanoma: European consensus-based interdisciplinary guideline. Eur J Cancer 2010;46:270–283.
25. Middleton M, Grob J, Aaronson N., et al. Randomized phase III study of temozolomide versus dacarbazine in the treatment of patients with advanced metastatic malignant melanoma. J Clin Oncol 2000;18: 158–166.
26. Garbe C, Eigentler T, Keilholz U, et al. Systematic review of medical treatment in melanoma: Current status and future prospects. Oncologist 2011;16:5–24.
27. Chapman P, Einhorn L, Meyers M, et al. Phase III multicenter randomized trial of the dartmouth regimen versus dacarbazine in patients with metastatic melanoma. J Clin Oncol 1999;17:2745–27451.
28. Hauschild A, Agarwala S, Trefzer U, et al. Results of a phase III, randomized, placebo-controlled study of sorafenib in combination with carboplatin and paclitaxel as second-line treatment in patients with unresectable stage III or stage IV melanoma. J Clin Oncol 2009;27:2823–2830.
29. Pflugfelder A, Eigentler E, Keim U, et al. Effectiveness of carboplatin and paclitaxel as first- and second-line treatment in 61 patients with metastatic melanoma. PLoS One 2011;6(2):e16882.
30. Papadopoulos N, Bedikian A, Ring S, et al. Phase I/II study of a cisplatin-taxol-dacarbazine regimen in metastatic melanoma. Am J Clin Oncol 2009;32:509–514.
31. Kottschade L, Suman V, Amatruda T, et al. A phase II trial of nab-paclitaxel (ABI-007) and carboplatin in patients with unresectable stage IV melanoma. Cancer 2011;117:1704–1710.
32. Weber J. Immunotherapy for melanoma. Curr Opin Oncol 2011;23: 163–169.
33. Jonasch E, Haluska F. Interferon in oncological practice: Review of interferon biology, clinical applications, and toxicities. Oncologist 2001;6:34–55.
34. Mocellin S, Pasquali S, Rossi C, Nitti D. Interferon alpha adjuvant therapy in patients with high-risk melanoma: A systematic review and meta-analysis. J Natl Cancer Inst 2010;102:493–501.
35. National Comprehensive Cancer Network. Melanoma Guidelines [Internet]. Available from: *http://www.nccn.org.*

36. Hauschild A, Gogas H, Tarhini A, et al. Practical guidelines for the management of interferon-a-2b side effects in patients receiving adjuvant treatment for melanoma. Expert opinion. Cancer 2008;112:982–994.

37. Atkins M, Lotze M, Dutcher J, et al. High-dose recombinant interleukin 2 therapy for patients with metastatic melanoma: Analysis of 270 patients treated between 1985 and 1993. J Clin Oncol 1999;17: 2105–2116.

38. Buzaid A, Atkins M. Practical guidelines for the management of biochemotherapy related toxicity in melanoma. Clin Can Res 2001;7:2611–2619.

39. Schwartzentruber D. Guidelines for the safe administration of high-dose interleukin-2. J Immunother 2001;24:287–293.

40. Boasberg P, Hamid O, O'Day S. Ipilimumab: Unleashing the power of the immune system through CTLA-4 blockade. Semin Oncol 2010;37:440–449.

41. Hodi F, O'Day S, McDermott D, et al. Improved survival with ipilimumab in patients with metastatic melanoma. N Engl J Med 2010; 363:711–723.

42. Kähler C, Hauschild A. Treatment and side effect management of CTLA-4 antibody therapy in metastatic melanoma. J Dtsch Dermatol Ges 2011;9:277–285.

43. Luke J, Hodi F. Vemurafenib and BRAF inhibition: A new class of treatment for metastatic melanoma. Clin Can Res 2012; 18(1):9–14.

44. Chapman P, Hauschild A, Robert C, Haanen J, Ascierto P, Larkin J, et al. Improved survival with vemurafenib in melanoma with BRAF V600E mutation. N Engl J Med 2010;364:2507–2516.

45. Fields R, Coit D. Evidence-based follow-up for the patient with melanoma. Surg Oncol Clin North Am 2011;20:181–200.

46. Madan V, Lear J, Szeimies R. Non-melanoma skin cancer. Lancet 2010;375:673–685.

47. Kwasniak L, Garcia-Zuazaga J. Basal cell carcinoma: Evidence-based medicine and review of treatment modalities. Int J Dermatol 2011;50:645–658.

48. LeBoeuf N, Schmults C. Update on the management of high-risk squamous cell carcinoma. Semin Cutan Med Surg 2011;30:26–34.

49. Galiczynski E, Vidimod A. Nonsurgical treatment of non melanoma skin cancer. Dermatol Clin 2011;29:293–309.

50. National Comprehensive Cancer Network. Basal Cell and Squamous Cell Skin Cancer. Version 1. 2012 [Internet]. Available from: *http://www.nccn.org.*

94 Ovarian Cancer

Judith A. Smith

INTRODUCTION

Ovarian cancer is relatively uncommon but is the most fatal gynecologic cancer. The primary reason for the high mortality rate associated with ovarian cancer is the nonspecific symptoms and difficulty for early detection or screening that result in patients presenting with advanced disease. The majority of ovarian cancers are of epithelial origin. Each time ovulation occurs, the epithelium of the ovary is broken followed by occurrence of cell repair. The *incessant ovulation hypothesis* proposes that the increasing number of times the ovary epithelium undergoes cell repair is associated with the increasing risk of mutations and ultimately ovarian cancer. Ovarian cancer is often denoted as the "silent killer" because although the majority of patients will achieve a complete response (CR) to primary surgery and chemotherapy, disease

Patient Encounter 1, Part 1

BN, a 63-year-old active woman, has been in good health up until recently (about 4 months or so). She has had significant indigestion after meals and feels "nausea" frequently throughout the day. Her general physician completed upper and lower GI series, which both had normal results. One month later, her symptoms persisted, so her physician ordered a CT scan, which came back positive for an abdominal mass and thickening of the omentum. Of note, she has been married for 35 years with only one sexual partner in her lifetime. They have one child who is now 20 years old. Her first menses was when she was 12 years old and menopause was at age 57 years. She denies any alcohol or tobacco use.

Based on the CT scan, what additional diagnostic tests would be recommended to complete her workup?

In the context of BN, discuss why ovarian cancer is often denoted the "silent killer" and what needs to be done for earlier diagnosis of ovarian cancer.

Compare and contrast the treatment options for BN after her initial surgery.

recurs in more than 50% of patients in the first 2 years after completion of primary treatment. Ovarian cancers often cause metastasis via the lymphatic and blood systems to the liver, and/or lungs. Common complications of advanced and progressive ovarian cancer include ascites and small bowel obstruction (SBO), which often are associated with the end of life.

EPIDEMIOLOGY AND ETIOLOGY

In 2012, there were an estimated 22,280 new cases of ovarian cancer diagnosed with an associated 15,500 deaths.[1] Ovarian cancer remains the number one gynecologic killer and the fifth leading cause of cancer-related death in women. Despite great efforts and extensive research, there has been little change in the mortality rate associated with ovarian cancer over the past 4 decades. The high mortality rate associated with ovarian cancer can be attributed to its insidious onset of nonspecific symptoms, resulting in the majority of patients not presenting until the cancer has progressed to stages III to IV disease.

As with many other disease states, a significant risk factor associated with ovarian cancer is aging. A woman's risk increases as her age advances from 40 to 79 years, with the mean age at diagnosis being 63 years and the majority of women being diagnosed between 55 and 64 years.[2]

❶ *Ovarian cancer is a sporadic disease; fewer than 10% of ovarian cancers can be attributed to heredity.* The majority of cases of ovarian cancer occur sporadically, thus making it difficult to screen and prevent. Although hereditary accounts for fewer than 10% of all ovarian cancer cases, when there is a family history, it appears to be an important risk factor in the development of ovarian cancer in some patients.[3] If

one family member has a diagnosis of ovarian cancer, the associated risk is about 9%, but this risk increases to greater than 50% if there are two or more first-degree relatives (i.e., mother and sister) with a diagnosis of ovarian cancer or multiple cases of ovarian and breast cancer.[3] Both breast cancer activator gene 1 (*BRCA1*) and breast cancer activator gene 2 (*BRCA2*) mutations have been associated with ovarian cancer. However, *BRCA1* is more prevalent, being associated with 90% of hereditary and 10% of sporadic cases of ovarian cancer.[3] Hereditary breast and ovarian cancer (HBOC) syndrome is one of the two different forms of hereditary ovarian cancer and is associated with germline mutations in *BRCA1* and *BRCA2*.[3,4] The hereditary nonpolyposis colorectal cancer (HNPCC) or Lynch syndrome is a familial syndrome with germline mutations causing defects in enzymes involved in DNA mismatch repair, which has been associated with up to 12% of hereditary ovarian cancer cases.[4]

Although it is not clearly defined, hormones and reproductive history are associated with the risk of developing ovarian cancer. Nulliparity, infertility, early menarche, or late menopause is associated with an increased risk of ovarian cancer.[5]

Ovarian cancer is associated with certain dietary and environmental factors as well. A diet that is high in galactose and animal fat and meat increases the risk of ovarian cancer, whereas a vegetable-rich diet is suggested to decrease the risk.[6] Although controversial, exogenous factors such as asbestos and talcum powder use on the perineal area have also been suggested to increase the risk of ovarian cancer.[6]

Screening and Prevention

▶ *Screening*

Currently there is no standard effective screening tool that is adequately predictive or sensitive for early detection.

Pelvic examinations are effective for detecting obvious tumors present with a sensitivity of 67% for detecting all tumors; however, minimal or microscopic disease cannot be detected on physical examination.[8] Pelvic examinations are noninvasive and well accepted, but they do not usually detect ovarian cancer until it is in advanced stage. Therefore, routine pelvic examinations will not improve earlier diagnosis or help decrease overall mortality.[8]

Serum cancer antigen-125 (CA-125) is the most extensively evaluated tumor marker for ovarian cancer. Unfortunately, CA-125 is nonspecific, and elevated levels can be associated with a number of other gynecologic and GI-related diseases. CA-125 levels in a woman without ovarian cancer are static or tend to decrease over time, but levels associated with malignancy continue to rise.[9,10] **❷** *Because CA-125 is a nonspecific marker, there is no standard recommendation for routine screening for prevention of ovarian cancer.*

Transvaginal ultrasound (TVUS) is a component of current screening practices. Typically, it is used in combination with CA-125 or could be used as a single modality. TVUS releases sonic sound waves that create an image of the ovary to evaluated the size and shape and detect the presence of cystic or solid masses. Limitations of this technique are lack

ST, a 34-year-old woman who has been in good health, presents to your clinic complaining of constipation and abdominal pain. She explains to you that she is concerned about her cancer risk because her 54-year-old mother had breast cancer and underwent surgery and chemotherapy approximately 20 years ago after the birth of her third child. Last month, her cousin was diagnosed with stage I ovarian cancer and underwent TAH-BSO and had genetic testing completed that revealed she was BRCA1 positive. She is requesting to check her CA-125 level today in clinic.

Explain the association between hereditary and ovarian cancer risk.

Discuss why monitoring CA-125 is not used as a screening tool for ovarian cancer.

Describe the potential advantages and disadvantages of using oral contraceptives for prevention of ovarian cancer for ST.

colon cancer.[13] Although observational studies have linked these to a reduction of ovarian carcinoma risk, evidence is still lacking. Potential mechanisms include effects on normal ovulation shed and inhibition of ovulation.[13] Other pharmacologic interventions that have been suggested but are still being evaluated include vitamin A, lutein, and other carotenoids.[14-15] The protective effect of these agents is associated with inhibition of cell growth as well as promotion of cellular differentiation.[14]

Prophylactic Surgery Surgical strategies are also used in the prevention of ovarian cancer. The goal is to remove healthy, at-risk organs and ultimately reduce the risk of developing cancer. These surgeries include prophylactic **bilateral salpingo-oophorectomy** (BSO) or tubal ligation (see Fig. 94–1).

Prophylactic oophorectomy should be considered in any woman with a high risk of developing ovarian cancer.[16] The criteria for defining high risk includes any woman with two or more first-degree relatives with epithelial ovarian carcinoma; a family history of multiple occurrences of **nonpolyposis** colon cancer, endometrial cancer, and ovarian cancer; and a family history of multiple cases of breast and ovarian cancer.[17] Patients undergoing prophylactic oophorectomy need to be made aware that complete protection is not guaranteed.[17-19] Although a 67% reduction in risk has been shown, a potential 2% to 5% risk of peritoneal **carcinomatosis** remains.[18-20]

Tubal ligation is another procedure that has shown potential for risk reduction. However, it is not recommended as a sole procedure in prophylaxis. Protective effect may be attributable to the limiting exposure of the ovary to environmental carcinogens. A case-control study conducted by Narod and colleagues[19] found that a history of tubal ligation in *BRCA*-positive women was associated with a statistically significant 63% reduction in risk.

Genetic Screening Genetic screening is another option available for high-risk patients. Patients can be screened for genes such as *BRCA1* and *BRCA2* or other genes such as those associated with HNPCC or the HBOC syndrome.[3,21] Patient

of specificity and an inability to detect peritoneal cancer or cancer in normal size ovaries.[2,9] Most prevention clinics use this multimodality approach to screen high-risk women and recommend yearly ultrasound in combination with CA-125 blood test every 6 months.

▶ *Prevention*

Ovulation is considered a hostile event to the ovarian epithelium, making it more susceptible to damage and cancer. Interventions or conditions that limit the number of ovulations in a woman's reproductive history, including multiparity, have a protective effect.

Chemoprevention Investigational chemoprevention strategies used for ovarian cancer include oral contraceptives (OCs), aspirin and nonsteroidal anti-inflammatory agents, and retinoids, although none of these is currently accepted as standard treatment for the prevention of ovarian cancer. The theory that OCs reduce the number of ovulatory events is a basic explanation of its protective effect. Recent studies have suggested that progestin-induced apoptosis of the ovarian epithelium is responsible for the chemopreventive effect of OCs. The theory is that cells that have genetic damage but are not yet neoplastic have an increased chance of undergoing apoptosis.[11] OCs decrease the relative risk to less than 0.4% in women that use OCs for longer than 10 years.[12] However, the maximum protective effect of OC use in women with *BRCA* mutations has been reported to be between 3 and 5 years.[12] At the same time, OC use has been associated with an increased risk of breast cancer.[11,13] Thus, women with a family history of breast cancer would not be ideal candidates for this preventive measure.

Nonsteroidal antiinflammatory agents, aspirin, and acetaminophen have been suggested for use in the prevention of different cancers, especially hereditary nonpolyposis

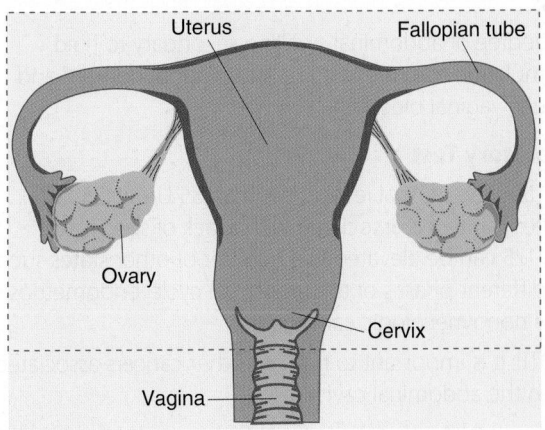

FIGURE 94–1. Diagram of female reproductive tract (uterus, fallopian tubes, ovaries, vagina). The *dashed line box* outlines what is removed during the total abdominal hysterectomy with bilateral salpingo-oophorectomy (TAH/BSO).

and family counseling and genetic counseling should be available for the patient and family to prepare and deal with the health and psychosocial implications of the genetic test results. Before this decision, the potential preventive options should be discussed, such as prophylactic BSO and/or total hysterectomy. Patients specifically positive for *BRCA1* or *BRCA2* may also consider a mastectomy to reduce the risk of breast cancer.[18-20] Cancer risk and patient's health need to be balanced, but typically surgery can be held off until after the childbearing years.[20,21]

PATHOPHYSIOLOGY

The three current theories are the incessant ovulation hypothesis, the pituitary gonadotropin hypothesis, and the chronic inflammatory processes hypothesis.[2] The incessant ovulation hypothesis proposes that the pathogenesis of ovarian cancer is connected to continual ovulation. Ovulation is considered a "hostile" event to the ovaries, perhaps with not enough time for adequate repair. Each time ovulation occurs, the ovary epithelium is disrupted, and cell damage occurs. Thus, repeated ovulations may lead to a greater number of repairs of the ovarian epithelium and

increase the possibility of aberrant repairs, mutation, and carcinogenesis.[22] The pituitary gonadotropin hypothesis associates the disease with elevations in gonadotropin and estrogen levels.[2] This leads to an increase in the number of follicles and therefore an increased risk of malignant changes. Finally, the chronic inflammatory processes may be involved with various environmental carcinogens to cause cancer.[2,13]

The three major pathologic categories of ovarian tumors include sex-cord stromal, germ cell, and epithelial. About 85% to 90% of ovarian cancers are of epithelial origin. Epithelial ovarian tumors are composed of cells that cover the surface of the ovary such as serous, mucinous, endometrioid, clear cell, and poorly differentiated adenocarcinomas. Germ cell tumors involve the precursors of ova with the most common type being dysgerminoma, which are most commonly diagnosed in women younger than the age of 40 years and generally have a better prognosis.[2] Sex-cord stromal tumors are indolent tumors that produce excess estrogen and androgens but also have a better overall prognosis.[2] Although the histologic type of the tumor is not a significant prognostic factor, it is important to know the histopathologic grade. Undifferentiated tumors are associated

Clinical Presentation and Diagnosis of Ovarian Cancer

General

③ *Ovarian cancer has often been denoted the "silent killer" because of the nonspecific signs and symptoms.* By the time symptoms become unrelenting and bothersome, patients most likely have advanced stage disease.

Symptoms

Patients may experience episodes or persistent symptoms such as abdominal pain, constipation or diarrhea, flatulence, urinary frequency, or incontinence.

Signs

The degree of abdominal swelling secondary to fluid accumulation may present like "pregnant abdomen" and irregular vaginal bleeding.

Laboratory Test

* *CA-125.* The normal level is less than 35 U/mL (35 kU/L). Note: This test is associated with a lack of specificity. CA-125 can be elevated in a number of other states such as different phases of the menstrual cycle, endometriosis, and nongynecologic cancers.
* NOTE: It is important to rule out other cancers associated with the abdominal cavity.
* *Carcinoembryonic antigen (CEA).* CEA is marker for colon cancer. A normal value is less than 3 ng/mL (3 mcg/L).
* *CA-19–9* is a marker for many GI tumors such as cholangiocarcinomas.

Chemistries With Liver Function Tests (LFTs)

* LFTs and serum creatinine might be suggestive of extent of disease. The majority of this information is needed to determine if patient is a surgical candidate. Laboratory study results should be within normal limits.

Complete Blood Count (CBC)

* Abnormalities in CBC are not associated with ovarian cancer; however, this information is needed to determine if patient is a surgical candidate. Laboratories should be within normal limits.

Other Diagnostic Tests

To characterize local disease, one or both of the following are completed:

* TVUS
* Abdominal ultrasound

To evaluate the extent of disease, only one of the following is completed:

* CT scan
* MRI
* PET scan

Chest x-ray is also often done as part of clearance for surgery.

with a poorer prognosis than lesions that are considered to be well or moderately differentiated.

Ovarian cancer is usually confined to the abdominal cavity, but spread can occur to the lung and liver and less commonly to the bone or brain. Disease is spread by direct extension, peritoneal seeding, lymphatic dissemination, or bloodborne metastasis. Lymphatic seeding is the most common pathway and frequently causes ascites.

Mechanisms of Resistance

The common mechanisms of drug resistance in ovarian cancer include (a) alteration of drug inactivation by agents such as glutathione S-transferase (GST), (b) enhanced DNA repair, (c) dysregulation of apoptotic pathways through activation of oncogenes or the loss of tumor suppressor gene functions, (d) *p*-glycoprotein (Pgp) multidrug resistance that leads to decreased drug accumulation, and (e) steroid xenobiotic receptor (SXR) that leads to enhanced drug metabolism. At this time, our understanding about the mechanism of drug resistance in ovarian cancer is incomplete and limited mostly to in vitro studies. Ongoing improvements in current technology have allowed development of in vivo studies to evaluate mechanisms of drug resistance in ovarian cancer. MDR has been one of the major limitations and is one of the ongoing challenges for the successful therapeutic treatment on recurrent and persistent ovarian cancer.

TREATMENT

Desired Outcomes

Health care providers use a multimodality approach, including surgery and chemotherapy, in initial treatment of patients with ovarian cancer with a curative intent, or restoring a normal life span. ❼ *Although the majority of patients initially achieve a complete response, disease will recur within the first 2 years in more than 50% of patients.*[2,23] CR to treatment is defined as no evidence of disease can be detected by physical examination or diagnostic tests and patient has a normalized CA-125.

The stage of disease at the time of diagnosis is the most important prognostic factor affecting overall survival in ovarian cancer patients.[24] The estimated 5-year survival rates of patients with localized, regional, distant, and unstaged ovarian cancer are 92.7%, 71.1%, 30.6%, and 26%, respectively.[24] The histology of the disease is another predominant prognostic factor influencing treatment outcomes. Clear cell and undifferentiated tumors do not respond as well to chemotherapy.[2] The extent of residual disease and tumor grade are also predictive of response to chemotherapy and overall survival.[2] There are other prognostic factors that may predict how well a patient will respond to adjuvant chemotherapy.

Generally, younger patients with a better performance status tolerate chemotherapy better than elderly patients. White women tend to have a worse prognosis and response to therapy compared to women of other ethnic backgrounds.[2,4,5]

The treatment goals shift when a patient presents with recurrent ovarian cancer. The desired outcomes focus on relief of symptoms such as pain or discomfort from ascites, slowing disease progression, and prevention of serious complications such as SBO. When a patient relapses, the prognostic factors are similar as after initial surgery except that the amount of time that has lapsed since the completion of chemotherapy should be considered to determine if drug resistance is emerging in the tumor. Recurrent platinum-sensitive ovarian cancer patients generally have a better prognosis than platinum-resistant patients.

Nonpharmacologic Therapy

❹ *Surgery is the primary treatment intervention for ovarian cancer.*[25-27] A total abdominal hysterectomy with BSO (TAH-BSO) (Fig. 94–1), omentumectomy, and lymphonectomy (or lymph node dissection) is the standard initial surgical treatment of ovarian cancer.[25] The objective of the surgery is to debulk the patient to less than 1 cm of residual disease remains. Residual disease less than 1 cm correlates with better CR rates to chemotherapy and better overall survival compared with patients with bulky residual disease (greater than 1 cm).[26,27] Indeed, the size of residual tumor masses after primary surgery is found to be another important prognostic factor in patients with advanced ovarian cancer.[27]

A thorough exploratory laparotomy is essential for the accurate staging of the patient.[25-27] ❺ *Ovarian cancer is staged surgically using the International Federation of Gynecology and Obstetrics (FIGO) staging algorithm* (Fig. 94–2). For certain patients with limited stage disease, surgery may be curative.

Other surgical procedures have been evaluated to improve overall survival. Debulking surgery is intended to relieve symptoms associated with complications such as SBO and help improve the patient's quality of life but does not have a curative intent. Interval debulking that is completed after two to three cycles of chemotherapy has not translated to an improved survival benefit. Often debated, the benefit of the "second-look laparotomy" to evaluate residual disease after the patient has completed chemotherapy remains controversial because it has been difficult to establish any impact on patients' overall survival. It has questionable benefit because although approximately 40% of patients with advanced disease have a negative second look, 50% still relapse.[2] The role of laparoscopic surgery is somewhat controversial for initial surgery but is more often considered in debulking of recurrent or advanced disease when the intent is palliative rather than curative.[25]

Pharmacologic Therapy

▶ First-Line Chemotherapy

❻ *After initial surgery, the gold standard of care is six cycles of taxane/platinum-containing regimen for patients with*

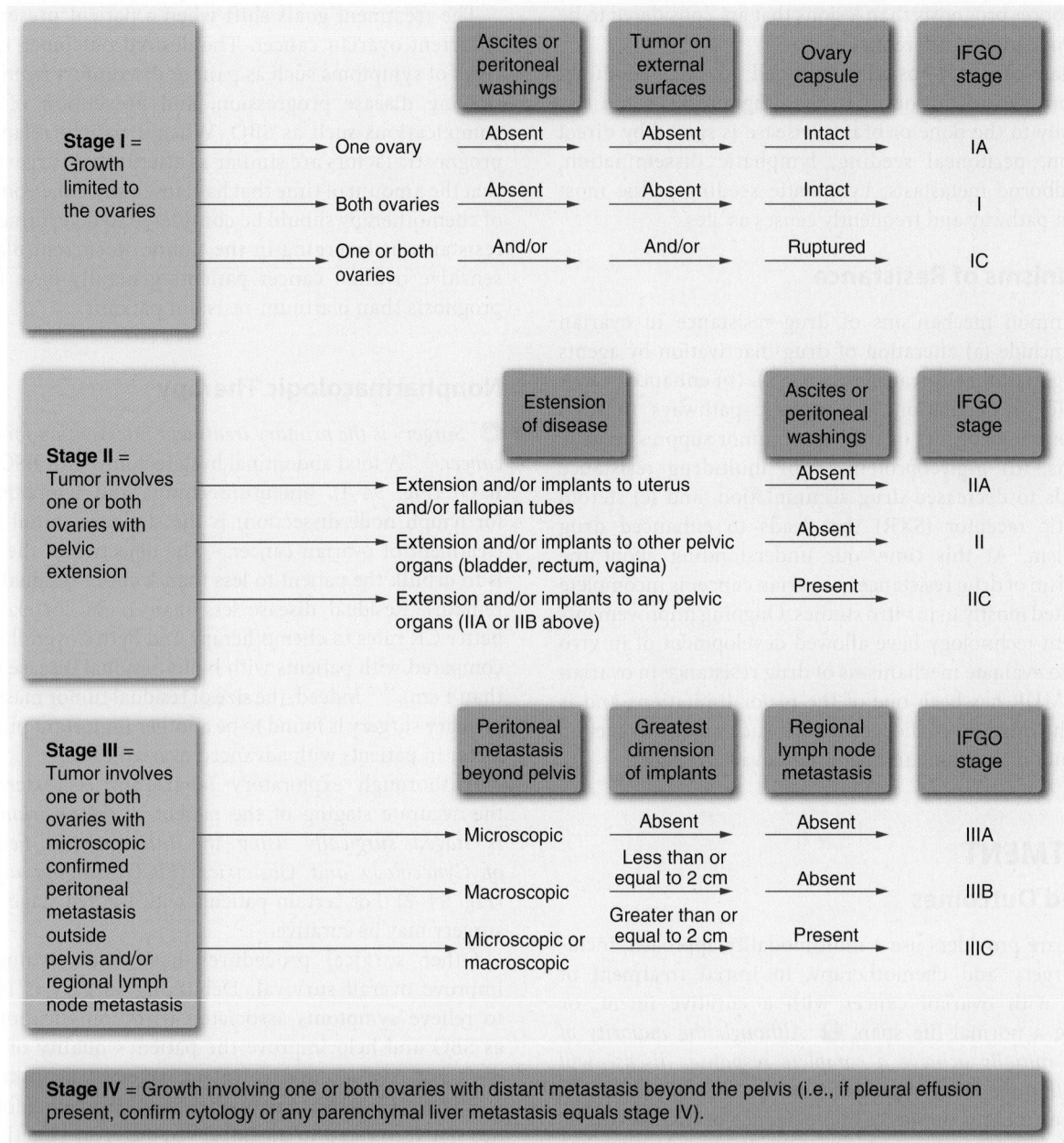

FIGURE 94–2. International Federation of Gynecology and Obstetrics (FIGO) staging algorithm for ovarian cancer.

advanced ovarian cancer.[28-30] Patients with limited disease will have observation alone after surgery (Fig. 94–3). Most often, paclitaxel is the taxane agent used in combination with carboplatin as the preferred platinum agent.[28-30] Depending on patients' preexisting comorbidities and how well they tolerate chemotherapy regimens, substitution with docetaxel or cisplatin might be considered. The route of administration should also be discussed. Although intravenous (IV) administration is often used, intraperitoneal (IP) administration has been shown to improve overall survival and should be considered for first-line treatment; however, patient selection for IP therapy is critical[31] (Table 94–1). Close monitoring of organ function, nausea/vomiting, myelosuppression, and neuropathies is necessary for all taxane/platinum regimens (Table 94–2).

▶ *Intraperitoneal Chemotherapy*

For more than 3 decades, numerous investigators have evaluated the IP route for administration of chemotherapy; however, it was not until the third report of an improvement in overall survival that brought its use to the forefront in the first-line setting.[32] The principal theory supporting IP administration is to increase drug concentration in the site of disease, specifically the abdominal cavity. Patient characteristics greatly influence response and tolerability of IP chemotherapy. To be selected to receive IP chemotherapy for first-line treatment of ovarian cancer, the patient should have tumor optimally debulked and no bowel resection with primary surgery, normal renal and liver function, younger age, and no significant comorbidities.

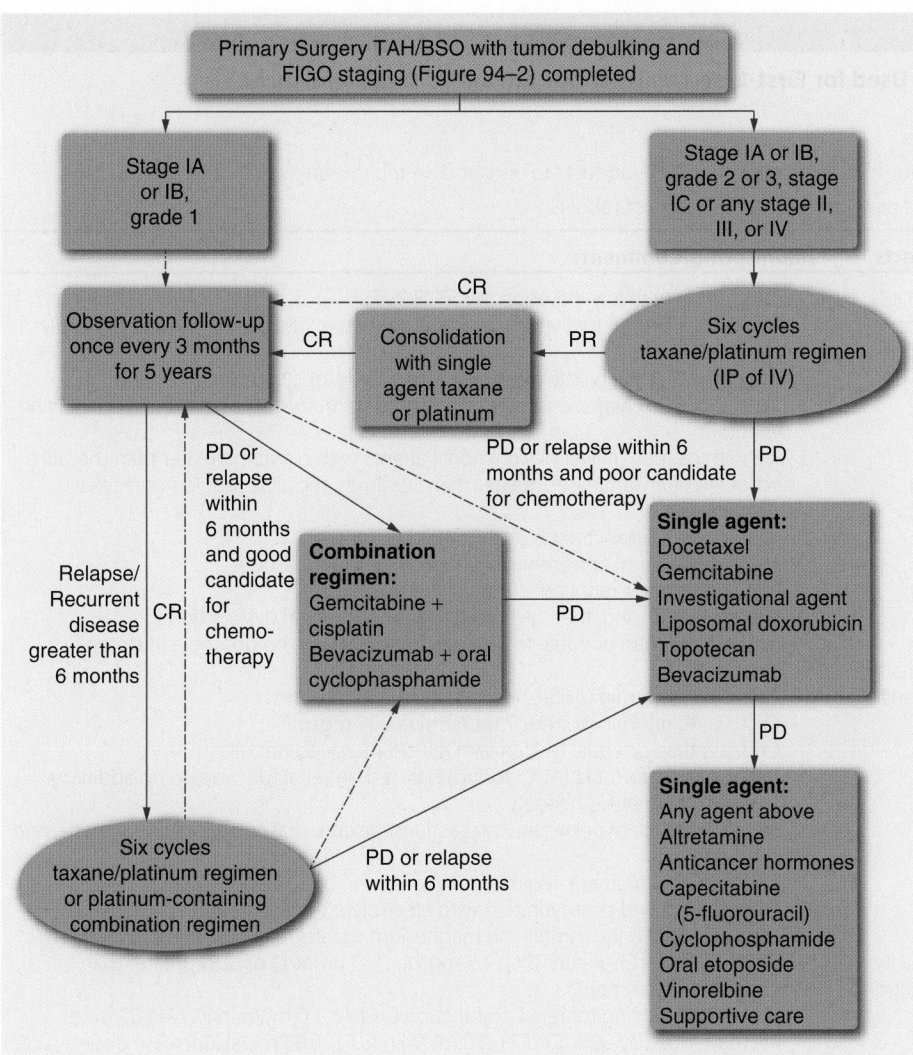

FIGURE 94–3. Summary of a chemotherapy treatment algorithm for epithelial ovarian cancer. (CR, complete response; FIGO, Federation of Gynecology and Obstetrics; PR, partial response; PD, progressive disease; TAH-BSO, total abdominal hysterectomy with bilateral salpingo-oophorectomy.)

Table 94–1

Summary of First-Line Chemotherapy Regimens for Advanced Ovarian Cancer

Gold standard first-line chemotherapy after initial surgery for treatment of ovarian cancer:
Paclitaxel 175 mg/m² IV infused over 3 hours + carboplatin AUC = 5 IV infused over 1 hour. Regimen is given once every 21 days × 6 cycles

Alternative first-line regimen: Paclitaxel IV with substitution of carboplatin IV with cisplatin IP and addition of paclitaxel IP therapy:
Patient selection is critical: must have optimally debulked disease (less than 1 cm) and no significant comorbidities; younger patients tolerate better
Day 1: paclitaxel 135 mg/m² IV infused over 24 hours + day 2: cisplatin 100 mg/m² IP infused over 1 hour + day 8: paclitaxel 60 mg/m² IP infused over 1 hour. Regimen is given once every 21 days × 6 cycles

Alternative first-line regimen: Dose density. Consider for patients with optimal debulking, no comorbidities, good performance status:
Paclitaxel 80 mg/m² IV infused over 1 to 3 hours once a week with carboplatin AUC = 6 IV infused over 1 hour on day 1 only of 21-day cycle.

Alternative first-line regimen: Substitution of cisplatin in place of carboplatin. Consider for patients experiencing difficulty with maintaining platelet counts:
Paclitaxel 135 mg/m² IV infused over 24 hours + day 2: cisplatin 75 mg/m² IV infused over 4 hours. Regimen is given once every 21 days × 6 cycles

Alternative first-line regimen: Substitution of docetaxel in place of paclitaxel. Consider for patients with preexisting or increased risk of neuropathies:
Docetaxel 75 mg/m² IV infused over 1 hour + carboplatin AUC = 5 IV infused over 1 hour. Regimen is given once every 21 days × 6 cycles

AUC, area under the curve; IV, intravenous.

Table 94–2

Summary of Chemotherapy Agents Used for First-Line Treatment of Advanced Ovarian Cancer

Mechanism of Action of First-Line Agents

Platinum analogues: Produce intra- and interstrand cross-links and DNA adducts to disrupt DNA replication

Taxanes agents: Stabilize microtubules and prevents depolymerization of tubulin

Agent	Common Adverse Effects	Monitoring/Comments
Paclitaxel	Peripheral neuropathy (DLT), nausea/vomiting, alopecia, hypersensitivity reactions	1. Use caution with any elevation in AST (SGOT) 2. Give proper dosing for liver dysfunction. At least a 50% dose reduction generally recommended 3. Do not give if total bilirubin is greater than 5 mg/dL (85 µmol/L) 4. Premedicate for hypersensitivity reactions: dexamethasone, diphenhydramine, and cimetidine
Docetaxel	Neutropenia (DLT) hyperlacrimation, fluid retention, nail disorders, myelosuppression	1. Use with caution in liver dysfunction. Patients with bilirubin greater than the ULN and/or liver transaminases greater than 1.5 times, the ULN should not receive docetaxel 2. Do not give if biliary tract is obstructed 3. Premedicate for hypersensitivity reactions: dexamethasone

Carboplatin	Myelosuppression (DLT), nephrotoxicity, nausea/vomiting, electrolyte wasting, diarrhea, stomatitis, hypersensitivity reactions	1. Prehydration not required
		2. If using BSA dosing, then give proper dosing for renal dysfunction
		   CrCl greater than or equal to 60 mL/min (1.00 mL/s): no dosage adjustment needed.
		   CrCl 41–59 mL/min (0.68-0.99 mL/s): give 250 mg/m^2
		   CrCl 16–40 mL/min (0.26-0.67 mL/s): give 200 mg/m^2
		   CrCl less than or equal to 15 mL/min (0.25 mL/s): do not give
		   NOTE: Calvert formula (AUC dosing) is based on renal function, so no additional dose adjustment is needed
		3. Premedicate for hypersensitivity reactions: dexamethasone, diphenhydramine, and cimetidine
		4. Appropriate antiemetic regimen for prevention of acute and delayed nausea

Cisplatin	Neurotoxicity (DLT), nausea/vomiting, ototoxicity, nephrotoxicity, myelosuppression, electrolyte wasting, diarrhea	1. Prehydration and posthydration with electrolyte replacement (i.e., potassium chloride 10 mEq [10 mmol] and magnesium sulfate 16 mEq [8 mmol]) required 2. Do not use if SrCr greater than 1.5 mg/dL (133 µmol/L) or BUN greater than 25 mg/dL (8.9 mmol/L) 3. Give proper dosing for renal dysfunction CrCl 46–60 mL/min (0.77–1.00 mL/s): decrease dose by 50%. CrCl 31–50 mL/min (0.51–0.83 mL/s): decrease dose by 75%. CrCl less than or equal to 30 mL/min (0.50 mL/s): do not use 4. Appropriate antiemetic regimen for prevention of acute and delayed nausea

AST, aspartate aminotransferase; AUC, area under the curve; BSA, body surface area; BUN, blood urea nitrogen; CrCl, creatinine clearance; DLT, dose-limiting toxicity; SrCr, serum creatinine; ULN, upper limit of normal.

If IP therapy is going to be considered, the placement of an IP catheter should occur at the time of surgery unless otherwise contraindicated. During IP administration, chemotherapy is delivered to the peritoneal space in 1 L of normal saline (NS) that has been warmed followed by another liter of NS to enhance drug distribution as tolerated.[33,34] In addition, it is recommend to alternate the position of patient every 15 minutes for the first hour after drug IP administration to ensure proper distribution.[33,34] The current standard IP regimen includes the administration of paclitaxel IV on day 1 followed by cisplatin IP on day 2 and then paclitaxel IP on day 8 given on a 21-day cycle for a total of six cycles (see Table 94–2). The most common toxicities associated with IP administration include abdominal pain, myelosuppression, neurotoxicity, and catheter-related infections. The substitution of carboplatin IP in place of cisplatin remains investigational and should not be recommended outside a clinical trial protocol.

▶ Neoadjuvant Chemotherapy

Neoadjuvant chemotherapy is first-line treatment for patients who are poor surgical candidates or patients with bulky or significant tumor burden.[23] For patients who are poor surgical candidates because of significant comorbidities, a combination of taxane with platinum agent is administered every 21 to 28 days as tolerated with the intent to relieve symptoms and slow progression of disease. In some cases, especially in elderly patients, single-agent carboplatin is used as palliative treatment instead. Chemotherapy alone has not been curative for patients with advanced ovarian cancer.[23]

In patients with bulky disease or significant tumor burden, neoadjuvant chemotherapy can be used to decrease tumor burden to increase the likelihood of optimal tumor debulking during surgery.[31] Typically, three cycles of the standard combination taxane/platinum regimen is administered once every 21 days. After surgery, patient will receive another three to six cycles depending on their response to chemotherapy.

▶ Consolidation and Maintenance Chemotherapy

Consolidation chemotherapy is the addition of cycles of the taxane/platinum regimen or the addition of single-agent platinum or single taxane after completion of first-line chemotherapy.[36] If the tumor has a partial response (PR) to first-line chemotherapy evident by a significant decline in CA-125 by greater than 50% presurgery level and/or tumor regression or decrease in size, then cancer is still considered taxane/platinum sensitive. Additional cycles of chemotherapy are given until CR is achieved (see Fig. 94–3). Maintenance chemotherapy is similar to consolidation chemotherapy except maintenance chemotherapy is given to patients who have achieved a clinically CR.[37] Maintenance chemotherapy is used to hopefully extend progression-free and overall survival by eliminating any microscopic disease present after completion of primary chemotherapy.

▶ Agents Used in First-Line, Consolidation, and Maintenance Chemotherapy of Ovarian Cancer

Taxanes

Paclitaxel. Paclitaxel is a taxane that is naturally derived from the bark of the yew tree. Paclitaxel is cytotoxic to cells by stabilizing microtubules to prevent depolymerization of tubulin, causing cell cycle arrest in the M-phase. The two most common regimens used in ovarian cancer is a 3-hour infusion of 175 mg/m^2 or a 24-hour infusion of 135 mg/m^2. In addition, dose-dense paclitaxel 80 mg/m^2 once a week is also becoming more common in practice.[35]

Paclitaxel is a water-insoluble drug, so an alcohol-based diluent, Cremophor, is used in the formulation and is associated with increase hypersensitivity reactions. Patients are pretreated with an H$_2$ blocker, diphenhydramine, and steroids. The dose-limiting toxicity (DLT) of paclitaxel is infusion dependent. For shorter infusion (e.g., 3 hours), the DLT is neuropathy, and for longer infusions, the DLT is myelosuppression. Additional common adverse effects can be found in Table 94–2.

Docetaxel. Docetaxel is another agent in the class of taxanes with a similar mechanism of action as paclitaxel but with differences in affinity for α-tubulin–binding sites and is hence more potent.

Because the experience with docetaxel in the treatment of ovarian cancer is limited, it is often considered a second-line option. However, ongoing clinical trials are comparing the efficacy and toxicity of docetaxel with paclitaxel in the combination with platinum agents for first-line treatment of ovarian cancer.[38] The dose of docetaxel typically used is 75 mg/m^2 given every 21 days and is reasonably well tolerated. To avoid severe fluid retention or hypersensitivity reactions, patients are premedicated with corticosteroids. The DLT associated with docetaxel primarily is neutropenia. Additional common adverse effects can be found in Table 94–2.

Platinum Analogues

Cisplatin. Cisplatin forms Platinum (Pt) DNA adducts that intercalate the DNA interrupting DNA synthesis.

The typical dose of cisplatin used for the treatment of ovarian cancer is 75 mg/m^2 when administered via the IV route or 100 mg/m^2 if administered via the IP route. Because cisplatin is nephrotoxic, regardless of route of administration, prehydration with 1 to 3 L of NS with replacement of electrolytes such as magnesium and potassium is required, which often requires an inpatient stay. The DLT of cisplatin is neurotoxicity that is nonreversible in many patients. Cisplatin is highly emetogenic but can be minimized with seratonin (5HT$_3$) antagonists and neurokinin 1 (NK1) receptor antagonist plus dexamethasone. Additional common adverse effects can be found in Table 94–2.

Carboplatin. Carboplatin has a similar mechanism of action as cisplatin, forming Pt-DNA adducts that intercalate the DNA interrupting DNA synthesis to ultimately cause cell death.

Carboplatin dose is determined using the Calvert formula: *Carboplatin dose (mg) = Target AUC * (CrCl + 25)*. The Calvert formula uses the calculated glomerular filtration rate (GFR) for the estimated creatinine clearance (CrCl) in this equation to individualize the dose and minimize dose-related toxicity. For the first-line treatment of ovarian cancer, the target area under the curve (AUC) is 5 to 7.5. Individualized dosing has decreased the incidence and degree of nephrotoxicity associated with carboplatin compared with cisplatin, eliminating the need for intensive prehydration, thus allowing for outpatient administration. Myelosuppression, primarily thrombocytopenia, is the DLT of carboplatin. Additional common adverse effects can be found in Table 94–2.

Recurrent Chemotherapy

In the recurrent setting, platinum sensitivity of the tumor is assessed first. If recurrence occurs in less than 6 months or disease progresses while the patient is receiving a platinum-based regimen, the cancer is considered platinum resistant (see Fig. 94–3). These parameters are also used to determine if tumors are taxane sensitive or resistant. However, patients resistant to paclitaxel may still respond to docetaxel.[39] If the treatment goal is palliative care, then often single therapy will be used, but curative care typically is an aggressive combination regimen (see Fig. 94–3 and Table 94–3). Sometimes an investigational agent may achieve responses equivalent or surpassing standard therapy, and should be considered for most patients.

▶ Platinum Sensitive

In patients who experienced a CR to first-line chemotherapy and have had greater than a 6-month platinum-free interval, retreatment with a platinum-containing regimen is appropriate. Current National Comprehensive Cancer Network (NCCN) guidelines recommend the combination of carboplatin with gemcitabine, liposomal doxorubicin, or

Table 94–3

Summary of Combination Chemotherapy Regimens Used for Treatment of Recurrent Ovarian Cancer

Drug(s)	Regimen Dosing	Drug Monitoring Comments[b]
Combination Regimens		
Platinum Sensitive		
Paclitaxel and carboplatin	175 mg/m² IV (3-hr infusion) AUC 5–7.5 IV every 21 days	• Monitor closely for hypersensitivity reactions
Paclitaxel and cisplatin	135 mg/m² IV (24-hr infusion) 75 mg/m² IV	• Monitor closely for hypersensitivity reactions
Docetaxel and carboplatin	75 mg/m² IV AUC 5 IV every 21 days	• Monitor closely for hypersensitivity reactions
Gemcitabine and carboplatin	800 mg/m² IV days 1 and 8 AUC 5 IV day 1 every 21 days	• Monitor platelet counts closely • Monitor closely for hypersensitivity reactions
Liposomal doxorubicin and carboplatin	30 mg/m² IV over 1–3 hr AUC 5 IV every 28 days	• Monitor closely for hypersensitivity reactions • Liposomal doxorubicin infusion start over 3 hr and decrease to 1 hr as tolerated • Counsel patient for PPE prevention
Platinum-Resistant[a]		
Gemcitabine and cisplatin	1000 mg/m² IV days 1 and 8 40 mg/m² IV days 1 and 8 every 21 days	• Monitor renal function closely • Monitor ANC closely, consider primary use of growth factor • Monitor closely for hypersensitivity reactions
Cyclophosphamide and bevacizumab	50 mg PO once daily 10 mg/kg IV once every 2 weeks every 28 days (continuous)	• Monitor for hypertension; hold therapy blood pressure greater than 140/90 mm Hg • Monitor urine-to-creatinine baseline and every two cycles; hold therapy if the ratio is greater than 2 • Use caution in patients with history of thrombosis

[a]*Platinum resistance* = disease progression while on platinum agent or recurrence within 6 months of completion of platinum-based therapy.

[b]See Table 94–2 for specific monitoring parameters.

ANC, absolute neutrophil count; AUC, area under the curve; IV, intravenous; PO, oral; PPE, palmar-plantar erythrodysesthesia.

paclitaxel for the treatment of platinum-sensitive recurrent ovarian cancer with a curative intent[31,40,41] (see Table 94–3). However, in patients who are unable to tolerate additional combination chemotherapy regimens, carboplatin alone or any one of the second-line agents would be appropriate[42] (see Table 94–2).

▶ Platinum Resistant

Recurrent or persistent ovarian cancer after platinum-based regimens has a discouraging prognosis. Second-line agents have not been successful to date, but any active agent that has not been used during initial treatment is available to use. ⑧ *Single-agent chemotherapy is standard practice for recurrent platinum-resistant ovarian cancer.* However, two combination regimens have demonstrated promising activity in the recurrent setting: (a) gemcitabine plus cisplatin because gemcitabine modulates platinum resistance allowing it to regain its cytotoxic activity, and (b) bevacizumab with metronomic oral cyclophosphamide.[43,44] Active agents include altretamine (formerly hexamethylmelamine), anastrozole, capecitabine (5-fluorouracil), cyclophosphamide, docetaxel, gemcitabine, liposomal doxorubicin, oral etoposide, vinorelbine, topotecan, bevacizumab, or investigational agents. Numerous ongoing

investigational studies are evaluating the benefit of addition of bevacizumab with other cytotoxic agent to improve outcomes in the recurrent ovarian cancer setting (see Fig. 94–3). ⑧ *Because the efficacy of the agents is similar, the selection of agent for treatment of recurrent platinum-resistant ovarian cancer is dependent upon residual toxicities, clinician preference, and patient convenience.* Table 94–4 gives a short summary of the adverse effects and monitoring parameters for chemotherapy agents commonly used for the treatment of recurrent ovarian cancer.

OUTCOME EVALUATION

Overall survival is impacted by success of initial surgery to debulk tumor to less than 1 cm of disease and response to first-line chemotherapy. The CA-125 level should be monitored with each cycle, and at least a 50% reduction in CA-125 after four cycles of taxane/platinum chemotherapy is related to an improved prognosis. Patients who achieve CR should have follow-up examinations once every 3 months, including CA-125, physical examination, and pelvic examination, and appropriate diagnostic scans (i.e., computed tomography [CT], magnetic resonance imaging

Table 94–4

Summary of Chemotherapy Single-Agent Regimens Used for Treatment of Progressive and Recurrent Platinum-Resistant Ovarian Cancer

Agent	Dose	Response Rate (%)	Common Adverse Effects	Monitoring/Comments
Docetaxel	75 mg/m² IV over 1 hour repeat every 21–28 days vs.	22	Neutropenia (DLT) hyperlacrimation, fluid retention, nail disorders, myelosuppression	1. Premedicate for hypersensitivity reactions with dexamethasone
	30–40 mg/m² IV over 1 hr once every week	NR		2. Use with caution in liver dysfunction. Patients with bilirubin greater than the ULN and/or liver transaminases greater than 1.5 times the ULN should not receive docetaxel
				3. Do not give if the biliary tract is obstructed
Gemcitabine	800 mg/m² IV infused over 30 minutes once a week on days 1, 8, and 15 followed by 1 week of rest	13.9–27	Myelosuppression (DLT), flulike symptoms, headache, somnolence, nausea/vomiting, stomatitis, diarrhea, constipation, rash	1. Use with caution in renal or liver dysfunction. No specific guidelines available
Liposomal doxorubicin	40 mg/m² IV infused over 3 hours cycle 1 and 2; then infused over 1 hr; thereafter repeat every 28 days	12.3–18	Myelosuppression, stomatitis, mucositis, alopecia, flushing, shortness of breath, hypotension, headaches, cardiotoxicity, hand–foot syndrome	1. Give proper dosing for liver dysfunction; total bilirubin 1.2–3 mg/dL (21–51 µmol/L): reduce dose by 50%; total bilirubin greater than or equal to 3 mg/dL (51 µmol/L): reduce dose by 75%
				2. Do not give if total bilirubin is greater than 5 mg/dL (86 µmol/L)
Topotecan	1.5 mg/m² IV infused over 30 minutes on days 1, 2, 3, 4, and 5; repeat every 21 days OR	6.5–17	Myelosuppression (DLT), nausea/vomiting, diarrhea, stomatitis, abdominal pain, alopecia, AST/ALT elevation	1. Give proper dosing for renal dysfunction; CrCl 40–60 mL/min (0.67–1.00 mL/s): no dosage adjustment needed; CrCl 20–39 mL/min (0.33–0.66 mL/s): reduce dose by 50%
	4 mg/m² IV infused over 30 minutes once a week for 3 consecutive weeks followed by 1-week rest	31		2. Do not give if CrCl less than 20 mL/min (0.33 mL/s)
Altretamine (Hexalen)	260 mg/m² PO daily for 14–21 days; repeat every 28 days	9.7	Nausea/vomiting, diarrhea, abdominal cramping, myelosuppression	1. Monitor for potential CYP450 drug interactions
Capecitabine	1,800–2,500 mg/m² PO as divided dose twice daily for 14 consecutive days followed by 1 week of rest	29	Myelosuppression, hand–foot syndrome, nausea/vomiting, edema, stomatitis, diarrhea, cardiotoxicity, rash	1. Monitor for PPE and recommend regular use of lotions on hands and feet
				2. Use with caution in renal dysfunction; CrCl greater than or equal to 51 mL/min (0.84 mL/s): no dose adjustment; CrCl 30–50 mL/min (0.50–0.83 mL/s): reduce dose by 25%; CrCl less than 30 mL/min (0.50 mL/s): do not give
				3. Use with caution in liver dysfunction; no specific guidelines available
Etoposide	50 mg/m²/day PO in divided doses given daily for 3 consecutive weeks followed by 1 week of rest	18	Myelosuppression, nausea/vomiting, anorexia, alopecia, headache, fever, hypotension	1. Give proper dosing for liver dysfunction; total bilirubin 1.5–3 mg/dL (26–51 µmol/L): decrease dose by 50%; total bilirubin 3–5 mg/dL (51–86 µmol/L): decrease dose by 75%
				2. Do not give if total bilirubin is greater than 5 mg/dL (85 µmol/L)
				3. Give proper dosing for renal dysfunction; CrCl 60–45 mL/min (1.00–0.75 mL/s): reduce dose by 15%; CrCl 44–30 mL/min (0.74–0.50 mL/s): reduce dose by 20%; CrCl less than 30 mL/min (0.50 mL/s): reduce dose by 25%
Letrozole	2.5 mg once daily	15	Headache, nausea, dyspepsia, skin rash	1. No protective effect on bone; recommend calcium supplementation
Tamoxifen	20 mg PO twice a day continuously until PD	10	Thrombocytopenia, anemia, thromboembolism, hot flashes, decreased libido, nausea/vomiting	1. Protective effect on bone and lipids
				2. Increased risk for endometrial cancer

(Continued)

Table 94–4

Summary of Chemotherapy Single-Agent Regimens Used for Treatment of Progressive and Recurrent Platinum-Resistant Ovarian Cancer (*Continued*)

Agent	Dose	Response Rate (%)	Common Adverse Effects	Monitoring/Comments
Vinorelbine	30 mg/m^2 IV infused over 15 minutes on days 1 and 8; repeat every 21 days	29	Constipation, neutropenia, anemia, thrombocytopenia, neurotoxicity	1. Consider bowel regimen to prevent constipation
Bevacizumab	15 mg/kg IV infused over 30–90 minutes every 21 days		Hypertension, proteinuria, infusion-related reactions, fluid retention, increase risk of thrombosis, myelosuppression	1. Monitor urine–to-creatinine baseline and every two cycles; hold therapy if ratio greater than 2 2. Use caution in patients with a history of thrombosis

CrCl, creatinine clearance; DLT, dose-limiting toxicity; IV, intravenous; NR, not reported; PD, progressive disease; PO, oral; PPE, palmar-plantar erythrodysesthesia; ULN, upper limit of normal.

Patient Encounter 1, Part 2: Completion of Primary Treatment

BN was optimally debulked. After surgery, she completed four cycles of paclitaxel IV plus cisplatin IP and IP paclitaxel on day 8 given every 21 days but then had to discontinue IP therapy because of catheter complications. To complete adjuvant chemotherapy she was give two cycles of paclitaxel IV plus carboplatin IV. Her CT scan findings were negative and CA-125 had decreased but was still above the normal range (48 U/mL [48 kU/L]) upon completion of her chemotherapy. She feels great and has no symptoms of ovarian cancer at this time.

Compare and contrast the possible advantages and disadvantages of consolidation chemotherapy versus "watchful waiting" for this patient.

Describe the role of second-look surgery for this patient.

Explain the challenges of using bevacizumab for consolidation treatment in this patient.

[MRI], positron emission tomography [PET] scan) should be evaluated for the detection of disease. Side effects while evaluating patient for resolution of any residual chemotherapy include neuropathies, nephrotoxicity, ototoxicity, myelosuppression, or nausea/vomiting. Younger patients with an active menstrual cycle before surgery will encounter "surgical menopause" and often experience intense hot flushes. Because there are concerns about potential of hormones in the pathogenesis of ovarian cancer, the use of hormone replacement therapy is controversial. The use of phytoestrogen supplements, such as black cohosh or soy, is also controversial. An effective alternative has been the use of the class of serotonin reuptake inhibitors such as venlafaxine controlled-released once daily.

In the PD or recurrent setting, CA-125 levels should still be monitored with each cycle, but no change in therapy is recommended until after minimum of three cycles of chemotherapy. In addition, appropriate diagnostic scans (i.e., CT scan, MRI, or PET scan) should be evaluated once every three cycles. Patients should also have routine physical examinations with each cycle of chemotherapy to evaluate for any physical toxicity associated with chemotherapy such as neuropathies, fluid retention, palmar-plantar erythrodysesthesia, myelosuppression, or nausea/vomiting.

Unfortunately, most patients will eventually progress through all chemotherapy options, and supportive care measures should be provided to maintain patient comfort and quality of life. Common complications while developing a plan for treatment of advanced or progressive ovarian cancer include ascites, uncontrollable pain, and SBO. ⑨ *Precaution should be used in removal of ascites because of the potential complications associated with rapid fluid shifts.* Liberal use of opioids to control pain is appropriate as ovarian cancer patients cope with PD and approaching end of life. Appropriate bowel regimens with laxatives and stool softeners should be used to prevent constipation. However, when a patient with a well-controlled bowel regimen presents with new onset of constipation, additional workup is required before altering the bowel regimen. ⑩ *In ovarian cancer patients, SBO is a common complication of progressive disease. In general, laxatives should not be used in patients with SBOs.* Before treating constipation, patients should have a physical examination and abdominal x-ray to rule out SBO. Often, palliative surgery is required to correct SBO and alleviate patient pain. Patients should not eat any solid or liquids until resolution of SBO. If inoperable SBO exists, then parenteral nutrition can be considered but weighed against ultimate treatment objectives. Overall, providing any measures needed to maintain patient comfort is the priority for patients with progressive ovarian cancer.

Patient Care and Monitoring

1. Assess patient history of nonspecific symptoms to determine if the patient should be evaluated by a gynecologist.

2. Determine if patient is at high risk for development of ovarian cancer and make appropriate recommendations for screening and prevention.

3. Evaluate patient comorbidities and medications to determine if additional workup is necessary before tumor debulking surgery. Do any medications need to be stopped or changed before surgery (i.e., aspirin, warfarin, nonsteroidal antiinflammatory agents)?

4. Develop a plan for preventing and treatment of nausea and vomiting for patient receiving emetogenic chemotherapy.

5. Monitor patient for signs of hypersensitivity reactions to taxane or platinum chemotherapy regimens.

6. Monitor appropriate laboratories to determine

   a. Changes in organ function: Adjust chemotherapy doses as indicated

   b. Electrolyte wasting: Replace and supplement electrolytes IV or oral as indicated.

7. Provide appropriate patient education on respective chemotherapy agents that will be given for treatment of recurrent ovarian cancer.

   a. What chemotherapy is and how it works

      i. Explain the plan for monitoring response to treatment.

   b. What side effects to expect during chemotherapy?

      i. Precautions to take to prevent infection when neutropenic.

      ii. Monitor for signs and symptoms of infection

   c. When to contact physician or clinic between cycles of chemotherapy

   d. Drug or food interactions with chemotherapy to avoid

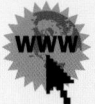 Self-assessment questions and answers are available at *http://www.mhpharmacotherapy.com/pp.html.*

Abbreviations Introduced in This Chapter

AUC	Area under the curve
BRCA1	Breast cancer activator gene 1
BRCA2	Breast cancer activator gene 2
BSO	Bilateral salpingo-oophorectomy
CA-125	Cancer antigen 125
CA-19	Cancer antigen 19
CEA	Carcinoembryonic antigen
CR	Complete response
CrCl	Creatinine clearance
DLT	Dose-limiting toxicity
FIGO	International Federation of Gynecology and Obstetrics
GFR	Glomerular filtration rate
GST	Glutathione S-transferase
HBOC	Hereditary breast and ovarian cancer
HNPCC	Hereditary nonpolyposis colorectal cancer
IP	Intraperitoneal
LFT	Liver function test
NCCN	National Comprehensive Cancer Network
NS	Normal saline
OC	Oral contraceptive
Pgp	*p*-Glycoprotein
PD	Progressive disease
PET	Positron emission tomography
PR	Partial response
SBO	Small bowel obstruction
SXR	Steroid xenobiotic receptor
TAH	Total abdominal hysterectomy
TVUS	Transvaginal ultrasound

REFERENCES

1. American Cancer Society, Cancer Fact & Figures 2012; Atlanta: American Cancer Society; 2012.

2. Cannistra SA. Cancer of the ovary. N Engl J Med 2004;351:2519–2529.

3. Lux MP, Fashing PA, Beckmann MW. Hereditary breast and ovarian cancer: Review and future perspectives. J Mol Med 2006;84(1):16–28.

4. Lu KH, Dinh M, Kohlmann W, et al. Gynecologic cancer as a "sentinel cancer" for women with hereditary nonpolyposis colorectal cancer syndrome. Obstet Gynecol 2005;105:569–574.

5. Colomob N, VanGorp T, Parma G, et al. Ovarian cancer. Crit Rev Oncol Hematol 2006;60:159–179.

6. Heintz APM, Odicino F, Maisonneuve P, et al. Carcinoma of the ovary. FIGO 6th annual report on the results of treatment in gynecological cancer. Int J Gynaecol Obstet 2006;95(Suppl):S161–S192.

7. Prentice RK, Thomson CA, Caan B, et al. Low-fat dietary pattern and cancer incidence in the Women's Health Initiative Dietary Modification randomized controlled trial. J Natl Cancer Inst 2007;99:1534–1543.

8. Krygiou M, Tsoumpou I, Martin-Hirsch P, et al. Ovarian cancer screening. Anticancer Res 2006;26:4793–4801.

9. Edwards BK, Brown ML, Wingo PA, et al. Annual report to the nation on the status of cancer 1975–2002, featuring population-based trends in cancer treatment. J Nat Cancer Inst 2005;97(19):1407–1427.

10. Bast RC, Brewer M, Zou, C, et al. Prevention and early detection of ovarian cancer: Mission impossible? Recent Results Cancer Res 2007;174:91–100

11. Whittemore AS, Balise RR, Pharoah PD, et al. Oral contraceptive use and ovarian cancer risk among carriers of BRCA1 or BRCA2 mutations. Br J Cancer 2004;91(11):1911–1915.

12. La Vecchia C. Oral contraceptives and ovarian cancer: an update, 1998–2004. Eur J Cancer Prev 2006;15:117–124.

13. McLaughlin JR, Risch HA, Lubinski J, et al. Reproductive risk factors for ovarian cancer in carriers of BRCA1 or BRCA2 mutations: A case control study. Lancet Oncol 2007;8:26–34.

14. Harris RE, Beebe-Donk J, Doss H, et al. Aspirin, ibuprofen, and other non-steroidal anti-inflammatory drugs in cancer prevention: A critical review of non-selective COX-2 blockade. Oncol Rep 2005;13:559–583.

15. Bertone ER, Hankinson SE, Newcomb PA, et al. A population-based case-control study of carotenoid and vitamin A intake and ovarian cancer. Cancer Causes Control 2001;12:83–90.

16. Meeuwissen PAM, Seynaeve C, Brekelmans CTM, et al. Outcome of surveillance and prophylactic salpingo-oophorectomy in asymptomatic women at high risk for ovarian cancer. Gynecol Oncol 2005;97(2):476–482.

17. DannJL, Zorn KK. Strategies for ovarian cancer prevention. Obstet Gynecol Clin North Am. 2007;34:667–686.

18. Finch A, Beiner M, Lubinski J, et al. Salpingo-oophorectomy and the risk of ovarian, fallopian tube, and peritoneal cancers in women with a BRCA1 or BRCA2 mutation. JAMA 2006;296:185–192.

19. Narod SA, Sun P, Ghadirian P, et al. Tubal ligation and risk of ovarian cancer in carriers of BRCA1 and BRCA2 mutations: A case control study. Lancet 2001;357:1467–1470.

20. Batista LI, Lu KH, Beahm EK, et al. Coordinated prophylactic surgical management for women with hereditary breast-ovarian cancer syndrome. BMC Cancer 2008;14(8):101–106.

21. Pavelka JC, Li AJ, Karlan BY. Hereditary ovarian cancer-assessing risk and prevention strategies. Obstet Gynecol Clin North Am 2007;34(4):651–665.

22. Klip H, Burger CW, Kenemans P, et al. Cancer risk associated with subfertility and ovulation induction: A review. Cancer Causes Control 2000;11:319–344.

23. Salzberg M, Thurlimann B, Bonnefois H, et al. Current concepts of treatment strategies in advanced or recurrent ovarian cancer. Oncology 2005;68:293–298.

24. National Cancer Institute. Cancer Stat Fact Sheets. Cancer of the Ovary, 2012 Available at: *http://seer.cancer.gov/statfacts/html/ovary.html*.

25. Cooper A, DePriest P. Surgical management of women with ovarian cancer. Semin Oncol 2007;34:226–23338.

26. Wimberger P, Lehmann N, Kimmig R, et al. Prognostic factors for complete debulking in advanced ovarian cancer and its impact on survival. An exploratory analysis of a prospectively randomized phase III study of the Arbeitsgemeinschaft Gynaekologishce Onkologie Ovarian Cancer Study Group (AGO-OVAR). Gynecol Oncol 2007;106:69–74.

27. Hoffman MS, Griffin D, Tebes S, et al. Sites of bowel resected to achieve optimal ovarian cancer cytoreduction: Implications regarding surgical management. Am J Obstet Gynecol 2005;193:582–588.

28. Ozols RF, Bundy BN, Greer BE, et al. Phase III trial of carboplatin and paclitaxel compared with cisplatin and paclitaxel in patients with optimally resected stage III ovarian cancer: A gynecologic oncology group study. J Clin Oncol 2003;21:3194–3200.

29. Neijt JP, Engelholm SA, Tuxen MK, et al. Exploratory phase III study of paclitaxel and cisplatin versus paclitaxel and carboplatin in advanced ovarian cancer. J Clin Oncol 2000;18:3084–3092.

30. National Comprehensive Cancer Network (NCCN) Practice Guidelines in Oncology—Ovarian Cancer—v.1. 2012, *http://www.nccn.org*.

31. Armstrong DK, Bundy B, Wenzel L, et al. Intraperitoneal cisplatin and paclitaxel in ovarian cancer. N Engl J Med 2006;354:34–43.

32. Rao G, Crispens M, Rothenberg ML. Intraperitoneal chemotherapy for ovarian cancer: Overview and perspective. J Clin Oncol 2007;25:2867–2872.

33. National Cancer Institute. NCI Clinical Announcement: Intraperitoneal Chemotherapy for Ovarian Cancer. January 5, 2006. Available at *http://ctep.cancer.gov/highlights/clin_annc_010506.pdf*.

34. Alberts DS, Bookman MA, Chen T, et al. Proceedings of a GOG workshop on intraperitoneal therapy for ovarian cancer. Gynecol Oncol 2006;103:783–792.

35. Katsumata N, Yasuda M, Takahashi F, Isonishi S, Jobo T, Aoki D, et al. Dose-dense paclitaxel once a week in combination with carboplatin every 3 weeks for advanced ovarian cancer: A phase 3, open-label, randomised controlled trial. Lancet 2009;374:1331–1338.

36. Gadducci A, Cosio S, Conte PF, et al. Consolidation and maintenance treatments for patients with advanced epithelial ovarian cancer in CR after first-line chemotherapy: A review of the literature. Crit Rev Oncol Hematol 2005;55:153–166.

37. Abaid LN, Goldstein BH, Micha JP, Rettenmaier MA, Brown JV 3rd, Markman M. Improved overall survival with 12 cycles of single-agent paclitaxel maintenance therapy following a complete response to induction chemotherapy in advanced ovarian carcinoma. Oncology 2010;78:389–393.

38. Vasey PA, Jayson GC, Gordon A, et al. Phase III randomized trial of docetaxel-carboplatin versus paclitaxel-carboplatin as first-line chemotherapy for ovarian carcinoma. J Natl Cancer Inst 2004;1796(22):1682–1691.

39. Rose PG, Blessing JA, Ball HG, et al. A phase II study of docetaxel in paclitaxel-resistant ovarian and peritoneal carcinoma: A Gynecologic Oncology Group study. Gynecol Oncol 2003;88:130–135.

40. Alberts DS, Liu PY, Wilczynski SP, et al. Randomized trial of pegylated liposomal doxorubicin (PLD) plus carboplatin versus carboplatin in platinum-sensitive (PS) patients with recurrent epithelial ovarian or peritoneal carcinoma after failure of initial platinum-based chemotherapy (Southwest Oncology Group Protocol S0200) Gynecol Oncol 2008;108:90–94.

41. Pfisterer J, Plante M, Vergote I, et al: Gemcitabine plus carboplatin compared with carboplatin in patients with platinum-sensitive recurrent ovarian cancer: An intergroup trial of the AGO-OVAR, the NCIC CTG, and the EORTC GCG. J Clin Oncol 2006;24:4699–4707.

42. Herzog TJ, Pothuri B. Ovarian cancer: A focus on management of recurrent disease. Nat Clin Pract Oncol 2006;3:604–611.

43. Boza G, Bamias A, Koutsoukou V, et al. Biweekly gemcitabine and cisplatin in platinum-resistant/refractory, paclitaxel-pre-treated, ovarian and peritoneal carcinoma. Gynecol Oncol 2007;104(3):580–585.

44. Garcia AA, Hirte H, Fleming G, et al. Phase II clinical trial of bevacizumab and low-dose metronomic oral cyclophosphamide in recurrent ovarian cancer: A trial of the California, Chicago, and Princess Margaret Hospital Phase II Consortia. J Clin Oncol 2008;26(1):76–82.

95 Acute Leukemia

Nancy Heideman and Richard Heideman

LEARNING OBJECTIVES

● **Upon completion of the chapter, the reader will be able to:**

1. Describe the pathogenesis of acute leukemia.

2. Compare the classification systems for acute lymphocytic leukemia (ALL) and acute myelogenous leukemia (AML).

3. Identify the risk factors associated with a poor outcome for the acute leukemias.

4. Explain the importance of minimal residual disease (MRD) and its implication on early bone marrow relapse.

5. Explain the role of induction, consolidation, and maintenance phases for acute leukemia.

6. Define the role of CNS preventive therapy for acute leukemia.

7. Recognize the treatment complications associated with therapy for acute leukemias.

8. Describe the late effects associated with the treatment of long-term survivors of acute leukemias.

KEY CONCEPTS

❶ The acute leukemias are hematologic malignancies of bone marrow precursors characterized by excessive production of immature hematopoietic cells. This proliferation of "blast" cells eventually replaces normal bone marrow and leads to the failure of normal hematopoiesis and the appearance of leukemia cells in peripheral blood as well as infiltration of other organs.

❷ Acute leukemias are classified according to their cell of origin. Acute lymphocytic leukemia (ALL) arises from the lymphoid precursors. Acute nonlymphocytic leukemia (ANLL) or acute myelogenous leukemia (AML) arises from the myeloid or megakaryocytic precursors.

❸ The goal is to match treatment to risk and minimize over- or undertreatment. Children and adults with leukemia are sorted into prognostic categories based on clinical and biological features that mirror their risk of relapse. Risk assessment is an important factor in the selection of treatment.

❹ Minimal residual disease (MRD) is a quantitative assessment of subclinical remnant of leukemic burden remaining at the end of the initial phase of treatment (induction) when a patient may appear to be in a complete morphologic remission. This measure has become one of the strongest predictors of outcome for patients with acute leukemia. The elimination of

MRD is a principal objective of postinduction leukemia therapy.

❺ The initial treatment for acute leukemias is called **induction**. The purpose of induction is to induce a **remission**, a state in which there is no identifiable leukemic cells in the bone marrow or peripheral blood with light microscopy.

❻ The current induction therapy for ALL typically consists of vincristine, L-asparaginase, and a steroid (prednisone or dexamethasone). An anthracycline is added for higher risk patients.

❼ Leukemic invasion of the CNS is considered to be an almost universal event in patients, even in those whose cerebrospinal fluid (CSF) cytology shows no apparent disease. Thus, all patients with ALL and AML receive intrathecal chemotherapy. Although this is often referred to as "prophylaxis," it more realistically represents treatment.

❽ Bone marrow relapse is the major form of treatment failure in 15% to 20% of patients with ALL. Most relapses have the same immunophenotype and cytogenetic changes seen in the original disease.

❾ The current induction therapy for AML usually consists of a combination of cytarabine and an anthracycline daunorubicin or idarubicin, with the frequent addition of a steroid and/or an antimetabolite such as 6-thioguanine. The second phase of treatment for AML is called consolidation. The purpose of this phase is to further enhance remission with more cytoreduction. This period is also a time to consider hematopoietic stem cell transplantation for patients in first remission.

⑩ Despite this significant increase in survival, many patients, particularly pediatric cancer survivors, have disease- or treatment-related disabilities. As many as 50% to 60% of these survivors are estimated to have at least one chronic or late-occurring complication of treatment.

INTRODUCTION

① *The acute leukemias are hematologic malignancies of bone marrow precursors characterized by excessive production of immature hematopoietic cells. This proliferation of "blast" cells eventually replaces normal bone marrow and leads to the failure of normal hematopoiesis and the appearance in peripheral blood as well as infiltration of other organs.* These blast cells proliferate in the marrow and inhibit normal cellular elements, resulting in anemia, neutropenia, and thrombocytopenia. Leukemia also may infiltrate other organs, including the liver, spleen, bone, skin, lymph nodes, testis and central nervous system (CNS). Virtually anywhere there is blood flow, the potential for extramedullary (outside the bone marrow) leukemia exists.

② *Acute leukemias are classified according to their cell of origin. Acute lymphocytic leukemia (ALL) arises from the lymphoid precursors. Acute nonlymphocytic leukemia (ANLL) or acute myelogenous leukemia (AML) arises from the myeloid or megakaryocytic precursors.* As a result of clinical trials defining various prognostic (risk) factors that helped guide treatment modifications, the outcomes of acute leukemias, especially ALL, has improved dramatically over the past 30 years.[1] Risk-based treatment strategies that consider multiple phenotypic and biological risk factors and attempt to match the aggressiveness of therapy with the presumed risk of relapse and death are now the standard of care.

EPIDEMIOLOGY AND ETIOLOGY

Epidemiology

Leukemia is a relatively uncommon disease overall. The current overall age-adjusted annual incidence of acute leukemia in the United States has remained relatively stable at 10 per 100,000 in children and 1 to 2 per 100,000 in adults.[2] It was projected that of the estimated 1.5 million new cancers diagnosed in 2010, only 1.2% would be acute leukemia, with 5,330 cases of ALL and about 12,330 cases of AML.[3,4]

In the pediatric population, leukemia is a common disease, accounting for almost one-third of all childhood malignancies. ALL accounts for 75% to 80% of all cases of childhood leukemia, whereas AML accounts for no more than 20%. Males generally are affected more often than females in all but the infant age group, and its incidence is higher in whites than among other racial groups.

The incidence of AML in children is bimodal: It peaks at 2 years of age, decreases steadily thereafter to age 9 years, and then increases again at around age 16.[4] The average age of diagnosis for AML is about 65 years and is a result of an increasing incidence of AML with age.

Etiology

The causes of the acute leukemias is unknown; multiple influences related to genetics, socioeconomics, infection, environment, hematopoietic development, and chance all may play a role.[4] Table 95–1 lists the major conditions that have been associated with the acute leukemias. In most cases, however, there is no identifiable cause of the leukemia.

Although leukemia is rarely a hereditary disease, some genetic associations are evident. For example, among identical twins, the concordance for ALL in the initially unaffected twin is 20% to 25% within 1 year. Although the incidence in fraternal twins is much less, there is still a fourfold increase in the risk of leukemia in the initially unaffected twin compared with the normal population. One explanation for this association may be a shared placental circulation, which allows for transmission of disease from one twin to the other. Additionally, leukemia is known to have an increased incidence in several chromosomally abnormal populations. Patients with Down's syndrome have a 20 times increased risk of developing leukemia compared with the rest of the population. Patients with Klinefelter's syndrome and Bloom's syndrome also have an increased incidence of leukemias.[4]

Exposure to environmental agents such as agricultural chemicals, pesticides, and radiation have also been periodically associated with leukemia, but none is conclusively related to the development of leukemia. An increased frequency of ALL is associated with higher socioeconomic status. It is

Table 95–1
Clinical Conditions Associated With an Increased Frequency of Acute Leukemias

Drugs Alkylating agents Epipodophyllotoxins	**Chemicals** Benzene

Genetic Conditions
Down's syndrome
Bloom's syndrome
Fanconi's anemia
Klinefelter's syndrome
Ataxia telangiectasia
Langerhans' cell histiocytosis
Shwachman's syndrome
Severe combined immunodeficiency
  syndrome
Kostmann's syndrome
Neurofibromatosis type 1
Familial monosomy 7
Diamond-Blackfan anemia
	Radiation
	Ionizing radiation
	
	Viruses
	Epstein-Barr virus
	Human T-lymphocyte
	  virus (HTLV-1 and
	  HTLV-2)
	
	Social Habits
	Cigarette smoking
	Maternal marijuana use
	Maternal ethanol use

Adapted from Pieters R, Carroll WL. Biology and treatment of acute lymphoblastic leukemia. Pediatr Clin North Am 2008;55(1):1–20

postulated that less social contact in early infancy and thus a late exposure to some common infectious agents may have some impact.[4]

Risk factors for the development of AML include exposure to environmental toxins, Hispanic ethnicity, and genetics.[5] Of greater concern is the increased prevalence of AML as a secondary malignancy, resulting from chemotherapy and radiation treatment for other cancers. Alkylating agents, such as ifosfamide and cyclophosphamide, and topoisomerase inhibitors, such as etoposide, are linked to an increased risk of AML and myelodysplastic syndrome (MDS).[5]

PATHOPHYSIOLOGY

Hematopoiesis is defined as the development and maturation of blood cells and their precursors. In utero, hematopoiesis may occur in the liver, spleen, and bone marrow; after birth, this process occurs exclusively in the bone marrow. All blood cells are generated from a common hematopoietic precursor, or *stem cell*. These stem cells are self-renewing and pluripotent and thus are able to commit to any one of the different lines of maturation that give rise to platelet-producing megakaryocytes, lymphoid, erythroid, and myeloid cells. The myeloid cell line produces monocytes, basophils, neutrophils, and eosinophils, whereas the lymphoid stem cell differentiates to form circulating B and T lymphocytes, natural killer (NK) cells, and dendritic cells. In contrast to the ordered development of normal cells, the development of leukemia seems to represent an arrest in differentiation at an early phase in the continuum of stem cell to mature cell.[1]

Both AML and ALL are presumed to arise from clonal expansion of these "arrested" cells. As these cells expand, they acquire one and often more chromosomal aberrations, including translocations, inversions, deletions, point mutations, and amplifications.[4] The translocation t(12;21) or *TEL–AML1* is found in approximately 25% of cases of pediatric ALL and is associated with a favorable prognosis.[6] This translocation is uncommon in adults. Another example is the t(9;22) translocation (Philadelphia chromosome, Ph⁺), which results in the *BCR–ABL* fusion protein. This translocation produces a novel kinase that leads to uncontrolled proliferation, survival, and self-renewal of cells. It is uncommon in childhood ALL and commonly found in adult ALL, especially in older patients.

Patients with MDS or AML as a secondary neoplasm are often characterized by having had prior alkylator-based or etoposide-based chemotherapy. Patients who have received treatment for Hodgkins disease or solid tumors are most at risk for this problem because they often treated with these agents. Patients with MDS have an abnormal bone marrow and a variety of cytopenias involving one or more of their marrow cell lines. They are at high risk of converting to overt leukemia over time. A variety of complex cytogentic findings and monosomies of chromosome 5 or 7, and 11q26 translocactions are often present in this population.[5]

Leukemia Classification

Classification methods for leukemia have evolved from simple schemes that were largely phenotypic and considered only age, gender, white blood cell (WBC) count, and blast morphology to now-complex methods that include biological features such as cell-surface receptors, DNA content (ploidy; more or less then normal chromosomal DNA content), and a variety of cytogenetic abnormalities.

For all newly diagnosed patients with leukemia, an aspirate of the liquid marrow and a bone marrow core biopsy are obtained. Analysis of the leukemic cell surface markers (immunophenotyping) establish three types of ALL, pre-B, mature B, and T-cell precursor ALL. There are eight subtypes of AML (M0 to M7) as classified by the French-American-British (FAB) scheme (Tables 95–2 and 95–3).

Immunophenotyping by flow cytometry has taken on an increasingly important role in the diagnosis of leukemia. Owing to the ease of application, sensitivity, and quantifiable results, flow cytometry is the preferred method for leukemic lineage as well as prognostic assignment.[7] This approach takes advantage of the development of diagnostic

---

Table 95–2				
Morphologic (FAB) Classification of AML				
			Frequency of FAB Subtype	
Subtype		**Adults (%)**	**Children Older Than 2 Years (%)**	**Children Younger Than 2 Years (%)**
M0	Acute myeloblastic leukemia without maturation	5	Low	Low
M1	Acute myeloblastic leukemia with minimal maturation	15	17	25
M2	Acute myeloblastic leukemia with maturation	25		27
M3	Acute promyelocytic leukemia	10		5
M4	Acute myelomonocytic leukemia	25	30	26
M5a	Acute monoblastic leukemia, poorly differentiated	5	52	16
M5b	Acute monoblastic leukemia, well differentiated	5		
M6	Acute erythroleukemia	5		2
M7	Acute megakaryoblastic leukemia	10		5–7

FAB, French-American-British.

Table 95–3

WHO Classification of AML

AML with recurrent genetic abnormalities:
AML with t(8;21)(q22;q22), (AML1/ETO)
AML with abnormal bone marrow eosinophils and inv(16)
  (p13q22) or t(16;16)(p13;q22), (CBFβ/MYH11)
Acute promyelocytic leukemia with t(15;17)(q22;q12), (PML/RARα)
  and variants
AML with 11q23 (MLL) abnormalities
AML with multilineage dysplasia
After MDS or MDS/MPD
Without antecedent MDS or MDS/MPD but with dysplasia in at
  least 50% of cells in two or more myeloid lineages
AML and MDSs, therapy related
Alkylating agent–or radiation-related type
Topoisomerase II inhibitor–related type (some may be lymphoid)

Others:
AML not otherwise categorized

Classify as:
AML, minimally differentiated
AML without maturation
AML with maturation
Acute myelomonocytic leukemia
Acute monoblastic/acute monocytic leukemia
Acute erythroid leukemia (erythroid/myeloid and pure
  erythroleukemia)
Acute megakaryoblastic leukemia
Acute basophilic leukemia
Acute panmyelosis with myelofibrosis
Myeloid sarcoma

AML, acute myeloid leukemia; MDS, myelodysplastic syndrome;
MPD, myeloproliferative disorders.

Adapted from Pieters R, Carroll WL. Biology and treatment of acute
lymphoblastic leukemia. Pediatr Clin North Am 2008;55(1):1–20.

monoclonal antibodies (MABs) to many cell-surface antigens
that are differentially expressed during hematopoietic
differentiation. The antigens are referred to as antibody
cluster determinants (CDs) that define cells at various stages
of development and can easily separate ALL from AML
and T-cell from pre–B-cell ALL.[4,7] The combined approach
of flow cytometric identification and cytogenetic DNA
content, much of which is also revealed by flow cytometry
and fluorescent in situ hybridization (FISH; microscopic,
fluorescence identification of chromosomal features) has
facilitated diagnosis and delineation of specific subtypes of
the acute leukemias. Common immunophenotypic markers
seen in AML and ALL are provided in Table 95–4.

Prognostic Factors

❸ *The goal of treatment is to match treatment to risk and
minimize over- or undertreatment. Patients with leukemia
are sorted into prognostic categories based on clinical and
biological features that mirror their risk of relapse. Risk
assessment is an important factor in the selection of treatment.*
Age, WBC, leukemic cell-surface markers, DNA content,
and specific cytogenetic abnormalities predict response to
therapy and are used to assign risk and associated treatment.[4]

Patient Encounter, Part 1

MV is a 8-year-old boy who presents to the pediatric
emergency department with his father with a history of
aches, chills, and fevers for the past 4 to 5 days. He has had
several colds over the past few weeks that do not seem
to be improving. He has also had diffuse body and bone
pain in his legs over the past couple of weeks. Physical
examination reveals pallor, cervical lymphadenopathy,
and hepatosplenomegaly. Electrolytes and uric acid are
within normal limits. A CBC shows a normochromic,
normocytic anemia with a hemoglobin of 7.0 g/dL
(70 g/L, 4.34 mmol/L; reference range, 11.7 to 15.7 g/dL,
7.26 to 9.74 mmol/L), hematocrit of 21% (0.21; reference
range, 35% to 47% or 0.35 to 0.47), and WBC count of 4.1 ×
10^3/mm³ (4.1 × 10^9/L). The differential on the WBC count
reveals 65% (0.65) lymphocytes (reference range, 20% to
40% or 0.2 to 0.4), 13% (0.13) neutrophils (reference range,
55% to 62% or 0.55 to 0.62), and 22% (0.22) lymphoblasts
(normal amount, 0%). Flow cytometry from the peripheral
blood is consistent with pre–B-cell ALL.

What information is consistent with the diagnosis of ALL?

What are the prognostic factors for MV?

What is the role of flow cytometry in identifying ALL?

On the basis of these prognostic variables, patients are
assigned to standard-, high-, or very-high-risk groups that
determine the aggressiveness of treatment.

▶ *Prognostic Factors in ALL*

● In both children and adults with ALL, clinical trials have
identified several risk factors that correlate with outcome
(Table 95–5). Prognostic features include age, WBC count,
cytogenetic abnormalities, ploidy (DNA content), leukemic cell
immunophenotype, and degree of initial response to therapy,
and minimal residual disease (MRD; the degree of subclinical
disease remaining at various times after starting treatment)[4,7,8]
When these factors are combined, they predict groups of
patients with varying degrees of risk for treatment failure.

Table 95–4

Common Immunophenotypes in Acute Leukemia

Leukemia	Common Immunophenotypes
AML	CD13, CD15, CD33, CD14, CD64, and C-KIT
B-cell ALL	CD19, CD20, CD10, and CD22
T-cell ALL	CD2, CD3, CD4, CD5, and CD7

ALL, acute lymphoblastic leukemia; AML, acute myeloid leukemia;
CD, cluster determinants.

Adapted from Pieters R, Carroll WL. Biology and treatment of acute
lymphoblastic leukemia. Pediatr Clin North Am 2008;55(1):1–20.

Table 95–5		
Prognostic Factors in ALL		
	Risk for Leukemic Relapse	
Factor	**Low**	**High**
Immunologic phenotype	Early pre–B cell	Null cell, T cell, pre–B cell, B cell
WBC count at diagnosis	Less than 10 × 10³/mm³ (10 × 10⁹/L)	Greater than 50 × 10³/mm³ (50 × 10⁹/L)
Platelets	Greater than 100 × 10³/mm³ (100 × 10⁹/L)	Less than 30 × 10³/mm³ (30 × 10⁹/L)
Patient age	3–7 years	Less than 1 year or greater than 10 years
Cytogenetics	Normal karyotype	t(9;22); t(4;11); −7; +8
Myeloid markers	Absent	Present
CNS leukemia	Absent	Present
Node/liver/spleen enlargement	Absent	Massive
Mediastinal mass	Absent	Present
Time to remission	Less than 4 weeks	Greater than 4 weeks

WBC, white blood cell.

Adapted from Pieters R, Carroll WL. Biology and treatment of acute lymphoblastic leukemia. Pediatr Clin North Am 2008;55(1):1–20.

The importance of age is seen is evident in both children and adults. Children younger than 1 year or older than 10 years of age have a poorer outcome than others. Likewise, in adults, there is a steady decline in the rate survival with increasing age.

Similar to age, the WBC count at presentation is a reliable indicator of complete response (CR) rate and outcome. The WBC count is indicative of tumor burden, although the underlying biological mechanisms that account for the unfavorable outcomes associated with an elevated WBC count are unclear. Patients with WBC counts of less than 50 × 10³/mm³ (50 × 10⁹/L) are considered being at standard risk and have a better outcome than those with a higher WBC counts at presentation, which is associated with higher risk of treatment failure (Table 95–5).

Specific chromosomal abnormalities in leukemic cells also possess prognostic significance. Blast cells with a translocation of parts of chromosome 12 and 21 (the *TEL–AML1* fusion) or trisomies of 4, 10, and 17 are considered to have favorable genetic features.[4] The presence of the Philadelphia chromosome (Ph⁺), the result of a specific translocation between chromosome 9 and 22, **t(9;22) (q34;q11.2)**, is a high-risk feature, which is present in about 5% of children but is much more common in adults with ALL. This translocation results in a novel tyrosine kinase that drives cell proliferation.[7,8]

Among children younger than 1 year of age, as many as 80% possess a poor prognostic genotype represented by the presence of the *MLL* (11q22) gene rearrangement. This finding is rare among older patients. Leukemias with the *MLL* gene rearrangement are highly resistant to the key antileukemic drugs such as glucocorticoids and L-asparaginase.[9]

The DNA content of blast cells, hyper-, hypo-, or diploid, corresponding to increased, decreased, or normal chromosome numbers, has been considered prognostic. Lower risk patients with hyperdiploidy (greater than 50 chromosomes per leukemic cell) generally include approximately 25% of children who have B-cell lineage ALL.[6] These children are between the ages of 1 and 9 years, but the higher risk patients with normal diploidy (50 chromosomes) generally are older.

Patients with cell-surface markers indicating that the blasts are early in the B-cell lineage (CD markers) are considered favorable and standard risk, whereas those with mature B-cell and T-cell blasts are considered high risk. T-cell ALL is found in approximately 15% of childhood ALL. Compared with B-lineage ALL, T-cell ALL is relatively resistant to different classes of drugs, including methotrexate and cytarabine.

Patients completing induction treatment and in apparent remission still harbor malignant cells in their bone marrow even though they appear disease free by peripheral blood and bone marrow morphology. Assuming that most patients present with about a 10¹¹ leukemic cell burden at diagnosis, at least 10⁹ cells remain after initial treatment. These residual leukemic cells are below the limits of detection using standard morphologic examination. Measurement of this population of cells has become an increasingly significant prognostic factor and a determinant of the aggressiveness of postinduction therapy. Through flow cytometric analysis and **polymerase chain reaction**, it is possible to detect one leukemic cell among 10⁶ normal cells, representing 1,000-fold greater sensitivity than morphologic examination.[10,11]

❹ Minimal residual disease *(MRD) is a quantitative assessment of subclinical remnant of leukemic burden remaining at the end of the initial phase of treatment (induction) when a patient may appear to be in a complete morphologic remission. This measure has become one of the strongest predictors of outcome for patients with acute leukemia. The elimination of MRD is a principal objective of postinduction leukemia therapy.* Several studies in children, in whom ALL is common, have evaluated disease levels at the end of induction and correlated these values with event-free survival (EFS). For a patient with detectable MRD less than 0.1% at the end of induction, EFS is 88% at 3 years. Conversely, a patient with high MRD (more than 1%) has a 3-year EFS of only 30%.[12] Assessment of MRD is also emerging as an important indicator of disease recurrence in the adult population and in patients with AML.

▶ Prognostic Factors in AML

The major prognostic factors in newly diagnosed AML are age, subtype, chromosome status, ethnicity, and body mass index.

Older adults with AML (older than 60 years), compared with younger patients with the same disease, have a dismal prognosis and represent a distinct population in terms of disease biology, treatment-related complications, and overall survival (OS). These older patients have a higher incidence of unfavorable chromosomal abnormalities, such as aberrations

---

Patient Encounter, Part 2

MV is admitted to the pediatric oncology service. A bone marrow biopsy and aspirate is done, which shows 85% replacement with precursor B-cell blasts. FISH analysis performed on the peripheral blood is positive for the BCR/ABL translocation (Ph⁺) in 5.5% of the cells examined. He is started on intravenous hydration with sodium bicarbonate and allopurinol. A diagnostic lumbar puncture (LP) is performed, which is negative for CNS leukemia. During the LP, MV receives IT cytarabine.

What is the role of CNS prophylaxis for MV?

What is the BCR/ABL translocation?

How does the presence of this chromosomal abnormality change MV's risk status?

---

of chromosomes 5, 7, or 8, and fewer abnormalities that are associated with a more favorable outcome, such as t(8;21) or inv(16) (see **Table 95–6**).[5,12]

Recent studies suggest that ethnicity may be an important predictor of outcome in children with AML. Investigators found that African Americans treated with chemotherapy had a significantly worse outcome than whites, perhaps suggesting race-related pharmacogenetic differences. Body mass index may also affect the prognosis of children with AML. Underweight patients and overweight patients were less likely to survive than normal weight patients because of a greater risk of treatment-related deaths.[13]

TREATMENT

Desired Outcome

The primary objective in treating patients with acute leukemia is to achieve a continuous complete remission (CCR). Remission is defined as the absence of all clinical evidence of leukemia with the restoration of normal hematopoiesis. For both ALL and AML, remission induction is achieved with the use of myelosuppressive chemotherapy that initially induces a state of bone marrow aplasia as the leukemic cells die followed by a slow return and proliferation of normal cells. After this period, hematopoiesis is restored. Failure to achieve remission in the first 7 to 14 days of therapy is highly predictive of later disease recurrence. This again represents the growing importance of MRD in prognosis and treatment.

Clinical Presentation and Diagnosis of ALL[3,6,11]

General

Typically, patients have symptoms for 1 to 3 months before presentation. These include fatigue, fever, and pallor, but patients generally are in no obvious distress.

Symptoms

- The patient may present with weakness, malaise, bleeding, and weight loss.
- Neutropenic patients are often febrile and highly susceptible to infection.
- Anemia usually presents as pallor, tiredness, and general fatigue.
- Patients with thrombocytopenia usually present with bruising, petechiae, and ecchymosis.
- Patients often present with bone pain secondary to expansion of the marrow cavity from leukemic infiltration.
- CNS involvement is common at diagnosis.

Signs

- Temperature may be elevated secondary to an infection associated with a low WBC count.
- Petechiae and bleeding are indicative of thrombocytopenia.
- Patients may present with organ involvement, such as peripheral adenopathy, hepatomegaly, and splenomegaly.
- T-lineage ALL may present with a mediastinal mass.

Laboratory Tests

- CBC with differential is performed.
- The anemia is usually normochromic and normocytic. Approximately 50% of children present with platelet counts of less than $50 \times 10^3/mm^3$ ($50 \times 10^9/L$). The WBC count may be normal, decreased, or high. About 20% of patients have WBC counts over $100 \times 10^3/mm^3$ ($100 \times 10^9/L$), which places them at risk for leukostasis.
- Uric acid is increased in approximately 50% of patients secondary to rapid cellular turnover.
- *Electrolytes:* Potassium and phosphorus often are elevated. Calcium usually is low.
- *Coagulation disorders:* Elevated prothrombin time, partial thromboplastin time, D-dimers; hypofibrinogenemia

Other Laboratory Tests

Flow cytometric evaluation of bone marrow and peripheral blood is performed to characterize the type of leukemia as well as to detect specific chromosomal rearrangements. The bone marrow at diagnosis usually is hypercellular, with normal hematopoiesis being replaced by leukemic blasts. At diagnosis, a lumbar puncture is performed to determine if CNS leukemia is present.

TABLE 95-6

Risk Category According to Cytogenetic Abnormalities Present

	Risk Category		
Disease	Good Risk	Intermediate Risk	High Risk
AML	t(8;21)(q22;q22); inv(16); t(15;17); t(9;11) trisomy 21	Normal karyotype; trisomy 8; 11q23; del(7q); del(9q); trisomy 22	Complex karyotype; −5; −7; del (5q); inv(3P)
Probability of relapse	Less than or equal to 25%	50%	Greater than 70%
4-Year survival	Greater than or equal to 70%	40%–50%	Less than or equal to 20%
ALL	Hyperdiploidy; t(10;14); or 6q		t(9;22); t(8;14); t(4;11); t(1;9)

ALL, acute lymphocytic leukemia; AML, acute myelogenous leukemia.

Adapted from Pieters R, Carroll WL. Biology and treatment of acute lymphoblastic leukemia. Pediatr Clin North Am 2008;55(1):1–20.

Nonpharmacologic Therapy

This year, roughly 1.6 million people will be diagnosed with cancer in the United States and Canada. With improvements in detection and treatment, approximately two-thirds of those diagnosed with the disease can expect to be alive in 5 years. With improving longevity, the cumulative adverse effects of both the disease and treatment are becoming an increasingly important issue. "Late-effects" data show that both adult and pediatric cancer survivors are at greater risk for developing second malignancies, cardiovascular disease, diabetes, and osteoporosis than those in the general population. With respect to the growing population of pediatric cancer survivors, data confirm that they are eight times more likely than their siblings to have a severe or life-threatening chronic health condition. For example, the survivors of pediatric ALL have an increased onset of obesity, osteopenia, and associated comorbidities. Thus, it is important to provide supportive care and intervention and counseling related to nutrition, smoking cessation, and exercise as a part of their active treatment. Health care professionals should think beyond the immediate treatment-related issues of their patients and provide appropriate, active assistance to promote healthy lifestyles and encourage patients to take active roles in pursuing general preventive health strategies.[14]

Pharmacologic Therapy: ALL

The treatment for ALL consists of four main elements: remission induction (the initial tumor reduction leading to morphologic remission), CNS-directed treatment, and intensive postremission consolidation regimens, followed by a prolonged maintenance phase (Table 95–7).

▶ Remission Induction

⑤ *The initial treatment for acute leukemias is called induction. The purpose of induction is to induce a remission, a state in which there is no identifiable leukemic cells in the bone marrow or peripheral blood with light microscopy.*
⑥ *Current induction therapy for ALL typically consists of vincristine, L-asparaginase, and a steroid (prednisone or dexamethasone). An anthracycline is added for higher risk*

patients. Although induction treatment produces 95% CR in children, it declines to no more than 60% in patients older than 60 years of age.

Adults, unlike children, are universally considered to be at high risk for relapse; therefore, their induction regimens include an anthracycline (daunorubicin or doxorubicin) in addition to the standard steroid and vincristine treatment that have been the backbone of treatment for this disease for the last 40 years.[14,15] Dexamethasone is often replacing prednisone as the steroid of treatment because of its longer half-life and better CNS penetration.[15] Even though dexamethasone possesses more favorable pharmacologic characteristics than prednisone, its use may be associated with more aseptic osteonecrosis of the femoral and humoral heads as well as an increase in life-threatening infections and septic deaths.[15]

▶ CNS Prophylaxis

⑦ *Leukemic invasion of the CNS is considered to be an almost universal event in patients even in those whose cerebrospinal fluid (CSF) cytology shows no apparent disease. Thus, all patients with ALL and AML leukemia receive intrathecal (IT) chemotherapy. Although this is often referred to as "prophylaxis," it more realistically represents treatment.* CNS prophylaxis relies on IT chemotherapy (e.g., methotrexate, cytarabine, and corticosteroids), systemic chemotherapy with dexamethasone and high-dose methotrexate, and craniospinal irradiation (XRT) in selected high-risk patients.[16] Cranial radiation was once a common intervention, but it is now reserved for only high-risk patients in whom IT treatment is inadequate. Its use has diminished substantially once the efficacy of IT treatment was evident, and the toxicities associated with radiation, learning disabilities, growth retardation, and secondary malignancies (particularly with the use of 6-mercaptopurine), were recognized. IT therapy has replaced cranial XRT as CNS prophylaxis for all except the very high-risk patients and those with T-cell ALL who are at higher risk of CNS disease.

Inexplicably, the treatment of CNS leukemia has not had the same remarkable impact on the OS of adults as it has for childhood ALL. With IT chemotherapy alone, the incidence of CNS relapse in adults is 9% to 13% compared with less than 3% in children.[5,11]

Clinical Presentation and Diagnosis of AML[3,6,11]

General

Patients may have symptoms of AML for 1 to 3 months before presentation. These include fatigue, fever, and pallor, but patients generally are in no obvious distress.

Symptoms

- The patient may present with weakness, malaise, bleeding, and weight loss.
- Neutropenic patients are often febrile and highly susceptible to infection.
- Anemia usually presents as pallor, tiredness, and general fatigue.
- Patients with thrombocytopenia usually present with bruising, petechiae, and ecchymosis.
- Chloromas (localized leukemic deposits named after their color) may be seen, especially in the periorbital regions and as skin infiltrates.
- Gum hypertrophy is indicative of AML M4 and AML M5 subtypes.
- Disseminated intravascular coagulation is common in AML M3 and is associated with generalized bleeding or hemorrhage.
- Lymphadenopathy, massive hepatosplenomegaly, and bone pain are not as common in AML as in ALL.

Signs

- Temperature may be elevated secondary to an infection associated with a low WBC count.

- Petechiae and bleeding are indicative of thrombocytopenia.

Laboratory Tests

- CBC with differential is performed.
- The anemia is usually normochromic and normocytic.
- Approximately 50% of children present with platelet counts of less than $50 \times 10^3/mm^3$ ($50 \times 10^9/L$).
- The WBC count may be normal, decreased, or high. About 20% of patients have WBC counts of over $100 \times 10^3/mm^3$ ($100 \times 10^9/L$), which places them at risk for leukostasis.
- Uric acid is increased in approximately 50% of patients secondary to rapid cellular turnover.
- *Electrolytes:* Potassium and phosphorus are often elevated. Calcium is usually low.
- *Coagulation disorders:* Elevated prothrombin time, partial thromboplastin time, D-dimers; hypofibrinogenemia

Other Diagnostic Tests

Flow cytometric evaluation of bone marrow and peripheral blood to characterize the type of leukemia, as well as to detect specific chromosomal rearrangements. The bone marrow at diagnosis usually is hypercellular, with normal hematopoiesis being replaced by leukemic blasts. The presence of greater than 20% blasts in the bone marrow is diagnostic for AML. At diagnosis, a lumbar puncture is performed to determine if CNS leukemia is present.

▶ *Postremission Consolidation Regimens*

Consolidation After completion of induction and restoration of normal hematopoiesis, patients begin consolidation. The goal of consolidation is to administer dose-intensive chemotherapy in an effort to further reduce the burden of residual leukemic cells. It is in this and subsequent treatment phases that the remaining leukemic burden is eliminated. Several regimens use agents and schedules designed to minimize the development of drug cross-resistance. Studies have demonstrated that this phase of treatment has proven to be an effective strategy in the prevention of relapse in children with ALL, but its benefits in adults are less clear.

In children, the intensity of the consolidation treatment is now determined not only by the child's risk classification but also by the degree of cytoreduction during induction (MRD). Patients who respond slowly to induction therapy (as determined by bone marrow examination early in induction) are at higher risk of relapse and are treated with more aggressive regimens.[16]

Delayed Intensification The Berlin-Frankfurt-Munster (BFM) Study Group introduced a treatment element called

delayed intensification (or *reinduction*) *therapy*. This therapy consisted of repetition of the initial remission induction therapy administered approximately 3 months after remission. This, similar to consolidation, has been adopted as a component of treatment for children by virtually all institutions.[13]

Intensification regimens may vary in their aggressiveness and the drugs they use depending on the patient's risk group and immunophenotype. For example, the use of high-dose methotrexate (5 g/m^2) appears to improve outcome in patients with T-cell ALL. The use of intensive asparaginase treatment in T-cell ALL patients also has improved outcomes significantly.[15]

▶ *Maintenance*

The purpose of maintenance therapy is to further eliminate leukemic cells and produce an enduring CCR. The two most important agents in maintenance chemotherapy are a combination of oral methotrexate and 6-mercaptopurine. Improved outcome has been associated with increasing 6-mercaptopurine doses to the limits of individual tolerance

Table 95–7

Representative Chemotherapy Regimens for Adult ALL

Remission Induction		CNS Prophylaxis		Consolidation		Maintenance
Drug and Dose	Days	Prophylaxis	Days	Drug and Dose	Days	Drug, Dose, and Timing

German or Hoelzer Regimen (Adult)[a]

PRED (PO) 60 mg/m²	1–28	Cranial irradiation		DEX (PO) 10 mg/m²	1–28	MP (PO) 60 mg/m² daily and
VCR (IV) 1.5 mg/m²[b]	1, 8, 15, 22	MTX (IT) 10 mg/m²[c]	31, 38, 45, 52	VCR (IV) 1.5 mg/m²[b]	1, 8, 15, 22	MTX (PO/IV) 20 mg/m² weekly, weeks 10–18
DNR (IV) 25 mg/m²	1, 8, 15, 22			DOX (IV) 25 mg/m²	1, 8, 15, 22	and 29–130
ASP (IV) 5,000 units/m²	1–14			CTX (IV) 650 mg/m²[d]	29	
CTX (IV) 650 mg/m²[d]	29, 43, 57			Ara-C (IV) 75 mg/m²	31–34, 38–41	
Ara-C (IV) 75 mg/m²	31–34, 38–41, 45–48, 52–55			TG (PO) 60 mg/m²	29–42	
MP (PO) 60 mg/m²	29–57					

CALGB 8811 (Adult)[e]

Course I

CTX (IV) 1,200 mg/m² 1
DNR (IV) 45 mg/m² 1, 2, 3
VCR (IV) 2 mg 1, 8, 15, 22
PRED (PO) 60 mg/m² 1–21
ASP (SC) 6,000 units/m² 5, 8, 11, 15, 18, 22

Induction chemotherapy for patients 60 years old or older, use:
CTX (IV) 800 mg/m² 1
DNR (IV) 30 mg/m² 1–3
PRED (PO) 60 mg/m² 1–7

Course III
Cranial irradiation

MTX (IT) 15 mg 1, 8, 15, 22, 29
MP (PO) 60 mg/m² 1–70
MTX (PO) 20 mg/m² 36, 43, 50, 57, 64

Course II: Early intensification
MTX (IT) 15 mg 1
CTX (IV) 1,000 mg/m² 1–14
MP (PO) 60 mg/m² 1–4, 8–11
Ara-C (SC) 75 mg/m² 15, 22
VCR (IV) 2 mg 15, 18, 22, 25
ASP (SC) 6,000 units/m²

Course IV: Late intensification
DOX (IV) 30 mg/m² 1, 8, 15
VCR (IV) 2 mg 1, 8, 15
DEX (PO) 10 mg/m² 1–14
CTX (IV) 1,000 mg/m² 29
TG (PO) 60 mg/m² 29–42
Ara-C (SC) 75 mg/m² 29–32, 36–39

Course V
VCR (IV) 2 mg day 1 monthly
PRED (PO) 60 mg/m² days 1–5 monthly
MTX (PO) 20 mg/m² days 1, 8, 15, 22 monthly
MP (PO) 60 mg/m² days 1–28 monthly

ASP, asparaginase; C, cytarabine; CALGB, Cancer and Leukemia Group B; CTX, cyclophosphamide; DEX, dexamethasone; DNR, daunorubicin; DOX, doxorubicin; IT, intrathecal; MP, mercaptopurine; MTX, methotrexate; PO, oral; PRED, prednisone; SC, subcutaneous; TG, thioguanine; VCR, vincristine.

[a]Holzer D, Thiel E, Ludwig WD, et al. Follow-up of the first two successive German multicentre trials for adult ALL (01/81 and 2/84). Leukemia 1993;7(Suppl 2):130–134.

[b]Maximum single dose, 2 mg.

[c]Maximum single dose, 15 mg.

[d]Maximum single dose, 1,000 mg.

[e]Larson RA, Dodge RK, Burns CP, et al. A five-drug remission induction regimen with intensive consolidation for adults with acute lymphocytic leukemia. Cancer and leukemia Group B study 8811. Blood 1995;85:2025–2037.

Adapted from Leather HL, Bickert B. Acute leukemias. In: DiPiro JT, Talbert RL, Yee GC, et al., eds. Pharmacotherapy: A Pathophysiologic Approach, 6th ed. New York: McGraw-Hill; 2005:2191–2213.

based on absolute neutrophil count (ANC). The benefit of adding intermittent "pulses" of vincristine and a steroid (usually dexamethasone) to the antimetabolite backbone remains unclear, but it is common practice in most modern treatment regimens.[15] The goal is to induce a moderate immunosuppression and leukemic cell kill.

6-Mercaptopurine is a key agent in maintenance therapy. It has a complex metabolism and is initially cleared by thiopurine methyltransferase (TPMT). TPMT activity is variable with about 90% of patients having normal activity, about 10% having intermediate activity, and fewer than 1% having very low or no activity. These enzymatic polymorphisms are inherited in an autosomal recessive fashion and have a profound influence on 6-mercaptopurine tolerance.[18,19]

TPMT screening is recommended for children starting therapy with 6-mercaptopurine. Children who possess alleles that have diminished activity require 6-mercaptopurine dose reductions of 50% to 90% to prevent severe immunosuppression and infection. Despite these reductions, these children have equivalent OS when compared with those receiving full-dose 6-mercaptopurine. The optimal duration of maintenance therapy in both children and adults is unknown, but most regimens are given for 2 to 3 years; extension of the regimen beyond 3 years has not shown any additional benefit.

ALL in Infants and Young Children

Infants and children younger than 1 year of age account for approximately 5% of all children with ALL and have the worst outcome of any group with this disease. These patients have several poor prognostic features at diagnosis, including hyperleukocytosis, hepatomegaly, splenomegaly, and CNS leukemia.[9]

A characteristic finding in up to 70% this group is a chromosomal translocation involving the *MLL* gene located at 11q23. There are multiple possible rearrangements of this gene with other chromosomes, and all confer a poor prognosis. In vitro, blasts these patients showed greater drug resistance to prednisolone and L-asparaginase than those from other patients, although they are more sensitive to cytarabine.[20] Based on this information, several studies are

testing the efficacy of intensified chemotherapy that includes high-dose cytarabine. Another achievement is the prevention of CNS relapse using IT cytarabine in conjunction with high-dose systemic cytarabine. This combination has eliminated the need for cranial XRT in this young population. Even with major advances in cure rates for the general pediatric ALL population, in whom survival is 80% or more, the long-term survival of infants is only about 40% (Tables 95–8 and 95–9).

ALL in Adolescents and Young Adults

As noted previously, age is an important prognostic factor in ALL. Adolescents and adult patients have generally been shown to have poorer survival than children. However, the group of patients between late adolescence and age 30 years (adolescents and young adults) has recently been shown to have a substantially better outcome than older adult patients. This appears to be the result of using treatment regimens that are the same as or closely resemble pediatric ALL regimens. Retrospective studies show that outcome is improved from the range of 30% to 40% with standard adult therapy to as high as 65% with pediatric protocols.[2,21] The reasons for this are not entirely clear, and multiple factors are likely to play a role. Among the likely explanations is that pediatric protocols use more aggressive and prolonged postremission consolidation therapy before maintenance. Other proposed explanations are the potential differences in disease biology in this versus older age patients, more intense CNS prophylaxis, and the greater degree of social support and better compliance fostered in a pediatric environment. Current and planed trials are focusing on the potential of extending this treatment approach to patients age 40 years and possibly older.

ALL in Adults

The incidence of ALL in adults ages 30 to 60 years is only two per 100,000 persons per year compared with almost 10 per 100,000 in children. The conventional risk factors such as high WBC counts, older age, and CNS disease hold true in adults as in children. However, the significance of cytogenetic and molecular markers that are so important in children seem to be less predictive of outcome in adults. An exception is the adverse prognostic factor, the presence of the *BCR-ABL* translocation (Ph$^+$) just as in childhood ALL. This occurs in 15% to 30% of adults and is even more common in patients older than 60 years of age.[21] The use of imatinib or dasatinib, both potent inhibitors of the Ph$^+$-associated BCR-ABL tyrosine kinase, has now become a standard of practice for all patient groups with Ph$^+$ disease.[7] Results show that the combination of these agents with conventional chemotherapy improves remission rates as well as OS compared with the use of conventional chemotherapy alone.[7,8,21]

Currently, the induction and consolidation regimens in adults is similar to the regimens in pediatric patients, but the more aggressive postinduction regimens are not as well tolerated in this population, particularly in elderly patients (age older than 60 years) and are associated with

Representative Chemotherapy Regimens for Pediatric ALL

Induction (1 month)
IT cytarabine on day 0

Prednisone 40 mg/m²/day or dexamethasone 6 mg/m²/day PO for 28 days

Vincristine 1.5 mg/m²/dose (maximum, 2 mg) IV weekly for 4 doses

Pegaspargase 2,500 units/m²/dose IM for 1 dose or asparaginase 6,000 units/m²/dose IM Monday, Wednesday, and Friday for 6 doses

IT methotrexate weekly for 2–4 doses

Consolidation (1 month)
Mercaptopurine 50–75 mg/m²/dose PO at bedtime for 28 days
Vincristine 1.5 mg/m²/dose (maximum, 2 mg) IV on day 0
IT methotrexate weekly for 1–3 doses
Patients with CNS or testicular disease may receive radiation

Interim Maintenance (1 or 2 cycles) (2 months)
Methotrexate 20 mg/m²/dose PO at bedtime weekly
Mercaptopurine 75 mg/m²/dose PO daily on days 0–49
Vincristine 1.5 mg/m²/dose (maximum, 2 mg) IV on days 0 and 28
Dexamethasone 6 mg/m²/day PO on days 0–4 and 28–32

Delayed Intensification (1 or 2 cycles) (2 months)
Dexamethasone 10 mg/m²/day PO on days 0–6 and 14–20
Vincristine 1.5 mg/m²/dose (maximum, 2 mg) IV weekly for 3 doses
Pegaspargase 2,500 units/m²/dose IM for 1 dose
Doxorubicin 25 mg/m²/dose IV on days 0, 7, and 14
Cyclophosphamide 1,000 mg/m²/dose IV on day 28
Thioguanine 60 mg/m²/dose PO at bedtime on days 28–41
Cytarabine 75 mg/m²/dose SC or IV on days 28–31 and 35–38
IT methotrexate on days 0 and 28

Consolidation Option (2- to 3-week intervals for 6 courses on weeks 5–24)
Mercaptopurine 50 mg/m²/dose PO at bedtime
Prednisone 40 mg/m²/day for 7 days on weeks 8 and 17
Vincristine 1.5 mg/m²/dose (maximum, 2 mg) IV on the first day of weeks 8, 9, 17, and 18
Methotrexate 200 mg/m²/dose IV + 800 mg/m²/dose over 24 hours on day 1 of weeks 7, 10, 13, 16, 19, and 22
IT methotrexate on weeks 5, 6, 9, 12, 15, and 18

Late Intensification (weeks 25–52)
Methotrexate 20 mg/m²/dose IM weekly or 25 mg/m²/dose PO every 6 hours for 4 doses every other week
Mercaptopurine 75 mg/m²/dose PO at bedtime
Prednisone 40 mg/m²/day PO for 7 days on weeks 25 and 41
Vincristine 1.4 mg/m²w/dose (maximum, 2 mg) IV on the first day of weeks 25, 26, 41, and 42
IT methotrexate on day 1 of weeks 25, 33, 41, and 49

Maintenance (12-week cycles)
Methotrexate 20 mg/m²/dose PO at bedtime or IM weekly with dose escalation as tolerated
Mercaptopurine 75 mg/m²/dose PO at bedtime on days 0–83
Vincristine 1.5 mg/m²/dose (maximum, 2 mg) IV on days 0, 28, and 56
Dexamethasone 6 mg/m²/day PO on days 0–4, 28–32, and 56–60
IT methotrexate on day 0

IM, intramuscular; IT, intrathecal; PO, oral; SC, subcutaneous.

Adapted from Leather HL, Bickert B. Acute Leukemias. In: DiPiro JT, Talbert RL, Yee GC, et al, eds. Pharmacotherapy: A Pathophysiologic Approach, 6th ed. New York: McGraw-Hill; 2005:2458–2511.

a much higher incidence of toxicity and treatment-related deaths.[7] Some investigators are studying "moderate-dose" consolidation regimens that are better tolerated. These studies are yet too early to have meaningful data. Even though remissions are achieved in 80% to 90% of adult patients, 5 years disease-free survivals are only in the 30% to 40% range. Among elderly patients, the outcome is even poorer with no more than 20% having long-term survival.

Relapsed ALL

Relapse is the recurrence of leukemic cells at any site after remission has been achieved. ❽ *Bone marrow relapse is the major form of treatment failure in 15% to 20% of patients with ALL. Most relapses have the same immunophenotype and cytogenetic changes seen of the original disease.* Bone marrow relapse is the principal form of treatment failure in patients with ALL. Extramedullary sites of relapse include the CNS and the testicles.[22] Extramedullary relapse, although once common, has decreased to 5% or less because of effective prophylaxis. Site of relapse and the length of the first remission are important predictors of second remission and OS. Marrow relapses occurring less than 18 to 24 months into first remission are associated with a poor survival, but longer periods of remission (greater than 36 months) have a much higher chance of survival.[22] Treatment strategies for relapsed ALL include chemotherapy or allogeneic hematopoietic stem cell transplant (allo-HSCT). Even though patients undergoing allo-HSCT are less likely to relapse, treatment-related toxicity leads to a higher incidence of morbidity and mortality compared with chemotherapy alone.[6] Clofarabine, a next-generation deoxyadenosine analog, has shown considerable activity in children and adults with refractory acute leukemias. Of interest, this is the only anticancer drug to receive primary indication for use in pediatrics in the past 10 years.[23]

Treatment of AML

As with ALL, the primary aim in treating patients with AML is to induce remission and thereafter prevent relapse. Treatment of AML is conventionally divided into two phases: induction and consolidation. Despite several strategies to increase the intensity of therapy, the OS rate has reached a plateau at 50% to 60%, suggesting that further intensification of therapy may not improve survival rates greatly; conventional treatment of AML already uses drug doses that are at or near those maximally tolerable.

❾ *The current induction therapy for AML usually consists of a combination of cytarabine and daunorubicin, with the frequent addition of a steroid and/or an antimetabolite such as 6-thioguanine. The second phase of treatment for AML is called* consolidation. *The purpose of this phase is to further enhance remission with more cytoreduction. This period is also a time to consider HSCT for patients in first remission.*

▶ Remission Induction

The goal of induction chemotherapy in AML is essentially identical to that in ALL—"empty" the bone marrow of

Table 95–9

Chemotherapy for the Acute Leukemias

Agent and Major Uses	Class and Mechanism	Major Side Effects	Drug Interactions
Asparaginase (L-asparaginase, Elspar) Pegaspargase (Oncaspar): ALL	Antitumor enzyme, hydrolyzes L-asparaginase in bloodstream, depriving tumor cells of the essential amino acid; results in inhibition of protein, DNA, and RNA synthesis and cell proliferation; derived from *Escherichia coli*	Hypersensitivity reactions (fever, hypotension, rash, dyspnea in 25%), much lower risk with polyethylene glycol form; low emetogenic potential; pancreatitis; decreased synthesis of proteins, clotting factors; CNS: lethargy	Increased toxicity has been noted when given concurrently with vincristine and prednisone; decreased metabolism when used with cyclophosphamide; increased hepatotoxicity when used with mercaptopurine
Cytarabine (Ara-C, cytosine arabinoside, Cytosar-U): ANLL, ALL, lymphomatous meningitis, NHL, MDS High-dose Ara-C (HiDAC) liposomal cytarabine (DepoCyt) for IT use for lymphomatous meningitis	Antipyrimidine antimetabolite; inhibits DNA polymerase with inhibition of DNA strand elongation and replication; activated in tumor cells in triphosphate form; competes with conversion of cytidine to deoxycytidine nucleotides, further blocking polymerization of DNA; leads to production of short DNS strands; cell-cycle specific (S phase): acts only on proliferating cells	Myelosuppression; alopecia; moderate emetogenic; worse with high dose (greater than 1 g/m^2) or IT administration; diarrhea; mucositis; flulike syndrome with fever and arthralgias; rash often followed by desquamation on palms and soles HiDAC toxicities; cerebellar direct neurotoxicity: ataxia, slurred speech, nystagmus; conjunctivitis (drug is excreted into tears and blocks corneal DNA synthesis)	Possible increased toxicity when given concurrently with alkylating agents, radiation, purine analogs, and methotrexate
Daunorubicin (daunomycin, Dauno, Cerubidine) Liposomal daunorubicin (DaunoXome): ANLL, ALL, KS	Antitumor antibiotic; topoisomerase II inhibitor; DNA intercalator; free radical formation (thought to be related to cardiac toxicity and tissue injury)	Myelosuppression (dose related); mucositis (worse with continuous infusion); moderate emetogenic potential; alopecia; vesicant: severe extravasation injury; cardiac toxicities: *acute*—not related to cumulative dose; arrhythmias, pericarditis; chronic—cumulative injury to myocardium (total dose greater than 550 mg/m^2; lower total cumulative doses cause damage to myocardium in children (e.g., 350 mg/m^2)	
Etoposide (VP-16, Vepesid), etoposide phosphate (Etopophos): testicular cancer, SCLC, NSCLC, ANLL, KS, HD, NHL, BMT preparative chemotherapy, gastric cancer	Plant alkaloid, epipodophyllotoxin; inhibits DNA binding activity of topoisomerase II, resulting in multiple DNA double-strand breaks	Myelosuppression; moderately emetogenic: may be worse with oral and high-dose regimens; alopecia; mucositis; hypotension: infusion rate related; etoposide phosphate can be given IV push without hypotension risk; hypersensitivity reactions: especially common in children	Substrate of MDR; cyclosporine may increase levels of etoposide
Gemtuzumab ozogamicin (Mylotarg)	Humanized antiCD33 antibody linked to calicheamicin, a potent toxin; binding to the CD33 receptor results in internalization of the antibody–antigen complex; calicheamicin is then released intracellularly and exerts cytotoxicity by causing DNA double-strand breaks, resulting in cell death	Infusion reactions: fevers, chills, nausea, vomiting, hypotension, dyspnea; myelosuppression may be severe and prolonged; tumor lysis syndrome: WBC counts should be reduced to less than 30 × 10^3/mm^3 (30 × 10^9/L) before administration, if possible, to decrease risk; increased liver function tests and bilirubin, hepatic veno-occlusive disease	
Imatinib mesylate (Gleevec, STI 571) CML (adults and children), GIST, Ph$^+$ALL	Tyrosine kinase inhibitor; relatively specific for the tyrosine kinase coded for by the BCR–abl translocation in CML patients	Moderate emetogenic potential: take with meals and a full glass of water; edema; periorbital edema is characteristic; pleural effusions, ascites, or pulmonary edema also occur; rash; diarrhea; neutropenia, thrombocytopenia (sometimes difficult to distinguish from CML-induced cytopenias); increased liver function tests	Drug interactions are minimal; substrate of CYP 3A4; serum concentrations of imatinib may be increased by drugs that inhibit CYP3A4

(Continued)

Table 95–9			
Chemotherapy for the Acute Leukemias (*Continued*)			
Agent and Major Uses	**Class and Mechanism**	**Major Side Effects**	**Drug Interactions**
6-Mercaptopurine (Purinethol, 6-MP): ALL	Antipurine antimetabolite; purine analog; inhibits DNA, RNA, protein synthesis; metabolized by xanthine oxidase	Myelosuppression: mild, anorexia, low emetogenic potential; dry skin rash, photosensitivity; hepatotoxicity: jaundice and hyperbilirubinemia occur after 1–2 months of therapy and may be dose limiting	Allopurinol can increase levels of mercaptopurine; aminosalicylates may inhibit TPMT
Methotrexate (MTX): ALL CNS leukemia (IT), breast cancer, NHL, osteosarcoma, head and neck cancer, bladder cancer, rheumatoid arthritis	Folic acid antagonist; inhibits DHFR; blocks reduction of folate to tetrahydrofolate; inhibits de novo purine synthesis; results in arrest of DNA, RNA, and protein synthesis / Leucovorin provides reduced folate to bypass the metabolic block	Myelosuppression: can be prevented with leucovorin rescue / Mucositis: can be prevented with leucovorin / Renal dysfunction: (high-dose regimens) caused by precipitation of drug in renal tubules; hydration (3 L/m^2/day) and alkalinization of urine	Salicylates, sulfonamides, probenecid, and high-dose penicillin may decrease clearance of methotrexate
Vincristine (VCR, Oncovin) ALL, HD, NHL, multiple myeloma, breast cancer, SCLC, KS, brain tumors, soft tissue sarcomas, osteosarcomas, neuroblastoma, Wilms' tumor	Antimicrotubule agent or vinca alkaloid; derived from periwinkle plant; disrupts formation of microtubules	Peripheral neuropathy: primary dose-limiting toxicity; motor sensory, autonomic, and cranial nerves may all be affected (paresthesias, ileus, urinary retention, facial palsies); may be irreversible; mild emetogenic; SIADH; vesicant: extravasation injury	Vincristine levels may be increased when given with drugs that inhibit cytochrome CYP3A enzyme (itraconazole)

ALL, acute lymphocytic leukemia; ANLL, acute nonlymphocytic leukemia; BMT, bone marrow transplant; C, cytarabine; CD, cluster determinants; CML, chronic myeloid leukemia; CNS, central nervous system; CYP, cytochrome; DHFR, dihydrofolate reductase; DNS, DNS strands; GIST, gastrointestinal stromal tumor; HD, Hodgkin's disease; HiDAC, high-dose Ara-C; IT, intrathecal; KS, Kaposi's sarcoma; MDS, myelodysplastic syndrome; MTX, methotrexate; NHL, non-Hodgkin's lymphoma; NSCLC, non–small cell lung cancer; Ph$^+$, Philadelphia chromosome; SIADH, syndrome of inappropriate antidiuretic hormone; SCLC, small cell lung cancer; VCR, vincristine; VP, etoposide.

Adapted from McManus Balmer C, Wells Valley A, Iannucci A. Cancer Treatment and Chemotherapy. In: DiPiro JT, Talbert RL, Yee GC, et al, eds. Pharmacotherapy: A Pathophysiologic Approach, 6th ed. New York: McGraw-Hill; 2005:2458–2511.

all hematopoietic precursors and allow repopulation with normal cells. The combination of an anthracycline (e.g., daunorubicin, doxorubicin, or idarubicin) and the antimetabolite cytarabine forms the backbone of AML induction therapy. The most common induction regimen (7 + 3) combines daunorubicin for 3 days with cytarabine on days 1 to 7.[12] The remission rate for this combination is approximately 80% in children and younger adults but declines to 40% to 50% in patients older than 60 years of age.[5,12] Despite studies that have used alternative anthracyclines or substituted high-dose for conventional-dose cytarabine and added etoposide and/or thioguanine, the 7 + 3 regimen remains the standard induction regimen. Paving the way for more innovative therapies, gemtuzumab ozogamicin, a humanized anti-CD33 antibody, has shown it improved the outcome of pediatric and younger adults patient (age younger than 60 years) when added to conventional 7 + 3 chemotherapy.[24,25]

▶ *Postremission Chemotherapy*

In AML, postremission chemotherapy is often referred to as *consolidation therapy*. Several cycles of intensive postremission chemotherapy combining non–cross-resistant

agents given every 4 to 6 weeks substantially improves DFS. Without postremission treatment, all patients would relapse within several weeks. This is analogous to the consolidation and other phases of postremission chemotherapy in ALL. One of three cytarabine-based regimens has been used in current treatment programs, either alone or in combination with L-asparaginase, mitoxantrone, or etoposide. The following cytarabine dosing schedule is used: 100 mg/m^2/day for 5 days by continuous infusion (standard-dose arm); 400 mg/m^2/day for 5 days by continuous infusion (intermediate-dose arm); or 3 g/m^2 twice daily over 3 hours on days 1, 3, and 5 (high-dose arm). The higher dose regimen for cytarabine can be tolerated only by younger patients (younger than 60 years of age). Although the optimal number of courses remains to be determined, at least three are probably required.[12]

Allogeneic Hematopoietic Stem Cell Transplantation

Allo-HSCT has been used in the treatment of pediatric AML in first complete remission. In HSCT, very high doses of chemotherapy with or without total-body irradiation (TBI) are given in an attempt to potentiate leukemia cell kill. Hematopoiesis is restored by the infusion of stem cells harvested from a human leukocyte antigen (HLA)–compatible donor, thereby rescuing the patient from the consequences of total aplasia.[5,6] It may be the most effective antileukemic therapy currently available.

The availability of HLA-matched sibling donors determined whether patients underwent HSCT as postremission treatment. To facilitate this process, it is important to obtain HLA typing on all younger patients and siblings shortly after diagnosis. Patients who do not have an HLA-matched sibling proceed to postremission therapy with chemotherapy alone.

Transplantations from nonidentical sources have many complications, including graft-versus-host disease (GVHD), delayed or incomplete engraftment, and an increased likelihood of opportunistic infections that substantially increase morbidity and mortality. A benefit of allo-HSCT is an immunologic effect of the donor marrow on residual host leukemic cells that seems to improve antileukemic activity. This is evidenced by the lower relapse rates in patients with GVHD.

Transplant-related mortality following matched-sibling allo-HSCT is 20% to 30% in most series. Complications from transplantation increase with age; therefore, patients older than 60 years of age are uncommonly considered to receive a myeloablative allo-HSCT. Because the average age of AML patients is 65 years, most patients with this disease are not candidates for this form of therapy. For older patients up to 70 years of age, a reduced-intensity (mini or nonmyeloablative allogeneic) transplant may be an option. These transplants use less intensive preparative regimens and rely on the allogeneic graft-versus-leukemia effect to eliminate their disease.[12]

HSCT in first remission is often recommended for patients with a matched-sibling donor because of the lower relapse rate with transplant versus postremission chemotherapy. However, only 30% of patients have an HLA-matched sibling. Some types of AML patients may be curable with conventional-dose chemotherapy alone. Thus indiscriminate use of allo-HSCT could reduce the rate and quality of survival in these individuals.

Autologous Hematopoietic Stem Cell Transplantation

Because the majority of AML patients lack a HLA-identical donor, investigators began to consider the use of the patient's own bone marrow, obtained while in CR, as a source of hematopoietic regeneration. However, relapse continues to be a problem secondary to the presence of residual disease in the graft. Despite the reduced morbidity and mortality associated with auto-HSCT, this type of transplant does not compare favorably to standard postremission chemotherapy.[12]

▶ CNS Therapy

The prevalence of CNS disease at diagnosis of AML ranges from 5% to 30% in various clinical series. Features associated with the risk of CNS leukemia include hyperleukocytosis, monocytic, or myelomonocytic leukemia (FAB M4 or M5), and young age. Adequate CNS prophylaxis is an essential component of therapy. Studies have shown that patients with CNS disease at diagnosis can be cured with IT therapy alone without the use of cranial XRT. In most cases, IT cytarabine with or without methotrexate and systemic high-dose cytarabine provide effective treatment.

AML in Infants

AML in infants younger than 12 months of age shows clinical and biological characteristics different from those of older children. The disease phenotype is more commonly monoblastic or myelomonoblastic (M4, M5), and the patients usually present with hyperleukocytosis. Extramedullary involvement is common, often involving skin and other organs. As in infant ALL, there is a high incidence of translocations involving the *MLL* gene in infant AML. The number of infant AML trials reported is limited, but the EFS of this population is similar to that of older children with AML. This is in marked contrast to the outcomes for infants with ALL for whom the EFS is much lower than in older children.[26]

AML in the Elderly

AML is the most common acute leukemia in the elderly. Compared with younger patients with the same disease, older adults have a poor prognosis and represent a distinct population with regard to the biology of their disease. Older adults have a lower incidence of favorable chromosomal aberrations and a higher incidence of unfavorable aberrations.[5,12] They also have a much higher incidence of comorbidities, such as type 2 diabetes, obesity, and other physiologic limitations. Thus, the poor prognostic significance of older age is only partly a result of unfavorable biology.

In older adults, in contrast to AML in children, AML is more likely to arise from a proximal bone marrow–stem cell disorder, such as MDS, or present as a secondary, prior treatment-related leukemia. These forms of AML are notoriously poorly responsive to conventional chemotherapy and thus have a lower CR rate and poorer survival.[27]

As previously noted, age is an important prognostic factor. Older adults are not as tolerant of or as responsive to remission induction and consolidation chemotherapy as younger patients. Using a standard induction regimen of cytarabine and anthracycline, patients older than 60 years of age have only a 38% to 62% probability of remission. In contrast, younger adults treated with a similar standard-induction regimen have approximately 70% probability of attaining a CR. Furthermore, long-term survival for patients older than 60 years is only 5% to 15% compared with 30% DFS for younger adults.[5,12]

Relapsed AML

Even though 75% to 85% of patients with AML achieve a remission, only about 50% survive. Patients who relapse usually respond poorly to additional treatment and have a shorter duration of remission. This is probably related to drug resistance induced during induction and certain chromosomal abnormalities.

Even though there is no standard therapy for relapse, most studies have shown that high-dose cytarabine-containing regimens have considerable activity in obtaining a second remission. Cytarabine has been used in combination with mitoxantrone, etoposide, fludarabine, 2-chlorodeoxyadenosine, and (more recently) clofarabine.[5,12] After a patient has achieved a second remission with conventional chemotherapy, allo-HSCT is the therapy of choice. For patients without an HLA-matched sibling, a matched unrelated donor (MUD) or cord blood transplant may be a reasonable alternative. The combination of myeloablative high-dose chemotherapy and the GVL effect is thought to offer the best chance of survival in AML.

Complications of Treatment

▶ *Tumor Lysis Syndrome*

Tumor lysis syndrome (TLS) is an oncologic emergency that is characterized by metabolic abnormalities resulting from the death of blast cells and the release of large amounts of purines, pyrimidines, and intracellular potassium and phosphorus. Uric acid, the ultimate breakdown product of purines, is poorly soluble in plasma and urine. Deposition of uric acid and calcium phosphate crystals in the renal tubules can lead to acute renal failure. Many patients with acute leukemia, especially those with a high tumor burden, are at risk for TLS during the first several days of chemotherapy. Measures to prevent TLS include aggressive hydration, alkalinization to help solubilize uric acid, and allopurinol to promote other purine metabolites other than uric acid. Hyperhydration and alkalinization is generally an effective method of dealing with this issue. However, on some occasions, the use of rasburicase is indicated. Rasburicase is an enzyme that catalyzes the oxidation of uric acid to allantoin, which is much more soluble than uric acid and excreted more easily.[28,29] Given its high cost, rasburicase generally is restricted to patients with high WBC counts (greater than 50×10^3/mm³, 50×10^9/L) and uric acid levels greater than 8 mg/dL (476 µmol/L).

▶ *Infection*

Infection is a primary cause of death in acute leukemia patients. Both the disease and aggressive chemotherapy cause severe myelosuppression, placing the patient at risk for sepsis.

The therapy for AML is extremely myelosuppressive. Children with AML have a 10% to 20% induction mortality rate secondary to infection and bleeding complications. Therefore, patients receiving induction therapy usually are hospitalized for the first 4 to 6 weeks of therapy. The induction therapy for ALL is far less myelosuppressive, and these patients recover their neutrophil counts quicker and usually do not require prolonged hospitalizations.[6]

It is important to recognize that symptoms and signs of infection may be absent in a severely immunosuppressed or neutropenic patient. Fever (greater than 38.3°C [100.9°F]) in a neutropenic patient is a medical emergency. Because the progression of infection in neutropenic patients can be rapid,

empirical antibiotic therapy should be administered quickly when fever is documented. Currently, the most commonly used initial antibiotic agent is cefepime, a fourth-generation cephalosporin that has good antipseudomonal coverage as well as adequate coverage against *Streptococcus viridans* and pneumococci.[30]

Trimethoprim–sulfamethoxazole is started in all patients with any acute leukemia for the prevention of *Pneumocystis jiroveci* pneumonia (PJP). Patients normally continue this therapy for 6 months after completion of treatment. The use of additional antibiotic prophylaxis is not encouraged because of concerns for antibiotic resistance.

Of note is that up to 10% of patients seem to exhibit excessive myelosuppression with trimethoprim–sulfa antibiotics (presumably the result of the antifolate trimethoprim in combination with other systemic cytotoxic agents). Changing to another anti-PJP agent such as dapsone or inhaled pentamidine may help to alleviate this problem.

▶ *Secondary Malignancies*

Secondary malignancies are a risk of the successful treatment of a prior cancer or the use of cytotoxic agents in a variety of autoimmune diseases. The chemotherapy agents used, especially alkylating agents and topoisomerase II inhibitors, predispose patients to secondary hematopoietic neoplasms. As the aggressiveness of treatment and the number of survivors of AML increase, the risk of secondary neoplasms also may rise. There are two different types of second malignancies: acute leukemia, which is generally myeloid in origin, or MDS. There are also reports of secondary solid tumors, especially within regions of prior radiation exposure. The latency period between the end of treatment and the development of a secondary leukemia is generally in the range of 5 to 10 years. For those patients who develop secondary solid malignancies, the latency may be as long as 10 to 20 years.

The incidence of second cancers attributed to alkylators peaks 4 to 6 years after exposure and plateaus after 10 to 15 years. Higher cumulative doses and older age at the time of treatment are risk factors for this type of cancer.

Epipodophyllotoxins (etoposide and others) can induce a second malignancy characterized by balanced chromosomal translocations and short latency periods (2 to 4 years). The risk of this leukemia is related to schedule (dose intensity) and the concomitant use of other agents (L-asparaginase, alkylating agents, and possibly antimetabolites). The prognosis for topoisomerase II inhibitor–related secondary leukemia is extremely poor. Only about 10% of these patients survive after salvage chemotherapy, and only 20% survive after HSCT.

Ionizing radiation therapy is also a cause of secondary malignancies. These secondary tumors generally develop within or adjacent to the previous radiation field. These cancers often have a prolonged latency, typically 15 or more years, but shorter latencies (5 to 14 years) are known. Higher doses of radiation and younger age are associated with an increased risk of secondary malignancy.

Unlike children, adults may have other factors that predispose them to secondary malignancies. Lifestyle choices such as tobacco use, alcohol use, and diet have been implicated in influencing the development of secondary neoplasms in the adult population.

Now that 80% or more of children survive their primary cancers, the incidence of secondary neoplasms may increase. Recognizing this potential, many treatment regimens for children are being modified appropriately to reduce exposure to alkylators, topoisomerase inhibitors, and radiation. Late effects clinics screen for secondary malignancies and other disease and treatment-related disabilities that accompany childhood cancer. Similar screening and educational opportunities are not as established in adult survivors. The Lance Armstrong Foundation focuses much of its efforts on these issues and the concerns of adult and pediatric cancer survivors.

▶ *Late Effects*

With increased success in pediatric clinical trials, the OS rate for pediatric cancers has increased markedly over the last 35 years. For some diseases (acute lymphoblastic leukemia, Wilms' tumor, low-grade and common germ cell tumors), the OS rate is now at or above 80%. ❿ *Despite this significant increase in survival, many patients, particularly pediatric cancer survivors, have disease- or treatment-related disabilities. As many as 50% to 60% of these survivors are estimated to have at least one chronic or late-occurring complication of treatment.*[31] In leukemia, the intensified use of methotrexate may be responsible for some sporadic neurotoxicity seen in children and adults. Likewise, the use of pharmacologic doses of glucocorticoids has been associated with avascular necrosis of bone in older children and adults. High cumulative doses of anthracyclines can cause irreversible cardiomyopathy. Cranial XRT is now less frequently used for CNS leukemia prophylaxis but can cause neuropsychological and neuroendocrine abnormalities that may lead to obesity, short stature, or precocious puberty.[4] As newer and more intensive treatments enter clinical trials, close observation for long-term side effects will assume even greater importance.

Supportive Care

Because of the need for repeated venous access, a central venous catheter or infusion port is placed before starting treatment. These devices are useful not only for delivery of chemotherapy but also to support patients during periods of myelosuppression. Infection and bleeding complications are the primary causes of mortality in patients with leukemia.

Platelet transfusions are a common tool to prevent hemorrhage. Patients with uncomplicated thrombocytopenia can be transfused when the platelet count falls below $10 \times 10^3/mm^3$ (10×10^9/L). Patients who are either highly febrile or actively bleeding may require transfusions at higher levels. Red blood cell transfusions generally are not necessary for a hemoglobin concentration greater than 8 g/dL (80 g/L, 4.97 mmol/L).

There is much controversy regarding the routine use of colony-stimulating factors (e.g., granulocyte colony-stimulating factor [G-CSF] and granulocyte-macrophage colony-stimulating factor [GM-CSF]) in neutropenic patients. Even though several clinical trials have shown the time to ANC recovery is decreased with a colony-stimulating factor, none have demonstrated that CSFs statistically influence infection-related mortality. At present, the use of colony-stimulating factors (G-CSF most commonly) generally is limited to those chemotherapy regimens that place the patient at highest risk for prolonged neutropenia.

OUTCOME EVALUATION

Developing strategies for the treatment and monitoring of acute leukemias begins with risk stratification. Understanding the likely risk of relapse determines the aggressiveness and length of therapy. Remission status and MRD after the induction phase of treatment must be closely observed. Failure to obtain morphologic bone marrow remission by day 28 is a very adverse prognostic sign and dictates further induction treatment. For those who have a morphologic remission, quantification of MRD has become an increasingly important prognostic factor. *Levels of residual less than 0.01% appear to be associated with better outcomes.*

A clinician is generally charged with developing a plan to educate patients and families about their drugs and doses. This is a critical responsibility; it is imperative that the patients and their families understand why they are receiving their medications and how to take them. Frank, open discussion (with the family or patient in possession of their prescriptions) go a long way toward

---

Patient Care and Monitoring

1. Evaluate the patient for response to therapy during induction, consolidation, and maintenance by following hematologic indices closely.

2. Review the treatment plan closely with the patient.

3. Educate the patient on potential adverse reactions and drug interactions.

4. Stress the importance of medication compliance.

5. Provide patient education regarding disease state and drug therapy:
   - Possible complications of leukemia, especially infections.
   - Potential side effects of drug therapy
   - Warning signs to report to the physician (e.g., temperature, bruising, or bleeding)

6. Based on WBC counts during ALL maintenance, is the patient receiving the appropriate dose of mercaptopurine?

7. Provide education regarding the long-term sequelae associated with the treatment for the acute leukemias.

preventing errors that occur as a result of "assuming" that they understand their medications. If modifications are necessary secondary to toxicity or inadequate response, establish a plan for treatment change. Remember that individual patients often do not fit the "average" patient profile, and dose modifications are frequently needed. The practitioner should be familiar with dosing ranges, WBC count, and other parameters that indicate appropriate treatment response. Based on response to prior phases of treatment, the clinician should recognize potential toxicities in subsequent phases of treatment with the same or different drugs at similar or different doses.

Abbreviations Introduced in This Chapter

ALL	Acute lymphocytic/lymphoblastic leukemia
allo-HSCT	Allogeneic hematopoietic stem cell transplantation
AML	Acute myelogenous leukemia
ANC	Absolute neutrophil count
ANLL	Acute nonlymphocytic leukemia
BFM	Berlin-Frankfurt-Munster
CCR	Continuous complete remission
CD	Cluster determinants
CML	Chronic myelogenous leukemia
CR	Complete remission
CSF	Cerebrospinal fluid
CSF	Colony-stimulating factor
DFS	Disease-free survival
EFS	Event-free survival
FISH	Fluorescent in situ hybridization
G-CSF	Granulocyte colony-stimulating factor
GM-CSF	Granulocyte-macrophage colony-stimulating factor
GVHD	Graft-versus-host disease
GVL	Graft-versus-leukemia
HLA	Human leukocyte antigen
HSCT	Hematopoietic stem cell transplantation
MAB	Monoclonal antibody
MDS	Myelodysplastic syndrome
MPD	Myeloproliferative disorder
MRD	Minimal residual disease
MUD	Matched unrelated donor
OS	Overall survival
Ph+	Philadelphia chromosome
TBI	Total-body radiation
TLS	Tumor lysis syndrome
XRT	Irradiation

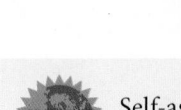

Self-assessment questions and answers are available at *http://mhpharmacotherapy. com/pp.html.*

REFERENCES

1. Pui CH, Relling MV, Downing JR. Acute lymphocytic leukemia. N Engl J Med 2004;350(15):1535–1548.
2. Ribera JM, Oriol A. Acute lymphoblastic leukemia in adolescents and young adults. Hematol Oncol Clin North Am 2009;23:1033–1042.
3. Jemal A, Siegel R, Xu J, Ward E. Cancer statistics, 2010. CA Cancer J Clin 2010;60:277–300.
4. Campana D, Pui CH. Childhood leukemia. In: Abeloff MD, Armitage JO, Niederhuber JE, et al, eds. Clinical Oncology, 4th ed. Philadelphia: Elsevier, 2008:2139–2169.
5. Applebaum FR. Acute myeloid leukemia in adults. In: Abeloff MD, Armitage JO, Niederhuber JE, et al, eds. Clinical Oncology, 4th ed. Philadelphia: Elsevier, 2008:2215–2134.
6. Pieters R, Carroll WL. Biology and treatment of acute lymphoblastic leukemia. Pediatr Clin North Am 2008;55(1):1–20.
7. Faderl SF, O'Brien S, Pui CH. et al. Adult acute lymphoblastic leukemia. Cancer 2010;116: 1165–1176.
8. Bassan R, Hoelzer D. Modern therapy of acute lymphoblastic leukemia. J. Clin Oncol 2011; 29:532–543.
9. Silverman LB. Acute lymphoblastic leukemia in infancy. Pediatr Blood Cancer 2007;49:1070–1073.
10. Mandrell BN, Pritchard M. Understanding the clinical implications of minimal residual disease in childhood leukemia. J Pediatr Oncol Nurs 2006;23:38–44.
11. Margolin JE, Rabin KR, Steuber CP, et al. Acute lymphoblastic leukemia. In: Pizzo R, Poplack DG, eds. Principles and Practice of Pediatric Oncology 6th ed. Philadelphia: Lippincott Williams & Wilkins, 2011:518–565.
12. Shipley JL, Butera JN. Acute myelogenous leukemia. Exp Hematol 2009;37:649–658.
13. Rubnitz JE, Gibson B, Smith FO. Acute myeloid leukemia. Pediatr Clin North Am 2008;55:21–51.
14. Hoelzer D, Gokbudet N. Acute lymphoid leukemia in adults. In: Abeloff MD, Armitage JO, Niederhuber JE, et al, eds. Clinical Oncology, 4th ed. Philadelphia: Elsevier, 2008:2191–2213.
15. Rabin KR, Poplack DG. Management strategies in acute lymphoblastic leukemia. Oncology 2011;15:328–347.
16. Pieters R, Carroll WL. Biology and treatment of acute lymphoblastic leukemia. Hematol Oncol Clin North Am 2010;24:1–18.
17. Pui CH, Campana D, et al. Treating childhood acute lymphoblastic leukemia without cranial irradiation. N Engl J Med 2009; 360:2730–2741.
18. Karran P, Attard N. Thiopurines in current medical practice: Molecular mechanisms and contributions to therapy related cancer. Nat Rev Cancer 2008;8:24–36.
19. Wang L, Weinshilboum R. Thiopurine S-methyltransferase pharmacogenetics; insights challenges and future directions. Oncogene 2006;25:1629–1638.
20. Pui CH, Relling MV, Campana D, et al. Childhood acute lymphoblastic leukemia. Rev Clin Exp Hematol 2002;6:161–180.
21. Larson S, Stock W. Progress in the treatment of adults with acute lymphoblastic leukemia. Curr Opin Hematol 2008;15:400–407.
22. Ribera JM, Oriol A. Acute lymphoblastic leukemia in adolescents and young adults. Hematol Oncol Clin North Am 2009;23:1033–1042.
23. Jeha S. Clofarabine for the treatment of acute lymphoblastic leukemia. Expert Rev Anticancer Ther 2007;7:113–118.
24. Cooper TM, Franklin J, Gerbing RB, et al. AAML03P1, a pilot study of the safety of gemtuzumab ozogamicin in combination with chemotherapy for newly diagnosed childhood acute myeloid leukemia: A report from the Children's Oncology Group. Cancer 2011;118(3): 761–769.
25. Burnett AK, Hills RK, Milligan D, et al. Identification of patients with acute myeloblastic leukemia who benefit from the addition of gemtuzumab ozogamicin: Results of the MRC AML15 trial. J Clin Oncol 2011;29:369–377.
26. Ishii E, Kawasaki H, Isoyama K, Eguchi-Ishimae M, Eguchi M. Recent advances in the treatment of infant acute myeloid leukemia. Leuk Lymphoma 2003;44:741–748.

27. Foran JM, Sekeres MA. Myelodysplastic syndromes. In: Abeloff MD, Armitage JO, Niederhuber JE, et al, eds. Clinical Oncology, 4th ed. Philadelphia: Elsevier, 2008:2235–2251.

28. Coiffier B, Altman A, Pui CH, et al. Guidelines for the management of pediatric and adult tumor lysis syndrome: An evidence-based review. J Clin Oncol 2008;26:2767–2778.

29. Davidson MB, Thakkar S, Hix JK, et al. Pathophysiology, clinical consequences, and treatment of tumor lysis syndrome. Am J Med 2004;116:546–554.

30. Hughes WT, Armstrong D, Bodey GP, et al. 2002 guidelines for the use of antimicrobial agents in neutropenic patients with cancer. Clin Infect Dis 2002;34:730–751.

31. Nathan PC, Wasilewski-Masker K, Janzen LA. Long term outcomes in survivors of childhood acute lymphoblastic leukemia. Hematol Clin North Am. 2009;23:1065–1082.

96

Chronic Leukemias and Multiple Myeloma

Amy M. Pick

LEARNING OBJECTIVES

● **Upon completion of the chapter, the reader will be able to:**

1. Explain the role of the Philadelphia chromosome in the pathophysiology of chronic myelogenous leukemia (CML).

2. Describe the natural history of CML.

3. Identify the clinical signs and symptoms associated with CML.

4. Discuss treatment options for CML with special emphasis on tyrosine kinase inhibitors.

5. Describe the clinical course of chronic lymphocytic leukemia (CLL).

6. Describe patients who may be observed without treatment and those who receive aggressive treatment for CLL.

7. Discuss the various treatment options available for CLL.

8. Describe the clinical presentation of multiple myeloma.

9. Discuss the treatment options available for multiple myeloma..

KEY CONCEPTS

❶ The Philadelphia chromosome (Ph) is a chromosomal translocation responsible for chronic myelogenous leukemia (CML).

❷ The Ph results in the formation of an abnormal fusion gene, *BCR-ABL*, which encodes an overly active tyrosine kinase.

❸ Allogeneic stem cell transplantation is the only curative treatment option for CML.

❹ Nearly all patients with CML are treated initially with a tyrosine kinase inhibitor (TKIs).

❺ Dasatinib and nilotinib are two second-generation TKIs that can overcome imatinib resistance or intolerance.

❻ Chronic lymphocytic leukemia (CLL) can have a variable disease course, but most patients survive for many years.

❼ Chemotherapy does not improve overall survival in early stage CLL.

❽ Fludarabine-based chemotherapy is commonly used as first-line therapy for younger patients with CLL.

❾ Autologous transplant either as a single or double transplant offers younger patients with myeloma longer disease-free survival.

❿ Newer therapies for multiple myeloma, including thalidomide, lenalidomide, and bortezomib in combination with dexamethasone, produce major responses.

INTRODUCTION

Several diseases comprise chronic leukemia. The two most common forms are chronic myelogenous leukemia (CML) and chronic lymphocytic leukemia (CLL). The slower progression of the disease contrasts it from acute leukemia, with the survival of chronic leukemia often lasting several years without treatment. This chapter covers CML and CLL. The chapter also discusses multiple myeloma and provides a brief discussion of Waldenström macroglobulinemia.

CHRONIC MYELOGENOUS LEUKEMIA

CML is a hematologic cancer that results from an abnormal proliferation of an early myeloid progenitor cell. The clinical course of CML has three phases: chronic phase, accelerated phase, and blast crisis.[1] Chemotherapy can be used to control white blood cell (WBC) counts in the chronic phase, but as CML slowly progresses, the cancer becomes resistant

Table 96–1		
Clinical Course of CML		
Phase	Characteristics	Median Duration (With Treatment)
Chronic	Elevated WBC Responsive to treatment	4–6 years[a]
Accelerated	Elevated WBC count Unresponsive to treatment Increased symptoms	6–9 months
Blast	Disease transformation to acute leukemia	3–6-month

[a]Before imatinib therapy.

CBC, complete blood count; WBC, white blood cell.

to treatment. Blast crisis resembles acute leukemia, and immediate aggressive treatment is required. Table 96–1 describes each of the phases of CML.

EPIDEMIOLOGY AND ETIOLOGY

It was estimated that 5,150 new cases of CML would be diagnosed in 2011, accounting for 12% of all adult leukemias.[2] The incidence of CML increases with age, with the median age of diagnosis being 67 years.[3,4] In most newly diagnosed cases, the etiology cannot be determined, but high doses of ionizing radiation and exposure to solvents such as benzene are recognized risk factors.

PATHOPHYSIOLOGY

Cell of Origin

CML arises from a defect in an early progenitor cell. The pluripotent (noncommitted) stem cell is implicated as the origin of the disease; therefore, multiple cell lineages of hematopoiesis may be affected, including myeloid, erythroid, megakaryocyte, and (rarely) lymphoid lineages. These cells remain functional in chronic phase CML, which is why patients in this phase are at low risk for developing infections.

Ph Chromosome

❶ *The Philadelphia chromosome (Ph) results from a translocation between chromosomes 9 and 22, leaving a shortened chromosome 22.* ❷ *The Ph results in the formation of an abnormal fusion gene between the breakpoint cluster region and the abelson proto-oncogene (BCR-ABL), which encodes an overly active tyrosine kinase. The loss of control of tyrosine kinase activity causes abnormal cellular proliferation and inhibition of apoptosis.*[1,4] Molecular tools such as quantitative and qualitative polymerase chain reaction (Q-PCR) and fluorescence in situ hybridization (FISH) are used in the detection and monitoring of CML.[5]

Clinical Presentation and Diagnosis of CML

Signs and Symptoms
- 30–50% are asymptomatic at diagnosis
- Symptoms may include fatigue, fever, weight loss, bleeding.
- Organomegaly consisting of splenomegaly and hepatomegaly

Diagnostic Procedures
- Peripheral blood smear
- Bone marrow biopsy (percentage of blasts)
- Cytogenetic studies
- Molecular testing (Q-PCR and FISH to detect *BCR-ABL* transcripts)

Laboratory Findings
Peripheral blood smear
- Leukocytosis (most present with WBC count more than 100×10^9/L, [100×10^3/mm³])
- Thrombocytosis (approximately 50% of patients in chronic phase)
- Anemia
- Presence of blasts
Bone marrow
- Hypercellularity with presence of blasts
- Presence of Ph

Poor Prognostic Factors
- Older age
- Splenomegaly
- High percent blasts in the blood
- High or low platelet count
- Increased eosinophils or basophils

TREATMENT

Desired Outcome

The primary goal in the treatment of CML is to eradicate the Ph positive clones. Elimination of the Ph is termed *cytogenetic complete remission*. If treatment produces Q-PCR–negative disease (no *BCR-ABL* transcripts detected), it is termed *molecular complete remission* and indicates a several log reduction over cytogenetic complete remission. An early goal of therapy is to achieve hematologic complete remission or to normalize peripheral blood counts. A cure from CML can only come from complete eradication of the Ph clone.

General Approach to Treatment

There have been significant advances in the treatment of CML since the discovery of the Ph in 1960. The success of therapy is partially dependent on the clinical phase of the disease. Treatment decisions are based on patient's age, phase of CML, comorbidities, and availability of a donor for transplant. Nearly all patients with CML are treated initially with a tyrosine kinase inhibitor (TKI). Three TKIs—imatinib, dasatinib, and nilotinib—are available for first-line therapy. Hydroxyurea may be used after diagnosis to rapidly reduce high WBC counts and prevent potentially serious complications (respiratory and neurologic) associated with large numbers of circulating neutrophils. Hydroxyurea, though, does not alter the disease process. TKIs can also reduce peripheral WBC counts over several weeks; therefore, many patients are started on a TKI alone. Before the development of imatinib, interferon-α (INF-α) was the treatment of choice. With the emergence of more effective therapies in CML, today INF-α's role is minimal. INF-α should be reserved for use in patients who do not respond to TKI therapy and do not enroll in a clinical trial. Although allogeneic stem cell transplant is the only curative therapy for CML, the effectiveness and survival benefit of TKIs have decreased the use of transplantation. Transplantation is reserved for patients with the T315I mutation (i.e., TKI resistance) or patients who have failed TKIs. **Figure 96–1** illustrates one common method of clinically managing newly diagnosed CML patients.

Nonpharmacologic Therapy

▶ *Hematopoietic Stem Cell Transplantation*

③ *Allogeneic stem cell transplantation is the only curative treatment option for CML.* The National Comprehensive Cancer Network (NCCN) recommends that allogeneic stem cell transplant be considered for patients with the ABL kinase domain mutation known as T315I, which confers resistance to the TKIs imatinib, dasatinib, and nilotinib. Transplant should also be considered for patients who progress on a TKI in accelerated phase or blast crisis.[3] Patients who undergo an allogeneic stem cell transplant require a human leukocyte antigen (HLA)–matched donor. Cure rates are superior when patients are transplanted in chronic phase within the first year of diagnosis and may be as high as 75%.[3] Unfortunately, only 30% to 40% of patients will be candidates for transplantation. Significant risks are associated with allogeneic transplant with a 10% to 20% early mortality rate or within 100 days of transplant.[6] Patients may also have a significant decline in quality of life from chronic graft-versus-host disease and other long-term complications associated with allogeneic stem cell transplantation. For patients who do not achieve a molecular complete remission or have a relapse after transplant, the infusion of donor lymphocytes may place the patient back into a durable remission.[3]

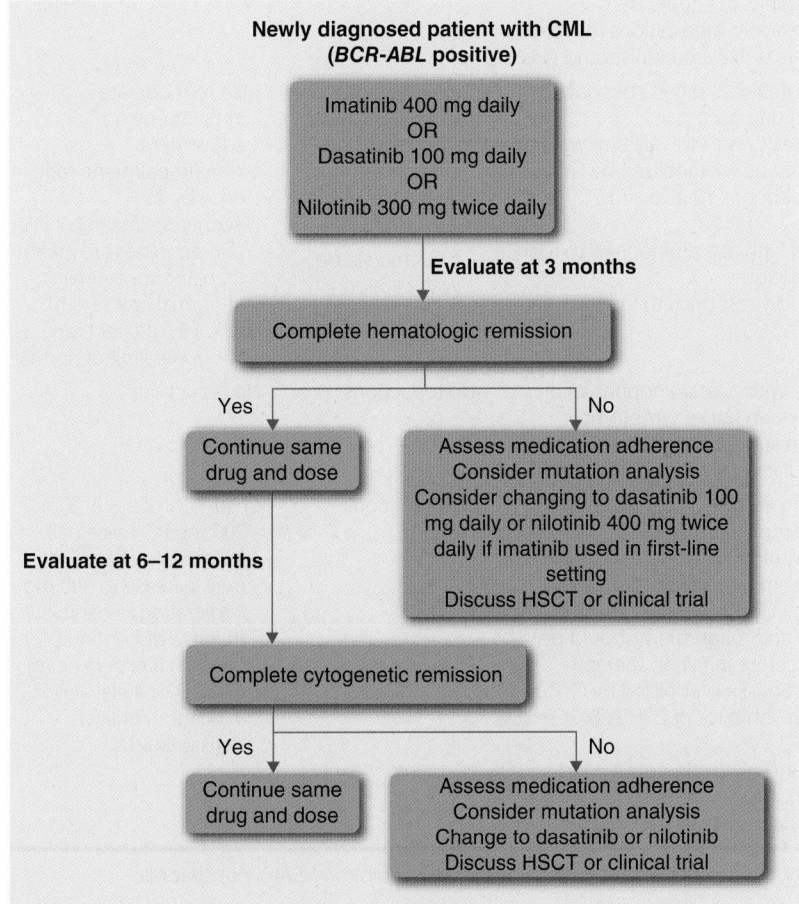

FIGURE 96–1. Algorithm for tyrosine kinase inhibitor therapy in newly diagnosed chronic myeloid leukemia (CML) patients. (HSCT, hematopoietic stem cell transplantation.)

Pharmacologic Therapy (Table 96–2)

The treatment of CML has dramatically changed since the introduction of the first- and second-generation TKIs. ❹ *Nearly all patients with CML are treated initially with TKIs.* These oral agents do not cure CML but are able to produce long-term disease control in the vast majority of patients.

▶ *Imatinib Mesylate (Gleevec)*

Imatinib mesylate (STI-571; Gleevec) was the first TKI to show efficacy in the treatment of CML. Imatinib inhibits phosphorylation of various proteins involved in cell proliferation. In CML, imatinib works by binding to the adenosine triphosphate–binding pocket of *BCR-ABL*.[4] Data show that the use of imatinib in chronic phase CML results in 88% of patients reaching 6-year survival.[7] The drug induces complete hematologic responses in more than 97% of patients and complete cytogenetic responses in about 87% of patients in chronic phase.[8] As expected with more aggressive disease, lower response rates are reported in accelerated phase and blast crisis.[9] Disease progression is typically attributed to imatinib primary or secondary resistance.[10] The ABL mutation T315I is one such mechanism of secondary resistance that results in reactivation of *BCR-ABL* activity. The T315I mutation renders imatinib and the second-generation TKIs ineffective; therefore, alternative therapy such as allogeneic

Table 96–2

Drugs Used in CML

Drug	Adverse Effects	Comments	Renal Dosing	Hepatic Dosing
Dasatinib (Sprycel)	Thrombocytopenia, neutropenia, headache, rash, edema, pleural effusions	Dose: 100 mg PO once daily for chronic phase CML or 140 mg PO daily for accelerated phase or blast crisis Avoid concomitant medications that prolong the QT-interval; low levels of potassium and magnesium should be corrected before initiating therapy Drug interactions: metabolized by CYP 3A4 (e.g., cyclosporine, erythromycin, itraconazole, phenytoin, St. John's wort) Dasatinib exhibits pH-dependent absorption; avoid medications that alter gastric pH (e.g., H2 antagonists and PPIs)	No reductions	No reductions
Imatinib mesylate (Gleevec, STI 571)	Neutropenia, thrombocytopenia, diarrhea, rash, nausea, edema, fatigue, arthralgias, myalgias, headache, increased liver function tests, congestive heart failure (rare)	Dose range: 400–800 mg PO per day depending on phase Take with meals and a full glass of water Drug interactions: metabolized by CYP 3A4; weak inhibitor of CYP 2D6 and 2C9 (e.g., warfarin) Avoid taking with acetaminophen to reduce hepatic toxicity Diarrhea usually responds to loperamide	CrCl 20–39 mL/min (0.33–0.66 mL/s): 50% reduction in dose CrCl less than 20 mL/min (0.33 mL/s): use with caution	Mild to moderate impairment: no adjustment Severe impairment: reduce dose by 25% Discontinue imatinib if liver transaminases are greater than 5 × upper limit of normal or if serum bilirubin greater than 3 × upper limit of normal
Interferon-α (Intron A, Roferon-A, IFN)	Flulike symptoms: fever, chills, myalgias, fatigue; depression; insomnia; thrombocytopenia	Premedicate with acetaminophen or an NSAID to lessen flulike symptoms Dose is given subcutaneously or intramuscularly daily	No reductions	No reductions
Nilotinib (Tasigna)	Thrombocytopenia, neutropenia, elevated bilirubin, elevated serum lipase	Dose: 400 mg PO twice daily Take on an empty stomach Black box warning for QT prolongation; avoid concomitant medications that prolong the QT interval; low levels of potassium and magnesium should be corrected before initiating therapy Drug interactions: metabolized by CYP 3A4; competitive inhibitor of CYP 2C8, 2C9, 2D6, and UGT1A1. Pharmacogenomic testing of UGT1A1 polymorphisms can be used to identify patients who may have hyperbilirubinemia	No reductions	Child-Pugh class A, B, or C: 200 mg PO twice daily for chronic phase CML; may increase to 300 mg if tolerating nilotinib therapy; discontinue nilotinib if experiencing grade 3 or 4 elevations in bilirubin or liver transaminases

CML, chronic myeloid leukemia; CrCl, creatinine clearance; IV, intravenous; PO, oral; PPI, proton pump inhibitor; NSAID, nonsteroidal anti-inflammatory drug.

stem cell transplant or clinical trials should be considered.[3,10] In addition, agents that circumvent this mutation are in clinical development.

Imatinib may be used as first-line therapy in patients with CML. Standard dosing of imatinib is 400 mg/day in chronic phase CML. Because lower response rates are seen with advanced disease, studies are investigating the use of 600 to 800 mg/day of imatinib in accelerated phase and blast crisis. Although these higher doses are used quite often in clinical practice, increased efficacy over standard dose imatinib has not been demonstrated.[11]

Therapy with imatinib is generally well tolerated. Common side effects include **myelosuppression** (phase and dose related), rash, gastrointestinal disturbances, edema, fatigue, arthralgias, myalgias, and headaches. Congestive heart failure is a rare but serious side effect (1.7% of patients) and requires careful monitoring in patients with preexisting cardiac conditions.[3] Imatinib is metabolized by CYP450 3A4, and possible drug interactions include agents that inhibit or induce 3A4, such as erythromycin, ketoconazole, and phenytoin.[12]

▶ Dasatinib (Sprycel) and Nilotinib (Tasigna)

⑤ *Dasatinib and nilotinib are two second-generation TKIs that can overcome imatinib resistance or intolerance.* These inhibitors are anywhere from 10 to 325 times more potent than imatinib in inhibiting *BCR-ABL* and are able to overcome most *BCR-ABL* mutations that lead to imatinib resistance.[10] The one exception is that neither drug can overcome the T315I mutation. Dasatinib and nilotinib were initially indicated for use in CML when patients failed imatinib therapy. Their indication has now expanded to include first-line therapy. Several phase II trials have compared dasatinib or nilotinib with imatinib. These study results suggest that dasatinib and nilotinib are comparable to, if not better than, imatinib.[13,14] Common side effects are similar to those of imatinib. A significant and potentially severe side effect of pleural effusions has been reported with the use of imatinib and dasatinib but not with the use of nilotinib. Additional side effects include QT prolongation (dasatinib and nilotinib) and increases in indirect bilirubin (nilotinib).[3,10]

▶ Interferon-α and Cytarabine

Before the introduction of TKIs, the combination of INF-α and low-dose cytarabine was the nontransplant treatment of choice for patients in chronic phase CML. The precise mechanism of action of INF-α remains unknown. The addition of cytarabine to INF-α improves the response compared with INF alone. This combination produces cytogenetic response rates of 30%, much lower than imatinib.[15] One of the major drawbacks, in addition to the low response rates, is INF's toxicity, including flulike symptoms, depression, and thrombocytopenia. Today, INF-α and cytarabine should only be considered in rare circumstances for patients who do not respond to any TKI and are not candidates for stem cell transplantation or a clinical trial.

OUTCOME EVALUATION

Successful treatment for CML depends on the elimination of the Ph. Nearly all newly diagnosed CML patients will initially be placed on a TKI. Although historically imatinib has been used as first-line therapy, dasatinib and nilotinib are also viable options, receiving their first-line indications in 2010. Which agent to use depends on several factors, including mutational status, disease risk score, age, comorbid conditions, and medication safety profile. Patients should be counseled on the importance of medication adherence. Patients should understand that poorer outcomes may result if they are not adherent to daily TKI therapy. If patients fail to obtain a cytogenetic response within 6 to 12 months, a change in therapy is recommended. If imatinib was used as first line, a change to dasatinib or nilotinib is recommended.[3] If dasatinib or nilotinib was chosen as first line, then a switch to the other second-generation TKI is recommended. If the T315I mutational status is present, the patient should consider transplantation or a clinical trial without trying another TKI. Patients who do not respond to a TKI and cannot be transplanted should be encouraged to enroll in a clinical trial. Some patients will not respond to treatment and will progress to blast crisis when they will receive treatment for acute leukemia. Although its use is limited, allogeneic

---

Patient Encounter 1

KC is a 32-year-old man who presents to his ophthalmologist with complaints of blurry vision when looking at a distance. KC's medical history consists of gastroesophageal reflux disease treated with twice daily famotidine and bipolar depression treated with ziprasidone. An eye examination reveals retinal infiltrates. A CBC is drawn and shows the following:

Total WBC: 225×10^9/L (225×10^3/mm^3), (4% [0.04] blasts, 86% [0.86] segs, 10% [0.10] lymphs)

HgB/HCT: 8.3 g/dL (83 g/L; 5.15 mmol/L)/25% (0.25)

Platelets: 65×10^9/L (65×10^3/mm^3)

KC is referred to an oncologist for further workup. A bone marrow biopsy is performed and reveals hypercellular marrow with 5% (0.05) blasts. FISH analysis is positive for Ph.

What are the first-line treatment options for chronic phase CML patient?

Which specific treatment do you recommend for this patient and why?

Identify your treatment goals for this patient.

If this patient has suboptimal response to your initial therapy, what would you recommend?

What factors may contribute to this patient's having a suboptimal response?

transplant offers the only cure for CML. Allogeneic stem cell transplantation may be discussed with the minority of patients who have a matched donor and are young enough to tolerate transplant.[3]

CHRONIC LYMPHOCYTIC LEUKEMIA

CLL is a cancer that results in the accumulation of functionally incompetent lymphocytes.[16] CLL is considered an indolent, incurable disease, and treatment should only be initiated when patients have symptoms. A subset of patients has

Clinical Presentation and Diagnosis of CLL

Signs and Symptoms (40% are asymptomatic at diagnosis)[16]

- Lymphadenopathy
- Organomegaly consisting of splenomegaly and hepatomegaly
- Fatigue, weight loss, night sweats, fevers
- Chronic infections caused by immature lymphocytes

Diagnostic Procedures

- Peripheral blood smear
- Bone marrow biopsy
- Cytogenetic studies
- Molecular testing

Laboratory Findings

Peripheral-blood

- Leukocytosis (WBC count more than 100×10^9/L [more than 100×10^3/mm³])
- Lymphocytosis (absolute lymph count more than 5×10^9/L, [more than 5×10^3/mm³])
- Anemia
- Thrombocytopenia
- Hypogammaglobinemia

Bone marrow

- Must have at least 30% (0.30) lymphocytes

Poor Prognostic Factors

- Lymphocytosis with accompanying:
  - Anemia (hemoglobin less than or equal to 11.0 g/dL [less than or equal to 110 g/L; less than or equal to 6.83 mmol/L])
  - Thrombocytopenia (platelets less than 100×10^9/L [less than 100×10^3/mm³])
- ZAP-70 and CD38 antigen expression
- Cytogenetics such as deletions of chromosomes 17p and 13q

aggressive disease, and these individuals need to be treated aggressively.

EPIDEMIOLOGY AND ETIOLOGY

CLL is the most common type of leukemia diagnosed in adults, accounting for 30% of all adult leukemias. It was estimated that in 2011, 14,570 new cases would be diagnosed in the United States.[2] The median age at diagnosis is the sixth decade of life with the incidence increasing with age. The etiology of CLL is unknown, but hereditary factors may have a role, with family members of CLL patients having a two- to sevenfold increased risk of CLL.[16]

PATHOPHYSIOLOGY

Cell of Origin

CLL is characterized by small, relatively incompetent B lymphocytes that accumulate in the blood and bone marrow over time. The lack of apoptotic mechanisms leads to the persistence and accumulation of B lymphocytes. The exact cell of origin is controversial but has been described as an antigen activated B lymphocyte.[16] Chromosomal abnormalities have been identified in 40% to 50% cases of CLL. Detection of some of these markers may predict clinical course and prognosis and may influence treatment decisions.[16,17]

Clinical Course

⑥ *CLL can have a variable clinical course with survival ranging from months to decades.* Low-risk disease is asymptomatic, and median survival times exceed 10 years. Intermediate risk is associated with lymphadenopathy and has median survival times of about 7 years. High-risk patients with anemia have median survival times of only 3 years.[18] The typical low-risk patient is an elderly patient without symptoms who is diagnosed on routine blood draw. The typical high-risk patient is a middle-aged patient in which symptoms have brought him or her to a physician.

PROGNOSTIC FACTORS

Two staging systems, Rai's and Binet's, have been developed to help practitioners determine the overall prognosis of patients with CLL. They are comparable systems and are useful when broadly determining good, intermediate, and poor prognostic disease.[16,17] Risk stratification criteria included in these systems are the presence of lymphadenopathy, splenomegaly, hepatomegaly, and cytopenias. Increasingly, a number of biological markers of the disease such as deletions of chromosome 17p and 13q and mutational status of immunoglobulin heavy chain variable region gene (IgVH) are being used to predict the likely clinical course.[18] These biological markers are not included in the Rai or Binet staging systems.

TREATMENT

Desired Outcomes

The primary goals in the treatment of CLL are to provide palliation of symptoms and improve overall survival. Because the current treatments for CLL are not curative, reduction in tumor burden and improvement in disease symptoms are reasonable end points, particularly in older patients. A complete response (CR) to therapy can be defined as a resolution of lymphadenopathy and organomegaly, normalization of peripheral blood counts, and elimination of lymphoblasts in the bone marrow.

Nonpharmacologic Therapy

❼ *Chemotherapy does not improve overall survival in early stage CLL.* In addition, deferring therapy until a patient becomes symptomatic does not alter overall survival.[19,20] For this reason, the notion of "watch and wait" (observation) is considered reasonable for older patients with indolent disease. Several factors will influence this approach, including the patient's life expectancy, disease characteristics, and the patient's ability to tolerate therapy.[21]

▶ *Hematopoietic Stem Cell Transplantation*

The use of hematopoietic stem cell transplantation (HSCT) in CLL is limited. Allogeneic transplantation offers longer disease-free remissions than autologous transplantation but is associated with high treatment morbidity and mortality. Several factors must be considered before allogeneic stem cell transplantation. The lack of a donor, older age, and poor performance status make transplant an uncommon procedure in this population. Allogeneic transplantation may be an option for younger patients who have aggressive disease. NCCN guidelines suggests that patients younger than 70 years of age with the deletion of chromosome 17p or who relapse after initial treatment consider allogeneic stem cell transplantation because these patients have a poor response to conventional therapies.[22] Although its use is currently limited, HSCT may someday be an important component in achieving a cure for CLL.[16]

Pharmacologic Therapy (Table 96–3)

Numerous agents can be used as initial therapy in the treatment of symptomatic or advanced CLL. The discussion below focuses on the common agents used in the treatment of CLL. Because many of these chemotherapy regimens have never been compared directly with one another, there is not one preferred regimen. Selection of the appropriate chemotherapy depends on the individual patient and practitioner's preference. Figure 96–2 illustrates one approach for initial therapy in newly diagnosed patients with CLL.

▶ *Single-Agent Chemotherapy*

Historically, chlorambucil (Leukeran), an alkylating agent, was considered the standard treatment for CLL. Today, the treatment for CLL has changed with the development of the purine analogs. There are three purine analogs used in the treatment of CLL: fludarabine (Fludara), pentostatin (Nipent), and cladribine (Leustatin) with fludarabine being the most studied. **❽** *Today, fludarabine-based chemotherapy is often used as first-line therapy for younger patients with CLL.* Randomized clinical trials have shown that fludarabine is superior to chlorambucil in achieving higher response rates and producing a longer duration of response (CR 20% versus 4%, respectively).[23] Fludarabine is effective in previously untreated patients as well as patients who have chlorambucil-resistant disease.[24] Although fludarabine is one of the most effective agents in the treatment of CLL, it is rarely used as a sole agent. Instead fludarabine is given in combination with other drugs.[16,22,23]

The most common dose for fludarabine is 20 mg/m^2 intravenously (IV) daily for 5 consecutive days, but chlorambucil can be taken daily as an oral tablet with the dose ranging from 4 to 10 mg/day.[24] Fludarabine is associated with more toxicities than chlorambucil, including myelosuppression and prolonged immunosuppression.[23] Resultant infectious complications may occur during the periods of prolonged immunosuppression. NCCN guidelines recommend that clinicians consider antibacterial and antiviral prophylaxis for *Pneumocystis* carinii and varicella zoster when using fludarabine-based therapy.[22] Today, chlorambucil remains a practical option for symptomatic elderly patients who require palliative therapy because of the ease of oral administration and limited side effects profile.

Bendamustine (Treanda) is an alkylating agent approved in 2008 for the treatment of CLL. As first-line therapy for CLL, bendamustine was shown to have superior overall response rates, CRs, and longer progression-free survival than chlorambucil.[22] The efficacy of bendamustine has not been compared to fludarabine-based combination therapy. NCCN guidelines suggest that bendamustine may be given as first-line therapy with rituximab.[22] The dosing for bendamustine is 100 mg/m^2 given IV on days 1 and 2 of a 28-day cycle. Table 96–3 lists some of the adverse effects seen with bendamustine.

▶ *Monoclonal Antibodies*

Rituximab (Rituxan) Rituximab is a naked chimeric monoclonal antibody directed against the CD20 antigen on B-lymphocytes.[25] Similar to other B-cell malignancies, CLL expresses CD20 antigens. Dose escalation studies suggest that higher doses are required than those used in non-Hodgkin's lymphoma.[25] The higher dose required in CLL is probably a combined effect of lower CD20 antigen expression and higher concentrations of soluble CD20 antigen than in non-Hodgkin's lymphoma.[16,25] Rituximab is typically given in combination with other therapies since these combinations result in higher CRs than rituximab alone.[26] The most commonly observed side effects of rituximab include infusion reactions consisting of fever, chills, hypotension, nausea, vomiting, and headache.[16] Premedication with diphenhydramine

Table 96–3

Drugs Used in CLL

Drug	Adverse Effects	Comments	Renal Dosing	Hepatic Dosing
Alemtuzumab (Campath)	Infusion reactions: fever, chills, nausea, vomiting; hypotension; prolonged immunosuppression (resulting in infectious complications)	Antiviral and PCP prophylaxis should be initiated during treatment Consider antifungal prophylaxis Premedicate with acetaminophen, diphenhydramine with or without a steroid to alleviate infusion-related reactions SC dosing may lessen acute toxicity	No reductions	No reductions
Bendamustine (Treanda)	Myelosuppression, fever, nausea, vomiting, infusion reactions, tumor lysis syndrome	Consider using allopurinol for tumor lysis syndrome during first few cycles of therapy	CrCl less than 40 mL/min (0.67 mL/s): do not use	Mild impairment: use with caution Moderate to severe impairment: do not use
Chlorambucil (Leukeran)	Myelosuppression; allergic reactions (skin rash); secondary malignancies	Take on an empty stomach because food decreases absorption Dose range: 4–10 mg PO daily	No reductions	No reductions
Fludarabine (Fludara)	Myelosuppression; prolonged immunosuppression, resulting in secondary infectious complications; edema; neurotoxicity	Dose: 20 mg/m² IV daily for 5 days Often given in combination	CrCl 30–70 mL/min (0.50–1.17 mL/s): 20% reduction of dose (IV and PO) CrCl less than 30 mL/min (0.50 mL/s): do not use IV; reduce dose of oral by 50%	No reductions
Ofatumumab (Arzerra)	Severe infusion-reactions: bronchospasm, edema, fever, chills, rigors, hypotension; prolonged myelosuppression	Premedicate with acetaminophen, IV antihistamine, and an IV steroid to alleviate infusion-related reactions Rate of infusion should be increased gradually to minimize reactions Monitor for reactivation of hepatitis B	No reductions	No reductions
Pentostatin (Nipent)	Myelosuppression; infectious complications	Fatal pulmonary toxicity when given with fludarabine	Hold dose if serum creatinine increases	No reductions
Rituximab (Rituxan)	Infusion reactions: fever, chills, rigors, hypotension	Premedicate with acetaminophen, diphenhydramine with or without a steroid to alleviate infusion related reactions Rate of infusion should be increased gradually to minimize reactions Monitor for reactivation of hepatitis B	No reductions	No reductions

CrCl, creatinine clearance; IV, intravenous; PO, oral; PCP, pneumocystits pneumonia; SC, subcutaneous.

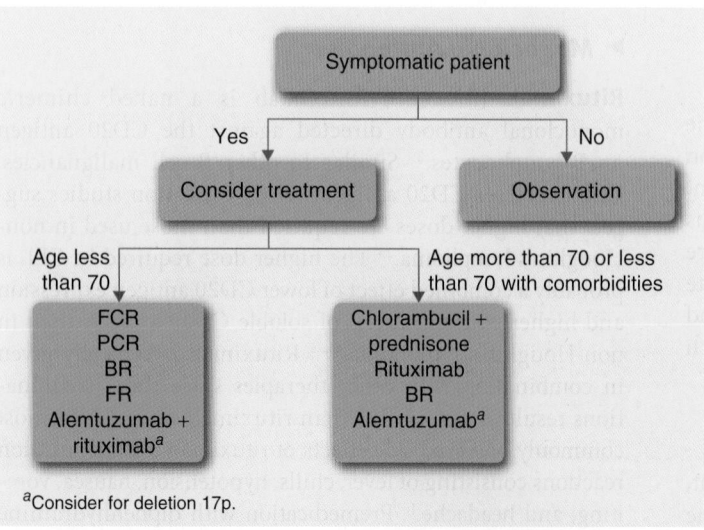

FIGURE 96–2. Algorithm for initial therapy in newly diagnosed chronic lymphocytic leukemia (CLL) patients. B, bendamustine; C, cyclophosphamide; F, fludarabine; P: pentostatin; R, rituximab.

and acetaminophen is recommended to minimize infusion reactions.

Ofatumumab (Arzerra) Ofatumumab is a newer CD20 antigen-directed monoclonal antibody that is approved in CLL patients who fail fludarabine and alemtuzumab.[22] Premedications are similar to rituximab with the addition of a corticosteroid to reduce the incidence of infusion reactions. The rate of infusion depends on patient tolerability of ofatumumab. Although it is currently used in refractory patients, its use in CLL may expand in the future. Table 96–3 lists some of the adverse effects seen with ofatumumab.

Alemtuzumab (Campath) Alemtuzumab is a humanized monoclonal antibody directed against the CD52 antigen.[27] CD52 antigen is expressed on the majority of B and T lymphocytes. Alemtuzumab is approved by the Food and Drug Administration for single-agent use in the treatment of CLL. Studies have shown alemtuzumab to be effective in fludarabine-resistant disease, in patients with the deletion of 17p, and as front-line therapy.[23] Infusion-related reactions can be significant and typically occur with the initial dose and lessen in severity with subsequent doses. To limit acute allergic reactions, subcutaneous administration may be given instead of IV dosing.[16,23] Premedication with oral antihistamines and acetaminophen is recommended. Alemtuzumab also suppresses the T cells, resulting in prolonged immunosuppression. Infectious complications may occur from the reactivation of cytomegalovirus and herpes virus and from infection with *Pneumocystis* carinii. These infections have been shown to occur with both the IV and subcutaneous routes of administrations. Guidelines recommend that patients receive trimethoprim–sulfamethoxazole and acyclovir or an equivalent antiviral to prevent these infections.[16,28]

● **Fludarabine-Based Combination Therapy** Fludarabine-based combination therapy may improve long-term disease-free survival. The combination of fludarabine, cyclophosphamide, and rituximab improves CR rates compared with fludarabine alone (70% versus 20%, respectively) but at the expense of increased infections.[28,29] The combination of fludarabine and alemtuzumab is also being investigated, with the hopes of improving overall survival.[16] No fludarabine-based regimen has been shown to be superior to another.[23]

OUTCOME EVALUATION

Successful outcomes depend on the appropriate treatment selection for a specific patient. A risk-versus-benefit analysis should be done in the treatment of older CLL patients.
● Because CLL is not curable, watch and wait is a reasonable approach for those with indolent disease. Treatment can then begin when the patient becomes symptomatic. Aggressive fludarabine-based therapy is often reserved for younger patients with high-risk CLL, with the goal being prolonged disease-free survival. A desirable response to therapy includes

---

Patient Encounter 2

JR is a 72-year-old man who is admitted to the hospital for fever, chills, and shortness of breath. His medical history includes chronic obstructive pulmonary disease, type 2 diabetes mellitus, and hypertension. A thorough workup is performed with the following results reported:

Chest x-ray: right upper lobe infiltrates and a right lung base nodule

Chest CT with contrast: stable noncalcified mass in the peripheral right lower lobe; bilateral airspace infiltrates in lower lobes compatible with pneumonia; stable mediastinal adenopathy; splenomegaly

Abdominal ultrasound: hepatosplenomegaly; prior cholecystectomy

Bone marrow biopsy: extensive bone marrow and peripheral blood involvement by chronic lymphocytic leukemia; CD20 essentially negative; cytogenetics report: deletions of 13q, 17p, and 11q

Peripheral blood smear: macrocytic anemia, marked thrombocytopenia, and marked absolute lymphocytosis with atypical lymphocytes and smudge cells consistent with chronic lymphocytic leukemia

What information supports the diagnosis of CLL?

Identify your treatment goals for this patient.

What treatment approach do you recommend?

Would your treatment options change if this patient were an otherwise healthy 46-year-old man? If so, what would be your new treatment?

---

a reduction in lymphocytes, decrease in stage of the disease, and resolution of symptoms.

MULTIPLE MYELOMA

Multiple myeloma is a malignancy of the plasma cell and is characterized by an abnormal production of a monoclonal protein in the bone marrow. Features of the disease include bone lesions, anemia, and renal insufficiency.[30] Multiple myeloma is an incurable disease; however, advancements in the treatment of myeloma have significantly extended survival.

EPIDEMIOLOGY AND ETIOLOGY

Multiple myeloma is the second most common hematologic malignancy. It is estimated that approximately 20,520 new cases of multiple myeloma would be reported in 2011, accounting for 1% to 2% of all cancers.[2] The median age at diagnosis is 70 years, and fewer than 2% are diagnosed before the age of 40 years.[30,31] The incidence of myeloma is highest in African Americans, lowest in Asians, and occurs more frequently in men than women.[31] The etiology of multiple myeloma is unknown.

PATHOPHYSIOLOGY

The pathogenesis of multiple myeloma is quite complex with multiple-step models created to postulate the process. Myeloma must be distinguished from a condition called monoclonal gammopathy of unknown significance (MGUS), which is characterized by a monoclonal immunoglobulin without malignant plasma cells. Yearly, about 1% of patients with MGUS will develop multiple myeloma. Chromosomal abnormalities and changes in gene expression lead to cell cycle dysregulation and appear to be involved early in the disease process.[30] The pathophysiology of multiple myeloma involves complex bone marrow microenvironment, and cytokine interactions. Interleukin-6, tumor necrosis factor, vascular endothelial growth factor, and stroma-derived factor-1 support the establishment and proliferation of myeloma cells.[30,31] The understanding of these interactions has led to novel agents used in the treatment of multiple myeloma.

PROGNOSTIC FACTORS

Prognostic factors for myeloma include extent of tumor burden and patient performance status. The International Staging System is used to predict outcomes after therapy. Staging is stratified based on the levels of serum β_2-microglobulinemia and serum albumin. High β_2-microglobulinemia and low albumin are poor prognostic factors and are indicative of high tumor load.[34] Although cytogenetic abnormalities are not included in the International Staging System, many abnormalities are associated with poor outcomes. Chromosomal changes are being used to predict high-risk patients with perhaps the most important being deletions of the long arm of chromosome 13 and translocation of chromosomes 4 and 14.[30,32,33] Older patients, renal impairment, and other comorbidities also predict for poorer outcomes.[34]

TREATMENT

Desired Outcomes

The primary goal in the treatment of multiple myeloma is to decrease tumor burden and minimize complications

---

Clinical Presentation and Diagnosis of Multiple Myeloma

Signs and Symptoms
- "CRAB"
  - "C"—hyper**C**alcemia
  - "R"—**R**enal failure (serum creatinine greater than 2 mg/dL [greater than 177 μmol/L])
  - "A"—**A**nemia (fatigue)
  - "B"—**B**one disease (pain, lesions, fractures)
- Weight loss
- Recurrent infections

Diagnostic Procedures
- Laboratory
  - CBC, chemistry panel, β_2 microglobulin
  - Peripheral blood smear
  - Serum protein electrophoresis and immunofixation
  - Urine protein electrophoresis and immunofixation
  - Serum free light chains
- Radiologic evaluation (MRI, bone densitometry)
- Bone marrow biopsy
  - Cytogenetic studies
  - Molecular testing

Laboratory Findings
- Peripheral blood
  - Monoclonal protein in serum (usually IgG or IgA)
  - High β_2 microglobulin
  - Low platelets and hemoglobin
  - High creatinine, urea, lactate dehydrogenase, C-reactive protein, and calcium
  - Rouleaux formation
- Urinalysis
  - Urinary free light chains (Bence-Jones Protein)
- Bone marrow
  - Plasma cells (10% or more)
  - Abnormal cytogenetics
- Radiologic findings
  - Bone lesions, fractures, osteoporosis

Poor Prognostic Factors
- High serum β₂-microglobulin and low serum albumin
- Elevated C-reactive protein
- Elevated lactate dehydrogenase
- IgA isotype
- Low platelet count
- Chromosome 13 deletions and other cytogenetic abnormalities

Patient Encounter 3

A 52-year-old woman presents with her health care provider with complaints of upper left leg and hip pain. Her medical history is irrelevant with the exception of a recent fall (2 months ago) while ice skating. Workup reveals:

Radiologic data:

X-ray of left hip: Osteolytic lesions

Laboratory data:

Hemoglobin: 6.7 g/dL (67 g/L; 4.16 mmol/L)

Platelets: 180×10^9/L (180×10^3/mm³)

Corrected calcium: 12.6 mg/dL (3.15 mmol/L)

Serum creatinine: 2.4 mg/dL (212 μmol/L)

Serum IgG: 3700 mg/dL (37 g/L) (normal, 620–1500 mg/dL [6.2–15 g/L])

Serum IgM: 100 mg/dL (1 g/L) (normal 50–200 mg/dL [0.5–2 g/L])

Bone marrow: 90% (0.90) plasma cell infiltrates

What information is suggestive of multiple myeloma?

What treatment options are available for this patient?

Assuming this patient is a candidate for autologous stem cell transplantation, what would be an appropriate induction regimen?

Assuming this patient is a not a candidate for autologous stem cell transplantation, what would be an appropriate induction regimen?

What may be used for maintenance therapy after an autologous stem cell transplantation?

---

associated with the disease. A watch and wait approach is an option for asymptomatic patients (smoldering myeloma) who have no lytic lesions in the bone. When symptoms occur, treatment is required. All patients should be evaluated to see it they are eligible candidates for transplant. Autologous stem cell transplantation prolongs overall survival in patients who can tolerate high-dose chemotherapy. Immunomodulators such as thalidomide should be incorporated into initial therapy to reduce tumor burden in patients with symptomatic disease. Almost all patients become refractory to initial treatment and require the use of salvage therapies. Maintenance therapy with immunomodulators or bortezomib is frequently being used to prolong the duration of response. Figure 96–3 illustrates possible treatment approaches for transplant-eligible and -ineligible patients.

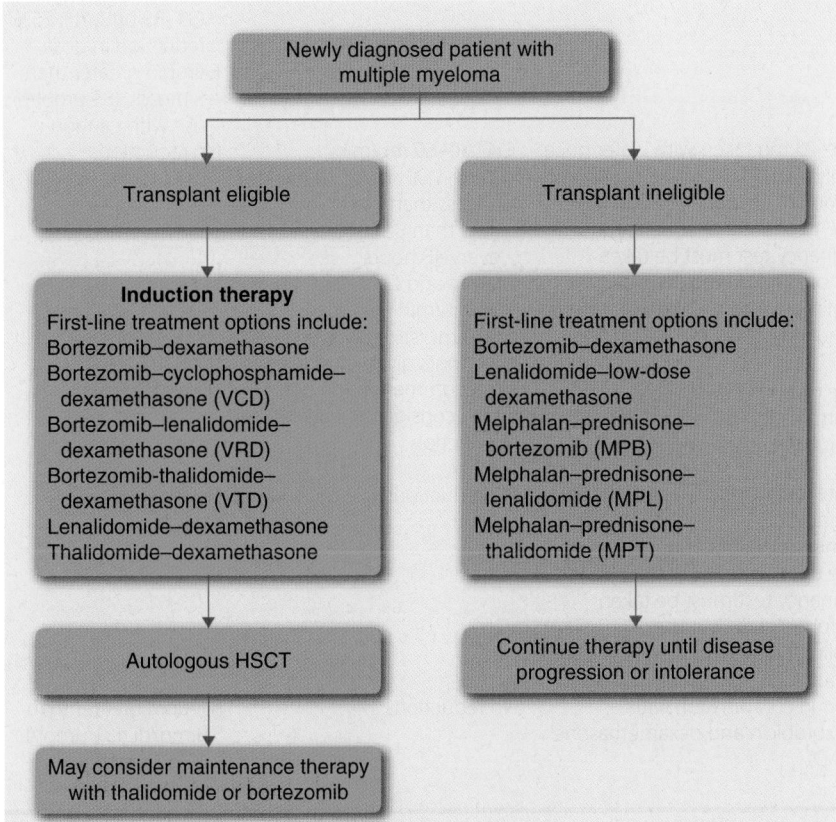

FIGURE 96–3. Possible approach for treatment in newly diagnosed patients with multiple myeloma. (HSCT, hematopoietic stem cell transplantation.)

Nonpharmacologic Therapy

▶ *Autologous Stem Cell Transplantation*

❾ *Autologous stem cell transplantation results in higher response rates and extends overall survival compared with those who receive conventional therapy such as vincristine–doxorubicin–dexamethasone (VAD).* Because overall median survival is prolonged from 42 to 54 months, stem cell transplant should be considered in all patients who can tolerate high-dose chemotherapy.[34,35] High-dose melphalan is the most common preparative regimen. Two sequential transplants (tandem transplants) improve overall survival in patients who do not have a good partial response after one transplant.[31] The use of maintenance therapy after autologous transplantation with thalidomide or bortezomib may be used in select patients to extend progression-free survival.[33] It should be noted that the studies supporting the use of transplant were done before the development of many of the novel agents used in the treatment of myeloma; thus, the future role of stem cell transplantation may evolve.

Pharmacologic Therapy (Table 96–4)

▶ *Conventional-Dose Chemotherapy*

When patients present with symptomatic disease, they are started on therapy. The use of conventional-dose chemotherapy

---

Table 96–4

Drugs Used in Multiple Myeloma

Drug	Adverse Effects	Comments	Renal Dosing	Hepatic Dosing
Bortezomib (Velcade)	Constipation; decreased appetite; asthenia; fatigue; fever; thrombocytopenia; dose related, reversible peripheral neuropathy	Dose: 1.3 mg/m² IV bolus twice weekly for 2 weeks; week 3 off; repeat SC administration is being studied Consider herpes zoster prophylaxis with daily acyclovir	No reductions	Bilirubin greater than 1.5 × the upper limit of normal: reduce dose to 0.7 mg/m²
Dexamethasone	Hyperglycemia, edema, adrenal cortical insufficiency	Dose given PO once daily	No reductions	No reductions
Doxorubicin (Adriamycin)	Myelosuppression; alopecia; cumulative dose-limiting toxicity: myocardium damage	Given in combination with VAD	No reductions	Bilirubin 1.2–3 mg/dL (21–51 μmol/L): 50% reduction in dose Bilirubin 3.1–5 mg/dL (53–85 μmol/L): 75% reduction in dose Bilirubin greater than 5 mg/dL (85 μmol/L): use with caution
Lenalidomide (Revlimid)	Possible birth defects (because it is an analogue of thalidomide), neutropenia, thrombocytopenia, DVT, PE, pruritus, fatigue	Dose: 25 mg taken with water once daily Women of childbearing age must use two forms of contraception Pregnancy test must be taken before and during use Enrollment into monitoring program required	CrCl 30–60 mL/min (0.50–1.00 mL/s): 10 mg/day CrCl less than 30 mL/min (less than 0.50 mL/s): 15 mg every 48 hours Dialysis and CrCl less than 30 mL/min (less than 0.50 mL/s): 5 mg every 24 hours given after dialysis	No reductions
Melphalan (Alkeran)	Myelosuppression, secondary malignancies, pulmonary fibrosis, sterility, alopecia	Dose given PO once daily IV formulation used for stem cell transplantation	No recommendation but may consider an initial dose reduction	No reductions
Thalidomide (Thalomid)	Severe birth defects, peripheral neuropathy, DVT, somnolence, constipation	Titrate initial doses; doses are taken nightly Women of childbearing age must use two forms of contraception Pregnancy test must be taken before and during use Enrollment into monitoring program required	No reductions	No reductions
Vincristine (Oncovin)	Dose-limiting toxicity: peripheral neuropathies; paresthesias, constipation, alopecia	Given in combination with doxorubicin and dexamethasone (VAD)	No reductions	Bilirubin greater than 3 mg/dL (51 μmol/L): 50% reduction in dose

DVT, deep venous thrombosis; IV, intravenous; PE, pulmonary embolism; PO, oral; SC, subcutaneous; VAD, vincristine–dexamethasone.

has declined with the advent of immunomodulators and bortezomib. The combination of melphalan and prednisone (MP) was once the most common initial treatment combination for myeloma. Today, MP is often used in combination therapy with immunomodulators as front-line therapy for patients who are not eligible for transplant. VAD is another combination chemotherapy regimen that was often used in patients with myeloma. VAD may be an alternative option for induction therapy in patients who are transplant eligible because it avoids the alkylating agent melphalan, thus minimizing the risk of secondary malignancies that are associated with chronic alkylating therapy.[32]

▶ *Thalidomide (Thalomid)*

Thalidomide as monotherapy or combination therapy is effective in the treatment of multiple myeloma. The precise mechanism of action of thalidomide is unknown, but its antimyeloma activity may be attributable to its antiangiogenic and anticytokine properties.[36] ⑩ *The combination of thalidomide, bortezomib, and dexamethasone has emerged as the one of the most commonly used induction regimens in the treatment of transplant-eligible patients with myeloma.* Thalidomide and steroid combinations produce responses in 60% to 80% of previously untreated patients.[37] Responses can be improved to 94% with the addition of a third agent, bortezomib, but adding a fourth agent does not further improve responses.[38,39] The addition of thalidomide to MP also improves overall response and overall survival in newly diagnosed patients.[40] This combination (MPT) can be used as initial therapy in patients who are not transplant eligible. Common side effects of thalidomide therapy include somnolence, constipation, peripheral neuropathy, and deep venous thrombosis (DVT). Standard dose warfarin or low-molecular-weight heparins are recommended to prevent DVT.[34,41] There are substantial teratogenic effects of thalidomide if it is used during pregnancy, so distribution of the drug is closely monitored through the STEPS program.

▶ *Lenalidomide (Revlimid)*

Lenalidomide is an immunomodulating agent related to thalidomide that is approved for the treatment of relapsed myeloma in combination with dexamethasone. ⑩ *Lenalidomide and dexamethasone with or without bortezomib may be used for induction therapy before a transplant.* Phase III trials showed that lenalidomide in combination with dexamethasone produced higher response rates and a longer time to progression than dexamethasone alone in relapsed and refractory myeloma.[34,42] Low-dose dexamethasone with lenalidomide offers improved overall survival compared with high-dose dexamethasone.[43] The combination of melphalan, prednisone, and lenalidomide (MPL) may be used as initial therapy in patients not eligible for transplant. The response rate appears to be quite high at 81% with 24% achieving a CR.[42] A randomized trial comparing MPL with MPT is currently underway. Lenalidomide has a more favorable safety profile over thalidomide because it

lacks the common side effects of somnolence, constipation, and peripheral neuropathy. Significant adverse effects of lenalidomide include myelosuppression and DVT. Similar to thalidomide–dexamethasone, DVT prophylaxis is recommended with lenalidomide–dexamethasone combinations.[34,41] Stem cells should be collected shortly after starting lenalidomide because CD34-positive stem cell counts tend to decrease with prolonged lenalidomide exposure.[34] In addition, maintenance lenalidomide after stem cell transplantation has been associated with an increased incidence of secondary malignancies, so alternatives such as thalidomide should be considered.[34]

▶ *Bortezomib (Velcade)*

Bortezomib is a proteosome inhibitor approved for the treatment of multiple myeloma. Proteosome inhibitors induce myeloma cell death by modulating nuclear factor kappa-B products, including inflammatory cytokines and adhesion molecules that support myeloma cell growth. Bortezomib also disrupts the myeloma microenvironment by inhibiting the binding of myeloma cells to the bone marrow stromal cells.[31] Initially approved in the treatment of relapsed disease, bortezomib produces response rates of 35% in heavily pretreated individuals.[44] ⑩ *Today, bortezomib is frequently given in combination with dexamethasone and thalidomide or lenalidomide as induction therapy before a transplant.* The response rates have been reported as high as 97% in newly diagnosed myeloma.[30] Bortezomib can also be given in combination with prednisone and melphalan (MPB) in patients who are not transplant eligible. Superior response rates and survival are seen with the combination of MPB compared with MP.[42] Side effects of bortezomib include fatigue, nausea, peripheral neuropathy, and hematologic effects.[42] The incidence of DVT is lower than the immunomodulators; thus, bortezomib does not routinely require prophylactic anticoagulation. However, prophylactic acyclovir should be considered to reduce the risk of herpes zoster infections.[34]

▶ *Bisphosphonates*

Bone disease is a common manifestation of multiple myeloma. Bisphosphonates should be initiated in symptomatic patients with bone lesions to slow osteopenia and reduce the fracture risk associated with the disease. Pamidronate 90 mg and zolendronic acid 4 mg have equivalent efficacy in the management of osteolytic lesions.[46] The use of zolendronic acid decreases pain and bone-related complications and improves quality of life. Osteonecrosis of the jaw is a major concern with bisphosphonate therapy. Risk factors are unclear, but osteonecrosis of the jaw is more common in patients receiving IV administration of bisphosphonates and having dental procedures performed. It is recommended that patients have dental restoration work before starting bisphosphonate therapy. Several consensus guidelines have been published on the use of bisphosphonates and myeloma. Recommendations on the duration of therapy and which bisphosphonate to use have largely been left up to the practitioner.[47,48]

Patient Care and Monitoring

Chronic Myeloid Leukemia

1. Patients are placed on a TKI at the time of diagnosis. Imatinib, dasatinib, and nilotinib are all viable options for first-line therapy. If patients do not have a complete cytogenetic response at 6 to 12 months, then either dasatinib or nilotinib should be tried if imatinib was used in the first line setting.

2. Patients should be monitored for a dose-dependent myelosuppression, gastrointestinal intolerance, edema, and rash. Drug interactions with CYP 3A4 inducers are clinically important and should be monitored.

3. Patients should avoid acid suppression while taking dasatinib, and the QT interval should be monitored while the patient is taking dasatinib and nilotinib.

4. HSCT may be considered when the patient fails to respond or is intolerant to TKIs. Ideal candidates include younger patients in chronic phase CML that have an HLA-matched related or unrelated donor.

Chronic Lymphocytic Leukemia

1. Observation is a reasonable approach if the patient is asymptomatic.

2. Monitor WBC count and monitor for signs of infection if the patient is receiving fludarabine-based chemotherapy.

3. Monitor for infusion reactions with rituximab, ofatumumab and alemtuzumab. Premedicate with acetaminophen and diphenhydramine to prevent these reactions. IV corticosteroid should also be used with ofatumumab. Titrating the rate of infusion may lessen the risk of severe reactions.

4. Prophylactic trimethoprim–sulfamethoxazole and an antiviral (acyclovir, famciclovir, or valacyclovir) are recommended for all patients receiving alemtuzumab. Consider adding an antifungal (fluconazole) if warranted.

Multiple Myeloma

1. During therapy, monitor myeloma monoclonal protein in urine and serum, renal function, hemoglobin, and platelets. Caution using NSAIDS in patients with renal dysfunction.

2. Monitor peripheral neuropathy with bortezomib, thalidomide and vincristine. Dose reduction may be necessary to prevent permanent neurologic damage.

3. Prophylactic anticoagulation is prescribed with thalidomide or lenalidomide with dexamethasone.

4. Bisphosphonates should be initiated in symptomatic patients. Renal function must be monitored. Patients may need pain medication for bone pain.

5. If a reduction in myeloma protein is not seen with one chemotherapy regimen, another regimen should be used

OUTCOME EVALUATION

Newly diagnosed, asymptomatic patients with myeloma may be observed without treatment. This asymptomatic period may last for months to a couple years. All patients with multiple myeloma become symptomatic, and when this occurs, treatment is required. All patients should be evaluated for an autologous stem cell transplant. For patients who are eligible for transplant, induction therapy often consists of thalidomide or lenalidomide, bortezomib, and dexamethasone. For those patients who are not transplant eligible, therapy may consist of MPT, MPB, or MPL. Nearly all patients progress at some point, and second-line therapy usually includes bortezomib. Monthly bisphosphonates should be given to patients who have bone lesions with the hope of reducing pain and fractures.

WALDENSTRÖM MACROGLOBULINEMIA

Waldenström macroglobulinemia is a rare immunoglobulin disorder that is associated with non-Hodgkin's lymphoma. Approximately 4 in 1 million individuals are affected with the disease. Waldenström macroglobulinemia is characterized by an elevation of serum immunoglobulin M and involvement of the lymph nodes, bone marrow, and spleen. Patients are typically asymptomatic at the time of diagnosis, with the disease being discovered by routine laboratory examination. Similar to indolent lymphomas, the watch and wait approach is used for asymptomatic patients. Symptomatic patients experience anemia, fatigue, hepatosplenomegaly, lymphadenopathy, and hyperviscosity syndrome.[49] When these symptoms arise, treatment is necessary with the goal being palliation. Systemic therapy includes alkylating agents, nucleoside analogs, rituximab, thalidomide, or bortezomib. Treatment is often continued until a desired response (reduction in symptoms) is achieved. Plasmapheresis may be required in addition to systemic therapies to alleviate symptoms associated with hyperviscosity syndrome.[50]

Abbreviations Introduced in This Chapter

CD	Cluster of differentiation
CLL	Chronic lymphocytic leukemia
CML	Chronic myelogenous leukemia
CR	Complete response
DVT	Deep venous thrombosis
FISH	Fluorescence in situ hybridization
HLA	Human leukocyte antigen

HSCT   Hematopoietic stem cell transplantation
MGUS   Monoclonal gammopathy of unknown significance
MP   Melphalan–prednisone
MPB   Melphalan–prednisone–bortezomib
MPL   Melphalan–prednisone–lenalidomide
MPT   Melphalan–prednisone–thalidomide
NCCN   National Comprehensive Cancer Network
Ph   Philadelphia chromosome
Q-PCR   Qualitative and quantitative polymerase chain
        reaction
TKI   Tyrosine kinase inhibitor
VAD   Vincristine–doxorubicin–dexamethasone
WBC   White blood cell

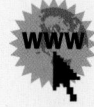

Self-assessment questions and answers are available at REF *http://www.hpharmacotherapy. com/pp.html.*

REFERENCES

1. Pinilla-Ibarz J, Bello C. Modern approaches to treating chronic myelogenous leukemia. Curr Oncol Rep 2008;10:365–371.
2. Siegel R, Ward E, Brawley O, et al. Cancer statistics, 2011. CA Cancer J Clin 2011;61:212–236.
3. National Comprehensive Cancer Network Clinical Practice Guidelines in Oncology [Internet]. Chronic Myelogenous Leukemia, version 2. 2011. Available from *http://www.nccn.org.*
4. Kantargian HM, Cortes J, La Rosee P, Hochhaus A. Optimizing therapy for patients with chronic myelogenous leukemia in chronic phase. Cancer 2010;116:1419–1430.
5. Aguayo A, Couban S. State-of-the-art in the management of chronic myelogenous leukemia in the era of the tyrosine kinase inhibitors: Evolutionary trends in diagnosis, monitoring and treatment. Leuk Lymphoma 2009;50(Suppl 2):1–8.
6. Faderl S, Talpaz M, Estrov Z, Kantarjian HM. Chronic myelogenous leukemia: Biology and therapy. Ann Intern Med 1999;131:207–219.
7. Kantarjian H, O'Brien S, Cortes J, et al. Therapeutic advances in leukemia and myelodysplastic syndrome over the past 40 years. Cancer 2008;113(Suppl 7):1933–1952.
8. Druker BJ, Guilhot F, O'Brien S, et al. Five year follow-up of patients receiving imatinib for chronic myelogenous leukemia. N Eng J Med 2006;355:2408–2417.
9. Martin M, Dipersio JF, Uy GL. Management of the advances phases of chronic myelogenous leukemia in the era of tyrosine kinase inhibitors. Leuk Lymphoma 2009;50(1):14–23.
10. Santos FPS, Ravandi F. Advances in treatment of chronic myelogenous leukemia-new treatment options with tyrosine kinase inhibitors. Leuk Lymphoma 2009;50(Suppl 2):16–26.
11. Gafter-Gvili A, Leader A, Gurion R, et al. High-dose imatinib for newly diagnosed chronic phase chronic myeloid leukemia patients: Systematic review and meta-analysis. Am J Hematol 2011;86:657–662.
12. Deininger MWN, O'Brien SG, Ford JM, Druker BJ. Practical management of patients with chronic myeloid leukemia receiving imatinib. J Clin Oncol 2003;21:1637–1647.
13. Kantarjian H, Shah NP, Hochhaus A, et al. Dasatinib versus imatinib in newly diagnosed chronic-phase chronic myeloid leukemia. N Engl J Med 2010;362:2260–2270.
14. Saglio G, Kim DW, Issaragrisil S, et al. Nilotinib versus imatinib for newly diagnosed chronic myeloid leukemia. N Engl J Med 2010;362:2251–2259.
15. O'Brien SG, Guilhot F, Larson RA, et al. Imatinib compared with interferon and low-dose cytarabine for newly diagnosed chronic-phase chronic myeloid leukemia. N Engl J Med 2003;348:994–1004.
16. Wierda WG, Keating MJ, O'Brien S. Chronic lymphocytic leukemias. In: Devita VT, Hellman S, Rosenberg SA, eds. Cancer: Principles and Practice of Oncology, 8th ed. Philadelphia: Lippincott, 2008:2278–2304.
17. Hallek M. Prognostic factors in chronic lymphocytic leukemia. Ann Oncol 2008;19:iv51–iv53.
18. Montserrat E. New prognostic markers in CLL. Hematology Am Soc Hematol Educ Program 2006;279–284.
19. Dighiero G, Maloum K, Desablens B, et al. Chlorambucil in indolent chronic lymphocytic leukemia. N Engl J Med 1998;338:1506–1514.
20. Chemotherapeutic options in chronic lymphocytic leukemia: A meta-analysis of the randomized trials. CLL Trialists' Collaborative Group. J Natl Cancer Inst 1999;91:861–868.
21. Shanafelt TD, Kay NE. Comprehensive management of the CLL patient: A holistic approach. Hematology Am Soc Hematol Educ Program 2007:324–331.
22. National Comprehensive Cancer Network Clinical Practice Guidelines in Oncology. Non-Hodgkin's Lymphoma, version 4. 2011, *http://www. nccn.org.*
23. Wierda WG. Current and investigational therapies for patients with CLL. Hematology Am Soc Hematol Educ Program 2006:285–294.
24. Flinn I, Neuberg D, Grever M, et al. Phase III trial of fludarabine plus cyclophosphamide compared with fludarabine for patients with previously untreated chronic lymphocytic leukemia: US Intergroup Trial E2997. J Clin Oncol 2007;25(7):793–798.
25. Hillmen P. Advancing therapy for chronic lymphocytic leukemia—The role of rituximab. Semin Oncol 2004;31(Suppl 2):22–26.
26. Byrd JC, Rai K, Peterson BL, et al. Addition of rituximab to fludarabine may prolong progression-free survival and overall survival in patients with previously untreated chronic lymphocytic leukemia: An updated retrospective comparative analysis of CALGB 9712 and CALGB 9011. Blood 2005;105:49–53.
27. Moreton P, Hillmen P. Alemtuzumab therapy in B-cell lymphoproliferative disorders. Semin Oncol 2003;30:493–501.
28. Keating MJ, O'Brien S, Albitar M, et al. Early results of a chemoimmunotherapy regimen of fludarabine, cyclophosphamide, and rituximab as initial therapy for chronic lymphocytic leukemia. J Clin Oncol 2005;23:4079–4088.
29. Wierda W, O'Brien S, Wen S, et al. Chemoimmunotherapy with fludarabine, cyclophosphamide, and rituximab for relapsed and refractory chronic lymphocytic leukemia. J Clin Oncol 2005;23:4070–4078.
30. Palumbo A, Anderson K. Multiple myeloma. N Engl J Med 2011;364:1046–1060.
31. Munshi NC, Anderson KC. Plasma cell neoplasms. In: Devita VT, Hellman S, Rosenberg SA, eds. Cancer: Principles and Practice of Oncology, 8th ed. Philadelphia: Lippincott, 2008:2305–2342.
32. National Comprehensive Cancer Network Clinical Practice Guidelines in Oncology [Internet]. Multiple Myeloma, version 1. 2012. Available from *http://www.nccn.org.*
33. Kumar S. Treatment of newly diagnosed multiple myeloma in transplant-eligible patients. Curr Hematol Malig Rep 2011;6:104–112.
34. Greipp PR, San Miguel J, Durie BGM, et al. International staging system for multiple myeloma. J Clin Oncol 2005;23:3412–3420.
35. Child JA, Morgan GJ, Davies FE, et al. High-dose chemotherapy with hematopoietic stem-cell rescue for multiple myeloma. N Engl J Med 2003;348:1875–1883.
36. Lacy MQ. New immunomodulatory drugs in myeloma. Curr Hematol Malig Rep 2011;6:120–125.
37. Weber D, Rankin K, Gavino M, et al. Thalidomide alone or with dexamethasone for previously untreated multiple myeloma. J Clin Oncol 2003;21:16–19.
38. Kaufman JL, Nooka A, Vrana M, et al. Bortezomib, thalidomide, and dexamethasone as induction therapy for patients symptomatic multiple myeloma: A retrospective study. Cancer 2010;116(13):3134–3151.
39. Palumbo A, Bringhen S, Rossi D, et al. Bortezomib-melphalan-prednisone-thalidomide followed by maintenance with bortezomib-thalidomide compared with bortezomib-melphalan-prednisone for initial treatment of multiple myeloma: a randomized controlled trial. J Clin Oncol 2010;28:5101–5109.

40. Facon T, Mary JY, Hulin C, et al. Melphalan and prednisone plus thalidomide versus melphalan and prednisone alone or reduced-intensity autologous stem cell transplantation in elderly patients with multiple myeloma (IFM 99–06): A randomized trial. Lancet 2007;370: 1209–1218.

41. Palumbo A, Rajkumar SV, Dimopoulous MA, et al. Prevention of thalidomide- and lenalidomide-associated thrombosis in myeloma. Leukemia 2008;22(2):414–423.

42. Kyle RA, Rajkumar SV. Multiple myeloma. Blood 2008;111(6): 2962–2972.

43. Rajkumar SV, Jacobus S, Callander NS, et al. Lenolidomide plus high-dose dexamethasone versus lenalidomide plus low-dose dexamethasone as initial therapy for newly diagnosed multiple myeloma: An open-label randomized controlled trial. Lancet Oncol 2010;11:29–37.

44. Richardson PG, Barlogie B, Berenson J, et al. A phase 2 study of bortezomib in relapsed, refractory myeloma. N Engl J Med 2003;348: 2609–2617.

45. Blade J, Cibeira MT, Rosinol L. Bortezomib: A valuable new antineoplastic strategy in multiple myeloma. Acta Oncologica 2005;44:440–448.

46. Rosen LS, Gordon D, Kaminski M, et al. Long-term efficacy and safety of zoledronic acid compared with pamidronate disodium in the treatment of skeletal complications in patients with advanced multiple myeloma or breast carcinoma: A randomized, double-blind, multicenter, comparative trial. Cancer 2003;98:1735–1744.

47. Lacy MQ, Dispenzieri A, Gertz MA, et al. Mayo clinic consensus statement for the use of bisphosphonates in multiple myeloma. Mayo Clin Proc 2006;81:1047–1053.

48. Kyle Ra, Yee GC, Somerfield MR, et al. American Society of Clinical Oncology 2007 clinical practice guideline update on the role of bisphosphonates in multiple myeloma. J Clin Oncol 2007;25: 2462–2472.

49. Dimopoulos MA, Kyle RA, Anagnostopoulos A, Treon SP. Diagnosis and management of Waldenstrom's macroglobulinemia. J Clin Oncol 2005;23:1564–1577.

50. National Comprehensive Cancer Network Clinical Practice Guidelines in Oncology [Internet]. Waldenstrom's Macroglobulinemia/ Lymphoplasmacytic Lymphoma, version 2. 2012. Available from *http:// www.nccn.org*.

97 Malignant Lymphomas

Keith A. Hecht and Susanne E. Liewer

LEARNING OBJECTIVES

● **Upon completion of the chapter, the reader will be able to:**

1. Discuss the underlying pathophysiologic mechanisms of the lymphomas and how they relate to presenting symptoms of the disease.

2. Differentiate the pathologic findings of Hodgkin's lymphoma (HL), follicular indolent non-Hodgkin's lymphoma (NHL), and diffuse aggressive NHL and how this information yields a specific diagnosis.

3. Describe the general staging criteria for the lymphomas and how it relates to prognosis; evaluate the role of the prognostic systems such as the International Prognostic Score for HL, the Follicular Lymphoma International Prognostic Index (FLIPI), and the International Prognostic Index (IPI) for diffuse, aggressive NHL.

4. Compare and contrast the treatment algorithms for early and advanced stage disease for HL.

5. Delineate the clinical course of follicular indolent and diffuse aggressive NHL and the implications for disease classification schemes and treatment goals.

6. Outline the general treatment approach to follicular indolent and diffuse aggressive NHL for localized and advanced disease.

7. Interpret the current role for monoclonal antibody therapy in NHL.

8. Assess the role of autologous hematopoietic stem cell transplantation (SCT) for relapsed lymphomas.

KEY CONCEPTS

① There are two broad classifications of lymphoma, Hodgkin's lymphoma (HL) and non-Hodgkin's lymphoma (NHL), and both contain numerous histologic subtypes that are pathologically distinct disease entities.

② Specific pathologic characteristics distinguishing HL from NHL include morphology, cell surface antigens, and chromosomal mutations.

③ Classic signs and symptoms of the lymphomas include lymphadenopathy and B symptoms (i.e., fever, night sweats, and weight loss).

④ The diagnosis of malignant lymphomas is established by tumor biopsy sample, analysis of the biopsy tissue, and determination of the extent of the disease in the patient.

⑤ The goal of treatment of HL is cure for all stages of disease and first relapse.

⑥ Initial treatment of HL includes combination chemotherapy, these regimens have demonstrated efficacy and have an acceptable long-term toxicity profile.

⑦ Follicular indolent NHL is incurable, so therapy goals focus on inducing and maintaining remission duration while minimizing treatment-related toxicities.

⑧ Diffuse, aggressive NHL centers on curative-intent therapy using anthracycline-based combination chemotherapy for initial treatment and high-dose chemotherapy with autologous stem cell transplantation for relapsed disease.

⑨ The recombinant monoclonal antibody rituximab is an effective treatment option for patients with B-cell origin CD20+ NHL as a single agent and enhances the efficacy of combination chemotherapy regimens.

INTRODUCTION

The malignant lymphomas are a clonal disorder of hematopoiesis with the primary malignant cells consisting of lymphocytes of B-, T-, or natural killer (NK) cell origin. These cells originate from a small population of lymphocytes that have undergone malignant transformation from a series of genetic mutations. Lymphoma cells predominate in the lymph nodes; however, they can infiltrate lymphoid and nonlymphoid tissues, such as the bone marrow, central nervous system (CNS), gastrointestinal (GI) tract, liver, mediastinum, skin, and spleen. An overview of the lymph node regions is depicted in **Figure 97–1**. ❶ *There are two broad classifications of lymphoma, Hodgkin's lymphoma (HL) and non-Hodgkin's lymphoma (NHL), and both contain numerous histologic subtypes that are pathologically distinct disease entities.* HL is distinguished from NHL by the presence of the pathognomonic Reed-Sternberg (RS) cell. Other lymphomatous disease entities are classified as types of NHL.

The clinical course varies widely among histologies of HL and NHL. More aggressive lymphoma subtypes are highly proliferating tumor cells that require aggressive therapeutic intervention with chemotherapy, radiation therapy, or both. By contrast, certain subtypes of NHL are characterized by a disease course that flares and remits intermittently over a period of years regardless of treatment.

EPIDEMIOLOGY AND ETIOLOGY

Hodgkin's Lymphoma

Approximately 8,830 new cases of HL were estimated to be diagnosed in the United States in 2011, with 1,300 deaths attributed to the disease.[1] The incidence of HL is bimodal, with its peaks occurring in the third decade of life and in patients older than 50 years of age.[2] The precise cause of HL is unknown, but certain associations have been reported and provide insight about into possible etiologic factors. Epstein-Barr virus (EBV) has been associated with HL in various studies. The viral genome has been detected in RS cells in up to 40% of cases in developed countries. Other viruses (cytomegalovirus, human herpesviruses, and adenoviruses) have been associated with HL; however, conflicting data have been reported regarding their association with HL.[2] The risk of HL has also been associated with HIV. However, the reason for this association remains unclear. Other possible risk factors identified include woodworking and a familial history of HL.

Non-Hodgkin's Lymphoma

Approximately 66,360 cases of NHL were estimated to be diagnosed in the United States in 2011, with an estimated 20,620 deaths. These figures represent a stabilization in the incidence of NHL since 1998 that follows a dramatic increase that had nearly doubled the number of cases in the United States since 1950.[1,3] The previous increase is thought to have been related to the development of aggressive NHL in young men with HIV, although the overall increase is independent of HIV disease, particularly for patients older than 65 years of age. The median age for diagnosis is 50 years, although children and young adults may also be affected. The etiology of certain aggressive NHL subtypes is related to specific endemic geographic factors. Follicular or low-grade lymphoma is more common in the United States and Europe and is relatively uncommon in the Caribbean, Far East, Middle East, or Africa. The human T-cell leukemia virus I induces T-cell lymphoma or leukemia in both Japan and the Caribbean. Kaposi's sarcoma–associated herpes virus, or human herpes virus 8, and hepatitis C have been implicated in inducing NHL. Lymphomas of the GI tract are more prevalent in patients with celiac sprue, inflammatory bowel disease, or *Helicobacter pylori* infection. The incidence of Burkitt's NHL is seven cases per 100,000 people in Africa compared with 0.1 per 100,000 in the United States. Malaria or EBV is thought to contribute to the chronic B-lymphocyte stimulation that leads to malignant transformation in Burkitt's NHL. EBV has been shown to transform lymphocytes in vitro to a monoclonal malignant

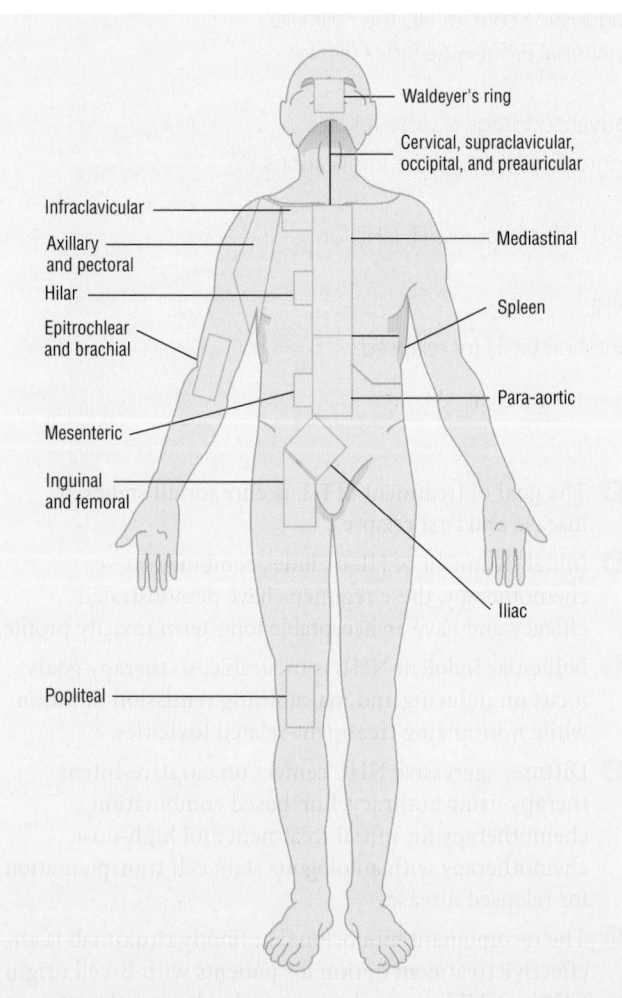

FIGURE 97–1. Representation of the anatomic regions used in the staging of Hodgkin disease. (From Rosenberg SA. Staging of Hodgkin disease. Radiology 1966;87:146.)

population, which is believed to drive the development of disease in patients who have received a solid organ transplant or bone marrow transplant or have other chronic immunosuppressed states. Patients with congenital diseases such as Wiskott-Aldrich syndrome, common variable hypogammaglobinemia; X-linked lymphoproliferative syndrome; and severe combined immunodeficiency, including drug-induced immunosuppression, are also at risk.[4] Environmental factors have been identified as contributing to the development of NHL. Certain occupations such as wood and forestry workers, butchers, exterminators, grain millers, machinists, mechanics, painters, printers, and industrial workers have a higher prevalence of disease. Industrial chemicals such as pesticides, herbicides, organic chemicals (e.g., benzene), solvents, and wood preservatives are also associated with NHL.

PATHOPHYSIOLOGY

Pluripotent stem cells in the bone marrow are able to differentiate to both lymphoid and myeloid progenitor cells. Lymphoid progenitor cells undergo gene rearrangement to yield either B-cell or T-cell lineage precursor cells. Normal maturation for naive B cells includes expression of cell surface antibody or the cells typically undergo apoptosis. These cells are differentiated from other B cells, such as memory cells, by virtue of cell surface antigen (CD5+ or CD5− and CD27−) and bound antibody (IgM+ and IgD+). When naive B cells recognize antigen with their cell surface antibody, they accumulate in the lymph nodes, spleen, or other lymphoid tissue. The DNA of these B cells is susceptible to three different types of genetic modification: receptor editing, somatic hypermutation, and class switching within the germinal center of the lymph node. Germinal centers are microanatomic structures located within lymph nodes that develop with clonal B-cell expansion secondary to antigen stimulation. Under normal circumstances, these genetic changes allow for adaptation of the immune system to the repeated exposure to environmental antigens.

Hodgkin's Lymphoma

The pathophysiology of HL is defined by the presence of the RS cell in a grouping of lymph nodes. The RS cell is a morphologically large cell with a multinucleated structure possessing pronounced eosinophilic nucleoli.[5] In the affected lymph nodes, the RS cells are contained in a reactive milieu of B cells, T cells, plasma cells, eosinophils, and mast cells. It is believed this microenvironment is essential for the survival of RS cells.[6]

RS cells are genetically derived preapoptotic germinal center B cells. The majority of these cells demonstrate numerous chromosome abnormalities.[7] Despite their origin, RS cells have lost the expression of most B-cell markers. Common cell-surface antigens expressed by RS cells include CD30 and CD15, but other common B-cell antigens, such as CD20 are inconsistently expressed.[8] The overexpression of a proliferative and antiapoptotic transcription factor nuclear

factor kappa-B (NF-κB) is believed to contribute to the expansion and survival of RS cells.[6]

HL is classified into disease subtypes based on the number and morphologic appearance of RS cells and the background cellular milieu. These are listed in the World Health Organization (WHO) classification of lymphoid neoplastic diseases in Table 97–1.[9] Nodular sclerosing is the most common form of HL, representing 70% of cases. It is more common in young adults and is marked by the presence of the RS variant cell, the lacunar cell. The second most common form of HL, accounting for approximately 20% of cases, is the mixed-cellularity variant, with others accounting for the

Table 97–1
WHO Classification of Lymphoid Neoplasms

B-Cell Neoplasms
Precursor B-cell neoplasm
Precursor B-lymphoblastic leukemia/lymphoma
Mature (peripheral) B-cell neoplasms
B-cell chronic lymphocytic leukemia/small lymphocytic lymphoma
B-cell prolymphocytic leukemia
Lymphoplasmacytic lymphoma
Splenic marginal zone B-cell lymphoma (+/− villous lymphocytes)
Hairy cell leukemia
Plasma cell myeloma/plasmacytoma
Extranodal marginal zone B-cell lymphoma of MALT type
Nodal marginal zone B-cell lymphoma (+/− monocytoid B cells)
Follicular lymphoma
Mantle cell lymphoma
Diffuse large B-cell lymphoma
Mediastinal large B-cell lymphoma
Primary effusion lymphoma
Burkitt's lymphoma/Burkitt's cell leukemia

T-Cell and NK-Cell Neoplasms
Precursor T-cell neoplasm
Precursor T-lymphoblastic lymphoma/ALL
Mature (peripheral) T-cell neoplasms
T-cell prolymphocytic leukemia
T-cell granular lymphocytic leukemia
Aggressive NK cell leukemia
Adult T-cell lymphoma/leukemia (HTLV1+)
Extranodal NK/T-cell lymphoma, nasal type
Enteropathy-type T-cell lymphoma
Hepatosplenic gamma-delta T-cell lymphoma
Subcutaneous panniculitis-like T-cell lymphoma
Mycosis fungoides/Sézary syndrome
Anaplastic large-cell lymphoma, T/null cell, primary cutaneous type
Peripheral T-cell lymphoma, not otherwise characterized
Angioimmunoblastic T-cell lymphoma
Anaplastic large-cell lymphoma, T/null cell, primary systemic type

HL
Nodular lymphocyte-predominant HL
Classical HL
Nodular sclerosis HL (grades 1 and 2)
Lymphocyte-rich classical HL
Mixed cellularity HL
Lymphocyte depletion HL

ALL, acute myeloid leukemia; HL, Hodgkin's lymphoma; MALT, mucosa-associated lymphoid tissue; NK, natural killer.

Table 97–2

Negative Prognostic Factors for HL

International Prognostic Score—Advanced HL
Albumin less than 4 g/dL (40 g/L)
Hemoglobin less than 10.5 g/dL (105 g/L; 6.52 mmol/L)
Male sex
Age older than 45 years
Stage IV disease
WBC greater than or equal to 15,000/mm³ (15 × 10⁹/L)
Lymphocytopenia (count less than 600/mm³ (0.6 × 10⁹/L),
  less than 8% (0.08) of WBC count, or both)

WBC, white blood cell.

remainder of cases.[8] Factors identified as negative disease prognostic indicators are listed in Table 97–2. Patients with advanced HL who have at least four of the criteria may warrant more aggressive treatment.[10]

Non-Hodgkin's Lymphoma

The pathophysiology of NHL is governed by numerous environmental and genetic events culminating with a monoclonal population of malignant lymphocytes. B cells represent the cells of origin in excess of 90% of cases of NHL. Figure 97–2 outlines normal B-cell maturation with accompanying cell-surface antigens. Evolving data are correlating chromosomal mutations with specific disease subtypes. Cytogenetic abnormalities involving translocations of antigen receptor genes are prevalent in NHL. These include T-cell receptor genes in T-cell lymphomas and immunoglobulin genes in B-cell lymphomas. The principal defect appears to be an error in the assembly of the regulatory gene segment of an antigen receptor gene, resulting in inappropriate binding to an oncogene. This results in dysregulation of cell growth and proliferation, leading to the malignant clone of lymphocytes. Oncogenes that have been identified in different lymphomatous diseases include

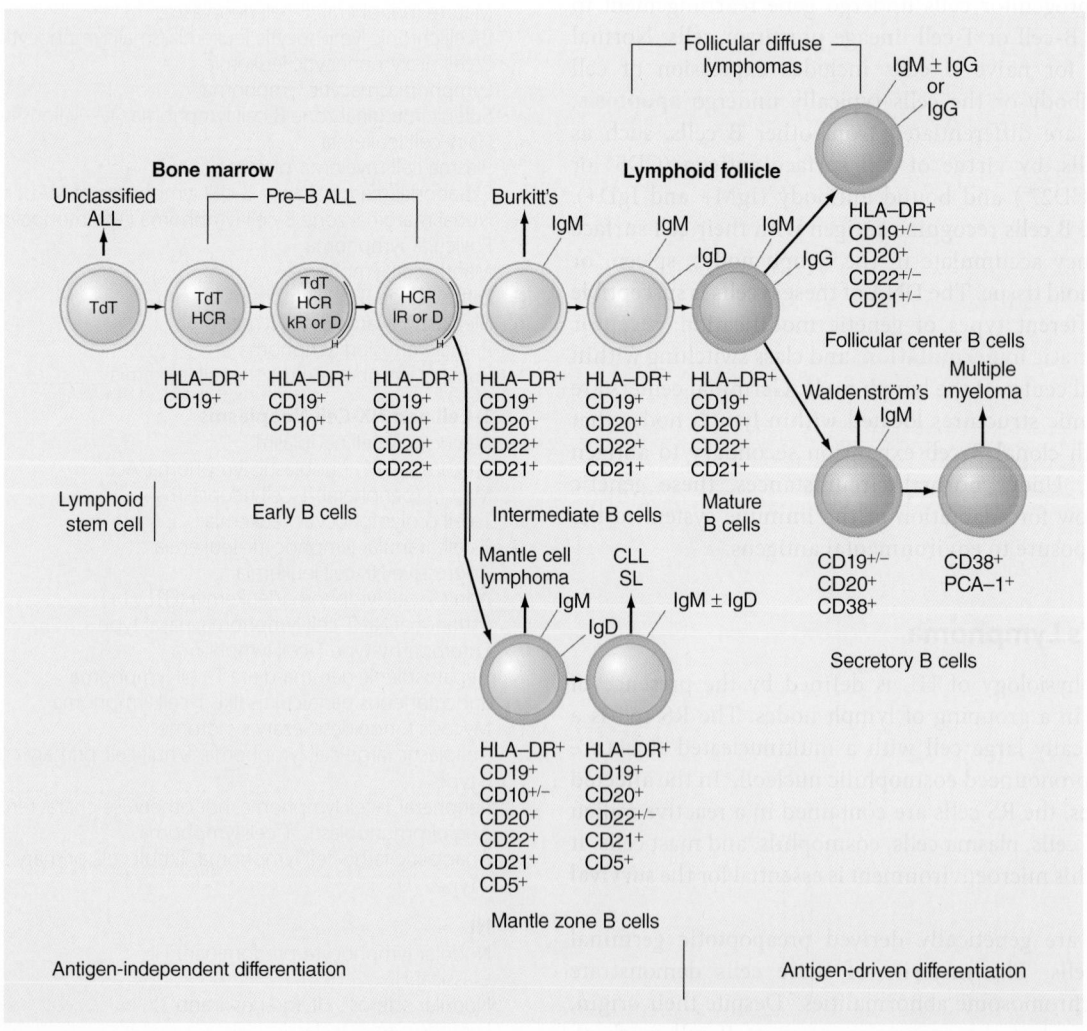

FIGURE 97–2. Pathway of normal B-cell differentiation and relationship to B-cell lymphocytes. (ALL, acute lymphoblastic leukemia; HLA, human leukocyte antigen; HCR, human chemokine receptor; Ig, immunoglobulin; TdT, terminal deoxynucleotidyl transferase.) (From Armitage JO, Longo DL. Malignancies in lymphoid cells. In: Kasper DL, Braunwald E, Fauci AS, et al., eds. Harrison's Principles of Internal Medicine, 16th ed. New York: McGraw-Hill, 2005:544.)

c-myc, a regulator of gene transcription; *bcl-1* important in the regulation of mitosis; *bcl-2*, a regulator of apoptosis; and *bcl-3*, *NF-κB*, and *bcl-6*, which regulate cell differentiation.[11] Classic translocations for NHL include t(8;14) in Burkitt's lymphoma, t(14;18) in follicular lymphomas, t(11;14) mantle cell lymphoma, and t(11;18)/t(1;14) in mucosa-associated lymphoid tissue (MALT).

❷ *Characterization of the morphology of the lymphocytes, the reactivity of the other cells in the lymph node, and the lymph node architecture is essential in obtaining a diagnosis and predicting disease course.* The nodal presentation of NHL is divided into two main categories: follicular, corresponding to low-grade disease, and diffuse, corresponding to aggressive disease. A follicular disease pattern in the inspected lymph node is indicative of a more indolent or low-grade progression that has survival measured in years if left untreated. In contrast, a diffuse pattern of lymph node infiltration is a marker of highly aggressive disease, resulting in death within weeks to months if untreated. Follicular NHL is the most common indolent subtype, comprising 22% of NHL cases, in which diffuse, large B-cell lymphoma is the most common aggressive histology, 31% of NHL. The cells of origin for follicular NHL tend to be more mature, nondividing lymphocytes, whereas aggressive NHL is derived from rapidly dividing lymphoid precursors, such as immunoblasts, lymphoblasts, and centroblasts. A unique feature of the biology of NHL is that follicular low-grade histologies can undergo further malignant transformation, transforming further into a diffuse, large B-cell lymphoma population. This syndrome, called *Richter's transformation*, may occur in up to 20% of follicular low-grade lymphoma patients and involves multiple genetic events, including abnormalities of chromosomes 11 and 12 and tumor suppressor genes. Richter's transformation may also occur in patients with chronic lymphocytic leukemia, which results in a transformation to diffuse lymphoma.[12]

The classification of NHL has undergone several revisions as the histology, molecular biology, and clinical course of the disease have been more precisely defined. Classification schemes such as the *Working Formulation* categorize disease on aggressiveness into three general categories: low grade—survival estimated in years without treatment, intermediate grade—survival estimated in months without treatment, and high grade—survival measured in days to weeks for untreated disease. This scheme is limited in its clinical applicability because the large number of distinct clinical diseases that are not categorized by this classification. The Working Formulation classification of NHL and diseases unclassifiable by that system are presented in Table 97–3. The WHO has updated a classification scheme published in 1994 by the International Lymphoma Study Group called the *Revised European American Classification of Lymphoid Neoplasms* (REAL) that broadly categorizes histologic subtypes into B- and T-cell subtypes. This newer classification incorporates immunologic morphologic and genetic and clinical attributes of various NHL histologies.

Prognostic factors present at diagnosis have been identified for NHL. Age, the presence of B symptoms, performance status,

---

Table 97–3

Working Formulation for NHL

Classification	Immunophenotype
Low Grade	
Small lymphocytic	100% B cell
Follicular, small cleaved cell	100% B cell
Follicular, mixed small cleaved cell and large cell	100% B cell
Intermediate Grade	
Follicular, large cell	100% B cell
Diffuse, small cleaved cell	75% B cell, 20% T cell, 5% null cell
Diffuse, mixed small and large cell	75% B cell, 20% T cell, 5% null cell
Diffuse, large cell	70% B cell, 20% T cell, 10% null cell
Diffuse, large cell	70% B cell, 20% T cell, 10% null cell
High Grade	
Immunoblastic	50% B cell, 50% T cell
Lymphoblastic	5% B cell, 95% T cell
Diffuse, small noncleaved cell	100% B cell

*ª*Lymphomas not included in the working formulation: *Mycosis fungoides*, mantle cell lymphoma, monocytoid B-cell lymphoma, mucosa-associated lymphoid tissue, anaplastic large cell lymphoma, angiocentric lymphoma, angioimmunoblastic lymphadenopathy, Castleman's disease, adult T-cell leukemia/lymphoma.

---

number of nodal and extranodal sites, lactate dehydrogenase (LDH) concentration, bulky disease (greater than 10 cm), advanced stage, and β_2-microglobulin concentration have been shown to be important prognostic features in NHL. Table 97–4 shows the International Prognostic Index (IPI), a predictive model for aggressive NHL to be treated with doxorubicin-containing chemotherapy regimens.[13] This index is used as a tool for selecting therapy for patients who may warrant a more intense treatment regimen based on known poor prognostic factors. Additionally, patients with diffuse aggressive B-cell lymphoma that is of germinal center type carry a better prognosis than other patients.[14] A model similar to the IPI, the Follicular Lymphoma International Prognostic Index (FLIPI), is used to help guide treatment decisions in follicular lymphoma.[15]

TREATMENT OF HL
Desired Outcome

Staging of HL with a standard classification is necessary to guide appropriate treatment. The number of involved sites, disease involvement on one or both sides of the diaphragm, localized or disseminated extranodal disease, and B symptoms are factors in assignment of stage. The Cotswold staging system, a revision of the original Ann Arbor classification, is outlined in Table 97–5.[16]

Table 97–4

Negative Prognostic Factors for NHL

International Prognostic Index—Diffuse, Aggressive NHL

Criteria	Risk Assessment	
Age 60 years or older	Risk group	Number of criteria
Stage III/IV disease	Low	0–1
Extranodal disease greater than one site	Low-intermediate	2
ECOG performance status 2 or greater	High-intermediate	3
Serum LDH greater than 1 × normal limit	High	4-5

Follicular Lymphoma International Prognostic Index

Criteria	Risk Assessment	
Age 60 years or older	Risk group	Number of criteria
Stage III/IV disease	Low	0-1
Hemoglobin less than 12.0 g/dL (120 g/L; 7.45mmol/L)	Intermediate	2
Serum LDH greater than 1 × normal limit	High	3 or more
Number of nodal sites greater than or equal to 5[a]		

[a]The nodal map used in the Follicular Lymphoma International Prognostic Index is different than the nodal map used in conventional staging.

Table 97–5

Cotswold Staging Classification for Hodgkin Disease (1989 Revision of Ann Arbor Staging)[a]

Stage	Description
I	Involvement of a single lymph node region or lymphoid structure (e.g., spleen, thymus, Waldeyer's ring)
II	Involvement of two or more lymph node regions on the same side of the diaphragm; the number of anatomic sites is indicated by a subscript
III	Involvement of lymph node regions or structure on both sides of the diaphragm
	III$_1$: With or without involvement of splenic, hilar, celiac, or portal nodes
	III$_2$: Involvement of para-aortic, iliac, or mesenteric
IV	Involvement of extranodal site(s) beyond that designated E

Designations Applicable to All Stages

A	No symptoms
B	Fever, night sweats, and weight loss
X	Bulky disease: greater than one-third the width of the mediastinum or greater than 10 cm maximal dimension of nodal mass
E	Involvement of a single extranodal site, contiguous or proximal to a known nodal site
CS	Clinical stage
PS	Pathologic stage

[a]Also used for non-Hodgkin's lymphoma.

Clinical Presentation and Diagnosis of Malignant Lymphomas

General

Nonspecific; can range from an asymptomatic patient with a less aggressive lymphoma to a patient who is gravely ill with advanced disease

❸ Symptoms

- Lymphadenopathy, generally in the cervical, axillary, supraclavicular, or inguinal lymph nodes
- Splenomegaly
- Shortness of breath, dry cough, chest pressure (patients with mediastinal mass)
- GI complications (nausea, vomiting, early satiety, constipation, and diarrhea)
- Back, chest, or abdominal pain

Signs

- Fever[a]
- Night sweats[a]
- Weight loss greater than 10% within last 6 months[a]
- Pruritus

Laboratory Tests

- LDH
- ESR

- Serum chemistries
- CBC with differential

❹ Other Diagnostic Tests

- Physical exam with careful attention to lymph node inspection
- Imaging—chest x-ray, chest CT, abdominal or pelvic CT; integrated PET and CT is recommended as part of the initial workup
- Bone marrow biopsy
- Biopsy of suspected lymph node(s)—either open lymph node biopsy(preferred) or core biopsy; fine-needle aspiration should only be performed if preferred biopsy methods are unobtainable
- Hematopathology evaluation of biopsy specimen—morphologic inspection, immunohistochemistry for cell surface antigens to characterize lymphoma cells, cytogenetic analysis

[a]Known collectively as B symptoms.

CBC, complete blood count; CT, computed tomography; ESR, erythroid sedimentation rate; LDH, lactate dehydrogenase; PET, positron emission tomography.

⑤ *The principal goal in treating HL is to cure the patient of the primary malignancy.* HL is sensitive to both radiation and chemotherapy, resulting in an 80% rate of cure with modern therapy. Treatment strategy is generally divided into approaches for early stage I/II localized disease and stage III /IV advanced disease. Patients with early stage I/II disease are further classified into favorable, unfavorable with bulky disease, and unfavorable with nonbulky disease. Regardless of the stage of the disease, all patients are treated with curative intent. Other goals during treatment include:

- Complete resolution of symptoms of disease

- Minimization of acute and long-term treatment-related toxicity

- Incorporation of supportive care measures to optimize quality of life during chemotherapy and/or radiation therapy

- Selection of palliative therapy for refractory disease.

Nonpharmacologic Therapy

Radiation therapy is an effective single agent in the treatment of HL and has cured patients of their disease. Historically, patients with favorable early stage I/II disease were treated with subtotal lymphoid radiation as the only modality of therapy. However, the long-term toxicities associated with the larger fields of irradiation have precluded the use of radiation therapy alone. Current treatment strategies combine radiation therapy with chemotherapy. This has been reported to reduce the irradiated volume and dose as well as the number of cycles of chemotherapy.

Historically in the treatment of HL, the radiation fields were large and often included the lungs, liver, heart, and breast. Today, the use of involved-field radiotherapy (IFRT) limits radiation to the involved area. It is estimated that compared with larger radiation areas such as total lymphoid irradiation, the involved field will reduce the volume by more than 80%. In addition to the smaller radiation volumes, other organs such as the breast, heart, and lungs have reduced exposure.[17]

Treatment with radiotherapy produces significant toxicity. Both acute and late effects of radiotherapy occur. Acute effects of mantle-field irradiation include nausea, vomiting, anorexia, xerostomia, dysgeusia, pharyngitis, dry cough, fatigue, diarrhea, and rash. Prophylaxis with antiemetics such as dexamethasone or prochlorperazine helps to prevent or treat nausea. These effects generally are transient and resolve shortly after completion of treatment. Delayed effects from radiotherapy are more concerning in that they may be permanent and present months to years after therapy is complete. Pneumonitis, pericarditis, hypothyroidism, infertility (with pelvic field irradiation), coronary artery disease, deformities in bone and muscle growth in adolescents and children, herpes zoster reactivation, Lhermitte's sign, and secondary malignancies are not uncommon. Patients cured with radiotherapy are at increased risk for breast cancer, lung cancer (particularly in smokers), stomach cancer, melanoma, and NHL depending on the involved radiation field.

Pharmacologic Therapy

▶ *Early Stage Disease*

⑥ *Initial treatment of HL includes combination chemotherapy, these regimens have demonstrated efficacy and have an acceptable long-term toxicity profile.* Combined modality therapy of ABVD (doxorubicin, bleomycin, vinblastine, and dacarbazine) (2–4 cycles) plus 20 to 30 Gy (Gray, the absorbed radiation dose) of IFRT or Stanford V chemotherapy (2 cycles) plus 30 Gy of IRFT is the preferred treatment of patients with favorable stage I/II HL. Patients with favorable disease have: an erythrocyte sedimentation rate (ESR) less than 50 mm/h, no extralymphatic lesions, and one or two lymph nodes involved. Only patients who are unable to tolerate combination chemotherapy because of comorbidities should be treated with radiation alone. Restaging should occur after a minimum of two cycles of chemotherapy. IFRT should be initiated within 3 weeks and is recommended for all patients who achieve a complete response (CR) or a partial response (PR). After completion of IFRT, no further treatment is necessary for patients with a CR, but further restaging is required for patients with PR to therapy.

ABVD or Stanford V followed by IFRT is recommended for patients with unfavorable, bulky disease. Two cycles of ABVD are given before restaging. For patients with a CR, an additional two to four more cycles of ABVD are given before IFRT without restaging between cycles. Patients with a PR will receive 2 cycles of chemotherapy followed by restaging for up to 6 total cycles of chemotherapy. If there is a chemotherapy response (CR or PR), patients then receive IFRT followed by end of treatment restaging to determine disease response. The use of the Stanford V regimen should

---

Table 97–6

Common Treatment Regimens in HL

MOPP—Every 28 Days
Mechlorethamine 6 m/m^2 IV × 1, days 1 and 8
Vincristine 1.4 mg/m^2 IV × 1, days 1 and 8
Procarbazine 100 mg/day PO, days 1–14
Prednisone 40 mg/day PO, days 1–14

ABVD—Every 28 Days
Doxorubicin 25 mg/m^2 IV × 1, days 1 and 15
Bleomycin 10 units IV × 1, days 1 and 15
Vinblastine 6 mg/m^2 × 1, days 1 and 15
Dacarbazine 375 mg/m^2 IV, days 1 and 15

MOPP/ABV Hybrid—Every 28 Days
Mechlorethamine 6 mg/m^2 IV × 1 day 1
Vincristine 1.4 mg/m^2 IV × 1; day 1
Procarbazine 100 mg orally daily, days 1–7
Prednisone 40 mg orally daily, days 1–14
Doxorubicin 35 mg/m^2 IV × 1 day 8
Bleomycin 10 units IV × 1 day 8
Vinblastine 6 mg IV × 1 day 8

Stanford V
Doxorubicin 25 mg/m^2 IV weeks 1, 3, 5, 7, 9, and 11
Vinblastine 6 mg/m^2 IV weeks 1, 3, 5, 7, 9, and 11
Mechlorethamine 6 mg/m^2 IV weeks 1, 5, and 9
Etoposide 60 mg/m^2 IV weeks 3, 7, and 11
Vincristine 1.4 mg/m^2 IV weeks 2, 4, 6, 8, 10, and 12
Bleomycin 5 mg/m^2 IV weeks 2, 4, 6, and 8
Prednisone 40 mg PO every other day for 12 weeks, start taper
  at week 10

BEACOPP (Escalated)—Every 21 Days
Bleomycin 10 mg/m^2 IV, day 8
Etoposide 200 mg/m^2 IV daily × days 1–3
Doxorubicin 35 mg/m^2, day 1
Cyclophosphamide 1,200 mg/m^2 IV, day 1
Vincristine 1.4 mg/m^2 IV, day 8
Procarbazine 100 mg/m^2 orally daily, days 1–7
Prednisone 40 mg orally daily, days 1–14

BCV (High-Dose with Autologous SCT)^a
Carmustine 400 mg/m^2 IV × 1 day
Etoposide 800 mg/m^2 IV daily × 3 days
Cyclophosphamide 1,800 mg/m^2 IV daily × 4 days

BEAM (High-Dose With Autologous SCT^a)
Carmustine 300 mg/m^2 IV × 1day
Etoposide 100–200 mg/m^2 IV every 12 hours × 4 days
Cytarabine 100–200 mg/m^2 IV every 12 hours × 4 day
Melphalan 140 mg/m^2 IV × 1 day

^{a}Used for both Hodgkin's lymphoma and non-Hodgkin's lymphoma.

IV, intravenous; PO, oral; SCT, stem cell transplantation

be considered for patients with mediastinal disease, bulky disease, B symptoms, or unfavorable nonbulky disease.[18] A listing of chemotherapy regimens used in HL is presented in Table 97–6.

▶ Advanced Disease

Treatment of advanced stage (bulky disease greater than 10 cm, presence of B symptoms and/or stage III/IV) HL has been associated with treatment failure rates as high as 40%.[19] Trials have focused on the use of multiagent chemotherapy for six to eight total cycles. The combination chemotherapy regimen MOPP (mechlorethamine, vincristine, procarbazine, and prednisone) is of historical significance because it was the first

chemotherapy regimen to cure HL when it was introduced in the 1960s. However, significant toxicity, including sterility and secondary leukemia, prompted investigators to evaluate other regimens. ABVD was compared with MOPP or ABVD–MOPP alternating.[20] This pivotal phase III Cancer and Leukemia Group B (CALGB) trial comparing these regimens in 361 patients with stage III/IV HL documented a higher CR in the ABVD containing arms (82% and 83%) versus MOPP (65%). There was increased hematologic toxicity in the MOPP arm. A recent update of the data shows the 18-year freedom from progression of 35% in the MOPP arm and 43% in the ABVD containing arms.[21] A survival advantage has yet to be demonstrated. ABVD is now considered standard therapy for initial treatment of stage III or IV HL. Further information on ABVD may be found in Table 97–7.

Additional regimens such as Stanford V and BEACOPP were developed to improve the outcomes of patients with advanced HL. The Stanford V regimen has demonstrated similar response rates to ABVD reported for event-free survival, overall survival, and toxicity. A dose-escalated regimen of BEACOPP (with colony-stimulating factor [CSF] support) was compared with a standard-dose of BEACOPP and also COPP (cyclophosphamide substituted for mechlorethamine for MOPP) alternating with ABVD. The dose-escalated BEACOPP was superior to the other arms in both freedom from treatment failure and overall survival at 10 years.[22] However, the escalated BEACOPP regimen has been associated with a higher number of cases of secondary leukemia and an increased risk of infertility. Currently, neither BEACOPP regimen is widely used in the United States but is considered for advanced stage HL with a high number of poor prognostic factors.

Despite the high success rate in treating HL, approximately 5% to 10% of patients will be refractory to initial treatment and 10% to 30% will have disease relapse after CR. Patients relapsing after treatment should be offered additional therapy as durable responses have been reported in these patients. The duration of remission after chemotherapy remains a vital prognostic factor for likelihood of response to future treatment.[23] For healthy patients, the definitive therapy after relapse is high-dose chemotherapy with autologous stem cell transplantation (SCT).[24] This treatment offers a cure rate of approximately 40%.

Several studies have reported the importance of giving conventional chemotherapy before SCT. The purpose of the initial treatment after relapse is to decrease the tumor bulk before the high-dose chemotherapy. High-dose chemotherapy given to patients who are in first relapse has provided encouraging results. A series of 58 patients had a progression-free survival (PFS) of over 60% with a median follow-up of 2.3 years. The safety profile of autologous SCT continues to improve as refinements in supportive care are realized. Current estimates of mortality from autologous SCT for HL are approximately 5%. Morbidity commonly associated with the preparative regimens in HL, aside from infectious and bleeding complications, includes the additive pulmonary toxicity of bleomycin coupled with carmustine, inducing potentially fatal pulmonary pneumonitis.

Table 97–7			
Practical Information for ABVD and CHOP			
Regimen	**Drug Class**	**Pharmacokinetics**	**Unique Toxicities**
ABVD			
Doxorubicin	Anthracycline	Hepatic metabolism[a]	Cardiomyopathy Maximum lifetime dose, 550 mg/m²
Bleomycin	Antitumor antibiotic	Renal clearance[a]	Pulmonary fibrosis Maximum lifetime dose, 400 mg
Vinblastine	Vinca alkaloid	CYP 3A4/5 metabolism[a]	Neuropathy, constipation
Dacarbazine	Alkylating agent	Hepatic metabolism[a]	Myelosuppression
CHOP			
Cyclophosphamide	Alkylating agent	Prodrug; CYP3A4/5, 2D6	Hemorrhagic cystitis
Doxorubicin	Anthracycline	Hepatic metabolism	Cardiomyopathy
Vincristine	Vinca alkaloid	CYP3A4/5	Neuropathy, constipation
Prednisone	Corticosteroid	100% oral bioavailability	Hyperglycemia, osteopenia See dose adjustments[a] (Chap. 88)

Patients who are not deemed candidates for high-dose chemotherapy with autologous SCT may receive standard multiagent salvage chemotherapy, such as etoposide, methylprednisolone, cytarabine, and cisplatin (ESHAP) or dexamethasone, cytarabine, and cisplatin (DHAP). Newer regimens such as GVD (gemcitabine, vinorelbine, and pegylated liposomal doxorubicin), IGEV (ifosfamide, gemcitabine, and vinorelbine) and GCD (gemcitabine, carboplatin, and dexamethasone) have also been effective for relapsed refractory HL. Recently, a new monoclonal antibody, brentuximab, was approved for the treatment of relapsed or refractory HL. This novel agent targets CD-30 and is linked to a microtubule-disrupting agent, monomethylauristatin E.[25]

TREATMENT OF NHL

Desired Outcome

Treatment of NHL depends primarily on histologic subtype (follicular low grade versus diffuse aggressive) and staging (local stage I/II versus advanced stage III/IV) to guide appropriate treatment strategy with observation, chemotherapy, radiotherapy, or chemotherapy and radiation. The Cotswold modification of the Ann Arbor staging system for HL is generally used in NHL as well.

Treatment goals depend on the patient's specific subtype of NHL. For follicular low-grade NHL, the disease is considered to be incurable with standard therapies. There is a small prospect for cure using allogeneic SCT owing to the graft-versus-lymphoma effect of donor T cells. Many patients with follicular low-grade NHL are older than 60 years of age, making allogeneic SCT impractical because of the high treatment-related mortality for older patients.

7 *The treatment goals for low-grade NHL include:*

- *Observation of the disease until the patient exhibits obvious progression that limits functional capacity or is life-threatening for low-grade NHL*

- Treatment that induces the disease into remission with resolution of disease symptoms and manageable toxicity

- Judicious selection of treatment options to avoid long-term toxicity

- Prevention of infectious complications of treatment

The intent of treatment for patients with aggressive histologies is cure of the malignancy. Some histologic subtypes exhibit an aggressive clinical course and are not considered to be curable. These patients are still treated with curative-intent chemotherapy or may be considered for a clinical trial.

Nonpharmacologic Therapy

For patients with low-grade follicular NHL, deferring initiation of therapy until progression of disease is a standard approach. The median survival time is 6 to 10 years. Some patients may be asymptomatic for several years after initial diagnosis, making observation a reasonable front-line therapy for most of these patients. Radiation therapy has a limited role in NHL relative to HL. NHL is more often a systemic disease, and radiation typically has been reserved for consolidation therapy after chemotherapy in patients presenting with a large extranodal mass. However, IFRT without systemic therapy is a treatment option for patients with stage I/II follicular lymphoma.

For early-stage diffuse, aggressive NHL, combined-modality therapy was tested versus a longer course of chemotherapy.[26] Overall survival favored the CHOP–radiation arm for 5 years (82% versus 72%). There was a trend toward increased toxicity, particularly hematologic and cardiac toxicity, in the CHOP alone arm. The results of this trial have established combined-modality therapy as first-line treatment for early stage NHL. Unique presentations of NHL, such as primary CNS disease, may incorporate radiation into treatment algorithms.[27]

Pharmacologic Therapy

▶ Follicular Low-Grade NHL

● The management of low-grade lymphomas is an area of controversy, especially in patients who present with early stage disease. In patients with localized disease, observation alone can be an appropriate treatment strategy. Typical indications for treatment in this population include cytopenias, recurrent infections, threatened end-organ function, disease progression over at least 6 months, or patient preference. In these patients, single-agent chemotherapy such as fludarabine or bendamustine, a unique alkylating agent with a novel chemical structure, is often offered initially. In patients in whom a more rapid response is desired, such as patients with advanced disease, multiagent chemotherapy such as CVP (cyclophosphamide, vincristine, and prednisone or prednisolone) or CHOP may be used. These regimens, detailed in Table 97–8, have not been associated with an improvement in overall survival, making it impossible to select an unequivocal first-line regimen.[28-30]

Rituximab has become an integral component in drug therapy for this disease. Rituximab is a chimeric monoclonal antibody that binds specifically to the antigen CD20 expressed on pre-B and mature B lymphocytes.[31] NHL of B-cell origin expresses CD20 in greater than 90% of cases. CD20 is believed to play a role in early differentiation and activation of the cell cycle. Rituximab exerts its activity through antibody-dependent cytotoxicity activation of complement and induction of apoptosis. The initial clinical experience with rituximab involved 166 patients with CD20+ low-grade lymphoma treated with four doses of 375 mg/m^2 of rituximab weekly.[32] The overall response rate was 48%, with CR in 6% of patients. The median follow-up of 12 months demonstrated a median time to progression of 13 months by intent-to-treat analysis. These data established the role of rituximab as a viable treatment option in patients with indolent follicular NHL and is added to chemotherapy in most patients. Additionally, rituximab was examined as maintenance therapy administered every 8 weeks for to 2 years after rituximab-containing multiagent chemotherapy. Compared with observation, rituximab increased 3-year PFS (74.9 versus 57.6 months).[33]

Novel strategies for treatment of low-grade lymphomas include the combination of monoclonal antibodies directed against CD20 with a radioactive moiety attached. Two such entities—ibritumomab-yttrium 90 and tositumomab-iodine[131]—are now approved by the Food and Drug Administration (FDA). The radiation component necessitates compounding both medications in a nuclear medicine pharmacy. Bendamustine has also been studied in a phase III trial of rituximab-refractory indolent lymphomas. Among 62 patients with follicular lymphoma, there was an overall response rate of 74% with a median duration of response of 9.2 months.[34] High-dose chemotherapy is being evaluated for low-grade follicular NHL, but its role is currently limited to clinical trials.

▶ Diffuse, Aggressive NHL

❽ *The mainstay of therapy for diffuse, aggressive NHL has been the administration of anthracycline-based combination chemotherapy, which generally consists of four or more drugs.* Therapy options for intermediate- and high-grade NHL generally are segregated between localized (stage I/II) and advanced (stage III/IV) disease. Combined-modality therapy with an abbreviated course of CHOP and local radiation is considered a standard of care for stage I/II disease.

The standard therapy for disseminated disease since the 1970s has been CHOP. This regimen conferred a response of 50% to 60%, with long-term survival of approximately 30%. However, the 1980s were notable for the development of newer combination chemotherapy regimens that incorporated increasing numbers of agents with varying schedules. More complex chemotherapy regimens were shown in phase II trials to have higher response rates than CHOP. The CALGB designed a phase III randomized four-arm trial to assess the impact on survival of three more intensive regimens compared with CHOP.[35] This trial randomized 899 patients with intermediate- or high-grade (Working Formulation classification) NHL to CHOP or one of the three more intensive advanced-generation regimens. There were no significant differences in response rate or overall survival, which was consistent among all subgroups. Severe toxicity and death were higher in the advanced-generation treatment programs relative to CHOP. This pivotal trial has cemented CHOP as first-line chemotherapy in diffuse NHL.

Rituximab has also come to play a vital role in treating diffuse, aggressive NHL. A French study randomized patients 60 to 80 years of age with newly diagnosed diffuse, large B-cell NHL to either CHOP for eight cycles or CHOP plus

---

Table 97–8

Chemotherapy Regimens for Low-Grade, Follicular NHL

Fludarabine/Rituximab
Fludarabine 25 mg/m^2 IV days 1–5 every 28 days
Rituximab 375 mg/m^2 IV, days 1 and 5 of week 1 and 26; single dose 72 hours before fludarabine cycles 2, 4, and 6

Bendamustine/Rituximab—Every 28 Days
Bendamustine 90 mg/m^2 IV days 1 and 2
Rituximab 375 mg/m^2 IV, day 1

rCVP—Every 21 Days
Rituximab 375 mg/m^2 IV, day 1
Cyclophosphamide 750 mg/m^2 IV, day 1
Vincristine 1.4 mg/m^2 IV, day 1
Prednisone 40 mg/m^2 PO daily, days 1–5

rCHOP—Every 21 Days
Rituximab 375 mg/m^2 IV, day 1
Cyclophosphamide 750 mg/m^2 IV, day 1
Doxorubicin 50 mg/m^2 IV, day 1
Vincristine 1.4 mg/m^2 IV, day 1
Prednisone 100 mg/day PO, days 1–5

IV, intravenous; PO, oral.

Table 97–9

Treatment Regimens for Diffuse, Aggressive NHL

CHOP—Every 21 Days
Cyclophosphamide 750 mg/m^2 IV, day 1
Doxorubicin 50 mg/m^2 IV, day 1
Vincristine 1.4 mg/m^2 IV, day 1
Prednisone 100 mg orally daily, days 1–5

rCHOP—Every 21 Days
Rituximab 375 mg/m^2 IV, day 1
Cyclophosphamide 750 mg/m^2 IV, day 1
Doxorubicin 50 mg/m^2 IV, day 1
Vincristine 1.4 mg/m^2 IV, day 1
Prednisone 100 mg/day PO, days 1–5

m-BACOD—Every 21 Days
Methotrexate 200 mg/m^2 IV, days 8 and 15
Bleomycin 4 mg/m^2 IV, day 1
Doxorubicin 45 mg/m^2, day 1
Cyclophosphamide 600 mg/m^2 IV, day 1
Vincristine 1.4 mg/m^2 IV, day 1
Dexamethasone 6 mg orally daily, days 1–5
Leucovorin 10 mg PO every 6 hours, 24 hours after
    methotrexate × 8 doses

ProMACE-CytaBOM—Every 28 Days
Prednisone 60 mg/day PO, days 1–14
Doxorubicin 25 mg/m^2 IV, day 1
Cyclophosphamide 650 mg/m^2 IV, day 1
Etoposide 120 mg/m^2 IV, day 1
Cytarabine 300 mg/m^2 IV, day 8
Bleomycin 5 units IV, day 8
Vincristine 1.4 mg/m^2 IV, day 8
Methotrexate 120 mg/m^2, day 8
Leucovorin 25 mg/m^2 IV every 6 hours, 24 hours after methotrexate
    × 5 doses

MACOP-B
Methotrexate 400 mg/m^2 IV, day 8
Doxorubicin 50 mg/m^2 IV, days 1 and 15
Cyclophosphamide 350 mg/m^2 IV, days 1 and 15
Vincristine 1.4 mg/m^2 IV, days 8 and 15

Prednisone 75 mg/day PO × 12 weeks
Bleomycin 10 units IV, day 28
Leucovorin 15 mg PO every 6 hours, 24 hours after methotrexate ×
    6 doses

Hyper-CVAD
Cyclophosphamide 300 mg/m^2 IV every 12 hours, days 1–3 (with
    Mesna)
Doxorubicin 50 mg/m^2 IV, day 1
Vincristine 1.4 mg/m^2 IV, days 1,11
Dexamethasone 40 mg/day PO, days 1–4 and 11–14
Methotrexate 15 mg intrathecal, day 2
Cytarabine 30 mg intrathecal, day 2
Hydrocortisone 15 mg intrathecal, day 2

Above Drugs Given on Courses 1, 3, 5, and 7
Methotrexate 1,000 mg/m^2 IV over 24 hours, day 1
Cytarabine 3,000 mg/m^2 IV every 12 hours, days 2 and 3
Leucovorin 25 mg IV × 1; then 25 mg PO every 6 hours for 7 doses
Methotrexate 15 mg intrathecal, day 2

Above Drugs Given on Courses 2, 4, 6, and 8
Relapsed Disease

ESHAP

Etoposide 40 mg/m^2 IV per day continuous infusion, days 1–4
Cisplatin 25 mg/m^2 IV per day continuous infusion, days 1–4
Cytarabine 2,000 mg/m^2 IV × 1, day 5
Methylprednisone 250 mg IV every 12 hours, days 1–4

DHAP

Dexamethasone 40 mg PO or IV daily, days 1–4
Cisplatin 100 mg/m^2 IV continuous infusion, day 1
Cytarabine 2,000 mg/m^2 IV every 12 hours for 2 doses on day 2

ICE

Etoposide 100 mg/m^2 IV daily, days 1–3
Carboplatin AUC 5 (maximum dose, 800 mg) IV, day 2
Ifosfamide 5,000 mg/m^2 IV continuous infusion × 1 on day 2 (with
    100% replacement with Mesna)

AUC, area under the curve; IV, intravenous; Mesna, 2-mercaptoethane sulfonate; PO, oral.

---

rituximab for eight cycles.[36] Initial 2-year follow-up showed that rituximab improved CR (76% versus 63%) and median event-free survival (57% versus 38%). Long-term follow-up also showed an increase in 10-year survival (43% versus 27.6%). Similar findings in younger patients have been reported recently, making CHOP plus rituximab first-line therapy for advanced-stage diffuse, aggressive NHL (Table 97– 9).

▶ Special Populations

There are certain histologic subtypes of diffuse, aggressive NHL that respond less well to treatment with conventional regimens such as CHOP. Burkitt's lymphoma, lymphoblastic lymphoma, mantle cell lymphoma, and primary CNS lymphoma are examples of disease that benefit from more intensive therapy. Regimens such as hyper-CVAD, which alternate cycles of hyperfractionated cyclophosphamide, doxorubicin, vincristine, and dexamethasone with high-dose cytarabine and methotrexate, may be substituted for CHOP.

Patients with CNS NHL have disease that is poorly responsive to therapy because of inadequate penetration of standard doses of chemotherapy across the blood–brain barrier. High-dose methotrexate, ranging from 2,500 to

Patient Encounter 1, Part 2

Based on the patient's diagnosis of stage III diffuse large B-cell lymphoma, the patient is to start treatment immediately.

What therapy (or therapies) is (are) most appropriate for this patient?

What other information (e.g., laboratory studies, diagnostic tests) is needed before the patient can start chemotherapy?

8,000 mg/m² is a mainstay of therapy. Treatment may also include direct instillation of intrathecal chemotherapy into the cerebrospinal fluid. Drugs that are commonly instilled intrathecally include methotrexate, cytarabine (conventional formulation and liposomal products), and corticosteroids.

The recent appreciation of the etiology of *Helicobacter pylori* in the etiology of peptic ulcer disease and the association between colonization and MALT has spurred the more aggressive treatment of this organism with antibiotics. In patients with localized disease, aggressive, combination therapy targeted at *H. pylori* has been shown to induce MALT remission. Patients with advanced disease may require combination chemotherapy, such as CHOP.

Mantle cell lymphoma, which comprises 6% of NHL cases, is defined by a chromosomal translocation of t(11;14)(q13;32). This translocation results in the overexpression of cyclin D1 coupled with NF-κB, which plays a critical role in intracellular protein regulation and protranscription factors leading to increased cell survival. Bortezomib, a novel proteosome inhibitor, disrupts the regulation and degradation of proteins required for cell cycle regulation. Bortezomib is approved by the FDA for the treatment of patients with mantle cell lymphoma who have failed prior chemotherapy. A study conducted in 155 patients demonstrated that bortezomib resulted in 31% overall response rate with a median survival of 9.3 months.[37] Bortezomib is well tolerated, with peripheral neuropathy, thrombocytopenia, neutropenia, and nausea reported most frequently.

With more than half of patients with NHL expected to relapse with disease, salvage therapy plays a major role in the attempt to cure patients with recurrence. Multiple drug regimens such as ESHAP and DHAP can induce a CR, but the long-term cure rate with these regimens is less than 10%. Salvage therapy can induce remissions with subsequent relapses; however, the chance for a CR and the duration of remission is further diminished.

High-dose chemotherapy with autologous SCT has been studied as an alternative to standard dose regimens in the setting of first relapse.[38] The best-studied indication for SCT is for patients with intermediate- or high-grade disease that fails to respond to first-line therapy. A 3- to 5-year survival of greater than 40% is achieved in patients who have good performance and disease that demonstrates a significant response to one or two cycles of salvage chemotherapy. The procedure-related mortality rate has ranged from 5% to 10% in published reports. However, as with HL, with more broad application of peripheral blood stem cells and improved

supportive care, the mortality rate continues to decline. The role of allogeneic SCT in this setting is limited because of donor availability, the older age of patients, and the high treatment-related morbidity and mortality. Additionally, outcomes between autologous and allogeneic transplant appear similar.

Patients with HIV-related lymphoma represent a therapeutic dilemma considering many have high-grade disease of B-cell origin. A common presentation is that of extranodal disease, frequently in the GI tract, CNS, and bone marrow. Therapy for this population thus far has fared poorly, with a median survival time of 6 to 12 months, which decreases to 3 months with CNS involvement.[39] It remains to be seen if improved antiretroviral therapy will have an impact on the incidence and treatment options for these patients. The addition of rituximab to chemotherapy has failed to improve overall survival in this patient population and is associated with increased infectious complications.[40]

OUTCOME EVALUATION

Treatment success in lymphoma is measured in successive stages, the first being inducing tumor regression and the degree of that regression: CR versus PR versus stable disease (SD) versus progressive disease (PD). The response evaluation criteria in solid tumors (RECIST) is a uniform criteria assessing tumor response developed by the National Cancer Institute is the standard methodology that physicians use to gauge treatment efficacy. HL and NHL may have residual masses after completion of treatment, adding to the difficulty in establishing a definitive remission from treatment. Clinical trials with limited numbers of patients have been published suggesting the value of positron emission tomography (PET) scans or gallium scans to rule out whether residual tumor masses after treatment contain viable tumor.[41] The National Comprehensive Cancer Network recommends using integrated PET–computed tomography (CT) scanning as part of the initial workup and to evaluate for residual disease at the end of treatment.[42]

Long-term follow-up monitors patients for continued disease remission or relapse with careful physical examination of the lymph nodes and sites of prior disease involvement and imaging studies. Patients will have routine chest x-rays and CT scans to screen for disease recurrence. Patients require long-term monitoring for toxicities of their primary treatment, either chemotherapy or radiation therapy.

Most patients treated for lymphoma with chemotherapy or radiation notice a regression of palpable lymphadenopathy within days. This is because of the high sensitivity of the rapidly proliferating malignant lymphocytes to chemotherapy and radiotherapy. This necessitates implementation of tumor lysis syndrome precautions with aggressive intravenous fluid resuscitation and allopurinol. Rasburicase should be considered for patients with moderate to high tumor burdens. Most chemotherapy treatments for lymphoma have a significant risk of infectious complications. Combination regimens for both HL and NHL are associated with rates of

Patient Encounter 1, Plan 3: Creating a Care Plan

Based on the information presented, create a care plan for this patient, including the goals of therapy, antineoplastic therapy plan, and necessary supportive care.

severe leukopenia and/or neutropenia ranging from 20% to 100% of patients. Consideration must be given to supportive care with prophylactic antibiotics and CSFs. Published guidelines recommend CSFs be used as primary prevention when the incidence of febrile neutropenia with chemotherapy is approximately 20% and no other equally effective and less myelosuppressive regimen is available or for secondary prevention where the patient already has experienced febrile neutropenia.[43] Effective antiemetic support is currently available that can control chemotherapy-induced nausea and vomiting reasonably well for most standard-dose regimens.[44]

Advances in the treatment of lymphoma have increased the number of long-term survivors. Identification of long-term side effects associated with lymphoma therapy are vital to patient follow-up and may influence treatment decisions in newly diagnosed patients. Outcomes associated with the treatment of HL make up the majority of data. However, advances in NHL treatment have provided more information regarding long-term toxicities. Two leading causes of death associated with HL are secondary malignancies and cardiovascular disease. Secondary malignancies after HL are classified into leukemia, NHL, and solid tumors. Several studies have reported that cardiac mortality is the leading cause of non–malignancy-related death in HL survivors. The use of combined modality of irradiation with doxorubicin-based therapy has been reported to increase the risk of cardiac dysfunction. Treatment-related pulmonary toxicity, hypothyroidism, and infertility have all been associated with HL therapy. The most common solid tumors include cancers of the breast, lung, and GI tract. NHL survivors have an increased risk for developing myelodysplasia, acute myelogenous leukemia, and various solid tumors. The most common non–malignancy-based toxicities associated with NHL includes cardiac disease, infertility, neuropathy, renal insufficiency, GI toxicities, and lung fibrosis.[45]

A limitation of rituximab is the severe, potentially fatal infusion-related reactions. Deaths have been reported resulting from the profound hypotension and circulatory collapse seen with the drug, particularly on the first dose. The package labeling recommends premedication with acetaminophen and diphenhydramine before each infusion. For the first infusion, the drug should be administered at 50 mg/h. The infusion rate may be increased by 50 mg/h every 30 minutes to a maximum of 400 mg/h if tolerated. If infusion-related reactions do occur, the infusion should be stopped temporarily until symptoms resolve. The infusion should be reinstituted at a rate that is one-half the previous rate. For subsequent infusions, the rate may commence at 100 mg/h and be increased at 100-mg/h increments every 30 minutes for a maximum of 400 mg/h as tolerated. Tumor lysis syndrome is reported frequently with rituximab, and patients with a high tumor burden should be considered for prophylaxis with allopurinol and hydration. Reactivation of hepatitis B infections have occurred in patients treated with rituximab, so patients at high risk for hepatitis B should be screened and monitored carefully for reactivation of hepatitis. If hepatitis occurs, rituximab should be discontinued, and

Patient Care and Monitoring

1. Verify chemotherapy regimen doses with a standardized reference and assess for dose adjustment for height, weight, and body surface area and organ dysfunction (renal or hepatic).

2. Assess appropriateness of supportive care for each chemotherapy regimens such as antiemetics or colony-stimulating factors.

3. Before initiation of treatment with chemotherapy, determine if tumor lysis syndrome precautions need to be implemented.

4. Take a thorough medication history with particular attention to nonprescription or herbal medications.

5. Provide patient education regarding common toxicities associated with chemotherapy such as nausea/vomiting, mucositis, myelosuppression, and alopecia.

6. For doxorubicin-containing regimens, total the cumulative dosage received by the patient to monitor for cardiac toxicity.

7. For bleomycin-containing regimens, total the cumulative dosage received by the patient to monitor for pulmonary fibrosis.

8. Educate patients regarding the short- and long-term complications associated with radiation therapy.

9. Monitor patient for signs and symptoms of response of tumor to chemotherapy.

10. Provide contact numbers for patient in the event of a fever and a response plan if the patient is considered to be at risk for neutropenic fever

patients should be treated with antivirals. Other associated toxicities of rituximab include fever, chills, headache, asthenia, nausea, vomiting, angioedema, bronchospasm, and skin reactions. ❾ *Rituximab is an effective treatment option for patients with various forms of NHL in combination with chemotherapy or as a single agent as long as patients are monitored appropriately.* Radiolabeled rituximab causes more myelosuppression than rituximab alone and, similar to combination cytotoxic chemotherapy regimens, has a long-term risk of inducing secondary leukemias.[46]

Abbreviations Introduced in This Chapter

Bcl-1	Important in the regulation of mitosis
Bcl-2	A regulator of apoptosis
Bcl-3	A regulator of nuclear transcription factor
Bcl-6	Regulates cell differentiation
c-myc	Regulator of gene transcription
ABVD	Doxorubicin, bleomycin, vinblastine, and dacarbazine

CALGB	Cancer and leukemia group B
CD	Cluster of differentiation
CHOP	Cyclophosphamide, doxorubicin, vincristine, and prednisone
CSFs	Colony-stimulating factors
CVP	Cyclophosphamide, vincristine, and prednisone or prednisolone
EBV	Epstein-Barr virus
ESR	Erythroid sedimentation rate
FLIPI	Follicular lymphoma international prognostic index
HL	Hodgkin's lymphoma
IPI	International Prognostic Index
IFRT	Involved field radiation therapy
LDH	Lactate dehydrogenase
MALT	Mucosa-associated lymphoid tissue
MOPP	Mechlorethamine, vincristine, procarbazine, and prednisone
NHL	Non-Hodgkin's lymphoma
PET	Positron emission tomography
RECIST	Response evaluation criteria in solid tumors
RS	Reed-Sternberg
SCT	Stem cell transplant

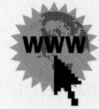 Self-assessment questions and answers are available at *http://www.mhpharmacotherapy.com/pp.html.*

REFERENCES

1. Siegel R, Ward E, Brawley O, Jemal A. Cancer statistics, 2011. CA Cancer J Clin 2011;61:212–236.
2. Caporaso NE, Lynn R, Goldin WF, et al. Current Insight on Trends, Causes and Mechanisms of Hodgkin Lymphoma. Cancer J 2009;15(2):117–123.
3. Fisher SG, Fisher RI. The epidemiology of non-Hodgkin lymphoma. Oncogene 2004;23:6524–6534.
4. Evans LS, Hancock BW. Non-Hodgkin lymphoma. Lancet 2003;362:139–146.
5. Kuppers R, Hansmann ML. The Hodgkin and Reed/Sternberg cell. Int J Biochem Cell Biol 2005;37:511–517.
6. Kuppers R. Molecular biology of Hodgkin lymphoma. Hematology Am Soc Hematol Educ Program 2009;491–496.
7. Brauninger A, Schmitz R, Bechtel D, et al. Molecular biology of Hodgkin and Reed/Sternberg cells in Hodgkin lymphoma. Int J Cancer 2006;118:1853–1861.
8. Eberle FC, Mani H, Jaffe ES. Histopathology of Hodgkin lymphoma. Cancer J 2009;15(2):129–137.
9. Campo E, Swerdlow SH, Harris NL, et al. The 2008 WHO classification of lymphoid neoplasms and beyond: Evolving concepts and practical applications. Blood 2011;117(19):5019–5032.
10. Hasenclever D, Diehl V. A prognostic score for advanced Hodgkin disease. N Engl J Med 1998;339:1506–1514.
11. Kuppers R, Klein U, Hansmann ML, Rajewsky K. Cellular origin of human B-cell lymphomas. N Engl J Med 1999;341:1520–1529.
12. Tsimberidou AM, Keating MJ. Richter syndrome: Biology, incidence and therapeutic strategies. Cancer 2005;103:216–228.
13. The International non-Hodgkin Lymphoma Prognostic Factors Project. A predictive model for aggressive non-Hodgkin lymphoma. N Engl J Med 1993;329:987–994.
14. van Imhoff GW, Boerma EJ, van der Holt B, et al. Prognostic impact of germinal center-associated proteins and chromosomal breakpoints in poor risk diffuse large B-cell lymphoma. J Clin Oncol 2006;24:4135–4142.
15. Solal-Celigny P, Roy P, Colombat P, et al. Follicular lymphoma international prognostic index. Blood 2004;104:1258–1265.
16. Lister TA, Crowther D, Sutcliffe SB, et al. Report of a committee convened to discuss the evaluation and staging of patients with Hodgkin disease: Cotswold meeting. J Clin Oncol 1989;7:1630–1636.
17. Yahalom J. Role of Radiation Therapy in Hodgkin Lymphoma. Caner J 2009;15(2):155–160.
18. Advani RH, Hoppe RT, Baer DM et al. Efficacy of abbreviated Stanford V chemotherapy and involved field radiotherapy in early stage Hodgkin disease: Mature results of the G4 trial. Blood 2009;114:1670a.
19. Kuruvilla J, Standard therapy of advanced Hodgkin lymphoma. Hematology Am Soc Hematol Educ Program 2009;497–506.
20. Canellos GP, Anderson JR, Propert KJ, et al. Chemotherapy of advanced Hodgkin disease with MOPP, ABVD, or MOPP alternating with ABVD. N Engl J Med 1992;327:1478–1484.
21. Canellos GP, Niedzwiecki D, Johnson JL. Long-Term Follow-up of Survival in Hodgkin lymphoma. N Engl J Med 2009;361:2390–2391.
22. Engert A, Diehl V, Franklin J, et al. Escalated-Dose BEACOPP in the treatment of patients with advance-stage Hodgkin lymphoma: 10 years of follow-up of the GHSG HD9 study. J Clin Oncol 2009;27:4548–4544.
23. Quddus F, Armitage JO. Salvage therapy for Hodgkin lymphoma. Cancer J 2009;15(2):161–163.
24. Linch DC, Winfield D, Goldstone AH, et al. Dose intensification with autologous bone-marrow transplantation in relapsed and resistant Hodgkin disease: Results of a BLNI randomised trial. Lancet 1993;341:1051–1054.
25. Chen R, Gopal AK, Smith SE. Results of a pivotal phase 2 study of brentuximabvedotin (SGN-35) in patients with relapsed or refractory Hodgkin lymphoma. ASH Annual Meeting Abstracts 2010;116:283.
26. Miller TP, Dahlberg S, Cassady JR, et al. Chemotherapy alone compared with chemotherapy plus radiotherapy for localized intermediate-and high-grade non-Hodgkin lymphoma. N Engl J Med 1998;339:21–26.
27. DeAngelis LM, Seiferheld W, Schold SC, Fisher B, Schultz CJ. Combination chemotherapy and radiotherapy for primary central nervous system lymphoma: Radiation Therapy Oncology Group Study 93–10. J Clin Oncol 2002;20:4643–4648.
28. Hagenbeek A, Eghbali H, Monfardini S, et al. Phase III intergroup study of fludarabine phosphate compared with cyclophosphamide, vincristine, and prednisone chemotherapy in newly diagnosed patients with stage III and IV low-grade malignant Non-Hodgkin lymphoma. J Clin Oncol 2006;24:1590–1596.
29. Marcus R, Imrie K, Belch A, et al. CVP chemotherapy plus rituximab compared with CVP as first-line treatment for advanced follicular lymphoma. Blood 2005;105:1417–1423.
30. Peterson BA, Petroni GR, Frizzera G, et al. Prolonged single-agent versus combination chemotherapy in indolent follicular lymphomas: A study of the cancer and leukemia group B. J Clin Oncol 2003;21:5–15.
31. McCune SL, Gockerman JP, Rizzieri DA. Monoclonal antibody therapy in the treatment of non-Hodgkin lymphoma. JAMA 2001;286:1149–1152.
32. McLaughlin P, Grillo-López AJ, Link BK, et al. Rituximab chimeric anti-CD20 monoclonal antibody therapy for relapsed indolent lymphoma: Half of patients respond to a four dose treatment program. J Clin Oncol 1998;16:2825–2833.
33. Salles G, Seymour JF, Offner F, et al. Rituximab maintenance for 2 years in patients with high tumor burden follicular lymphoma responding to rituximab plus chemotherapy (PRIMA). Lancet 2010;377:42–51.
34. Kahl BS, Bartlett NL, Leonard JP, et al. Bendamustine is effective therapy in patients with rituximab-refractory, indolent B-cell non-Hodgkin lymphoma: Results from a multicenter study. Cancer 2010;116:106–114.
35. Fisher RI, et al. Comparison of standard regimen (CHOP) with three intensive chemotherapy regimens for advanced non-Hodgkin lymphoma. N Engl J Med 1993;328:1002–1006.

36. Coiffer B, Thieblemont C, Van Den Neste E, et al. Long-term outcome of patients in the LNH-98.5 trial, the first randomized study comparing rituximab-CHOP to standard CHOP chemotherapy in DLBCL patients: A study by the Groupe d'Etudes des Lymphomes de l'Adulte. Blood 2010;116:2040–2045.

37. Kane RC, Dagher R, Farrell A, et al. Bortezomib for the treatment of mantle cell lymphoma. Clin Cancer Res 2007;13:5291–5294.

38. Stebbing J, Marvin V, Bower M. The evidence-based treatment of AIDS-related non-Hodgkin lymphoma. Cancer Treat Rev 2004;30:249–253.

39. Thierry P, Guglielmi C, Hagenbeek A, et al. Autologous bone marrow transplant as compared with salvage chemotherapy in relapses of chemotherapy-sensitive non-Hodgkin lymphoma. N Engl J Med 1995;333:1540–1545.

40. Kaplan LD, Lee JY, Ambinder RF, et al. Rituximab does not improve clinical outcome in a randomized phase III trial of CHOP with or without rituximab in patients with HIV-associated non-Hodgkin lymphoma: AIDS-Malignancies Consortium Trial 010. Blood 2005;106:1538–1543.

41. Juweid ME, Wiseman GA, Vose JA, et al. Response assessment of aggressive non-Hodgkin lymphoma by Integrated International Workshop Criteria and fluorine-18-fluorodeoxyglucose positron emission tomography. J Clin Oncol 2005;21:4652–4661.

42. Podoloff DA, Advani RH, Allred C, et al. NCCN task force report: positron emission tomography (PET)/computed tomography (CT) scanning in cancer. J Natl Compr Canc Netw 2007;5(Suppl 1):S1–S22.

43. Smith TJ, Khatcheressian J, Lyman GH, et al Update of recommendations for the use of white blood cell. growth factors: An evidence-based clinical practice guideline. J Clin Oncol 2006;24(19):3187–3205.

44. Kris MG, Hesketh PJ, Somerfield MR, et al. American Society of Clinical Oncology guideline for antiemetics in oncology: Update 2006. J Clin Oncol 2006;17:2971–2994.

45. Ng AK, LaCasce A, Travis LB. Long-term complications of lymphoma and its treatment. J Clin Oncol 2011; 29:1885–1892.

46. Armitage JO, Carbone PP, Connors JM, Levine A, Bennett JM, Kroll S. Treatment-related myelodysplasia and acute leukemia in non-Hodgkin lymphoma patients. J Clin Oncol 2003;21:897–906.

98 Hematopoietic Stem Cell Transplantation

Amber P. Lawson

LEARNING OBJECTIVES

● **Upon completion of the chapter, the reader will be able to:**

1. Explain the rationale for using hematopoietic stem cell transplant (HSCT) to treat cancer.

2. Compare the different types of HSCTs, specifically (a) the types of donors (i.e., autologous and allogeneic), (b) the source of hematopoietic cells (i.e., umbilical cord, peripheral blood progenitor cells [PBPCs], and bone marrow), and (c) the type of preparative regimen (i.e., myeloablative and nonmyeloablative).

3. List the nonhematologic toxicity to high-dose chemotherapy used in myeloablative preparative regimens, specifically busulfan-induced seizures, hemorrhagic cystitis, GI toxicities, and sinusoidal obstruction syndrome.

4. Develop a plan for monitoring and managing engraftment of hematopoiesis.

5. Explain graft-versus-host disease (GVHD).

6. Recommend a prophylactic and treatment regimen for GVHD.

7. Choose an appropriate regimen to minimize the risk of infectious complications in HSCT patients.

8. Evaluate the long-term health care of HSCT survivors.

KEY CONCEPTS

❶ Hematopoietic stem cell transplantation (HSCT) is a procedure used mainly to treat hematologic malignancies via high-dose chemotherapy and/or a graft-versus-tumor effect.

❷ An autologous HSCT involves the infusion of a patient's own hematopoietic cells and allows for the administration of higher doses of chemotherapy, radiation, or both to treat the malignancy. Infusion of another's hematopoietic cells is an allogeneic HSCT; these cells can be from donors related or unrelated to the recipient.

❸ Umbilical cord blood, peripheral blood progenitor cells (PBPCs), and bone marrow can serve as the source of hematopoietic cells. The optimal cell source differs based on the donor and recipient characteristics.

❹ A myeloablative preparative regimen involves the administration of sublethal doses of chemotherapy to the recipient to eradicate residual malignant disease. The recipient will not regain his or her own hematopoiesis and will be at risk for substantial life-threatening nonhematologic toxicity.

❺ A nonmyeloablative preparative regimen is less toxic than a myeloablative regimen in hopes of being able to offer the benefits of an allogeneic HSCT to more patients. A nonmyeloablative HSCT is based on the concept of donor immune response having a graft-versus-tumor effect.

❻ Nonhematologic toxicity differs based on the preparative regimen administered.

❼ Engraftment is the reestablishment of functional hematopoiesis. It is commonly defined as the point at which a patient can maintain a sustained absolute neutrophil count (ANC) of greater than 500 cells/mm³ (0.5×10^9/L) and a sustained platelet count of greater 20,000/mm³ (20×10^9/L) lasting for 3 or more consecutive days without transfusions.

❽ Graft-versus-host disease (GVHD) is caused by the activation of donor lymphocytes, leading to immune damage to the skin, gut, and liver in the recipient. An immunosuppressive regimen is administered to prevent GVHD in recipients of an allogeneic graft; this regimen is based on the type of preparative regimen and the source of the graft.

❾ Recipients of HSCT are at higher risk of bacterial, viral, and fungal infections and usually receive a prophylactic or preemptive regimen to minimize the morbidity and mortality owing to infectious complications.

⑩ Long-term survivors of HSCT should be monitored closely, particularly for infections and secondary malignant neoplasms.

INTRODUCTION

Hematopoietic stem cell transplantation (HSCT) is a procedure used mainly to treat hematologic malignancies via high-dose chemotherapy and/or a graft-versus-tumor effect. An essential component of this procedure is the infusion of hematopoietic cells into the recipient to facilitate an immunologic response against the residual malignancy and/or restore normal hematopoiesis and lymphopoiesis. The first HSCTs were performed using allogeneic bone marrow, which involved administration of high-dose chemotherapy and/or radiation aimed at eradicating residual malignant disease followed by transplantation of bone marrow from one individual to another to "rescue" the recipient's immune system from the myelotoxic effects of the treatment. Bone marrow contains pluripotent stem cells and postthymic lymphocytes, which are responsible for long-term hematopoietic reconstitution, immune recovery, and its associated graft-versus-host disease (GVHD). Subsequently, the dose-intensity concept for cancer treatment was expanded to using myeloablative preparative regimens followed by autologous HSCT.

The type of HSCT performed depends on a number of factors, including the type and status of disease, availability of a compatible donor, patient age, performance status, and organ function. In addition to bone marrow, hematopoietic stem cells may be obtained from the peripheral blood progenitor cells (PBPCs) and umbilical cord blood. The essential properties of the hematopoietic cells are their ability to engraft, the speed of engraftment, and the durability of engraftment.

Examples of diseases treated with HSCT are listed in Table 98–1. ❷ *Autologous HSCT, or infusion of a patient's own hematopoietic cells, allows for the administration of higher doses of chemotherapy, radiation, or both to treat the malignancy or autoimmune disorder.* In this setting, the hematopoietic cells "rescue" the recipient from otherwise dose-limiting hematopoietic toxicity. Autologous HSCT is used to treat intermediate- and high-grade non-Hodgkin's lymphoma (NHL), multiple myeloma (MM), autoimmune diseases, and relapsed or refractory Hodgkin's disease.[1] ❷ *Allogeneic HSCT involves the transplantation of hematopoietic cells obtained from a different person's (donor) bone marrow, peripheral blood, or umbilical cord blood to the recipient.* Unless the donor and the recipient are identical twins (referred to as a *syngeneic HSCT*), they are dissimilar genetically. Allogeneic HSCT is used to treat both nonmalignant conditions and hematologic malignancies such as acute and chronic leukemias.[1]

The infusion of hematopoietic cells follows the administration of a combination of chemotherapy and/or radiation, termed the *conditioning* or *preparative regimen.* ❹ *A myeloablative preparative regimen involves the administration of sublethal doses of chemotherapy to the recipient to eradicate residual malignant disease. The recipient will not regain his or her own hematopoiesis and will be at risk for substantial*

	Table 98–1	
Diseases Commonly Treated With HSCT		
	Autologous Graft	**Allogeneic Graft**
Cancers	Multiple myeloma	Acute myeloid leukemia
	Non-Hodgkin's lymphoma	Acute lymphoblastic leukemia
	Hodgkin's disease	Chronic myeloid leukemia
	Neuroblastoma	Myelodysplastic syndrome
	Germ cell tumors	Myeloproliferative disorders
		Non-Hodgkin's lymphoma
		Hodgkin's disease
		Chronic lymphocytic leukemia
		Multiple myeloma
Other diseases	Autoimmune diseases	Aplastic anemia
	Amyloidosis	Paroxysmal nocturnal hemoglobinuria
		Fanconi's anemia
		Thalassemia major
		Sickle cell anemia
		Severe combined immunodeficiency
		Inborn errors of metabolism

life-threatening nonhematologic toxicity. For those undergoing an autologous HSCT, their hematopoietic cells must be harvested and stored before the myeloablative preparative regimen is administered. After the administration of the myeloablative preparative regimen, these hematopoietic cells serve as a rescue intervention to reestablish bone marrow function and avoid long-lasting, life-threatening bone marrow aplasia. In the setting of an allogeneic HSCT, the preparative regimen is designed to suppress the recipient's immunity, eradicate residual malignancy, or create space in the marrow compartment. Improved survival outcomes have been observed with both autologous and allogeneic HSCT when the hematologic malignancy is in complete remission at the time of HSCT.[2] At most HSCT centers, age younger than 65 years and normal renal, hepatic, pulmonary, and cardiac function are considered eligibility requirements for myeloablative allogeneic HSCT. A myeloablative or nonmyeloablative preparative regimen may be used for allogeneic HSCT; only myeloablative preparative regimens are used for autologous HSCT. Allogeneic HSCT offers the potential for a graft-versus-tumor effect in which immune effector cells from the donor recognize and eliminate residual tumor in the recipient.[1]

The recognition of graft-versus-tumor effect, which likely is caused by cytotoxic T lymphocytes in the donor stem cells, led to investigations with nonmyeloablative transplants, in which less toxic preparative regimens are used in the hope of expanding the availability of HSCT to recipients whose medical condition or age prohibits use of myeloablative regimens.

EPIDEMIOLOGY AND ETIOLOGY

Each year, the number of allogeneic HSCTs is less than the number of autologous HSCTs. Worldwide, approximately 35,000 autologous HSCTs and 25,000 allogeneic HSCTs are performed per year, with approximately one-third of allogeneic HSCTs using reduced-intensity preparative regimens. In the late 1990s, the number of allogeneic HSCTs reached a plateau, most likely related to the introduction of imatinib (Gleevec) for treatment of newly diagnosed chronic-phase chronic myelogenous leukemia (CML). Furthermore, the limited availability of suitable donors may have contributed to the plateau effect. Recently, however, the number of allogeneic transplants for hematologic malignancies other than CML appears to be increasing.[2]

Autologous PBPC use has increased and essentially has replaced bone marrow as a graft source in many transplant centers. From years 2004 through 2008, approximately 98% of autologous HSCTs in adults and 91% in children used PBPCs as the source of hematopoietic cells.[2] Patients do not benefit from an immunologic graft-versus-tumor effect while undergoing an autologous transplant; instead, the administration of high-dose chemotherapy followed by an autologous stem cell transplant in chemotherapy-sensitive malignancies relies on the preparative regimen alone to eradicate the malignant disease. Autologous HSCT is used to treat a variety of malignancies; Hodgkin's lymphoma, NHL, and MM are the most common indications for this procedure.[2] Autologous HSCT circumvents the need for histocompatible donors, is associated with a lower mortality rate, and is not restricted to younger patients.[3] The use of allogeneic PBPCs is increasing; from years 2004 through 2008, 80% of allogeneic HSCTs performed worldwide used PBPCs as the source of hematopoietic cells rather than bone marrow in adult patients.[3]

PATHOPHYSIOLOGY

For an allogeneic HSCT, the recipient and the donor are dissimilar genetically unless they are identical twins (a transplant between twins is referred to as a *syngeneic HSCT*). The transplanted tissue is immunologically active, and thus there is potential for bidirectional graft rejection. In the first scenario, cytotoxic T cells and natural killer (NK) cells belonging to the host (recipient) recognize minor histocompatibility (MHC) antigens of the graft (donor hematopoietic stem cells) and lead to a rejection response. In the second scenario, immunologically active cells in the graft recognize host MHC antigens and elicit an immune response. The former is referred to as *host-versus-graft disease,* and the latter is referred to as GVHD. Host-versus-graft effects are more common in solid-organ transplantation. When host-versus-graft effects occur in allogeneic HSCT, they are referred to as *graft failure* or *rejection,* which results in ineffective hematopoiesis (i.e., adequate ANC and/or platelet counts were not obtained). ❼ *Engraftment is defined as the point at which a patient can maintain a sustained absolute neutrophil count (ANC) of greater than 500 cells/mm³ (0.5 × 10⁹/L) and a sustained platelet count of greater than or equal to 20,000/mm³ (20 × 10⁹/L) lasting greater than or equal to 3 consecutive days without transfusions.*[4] Therefore, an essential first step for patients eligible for HSCT is finding a human leukocyte antigen (HLA)–compatible graft with an acceptable risk of graft failure and GVHD.

Histocompatibility

Histocompatibility differences between the donor and the recipient necessitate immunosuppression after an allogeneic HSCT because considerable morbidity and mortality are associated with graft failure and GVHD. Rejection is least likely to occur with a syngeneic donor, meaning that the recipient and host are identical (monozygotic) twins. In patients without a syngeneic donor, initial HLA typing is conducted on family members because the likelihood of complete histocompatibility between unrelated individuals is remote. Siblings are the most likely individuals to be histocompatible within a family. The chance for complete histocompatibility occurring in an individual with only one sibling is 25%. Approximately 40% of patients with more than one sibling will have an HLA-identical match. Having a matched-sibling donor is no longer a requirement for allogeneic HSCT because improved immunosuppressive regimens and the National Marrow Donor Program have allowed an increase in the use of unrelated or related matched or mismatched HSCTs. The use of alternative sources of allogeneic hematopoietic cells, such as related donors mismatched at one or more HLA loci or phenotypically (i.e., serologically) matched unrelated donors, has been evaluated.[5] Establishment of the National Marrow Donor Program has helped to increase the pool of potential donors for allogeneic HSCT. Through this program, an HLA-matched unrelated volunteer donor might be identified. Recipients of an unrelated graft are more likely to experience graft failure and acute GVHD relative to recipients of a matched-sibling donor. Determination of histocompatibility between potential donors and the patient is completed before allogeneic HSCT. Initially, HLA typing is performed using blood samples and compatibility for class I MHC antigens (i.e., HLA-A, HLA-B, and HLA-C) is determined through serologic and DNA-based testing methods. In vitro reactivity between donor and recipient also can be assessed in mixed-lymphocyte culture, a test used to measure compatibility of the MHC class II antigens (i.e., HLA-DR, HLA-DP, and HLA-DQ). Currently, most clinical and research laboratories are also performing molecular DNA typing using polymerase chain reaction (PCR) methodology to determine the HLA allele sequence.[6]

The preparative regimen or GVHD prophylaxis may be altered based on the mismatch between the donor and the recipient. The risk of graft failure decreases with better matches such that those with a class I (i.e., HLA-A, -B, or -C) antigen mismatch have the highest risk of rejection; those with just one class I allele mismatch have a minimal risk. Graft failure does not appear to be associated with mismatch at a single class II antigen or allele.[6] GVHD and survival have been associated with disparity for classes I and II antigens and alleles.[7]

Stem Cell Sources

Autologous hematopoietic stem cells are obtained from bone marrow or peripheral blood. The technique for harvesting autologous hematopoietic cells depends on the anatomic source (i.e., bone marrow or peripheral blood). A surgical procedure is necessary for obtaining bone marrow. Multiple aspirations of marrow are obtained from the anterior and posterior iliac crests until a volume with a sufficient number of hematopoietic stem cells is collected (i.e., 600 to 1,200 mL of bone marrow). The bone marrow then is processed to remove fat or marrow emboli and usually is infused intravenously into the patient similar to a blood transfusion.

The shift to the use of PBPCs over bone marrow for autologous HSCT is primarily because of the more rapid engraftment and decreased health care resource use. Because the harvest occurs before administering the preparative regimen, autologous hematopoietic cells must be cryopreserved and stored for future use.

Transplantation with PBPCs essentially has replaced bone marrow transplantation (BMT) as autologous rescue after myeloablative preparative regimens. Autologous PBPCs are obtained by administering a mobilizing agent(s) followed by apheresis, which is an outpatient procedure similar to hemodialysis. Hematopoietic growth factors (HGFs) alone or in combination with myelosuppressive chemotherapy are used for mobilization of autologous PBPCs with similar results. The HGFs granulocyte-macrophage colony-stimulating factor (sargramostim, Leukine) and granulocyte colony-stimulating factor (filgrastim, Neupogen) are used as mobilizing agents. The use of pegylated granulocyte colony-stimulating factor (pegfilgrastim, Neulasta) for mobilization of PBPCs appears more convenient and is promising as a mobilization agent; however, further data are needed regarding graft composition, HSCT outcomes, and donor safety in allogeneic donations before widespread use of this agent can be recommended.

The combination of chemotherapy with an HGF enhances PBPC mobilization relative to HGF alone.[1] In addition to treating the underlying malignancy, this approach lowers the risk of tumor cell contamination and the number of apheresis collections required, but there is a greater risk of neutropenia and thrombocytopenia. The HGF is initiated after completion of chemotherapy and is continued until apheresis is complete. Many centers monitor the number of cells that express the CD34 antigen (i.e., CD34+ cells) to determine when to start apheresis. The CD34 antigen is expressed on almost all unipotent and multipotent colony-forming cells and on precursors of colony-forming cells but not on mature peripheral blood cells. Apheresis is continued daily until the target number of PBPCs per kilogram of the recipient's weight is obtained. For adult recipients, the number of CD34+ cells correlates with time to engraftment. Lower yield of CD34+ cells is associated with administration of stem cell toxic drugs (e.g., carmustine and melphalan) and intensive prior chemotherapy or radiotherapy.

If patients are unable to obtain an adequate yield of CD34+ cells per kilogram after mobilization attempts fail, then allogeneic transplant may be considered as an alternative. Plerixafor (Mobozil) is approved by the Food and Drug Administration (FDA) for use in combination with granulocyte colony-stimulating factor to mobilize PBPCs for collection and subsequent autologous transplantation

in patients with NHL and MM. Plerixafor is an inhibitor of the CXCR4 chemokine receptor that results in more circulating PBPCs in the peripheral blood because of the inability of CXCR4 to assist in anchoring hematopoietic stem cells to the bone marrow matrix. Because administration of plerixafor with granulocyte colony-stimulating factor results in increased yield of CD34+ cells per kilogram compared to granulocyte colony-stimulating factor alone, this combination may serve as an alternative mobilization strategy in patients deemed to be at risk for mobilization failure with conventional methods.

TREATMENT

Desired Outcome

The desired outcome with HSCT is to cure the patient of his or her underlying disease while minimizing the short- and long-term morbidity associated with HSCT.

Nonpharmacologic Therapy

▶ Harvesting, Preparing, and Transplanting Allogeneic Hematopoietic Cells

③ Bone marrow, PBPCs, and umbilical cord blood can serve as the source of hematopoietic cells. The optimal cell source differs based on the donor and recipient characteristics.

Bone Marrow Harvesting the bone marrow from an allogeneic donor is conducted via the same process as for an autologous HSCT. The harvest occurs on day 0 of the HSCT such that it is infused into the recipient immediately after processing. The bone marrow may need additional processing if the donor and recipient are ABO incompatible, which occurs in up to 30% of HSCTs. Red blood cells (RBCs) may need to be removed before infusion into the recipient to prevent immune-mediated hemolytic anemia and thrombotic microangiopathic syndromes.

Peripheral Blood Progenitor Cells The allogeneic donor first undergoes mobilization therapy with an HGF to increase the number of hematopoietic cells circulating in the peripheral blood. The most commonly used regimen to mobilize allogeneic donors is a 4- to 5-day course of filgrastim, 10 to 16 mcg/kg/day, administered subcutaneously followed by leukophereses on the fourth or fifth days when peripheral blood levels of CD34+ cells peak. An adequate number of hematopoietic cells usually are obtained with one to two apheresis collections, with the optimal number of CD34+ collected being a minimum of 5×10^6 cells/kg of recipient body weight. Higher numbers of CD34+ cells are associated with more rapid neutrophil and platelet engraftment; patients who receive less than 2×10^6/kg CD34+ cells experience a higher mortality rate and a decreased overall survival than patients who receive at least 2×10^6/kg CD34+ cells.[8] Hematopoietic stem cells obtained from the peripheral blood are processed like bone marrow–derived stem cells and may be infused immediately into the recipient or frozen for future use. Compared with bone marrow donation, allogeneic PBPC donation leads to quicker hematopoietic recovery. Neutrophil engraftment occurs 2 to 6 days earlier, and platelet engraftment occurs approximately 6 days earlier with PBPC grafts than bone marrow grafts.[9] The donor may experience musculoskeletal pain, headache, and mild increases in hepatic enzyme or lactate dehydrogenase levels related to filgrastim administration. Hypocalcemia may also occur owing to citrate accumulation, which decreases ionized calcium concentrations during apheresis.

Allogeneic PBPC grafts contain approximately 10 times more T and B cells than bone marrow grafts. Historically, there has been significant concern that the greater T- and B-cell content of PBPCs could increase the risk of acute and/or chronic GVHD. In patients with a hematologic malignancy who have an HLA-matched sibling donor, a PBPC graft is optimal relative to bone marrow graft because the PBPC graft is associated with quicker neutrophil and platelet engraftment and potentially improved disease-free survival rates.[10] Grafts from PBPCs are likely associated with a higher incidence of acute GVHD and an approximately 20% increase in the incidence of extensive-stage and overall chronic GVHD.[10] Similar trends for engraftment and GVHD have been found with unrelated donors.[11]

Umbilical Cord Blood Transplant with umbilical cord blood offers an alternative stem cell source to patients who do not have an acceptable matched related or unrelated donor. When allogeneic hematopoietic cells are obtained from umbilical cord blood, the cord blood is obtained from a consenting donor in the delivery room after birth and delivery of the placenta. The cord blood is processed, a sample is sent for HLA typing, and the cord blood is frozen and stored for future use. Numerous umbilical cord blood registries exist, with the goal of providing alternative sources of allogeneic stem cells. One potential limitation to the use of umbilical cord blood transplants is the inability to use donor-lymphocyte infusions in the event of relapse. Engraftment is slower in umbilical cord blood transplants, with a potential lower risk of GVHD and similar survival rates relative to BMT.[1,12] In children receiving an umbilical cord blood graft from an unrelated donor, cell dose (e.g., nucleated cells) is related to engraftment, transplant-related morbidity, and survival.[13] Although there were initial concerns regarding whether a umbilical cord blood transplant could provide enough nucleated cells to engraft adequately within an adult, there is growing experience to indicate that a umbilical cord blood transplant is feasible when at least 1×10^7 nucleated cells per kilogram of recipient body weight are administered.[13] The prospective use of dual umbilical cord units and ex vivo expansion of umbilical cord units to obtain adequate engraftment are methods currently under exploration.

T-Cell Depletion Immunocompetent T lymphocytes may be depleted from the donor bone marrow ex vivo before infusion (referred to as *T-cell–depleted hematopoietic cells*) into the recipient as a means of preventing GVHD. Depletion of T lymphocytes in donor hematopoietic cells is completed ex vivo using physical (e.g., density-gradient fractionation) and/or immunologic (e.g., antithymocyte globulin [ATG]

antibodies) methods. Functional recovery of T cells in the recipient is delayed, and the risk of Epstein-Barr virus–associated lymphoproliferative disorders is higher with the use of T-cell–depleted bone marrow. The use of T-cell–depleted grafts reduces the incidence of GVHD, but graft failure and relapse are more common. The use of donor lymphocyte infusion in patients who relapse after receiving a T-cell–depleted HSCT is being investigated.

Engraftment After chemotherapy and radiation, pancytopenia lasts until the infused stem cells reestablish functional hematopoiesis. The median time to engraftment is a function of several factors, including the source of stem cells such as PBPCs, which can result in earlier engraftment than bone marrow.[9] Myeloablative preparative regimens have significant regimen-related toxicity and morbidity and thus usually are limited to healthy, younger (i.e., usually younger than 50 years) patients. Alternatively, nonmyeloablative transplants are being performed with the hope of curing more patients with cancer by increasing the availability of HSCT with less regimen-related toxicity and by using the graft-versus-tumor effect.[1]

A delicate balance exists between host and donor effector cells in the bone marrow environment. Residual host-versus-graft effects may lead to graft failure, which is also known as graft rejection. *Graft failure* is defined as the lack of functional hematopoiesis after HSCT and can occur early (i.e., lack of initial hematopoietic recovery) or late (i.e., in association with recurrence of the disease or reappearance of host cells after initial donor cell engraftment). Engraftment usually is evident within the first 30 days in patients undergoing an HSCT; however, rejection can occur after initial engraftment. Therapeutic options for the treatment of graft rejection are limited; a second HSCT is the most definitive therapy, although the toxicities are formidable.[14]

▶ *Graft-Versus-Tumor Effect*

A graft-versus-tumor effect occurs owing to the donor lymphocytes, as supported by three observations after myeloablative allogeneic HSCT; namely, (a) lower relapse rates in patients with GVHD relative to those who did not have GVHD; (b) a higher rate of leukemia relapse after T-cell–depleted, autologous, or syngeneic HSCT; and (c) the effectiveness of donor lymphocyte infusions in reinducing a remission in patients who relapsed after allogeneic HSCT. Rapid taper of immunosuppression in patients with residual disease may induce a graft-versus tumor effect. In donor lymphocyte infusion, lymphocytes are collected from the peripheral blood of the donor and administered to the recipient. Eradication of the recurrent malignancy is caused by either specific targeting of the tumor antigens or GVHD, which may affect cancer cells preferentially. Patients with hematologic malignancies (e.g., CML and acute myelogenous leukemia [AML]) and certain solid tumors (e.g., renal cell carcinoma) appear to benefit from a graft-versus-tumor effect. These data gave rise to the use of nonmyeloablative preparative regimens.

Patient Encounter, Part 1

ZN is a 52-year-old woman diagnosed with acute myeloid leukemia with complex cytogenetics. The patient achieved complete remission with induction therapy and is now being evaluated for an allogeneic stem cell transplant with a peripheral blood stem cell graft from a full HLA-matched sibling. She has no other siblings. Her preparative regimen consists of busulfan and cyclophosphamide (BU-CY) and her GVHD prophylaxis consists of tacrolimus and methotrexate.

What nonhematologic toxicities are associated with the preparative regimen?

What are the advantages and disadvantages of obtaining and infusing hematopoietic stem cells from a peripheral blood stem cell source as opposed to a bone marrow source?

What are the implications for ZN if the sibling was not an HLA match?

Pharmacologic Therapy

▶ *Preparative Regimens for HSCT*

Examples of commonly used preparative regimens are included in Table 98–2. ❻ *The nonhematologic toxicity differs based on the preparative regimen administered.*

● **Myeloablative Preparative Regimens** In both autologous and allogeneic HSCT, infusion of stem cells circumvents dose-limiting myelosuppression, maximizing the potential value of the steep dose–response curve to alkylating agents

and radiation, suppressing the host immune system, and creating space in the marrow compartment to facilitate engraftment. The preparative regimen is designed to eradicate immunologically active host tissues (lymphoid tissue and macrophages) and to prevent or minimize the development of host-versus-graft reactions. Most allogeneic preparative regimens for the treatment of hematologic malignancies contain cyclophosphamide, radiation, or both. The combination of cyclophosphamide and total-body irradiation (TBI) was one of the first preparative regimens developed and is still used widely today. This regimen is immunosuppressive and has inherent activity against hematologic malignancies (e.g., leukemias and lymphomas). TBI has the added advantage of being devoid of active metabolites that might interfere with the activity of donor hematopoietic cells. In addition, TBI eradicates residual malignant cells at sanctuary sites such as the central nervous system. Modifications of the cyclophosphamide–TBI preparative regimen include replacing TBI with other agents (e.g., busulfan) or adding other chemotherapeutic or monoclonal agents to the existing regimen in hopes of minimizing long-term toxicities. In the case of a mismatched allogeneic HSCT with a substantially increased chance of graft rejection, ATG also may be added to the preparative regimen to further immunosuppress the recipient.

The optimal myeloablative preparative regimen remains elusive. The long-term outcomes of busulfan–cyclophosphamide (BU-CY) and cyclophosphamide–TBI (CY-TBI) in patients with AML and CML, the more common indications for allogeneic HSCT, have been compared in a meta-analysis of four clinical trials.[18] Equivalent rates of long-term complications were present between the two preparative regimens except that there was a greater risk of cataracts with CY-TBI and alopecia with BU-CY. Overall and disease-free survivals were similar in patients with CML, but there was a

Table 98–2

Commonly Used Preparative Regimens for HSCT[a]

Type of HSCT	Preparative Regimen	Dose and Schedule for Adults	Dose and Schedule for Pediatric Patients
Allogeneic[15]	Myeloablative CY-TBI	CY 60 mg/kg/day IV on 2 consecutive days before TBI 1,000–1,575 rads (10–15.75 Gy) fractionated over 1–7 days	CY 60 mg/kg/day IV on 2 consecutive days before TBI 1,000–1,575 rads (10–15.75 Gy) fractionated over 1–7 days
Allogeneic, autologous[16]	Myeloablative BU-CY	BU 1 mg/kg per dose PO or 0.8 mg/kg per dose IV every 6 hours × 16 doses; CY 60 mg/kg/day IV daily × 2 days after BU	BU 1 mg/kg per dose PO or 0.8 mg/kg per dose IV every 6 hours × 16 doses; CY 120–200 mg/kg IV given over 2–4 days after BU
Autologous[17]	Myeloablative BEAM (carmustine/etoposide/-cytarabine/melphalan)	Carmustine 300 mg/m² IV Etoposide 400–800 mg/m² IV given over 4 days Cytarabine 400–1,600 mg/m² IV given over 4 days Melphalan 140 mg/m² IV	Carmustine 300 mg/m² IV Etoposide 400–800 mg/m² IV given over 4 days Cytarabine 400–1,600 mg/m² IV given over 4 days Melphalan 140 mg/m² IV
Allogeneic[3]	Nonmyeloablative BU-FLU	Fludarabine 30 mg/m²/day IV on day –10 to day –5 followed by busulfan 1 mg/kg/dose PO every 6 hours × 8 doses on days –6 and –5	Fludarabine 30 mg/m²/day IV on day –10 to day –5 followed by busulfan 1 mg/kg/dose PO every 6 hours × 8 doses on days –6 and –5

BEAM, carmustine, etoposide, cytarabine, and melphalan; BU-CY, busulfan and cyclophosphamide; BU-FLU, busulfan and fludarabine; CY-TBI, cyclophosphamide–total-body irradiation; IV, intravenous; PO, oral; TBI, total-body irradiation.

trend for improved disease-free survival with CY-TBI in AML patients. Thus, the preparative regimen can be tailored to the primary disease and to the degree of HLA compatibility.

Nonmyeloablative Preparative Regimens ⑤ *A nonmyeloablative preparative regimen is less toxic than a myeloablative regimen in the hope of being able to offer the benefits of an allogeneic HSCT to more patients. A nonmyeloablative HSCT is based on the concept of donor immune response having a graft-versus-tumor effect.*

Because of the severe regimen-related toxicity of a myeloablative preparative regimen, the use of HSCT traditionally was limited to younger patients with minimal comorbidities. Most patients diagnosed with cancer are elderly; therefore, myeloablative HSCT could not be offered to a substantial portion of cancer patients. The concept of donor immune response having a graft-versus-tumor effect gave rise to the theory that a strongly immunosuppressive, but not myeloablative, preparative regimen (i.e., a nonmyeloablative transplant may result in a state of chimerism in which the recipient and donor are coexisting). The toxicity and efficacy of nonmyeloablative transplants are being evaluated in patients with malignant and nonmalignant conditions who are not eligible for a myeloablative HSCT.

A nonmyeloablative preparative regimen allows for development of mixed chimerism (defined as 5% to 95% peripheral donor T cells) between the host and recipient to allow for a graft-versus-tumor effect as the primary form of therapy (Fig. 98–1). Chimerism is assessed within peripheral blood T cells and granulocytes and bone marrow using conventional (e.g., using sex chromosomes for opposite-sex

donors) and molecular (e.g., variable number of tandem repeats) methods for same-sex donors.

The nonmyeloablative preparative regimen does not completely eliminate host normal and malignant cells. Donor cells eradicate residual host hematopoiesis, and the graft-versus-tumor effects generally occur after the development of full donor T-cell chimerism. After engraftment, mixed chimerism should be present and is shown by the presence of both donor- and recipient-derived cells. Autologous recovery should occur promptly if the graft is rejected. The intensity of immunosuppression required for engraftment depends on the immunocompetence of the recipient and the histocompatibility and composition of the HSCT.[19] More intensive conditioning regimens that are required for engraftment in the setting of unrelated-donor- or HLA-mismatched-related HSCT have been termed *reduced-intensity myeloablative transplants*. After chimerism develops, donor-lymphocyte infusion can be administered safely in patients without GVHD to eradicate malignant cells.

Nonmyeloablative preparative regimens typically consist of a purine analog (e.g., fludarabine) in combination with an alkylating agent or low-dose TBI. Adverse effects in the early posttransplant period are decreased because of the lower intensity preparative regimen, thus making HSCT available to patients who in the past were not healthy or young enough to receive a myeloablative preparative regimen. The risk of GVHD remains with nonmyeloablative transplant; the GVHD prophylaxis regimens are reviewed in the GVHD section below. Presently, nonmyeloablative transplant is not indicated as first-line therapy for any malignant or nonmalignant conditions, although research is ongoing.

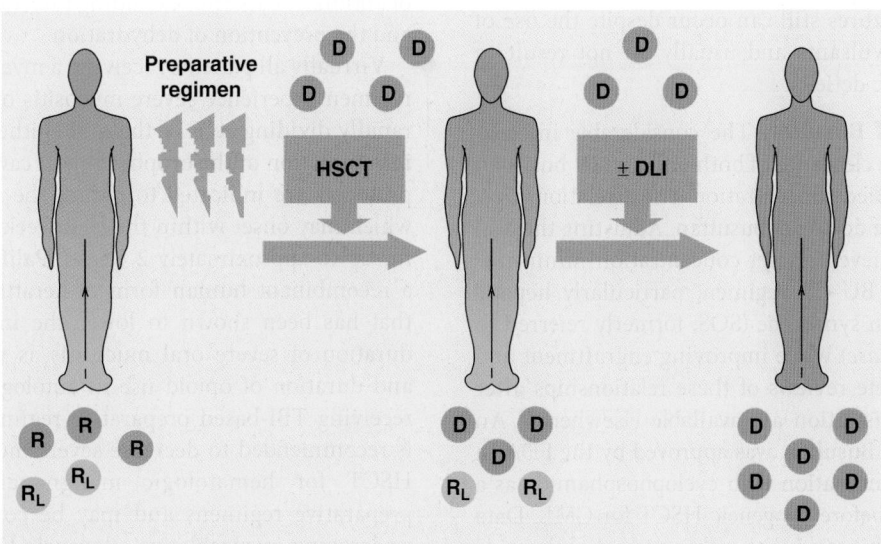

FIGURE 98–1. Schema for nonmyeloablative transplantation. Recipients (R) receive a nonmyeloablative preparative regimen and an allogeneic hematopoietic stem cell transplantation (HSCT). Initially, mixed chimerism is present with the coexistence of donor (D) cells and recipient-derived normal and leukemia or lymphoma (R$_L$) cells. Donor-derived T cells mediate a graft-versus-host hematopoietic effect that eradicates residual recipient-derived normal and malignant hematopoietic cells. Donor-lymphocyte infusions (DLIs) may be administered to enhance graft-versus-tumor effects. (From Champlin R, Khouri I, Anderlini P, et al. Nonmyeloablative preparative regimens for allogeneic hematopoietic transplantation. Biology and current indications. Oncology (Williston Park) 2003;17:94–100; discussion 103–107.)

Nonmyeloablative transplantation is being evaluated for cancers sensitive to a graft-versus-tumor effect (e.g., CML and AML), in older patients, or for those with comorbidities who would not be able to tolerate a myeloablative HSCT.

Toxicities and Management of Preparative Regimens

Myelosuppression is a frequent dose-limiting toxicity for antineoplastics when administered in the conventional doses used to treat cancer. However, because myelosuppression is circumvented with hematopoietic rescue in the case of patients receiving HSCT, the dose-limiting toxicities of these myeloablative preparative regimens are nonhematologic and vary with the preparative regimen used. Most patients undergoing HSCT experience toxicities commonly associated with chemotherapy (e.g., alopecia, mucositis, nausea and vomiting, and infertility), albeit these toxicities are magnified in the HSCT population.

Busulfan Seizures Seizures have been reported in both adult and pediatric patients receiving high-dose busulfan for HSCT preparative regimens. Anticonvulsants are used to minimize the risk of seizures. Anticonvulsants are begun shortly before busulfan, with the loading dose completed at least 6 hours before the first busulfan dose. Oral loading and maintenance regimens generally are sufficient because target phenytoin concentrations of 10 to 20 mcg/mL (10 to 20 mg/L; 40 to 79 μmol/L) can be achieved by the peak time of seizure risk. If patients are experiencing significant vomiting or have difficulty maintaining therapeutic phenytoin concentrations, intravenous (IV) phenytoin should be substituted. Benzodiazepines such as lorazepam or clonazepam also have been used for seizure prophylaxis during high-dose busulfan therapy before HSCT. Antiseizure medications usually are discontinued 24 to 48 hours after administration of the last dose of busulfan. Seizures still can occur despite the use of prophylactic anticonvulsants and usually do not result in permanent neurologic deficits.

Adaptive Dosing of Busulfan The considerable interpatient variability in the clearance of both oral and IV busulfan along with the identified concentration–effect relationships, has led to the adaptive dosing of busulfan. Adjusting the oral busulfan dose to achieve a target concentration minimizes the toxicities of the BU-CY regimen, particularly hepatic sinusoidal obstruction syndrome (SOS; formerly referred to as *veno-occlusive disease*) while improving engraftment and relapse rates. Complete reviews of these relationships after oral busulfan administration are available elsewhere.[20] An IV busulfan product, Busulfex, was approved by the FDA in February 1999 in combination with cyclophosphamide as a preparative regimen before allogeneic HSCT for CML. Data with Busulfex in combination with either cyclophosphamide or fludarabine suggest that therapeutic drug monitoring may be needed.[21]

Hemorrhagic Cystitis High-dose cyclophosphamide causes moderate to severe hemorrhagic cystitis; acrolein, a metabolite of cyclophosphamide, is the putative bladder toxin. Preventive measures to lower the risk of hemorrhagic cystitis include vigorous hydration, continuous bladder irrigation,

or concomitant use of the uroprotectant mesna. The American Society of Clinical Oncology (ASCO) Guidelines for the Use of Chemotherapy and Radiotherapy Protectants recommends the use of Mesna (2-mercaptoethane sulfonate) plus saline diuresis or forced saline diuresis to lower the incidence of urothelial toxicity with high-dose cyclophosphamide in the setting of HSCT.[22]

Chemotherapy-Induced Gastrointestinal Effects Preparative regimens for myeloablative HSCT result in other end-organ toxicities, such as renal failure and idiopathic pneumonia syndrome. In addition, recipients of myeloablative preparative regimens are at risk for severe gastrointestinal (GI) toxicity, specifically chemotherapy-induced nausea and vomiting (CINV), diarrhea, and mucositis. CINV can be caused by administration of highly emetogenic chemotherapy over several days, TBI, and poor control of CINV before HSCT. Thus, patients who are undergoing a myeloablative HSCT should receive a prophylactic corticosteroid with a serotonin antagonist, with higher doses of serotonin antagonists potentially being needed in this patient population. In addition, these patients are at high risk for delayed CINV in the immediate posttransplant period, and these issues should be addressed accordingly as per published clinical practice guidelines.[23]

Diarrhea is also an adverse effect experienced by a majority of patients undergoing HSCT. Chemotherapy-induced diarrhea occurs because of the effects of the preparative regimen, which results in inflammation and damage to the cells lining the GI tract. Diarrhea caused by the preparative regimen is usually apparent within the first week after the initiation of chemotherapy and/or radiation. Treatment strategies for chemotherapy-induced diarrhea include the administration of antidiarrheals after excluding infectious causes of diarrhea and the prevention of dehydration.

Virtually all patients receiving a myeloablative preparative regimen experience severe mucositis owing to its effects on rapidly dividing cells of the oral epithelium and subsequent inflammation of the oropharyngeal cavity. Routine oral care protocols are indicated to reduce the severity of mucositis, which may onset within the first week of HSCT and persist for up to approximately 2 weeks. Palifermin (Kepivance) is a recombinant human form of keratinocyte growth factor that has been shown to lower the incidence and average duration of severe oral mucositis as well as the incidence and duration of opioid use in autologous HSCT recipients receiving TBI-based preparative regimens.[24] Palifermin use is recommended to decrease severe mucositis in autologous HSCT for hematologic malignancies with TBI-based preparative regimens and may be considered for patients undergoing myeloablative allogeneic HSCT with TBI-based preparative regimens, although data are limited in the allogeneic setting.[22] Patients still may require parenteral opioid analgesics for pain relief owing to mucositis, and total parenteral nutrition may be necessary to prevent the development of nutritional deficiencies.

Sinusoidal Obstruction Syndrome Hepatic SOS is a life-threatening complication that may occur secondary to preparative regimens or radiation. The pathogenesis of SOS is not understood completely, but several mechanisms have been proposed. The key event appears to be endothelial damage caused by the preparative regimen. The primary site of the toxic injury is the sinusoidal endothelial cells; the endothelial damage initiates the coagulation cascade, induces thrombosis of the hepatic venules, and eventually leads to fibrous obliteration of the affected venules.[25]

The clinical manifestations of SOS are hyperbilirubinemia, jaundice, fluid retention, weight gain, and right upper quadrant abdominal pain. To make a clinical diagnosis of SOS, these features must occur in the absence of other causes of posttransplant liver failure, including GVHD, viral hepatitis, fungal abscesses, or drug reactions. Most cases of SOS occur within 3 weeks of HSCT, and the clinical diagnosis can be confirmed histologically via liver biopsy.

Patients with mild SOS have an excellent prognosis, but those with more severe disease (i.e., bilirubin greater than 20 mg/dL [342 μmol/L] or weight gain greater than 15%) have a high mortality rate. Pretransplant risk factors for SOS include a mismatched or unrelated graft, increased age, prior abdominal radiation or stem cell transplant, and increased transaminases before HSCT.[25] Interpatient variability in the metabolism and clearance of the chemotherapy (i.e., busulfan and cyclophosphamide) used within the preparative regimen also may be associated with a poor outcome, although the relationships vary within the various preparative regimens.[20] The association of SOS with busulfan concentrations is discussed in the section on adaptive dosing of busulfan. Preliminary data suggest that IV busulfan may be associated with a lower risk of SOS, although more data are needed.[26] Use of ursodiol, unfractionated heparin, or low-molecular-weight heparin has been associated with a lower incidence of SOS in a limited number of small, randomized studies and may be recommended for SOS prophylaxis.[25]

The mainstay of treatment for established SOS is supportive care aimed at sodium restriction, increasing intravascular volume, decreasing extracellular fluid accumulation, and minimizing factors that contribute to or exacerbate hepatotoxicity and encephalopathy. Recombinant tissue plasminogen activator administered with or without heparin has been investigated for treatment of SOS, but the life-threatening risk of bleeding precludes any potential benefit.[25] Defibrotide, an oligonucleotide with antithrombotic, anti-ischemic, and anti-inflammatory activity, has shown promising results in the treatment of SOS in clinical trials.[25]

Myelosuppression and Hematopoietic Growth Factor Use Hematopoietic growth factors (HGFs) may be administered to mobilize PBPCs before an HSCT, to hasten hematopoietic recovery during the period of aplasia after an autologous HSCT, and to stimulate hematopoietic recovery when the patient fails to engraft.[27]

Autologous HSCT is associated with profound aplasia owing to the myeloablative preparative regimen. Aplasia typically lasts 7 to 14 days after an autologous PBPC transplant. During this period of aplasia, patients are at high risk for complications such as bleeding and infection. Filgrastim and sargramostim exert their effects by stimulating the proliferation of committed progenitor cells and accelerating recovery on hematopoiesis. Once engraftment occurs, HGFs may be discontinued. The anatomic source of hematopoietic cells predicts the degree of benefit, with the greatest benefit reached when bone marrow is the graft source. With autologous PBPC transplant, the effect of HGF on neutrophil recovery is variable.

The use of HGF after allogeneic HSCT—whether from bone marrow or PBPC grafts—is controversial. The amount of data with sargramostim is limited in this setting; data with filgrastim have shown more rapid neutrophil but slower platelet engraftment in those receiving grafts from bone marrow or PBPCs.[28] The effects of post-HSCT filgrastim use on acute and chronic GVHD have been conflicting, with either no effect or increases in both the incidence of acute

Clinical Presentation and Diagnosis of Sinusoidal Obstructive Syndrome

General

- Sinusoidal obstructive syndrome (SOS) usually occurs within the first 3 weeks after HSCT
- Busulfan, cyclophosphamide, pretransplant exposure to gemtuzumab, TBI-containing preparative regimens, and pretransplant abnormalities in liver function tests may increase the risk for SOS

Symptoms

- Patients may complain of weight gain and abdominal pain

Signs

- Fluid retention: Weight gain caused by ascites greater than 2% compared with pretransplant weight

- Hepatomegaly: May result in right upper quadrant pain
- Hepatic: Jaundice caused by hyperbilirubinemia defined as a bilirubin greater than 2 mg/dL (34.2 μmol/L)

Laboratory Tests

- Hepatic: Elevation of bilirubin, alkaline phosphatase, and γ-glutamyltransferase (GGT)
- Hematologic: Complete blood count with differential may reveal thrombocytopenia, elevated plasminogen activator-1 levels, decreased antithrombin III, protein C, and protein S

Other Diagnostic Tests

- Reversal of blood flow in portal and hepatic veins on Doppler ultrasonography
- Liver biopsy for pathologic review

and chronic GVHD and treatment-related mortality.[28] Thus, there is little reason to treat allogeneic BMT with filgrastim as prophylaxis after HSCT.

Graft Failure A delicate balance between host and donor effector cells in the bone marrow is necessary to ensure adequate engraftment because residual host-versus-graft effects may lead to graft rejection. The incidence of graft rejection is higher in patients with aplastic anemia and those undergoing HSCT with histoincompatible marrow or T-cell–depleted marrow.[1] Graft rejection is uncommon in leukemia patients receiving myeloablative preparative regimens with a histocompatible allogeneic donor.

Therapeutic options for the treatment of graft rejection or graft failure are limited. A second HSCT is the most definitive therapy, although the associated complications and toxicities may preclude its use. Graft rejection is best managed with immunosuppressants such as ATG. Primary graft failure occasionally can be treated successfully using HGFs, although patients who received purged autografts are less likely to respond.

Patient Encounter, Part 2

PMH: Coronary artery disease, hypertension, type 2 diabetes, hyperlipidemia, hypothyroidism, sleep apnea, and gout

FH: Father died at age of 56 years of myocardial infarction. Mother has history of hypertension. One younger sister with a history of hypertension.

SH: She is a high school teacher and is married with no children. She drinks alcohol occasionally and does not smoke or use illicit drugs.

Allergies: NKDA

Medications:

- Metformin 500 mg by mouth twice daily
- Lisinopril 20 mg by mouth once daily
- Carvedilol 12.5 mg by mouth twice daily
- Clopidogrel 75 mg by mouth once daily
- Aspirin 81 mg by mouth once daily
- Atorvastatin 40 mg by mouth once nightly at bedtime
- Levothyroxine 75 μg by mouth once daily
- Allopurinol 300 mg by mouth once daily

ROS: (+) fatigue

PE:

VS: 134/82, P 69, RR 18, T 37.6°C

Physical exam reveals no acute findings.

Laboratory analysis is within normal limits except for serum creatinine of 1.3 g/dL (115 μmol/L) and hemoglobin of 10.2 g/dL (102 g/L; 6.33 μmol/L).

Given this additional information, what is your assessment of the planned preparative regimen?

▶ Graft-Versus-Host Disease

❽ *GVHD is caused by the activation of donor lymphocytes, leading to immune damage to the skin, gut, and liver in the recipient.* Immune-mediated destruction of tissues, a hallmark of GVHD, disrupts the integrity of protective mucosal barriers and thus provides an environment that favors the establishment of opportunistic infections. ❽ *An immunosuppressive regimen is administered to prevent GVHD in recipients of an allogeneic graft; this regimen is based on the type of preparative regimen and the source of the graft.* The combination of GVHD and infectious complications are leading causes of mortality for allogeneic HSCT patients. GVHD is divided into two forms (i.e., acute and chronic) based on clinical manifestations. Traditionally, the boundary between acute and chronic GVHD was set at 100 days after HSCT; however, more recent definitions hinge upon different clinical symptoms rather than the time of onset.[29]

Acute GVHD The degree of histocompatibility between donor and recipient is the most important factor associated with the development of acute GVHD. The pathophysiology for acute GVHD is a multistep phenomenon, including (a) the development of an inflammatory milieu that results from host tissue damage induced by the preparative regimen; (b) both recipient and donor antigen-presenting cells and inflammatory cytokines triggering activation of donor-derived T cells; and (c) the activated donor T cells mediate cytotoxicity through a variety of mechanisms, which leads to tissue damage characteristic of acute GVHD.[30]

Clinically relevant grades II to IV acute GVHD occurs in up to 30% of HLA-matched sibling grafts and 50% to 80% of HLA-mismatched sibling or HLA-identical unrelated donors.[30] Other factors that increase the risk of acute GVHD include increasing recipient or donor age (older than 20 years), female donor to a male recipient, and mismatches in minor histocompatibility antigens in HLA-matched transplants.[30] T-cell depletion or receipt of an umbilical cord blood graft appears to lower the risk of acute GVHD.[1]

Clinical Presentation and Staging of Acute GVHD Acute GVHD must be distinguished accurately from other causes of skin, liver, or GI toxicity in HSCT patients. Other causes of toxicities affecting the skin, liver, or GI tract may include a drug reaction or an infectious process. A staging system based on clinical criteria is used to grade acute GVHD (**Fig. 98–2**). The severity of organ involvement is scored on an ordinal scale from 0 (no symptoms) to IV (severe symptoms), and then an overall grade is established based on the number and extent of involved organs.

Immunosuppressive Prophylaxis of Acute GVHD GVHD is a leading cause of morbidity and mortality after allogeneic HSCT and thus, efforts have focused on preventing acute GVHD. The donor graft and preparative regimen influence the prophylactic regimen for acute GVHD, with two approaches having been taken by clinicians over time. One approach involves T-cell depletion, which was discussed more fully in the section on T-cell depletion earlier.

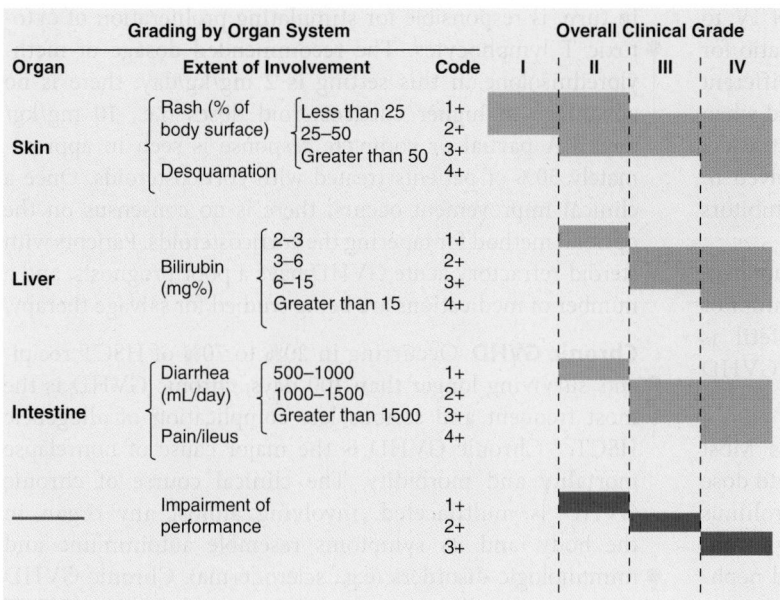

FIGURE 98–2. Clinical grading of acute graft-versus-host disease. The left *panel* summarizes the grading of one organ system; the *right panel* shows the overall clinical grade. With grade I, only the skin can be involved. With more extensive involvement of the skin or involvement of liver and intestinal tract and impairment of the clinical performance status, either alone or in any combination, the severity grade advances from II to IV. (From Perkins JB, Yee GC. Hematopoietic stem cell transplantation. In: DiPiro JT, Talbert RL, Yee GC, et al, eds. Pharmacotherapy: A Pathophysiologic Approach, 6th ed. New York: McGraw-Hill; 2005:2552.)

Clinical Presentation and Diagnosis of Acute Graft-Versus-Host Disease

General

- Patients may present with any or all of the following: skin rash, GI complaints, or jaundice
- Signs and symptoms present after engraftment when donor lymphoid elements begin to proliferate

Symptoms

- Patients may complain of nausea, vomiting, bloody diarrhea, or itching from skin rash

Signs

- Skin: Maculopapular skin rash on the face, truck, extremities, palms, soles, and ears, which may progress to generalized total-body erythroderma, bullous formation, and skin desquamation

- GI: Ileus, malnutrition, dehydration, and electrolyte abnormalities caused by nausea, vomiting, and diarrhea
- Hepatic: Jaundice caused by hyperbilirubinemia

Laboratory Tests

- Hepatic: Elevation of bilirubin, alkaline phosphatase, and hepatic transaminases
- GI: send stool for bacterial, viral, and parasitic cultures to rule out infectious causes

Other Diagnostic Tests

- Biopsy of affected site for pathologic review

The more common method is to use two-drug immunosuppressive therapy that typically consists of a calcineurin inhibitor (i.e., cyclosporine or tacrolimus) with methotrexate after myeloablative HSCT and a calcineurin inhibitor with mycophenolate mofetil after nonmyeloablative HSCT.

After myeloablative conditioning, acute GVHD rates have been similar or lower with triple-drug regimens, but infectious complications are higher and overall survival is similar to that with two-drug regimens.[31] With the two-drug regimen, a short-course of low-dose methotrexate (e.g., on days +1, +3, +6, and day +11) is used and thus, can delay engraftment, increase the incidence and severity of mucositis, and cause liver function test (LFT) elevations. The methotrexate dose is reduced in the setting of renal or liver impairment. The calcineurin inhibitors (i.e., cyclosporine and tacrolimus) should be initiated before

donor cell infusion (e.g., day –1) when used for GVHD prophylaxis. This schedule is recommended because of the known mechanism of action of cyclosporine, which entails blocking the proliferation of cytotoxic T cells by inhibiting production of T helper cell–derived interleukin-2 (IL-2). Administering cyclosporine before the donor cell infusion allows inhibition of IL-2 secretion to occur before a rejection response has been initiated. Studies comparing cyclosporine and tacrolimus in combination with methotrexate have shown that tacrolimus administration is associated with a lower incidence of grade II to IV acute GVHD and a similar incidence of chronic GVHD but variable effects on overall survival.[32,33] Because of the mucosal toxicity from myeloablative preparative regimens, the calcineurin inhibitors are administered IV until the GI toxicity from a myeloablative preparative regimen has resolved (e.g., for 7 to 21 days).

Most centers use a 1:2 to 1:3 ratio for conversion of IV to oral cyclosporine with the Neoral formulation; the ratio for tacrolimus conversion from IV to oral is often 1:4. Different conversion ratios for IV to oral regimens may be used when patients are receiving concomitant medications that affect CYP 3A or p-glycoprotein; these pathways are involved in the metabolism and transport of the calcineurin inhibitors (e.g., voriconazole).

Prophylaxis of acute GVHD for nonmyeloablative preparative regimens is varied, but a calcineurin inhibitor with either methotrexate or mycophenolate mofetil is used.[3] To date, trials evaluating the optimal acute GVHD prophylaxis regimen have not been conducted.

Adaptive Dosing of the Calcineurin Inhibitors Most HSCT centers have their own standardized approach to dose adjust the calcineurin inhibitors cyclosporine and tacrolimus to target concentration ranges. Cyclosporine trough concentrations are associated with the acute GVHD and nephrotoxicity. Cyclosporine trough concentrations usually are maintained between 150 and 400 ng/mL (125 to 333 nmol/L) in patients undergoing allogeneic HSCT. Tacrolimus trough concentrations are targeted to a range of 10 to 20 ng/mL (10 to 20 mcg/L; 12.4 to 24.8 nmol/L).[34] Dosage adjustments to either calcineurin inhibitor also should be made for elevated serum creatinine (SCr) regardless of their serum concentrations. Nephrotoxicity can occur despite low or normal concentrations of the calcineurin inhibitor cyclosporine and may be a consequence of other drug- or disease-related factors known to influence the development of nephrotoxicity (e.g., genetic risk factors, concurrent use of other nephrotoxic agents, and sepsis). Careful monitoring for drug interactions via CYP 3A4 and p-glycoprotein is also warranted. The calcineurin inhibitor doses are adjusted based on serum drug levels and the calculated creatinine clearance. Common adverse effects to these agents include neurotoxicity, hypertension, hyperkalemia, hypomagnesemia, and/or nephrotoxicity (which may lead to an impaired clearance of methotrexate).

Tapering schedules for the calcineurin inhibitors after myeloablative HSCT vary widely. In patients without GVHD, the calcineurin inhibitor doses usually are stable to day +50 and then are tapered slowly with the intent of discontinuing all immunosuppressive agents by 6 months after HSCT. By this time, immunologic tolerance has developed, and patients no longer require immunosuppressive therapy. There is a paucity of information regarding the optimal duration of GVHD prophylaxis after nonmyeloablative HSCT, with data suggesting that a 2-month duration of cyclosporine with a 4-month taper lowers the rate of severe acute GVHD.[35]

Treatment of Acute GVHD The most effective way to treat GVHD is to prevent its development. Corticosteroids, usually in combination with a calcineurin inhibitor, are the first-line therapy for treatment of established acute GVHD. Corticosteroids indirectly halt the progression of immune-mediated destruction of host tissues by blocking macrophage-derived IL-1 secretion. IL-1 is a primary stimulus for T helper cell–induced secretion of IL-2, which,

in turn, is responsible for stimulating proliferation of cytotoxic T lymphocytes. The recommended dosage of methylprednisolone in this setting is 2 mg/kg/day; there is no advantage to higher corticosteroid doses (i.e., 10 mg/kg/day).[30] A partial or complete response is seen in approximately 50% of patients treated with corticosteroids. Once a clinical improvement occurs, there is no consensus on the optimal method for tapering the corticosteroids. Patients with steroid-refractory acute GVHD have a poor prognosis, and a number of medications are being studied for salvage therapy.

Chronic GVHD Occurring in 20% to 70% of HSCT recipients surviving longer than 100 days, chronic GVHD is the most frequent and serious late complication of allogeneic HSCT.[36] Chronic GVHD is the major cause of nonrelapse mortality and morbidity. The clinical course of chronic GVHD is multifaceted, involving almost any organ in the body, and its symptoms resemble autoimmune and immunologic disorders (e.g., scleroderma). Chronic GVHD symptoms usually present within 3 years of allogeneic HSCT and often are preceded by acute GVHD.[29] Traditionally, the boundary between acute and chronic GVHD was set at 100 days after HSCT; however, more recent definitions hinge on different clinical symptoms rather than the time of onset.[36] A consensus document regarding the diagnosis and scoring of chronic GVHD has been published that proposes a clinical scoring system to describe chronic GVHD as opposed to historical descriptions of chronic GVHD, which described the phenomenon as being "limited" versus "extensive" in nature.[29] The diagnosis of chronic GVHD requires (a) distinction from acute GVHD, (b) the presence of at least one diagnostic clinical sign of chronic GVHD or presence of at least one distinctive manifestation confirmed by pertinent biopsy or other relevant tests, and (c) exclusion of other possible diagnoses.

Prevention and Treatment of Chronic GVHD Chronic GVHD is not a continuation of acute GVHD, and separate approaches are needed for its prevention and management. Prevention of chronic GVHD through prolonged use of immunosuppressive medications has been unsuccessful.[36] Thus, its prevention is focused on minimization of factors associated with higher rates of chronic GVHD. Several recipient, donor, and transplant factors are relevant. Recipient risk factors that are not modifiable include older age, certain diagnoses (e.g., chronic myeloid leukemia), and lack of an HLA-matched donor. Modifiable factors that may lower the risk of chronic GVHD include selection of a younger donor, avoidance of a multiparous female donor, use of umbilical cord blood or bone marrow grafts rather than PBPCs, and limitation of CD34+ and T-cell dose infused.[36] Development of acute GVHD is a major predictor for chronic GVHD, with 70% to 80% of those with grade II to IV acute GVHD developing chronic GVHD.[36]

Relative to no treatment, survival in those with chronic GVHD is improved by extended corticosteroid therapy; however, multiple long-term adverse effects are associated with corticosteroid use. The prednisone dosage is 1 mg/kg/day administered orally in divided doses for 30 days and then slowly converted to an alternate-day therapy by increasing the "on day" and decreasing the "off day" dose until a total of 2 mg/kg/day on alternate days is administered. Once therapy is initiated, 1 to 2 months may pass before an improvement in clinical symptoms is noted, and therapy usually is continued for 9 to 12 months. Therapy can be tapered slowly after resolution of signs and symptoms of chronic GVHD. If a flare of chronic GVHD occurs during the tapering schedule or after therapy is discontinued, immunosuppressive therapy is restarted. Other potential approaches for patients who are refractory to initial therapy include etanercept (Enbrel), infliximab (Remicade), mycophenolate mofetil (Cellcept), rituximab (Rituxan), extended use of calcineurin inhibitors, or extracorporeal photochemotherapy.[36] When immunosuppressive therapy is administered for long periods, the patient must be monitored closely for chronic toxicity. Cushingoid effects, aseptic necrosis of the joints, and diabetes can develop with long-term corticosteroid use. Other severe complications include a high incidence of infection with encapsulated organisms and atypical pathogens such as *Pneumocystis jiroveci*, cytomegalovirus (CMV), and varicella zoster virus (VZV).

▶ Infectious Complications

⑨ *Recipients of HSCT are at higher risk of bacterial, viral, and fungal infections and usually receive a prophylactic or preemptive regimen to minimize the morbidity and mortality owing to infectious complications.* After myeloablative and nonmyeloablative HSCT, opportunistic infections are a major source of morbidity and mortality. There are three periods of infectious risks, early (days 0–30), middle (engraftment to day +100), and late (after day +100). From days 0 to 30 after HSCT, particularly for patients undergoing myeloablative HSCT, the primary pathogens are aerobic bacteria, *Candida* spp., and herpes simplex virus (HSV). Respiratory viruses such as respiratory syncytial virus (RSV), influenza, adenovirus, and parainfluenza virus are recognized increasingly as pathogens causing pneumonia, particularly during community outbreaks of infection with these organisms. To reduce potential exposure of HSCT recipients to such respiratory viruses, visitors and staff members with respiratory signs and symptoms of a viral illness may not be allowed direct contact with patients.

The second period of infectious risk occurs after engraftment to posttransplant day +100. Bacterial infections are still of concern, but pathogens such as CMV, adenovirus, and *Aspergillus* spp. are common. A common manifestation of infection is interstitial pneumonitis (IP), which can be caused by CMV, adenovirus, *Aspergillus*, and *P. jiroveci*. Suppression of the immune system from acute GVHD and corticosteroids contributes to the risk of such infections during this period. Therefore, patients undergoing nonmyeloablative transplant who are receiving corticosteroids to treat GVHD can be expected to have a similar risk for infection as those undergoing myeloablative HSCT.[37] Invasive fungal infections over the first year after HSCT occur at a similar rate in nonmyeloablative transplant

compared with historical control participants receiving a myeloablative preparative regimen.[38]

During the late period (after day +100), the predominant organisms are the encapsulated bacteria (e.g., *Streptococcus pneumoniae*, *Haemophilus influenzae*, and *Neisseria meningitidis*), fungi, and VZV. The encapsulated organisms commonly cause sinopulmonary infections. The risk of infection during this late period is increased in patients with chronic GVHD as a result of prolonged immunosuppression.

Prevention and Treatment of Bacterial and Fungal Infections Because of the need to administer chemotherapy, blood products, antibiotics, and other adjunctive medications, the placement of a semipermanent double- or triple-lumen central venous catheter is necessary before HSCT. However, the indwelling IV central catheters put HSCT recipients at increased risk for *Staphylococcus* infections.

Between the time of administration of the preparative regimen and successful engraftment, allogeneic myeloablative HSCT patients undergo a period of pancytopenia that can last from 2 to 6 weeks. During this time, multiple transfusions of blood and platelet products are needed to support the patient through the pancytopenic period. Transfusions with multiple blood products place patients at risk for blood product–derived infection (e.g., CMV and hepatitis) and sensitization to foreign leukocyte HLA antigens (i.e., alloimmunization), which can lead to immune-mediated thrombocytopenia. Thus, blood product support in myeloablative allogeneic HSCT patients must incorporate strategies that reduce the risk of viral infection and alloimmunization by minimizing the number of pretransplant infusions, using of single-donor (rather than pooled-donor) blood products, irradiating blood products to inactivate T cells in the product, or filtering blood products with leukocyte-reduction filters. The risk of infection in autologous and allogeneic myeloablative HSCT patients is minimized through a variety of measures. Private reverse isolation rooms equipped with positive-pressure HEPA filters and adherence to strict hand hygiene techniques reduce the incidence of bacterial and fungal infections.[4] To reduce exposure to exogenous sources of bacteria, immunosuppressed-patient (low-microbial) diets are used, and live plants or flowers are not allowed in the patient's room. Chemotherapy-induced mucosal damage serves as a portal of entry for many organisms (e.g., *Streptococcus viridans*, aerobic gram-negative bacteria, and fungi) into the bloodstream. The mouth should be kept clean by using frequent (at least four to six times daily) mouth rinses with sterile water, normal saline, or sodium bicarbonate.[4] Soft toothbrushes may be used for oral hygiene during periods of neutropenia and thrombocytopenia. The risk of infection is also reduced by aggressive use of antibacterial, antifungal, and antiviral therapy both prophylactically and for the treatment of documented infection. The antibacterial prophylactic regimens vary substantially among HSCT centers. Some HSCT centers use a prophylactic fluoroquinolone (e.g., levofloxacin) on admission for HSCT and then switch to a broad-spectrum IV antibiotic (e.g., meropenem) when the patient experiences his or her first neutropenic fever. Although fluoroquinolones reduce the incidence of gram-negative bacteremia, they have not been shown to affect mortality; the possibility of developing clostridium difficile-associated diarrhea exists with fluoroquinolone use and infectious causes should be ruled out if diarrhea occurs.[4] Concerns with fluoroquinolone use in the prophylactic setting during HSCT include the emergence of resistant organisms and an increased risk for streptococcal infection.[4] Broad-spectrum IV antibiotics should be initiated immediately at the time of the first neutropenic fever under the treatment guidelines endorsed by the Infectious Disease Society of America for management of fever of unknown origin in the neutropenic host.[39]

Prevention of HSV and VZV Patients who are HSV antibody seropositive before HSCT are at high risk for reactivation of their HSV infection. Acyclovir is highly effective in preventing HSV reactivation, and thus, prophylactic acyclovir is used commonly in HSV-seropositive patients who are undergoing an allogeneic or autologous HSCT.[4] In the setting of HSV prophylaxis, dosing regimens for prophylactic acyclovir vary widely and most centers discontinue acyclovir at the time of hematopoietic recovery.[4] Valacyclovir (Valtrex), a prodrug of acyclovir with improved bioavailability, may allow for adequate serum concentrations to prevent HSV in patients undergoing HSCT as well.

In those with a history of VZV infection, VZV disease occurs in 30% of allogeneic HSCT recipients.[40] The appropriate duration of VZV prophylaxis is controversial. Although VZV infections are reduced by prophylactic acyclovir administered from 1 to 2 months until 1 year after HSCT, the risk of VZV persists in those on continued immunosuppression.[40]

Prevention and Preemptive Therapy of CMV Disease
After allogeneic HSCT, CMV disease is common and has high morbidity and mortality rates. Allogeneic patients are at greater risk than autologous recipients primarily because the latter more efficiently reconstitute their immune system after transplantation. However, autologous HSCT recipients who are CMV seropositive before HSCT are at risk for CMV infection, and prophylaxis should be considered in a select minority of patients.[4] Infection caused by CMV is usually asymptomatic and develops when CMV replication occurs primarily in body fluids such as the blood (viremia), bronchoalveolar fluid, or urine (viruria). Cytomegalovirus disease is symptomatic and occurs when the virus invades an organ or tissue. Pneumonia and gastritis are the most common types of CMV disease after allogeneic HSCT. The presence of a CMV infection substantially increases the risk for developing invasive CMV disease. Strategies to prevent CMV infection have resulted in dramatic reductions in the incidence of CMV disease.

Primary CMV can be prevented with CMV seromatching, which includes transplanting PBPCs or bone marrow from CMV-seronegative donors and infusing CMV-negative blood products to CMV-negative recipients. Antivirals are essential in those who are CMV seropositive or have a CMV-seropositive graft, with two available approaches to minimize the morbidity associated with CMV. The first is universal prophylaxis, in which ganciclovir is begun at the time of engraftment and is continued until approximately day +100. The second approach is called preemptive therapy, for which ganciclovir is selectively administered based on detection of CMV reactivation.

Preemptive therapy is the most commonly used strategy for preventing CMV disease after allogeneic HSCT because ganciclovir is used only in patients at highest risk for developing CMV disease. This approach minimizes administration of ganciclovir, thus lowering the risk of ganciclovir-induced neutropenia with its subsequent increased risk of invasive bacterial and fungal infections. With a decreased risk of ganciclovir-induced neutropenia, fewer interruptions of ganciclovir therapy because of myelosuppression may occur with a preemptive approach and the subsequent use of filgrastim to maintain adequate neutrophil counts may be limited. Preemptive therapy hinges on the ability to detect early reactivation of CMV using shell vial cultures, assays of blood for CMV antigens (such as pp65), or viral nucleic acids using PCR. Antigenemia-based preemptive therapy has similar efficacy in preventing CMV disease as universal ganciclovir prophylaxis, and preemptive therapy also has been associated with a significant reduction in CMV mortality. Preemptive strategies typically use an induction course of ganciclovir for 7 to 14 days followed by a maintenance course until 2 or 3 weeks after the last positive antigenemia result or until day +100 after HSCT.[4] Oral valganciclovir (Valcyte) is an orally bioavailable prodrug of ganciclovir that is converted to ganciclovir in vivo after intestinal absorption and has been used for preemptive therapy. Foscarnet may be given as an alternative to ganciclovir to prevent CMV disease, although its use is complicated by nephrotoxicity and electrolyte wasting.

Fungal Infections

Prevention of Fungal Infections. The widespread use of fluconazole prophylaxis since the early 1990s has led to a significant decline in the morbidity and mortality associated with invasive candidiasis in HSCT recipients. However, invasive aspergillosis (IA); zygomycetes; and fluconazole-resistant *Candida* spp., such as *Candida krusei* and *Candida glabrata,* have increased markedly in incidence.[41] Itraconazole, another azole antifungal agent, has better in vitro activity against fluconazole-resistant fungi (e.g., *Aspergillus* and some *Candida* spp.) and is more effective than fluconazole for long-term prophylaxis of invasive fungal infections after allogeneic HSCT; however, itraconazole is used less often because of frequent GI side effects and concern for potential drug interactions.[42] Posaconazole (Noxafil) is a triazole antifungal that has been approved by the FDA for prophylaxis against IA in HSCT patients with GVHD and is now the recommended prophylactic agent for this subset of HSCT patients on immunosuppression.[43] Posaconazole should be given with food for adequate absorption. Micafungin (Mycamine), an agent of the newer class of antifungals known as the echinocandins, has been FDA approved for prophylaxis of *Candida* infections in patients undergoing HSCT.

Risk Factors for Invasive Mold Infections. Invasive mold infections (e.g., *Aspergillus* spp., *Fusarium* spp., *Zygomycetes,* and

Scedosporium spp.) are an increasing cause of morbidity and death after allogeneic and autologous HSCT. It has been estimated that up to one-third of febrile neutropenic patients who do not respond to antibiotic therapy after 1 week are harboring a fungal infection.[39] In HSCT recipients, risk factors for invasive fungal infections include (a) previous history of IA; (b) recipient factors, including older age, CMV seropositivity, and type of stem cell transplant; (c) treatment factors (e.g., a fludarabine-based preparative regimen); (d) transplant complications (e.g., prolonged neutropenia, graft failure, and higher grade GVHD); and (e) host factors (e.g., diabetes, iron overload).[44] Infections with *Aspergillus* spp. remain the most common mold infections diagnosed in the HSCT population and optimal treatment must be promptly initiated if indicated.

Treatment of Invasive Aspergillosis. Early diagnosis and initiation of appropriate therapy may reduce the high mortality rate of IA. Outcomes also depend on recovery of the recipient's immune system and reduction of immunosuppression. Diagnosis is difficult with the use of computed tomography scans and cultures. Research is ongoing to evaluate the benefit of using nonculture-based methods, such as galactomannan and (1,3)-β-D-glucan antigen detection, which are components of the fungal cell wall that can be detected by commercially available assays.

Practice guidelines are available for the treatment of invasive *Aspergillus* infections in immunocompromised patients.[43] Available mold-active agents include triazole antifungals (itraconazole, voriconazole, and posaconazole), echinocandins (caspofungin, micafungin, and anidulafungin), and amphotericin B formulations. Historically, conventional amphotericin B (c-AmB) has been considered the "gold standard" antifungal therapy for any IA infection, although the majority of responders eventually died of their infection. Significant toxicity occurs with c-AmB administration, with nephrotoxicity, electrolyte wasting (e.g., potassium and magnesium), and infusion-related reactions being the most troublesome side effects. Lipid analogs of amphotericin B were developed with the specific intent of reducing nephrotoxicity associated with conventional amphotericin B while retaining therapeutic efficacy, albeit at a higher acquisition cost.[45] These products include amphotericin B lipid complex (Abelcet, ABLC), liposomal amphotericin B (Ambisome, L-Amb), and amphotericin B colloidal dispersion (Amphotec, ABCD).

With significant toxicity limiting the overall utility of conventional amphotericin B, voriconazole (Vfend) was compared with c-AmB for treatment of IA. For initial therapy of IA, voriconazole had higher response and survival rates than c-AmB and is now considered the primary option for patients with IA.[46] An advantage of voriconazole is its 96% oral bioavailability, making use of this oral drug an attractive alternative. Common toxicities reported with voriconazole include infusion-related reactions, transient visual disturbances, skin reactions, elevations in hepatic transaminases and alkaline phosphatase, nausea, and headache. In addition, voriconazole increases the serum concentrations of medications cleared by cytochrome P-450

2C9, 2C19, and 3A4 (e.g., cyclophosphamide and calcineurin inhibitors); concomitant use of voriconazole and sirolimus should be carefully monitored. Because of pharmacokinetic and pharmacodynamic relationships, antifungal therapy with triazole antifungals such as voriconazole may be optimized for efficacy and toxicity through the practice of therapeutic monitoring of serum levels of these agents.[43]

In patients who have failed initial therapy (i.e., salvage), lipid formulations of amphotericin products, itraconazole, posaconazole or an agent from the echinocandin class may be used. The echinocandins have a unique target for their antifungal activity—specifically, β-1,3-glucan synthase, an enzyme that produces an important component of the fungal cell wall. Three agents in the echinocandin class (caspofungin, micafungin, and anidulafungin) are currently FDA approved and are only available as IV formulations. Caspofungin (Cancidas) is the only member of the echinocandin class approved for use in pediatric patients, for patients with persistent neutropenic fever, and for patients with probable or proven IA that is refractory to or intolerant of other approved therapies. The most common adverse effects observed include increased liver aminotransferase enzyme levels; mild to moderate infusion reactions; and headache, with a smaller number of patients experiencing dermatologic reactions related to histamine release (e.g., flushing, erythema, and wheals).

The optimal duration of appropriate antifungal therapy for treating IA is individualized to the reconstitution of the patient's immune system and his or her response to antifungal treatment. Most clinicians continue aggressive antifungal therapy until the infection has stabilized radiographically and may continue with less aggressive "maintenance" therapy (e.g., oral voriconazole) until immunosuppression is lessened or completed. In general, it is common to require several months of antifungal therapy to treat IA.

Pneumocystis jiroveci. After allogeneic HSCT, prophylaxis for *P. jiroveci* (formerly *P. carinii*) pneumonia (PCP) is used because *Pneumocystis* is a common infection with a high mortality rate if left untreated. The optimal prophylactic regimen in this setting is unclear, with most centers using cotrimoxazole for 6 to 12 months after HSCT.[4] Aerosolized or IV pentamidine and oral dapsone are alternatives for patients who are allergic to sulfa drugs or who do not tolerate cotrimoxazole. Because PCP most often occurs after engraftment, cotrimoxazole usually is begun after neutrophil recovery because of its myelosuppressive effects. Patients receiving prophylactic cotrimoxazole should be monitored closely for rash and unexplained neutropenia or thrombocytopenia. Cotrimoxazole usually is avoided on days of methotrexate administration because the sulfonamides can displace methotrexate from plasma binding sites and decrease renal methotrexate clearance, resulting in higher methotrexate concentrations. Autologous HSCT patients do not receive posttransplant immunosuppression, and thus, their risk of developing PCP is lower.[4] PCP prophylaxis is used often after autologous HSCT in patients with a hematologic malignancy.

Patient Encounter, Part 3

ZN is admitted for allogeneic HSCT with a reduced-intensity preparative regimen consisting of fludarabine and melphalan. Her hospital course was complicated for neutropenic fever and gastrointestinal toxicities associated with melphalan. Neutrophil engraftment occurred on day +12 after HSCT, and the patient was discharged from the hospital on day +14 with minimal complaints. She presents to the transplant clinic on day +22 complaining of several watery stools in the past 24 hours. She does not report nausea, vomiting, or any other symptoms.

What is the differential diagnosis for the patient's current condition?

It is determined that ZN has 1600 mL of liquid stool output in a 24-hour period. How should ZN be managed until a diagnosis is made?

▶ *Issues of Survivorship After HSCT*

The number of long-term HSCT survivors is increasing as 5-year disease-free survival rates improve. Because nonmyeloablative preparative regimens were developed over the past decade, the late effects reported in HSCT survivors describe those resulting from myeloablative preparative regimens.[47] HSCT recipients—with either an autologous or an allogeneic graft—have a higher mortality rate than the general population.[48] ❿ *Long-term survivors of HSCT should be monitored closely, particularly for infections and secondary malignant neoplasms.*

Survivors of HSCT are at higher risk for secondary malignant neoplasms.[47] Long-term impairment of end-organ function, including the kidneys, liver, and lungs, may be caused by the preparative regimen, infectious complications, and/or posttransplant immunosuppression. Many HSCT recipients experience endocrine dysfunction, such as hypothyroidism from TBI, adrenal insufficiency from long-term corticosteroids to treat GVHD, and infertility from radiation and/or high doses of alkylating agents in myeloablative preparative regimens. Osteopenia has been found in more than half of HSCT recipients, most likely from gonadal dysfunction and/or corticosteroid administration.

Close monitoring of HSCT recipients for infections is necessary because recovery of immune function is slow, sometimes requiring more than 2 years, even in the absence of immunosuppressants.[47] Fevers should be assessed and treated rapidly to minimize the likelihood of a fatal infection. HSCT recipients—both autologous and allogeneic—lose protective antibodies to vaccine-preventable diseases; international guidelines been published regarding recommendations for reimmunization of HSCT recipients.[49]

Survivors of HSCT should be monitored routinely for signs of relapse and, if an allogeneic graft was used, chronic GVHD. They should be advised regarding revaccination and obtaining prompt medical care for fevers or signs of infection. Routine evaluations of organ function (i.e., renal, hepatic, thyroid, and ovarian) and osteopenia should occur and the appropriate management strategies initiated if necessary.

OUTCOME EVALUATION

Monitor for symptoms and signs of the disease that is being treated by HSCT to assess the effectiveness of the HSCT. For example, the monitoring plan for a patient with CML would be to monitor disease response by PCR of the *BCR-ABL* transcript. The actual clinical outcome monitored, along with the frequency of monitoring, is based on the underlying disease.

Monitor for nonhematologic toxicity of the preparative regimen during its administration. Monitor these symptoms at least daily, with more frequent monitoring if the patient is experiencing these nonhematologic effects. The goal is to prevent or minimize these adverse effects. Specifically:

- *Busulfan:* Seizures, busulfan concentrations if being used with the BU-CY preparative regimen, number of vomiting episodes, and nausea by patient self-report, total bilirubin, and sudden weight changes (SOS)
- *Cyclophosphamide:* Electrocardiography during IV administration, RBCs in urine, frequency of urination, pain on urination, urinary output, number of vomiting episodes, and nausea by patient self-report, total bilirubin, and sudden weight changes (SOS)
- *Etoposide:* Blood pressure, respiratory rate, serum pH, serum bicarbonate with arterial blood gases, and evaluation of anion gap if necessary
- *Total-body irradiation:* Number of vomiting episodes, nausea by patient self-report, sudden weight changes (SOS), total bilirubin, and skin assessment for the presence of irritation or blister formation

Until the patient has achieved engraftment, monitor the patient for engraftment with at least daily complete blood counts with differentials; these tests may be needed more often if the patient is critically ill or had a prior low hemoglobin. Patients will require transfusion support with blood products and platelets until engraftment occurs if hemoglobin and/or platelets drop below unsafe levels. Transfusion parameters may differ for individual patients, but typically patients are transfused if the hemoglobin drops below 8.0 g/dL (80 g/L; 4.97 mmol/L); platelets are maintained at least above 10,000/mm³ (10 × 10⁹/L) to prevent spontaneous bleeding.

Until engraftment has occurred, monitor the patient's temperature every 4 to 8 hours for signs of infection. Also guide monitoring signs of focal point of infection based on clinical symptoms. For example, if the patient develops shortness of breath, then imaging of the lungs should occur to assess pulmonary infection. Monitor for the toxicity of prophylaxis and/or treatment of bacterial, fungal, or viral infections.

Patient Care and Monitoring

1. Assess the patient regarding the indication for HSCT, the type of preparative regimen, and the type of donor. Determine the nonhematologic toxicity of the preparative regimen, the expected timing of engraftment after the graft is infused, and the need for GVHD prophylaxis.

2. Determine the supportive care needs during administration of the preparative regimen, including use of indwelling central venous catheters; blood product support; and pharmacologic management of CINV, mucositis, and pain.

3. After the graft is infused, monitor the complete blood count with differential at least daily to evaluate engraftment. Allogeneic HSCT patients experience an initial period of pancytopenia followed by a more prolonged period of immunosuppression, which substantially increases the risk of bacterial, fungal, viral, and other opportunistic infections.

4. Counsel the patient regarding adherence to prophylactic antibiotic, antifungal, and antiviral regimens. Evaluate the patient for infection and adverse drug reactions to antibiotics, antifungals, and antivirals. Ensure that the patient is appropriately immunized after recovery from HSCT.

5. Counsel the patient regarding adherence to GVHD prophylaxis and treatment. Monitor and manage for adverse drug reactions.

Monitor for acute nonhematologic toxicity to the preparative regimen to approximately day +30. Specifically,

- Monitor the inside of the mouth and assess the patient's mouth pain for signs and symptoms of mucositis.

- Monitor weight and skin color daily to observe sudden weight changes suggesting SOS. Obtain a total bilirubin determination at least twice weekly or more frequently if SOS is suspected based on weight change.

Monitor for signs of acute GVHD at least daily during engraftment and more often if GVHD is suspected or diagnosed. The patient and his or her caregivers should be educated regarding the signs and symptoms to self-monitor for GVHD. The signs and symptoms for acute GVHD that occur between day +0 and day +100 are rash, nausea, diarrhea, jaundice, elevated liver function test results, and elevated bilirubin.

Abbreviations Introduced in This Chapter

AML	Acute myelogenous leukemia
ANC	Absolute neutrophil count
ASCO	American Society of Clinical Oncology
ATG	Antithymocyte globulin
BMT	Bone marrow transplantation
BU-CY	Busulfan–cyclophosphamide
CINV	Chemotherapy-induced nausea and vomiting
CML	Chronic myelogenous leukemia
CMV	Cytomegalovirus
CY-TBI	Cyclophosphamide–total-body irradiation
GVHD	Graft-versus-host disease
HGF	Hematopoietic growth factors
HLA	Human leukocyte antigen
HSCT	Hematopoietic stem cell transplant
IA	Invasive aspergillosis
IL-2	Interleukin-2
MHC	Minor histocompatibility
MM	Multiple myeloma
NHL	Non-Hodgkin's lymphoma
NK	Natural killer
PBPC	Peripheral blood progenitor cells
PCP	Pneumocystis pneumonia
SOS	Sinusoidal obstruction syndrome
SCr	Serum creatinine
TBI	Total-body irradiation
VZV	Varicella zoster virus

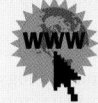 Self-assessment questions and answers are available at *http://www.mhpharmacotherapy.com/pp.html.*

REFERENCES

1. Copelan EA. Hematopoietic stem-cell transplantation. N Engl J Med 2006;354:1813–1826.
2. Pasquini MC, Wang Z, Horowitz MM, Gale RP. Milwaukee, WI: 2010 report from the Center for International Blood and Marrow Transplant Research (CIBMTR): Current use and outcome of hematopoietic stem cell transplantation. Clin Transpl 2010;87–105.
3. Baron F, Sandmaier BM. Current status of hematopoietic stem cell transplantation after nonmyeloablative conditioning. Curr Opin Hematol 2005;12:435–443.
4. Centers for Disease Control and Prevention; Infectious Disease Society of America; American Society of Blood and Marrow Transplantation. Guidelines for preventing opportunistic infections among hematopoietic stem cell transplant recipients. MMWR Recomm Rep 2000;49:1–125, CE1-7.
5. Davies SM, Kollman C, Anasetti C, et al. Engraftment and survival after unrelated-donor bone marrow transplantation: A report from the national marrow donor program. Blood 2000;96:4096–4102.
6. Petersdorf EW, Hansen JA, Martin PJ, et al. Major-histocompatibility-complex class I alleles and antigens in hematopoietic-cell transplantation. N Engl J Med 2001;345:1794–1800.
7. Morishima Y, Sasazuki T, Inoko H, et al. The clinical significance of human leukocyte antigen (HLA) allele compatibility in patients receiving a marrow transplant from serologically HLA-A, HLA-B, and HLA-DR matched unrelated donors. Blood 2002;99:4200–4206.
8. Kessinger A, Sharp JG. The whys and hows of hematopoietic progenitor and stem cell mobilization. Bone Marrow Transplant 2003;31:319–329.
9. Schmitz N. Peripheral blood hematopoietic cells for allogeneic transplantation. In: Blume KG, Forman SJ, Thomas ED, eds. Hematopoietic Cell Transplantation, 3rd ed. Malden, MA: Blackwell Science, 2004:588–598.

10. Stem Cell Trialists' Collaborative Group. Allogeneic peripheral blood stem-cell compared with bone marrow transplantation in the management of hematologic malignancies: An individual patient data meta-analysis of nine randomized trials. J Clin Oncol 2005;23:5074–5087.

11. Remberger M, Ringden O, Blau IW, et al. No difference in graft-versus-host disease, relapse, and survival comparing peripheral stem cells to bone marrow using unrelated donors. Blood 2001;98:1739–1745.

12. Barker JN, Davies SM, DeFor T, et al. Survival after transplantation of unrelated donor umbilical cord blood is comparable to that of human leukocyte antigen-matched unrelated donor bone marrow: Results of a matched-pair analysis. Blood 2001;97:2957–2961.

13. Rocha V, Gluckman E. Clinical use of umbilical cord blood hematopoietic stem cells. Biol Blood Marrow Transplant 2006;12:34–41.

14. Wolff SN. Second hematopoietic stem cell transplantation for the treatment of graft failure, graft rejection or relapse after allogeneic transplantation. Bone Marrow Transplant 2002;29:545–552.

15. Clift RA, Buckner CD, Thomas ED, et al. Marrow transplantation for patients in accelerated phase of chronic myeloid leukemia. Blood 1994;84:4368–4373.

16. Woods WG, Neudorf S, Gold S, et al.; Children's cancer group. A comparison of allogeneic bone marrow transplantation, autologous bone marrow transplantation, and aggressive chemotherapy in children with acute myeloid leukemia in remission. Blood 2001;97:56–62.

17. Bierman PJ, Freedman AS. Autologous hematopoietic stem cell transplantation for non-Hodgkin lymphoma. In: Atkinson K, Champlin R, Ritz J, Fibbe WE, Ljungman P, Brenner MK, eds. Clinical Bone Marrow and Blood Stem Cell Transplantation, 3rd ed. New York: Cambridge University Press, 2004:524.

18. Socie G, Clift RA, Blaise D, et al. Busulfan plus cyclophosphamide compared with total-body irradiation plus cyclophosphamide before marrow transplantation for myeloid leukemia: Long-term follow-up of 4 randomized studies. Blood 2001;98:3569–3574.

19. Champlin R, Khouri I, Anderlini P, et al. Nonmyeloablative preparative regimens for allogeneic hematopoietic transplantation. Biology and current indications. Oncology (Williston Park) 2003;17:94–100; discussion 103–107.

20. McCune JS, Gibbs JP, Slattery JT. Plasma concentration monitoring of busulfan: Does it improve clinical outcome? Clin Pharmacokinet 2000;39:155–165.

21. Grochow LB. Parenteral busulfan: Is therapeutic monitoring still warranted? Biol Blood Marrow Transplant 2002;8:465–467.

22. Hensley ML, Hagerty KL, Kewalramani T, et al. American Society of Clinical Oncology 2008 clinical practice guideline update: Use of chemotherapy and radiation therapy protectants. J Clin Oncol 2008;27(1):127–145.

23. Kris MG, Hesketh PJ, Somerfield MR, et al. American Society of Clinical Oncology guideline for antiemetics in oncology: Update 2006. J Clin Oncol 2006;24(18):2932–2947.

24. Radtke ML, Kolesar JM. Palifermin (Kepivance) for the treatment of oral mucositis in patients with hematologic malignancies requiring hematopoietic stem cell support. J Oncol Pharm Pract 2005;11:121–125.

25. Ho VT, Revta C, Richardson PG. Hepatic veno-occlusive disease after hematopoietic stem cell transplantation: Update on defibrotide and other current investigational therapies. Bone Marrow Transplant 2008;41:229–237.

26. Kashyap A, Wingard J, Cagnoni P, et al. Intravenous versus oral busulfan as part of a busulfan/cyclophosphamide preparative regimen for allogeneic hematopoietic stem cell transplantation: Decreased incidence of hepatic venoocclusive disease (HVOD), HVOD-related mortality, and overall 100-day mortality. Biol Blood Marrow Transplant 2002;8:493–500.

27. Smith TJ, Khatcheressian J, Lyman GH, et al. 2006 update of recommendations for the use of white blood cell growth factors: An evidence-based clinical practice guideline. J Clin Oncol 2006;24(19):3187–3205.

28. Ringden O, Labopin M, Gorin NC, et al. Treatment with granulocyte colony-stimulating factor after allogeneic bone marrow transplantation for acute leukemia increases the risk of graft-versus-host disease and death: A study from the Acute Leukemia Working Party of the European Group for Blood and Marrow Transplantation. J Clin Oncol 2004;22:416–423.

29. Filipovich AH, Weisdorf D, Pavletic S, et al. National Institutes of Health consensus development project on criteria for clinical trials in chronic graft-versus-host disease: I. Diagnosis and staging working group report. Biol Blood Marrow Transplant 2005;11:945–956.

30. Couriel D, Caldera H, Champlin R, Komanduri K. Acute graft-versus-host disease: Pathophysiology, clinical manifestations, and management. Cancer 2004;101:1936–1946.

31. Chao NJ, Schmidt GM, Niland JC, et al. Cyclosporine, methotrexate, and prednisone compared with cyclosporine and prednisone for prophylaxis of acute graft-versus-host disease. N Engl J Med 1993;329:1225–1230.

32. Ratanatharathorn V, Nash RA, Przepiorka D, et al. Phase III study comparing methotrexate and tacrolimus (prograf, FK506) with methotrexate and cyclosporine for graft-versus-host disease prophylaxis after HLA-identical sibling bone marrow transplantation. Blood 1998;92:2303–2314.

33. Nash RA, Antin JH, Karanes C, et al. Phase 3 study comparing methotrexate and tacrolimus with methotrexate and cyclosporine for prophylaxis of acute graft-versus-host disease after marrow transplantation from unrelated donors. Blood 2000;96:2062–2068.

34. Leather HL. Drug interactions in the hematopoietic stem cell transplant (HSCT) recipient: What every transplanter needs to know. Bone Marrow Transplant 2004;33:137–152.

35. Burroughs L, Mielcarek M, Leisenring W, et al. Extending postgrafting cyclosporine decreases the risk of severe graft-versus-host disease after nonmyeloablative hematopoietic cell transplantation. Transplantation 2006;81:818–825.

36. Lee SJ. New approaches for preventing and treating chronic graft-versus-host disease. Blood 2005;105:4200–4206.

37. Junghanss C, Boeckh M, Carter RA, et al. Incidence and outcome of cytomegalovirus infections following nonmyeloablative compared with myeloablative allogeneic stem cell transplantation, a matched control study. Blood 2002;99:1978–1985.

38. Fukuda T, Boeckh M, Carter RA, et al. Risks and outcomes of invasive fungal infections in recipients of allogeneic hematopoietic stem cell transplants after nonmyeloablative conditioning. Blood 2003;102:827–833.

39. Freifeld AG, Bow EJ, Sepkowitz KA, et al. Clinical practice guideline for the use of antimicrobial agents in neutropenic patients with cancer: 2010 update by the Infectious Diseases Society of America. Clin Infect Dis 2011;52(4):56–93.

40. Boeckh M, Kim HW, Flowers ME, et al. Long-term acyclovir for prevention of varicella zoster virus disease after allogeneic hematopoietic cell transplantation—A randomized double-blind placebo-controlled study. Blood 2006;107:1800–1805.

41. Richardson M, Lass-Flörl C. Changing epidemiology of systemic fungal infections. Clin Microbiol Infect 2008;(Suppl 4):5–24.

42. Winston DJ, Maziarz RT, Chandrasekar PH, et al. Intravenous and oral itraconazole versus intravenous and oral fluconazole for long-term antifungal prophylaxis in allogeneic hematopoietic stem-cell transplant recipients. A multicenter, randomized trial. Ann Intern Med 2003;138:705–713.

43. Walsh TJ, Anaissie EJ, Denning DW, et al. Treatment of aspergillosis: Clinical Practice Guidelines of the Infectious Diseases Society of America. Clin Infect Dis 2008;46(3):327–360.

44. Garcia-Vidal C, Upton A, Kirby KA, Marr KA. Epidemiology of invasive mold infections in allogeneic stem cell transplant recipients: Biological risk factors for infection according to time after transplantation. Clin Infect Dis 2008;47:1041–1050.

45. Dupont B. Overview of the lipid formulations of amphotericin B. J Antimicrob Chemother 2002;49(Suppl 1):31–36.

46. Herbrecht R, Denning DW, Patterson TF, et al. Voriconazole versus amphotericin B for primary therapy of invasive aspergillosis. N Engl J Med 2002;347:408–415.

47. Antin JH. Clinical practice. Long-term care after hematopoietic-cell transplantation in adults. N Engl J Med 2002;347:36–42.

48. Bhatia S, Robison LL, Francisco L, et al. Late mortality in survivors of autologous hematopoietic-cell transplantation: Report from the Bone Marrow Transplant Survivor Study. Blood 2005;105:4215–4222.

49. Tomblyn, M, Chiller, T, Einsele, H, et al. Guidelines for preventing infectious complications among hematopoietic cell transplantation recipients: A global perspective. Biol Blood Marrow Transplant 2009;15:1143–1238.

99 Supportive Care in Oncology

Sarah L. Scarpace

● **Upon completion of the chapter, the reader will be able to:**

1. Describe the impact of various supportive care interventions on the prognosis of patients with cancer.

2. Discuss the scientific basis for providing various supportive care interventions in the oncology patient population.

3. Identify patient-related and disease-related risk factors in defining a population for whom supportive care interventions would be of benefit.

4. Recognize typical presenting signs and symptoms of common complications and emergencies that require supportive care interventions.

5. Outline an appropriate prevention and management strategies for various supportive care interventions.

6. Prepare a monitoring plan to evaluate the efficacy and toxicity of pharmacotherapy interventions for supportive care problems.

KEY CONCEPTS

❶ The optimal method of managing chemotherapy-induced nausea/vomiting (CINV) is to provide adequate pharmacologic prophylaxis given a patient's risk level for emesis.

❷ The fundamental approach to lessen the severity of mucositis begins with basic, good oral hygiene.

❸ A risk assessment should be performed at presentation of febrile neutropenia (FN) to identify low-risk patients for potential outpatient treatment. Patients who do not meet low-risk criteria should be hospitalized for immediate parenteral administration of broad-spectrum antibacterials before culture results are obtained.

❹ The primary goal of treatment of superior vena cava syndrome (SVCS) is to relieve obstruction of the superior vena cava (SVC) by treating the underlying malignancy.

❺ Because patients with spinal metastases are generally incurable, the primary goal of treatment of spinal cord compression is palliation. The most important prognostic factor for patients presenting with spinal cord compression is the underlying neurologic status.

❻ The goals of treatment of brain metastases are to manage symptoms and improve survival by reducing cerebral edema, treating the underlying malignancy both locally and systemically.

❼ The use of effective prevention strategies can decrease the incidence of hemorrhagic cystitis to less than 5% in patients receiving cyclophosphamide or ifosfamide. There are three methods to reduce the risk: administration of Mesna, hyperhydration, and bladder irrigation with catheterization.

❽ The primary goal of treatment for hypercalcemia is to control the underlying malignancy. Therapies directed at lowering the calcium level are temporary measures that are useful until anticancer therapy begins to work.

❾ The primary goals of management of tumor lysis syndrome (TLS) are (a) prevention of renal failure and (b) prevention of electrolyte imbalances. Thus, the best treatment for TLS is prophylaxis to enable delivery of cytotoxic therapy for the underlying malignancy.

❿ Chemotherapy extravasation may be avoided in many cases by the use of successful prevention strategies. The most important preventative measure is proper patient education.

INTRODUCTION

Patients with cancer are at risk for serious adverse events that result from their treatment, the cancer, or both.

The management of these complications is generally referred to as supportive care (or symptom management). Treatment-related complications include chemotherapy-induced nausea and vomiting (CINV), febrile neutropenia (FN), extravasation, hemorrhagic cystitis, mucositis, and tumor lysis syndrome (TLS). Tumor or cancer-related complications include superior vena cava (SVC) obstruction, spinal cord compression, and hypercalcemia and brain metastases. In some cases, these events can be life threatening. SVC obstruction, spinal cord compression, TLS, and hypercalcemia have traditionally been defined as oncologic emergencies. Although some of these conditions are not imminently life threatening (i.e., chemotherapy extravasation), as a group of treatment- and disease-related complications in the oncology population, they do require rapid assessment and supportive care interventions and treatment. The onset of oncologic emergencies may herald the onset of an undiagnosed malignancy or progression or relapse of a preexisting malignancy. Optimal management of patients with various oncologic emergencies and complications requiring supportive care interventions can significantly decrease morbidity and mortality in patients with cancer. This chapter provides an overview of these issues. First, an overview of the management of common side effects of treatment is given. Later, a summary of common oncologic emergencies is presented.

CHEMOTHERAPY-INDUCED TOXICITIES: NAUSEA/VOMITING

Nausea and vomiting are among the most commonly feared toxicities by patients undergoing chemotherapy. One study demonstrated that both nausea and vomiting ranked in the top five bothersome side effects of chemotherapy.[1] ❶ *The optimal method of managing CINV is to provide adequate pharmacologic prophylaxis given a patient's risk level for emesis.* Studies have demonstrated that insufficient control during the first cycle of chemotherapy leads to more difficulty in controlling emesis for subsequent cycles.[2]

EPIDEMIOLOGY AND ETIOLOGY

Although it is widely known that chemotherapy causes nausea and vomiting, the rate of emesis varies depending on individual patient risk factors and drug therapy regimen. Therefore, cancer treatments are stratified into varying risk levels: high, moderate, low, and minimal. Agents with a "high" emetic risk cause emesis in more than 90% of cases if not given any prophylaxis. The rates of emesis for "moderate," "low," and "minimal" are 30% to 90%, 10% to 30%, and less than 10%, respectively. Table 99–1 lists the individual agents and their risk category.[3] With proper prophylaxis using antiemetics, the rate of emesis when receiving a highly emetogenic regimen can decrease to about 30%.[4]

PATHOPHYSIOLOGY

The pathophysiology of nausea and vomiting is described in Chapter 20. Specific to CINV, the key receptors include

Table 99–1

Emetogenic Potential of Chemotherapy

Risk	Agent
High emetic risk (more than 90% of patients will vomit without appropriate antiemetics)	Altretamine
	Carmustine greater than 250 mg/m²
	Cisplatin equal to or greater than 50 mg/m²
	Cyclophosphamide greater than 1,500 mg/m²
	Dacarbazine
	Mechlorethamine
	Streptozocin
Moderate emetic risk (30–90%)	Aldesleukin greater than 12–15 million units/m²
	Amifostine greater than 300 mg/m²
	Arsenic trioxide
	Azacitidine
	Bendamustine
	Busulfan greater than 4 mg/m²
	Carboplatin
	Carmustine less than or equal to 250 mg/m²
	Cisplatin less than 50 mg/m²
	Cyclophosphamide less than or equal to 1,500 mg/m²
	Cyclophosphamide (oral)
	Cytarabine greater than 1 g/m²
	Dactinomycin
	Daunorubicin
	Doxorubicin
	Epirubicin
	Etoposide (PO)
	Idarubicin
	Ifosfamide
	Irinotecan
	Imatinib (PO)
	Lomustine
	Melphalan
	Methotrexate greater than 1,000 mg/m²
	Oxaliplatin greater than 75 mg/m²
	Temozolamide (PO)
	Vinorelbine (PO)
Low emetic risk (10–30%)	Amifostine less than 300 mg/m²
	Bexarotene
	Capecitabine
	Docetaxel
	Etoposide
	Fludarabine (PO)
	5-Fluorouracil less than 1,000 mg/m²
	Gemcitabine
	Ixabepilone
	Methotrexate greater than 50 mg/m² and less than 250 mg/m²
	Mitomycin
	Nilotinib
	Paclitaxel
	Pemetrexed
	Topotecan
	Vorinostat
Minimal risk (less than 10%)	Most other agents

From Hesketh PJ. Chemotherapy-induced nausea and vomiting. N Engl J Med 2008;358:2482–2494.

serotonin (5-HT₃) receptors (located in the chemoreceptor trigger zone, emetic center of the medulla, and gastrointestinal [GI] tract) and neurokinin-1 (NK1) receptors (located in the emetic center of the medulla). Serotonin plays an important role in the genesis of acute vomiting because some cancer drug therapies can stimulate a release of serotonin from enterochromaffin cells in the GI tract. Serotonin then activates the emetic response by binding to $5HT_3$ receptors in the emetic center. This short-lived release of serotonin likely explains why serotonin antagonists are more beneficial for preventing acute versus delayed vomiting.[5] Other sites that are targeted by antiemetics include dopamine, muscarinic (acetylcholine), histamine, and cannabinoid receptors.

CLINICAL PRESENTATION AND DIAGNOSIS

CINV, although frequently discussed as one syndrome, includes two distinct clinical entities. Nauseous patients may present with general GI upset and reflux and may report a sensation or desire to vomit without being able to do so (patients may describe this as having "dry heaves"). Patients with chemotherapy-induced vomiting may experience vomiting with the first 24 hours of chemotherapy administration ("acute" nausea/vomiting) or several days after chemotherapy ("delayed" nausea/vomiting).[3] Patients may additionally experience nausea/vomiting before chemotherapy administration ("anticipatory" nausea/vomiting).[3] In all cases, it is important that other causes of nausea and vomiting are ruled out before diagnosing chemotherapy as the source.[6] Other causes of nausea and vomiting may include bowel obstruction, opioids, electrolyte imbalances, brain metastases, and vestibular dysfunction.[6]

Clinical Presentation and Diagnosis of CINV

Acute Nausea/Vomiting

- Occurs within the first 24 hours after chemotherapy administration

Delayed Nausea/Vomiting

- Occurs between 24 hours and 5 days after chemotherapy administration

Anticipatory Nausea/Vomiting

- A learned, conditioned reflex response to a stimulus (sight, sound, smell) often associated with poor emetic control in a previous cycle of chemotherapy

Breakthrough Nausea/Vomiting

- Occurs despite prophylaxis with an appropriate antiemetic regimen

Differential Diagnosis

- Surgery, radiation
- Gastric outlet or bowel obstruction, constipation
- Hypercalcemia, hyperglycemia, hyponatremia, uremia
- Other drugs (opioids)

TREATMENT

Desired Outcomes

The desired outcome is to completely prevent or minimize the severity of nausea, vomiting, and the use of breakthrough antiemetic medications. In clinical trials, a common end point is "complete response," defined as having no emesis and no breakthrough medication use within a defined period of time. If patients experience nausea or emesis, the goal is to quickly relieve the episode and prevent future nausea or vomiting, whether in the next few days or for the next cycle of chemotherapy.

General Approach to Treatment

Treatment-related factors and patient-related factors can help define a patient population at risk for developing CINV. Treatment-related factors include those chemotherapy agents with high levels of emetogenicity (see Table 99–1 for a complete listing). CINV is typically a cyclical occurrence. Although this section focuses on CINV, it can be helpful for practitioners to remember that patients undergoing concomitant radiation therapy and chemotherapy are at risk for more severe nausea and vomiting. Radiation (particularly total-body irradiation as part of a conditioning regimen for stem cell transplant) can cause a more cumulative (versus cyclical) nausea/vomiting phenomenon.

Specific patient-related factors such as female gender, age (children), history of motion sickness, pregnancy-induced nausea or vomiting, and poor emetic control in previous chemotherapy cycles increase the risk of emesis. Interestingly, patients with a history of alcohol abuse have a reported decreased risk of emesis.[3] It is important to design an antiemetic regimen with consideration of these patient-specific risk factors.

A well-designed regimen includes a prophylactic regimen and a breakthrough antiemetic drug "as needed." Although many drugs are recommended as "breakthrough" drugs, choose a drug with a different mechanism of action compared with the drugs used for prophylaxis.[6]

▶ Nonpharmacologic Therapy

Nonpharmacologic therapy for nausea and vomiting can be useful adjuncts to drug therapy, particularly in the setting of anticipatory nausea and vomiting. The National Comprehensive Cancer Network (NCCN) recommends behavior therapies such as relaxation, guided imagery, and music therapy as well as acupuncture or acupressure as useful in this setting.[6] Other general measures that can be taken include ensuring adequate sleep before treatment, eating smaller meals, and avoiding greasy foods and foods with strong odors.[7] Nonprescription medications such as antacids, histamine-2-receptor blockers, and proton pump inhibitors can be helpful in reducing gastroesophageal reflux associated with some cancer treatments that may trigger or exacerbate CINV.[8]

Nonprescription antihistamines marketed for nausea associated with motion sickness are not usually helpful in managing CINV.

▶ *Pharmacologic Therapy*

According to the American Society of Clinical Oncology's antiemesis guidelines, three drug classes have a "high therapeutic index" to treat CINV: corticosteroids (dexamethasone), serotonin receptor antagonists, and NK1 receptor antagonists (aprepitant or fosaprepitant).[9] A drug in these three classes will be used either in combination with drugs from the other classes or as a single agent for prophylaxis, depending on the emetic risk level (Table 99–2). Dexamethasone, serotonin antagonists, and fosaprepitant are usually administered 30 minutes before chemotherapy, and oral aprepitant is administered 60 minutes before chemotherapy. Dexamethasone is the preferred agent to prevent CINV in the delayed setting and is recommended to be scheduled at a dose of 4 mg orally twice daily (or 8 mg once daily) for 3 to 4 days after chemotherapy to prevent delayed nausea vomiting. In some cases, the serotonin antagonists may also be continued orally for 3 to 4 days after chemotherapy. For patients in whom aprepitant is used prechemotherapy (as either 125 mg orally or 115 mg intravenously as fosaprepitant), the aprepitant is continued as 80 mg orally once daily on days 2 and 3 of the chemotherapy cycle. The other antiemetics are usually prescribed "as needed" for breakthrough nausea or vomiting. The dopamine antagonists prochlorperazine and metoclopramide are usually recommended because they antagonize a different receptor than the drugs already given for prophylaxis. However, the NCCN guidelines state that other drugs, including serotonin receptor antagonists, cannabinoids, dexamethasone, scopolamine, or olanzapine, may be used.[6] For those in any risk group who experience anticipatory nausea and vomiting, the addition of lorazepam for prophylaxis and breakthrough is recommended for its antiemetic and antianxiety properties. Table 99–3 lists the doses of the antiemetic agents for prophylaxis and breakthrough use.

A prophylactic antiemetic regimen for high emetic risk levels should be with a triple-drug combination using dexamethasone, aprepitant, and 5-HT₃ antagonist to prevent both acute and delayed emesis. Dexamethasone should be continued until day 4, and aprepitant is also administered on days 2 and 3 if the oral formulation is used. When fosaprepitant150 mg intravenous (IV) is administered on day 1, no oral aprepitant is needed on days 2 and 3 of therapy. If fosaprepitant 115 mg IV is administered on day 1, then oral aprepitant 80 mg once daily on days 2 and 3 is needed.

For moderately emetogenic regimens, acute emesis is still of major concern, but the incidence of delayed emesis is less. Therefore, dexamethasone plus a 5-HT₃ antagonist should be given on day 1. On days 2 to 4, choose to continue either the dexamethasone or the 5-HT₃ antagonist to prevent delayed emesis. One exception is when palonosetron is given as the 5-HT₃ antagonist on day 1. Because its half-life is long, no redosing is necessary on subsequent days. Aprepitant and fosaprepitant 115 mg IV are also approved by the Food and Drug Administration (FDA) for the prevention of CINV in the moderate setting and can be prescribed as a 3-day regimen. Of note, fosaprepitant 150 mg is not FDA approved for use in the moderately emetogenic setting. For patients with additional risk factors or who had uncontrolled emesis with previous chemotherapy cycles, the same regimen for "high-" risk levels may be used.

For low emetic risk regimens, single antiemetic prophylaxis with either dexamethasone or a dopamine antagonist

Table 99–2

Recommended Therapy by Emetic Risk

Emetic Risk Category (Incidence of Emesis Without Antiemetics)	Antiemetic Regimens and Schedules
High (greater than 90%)	5-HT₃ serotonin receptor antagonist: day 1 Dexamethasone: days 1–4 Aprepitant: days 1, 2, 3 or fosaprepitant 150 mg IV day 1 only
Moderate (30–90%)	5-HT₃ serotonin receptor antagonist: day 1 Dexamethasone: day 1
Moderate (30–90%) but getting anthracycline, carboplatin, cisplatin, irinotecan cyclophosphamide, methotrexate	5-HT₃ serotonin receptor antagonist: day 1 Dexamethasone: days 1, 2, and 3 Aprepitant: days 1, 2, and 3
Low (10–30%)	Dexamethasone: day 1
Minimal (less than 10%)	As needed

From Kris MG, Hesketh PJ, Somerfield MR, et al. American Society of Clinical Oncology Guidelines for Antiemesis in Oncology: Update 2006. J Clin Oncol 2006;24:2932–2947.

Table 99–3

Antiemetic Dosing

Antiemetic	Single Dose Administered Before Chemotherapy	Daily Schedule
5-HT₃ Serotonin Receptor Antagonists		
Dolasetron	PO: 100 mg IV: 100 mg or 1.8 mg/kg	100 mg PO daily
Granisetron	PO: 2 mg IV: 1 mg or 0.01 mg/kg Topical: 34.3-mg patch (apply 24–48 hours before chemotherapy, leave on for 7 days)	1–2 mg PO daily or 1 mg two times a day
Ondansetron	PO: 16–24 mg IV: 8 mg or 0.15 mg/kg	8 mg PO two times a day or 16 mg PO daily
Palonosetron	IV: 0.25 mg PO: 0.5 mg	
Others		
Aprepitant	PO: 125 mg	80 mg PO days 2 and 3
Fosaprepitant	IV: 150 mg	No aprepitant on days 2 or 3
Dexamethasone	PO: 12 mg	12 mg PO days 2–4

From Kris MG, Hesketh PJ, Somerfield MR, et al. American Society of Clinical Oncology Guidelines for Antiemesis in Oncology: Update 2006. J Clin Oncol 2006;24:2932–2947.

(prochlorperazine, metoclopramide) is recommended. For minimal emetic risk groups, guidelines do not recommend routine prophylaxis with antiemetics; instead, patients should be provided something as needed for nausea and vomiting. Table 99–2 summarizes the NCCN guidelines for antiemetic prophylaxis for the different risk levels.

OUTCOME EVALUATION

It is often difficult to evaluate nausea and vomiting when chemotherapy is given as an outpatient. After drug

Patient Encounter 1: CINV

RK is a 62-year-old man who presents to the clinic today to receive his first dose of cisplatin 100 mg/m² with concurrent radiation for his aggressive head and neck supraglottic squamous cell carcinoma. He is status post laryngectomy for pathological T4aN2C. He had disease progression soon after resection. He appears to be tolerating radiation very well with no obvious adverse side effects. He has a poor appetite and has difficulty swallowing, but he is keeping very well with his nutrition via percutaneous endoscopic gastrostomy (PEG) tube. He takes all of his regular medication through the PEG tube. He has some secretion from the tracheostomy tube. He denies any worsening shortness of breath, cough, hemoptysis, and palpitations. RK also denies any abdominal pain, melena, diarrhea, or constipation. He denies any dysuria, hematuria, or change in frequency of urine.

How would you approach the prevention and monitoring of RK for CINV?

Patient Care and Monitoring: CINV

Monitoring

- Using a visual analogue or numerical rating scale (0–10), have the patient rate the severity of nausea (assess nausea first; then move on to emesis)
- Daily, ask about the number of emesis episodes in the last 24 hours
- Assess scheduled and breakthrough medication adherence

Counsel the patient regarding his or her antiemetics

- Explain which drugs are taken as prophylaxis to prevent nausea and vomiting and which are taken as needed to treat it.
- Have the patient journal when a dose is taken in relation to the chemotherapy. Encourage journaling the severity and frequency of nausea, vomiting, diet, and antiemetic adherence.
- Discuss expected or common side effects of antiemetic medications.

administration, patients return home and may or may not report inadequate control of emesis. Subsequent chemotherapy cycles may also be poorly controlled, especially if patients do not state their experience with the previous cycle. To ameliorate this problem, patients' experiences with CINV should be assessed, particularly after the first and second cycles of chemotherapy. Patients should be asked about their previous emesis control with subsequent cycles of chemotherapy, and a prophylaxis regimen may need to be adjusted. Patients should also be encouraged to self-report poor control of emesis while at home. Side effects of the antiemetic regimen should also be assessed and reported.

MUCOSITIS

Mucositis is the degradation of mucosal lining in the oral cavity and GI tract caused by damage from radiation or chemotherapy.[10] Mucositis is a common supportive care issue that deserves attention and is associated with many negative health consequences, including pain, inadequate nutritional intake, and risk for infection. Patients with mucositis often require parenteral analgesics, nutrition supplementation, and antiinfectives to treat concomitant bacterial, fungal, or viral infections. Furthermore, mucositis is associated with economic consequences, primarily increased lengths of hospital stay.[11] An understanding of the current guidelines for prevention and treatment of mucositis can help improve patient outcomes.

EPIDEMIOLOGY AND ETIOLOGY

The incidence of chemotherapy or radiation-induced mucositis depends mostly on the type and area of radiation, the type of chemotherapy, and the specific cancer. Studies have reported an incidence of about 80% in head and neck cancer patients receiving chemoradiation.[12] The World Health Organization estimates that approximately 75% of patients who are treated with high-dose chemotherapy for stem cell transplantation developed oral mucositis.[10] Specific chemotherapy agents associated with mucositis include taxanes, anthracyclines, platinum analogues, methotrexate, and the fluoropyrimidines.

PATHOPHYSIOLOGY

The classical concept of mucositis pathophysiology asserts that direct cytotoxicity from chemotherapy or radiation to basal epithelial cells results in ulcerative lesions caused by a lack of regeneration. These lesions are further complicated by trauma or microorganism growth. However, the most recent theory of mucositis pathophysiology is more detailed and involves a multistage, dynamic process that builds upon the historical model.[13] According to this theory, there are five stages of mucositis: initiation, primary damage response, signal amplification, ulceration, and healing. It is important to note that these stages do not occur sequentially. Rather, they are dynamic and may overlap.

CLINICAL PRESENTATION AND DIAGNOSIS

● Patients with mucositis may present along a continuum of mild, painless, erythematous ulcers to those that are painful and/or bleeding that may interfere with eating and swallowing or that may require treatment with hydration, antibiotics, or even parenteral nutrition in its most severe forms.[13]

TREATMENT

Nonpharmacologic Treatment

The goal of nonpharmacologic measures to prevent mucositis is to reduce the bacterial load of organisms in the mouth to prevent infection of the inflamed mucosa. Prevention of mucositis with good basic oral hygiene (brushing with a soft-bristled toothbrush at least twice daily, flossing, bland rinses, and saline substitutes) is key. ❷ *The fundamental approach to lessen the severity of mucositis begins with basic, good oral hygiene.*[10,13,14]

Pharmacologic Treatment

In the setting of radiation therapy, amifostine at doses equal to or greater than 340 mg/m² IV before each dose of radiation therapy may be considered.[14] Cryotherapy, such as with ice chips, is recommended as a prophylactic measure for patients treated with both standard-dose and high-dose chemotherapy regimens.[14] Antimicrobial lozenges, sucralfate and chlorhexidine rinses, and "magic-mouthwash" compounded rinses are not generally recommended by clinical practice guidelines for mucositis prevention even though they are sometimes used in practice.[10,13,14]

Unfortunately, little evidence is available to recommend specific treatments for mucositis. Pain assessment and appropriate management are important.[10,13,14] Pain management may be achieved with oral morphine, topical anesthetic products, and compounded rinses that incorporate

---

Clinical Presentation and Diagnosis of Mucositis

- Painful, erythematous ulcers develop on the lips, cheeks, soft palate, floor of mouth.
- Asses mucositis using validated scales, either oral mucositis assessment scale (OMAS) or University of Nebraska oral assessment score (MUCPEAK).
- Symptoms appear within 5 to 7 days after chemotherapy and resolve in 2 to 3 weeks.
- Pain may affect ability to swallow and eat.
- The patient may have concomitant localized or systemic infection.
- Diarrhea can lead to electrolyte imbalances.

---

lidocaine.[10,13,14] In more severe cases in which infection of the oral mucosa is suspected, appropriate antibiotic therapy is necessary to prevent systemic infection.[10,13,14]

● Palifermin is FDA approved for the prevention and treatment of mucositis in patients receiving high-dose chemotherapy for stem cell transplant or leukemia induction. Palifermin is administered as an IV bolus injection at a dosage of 60 mcg/kg/day for 3 consecutive days before and three consecutive days after myelotoxic therapy for a total of six doses. Administering Palifermin within 24 hours of chemotherapy can result in an increased sensitivity of rapidly dividing epithelial cells to the cytotoxic agent. For this reason, Palifermin should not be administered for 24 hours before, 24 hours after, or during the infusion of myelotoxic chemotherapy to avoid increasing the severity and the duration of oral mucositis.

OUTCOME EVALUATION

Based on these goals, outcomes measured in clinical trials often assess the incidence, duration, and severity of mucositis with a given intervention intended to prevent or treat mucositis. Agents that are intended to palliate the symptoms of mucositis are usually assessed by measures in pain scales and the ability to eat or drink.

HEMATOLOGIC COMPLICATIONS: FN

INTRODUCTION

● FN is a common adverse effect after administration of cytotoxic chemotherapy. The mortality rate in neutropenic patients caused by infectious complications currently remains between 5% and 10%; therefore, FN is considered a true oncologic emergency. Patients frequently require hospitalization for prompt administration of broad-spectrum antibiotics that are critical to avoid morbidity and mortality.

EPIDEMIOLOGY AND ETIOLOGY

The microorganisms responsible for infections in neutropenic patients have changed significantly in the last 50 years. From the 1960s through the mid-1980s, gram-negative organisms were the most common bacteria isolated. This pattern shifted to the gram-positive organisms in the late 1980s, which remain the most common isolates. Recent data indicate that gram-positive organisms account for 62% to 76% of all bloodstream infections.[15] The causes of this change are attributed to the widespread use of central venous catheters and more aggressive chemotherapy regimens as well as the use of prophylactic antibiotics with relatively poor gram-positive coverage (quinolones). Commonly isolated pathogens are shown in Table 99–4. Although gram-negative infections are less common, they cause the majority of infections in sites other than the blood and are particularly virulent. It should be noted that isolates vary considerably among institutions; thus, attention to institutional isolation patterns is prudent.

In addition, *Aspergillus* spp. are important pathogens in patients with prolonged and severe neutropenia.

PATHOPHYSIOLOGY

The neutrophils are the primary defense mechanism against bacterial and fungal infection. Most infections in neutropenic patients are a result of organisms contained in endogenous flora, both on the skin and within the GI tract. These organisms are provided access to the bloodstream through breakdowns in host defense barriers (**mucositis**, use of central venous catheters). Mucositis in particular is a significant risk factor for sepsis and is increasingly more common because of the widespread use of aggressive chemotherapy regimens.[18]

Neutropenia is defined as an absolute neutrophil count (ANC) less than 500/µL (0.50×10^9/L) cells or an ANC less than 1,000/µL (1.00×10^9/L) cells with a predicted decrease to less than 500/µL (0.50×10^9/L) cells. The ANC is calculated by multiplying the total WBC by the percentage of neutrophils (segmented neutrophils plus "bands"). Fever is defined as a single oral temperature greater than or equal to 38.3°C (101°F) or a temperature greater than or equal to 38.0°C (100.4°F) for at least 1 hour. The combination of these two factors defines FN.[19] The risk of infection during the period of neutropenia depends primarily on two factors:

- The duration of the neutropenia (time period of ANC less than 500/µL (0.50×10^9/L) cells)
- The severity of the neutropenia (lowest ANC level reached [nadir])

A multitude of other risk factors for FN have been identified (Table 99–5). Many of these are also risk factors for poor outcome in patients who experience FN. Cancer drug therapy regimens are also categorized as being high

---

Patient Encounter 2: FN

NB is a 73-year-old man with a history of AML in remission s/p first of two cycles of cytarabine consolidation, dose adjusted based on renal function. He presents today 8 days later for follow-up and laboratory check. Relevant laboratory study results include WBC count, 0.7×10^3/mL (3×10^9/L); HgB 9.0 g/dL (0.09 g/L); HCT 26.6% (0.266); PLT, 6×10^3/mL (6×10^9/L); serum chemistries within normal limits except; SCr, 1.3 mg/dL (115 mmol/L); and estimated GFR 54 mL/min. Vitals: temperature, 98.2°F (36.6°C); pulse, 71 beats/min; respiratory rate, 18 breaths/min; BP 116/64 mm Hg. NB has no known drug allergies.

What risk factors for FN does this patient have?

How would you approach NB?

Fungal infections caused by *Candida* spp. (especially *Candida albicans*) have emerged as significant pathogens, especially in patients with hematologic malignancies and those undergoing bone marrow transplantation (BMT).

Table 99–4
Commonly Isolated Pathogens in Patients With FN

Type of Organism	Comments
Bacteria	
Gram-positive organisms	Most common isolates in FN
Coagulase-negative staphylococci (i.e., *Staphylococcus epidermidis*)	Between 70% and 90% resistant to methicillin; indolent course with low mortality
	Some centers report greater than 50% resistance to methicillin
Staphylococcus aureus	Resistance to vancomycin greater than or equal to 30%
Enterococcus spp.	
Viridans streptococcus	Increasing resistance to penicillin; result of fluoroquinolone prophylaxis; associated with mucositis
Gram-negative organisms	Infections rapidly fatal
Pseudomonas aeruginosa	High mortality rate; increasing resistance to quinolones
Escherichia coli	Increased incidence of β-lactamase–producing strains
Klebsiella spp.	Increased incidence of β-lactamase–producing strains
Enterobacter spp.	
Fungi	Occur primarily after prolonged neutropenia (longer than 1 week)
Yeasts	
Candida albicans	Increasing incidence (~10%); high mortality rate
Non-*albicans Candida* (*Candida krusei, Candida glabrata*)	Resistant to fluconazole; high mortality rate
Molds	Resistant to fluconazole; high mortality
Aspergillus spp.	Pulmonary infection common
Fusarium spp.	Emerging pathogen
Scedosporium spp.	Emerging pathogen

FN, febrile neutropenia.
From Refs. 16 and 17.

Table 99–5
Risk Factors for FN

Patient Related	Therapy Related
Age 60 years or older	History of extensive chemotherapy
Poor **performance status**	Planned full **dose intensity** of chemotherapy
Bone marrow involvement by tumor	High-dose chemotherapy (i.e., bone marrow transplant)
Poor nutritional status	
Hematologic malignancy	Greater than 20% incidence of FN reported in clinical trials with treatment regimen
Elevated LDH	
Decreased hemoglobin level	
Baseline or first-cycle low neutrophil counts	10% to 20% incidence of FN reported in clinical trials with treatment regimen plus presence of patient-specific risk factors
History of previous FN	
Uncontrolled or advanced stage cancer	

FN, febrile neutropenia; LDH, lactate dehydrogenase.

From Lyman GH, Lyman CH, Agboola O. Risk models for predicting chemotherapy-induced neutropenia. Oncologist 2005;10:427–437.

Table 99–6

MASCC Risk-Index for Identifying Low-Risk Patients With FN[a]

Characteristic	Score
Burden of illness[b]	
No symptoms	5
Mild symptoms	5
Moderate symptoms	3
No hypotension	5
No COPD	4
Solid tumor or hematologic malignancy without fungal infection	4
	3
No dehydration	3
Outpatient onset of fever	3
Age less than 60 years[c]	2

[a]Note: A risk-index score of 21 or higher indicates that the patient is likely to be at low risk for complications and morbidity.

[b]Choose one item only.

[c]Does not apply to patients 16 years of age or younger.

COPD, chronic obstructive pulmonary disease; FN, febrile neutropenia; MASCC, Multinational Association for Supportive Care in Cancer.

From Klastersky J, Paesmans M, Rubenstein EB, et al. The Multinational Association for Supportive Care in Cancer risk index: A multinational scoring system for identifying low-risk febrile neutropenic patients. J Clin Oncol 2000;18:3038–3051.

risk (greater than 20% incidence of FN reported in clinical trials) or intermediate risk (10% to 20% risk of FN reported in clinical trials). Similar to the approach to the prevention of CINV, it is important to consider both the regimen and patient-specific risk factors when determining whether a patient should receive prophylactic therapy for FN.

It is clear that patients with FN represent a heterogenous group. Some patients are at lower risk and could potentially be treated as outpatients, thereby avoiding the risk and cost of hospitalization. The Multinational Association for Supportive Care in Cancer (MASCC) has validated a risk assessment tool that assigns a risk score to patients presenting with FN (Table 99–6).[21] Patients with a risk-index score greater than or equal to 21 are identified as low-risk and are candidates for outpatient therapy (discussed under Treatment).

CLINICAL PRESENTATION AND DIAGNOSIS

Patients with suppressed immune systems are often unable to mount the same response to infection as normal individuals, thus limiting the expression of typical presenting signs and symptoms.[22] Often fever is the only indicator of infection, and diagnosis is made empirically based on the patient's temperature; ANC; and coexisting risk factors for infection such as presence of an indwelling catheter, inpatient status, history of chemotherapy or radiotherapy, peripheral blood stem cell or bone marrow transplant, renal or hepatic compromise, and older age.[22,23]

PREVENTION

Three primary modalities for preventing infection in patients who are expected to become neutropenic have used utilized, the first of which is the least expensive and simplest:

- Vigilant hand hygiene
- Prophylactic antibiotics
- Colony-stimulating factors (CSFs)

The advantages and disadvantages of these strategies are discussed individually in the following section.

Hand Hygiene

As previously discussed, most infections in neutropenic patients are a result of endogenous flora; however, prevention of further acquisition of environmental pathogens is also important. Patients who are or will become neutropenic should practice careful handwashing and avoid contact with people who neglect hand hygiene. In addition, ingestion of certain fresh fruits and vegetables as well as unprocessed dairy products should be avoided during the neutropenic period.

Prophylactic Antibiotics

Routine antibacterial prophylaxis is controversial and has been attempted primarily with sulfamethoxazole–trimethoprim (SMZ-TMP) and quinolones. SMZ-TMP offers improved prophylaxis for gram-positive organisms compared with quinolones; quinolones are more effective prophylaxis against gram-negative infections. The 2010

Clinical Presentation and Diagnosis of FN

General

- Only 50% of patients with FN have a clinically documented infection.
- Only 25% of patients with FN have a microbiologically documented infection.

Signs and Symptoms

- Fever is typically the only sign of infection, although septic patients may have chills.
- Infected catheter sites may be erythematous and tender to the touch.

Laboratory Tests

- CBC with differential
- Two blood cultures from each access site (peripheral and central), urinalysis, urine culture, chest x-ray, sputum cultures

Other Diagnostic Tests

- Detailed physical exam of the oral mucosa, sinuses, skin, catheter access sites, perineal area (no rectal examination because of the risk of bacteremia)

Infectious Diseases Society of America (IDSA) guidelines recommend fluoroquinolone prophylaxis in patients who are at high risk for "prolonged and profound" neutropenia.[19] The IDSA does not recommend routine antibiotic prophylaxis for low-risk patients because of the lack of a clear benefit on mortality rates and concerns regarding increasing antibiotic resistance. One exception is that SMZ-TMP is recommended for prophylaxis of *Pneumocystis jiroveci* (formerly *Pneumocystis carinii*) pneumonitis (PCP) in all at-risk patients (i.e., bone marrow transplant recipients, AIDS), regardless of the presence of neutropenia.

Two recent meta-analyses add fuel to the controversy of routine antibiotic prophylaxis.[24,25] Decreases in infection-related mortality and gram-negative bacteremia were demonstrated with the use of quinolones; however, overall adverse events were higher, and most of the studies were conducted in patients with hematologic malignancies (an inherently high-risk group). Although two additional randomized trials in patients with both solid tumors and hematologic malignancies demonstrated lower rates of FN, infection, and hospitalization with oral prophylactic levofloxacin compared with placebo, both the NCCN and IDSA only recommend prophylactic levofloxacin for patients with expected duration of neutropenia (defined as an ANC less than 1,000/μL [1.00×10^9/L]) for more than 7 days because of the:

- Unknown long-term consequences on the development of resistant organisms
- Emergence of *Clostridium difficile* and methicillin-resistant *Staphylococcus aureus* (MRSA) from fluoroquinolone overuse
- Ability to treat lower risk patients on an outpatient basis[26–28]

Therefore, the use of prophylactic quinolones in patients who are at high risk for infection (i.e., hematologic malignancies) is reasonable; however, use should not be routine for low-risk patients. If prophylactic quinolone use is adopted, changes in local patterns of resistance should be closely monitored.

Colony-Stimulating Factors

The CSFs stimulate the maturation and differentiation of neutrophil precursors. Three agents are currently approved for use in the United States (Table 99–7). The prophylactic use of these agents decreases days of hospitalization and use of empiric antibiotics by shortening the duration of severe neutropenia (defined as ANC less than 500/μL [0.50×10^9/L]). There is little to no effect on the depth of neutrophil nadir. A recent meta-analysis found that the use of prophylactic granulocyte CSF (either filgrastim or pegfilgrastim) results in a 46% risk reduction of FN and a 48% risk reduction in infectious mortality, although absolute differences are small (3.3% versus 1.7%).[29] It is critical to note that patients who receive these agents may still experience FN despite the risk reduction. The primary limitation of the use of these agents is cost. Clinical practice guidelines for the use of CSFs have been developed by the NCCN.[23] These guidelines recommend the use of CSFs beginning with the first cycle (primary prophylaxis) of chemotherapy when the risk of FN is greater than or equal to 20%, regardless if the goal of therapy is curative or palliative. This is the point where the use of CSFs is cost effective when balanced against the cost of hospitalization and antimicrobials. Secondary prophylaxis refers to the subsequent prophylactic use of a CSF after a

Table 99–7

Overview of CSF

Agent	Effector Cell(s)	Dosage	Common Adverse Effects	Comments[a]
Filgrastim (Neupogen GCSF)	Neutrophil	5 mcg/kg/day SC or IV or round to 300- or 480-mcg vial size	Bone pain (approximately 25%)	Begin 1–3 days after chemotherapy
Pegfilgrastim (Neulasta)	Neutrophil	6 mg SC once	Bone pain (approximately 25%)	Self-mediated clearance via neutrophils Once per cycle dosing Administer 1–3 days after chemotherapy
Sargramostim (Leukine GM-CSF)	Neutrophil, eosinophil, macrophage	250 mcg/m²/day SC or IV or round to 250- or 500-mcg vial size	First dose effect (hypotension, flushing) Low-grade fever Bone pain Injection-site skin reaction	Indicated for use after induction chemotherapy in older patients with AML Limited experience and lack of FDA approval for prevention of FN

AML, acute myeloid leukemia; FDA, Food and Drug Administration; FN, febrile neutropenia; GC-SF, granulocyte-colony stimulating factor; GM-CSF, granulocyte-macrophage colony stimulating factor; SC, subcutaneous.

[a]No renal or hepatic dose adjustments are required for any product listed in this table.

From National Comprehensive Cancer Network [Internet]. Fort Washington, PA: National Comprehensive Cancer Network. Clinical practice guidelines in oncology: Myeloid growth factors. version, v.1.2011, accessed 10/4/2011. Available at: http://www.nccn.org/professionals/physician_gls/PDF/myeloid_growth.pdf.

patient has had an episode of FN. This strategy should be used especially when the chemotherapy is being given in patients with the intention of cure (i.e., Hodgkin's lymphoma, early breast cancer). In this circumstance, administration of full doses of chemotherapy on time without delays has been shown to improve patient outcomes.

Although generally well tolerated, CSFs may cause bone pain in around 25% of patients. This may be managed with acetaminophen or nonsteroidal anti-inflammatory drugs (NSAIDs), although attention to the platelet count is warranted with the use of NSAIDs. Sargramostim in particular may result in low-grade fever and myalgias, perhaps as a result of its wider pattern of effector cell stimulation.

TREATMENT

Desired Outcomes

Because rapid death may occur with certain infections in neutropenic patients, prompt and emergent treatment is indicated. The primary goal is to prevent morbidity and mortality during the neutropenic period. This is accomplished by effectively treating subclinical or established infections.

General Approach to Treatment

❸ *A risk assessment should be performed at presentation of FN to identify low-risk patients for potential outpatient treatment (see Table 99–6). Patients who do not meet low-risk criteria should be hospitalized for parenteral administration of broad-spectrum antibacterials.* The IDSA has published evidence-based guidelines for the management of FN (Fig. 99–1).[19,30] The choice of initial antimicrobial agent(s) depends on the following factors:

- Presence of a central venous catheter
- Drug allergies
- Concurrent renal dysfunction or use of nephrotoxic agents
- Use of prophylactic antibiotics
- Institutional and/or community susceptibility patterns
- Cost

❸ *The administration of empiric therapy should begin immediately after cultures are taken. Therapy should not be withheld until after culture results are obtained.*

As illustrated in Figure 99–1, specific criteria exist for the addition of vancomycin for coverage of resistant gram-positive organisms or agents for coverage of fungal infections. Additional agents are necessary in the setting of continued fever or declining clinical status in neutropenic patients. In general, all empiric therapy is continued until recovery of the ANC to levels above 500/μL (0.500 × 10⁹/L) cells in patients with negative culture results. If a specific etiology is identified, appropriate therapy should be continued until 7 days after neutropenia resolves. Specific regimens with recommended dosages are summarized in Table 99–8.

▶ Nonpharmacologic Therapy

Prevention of infection is key. Handwashing is critical in the prevention of disease transmission.[26] It is also important to ensure that patients receive annual influenza vaccines and have had a pneumonia vaccine, and neutropenic patients should avoid individuals with active respiratory infections.[31] Plants and animal secretions are also sources of infection and should be avoided.[31] Indwelling catheters are often sources of infection; however, the Infectious Disease Society of America acknowledges that catheters do not always need to be removed. Catheters should be removed in the following circumstances: established tunnel infection (subcutaneous tunnel or periport infection, septic emboli, hypotension associated with catheter use, or a nonpatent catheter), recurrent infection, or no response to antibiotics within 2 or 3 days.[19] Wound debridement should also be performed upon catheter removal. In the setting of peripheral blood stem cell or bone marrow transplant, the Centers for Disease Control and Prevention recommends the use of high-efficiency particulate air (HEPA) filtration systems in patient rooms, and the NCCN suggests that HEPA filters are reasonable to be considered for other patients who experience prolonged neutropenia.[26] HEPA filters are likely to be most useful in preventing mold infections. Although several small studies have attempted to evaluate the effectiveness of isolation of neutropenic patients as a mechanism for infection prevention, no clear data are available to support this practice.[31]

▶ Pharmacologic Therapy

There are two primary choices for the initial management of high-risk FN: monotherapy and dual therapy (see Fig. 99–1). Both regimens have been shown to be equivalent in randomized studies and meta-analyses. Monotherapy avoids the nephrotoxicity of the aminoglycosides and is potentially less expensive but lacks significant gram-positive coverage and may increase selection of resistant organisms. Dual therapy provides synergistic activity, decreased resistance, and dual coverage of *Pseudomonas aeruginosa* but requires therapeutic monitoring for aminoglycosides.

Vancomycin adds broad-spectrum gram-positive coverage; however, the increasing emergence of vancomycin-resistant organisms (i.e., *Enterococcus* spp.) prompts conservative use of this medication. Furthermore, the European Organization for the Research and Treatment of Cancer (EORTC) found that although empiric vancomycin decreased the number of days of fever, it did not improve survival, and it resulted in increased renal and hepatic toxicities.[32] Thus, vancomycin should only be included as part of the initial therapy in the following cases:

- Severe mucositis
- Soft tissue infection
- Quinolone or TMP-SMX prophylaxis
- Hypotension or septic shock
- Colonization with resistant gram-positive organisms (i.e., MRSA)
- Evidence of central venous catheter infection

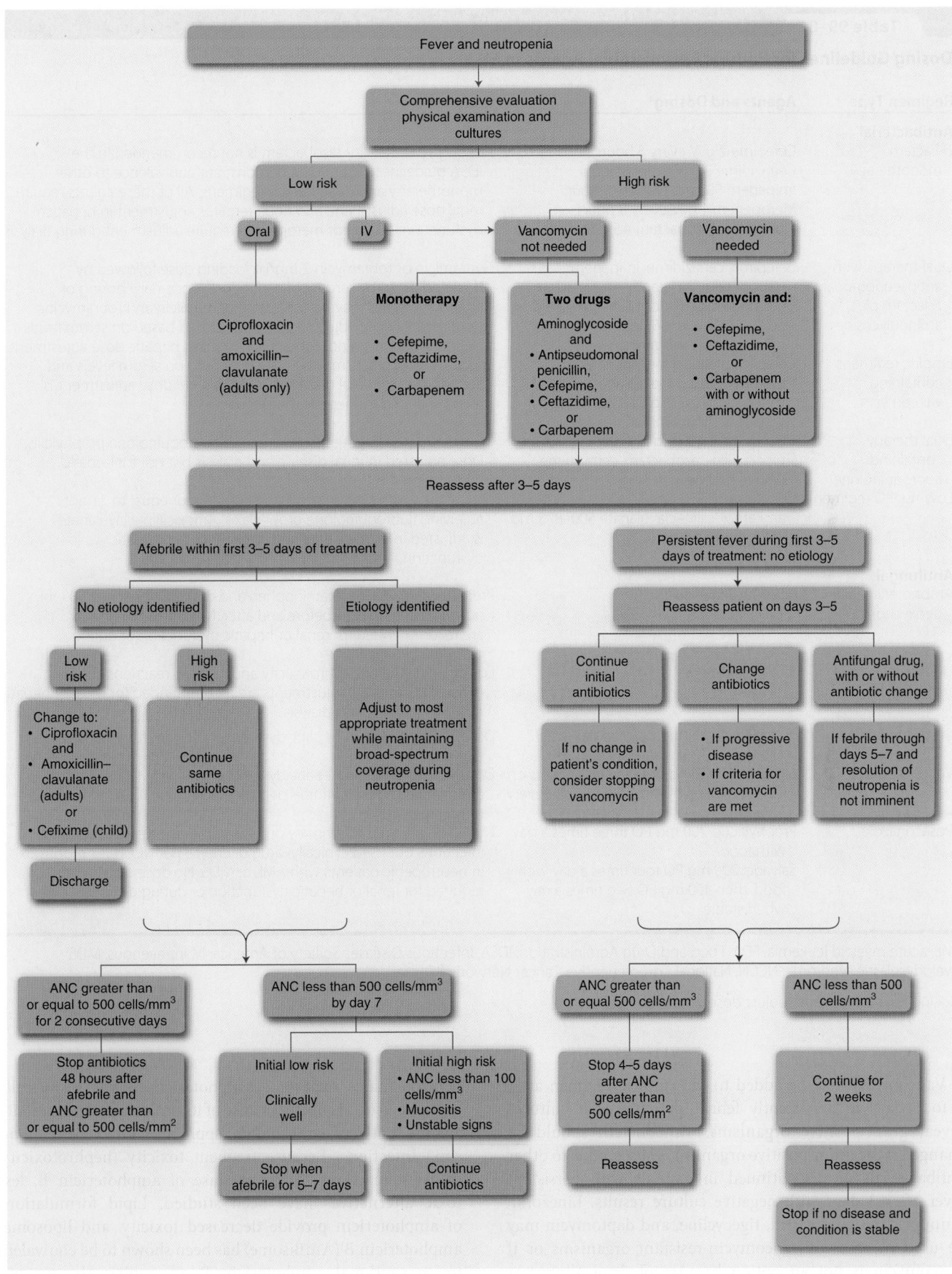

FIGURE 99–1. Management of febrile episodes in neutropenic cancer patients. (ANC, absolute neutrophil count.) (From Refs. 5 and 12.)

Table 99–8

Dosing Guidelines for Empiric Antimicrobial Agents in FN

Regimen Type	Agents and Dosing[a]	Comments
Antibacterial		
β-Lactam monotherapy	Cefepime 2 g IV every 8 hours Ceftazidime 2 g IV every 8 hours Imipenem 500 mg IV every 6 hours Meropenem 1 g IV every 8 hours Piperacillin–tazobactam 4.5 g IV every 8 hours	Although piperacillin–tazobactam is not recommended in the IDSA guidelines, recent data demonstrate equivalence to other monotherapy and dual therapy regimens. All of these agents require renal dose adjustment, and none requires adjustment in hepatic dysfunction. All except meropenem require adjustment during dialysis.
Dual therapy with antipseudomonal β-lactam plus aminoglycoside	Cefepime, ceftazidime, imipenem, meropenem, piperacillin–tazobactam (above dosages), ticarcillin–clavulanic acid 3.1 g IV every 6 hours and gentamicin or tobramycin	Gentamicin or tobramycin 2 mg/kg loading dose followed by doses adjusted by serum concentrations; once-daily dosing of aminoglycosides may be used. Both gentamicin and tobramycin require renal dose adjustment but are dosed based on serum levels. Neither gentamicin nor tobramycin requires hepatic dose adjustment.
Empiric regimens containing vancomycin	Cefepime, ceftazidime, imipenem, meropenem (above dosages) and vancomycin 0.5–1 g every 6–12 hours with or without aminoglycoside	Vancomycin dosages may be adjusted based on serum levels and are adjusted for renal disease and dialysis. No dose adjustment is recommended for hepatic dysfunction.
Dual therapy containing fluoroquinolone	Ciprofloxacin 400 mg IV every 8 hours and piperacillin–tazobactam, ceftazidime (above dosages)	Cannot be used in patients who receive fluoroquinolone prophylaxis. Dose adjusted in renal disease and dialysis but not for hepatic dysfunction.
Low-risk PO regimen	Ciprofloxacin 750 mg PO every 12 hours and amoxicillin–clavulanate 500–875 mg PO every 12 hours	For patients with MASCC scores greater than or equal to 21 not receiving fluoroquinolone prophylaxis. Amoxicillin–clavulanate is adjusted in renal disease and dialysis but not hepatic dysfunction.
Antifungal		
Amphotericin B deoxycholate	0.5–1 mg/kg IV daily	Premedication with acetaminophen and diphenhydramine; 500 mL normal saline boluses before and after. No dose adjustments are recommended for renal or hepatic dysfunction or during dialysis.
Liposomal amphotericin B	3 mg/kg IV daily	Lower incidence of nephrotoxicity and infusion reactions; more expensive. No dose adjustments are recommended for renal or hepatic dysfunction or during dialysis.
Caspofungin	70 mg/kg IV loading dose on day 1 followed by 50 mg/kg IV daily	Dosage adjustment in hepatic dysfunction but not for renal disease or dialysis.
Voriconazole	6 mg/kg IV loading dose every 12 hours on day 1 followed by 4 mg/kg PO or IV every 12 hours	Dosage adjustment in hepatic dysfunction; IV formulation contraindicated if creatinine clearance less than 50 mL/min; multiple drug interactions.
Posaconazole	Prophylactic: 200 mg PO three times a day with food Salvage: 200 mg PO four times a day with food; then 400 mg PO two times a day when stable	Not FDA approved for primary or salvage therapy for invasive fungal infections but used clinically; drug of choice per NCCN for prophylaxis in neutropenic patients with AML or MDS. No dose adjustments required for renal or hepatic dysfunction or during dialysis.

AML, acute myeloid leukemia; FDA, Food and Drug Administration; IDSA, Infectious Diseases Society of America; IV, intravenous; MDS; myelodysplastic syndrome; NCCN, National Comprehensive Cancer Network; PO, oral.

[a]Dosing for adult patients; adjust doses for renal dysfunction.

Vancomycin may be added to the empiric regimen after 3 to 5 days in persistently febrile patients or if cultures reveal gram-positive organisms. Vancomycin should be changed if the gram-positive organism is susceptible to other antibacterials or discontinued in patients with persistent fever after 3 days with negative culture results. Linezolid, quinupristin–dalfopristin, tigecycline, and daptomycin may be used in cases of vancomycin-resistant organisms or if vancomycin is not an option because of drug allergy or intolerance.

Empiric antifungal agents are typically added in persistently febrile patients after 5 to 7 days, especially if continued neutropenia is expected. Amphotericin B has historically been the drug of choice because of its broad-spectrum activity against both yeast (*Candida* spp.) and mold (*Aspergillus* spp.) infections. Because frequent toxicity (nephrotoxicity, infusion reactions) limits the use of amphotericin B, less toxic alternatives have been studied. Lipid formulations of amphotericin provide decreased toxicity, and liposomal amphotericin B (AmBisome) has been shown to be equivalent to conventional amphotericin B as empiric therapy but is significantly more expensive. The role of voriconazole is unclear at this time; however, caspofungin has been shown to be equivalent with less toxicity compared with liposomal amphotericin B in a randomized trial and is FDA approved for this indication.[33] Itraconazole has also been used in some institutions, but its use is complicated by poor bioavailability of oral preparations and numerous drug interactions. Posaconazole is a newer azole that is preferred by the NCCN for prophylactic use in neutropenic patients with acute myeloid leukemia or myelodysplastic syndrome and for patients with graft-versus-host disease while receiving intensive immunosuppressive therapy. It is not FDA approved as primary or salvage therapy for the treatment of invasive fungal infections but it is approved by the European Union for invasive aspergillosis and other fungal infections that are refractory to standard antifungal agents.

As stated earlier, low-risk patients fulfilling the MASCC criteria (see Table 99–6) may be treated empirically as an outpatient with a regimen combining amoxicillin–clavulanic acid and ciprofloxacin. Ciprofloxacin and clindamycin are reasonable alternatives for penicillin-allergic patients.

The CSF should not routinely be used for treatment of FN in conjunction with antimicrobial therapy.[19] However, the use of CSFs in certain high-risk patients with hypotension, documented fungal infection, pneumonia, or sepsis is reasonable. A recent meta-analysis demonstrated that hospitalization and neutrophil recovery are shortened and

infection-related mortality is marginally improved.[34] As with prophylactic use of these agents, cost considerations limit their use to high-risk patients.

OUTCOME EVALUATION

The success of the treatment of FN depends on the adequate recovery of the ANC and either optimal antimicrobial coverage of identified organisms or empiric coverage of unidentified organisms. Monitor the complete blood count (CBC) with differential and T_{max} (maximum temperature during previous 24 hours) daily. Assess renal and hepatic function at least twice weekly, especially in patients receiving nephrotoxic agents. Vital signs should be taken every 4 hours. Follow-up on blood and urine culture results daily because many cultures do not become positive for several days. Assess the patient daily for pain that may indicate an infectious source. Conduct daily physical examination of common sites of infection. Repeat cultures and chest x-ray in persistently febrile patients and culture developing sources of infection (i.e., stool cultures for diarrhea).

CARDIOVASCULAR COMPLICATIONS: SVCS

INTRODUCTION

Superior vena cava syndrome (SVCS) is a relatively rare complication that, although nonmalignant, may occur in patients with cancer. SVCS is rarely immediately life threatening except in patients with airway compromise and/ or laryngeal or cerebral edema. However, rapid recognition of typical presenting symptoms facilitates referral for tissue diagnosis (if unknown) and treatment.

EPIDEMIOLOGY AND ETIOLOGY

SVCS occurs in around 15,000 patients per year, 90% of which are caused by malignancy. Specific cancers most commonly associated with SVCS are listed in Table 99–9. Lung cancer is the most frequent cause, of which small cell lung cancer (SCLC) is the most frequent subtype associated

Patient Care and Monitoring: FN

1. Counsel patients receiving cytotoxic chemotherapy or alemtuzumab to promptly report fever. Provide patients with a diet to use during the neutropenic period. Counsel patients to avoid close contact with sick friends and relatives and remind patients and caregivers of the importance of handwashing.

2. If FN occurs, patient history is important:
   a. What chemotherapy did the patient receive and when? Is the ANC on the way down (before nadir) or on the way up (after nadir)? Was the patient receiving prophylactic antibiotics, filgrastim, sargramostim, or pegfilgrastim?
   b. Did the patient have previous episodes of FN? What were the previous culture results to determine colonization status?

3. Assess the patient daily for any new signs or symptoms of infection. Evaluate the patient for adverse drug reactions, drug allergies, and interactions. Have all antibiotics been dose adjusted for renal or hepatic dysfunction?

4. For patients receiving oral antibiotics either prophylactically or as treatment of FN: Counsel patients that initial or persistent fever should be promptly reported and that compliance with the regimen is critical. Patients should also have easy access to medical care and adequate caregiver support. Provide information on drug interactions and adverse effects.

Table 99–9

Tumors Most Commonly Associated With SVCS

Cause	Frequency (%)
Non–small cell lung cancer	50
Small cell lung cancer	22
Lymphoma	12
Metastatic cancer (especially breast)	9
Germ cell tumor	3
Thymoma	2
Mesothelioma	1

From Wilson LD, Detterbeck FC, Yahalom J. Superior vena cava syndrome with malignant causes. N Engl J Med 2007;356(8):1862–1869.

with SVCS. This is thought to be because of its predilection for the central and perihilar areas of the lung. Interestingly, right-sided lung cancers are four times more likely than left-sided lesions to cause SVCS. Mediastinal masses from lymphomas are the second most common cause.

The most common nonmalignant etiology of SVCS is catheter-related thrombosis, primarily caused by the increasing use of central access devices. Other causes include benign teratoma, tuberculosis, silicosis, and sarcoidosis.

PATHOPHYSIOLOGY

The SVC is the primary drainage vein for blood return from the head, neck, and upper extremities. It is a relatively thin-walled vein that is particularly vulnerable to obstruction from adjacent tumor invasion or thrombosis. The obstruction leads to elevated venous pressure, although collateral veins partially compensate. This is one reason for the relatively slow onset of the classic symptoms of SVCS. In fact, 75% of patients have signs and symptoms for more than 1 week before seeking medical attention.[35]

CLINICAL PRESENTATION AND DIAGNOSIS

Visible swelling of the face, neck, chest, and upper limbs with obvious venous distention are the usual presenting symptoms of SVCS.[35] Patients may also report coughing, hoarseness, sleep disturbances, dyspnea, headache, and confusion.[35] Diagnosis is made with consideration of these symptoms in conjunction with imaging studies that show unusual narrowing of the upper airway.[35]

TREATMENT

Desired Outcomes

④ *The primary goal of treatment of SVCS is to relieve the obstruction of the SVC by treating the underlying malignancy.* In the case of SVCS caused by thrombosis, the goal is to eliminate the thrombus and prevent further clot formation. Resolution of the obstruction will rapidly relieve symptoms and restore normal SVC function. The final goal of therapy is to avoid potentially fatal complications of SVCS such as cerebral edema from rapid increases in intracranial pressure (ICP) and intracranial thrombosis or bleeding.

General Approach to Treatment

Because the majority of SVCS is not immediately life threatening, a tissue diagnosis (if malignancy is unknown) to specifically identify the cancer origin is critical because treatment approaches vary considerably according to tumor histology. Thus, therapy can typically be withheld until a definitive tissue diagnosis is established. While biopsy results are pending, supportive measures such as head elevation, diuretics, corticosteroids, and supplemental oxygen may be used.

Clinical Presentation and Diagnosis of SVCS

General

- Presentation depends on the degree of SVCS obstruction
- Almost complete obstruction is necessary to demonstrate classic symptoms

Signs and Symptoms

- Most common: face, neck, and upper extremity edema; dyspnea; cough; dilated upper extremity veins; orthopnea
- Less common: hoarseness, dysphagia, dizziness, headache, lethargy, chest pain
- Patients with elevated ICP may have mental status changes.
- Patients with airway obstruction may have shortness of breath.

Diagnostic Tests

- Tissue biopsy to determine underlying malignancy (if unknown), chest x-ray, CT scan, bronchoscopy, mediastinoscopy

---

▶ *Nonpharmacologic Therapy*

Radiation therapy is the treatment of choice for chemotherapy-resistant tumors such as NSCLC or in chemotherapy-refractory patients with SVCS. Between 70% and 90% of patients experience relief of symptoms. Radiation therapy may also be combined with chemotherapy for chemotherapy-sensitive tumors such as SCLC and lymphoma. In the rare emergency situations of airway obstruction or elevated ICP, empiric radiotherapy before tissue diagnosis should be used. In most patients, symptoms resolve within 1 to 3 weeks.

Surgical options for the management of SVCS include stent placement and surgical bypass. SVC stenting may provide longer term relief of symptoms than radiotherapy, so it is often used in the palliative care setting when chemotherapy has failed.[36] One disadvantage of SVC stenting is the need for anticoagulation, especially in patients at high risk for thrombosis. The role of surgical bypass is limited to patients with complete SVC obstruction or patients who are refractory to chemotherapy and radiotherapy; thus, it is rarely indicated.

▶ *Pharmacologic Therapy*

Cytotoxic chemotherapy is the treatment of choice for chemotherapy-sensitive tumors such as SCLC and lymphoma. As indicated earlier, chemotherapy may also be combined with radiotherapy, especially in patients with lymphoma who have bulky mediastinal lymphadenopathy.

Corticosteroids play a key role in the management of SVCS, particularly in cases of lymphoma, because these tumors inherently respond to corticosteroid therapy. They are also helpful in the setting of respiratory compromise. Corticosteroids benefit patients who are receiving radiation therapy by reduction of local radiation-induced inflammation and patients with increased ICP. Dexamethasone 4 mg IV or by mouth every 6 hours is a frequently used regimen. The dosage should be tapered upon completion of radiation therapy or resolution of symptoms.

The role of diuretics in the management of SVCS is controversial. Although patients may derive symptomatic relief from edema, complications such as dehydration and reduced venous blood flow may exacerbate the condition. If diuretics are used, furosemide is most frequently used with diligent monitoring of the patient's fluid status and blood pressure.

In the case of thrombosis-related SVCS, anticoagulation is controversial because there is a lack of survival benefit. However, thrombolytics (i.e., alteplase) and anticoagulation with heparin and warfarin may be beneficial in patients with thrombosis caused by indwelling catheters if used within 7 days of onset of symptoms, although catheter removal may be required.

OUTCOME EVALUATION

The major measure of outcome of treatment of SVCS is the relief of symptoms, regardless of the therapy used.

NEUROLOGIC COMPLICATIONS: SPINAL CORD COMPRESSION

INTRODUCTION

Although not typically life threatening, spinal cord compression is a true oncologic emergency because delays in treatment by mere hours may lead to permanent neurologic dysfunction. Practitioners must quickly recognize the signs and symptoms of this condition to facilitate rapid management strategies.

EPIDEMIOLOGY AND ETIOLOGY

Around 20,000 cancer patients experience spinal cord compression in the United States every year, most of which involves the thoracic spine (approximately 70%). Cancers that inherently metastasize to the bone (i.e., breast, prostate, and lung) are the most frequent underlying malignancies associated with this complication. Most spinal cord compression occurs in patients with a known malignancy; however, 8% to 34% of cases occur as the initial presentation of cancer, especially in patients with non-Hodgkin's lymphoma, multiple myeloma, and lung cancer.[37]

PATHOPHYSIOLOGY

The spinal cord emerges from the brain stem at the base of the skull and terminates at the second lumbar vertebra. The thoracic spine is most vulnerable to cord compression because of natural kyphosis and because the width of the thoracic spinal canal is the smallest among the vertebrae. Most spinal cord compression is caused by adjacent vertebral metastases that compress the spinal cord or from pathologic compression fracture of the vertebra. This results in significant edema and inflammation in the affected area.

Patients with spinal cord compression are in acute, severe back and/or neck pain and may present to the emergency department for evaluation. Diagnosis is made based on symptoms and imaging studies that show fractured vertebrae.

TREATMENT

Desired Outcomes

⑤ *Because patients with spinal metastases are generally incurable, the primary goal of treatment of spinal cord compression is palliation. The most important prognostic factor for patients presenting with spinal cord compression is the degree of underlying neurologic dysfunction.* Only around 10% of patients who present with paralysis are able to ambulate after treatment.[37] Therefore, the goals of treatment are recovery of normal neurologic function, local tumor control, pain control, and stabilization of the spine. Therapeutic options depend primarily on the following factors:

- Underlying malignancy
- Prior therapies
- Stability of the spine at presentation
- Overall patient prognosis

▶ Nonpharmacologic Therapy

Radiation therapy is generally considered to be the treatment of choice for most patients. Exceptions to this include patients with prior radiation to the treatment site and patients with inherently radio-resistant tumors (i.e., melanoma, renal cell carcinoma). The radiation field should include two vertebral bodies above and below the involved area.

Surgery for spinal cord compression typically involves either laminectomy for posterior lesions or decompression with fixation. Surgery is the treatment of choice for the following patients: (a) patients with unstable spine requiring stabilization, (b) immediately impending sphincter dysfunction requiring rapid spinal decompression, (c) patients who do not respond to or have received their maximum dose of radiotherapy, and (d) direct compression of the spinal cord caused by spinal bony fragments.[37] Recent evidence suggests that surgery followed by radiation therapy may be superior to radiotherapy alone in terms of increased ambulation time after treatment, maintenance of continence, and rates of nonambulatory patients becoming ambulatory.[38] Surgery is also useful for establishing a tissue diagnosis in cases of unknown malignancy. Overall, the risks and benefits of surgery must be weighed against the expected prognosis of the patient in light of the significant rehabilitation required after surgery.

▶ Pharmacologic Therapy

Corticosteroids play a vital role in the management of spinal cord compression. Dexamethasone is most frequently used to reduce edema, inhibit inflammation, and delay the

---

> ### Patient Care and Monitoring: Spinal Cord Compression
>
> Monitor patients for:
>
> 1. Improved symptoms of sensory loss using physical exam every 4 hours until symptoms improve then daily
> 2. Improved autonomic system function, including urine and bowel control, every 4 hours until symptoms improve; then daily
> 3. Improved pain control using detailed pain assessment every 2 to 4 hours during initial titration then daily thereafter
> 4. For corticosteroid use: serum glucose, insomnia, fluid retention, GI upset, mental status changes, signs and symptoms of infection daily

---

onset of neurologic complications. Dexamethasone has been shown to improve ambulation in combination with radiation compared with radiation alone.[39] Significant controversy exists regarding the optimal dosing of dexamethasone. Oral loading doses of 10 to 100 mg followed by 4 to 24 mg orally four times daily have been used. Higher doses may be used in cases of rapidly progressing symptoms, but adverse effects, including GI bleeding and psychosis, are more severe. Steroids should be continued during radiation therapy and then tapered appropriately.

Pain management is also of critical importance in patients with spinal cord compression. Although dexamethasone will provide some benefit, opioid analgesics should also be used and titrated rapidly to achieve adequate pain control.

OUTCOME EVALUATION

Patients who receive definitive treatment with radiation and/ or surgery generally derive benefit within days.

COMPLICATIONS OF BRAIN METASTASES

INTRODUCTION

Brain metastases are among the most feared complications of cancer and generally carry a poor prognosis. One serious consequence of brain metastases is elevated ICP, which can rapidly lead to fatal intracranial herniation and death. Rapid identification of the signs and symptoms of brain metastases is critical to improve long-term outcome and avoid mortality. The signs and symptoms of brain metastasis can be confused with common psychological distress or other neurologic problems (e.g., headaches) that may go unrecognized. It is important that patients who are suspected to have brain metastasis are quickly referred for appropriate management.

EPIDEMIOLOGY AND ETIOLOGY

Brain metastasis is the most common neurologic complication seen in patients with cancer. Approximately 170,000 patients develop brain metastases in the United States each year.[40] Many malignancies are frequently associated with brain metastases (Table 99–10). Although melanoma is the tumor type most likely to metastasize to the brain, brain metastases caused by lung and breast cancer are seen more often because they are among the most common cancers. In addition, brain metastases may be diagnosed at the same time as the primary malignancy in around 20% of cases.[41] Around 80% of brain metastases occur in the cerebral hemispheres, 15% in the cerebellum, and 5% in the brain stem.

PATHOPHYSIOLOGY

A delicate balance of normal pressure is maintained in the brain and spinal cord by brain, blood, and cerebrospinal fluid. Because the brain is contained within a confined space (skull), any foreign mass contained within that space causes adverse sequelae. This results in either destruction or displacement of normal brain tissue with associated edema. Most brain metastases occur through hematogenous spread of the primary tumor and around 80% of patients have multiple sites of metastases within the brain.

CLINICAL PRESENTATION AND DIAGNOSIS

Patients with brain metastases may have no symptoms. Alternatively, they may have severe headaches, vision changes, and personality or mood disturbances depending on the location of the metastasis. Diagnosis is made based on physical signs and symptoms and brain computed tomography (CT) or magnetic resonance imaging (MRI) indicating a mass.

TREATMENT

Desired Outcomes

Therapeutic modalities used for the management of brain metastases may be divided into symptomatic management

Table 99–10

Cancers Most Frequently Associated With Brain Metastases

Type of Cancer	Frequency (%)
Lung cancer	18–64
Breast cancer	2–21
Melanoma	4–16
Colorectal cancer	2–11
Hematologic malignancies (i.e., leukemia)	Approximately 10 (primarily caused by leptomeningeal spread)

From Lassman AB, DeAngelis LM. Brain metastases. Neurol Clin North Am 2003;21:1–23.

Clinical Presentation and Diagnosis of Brain Metastasis

General

- Almost all patients with brain metastases are symptomatic.
- New cerebral neurologic symptoms in a cancer patient should initiate evaluation for brain metastases.
- Other causes of brain lesions, including hemorrhage, infection, and infarct, should be ruled out.

Signs and Symptoms

- Mental status changes (most common): loss of consciousness, irritability, confusion
- Hemiparesis, aphasia, papilledema, weakness, seizure, nausea, and vomiting
- Headache: may be of gradual onset or sudden in the case of hemorrhage

Diagnostic Tests

- MRI with contrast enhancement is the gold standard.
- CT scans may be used in patients with pacemakers, but may miss small metastases.

---

and definitive management. ❻ *The goals of treatment of brain metastases are to manage symptoms by reducing cerebral edema, treat the underlying malignancy both locally and systemically, and improve survival.*

General Approach to Treatment

Patients with brain metastases have a poor prognosis. Untreated patients generally have a median survival of 1 month. The choice of treatment depends primarily on the status of the patient's underlying malignancy and the number and sites of brain metastases. The primary definitive treatments for brain metastases are surgery and radiation therapy. Pharmacologic modalities are primarily used to control symptoms, although cytotoxic chemotherapy plays a limited role in the management.

▶ Nonpharmacologic Therapy

Radiation therapy is the treatment of choice for most patients with brain metastases. Most patients receive whole-brain radiation because the majority of brain metastases are multifocal. Another method known as stereotactic radiosurgery provides intense focal radiation, typically using a **linear accelerator** or **gamma knife**, in patients who cannot tolerate surgery or have lesions that are surgically inaccessible (i.e., brain stem). Because brain metastases can occur in up to 50% of patients with small cell lung cancer, prophylactic cranial irradiation is recommended in patients with good performance status who at least partially respond to chemotherapy to both prevent the development of brain metastases and to prolong survival.[42] Although other cancers can metastasize to the brain, the benefits of routine prophylactic cranial irradiation have only been demonstrated in studies conducted in patients with small cell lung cancer.[42]

Surgery plays a key role in the management of patients with brain metastases, particularly in patients whose systemic disease is well controlled and in patients with solitary lesions. Surgery may also benefit patients with multiple metastatic sites who have a single dominant lesion with current or impending neurologic sequelae.

In cases of elevated ICP caused by cerebral herniation, mechanical hyperventilation to decrease the arterial P_{CO_2} down to 25 mm Hg (3.33 kPa) acutely decreases ICP by causing cerebral vasoconstriction. Elevation of the patient's bed may also quickly reduce the ICP. It should be noted that these strategies only relieve symptoms, and definitive therapy is still required.

▶ Pharmacologic Therapy

Corticosteroids are a mainstay in the management of brain metastases. They reduce edema that typically surrounds sites of metastases thereby reducing ICP. A loading dose of dexamethasone 10 mg IV followed by 4 mg by mouth or IV every 6 hours is typically used. Symptom relief may occur shortly after the loading dose, although the maximum benefit may not be seen for several days (after definitive therapy).

Mannitol is an agent that may be used in patients with impending cerebral herniation. Mannitol is an osmotic diuretic that shifts brain osmolarity from the brain to the blood. Doses of 100 g (1 to 2 g/kg) as an IV bolus should be used. Repeated doses are typically not recommended because mannitol may diffuse into brain tissue, leading to rebound increased ICP.[43]

Twenty percent of patients with brain metastases may present with seizures and require anticonvulsant therapy. Phenytoin is the most frequently used agent with a loading

dose of 15 mg/kg followed by 300 mg by mouth daily (titrated to therapeutic levels between 10 and 20 mcg/mL [40 and 79 μmol/L]). Diazepam 5 mg IV may be used for rapid control of persistent seizures. Prophylactic anticonvulsants have frequently been used; however, a recent metaanalysis did not support their use.[44] Thus, because adverse effects and drug interactions are common, the routine use of prophylactic anticonvulsants is not recommended.

OUTCOME EVALUATION

The success of therapy is based on the ability to decrease symptoms, treat the underlying sites of disease within the brain, and prolong survival.

UROLOGIC COMPLICATIONS: HEMORRHAGIC CYSTITIS

INTRODUCTION

Hemorrhagic cystitis is defined as acute or insidious bleeding from the lining of the bladder. Although therapy with certain medications is the most common cause, it is also the most preventable. Once it occurs, hemorrhagic cystitis causes significant morbidity and mortality rates between 2% and 4%. This section focuses on preventive strategies for chemotherapeutic agents, which rely heavily on pharmacotherapeutic approaches.

EPIDEMIOLOGY AND ETIOLOGY

Numerous etiologies have been linked to hemorrhagic cystitis (Table 99–11).[45] Of these, the oxazaphosphorine alkylating agents (cyclophosphamide and ifosfamide) are most frequently implicated. Incidence rates vary considerably but generally range between 18% and 40% with ifosfamide and 0.5% to 40% with high-dose cyclophosphamide in the absence of prophylactic measures.[46] Chronic, low-dose oral cyclophosphamide as typically used in autoimmune disorders and chronic lymphocytic leukemia is also infrequently associated with hemorrhagic cystitis.

Patient Care and Monitoring: Brain Metastasis

1. Assess the patient's symptoms for prompt referral for radiation or surgery.

2. For patients receiving corticosteroids, monitor for adverse effects and drug interactions. Does the patient need GI prophylaxis for long-term treatment? Slowly taper once symptoms improve and/or radiation or surgery is completed.

3. Evaluate the patient for drug interactions, allergies, and adverse effects with phenytoin or corticosteroid therapy.

4. Instruct patients receiving phenytoin about symptoms of elevated serum concentrations (nystagmus, blurred vision, dizziness, drowsiness, lethargy).

5. Provide patient education regarding when to take medications and the importance of compliance and to promptly report symptoms of recurrence (mental status changes, seizures).

Table 99–11	
Primary Causes of Hemorrhagic Cystitis	
Pharmacologic	**Nonpharmacologic**
Cyclophosphamide	Pelvic irradiation
Chronic low doses	Viral infection
High-doses used in BMT	CMV
Ifosfamide	Papovavirus
Intravesicular thiotepa	Herpes simplex virus
Chronic oral busulfan	Adenovirus
Anabolic steroids	

BMT, bone marrow transplantation; CMV, cytomegalovirus.

From West NJ. Prevention and treatment of hemorrhagic cystitis. Pharmacotherapy 1997;17:696–706.

Twenty percent of patients receiving pelvic irradiation may experience hemorrhagic cystitis, especially with concurrent cyclophosphamide. Viral infections commonly associated with this condition most frequently occur in bone marrow transplant recipients who may also receive cyclophosphamide.

PATHOPHYSIOLOGY

Cyclophosphamide- or ifosfamide-induced damage to the bladder wall is primarily caused by their shared metabolite known as acrolein. Acrolein causes sloughing and inflammation of the bladder lining, leading to bleeding and hemorrhage. This is most common when urine output is low because higher concentrations of acrolein come into contact with the bladder urothelium for longer periods of time.

CLINICAL PRESENTATION AND DIAGNOSIS

● Patients with hemorrhagic cystitis from treatment may present with dysuria, anuria, or hematuria. Diagnosis is made based on symptoms and urinalysis, which shows the presence of red blood cells in the urine.

PREVENTION

❼ *The use of effective prevention strategies can decrease the incidence of hemorrhagic cystitis to fewer than 5% in patients receiving cyclophosphamide or ifosfamide. Three methods are used to reduce the risk: administration of Mesna (2-mercaptoethane sulfonate), hyperhydration, and bladder irrigation with catheterization.* Mesna is the primary method used with ifosfamide; all three strategies are used with cyclophosphamide.

Mesna is a thiol compound that is rapidly oxidized in the bloodstream after administration to dimesna, which is inactive. However, after being filtered through the kidneys, dimesna is reduced back to Mesna, which binds to acrolein, leading to inactivation and excretion. The American Society of Clinical Oncology (ASCO) has published evidence-based guidelines for the dosing and administration of Mesna (Table 99–12).[46] The dose of oral Mesna must be double the IV dose because of oral bioavailability between 40% and 50%. Because the half-life of Mesna (approximately 1.2 hours) is much shorter than that of ifosfamide or cyclophosphamide, prolonged administration of Mesna beyond the end of the chemotherapy infusion is critical (Fig. 99–2). Patients should receive at least 2 L of IV fluids beginning 12 to 24 hours before and ending 24 to 48 hours after the last dose of chemotherapy.

Hyperhydration with normal saline at 3 L/m²/day with IV furosemide to maintain urine output greater than 100 mL/h has also been used with cyclophosphamide. Continuous bladder irrigation by catheterization uses normal saline at 250 to 1,000 mL/h to flush acrolein from the bladder. Mesna is equivalent to both strategies in patients receiving high-dose cyclophosphamide and avoids the discomfort and infection risk with catheterization and the intensity of hyperhydration. Thus, Mesna is the preventive method of choice.

TREATMENT

Desired Outcomes

If hemorrhagic cystitis occurs, the goals of treatment are to decrease exposure to the offending etiology, establish and maintain urine outflow, avoid obstruction and renal compromise, and maintain blood and plasma volume. Restoration of normal bladder function is the ultimate goal following acute treatment.

General Approach to Treatment

The treatment of hemorrhagic cystitis first involves discontinuation of the offending agent. Agents such as anticoagulants and inhibitors of platelet function should also be discontinued. IV fluids should be aggressively administered to irrigate the bladder. Blood and platelet transfusions may be necessary to maintain normal hematologic values. Pain should be managed with opioid analgesics. Local intravesicular therapies may be necessary if hematuria does not resolve (Fig. 99–3).

► Nonpharmacologic Therapy

A large-diameter, multihole urethral catheter should be inserted to facilitate saline lavage and evacuation of blood clots. Surgical removal of blood clots under anesthesia may be required if saline lavage is ineffective. Active bleeding

---

Clinical Presentation and Diagnosis of Urologic Complications

General

- Presentation may be mild (microscopic hematuria) or severe (massive hemorrhage) and develops during or shortly after chemotherapy infusion.

Signs and Symptoms

- Suprapubic pain and cramping, urinary urgency and frequency, dysuria and burning, hematuria
- Urinary retention leading to hydronephrosis and renal failure may occur if large blood clots obstruct the ureters or bladder outlet.

Laboratory Tests

- Urine dipsticks for blood
- Urinalysis reveals more than 3 RBCs per high-power field: microscopic hematuria
- CBC with differential, prothrombin time or international normalized ratio, activated partial thromboplastin time, blood urea nitrogen, creatinine

Table 99–12

ASCO Guidelines for the Use of Mesna With Ifosfamide and High-Dose Cyclophosphamide

Chemotherapy Schedule	Dosing Schedule for Mesna	Comments
Low-dose ifosfamide 2 g/m²/day	Oral: 100% of total daily dose of ifosfamide given 20% IV 15 minutes before and 40% PO 2 and 6 hours after start of ifosfamide	Available in 400-mg tablets Peak urinary thiol concentrations with oral Mesna is at 3 hours If patient vomits within 2 hours of administration, repeat dose PO or IV
Standard-dose ifosfamide 2.5 g/m²/day	Bolus: 60% of total daily dose of ifosfamide given IV in 20% increments 15 minutes before and 4 and 8 hours after start of ifosfamide Infusion: 60% of total daily dose of ifosfamide given 20% IV 15 minutes before and 40% by continuous infusion during and for 12–24 hours after end of ifosfamide	Peak urinary thiol concentrations with IV Mesna is at 1 hour Compatible with ifosfamide and cyclophosphamide by Y-site administration or when admixed in the same bag
High-dose ifosfamide greater than 2.5 g/m²/day	Lack of evidence for dosing, but higher doses for longer duration recommended based on longer half-life of ifosfamide at high doses	
Standard-dose cyclophosphamide	Use of Mesna is not routinely necessary	Should be combined with saline diuresis (1.5 L/m²/day of normal saline)
High-dose cyclophosphamide (BMT)	Bolus: 40% of cyclophosphamide dose given IV at hours 0, 3, 6, and 9 after cyclophosphamide Infusion: 100% of cyclophosphamide dose given by continuous infusion until 24 hours after cyclophosphamide	

ASCO, American Society of Clinical Oncology; BMT, bone marrow transplantation; IV, intravenous; Mesna, 2-mercaptoethane sulfonate; PO, oral.

From Schuchter LM, Hensley ML, Meropol NJ, et al. 2002 Update of recommendations for the use of chemotherapy and radiotherapy protectants: Clinical practice guidelines of the American Society of Clinical Oncology. J Clin Oncol 2002;20:2895–2903.

from isolated areas may be cauterized with an electrode or laser. In severe cases that are unresponsive to local or systemic pharmacologic intervention, urinary diversion with percutaneous nephrostomy or surgical removal of the bladder may be required.

▶ Pharmacologic Therapy

A number of local or systemic agents are used in the treatment of hemorrhagic cystitis.[45] Local (direct instillation into the bladder), one-time administration of hemostatic agents

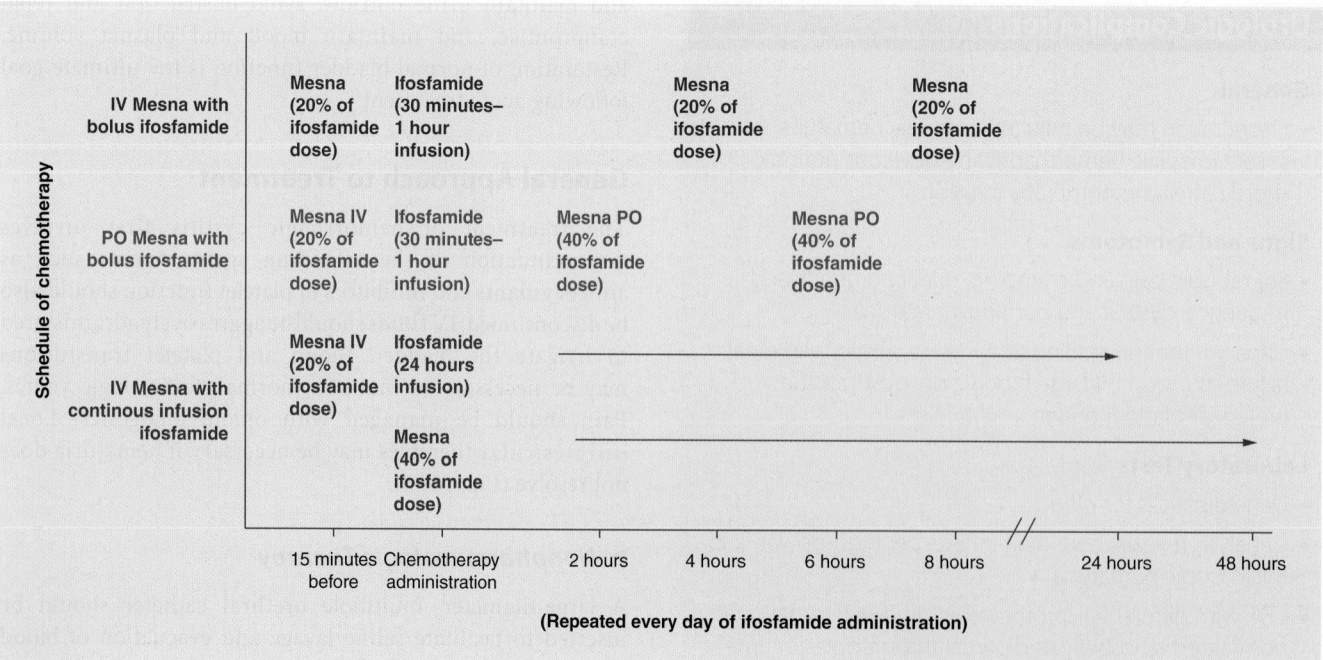

FIGURE 99–2. Examples of Mesna (2-mercaptoethane sulfonate) administration with ifosfamide. (IV, intravenous; PO, oral.)

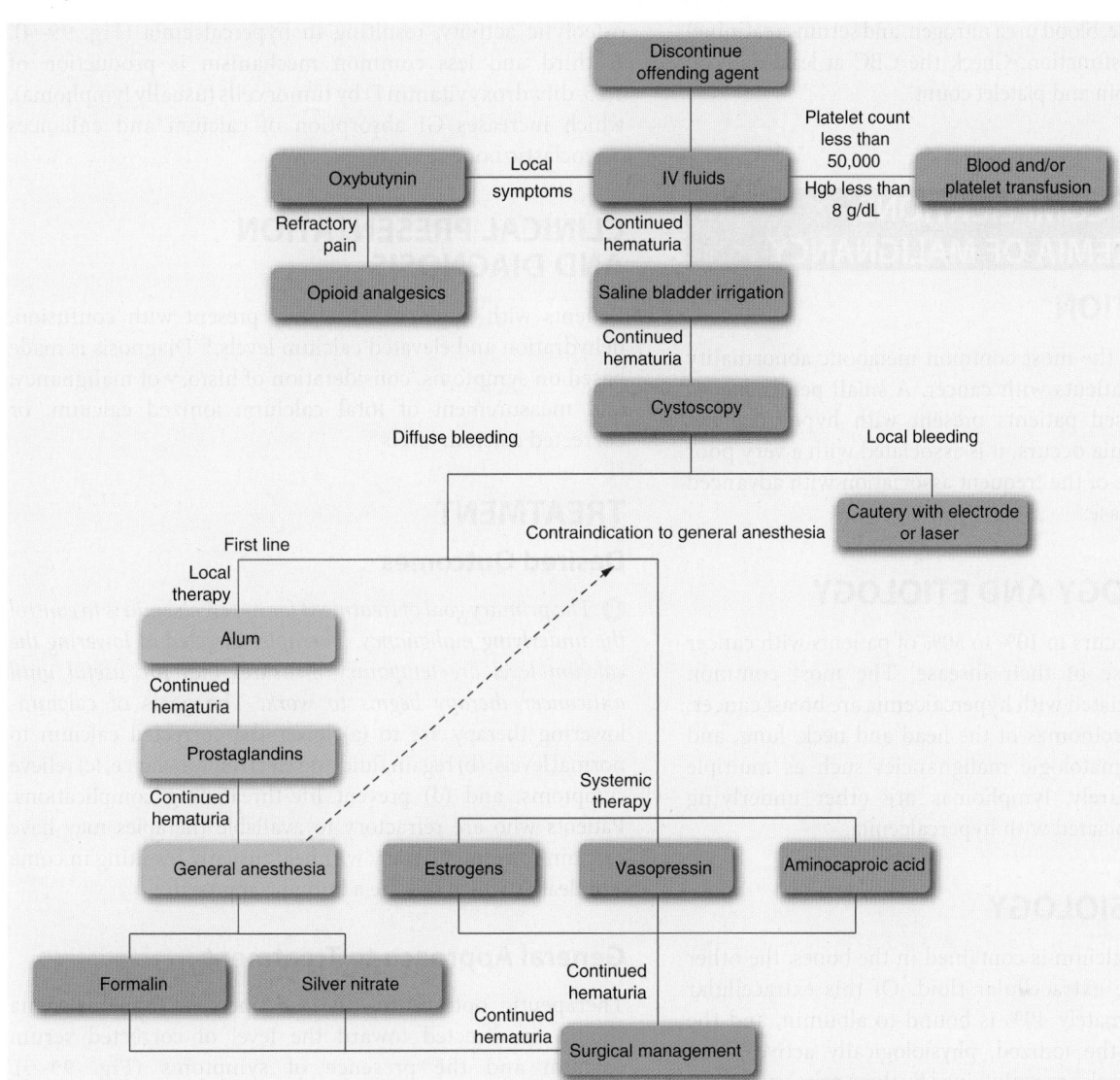

FIGURE 99–3. Treatment of hemorrhagic cystitis. (From Bucavene G, Micuzzi A, Menichetti F, et al. Levofloxacin to prevent bacterial infection in patients with cancer and neutropenia. N Engl J Med 2005;353: 977–987.)

such as alum, prostaglandins, silver nitrate, and formalin may be used; however, general anesthesia is required, especially with formalin, because of pain. Systemic agents, including estrogens, vasopressin, and aminocaproic acid, may be used in patients who are refractory to local therapy, although they introduce the risk of systemic side effects. These agents should be continued until bleeding stops.

Antispasmodic agents such as oxybutynin 5 mg by mouth two to three times daily may be used for bladder spasms. In patients with refractory pain, opioid analgesics should be titrated to adequate pain control.

OUTCOME EVALUATION

The goal of treatment is resolution of bladder symptoms and appropriate pain management.

Monitor the patient for resolution of hematuria after each successive therapeutic intervention. The frequency of monitoring is based on the severity of hemorrhaging. Monitor urinary output and serum chemistries (including sodium,

---

Patient Care and Monitoring: Urologic Complications

1. Assess the patient receiving ifosfamide or cyclophosphamide at least daily for the development of hematuria.

2. Ensure administration of adequate hydration and proper doses of Mesna.

3. Counsel patient receiving oral Mesna on the importance of compliance, when to take doses, and to immediately report any episodes of vomiting for IV readministration.

4. Assess the quantity of urinary bleeding and promptly refer to a urologist for local or surgical management.

5. Patients receiving systemic treatment should be monitored every 4 hours for resolution of hematuria. Promptly refer to urologist for refractory hematuria.

6. Evaluate the patient for drug interactions, allergies, and adverse effects with chemotherapy, Mesna, or systemic therapies for management.

potassium, chloride, blood urea nitrogen, and serum creatinine) daily for renal dysfunction. Check the CBC at least daily to monitor hemoglobin and platelet count.

METABOLIC COMPLICATIONS: HYPERCALCEMIA OF MALIGNANCY

INTRODUCTION

Hypercalcemia is the most common metabolic abnormality experienced by patients with cancer. A small percentage of as yet undiagnosed patients present with hypercalcemia. Once hypercalcemia occurs, it is associated with a very poor prognosis because of the frequent association with advanced or metastatic disease.[47]

EPIDEMIOLOGY AND ETIOLOGY

Hypercalcemia occurs in 10% to 30% of patients with cancer during the course of their disease. The most common tumor types associated with hypercalcemia are breast cancer; squamous cell carcinomas of the head and neck, lung, and renal cancer. Hematologic malignancies such as multiple myeloma and, rarely, lymphomas are other underlying malignancies associated with hypercalcemia.

PATHOPHYSIOLOGY

Around 99% of calcium is contained in the bones; the other 1% resides in the extracellular fluid. Of this extracellular calcium, approximately 40% is bound to albumin, and the remainder is in the ionized, physiologically active form. Normal calcium levels are maintained by three primary factors: parathyroid hormone (PTH), 1,25-dihydroxyvitamin D, and calcitonin. PTH increases renal tubular calcium resorption and promotes bone resorption. The active form of vitamin D, 1,25-dihydroxyvitamin D, regulates absorption of calcium from the GI tract. Calcitonin serves as an inhibitory factor by suppressing osteoclast activity and stimulating calcium deposition into the bones.

The delicate balance maintained by these factors is altered in patients with cancer by two principal mechanisms: tumor production of humoral factors that alter calcium metabolism (humoral hypercalcemia) and by local osteolytic activity from bone metastases.[48] Humoral hypercalcemia causes around 80% of all hypercalcemia cases and is primarily mediated by systemic secretion of PTH-related protein (PTHrP). This protein mimics the action of endogenous PTH on bones. Local osteolytic activity causes 20% to 30% of hypercalcemia cases, although local osteolytic activity may also have a humoral component. Local production of various factors directly stimulates osteoclastic bone resorption, which releases growth factors and cytokines (i.e., transforming growth factor-β) that are necessary for tumor growth. Thus, these metastatic tumors perpetuate their own growth through this mechanism. Calcium is also released by the

osteolytic activity, resulting in hypercalcemia (Fig. 99–4). A third and less common mechanism is production of 1,25-dihydroxyvitamin D by tumor cells (usually lymphoma), which increases GI absorption of calcium and enhances osteoclastic bone resorption.

CLINICAL PRESENTATION AND DIAGNOSIS

Patients with hypercalcemia may present with confusion, dehydration and elevated calcium levels.[47] Diagnosis is made based on symptoms, consideration of history of malignancy, and measurement of total calcium, ionized calcium, or corrected calcium levels.[47]

TREATMENT
Desired Outcomes

❽ *The primary goal of treatment for hypercalcemia is to control the underlying malignancy. Therapies directed at lowering the calcium level are temporary measures that are useful until anticancer therapy begins to work.* The goals of calcium-lowering therapy are to (a) lower the corrected calcium to normal levels, (b) regain fluid and electrolyte balance, (c) relieve symptoms, and (d) prevent life-threatening complications. Patients who are refractory to available therapies may have calcium-lowering therapy withheld (usually resulting in coma and death), which may be a humane approach.[47]

General Approach to Treatment

Therapeutic options for the treatment of hypercalcemia should be directed toward the level of corrected serum calcium and the presence of symptoms (Fig. 99–5). Hypercalcemia may be classified as mild (corrected calcium equal to 10.5 to 11.9 mg/dL [2.6 to 3.0 mmol/L]), moderate (12 to 13.9 mg/dL [3.0 to 3.5 mmol/L]), and severe (greater than 14 mg/dL [3.5 mmol/L]).[47] Adequate treatment of mild or asymptomatic hypercalcemia may be achieved on an outpatient basis with nonpharmacologic measures. Moderate to severe or symptomatic hypercalcemia almost always requires pharmacologic intervention.

▶ Nonpharmacologic Therapy

Calciuric therapy in the form of hydration is a key component in the treatment of hypercalcemia, regardless of severity or presence of symptoms.[49] Mild or asymptomatic patients may be encouraged to increase their oral fluid intake (3 to 4 L/day). Patients with moderate to severe or symptomatic hypercalcemia should receive normal saline at 200 to 500 mL/h according to their dehydration and cardiovascular status. Patients should be encouraged to ambulate as much as possible because immobility enhances bone resorption. Although calcium should be discontinued from parenteral feeding solutions, oral calcium supplementation minimally contributes to hypercalcemia unless it is mediated by vitamin D. In these cases, oral calcium should be discontinued. Finally,

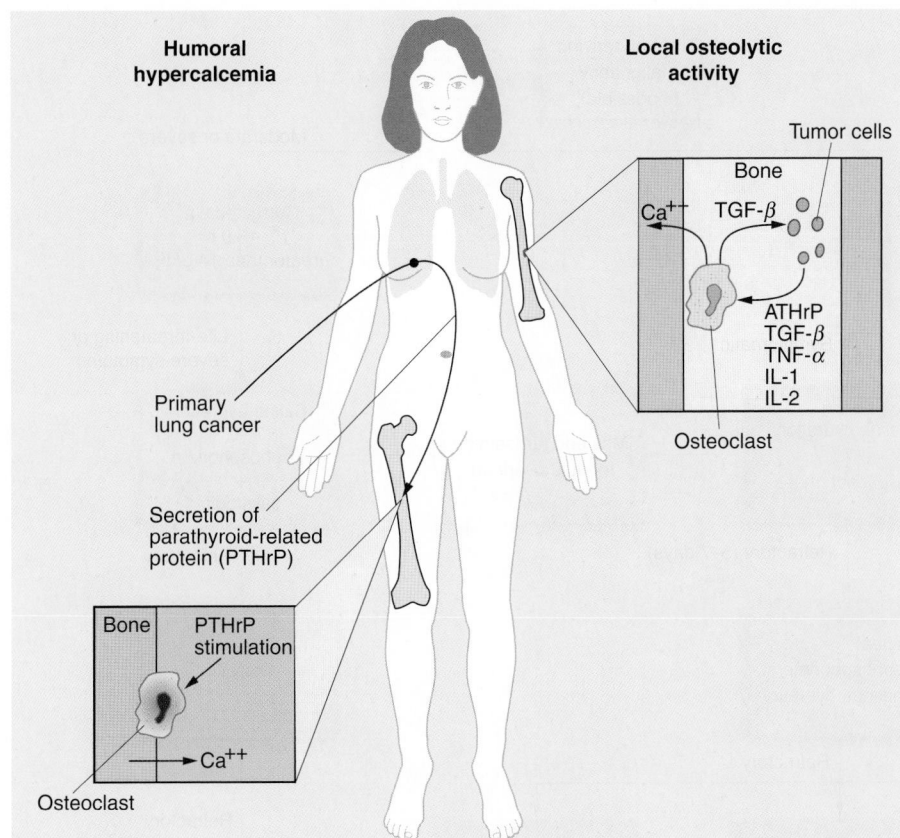

FIGURE 99–4. Pathophysiology of the hypercalcemia of malignancy. (Ca^{2+}, calcium; IL-1, interleukin-1; IL-2, interleukin-2; PTHrP, parathyroid hormone–related protein; TGF-β, transforming growth factor β; TNF-α, tumor necrosis factor α.)

agents that may contribute to hypercalcemia (thiazide diuretics, vitamin D, lithium) or decrease renal function (NSAIDs) should be discontinued. Dialysis may be used in refractory cases or patients who cannot tolerate aggressive saline hydration.

► Pharmacologic Therapy

Multiple pharmacologic interventions are available for the treatment of hypercalcemia (Table 99–13). Furosemide 20 to 40 mg/day may be added to hydration after rehydration has been achieved to avoid fluid overload and enhance renal

Clinical Presentation and Diagnosis of Hypercalcemia

General

- Presence of symptoms depends not only on the calcium level but the rapidity of onset
- Normal calcium level is 8.5 to 10.5 g/dL (2.1–2.6 mmol/L) (varies by lab)
- Serum calcium level *must* be corrected for albumin level using the following formula:

Corrected calcium = Serum calcium + 0.8 (4 – Serum albumin)

Signs and Symptoms

- Five primary organ systems may be affected:
  - GI: anorexia, nausea, vomiting, constipation
  - Musculoskeletal: weakness, bone pain, fatigue, ataxia
  - CNS: confusion, headache, lethargy, seizures, coma
  - Genitourinary: polydipsia, polyuria, renal failure
  - Cardiac: Bradycardia, ECG abnormalities, arrhythmias

Laboratory Tests

- Elevated corrected serum calcium level (greater than or equal to 10.5 g/dL [2.6 mmol/L]), serum albumin, low to normal serum phosphate
- Patient may have elevated blood urea nitrogen and serum creatinine
- Elevated alkaline phosphatase may indicate bone destruction
- ECG may indicate prolonged PR interval, shortened QT interval, widened T wave

Other Diagnostic Tests

- Rule out other causes of hypercalcemia, including primary hyperparathyroidism, hyperthyroidism, vitamin D intoxication, chronic renal failure

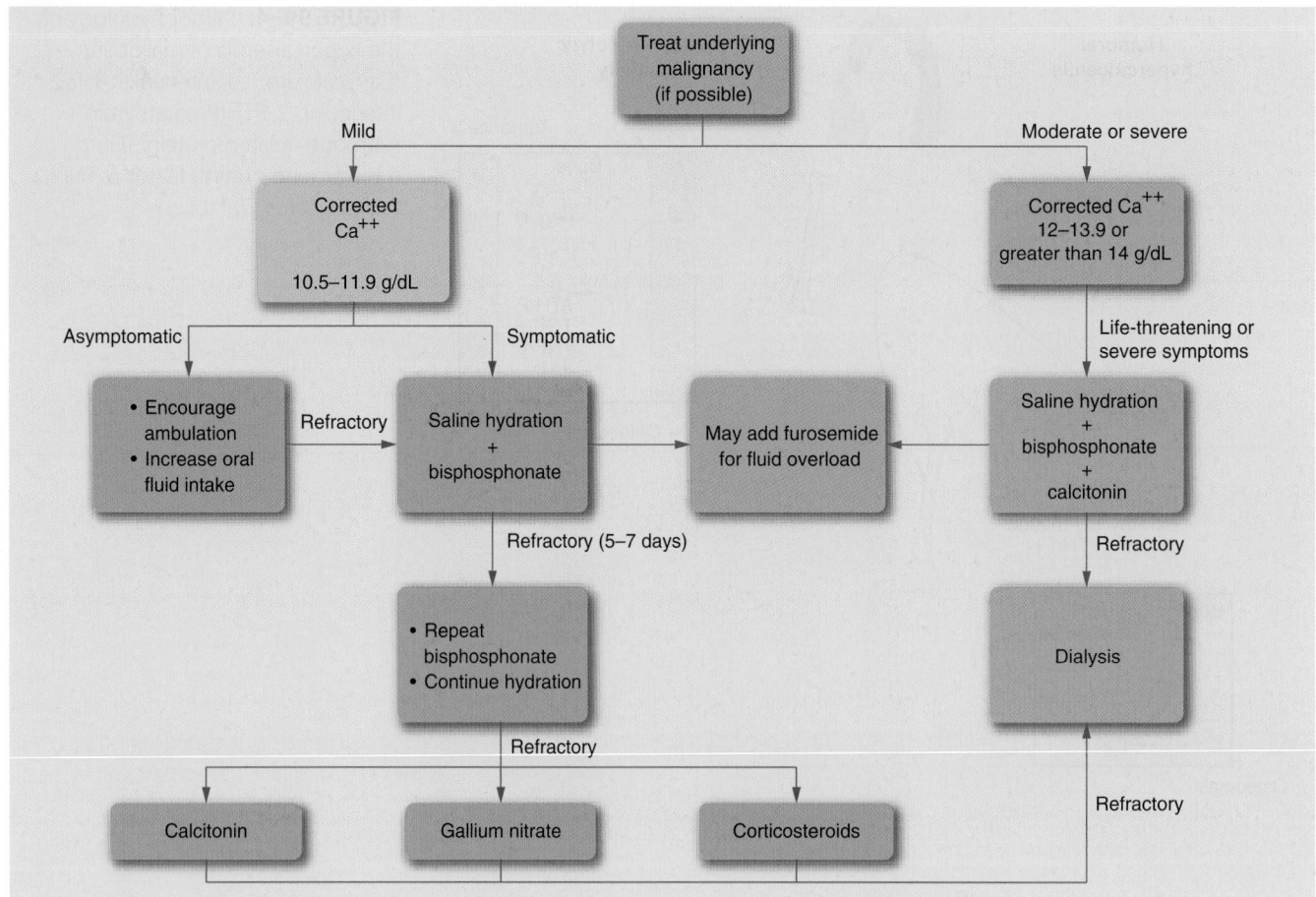

FIGURE 99–5. Treatment algorithm for the hypercalcemia of malignancy.

Table 99–13

Treatment Options for Hypercalcemia of Malignancy

	Agent	Dosage	Onset	Duration	Reduction in Serum Calcium Concentration	Comments
Calciuric therapy	IV normal saline	200–500 mL/h	24–48 hours	2–3 days	0.5–2 mg/dL	Avoid fluid overload, monitor electrolytes
	Furosemide	20–40 mg IV	4 hours	2–3 days	—	Monitor for hypokalemia, dehydration
Antiresorptive therapy	Pamidronate	60–90 mg IV over 2–24 hours[a]	24–72 hours	3–4 weeks	Greater than 1 mg/dL	Nadir not seen until after 4–7 days; may cause fever, renal dysfunction; pamidronate less expensive
	Zoledronic acid	4 mg IV over 15 minutes	24–48 hours	4+ weeks	Greater than 1 mg/dL	
	Corticosteroids	Prednisone (or equivalent) 50–100 mg/day	5–7 days	3–4 days	0.5–3 mg/dL	Monitor for hyperglycemia, insomnia, immunosuppression
	Calcitonin	4–8 IU/kg SC or IM every 6–12 hours	2–4 hours	1–3 days	2–3 mg/dL	Salmon-derived formulation preferred; 1-unit test dose recommended; can be given in renal failure; may cause flushing, nausea
	Gallium nitrate	100–200 mg/m² CIV daily for 5 days	24–48 hours	—	—	Do not administer if creatinine greater than 2.5 mg/dL; may cause renal failure

CIV, continuous intravenous infusion; IM, intramuscular; IV, intravenous; SC, subcutaneous.

[a]60 mg of pamidronate may be used in smaller patients or in patients with mild hypercalcemia or renal dysfunction. May use longer infusion time in patients with renal dysfunction.

From Refs. 47and 49.

excretion of calcium. Although effective in relieving symptoms, hydration and diuretics are temporary measures that are useful until the onset of antiresorptive therapy; thus, hydration and antiresorptive therapy should be initiated simultaneously.

The antiresorptive therapy of choice for hypercalcemia of malignancy is a bisphosphonate. Because of poor oral bioavailability, only IV agents should be used. Pamidronate and zoledronic acid are most commonly used and are potent inhibitors of osteoclast activity.[50] The choice of bisphosphonate is a difficult one; zoledronic acid is more efficacious in terms of response rate and longer duration of normocalcemia but is approximately four times more expensive.[51] Regardless of selection, the bisphosphonates should be administered at diagnosis because of their delayed onset of action.

Calcitonin is the drug of choice in cases of emergent hypercalcemia (patients with life-threatening electrocardiographic (ECG) changes, arrhythmias, or central nervous system [CNS] effects) because of its rapid onset of action. Calcitonin inhibits osteoclast activity and decreases renal tubular calcium resorption. Corticosteroids are useful in patients with steroid-responsive malignancies,

---

Patient Encounter 3: Hypercalcemia of Malignancy

LP is a 79-year-old man with stage IV moderately differentiated adenocarcinoma with features suggestive of a combined hepatocellular cholangiocarcinoma. The patient feels well but is fatigued and has a headache. He presents today to discuss treatment options for his disease. Relevant labs today are: calcium, 11.1 mg/dL (2.76 mmol/L) and albumin, 3.2 g/dL (32 g/L).

What is LP's corrected calcium level?

How would you approach LP's hypercalcemia?

---

such as lymphomas or multiple myeloma, and may delay tachyphylaxis to calcitonin. Gallium nitrate was also recently reapproved for treatment, although the 5-day administration regimen and risk of nephrotoxicity limit its use.

OUTCOME EVALUATION

The long-term success of therapy for hypercalcemia is determined primarily by the success of treatment of the underlying malignancy. The goal of treatment is to reduce serum calcium levels to normal range and to relieve patient symptoms if present.

METABOLIC COMPLICATIONS: TLS

INTRODUCTION

Although not as common as hypercalcemia, TLS may cause significant morbidity and mortality if adequate prophylaxis and treatment are not instituted. TLS is the result of rapid destruction of malignant cells with subsequent release of intracellular contents into the circulation.

EPIDEMIOLOGY AND ETIOLOGY

The overall incidence of TLS is unknown but has been linked to a number of patient- and tumor-related risk factors (Table 99–14).[52] TLS typically occurs in malignancies with high tumor burdens or high proliferative rates. Because of this, children are most frequently affected because they frequently have aggressive malignancies. TLS is typically induced by cancer treatment modalities, including chemotherapy, hormonal therapy, radiation, biologic therapy, or corticosteroids, although some patients may present spontaneously before treatment.

PATHOPHYSIOLOGY

Patients with TLS experience a wide range of metabolic abnormalities. The massive cell lysis that occurs leads to the release of intracellular electrolytes, resulting in hyperkalemia

---

Patient Care and Monitoring: Hypercalcemia

1. Determine the disease status of the patient: Is the patient newly diagnosed or has the patient had multiple episodes of hypercalcemia and is becoming refractory to calcium-lowering therapy?

2. Assess the patient's symptoms and serum calcium level to determine appropriate therapy. Is the patient taking any medications that may elevate the calcium level, inhibit its excretion, or affect renal function?

3. Educate the patient regarding the importance of oral hydration and ambulation if an outpatient. Counsel to immediately report any worsening signs or symptoms.

4. Develop a plan to maintain normocalcemia chronically using monthly bisphosphonates.

   • Monitor patients for relief of symptoms and restoration of fluid balance.

   • Monitor the serum calcium level, serum albumin, serum blood urea nitrogen and creatinine, and electrolytes daily during therapy.

   • Assess the fluid balance by daily input and output, weights, and signs of fluid overload.

   • Monitor the ECG in patients with cardiac manifestations until normalized.

   • Repeat doses of bisphosphonate after 5 to 7 days if the patient does not become normocalcemic.

   • Reassess patient status in terms of refractoriness to treatment to determine if treatment should be changed.

5. Evaluate the patient for drug interactions, allergies, and adverse effects with calcium-lowering therapy.

Table 99–14

Risk Factors for TLS

Disease Related

High risk

Acute lymphoblastic leukemia

High-grade non-Hodgkin's lymphoma (i.e., Burkitt's lymphoma)

Intermediate risk

Chronic lymphocytic leukemia (especially bulky lymphadenopathy)

Acute myeloid leukemia (especially WBC count greater than 50,000 $10^3/\mu L$ ($500 \times 10^9/L$)

Multiple myeloma

Low risk

Low- and intermediate-grade non-Hodgkin's lymphoma

Hodgkin's disease

Chronic myeloid leukemia (blast crisis)

Rare

Breast cancer

Small cell lung cancer

Testicular cancer

Patient Related

Decreased urinary output, dehydration, or renal failure

Preexisting hyperuricemia

Acidic urine

WBC count greater than 50,000 $10^3/\mu L$ ($500 \times 10^9/L$)

LDH levels greater than 1500 IU/L (1500 units/L)

High tumor sensitivity to treatment modalities

LDH, lactate dehydrogenase; WBC, white blood cell.

From Refs. 52 and 54.

and hyperphosphatemia. High concentrations of phosphate bind to calcium, leading to hypocalcemia and calcium phosphate precipitation in the renal tubule. Purine nucleic acids are also released, which are subsequently metabolized to uric acid through multiple enzyme-mediated steps (Fig. 99–6). Uric acid is poorly soluble at urinary acidic pH, leading to crystallization in the renal tubule. The precipitation of uric acid and calcium phosphate leads to metabolic acidosis, facilitating further uric acid crystallization. Acute renal failure may be the end result.

Clinical Presentation and Diagnosis of TLS

General

- Patients present primarily with laboratory abnormalities.
- Normal uric acid is equal to 2 to 8 mg/dL (119–476 μmol/L).
- Most often occurs within 12 to 72 hours of initiation of cytotoxic therapy

Signs and Symptoms

- Most patients are asymptomatic.
- Patients may develop edema, fluid overload, and oliguria, which may progress to anuria with acute renal failure.
- Some patients with hyperuricemia may have nausea, vomiting, and lethargy.
- Hyperkalemia: lethargy, muscle weakness, **paresthesia**, ECG changes, bradycardia
- Hypocalcemia: muscle cramps, **tetany**, irritability, paresthesias, arrhythmias

Laboratory Tests (Adults)

- Serum uric acid level greater than 8 mg/dL (476 μmol/L)
- Serum potassium greater than 6 mEq/L (6 mmol/L)
- Serum phosphorus greater than 4.5 mg/dL (1.45 mmol/L)
- Serum calcium less than 7 mg/dL (1.75 mmol/L)
- Elevated blood urea nitrogen and creatinine once renal dysfunction develops

or

- A change of greater than 25% from baseline in the above lab values[35]

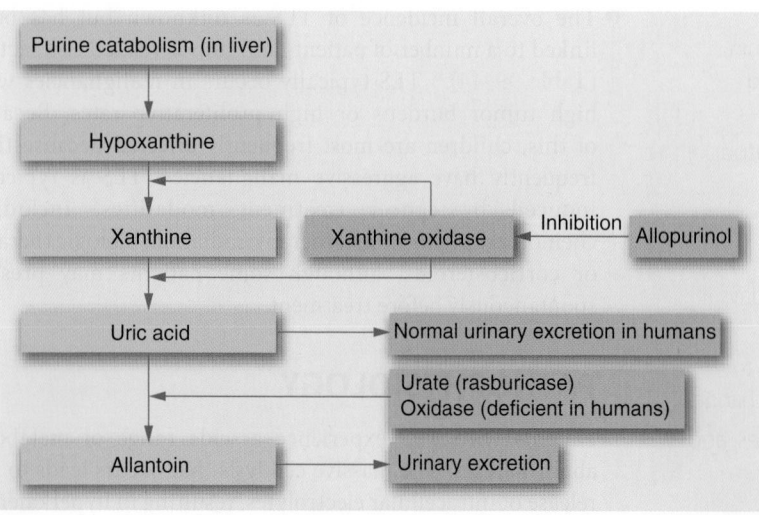

FIGURE 99–6. The role of allopurinol and rasburicase in the enzymatic degradation of purine nucleic acids.

CLINICAL PRESENTATION AND DIAGNOSIS

Patients with TLS are diagnosed based on laboratory monitoring indicating hyperuricemia, hyperkalemia, hyperphosphatemia, hypocalcemia, and renal dysfunction.[53] As a result of these electrolyte abnormalities, patients may present with uremia, visual disturbances, muscle cramping, edema, hypertension, cardiac arrhythmias, seizures, and even sudden death.[53]

TREATMENT

Desired Outcomes

9 *The primary goals of management of TLS are (a) prevention of renal failure and (b) prevention of electrolyte imbalances. Thus, the best treatment for TLS is prophylaxis to enable delivery of cytotoxic therapy for the underlying malignancy.* For patients who present with or develop TLS despite prophylaxis, treatment goals include (a) decreasing uric acid levels, (b) correcting electrolyte imbalances, and (c) preventing compromised renal function. These goals should be achieved in a cost-effective manner.

General Approach to Treatment

Prevention of TLS is generally achieved by increasing the urine output and preventing accumulation of uric acid. Prophylactic strategies should begin immediately upon presentation, preferably 48 hours prior to cytotoxic therapy. Treatment modalities primarily increase uric acid solubility, maintain electrolyte balance, and support renal output.

► Nonpharmacologic Therapy

Vigorous IV hydration with dextrose 5% in water with ½ normal saline at 3 L/m²/day to maintain a urine output greater than or equal to 100 mL/m²/h is necessary unless the patient presents with acute renal dysfunction. Alkalinization of the urine to a pH greater than or equal to 7.0 with 50 to 100 mEq/L (50 to 100 mmol/L) of sodium bicarbonate has been used to promote uric acid solubility for excretion. This measure is controversial because xanthine and hypoxanthine are less soluble at alkaline pH, potentially leading to crystallization, especially during and after allopurinol therapy (see Fig. 99–6).[54] Medications that increase serum potassium (angiotensin-converting enzyme inhibitors, spironolactone) or block tubular resorption of uric acid (probenecid, thiazides) should be discontinued. Nephrotoxic agents such as amphotericin B or aminoglycosides should also be avoided. Hemodialysis may be required in patients who develop anuria or uncontrolled hyperkalemia, hyperphosphatemia, hypocalcemia, acidosis, or volume overload.

► Pharmacologic Therapy

Pharmacologic prevention strategies for TLS are aimed at low- and high-risk patients (Fig. 99–7). Allopurinol is a xanthine oxidase inhibitor that is used for prevention only because it has no effect on pre-existing elevated uric acid. Rasburicase is a recombinant form of urate oxidase that is useful for both prevention and treatment, but is extremely expensive (Table 99–15). Although the approved dose is 0.2 mg/kg/day for 5 days, recent studies using abbreviated courses (1–3 days) and/or lower doses (0.05–0.1 mg/kg/day) may be equally efficacious with significantly reduced cost.[54]

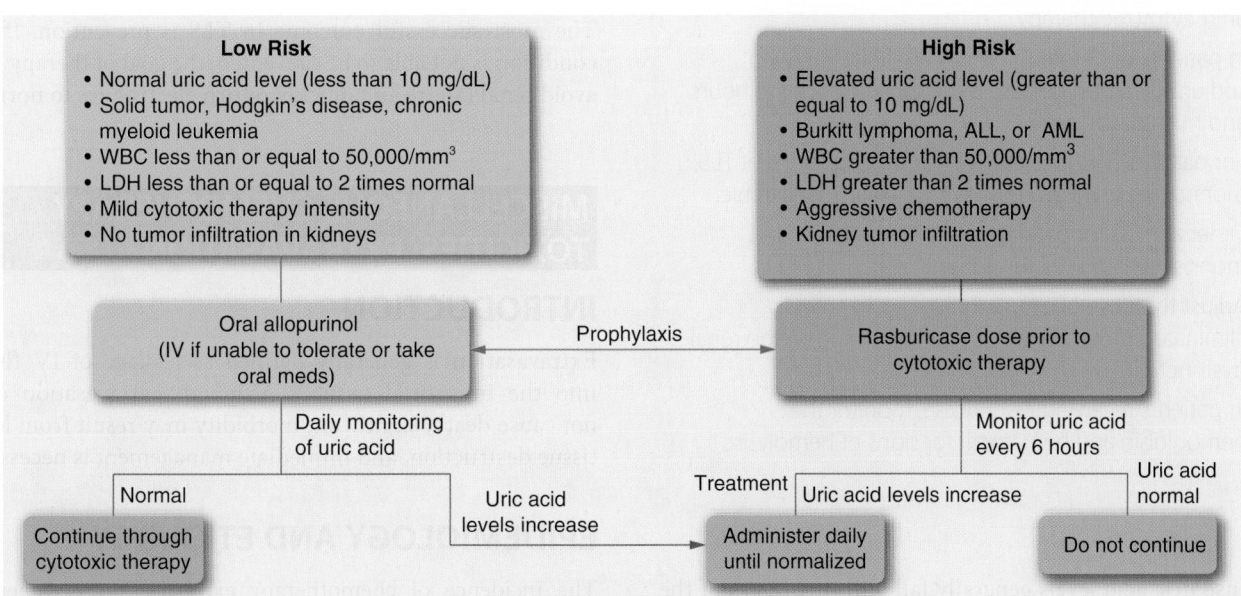

FIGURE 99–7. Prophylaxis and treatment of hyperuricemia associated with tumor lysis syndrome. (ALL, acute lymphoblastic leukemia; AML, acute myelogenous leukemia; IV, intravenous; LDH, lactate dehydrogenase; WBC, white blood cell.) (From Refs. 35 and 36.)

Table 99–15

Comparison of Allopurinol and Rasburicase in TLS

Drug	Dosing	AWP[a]	Comments
PO allopurinol (Zyloprim)	Adult: 600–800 mg/day in 2–3 divided doses Pediatric: 10 mg/kg/day or 200–300 mg/m²/day	$0.48/day (generic)	Adjust dose for renal impairment Avoid drug interactions (mercaptopurine) Monitor for skin rash
IV allopurinol (Aloprim)	Adult: 200–400 mg/m²/day Pediatric: 200 mg/m²/day	$625–$1,250/day	As above Reserve for patients who cannot tolerate or take oral medications Maximum dose = 600 mg/day
Rasburicase (Elitek)	0.2 mg/kg/day for up to 5 days	$12,000/day	Lower doses and abbreviated schedules may be used to decrease cost (0.05–0.1 mg/kg/day) May rarely cause nausea and vomiting Contraindicated in patients with G6PD deficiency → hemolytic anemia Rare cases of hypersensitivity and antibody formation

AWP, average wholesale price; G6PD, glucose-6-phosphate dehydrogenase; PO, oral.

[a]Normalized for 70-kg patient or body surface area = 1.73 m²; all costs are estimated and may vary.

From Yim BT, Sims-McCallum RP, Chong PH. Rasburicase for the treatment and prevention of hyperuricemia. Ann Pharmacother 2003;37:1047–1054.

Patient Care and Monitoring: TLS

1. Monitor daily at-risk patients who present with normal laboratory values daily for serum uric acid, electrolytes (Na, K, Ca, Mg, Cl, PO₄), blood urea nitrogen, creatinine, and urine output.

2. Monitor for signs of fluid overload during aggressive hydration.

3. Continue hydration and prophylaxis until 2 to 3 days after cytotoxic therapy.

4. In patients undergoing urinary alkalinization with sodium bicarbonate, assess the urine pH every 6 hours and maintain above 7.

5. For patients who present with or develop signs of TLS, monitor these parameters every 6 hours until stable.

6. Order an ECG for patients with hyperkalemia and monitor serially until resolution.

7. Adjust the dose of allopurinol and other renally eliminated medications for patients who develop renal dysfunction.

8. In patients receiving rasburicase, monitor the hemoglobin and hematocrit for signs of hemolysis.

Because uric acid levels generally fall within 4 hours of the first dose, one dose may be administered with frequent, serial monitoring of the uric acid level for repeat dosing if necessary (Fig. 99–7). Of note, rasburicase continues to break down uric acid in blood samples drawn from patients.

This can be avoided by immediately placing the sample in an ice bath for processing to avoid falsely lowered uric acid levels.

Electrolyte disturbances that develop in patients with TLS should be aggressively managed to avoid renal failure and cardiac sequelae. One exception pertains to the use of IV calcium for hypocalcemia. Adding calcium may cause further calcium phosphate precipitation in the presence of hyperphosphatemia and should be used cautiously.

OUTCOME EVALUATION

The most successful outcome in TLS is prevention. If the condition is not able to be prevented, the goal of therapy is to avoid renal failure and quickly return electrolytes to normal.

MISCELLANEOUS CHEMOTHERAPY TOXICITIES: EXTRAVASATION

INTRODUCTION

Extravasation is generally defined as leakage of IV fluids into the interstitial tissue.[56] Although extravasation does not cause death, significant morbidity may result from local tissue destruction, and immediate management is necessary.

EPIDEMIOLOGY AND ETIOLOGY

The incidence of chemotherapy extravasation is generally reported to be between 0.5% and 6% of all chemotherapy-related adverse events.[57] A number of risk factors have been identified for chemotherapy extravasation (Table 99–16). Chemotherapy agents are generally classified into three groups: vesicants,

Table 99–16

Risk Factors for Chemotherapy Extravasation

Presence of multiple venipunctures (common in cancer patients)

Poor needle insertion technique

Poor catheter location (dorsum of the hand, antecubital fossa)

Inability to communicate symptoms (children, sedated patients, language barrier between patient and nurse)

Presence of peripheral neuropathy

Nurse experience and training

Young age or elderly patients (small or fragile veins)

Gross obesity

Clinical Presentation and Diagnosis of Extravasation

General

- Anthracycline, mechlorethamine, and vinca alkaloid extravasations typically cause immediate pain.
- Patients may be asymptomatic at the time of extravasation but return within days to weeks with signs of tissue damage (particularly with mitomycin C).
- Exposure to ultraviolet light may worsen some lesions.

Signs and Symptoms

- Local pain (burning, tingling, stinging), swelling, erythema, induration
- Lack of blood return
- Ulceration may not develop until after 1 to 2 weeks or longer.

Diagnostic Tests

- Usually based on clinical history and presenting symptoms, but tissue biopsy may reveal definitive findings

irritants, and nonvesicants (Table 99–17).[58] Either vesicants or irritants may cause local symptoms, however vesicants cause local tissue necrosis upon extravasation whereas irritants do not. The degree of tissue injury depends on the concentration and amount of fluid extravasated. It is important to note that some agents are well-known vesicants; however, for many agents, only isolated case reports of tissue necrosis exist. Therefore, it is imperative to use caution when administering any chemotherapeutic agent, especially new or investigational agents that have unknown vesicant properties.

PATHOPHYSIOLOGY

The mechanism of tissue injury is related to the pharmacodynamic characteristics of the extravasated drug. These agents may be classified into DNA binding and non–DNA binding. Examples of DNA-binding agents include the anthracyclines, mechlorethamine, and mitomycin C. These agents first cause cell death through interactions with DNA and are then released into the surrounding tissue and taken up by adjacent cells. This repeating cycle is perpetuated by the lipophilic nature of these drugs, resulting in chronic, slow-healing tissue injury because of long tissue retention. Doxorubicin in particular may remain in tissues for weeks to months.[58]

Non–DNA-binding agents include the vinca alkaloids and etoposide. These agents tend to cause injury in the pattern of a thermal burn and are more easily cleared from interstitial spaces. Thus, they are more readily neutralized and tend to have a better healing prognosis.

CLINICAL PRESENTATION AND DIAGNOSIS

Patients who experience extravasation report burning pain and discomfort in the limb of the infusion site, which can be severe. The area may be erythematous at first. If not quickly treated, the tissue will become necrotic and require amputation. Diagnosis is made based on symptoms.

Table 99–17

Chemotherapeutic Agents With Vesicant or Irritant Properties

Vesicants	Irritants
Common	Camptothecins
Anthracyclines	Carmustine
Daunorubicin	Cyclophosphamide
Doxorubicin	Dacarbazine
Epirubicin	Epipodophyllotoxins
Idarubicin	Etoposide
Dactinomycin	Fluorouracil
Mechlorethamine	Gemcitabine
Mitomycin C	Ifosfamide
Vinca alkaloids	Irinotecan
Vincristine	Melphalan
Vinblastine	Pentostatin
Vinorelbine	Streptozocin
Rare[a]	Teniposide
Cisplatin	Topotecan
Liposomal doxorubicin	
Mitoxantrone	
Oxaliplatin	
Taxanes	
Docetaxel	
Paclitaxel	

[a]Agents for which there are isolated case reports of local tissue necrosis.

From Ener RA, Meglathery SB, Styler M. Extravasation of systemic hemato-oncological therapies. Ann Oncol 2004;15:858–862.

Table 99–18

Prevention Strategies for Chemotherapy Extravasation

Central venous catheters should be placed for vesicant administration whenever possible, especially in high-risk patients.
Avoid the dorsum of the hand, antecubital fossa, and limbs with significant lymphedema.
Use uncovered plastic cannulas or a butterfly needle for peripheral administration.
Always test the line with IV fluids before chemotherapy administration and observe site for swelling.
Check for blood return before and frequently during administration.
If venipuncture is repeated, should be proximal to before needle insertion site.
Vesicants given via peripheral vein should be given by IV push rather than by infusion to enable immediate cessation and withdrawal of fluids if extravasation occurs.

IV, intravenous.

From Oncology Nursing Society. Cancer Chemotherapy and Biotherapy Guidelines and Recommendations for Practice: Module XXII. Pittsburgh, PA: Oncology Nursing Press, 2002.

PREVENTION

⑩ *Chemotherapy extravasation may be avoided in many cases by the use of successful prevention strategies. The most important preventive measure is proper patient education.*

Patients must be instructed to promptly report any local symptoms not only during administration but also days to weeks later. Another key factor is the exclusive use of highly trained personnel who are trained to administer chemotherapeutic drugs. The Oncology Nursing Society has developed guidelines for the administration of vesicant drugs as summarized in Table 99–18.[59] Although placement of a central venous catheter is recommended, extravasations may still occur because of dislodged or poorly placed needles or nicked catheters.

TREATMENT

Desired Outcomes

Once extravasation occurs, the primary goals of treatment are to (a) avoid further tissue damage by using appropriate nonpharmacologic and pharmacologic strategies and (b) promptly refer patients for surgery if required. Optimal pharmacologic and nonpharmacologic treatment of the extravasation allows the cancer patient to continue with chemotherapy (Table 99–19).

▶ *Nonpharmacologic Therapy*

If extravasation occurs, the infusion should be stopped immediately with aspiration of fluid from the site, needle, and tubing as much as possible. The affected limb or area should be elevated (if possible). The site should be documented photographically, as should the time, date, site,

---

Table 99–19

Management of Chemotherapy Extravasation

Drug	Application of Heat or Cold	Pharmacologic Antidote	Dose	Comments
Anthracyclines	Cold packs	DMSO 50–99% Alternative: dexrazoxane	Apply 1–2 mL to area of skin twice the size of lesion every 6–8 hours for 7–14 days 1,000 mg/m² IV within 5 hours of extravasation followed by 1,000 mg/m² on day 2 and 500 mg/m² on day 3	Allow to air dry Do not cover Promising new agent; expensive and may not be reimbursed by payors
Mitomycin C	Cold packs	DMSO 50%–99%	As above	
Mechlorethamine; concentrated cisplatin	Cold packs	Sodium thiosulfate	Prepare 1/6M solution by adding 4 mL of 10% solution to 6 mL of sterile water; inject 2 mL for each mg of mechlorethamine. Follow with 1 mL SC (0.1-mL doses clockwise around area); may repeat every 3–4 hours if needed	Sodium thiosulfate must be diluted before administration
Vinca alkaloids	Hot packs	Hyaluronidase	Inject 1–6 mL of 150 units/mL concentration (150–900 units) through IV line or SC if removed; may repeat every 3–4 hours if needed	Dilute with normal saline
Paclitaxel	Cold packs	Hyaluronidase	As above	Hot packs paradoxically shown to worsen lesions in some case reports

DMSO, dimethylsulfoxide; IV, intravenous; SC, subcutaneous.

From Ener RA, Meglathery SB, Styler M. Extravasation of systemic hemato-oncological therapies. Ann Oncol 2004;15:858–862.

patient complaints, and estimated volume of extravasated drug.[58] Both hot and cold packs have been used to manage extravasations; however, the use of the proper therapy for certain agents is critical. For example, warm compresses have been shown to worsen doxorubicin extravasations, but cold packs may exacerbate vinca alkaloid lesions. Pressure should not be applied to the area because this may facilitate spread. Finally, patients should be referred to a plastic surgeon if pain persists or ulceration develops despite treatment.

▶ *Pharmacologic Therapy*

Therapeutic modalities to treat extravasation events consist of specific antidotes to halt or decrease the severity of local tissue necrosis. It should be noted that only one-third of extravasation events lead to local tissue necrosis, and most studies of antidotes are in animal models or isolated case reports. Antidotes either disperse or bind the chemotherapy agent and accelerate the removal of the agent from the tissues. Specific antidotes and their uses are presented in Table 99–19.

Dimethylsulfoxide (DMSO) is the antidote of choice for anthracycline and mitomycin C extravasations. It readily penetrates tissues and increases diffusion in the tissue area. In addition, DMSO is a free radical scavenger that functions to block this principle mechanism of anthracycline and mitomycin C–mediated tissue injury. DMSO is generally well tolerated but may cause some mild burning and redness. Dexrazoxane is a free-radical scavenger typically used for cardioprotection from anthracyclines. A special formulation of dexrazoxane (Totect) is the only commercially available product that is FDA approved to treat doxorubicin extravasation, although much controversy exists surrounding whether generic dexrazoxane may be equally efficacious than the newer, more expensive alternative.

Hyaluronidase is the antidote of choice for vinca alkaloid and high-concentration epipodophyllotoxin extravasations. Hyaluronidase breaks down hyaluronic acid, which functions as "tissue cement." This promotes the absorption of the extravasated drug away from the local site. Hyaluronidase may also be used for paclitaxel extravasations; however, there are conflicting reports regarding its efficacy.[60] Hyaluronidase should not be used with anthracycline extravasations because enhancement of local spread may occur.

The antidote of choice for mechlorethamine extravasations is sodium thiosulfate. This agent binds alkylating agents, resulting in neutralization to inactive compounds that are then excreted. Sodium thiosulfate may also be effective for high-concentration cisplatin or dacarbazine extravasations.

OUTCOME EVALUATION

The primary outcome is the prevention of extravasation events using proper administration techniques. Instruct patients to promptly report any symptoms of extravasation. If extravasation occurs, select the proper antidote and thermal application for immediate administration. Promptly refer the patient for plastic surgery if pain persists or ulceration develops.

Patient Care and Monitoring: Extravasation

1. Upon diagnosis, determine the need for administration of chemotherapy with vesicant properties. Refer the patient for surgical placement of a central access device.

2. Insure proper training and certification of all personnel in institution who administer chemotherapeutic agents.

3. Educate the patient regarding signs and symptoms of extravasation and instruct to immediately relate to caregiver.

4. Educate the patient to promptly report increasing pain, spread of the lesion or ulceration.

5. Educate the patient regarding proper application of hot or cold packs as well as topical antidotes. Should the area be allowed to air dry or be covered?

6. Evaluate the patient for allergies and adverse effects of pharmacologic antidotes.

Abbreviations Introduced in This Chapter

ANC	Absolute neutrophil count
AWP	Average wholesale price
BMT	Bone marrow transplantation
BUN	Blood urea nitrogen
CIV	Continuous intravenous infusion
CSF	Colony-stimulating factor
DMSO	Dimethylsulfoxide
G6PD	Glucose-6-phosphate dehydrogenase
ICP	Intracranial pressure
LDH	Lactate dehydrogenase
NSAID	Nonsteroidal anti-inflammatory drug
NSCLC	Non–small cell lung cancer
PCP	*Pneumocystis jiroveci* pneumonitis (formerly *Pneumocystis carinii*)
PTHrP	Parathyroid hormone–related protein
SCLC	Small cell lung cancer
SVCS	Superior vena cava syndrome

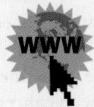

Self-assessment questions and answers are available at http://www.mhpharmacotherapy.com/pp.html.

REFERENCES

1. deBoer-Dennert M, deWit R, Schmitz PI, et al. Patient perceptions of the side effects of chemotherapy: The influence of 5HT3 antagonists. Br J Cancer 1997;76:1055–1061.

2. Roscoe JA, Bushnnow P, Morrow GR, et al. Patient experience is a strong predictor of severe nausea after chemotherapy: A University of Rochester Community Clinical Oncology Program study of patients with breast carcinoma. Cancer 2004;101:2701–2708.

3. Hesketh PJ. Chemotherapy-induced nausea and vomiting. N Engl J Med 2008;358:2482–2494.

4. Hesketh PJ, Grunberg SM, Gralla RJ, et al. The neurokinin-1 antagonist aprepitant for the prevention of chemotherapy-induced nausea and vomiting: A multinational, randomized, double-blind, placebo-controlled trial in patients receiving high-dose cisplatin—The Aprepitant Protocol 052 Study Group. J Clin Oncol 2003;21:4112–4119.

5. Geling O, Eichler HG. Should 5-hydroxytryptamine-3-receptor antagonists be administered beyond 24 hours after chemotherapy to prevent delayed emesis? Systematic re-evaluation of clinical evidence and drug cost implications. J Clin Oncol 2005;23:1289–1294.

6. National Comprehensive Cancer Network [Internet]. Fort Washington, PA: National Comprehensive Cancer Network. Clinical practice guidelines in oncology: Antiemesis. version v.1.2012, accessed 10/4/2011. Available from: http://www.nccn.org/professionals/physician_gls/PDF/antiemesis.pdf.

7. Polovich M, White JM, Kelleher LO, eds. Chemotherapy and Biotherapy Guidelines and Recommendations for Practice, 2nd ed. Pittsburgh, PA: Oncology Nursing Society, 2005.

8. Berardi RR, Kroon LA, McDermott JH, et al. Handbook of Nonprescription Drugs, 15th ed. Washington, DC: American Pharmacists Association, 2006.

9. Kris MG, Hesketh PJ, Somerfield MR, et al. American Society of Clinical Oncology Guidelines for Antiemesis in Oncology: Update 2006. J Clin Oncol 2006;24:2932–2947.

10. Peterson DE, Bensadoun RJ, Roila F. Management of oral and gastrointestinal mucositis: ESMO clinical recommendations. Ann Oncol 2008;19(Suppl 2):ii122–ii125.

11. Nonzel NJ, Dandade NA, Markossia T, et al. Evaluating the supportive care costs of severe radiochemotherapy-induced mucositis and pharyngitis: Results from a Northwestern University costs of cancer program pilot study with head and neck and non-small cell lung cancer patients who received care at a county hospital, a Veterans Administration hospital, and a comprehensive care center. Cancer 2008;113:1446–1452.

12. Troth A, Bellm LA, Epstein JB, et al. Mucositis incidence, severity, and associated outcomes in patients with head and neck cancer receiving radiotherapy with or without chemotherapy: A systematic literature review. Radiother Oncol 2003;66:253–262.

13. Saadeh CE. Chemotherapy- and radiotherapy-induced oral mucositis: Review of preventative strategies and treatment. Pharmacotherapy 2005;25:540–544.

14. Keefe DM, Schubert MM, Elting LS. Updated clinical practice guidelines for the prevention and treatment of mucositis. Cancer 2007;109:820–831.

15. Wisplinghoff H, Seifert H, Wenzel RP, Edmond MB. Current trends in the epidemiology of nosocomial bloodstream infections in patients with hematological malignancies and solid neoplasms in hospitals in the United States. Clin Infect Dis 2003;36:1103–1110.

16. Rolston KVI. Challenges in the treatment of infections caused by gram-positive and gram-negative bacteria in patients with cancer and neutropenia. Clin Infect Dis 2004;40(Suppl):S246–S252.

17. Picazo JJ. Management of the febrile neutropenic patient: A consensus conference. Clin Infect Dis 2004;39(Suppl):S1–S6.

18. Elting L, Cooksley C, Chambers M, et al. The burdens of cancer therapy: Clinical and economic outcomes of chemotherapy-induced mucositis. Cancer 2003;98:1531–1539.

19. Freifeld AG, Bow EJ, Sepkowitz KA, et al. Clinical practice guidelines for the use of antimicrobial agents in neutropenic patients with cancer: 2010 update by the Infectious Disease Society of America. Clin Infect Dis 2011;52:e56–e93.

20. Lyman GH, Lyman CH, Agboola O. Risk models for predicting chemotherapy-induced neutropenia. Oncologist 2005;10:427–437.

21. Klastersky J, Paesmans M, Rubenstein EB, et al. The Multinational Association for Supportive Care in Cancer risk index: A multinational scoring system for identifying low-risk febrile neutropenic patients. J Clin Oncol 2000;18:3038–3051.

22. Greil R, Psenak O, Roila F, et al. Hematopoietic growth factors: ESMO recommendations for the applications. Ann Oncol 2008;2:16–18.

23. National Comprehensive Cancer Network [Internet]. Fort Washington, PA: National Comprehensive Cancer Network. Clinical practice guidelines in oncology: Myeloid growth factors. version, v.1.2011, accessed 10/4/2011. Available at : http://www.nccn.org/professionals/physician_gls/PDF/myeloid_growth.pdf.

24. Gafter-Gvili A, Fraser A, Paul M, et al. Meta-analysis: Antibiotic prophylaxis reduces mortality in neutropenic patients. Ann Intern Med 2005;142:979–995.

25. van de Wetering MD, de Witte MA, Kremer LCM, et al. Efficacy of oral prophylactic antibiotics in neutropenic afebrile oncology patients: A systematic review of randomized controlled trials. Eur J Cancer 2005;41:1372–1382.

26. The National Comprehensive Cancer Network [Internet]. Fort Washington, PA: National Comprehensive Cancer Network. Clinical practice guidelines in oncology: Prevention and treatment of cancer-related infections. version v.2.2011, accessed 10/4/2011. Available at: http://www.nccn.org/professionals/physician_gls/PDF/infections.pdf.

27. Bucavene G, Micuzzi A, Menichetti F, et al. Levofloxacin to prevent bacterial infection in patients with cancer and neutropenia. N Engl J Med 2005;353:977–987.

28. Cullen M, Steven N, Billinham L, et al. Antibacterial prophylaxis after chemotherapy for solid tumors and lymphomas. N Engl J Med 2005;353:988–998.

29. Kuderer NM, Crawford J, Dale DC, et al. Meta-analysis of prophylactic granulocyte colony-stimulating factor in cancer patients receiving chemotherapy. J Clin Oncol 2005;23(Suppl):758S.

30. Fish DN, Goodwin SD. Infections in immunocompromised patients. In: Dipiro JT, Talbert RL, Yee GC, et al, eds. Pharmacotherapy: A Pathophysiologic Approach, 6th ed. New York: McGraw-Hill, 2005:2191–2215.

31. Oncology Nursing Society [Internet]. Pittsburgh, PA: Oncology Nursing Society. ONS putting evidence into practice: Prevention of infection. version v.2.2011, accessed 10/4/2011. Available at: http://www.ons.org/outcomes/volume1/prevention/pdf/INFECTION-Detailed-PEPCard4–06.pdf.

32. National Comprehensive Cancer Network [Internet]. Fort Washington, PA: National Comprehensive Cancer Network. Clinical Practice Guidelines in Oncology: Small Cell Lung Cancer. version v.2.2009, accessed 10/4/2011. Available at: http://www.nccn.org/professionals/physician_gls/PDF/sclc.pdf.

33. Walsh TJ, Teppler H, Donowitz GR, et al. Caspofungin versus liposomal amphotericin B for empirical antifungal therapy in patients with persistent fever and neutropenia. N Engl J Med 2004;351:1391–1402.

34. Clark OAC, Lyman GH, Castro AA, et al. Colony-stimulating factors for chemotherapy-induced febrile neutropenia: A meta-analysis of randomized controlled trials. J Clin Oncol 2005;23:4198–4214.

35. Wilson LD, Detterbeck FC, Yahalom J. Superior vena cava syndrome with malignant causes. N Engl J Med 2007;356(8):1862–1869.

36. Kvale PA, Simoff M, Prakash UB. Lung cancer. Palliative care. Chest 2003;123(Suppl 1):284S–311S.

37. Prasad D, Schiff D. Malignant spinal-cord compression. Lancet Oncol 2005;6:15–24.

38. Patchell RA, Tibbs PA, Regine WF, et al. Direct decompressive surgical resection in the treatment of spinal cord compression caused by metastatic cancer: A randomized trial. Lancet 2005;366:643–648.

39. Loblaw DA, Perry J, Chambers A, et al. Systematic review of the diagnosis and management of malignant extradural spinal cord compression: The Cancer Care Ontario Practice Guidelines Initiative's Neuro-Oncology Disease Site Group. J Clin Oncol 2005;23:2028–2037.

40. Langer CJ, Mehta MP. Current management of brain metastases, with a focus on systemic options. J Clin Oncol 2005;23:6207–6219.

41. Patchell RA. The management of brain metastases. Cancer Treat Rev 2003;29:533–540.

42. Slotman B, Faivre-Finn C, Kramer G, et al. Prophylactic cranial-irradiation in extensive small cell lung cancer. N Engl J Med 2007;357:664–672.

43. Lassman AB, DeAngelis LM. Brain metastases. Neurol Clin North Am 2003;21:1–23.

44. Glantz MJ, Cole BF, Forsyth PA, et al. Practice parameter: Anticonvulsant prophylaxis in patients with newly diagnosed brain tumors. Report of the Quality Standards Subcommittee of the American Academy of Neurology. Neurology 2000;54:1886–1893.

45. West NJ. Prevention and treatment of hemorrhagic cystitis. Pharmacotherapy 1997;17:696–706.
46. Schuchter LM, Hensley ML, Meropol NJ, et al. 2002 Update of recommendations for the use of chemotherapy and radiotherapy protectants: Clinical practice guidelines of the American Society of Clinical Oncology. J Clin Oncol 2002;20:2895–2903.
47. Stewart AF. Hypercalcemia associated with cancer. N Engl J Med 2005;352:373–379.
48. Solimando DA. Overview of hypercalcemia of malignancy. Am J Health Syst Pharm 2001;58(Suppl 3):S4–S7.
49. Davidson TG. Conventional treatment of hypercalcemia of malignancy. Am J Health Syst Pharm 2001;58(Suppl 3):S8–S15.
50. Berenson JR. Treatment of hypercalcemia of malignancy with bisphosphonates. Semin Oncol 2002;29(Suppl 21):12–18.
51. Major P, Lortholary A, Hon J, et al. Zoledronic acid is superior to pamidronate in the treatment of hypercalcemia of malignancy: A pooled analysis of two randomized, controlled clinical trials. J Clin Oncol 2001;19:558–567.
52. Davidson MB, Thakkar S, Hix JK, et al. Pathophysiology, clinical consequences, and treatment of tumor lysis syndrome. Am J Med 2004;116:546–554.
53. Hochberg J, Cairo MS. Tumor lysis syndrome: Current perspective. Haematologica 2008;93:9–13.
54. Cairo MS, Bishop M. Tumor lysis syndrome: New therapeutic strategies and classification. Br J Hematol 2004;127:3–11.
55. Yim BT, Sims-McCallum RP, Chong PH. Rasburicase for the treatment and prevention of hyperuricemia. Ann Pharmacother 2003;37:1047–1054.
56. National Cancer Institute [Internet]. Washington, DC: National Cancer Institute Dictionary of Cancer Terms. Accessed 10/4/2011. Available at: http://www.cancer.gov/dictionary/.
57. Kassner E. Evaluation and treatment of chemotherapy extravasation injuries. J Pediatr Oncol Nurs 2000;17:135–148.
58. Ener RA, Meglathery SB, Styler M. Extravasation of systemic hemato-oncological therapies. Ann Oncol 2004;15:858–862.
59. Oncology Nursing Society. Cancer Chemotherapy and Biotherapy Guidelines and Recommendations for Practice: Module XXII. Pittsburgh, PA: Oncology Nursing Press, 2002.
60. Stanford BL, Hardwicke F. A review of clinical experience with paclitaxel extravasations. Support Care Cancer 2003;11:270–277.

100

Parenteral Nutrition

Michael D. Kraft, Imad F. Btaiche,
and Melissa R. Pleva

LEARNING OBJECTIVES

● **Upon completion of the chapter, the reader will be able to:**

1. List appropriate indications for the use of parenteral nutrition (PN) in adult patients.

2. Describe the components of PN and their role in nutrition support therapy.

3. List the elements of nutrition assessment and factors considered in assessing an adult patient's nutritional status and nutritional requirements.

4. Explain the pharmaceutical and compounding issues with PN admixtures.

5. Develop a plan to design, initiate, and adjust a PN formulation for an adult patient based on patient-specific factors.

6. Describe the etiology and risk factors for PN macronutrient-associated complications, including hyperglycemia, hypoglycemia, hyperlipidemia, and azotemia, in adult patients receiving PN.

7. Describe the etiology and risk factors for the refeeding syndrome.

8. Describe the etiology and risk factors for liver complications and metabolic bone disease in adult patients receiving PN.

9. Design a plan to monitor and correct fluid, electrolyte, vitamin, and trace element abnormalities in adult patients receiving PN.

10. Design a plan to assess the efficacy and monitor the safety of PN therapy.

KEY CONCEPTS

① Parenteral nutrition (PN), also called total parenteral nutrition (TPN), is the intravenous (IV) administration of fluids, macronutrients, electrolytes, vitamins, and trace elements for the purpose of weight maintenance or gain, to preserve or replete lean body mass and visceral proteins, and to support anabolism and nitrogen balance *when the oral or enteral route is not feasible or adequate.*

② Amino acids are provided in PN to preserve or replete lean body mass and visceral proteins, to promote protein anabolism and wound healing, and as an energy source.

③ Dextrose (D-glucose) is the major immediate energy source in PN and is vital for cellular metabolism, body protein preservation, tissue formation, and cellular growth.

④ IV lipid emulsions are used as an energy source in PN and to prevent or treat essential fatty acid deficiency.

⑤ PN should not be used to treat acute fluid and electrolyte abnormalities. Rather, PN should be adjusted to meet maintenance requirements and to minimize worsening of underlying fluid and electrolyte disturbances.

⑥ Electrolytes, vitamins, and trace elements are essential for numerous biochemical and metabolic functions and should be added to PN daily unless otherwise not indicated.

⑦ PN can be administered via a small peripheral vein [as peripheral PN (PPN)] or via a larger central vein (as central PN).

⑧ PN admixtures can be prepared by mixing all components into one bag [3-in-1 admixture or a total nutrient admixture (TNA)] or by mixing and infusing dextrose, amino acids, and all other components together and infusing IV lipid emulsion separately (2-in-1 admixture).

⑨ PN is associated with significant complications with both short- and long-term therapy.

⑩ Patients receiving PN should have specific laboratory parameters periodically monitored as indicated clinically. These mainly include fluid and electrolyte status, organ function, nutritional status, and micronutrient levels.

INTRODUCTION

Malnutrition in hospitalized patients is associated with significant complications, including increased infection risk, poor wound healing, prolonged hospital stays, and increased mortality, especially in surgical and critically ill patients.[1] Maintaining adequate nutritional status, especially during periods of illness and metabolic stress, is an important part of patient care. *Nutrition support therapy* refers to the administration of nutrients via the oral, enteral, or parenteral route for therapeutic purposes.[1] ❶ *Parenteral nutrition (PN), also called total parenteral nutrition (TPN), is the intravenous (IV) administration of fluids, macronutrients, electrolytes, vitamins, and trace elements for the purpose of weight maintenance or gain, to preserve or replete lean body mass and visceral proteins, and to support anabolism and nitrogen balance when the oral or enteral route is not feasible or adequate.* PN is a potentially lifesaving therapy in patients with intestinal failure but can be associated with significant complications.

Desired Outcomes and Goals

The goals of nutrition support therapy include:

- Correction or avoidance of nutritional deficiencies
- Weight maintenance (or weight gain in malnourished patients and growing children)
- Preservation or repletion of lean body mass and visceral proteins
- Support of anabolism and nitrogen balance and improvement of healing
- Correction or avoidance of fluid and electrolyte abnormalities
- Correction or avoidance of vitamin and trace element abnormalities
- Improving clinical outcomes

Indications for PN

PN can be a lifesaving therapy in patients with intestinal failure, but the oral or enteral route is preferred when providing nutrition support therapy ("when the gut works, use it"). Compared with PN, enteral nutrition is associated with a lower risk of hyperglycemia and fewer infectious complications (e.g., pneumonia, intra-abdominal abscess, catheter-related infections).[1-3] However, if used appropriately, PN can be safe and effective and can improve nutrient delivery. Indications for PN are listed in Table 100–1.[1,2] In general, PN should be reserved for patients with altered intestinal function or absorption or when the gastrointestinal (GI) tract cannot be used. In addition, the anticipated duration of adequate PN therapy should be at least 5 to 7 days because shorter durations of therapy are unlikely to have a beneficial effect on a patient's clinical and nutritional outcomes but may increase infection risk.[1,2]

Table 100–1

Indications for Parenteral Nutrition in Adults[1,2,a]

- Bowel obstruction
  - Physical or mechanical (e.g., tumor compressing intestinal lumen)
  - Functional (e.g., ileus, colonic pseudo-obstruction)
- Major small bowel resection (e.g., short-bowel syndrome)
  - Adult patients with less than 100 cm of small bowel distal to the ligament of Treitz without a colon
  - Adult patients with less than 50 cm of small bowel if the colon is intact
- Diffuse peritonitis
- Intestinal fistulas if EN cannot be provided above or below the fistula
- Pancreatitis—if patients have failed EN beyond the ligament of Treitz or cannot receive EN (e.g., because of intestinal obstruction)
- Severe intractable vomiting
- Severe intractable diarrhea
- Preoperative nutrition support in patients with moderate to severe malnutrition who cannot tolerate EN and in whom surgery can be delayed safely for at least 7 days
- In critically ill patients without malnutrition who cannot receive oral or EN in the first 7 days of ICU admission, PN should only be initiated after the first 7 days of admission and if oral or EN is still not feasible

*a*When adequate oral or enteral nutrition will not be possible for ~5 to 10 days in patients with malnutrition or for ~7 to 14 days in most other cases, unless noted otherwise; anticipated duration of PN should be at least 5 to 7 days.

EN, enteral nutrition; ICU, intensive care unit; PN, parenteral nutrition.

PN COMPONENTS

PN should provide a *balanced* nutrition formula, including macronutrients, micronutrients, fluids, and electrolytes. Macronutrients, including amino acids, dextrose, and IV lipid emulsions, are important sources of structural and energy-yielding substrates. Total daily calories in a balanced PN formulation for adult patients are typically provided as 10% to 20% from amino acids, 50% to 60% from dextrose, and 20% to 30% from IV lipid emulsion. Amino acids may provide more than 20% of the total daily calories in patients with conditions that increase protein requirements (e.g., severe thermal injury, healing wounds, cachexia, treatment with continuous renal replacement therapy, hypocaloric feeding—discussed later). Electrolytes and micronutrients, including vitamins and trace elements, are required to support essential biochemical reactions. PN also provides a significant source of fluid. Patients require individual adjustments of PN components based on their nutritional status, nutritional requirements, underlying disease state(s), level of metabolic stress, clinical status, and organ functions.

Patient Encounter, Part 1

WS is a 26-year-old woman admitted to the hospital with chief complaints of constipation, abdominal pain, abdominal distention, nausea, and vomiting for 4 days. She also reports decreased appetite and decreased oral intake for the past 3 to 4 days and gradual unintentional weight loss of about 10 lb (4.5 kg) over the past month. WS reports a history of chronic constipation and chronic abdominal pain and that she has had several abdominal surgeries in the past due to obstructions and severe constipation. She also states that she usually "doesn't eat much" because she starts to "feel full" quickly. She has had multiple hospital admissions over the past 2 or 3 years for abdominal pain, constipation, and intestinal obstructions.

Medical History

Possible Hirschsprung's disease, chronic constipation, chronic abdominal pain, recurrent bowel obstructions, malnutrition

Surgical History

Colon resection with colostomy and mucus fistula, colostomy takedown with anastomosis, two small bowel resections for obstruction and lysis of adhesions (greater than 100 cm of small intestine remaining, ileocecal valve intact, part of the colon remaining)

Family History

Grandmother with chronic constipation and presumed Hirschsprung's disease

Social History

Nonsmoker; patient reports only occasional alcohol; no recreational drugs but does require chronic prescription opioid therapy for chronic abdominal pain

Medications Before Admission

Hydrocodone—acetaminophen 5/325, 1 tablet every 4 to 6 hours as needed for abdominal pain (patient states taking 1 tablet about every 4 to 5 hours around the clock)

Docusate 100 mg PO twice daily

Polyethylene glycol 3,350, 17 g PO once daily

Physical Exam

Height, 163 cm (~5 ft, 4 in); actual body weight, 41 kg (90 lb); ideal body weight, 54.5 kg (120 lb); temperature 36.7°C (98°F); heart rate, 95 beats/min; blood pressure, 100/62 mm Hg; respiratory rate 25 breaths/min; alert and oriented × 3; mucous membranes and skin appear cool and dry; tachycardic; tachypneic; lungs clear

Abdomen: Tense, distended, diffuse crampy abdominal pain, bowel sounds absent

Diagnoses

Likely recurrent intestinal obstruction related to chronic constipation or possibly Hirschsprung's disease, mild dehydration, and malnutrition

Plan

Admit to the hospital (non-ICU) for fluid resuscitation and treatment; evaluate for possible surgical intervention (exploratory laparotomy).

Is PN therapy indicated in this patient? Why or why not?

Amino Acids

Amino acids are the building blocks of proteins and an essential component of PN admixtures. ❷ *Amino acids are provided to preserve or replete lean body mass and visceral proteins, to promote protein anabolism and wound healing, and as a source of energy.* Amino acids have a caloric value of 4 kcal/g (17 kJ/g).

Parenteral crystalline amino acid solutions are supplied by various manufacturers in various concentrations (e.g., 7%, 8%, 8.5%, 10%, 15%, and others). Different formulations are tailored for specific age groups (e.g., adults, infants) and disease states (e.g., kidney or liver dysfunction). Specialized formulations for patients with acute kidney injury contain higher proportions of essential amino acids. Formulations for patients with hepatic encephalopathy contain higher amounts of branched-chain and lower amounts of aromatic amino acids. However, these specialized formulations have not been clearly shown to improve patient outcomes and therefore are not routinely used in clinical practice. Crystalline amino acid solutions have an acidic pH (pH ≈ 5 to 7) and may contain inherent electrolytes (e.g., sodium, potassium, acetate, phosphate).

Dextrose

❸ *Dextrose (D-glucose) is the major energy source, and it is vital for cellular metabolism, body protein preservation, and cellular growth.* Body tissues that depend primarily on dextrose as a source of energy include the central nervous system, red blood cells, and the renal medulla.

Typically, a 70% (70 g/100 mL) parenteral dextrose (hydrous dextrose) stock solution is used in PN compounding (a 50% stock solution is also available). Hydrous dextrose provides 3.4 kcal/g (14.2 kJ/g). A dextrose infusion rate of 2 mg/kg/min in adult patients is typically sufficient to suppress gluconeogenesis and spare body proteins from being used for energy.[4] Dextrose infusion rate in hospitalized adult patients generally should not exceed 4 to 5 mg/kg per minute.[5,6]

Intravenous Lipid Emulsions

④ *Intravenous lipid emulsions have two main clinical uses, which are to prevent or treat essential fatty acid deficiency and provide an energy source.* IV lipid emulsions marketed in the United States consist of long-chain triglycerides. Lipid particles consist of a triglyceride core surrounded by a layer of egg phospholipids (emulsifiers). These particles carry a negative charge on their surface that creates repulsive electrostatic forces between droplets and maintains the stability of the emulsion. Glycerol is added to adjust the tonicity, and water is the solvent. The negative charges on the surface of lipid particles can be disrupted by cations, especially divalent cations, such as calcium, magnesium, and iron,[7] and extreme pH changes, particularly acidic pH. Creaming of the emulsion occurs when lipid particles begin to aggregate and migrate to the surface of the emulsion but can be reversed with mild agitation. If these particles continue to aggregate, coalescence may occur and destabilize the emulsion. A coalesced emulsion should not be infused into a patient because this can result in fat emboli. If coalescence continues, irreversible separation of the emulsion can occur (oiling out, also called "breaking" or "cracking" of the emulsion). If there is any apparent disruption to a lipid emulsion, it should *not* be infused into a patient.

Intravenous lipid emulsions differ in their concentration (10%, 20%, and 30%), caloric density by volume, natural source of lipids, and ratio of phospholipids to triglycerides (PL:TG ratio). Table 100–2 shows a comparison of commercially available IV lipid emulsions in the United States. Because of the addition of phospholipid emulsifiers and glycerol, the caloric density of IV lipid emulsions by weight is approximately 10 kcal/g (42 kJ/g; dietary fat is ~ 9 kcal/g [38 kJ/g]). Compared with the 10% lipid emulsion, 20% and 30% lipid emulsions have a lower PL:TG ratio and lower phospholipid content; this translates to better plasma clearance of the 20% and 30% lipid emulsions compared with the 10% lipid emulsion.[8] The 30% lipid emulsion is only approved by the Food and Drug Administration (FDA) for infusion in a total nutrient admixture (TNA) and should not be infused directly into patients nor via Y-site injection.

Lipid particles are hydrolyzed in the bloodstream by lipoprotein lipase to release free fatty acids and glycerol. Fatty acids are taken up into adipose tissue for storage (triglycerides), oxidized to energy in various tissues (e.g., skeletal muscles), or recycled in the liver to make lipoproteins. The typical daily dose of IV lipid emulsions in adults is about 0.5 to 1 g/kg/day. The maximum dose is 2.5 g/kg/day[6] or 60% of total daily calories, although doses this high are rarely used in practice and should be avoided to prevent complications.

The essential fatty acids that cannot be produced endogenously in humans are linoleic acid (C18:2 n-6) and α-linolenic acid (C18:3 n-3). Arachidonic acid (C20:4 n-6) is also essential but can be synthesized in vivo from linoleic acid. Adult patients should receive a minimum of 2% to 4% of total daily calories as linoleic acid and 0.25% to 0.5% of total daily calories as α-linolenic acid to prevent essential fatty acid deficiency.[6] This can be achieved by providing a minimum of about 500 mL of 20% (100 g) IV lipid emulsion once a week (or 250 mL twice a week on separate days) for most adult patients. Biochemical evidence of essential fatty acid deficiency (e.g., decreased serum linoleic acid, α-linolenic acid, and arachidonic acid concentrations; elevated mead acid concentrations; elevated triene-to-tetraene ratio) can develop in nonmalnourished adult patients within about 2 to 4 weeks of receiving lipid-free PN, and clinical manifestations (e.g., dry skin, skin desquamation, hair loss, hepatomegaly, anemia, thrombocytopenia, poor wound healing) may appear after an additional 1 to 2 weeks, although skin changes may take longer to develop.[9]

Complications and safety concerns related to the administration of IV lipid emulsions include severe hypertriglyceridemia, systemic infection, anaphylactic reactions, and infusion-related reactions. Patients with a history of hypertriglyceridemia, acute kidney injury, chronic kidney disease, hepatic dysfunction, severe

Table 100–2
Comparison of Intravenous Lipid Emulsions

Brand Names	Liposyn II		Liposyn III			Intralipid		
Source	Soybean and safflower oil		Soybean oil			Soybean oil		
Concentration (%)	10	20	10	20	30	10	20	30
Linoleic acid (%)	65.8	65.8	54.5	54.5	54.5	44 – 62	44 – 62	44 – 62
Linolenic acid (%)	4.2	4.2	8.3	8.3	8.3	4 – 11	4 – 11	4 – 11
Phospholipids (egg yolk) (%)	1.2	1.2	1.2	1.2	1.8	1.2	1.2	1.2
PL:TG ratio	0.12	0.06	0.12	0.06	0.06	0.12	0.06	0.04
Caloric density[a] (kcal/mL)	1.1	2	1.1	2	3	1.1	2	3
Approximate osmolarity (mOsm/L)	276	258	284	292	293	300	350	310
Approximate mean pH (range)	8.0 (6.0–9.0)	8.3 (6.0–9.0)	8.3 (6.0–9.0)		8.4 (6.0–9.0)	8.0 (6.0–8.9)		

PL, phospholipid; TG, triglyceride.

[a]One kcal/mL is equivalent to 4.19 kJ/mL.

metabolic stress, or **pancreatitis** (particularly if caused by hypertriglyceridemia) may have reduced lipid clearance and be at risk of developing hypertriglyceridemia. IV lipid emulsions should be withheld in adult patients with serum triglyceride concentrations exceeding 400 mg/dL (4.52 mmol/L).

Intravenous lipid emulsions support the growth of bacterial and fungal pathogens, but bacterial growth is slower in TNAs than in IV lipid emulsions alone.[10,11] This is because of the acidic pH of amino acid solutions and higher osmolarity of PN formulations. The Centers for Disease Control and Prevention (CDC) recommends that infusion of IV lipid emulsions separately from PN (i.e., 2-in-1) be completed within 12 hours of initiation (e.g., two lipid containers can be used with each container infused over 12 hours). If fluid or volume considerations prohibit a reduced infusion time, the lipid infusion can be completed within 24 hours, although there is debate about the appropriateness of this approach. Because TNAs support microbial growth at a slower rate than IV lipid emulsions, the CDC recommends that TNA infusion be completed within 24 hours of initiation. A 0.22-micron bacterial retention filter cannot be used on the TNA infusion line; the average size of lipid particles is approximately 0.4 to 0.5 microns, which cannot pass through the smaller filter intact. Strict aseptic technique must be used when handling IV lipid emulsions to minimize the risk of PN contamination and possible infectious complications.

Patients with an allergy to eggs or specific legumes (e.g., soy beans, broad beans, lentils) may develop cross-allergic reactions to IV lipid emulsions. Rarely, infusion-related adverse effects may occur with rapid infusion, including fever, chills, headache, palpitations, dyspnea, chest tightness, and nausea. Extending the IV lipid infusion time (e.g., over 12 to 24 hours) can minimize infusion-related adverse events and improves lipid clearance. Infusion rate of IV lipid emulsions should not exceed 0.12 g/kg/h.[6]

Fluid

⑤ *Parenteral nutrition should not be used to treat acute fluid abnormalities. PN should be adjusted to provide maintenance fluid requirements and to minimize worsening of underlying fluid disturbances, taking into account other fluids the patient is receiving.* Daily maintenance fluid requirements for adults can be estimated with the following equation:

$$\text{Total daily maintenance fluid requirements} = 1{,}500 \text{ mL} + (20 \text{ mL/kg} \times [\text{Wt (kg)} - 20])^*$$

For patients with significant fluid deficits, it is safer and more cost effective to correct fluid abnormalities using standard IV fluids (e.g., 0.9% sodium chloride in water, dextrose 5% and sodium chloride 0.45% in water, lactated Ringer's solution). Minimizing PN fluid volume may be indicated in patients with fluid overload, such as those who receive large volumes of resuscitation fluid and/or multiple IV medications (e.g., critically ill, bone marrow transplant),

patients with oliguric (urine output less than 400 mL/day, or less than 0.5 mL/kg/h) or anuric (urine output less than 50 mL/day) acute kidney injury, or those with congestive heart failure or symptomatic pleural effusion. It is reasonable to provide total daily fluid requirements (maintenance requirements and replacement for GI or other abnormal losses) in the PN admixture in patients who depend on long-term PN. However, caution should be exercised when the PN admixture is diluted to an extent that may alter the stability and compatibility of the components. Diluting a PN admixture may affect its physical and chemical properties (e.g., pH, which could affect lipid emulsion stability and calcium–phosphate compatibility); therefore, stability and compatibility data should first be confirmed.

Electrolytes

⑥ *Electrolytes are essential for many metabolic and homeostatic functions, including enzymatic and biochemical reactions, maintenance of cell membrane structure and function, neurotransmission, hormone function, muscle contraction, cardiovascular function, bone composition, and fluid homeostasis.* The causes of electrolyte abnormalities in patients receiving PN may be multifactorial, including altered absorption and distribution; excessive or inadequate intake; altered hormonal, neurologic, and homeostatic mechanisms; altered excretion and losses via the GI tract and kidneys; changes in fluid status and fluid shifts; and medication therapies. PN should not be used to treat acute electrolyte abnormalities but should be adjusted to meet maintenance requirements and to minimize worsening of underlying electrolyte disturbances.

Electrolytes that are included routinely in PN admixtures include sodium, potassium, phosphorus (as phosphate), calcium, magnesium, chloride, and acetate. Always assess the patient's kidney function when determining electrolytes in PN admixtures. Typical daily electrolyte maintenance requirements for adults with normal kidney function are listed in Table 100–3.

▶ Sodium

Sodium is the most abundant extracellular cation in the body and is the major osmotically active ion in the extracellular fluid. Sodium concentration determines distribution of water in extracellular space, and sodium disorders can be caused by many factors. Patients with abnormal GI losses (e.g., gastric, diarrhea, **ostomy**, enterocutaneous **fistula**) have increased sodium requirements. Patients with fluid overload and hypervolemic hypotonic hyponatremia may require sodium and fluid restriction. Sodium in PN can be provided in the forms of chloride, acetate, and phosphate salts (see Table 100–3). Total sodium concentration in PN should not exceed 154 mEq/L (154 mmol/L, the equivalent of normal saline).

▶ Potassium

Potassium is the most abundant intracellular cation in the body. Potassium has many important physiologic functions, including regulation of cell membrane electrical

---

*For elderly patients (e.g., greater than 60 years old), use 15 mL/kg for every kilogram above 20 kg.

Table 100–3

Approximate Daily Maintenance Electrolyte Requirements for Adults[6]

Electrolyte	Approximate Daily Maintenance Requirements[a]	Electrolyte Salts Used in PN
Sodium	1–2 mEq/kg	Chloride, acetate, phosphate
Potassium	1–2 mEq/kg	Chloride, acetate, phosphate
Phosphorus	20–40 mmol	Sodium phosphate, potassium phosphate
Calcium	10–15 mEq	Gluconate
Magnesium	8–20 mEq	Sulfate
Chloride	[b]	Sodium, potassium
Acetate	[b]	Sodium, potassium
Conversions	1 mmol potassium phosphate = 1.47 mEq potassium	
	1 mmol sodium phosphate = 1.33 mEq sodium	

[a]Electrolyte requirements are adjusted based on serum electrolyte concentrations and vary depending on kidney function, gastrointestinal losses, nutritional status, specific metabolic and endocrine functions, and medication therapy that affect electrolyte losses or retention.

[b]As needed to maintain acid–base balance; linked to amounts of sodium and potassium provided (as chloride and acetate salts).

action potential, muscular function, cellular metabolism, and glycogen and protein synthesis. Potassium in PN can be provided as chloride, acetate, and phosphate salts (see Table 100–3). Generally, concentrations of potassium in PN admixtures should not exceed 120 mEq/L (120 mmol/L) for safety reasons and to avoid excessive potassium infusion. This may also decrease the risk of **thrombophlebitis** when administered as peripheral PN (PPN) via a peripheral vein (refer to the section Route of PN Administration). In addition, when admixed with IV lipid emulsion, high concentrations of cations can destabilize the emulsion (refer to the section Types of PN Formulations).[6] IV potassium should be infused at a maximum of 10 mEq/h (10 mmol/h) via a peripheral vein in patients who are not on a cardiac monitor, and 20 mEq/h (20 mmol/h) via a central vein if the patient is on a cardiac monitor (nonemergent situations). Patients with abnormal potassium losses (e.g., loop or thiazide diuretic therapy, diarrhea) may have higher potassium requirements, and patients with acute kidney injury or chronic kidney disease or those who receive medications that can cause potassium retention (e.g., spironolactone, tacrolimus) may require potassium restriction.

▶ *Calcium and Phosphorus*

Calcium and phosphorus are essential electrolytes for many physiologic processes and biochemical reactions. Phosphorus in PN is provided as sodium or potassium phosphate (see Table 100–3), and phosphate is essential for energy and adenosine triphosphate (ATP). Approximately 10 to 15 mmol of phosphate is needed per 1,000 kilocalories (4,186 kJ) to maintain normal serum phosphorus concentrations in well-nourished adult patients (with normal kidney function).[12] Patients with impaired kidney function typically require phosphorus restriction.

The FDA published a safety alert in response to two deaths associated with calcium–phosphate precipitation in PN.[13] Autopsy reports from these patients revealed diffuse **microvascular pulmonary emboli** containing calcium-phosphate precipitates. Because calcium and phosphate can bind and precipitate in solution, caution must be exercised

when mixing these two electrolytes in PN admixtures. Several factors can affect calcium–phosphate solubility, including:

- *pH.* Largely affected by the final amino acid concentration, to a lesser extent by the dextrose concentration (unless the final amino acid concentration is very low); the lower the solution pH, the less chance for calcium–phosphate precipitation. Monobasic phosphates predominate at low pH, leaving fewer free dibasic phosphates for precipitation with divalent calcium; monobasic calcium phosphate is more soluble than dibasic calcium phosphate.

- *Amino acid concentration.* Primary factor that affects pH of the PN admixture. The pH of amino acid stock solutions may vary between commercial products and thus differently affects the final pH of PN admixtures, but in general, the higher the final amino acid concentration, the lower the pH of the final admixture. Phosphates can also bind with amino acids, leaving fewer phosphates available to bind with calcium.

- *Calcium salt.* Calcium gluconate is the preferred calcium salt in PN because it has a low dissociation constant in solution with less free calcium available at a given time to bind phosphate (as opposed to calcium chloride, which dissociates rapidly in solution). One gram of calcium gluconate provides 4.5 mEq (2.2 mmol) of elemental calcium.

- *Time.* The longer calcium and phosphate are in solution, the more calcium and phosphate will dissociate over time and increase the risk for calcium–phosphate precipitation.

- *Temperature.* As temperature increases, more calcium and phosphate dissociate and increase the risk of calcium-phosphate precipitation.

- *Order of mixing.* Calcium and phosphate should not be added simultaneously or consecutively when compounding PN admixtures (e.g., add phosphate first, then add other PN components, and then add calcium near the end of compounding). The volume in the PN admixture at the time calcium is added (not necessarily the final volume) must be used to determine the maximum calcium that can be added.

When compounding PN admixtures, specific calcium–phosphate solubility curves must be used to determine safe and appropriate calcium and phosphate concentration limits.

▶ *Magnesium*

● Magnesium is the second most abundant intracellular cation after potassium. Magnesium is an essential cofactor for numerous enzymes and in many biochemical reactions, including reactions involving ATP.[14] Magnesium disorders are multifactorial and can be related to kidney function, GI losses, disease states, and medication therapy. Magnesium in PN is typically provided as magnesium sulfate. One gram of magnesium sulfate provides 8.1 mEq (4.0 mmol) of elemental magnesium.

▶ *Chloride and Acetate*

Concentration limits for chloride and acetate in PN typically are linked to limitations of sodium and potassium. The usual ● ratio of chloride to acetate in PN is about 1:1 to 1.5:1. Chloride and acetate play a role in acid–base balance. Serum chloride concentrations that exceed 130 mEq/L (130 mmol/L) may cause hyperchloremic acidosis. Acetate is converted to bicarbonate at a 1:1 molar ratio, and this conversion appears to occur mostly outside the liver. Acetate conversion to bicarbonate is rapid, but not immediate, and thus acetate salts should not be used to correct acute severe acidemia. Bicarbonate should *never* be added to or co-infused with PN admixtures. This can lead to the release of carbon dioxide and result in the formation of insoluble calcium or magnesium carbonate salts.

Vitamins

● ⑥ *The water-soluble and fat-soluble vitamins in the parenteral multivitamin mix are essential cofactors for numerous biochemical reactions and metabolic processes. Parenteral multivitamins are added daily to the PN admixture.* Patients with chronic kidney disease are at risk for vitamin A accumulation and potential toxicity. Serum vitamin A concentrations should be measured in patients with chronic kidney disease when vitamin A accumulation is a concern. Previously, vitamin K was administered either daily or once weekly because IV multivitamin formulations did not contain vitamin K. However, reformulated parenteral multivitamin products contain 150 mcg of vitamin K in accordance with FDA recommendations. A parenteral adult multivitamin formulation is available without vitamin K (e.g., for patients who require warfarin therapy), but standard compounding of PN formulations should include a parenteral multivitamin that contains vitamin K unless otherwise clinically indicated. Water-soluble vitamins, with the exception of vitamin B_{12}, are generally readily excreted and not stored in the body in significant amounts. Deficiencies of water-soluble vitamins can occur rapidly in the absence of adequate vitamin supplementation in PN. For example, severe refractory lactic acidosis and deaths were reported in patients who received PN without added thiamine. Thiamine is an essential cofactor in carbohydrate metabolism, specifically a cofactor of the pyruvate dehydrogenase enzyme that is involved in the aerobic metabolism of pyruvate to acetyl-CoA (via the tricarboxylic acid cycle). Deficiency of thiamine pyrophosphate prevents the formation of acetyl-CoA from pyruvate, which is instead converted to lactate via anaerobic metabolism, resulting in lactic acidosis.

Trace Elements

● ⑥ *Trace elements are essential cofactors for numerous biochemical processes. Trace elements added routinely to PN include zinc, selenium, copper, manganese, and chromium* (Table 100–4). Various individual and multi-ingredient parenteral trace element formulations can be added to PN admixtures. Trace element supplementation in PN should be individualized, especially for long term PN-dependent patients, rather than using a fixed dose of multi-trace element products.[15] Zinc is important for wound healing, and patients with high-output enterocutaneous fistulas, diarrhea, burns, and large open wounds may require additional zinc supplementation. Patients may lose as much as 12 to 17 mg zinc per liter of GI output (e.g., diarrhea, enterocutaneous fistula); however, 12 mg/day may be adequate to maintain these patients in positive zinc balance.[16] Patients with chronic severe diarrhea, malabsorption, high-output enterocutaneous fistula, or short-bowel syndrome may also have increased selenium losses and may require additional selenium supplementation. Chromium is a cofactor for glucose metabolism, and patients with chromium deficiency may exhibit glucose intolerance; however, chromium deficiency is a rare cause of hyperglycemia. Patients who are chronically dependent on PN may accumulate chromium[6] and manganese, resulting in high serum levels because these are known contaminants of parenteral products that are used in

Table 100–4				
Approximate Daily Maintenance Trace Element Requirements for Adults[6,a]				
Zinc (Zn)	Selenium (Se)	Copper (Cu)	Manganese (Mn)	Chromium (Cr)
2.5–5 mg	20–60 mcg	0.3–0.5 mg	0.06–0.1 mg	10–15 mcg

[a] Trace element requirements may vary based on patients' trace element levels, kidney function, liver function, gastrointestinal losses, nutritional status, specific metabolic and endocrine functions, and medication therapy. In addition, contamination of some parenteral nutrition (PN) ingredients with trace elements (e.g., chromium, manganese) can contribute significantly to the total amount the patient receives. Serum trace element levels should be monitored in patients receiving long-term PN therapy.

the making of PN.[6,15] Patients with cholestasis (serum direct bilirubin concentrations that exceed 2 mg/dL [34.2 μmol/L]) should have manganese and possibly copper restricted to avoid accumulation and possible toxicity because both elements undergo biliary elimination. Manganese-induced neurotoxicity has been reported in PN patients with cholestasis and those receiving chronic PN. However, copper deficiency resulting in anemia, pancytopenia, and death has occurred in PN-dependent patients when copper was omitted from the PN admixture. Because copper deficiency has been reported to occur anywhere between 6 weeks and 12 months after copper elimination from PN,[17] serum copper concentrations need to be regularly monitored (e.g., every 6 weeks at first and then every 2 to 3 months thereafter) when copper is omitted from PN admixtures. Trace element status should initially be monitored periodically (e.g., every 3 months) in patients at risk for trace element deficiency or accumulation. When stable, serum trace element concentrations can be monitored less frequently (e.g., every 6 to 12 months).

PN Additives

▶ Heparin

Heparin (0.5 to 1 unit/mL of final PN volume) may be added to PN admixtures for three reasons:

- Maintain catheter patency (although this effect is debated)
- Reduce thrombophlebitis (with PPN infusion)
- Enhance lipid particle clearance as a cofactor for the lipoprotein lipase enzyme

The benefits and necessity of adding heparin to PN are unclear. Although practices vary, the addition of heparin to PN admixtures for adult patients is becoming less common. There are also concerns about the stability and compatibility of IV lipid emulsions with heparin added at concentrations above 1 unit/mL. Heparin should be omitted in patients with active bleeding, thrombocytopenia, heparin-induced thrombocytopenia (HIT), or heparin allergy.

▶ Regular Insulin

Regular insulin may be added to PN admixtures for glycemic control. The dose depends on the severity of hyperglycemia, predisposing factors for hyperglycemia, renal function, and daily insulin requirements. Generally, after the patient is receiving his or her goal dextrose dose in PN, about 50% to 70% of the total insulin doses administered over the previous 24 hours as sliding scale or continuous infusion can be added to the next PN admixture. The insulin dose should be adjusted based on frequent capillary blood glucose evaluation. Caution should be used when insulin is added to PN to avoid hypoglycemia, especially when reversible causes of hyperglycemia have resolved (e.g., stress, acute pancreatitis, corticosteroids therapy) or more than one form of insulin therapy is concurrently used. Adding insulin to PN rather than administering as a continuous IV infusion does not provide the flexibility of frequent titration of the insulin dose to the desired target blood glucose concentration.

As such, severe uncontrolled hyperglycemia is best treated with a continuous insulin infusion.

▶ Histamine-2 Receptor Antagonists

Intravenous histamine-2 receptor antagonists such as ranitidine, famotidine, and cimetidine are compatible with PN and can be added to the daily PN when indicated (e.g., prevention of stress-related mucosal damage). This provides continuous acid suppression and reduces pharmacy and nursing time by avoiding intermittent scheduled infusions.

▶ Human Albumin

Human albumin is a colloid used as a plasma volume expander and *not* a source of nutrition. Albumin should not be added to the PN admixture and should be administered separately from PN because it may increase microbial growth and infectious risk when mixed in the PN admixture. Furthermore, co-infusion of human albumin at the Y-site injection of IV lipid emulsion and TNAs may cause disruption and creaming of the IV lipid emulsion.

▶ Parenteral Iron

Iron-deficiency anemia in chronic PN-dependent patients may be caused by underlying clinical conditions and the lack of regular iron supplementation in PN. Parenteral iron therapy becomes necessary in iron-deficient patients who cannot absorb or tolerate oral iron. Parenteral iron should be used with caution owing to its infusion-related adverse effects. A test dose of 25 mg of iron dextran should be administered first, and the patient should be monitored for adverse effects for at least 60 minutes. Iron dextran then may be added to lipid-free PN at a daily dose of 100 mg until the total iron dose is given. Iron dextran is not compatible with IV lipid emulsions and can cause oiling out of the emulsion. Other parenteral iron formulations (e.g., iron sucrose, ferric gluconate) have not been evaluated for compounding in PN and should NOT be added to PN admixtures.

NUTRITION ASSESSMENT AND NUTRIENT REQUIREMENTS

The first step before delivering nutrition support therapy is to perform a nutrition assessment and determine nutrient requirements based on the patient's nutritional status and clinical conditions. Collect subjective and objective data of dietary intake, functional capacity, anthropometrics, weight changes, GI function, medical history, medication therapy, and laboratory data to determine a patient's nutritional status, identify patients with malnutrition or at risk for malnutrition, identify risk factors that may put a patient at risk for nutrition-related problems, and identify or rule out specific nutrient deficiencies.[1] A nutrition assessment should include:[1,18]

- Patient history
- Physical assessment including height, weight, ideal body weight (IBW), body mass index (BMI = weight [kg]/height [m²]), and recent weight loss (intentional or unintentional)

BMI relates a person's body weight to height and is a vague indicator of total body fat mass in adults. BMI categories do not account for frame size, muscle mass, bone, and water weight. Furthermore, BMI is not an indicator of body nutrient stores. Classifications of weight status in relation to BMI are underweight, less than 18.5 kg/m^2; normal, 18.5 to 24.9 kg/ m^2; overweight, 25 to 29.9 kg/ m^2; obese, greater than or equal to 30 kg/ m^2.

- Physical examination of the musculoskeletal system (e.g., biceps, triceps, quadriceps, temporalis, deltoid, and interosseus muscles) for loss of muscle mass, and examination of the skin and mucous membranes for abnormalities (e.g., noting dry or flaky skin, bruising, edema, ascites, poorly healing wounds) and loss of subcutaneous fat (e.g., triceps, chest)

- Changes in eating habits and GI function and associated GI symptoms

- Presence and severity of underlying and concurrent disease(s)

- Serum visceral protein concentrations (e.g., albumin, prealbumin). Hypoalbuminemia at baseline or before hospitalization may be indicative of malnutrition, and severe hypoalbuminemia may be associated with poor patient outcome. Serum albumin and prealbumin are negative acute phase proteins and therefore are not sensitive or specific indicators of nutritional status and protein stores in hospitalized patients under metabolic stress (e.g., postsurgery, organ failure, severe burns, trauma, sepsis). Synthesis and distribution of these proteins may be altered, and serum concentrations are affected by non-nutritional factors, including hydration status, kidney function, and liver function. Because prealbumin has a shorter half-life (~2 days) than albumin (~20 days), serum prealbumin concentrations are measured usually once weekly to help evaluate the net anabolism in response to nutrition support therapy.

- Serum concentrations of vitamins, trace elements, and iron studies as indicated

Several methods may be used to conduct a nutrition assessment, but one validated approach in adult patients is the Subjective Global Assessment (SGA).[1] Application of the SGA requires gathering the data listed above and assessing these parameters (i.e., weight change, dietary changes, GI symptoms, functional capacity, and physical examination) and then assigning a subjective rating (A = well nourished, B = moderately malnourished or suspected of being malnourished, and C = severely malnourished).[18]

After performing a nutrition assessment, estimate the patient's daily energy and protein requirements (Table 100–5). Indirect calorimetry involves measuring the volumes of oxygen consumption (VO$_2$) and carbon dioxide production (VCO$_2$) to determine the resting metabolic rate (RMR) or resting energy expenditure (REE) and respiratory quotient (RQ = VCO$_2$/VO$_2$). The REE or RMR is the amount of calories required during 24 hours by the body in a non-active state and is approximately 10% higher than the basal energy expenditure (BEE, metabolic

activity required to maintain life) as it adjusts for the thermic effect of food and awake state. Because critically ill patients may have variable energy expenditure (EE), indirect calorimetry is a valuable tool in assessing EE in mechanically ventilated patients with multiple and changing clinical conditions. Indirect calorimetry requires expensive equipment and trained personnel to use and therefore is not feasible in all institutions. More than 200 equations have been developed to predict EE for adults. The Harris-Benedict equations, Penn State equations (for non-obese critically ill patients), and Mifflin-St. Jeor equations (for obese noncritically ill patients) are some of the most widely used. Harris-Benedict equations take into account a patient's sex, weight, height, and age to determine the BEE. A "stress" or "injury" factor is then applied to estimate the daily total EE (TEE). Daily energy requirements are about 100% to 130% of the RMR with adequate protein intake. Alternatively, EE can be estimated based on EE per body weight (i.e., kilocalories per kilogram or in kilojoules per kilogram). However, dry weight or hospital admission weight should be used, and this estimation may not be appropriate in obese or elderly patients. There is debate over the best method to estimate energy requirements for obese patients. Indirect calorimetry would be the preferred method to estimate energy requirements for obese patients but may not always be available. Several equations have been developed to estimate EE in obese patients. Although there is no consensus on the weight used to estimate EE in obese patients, it is reasonable to use an adjusted body weight (AdjBW) in obese patients to avoid overfeeding. AdjBW can be calculated with 25% to 50% of the difference between the actual weight and IBW added to the IBW. Using a 25% difference in calculating the AdjBW further avoids overfeeding when estimating energy requirements:

$$AdjBW = IBW + (0.25 \times [Actual\ weight - IBW])$$

Amino acid requirements are based on the patient's nutritional status, clinical condition(s), kidney function, and liver function. Amino acids are needed in adequate amounts to facilitate anabolism, restore lean body mass, or promote wound healing while avoiding adverse effects from excessive amino acid loading (e.g., azotemia). No evidence-based data are available on the optimal body weight (actual, ideal, or adjusted) to use for dosing amino acids in adult patients. It is, however, suggested to dose amino acids based on actual body weight for normal body sized or malnourished adult patients (i.e., when actual weight is at or below IBW) and based on IBW for obese patients.

Hypocaloric nutrition support therapy for obese patients (BMI greater than or equal to 30 kg/m^2 or actual weight greater than 130% of IBW) is a promising approach. Hypocaloric feeding involves providing high amounts of protein (greater than or equal to 2 to 2.5 g/kg IBW/day) to support anabolism with lower amounts of total calories (average ~11 to 14 kcal/ kg actual weight/day [~46 to 59 kJ/kg actual weight/day] or ~22 to 25 kcal/kg IBW/day [~92 to 105 kJ/kg IBW/day]) with primary goals to promote net protein anabolism and avoid hyperglycemia or exacerbation of metabolic stress in critically ill patients.[2,19] Secondary benefits of hypocaloric feeding could be avoiding fat weight gain or possibly promoting fat

Table 100–5

Estimating Daily Nutritional Requirements in Adults[1,6,18]

Determining Energy Expenditure:

Harris-Benedict equations	Men: BEE = 66.42 + 13.75 (W) + 5 (H) – 6.78 (A) Women: BEE = 655.1 + 9.65 (W) + 1.85 (H) – 4.68 (A) W = weight in kg, H = height in cm, A = age in years Energy expenditure should then be multiplied by a stress factor. To estimate the TEE: Bed rest ≈ 1.2 × BEE Ambulatory ≈ 1.3 × BEE Anabolic ≈ 1.5 × BEE Energy requirements should also be increased ~12% with each degree of fever above 37°C (98.6°F).
Penn State equations (for critically-ill non-obese adult patients)	$RMR = (0.85 \times BEE^a) + (33 \times V_E) + (175 \times T_{max}) - 6,433$ $RMR = (0.96 \times BMR^b) + (31 \times V_E) + (167 \times T_{max}) - 6,212$
Mifflin-St. Jeor equations (for non-obese, overweight and obese noncritically ill adult patients)	Men BMR = (10 × Wt) + (6.25 × Ht) – (5 × Age) + 5 Women BMR = (10 × Wt) + (6.25 × Ht) – (5 × Age) – 161
Energy expenditure per body weight (i.e., kcal/kg)[c]	Range of ~20–30 kcal/kg/day, possibly up to 35 kcal/kg/day Maintenance ~20–25 kcal/kg/day Repletion, postoperative wound healing, critical illness, sepsis, severe trauma, severe burns ~25–30 kcal/kg/day, possibly up to 35 kcal/kg/day

Determining Amino Acid Requirements

Patient Clinical Condition	Daily Amino Acid Requirements[d] (g/kg)
Maintenance or nonstressed	0.8–1
Repletion	1.3–2
Trauma, burns, sepsis, critical illness, wound healing	1.5–2
Hepatic failure with encephalopathy	0.8–1
Acute kidney injury, predialysis	0.8–1
Acute kidney injury receiving IHD	1.2–1.5
Chronic kidney disease receiving CAPD	1.2–1.5
Acute kidney disease receiving CRRT	1.5–2.5

BMR, basal metabolic rate; CAPD, continuous ambulatory peritoneal dialysis; CRRT, continuous renal replacement therapy; Ht, height (cm); IHD, intermittent hemodialysis; RMR, resting metabolic rate; TEE, total energy expenditure; T_{max}, maximum body temperature in degrees Celsius; V_E, minute ventilation in liters per minute; Wt, weight (kg).

[a]BEE calculated using the Harris-Benedict equation.

[b]BMR calculated using Mifflin-St. Jeor equation.

[c]One kcal/kg is equivalent to 4.186 kJ/kg.

[d]Amino acid requirements are based on actual body weight for normal body sized or malnourished adult patients and on ideal body weight (IBW) for obese patients.

weight loss. The role of hypocaloric feeding in patients with kidney dysfunction or in patients with end-stage liver disease and hepatic encephalopathy is unknown. Also, the optimal safe duration of hypocaloric feeding in critically ill obese patients is unknown.

Permissive underfeeding refers to providing a lower calorie nutrition support regimen to critically ill adult patients for a short period of time during the initial phase of high metabolic stress. The aims of permissive underfeeding are to avoid the burden of caloric intake on worsening metabolic stress and the negative effects of carbohydrate loading and associated hyperglycemia, increased carbon dioxide production, and fat accumulation. Typically, a permissive underfeeding PN regimen provides about 60% to 80% of daily energy requirements. Because the optimal amounts of calories for critically ill patients is not well defined, strong clinical evidence to support the use

of permissive underfeeding is also lacking. Furthermore, severe underfeeding should be avoided because it can result in energy deficit to the patient with the consequences of increased infectious complications with negative patient outcomes.

Special Patient Considerations: Ethical and Personal Beliefs

When assessing a patient for PN, attention should be given to patients with special personal dietary choices (e.g., vegetarians, vegans) or religious beliefs (e.g., Jehovah's Witness). These situations may present unique challenges for clinicians. Most nutrients used in PN formulations are usually from synthetic sources (e.g., crystalline amino acids) or vegetable sources (e.g., triglycerides used in IV lipid emulsions), with the only exception usually being egg phospholipids used in IV lipid emulsions. Discuss these issues for patients with specific needs who require PN so that a plan can be developed to provide appropriate nutrition support therapy.

AMERICAN SOCIETY FOR PARENTERAL AND ENTERAL NUTRITION SAFE PRACTICES FOR PN

Because serious and sometimes fatal adverse events have occurred with inappropriate use of PN, the American Society for Parenteral and Enteral Nutrition (A.S.P.E.N.) has published updated safe practice guidelines for PN.[6] These practice guidelines provide a tool and reference for health professionals for the safe and efficacious use of PN. The guidelines represent the standards of practice as they relate to PN prescribing, compounding, stability, compatibility, labeling, administration, and quality assurance. Although application of these guidelines is voluntary, pharmacists who handle PN should review and apply them to their practice sites whenever possible.

PREPARING THE PN PRESCRIPTION: ADMINISTRATION, COMPOUNDING, AND PHARMACEUTICAL ISSUES

After performing a nutrition assessment and estimating nutritional requirements, determine the optimal route to provide nutrition support therapy (e.g., oral, enteral, or parenteral). If PN is deemed necessary, venous access (i.e., peripheral or central; see below) for PN infusion must be obtained. Finally, formulate a PN prescription and administer PN according to safety guidelines.

Route of PN Administration: Peripheral versus Central Vein Infusion

❼ *PN can be administered via a smaller peripheral vein (e.g., cephalic or basilic vein) or via a larger central vein (e.g., superior vena cava)* (Fig. 100–1). Peripheral PN (PPN) is infused via a peripheral vein and generally is reserved for short-term administration (up to 7 days) when central venous access is not available. PN formulations are hyperosmolar, and PN infusion via a peripheral vein can cause thrombophlebitis. Factors that increase the risk of phlebitis include high solution osmolarity, extreme pH, rapid infusion rate, vein properties, catheter properties (e.g., diameter, material), and infusion time via the same vein.[20] The osmolarity of PPN admixtures should be limited to 900 mOsm/L or less to minimize the risk of phlebitis. The approximate osmolarity of a PN admixture can be calculated from the osmolarity of the individual components:

- Amino acids ~10 mOsm/g (or 100 mOsm/L% final concentration in PN)
- Dextrose ~5 mOsm/g (or 50 mOsm/L% final concentration in PN)
- Sodium (chloride, acetate, and phosphate) = 2 mOsm/mEq
- Potassium (chloride, acetate, and phosphate) = 2 mOsm/mEq
- Calcium gluconate = 1.4 mOsm/mEq
- Magnesium sulfate = 1 mOsm/mEq

PPN admixtures should be co-infused with IV lipid emulsion when using the two-in-one PN because this may decrease the risk of phlebitis caused by the iso-osmolarity and near-neutral pH of IV lipid emulsions (see Table 100–2). Infectious and mechanical complications may be lower with

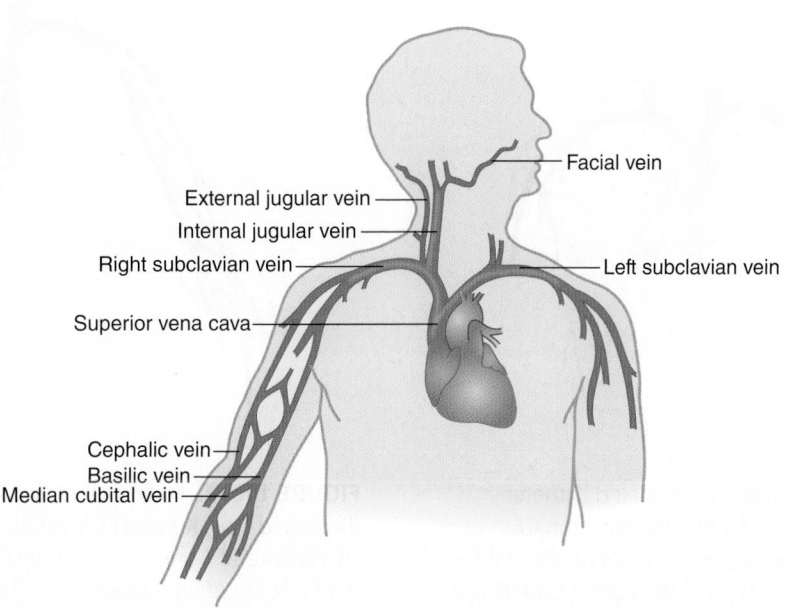

FIGURE 100–1. Selected vascular anatomy. (Reprinted from Krzywda EA, Andris DA, Edmiston CE, Wallace JR. Parenteral Access Devices. In: Gottschlich MM, ed. *The A.S.P.E.N. Nutrition Support Core Curriculum: A Case-Based Approach—The Adult Patient.* Silver Spring, MD: American Society for Parenteral and Enteral Nutrition, 2007:300–322 with permission from the American Society for Parenteral and Enteral Nutrition (A.S.P.E.N.). A.S.P.E.N. does not endorse the use of this material in any form other than its entirety.)

PPN compared with central venous PN administration. However, because of the risk of phlebitis and osmolarity limit, PPN admixtures have low macronutrient concentrations and therefore usually require large fluid volumes to meet a patient's nutritional requirements. Given these limitations, every effort should be made to obtain central venous access and initiate central PN in patients who have an indication for PN (see Table 100–1).

Central PN refers to the administration of PN via a large central vein, and the catheter tip must be positioned in the superior vena cava (**Fig. 100–2**). Central PN allows the infusion of a highly concentrated, hyperosmolar nutrient admixture. The typical osmolarity of a central PN admixture is about 1,500 to 2,000 mOsm/L. Central veins have much higher blood flow and the PN admixture is diluted rapidly on infusion, so phlebitis is usually not a concern. Patients who require PN therapy for longer periods of time (greater than 7 days) should receive central PN. One limitation of central PN is the need for placing a central venous catheter and an x-ray to confirm placement of the catheter tip. A commonly used central catheter for PN infusion is a peripherally inserted central venous catheter (PICC), which is inserted into a peripheral vein but the catheter tip is placed in the superior vena cava (**Fig. 100–3**). Central venous catheter placement may be associated with complications, including **pneumothorax**, arterial injury, **air embolus**, venous thrombosis, infection, **chylothorax**, and **brachial plexus** injury.[1,20]

Types of PN Formulations: 3-in-1 versus 2-in-1

❽ *PN admixtures can be prepared by mixing all components into one bag, or instead, IV lipid emulsion may be infused separately (via a Y-site infusion or through a separate IV catheter or lumen). When all components are mixed together, it is referred to as a 3-in-1 admixture or a TNA.[21] When dextrose, amino acids, and all other PN components are mixed together without IV lipid emulsion, this is referred to as a 2-in-1 PN admixture.* There are various advantages and disadvantages to using either 3-in-1 or 2-in-1 PN admixtures (**Table 100–6**). With a 2-in-1 PN admixture, IV lipid emulsion can be infused separately on a daily or intermittent basis. When lipid emulsion is mixed in the PN, the 3-in-1 admixture becomes an emulsion with respect to physical and chemical characteristics. The final concentration of IV lipid emulsion in a 3-in-1 admixture should be greater than or equal to 2% (20 g/L) to prevent compromising the stability of the emulsion.[21]

A primary concern when administering PN is safety, as described throughout this chapter (e.g., calcium–phosphate solubility). The FDA has provided recommendations for safe infusion of PN admixtures containing calcium and phosphate:

- A 0.22-micron air-eliminating in-line filter should be used for infusion of non–lipid-containing PN.
- A 1.2-micron in-line filter should be used for the infusion of 3-in-1 PN (i.e., a TNA) because it can remove large and unstable lipid droplets and particulate matter.[22]

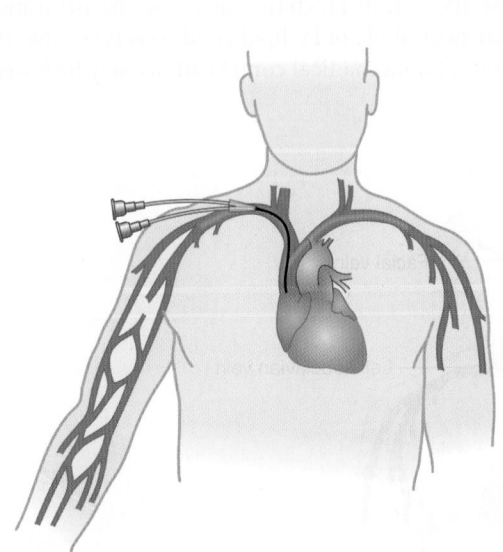

FIGURE 100–2. Percutaneous nontunneled catheter. (Reprinted from Krzywda EA, Andris DA, Edmiston CE, Wallace JR. Parenteral Access Devices. In: Gottschlich MM, ed. *The A.S.P.E.N. Nutrition Support Core Curriculum: A Case-Based Approach—The Adult Patient.* Silver Spring, MD: American Society for Parenteral and Enteral Nutrition, 2007:300–322 with permission from the American Society for Parenteral and Enteral Nutrition (A.S.P.E.N.). A.S.P.E.N. does not endorse the use of this material in any form other than its entirety.)

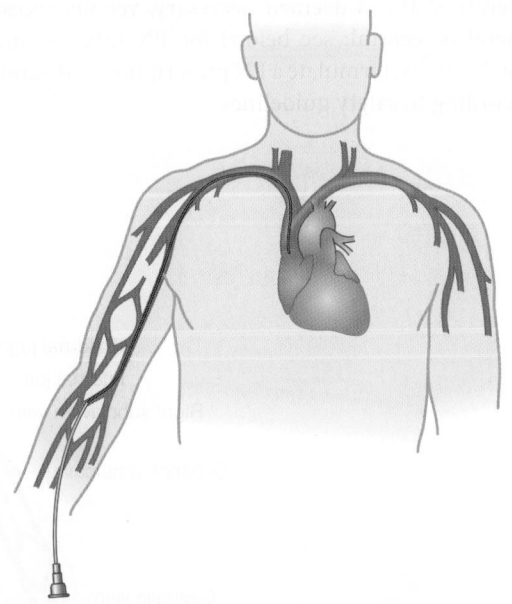

FIGURE 100–3. Peripherally inserted central venous catheter. (Reprinted from Krzywda EA, Andris DA, Edmiston CE, Wallace JR. Parenteral Access Devices. In: Gottschlich MM, ed. *The A.S.P.E.N. Nutrition Support Core Curriculum: A Case-Based Approach—The Adult Patient.* Silver Spring, MD: American Society for Parenteral and Enteral Nutrition, 2007:300–322 with permission from the American Society for Parenteral and Enteral Nutrition (A.S.P.E.N.). A.S.P.E.N. does not endorse the use of this material in any form other than its entirety.)

	Table 100–6	
	Advantages and Disadvantages of Using 3-in-1 (TNA) or 2-in-1 PN Admixtures	
	3-in-1 (TNA)	**2-in-1**
Advantages	Simplified regimen for patient	Improved stability compared with TNA
	Increased patient compliance at home	Increased number of compatible medications
	Decreased labor (less nursing time)	Decreased bacterial growth (in dextrose–amino acid
	Decreased costs (fewer supplies and equipment needed)	component) compared with TNA
	Decreased risk of contamination (caused by less manipulation	Easier visual inspection
	and all components aseptically compounded)	Can use 0.22-micron bacterial retention filter
	Inhibited bacterial growth vs. separate IV lipid emulsion	Cost savings if unused (i.e., not spiked or opened) IV
	Minimize infusion-related reactions from IV lipid emulsions and	lipid emulsion can be reused
	possibly improved lipid clearance (if infused over 12 hours)	
	Decreased vein irritation (with PPN)	
Disadvantages	Decreased stability compared to 2-in-1 PN	Increased labor and costs (if IV lipid emulsion
	Cannot use 0.22-micron bacterial retention filter; must	infused separately)
	use 1.2-micron filter	
	Increased bacterial growth compared with 2-in-1 PN	Increased vein irritation, especially if PPN is not
	Visual inspection is difficult	co-infused with IV lipid emulsion
	Limited compatibility with medications	

PN, parenteral nutrition; PPN, peripheral parenteral nutrition; TNA, total nutrient admixture.

Another concern is the co-infusion of IV medications with PN admixtures. Many IV medications have limited compatibility with 3-in-1 formulations but may be co-infused with a 2-in-1 formulation.[23,24] Some medications can be co-infused at the Y-site, few medications can be mixed directly into the PN admixture or co-infused with IV lipid emulsion, and some cannot be mixed or co-infused with the PN admixture.[23,24] *Always* consult compatibility data before adding a medication to a PN admixture or co-infusing it with PN. Medications should only be added to or co-infused with PN if there is evidence documenting compatibility and if it reasonable and safe (i.e., based on toxicity profile, pharmacokinetic and pharmacodynamic considerations).

United States Pharmacopeia, Chapter <797>

The U.S. Pharmacopeia, Chapter <797> (USP <797>) is a document that provides guidelines and best practices for pharmaceutical compounding of sterile products.[25] These guidelines address many aspects of compounded sterile preparations (CSPs), including (but not limited to) appropriate training of personnel; appropriate environments for compounding; appropriate storage, handling, and labeling of ingredients and final products; and quality assurance. The purpose of USP <797> is to prevent patient harm from CSPs as a result of contamination (including physical, chemical, and bacterial or fungal pathogens); inappropriate ingredients (variability in strength or quality); or inappropriate preparation, compounding, handling, transportation, or storage. CSPs are classified either as low-, medium-, or high-risk level or for immediate use. CSPs are also assigned an appropriate beyond-use date (BUD), which is the date or time after which a CSP shall not be stored or transported, and it is determined from the date or time the

CSP is compounded. PN admixtures are usually classified as medium-risk products, and they are assigned a BUD of 30 hours at controlled room temperature or 9 days at a cold (refrigerated) temperature. The full details of USP <797> are beyond the scope of this chapter. Pharmacists and other healthcare professionals involved in the preparation of CSPs should review this document along with institutional policies and procedures regarding CSPs.

Standardized, Commercially Available (Premixed) PN Formulations

A standardized, commercially available PN formulation (also referred to as premixed PN) is a product available from a manufacturer that requires fewer compounding steps before administration.[26] These products usually contain amino acids and dextrose in a two-chamber bag, with or without electrolytes. Vitamins and trace elements must be manually added. Lipids can be added to create a TNA or infused separately. Potential advantages to the use of premixed PN include improvements in safety (both decreased compounding errors and microbiologic contamination) and reduced costs.[26] The safety advantages are logically related to fewer manual manipulations of the system but remain theoretical with no clinical trial confirmation. Cost advantages have been demonstrated in some trials, with others finding no difference or increased costs. Limitations with the use of premixed PN in the United States are related to the limited number of products available, including a lack of formulations containing lipids (in a three-chamber bag), relatively low amino acid concentration, only 1- and 2-L volumes, limited variability in electrolyte content, and no formulations available for neonatal patients (less than 1 year old).[26] These limitations may make premixed PN less appropriate for critically ill patients, obese patients, or those who have organ dysfunction or require fluid restriction.

Patient Encounter, Part 2

WS was diagnosed with recurrent intestinal obstruction related to chronic constipation or possible Hirschsprung's disease, mild dehydration, and malnutrition. A nasogastric (NG) tube was placed for intestinal decompression and to relieve symptoms; the tube initially drained approximately 1,000 mL of gastric or bilious fluid and then remained in place on low continuous suction.

Laboratory Data

Na = 135 mEq/L (135 mmol/L), K = 3.4 mEq/L (3.4 mmol/L), Cl = 96 mEq/L (96 mmol/L), HCO_3 = 27 mEq/L (27 mmol/L), BUN = 15 mg/dL (5.4 mmol/L), serum creatinine = 0.5 mg/dL (44 µmol/L), blood glucose = 78 mg/dL (4.3 mmol/L), total Ca = 8.1 mg/dL (2.03 mmol/L)], ionized Ca = 2.28 mEq/L (1.14 mmol/L), Mg = 1.6 mg/dL (0.66 mmol/L), phosphorus = 2.2 mg/dL (0.71 mmol/L), TG = 141 mg/dL (1.59 mmol/L), albumin = 2.7 g/dL (27 g/L), WBC count = 7,700/mm^3 (7.7 × 10^9/L), hemoglobin = 11.2 mg/dL (112 g/L or 6.95 mmol/L), hematocrit = 32.9% (0.33), and platelets = 188,000/mm^3 (188 × 10^9/L)

The surgical team decided to manage WS conservatively (NG tube, plan to manage pain and wean opioids, antiemetic therapy as needed, nutrition support) given her medical condition, medical and surgical histories (chronic constipations, multiple bowel obstructions and abdominal surgeries), and high risk for complications. Because of these factors and possible need for surgical intervention, a peripherally inserted central catheter (PICC) was placed, and the team decided to initiate central PN.

Determine appropriate nutritional goals for WS (calorie and protein requirements).

What other patient data should be collected to help formulate a PN prescription?

Patient Encounter, Part 3

The surgical team plans to initiate the PN, and they ask for your recommended for WS.

Develop a plan for a complete and balanced PN prescription for amino acids (including fluid, total calories, dextrose, amino acids, lipid emulsion, electrolytes, vitamins, trace elements, and any additives) and explain the rationale supporting your PN formulation and plan.

How should this PN admixture be initiated and titrated to goal?

Would you recommend any other treatments before initiating PN? (Hint: Is this patient at risk for refeeding syndrome?)

control is maintained and the patient does not experience any significant fluid or electrolyte abnormalities. Monitor electrolytes daily and correct as needed. Patients with severe malnutrition should have their PN advanced to goal more slowly and cautiously, and they should be monitored for refeeding syndrome (see Complications of PN).

Cycling PN

PN should be administered over 24 hours in most hospitalized patients to minimize glucose, fluid, and electrolyte abnormalities. However, administering PN via a cyclic infusion over less than 24 hours, or *cycling PN*, may be advantageous in certain patients and situations. Cycling PN typically involves administering the same PN volume over a goal infusion time, usually over 12 hours rather than over 24 hours. Begin with PN infusion over 24 hours; then taper the PN infusion to the goal cycle over 2 to 4 days (e.g., 24 hours, then 18 to 20 hours the next day, then 14 to 16 hours the next day, and then 12 hours the next day). Titrate the PN infusion rate up over 1 to 2 hours to goal rate to avoid hyperglycemia and taper down over 1 to 2 hours at the end of the cycle to avoid reactive hypoglycemia. Most home infusion pumps can be programmed to cycle a given PN volume automatically over a given time. However, the pharmacist may have to develop an appropriate PN cycle if the infusion pump cannot be programmed for an automatic cycle.

Cyclic PN has the following advantages:

- It helps prevent and alleviate PN-associated liver disease by avoiding continuous compulsive nutrient overload on the liver.[27]

- It improves the quality of life of patients receiving home PN by allowing the patient time off of PN to engage in normal activities of daily living.

Concerns with cycling PN include hyperglycemia with high infusion rates, reactive hypoglycemia when PN infusion is stopped, and fluid and electrolyte abnormalities (refer to the Complications of PN section for more information). Random capillary blood glucose concentrations should be checked 4 hours into the PN cycle (~2 hours after reaching

Formulating a PN Admixture and Regimen

After completing a full nutrition assessment (e.g., SGA)[1,18]; estimating the patient's daily fluid, energy, and protein requirements (see Table 100–5); and determining if PN is indicated (see Table 100–1), develop an appropriate PN prescription.

Initiating PN

Exercise caution when initiating PN to avoid hyperglycemia and fluid and electrolyte abnormalities. After the goal daily PN volume has been determined, infuse the PN admixture first over 24 hours. For safety, initiate PN at a lower infusion rate (e.g., ~50% of goal for anywhere from ~12 to 24 hours) on day 1 with no more than 150 to 200 g of dextrose per day (or a maximum dextrose infusion rate of ~2 mg/kg per minute for the first 24 hours). Then increase PN to goal over about the following 12 to 24 hours, provided that glycemic

goal rate), 15 to 60 minutes after PN stops, and intermittently during the PN cycle as needed for glycemic control. During cyclic PN infusion, the potassium infusion rate should not exceed 10 mEq/h (10 mmol/h) if the patient is not on a cardiac monitor. If nocturnal cyclic PN infusion interferes with patient's sleep pattern by causing overdiuresis, the PN cycle can be extended over a longer infusion time or PN can be infused during other times of the day that are most convenient to the patient.

Transition to Oral or Enteral Nutrition

The goal is to transition the patient to enteral or oral nutrition and taper off PN as soon as indicated clinically. After initiation of enteral or oral nutrition, monitor the patient for glucose, fluid, and electrolyte abnormalities. When oral nutrition intake is inconsistent, perform calorie counts to determine the adequacy of nutrition via the oral route. When the patient is tolerating more than 50% of total estimated daily calorie and protein requirements via the oral or enteral route, wean PN by about 50%. PN can be stopped when the patient is tolerating at least 75% of total daily calorie and protein requirements via the oral or enteral route, assuming that intestinal absorption is maintained.

COMPLICATIONS OF PN

⑨ *PN therapy is associated with significant complications, both with short- and long-term therapy.* Many complications are related to overfeeding (Table 100–7). Metabolic complications include hyperglycemia, hypoglycemia, hyperlipidemia, hypercapnia, electrolyte abnormalities, refeeding syndrome, and acid–base disturbances. Long-term metabolic complications include liver toxicity, vitamin abnormalities, trace element abnormalities, and metabolic bone disease. Other complications include infectious and mechanical complications that relate to venous catheters.

Hyperglycemia

Hyperglycemia is one of the most common complications associated with PN therapy. The rate of dextrose oxidation

Table 100–7

Consequences of Overfeeding

Source of Overfeeding	Consequences
Dextrose	Hyperglycemia, hypertriglyceridemia, hepatic steatosis, hypercapnia; hyperglycemia may cause fluid and electrolyte disturbances and increased infection risk
IV lipid emulsions	Hypertriglyceridemia, hyperlipidemia, hepatic steatosis
Amino acids	Azotemia
Total calories	Hepatic steatosis, cholestasis, hypercapnia

may be reduced in patients with stress and hypermetabolism, patients with diabetes or acute pancreatitis, and patients receiving certain medications (e.g., corticosteroids, vasopressors, octreotide, and tacrolimus).[28,29] Uncontrolled hyperglycemia can lead to fluid and electrolyte disturbances, hyperglycemic hyperosmolar nonketotic syndrome, hypertriglyceridemia, and an increased risk of infection.[30]

Hyperglycemia in critically ill patients may be more a reflection of illness severity than from dextrose infusions, provided that the patient is not being overfed with dextrose.[31] Critical illness is associated with increased endogenous glucose production (caused by increased glycogenolysis and gluconeogenesis) and insulin resistance. Therefore, critically ill patients have lower tolerance for dextrose infusion compared with nonstressed patients. In patients with hyperglycemia, it is reasonable to initiate PN with a continuous dextrose infusion rate of approximately 2 mg/kg/min until glycemic control is achieved and then advance to goal.[4] Dextrose infusion rate typically ranges between approximately 2 and 4 mg/kg per minute but should not exceed 5 mg/kg/min in adult patients.[1,5] Use AdjBW rather than actual weight in obese patients when calculating the dextrose infusion rate. A portion of daily calories (~20% to 30%) can be administered with IV lipid emulsion to help decrease hyperglycemia, provided that the patient does not have hypertriglyceridemia. Overfeeding (with dextrose and with total calories) always must be avoided.

Hyperglycemia can impair cellular and humoral host defenses and can lead to the development of nosocomial and wound infections.[30] Historically, hyperglycemia was defined as blood glucose concentrations of more than 200 to 220 mg/dL (11.1 to 12.2 mmol/L), and concentrations of 150 to 200 mg/dL (8.3 to 11.1 mmol/L) were considered "acceptable" in critically ill patients. Early clinical evidence evaluating tight glucose control (e.g., 80 to 110 mg/dL or 4.4 to 6.1 mmol/L) with intensive insulin therapy using continuous insulin infusion in surgical critically ill patients appeared to be associated with reduced infection rates, patient comorbidities, and mortality.[32,33] However, these results were not replicated in later studies of critically ill medical intensive care unit (ICU) patients[34] and mixed medical and surgical ICU patients,[35] and tight glycemic control was associated with increased mortality.[35] The higher mortality rate may have been related to a higher incidence of hypoglycemia (blood glucose concentrations less than or equal to 40 mg per dL [less than or equal to 2.2 mmol/L]).[35] These data suggest that more moderate glucose control is indicated in critically ill patients (e.g., capillary glucose concentrations between ~140 and 180 mg per dL [8.0 and 10.0 mmol/L]).[35]

The use of regular insulin as a continuous infusion rather than adding insulin to PN reduces the risk of prolonged hyperglycemia or hypoglycemia because the insulin drip can be readily titrated as insulin requirements change. In patients with diabetes, IV insulin doses in the PN admixture to maintain euglycemia range from 0.05 to 0.2 unit of insulin per each gram of dextrose in PN. Starting with a low insulin dose and adjusting the dose daily based on capillary blood glucose concentrations is indicated in order to avoid hypoglycemia. Careful adjustments or reductions should be made to the insulin dose as guided by frequent capillary blood glucose monitoring when metabolic stress decreases, acute pancreatitis resolves or when corticosteroid doses are tapered off or discontinued.

Hypoglycemia

Hypoglycemia can occur in patients when PN is interrupted suddenly (reactive hypoglycemia), especially when patients are treated with insulin or as a result of insulin overdosing in PN.[1] It is essential to prevent hypoglycemia and, if it occurs, identify and treat it promptly. Reactive hypoglycemia typically is rare and usually can be avoided by tapering PN over 1 to 2 hours before discontinuation rather than abruptly stopping the infusion (especially if the patient is receiving insulin in PN or if the patient is not receiving oral or enteral nutrition). Reactive hypoglycemia generally occurs within 15 to 60 minutes after stopping PN (especially in neonatal patients), although it can occur later than this after discontinuing PN.[1] Capillary blood glucose concentrations should be monitored about 15 to 60 minutes after stopping PN infusion to detect any potential hypoglycemia. If PN is interrupted abruptly (e.g., because of lost IV access), infusing dextrose 10% in water at the same rate as PN should prevent hypoglycemia. In patients with poor venous access, reduce the PN infusion rate by 50% for 1 hour before discontinuing. Another alternative to prevent reactive hypoglycemia is to provide a glucose source via the oral route (by mouth or sublingually) when feasible. Monitor capillary blood glucose concentrations regularly in patients receiving insulin in PN and adjust insulin doses accordingly.

Hyperlipidemia

Patients receiving IV lipid emulsion may be at risk for hyperlipidemia and hypertriglyceridemia. Hyperlipidemia in patients receiving PN may lead to a reduction in pulmonary gas diffusion and pulmonary vascular resistance (especially in patients with underlying pulmonary and vascular disease).[36] Severe hypertriglyceridemia (especially when serum triglyceride concentrations exceed 1,000 mg/dL or 11.30 mmol/L) can precipitate acute pancreatitis.[37] Hypertriglyceridemia may develop as a result of increased fatty acid synthesis caused by hyperglycemia or impaired lipid clearance or in patients with history of hyperlipidemia, obesity, diabetes, alcoholism, kidney failure, liver failure, multiorgan failure, sepsis, or pancreatitis or as a result of medications (e.g., propofol, corticosteroids, cyclosporine, and sirolimus).[38] Hyperglycemia is probably the most common cause of hypertriglyceridemia in patients receiving PN. Propofol is formulated in a 10% lipid emulsion and may lead to hypertriglyceridemia. It also has been proposed that propofol could have direct effects on lipid metabolism, given that hypertriglyceridemia associated with propofol infusion has been observed with lipid doses that are lower than those typically given in PN.[38,39]

A higher PL:TG ratio in the 10% lipid emulsion has been proposed to cause the appearance of the abnormal lipoprotein X particles (rich in phospholipids [~60%] and cholesterol [~25%], small amounts of triglycerides) in the blood.[8,38] Lipoprotein X may compete with lipid particles for metabolism by lipoprotein lipase. Therefore, it is preferred to use IV lipid emulsions with a lower PL:TG ratio (i.e., 20% or 30% lipid emulsions), especially in patients with hypertriglyceridemia, because they have improved clearance compared with emulsions with a higher PL:TG ratio (i.e., 10% lipid emulsion).[8,38]

Monitor serum triglyceride concentrations regularly during PN therapy (e.g., at the initiation of PN, then once per week initially, and monthly thereafter depending on clinical condition). If a patient develops hypertriglyceridemia, identify and correct the underlying cause(s) if possible (e.g., treatment of hyperglycemia or reduction of dextrose and/or lipid dose). Prolonging the infusion of IV lipid emulsion (e.g., over 24 hours) may improve lipid clearance; however, this may require hanging two containers daily because each container of lipid emulsion should infuse for only 12 hours based on USP <797> and infection control policies and practices. If a patient is receiving propofol, take into account the calories administered from the 10% lipid emulsion in propofol (1.1 kcal/mL or 4.6 kJ/mL). For safety reasons, IV lipid emulsion should be withheld in patients receiving propofol. It also should be held when the serum is lipemic or when serum triglyceride concentrations are greater than 400 mg/dL (4.52 mmol/L). When this occurs, restart IV lipid emulsions when the serum triglyceride concentration is approximately 200 to 400 mg/dL (2.26 to 4.52 mmol/L) (or less) and administer only two to three times per week to prevent essential fatty acid deficiency.

Hypercapnia

Hypercapnia (abnormally high concentration of carbon dioxide in the blood) can develop as a result of overfeeding with dextrose and/or total calories.[1,40] Excess carbon dioxide production and retention can lead to acute respiratory acidosis. The excess carbon dioxide will also stimulate compensatory mechanisms, resulting in an increase in respiratory rate in order to eliminate the excess carbon dioxide via the lungs. This increase in respiratory workload can cause respiratory insufficiency that may require mechanical ventilation. Reducing total calorie and dextrose intake would result in resolution of hypercapnia if due to overfeeding.

Acid–Base Disturbances

Acid–base disturbances associated with PN are usually related to the patient's underlying condition(s). However, acid–base abnormalities may develop as a result of changes in chloride or acetate concentrations in PN admixtures. Because acetate is converted to bicarbonate in the body, excessive acetate salts in PN can lead to metabolic alkalosis;

excessive chloride salts in PN can lead to hyperchloremic metabolic acidosis. PN should not be used to treat or correct acute underlying acid–base disorders. However, adjusting chloride or acetate salts in the PN admixture may help to prevent or minimize exacerbation of acid–base disorders.

Liver Complications

The incidence of liver complications associated with PN ranges from approximately 7% to 84%, and end-stage liver disease develops in as many as 15% to 40% of adult patients on long-term PN.[38] Patients may develop a mild increase in liver transaminases within 1 to 2 weeks of initiating PN, but this generally resolves as PN continues, provided overfeeding is avoided. Severe liver complications include hepatic steatosis, steatohepatitis, cholestasis, and cholelithiasis.[38]

Hepatic steatosis usually is a result of excessive administration of carbohydrates or lipids, but deficiencies of carnitine, choline, and essential fatty acids also may contribute. Hepatic steatosis can be minimized or reversed by avoiding overfeeding, especially from dextrose and lipids.[38] Carnitine is an important amine that transports long-chain triglycerides into the mitochondria for oxidation, but carnitine deficiency in adults is extremely rare and is mostly a problem in premature infants and patients receiving chronic dialysis. Choline is an essential amine required for synthesis of cell membrane components such as phospholipids. Although a true choline deficiency is rare, preliminary studies of choline supplementation to adult patients' PN caused reversal of steatosis. Compelling evidence for routine carnitine or choline supplementation to prevent or treat steatosis in PN patients is lacking.

Cholestasis is a common and potentially serious complication in PN-dependent patients. Factors that predispose PN patients to cholestasis include overfeeding, bowel rest (decrease in cholecystokinin secretion), long duration of PN, short-bowel syndrome, bacterial overgrowth and translocation, and sepsis.[38] Patients may exhibit increased liver transaminases, increase alkaline phosphatase and gamma-glutamyl transferase concentrations, and mainly increased bilirubin concentrations with jaundice. The most sensitive marker of cholestasis is increased serum conjugated bilirubin concentration of greater than 2 mg/dL (34.2 μmol/L).[38] Cholestasis generally is reversible if PN is discontinued before permanent liver damage occurs. Serum liver function tests may take up to 3 months to return to normal after discontinuing PN. Steps to prevent cholestasis associated with PN include early enteral or oral feedings, using a balanced PN formulation, avoiding overfeeding, using cyclic PN infusion, and treating and avoiding sepsis.[38] Limiting soy-based IV lipid emulsion infusion to one or two times weekly at a dose no less than that required to prevent essential fatty acid deficiency may also decrease serum bilirubin concentrations and improve cholestasis.[41] The use of ω-3-fatty acid-rich fish oil-based IV lipid emulsions may hold promise in preventing or reversing PN-associated cholestasis.[42] However, these formulations

are not yet commercially available in the United States. Pharmacologic treatments include ursodeoxycholic acid (ursodiol), which may improve bile flow and reduce the signs and symptoms of cholestasis. However, ursodiol is only available in an oral dosage form, and absorption may be limited in patients with intestinal resections. If other measures are not successful and bacterial overgrowth is thought to be contributing to cholestasis, courses of oral metronidazole, oral gentamicin, or oral neomycin have been used to reduce bacterial overgrowth.

Cholelithiasis can develop as a result of decreased gallbladder contractility, especially in the absence of enteral or oral intake. Lack of intestinal stimulation reduces secretion of cholecystokinin, a peptide hormone secreted in the duodenum that induces gallbladder contractility and emptying. The best prevention of cholelithiasis is early initiation of enteral or oral feeding (to stimulate secretion of cholecystokinin and intestinal motility). Pharmacologic treatment with cholecystokinin–octapeptide (sincalide) to stimulate gallbladder contraction and bile flow does not prevent PN-associated cholestasis or improve serum conjugated bilirubin concentrations.

Monitor liver function tests, including serum aspartate aminotransferase (AST), alanine aminotransferase (ALT), alkaline phosphatase, total bilirubin, conjugated bilirubin, unconjugated bilirubin, and γ-glutamyl transferase at the initiation of PN therapy and regularly thereafter during PN therapy. The frequency of monitoring liver function tests depends on the presence or absence of liver disease. This varies from one to two times weekly in the acute setting to once weekly to once monthly in stable home PN patients.

Manganese Toxicity

Manganese is a trace element that serves as a coenzyme in multiple biochemical reactions. Manganese accumulation can occur in patients with cholestasis or in patients receiving long-term PN therapy. The most common toxicity is neurotoxicity, but liver toxicity also may occur. Neurologic symptoms associated with manganese toxicity include headache, somnolence, weakness, confusion, tremor, muscle rigidity, altered gait, and masklike face (a Parkinson's-like syndrome).[38] Conversely, some patients with hypermagnesemia may not exhibit symptoms of toxicity. Periodically monitor blood manganese concentrations in patients on long-term PN. Patients with cholestasis receiving PN may require restriction of manganese in PN to prevent its accumulation and possible toxicity.

Metabolic Bone Disease

Metabolic bone disease is a condition of bone demineralization leading to osteomalacia, osteopenia, or osteoporosis in patients receiving long-term PN. Metabolic bone disease may occur to some degree in as many as 40% to 100% of patients receiving long-term PN.[38] Often patients are asymptomatic, although symptoms can include bone pain, back pain, and fractures. Patients often have increased serum alkaline phosphatase concentrations, low to normal parathyroid hormone (PTH) concentrations, normal 25-hydroxyvitamin D and low 1,25 dihydroxyvitamin D concentrations, hypercalcemia or hypocalcemia, and hypercalcuria.[43] Because patients may be asymptomatic, diagnosis can be incidental. Radiographic techniques commonly used in diagnosing bone disease include quantitative computed tomography (CT) and bone mineral density.[43]

Factors that can predispose patients to developing metabolic bone disease include deficiencies of phosphorus, calcium, and vitamin D; aluminum toxicity; amino acids and hyperosmolar dextrose infusions; chronic metabolic acidosis; corticosteroid therapy; and lack of mobility.[38,43] Calcium deficiency (caused by decreased intake or increased urinary excretion) is one of the major causes of metabolic bone disease in patients receiving PN. Provide adequate calcium and phosphate with PN to improve bone mineralization and help to prevent metabolic bone disease. Administration of amino acids and chronic metabolic acidosis also appear to play an important role. Provide adequate amounts of acetate in PN admixtures to maintain acid–base balance.

Aluminum toxicity appears to play a role in the development of metabolic bone disease in patients on long-term PN, possibly by impairing calcium bone fixation, inhibiting the conversion of 25-hydroxyvitamin D to the active 1,25-dihydroxyvitamin D, and/or reducing PTH secretion.[38,43] Measure serum aluminum concentrations in PN patients with suspected metabolic bone disease to rule out aluminum toxicity. The FDA has investigated aluminum contamination in parenteral products and issued a rule specifying acceptable aluminum concentrations in large-volume parenterals in 2000.[44] The rule further stated that the package insert ("Precautions") for large-volume parenterals used in making PN should indicate that the product contains no more than 25 mcg/L (0.93 μmol/L) of aluminum and defined a safe upper limit for parenteral aluminum intake at less than 4 to 5 mcg/kg/day. This has required a great amount of effort by manufacturers to meet these limits and requires pharmacy policies for monitoring aluminum concentrations in PN admixtures. Pharmacies should use products with the lowest labeled aluminum content for the making of PN. Patients who are chronically dependent on PN should have their serum aluminum concentrations routinely monitored or whenever metabolic bone disease is suspected or diagnosed.

Encourage patients on long-term PN to engage in regular low-intensity exercise. Yearly bone density measurements also should be performed on patients on long-term PN and when metabolic bone disease is suspected.

Refeeding Syndrome

Refeeding syndrome describes the metabolic derangements that occur during nutritional repletion of patients who are starved, underweight, or severely malnourished.[45] Hypophosphatemia and hypokalemia (along with associated complications) are the classic signs and symptoms, but refeeding syndrome encompasses a constellation of fluid and electrolyte abnormalities affecting neurologic, cardiac, hematologic, neuromuscular, and pulmonary systems. The most severe cases of refeeding syndrome have resulted in cardiac failure, seizures, coma, and death.[45] The reintroduction of energy substrates, especially carbohydrates or glucose, increases metabolism and the utilization of glucose as the predominant fuel source. This increases insulin secretion and the demand for phosphorylated intermediates of glycolysis (e.g., ATP and 2,3-diphosphoglycerate [2,3-DPG]), inhibits fat metabolism, and causes an intracellular shift of phosphorus, potassium, and magnesium. These changes, in combination with preexisting low total body stores of phosphorus, potassium, and magnesium and enhanced cellular uptake of phosphorus during anabolic refeeding, result in hypophosphatemia, hypokalemia, and hypomagnesemia. Vitamin deficiencies (e.g., thiamine) also may exist or be precipitated during refeeding. High carbohydrate intake increases the demand for thiamine, which can precipitate thiamine deficiency and cause lactic acidosis and neurologic abnormalities,[45] as well as myocardial dysfunction and congestive heart failure. Other metabolic alterations that may occur include expansion of the extracellular water compartment and fluid intolerance.

The primary goal is preventing refeeding syndrome when initiating PN in high-risk patients (e.g., prolonged lack of adequate nutritional intake, significant weight loss, or moderate to severe malnutrition). When initiating nutrition support, the rule of thumb to prevent refeeding syndrome is to "start low and go slow." Initiate PN cautiously (e.g., ~25% of estimated nutritional requirements on day 1) and gradually increase to goal over 3 to 5 days. Correct electrolyte abnormalities (e.g., hypophosphatemia, hypokalemia, and hypomagnesemia) before initiating PN and provide supplemental phosphate, potassium, and magnesium in or outside of PN (if the patient has normal kidney function). Well-nourished patients require 10 to 15 mmol of phosphate per 1,000 kcal (4,186 kJ) to avoid hypophosphatemia,[12] but patients with moderate to severe malnutrition who are at risk for refeeding syndrome require more aggressive supplementation. Doses of IV phosphate up to 0.64 to 1 mmol/kg may be used to treat severe hypophosphatemia (in patients with normal kidney function), and doses can be repeated as needed until serum phosphorus concentration has normalized.[46] Provide vitamin supplementation in addition to the multivitamin administered in PN (e.g., provide supplemental oral or IV thiamine 100 mg/day and folic acid 1 mg/day for about 1 week). In addition, minimize fluid and sodium intake during the first few days of PN (e.g., total fluid of 1,000 mL/day or less).[45] Assess patients for fluid balance, signs of edema, fluid overload, and weight gain because any gain of more than 1 kg per week likely represents fluid retention. Monitor patients closely for signs and symptoms of refeeding syndrome until they are tolerating PN at goal for a few days:

- Monitor vital signs (i.e., heart rate, blood pressure, and respiratory rate), mental status, and neurologic and neuromuscular function routinely (e.g., at least every 4–8 hours).

- Monitor pulse oximetry and any electrocardiographic changes when indicated clinically.
- Monitor serum laboratory values (including basic metabolic panel, phosphorus, and magnesium) at least once a day.

Infectious Complications

Patients receiving central PN are at increased risk of developing infectious complications caused by bacterial and fungal pathogens.[1,47] In addition, patients without malnutrition who receive early PN (e.g., within 48 hours of ICU admission) may have a higher incidence of infectious complications than patients who do not receive PN or receive late PN initiation (e.g., greater than 7 days after ICU admission).[2,10] Infections may be related to several factors, including placement of a central venous catheter, contamination of a central venous catheter or IV site (catheter-related infection), persistent hyperglycemia, and lack of stimulation of the intestinal tract. Strict aseptic techniques must be used when placing the catheter along with continuous care of the catheter and infusion site. Catheter-related bloodstream infections are a common complication in long-term PN patients, often requiring hospital admission for parenteral antimicrobial therapy and/or removal of the catheter. Contamination of the PN admixture is possible but rare if protocols are followed for aseptic preparation of PN admixtures. Lack of use of the intestinal tract also may increase the risk of infection possibly by reducing gut immunity, leading to intestinal bacterial overgrowth and subsequent systemic bacterial translocation.

Mechanical Complications

Mechanical complications of PN are related to venous catheter placement and the equipment used to administer PN. A central venous catheter must be placed by a trained professional, and risks associated with placement include pneumothorax, arterial puncture, bleeding, hematoma formation, venous thrombosis, and air embolism.[1] Over time, the venous catheter may require replacement. Problems with the equipment include malfunctions of the infusion pump, IV tubing sets, and filters.

MONITORING PN THERAPY

⑩ When initiating PN, patients should have important baseline laboratory values checked to assess electrolyte status, organ function, and nutritional status (Table 100–8). Baseline laboratory monitoring should include:

- Basic metabolic panel (i.e., serum sodium, potassium, chloride, bicarbonate, blood urea nitrogen, creatinine, glucose, and calcium), serum phosphorus, and magnesium
- Liver function, including AST, ALT, alkaline phosphatase, lactate dehydrogenase (LDH), total and conjugated bilirubin; a comprehensive metabolic panel can be ordered (i.e., serum sodium, potassium, chloride, bicarbonate, blood urea nitrogen, creatinine, glucose, calcium, AST, ALT, alkaline phosphatase, albumin, and total bilirubin), but phosphorus, magnesium, and fractionated or conjugated bilirubin are not included on this panel and must be ordered separately

Table 100–8

Suggested Frequency of Monitoring Parameters in Hospitalized Patients Receiving PN

Parameters	Initial	Daily (Unstable)	2–3 × Weekly (Stable)	Weekly	As Indicated
BUN, creatinine	X	X	X		
Sodium, potassium, chloride, bicarbonate	X	X	X		
Glucose	X	X	X		
Calcium, phosphorus, magnesium albumin, AST, ALT, LDH, alkaline phosphatase, total bilirubin	X	X	X		
Conjugated bilirubin	X			X	X
Prealbumin	X			X	X (once weekly)
Triglycerides	X			X	X
RBC count, hemoglobin, hematocrit, WBC count ± differential, platelets, PTT	X				X
PT or INR				X	X
Nitrogen balance					X
Zinc, selenium, chromium, copper, manganese, iron					X
TIBC, ferritin					X
Vitamin concentrations					X
Ammonia					X
Blood cultures					X
Body weight	X	X	X		

ALT, alanine aminotransferase; AST, aspartate aminotransferase; BUN, blood urea nitrogen; INR, international normalized ratio; LDH, lactate dehydrogenase; PT, prothrombin time; PTT, partial thromboplastin time; RBC, red blood cell; TIBC, total iron-binding capacity; WBC, white blood cell.

Patient Encounter, Part 4

The surgical team plans to initiate PN for WS per your recommendations. Laboratory data were listed previously.

What monitoring parameters related to PN therapy should you follow in WS after initiating PN? List monitoring parameters and frequency.

What potential complications of PN should you monitor for in WS?

What special considerations must be made when developing a plan for nutrition support therapy and a PN formulation for patients with severe malnutrition?

- Serum albumin, prealbumin, and triglycerides
- Complete blood count (including hemoglobin, hematocrit, red blood cell count, and white blood cell count) with differential and platelets

⑩ *Thereafter, these and other nutritional parameters should be monitored routinely or as indicated* (see Table 100–8). Random capillary blood glucose concentrations also should be monitored every 6 to 8 hours when initiating PN, and regular insulin should be administered to control blood glucose concentrations as needed.

SUMMARY AND CONCLUSION

PN is an effective and potentially lifesaving method of administering nutrition support therapy in patients who cannot receive adequate oral or enteral nutrition. Preparation and administration of PN are associated with significant adverse effects and metabolic, infectious, and mechanical complications. Optimal design, compounding, and administration of a PN regimen is essential to minimize the risk of adverse effects and complications, and patients must be monitored closely while receiving PN to optimize outcomes.

Abbreviations Introduced in This Chapter

ALT	Alanine aminotransferase
ASPEN	American Society for Parenteral and Enteral Nutrition
AST	Aspartate aminotransferase
ATP	Adenosine triphosphate
CT	Computed tomography
2,3-DPG	2,3-Diphosphoglycerate
FDA	Food and Drug Administration
GI	Gastrointestinal
HIT	Heparin-induced thrombocytopenia
IBW	Ideal body weight
kcal	Kilocalorie(s)
kJ	Kilojoule(s)

LDH	Lactate dehydrogenase
mEq	Milliequivalents
mmol	Millimoles
mOsm	Milliosmoles
PL	Phospholipid(s)
PN	Parenteral nutrition
PPN	Peripheral parenteral nutrition
PTH	Parathyroid hormone
TG	Triglyceride
TNA	Total nutrient admixture
TPN	Total parenteral nutrition

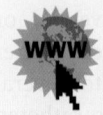 Self-assessment questions and answers are available at *http://www.mhpharmacotherapy. com/pp.html.*

REFERENCES

1. American Society for Parenteral and Enteral Nutrition Board of Directors and the Clinical Guidelines Task Force. Guidelines for the use of parenteral and enteral nutrition in adult and pediatric patients. JPEN J Parenter Enteral Nutr 2002;26:1SA–138SA.
2. McClave SA, Martindale RG, Vanek VW, et al., and the A.S.P.E.N. Board of Directors; American College of Critical Care Medicine; Society of Critical Care Medicine. Guidelines for the Provision and Assessment of Nutrition Support Therapy in the Adult Critically Ill Patient: Society of Critical Care Medicine (SCCM) and American Society for Parenteral and Enteral Nutrition (A.S.P.E.N.). JPEN J Parenter Enteral Nutr 2009;33:277–316.
3. Peter JV, Moran JL, Phillips-Hughes J. A metaanalysis of treatment outcomes of early enteral versus early parenteral nutrition in hospitalized patients. Crit Care Med 2005;33:213–220.
4. Wolfe RR, Allsop JR, Burke JF. Glucose metabolism in man: Responses to intravenous glucose infusion. Metabolism 1979;28:210–220.
5. Rosmarin DK, Wardlaw GM, Mirtallo J. Hyperglycemia associated with high, continuous infusion rates of total parenteral nutrition dextrose. Nutr Clin Pract 1996;11:151–156.
6. The American Society for Parenteral and Enteral Nutrition. Task Force for the Revision of Safe Practices for Parenteral Nutrition. Safe practices of parenteral nutrition. JPEN J Parenter Enteral Nutr 2004;28(Suppl):S39–S70.
7. Driscoll DF, Bhargava HN, Li L, et al. Physicochemical stability of total nutrient admixtures. Am J Health Syst Pharm 1995;52:623–634.
8. Ferezou J, Bach AC. Structure and metabolic fate of triacylglycerol- and phospholipid-rich particles of commercial parenteral fat emulsions. Nutrition 1999;15:44–50.
9. Hamilton C, Austin T, Seidner DL. Essential fatty acid deficiency in human adults during parenteral nutrition. Nutr Clin Pract 2006;21:387–394.
10. Crocker KS, Noga R, Filibeck DJ, et al. Microbial growth comparisons of five commercial parenteral lipid emulsions. JPEN J Parenter Enteral Nutr 1984;8:391–395.
11. D'Angio R, Quercia RA, Treiber NK, et al. The growth of microorganisms in total parenteral nutrition admixtures. JPEN J Parenter Enteral Nutr 1987;11:394–397.
12. Sheldon GF, Grzyb S. Phosphate depletion and repletion: relation to parenteral nutrition and oxygen transport. Ann Surg 1975;182:683–689.
13. Food and Drug Administration. Safety alert: Hazards of precipitation associated with parenteral nutrition. Am J Hosp Pharm 1994;51:1427–1428.
14. Tong GM, Rude RK. Magnesium deficiency in critical illness. J Intensive Care Med 2005;20:3–17.

15. Btaiche IF, Carver PL, Welch KB. Dosing and monitoring of trace elements in long-term home parenteral nutrition patients. JPEN J Parenter Enteral Nutr 2011;35(6):736–747.

16. Jeejeebhoy K. Zinc: An essential trace element for parenteral nutrition. Gastroenterology 2009;137(5 Suppl):S7–S12.

17. Shike M. Copper in parenteral nutrition. Gastroenterology 2009;137(5 Suppl):S13–S17.

18. Keith JN. Bedside nutrition assessment past, present and future: A review of the Subjective Global Assessment. Nutr Clin Pract 2008;23:410–416.

19. Dickerson RN. Specialized nutrition support in the hospitalized obese patient. Nutr Clin Pract 2004;19:245–254.

20. Gura KM. Is there still a role for peripheral parenteral nutrition? Nutr Clin Pract 2009;24:709–717.

21. Driscoll DF. Lipid injectable emulsions: 2006. Nutr Clin Pract 2006;21:381–386.

22. Driscoll DF, Bacon MN, Bistrian BR. Effects of in-line filtration on lipid particle size distribution in total nutrient admixtures. JPEN J Parenter Enteral Nutr 1996;20:296–301.

23. Trissel LA, Gilbert DL, Martinez JF, et al. Compatibility of parenteral nutrient solutions with selected drugs during simulated Y-site administration. Am J Health Syst Pharm 1997;54:1295–1300.

24. Trissel LA, Gilbert DL, Martinez JF, et al. Compatibility of medications with three-in-one parenteral nutrition admixtures. JPEN J Parenter Enteral Nutr 1999;23:67–74.

25. (797) Pharmaceutical Compounding—Sterile Preparations. United States Pharmacopeial Convention, Revision Bulletin 2008;1–61.

26. Miller SJ. Commercial premixed parenteral nutrition: Is it right for your institution? Nutr Clin Pract 2009;24:459–469.

27. Stout SM, Cober MP. Metabolic effects of cyclic parenteral nutrition infusion in adults and children. Nutr Clin Pract 2010;25:277–281.

28. Watters JM, Norris SB, Kirkpatrick SM. Endogenous glucose production following injury increases with age. J Clin Endocrinol Metab 1997;82:3005–3010.

29. Campbell IT. Limitations of nutrient intake. The effect of stressors: trauma, sepsis and multiple organ failure. Eur J Clin Nutr 1999;53(Suppl 1):S143–S147.

30. Butler SO, Btaiche IF, Alaniz C. Relationship between hyperglycemia and infection in critically ill patients. Pharmacotherapy 2005;25:963–976.

31. Atkinson M, Worthley LI. Nutrition in the critically ill patient: Part I. Essential physiology and pathophysiology. Crit Care Resusc 2003;5:109–120.

32. Van Den Berghe G, Wouters PJ, Weekers F, et al. Intensive insulin therapy in critically ill patients. N Engl J Med 2001;345:1359–1367.

33. Van Den Berghe G, Wouters PJ, Bouillon R, et al. Outcome benefit of intensive insulin therapy in the critically ill: Insulin dose versus glycemic control. Crit Care Med 2003;31:359–366.

34. Van den Berghe G, Wilmer A, Hermans G, et al. Intensive insulin therapy in the medical ICU. N Engl J Med 2006;354:449–461.

35. The NICE-SUGAR Study Investigators. Intensive versus conventional glucose control in critically Ill patients. N Engl J Med 2009;360:1283–1297.

36. Suchner U, Katz DP, Fürst P, et al. Effects of intravenous fat emulsions on lung function in patients with acute respiratory distress syndrome or sepsis. Crit Care Med 2001;29:1569–1574.

37. National Cholesterol Education Program (NCEP) Expert Panel on Detection, Evaluation, and Treatment of High Blood Cholesterol in Adults (Adult Treatment Panel III). Third Report of the National Cholesterol Education Program (NCEP) Expert Panel on Detection, Evaluation, and Treatment of High Blood Cholesterol in Adults (Adult Treatment Panel III) final report. Circulation 2002;106:3143–3421.

38. Btaiche IF, Khalidi N. Metabolic complications of parenteral nutrition in adults, part 1 and part 2. Am J Health Syst Pharm 2004;61:1938–1949, 2050–2059.

39. Devlin JW, Lau AK, Tanios MA. Propofol-associated hypertriglyceridemia and pancreatitis in the intensive care unit: An analysis of frequency and risk factors. Pharmacotherapy 2005;25:1348–1352.

40. McClave SA, Lowen CC, Kleber MJ, McConnell JW, Jung LY, Goldsmith LJ. Clinical use of the respirator quotient obtained from indirect calorimetry. JPEN J Parenter Enteral Nutr 2003;27:21–26.

41. Cober MP, Teitelbaum DH. Prevention of parenteral nutrition-associated liver disease: lipid minimization. Curr Opin Organ Transplant 2010;15:330–333.

42. Le HD, de Meijer VE, Robinson EM, et al. Parenteral fish-oil-based lipid emulsion improves fatty acid profiles and lipids in parenteral nutrition-dependent children. Am J Clin Nutr 2011;94:749–758.

43. Ferrone M, Geraci M. A review of the relationship between parenteral nutrition and metabolic bone disease. Nutr Clin Pract 2007;22:329–339.

44. Department of Health and Human Services, Food and Drug Administration. Aluminum in large and small volume parenterals used in total parenteral nutrition. Fed Regist 2000(Docket No. 90N-0056);65:4103–4111.

45. Kraft MD, Btaiche IF, Sacks GS. Review of the refeeding syndrome. Nutr Clin Pract 2005;20:625–633.

46. Brown KA, Dickerson RN, Morgan LM, et al. A new graduated dosing regimen for phosphorus replacement in patients receiving nutrition support. JPEN J Parenter Enteral Nutr 2006;30:209–214.

47. Beghetto MG, Victorino J, Teixeira L, de Azevedo MJ. Parenteral nutrition as a risk factor for central venous catheter-related infection. JPEN J Parenter Enteral Nutr 2005;29:367–373.

101

Enteral Nutrition

Sarah J. Miller

KEY CONCEPTS

❶ EN is the preferred route if the gut can be used safely in a patient who cannot meet nutritional requirements by oral intake.

❷ EN is associated with fewer infectious complications than PN.

❸ For patients intolerant of gastric feedings or in whom the risk of aspiration is high, feedings delivered with the tip of the tube in the jejunum are preferred.

❹ Standard EN formulas are polymeric formulas; these are appropriate for most patients.

❺ When choosing an EN formula, the patient's fluid status should dictate the caloric density selected.

❻ Robust clinical trial data supporting the use of specialty formulas in niche populations typically remain lacking in terms of improved patient outcomes.

❼ Acceptance of enteral immunonutrition in certain clinical settings is gaining momentum.

❽ Gastrointestinal complications are the most common complications of EN limiting the amount of feeding patients receive.

❾ An important practice to help prevent medication-related occlusion is adequate water flushing of the tube before, between, and after each medication is given through the tube.

❿ Compatibility of medications with an EN formula is of concern when administering medications through feeding tubes.

Enteral nutrition (EN) is broadly defined as delivery of nutrients via the gastrointestinal (GI) tract. This includes normal oral feeding as well as delivery of nutrients in liquid form by tube. Sometimes when the term *enteral nutrition* is used, only tube feedings are included; hence, the terms *enteral nutrition* and *tube feedings* are often used synonymously. The bulk of this chapter includes information regarding delivery of feedings via tubes. Formulas for EN usually are delivered in the form of commercially prepared liquid preparations, although some products are produced as powders for reconstitution. Modern techniques for enteral access, both placement of the tubes and the materials for making pliable, comfortable tubes, were developed in the 1960s to 1980s. Nonvolitional feedings in patients who cannot meet nutritional requirements by oral intake include EN and **parenteral nutrition** (PN), which are collectively known as *specialized nutrition support* (SNS).

Several organizations have issued clinical guidelines on the use of EN. These include the American Society for Parenteral and Enteral Nutrition (A.S.P.E.N.), European Society for Clinical Nutrition and Metabolism (ESPEN), and Canadian team known as Critical Care Nutrition.[1-4] A.S.P.E.N. and the Society for Critical Care Medicine (SCCM) have jointly issued guidelines for SNS in critically ill patients.[5]

GI TRACT STRUCTURE AND FUNCTION

Anatomy and Absorptive Function

With normal volitional feeding, food is ingested via the mouth. There, the process of breaking down complex foodstuffs into simpler forms that can be absorbed by the small bowel begins.

Table 101–1	
Length of the Small Bowel in Adults	
Segment	Length (ft)^a
Total	12–20
Duodenum	1
Jejunum	5–8
Ileum	7–12

^{a}One ft is equivalent to approximately 0.31 m.

Solid food is chewed in the mouth, and enzymes begin digestion. The trigger for release of many enzymes and GI hormones is the presence of food in specific regions of the GI tract. Food is swallowed and passes through the esophagus and the esophageal sphincter to the stomach, where additional digestive enzymes and acids further break it down. The stomach also serves a mixing and grinding function.

The food, now in a liquid form known as *chyme*, passes through the pyloric sphincter into the duodenum, where stomach acid is neutralized. There is wide variation in lengths of the components of the small intestine (i.e., duodenum, jejunum, and ileum) among individuals (Table 101–1). Most absorption of digested carbohydrate and protein occurs within the jejunum. Most fat absorption occurs within the jejunum and ileum. In the small bowel, breakdown of macronutrients (i.e., carbohydrate, protein, and fat) occurs both within the lumen and at the intestinal mucosal membrane surface. The absorptive units on the intestinal mucosal membrane are infoldings known as *villi*. These villi are made up of epithelial cells called *enterocytes*. Projections (striations) from these enterocytes called *microvilli* increase the surface area of the small bowel and make up what is known as the *brush-border membrane.*

Digestive substances secreted by the pancreas play a role in food breakdown. The pancreas secretes large amounts of sodium bicarbonate that neutralize stomach acid. These substances flow from the pancreas through the pancreatic duct. The pancreatic duct typically joins the hepatic duct to become the common bile duct that empties through the sphincter of Oddi into the duodenum. Bile secreted by the liver does not contain digestive enzymes, but bile salts help to emulsify fat and facilitate fat absorption. Bile flows through bile ducts into the hepatic duct and common bile duct. Bile is stored in the gallbladder until needed in the gut to aid fat digestion, at which time it empties through the cystic duct to the common bile duct to the duodenum. Pathways through which carbohydrate, protein, and fat are digested and absorbed through the small bowel are illustrated in Figure 101–1.

After absorption in the small bowel, remaining undigested food passes from the ileum through the ileocecal valve to the colon. A major role of the colon is fluid absorption. Some of the water and sodium absorption achieved by the colon is facilitated by short-chain fatty acids (SFCAs) formed from digestion of certain dietary fibers by colonic bacterial enzymes.

Gut Immune Function

In addition to roles in digestion and absorption, the gut plays significant immune roles. The distal small bowel and colon host many bacteria and their endotoxins, and it is important that these organisms not gain access to the internal systems of the body. This function is known globally as the *gut barrier*

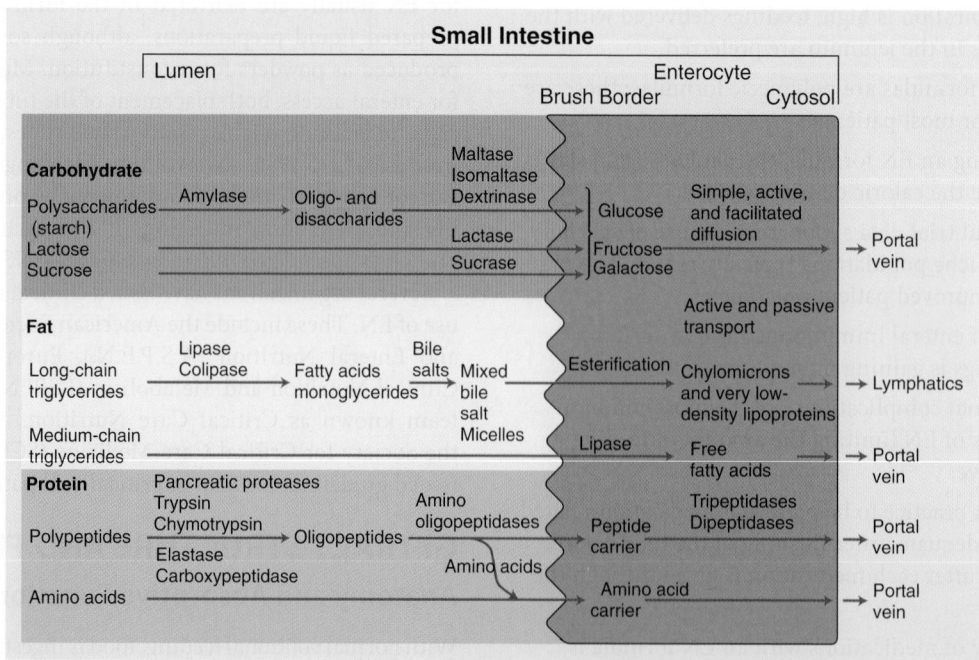

FIGURE 101–1. Schematic of carbohydrate, fat, and protein digestion. (From Kumpf VJ, Chessman KH. Enteral nutrition. In: DiPiro JT, Talbert RL, Yee GC, et al, eds. *Pharmacotherapy: A Pathophysiologic Approach*, 8th ed. New York: McGraw-Hill, 2011:2528.)

function and can be divided into several components.[6] Normal flora of the gut comprise one component. The normal flora, particularly some anaerobes, help to prevent overgrowth of potential pathogens. A second component involves mechanical factors. These include an epithelial mucus gel layer that prevents adherence of bacteria and peristalsis of the small bowel that prevents stasis of bacteria. **Gut-associated lymphoid tissue** (GALT) and **mucosa-associated lymphoid tissue** (MALT), prominent in the small bowel, serve as local immune systems. Secretory immunoglobulin A produced at the mucosal surface in response to food in the gut prevents bacteria from invading the surface. Bile salts and the **reticuloendothelial system** of the liver are believed to bind bacterial endotoxin and help clear it from the blood if it is absorbed into the portal circulation.

PATIENT SELECTION

In general, ❶ *EN is the preferred route if the gut can be used safely in patients who cannot meet nutritional requirements by oral intake.* If the gut functions, EN is usually preferred over PN. The timing of SNS (either EN or PN) is controversial, but definitive guidelines for these therapies state that SNS should be started when intake has been inadequate for 7 to 14 days or if inadequate oral intake is anticipated to last at least 7 to 14 days.[1] The prior nutritional status of the patient should be considered. Previously well-nourished patients can better afford not being fed for longer periods than previously poorly nourished patients. Patients in the intensive care unit (ICU) setting probably benefit from early EN started within 24 to 48 hours of admission to the ICU.[3,5] Ethical questions sometimes come into play when consideration is given to starting (or stopping) EN in seemingly futile situations. Methods for assessing nutritional status and designing SNS regimens are covered in Chapter 100. In general, non-obese hospitalized patients require 20 to 35 total kcal/kg of body weight/day (84 to 147 kJ/kg body weight/day) and 1 to 2 g protein/kg of body weight/day.

Indications

Many potential indications for EN exist (Table 101–2). PN was used extensively in the past for many of these conditions. Advances in EN technology now allow many patients with these conditions to receive EN. EN is administered in both institutional and home settings.

Contraindications and Precautions

EN should not be used or should be used with extreme caution in certain conditions (Table 101–3). It is possible to use EN in some patients with these conditions depending on severity of illness, location of abnormality, and experience of practitioners delivering care. Controversy surrounds some of these contraindications and precautions. For example, whereas some clinicians deliberately avoid enteral feedings in the hemodynamically unstable patient for fear of worsening intestinal ischemia, others believe that early feeding may

Table 101–2
Potential Indications for EN

Neoplastic Disease	**GI Disease**
Chemotherapy	IBD
Radiation therapy	Short-bowel syndrome
Upper GI tumors	Esophageal motility disorder
Cancer cachexia	Pancreatitis
Organ Failure	Fistulas
Hepatic	Gastroesophageal reflux disease
Renal	Esophageal atresia
Cardiac cachexia	**Neurologic Impairment**
Pulmonary	Comatose state
Bronchopulmonary	Cerebrovascular accident
dysplasia	Demyelinating disease
Congenital heart disease	Severe depression
Hypermetabolic States	Failure to thrive
Closed head injury	Cerebral palsy
Burns	**Other Indications**
Trauma	AIDS
Postoperative major	Anorexia nervosa
surgery	Complications during pregnancy
Sepsis	Geriatric patients with multiple
	chronic disease
	Organ transplantation
	Inborn errors of metabolism
	Cystic fibrosis
	Extreme prematurity

IBD, inflammatory bowel disease.

From Kumpf VJ, Chessman KH. Enteral nutrition. In DiPiro JT, Talbert RL, Yee GC, et al, eds. *Pharmacotherapy: A Pathophysiologic Approach*, 8th ed. New York: McGraw-Hill, 2011.

facilitate intestinal perfusion and is beneficial.[5,7-9] Still others might avoid jejunal feedings in this setting but would proceed with cautious gastric feedings.

Enteral Versus Parenteral Feeding

With the advent of the technique of PN by a large central vein in the late 1960s, this modality of feeding quickly became popular. PN was used originally in patients with inflammatory bowel disease (IBD) or congenital bowel abnormalities but was incorporated quickly into care of

Table 101–3
Contraindications and Precautions for EN

Severe hemorrhagic pancreatitis
Severe necrotizing pancreatitis
Necrotizing enterocolitis
Diffuse peritonitis
Small bowel obstruction
Paralytic ileus
Severe hemodynamic instability
Enterocutaneous fistulae
Severe diarrhea
Severe malabsorption
Severe GI hemorrhage
Intractable vomiting

other types of patients such as critically ill patients. The relative ease of PN administration, along with the perception that critically ill patients had prolonged high-energy expenditures, led to complications of overfeeding. In the United States, where no intravenous (IV) fat emulsion was available commercially for several years during the 1970s, the impact of dextrose overfeeding was observed. Complications included hyperglycemia, carbon dioxide overproduction leading to delays in weaning from mechanical ventilation, and liver abnormalities owing to hepatic steatosis.

The pendulum began to swing toward EN in the late 1980s and early 1990s as clinical studies showed better clinical outcomes with EN compared with PN. Some of the potential advantages of EN over PN are included here. First, EN is expected to preserve the gut barrier function better than PN. This could prevent translocation of bacteria and endotoxin from the gut lumen into the lymphatic system and systemic circulation, thus preventing infections. Studies from the same era support that ❷ *EN is associated with fewer infectious complications than PN.* EN is cited frequently as having a better overall safety profile than PN. Whereas PN is associated with more severe complications, such as pneumothorax and catheter sepsis, EN is associated with more nuisance complications, such as GI side effects that delay or limit delivery of nutrients. Another major frequently cited advantage of EN over PN is that EN is less expensive. It is true that EN formulas typically are cheaper and less labor intensive to prepare than PN, although some specialty EN formulas approach the cost of PN formulas. Depending on the method of feeding tube placement, EN costs can mount if the tube must be placed by a radiologist or gastroenterologist rather than a nurse or if the tube must be replaced for some reason.

Arguments in support of EN over PN have been questioned. Part of this questioning relates to the question of whether EN is beneficial compared with PN or whether PN as commonly administered may be detrimental. Overfeeding and hyperglycemia occur easily with PN administration, and the potential harm of hyperglycemia, especially in critical care populations, has been demonstrated poignantly, although the exact range optimal for glycemic control in ICU patients remains controversial.[10,11] A study published in 1991 demonstrated in a mildly malnourished perioperative population that there were more infectious complications in patients randomized to receive PN compared with those randomized to receive no SNS; there was no difference in noninfectious complications between the two groups.[12] Only in severely malnourished perioperative patients were fewer noninfectious complications seen with PN; in these patients, no difference in infectious complications was seen between groups. Whether EN truly prevents infections and improves clinical outcomes or whether PN is detrimental continues to be debated and probably depends on the specific patient population. However, at present, EN is preferred by most experts over PN when the gut is functional. In Europe (more so than in North America), PN has been used to supplement EN during the first week of intensive care therapy when EN is not yet being tolerated at full rates.[2] This approach

is currently discouraged by the American and Canadian ICU guidelines and the A.S.P.E.N./SCCM guidelines for SNS in critically ill patients, and a recent randomized controlled trial from Europe corroborates the prudence of this recommendation.[3,4,13] One meta-analysis did indicate that PN may be superior to delayed EN in critical care.[14] The Algorithms for Critical-Care Enteral and Parenteral Therapy (ACCEPT) trial showed that use of an evidence-based algorithm for SNS in critical care patients in community and teaching hospitals improved provision of EN and was associated with reduced hospital stays.[15] A more recent study showed that although feeding guidelines resulted in earlier and more successful feeding, they did not result in decreases in mortality or hospital length of stay.[16]

ROUTES OF ACCESS[17]

There are several access sites for EN (Fig. 101–2). Nasogastric (NG), orogastric (OG), nasoduodenal (ND), and nasojejunal (NJ) routes generally are for short-term use (less than 1 month), whereas gastrostomy, percutaneous endoscopic gastrostomy (PEG), jejunostomy, and percutaneous endoscopic jejunostomy (PEJ) tubes are preferred for longer term treatment. Esophagostomy or pharyngostomy is used rarely. Both advantages and disadvantages exist for each EN route (Table 101–4).

Gastric Feeding

Gastric feedings are used commonly. They require an intact gag reflex and normal gastric emptying for safety and success. Certain patients, such as those who have suffered head trauma, may not empty their stomachs efficiently and therefore may not be good candidates for gastric feedings. In these patients, it may be impossible to achieve a gastric tube feeding rate to provide adequate nutrients. In addition, pooling of formula in the stomach could increase risk of aspirating feeding formula into the lungs.

The NG route is used most commonly for short-term (less than 1 month) enteral access. The major advantage of this route is that the tube can be placed quickly and inexpensively by the nurse at the bedside.

Gastrostomy tubes, in which an incision is made directly through the abdominal wall, are indicated for patients who can tolerate gastric feedings but in whom long-term (longer than 1 month) feedings are anticipated. The most commonly placed gastrostomy tubes are PEG tubes placed endoscopically. Gastrostomy tubes also can be placed laparoscopically or during an open procedure by a surgeon. Placement of a gastrostomy tube either endoscopically or surgically is more expensive than bedside OG or NG placement but can result in placement of a larger bore tube.

An advantage of feeding into the stomach is that the feedings can be delivered either intermittently or continuously. This is unlike feeding directly into the small bowel, where continuous feedings must be used. Intermittent feedings into the small bowel result in GI intolerance in most patients.

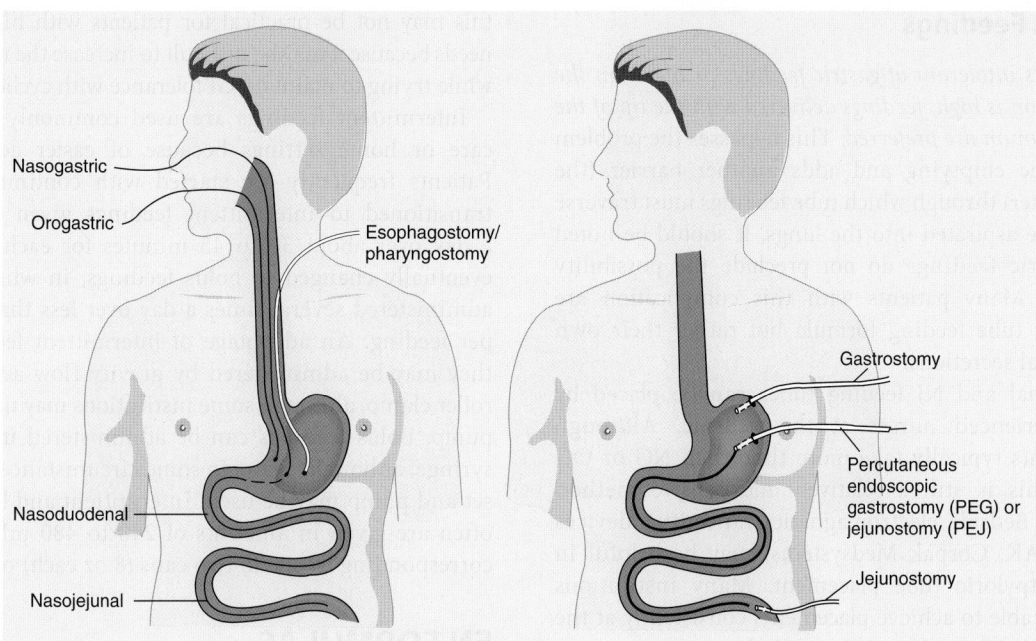

FIGURE 101–2. Access sites for tube feeding. (From Kumpf VJ, Chessman KH. Enteral nutrition. In DiPiro JT, Talbert RL, Yee GC, et al, eds. *Pharmacotherapy: A Pathophysiologic Approach*, 8th ed, New York: McGraw-Hill, 2011:2531.)

Table 101–4

Options and Considerations in the Selection of Enteral Access

Access	Indications	Tube Placement Options	Advantages	Disadvantages
Nasogastric or orogastric	Short term Intact gag reflex Normal gastric emptying	Manually at bedside	Ease of placement Allows for all methods of administration Inexpensive Multiple commercially available tubes and sizes	Potential tube displacement Potential increased aspiration risk
Nasoduodenal or nasojejunal	Short term Impaired gastric motility or emptying High risk of GER or aspiration	Manually at bedside Fluoroscopically Endoscopically	Potential reduced aspiration risk Allows for early postinjury or postoperative feeding Multiple commercially available tubes and sizes	Manual transpyloric passage requires greater skill Potential tube displacement or clogging Bolus or intermittent feeding not tolerated
Gastrostomy	Long term Normal gastric emptying	Surgically Endoscopically Radiologically Laparoscopically	Allows for all methods of administration Large-bore tubes less likely to clog Multiple commercially available tubes and sizes Low-profile buttons available	Attendant risks associated with each type of procedure Potential increased aspiration risk Requires stoma site care
Jejunostomy	Long term Impaired gastric motility or gastric emptying High risk of GER or aspiration	Surgically Endoscopically Radiologically Laparoscopically	Allows for early postinjury or postoperative feeding Potential reduced aspiration risk Multiple commercially available tubes and sizes	Attendant risks associated with each type of procedure Bolus or intermittent feeding not tolerated Requires stoma site care

GER, gastroesophageal reflux.

From Kumpf VJ, Chessman KH. Enteral nutrition. In DiPiro JT, Talbert RL, Yee GC, et al, eds. *Pharmacotherapy: A Pathophysiologic Approach*, 8th ed. New York: McGraw-Hill, 2011.

Postpyloric Feedings

❸ *For patients intolerant of gastric feedings or in whom the risk of aspiration is high, feedings delivered with the tip of the tube in the jejunum are preferred.* This bypasses the problem of poor gastric emptying and adds another barrier (the pyloric sphincter) through which tube feedings must traverse before they are aspirated into the lungs. It should be noted that postpyloric feedings do not preclude the possibility of aspiration. Many patients with this complication are not aspirating tube feeding formula but rather their own nasopharyngeal secretions.

Nasoduodenal and NJ feeding tubes can be placed by trained, experienced nurses at the bedside. Although such placements typically take more time than NG or OG placements, this is still a relatively inexpensive method of placement. Bedside electromagnetic transmitter devices (e.g., CORTRAK, Corpak Medsystems) may be helpful in attaining postpyloric tube placement. Many institutions have not been able to achieve placements consistently at the bedside. In some institutions, ND or NJ placements are done in radiology by a radiologist using fluoroscopy to visualize tube advancement. This procedure increases the cost of EN therapy. NJ tubes generally are preferred over ND tubes; placement of the tip of the tube distal to the ligament of Treitz (located near the junction of the duodenum and the jejunum) may reduce risk of aspiration. Alternatively, during a laparotomy, the surgeon can place an ND or NJ tube.

Surgically placed jejunostomy tubes are an option; similar to surgically placed gastrostomy tubes, they are placed through an incision in the abdominal wall, precluding the need for a tube down the nose or mouth. These tubes frequently are placed during laparotomy following abdominal trauma. Alternatively, jejunal access can be obtained by placing a jejunal extension through a PEG tube; the resulting tube is sometimes referred to as a *PEGJ tube* or *G-J tube*. Another option is to place a PEJ tube directly; this is more technically difficult than PEG placement. Tubes with both gastric and jejunal lumens are sometimes used, the gastric lumen for suctioning stomach contents and the jejunal lumen for delivery of feedings.

METHODS OF DELIVERY

Enteral feedings are delivered by several different methods. Continuous infusion must be used when duodenal or jejunal feedings are administered. For gastric feedings, bolus or intermittent feedings could be administered instead of continuous feedings. Each method has advantages and disadvantages.

In many hospitals, EN is delivered most commonly as a continuous infusion over 24 hours at a constant rate regulated by an infusion pump. A variation of continuous infusion is cyclic feeding, in which a constant rate is maintained by a pump over a certain number of hours daily. This method of administration is used commonly in long-term care or home settings. Often EN is administered overnight, giving the patient "freedom" from the infusion pump during the day, although

this may not be practical for patients with high nutritional needs because it may be difficult to increase the rate of feedings while trying to maintain GI tolerance with cyclic feeding.

Intermittent feedings are used commonly in long-term care or home settings because of easier administration. Patients frequently are started with continuous feedings; transitioned to intermittent feedings given several times a day over about 30 to 45 minutes for each feeding; and eventually changed to bolus feedings, in which feeding is administered several times a day over less than 10 minutes per feeding. An advantage of intermittent feedings is that they may be administered by gravity flow adjusted with a roller clamp, although some institutions may use an infusion pump. Bolus feedings can be administered using a 60-mL syringe, although, again, in some circumstances, an infusion set and pump may be used. Intermittent and bolus feedings often are given in amounts of 240 to 480 mL per feeding, corresponding to one to two cans (8 oz each) of formula.

EN FORMULAS

One advantage of EN over PN is the availability in the United States of certain nutrients in some EN formulations (e.g., glutamine, fish oils) that are not available for parenteral use. A number of EN formulas are marketed commercially. Hospitals and long-term care facilities usually limit formularies of EN formulas, stocking only a limited number of products.

Polymeric versus Oligomeric Formulas

A major criterion for categorizing EN products is whether they contain more intact (polymeric) macronutrients (particularly the protein component) or their macronutrient ingredients are present in simpler forms (oligomeric). **❹** *Standard EN formulas are polymeric formulas; these are appropriate for most patients.* Oligomeric formulas should be reserved for patients with GI dysfunction.

Polymeric formulas typically contain intact proteins (most commonly casein). They have low osmolality of 300 to 500 mOsm/kg (300 to 500 mmol/kg). These formulas usually supply essential vitamins and minerals in amounts similar to the Adequate Intakes (AI) or Recommended Dietary Allowances (RDA) for these nutrients when the formula is delivered in amounts adequate to meet macronutrient requirements of most patients. Many polymeric formulas are inexpensive relative to oligomeric formulas. Most polymeric formulas are lactose free and gluten free, as are most modern tube feeding products. Products designed to be used as oral supplements generally are polymeric and often have sucrose or other simple sugars added to improve taste.

The oligomeric formulas are also known as *chemically defined formulas.* These can be subcategorized based on whether the formula contains all free amino acids (elemental formulas) or peptides (peptide based) as the protein source. Some formulas contain a combination of free amino acids and small peptides. Dipeptides and tripeptides are absorbed more efficiently than free amino acids. Oligomeric formulas may be better tolerated than polymeric formulas for patients with defects in GI function and may be particularly useful with severe pancreatic dysfunction or significantly decreased GI surface area (e.g., short-bowel syndrome).

Oligomeric formulas typically are more expensive than polymeric formulas and have higher osmolality because they contain more osmotically active particles. However, the osmolality of these products usually does not exceed 700 mOsm/kg (700 mmol/kg), a value less than that of many oral medications or a regular diet. In the past, there was concern that higher osmolality EN formulas could cause GI intolerance, particularly diarrhea. This led to dilution of formulas and gradually increasing both the strength and rate of formula administration. This practice is unnecessary and serves only to delay attainment of goal nutritional support. Sometimes enteral feedings are diluted to deliver extra water required by the patient; this practice generally is discouraged because of potential risk of formula contamination. Instead, it is better to give extra water as boluses through the tube. If medications are administered through the feeding tube, generous amounts of water should be used to flush the tube before and after each medication; this practice helps provide extra fluid and prevent problems with occlusion of the tube.

Oligomeric formulas usually are less palatable than polymeric formulas and are not designed for use as oral supplements. Many of the oligomeric formulas provide some fat calories as medium-chain triglycerides (MCTs), a fat source that is more readily absorbed and metabolized than long-chain triglycerides (LCTs) typically found in polymeric formulas. The MCTs do not require bile salts or pancreatic enzymes for absorption. Some of the elemental formulas contain a low proportion of fat (less than 10% of total calories), which makes them useful in certain situations where fat needs to be restricted. The carbohydrate source in oligomeric formulas is also less complex than in polymeric formulas, consisting of oligosaccharides rather than hydrolyzed starch.

Fiber Content

Another distinguishing factor of enteral formulas is whether or not they contain fiber. Both soluble and insoluble fibers may be included in the formula. Insoluble fiber exerts an effect on gut motility by drawing water into the intestine and decreasing transit time, thus preventing constipation. Soluble fiber can help to lower blood cholesterol levels, regulate blood sugar, and prolong gastric emptying. Soluble fiber may also help control diarrhea. Cellulose gum is an example source of insoluble fiber. Oat fiber and guar gum provide primarily soluble fiber. Soy fiber provides primarily insoluble fiber but also some soluble fiber and is the most commonly used fiber source in tube feeding products. Fiber has been useful for regulating gut motility in some but not all clinical studies; it certainly can be useful in selected patients.[18] Some patients may experience GI discomfort secondary to gas production with introduction of fiber-containing formulas.

Fructooligosaccharides (FOS) are a form of fiber that pass through the stomach and small bowel undigested and are fermented by colonic bacteria to the SCFA butyrate,

propionate, and acetate. The SCFAs serve as a major fuel source for colonocytes and facilitate water and sodium reabsorption in the colon.[19] The FOS are thus *prebiotics* that serve as fermentable substrates for the normal flora of the colon. The SCFAs are not added directly to EN products because they would be absorbed completely before reaching the colon; rather, FOS are added, allowing bacterial degradation to form SCFAs.

Caloric Density

Enteral feeding formulas can be categorized based on caloric density. Standard caloric density is 1 to 1.3 kcal/mL (4.2 to 5.4 kJ/mL). More calorically dense formulas containing 1.5 to 2 kcal/mL (6.3 to 8.4 kJ/mL) are available and have a higher osmolality. **⑤** *When choosing an EN formula, the patient's fluid status should dictate the caloric density selected.* Fluid-overloaded patients may benefit from more calorically dense formulas. As caloric content of a formula increases, the amount of free water decreases. For example, whereas 1-kcal/mL (4.2 kJ/mL) formulas contain about 850 mL of free water/L, the 2-kcal/mL (8.4 kJ/mL) formulas contain about 710 mL of free water/L.[20]

Protein Content

Protein content is an important factor in choosing an EN formula. Standard protein content in EN formulas is up to about 15% of total calories as protein. High-protein formulas containing up to 25% of total calories as protein are available for highly stressed patients with elevated protein needs. So are low-nitrogen formulas containing less than 10% of total calories as protein for use in patients requiring protein restriction. A wide range of protein is available, from about 35 to 85 g/L.

Carbohydrate Content

The most common carbohydrate source in tube feeding products is maltodextrin, a partially hydrolyzed starch that is easily digestible. Corn syrup solids are another hydrolyzed starch found in many products. Products containing simple sugars (often those intended for oral use) tend to be higher in osmolality.

Fat Content

Both MCTs and LCTs are used in tube feeding products. Corn, soy, and safflower oils have been the mainstay sources of fat, providing mainly ω-6 polyunsaturated fatty acids (PUFAs). Some newer EN products contain higher quantities of ω-3 PUFAs from sources such as fish oil (i.e., docosahexanoic acid [DHA] and eicosapentaenoic acid [EPA]). Other formulas contain higher quantities of monounsaturated fatty acids (MUFAs) from canola oil and high-oleic safflower or sunflower oils. The essential fatty acid (EFA) content (mainly linoleic acid) of EN formulas is important because EFA deficiency can be induced if at least 1% to 4% of total calories are not supplied as EFAs. MCT oil does not contain any EFAs.

Vitamin, Mineral, and Electrolyte Content

Most EN products contain vitamins and minerals, including the major electrolytes, in amounts adequate to deliver the RDA or AI when a standard volume of the formula is delivered daily. Some of the specialty formulas (e.g., renal formulas) may have altered amounts of certain micronutrients.

Specialty Formulas

Specialty formulas designed for use in specific clinical situations generally are much more expensive than standard polymeric formulas. ❻ *Robust clinical trial data supporting use of these specialty formulas in niche populations typically remain lacking in terms of improved patient outcomes.*

▶ Stress and Trauma Formulas

Historically, formulas aimed specifically for highly stressed, critically ill patients, including those who have sustained significant trauma and those undergoing major surgical procedures, were enriched with branched-chain amino acids (BCAAs). The rationale was that skeletal muscle BCAAs are preferentially used for energy in critical illness. Provision of BCAAs might limit breakdown of muscle in these patients. Clinical data failed to support or refute benefit of these formulas unequivocally in terms of clinical outcomes.[3]

The newer generation of enteral feeding formulas marketed for use in these populations covers a broad spectrum of characteristics (Table 101–5). Whereas some are polymeric, others are oligomeric to address malabsorption that may accompany high stress. Some formulas marketed for use in critical illness are calorically dense (1.5 to 2 kcal/mL [6.3 to 8.4 kJ/mL]) to address fluid restrictions seen in this population, and others are less calorically dense. Most products contain generous amounts of protein to address requirements of highly stressed patients (nonprotein kilocalorie to nitrogen ratios typically between 75:1 and 125:1). Many products contain ingredients purported to increase immune function; the term *immunonutrition* is sometimes attached to these products.

Immune-enhancing ingredients present in some enteral feeding products include arginine, glutamine, ω-3 fatty acids, nucleic acids, and antioxidants. Few products contain all of these (see Table 101–5). Arginine is an important substrate for nitric oxide (NO) synthesis, and small amounts of NO have beneficial effects on immune function under certain conditions. Arginine has been purported to have a positive influence on lymphocyte and macrophage function. Glutamine is considered to be conditionally essential in critical illness. This amino acid is a preferred fuel source for enterocytes of the small bowel. Supplementation with glutamine, either parenterally or enterally, may help to maintain the integrity of the gut mucosa, preventing translocation of bacteria and endotoxin from the gut lumen into the lymphatic system and systemic circulation. However, the importance of translocation in humans remains controversial. The ω-3 fatty acids, primarily from fish oils, are included in many immunonutrition products.

Metabolites of ω-6 fatty acids include mediators such as prostaglandins, leukotrienes, and thromboxanes that are primarily proinflammatory and increase coagulation. On the other hand, mediators produced from ω-3 fatty acids are less proinflammatory and decrease coagulation. Thus ω-3 fatty acids may help preserve the antimicrobial capacity of critically ill patients by downregulating inflammation.[21] Limited data support nucleic acids as immunomodulators. Quantities of antioxidants (particularly vitamin C, vitamin E, and β-carotene) higher than those traditionally found in standard enteral formulas are added to some immunonutrition formulas to protect body systems, including the immune system, from damage by oxygen-free radicals.[22] Oxygen-free radicals may be produced in high quantities in the setting of injury or infection.

❼ *Acceptance of enteral immunonutrition in certain clinical settings is gaining momentum.* Several meta-analyses of the commercial immunonutrition products and/or specific ingredients (e.g., arginine and glutamine) found in these products have been conducted.[3,23] In general, these analyses have found no benefit in terms of mortality rates. However, several have concluded that infection rates, length of stay, and length of time on a ventilator may be decreased with these products. The 2009 A.S.P.E.N./SCCM ICU Guidelines support use of these formulas in major elective surgery, trauma, burns, head and neck cancer, and mechanically ventilated patients.[5] The best timing (initiation and duration) of delivery remains to be determined. There is some concern that supplementation with arginine may be detrimental in septic patients.[3]

▶ Pulmonary Formulas

Enteral feeding formulas designed for use in patients with chronic obstructive pulmonary disease or receiving mechanical ventilation contain higher amounts of fat (40% to 55% of total kilocalories) than most formulas. The rationale for high fat content is that burning of fat for energy is associated with less carbon dioxide production compared with burning of carbohydrate. Less carbon dioxide production theoretically would be advantageous in patients with retention of this substance and might facilitate weaning from mechanical ventilation. Because part of the market targeted by the manufacturers of these products comprises mechanically ventilated patients, these products are included in Table 101–5. Carbon dioxide retention owing to carbohydrate administration was a problem previously when feeding was overzealous. However, at conservative calorie levels, even standard enteral formulas usually can be given without fear of excess carbon dioxide production.

One formula, Oxepa (Nestle), has been studied specifically in critically ill patients with acute respiratory distress syndrome (ARDS), acute lung injury (ALI), and sepsis. This formula contains high quantities of the ω-3 fatty acids (EPA) and γ-linolenic acid (GLA). GLA is metabolized to a prostaglandin with vasodilatory properties. EPA is converted to prostaglandins and leukotrienes with primarily an anti-inflammatory profile. This formula contains large quantities of antioxidants. Patients receiving this formula had improved

Table 101–5

Selected Enteral Feeding Formulas Marketed for Use in High-Stress, Pulmonary Disease and Ventilator-Dependent, and Trauma Patients[a]

Product Name/Manufacturer	kcal/mL	Protein (g/L)	Enriched Ingredients[b]	Selected Specialized Indications
Polymeric[c]				
Impact/Nestle	1	56	Arginine, nucleotides, ω-3 fatty acids	HS, TR, PD, CI
Impact 1.5/Nestle	1.5	84	Arginine, nucleotides, ω-3 fatty acids, MCT	HS, TR, PD, CI
Impact with Fiber/Nestle	1	56	Arginine, nucleotides, ω-3 fatty acids	HS, TR, PD, CI
Nutren Pulmonary/Nestle	1.5	68	55% total kcal as fat	PD, CI
Pulmocare/Abbott	1.5	62.4	55% total kcal as fat	PD
Oxepa/Abbott	1.5	62.4	55% total kcal as fat; ω-3 fatty acids	PD, CI
Isosource 1.5 Cal/Nestle	1.5	68	38% total kcal as fat	PD
Two Cal HN/Abbott	2	84		HS
Oligomeric/Monomeric[c]				
Impact Glutamine/Nestle	1.3	78	Arginine, nucleotides, ω-3 fatty acids, glutamine	HS, TR, PD, CI
Impact Peptide 1.5/Nestle	1.5	94	Arginine, ω-3 fatty acids, MCT	HS, TR, PD, CI
Crucial/Nestle	1.5	94	Arginine, ω-3 fatty acids, MCT	HS, TR, PD, CI
Pivot 1.5 Cal/Abbott	1.5	93.8	Arginine, ω-3 fatty acids	HS, TR
Optimental/Abbott	1	51.5	ω-3 fatty acids	HS, TR
Vivonex Plus/Nestle	1	45	Glutamine	CI
Vivonex RTF/Nestle	1	50	MCT	CI
Vivonex T.E.N./Nestle	1	38		CI
Peptamen 1.5/Nestle	1.5	67.6	MCT	CI
Peptamen AF/Nestle	1.2	75.6	MCT, ω-3 fatty acids	HS, CI, PD
Perative/Abbott	1.3	66.7	MCT	HS, TR
Vital AF 1.2 Cal/Abbott	1.2	75	ω-3 fatty acids, MCT	HS

CI, critical illness; EPA, eicosapentaenoic acid; GLA, γ-linolenic acid; HS, high stress; MCT, medium-chain triglycerides; PD, pulmonary disease/ventilator dependent; TR, trauma

[a]One kcal is equivalent to 4.186 kJ.

[b]Formula considered enriched if following criteria met: arginine—greater than 10 g/1,500 kcal (6,279 kJ); glutamine—greater than 10 g/1,500 kcal (6,279 kJ); MCT—greater than 30% of total fat; and ω-3 fatty acid—ratio of ω-6 to ω-3 less than or equal to 2:1 or greater than 1.5 g/L ω-3 fatty acids.

[c]Polymeric vs. oligomeric/monomeric designation based on protein content.

outcomes, including fewer days of mechanical ventilation, compared with patients receiving a high-fat enteral feeding product as a control.[24] A more recent study using a standard enteral feeding product as a control did not show clear benefit in septic patients with ARDS or ALI.[25] However, another recent study demonstrated benefit from Oxepa in patient with early sepsis even when using a standard enteral feeding control product.[26] The timing and duration of use of this product for optimum benefit in these populations remains to be determined.

▶ Diabetic Formulas

Similar to pulmonary formulas, formulas designed for patients with diabetes or stress-induced hyperglycemia are relatively high in fat and low in carbohydrates (Table 101–6). The macronutrient content of these products does not follow the recommendations of the American Diabetes Association for patients with diabetes (lower carbohydrate content and higher fat content than recommended), which could be an issue if used for a long period of time. These formulas

Table 101–6

Selected Enteral Feeding Formulas Marketed for Use in Diabetes and Stress-Induced Hyperglycemia[a]

Product Name/Manufacturer	kcal/mL	% kcal as Fat	% kcal as Carbohydrate	Fiber (g/L)
Nutren Glytrol/Nestle Nutrition	1	42	40	15.2
Glucerna 1.0 Cal/Abbott	1	49	34.3	14.4
Glucerna 1.2 Cal/Abbott	1.2	45	35	16
Glucerna 1.5 Cal/Abbott	1.5	45	33	16
Diabetisource AC/Nestle Nutrition	1.2	44	36	15

[a]One kcal is equivalent to 4.186 kJ.

typically contain fiber (primarily soluble) because it plays some role in glycemic control. They also may contain fructose and MUFAs. Data support improved blood sugar control with use of these formulas in patients with diabetes.[27] Whether or not a diabetic EN formula is chosen, avoidance of overfeeding and maintenance of good glycemic control with insulin or other hypoglycemic medications are important in these populations.

▶ Renal Formulas

Products designed for use in renal failure have high caloric density (1.8 to 2 kcal/mL [7.5 to 8.4 kJ/mL]) to decrease administered fluid (Table 101-7). The products vary in amounts of nutrients of interest in renal failure patients such as protein, potassium, phosphorus, and magnesium. Products low in protein (20 to 35 g/L) may be appropriate in chronic renal failure patients not yet receiving dialysis. On the other hand, removal of nitrogen by dialysis, coupled with the hypercatabolic, hypermetabolic condition seen in many acute renal failure patients, makes use of higher protein formulas (70 to 85 g/L) appropriate in these situations. Potassium, phosphorus, and magnesium contents of EN formulas designed for use in renal failure tend to be lower than standard formulas because these renally excreted electrolytes accumulate during renal failure.

Historically, elemental formulas designed for renal failure were enriched with essential amino acids (EAAs) and contained lesser amounts of nonessential amino acids (NEAAs) than standard formulas. Theoretically, EAAs could combine with urea nitrogen in the synthesis of NEAAs, leading to a decrease in blood urea nitrogen (BUN). The only situation in which such formulas may be appropriate is in patients with chronic renal failure who are not candidates for dialysis. Even in this setting, use of these products should be limited to no more than 2 or 3 weeks owing to the risk of increased serum ammonia levels.[1] These EAA-enriched formulas have been supplanted largely by polymeric formulas with protein content similar to standard EN formulas. Many dialysis patients tolerate standard, high-protein EN formulas, although electrolytes must be monitored closely.

▶ Hepatic Formulas

Specialized formulas for patients with hepatic insufficiency are limited in number. These are enriched with BCAAs while containing a reduced quantity of aromatic amino acids (AAAs) and methionine compared with standard enteral formulas. These changes address the high levels of AAAs and low levels of BCAAs found in the blood of patients with hepatic insufficiency. Theoretically, these products might help patients with hepatic encephalopathy (HE). One of the mechanisms postulated as a cause of HE is the "false neurotransmitter" hypothesis. According to this hypothesis, high levels of AAA in the blood allow large quantities of these amino acids to cross the blood–brain barrier and form false neurotransmitters. Administration of high amounts of BCAAs could competitively inhibit some AAAs from crossing the blood–brain barrier, thus decreasing formation of false neurotransmitters. Hepatic formulas have low AAA content, and this distinguishes them from the BCAA-enriched formulas historically used in patient with critical illness and stress. Improvement in mortality attributable to these products has not been consistent.[1]

The A.S.P.E.N./SCCM guidelines for the ICU recommend against the use of protein restriction to reduce risk of development of hepatic encephalopathy.[5] These guidelines recommend use of standard EN formulas for ICU patients with acute or chronic liver disease but state that the hepatic specialty formulas may be useful in improving coma grade in HE patients refractory to standard treatment with locally acting antibiotics and lactulose. An example of a specialized hepatic formula is Hepatic-Aid II, a product supplied as a powder for reconstitution that requires vitamin, mineral, and electrolyte supplementation. A second product is NutriHep (Nestle), supplied as a liquid formula containing the recommended amounts of key vitamins, minerals, and electrolytes.

▶ Wound Healing Formulas

Tube feeding and oral supplement formulas designed for use in patients with wounds or decubitus ulcers typically supply high amounts of protein and calories. The antioxidant vitamins A, C, and E are frequently also found in high quantities as is zinc.

Table 101–7

Selected Enteral Feeding Products Designed for Use in Renal Failure

Product Name/Manufacturer	Protein/L	Characteristics
Renalcal/Nestle	34.4	Enriched with EAAs, arginine, histidine; incomplete[a] formula because of negligible electrolytes and lack of fat-soluble vitamins
Nepro with Carb Steady/Abbott	80.6	Complete formula[b] similar to Novasource Renal
Novasource Renal/Nestle	74	Complete formula similar to Nepro with Carb Steady
Suplena with Carb Steady/Abbott	44.7	Complete formula with low amounts of protein for patients not yet receiving dialysis

[a]Incomplete formula—contains insufficient amounts of one or more essential nutrients.

[b]Complete formula—contains all nutrients in amounts sufficient to meet needs of most patients in a volume equal to or less than that usually administered.

EAA, essential amino acid.

Patient Encounter, Part 1

FH is a 40-year-old paraplegic woman admitted to the hospital with increasing shortness of breath, fever, and hypotension. She is intubated and placed on mechanical ventilation in the ICU. A diagnosis of sepsis and septic shock is made; her lactic acid level is elevated, as is her white blood cell count. Several sources of the sepsis are possible; in addition to pneumonia, she also has a significant sacral ulcer and a suprapubic catheter with urinalysis positive for leukocyte esterase and a few white blood cells. She is placed on a sepsis protocol to include fluid resuscitation, pressors, antibiotics, and stress-dose corticosteroids. She is given propofol for sedation while on the ventilator and is receiving an insulin drip.

FH responds well to treatment of her sepsis and by day 2 of hospitalization is receiving a stable low dose of pressors. A decision is then made to start EN. Her current weight is 57 kg, her height is 67 inches (170 cm), and her body mass index is 19.5 kg/m².

Is there any concern regarding starting EN at this time?

How does the propofol that the patient is receiving affect the EN prescription?

Design an enteral feeding regimen appropriate for this patient at this time.

What are this patient's risk factors for hyperglycemia, and is the insulin drip a good method of management?

Is there any indication for additional micronutrient supplementation for this patient beyond what is included in the EN formula?

▶ Modular Components

Single nutrient components are frequently administered through feeding tubes to augment the composition of the EN formula. Protein modules are probably the most commonly used. These may be supplied by the manufacturer as a powder that must be reconstituted with water or as a liquid product. Other commonly used modular components include fiber and glutamine supplements.

MONITORING AND COMPLICATIONS

Although complications of EN generally are considered less serious than those of PN, some complications nevertheless can be dangerous or can lead to impaired delivery of desired nutrient load. Complications of EN can be divided into four categories: GI, technical, infectious, and metabolic. The first three of these categories, along with common causes, are listed in Table 101–8. Patients on EN must be monitored for prevention of complications (Table 101–9). Note that monitoring of many parameters can become less frequent as the patient's condition stabilizes. Monitoring for efficacy of EN is also important.

Table 101–8
Complications of Tube Feeding

Complication	Causes
GI	
Diarrhea	Drug related
	Antibiotic-induced bacterial overgrowth
	Hyperosmolar medications administered via feeding tubes
	Antacids containing magnesium
	Malabsorption
	Hypoalbuminemia or gut mucosal atrophy
	Pancreatic insufficiency
	Inadequate GI tract surface area
	Rapid GI tract transit
	Radiation enteritis
	Tube feeding related
	Rapid formula administration
	Formula hyperosmolality
	Low residue (fiber) content
	Lactose intolerance
	Bacterial contamination
Nausea and vomiting	Gastric dysmotility (surgery, anticholinergic drugs, diabetic gastroparesis)
	Rapid infusion of hyperosmolar formula
Constipation	Dehydration
	Drug induced (anticholinergics)
	Inactivity
	Low residue (fiber) content
	Obstruction or fecal impaction
Abdominal distention or cramping	Too rapid formula administration
Technical	
Occluded feeding tube lumen	Insoluble complexation of enteral formula and medication(s)
	Inadequate flushing of feeding tube
	Undissolved feeding formula
Tube displacement	Self-extubation
	Vomiting or coughing
	Inadequate fixation (jejunostomy)
Aspiration	Improper patient position
	Gastroparesis or atony causing regurgitation
	Feeding tube malpositioned
	Compromised lower esophageal sphincter
	Diminished gag reflex
Peristomal excoriation	Improper skin and tube care
	GI tract secretions leaking peristomally
Infectious	
Aspiration pneumonia	Same as technical—aspiration comments
	Prolonged use of large-bore polyvinylchloride tube

GI, gastrointestinal.

From Janson DD, Chessman KH. Enteral nutrition. In DiPiro JT, Talbert RL, Yee GC, et al, eds. *Pharmacotherapy: A Pathophysiologic Approach*, 5th ed. New York: McGraw-Hill, 2005.

GI Complications

8 *GI complications are the most common complications of EN limiting the amount of feeding that patients receive.* Although diarrhea frequently is blamed on the tube feeding formula or the method of EN administration, other possible causes of diarrhea usually exist (see Table 101–8).

Table 101–9

Suggested Monitoring for EN Patients to Prevent the Development of Complications

Parameter	During Initiation of EN Therapy	During Stable EN Therapy
Vital signs	Every 4–6 hours	As needed with suspected change (i.e., fever)
Clinical assessment		
Weight	Daily	Weekly
Length and height (children)	Weekly–monthly	Monthly
Head circumference (less than 3 years of age)	Weekly–monthly	Monthly
Total intake or output	Daily	As needed with suspected changed in intake or output
Tube feeding intake	Daily	Daily
Enterostomy tube site assessment	Daily	Daily
GI tolerance		
Stool frequency and volume	Daily	Daily
Abdomen assessment	Daily	Daily
Nausea or vomiting	Daily	Daily
Gastric residual volumes	Every 4–8 hours (varies)	As needed when delayed gastric emptying is suspected
Tube placement	Before starting; then ongoing	Ongoing
Laboratory		
Electrolytes, BUN/S_{cr}, glucose	Daily	Every 1–3 months
Calcium, magnesium, phosphorus	3–7 times/week	Every 1–3 months
Liver function tests	Weekly	Every 1–3 months
Trace elements, vitamins	If deficiency or toxicity is suspected	If deficiency or toxicity is suspected

BUN, blood urea nitrogen; EN, enteral nutrition; S_{cr}, serum creatinine.

From Knopf VS, Chessman KH. Enteral nutrition. In DiPiro JT, Talbert RL, Yee GC, et al, eds. *Pharmacotherapy: A Pathophysiologic Approach*, 8th ed. New York: McGraw-Hill, 2011.

In the inpatient setting, patients receiving EN frequently are some of the sickest patients. Along these lines, *Clostridium difficile* colitis must be considered as a possible cause of diarrhea, especially in patients who have been receiving antimicrobial therapy or proton pump inhibitors.[28-30] Antibiotic therapy is a major cause of diarrhea in acutely ill patients, including those receiving EN. A medication-related cause of diarrhea is the sorbitol content of medications.[31] Large quantities of this substance present in many oral liquid medications (often considered the dosage form of choice for administration through a feeding tube) can cause diarrhea. Unfortunately, the sorbitol content of many medications is not listed on their labeling, and some manufacturers frequently reformulate these preparations to contain varying amounts of excipients, such as sorbitol.

Determining the cause of the diarrhea is important to know how to address the problem. Whereas *C. difficile* colitis should be treated with metronidazole or vancomycin, sorbitol- or other medication-induced diarrhea can be addressed by removal of the offending agent. Likewise, diarrhea secondary to malabsorption sometimes can be addressed by changing to an oligomeric EN formula. Antiperistaltic agents such as loperamide may be useful in some cases of noninfectious diarrhea.

On the other hand, constipation may occur in some patients receiving tube feedings, especially the elderly. Increased provision of fluid or fiber may be useful in attaining bowel regularity. Constipation may be drug related, in which case discontinuation or replacement of the offending drug may help alleviate the problem.

Impaired gastric emptying is seen commonly in EN patients receiving gastric feedings and may be associated with nausea and vomiting. Impaired gastric emptying may be related to a disease process (e.g., diabetic gastroparesis or sequelae to head injury) or to drug therapy, most notably narcotics. Gastric residual checks frequently are measured in patients receiving gastric feedings (see Table 101–9). To accomplish such a check, a syringe is attached to the feeding device, and as much liquid as possible is aspirated into the syringe. Debate is ongoing as to what constitutes a significant gastric aspirate, with numbers between 100 and 500 mL most commonly defended; some experts would even argue that residual checks are not necessary.[4,32-34] Approaches to the patient with delayed gastric emptying might include changing to an enteral formula containing less fat because dietary fat is associated with slower gastric emptying. Metoclopramide often is given to patients receiving gastric feedings to facilitate gastric emptying. Erythromycin is an alternative medication that may be useful in stimulating gastric motility, although it can be associated with drug–drug interactions. Feedings by a PEG tube may be associated with a decreased risk of aspiration compared with NG feedings.[32] Patients with consistently high gastric aspirates are considered to be at higher risk of aspirating feedings into their lungs and should be considered for transition to postpyloric feedings. Postpyloric feedings may help relieve EN-related nausea and vomiting and are preferred for patients without an intact gag reflex.

An important practice to help prevent aspiration is elevation of the head of the bed to at least 30 degrees during continuous feedings and during and for 30 to 60 minutes after intermittent and bolus feedings.

Technical Complications

Technical or mechanical complications are encountered frequently in EN patients. Tube occlusion most commonly is related to formula occlusion or medication administration through the tube. ⑨ *An important practice to help prevent medication-related occlusion is adequate water flushing of the tube before, between, and after each medication is given through the tube.* If intermittent feedings are used, water flushing after each feeding is recommended. Tube occlusion can increase cost of EN significantly if the tube has to be removed and replaced. Clearing of the occlusion using water or pancreatic enzymes plus sodium bicarbonate can be attempted, and special devices and kits (e.g., DeClogger, Bionix) are available for this purpose.[35]

Tube displacement is a potentially significant complication of EN. This may be seen secondary to an agitated patient pulling at the tube, or in some cases, the tip of the tube migrates spontaneously. The danger of this complication arises if the tip of the tube is positioned in the tracheobronchial tree and feeding is delivered to this area, potentially leading to pneumonia, pneumothorax, and other problems. Location of the tip of the feeding tube should be confirmed initially by chest radiograph after placement and before use. For ongoing assessment of tube placement, auscultation and measurement of aspirate pH can be used.

Endoscopic and surgical feeding tubes can be complicated by erosion of the exit site caused by leakage of gastric or intestinal contents onto the skin. This complication must be addressed by good wound care and repair or replacement of the access device. Similarly, NG, ND, and NJ tubes can be complicated by nasopharyngeal irritation or necrosis. This is one reason why such tubes should be considered for short-term use only.

Infectious Complications

Infectious complications of EN include aspiration pneumonia and infections related to delivery of contaminated EN formula. Aspiration is a complication with GI, mechanical, and infectious implications. Although GI infections owing to contamination of enteral formulas have been reported uncommonly, there is ample opportunity for these formulas to be seeded with organisms during the processes of transferring from the can to the delivery bag with ready-to-use formulas and during the process of reconstitution with powdered formulas. The so-called closed systems of delivery, wherein the formulas come from the manufacturer premixed in a delivery bag, should help to decrease the chance of formula contamination. Practice recommendations from A.S.P.E.N. state that sterile water should be used for formula reconstitution, medication dilution, tube flushing, and additional water provision in acute or chronically ill patients requiring EN.[4] This recommendation can be difficult to implement into practice, especially in the home care setting.

Metabolic Complications

Metabolic complications of EN most commonly include disorders of fluid and electrolyte homeostasis and hyperglycemia. More severely ill patients require more frequent monitoring (see Table 101–9). Both dehydration and fluid overload can occur with tube feeding. Careful monitoring of fluid inputs and outputs as well as body weight is important. Dehydration may be caused by either excessive fluid losses or inadequate fluid intake. The trend in the ratio of BUN to serum creatinine can be useful in helping monitor for this complication; a ratio of greater than about 15:1 may be an indicator of dehydration. Attention should be paid to the free-water content of EN formulas. Free-water content of EN formulas varies from about 65% to 85%, with the percentage of free water typically dropping as caloric density of the formula rises. If dehydration develops, switching to a less calorically dense formula or using more water flushes may be appropriate. Fluid overload is reflected by increases in weight, lower extremity edema, and pulmonary rales and particularly may be a problem in patients with renal or cardiac insufficiency. Use of an EN formula that is more calorically dense may be helpful, and diuretic therapy may be necessary. Fluid imbalances often are associated with abnormalities of sodium homeostasis that should be addressed in concert with fluid imbalance.

Hypokalemia, hypomagnesemia, and hypophosphatemia are some of the most common electrolyte abnormalities in sick, hospitalized patients. These can occur in the context of the so-called refeeding syndrome. This syndrome occurs in chronically malnourished patients when they are aggressively started on a feeding regimen. Although more classically associated with PN, refeeding syndrome can also occur with aggressive EN. Careful monitoring of these electrolytes, coupled with a feeding regimen increased gradually to goal rate over a period of several days to a week, should help protect at-risk patients from this potentially harmful complication. Hypokalemia and hypomagnesemia also may be associated with excessive losses through the GI tract or urine and may be associated with various medication therapies, including diuretics. Repletion of these conditions may be accomplished enterally in nonsymptomatic patients or parenterally if the patient is symptomatic or the abnormality is severe. Enteral repletion with magnesium and phosphate can be associated with diarrhea. Hyperkalemia, hypermagnesemia, and hyperphosphatemia are encountered less commonly and usually are associated with renal insufficiency and decreased excretion. Hyperkalemia also is associated with several medications, including potassium-sparing diuretics, angiotensin-converting enzyme inhibitors, and angiotensin receptor blockers.

Although hyperglycemia is less common with EN than with PN, it can occur. Many severely ill patients (e.g., septic, highly stressed) receiving EN have a metabolic milieu promoting hyperglycemia. For ICU patients with hyperglycemia receiving continuous EN, an IV insulin drip may be the most effective way to achieve good glycemic control. Administration of scheduled intermediate or long-acting insulin is preferred over sliding-scale insulin alone in patients requiring insulin after they have been stabilized on their enteral feeding regimen.[36,37] Administration of a higher fat, lower carbohydrate EN formula may be useful in selected patients.

Monitoring for Efficacy and Outcome Evaluation

● The most useful physical measurement of efficacy of EN in the long-term patient is typically body weight. Depending on the clinical situation, the goal may be weight gain, weight maintenance, or weight loss. Whereas day-to-day fluctuations in weight generally reflect fluid changes, week-to-week variations are more useful in determining if caloric provision is appropriate.

The amount of EN actually administered is often less than the amount ordered owing to interruptions in therapy, especially in hospitalized patients. It is imperative to monitor volume of feedings actually received and to make adjustments in rates or amounts of EN as necessary.

Biochemical markers have been used historically to help interpret the adequacy of EN. However, use of visceral proteins such as albumin or prealbumin is limited by the effects of inflammation on serum levels of these biomarkers. In the acute phase of illness characterized by a proinflammatory state, proteins known as *acute-phase reactants* are preferentially synthesized. One of these acute-phase reactants measured clinically is C-reactive protein (CRP). In some patients with significant illness, prealbumin may not rise, even though the patients are receiving appropriate EN, until CRP begins to fall. Collection of urine to measure nitrogen balance can help analyze the adequacy of caloric and protein provision.

In patients with wounds (e.g., decubitus ulcers), a goal of nutritional therapy is to facilitate wound healing. Monitoring status of the wound becomes part of the ongoing nutritional assessment. In debilitated patients, particularly those on long-term EN, measures of functional status such as grip strength and ability to perform activities of daily living become important components of nutritional assessment.

MEDICATION ADMINISTRATION IN PATIENTS RECEIVING EN

Medication Administration Through Feeding Tubes

If a patient receiving EN is alert and can swallow oral medications, then medications should be given by mouth. Many patients are not able to receive medications by this route, and the feeding tube may be considered as a delivery route. Although used widely, the effects of medication administration through feeding tubes on the delivery of

---

> ## Patient Encounter, Part 2
>
> FH is extubated and transferred out of the intensive care unit on day 4 of hospitalization. The tube feeding is changed to a nocturnal feeding only, and a general diet including protein shakes is ordered. Unfortunately, FH's respiratory status deteriorates on the morning of day 5, prompting readmission to the ICU and reintubation with suspicion of adult respiratory distress syndrome; propofol is restarted. She has also developed loose stools and been found to be positive for *Clostridium difficile* toxin. The tube feeding is changed back to a continuous feeding around the clock.
>
> *What is the rationale for nocturnal tube feedings?*
>
> *Should any changes be made to the tube feeding regimen based on the patient's current status?*
>
> *Is Clostridium difficile infection a contraindication to EN?*
>
> *Would this patient benefit from glutamine supplementation?*

both the drug and the EN formula nutrients have been inadequately studied.[38]

🔟 *Compatibility of medication with an EN formula is of concern when administering medications through feeding tubes.* An important technical complication of EN is tube occlusion, which is related most commonly to medication administration. Not only must compatibility of the medication and the EN formula be considered, but interactions between these components and the feeding tube itself must be considered. Because either medication or EN formula or some combination thereof can physically stick to the tube itself, strict protocols for flushing the tube before, between, and after administration of medications are important.[5] The best fluid for flushing feeding tubes is warm water. Carbonated beverages and fruit juices are not recommended. Between 10 and 30 mL of water should be used as a flush before and after any medication administration through a feeding tube. Medications should be administered one at a time sequentially rather than being mixed together for simultaneous administration down the tube; about 5 mL of water should be used as a flush between each medication. This should help prevent interactions between drugs within the feeding tube itself that could lead to tube occlusion.

Different dosage forms present unique challenges for administration through feeding tubes. Certain solid dosage forms should not be crushed because crushing would alter release characteristics.[39] For example, controlled-release, extended-release, and sustained-release preparations should not be crushed. Sublingual dosage forms should not be crushed. Enteric-coated dosage forms generally are designed to protect acid-labile medications from stomach acid; when these dosage forms reach the small bowel with its higher pH, the drug then is released into an environment in which it is more stable. Alternatively, enteric-coated dosage forms protect the stomach from medications that could cause irritation. Thus, crushing of the enteric coating defeats the purpose of the dosage form and could lead to decreased efficacy or increased adverse events.

Medications available commercially as compressed tablets can be crushed for administration through feeding tubes. After such a tablet is crushed into a fine powder, it should be mixed with 10 to 30 mL of fluid (usually warm water) for administration. A powdered dosage form inside a hard-gelatin capsule similarly can be poured out and mixed with water for administration through feeding tubes. Soft-gelatin capsules can be dissolved in warm water. Some enteric-coated and delayed-release microencapsulated products can be opened, and the individually coated particles can be administered through the tube without crushing if the tube has a large enough diameter.

If a liquid dosage form of a medication exists, it would seem rational to use this dosage form for administration through a feeding tube. This may decrease the potential for tube clogging but may in some instances decrease tolerability of medication administration. Sorbitol is an excipient found in many liquid medications in amounts sufficient to cause diarrhea. If diarrhea secondary to sorbitol in a liquid medication is suspected, contact with the manufacturer to ascertain sorbitol content may be necessary.

Another potential problem with administration of liquid medications through feeding tubes is high osmolality of some products. Dilution of hypertonic medications with 30 to 60 mL of water (depending on osmolality of the medication and dosage volume of the undiluted medication) or administration of smaller dosages more frequently may help prevent diarrhea. Although administration of IV medications through feeding tubes sometimes may be entertained, these dosage forms frequently are hypertonic and contain excipients that can be problematic when given via the GI tract.

It is generally not recommended to mix medications directly into the EN formula because of concerns that physical incompatibilities might lead to tube occlusion. There is some evidence that polymeric formulas are more likely to demonstrate physical incompatibility with medications compared with monomeric formulas, although most of the work in this area has used casein or caseinate-based formulas, and other proteins may act differently.[38] Limited data currently available indicate that acidic syrups and elixirs may be most harmful, causing physical incompatibility when admixed with EN formulas. This incompatibility may be caused by changes in the protein structure after exposure to acid or alcohol.[38]

It would seem logical that medications considered being absorbed to a greater extent in the fasted state either should be given between feedings on an intermittent feeding schedule or the feedings should be held before and after medication administration. However, results of one provocative study with the antihypertensive medication hydralazine indicated that continuous feeding into the stomach resulted in a situation mimicking fasting in terms of rate of gastric emptying and drug absorption.[38] This issue deserves further study.

The location of the tip of the feeding tube is important when considering medication administration down a feeding tube. This is particularly true if the medication acts locally in the GI tract. For example, sucralfate and antacids act locally in the stomach; therefore, administration through a duodenal or jejunal tube is illogical. Likewise, for medications that require acid for best absorption, administration directly into the duodenum or jejunum would be expected to result in suboptimal absorption. Absorption of drugs when administered directly into the small bowel, especially the jejunum, is a topic where more research would be useful.

Problem Medications

▶ *Phenytoin*

Certain medications present specific challenges when administered through feeding tubes. The medication studied most thoroughly is phenytoin. Most studies have shown significant decreases in phenytoin absorption when the medication was administered enterally to patients receiving EN. Several mechanisms have been proposed for this apparent interaction. Many institutions have adopted a policy of holding tube feedings for 1 or 2 hours before and after administration of phenytoin to decrease the interaction, although some EN patients subjected to this routine still will require relatively high dosages of phenytoin to achieve therapeutic serum concentrations. Holding the feeding around medication administration can make meeting nutritional requirements difficult with continuous feedings, especially if the phenytoin is administered several times daily. Diligent monitoring of phenytoin serum concentrations is necessary for the patient on EN receiving this medication. In some cases, use of IV phenytoin or another anticonvulsant medication may be prudent.

▶ *Warfarin*

EN formulas contain vitamin K, which can antagonize the pharmacologic activity of warfarin. Vitamin K content of EN formulas generally has been adjusted down over the past several decades, resulting in products today that contain amounts of vitamin K unlikely to affect anticoagulation by warfarin significantly. However, inadequate warfarin anticoagulation in EN patients receiving formulas containing minimal vitamin K has been reported. There is some thought that a component of certain tube feedings, perhaps protein, may bind warfarin and result in suboptimal activity. One small study indicated a better response in terms of the international normalized ratio (INR) when feedings were held for 1 hour before and after warfarin administration compared with administration of the drug without holding the feedings.[40] When tube feedings are started, changed, or discontinued, the INR should be monitored closely.

Patient Encounter, Part 3

FH is extubated on day 9 but remains in the ICU because of difficulty clearing respiratory secretions. She is finally transferred out of the ICU on hospital day 11.

How should the transition from EN to oral feedings be accomplished?

▶ *Fluoroquinolones*

Absorption of antimicrobial agents such as fluoroquinolones and tetracyclines that can be bound by divalent and trivalent cations potentially could be compromised by administration with EN formulas containing these cations. The fluoroquinolones (e.g., levofloxacin and ciprofloxacin) have been best studied in this regard, and results of studies are not consistent.[41,42] Some institutions hold tube feedings for 30 to 60 minutes or more before and after enteral dosages of fluoroquinolones. Because ciprofloxacin absorption has

been shown to be decreased with jejunal administration, this drug probably should not be given by jejunal tube.[42]

SUMMARY AND CONCLUSION

EN is an important method of feeding patients who cannot or should not eat enough to meet nutrient requirements for a prolonged time. When the GI tract can be used safely, EN is preferred over PN. Various types of enteral access devices are available. Whereas tubes inserted through the nose often are adequate for patients expected to receive EN for a short time, more permanent devices (endoscopically or surgically placed) are preferred for longer term patients. The choice of whether to feed into the stomach or postpylorically is patient specific. Although numerous EN formulas are available commercially, many products are very similar, making a limited formulary feasible. Data supporting many of the specialized types of EN formulas are limited. Although complications of EN tend to be less serious than those of PN, the adverse effects encountered can be significant, and diligent ongoing monitoring is necessary. Although medications can be administered through feeding tubes, various factors must be taken into account in each individual patient.

Patient Care and Monitoring

1. Assess the patient's condition to estimate the amount of time he or she is expected to be unable to eat adequately to meet nutritional requirements. If inadequate intake has occurred or is anticipated for 7 to 14 days, start SNS. The threshold for starting SNS is lower for previously malnourished patients than for previously well-nourished patients. Also, critically ill patients should generally be started on EN within 24 to 48 hours of ICU admission.

2. Assess whether the GI tract is functional. If not, then PN is the SNS therapy of choice. If the GI tract is functional and no contraindication to EN exists, then EN is the SNS therapy of choice.

3. Does the patient have any condition precluding gastric feeding? If so, then postpyloric feeding should be initiated.

4. Choose the appropriate type of enteral access device based on the expected duration of SNS.

5. Choose an appropriate feeding formula based on patient-specific factors. This necessitates assessing nutritional requirements. Standard polymeric formulas are appropriate for the majority of patients.

6. Choose the method of feeding administration (e.g., intermittent or continuous) based on the type of feeding access (i.e., gastric versus postpyloric) and other patient factors. For example, in a patient with a gastric access, starting with or later transitioning to intermittent feedings may be preferred if it is anticipated that the patient still receiving these feedings will be discharged to a long-term care facility or to home.

7. Develop a plan to include monitoring at appropriate intervals for metabolic, GI, technical, and infectious complications.

8. Start the tube feeding at full strength and at a low rate and increase the rate as tolerated to the goal that will meet the patient's nutritional requirements.

9. Develop a monitoring plan for adequacy of the nutritional regimen.

10. If the patient is to be discharged to home on EN, educate the patient or caregiver on

   • Enteral access device care

   • Feeding delivery

   • Troubleshooting

   • Complications to observe for (e.g., fluid overload, dehydration)

Abbreviations Introduced in This Chapter

ALI	Acute lung injury
AI	Adequate intake
AAA	Aromatic amino acid(s)
ACCEPT	Algorithms for Critical-Care Enteral and Parenteral Therapy
ARDS	Acute respiratory distress syndrome
ASPEN	American Society for Parenteral and Enteral Nutrition
BCAA	Branched-chain amino acid(s)
BUN	Blood urea nitrogen
CRP	C-Reactive protein
DHA	Docosahexanoic acid
EAA	Essential amino acid(s)
EFA	Essential fatty acid(s)
EN	Enteral nutrition
EPA	Eicosapentaenoic acid
ESPEN	European Society for Clinical Nutrition and Metabolism
FOS	Fructooligosaccharide
GALT	Gut-associated lymphoid tissue
GI	Gastrointestinal
GLA	γ-Linolenic acid
HE	Hepatic encephalopathy
IBD	Inflammatory bowel disease
ICU	Intensive care unit
INR	International normalized ratio
LCT	Long-chain triglyceride
MALT	Mucosa-associated lymphoid tissue
MCT	Medium-chain triglyceride
MUFA	Monounsaturated fatty acid
ND	Nasoduodenal
NEAA	Nonessential amino acid
NG	Nasogastric
NJ	Nasojejunal
NO	Nitric oxide
OG	Orogastric
PEG	Percutaneous endoscopic gastrostomy
PEJ	Percutaneous endoscopic jejunostomy
PN	Parenteral nutrition
PUFA	Polyunsaturated fatty acid
RDA	Recommended Dietary Allowance
SCFA	Short-chain fatty acid
SCCM	Society for Critical Care Medicine
SNS	Specialized nutrition support

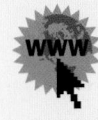

Self-assessment questions and answers are available at *http://www.mhpharmacotherapy.com/pp.html.*

REFERENCES

1. American Society for Parenteral and Enteral Nutrition Board of Directors. Guidelines for the use of parenteral and enteral nutrition in adult and pediatric patients. JPEN J Parenter Ent Nutr 2002;26(Suppl):1SA–138SA.
2. The European Society for Clinical Nutrition and Metabolism. ESPEN Guidelines on Adult Enteral Nutrition. Clin Nutr 2006;25:175–360.
3. Clinical Practice Guidelines. Critical Care Nutrition; 2009 [Internet]. Kingston, ON, Canada: Critical Evaluation Research Unit. 2009 [cited 2011 Oct 27]. Available from: http://www.criticalcarenutrition.com/index.php?option=com_content&view=article&id=18&Itemid=10.
4. Bankhead R, Boullata J, Brantley S, et al. Enteral nutrition practice recommendations. JPEN J Parenter Enter Nutr 2009;33:122–167.
5. McClave SA, Martindale RG, Vanek VW, et al. Guidelines for the provision and assessment of nutrition support therapy in the adult critically ill patient. JPEN J Parenter Ent Nutr 2009;33:277–316.
6. Magnotti LJ, Deitch EA. Mechanisms and significance of gut barrier function and failure. In: Rolandelli RH, Bankhead R, Boullata JI, Compher CW, eds. Enteral and Tube Feeding, 4th ed. Philadelphia: Elsevier, 2005:23–31.
7. Kudsk KA. Enteral feeding and bowel necrosis: An uncommon but perplexing problem. Nutr Clin Pract 2003;18:277–278.
8. McClave SA, Chang WK. Feeding the hypotensive patient: Does enteral feeding precipitate or protect against ischemic bowel? Nutr Clin Pract 2003;18:279–284.
9. Zaloga GP, Roberts PR, Marik P. Feeding the hemodynamically unstable patient: A critical evaluation of the evidence. Nutr Clin Pract 2003;18:285–293.
10. van den Berghe G, Wouters P, Weekers F, et al. Intensive insulin therapy in the critically ill patients. N Engl J Med 2001;345:1359–1367.
11. The NICE-SUGAR Study Investigators. Intensive versus conventional glucose control in critically ill patients. N Engl J Med 2009;360;1283–1297.
12. Veterans Affairs Total Parenteral Nutrition Cooperative Study Group. Perioperative total parenteral nutrition in surgical patients. N Engl J Med 1991;325:525–532.
13. Casaer MP, Mesotten D, Hermans G, et al. Early versus late parenteral nutrition in critically ill adults. N Engl J Med 2011;365:506–517.
14. Simpson F, Doig GS. Parenteral vs. enteral nutrition in the critically ill patient: A meta-analysis of trials using the intention to treat principle. Intensive Care Med 2005;31:12–23.
15. Martin CM, Doig GS, Heyland DK, et al. Multicentre, cluster-randomized clinical trial of algorithms for critical-care enteral and parenteral therapy (ACCEPT). Can Med Assoc J 2004;170:197–204.
16. Doig GS, Simpson F, Finfer S, et al. Effect of evidence-based feeding guidelines on mortality of critically ill adults: A cluster randomized controlled trial. JAMA 2008;300:2731-41.
17. Byrne KR, Fang JC. Endoscopic placement of enteral feeding catheters. Curr Opin Gastroenterol 2006;22:546–550.
18. Elia M, Engfer MB, Green CJ, Silk DBA. Systematic review and meta-analysis: The clinical and physiological effects of fibre-containing enteral formulae. Aliment Pharmacol Ther 2008;27:120–145.
19. Roy CC, Kien CL, Bouthillier L, Levy E. Short-chain fatty acids: Ready for prime time? Nutr Clin Pract 2006;21:351–366.
20. Charney P, Russell M. Enteral formulations. In: Rolandelli RH, Bankhead R, Boullata JI, Compher CW, eds. Enteral and Tube Feeding, 4th ed. Philadelphia: Elsevier, 2005:216–223.
21. Heyland DK, Dhaliwal R, Suchner U. Immunonutrition. In: Rolandelli RH, Bankhead R, Boullata JI, Compher CW, eds. Enteral and Tube Feeding, 4th ed. Philadelphia: Elsevier, 2005:224–242.
22. Heyland DK, Dhaliwal R, Day AG, et al. Reducing Deaths due to Oxidation Stress (The REDOXS Study): Rationale and study design for a randomized trial of glutamine and antioxidant supplementation in critically-ill patients. Proc Nutr Soc 2006;65:250–263.
23. Marik PE, Zaloga GP. Immunonutrition in critically ill patients: A systematic review and analysis of the literature. Intensive Care Med 2008;34:1980–1990.

24. Pontes-Arruda A, Demichele S, Seth A, Singer P. The use of an inflammation-modulating diet in patients with acute lung injury or acute respiratory distress syndrome: A meta-analysis of outcome data. JPEN J Parenter Ent Nutr 2008;32:596–605.

25. Grau-Carmona T, Moran-Garcia V, Garcia-de-Lorenzo A, et al. Effect of an enteral diet enriched with eicosapentaenoic acid, gamma-linolenic acid and anti-oxidants on the outcome of mechanically ventilated, critically ill, septic patients. Clin Nutr 2011;30(5):578–584.

26. Pontes-Arruda A, Ferreira Martins L, Maria de Lima S, et al. Enteral nutrition with eicosapentaenoic acid, γ-linolenic acid and antioxidants in the early treatment of sepsis: Results from a multicenter, prospective, randomized, double-blinded, controlled study: The INTERSEPT Study. Crit Care 2011;15(3):R144.

27. Elia M, Ceriello A, Laube H, et al. Enteral nutritional support and use of diabetes-specific formulas for patients with diabetes. Diabetes Care 2005;28:2267–2279.

28. Howell MD, Novack V, Grgurich P, et al. Iatrogenic gastric acid suppression and the risk of nosocomial *Clostridium difficile* infection. Arch Intern Med 2010;170:784–790.

29. Dial S, Delaney JA, Barkun AN, Suissa S. Use of gastric acid-suppressive agents and the risk of community-acquired *Clostridium difficile*-associated disease. JAMA 2005;294:2989–2995.

30. Jayatilaka S, Shakov R, Eddi R, et al. *Clostridium difficile* infection in an urban medical center: Five-year analysis of infection rates among adult admissions and association with the use of proton pump inhibitors. Ann Clin Lab Sci 2007;37:241–247.

31. Edes TE, Walk BE, Austin JL. Diarrhea in tube-fed patients: Feeding formula not necessarily the cause. Am J Med 1990;88:91–93.

32. McClave SA, Lukan JK, Stefater JA, et al. Poor validity of residual volumes as a marker for risk of aspiration in critically ill patients. Crit Care Med 2005;33:324–330.

33. Poulard F, Dimet J, Martin-Lefevre L, et al. Impact of not measuring residual gastric volume in mechanically ventilated patients receiving early enteral feeding: A prospective before-after study. JPEN J Parenter Ent Nutr 2010;34:125–130.

34. DeLegge MH. Managing gastric residual volumes in the critically ill patient: an update. Curr Opin Clin Nutr Metab Care 2011;14:193–196.

35. Lord LM. Restoring and maintaining patency of enteral feeding tubes. Nutr Clin Pract 2003;18:422–426.

36. Braithwaite SS. Inpatient insulin therapy. Curr Opin Endocrinol Diabetes Obes 2008;15:159–166.

37. Grainger A, Eiden K, Kemper J, Reeds D. A pilot study to evaluate the effectiveness of glargine and multiple injections of lispro in patients with type 2 diabetes receiving tube feedings in a cardiovascular intensive care unit. Nutr Clin Pract 2007;22:545–552.

38. Rollins C, Thomson C, Crane T. Pharmacotherapeutic issues. In: Rolandelli RH, Bankhead R, Boullata JI, Compher CW, eds. Enteral and Tube Feeding, 4th ed. Philadelphia: Elsevier, 2005:291–305.

39. Mitchell JF. Oral Dosage Forms That Should Not Be Crushed [Internet]. Horsham (PA): Institute for Safe Medication Practices; 2011. [1 Oct 2011; cited 27 Oct 2011]. Available from: http://www.ismp.org/tools/donotcrush.pdf.

40. Dickerson RN, Garmon WM, Kuhl DA, et al. Vitamin K-independent warfarin resistance after concurrent administration of warfarin and continuous enteral nutrition. Pharmacotherapy 2008;28:308–313.

41. Rollins CJ. Drug-nutrient interactions. In: Gottschlich MM, ed. The A.S.P.E.N. Nutrition Support Core Curriculum. Silver Spring, MD: A.S.P.E.N., 2007:340–359.

42. Nyffeler MS, Frankel E, Hayes E, Mighdoll S. Drug-nutrient interactions. In: Merritt R, ed. The A.S.P.E.N. Nutrition Support Practice Manual, 2nd ed. Silver Spring, MD: A.S.P.E.N., 2005:118–137.

102

Overweight and Obesity

Maqual R. Graham and Cameron C. Lindsey

● **Upon completion of the chapter, the reader will be able to:**

1. Explain the underlying causes of overweight and obesity.

2. Identify parameters used to diagnose obesity and other objective information that indicates the severity of disease.

3. Identify desired therapeutic goals for patients who are overweight or obese.

4. Recommend appropriate nonpharmacologic and pharmacologic therapeutic interventions for overweight or obese patients.

5. Implement a monitoring plan that will assess both the efficacy and safety of therapy initiated.

6. Educate patients about the disease state and associated risks, appropriate lifestyle modifications, drug therapy, and surgical options necessary for effective treatment.

KEY CONCEPTS

❶ Body mass index (BMI), waist circumference, comorbidities, and readiness to lose weight are used in the assessment of overweight or obese patients.

❷ The presence of comorbidities (coronary heart disease [CHD], atherosclerosis, type 2 diabetes mellitus, and sleep apnea) and cardiovascular risk factors (cigarette smoking, hypertension, elevated low-density lipoprotein cholesterol, low high-density lipoprotein cholesterol, impaired fasting glucose, family history of premature CHD, and age) requires identification and aggressive management for overall effective treatment of the overweight or obese patient.

❸ The treatment goals for overweight and obesity are to prevent additional weight gain, reduce and maintain a lower body weight, and control related risks.

❹ Weight loss is indicated for patients with a BMI of 25 to 29.9 kg/m^2 or a high-risk waist circumference with two or more comorbidities or for any patient with a BMI of 30 kg/m^2 or greater.

❺ Weight maintenance occurs after successful achievement of weight loss.

❻ Treatment of obesity includes lifestyle changes (e.g., dietary modification, enhanced physical activity, and behavioral therapy), pharmacologic treatment, surgical intervention, or a combination of modalities.

❼ Pharmacotherapy, in addition to lifestyle modifications, is reserved for patients with a BMI of 30 kg/m^2 or greater or a BMI of 27 kg/m^2 or greater with other obesity-related risk factors.

❽ Weight likely will be regained if lifestyle changes are not continued indefinitely.

❾ Surgery is warranted when other treatment attempts have failed in severely obese patients (BMI of 40 kg/m^2 or greater, or 35 kg/m^2 or greater with other obesity-related risk factors).

Overweight and obesity are terms used to describe weight measurements greater than what is considered healthy for a given height.[1] ❶ *Body mass index (BMI), waist circumference, comorbidities, and readiness to lose weight are used in the assessment of overweight or obese patients.* The primary modality in defining overweight and obesity is the BMI, a measure of body fat based on height and weight that applies to both adult men and women. BMI does not reflect distribution of body fat; therefore, the measurement of **waist circumference** is a more practical method to evaluate abdominal fat before and during weight loss treatment. Abdominal fat poses a greater health risk over peripheral fat and may be an independent risk predictor when BMI is not elevated significantly.[2,3] Both BMI and waist circumference should be used in the diagnosis and management of weight loss. Evaluation of the patient's risk status involves not only calculation of the BMI and measurement of waist circumference but also determination of comorbidities or the presence of cardiovascular disease (CVD) risk factors. ❷ *The presence of comorbidities (coronary heart disease [CHD], atherosclerosis, type 2 diabetes mellitus, and sleep apnea) and cardiovascular risk factors (cigarette smoking, hypertension, elevated low-density lipoprotein cholesterol, low high-density lipoprotein cholesterol, impaired fasting glucose, family history of premature CHD, and age) requires identification and aggressive management for overall effective treatment of the overweight or obese patient.* Obese patients may be at very high risk for mortality if concomitant risk factors exist; therefore, high-risk patients require aggressive modification of risk factors in addition to obesity treatment.[4]

ETIOLOGY AND EPIDEMIOLOGY

Obesity is a multifactorial, complex disease that occurs because of an interaction between genotype and the environment. Although the etiology is not known completely, it involves overlapping silos of social, behavioral, and cultural influence; pathophysiology; metabolism; and genetic composition.[5] The majority of overweight or obese individuals are adults, but these diseases are also prevalent in children between 2 and 19 years of age. Approximately 34% of adults 20 years of age and older are considered obese. Almost 6% meet the criteria for extreme obesity. The prevalence of obesity in men and women of various racial and ethnic origins differ. Thirty-three percent of non-Hispanic white adults are considered obese, where approximately 39% of Mexican Americans and 44% of non-Hispanic black Americans are obese.[6]

Among children and adolescents, 17% are obese where 32% are considered overweight.[7] Overweight children typically mature to overweight adults, but most obese adults were not overweight as children.[8] Overweight and obesity, when present in young adults, may be a better predictor of prevalence.[8] Additionally, adulthood overweight and obesity contribute to an increased risk of death in the presence of hypertension, hyperlipidemia, diabetes mellitus, coronary artery disease (CAD), stroke, sleep apnea, gallbladder disease, osteoarthritis, and certain cancers.[4] Psychosocial functioning also may be hindered because obese patients may be at risk for discrimination if negatively stereotyped.[4] Pediatric obesity is also associated with significant health-related problems and thus is a risk factor for much of the adult morbidity and mortality discussed previously.[9,10] Cardiovascular (e.g., dyslipidemia and hypertension), endocrine (e.g., hyperinsulinemia, impaired glucose tolerance, type 2 diabetes mellitus, and menstrual irregularities), and mental (e.g., low self-esteem and depression) health problems exist for obese children and adolescents.[11]

PATHOPHYSIOLOGY

Although a correlation between body weight in parents and children exists, the specific gene or genes contributing to obesity are unknown.[12] Syndromes in which obesity is a major

component collectively contribute very little to the incidence of obesity.[13] The key factor in the development of overweight and obesity is the imbalance that occurs between energy intake and energy expenditure. The extent of obesity is determined by the length of time this imbalance has been present. Energy intake is affected by environmental influences, including social, behavioral, and cultural factors, whereas genetic composition and metabolism affect energy expenditure.[14]

Energy Intake

Food intake is regulated by various receptor systems. Direct stimulation of serotonin 1A subtype (5-HT$_{1A}$) and noradrenergic α_2-receptors increases food intake, serotonin 2C subtype (5-HT$_{2C}$) and noradrenergic α_1- or β_2-receptor activation decreases food intake. Stimulation of histamine receptor subtypes 1 and 3 and dopamine receptors 1 and 2 results in lower food consumption. Recently, the cannabinoid receptor (CB1), which is a G protein–coupled receptor in the endocannabinoid system, has been identified and associated with food intake and regulation of energy homeostasis.[15,16] Inhibition of CB1 is shown to decrease the craving for food, resulting in weight loss when coupled with dietary and lifestyle modifications.[17] In addition to receptor-modulated food consumption, higher levels of the protein leptin are associated with decreased food intake.[18] In contrast, elevated levels of neuropeptide Y increase food intake.[18]

It is debatable whether obesity is related to total calorie intake or composition of macronutrients. Of the three macronutrients (i.e., carbohydrate, protein, and fat), fat has received the most attention, given its desirable texture and its ability to augment the flavor of other foods. Food high in fat promotes weight gain, in comparison with the other macronutrients, because fat is more energy dense. When compared with carbohydrate and protein, more than twice as many calories per gram are contained in fat. In addition, fat is stored more easily by the body compared with protein and carbohydrate.[19]

Energy Expenditure

A person's metabolic rate is the primary determinant of energy expenditure. The metabolic rate is enhanced after food consumption and is directly related to the amount and type.[13] Physical inactivity may predispose an individual to overweight and obesity. In addition, endocrine-related disorders (e.g., hypothyroidism and Cushing's syndrome) may lower the metabolic rate, further contributing to the development of overweight and obesity.

CLINICAL PRESENTATION AND DIAGNOSIS

Any interaction between a patient and a healthcare provider presents an opportunity to evaluate the patient's height and weight. From these parameters, the BMI should be determined as well as waist circumference and the presence of comorbidities or associated risks. ❶ *BMI, waist circumference, comorbidities, and readiness to lose weight are used in the*

Table 102–1

BMI Classification

Adult

Underweight	Less than 18.5 kg/m^2
Normal weight	18.5–24.9 kg/m^2
Overweight	25–29.9 kg/m^2
Obesity (class 1)	30–34.9 kg/m^2
Obesity (class 2)	35–39.9 kg/m^2
Extreme obesity (class 3)	Greater than or equal to 40 kg/m^2

Children (Does Not Pertain to Those Less Than 2 Years of Age[a])

Underweight	Less than 5th percentile
Healthy weight	5th–84th percentiles
Overweight	85th–94th percentiles
Obesity	Greater than or equal to the 95th percentile

[a]Weight for height values should be plotted and monitored over time for children younger than 2 years of age.

From Refs. 4 and 19.

---

assessment of overweight or obese patients. The BMI is calculated using the measured weight in kilograms divided by the height in meters squared (kg/m^2) for all adult patients regardless of gender. The BMI distribution changes with age for children just as height and weight. Percentiles specific for age and gender are used to classify pediatric patients as overweight and obese as well as healthy and underweight. The BMI is classified according to Table 102–1. Waist circumference should also be determined for adult patients by placing a measuring tape at the top of the right iliac crest and proceeding around the abdomen, ensuring that the tape is tight but not constricting the skin. The value is measured after normal expiration.[4] Table 102–2 defines high-risk waist circumference.[4] Measurement of waist circumference is not recommended for children and adolescents because reference values identifying risk are unavailable.[20] After obtaining patient appropriate parameters, further assess the adult patient for the presence of comorbidities and cardiovascular risk factors. ❷ *The presence of comorbidities (CHD, atherosclerosis, type 2 diabetes mellitus, and sleep apnea) and cardiovascular risk factors (cigarette smoking, hypertension, elevated low-density lipoprotein cholesterol, low high-density lipoprotein cholesterol, impaired fasting glucose, family history*

Table 102–2

High-Risk Waist Circumference

Adult

Men	Greater than 40 in (102 cm)
Women	Greater than 35 in (89 cm)

From U.S. Department of Health and Human Services, NIH-NHLBI. Clinical guidelines on the identification, evaluation and treatment of overweight and obesity in adults. NIH publication no. 00-4084. Bethesda, MD: National Institutes of Health, 2000.

Table 102–3

Risk Factors

- Cigarette smoking
- Hypertension (systolic blood pressure greater than or equal to 140 mm Hg or diastolic blood pressure greater than or equal to 90 mm Hg) or current use of blood pressure–lowering medication(s)
- LDL cholesterol greater than or equal to 160 mg/dL (4.14 mmol/L)
- LDL cholesterol greater than or equal to 130–159 mg/dL (3.36–4.11 mmol/L) plus two additional risk factors
- HDL cholesterol less than 40 mg/dL (1.03 mmol/L)
- Impaired fasting glucose (fasting blood glucose, 100–125 mg/dL [5.6–6.9 mmol/L])
- Family history of premature CHD (first-degree male relative less than 55 years of age or first-degree female relative less than 65 years of age)
- Men 45 years or older
- Women 55 years or older

CHD, coronary heart disease; HDL, high-density lipoprotein; LDL, low-density lipoprotein

From U.S. Department of Health and Human Services, NIH-NHLBI. Clinical guidelines on the identification, evaluation and treatment of overweight and obesity in adults. NIH publication no. 00-4084. Bethesda, MD: National Institutes of Health, 2000.

---

of premature CHD, and age) requires identification and aggressive management for overall effective treatment of the overweight or obese patient. A patient is at very high absolute risk if diagnosed with CHD or other atherosclerotic diseases, type 2 diabetes mellitus, or sleep apnea or if three or more of the risk factors listed in Table 102–3 are present.[4] Aggressive disease management should be initiated and not limited to weight loss. If the patient is a child or adolescent and the BMI is greater than the 85th percentile, determine the patient's risk for future obesity-related problems or presence of obesity-related medical problems such as sleep, respiratory, gastrointestinal (GI), endocrine, cardiovascular, and psychiatric disorders.[20,21]

TREATMENT

Desired Outcome

General management of obesity in adult patients is directed at weight reduction, maintenance of weight loss, and prevention of weight regain. ❸ *The treatment goals for overweight and obesity are to prevent additional weight gain, reduce and maintain a lower body weight, and control related risks.* A 10% weight loss as derived from the patient's current weight is the initial goal of obesity management because favorable outcomes on the negative effects of obesity have been documented.[4,22] Weight loss should occur at a rate of 0.45 to 0.9 kg (1–2 lb) per week, meeting the initial goal within the first 6 months of therapy. Overweight patients should lose weight at a rate of 0.23 kg (0.5 lb) per week. ❹ *Weight loss is indicated for patients with a BMI of 25 to 29.9 kg/m^2 or an elevated waist circumference with two or more comorbidities or for any patient with a BMI of 30 kg/m^2 or greater.* Weight then

Patient Encounter 1, Part 1

A 45-year-old woman presents to your clinic wanting to lose weight. She reports not currently following any specific diet but has enrolled at Slim-4-Life in the past, which resulted in significant weight loss. However, the products used in the program are expensive, and thus she prefers to lose weight the "old fashion way." She admits to eating foods high in sugar content such as sweetened beverages and candy bars, as well as foods that contain large amounts of starch (potatoes, bread, and chips). This patient is not currently exercising but has adhered to a daily walking regimen in the past. The patient does not smoke but consumes alcohol, 1 to 2 glasses of wine on the weekend. Her BMI is 30.8 kg/m², and her waist circumference is 42 in (107 cm).

What classification of overweight and obesity is appropriate for this patient?

Does this patient have a high-risk waist circumference?

Does she have other risk factors that may contribute to morbidity or mortality?

What are the treatment goals for the patient?

What additional information do you need to know before creating a treatment plan for this patient?

should be maintained (minimal regain of less than 3 kg [6.6 lb] and reduction in waist circumference of 1.6 in [4 cm]) sustained. If weight loss has been achieved and/or maintained for 6 months, therapy promoting further weight loss may be considered. When maximal weight loss has been attained, any therapy used to promote the weight loss must be continued in order to prevent weight regain.[4] **5** *Weight maintenance occurs after successful achievement of weight loss.*

It is desirable to achieve a goal of improved long-term physical health for a child or adolescent. A BMI below the 85th percentile is warranted but is difficult to assess in frequent or short time periods. Thus, serial weight measurements may better quantify energy balance. Goals are most likely accomplished through adaptation of lifelong healthy lifestyle habits. In doing so, weight loss or maintenance can be attained for some children. Others may need to incorporate changes that result in a negative energy balance or energy input less than energy output.[20,21]

General Approach to Treatment

Because the goals for obesity management in the adult population are multifactorial, it should be considered a chronic illness in which treatment is maintained for life. Any implemented therapy promoting weight loss should focus on behavior modification directed toward both dietary restriction and increased activity in conjunction with the selective use of pharmacologic or surgical intervention. Before initiating therapy, secondary causes of obesity

(e.g., hypothyroidism and Cushing's syndrome) must be considered. Current treatment with medications that negatively alter weight should be determined and if present, alternative therapies should be suggested.[23-25] Table 102–4 provides a list of drugs commonly associated with weight gain. If no secondary cause exists, the presence of other cardiovascular risk factors and comorbidities must be determined to guide clinical decisions. **2** *The presence of comorbidities (CHD, atherosclerosis, type 2 diabetes mellitus, and sleep apnea) and cardiovascular risk factors (cigarette smoking, hypertension, elevated low-density lipoprotein cholesterol, low high-density lipoprotein cholesterol, impaired fasting glucose, family history of premature CHD, and age) requires identification and aggressive management for overall effective treatment of the overweight or obese patient.* Therapy implemented to minimize associated risk(s) may not enhance weight loss, but weight loss will positively address risk factors. Weight loss should not be initiated in pregnant or lactating patients, decompensated psychiatric patients, or patients in whom reduced caloric intake can exacerbate an acute, serious illness.[4] **6** *Treatment of obesity includes lifestyle changes (dietary modification, enhanced physical activity, and behavioral therapy), pharmacologic treatment, surgical intervention, or a combination of modalities.*

Four stages have been suggested for the treatment of obesity in children and adolescents. Stage 1 or Prevention Plus is the first step for overweight or obese patients and includes adherence to healthy eating and activity habits. Patients should be encouraged to eat more than or equal to five servings of fruits and vegetables daily, limit consumption of sweetened drinks, decrease television or other screen time behaviors, and increase physical activity to greater than or

Table 102–4
Drugs Contributing to Weight Gain

Anticonvulsants and mood stabilizers
  Carbamazepine
  Gabapentin
  Valproic acid
  Lithium
Antidepressants
  Monoamine oxidase inhibitors (phenelzine)
  Presynaptic α-2 antagonist (mirtazapine)
  Selective serotonin reuptake inhibitors
  Tricyclics (amitriptyline, imipramine, nortriptyline)
Antidiabetics
  Insulin
  Meglintinides
  Sulfonylureas (glyburide, glipizide)
  Thiazolidinediones
Antipsychotics
  Atypical (clozapine, olanzapine, risperidone, paliperidone, quetiapine)
Others
  Antihistamines
  Corticosteroids
  Hormonal Contraceptives (depot injections)

From Refs. 23 to 25.

equal to 1 h/day. Stage 2 or Structured Weight Management incorporates Prevention Plus habits while setting specific eating and activity goals. Responsibilities include meal planning, observed physical activity or play daily for 1 hour, and documentation of energy consumption and expenditure.

- Comprehensive Multidisciplinary Interventions (stage 3) is directed at increasing the intensity of healthy behaviors. To accomplish goals, the child or adolescent should work closely with the primary care provider, registered dietician, exercise specialist, and behavioral counselor. Stage 4, Tertiary Care Intervention, may be needed for severely obese adolescents. A very low-calorie diet (LCD), medication or weight control surgery may be warranted.[26,27]

Nonpharmacologic Therapy

▶ *Dietary*

- An LCD is essential for weight-loss management in overweight and obese patients. The Step-1 Diet (Table 102–5) is an LCD recommended as part of an obesity education initiative from the National Heart, Lung, and Blood Institute.[4] In general, the Step-1 Diet restricts daily calories to a range of 1,000 to 1,200

kcal (4,186–5,023 kJ/day) for women weighing less than 75 kg (165 lb) and 1,400 to 1,600 kcal (5,860–6,697 kJ/day) for all others. However, this daily limit should be considered after assessing a patient's normal daily caloric intake and ensuring that the initial caloric restriction does not exceed 500 to 1,000 kcal (2,093–4,186 kJ/day). For example, a male patient who consumes 3,000 kcal (12,557 kJ/day) should not reduce his daily caloric intake to less than 2,000 kcal (8,372 kJ/day) when initially implementing a dietary program. Further reduction to the target of 1,600 kcal (6,697 kJ/day) can be attempted when the patient has reduced calories successfully as initially recommended for a period agreeable by the provider and the patient.[4] Diets that are too restrictive in calorie reduction are successful initially but fail in the long term because compliance is difficult to sustain.[26] Therefore, this less aggressive approach promotes gradual weight loss and weight maintenance.

Dietary consumption should be balanced in carbohydrates, protein, and fat. Several diet plans exist that promote weight loss through strict limitation or overabundance of only one macronutrient (e.g., low-fat, low-carbohydrate, or high-protein diets); however, overall energy consumption and expenditure will determine the amount of weight alteration. Consultation

Table 102–5

Low-Calorie Step I Diet

Nutrient	Recommended Intake
Calories[a]	~500–1,000 kcal/day (2,093–4,186 kJ/day) reduction from usual intake
Total fat[b]	30% or less of total calories
Saturated fatty acids[c]	8–10% of total calories
Monounsaturated fatty acids	Up to 15% of total calories
Polyunsaturated fatty acids	Up to 10% of total calories
Cholesterol[c]	Less than 300 mg/day
Protein[d]	~15% of total calories
Carbohydrate[e]	55% or more of total calories
Sodium chloride	No more than 100 mmol/day (~2.4 g of sodium or ~6 g of sodium chloride)
Calcium[f]	1,000–1,500 mg/day
Fiber[e]	20–30 g/day

[a]A reduction in calories of 500–1,000 kcal/day (2,093–4,186 kJ/day) will help achieve a weight loss of 1–2 lb/wk (~0.5–0.9 kg/wk). Alcohol provides unneeded calories and displaces more nutritious foods. Alcohol consumption not only increases the number of calories in a diet but also has been associated with obesity in epidemiologic studies as well as in experimental studies. The impact of alcohol calories on a person's overall caloric intake needs to be assessed and appropriately controlled.

[b]Fat-modified foods may provide a helpful strategy for lowering total fat intake but will only be effective if they are also low in calories and if there is no compensation by calories from other foods.

[c]Patients with high blood cholesterol levels may need to use the Step II diet to achieve further reductions in LDL cholesterol levels; in the Step II diet, saturated fats are reduced to less than 7% of total calories, and cholesterol levels to less than 200 mg/day. All of the other nutrients are the same as in Step I.

[d]Proteins should be derived from plant sources and lean sources of animal protein.

[e]Complex carbohydrates from different vegetables, fruits, and whole grains are good sources of vitamins, minerals, and fiber. A diet rich in soluble fiber, including oat bran, legumes, barley, and most fruits and vegetables, may be effective in reducing blood cholesterol levels.[5] A diet high in all types of fiber may also aid in weight management by promoting satiety at lower levels of calorie and fat intake. Some authorities recommend 20–30 g of fiber daily with an upper limit of 35 g.

[f]During weight loss, attention should be given to maintaining an adequate intake of vitamins and minerals. Maintenance of the recommended calcium intake of 1,000–1,500 mg/day is especially important for women who may be at risk for osteoporosis.

From U.S. Department of Health and Human Services, NIH-NHLBI. Clinical guidelines on the identification, evaluation and treatment of overweight and obesity in adults. NIH publication no. 00-4084. Bethesda, MD: National Institutes of Health, 2000.

with a dietician is recommended when implementing a healthy meal plan tailored to the individual's nutritional needs.

▶ Exercise

Although diet and exercise contribute to weight loss, combining an LCD with physical activity results in greater weight loss compared with either therapy alone.[22] In addition, physical activity can help to prevent weight regain and reduce related cardiovascular risks.[4] Slow titration of both the amount and intensity of physical activity is recommended for most overweight and obese patients.[4] A program that incorporates daily walking is a viable option for most patients (Table 102–6). Consider 10 min/day 3 days/week with a target of 30 to 45 minutes most days, if not every day.[4] This type and amount of activity equate to a 100 to 200 kcal (419–837 kJ/day) caloric expenditure.[4]

▶ Behavioral

Nonadherence with recommended lifestyle changes may result in unsuccessful weight loss for adults.[4,22] Therefore, eliminating these barriers through behavior modification is necessary to gain maximal benefit from both dietary modification and exercise. Components of successful behavioral modification include, but are not limited to, the following steps:[4]

- Determine the patient's readiness to lose weight and willingness to implement a weight-loss plan.
- Build and nurture the patient–provider partnership.
- Restructure cognitive abilities.
- Set achievable goals.
- Contact the patient frequently.
- Instruct the patient on the importance and technique of self-monitoring.

- Control stimuli that negatively affect weight loss or weight maintenance.
- Reward the patient for any amount of weight loss or avoidance of weight regain.

Targeted behaviors should be recommended to pediatric patients and their families because healthy habits help prevent excessive weight gain. These include, but are not limited to:[20,21]

- Limit the consumption of sugar-sweetened beverages.
- Meet daily fruit and vegetable requirements set forth by the U.S. Department of Agriculture.
- Limit the amount of time watching television to 2 hours or less. Other screen time activities, such as computer play, should also be limited.
- Consume a healthy breakfast daily.
- Limit the number of times the family eats at restaurants, especially those that serve fast food.
- Parents should eat dinner with their children and limit portion size when preparing and serving meals.

Pharmacologic Therapy

Pharmacotherapy is not recommended for individuals with BMIs of less than 27 kg/m². If lifestyle changes do not result in a 10% weight loss after 6 months, drug therapy in addition to a healthy lifestyle is warranted for overweight individuals with other related risks and for obese patients. ❼ *Pharmacotherapy in addition to lifestyle modification is reserved for patients with a BMI of 30 kg/m² or greater, or a BMI of 27 kg/m² or greater with other obesity-related risk factors.* Pharmacologic products promoting weight loss are classified according to their mechanisms of action,

Table 102–6

Examples of Moderate Physical Activity

Common Chores[a,b]	Sporting Activities[a,b]
Washing and waxing a car for 45–60 minutes	Playing volleyball for 45–60 minutes
Washing windows or floors for 45–60 minutes	Playing touch football for 45 minutes
Gardening for 30–45 minutes	Walking 1¾ miles in 35 minutes (20 min/mile [~12 min/km])
Wheeling self in wheelchair for 30–40 minutes	Basketball (shooting baskets) for 30 minutes
Pushing a stroller 1½ miles (2.4 km) in 30 minutes	Bicycling 5 miles (8 km) in 30 minutes
Raking leaves for 30 minutes	Dancing fast (social) for 30 minutes
Walking 2 miles in 30 minutes (15 min/mile [9.3 min/km])	Water aerobics for 30 minutes
Shoveling snow for 15 minutes	Swimming laps for 20 minutes
Stair walking for 15 minutes	Basketball (playing a game) for 15–20 minutes
	Jumping rope for 15 minutes
	Running 1½ miles (2.4 km) in 15 minutes (15 min/mile)

[a]A moderate amount of physical activity is roughly equivalent to physical activity that uses approximately 150 calories of energy/day (628 J/day) or 1,000 calories/week (4186 J/week).

[b]Some activities can be performed at various intensities; the suggested durations correspond to expected intensity of effort.

From U.S. Department of Health and Human Services, NIH-NHLBI. Clinical guidelines on the identification, evaluation and treatment of overweight and obesity in adults. NIH publication no. 00-4084. Bethesda, MD: National Institutes of Health, 2000.

Table 102–7			
Summary of Approved Pharmacologic Weight Loss Agents			
Drug	Class	Daily Dose (mg)	Duration of Therapy
Orlistat	Lipase inhibitor	360	More than 3 months[a]
Phentermine	Noradrenergic agent	15–37.5	Up to 6 months
Diethylpropion	Noradrenergic agent	75	Up to 12 months

[a]Efficacy and safety have not been determined beyond 4 years of use.

From U.S. Department of Health and Human Services, NIH-NHLBI. Clinical guidelines on the identification, evaluation and treatment of overweight and obesity in adults. NIH publication no. 00–4084. Bethesda, MD: National Institutes of Health, 2000.

including the suppression of appetite and the suppression of fat absorption (Table 102–7). Pharmacotherapy was indicated previously for short-term use; however, because obesity-related risks resurface with weight regain, long-term treatment is recommended to minimize these sequelae. ❽ *Weight likely will be regained if lifestyle changes are not continued indefinitely.* Prolonged use of both fenfluramine and dexfenfluramine monotherapy and fenfluramine and phentermine in combination resulted in cardiac valvular disease.[27] Long-term treatment with sibutramine resulted in an increased risk for nonfatal heart attacks and nonfatal strokes in patients with preexisting cardiovascular disease.[28] Therefore, orlistat is the only drug currently approved for long-term use in promoting weight loss and preventing weight regain.

▶ *Orlistat*

Orlistat promotes and maintains weight loss by acting locally in the GI tract. Orlistat is a chemically synthesized derivative of lipstatin, a natural product of *Streptomyces toxytricini* that inhibits pancreatic and gastric lipases, as well as triglyceride hydrolysis. As a result, undigested triglycerides are not absorbed, causing a caloric deficit and weight loss.[29]

Several studies have reported significant weight loss for patients receiving orlistat 120 mg three times a day compared with placebo.[30,31] Weight maintenance or prevention of weight regain also has been documented with continued orlistat use.[30,32] After 1 year of treatment, 57% of orlistat-treated patients lost at least 5% of their baseline weight.[29] The long-term weight-loss effect on one obesity-related comorbidity was assessed in a large placebo-controlled study. In 3,000 obese patients, 21% had impaired glucose tolerance at enrollment. After 4 years, weight loss was greater and the incidence of new diabetes was lower in patients receiving orlistat.[33]

One study evaluated the longer term effect of orlistat in adolescents. In a group of 12- to 16-year-old individuals, orlistat (120 mg three times daily) in combination with diet, exercise, and behavior modification resulted in a significant reduction in BMI and waist circumference compared with placebo. In addition, orlistat-treated subjects exhibited minimal weight increase after 1 year (0.53 kg) compared with placebo-treated patients (3.14 kg). Common adverse reactions observed were fatty or oily stools, oily spotting, oily evacuation, or abdominal pain and/or flatulence with bowel movements. Soft stools, nausea, increased defecation, and fecal incontinence also were noted.[34]

The safety and efficacy of orlistat have not been determined beyond 4 years of use. Minimal systemic effects exist because orlistat acts locally in the GI tract. Thus, common side effects reported include oily spotting, flatus with discharge, fecal urgency, fatty or oily stools, oily evacuation, increased defecation, and fecal incontinence.[29] Other adverse events include bloating, abdominal pain, dyspepsia, nausea, vomiting, diarrhea, and headache.[35] Thirty-two reports of severe liver injury have been reported to the Food and Drug Administration (FDA), including six cases of liver failure.[36] After a complete review by the FDA, 13 reports of severe liver injury were identified. Of the 13 cases, only 1 occurred within the United States. Although a cause-and-effect relationship has not been established, the FDA has added serious liver injury information to orlistat's product label that includes signs, symptoms, and when to seek medical attention for severe liver disease. Signs and symptoms include itching, yellowing of the eyes or skin, dark urine, decreased appetite and light-colored stools. Orlistat should be stopped if the patient complains of these signs and symptoms. In addition, liver function tests, including aspartate transaminase (AST) and alanine aminotransferase (ALT), should be assessed.[37]

Orlistat reduces the absorption of some fat-soluble vitamins and β-carotene. Daily intake of a multivitamin containing fat-soluble vitamins, as well as β-carotene, is recommended. Patients should take the multivitamin 2 hours before or after the dose of orlistat.[29] Because the availability of vitamin K may decline in patients receiving orlistat therapy, close monitoring of coagulation status should occur with concomitant administration of warfarin.[29] Hypothyroidism has been observed in patients taking both orlistat and levothyroxine. Patients taking both medications should separate the drug doses by 4 hours (administer levothyroxine 4 hours before or after the orlistat dose). These patients should also be monitored for changes in thyroid function. Administration of orlistat in conjunction with cyclosporine can result in decreased cyclosporine plasma levels. To avoid this interaction, cyclosporine should be taken 2 hours before or after the dose of orlistat. Additionally, cyclosporine levels should be monitored more frequently.[29]

Pregnant or lactating women should not take orlistat because no data exist to establish safety. Orlistat is contraindicated in patients with chronic malabsorption syndrome or cholestasis.[29]

Initiate orlistat 120 mg three times a day with a well-balanced but reduced-caloric meal containing no more than 30% of calories from fat. Orlistat may be taken during or up to 1 hour after the meal. If a meal is missed or contains little fat, the dose of orlistat may be omitted. Doses above 360 mg/day provide no greater benefit and thus are not recommended.[29]

▶ Sibutramine

Sibutramine and its two active metabolites (M_1 and M_2) induce weight loss by inhibiting the reuptake of serotonin, norepinephrine, and dopamine.[38] Appetite becomes suppressed because patients feel a sense of satiety.

The Sibutramine Cardiovascular Outcomes (SCOUT) trial was designed to evaluate the long-term, cardiovascular event rate, including death, in patients with preexisting cardiovascular disease, type 2 diabetes mellitus or both. An increased risk for nonfatal myocardial infarction (MI) and nonfatal stroke was observed for sibutramine-treated patients.[28] Results from the study prompted the FDA to ask Abbott Laboratories to withdraw sibutramine from the U.S. market.[39]

▶ Phentermine

Phentermine decreases food intake, and hence weight, by increasing norepinephrine and dopamine release in the central nervous system (CNS). This drug is indicated for short-term use—no more than a few weeks—in addition to lifestyle modifications in obese patients with a BMI of 30 kg/m² or greater, or a BMI of 27 kg/m² or greater in the presence of other risk factors.[40]

A recent meta-analysis evaluated patients at doses of 15 and 30 mg/day. Patients were analyzed for periods of 2 to 24 weeks. The majority of patients enrolled were female, and more than 80% of the patients evaluated received adjunctive modification in lifestyle. An average weight loss of 3.6 kg (7.9 lb) was demonstrated for patients treated with phentermine compared with placebo. Although modest in amount, this value was statistically significant.[35]

Safety and efficacy have not been determined in pediatric patients less than 16 years of age.[40]

Common adverse reactions seen with phentermine use include heart palpitations, tachycardia, elevated blood pressure, stimulation, restlessness, dizziness, insomnia, euphoria, dysphoria, tremor, headache, dry mouth, constipation, and diarrhea. Phentermine should be avoided in patients with unstable cardiac status, hypertension, hyperthyroidism, agitated states, or glaucoma. In combination with fenfluramine or dexfenfluramine, primary pulmonary hypertension and valvular heart disease have been reported. The risk of developing either serious adverse effect cannot be ruled out with use of phentermine alone. Because phentermine is related to the amphetamines, the potential for abuse is high; thus, this should be kept in mind when selecting this agent as an aid for weight loss.[40]

Phentermine use should be avoided in patients concomitantly receiving or having received a monoamine oxidase inhibitor (MAOI) within the preceding 14 days. Combination therapy with any stimulant or MAOI has the potential for causing hypertensive crisis. Alcohol is not recommended for patients prescribed phentermine.[40]

Because no studies have been conducted in pregnant women, phentermine should be administered only when clearly indicated. Owing to the potential for severe adverse effects in nursing infants, a decision to stop the drug or discontinue nursing must be made.[40]

Phentermine is available as an immediate- and a sustained-release product. In conjunction with a healthy lifestyle, 30 to 37.5 mg of phentermine is administered once daily, typically before breakfast or 1 to 2 hours after the morning meal. The dosage should be individualized; some patients may be managed adequately at 15 to 18.75 mg/day, but a dose of 18.75 mg twice daily may be used to minimize side effects, excluding insomnia. To lessen the risk of insomnia, dosing phentermine in the evening should be avoided. Timed-release preparations of phentermine are not recommended because phentermine's half-life is approximately 20 hours.[41]

▶ Diethylpropion

This sympathomimetic amine exudes similar pharmacologic activity as the amphetamines, resulting in CNS stimulation and appetite suppression. This drug is indicated for short-term use in conjunction with a reduced-calorie diet and exercise in obese patients with BMIs of 30 kg/m² or greater after failed attempts of diet and exercise alone.[42]

One meta-analysis reviewed patients receiving doses of 75 mg/day during periods of 6 to 52 weeks. Similar to study characteristics for phentermine, the majority of patients enrolled were female, and all patients implemented adjunctive lifestyle modifications. The average additional weight loss observed was 3 kg (6.6 lb) compared with diet and exercise alone, resulting in a borderline statistically significant difference.[35]

The safety and effectiveness of diethylpropion have not been established in patients under the age of 16; therefore, its use is not recommended.[42]

Use of diethylpropion for a period longer than 3 months is associated with an increased risk for development of pulmonary hypertension. When used as directed, reported common CNS adverse effects included overstimulation, restlessness, dizziness, insomnia, euphoria, dysphoria, tremor, headache, jitteriness, anxiety, nervousness, depression, drowsiness, malaise, mydriasis, and blurred vision. In addition, diethylpropion can decrease the seizure threshold, subsequently increasing a patient's risk for an epileptic event. Other organ systems also can adversely be affected, resulting in tachycardia, elevated blood pressure, palpitations, dry mouth, abdominal discomfort, constipation, diarrhea, nausea, vomiting, impotence or change in libido, gynecomastia, bone marrow suppression, agranulocytosis, and leukopenia. Diethylpropion is contraindicated in patients with pulmonary hypertension, advanced arteriosclerosis, severe hypertension, hyperthyroidism, agitated states, or glaucoma. Because diethylpropion is related to the amphetamines, the potential for abuse is high; therefore, its use is contraindicated in patients with a history of substance abuse.[42]

As with phentermine, use of diethylpropion should be avoided in patients concomitantly receiving or having received an MAOI within the preceding 14 days to prevent hypertensive crisis. Combination with other anorectic agents should be avoided.[42]

No adequate studies have been conducted using diethylpropion in pregnant women; therefore, the drug should be used only if the benefit outweighs potential fetal risk. Use with caution in nursing mothers because the drug is excreted in breast milk.[42]

Diethylpropion is available as both an immediate- and a controlled-release product. In conjunction with a reduced-calorie diet and/or exercise, dose diethylpropion (immediate release) 25 mg three times a day before meals or 75 mg (controlled release) once a day, usually midmorning.[42]

▶ Other Pharmacologic Therapy

Rimonabant diminishes food cravings by selectively inhibiting the cannabinoid (CB1) receptor.[16,19] Taranabant is another drug with a mechanism of action similar to rimonabant. Unfortunately, the increased neuropsychiatric risk (suicide) demonstrated during clinical trials halted the anticipated use of the CB1 receptor antagonists.[46,47]

Noradrenergic agents not approved by the FDA and subsequently not recommended for weight loss include amphetamine salts (e.g., ephedrine and phenylpropanolamine), methamphetamine, and benzphetamine. Although the selective serotonin reuptake inhibitors (e.g., fluoxetine and sertraline) appear to promote weight loss, further study is warranted given the inconsistent results available to date. Dietary supplements containing ephedra or ephedrine alkaloids are banned from sale following the FDA's final ruling.[48] However, ephedrine is available in nonprescription and prescription formulations for the treatment of bronchospasm, nasal congestion, hypotension or shock, and cardiac arrhythmias. Herbal products lack consistency in labeling, vary in effect, and present potentially dangerous health risks. Herbal products for weight loss are not recommended.

▶ Surgical Intervention

Weight reduction (bariatric) surgery is an option for patients whose BMIs are 40 kg/m² or greater, or 35 kg/m² or greater in the presence of other comorbid conditions and who have failed more conventional approaches to weight loss.[4,49] ❾
Surgery is warranted when other treatment attempts have

> ### Patient Encounter 1, Part 2: Medical History, Physical Exam, and Diagnostic Tests
>
> **PMH:** Occasional headaches, occasional heartburn
>
> **FH:** Father alive and 68 years of age. Mother also alive with history of obesity and CVD (MI in 2008).
>
> **SH:** (-) Tobacco, (+) alcohol, 1 to 2 drinks on the weekend
>
> **Meds:** Ibuprofen 400 mg PO as needed, ranitidine 75 mg PO as needed
>
> **ROS:** (+) Heartburn, regurgitation; (−) chest pain, nausea, vomiting, diarrhea, change in appetite, shortness of breath, or cough
>
> **PE:**
>
> **VS:** BP 124/82 mm Hg, P 72 beats/min, RR 16 breaths/min, T 98.6° F (37° C)
>
> **Weight:** 185 lb (84 kg); ht: 65 in (165 cm)
>
> **Waist circumference:** 42 in (107 cm)
>
> **Cardiovascular:** Normal S_1S_2; no murmurs, rubs, gallops
>
> **Abdominal:** Obese, soft, nontender, nondistended; (+) bowel sounds
>
> **Extremities:** (−) Edema
>
> **Labs:** All values are within normal limits.
>
> **ECG:** No evidence of past ischemia
>
> *Given this additional information, do you recommend weight loss? If so, how much weight should the patient lose and how fast?*
>
> *What nonpharmacologic and pharmacologic alternatives are available for the patient?*

---

failed in severely obese patients (BMI of 40 kg/m² or greater, or 35 kg/m² or greater with obesity-related risk factors). There are two basic surgical techniques: (a) **gastric bypass**—the full partitioning of the proximal gastric segment into a jejunal loop of the intestine—whereby weight loss is induced through both malabsorption of food and limited gastric capacity, and (b) **gastroplasty**—incomplete partitioning at the proximal gastric segment with the placement of a gastric outlet stoma of set diameter—which promotes weight loss by limiting gastric capacity.[4,49]

A meta-analysis of surgical options for obesity reported that surgical treatment produces a weight loss of 20 to 30 kg (44–66 lb) that is maintained for 5 to 10 years. Additionally, favorable outcomes for comorbid conditions are observed after surgery. When evaluating the various types of surgery available, pooled data concluded that gastric bypass produces a 10-kg (22-lb) greater weight loss at 12 and 36 months than gastroplasty procedures. Complications are inherent to any surgical procedure. The more common bariatric surgery complications are respiratory problems, wound formation, wound infections, hernia development, deep venous thrombosis, and pulmonary embolism. No differences were observed in mortality rates among various surgical procedures. Postoperative weight loss is much greater compared with pharmacologic therapies, but no comparative trials exist.[50]

Gastric surgery, either banding or bypass, is an alternative offered to adolescents because it results in substantial weight loss and medical health improvement. Patients with a BMI greater than or equal to 40 kg/m^2 and an associated medical condition or BMI greater than or equal to 50 kg/m^2 at or after the age of 13 and 15 years for girls and boys, respectively; display emotional and cognitive maturity; and have implemented a behavioral-based weight-loss program are candidates for surgery.[19]

All patients undergoing bariatric surgery should be part of an integrated program of health education, diet, exercise, and behavioral modification before and after surgery.[4] Patients must understand and commit to a substantial change in eating patterns to maintain long-term weight reduction.[19,50]

SPECIAL POPULATION CONSIDERATION

Elderly Patients with Obesity

The majority of obese female patients are 40 to 59 years of age where more male patients aged 60 and older are considered obese.[6] Therefore, it should not be surprising that more cardiovascular risk factors are present in this group of individuals. Additionally, obesity is a major predictor of functional limitation and mobility problems in older persons. Age alone should not prejudice clinicians from treating geriatric patients; instead, the benefits of cardiovascular health and functionality should be considered. Treatments should be initiated that minimize adverse effects on bone health and nutritional status and should include dietary and activity modifications.[4]

OUTCOME EVALUATION

Successful management of overweight and obesity is determined by the ability the treatment plan has to (a) prevent weight gain, (b) reduce and maintain a lower body weight, and (c) decrease the risk of obesity-related comorbidities. Because weight is necessary to calculate the BMI, the patient's weight as well as the waist circumference should be determined. Obesity management may encompass more than weight loss or maintenance in the presence of other conditions; other pertinent parameters should be assessed at baseline. The presence of hypertension, type 2 diabetes mellitus, hyperlipidemia, CAD, sleep apnea, hypothyroidism, osteoarthritis, gallbladder disease, gout, or cancer should be determined. Blood pressure and heart rate should be measured before implementation of any therapy. Certain laboratory parameters also should be assessed. A basic metabolic panel, liver function tests, complete blood count, fasting lipid profile,

full thyroid function tests, and other laboratory studies as deemed necessary should be obtained. An electrocardiogram should be performed if recent results are unknown.[4]

The patient should be assessed in 2 to 4 weeks after the implementation of therapy to determine effectiveness of and intolerance to treatment. Monthly visits are encouraged during the first 3 months. More frequent follow-up may be necessary in the presence of other medical conditions. Less frequent follow-up occurs after 6 months of effective weight loss therapy.[4]

At each follow-up visit, compliance with a healthy lifestyle should be determined, as well as measurement of physical parameters, including weight, blood pressure, and heart rate. Waist circumference should be measured intermittently. A complete assessment also includes identification of adverse drug reactions or drug interactions if weight loss medications have been initiated.[4]

When the patient has achieved the recommended weight loss, he or she then enters the weight maintenance phase, which includes continued contact for education, guidance, and risk factor assessment. If weight loss is not attained, further assessment is required to determine why the goals of therapy have not been met. The interaction should be directed toward determining the motivation to lose weight, balance between caloric intake and physical activity, adherence to behavioral therapy, and determination of psychological stressors present.[4]

Patient Encounter 2, Part 1

A 54-year-old white man presents to your CVD Risk Reduction Clinic. The patient currently denies chest pain, shortness of breath, dizziness, and lightheadedness. Upon review of progress notes, you discover that the patient's blood pressure has been elevated during the past three office visits. As an electrician, he frequently eats fast food for lunch. Evenings are spent at a nearby country club, where he eats dinners that vary from steak and potatoes to fried chicken to occasional fish. He reports playing golf two days a week (Saturday and Sunday). The patient's BMI is 32.6 kg/m^2, and his waist circumference is 47 in (119 cm).

What classification of overweight and obesity is appropriate for this patient?

Does this patient have a high-risk waist circumference?

Does he have other risk factors that may contribute to morbidity or mortality?

What are the treatment goals for the patient?

What additional information do you need to know before creating a treatment plan for this patient?

Patient Encounter 2, Part 2: Medical History, Physical Exam, and Diagnostic Tests

PMH: Hypertension diagnosed 4 years ago

FH: Father alive and 78 years of age. Mother also alive and 77 years of age.

SH: Drinks alcohol most days (socially) but denies any alcohol-related problems

Meds: Hydrochlorothiazide 12.5mg PO every morning

ROS: (-) Heartburn, regurgitation; (–) chest pain, nausea, vomiting, diarrhea, change in appetite, shortness of breath, or cough

VS: BP 154/92 mm Hg, P 76 beats/min, RR 15 breaths/min, T 98.7° F (37.1° C)

Weight: 208 lb (94.5 kg)

Height: 67 in (170 cm)

Waist circumference: 47 in (119 cm)

PE:

General: Well developed, in no acute distress

HEENT: Conjunctiva clear

CV: Regular rhythm, no S_3 or S_4 noted

Lungs: Clear to auscultation (CTA) bilaterally

Abd: Obese, soft, nontender, nondistended; (+) bowel sounds

Neuro: Normal gait, normal speech

Ext: (–) Edema

Labs:

Na: 142 mEq/L (142 mmol/L); K: 4.6 mEq/L (4.6 mmol/L); Cl: 107 mEq/L (107 mmol/L); CO_2: 23 mEq/L (23 mmol/L); BUN: 18 mg/dL (6.4 mmol/L); creatinine: 0.9 mg/dL (80 μmol/L); glucose: 72 mg/dL (4.0 mmol/L)

TC: 213 mg/dL (5.51 mmol/L); LDL: 153 mg/dL (3.96 mmol/L);

HDL: 30 mg/dL (0.78 mmol/L); TG: 152 mg/dL (1.72 mmol/L)

AST: 24 U/L (0.40 μkat/L); ALT: 30 U/L (0.50 μkat/L)

Given this additional information, do you recommend weight loss? If so, how much weight should the patient lose and how fast?

What nonpharmacologic and pharmacologic alternatives are available for the patient?

Patient Encounter 2, Part 3: CVD Risk Reduction 6-Month Follow-up Clinic Visit

The patient present for his 6-month follow-up visit in the CVD Risk Reduction Clinic. He states that he has been adhering to the Step 1 diet and currently jogs on a treadmill 30 minutes a day 5 days a week.

SH: Continues to drink 3 to 4 beers nightly

Meds: Hydrochlorothiazide 12.5 mg PO every morning, lisinopril 20 mg PO every morning, and aspirin 81 mg PO daily

ROS: (–) Heartburn, regurgitation; (–) chest pain, nausea, vomiting, diarrhea, change in appetite, shortness of breath, or cough

VS: BP 126/74 mm Hg, P 76 beats/min, RR 16 breaths/min, T 98.5° F (36.9° C)

Wt: 199 lb (90 kg)

Ht: 67 in (170 cm)

Waist circumference: 45 in (114)

PE:

General: Well developed, in no acute distress

HEENT: Conjunctiva clear

CV: Regular rhythm, no S_3 or S_4 noted

Lungs: CTA bilaterally

Abd: Obese, soft, nontender, nondistended; (+) bowel sounds

Neuro: normal gait, normal speech

Ext: (–) Edema

Labs:

Na: 142 mEq/L (142 mmol/L); K: 4.7 mEq/L (4.7 mmol/L); Cl: 107 mEq/L (107 mmol/L); CO_2: 23 mEq/L (23 mmol/L); BUN: 18 mg/dL (6.4 mmol/L); creatinine: 1.0 mg/dL (88 μmol/L); glucose: 84 mg/dL (4.7 mmol/L)

TC: 218 mg/dL (5.64 mmol/L); LDL: 155 mg/dL (4.01 mmol/L); HDL: 34 mg/dL (0.88 mmol/L); TG: 145 mg/dL (1.64 mmol/L)

AST: 20 U/L (33 μkat/L), ALT: 32 U/L (0.53 μkat/L)

Calculate the patient's BMI.

What is the best weight loss therapeutic option for the patient?

Should any other medication(s) be implemented?

Patient Care and Monitoring

1. Determine if history of BMI greater than or equal to 25 kg/m². If unavailable or BMI unknown, obtain weight, height, and waist circumference. Calculate the BMI. Assess the patient's willingness to lose weight.

2. If the BMI is greater than 25 kg/m² or waist circumference greater than 35 in for females or 40 in for male patients, determine the presence of risk factors.

3. Prevention of weight gain is recommended in all patients with a BMI greater than or equal to 25 kg/m². Weight loss is indicated for patients with a BMI 25 to 29.9 kg/m², or an elevated waist circumference with two or more risk factors, or for any patient with a BMI greater than or equal to 30 kg/m².

4. Educate the patient regarding a healthy lifestyle, one that includes a balance between caloric intake and energy expenditure as well as suggest methods to modify behavior.

5. If the patient presents with a desire to lose weight, develop treatment goals and weight loss strategies (nonpharmacologic, drug therapy, or surgical intervention), including control of associated risks.

6. Close monitoring should follow to assess weight, BMI, waist circumference, and the presence of complications related to the treatment plan. If weight loss goals are not attained, determine reasons for failure.

Abbreviations Introduced in This Chapter

AST	Aspartate transaminase
ALT	Alanine transaminase
BMI	Body mass index
CAD	Coronary artery disease
CB1	Cannabinoid receptor
CHD	Coronary heart disease
CNS	Central nervous system
CVD	Cardiovascular disease
FDA	Food and Drug Administration
5-HT_{1A}	Serotonin 1A subtype
5-HT_{2C}	Serotonin 2C subtype
GI	Gastrointestinal
LCD	Low-calorie diet
MAOI	Monoamine oxidase inhibitor
MI	Myocardial infarction
NIH-NHLBI	National Institute of Health-National Heart Lung and Blood Institute
SCOUT	Sibutramine Cardiovascular Outcomes

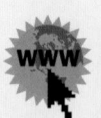 Self-assessment questions and answers are available at *http://www.mhpharmacotherapy. com/pp.html.*

REFERENCES

1. CDC: Centers for Disease Control and Prevention. [Internet]. Atlanta, GA: Centers for Disease Control and Prevention. Defining Overweight and Obesity; 2010 Jun 21 [cited 2011 Oct 2]; [1 screen]. Available from: http://www.cdc.gov/nccdphp/dnpa/obesity/defining.htm.

2. Dowling HJ, Pi-Sunyer FX. Race-dependent health risks of upper body obesity. Diabetes 1993;42:537–543.

3. Kissebah AH, Vydelingum N, Murray R, et al. Relation of body fat distribution to metabolic complications of obesity. J Clin Endocrinol Metab 1982;54:254–260.

4. U.S. Department of Health and Human Services, NIH-NHLBI. Clinical guidelines on the identification, evaluation and treatment of overweight and obesity in adults. NIH publication no. 00–4084. Bethesda, MD: National Institutes of Health, 2000.

5. Lew EA, Garfinkel L. Variations in mortality by weight among 750,000 men and women. J Chronic Dis 1979;23:563–576.

6. Flegal KM, Carroll MD, Ogden CL, Curtin LR. Prevalence and trends in obesity among US adults, 1999–2008. JAMA 2010;303:235–241.

7. Ogden CL, Carroll MD, Curtin LR, Lamb MM, Flegal KM. Prevalence of high body mass index in US children and adolescents, 2007–2008. JAMA 2010;303:242–249.

8. Power C, Lake JK, Cole TJ. Body mass index and height from childhood to adulthood in the 1958 British born cohort. Am J Clin Nutr 1997;66:1094–1101.

9. Freedman DS, Dietz WH, Srinivasan SR, et al. The relation of overweight to cardiovascular risk factors among children and adolescents: The Bogalusa heart study. Pediatrics 1999;103:1175–1182.

10. Must A, Jacques PF, Dallal GE, et al. Long-term morbidity and mortality of overweight adolescents. A follow-up of the Harvard Growth Study of 1922 to 1935. N Engl J Med 1992;327:1350–1355.

11. American Academy of Pediatrics Committee on Nutrition. Prevention of pediatric overweight and obesity. Pediatrics 2003;112(2):424–430.

12. Comuzzie AG, Allison DB. The search for human obesity genes. Science 1998;280:1374–1377.

13. Flier JS, Foster DW. Eating disorders: Obesity, anorexia nervosa, bulimia, nervosa. In: Wilson JD, Foster DW, Kronenberg HM, Larsen PR, eds. Williams' Textbook of Endocrinology, 9th ed. Philadelphia: WB Saunders, 1998:1061–1097.

14. National Research Council. Committee on Diet and Health. Implications for reducing chronic disease risk. Washington, DC: National Academies Press, 1989.

15. Di Marzo V, Bifulco M, De Petrocellis L. The endocannabinoid system and its therapeutic exploitation. Nat Rev Drug Discov 2004;3:771–784.

16. Bensaid M, Gary-Bobo M, Esclangon A, et al. The cannabinoid CB1 receptor antagonist SR141716 increases Acrp30 mRNA expression in adipose tissue of obese fa/fa rats and in cultured adipocyte cells. Mol Pharmacol 2003;6:908–914.

17. Van Gaal L, Rissanen A, Scheen A, et al. Effects of the cannabinoid-1 receptor blocker rimonabant on weight reduction and cardiovascular risk factors in overweight patients: 1-year experience from the RIO-Europe study. Lancet 2005;365:1389–1397.

18. Woods SC, Seeley RJ, Porte DJ, et al. Signals that regulate food intake and energy homeostasis. Science 1998;280:1378–1383.

19. Lissner L, Levitsky DA, Strupp BJ, et al. Dietary fat and the regulation of energy intake in human subjects. Am J Clin Nutr 1987;46:886–892.

20. Spear BA, Barlow SE, Ervin C, et al. Recommendations for treatment and adolescent overweight and obesity. Pediatrics. 2007;120(Suppl): S254–S288.

21. NICHQ: National Initiative for Children's Healthcare Quality. [Internet]. National Initiative for Children's Healthcare Quality. Expert committee recommendations on the assessment, prevention and treatment of child and adolescent overweight and obesity, dates unavailable [cited 2011 Oct 2]. Available from http://www.nichq.org/documents/coan-papers-and-publications/COANImplementationGuide62607FINAL.pdf.

22. Orzano AJ, Scott JG. Diagnosis and treatment of obesity in adults: An applied evidence-based review. J Am Board Fam Pract 2004;17(5):359–369.

23. Malone M. Medications associated with weight gain. Ann Pharmacother 2005;39:2046–2055.

24. Janssen, Division of Ortho-McNeil-Janssen Pharmaceuticals, Inc. Invega (Paliperidone) Package Insert. Titusville, NJ: Janssen, Division of Ortho-McNeil-Janssen Pharmaceuticals, Inc., 2007.

25. AstraZeneca Pharmaceuticals LP. Seroquel (Quetiapine) package insert. Wilmington, DE: AstraZeneca Pharmaceuticals LP, 2008 (July).

26. Wadden TA, Foster DD, Letizia KA. One-year behavioral treatment of obesity: comparison of moderate and severe caloric restriction and the effects of weight maintenance therapy. J Consult Clin Psychol 1994;62:165–171.

27. Connolly HM, Crary JL, McGoon MD, et al. Valvular heart disease associated with fenfluramine-phentermine. N Engl J Med 1997;337: 581–588.

28. James WP, Caterson ID, Coutinho W, et al. Effect of sibutramine on cardiovascular outcomes in overweight and obese subjects. N Engl J Med 2010;363(10):905–917.

29. Roche Laboratories. Xenical (Orlistat) package insert. Nutley, NJ: Roche Laboratories, 2009 (January).

30. Sjöström L, Rissanen A, Andersen T, et al. Randomized placebo-controlled trial of orlistat for weight loss and prevention of weight regain in obese patients. Lancet 1998;352:167–173.

31. Davidson MH, Hauptman J, DiGirolamo M, et al. Weight control and risk factor reduction in obese subjects treated for 2 years with orlistat. JAMA 1999;281:235–242.

32. Hill JO, Hauptman J, Anderson JW, et al. Orlistat, a lipase inhibitory, for weight maintenance after conventional dieting: A 1-year study. Am J Clin Nutr 1999;69:1108–1116.

33. Torgerson JS, Hauptman J, Boldrin MN, et al. XENical in the prevention of diabetes in obese subjects (XENDOS) study: A randomized study of orlistat as an adjunct to lifestyle changes for the prevention of type 2 diabetes in obese patients. Diabetes Care 2004;27:155–161.

34. Chapione JP, Hampl S, Jensen C, et al. Effect of orlistat on weight and body composition in obese adolescents: A randomized controlled trial. JAMA 2005;293:2873–2883.

35. Li Z, Maglione M, Tu W, et al. Meta-analysis: Pharmacologic treatment of obesity. Ann Intern Med 2005;142:532–546.

36. FDA: Food and Drug Administration. [Internet]. Silver Spring, MD: Food and Drug Administration. Early Communication about an Ongoing Safety Review Orlistat (marketed as Alli and Xenical); 2009 Aug 24 [cited 2011 Oct 2] [1 screen]. Available from: http://www.fda.gov/Drugs/DrugSafety/PostmarketDrugSafetyInformationforPatientsandProviders/DrugSafetyInformationforHeathcareProfessionals/ucm179166.htm.

37. FDA: Food and Drug Administration. [Internet]. Silver Spring, MD: Food and Drug Administration. FDA Drug Safety Communication: Completed safety review of Xenical/Alli (orlistat) and severe liver injury; 2010 May 26 [cited 2011 Oct 2]; [1 screen]. Available from: http://www.fda.gov/Drugs/DrugSafety/PostmarketDrugSafetyInformationforPatientsandProviders/ucm213038.htm.

38. Abbott Laboratories. Meridia (Sibutramine) package insert. North Chicago, IL: Abbott Laboratories, 2007 (October).

39. FDA: Food and Drug Administration. [Internet]. Silver Spring, MD: Food and Drug Administration. Follow-Up to the November 2009 Early Communication about an Ongoing Safety Review of Sibutramine, Marketed as Meridia; 2010 Jan 1 [cited 2011 Oct 2]; [1 screen]. Available from http://www.fda.gov/Drugs/DrugSafety/PostmarketDrugSafetyInformationforPatientsandProviders/DrugSafetyInformationforHealthcareProfessionals/ucm198206.htm.

40. Gate Pharmaceuticals. Adipex-P (Phentermine) package insert. Sellersville, PA: Gate Pharmaceuticals, 2005 (July).

41. Thompson Healthcare Products. MICROMEDEX Healthcare Series. www.micromedex.com/products/hcs.

42. Merrell Pharmaceuticals. Tenuate (Diethylpropion) package insert. Bridgewater, NJ: Merrell Pharmaceuticals, 2003 (November).

43. Christensen R, Kristensen PK, Bartels EM, Bliddal H, Astrup A. Efficacy and safety of the weight loss drug rimonabant: A meta-analysis of randomized trials. Lancet 2007;370:1706–1711.

44. Padwal RS, Majumdar SR. Drug treatments for Obesity: Orlistat, sibutramine and rimonant. Lancet 2007;369:71–77.

45. Topol EJ, Bousser M-G, Fox KAA, et al. Rimonabant for prevention of cardiovascular events (CRESCENDO): A randomized, multicenter, placebo-controlled trial. Lancet 2010;376:517–523.

46. European Medicines Agency: Sciences Medicine and Health. [Internet]. London: European Medicines Agency; c 1995-2012. The European Medicines Agency recommends suspension of the marketing authorisation of Acomplia; 2008 Oct 23 [cited 2011 Oct 2]. Available from: http://www.ema.europa.eu/docs/en_GB/document_library/Press_release/2009/11/WC500014774.pdf.

47. Merck Be Well [Internet]. Whitehouse Station, NJ: Merck Sharp and Dohme Corporation; c 2009-2011. Annual Report Pursuant to Section 13 or 15(d) of the Securities Exchange Act of 1934 For the Fiscal Year Ended December 31, 2008; 2009 Feb 27 [cited 2011 Oct 2]. Available from http://www.merck.com/finance/proxy/2008_form_10-k.pdf.

48. FDA: US Food and Drug Administration. [Internet]. Silver Spring, MD: U.S. Department of Health and Human Services Food and Drug Administration Center for Food Safety and Applied Nutrition. Guidance for Industry Final Rule Declaring Dietary Supplements Containing Ephedrine Alkaloids Adulterated Because They Present an Unreasonable Risk; 2011 Jun 6 [cited 2012 Feb 8]; [1 screen]. Available from: http://www.fda.gov/Food/GuidanceComplianceRegulatoryInformation/GuidanceDocuments/DietarySupplements/ucm072997.htm.

49. Snow V, Barry P, Fitterman N, et al. Pharmacologic and surgical management of obesity in primary care: A clinical practice guideline from the American College of Physicians. Ann Intern Med 2005;142:525–531.

50. Maggard MA, Shugarman LR, Suttorp M, et al. Meta-analysis: Surgical treatment of obesity. Ann Intern Med. 2005;142:547–559.

Appendix A: Conversion Factors and Anthropometrics*

CONVERSION FACTORS

SI Units

SI (*le Systéme International d'Unités*) units are used in many countries to express clinical laboratory and serum drug concentration data. Instead of using units of mass (e.g., micrograms), the SI system uses moles (mol) to represent the amount of a substance. A molar solution contains 1 mole (the molecular weight of the substance in grams) of the solute in 1 L of solution. The following formula is used to convert units of mass to moles (mcg/mL to μmol/L or, by substitution of terms, mg/mL to mmol/L or ng/mL to nmol/L).

▶ Micromoles per Liter

Micromoles per liter (μmol/L)

$$= \frac{\text{drug concentration (mcg/mL)} \times 1{,}000}{\text{molecular weight of drug (g/mol)}}$$

▶ Milliequivalents

An equivalent weight of a substance is the weight that will combine with or replace 1 g of hydrogen; a milliequivalent is 1/1,000 of an equivalent weight.

Milliequivalents per Liter

Milliequivalents per liter (mEq/L)

$$= \frac{\text{weight of salt (g)} \times \text{valence of ion} \times 1{,}000}{\text{molecular weight of salt}}$$

$$\text{Weight of salt (g)} = \frac{\text{mEq/L} \times \text{molecular weight of salt}}{\text{valence of ion} \times 1{,}000}$$

Approximate Milliequivalents: Weight Conversions for Selected Ions

Salt	mEq/g Salt	mg Salt/ mEq
Calcium carbonate ($CaCO_3$)	20.0	50.0
Calcium chloride ($CaCl_2 \cdot 2H_2O$)	13.6	73.5
Calcium gluceptate ($Ca[C_7H_{13}O_8]_2$)	4.1	245.2
Calcium gluconate ($Ca[C_6H_{11}O_7]_2 \cdot H_2O$)	4.5	224.1
Calcium lactate ($Ca[C_3H_5O_3]_2 \cdot 5H_2O$)	6.5	154.1
Magnesium gluconate ($Mg[C_6H_{11}O_7]_2 \cdot H_2O$)	4.6	216.3
Magnesium oxide (MgO)	49.6	20.2
Magnesium sulfate ($MgSO_4$)	16.6	60.2
Magnesium sulfate ($MgSO_4 \cdot 7H_2O$)	8.1	123.2
Potassium acetate ($K[C_2H_3O_2]$)	10.2	98.1
Potassium chloride (KCl)	13.4	74.6
Potassium citrate ($K_3[C_6H_5O_7] \cdot H_2O$)	9.2	108.1
Potassium iodide (KI)	6.0	166.0
Sodium acetate ($Na[C_2H_3O_2]$)	12.2	82.0
Sodium acetate ($Na[C_2H_3O_2] \cdot 3H_2O$)	7.3	136.1
Sodium bicarbonate ($NaHCO_3$)	11.9	84.0
Sodium chloride ($NaCl$)	17.1	58.4
Sodium citrate ($Na_3[C_6H_5O_7] \cdot 2H_2O$)	10.2	98.0
Sodium iodide (NaI)	6.7	149.9
Sodium lactate ($Na[C_3H_5O_3]$)	8.9	112.1
Zinc sulfate ($ZnSO_4 \cdot 7H_2O$)	7.0	143.8

Valences and Atomic/Molecular Weights of Selected Ions

Substance	Electrolyte	Valence	Atomic/Molecular Weight
Calcium	Ca^{2+}	2	40.1
Chloride	Cl^-	1	35.5
Magnesium	Mg^{2+}	2	24.3
Phosphate	HPO_4^- (80%)	1.8	96.0^a
(pH = 7.4)	$H_2PO_4^-$ (20%)		97.0
Potassium	K^+	1	39.1
Sodium	Na^+	1	23.0
Sulfate	SO_4^-	2	96.0^a

^{a}The atomic/molecular weight of phosphorus is only 31; that of sulfur is only 32.1.

*This appendix contains information from Appendices 1 and 2 of Smith KM, Riche DM, Henyan NN (eds). Clinical Drug Data, 11th ed. New York: McGraw-Hill, 2010:1239–1246; With permission.

Anion Gap

The anion gap is the concentration of plasma anions not routinely measured by laboratory screening. It is useful in the evaluation of acid–base disorders. The anion gap is greater with increased plasma concentrations of endogenous species (e.g., phosphate, sulfate, lactate, and ketoacids) or exogenous species (e.g., salicylate, penicillin, ethylene glycol, ethanol, and methanol). The formulas for calculating the anion gap are as follows:

$$\text{Anion gap} = (Na^+ + K^+) - (Cl^- + HCO_3^-)$$

or

$$\text{Anion gap} = Na^+ - (Cl^- + HCO_3^-)$$

where the expected normal value for the first equation is 11 to 20 mmol/L and for the second equation is 7 to 16 mmol/L. Note that there is a variation in the upper and lower limits of the normal range.

Temperature

Fahrenheit to Centigrade: (°F − 32) × 5/9 = °C
Centigrade to Fahrenheit: (°C × 9/5) + 32 = °F
Centigrade to Kelvin: °C + 273 = °K

Calories

1 calorie = 1 kilocalorie = 1,000 calories = 4.184 kilojoules (kJ)
1 kilojoule = 0.239 calories = 0.239 kilocalories = 239 calories

Weights and Measures

▶ Metric Weight Equivalents

1 kilogram (kg) = 1,000 grams
1 gram (g) = 1,000 milligrams
1 milligram (mg) = 0.001 gram
1 microgram (mcg, μg) = 0.001 milligram
1 nanogram (ng) = 0.001 microgram
1 picogram (pg) = 0.001 nanogram
1 femtogram (fg) = 0.001 picogram

▶ Metric Volume Equivalents

1 liter (L) = 1,000 milliliters
1 deciliter (dL) = 100 milliliters
1 milliliter (mL) = 0.001 liter
1 microliter (μL) = 0.001 milliliter
1 nanoliter (nL) = 0.001 microliter
1 picoliter (pL) = 0.001 nanoliter
1 femtoliter (fL) = 0.001 picoliter

▶ Apothecary Weight Equivalents

1 scruple (℈) = 20 grains (gr)
60 grains (gr) = 1 dram (ʒ)
8 drams (ʒ) = 1 ounce (℥)
1 ounce (℥) = 480 grains (gr)
12 ounces (℥) = 1 pound (lb)

▶ Apothecary Volume Equivalents

60 minims (m) = 1 fluidram (fl ʒ)
8 fluidrams (fl ʒ) = 1 fluid ounce (fl ℥)

1 fluid ounce (fl ℥) = 480 minims (m)
16 fluid ounces (fl ℥) = 1 pint (pt)

▶ Avoirdupois Equivalents

1 ounce (oz) = 437.5 grains
16 ounces (oz) = 1 pound (lb)

▶ Weight/Volume Equivalents

1 mg/dL = 10 mcg/mL
1 mg/dL = 1 mg%
1 ppm = 1 mg/L

▶ Conversion Equivalents

1 gram (g) = 15.43 grains (gr)
1 grain (gr) = 64.8 milligrams (mg)
1 ounce (℥) = 31.1 grams (g)
1 ounce (oz) = 28.35 grams (g)
1 pound (lb) = 453.6 grams (g)
1 kilogram (kg) = 2.2 pounds (lb)
1 milliliter (mL) = 16.23 minims (m)
1 minim (m) = 0.06 milliliter (mL)
1 fluid ounce (fl oz) = 29.57 milliliters (mL)
1 pint (pt) = 473.2 milliliters (mL)
1 US gallon = 3.78 liters (L)
1 Canadian gallon = 4.55 liters (L)
0.1 milligram = 1/600 grain
0.12 milligram = 1/500 grain
0.15 milligram = 1/400 grain
0.2 milligram = 1/300 grain
0.3 milligram = 1/200 grain
0.4 milligram = 1/150 grain
0.5 milligram = 1/120 grain
0.6 milligram = 1/100 grain
0.8 milligram = 1/80 grain
1 milligram = 1/65 grain

▶ Metric Length Conversion Equivalents

2.54 cm = 1 inch
30.48 cm = 1 foot
1 m = 3.28 feet
1.6 km = 1 mile

ANTHROPOMETRICS

Creatinine Clearance Formulas

▶ Formulas for Estimating Creatinine Clearance in Patients with Stable Renal Function

Cockcroft-Gault Formula
Adults (age 18 years and older)[1]:

$$CrCl\ (men) = \frac{(140 - age) \times weight}{SCr \times 72}$$

$$CrCl\ (women) = 0.85 \times above\ value^*$$

where CrCl is creatinine clearance (in mL/min), SCr is serum creatinine (in mg/dL [or µmol/L divided by 88.4]), age is in years, and weight is in kilograms.

* Some studies suggest that the predictive accuracy of this formula for women is better *without* the correction factor of 0.85.

Traub-Johnson Formula

Children (age 1–18 years)[2]:

$$CrCl = \frac{0.48 \times height \times BSA}{SCr \times 1.73}$$

where BSA is body surface area (in m²), CrCl is creatinine clearance (in mL/minute), SCr is serum creatinine (in mg/dL [or µmol/L divided by 88.4]), and height is in centimeters.

▶ Formula for Estimating Creatinine Clearance From a Measured Urine Collection

$$CrCl\,(mL/minute) = \frac{U \times V}{P \times T}$$

where U is the concentration of creatinine in a urine specimen in mg/dL, V is the volume of urine in mL, P is the concentration of creatinine in serum at the midpoint of the urine collection period in mg/dL, and T is the time of the urine collection period in minutes (e.g., 6 hours = 360 minutes; 24 hours = 1,440 minutes). Procedures for obtaining urine specimens should stress the importance of complete urine collection during the collection time period.

▶ MDRD Formula for Estimating Glomerular Filtration Rate (From the Modification of Diet in Renal Disease Study)[3]

Conventional calibration MDRD equation (used only with those creatinine methods that have *not* been recalibrated to be traceable to isotope dilution mass spectrometry [IDMS]) For creatinine in mg/dL:

$$X = 186 \text{ creatinine}^{-1.154} \times \text{age}^{-0.203} \times \text{constant}$$

For creatinine in µmol/L:

$$X = 32,788 \times \text{creatinine}^{-1.154} \times \text{age}^{-0.203} \times \text{constant}$$

where X is the glomerular filtration rate (GFR), constant for white men is 1 and for women is 0.742, and constant for African Americans is 1.21. Creatinine levels in µmol/L can be converted to mg/dL by dividing by 88.4.

▶ IDMS-Traceable MDRD Equation (Used Only With Creatinine Methods That Have Been Recalibrated to Be Traceable to IDMS)

For creatinine in mg/dL:

$$X = 175 \times \text{creatinine}^{-1.154} \times \text{age}^{-0.203} \times \text{constant}$$

For creatinine in µmol/L:

$$X = 175 \times (\text{creatinine}/88.4)^{-1.154} \times \text{age}^{-0.203} \times \text{constant}$$

where X is the GFR, constant for white men is 1 and for women is 0.742, and constant for African Americans is 1.21.

Ideal Body Weight

IBW is the weight expected for a nonobese person of a given height. The IBW formulas below and various life insurance tables can be used to estimate IBW. Dosing methods described in the literature may use IBW as a method in dosing obese patients.

Adults (age 18 years and older)[4]:

IBW (men) = 50 + (2.3 × height in inches over 5 ft)
IBW (women) = 45.5 + (2.3 × height in inches over 5 ft)

where IBW is in kilograms.

Children (age 1–18 years)[2] under 5 feet tall:

$$IBW = \frac{height^2 \times 1.65}{1,000}$$

where IBW is in kilograms and height is in centimeters.

Children (age 1–18 years) 5 feet or taller:

IBW (males) = 39 + (2.27 × height in inches over 5 ft)
IBW (females) = 42.2 + (2.27 × height in inches over 5 ft)

where IBW is in kilograms.

REFERENCES

1. Cockcroft DW, Gault MH. Prediction of creatinine clearance from serum creatinine. Nephron 1976;16:31–41.
2. Traub SI, Johnson CE. Comparison of methods of estimating creatinine clearance in children. Am J Hosp Pharm 1980;37:195–201.
3. Levey AS, Bosch JP, Lewis JB, et al. A more accurate method to estimate glomerular filtration rate from serum creatinine: A new prediction equation. Modification of Diet in Renal Disease Study Group. Ann Intern Med 1999;130:461–470.
4. Devine BJ. Gentamicin therapy. Drug Intell Clin Pharm 1974;8:650–655.

Appendix B: Common Laboratory Tests

The following table is an alphabetical listing of some common laboratory tests and their reference ranges for adults as measured in plasma or serum (unless otherwise indicated). Reference values differ among laboratories, so readers should refer to the published reference ranges used in each institution. For some tests, both the Système International Units and Conventional Units are reported.

Laboratory Test	Conventional Units	Conversion Factor	Système International Units
Acid phosphatase			
Male	2–12 U/L	16.7	33–200 nkat/L
Female	0.3–9.2 U/L	16.7	5–154 nkat/L
Activated partial thromboplastin time (aPTT)	25–40 sec		
Adrenocorticotropic hormone (ACTH)	15–80 pg/mL or ng/L	0.2202	3.3–17.6 pmol/L
Alanine aminotransferase (ALT, SGPT)	7–53 U/L	0.01667	0.12–0.88 μkat/L
Albumin	3.5–5.0 g/dL	10	35–50 g/L
Albumin:creatinine ratio (urine)		0.113	
Normal	Less than 30 mg/g creatinine		Less than 3.4 mg/mmol creatinine
Microalbuminuria	30–300 mg/g creatinine		3.4–34 mg/mmol creatinine
Proteinuria	Greater than 300 mg/g creatinine		Greater than 34 mg/mmol creatinine
or	or		
Normal			
Male	Less than 18 mg/g creatinine	0.113	Less than 2.0 mg/mmol creatinine
Female	Less than 25 mg/g creatinine	0.113	Less than 2.8 mg/mmol creatinine
Microalbuminuria			
Male	18–180 mg/g creatinine	0.113	2.0–20 mg/mmol creatinine
Female	25–250 mg/g creatinine	0.113	2.8–28 mg/mmol creatinine
Proteinuria			
Male	Greater than 180 mg/g creatinine	0.113	Greater than 20 mg/mmol creatinine
Female	Greater than 250 mg/mmol creatinine	0.113	Greater than 28 mg/mmol creatinine
Alcohol			
See under Ethanol			
Aldosterone			
Supine	Less than 16 ng/dL	27.7	Less than 444 pmol/L
Upright	Less than 31 ng/dL	27.7	Less than 860 pmol/L
Alkaline phosphatase			
10–15 years	130–550 IU/L	0.01667	2.17–9.17 μkat/L
16–20 years	70–260 IU/L	0.01667	1.17–4.33 μkat/L
Greater than 20 years	38–126 IU/L	0.01667	0.63–2.10 μkat/L
α-Fetoprotein (AFP)	Less than 15 ng/mL	1	Less than 15 mcg/L
α-1-Antitrypsin	80–200 mg/dL	0.01	0.8–2.0 g/L
Amikacin, therapeutic			
Peak	15–30 mg/L	1.71	25.6–51.3 μmol/L
Trough	Less than or equal to 8 mg/L	1.71	Less than or equal to 13.7 μmol/L
Amitriptyline	80–200 ng/mL or mcg/L	3.605	288–721 nmol/L
Ammonia (plasma)	15–56 mcg NH_3/dL	0.5872	9–33 μmol NH_3/L
Amylase	25–115 U/L	0.01667	0.42–1.92 μkat/L
Androstenedione	50–250 ng/dL	0.0349	1.7–8.7 nmol/L
Angiotensin-converting enzyme	15–70 units/L	16.67	250–1167 nkat/L
Anion gap	7–16 mEq/L	1	7–16 mmol/L
Anti–double-stranded DNA (anti-ds DNA)	Negative		
Anti-HAV	Negative		

(Continued)

Laboratory Test	Conventional Units	Conversion Factor	Système International Units
Anti-HBc	Negative		
Anti-HBs	Negative		
Anti-HCV	Negative		
Anti-Sm antibody	Negative		
Antinuclear antibody (ANA)	Negative		
Apolipoprotein A-1			
Male	95–175 mg/dL	0.01	0.95–1.75 g/L
Female	100–200 mg/dL	0.01	1.0–2.0 g/L
Apolipoprotein B			
Male	50–110 mg/dL	0.01	0.5–1.10 g/L
Female	50–105 mg/dL	0.01	0.5–1.05 g/L
Aspartate aminotransferase (AST, SGOT)	11–47 IU/L	0.01667	0.18–0.78 μkat/L
β_2-Microglobulin	Less than 0.2 mg/dL	10	Less than 2 mg/L
Bicarbonate	22–26 mEq/L	1	22–26 mmol/L
Bilirubin			
Total	0.3–1.1 mg/dL	17.1	5.1–18.8 μmol/L
Direct	0–0.3 mg/dL	17.1	0–5.1 μmol/L
Indirect	0.1–1.0 mg/dL	17.1	1.7–17.1 μmol/L
Bleeding time	3–7 minutes	60	180–420 seconds
Blood gases (arterial)			
pH	7.35–7.45	1	7.35–7.45
Po_2	80–105 mm Hg	0.133	10.6–14.0 kPa
Pco_2	35–45 mm Hg	0.133	4.7–6.0 kPa
HCO_3	22–26 mEq/L	1	22–26 mmol/L
O_2 saturation	Greater than or equal to 95%	0.01	Greater than or equal to 0.95
Blood urea nitrogen (BUN)	8–25 mg/dL	0.357	2.9–8.9 mmol/L
B-type natriuretic peptide (BNP)	0–99 pg/mL	1	0–99 ng/L
		0.289	0–29 pmol/L
BUN-to-creatinine ratio	10:1–20:1		
C-peptide	0.51–2.70 ng/mL	331	170–894 pmol/L
		0.331	0.17–0.89 nmol/L
C-reactive protein	Less than 0.8 mg/dL	10	Less than 8 mg/L
CA-125	Less than 35 units/mL	1	Less than 35 kU/L
CA 15–3	Less than 30 units/mL	1	Less than 30 kU/L
CA 19–9	Less than 37 units/mL	1	Less than 37 kU/L
CA 27.29	Less than 38 units/mL	1	Less than 38 kU/L
Calcium			
Total	8.6–10.3 mg/dL	0.25	2.15–2.58 mmol/L
	4.3–5.16 mEq/L	0.50	2.15–2.58 mmol/L
Ionized	4.5–5.1 mg/dL	0.25	1.13–1.28 mmol/L
	2.26–2.56 mEq/L	0.50	1.13–1.28 mmol/L
Carbamazepine, therapeutic	4–12 mg/L	4.23	17–51 μmol/L
Carboxyhemoglobin (nonsmoker)	Less than 2%	0.01	Less than 0.02
Carcinoembryonic antigen (CEA)			
Nonsmokers	Less than 2.5 ng/mL	1	Less than 2.5 mcg/L
Smokers	Less than 5 ng/mL	1	Less than 5 mcg/L
CD4 lymphocyte count	31–61% of total lymphocytes	0.01	0.31–0.61 of total lymphocytes
CD8 lymphocyte count	18–39% of total lymphocytes	0.01	0.18–0.39 of total lymphocytes
Cerebrospinal fluid (CSF)			
Pressure	75–175 mm H_2O		
Glucose	40–70 mg/dL	0.0555	2.2–3.9 mmol/L
Protein	15–45 mg/dL	0.01	0.15–0.45 g/L
White blood cell (WBC) count	Less than 10/mm³	1	Less than 10×10^6/L
Ceruloplasmin	18–45 mg/dL	10	180–450 mg/L
Chloride	97–110 mEq/L	1	97–110 mmol/L
Cholesterol			
Desirable	Less than 200 mg/dL	0.0259	Less than 5.18 mmol/L
Borderline high	200–239 mg/dL	0.0259	5.18–6.19 mmol/L
High	Greater than or equal to 240 mg/dL	0.0259	Greater than or equal to 6.2 mmol/L
Chorionic gonadotropin (β-hCG)	Less than 5 mIU/mL	1	Less than 5 IU/L
Clozapine, minimum trough	300–350 ng/mL or mcg/L	3.06	918–1,071 nmol/L
		0.00306	0.92–1.07 μmol/L
CO_2 content	22–30 mEq/L	1	22–30 mmol/L
Complement component 3 (C3)	70–160 mg/dL	0.01	0.70–1.60 g/L
Complement component 4 (C4)	20–40 mg/dL	0.01	0.20–0.40 g/L
Copper	70–150 mcg/dL	0.157	11–24 μmol/L
Cortisol (fasting, morning)	5–25 mcg/dL	27.6	138–690 nmol/L

(Continued)

Laboratory Test	Conventional Units	Conversion Factor	Système International Units
Cortisol (free, urinary)	10–100 mcg/d	2.76	28–276 nmol/day
Creatine kinase			
Male	30–200 IU/L	0.01667	0.50–3.33 μkat/L
Female	20–170 IU/L	0.01667	0.33–2.83 μkat/L
MB fraction	0–7 IU/L	0.01667	0.0–0.12 μkat/L
Creatinine clearance (CrCl) (urine)	85–135 mL/min/1.73 m^2	0.00963	0.82–1.30 mL/s/m^2
Creatinine			
Male 4–20 years	0.2–1.0 mg/dL	88.4	18–88 μmol/L
Female 4–20 years	0.2–1.0 mg/dL	88.4	18–88 μmol/L
Male (adults)	0.7–1.3 mg/dL	88.4	62–115 μmol/L
Female (adults)	0.6–1.1 mg/dL	88.4	53–97 μmol/L
Cyclosporine			
Renal, cardiac, liver, or pancreatic transplant	100–400 ng/mL or mcg/L	0.832	83–333 nmol/L
Cryptococcal antigen	Negative		
D-dimers	Less than 250 ng/mL	1	Less than 250 mcg/L
Desipramine	75–300 ng/mL or mcg/L	3.75	281–1125 nmol/L
Dexamethasone suppression test (DST) (overnight), 8:00 am cortisol	Less than 5 mcg/dL	27.6	Less than 138 nmol/L
DHEAS (dehydroepiandrosterone sulfate)			
Male	170–670 mcg/dL	0.0272	4.6–18.2 μmol/L
Female			
Premenopausal	50–540 mcg/dL	0.0272	1.4–14.7 μmol/L
Postmenopausal	30–260 mcg/dL	0.0272	0.8–7.1 μmol/L
Digoxin, therapeutic (heart failure)	0.5–0.8 ng/mL or mcg/L	1.28	0.6–1.0 nmol/L
Therapeutic (atrial fibrillation)	0.8–2.0 ng/mL or mcg/L	1.28	1.0–2.6 nmol/L
Erythrocyte count (blood)			
See under red blood cell (RBC) count			
Erythrocyte sedimentation rate (ESR)			
Westergren			
Male	0–20 mm/h		
Female	0–30 mm/h		
Wintrobe			
Male	0–9 mm/h		
Female	0–15 mm/h		
Erythropoietin	2–25 mIU/mL	1	2–25 IU/L
Estradiol			
Male	10–36 pg/mL	3.67	37–132 pmol/L
Female	34–170 pg/mL	3.67	125–624 pmol/L
Ethanol, legal intoxication (depends on location)	Greater than or equal to 50–100 mg/dL	0.217	Greater than or equal to 10.9–21.7 mmol/L
	Greater than or equal to 0.05–0.1%	217	Greater than or equal to 10.9–21.7 mmol/L
Ethosuccimide, therapeutic	40–100 mg/L or mcg/mL	7.08	283–708 μmol/L
Factor VIII or factor IX			
Severe hemophilia	Less than 1 IU/dL	0.01	Less than 0.01 IU/mL
Moderate hemophilia	1–5 IU/dL	0.01	0.01–0.05 IU/mL
Mild hemophilia	Greater than 5 IU/dL	0.01	Greater than 0.05 IU/mL
Usual adult levels	60 to 140 IU/dL	0.01	0.60–1.40 IU/mL
Ferritin			
Male	20–250 ng/mL	1	20–250 mcg/L
Female	10–150 ng/mL	1	10–150 mcg/L
Fibrin degradation products (FDP)	2–10 mg/L		
Fibrinogen	200–400 mg/dL	0.01	2.0–4.0 g/L
Folate (plasma)	3.1–12.4 ng/mL	2.266	7.0–28.1 nmol/L
Folate (RBC)	125–600 ng/mL	2.266	283–1,360 nmol/L
Follicle-stimulating hormone (FSH)			
Male	1–7 mIU/mL	1	1–7 IU/L
Female			
Follicular phase	1–9 mIU/mL	1	1–9 IU/L
Midcycle	6–26 mIU/mL	1	6–26 IU/L
Luteal phase	1–9 mIU/mL	1	1–9 IU/L
Postmenopausal	30–118 mIU/mL	1	30–118 IU/L
Free thyroxine index (FT$_4$I)	6.5–12.5		
Gamma glutamyltransferase (GGT)	0–30 IU/L	0.01667	0–0.50 μkat/L
Gastrin (fasting)	0–130 pg/mL	1	0–130 ng/L
Gentamicin, therapeutic (traditional dosing)			
Peak	4–10 mg/L	2.09	8.4–21 μmol/L
Trough	Less than or equal to 2 mg/L	2.09	Less than or equal to 4.2 μmol/L

(Continued)

Laboratory Test	Conventional Units	Conversion Factor	Système International Units
Globulin	2.3–3.5 g/dL	10	23–35 g/L
Glucose (fasting, plasma)	65–109 mg/dL	0.0555	3.6–6.0 mmol/L
Glucose, 2-hour postprandial blood (PPBG)	Less than 140 mg/dL	0.0555	Less than 7.8 mmol/L
Granulocyte count	1.8–6.6 × 10³/mm³	10⁶	1.8–6.6 × 10⁹/L
Growth hormone (fasting)			
Male	Less than 5 ng/mL	1	Less than 5 mcg/L
Female	Less than 10 ng/mL	1	Less than 10 mcg/L
Haptoglobin	60–270 mg/dL	0.01	0.6–2.7 g/L
Hepatitis B surface antigen, extracellular form (HBeAg)	Negative		
Hepatitis B surface antigen (HbsAg)	Negative		
Hepatitis B virus (HBV) DNA	Negative		
Hematocrit			
Male	40.7–50.3%	0.01	0.407–0.503
Female	36.1–44.3%	0.01	0.361–0.443
Hemoglobin (blood)			
Male	13.8–17.2 g/dL	10	138–172 g/L
		0.621	8.56–10.68 mmol/L
Female	12.1–15.1 g/dL	10	121–151 g/L
		0.621	7.51–9.36 mmol/L
Hemoglobin A1c	4.0–6.0%	0.01	0.04–0.06
		[a]	20–42 mmol/mol hemoglobin
Heparin			
Via protamine titration method	0.2–0.4 units/mL		
Via antifactor Xa assay	0.3–0.7 units/mL		
High-density lipoprotein (HDL) cholesterol	Greater than 35 mg/dL	0.0259	Greater than 0.91 mmol/L
Homocysteine	3.3–10.4 µmol/L		
Ibuprofen			
Therapeutic	10–50 mcg/mL	4.85	49–243 µmol/L
Toxic	Greater than or equal to 100 mcg/mL	4.85	Greater than or equal to 485 µmol/L
Imipramine, therapeutic	100–300 ng/mL or mcg/L	3.57	357–1,071 nmol/L
Immunoglobulin A (IgA)	85–385 mg/dL	0.01	0.85–3.85 g/L
Immunoglobulin G (IgG)	565–1,765 mg/dL	0.01	5.65–17.65 g/L
Immunoglobulin M (IgM)	53–375 mg/dL	0.01	0.53–3.75 g/L
Insulin (fasting)	2–20 µU/mL or mU/L	7.175	14.35–143.5 pmol/L
International normalized ratio (INR), therapeutic	2.0–3.0 (2.5–3.5 for some indications)		
Iron			
Male	45–160 mcg/dL	0.179	8.1–28.6 µmol/L
Female	30–160 mcg/dL	0.179	5.4–28.6 µmol/L
Iron-binding capacity (total)	220–420 mcg/dL	0.179	39.4–75.2 µmol/L
Iron saturation	15–50%	0.01	0.15–0.50
Itraconazole			
Trough, therapeutic	0.5–1 mcg/mL	1	0.5–1 mg/L
Lactate (plasma)	0.7–2.1 mEq/L	1	0.7–2.1 mmol/L
	6.3–18.9 mg/dL	0.111	0.7–2.1 mmol/L
Lactate dehydrogenase (LDH)	100–250 IU/L	0.01667	1.67–4.17 µkat/L
Lead	Less than 25 mcg/dL	0.0483	Less than 1.21 µmol/L
Leukocyte count	3.8–9.8 × 10³/mm³	10⁶	3.8–9.8 × 10⁹/L
Lidocaine, therapeutic	1.5–6.0 mcg/mL or mg/L	4.27	6.4–25.6 µmol/L
Lipase	Less than 100 IU/L	0.01667	1.67 µkat/L
Lithium, therapeutic	0.5–1.25 mEq/L	1	0.5–1.25 mmol/L
Low-density lipoprotein (LDL) cholesterol			
Target for very high-risk patients	Less than 70 mg/dL	0.0259	Less than 1.81 mmol/L
Target for high-risk patients (optimal)	Less than 100 mg/dL	0.0259	Less than 2.59 mmol/L
Desirable	Less than 130 mg/dL	0.0259	Less than 3.36 mmol/L
Borderline high risk	130–159 mg/dL	0.0259	3.36–4.11 mmol/L
High risk	Greater than or equal to 160 mg/dL	0.0259	Greater than or equal to 4.14 mmol/L
Luteinizing hormone (LH)			
Male	1–8 mIU/mL	1	1–8 IU/L
Female			
Follicular phase	1–12 mIU/mL	1	1–12 IU/L
Midcycle	16–104 mIU/mL	1	16–104 IU/L
Luteal phase	1–12 mIU/mL	1	1–12 IU/L
Postmenopausal	16–66 mIU/mL	1	16–66 IU/L
Lymphocyte count	1.2–3.3 × 10³/mm³	10⁶	1.2–3.3 × 10⁹/L
Magnesium	1.3–2.2 mEq/L	0.5	0.65–1.10 mmol/L
	1.58–2.68 mg/dL	0.411	0.65–1.10 mmol/L
Mean corpuscular volume (MCV)	80.0–97.6 µm³	1	80.0–97.6 fL
Mononuclear cell count	0.2–0.7 × 10³/mm³	10⁶	0.2–0.7 × 10⁹/L

(Continued)

Laboratory Test	Conventional Units	Conversion Factor	Système International Units
Nortriptyline, therapeutic	50–150 ng/mL or mcg/L	3.797	190–570 nmol/L
Osmolality (serum)	275–300 mOsm/kg	1	275–300 mmol/kg
Osmolality (urine)	250–900 mOsm/kg	1	250–900 mmol/kg
Parathyroid hormone (PTH), intact	10–60 pg/mL or ng/L	0.107	1.1–6.4 pmol/L
PTH, N-terminal	8–24 pg/mL or ng/L		
PTH, C-terminal	50–330 pg/mL or ng/L		
Phenobarbital, therapeutic	15–40 mcg/mL or mg/L	4.31	65–172 µmol/L
Phenytoin, therapeutic	10–20 mcg/mL or mg/L	3.96	40–79 µmol/L
Phosphate	2.5–4.5 mg/dL	0.323	0.81–1.45 mmol/L
Platelet count	140–$440 \times 10^3/mm^3$	10^6	140–$440 \times 10^9/L$
Potassium (plasma)	3.3–4.9 mEq/L	1	3.3–4.9 mmol/L
Prealbumin (adult)	19.5–35.8 mg/dL	10	195–358 mg/L
Primidone, therapeutic	5–12 mcg/mL or mg/L	4.58	23–55 µmol/L
Procainamide, therapeutic	4–10 mcg/mL or mg/L	4.25	17–42 µmol/L
Progesterone			
Male	13–97 ng/dL	0.0318	0.4–3.1 nmol/L
Female			
Follicular phase	15–70 ng/dL	0.0318	0.5–2.2 nmol/L
Luteal phase	200–2,500 ng/dL	0.0318	6.4–79.5 nmol/L
Prolactin	Less than 20 ng/mL	1	Less than 20 mcg/L
Prostate-specific antigen (PSA)	Less than 4 ng/mL	1	Less than 4 mcg/L
Protein, total	6.0–8.0 g/dL	10	60–80 g/L
Prothrombin time (PT)	10–12 second		
Quinidine, therapeutic	2–5 mcg/mL or mg/L	3.08	6.2–15.4 µmol/L
Radioactive iodine uptake (RAIU)	Less than 6% in 2 hours		
Red blood cell (RBC) count (blood)			
Male	4–$6.2 \times 10^6/mm^3$	10^6	4–$6.2 \times 10^{12}/L$
Female	4–$6.2 \times 10^6/mm^3$	10^6	4–$6.2 \times 10^{12}/L$
Pregnant			
Trimester 1	4–$5 \times 10^6/mm^3$	10^6	4–$5 \times 10^{12}/L$
Trimester 2	3.2–$4.5 \times 10^6/mm^3$	10^6	3.2–$4.5 \times 10^{12}/L$
Trimester 3	3–$4.9 \times 10^6/mm^3$	10^6	3–$4.9 \times 10^{12}/L$
Postpartum	3.2–$5 \times 10^6/mm^3$	10^6	3.2–$5 \times 10^{12}/L$
Red blood cell distribution width (RDW)	11.5–14.5%	0.01	0.115–0.145
Reticulocyte count			
Male	0.5–1.5% of total RBC count	0.01	0.005–0.015
Female	0.5–2.5% of total RBC count	0.01	0.005–0.025
Retinol-binding protein (RBP)	2.7–7.6 mg/dL	10	27–76 mg/L
Rheumatoid factor (RF) titer	Negative		
Salicylate, therapeutic	150–300 mcg/mL or mg/L	0.00724	1.09–2.17 mmol/L
	15–30 mg/dL	0.0724	1.09–2.17 mmol/L
Sirolimus (renal transplant)	4–20 ng/mL	1	4–20 mcg/L
		1.094	4–22 nmol/L
Sodium	135–145 mEq/L	1	135–145 mmol/L
Tacrolimus			
Renal, cardiac, liver, or pancreatic	5–20 ng/mL	1	5–20 mcg/L
transplant		1.24	6.2-24.8 nmol/L
Testosterone (total)			
Men	300–950 ng/dL	0.0347	10.4–33.0 nmol/L
Women	20–80 ng/dL	0.0347	0.7–2.8 nmol/L
Testosterone (free)			
Men	9–30 ng/dL	0.0347	0.31–1.04 nmol/L
Women	0.3–1.9 ng/dL	0.0347	0.01–0.07 nmol/L
Theophylline			
Therapeutic	5–15 mcg/mL or mg/L	5.55	28–83 µmol/L
Toxic	20 mcg/mL or mg/L or more	5.55	111 µmol/L or more
Thiocyanate	Toxic level unclear; units are mcg/mL or mg/L	17.2	µmol/L
Thrombin time	20–24 second		
Thyroglobulin	Less than 42 ng/mL	1	Less than 42 mcg/L
Thyroglobulin antibodies	Negative		
Thyroxine-binding globulin (TBG)	1.2–2.5 mg/dL	10	12–25 mcg/L
Thyroid-stimulating hormone (TSH)	0.35–6.20 µIU/mL	1	0.35–6.20 mIU/L
TSH receptor antibodies (TSHRab)	0–1 units/mL		
Thyroxine (T_4)			
Total	4.5–12.0 mcg/dL	12.87	58–154 nmol/L
Free	0.7–1.9 ng/dL	12.87	9.0–24.5 pmol/L
Thyroxine index, free (FT_4I)	6.5–12.5		
TIBC—see Iron binding capacity (total)			

(Continued)

Laboratory Test	Conventional Units	Conversion Factor	Système International Units
Tobramycin, therapeutic			
Peak	4–10 mcg/mL or mg/L	2.14	8.6–21.4 µmol/L
Trough	Less than or equal to 2 mcg/mL or mg/L	2.14	Less than or equal to 4.3 µmol/L
Transferrin	200–430 mg/dL	0.01	2.0–4.3 g/L
Transferrin saturation	30–50%	0.01	0.30–0.50
Triglycerides (fasting)	Less than 160 mg/dL	0.0113	Less than 1.81 mmol/L
Triiodothyronine (T_3)	45–132 ng/dL	0.0154	0.0.69–2.03 nmol/L
Triiodothyronine (T_3) resin uptake	25–35%		
Uric acid	3–8 mg/dL	59.48	178–476 µmol/L
Urinalysis (urine)			
pH	4.8–8.0		4.8–8.0
Specific gravity	1.005–1.030		
Protein	Negative		
Glucose	Negative		
Ketones	Negative		
RBC	1–2 per low-power field		
WBC	Less than 5 per low-power field		
Valproic acid, therapeutic	50–100 mcg/mL or mg/L	6.93	346–693 µmol/L
Vancomycin, therapeutic			
Peak	20–40 mcg/mL or mg/L	0.690	14–28 µmol/L
Trough	10–20 mcg/mL or mg/L	0.690	7–14 µmol/L
Trough for central nervous system infections	15–20 mcg/mL or mg/L	0.690	10–14 µmol/L
Vitamin A (retinol)	30–95 mcg/dL	0.0349	1.05–3.32 µmol/L
Vitamin B_{12}	180–1,000 pg/mL	0.738	133–738 pmol/L
Vitamin D_3, 125-dihydroxy	20–76 pg/mL	2.4	48–182 pmol/L
Vitamin D_3, 25-hydroxy	10–50 ng/mL	2.496	25–125 nmol/L
Vitamin E (a-tocopherol)	0.5–2.0 mg/dL	23.22	12–46 µmol/L
WBC count	$4–10 \times 10^3/mm^3$	10^6	$4–10 \times 10^9/L$
WBC differential (peripheral blood)			
Polymorphonuclear neutrophils (PMNs)	50–65%	0.01	0.50–0.65
Bands	0–5%	0.01	0–0.05
Eosinophils	0–3%	0.01	0–0.03
Basophils	1–3%	0.01	0.01–0.03
Lymphocytes	25–35%	0.01	0.25–0.35
Monocytes	2–6%	0.01	0.02–0.06
WBC differential (bone marrow)			
PMNs	3–11%	0.01	0.03–0.11
Bands	9–15%	0.01	0.09–0.15
Metamyelocytes	9–25%	0.01	0.09–0.25
Myelocytes	8–16%	0.01	0.08–0.16
Promyelocytes	1–8%	0.01	0.01–0.08
Myeloblasts	0–5%	0.01	0–0.05
Eosinophils	1–5%	0.01	0.01–0.05
Basophils	0–1%	0.01	0–0.01
Lymphocytes	11–23%	0.01	0.11–0.23
Monocytes	0–1%	0.01	0–0.01
Zinc	60–150 mcg/dL	0.153	9.2–23.0 µmol/L

[a]Hemoglobin A1c (mmol/mol hemoglobin) = (Hemoglobin A1c (%) − 2.15) × 10.929.

This table is a modification of the Medical Algorithms Project (Chapter 40), unit conversions of the following Excel worksheets: Conversion of Conventional to SI units: Blood Chemistries; Conversion of Conventional to SI units: Urine Chemistries; Conversion of Conventional to SI units: Hematology and Coagulation; and Conversion of Conventional to SI units: Therapeutic Drug Monitoring.

Other references (conventional and SI units from the preceding table were double-checked against the following references and modified as needed):

A–Z Health Guide from WebMD. Medical Tests: Brain Natriuretic Peptide (BNP) Test. Available at http://www.webmd.com/heart-disease/brain-natriuretic-peptide-bnp-test?page=2; accessed October 28, 2011.

proBNP ©2005 Roche Diagnostics Roche Diagnostics GmbH, D-68298 Mannheim.

Jacobs, D.S., Oxley, D.K., DeMott, W.R. (Eds.). (2001) Laboratory Test Handbook (5th ed.). Hudson OH: Lexi-Comp, Inc.

Young, D.S., Huth, E.J. (Eds.). (1998) SI units for clinical measurement. Philadelphia, PA: American College of Physicians.

Reviewed and updated by: Edward W. Randell.

Appendix C: Common Medical Abbreviations

These are the abbreviations used commonly in medical practice both in verbal communication and in the medical record.

A&O	alert and oriented
A&O×3	awake (or alert) and oriented to person, place, and time
A&O×4	awake (or alert) and oriented to person, place, time, and situation
A&P	active and present; anterior and posterior; assessment and plans; auscultation and percussion
A&W	alive and well
A1c	hemoglobin A1c
AA	aplastic anemia; alcoholics anonymous
AAA	abdominal aortic aneurysm
AAO	awake, alert, and oriented
AAO×3	awake and orientated to time, place, and person
ABC	absolute band counts; absolute basophil count; apnea, bradycardia, and cytology; aspiration, biopsy, and cytology; artificial beta cells
Abd	abdomen
ABG	arterial blood gases
ABO	blood group system (A, AB, B, and O)
ABP	arterial blood pressure
ABW	actual body weight
ABx	antibiotics
AC	before meals (*ante cibos*)
ACE	angiotensin-converting enzyme
ACE-I	angiotensin-converting enzyme inhibitor
ACLS	advanced cardiac life support
ACS	acute coronary syndromes
ACTH	adrenocorticotropic hormone
AD	Alzheimer's disease; right ear (*auris dextra*)
ADA	American Diabetes Association; adenosine deaminase
ADE	adverse drug effect (or event)
ADH	antidiuretic hormone
ADHD	attention-deficit hyperactivity disorder
ADL	activities of daily living
ADR	adverse drug reaction
AF	atrial fibrillation
AFB	Acid-fast bacillus; aortofemoral bypass; aspirated foreign body

AFEB	afebrile
AI	aortic insufficiency
AIDS	acquired immune deficiency syndrome
AKA	above-knee amputation; alcoholic ketoacidosis; all known allergies; also known as
AKI	acute kidney injury
ALFT	abnormal liver function test
ALL	acute lymphoblastic leukemia; acute lymphocytic leukemia
ALP	alkaline phosphatase
ALS	amyotrophic lateral sclerosis
ALT	alanine transaminase (SGPT); alanine aminotransferase
AMA	against medical advice; American Medical Association; antimitochondrial antibody
AMI	acute myocardial infarction
AML	acute myelogenous leukemia
Amp	ampule
ANA	antinuclear antibody
ANC	absolute neutrophil count
ANLL	acute nonlymphocytic leukemia
AODM	adult-onset diabetes mellitus
AOM	acute otitis media
AP	anteroposterior
APAP	acetaminophen (acetyl-*p*-aminophenol)
aPTT	activated partial thromboplastin time
ARB	angiotensin receptor blocker
ARC	AIDS-related complex
ARD	acute respiratory disease; adult respiratory disease; antibiotic removal device; aphakic retinal detachment
ARDS	adult respiratory distress syndrome
ARF	acute renal failure; acute respiratory failure; acute rheumatic fever
AROM	active range of motion
AS	left ear (*auris sinistra*)
ASA	aspirin (acetylsalicylic acid)
ASCVD	arteriosclerotic cardiovascular disease
ASD	atrial septal defect
ASH	asymmetric septal hypertrophy
ASHD	arteriosclerotic heart disease

AST	aspartate transaminase (SGOT); aspartate aminotransferase
ATG	antithymocyte globulin
ATN	acute tubular necrosis
AU	each ear (*auris uterque*)
AV	arteriovenous; atrioventricular; auditory visual
AVR	aortic valve replacement
BBB	bundle branch block; blood–brain barrier
BC	blood culture
BCOP	Board Certified Oncology Pharmacist
BCP	birth control pill
BCPP	Board Certified Psychiatric Pharmacist
BCPS	Board Certified Pharmacotherapy Specialist
BE	barium enema
BG	blood glucose
bid	twice daily (*bis in die*)
BKA	below-knee amputation
BM	bone marrow; bowel movement; an isoenzyme of creatine phosphokinase
BMC	bone marrow cells
BMD	bone mineral density
BMI	body mass index
BMP	basic metabolic panel
BMR	basal metabolic rate
BMT	bone marrow transplantation
BP	blood pressure
BPD	bronchopulmonary dysplasia
BPH	benign prostatic hyperplasia
bpm	beats per minute
BR	bed rest
BS	bowel sounds; breath sounds; blood sugar
BSA	body surface area
BUN	blood urea nitrogen
Bx	biopsy
C&S	culture and sensitivity
CA	cancer; calcium
CABG	coronary artery bypass grafting
CAD	coronary artery disease
CAH	chronic active hepatitis
CAM	complementary and alternative medicine
CAPD	continuous ambulatory peritoneal dialysis
CBC	complete blood count
CBD	common bile duct
CBG	capillary blood gas; corticosteroid-binding globulin
CC	chief complaint
CCA	calcium channel antagonist
CCB	calcium channel blocker
CCE	clubbing, cyanosis, edema
CCK	cholecystokinin
CCU	coronary care unit
CF	cystic fibrosis
CFS	chronic fatigue syndrome
CFU	colony-forming unit
CHD	coronary heart disease
CHF	congestive heart failure; chronic heart failure
CHO	carbohydrate
CI	Cardiac index

CIWA	Clinical Institute Withdrawal Assessment
CK	creatine kinase
CKD	chronic kidney disease
CLL	chronic lymphocytic leukemia
CM	costal margin
CMG	cystometrogram
CML	chronic myelogenous leukemia
CMV	cytomegalovirus
CN	cranial nerve
CNS	central nervous system
C/O	complains of
CO	cardiac output; carbon monoxide
COLD	chronic obstructive lung disease
COPD	chronic obstructive pulmonary disease
CP	chest pain; cerebral palsy
CPAP	continuous positive airway pressure
CPK	creatine phosphokinase (BB, MB, and MM are isoenzymes)
CPP	cerebral perfusion pressure
CPR	cardiopulmonary resuscitation
CrCl	creatinine clearance
CRF	chronic renal failure; corticotropin-releasing factor
CRH	corticotropin-releasing hormone
CRI	chronic renal insufficiency; catheter-related infection
CRNA	Certified Registered Nurse Anesthetist
CRNP	Certified Registered Nurse Practitioner
CRP	C-reactive protein
CRTT	Certified Respiratory Therapy Technician
CSF	cerebrospinal fluid; colony-stimulating factor
CT	computed tomography; chest tube
cTnI	cardiac troponin I
CTZ	chemoreceptor trigger zone
CV	cardiovascular
CVA	cerebrovascular accident
CVC	central venous catheter
CVP	central venous pressure
Cx	culture; cervix
CXR	chest x-ray
CYP	cytochrome P450
D&C	dilatation and curettage
D_5W	5% dextrose in water
DBP	diastolic blood pressure
D/C	discontinue; discharge
DCC	direct-current cardioversion
DI	diabetes insipidus
DIC	disseminated intravascular coagulation
Diff	differential
DJD	degenerative joint disease
DKA	diabetic ketoacidosis
dL	deciliter
DM	diabetes mellitus
DNA	deoxyribonucleic acid
DNR	do not resuscitate
DO	Doctor of osteopathy
DOA	dead on arrival; date of admission; duration of action

DOB	date of birth
DOE	dyspnea on exertion
DOT	directly observed therapy
DPGN	diffuse proliferative glomerulonephritis
DPI	dry powder inhaler
DRE	digital rectal examination
DRG	diagnosis-related group
DS	double strength
d/t	due to
DTP	diphtheria–tetanus–pertussis
DTR	deep tendon reflex
DVT	deep vein thrombosis
Dx	diagnosis
EBV	Epstein-Barr virus
EC	enteric coated
ECF	extracellular fluid
ECG	electrocardiogram
ECHO	echocardiogram
ECT	electroconvulsive therapy
ED	emergency department
EEG	electroencephalogram
EENT	eyes, ears, nose, throat
EF	ejection fraction
EGD	esophagogastroduodenoscopy
EIA	enzyme immunoassay
ECG	electrocardiogram
EMG	electromyogram
EMT	Emergency Medical Technician
Endo	endotracheal, endoscopy
EOMI	extraocular movements (or muscles) intact
EPO	erythropoietin
EPS	extrapyramidal symptoms
ER	emergency room
ERCP	endoscopic retrograde cholangiopancreatography
ERT	estrogen replacement therapy
ESKD	end-stage kidney disease
ESLD	end-stage liver disease
ESR	erythrocyte sedimentation rate
ESRD	end-stage renal disease
ET	endotracheal
EtOH	ethanol
FB	finger breadth; foreign body
FBS	fasting blood sugar
FDA	Food and Drug Administration
FEF	forced expiratory flow rate
FEV_1	forced expiratory volume in 1 second
FFP	fresh-frozen plasma
FH	family history
FiO_2	fraction of inspired oxygen
FOBT	fecal occult blood test
FPG	fasting plasma glucose
FPIA	fluorescence polarization immunoassay
FSH	follicle-stimulating hormone
FTA	fluorescent treponemal antibody
FT_4	free thyroxine
F/U	follow-up
FUO	fever of unknown origin
Fx	fracture

g	gram
G-CSF	granulocyte colony-stimulating factor
G6PD	glucose-6-phosphate dehydrogenase
GB	gallbladder
GBS	group B *Streptococcus*; Guillain-Barré syndrome
GC	gonococcus
GDM	gestational diabetes mellitus
GE	gastroesophageal; gastroenterology
GERD	gastroesophageal reflux disease
GFR	glomerular filtration rate
GGT	γ-glutamyl transferase
GGTP	γ-glutamyl transpeptidase
GI	gastrointestinal
GM-CSF	granulocyte-macrophage colony-stimulating factor
GN	glomerulonephritis; graduate nurse
gr	grain
GT	gastrostomy tube
gtt	drops (*guttae*)
GTT	glucose tolerance test
GU	genitourinary
GVHD	graft-versus-host disease
GVL	graft-versus-leukemia
Gyn	gynecology
H&H, H/H	hemoglobin and hematocrit
H&P	history and physical examination
HA	headache
HAART	highly active antiretroviral therapy
HAMD	Hamilton Rating Scale for Depression
HAV	Hepatitis A virus
Hb, hgb	hemoglobin
HbAlc	glycosylated hemoglobin (hemoglobin Alc)
HBIG	hepatitis B immune globulin
HBP	high blood pressure
HBsAg	hepatitis B surface antigen
HBV	hepatitis B virus
HC	hydrocortisone, home care
HCG	human chorionic gonadotropin
HCO_3	bicarbonate
Hct	hematocrit
HCTZ	hydrochlorothiazide
HCV	hepatitis C virus
HD	Hodgkin's disease; hemodialysis
HDL	high-density lipoprotein
HEENT	head, eyes, ears, nose, and throat
HF	heart failure
HFA	hydrofluoroalkane
H flu	*Hemophilus influenzae*
HGH	human growth hormone
HH	hiatal hernia
Hib	*Hemophilus influenzae* type b
HIT	heparin-induced thrombocytopenia
HIV	human immunodeficiency virus
HJR	hepatojugular reflux
HLA	human leukocyte antigen; human lymphocyte antigen
HMG-CoA	hydroxy-methylglutaryl coenzyme A

H/O	history of	kcal	kilocalorie
HOB	head of bed	KCl	potassium chloride
HPA	hypothalamic–pituitary axis	KOH	potassium hydroxide
hpf	high-power field	KUB	kidney, ureter, and bladder
HPI	history of present illness	KVO	keep vein open
HR	heart rate	L	liter
H_2RA	H_2 receptor antagonist	LABA	long-acting beta agonist
HRSD	Hamilton Rating Scale for Depression	LAD	left anterior descending; left axis deviation
HRT	hormone-replacement therapy	LAO	left anterior oblique
HS	at bedtime (*hora somni*)	LBBB	left bundle branch block
HSV	herpes simplex virus	LBP	low-back pain
HTN	hypertension	LDH	lactate dehydrogenase
Hx	history	LDL	low-density lipoprotein
I&D	incision and drainage	LE	lower extremity
I&O, I/O	intake and output	LES	lower esophageal sphincter
IBD	inflammatory bowel disease	LFT	liver function test
IBW	ideal body weight	LHRH	luteinizing hormone-releasing hormone
ICD	implantable cardioverter defibrillator	LLE	left lower extremity
ICP	intracranial pressure	LLL	left lower lobe
ICS	intercostal space; inhaled corticosteroid	LLQ	left lower quadrant (abdomen)
ICU	intensive care unit	LMD	local medical doctor
ID	identification; infectious disease	LMP	last menstrual period
IDDM	insulin-dependent diabetes mellitus	LMWH	low-molecular-weight heparin
IFN	interferon	LOS	length of stay
Ig	immunoglobulin	LP	lumbar puncture
IgA	immunoglobulin A	LPN	Licensed Practical Nurse
IgD	immunoglobulin D	LPT	Licensed Physical Therapist
IHD	ischemic heart disease	LR	Lactated Ringer's
IJ	internal jugular	LS	lumbosacral
IM	intramuscular; infectious mononucleosis	LT_4	levothyroxine
INH	isoniazid	LUE	left upper extremity
INR	international normalized ratio	LUL	left upper lobe
IOP	intraocular pressure	LUQ	left upper quadrant
IP	intraperitoneal	LUTS	lower urinary tract symptoms
IPG	impedance plethysmography	LVH	left ventricular hypertrophy
IPN	interstitial pneumonia	MAP	mean arterial pressure
IRB	institutional review board	MAR	medication administration record
ISA	intrinsic sympathomimetic activity	MB-CK	a creatine kinase isoenzyme
ISH	isolated systolic hypertension	mcg	microgram
IT	intrathecal	MCH	mean corpuscular hemoglobin
ITP	idiopathic thrombocytopenic purpura	MCHC	mean corpuscular hemoglobin concentration
IU	international units (this can be dangerous abbreviation because it may be read as "IV" for "intravenous")	MCV	mean corpuscular volume
		MD	Medical Doctor
		MDI	metered-dose inhaler
IUD	intrauterine device	MDRD	modification of diet in renal disease
IV	intravenous; Roman numeral four; symbol for class 4 controlled substances	MEFR	maximum expiratory flow rate
		mEq	milliequivalent
IVC	inferior vena cava; intravenous cholangiogram	mg	milligram
		MHC	major histocompatibility complex
IVDA	intravenous drug abuse	MI	myocardial infarction; mitral insufficiency
IVDU	injection drug use; intravenous drug use	MIC	minimum inhibitory concentration
IVF	intravenous fluids	mL	milliliter
IVIG	intravenous immunoglobulin	MM	multiple myeloma; an isoenzyme of creatine phosphokinase
IVP	intravenous pyelogram; intravenous push		
JODM	juvenile-onset diabetes mellitus		
JRA	juvenile rheumatoid arthritis	MMR	measles–mumps–rubella; midline malignant reticulosis
JVD	jugular venous distension		
JVP	jugular venous pressure	MOM	milk of magnesia
K	potassium	MPV	mean platelet volume

m/r/g	murmur/rub/gallop
MRI	magnetic resonance imaging
MRSA	methicillin-resistant *Staphylococcus aureus*
MRSE	methicillin-resistant *Staphylococcus epidermitis*
MS	mental status; mitral stenosis; musculoskeletal; multiple sclerosis; morphine sulfate
MSE	mental status exam
MSW	Master of Social Work
MTD	maximum tolerated dose
MTX	methotrexate
MVA	motor vehicle accident
MVI	multivitamin
MVR	mitral valve replacement; mitral valve regurgitation
MVS	mitral valve stenosis; motor, vascular, and sensory
N&V	nausea and vomiting
NAD	no acute (or apparent) distress
N/C	noncontributory; nasal cannula
NG	nasogastric
NGT	nasogastric tube; normal glucose tolerance
NIDDM	non–insulin-dependent diabetes mellitus
NIH	National Institutes of Health
NKA	no known allergies
NKDA	no known drug allergies
NHDA	nonketotic hyperosmolar acidosis
NL	normal
NOS	not otherwise specified
NPN	nonprotein nitrogen
NPO	nothing by mouth (*nil per os*)
NS	normal saline solution (0.9% sodium chloride solution); neurosurgery
NSAID	nonsteroidal antiinflammatory drug
NSR	normal sinus rhythm
NSS	normal saline solution
NTG	nitroglycerin
NT/ND	nontender, nondistended
NVD	nausea/vomiting/diarrhea; neck vein distension; neovascularization of the disk; neurovesicle dysfunction; nonvalvular disease
N&V	nausea and vomiting
NYHA	New York Heart Association
O&P	ova and parasites
OA	osteoarthritis
OB	obstetrics
OCD	obsessive-compulsive disorder
OD	right eye (*oculus dexter*)
OGTT	oral glucose tolerance test
OPV	Oral poliovirus vaccine
OR	operating room
OR×1	oriented to time
OR×2	oriented to time and place
OR×3	oriented to time, place, and person
OS	left eye (*oculus sinister*)
OSA	obstructive sleep apnea
OT	occupational therapy
OTC	over the counter
OU	each eye (*oculus uterque*)

P	pulse; plan; percussion; pressure
P&A	percussion and auscultation
P&T	peak and trough
PA	physician assistant; posteroanterior; pulmonary artery
PAC	premature atrial contraction
$Paco_2$	arterial carbon dioxide tension
Pao_2	arterial oxygen tension
PAOP	pulmonary artery occlusion pressure
PC	after meals (*post cibum*)
PCA	patient-controlled analgesia
PCI	percutaneous coronary intervention
PCKD	polycystic kidney disease
PCN	penicillin
PCP	*Pneumocystis carinii* pneumonia (also known as *Pneumocystis jirovecii* pneumonia); pneumocystis pneumonia; primary care physician; phencyclidine
PCWP	pulmonary capillary wedge pressure
PDE	paroxysmal dyspnea on exertion
PE	physical examination; pulmonary embolism
PEEP	positive end-expiratory pressure
PEFR	peak expiratory flow rate
PEG	percutaneous endoscopic gastrostomy; polyethylene glycol
Peg-IFN	pegylated interferon
PERL	pupils equal, react to light
PERRLA	pupils equal, round, and reactive to light and accommodation
PERRRLA	pupils equal, round, regular, and react to light and accommodation
PET	positron emission tomography
PFT	pulmonary function test
pH	hydrogen ion concentration
PH	past history; personal history; pinhole; poor health; pubic hair; public health
PHx	past history
PharmD	Doctor of Pharmacy
PID	pelvic inflammatory disease
PJD	*Pneumocystis jirovecii* pneumonia (also known as *Pneumocystis carinii* pneumonia)
PKU	phenylketonuria
PMH	past medical history
PMI	past medical illness; point of maximal impulse
PMN	polymorphonuclear leukocyte
PMS	premenstrual syndrome
PND	paroxysmal nocturnal dyspnea
Po	by mouth (*per os*)
Po_2	partial pressure of oxygen
POAG	primary open-angle glaucoma
POD	postoperative day
PPBG	postprandial blood glucose
ppd	packs per day
PPI	proton pump inhibitor
PPN	peripheral parenteral nutrition
PR	per rectum
PRBC	packed red blood cell

PRERLA	pupils round, equal, react to light and accommodation
PRN	when necessary, as needed (*pro re nata*)
PSA	prostate-specific antigen
PSH	past surgical history
PST	paroxysmal supraventricular tachycardia
PSVT	paroxysmal supraventricular tachycardia
PT	prothrombin time; physical therapy; patient
PTA	prior to admission; percutaneous transluminal angioplasty
PTCA	percutaneous transluminal coronary angioplasty
PTE	pulmonary thromboembolism
PTH	parathyroid hormone
PTSD	posttraumatic stress disorder
PTT	partial thromboplastin time
PUD	peptic ulcer disease
PVC	premature ventricular contraction
PVD	peripheral vascular disease
PVR	peripheral vascular resistance
PVT	paroxysmal ventricular tachycardia
q	every (*quaque*)
QA	quality assurance
qday	every day (*quaque die*)
QI	quality improvement
qid	four times daily (*quater in die*)
QNS	quantity not sufficient
qod	every other day
QOL	quality of life
QS	quantity sufficient
QTc	corrected QT interval
R&M	routine and microscopic
R&R	rate and rhythm
RA	rheumatoid arthritis; right atrium
RAAS	renin–angiotensin–aldosterone system
RBC	red blood cell
RCA	right coronary artery
RCM	right costal margin
RDA	Recommended Daily Allowance
RDS	respiratory distress syndrome
RDW	red blood cell distribution width
REM	rapid eye movement; recent event memory
RES	reticuloendothelial system
RF	rheumatoid factor; renal failure; rheumatic fever
Rh	rhesus factor in blood
RHD	rheumatic heart disease
RLE	right lower extremity
RLL	right lower lobe
RLQ	right lower quadrant
RML	right middle lobe
RN	Registered Nurse
RNA	ribonucleic acid
R/O	rule out
ROM	range of motion
ROS	review of systems
RPh	Registered Pharmacist
RR	respiratory rate; recovery room
RRR	regular rate and rhythm
RRT	Registered Respiratory Therapist
RSV	respiratory syncytial virus
RT	radiation therapy
RUE	right upper extremity
RUL	right upper lobe
RUQ	right upper quadrant
RVH	right ventricular hypertrophy
S_1	first heart sound
S_2	second heart sound
S_3	third heart sound (ventricular gallop)
S_4	fourth heart sound (atrial gallop)
SA	sinoatrial
SABA	short-acting beta agonist
SAD	seasonal affective disorder
SAH	subarachnoid hemorrhage
Sao_2	arterial oxygen percent saturation
SBE	subacute bacterial endocarditis
SBFT	small bowel follow-through
SBGM	self-blood glucose monitoring
SBO	small bowel obstruction
SBP	systolic blood pressure
SC	subcutaneous; subclavian
SCr	serum creatinine
SEM	systolic ejection murmur
SG	specific gravity
SGOT (AST)	serum glutamic oxaloacetic transaminase (aspartate transaminase)
SGPT (ALT)	serum glutamic pyruvic transaminase (alanine transaminase)
SH	social history
SIADH	syndrome of inappropriate antidiuretic hormone secretion
SIDS	sudden infant death syndrome
SJS	Stevens-Johnson syndrome
SL	sublingual
SLE	systemic lupus erythematosus
SMA-6	sequential multiple analyzer for sodium, potassium, CO_2, chloride, glucose, and BUN
SMA-7	sequential multiple analyzer for sodium, potassium, CO_2, chloride, glucose, BUN, and creatinine
SMA-12	sequential multiple analyzer for glucose, BUN, uric acid, calcium, phosphorous, total protein, albumin, cholesterol, total bilirubin, alkaline phosphatase, SGOT, and LDH
SMA-23	includes the entire SMA-12 plus sodium, potassium, CO_2, chloride, direct bilirubin, triglyceride, SGPT, indirect bilirubin, R fraction, and BUN/creatinine ratio
SMBG	self-monitoring of blood glucose
SNF	skilled nursing facility
SNS	sympathetic nervous system
SOB	shortness of breath; see order book; side of bed
S/P	status post
SPF	sun protection factor
SQ	subcutaneous

SSKI	saturated solution of potassium iodide		TOD	target organ damage
SSRI	selective serotonin reuptake inhibitor		TPN	total parenteral nutrition
STAT	immediately; at once		TPR	temperature, pulse, respiration
STEMI	ST-segment elevated myocardial infarction		T PROT	total protein
STD	sexually transmitted disease		TSH	thyroid-stimulating hormone
SV	stroke volume		TURP	transurethral resection of the prostate
SVC	superior vena cava		Tx	treat, treatment
SVRI	systemic vascular resistance index		UA	urinalysis, uric acid
SVR	supraventricular rhythm; systemic vascular resistance		UC	ulcerative colitis
			UE	upper extremity
SVT	supraventricular tachycardia		UFH	unfractionated heparin
SW	social worker		UGI	upper gastrointestinal
Sx	signs		UOQ	upper outer quadrant
T	temperature		UPT	urine pregnancy test
T_3	triiodothyroxine		URI	upper respiratory infection
T_4	thyroxine		USP	United States Pharmacopeia
T&A	tonsillectomy and adenoidectomy		UTI	urinary tract infection
T&C	type and crossmatch		UV	ultraviolet
TB	tuberculosis		VF	ventricular fibrillation
TBG	thyroid-binding globulin		VLDL	very low-density lipoprotein
TBI	total-body irradiation; traumatic brain injury		VO	verbal order
TBW	total body weight		VOD	veno-occlusive disease
T bili	total bilirubin		V_A/Q	ventilation–perfusion
TCA	tricyclic antidepressant		VRE	vancomycin-resistant Enterococcus
TCN	tetracycline		VS	vital signs
Tdap	tetanus, diphtheria, acellular pertussis vaccine		VSS	vital signs stable
			VT	ventricular tachycardia
TEE	transesophageal echocardiogram		VTE	venous thromboembolism
TFT	thyroid function test		WA	while awake
TG	triglyceride		WBC	white blood cell (count)
TIA	transient ischemic attack		W/C	wheelchair
TIBC	total iron-binding capacity		WDWN	well-developed, well-nourished
tid	three times daily (*ter in die*)		WHO	World Health Organization
TLC	therapeutic lifestyle changes		WNL	within normal limits
TMJ	Temporomandibular joint		W/U	workup
TMP-SMX	trimethoprim–sulfamethoxazole		yo	year old
TNTC	too numerous to count		y	year

Acanthosis nigricans: Increased thickness and hyperpigmentation of the outer cell layers of the skin; typically observed at areas of flexure.

Acaricide: A chemical that kills mites and ticks.

Acetaldehyde: Metabolic by-product of alcohol; hepatotoxic.

Acetylcholine: Neurotransmitter responsible for transmitting messages between certain nerve cells in the brain.

Achalasia: Disorder in which the esophageal sphincter is impaired, preventing normal swallowing and often causing reflux of contents and a feeling that something is caught in the throat.

Achlorhydria: Absence of free hydrochloric acid in the stomach.

Acidemia: An increase in the hydrogen ion concentration of the blood or a fall below normal in pH.

Acidosis: Any pathologic state that leads to acidemia.

Acinar cells: Exocrine glands of the pancreas that secrete digestive enzymes.

Acromegaly: A pathologic condition characterized by excessive production of growth hormone during adulthood after epiphyseal (long bone) fusions have completed.

Action potential: A rapid change in the polarity of the voltage of a cell membrane from negative to positive and back to negative; a wave of electrical discharge that travels across a cell membrane.

Acute coronary syndromes: Ischemic chest discomfort at rest most often accompanied by ST-segment elevation, ST-segment depression, or T-wave inversion on the 12-lead electrocardiogram; further, it is caused by plaque rupture and partial or complete occlusion of the coronary artery by thrombus. Acute coronary syndromes include myocardial infarction and unstable angina. Former terms used to describe types of acute coronary syndromes include Q-wave myocardial infarction, non–Q-wave myocardial infarction, and unstable angina.

Acute disorder: An acid-base disturbance that has been present for minutes to hours.

Acute kidney injury: Spectrum of acute changes in kidney function ranging from minor changes to those requiring renal replacement therapy.

Acute otitis media: Inflammation of the middle ear accompanied by fluid in the middle ear space and signs or symptoms of an acute ear infection.

Acute tubular necrosis: Form of acute kidney injury that results from toxic or ischemic injury to the cells in the proximal tubule of the kidney.

Adenoma: A nonmalignant tumor of the epithelial tissue that is characterized by glandular structures.

Adenomatous polyposis coli gene: A tumor suppressor gene (see definition) that is one of the first genes mutated in the development of colon cancer. Patients with familial adenomatous polyposis are born with this gene mutated.

Adjuvant chemotherapy: Treatment given after the primary treatment that is designed to eliminate any remaining cancer cells that are undetectable with the goal of improving survival. Adjuvant therapy for cancer usually refers to surgery followed by chemotherapy or radiation.

Adjuvant therapy: Treatment which follows the primary modality with the intent of reducing the risk of disease relapse and prolonging survival. The ultimate goal is to cure patients who would not otherwise be cured by the primary modality alone.

Adnexal: Adjacent or appending as the fallopian tubes and ovaries are to the uterus.

Adrenalectomy: Surgical removal of an adrenal gland.

Adrenocorticotropic hormone: A hormone secreted by the anterior pituitary that controls secretion of cortisol from the adrenal glands. Also referred to as corticotropin.

Adverse drug reaction: Any unexpected, unintended, undesired, or excessive response to a medication that may require discontinuing the medication, changing the medication, or modifying the dose (except for minor dosage adjustments); necessitates admission to the hospital; prolongs stay in a healthcare facility; necessitates supportive treatment; significantly complicates diagnosis; negatively affects prognosis; or results in temporary or permanent harm, disability, or death.

Aeroallergen: An airborne substance that causes an allergic response.

Afterload: The force against which a ventricle contracts that is contributed to by the vascular resistance, especially of the arteries, and by the physical characteristics (mass and viscosity) of the blood.

Ageism: Discrimination against aged persons.

Air embolus: An obstruction in a small blood vessel caused by air that is introduced into a blood vessel and is carried through the circulation until it lodges in a smaller vessel.

Aldosterone: A hormone produced in and secreted by the zona glomerulosa of the adrenal cortex. Aldosterone acts on the kidneys to reabsorb sodium and excrete potassium. It is also a part of the renin-angiotensin-aldosterone system that regulates blood pressure and blood volume.

Alkalemia: A decrease in the hydrogen ion concentration of the blood or a rise above normal in pH.

Alkalosis: Any pathologic state that leads to alkalemia.

Allogeneic: A transplant taking cells from one person and donating them to another.

Allogeneic HSCT: In the setting of stem cell transplantation, the scenario in which the donor is genetically similar but not identical to the recipient. The donor is usually a sibling or a matched related donor.

Allograft: Tissue or organ transplanted from a donor of the same species but different genetic makeup; recipient's immune system must be suppressed to prevent rejection of the graft.

Allograft survival: After the transplant procedure, when the transplanted organ continues to have some degree of function, from excellent to poor.

Allorecognition: Recognition of the foreign antigens present on the transplant organ or the donor's antigen presenting cells.

Alopecia: Hair loss.

Amenorrhea: Abnormal cessation or absence of menses.

Ampulla of Vater: Dilation of the duodenal wall at the opening of the fused pancreatic and common bile ducts.

Amyloid: Any of a group of chemically diverse proteins which are composed of linear nonbranching aggregated fibrils.

Anaphylactic/anaphylaxis: Immediate, severe, potentially fatal hypersensitivity reaction induced by an antigen.

Anaphylactoid: An anaphylactic-like reaction, similar in signs and symptoms but not mediated by IgE. The drug causing this reaction produces direct release of inflammatory mediators by a pharmacologic effect.

Anastomosis: The connection of two hollow organs to restore continuity after resection.

Androgen: A steroid hormone, such as testosterone or androsterone, that controls the development and maintenance of masculine characteristics.

Anemia: A reduction below normal in the concentration of hemoglobin in the body that results in a reduction of the oxygen-carrying capacity of the blood.

Anemia of chronic kidney disease: A decline in red blood cell production caused by a decrease in erythropoietin production by the progenitor cells of the kidney. As kidney function declines in chronic kidney disease, erythropoietin production also declines, resulting in decreased red blood cell production. Other contributing factors include iron deficiency and decreased red blood cell life span caused by uremia.

Anergy: A reduction or lack of an immune response to a specific antigen.

Angina: Discomfort in the chest or adjacent areas caused by decreased blood and oxygen supply to the myocardium (myocardial ischemia).

Angina pectoris: Severe constricting pain in the chest, often radiating from the precordium to a shoulder (usually left) and down the arm, due to ischemia of the heart muscle usually caused by a coronary disease.

Angioedema: Swelling similar to urticaria (hives), but the swelling occurs beneath the skin instead of on the surface. Angioedema is characterized by deep swelling around the eyes and lips and sometimes of the hands and feet. If it proceeds rapidly, it can lead to airway obstruction and suffocation, and it should therefore be treated as a medical emergency.

Angiogenesis: The formation of new blood vessels; tumors require angiogenesis to grow and spread. Antiangiogenesis drugs attempt to block this process, thereby preventing tumor growth.

Angiography: Examination of the blood vessels using x-rays after injection of a radiopaque substance.

Anorexia: The loss of appetite, especially as a result of disease.

Antiangiogenic: Preventing or inhibiting the formation and differentiation of blood vessels.

Anticoagulant: Any substance that inhibits, suppresses, or delays the formation of blood clots. These substances occur naturally and regulate the clotting cascade. Several anticoagulants have been identified in a variety of animal tissues and have been commercially developed for medicinal use.

Antimicrobial prophylaxis: Use of an antimicrobial to prevent an infection.

Antiproteinase: A substance that inhibits the enzymatic activity of a proteinase.

Anuria: Urine output of less than 50 mL over 24 hours.

Apoptosis: Programmed cell death as signaled by the nuclei in normally functioning cells when age or state of cell health and condition dictates.

Arcuate scotoma: An arc-shaped area of blindness in the field of vision.

Arthrocentesis: Puncture and aspiration of a joint. Certain drugs can be injected into the joint space for a local effect.

Arthus reaction: Local inflammatory response due to deposition of immune complexes in tissues.

Articular: Related to a joint or joints.

Ascites: Accumulation of fluid within the peritoneal cavity.

Asterixis: A flapping tremor of the arms and hands that is seen in patients with end-stage liver disease.

Astringent: A substance that causes tissues to constrict, resulting in a drying effect of the skin.

Atelectasis: Decreased or absent air in a partial or entire lung, with resulting loss of lung volume.

Atherosclerosis: Accumulation of lipids, inflammatory cells, and cellular debris in the subendothelial space of the arterial wall.

Atopy: A genetic predisposition to develop type I hypersensitivity reactions against common environmental antigens. Commonly seen in patients with allergic rhinitis, asthma, and atopic dermatitis.

Atresia: Congenital absence of a normal opening or normally patent lumen.

Attenuate: Render less virulent.

Auto-induction: The process of a drug increasing or inducing its own metabolism.

Autologous: A transplant using one's own stem cells.

Autologous HSCT: In the setting of stem cell transplantation, the scenario in which the donor and recipient are the same person.

Automaticity: Ability of a cardiac fiber or tissue to spontaneously initiate depolarizations.

Azoospermic: Having no living spermatozoa in the semen, or failure of spermatogenesis.

B2 microglobulin: A low-molecular-weight protein that may be elevated in multiple myeloma.

Bacille Calmette-Guérin: A tuberculosis vaccine prepared from an attenuated strain of the closely related species *Mycobacterium bovis*, used for immunization against tuberculosis in many countries, but not in the United States.

Bacteriuria: Presence of bacteria in urine.

Barium enema: A diagnostic test using an x-ray examination to view the lower gastrointestinal tract (colon and rectum) after rectal administration of barium sulfate, a chalky liquid contrast medium.

Barrett's esophagus: Disorder in which the cells of the lower esophagus are damaged, most often a result of long-standing reflux.

Bence-Jones proteins: Free light chains of immunoglobulins found in the urine.

Bilateral salpingo-oophorectomy: Surgical excision (removal) of both ovaries.

Bile acids: The organic acids in bile. Bile is the yellowish-brown or green fluid secreted by the liver and discharged into the duodenum where it aids in the emulsification of fats, increases peristalsis, and retards putrefaction; contains sodium glycocholate and sodium taurocholate, cholesterol, biliverdin and bilirubin, mucus, fat, lecithin, and cells and cellular debris.

Biliary sludge: A deposit of tiny stones or crystals made up of cholesterol, calcium bilirubinate, and other calcium salts. The cholesterol and calcium bilirubinate crystals in biliary sludge can lead to gallstone formation.

Biopsy: A procedure that involves obtaining a tissue specimen for microscopic analysis to establish a precise diagnosis.

Bladder hypotonicity: Inability of the detrusor muscle of the bladder to contract when the bladder is full.

Blast: An immature cell.

Blastopore: A fungal spore produced by budding.

Blood dyscrasias: Any abnormality in the blood or bone marrow's cellular components such as low white or red blood cell count or low platelets.

Blood urea nitrogen (BUN): A waste product in the blood produced from the breakdown of dietary proteins. The kidneys filter blood to remove urea and maintain homeostasis; a decline in kidney function results in an increase in BUN.

Body mass index: A calculation utilized to correct weight changes for height and is a direct calculation regardless of gender. It is the result of the weight in kilograms divided by the height in meters squared. If nonmetric measurements are used, it is the result of the weight in pounds multiplied by 703 and then that quantity divided by the product of height in inches squared.

Bone remodeling: The constant process of bone turnover involving bone resorption followed by bone formation.

Bouchard's nodes: Hard, bony enlargement of the proximal interphalangeal (middle) joint of a finger or toe.

Brachial plexus: Collection of nerves that arises from the spine at the base of the neck from nerves that supply parts of the shoulder, arm, forearm, and hand.

Brachytherapy: A procedure in which radioactive material sealed in needles, seeds, wires, or catheters is placed directly into or near a tumor. Also called internal radiation, implant radiation, or interstitial radiation therapy.

Bronchiectasis: Chronic condition of one or more bronchi or bronchioles marked by irreversible dilatation and destruction of the bronchial walls.

Bronchoalveolar lavage: Diagnostic procedure in which a scope is passed through the nose or mouth into the lungs and fluid is squirted into an area of lung, then recollected for examination.

Bullectomy: Surgical removal of one or more bullae (air spaces in the lung measuring more than 1 cm in diameter in the distended state).

Bursitis: An inflammation of the bursa, the fluid-filled sac near the joint where tendons and muscles pass over bone.

Cachexia: Weight loss, wasting of muscle, loss of appetite, and general debility that can occur with cancer. Anorexia may or may not be present.

Capillary leak: Loss of intravascular volume into the interstitial space within the body.

Carcinoembryonic antigen: A protein normally seen during fetal development. When elevated in adults, it suggests the presence of colorectal and other cancers. Normal level range is less than 2.5 ng/mL (less than 2.5 mcg/L) in nonsmokers but can be elevated in smokers and other nonmalignant conditions such as pancreatitis.

Carcinogenesis: Production or origin of cancer.

Carcinoma: A malignant growth that arises from epithelium, found in skin or the lining of body organs. Carcinomas tend to infiltrate into adjacent tissue and spread to distant organs.

Carcinomatosis: Condition of having widespread dissemination of carcinoma (cancer) in the body.

Cardiac cachexia: Physical wasting with loss of weight and muscle mass caused by cardiac disease; a wasting syndrome that causes weakness and a loss of weight, fat, and muscle.

Cardiac index: Cardiac output normalized for body surface area (cardiac index = cardiac output/body surface area).

Cardiac output: The volume of blood ejected from the left side of the heart per unit of time [cardiac output (L/min) = stroke volume × heart rate].

Cardiac remodeling: Genome expression resulting in molecular, cellular, and interstitial changes and manifested clinically as changes in size, shape, and function of the heart resulting from cardiac load or injury.

Carotid: The two main arteries in the neck.

Carotid bruit: Abnormal sound heard when auscultating a carotid artery caused by turbulent blood flow usually due to the presence of atherosclerotic plaques.

Carotid intima-media thickness: A measurement of the surface between the intima and media. This is a well-validated measure of the progression of atherosclerosis. Increasing measurements over time correlate with increasing atherosclerosis, whereas a decrease in the measurement is indicative of atherosclerotic regression.

Caseating granulomas: A central soft, dry, crumbly cheeselike necrotic mass bordered by giant multinucleated cells, and surrounded by epithelioid cell aggregates, lymphocytes, and fibroblasts.

Cavitary lesions: A spherical, air-containing lesion found on radiograph or computer tomography. The lesion usually has a thick wall and can be found within an area of a surrounding infiltrate or mass.

CCR5 inhibitor: A drug that prevents the binding of HIV to the coreceptor CCR5 on the host cell surface, thereby inhibiting viral entry into the cell.

Cephalic: Of or relating to the head.

Cervicitis: Inflammation of the cervix.

Chemoprevention: The use of drugs, vitamins, or other agents to reduce the risk of, or delay the development or recurrence of, cancer.

Chemoreceptor trigger zone: Located in the area postrema of the fourth ventricle of the brain, it is exposed to cerebrospinal fluid and blood and is easily stimulated by circulating toxins to induce nausea and vomiting.

Chemosis: Edema of the bulbar conjunctiva.

Cheyne-Stokes respiration: Pattern of breathing with gradual increase in depth (and sometimes in rate) to a maximum, followed by a decrease resulting in apnea; the cycles ordinarily are 30 seconds to 2 minutes in duration, with 5 to 30 seconds of apnea.

Chimeric: Composed of parts from different origins.

Chloasma: Melasma characterized by irregularly shaped brown patches on the face and other areas of the skin, often seen during pregnancy or associated with the use of oral contraceptives.

Cholecystitis: Inflammation of the gallbladder.

Cholelithiasis: Formation of stones in the gallbladder.

Cholestasis: Reduced or lack of flow of bile, or obstruction of bile flow.

Cholesteatoma: A mass of keratinized epithelial cells and cholesterol resembling a tumor that forms in the middle ear or mastoid region.

Cholinesterase inhibitors: A class of medications used in the treatment of Alzheimer's disease which prevent the breakdown of acetylcholine.

Chronic disorder: An acid-base disturbance that has been present for hours to days.

Chronic kidney disease: A progressive, irreversible decline in kidney function that occurs over a period of several months to years.

Chronic stable angina: Manifestation of ischemic heart disease that typically results when an atherosclerotic plaque progresses to occlude at least 70% of a major coronary artery. Patients typically present with a sensation of chest pressure or heaviness that is provoked by exertion and relieved with rest or sublingual nitroglycerin.

Chronotropic: Pertaining to the heart rate.

Chvostek's sign: A tap on the patient's facial nerve adjacent to the ear produces a brief contraction of the upper lip, nose, or side of the face.

Chylothorax: The presence of lymphatic fluid (chyle) in the pleural cavity.

Circulatory shock: A condition wherein the circulatory system is inadequately supplying oxygen and vital metabolic substrates to cells throughout the body.

Cirrhosis: Progressive scarring of the liver resulting in nonfunctional hepatocytes.

Clinical cure: Resolution of signs and symptoms of a disease.

Clonal expansion: An immunologic response in which lymphocytes stimulated by antigen proliferate and amplify the population of relevant cells.

Closed comedo: A plugged follicle of sebum, keratinocytes, and bacteria that remains beneath the surface of the skin. Also referred to as a "whitehead."

Clotting cascade: A series of enzymatic reactions by clotting factors leading to the formation of a blood clot. The clotting cascade is initiated by several thrombogenic substances. Each reaction in the cascade is triggered by the preceding one and the effect is amplified by positive feedback loops.

Clotting factor: Plasma proteins found in the blood that are essential to the formation of blood clots. Clotting factors circulate in inactive forms but are activated by their predecessor in the clotting cascade or a thrombogenic substance. Each clotting factor is designated by a Roman numeral (e.g., Factor VII) and by the letter "a" when activated (e.g., Factor VIIa).

Clubbing: Proliferation of soft tissues, especially in the nail bed, which results in thickening and widening of finger and toe extremities.

Coalesence: Fusion of smaller lipid emulsion particles forming larger particles, resulting in destabilization of the emulsion.

Coitus: Sexual intercourse.

Collateral damage: Use of an antimicrobial agent that leads to an increase in colonization and infections with multidrug-resistant organisms in a population setting.

Colloids: Intravenous fluids composed of water and large-molecular-weight molecules used to increase volume in patients with hypovolemic shock via increased intravascular oncotic pressure.

Colon cancer: A disease in which cells in the lining of the colon become malignant and proliferate without control. Often referred to as colorectal cancer to include cancer cells found in the rectum.

Colonoscopy: A visual examination of the colon using a lighted, lens-equipped, flexible tube (colonoscope) inserted into the rectum.

Colony-forming units: The number of microorganisms that form colonies when cultured and is indicative of the number of viable microorganisms in a sample.

Combined modality: Use of two or more different treatment strategies such as systemic chemotherapy (i.e., cyclophosphamide plus doxorubicin; recently, non–anthracycline-containing regimens have also been shown to be effective) plus radiation to "consolidate" local-regional control of the tumor, and surgery such as modified radical mastectomy (breast conserving surgery has been performed with good results but established guidelines are limited by small numbers, lack of randomized trials, and absence of long-term follow-up).

Comedolytic: An agent that is able to break up or destroy a comedo.

Comorbidities: Multiple disease states occurring concurrently in one patient.

Compartment syndrome: The compression of nerves and blood vessels within an enclosed space.

Complete remission: Disappearance of all previously identifiable disease.

Complete response: In cancer, disappearance of all targeted lesions.

Complex regimen: Taking medications 3 or more times per day, or 12 or more doses per day.

Complicated disorder: The presence of two or more distinct acid-base disorders.

Congenital adrenal hyperplasia: A rare inherited condition resulting from a deficiency in cortisol and aldosterone synthesis with resulting excess androgen production. The clinical presentation depends on the variant of the condition but typically manifests as abnormalities in sexual development and/or adrenal insufficiency.

Conjunctivitis: Inflammation of the conjunctiva.

Conjunctivitis medicamentosa: A drug-induced form of allergic conjunctivitis resulting from overuse of topical ocular vasoconstrictors.

Consolidation: A type of high-dose chemotherapy given as the second phase (after induction) of a treatment regimen for leukemia.

Contiguous: Describes two structures that are in close contact, or located next to each other.

Convection: The movement of dissolved solutes across a semipermeable membrane by applying a pressure gradient to the fluid transport.

Convulsion: Uncontrolled muscle movement that may or may not result from abnormal electrical activity in the brain.

Cor pulmonale: Right-sided heart failure caused by lung disease.

Corneal arcus: Accumulation of lipid on the cornea.

Coronary artery bypass graft: Surgical intervention to improve coronary blood flow by removing a vein from the leg and attaching one end to the aorta and the other end to the coronary artery distal to the atherosclerotic plaque. Alternatively, an artery from the inside of the chest wall may be used to bypass the coronary occlusion.

Coronary artery disease: Narrowing of one or more of the major coronary arteries, most commonly by atherosclerotic plaques. May be referred to as coronary heart disease.

Coronary heart disease: Narrowing of one or more of the major coronary arteries, most commonly by atherosclerotic plaques. May be referred to as coronary artery disease.

Corpus luteum: The small yellow endocrine structure that develops within a ruptured ovarian follicle and secretes progesterone and estrogen.

Corticotropin-releasing hormone: A hormone released by the hypothalamus that stimulates release of adrenocorticotropic hormone by the anterior pituitary gland.

Cortisol: An adrenal gland hormone responsible for maintaining homeostasis of carbohydrate, protein, and fat metabolism.

Cosyntropin: A synthetic version of adrenocorticotropic hormone.

Counterirritant: A substance that elicits a superficial inflammatory response with the objective of reducing inflammation in deeper, adjacent structures.

Creaming: Aggregation of lipid emulsion particles that then migrate to the surface of the emulsion; can be reversed with mild agitation.

Creatine kinase, creatine kinase myocardial band: Creatine kinase (CK) enzymes are found in many isoforms, with varying concentrations depending on the type of tissue. Creatine kinase is a general term used to describe the nonspecific total release of all types of CK, including that found in skeletal muscle (MM), brain (BB), and heart (MB). Creatine kinase MB is released into the blood from necrotic myocytes in response to infarction and is a useful laboratory test for diagnosing myocardial infarction. If the total CK is elevated, then the relative index (RI), or fraction of the total that is composed of CK-MB, is calculated as follows:

$$RI = (CK\text{-}MB/CK\ total) \times 100$$

A RI greater than 2 is typically diagnostic of infarction.

Creatinine: A waste product in the blood produced from the breakdown of protein by-products generated by muscle in the body or ingested in the diet. The kidneys filter blood to remove creatinine and maintain homeostasis; a decline in kidney function results in an increase in creatinine.

Creatinine clearance: Rate at which creatinine is filtered across the glomerulus; estimate of glomerular filtration rate.

Crepitus: A grating sound or sensation typically produced by friction between bone-on-cartilage or bone-on-bone contact.

Cross-allergenicity: Sensitivity to one drug and then reacting to a different drug with a similar chemical structure.

Crypt abscess: Neutrophilic infiltration of the intestinal glands (Crypts of Lieberkuhn); a characteristic finding in patients with ulcerative colitis.

Crystalloids: Intravenous fluids composed of water and electrolytes (e.g., sodium chloride, etc.) used as intravascular volume expanders for patients with hypovolemic shock.

Culture-negative IE: Implies acute endocardial damage with negative blood cultures. It is common in patients treated with antibiotics before blood cultures are obtained.

Cure: Disease-free period, which may vary by tumor type or disease state, exceeding an arbitrary duration of time. For breast cancer, this period exceeds 15 years from the end of treatment; for acute leukemia, the period is 5 years. [Note: By this definition, dormant viable tumor cells may still be present even in patients who are deemed cured.]

Cutis laxa: Hypereflacidity of the skin with loss of elasticity.

Cyanosis: Bluish discoloration of the skin and mucous membranes due to lack of oxygenation.

Cyclic citrullinated peptide: A circular peptide (a ring of amino acids) containing the amino acid citrulline. Autoantibodies directed against cyclic citrullinated peptide provide the basis for a test of importance in rheumatoid arthritis.

Cyclooxygenase: An enzyme that catalyzes the conversion of arachidonic acid to prostaglandins and consists of two isoforms, generally abbreviated COX-1 and COX-2.

Cystitis: Inflammation of urinary bladder.

Cystocele: Hernial protrusion of the bladder, usually through the vaginal wall.

Cytokines: Regulatory proteins, such as interleukins and lymphokines, that are released by cells of the immune system and act as intercellular mediators in the generation of an immune response. Soluble glycoproteins released by the immune system which act through specific receptors to regulate immune responses.

Cytomegalovirus (CMV) disease: This is the term used when patients who are already infected with CMV present with the classic associated symptoms that resemble a viral infection and may include fever, malaise, arthralgias and others.

Cytomegalovirus (CMV) infection: This is the term used when a patient has anti-CMV antibodies in the blood, when CMV antigens are detected in infected cells, or when the virus is isolated from a culture.

Deep vein thrombosis: A disorder of thrombus formation causing obstruction of a deep vein in the leg, pelvis, or abdomen.

Delirium: Transient brain syndrome presenting as disordered attention, cognition, psychomotor behavior, and perception.

Dementia: Loss of brain function that occurs with certain diseases. It affects memory, thinking, judgment, and behavior.

Dennie-Morgan line: A line or fold below the lower eyelids; associated with atopy.

Dermatophytes: Any microscopic fungus that grows on the skin, scalp, nails, or mucosa but does not invade deeper tissues.

Desensitization: A method to reduce or eliminate an individual's negative reaction to a substance or stimulus.

Desquamation: Peeling or shedding of the epidermis (superficial layer of the skin) in scales or flakes.

Detumescence: The return of the penis to a flaccid state.

Dialysate: The physiologic solution used during dialysis to remove excess fluids and waste products from the blood.

Dialysis: The process of removing fluid and waste products from the blood across a semipermeable membrane to maintain fluid, electrolyte, and acid-base balance in patients with kidney failure.

Diaphoresis: Perspiration.

Diarthrodial joint: A freely moveable joint (e.g., knee, shoulder). Contrast with amphiarthrodial joint (a slightly movable joint; e.g., vertebral joint) and synarthrodial joint (an unmovable joint; e.g., fibrous joint).

Diastolic dysfunction: Abnormal filling of the ventricles during diastole.

Diffusion: The movement of a solute across the dialyzer membrane from an area of higher concentration (usually the blood) to a lower concentration (usually the dialysate).

2,3-Diphosphoglycerate: A compound in red blood cells that affects oxygen binding to and release from hemoglobin.

Direct current cardioversion: The process of administering a synchronized electrical shock to the chest, the purpose of which is to simultaneously depolarize all of the myocardial cells, resulting in restoration of normal sinus rhythm.

Directly observed therapy: Directly observing patients while taking their anti-tuberculosis medication to ensure compliance.

Disease-free survival: Length of time after treatment during which no disease is found.

Disease progression: In cancer, at least a 20% increase in the sum of the longest diameter of target lesions from baseline, including new lesions discovered during treatment.

Disseminated idiopathic skeletal hyperostosis: Excessive bone formation at skeletal sites subject to stress, generally where tendons and ligaments attach to bone.

DNA mismatch repair genes: Genes that identify and correct errors in DNA base pairs during DNA replication. Mutations in the genes can lead to cancer by allowing abnormal cells to continue to grow.

Down-regulation: The process of reducing or suppressing a response to a stimulus.

Drusen: Tiny yellow or white deposits of extracellular material in the eye.

Ductus arteriosus: Shunt connecting the pulmonary artery to the aortic arch that allows most of the blood from the right ventricle to bypass fetal lungs.

Duodenal: The first of three parts of the small intestine.

Dysarthria: Speech disorder due to weakness or incoordination of speech muscles; speech is slow, weak, and imprecise.

Dyslipidemia: Elevation of the total cholesterol, low-density lipoprotein cholesterol, or triglyceride concentrations or a decrease in high-density lipoprotein cholesterol concentration in the blood.

Dysmenorrhea: Crampy pelvic pain occurring with or just prior to menses. "Primary" dysmenorrhea implies pain in the setting of normal pelvic anatomy, while "secondary" dysmenorrhea is secondary to underlying pelvic pathology.

Dyspareunia: Pain during or after sexual intercourse.

Dysphagia: Difficulty in swallowing.

Dysphonia: Impairment of the voice or difficulty speaking.

Dysphoria: An unhappy or depressed feeling.

Dyspnea: Shortness of breath or difficulty breathing.

Dyssynergic defecation: A lack of coordination between the pelvic floor muscles and the anal sphincter.

Dysuria: Difficulty or pain in urination.

Ebstein's anomaly: Congenital heart defect in which the opening of the tricuspid valve is displaced toward the apex of the right ventricle of the heart.

Eburnation: A condition in which bone or cartilage becomes hardened and denser.

Ecchymosis: Passage of blood from ruptured blood vessels into subcutaneous tissue causing purple discoloration of the skin.

Ectopic pregnancy: Presence of a fertilized ovum outside of the uterine cavity.

Effector cells: Cells that become active in response to initiation of the immune response.

Ejection fraction: The fraction of the volume present at the end of diastole that is pushed into the aorta during systole.

Electrocardiogram: A noninvasive recording of the electrical activity of the heart.

Electroencephalogram: A test that measures and records electrical activity in the brain.

Embolectomy: Surgical removal of a clot or embolism.

Embolism: The sudden blockage of a vessel caused by a blood clot or foreign material which has been brought to the site by the flow of blood.

Embolization: The process by which a blood clot or foreign material dislodges from its site of origin, flows in the blood, and blocks a distant vessel.

Emesis: See vomiting.

Endarterectomy: Removal of a thrombus from the carotid artery.

Endometritis: Inflammation of the endometrium.

Endoscopic evaluation: General term used to describe the visual inspection of the inside of hollow organs with an endoscope; used mainly for diagnostic purposes; refers to procedures such as gastroscopy, duodenoscopy, colonoscopy, sigmoidoscopy, and others.

Endoscopy: A diagnostic tool used to examine the inside of the body using a lighted, flexible instrument called an endoscope.

Endothelial cell: A single layer of cells surrounding the lumen of arteries.

End-stage liver disease: Liver failure that is usually accompanied by complications such as ascites or hepatic encephalopathy.

Engraftment: The process by which transplanted stem cells begin to grow and reproduce in the recipient to produce functioning leukocytes, erythrocytes, and platelets.

Enteral nutrition: Delivery of nutrients via the gastrointestinal tract, either by mouth or by feeding tube.

Enterobacteriaceae: A family of enteric gram-negative bacilli, e.g., *Escherichia coli* or *Klebsiella pneumoniae*.

Enterocytes: Cells lining the small intestine.

Enthesitis: Inflammation of the sites where tendons, ligaments, or fascia attach to bone.

Enuresis: Incontinence at night.

Enzyme-linked immunosorbent assay: A solid phase in the form of a microtiter plate or bead to which HIV antigen is attached. The antigen may be either a preparation of lysed whole virus or a combination of recombinant viral antigens.

Epilepsy: The propensity for a patient to have repeated, unprovoked seizures.

Epistaxis: A nosebleed.

Erectile dysfunction: Condition defined as the inability to achieve or maintain an erection sufficient for sexual intercourse.

Erythema multiforme: A rash characterized by papular (small raised bump) or vesicular lesions (blisters), and reddening or discoloration of the skin often in concentric zones about the lesion.

Erythematous: Flushing of the skin caused by dilation of capillaries. Erythema is often a sign of inflammation and infection.

Erythropoiesis stimulating agents: Agents developed by recombinant DNA technology that have the same biologic activity as endogenous erythropoietin to stimulate erythropoiesis (red blood cell production) in the bone marrow. The currently available agents in the United States are epoetin alfa and darbepoetin alfa.

Erythropoietin: A hormone primarily produced by the progenitor cells of the kidney that stimulates red blood cell production in the bone marrow. Lack of this hormone leads to anemia.

Esophageal varices: Dilated blood vessels in the esophagus.

Essential fatty acid deficiency: Deficiency of linoleic acid, linolenic acid, and/or arachidonic acid, characterized by hair loss, thinning of skin, and skin desquamation. Long-chain fatty acids include trienes (containing 3 double-bonds [e.g., 5,8,11-eicosatrienoic acid {or Mead acid}, trienoic acids]) and tetraenes (containing 4 double-bonds [e.g., arachidonic acid]). Biochemical evidence of essential fatty acid deficiency includes a triene-to-tetraene ratio greater than 0.2 and low linoleic or arachidonic acid plasma concentrations.

Euphoria: A feeling of happiness and excitement.

Event-free survival: This term refers to the length of time after treatment that a person remains free of certain negative events.

Evoked potential testing: A procedure in which sensory nerve pathways are stimulated, and the time lapse to electrical response in the corresponding area of the brain is measured.

Exanthem: Eruption of the skin.

Exfoliative dermatitis: Severe inflammation of the entire skin surface due to a reaction to certain drugs.

Exploratory laparotomy: Surgical incision into the abdominal cavity, performed to examine the abdominal organs and cavity in search of an abnormality and diagnosis.

External beam radiotherapy: Treatment by radiation emitted from a source located at a distance from the body. Also called beam therapy and external beam therapy.

Extra-abdominal: Outside of the abdominal cavity.

Extraction ratio: Fraction of the drug entering the liver in the blood which is irreversibly removed.

Extrapyramidal symptoms: Adverse drug effects of medications such as phenothiazines; includes dystonia (involuntary muscle contractions), tardive dyskinesia (repetitive, involuntary movements), and akathisia (motor restlessness or anxiety).

Facultative: Biologic term meaning "optional." A facultative intracellular pathogen can optionally survive intracellularly even if it is typically an extracellular pathogen.

Facultative anaerobe: An organism that makes adenosine triphosphate by aerobic respiration if oxygen is present, but switches to fermentation under anaerobic conditions.

Felty's syndrome: An extraarticular manifestation of rheumatoid arthritis associated with splenomegaly and neutropenia.

Fibrin: An insoluble protein that is one of the principal ingredients of a blood clot. Fibrin strands bind to one another to form a fibrin mesh. The fibrin mesh often traps platelets and other blood cells.

Fibrinolysis: A normal ongoing process that dissolves fibrin and results in removal of small blood clots; hydrolysis of fibrin.

Fibroadenoma: A benign neoplasm which commonly occurs in breast tissue and is derived from glandular epithelium.

Fibrosis: Formation of tissue containing connective tissues formed by fibroblasts as part of tissue repair or as a reactive process.

Fistula: Abnormal connection between two internal organs (e.g., arteriovenous fistula is a connection between an artery and a vein), or between an internal organ and the exterior or skin (e.g., enterocutaneous fistula is a connection between the intestine and the skin).

Floppy iris syndrome: Alpha-adrenergic antagonists cause relaxation of the iris and papillary constriction. This complicates cataract surgery. Also known as the small pupil syndrome.

Flow cytometry: A technology used to study characteristics of individual cells in a suspension.

Fluorescence in situ hybridization: A laboratory technique used to look at genes or chromosomes in cells and tissues. Pieces of DNA that contain a fluorescent dye are made in the laboratory and added to cells or tissues on a glass slide. When these pieces of DNA bind to specific genes or areas of chromosomes on the slide, they light up when viewed under a microscope with a special light.

Foam cell: Lipid-laden white blood cell.

Forced expiratory volume in 1 second: The volume of air that a patient can blow out in the first second of forced exhalation after taking a maximal breath.

Forced vital capacity: The maximum volume of air that can be forcibly exhaled after taking a maximal breath.

Fragility fracture: A fracture resulting from a fall from standing height or less amount of trauma.

Frailty: Excess demand imposed on reduced capacity; a common biologic syndrome in the elderly.

Frank-Starling mechanism: One of the mechanisms by which the heart can increase cardiac output.

Fremitus: A palpable vibration, as felt by the hand placed on the chest during coughing or speaking.

Friable: Easily crumbled, pulverized, or reduced to powder.

Friction: Risk factor for pressure ulcers that is created when a patient is dragged across a surface, which can lead to superficial skin damage.

Fructooligosaccharides: Polymers of fructose that reach the colon undigested and are broken down there to short-chain fatty acids by bacterial enzymes.

Functional gastrointestinal disorder: A term used to describe symptoms occurring in the gastrointestinal tract in the absence of a demonstrated pathologic condition; the clinical product of psychosocial factors and altered intestinal physiology involving the brain–gut interrelationship.

Gadolinium: An intravenous contrast agent used with magnetic resonance imaging.

Gallstone (cholelithiasis): A solid formation in the gallbladder or bile duct composed of cholesterol and bile salts.

Gastrectomy: Surgical excision of part or all of the stomach.

Gastric bypass: A surgical procedure for weight loss that elicits its effectiveness through malabsorption and volume limitation. The procedure involves full partitioning of the proximal gastric segment into a jejunal loop.

Gastritis: Chronic or acute inflammation of the lining of the stomach.

Gastroenteritis: Inflammation of the gastrointestinal tract causing nausea, vomiting, diarrhea, and fever; sometimes referred to as the stomach flu although not related to influenza.

Gastroplasty: A surgical procedure for weight loss that elicits its effectiveness through gastric volume limitation. The procedure involves partial partitioning at the proximal gastric segment with the placement of a gastric outlet stoma of fixed diameter.

Gastroschisis: Inherited congenital abdominal wall defect in which the intestines and sometimes other organs develop outside the fetal abdomen through an opening in the abdominal wall.

Gastrostomy: Operative placement of a new opening into the stomach, usually associated with feeding tube placement.

Geniculate nucleus: The portion of the brain that processes visual information from the optic nerve and relays it to the cerebral cortex.

Genotype: The genetic constitution of an individual.

Geriatric syndrome: Age-specific presentations or differential diagnoses, including visual and hearing impairment, malnutrition and weight loss, urinary incontinence, gait impairment and falls, osteoporosis, dementia, delirium, sleep problems, and pressure ulcers; commonly seen conditions in elder patients.

Gigantism: A condition of abnormal size or overgrowth of the entire body or of any of its parts.

Glasgow Coma Scale: A scale for evaluating level of consciousness after central nervous system injury (evaluates eye opening and verbal and motor responsiveness).

Glomerular filtration rate: The volume of plasma that is filtered by the glomerulus per unit time, usually expressed as mL/min or mL/min/1.73 m^2, which adjusts the value for body surface area. This is the primary index used to describe overall renal function.

Glomerulonephritis: Glomerular lesions that are characterized by inflammation of the capillary loops of the glomerulus. These lesions are generally caused by immunologic, vascular or other idiopathic diseases. Leads to high blood pressure and possible loss of kidney function.

Glutamate: Primary excitatory neurotransmitter in the central nervous system involved in memory, learning, and neuronal plasticity.

Gonioscopy: Examination of the anterior chamber angle. A gonioprism or Goldman lens are used to perform gonioscopic evaluation.

Graft versus host disease: A complication of stem cell transplantation where the donor's cells attack the host's tissue.

Graft versus tumor effect: The phenomenon by which transplanted donor cells recognize host malignant cells as foreign and thus eradicate the malignant cells through immunologic mechanisms.

Granulomas: Unique inflammatory response composed of macrophages, giant cells and other cells of the immune response to wall off infectious pathogens perceived as foreign but cannot be eliminated.

Gummatous: A tumor of rubbery consistency that is characteristic of the tertiary stage of syphilis.

Gut-associated lymphoid tissue: Lymphoid tissue, including Peyer's patches, found in the gut that are important for providing localized immunity to pathogens.

Haptenation: The process where a drug, usually of low molecular weight, is bound to a carrier protein or cell and becomes immunogenic.

Health literacy: Degree to which individuals have the capacity to obtain, process, and understand basic health information and services needed to make appropriate health decisions.

Heberden's nodes: Hard, bony enlargement of the distal interphalangeal (terminal) joint of a finger or toe.

Hemarthrosis: Blood in the joint space.

Hematemesis: The vomiting of blood.

Hematochezia: Bright red blood per rectum.

Hematogenous: Spread through the blood.

Hematuria: Presence of blood or red blood cells in urine.

Hemiparesis: Weakness on one side of the body.

Hemisensory deficit: Loss of sensation on one side of the body.

Hemithorax: A single side of the trunk between the neck and the abdomen in which the heart and lungs are situated.

Hemoptysis: The expectoration of blood or blood-tinged sputum from the larynx, trachea, bronchi, or lungs.

Hemorrhagic conversion: Conversion of an ischemic stroke into a hemorrhagic stroke.

Hemostasis: Cessation of bleeding through natural (clot formation or construction of blood vessels), artificial (compression or ligation), or surgical means.

Heparin-induced thrombocytopenia: A clinical syndrome of IgG antibody production against the heparin-platelet factor 4 complex occurring in approximately 1% to 5% of patients exposed to either heparin or low-molecular-weight heparin. Heparin-induced thrombocytopenia results in excess production of thrombin, platelet aggregation, and thrombocytopenia (due to platelet clumping), often leading to venous and arterial thrombosis, amputation of extremities, and death.

Hepatic encephalopathy: Confusion and disorientation experienced by patients with advanced liver disease due to accumulation of ammonia in the bloodstream.

Hepatic steatosis: Accumulation of fat in the liver.

Hepatocellular carcinoma: Cancer of the liver.

Hepatojugular reflex: Distention of the jugular vein induced by pressure over the liver; it suggests insufficiency of the right heart.

Hepatorenal syndrome: Acute kidney injury resulting from decreased perfusion in cirrhosis.

Hepatosplenomegaly: An enlarged liver and spleen secondary to leukemic infiltration.

Hepatotoxicity: Toxicity to the liver causing damage to liver cells.

Herniation: Protrusion of the brain through the cranial wall.

Heterotopic: Placing a transplanted organ into an abnormal anatomic location.

Heterozygous: Having different alleles at a gene locus.

Hirschsprung's disease: A congenital abnormality where the ganglia in sections of the large intestine do not develop, resulting in chronic constipation and possibly obstruction; the severity of the condition can range from mild to severe.

Hirsutism: Excessive body and facial hair, especially in the female.

Histocompatibility: The examination of human leukocyte antigen differences between a donor and a recipient in order to determine if the recipient is more likely to accept, rather than reject, a graft from that particular donor.

HIV genotype: A type of resistance testing for HIV where a patient's blood sample is obtained, their HIV RNA is sequenced, and mutations that have developed which may confer resistance to antiretrovirals are reported.

HIV phenotype: A type of resistance testing for HIV where a patient's blood sample is obtained, and the patient's HIV genes that encode for reverse transcriptase and protease are removed and placed in an HIV viral vector. This viral vector is replicated in a cell culture system with varying concentrations of antiretrovirals. A drug concentration-viral inhibition curve is developed and the concentration needed to inhibit 50% of the patient's virus is reported. This is used to predict resistance versus susceptibility.

HIV virtual phenotype: A database of matching HIV genotypes and phenotypes is developed. When an HIV genotype for a patient is obtained, the database is used to predict the patient's phenotype based on their actual genotype using matches that occur in the database.

Homeostenosis: Impaired capability to withstand stressors and decreased ability to maintain physiologic and psychosocial homeostasis; a state commonly found in the elderly.

Homozygous: Having identical alleles at a gene locus.

Hormone-receptor positive breast cancer: Tumors that appear to grow in the presence of estrogens; likewise, anti-estrogen therapy or estrogen deprivation strategies lead to tumor regression.

Hospice: The provision of palliative care during the last 6 months of life as defined by federal guidelines.

Hot flashes: A feeling of warmth that is commonly accompanied by skin flushing and mild to severe perspiration.

Human leukocyte antigens (HLA): Groups of genes found on the major histocompatibility complex which contain cell-surface antigen presenting proteins. The body uses HLA to distinguish between self cells and nonself cells.

Humoral: Products secreted into the blood or body fluids.

Hydramnios: Increased amniotic fluid.

Hyperalgesia: An exaggerated intensity of pain sensation.

Hypercalcemia: Excessive amount of calcium in the blood.

Hypercalciuria: Excessive amount of calcium in the urine.

Hypercapnia: Abnormally high concentration of carbon dioxide in the blood.

Hypercoagulable state: A disorder or state of excessive or frequent thrombus formation; also known as thrombophilia.

Hyperemesis gravidarum: A rare disorder of severe and persistent nausea and vomiting during pregnancy that can result in dehydration, malnutrition, weight loss, and hospitalization.

Hyperglycemic hyperosmolar nonketotic syndrome: Severe increase in serum glucose concentration without the production of ketones, leading to an increase in serum osmolality and symptoms such as increased thirst, increased urination, weakness, fatigue, confusion, and in severe cases, convulsions and/or coma.

Hyperopia: Farsightnedness.

Hyperpigmentation: A common darkening of the skin which occurs when an excess of melanin forms deposits in the skin.

Hyperplasia: An abnormal or unusual increase in the cells of a body part.

Hyperprolactinemia: A medical condition of elevated serum prolactin characterized by prolactin serum concentrations greater than 20 ng/mL (20 mcg/L) in men or 25 ng/mL (25 mcg/L) in women.

Hypertrichosis: Excessive growth of hair.

Hypertrophy: An increase in the size of the cells in a tissue or organ.

Hypogammaglobinemia: Reduced levels of antibodies.

Hypogonadism: A medical condition resulting from or characterized by abnormally decreased functional activity of the gonads, with retardation of growth and sexual development. Associated with testosterone deficiency resulting from either testicular or pituitary/hypothalamic diseases. Presenting symptoms differ according to the timing of disease onset in relation to puberty.

Hypopituitarism: A clinical disorder characterized by complete or partial deficiency in pituitary hormone production.

Hypovolemic shock: Circulatory shock caused by severe loss of blood volume and/or body water.

Hypoxemia: Deficiency of oxygen in the blood.

Hysterectomy: Excision of the uterus.

Immune reconstitution inflammatory syndrome: A condition in AIDS patients or other types of immunosuppression where paradoxical worsening of the infection is observed as the immune system begins to recover due to increasing inflammation at the site of infection.

Immunogenicity: The property that gives a particular substance the ability to provoke an immune response.

Immunoglobulin G index: The ratio of immunoglobulin G to protein in the serum or cerebrospinal fluid.

Immunophenotype: The process of identification and quantitation of cellular antigens through flourochrome-labeled monoclonal antibodies.

Immunotherapy: Treatment of a disease by stimulating the body's own immune system.

Impedance pH monitoring: Detects gastroesophageal reflux based on changes in resistance to electrical current flow between two electrodes when a liquid and/or gas bolus moves between them. It can detect both acid and nonacid reflux.

Implantable cardioverter-defibrillator: A device implanted into the heart transvenously with a generator implanted subcutaneously in the pectoral area that provides internal electrical cardioversion of ventricular tachycardia or defibrillation of ventricular fibrillation.

Index patient: The patient originally diagnosed with a disease.

Indirect immunofluorescence assay: HIV-infected T-lymphocytes are fixed onto a microscope slide, covered with the blood sample to be tested, incubated under heat, and washed. If antibodies to HIV are bound to the fixed viral antigens, they will remain on the slide. FITC-conjugated anti-human globulin is then added, incubated, and washed. If the sample contains antibodies to HIV, the cells will show a bright, fluorescent membrane under the microscope.

Induction: Treatment designed to be used as the first step in eliminating the leukemic burden.

Infarction: The formation of an infarct, an area of tissue death due to a local lack of oxygen.

Initiation: It occurs in cancer when a carcinogenic substance encounters a normal cell to produce genetic damage, and results in a mutated cell.

Inotropic: Relating to or influencing the force of muscular contractions.

Insulin-like growth factor-I: An anabolic peptide that acts as a direct stimulator of cell proliferation and growth in all body cells.

Integrase strand transfer inhibitor: A drug that prevents the enzyme integrase from allowing the HIV RNA to incorporate into the host cell genome.

International normalized ratio (INR): The ratio of the patient's clotting time to the clinical laboratory's mean reference value; normalized by raising it to the international sensitivity index (ISI) power to account for differences in thromboplastin reagents. Therefore: INR = (Patient's prothrombin time/laboratory's mean normal prothrombin time)^{ISI}.

Intima: The inner layer of the wall of an artery or vein.

Intraarticular: Administered to or occurring in the space within joints.

Intraabdominal: Within the abdominal cavity.

Intraperitoneal: Within the peritoneal cavity.

Intrathecal: Within the meninges of the spinal cord.

Intravenous pyelogram: After intravenous administration of radiocontrast media, an x-ray of kidneys, ureters, bladder, and urethra is performed, which provides information on anatomic aspects (size, shape, location, axis) and function of these organs.

Intravesicular: Administration directly into the bladder through the urethra.

Intussusception: The prolapse of one part of the intestine into the lumen of an immediately adjoining part.

Iontophoresis: Introduction of a medication into tissue through use of an electric current.

Ipsilateral: Occurring on the same side.

Ischemic heart disease: Imbalance between myocardial oxygen supply and oxygen demand.

Jejunal: A section of the small intestine connecting the duodenum to the ileum.

Jejunostomy: Operative placement of a new opening into the jejunum, usually associated with feeding tube placement.

Kegel exercises: Specific exercises that strengthen the pelvic floor muscles and help to prevent and treat stress incontinence.

Keratinization: The sloughing of epithelial cells in the hair follicle.

Keratinocyte: The epidermal cell that synthesizes keratin; makes up 95% of all epidermal cells; commonly called "skin cells."

Keratitis: Infection of the cornea.

Keratoconjunctivitis sicca: Ocular surface disease caused by dysfunctional tear film; also known as Sjogren's syndrome or dry eye syndrome.

Kindling: A process of inducing epilepsy in a laboratory animal by repeated, low-level electrical stimulation of specific areas of the brain.

Koebner phenomenon: The occurrence of psoriatic lesions due to skin trauma.

Korotkoff sounds: The noise heard over an artery by auscultation when pressure over the artery is reduced below the systolic arterial pressure.

KRAS: Protein involved in normal cell signaling processes (product of KRAS gene).

Kyphosis: Abnormal curvature of the spine resulting in protrusion of the upper back; hunchback.

β-Lactam allergy: Allergy to the β-lactam family, namely penicillins and cephalosporins, but may also include carbapenems.

Lactose intolerance: An inability to digest milk and some dairy products, resulting in abnormal bloating, cramping, and diarrhea; caused by enzymatic lactase deficiency.

Lag-ophthalmos: Poor closure of the upper eyelid.

Lamina cribrosa: A series of perforated sheets of connective tissue that the optic nerve passes through as it exits the eye.

Laminectomy: Excision of the posterior arch of a vertebra to relieve pressure on the spinal cord.

Laparoscopic: Abdominal exploration or surgery employing a type of endoscope called laparoscope.

Laparotomy: Surgical opening of the abdominal cavity.

Latent tuberculosis (TB) infection: Infection with *Mycobacterium tuberculosis* has occurred but the disease is not active. Patients with latent tuberculosis are not infectious, and it is not possible to get TB from someone with latent tuberculosis.

Lentigines: Plural of lentigo—a small, flat, tan to dark brown or black, macular melanosis on the skin which looks like a freckle but is histologically distinct. Lentigines do not darken on exposure to sunlight, freckles do.

Leukocytoclastic: The breaking up of white blood cells.

Leukopenia: A condition where the number of circulating white blood cells are abnormally low due to decreased production of new cells, possibly in conjunction with medication toxicities.

Leukostasis: An abnormal intravascular leukocyte aggregation and clumping seen in leukemia patients. The brain and the lungs are the two most frequent organs involved.

Lhermitte's sign: Tingling or shock-like sensation passing down the arms or trunk when the neck is flexed.

Libido: Conscious or unconscious sexual desire.

Ligament of Treitz: Landmark in the proximal portion of the jejunum beyond which it is preferred that postpyloric feedings be delivered for minimization of aspiration.

Light chain assay: A highly sensitive assay that determines the ratio of serum free light chain kappa to lambda.

Linea nigra: Dark vertical line that appears on the abdomen during pregnancy.

Lipoprotein lipase: Enzyme located in the capillary endothelium involved in the breakdown of intravenous lipid emulsion particles.

Liver biopsy: A procedure whereby tissue is removed from the liver and used to determine the severity of liver damage.

Luteolysis: Death of the corpus luteum.

Lymphadenectomy: Surgical excision of lymph nodes.

Lymphangitis: Inflammation of lymphatic channels.

Lymphatic: The network of vessels carrying tissue fluids.

Lymphoproliferative: Of or related to the growth of lymphoid tissue.

Maceration: The softening or breaking down of a solid by leaving it immersed in a liquid.

Macrophages: Large scavenger cell.

Macula: The central portion of the retina.

Maculopapular: A rash that contains both macules and papules. A macule is a flat discolored area of the skin, and a papule is a small raised bump. A maculopapular rash is usually a large area that is red, and has small, confluent bumps.

Major malformation: A defect that has either cosmetic or functional significance to the child.

Mastalgia: Tenderness of the breast.

Matrix metalloproteinases: Any of a group of enzymes, normally located in the extracellular space of tissue, that function to break down proteins (e.g., collagen), and require zinc or calcium atoms as cofactors for enzymatic activity.

Meatal stenosis: Abnormal narrowing or closing of the urethral opening, which slows urination or causes a change in the direction of the urinary stream.

Meconium: The first intestinal discharge or "stool" of a newborn infant, usually green in color and consisting of epithelial cells, mucus, and bile.

Media: The middle layer of the wall of an artery or vein.

Melanosis: Excessive pigmentation of the skin due to a disturbance in melanin pigmentation; also called melanism.

Melasma: Dark skin discoloration.

Melena: Abnormally dark black, tarry feces containing blood (usually from gastrointestinal bleeding).

Menarche: The onset of cyclic menstrual periods in a woman.

Meninges: Covering of the brain consisting of three layers.

Menopause: Permanent cessation of menses following the loss of ovarian follicular activity.

Menorrhagia: Menstrual blood loss of greater than 80 mL per cycle or menstrual cycles lasting greater than 7 days.

Mesothelioma: A benign or malignant tumor affecting the lining of the chest or abdomen. Commonly caused by exposure to asbestos fibers.

Metabolic acidosis: A condition in the blood and tissues that is a consequence of an accumulation of lactic acid resulting from tissue hypoxia and anaerobic metabolism.

Metabolic alkalosis: Alkalosis that is caused by an increase in the concentration of alkaline compounds (typically bicarbonate).

Metabolic syndrome: Constellation of cardiovascular risk factors related to hypertension, abdominal obesity, dyslipidemia, and insulin resistance diagnosed by the presence of at least three of the following criteria: increased waist circumference, elevated triglyceride concentrations, decreased high-density lipoprotein (HDL) cholesterol or active treatment to raise HDL cholesterol, elevated blood pressure or active treatment with antihypertensive therapy, or elevated fasting glucose or active treatment for diabetes.

Metastasis: Plural is metastases. Cancer that has spread from the original site of the tumor.

Micelles: A microscopic particle of digested fat and cholesterol.

Microalbuminuria: Urinary excretion of small but abnormal amounts of albumin. Confirmed spot urine albumin to creatinine ratio of 30 to 300 mg/g (3.4 to 34 mg/mmol creatinine) is consistent with microalbuminuria. Considered an early sign of chronic kidney disease.

Micrognatia: Abnormal smallness of the jaws.

Micrometastasis: Deposits of tumor cells in distant organs that cannot be detected by any imaging techniques available.

Microsatellite instability: Unstable sequences of repeating DNA caused by deficiencies in the normal DNA repair process.

Microvascular pulmonary emboli: An obstruction in the small blood vessels in the lung caused by material (e.g., blood clot, fat, air, foreign body) that is carried through the circulation until it lodges in another small vessel.

Minimal residual disease: A quantitative assessment of subclinical remnant of leukemic burden remaining at the end of the initial phase of treatment (induction) when a patient may appear to be in a complete morphologic remission.

Minimum inhibitory concentration: The lowest concentration of an antimicrobial agent that inhibits visible bacterial growth after approximately 24 hours.

Minor malformation: A defect that has neither cosmetic nor functional significance to the child.

Mixed disorder: See Complicated disorder.

Miosis: Pupil constriction.

Mobilization: The release of stem cells into the peripheral blood from the bone marrow compartment for the purposes of collecting these stem cells (in anticipation of stem cell transplantation).

Mobitz type I: A type of second-degree AV nodal blockade.

Mobitz type II: A type of second-degree AV nodal blockade.

Moebius syndrome: Extremely rare congenital neurologic disorder which is characterized by facial paralysis and affects eye movement.

Monocytes: A variety of white blood cells.

Monoparesis: Slight or incomplete paralysis affecting a single extremity or part of one.

Monosodium urate: A crystallized form of uric acid that can deposit in joints leading to an inflammatory reaction and the symptoms of gout.

Morphology: The science of structure and form of cells without regard to function.

Mucosa-associated lymphoid tissue: Lymphoid tissue in the gut that samples luminal antigens and delivers them to the systemic lymph system.

Mucositis: Inflammation of mucous membranes, typically within the oral and esophageal mucosa. Usually associated with certain chemotherapy agents and radiation therapy involving mucosal area.

Mucous colitis: A condition of the mucous membrane of the colon characterized by pain, constipation, or diarrhea (sometimes alternating), and passage of mucus or mucous shreds.

Muscularis mucosa: The thin layer of smooth muscle found in most parts of the gastrointestinal tract.

Mydriasis: Pupil dilation.

Myelin: A protein and phospholipid sheath that surrounds the axons of certain neurons. Myelinated nerves conduct impulses more rapidly than nonmyelinated nerves.

Myeloablative preparative regimen: Radiation and/or chemotherapy that destroys bone marrow activity in preparation for a stem cell transplant. Patients will not likely recover bone marrow function without an infusion of "rescue" autologous or allogeneic stem cells.

Myelodysplastic syndrome: A disease in which the bone marrow does not function properly.

Myelosuppression: Reduction in white blood cells, red blood cells, and platelets caused by bone marrow suppression.

Myocarditis: Inflammation of the muscular wall of the heart.

Myoglobinuria: The presence of myoglobin in urine.

Myonecrosis: Necrotic damage to muscle tissue.

Myopathy: Any disease of the muscle causing weakness, pain, and tenderness.

Myringotomy: A surgical incision in the tympanic membrane to relieve pressure and drain fluid from the middle ear.

Nasal scotoma: An area of blindness in the nasal portion of peripheral vision.

Nascent: Immature.

Nasolacrimal occlusion: The closing of the tear duct to decrease systemic absorption of a drug.

Nausea: The subjective feeling of a need to vomit.

Necrosectomy: Surgical excision of necrotic tissue; debridement.

Necrotizing enterocolitis: Medical condition primarily seen in premature infants, where portions of the bowel undergo necrosis Nelson syndrome: A condition characterized by the aggressive growth of a pituitary tumor and hyperpigmentation of the skin.

Neoadjuvant chemotherapy: Chemotherapy or radiation therapy given prior to primary surgical treatment. In cancer, it is often used to downstage the tumor to a resectable stage.

Neoadjuvant therapy: Therapeutic strategy that precedes primary treatment modality (usually surgery). The goals are to "down-stage" tumors so that the surgical field is smaller or to transform a patient from a nonsurgical candidate to one that is. Neoadjuvant therapy may improve overall survival. Strategies usually involve the use of systemic therapy with or without radiation.

Neovascular maculopathy: Proliferation of blood vessels in the macula.

Nephrolithiasis: A condition marked by the presence of renal calculi (stones) in the kidney or urinary system.

Nephron: The working unit of the kidney that filters blood to remove fluid, toxins, and drugs. Each kidney contains approximately 1 million nephrons.

Nephrostomy: Insertion of a catheter through the skin into the renal pelvis to bypass ureteral obstruction and facilitate urine drainage.

Neuralgia: Pain which extends along the course of one or more nerves.

Neuritis: Inflammation of a nerve.

Neutralizing antibodies: Antibodies that develop in response to a therapeutic agent that decrease the efficacy of the agent.

Nidus: A central point or focus consisting of a fibrin matrix (in the case of infective endocarditis), where bacteria are able to accumulate and multiply, allowing for formation of an infected vegetation.

Nitric oxide: An endogenous vasodilator.

NMDA-receptor antagonist: A medication used in the treatment of Alzheimer's disease. It blocks the *N*-methyl-D-aspartate receptors and protects cells against excess glutamate.

Nociceptors: Receptors for pain caused by injury from physical stimuli (mechanical, electrical, or thermal) or chemical stimuli (toxins); located in the skin, muscles, or in the walls of the viscera.

Nocturia: Excessive urination at night.

Nodules: When seen with rheumatoid arthritis, nodules are subcutaneous knobs over bony prominences or extensor surfaces.

Nonbacterial thrombotic endocarditis: Endocarditis caused by noninfectious vegetations.

Nonmyeloablative preparative regimen: Radiation and/or chemotherapy that does not completely eradicate host bone marrow activity; host bone marrow activity is suppressed but may recover after approximately 4 weeks, even in the absence of "rescue" allogeneic stem cells.

Nonnucleoside reverse transcriptase inhibitor (NNRTI): A noncompetitive inhibitor of the viral reverse transcriptase enzyme by binding to the active site of the enzyme itself, rather than by terminating the enzymatic product. NNRTIs are only active against HIV-1.

Nonpolyposis: Absence of polyps.

Nonprotein kilocalorie-to-nitrogen ratio: Numerical value derived from dividing kilocalories from carbohydrate plus fat by the number of grams of nitrogen in the diet.

Non–ST-segment elevation: A type of myocardial infarction (MI) that is limited to the subendocardial myocardium and is smaller and less extensive than an ST-segment MI, and usually there is no pathologic Q wave on the electrocardiogram.

Normochromic: Being normal in color; referring especially to red blood cells.

Normocytic: Normal size especially referring to red blood cells.

Nuchal rigidity: Neck stiffness.

Nuclear factor kappa B (Nf-kappa-B): Regulates cytokine production.

Nucleoside reverse transcriptase inhibitor (NRTI)/nucleotide reverse transcriptase inhibitor (NtRI): A modified version of a naturally occurring nucleoside or nucleotide that prevents HIV replication by interfering with the function of the viral reverse transcriptase enzyme. The nucleoside/nucleotide analog causes early termination of the proviral DNA chain. For activity, an NRTI requires three phosphorylation steps once inside the cell, whereas a NtRI has a phosphate group attached and needs only two phosphorylation steps inside the cell for activity.

Nulliparity: Condition of not having given birth to a child.

Nystagmus: Rapid involuntary eye movement.

Obliterative bronchiolitis: Inflammation of the bronchioles (the small elements of the tracheobronchial tree) characterized by obliteration and/or permanent narrowing of the airways.

Off-label use: Use of a medication outside the scope of its approved, labeled use.

Oiling out: Continued coalescence of lipid emulsion particles, resulting in irreversible separation of the emulsion (also called "breaking" or "cracking" of the emulsion).

Oligoanovulation: The condition of having few to no ovulatory menstrual cycles.

Oligoclonal bands: Small discrete bands in the γ-globulin region of fluid electrophoresis.

Oligohydramnios: Decreased amniotic fluid.

Oligomenorrhea: Abnormally light or infrequent menstruation.

Oliguria: Reduced urine output; usually defined as less than 400 mL in 24 hours or less than 0.5 mL/kg/h.

Omentumectomy: Excision of the double fold of peritoneum attached to the stomach and connecting it with abdominal viscera (omentum).

Oncogene: Genes that cause transformation of normal cells into cancer cells by promoting uncontrolled cell growth and multiplication leading to tumor formation.

Open comedo: A plugged follicle of sebum, keratinocytes, and bacteria that protrudes from the surface of the skin and appears black or brown in color. Also referred to as a "blackhead."

Opsonization: The process by which an antigen is altered so as to become more readily and more efficiently engulfed by phagocytes.

Optic neuritis: Usually monocular central visual acuity loss and ocular/periorbital pain caused by demyelination of the optic nerve.

Oral rehydration solution: A liquid preparation, commercially prepared or made at home using common ingredients according to a formula developed by the World Health Organization, designed to replace fluid loss in persons with diarrhea.

Orchiectomy: The surgical removal of the testicles.

Orthopnea: Difficulty in breathing that occurs when lying down and is relieved upon changing to an upright position.

Orthostasis: Characterized by a drop in blood pressure when standing up from sitting or lying down, often causing lightheadedness and dizziness.

Orthotopic: Placing a transplanted organ into the normal anatomic location.

Osmolality: A measure of the number of osmotically active particles per unit solution, independent of the weight or nature of the particle.

Osmolar gap: The difference between the measured serum osmolality and the calculated serum osmolality.

Osteoblasts: Cells involved in bone formation; "builders of bone."

Osteoclasts: Cells involved in bone resorption; "creators of cavities."

Osteomalacia: Softening of the bones.

Osteonecrosis: Death of bone tissue.

Osteopenia: Reduced bone density or mass, which can lead to osteoporosis.

Osteophytes: Bony outgrowths (also called bone spurs) into the joint space.

Osteoporosis: Disease of the bones characterized by a loss of bone tissue, resulting in brittle, weak bones that are susceptible to fracture (porous bones).

Ostomy: Surgical operation where part of the abdominal wall is opened and part of the intestine is connected to the opening for intestinal draining (e.g., colostomy, ileostomy)

Otitis media with effusion: Fluid in the middle ear space with no signs or symptoms of an acute infection.

Ovulation: Periodic ripening and rupture of mature follicle and the discharge of ovum from the cortex of the ovary.

Pacemaker: A mass of fibers that possess actual or potential automaticity which initiates and determines the rate of spontaneous depolarizations.

Palliative care: The active, total care of patients whose disease is not responsive to curative treatment.

Palliative chemotherapy: Treatment given to control the symptoms of an incurable cancer.

Pancolitis: Inflammation that involves the majority of the colon in patients with inflammatory bowel disease.

Pancreatic pseudocysts: A cyst-like space not lined by epithelium and contained within the pancreas.

Pancreatitis: Inflammation of the pancreas.

Panhypopituitarism: A state in which the secretion of all anterior pituitary hormones is inadequate or absent.

Pannus: Inflamed synovial tissue that invades and destroys articular structures.

Paracentesis: Removal of (ascitic) fluid from the peritoneal space.

Paracentral scotoma: Blind spots near the center of the visual field.

Parenchyma: Specific cells or tissue of an organ.

Parenteral nutrition: Delivery of nutrients via the intravenous route.

Paroxysmal: Intermittent occurrence, initiating suddenly and spontaneously, lasting minutes to hours, and terminating suddenly and spontaneously.

Partial response: In cancer, at least a 30% decrease in the sum of the longest diameter of target lesions from baseline.

Patient survival: After the transplant procedure, the survival of the transplant recipient, without regard to the function or survival of the allograft.

Peak expiratory flow: The maximum flow rate of air leaving the lungs upon forced exhalation.

Pelvic inflammatory disease: Inflammation of the endometrium, uterine tubes, and pelvic peritoneum; often due to a sexually transmitted infection.

Percutaneous coronary intervention: A minimally invasive procedure whereby access to the coronary arteries is obtained through the femoral artery up the aorta to the coronary os. Contrast media is used to visualize the coronary artery stenosis using a coronary angiogram. A guidewire is used to cross the stenosis and a small balloon is inflated and/or stent is deployed to break up atherosclerotic plaque and restore coronary artery blood flow. The stent is left in place to prevent acute closure and restenosis of the coronary artery. Newer stents are coated with antiproliferative drugs, such as paclitaxel and sirolimus, which further reduce the risk of restenosis of the coronary artery.

Percutaneous endoscopic gastrostomy: Gastric feeding tube placed via endoscopic technique.

Percutaneous endoscopic jejunostomy: Jejunal feeding tube placed via endoscopic technique.

Performance status: An attempt to quantify the ability of a cancer patient to perform daily activities. This is used to determine if and how much chemotherapy they can receive. Patients with good performance status can tolerate more aggressive chemotherapy.

Perihilar: The area surrounding the depression in the medial surface of a lung that forms the opening through which the bronchus, blood vessels, and nerves pass.

Perimenopause: Also known as the climacteric, it is the period of time prior to menopause when hormonal and biologic changes and physical symptoms begin to occur and usually last for 1 year after the last menstrual period. The perimenopausal period may last for an average of 3 to 5 years.

Perimetry: Measurement of the field of vision.

Peripheral artery disease: Atherosclerosis of the peripheral arteries.

Peripheral resistance: The sum of resistance to blood flow offered by systemic blood vessels.

Peritonitis: An acute inflammatory reaction of the peritoneal lining to microorganisms or chemical irritation.

Petechiae: Tiny localized hemorrhages from the small blood vessels just beneath the surface of the skin.

PET scan: A scan that produces images of the body after the injection of a radioactive form of glucose. The scan is often used to detect cancer since tumors use more sugar than normal cells. PET scans may also be used to see how well the tumor is responding to treatment.

Phagocytic cell: A cell that absorbs waste material, harmful microorganisms, or other foreign bodies in the bloodstream and tissues.

Phagocytosis: The process of engulfing and ingesting an antigen by phagocytes.

Pharmacogenomic: The influence of genetic variation on drug response in patients and is used to correlate gene expression with a drug's efficacy or toxicity.

Pharyngitis: Inflammation and/or infection of the pharynx that causes throat pain.

Pheochromocytoma: A tumor arising from chromaffin cells, most commonly found in the adrenal medulla. The tumor causes the adrenal medulla to hypersecrete epinephrine and norepinephrine resulting in hypertension and other signs and symptoms of excessive sympathetic nervous system activity. The tumor is usually benign but may occasionally be cancerous.

Phenotype: The visible properties of an organism that are produced by the interaction of the genotype and the environment.

Phlebitis: Inflammation of a blood vessel (e.g., vein).

Photochemotherapy: The use of phototherapy together with topical or systemic drugs in the treatment of psoriasis.

Photodynamic therapy: Cancer treatment that uses interaction between laser light and a substance that makes the cells more sensitive to light. When light is applied to cells that have been treated with this substance, a chemical reaction occurs and destroys cancer cells.

Photophobia: Intolerance to bright light.

Phototherapy: The use of ultraviolet light applied to the skin, for example in treating psoriasis or neonatal hyperbilirubinemia.

Pilosebaceous unit: A hair follicle and the surrounding sebaceous glands.

Plaques: Extracellular protein deposits of fibrils and amorphous aggregates of b-amyloid protein.

Plasma cell: Antibody producing cells.

Plasmapheresis: A process of separating cells out from the plasma. This process is used to remove the monoclonal antibodies from the blood.

Pleocytosis: A transient increase in the number of leukocytes in a body fluid.

Pleuritis: Inflammation of the lining around the lungs.

Pneumatic otoscopy: A diagnostic technique involving visualization of the tympanic membrane for transparency, position, and color, and its response to positive and negative air pressure to assess mobility.

Pneumothorax: The presence of air in the pleural cavity, often causing part of the lung to collapse.

Podocyte: The epithelial cells that surround the capillaries in the Bowman's capsule and are responsible for filtering blood in the glomerulus of the nephron.

Polycythemia: An abnormal increase in the number of erythrocytes in the blood.

Polypharmacy: Taking multiple medications concurrently.

Polyps: A growth from a mucous membrane commonly found in organs such as the colon, rectum, and the nose. Usually not malignant, these can develop into cancer and require removal once found.

Polyuria: Excessive excretion of urine resulting in profuse micturition.

Portal hypertension: Increased pressure in vessel leading to liver; usually a result of cirrhosis.

Postpyloric feeding: Delivery of nutrients via a tube placed with its tip past the pyloric sphincter separating the stomach from the duodenum.

Prader-Willi syndrome: A genetic disorder characterized by short stature, mental retardation, low muscle tone, abnormally small hands and feet, hypogonadism, and excessive eating leading to extreme obesity.

Predictive factors: Any measurements associated with response to therapy (e.g., over-expression of HER2 increases the likelihood of response to agents targeting the receptor; the same is true for ER).

Preload: The stretched condition of the heart muscle at the end of diastole just before contraction; volume in the left ventricle at the end of diastole estimated by the pulmonary artery occlusion pressure (also known as the pulmonary artery wedge pressure or pulmonary capillary wedge pressure).

Preparative regimen (conditioning regimen): Radiation and/or chemotherapy given to stem cell transplant patients in order to kill malignant cells, create space in the bone marrow compartment, and suppress the immune system of the host in order to prevent graft rejection.

Priapism: A prolonged, painful erection lasting more than 4 hours. Considered a medical emergency.

Primary amenorrhea: Absence of menses by age 15 in the presence of normal secondary sexual development or absence of menses within 5 years of breast development (if occurring prior to age 10).

Primary prevention: The removal or reduction of risk factors before the development of disease.

Prinzmetal's angina: Vasospasm or contraction of the coronary arteries in the absence of significant atherosclerosis. Also referred to as variant angina.

Probiotics: Dietary supplements containing potentially beneficial bacteria that promote health by stimulating optimal mucosal immune responses.

Proctitis: Inflammation confined to the rectum in patients with inflammatory bowel disease.

Progenitor: A primitive cell.

Prognostic factors: Biologic or clinical indicators associated with survival independent of therapy (e.g., over-expression of HER2 is associated with increased risk of relapse and shorter survival).

Progression: In cancer, cell proliferation takes over and the tumor spreads or develops metastases.

Progression-free survival: Length of time that a disease remains stable following treatment.

Progressive primary disease: Tuberculosis infection in which the immune response fails to control multiplication of the tubercle bacilli. The primary focus in the lung enlarges rapidly and spreads. This occurs in less than 10% of normal adults, but it is more common in children younger than 5 years, and in patients with suppressed immunity.

Prolapse: Protrusion of an organ or part of an organ through an opening, e.g., uterine prolapse occurs when the uterus is displaced downward such that the cervix is within the vaginal opening (first degree), the cervix is outside the opening (second degree), or the entire uterus is outside the opening (third degree).

Promotion: Reversible process in cancer, the environment is altered by carcinogens or other factors to favor the growth of the mutated cell over the normal cell.

Prostaglandin: Any of a large group of biologically active, carbon-20, unsaturated fatty acids that are produced by the metabolism of arachidonic acid through the cyclooxygenase pathway.

Prostatectomy: Surgical removal of the prostate.

Prostatic hyperplasia: Enlargement of the prostate.

Prosthetic-valve endocarditis: Endocarditis that occurs in patients with bioprosthetic or synthetic implanted heart valves.

Protease inhibitor: A drug that acts by inhibiting the viral protease enzyme, which prevents long strands of protein from being cleaved into the smaller proteins that the virus requires for assembly.

Protectant: An agent that forms an occlusive barrier between the skin and surrounding moisture.

Protected specimen brush: Used in bronchoscopy, a brush in the lumen of a tube inside the bronchoscope. The brush is extended into the lung to obtain a sample, then retracted back into the tube for removal from the lung.

Proteinase: Any of numerous enzymes that catalyze the breakdown of proteins (also called protease).

Proteinuria: The presence of measurable amounts of protein (greater than 150 mg/day) in the urine, which is often indicative of glomerular or tubular damage in the kidney.

Proteoglycans: Glycosaminoglycans (mucopolysaccharides) bound to protein chains in covalent complexes. Proteoglycans are present in the extracellular matrix of connective tissue.

Proteolysis: The degradation of proteins in damaged tissue.

Proteosome: An enzyme complex that degrades intracellular proteins.

Prothrombin: A clotting factor that is converted to thrombin; also known as Factor II.

Prothrombin time: A measure of coagulation representing the amount of time required to form a blood clot after the addition of thromboplastin to the blood sample; also known as Quick's test.

Prothrombotic state: A state of high coagulation of the blood.

Protooncogenes: Normal genes that are present in all normal cells and regulate cell function and replication, and through some genetic alteration caused by carcinogens, change into oncogenes.

Pseudohyphae: Elongated forms created by replicating yeast that form buds but do not detach from one another.

Pseudophakic: Presence of an artificial lens placed after cataract extraction.

Pseudopolyps: An area of hypertrophied gastrointestinal mucosa that resembles a polyp and contains nonmalignant cells.

Pulmonary artery catheter: An invasive device used to measure hemodynamic parameters directly, including cardiac output and pulmonary artery occlusion pressure; calculated parameters include stroke volume and systemic vascular resistance.

Pulmonary artery occlusion pressure: A hemodynamic measurement obtained via a catheter placed into the pulmonary artery used to evaluate patient volume status within the left ventricle.

Pulmonary embolism: A disorder of thrombus formation causing obstruction of a pulmonary artery or one of its branches and resulting in pulmonary infarction.

Pulsus paradoxus: A large fall in systolic blood pressure and pulse volume during inspiration or an abnormal variation in pulse volume during respiration in which the pulse becomes weaker with inspiration and stronger with expiration.

Purkinje fiber: Specialized myocardial fibers that conduct impulses from the atrioventricular node to the ventricles.

Purified protein derivative: A mixture of antigens obtained from the culture of M. tuberculosis that can be injected intracutaneously to stimulate the immune system to produce a measurable response.

Purpura: A small hemorrhage of the skin, mucous membrane, or serosal surface.

Purulent: Containing, consisting of, or being pus.

Pyelonephritis: Inflammation of a kidney.

Pyuria: Presence of pus in urine when voided.

Quality indicators: A list of indicator used by long-term care facility administrators and government overseers to identify potential problems in patient care.

Quality of life: Perceived physical and mental health over time.

Radiofrequency catheter ablation: Procedure during which radiofrequency energy is delivered through a catheter positioned at the atrioventricular node for the purpose of destroying one pathway of a reentrant circuit.

Receptor editing: The process by which cells proofread, alter, and reexpress modified receptors to become non-autoreactive.

Recombinant activated factor VII: A clotting factor manufactured via recombinant technology used off-label (non–Food and Drug Administration approved) to foster clotting in hemorrhagic shock patients with massive hemorrhage refractory to conventional therapies such as fresh frozen plasma.

Rectal prolapse: Sinking of the rectum through the anal sphincter so that it is visible externally.

Reentry: Circular movement of electrical impulses, a mechanism of many arrhythmias.

Refractory period: The period of time after an impulse is initiated and conducted during which cells cannot be depolarized again.

Regurgitation: A passive process without involvement of the abdominal wall and the diaphragm wherein gastric or esophageal contents move into the mouth.

Remission: An inability to detect the presence of disease.

Renal osteodystrophy (ROD): Altered bone turnover that results from sustained metabolic conditions that occur in chronic kidney disease, including secondary hyperparathyroidism, hyperphosphatemia, hypocalcemia, and vitamin D deficiency. The disease can be characterized by high bone turnover, low bone turnover, or adynamic disease, or may be a mixed disorder.

Renin-angiotensin-aldosterone system: The hormonal system controlled mainly by the kidneys and adrenal glands that regulates blood pressure, blood volume, and electrolyte balance.

Replication capacity: This term is often used interchangeably with the term "viral fitness" and refers to how quickly HIV reproduces or replicates. The slower HIV replicates, the less likely a patient is to have disease progression. A replication capacity may be reported on a resistance test. It is reported as a percentage of the median replication rate for drug-sensitive (wild-type) HIV strains.

Resorption: The process of bone breakdown by osteoclasts.

Respiratory acidosis: Acidosis that is caused by an accumulation of carbon dioxide.

Respiratory alkalosis: Alkalosis that is caused by a loss of carbon dioxide.

Restenosis: Renarrowing of the coronary artery after a percutaneous intervention to improve coronary blood flow.

Retching: A process that follows nausea and consists of diaphragm, abdominal wall, and chest wall contractions and spasmodic breathing against a closed glottis.

Reticulocytes: Immature blood cells that mature into erythrocytes.

Reticuloendothelial system: Phagocytic cells excluding granulocytes; widely distributed throughout the body.

Retrograde ejaculation: Flow of ejaculate into the bladder instead of antegrade out of the urethra.

Rhabdomyolysis: Destruction of skeletal muscle.

Rheumatic fever: An acute inflammatory disease involving the joints, heart, skin, brain, and other tissues caused by an immune response to streptococcal infection in genetically susceptible people, particularly in children.

Rheumatoid factors: Antibodies reactive with the Fc region of IgG.

Rhinosinusitis: Inflammation of the mucous membranes in the nose and sinuses.

Rhonchi: Abnormal, rumbling sounds heard on auscultation of an obstructed airway. They are more prominent during expiration and may clear somewhat on coughing.

Rouleaux formation: The stacking of red blood cells on a peripheral smear when diluted.

Rubefacients: A substance that produces redness of the skin.

Salicylism: A toxic syndrome caused by excessive doses of acetylsalicylic acid (aspirin), salicylic acid, or any other salicylate product. Signs and symptoms may include severe headache, nausea, vomiting, tinnitus (ringing in the ears), confusion, increased pulse, and increased respiratory rate.

Scarlatiniform rash: Bright, scarlet-colored skin eruption that occurs in patches over the entire body with eventual peeling as a result of streptococcal infection.

Scleritis: Inflammation of the outer layer of the eyeball.

Scoliosis: A congenital lateral curvature of the spine.

Secondary amenorrhea: Absence of menses for 3 cycles or 6 months in a previously menstruating woman.

Secondary hyperparathyroidism: Increased secretion of parathyroid hormone from the parathyroid glands caused by hyperphosphatemia, hypocalcemia, and vitamin D deficiency that results from decreased kidney function. Secondary hyperparathyroidism can lead to bone disease (renal osteodystrophy).

Secondary transmission: Transferring a disease from the primary source to another person.

Seizure: A sudden electrical disturbance in the brain that results from a population of neurons rapidly and repetitively firing in a rhythmic and synchronous pattern for seconds to minutes.

Semiology: The clinical symptoms and presentation of a seizure.

Sentinel lymph node: Refers to the first (axillary) node that picks up dye injected into the tumor.

Sera: Pertaining to human serum.

Seropositive: Showing a positive reaction to a test on blood serum for a disease.

Serum sickness: A group of symptoms caused by a delayed immune response to certain medications. Arthralgias, fever, malaise, and urticaria may develop usually 7 to 14 days after exposure to the causative antigen.

Shear stress: Risk factor for pressure ulcers that is generated when the head of a patient's bed is elevated and can cause deeper blood vessels to crimp, leading to ischemia.

Sick sinus syndrome: Idiopathic sinus node dysfunction leading to symptomatic sinus bradycardia.

Sigmoidoscopy: A visual inspection of the sigmoid colon and rectum with a flexible tube called a sigmoidoscope.

Simple disorder: The presence of a single acid-base disorder, with or without compensation.

Sjögren's syndrome: A chronic autommimune disease characterized by dry eyes and dry mouth.

Sleep apnea: The temporary stopping of breathing during sleep; can be caused by narrowing of the airways resulting from swelling of soft tissue.

Slit-lamp biomicroscope: An instrument that allows for the microscopic examination of the cornea, anterior chamber lens, and posterior chamber.

Somatic hypermutation: The occurrence of multiple point mutations.

Somatotrope: Growth hormone producing cells in the anterior pituitary

Spastic colon: A synonym for irritable bowel syndrome.

Spasticity: A motor disorder characterized by an increase in muscle tone with exaggerated tendon jerks, resulting from hyperexcitability of the stretch reflex.

Spectrum of activity: A qualitative term that describes the number of different bacterial species that are susceptible to an antimicrobial regimen. Generally, broad-spectrum activity refers to regimens that possess activity against many bacterial species, whereas narrow-spectrum therapy refers to activity against a few bacterial species.

Sphincter of Oddi: Structure through which the common bile duct empties bile and pancreatic secretions into the duodenum.

Spirometry: Measurement by means of a spirometer of the air entering and leaving the lungs.

Splenomegaly: An enlarged spleen secondary to leukemic infiltration.

Sprain: An overstretching of supporting ligaments that results in a partial or complete tear of the ligament.

Sputum culture: A sputum sample obtained from the lower respiratory tract is placed into a container that contains substances to promote, in this case, mycobacterial growth. Positive results indicate live mycobacteria, which can be tested for susceptibility to drugs.

Sputum smear: A sputum sample obtained from the lower respiratory tract, spread on a glass slide, and stained for examination under a microscope. Used to identify the presence of microorganisms.

Stable disease: In cancer, neither sufficient shrinkage to qualify for partial response nor sufficient increase to qualify for progressive disease.

Staging: Analysis that provides a semiquantitative estimate of tumor burden, which is not only of prognostic importance, but also has important implications regarding appropriate treatment options.

Steatohepatitis: A severe form of liver disease caused by fat deposition in the liver, characterized by hepatic inflammation that may rapidly progress to liver fibrosis and cirrhosis.

Steatorrhea: Excessive loss of fat in stool.

Steatosis: Excessive fat accumulation. Fat deposition in liver.

Stenosis: Blockage of an artery.

Stenting: Placement of a stent to allow blood flow through an artery.

Stereotactic radiosurgery: Radiation technique that uses a large number of narrow, precisely aimed, highly focused beams of ionizing radiation. The beams are aimed from many directions circling the head and meet at a specific point.

Stevens-Johnson syndrome: A severe expression of erythema multiforme (also known as erythema multiforme major). It typically involves the skin and the mucous membranes with the potential for severe morbidity and even death.

Stomatitis: Inflammation of mucous membranes in the mouth.

Strain: Damage to the muscle fibers or tendon without tearing of the ligament.

Striae: Linear, atrophic, pinkish or purplish, scarlike lesions that later become white (striae albicantes, lineae albicantes), which may occur on the abdomen, breasts, buttocks, and thighs. They are due to weakening of the elastic tissues; commonly called stretch marks.

Stricture: An area of narrowing or constriction in the gastrointestinal tract due to buildup of fibrotic tissue; often a result of long-standing inflammation.

Stroke volume: The amount of blood ejected from the heart during systole.

ST-segment elevation: A type of myocardial infarction that typically results in an injury that transects the thickness of the myocardial wall. Following an ST-elevation myocardial infarction, pathologic Q waves are frequently seen on the electrocardiogram, indicating transmural myocardial infarction.

Subchondral: Situated beneath and supporting cartilage.

Subtrochanteric: Below the trochanter (the bony protrusion at the end of the femur where the hip and thigh muscles attach).

Surgical site infection: Infections occurring at or near the surgical incision within 30 days of the operation; up to 1 year if a prosthesis is implanted.

Suspending agent: An additive used in the compounding of oral liquid medications to suspend drug particles throughout a liquid and enables resuspension of particles by agitation (e.g., shaking well).

Synechia: Adhesions or the abnormal attachment of the iris to another structure. Peripheral anterior synechia refers to occurrence of synechia with the trabecular meshwork.

Synovitis: Inflammation of the synovial membrane, often in combination with pain and swelling of the affected joint.

Synovium: The membrane lining the internal surfaces of the joint.

Systolic dysfunction: An abnormal contraction of the ventricles during systole.

Tachycardia: Abnormally fast heart rate.

Tachyphylaxis: Rapid decreasing response to a drug or other physiologically active agent after a few doses.

Tachypnea: Abnormally fast respiratory rate.

Tangles: Twisted fibers of a protein, tau, that build up inside cells.

Telangiectasia: Permanent dilation of preexisting small blood vessels (capillaries, arterioles, venules), usually in the skin or mucous membranes which presents as a coarse or fine red line.

Tendonitis: Inflammation of the tendon.

Tenesmus: Difficulty with bowel evacuation despite the urgency to defecate.

Tenosynovitis: Inflammation of the tendon sheath.

Teratogenic potential: The ability of an agent to cause harm or malformations to a fetus or embryo. Medications are assigned pregnancy categories based on their teratogenic potential.

Terminal secretions: The noise produced by the oscillatory movements of secretions in the upper airways in association with the inspiratory and expiratory phases of respiration. It is also known as "death rattle."

Thelarche: The onset of breast development in women.

Third spacing: Fluid accumulation in the interstitial space disproportionate to the intracellular and extracellular fluid spaces.

Thoracentesis: Removal of fluid that is present in the pleural space. Common procedure to determine what caused the fluid accumulation.

Thrombin: An enzyme formed from prothrombin which converts fibrinogen to fibrin. It is the principal driving force in the clotting cascade.

Thrombocytopenia: A condition where the number of circulating platelets are abnormally low due to decreased production of new cells, possibly secondary to medication toxicities.

Thrombocytosis: Increased number of platelets in the blood.

Thrombogenesis: The process of forming a blood clot.

Thrombolysis: The process of enzymatically dissolving or breaking apart a blood clot.

Thrombolytic: An enzyme that dissolves or breaks apart blood clots.

Thrombophlebitis: Inflammation of a blood vessel (e.g., vein) associated with the stimulations of clotting and formation of a thrombus (or blood clot).

Thromboplastin: A substance that triggers the coagulation cascade. Tissue factor is a naturally occurring thromboplastin and is used in the prothrombin time test.

Thrombosis: A condition in which blood changes from a liquid to a solid state and produces a blood clot.

Thrombotic thrombocytopenic purpura: Condition characterized by formation of small clots within the circulation resulting in the consumption of platelets and a low platelet count.

Thrombus: Blood clot attached to the vessel wall and consisting of platelets, fibrin, and clotting factors. A thrombus may partially or completely occlude the lumen of a blood vessel compromising blood flow and oxygen delivery to distal tissue.

Thyroiditis: Inflammation of the thyroid gland.

Tocolytic: Medication used to suppress premature labor.

Tonometry: A method by which the cornea is indented or flattened by an instrument. The pressure required to achieve corneal indentation or flattening is a measure of intraocular pressure.

Topoisomerase: Enzymes that temporarily alter supercoiled DNA by cutting the DNA, causing the DNA to relax the supercoil during DNA replication. Topoisomerase inhibitors prevent the DNA from sealing the cut which causes DNA strand breakage.

Torsade de pointes: Very rapid ventricular tachycardia characterized by a gradually changing QRS complex in the ECG; may change into ventricular fibrillation.

Toxic epidermal necrolysis: A life-threatening skin disorder characterized by blistering and peeling of the top layer of skin.

Toxoid: A modified bacterial exotoxin that has lost toxicity.

Tracheal aspirate: Suctioning of secretions from the trachea.

Transesophageal echocardiogram: Procedure used to generate an image of the heart via sound waves, via a probe introduced into the esophagus (rather than the traditional transthoracic view) in order to obtain a better image of the left atrium.

Transformation (conversion): Mutated cell becomes malignant.

Transient ischemic attack: Focal neurologic deficit lasting less than 24 hours where symptoms resolve completely.

Translocation: Movement of bacteria and endotoxin from the intestinal lumen through the gut mucosa and into the lymphatic and systemic circulation.

Transmural: Across the wall of an organ or structure; in the case of Crohn's disease, inflammation may extend through all four layers of the intestinal wall.

Tubal ligation: Surgical process of tying up the fallopian tubes to prevent passage of ova from the ovaries to the uterus.

Tumor suppressor genes: Genes that normally restrain cell growth but, when missing or inactivated by mutation, allow cells to grow uncontrolled and tumors to form.

Tuberoeruptive xanthomas: Small yellow-red raised papules usually presenting on the elbows, knees, back, and buttocks.

Tubulointerstitial: Involving the tubules or interstitial tissue of the kidneys.

Tumor lysis syndrome: A syndrome resulting from cytotoxic therapy, occurring generally in aggressive, rapidly proliferating lymphoproliferative disorders. It is characterized by combinations of hyperuricemia, lactic acidosis, hyperkalemia, hyperphosphatemia, and hypocalcemia.

T2-weighted magnetic resonance imaging: A setting of the magnetic resonance imaging machine that shows water as a bright signal.

Tympanocentesis: Puncture of the tympanic membrane with a needle to aspirate middle ear fluid.

Tympanostomy tube: Small plastic or metal tube inserted in the eardrum to keep the middle ear aerated and improve hearing in patients with chronic middle ear effusion.

Uhthoff's phenomenon: Acute worsening of multiple sclerosis symptoms on exposure to heat because high body temperatures may exceed the capacitance of the demyelinated nerve and conduction may fail.

Ultrafiltration: The movement of plasma water across a semipermeable membrane.

Uncomplicated disorder: See Simple disorder.

Uremia: A condition that results from accumulation of metabolic waste products and endogenous toxins in the body resulting from impaired kidney function. Symptoms of uremia include nausea, vomiting, weakness, loss of appetite, and mental confusion.

Urethral stricture: Narrowing of the urethral lumen by scar tissue. This could result from trauma, inflammation, infection, or instrumentation.

Uricosuric: Pertaining to, characterized by, or promoting renal excretion of uric acid.

Urosepsis: Sepsis resulting from a urinary source.

Urticaria: Itchy, raised, swollen areas on the skin. Also known as hives.

Uveitis: An inflammation of the uvea. Uveal structures include the iris, the ciliary body, and the choroids.

Vagal maneuvers: Stimulate the activity of the parasympathetic nervous system, which inhibits atrioventricular nodal conduction. Examples of vagal maneuvers include cough, carotid sinus massage, and Valsalva.

Vagotomy: A surgical procedure that blocks vagal (cholinergic) stimulation to the stomach.

Valsalva maneuver: Vagal maneuver; patient bears down against a closed glottis, as if they were having a bowel movement.

Variceal bleeding: Varices are weak collateral blood vessels that are friable and rupture easily; often observed in the esophagus or stomach.

Vasculitis: Inflammation of the walls of blood vessels.

Vasomotor symptoms: Menopausal symptoms that include both hot flashes and night sweats.

Vasopressors: Medications that cause constriction of blood vessels, increase in vascular resistance, and increase in blood pressure.

Vasospasm: Narrowing (constriction) of a blood vessel causing a reduction in blood flow.

Ventilation/perfusion ratio (V_A/Q): A comparison of the proportion of lung tissue being ventilated by inhaled air to the rate of oxygenation of pulmonary blood.

Ventricular depolarization: Change in the membrane potential of a ventricular myocyte, resulting in loss of polarization. Under normal conditions, depolarization of ventricular myocytes is followed by ventricular contraction.

Vertigo: Sensation of spinning or feeling out of balance.

Vesicants: A chemical or agent that causes significant tissue damage if extravasation occurs during IV administration.

Virilization: Production or acquisition of virilism, which is masculine characteristics.

Volvulus: Twisting of the intestine causing obstruction and possible necrosis.

Vomiting: A reflexive rapid and forceful oral expulsion of upper gastrointestinal contents due to powerful and sustained contractions in the abdominal and thoracic musculature.

Waist circumference: A practical tool to measure the abdominal fat in patients with a BMI of less than 35.

Western blot analysis: The "gold standard" for HIV diagnostic testing. Disrupted virus is purified, gel-electrophoresed to separate by molecular weight to form bands corresponding to the nine HIV antigens, and blotted onto a membrane support. HIV serum antibodies from the patient are allowed to bind to proteins in the membrane support. If HIV antibodies from the patient are bound, the bands will change color. The test is considered reactive if 2 of the 3 major bands (p24, gp41, and/or gp120/160) change color. The test is nonreactive if no viral bands are visible.

White coat hypertension: A persistently elevated average office blood pressure of greater than 140/90 mm Hg and an average awake ambulatory reading of less than 135/85 mm Hg.

Wilson's disease: A disorder of copper metabolism, characterized by cirrhosis of the liver and neurologic manifestations.

Xanthoma: Firm raised nodules composed of lipid-containing histocytes.

Xerostomia: Dry mouth resulting from decreased salivary secretion.

ZAP-70 expression: An intracellular tyrosine kinase found in CLL B-cells.

Zymogen: An inactive protein precursor of an enzyme that is converted into an active form.

Appendix E: Prescription Writing Principles

Julie Haase, Kim Hawkins, Jill Isaacs, Emily Knezevich, and Jon Knezevich

According to the International Monetary Systems (IMS) Health Report, 3.9 billion prescriptions were written and dispensed in the United States in 2009. This demonstrated an increase of 5.1% from 2008 and reflects a need for prescribers and dispensers to fully understand prescriptive privileges and rational prescribing.[1] The following outlines principles of pharmacotherapy, including obtaining prescriptive privileges, rational prescribing of medications, electronic prescribing, safe prescribing practices, adverse event reporting, and medication education.

It is essential that the prescriber and dispenser familiarize themselves with the professional guidelines, state laws, and federal laws. In addition, they must also understand the components of rational prescribing. Table E–1 below provides key elements a prescriber should understand as well as useful resources.

TYPES OF PRESCRIPTION ORDERS

Prescription orders can be provided in a variety of ways by authorized prescribers. Outpatient prescriptions may be written, verbally authorized by phone, faxed, or provided via electronic means. All outpatient prescriptions are subject to federal regulations and contain the same basic components. Laws and regulations for outpatient prescription requirements can vary from state to state, so prescribers should be knowledgeable of all applicable laws. The basic components of a prescription are listed below as well as numbered in Figure E–1.[2]

1. Prescriber information: name, address, and phone number

2. Prescriber's signature and prescriptive authority number or Drug Enforcement Administration (DEA) number (if applicable)

3. Patient information: full name and address, and weight and age if appropriate

4. Date the prescription was written

5. Superscription (Rx symbol), meaning "you take" or "recipe"

6. Inscription: medication being prescribed (name of medication, strength, and dose)

7. Signa, sig, or signature: directions to the patient (e.g., take one tablet daily)

8. Subscription: dispensing instructions to the pharmacist (number, quantity, or volume to dispense)

9. Number of refills allowed

10. Generic substitution requirement: "DAW (dispense as written)" or "no substitution" if brand name medication only is desired

Further regulations are in place for prescriptions written for controlled substances. In addition to the above elements, prescriptions for controlled substances must also include the patient's full name and address as well as the full name, address, and DEA number of the prescriber. Stricter regulations exist for Schedule II controlled substances compared with Schedule III-V. Schedule II prescriptions must be written and can only be provided orally in an emergency situation. Refills are prohibited with Schedule II prescriptions.[3]

Chart orders, orders written for hospital inpatients, are not considered prescriptions and are not subject to the same requirements. Typically chart orders include:

- Patient identifiers including name, account number

- Physician name

- Medication name, dose, route, and frequency of administration

- Date and time of order

- Physician signature

- If the order was given verbally, the person reducing the order to writing must sign the order and the ordering physician countersign

Electronic prescribing has become common practice because of government incentives aimed at moving health records to electronic databases.[4] Principles discussed previously in regard to requirements of a prescription hold true for electronic orders; however, additional considerations must be taken to ensure safe prescribing habits occur. A brief list of potential risks and benefits is summarized in Table E–2.

Electronic prescribing is no longer a projection of the future but instead is becoming the norm amongst prescribers and clinical staff. Careful thought should be placed into the

Table E–1

Pharmacotherapy Principles

Pharmacotherapy Principle	Description	Online Resources
Prescriptive privileges	Dictated by federal and state law Scope of practice and formularies vary by profession. Physicians, nurse practitioners, physician assistants, and dentists all have varying scopes of practice, which may include formularies or supervising prescribers. Each provider must become familiar with his or her profession's scope of practice. Pharmacology courses in program of study and Continuing Education required Prescribing legend drugs requires board examination and National Provider Identifier (NPI) Prescribing controlled substances requires DEA registration number	*https://nppes.cms.hhs.gov/NPPES/Welcome.do* *http://www.justice.gov/dea/*

Rational prescribing	Ensure necessity of medication
	Obtain pertinent history
	• Health history: comorbidities or contraindications (i.e. pregnancy, hepatic failure, or renal failure)
	• Medication history: prior and current prescription, OTC, or herbal use; drug allergies or sensitivities; compliance issues
	• Family and social history
	Select correct medication
	• It is important to know the following components of each medication when prescribing or dispensing:
	  • Pharmacokinetics
	  • Pharmacodynamics
	  • Drug interactions
	  • Drug-disease interactions
	  • Interdisciplinary collaboration when necessary
		http://www.jointcommission.org/

DEA, Drug Enforcement Administration; OTC, over the counter.

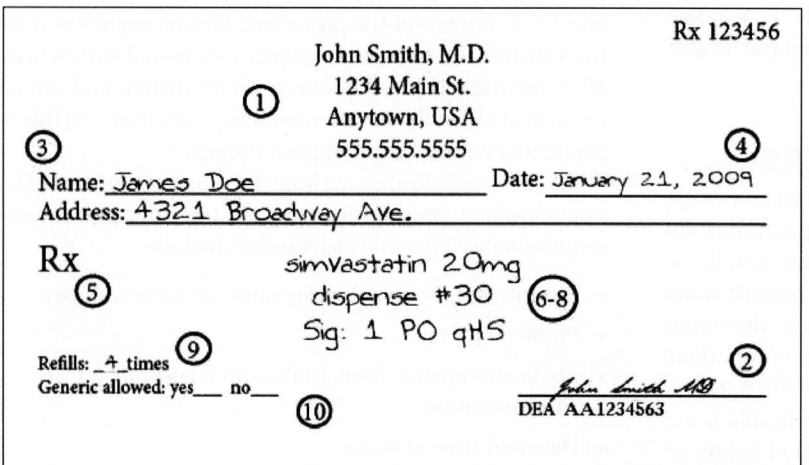

FIGURE E–1. Example of a prescription.

Table E–2

Electronic Prescribing[4-6]

Benefits	Risks
Reduce medication errors	Cost of software programs
Reduce adverse drug events	Lack of financial benefit seen immediately
Improves efficiency	Lack of software standardization
Improved recognition of drug–drug and drug–disease interactions	Indirect costs: training personnel, reduced patient visits during training period
Improved recognition of medication allergy cross-sensitivity	Clinician resistance: worry of worsening relationship with patient, negative impact on workflow, and fears of restrictions on prescribing habits
Enhanced prescriber knowledge of patient adherence	
Enhanced prescriber knowledge of insurance coverage for medications	

implementation process to ensure that patient care is not compromised. With appropriate use of this technology, patients are provided ultimately with safer and more efficient care.

Omission of any of the above-discussed elements on a prescription order can be considered erroneous and poses a danger to patient care. Responsibility lies with the prescriber as well as the pharmacist dispensing the medication to ensure the prescriptions are not only accurate but also appropriate for the given patient.

SAFE PRESCRIBING PRACTICES

Safe prescribing should be a priority of all healthcare providers. To avoid inappropriate use of medications in patients, prescribers should take careful consideration in writing clear and descriptive prescriptions. This ensures appropriate communication among all interdisciplinary healthcare providers.

A thorough understanding of the medication prescribed, including its expected risks and benefits, should be realized by the prescriber ensuring appropriate drug selection. Providers should be aware of common errors related to prescription writing. These errors include: sound-alike/look-alike medications and inappropriate use of shorthand language and abbreviations. The Joint Commission, as well as the Institute for Safe Medication Practices (ISMP), has collected common examples of these errors seen during the ordering process. Common examples are described in Tables E–3 and E–4.

Table E–3
Sound-Alike/Look-alike Medications[7,a]

Medication Name	Misinterpreted Medication Name
acetoHEXAMIDE	acetaZOLAMIDE
chlordiazePOXIDE	chlorproMAZINE
CISplatin	CARBOplatin
ePHEDrine	EPINEPHrine
hydrALAZINE	hydrOXYzine
LORazepam	ALPRAZolam
NIFEdipine	niCARdipine
RABEprazole	ARIPiprazole
risperiDONE	rOPINIRole
sulfADIAZINE	sulfaSALAzine
valACYclovir	valGANciclovir
Zantac	Xanax

[a]For additional information, please see *http://www.ismp.org/tools/confuseddrugnames.pdf.*

Table E–4
Error-Prone Abbreviations[8,a]

Abbreviation	Anticipated Meaning	Misinterpretation	Correction
µg	Microgram	Mistaken as "mg"	Use "mcg"
IJ	Injection	Mistaken as "IV" or "intrajugular"	Use "injection"
q.d. or QD	Every day	Mistaken as q.i.d., especially if the period after the "q" or the tail of the "q" is misunderstood as an "i"	Use "daily"

Dose Designation	Anticipated Meaning	Misinterpretation	Correction
Trailing zero after decimal point (e.g., 4.0 mg)	4 mg	Mistaken as 40 mg if the decimal point is not seen	Do not use trailing zeros for doses expressed in whole numbers
No leading zero before a decimal point (e.g., .8 mg)	0.8 mg	Mistaken as 8 mg if the decimal point is NOT seen	Use zero before a decimal point when the dose is less than a whole unit
Large doses without properly placed commas (e.g., 100000 units; 1000000 units)	100,000 units 1,000,000 units	100000 has been mistaken as 10,000 or 1,000,000; 1000000 has been mistaken as 100,000	Use commas for dosing units at or above 1,000 or use words such as 100 "thousand" or 1 "million" to improve readability

Drug Name Abbreviation	Anticipated Meaning	Misinterpretation	Correction
AZT	Zidovudine (Retrovir)	Mistaken as azathioprine or aztreonam	Use complete drug name
MS, MSO_4	Morphine sulfate	Mistaken as magnesium sulfate	Use complete drug name
PCA	Procainamide	Mistaken as patient-controlled analgesia	Use complete drug name
T3	Tylenol with codeine No. 3	Mistaken as liothyronine	Use complete drug name

Stemmed Drug Names	Anticipated Meaning	Misinterpretation	Correction
"Nitro" drip	Nitroglycerin infusion	Mistaken as sodium nitroprusside infusion	Use complete drug name
"IV Vanc"	Intravenous vancomycin	Mistaken as Invanz	Use complete drug name

Symbol	Anticipated Meaning	Misinterpretation	Correction
x3d	For three days	Mistaken as 3 doses	Use "for three days"
&	And	Mistaken as "2"	Use "and"
°	Hour	Mistaken as a zero (e.g., q2° seen as q 20)	Use "hr," "h," or "hour"

[a]For additional information, please see ISMP/Joint Commission List of Error Prone Abbreviations.

Table E–5

Frequently Used Abbreviations[2]

Abbreviation or Shorthand	Meaning	Abbreviation or Shorthand	Meaning
QD	Daily	PO	By mouth
BID	Twice daily	PR, rect	Per rectum
TID	Three times daily	gtt	Drop
QID	Four times daily	subQ	Subcutaneously
HS	At bedtime	V, PV	Vaginally
PRN	As needed	supp	Suppository
WM	With meals	SL	Sublingual
q4h, q6h, etc.	Every 4 hours, every 6 hours, etc.	ou	Each eye
qAM	Every morning	od	Right eye
qPM	Every evening	os	Left eye
QS	Quantity sufficient	pc	After a meal
au	Each ear	ac	Before a meal
ad	Right ear	HCTZ	Hydrochlorothiazide
as, al	Left ear		

Other abbreviations are commonly used in prescription writing. Examples are included in Table E–5.

Adverse Event Reporting

If adverse events related to medication use are determined, the healthcare provider who discovers the event is responsible for reporting it. The Food and Drug Administration's reporting system for such adverse events is MedWatch *http://www.fda.gov/Safety/MedWatch/default.htm*.[9] This online database archives medication-related adverse events, and providers are able to report errors seen in clinical practice through this same system.

Medication Education

After a prescription has been written, counseling patients on newly prescribed therapies is an essential responsibility of the prescriber as well as the pharmacist dispensing the medication. The patient should be made aware of the rationale for drug use, the dose, route, and frequency at which they should administer the medication and expectations of the prescribed drug. Expectations should include risks and benefits to avoid patient confusion about side effects or efficacy measures. Thorough discussion of medication therapy selected with the patient may identify contraindications previously unknown or a patient history of failure or success with the selected agent in the past.

CONCLUSION

Multiple principles must be exercised for appropriate drug delivery from the bedside to the patient. As a healthcare provider, understanding these processes helps to ensure safe medication prescribing, as outlined in this appendix.

REFERENCES

1. Sullivan D. Prescription writing and electronic prescribing. In: Sullivan D, ed. Guide to Clinical Documentation. Philadelphia, PA: FA Davis; 2012:207–217.
2. Ansel HC. The prescription. In: Troy DB, ed. Remington: The Science and Practice of Pharmacy. Philadelphia, PA: Lippincott Williams & Wilkins; 2005:1828–1841.
3. Section V–Valid Prescription Requirements [Internet]. Office of Diversion Control. [cited 2012 Jan 10]. Available from: *http://www.deadiversion.usdoj.gov/pubs/manuals/pract/section5.htm*.
4. Cusack CM. Electronic health records and electronic prescribing: Promise and pitfalls. Obstet Gynecol Clin North Am 2008;35:63–79.
5. Lapane KL, Rosen RK, Dube C. Perceptions of e-prescribing efficiencies and inefficiencies in ambulatory care. Intern J Med Informatics 2011;80 39–46.
6. Ammenwerth E, Schnell-Inderst P, Machan C, Siebert U. The effect of electronic prescribing on medication errors and adverse drug events: A systematic review. J Am Med Informatics Assn 2008;15:585–600.
7. ISMP's List of Confused Drug Names [Internet]. Horsham (PA): Institute of Safe Medication Practices:c2001 [updated 2011; cited 2011 Sept 28]. Available from: *http://ismp.org/tools/confuseddrugnames.pdf*.
8. ISMP's List of Error-Prone Abbreviations, Symbols, and Dose Designations [Internet]. Horsham (PA): Institute of Safe Medication Practices:c2001 [updated 2010; cited 2011 Sept 28]. Available from: *http://ismp.org/tools/errorproneabbreviations.pdf*.
9. MedWatch: The FDA Safety Information and Adverse Event Reporting Program [Internet]. Bethesda (MD): The U.S. Food and Drug Administration. C2011 [updated 2011; cited 2011 Sept 28]. Available from: *http://www.fda.gov/Safety/MedWatch/default.htm*.

Page numbers followed by *f*, *t*, and *a* refer to figures, tables, and algorithms, respectively.